CURRENT SURGICAL THERAPY

CURRENT SURGICAL THERAPY

9th EDITION

JOHN L. CAMERON,
MD, FACS, FRCS (Eng) (hon); FRCSI (hon)

The Alfred Blalock Distinguished Service Professor
Department of Surgery
The Johns Hopkins Medical Institutions
Baltimore, Maryland

MOSBY

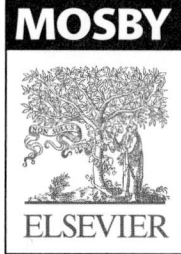

ELSEVIER

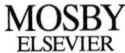

MOSBY
ELSEVIER

1600 John F. Kennedy Blvd.
Ste 1800
Philadelphia, PA 19103–2899

CURRENT SURGICAL THERAPY   ISBN: 978-1-4160-3497-1
NINTH EDITION

Notice

Knowledge and best practice in this field are constantly changing. As new research and experience broaden our knowledge, changes in practice, treatment and drug therapy may become necessary or appropriate. Readers are advised to check the most current information provided (i) on procedures featured or (ii) by the manufacturer of each product to be administered, to verify the recommended dose or formula, the method and duration of administration, and contraindications. It is the responsibility of the practitioner, relying on their own experience and knowledge of the patient, to make diagnoses, to determine dosages and the best treatment for each individual patient, and to take all appropriate safety precautions. To the fullest extent of the law, neither the Publisher nor the Authors assume any liability for any injury and/or damage to persons or property arising out of or related to any use of the material contained in this book.

The Publisher

Previous editions copyrighted 1984, 1986, 1989, 1992, 1995, 1998, 2001, 2004

Library of Congress International Standard Serial Number ISSN 0835-3689

Acquisitions Editor: Scott Scheidt
Developmental Editor: Faith Voit
Senior Project Manager: David Saltzberg
Design Direction: Steve Stave

Printed in the United States of America

Last digit is the print number: 9 8 7 6 5 4 3 2 1

CONTRIBUTORS

Herand Abcarian, MD
Turi Josefsen Professor and Head
University of Illinois at Chicago
Department of Surgery
Chicago, Illinois
FECAL INCONTINENCE

Michel B. Aboutanos, MD
Assistant Professor of Surgery
Virginia Commonwealth University
VCU Medical Center
Richmond, Virginia
THE ABDOMEN THAT WON'T CLOSE

Ali F. AbuRahma, MD
Professor of Surgery
Robert C. Byrd Health Sciences Center
West Virginia University
Charleston Area Medical Center
Charleston, West Virginia
BRACHIOCEPHALIC RECONSTRUCTION

David B. Adams, MD
Medical University of South Carolina
Charleston, South Carolina
PANCREATIC ABSCESS

Reid B. Adams, MD, FACS
University of Virginia Health System
Department of Surgery
Charlottesville, Virginia
CYSTIC DISEASE OF THE LIVER

Samuel S. Ahn, MD
PERIPHERAL ARTERIAL OCCLUSIVE DISEASE:
ANGIOPLASTY, STENTING, AND
ENDOVASCULAR GRAFT TREATMENT

Steven A. Ahrendt, MD
Associate Professor of Surgery
University of Pittsburgh;
UPMC Cancer Center
Pittsburgh, Pennsylvania
GALLSTONE ILEUS

Nita Ahuja, MD
Department of Surgery
The Johns Hopkins Hospital
Baltimore, Maryland
RECTAL CANCER

Matthew J. Alef, MD
ENDOSCOPIC TREATMENT OF BARRETT'S
ESOPHAGUS

Luz P. Angel, MD
CHRONIC ULCERATIVE COLITIS

Aravind Arepally, MD
Assistant Professor of Radiology
and Surgery
Division of Interventional Radiology
The Johns Hopkins Hospital
Baltimore, Maryland
TRANSJUGULAR INTRAHEPATIC
PORTOSYSTEMIC SHUNTS (TIPS)

Meghan A. Arnold, MD
Department of Surgery
Sinai Hospital of Baltimore
Baltimore, Maryland
SURGICAL SITE INFECTIONS

Stanley W. Ashley, MD
Department of Surgery
Brigham and Women's Hospital
Boston, Massachusetts
ACUTE PANCREATITIS

Jennifer M. Ayscue, MD
Washington Hospital Center
Washington, D.C.
TUMORS OF THE ANAL REGION

Marshall S. Baker, MD, MBA
Assistant Professor of Surgery
Division of Surgical Oncology
Feinberg School of Medicine
Northwestern University
Evanston, Illinois
BENIGN BILIARY STRICTURES

Leora B. Balsam, MD
Stanford University School of Medicine
Department of Cardiothoracic Surgery
Palo Alto, California
PRIMARY CHEST WALL TUMORS

Dennis F. Bandyk, MD
Professor of Surgery;
Director, Division of Vascular and
Endovascular Surgery
University of South Florida College
of Medicine
Tampa, Florida
DIABETIC FOOT

Adrian Barbul, MD
Department of Surgery
Sinai Hospital of Baltimore
Baltimore, Maryland
SURGICAL SITE INJECTIONS

Philip S. Barie, MD, MBA
Professor of Surgery and Public Health;
Chief, Division of Critical Care and Trauma
Weill Medical College of Cornell University
New York, New York
FLUID AND ELECTROLYTE THERAPY

John G. Bartlett, MD
The Johns Hopkins University School
of Medicine
Baltimore, Maryland
OCCUPATIONAL EXPOSURE TO HIV AND
OTHER BLOOD-BORNE PATHOGENS

Robert Bartlett, MD
Professor of Surgery, Emeritus
Department of Surgery
University of Michigan
Ann Arbor, Michigan
EXTRACORPOREAL LIFE SUPPORT FOR
RESPIRATORY FAILURE

Todd W. Bauer, MD
Assistant Professor of Surgery,
Hepatobiliary, and Pancreatic Surgery
University of Virginia Health System
Charlottesville, Virginia
CYSTIC DISEASE OF THE LIVER

Robert W. Beart, Jr., MD, FACS
Professor and Chairman
Department of Colorectal Surgery
Keck School of Medicine
University of Southern California
Los Angeles, California
POSTOPERATIVE ILEUS

Jean Pierre Becquemin, MD
Professor, Vascular Surgery;
Chief, Division of Vascular Surgery
Hospital Henri Mondor
Paris, France
BALLOON ANGIOPLASTY AND STENTS IN
CAROTID ARTERY OCCLUSIVE DISEASE

Kevin E. Behrns, MD
Robert H. Hux Professor;
Chief of General and Gastrointestinal
Surgery
University of Florida
Gainesville, Florida
PANCREATIC PSEUDOCYSTS

Avraham Belizon, MD
Surgical Resident
North Shore/Long Island Jewish
Medical Center
New Hyde Park, New York
LAPAROSCOPIC APPENDECTOMY

Sean Berenholtz, MD, MHS, FCCM
Adult Critical Care Medicine
The Johns Hopkins University School
of Medicine
Baltimore, Maryland
*ENDOCRINE CHANGES WITH CRITICAL
ILLNESS*

Douglas Bernstein, MD
DIVERTICULOSIS OF THE SMALL BOWEL

Parag Bhanot, MD
GASTROESOPHAGEAL REFLUX DISEASE

Anton J. Bilchik, MD, PhD, FACS
Director, Gastrointestinal Program
John Wayne Cancer Institute
Santa Monica, California
*COLORECTAL CANCER METASTATIC TO THE
LIVER: RADIOFREQUENCY ABLATION*

James H. Black, III, MD
Division of Vascular and Endovascular
Surgery
The Johns Hopkins Hospital
Baltimore, Maryland
*THORACIC AND THORACOABDOMINAL
AORTIC ANEURYSMS*

Kirby I. Bland, MD
Chairman, Department of Surgery
University of Alabama at Birmingham
Birmingham, Alabama
*CELLULAR, BIOCHEMICAL, AND MOLECULAR
TARGETS IN BREAST CANCER*

John M.A. Bohnen, MD, FRCSC, FACS
Division of General Surgery
St. Michael's Hospital;
Professor and Vice-Chair of Education
Department of Surgery;
Vice-Dean, Clinical Affairs
Faculty of Medicine
University of Toronto
Toronto, Ontario, Canada
ANTIBIOTICS FOR CRITICALLY ILL PATIENTS

Anne-Marie Boller, MD, MA
Fellow
Mayo Clinic
Division of Colon and Rectal Surgery
Rochester, Minnesota
LARGE BOWEL OBSTRUCTION

Kevin N. Boykin, MD
Assistant Professor of Surgery
Louisiana State University School
of Medicine
Shreveport, Louisiana
*ESOPHAGEAL ATRESIA AND
TRACHEOESOPHAGEAL FISTULA*

Steven B. Brandes, MD
Associate Professor of Surgery
Division of Urologic Surgery
Washington University School of Medicine
St. Louis, Missouri
*RETROPERITONEAL INJURIES: KIDNEY AND
URETER*

**Cedric G. Bremner, MB, BCh, MCh,
FRCS (ret)**
Johannesburg, South Africa
ESOPHAGEAL FUNCTION TESTS

Murray F. Brennan, MD
Memorial Sloan-Kettering Cancer Center
New York, New York
GASTRIC ADENOCARCINOMA

L.D. Britt, MD, MPH
Eastern Virginia Medical School
Norfolk, Virginia
PENETRATING ABDOMINAL TRAUMA

Malcolm V. Brock, MD
Associate Professor of Surgery and
Oncology
The Johns Hopkins University School of
Medicine
Baltimore, Maryland
ESOPHAGEAL STENTS

F. Charles Brunicardi, MD, FACS
DeBakey/Bard Professor and Chairman
Michael E. DeBakey Department of Surgery
Baylor College of Medicine
Houston, Texas
BENIGN GASTRIC ULCER

L. Michael Brunt, MD
Department of Surgery
Washington University School of Medicine
St. Louis, Missouri
ADRENAL INCIDENTALOMA

Robert F. Buckman, Jr., MD
Langhorne, Pennsylvania
*RETROPERITONEAL INJURIES: KIDNEY AND
URETER*

John R. Burton, MD
Mason F. Lord Professor of Medicine
Division of Geriatric Medicine and
Gerontology
The Johns Hopkins University School of
Medicine
Baltimore, Maryland
*PREOPERATIVE ASSESSMENT OF THE
ELDERLY PATIENT*

Ronald W. Busuttil, MD, PhD
Professor and Chairman
Department of Surgery
The David Geffen School of Medicine at
UCLA
University of California at Los Angeles
Los Angeles, California
*PORTAL HYPERTENSION: ROLE OF LIVER
TRANSPLANTATION*

John Byrne, MCh, FRCSI (Gen)
DEEP VENOUS THROMBOSIS

Frank J. Caliendo, MD
Department of Colon and Rectal Surgery
North Shore University Hospital
Great Neck, New York
CHRONIC ULCERATIVE COLITIS

Andrew M. Cameron, MD, PhD
Department of Surgery
The David Geffen School of Medicine
at UCLA
University of California at Los Angeles
Los Angeles, California
*PORTAL HYPERTENSION: ROLE OF LIVER
TRANSPLANTATION*

Kurtis A. Campbell, MD
Associate Professor
Department of Surgery
The Johns Hopkins Medical Institutions
Baltimore, Maryland
*SMALL BOWEL OBSTRUCTION; INCISIONAL,
EPIGASTRIC, AND UMBILICAL HERNIAS*

Robert J. Canter, MD
Sarcoma Disease Management Program
Department of Surgery
Memorial Sloan-Kettering Cancer Center
New York, New York
SOFT-TISSUE SARCOMA

David J. Caparrelli, MD
Fellow, Division of Cardiac Surgery
The Johns Hopkins Medical Institutions
Baltimore, Maryland
THORACIC OUTLET SYNDROMES

John G. Carson, MD
Department of Surgery
The University of Chicago
Chicago, Illinois
ANORECTAL STRICTURE

Eric T. Castaldo, MD
Resident, Department of Surgery
Vanderbilt University Medical Center
Nashville, Tennessee
*HEPATIC MALIGNANCY: RESECTION VERSUS
TRANSPLANTATION*

Peter A. Cataldo, MD
General Surgery/Urology
Fletcher Allen Health Care
Burlington, Vermont
ANAL FISSURES

Rabih A. Chaer, MD
Vascular Surgery Fellow
New York Presbyterian Hospital
Weill Medical College of Cornell University
Columbia University College of Physicians
and Surgeons
New York, New York
AORTOILIAC OCCLUSIVE DISEASE

Santiago Chahwan, MD
Senior Vascular Resident
Jobst Vascular Center
The Toledo Hospital
Toledo, Ohio
*PERIPHERAL ARTERIAL AND BYPASS GRAFT
OCCLUSION: THROMBOLYTIC THERAPY*

Elliot L. Chaikof, MD, PhD
John E. Skandalakis Professor;
Chief, Division of Vascular Surgery and
Endovascular Therapy
Department of Surgery
Emory University
Atlanta, Georgia
*MANAGEMENT OF PERIPHERAL ARTERIAL
EMBOLISM*

William C. Chapman, MD
Professor and Chief
Section of Transplantation
Washington University in St. Louis
St. Louis, Missouri
BENIGN LIVER LESIONS

Herbert Chen, MD, FACS
Chief, Endocrine Surgery
University of Wisconsin Comprehensive
Cancer Center
Madison, Wisconsin
*MANAGEMENT OF PANCREATIC
ISLET CELL TUMORS EXCLUDING
GASTRINOMA*

Edward H. Chin, MD
Clinical Fellow in Laparoscopic Surgery
Department of Surgery
Mount Sinai School of Medicine
New York, New York
LAPAROSCOPIC NISSEN FUNDOPLICATION

Clifford S. Cho, MD
Department of Surgery
University of Wisconsin School of Medicine
and Public Health
Madison, Wisconsin
GASTRIC ADENOCARCINOMA

Michael A. Choti, MD, MBA, FACS
Jacob C. Handelsman Professor of Surgery
Department of Surgery
The Johns Hopkins University School
of Medicine
Baltimore, Maryland
COLON CANCER

Colleen Christmas, MD
Assistant Professor of Medicine
Division of Geriatric Medicine and
Gerontology
The Johns Hopkins University School of
Medicine
Baltimore, Maryland
*PREOPERATIVE ASSESSMENT OF THE
ELDERLY PATIENT*

James M. Church, MD
Department of Colorectal Surgery
University of Cincinnati
Cleveland, Ohio
SURGERY OF THE POLYPOSIS SYNDROMES

Robert R. Cima, MD, FACS, FASCRS
Assistant Professor of Surgery
Division of Colon and Rectal Surgery
Mayo Clinic
Rochester, Minnesota
STRICTUREPLASTY IN CROHN'S DISEASE

G. Patrick Clagett, MD
Professor and Chairman
Division of Vascular and Endovascular
Surgery
University of Texas Southwestern Medical
Center
Dallas, Texas
PULMONARY THROMBOEMBOLISM

Orlo H. Clark, MD
Department of Surgery
University of California at San Francisco;
Comprehensive Cancer Center at Mount
Zion Medical Center
San Francisco, California
THYROID CANCER

James I. Cohen, MD
Professor, Head and Neck Surgery;
Director of Thyroid/Parathyroid Surgery
Program
Department of Otolaryngology/Head and
Neck Surgery
Oregon Health and Sciences University
Portland, Oregon
*MANAGEMENT OF PHARYNGOESOPHAGEAL
(ZENKER'S) DIVERTICULA*

Paul M. Colombani, MD
Professor of Surgery
The Johns Hopkins Hospital
Baltimore, Maryland
*ESOPHAGEAL ATRESIA AND
TRACHEOESOPHAGEAL FISTULA*

Steven Colquhoun, MD
Director of Liver Transplantation
Cedars-Sinai Medical Center
Beverly Hills, California
BUDD-CHIARI SYNDROME

Anthony J. Comerota, MD, FACS
Jobst Vascular Center
Toledo, Ohio
*PERIPHERAL ARTERIAL AND BYPASS GRAFT
OCCLUSION: THROMBOLYTIC THERAPY*

John J. Como, MD
Assistant Professor of Surgery
Case Western Reserve University;
Division of Trauma
MetroHealth Medical Center
Cleveland, Ohio
*ABNORMAL OPERATIVE AND
POSTOPERATIVE BLEEDING*

Michael S. Conte, MD
Division of Vascular and Endovascular
Surgery
Brigham and Women's Hospital
Boston, Massachusetts
CAROTID ENDARTERECTOMY

Zara Cooper, MD, MSc
Chief Resident in Surgery
Brigham and Women's Hospital
Boston, Massachusetts
ACUTE PANCREATITIS

**Edward E. Cornwell, III, MD, FACS,
FCCM**
Professor of Surgery;
Associate Professor of Anesthesia and
Critical Care Medicine and Department of
Health Policy and Management;
Chief, Adult Trauma Service
The Johns Hopkins Hospital
Baltimore, Maryland
*SPLENIC SALVAGE PROCEDURES:
THERAPEUTIC OPTIONS*

Michael J. Costanza, MD
Assistant Professor of Surgery and
Radiology
State University of New York Upstate
Medical University
College of Medicine
Syracuse, New York
VASCULAR ACCESS

Meagan M. Costedio, MD
Fletcher Allen Health Care
Burlington, Vermont
ANAL FISSURES

Sarah M. Cowgill, MD
Department of Surgery
Tampa General Hospital
Tampa, Florida
*LAPAROSCOPIC REPAIR OF
PARAESOPHAGEAL HERNIAS*

Paul R. Crisostomo
CARDIOVASCULAR PHARMACOLOGY

Martin A. Croce, MD
Professor of Surgery
University of Tennessee
Health Science Center
Memphis, Tennessee
THE MANAGEMENT OF VASCULAR TRAUMA

H. Gill Cryer, III, MD, PhD
Professor of Surgery
Department of Surgery
David Geffen School of Medicine at UCLA
University of California at Los Angeles
Los Angeles, California
PELVIC FRACTURES

Steven C. Cunningham, MD
Resident, Surgery Department
University of Maryland Hospital
Baltimore, Maryland
LIVER HEMANGIOMA; BILE DUCT CANCER

Michael A. Curi, MD, MPA
Assistant Professor of Surgery
University of Maryland School of Medicine
Baltimore, Maryland
ABDOMINAL AORTIC ANEURYSM: OPEN REPAIR

Steven A. Curley, MD
University of Texas M.D. Anderson Cancer Center
Department of Surgical Oncology
Houston, Texas
FACTORS AFFECTING MORBIDITY AND MORTALITY AFTER LIVER RESECTION

Melissa M. Cushing, MD
Transfusion Medicine Fellow
The Johns Hopkins Hospital
Baltimore, Maryland
BLOOD TRANSFUSION THERAPY

Gregory Czuczman, BS
The Johns Hopkins University School of Medicine
Baltimore, Maryland
TRANSJUGULAR INTRAHEPATIC PORTOSYSTEMIC SHUNTS (TIPS)

Alan P. B. Dackiw, MD
Department of Surgery
Division of Endocrine and Oncologic Surgery
Section of Endocrine Surgery
The Johns Hopkins Hospital
Baltimore, Maryland
THYROIDITIS

R. Clement Darling, III, MD
DEEP VENOUS THROMBOSIS

Sebastian G. de la Fuente, MD
General Surgery Resident
Department of Surgery
Duke University
Durham, North Carolina
PALLIATIVE THERAPY FOR PANCREATIC CANCER

A. Lee Dellon, MD
Professor of Plastic Surgery and Neurosurgery
The Johns Hopkins University
Baltimore, Maryland;
Clinical Professor of Plastic Surgery, Neurosurgery, and Anatomy
University of Arizona
Tucson, Arizona
NERVE INJURY AND REPAIR

Ronald P. DeMatteo, MD, FACS
Vice Chair, Department of Surgery;
Chief, Division of General Surgical Oncology
Memorial Sloan-Kettering Cancer Center
New York, New York
SURGERY FOR COLORECTAL LIVER METASTASES

Steven R. DeMeester, MD
Associate Professor
Department of Cardiothoracic Surgery
University of Southern California
Los Angeles, California
ESOPHAGEAL PERFORATION

Tom R. DeMeester, MD
Professor and Chairman
Department of Surgery
Keck School of Medicine
University of Southern California
Los Angeles, California
MANAGEMENT OF ESOPHAGEAL TUMORS

Daniel T. Dempsey, MD
George and Louise Peters Professor and Chairman
Department of Surgery
Temple University
Philadelphia, Pennsylvania
MALLORY-WEISS SYNDROME

Christopher J. Dente, MD
Emory University School of Medicine
Department of Surgery
Atlanta, Georgia
THE SURGEON'S USE OF ULTRASOUND IN THORACOABDOMINAL TRAUMA

Brian G. DeRubertis, MD
Division of Vascular Surgery
New York Presbyterian Hospital
Weill Medical School of Cornell University and Columbia University College of Physicians and Surgeons
New York, New York
RUPTURED ABDOMINAL AORTIC ANEURYSM; AORTOILIAC OCCLUSIVE DISEASE

Joseph DeSimone, MD
Division of Thoracic Surgery
Department of Surgery
The Johns Hopkins Medical Institutions
Baltimore, Maryland
DISORDERS OF ESOPHAGEAL MOTILITY

E. Gene Deune, MD
Associate Professor;
Director, Hand Surgery Section
The Johns Hopkins Hospital Division of Plastic Surgery
Baltimore, Maryland
LYMPHEDEMA

Karen E. Deveney, MD
Professor of Surgery;
Program Director, General Surgery Residency
Oregon Health and Science University
Portland, Oregon
CLOSTRIDIUM DIFFICILE COLITIS

David W. Dietz, MD
Department of Colon and Rectal Surgery
Washington University School of Medicine
St. Louis, Missouri
ANORECTAL ABSCESS AND FISTULA

Matthew R. Dixon, MD
Clinical Fellow
University of Minnesota Medical School
St. Paul, Minnesota
DIVERTICULAR DISEASE OF THE COLON

Todd Dorman, MD
Associate Professor
Department of Anesthesiology and Critical Care Medicine and Surgery
The Johns Hopkins University
Baltimore, Maryland
POSTOPERATIVE RESPIRATORY FAILURE

Thérèse M. Duane, MD
Assistant Professor of Surgery
Virginia Commonwealth University
VCU Medical Center
Richmond, Virginia
THE ABDOMEN THAT WON'T CLOSE

Mark D. Duncan, MD
Associate Professor of Surgery and Oncology
The Johns Hopkins University School of Medicine
Baltimore, Maryland
ACUTE APPENDICITIS

Geoffrey P. Dunn, MD, FACS
Erie, Pennsylvania
SURGICAL PALLIATIVE CARE

Christy Dunst, MD
Foregut Surgery Service
Legacy Health System
Portland, Oregon
MINIMALLY INVASIVE ESOPHAGECTOMY

Soumitra R. Eachempati, MD
Associate Professor of Surgery and Public Health
Weill Medical College of Cornell University
New York, New York
FLUID AND ELECTROLYTE THERAPY

Ignacio A. Echenique
Memorial Sloan-Kettering Cancer Center
New York, New York
THE USE OF ^{18}F-FLUORODEOXYGLUCOSE POSITRON EMISSION TOMOGRAPHY IN THE MANAGEMENT OF COLORECTAL CANCER

Aaron Eckhauser, MD
Surgical Resident, Department of Surgery
Vanderbilt University Medical Center
Nashville, Tennessee
COMPLICATIONS OF LAPAROSCOPIC CHOLECYSTECTOMY

Frederic E. Eckhauser, MD
Professor of Surgery;
Chief, Ravitch Division of General Surgery;
Chief of Clinical Operations
Department of Surgery
The Johns Hopkins Hospital
Baltimore, Maryland
DIVERTICULOSIS OF THE SMALL BOWEL

Rebecca D. Edmonds, MD
Resident in Surgery
University of Pittsburgh
Pittsburgh, Pennsylvania
INJURY TO THE SPLEEN

David T. Efron, MD
Department of Surgery
The Johns Hopkins Hospital
Baltimore, Maryland
GASTROINTESTINAL STROMAL TUMORS

Jennifer Eldred, MB, BS, RD, LD, CNSD
Clinical Dietitian Specialist
The Johns Hopkins Bayview Medical Center
Baltimore, Maryland
FLUID MANAGEMENT AND NUTRITIONAL SUPPORT OF THE BURN PATIENT

C. Neal Ellis, MD
Associate Professor of Surgery
University of South Alabama
Mobile, Alabama
ISCHEMIC COLITIS

E. Christopher Ellison, MD
Associate Vice President for Health Sciences;
Vice Dean of Clinical Affairs;
Robert M. Zollinger Professor and Chair
Department of Surgery
The Ohio State University Medical Center
Columbus, Ohio
DUODENAL ULCER

Nestor F. Esnaola, MD, MPH
Section of Surgical Oncology
Department of Surgery
Medical University of South Carolina
Charleston, South Carolina
FACTORS AFFECTING MORBIDITY AND MORTALITY AFTER LIVER RESECTION

Jesus Esquivel, MD
Director, Peritoneal Surface Malignancy Center
Surgical Oncology
St. Agnes Hospital
Baltimore, Maryland
MANAGEMENT OF PERITONEAL SURFACE MALIGNANCY: THE SURGEON'S ROLE

Douglas B. Evans, MD
The University of Texas M.D. Anderson Cancer Center
Houston, Texas
UNUSUAL PANCREATIC TUMORS

B. Mark Evers, MD
Professor and Robertson Poth Distinguished Chair in General Surgery
Department of Surgery
The University of Texas Medical Branch
Galveston, Texas
SMALL BOWEL CARCINOID TUMORS

Kathryn Evers, MD
Fox Chase Cancer Center
Philadelphia, Pennsylvania
THE ROLE OF STEREOTACTIC BREAST BIOPSY IN THE MANAGEMENT OF BREAST DISEASE

Timothy C. Fabian, MD
University of Tennessee-Memphis
Memphis, Tennessee
RECTAL INJURIES

Katherine Facklis, MD, FACS, FASCRS
Chief, Division of Colon and Rectal Surgery
Cedars-Sinai Medical Center
Los Angeles, California
CONDYLOMA ACUMINATA

Robert Fang, MD
Resident in General Surgery
Mt. Sinai Hospital
Chicago, Illinois
LAPAROSCOPIC REPAIR OF RECURRENT INGUINAL HERNIAS

Mark B. Faries, MD
John Wayne Cancer Institute
Santa Monica, California
CUTANEOUS MELANOMA

Peter L. Faries, MD, FACS
Chief of Vascular Surgery and Professor of Surgery
Mount Sinai School of Medicine
New York, New York
RUPTURED ABDOMINAL AORTIC ANEURYSM

Daniel L. Feingold, MD, FACS
Assistant Professor of Surgery
Section of Colorectal Surgery
Columbia University
New York, New York
LAPAROSCOPIC APPENDECTOMY

David V. Feliciano, MD
Professor of Surgery
Emory University School of Medicine
Chief of Surgery
Grady Memorial Hospital
Atlanta, Georgia
THE MANAGEMENT OF EXTREMITY COMPARTMENT SYNDROME

Charles M. Ferguson, MD
Associate Professor of Surgery
Harvard Medical School
Surgical Residency Program Director
Massachusetts General Hospital
Department of Surgery
Boston, Massachusetts
MESENTERIC VASCULAR DISEASE OF THE SMALL BOWEL

Aaron S. Fink, MD
Professor of Surgery
Emory University School of Medicine
Atlanta;
Manager, Surgical and Perioperative Care
Atlanta Veterans Administration Medical Center
Decatur, Georgia
COLONIC VOLVULUS

Anne C. Fischer, MD, PhD
Pediatric Surgery
The Johns Hopkins Hospital
Baltimore, Maryland
CHEMICAL ESOPHAGEAL INJURIES

Josef E. Fischer, MD, FACS
William V. McDermott Professor of Surgery
Harvard Medical School;
Chairman, Department of Surgery;
Surgeon-in-Chief
Beth Israel Deaconess Medical Center
Boston, Massachusetts
SMALL BOWEL TUMORS

William E. Fischer, MD, FACS
Associate Professor
Michael E. DeBakey Department of Surgery;
Director, the Pancreas Center
Baylor College of Medicine
Houston, Texas
BENIGN GASTRIC ULCER

Elliot K. Fishman, MD
Professor of Radiology
Department of Radiology
The Johns Hopkins Medical Institutions
Baltimore, Maryland
VIRTUAL COLONOSCOPY

Jason B. Fleming, MD
Department of Surgical Oncology
The University of Texas M.D. Anderson Cancer Center
Houston, Texas
UNUSUAL PANCREATIC TUMORS

Phillip Fleshner, MD
Clinical Professor of Surgery
University of California at Los Angeles
School of Medicine;
Program Director, Colorectal Surgery
Residency
Cedars-Sinai Medical Center
Los Angeles, California
CONDYLOMA ACUMINATA

Yuman Fong, MD
Murray F. Brennan Chair in Surgery
Department of Surgery
Memorial Sloan-Kettering Cancer Center
New York, New York
NEWER TECHNIQUES IN LIVER SURGERY

Mehran Fotoohi, MD
*PANCREATIC DUCTAL DISRUPTIONS
LEADING TO PANCREATIC FISTULA,
PANCREATIC ASCITES, OR PLEURAL
EFFUSION*

Paul Freeswick, MD, FACS
Department of Surgery
The Johns Hopkins Bayview Medical Center
Baltimore, Maryland
*CHEST WALL TRAUMA; NECROTIZING SKIN
AND SOFT-TISSUE INFECTIONS*

Julie A. Freischlag, MD
The William Stewart Halsted Professor;
Chair, Department of Surgery;
Surgeon-in-Chief
The Johns Hopkins Medical Institutions
Baltimore, Maryland
THORACIC OUTLET SYNDROMES

Charles M. Friel, MD
Assistant Professor of Surgery
Section of Colon and Rectal Surgery
University of Virginia
*SURGICAL MANAGEMENT OF
CONSTIPATION*

Donald E. Fry, MD, FACS
Professor Emeritus
Department of Surgery
University of New Mexico School of
Medicine
Albuquerque, New Mexico;
Executive Vice-President
Michael Pine and Associates
Chicago, Illinois
ANTIBIOTIC SELECTION IN BILIARY SURGERY

Robert D. Fry, MD
Emilie and Roland deHellebranth Professor
of Surgery;
Chief, Division of Colon and Rectal Surgery
University of Pennsylvania Health System
Philadelphia, Pennsylvania
*RADIATION INJURY TO THE SMALL AND
LARGE BOWEL*

James K. Fullerton, MD
Surgical Endoscopy Fellow
Department of Surgery
University of Louisville School of Medicine
Louisville, Kentucky
CHRONIC PANCREATITIS

Vivian Gahtan, MD
Professor of Surgery
State University of New York Upstate
Medical University
College of Medicine
Syracuse, New York
VASCULAR ACCESS

Susan Galandiuk, MD
Department of Surgery
University of Louisville
Louisville, Kentucky
CROHN'S COLITIS

Richard L. Gamelli, MD, FACS
The Robert J. Freeark Professor and
Chairman
Department of Surgery
Loyola University Medical Center
Maywood, Illinois
BURN WOUND MANAGEMENT

Robert Garvin, MD
General Surgery Resident
The Western Pennsylvania Hospital;
Temple University School of Medicine
Pittsburgh, Pennsylvania
*ACUTE AORTIC DISSECTION AND ITS
COMPLICATIONS*

Robert A. Garwood, MD
Harrisonburg Surgical Associates
Harrisonburg, Virginia
ASYMPTOMATIC (SILENT) GALLSTONES

Colleen B. Gaughan, MD
ESOHAGEAL ACHALASIA

Susan L. Gearhart, MD
Department of Surgery
The Johns Hopkins Hospital
Baltimore, Maryland
*RECTAL PROLAPSE AND OBSTRUCTED
DEFECATION*

Christos S. Georgiades, MD, PhD
Assistant Professor of Radiology and
Surgery
Fellowship Program Director,
Vascular and Interventional Radiology
The Johns Hopkins Hospital
Baltimore, Maryland
*TRANSHEPATIC INTERVENTIONS FOR
OBSTRUCTIVE JAUNDICE; INFERIOR VENA
CAVA FILTERS*

Henning Gerke, MD
Assistant Professor
Division of Gastroenterology and
Hepatology
Department of Internal Medicine
University of Iowa Hospitals and Clinics
Iowa City, Iowa
BARRETT'S ESOPHAGUS

Jean-Francois Geschwind, MD
Associate Professor of Radiology, Surgery,
and Oncology;
Director, Vascular and Interventional
Radiology
The Johns Hopkins University School of
Medicine
Baltimore, Maryland
*TRANSHEPATIC INTERVENTIONS FOR
OBSTRUCTIVE JAUNDICE*

Bruce L. Gewertz, MD
Surgeon-in-Chief;
Chair, Department of Surgery;
Vice-President for Interventional Services
Cedars-Sinai Health System
Los Angeles, California
*BUERGER'S DISEASE (THROMBOANGIITIS
OBLITERANS)*

B. Robert Gibson, MD
The Johns Hopkins Hospital
Baltimore, Maryland
CHEST WALL TRAUMA

Michael K. Gibson, MD
University of Pittsburgh Medical
Center Cancer Pavilion
Pittsburgh, Pennsylvania
*NEOADJUVANT AND ADJUVANT THERAPY
OF ESOPHAGEAL CANCER*

Armando E. Giuliano, MD
Chief of Science and Medicine
John Wayne Cancer Institute
Santa Monica;
Clinical Professor of Surgery
University of California at Los Angeles
Los Angeles, California
*DUCTAL AND LOBULAR CARCINOMA IN SITU
OF THE BREAST*

Sean C. Glasgow, MD
ANORECTAL ABSCESS AND FISTULA

Jerry Goldstone, MD
Professor of Surgery
Case Western Reserve University School of
Medicine;
Chief, Division of Vascular and
Endovascular Surgery
University Hospitals Case Medical Center
Cleveland, Ohio
*MANAGEMENT OF ANEURYSMS OF THE
EXTRACRANIAL CAROTID AND VERTEBRAL
ARTERIES*

Clive S. Grant, MD
Professor of Surgery
Mayo College of Medicine
Rochester, Minnesota
HYPERTHYROIDISM;
PHEOCHROMOCYTOMA

Keith D. Gray, MD
University of Tennessee
Knoxville, Tennessee
MALIGNANT LIVER TUMORS

Sharon G. Gregorcyk, MD, FACS, FASCRS
Attending Colorectal Surgeon
Medical City Dallas Hospital
Dallas, Texas
HEMORRHOIDS

Russell L. Gruen, MBBS, PhD
Fellow in Trauma and Surgical
Critical Care
Harborview Medical Center
University of Washington
Seattle, Washington
HEMOTHORAX

José G. Guillem, MD, MPH
Professor of Surgery
Memorial Sloan-Kettering Cancer Center
New York, New York
THE USE OF ^{18}F-FLUORODEOXYGLUCOSE
POSITRON EMISSION TOMOGRAPHY IN
THE MANAGEMENT OF COLORECTAL
CANCER

Vinay K. Gupta, MD
Department of Surgery
Union Memorial Hospital
Baltimore, Maryland
COMPLICATIONS OF ESOPHAGEAL
SURGERY

Jonathan Haft, MD
Assistant Professor of Surgery
Department of Surgery
University of Michigan
Ann Arbor, Michigan
EXTRACORPOREAL LIFE SUPPORT FOR
RESPIRATORY FAILURE

Jeffrey A. Hagen, MD
Associate Professor of Clinical Surgery
Keck School of Medicine
University of Southern California
Los Angeles, California
ESOPHAGEAL ACHALASIA

Adil H. Haider, MD, MPH
Department of Surgery
The Johns Hopkins University School of
Medicine
Baltimore, Maryland
SPLENIC SALVAGE PROCEDURES:
THERAPEUTIC OPTIONS

Jason F. Hall, MD
Massachusetts General Hospital
Department of Surgery
Boston, Massachusetts
MESENTERIC VASCULAR DISEASE OF THE
SMALL BOWEL

Amy L. Halverson, MD
Assistant Professor of Surgery
Northwestern University
Feinberg School of Medicine
Division of Surgical Oncology
Chicago, Illinois
ACUTE COLONIC PSEUDO-OBSTRUCTION
(OLGILVIE'S SYNDROME)

David C. Han, MD
Division of Vascular Surgery
Pennsylvania State University
Milton S. Hershey Medical Center
Pennsylvania State College of Medicine
Hershey, Pennsylvania
FALSE ANEURYSM AND ARTERIOVENOUS
FISTULA

John B. Hanks, MD
Department of Surgery
University of Virginia Health System
Charlottesville, Virginia
ASYMPTOMATIC (SILENT) GALLSTONES

Sean P. Harbison, MD
Professor of Surgery
Temple University
Philadelphia, Pennsylvania
MALLORY-WEISS SYNDROME

Alden H. Harken, MD
Department of Surgery
University of California at San Francisco-
East Bay
Oakland, California
CARDIOVASCULAR PHARMACOLOGY

John W. Harmon, MD
Department of Surgery
The Johns Hopkins Bayview Medical Center
Baltimore, Maryland
NECROTIZING SKIN AND SOFT-TISSUE
INFECTIONS

Heitham T. Hassoun, MD
Assistant Professor of Surgery
Division of Vascular and Endovascular
Surgery
The Johns Hopkins University School of
Medicine
Baltimore, Maryland
ACUTE MESENTERIC ISCHEMIA

Elliott R. Haut, MD
Assistant Professor of Surgery
Division of Trauma Surgery and Clinical
Care
Department of Surgery
The Johns Hopkins Hospital
Baltimore, Maryland
BLUNT CARDIAC INJURY

David Hazzan, MD
Attending Surgeon
Department of Surgery
Carmel Medical Center
Haifa, Israel
LAPAROSCOPIC NISSEN FUNDOPLICATION

Richard F. Heitmiller, MD
Chief of Surgery
Union Memorial Hospital
Baltimore, Maryland
COMPLICATIONS OF ESOPHAGEAL SURGERY

J. Michael Henderson, MD
The Cleveland Clinic
Department of General Surgery
Cleveland, Ohio
HEPATIC ABSCESS

Peter W. Henderson, MD
Research Assistant, Department of Surgery
Weill Medical College of Cornell University
New York, New York
LYMPHATIC MAPPING AND SENTINEL
LYMPHADENECTOMY

B. Todd Heniford, MD
Chief, Division of Gastrointestinal and
Minimally Invasive Surgery
Department of Surgery
Carolinas Medical Center
Charlotte, North Carolina
LAPAROSCOPIC GASTRIC SURGERY

H. Franklin Herlong, MD
Division of Hepatology/Gastroenterology
The Johns Hopkins Bayview Medical Center
Baltimore, Maryland
REFRACTORY ASCITES

David N. Herndon, MD
Shriners Burn Institute
Galveston, Texas
NUTRITIONAL SUPPORT IN THE
CRITICALLY ILL

Jonathan R. Hiatt, MD
Dumont-UCLA Transplant Center
Department of Surgery
The David Geffen School of Medicine at
UCLA
University of California at Los Angeles
Los Angeles, California
PORTAL HYPERTENSION: ROLE OF LIVER
TRANSPLANTATION

O. Joe Hines, MD
Department of Surgery
David Geffen School of Medicine at UCLA
University of California at Los Angeles
Los Angeles, California
PERIAMPULLARY CANCER

Horacio Hojman, MD
Assistant Professor of Surgery
Section of Trauma and Surgical Critical Care
Yale University School of Medicine
New Haven, Connecticut
ABDOMINAL COMPARTMENT SYNDROME

Michael Holzman, MD, MPH
SPIGELIAN, LUMBAR, AND OBTURATOR HERNIATION

Kelvin Hong, MD
Vascular and Interventional Radiology
The Johns Hopkins Hospital
Baltimore, Maryland
INFERIOR VENA CAVA FILTERS

Karen M. Horton, MD
Associate Professor of Radiology
Department of Radiology
The Johns Hopkins Medical Institutions
Baltimore, Maryland
VIRTUAL COLONOSCOPY

Thomas J. Howard, MD
Professor of Surgery
Indiana University School of Medicine
Indianapolis, Indiana
MANAGEMENT OF GALLSTONE PANCREATITIS

Philip J. Huber, Jr., MD, FACS, FASCRS
Attending Colorectal Surgeon
Medical City Dallas Hospital
Dallas, Texas
HEMORRHOIDS

John G. Hunter, MD, FACS
Mackenzie Professor and Chair
Department of Surgery
Oregon Health and Science University
Portland, Oregon
LAPAROSCOPIC SPLENECTOMY

Jared M. Huston, MD
Resident in General Surgery
Weill Medical College of Cornell University
New York, New York
FLUID AND ELECTROLYTE THERAPY

David F. Hutcheon, MD
Lutherville, Maryland
OBSTRUCTIVE JAUNDICE: ENDOSCOPIC THERAPY

Mark D. Iannettoni, MD
The Johann L. Ehrenhaft Professor and Chairman
Department of Cardiothoracic Surgery
University of Iowa Hospitals and Clinics
Iowa City, Iowa
BARRETT'S ESOPHAGUS

Kenji Inaba, MD
COAGULOPATHY IN THE TRAUMA PATIENT

Jeff Infante, MD
Gastrointestinal Oncology
Sidney Kimmel Comprehensive Cancer Center at Johns Hopkins
Baltimore, Maryland
ADJUVANT TREATMENT FOR COLORECTAL CANCER

Corey W. Iqbal, MD
Resident, Department of Surgery
Mayo Clinic College of Medicine
Rochester, Minnesota
MOTILITY DISORDERS OF THE STOMACH AND SMALL BOWEL

Rao R. Ivatury, MD
Professor and Chair
Department of Surgery
Virginia Commonwealth University
Richmond, Virginia
THE ABDOMEN THAT WON'T CLOSE

Lindsey N. Jackson, MD
Department of Surgery
The University of Texas Medical Branch
Galveston, Texas
SMALL BOWEL CARCINOID TUMORS

Lisa K. Jacobs, MD, FACS
Assistant Professor of Surgery
Division of Surgical Oncology
Department of Surgery
The Johns Hopkins Hospital
Baltimore, Maryland
SCREENING FOR BREAST CANCER

Badar U. Jan, MD
University of Medicine and Dentistry of New Jersey
Department of Surgery
Robert Wood Johnson School of Medicine
New Brunswick, New Jersey
THE SEPTIC RESPONSE

Juan Carlos Jimenez, MD
Los Angeles, California
PERIPHERAL ARTERIAL OCCLUSIVE DISEASE: ANGIOPLASTY, STENTING, AND ENDOVASCULAR GRAFT TREATMENT; GANGRENE OF THE FOOT

Blair A. Jobe, MD
Oregon Health and Science University
Department of Surgery
Portland, Oregon
LAPAROSCOPIC TREATMENT OF ESOPHAGEAL MOTILITY DISORDERS

Kaj H. Johansen, MD, PhD
Director of Vascular Surgical Services
Heart and Vascular Institute
Swedish Medical Center
Seattle, Washington
MANAGEMENT OF CHRONIC MESENTERIC ISCHEMIA

Gregory J. Jurkovich, MD
Professor of Surgery and Director of Trauma
Harborview Medical Center
University of Washington
Seattle, Washington
HEMOTHORAX

Andreas M. Kaiser, MD, FACS
Associate Professor
Department of Colorectal Surgery
Keck School of Medicine
University of Southern California
Los Angeles, California
POSTOPERATIVE ILEUS

Larry R. Kaiser, MD
The John Rhea Barton Professor and Chairman
Department of Surgery
Hospital of the University of Pennsylvania
Philadelphia, Pennsylvania
VIDEO-ASSISTED THORACIC SURGERY

Anthony N. Kalloo, MD
Chief, Division of Gastroenterology and Hepatology
The Johns Hopkins Hospital
Baltimore, Maryland
ENDOSCOPIC THERAPY FOR ESOPHAGEAL VARICEAL HEMORRHAGE

Michael S. Kasparek, MD
Research Fellow, Department of Surgery
Mayo Clinic College of Medicine
Rochester, Minnesota
MOTILITY DISORDERS OF THE STOMACH AND SMALL BOWEL

Edmund S. Kassis, MD
Chief Resident in Surgery
The Johns Hopkins University School of Medicine
Baltimore, Maryland
ENTEROCUTANEOUS FISTULA

Stephen M. Kavic, MD
LAPAROSCOPIC VENTRAL AND INCISION HERNIA REPAIR

Rebecca Kazin, MD
Johns Hopkins Dermatology and Cosmetic Center at Greenspring Station
Lutherville, Maryland
SKIN LESIONS: EVALUATION, DIAGNOSIS, AND MANAGEMENT

Kevin P. Keating, MD
Surgical and Critical Care Department
Hartford Hospital
Hartford, Connecticut
PREOPERATIVE AND POSTOPERATIVE NUTRITIONAL SUPPORT IN THE CRITICALLY ILL

Electron Kebebew, MD, FACS
Associate Professor of Surgery in Residence
University of California at San Francisco
Department of Surgery and UCSF
Comprehensive Cancer Center
San Francisco, California
ADRENOCORTICAL TUMORS

E. Lynne Kelley, MD
Medical Director
Vascular Surgery
Peripheral Interventions
Boston Scientific
Natick, Massachusetts
BALLOON ANGIOPLASTY AND STENTS IN CAROTID ARTERY OCCLUSIVE DISEASE

Dwight C. Kellicut, MD
MANAGEMENT OF TIBIOPERONEAL ARTERIAL OCCLUSIVE DISEASE

K. Craig Kent, MD
Chief of Vascular Surgery
New York Presbyterian Hospital
Weill Medical College of Cornell University
and Columbia University College of
Physicians and Surgeons
New York, New York
AORTOILIAC OCCLUSIVE DISEASE

Christopher Kenyon, MD, FRCSC
Colorectal Surgery Fellow
Department of Surgery
University of Calgary
Calgary, Alberta, Canada
PRURITUS ANI

Kenneth A. Kern, MD, MPH, FACS, FSSO
Director, Oncology Clinical Development
Pfizer Global Research and Development
La Jolla Laboratories
Pfizer, Inc.
San Diego, California
MALE BREAST CANCER

Kenneth A. Kesler, MD
Professor of Surgery
Department of Surgery
Thoracic Division
Indiana University School of Medicine
Indianapolis, Indiana
PRIMARY TUMORS OF THE THYMUS

Leena Khaitan, MD
GROIN HERNIA

H. Alden Kirk, MD
NONOPERATIVE TREATMENT OF CLAUDICATION

Andrew S. Klein, MD, MBA
Director, Comprehensive Transplant Center
Cedars-Sinai Medical Center
Beverly Hills, California
BUDD-CHIARI SYNDROME

V. Suzanne Klimberg, MD
Department of Surgery
Division of Breast Surgical Oncology
University of Arkansas for Medical Sciences
Little Rock, Arkansas
ABLATIVE TECHNIQUES IN THE TREATMENT OF BENIGN AND MALIGNANT BREAST DISEASE

Wayne M. Koch, MD
Department of Otolaryngology-Head and
Neck Surgery
The Johns Hopkins Medical Institutions
Baltimore, Maryland
MANAGEMENT OF THE ISOLATED NECK MASS

Richard A. Kozarek, MD
PANCREATIC DUCTAL DISRUPTIONS LEADING TO PANCREATIC FISTULA, PANCREATIC ASCITES, OR PLEURAL EFFUSION

Helen Krontiras, MD
Assistant Professor of Surgery
Section of Surgical Oncology
University of Alabama at Birmingham
Birmingham, Alabama
CELLULAR, BIOCHEMICAL, AND MOLECULAR TARGETS IN BREAST CANCER

William C. Krupski, MD
Department of Surgery
University of California at San Francisco
San Francisco, California
POPLITEAL AND FEMORAL ARTERY ANEURYSMS

David P. Kuwayama, MD
ABDOMINAL AORTIC ANEURYSM AND UNEXPECTED ABDOMINAL PATHOLOGY

Nicos Labropoulos, PhD
Vascular Surgery
Department of Surgery
University of Medicine and Dentistry of
New Jersey
Newark, New Jersey
DIAGNOSIS OF VENOUS DISEASE

Daniela P. Ladner, MD
GALLBLADDER CANCER

Edward C. S. Lai, MS, FRCS (Ed.), FRACS, FHKCS, FHKAM (Surgery), FACS
Pedder Clinic
Hong Kong S.A.R.
LAPAROSCOPIC HEPATECTOMY

Jeffrey Lamont, MD
MORBID OBESITY

Julie R. Lange, MD, ScM
Department of Surgery
The Johns Hopkins Medical Institutions
Baltimore, Maryland
BENIGN BREAST DISEASE

Peter F. Lawrence, MD, FACS
Director, Gonda (Goldschmied) Vascular
Center
University of California at Los Angeles
Los Angeles, California
GANGRENE OF THE FOOT

Anna M. Ledgerwood, MD
Wayne State University School of Medicine
Detroit, Michigan
BLUNT ABDOMINAL TRAUMA; APPROACH TO LOWER GASTROINTESTINAL BLEEDING

James A. Lee, MD
Fellow in Endocrine Surgery
Department of Surgery
University of California at San Francisco
San Francisco, California
ADRENOCORTICAL TUMORS

Tobias Leibold, MD
Research Fellow, Department of Surgery
Colorectal Service
Memorial Sloan-Kettering Cancer Center
New York, New York
THE USE OF ^{18}F-FLUORODEOXYGLUCOSE POSITRON EMISSION TOMOGRAPHY IN THE MANAGEMENT OF COLORECTAL CANCER

Mark Li, MD, PhD
SPINE AND SPINAL CORD INJURIES

Eleni Liapi, MD
Division of Interventional Radiology
The Johns Hopkins Hospital
Baltimore, Maryland
TRANSHEPATIC INTERVENTIONS FOR OBSTRUCTIVE JAUNDICE

Siong-Seng Liau, MB, ChB Ed, MRCS Ed
IHPBA Kenneth W. Warren Fellow
Department of Surgery
Brigham and Women's Hospital
Harvard Medical School
Boston, Massachusetts
ACUTE CHOLANGITIS

Jane M. Liaw, MD
Transplant Surgery Research Fellow
Department of Surgery
Section of Transplantation
Washington University School of Medicine
St. Louis, Missouri
BENIGN LIVER LESIONS

Anne Lidor, MD, MPH
Department of Surgery
The Johns Hopkins Hospital
Baltimore, Maryland
LAPAROSCOPIC CHOLECYSTECTOMY

Keith D. Lillemoe, MD
Jay L. Grosfeld Professor and Chairman
Department of Surgery
Indiana University School of Medicine
Indianapolis, Indiana
BENIGN BILIARY STRICTURES

Pamela A. Lipsett, MD, FACS, FCCM
Professor of Surgery, Anesthesiology and
Critical Care Medicine and Nursing
The Johns Hopkins University Schools of
Medicine and Nursing
Baltimore, Maryland
CYSTIC DISORDERS OF THE BILE DUCTS

Evan C. Lipsitz, MD
Associate Professor of Surgery
Montefiore Medical Center
Albert Einstein College of Medicine
Bronx, New York
AXILLOFEMORAL BYPASS

Jayme E. Locke, MD
Fellow, Department of Surgery
The Johns Hopkins University School of
Medicine
Baltimore, Maryland
CYSTIC DISORDERS OF THE BILE DUCTS

Ann C. Lowry, MD
Adjunct Professor of Surgery
Division of Colon and Rectal Surgery
University of Minnesota
Edina, Minnesota
SURGICAL MANAGEMENT OF CONSTIPATION

Stephen F. Lowry, MD
College of Medicine and Dentistry of New
Jersey
Robert Wood Johnson School of Medicine
Department of Surgery
New Brunswick, New Jersey
THE SEPTIC RESPONSE

Charles E. Lucas, MD
Department of Surgery
Detroit Receiving Hospital
Detroit, Michigan
*BLUNT ABDOMINAL TRAUMA; APPROACH
TO LOWER GASTROINTESTINAL
BLEEDING*

James D. Luketich, MD
Chief, Division of Thoracic and Foregut
Surgery
University of Pittsburgh Medical Surgery
Pittsburgh, Pennsylvania
*ENDOSCOPIC TREATMENT OF BARRETT'S
ESOPHAGUS*

Alan B. Lumsden, MD, ChB
Professor of Surgery
Division of Vascular Surgery and
Endovascular Therapy
Michael E. DeBakey Department of Surgery
Baylor College of Medicine
Houston, Texas
*PREVENTION OF VENOUS
THROMBOEMBOLISM*

William R. Lynch, MD
Assistant Professor of Thoracic Surgery
Department of Cardiothoracic Surgery
University of Iowa Hospitals and Clinics
Iowa City, Iowa
BARRETT'S ESOPHAGUS

Helen Mabry, MD
John Wayne Cancer Institute
Santa Monica, California
*DUCTAL AND LOBULAR CARCINOMA IN SITU
OF THE BREAST*

David Maccabee, MD, FACS
General Surgery
Hood River, Oregon
LAPAROSCOPIC SPLENECTOMY

Bruce V. MacFadyen, MD, FACS
Moretz Mansberger Professor and
Chairman of Surgery
Medical College of Georgia
Augusta, Georgia
*LAPAROSCOPIC COMMON BILE DUCT
EXPLORATION*

Robert C. Mackersie, MD, FACS
Professor of Surgery
San Francisco General Hospital
San Francisco, California
*AIRWAY MANAGEMENT IN THE TRAUMA
PATIENT*

Anthony R. MacLean, MD
Clinical Assistant Professor
Department of Surgery
University of Calgary;
Faculty Foothills Medical Centre
Calgary, Alberta, Canada
PRURITUS ANI

Priscilla Magno, MD
Division of Gastroenterology and
Hepatology
The Johns Hopkins Medical Institutions
Baltimore, Maryland
*ENDOSCOPIC THERAPY FOR ESOPHAGEAL
VARICEAL HEMORRHAGE*

Thomas Magnuson, MD
*LAPAROSCOPIC SURGERY FOR MORBID
OBESITY*

Najjia N. Mahmoud, MD
Assistant Professor of Surgery
Division of Colon and Rectal Surgery
University of Pennsylvania Health System
Philadelphia, Pennsylvania
*RADIATION INJURY TO THE SMALL AND
LARGE BOWEL*

Ronald V. Maier, MD, FACS
Jane and Donald D. Trunkey Professor and
Vice Chair of Surgery
University of Washington;
Surgeon-in-Chief
Harborview Medical Center
Seattle, Washington
ACID-BASE PROBLEMS

Martin A. Makary, MD, MPH
Assistant Professor of Surgery and Health
Policy and Management
Department of Surgery
The Johns Hopkins University School of
Medicine
Baltimore, Maryland
*ENTEROCUTANEOUS FISTULA;
PREOPERATIVE ASSESSMENT OF THE
ELDERLY PATIENT; DIVERTICULOSIS OF THE
SMALL BOWEL*

Mahmoud B. Malas, MD
Chief of Endovascular Surgery
The Johns Hopkins Bayview Medical Center
Baltimore, Maryland
*ENDOVASCULAR TREATMENT OF
ABDOMINAL AORTIC ANEURYSMS*

Ashkan A. Malayeri, MD
Research Associate
Division of Cardiovascular and
Interventional Radiology
The Johns Hopkins Medical Institutions
Baltimore, Maryland
*TRANSJUGULAR INTRAHEPATIC
PORTOSYSTEMIC SHUNTS (TIPS)*

Ajai K. Malhotra, MD
Assistant Professor of Surgery
Virginia Commonwealth University
VCU Medical Center
Richmond, Virginia
THE ABDOMEN THAT WON'T CLOSE

Michele A. Manahan, MD
*NECROTIZING SKIN AND SOFT-TISSUE
INFECTIONS; BREAST RECONSTRUCTION
FOLLOWING MASTECTOMY: INDICATIONS,
TECHNIQUES, AND RESULTS*

Gregory J. Mancini, MD
Department of Surgery
Division of General Surgery
University of Missouri-Columbia
Columbia, Missouri
*THE MANAGEMENT OF RECURRENT
INGUINAL HERNIA*

George Manis, MD
Vascular Surgery
Department of Surgery
University of Medicine and Dentistry of
New Jersey
Newark, New Jersey
DIAGNOSIS OF VENOUS DISEASE

Paul N. Manson, MD
Professor of Surgery
The Johns Hopkins Medical Institutions
Baltimore, Maryland,
LYMPHEDEMA; FACIAL INJURIES

David A. Margolin, MD
Department of Colon and Rectal Surgery
The Ochsner Clinic Foundation
New Orleans, Louisiana
PREOPERATIVE BOWEL PREPARATION

Michael R. Marohn, DO
Department of Surgery
The Johns Hopkins Hospital
Baltimore, Maryland
SPLENECTOMY FOR HEMATOLOGIC DISORDERS

John C. Marshall, MD
St. Michael's Hospital
Toronto, Ontario, Canada
INTRA-ABDOMINAL INFECTIONS

William Marshall, DO
Director of Trauma;
Associate Director of SICU
St. Francis Hospital and Medical Center
Hartford, Connecticut
NUTRITIONAL SUPPORT IN THE CRITICALLY ILL

Elizabeth A. Martinez, MD
Department of Anesthesiology/Critical Care Medicine
The Johns Hopkins Hospital
Baltimore, Maryland
PERIOPERATIVE CARE AND MONITORING OF THE SURGICAL PATIENT: EVIDENCE-BASED PERFORMANCE PRACTICES

Douglas J. Mathisen, MD
MANAGEMENT OF TRACHEAL STENOSIS

Brent D. Matthews
Section of Hepatobiliary-Pancreatic and Gastrointestinal Surgery
Washington University
St. Louis, Missouri
MANAGEMENT OF COMMON DUCT STONES

Todd M. McCarty, MD
Dallas, Texas
MORBID OBESITY

David A. McClusky, III, MD, FACS
COLONIC VOLVULUS

David W. McFadden, MD, FACS
Stanley S. Fieber Professor and Chair
Department of Surgery;
Surgical Service Leader
Fletcher Allen Health Care
Burlington, Vermont
POSTGASTRECTOMY SYNDROMES

Christopher R. McHenry, MD
Department of Surgery
MetroHealth Medical Center
Cleveland, Ohio
MANAGEMENT OF THYROID NODULES

Thomas McIntyre, MD
Assistant Professor of Surgery
State University of New York Downstate Medical Center
Brooklyn, New York
CYSTS, TUMORS, AND ABSCESSES OF THE SPLEEN

J. Barry McKernan, MD, PhD
Clinical Professor of Surgery
Medical College of Georgia
Augusta;
Center for Videoscopic and Laser Surgery
Woodstock, Georgia
GROIN HERNIA

Norman E. McSwain, Jr., MD, FACS
Professor of Surgery
Tulane University School of Medicine
New Orleans, Louisiana
INITIAL ASSESSMENT AND RESUSCITATION OF TRAUMA PATIENTS: A PRACTICAL, EFFICIENT, AND EVIDENCE-BASED MEDICINE APPROACH

Joseph Keith Melancon, MD
Division of Transplant Surgery
The Johns Hopkins Hospital
Baltimore, Maryland
TRANSPLANTATION OF THE PANCREAS

Daniel R. Meldrum
CARDIOVASCULAR PHARMACOLOGY

John D. Mellinger, MD, FACS
Associate Professor of Surgery
Medical College of Georgia
Augusta, Georgia
LAPAROSCOPIC COMMON BILE DUCT EXPLORATION

Genevieve B. Melton, MD
Fellow in Colorectal Surgery
The Cleveland Clinic
Cleveland, Ohio
ACUTE APPENDICITIS

W. Scott Melvin, MD
Department of Surgery
The Ohio State University
Columbus, Ohio
LAPAROSCOPIC ADRENALECTOMY

Jay Menaker, MD
EMERGENCY DEPARTMENT THORACOTOMY

Pedro Alejandro Mendez-Tellez, MD
Assistant Professor
Department of Anesthesiology and Critical Care Medicine
Department of Surgery
The Johns Hopkins University School of Medicine
Baltimore, Maryland
POSTOPERATIVE RESPIRATORY FAILURE

Robert E. Merritt, MD
Cardiothoracic Surgery Resident
Thoracic Surgery
Massachusetts General Hospital
Boston, Massachusetts
MANAGEMENT OF TRACHEAL STENOSIS

Wells Messersmith, MD
Director, Gastrointestinal Medical Oncology Program;
Visiting Associate Professor
Division of Medical Oncology
University of Colorado Cancer Center
Aurora, Colorado
ADJUVANT TREATMENT FOR COLORECTAL CANCER

Anthony Meyer, MD, PhD
Collin G. Thomas, Jr., MD, Distinguished Professor and Chairman of Surgery
The University of North Carolina School of Medicine
Chapel Hill, North Carolina
ELECTROLYTE DISORDERS

Stephen M. Milner, MB, BS, BDS, FRCS (Ed), FACS
Professor of Plastic Surgery
Department of Surgery
The Johns Hopkins Bayview Medical Center
Baltimore, Maryland
FLUID MANAGEMENT AND NUTRITIONAL SUPPORT OF THE BURN PATIENT; NECROTIZING SKIN AND SOFT-TISSUE INFECTIONS

Yoav Mintz, MD
Surgical Fellow
Department of Surgery
University of California at San Diego
San Diego, California
CROHN'S DISEASE OF THE SMALL BOWEL

John D. Mitchell, MD
Associate Professor of Surgery
Chief, Section of General Thoracic Surgery
University of Colorado Hospital at Denver and Health Sciences Center, Division of Cardiothoracic Surgery
Denver, Colorado
MEDIASTINAL MASSES

Mack C. Mitchell Jr., MD, FACP, FACG
Director of Gastroenterology
The Johns Hopkins Bayview Medical Center
Baltimore, Maryland
HEPATIC ENCEPHALOPATHY

Elizabeth A. Mittendorf, MD
Department of Surgical Oncology
The University of Texas M.D. Anderson
Cancer Center
Houston, Texas
*PERSISTENT OR RECURRENT
HYPERPARATHYROIDISM;
MANAGEMENT OF THYROID NODULES*

Robert C. Moesinger, MD
Intermountain Health Care
McKay-Dee Hospital
Northern Utah Surgeons
Ogden, Utah
LIVER HEMANGIOMA

Daniela Molena, MD
Resident, Department of Surgery
University of Rochester Medical Center
Rochester, New York
ACHALASIA OF THE ESOPHAGUS

Jeffrey F. Moley, MD
Department of Surgery
Washington University School of Medicine
St. Louis, Missouri
ADRENAL INCIDENTALOMA

Frederick A. Moore, MD, FACS
Head, Division of Surgical Critical Care and
Acute Care Surgery
The Methodist Hospital
Houston, Texas
PNEUMOTHORAX

Kevin A. Moreman, MD
REFRACTORY ASCITES

Katherine A. Morgan, MD
Assistant Professor of Surgery
Medical University of South Carolina
Charleston, South Carolina
PANCREATIC ABSCESS

Monica Morrow, MD
Chairman, Department of Surgical
Oncology;
G. Willing Pepper Chair in Cancer Research
Fox Chase Cancer Center
Philadelphia, Pennsylvania
*THE ROLE OF STEREOTACTIC BREAST
BIOPSY IN THE MANAGEMENT OF
BREAST DISEASE*

Donald L. Morton, MD
Director, Melanoma Programs
John Wayne Cancer Institute
Santa Monica, California
CUTANEOUS MELANOMA

Richard J. Mullins, MD
Chief, Trauma/Critical Care Section
Division of General Surgery
Oregon Health and Science University
Portland, Oregon
ACUTE RENAL FAILURE

Peter Muscarella, II, MD
Assistant Professor
Department of Surgery
Division of General and Gastrointestinal
Surgery
The Ohio State University
Columbus, Ohio
GAS GANGRENE OF THE EXTREMITY

Deborah Nagle, MD
Beth Israel Deaconess Hospital
Boston, Massachusetts
LAPAROSCOPIC COLORECTAL SURGERY

Deepak Nair, MD
Division of Vascular Surgery and
Endovascular Therapy
Department of Surgery
Emory University
Atlanta, Georgia
*MANAGEMENT OF PERIPHERAL ARTERIAL
EMBOLISM*

Attila Nakeeb, MD
Associate Professor of Surgery
University of Indiana Medical School
Indianapolis, Indiana
LAPAROSCOPIC PANCREATIC RESECTIONS

**Lena M. Napolitano, MD, FACS,
FCCP, FCCM**
Professor of Surgery
University of Michigan School of Medicine
Ann Arbor, Michigan
*MULTIPLE ORGAN DYSFUNCTION AND
FAILURE*

Vimal K. Narula, MD
Clinical Assistant Professor
Center for Minimally Invasive Surgery
The Ohio State University
Columbus, Ohio
LAPAROSCOPIC ADRENALECTOMY

Rahima Nenshi, MD
Department of Surgery
St. Michael's Hospital
Toronto, Ontario, Canada
INTRA-ABDOMINAL INFECTIONS

Paul M. Ness, MD
Department of Pathology
The Johns Hopkins Hospital
Baltimore, Maryland
BLOOD TRANSFUSION THERAPY

Mark A. Newell, MD, FACS
Assistant Professor of Surgery, Trauma, and
Surgical Critical Care
The Brody School of Medicine at Eastern
Carolina University
Greenville, North Carolina
PANCREATIC AND DUODENAL INJURIES

Lisa A. Newman, MD, MPH, FACS
Associate Professor of Surgery;
Director, Breast Care Center
University of Michigan
Ann Arbor, Michigan
*ADVANCES IN ADJUVANT AND
NEOADJUVANT THERAPY FOR BREAST
CANCER*

Louis L. Nguyen, MD, MBA, MPH
Division of Vascular and Endovascular
Surgery
Brigham and Women's Hospital
Boston, Massachusetts
CAROTID ENDARTERECTOMY

William B. Norbury
*NUTRITIONAL SUPPORT IN THE
CRITICALLY ILL*

Jeffrey A. Norton, MD
Professor of Surgery
Stanford University
Palo Alto, California
ZOLLINGER-ELLISON SYNDROME

Charles S. O'Mara, MD
Mississippi Baptist Medical Center
Associate Professor of Surgery
University Medical Center
Jackson, Mississippi
*NONOPERATIVE TREATMENT OF
CLAUDICATION*

Raymond P. Onders, MD
Director of Minimally Invasive Surgery
University Hospitals of Cleveland;
Associate Professor
Case Western Reserve University School of
Medicine
Cleveland, Ohio
LAPAROSCOPIC INGUINAL HERNIA

Adrian W. Ong, MD, FACS
Assistant Professor of Surgery;
Attending Surgeon
Allegheny General Hospital
Pittsburgh, Pennsylvania
*DAMAGE CONTROL IN THE TRAUMA
PATIENT*

Robert W. O'Rourke, MD
Oregon Health and Science University
Portland, Oregon
*LAPAROSCOPIC TREATMENT OF
ESOPHAGEAL MOTILITY DISORDERS*

H. Leon Pachter, MD, FACS
George David Stewart Professor of Surgery;
Chair, Department of Surgery
New York University Medical Center
New York, New York
DIAPHRAGMATIC INJURIES

Jimmy Pak, MD
Vascular Surgery Fellow
Stanford University Medical Center
Palo Alto, California
PROFUNDA FEMORIS RECONSTRUCTION

Peter J. Pappas, MD
Vascular Surgery
Department of Surgery
University of Medicine and Dentistry of
New Jersey
Newark, New Jersey
DIAGNOSIS OF VENOUS DISEASE

Sam G. Pappas, MD
Surgical Oncology Fellow
Department of Surgery
University of Pittsburgh
Pittsburgh, Pennsylvania
GALLSTONE ILEUS

Theodore N. Pappas, MD
Professor of Surgery
Department of Surgery
Duke University
Durham, North Carolina
*PALLIATIVE THERAPY FOR PANCREATIC
CANCER*

Sanjiv Parikh, MD
Director of Interventional Radiology, Heart
and Vascular Institute
Swedish Medical Center
Seattle, Washington
*MANAGEMENT OF CHRONIC MESENTERIC
ISCHEMIA*

Adrian Park, MD
Campbell and Jeannette Plugge Professor of
Surgery
University of Maryland School of Medicine
Baltimore, Maryland
*LAPAROSCOPIC VENTRAL AND INCISION
HERNIA REPAIR*

Julie E. Park, MD
LYMPHEDEMA

Michael D. Pasquale, MD, FACS
Department of Surgery
Division of Trauma/Surgical Critical Care
Lehigh Valley Hospital
Allentown, Pennsylvania
SPINE AND SPINAL CORD INJURIES

Timothy M. Pawlik, MD, MPH
Department of Surgery
Johns Hopkins Hospital
Baltimore, Maryland
ECHINOCOCCAL DISEASE OF THE LIVER

Jonathan Pearl, MD
Clinical Instructor in Surgery
Case Medical Center
Cleveland, Ohio
LAPAROSCOPIC INGUINAL HERNIA

Eric Peden, MD
Assistant Professor of Surgery
Division of Vascular Surgery and
Endovascular Therapy
Michael E. DeBakey Department of Surgery
Baylor College of Medicine
Houston, Texas
*PREVENTION OF VENOUS
THROMBOEMBOLISM*

Andrew B. Peitzman, MD
Professor of Surgery;
Vice-Chairman, Department of Surgery;
Chief, General Surgery
University of Pittsburgh Medical Center
Pittsburgh, Pensylvania
INJURY TO THE SPLEEN

John H. Pemberton, MD
Professor of Surgery
Mayo Clinic College of Medicine;
Consultant, Colon and Rectal Surgery
Rochester, Minnesota
*STRICTUREPLASTY IN CROHN'S
DISEASE*

Bruce A. Perler, MD
Julius H. Jacobson II Professor of Surgery
Chief, Division of Vascular Surgery
The Johns Hopkins Hospital
Baltimore, Maryland
*MANAGEMENT OF INFECTED VASCULAR
GRAFT*

Nancy D. Perrier, MD, FACS
Associate Director, Multidisciplinary
Endocrine Center
Associate Professor of Surgery
Department of Surgical Oncology
The University of Texas M.D. Anderson
Cancer Center
Houston, Texas
*PERSISTENT OR RECURRENT
HYPERPARATHYROIDISM*

Jeffrey H. Peters, MD
Chairman, Department of Surgery
University of Rochester Medical Center
Rochester, New York
ACHALASIA OF THE ESOPHAGUS

Christian G. Peyré, MD
Esophageal Research Fellow
Department of Surgery
Division of Thoracic and Foregut Surgery
Keck School of Medicine
University of Southern California
Los Angeles, California
*MANAGEMENT OF ESOPHAGEAL
TUMORS*

Kacy Phillips, MD
The University of Texas M.D. Anderson
Cancer Center
Houston, Texas
UNUSUAL PANCREATIC TUMORS

Allan S. Philp, MD
University of Maryland Hospital
Baltimore, Maryland
*TRACHEOSTOMY: TIMING, TECHNIQUES,
AND OUTCOMES*

Vincent J. Picozzi, MD, MMM
Virginia Mason Medical Center
Seattle, Washington
*NEOADJUVANT AND ADJUVANT THERAPY
OF PANCREATIC CANCER*

C. Wright Pinson, MD, MBA
H. William Scott Professor of Surgery
Department of Surgery
Division of Hepatobiliary Surgery and Liver
Transplantation
Vanderbilt University Medical Center
Nashville, Tennessee
*HEPATIC MALIGNANCY: RESECTION VERSUS
TRANSPLANTATION*

Henry A. Pitt, MD
Professor of Surgery
Indiana University School of Medicine
Indianapolis, Indiana
PRIMARY SCLEROSING CHOLANGITIS

Madeleine Poirier, MD
Clinical Instructor
University of Illinois at Chicago
Department of Surgery
Chicago, Illinois
FECAL INCONTINENCE

Todd A. Ponsky, MD
Fellow in Pediatric Surgery
Children's National Medical Center
Washington, D.C.
ACUTE CHOLECYSTITIS

Benjamin K. Poulose, MD, MPH
Chief Resident in General Surgery
Vanderbilt University Medical Center
Nashville, Tennessee
*ENDOLUMINAL APPROACHES TO
GASTROESOPHAGEAL REFLUX DISEASE*

Vitaliy Y. Poylin, MD
Department of Surgery
Beth Israel Deaconess Medical Center
Boston, Massachusetts
SMALL BOWEL TUMORS

John A. Procaccino, MD
Chief, Division of Colon and Rectal Surgery
Department of Surgery
North Shore University Hospital
Manhasset, New York
CHRONIC ULCERATIVE COLITIS

Reuven Rabinovici, MD, FACS
Professor and Chief, Division of Trauma
Tufts-New England Medical Center
Boston, Massachusetts
ABDOMINAL COMPARTMENT SYNDROME

Janice F. Rafferty, MD
Associate Professor;
Chief, Division of Colon and Rectal Surgery
University of Cincinnati Department of
Surgery
Cincinnati, Ohio
SOLITARY RECTAL ULCER SYNDROME

Jan Rakinic, MD, FACS, FASCRS
Associate Professor of Surgery
Southern Illinois University School of
Medicine
Springfield, Illinois
*MODERN MANAGEMENT OF PILONIDAL
DISEASE*

Bruce Ramshaw, MD, FACS
Associate Professor;
Chief, Division of General Surgery
University of Missouri-Columbia
Columbia, Missouri
*THE MANAGEMENT OF RECURRENT
INGUINAL HERNIA*

Thomas Rauth, MD, MPH
*SPIGELIAN, LUMBAR, AND OBTURATOR
HERNIATION*

Thomas E. Read, MD
Department of Surgery
Western Pennsylvania Hospital
Pittsburgh, Pennsylvania,
*LAPAROSCOPIC MANAGEMENT OF
CROHN'S DISEASE*

Howard A. Reber, MD
Section of Gastrointestinal Surgery
Department of Surgery
David Geffen School of Medicine at UCLA
University of California at Los Angeles
Los Angeles, California
PERIAMPULLARY CANCER

Richard J. Redett, MD
Assistant Professor, Plastic and
Reconstructive Surgery
The Johns Hopkins Hospital
Baltimore, Maryland
HAND INFECTIONS

Thomas Reifsnyder, MD
Assistant Professor of Surgery
The Johns Hopkins Bayview Medical Center
Baltimore, Maryland
*ACUTE AORTIC DISSECTION AND ITS
COMPLICATIONS*

Patrick M. Reilly, MD, FACS
Associate Professor
Division of Traumatology and Surgical
Critical Care
Department of Surgery
University of Pennsylvania School of
Medicine
Philadelphia, Pennsylvania
PENETRATING NECK TRAUMA

Peter Rhee, MD, MPH
Director of NRRC;
Professor of Surgery/Molecular Cellular
Biology
Los Angeles, California
*COAGULOPATHY IN THE TRAUMA
PATIENT*

Taylor S. Riall, MD
Assistant Professor
Department of Surgery
University of Texas Medical Branch
Galveston, Texas
*INTRADUCTAL PAPILLARY MUCINOUS
NEOPLASMS OF THE PANCREAS*

Dario Ribero, MD
Department of Surgical Oncology
The University of Texas M.D. Anderson
Cancer Center
Houston, Texas
MALIGNANT LIVER TUMORS

Samuel E. Rice-Townsend, MD
ZOLLINGER-ELLISON SYNDROME

William O. Richards, MD
Director of Laparoscopic Surgery
Vanderbilt University Medical Center
Nashville, Tennessee
*ENDOLUMINAL APPROACHES TO
GASTROESOPHAGEAL REFLUX DISEASE*

J. David Richardson, MD
Department of Surgery
University of Louisville
Louisville, Kentucky
INJURIES TO THE SMALL AND LARGE BOWEL

Layton F. Rikkers, MD
A.R. Curreri Professor;
Chairman, Department of Surgery
University of Washington School of
Medicine and Public Health
Madison, Wisconsin
*PORTAL HYPERTENSION: THE ROLE OF
SHUNTING PROCEDURES*

Sean P. Roddy, MD
The Vascular Group, PLLC
Albany, New York
DEEP VENOUS THROMBOSIS

Aurelio Rodriguez, MD, FACS
Chief, Division of Trauma Surgery
Allegheny General Hospital
Pittsburgh, Pennsylvania
*DAMAGE CONTROL IN THE TRAUMA
PATIENT*

Sanziana A. Roman, MD, FACS
Chief, Division of Endocrine Surgery;
Assistant Professor of Surgery
Yale University School of Medicine
New Haven, Connecticut
*SECONDARY AND TERTIARY
HYPERPARATHYROIDISM; PRIMARY
HYPERPARATHYROIDISM*

Glen S. Roseborough, MD
Assistant Professor of Surgery
Division of Vascular Surgery
The Johns Hopkins Hospital
Baltimore, Maryland
*ABDOMINAL AORTIC ANEURYSM AND
UNEXPECTED ABDOMINAL PATHOLOGY:
HOW TO MAKE THE RIGHT DECISION*

Frank Rosemeier, MD, MRCP
*ENDOCRINE CHANGES WITH CRITICAL
ILLNESS*

Alexander S. Rosemurgy, II, MD
Professor of Surgery
University of South Florida
Tampa General Hospital
Tampa, Florida
*LAPAROSCOPIC REPAIR OF
PARAESOPHAGEAL HERNIAS*

Michael Rosen, MD
Assistant Professor of Surgery;
Director of Case Comprehensive Hernia
Center
Case Medical Center
Cleveland, Ohio
LAPAROSCOPIC INGUINAL HERNIA

David Rosenthal, MD
Program Director, Department of General
Surgery;
Chief of Vascular Surgery
Atlanta Medical Center
Atlanta, Georgia
FEMOROPOPLITEAL OCCLUSIVE DISEASE

Robert H. Rosenwasser, MD
Professor and Chairman
Department of Neurosurgery
Thomas Jefferson University
Philadelphia, Pennsylvania
*MANAGEMENT OF RECURRENT CAROTID
STENOSIS*

Gedge D. Rosson, MD
Assistant Professor
Division of Plastic Surgery
The Johns Hopkins University School of
Medicine;
Johns Hopkins Outpatient Center
Baltimore, Maryland
NERVE INJURY AND REPAIR

Michael F. Rotondo, MD
Greenville, North Carolina
PANCREATIC AND DUODENAL INJURIES

Grace S. Rozycki, MD, RDMS, FACS
Department of Surgery
Emory University School of Medicine
Atlanta, Georgia
*THE SURGEON'S USE OF ULTRASOUND IN
THORACOABDOMINAL TRAUMA*

Brian G. Rubin, MD
Professor of Surgery
Washington University School of Medicine
St. Louis, Missouri
ABDOMINAL AORTIC ANEURYSM: OPEN REPAIR

Udo Rudloff, MD
Department of Surgery
New York University Medical Center
New York, New York
DIAPHRAGMATIC INJURIES

G.D. Rushing, MD
PENETRATING ABDOMINAL TRAUMA

Barry A. Salky, MD, FACS
Franz W. Sichel Professor of Surgery
The Mount Sinai Medical Center
New York, New York
LAPAROSCOPIC NISSEN FUNDOPLICATION

Michael G. Sarr, MD
James C. Masson Professor of Surgery
Mayo Clinic College of Medicine
Rochester, Minnesota
MOTILITY DISORDERS OF THE STOMACH AND SMALL BOWEL

Thomas M. Scalea, MD, FACS
Physician-in-Chief, Shock Trauma Center
University of Maryland School of Medicine
Baltimore, Maryland
EMERGENCY DEPARTMENT THORACOTOMY; TRACHEOSTOMY: TIMING, TECHNIQUES, AND OUTCOMES

Carol R. Schermer, MD, MPH, FACS
Associate Professor of Surgery
Division of Trauma
Surgical Critical Care and Burns
Loyola University Medical Center
Maywood, Illinois
CATHETER SEPSIS IN THE INTENSIVE CARE UNIT

Matthew J. Schuchert, MD
ENDOSCOPIC TREATMENT OF BARRETT'S ESOPHAGUS

Richard D. Schulick, MD, FACS
Chief, Cameron Division of Surgical Oncology;
Associate Professor of Surgery, Oncology, and Obstetrics and Gynocology;
John L. Cameron Endowed Chair in Surgery
The Johns Hopkins Medical Institutions
Baltimore, Maryland
BILE DUCT CANCER

Michael Schweitzer, MD, FACS
Assistant Professor of Surgery
The Johns Hopkins University School of Medicine;
Director of Minimally Invasive Bariatric Surgery
The Johns Hopkins Bayview Medical Center
Department of Surgery
Baltimore, Maryland
LAPAROSCOPIC SURGERY FOR MORBID OBESITY

Molly L. Sebastian, MD
Minimally Invasive Surgery Fellow
The Johns Hopkins Hospital
Baltimore, Maryland
SPLENECTOMY FOR HEMATOLOGIC DISORDERS

Anthony J. Senagore, MD, MS, MBA
Vice President of Research and Education
Spectrum Health
Grand Rapids, Michigan
COLORECTAL POLYPS

Anna Serur, MD
CHRONIC ULCERATIVE COLITIS

Kenneth W. Sharp, MD
Professor of Surgery;
Chief, Division of General Surgery
Vanderbilt University Medical Center
Nashville, Tennessee
COMPLICATIONS OF LAPAROSCOPIC CHOLECYSTECTOMY

Alexander D. Shepard, MD
Program Director, Surgery Residency
Department of Surgery
Henry Ford Hospital
Detroit, Michigan
UPPER EXTREMITY ARTERIAL OCCLUSIVE DISEASE

Brett C. Sheppard, MD
Division of General Surgery
Department of Surgery
Oregon Health and Science University
Portland, Oregon
LAPAROSCOPIC MANAGEMENT OF PANCREATIC PSEUDOCYST

Michele A. Shermak, MD
Assistant Professor
Division of Plastic Surgery and Reconstructive Surgery
The Johns Hopkins Bayview Medical Center
Baltimore, Maryland,
SKIN LESIONS: EVALUATION, DIAGNOSIS, AND MANAGEMENT

J. Timothy Sherwood, MD
Virginia Cardiovascular and Thoracic Surgery, Inc.;
Mary Washington Hospital
Fredericksburg, Virginia
MEDIASTINAL MASSES

Gregorio A. Sicard, MD
Washington University School of Medicine
St. Louis, Missouri
REYNAUD'S SYNDROME

Adnan H. Siddiqui, MD, PhD
Assistant Professor
Department of Neurosurgery
State University of New York at Buffalo
Neurosurgery, Inc.
Buffalo, New York
MANAGEMENT OF RECURRENT CAROTID STENOSIS

Kristen C. Sihler, MD, MS
University of Michigan Health System
Ann Arbor, Michigan
ACID-BASE PROBLEMS

Geoffrey M. Silver, MD
BURN WOUND MANAGEMENT

Rache M. Simmons, MD, FACS
Associate Professor of Surgical Oncology
Weill Medical College of Cornell University
New York, New York
LYMPHATIC MAPPING AND SENTINEL LYMPHADENECTOMY

Brett A. Simon, MD, PhD
Associate Professor;
Vice Chair for Faculty Development;
Chief, Division of Adult Anesthesia
Johns Hopkins Department of Anesthesiology/Critical Care Medicine
The Johns Hopkins Hospital
Baltimore, Maryland
PERIOPERATIVE CARE AND MONITORING OF THE SURGICAL PATIENT: EVIDENCE-BASED PERFORMANCE PRACTICES

Conrad H. Simpfendorfer, MD
The Cleveland Clinic
Department of General Surgery
Cleveland, Ohio
HEPATIC ABSCESS

Carrie A. Sims, MD
Assistant Professor
Division of Traumatology and Surgical
Critical Care
Department of Surgery
University of Pennsylvania School of
Medicine
Philadelphia, Pennsylvania
PENETRATING NECK TRAUMA

Samuel Singer, MD
Chief, Sarcoma Disease Management Team;
Associate Professor of Surgery
Weill Medical College of Cornell University;
Associate Attending
Department of Surgery
Memorial Sloan-Kettering Cancer Center
New York, New York
SOFT-TISSUE SARCOMA

Navin Singh, MD, MBA, FACS
Director of Breast Reconstruction;
Program Director, Plastic Surgery Residency
The Johns Hopkins Hospital
Baltimore, Maryland
*BREAST RECONSTRUCTION FOLLOWING
MASTECTOMY: INDICATIONS, TECHNIQUES,
AND RESULTS*

Vijay A. Singh, MD
Burn Fellow
Johns Hopkins Burn Center
Baltimore, Maryland
*FLUID MANAGEMENT AND NUTRITIONAL
SUPPORT OF THE BURN PATIENT*

Sunil Singhal, MD
Senior Resident, Cardiothoracic Surgery
Hospital of the University of
Pennsylvania
Philadelphia, Pennsylvania
VIDEO-ASSISTED THORACIC SURGERY

S. Eva Singletary, MD, FACS
Department of Surgical Oncology
The University of Texas M.D. Anderson
Cancer Center
Houston, Texas
INFLAMMATORY BREAST CANCER

Esther Situ
NUTRITIONAL SUPPORT IN THE CRITICALLY ILL

Robert R. Slater, MD
Administrative Chief Resident
Department of Surgery
Henry Ford Hospital
Detroit, Michigan
*UPPER EXTREMITY ARTERIAL OCCLUSIVE
DISEASE*

C. Daniel Smith, MD, FACS
Professor and Chair, Department of Surgery
Mayo Clinic
Jacksonville, Florida
PARAESOPHAGEAL HIATAL HERNIA

Dane E. Smith, MD
*MANAGEMENT OF TIBIOPERONEAL
ARTERIAL OCCLUSIVE DISEASE*

Lee E. Smith, MD
Washington, D.C.
TUMORS OF THE ANAL REGION

Stephen T. Smith, MD
Assistant Professor
Division of Vascular and Endovascular
Surgery
Department of Surgery
University of Texas Southwestern Medical
Center
Dallas, Texas
PULMONARY THROMBOEMBOLISM

Joseph S. Solomkin, MD
Department of Surgery
Division of Trauma and Critical Care
University of Cincinnati
College of Medicine
Cincinnati, Ohio
*ANTIFUNGAL THERAPY IN THE SURGICAL
PATIENT*

Christopher J. Sonnenday, MD, MHS
Transplant Surgery Fellow;
Clinical Lecturer
University of Michigan School of Medicine
Ann Arbor, Michigan
LIVER INJURY

Nathaniel J. Soper, MD
Vice Chair of Clinical Affairs
Northwestern University
Chicago, Illinois
GASTROESOPHAGEAL REFLUX DISEASE

Julie Ann Sosa, M.A, MD, FACS
Assistant Professor of Surgery and Clinical
Epidemiology
Yale University School of Medicine
New Haven, Connecticut
*SECONDARY AND TERTIARY
HYPERPARATHYROIDISM*

Robert J. Spence, MD, FACS
The Johns Hopkins Bayview Medical Center
Baltimore, Maryland
*COLD INJURY; ELECTRICAL AND LIGHTNING
INJURIES*

Michael J. Stamos, MD
Professor of Surgery;
Chief, Division of Colon and Rectal
Surgery;
Vice-Chair, Department of Surgery
University of California at Irvine School of
Medicine
Orange, California
ANORECTAL STRICTURE

Kimberly Steele, MD
LAPAROSCOPIC CHOLECYSTECTOMY

James A. Stefater
Department of Surgery
Division of Endocrine and Oncologic
Surgery
Section of Endocrine Surgery
The Johns Hopkins Hospital
Baltimore, Maryland
THYROIDITIS

Hugo St-Hilaire, MD, DDS
Fellow, Division Plastic and Reconstructive
Surgery
Department of Surgery
Louisiana State University
New Orleans, Louisiana
HAND INFECTIONS

Patrick A. Stone, MD
Assistant Professor of Surgery
Department of Vascular Surgery
West Virginia College of Medicine
Charleston, West Virginia
*DIABETIC FOOT; BRACHIOCEPHALIC
RECONSTRUCTION*

Steven M. Strasberg, MD
Washington University
St. Louis, Missouri
*MANAGEMENT OF COMMON DUCT
STONES*

Michael B. Streiff, MD
Assistant Professor of Medicine and
Pathology
The Johns Hopkins Medical Institutions
Baltimore, Maryland
*COAGULOPATHY IN THE CRITICALLY
ILL PATIENT*

Paul H. Sugarbaker, MD, FACS, FRCS
Washington Cancer Institute
Washington, D.C.
*MANAGEMENT OF PERITONEAL SURFACE
MALIGNANCY: THE SURGEON'S ROLE*

Choichi Sugawa, MD
*APPROACH TO LOWER GASTROINTESTINAL
BLEEDING*

Magesh Sundaram, MD, FACS
POSTGASTRECTOMY SYNDROMES

Lee L. Swanstrom, MD
Division of Minimally Invasive Surgery
Legacy Health System
Portland, Oregon
MINIMALLY INVASIVE ESOPHAGECTOMY

Mark A. Talamini, MD
Professor and Chairman
Department of Surgery
University of California at San Diego
San Diego, California
CROHN'S DISEASE OF THE SMALL BOWEL

Eric P. Tamm, MD
The University of Texas M.D. Anderson
Cancer Center
Houston, Texas
UNUSUAL PANCREATIC TUMORS

Miguel Tan, MD, CM, MSc, FRCS
Assistant Professor of Surgery
The Johns Hopkins University School
of Medicine
Baltimore, Maryland
TRANSPLANTATION OF THE PANCREAS

Julin F. Tang, MD, MS
*AIRWAY MANAGEMENT IN THE TRAUMA
PATIENT*

John Tarpley, MD
Professor of Surgery
Vanderbilt University Medical Center
Nashville, Tennessee
*SPIGELIAN, LUMBAR, AND OBTURATOR
HERNIATION*

Kevin E. Taubman, MD
Fellow in Vascular Surgery
Pennsylvania State University
Milton S. Hershey Medical Center
Hershey, Pennsylvania
*FALSE ANEURYSM AND ARTERIOVENOUS
FISTULA*

Rebecca Taylor, MD
Clinical Fellow
Memorial Sloan-Kettering Cancer Center
New York, New York
NEWER TECHNIQUES IN LIVER SURGERY

Spence M. Taylor, MD
Academic Department of Surgery
Greenville Hospital System University
Medical Center
Greenville, South Carolina
*MANAGEMENT OF TIBIOPERONEAL
ARTERIAL OCCLUSIVE DISEASE*

Swee H. Teh, MD
Department of Surgery
Oregon Health and Science University
Portland, Oregon
*LAPAROSCOPIC MANAGEMENT OF
PANCREATIC PSEUDOCYST*

Geoffrey B. Thompson, MD
Professor of Surgery
Mayo Clinic College of Medicine;
Consultant, Division of Gastroenterologic
and General Surgery
Mayo Clinic
Rochester, Minnesota
*HYPERTHYROIDISM;
PHEOCHROMOCYTOMA*

Jon S. Thompson, MD
Department of Surgery
University of Nebraska Medical Center
Omaha, Nebraska
*MANAGEMENT OF THE SHORT BOWEL
SYNDROME*

Robert W. Thomsen, MD
Department of Anesthesiology
The Johns Hopkins Hospital
Baltimore, Maryland
*PERIOPERATIVE CARE AND MONITORING OF
THE SURGICAL PATIENT: EVIDENCE-BASED
PERFORMANCE PRACTICES*

Alan G. Thorson, MD, FACS
Omaha, Nebraska
RECTOVAGINAL FISTULA

S. Rob Todd, MD, FACS
Surgical Critical Care and Acute Care
Surgery
The Methodist Hospital
Houston, Texas
PNEUMOTHORAX

N. Anh Tran, MD
Resident in Colon and Rectal Surgery
Creighton University School of Medicine
Omaha, Nebraska
RECTOVAGINAL FISTULA

L. William Traverso, MD
Clinical Professor of Surgery
University of Washington;
Director of Digestive Disease Institute
(Pancreas)
Virginia Mason Medical Center
Seattle, Washington
*PANCREATIC DUCTAL DISRUPTIONS
LEADING TO PANCREATIC FISTULA,
PANCREATIC ASCITES, OR PLEURAL
EFFUSION*

**Judith L. Trudel, MD, MSc, MHPE,
FRCSC, FACS**
Adjunct Associate Professor of Surgery
University of Minnesota Medical School
St. Paul, Minnesota
DIVERTICULAR DISEASE OF THE COLON

Theodore N. Tsangaris, MD, FACS
Associate Professor of Surgery;
Chief of Breast Surgery
Division of Oncology;
Director, Johns Hopkins Avon Breast Center
The Johns Hopkins Medical Institutions
Baltimore, Maryland
*THE MANAGEMENT OF RECURRENT
AND DISSEMINATED BREAST CANCER*

Anthony P. Tufaro, DDS, MD, FACS
*INCISIONAL, EPIGASTRIC, AND UMBILICAL
HERNIAS*

David E. Tunkel, MD
Department of Otolaryngology-Head and
Neck Surgery
The Johns Hopkins Medical Institutions
Baltimore, Maryland
*MANAGEMENT OF THE ISOLATED NECK
MASS*

Robert Udelsman, MD, MBA
Lampman Professor of Surgery and
Chairman
Department of Surgery
Yale University School of Medicine
New Haven, Connecticut
PRIMARY HYPERPARATHYROIDISM

Marshall M. Urist, MD
University of Alabama at Birmingham
Birmingham, Alabama
BREAST CANCER: SURGICAL THERAPY

Anatolie Usatii, MD
Clinical Instructor House Staff
Department of Surgery
The Ohio State University Health Sciences
Center
Columbus, Ohio
DUODENAL ULCER

Thomas Vargish, MD
Chairman, Department of Surgery
Mt. Sinai Hospital
Chicago, Illinois
*LAPAROSCOPIC REPAIR OF RECURRENT
INGUINAL HERNIAS*

Jean-Nicolas Vauthey, MD
Department of Surgical Oncology
The University of Texas M.D.
Anderson Cancer Center
Houston, Texas
MALIGNANT LIVER TUMORS

Ravi Veeraswamy, MD
Assistant Professor of Surgery
Emory University
Atlanta, Georgia
REYNAUD'S SYNDROME

Gary A. Vercruysse, MD
Assistant Professor of Surgery, General
Surgery, Trauma, and Surgical Critical Care
Emory University School of Medicine
Atlanta, Georgia
PNEUMOTHORAX

Gary C. Vitale, MD
Professor of Surgery
University of Louisville
Health Sciences Center
Louisville, Kentucky
CHRONIC PANCREATITIS

Carl-Magnus Wahlgren, MD
Fellow, Department of Surgery
University of Chicago
Chicago, Illinois
*BUERGER'S DISEASE (THROMBOANGIITIS
OBLITERANS)*

Brett Waibel, MD
Assistant Professor of Surgery
East Carolina University
The Brody School of Medicine
Greenville, North Carolina
ELECTROLYTE DISORDERS

Andrew L. Warshaw, MD
W. Gerald Austen Professor of Surgery
Harvard Medical School;
Surgeon-in-Chief and Chairman
Department of Surgery
Massachusetts General Hospital
Boston, Massachusetts
*PANCREAS DIVISUM AND OTHER VARIANTS
OF DOMINANT DORSAL DUCT ANATOMY*

William C. Watson
GAS GANGRENE OF THE EXTREMITY

Jordan A. Weinberg, MD
Assistant Professor
Department of Surgery
Section of Trauma, Burns, and Surgical
Critical Care
University of Alabama at Birmingham
Birmingham, Alabama
RECTAL INJURIES

Jon David Weingart, MD
Department of Neurosurgery
The Johns Hopkins Hospital
Baltimore, Maryland
HEAD INJURIES

Edward E. Whang, MD
Associate Professor of Surgery
Division of General and Gastrointestinal
Surgery
Brigham and Women's Hospital
Boston, Massachusetts
ACUTE CHOLANGITIS

**Richard L. Whelan, MD, FACS,
FASCRS**
Department of Surgery
New York Presbyterian Hospital
New York, New York
LAPAROSCOPIC APPENDECTOMY

Charles B. Whitlow, MD
Department of Colon and Rectal Surgery
Ochsner Clinic Foundation
New Orleans, Louisiana
PREOPERATIVE BOWEL PREPARATION

Richard I. Whyte, MD, MBA
Stanford University School of Medicine
Department of Cardiothoracic Surgery
Palo Alto, California
PRIMARY CHEST WALL TUMORS

G. Melville Williams, MD
Department of Surgery
The Johns Hopkins Hospital
Baltimore, Maryland
*TRANSPERITONEAL VERSUS
RETROPERITONEAL APPROACH TO THE AORTA*

Valerie A. Williams, MD
Thoracic/Foregut Research Fellow
Department of Surgery
University of Rochester Medical Center
Rochester, New York
ACHALASIA OF THE ESOPHAGUS

Brian J. Winkleman, MD
Clinical Instructor House Staff
Department of Surgery
The Ohio State University Health Sciences
Center
Columbus, Ohio
DUODENAL ULCER

Brad Winters, MD
Department of Anesthesiology
and Critical Care Medicine
The Johns Hopkins Hospital
Baltimore, Maryland
*ANALGESIA AND SEDATION IN CRITICAL
CARE MEDICINE*

Bruce G. Wolff, MD
Professor of Surgery
Mayo Clinic College of Medicine;
Chair, Division of Colon and Rectal Surgery
Rochester, Minnesota
LARGE BOWEL OBSTRUCTION

Virginia L. Wong, MD
Division of Vascular and Endovascular
Surgery
University Hospitals Case Medical Center
Cleveland, Ohio
*MANAGEMENT OF ANEURYSMS OF THE
EXTRACRANIAL CAROTID AND VERTEBRAL
ARTERIES*

Kenneth J. Woodside, MD
Chief Resident
Department of Surgery
University of Texas Medical Branch
Galveston, Texas
*INTRADUCTAL PAPILLARY MUCINOUS
NEOPLASMS OF THE PANCREAS*

Sherry M. Wren, MD
Professor of Surgery
Stanford University Department of Surgery;
Chief, General Surgery
Palo Alto Veterans Hospital
Palo Alto, California
GALLBLADDER CANCER

Cameron D. Wright, MD
Massachusetts General Hospital
Boston, Massachusetts
*THE MANAGEMENT OF ACQUIRED
ESOPHAGEAL RESPIRATORY TRACT FISTULA*

Stephen C. Yang, MD
Chief of Thoracic Surgery
The Johns Hopkins Medical Institutions
Baltimore, Maryland
DISORDERS OF ESOPHAGEAL MOTILITY

Jerry R. Youkey, MD
*MANAGEMENT OF TIBIOPERONEAL
ARTERIAL OCCLUSIVE DISEASE*

Charles J. Yowler, MD
Associate Professor of Surgery
MetroHealth Medical Center
Cleveland, Ohio
*ABNORMAL OPERATIVE AND
POSTOPERATIVE BLEEDING*

Christopher K. Zarins, MD
Chidester Professor of Surgery
Department of Surgery
Stanford University Medical Center
Palo Alto, California
PROFUNDA FEMORIS RECONSTRUCTION

Rasa Zarnegar, MD
Department of Surgery
University of California at San Francisco
Comprehensive Cancer Center at Mount
Zion Medical Center
San Francisco, California
THYROID CANCER

Ben L. Zarzaur, MD, MPH
Department of Surgery
University of Tennessee, Health Science
Center
Memphis, Tennessee
*CATHETER SEPSIS IN THE INTENSIVE CARE
UNIT; THE MANAGEMENT OF VASCULAR
TRAUMA*

Martha A. Zeiger, MD
Department of Surgery
The Johns Hopkins Hospital
Baltimore, Maryland
NONTOXIC GOITER

Harry Zemon, MD
Hudson Valley Surgical Group
Sleepy Hollow, New York
ACUTE CHOLECYSTITIS

Michael E. Zenilman, MD
Department of Surgery
State University of New York Downstate
Medical Center
Brooklyn, New York
*CYSTS, TUMORS, AND ABSCESSES OF THE
SPLEEN*

R. Eugene Zierler, MD
University of Washington
Department of Surgery
Seattle, Washington
*ATHEROSCLEROTIC RENOVASCULAR
DISEASE*

Nicholas J. Zyromski, MD
Assistant Professor of Surgery
Indiana University School of Medicine
Indianapolis, Indiana
PRIMARY SCLEROSING CHOLANGITIS

PREFACE

I wrote the Preface for the first edition of *Current Surgical Therapy* in January 1984, more than 23 years ago. The book has become more popular and more widely distributed with each edition. The ability to open a book and quickly find a concise description of the current therapy for a surgical disease, often with operative drawings, has led to a large following of residents, fellows, and attending surgeons. The book clearly has found a niche. Besides serving a need, a major benefit to me is the ability to review what surgeons throughout the United States, including some international surgeons, consider to be the most important and up-to-date current therapy in their areas of expertise. I continue to be active surgically, and operate 5 days a week. Editing this textbook every 3 years has allowed me to continue to remain current in virtually all areas of general surgery. This book has provided that same opportunity to thousands of surgeons over the last 20-plus years.

The ninth edition contains approximately 270 chapters, with virtually all new authors. In only two or three instances are the authors for this edition the same as for the eighth edition. In those exceptions I could not find another author to agree to write the chapter because they felt the chapter from the eighth edition could not be improved upon. This edition should not be used as the only source for reviewing current surgical therapy for a specific surgical disease. Unlike many excellent general surgical textbooks, which contain complete discussions of presentation, pathophysiology, and diagnosis, as well as many treatment options, this book concentrates primarily on a specific treatment by a recognized expert in the field. Thus, the treatment may be very individualized, as I have asked each author to describe what he or she feels personally is the most appropriate therapy for a given disease. Therefore, one or two other editions of *Current Surgical Therapy* should also be reviewed, to give the reader a broad overview of the therapy for that disease.

Current Surgical Therapy is written and meant primarily for surgical residents, fellows, and fully trained surgeons either in private practice or in an academic setting. I have been in full-time academic practice for my entire career, and a week never goes by without my picking up *Current Surgical Therapy* to review a topic. Medical students have also told me they find the book of value, but it is not written principally for medical students, and I think they are often better served reviewing a surgical disease in a larger, more classic surgical textbook. As with past editions, some topics from the eighth edition have been deleted and new ones added. We have continued to try to encourage illustrations, particularly operative drawings, so that the surgeon prior to going to the operating room might have a quick review by reading a brief chapter and looking at operative illustrations. Again, this book concentrates principally on treatment. The introduction tends to be brief in each chapter, with only a short reference to presentation, pathophysiology, and diagnosis. The emphasis is clearly on surgical therapy.

I am indebted to the many surgeons throughout the country, indeed throughout the world, who have continued to participate in this textbook. In addition, I have been supported by a dedicated group of individuals at Hopkins in the preparation of this text. Ms. Irma Silkworth has been the key individual in preparing this and previous texts, and my secretary, Ms. Bonnie Bowling, has also been of immense help. Ms. Fran Goldsborough has also contributed. I have decided to edit one more edition of *Current Surgical Therapy*, 3 years from now. That will make 10 editions of *Current Surgical Therapy* that I have compiled. I will perhaps recruit a co-editor for the tenth edition, so someone will be prepared to carry on this textbook, which I feel has provided a substantial service to the surgical community in this country. Finally, I would like to dedicate this edition to the surgical house staff at the Johns Hopkins Hospital, who are "the best of the best."

JOHN L. CAMERON, MD
May 2007

CONTENTS

Color Section Follows Table of Contents

PORTAL HYPERTENSION

GALLBLADDER AND BILIARY TREE

THE PANCREAS

COLOR SECTION

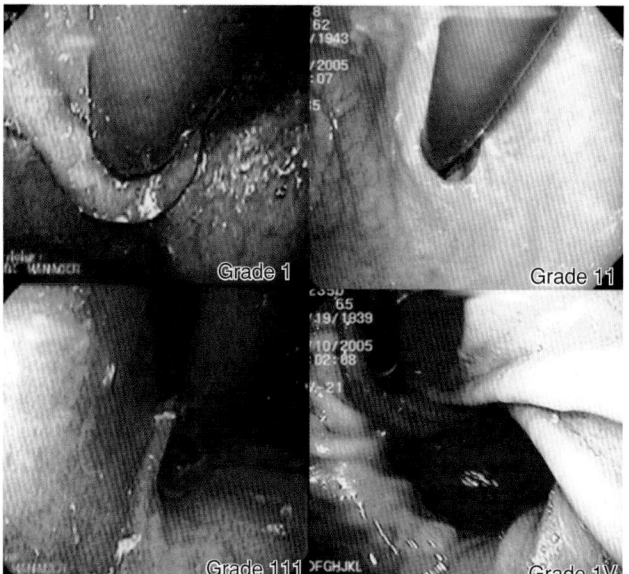

Figure 1 Hill's endoscopic grading of the retroflexed view of the cardia. Grade I valve: A ridge of tissue 3 to 4 cm long on the lesser curve is closely applied to the endoscope. Grade II valve: The ridge is less well defined than in grade I, and it opens occasionally with respiration but closes promptly. Grade III valve: The ridge is barely present, and there is often failure to close around the endoscope. It is nearly always accompanied by a hiatal hernia and esophagitis. Grade IV valve: There is no muscular ridge. The gastroesophageal junction remains open all the time, and the squamous epithelium can often be seen from this retroflexed position. A hiatal hernia is always present. *From Hill LD, Kozarek RA:* J Clin Gastroenter *28:194, 1999.*

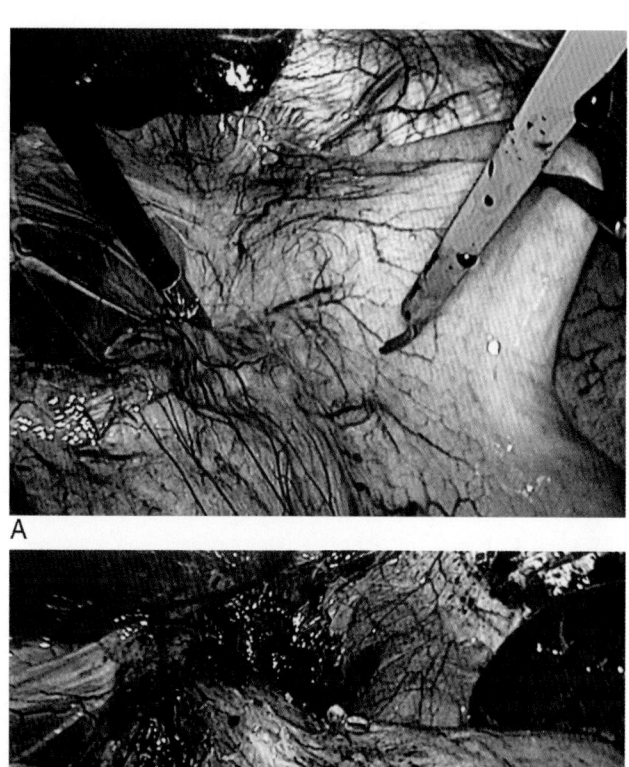

Figure 2 Dissection of the gastroesophageal fat pad to expose the gastroesophageal junction.

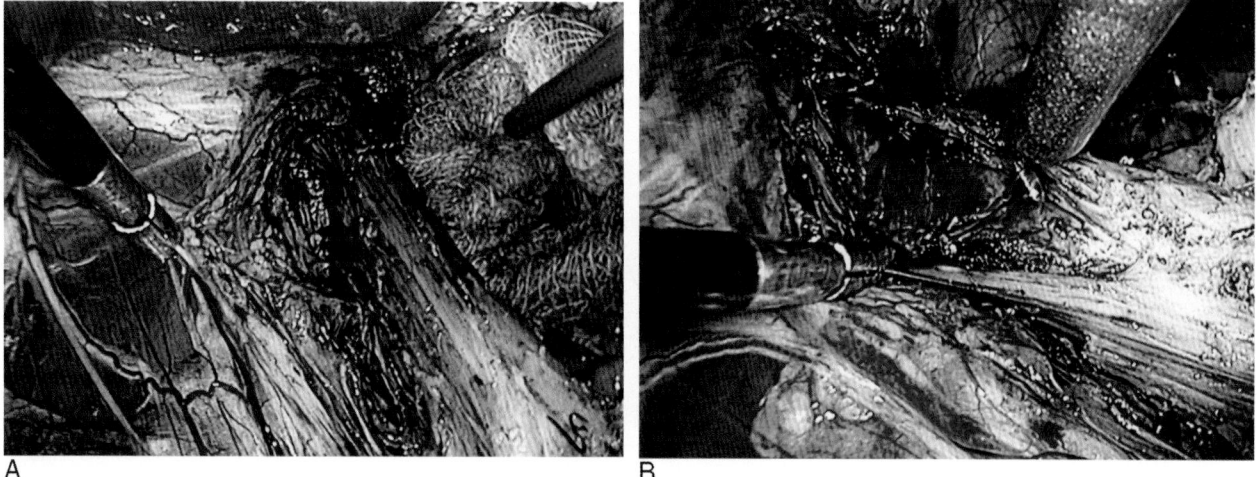

Figure 3 Mobilized esophagus **(A)** and creation of an esophageal myotomy by separation of the muscle edges down to esophageal mucosa and then proximally onto the esophagus and distally onto the stomach **(B)**.

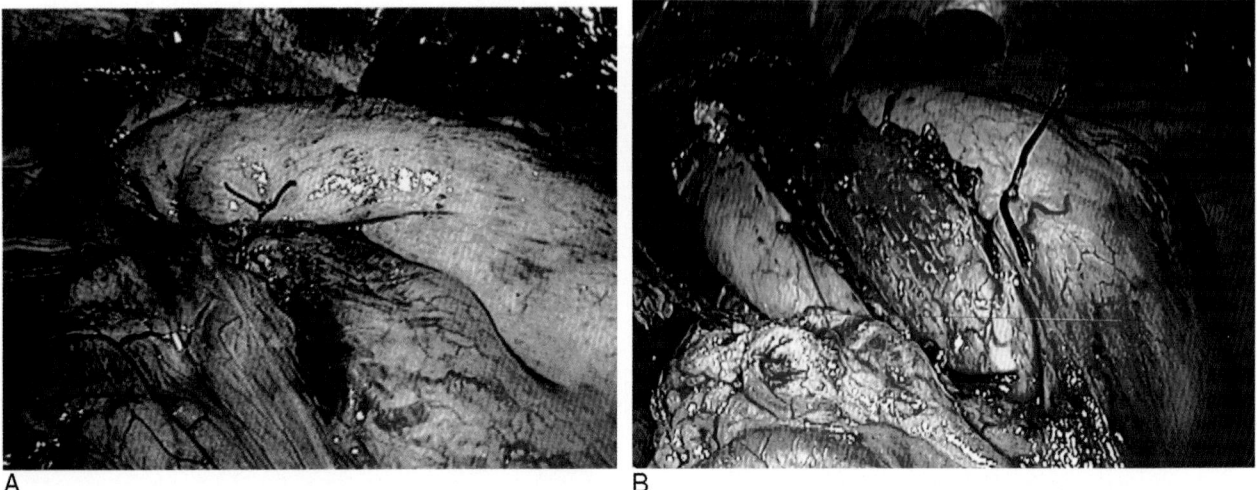

Figure 4 Ninety- to 180-degree Dor fundoplication positioned anteriorly to Heller myotomy **(A)** and 270-degree Toupet fundoplication positioned posteriorly **(B)**.

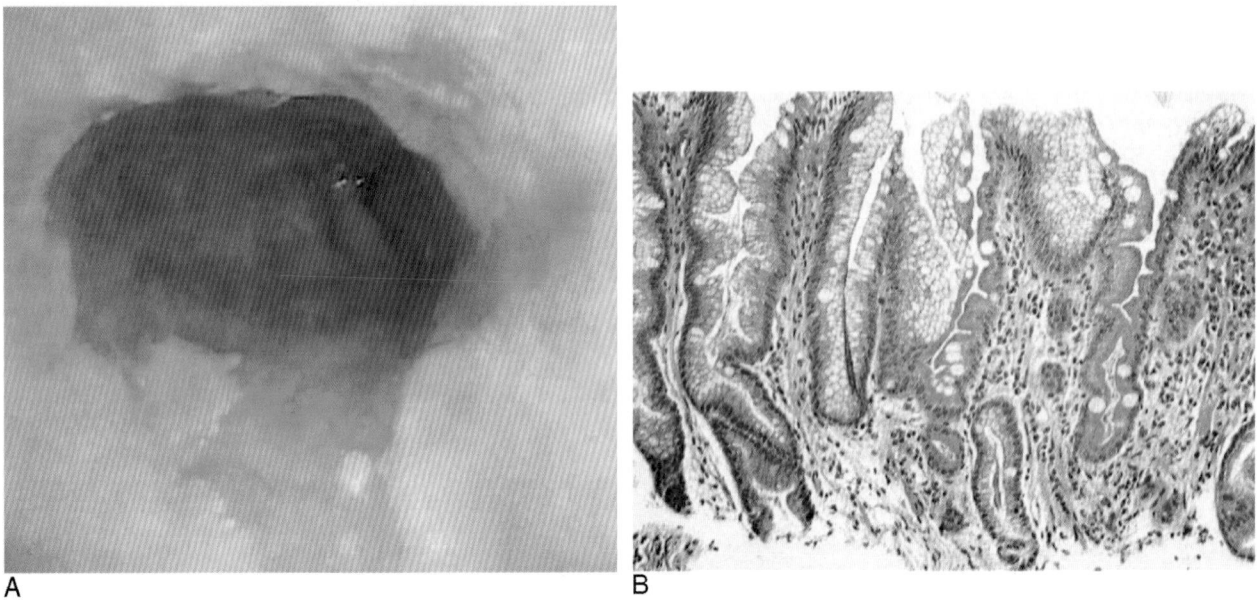

Figure 5 Barrett's esophagus. **(A)** Salmon-colored Barrett's mucosa is seen extending above the proximal extent of the gastric folds. **(B)** Microscopic features of Barrett's mucosa highlighting metaplastic columnar epithelium containing mucin-producing goblet cells.

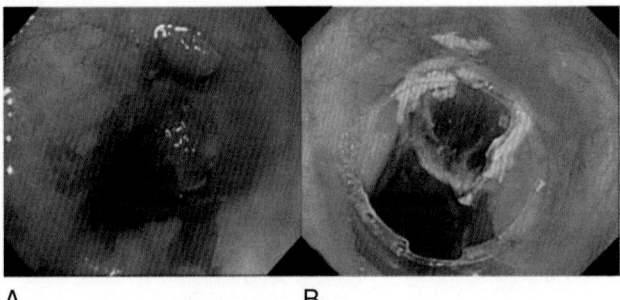

Figure 6 Endoscopic mucosal resection **(A)**, before; **(B)**, after.

From Peters FP, Kara MA, Rosmolen WD, and others: Gastrointest Endosc 61:506, 2005.

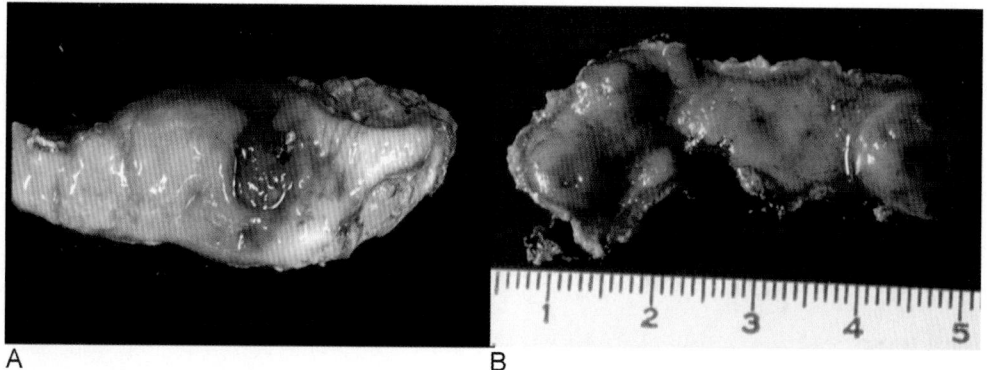

Figure 7 **(A)** Solitary duodenal gastrinoma in a sporadic patient vs. **(B)** Multiple duodenal gastrinomas in a multiple endocrine neoplasia syndrome type 1 patient.

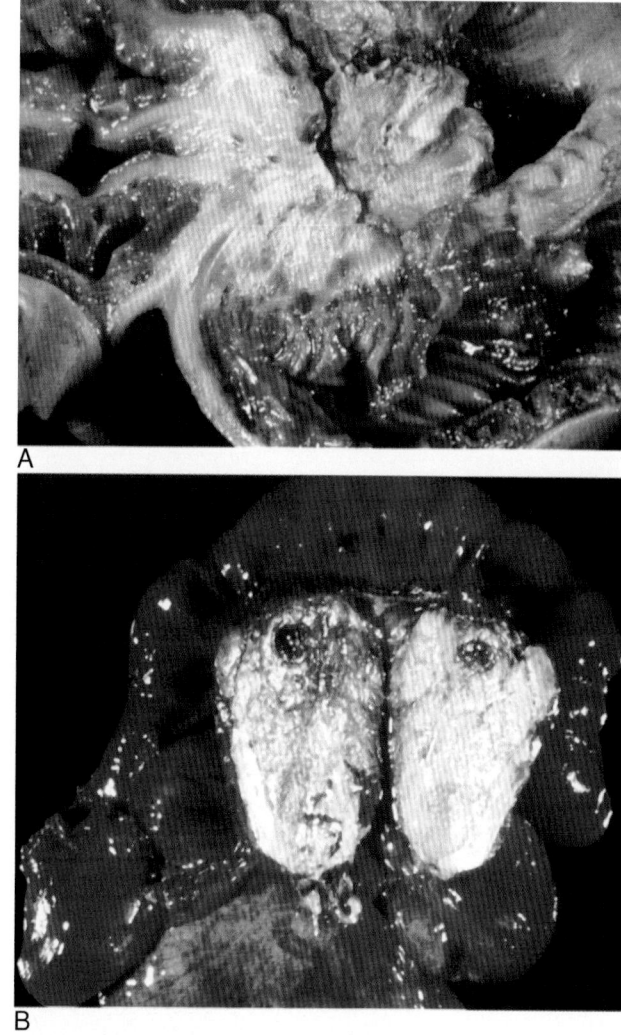

Figure 9 Gross pathologic characteristics of a small bowel carcinoid tumor. **(A)** Carcinoid tumor of the distal ileum with an intense desmoplastic reaction and fibrosis of the bowel wall. **(B)** Mesenteric metastases from a carcinoid tumor of the small bowel. *From Evers BM, Townsend CM Jr, Thompson JC, in Schwartz SI, editor: Principles of surgery, New York, 1999, McGraw-Hill, p. 1217.*

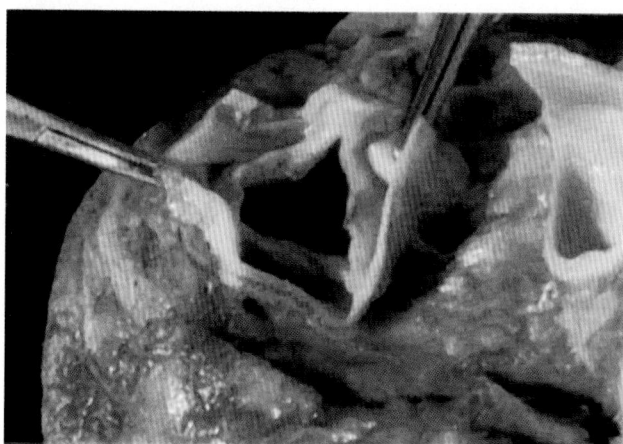

Figure 8 Fibrotic pulmonary valve from a patient with carcinoid heart disease. *Courtesy James R. Stone, MD, PhD, Department of Pathology, Brigham and Women's Hospital, Boston.*

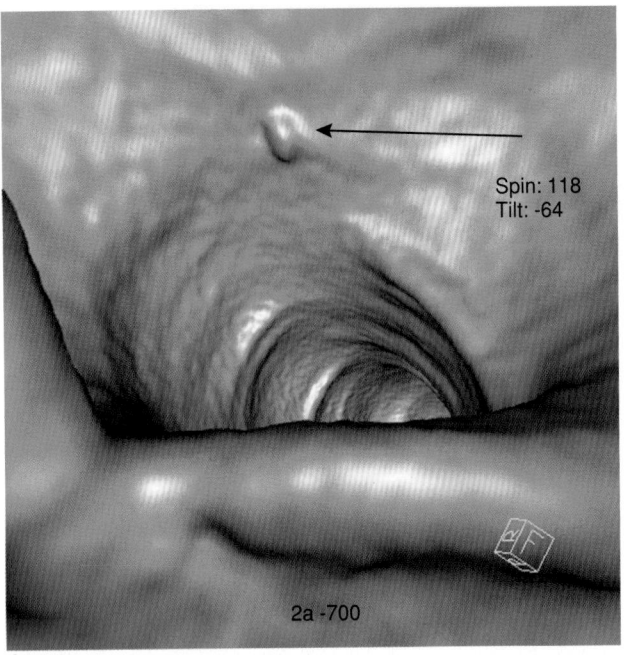

A

Figure 10 **(A)** Endoluminal view demonstrating a small polypoid lesion in the colon. When lesions are detected on the three-dimensional (3D) endoluminal views, they must be correlated with the axial or multiplaner reconstruction.

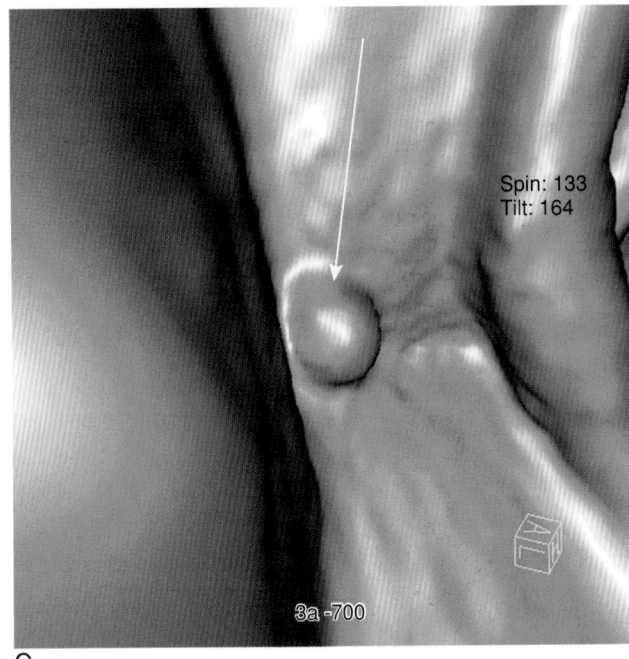

C

Figure 12 Polyp of 8 mm in the ascending colon. Small polyps can be a challenge during virtual colonoscopy but with careful review can be detected reliably. This small polyp is seen in the ascending colon on the three-dimensional endoluminal view **(C)**.

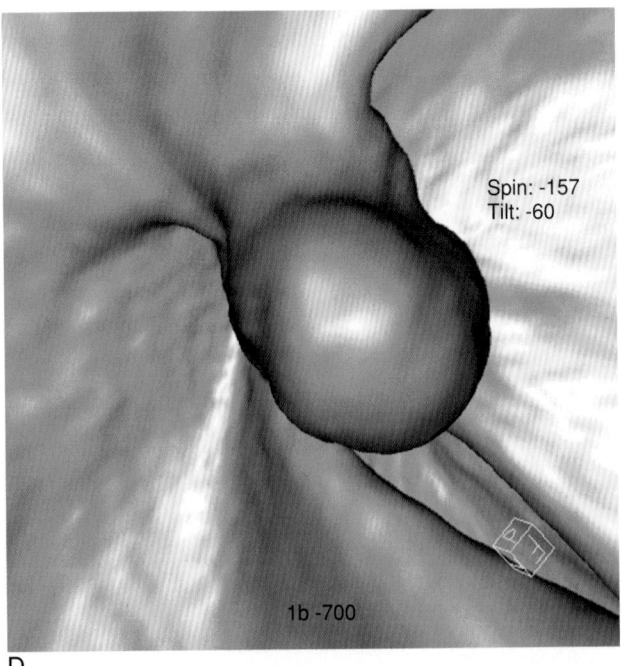

D

Figure 11 A villous adenoma (2.5 cm) in the rectum. **(D)** The three-dimensional endoluminal view.

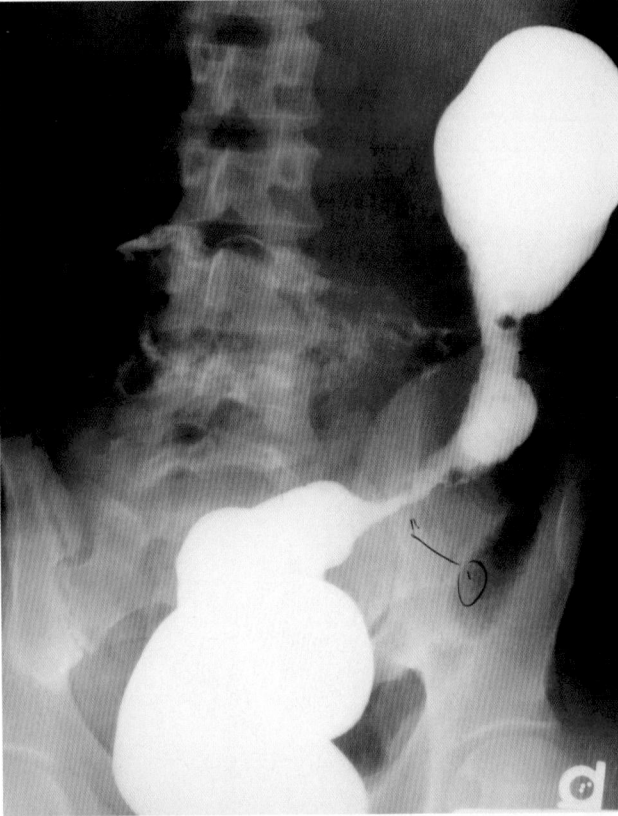

Figure 13 Radiographic contrast study showing sigmoid colon stricture secondary to Crohn's disease. This stricture caused symptoms of severe abdominal pain and diarrhea and was refractory to medical therapy.

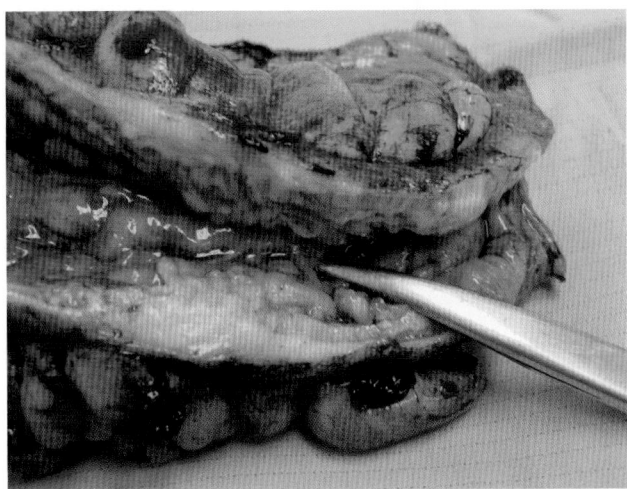

Figure 14 Sigmoid colon stricture with associated fistula indicated at tip of Mayo scissors. This stricture also was refractory to steroid and antimetabolite therapy and required segmental sigmoid resection.

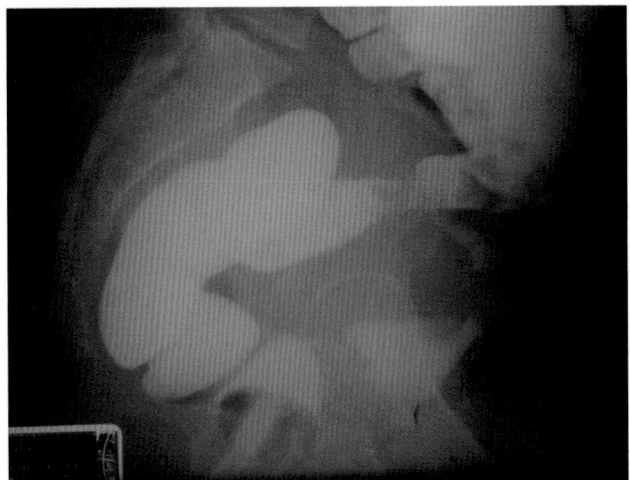

Figure 15 Gastrografin enema demonstrating large enterovesical fistula in patient with Crohn's colitis. This patient developed recurrent urinary tract infections despite continued antibiotic suppression, had severe associated bladder spasm, and required surgical resection and repair.

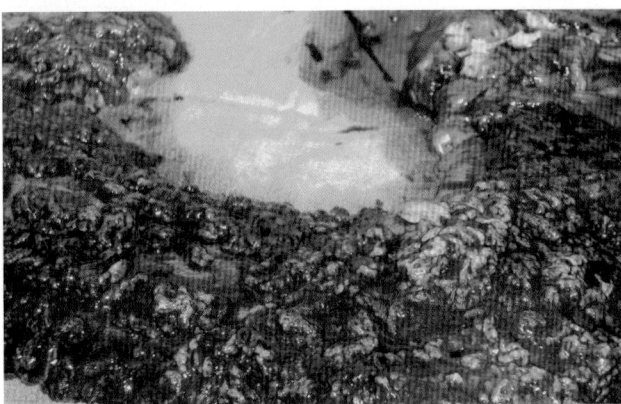

Figure 16 Endoluminal appearance of a colectomy specimen shortly after resection in a patient with toxic megacolon. Note the almost "autolytic" appearance of the colon, which was close to perforation.

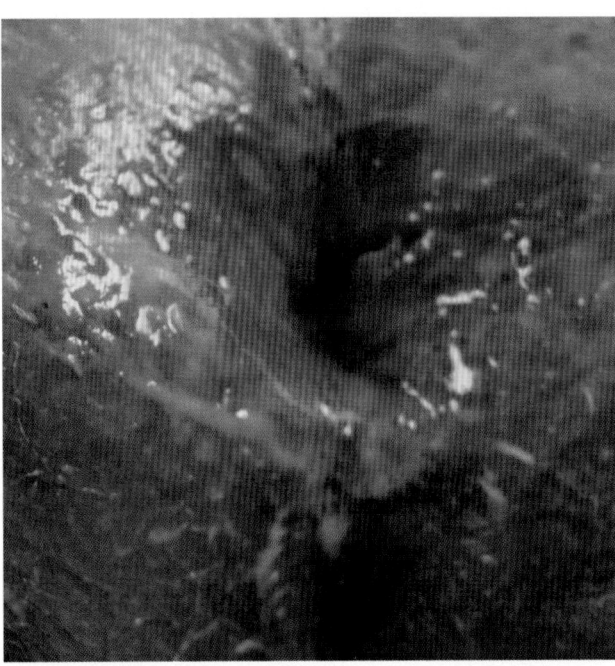

Figure 17 Severe perianal Crohn's disease stricture resulting in severe diarrhea, perianal excoriation, and small fistula right posteriolaterally. Note purulent discharge from anal canal.

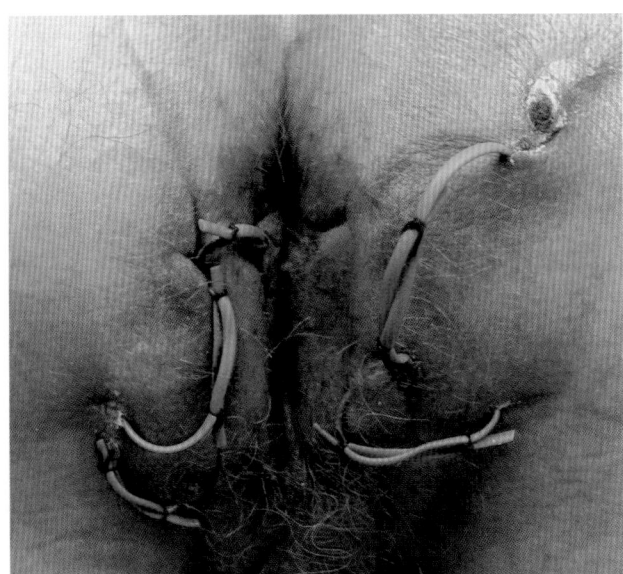

Figure 18 Perianal Crohn's disease resulting in recurrent abscesses and fistulae. The patient underwent placement of multiple setons. Here, blue vessel loops were used for this purpose to prevent abscesses from forming and to provide for continued drainage of the fistula tracts.

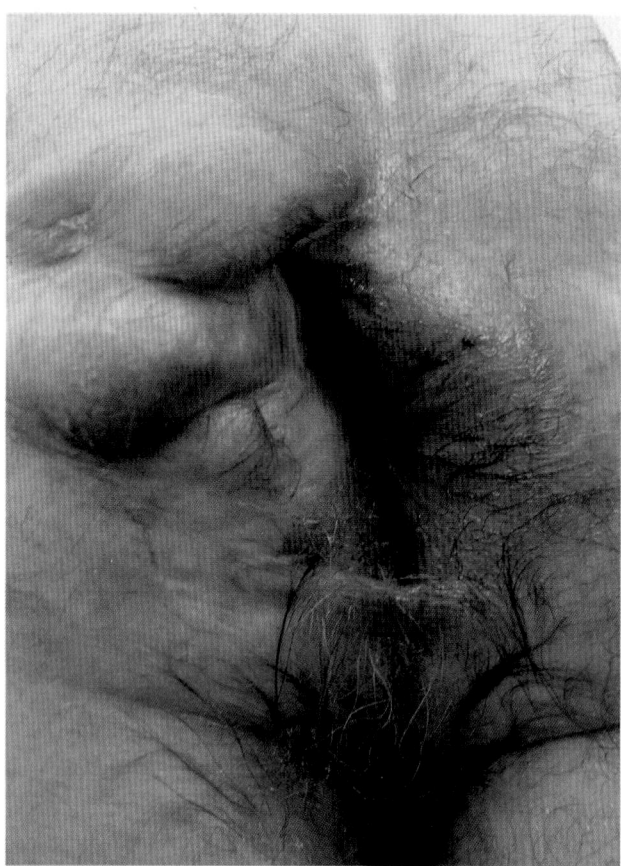

Figure 19 Severe deformity of the anal canal in a patient who has undergone multiple and extensive prior fistulotomies and abscess drainage procedures that have resulted in incontinence.

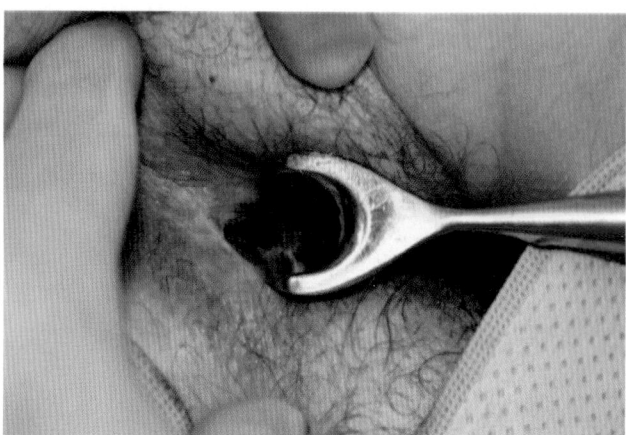

Figure 21 Chronic posterior anal fissure.

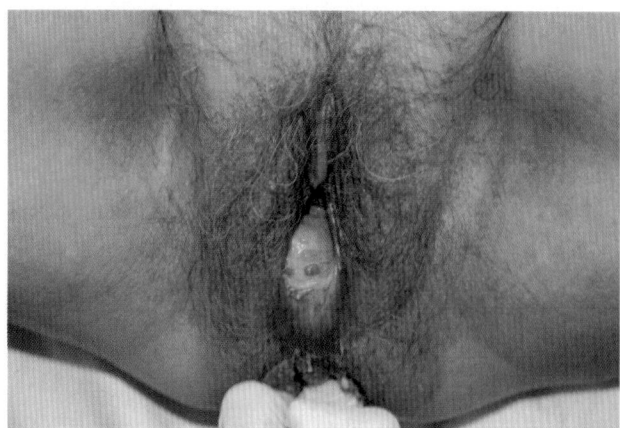

Figure 20 Rectocele repair using an implant to reinforce rectal vaginal septum.

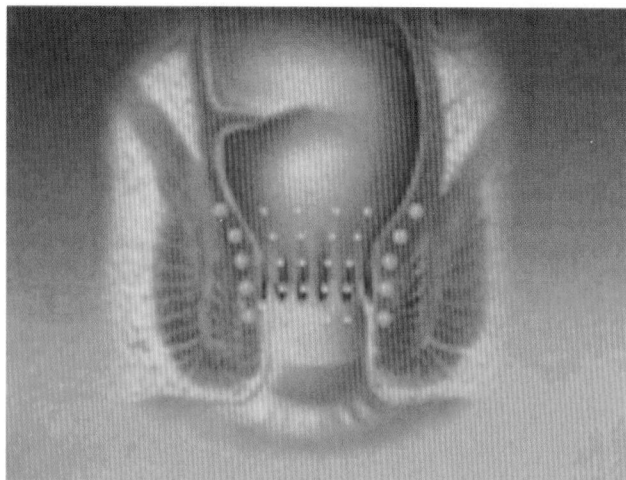

Figure 22 Secca procedure. Thermal lesions are delivered in a stepwise manner to all quadrants of the anal canal, beginning just distal to the dentate line and progressing proximally. *From Takahashi T, Garcia-Osogobio S, Valdovinos MA, and others: Dis Colon Rectum 46:711.*

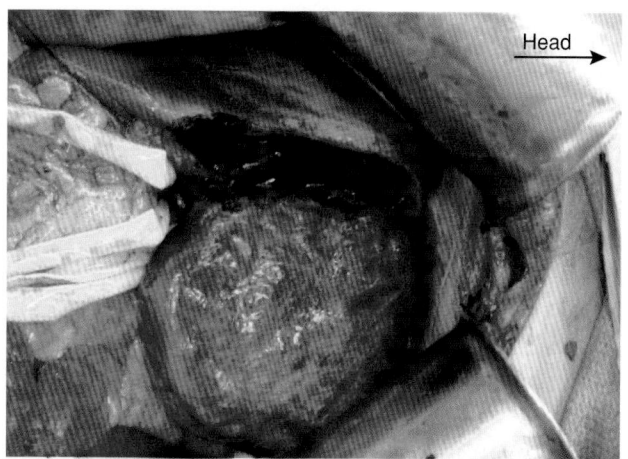

Figure 23 Intraoperative photograph. The patient's head is to the right. A large hemangioma in segments II, III, and IV is being enucleated. *Courtesy Richard Schulick, MD, Department of Surgery, Johns Hopkins Hospital.*

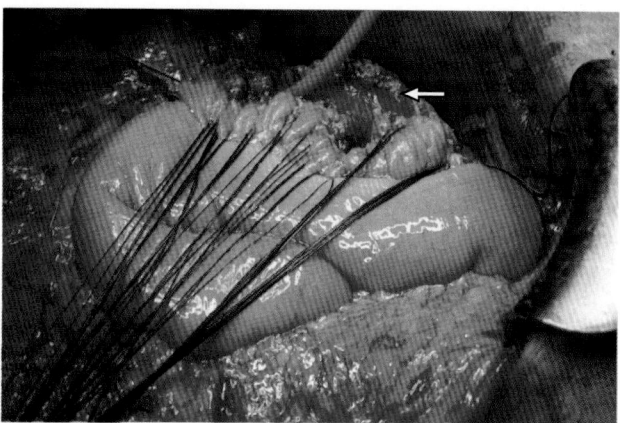

Figure 25 Lateral pancreaticojejunostomy demonstrating an anastomosis between the opened pancreatic duct *(arrow)* and Roux-en-Y limb of jejunum.

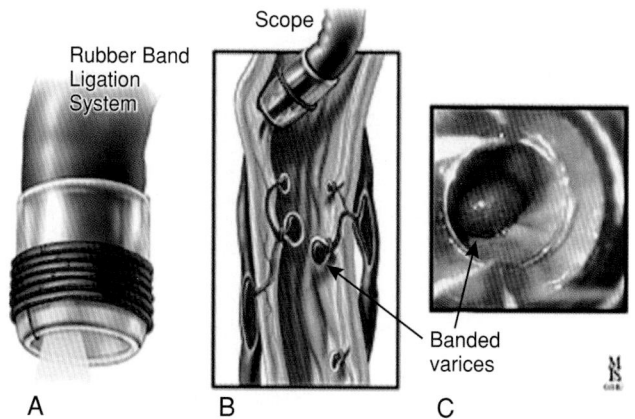

Figure 24 Endoscopic band ligation. **(A)** The multishot band device has 6 to 8 "O" elastic bands stretched and preloaded onto a transparent cylinder attached to the tip of an end-viewing endoscope. **(B)** The varix is suctioned into the banding device and ensnared by a firing mechanism that deploys the band at the base of the varix. **(C)** The strangulated varix is dislodged from the banding device, undergoing necrosis and sloughing of the thrombosed varix and band approximately 1 week later. *Used with permission from www.hopkins-gi.org.*

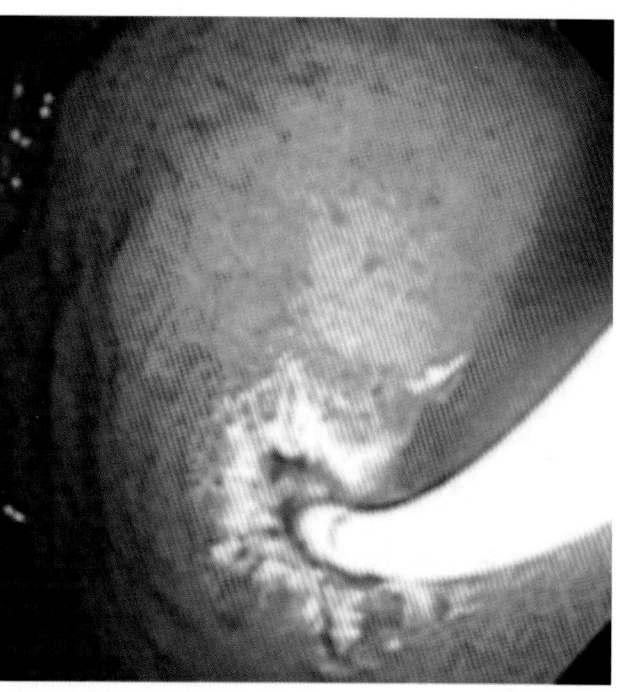

Figure 26 Endoscopic drainage of pancreatic pseudocyst. Cystotome is used to create the cystgastrostomy.

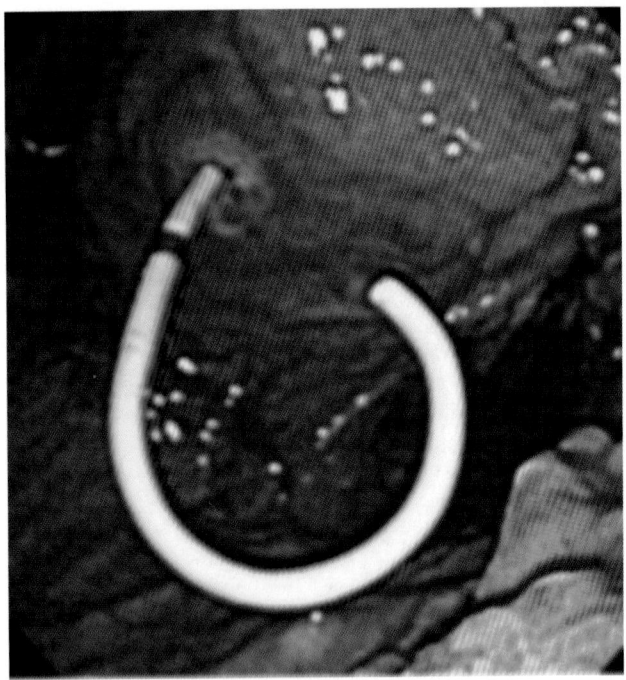

Figure 27 Endoscopic drainage of pancreatic pseudocyst. A 10-F pigtail stent is placed to maintain drainage of the pseudocyst.

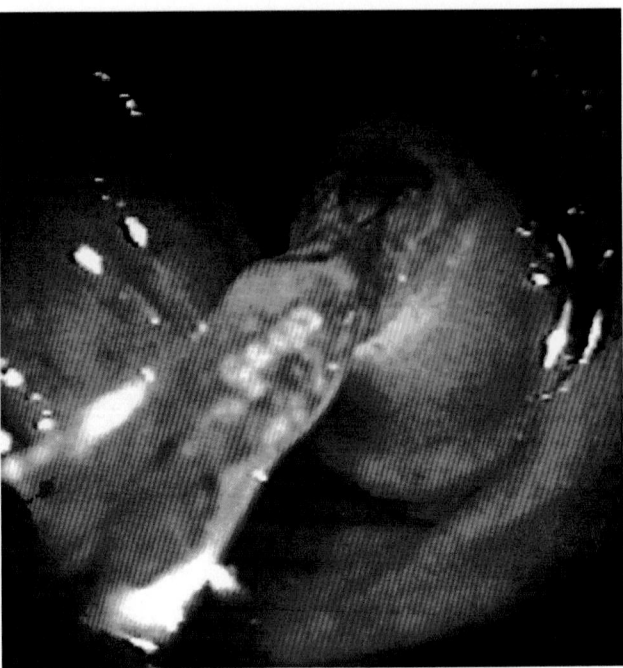

Figure 29 Patulous bulging ampulla with extruding mucin seen at endoscopy. *From Conlon KC: J Clin Oncol 23:4518, 2006. Used with permission from the American Society of Clinical Oncology.*

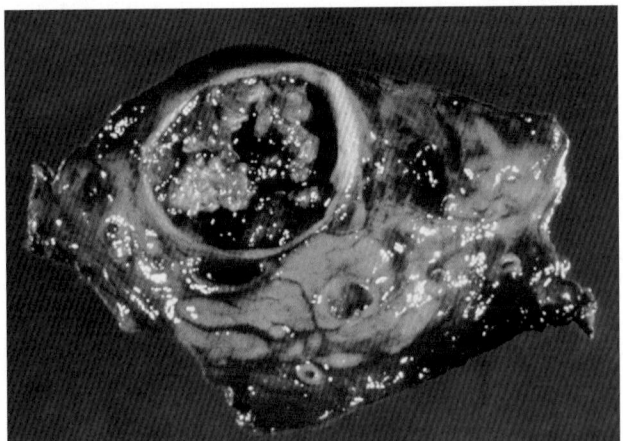

Figure 28 Gross photograph of a main duct intraductal papillary mucinous neoplasm demonstrating a cross section of the gland through the main pancreatic duct. The main pancreatic duct is massively dilatated with papillary fronds growing within the duct itself.

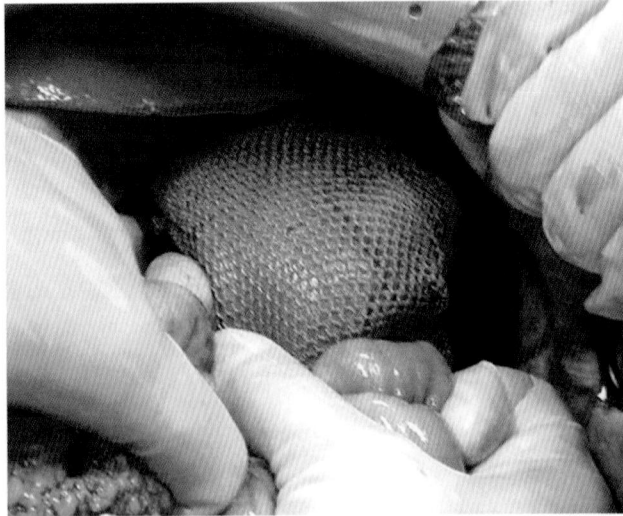

Figure 30 Mesh splenorrhaphy in situ with Surgicel placed directly over the injured portion of the spleen, before suturing to secure the mesh. *Photo Credit: Horacio A. Massotto, MD, Costa Rica. Reproduced with permission from www.trauma.org.*

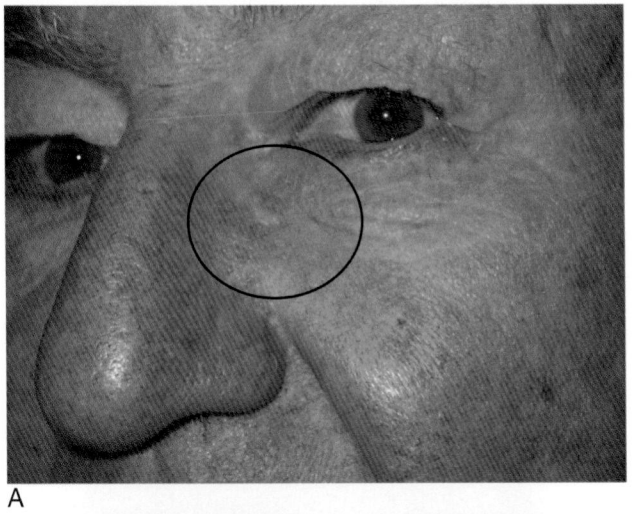

A

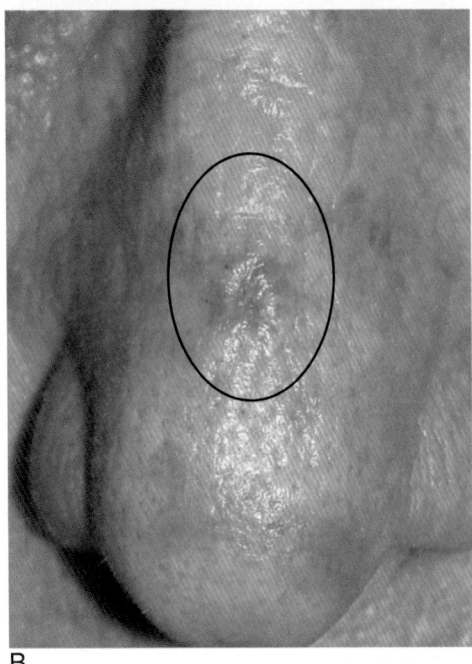

B

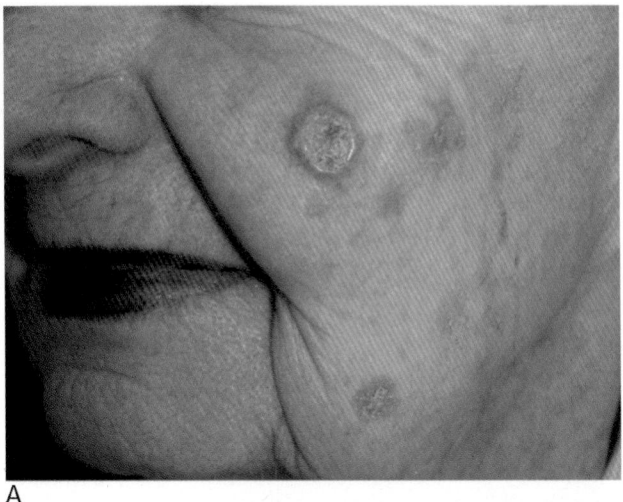

A

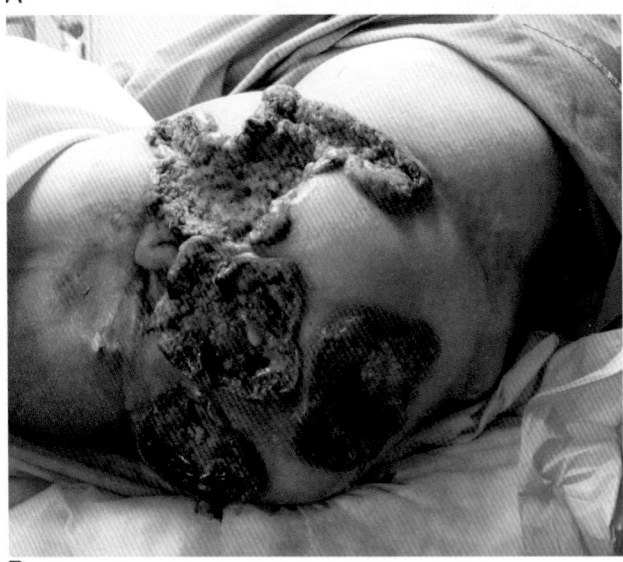

B

Figure 44 Nodular basal cell cancer, the most common form, presents as dome-shaped, "pearly" papules with a telangiectatic surface and a rolled, raised border on sun-exposed parts of the body, often on the head and neck. The basal cancers here are on the **A)** face and **B)** nasal dorsum.

Figure 45 **(A)** Squamous cell carcinoma (SCCA) is associated with sun exposure, and is shown on the face with characteristics including hyperkeratosis and ulceration. **(B)** Marjolin's ulcers are chronic wounds that develop SCCA over the long term.

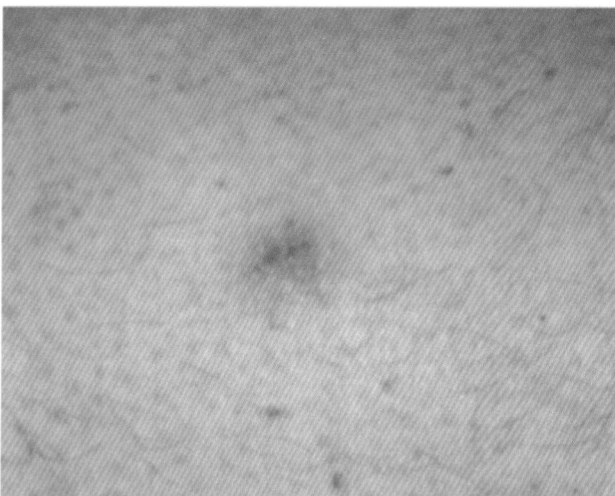

Figure 39 Dermatofibromas are firm, dome-shaped papules often found on the lower extremities.

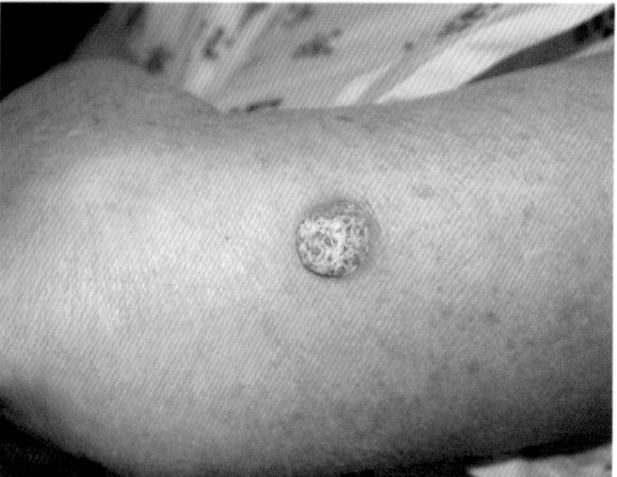

Figure 40 Keratoacanthomas are typically solitary neoplasms on sun-exposed skin that rapidly enlarge and spontaneously involute. Because of an appearance resembling squamous cell cancer, biopsy is recommended.

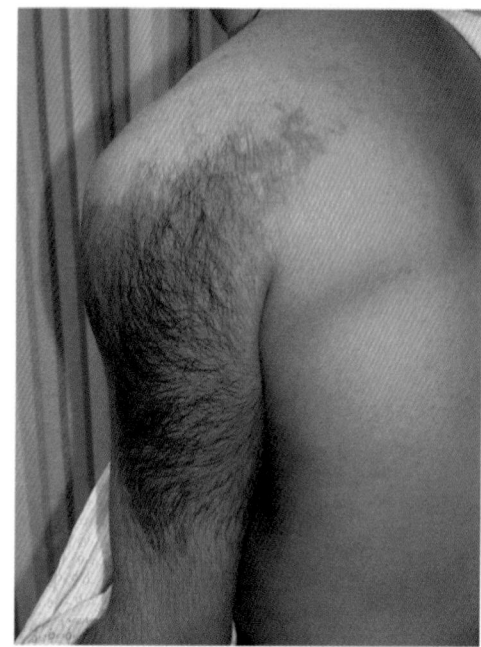

Figure 42 Becker's nevus occurs predominantly in males and presents as an irregularly shaped tan-to-brown patch, typically located over the shoulder, upper chest, or back.

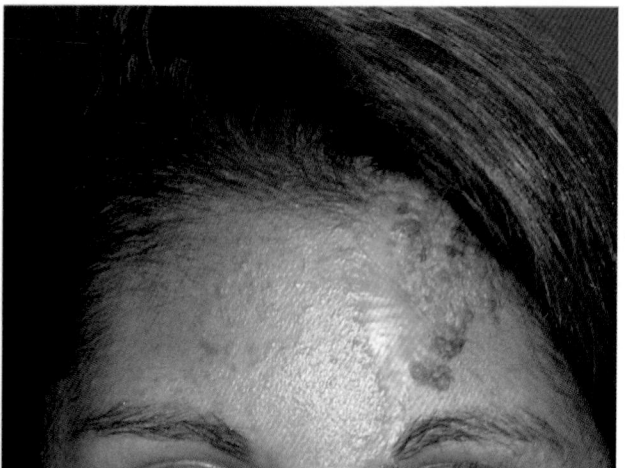

Figure 41 Nevus sebaceous is often diagnosed in children; it is found on the head and neck region and is reported to convert to basal cell cancer. In this case, serial excision was necessary because of the extensive surface area involved.

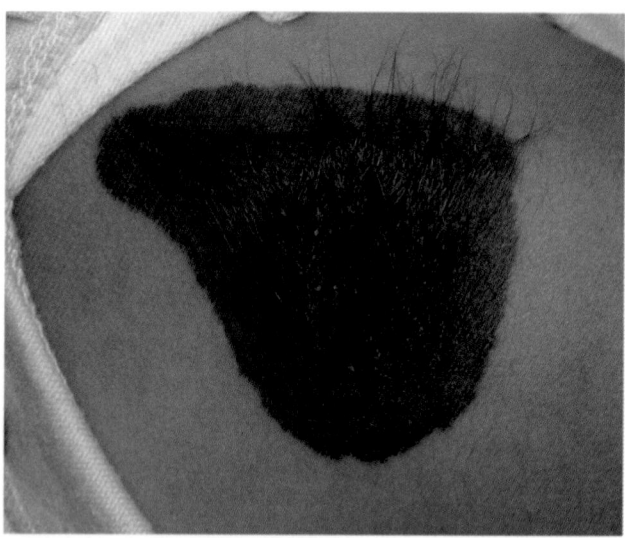

Figure 43 Giant congenital nevi present during childhood. Excision is recommended because of the risk of malignant transformation.

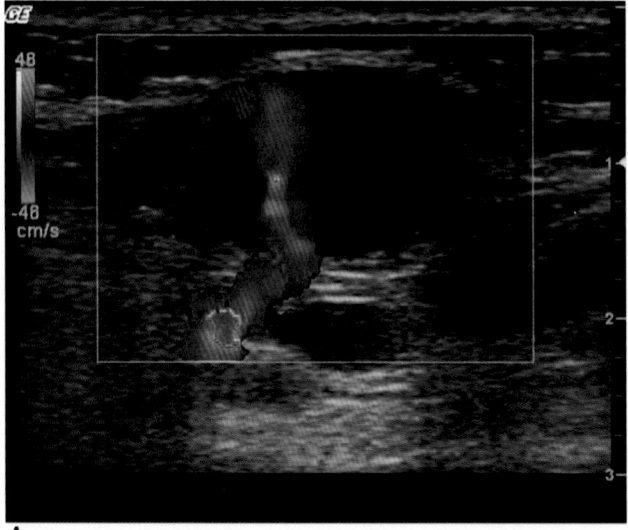

A

Figure 35 **(A)** Duplex ultrasound of femoral pseudoaneurysm.

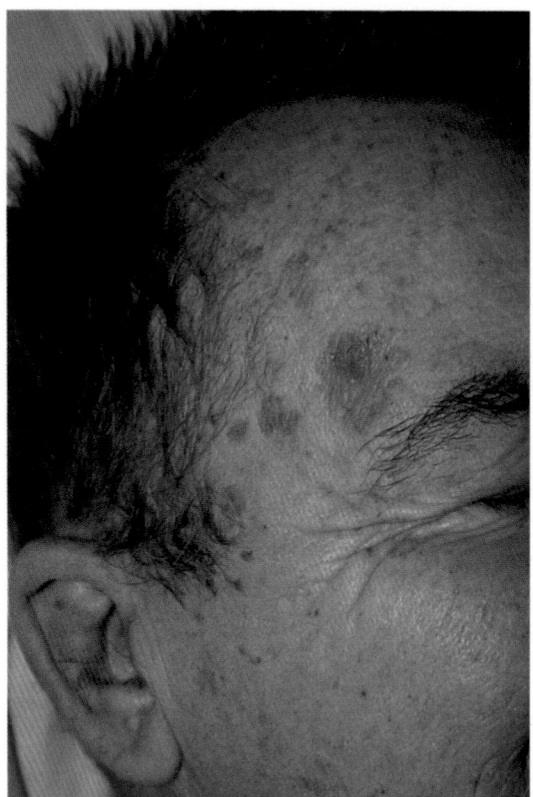

Figure 37 Seborrheic keratosis (SK) is often seen in large numbers, especially on the trunk, face, and arms of individuals older than 30 years of age. The SK typically presents as a sharply circumscribed, waxy, papillomatous plaque with a friable, hyperkeratotic surface, most often described as having a "stuck-on" appearance.

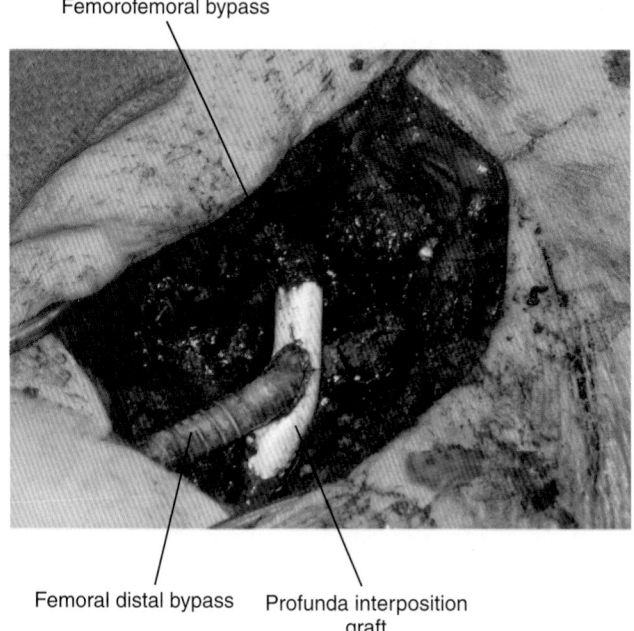

Femorofemoral bypass

Femoral distal bypass   Profunda interposition graft

Figure 36 An interposition graft to the left profunda femoris artery provides outflow for a femorofemoral bypass and serves as the inflow source for a left femorotibial bypass graft.

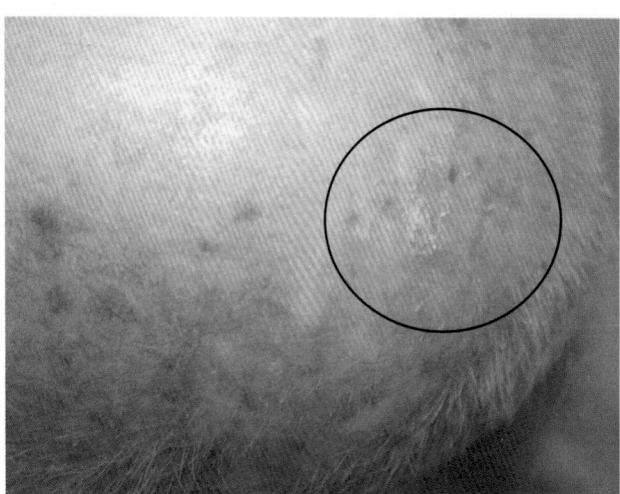

Figure 38 Actinic keratoses (AKs) are found primarily on exposed surfaces as rough adherent hyperkeratosis that are skin-colored, yellow-brown or brown, possibly with a reddish tinge. They are often numerous in older adults.

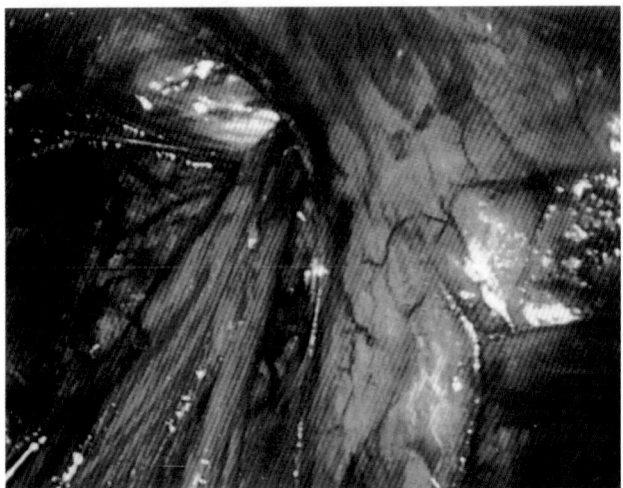

Figure 31 Dissection begins at the pubis and is carried laterally along Cooper's ligament to the iliac vein.

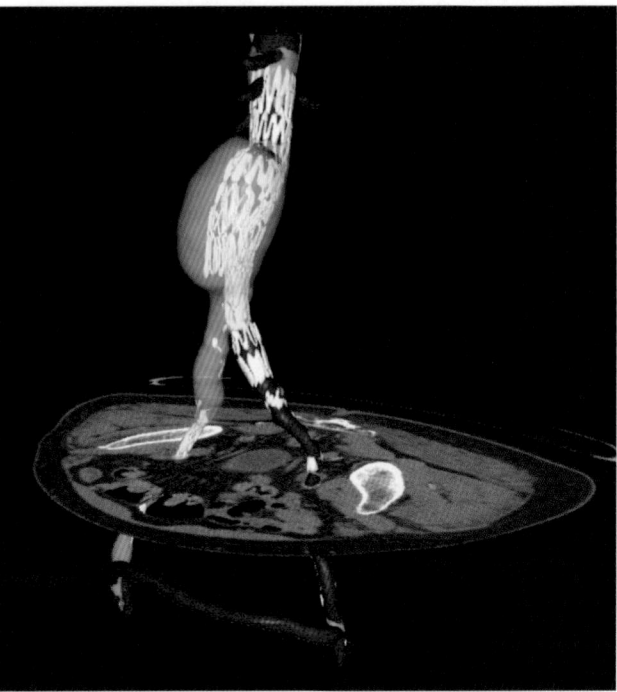

Figure 33 Repair of migrating endograft with resulting large type I endoleak. Three-dimensional model shows an aorto-uni-iliac endograft placed through the left iliacs. Left to right femorofemoral bypass is performed. *From M2S the fusion of clinical data and 3D imaging, West Lebanon, NH.*

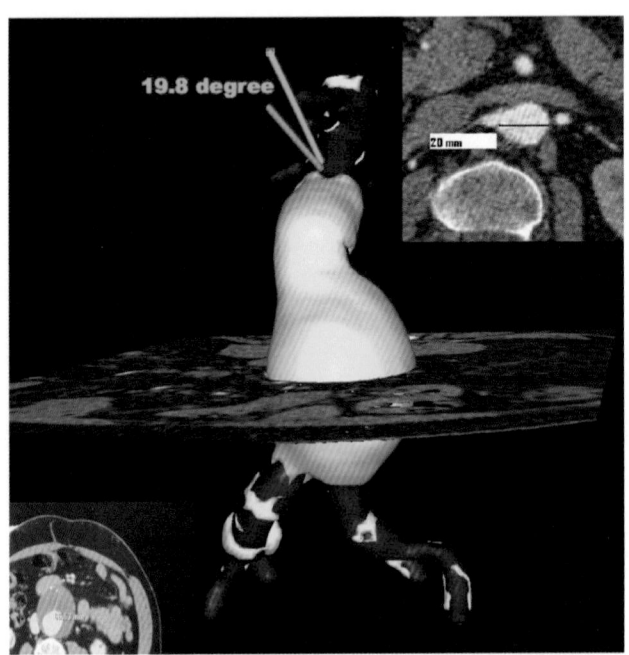

Figure 32 The benefits of three-dimensional (3D) computed tomography scan reconstruction in preoperative planning. Accurate measurement of aortic neck diameter and angulation with centerline technique by using 3D imaging along with axial slices. *From M2S the fusion of clinical data and 3D imaging, West Lebanon, NH.*

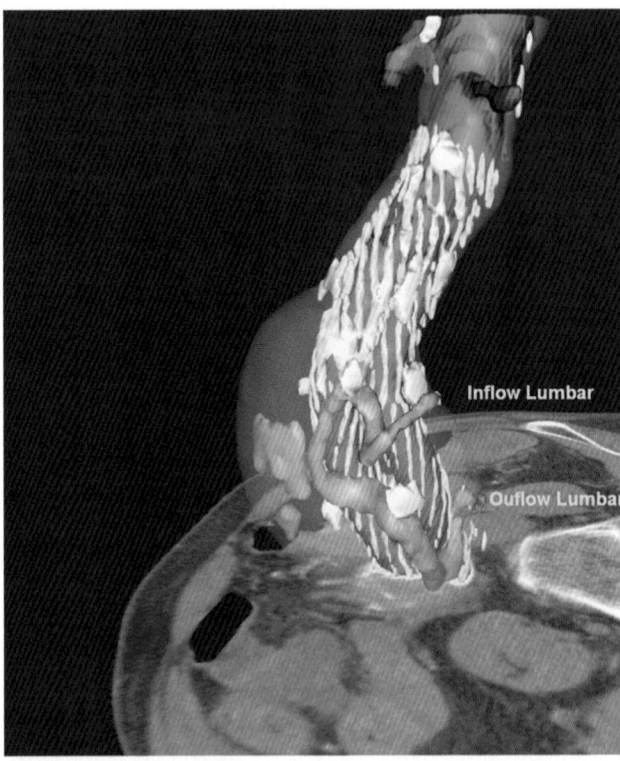

Figure 34 Three-dimensional model of type II endoleak with two lumbar arteries, one acting as inflow and the second as the outflow channel. *From M2S the fusion of clinical data and 3D imaging, West Lebanon, NH.*

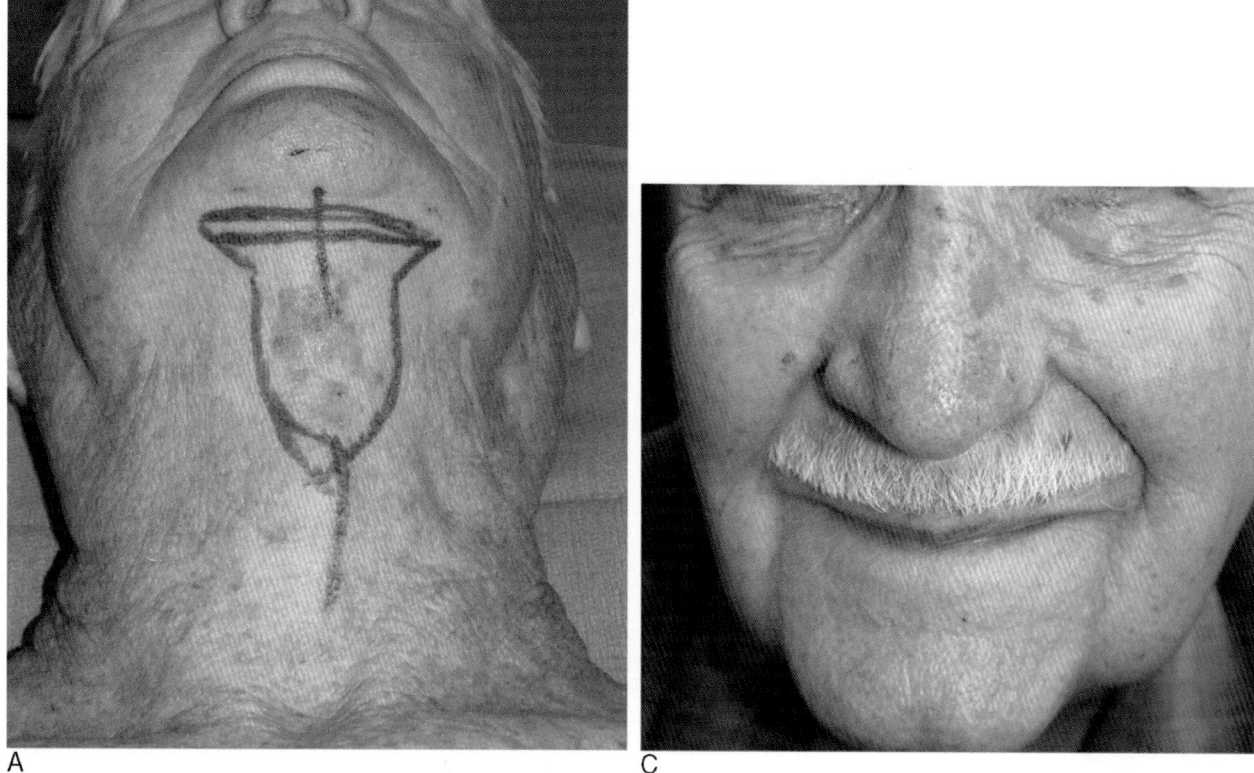

Figure 46 Squamous cell carcinoma in situ (SCCis), Bowen's disease, presents as poorly defined, scaly, erythematous plaques and is most common on the head and neck. Preoperative photograph of SCCis on the neck **(A)**, and lateral **(C)** views after excision with advancement of lateral skin and working out of "dog ears" superiorly and inferiorly.

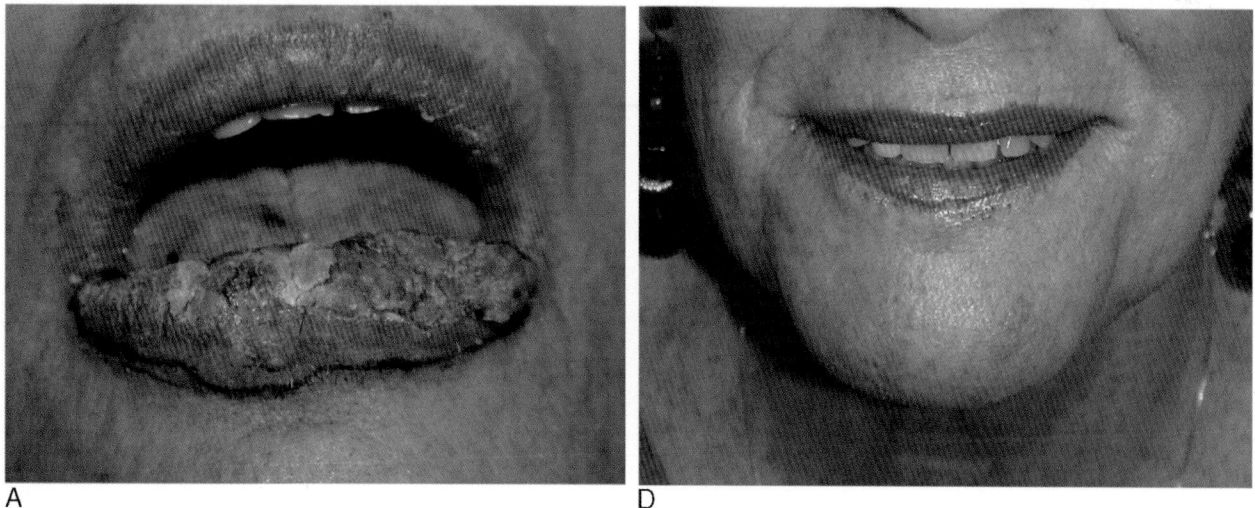

Figure 47 **(A)** Female patient in her 60s presents with squamous cell carcinoma of the vermilion of the lower lip. **(D)** Postoperative result 1 year later.

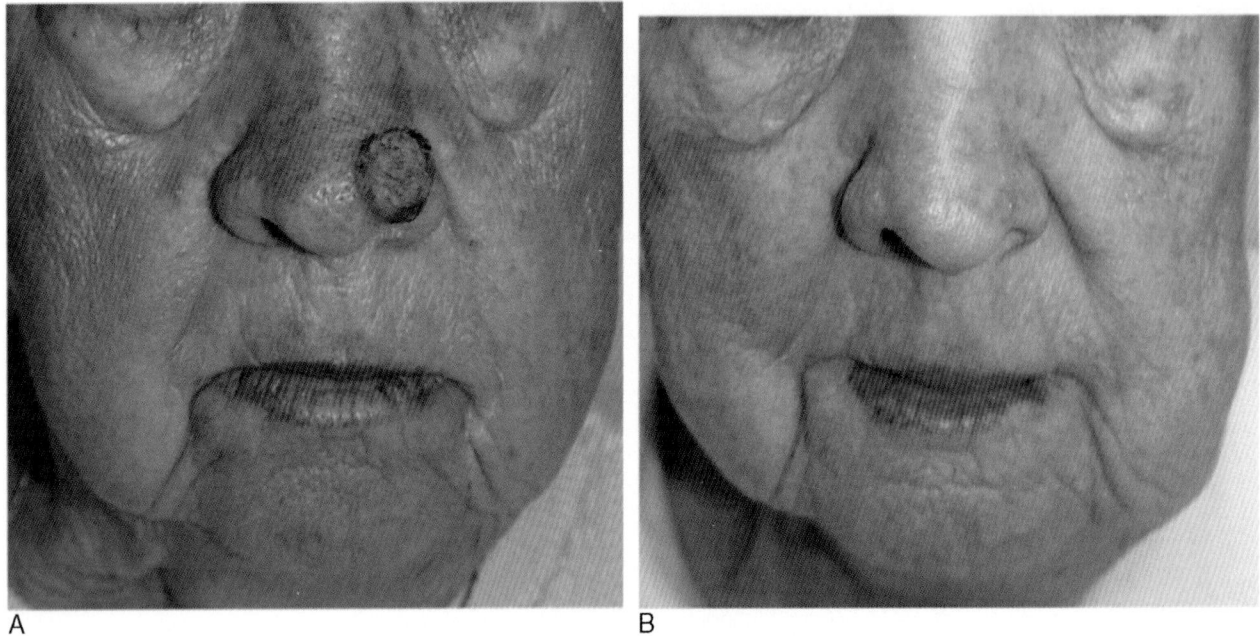

A B

Figure 48 Full-thickness skin grafts (FTSGs) are useful in older patients and may be taken from around the ear or clavicle. **(A)** Squamous cell carcinoma of the left nasal ala. **(B)** Cosmetic result of FTSG reconstruction is satisfactory 6 months later.

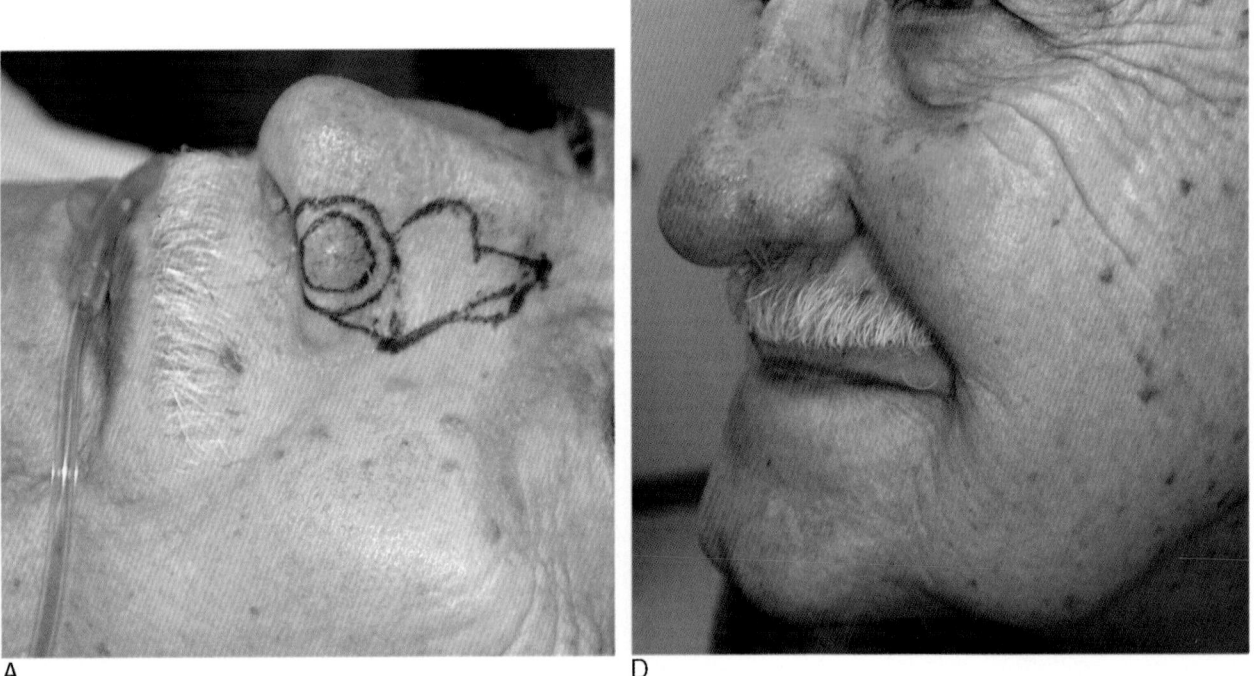

A D

Figure 49 **(A)** Basal cell carcinoma of the left nasal ala, with markings designated for the Zitelli modification of the bilobed flap. This is a random rotation flap. Lateral **(D)** views demonstrates satisfactory aesthetic result.

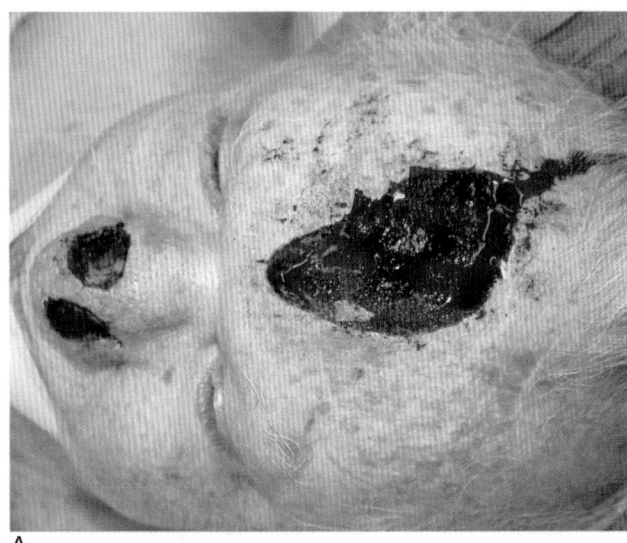

A

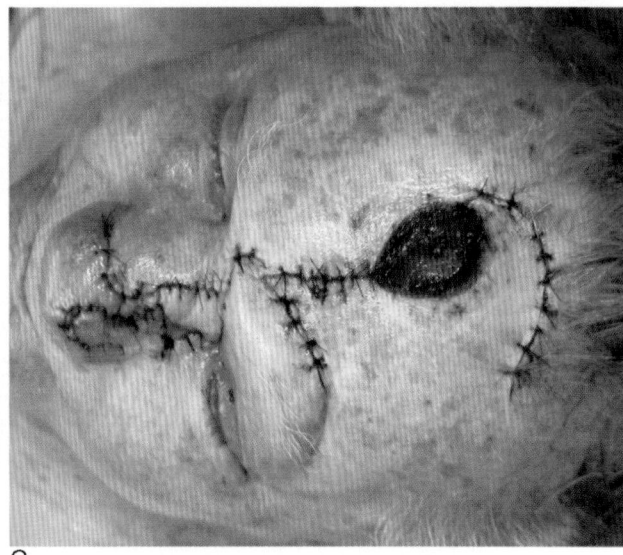

C

Figure 50 **(A)** Patient referred for reconstruction on the same day as her Mohs surgery, with defects of forehead, dorsal nose, and left ala. **(C)** Flaps are advanced and closed. An advancement of forehead skin was also performed along the brow and hairline, leaving the rest of the frontal defect to heal in secondarily.

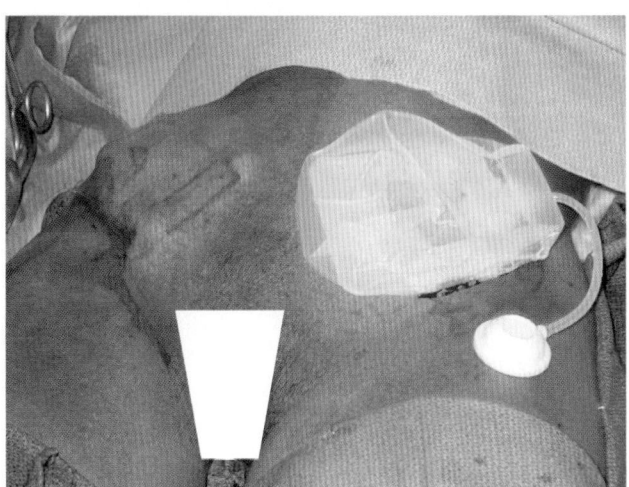

Figure 51 Tissue expander placement in the inguinal region to prepare full-thickness skin grafts. The right expander is already placed within its subcutaneous pocket.

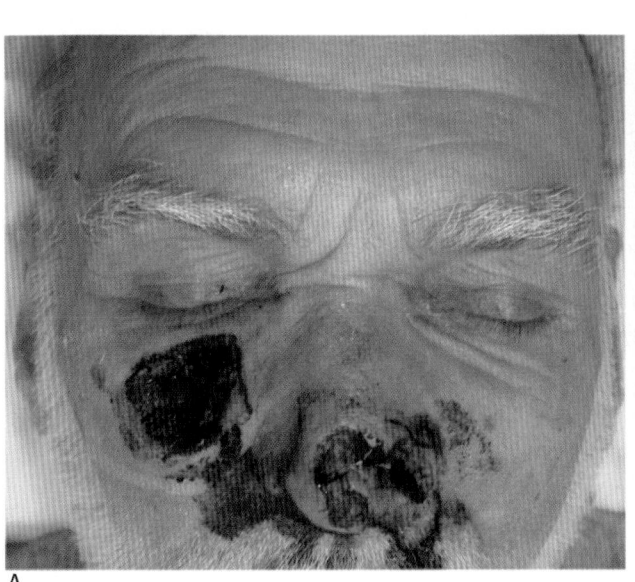

A

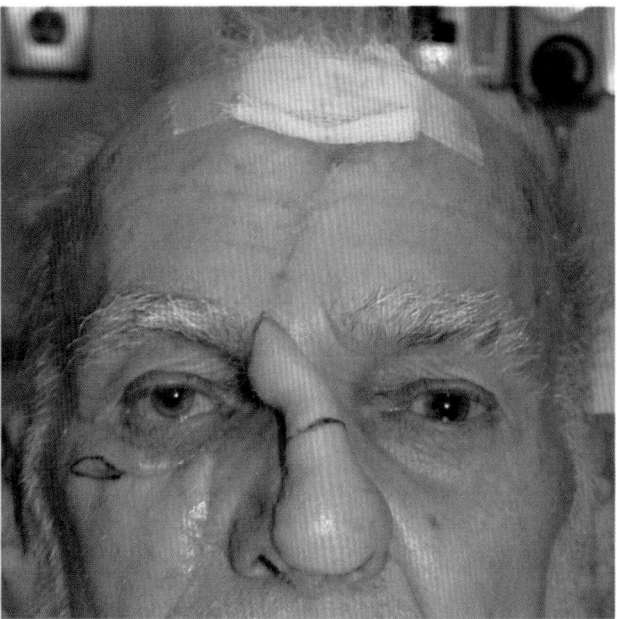

D

Figure 52 **(A)** Patient referred after Mohs surgery with dorsal nasal defect and right cheek defect. **(D)** Nasal flap just before division of pedicle 1 month later with forehead healing secondarily. "Dog ear" excision planned for cheek below the right eye.

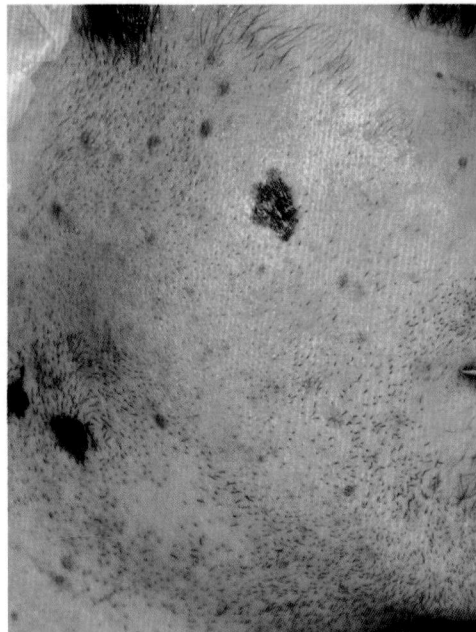
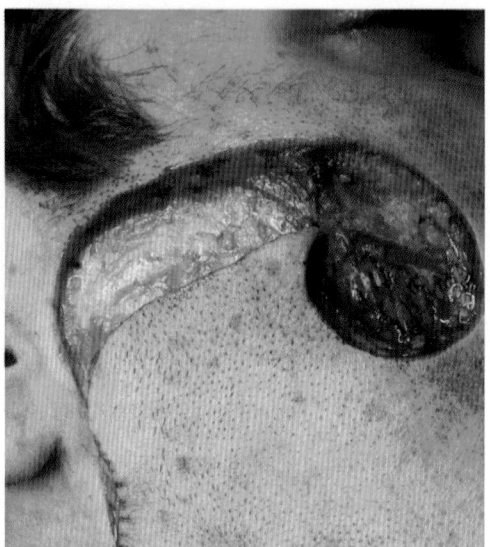
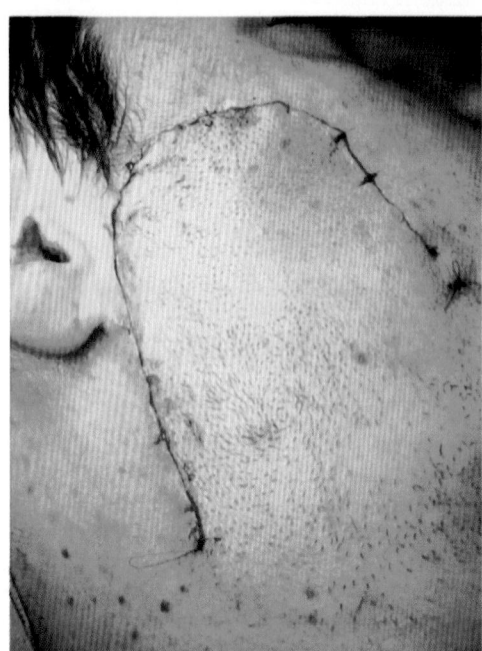

Figure 53 Rotational flap closure of cheek defect. *Top right:* The upper edge of the wide local excision line is extended laterally toward the ear and then inferiorly. The flap is created with dissection along the so-called facelift plane. Care must be taken to avoid penetrating too deeply and risking injury to the facial nerve. *Bottom:* The flap is then rotated into position, and any redundant skin at the inferomedial edge of the suture line removed. One potential difficulty with this reconstruction is downward tension on the lower eyelid. To avoid this, deep sutures can be used to secure the flap to underlying periosteum.

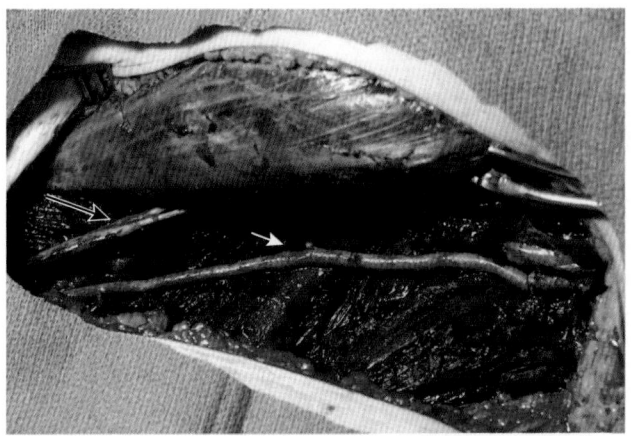

B

Figure 54 **(B)** Intraoperative photograph following en bloc resection of proximal thigh sarcoma with the superficial femoral artery and vein. The artery was reconstructed with a reversed saphenous bypass graft *(thick arrow)*. The femoral nerve was skeletonized, and branches to the vastus lateralis muscle were preserved *(thin arrow)*. Tumor extended to this margin, but postoperative external beam radiotherapy was administered, and excellent limb function was maintained.

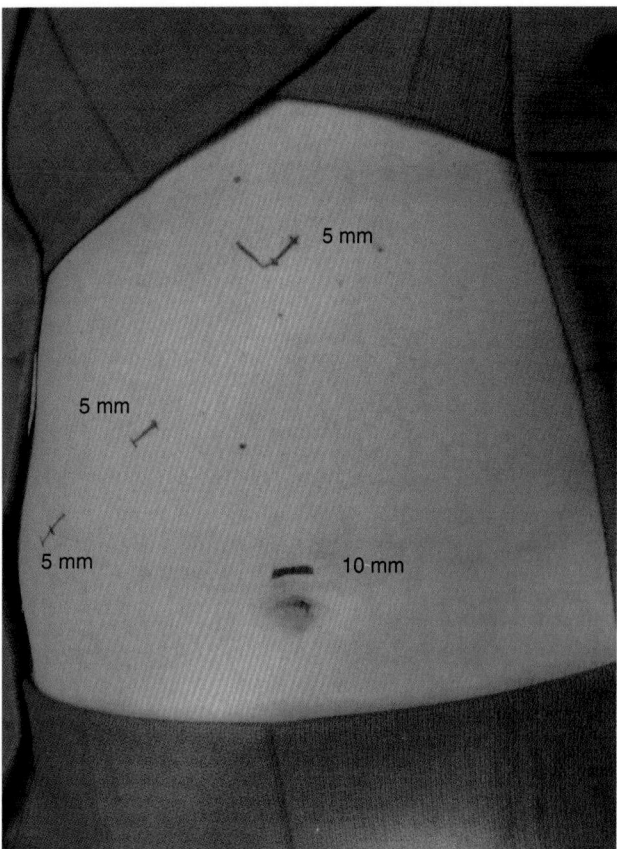

Figure 55 Common trocar size and placement for laparoscopic cholecystectomy. The umbilical trocar is almost always 10 mm, whereas the size and location of the remaining trocars may vary (2–10 mm), depending on surgeon preference and the availability of smaller instrumentation.

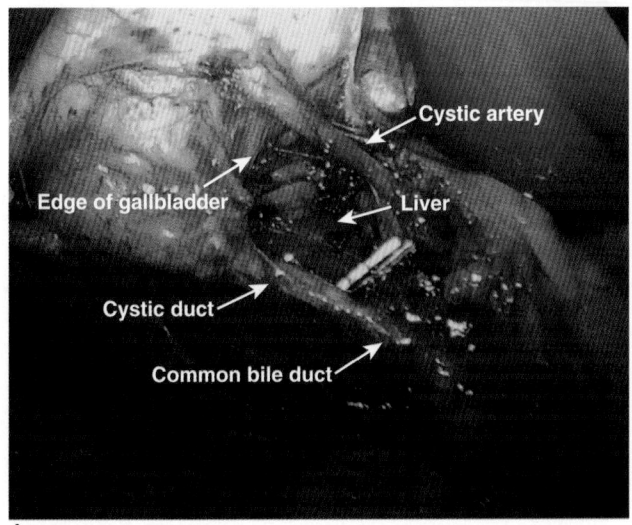

A

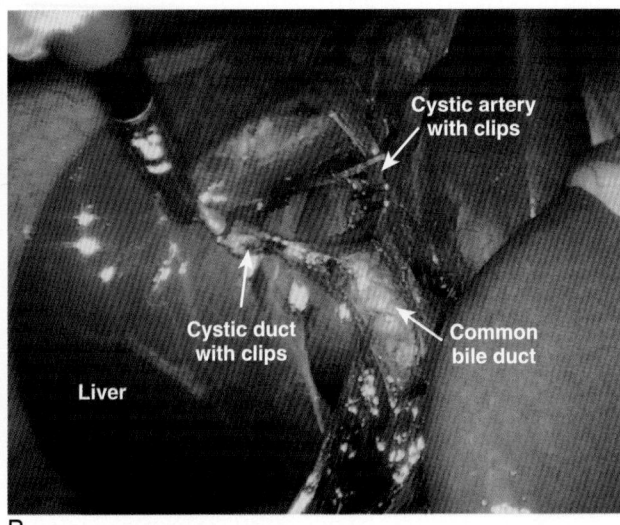

B

Figure 56 **(A)** Calot's triangle, defined superiorly by the inferior border of the liver, inferolaterally by the cystic duct, and medially by the common hepatic duct, is clearly identified. **(B)** The "critical view" affords unobstructed visualization of the liver posterior to the structures in Calot's Triangle, allowing the surgeon to safely place clips proximally and distal on the cystic duct and cystic artery before transaction. Failure to achieve this critical view risks potential injury to the common bile duct.

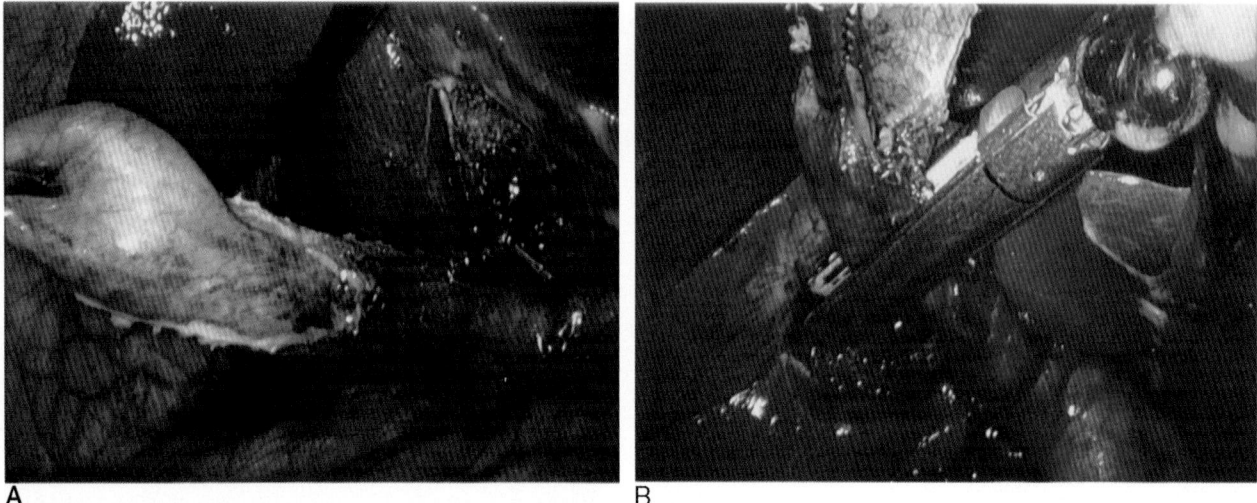

A   B

Figure 57 **(A)** "Dome down technique." Note that the gallbladder has been dissected free from the liver bed and is attached only to the cystic duct. **(B)** The thickened inflamed cystic duct is transected with the use of an endostapler.

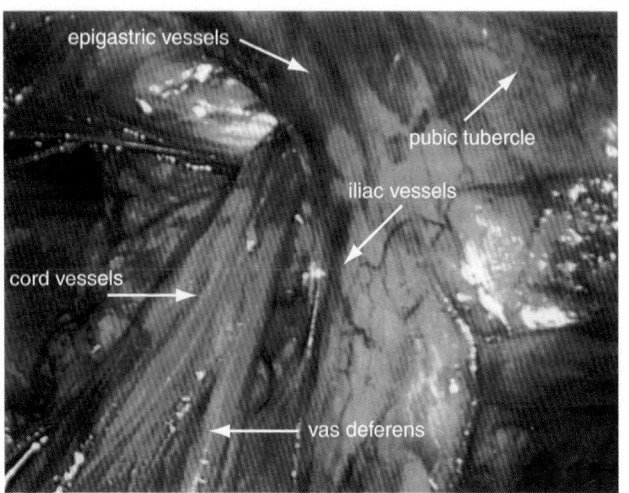

epigastric vessels

pubic tubercle

iliac vessels

cord vessels

vas deferens

Figure 58 Completed dissection during the totally extraperitoneal (TEP) approach (left sided).

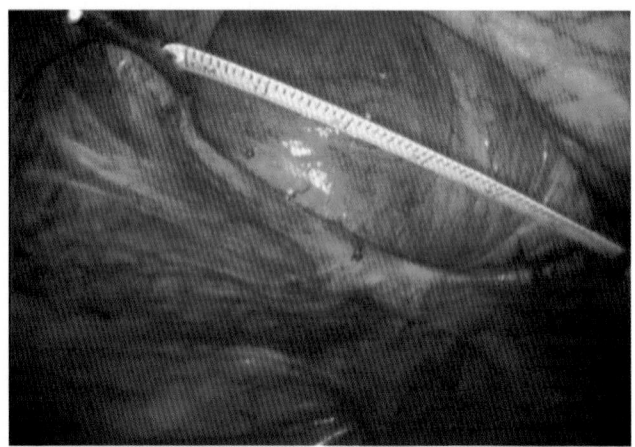

Figure 60 Measurement of the exposed hernia defect.

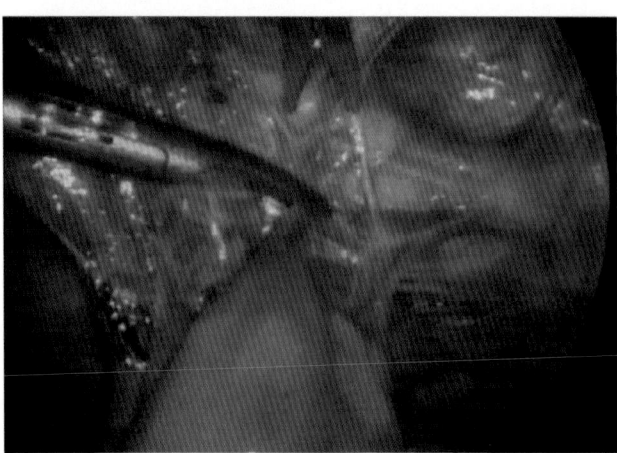

Figure 59 Adhesiolysis, performed with sharp dissection and judicious use of electrocautery.

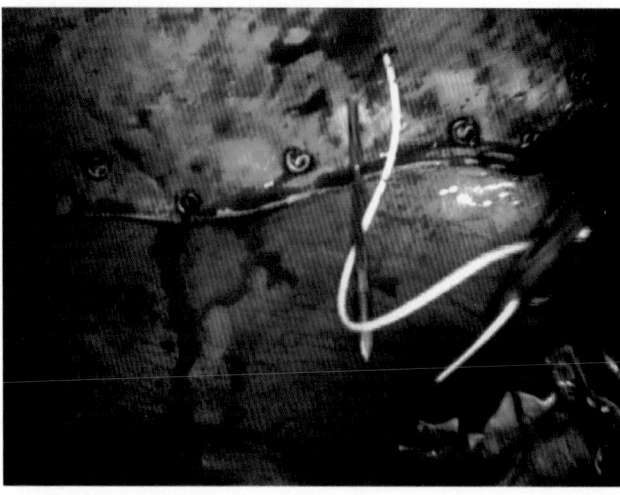

Figure 61 Use of the suture passer device to retrieve the ends of the transfascial sutures.

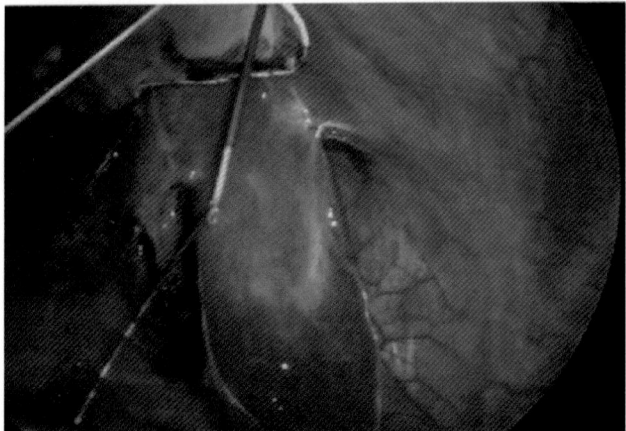

Figure 62 Use of the Keith needle and spinal cannula as an alternate means of placing transfascial sutures.

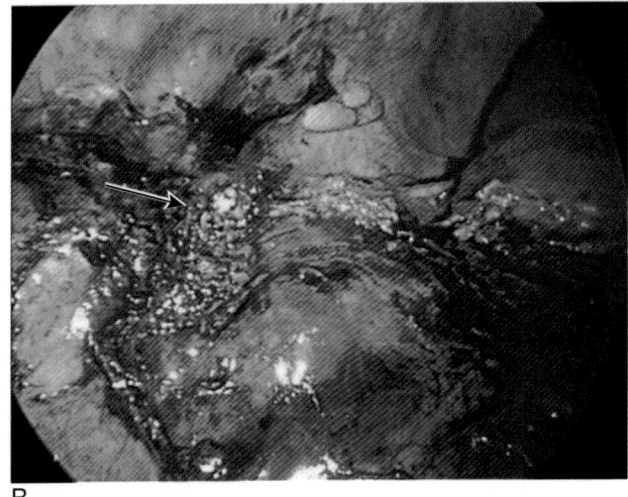

B

Figure 65 Complicated ileocolic Crohn's with fistula through retroperitoneum. **(B)** Retroperitoneum after laparoscopic mobilization of terminal ileum and right colon demonstrating fistula.

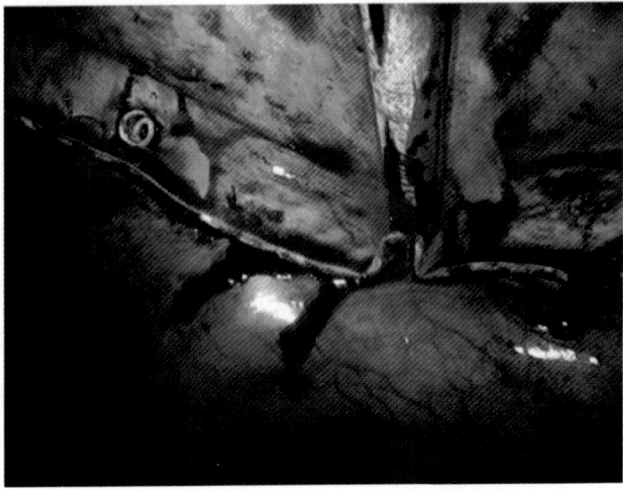

Figure 63 The mesh is secured by means of stapling device.

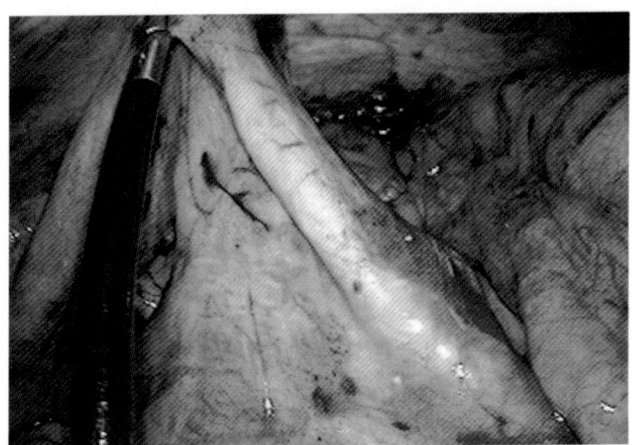

Figure 64 The ileocolic artery is identified by elevating the cecum at the junction of the bowel and the mesentery.

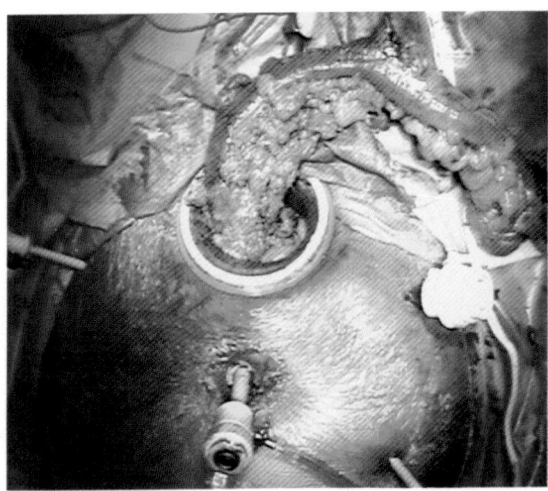

Figure 66 Extraction of the colon via the base of the Gelport hand-assist device. *Applied Medical Resources, Rancho Santo Margarita, CA.*

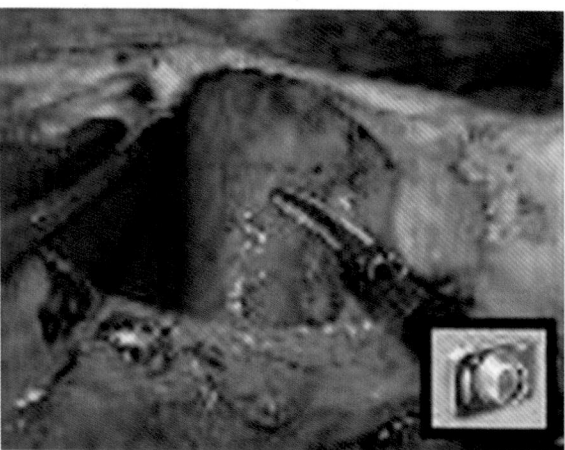

Figure 67 The gastrohepatic ligament is widely opened to expose the right crus of the diaphragm.

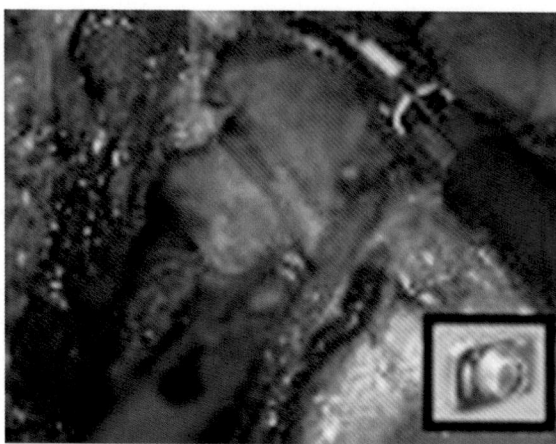

Figure 70 The posterior vagal trunk is identified.

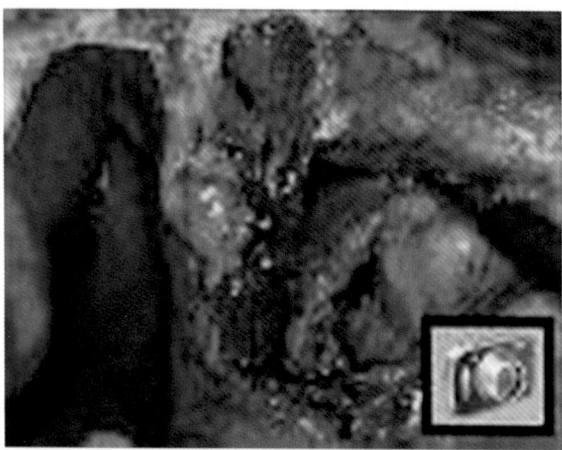

Figure 68 The dissection continues anteriorly across the esophagus until the left crus of the diaphragm is identified.

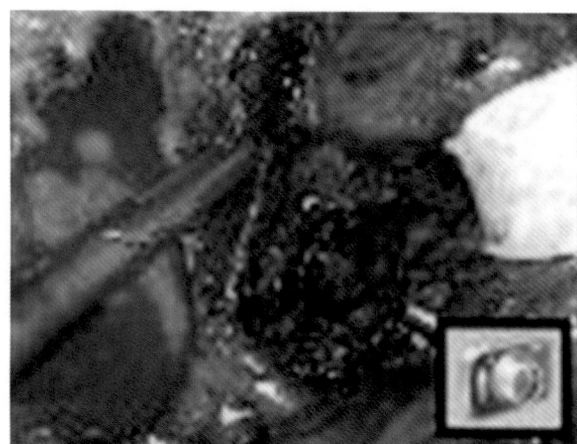

Figure 71 After an adequate window is created behind the esophagus, a Penrose drain is used to encircle the distal esophagus and both vagal trunks.

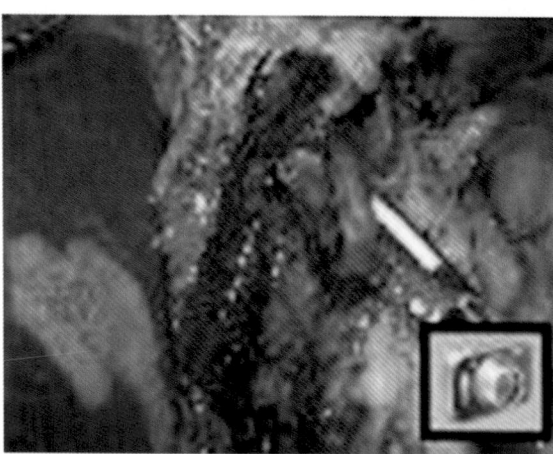

Figure 69 The anterior vagal trunk is identified and preserved.

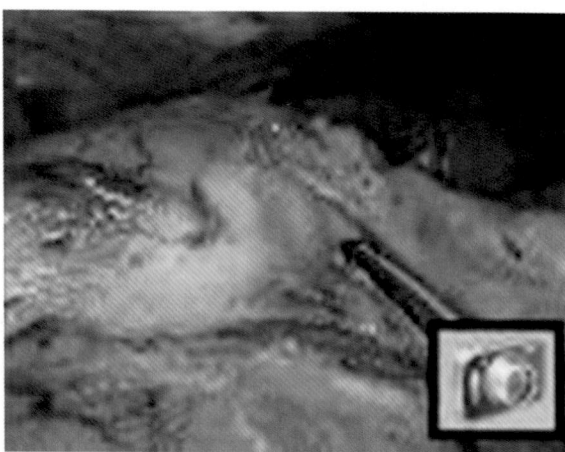

Figure 72 After the esophagus is completely mobilized and the right and left crus have been fully exposed, the short gastric vessels are divided completely.

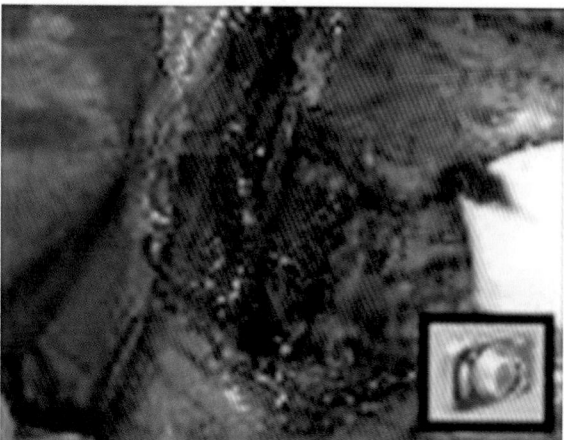

Figure 73 The size of the hiatal defect dictates the number of sutures placed, typically two or three. Excessive narrowing of the hiatus leads to postoperative dysphagia. A 5-mm telescope is used for this portion of the operation, as sutures are passed through the 10-mm port.

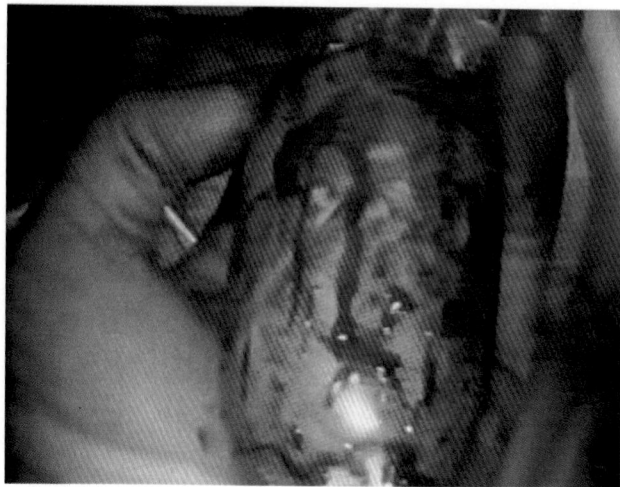

Figure 76 Extraction of the adrenal gland in an impermeable bag.

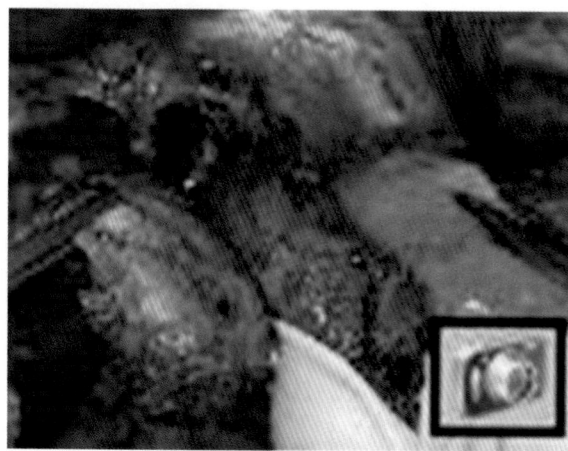

Figure 74 A short, floppy fundoplication is then performed with two sutures of 2-0 silk, placed 3 to 4 cm apart. See also Fig. 75.

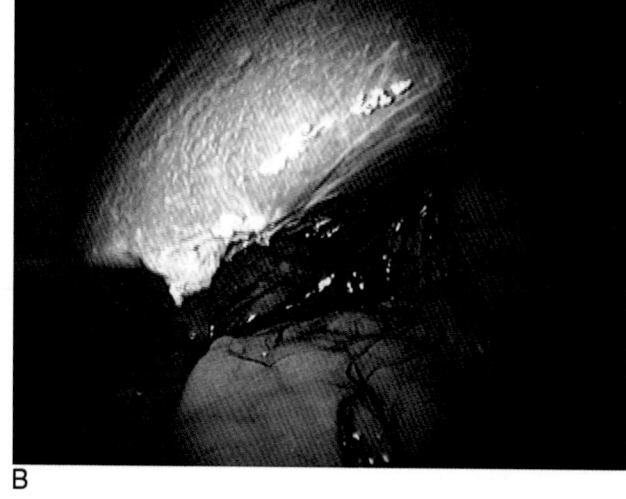

B

Figure 77 Right adrenal gland. **(B)** Laparoscopic view.

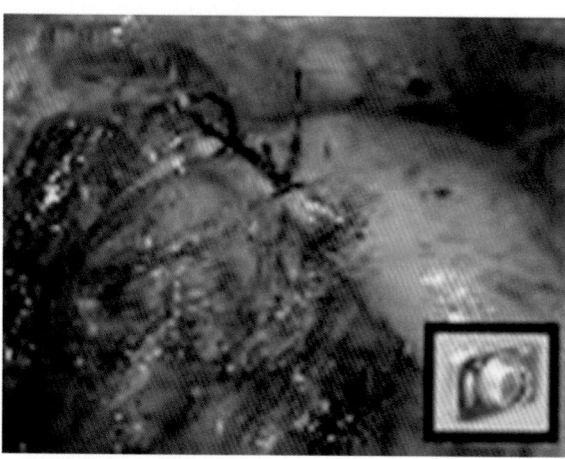

Figure 75

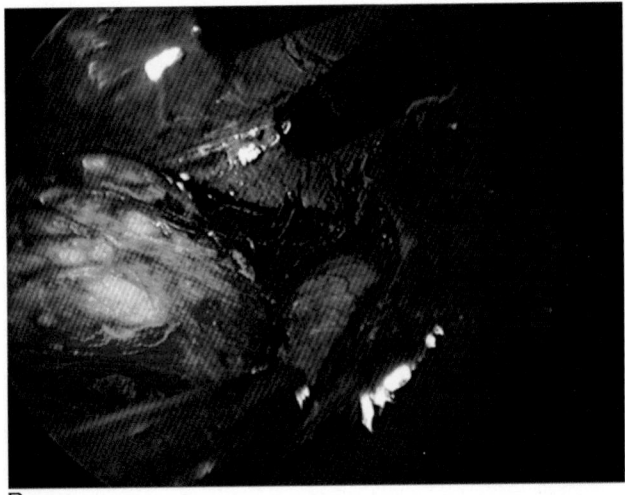

B

Figure 78 Dissection of the right adrenal gland. **(B)** Laparoscopic view.

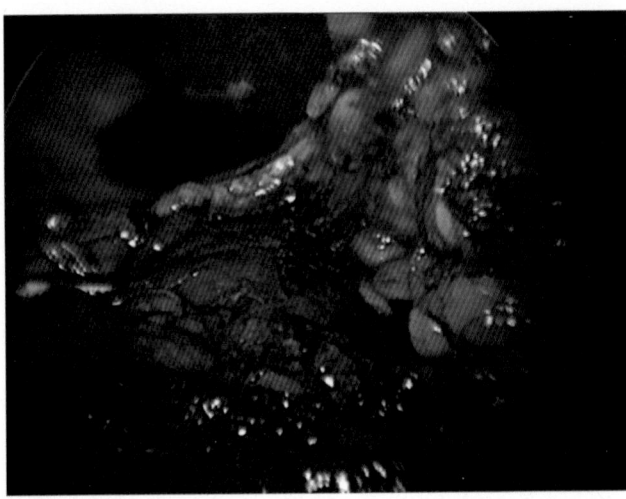

Figure 79 Laparoscopic view of the inferomedial dissection of the right adrenal gland.

ESOPHAGUS

ESOPHAGEAL FUNCTION TESTS

Cedric G. Bremner, MB, BCh, MCh

Esophageal function tests are used to evaluate patients with suspected esophageal motility disorders and gastroesophageal reflux disease, as well as to plan treatment. There are many ways to investigate the esophagus. The selection of tests used is related to the type of disorder investigated and the need to adjust surgical treatment to the motor capacity of the esophagus. Cineradiologic studies detect organic lesions fairly accurately but are less sensitive for functional disorders. Endoscopy is necessary in most disorders to view and biopsy mucosal lesions, especially Barrett's mucosa. Endoscopic ultrasonography has been used to detect the depth of invasion of malignant lesions and to detect metastatic nodes. Endoscopic mucosal resection (EMR) is a practical method for histologic staging of early cancers. pH monitoring is now routinely used to detect or confirm esophageal acid exposure. The detection of bilirubin in the stomach and esophagus has been used mainly as a research tool but has added insight into the pathogenesis of intestinalization and adenocarcinoma in Barrett's mucosa. Esophageal impedance studies have been introduced more recently and have an advantage in the evaluation of bolus movement and the detection of nonacid gastroesophageal reflux.

CINERADIOLOGY OF THE ESOPHAGUS

General indications for a video-esophagram are the following:

Globus sensation
Dysphagia
Regurgitation
Gastroesophageal reflux disease
Noncardiac chest pain
Esophageal neoplasm
Suspected postoperative complications

The act of swallowing is a dynamic process and cannot be assessed by static films. All studies should therefore include a videotape recording. The overall sensitivity for detecting esophageal disorders by video-esophagram is 55%. A video-esophagram is sensitive for detecting achalasia (94%) and scleroderma (100%); however, it is relatively insensitive for detecting nonspecific motility disorders.

Radiology will give a "road map" to guide the endoscopist to the site and nature of obstructing lesions of the esophagus. Radiology is often excluded from the investigation, and this may have serious consequences when dysphagia is being investigated. A cricopharyngeal bar, esophageal web, early achalasia, and even small diverticula may not be evident on endoscopy alone. A video-esophagram is therefore recommended as the first test in any patient who presents with dysphagia.

ESOPHAGEAL ENDOSCOPY

Endoscopic evaluation is necessary to confirm or establish a diagnosis in most esophageal disorders.

Specific Indications

Specific indications for endoscopy have been recommended by the American Society for Gastrointestinal Endoscopy (Consensus Statement. *Gastrointest Endosc* 52: 831–837, 2001). A modification of these indications that applies to surgical practice is as follows:

A. Upper abdominal symptoms that persist despite an appropriate trial of therapy
B. Upper abdominal symptoms associated with other symptoms or signs suggesting serious organic disease (e.g., anorexia and weight loss) or in patients older than 45 years
C. Dysphagia, odynophagia, aspiration, unexplained laryngeal symptoms, unexplained chronic cough, or asthma
D. Esophageal reflux symptoms that are persistent or recurrent despite appropriate therapy
E. Other diseases in which the presence of upper GI pathology might modify other planned management (e.g., patients who have a history of ulcer or GI bleeding who are scheduled for organ transplantation, long-term anticoagulation or chronic nonsteroidal anti-inflammatory drug therapy for arthritis, and those with cancer of the head and neck)
F. For confirmation and specific histologic diagnosis of radiologically demonstrated ulcers, strictures, and neoplastic lesions
G. Upper gastrointestinal bleeding
H. To assess acute injury after caustic ingestion
I. Removal of foreign bodies
J. Removal of selected polypoid lesions
K. Placement of feeding or drainage tubes (per oral, percutaneous endoscopic gastrostomy, percutaneous endoscopic jejunostomy)
L. Dilatation of stenotic lesions (e.g., with transendoscopic balloon dilators or dilatation systems employing guidewires)
M. Palliative treatment of stenosing neoplasms (e.g., laser, multipolar electrocoagulation, stent placement)

Normal Anatomy

Evaluation of the esophagus starts with a good view of the vocal cords and aryepiglottic folds. High gastroesophageal reflux is suspected in symptomatic patients who have inflammation of the posterior wall of the pharynx. The position of the crico-pharyngeal sphincter is best assessed on the final withdrawal of the endoscope and is noted by an encroachment on the lumen as the scope is withdrawn. On entering the esophagus, the scope shows that the mucosa is whitish, and fine vessels may be seen on the surface, especially at the lower end. The aortic arch causes a wall indentation usually at or beyond the 20-cm mark. The squamocolumnar junction is usually seen just proximal to the hiatus. It has a regular margin. There should not be any food residue in the esophagus.

The diaphragmatic crura cause a narrowing at the lower end of the esophagus and can be identified by asking the patient to sniff, whereupon the lumen of the esophagus narrows further. The gastroesophageal junction is identified as the site at which the gastric mucosal folds meet the tubular esophagus. On entering the stomach, the scope should indicate that there is a minimal amount of clear secretion. The gastric mucosa is carefully inspected, and its distensability is noted. The endoscope is advanced into the duodenal bulb and second part of the duodenum to exclude other pathology. When the endoscope is retracted to the incisura level, it is retroflexed to give a view of the gastroesophageal junction. The normal anatomy of the junction is noted, and the stomach is insufflated to assess the competency of the lower esophageal sphincter and to grade the sphincter according to Hills's grading (Fig. 1). The lesser and greater curvatures and the anterior and posterior aspects of the mucosa are systematically and carefully inspected for any abnormalities. The stomach is deflated before the instrument is retracted for a final viewing of the esophagus.

Biopsies from the retroflexed view of the squamocolumnar junction and the esophagus are recommended in patients with a history

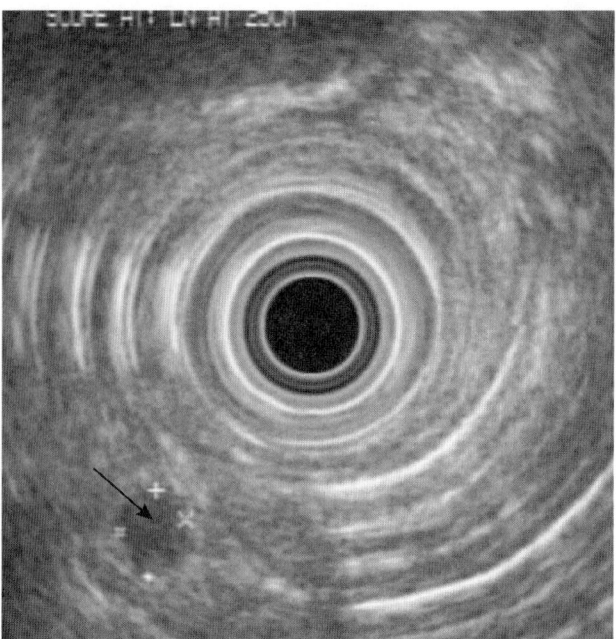

Figure 2 Endoscopic esophageal ultrasonography shows five esophageal layers. A lymph node is evident on this study. *From Rice TW, Blackstone EH, Rybicki LA, and others: J Thorac Cardiovasc Surg 125:1103, 2003.*

of gastroesophageal reflux disease (GERD), especially if there is a history of GERD of more than 5 years, to exclude Barrett's epithelium. Microscopic evidence of GERD may be present even in the absence of macroscopic esophagitis. It is routine in many clinics to biopsy the antrum for evidence of *Helicobacter pylori* infection. Any suspicious areas should also be biopsied.

ENDOSCOPIC ULTRASONOGRAPHY

Endoscopic ultrasonography combines endoscopy and 5–12 MHz frequency ultrasonography to evaluate the different layers of the esophageal wall and adjacent structures outside the wall. The presence of nodal metastases increases with the depth of tumor invasion (Fig. 2). If the tumor is confined to the mucosa, nodal metastases are unlikely, but they are likely to be present in nearly 90% of patients who have disease eroding through the wall. The technique requires training, however, and is used mostly in centers dedicated to the treatment of esophageal cancer. A more practical method of assessing the depth of early tumors is by endoscopic mucosal resection.

ENDOSCOPIC MUCOSAL RESECTION

Endoscopic mucosal resection (EMR) for small lesions is proving to be invaluable in the assessment of the depth of small lesions. This technique is suitable only for lesions that are small, flat, or only slightly raised, and in which it appears that there is a good chance that the mucosal resection will be a complete resection of the tumor. The lesion is first raised from the submucosa by endoscopic injection of saline. The lesion is drawn into a cap applied to the lower end of the endoscope using suction and is then snared from its attachment for retrieval. If the lesion is malignant and the EMR demonstrates a complete resection, there is a minimal chance of nodal metastases, and an esophageal resection without node removal should be curative. However, if the EMR demonstrates deeper infiltration beyond the muscularis mucosa, nodal metastases are more likely and an en bloc resection may offer a better prognosis. At present, we do not believe that EMR alone should be the definitive treatment of esophageal adenocarcinoma, as is practiced in some centers.

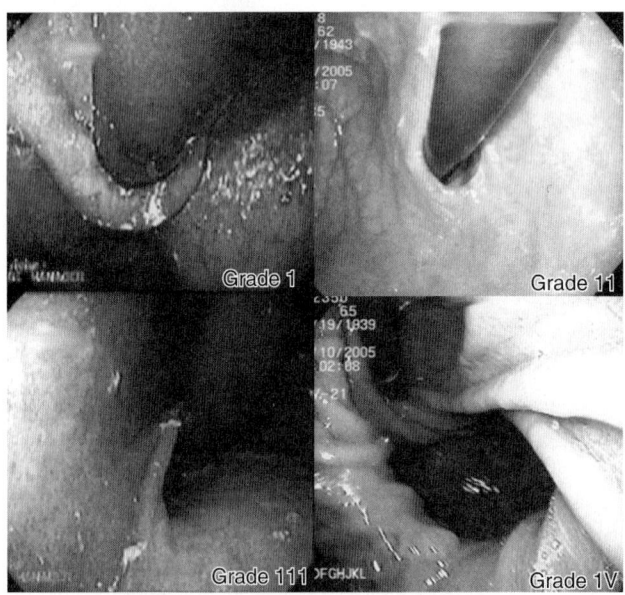

Figure 1 Hill's endoscopic grading of the retroflexed view of the cardia. Grade I valve: A ridge of tissue 3 to 4 cm long on the lesser curve is closely applied to the endoscope. Grade II valve: The ridge is less well defined than in grade I, and it opens occasionally with respiration but closes promptly. Grade III valve: The ridge is barely present, and there is often failure to close around the endoscope. It is nearly always accompanied by a hiatal hernia and esophagitis. Grade IV valve: There is no muscular ridge. The gastroesophageal junction remains open all the time, and the squamous epithelium can often be seen from this retroflexed position. A hiatal hernia is always present. *From Hill LD, Kozarek RA. J Clin Gastroenter 28:194–197, 1999.* (See *color insert Figure 1.*)

ESOPHAGEAL MANOMETRY

Esophageal manometry is used to evaluate the resting pressures in the esophageal body and upper and lower sphincters and the response to swallowing. The various systems available use a flexible catheter that is either water perfused or that incorporates solid-state transducers. Software programs are used to give an accurate assessment of pressures generated. It is important to refer to normal values generated by previous researchers or to generate a new set of values for the given equipment.

The indications for esophageal manometry are as follows.

Diagnostic

1. Motility disorders: achalasia, hypertensive lower esophageal sphincter, nutcracker esophagus, inadequate esophageal motility (IEM; includes scleroderma and diffuse esophageal spasm), nonspecific esophageal motor disorder
2. Dysphagia: assessment of the cause of functional obstruction
3. Chest pain: assessment of the cause and relation to gastroesophageal reflux
4. Respiratory disorders (especially chronic cough): a motility disorder may be associated with gastroesophageal reflux responsible for the cough

Preoperative Assessment

1. Verify the correct diagnosis and suitability for surgery.
2. Avoid postoperative dysphagia.

Postoperative Assessment

1. Assessment of the response to surgery.
2. Confirmation of the effect of treatment on the lower esophageal sphincter (e.g., for achalasia).
3. Assess the cause of failed surgery.

Technical Considerations

A solid-state or water-perfused catheter system is used.

It is important to use a water-perfused catheter system that maintains a steady rate of flow.

Pressures recorded may vary according to the equipment used, and it is therefore important for each esophageal function laboratory either to develop its own normal values or to use normal values published in the literature and generated from comparable equipment and techniques.

Motility is usually assessed in a resting state and during swallowing. The manometry catheter is swallowed until all of the sensor sites are in the stomach. The catheter is then pulled back in increments of 0.5 to 1 cm to measure the resting pressures of the lower esophageal sphincter, the esophageal body, and the cricopharyngeal sphincter (Fig. 3).

A swallow study of 10 consecutive swallows each of a 5-ml bolus of water is then performed. This will assess the relaxation of the two sphincters and the esophageal body contractions (Figs. 4–7).

A newer device, the Manoscan (Sierra Scientific Instruments, San Diego, CA), incorporates 32 solid-state transducers into one tube so that a pull-through is unnecessary. Ambulatory manometry is also available

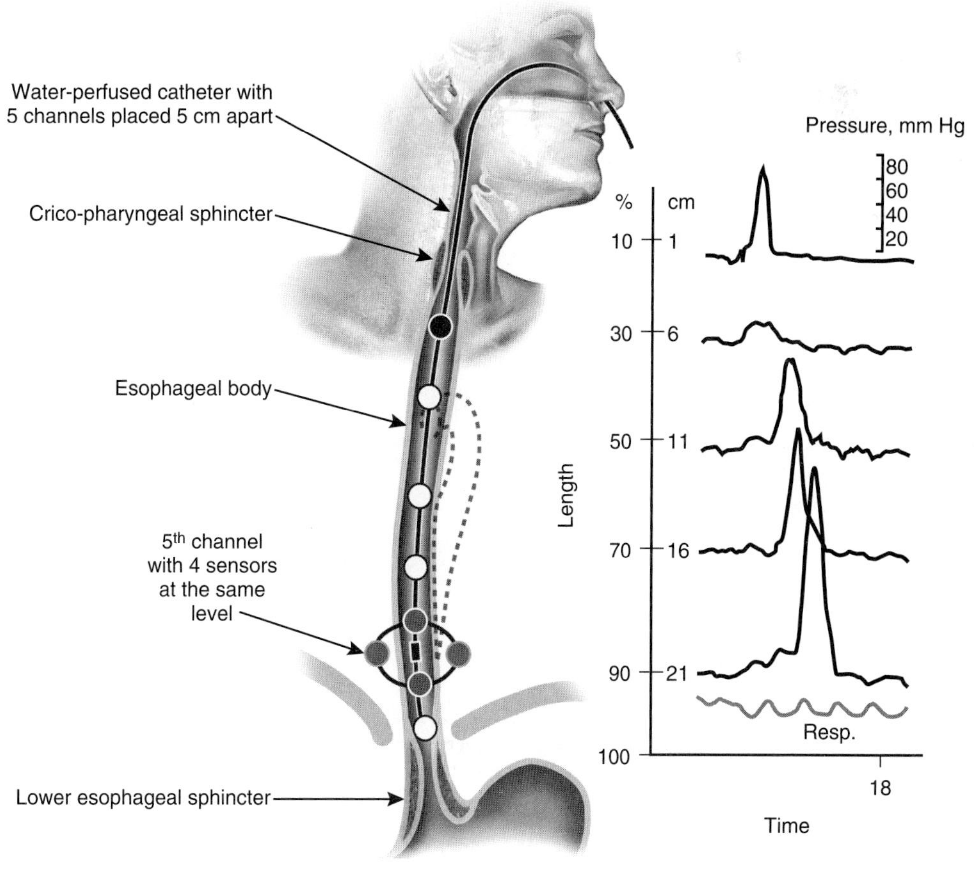

Figure 3 Esophageal manometry: a water-perfused or solid-state catheter is positioned in the esophagus. The sensors are 5 cm apart, and in this catheter, there are four radially placed sensors at the same level to measure the lower esophageal sphincter.

Water-perfused catheter with 5 channels placed 5 cm apart

Crico-pharyngeal sphincter

Esophageal body

5th channel with 4 sensors at the same level

Lower esophageal sphincter

Pressure, mm Hg

Length

Resp.

Time

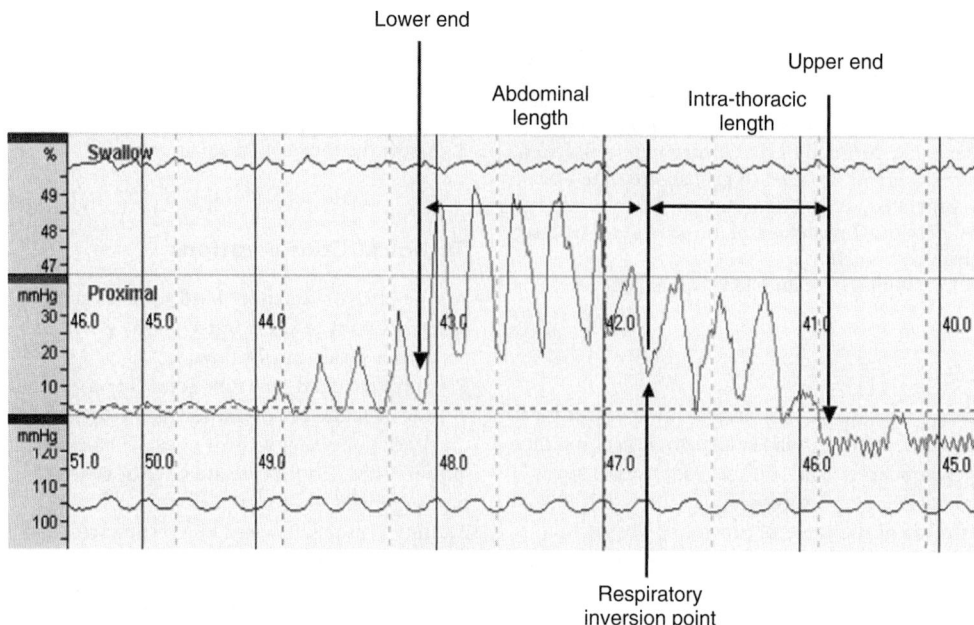

Figure 4   A normal lower esophageal sphincter. The total length is divided into a thoracic and abdominal segment at the respiratory inversion point. Baseline pressures in the stomach are measured at the end-expiratory phase of respiration. Note that the pressure in the thoracic esophagus is negative.

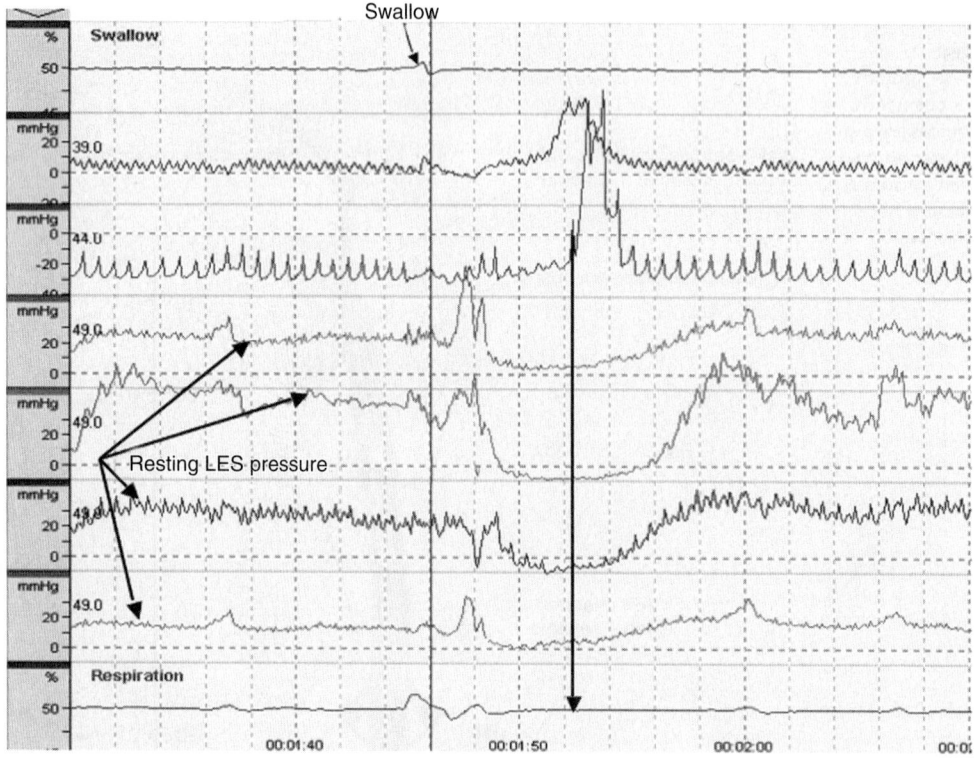

Figure 5   A relaxation study of the lower esophageal sphincter *(LES)*. Four probes are positioned at the same level in the lower esophageal sphincter. Following a swallow of 5 ml water, the sphincter pressure drops to baseline, demonstrating complete relaxation. The uppermost probe, 5 cm above the LES, shows a contraction response to a swallow.

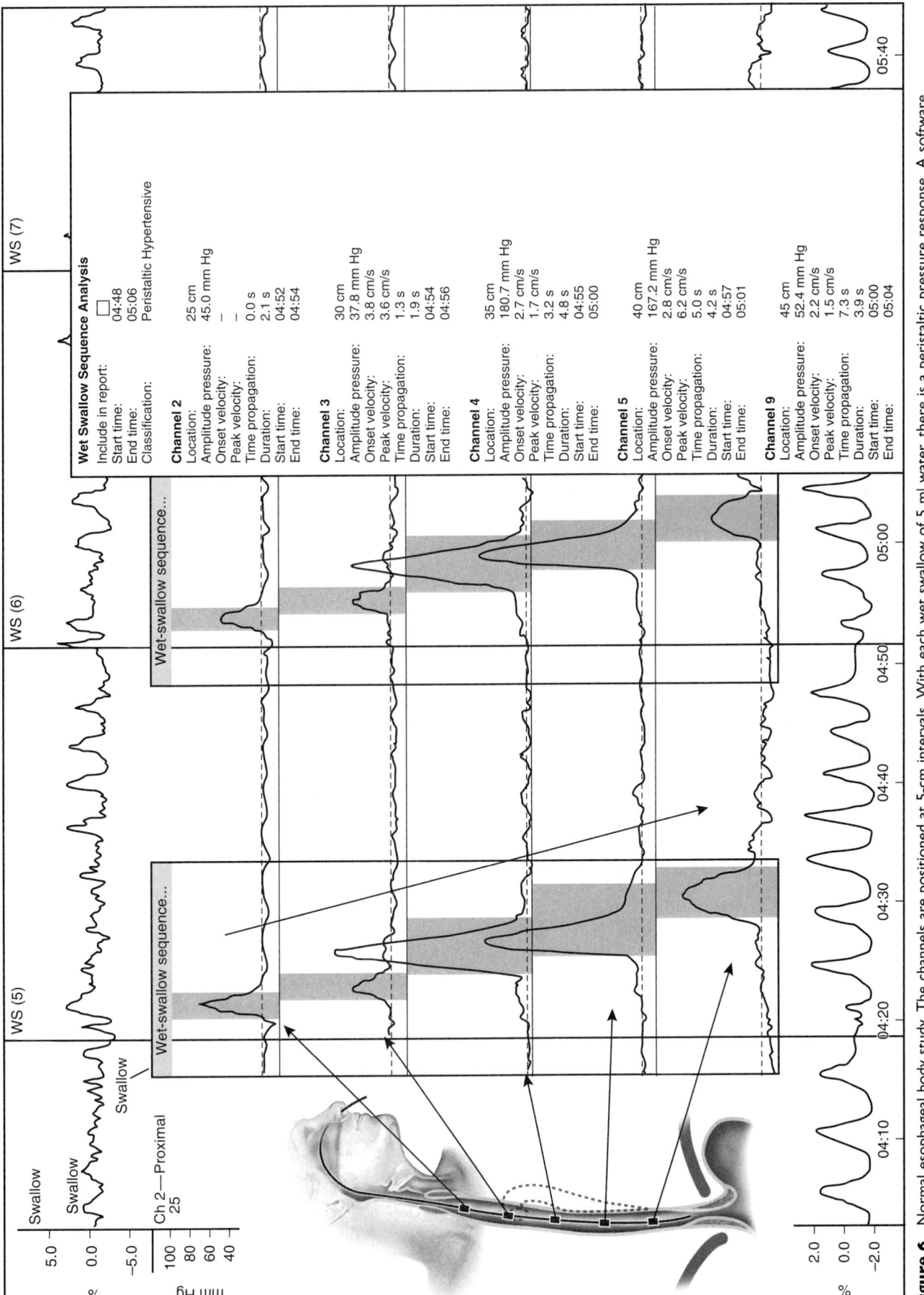

Figure 6 Normal esophageal body study. The channels are positioned at 5-cm intervals. With each wet swallow of 5 ml water, there is a peristaltic pressure response. A software program calculates the height, duration, and propagation of each swallow response.

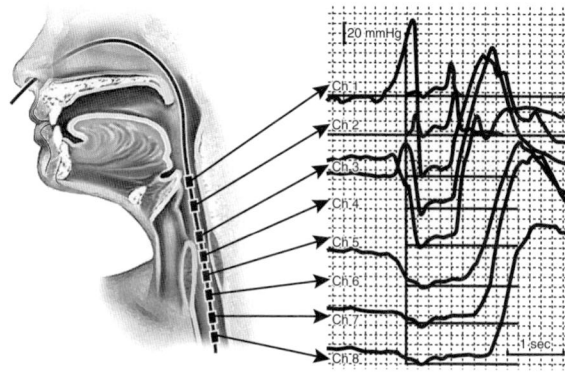
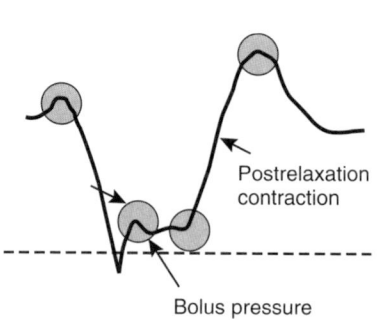

Figure 7 Normal cricopharyngeal sphincter *(CPS)* swallow study using an 8-channel catheter. The channels are 1 cm apart. In the diagram on the left, two channels are in the pharynx, three in the CPS, and three in the esophagus. On swallowing, the resting CPS pressure falls precipitously (see also diagram on the right). This pressure drop is followed by a brief bolus pressure rise before a postrelaxation contraction. Channel 5 demonstrates that the relaxation of the lower part of the sphincter occurs before the relaxation of the upper part of the sphincter.

and used when the results of the stationary assessment are indefinite. The stationary method assesses only 10 swallows, compared with approximately 1000 swallows that accumulate in a 24-hour ambulatory period.

The normal lower esophageal sphincter (LES) high-pressure zone is composed of both the hiatal pressure and the intrinsic lower esophageal sphincter. Approximately one third of the LES lies within the thoracic cavity, and two thirds within the abdominal cavity. The manometric division between the thoracic and abdominal portions is marked by the pressure inversion point (also termed respiratory inversion point [RIP]), the point at which the inspiratory upstroke becomes a respiratory downstroke (see Figs. 4–7).

Normal values for the lower esophageal sphincter, the esophageal body, and the cricopharyngeal sphincter are listed in Tables 1, 2, and 3.

Normal relaxation of the LES in response to a swallow is demonstrated in Figure 5.

Mechanically Defective Lower Esophageal Sphincter

A lower esophageal sphincter is considered to be mechanically defective when one or more of the components is abnormal (pressure <6 mm Hg, total length <2 cm, abdominal length <1 cm). The chance of gastroesophageal reflux is 74% when one component is defective, 75% with two components, and 92% with three components.

Hypertensive Lower Esophageal Sphincter

Definition

A hypertensive LES has a sphincter pressure above the 95th percentile of normal. The value will differ according to the method used

for measurement. This is the second most common motility disorder.

1. Pressure measurement at the point of respiratory reversal according to DeMeester: mean >26 mm Hg ± 2 SD (Fig. 8).
2. Pressure measurement at the midrespiratory pressure level of the highest peaks according to Castell: mean >40 mm Hg ± 3 SD.

A hypertensive lower esophageal sphincter can be diagnosed only by manometry, and failure to perform manometry on patients with undiagnosed chest pain and/or dysphagia may miss the diagnosis. A hypertensive lower esophageal sphincter may cause outflow obstruction not evident on radiologic studies.

Achalasia

Definition: The most common motility disorder in which the LES does not relax adequately and in which there is absent peristalsis in the esophageal body. The LES in achalasia is hypertensive in approximately 50% of patients and characteristically fails to relax adequately. There is pressurization (intrathoracic pressures that are normally negative become positive) in approximately 60% of studies (Figs. 9 and 10). The most diagnostic feature of achalasia is absence of peristalsis in 100% of swallow responses (Fig. 11).

Table 4 gives distinguishing features between a hypertensive lower esophageal sphincter and achalasia, which may also have a high sphincter pressure.

Hypercontractile Esophagus ("Nutcracker Esophagus")

Definition: The mean height of swallow responses in either of the two distal channels exceeds the upper limit of normal (180 mm Hg) or the duration of swallow responses exceeds 7 seconds in patients who have either chest pain or dysphagia (Fig. 12).

Table 1: Normal Lower Esophageal Sphincter Parameters in 50 Healthy Volunteers (after Zaninotto and DeMeester 1988)

LES Measurements	Mean	SD	Median	Maximum	Minimum	Percentile	
						2.5	5
Pressure (mm Hg)	14.87	5.14	13.8	25.6	5.2	6.1	8
Abdominal length (cm)	2.18	0.72	2.2	5	0.8	0.89	1.1
Overall length (cm)	3.65	0.68	3.5	5.5	2.4	2.4	2.6

Table 2: Normal Values for Swallow Responses in the Esophageal Body: Medians (5th and 95th Percentiles)

		Wet Swallows	Dry Swallows
Amplitude (mm Hg)			
	Level I	88 (40–177)	74 (26–154)
	Level II	40 (14–94)	28 (14–74)
	Level III	76 (30–164)	52 (26–142)
	Level IV	93 (38–180)	61 (20–148)
	Level V	93 (36–190)	78 (22–172)
Duration (s)			
	Level I	2.3 (1.5–4.3)	2.3 (1.4–3.9)
	Level II	3.1 (1.8–4.8)	2.8 (1.0–4.5)
	Level III	3.3 (2.4–5.2)	3.1 (1.8–4.6)
	Level IV	3.6 (2.6–5.7)	3.4 (2.0–5.6)
	Level V	3.7 (2.4–7.0)	3.6 (2.4–6–4)
Slope (mm Hg/s)			
	Level I	99 (22–222)	72 (25–153)
	Level II	30 (9–61)	22 (6–61)
	Level III	52 (20–117)	40 (14–96)
	Level IV	66 (25–120)	45 (14–102)
	Level V	62 (23–120)	47 (16–104)
Propagation speed (cm/sec)			
	Level I	2.4 (1.5–4.6)	2.8 (1.6–6.2)
	Level II–III	2.8 (1.9–6.2)	3.1 (1.9–8.3)
	Level III–IV	3.8 (1.9–8.3)	4.5 (1.8–8.3)
	Level IV–V	2.6 (1.3–8.3)	3.5 (1.7–12)
	Level I–IV	2.9 (2.2–3.7)	3.3 (2.3–4.4)
	Level I–V	2.9 (2.1–4)	3.4 (2.2–5)

From Costantini M, Bremner RM, Hoeft SF, and others. *Gastroenterology* 103:A 1407, 1992.

Table 3: Normal Swallow Responses for the Cricopharyngeal Sphincter

	Median	5th Percentile	95th Percentile
Length of UES (cm)	5.0	4.1	5.1
Resting pressure (mm Hg)	61.0	40.0	87.0
Bolus pressure (mm Hg)	13.3	11.2	15.7
Pharyngeal pressure (mm Hg)	52.0	46.4	56.5
Minimal residual pressure (mm Hg)	0.5	−2.3	3.2
Maximal residual pressure (mm Hg)	11.3	8.9	14.5
Relaxation time (s)	0.58	0.546	0.60
Time of initiation of relaxation (s)			
Upper UES	−0.10	0.19	−0.43
Lower UES	−0.28	−0.401	−0.19

UES, upper esophageal sphincter.
1. Station pull-through study: Length 5 cm (4.1–5.1); resting pressure 62.9 mm Hg (41.3–87.2).

Ineffective Esophageal Motility (IEM)

Definition: A distinct manometric entity characterized by a hypocontractile esophagus in which the distal esophageal amplitudes are <30 mm Hg or the contractions are nontransmitted in >30% of the wet swallows (Fig. 13). IEM incorporates scleroderma of the esophagus and end-stage reflux disease.

Diffuse Esophageal Spasm

Definition: A clinical syndrome characterized by symptoms of substernal chest pain, dysphagia, or both; the radiographic appearance of localized nonprogressive waves (tertiary contractions); and an increased incidence of nonperistaltic contractions recorded by intraluminal manometry (Fig. 14). Because the abnormal contractions are usually seen in the distal esophagus, Castell has suggested that the term "distal esophageal spasm" is more appropriate. Note that the disorder relates more to uncoordinated contractions than to high-pressure contractions.

This is an uncommon condition, accounting for 3% to 10% of all motility abnormalities.

Nonspecific Esophageal Motor Disorder (NSEMD)

Definition: An esophageal motility disorder that does not have features of a named motility disorder. Many of the features of NSEMD described in older classifications have been incorporated into the

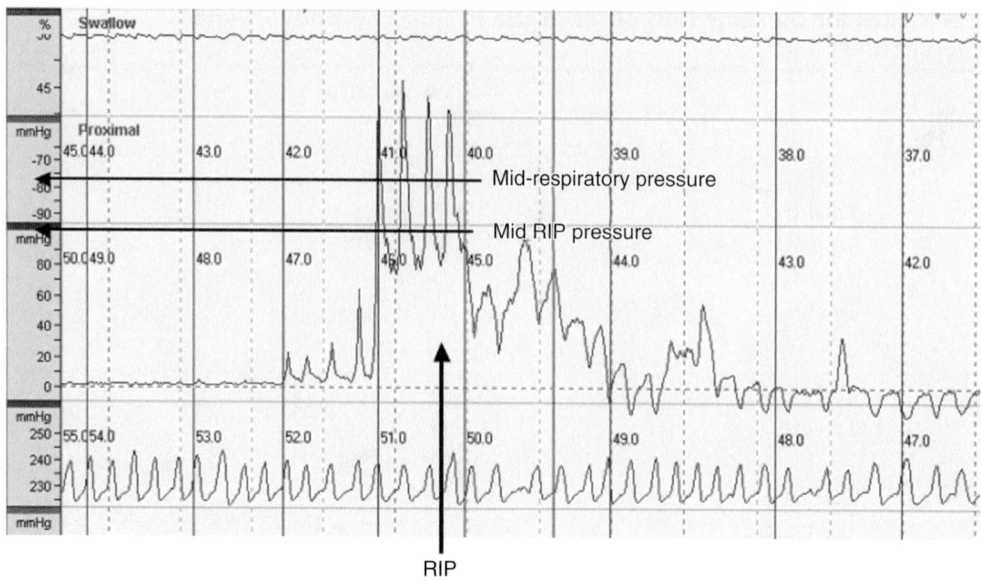

Figure 8 A hypertensive lower esophageal sphincter with resting pressures >26 mm Hg measured at the respiratory inversion point.

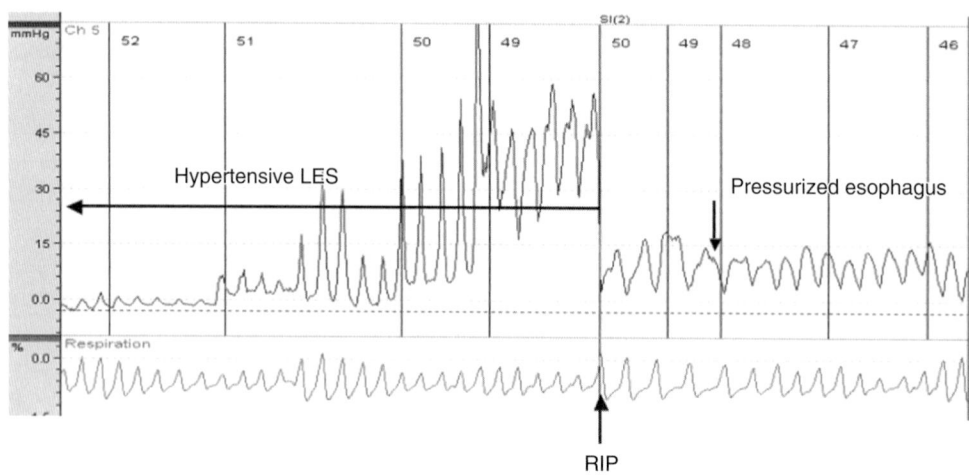

Figure 9 Achalasia. The lower esophageal sphincter is hypertensive in approximately 50% of studies, and the esophagus is pressurized in approximately 60% of studies.

category of ineffective esophageal motility. However, some unnamed features are still encountered and are included as NSEMD (e.g., triple-peaked contractions, retrograde contractions).

Hiatal Hernia

Manometric features of a hiatal hernia are well described. The lower esophageal sphincter is displaced away from the diaphragm so that two pressure profiles ("double hump" with an intervening "plateau") are recorded (Fig. 15).

Pharyngeal Manometry

Because of the short length and rapid sequences of the swallow responses, pharyngeal manometry requires experience and a deeper understanding of the swallow events. Although some laboratories have not been successful using water-perfused systems, we have been successful with a special catheter in which the sensor sites are only 1 cm apart.

The important sequences of both the water-perfused and solid-state systems are the same and will detect the important essentials of pharyngeal pressure, failed relaxation, and an increase in bolus pressures (see Fig. 7).

ESOPHAGEAL pH MEASUREMENTS

Indications for pH Monitoring

1. Symptomatic patients with normal endoscopy for surgical consideration
2. Failed antireflux surgery evaluation
3. Symptoms refractory to proton pump inhibitor therapy
4. Chest pain evaluation
5. Otorhinolaryngolic symptoms
6. Nonallergic asthma and chronic undiagnosed cough

Acid exposure to the esophagus is measured using an intraluminal pH probe. Two methods are available: an intraluminal tube method

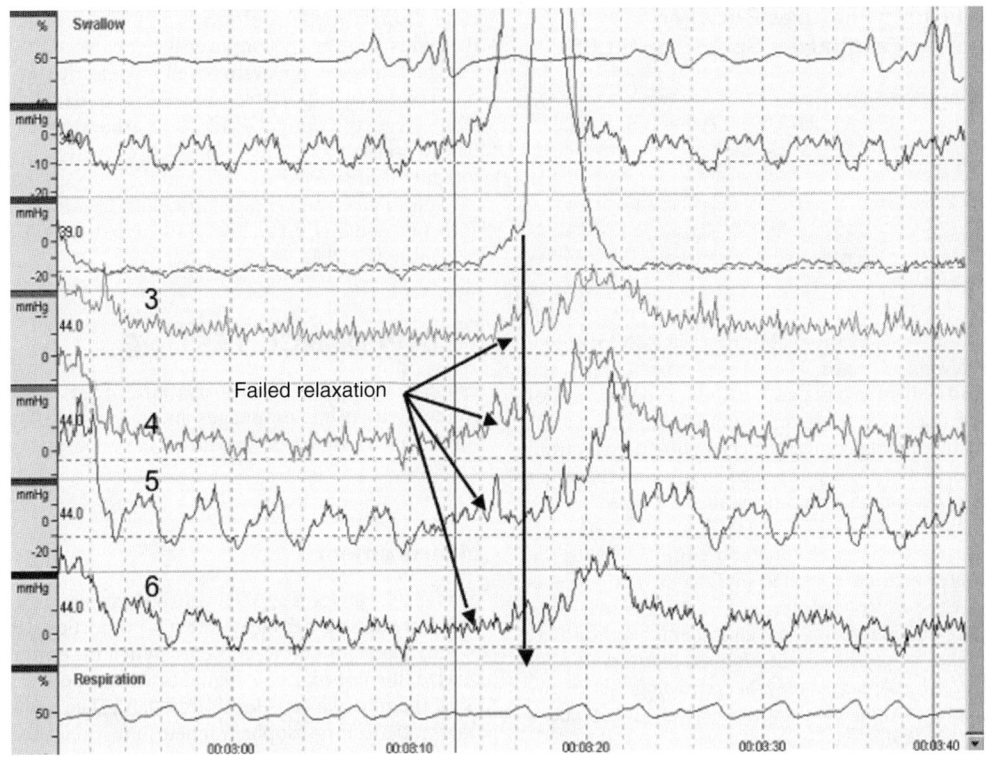

Figure 10   Achalasia. A swallow study shows incomplete relaxation of the lower esophageal sphincter.

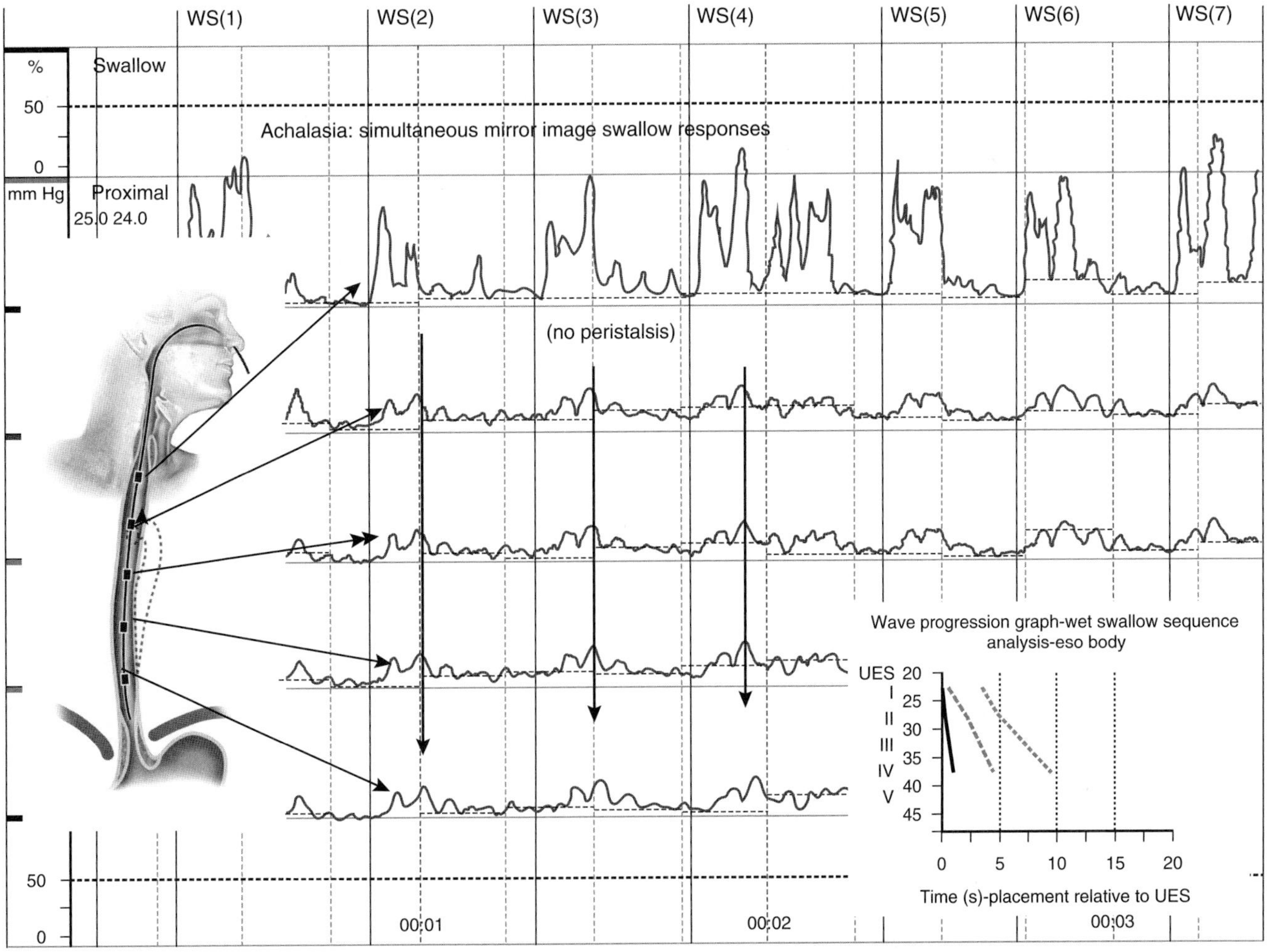

Figure 11   Achalasia. A swallow study in the esophageal body demonstrates mirror-image swallow responses (simultaneous responses).

Table 4: Distinguishing Features Between a Hypertensive Lower Esophageal Sphincter HLES and Achalasia

	HLES	Achalasia
Relaxation of LES	Usual	Fails or incomplete
Negative intrathoracic pressure	+	Usually positive
Peristaltic swallow responses	+	Never

LES, lower esophageal sphincter.

and a tubeless "Bravo" probe (Medtronic, Minneapolis, MN) method. Both methods provide similar results. The tubeless probe (Bravo) is a more comfortable and patient-acceptable method. A comparison of the normal values for the Bravo probe measurement and the values from the conventional nasoesophageal catheter method derived from 50 healthy volunteers with the probe positioned 5 cm above the upper border of the LES as measured manometrically are listed in the Table 5.

Normal values for the Bravo probe method compared with the nasopharyngeal catheter method are listed in Table 5. The probe is also placed 5 cm above the upper border of the LES as measured manometrically or as judged at endoscopy. The endoscopic method may lack accuracy at present, but studies are in progress to assess this.

Acid exposure of the esophagus may be physiological, in the supine position, erect position, or postprandial, or it may be a combined exposure (Fig. 16).

The percentage time pH <4 in the 2-hour postprandial period in normal subjects (*n* = 94) is 8.43 (95th percentile).

BILITEC MONITORING

The bilirubin concentration in a solution can be directly measured by spectrophotometry, based on specific absorption at a wavelength of 453 nm. Measurement of bilirubin in the stomach and esophagus

is an indirect method of measuring bile, a frequent constituent of the refluxate in gastroesophageal reflux (see Fig. 17).

The Bilitec, an apparatus used to measure the presence of bilirubin, consists of a portable optoelectronic data logger, which can be strapped to the patient's side, and a fiber-optic probe that can be passed transnasally and positioned anywhere in the lumen of the foregut (Bilitec; Medtronic).

The median percentage time with absorbance >0.2 is 0%, the 75th percentile is 0.1%, the 95th percentile is 1.7%, and the 99th percentile is 6.7%.

IMPEDANCE TESTING

Esophageal impedance is a measure of the resistance to electrical conductivity of the esophagus and its contents and is used to measure bolus transport. Impedance is inversely proportional to electrical conductivity.

Measurement

A small AC voltage is applied to two electrodes on a catheter assembly. This generates a small current that is proportional to the conductivity of the esophagus and its contents. When the esophagus is empty and relaxed, the impedance is high, but when a bolus expands the esophagus, the impedance is low. The electrical current is so small that it does not affect the esophageal neuromuscular mechanism.

Esophageal Impedance Combined with Motility and Reflux Monitoring

A single catheter incorporates electrodes for impedance measurement, transducers for pressure measurement, and a pH probe (Multi-channel Intra-luminal Impedance-MII; Sandhill, Highlands Ranch, CO).

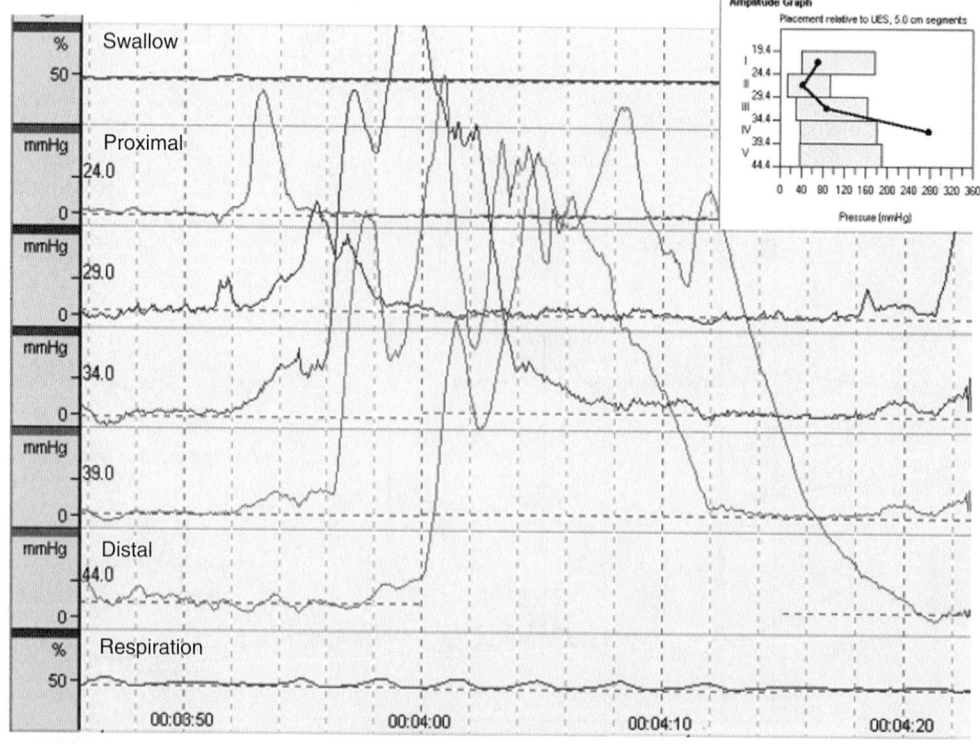

Figure 12 A hypercontracting esophageal body that is designated a "nutcracker esophagus" if the pressures are >180 mm Hg and if the patient complains of chest pain or dysphagia.

Figure 13 Ineffective esophageal motility. Thirty percent or more of the contractions are below 30 mm Hg pressure, and/or >30% of the contractions are nonpropulsive.

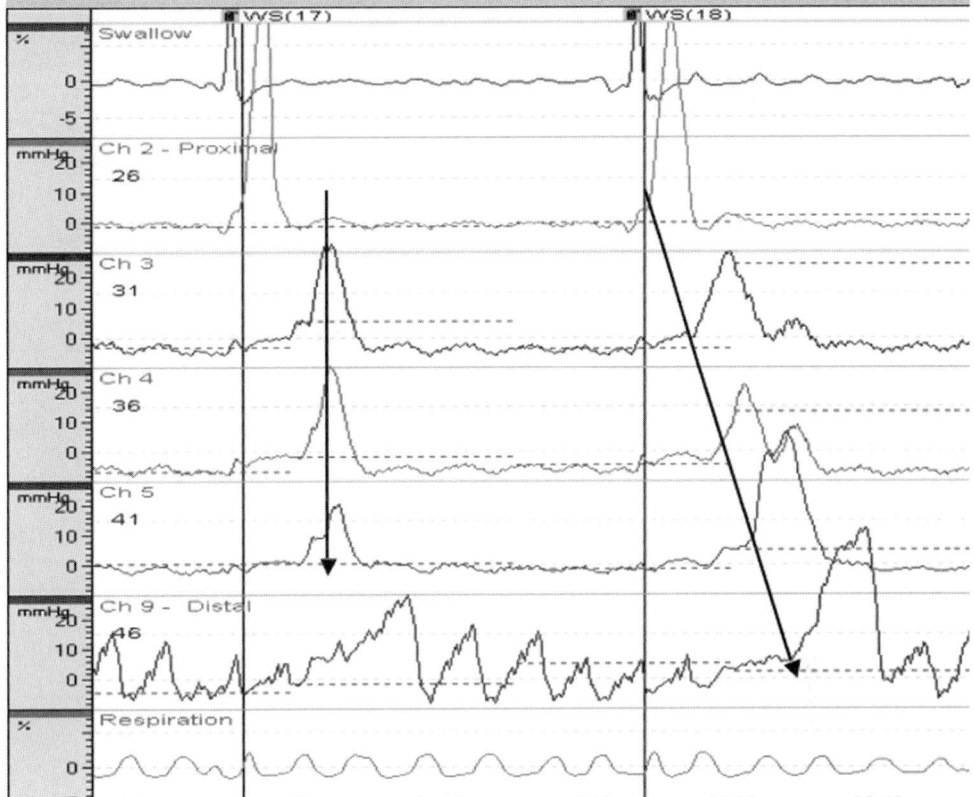

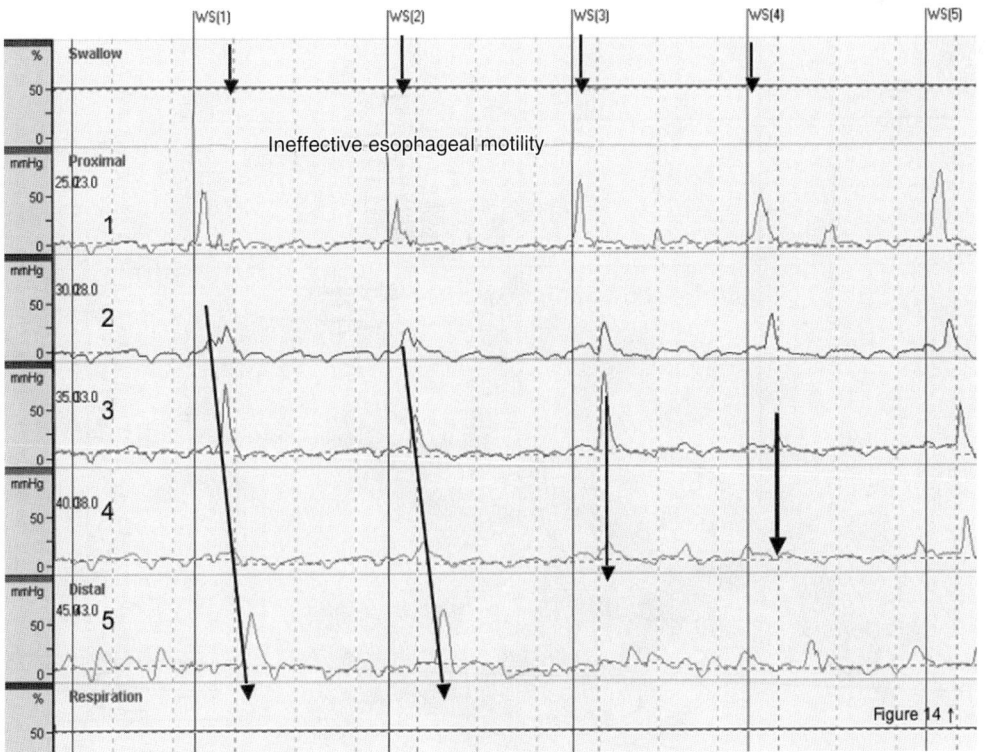

Figure 14 Diffuse esophageal spasm. More than 30% of the swallow responses are simultaneous, and the remaining responses are peristaltic.

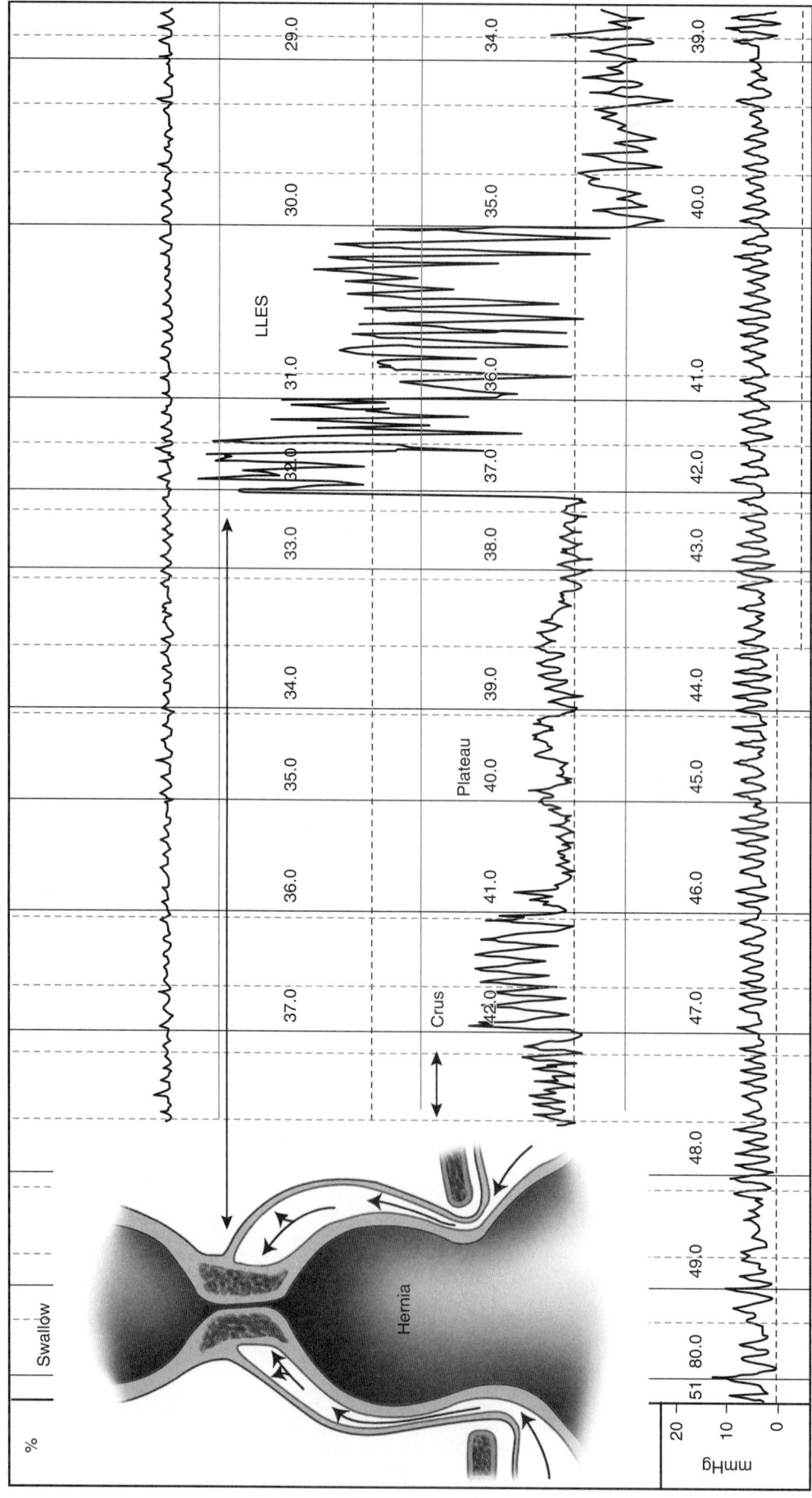

Figure 15 Manometric features of a hiatal hernia. There is a "double hump": hiatal pressure "hump" and lower esophageal sphincter "hump" with an intervening plateau of pressure. The diagram on the left demonstrates the origin of the two humps from the crura and the intrinsic lower esophageal sphincter.

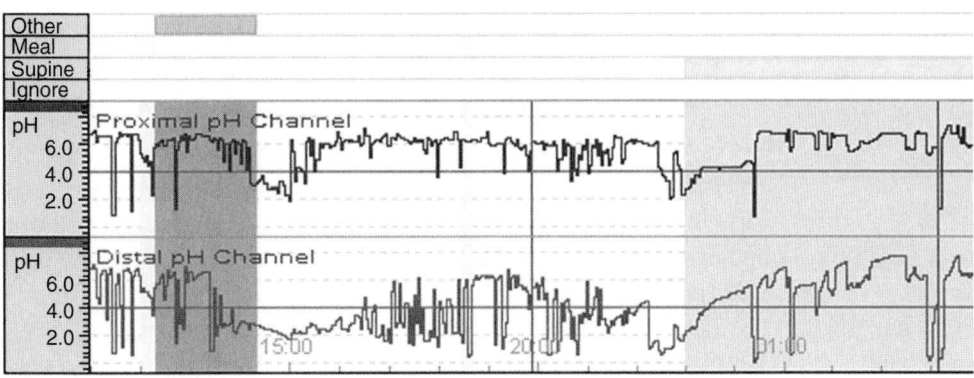

Reflux Table - Proximal

	Total	Meal	Supine	Upright	PostPr	Other
Duration of period (HH:MM)	21:11	00:30	06:59	14:11	03:59	02:00
Number of refluxes	40	1	6	35	11	9
Number of long refluxes (>5 [min])	3	0	1	3	0	0
Duration of longest reflux (min)	30	0	8	30	1	1
Time pH <4 ([min])	74	0	14	60	5	4
Fraction time pH <4 ([%])	5.9	0.2	3.4	7.1	2.1	4.1

DeMeester score-proximal
Total score = 21.3, DeMeester normals less than 14.72 (95th percentile)

Figure 16 Esophageal pH measurement. Dual pH probes (placed 15 cm apart) have recorded the 24-hour acid exposure to the esophagus. Acid exposure is abnormal at both sites. The software program has reported six parameters of measurement and has calculated a mathematical score from the components (DeMeester score), which is abnormal for the upper probe recording (lower probe results not included here).

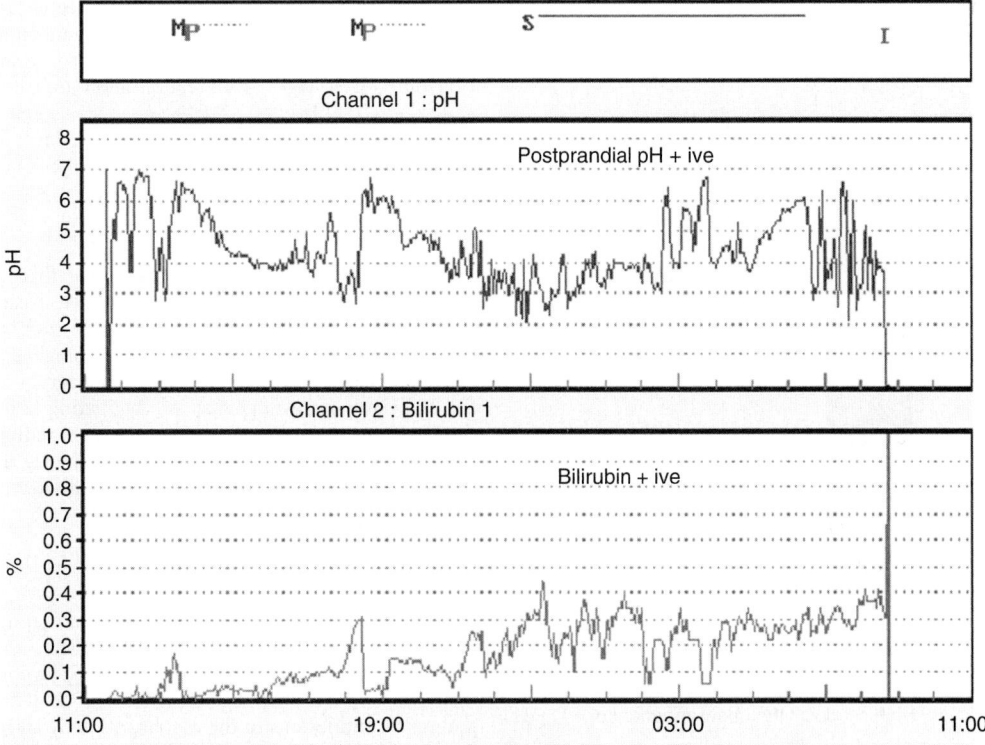

Figure 17 Bilirubin (Bilitec) and pH made simultaneously.

Table 5: Esophageal Acid Exposure Measured with the Bravo pH Capsule During the First 24 Hours in 50 Asymptomatic Subjects Compared with Reported Values for the Nasoesophageal pH Catheter

Component	Bravo pH Capsule (n = 50)			Nasoesophageal pH Catheter (n = 50)*		
	Mean (± SD)	Median	95th perc.	Mean (± SD)	Median	95th perc.
% total time pH <4	1.79 (2.16)	1.08	5.89	1.51 (1.36)	1.2	4.45
% upright time pH <4	2.45 (3.14)	1.26	7.81	2.34 (2.34)	2.3	8.42
% supine time pH <4	0.37 (1.18)	0	1.58	0.63 (1.0)	1.0	3.45
No. reflux episodes	21.22 (18.6)	15	55.30	19.00 (12.8)	16.0	46.9
No. reflux episodes ≥5 min	0.62 (1.21)	0	3.55	0.84 (1.18)	0	3.45
Longest reflux episode (min)	3.79 (4.31)	2.74	11.23	6.74 (7.85)	4.0	19.8
Composite pH score	6.02 (4.82)	4.45	15.93	6.00 (4.40)	5.0	14.74

From Jamieson JR and others: Am J Gastroenterol 87:1102–1111, 1992.

Clinical Uses

1. Measurement of all types of gastroesophageal reflux (i.e., acid and nonacid refluxates, liquid or gas and mixed refluxates; [Figs. 18–21]).
2. Assessment of high gastroesophageal reflux
3. Measurement of swallow function by bolus transport
4. Assessment of patients for GERD therapy (i.e., suitability for endoscopic or operative antireflux procedure)
5. Identification of patients "at risk" for 360-degree fundoplication because of poor bolus transport
6. Assessment of patients with dysphagia, IEM, and precordial chest pain
7. Assessment of recurrent symptoms after antireflux surgery

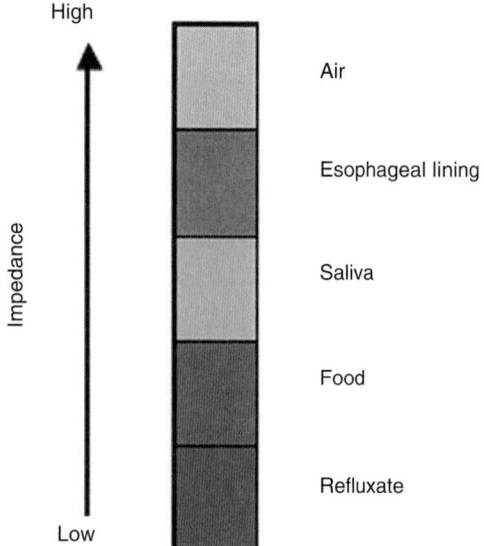

Low conductivity = High impedance

High

Impedance

Air

Esophageal lining

Saliva

Food

Refluxate

Low

High conductivity = Low impedance

Figure 18 Diagram illustrating the range of impedance measurements with different refluxates.

The software includes an Auto SCAN component that 1) locates waveform areas with retrograde bolus movements, 2) determines bolus entry and clearance points when reflux occurs, and 3) analyzes the pH channel to determine when the pH drops below 4.

Clinical Application of Esophageal Function Tests

The selection of tests used varies according to the patient's symptoms and possible diagnosis.

Gastroesophageal Reflux Disease

It is recommended that surgeons who are contemplating antireflux surgery complete the investigation of patients with suspected GERD by doing a video-esophagram, endoscopy with biopsies, manometry, and pH measurements. Failure to appreciate fully the physiology of the patient's deficit may result in inappropriate surgery (e.g., fundoplication for achalasia, 360-degree fundoplication for scleroderma). Although the esophageal team at the University of Southern California has demonstrated that serious symptoms of heartburn, dysphagia, and regurgitation together with grade III endoscopic esophagitis is 100% predictive of a positive pH test, the clinical combination is unusual today, probably because patients who present to the clinician are already on treatment.

Dysphagia

A video-esophagram is the appropriate first investigation for patients with dysphagia. Radiology will detect causes of dysphagia that are not evident on endoscopy alone, such as a cricopharyngeal bar or small Zenker diverticulum, small epiphrenic diverticula, and early achalasia. A video-esophagram will also provide the clinician with a road map of obstructing lesions such as strictures and cancers and allow for the preparation of the patient should dilatation be necessary. Dysphagia may also be related to a motility disorder or GERD, and appropriate tests are necessary to make a diagnosis.

Oropharyngeal Dysphagia

A video-esophagram is the appropriate first examination to exclude a cricopharyngeal bar or Zenker diverticulum. This study will also assess pooling in the hypopharynx and aspiration of the contrast medium. Cervical dysphagia may also be related to gastroesophageal reflux and lesions in the esophageal body and gastroesophageal junction. It is important, therefore, to do a complete assessment of the whole esophagus because dual pathology may also be present.

Figure 19 The upper diagram illustrates the pattern of impedance when a bolus is swallowed. An initial impedance rise signifies the swallowing of air prior to the bolus passage. The duration of the bolus in the esophagus is demonstrated. The diagram below is a manometry recording taken simultaneously and demonstrates the esophageal contraction.

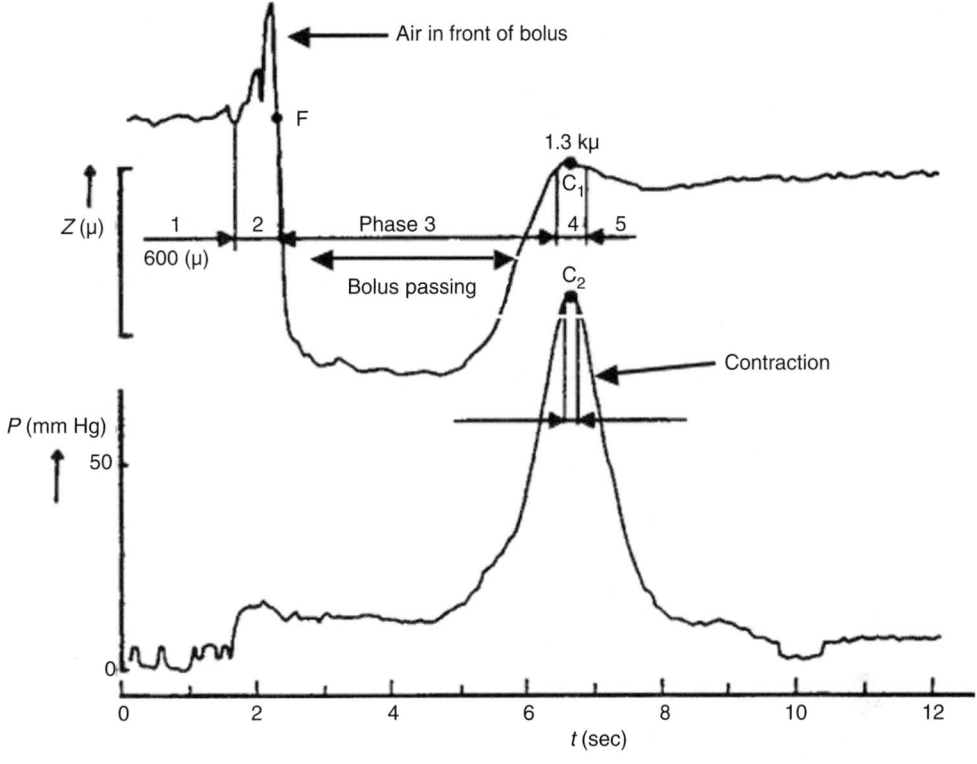

Figure 20 Impedance study showing anterograde and retrograde movements of a swallowed bolus.

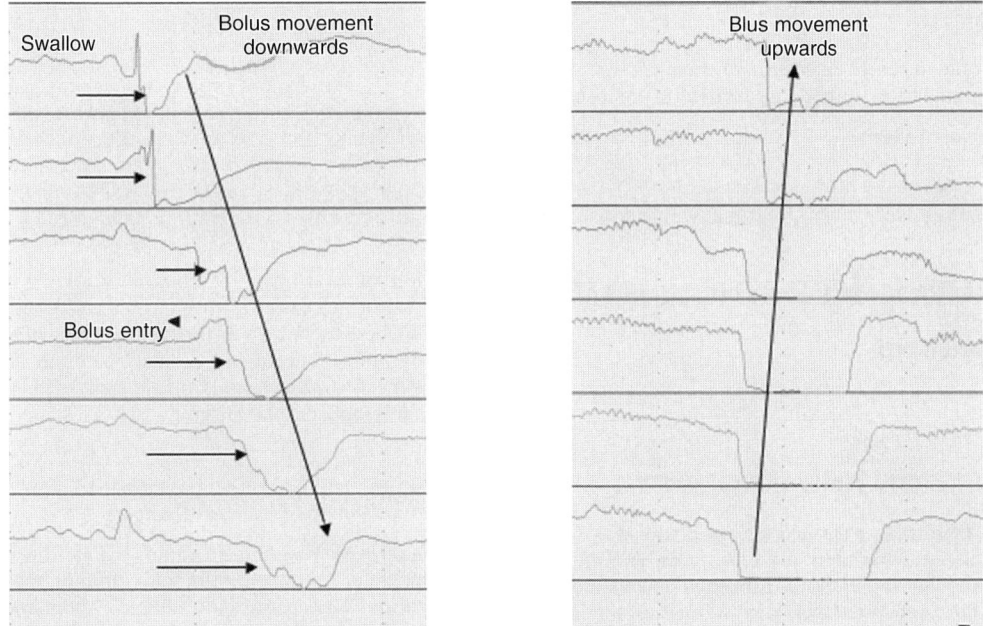

In the absence of a structural abnormality in the cervical esophagus, manometric and pH studies are necessary. Abnormal cricopharyngeal function may not be detected by radiology, and a detailed cricopharyngeal manometric study may be compelling when no other esophageal abnormality has been demonstrated.

Important values are the cricopharyngeal swallow pressures, which may be weak (especially in the aged), the opening pressure of the sphincter, and the bolus pressure.

Failure of the cricopharyngeal sphincter to open adequately to accommodate the food bolus will result in an increase in the bolus pressure and may indicate a need for a cricopharyngeal myotomy.

Undiagnosed Chest Pain

Chest pain may also be related to a motility disorder or GERD, and a video-esophagram, endoscopy, manometry, and pH testing are recommended.

Undiagnosed Laryngitis, Chronic Cough and Nonallergic Asthma

These symptoms may be related to gastroesophageal reflux, sometimes in association with a motility deficit, and a full investigation as for GERD is recommended. A dual pH probe is used for pH assessment.

Non-acid reflux

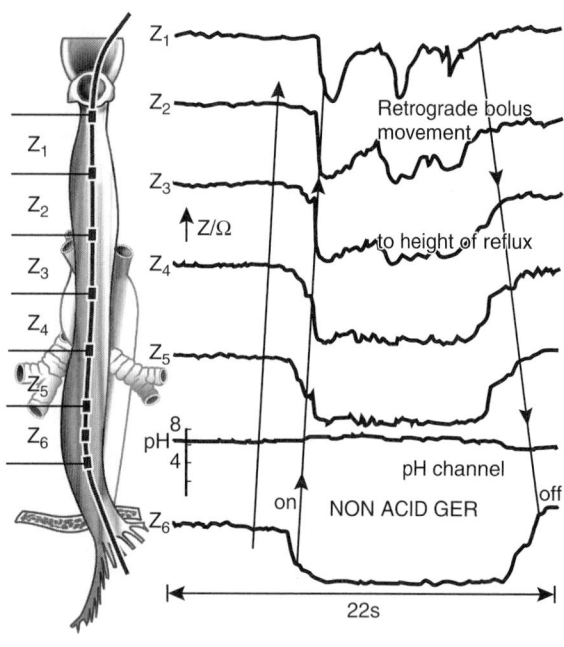

Figure 21 An impedance study demonstrating retrograde bolus movement. An attached pH probe has not detected any fall in the pH, demonstrating nonacid reflux.

Therapeutic pH studies

pH studies are the only means to determine whether acid reflux has been controlled or not. The pH probe may be used in combination with an impedance study, which will assess reflux whether the refluxate is acid or not. Such studies are becoming more important in the management of Barrett's esophagus when control of all reflux may be an important issue.

SUGGESTED READINGS

Bremner CG, DeMeester TR, Huprich J, and others: *Esophageal disease and testing*, New York, London, 2005, Taylor and Francis.

Bremner RM, Bremner CG, DeMeester TR: Gastroesophageal reflux: the use of pH monitoring, *Curr Probl Surg* 6:429, 1995.

Gockel I, Lord RVN, Bremner CG, and others: The hypertensive lower esophageal sphincter: a motility disorder with manometric features of outflow obstruction, *J Gastrointest Surg* 7:692, 2003.

Hill Lucius D, Kozarek RA: The gastro-esophageal flap valve, *J Clin Gastro-enterol* 28:194, 1999.

Sperandio M, Tutuian R, Gideon RM, and others: Diffuse esophageal spasm: not diffuse but distal esophageal spasm, *Dig Dis Sci* 48(7):1380–1384, 2003.

Tutuian R, Castell DO: Clarification of the esophageal function defect in patients with manometric ineffective esophageal motility: studies using combined impedance-manometry, *Clin Gastroenterol Hepatol* 2:230, 2004.

Vieth M, Gossner C, May L, and others: Histological analysis of endoscopic resection specimens from 326 patients with Barrett's esophagus and early neoplasia, *Endoscopy* 36:776, 2004.

Zaninotto G, DeMeester TR: The lower esophageal sphincter in health and disease, *Am J Surg* 155:104–111, 1988.

ESOPHAGEAL PERFORATION

Steven R. DeMeester, MD

INTRODUCTION AND ETIOLOGY

In 1724, Hermann Boerhaave published a classic treatise in which he described in exacting detail the symptoms, signs, and autopsy findings related to the illness and death from spontaneous esophageal perforation in Lord van Wassenaer, High Admiral of the Dutch navy. Not until more than 200 years later were the first successful repairs for spontaneous esophageal perforation reported by Barrett, Olsen, and Claggett. Although spontaneous esophageal rupture is uncommon, the incidence of iatrogenic esophageal perforation has increased in tandem with the increased use of endoscopy for the diagnosis and treatment of gastrointestinal diseases. Fortunately, advances in medical, surgical, and endoscopic therapies have dramatically reduced the mortality associated with this condition.

A list of the potential causes for esophageal perforation is shown in Table 1. The most common cause is iatrogenic injury, typically related to instrumentation of the esophagus. The risk of perforation during routine upper endoscopy using modern flexible endoscopes is extremely small but increases considerably with the addition of therapeutic interventions, such as disimpaction of a food bolus or dilatation of a stricture or tumor, or of the lower esophageal sphincter for achalasia. Iatrogenic injuries occur most commonly in areas where the lumen of the esophagus is narrowed, either from pathology or at one of the normal anatomic sites of narrowing, such as the cricopharyngeous, aortic arch, left mainstem bronchus, and gastroesophageal junction.

PATHOPHYSIOLOGY

Intrathoracic esophageal perforation is a life-threatening condition, and successful therapy begins with prompt diagnosis and rapid intervention. One reason intrathoracic esophageal perforation is so lethal is that negative intrathoracic pressure sucks esophageal and gastric contents out of the site of perforation and into the mediastinum. Leaking gastric juice induces a chemical burn, and saliva, oral bacteria, and digestive enzymes initiate a mixed necrotizing superinfection adjacent to vital organs in the mediastimun and upper abdomen. This combination of chemical injury and bacterial infection causes rapid tissue destruction and severe sepsis.

CLINICAL FEATURES

The presentation of esophageal perforation depends on three main factors: the location of the perforation, degree of containment, and elapsed time since injury. Cervical perforation typically presents

Table 1: Causes of Esophageal Perforation

1. Iatrogenic
   a. Intraluminal
      i. Esophagoscopy, particularly with dilatation
      ii. Endoscopic or transesophageal ultrasound
      iii. Endoscopic antireflux procedures
      iv. Endoscopic mucosal resection or ablation
      v. Esophageal intubation with a tube (nasogastric, Sengstaken–Blakemore) or bougie (for antireflux surgery or dilatation)
      vi. Misplaced endotracheal tube during intubation
   b. Extraluminal
      i. Intraoperative injury during neck, mediastinal, thoracic, or upper abdominal procedures
      ii. Radiation therapy for esophageal tumor
2. Trauma
   a. Penetrating or blunt injury
   b. Barotrauma (seizure, weightlifting, postemetic or Boerhaave's syndrome)
   c. Foreign body or caustic ingestion
      i. Fish bones
      ii. Food or solid objects (coins, nails, pins)
      iii. Acid or alkaline material
3. Malignancy
4. Inflammation
   a. Crohn's disease of the esophagus
   b. Gastroesophageal reflux and ulceration
5. Infection

with neck tenderness, odynophagia, and subcutaneous emphysema. Iatrogenic perforation of the intrathoracic esophagus usually presents shortly after the procedure with dysphagia, pain, tachycardia, and fever. If left untreated, it progresses rapidly to hypoxia, sepsis, and shock. Spontaneous perforation is typically associated with an episode of emesis, and patients present with chest pain and shortness of breath. The differential diagnosis includes myocardial infarction, peptic ulcer disease, pancreatitis, aortic dissection, spontaneous pneumothorax, or pneumonia. Most commonly, the perforation is in the distal esophagus toward the left chest. A left-sided pleural effusion or hydropneumothorax may be present by the time patients present for evaluation and should be an indication of the correct diagnosis. Crepitance in the neck or mediastinal air on chest x-ray or computed tomographic (CT) scan also suggest the diagnosis. Intraabdominal perforations usually present with peritonitis, and free air may be present on upright chest x-ray, mimicking other forms of gastrointestinal perforation.

DIAGNOSIS

An antecedent history of esophageal instrumentation or vomiting can be elicited from most patients with esophageal perforation. A chest x-ray may show pneumomediastinum, subcutaneous emphysema, or air under the diaphragm within the first hour of perforation, but a pleural effusion often takes several hours to develop. Therefore a normal chest film, especially soon after the injury, should not exclude the diagnosis. When an esophageal perforation is suspected, the initial test in most circumstances should

be a water-soluble (gastrograffin) contrast swallow. The study should be done in the right lateral decubitus position to avoid rapid transit of contrast into the stomach, and if no leak is seen with gastrograffin, then thin barium should be used because this may show a small leak missed by gastrograffin. Using these techniques, a leak will be identified in the majority of patients, but again a negative contrast swallow study does not definitively rule out esophageal perforation. If the diagnosis remains unclear, a CT scan of the chest can be helpful, and it should be done immediately after the contrast swallow because even very small leaks will be apparent with the resolution offered by a CT scan. In addition, mediastinal inflammation and emphysema are also well visualized on CT scan. Lastly, upper endoscopy is a valuable adjunct for making or confirming the diagnosis of esophageal perforation and for planning therapy. In my opinion, flexible endoscopy should be performed in most patients with perforations distal to the cervical esophagus. Small mucosal tears or perforations that are not seen well by radiographic studies can be detected with the excellent visualization offered by modern endoscopes. However, the injury may be subtle and appear only as a slight bruise or area of discoloration. Look for slight fluttering of the mucosa during air insufflation as a clue to the location of the injury. Concerns regarding making the hole larger are unfounded because the size of the hole is irrelevant in terms of prognosis; nonetheless, reasonable care should be taken to avoid excessive air insufflation that might spread the mediastinal contamination. In my experience, careful endoscopic evaluation of an injury has not turned a contained perforation into an uncontained perforation, nor has an uncontained perforation been made worse by endoscopic evaluation.

THERAPY

Initial Resuscitation

Treatment for esophageal perforation begins with aggressive fluid resuscitation and administration of broad-spectrum antibiotics covering gram-positive and gram-negative organisms, as well as anaerobes. I avoid aminoglycosides or other nephrotoxic antibiotics in these patients because sepsis and intravascular volume depletion increase the risk of renal insufficiency. In patients on chronic acid-suppression medications, antifungal therapy is also appropriate. A nasogastric tube to decompress the stomach is important but must be placed carefully; it may be best inserted immediately after the contrast swallow with the aid of fluoroscopy or during the endoscopic evaluation of the esophagus. A chest tube should be placed to drain an associated pleural effusion or hydropneumothorax. The following sections consider the factors influencing the decision to operate and the type of operation.

Resection or Repair of the Esophagus

Following stabilization and resuscitation of the patient with an esophageal perforation, the critical next step is to decide how best to manage the injury. Although a number of factors are important, none is as critical as an understanding of the location and cause of the injury and any underlying pathology in the esophagus. The decision tree starts with obtaining a careful history from the patient or immediate family. Patients with a history of significant esophageal pathology such as malignancy, long-segment Barrett's esophagus, or a severe stricture that has required repeated dilatations should be considered for esophagectomy rather than esophageal preservation or conservative therapy. Likewise, patients with symptoms indicating a significant problem with esophageal function such as long-standing dysphagia or severe reflux with regurgitation and aspiration events also should be considered for esophagectomy because these problems are likely to be even worse if the perforation is repaired or managed conservatively. It makes no sense to preserve the esophagus in a patient with a perforation at a stricture that has required repeated dilatations because the stricture will recur and place the patient at risk for another perforation with subsequent dilatations. Likewise, the scarring and fixation of the esophagus that occurs with mediastinitis will make subsequent antireflux surgery difficult or impossible in patients with a thoracic esophageal perforation and a history of severe reflux disease.

In patients with an intra-abdominal esophageal perforation and severe reflux, esophageal preservation may be possible because an antireflux procedure may be added to buttress the repair and allow both conditions to be addressed simultaneously. A perforation during balloon dilatation for achalasia is another condition in which repair is warranted despite significant esophageal pathology, unless there is end-stage achalasia with sigmoid-shaped esophagus, in which case resection is probably a better choice. In my opinion, an esophageal exclusion and diversion procedure is rarely necessary or appropriate, considering the number of options currently available. Moreover, stapling off of the distal esophagus almost always leads to breakdown of the closure, with formation of a salivary fistula or abscess and a protracted illness that complicates subsequent efforts to reestablish gastrointestinal continuity.

Esophagectomy

If esophagectomy is appropriate, the next decision is whether to reconstruct immediately or plan for delayed reconstruction. I rarely think that immediate reconstruction is advisable because most patients have extensive mediastinal inflammation and infection and often are becoming ill by the time they are in the operating room. In this circumstance, I scope the patient in the operating room, place a percutaneous gastrostomy tube, and then perform a thoracotomy on the side with the pleural effusion (or the right side if both sides are involved) and debride the mediastinum while mobilizing the esophagus up to the thoracic inlet. The gastroesophageal junction is divided with a gastrointestinal anstomosis (GIA) stapler, and the pleural cavity and mediastinum are extensively drained. The patient is repositioned supine and the left neck opened; an end cervical esophagostomy is then created. I retain as much normal esophagus as possible to facilitate subsequent reconstruction, and this also allows the esophagostomy to be placed on the anterior chest below the clavicle. An esophagostomy in this position permits the stoma bag to lie nicely under a shirt and minimizes leaks from around the edges of the bag because it lies flat on the chest wall rather than on the neck or near the clavicle. If a percutaneous endoscopic gastronomy tube cannot be placed, a feeding jejunostomy tube or open gastrostomy should be performed to provide alimentary tract access for nutrition and medications. If immediate reconstruction is planned, consideration should be given to bringing the graft substernally away from the infected posterior mediastinum; however, if the patient is ill, this will potentially compromise graft healing, and a leaking anastomosis or an ischemic graft can be an insult from which the patient is unable to recover. Thus restraint from the inclination to reconstruct is appropriate in most cases despite the temporary inconvenience of an esophagostomy for the patient.

Esophageal Repair versus Nonoperative Therapy

In the absence of an indication to remove the esophagus, other factors take on increased significance. These include the location of the injury, the time since the perforation occurred, whether the leak is contained or free, and the clinical status of the patient. Most cervical esophageal perforations can be managed conservatively, but intrathoracic and intra-abdominal perforations are more likely to require an intervention. The time since the perforation occurred is an important consideration because evaluation of the patient's clinical status may not be informative, depending on the elapsed time since the injury. Although perforation should be suspected in any patient who complains of significant pain after an endoscopy, particularly when a dilatation has been performed, it generally takes several hours before systemic signs of infection become apparent. Rather than wait, a contrast swallow is warranted in any patient suspected of having a perforation because early intervention for perforation offers the opportunity to address the injury before the onset of septic physiologic changes. Thoracic esophageal perforations that are diagnosed early can potentially be treated endoscopically. One option in the absence of a perforated cancer or stricture is endoscopic clipping of the mucosal defect. This is best done with a double channel endoscope, and clips available from several companies can be used to reapproximate the mucosal edges of the defect securely and avoid further mediastinal contamination. In patients with a perforated cancer or stricture, mucosal clipping is not likely to be successful, but stenting the injury is an option. Permanent, coated, self-expanding metal stents are appropriate only for patients with malignancy, but recently temporary, removable, coated stents have been developed that are suitable for perforations in the setting of benign disease. These tend to migrate more frequently than metallic stents but can be effective particularly in patients with a stricture.

Esophageal Repair: Intrathoracic Perforation

In patients already septic from their perforation, urgent intervention is required. Because most patients with a thoracic esophageal perforation and sepsis have an extensive mediastinal phlegmon, endoscopic therapy alone is unlikely to be adequate. The treatment principles for esophageal perforation in patients exhibiting sepsis are outlined in Table 2. Traditional therapy is left or right

Table 2: Treatment Principles for Esophageal Perforation Requiring Surgical Intervention

1. Evaluation of the esophagus including the site and severity of the injury (flexible esophagoscopy)

2. Decision to either resect or repair the esophagus

3. Placement of a percutaneous endoscopic gastronomy tube before esophageal repair or planned resection without reconstruction

4. Complete debridement of infected and necrotic tissues with wide drainage (obtain cultures in the operating room to guide selection of antibiotics or antifungal medications)

5. Precise two-layer closure of the perforation followed by buttressing of the closure with adjacent healthy tissue (pleura, diaphragm, intercostal muscle, gastric fundus) in patients in whom repair is appropriate or esophagectomy with immediate or delayed reconstruction

6. Establishment of enteral access if not done before repair or resection

thoracotomy with debridement of necrotic and infected tissue, extensive drainage, and precise closure of the injury. Perforations of the middle third of the esophagus are best approached through a right thoracotomy, whereas a left thoracotomy is best for perforations of the lower esophagus. As a general rule, however, the perforation should be approached through the side with pleural contamination. To achieve precise closure of the injury, the esophageal muscle layers must be opened above and below the injury to allow complete exposure of the mucosal defect. The mucosa is then reapproximated with fine (4–0) absorbable monofilament sutures, and the muscle layers are closed over the mucosa with 2–0 silk or an absorbable suture. Lastly the entire closure is buttressed with adjacent normal tissue. Intrathoracic perforations are best buttressed with pleura, a strip of diaphragm, or intercostal muscle.

Reports in the past have stressed that primary closure should be considered only in patients with a recent (within 24–48 hours) perforation, but current series suggest that even with delayed presentation, primary closure is still feasible in many patients. In a severely ill and unstable patient or when there is such extensive tissue inflammation that primary closure is not a good option, placement of a large T-tube into the defect that is brought out the chest wall to create a controlled fistula should be considered. In most patients, the T-tube can be removed after establishment of a secure fibrotic tract, similar to a T-tube for the biliary tree. Debridement and drainage are necessary in addition to placement of the T-tube, but the procedure is faster and potentially safer given the likelihood and significant consequences of a breakdown of the repair in an ill patient. Advances in endoscopic therapies will perhaps make hybrid procedures combining thoracoscopic debridement and drainage with simultaneous endoscopic stenting or repair of the perforation feasible, and this may further reduce the operative insult in an unstable patient.

Esophageal Repair: Intra-abdominal Perforation

Intra-abdominal perforations are approached via a laparotomy; in some situations, a laparoscopic approach can be considered. The goals of the operation are identical to those for an intrathoracic perforation, namely, debridement of infected tissue, drainage, and precise closure of the injury in two layers with a buttress over the closure. In most circumstances, a Nissen or partial fundoplication can be used to buttress an intra-abdominal perforation because it is likely to be at or near the gastroesophageal junction. If the perforation is secondary to balloon dilatation for achalasia, then the appropriate therapy includes precise two-layer closure of the perforation with a myotomy on the opposite side of the esophagus and a partial fundoplication to cover the site of the perforation, if possible. It is important to carry the myotomy 3 cm down onto the stomach to ensure complete division of the dysfunctional lower esophageal sphincter because even with a full perforation, the balloon dilatation may not have been adequate distally to relieve the outflow obstruction of the esophagus and palliate the achalasia adequately. Everything possible should be done to avoid the need for later reintervention in such a patient.

Nonoperative Management

Another important issue is whether the leak is contained on contrast swallow. If it is and the patient is not exhibiting any signs of sepsis, then a trial of conservative therapy with intravenous antibiotics, no oral intake, and parenteral nutrition may be appropriate. An intravenous proton pump inhibitor is appropriate for patients with injuries in the distal esophagus or those with a history of reflux. When the injury is in the thoracic esophagus, I prefer to endoscope the esophagus to understand the nature of the injury and the status of the remainder of the esophagus. I then follow healing and resolution of the injury with an endoscopy in 7 to 10 days. If the patient does well for 72 hours and the defect appears to be a small mucosal injury, I usually allow the patient to begin a liquid diet. Evidence of sepsis during conservative therapy should prompt consideration of surgical intervention for the injury.

Nonoperative therapy is most apt to be successful in patients with a cervical esophageal perforation. This injury typically heals with a short course of nothing per os (NPO), oral suctioning of secretions, and intravenous antibiotics, but if a cervical abscess develops, it should be drained. When draining an abscess, it is not necessary to identify and close the esophageal perforation because drainage of the abscess is usually all that is necessary unless the perforation is within a Zenker's diverticulum. In this situation, the diverticulum should be excised and a cricopharyngeal myotomy performed. In rare cases, cervical perforations can track into the mediastinum via the thoracic inlet and require mediastinal drainage. Often this can be accomplished through the neck by opening the retroesophageal plane down into the mediastinum and placing closed suction drains in this space. A similar approach is useful for oral-pharyngeal abscesses that track down into the upper mediastinum.

Cameron and more recently Altorjay have listed criteria for selecting patients for nonoperative therapy. These include (1) intraluminal dissection, (2) transmural perforation that drains back into the esophagus, (3) no associated distal obstruction, (4) a perforation that is not in the abdominal cavity, and (5) no evidence of systemic sepsis. I would add to these that no malignancy or other compelling reason for esophagectomy be present. Intraluminal dissections are most often seen with passage of a nasogastric or similar tube and usually start in the posterior pharynx or cervical esophagus and reenter the esophageal lumen distally. The offending tube should be removed, and typically the injury heals without sequelae. Perforations that drain back into the esophagus are appropriate to consider for nonoperative management, but the size and degree of dependency of the cavity should be considered. If a large cavity is present, healing may be faster if the injury is endoscopically clipped or stented and the cavity drained with a CT-guided pigtail catheter. An algorithm of the suggested management of an esophageal perforation is shown in Figure 1.

SUMMARY

Esophageal perforation remains a diagnostic and therapeutic challenge and is associated with substantial mortality if not treated promptly and effectively. Instrumentation has replaced spontaneous rupture as the leading cause of esophageal perforation. Nonoperative management is appropriate in select patients, but patients with evidence of systemic illness require prompt intervention. In the absence of cancer or an undilatable stricture, reinforced primary repair is the preferred treatment for most patients who require an operation. However, treatment must be individualized and take into account many variables, including cause, duration, underlying esophageal disease, and the condition of the patient. Esophagectomy may be the best therapy in patients with significant underlying esophageal pathology, and in most circumstances, reconstruction should be delayed to allow the patient to recover from the perforation. With appropriate therapy, the mortality of this lethal condition can be minimized, and currently most patients are successfully discharged from the hospital.

ESOPHAGEAL PERFORATION

Figure 1 Algorithm for the management of an esophageal perforation. *NPO,* no food by mouth.

SUGGESTED READINGS

Altorjay A, Kiss J, Voros A, Bohak A: Nonoperative management of esophageal perforations. Is it justified? *Ann Surg* 225:415, 1997.

Barrett N: Spontaneous perforation of the esophagus: review of the literature and a report of three new cases, *Thorax* 1:48, 1946.

Barrett N: Report of a case of spontaneous rupture of the esophagus successfully treated by operation, *Br J Surg* 35:216, 1947.

Cameron JL, Kieffer RF, Hendrix TR, and others: Selective nonoperative management of contained intrathoracic esophageal disruptions, *Ann Thorac Surg* 27:404, 1979.

Salo JA, Isolauri JO, Heikkila LJ, and others: Management of delayed esophageal perforation with mediastinal sepsis. Esophagectomy or primary repair? *J Thorac Cardiovasc Surg* 106:1088, 1993.

Whyte RI, Iannettoni MD, Orringer MB: Intrathoracic esophageal perforation. The merit of primary repair, *J Thorac Cardiovasc Surg* 109:140; discussion 144, 1995.

Wang N, Razzouk AJ, Safavi A, and others: Delayed primary repair of intrathoracic esophageal perforation: is it safe? *J Thorac Cardiovasc Surg* 111:114; discussion 121. 1996.

Urbani M, Mathisen DJ, and others: Repair of esophageal perforation after treatment for achalasia. *Ann Thorac Surg* 69:1609, 2000.

ACHALASIA OF THE ESOPHAGUS

Valerie A. Williams, MD, Daniela Molena, MD, and Jeffrey H. Peters, MD

INTRODUCTION

Achalasia is a primary esophageal motility disorder of unclear etiology. It is an uncommon disease affecting approximately 1 in 100,000 individuals per year. Occurring equally in male and female patients, it is an acquired condition usually diagnosed between 20 and 50 years of age but can occur at any age. Achalasia is characterized by a nonrelaxing lower esophageal sphincter (LES) and aperistalsis of the esophageal body and is thought to result from an absence of inhibitory ganglion cells in the myenteric plexus of the esophagus. This loss creates an imbalance between excitatory and inhibitory neurons, causing failure of the LES to relax. An infectious agent, such as a virus, and its subsequent immune response is thought to be the cause of ganglion loss, but the exact etiology is unknown.

PRESENTATION AND DIAGNOSIS

Achalasia is a slowly progressive disease. As a consequence, patients often present late in the course of this disease, when their symptoms and anatomic abnormalities have become prominent.

Diagnosis earlier in the disease process is possible, however, with conscientious attention to patients' esophageal complaints and a high degree of suspicion. Clinical symptoms include slowly progressive dysphagia for both solids and liquids, regurgitation of bland undigested food, chest pain, and weight loss. Patients may also have a history suggestive of aspiration, including recurrent pneumonia or chronic cough. A simple chest radiograph may provide the diagnosis by the absence of a gastric bubble and the presence of a dilated, fluid-filled esophagus, generally seen as a right-sided posterior mediastinal shadow. Upper endoscopy should be performed in all patients to exclude obstruction caused by tumor or stricture. Findings commonly include retention of saliva and undigested food associated with a dilated esophagus but can be normal. A barium swallow is often diagnostic, showing the presence of an air-fluid level or a characteristic "bird's beak" appearance created by a nonrelaxing LES (Fig. 1). Careful examination of the fluoroscopic or video images will reveal a flaccid nonperistaltic esophagus, devoid of the usual "stripping" waves. Depending on the chronicity of the disease, the esophageal body is usually dilated but may occasionally be normal. The gold standard for diagnosis of achalasia is esophageal manometry. There are four classic manometric characteristics (Table 1): (1) a hypertensive LES, present in approximately 50% of patients; (2) a nonrelaxing LES; (3) esophageal aperistalsis; and (4) an elevated lower esophageal baseline pressure.

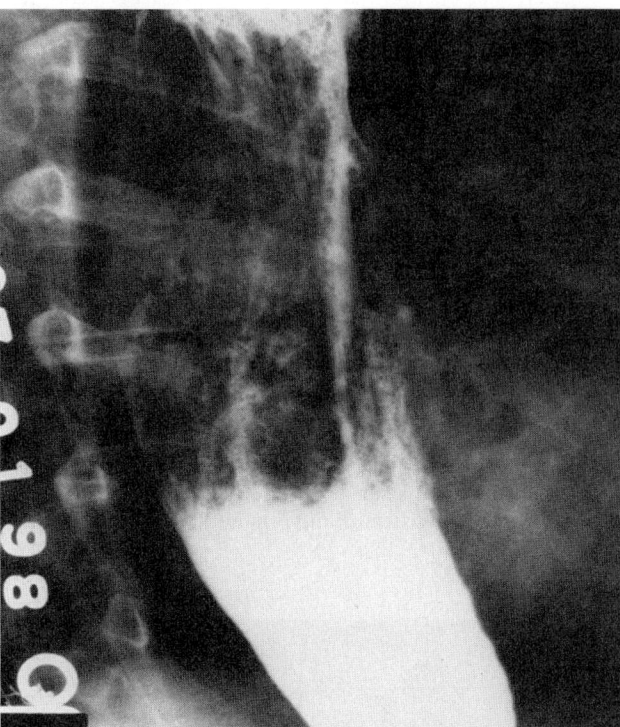

Figure 1 Barium esophagogram in a patient with achalasia. Note the esophageal air-fluid level and characteristic "bird's beak" narrowing created by a nonrelaxing lower esophageal sphincter.

Table 1: Manometric Characteristics of Achalasia

- Hypertensive LES resting pressure
- Incomplete or nonrelaxing LES
- Aperistalsis of the esophageal body
- Esophageal pressurization: elevated lower esophageal baseline pressure

LES, lower esophageal sphincter.

A subset of achalasia patients may have simultaneous contraction waves of variable amplitudes, consistent with preserved muscle function, and this is termed *vigorous achalasia.*

TREATMENT

Achalasia is an incurable disease, and thus treatment is focused on relief of symptoms. The goal of both surgical and nonsurgical treatment is to eliminate the outflow obstruction afforded by a nonrelaxing sphincter, relieve dysphagia, and maintain a barrier against gastroesophageal reflux when possible. Nonsurgical treatment includes calcium channel blockers and nitrates, injection of botulinum toxin into the LES, and large-caliber (30–40 mm) pneumatic dilatation of the LES. Surgical treatment includes division of the muscle fibers of the LES and proximal cardia. Although pharmacologic treatments such as calcium channel blockers, nitrates, and sildenafil have been shown to have physiologic effects on esophageal function, they rarely result in meaningful clinical improvement. With the advent of minimally invasive surgery, laparoscopic myotomy has slowly shifted the treatment of achalasia toward the greater use of surgical therapy.

Nonsurgical Treatment

Pharmacologic treatments of achalasia, such as oral nitrates and calcium channel blockers, act to inhibit intramural neurons. These drugs attempt to re-create a balance between stimulatory and inhibitory nerve fibers to decrease the resting and residual pressure of the LES. Their effect, however, is sporadic and has shown only short-term success. Given their poor outcomes and potentially harmful systemic effects, these agents are unreliable and unrealistic modalities for long-term symptom relief.

Endoscopic injection of botulinum toxin into the LES aims to block the release of acetylcholine from cholinergic neurons in an effort to lower both basal and residual LES pressures. This treatment is short-lived, rarely results in significant reduction in LES pressure, and, although it may improve dysphagia, it often requires repeat injections for continued relief. In a prospective randomized controlled trial comparing injection of Botox (Allergan, Irvine, CA) ($n = 40$) to laparoscopic myotomy and partial fundoplication ($n = 40$), Zaninotto and colleagues found that although patients in both groups showed initial improvement in symptoms, 6 months following treatment, dysphagia and regurgitation recurred in nearly half (45%) of those treated with Botox. Furthermore, they determined that the probability of being symptom free at 2 years was significantly higher following myotomy (87.5%) than following Botox injection (34%). It is also now recognized that Botox injection creates an inflammatory reaction at the LES with consequent submucosal fibrosis, which has been found to make subsequent surgical myotomy more difficult. Although commonly tried as a short-term treatment option, we believe Botox should be reserved for those who are not surgical candidates or should be abandoned altogether.

Pneumatic balloon dilatation decreases esophageal outflow resistance by forceful "tearing" of the LES muscle fibers. Although the technique has been found to have a more lasting effect on dysphagia than Botox injection, it has not demonstrated the longer-lasting outcomes seen with surgical myotomy. In a prospective randomized trial comparing pneumatic dilatation to surgical myotomy, Csendes and colleagues found that 100% of patients treated with myotomy ($n = 18$) had only mild or no dysphagia at a mean of 3.5 years compared with only 61% of those treated with dilatation ($n = 20$). Similarly, in a more recent retrospective evaluation of 125 achalasia patients followed prospectively for more than 5 years after pneumatic dilatation, West and colleagues found that only 50% of patients had no or occasional (less than once per week) dysphagia at 5 years and only 40% at 15 years.

Surgical Treatment

Esophageal myotomy for achalasia was first described by Ernest Heller in 1913. In this operation, both the anterior and posterior LES muscle fibers were disrupted. A modified version of this procedure, referred to today as the *Heller myotomy*, consists of a single, anterior, longitudinal myotomy and has become the standard operative technique. Once performed only through a thoracotomy or laparotomy, esophageal myotomy can now be performed through a thoracoscopic or laparoscopic approach. Outcomes of thoracoscopic myotomy, however, have been shown to be inferior. Laparoscopic myotomy has become the standard surgical approach for the treatment of achalasia today and is described here.

Technique: Laparoscopic Esophageal Myotomy and Partial Fundoplication

The patient is placed on the table in the modified lithotomy position. The lower extremities are abducted in specialized leg holders with the knees slightly flexed. The table is placed in the reverse Trendelenburg position to allow the transverse colon and small bowel to fall toward the pelvis out of the visual and operative field. The surgeon stands between the patient's legs. The assistant on the left controls the video camera, and the assistant on the right retracts the stomach and gastroesophageal (GE) junction.

We prefer an open technique to establish the pneumoperitoneum. A cm incision is made at one third of the distance between the umbilicus and the xiphoid, just to the left of the midline. Soft tissues are dissected bluntly down to the anterior rectus fascia. The fascia is opened, and the muscle is split laterally. The posterior fascia is then opened, and the abdominal cavity is opened under direct vision. Sutures are placed on both sides of the rectus facia, and a Hassan trocar is secured in place. Pneumoperitoneum is established, and four additional ports are placed under video laparoscopic control. A 5- to 10-mm laparoscopic port for retraction of the stomach is placed in the left midabdomen at or just above the level of the umbilicus. The surgeon's right-handed port is placed just below the costal margin in the left midclavicular line and his or her left-handed port just to the right of the midline in the subxiphoid area. Finally a 5- to 10-mm liver retraction port is placed in the right midclavicular line approximately even with the umbilicus.

The left lateral segment of the liver is retracted upward and rightward with a fan liver retractor placed through the right lower trocar. We prefer a table-mounted retractor holder to keep it in place. The dissection begins by freeing the upper third of the gastric fundus in preparation for later Dor anterior hemifundoplication. This is best done by suspending the gastrosplenic omentum anteroposteriorly in a clothesline fashion via two Babcock forceps and opening into the lesser sac approximately one third of the distance down the greater curvature of the stomach. The short gastric vessels can then be sequentially dissected and divided with the aid of ultrasonic shears. In contrast to a Nissen fundoplication for gastroesophageal reflux disease, the posterior attachments and pancreaticogastric branches should not be divided so as to preserve as much of the normal posterior gastroesophageal anatomy as possible. If a Toupet posterior hemifundoplication is planned, a posterior dissection is necessary. This would be the preferred approach in the small (4%–5%) subset of patients who present with a concomitant hiatal hernia.

The GE junction is then exposed by dissecting the gastroesophageal fat pad and retracting it laterally. This is done in a fashion analogous to a localized, highly selective vagotomy. The dissection begins on the lesser curve slightly below the GE junction and continues obliquely toward the angle of His. The gastroesophageal fat pad is dissected obliquely from right to left, progressively rolling the anterior vagus nerve rightward (Fig. 2). Large venous branches common at the GE junction can be divided using the ultrasonic shears. The GE junction is cleared for 6 to 8 cm in preparation for the myotomy. A vessel loop can be placed around this tissue bundle, which includes the anterior vagus nerve, and brought out through the subxiphoid trocar if necessary. Unless a posterior fundoplication is being performed, dissection behind the esophagus is not necessary.

Esophageal Myotomy

Once the esophagus is mobilized and GE junction exposed, the myotomy is performed with a combination of scissors and hook-type electrocautery (Fig. 3). Using cautery, the site of the myotomy is marked out on the anterior aspect of the esophagus. It should extend from the upper limit of the anterior extension of the esophageal hiatus down across the GE junction to ensure that the clasp fibers are divided and onto the anterior wall of the fundus of the stomach for 2 to 3 cm. The esophageal longitudinal and circular muscles are divided down to the mucosa starting above the GE junction. The myotomy is extended superiorly with the scissors and inferiorly with the cautery hook sponge. When the esophageal mucosa is clearly identified, the myotomy is carried both proximally and distally for a total distance of 4 to 6 cm and for 2.5 to 3 cm onto the surface of the anterior stomach. It may be helpful to visualize the distal extent of the myotomy with an intraluminal

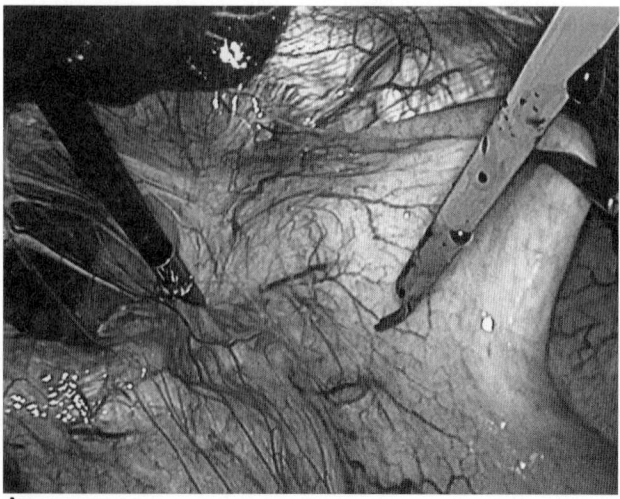
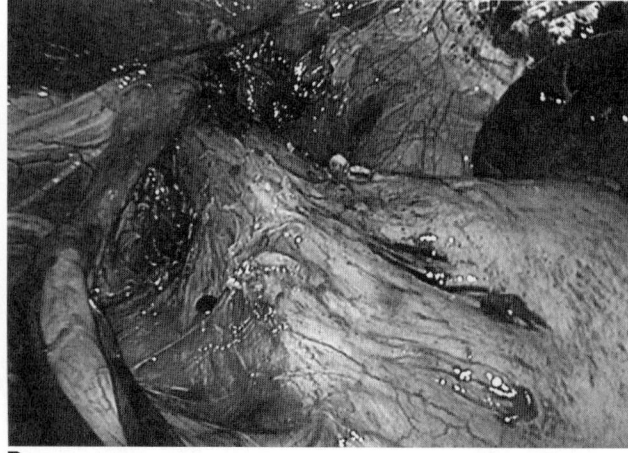

A   B

Figure 2 Dissection of the gastroesophageal fat pad to expose the gastroesophageal junction. (*See color insert Figure 2.*)

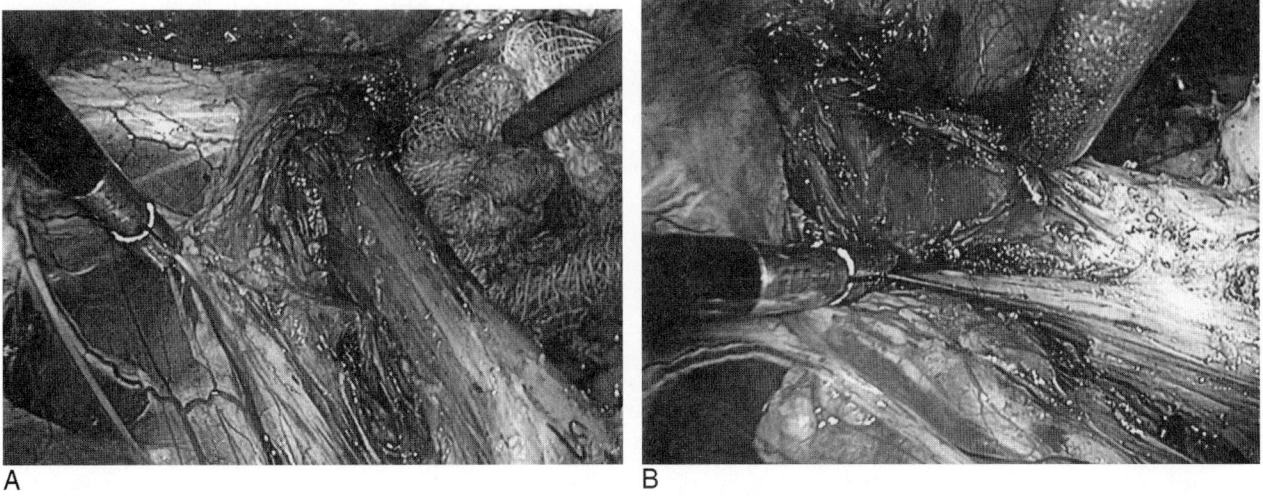

Figure 3   Mobilized esophagus **(A)** and creation of an esophageal myotomy by separation of the muscle edges down to esophageal mucosa and then proximally onto the esophagus and distally onto the stomach **(B)**. (*See color insert Figure 3.*)

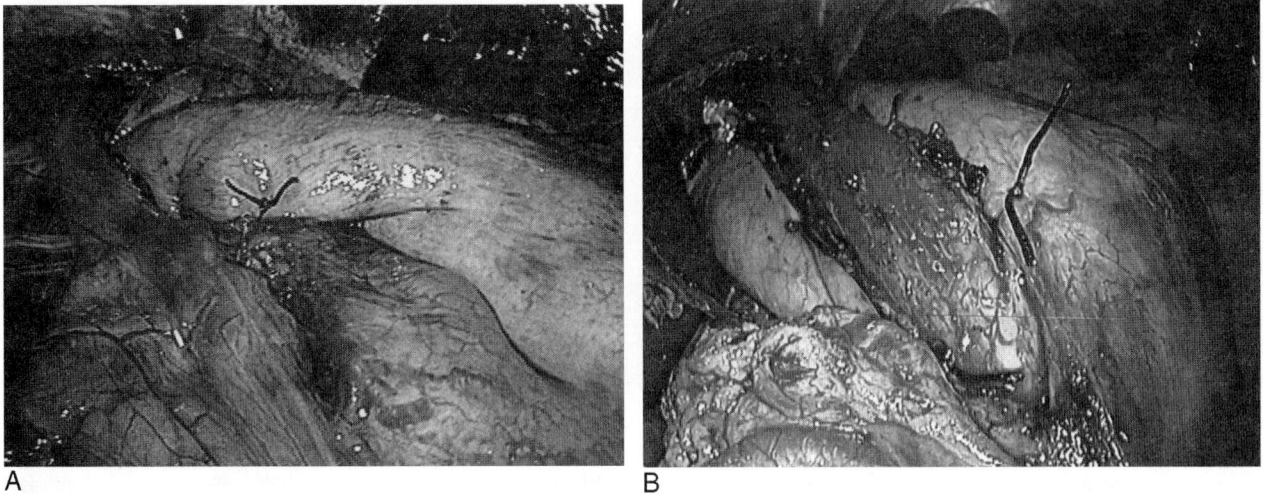

Figure 4   Ninety- to 180-degree Dor fundoplication positioned anteriorly to Heller myotomy **(A)** and 270-degree Toupet fundoplication positioned posteriorly **(B)**. (*See color insert Figure 4.*)

endoscope. The edges of the myotomy are carefully separated from the underlying mucosa for 40% to 50% of the esophageal circumference. Violation of the mucosa can occur and, given the surgeon's experience, can be repaired laparoscopically by gently and carefully placing interrupted sutures of 5–0 polypropylene. The procedure is completed by fashioning an anterior (Dor) or posterior (Toupet) partial fundoplication (Fig. 4). A partial fundoplication is used in preference to a 360-degree fundoplication to avoid long-term esophageal dysfunction secondary to outflow obstruction afforded by the fundoplication itself.

Fundoplication

An anterior partial fundoplication of the Dor type is the most commonly performed antireflux barrier created following myotomy for achalasia. After fundic mobilization the anterior fundus is laid over the myotomy site, and the left fundic edge is sewn to the left cut edge of the esophageal myotomy with three or four interrupted sutures of 2–0 silk. Each suture must be carefully passed through the tissues to prevent tearing of the muscle. The highest stitch is taken through the left crural pillar as an anchor to prevent torsion of the fundus. The fundus is then sewn to the right edge of the cut

esophageal muscle similarly, again using three or four interrupted sutures of 2–0 silk and taking the highest stitch through the right crural pillar to prevent torsion. A dilator is not necessary to calibrate this partial wrap.

DATA SUPPORTING TECHNICAL COMPONENTS

Extent of Myotomy

Recent data show that both the proximal and distal extent of esophageal myotomy are important. Chen and colleagues reported that up to 67% of patients followed 7 to 16 years postmyotomy and fundoplication develop an epiphrenic pseudo-diverticulum. This is likely caused by an absence of coverage by the fundoplication over the proximal extent of the myotomy. This increased recognition of the potential for diverticulum formation has led many to limit the proximal extent of the myotomy to that which can be covered by a fundoplication.

Relief of dysphagia may be better when lengthening the distal extent of myotomy. Oelschlager and colleagues reported better symptomatic improvement and a lower incidence of recurrent dysphagia by increasing the distal extent of myotomy onto the proximal stomach from 1.5 to 3 cm. They compared the outcomes of 52 patients treated with a standard myotomy of 1.5 cm onto the proximal stomach with the outcomes of 58 patients treated with an extended myotomy of 3 cm. Postoperative LES pressures were significantly lower (9.5 mm Hg with extended vs. 15.8 mm Hg with standard myotomy), and postoperative dysphagia improved following the longer myotomy. Importantly, postoperative 24-hour pH data showed that extension of the distal aspect of the myotomy did not result in a higher prevalence of gastroesophageal reflux.

Addition of Fundoplication

Although myotomy effectively lowers esophageal outflow resistance and improves esophageal emptying, it also increases the propensity for the development of gastroesophageal reflux. The importance of the addition of a fundoplication to the myotomy has, until recently, been debated. A recent prospective randomized study has put this issue to rest. Richards and colleagues reported on 43 achalasia patients randomized to laparoscopic Heller myotomy with and without Dor fundoplication. Gastroesophageal reflux, defined by 24-hour distal esophageal acid exposure time greater than 4.2%, was present in 47.5% of patients undergoing Heller myotomy alone, compared with 9.1% of patients undergoing Heller myotomy with partial fundoplication. Importantly, there was no significant difference in postoperative LES pressures or dysphagia scores between the two groups. Similarly, a retrospective evaluation of 149 patients who underwent laparoscopic Heller myotomy with ($n = 88$) or without ($n = 61$) Dor fundoplication by Rice and colleagues found that pH-proven gastroesophageal reflux occurred significantly less often following the addition of a partial fundoplication. Furthermore, the addition of Dor fundoplication to Heller myotomy did not decrease esophageal emptying when assessed by barium esophagography.

In the presence of an aperistaltic, often dilated and tortuous esophagus, virtually all authors agree that a complete fundoplication should be avoided. On the other hand, the precise degree (180°, 270°) and location (anterior, posterior) of a partial fundoplication is unclear. Current data suggest a minimal difference between a posterior 270-degree (Toupet) fundoplication and an anterior 90- to 180-degree (Dor) fundoplication. For example, Arain and colleagues found no difference in the relief of symptoms including dysphagia, heartburn, or chest pain or the need for proton pump inhibitors when comparing myotomy with Dor to myotomy with Toupet. Given the preservation of natural posterior attachments and the easier technical construction of Dor fundoplication, most centers have migrated toward its routine use.

OUTCOMES

The outcomes of laparoscopic Heller myotomy have now been studied for well over a decade. The data show that surgical myotomy is more effective than nonsurgical treatments at providing long-term relief of dysphagia, regurgitation, and chest pain while promoting weight gain and patient satisfaction. Therefore many surgeons and gastroenterologists believe that surgical myotomy should be recommended as primary therapy for virtually all patients with achalasia.

The medium-term outcomes of laparoscopic myotomy have been reported from centers around the world (Table 2). Assessed 2 to 5 years after surgery, more than 90% of patients have either complete relief or only mild persistent dysphagia. Investigators from Padua, Italy, have provided some of the longest-term data. Zaninotto and colleagues reported outcomes for 113 patients who underwent laparoscopic Heller myotomy from 1992 to 1999. More than 90% (91.2%) were symptom free at a median of 2-year follow-up, with Kaplan–Meier analysis showing a 90% probability of remaining asymptomatic at 5 years. Most published results report similar improvement. However, the degree of improvement may not be the same with all symptoms. Arain and colleagues found that the most marked improvement occurred for the symptom of regurgitation (74% complete relief). Moderate relief was seen for dysphagia (33% complete relief), and the least relief was observed for chest pain (18% complete relief). The difficulty in relieving chest pain has also been reported following pneumatic dilatation.

Complications are infrequent, averaging 10% to 15%, and generally mild. Mortality is uncommon, with no deaths reported in most large published series. Inadvertent violation of the esophageal mucosa occurs in 5% to 10% of procedures; when recognized and repaired, it is rarely of clinical consequence. Unrecognized mucosal perforation will present as acute abdominal or chest pain in the early postoperative period and has been treated both operatively and nonoperatively. Conversion from a laparoscopic operation to open laparotomy is infrequent at experienced laparoscopic centers and is caused by esophageal perforation, uncontrolled hemorrhage, or adhesions.

Postoperative assessment via contrast esophagography, manometry, and pH monitoring has shown that esophageal outflow obstruction improves and esophageal diameter decreases, as does resting and residual LES pressure, following surgery. Zaninotto and colleagues reported pH data on 84 of 113 patients who underwent postoperative 24-hour pH monitoring. Only 5 of the 84 (6%) had tracings consistent with gastroesophageal reflux; 3 of these reported mild heartburn, and 1 had erosive esophagitis at endoscopy. Long-term follow-up data from the era of open myotomy suggest, however, that gastroesophageal reflux is a common cause of recurrent symptoms, with a significant minority of patients developing progressive regurgitation, heartburn

Table 2: Outcomes Following Laparoscopic Heller Myotomy

Author	Year	Patients	Follow-up (median months/ranges)	Relief of Dysphagia (%)	Length of Stay (median days/ranges)	Perforations (%)	Reflux (%)
Portale	2005	248	43 (1–131)	88	5 (3–11)	4.0	7*
Bonatti	2005	75	64 (10–131)	84	2 (1–6)	4.0	11
Khajanchee	2005	121	9 (6–48)	91	1.7 (na)	6.6	13*
Arain	2004	78	24 (6–100)	77	na	0	17
Perrone	2004	100	26 (6–72)	96	1.2 (1–4)	3.0%	na
Oelschlager	2003	110	26 (1–85)	90	na	na	23
Donahue	2002	81	45 (1–70)	84	1 (na)	14.0%	4
Sharp	2002	100	11 (na)	93	1.5 (na)	8.0%	4
Patti	2001	102	25 (na)	89	1.5 (na)	5.0%	na
Zaninotto	2001	113	24 (1–83)	91	na	na	6
Patti	1999	133	23 (na)	89	2	5.0%	17

*Based on postoperative 24-hour pH monitoring. *na,* Not applicable.

or chest pain, erosive esophagitis, and Barrett's esophagus. Whether this will also be true in the laparoscopic era remains to be determined.

Outcome Predictors

Several factors have been proposed as outcome predictors following treatment for achalasia. The degree of improvement in resting LES pressure has been reported by several authors to affect significantly the long-term success of pneumatic dilatation. Patients in whom the LES pressure was reduced to ≤10 mm Hg had long-lasting (5 years or more) relief of dysphagia, whereas those with persistent LES pressures >20 mm Hg developed recurrent dysphagia within the first 12 to 24 months following surgery (Fig. 5). This principle is likely as true for surgical myotomy as it is for pneumatic dilatation, although lowering resting LES pressure to near 10 mm Hg is much more reproducible with myotomy. Young patients (<40 years), male patients, and those with a nondilated esophagus have also been shown to respond less well to pneumatic dilatation and thus are good candidates for primary myotomy.

Several factors have been suggested to affect the outcome of laparoscopic myotomy. These include (1) the magnitude of preoperative LES resting pressure, (2) the degree of preoperative esophageal dilatation or tortuosity, and (3) the presence or absence of prior nonoperative interventions.

Evaluating the outcomes of 78 consecutive achalasia patients treated with laparoscopic myotomy, Arain and colleagues found that a high preoperative resting LES pressure was an independent predictor of the relief of dysphagia. This was confirmed in a recent series of 200 consecutively treated achalasia patients by investigators at Vanderbilt University. They found that patients with a preoperative LES resting pressure >35 mm Hg were 21.3 times more likely to have relief of dysphagia than those with preoperative LES pressures <35 mm Hg. These authors also reported that the greater the decrease in LES pressure following surgery, the greater the improvement in postoperative dysphagia (Fig. 6).

The benefit of surgical myotomy in patients with a dilated and tortuous esophagus is unclear. In this setting in which the esophagus is not only massively dilated but sigmoid-shaped, bolus flow is impaired by the shape of the esophagus in addition to LES spasm. Even in these circumstances, patients may perceive benefits, however. Patti and colleagues, evaluating 66 patients with varying degrees of dilatation, found that all 7 patients with esophageal diameters >6 cm and tortuosity had a satisfactory outcome. In contrast, a case-controlled study by Pechlivanides and colleagues found that

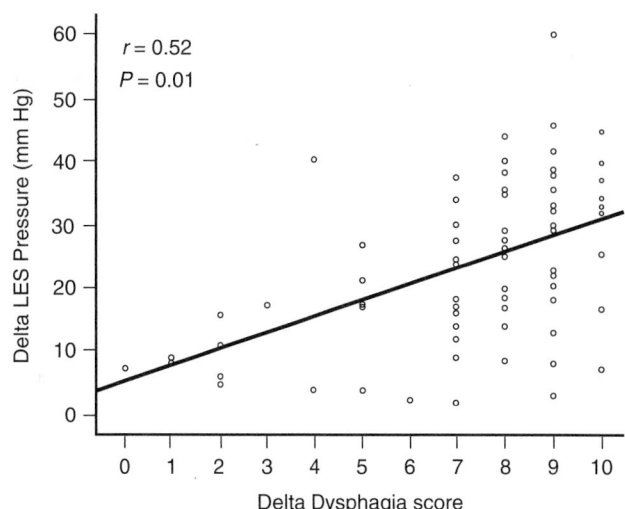

Figure 6 Correlation between the change in lower esophageal sphincter pressure and change in dysphagia score following Heller myotomy. *From Torquati A, Richards WO, Holzman MD, Sharp KW: Ann Surg 243:587, 2006.*

esophageal diameter decreased in all patients with esophageal dilatation, but only patients with a postoperative diameter of <4 cm experienced excellent results. Given these data and the low morbidity and mortality associated with laparoscopic Heller myotomy compared with esophagectomy, myotomy is often chosen as the first line of treatment regardless of the extent of dilatation.

Endoscopic interventions performed in achalasia patients before surgical intervention likely influence the success of surgical myotomy. Several studies have shown that patients treated endoscopically, particularly with Botox injection before myotomy, have a higher incidence of intraoperative mucosal violation. Smith and colleagues recently reported that previously given treatment may also affect symptomatic outcome. Patients with (n = 154) or without (n = 55) a history of prior balloon dilatation or Botox injection were compared. Defined as persistent or recurrent symptoms or the need for further treatment, the failure rate of those with prior interventions was found to be almost twice that of those who had no prior intervention (19.5% vs. 10.1%). In addition, patients with previous endoscopic therapies were found to have more difficult dissection planes, increased mediastinal scarring that resulted in a higher incidence of intraoperative mucosal perforations, and longer postoperative recovery than those without prior treatment. These findings support the use of surgical myotomy as the initial treatment method for achalasia and suggest that endoscopic interventions should be reserved for the rare patient who is not a surgical candidate.

Persistent or Recurrent Symptoms

Long-term outcome data suggest that a properly performed laparoscopic myotomy and partial fundoplication will be the only therapeutic intervention required in up to 80% of patients with achalasia. Mild to moderate symptoms of dysphagia, regurgitation, heartburn, and chest pain recur over time in up to 40% to 50% of patients, but few of these require further intervention beyond lifestyle and behavioral changes or proton-pump inhibitor therapy. Mechanisms of failure include (1) inadequate myotomy, (2) scarring or anatomic distortion of the GE junction, (3) complications of gastroesophageal reflux disease, and (4) progressive esophageal dilatation or distortion, usually secondary to persistent outflow resistance. Early failures are usually caused by failure to extend the myotomy far enough into the stomach, anatomic distortion, or both. Late failures occur secondary to the development of complicated gastroesophageal reflux with stricturing or Barrett's changes and

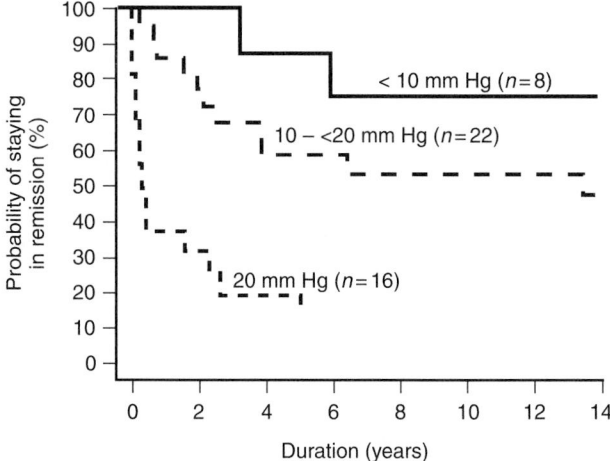

Figure 5 Kaplan–Meier curve demonstrating time to symptom recurrence following lower esophageal sphincter pneumatic dilatation to pressures of <10 mm Hg, 10 to <20 mm Hg, and ≥20 mm Hg. *From Eckardt VF, Gockel I, Bernhard G: Gut 53:629, 2004.*

disease progression. The development of a distal esophageal diverticulum, thought to be secondary to proximal extension of the myotomy into the lower posterior mediastinum, is also an increasingly recognized occurrence. The predisposing factors and symptomatic significance of this are as yet unclear, however.

Recurrent dysphagia following surgical myotomy should be investigated by upper endoscopy to exclude an obstructing lesion, by contrast esophagography to assess for esophageal dilatation or tortuosity, and by repeat manometry to assess for high persistent LES resting pressure (>10–15 mm Hg). Management options include pneumatic dilatation or remyotomy for suspected incomplete or scarred myotomy, and esophagectomy for those with end-stage dilatation and tortuosity, stricture, or cancer. Pneumatic dilatation, once felt to be contraindicated following myotomy, may be an attractive option for early persistent dysphagia. In a retrospective analysis of 113 patients treated with myotomy for achalasia, Zaninotto and colleagues found that most (78%) of the 10 patients with recurrent dysphagia could be effectively treated with pneumatic dilatation. They concluded that pneumatic dilatation should be considered as the first-line treatment for patients with persistent dysphagia and that reoperation should be reserved for those who do not respond.

CONCLUSION

Laparoscopic Heller myotomy has become the initial primary treatment and standard surgical approach for patients with achalasia. Several studies have shown surgical myotomy to provide superior long-term symptom relief compared with nonsurgical interventions such as Botox injection or pneumatic dilatation. Extended distal myotomy with a partial fundoplication has been found to provide greater dysphagia relief with minimal development of gastroesophageal reflux. A high preoperative LES pressure portends a better symptomatic outcome following surgery, as does the absence of prior nonoperative interventions. Persistent or recurrent symptoms following surgical myotomy that do not respond to lifestyle changes can be treated effectively with pneumatic dilatation.

SELECTED READING

Arain MA, Peters JH, Tambanker AP, and others: Preoperative lower esophageal sphincter pressure affects outcome of laparoscopic esophageal myotomy for achalasia, *J Gastrointest Surg* 8:328–334, 2004.

Bonatti H, Hinder RA, Klocker J, and others: Long-term results of laparoscopic Heller myotomy with partial fundoplication for the treatment of achalasia, *Am J Surg* 190:874–878, 2005.

Chen LQ, Chughtai T, Sideris L, and others: Long-term effects of myotomy and partial fundoplication for esophageal achalasia, *Dis Esoph* 15:171–179, 2002.

Csendes A, Velasco N, Graghetto I, Henriquez A: A prospective randomized study comparing forceful dilatation and esophagomyotomy in patients with achalasia of the esophagus, *Gastroenterology* 80:789–795, 1981.

Donohue PE, Horgan S, Liu KJ, Madura JA: Floppy Dor fundoplication after asophagocardiomyotomy for achalasia, *Surgery* 132:716–722; discussion 722–723, 2002.

Eckardt VF, Gockel I, Bernhard G: Pneumatic dilatation for achalasia: late results of a prospective follow up investigation, *Gut* 53:629, 2004.

Khajanchee YS, Kanneganti S, Leatherwood AE, and others: Laparoscopic Heller myotomy with Toupet fundoplication: outcomes predictors in 121 consecutive patients, *Arch Surg* 140:827–833; discussion 833–834, 2005.

Oelschlager BK, Chang L, Pellegrini CA: Improved outcome after extended gastric myotomy for Achalasia, *Arch Surg* 138:490–495; discussion 495–497, 2003.

Patti MG, Feo CV, Diener U, and others: Laparoscopic Heller myotomy relieves dysphagia in achalasia when the esophagus is dilated, *Surg Endo* 13:843–847, 1999.

Patti MG, Molena D, Fisichella PM, and others: Laparoscopic Heller myotomy and Dor fundoplication for achalasia: analysis of successes and failures, *Arch Surg* 136:870–877, 2001.

Patti MG, Pellegrini CA, Horgan S, and others: Minimally invasive surgery for achalasia: an 8-year experience with 168 patients, *Ann Surg* 230:587–593; discussion 593–594, 1999.

Pechlivanides G, Chrysos E, Athanasakis E, and others: Laparoscopic Heller cardiomyotomy and Dor fundoplication for esophageal achalasia: possible factors predicting outcome, *Arch Surg* 136:1240–1243, 2001.

Perrone JM, Frisella MM, Desai KM, Soper NJ: Results of laparoscopic Heller-Toupet operation for achalasia, *Surg Endosc* 18:1565–1571, 2004.

Portale G, Costantini M, Rizzetto C, and others: Long-term outcome of laparoscopic Heller-Dor surgery for esophageal achalasia: possible detrimental role of previous endoscopic treatment, *J Gastrointest Surg* 9:1332–1339, 2005.

Rice TW, McKelvey AA, Richter JE, and others: A physiologic clinical study of achalasia: Should Dor fundoplication be added to Heller myotomy? *J Thorac Cardiovasc Surg* 130(6):1593–1600, 2005.

Richards WO, Torquati A, Holzman MD, and others: Heller myotomy versus Heller myotomy with Dor fundoplication for achalasia: a prospective randomized double-bline clinical trial, *Ann Surg* 240(3):405–415, 2004.

Sharp KW, Khaitan L, Scholz S, and others: 100 consecutive minimally invasive Heller myotomies: lessons learned, *Ann Surg* 235:631–638; discussion 638–639, 2002.

Smith CD, Stival A, Howell L, Swafford V: Endoscopic therapy for achalasia before Heller myotomy results in worse outcomes than Heller myotomy alone, *Ann Surg* 243:579–586, 2006.

Torquati A, Richards WO, Holzman MD, Sharp KW: Laparoscopic myotomy for achalasia: predictors of successful outcome after 200 cases, *Ann Surg* 243:587, 2006.

West RL, Hirsch DP, Bartelsman WM, and others: Long term results of pneumatic dilatation in achalasia followed for more than 5 years, *Am J Gast* 97:1326–1351, 2002.

Zaninotto G, Annese V, Costantini M, and others: Randomized controlled trial of botulinum toxin versus laparoscopic Heller myotomy for esophageal achalasia, *Ann Surg* 239:364, 2004.

Zaninotto G, Constantini M, Portale G, and others: Etiology, diagnosis, and treatment of failures after laparoscopic Heller myotomy for achalasia, *Ann Surg* 235:186–192, 2002.

DISORDERS OF ESOPHAGEAL MOTILITY

Joseph DeSimone, MD, and Stephen C. Yang, MD

INTRODUCTION

In 1892, William Osler first described esophageal spasms in what he referred to as "hypochondriac patients with unexplained chest pain." Retrosternal chest pain and dysphagia are the two most common complaints of patients presenting with an esophageal motility disorder. However, the majority of noncardiac chest pain is due to gastroesophageal reflux disease (GERD). Furthermore, of patients who present with either dysphagia or chest pain, only approximately 3% of cases are the result of a motility disorder. Covered in this chapter are the presenting symptoms as well as treatment for the following disorders: achalasia; vigorous achalasia; diffuse esophageal spasm (DES); high-amplitude peristaltic contractions (HAPC, or "nutcracker esophagus"); hypertensive lower esophageal sphincter (LES); and ineffective esophageal motility (IEM).

CLASSIFICATION

The 2001 review by Spechler and Castell is adopted here as the classification system for the various esophageal motility disorders.

Table 1: Manometric Classification of Esophageal Motility Disorders

Inadequate lower esophageal sphinchter relaxation
Achalasia
Vigorous achalasia
Epiphrenic diverticulum with spasm
Uncoordinated esophageal contraction
Diffuse esophageal spasm
Hypercontraction
High-amplitude peristaltic contraction or nutcracker esophagus
Hypertensive lower esophageal sphincter
Hypocontraction
Ineffective esophageal motility

The pathology is organized manometrically into four patterns (Table 1). The category of inadequate LES relaxation comprises achalasia, the vigorous form with an epiphrenic diverticulum and spasm, uncoordinated esophageal contraction including DES, hypercontraction of the esophagus presenting as HAPC and HLES, and hypocontraction of the esophagus including IEM.

INADEQUATE LOWER ESOPHAGEAL SPHINCTER RELAXATION

The term *achalasia* means failure to relax. This is the most common esophageal motility disorder. The two subtypes are primary achalasia and secondary. The cause of primary achalasia is unknown; however, various hypotheses suggest hereditary, degenerative, autoimmune, or infectious causes as the source. The pathologic change that occurs in these patients is an inflammatory reaction with the loss of ganglion cells of the myenteric (Auerbach's) plexus. This results in the failure of the LES to relax. In classic achalasia, the nonperistaltic tertiary contractions in the body of the esophagus are of low amplitude; in the vigorous form, these contractions are of high amplitude. Secondary achalasia is the result of another existing pathology, including Chagas's disease, idiopathic pseudo-obstruction, postvagotomy, infiltrative disorders (sarcoidosis, amyloidosis), scleroderma, and diabetes mellitus. This should not be confused with pseudo-achalasia resulting from an obstructing or near-obstructing tumor at the gastroesophageal (GE) junction.

Patients may present with dysphagia to both liquid and solids, but pain is not typical, as it is with other esophageal spasm disorders. It is usually postprandial, particularly after a full meal, and often relieved with regurgitation. The workup of a suspected diagnosis begins with a barium swallow that has a smooth tapering of the LES resembling a bird's beak. There can also be an air-fluid level of retained food within the dilated esophagus. Alternatively, a video cine-esophagogram not only will demonstrate the anatomic abnormality but can also show the functional motor disorder in real time. Confirmation is established with esophageal manometry revealing any of the following possibilities: (1) lack of, or abnormal relaxation of a normal or hypertensive LES, although if there is normal relaxation (the minority of patients), it is for a brief period of time; (2) aperistalsis in the body of the esophagus; or (3) nonfunctional contractions, typically of low amplitude but in some circumstances normal or even high amplitude (vigorous achalasia). The workup should finally include an esophagoscopy/endoscopic ultrasound (EGD/EUS) to look for any evidence of a tumor (pseudo-achalasia).

The treatment of achalasia is palliative, and at present there is no treatment to restore any muscular activity. The primary goals are to relieve the obstruction of the dysfunctioning LES and allow gravity to empty the esophagus, thus preventing an end-stage situation (megaesophagus) that would require esophagectomy. Successful treatment usually requires multiple disciplines. Unfortunately, randomized trials are lacking, and most therapeutic practices are based on patient and physician preferences and little evidence-based data.

Dilatation of the LES is the oldest form of treatment for achalasia, dating back more than 300 years to Thomas Willis, who performed it with a whalebone. The rupture of smooth muscle fibers of the LES caused by pneumatic dilatation has a lasting effect, as opposed to the ineffective stretching that occurs with a bougie dilator. Endoscopically guided balloons are placed across the LES and are progressively inflated. This is the most cost-effective and successful nonsurgical form of treatment, with only approximately 30% of patients needing further intervention. The primary problem with pneumatic dilatation is that each treatment carries a 2% risk of perforation.

Botulinum toxin type A (Botox; Allergan, Irvine, CA) injection inhibits acetylcholine release from nerve endings, resulting in the decreased stimulation of LES smooth muscle. The endoscopically guided injection at the LES is an effective treatment initially but loses its efficacy over time. More than 50% of patients will have recurrent symptoms in 6 months. Most important to the surgeon is the scarring that can occur from the multiple injections (and likely many pneumatic dilatations) in the submucosal plane, making the dissection during myotomy more dangerous and potentially less effective. Patients who are poor surgical candidates (older age and comorbidities), as well as those with vigorous achalasia, are likely the best candidates for Botox.

Surgical esophagomyotomy is considered the gold standard of therapy. The indication for surgery is generally the failure of conservative management, usually indicated by the return of symptoms following two or three attempts at dilatation or Botox injection (or both). Preoperatively, the patient should be on a clear liquid diet for several days to allow for better clearing of undigested food from the esophagus. A number of options and controversies exist regarding the optimal technique for the Heller myotomy. These include the approach (chest or abdomen), the extent (open vs. minimally invasive), the proper proximal and distal extent of the myotomy, and whether an antireflux maneuver is added (and which one). Many of these decisions made on the basis of surgeon experience and comfort level. Irrespective of the technique, when done properly the myotomy establishes a reliable opening for food to pass. There are differing opinions as to how far to extend onto the stomach, balancing the risk of continued dysphagia with the risk of severe reflux. Advantages of the thoracic approach include the ability to extend the myotomy more proximally when severe tertiary contractions or spasms coexist with achalasia, and a lower incidence of GER compared with an abdominal approach. More extensive dissection of the esophageal hiatus is required with an abdominal technique, and thus there is a higher likelihood of GER. To reduce reflux, there are several options for a partial fundoplication, but not all surgeons perform this. An anterior Dor hemifundoplication covers the myotomy, or a posterior 180-degree Toupet hemifundoplication can be performed.

Given the advantages of minimally invasive surgery such as laparoscopy, video-assisted thoracic surgery (VATS), and even robotic technology, earlier referrals for surgery are made at an increasing rate. For patients with classic achalasia, the laparoscopic approach is a safe, reasonable, and effective approach. A complete myotomy can be performed, as well as fundoplication, with excellent visualization. With long-standing achalasia and larger esophageal lumens, a nasogastric tube should be inserted first to prevent aspiration after induction of general anesthesia. It is good practice to perform flexible esophagoscopy to get an idea of the caliper of the esophageal lumen and to suction out remaining retained food and saliva. It is suggested that the scope be left in place during the operative portion to help with identification of the esophagus, to aid in staying outside the mucosal layer, and to allow later access if the mucosal layer has been violated during the myotomy. Usually four or five laparoscopic port sites are placed, as shown in Figure 1A. Dissection is performed down to the mucosal layer along the anterior portion of the esophagus, staying to the left of the anterior vagus nerve. A hook cautery on low voltage is used to divide the outer longitudinal and circular muscle layers, extending 6 to 8 cm proximally on the

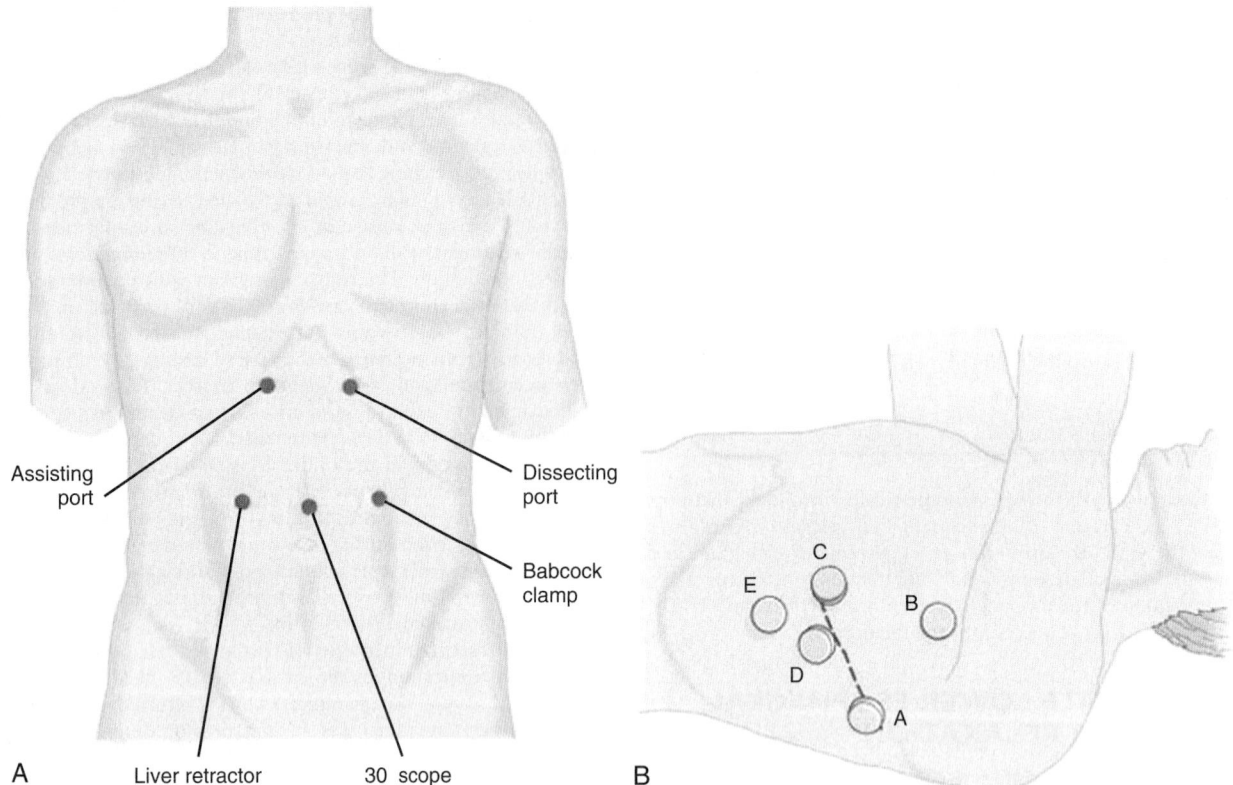

Figure 1 **(A)** Laparoscopic port placement for Heller myotomy. **(B)** Video-assisted thoracic surgery port placement for Heller myotomy. *Port A,* cautery; *port B,* retraction; *port C,* grasper; *port D,* optional utility; *port E,* camera. *From Patti M, Fisichella P. In Wilmore D, Cheung L, Harken A, and others, editors: ACS Surgery, New York, 2003, WebMD, p. 705.*

esophagus and 1 to 2 cm past the GE junction on the gastric side. As stated previously, the myotomy is more difficult than usual if the patient has undergone multiple prior Botox injection or dilatation procedures. The submuscular plane is difficult to distinguish from the mucosal layer, and a mucosal tear can easily occur. If this happens, the defect should be closed (with 4–0 Vicryl), the muscle reapproximated, and myotomy reperformed on the opposite wall, draining the area well. However, if no obvious mucosal violation has occurred, the indwelling esophagoscope is used to insufflate the esophagus and stomach under saline to check for leaks. The muscle layer is sharply dissected away from the mucosal layer approximately 50% around circumferentially to allow for a better myotomy affect. A Dor or Toupet partial fundoplication is added to minimize GER and to cover the exposed mucosa in case mucosal violations exist that are not evident.

As stated previously, a VATS or thoracic approach has the advantage of a longer proximal myotomy in cases with associated severe spasm but has the disadvantage of slightly more pain and difficulty in doing a partial fundoplication, such as a loose Belsey Mark IV. Port placement is critical, again using 4–5 trocars (Fig. 1.4-1, *B*), and should be not too far posterior, where the intercostal spaces are narrow. The procedure is performed similarly to the laparoscopic technique, but the myotomy is carried out anterior to the left vagus nerve. In the rare patient who has a hiatal hernia, a diaphragmatic crural repair is added to the myotomy with a hemifundoplication procedure during either the abdominal or thoracic approach. With the minimally invasive techniques, the patient's hospital stay is limited to approximately 48 hours, and more than 90% of patients report good to excellent results.

An epiphrenic diverticulum occurs in conjunction with achalasia in approximately 10% of cases. These are considered pulsion in etiology and do not contain all layers of the esophageal wall ("false" diverticulum). Although achalasia is the most common abnormality associated with epiphrenic diverticula, other esophageal motility disorders should be considered; these are usually

identified with esophagography, manometry, or both. The defect nearly always occurs on the right side of the esophagus, but despite this the surgical approach to address these diverticula should be via the left chest. Smaller (<1 cm), wide-based diverticula can be simply inverted by dissecting out the diverticular wall and closing the esophageal muscle wall, dunking the diverticulum with interrupted 3–0 silk sutures in a Lembert fashion. Tethering or performing a diverticulopexy is rarely done and should not be considered in patients with narrow necks. Surgical resection is the standard therapy and should be combined with myotomy and partial fundoplication. The distal esophagus is exposed via the left chest, and the diverticulum is dissected down to the base along the esophageal wall. A transabdominal (TA) stapler is positioned at the diverticulum neck and fired with a 50-F Maloney dilator in place to prevent narrowing of the esophageal lumen. Occasionally, the diverticulum is partly opened at the top to remove retained food and allow better closure of the staples. After the stapler has been fired and the diverticulum cut away, the muscle layer is closed over the staple line with interrupted 3–0 silk sutures. A long, 10-cm myotomy across the GE junction is performed on the esophageal wall opposite the diverticulum, and a partial fundoplication is performed.

Finally, esophagectomy is reserved for patients with end-stage achalasia, manifested by a megaesophagus, recurring aspiration, or failure of a prior myotomy. The techniques (described elsewhere in this book) include the transhiatal, Ivor Lewis, and three-incision approaches. Most prefer an Ivor Lewis esophagectomy because mobilization of the intrathoracic esophagus is easier, given the tortuous nature of the esophagus and the thick and vascular adhesions.

DIFFUSE ESOPHAGEAL SPASM

DES is a motility disorder in which normal peristalsis is periodically interrupted by simultaneous, high-amplitude disordered contractions, although strict criteria are not widely accepted. The precise etiology is unknown. The esophagus is sensitive to certain stimuli (stretch, pentagastrin, cholinergic) that produce symptoms. Degeneration of the esophageal vagal branches has been observed but are not consistent. Anxiety disorders should also be excluded. Patients with DES complain of chest pain, as well as dysphagia with both liquids and solids.

Patients present with cardiac-like chest pain that varies in location, quantity, and quality. The pain can be related to rapid eating, carbonated beverages, or liquids of extreme temperature and is almost never exertional. A contrast esophagogram can reveal a corkscrew appearance or segmentation; many of the studies, however, appear normal. The diagnosis is made by manometry, which typically shows that more than 20% of wet swallows have simultaneous contractions with amplitudes of 30 mm Hg or more. Patients less often have repetitive spontaneous contractions, as well as inconsistent findings of LES dysfunction.

Once the diagnosis of DES is established in symptomatic patients, treatment should begin with patient reassurance. Following this first-line treatment, many medications directed at smooth-muscle relaxation (nitrates, calcium-channel blockers, and phosphodiesterase inhibitors) are available. Tricyclic antidepressants and serotonin reuptake inhibitors also have been shown to work. Local therapies are ineffective because of the diffuse nature of the disorder. Recently, Botox seems to be the most popular reported treatment, especially when directed at DES with associated LES dysfunction. Again, bougie dilatation has little effect, whereas pneumatic dilatation can be effective in patients with documented LES emptying problems. Patients who do not improve following the earlier-mentioned treatments and who continue to have pain and dysphagia should be considered for surgery. Additionally, symptomatic patients who have been diagnosed with DES and whose diagnoses are complicated with hiatal hernias or diverticula are candidates for surgery.

The left chest is entered either by VATS or limited open thoracotomy. A long myotomy is performed on the esophagus from the level of the aortic arch down to the LES with electrocautery, carefully preserving the integrity of the mucosal layer. As described previously, we prefer to keep the esophagoscope in and insufflate the esophagus at this point to check for mucosal air leaks. The muscle layer is then dissected away from the mucosal layer from both edges of the muscle along the length of the myotomy not more than half of the esophageal circumference. If there is LES dysfunction, the myotomy is extended on to the stomach, and a partial fundoplication, such as a modified Belsey Mark IV, should be constructed to minimize GER, although this is more difficult to do by VATS.

ESOPHAGEAL HYPERCONTRACTION

The majority of patients with abnormal hypercontraction of the esophagus present with HAPC, or "nutcracker esophagus." The contractions that occur are coordinated and exist in the body of the esophagus. HAPC is defined as distal esophageal contractions that are two standard deviations higher than the mean amplitude of a large number of normal patients at any given manometry lab or, alternatively, contractions with peak amplitudes >180 mm Hg. The common presenting symptom is chest pain of unclear etiology, and dysphagia is present only approximately 10% of the time. Approximately 30% of patients fulfill criteria for psychiatric disorders, especially anxiety diagnoses, and have profiles similar to patients with irritable bowel syndromes.

HAPC disorders are best diagnosed with manometry; esophagography is usually normal and therefore offers no additional benefit. The algorithm for treatment of these disorders is similar to that of DES. No evidence supports the use of bougie or pneumatic

dilatation. The patients who fail medical therapy are candidates for a long myotomy with or without an antireflux procedure; however, results have been inconsistent.

Less often, patients can present with hypertensive LES (HLES). This is defined as a resting LES pressure >45 mm Hg with normal relaxation, in contrast to the lack of relaxation of the LES seen in achalasia. These patients present with dysphagia rather than chest pain, and treatment follows the algorithm of DES therapy. However, when medical treatment fails, a Heller myotomy with fundoplication may be indicated.

ESOPHAGEAL HYPOCONTRACTION

IEM is typically a secondary motility disorder as a result of other systemic illnesses such as scleroderma, rheumatoid arthritis, diabetes mellitus, multiple sclerosis, systemic lupus erythematosis (SLE), and alcoholism. Patients typically present with GERD symptoms and rarely with dysphagia. These dysmotility issues are characterized by an esophagus that generates abnormally low-amplitude (<30 mm Hg) contractions. Some contractions are simultaneous and dyscoordinated, resulting in ineffective peristalsis in the distal esophagus. The contractions that are coordinated have been shown to be too weak to push along a bolus of barium during contrast cine. Despite a normally functioning LES, patients with IEM suffer from GERD because of the lack of peristalsis in the esophagus. In these patients, symptoms of heartburn and reflux are more common than dysphagia.

The diagnosis of esophageal involvement in the diseases described previously should always be suspected. Diagnostic studies should include contrast esophagograms, endoscopy to exclude mechanical obstruction or malignant disorders, and manomety. Manometry typically reveals weak or absent peristalsis in the distal two thirds of the esophagus with decreased LES pressure. Patients who have symptoms of reflux should also have a 24-hour pH probe study.

Treatment should be directed at the GERD symptoms, and as dysphagia becomes a problem, the therapy should be directed toward the anatomic abnormality (peptic stricture, tumor). Medications to increase esophageal motility are no longer available. Mechanical bougienage should be offered if distal esophageal strictures occur. Drugs to slow the hypocontraction process, such as D-penicillamine therapy, are generally ineffective. Surgical antireflux procedures are offered to patients with severe or refractory GERD; these should be partial fundoplication wraps such as the Dor or Toupet techniques and should be approached by laparoscopy. Patients with better access through the left chest are offered Belsey Mark IV fundoplication. Care is taken not to make the wrap too tight because this would cause a functional obstruction; thus these repairs are performed over a 50-F Maloney dilator. Finally, esophagectomy should be considered only in the most extreme cases in which patients have failed a prior antireflux procedure and continue to have persistent severe symptoms or develop secondary problems such as undilatable strictures or cancer.

SUGGESTED READINGS

Horgan S, Galvani C, Gorodner M, and others: Robotic-assisted Heller myotomy versus laparoscopic Heller myotomy for the treatment of esophageal achalasia: multicenter study, *J Gastroint Surg* 9:1020, 2005.

Patti M, Gorodner M, Galvani C, and others: Spectrum of esophageal motility disorders: implications for diagnosis and treatment, *Arch Surg* 140:442, 2005.

Spechler SJ, Castell DO: Classification of oesophageal motility abnormalities, *Gut* 49:145, 2001.

Tedesco P, Fisichella F, Way L, Patti M: Cause and treatment of epiphrenic diverticula, *Am J Surg* 190:891, 2005.

MANAGEMENT OF PHARYNGOESOPHAGEAL (ZENKER'S) DIVERTICULA

James I. Cohen, MD

INTRODUCTION

The most common esophageal diverticulum, the Zenker's diverticulum, occurs at the junction of the hypopharynx and cervical esophagus and is due to a natural weakness in the buttressing muscular layer that occurs between the inferior aspect of the inferior pharyngeal constrictor and the cricopharyngeus muscle (Fig. 1). Its etiology is at least in part due to the prolonged effects of the patient's swallowing against the relative obstruction of a cricopharyngeus muscle, which does not relax appropriately (either in degree or in timing) with swallowing. Support for this theory comes from longitudinal studies of patients with untreated diverticula that show a gradual growth and extension of the diverticulum with increasing cricopharyngeal spasm and cervical esophageal obstruction.

An understanding of the etiologic role of the cricopharyngeus in the management of Zenker's diverticulum is important because failure to address the cricopharyngeus muscle, regardless of how the diverticulum is dealt with, results in inevitable recurrence of the diverticulum. In addition, the realization that the diverticulum is a pulsion pseudo-diverticulum that is not surrounded by muscular layers but consists only of mucosa and serosa can aid in the surgical identification of its true "neck," where it joins the hypopharyngeal

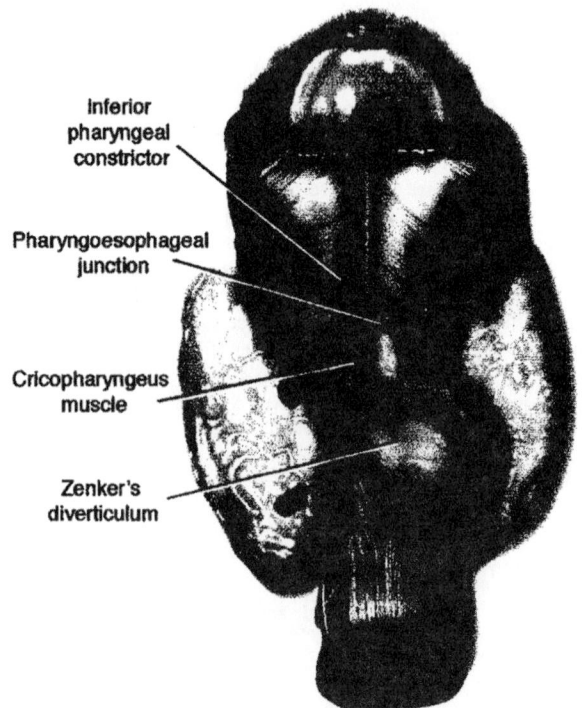

Figure 1   Pharyngoesophageal junction from posterior aspect with Zenker's diverticulum emerging between the inferior pharyngeal constrictor and cricopharyngeus muscles.

esophageal junction, and prevent a stricture from overzealous resection during an external approach.

What is much less well understood is the etiology of the cricopharyngeal spasm, tightening, and hypertrophy. Although there is clearly a strong association between this phenomenon and gastroesophageal reflux as documented by pH probe studies and the higher incidence of Zenker's diverticulum in individuals with a known hiatal hernia than in a general population, the correlation is not universal. In addition, theories that support neuromuscular dyscoordination as the primary etiology also exist.

DIAGNOSIS AND PATIENT SELECTION

Although classically patients with a Zenker's diverticulum will have the perception of food sticking in their throat with latent regurgitation (often hours to days later), this symptom is by no means universal. As the degree of cricopharyngeal obstruction varies, so too will the symptoms. In those with significant obstruction, the predominant symptoms may be difficulty with swallowing and weight loss. By contrast, in patients with a relatively open esophageal introitus, the predominant symptoms may be due to regurgitation of the sac contents with associated cough, microaspiration, and throat clearing.

Ultimately, the diagnosis needs to be established radiologically. A modified barium swallow, rather than a barium swallow alone, is fundamental to the diagnosis of this disease. Unlike a routine barium swallow, which tends to focus on the esophagus distal to the cricopharyngeus muscle, a modified barium swallow focuses on the swallowing mechanisms of the upper aerodigestive tract, not only with liquid barium but with other consistencies as well. There is a relatively high incidence of associated problems in the swallowing mechanism in patients with Zenker's diverticulum, both in terms of the pharyngeal phases of swallowing and with secondary and tertiary contractions of the esophagus. Understanding that these exist and the relative contribution that they make to the overall swallowing problem that the patient is having is a fundamental part of preoperative counseling in terms of reasonable expectations from the operation itself. By personally reviewing the video swallow and correlating what is seen with the patient's symptoms, the surgeon can best understand whether the operation will be of benefit. This is particularly true in reoperative situations.

The lateral views of the modified barium swallow are most important in terms of understanding the size of the diverticulum and confirming its location as being just proximal to the cricopharyngeus (Fig. 2). Placement of a radio-opaque object of known dimensions, such as a penny, on the lateral neck of the patient at the time of radiological examination will help to determine the true vertical dimension of the diverticulum, a key issue in selection of the surgical approach. The spectrum of Zenker's diverticulum will vary from cricopharyngeal spasm alone with minimal redundancy of the mucosa above the muscle (the cricopharyngeal bar) to diverticula of varying lengths from 1 to 15 cm. The presence of associated gastroesophageal reflux, if seen on modified barium swallow or barium swallow, is important for patient counseling because release of the cricopharyngeal sphincter may worsen laryngopharyngeal symptoms.

SURGICAL STRATEGIES

The traditional management of a Zenker's diverticulum has consisted of an open approach during which the sac is removed and the cricopharyngeus muscle is sectioned in its entirety to restore

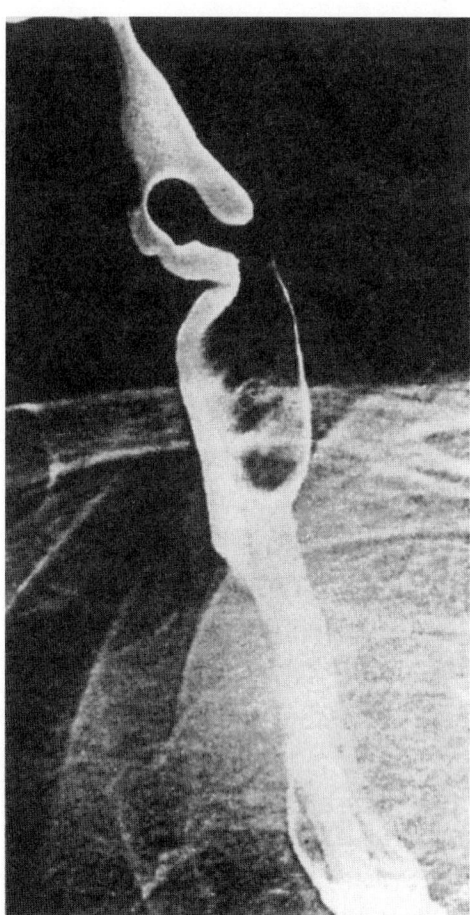

Figure 2 Pharyngoesophageal diverticulum with prominent cricopharyngeal bar. *From Ferguson MK: Diverticula of the esophagus. In Cameron JL, editor: Current surgical therapy, ed 7, St. Louis, 2001, Mosby.*

free passage of food into the cervical esophagus. In the days before stapling devices, when secure closure of the pharyngeal defect left after diverticulectomy was technically more difficult, the risk of fistula and mediastinitis was relatively high. This was especially true if the cricopharyngeal myotomy was incomplete because any residual obstruction caused by the remaining fibers served to increase pressure on the suture line generated by swallowing. As a result, alternate strategies that avoided the need for pharyngotomy were devised for high-risk patients, such as sac inversion or superior suspension ("pexy") to the prevertebral fascia. With stapling devices, however, these approaches are of historic interest only.

In recent years, transoral management of Zenker's diverticulum has superseded the open approach for the majority of patients. The concept of this operation is that the party wall between the Zenker's diverticulum and the esophagus contains the cricopharyngeus muscle (Fig. 3, A and B). If this party wall can be divided over a length of at least 2.0 to 2.5 cm, division of the cricopharyngeus muscle is ensured, and the Zenker's diverticulum, although not removed, will now empty into the esophagus rather than the hypopharynx, where it will be asymptomatic. Although this concept is not new and has been understood since the early 1900s, the risk of fistula with division of the party wall was too high in the days before operative laryngoscopes and endoscopes made adequate visualization possible and endoscopic stapling devices allowed sealing of the cut mucosal edges.

In patients who have predominantly cricopharyngeal spasm with minimal (<1.5–2.0 cm) mucosal redundancy proximal to it, an open approach with cricopharyngeal myotomy alone is generally sufficient because this redundancy will disappear with release of the cricopharyngeus muscle. For sacs that are greater than 2.0 to 2.5 cm in length, an endoscopic approach is recommended because there should be sufficient party wall length to allow for complete division of the cricopharyngeus muscle and the overall operative morbidity is lower. In the limited number of remaining patients with insufficient mouth opening or neck mobility to allow for adequate transoral exposure of the sac, a traditional open approach with cricopharyngeal myotomy and diverticulectomy still needs to be performed. Management of extremely large sacs (>7 cm) remains controversial; some believe that the patulous nature of the resulting

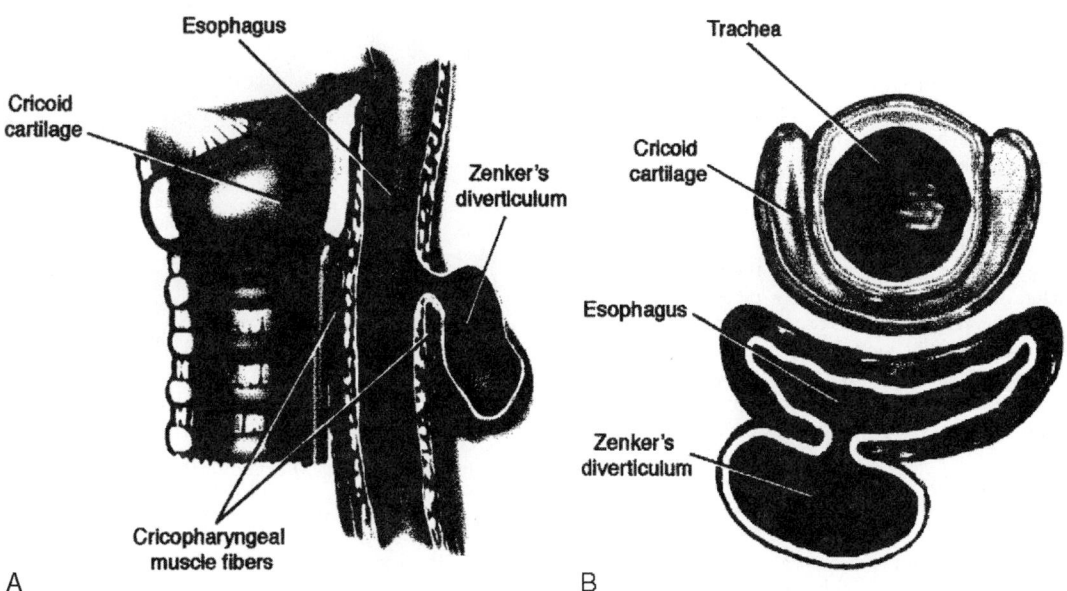

Figure 3 **(A)** Sagittal section through Zenker's diverticulum and esophagus showing party wall composed primarily of cricopharyngeal fibers covered by mucosa. **(B)** "Operative view" axial section through Zenker's diverticulum and esophagus demonstrating two lumens with intervening party wall containing the cricopharyngeus muscle.

hypopharyngeal-esophageal complex created after endoscopic division of the party wall still allows for such significant food retention that symptoms may persist, and therefore open diverticulectomy might be preferred.

OPERATIVE TECHNIQUE

Endoscopic Approach

Adequate sac length (>2.5 cm), mouth opening, and neck mobility are prerequisites for this procedure, which is usually performed on an outpatient basis. Perioperative antibiotics are given because of the theoretical risk of perforation but are not continued beyond the procedure itself.

The patient is intubated with a small endotracheal tube to allow maximal working room in the hypopharynx. Problems with chipping of upper incisors, one of the most common minor complications of the procedure, can be avoided by the use of a tooth guard. Under direct vision, the bivalved diverticuloscope is introduced into the hypopharynx, and the larynx is suspended forward with exposure of the mouth of the sac, the introitus of the esophagus, and the party wall between them. This is often the most difficult part of the procedure because the tightness of the cricopharyngeus around the esophageal opening minimizes its opening and places it in an anterior location. If possible, the anterior blade of the diverticuloscope is introduced sufficiently into the cervical esophagus to stabilize the laryngopharyngeal complex anteriorly as the diverticuloscope is suspended on a Mayo stand placed over the patient's chest.

Once adequate exposure has been obtained, the bivalved diverticuloscope is opened proximally to allow for introduction of a telescope down the side for distal viewing and distally to allow sufficient working room for the endoscopic stapler (Fig. 4, A and B). A 16-F nasogastric tube is placed into the esophageal introitus and advanced to confirm proper orientation. It is then removed with the endoscopic gastrointestinal anastomois (GIA) stapler (3.5 cm in length), introduced under endoscopic visual control, and opened; its jaws are then advanced over the party wall. The jaw containing the staples and cutting blade is longer, and therefore to maximize division of the party wall it should be introduced into the esophageal introitus where sac length will not limit its advance (Fig. 5). The anterior location of the esophageal introitus and the straight nature of the endoscopic stapler can make it difficult to angle the stapler far enough forward to engage the esophageal introitus. This can be facilitated by posterior traction on the party wall with a second grasping device or a stitch.

After the party wall has been engaged, the stapler is advanced over it as far as possible, with care taken not to push so hard against the distal end of the sac that a perforation occurs (Fig. 6). It is then closed, its position confirmed by gentle traction and rotation, and fired. With its removal, the edges of the cut party wall should be seen to separate as they are pulled apart by the divided cricopharyngeal sphincter, and a common lumen is established. If there is significant party wall remaining, the procedure can be repeated as necessary to marsupialize the sac fully.

If the procedure has been uncomplicated, patients are allowed to eat as tolerated in the immediate postoperative period. Repeat modified barium swallows are not performed unless residual or recurrent symptoms are present; there will always be some residual distal sac seen, and this does not necessarily correlate with the presence of symptoms. Patients should be counseled about this in terms of what can be expected to be seen on future barium swallow examinations if they are performed elsewhere.

In younger patients and those with significant gastroesophageal reflux symptoms, pH probe studies should be performed at follow-up. If significant disease is present, it should be managed appropriately, because there seems to be an association between recurrence of sac symptoms and the presence of reflux.

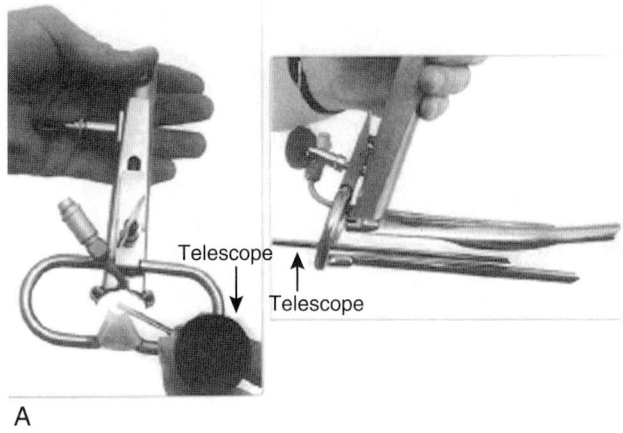

A

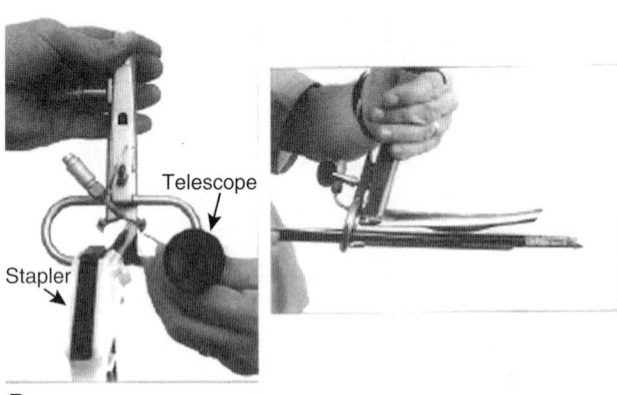

B

Figure 4 **(A)** Diverticuloscope demonstrating proximal and distal opening capability with telescope placement. **(B)** Telescope and linear endoscopic stapler in place in diverticuloscope.

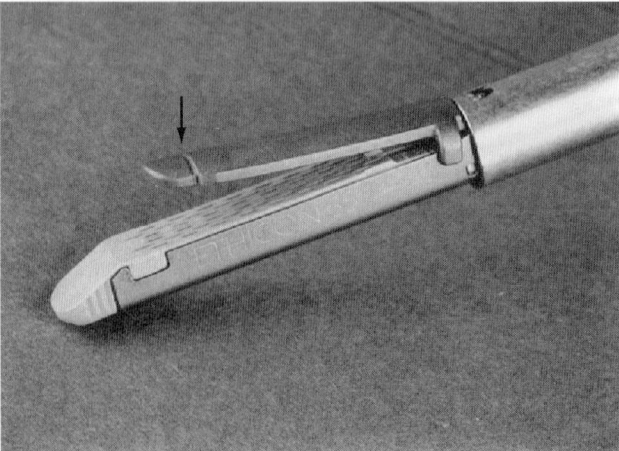

Figure 5 Endoscopic linear stapler showing discrepancy between the two jaw lengths. The longer jaw is inserted into the esophagus.

Open Approach

After the induction of general anesthesia, direct laryngoscopy is performed first with a twofold purpose. The sac is packed with NuGauze (Johnson & Johnson, New Brunswick, NJ), the end of which is brought out through the mouth to facilitate intraoperative removal. This creates a mass effect in the sac that facilitates intraoperative sac identification and dissection. In addition, a

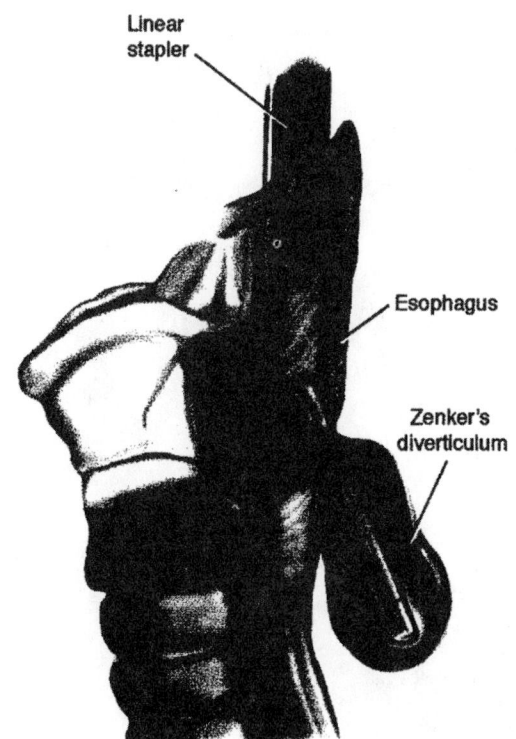

Linear stapler

Esophagus

Zenker's diverticulum

Figure 6 Endoscopic treatment of pharyngoesophageal diverticulum is performed by cutting the septum between the esophagus and the diverticulum using a linear stapler. *From Ferguson MK: Diverticula of the esophagus. In Cameron JL, editor: Current surgical therapy, ed 7, St. Louis, 2001, Mosby.*

small endotracheal tube (5.5 or 6 F) is placed into the cervical esophagus. Placement of this tube can be difficult because the introitus can be tight and anterior. Initial use of an intubating bougie over which the tube is advanced can be helpful. To prevent intraoperative confusion with the airway endotracheal tube, the airway circuit connector should be removed from this second tube and a syringe attached to the pilot balloon. This second tube is prepped into the field with the syringe in place.

The patient is positioned on a shoulder roll with the neck extended and turned to the right side. In general terms, the sac is approached from the left because the recurrent laryngeal nerve is longer on the left side and remains in the tracheoesophageal groove over its entire cervical course as it is descends into the chest. These factors serve to protect it from a direct or stretch injury that can occur with the rotation and manipulation of the laryngotracheal complex that occurs with this procedure.

Perioperative antibiotics are given to guard against the possibility of perforation but are immediately discontinued postoperatively if the procedure goes smoothly.

From a cosmetic standpoint, a horizontal incision is preferred over one that runs along the anterior border of the sternocleidomastoid and gives adequate exposure. It is generally centered at approximately the level of the cricoid cartilage in terms of its superior-inferior location. Subplatysmal skin flaps are raised for a short distance superiorly and inferiorly, and the fascia along the anterior border of the sternocleidomastoid muscle is incised. The muscle is retracted laterally, and the sternohyoid and sternothyroid muscles retracted medially to expose the carotid sheath. The middle layer of the deep cervical fascia where it runs between the tracheoesophageal complex and the carotid sheath is incised. The middle thyroid vein is taken, and, in some circumstances, the inferior thyroid

artery should be divided to prevent lateral traction on it from pulling the recurrent laryngeal nerve out of the groove and exposing it to a higher risk for injury. If necessary, the anterior belly of the omohyoid can be divided to facilitate rotation of the laryngotracheal complex, although it is usually just retracted superiorly.

The retropharyngeal space is thus entered, and the sac, packed with Nugauze, can then be palpated. The sac is then gradually dissected free of the surrounding fascia down to its neck and is retracted superiorly. Dissecting the sac completely free as the initial step in the procedure is critical to full exposure of the cricopharyngeus muscle, particularly the upper fibers that are critical to the performance of an adequate myotomy. These are the ones that are most commonly missed in cases of recurrence because of their proximity to the neck of the sac, where the dissection can be most difficult. With the sac fully dissected and the posterior cricopharyngeus muscle and cervical esophagus exposed, the packing is removed from the sac. The balloon on the endotracheal tube that is in the esophagus is then inflated so that it distends the esophagus to a moderate degree. The tube is gradually retracted superiorly so that the balloon distends the muscular fibers of the upper cervical esophagus and cricopharyngeus. Beginning inferior to the cricopharyngeus muscle in the posterior midline, where the plane is easiest to find, these muscle fibers under tension are sharply divided down to the underlying mucosa. This is continued superiorly all the way to the neck of the sac so that there are no remaining crossing fibers and a continuous strip of mucosa is exposed. After the myotomy has been completed, a linear endoscopic GIA stapler is used to remove the sac (Fig. 7). If the sac is removed before the myotomy, the upper cricopharyngeal fibers may be included in the staple line and not effectively divided. Keeping the endotracheal tube within the hypopharynx during diverticulectomy guards against stricture of the hypopharynx, which can occur if too much mucosa is removed.

Alternate methods of division of the cricopharyngeus muscle include placing the muscle under tension using a right-angle clamp slipped between the muscle and underlying mucosa. One must be careful in this circumstance not to imbricate the mucosa over the end of the clamp and cause a perforation. Similarly, instead of an endotracheal tube, a large bougie dilator can be placed in the esophagus to facilitate the myotomy. However, this can be difficult to place because the esophageal introitus is tight, and the stiffness of a dilator of sufficient size can make it difficult to achieve full rotation of the laryngotracheal complex that is needed to expose the posterior midline.

Drains are not necessary unless there have been problems with the procedure itself. The patient is fed in the immediate postoperative period as tolerated.

Revision Cases

The need for revision surgery should be premised on a strong correlation between recurrent symptoms and what is seen radiographically and not just the presence of a sac itself. This is particularly true in cases in which the sac was initially managed endoscopically, because there will always be a residual sac present on modified barium swallow, although it may not be symptomatic. It is also important to make sure that associated problems and dysmotility in the pharyngeal and esophageal phases of swallowing, rather than the diverticulum itself, are not primarily responsible for symptoms.

If after careful study with a modified barium swallow it becomes clear that the sac or recurrent cricopharyngeal spasm are the source of the problems, reoperation should be considered, using the same criteria as for the first operation. If despite adequate party wall division the patulous nature of the residual lumen is the cause for retained secretions, excision from an external approach should be considered. On the other hand, if after an external procedure it is clear that the upper fibers of the cricopharyngeus were not completely divided and there is a residual party wall, a transoral approach may be ideal for approaching these fibers.

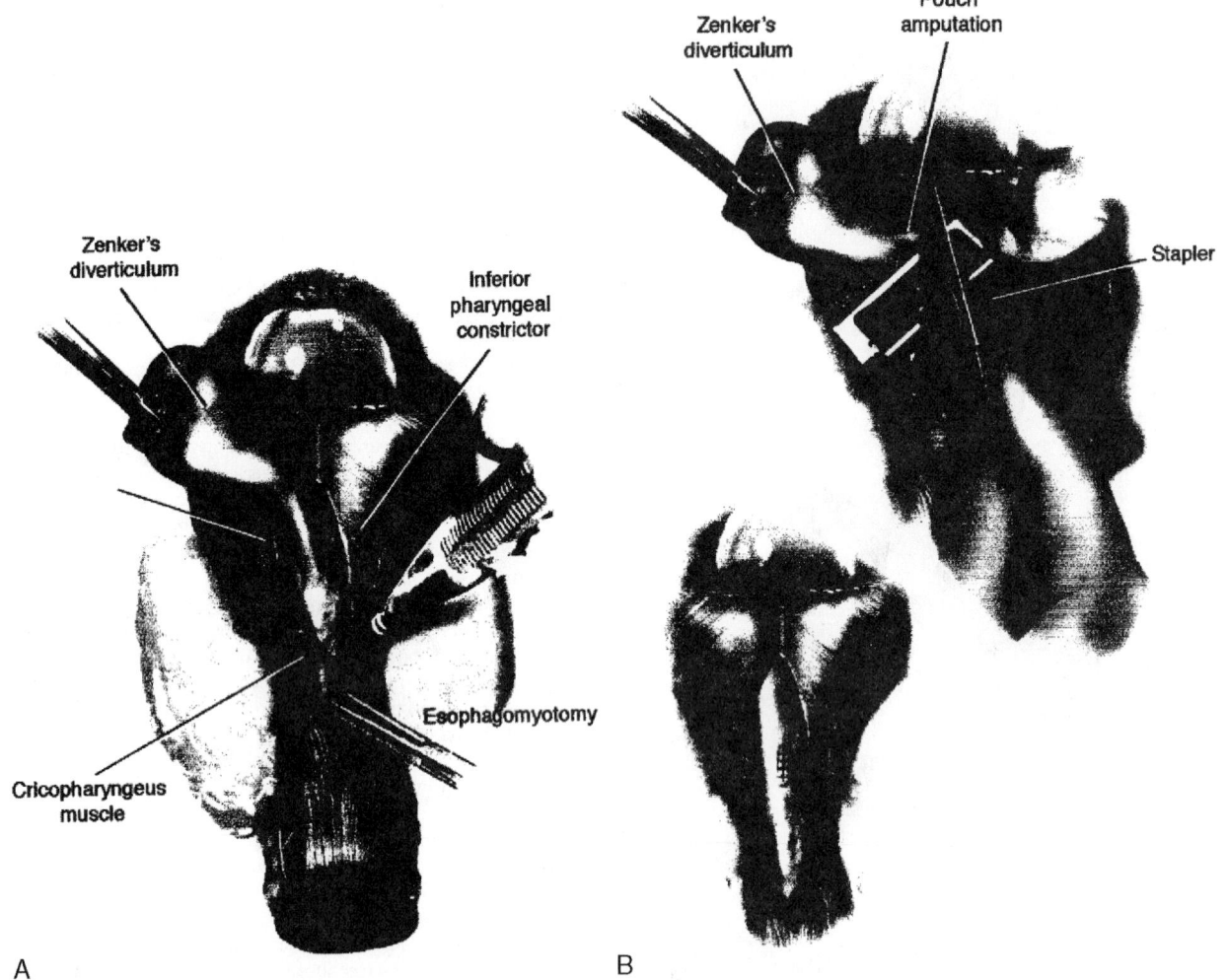

Figure 7 Pharyngoesophageal diverticulum treatment includes a cervical esophagomyotomy and pouch resection.
(A) An esophagomyotomy is performed for several centimeters in either vertical direction. **(B)** The pouch is amputated at its base using a stapler. *From Orringer MB: The esophagus. In Textbook of surgery, ed 15, Philadelphia, 1997, WB Saunders.*

SUGGESTED READINGS

Adams J, Sheppard B, Andersen P, and others: Zenker's diverticulostomy with cricopharyngeal myotomy: the endoscopic approach, *Surg Endosc* 15:34, 2001.

Chang CY, Payyapilli RJ, Scher RL: Endoscopic staple diverticulostomy for Zenker's diverticulum: review of literature and experience in 159 consecutive cases, *Laryngoscope* 113:957, 2003.

Cohen JI, Andersen PE, Veenker E: Cricopharyngeal spasm and Zenker's diverticulum, *Head Neck* 25:681, 2003.

Gross ND, Cohen JI, Andersen PE: Outpatient endoscopic Zenker's diverticulotomy, *Laryngoscope* 114:208, 2004.

Richtsmeier J: Endoscopic management of Zenker diverticulum: the staple-assisted approach, *Am J Med* 115 (suppl 3A), 175S, 2003.

Veenker E, Cohen JI: Current trends in management of Zenker diverticulum, *Curr Opin Otolaryngol Head Neck Surg* 11:160, 2003.

GASTROESOPHAGEAL REFLUX DISEASE

Parag Bhanot, MD, and Nathaniel J. Soper, MD

INTRODUCTION

Gastroesophageal reflux disease (GERD) is a disorder in which gastric contents reflux into the esophagus, causing heartburn and other symptoms. In the United States, it is estimated that GERD affects more than 40% of the population at least once per month, 20% once per week, and 7% daily. Medical treatment of GERD results in a cost of at least $6 billion a year.

Besides lifestyle modifications, patients with GERD primarily have two treatment options: lifelong medication or procedural therapy. The best treatments in these categories consist of proton pump inhibitors (PPIs) or laparoscopic antireflux surgery (LARS). More recently, endoscopic techniques aimed at treating GERD have been introduced clinically; the impact of these endoluminal procedures remains to be determined. Several prospective randomized trials comparing medical and surgical treatment for GERD have shown surgical therapy to be more effective.

In 1954, Dr. Rudolf Nissen performed the first fundoplication for a patient with reflux esophagitis. In 1987, approximately 12,000 traditional ("open") antireflux procedures were performed in the United States. DeMeester reported his results of 100 consecutive patients who underwent an open Nissen fundoplication for GERD showing an initial 1% mortality and 13% morbidity rate with an overall 91% success rate at 10-year follow-up. The introduction of minimally invasive procedures, with the first laparoscopic Nissen fundoplication (LNF) reported in 1991, greatly increased the frequency of these operations. This development in laparoscopic techniques has led to an increase in the number of antireflux procedures, with approximately 64,000 LNFs performed in 2003. The continued acceptance and long-term success of this procedure require an understanding of the pathophysiology of GERD, appropriate patient selection, sound surgical technique, and excellent postoperative care.

CLINICAL MANIFESTATIONS OF GASTROESOPHAGEAL REFLUX DISEASE

Patients with GERD can present with a variety of typical symptoms or with complications from long-standing disease (Table 1). There are also extra-esophageal symptoms caused by GERD (Table 2). It is important to realize that patients can present with these latter complaints without exhibiting typical symptoms.

Heartburn is described as a retrosternal burning sensation. Patients with regurgitation complain of food or stomach juice refluxing into their throat or having a sour taste in their mouth.

Table 1: Typical Symptoms and Complications of Gastroesophageal Reflux Disease

Symptoms
Heartburn
Regurgitation
Waterbrash
Dysphagia
Complications
Esophagitis and ulcers
Esophageal strictures
Barrett's disease
Anemia

Table 2: Extra-Esophageal Manifestations of Gastroesophageal Reflux Disease

Dental
Erosions
Laryngeal
Laryngitis
Polyps
Cancer
Hoarseness
Stenosis
Pulmonary
Chronic cough
Asthma
Bronchitis
Fibrosis

Waterbrash is the spontaneous appearance in the mouth of a slightly sour or salty fluid. These symptoms are particularly prevalent after the consumption of large meals. There may be an association with fatty foods, chocolate, coffee, peppermint, alcohol, tobacco, and other products that are associated with transient lowering of the lower esophageal sphincter (LES) pressure. Some degree of symptom relief is often achieved with antacids.

Before considering procedural intervention for GERD, it is important to both prove its existence and exclude other etiologies that may have similar symptoms, such as peptic ulcer disease, gastritis, biliary disease, esophageal motility disorders, and cardiopulmonary disease.

DIAGNOSIS AND PREOPERATIVE EVALUATION

A complete and accurate patient history alone may be adequate to establish the diagnosis of GERD with a high degree of likelihood. Empiric medical therapy with PPIs can be initiated at this time. However, in patients in whom the diagnosis is unclear because of atypical symptoms or those for whom procedural therapy is being considered, additional testing is required. Symptoms thought to be indicative of GERD are not 100% specific. Further evaluation can be divided into anatomic and physiologic tests (Table 3). In patients with typical symptoms, at least one additional piece of objective evidence of reflux is required to make the diagnosis. For patients with atypical symptoms, at least two corroborative tests are required.

Although endoscopy may be normal in 70% of patients with GERD, it is still an essential part of the evaluation. It can determine the extent and severity of existing esophagitis or exclude Barrett's disease and malignancy. Approximately 10% of patients with long-standing GERD will have biopsy-proved Barrett's disease. This is important given the known relationship of Barrett's esophagus and adenocarcinoma.

Radiologic studies include an upper gastrointestinal series (UGI) and gastric emptying study. A UGI series is useful to detect hiatal hernias, to localize the gastroesophageal junction (GEJ) in relation to the hiatus, and to assess qualitatively the adequacy of esophageal peristalsis. It can also identify complications of GERD such as strictures or esophageal shortening.

The 24-hour pH test is considered the gold standard for the diagnosis of GERD. It quantifies the number and duration of reflux episodes, differentiates upright and supine reflux events, and correlates these events with subjective symptoms. The BRAVO wireless transducer (Medtronic, North Shoreview, MN) is an option that obviates the need for an indwelling nasoesophageal tube.

Esophageal manometry should be performed in every patient considering antireflux surgery. It is a test of esophageal function assessing esophageal peristalsis and LES pressure. With this test,

Table 3: Diagnostic Tests for Suspected Gastroesophageal Reflux Disease

Anatomic
Esophagogastroduodenoscopy ($\pm$ biopsy)
Upper gastrointestinal series
Physiologic
24-hour pH test
Esophageal manometry
Impedance monitoring
Gastric emptying test
Bernstein acid test

the length, location, and tone of the LES are characterized. Manometry may also be useful to diagnose individuals with a primary motility disorder.

Impedance monitoring is an additional method to evaluate esophageal motility and function, assessing directional bolus transit within the esophagus. This test may be particularly useful in evaluating patients suspected of nonacidic reflux.

In patients with a history of diabetes, severe nausea or vomiting (or both) or postprandial bloating, a gastric emptying test should be considered. If abnormal, an additional procedure such as a pyloroplasty may be required.

INDICATIONS AND CONTRAINDICATIONS

The most common indications for antireflux surgery are listed in (Table 4). Ideal patients exhibit abnormal 24-hour pH test, manometry-proved incompetent LES, and symptoms that are responsive to PPIs.

There are few absolute contraindications to LARS (Table 5). A number of conditions that make LARS more difficult do exist and can be considered relative contraindications. These conditions may be specific to this procedure, such as severe inflammation, stricture, or esophageal shortening, or may be inclusive to all laparoscopic procedures. Patients with GERD who are morbidly obese may be best treated with a gastric bypass rather than a traditional antireflux procedure.

Table 4: Indications for Laparoscopic Antireflux Surgery

Chronic GERD requiring continuous PPI use in patients desiring discontinuation of medical therapy (because of, e.g., financial burden, side effects)
GERD symptoms (e.g., respiratory symptoms) interfering with lifestyle despite medical therapy and lifestyle modifications
High-volume reflux not managed effectively with PPIs
Complications of GERD (e.g., esophagitis, stricture, Barrett's esophagus) not responding to medical therapy
Paraesophageal hernia with GERD
Pediatric population with GERD-associated esophagitis, pulmonary compromise, or failure to thrive

GERD, gastroesophageal reflux disease; PPI, proton pump inhibitor.

Table 5: Contraindications to Laparoscopic Antireflux Surgery

Absolute	Relative
Surgeon inexperience	Previous upper abdominal surgery
Inability to tolerate general anesthesia	Severely shortened esophagus
Inability to tolerate laparotomy	Morbid obesity
Advanced cardiac-pulmonary disease	
Uncorrectable coagulopathy	
Portal hypertension	

MANAGEMENT

The management of patients with GERD can be divided into three phases: (1) diagnosis and severity assessment, (2) symptom control, and (3) selection of a long-term management plan. All patients should have a trial of medical therapy before considering an antireflux operation. The majority of patients can be managed medically. In patients with mild reflux, diet and lifestyle modifications should be instituted. The initial treatment of reflux disease should be with PPIs. This class of antacids is more effective than histamine receptor antagonists and can heal esophagitis in 85% of patients. If the initial treatment is not effective, the surgeon should make certain that the diagnosis of GERD is correct. If the diagnosis is confirmed, the dosage can be increased or a second antacid can be added to the regimen. Patients at this point are placed on maintenance therapy.

Most patients find it difficult to maintain lifestyle changes. Furthermore, patients may require escalating doses of PPIs, relapse when the medication is discontinued or reduced, or desire to be medication free. These patients are ideal candidates for LARS.

Several operations have been described for the treatment of GERD and differ in the approach used and the type of fundoplication constructed. The approach to the repair can be abdominal (open or laparoscopic), thoracic (open or video assisted), or thoracoabdominal. Antireflux procedures can generally be divided into partial fundoplications (Belsey Mark IV, Dor, or Toupet) or total fundoplications (Nissen or Nissen–Rosetti). The Hill repair is unique in that it does not include a formal fundoplication. No single approach or procedure is ideal for every patient, and there has been no large-scale comparison of the various procedures. It is important to select the correct procedure through appropriate preoperative evaluation to ensure an optimal outcome. Nevertheless, the primary operation currently used to treat GERD is the laparoscopic Nissen fundoplication.

SURGICAL TECHNIQUE

Many technical variations are associated with LARS. The following is a stepwise description of the technique of LNF as we practice it.

Patient Preparation and Operating Room Layout

The patient is placed in a supine position with the legs abducted on flat, padded boards. This positioning is preferable to stirrups to minimize the possibility of lower extremity neurovascular injury. The right arm is tucked and protected at the side to allow space for the table-mounted liver retractor. A vacuum beanbag is used to prevent patient movement when placed in steep reverse Trendelenburg position, which allows gravity to displace the abdominal viscera from the hiatus. Preoperative antibiotics should be administered, and compression boots should be used. A temporary orogastric tube is placed to decompress the stomach. A Foley catheter is not necessary if the patient voids immediately preoperatively.

The operating room equipment is arranged to allow the surgeon to stand between the patient's legs, the assistant to the patient's right, and camera holder on the opposite side. Video monitors are positioned at the head of the table to allow adequate inline visualization for the operating surgeon and assistants (Fig. 1).

Abdominal Access and Port Placement

An open or closed technique may be used to access the peritoneal cavity. We prefer the closed technique with a Veress needle because the first port is generally placed superior to the umbilicus and to the left of midline. The first four of the five ports are placed in least 15 cm from the xiphoid process and 2 cm below the right costal margin. An additional 5-mm port is placed midway between these first two ports. The fourth port is placed 10 cm from the xiphoid process and 2 cm below the left costal margin. This port is for the surgeon's right-hand instruments; we use a 10-mm port to allow the insertion of SH-sized needles. The last port is placed in the right paramedian location below the retracted liver edge. This port arrangement allows optimal "triangulated" access to the hiatus and maximizes the range of motion of the instruments.

Dissection and Esophageal Mobilization

The first maneuver is dividing the gastrohepatic ligament beginning at the pars flaccida using the ultrasonic shears (Fig. 3). The assistant grasps the gastroesophageal fat pad for countertraction. The hepatic branch of the vagus nerve may be divided. However, the surgeon must be aware of the possibility of a replaced left hepatic artery. The gastrohepatic ligament is divided up to the level of the medial border of the right crus of the diaphragm.

The phrenoesophageal membrane is divided in a transverse direction approaching the left crus. Limited blunt dissection should be used to prevent injury to the underlying esophagus and anterior vagus nerve. With the gastric fundus pulled inferiorly and to the right, the gastrophrenic ligament is divided to mobilize the gastric cardia.

The initial hiatal dissection is carried out with attention to mediastinal structures. A plane is first developed between the medial border of the right crus and the esophagus. The assistant grasps the epiphrenic fat pad and retracts inferiorly. The dissection consists mainly of blunt dissection except for small vessels, which can be divided with the ultrasonic shears. It is important to visualize the posterior vagus nerve and maintain its position alongside the esophagus. The mediastinal attachments are dissected from the esophagus using blunt instruments in broad sweeps. The tissue attached to the base of the right crus is divided until the junction with the left crus is seen. Once the right side of the esophagus has been mobilized several centimeters above the diaphragm, the dissection of the left crus is performed (Fig. 4). The anterior vagus nerve is identified and spared, also maintaining its position on the surface of the esophagus. A plane is developed between the esophagus and the underlying aorta.

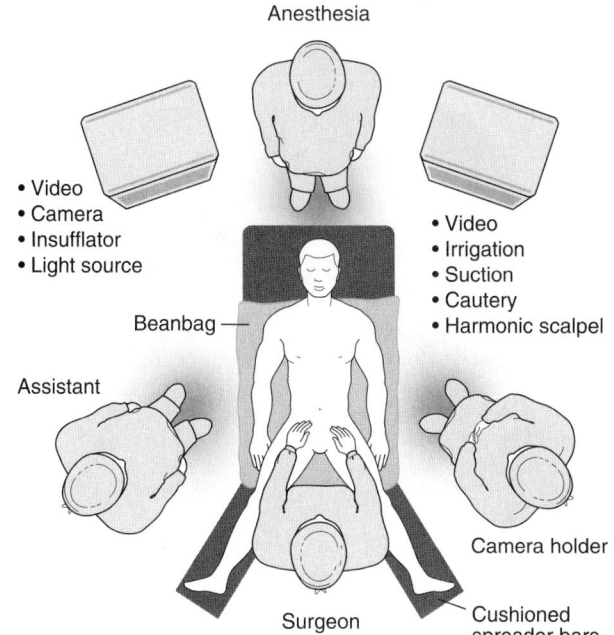

Anesthesia

- Video
- Camera
- Insufflator
- Light source

- Video
- Irrigation
- Suction
- Cautery
- Harmonic scalpel

Beanbag

Assistant

Camera holder

Surgeon

Cushioned spreader bars

Figure 1 Layout of operating room. The surgeon is situated comfortably between the patient's legs. *From Baker RJ, Fischer JE, editors: Mastery of surgery, ed 4, Philadelphia, 2001, Lippincott Williams & Wilkins, p. 793.*

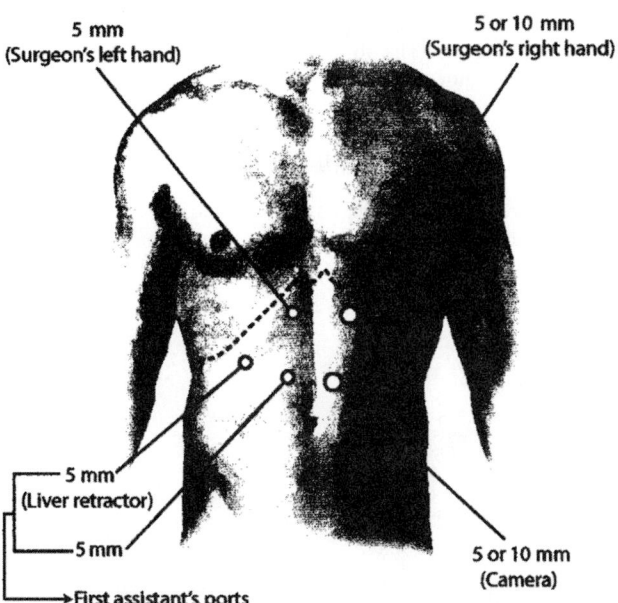

5 mm
(Surgeon's left hand)

5 or 10 mm
(Surgeon's right hand)

5 mm
(Liver retractor)

5 mm

5 or 10 mm
(Camera)

First assistant's ports

Figure 2 Port placement. The xiphoid process is the landmark used for the gastroesophageal junction. *From Baker RJ, Fischer JE, editors: Mastery of surgery, ed 4, Philadelphia, 2001, Lippincott Williams & Wilkins, p. 793.*

a standard fashion using the xiphoid process as a landmark for the GEJ (Fig. 2). The last port is placed after the left lateral segment of the liver is retracted. A 5- or 10-mm camera can be used, depending on the surgeon's preference. After the abdomen is insufflated to a pressure of 15 mm Hg, the camera port is placed 12 cm caudal to the xiphoid just left of the midline. In most patients, the placement of the camera at the umbilicus will be too low. The rest of the ports are placed under direct visualization using a 30-degree laparoscope. The 5-mm port used for the self-retaining liver retractor is placed at

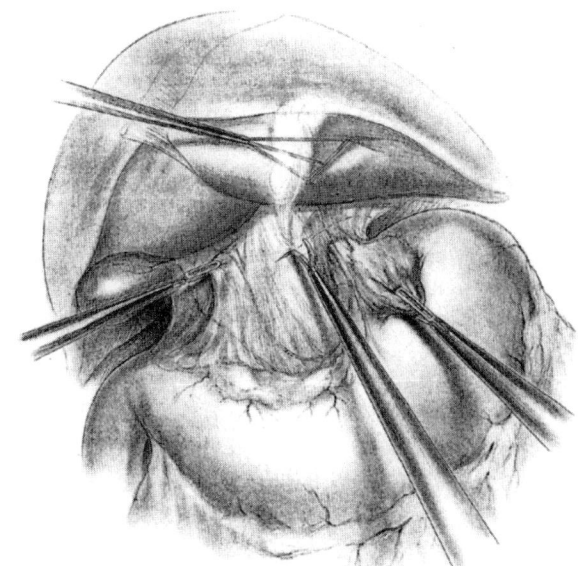

Figure 3 Division of gastrohepatic ligament. The dissection begins in the pars flaccida. *From Soper NJ, Swanstrom LL, Eubanks WS, editors: Mastery of endoscopic and laparoscopic surgery, ed 2, Philadelphia, 2005, Lippincott Williams & Wilkins, p. 198.*

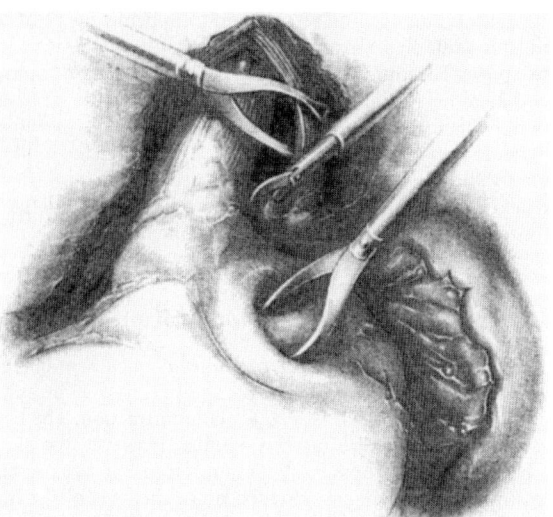

Figure 4   Dissection of left crus. The esophagus is gently retracted to the right using a blunt instrument.   *From Cameron JL:* Current surgical therapy, *ed 8, Philadelphia, 2004, Elsevier Mosby, p. 29.*

The gastric fundus is mobilized by dividing the short gastric vessels starting at the inferior pole of the spleen (Fig. 5). The assistant grasps the fundus, and the surgeon grasps the gastrosplenic ligament. With a small amount of blunt dissection, the lesser sac is entered. We prefer the ultrasonic shears to perform this task. All structures that prevent complete mobilization of the fundus, including the posterior gastric vessels, are also divided. The dissection eventually parallels the medial border of the left crus and is carried to the angle of His. This allows visualization of the retroesophageal space from the left side and creation of a large window to allow passage of the fundus.

After tension on the mobilized proximal stomach is released, the length of the intraabdominal esophagus is determined; it should be at least 3 cm. If that is not the case, further esophageal mobilization must be performed within the mediastinum, or an esophageal lengthening procedure should be performed.

A Babcock clamp is placed through the retroesophageal window by the assistant from right to left in front of both crura so that the fundus can be pulled behind the esophagus. The surgeon retracts the gastroesophageal fat pad inferiorly to expose the tip of the

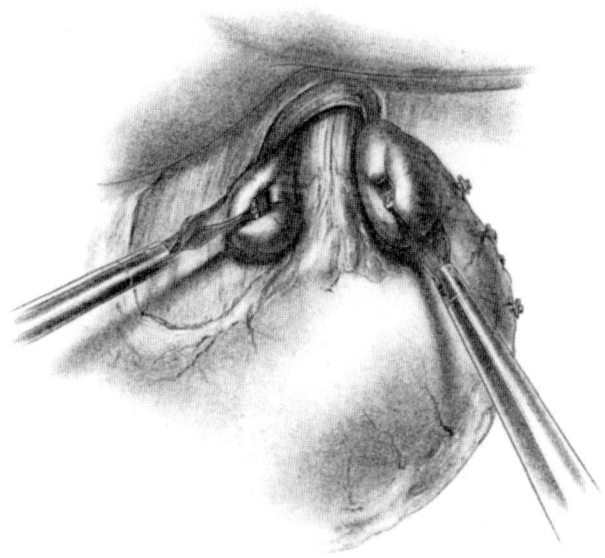

Figure 6   Performing the "shoeshine maneuver." This wrap is visualized before placement of sutures.   *From* Mastery of endoscopic and laparoscopic surgery, *ed 2, p. 200.*

instrument. Once the fundus has been pulled to the right of the esophagus, it is checked for tension. If it retracts back to the left after release, an excessive amount of tension is present, and further dissection is necessary. Once fully mobilized, both sides of the fundus are grasped and manipulated to perform the "shoeshine maneuver" (Fig. 6). The fundus is retracted back and forth to ensure that it is not twisted and is in continuity.

Crural Closure and Fundoplication

The crura are reapproximated posterior to the esophagus using 2–0 gauge nonabsorbable, braided polyester sutures on an SH needle (Fig. 7). Exposure of the retroesophageal space may be provided by retraction on a Penrose drain sling or by retracting the wrapped

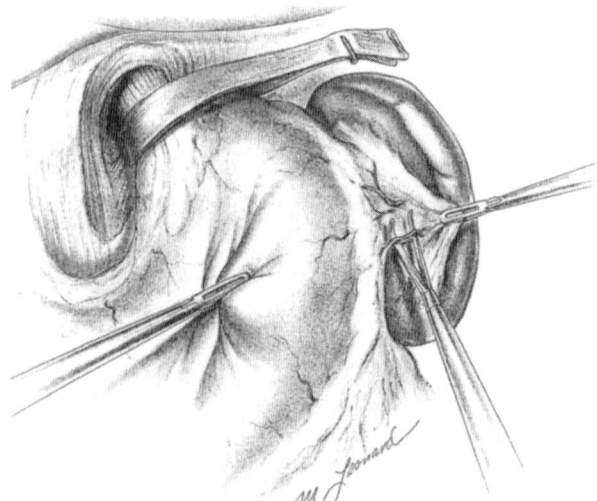

Figure 5   *Division of gastrosplenic ligament.* The division of the short gastric vessels allows for complete fundic mobilization.   *From* Mastery of endoscopic and laparoscopic surgery, *ed 2, p. 199.*

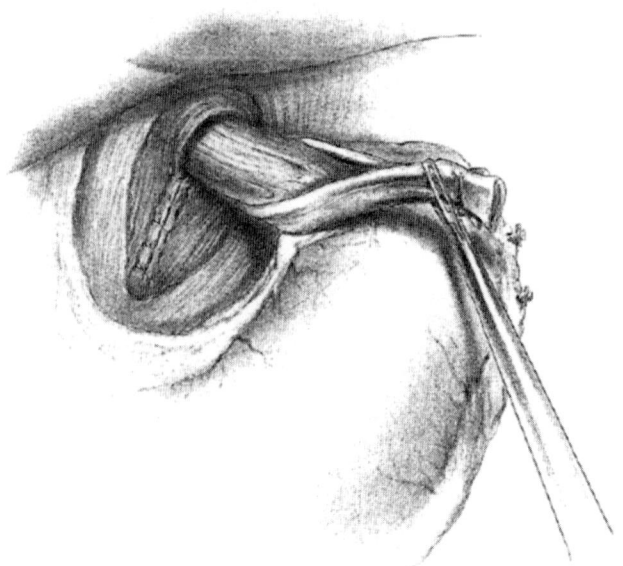

Figure 7   Closure of the crura. A posterior hiatal closure is performed with interrupted sutures.   *From* Mastery of endoscopic and laparoscopic surgery, *ed 2, p. 200.*

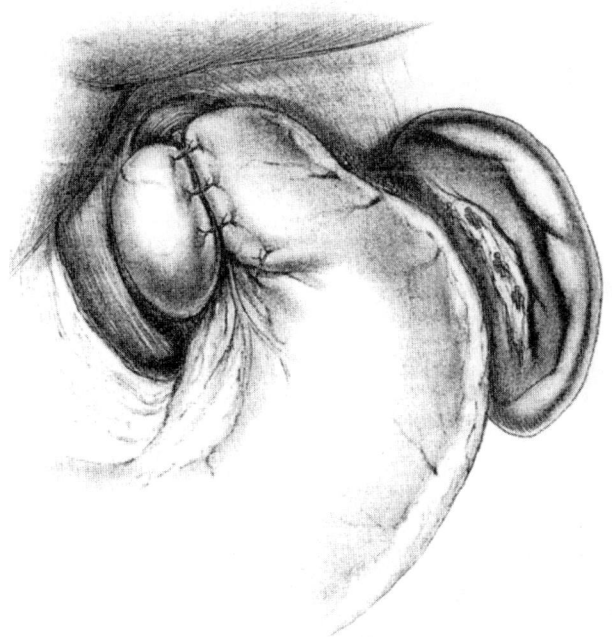

Figure 8 Completed fundoplication. The completed wrap lies to the right of the anterior midline. *From* Mastery of endoscopic and laparoscopic surgery, *ed 2, p. 201.*

fundus to the left. Additional sutures can be placed anterior to the esophagus if needed to prevent excessive angulation. The crura are closed until they touch the empty esophagus. An esophageal dilator is not used at this stage because its presence may limit exposure. If the crura cannot be approximated without tension, a bioprosthetic mesh patch may be applied.

After closing the crura but before constructing the fundoplication, we serially pass 50-F and 60-F Maloney dilators. The risk of esophageal perforation by the dilator can be reduced with control of the GEJ by the surgeon. During passage of the dilators, communication is maintained between the individual inserting the dilator and the surgeon. The fundoplication is performed with either a 50-F or 60-F dilator in place.

A "short floppy" wrap of 2 cm is created with three interrupted sutures (Fig. 8). Again, 2–0 gauge, nonabsorbable, braided polyester sutures on an SH needle are used. The first suture opposes fundus to fundus with seromuscular bites, without incorporating the esophageal wall. This allows the wrap to be repositioned just proximal to the GEJ. The next two sutures incorporate the muscularis layer of the esophagus to prevent slippage of the wrap. The final orientation of the wrap should be to the right of the midline. The dilator is then removed. The wrap should be loose enough to allow the tip of a blunt instrument between it and the esophagus.

Conclusion of Procedure

The liver retractor is removed, and the undersurface of the liver is examined for bleeding. After hemostasis is obtained, the ports are removed. The abdomen is exsufflated fully by the anesthetist's administering vital capacity breaths. The incisions are then infiltrated with bupivacaine. With the use of radially dilating trocars, the fascial defects generally do not require closure. The skin incisions are closed with 4–0 gauge absorbable sutures. Appropriate dressings are placed. A nasogastric tube is not routinely used postoperatively.

INTRAOPERATIVE COMPLICATIONS

Esophageal perforation occurs in less than 1% of cases. If perforation occurs, intraoperative recognition and repair is critical to prevent sepsis or death. The incidence of perforation can be minimized by not directly grasping the esophagus for retraction but rather using the gastroesophageal fat pad or Penrose drain. Simple perforations are repaired using absorbable interrupted sutures and coverage by the fundoplication.

Pleural injury with resulting pneumothorax can occur during the mediastinal dissection and rarely causes untoward sequelae. If mediastinal dissection is tolerated poorly by the patient, positive pressure ventilation can be used, intra-abdominal pressure can be decreased, or both can be done. A chest tube is rarely necessary with a pleural tear. A postoperative chest x-ray is not necessary unless clinically indicated.

Bleeding is an uncommon complication that can usually be controlled with the harmonic scalpel or clips. Severe hemorrhage can occur from a hepatic or splenic injury, which may require conversion to an open procedure.

POSTOPERATIVE CARE

Patients are generally admitted overnight for observation. Ketorolac and ondansetron are administered intravenously at regular intervals to diminish postoperative pain and nausea. Narcotics are administered as needed for additional pain control. All antireflux medications may be discontinued. Clear liquid diet is started the evening of surgery and continued the following morning. If tolerated, a soft diet is given for lunch and the patient is discharged. Early postoperative complications include ileus, urinary retention, dysphagia, and bloating. If the patient experiences severe postoperative pain or emesis, a UGI series is obtained to rule out disruption of the fundoplication (using barium) or a missed perforation (using gastrograffin). Other signs of a missed injury include fever, tachycardia, and leukocytosis.

The patient can be discharged on the first postoperative day if no issues arise. A soft diet is followed for 2 to 4 weeks to allow esophageal edema to reside. Rapid resumption of full activity is encouraged. The only physical limitation is avoidance of excessively heavy lifting, that which strains the diaphragm, for 4 to 6 weeks. The patient is seen in clinic 2 to 4 weeks postoperatively.

OUTCOMES

There have been several long-term studies published by experienced surgeons demonstrating the efficacy of LARS. The results consistently show low rates of perioperative morbidity and mortality, with conversion rates less than 5%. Relief of typical symptoms, such as heartburn, regurgitation, and dysphagia, occurs in more than 90% of patients. New-onset dysphagia is present in approximately 10% of patients but usually resolves by 12 months. The fraction of patients requiring antacids ranges between 5% and 25%, with greater than 90% patient satisfaction and an overall improvement in quality of life. LARS reduces postoperative pain, shortens the hospital stay, reduces recovery time, and improves cosmesis compared with "open" antireflux procedures.

The learning curve for LARS is approximately 40 to 50 cases as reflected by operative time and complication rate. The failure rate is approximately 1% per year in most series. Dallemagne and colleagues published a series of 100 patients with GERD who had undergone either a Nissen or Toupet fundoplication and had 10-year follow-up. The overall success rate at 10 years was 90%. They reported that 33% of patients with a Toupet fundoplication had intrathoracic

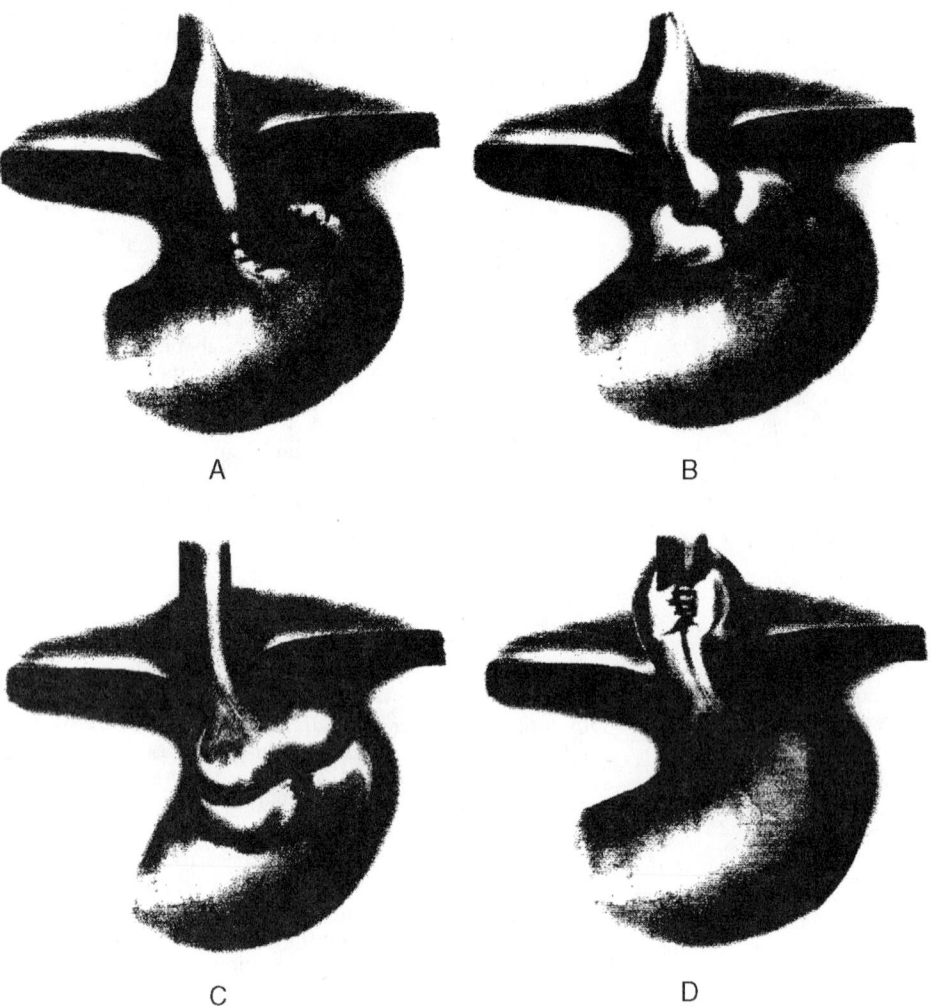

A

B

C

D

Figure 9 Patterns of failed fundoplications. **(A)** Completed disrupted wrap, "missing" Nissen. **(B)** Sliding hiatal hernia. **(C)** Wrap slipped onto proximal stomach. **(D)** Intrathoracic migration of wrap. *From Mastery of endoscopic and laparoscopic surgery, ed 2, p. 202.*

migration of their wrap compared with 0% in the Nissen cohort. Overall, 4% of patients required a revisional procedure.

There are several types of failed fundoplications (Fig. 9). The "slipped" Nissen down onto the stomach is more common with the open approach. In the laparoscopic approach, the migration of the wrap through the hiatus is more frequent. The management of these failures is complex and should be performed by an experienced surgeon. A thorough preoperative evaluation should be conducted, repeating the initial workup already described. The rates of complications and conversions are higher with reoperations. In repeat failures, esophagectomy, gastrectomy, or Roux-en-Y bypass may be viable options.

ENDOLUMINAL THERAPY OF GERD

Although several long-term studies have shown excellent results with LARS, there has been ongoing research into an even less invasive approach for GERD using incisionless procedures. Since 2001, the U.S. Food and Drug Administration (FDA) has approved four endoscopic procedures for the management of GERD: Stretta (Curon Medical, Fremont, CA), Endocinch (CR Bard, Murray Hill, NJ), Endoscopic Full-Thickness Plicator (NDO Surgical, Mansfield, MA), and Enteryx (Boston Scientific, Natick, MA). With the exception of Enteryx, which was recently withdrawn by the FDA for patient safety issues, early results from small groups of treated patients demonstrate these procedures to be safe, with up to 80% of patients achieving control of their symptoms. However, true

control of reflux as evidenced by normal postprocedure esophageal pH tests is uncommon. There is currently no randomized controlled study comparing endoluminal therapies with LARS or PPI therapy. Until these data, including long-term follow-up, are available, the use of endoluminal procedures for management of GERD should be cautiously applied.

CONCLUSION

GERD is a complex disease, the therapy for which should be provided by a foregut specialist who can offer a comprehensive approach. Surgical therapy is an excellent option for the appropriate patient and offers superb long-term results. The laparoscopic approach has lowered the threshold of surgical intervention. To maintain physician and patient acceptance of LARS, this procedure should be performed only by experienced surgeons who are able to offer long-term follow-up and manage associated complications. Endoluminal treatment of GERD is promising but has not achieved acceptance by most physicians.

SUGGESTED READINGS

Dallemagne B, Weerts J, Markiewicz S, and others: Clinical results of laparoscopic fundoplication at ten years after surgery, *Surg Endosc* 20:159, 2006.
DeMeester TR, Bonavina C, Albertucci M: Nissen fundoplication for gastroesophageal reflux disease. Evaluation of primary repair in 100 consecutive patients, *Ann Surg* 204(1):9–20, 1986.

Desai KM, Soper NJ, Frisella MM, and others: Efficacy of laparoscopic antireflux surgery in patients with Barrett's esophagus, *Am J Surg* 186:652, 2003.

Lundell L, Miettinen P, Myrvold HE, and others: Continued follow-up of a randomized clinical study comparing antireflux surgery and omeprazole in GERD, *J Am Coll Surg* 192:172, 2001.

Peters JH, DeMeester TR, Crookes P, and others: The treatment of GERD with laparoscopic Nissen fundoplications: prospective evaluation of 100 patients with typical symptoms, *Ann Surg* 248:40, 1998.

Smith CD, McClusky DA, Rajad MA, and others: When fundoplication fails: redo? *Ann Surg* 241:861, 2005.

ENDOLUMINAL APPROACHES TO GASTROESOPHAGEAL REFLUX DISEASE

Benjamin K. Poulose, MD, MPH, and William O. Richards, MD

INTRODUCTION

Endoluminal transoral procedures offer an exciting new treatment modality for select patients with symptomatic gastroesophageal reflux disease (GERD). These procedures offer outpatient therapy for those seeking an alternative to chronic proton pump inhibitor (PPI) use or laparoscopic fundoplication. Initial results are promising, but there are few long-term studies, and the precise role of these novel procedures in the treatment of GERD remains to be determined.

INDICATIONS AND CONTRAINDICATIONS

Patients with symptomatic GERD are potential candidates for endoluminal therapy. The standard preoperative workup for operative intervention of GERD should be performed, including endoscopy, esophageal manometry, and 24-hour pH monitoring to confirm the pathologic acid exposure in the esophagus. Relative contraindications to performing these procedures include grade 2 or higher esophagitis, hiatal hernia greater than 3 cm in size, and Barrett's esophagus.

Special consideration should be given to those patients who have refractory GERD after fundoplication or after gastric bypass. Although fundoplication is effective at controlling symptoms in 90% of patients long term, redo fundoplication has been associated with higher perioperative morbidity and mortality. At best, symptomatic outcomes are worse and morbidity higher than that for the first fundoplication. Similarly, patients after gastric bypass who have continued symptoms have limited surgical options for treatment. Barring correctable mechanical failure, select patients with recurrent GERD after fundoplication or gastric bypass may be ideal candidates for an endoluminal approach.

TECHNIQUE

Currently approved endoluminal therapies for GERD are based on either application of radio frequency (RF) energy or mechanical suturing of the gastroesophageal junction. In general, these procedures can be performed with a level of sedation slightly greater than standard upper endoscopy. Monitored anesthesia care should be administered for those patients with Mallampati class I or II airways. Those with higher-risk airways (class III or IV) should undergo general anesthesia.

Radio Frequency Energy

The Stretta system (Curon Medical, Fremont, CA) uses RF energy to deliver controlled cautery to the gastroesophageal junction. The mechanism of action is partially mechanical (heat-induced thickening of the GE junction musculature), reducing compliance of the lower esophageal sphincter (LES), and through reduction in the frequency of transient LES relaxations.

The components of the Stretta system include the RF generator and catheter (Fig. 1). The catheter consists of a bougie tip, a balloon-basket assembly, and four radially oriented electrode delivery sheaths. The patient is placed in the left lateral decubitus position, and upper endoscopy is performed. The distance from the incisors to the squamocolumnar junction (SCJ) is measured, a guidewire is placed, and the endoscope is removed. The Stretta catheter is then inserted transorally over the guidewire to a target electrode deployment 1 cm above the SCJ. The balloon is inflated, and the electrodes are deployed into the muscle. RF energy is delivered with active tissue impedance monitoring to confirm appropriate deployment of the electrodes into the muscle. The RF generator maintains muscle tissue temperature at 85 °C and mucosal temperature below 50 °C through delivery of chilled water. After 1.5 minutes of RF energy delivery, the electrodes are retracted and the balloon deflated. The catheter is rotated 45 degrees, and the RF energy delivery process is repeated. The catheter is then moved 0.5 cm distally, and eight more lesions are created in a similar fashion until four rings of eight lesions have been created. The catheter is then advanced into the stomach and the balloon reinflated with 25 ml of air and pulled back until resistance is met. The needles are deployed and RF energy administered. RF delivery is performed twice more at the same level, turning the catheter 30 and 60 degrees to the right original position. After balloon deflation, the catheter is advanced into the stomach, the balloon is inflated with 22 ml of air, and the catheter is pulled back to resistance. Three more sets of lesions are created at this level. At the conclusion of the procedure, there are six rings with a total of 56 lesions (Fig. 2). Key technical points to success include precise measurements and positioning of the catheter itself, close monitoring of muscle and mucosal temperatures, impedance monitoring, and correct balloon inflation volumes.

At the conclusion of the procedure, repeat upper endoscopy is performed to confirm placement of the lesions. The patient is

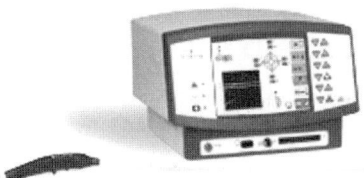

Figure I Stretta radiofrequency generator and catheter system.

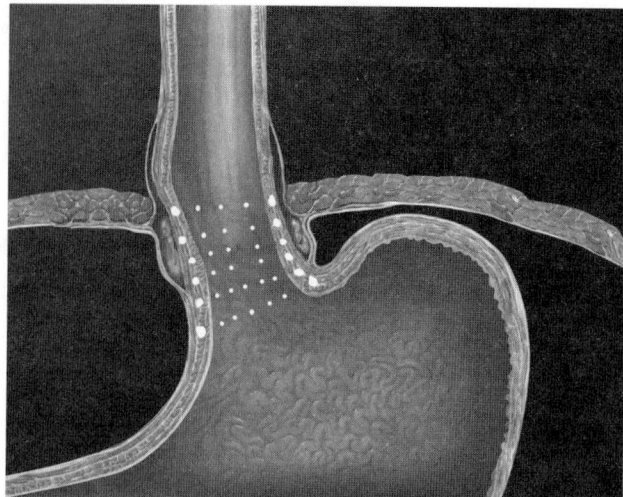

Figure 2 Completed delivery of radiofrequency energy to lower esophagus using the Stretta system.

discharged the same day with continued acid-suppression medication for 1 month and is then weaned from the medications.

Endoluminal Gastroplication (EG)

Currently used transoral gastroplication systems place a variable number of sutures near the LES under direct endoscopic visualization. The Bard Endocinch procedure (Bard Endoscopic Technologies, Billerica, MA) is performed under deep sedation. The patient is placed in the left lateral decubitus position. Upper endoscopy is performed, and an overtube is placed. The Endocinch suturing device is attached to a 9-mm endoscope and advanced to 2.5 cm below the SCJ, where a fold of tissue is sucked into a capsule, and a needle is advanced through the "grasped" tissue. A suture is passed through the needle, placing the stitch to begin the plication. The device is rotated, and a second bite of tissue is taken 1-2 cm away from the first bite. The sutures are secured together using a ceramic plug and cut by the device, completing the plication (Fig. 3). A helical configuration of four separate plications between 0.5 and 2.5 cm below the SCJ has been used with success. The endoscope must be inserted and removed for each complete plication.

The NDO Full-Thickness Plicator (NDO Medical, Mansfield, MA) relies on taking full-thickness bites, creating a serosa-to-serosa union and restoring the valvular mechanism of the LES. This is accomplished under direct vision of a slim, 6-mm gastroscope that goes through a separate channel of the instrument. With the scope and plicator retroflexed, the corkscrew tissue retractor is inserted into the gastric wall near the LES, and then the tissue is retracted toward the instrument. The arms are then closed, and the implant (consisting of pretied 2–0 polypropylene sutures, two expanded polytetrafluoroethylene bolsters, and two titanium retention bridges) is deployed creating a full-thickness plication (Fig. 4).

Patients are discharged the same day of the procedure and are instructed to restrict their diet to liquids (avoiding carbonated beverages) for the first week after plication.

■ OUTCOMES AND SAFETY

Most endoscopic approaches to GERD have been found to be safe with very few serious side effects; however, at least one technique (Enteryx; Boston Scientific, Natick, MA) has been abandoned because of deaths and serious morbidity associated with injection of Enteryx outside of the esophagus. The Stretta and EG procedures, on the other hand, has been performed in nearly 20,000

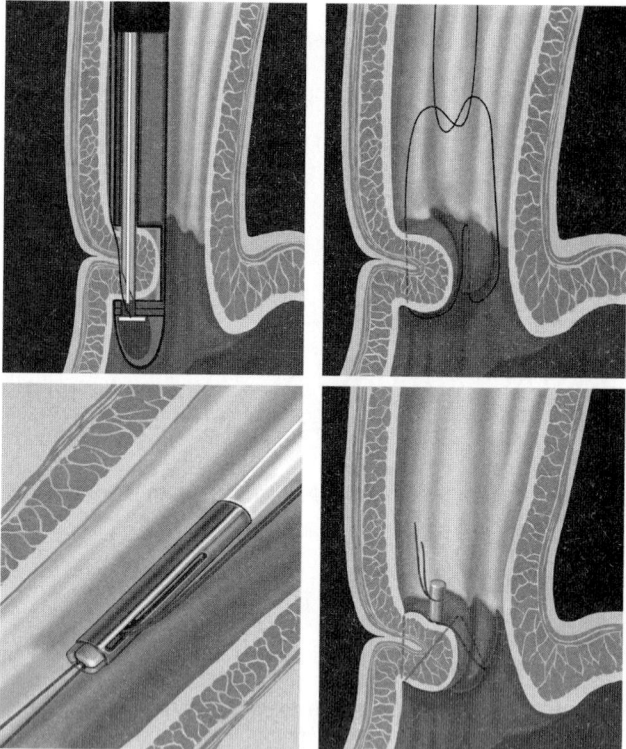

Figure 3 Endocinch suturing system. Two separate endoscopic "bites" of tissue are taken and secured with the device, creating an endoluminal plication.

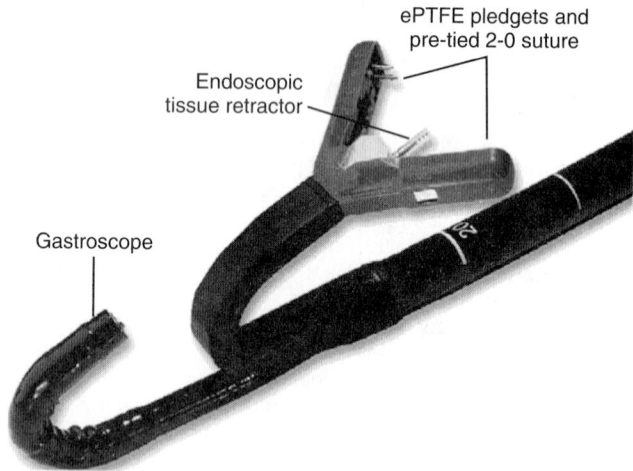

Figure 4 Full-thickness plicator. Note helical endoscopic tissue retractor and pretied sutures and pledgets.

patients, and estimates of the current rate of complications are approximately 0.2%. The safety profile of the NDO surgical plicator has been assessed in a limited number of patients but to date appears to have a safety record similar to other endoscopic suturing techniques. One advantage of all the endoscopic treatments of GERD over laparoscopic fundoplication appears to be the virtual absence of gas bloat and dysphagia sometimes seen after laparoscopic Nissen fundoplication.

Three randomized trials of endoscopic versus sham therapy have shown the endoscopic treatments to be efficacious. The sham versus Stretta trial showed that the Stretta treatment group had significantly improved GERD symptoms (the primary endpoint), whereas the sham group had no improvement. The study also demonstrated no significant difference in 24-hour acid exposure between the sham- or Stretta-treated groups. Favorable long-term results after the Stretta procedure have been observed by Lutfi and colleagues, who studied 77 patients for 2 years after intervention. Sixty percent of patients no longer required antisecretory therapy or had their dose reduced by at least 50%. Mean DeMeester score was reduced from 40 to 30 with normal acid exposure time (pH <4%) achieved in 42% of patients who were studied with pH monitoring.

The only randomized sham versus EG study reported in abstract form showed the EG treatment arm had fewer episodes of heartburn and reduced esophageal acid exposure compared with the sham-treated patients. This trial has not yet been published and was done in only a small number of cases ($N = 34$), thereby limiting enthusiasm for this modality. In a prospective case series of 85 patients undergoing the Endocinch procedure, the majority showed resolution of heartburn (52%) and regurgitation (77%) 2 years after intervention. Only one patient (1.1%) experienced significant dysphagia warranting stitch removal. However, a separate 70-patient prospective series of the same procedure revealed only 20% success of either symptom relief or reduction in PPI use at 18 months. In fact, sutures were not detected in 26% of patients by surveillance endoscopy. In addition, no changes in 24-hour pH testing or LES pressure could be detected after Endocinch plication.

Favorable short-term results have been obtained with the NDO Full-Thickness Plicator. In a sham-controlled, randomized trial, 78 patients received plication, and 81 patients underwent sham procedure. At 12 months, 65% of intervention patients showed >50% improvement in GERD health-related quality of life scores compared with 20% in the sham group. Fifty-seven percent of patients achieved complete PPI cessation compared with 25% of sham patients. In addition, median time of esophageal acid exposure was significantly reduced in the plication group.

Comparative trials evaluating EG ($n = 47$) and laparoscopic fundoplication (LF; $n = 40$) have shown that LF is more reliable than EG in reducing antisecretory medication use (32% of EG and 13% of LF at 7 months) and has better patient satisfaction (93%) than EG (66%). Complications of hypoxia or bleeding occurred in 0.6% of Endocinch patients.

CONCLUSION

The minimally invasive management of GERD continues to evolve with the advent of endoluminal therapies. These interventions offer outpatient treatment with a good chance of symptom relief without medication in the short term for patients who have limited early-stage disease. Studies to evaluate long-term outcome and to compare endoluminal therapies with laparoscopic fundoplication and medical therapy are necessary. Importantly, additional studies examining the role of these novel procedures in patients with recurrent symptoms after fundoplication or gastric bypass should be explored. These results will help identify those patients who will benefit the most from an endoluminal approach.

SUGGESTED READINGS

Chadalavada R, Lin E, Swafford V, and others: Comparative results of endoluminal gastroplasty and laparoscopic antireflux surgery for the treatment of GERD, *Surg Endosc* 18:261, 2004.

Corley DA, Katz P, Wo JM, and others: Improvement in gastroesophageal reflux symptoms after radiofrequency energy: a randomized sham-controlled trial, *Gastroenterology* 125:668, 2003.

Lutfi R, Torquati A, Kaiser J, and others: Three year's experience with the Stretta procedure: did it really make a difference? *Surg Endosc* 19:289, 2005.

Mattar SG, Qureshi F, Taylor D, Schauer PR: Treatment of refractory gastroesophageal reflux disease with radiofrequency energy (Stretta) in patients after Roux-en-Y gastric bypass, *Surg Endosc* 20:850, 2006.

Rothstein R, Filipi C, Caca K, and others: Endoscopic full-thickness plication for the treatment of GERD: a randomized, sham-controlled trial, *Gastroenterology* 131:704, 2006.

BARRETT'S ESOPHAGUS

William R. Lynch, MD, Henning Gerke, MD, and Mark D. Iannettoni, MD

INTRODUCTION

Barrett's esophagus is characterized by the replacement of the stratified squamous epithelium that lines the distal esophagus with specialized columnar epithelium-containing goblet cells. Histologically, the columnar lining of Barrett's may have features of gastric, small intestinal, and colonic epithelia. This lining is called "specialized columnar epithelium" or "specialized intestinal metaplasia." Barrett's is seen as a complication of gastroesophageal reflux disease (GERD) and is considered to be a premalignant condition. Diagnosis requires endoscopy and biopsy.

Endoscopically, Barrett's mucosa has a salmon-colored appearance indistinguishable from gastric mucosa, in contrast to the white-appearing squamous epithelium of the normal esophagus. The intestinal metaplasia starts distally at the gastroesophageal junction, and the proximal extent is variable. The clinical relevance of Barrett's esophagus lies in the potential progression to adenocarcinoma. The development of adenocarcinoma is believed to follow a sequence of histologic alterations from low-grade to high-grade dysplasia and finally to invasive cancer. This proposed sequential evolution from metaplasia to invasive cancer is the basis for endoscopic surveillance. Current guidelines recommend that four quadrant biopsies should be taken at 2-cm intervals beginning 1 cm below the esophagogastric junction and extending to 1 cm above the squamocolumnar junction. The risk for adenocarcinoma is considered to be low if no dysplastic changes are present, and surveillance endoscopies with biopsies are recommended in 3-year intervals. In the presence of low-grade dysplasia, endoscopic surveillance should be performed at 6-month intervals for the first year and then every year if no progression is detected. High-grade dysplasia in Barrett's esophagus describes severe architectural and cellular alteration of the specialized intestinal epithelium. Diagnosis of high-grade dysplasia must be confirmed by a second, independent, experienced pathologist. In approximately 10% to 30% of patients with high-grade dysplasia, the disease will progress to cancer within 5 years. Although the number of these patients is small, this group has a 30- to 125-fold increased risk for invasive adenocarcinoma of the esophagus, warranting an aggressive approach for diagnosis, as well as treatment.

BARRETT'S MANAGEMENT AND TREATMENT

The management goals of Barrett's equate to those for GERD: provide long-term relief of symptoms and promote healing of reflux-induced esophageal mucosal injury, including stricture formation. More specific to Barrett's, treatment strategies should prevent progression to more advanced mucosal injury, dysplastic change, and carcinoma. In addition, treatment should offer potential regression of dysplastic Barrett's to nondysplastic pathology. Most patients with Barrett's esophagus are treated with lifelong proton pump inhibitors for symptom relief and to control esophagitis and stricture. Symptom control has historically been the endpoint of treatment; however, some evidence suggests that reflux control may lead to regression of dysplastic and nondysplastic segments of Barrett's and may prevent the development of adenocarcinoma. Long-term success in treating Barrett's is challenging. It represents severe GERD and is often associated with large hiatal hernias. Acid suppression therapy in this group of patients is increasingly ineffective, leaving antireflux surgery as a superior treatment option.

Antireflux surgery can be a successful treatment option for many patients with Barrett's. Barrett's is often associated with severe reflux that is exacerbated by anatomic aberrations such as large hiatal hernia, shortened esophagus, stricture, and dysmotility. These anomalies must be recognized and incorporated into the surgical strategy. These anatomic and physiologic features have bearing on the approach, as well as the type of antireflux procedure offered. Most typically, the 360-degree Nissen fundoplication is the operation of choice for medically refractory GERD. When there is severe dysmotility of the esophageal body, a partial fundoplication (Toupet, Dor, or Belsey) can offer protection from reflux while minimizing postoperative dysphagia. A relatively loose and short Nissen fundoplication is an alternate strategy to minimize dysphagia while affording reflux protection. These approaches can be successfully offered laparoscopically. When there is a large (>5 cm) hiatal hernia or associated stricture, esophageal shortening is commonly present. A shortened esophagus makes accomplishing a tension-free repair with a sufficient intra-abdominal length of esophagus unlikely, diminishing the likelihood of long-term surgical success. A Collis gastroplasty (as an esophageal lengthening procedure) associated with a Nissen fundoplication enhances the chances of a long-term surgical success. This procedure is also being performed laparoscopically.

RESULTS OF ANTIREFLUX SURGERY IN BARRETT'S ESOPHAGUS

Several studies focused on symptom control as the outcome measure after antireflux surgery describe good to excellent results in 72% to 95% of patients at 5 years. One study compared medical to surgical treatment, and antireflux surgery was superior in immediate and long-term control of symptoms. Recurrence of heartburn or dysphagia was 88% in medical treatment group and 21% in the surgical group. The complication of a reflux-related stricture occurred more often in the medically treated group: 38% versus 16%. Other studies suggest that there is little difference in symptom control between medical treatment with proton pump inhibitors and antireflux surgery. There did seem to be an increased incidence of persistent esophagitis or stricture (or both) in the medically treated group. Some reports have shown a higher prevalence of anatomic failures requiring reoperation in patients with Barrett's compared with non-Barrett's patients with reflux.

Dysplasia in Barrett's esophagus is the first step in the neoplastic process. The histologic grade correlates with the potential for developing adenocarcinoma. Surveillance strategies are based on this relationship between dysplasia grade and the evolution of adenocarcinoma. Risk of this evolution can be stratified by patient age, gender, length of the Barrett's segment, size of hiatal hernia, and the histologic grade. There is an increasing body of evidence suggesting that the metaplasia-dysplasia-carcinoma sequence may be interrupted or even reversed by antireflux surgery. There are studies that have suggested that reducing reflux seems to decrease the likelihood of developing Barrett's esophagus. When Barrett's exists, reflux control, although necessary for control of symptoms, appears to diminish the transition to dysplasia. When dysplastic change is already present in Barrett's esophagus, reflux control may reverse these changes. There is evidence that controlling the reflux of duodenal contents, along with acid, is important to protect against dysplastic change and promote regression of these histologic changes. These goals are best achieved with antireflux surgery. It is clear that for symptom relief in patients with Barrett's esophagus, antireflux surgery is safe and effective. It is less clear that antireflux surgery will alter the disease progression from metaplasia to carcinoma. For this reason, patients with Barrett's esophagus who are treated with antireflux surgery must continue with endoscopic surveillance.

BARRETT'S ESOPHAGUS WITH DYSPLASIA

Dysplasia is classified into four categories:

1. No dysplasia; intestinal metaplasia
2. Indefinite for dysplasia
3. Low-grade dysplasia
4. High-grade dysplasia

A diagnosis of high-grade dysplasia must be confirmed by at least two pathologists experienced in the field before definitive therapy is offered. Distinguishing between high-grade dysplasia and well-differentiated intramucosal adenocarcinoma can be difficult. High-grade dysplasia is neoplastic change involving the epithelium but not extending into the lamina propria. Neoplasia involving the epithelium and lamina propria is intramucosal adenocarcinoma. The prevalence of low-grade dysplasia in Barrett's is 15% to 25%, whereas that of high-grade dysplasia is approximately 5%. The incidence of developing dysplasia in Barrett's is approximately 5% per year.

High-grade dysplasia is considered a malignant condition limited to the mucosal layer, and three treatment strategies are advocated: surveillance until carcinoma is identified, mucosal ablative techniques, and esophagectomy. Esophagectomy is typically offered when the patient is considered a surgical candidate. The likelihood of finding invasive carcinoma in specimens resected for high-grade dysplasia is almost 40%. Twenty-five percent of patients followed with surveillance have carcinoma at 18 months, 50% at 3 years, and almost 80% at 8 years. Most patients with high-grade dysplasia will have invasive adenocarcinoma within 5 to 10 years. A strategy that employs regular surveillance with esophagectomy can result in detection of early-stage cancers and high overall survival. Five-year survival can approach 90% in this setting.

Esophagectomy removes all Barrett's epithelium and associated adenocarcinoma. The transhiatal approach is favored in most experienced centers, and mortality should be less than 1%. The anastomosis in the neck minimizes the disabling reflux that can be associated with intrathoracic anastomosis. Recovery is described as good to excellent by most patients. Although esophagectomy can offer significant morbidity and mortality risks and can be a challenge to recover from, many patients prefer to accept these risks in exchange for a chance to be cured of a likely cancer.

ENDOSCOPIC MANAGEMENT OF BARRETT'S ESOPHAGUS WITH HIGH-GRADE DYSPLASIA OR EARLY ADENOCARCINOMA

Traditionally, esophagectomy has been considered standard of care in patients with high-grade dysplasia. However, given the surgical morbidity and mortality, endoscopic techniques have been evaluated to ablate the Barrett's mucosa and even to treat early adenocarcinoma. Although these techniques were initially reserved for poor operative candidates, data are emerging to support their broader application as a less invasive alternative to esophagectomy. Advanced tumors (T2) and metastatic lymphadenopathy are contraindications for endoscopic therapy and should be ruled out by endoscopic ultrasound. Endoscopic treatment modalities that have been used to ablate Barrett's mucosa include photodynamic therapy (PDT), argon plasma coagulation, and cryoablation. The best data are available for PDT. This method consists of intravenous application of a photosensitizing drug followed by illumination of the Barrett's mucosa with a laser probe during endoscopy. Barrett's mucosa that is successfully ablated in this manner will be replaced by normal squamous epithelium. Problems with PDT include incomplete ablation of the Barrett's area in 20% of patients, phototoxic side effects, and formation of esophageal strictures requiring dilatation in approximately 30% of patients.

Early adenocarcinomas within the Barrett's mucosa and areas that are suspicious by their endoscopic appearance can be removed with endoscopic mucosal resection (EMR). EMR achieves focal removal of the esophageal lining up to the submucosal level. Several technical variations of EMR are available. A common method to perform EMR uses a special cap that is attached to the tip of the endoscope. The cap contains a distal rim in which an electrocautery snare is fitted (Fig. 1). The target area is suctioned into the cap to create a pseudopolyp that is then resected with the electrocautery snare (Fig. 2). Submucosal injection of normal saline or epinephrine solution is usually performed before EMR to lift the mucosa and minimize the risk of perforation. Larger Barrett's areas can be resected by repeating this method at adjacent areas (Fig. 3). Whether early adenocarcinoma is curable by EMR depends on the depth of invasion,

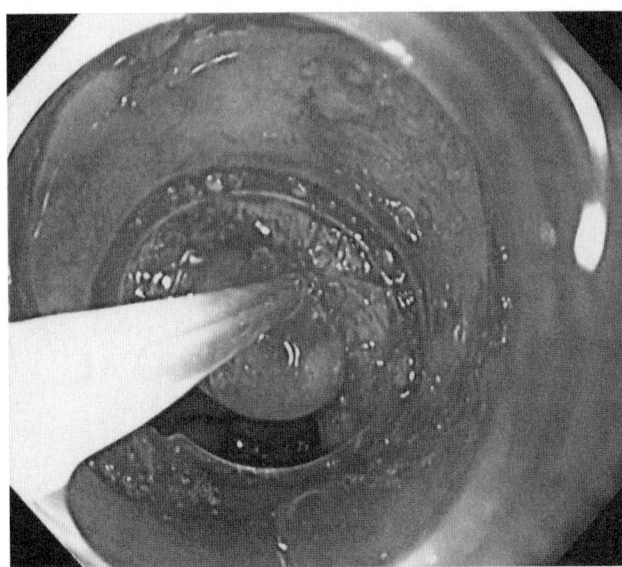

Figure 2 The snare is closed around the mucosa.

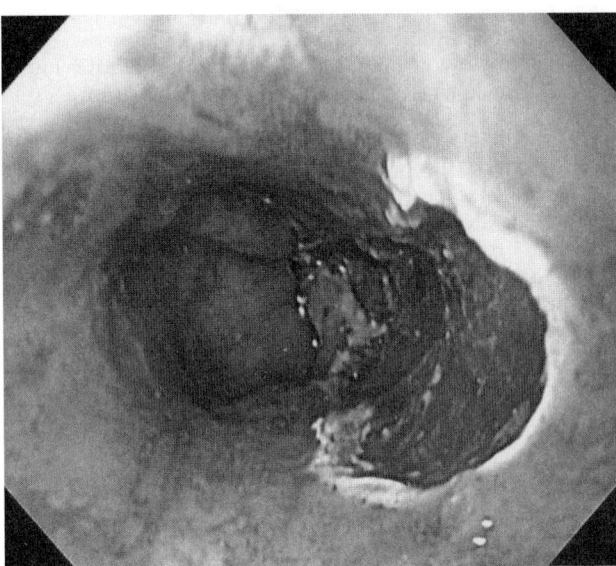

Figure 3 Status post–mucosal resection.

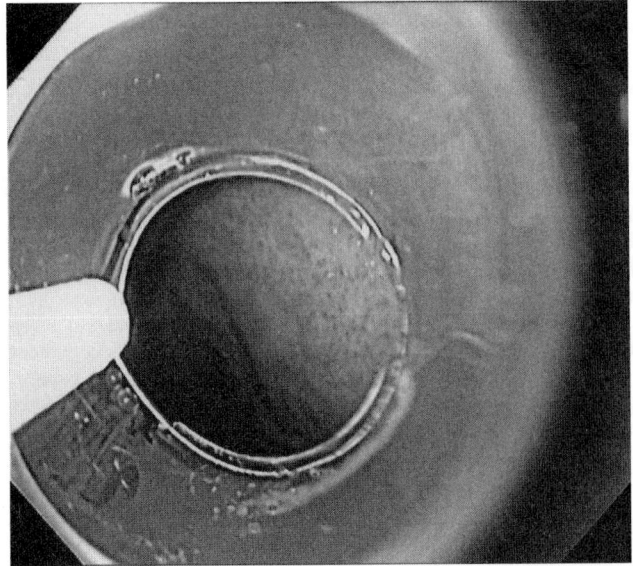

Figure 1 Endoscopic view through with attached cap. A snare is fitted in the cap.

which can be accurately determined by histologic assessment of the EMR specimen. If the cancer invades beyond the mucosa into the submucosal layer, endoscopic therapy alone is unlikely curative because of the high risk of lymphatic spread, and these patients should be offered esophagectomy. Following EMR for early adenocarcinoma, complete ablation of the residual Barrett's mucosa is warranted to avoid the development of metachronous cancer. This can be achieved by combining EMR with PDT. However, stepwise circumferential resection of the entire Barrett's mucosa by EMR techniques alone is under investigation. Long-term follow-up data of endoscopic therapy for high-grade dysplasia and early adenocarcinoma are still limited, and continuation of endoscopic surveillance is necessary following these techniques.

Close endoscopic surveillance at 3-month intervals is an alternative strategy to endoscopic therapy in poor surgical candidates with Barrett's esophagus and high-grade dysplasia. If mucosal adenocarcinoma occurs during surveillance, EMR may be an option.

Suggested Readings

Duranceau A, Pera M: Barrett's Esophagus, *Chest Surg Clin North Am* 12:1, 2002.

Larghi A, Waxman I: Endoscopic mucosal resection: treatment of neoplasia, *Gastrointest Endosc Clin N Am* 15:431, viii, 2005.

Pacifico RJ, Wang KK, Wongkeesong LM, and others: Combined endoscopic mucosal resection and photodynamic therapy versus esophagectomy for management of early adenocarcinoma in Barrett's esophagus, *Clin Gastroenterol Hepatol* 1:252, 2003.

Peters JH, Hagen JA, DeMeester SR: Barrett's esophagus, *J Gastrointest Surg* 8:1, 2004.

Spechler SJ: Dysplasia in Barrett's esophagus: limitations of current management strategies, *Am J Gastroenterol* 100:927, 2005.

Paraesophageal Hiatal Hernia

C. Daniel Smith, MD

INTRODUCTION

The terms *paraesophageal hernia* and *hiatal hernia* are often intermixed and used synonymously to describe enlargement of the esophageal hiatus and the subsequent transdiaphragmatic migration of intraabdominal content, most commonly the gastric cardia and fundus. Although this exchange of terms is reasonable for health care providers who primarily diagnose the anatomically enlarged esophageal hiatus, the distinction between paraesophageal and hiatal hernia becomes important when considering how patients with this defect should be managed. Hiatal hernia describes all types of defects involving the esophageal hiatus, of which a subset are known as paraesophageal hernias. The anatomic differences help predict the natural history and guide decisions about management. This chapter discusses all hiatal hernias, including the paraesophageal hiatal hernia.

PATHOPHYSIOLOGY AND CLASSIFICATION

Although the exact etiology of this anatomic defect is unknown, what is clear is that attenuation of the phrenoesophageal membrane allows the gastroesophageal junction (GEJ) to migrate through a patulous hiatus into the chest or the gastric fundus to herniate alongside the GEJ and into the chest. The nature of these defects remains unknown, but all types of hiatal hernias are more common in older individuals, and recent studies suggest hiatal hernia is more common among the obese and those with delayed gastric emptying. All of this suggests an acquired weakness of tissue as a result of aging or excess strain on the diaphragm.

There is a well-described familial occurrence of hiatal hernias believed to represent an autosomal-dominant link with variable clinical expression. Younger siblings of children who have a hiatal hernia are 20 times more likely to have a hiatal hernia. Some have suggested that any hiatal hernia in a young patient indicates an underlying congenital problem. Clearly, confounding data are available from which to guess about etiology.

Hiatal hernias are classified according to the anatomic position of the GEJ and the extent of herniated stomach (Table 1). A type I hiatal hernia, also known as a "sliding hiatal hernia," consists of a simple herniation of the gastroesophageal junction into the chest. The phrenoesophageal ligament is attenuated, and there is no true hernia sac. This is the most common of the hiatal hernias; it is more common in women and in the fifth and sixth decades of life.

Table 1: Classification of Hiatal Hernias

Hernia Type	Location of Gastroesophageal Junction	Hernia Contents
I (Sliding)	Intrathoracic	Gastric cardia ± fundus
II (True paraesophageal)	Intraabdominal	Gastric fundus ± body
III (combination I and II)	Intrathoracic	Gastric fundus and body
IV	Intrathoracic	Gastric fundus, body and other abdominal organs (e.g., colon).

With a type II hiatal hernia, commonly referred to as a "true paraesophageal hernia," the GEJ remains at the esophageal hiatus, and the gastric fundus herniates alongside the esophagus into the chest. The type III hiatal hernia is a combination of type I and type II hernias, with the GEJ being displaced into the chest along with the gastric fundus and body. Paraesophageal hernias (types II and III) have a true hernia sac accompanying the herniated stomach. This becomes important when surgical repair is undertaken because the sac must be excised. Finally, some have characterized a type IV hernia as an advanced stage of hiatal hernia in which the entire stomach and other intraabdominal content (e.g., colon, spleen) are herniated into the chest. Use of this fourth classification is not widely accepted.

INCIDENCE

Although the exact prevalence of hiatal hernia remains unknown, it is clear that it is a relatively common abnormality and is the most common finding reported on barium studies of the upper gastrointestinal tract. The difficulty in establishing the incidence of hiatal hernia lies in the fact that a large number of patients with hiatal hernia are asymptomatic, and the diagnosis is often made incidentally during investigation of other gastrointestinal problems.

In contrast to all hiatal hernias, paraesophageal hernia is a very rare type of hiatal hernia. In a series of 46,236 Mayo Clinic patients with hiatal hernias, only 147 (0.32%) were type II or true paraesophageal hernias, with women twice as likely to have this type of hernia as men. The frequency of paraesophageal hernia increases with advancing age.

SYMPTOMS AND PRESENTATION

Most type I and III hiatal hernias are diagnosed incidentally during a contrast upper GI or during upper endoscopy performed for

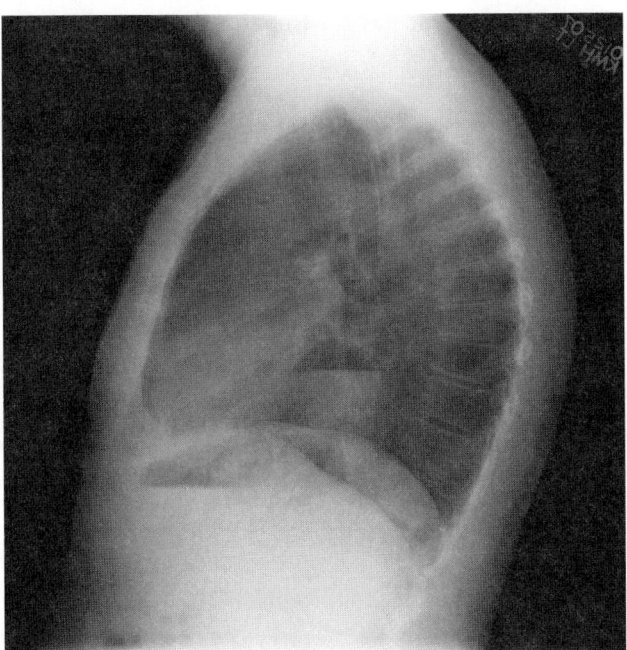

Figure 1   Chest x-ray showing air-fluid levels from the herniated stomach.

other reasons. Type II hernias can be similarly diagnosed but are also frequently found on a radiograph of the chest showing an air-fluid level in the mediastinum or the left chest (Fig. 1). Occasionally, the inability to pass a nasogastric tube followed by a contrast study reveals a twisted intrathoracic stomach, or a contrast study of the colon reveals colon in the chest, leading to the diagnosis of a type IV hernia.

When symptoms are present, sliding hernias have a different presentation from paraesophageal hernias. Type I hernias are frequently accompanied by symptoms of gastroesophageal reflux (GERD), most commonly heartburn or regurgitation. Type II and III hernias tend to produce symptoms that are more mechanical in nature because of the anatomic consequence of the hiatal outflow restriction. Typical symptoms include epigastric pain, postprandial fullness or discomfort in the chest, dysphagia, abdominal bloating, and respiratory problems. Again, these symptoms are caused by hiatal outflow restriction, altered gastric anatomy, and distension of the intrathoracic portion of the stomach with esophageal or pulmonary compression. Interestingly, patients often report a remote history of GERD-type symptoms that abruptly abate and are replaced by obstructive symptoms; this is thought to occur as the hernia enlarges and the esophageal outlet becomes obstructed.

Acute symptoms may develop as a consequence of complete obstruction or strangulation of the stomach within the chest, mimicking myocardial infarction. Type II hernias are at particular risk for incarceration with obstruction, strangulation, and perforation of the herniated stomach. Borchardt's triad comprises chest pain, retching with inability to vomit, and inability to pass a nasogastric tube and is indicative of an incarcerated hernia, and is a surgical emergency.

An often-overlooked presentation is anemia from chronic GI blood loss. This occurs in one third of patients with type II hernias and prompts an often exhaustive evaluation for cause. This anemia is caused by linear ulcerations of the gastric cardia resulting from the proximal stomach's repetitive movement across the diaphragm. Ninety-two percent of patients will have their anemia resolve after surgical correction of the hernia.

MANAGEMENT

Although most hiatal hernias are asymptomatic, the diagnosis is rarely in question when patients present with symptoms as outlined earlier and a chest x-ray or contrast esophagram confirms the defect. An esophagogastroduodenoscopy (EGD) should be attempted in all patients to assess the distal esophagus and stomach for concomitant pathology, with caution exercised not to overinflate the stomach, which may be incarcerated in the chest. Although motility studies may help identify the patient with esophageal motor abnormality and direct the type of fundoplication used in repair, the distortion of the GEJ and distal esophagus makes motility studies difficult to acquire and interpret. For this reason, motility studies are not useful for most type II and III hernias. The same is true of 24-hour pH or gastric-emptying studies. These studies can be difficult to interpret and rarely change the decisions regarding management. A computed tomography scan of the chest and abdomen may help confirm the extent of the hernia but is not necessary for straightforward cases.

Because hiatal hernia is a purely mechanical abnormality, there is no nonoperative treatment. Currently there is controversy about which patients should undergo repair. Traditionally it has been held that all patients with type II or II hernias should undergo surgical repair regardless of symptoms. This has been based on a report in 1967 documenting a mortality rate of 30% in patients with paraesophageal hernia (6 of 21 patients died secondary to complications of their hernia). More recently, a series of 23 patients with a paraesophageal hernia was followed for a median of 78 months; no life-threatening complications developed in this group, and symptoms remained unchanged in 83% of these patients. This has led many to recommend repair in only select asymptomatic patients. In contrast, those with symptoms, esophageal mucosal damage (esophagitis or Barrett's), or anemia should undergo elective repair.

Similarly, a significant number of patients with type I hiatal hernias are asymptomatic and remain so throughout their lives. Therefore, the presence of a sliding hiatal hernia alone does not mandate intervention. However, those patients with a type I hernia and gastroesophageal reflux, chest pain, dysphagia, regurgitation, or other symptoms referable to their hernia should undergo symptom-specific workup and may be best served with an operative repair.

Operative Technique

Operative correction of esophageal hiatal hernia, regardless of technique, should (1) return the herniated content to its anatomically correct position below the diaphragm, (2) resect the hernia sac, (3) establish adequate esophageal length and return the GEJ to an intra-abdominal position, (4) repair the hernia defect, and (5) prevent recurrence while minimizing associated morbidity. A number of operations can be performed through the chest or abdomen to accomplish these goals.

Currently, the most common approach to hiatal hernia repair is transabdominal using laparoscopy, although many advocate the open transabdominal approach. Debate continues over whether a laparoscopic approach compromises the long-term outcome of the repair (see Controversies). Although most would agree that the laparoscopic approach is preferred because of the associated enhanced recovery, especially in this typically more elderly patient population, it is clear that the laparoscopic approach is more technically challenging and, if performed by inexperienced surgeons, may lead to a higher incidence of perioperative complications or long-term failure. On the other hand, when performed by an experienced laparoscopist and foregut surgeon, the technique of the operation should not differ from that performed open and therefore should lead to no differential outcome.

Historically, the thoracic approach has been preferred for larger hernias and those with suspected esophageal shortening.

The relative ease of dissecting the hernia sac and mobilizing the esophagus makes this approach appealing in select settings. However, the morbidity associated with a thoracotomy, both immediately postoperatively and long-term with chronic incisional problems, makes this approach appealing in only a small subset of patients.

OUTCOMES

The outcomes of hiatal hernia repair can be broken into symptomatic outcomes and anatomic outcomes. When considering symptomatic response to operative repair, 88% of patients after hiatal hernia repair report a significant improvement or resolution of their preoperative symptoms. This response appears durable, with sustained symptom improvement for up to 4 years after surgery. Ninety-two percent of those with anemia have resolution after hernia repair. On the other hand, anatomic failure after hernia repair remains high, with up to 41% of patients demonstrating recurrent hernia an average of 4 years after repair. Some have suggested that this rate of anatomic failure is lower when the repair is performed open (see Controversies). Regardless, the significance of these anatomic failures remains debated. A small transdiaphragmatic migration of the wrap or GEJ, essentially an asymptomatic type I hernia, is clinically inconsequential. To aspire to a higher rate of anatomic success risks overtreatment and potentially profound complications, especially when mesh is used in the repair (see Controversies).

CONTROVERSIES

Should an Antireflux Procedure Accompany All Hiatal Hernia Repairs?

Whether to include an antireflux procedure with all hiatal hernia repairs remains controversial, especially when dealing with a type II paraesophageal hernia (Fig. 2). Because most sliding-type hernias are repaired on the basis of symptoms, adding an antireflux procedure seems more straightforward because of the prevalence of reflux symptoms in type I and III hernias. In contrast, most patients who have type II hernias do not have reflux symptoms, and adding an antireflux operation in these patients may add little to the outcome. However, with careful questioning, many patients with type II hernias give a history of GERD symptoms that spontaneously abated, suggesting that an anatomic change (perhaps hernia development) led to this resolution of symptoms. Recent data from small series are suggesting that GERD may be more prevalent in type II hernia than earlier recognized, and as many as 30% of patients without GERD preoperatively will have GERD unmasked after hiatal hernia repair.

The role of fundoplication in patients with type II paraesophageal hernia remains controversial. Conventional thinking suggests that because the lower esophageal sphincter is located within the abdomen, it is competent and fundoplication is unnecessary. On the other hand, a key principle in repairing a hiatal hernia is to anchor the stomach within the abdomen to help prevent recurrence, and some surgeons are now using a fundoplication to serve as this anchor (the wrap buttresses against the hernia repair and holds the distal esophagus and stomach intra-abdominally). In as many as one third of patients, adding fundoplication may avert the unmasking of GERD following repair. This rationale is leading many surgeons to use fundoplication routinely for all hiatal hernia repairs. Early data suggest that this is a safe and effective means to manage paraesophageal hernias. However, few studies have objectively evaluated addition of an antireflux procedure to hiatal hernia repair, and there are limited data available to definitively answer this question.

Should Hiatal Hernias Be Repaired Laparoscopically?

The role of laparoscopy in repairing hiatal hernias has recently been challenged. Anecdotal data suggest that the risk of esophageal or gastric perforation and hernia recurrence is higher following laparoscopic repair than after traditional open hiatal hernia repair. The proposed basis for this is increased technical demands with a laparoscopic approach, the difficulty of closing the attenuated esophageal hiatus laparoscopically, and the relative absence of intra-abdominal adhesions that accompanies laparoscopic hernia repair compared with open operations. The absence of these adhesions to anchor the stomach and distal esophagus allows the stomach to "slip" back more readily through the esophageal hiatus and into the chest than would be the case with the adhesions associated with open repairs. These anecdotal experiences need further investigation before any conclusions regarding route of abdominal access for repair of hiatal hernia can be made, and most would agree that a laparoscopic repair performed by a skilled laparoscopic foregut surgeon should not have any higher rate of complications or failure.

Should Mesh Be Used to Repair All Hiatal Hernias?

The high rate of anatomic failure of hiatal hernia repairs has led many to suggest that some sort of prosthetic should be used to reduce these failures. Many argue that the principle of "tension-free" repair embraced for abdominal wall hernias is generalizable to hiatal hernias as well. Over the past several years, many types of prosthetic material have been used empirically for reinforcement of the crural repair or hiatal reconstruction for the crura that cannot be approximated. A nonrandomized prospective study suggested a lower recurrence rate without any increase in dysphagia in a series of patients in which permanent mesh (polypropylene) was used in all those undergoing laparoscopic Nissen fundoplication. A more recent collection of experience from several experienced foregut surgeons identified more than 20 patients in whom mesh was used to reconstruct the esophageal hiatus and subsequently eroded into the esophagus; this led to significant complications, including progression to esophagectomy in several patients. In the only prospective randomized study

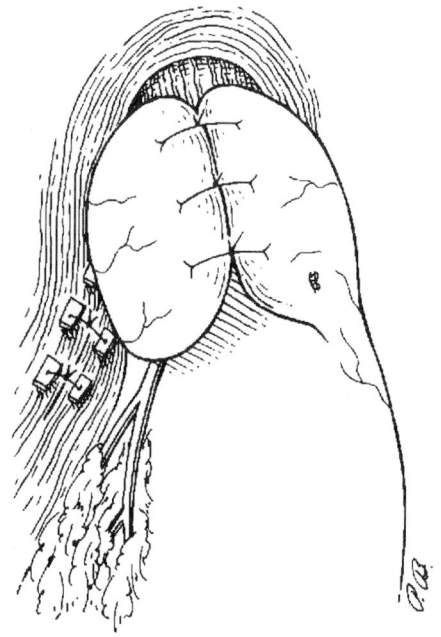

Figure 2 Nissen fundoplication.

comparing repair with a biomesh (reabsorbed) versus no mesh, a significant reduction in hernia recurrence was found in the biomesh group at 6 months postsurgery, suggesting a benefit to mesh without the associated risk of long-term mesh erosions or complications. This study looked at only short-term results, leaving the role of mesh in preventing long-term failure unanswered. Today most would advocate the cautious use of mesh for hiatal hernia repair until long-term studies with biomesh can be completed or until the long-term behavior of mesh on the diaphragm and adjacent to the esophagus can be evaluated.

SUGGESTED READINGS

El Sherif A, Yano F, Mittal S, Filipi CJ: Collagen metabolism and recurrent hiatal hernia: cause and effect? *Hernia* 10:511, 2006.

Lin E, Swafford V, Chadalavada R, and others: Disparity between symptomatic and physiologic outcomes following esophageal lengthening procedures for antireflux surgery, *J Gastrointest Surg* 8:31; discussion 38, 2004.

Mattar SG, Bowers SP, Galloway KD, and others: Long-term outcome of laparoscopic repair of paraesophageal hernia, *Surg Endosc* 16:745, 2002.

Oelschlager BK, Pellegrini CA, Hunter J, and others: Biologic prosthesis reduces recurrence after laparoscopic paraesophageal hernia repair: a multicenter, prospective, randomized trial, *Ann Surg* 244:481, 2006.

Skinner DB, Belsey RH: Surgical management of esophageal reflux and hiatus hernia. Long-term results with 1,030 patients, *J Thorac Cardiovasc Surg* 53:33, 1967.

Smith CD, McClusky DA, Rajad MA, and others: When fundoplication fails: redo? *Ann Surg* 241:861; discussion 869, 2005.

Terry M, Smith CD, Branum GD, and others: Outcomes of laparoscopic fundoplication for gastroesophageal reflux disease and paraesophageal hernia, *Surg Endosc* 15:691, 2001.

CHEMICAL ESOPHAGEAL INJURIES

Anne C. Fischer, MD, PhD

The ingestion of caustic agents can potentially induce a rapidly progressive, often devastating injury to the esophagus and contiguous mediastinal structures. Approximately 34,000 caustic injuries occur annually in the United States; these are the leading toxic exposure in children, as well as the second most common toxic ingestion in adults after analgesic ingestions. The former are usually accidental, typically in children aged younger than 5; the latter are generally suicide attempts. Historically, lye was crystalline, and the dry crystals localized to the oropharynx because of their adherence to the mucosa. The dry crystals elicited immediate, intense pain with the oropharyngeal burns, which in turn induced a protective, rapid expulsion of the crystals, limiting esophageal penetration. Only 10% to 25% of crystalline ingestions ever resulted in esophageal injury. The 1960s heralded the introduction of commercially available liquid lye, which correlated with the increase in severity and incidence of esophageal injuries. Ingestions of liquid lye, tasteless and odorless, circumvent the protective emetic reflexes invoked by crystalline ingestion. Legislative efforts successfully reduced the concentration of liquid lye from 35% to 5% sodium hydroxide and mandated childproof containers. However, the erroneous practice of storing liquid chemicals in reusable milk jugs or soda bottles continues to result in toxic ingestions. Finland's governmental ban on all liquid alkalis successfully decreased the actual incidence of severe esophageal burns.

MECHANISM OF INJURY

The extent of injury depends on the type of chemical ingested, its concentration, quantity, and duration of contact. Table 1 lists commonly ingested toxic chemicals. The concentration, or "strength," of the acid base determines the degree of injury. Mild caustic agents, such as household bleach, liquid laundry detergents, and dilute ammonia, result in mild injuries because they are weak bases at low concentrations. Most mortalities are associated with ingestions of strong alkalis such as liquid lye, solid Clinitest tablets, or button batteries because they are the most concentrated strong bases available. The most significant injuries occur at higher pHs ($\geq$11). The high

Table 1: Common Chemical Exposures

Chemicals	Source
Alkaline	
Sodium hypochlorite (weak base)	Bleaches
Ammonia Base (weak base)	Toilet bowl cleaners, hair dyes, floor strippers, glass cleaners
Sodium hydroxide (weak base)	Clinitest tablets, detergents, laundry powders, paint removers, drain cleaners, button batteries
Sodium borates, carbonates, phosphates	Detergents, electric dishwashers, water softeners
Acid	
Hydrochloric acid	Swimming pool cleaners, metal and toilet bowl cleaners
Hydrofluoric acid	Antirust products
Sulfuric acid	Car battery fluids

viscosity translates into a slow transit time with prolonged exposure and rapid deep tissue penetration, causing liquefactive necrosis. In contrast, acids cause a coagulation necrosis, which forms a superficial eschar on the esophageal surface, limiting the extension of further mucosal penetration. The lack of viscosity of acids is associated with a rapid transit time with relative esophageal sparing. The odor and bitter taste of strong acids initially induce a rapid protective emetic response, and thus acids usually spare the oropharynx and esophagus, causing skip lesions with a higher incidence of distal perforations. A caveat is that the ingestion of highly concentrated sulfuric or hydrochloric acid can cause esophageal injury in 50% of cases.

PRESENTATION

The most common features of ingestions are oropharyngeal pain, odynophagia or dysphagia, salivation, and chest pain. Unfortunately, clinical symptoms are poor predictors of the degree of injury. Stridor and hoarseness indicate laryngeal and epiglottal edema, requiring orotracheal intubation. Dysphagia and hematemesis, secondary to the sloughing of esophageal mucosa, are markers for esophageal injury. Ominous findings such as retrosternal pain radiating to the back and acute epigastric pain herald a full-thickness injury, either esophageal or gastric in origin, respectively, with a potential for perforation and impending mediastinitis. A coincident pleural effusion and acidotic serum (pH <7.2) correlates with the severity of injury. Worsening hemodynamic instability or systemic signs such as a change in mental status, fever, or tachycardia typically follow massive ingestions. In summary, no single symptom or combination of symptoms can identify all patients with an esophageal injury. Studies have shown that all asymptomatic patients typically have normal findings on endoscopy, whereas all patients with clinically significant injury (grades II and III) are symptomatic at initial assessment.

Except for massive and rapidly fatal ingestions, significant tissue destruction is noted within 24 hours. Phase I injury occurs within seconds, with erythema and edema evolving into shallow ulcers. Phase II is often the progression of injury. Vascular thrombosis results in further necrosis and mucosal sloughing in 2 to 4 days, followed by a period of granulation for 3 to 4 weeks, the critical window of esophageal wall weakness. Phase III begins with fibroblast proliferation, cicatrisation, and stricture formation over weeks to months. Scar formation is complete within 8 weeks in 80% of patients but often continues for 6 to 8 months.

IMMEDIATE THERAPY

The key to successful management of chemical ingestions is to identify the severity of injury and minimize its extension. The type and amount of ingestion should be readily identified. Airway assessment is the initial primary goal, followed by standard Advanced Trauma Life Support protocol. Stridor is the sine qua non of laryngeal insult and requires orotracheal intubation. Direct visualization of the oropharynx and a laryngoscopic examination are the initial steps in evaluating the extent of injury. The airway should be directly visualized with a fiber-optic nasopharyngoscope.

Immediately on the patient's arrival at the hospital, all oral intake should be prohibited and intravenous fluid resuscitation initiated. Chest and abdominal films can readily identify pneumomediastinum, pneumoperitoneum, and pleural effusions, all associated with full-thickness injury and necessitating immediate operative intervention. Blind passages of nasogastric tubes or blind nasopharyngeal intubation are contraindicated. Measures to dilute or neutralize the corrosive agent are contraindicated to avoid inducing emesis and thus reexposure of the esophagus to the caustic agent. Attempts to neutralize acids or alkalis also cause an exothermic reaction, further injuring surrounding tissue.

The indications for endoscopy are any patient with stridor, all intended suicidal ingestions, and any symptomatic children (vomiting, drooling) or those with oropharyngeal burns. Early endoscopy is the gold standard for the evaluation of caustic injuries and should occur within the first 12 to 24 hours. Most perforations occur in a delayed fashion on the second to third day after injury, when the burn weakens with friable granulation tissue; hence the mandate for early endoscopy. The most frequent exposures in children are inadvertent ingestions of mild alkalis, such as household bleach; endoscopy is not necessary in such a mild injury if the child is asymptomatic and the ingestion is unintended. Clinical observation for 24 hours to ensure normal esophageal function and endoscopy in symptomatic cases with dysphagia or drooling (Fig. 1) is standard.

Caustic injuries are classified endoscopically in the same manner as surface thermal injuries (see Table 2). The grade of mucosal injury at endoscopy has been shown to be the strongest predictive factor for the occurrence of systemic and GI complications and mortality. First-degree injuries are superficial, and the mucosa sloughs without scar or stricture. Second-degree injuries penetrate through the mucosa to the muscular layer with thrombosis, and within days the sloughing causes deep ulcerations. Second-degree injuries can be subclassified by the presence of circumferential injury as opposed to linear or patchy areas. Third degree is a full-

Caustic Ingestion Algorithm

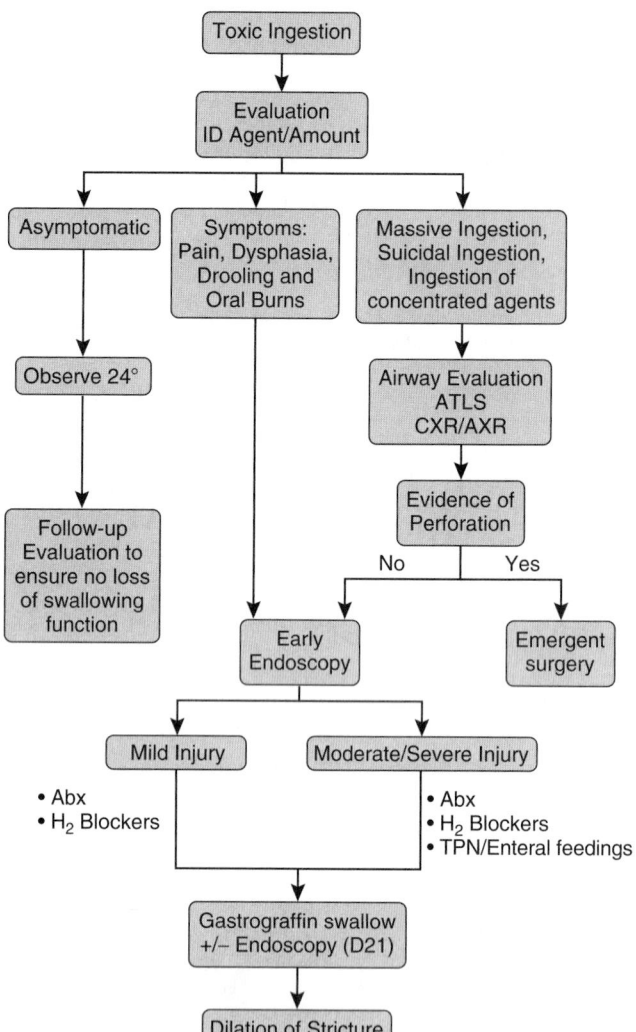

Figure 1 Management algorithm based on presence of symptoms and degree of injury. Treatment algorithm for management of patients who have swallowed a caustic agent. This algorithm stratifies treatment based on (+/-) symptoms or massive quantity of ingestion. *Modified from Fischer AC, Haller, AJ Jr. In Cameron JL: Current surgical therapy, ed 7, Philadelphia, 2001, Elsevier Mosby, and from Colombani PM. In Cameron JL: Current Surgical Therapy, ed 8, Philadelphia, 2004, Elsevier Mosby.*

Table 2: Classification of Injury

Grade	Degree of Injury	Endoscopic Findings
I	Superficial mucosal burn	Mucosal edema and hypermia
IIA	Transmucosal injury	Patchy ulcerations, exudates, sloughing mucosa
IIB	Transmucosal injury	Circumferential injury
III	Transmural injury + Periesophageal or perigastric extension	Deep ulcerations. Black or gray discoloration, full-thickness necrosis

Modified classification from Estrera A, Taylor W, Mills LJ, and others: Ann Thorac Surg 41:276, 1986.

thickness penetration with mediastinitis or peritonitis occurring usually within 48 hours. Grades I and IIA do not evoke strictures. All grade III injuries and more than 70% of grade IIB injuries will have variable progression to strictures. The limitations of endoscopy are (1) the presence of circumferential burns that preclude full visualization, (2) the unrecognized progression of injuries resulting in delayed perforation at 7 to 14 days, and (3) the difficulty in reliably distinguishing grade IIB from grade III. Differentiation between second- and third-degree injury may be difficult, but third-degree injury is often indicated by the presence of gray friable tissue, thrombosed submucosal vessels, and extensive black eschar. Endoscopy up to the site of maximal esophageal injury provides the ideal evaluation for directed therapy (see Fig. 1) and minimizes the risks of iatrogenic perforation. Contrast radiography, performed first with water-soluble contrast followed by thin barium contrast, can identify grade III injuries. Extravasation is diagnostic for perforation.

If mild injury (grades I and IIA) is found, the patient should be started on liquids, progressing to regular diet in 24 to 48 hours, and a follow-up contrast study to ensure no stricture formation should be performed at approximately 3 weeks. Grade IIB and III injuries should be observed at a minimum of 48 hours to 1 week, with hyperalimentation for nutrition. A high index of suspicion is essential to detect a delayed perforation or progression to full-thickness injury. For nutrition, intravenous alimentation or enteric feedings are essential. Gastrostomies are placed in severe injuries for an enteral conduit and retrograde dilatations.

Most investigators recommend the judicious use of prophylactic antibiotics such as ampicillin or clindamycin to cover the oropharyngeal flora for 3 weeks. At 1 to 2 weeks postingestion, the height of tissue remodeling occurs and correlates within this window with the timing of a potential delayed perforation. Gastric acid suppression with histamine (H2) blockers is empirically recommended to decrease acid reflux secondary to the esophageal dysmotility and theoretically decrease stricture rates. The therapeutic role of corticosteroids is controversial in preventing strictures. A controlled trial has shown no proven benefit. Grade I and IIA injuries do not result in strictures, and thus steroids provide no potential benefit; grade III injuries evolve into strictures regardless of therapy. Steroids may actually be detrimental in masking an evolving perforation. No clinical studies have evaluated collagen synthesis inhibitors, such as N-acetylcysteine, which are experimental lathyrogenic compounds designed to inhibit stricture formation.

SURGICAL INTERVENTION

The extent of tissue injury dictates management. Early surgical exploration is essential for visceral perforation or necrosis of surrounding structures. Estrera and associates showed that three of eight grade IIB patients actually had full-thickness injuries (grade III) requiring immediate surgery. Because endoscopy is limited to superficial mucosal evaluation, laparoscopy can assist in documenting full-thickness injury, except for the posterior serosal aspect of the stomach. Some surgeons advocate routine laparoscopy or laparotomy for all patients with grade IIB and III burns of the esophagus for evaluation of serosal surfaces to determine a full-thickness injury.

The severity of the endoscopic grade of injury correlates with the expected incidence of subsequent strictures, as shown by Webb in 1970. Endoscopic grades of injury exceeding grade IIA are associated with the complications of esophageal perforation and stricture and mandate a follow-up contrast study in 3 weeks. All areas of anatomic esophageal indentation—the regions of the cricopharyngeus, the aortic arch, and lower esophageal sphincter (LES)—are potential areas where the ingestion can pool, causing a circumferential burn with delayed strictures. Marchand reported that 95% of severe strictures were usually situated in the distal esophagus, sparing the constricted LES.

Early identification of patients with full-thickness injuries to the upper digestive tract is critical for immediate resection of devitalized organs and limiting injury extension. The decision to perform emergent surgery is dictated by radiographic signs of perforation,

the presence of peritoneal signs, or endoscopic stigmata of a full-thickness injury. No single criterion can identify those patients without an obvious perforation who require surgery. A depressed or agitated mental status, shock, persistent acidemia, or coagulation disorders are usually correlated with severe intraoperative findings. Delaying surgery has been correlated with increased morbidity and mortality. Identifying the subtle progression of injuries in patients who have not initially manifested evidence of significant tissue damage is challenging. The overall mortality rate is high but has been reduced from 20% to 3% over the past 20 years because of improved and timely surgery and the early introduction of hyperalimentation and antibiotics. The morbidity for full-thickness esophageal necrosis remains high at 100% with a prohibitive 20% mortality.

The operative field should span from the mandible to the pelvis to accommodate cervical, thoracic, and abdominal approaches. Emergent operative intervention is best approached through the abdomen with complete visualization of the stomach and contiguous structures. Black eschar and thrombosis of the submucosal vessels indicate full-thickness gastric injury and warrant consideration of a total gastrectomy. Severe gastric injury is often associated with an equally severe esophageal injury. Patients can be managed with an esophagectomy, cervical esophagostomy, and feeding gastrostomy and jejunostomy, or alternatively with an esophagectomy with transhiatal gastric transposition. An emergent esophageal resection can be completed by a transhiatal approach, necessitating a cervical esophagostomy and avoiding a thoracotomy. This transhiatal dissection is actually facilitated by the accompanying extensive periesophageal edema. Delaying resection in the setting of third-degree burns and perforation is associated with 100% mortality. Tracheoesophageal fistulae can occur within the first week of injury, particularly with battery injuries, and necessitate a tracheostomy, a cervical esophagostomy to exclude the thoracic esophagus, and a gastrostomy. After immediate and urgent resection, the reconstruction is delayed for several months until full recovery.

Limiting the severity of injury is important because esophageal replacement can be problematic and less satisfactory than retention of a scarred, damaged but functional esophagus. The reconstruction of a destroyed esophagus is challenging and may require a substernal isoperistaltic colon interposition with the right or transverse colon or a reversed gastric tube. A colon interposition is the most widely used anatomic reconstruction. It provides a similar anatomic reservoir and dependable blood supply. Redundancy and stasis may present as late complications. Gastric tubes may be of inadequate length, usually because of the original injury and associated stricture; furthermore, an emergently placed gastrostomy may limit a gastric tube reconstruction. Other disadvantages are dumping symptoms following the usual pyloroplasty and reflux esophagitis occurring above the esophagogastric anastomosis. Microvascularized free tissue jejunal grafts are excellent reconstructive bridges for minimal defects, particularly those in the hypopharynx, and are used in conjunction with the previously described surgical techniques.

LATE SEQUELAE

The most serious complication from a caustic ingestion is an esophageal stricture and its potential malignant transformation. Corticosteroid therapy was thought to prevent esophageal stricture and severe scarring. The use of steroids in the acute caustic burn remains highly controversial. Anderson's controlled trial demonstrated that strictures did not occur in patients with grade I injuries, whereas they typically did occur in grade III injuries regardless of steroids. In grade II injuries, 1 of 15 patients treated with steroids developed strictures compared with 0 of 5 patients in the control group. A European retrospective review of all clinical studies also showed no benefit of systemic steroids, which actually led to adverse effects. Worsening dysphagia usually implicates a stricture, which can be documented radiographically. Bougienage is useful in the setting of a documented stricture no less than 4 weeks postingestion. Earlier dilations have a nontrivial risk of iatrogenic perforations. Dilatation should be performed on alternative weeks, aiming for a passage of a 46- to 50-F dilator in adults to a 32- to 36-F dilator in toddlers. Intractable strictures require a bypass, resection or esophagoplasty. Persistent strictures or iatrogenic perforation may require an esophagectomy with an esophagogastrostomy or a colon interposition.

An esophageal bypass leaves the native esophagus in situ with the reconstruction of a new esophageal conduit and risks the formation of a mucocele in the isolated segment. A mucocele can be a potential source of abscess formation, but the risk of this is probably negligible given the absence of functional mucosa following a severe corrosive injury. In general, chronic strictures following esophageal burns are regarded as premalignant. The risk of carcinomatous degeneration in a stricture of the residual esophagus is said to be up to 1000-fold higher than the expected frequency in the general population. In 1955, Marchand was unable to document any cases of carcinoma in follow-up of 133 patients; however, the interval between injury and the development of cancer typically is greater than 40 years. The location of the cancer is at the site of the stricture, usually in the midesophagus, and often a squamous cell. Long-term annual follow-up of grade IIB and III injuries is warranted given this high incidence of cicatrical cancer. Continuing or recurrent dysphagia after a caustic ingestion should be evaluated serially with both endoscopy and periodic brushings and radiographic barium swallow annually.

In summary, the ingestion of toxic chemicals continues to require emergent medical and surgical intervention despite preventive strategies. The initiation of broad-based prevention strategies can increase public awareness and reduce the incidence of severe injuries. Early recognition of the extent of injury, aggressive management, and early surgical intervention correlate with the lowest morbidity and mortality.

INJURY FROM UNCOMMON AGENTS

Unusual ingestions bear comment. Button batteries, such as those in hearing aids, watches, and computer games, are solid caustic ingestions common to children. Each contains concentrated caustic alkalis, similar to crystalline lye, with a potential for significant burns, leakage, and pressure necrosis. Intact batteries, which pass the pylorus in asymptomatic patients, can be followed with serial stool examinations for up to 7 days. In children aged younger than 6 years, batteries greater than 15 mm are not likely to pass the pylorus spontaneously. Failure to pass the pylorus within 48 hours requires retrieval by endoscopy. A thorough evaluation is mandatory because a delay in diagnosis can result in an aortoesophageal perforation or tracheal esophageal perforation.

Notably, the ingestion of concentrated hydrofluoric acid (HF) unexpectedly produces liquefactive necrosis and fatal systemic absorption with life-threatening disturbance of calcium metabolism. The risk of perforation by passage of a nasogastric tube is markedly lower than the risk of death by systemic absorption of HF. Unique only to this exposure, blind nasogastric decompression to evacuate the stomach is acceptable because these exposures are otherwise universally fatal.

SUGGESTED READINGS

Anderson KD, Rouse TM, Randolph JG: A controlled trial of corticosteroids in children with corrosive injury of the esophagus, *N Engl J Med* 323:637, 1990.

Cattan P, Munoz-Bangrand N, Berney T, and others: Extensive abdominal surgery after caustic ingestion, *Ann Surg* 231:519, 2000.

Estrera A, Taylor W, Mills LJ, and others: Corrosive burns of the esophagus and stomach: a recommendation for an aggressive surgical approach, *Ann Thorac Surg* 41:276, 1986.

Haller JA, Andrews HG, White JJ: Pathophysiology and management of acute corrosive burns of the esophagus: results and treatment in 285 children, *J Pediat Surg* 6:578, 1971.

Hugh TB, Kelly MD: Corrosive ingestion and the surgeon, *J Am Coll Surg* 189:508, 1999.

Kim YT, Sung SW, Kim JH: Is it necessary to resect the diseased esophagus in performing reconstruction for corrosive esophageal stricture? *Eur J Cardiothorac Surg* 20:1, 2001.

Marchand P: Caustic strictures of esophagus, *Thorax* 10:171, 1956.

Sugawa C, Lucas CF: Caustic injury of the upper gastrointestinal tract in adults: a clinical and endoscopic study, *Surgery* 106:802, 1989.

Webb WR, Koutras P, Ecker RR, and others: An evaluation of steroids and antibiotics in caustic burns of the esophagus, *Ann Thorac Surg* 9:95, 1970.

MANAGEMENT OF ESOPHAGEAL TUMORS

Christian G. Peyré, MD, and Tom R. DeMeester, MD

INTRODUCTION

The incidence of esophageal cancer is on the rise in the United States and accounts for approximately 4% of cancers diagnosed each year. It frequently presents as advanced disease and accordingly has an overall poor rate of survival. Historically, squamous cell carcinoma predominated, but the incidence of adenocarcinoma has risen sixfold over the last quarter century; it now represents the most common histologic type of esophageal cancer, accounting for 55% of all diagnoses in the United States. Although smoking and alcohol use are the most important risk factors for squamous cell carcinoma, Barrett's esophagus (BE) and long-standing gastroesophageal reflux disease (GERD) are the predominant risk factors in the development of esophageal adenocarcinoma.

GERD affects nearly 20 million Americans. Reflux of gastroduodenal contents into the distal esophagus initiates a sequence of epithelial changes in response to cellular injury from normal squamous mucosa to cardiac-type mucosa to intestinal metaplasia to dysplasia and ultimately to invasive adenocarcinoma. Greater understanding of the relationship among reflux, intestinal metaplasia, and adenocarcinoma; liberal use of diagnostic flexible endoscopy; and widespread adoption of surveillance programs for BE have resulted in increased detection of esophageal tumors at early stages.

PRESENTATION

Dysphagia is the most common presentation of esophageal cancer, accounting for nearly half of patients. One fourth of patients are discovered at endoscopy performed for chronic GERD symptoms or BE surveillance. Other common presentations include bleeding (anemia or hematemesis) and chest or abdominal pain.

Typically, patients presenting with dysphagia are more likely to have locally advanced disease with nodal metastasis. Patients diagnosed without dysphagia because of GERD assessment or BE surveillance are more likely to have limited early disease. Correspondingly, we have found that approximately a third of our patients who go to surgery have early disease limited to intramucosal or submucosal layers (T1 disease).

PREOPERATIVE EVALUATION

Preoperative assessment of patients with esophageal tumors is directed at confirmation of diagnosis, determining extent of disease, and evaluating a patient's physiologic status in preparation for surgery. Initial consultation should include a thorough history and physical examination in search of comorbid factors that may influence operative strategy. Particular attention must be paid to the cardiac and pulmonary systems, the most common source of postoperative complications. Furthermore, some patients may have significant weight loss and poor nutritional status that must be evaluated and addressed. Noninvasive cardiac stress evaluation and pulmonary function tests are necessary to determine cardiopulmonary reserve.

Appropriate patient selection for therapeutic resection requires a detailed evaluation of the local, regional, and systemic extent of disease. Currently, the two most important studies include the flexible upper endoscopy and computed tomography (CT) of chest and abdomen. Upper endoscopy should be performed to locate the tumor precisely, evaluate for existence and extent of BE, and perform biopsy to confirm diagnosis. CT is most useful to identify distant metastasis, most commonly hepatic or pulmonary. It underestimates tumor depth in approximately 40% of patients and has been found to have an accuracy of 55% to 63% in detecting regional disease, relegating its utility to the detection of systemic metastatic disease. Positron emission tomography (PET) and combined PET-CT are gaining favor as newer modalities with increased sensitivity over CT alone for the detection of metastatic disease.

Endoscopic ultrasound (EUS) is gaining acceptance as the modality of choice for the staging of esophageal cancer, particularly to evaluate depth of tumor penetration and nodal involvement. However, the utility of EUS is somewhat limited by incorrectly classifying tumor depth in 10% to 20% of patients and nodal status in 25% to 30%. Detection of nodal disease is likely to improve with the introduction of EUS-guided fine-needle aspiration. Accurate differentiation between intramucosal and submucosal tumor involvement is limited using EUS, with one report documenting accuracy as low as 14% for tumors located near the gastroesophageal junction, likely because of the inability to differentiate tumor from localized edema.

We have begun to use endoscopic mucosal resection (EMR) for early lesions to determine the depth of tumor penetration. It is used to sample an area of BE or a lesion limited to 20 mm in diameter. The depth of the resection is often into the muscularis propria and thus allows more accurate determination of tumor depth by histologic analysis.

SURGICAL THERAPY

Esophagectomy is the standard of care for the management of nonmetastatic esophageal cancer, with the primary goal of complete resection (R_0) of the tumor and surrounding lymph nodes to maximize the opportunity for cure and minimize the incidence of local recurrence. There are several approaches to resection of the esophagus, and one is selected on consideration of patient's medical condition, surgeon's expertise, and hospital support systems. The

transhiatal approach is performed from the abdomen with blind dissection in the chest and a cervical esophagogastrostomy. The Ivor-Lewis approach is a combined abdominal and thoracic dissection with intrathoracic esophagogastrostomy. The en bloc esophagectomy is an abdominal and thoracic dissection with complete upper abdominal and thoracic-mediastinal lymphadenectomy (two field) and a cervical esophagogastrostomy. Some surgeons extend the lymphadenectomy to include the cervical region (three field). More recently, a minimally invasive (laparoscopic ± thoracoscopic) approach has been described. Vagal-sparing esophagectomy preserves vagal integrity and omits a lymphadenectomy; it was introduced as a resectional technique for early tumor confined to the lamina propria. This method preserves gastrointestinal tract innervation and function, and, by keeping the left gastric artery intact, provides improved blood supply to the gastric pull-up.

Reconstruction can be performed with the tubularized stomach, whole stomach, colon, or small intestine. The gastric tube remains the most popular method of reconstruction because it is the easiest approach, requires only a single anastomosis, has enough length to reach the neck, and serves as an effective alimentary conduit. Its deficiency is the reliability of the blood supply for performing a neck anastomosis. Colon is typically used in those patients with unusable stomach resulting from previous surgery or extensive involvement with tumor. Small intestine interposition is the most complex method of reconstruction requiring microvascular and multiple intestinal anastomoses. Consequently it is reserved for those patients without suitable gastric or colonic conduits.

Our approach to the surgical management of esophageal cancer has evolved and depends on stage of disease and the patient's physiologic status and overall medical condition. We have begun to limit the extent of surgical resection in favor of a more physiologic outcome in the earliest of lesions but advocate extended lymphadenectomy for those patients with more advanced locoregional disease and good cardiopulmonary reserve (Fig. 1).

Early Disease (High-Grade Dysplasia, Intramucosal Adenocarcinoma)

An increasing number of patients are referred to surgery with early disease detected on diagnostic or surveillance endoscopy. We recommend that patients with BE undergo endoscopies at regular intervals, with biopsies performed every 1 to 2 cm, with four quadrant biopsies at each level. The detection of high-grade dysplasia (HGD) is an indication for esophagectomy because HGD is a marker for occult adenocarcinoma or the future development of adenocarcinoma. Several series of esophagectomies for HGD reported in the literature document the presence of occult adenocarcinoma in the resected specimen to range from 30% to 50%. Others have advocated aggressive endoscopic surveillance for HGD despite reports that identify adenocarcinoma in 25% of patients at 1.5 years, 50% at 3 years, and 80% at 8 years with this type of expectant management strategy. Furthermore, overall survival is significantly worse for those patients who postpone esophagectomy until biopsy-proved adenocarcinoma when compared with patients who undergo definitive surgical intervention at the time of the diagnosis of high-grade dysplasia. This questions the wisdom behind the delayed expectant approach.

For patients with HGD or occult adenocarcinoma detected only on biopsy, we recommend a vagal-sparing esophagectomy as initially described by Akiyama. Our experience indicates that this type of resection, which preserves vagal integrity and maintains better gastric blood supply, can be accomplished with lower morbidity and mortality, shorter hospital stay, and improved gastrointestinal function than traditional esophagectomy. These patients have less diarrhea, less dumping, improved gastric emptying, and improved alimentation. It is a more physiologic approach to the management of early disease limited to the lamina propria of the esophageal mucosa (Fig. 2).

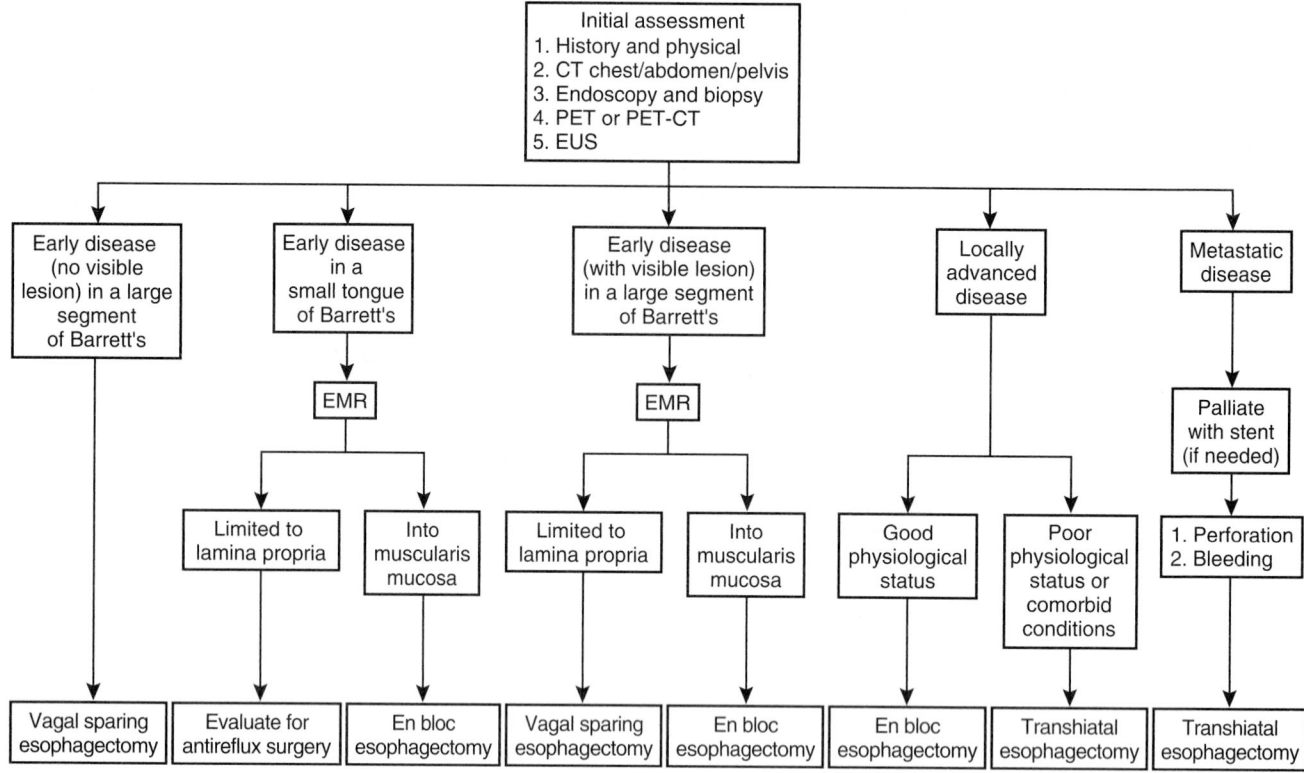

Figure 1 Algorithm for the management of esophageal cancer.

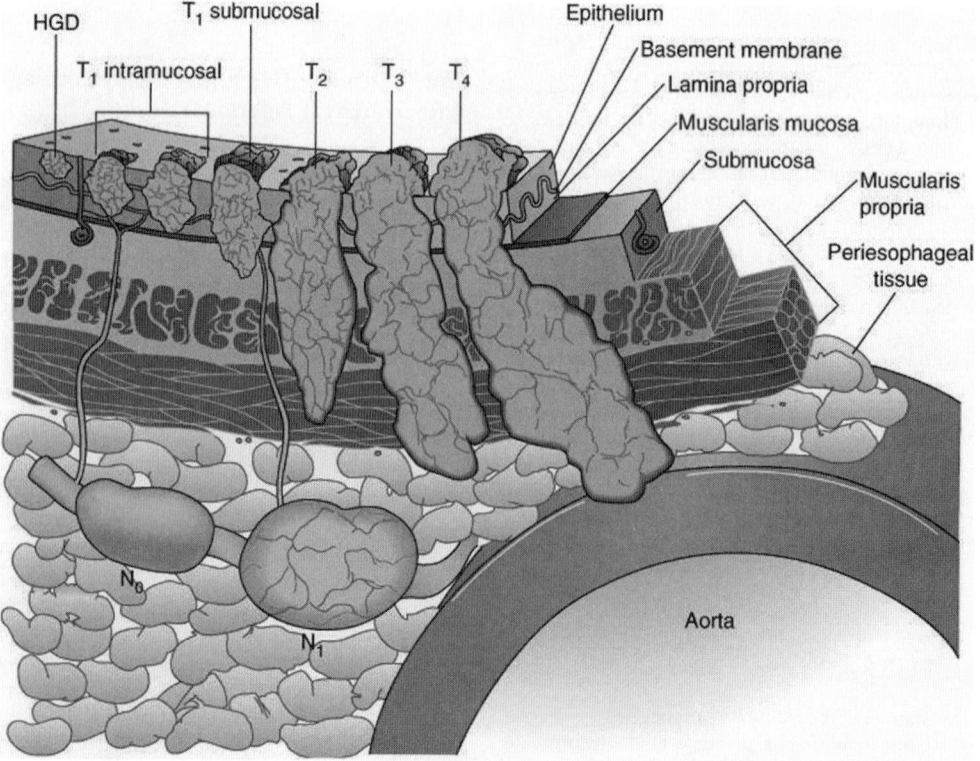

Figure 2 Primary tumor status *(T)* is defined by depth of tumor invasion. Regional lymph node *(N)* status is defined by the absence *(N0)* or presence *(N1)* of regional nodal metastases. *HGD,* high-grade dysplasia. *From Rice TW: Esophageal carcinoma: diagnosis and staging of esophageal carcinoma. In Pearson FG, Cooper JD, Deslauriers J, and others, editors:* Esophageal surgery, *ed 2, Philadelphia, 2002, Churchill Livingstone, p. 687.*

For those patients with early disease yet small, visible mucosal lesions, we initially perform EMR to determine tumor depth accurately and guide surgical therapy. EMR alone is adequate therapy for an area of BE <20 mm in diameter in which the cancer is confined to the lamina propria, is excised with clear margins and does not touch the muscularis mucosa. Tumors limited to the lamina propria and arising within a Barrett segment too large for total removal by EMR undergo esophagectomy by the vagal-sparing approach. Tumors that touch or invade the muscularis mucosa or that extend into the submucosa are treated as locally advanced disease with an en bloc esophagectomy. At present, EUS does not accurately determine depth of invasion in these early lesions, necessitating EMR.

Our current understanding of nodal metastasis suggests that nodal disease is exceedingly rare in cancer limited to the lamina propria and increases in incidence with deeper penetration (Fig. 3). In a recent analysis of 23 of our patients who had a complete lymphadenectomy (en bloc transthoracic esophagectomy) for intramucosal carcinoma, a total of 1020 lymph nodes were examined. Only one lymph node (0.09%) in one patient (4%) was detected with metastatic disease on hematoxylin and eosin staining, suggesting the incidence of nodal metastasis in intramucosal carcinomas to be rare. Subdividing this cohort of patients limited to the lamina propria or those penetrating superficially into the muscularis mucosa found an incidence of nodal metastasis of 0 of 13 (0%) and 1 of 10 (10%), respectively. Similarly, others have reported lymph node metastasis in intramucosal tumors to occur in 3% to 6% of patients. In contrast, more than 30% of patients with submucosal tumor penetration are found to have nodal metastasis. Consequently, we recommend that lymphadenectomy be performed for all tumors invading into the muscularis mucosa but that tumors limited to the lamina propria be approached by the more physiologic vagal-sparing operation. This difference in nodal metastasis between intramucosal and submucosal tumors underscores the importance of accurate assessment of tumor depth in early disease to guide surgical therapy.

There is emerging interest in performing endoscopic mucosal ablation or mucosal resection as definitive therapy for these early lesions in patients with large segments of BE. At present, it is our opinion that esophagectomy is the best choice for their management. Esophagectomy is the most effective treatment for the elimination of all dysplastic and cancerous cells. Furthermore, it eradicates any residual intestinal metaplasia elsewhere in the esophagus that is at risk of malignant transformation and any metachronous occult cancer at its earliest stage with the greatest likelihood of cure. Trials of ablative therapy of dysplastic BE have demonstrated some reduction in cancer risk, but the technology remains unproved because a significant number of patients progress to adenocarcinoma. In addition, EMR does not effectively address multifocal disease and fails to treat occult residual cancer in the Barrett's segment. It is our position that endoscopic ablation and EMR are inferior therapeutic strategies to esophagectomy in patients with HGD or intramucosal carcinoma in a large segment of BE.

Locally Advanced, Nonmetastatic Disease

Controversy exists over the best surgical approach for resection of locally advanced, nonmetastatic cancer of the esophagus. As previously mentioned, there are several popular options in current practice. Balancing the risks of morbidity and the oncologic benefit of each type of resection, we believe the en bloc esophagectomy is the best operation for such patients in good medical condition with adequate cardiopulmonary reserve. In our practice, the transhiatal approach is reserved for patients with comorbid conditions and diminished reserve who in our estimation are at increased risk for morbidity and mortality if a more extensive operation is performed.

Complete (R_0) resection, a guiding principle of surgical oncology, represents the best opportunity for cure. To ensure removal of all disease and to minimize local recurrence in esophageal cancer necessitates resection of the diseased organ and its extensive lymph node basin. The unique lymphatic anatomy of the esophagus results in unpredictable drainage that typically involves both upper abdominal and mediastinal lymph nodes and may occasionally even extend into cervical nodes. The en bloc esophagectomy represents the best oncologic operation that removes all nodal tissue in the mediastinum and upper abdomen (two field) and has been routinely extended into the cervical region (three field) by some surgeons.

Figure 3 Prevalence of nodal metastases and 5-year survival by depth of tumor penetration. *Data from Hagen JA, DeMeester SR, Peters JH, and others: Ann Surg 234:520, 2001.*

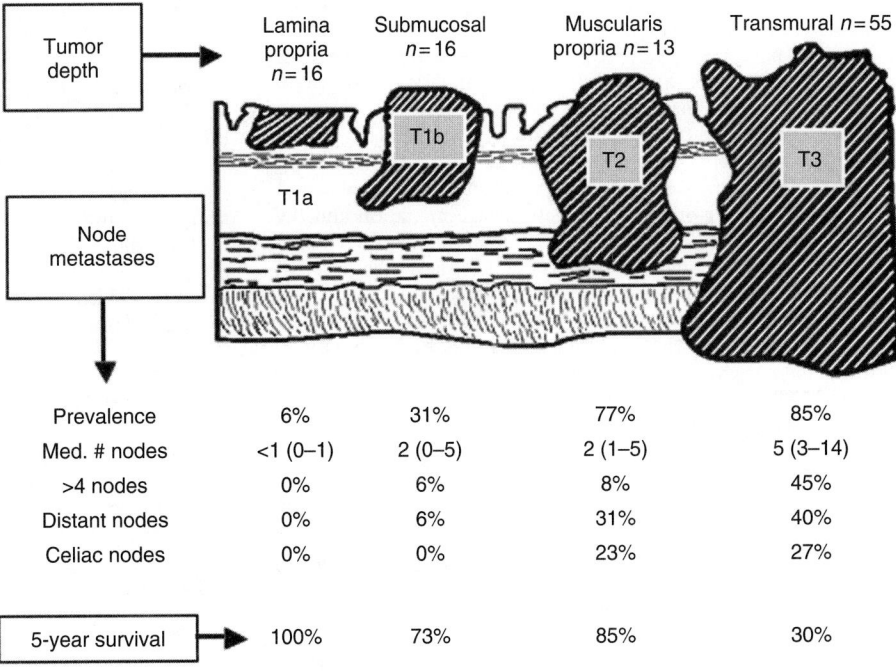

	Lamina propria $n=16$	Submucosal $n=16$	Muscularis propria $n=13$	Transmural $n=55$
Prevalence	6%	31%	77%	85%
Med. # nodes	<1 (0–1)	2 (0–5)	2 (1–5)	5 (3–14)
>4 nodes	0%	6%	8%	45%
Distant nodes	0%	6%	31%	40%
Celiac nodes	0%	0%	23%	27%
5-year survival	100%	73%	85%	30%

This is in stark contrast to the transhiatal approach, which has only an abdominal lymphadenectomy, often narrower in scope, with minimal removal of mediastinal lymphatic tissue. In comparing the en bloc with the transhiatal approach, data from the literature suggest that the en bloc esophagectomy can be performed with similar morbidity and mortality rates and is superior in control of local recurrence. Most important, extended lymphadenectomy offers a greater overall absolute survival from esophageal cancer.

En bloc esophagectomy demands appropriate patient selection and diligent postoperative care, with particular attention to the cardiac and pulmonary systems to minimize the morbidity and mortality of this operation and maximize the oncologic benefit. The en bloc approach is traditionally thought to carry a higher risk of complications than transhiatal esophagectomy, but improvements in intensive care and postoperative pain control with epidural analgesia have brought the complication rate to a level similar to that of the transhiatal approach. Comparison of large published series of esophagectomies over the past decade shows a mortality and morbidity rate for the en bloc procedure ranging from 2.5% to 10% and 24% to 75%, respectively. Similarly, the transhiatal approach has a mortality and morbidity rate of 2% to 11% and 26% to 69%, respectively. With appropriate support from anesthesia, surgical intensivists, critical care nursing, and interventional radiologists, en bloc esophagectomy can be performed safely.

Local recurrence is the most common pattern of failure after transhiatal resection, with a published rate that ranges from 14% to 47%. The rate of locoregional recurrence reported after en bloc resection ranges from 1% to 12%. In our own experience, we analyzed 100 consecutive en bloc operations with complete 5-year follow-up and found that only 1 patient (1%) suffered from local recurrence, indicating that the en bloc esophagectomy offers improved local control over the transhiatal approach.

Similarly, the en bloc approach has a greater impact on absolute survival than transhiatal esophagectomy. Several large series document the overall survival after en bloc esophagectomy to range from 39% to 50% for all stages. At our own institution, even stage IV disease had an overall survival of 27% at 5 years. The data from the transhiatal experience is less impressive, with overall survival reported from 23% to 29% for all stages and stage IV disease results in the single digits.

Recently, a randomized clinical trial was performed in Europe comparing en bloc and transhiatal esophagectomy. Overall, 5-year survival rates were 39% and 29%, respectively. Although not statistically different, close analysis of the data suggests that this difference might have been tempered by an increased percentage of patients in the en bloc group with stage III and IV disease (69% vs. 57%) and half as many patients with stage II disease (15% vs. 30%). Of note in this trial, hospital mortality was similarly low in both groups, 4% versus 2%, respectively.

A major criticism of any outcome studies between en bloc and transhiatal esophagectomy is the effect of stage migration and the comparison of dissimilar groups. One could argue that the en bloc operation more accurately classifies nodal status because of increased nodal sampling, and accordingly this selection bias would have improved survival stage for stage compared with the transhiatal approach. We performed a retrospective matched comparison between these two surgical approaches, looking specifically at T_3N_1 disease in patients with similar tumor size, more than 20 lymph nodes removed, and without neoadjuvant or adjuvant chemoradiotherapy. In these two groups matched for locally advanced tumor stage, a significant survival benefit was seen in those patients undergoing en bloc resection over the transhiatal approach when fewer than nine lymph nodes were involved with tumor. There was no difference in survival between the procedures when nine or more lymph nodes were involved.

Interestingly, there are data to indicate that a more extensive lymphadenectomy offers a survival advantage even when adjusted for the influence of T and N stage. This observation was recently reported in the literature with regard to gastric adenocarcinoma, and analysis of our own experience in esophageal cancer found similar results. Our study group consisted of patients who underwent esophagectomy alone, en bloc or transhiatal, without neoadjuvant or adjuvant chemoradiotherapy for nonmetastatic adenocarcinoma and followed until death or at least 5 years after surgery. As expected, tumor penetration and nodal involvement were the two most important prognostic factors for survival. Number of nodes removed, even when adjusted for T stage and N stage, was the next most important prognostic variable. We found that a survival benefit was seen with more nodes removed, and a receiver operator curve (ROC) analysis suggested that a threshold of 47 lymph nodes resected was necessary to see maximal survival benefit. En bloc operations typically remove at least 50 nodes, whereas the transhiatal approach is often limited to fewer than 28. Again, this finding adds to the mounting data suggesting a survival benefit of the en bloc approach with extended lymphadenectomy over the transhiatal approach.

Metastatic Disease

With improvements in endoscopic stenting and dilatation, there is less of a need for palliative resection in metastatic esophageal tumors. The most common indication for a palliative procedure is management of severe dysphagia, which can often be successfully relieved with endoscopic dilatation and stenting. Indications for surgical intervention include esophageal perforation, bleeding, and, rarely, unsuccessful stent placement. In these situations, the goal of operative therapy is removal of the primary tumor and restoration of intestinal continuity. The transhiatal approach is appropriate for most palliative resections except if invasion into vital mediastinal structures is suspected and careful dissection under direct vision is necessary. The esophageal bypass procedure is rarely indicated.

Follow-Up and Postoperative Chemotherapy

Patients are followed and investigated at regular intervals for the development of locoregional recurrence and metastatic disease. During the first 3 years, patients are seen every 3 months and then subsequently every 4 to 6 months. Each visit should include a history and physical, complete blood count and liver panel, and computed tomography of the chest and abdomen. Radiographic evidence of possible recurrence warrants biopsy to confirm diagnosis and can often be accomplished through interventional radiologic techniques.

Chemotherapy is reserved for those patients with four or more positive lymph nodes on histology of the surgical specimen or who have developed recurrence during follow-up. The toxicity of chemotherapy and the high prevalence of nonresponders to traditional 5-flourouracil-based chemotherapy regimens do not justify routine adjuvant chemotherapy. After en bloc esophagectomy, four or more positive lymph nodes has a significant negative impact on survival and consequently those patients may potentially benefit from chemotherapy.

ROLE OF NEOADJUVANT THERAPY

The perceived poor overall survival associated with esophageal cancer has spurred interest in multimodal therapy. The role of neoadjuvant therapy for esophageal cancer is controversial, and the data in the literature are mixed. Proponents argue that neoadjuvant therapy can downstage tumors and increase the likelihood of R_0 resection; some reports suggest an increased survival for surgery alone. Arguments against neoadjuvant therapy include the inherent harm of delaying surgery, the negative immunologic impact of preoperative chemotherapy during the perioperative period, and the unnecessary exposure and harm to nonresponders. Furthermore, the validity of existing trials must be scrutinized because the surgical arms often have poor results that do not compare with the results reported for en bloc esophagectomy or even transhiatal resection. In addition, with 5-year survival rates of stage I and II disease after en bloc esophagectomy in the 60% to 90% range, there is little benefit from neoadjuvant therapy in these early stages. The role of neoadjuvant therapy remains unclear, and criteria should be developed for appropriate patient selection as opposed to routine use. Chemoprediction, the assessment of a tumor's genetic makeup to predict response to a particular chemotherapy agent, will likely play a role in identifying those individuals best suited to receive neoadjuvant therapy.

SUMMARY

Esophageal cancer continues to be a devastating disease. The greatest impact on survival is the detection of early disease followed by complete removal of the tumor. Endoscopic surveillance for Barrett's esophagus and the low threshold for upper endoscopy of GERD patients has increased the detection of early disease and should continue to be encouraged. For those patients with advanced disease, en bloc esophagectomy represents the most complete oncologic operation. Multimodal therapy may be beneficial in selected patients, and further studies are necessary to identify appropriate patient populations.

SUGGESTED READINGS

Akiyama H, Tsurumaru M, Onon Y, and others: Esophagectomy without thoracotomy with vagal preservation, J Am Coll Surg 178(1):83–85, 1994.

Altorki N, Skinner D: Should en bloc esophagectomy be the standard of care for esophageal carcinoma? Ann Surg 234:581, 2001.

Banki F, Mason RJ, DeMeester SR, and others: Vagal-sparing esophagectomy: a more physiologic alternative, Ann Surg 236:324, 2002.

Hagen JA, DeMeester SR, Peters JH, and others: Curative resection for esophageal adenocarcinoma analysis of 100 en bloc esophagectomies, Ann Surg 234:520, 2001.

Johansson J, DeMeester SR, Hagen JA, and others: En bloc vs transhiatal esophagectomy for stage T3 N1 adenocarcinoma of the distal esophagus, Arch Surg 139:627, 2004.

Oh DS, Hagen JA, Chandrasoma PT, and others: Clinical biology and surgical therapy of intramucosal adenocarcinoma of the esophagus, J Am Coll Surg 203:152, 2006.

Peyre CG, DeMeester SR, Rizzetto C, and others: Vagal-sparing esophagectomy: The ideal operation for intramucosal adenocarcinoma and Barrett's with high grade dysplasia, Ann Surg 246(4):665, 2007.

Portale G, Hagen JA, Peters JH, and others: Modern 5-year survival of resectable esophageal adenocarcinoma: single institution experience with 263 patients, J Am Coll Surg 202:588, 2006.

Romagnoli R, Collard JM, Gutschow C, and others: Outcomes of dysplasia arising in Barrett's esophagus: a dynamic view, J Am Coll Surg 197:365, 2003.

ESOPHAGEAL STENTS

Malcolm V. Brock, MD

INTRODUCTION

More than 16,000 patients in the United States will present this year with esophageal cancer. The disease has now become the seventh leading cause of cancer death in men, and worldwide it is the eighth most common cancer. The two main histologic types of squamous cell and adenocarcinoma are thought to be associated with somewhat separate etiologies, with the former more related to tobacco and alcohol exposure and the latter believed to be related to the high prevalence of Barrett's esophagus in the Western world. The incidence of esophageal adenocarcinoma cancer in patients with Barrett's esophagus is approximately 0.5% per year. Since the early 1990s at the Johns Hopkins Hospital, patients with esophageal adenocarcinoma have outnumbered those with squamous esophageal cancer. Although the epidemiologic reasons remain uncertain, distal esophageal adenocarcinoma is most likely related to factors such as chronic gastroesophageal reflux disease (GERD), obesity, and male gender.

Complete tumor resection at surgery is the mainstay of therapy for early stage esophageal cancer. Unfortunately, in both histologic types of esophageal cancer, the majority of patients present to their clinicians with advanced disease that is not curative by surgery. Because the median survival of such patients is less than 6 months, palliative surgery has been replaced by nonsurgical techniques, primarily chemoradiation, brachytherapy, and endoscopic therapy.

Esophageal stenting is primarily a palliative procedure geared to treating the complications of advanced esophageal cancer—namely, esophageal dysphagia, esophageal fistulae, and esophageal bleeding. Although esophageal stent technology is still rapidly evolving, it is informative to consider briefly the development of modern esophageal stenting.

HISTORY OF ESOPHAGEAL STENTS

Although there is some debate about the origin of the word stent, the most plausible explanation is that it originates from the surname of Dr. Charles Stent (1807–1885), an English dentist who invented in 1856 a compound to cast dental models and splints. Although he used the compound to enable him to secure better and more accurate impressions of the mouth and oral structures, his name is now synonymous with any material or device that can hold tissue in place or provide support for biologic materials. Probably the earliest mention of stents in the medical literature was in 1916 by a Dutch plastic surgeon who commented that the use of "the mould of dental mass," which he later referred to as "stents mould," was instrumental in repairing the catastrophic facial injuries so prominent among soldiers in the World War I trenches.

The first stents widely used in the esophagus were constructed from silicon rubber (Silastic; Dow Corning, Midland, MI). In 1959, Celestin described the use of a plastic endoprosthesis introduced at laparotomy via an open gastrotomy to palliate an esophageal stricture. In the 1970s, Atkinson introduced an endoscopically inserted plastic prosthesis, with a much reduced complication rate. The Atkinson tube became particularly popular with gastroenterologists and surgeons over the years despite its small internal diameter, which resulted in many patients being unable to resume a normal diet after placement. In 1983, the modern era of esophageal stent innovation was ushered in when Frimberger published in Endoscopy the first description of the endoscopic placement of an expanding metallic spiral stent for a patient with a malignant esophageal stricture.

MODERN ESOPHAGEAL STENTING

Today, stents are made of either metal or plastic. The conventional plastic stents were nonexpandable, semirigid plastic esophageal stents and were employed mainly to palliate malignant dysphagia. Technically, they often were difficult to place. This was largely because these conventional plastic stents had a fixed external and internal diameter, and so the lesion had to conform to the stent. This meant that aggressive dilatation often was necessary for the stent to seat correctly. Perforation rates upward of 20% were observed, especially if tight, angulated malignant strictures were encountered. Once placed, many stents dislodged easily (migration), and malposition became a constant problem. Furthermore, optimal functional relief from dysphagia was difficult to achieve if the residual fixed internal diameter of a plastic stent was less than 12 mm.

Expandable metal stents have largely resolved many of the old problems. These stents, known as self-expanding metal stents (SEMs), were introduced in the 1990s, and despite their more expensive initial costs, they have rapidly supplanted the conventional plastic stents in the palliation of patients with esophageal cancer. Their internal diameter, once fully deployed, varies from 18 to 22 mm, making them ideally suited to relieve dysphagia. Recently, the authors of a randomized study comparing plastic and self-expanding metal stents concluded that SEMs improved a patient's quality of life. Furthermore, it was also found that the high, initial placement costs for SEMs over plastic stents were eliminated after 4 weeks of follow-up. In two large prospective trials that compared conventional plastic with expandable metal stents, it was found that expandable metal stents were far less likely to have complications. The complications of the conventional rigid plastic stents resulted in longer hospitalizations and higher costs associated with treating the complications. Although conventional rigid plastic stents are now largely of only historic value, there is a new plastic self-expandable stent known as Polyflex that is very much in clinical use. Figures 1 and 2 show examples of uncovered and covered SEMs.

There are four commercially available SEMs in the United States—the Ultraflex, the Esophacoil, the Z Stent, and the Wallstent—as well as one self-expandable plastic stent, Polyflex (see Table 1). The SEMs are composed of either stainless steel or Nitinol (a nickel-titanium alloy) that is tightly wound as wire coils or mesh around a small delivery device. Although these metals in stents are made to be inert, resistant to corrosion, and nonallergenic even in patients who are allergic to nickel, when the stent coils embed into the esophageal mucosa or submucosa, they do trigger a mild inflammatory response with fibrosis that reduces the risk of stent migration. The nitinol stents (Esophacoil and Ultraflex; see Table 1)

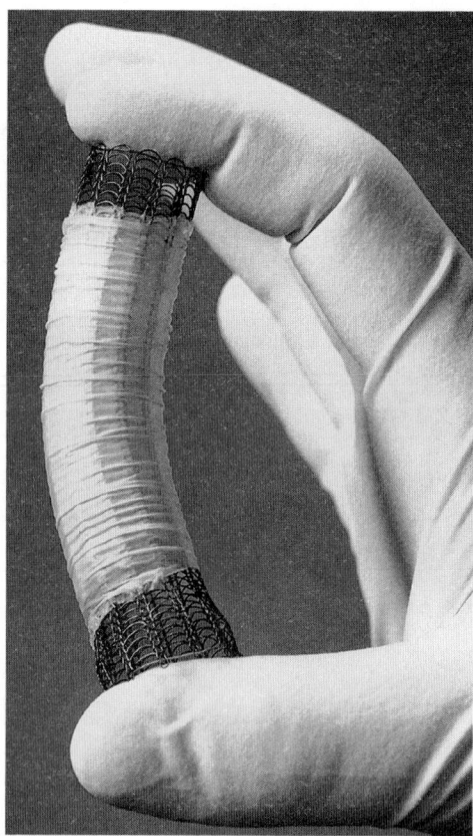

Figure 2 Expandable covered metal stent.

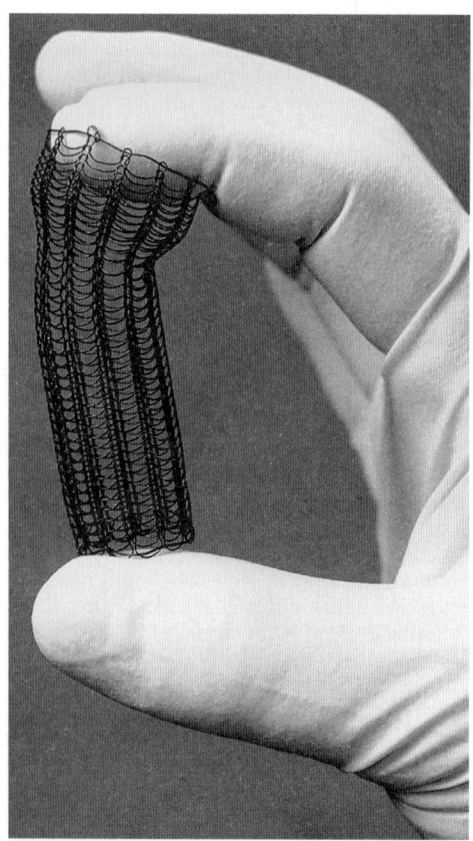

Figure 1 Expandable noncovered metal stent.

Table 1: Popular Esophageal Stents in Commercial Use in the United States

Stent Name	Manufacturer	Material	Covered Design
Esophacoil	Medtronic (Minneapolis, MN)	Nitinol	Uncovered
Wallstent	Boston Scientific (Natick, MA)	Stainless steel	Partially covered on the inside
Ultraflex	Boston Scientific	Nitinol	Partially covered or uncovered
Z-Stent	Wilson-Cook (Winston-Salem, NC)	Stainless steel	Fully covered
Polyflex	Boston Scientific	Plastic	Polyester netted lined with silicone

are made from a single wire and can be easily removed. The advantage of nitinol is that this alloy has thermal shape memory characteristics that enable it to expand at body temperature to fit the shape of a particular lesion. Covered designs are available for most SEMS, with a covering of polyurethrane or silicone. Most covered stents have "flared" proximal and distal ends that remain bare and uncovered to provide additional luminal anchorage. Covered stents are believed to have less tumor ingrowth but can potentially be more susceptible to stent migration, especially in high-risk areas such as the distal esophagus. Additional security of placement is provided by the radial expansive force of the stent after deployment that allows it to expand to its final shape and diameter. Today most stents that are placed have a covered design. Stents are available in a wide variety of diameters and lengths to fit various strictures. The most commonly employed stent is probably the 10 cm long, 17 to 23 mm diameter, covered SEM.

INDICATIONS—WHO SHOULD RECEIVE AN ESOPHAGEAL STENT?

In general, esophageal stents are placed when the dilatation becomes ineffective or the risk of esophageal perforation via dilatation becomes too high. The nature of the esophageal lesion itself often dictates whether esophageal stenting is the appropriate treatment. Table 2 describes the lesions that most often require stent placement. Relative contraindications include soft or noncircumferential stenoses, as well as markedly angulated strictures that may prevent adequate anchoring of the SEMs.

An often quoted surgical dictum is "no one with benign disease should receive an esophageal stent." Although this is still taught to most medical students and residents, the advent of easily introduced and retrievable temporary stents has allowed some compromise to this teaching, and patients with benign disease do undergo esophageal stent placement. Even now, however, esophageal stenting is primarily a palliative procedure indicated for dysphagia caused by a malignant esophageal stricture. Clinical judgment as to the timing of esophageal stent placement is important and must not be dismissed. A stent placed at either extreme of malignant esophageal dysphagia is inappropriate. A patient with mild dysphagia will not derive sufficient clinical benefit from an esophageal stent and may be more effectively palliated with other endoscopic measures, such as balloon dilatation. A moribund patient with only a few weeks to live is best placed in hospice care. In our experience, however, those inoperable patients with malignant disease who are in need of relief from dysphagia can be some of the most grateful patients once they receive a palliative stent and are able to swallow and enjoy gastronomic pleasures before their demise.

Benign patients with bronchoesophageal fistulae and refractory, nonmalignant strictures are also eligible to receive esophageal stents. Even in the early 1970s, there were reports of clinicians using Celestin tubes, often fixed transnasally for anchorage, to treat esophageal leaks, perforations, and resulting bronchoesophageal fistulae. In recent years, however, SEMs have increasingly been used to treat these conditions. In fact, SEMs have been used successfully to close both acute esophageal perforations immediately after they occur and chronic esophageal fistulae in patients who have failed conventional therapy of chest drainage, antibiotics, and hyperalimentation. Only covered stents should be used to treat bronchoesophageal fistulae and perforations. Esophageal stenting should be used only in a select group of patients with esophageal perforation and leaks. Some of the patients who could be considered are (1) those with a perforation in a normal or benignly diseased esophagus but with a medical condition too precarious for a major operative procedure, (2) those with a perforation of the esophagus that was diagnosed late in the course and in whom operative closure is not feasible, (3) those with a perforation of an esophageal carcinoma when surgery is precarious; (4) those with an anastomotic leak following esophagogastrectomy, and (5) those in whom there is immediate recognition of instrumental perforation during endoscopy.

The size of the perforations in published series has ranged from a few millimeters to several centimeters; even cases of rupture of 50% of a surgical anastomosis have been successfully managed with esophageal stents. When stenting any benign esophageal leak or stricture, one of the most important considerations is the length of time of stent placement because the stent must be *in situ* long enough for sufficient healing but not too long to cause fibrosis and late stricture recurrence. New SEMs, such as the Nitinol-covered retrievable stents, have made this treatment possible. In the management of esophageal perforations, most stents are left for approximately 2 to 3 months, with stent migration and tissue overgrowth having a higher complication rate than in patients with malignant esophageal strictures. These complications are due to the difficulty of anchoring these stents in place in the benign esophagus.

Because most benign strictures can be treated with dilatation, esophageal stenting for refractory benign strictures has been relatively uncommon, and until recently, there were only limited published reports. Corrosive strictures that are long and multiple are notoriously difficult to treat with dilatation. Placement of the fully covered retrievable devices, such as the Ultraflex or the Polyflex stent, for 1 to 2 months, followed by their removal, has resulted in high rates of success even in benign strictures caused by corrosive disease. With the Polyflex stent in particular, study patients are experiencing long-term relief without having to undergo further dilatation or surgery. As with esophageal leaks and bronchoesophageal fistulae, stent migration with these covered stents remains a problem.

Table 2: Lesions Amenable to Esophageal Stenting

Long, circumferential stenoses
Rapidly growing tumors
Extraluminal neoplasms resulting in compression of the esophageal lumen
Recurrent stenosis following
Chemoradiotherapy
Laser photocoagulation
Surgery—usually at anastomosis
Esophagotracheal fistula—requires placement of a covered self-expanding metal stent
Primary and secondary tumors within the mediastinum causing extrinsic compression
Esophageal perforation
Treatment of symptomatic gastroesophageal anastomotic leaks
Benign esophageal strictures

Modified from Jagannath S, Canto M: Endoscopic therapy for advanced esophageal cancer, unpublished manuscript.

WHICH ESOPHAGEAL STENT TO USE

Knowing the important, distinguishing properties of each stent is critical for any clinician placing them because it allows the selection of the most appropriate stent for the particular characteristics of a patient's malignant stricture. The physical properties of the most commonly used SEMs in the United States have been studied head to head because these esophageal stents differ according to clinically important variables such as rigidity, radial expansive force, absence or presence of shortening during expansion, radiologic markers, and the type of introducer. In summary, the choice of particular SEMs is determined by the physician's experience and preference.

Esophagocoil

In general, the *Esophacoil* has been reported to be the strongest of all the esophageal stents in withstanding compressive and angulation forces. *It* also had the greatest expansile force, and this may explain why many patients often complain of chest pain after receiving this stent. Cost is approximately $1500. These stents have not been widely used in the United States but are popular in Europe.

Wallstent or Flamingo Wallstent

This stent is manufactured by Boston Scientific as a crosshatched (woven) stainless steel wire in a double-wall configuration, with an occluding material between the two layers of the stent. It is now almost always covered, with only polyurethane on the inside. The Flamingo version is a tapered stent. Cost is approximately $1800. Once deployed, these stents are not removable. They are ideally suited for complex lesions because of their high radial force (second in expansile force after Esophagocoil), which makes them effective for the relief of dysphagia.

Ultraflex

Manufactured by Boston Scientific, this stent is made from a knitted nitinol mesh and is quite flexible. This ability to navigate tortuous strictures makes it ideal for upper-third esophageal strictures and therefore ideal for proximal esophageal lesions. Cost is approximately $1300. The *Ultraflex* has little expansile force compared with the other stents. Because Ultraflex stents have no bare metal ends, they are theoretically less traumatic to the mucosa and removable. Ultraflex stents are available both coated and uncoated, but the uncoated stent is susceptible to tissue ingrowth.

Gianturco-Zigzag Stent or Simply Z-Stent

This SEM is manufactured in the United Kingdom by Cook. It is made from stainless steel (bent in a zigzag shape) and a polyethylene covering with barbs on the outside or uncoated flared ends to prevent migration. Retraction percentage (or shortening properties) is low with this stent. Cost is approximately $1100. When positioning across the gastroesophageal junction is necessary, the stent is available with an antireflux distal valve, called the Dua.

Polyflex

This is a plastic, fully covered, self-expanding, silicone-coated, temporary esophageal stent (Polyflex, Microvasive; Boston Scientific, Natick, MA) with a cost of $400. In general, it causes less trauma to the surrounding tissue than metal stents and is removable. Polyflex stents have recently been shown to be effective as an alternative to serial dilatations at anastomotic strictures after transhiatal esophagectomy surgery.

Stent Selection

In the distal esophagus, an uncovered stent, such as the Wallstent or the Z-Stent, is the best choice to avoid any distal stent migration. Stent migration in this area often leads to severe gastroesophageal reflux symptoms and even to frank aspiration. In the proximal upper third of the esophagus, any stent can precipitate a persistent foreign-body sensation in the patient, especially if it transverses the cricopharyngeus muscle. The weakly expansile, flexible Ultraflex stent is preferred in the proximal esophagus because there is less of a propensity for patients to have a foreign body sensation with this stent in place. In the cervical esophagus, SEMs are generally not used because of all the potential risks, including tracheal compression and proximal migration.

HOW TO DEPLOY STENTS

Esophageal stent placement, therefore, should include endoscopic assessment, fluoroscopic guidance, guidewire insertion, tumor dilatation, and stent deployment. Esophageal dilatation is generally done before stent insertion. Although precise requirements for dilatation generally depend on the stent type, dilatation to no more than 12 mm is recommended. Proximal and distal borders of the tumor are marked using radio-opaque markers, endoclips, or contrast while the patient is lying supine. This position is critical because it is the same position used when the stent is deployed. SEM deployment is performed over a guidewire, with the stent introducer advanced until its tip is in the stomach. The introducer is then pulled back until the markings on the stent are placed within a 2-cm or more margin proximal and distal to marked proximal and distal tumor borders. Because full deployment to the maximum stent diameter predisposes to stent migration, most stents are only partially deployed to impart adequate tension against the obstruction. A 10- or 15-cm stent is usually sufficient to cover most malignant strictures completely. Final minor adjustments are made under fluoroscopy to ensure that the stent adequately covers the tumor markings. Endoscopic assessment alone often fails to identify accurately the most distal aspect of the tumor. Chest x-ray and barium esophagogram are often obtained postprocedure.

In consideration of the specific deployment of various stents, Ultraflex stents are deployed from a compressed state by gradually removing a suture that secures the stent. Once deployed, these stents, with their weak expansile force, often must be dilated because of incomplete expansion against a more rigid malignant stricture. For a Z stent, the delivery catheter is quite rigid and requires a relatively complicated loading process before fitting over a guidewire for stenting. Finally, Wallstents are deployed by pulling back a plastic catheter that constrains the actual stent. The manufacturer notes that the Wallstent can be reconstrained after approximately 50% of it has been deployed, but after this point, the stent must be fully deployed and placed or removed.

HOW TO REMOVE A STENT

Stents placed for benign conditions must be removed after the leak or fistula has healed. This can be especially challenging and technically demanding, depending on the type of stent originally employed. Of all the current stents, the most difficult to remove is the Wallstent because of its open-wire technology. The Ultraflex has the design most compatible with easy stent retrieval. It can be grasped at its most distal edge and then pulled proximally so that it invaginates and is then pulled into an overtube. Z-stents, on the other hand, are grasped proximally and invaginated into an overtube that is advanced distally. Polyflex plastic stents are extracted by use of a special wire loop, traction, and a twisting technique.

RESULTS

In most series over the past decade, the experience with SEMs has been largely favorable. The stents were correctly deployed and seated in almost all cases, and the mean dysphagia scores of patients improved after the stents were placed. As a reminder that esophageal stenting is a palliative procedure in patients with advanced cancer, the median survival from stent placement to patient death is 80 to 170 days.

COMPLICATIONS

Early Complications

Typically early complications are those that occur within 30 days of stent deployment. Early chest pain is the main complaint immediately after stent deployment. All patients should be given adequate pain medication before discharge. Chest pain is usually short in duration; prolonged pain occurs only in approximately 10% of patients. Pain tends to be more severe in those patients with proximal strictures that require a large-diameter stent. Other problems include bleeding, aspiration, perforation, fistulae, and fever. Stent migration is a particular problem with covered stents and those placed in the distal esophagus. Large-diameter stents are associated with less stent migration. In a prospective study of Ultraflex, Wallstent, and Z-Stents, stent migration was associated almost invariably with smaller-diameter stents. Other early complications include stent obstruction, aspiration pneumonia, bleeding, and perforation.

To avoid food impaction, patients should be advised to have only liquids for the first 24 hours to allow the stent to be fully deployed. Gradually, the diet can be advanced to a soft mechanical diet and then a regular diet. Still, all patients with esophageal stents should be cautioned to chew all foods properly and to avoid dense, fibrous foods (such as large pieces of meat).

Late Complications

Late complications typically are defined as those appearing after 30 days and are related primarily to tumor progression. Particularly with uncovered stents, tumor ingrowth can occur in up to 35% of cases. With covered stents, however, tumor ingrowth is not a common occurrence. Another common late problem is tumor overgrowth, which often leads to dysphagia. Occasionally, the overgrowth in the esophagus is not due to malignancy but is a benign, reactive epithelial hyperplasia, granulation tissue, or fibrosis attributable to chronic stent placement. Less common occurrences involve bleeding (3% to 10%), esophageal ulceration (7%), esophageal perforation or fistula (5%), stent migration (5%), and stent fracture (2%). Life-threatening complications are far more common when stenting of lesions in the upper third of the esophagus occurs, with the Ultraflex stent having the fewest complications compared with the other esophageal stents.

Chemoradiation Therapy

Finally, patients during chemoradiation therapy may have a higher incidence of life-threatening complications and stent-related mortality when an esophageal stent is in place. It is our practice not to place esophageal stents in patients who are about to undergo chemoradiation or who are under chemoradiation therapy. We believe that pressure necrosis on the esophageal wall from SEMs increases the likelihood of esophageal wall thinning and occasional perforation.

SUMMARY

In summary, SEMs have rapidly become an increasingly important part of the armamentarium to combat both malignant and benign esophageal strictures. As technology continues to evolve, so will indications for stents and their effect on the field.

SUGGESTED READINGS

De Palma GD, di Matteo E, Romano G, and others: Plastic prosthesis versus expandable metal stents for palliation of inoperable esophageal thoracic carcinoma: a controlled prospective study, *Gastrointest Endosc* 43:478, 1996.

Knyrim K, Wagner HJ, Bethge N, and others: A controlled trial of an expansile metal stent for palliation of esophageal obstruction due to inoperable cancer, *N Engl J Med* 329:1302, 1993.

Roseveare CD, Patel P, Simmonds N, and others: Metal stents improve dysphagia, nutrition and survival in malignant esophageal stenosis: a randomized controlled trial comparing modified Gianturco Z-stents with plastic Atkinson tubes, *Eur J Gastroenterol Hepatol* 10:653, 1998.

Siersema PD, Hop WC, Dees J, and others: Coated self-expanding metal stents versus latex prostheses for esophagogastric cancer with special reference to prior radiation and chemotherapy: a controlled, prospective study, *Gastrointest Endosc* 47:113, 1998.

NEOADJUVANT AND ADJUVANT THERAPY OF ESOPHAGEAL CANCER

Michael K. Gibson, MD

INTRODUCTION

Esophageal cancer is the eighth most common cancer worldwide, with the majority consisting of squamous cell carcinoma (SCC), and the sixth leading cause of cancer death. Although rare in the United States, it is highly fatal, occupying a position as the seventh leading cause of cancer death in U.S. men. It is much more common in men, particularly African Americans, than women. The shift in epidemiology from squamous cell to adenocarcinoma (AC) histology in countries such as the United States, the United Kingdom, and Australia is in contrast to the worldwide preponderance of SCC. Although gastric adenocarcinoma rates continue to decline, adenocarcinomas of the distal esophagus and gastroesophageal junction (GEJ) are steadily rising, particularly among white men.

Although it comprises a small percentage (1.5%) and low incidence (14,000) of total cancer cases in the United States, mortality remains high. Approximately 50% of patients present with unresectable, metastatic disease and are thus incurable. For those with locally advanced, nonmetastatic disease, cure is achieved in up to 40% of patients when multimodality therapy is used. As such, at most 20% of all patients presenting with esophageal cancer are cured. This high mortality rate is historically attributed to anatomic factors that lead to delayed diagnosis and early dissemination of disease. These factors include the intrathoracic location of the esophagus and the propensity for invasion of adjacent structures, the lack of a serosal membrane, the presence of an extensive network of lymphatics (Fig. 1), and the properties of a distensible tube that mask symptoms until disease is advanced.

The goals of this chapter are to review the current options for treatment of locally advanced, resectable esophageal cancer. These include surgery alone, preoperative and postoperative chemotherapy, postoperative concomitant chemoradiotherapy (CRT), and neoadjuvant concomitant CRT. Although the options are numerous, with some considered standard of care and others remaining investigational, it is often difficult to select the most appropriate treatment for a given patient. Nevertheless, a shared feature is the continued application of multimodality care with the goal of improving results achieved by the historic standard of surgery alone.

SURGERY ALONE

The initial and current mainstay of treatment for resectable esophageal cancer remains surgery, with the goal of achieving an R0 resection. Esophagectomy was the first curative therapy for esophageal cancer and remains one standard of care for treatment of locally advanced, resectable disease. Several approaches to resection are available, including minimally invasive surgery and the transthoracic (Ivor–Lewis), transhiatal, and en bloc methods. Selection of method is determined by the surgeon on the basis of technical experience, patient factors, and location of tumor. Major differences in these approaches include location and number of lymph nodes removed, as well as surgical morbidity and mortality.

Extensive data from a number of groups demonstrate that survival is directly related to pathologic stage. In a large series that was published by Orringer and colleagues in 1999, 800 patients with carcinoma of the intrathoracic esophagus underwent transhiatal esophagectomy. Both major histologies were represented (69% adenocarcinoma/28% squamous), and 234 patients underwent radiation before surgery. A second case series was published by the group at the Cleveland Clinic (see Rice and colleagues), where 480 patients underwent esophagectomy without induction therapy. Survival by pathologic stage as defined by American Joint Commission on Cancer system is shown in Figure 2. A common feature of both cohorts was the poor survival overall, with the Orringer study reporting an overall 5-year survival of 23%. A multitude of factors explains why, although surgery remains the mainstay of treatment for operable disease, local and distant recurrences after surgery alone are common. One in particular is the lymphatic anatomy that enables early distant spread of even stage T2 cancers, thus resulting in the presence of subclinical micrometastatic disease in the earliest stage patients (Fig. 1). As a result, approaches that combine surgery with radiation, chemotherapy, or both are increasingly used.

NEOADJUVANT AND ADJUVANT CHEMOTHERAPY

One approach to controlling the early spread of systemic micro-metastatic disease is to combine chemotherapy with surgery. Two large, randomized trials of preoperative and postoperative chemotherapy in patients with both adenocarcinoma and SCC of the esophagus provide conflicting results. In the U.S. study led by Kelsen, patients were randomized to either three cycles of preoperative 5-FU and

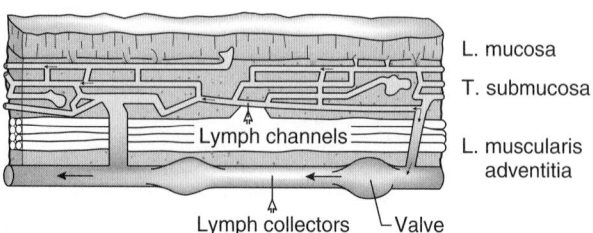

Figure 1 Lymphatic drainage of the esophageal wall.

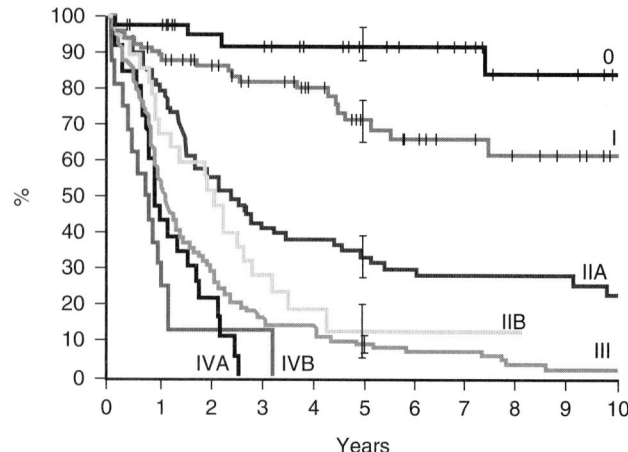

Figure 2 Survival after esophagectomy stratified by pathologic stage. *From Rice TW, Blackstone EH, Rybicki LA, and others: J Thorac Cardiovasc Surg 125:1103, 2003.*

cisplatin followed by surgery and two more cycles of postoperative chemotherapy or surgery alone. There was no difference in 3-year survival (23% vs. 26%). The UK Medical Research Council (MRC) study, led by Cunningham, evaluated two cycles of 5-FU and cisplatin followed by surgery versus surgery alone. In contrast to the U.S. study, the MRC trial found a better 3-year survival with the addition of preoperative chemotherapy to surgery (32% vs. 25%). There was a similar rate of R0 resection (59% Kelsen, 54% MRC) in each study, but patients in the U.S. study received more chemotherapy.

More recently, investigators with the U.K. MRC conducted a second study of preoperative chemotherapy. In contrast to the previously mentioned MRC study, which involved only esophageal cancer, the majority of patients in the second study had resectable gastric (74%) and gastroesophageal junction (12%) cancers. Distal esophageal adenocarcinomas accounted for only 14% of the tumors. Treatment consisted of three preoperative and three postoperative cycles of ECF (epirubicin, cisplatin, and infusional 5-FU) chemotherapy. Whereas 86% of patients completed preoperative chemotherapy, a slightly lower portion, 75.9%, of those who started postoperative therapy completed three cycles of ECF. Curative resection was higher in the chemotherapy group (69.3% vs. 66.4%), pathologic stage was lower in the chemotherapy group, and there was better survival in the patients treated with chemotherapy. Generalization of these results to esophageal adenocarcinoma must be made with care, as only 26% of patients had this disease.

Another approach to combining surgery with chemotherapy is to give the chemotherapy postoperatively (adjuvant chemotherapy) only. Several trials by the Japan Clinical Oncology Group randomized patients with intrathoracic SCC to esophageal resection with extended lymphadenectomy alone or followed by chemotherapy. In the earlier study in which adjuvant chemotherapy consisted of two cycles of cisplatin and vindesine, there was no difference in 5-year survival. The latter study updated the adjuvant chemotherapy to two cycles of cisplatin and infusional 5-FU for patients with an R0 transthoracic resection of intrathoracic SCC. At a median follow-up time of 62.8 months, the 5-year disease-free survival favored the combined therapy group, mostly for patients with node-positive disease. There was a statistically nonsignificant trend toward better overall survival as well.

A more recent study was carried out by the Eastern Cooperative Oncology Group (see Armanios and colleagues) in patients with adenocarcinoma. This phase II trial (E8296) evaluated adjuvant cisplatin and paclitaxel every 3 weeks for four courses in patients with completely resected adenocarcinoma of the esophagus, gastroesophageal junction, and cardia. Eligible patients had surgically staged T2 node-positive to T3-4, any node status, margin negative disease, and had not undergone preoperative therapy. A total of 55 eligible patients were analyzed, of which 49 (89%) had lymphnode involvement. The regimen was tolerable, and 46 (84%) of patients completed all four cycles of chemotherapy. After a median follow-up for surviving patients of 2.9 years (minimum follow-up of 2 years), the actual 2-year survival rate was 60%. The results are encouraging and favorable when compared with historical control patients treated with surgery alone.

CHEMORADIOTHERAPY FOLLOWED BY SURGERY

Given the encouraging but not overwhelming survival results obtained with surgery alone or with chemotherapy plus surgery, the logical subsequent combination is providing combined chemoradiotherapy (CRT) followed by surgery. Although not reviewed in this chapter, CRT without surgery in (mostly) SCC achieved cure rates approaching 27%, with failures involving a mixture of locally persistent disease and subsequent distant metastases. Escalating the

RT dose did not improve local control, so subsequent studies added esophagectomy after CRT to remove residual tumor. An additional benefit of surgery is the availability of a pathologic specimen, which provides the gold standard for response to neoadjuvant therapy. Chemotherapy, in addition to providing radiosensitization, may also reduce systemic, micrometastatic disease.

Phase II studies that used cisplatin/5-FU-based regimens demonstrated an encouraging pathologic complete response rate (pCR) of approximately 25% and survival approaching 40% (see Forastiere and colleagues). There was often an apparent improvement in survival and local control compared to historical control patients treated with surgery alone. In addition, pathologic response became a surrogate for postoperative survival. Of the 25% of patients with a pCR, 70% were cured, whereas in those with residual disease, survival was 30%.

Given these findings that surgical stage is the strongest predictor of survival in patients with locally advanced esophageal cancer treated with primary surgery and that better pathologic response portends higher survival, our research group aimed to evaluate the impact of preoperative chemoradiotherapy on disease stage and survival. Patients ($n = 42$) were treated with infusional cisplatin and 5-FU combined with daily radiotherapy (RT) followed by esophagectomy. Pretreatment stage was determined by combining results of endoscopic ultrasound (EUS), CT scan, and laparoscopy. Posttreatment pathologic stage was determined in the resected specimen. Pretreatment and posttreatment stages were compared in each patient to determine the effect of treatment on stage (downstaging, no change, progression). Logistic regression and survival analysis were used to evaluate the relationship between stage and survival, and these data were compared to historical information.

Median survivals for each pathologic stage were stage 0 (7 years), stage I (not reached), stage IIA (1.9 years), stage IIB (1 year), stage III (2.2 years), and stage IV (0.8 year). Higher pathologic stage (adjusted for clinical covariates) correlated with worse survival (hazard ratio 1.56; 95% confidence interval [CI] 1.16–2.1). The distribution of survivors by pathologic stage was as follows: stage 0 ($n = 5$), stage I ($n = 2$), stage IIA ($n = 2$), stage IIB ($n = 1$), stage III ($n = 0$), and stage IV ($n = 0$). On the basis of these data, neoadjuvant chemoradiotherapy for resectable esophageal cancer seems to affect the natural history of disease. The majority of patients were downstaged, and lower pathologic stage correlated with better survival. Survival stratified by pathologic stage was similar to that previously observed with similarly staged patients undergoing primary surgery alone. Similar results for patients treated with taxane-based preoperative chemoradiotherapy are presented in Figure 3. Subsequent randomized trials

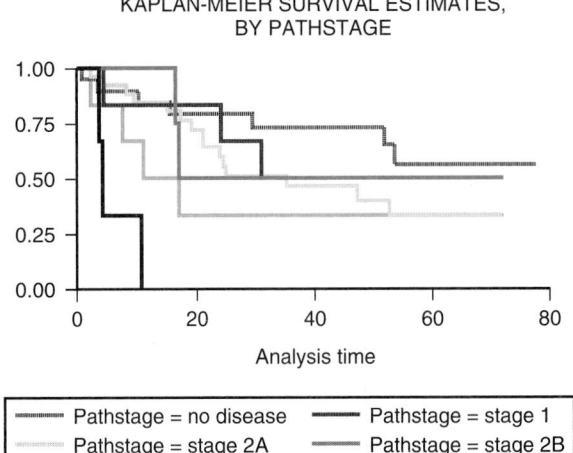

Figure 3 Survival by pathologic stage after treatment with taxane-based neoadjuvant chemoradio therapy.

assessing the value of preoperative cisplatin/5-FU/RT versus surgery alone, however, showed disparate results.

RANDOMIZED TRIALS OF PREOPERATIVE CHEMORADIOTHERAPY VERSUS SURGERY ALONE

There are at least six randomized trials of preoperative chemoradiotherapy versus surgery alone. They are summarized in Table 1. The trials by Urba, Walsh, and Tepper showed benefit, whereas the three by LePrise, Bosset, and Burmeister did not. Although the results are conflicting, no trial is considered definitive or without fault.

In the trial by Walsh and colleagues, 113 patients with adenocarcinoma were randomized to surgery alone or surgery combined with preoperative chemoradiotherapy. Radiation involved 40 Gy in 15 fractions. Chemotherapy, which began on the first day of radiotherapy, consisted of 5-FU 15 mg/kg by continuous infusion days 1–5 and cisplatin 75 mg/m day 1. Each drug was repeated during week 6 after the completion of RT. The pathologic complete response rate to neoadjuvant therapy was 25%, and the incidence of positive nodes in the surgical specimen was reduced from 82% to 42% ($p < .001$). The median survival was improved from 11 months to 16 months ($p = .01$). Survival at 1, 2, and 3 years improved from 44% to 52%, 26% to 37%, and 6% to 32%, respectively. Despite the striking results, the trial was criticized for the unexpectedly poor results achieved with surgery alone and the relatively small sample size.

At the University of Michigan study by Urba, 100 patients (68% adenocarcinoma) were randomized to surgery alone or neoadjuvant cisplatin, 5-FU, and vinblastine concomitant with 45 Gy of radiotherapy. The pathologic complete response rate was 28% (24% for adenocarcinoma). Median survival was 17.6 months with neoadjuvant therapy and 16.9 months with surgery alone. Three-year survival reached 30% versus 16% ($p = .18$). Unfortunately, this study did not have the statistical power to detect a modest but clinically significant improvement in survival. It is noteworthy, however, that the improvement in 3-year survival was similar to the outcome observed in the trial reported by Walsh.

A French multicenter randomized trial led by Bosset examined the role of preoperative chemoradiotherapy in 282 patients with stage I and II SCC. Although no survival benefit was seen, disease-free survival and local recurrence-free survival were prolonged. Several issues may explain the negative result. The radiotherapy regimen was unconventional, given as 18.5 Gy in 5 fractions over 1

week and repeated after a 2-week break for a total dose of only 37 Gy. Furthermore, single-agent cisplatin (80 mg/m^2 given 0–2 days before each week of RT) was given nonconcurrently with RT.

The study by LePrise and colleagues randomized 86 patients with SCC to two cycles of sequential 5-FU and cisplatin interrupted by radiotherapy to 20 Gy over 10 fractions. Median survival was no different between the two groups in these patients treated with a substandard dose of radiotherapy.

Two additional randomized studies were completed, each reaching a different conclusion. The Trans-Tasman Radiation Oncology Group and the Australasian Gastro-Intestinal Trials Group completed a study that examined one cycle of chemotherapy concurrently with 35 Gy of radiotherapy followed by surgery versus surgery alone in 256 patients with resectable SCC and adenocarcinoma. No difference was seen in either progression-free or overall survival. More recently, Tepper and colleagues published (in abstract form) the results of CALGB 9781. The addition of two cycles of chemotherapy and 50.4 Gy of radiotherapy to surgery in a total of 56 randomized patients improved median survival from 1.8 years to 4.5 years. Although these six studies differ greatly, a unified result is the achievement of a pCR rate no greater than 30% and long-term survival no greater than 40%, leaving a great need for improvement.

There are several possible explanations for these conflicting results. Comparing the six studies is difficult because of differences in factors that include sequencing of chemotherapy and radiation; doses, types, and schedules of chemotherapy; and radiation and surgical outcome. Although the results of these trials and other phase II studies have led to adoption of preoperative chemoradiotherapy as accepted treatment within community practice, the results are mixed. This approach cannot be considered standard of care and is best used in the confines of a clinical trial.

META-ANALYSES

There are two recently published meta-analyses of randomized controlled trials comparing neoadjuvant chemoradiation followed by surgery with surgery alone. The first study evaluated 1,116 patients enrolled on nine trials. When compared with surgery alone, the odds ratios showed a nonsignificant trend toward improved survival with neoadjuvant chemoradiotherapy (0.79, 0.77, and 0.66 for 1-, 2-, and 3-year survival, respectively); however, the improvement in 3-year survival reached the level of statistical significance only when the analysis was restricted to those trials using concurrent chemotherapy and radiation (odds ratio [OR] 0.45, 95% CI, 0.26–0.79).

Table 1: Randomized Studies of Preoperative Chemoradiotherapy

Ref	RO Resection Surgery Only Arm	3-year Surv., Surg.	3-year Surv., CMT	Median Follow-Up for Survivors	Histology	Schedule
Preoperative Chemoradiotherapy						
Le Prise	Not available ($n = 86$)	47%*	47%*	Not available	Squamous	Sequential to 20 Gy
Bosset	69% (94/137)	34%	36%	55.2 months	Squamous	Sequential, Interrupted (no 5-FU) to 37 Gy
Urba	88% (44/50)	16%	30%	8.2 years	Both	Concurrent to 45 Gy
Walsh	Not available ($n = 113$)	6%	32%	>5 years	Adeno	Concurrent to 40 Gy
Burmeister	59% (76/128)	19.3 mo	22.2 mo	> 5 years	Both	Concurrent to 35 Gy
Tepper	Not available ($n = 26$)	1.8 yr[†]	4.5 yr[†]	Not available	Both	Concurrent to 50.4 Gy

CMT, combined modality therapy; Surg., surgery, Surv., survival.

*Survival at 1 year (3-year results not available).

[†]Median survival.

The second study evaluated six randomized controlled trials of 764 patients (all were included in the previous analysis as well) that compared preoperative chemoradiotherapy plus surgery versus surgery alone. Most patients had squamous cell carcinoma, and in at least four of the six trials, radiation and chemotherapy were given concurrently. When compared with surgery alone, preoperative chemoradiotherapy again significantly improved 3-year survival (OR 0.53, 95% CI 0.31–0.93).

Starting with early studies of radiotherapy and surgery alone for the curative treatment of esophageal cancer, several decades of trials involving chemoradiotherapy confirmed the pathologic and clinical efficacy of this combined modality approach. Future challenges and opportunities involve developing a better understanding of the molecular basis for chemoradiotherapy that, it is hoped, will lead to a more rationale approach to combining chemotherapy and radiotherapy. The potential for translating this knowledge into clinical benefit through ongoing and future trials supports the expectation that the cure rate for esophageal cancer will continue to increase.

Suggested Readings

Allum W, Cunningham D, Weeden S: Perioperative chemotherapy in operable gastric and lower oesophageal cancer: a randomized, controlled trial (the MAGIC trial, ISRCTN 93793971). Proceedings of the American Society of Clinical Oncology Annual Meeting abstract, 998, 2003.

Ando N, Iizuka T, Ide H, and others: Surgery plus chemotherapy compared with surgery alone for localized squamous cell carcinoma of the thoracic esophagus: a Japan Clinical Oncology Group Study—JCOG9204, *J Clin Oncol* 21:4592, 2003.

Ando N, Iizuka T, Kakegawa T, and others: A randomized trial of surgery with and without chemotherapy for localized squamous carcinoma of the thoracic esophagus: the Japan Clinical Oncology Group Study, *J Thorac Cardiovasc Surg* 114:205, 1997.

Armanios M, Xu R, Forastiere A, and others: Phase II adjuvant chemotherapy for resected adenocarcinoma of the esophagus, gastro-esophageal (GE) junction and cardia (E8296): a trial of the Eastern Cooperative Oncology Group. Proceedings of the American Society of Clinical Oncology Annual Meeting, 2003.

Bosset JF, Gignoux M, Triboulet JP, and others: Chemoradiotherapy followed by surgery compared with surgery alone in squamous-cell cancer of the esophagus, *N Engl J Med* 337:161, 1997.

Brown LM, Devesa SS: Epidemiologic trends in esophageal and gastric cancer in the United States, *Surg Oncol Clin N Am* 11:235, 2002.

Burmeister BH, Smithers BM, Gebski V, and others: Surgery alone versus chemoradiotherapy followed by surgery for resectable cancer of the oesophagus: a randomised controlled phase III trial, *Lancet Oncol* 6:659, 2005.

Chan KW, Chan EY, Chan CW: Carcinoma of the esophagus. An autopsy study of 231 cases, *Pathology* 18:400, 1986.

Cunningham D, Allum WH, Stenning SP, and others: Perioperative chemotherapy versus surgery alone for resectable gastroesophageal cancer, *N Engl J Med* 355:11, 2006.

Devesa SS, Blot WJ, Fraumeni JF Jr.: Changing patterns in the incidence of esophageal and gastric carcinoma in the United States, *Cancer* 83:2049, 1998.

el-Serag HB: The epidemic of esophageal adenocarcinoma, *Gastroenterol Clin North Am* 31:421, viii, 2002.

Fiorica F, Di Bona D, Schepis F, and others: Preoperative chemoradiotherapy for oesophageal cancer: a systematic review and meta-analysis, *Gut* 53:925, 2004.

Forastiere A, Gibson M, Choi N: Radiation therapy, chemoradiotherapy, and neoadjuvant approaches for localized esophageal cancer, *UpToDate* 14.1, March 2007.

Forastiere AA, Heitmiller RF, Lee DJ, and others: Intensive chemoradiation followed by esophagectomy for squamous cell and adenocarcinoma of the esophagus, *Cancer J Sci Am* 3:144, 1997.

Forastiere AA, Orringer MB, Perez-Tamayo C, and others: Preoperative chemoradiation followed by transhiatal esophagectomy for carcinoma of the esophagus: final report, *J Clin Oncol* 11:1118, 1993.

Jemal A, Tiwari RC, Murray T, and others: Cancer statistics, 2004. *CA Cancer J Clin* 54:8, 2004.

Kelsen DP, Ginsberg R, Pajak TF, and others: Chemotherapy followed by surgery compared with surgery alone for localized esophageal cancer, *N Engl J Med* 339:1979, 1998.

Le Prise E, Etienne PL, Meunier B, and others: A randomized study of chemotherapy, radiation therapy, and surgery versus surgery for localized squamous cell cancer of the esophagus, *Cancer* 73:1779, 1994.

Medical Research Council Oesophageal Cancer Working Group: Surgical resection with or without preoperative chemotherapy in oesophageal cancer: a randomised controlled trial, *Lancet* 359:1727, 2002.

Orringer MB, Marshall B, Iannettoni MD: Transhiatal esophagectomy for treatment of benign and malignant esophageal disease, *World J Surg* 25:196–203, 2001.

Pisani P, Parkin DM, Bray F, and others: Estimates of the worldwide mortality from 25 cancers in 1990, *Int J Cancer* 83:18, 1999.

Rice TW, Blackstone EH, Rybicki LA, and others: Refining esophageal cancer staging, *J Thorac Cardiovasc Surg* 125:1103, 2003.

Schrump D, Altorki N, Forastiere A, and others Cancer of the esophagus. In DeVita V, Hellman J, Rosenberg S, *Cancer principles and practice of oncology*, ed 6, Baltimore, 2001, Williams & Wilkins.

Tepper J, Krasna MJ, Niedzwiecki D, and others: Superiority of trimodality therapy to surgery alone in esophageal cancer: Results of CALGB, 9781. Proceedings of the American Society of Clinical Oncology Annual Meeting, (abstract 4012) 2006.

Urba SG, Orringer MB, Turrisi A, and others: Randomized trial of preoperative chemoradiation versus surgery alone in patients with locoregional esophageal carcinoma, *J Clin Oncol* 19:305, 2001.

Urschel JD, Vasan H: A meta-analysis of randomized controlled trials that compared neoadjuvant chemoradiation and surgery to surgery alone for resectable esophageal cancer, *Am J Surg* 185:538, 2003.

Walsh TN, Noonan N, Hollywood D, and others: A comparison of multimodal therapy and surgery for esophageal adenocarcinoma, *N Engl J Med* 335:462, 1996.

Endoscopic Treatment of Barrett's Esophagus

Matthew J. Alef, MD, Matthew J. Schuchert, MD, and James D. Luketich, MD

INTRODUCTION

Barrett's esophagus (BE) represents the replacement of the normal squamous epithelium of the distal esophagus with metaplastic, intestinal-type columnar epithelium containing goblet cells (Fig. 1). There is a well-established relationship between BE and chronic gastroesophageal reflux disease (GERD). Barrett's esophagus is found in 5% to 10% of patients undergoing endoscopy for reflux symptoms. Patients with BE have a 30-fold increased risk of developing adenocarcinoma of the esophagus (0.5% per year). The incidence of esophageal adenocarcinoma has increased by 5% to 10% over the past 3 decades, representing the greatest increase in incidence of all cancers. Despite advances in diagnosis and treatment, the overall 5-year survival rate in patients with esophageal cancer is dismal at 10% to 15%.

It is thought that esophageal adenocarcinoma arises in a stepwise fashion from Barrett's metaplasia to low-grade dysplasia (LGD), to high-grade dysplasia (HGD), and ultimately to intramucosal carcinoma. Theoretically, the eradication of BE would reduce and even eliminate this cancer risk. Currently, those patients with no dysplasia are recommended to undergo surveillance endoscopy with

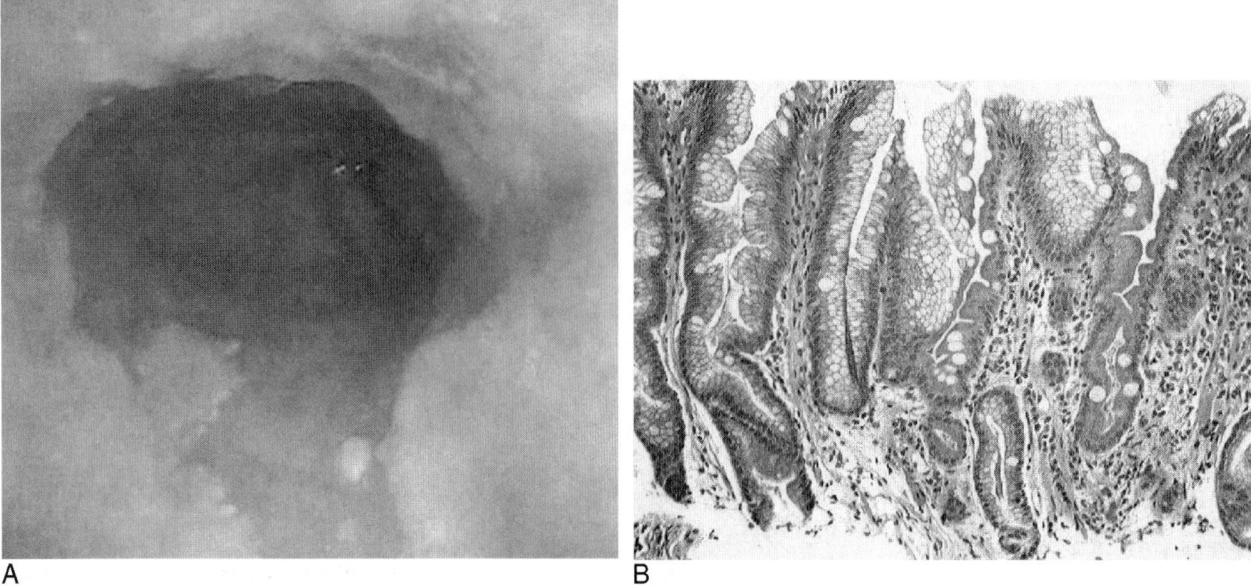

Figure 1 Barrett's esophagus. **(A)** Salmon-colored Barrett's mucosa is seen extending above the proximal extent of the gastric folds. **(B)** Microscopic features of Barrett's mucosa highlighting metaplastic columnar epithelium containing mucin-producing goblet cells. (*See color insert Figure 5.*)

biopsy every 2 to 3 years, and yearly for patients with low-grade dysplasia. HGD is a high-risk lesion and, if detected, should be confirmed by a second pathologist because of the substantial interobserver variation in establishing the diagnosis. When HGD is confirmed, patients have three options: intensive endoscopic surveillance, esophageal resection, and endoluminal ablative therapy.

Intensive endoscopic surveillance using the Seattle protocol (four quadrant biopsies using jumbo forceps at 1-cm intervals every 3 months) is designed to identify patients who progress from HGD to adenocarcinoma. Proponents of this technique argue that not all patients with HGD develop cancer. The cumulative incidence of progression of high-grade dysplasia to esophageal cancer ranges from 16% to 59% in published studies spanning 5 to 8 years of follow-up. Pathologic examination of esophagectomy specimens for BE with HGD, however, has shown unrecognized cancer in 38% to 73% of patients despite endoscopic biopsy protocols. In addition, adenocarcinoma and dysplasia can be multifocal and scattered, further complicating the accuracy of preoperative pathologic diagnosis.

Esophagectomy is the most definitive treatment for high-grade dysplasia by virtue of the complete removal of all Barrett's epithelium and should be considered the standard of therapy. Proponents of this approach highlight the substantial incidence of unsuspected intramucosal carcinoma in more than one third of patients with HGD. Critics point to the potentially high morbidity and mortality of esophagectomy and the fact that many patients may not have any cancer at the time of resection. However, high-volume surgical centers can achieve mortality rates as low as 1% to 5%, with associated low morbidity rates. In our recent review of 222 consecutive minimally invasive esophagectomies at the University of Pittsburgh Medical Center, the 30-day operative mortality was 1.4%. In carefully selected patients with high-grade dysplasia, esophagectomy can be performed with reasonably low morbidity and mortality rates and affords the best chance of cure in those patients who have progressed to carcinoma.

More recently, endoscopic ablative approaches have been developed in an effort to eradicate BE, HGD, and focal carcinoma in patients either unable or unwilling to undergo esophagectomy or intensive endoscopic surveillance. The main issue with these newer ablative strategies is limited experience, short and incomplete follow-up, potential incomplete ablation, and cancer recurrence.

PRINCIPLES OF ENDOSCOPIC ABLATION

The goals of endoscopic ablation include obliteration or removal of the abnormal Barrett's epithelium while preserving the overall integrity of the esophagus, minimizing morbidity, and offering a better quality of life for the patient. Groundbreaking work by Berensen and Sampliner demonstrated that when Barrett's mucosa is thermally damaged, it may be replaced by normal squamous epithelium, particularly in an acid-free environment. These observations spawned the development of multiple techniques designed to eradicate Barrett's mucosa selectively in an effort to minimize the risk of progression to cancer.

Although mucosal ablation techniques are less morbid than surgery, their efficacy remains to be proven in controlled trials, with the vast majority of available literature derived from single-institution, retrospective series. Although ablation appears effective in eliminating HGD in many patients (59%–98.6%), it is less efficient at eradicating the underlying BE (13%–88%; Table 1). All described ablative techniques have revealed a cohort of patients who have residual subsquamous Barrett's epithelium (Fig. 2). Subsquamous Barrett's epithelium remains at risk for progression to adenocarcinoma and complicates surveillance endoscopy because the metaplastic mucosa is difficult to identify and biopsy. Currently published ablation techniques have rates of residual subsquamous BE ranging from <2% to 69% (see Table 1). These rates loosely correlate with the depth of mucosal ablation, with more superficial penetration being associated with a higher rate of residual subsquamous mucosa.

METHODS OF ENDOSCOPIC TREATMENT

A number of strategies have been used to ablate Barrett's epithelium. Described techniques include laser ablation, argon plasma coagulation, multipolar electrocoagulation, and photodynamic therapy (PDT). Various techniques of endoscopic mucosal resection have also been reported. In addition, studies evaluating cryotherapy, heater probes, ultrasonic energy, and radiofrequency ablation are also under way.

Table 1: Endoscopic Ablative Modalities in the Treatment of Barrett's Esophagus

Modality	HGD Resolved	BE Resolved	Recurrence Rate	Subsquamous BE Rate	Stricture Rate	Complication Rate	Advantages	Disadvantages
KTP/YAG Laser	—	55%-88%	13%	20%-69%	12%	14%-33%	Noncontact	Many sessions, variable depth of penetration
APC	67%-98.6%	38%-98.%	33%-68% low power	25%-45% low power 0%-30% high power	4%-10%	24% low power 40%-60% high power	Noncontact, technically simple	Requires several treatment sessions
MPEC	—	25%-88%	7%	7%	2%	41%-43%	Noncontact, technically simple, relatively inexpensive, readily available	Requires several treatment sessions
PDT	77-88%	13%	5%-11%	2%-24%	4.8%-53%	4.8%-53%	Easy to perform; Only FDA-approved ablation method for treatment of precancerous lesions in BE	Photosensitivity, relatively high stricture rate
PDT + YAG/APC	77%-96%	42%-73%	13%	51.5%	4.8%-53%	94%		
EMR	59%-97%	53%	4%-30%	—	3%-30%	12%-60%	Histologic assessment; complete removal of circumferential short-segment BE; 1-2 sessions	Difficulty treating long-segment BE

BE, Barrett's esophagus; *FDA*, U.S. Food and Drug Administration; *HGD*, high-grade dysplasia.

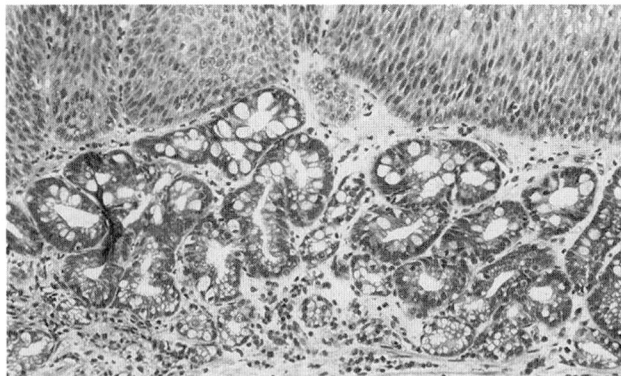

Figure 2 Subsquamous Barrett's epithelium cells. *From Hornick JL, Blount PL, Sanchez CA, and others: Am J Surg Path 29:372, 2005.*

Laser Therapy

Several lasers have been used in attempts to ablate BE, including the potassium titanyl phosphate (KTP) laser, and the neodymium: yttrium-aluminum-garnet (Nd:YAG) laser. Lasers generate an intense beam of light energy that thermally vaporizes the targeted tissue. The KTP laser (532 nm) penetrates to a depth of approximately 1 mm; the Nd:YAG laser (1064 nm) penetrates to a depth of approximately 4 mm. Both have shown limited promise in ablating BE but also have drawbacks related to their depth of penetration. The KTP laser tends to have a higher rate of residual subsquamous Barrett's epithelium because of its shallower depth of penetration, whereas the Nd:YAG laser has a higher rate of esophageal stricture because of its deeper level of penetration. In studies at four institutions, 35 patients were treated solely with the KTP laser for the ablation of BE. Although initial ablation rates were reportedly as high as 100%, 18% to 69% were ultimately found to have residual subsquamous Barrett's epithelium. The Nd:YAG laser was used exclusively on 31 patients from three institutions to ablate BE. After 1 to 6 laser sessions, there was an initial complete ablation in 100% of the patients, although recurrence was observed in 13% of this population. A fundamental problem encountered with laser therapy is the difficulty of providing homogeneous ablation and the need for repeated sessions in many patients (some requiring as many as six sessions for complete ablation). Odynophagia, chest pain, and dysphagia were observed in 33.3% of the cases, and esophageal stricture requiring dilatation has been observed in up to 12% of the patients. Although perforation and death have been reported, these outcomes are rare. Thus, the current data on laser therapy demonstrates complete elimination of BE in 55% to 88% of patients. There has been a 13% recurrence rate observed, and subsquamous Barrett's intestinal epithelium occurs in 20% to 69% of the patients treated with lasers.

Argon Plasma Coagulation

Argon plasma coagulation (APC) uses a high-frequency monopolar electrical current conducted to tissue via ionized argon gas. This treatment induces tissue surface coagulation, the depth of which typically ranges from 1 to 3 mm. However, the depth may reach 6 mm by varying the power, distance, gas flow, and duration of treatment. This technology is widely available, easy to use, and relatively inexpensive. Berenson first reported the use of APC to ablate BE in 1993 on 10 patients. These experiments demonstrated that regeneration of a neosquamous epithelium improved when the extent of ablation was contiguous with normal squamous epithelium. At least 12 centers have evaluated APC treatment on 444 patients with BE. Elimination of BE was reported in 38% to 88% of patients after follow-up ranging from 12 to 51 months. However,

long-term relapse of intestinal metaplasia was as high as 68% in this group of patients. Low-power-setting APC (30–60 watts) has been compared with high-power-setting APC (70–90 watts). Low-power APC studies have showed the development of subsquamous Barrett's in 25% to 45%, and an overall relapse rate of BE in nearly 60%. Complications of low-power APC occur with an incidence as high as 24% and include pain, ulceration, stricture, bleeding, perforation, pneumatosis, pneumoperitoneum, perforation, and even death. Limited studies with high-power-setting APC reported 98.6% ablation with no subsquamous BE. However, there was an increased incidence of adverse reactions, including chest pain and odynophagia in 40% to 60% of the cases, and esophageal strictures requiring dilatation in 4% to 10% of the cases. Subsquamous Barrett's epithelium was seen in 0% to 30% of these patients treated with high-power APC. Hence, studies to date suggest that HGD can be successfully eliminated in 67.0% to 98.6% of patients. In addition, the complete ablation of BE can be achieved in 38.0% to 98.6% of patients treated with APC with an associated recurrence rate of 33% to 68%.

Multipolar Electrocoagulation

Multipolar electrocoagulation (MPEC) delivers thermal energy to tissue by completing an electrical circuit between two or more electrodes on the probe tip. It is also a widely available, simple, and inexpensive means of ablating BE. Sampliner examined 58 patients with less than 6 cm of BE without dysplasia. One to six sessions (mean 3.5) were performed, resulting in 78% visual and histologic elimination of BE. Montes and associates used MPEC on 14 patients following laparoscopic fundoplication. All 14 were ablated successfully, with persistence of the neosquamous epithelium after a mean follow-up of 21 months. Kovacs reported the use of MPEC on 27 patients without dysplasia. After 18 weeks, 5 patients were found to have residual Barrett's epithelium. Adverse effects in these studies included dysphagia, odynophagia, and chest pain in up to 43% of patients. Esophageal strictures, however, were only seen in 2% of patients. Drawbacks to MPEC include the need for multiple treatment sessions and the fact that the success of ablation decreased significantly when the length of BE exceeded 4 cm. There was only a 25% eradication rate at this length or longer. Current literature demonstrates elimination of BE in 25% to 88% of patients treated with MPEC. Subsquamous BE has been seen in 7% of patients, and the reported recurrence rate is 7%.

Photodynamic Therapy

PDT employs a photosensitizing drug that is absorbed and retained at higher concentrations in neoplastic tissue. Light of the proper wavelength (630 nm for porfimer sodium) delivered at the time of endoscopy to the targeted tissue produces an oxidative photochemical reaction that elaborates singlet oxygen and reactive oxygen species, resulting in mucosal destruction. Probes ranging from 2 to 5 cm are centered in the esophageal lumen to ensure a uniform treatment effect. Balloon centering devices are now available that further enhance the homogenous distribution of the light source.

Several photosensitizing agents are currently being used: meta-tetrahydroxyphenyl chlorine, benzoporphyrin-derivative monoacid ring A, 5-aminolevulinic acid (ALA), and porfimer sodium (Photofrin). The only approved photosensitizer in North America, Japan, and Europe is Photofrin. In fact, PDT with Photofrin is the only ablative therapy approved by the U.S. Food and Drug Administration for treatment of precancerous lesions in BE. It is injected 24 to 72 hours prior to treatment at a dose of 2 mg/kg and is activated by red light at 630 nm. Photofrin is retained selectively in the tumor cells at the submucosal or muscularis level. Thus, treatments can produce a deeper level of tissue ablation compared with the other ablative strategies listed earlier. In addition, skin photosensitivity lasts from 4 weeks to 3 months because of its accumulation within skin macrophages.

Wang and coworkers from the Mayo Clinic reported their updated series of 146 patients with BE and pathology ranging from no dysplasia to cancer who were followed for a 2-year period. At the time of last surveillance, nearly one half the total population of patients had complete ablation of BE, whereas others had varying degrees of residual BE. During the 2-year follow-up, only 4 patients (2.7%) went on to develop cancer. Overholt and coworkers have presented their preliminary results of an international, multicenter, randomized, partially blinded trial of PDT and omeprazole ($n = 138$) versus omeprazole ($n = 70$) alone in 208 patients with BE with HGD. In the PDT/Omeprazole group, 77% of patients achieved complete ablation of HGD, compared with 39% in the omeprazole group ($p <.0001$). In addition, 52% of PDT/omeprazole patients achieved complete replacement of all Barrett's metaplasia/dysplasia compared with only 7% in the omeprazole group ($p <.0001$). Although cancer-free survival was substantially improved in the PDT/omeprazole group ($p <0.0014$), 13% of these patients advanced to adenocarcinoma during a mean follow-up of 24.2 months. Strictures occurred in 36% of patients. Common complications following PDT include cutaneous photosensitivity, chest pain, nausea, pleural effusions, candida esophagitis, atrial fibrillation, and odynophagia. The primary long-term side effect, especially with porfimer sodium, is formation of esophageal strictures, which occurs in 4.8% to 53% of patients. Such strictures are usually responsive to endoscopic dilatation. It has been hypothesized that oral steroids might reduce stricture formation, but Panjehpour found no statistical significance between using oral steroids and not using steroids in the formation of strictures. Virtually all studies using PDT report subsquamous intestinal metaplasia, with detailed pathologic studies reporting a prevalence as high as 51.5%. In addition, esophageal perforation and tracheoesophageal fistulae have been reported but are rare (<1% in most large studies). The University of Pittsburgh experience includes 50 high-risk patients with either HGD or localized esophageal cancer, with a mean follow-up of 28.1 months. Sixteen patients (32%) are alive and without evidence of disease, 30% are alive with residual or recurrent disease, and 38% have died with recurrent disease. The overall survival at 36 months was 31%. Strictures occurred in 42% of patients. The intent-to-treat success rate was 38% in HGD and 30% in cases of focal carcinoma.

Comparing Techniques

Multiple studies comparing ablation modalities and using multiple modalities have been performed. Wolfsen and coworkers from the Mayo Clinic in Jacksonville reported a series of 60 patients with HGD and 30 patients with cancer who were treated with Photofrin PDT and adjunct argon plasma coagulation (APC) for residual areas of BE. At a median follow-up of 1.6 years, complete ablation was seen in 52% of the patients with HGD and 73% of the patients with cancer.

Kelty and colleagues performed a prospective randomized controlled trial of ALA-PDT versus APC in 68 patients with BE. At a median follow-up of 12 months, patients showed a reduction in the area of BE (97% in the APC group vs. 50% in PDT). Subsquamous glandular mucosa was seen in 24% of the PDT versus 21% of the APC group. Hage and collaborators also compared ALA-PDT as a single dose and ALA-PDT as a fractionated dose versus APC in a randomized trial of 33 patients. Histologic ablation was completed in 8%, 33%, and 36%, respectively. APC was used to treat the remaining BE. At 12 months, complete ablation was seen in 82%, 90%, and 67%. Because of the lack of complete ablation, the authors did not recommend these techniques for prophylactic ablation of BE. Finally, Dulai and associates performed a randomized, partially

blinded trial of APC versus MPEC. The number of treatments to completely ablate BE was 2.9 treatments using MPEC and 3.8 treatments with APC, and the proportion of patients in whom complete ablation was achieved was 88% in the MPEC group versus 81% in the APC group.

Endoscopic Mucosal Resection

Endoscopic mucosal resection (EMR) was introduced in 1984 and has shown early outcomes comparable with to surgery in preliminary, nonrandomized studies evaluating patients with superficial squamous-cell carcinomas and early intramucosal esophageal and gastric adenocarcinoma. The technique involves raising the mucosal–submucosal target area by intramural saline or suction (or both) and subsequent endoscopic snare resection (Fig. 3). Candidates for EMR must have a preliminary endoscopic ultrasound to assess the depth of penetration and lymph node status. The lesion may be removed en bloc or in several fragments. En bloc resection is preferred because of the better assessment of the resection margins; however, most en bloc resections are limited to a small area (~1.5–2.0 cm). Thus, the elimination of all BE is difficult in most cases, although attempts to remove strips up to 5 cm have been successfully achieved in animals.

The safety of this procedure was evaluated by Seewald and coworkers, who performed EMR on five patients with multifocal HGD or cancer and seven patients with HGD. Complete resections were achieved, averaging 30 to 40 mm in length and 20 mm circumference. There were no recurrences in 9 months, although two patients had strictures that were treated with dilatation. Giovannini and associates also achieved complete, circumferential resection in 18 of 21 patients with HGD or cancer. All were disease free after 24 months except for two local recurrences that were again treated with EMR. May and coworkers evaluated the results of EMR in the treatment of 115 patients with HGD or early adenocarcinoma. Complete local remission was achieved in 98% of patients, with an associated 3-year survival rate of 88%. Interestingly, a 30% rate of metachronous lesions was observed during the follow-up period, and all but one were treated successfully with repeat EMR. This finding underscores the need for close endoscopic follow-up in patients undergoing local ablative approaches for BE and associated dysplasia and/or focal intraepithelial carcinoma. Buttar and associates combined EMR with PDT in treating 17 patients with superficial cancer. Importantly, cancer was seen at the margins of resection in 3 of 17 (18%) of the patients. Sixteen (94%) of the patients, however, achieved and remained in remission at a median follow-up of 13 months. EMR improved staging in 47% of the patients, and esophageal strictures were seen in 30% of the patients after EMR/PDT. The most common complication of EMR is bleeding (30%–50%). Esophageal stricture (especially when combined with PDT) is a late complication and is reported in up to 30% of cases. Perforation risk is less than 1%.

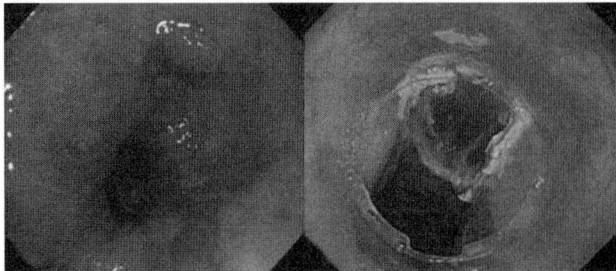

A   B

Figure 3 Endoscopic mucosal resection **(A),** before; **(B),** after. *From Peters FP, Kara MA, Rosmolen WD, and others:* Gastrointest Endosc *61:506, 2005. **(See color insert Figure 6.)***

Other Ablation Techniques

Sharma and colleagues published their preliminary data using radiofrequency ablation in pigs and cancer patients scheduled to undergo esophagectomy. This technique used sizing balloons to determine the inner diameter of the targeted portion of the esophagus, followed by placement of a balloon-based electrode with a 3-cm-long treatment area that incorporates tightly spaced, bipolar electrodes that alternate in polarity. The amount of energy used correlated with the depth of tissue destruction. In the four human patients undergoing this technique, there were no strictures reported, or residual subsquamous Barrett's epithelium at 1 month. However, no long-term follow-up data are available.

Cryotherapy, performed via application of a liquid-nitrogen-cooled probe, is a technique capable of inducing controlled superficial mucosal necrosis. Johnston and colleagues reported their pilot study data on 11 patients with disease ranging from no dysplasia to multifocal HGD. There was complete ablation in 82% of patients with no residual subsquamous Barrett's epithelium reported at 6 months. Sound-wave (ultrasonic energy) ablation has also been used in preliminary testing on 11 pigs with the encouraging finding of no resulting strictures. Heater probes have also been employed to ablate 13 patients with BE and no evidence of dysplasia. All 13 patients were ablated in 1 to 5 treatment sessions; however, three (23%) were found with subsquamous Barrett's epithelium on biopsy.

CONCLUSION

A number of techniques have been developed that demonstrate some success in ablating BE with or without HGD. However, a significant fraction of patients do not show complete regression of HGD or BE during longer periods of follow-up, and all techniques have been shown to result in a rate of residual subsquamous BE. In contradistinction, esophagectomy achieves the removal of all metaplastic epithelium, and thus remains the gold standard in patients with HGD. Endoscopic ablation for BE is only appropriate for those patients with HGD who are unwilling or unable to undergo esophagectomy. As techniques and technologies improve, it is likely that ablative strategies will become an important part of the armamentarium in the treatment of Barrett's esophagus. Prospective, controlled studies will be necessary to define the optimal role of ablative therapy in this setting.

SUGGESTED READINGS

Abbas G, Pennathur A, Keeley SB, and others: Laser ablation therapies for Barrett's esophagus, *Semin Thorac Cardiovasc Surg* 17:313, 2005.

Ackroyd R, Brown NJ, Davis MF, and others: Photodynamic therapy for dysplastic Barrett's esophagus: a prospective, double blind, randomized, placebo controlled trial, *Gut* 47:612, 2000.

Alikhan M, Rex D, Kahn A, and others: Variable pathologic interpretation of columnar lined esophagus by general pathologists in community practice, *Gastrointest Endosc* 50:23, 1999.

Barham CP, Jones RL, Biddleston LR, and others: Photothermal laser ablation of Barrett's esophagus: endoscopic and histological evidence of squamous re-epithelialization, *Gut* 41:281, 1997.

Biddlestone LR, Barham CP, and others: The histopathology of treated Barrett's esophagus: squamous reepithelialization after acid suppression and laser and photodynamic therapy, *Am J Surg Pathol* 22:239, 1998.

Brown LM, Devesa SS: Epidemiologic trends in esophageal and gastric cancer in the United States, *Surg Oncol Clin N Am* 11:235, 2002.

Buttar NS, Wang KK, Lutzke LS, and others: Combined endoscopic mucosal resection and photodynamic therapy for esophageal neoplasia within Barrett's esophagus, *Gastroinest Endosc* 54:682, 2001.

Cameron AJ, Carpenter HA: Barrett's esophagus, high-grade dysplasia, and early adenocarcinoma: a pathologic study, *Am J Gastroenterol* 92:586, 1997.

Clayton PE, Ackroyd R: Argon plasma coagulation ablation of Barrett's esophagus, *Scand J Gastroenterol* 40:617, 2005.

Collard JM: High-grade dysplasia in Barrett's esophagus: the case for esophagectomy, *Chest Surg Clin N Am* 12:77, 2002.

Conio M, Cameron AJ, Chak A, and others: Endoscopic treatment of high-grade dysplasia and early cancer in Barrett's oesophagus, *Lancet Oncol* 6:311, 2005.

Conio M, Cameron AJ, Romero Y, and others: Secular trends in the epidemiology and outcome of Barrett's esophagus in Olmsted County, Minnesota, *Gut* 48:304, 2001.

Dimick JB, Pronovost PJ, and others: Surgical volume and quality of care for esophageal resection: do high-volume hospitals have fewer complications? *Ann Thoracic Surg* 75:337, 2003.

Drewitz DJ, Sampliner RE, Garewal HS: The incidence of adenocarcinoma in Barrett's esophagus—a prospective study of 170 patients followed 4.8 years, *Am J Gastroenterol* 92:212, 1997.

Dulai GS, Jensen DM, Cortina G, and others: Randomized trial of argon plasma coagulation versus multipolar electrocoagulation for ablation of Barrett's esophagus, *Gastrointest Endosc* 61:232, 2005.

Eisen GM: Ablation therapy for Barrett's esophagus, *Gastrointest Endosc* 58:760, 2003.

Ell C, May A, Gossner L, and others: Endoscopic mucosal resection of early cancer and high-grade dysplasia in Barrett's esophagus, *Gastroenterology* 118:670, 2000.

Faybush EM, Sampliner RE: Randomized trials in the treatment of Barrett's esophagus, *Dis Esophagus* 18:291, 2005.

Giovannini M, Bories E, Pesenti C, and others: Circumferential endoscopic mucosal resection in Barrett's esophagus with high-grade intraepithelial neoplasia or mucosal cancer: preliminary results in 21 patients, *Endoscopy* 36:782, 2004.

Grant WE, Hopper C, MacRobert AJ, and others: Photodynamic therapy of oral cancer: photosensitization with systemic with aminolevulinic acid, *Lancet* 342:147, 1993.

Hage M, Siersema PD, and others: 5-aminolevulinic acid photodynamic therapy versus argon plasma coagulation for ablation of Barrett's esophagus: a randomized trial, *Gut* 53:785, 2004.

Heitmiller RF, Redmond M, Hamilton SR: Barrett's esophagus with high-grade dysplasia. An indication for prophylactic esophagectomy, *Ann Surg* 224:66, 1996.

Kelty C, Ackrod R, Brown NJ, and others: Endoscopic ablation of Barrett's esophagus: a randomized-controlled trial of photodynamic therapy vs. argon plasma coagulation, *Aliment Pharmacol Ther* 20:1289, 2004.

Luketich JD, Alvelo-Rivera M, Buenaventura PO, and others: Minimally invasive esophagectomy: outcomes in 222 patients, *Ann Surg* 238:486, 2003.

Luketich JD, Christie NA, Lovas KE, and others: Photodynamic therapy: results of curative intent for esophageal cancer and Barrett's with high-grade dysplasia in high-risk patients, *Proc SPIE* 4248:28, 2001.

May A, Gossner L, Gunter E, and others: Local treatment of early cancer in short Barrett's esophagus by means of argon plasma coagulation: initial experience, *Endoscopy* 31:497, 1999.

Morris CD, Byrne JP, Armstrong GR, Attwood SE, and others: Prevention of the neoplastic progression of Barrett's esophagus by endoscopic argon beam plasma ablation, *Br J Surg* 88:1357, 2001.

Overholt BF, Lightdale C, Wang KK, and others: Photodynamic therapy with porfimer sodium for ablation of high-grade dysplasia in Barrett's esophagus: international, partially blinded, randomized phase III trial, *Gastrointest Endosc* 62:488, 2005.

Reid BJ, Levine DS, Longton G, and others: Predictors of progression to cancer in Barrett's esophagus: baseline histology and flow cytometry identify low and high-risk patient subsets, *Am J Gastroenterol* 95:1669, 2000.

Sampliner RE: Practice guidelines on the diagnosis, surveillance, and therapy of Barrett's esophagus. The Practice Parameters Committee of the American College of Gastroenterology, *Am J Gastroenterol* 93:1028, 1998.

Sampliner RE, Faigel D, Fennerty MB, and others: Effective and safe endoscopic reversal of nondysplastic Barrett's esophagus with thermal electrocoagulation combined with high-dose acid inhibition: a multicenter study, *Gastrointest Endosc* 6:554, 2001.

Sampliner RE, Faigel D, Fennerty MB, and others: Effective and safe endoscopic reversal of nondysplastic Barrett's esophagus with thermal electrocoagulation combined with high-dose acid inhibition: a multicenter study, *Gastrointest Endosc* 6:554, 2001.

Schnell TG, Sontag SJ, Chejfek G, and others: Long-term nonsurgical management of Barrett's esophagus with high-grade dysplasia, *Gastroenterology* 120:1607, 2001.

Seewald S, Akaraviputh T, Seitz U, and others: Circumferential EMR and complete removal of Barrett's epithelium: a new approach to management of Barrett's esophagus containing high-grade intraepithelial neoplasia and intramucosal carcinoma, *Gastrointest Endosc* 57:854, 2003.

Shaheen NJ, Crosby MA, Bozymski EM: Is there publication bias in the reporting of cancer risk of Barrett's esophagus? *Gastroenterology* 119:333, 2000.

Sharma P, Jaffe PE, Bhattacharyya A: Laser and multipolar electrocoagulation ablation of early Barrett's adenocarcinoma: long-term follow-up, *Gastroinest Endosc* 49:442, 1999.

Sihvo EI, Luostarinen ME, Salo JA: Fate of patients with adenocarcinoma of the esophagus and the esophagogastric junction: a population-based analysis, *Am J Gastroenterol* 99:419–424, 2004.

Van Laetherm JL, Jagodzinski R, and others: Argon plasma coagulation in the treatment of Barrett's high grade dysplasia and in situ adenocarcinoma, *Endoscopy* 33:257, 2001.

Van Sandick JW, van Lanschot JJ, Kuiken BW, and others: Impact of endoscopic biopsy surveillance on pathological stage and clinical outcome of Barrett's carcinoma, *Gut* 43:216, 1998.

Wang KK: Photodynamic therapy of Barrett's esophagus, *Gastrointest Endosc Clin N Am* 10:409, 2000.

Weston AP, Sharma P: Neodymium: yttrium-aluminum garnet contact laser ablation of Barrett's high grade dysplasia and early carcinoma, *Am J Gastroenterol* 97:2998, 2002.

ESOPHAGEAL ATRESIA AND TRACHEOESOPHAGEAL FISTULA

Kevin N. Boykin, MD, and Paul M. Colombani, MD

The first successful primary repair of esophageal atresia (EA) with tracheoesophageal fistula (TEF) was accomplished by Dr. Cameron Height at the University of Michigan on March 15, 1941. Over the past 6 decades, advances in surgical technique, pediatric anesthesia, neonatal intensive care, and nutrition have increased the survival rate following reconstruction from universally fatal to approximately 95%.

Although EA and TEF may exist independently of each other, they are most commonly encountered together. EA with or without TEF represents the most common life-threatening congenital anomaly of the esophagus. EA/TEF occurs in 1 in every 4500 live births in the United States. Males are more commonly affected than females. Although most cases are sporadic, a parent with EA/TEF has approximately a 3% chance of having an affected child. Parents with one affected child have a 2% risk of having another child with EA/TEF.

The exact etiology of EA/TEF remains undetermined. At 22 to 24 days of gestation, the esophagus and trachea are a common diverticulum off of the primitive foregut. By 36 days of gestation, they have completed their separation. A disruption of embryogenesis during this fourth week of gestation is believed to account for the high incidence of

other disorders seen with EA/TEF. To date, no single unifying theory can explain all of the variations of EA and TEF that are encountered.

The most commonly used classification system is shown in Figure 1. Six types account for the vast majority of cases of EA/TEF. The most common form is a proximal EA with a distal TEF, occurring in 85% of cases. The second most common form is known as "pure" EA without TEF.

Associated anomalies can occur in 50% of patients with EA/TEF. Patients with pure EAs have an even higher risk. The most common abnormalities encountered are cardiac, genitourinary, and gastrointestinal. The VACTERL association is commonly associated with EA/TEF and comprises vertebral, anal, cardiac, tracheoesophageal, renal, and limb abnormalities. Likewise, EA/TEF can be seen with a variety of chromosomal or genetic disorders such as trisomy 13, trisomy 18, trisomy 21, DiGeorge sequence, polysplenia sequence, CHARGE association (coloboma, heart anomalies, choanal atresia, mental retardation, and genital/ear anomalies), and the Pierre–Robin sequence.

DIAGNOSIS

With the widespread use of fetal ultrasonography, prenatal diagnosis of EA/TEF is common. Patients with pure EA may have polyhydramnios, a blind ending esophageal pouch, and a small or absent gastric bubble on ultrasonography. In contrast, patients with a distal TEF may have a variable amount of amniotic fluid because the fistula may allow a path for the amniotic fluid to reach the gastrointestinal tract. Despite ultrasonography, most patients are diagnosed only after birth.

Within the first few hours after birth, most patients with EA/TEF will have excessive drooling and salivation. As secretions pool in a distended and atretic proximal esophageal pouch, the child

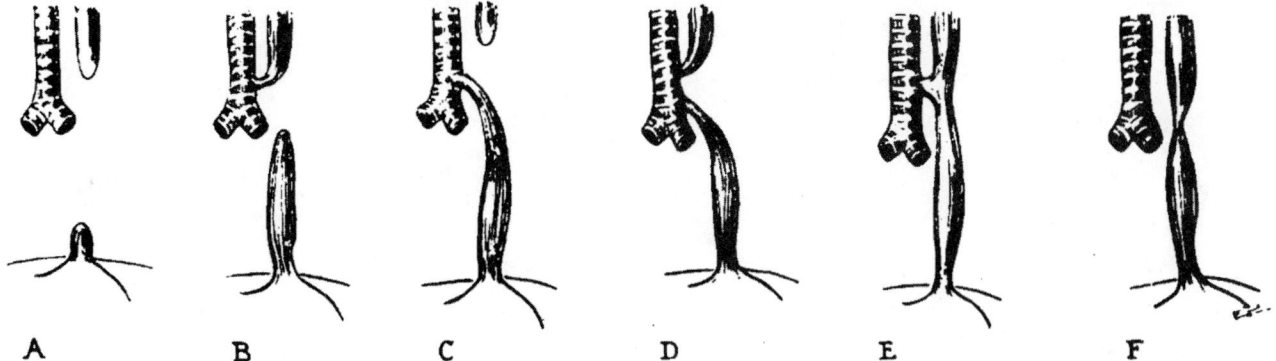

Figure I Vogt–Gross Classification System. **(A)** Isolated esophageal atresia; **(B)** esophageal atresia with proximal tracheoesophageal fistula (TEF); **(C)** esophageal atresia with distal TEF; **(D)** esophageal atresia with double (proximal and distal) TEF; **(E)** H-type tracheoesophageal fistula; **(F)** esophageal stenosis.

begins to aspirate saliva. The presence of a TEF may allow direct aspiration of saliva (from a proximal fistula) or gastric secretions (from a distal fistula), which may cause a severe chemical pneumonitis. If the diagnosis is not evident at birth, the child will typically experience coughing, choking, and regurgitation with its first feeding.

The diagnosis of EA can be easily accomplished at the bedside. Passage of a 10-F Replogle sump tube (or other firm catheter) from the oropharynx will usually be arrested 10 cm from the lips in affected patients. After injection of a small amount of air through the tube, a lateral chest x-ray will show the tube stopping or curling upon itself within the pouch (Fig. 2). The presence of bowel gas supports the finding of an associated distal TEF. In contrast, the presence of a scaphoid abdomen and lack of distal bowel gas would suggest a pure EA without an associated TEF. Contrast studies should be avoided, given the high risk of aspiration. If one is absolutely necessary, an experienced radiologist should perform the study with a small amount (1–2 ml) of water-soluble contrast. Figure 3 demonstrates a contrast study performed to demonstrate the presence of a proximal pouch TEF.

Patients with "H"-type TEF without EA usually present out of the newborn period with recurrent pneumonias or reactive airway disease. Because the esophagus is in continuity, these abnormalities are seldom suspected until the patient becomes symptomatic. Bronchoscopy, in addition to contrast studies of the esophagus, may be necessary to diagnose this rare type of TEF. Figure 4 demonstrates an H-type TEF noted on barium swallow.

PREOPERATIVE MANAGEMENT

The main goals of preoperative therapy in patients with EA/TEF are the avoidance of pneumonitis and the identification of other associated anomalies. Patients born outside of tertiary pediatric surgery centers should be transferred promptly.

Immediately after birth, these patients should undergo placement of a 10-F Replogle sump tube placed into the upper pouch and continuously suctioned to prevent aspiration. An H_2-blocker and broad spectrum antibiotics should be started immediately. The child is placed in a reverse Trendelenburg position to prevent reflux of gastric contents through the fistula. Positive pressure ventilation must be avoided in these patients because a distal TEF may allow air to escape into the GI tract, causing abdominal distension, worsening pulmonary compliance, and possible compartment syndrome or gastric perforation.

An echocardiogram and renal ultrasound should be performed to rule out cardiac or renal abnormalities. The side of the aortic arch should be documented. The presence of a right-sided aortic arch would mandate a left posterolateral thoracotomy instead of the traditional right-sided approach. Severe cardiac or renal abnormalities may have to be addressed before attempting repair of the EA/TEF. The perineum should be inspected to look for associated anorectal malformations.

The timing of surgery is mandated by the infant's condition, the type of EA/TEF encountered, birth weight, and severity of

Figure 2   Lateral chest x-ray demonstrating coiled nasogastric tube in proximal pouch of a patient with a Vogt-Gross type-C esophageal atresia/tracheoesophageal fistula (TEF).

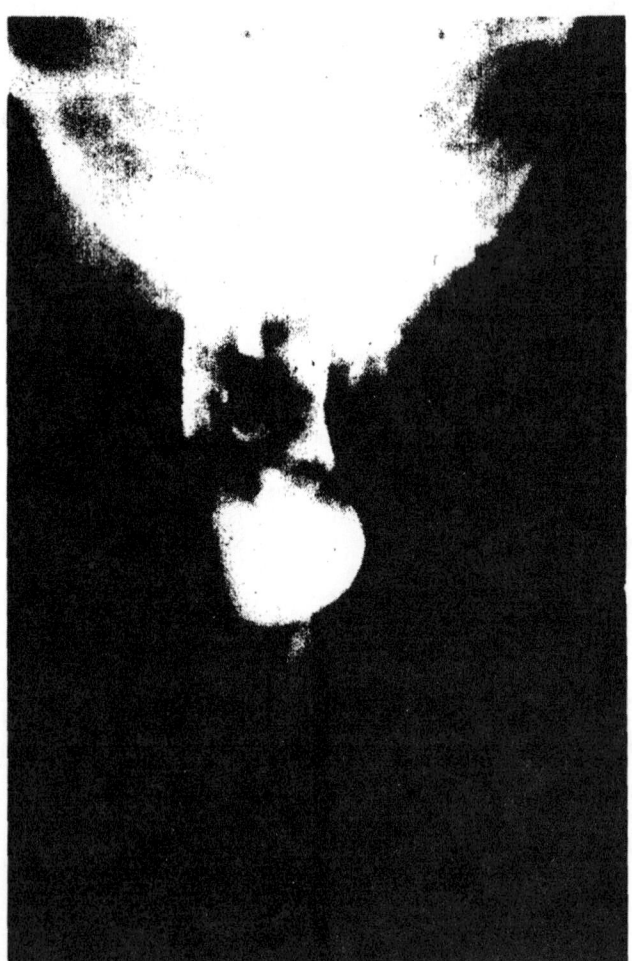

Figure 3   Limited barium study documenting blind ending proximal pouch with proximal fistula Vogt-Gross type B.

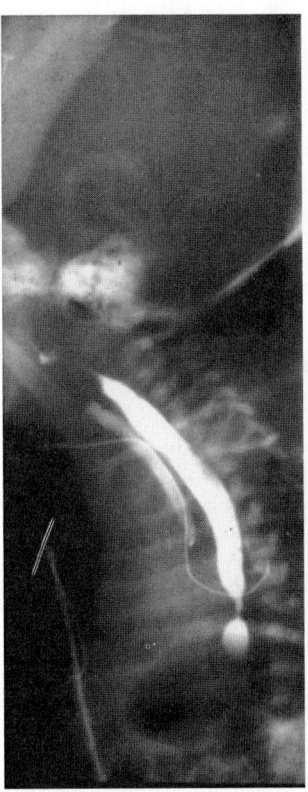
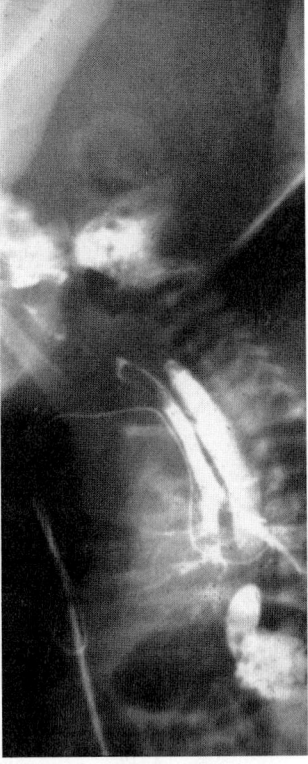

Figure 4 Barium swallow contrast study demonstrating H-type tracheoesophageal fistula. Note that the course of the fistula is craniocaudad from trachea to esophagus.

Table 1: Spitz Classification

Group	Description	Survival (%)
I	Birthweight >1500 g *without* major congenital cardiac defect	97
II	Birthweight <1500 g *or* major congenital cardiac defect	59
III	Birthweight <1500 g *and* major cardiac defect	22

associated abnormalities. Table 1 shows the most commonly used system to stratify risk in these patients. In most cases, repair can be performed within 24 to 48 hours. Delayed repair may be necessary in patients with long gap EA, extreme prematurity, or severe pneumonitis, or in whom other congenital anomalies must be addressed first.

█ OPERATIVE REPAIR

The type of repair depends on the type of EA/TEF encountered. Traditionally, a right posterolateral thoracotomy can be used for most types except an H-type fistula, which is usually approached via a right-sided, low cervical incision.

Traditional Approach: Esophageal Atresia with Distal Tracheoesophageal Fistula

Primary repair of EA/TEF follows three steps: fistula ligation, esophageal mobilization, and anastomosis. The standard approach for the most common type of EA/TEF is described.

The patient is intubated and gently ventilated or allowed to breathe spontaneously until the fistula is ligated. Bronchoscopy may be performed to identify the site of TEF and rule out a second fistula. The child is then placed in position for a standard right posterolateral thoracotomy with the right arm extended above the head. After incision and subcutaneous dissection, a muscle-sparing technique is used to identify the fourth intercostal space. The intercostal muscles are carefully cauterized, protecting the thin pleura underneath. An extrapleural dissection is used to "push" the lung away from the chest wall. This approach may prevent empyema formation in the event of an anastomotic leak. Once the lung is fully retracted, the azygous vein is identified and divided. At this point, the trachea, vagus nerve, and proximal and distal esophageal segments all must be correctly identified. The distal fistula is then dissected off the back wall of the trachea below its origin and encircled with a vessel loop to occlude the lumen and minimize loss of tidal volume. Care must be taken not to injure the thin-walled trachea at this point. The fistula is then ligated with 5–0 monofilament suture. The anesthesiologist may fully control the patient's ventilation at this point because the fistula has been ligated, and air can no longer escape into the gastrointestinal tract.

Mobilization of the proximal esophageal pouch is then performed. The anesthesiologist may gently push on the Replogle tube to extend the esophagus. A traction suture is placed through the tip of the pouch to allow the surgeon to manipulate the proximal pouch without grasping the esophagus directly. The blood supply to the proximal esophagus is excellent, and this segment tolerates circumferential dissection and mobilization up through the thoracic inlet. Dissection is often carried up into the thoracic inlet to gain enough length. Mobilization of the distal esophageal segment should be limited.

Esophageal anastomosis is begun with two corner stitches of 5–0 monofilament suture. In the posterior row, sutures are placed with the knots on the inside of the lumen. The mucosa and submucosa and muscularis must be included in each stitch. Once the back row is completed, the nasogastric (NG) tube is advanced into the stomach. The anterior row is then placed in a standard fashion. At this point a chest tube or drain is placed in proximity of the repair. Closure of the chest then follows in a standard fashion.

Thoracoscopic Approach: Esophageal Atresia with Distal Tracheoesophageal Fistula

As enthusiasm and experience with minimally invasive techniques in children has advanced in recent years, more centers have begun repairing EA/TEF through a thoracoscopic approach. Perhaps the best argument for thoracoscopic repair is the avoidance of complications associated with thoracotomy in children: scoliosis, winged scapula, shoulder girdle weakness, and chest-wall asymmetry. The thoracoscopic EA/TEF repair proceeds in a fashion similar to the open procedure: identification and ligation of the fistula, mobilization of the esophageal segments, and end-to-end anastomosis.

The patient is placed in a 45-degree prone position to allow separation of the lung from the posterior mediastinum. Two 3.0-mm ports and one 5.0-mm port are used to gain access to the thoracic cavity and collapse the lung by CO_2 insufflation. A 30-degree wide-angle telescope is used for visualization. Dissection is undertaken with 3-mm instruments. The azygos vein is divided with hook cautery, exposing the fistula, which is usually in close proximity. A 5-mm titanium endoclip is used to ligate the fistula.

The upper pouch is mobilized with a combination of sharp and blunt dissection. The surgeon should be careful while dissecting the proximal pouch near the membranous portion of the trachea. In addition, search for an upper-pouch fistula should be made during this dissection. A very small upper pouch (not dilated) may indicate an upper-pouch TEF. As with the open technique, a gentle push by the anesthesiologist on the NG tube helps to extend the esophagus during dissection. After the mobilization has reached the thoracic inlet, the distal tip of the pouch is resected.

Anastomosis is then performed with interrupted 5–0 monofilament absorbable sutures in a manner identical to the open technique. The back row of sutures is placed with the knots on the inside of the lumen. The NG tube is advanced into the stomach, and the anterior row is then completed. Adequate bites of mucosa must be taken to prevent tearing of sutures. Once the anastomosis is completed, a chest tube is placed using the lower trocar site. Postoperative care for thoracoscopic repair is no different from that for the open technique.

As of 2007, no randomized trials comparing open versus thoracoscopic repair have been completed. Retrospective analysis of patients undergoing thoracoscopic repair reveal comparable rates of postoperative complications. Because the technique was originally reported in the late 1990s, long-term data have not yet been generated.

Long Gap Esophageal Atresia

Patients with "pure" EA without a concomitant TEF or patients with EA/TEF with a "long" segment of absent esophagus present a dilemma to the surgeon. In this circumstance, a one-stage primary repair may be difficult. Most surgeons faced with a "pure" esophageal atresia will perform a gastrostomy tube for feeding followed by observation and a delayed repair 1 to 3 months later. During this interval, the proximal pouch will often lengthen with or without active stretching. Figure 5 shows an anteroposterior chest x-ray showing a dilator in the proximal pouch and a Bakes dilator passed through the gastrostomy tube site up into the distal blind esophagus. Note that the tips of the dilators come close to touching, indicating that, at surgical exploration, a primary repair can be performed.

Numerous open and closed techniques have been employed to lengthen the esophagus during the operation, either through stretching the segments toward each other or by performing myotomies to lengthen the upper segment. The majority of patients can be repaired primarily.

When a primary anastomosis is not technically possible, a number of esophageal replacement techniques can be used. Most

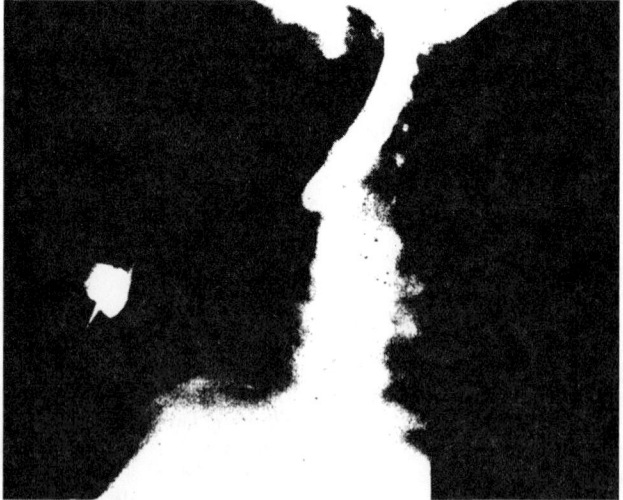

Figure 5 Plain radiograph of patient with isolated esophageal atresia (Vogt–Gross type A) with Maloney dilator in proximal pouch and Bakes biliary dilator passed through gastrostomy site retrograde into distal blind ending esophagus. Note that tips of dilators are almost apposed, indicating that the patient is ready for primary anastomosis.

commonly, a gastric pull-up procedure can be performed, mobilizing the stomach up into the right chest cavity and performing an esophagogastric anastomosis. Alternatives include reversed gastric tube and colon interpositions.

H-Type Tracheoesophageal Fistula

Bronchoscopy can be useful in diagnosing this rare type of fistula, and a small catheter can be placed through the fistula to aid in identification at time of dissection. A right-sided, low cervical incision is most commonly used to gain exposure to the tracheoesophageal groove. The esophagus is encircled with small vessel loops, and the fistula is identified. The recurrent laryngeal nerves must be avoided during this dissection. The fistula is divided with 5–0 monofilament suture. The two suture lines are separated by a small flap of adjacent muscle tissue to prevent fistula recurrence.

POSTOPERATIVE CARE

The chest drain is left on waterseal postoperatively. Antibiotics are continued until no leak is present on contrast examination and the chest drain has been removed. Patients should be extubated as soon as feasible. Careless reintubation may lead to anastomotic disruption if the esophagus is intubated by mistake. Because gastroesophageal reflux is common in these infants, acid suppression therapy should be continued postoperatively.

At 7 days postsurgery, a water-soluble contrast study is performed. The radiologist can place a small feeding tube just proximal to the anastomosis and inject a small amount of contrast. If no leak is present, the chest tube is removed, antibiotics are discontinued, the feeding tube is removed, and the infant is allowed to take feedings by mouth.

COMPLICATIONS

Anastomotic Leak

Up to 15% of all patients will have some form of anastomotic leak. The presence of a previously unrecognized pneumothorax or saliva-like drainage from the chest drain are suggestive of an anastomotic leak. Small leaks identified on contrast examination are best treated conservatively with continued antibiotics and chest drainage. A repeat study in 5 to 7 days usually shows resolution of the leak. Large or persistent leaks may require additional chest drains or even reexploration. Patients with anastomotic leaks are at higher risk of developing esophageal strictures.

Dysphagia

The vast majority of patients with EA have abnormal esophageal motility. The development of EA/TEF inhibits the normal formation of the myenteric plexus, thereby impairing esophageal peristalsis and sphincter function. Motility studies may illustrate a discoordinated esophageal contraction or an immobile segment of esophagus. Later in life, these patients may have difficulty swallowing solid foods or may require removal of impacted esophageal foreign bodies. Approximately 15% of adult patients will complain of dysphagia on a daily basis.

Esophageal Stricture

Strictures may form in up to one third of patients with EA/TEF. Contrast examination of the esophagus may be misleading: the anastomosis will look stenotic because of the dilated proximal pouch and small esophageal segment. A stricture is considered only if the patient is symptomatic. The longer the original gap between the proximal pouch and distal esophageal lumen, the higher the expected rate of stricture. This is believed to be secondary to the increased amount of tension required for primary anastomosis. A gap distance of >2.5 cm is associated with a higher rate of stricture formation. The cause of the stricture is felt to be ischemia, most likely from a poorly perfused distal segment. This reinforces the belief that mobilization of the distal segment should be performed with caution. Anastomotic leaks and severe gastroesophageal reflux increase the risk of stricture formation. Most strictures are treated by repeated esophageal dilatation.

Gastroesophageal Reflux

Approximately 50% of patients with EA/TEF will have gastroesophageal reflux disease (GERD). Reduced esophageal clearance of gastric secretions, a poorly functioning lower esophageal sphincter, and a shortened abdominal esophagus are some of the proposed mechanisms of GERD in patients with EA/TEF. Acid reflux may lead to other complications, such as stricture formation, aspiration pneumonia, reactive airway disease, apnea, or failure to thrive. If the patient is not responsive to medical therapy, a fundoplication may be required.

Tracheomalacia

Tracheomalacia will be seen on intraoperative bronchoscopy in many infants with EA/TEF but is usually not clinically significant. Patients with significant episodes of apnea, cyanosis, recurrent pneumonia, or worsening of stridor may be candidates for aortopexy.

Recurrence

Recurrence of a TEF may occur in 10% of patients. This may be caused by an anastomotic leak or an injury to the thin-walled trachea or may represent a second fistula not appreciated at the time of initial surgery. If recurrence is persistent, repeat surgery may be required. Bronchoscopy or esophagography may be required to diagnose recurrence.

SUGGESTED READINGS

Holcomb GW 3rd, Rothenberg S, Bax KM, and others: Thoracoscopic repair of esophageal atresia and tracheoesophageal fistula: a multi-institutional analysis, *Ann Surg* 242:422, 2005.
Kluth D, Fiegel H: The embryology of the foregut, *Semin Pediatr Surg* 12:3, 2003.
Kovesi T, Rubin S: Long-term complications of congenital esophageal atresia and/or tracheoesophageal fistula, *Chest* 126:915, 2004.
Rothenberg S: Thoracoscopic repair of esophageal atresia and tracheoesophageal fistula, *Semin Pediatr Surg* 14:2, 2005.
Spitz L: Esophageal atresia: past, present, and future, *J Pediatr Surg* 31:19, 1996.

COMPLICATIONS OF ESOPHAGEAL SURGERY

Vinay K. Gupta, MD, and Richard F. Heitmiller, MD

INTRODUCTION

A chapter devoted to complications of esophageal surgery is new to this edition of *Current Surgical Therapy*. We believe that this is an important addition for two reasons. The first is that the majority of esophagectomy complications occur not during but following surgery. These complications have the potential to dramatically affect morbidity, mortality, quality of life, length of hospital stay, and cost of therapy. The second reason is that postesophagectomy complications are so prevalent as to be considered almost inevitable. It is important for the esophageal surgeon to have an operative and postoperative patient care plan that anticipates these complications so that they can be managed promptly to minimize their impact on procedural outcome and cost. Doing so will yield safe esophagectomy results despite the 30% to 50% reported complication rates.

In this chapter, we discuss what we believe are the most important complications of esophageal surgery, their significance, incidence, and etiology, and how to identify, manage, and avoid them.

The likelihood and consequence of complications is related to esophagectomy technique. Therefore the various esophagectomy methods are briefly discussed.

ESOPHAGECTOMY TECHNIQUES

The operation generally referred to as esophagectomy involves removing some, but not all, of the esophagus, and usually a small proximal segment of stomach. As a result, the procedure is technically called a *partial esophagogastrectomy*. The four steps of this operation are 1) esophageal resection, 2) preparation of the replacement conduit, 3) esophageal reconstructive anastomosis, and 4) placement of adjuvant feeding jejunostomy. The surgical approaches for esophagectomy can be classified as either *thoracotomy* or *nonthoracotomy* techniques. The Ivor–Lewis (midline laparotomy and right thoracotomy), three-incision (right or left thoracotomy, midline laparotomy, left or right neck incisions), and left thoracoabdominal (LTA) approaches make up the thoracotomy group. Transhiatal esophagectomy (THE) primarily comprises the nonthoracotomy methods. Minimally invasive methods use laparoscopic, thoracoscopic, and cervical incisions that parallel their open-technique counterparts. Selection of esophagectomy technique involves many factors, including the balance of risk–benefit regarding the probability and consequences of potential complications.

COMPLICATIONS

Complications of esophagectomy are discussed roughly in the order in which they might be encountered during and after surgery. As mentioned earlier, most complications occur after surgery. However, a few notable complications may arise during surgery, and these will be covered first. For each complication, the etiology, reported incidence, methods of prevention, and management are discussed. Table 16.1-1 lists all of the complications covered in this chapter. Despite improvements in anesthesia, surgical technique,

Table 1: Esophagectomy Complications

Operative
Bleeding
Airway injury
Insufficient conduit length
Thoracic duct injury
Postoperative
Respiratory (pneumonia)
Esophageal conduit necrosis
Anastomotic leak
Anastomotic stricture
Hoarseness
Chylothorax
Transhiatal herniation of abdominal contents

and postoperative care, respiratory and anastomotic complications continue to be the two most devastating complications of esophagectomy.

Operative Complications

Bleeding

The esophagus has a rich blood supply and lies in very close proximity to large central vascular structures, so bleeding complications may be recognized at operation or early in the postoperative setting. Vessels most commonly injured include the pulmonary artery and veins, aorta, intrathoracic esophageal arteries, short gastric vessels, and the left gastric artery and vein. Bleeding occurs from blunt or sharp operative trauma. The incidence and severity of surgical bleeding is related to the operative approach. Open methods permit direct visualization of the operative field for dissection, control of vascular injury, and its repair. The use of standard surgical principles should minimize the risk of significant intrathoracic bleeding. Intrathoracic bleeding can be a much more challenging problem during a transhiatal mediastinal dissection. The overall reported incidence of significant operative bleeding is approximately 0.3% to 4.0%.

If bleeding is encountered in the chest during open thoracotomy, standard methods of proximal and distal vascular control and primary repair with nonabsorbable suture are used. When transhiatal esophagectomy is performed, the key to minimizing significant intrathoracic bleeding is to stay close to the esophageal wall while performing blunt dissection. Grey–Turner was the first to describe this "bloodless" paraesophageal plane, which he termed the "esophageal bursa." Later Liebermann-Meffert and colleagues documented the anatomic basis for this clinical observation (see Suggested Reading). We prefer to have a nasogastric tube within the esophagus during intrathoracic esophageal mobilization so that tactile feedback is constantly present to ensure that the dissection is in close proximity to the esophagus. If serious bleeding is encountered at surgery, knowledge of which vessel is injured is critical to deciding how to proceed. The surgeon makes this determination on the basis of where the dissection was located. The mediastinum should be packed and the anesthesia personnel alerted to prepare for blood loss. The surgeon then proceeds with left or right thoracotomy, depending on what vessel appears to be injured. In a relatively controlled situation, the abdominal incision can be closed rapidly and the patient repositioned. Median sternotomy is a terrible incision for visualizing and controlling posterior mediastinal

vascular structures. Once the injured vessel is visualized, standard surgical methods of control and repair are used.

Prevention of significant operative bleeding starts preoperatively. Imaging studies delineate the tumor extent and aid in selecting the appropriate surgical approach. If the esophageal pathology is close to a vascular structure, an open technique that will allow the surgeon to see, control, and repair a potential vascular injury should be considered. In the nonthoracotomy approach, it is important to stay in the "bloodless plane" to avoid significant bleeding. However, in cases in which this paraesophageal plane is not present because of previous surgery, radiation, inflammation, or an infiltrative disease process, choosing an open thoracotomy method should help to prevent significant operative bleeding.

The risk of abdominal bleeding is similar regardless of method selected because this part of the operation is the same for all techniques. Most significant bleeding comes from the short gastric and left gastric vessels and is related to poor exposure. The use of mechanical retraction devices helps greatly with exposure. Application of minimally invasive tools for ligation, coagulation, or vascular stapling also leads to secure vascular control when approaching vessels in deep spaces.

Airway Injury

The membranous wall of the trachea and the mainstem bronchi lie immediately adjacent to the esophagus. In addition, the endotracheal tube cuff focally distends and thins the soft, pliable membranous wall, increasing its risk for operative injury. Therefore the etiology of airway injury is operative trauma. With open esophagectomy methods, airway injury occurs when encircling the esophagus or when attempting to separate proximal esophageal pathology from the airway. With THE, the airway is most commonly injured when encircling the esophagus in the neck or during blunt dissection in the region of the left mainstem bronchus. The incidence of airway injury during esophagectomy has been reported to be between 0.8 and 6.0%. During open esophagectomy, this type of injury can be prevented by sharp dissection while pulling the esophagus away from the airway rather than bluntly encircling the esophagus. During THE, it is important to dissect close to the esophageal wall to avoid airway injury.

The two principles of managing an airway injury are first to address respiration and then to manage any air leak until the repair is complete. Respiration issues are related to whether the injury is proximal or distal to the endotracheal tube (ETT) cuff. If it is proximal, expose the injury site, close it with sutures, and reinforce with soft tissue patch (pleura, mediastinal fat or gastric serosa). Respiration should not be affected. If the injury is distal to the ETT cuff, then either advance the ETT beyond the injury or have the anesthesiologist employ a low-volume, high-frequency ventilation technique for respiration. Close the airway as described earlier. With open methods, the airway is already exposed and there is no concern with air leak leading to tension pneumothorax. When using THE, cervical tracheal injuries are managed as described earlier. If additional exposure is needed, a partial upper sternotomy can be used easily and quickly. For intrathoracic airway injury, place bilateral chest tubes, switch to a high-frequency-type ventilation, and perform thoracotomy (usually right sided) to expose and manage airway injury.

Insufficient Conduit Length

The stomach is the most commonly used esophageal replacement conduit. Properly mobilized it will reach to the neck without tension; it has excellent blood supply and is durable. In some patients, during THE, the stomach does not reach easily through the thoracic outlet to the neck. The etiology is usually that the thoracic outlet is not large enough to permit the stomach to pass easily into the neck. When this occurs, rather than attempting to pull the stomach harder or to abandon the stomach as a conduit, extend

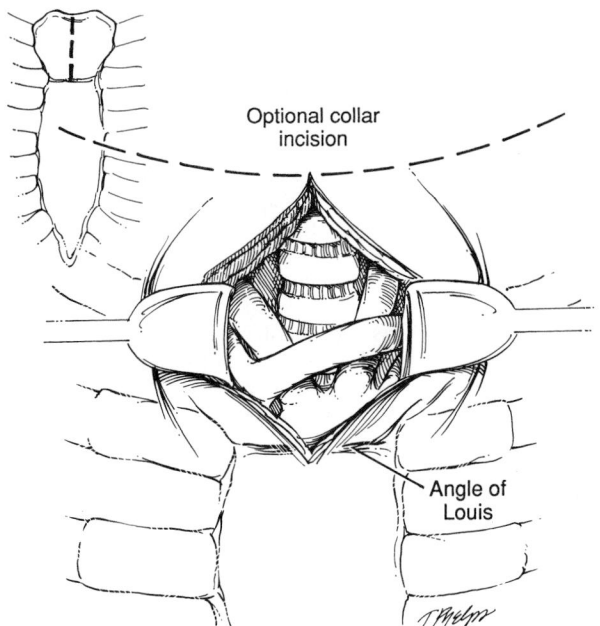

Figure I A partial sternotomy to the angle of Louis is shown, exposing the great vessels and the superior mediastinal trachea and esophagus. This approach widens the thoracic outlet and facilitates an esophagogastric anastomosis in the low neck reducing the risk for insufficient conduit length, conduit necrosis and anastomotic leak. *From Heitmiller RF: Thoracic incisions. In Baue AE, Geha AS, Hammond GL, and others, editors: Glenn's thoracic and cardiovascular surgery, ed 6, Stamford, CT, 1996, Appleton & Lange. Reprinted with permission.*

the cervical incision inferiorly and add a partial upper sternotomy (Fig. 1). This cervicomediastinal exposure widely opens the thoracic outlet and now permits esophagogastric anastomosis 2 to 4 cm lower than with neck incision alone.

Thoracic Duct Injury

The thoracic duct runs in close approximation to the esophagus within the chest and can be injured with dissection. Although a duct injury is recognized postoperatively with high volumes of serous drainage, the etiology is operative trauma. Administration of milk or cream through the jejunostomy will yield a milky drainage with a triglyceride level >100 mg/dL and thereby confirm the diagnosis. The reported incidence of chyle leak is 3.7%. With the THE method, dissection on the esophageal wall minimizes duct injury. With open thoracotomy methods, a more extensive mediastinal dissection is usually employed, and consequently there is an increased risk for duct injury. We attempt to minimize this problem and enable the nodal and esophageal dissection to proceed as planned. It is our practice to ligate the thoracic duct prophylactically low in the chest every time a right thoracotomy esophagectomy technique is used.

Postoperative Complications

Respiratory Complications

Historically, respiratory problems have been the most significant postoperative complication after esophagectomy because of their impact on length of stay, cost, and mortality rates. This is still true today, and thus prevention remains the key. After serious respiratory problems arise, there is no easy way to resolve them. We classify respiratory problems as either major or minor. Major respiratory complications require some change in the expected course of an uncomplicated esophagectomy patient, such as need

for mechanical ventilation, drainage of pleural fluid, initiation of intravenous antibiotics, or bronchoscopy. Examples of major respiratory problems include pneumonia, tracheobronchitis, respiratory failure, and large pleural effusion. Minor respiratory complications include small pleural effusions, basilar atelectasis, cough, and some increase in respiratory secretions. These complications generally can be managed easily without affecting the expected patient care plan or length of hospital stay.

Pneumonia is the main benchmark of major respiratory complications, and the etiology is primarily a result of aspiration. Reported incidence of postesophagectomy pneumonia rates vary from 2.9% to 50%. On the other hand, minor respiratory complications are a consequence of the extensive surgery compounded by the almost inevitable patient comorbidities and nutritional impairments. Consequently, minor respiratory complications, as we have previously shown, are almost universal (see Suggested Reading).

To minimize respiratory complications, several strategies have proven effective. These include optimizing a patient's preoperative medical and nutritional status, the use of regional anesthesia for postoperative pain control when possible, precise surgical technique, and protection of recurrent laryngeal nerve function. Two different methods of managing a patient's airway and ventilation in the early postoperative period have developed. One patient care plan leaves patients intubated, sedated, on mechanical ventilation, and under intensive care monitoring after surgery. Patients are extubated "late," usually the day after surgery. The other patient care plan targets "early" extubation in the operating room, with or without intensive care postoperative monitoring. We support and use the former, or late extubation method. The reason for this is not because patients cannot be extubated early and not to avoid respiratory failure, but to prevent pneumonia. Postesophagectomy pneumonia is a consequence of aspiration. There are two times after surgery when patients are at increased risk for aspiration. The first is early after surgery when they are sedated, supine, often with diminished airway defense from aspiration secondary to vocal cord dysfunction. Keeping patients intubated during this period further protects the airway from aspiration. The early postoperative period can be used to optimize fluid status, treat comorbidities, and manage atelectasis or pleural effusions before extubation. By the time patients are extubated, they are stable, with clear chest films, awake, and able to sit up. The second time patients are at risk for aspiration is when they resume oral feedings. We perform contrast video esophagograms before starting oral feedings to identify patients who might have a tendency for occult aspiration. The study also confirms no anastomotic leakage. We routinely use a postesophagectomy patient care pathway that incorporates the principles of late extubation and contrast swallow studies before oral feeding. Even in a community hospital setting, we have been able to establish a high-volume esophagectomy practice with a pneumonia rate of 4.2%, length of stay of 7.4 days, and an overall cost of surgical care that is less than or equal to state averages over the past 5 years.

The best management plan for respiratory complications is prevention. Management of postesophagectomy atelectasis, significant pleural effusions, and pneumonia is no different from how it would be managed for patients undergoing other major surgery. All major respiratory complications must be managed early and aggressively. We routinely place an adjuvant feeding jejunostomy tube at surgery. We have previously reported that if significant, occult aspiration is demonstrated on postoperative contrast swallow, this will dramatically improve or resolve in approximately 4 weeks (see Suggested Reading). These patients should be sent home on full jejunostomy tube feedings for this time. Feeding patients who have documented aspiration risks the development of pneumonia.

Esophageal Conduit Necrosis

The reconstructive component of esophagectomy is frequently the most challenging aspect of the surgery and the part that most directly affects swallowing function and therefore quality of life. Stomach, jejunum, and colon have all been used as an esophageal replacement conduit. The stomach is the most common choice because there is no need for preoperative studies or bowel preparation. It is easy to mobilize and results in a single reconstructive anastomosis. It permits "long segment" esophageal replacement, has the lowest rate of conduit ischemia and necrosis, and is durable. The etiology for most cases of conduit ischemia occurs secondary to the selection, preparation, and mobilization of the selected conduit. Preoperative surgeries or feeding tube insertion, comorbidities that affect visceral vasculature, and perioperative hemodynamics all contribute to the risk of conduit ischemia and necrosis. In a recent publication, Heitmiller reported that the average conduit necrosis rates for stomach, colon, and jejunum are 4.0%, 9.0%, and 5.6%, respectively (see Suggested Reading).

The best means to avoid this complication is careful preoperative patient preparation to optimize the medical status; selection of stomach as a replacement conduit whenever possible; careful technical conduit preparation; mobilizing the conduit without jeopardizing its blood supply; and close patient monitoring postoperatively. Operative techniques have been described that augment (also known as "supercharging") the blood supply of the conduit using microvascular grafting methods. For long-segment small and large bowel grafts, this method is believed to reduce the incidence of ischemic complications.

Prevention is key. Management is more damage control than salvage. It is essential to consider conduit ischemia or necrosis for all postesophagectomy patients who have persistent high fevers, leukocytosis, elevated potassium levels, or acidosis, especially when there is no other obvious source to explain these findings. Sometimes the findings are subtle, with only minimal blood test abnormalities in a patient not progressing as expected. If the diagnosis of conduit necrosis is suspected, it must be aggressively pursued to confirm it before there is transmural or anastomotic leakage. Select patients may be candidates for endoscopic assessment of mucosal viability, whereas others require cervical or thoracic exploration to directly view the graft. There are no data to suggest that steroids, anticoagulants, or vasoreactive medications will improve the chance of graft salvage.

Anastomotic Leak

Problems with anastomotic healing have historically been one of the most significant complications of esophagectomy, and remain so today. Anastomotic leakage in particular is associated with prolonged hospital stay, delay in oral feedings, late anastomotic strictures, and death. Anastomotic leak rates have also become an assessment of quality in assessing an esophagectomy practice. Factors thought to contribute to leaks include conduit ischemia, anastomotic tension, and technique. Some believe that anastomotic level (neck, upper chest, lower chest) influences leak rates. We have not found this to be the case.

The reported incidence of esophagogastric anastomotic leak ranges from 0% to 14%. Most high-volume practices are able consistently to yield leak rates of 3% to 5% or less. It is generally believed that the higher or more proximal the level of esophagogastric anastomosis, the greater the chance of leakage. In the past, many have felt that a cervical esophagogastric anastomotic leak was almost inevitable. We now do not believe this to be the case. In an earlier publication, we reviewed 262 transhiatal esophagectomy cases using a two-layered hand-sewn anastomotic technique and reported a cervical leak rate of 0.8%. More recently, stapled anastomotic techniques have reported cervical leak rates of 2.7% to 5%, so there is no reason to avoid cervical anastomoses on the basis of leak risk.

Prevention of anastomotic leaks involves avoiding conduit ischemia and tension at the anastomosis. Use the stomach as the esophageal replacement conduit whenever possible. Anastomoses

may be hand sewn (one or two layered) or stapled. We have routinely used a two-layered hand-sewn method and have previously reported cervical leak rates less than 1% in a large series. Others have demonstrated the security of this technique when used for intrathoracic anastomoses. More recently, reports have emerged that have demonstrated excellent results using a combination linear stapled and hand-sewn method. Although we do not use this method, many find that this approach gives superior results to hand-sewn and other stapled techniques. We advocate using a cervical esophageal anastomosis when possible because this greatly diminishes the morbidity and mortality of a leak if it occurs.

Management of leaks is primarily determined by location. If a cervical leak is suspected, the neck incision should be widely opened. It is generally possible to do this at the bedside. No attempt should be made to close the wound loosely around soft drains. The better the wound is drained, the less the chance of mediastinitis and the quicker the leak will resolve. Antibiotics are necessary only to treat cervical wound cellulitis. If there is concern about the viability of the conduit, drainage should be performed in the operating room, where the neck wound can be more aggressively explored to visualize the conduit. Hold oral feedings and advance enteral tube feedings to goal. Cervical dressings are initially dry dressings designed to collect the salivary output. Once the leak seals, cervical drainage abruptly lessens. Wet to dry saline dressings should then be started stimulate clean closure of the neck wound. Patients may be sent home during this process, on tube feedings in select cases.

If the anastomotic leak is in the chest, this is a much more difficult and dangerous problem. Operative anastomotic revision or reinforcement may be considered if the leak develops early and is detected without delay. Usually, this is not the case. Management options then include making the patient nil per os (NPO), administering intravenous antibiotics to combat oral flora bacteria, and reinitiating enteral tube feedings. Then either the mediastinum is drained with a generous-sized chest tube or salivary flow is diverted proximally. If the former approach is used (drainage), it can often take some time for healing, during which patients are quite sick. In the latter case (diversion), sepsis is more rapidly controlled or prevented; however, reconstruction becomes problematic. The surgeon must resist the temptation to "protect" the reconstruction at the risk of continued sepsis and multisystem organ failure.

Anastomotic Stricture

Anastomotic stricture, if it occurs, presents within the first 6 months after surgery. Patients complain of progressive solid food dysphagia. The diagnosis is usually clear clinically, but it can easily be confirmed with a contrast swallowing study. The impact of stricture formation is a diminished quality of life because patients cannot eat normally. In addition, there is a potential for dehydration and malnutrition and an increased risk for "overflow" aspiration.

Risk factors for stricture include conduit ischemia, associated leak with healing, anastomotic technique, anastomotic level, and tension. Some patients have none of these risk factors and still develop strictures, perhaps related to individual variability in wound healing. Reported incidence rates vary from near zero to approximately 25%. The risk of stricture formation is believed to increase the higher (toward the neck) the anastomosis is placed.

We believe that the safety and benefits of cervical anastomosis outweigh any potential increase in risk of stricture formation. Recent reports suggest that the linear staple anastomotic method, because it generates a larger anastomosis, may result in fewer postoperative strictures than other anastomotic methods.

If a stricture develops, it is usually clear by clinical assessment. Postoperative strictures develop within the first 6 months. Apparent late strictures should be evaluated carefully for recurrent tumor if the original operation was for cancer. Benign strictures are soft and dilateeasily. If the stricture is dilated to maximal diameter

Table 2: Anastomotic Stricture—Guidelines for Dilatation

- Dilatate the stricture in multiple stages.
- Follow dilatation schedule. Do not wait for recurrent symptoms.
- Use rigid dilators whenever possible.
- After anastomosis is fully opened, consider additional dilatation(s) to keep anastomosis open.
- Follow patient by symptoms.

Table 3: Chylous Effusion—Characteristic Findings

- Fluid is turbid and milky white
- Specific gravity is 1.020–1.030
- Protein content is 3–4 g/100 ml
- Fat content is 1–4 g/100 ml
- Triglyceride content is >110 mg/dl

at one time, the stricture will invariably recur ("rebound" stricture). Rebound structuring leads to great frustration for the patient and treating physician. The guidelines for dilatation that we have learned by our experience are listed in Table 2. They include the following: Dilatatestrictures in stages even though they could easily be stretched fully open in one session. Prepare the patient to undergo at least two or three dilatations. Rigid dilators are more effective than balloon dilators for keeping strictures open. Even after maximal dilatation is achieved, an additional "maintenance" dilatation seems to keep the anastomosis open.

Hoarseness

Significant hoarseness after esophageal surgery refers to vocal fold dysfunction as a consequence of recurrent laryngeal nerve (RLN) injury. Postoperative hoarseness leads to a "breathy" voice, increased work for speaking, less effective cough, and impaired airway protection against aspiration. Hoarseness can result only when esophagectomy methods are used in which the operative field includes the RLN, such as the three-incision and transhiatal methods. The reported incidence of hoarseness following transhiatal esophagectomy remains at 10% to 15% of patients. Studies in which vocal fold function is visually inspected for all patients after THE suggest that some degree of clinically silent ipsilateral vocal fold dysfunction may be present in an even higher percentage of patients.

The cause of nerve dysfunction is surgical injury. During transhiatal esophagectomy, the RLN is exposed to retraction injury during cervical esophageal mobilization. Avoid using a rigid retractor to pull the trachea medially because this will result in RLN dysfunction in a high percentage of cases. Knowledge of RLN anatomy, careful dissection in the region of the nerve, and avoidance of cervical tracheal retraction will minimize the risk of hoarseness secondary to RLN injury. In the majority of cases, the degree of hoarseness is mild and resolves spontaneously. If it is severe, especially if associated with aspiration, patients should be referred to an otolaryngologist to consider temporary or permanent vocal fold medialization.

Chylothorax

Historically, chylothorax was an ominous postesophagectomy complication associated with a high mortality secondary to dehydration, malnutrition, and immune deficiency. The introduction of intravenous alimentation and minimally invasive approaches to the thoracic duct have lessened the impact of a postoperative chylous leak; however, it still is a serious complication that will lengthen the hospital stay. Chylothorax results from surgical injury to the thoracic duct or its tributaries. The reported incidence of chylothorax as a complication of esophageal surgery is 3.7%.

Esophagectomy methods that use a right thoracotomy approach, mid- to upper-esophageal tumor locations, and intrathoracic lymph node dissections all increase the risk of postoperative chylothorax. Most often, chylothorax presents as a right pleural effusion but may present as a left-sided fluid collection, depending on the esophagectomy technique used.

It is not always possible to avoid thoracic duct injury at surgery. Complete resection of an esophageal malignancy, with or without nodal dissection, is more important than avoiding lymphatic duct injury. Duct injury is usually detected at right thoracotomy. The duct is visualized, and opening it releases fairly characteristic clear fluid. For all right thoracotomy esophagectomy patients, we routinely ligate the thoracic duct near the hemidiaphragm. When using a THE method, intrathoracic dissection close to the esophageal wall minimizes the risk of significant chylous leaks.

Early diagnosis helps to minimize the impact of this complication. If a thoracotomy approach was used for esophagectomy, leave the chest tube in place until some enteral feeding occurs because this will increase thoracic duct flow and turn the chyle whitish, thereby unmasking a chylous leak. We routinely place an adjuvant jejunostomy tube at esophagectomy. On postoperative day 3, low rate (10–30 ml/hr maximum) tube feedings are initiated. Even at this low rate, if there is a chylous leak, it will be apparent early. A high-volume whitish pleural drainage makes the clinical diagnosis easy. To confirm the diagnosis, fluid should be sent for evaluation. The characteristic findings of chyle are listed in Table 3. Management depends on chest tube output as follows:

<500 ml/24 hours: continue nonoperative management because these should stop spontaneously.

>500 but <1000 ml/24 hours: initial nonoperative management. If not resolved or significantly reduced in 5 to 7 days, proceed with operative duct ligation

>1000 ml/24 hours: early operative intervention for duct ligation.

Beware: the THE method does not open the mediastinal pleura, and therefore chylous leaks lead to postoperative mediastinal fluid collections. These are radiographically apparent but usually are not clinically significant.

Transhiatal Herniation of Abdominal Structures

The esophageal hiatus is widened at surgery to allow for unrestricted passage of the replacement conduit without risk of graft ischemia. It is possible, therefore, for postesophagectomy herniation of abdominal structures up into the mediastinum to occur. It is not common, especially in its acute presentation. Clinically, reports indicate that this complication presents in two forms—early and late. Early herniation occurs soon after surgery, while the patient is still hospitalized. Generally these patients are acutely symptomatic, with some chest discomfort and shortness of breath. A chest film demonstrates air-filled loops of bowel in the chest. Late herniation is detected on chest films obtained to watch for recurrent tumor. Most of the time a segment of transverse colon passes up through the widened hiatus. Aside from a tendency for constipation, patients are completely asymptomatic.

Options for prevention include the following. At surgery, widen the hiatus only as much as needed to accomplish the mediastinal dissection and to pass the esophageal conduit freely. Sometimes the hiatus must be narrowed slightly before abdominal closure. We do not tack the stomach to the hiatal rim because this may lead to serosal tearing or compromise of conduit blood supply. The residual omentum can sometimes be used as a "dam," tacking it around the hiatus. Patients who present acutely need immediate transabdominal reexploration, reduction of the herniated contents to the abdominal cavity, and the omentum sewn in the hiatus to prevent reherniation. Patients found to have herniation incidentally but who are asymptomatic can be followed for any worsening of symptoms.

Suggested Readings

Gillinov AM, Heitmiller RF: Strategies to reduce pulmonary complications after transhiatal esophagectomy, *Dis Esophagus* 11:43, 1998.

Heitmiller RF: Thoracic Incisions. In Baue AE, Geha AS, Hammond GL, and others, editors, *Glenn's thoracic and cardiovascular surgery*, ed 6, Stamford, CT, Appleton & Lange, 1996, p. 73.

Heitmiller RF, Fischer A, Liddicoat JR: Cervical esophagogastric anastomosis: results following esophagectomy, *Dis Esophagus* 12:264, 1999.

Heitmiller RF, Jones B: Transient diminished airway protection following transhiatal esophagectomy, *Am J Surg* 162:442, 1991.

Liebermann-Meffert DMI, Luescher U, Neff U, and others: Esophagectomy without thoracotomy: Is there a risk of mediastinal bleeding? *Ann Surg* 206:643, 1987

Orringer MB, Marshall B, Iannettoni MD: Eliminating the cervical esophagogastric anastomotic leak with side to side stapled anastomosis, *J Thorac Cardiovasc Surg* 119:277, 2000.

Turner GG: Some experience in the surgery of the oesophagus, *N Engl J Med* 205:657, 1991.

Wormuth JK, Heitmiller RF: Esophageal conduit necrosis, *Thorac Surg Clin* 16:11, 2006.

THE STOMACH

BENIGN GASTRIC ULCER

William E. Fisher, MD, and F. Charles Brunicardi, MD

The discovery of effective antacids in the 1970s eliminated 80% of the surgeries that were previously required to address complications of gastric ulcers. Nevertheless, benign gastric ulcers are still commonly encountered by practicing general surgeons. Although control of acid secretion is now addressed, *Helicobacter pylori* infection and the use of aspirin and nonsteroidal anti-inflammatory drugs (NSAIDs) remain as the two major etiological factors (Fig. 1). Cigarette smoking also inhibits the gastric mucosal defense barrier. Patients classically present with pain occurring shortly after meals. Pain boring through to the back suggests a posterior penetrating gastric ulcer. On physical exam, pain with palpation of the epigastrium may or may not be present. Distension and a succession splash are indicative of gastric outlet obstruction. A palpable mass should raise the suspicion of advanced gastric malignancy. Involuntary guarding is indicative of peritonitis and gastric perforation. A rectal exam should be performed to detect melena, which is indicative of a bleeding gastric ulcer. Laboratory evaluation includes a complete blood count and coagulation studies. Upper endoscopy is the best diagnostic test and allows for biopsy and therapy of bleeding ulcers. Benign ulcers are usually found on the lesser curve and have a smooth base and radiating folds extending out from the ulcer, whereas malignant ulcers usually have irregular, heaped overhanging margins. Multiple (eight) biopsies should be performed to assess for malignancy and the presence of *H. pylori*. Medical treatment includes cessation of the use of NSAIDs and antacids and eradication of *H. pylori* infection. Different combinations of antacids (H_2-receptor blockers or proton pump inhibitors), bismuth, and antibiotics (metronidazole, tetracycline, amoxicillin, clarithromycin) can be used to eliminate *H. pylori*. Endoscopy is repeated in 6 weeks to ensure healing of the gastric ulcer. Failure of the ulcer to heal may indicate malignancy.

INDICATIONS FOR SURGICAL TREATMENT AND TECHNIQUE

Although the frequency of surgical therapy for gastric ulcers has decreased, the indications have not changed and include the following: intractability, bleeding, perforation, and obstruction. In contrast to duodenal ulcers, most gastric ulcers are treated with resection, ideally with antrectomy. Not all gastric ulcers are associated with acid hypersecretion, and the location of the ulcer is an important factor in determining the proper surgical technique.

Gastric ulcers are separated into five types on the basis of their location and the importance of acid hypersecretion in their pathogenesis (Fig. 2). Type I gastric ulcers are the most common and occur along the lesser curve of the stomach, usually at the incisura. In type II gastric ulcers, there are two ulcers. One ulcer is in the body of the stomach, usually around the incisura, and another is in the duodenum. The ulcer in the duodenum can be active or healed. A type III gastric ulcer is prepyloric. Only type II and type III gastric ulcers are associated with acid hypersecretion and require an acid-reducing operation. A type IV gastric ulcer occurs high on the lesser curve, near the gastroesophageal junction. A type V gastric ulcer is caused by medications such as NSAIDs. Type V gastric ulcers respond to cessation of the offending medication (NSAIDs) when this is possible.

INTRACTABILITY OR NONHEALING

Intractability is a rare indication for gastric ulcer surgery today, and the surgeon should carefully consider operation for this reason. Traditionally, "intractable" was defined as an ulcer that failed to heal after 12 weeks of medical therapy. However, most patients are currently given more than twice this time before surgical consultation. Because acid suppression is now so effective, the surgeon must consider the reasons a gastric ulcer might fail to heal (Table 1). The presence of cancer is always high on the list. Persistent, resistant *H. pylori* infection or a patient who failed to comply with the multidrug regimen should be considered. Occult use of NSAIDs, motility disorders, and Zollinger-Ellison syndrome are additional reasons a gastric ulcer might fail to heal. Surgery should be approached cautiously in thin or marginally nourished patients. To avoid chronic problems associated with irreversible operations, a conservative approach is prudent.

Type II and type III ulcers are associated with acid hypersecretion, and traditional surgical treatment includes an acid-reducing component of the operation, such as antrectomy including the gastric ulcer with the addition of a truncal vagotomy. Type I and type IV gastric ulcers are not associated with acid hypersecretion, and successful surgical treatment does not require an acid-reducing operation. For type I gastric ulcers, an antrectomy including the ulcer is sufficient. Some surgeons would favor a wedge resection with (type II, III) or without (type I, IV) highly selective vagotomy in thin or frail patients who might not respond well to a major resection.

Given that surgical treatment of type IV ulcers is more complicated because of their location near the gastroesophageal junction, it is fortunate that these are the least common gastric ulcers. The surgeon must consider the distance from the gastroesophageal

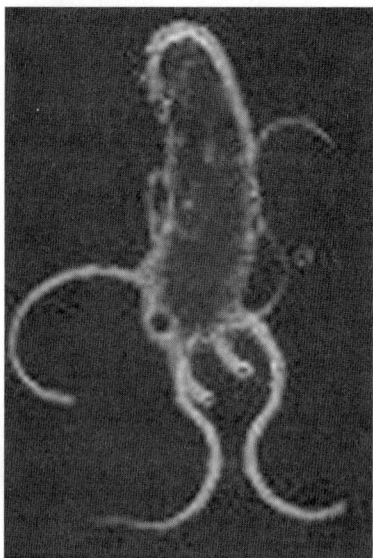

Figure 1 *Helicobacter pylori* (http://blogs.warwick.ac.uk/teampylori/2005/11/22/helicobacter_pylori_pic.jpg.warwickblogs; accessed June 12, 2007).

Table 1: Differential Diagnosis in Intractable Gastric Ulcer

- Cancer
- Persistent *Helicobacter pylori*
  - Resistant organisms
  - Poor patient compliance
- Occult use of nonsteroidal anti-inflammatory drugs/acetylsalicylic acid
- Motility disorder
- Zollinger-Ellison syndrome

junction, the size of the ulcer, and the extent of surrounding inflammation. Antrectomy with extension of the resection along the lesser curvature to include the ulcer (Pauchet procedure) can be performed if the stomach can be securely closed without narrowing the gastric inlet (if ulcer and severe inflammation ends 2–5 cm below the gastroesophageal junction) (Fig. 3). For rare type IV gastric ulcers located within 2 cm of the gastroesophageal junction, resection of the gastric antrum and body up to the gastroesophageal junction and reconstruction with a Roux-en-Y limb of jejunum (Csendes procedure) may be required (Fig. 3).

Sometimes a large gastric ulcer is encountered that is not truly a type IV ulcer but is so large that the ulcer and surrounding inflammation extend toward the gastroesophageal junction. A subtotal gastrectomy with truncal vagotomy and a Roux-en-Y reconstruction is an option in such a case. However, another option is to perform an antrectomy with truncal vagotomy, leaving the ulcer in place (Kelling-Madlener procedure) (Fig. 3). Multiple biopsies of the ulcer must be taken to rule out malignancy, and the ulcer bed should then be cauterized. Giant gastric ulcers are defined as

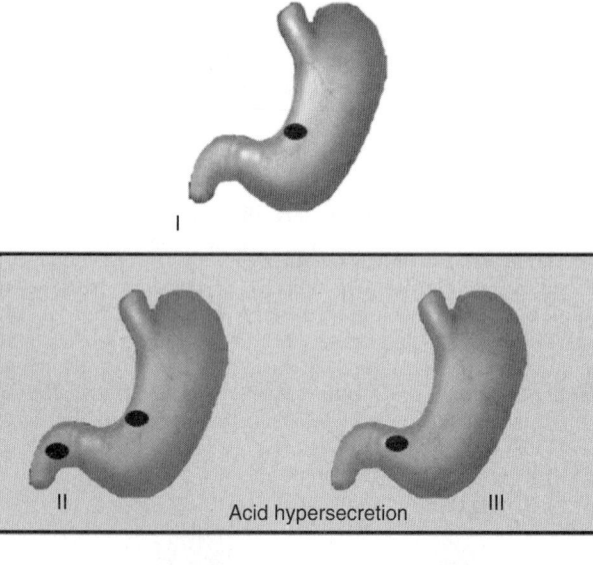

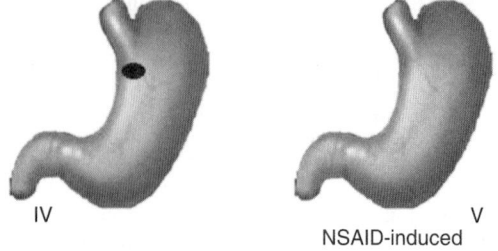

Figure 2 Modified Johnson classification of gastric ulcers. (**I**) Lesser curve, incisura. (**II**) Body of stomach, incisura + duodenal ulcer (active or healed). (**III**) Prepyloric. (**IV**) High on lesser curve, near gastroesophageal junction. (**V**) Medication induced (nonsteroidal anti-inflammatory drugs/acetylsalicylic acid), anywhere in stomach.

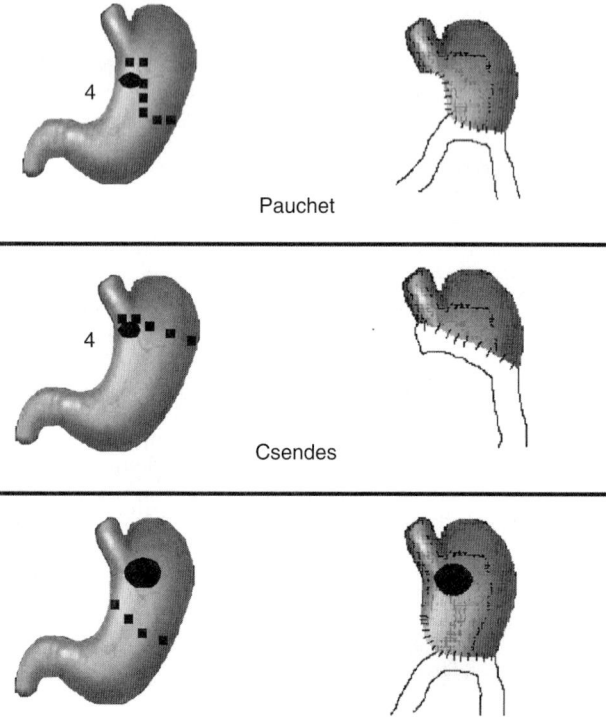

Pauchet

Csendes

Kelling-Madlener

Figure 3 Special surgical procedures for gastric ulcers.

ulcers >3 cm in diameter. As many as one third of these ulcers are actually ulcerated gastric cancers. Sometimes penetration of the ulcer into adjacent organs (pancreas, liver) precludes safe resection. A conservative technique is to incise the gastric wall circumferentially around the ulcer, leaving it in place and closing the gastric wall in two layers. Again, the ulcer is biopsied multiple times, and the mucosal surface is then cauterized. An omental patch can be sutured to the ulcer surface.

BLEEDING

Bleeding gastric ulcers tend to occur in older patients with multiple comorbidities, which increase the operative risk. Mortality for patients with bleeding gastric ulcers is approximately 10%. Endoscopy with the use of heater probe coagulation or injection therapy (or both) can usually stop the active bleeding and allow stabilization of the patient. In this setting, a semi-elective operation in a fully resuscitated patient is associated with a better outcome than an emergent operation in a patient who is in shock from recurrent bleeding. However, if the patient can be stabilized and the factors producing the ulcer (acid, *H. pylori*, NSAIDs) can be controlled, a major operation in a high-risk patient may be avoided altogether. Therefore assessing the likelihood of recurrent bleeding is important in surgical decision making. Unfortunately, there is no perfect method of predicting which patients will bleed again. Stigmata of recent bleeding, nonpulsatile bleeding, or an adherent clot seen at endoscopy are associated with a low risk of rebleeding. The two characteristics at endoscopy that predict a high rebleeding risk (50% to 80%) are active pulsatile bleeding or a visible vessel. However, the risk may be decreased after successful endoscopic therapy. Close communication between the endoscopist and the surgeon is critically important, and presence of the surgeon at the time of endoscopy is ideal.

Distal gastric resection to include the ulcer is the ideal procedure for bleeding gastric ulcers. In extremely high-risk patients, a second choice is gastrotomy with excision through the gastric lumen or oversewing and biopsy of the ulcer. Vagotomy and drainage or long-term acid suppression is also required for type II and type III gastric ulcers because these are associated with acid hypersecretion. Patients should also be tested for *H. pylori*, which should be eradicated if present.

PERFORATION

In the setting of perforation, surgery is almost always indicated. Nonsurgical treatment can occasionally be successful in a stable patient without peritonitis in whom radiologic studies document a sealed perforation. As with bleeding gastric ulcers, perforated gastric ulcers occur in elderly debilitated patients, and the mortality rate is reported to be 10% to 40%. Perforated gastric ulcers are commonly associated with NSAID use (type V). The ideal surgical option is distal gastric resection, particularly in hemodynamically stable patients with a long history of peptic ulcer disease or a failed previous vagotomy and drainage procedure. Vagotomy is added or revisited only in the setting of type II and type III ulcers that are associated with acid hypersecretion. Preoperative shock, a delay in surgery, and comorbid factors must be considered. In severely ill patients, who constitute the majority, lesser procedures such as local excision or biopsy and omental patch closure, with or without truncal vagotomy and drainage, are commonly practiced alternatives. Gastric ulcers should always be biopsied if not excised to rule out cancer. All patients should be tested for *H. pylori* and treated if positive. Some surgeons advocate more conservative procedures when patients are known to be *H. pylori* positive before surgical intervention. However, many patients with

perforated gastric ulcers are *H. pylori* negative. In the absence of resection, repeat endoscopy should be performed in approximately 6 weeks to ensure healing of the ulcer and eradication of *H. pylori*; biopsy should be performed to rule out cancer if the ulcer is not completely healed.

OBSTRUCTION

Obstruction is the least common indication for surgery in gastric ulcers. Antrectomy is the procedure of choice. In this setting, it is important for the surgeon to assess the duodenal stump before transaction of the duodenum. Scarring often precludes a Billroth I reconstruction and may also make a Billroth II reconstruction dangerous because of the risk of a duodenal stump leak. If there is concern about safe closure of the duodenal stump, a safe and conservative alternative is to perform a vagotomy and gastrojejunostomy. As with all gastric ulcers, a high vigilance for the presence of gastric cancer must be maintained.

A summary of the options for the surgical management of gastric ulcers is provided in Table 2. Although antrectomy to include the ulcer is the ideal treatment for all indications, there are acceptable alternatives in compromised patients. These should be considered in emergency situations.

STRESS GASTRITIS

Stress gastritis usually develops within 2 days of a major traumatic event or insult. Common predisposing clinical conditions include multiple traumas, often with hypotension and massive transfusion; sepsis, often with acute respiratory distress syndrome or systemic inflammatory response syndrome; and multiple organ failure. A large body of literature supports the concept that stress gastritis can be reduced with early prophylaxis using antacids, sucralfate, and prostaglandin-synthesis promoters. Stress gastritis usually begins in the proximal stomach but can involve the entire stomach. Bleeding can be slow or rapid enough to produce hemorrhagic shock. After lavage of the stomach, endoscopic measures confirm the diagnosis, establish the extent of disease, and offer an opportunity to stop the bleeding with heater probe coagulation and injection. When this fails, angiographic embolization or infusion of vasopressin is typically the next step and has been reported to decrease transfusion requirements but not mortality. When these measures are not effective, the last resort, surgical therapy,

Table 2: Surgical Treatment of Gastric Ulcers

Indication	Ideal Treatment*	Alternative Treatment
Intractability	Antrectomy to include ulcer	Local excision ● Add TV or HSV for II, III
Bleeding	Antrectomy to include ulcer	Local excision or gastrotomy with oversew ● Add TV for II, III
Perforation	Antrectomy to include ulcer	Local excision or biopsy and omental patch closure ● Add TV for II, III
Obstruction	Antrectomy to include ulcer	Gastrojejunostomy (if duodenum scarred) and TV

HSV, highly selective vagotomy; *TV*, truncal vagotomy

*Add truncal vagotomy for type II and type III ulcers.

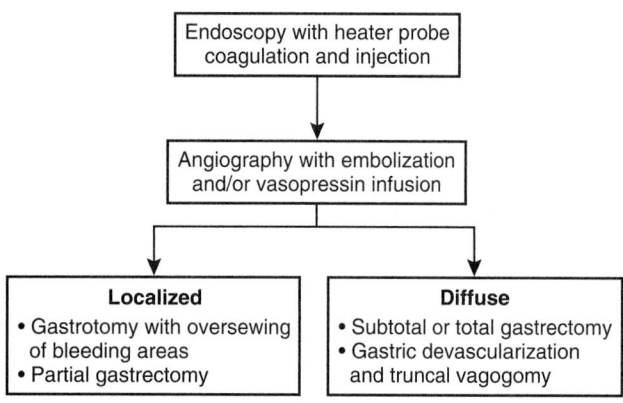

Figure 4 Management of stress gastritis.

is indicated. Endoscopic evaluation of the location of bleeding provides important information for the surgeon. If possible, a gastrotomy with oversewing of the bleeding areas is indicated.

In cases in which this is not effective but the bleeding is localized, a partial gastrectomy is recommended. When the entire gastric mucosa is bleeding, a subtotal or total gastrectomy has been advocated, but the mortality rate is high. Recently, gastric devascularization (ligation of all arterial blood supply except for the short gastric vessels) and truncal vagotomy have been recommended. This results in a rebleeding rate of 10% but may be associated with a lower mortality than total gastrectomy. An algorithm for the management of bleeding stress gastritis is provided in Fig. 4.

SUGGESTED READINGS

Csendes A and others: Type IV gastric ulcer: a new hypothesis, *Surgery* 101:361, 1987.

Dempsey DT: Stomach. In Brunicardi FC, Andersen DK, Billiar TR, and others, editors: *Schwartz's principles of surgery,* ed 8, New York, 2005, McGraw-Hill, p 1221.

Mulholland MW. Peptic ulcer disease. In Bell RH, Rikkers LF, Mulholland MW, editors: *Digestive tract surgery: a text and atlas,* Philadelphia, 1996, Lippincott-Raven Publishers, p 167.

DUODENAL ULCER

Brian J. Winkleman, MD, Anatolie Usatii, MD, and
E. Christopher Ellison, MD

The pathophysiology of duodenal ulcer has shifted in recent years from acid hypersecretion to *Helicobacter pylori* infection. Approximately 90% of patients with duodenal ulcer have *H. pylori* infection of the antral mucosa. The proportion of duodenal ulcers caused by nonsteroidal anti-inflammatory drug (NSAID) use is increasing, particularly in the elderly population. Lifetime risk for duodenal ulcer is approximately 10%. Current medical therapy (Table 1), including antibiotics, histamine receptor antagonists,

and proton pump inhibitors, has proved effective in eradicating *H. pylori* infection and reducing ulcer recurrence rates. Over the past 2 decades, the necessity for surgical intervention has declined significantly. Despite this trend, surgeons must remain familiar with the current surgical management of duodenal ulcer.

INDICATIONS FOR SURGERY

Although the frequency of operation for duodenal ulcer has decreased, the surgical indications have remained the same: bleeding, perforation, obstruction, and intractability. Bleeding or perforation account for nearly 90% of surgical procedures for duodenal ulcer. Table 2 shows the indications, preferred operations, and risk of ulcer recurrence.

Bleeding

Bleeding is the most common complication of duodenal ulcer and is the most common cause of ulcer-related death. The incidence of bleeding is 55 in 1000 person-years in recent long-term studies and has remained constant. Patients with bleeding duodenal ulcer may have a variety of presentations, ranging from melena or occult heme-positive stools to massive hematemesis resulting in hemorrhagic shock. Initial management consists of establishing large-bore

Table 1: Treatment Regimens for *Helicobacter pylori* Eradication

Triple Therapies

Bismuth subsalicylate 525 mg QID +
Metronidazole 250 mg QID +
Tetracycline 500 mg QID

Proton pump inhibitor BID +
Amoxicillin 1000 mg BID +
Clarithromycin 500 mg BID

Quadruple Therapy

Bismuth subsalicylate 525 mg QID +
Proton pump inhibitor BID +
Metronidazole 250 mg QID +
Tetracycline 500 mg QID

Note: Treatment for 10–14 days recommended. *BID,* twice daily; *QID,* four times daily.

Table 2: Indications, Preferred Operation, and Risk of Recurrence in Duodenal Ulcer Surgery

Indication	Preferred Operation	Risk of Recurrence
Acute bleeding	Oversewing of ulcer, pyloroplasty, ± truncal vagotomy	5%
Chronic bleeding	Truncal vagotomy and antrectomy	2%
Perforation	Closure with omental patch ± proximal gastric vagotomy	10%–20%
Obstruction	Truncal vagotomy and antrectomy	2%
Intractability	Proximal gastric vagotomy	10%–20%

intravenous access, resuscitation with isotonic crystalloid and blood products, and reversal of anticoagulation if necessary. A nasogastric tube should be inserted and the stomach lavaged with saline. Upper endoscopy will establish the diagnosis and exclude other sources of bleeding, including Mallory-Weiss tear, Dieulafoy ulcer, esophageal or gastric varices, inflammation, or neoplasm. Endoscopic therapy consisting of epinephrine injection, heater probe, or both may be sufficient to control bleeding. Findings of active bleeding or a visible vessel in the ulcer bed on initial endoscopy is associated with a 50% risk of rebleeding. Most patients with bleeding duodenal ulcer are treated successfully with a combination of endoscopic therapy and proton pump inhibitors. In selected cases, bleeding can be controlled in angiography with embolization. Factors predicting failure of nonoperative management include ongoing hemodynamic instability, significant comorbidities, and transfusion requirement exceeding 4 to 6 units in 24 hours (Table 3). Endoscopic findings of active bleeding, a visible vessel, adherent clot, or an ulcer >2 cm also predict failure of conservative therapy. Early surgical intervention after initial resuscitation should be considered in elderly patients with atherosclerotic coronary heart disease or hemorrhagic shock. Delay in operation may increase morbidity and mortality in this high-risk group.

Perforation

Perforation is the second most common complication of duodenal ulcer. The incidence of perforation has decreased in recent long-term studies from 14 in 1000 to 8 in 1000 person-years. Patients with free perforation usually present with sudden onset of severe, unrelenting abdominal pain. Fever, nausea, and vomiting are common, and physical examination often reveals peritonitis. Presentation may be more subtle, however, in elderly or debilitated patients. Upright chest radiograph shows pneumoperitoneum in approximately 80% of patients. The absence of free air, however, does not exclude the diagnosis. Essentially all patients with duodenal perforation require operation. Nonsurgical treatment has been advocated for patients when perforation is suspected to have occurred more than 24 hours before presentation and when a radiologic contrast study has documented a sealed perforation. This approach is not applicable to patients with hemodynamic instability or clinical peritonitis.

Obstruction

Modern medical therapy has reduced the incidence of gastric outlet obstruction secondary to duodenal ulcer to less than 5%. Patients with obstruction typically present with nausea and nonbilious vomiting and may have significant weight loss. A hypokalemic hypochloremic metabolic alkalosis may develop. Initial management includes nasogastric decompression, intravenous hydration, electrolyte repletion, and antisecretory medication. Obstruction is confirmed by endoscopy, and biopsies should be performed to exclude malignancy.

Table 3: Factors Predicting Failure of Nonoperative Management of Bleeding Duodenal Ulcer

Hemodynamic instability
Significant comorbid conditions
Transfusion requirements greater than 4–6 units in 24 hours
Endoscopic features of the ulcer
Actively bleeding vessel
Visible vessel
Adherent clot
Size >2 cm

Endoscopic balloon dilatation may transiently improve obstructive symptoms in up to 80% of patients, but long-term success is estimated at less than 50%. Most patients will ultimately require surgery for definitive management of gastric outlet obstruction.

Intractability

Intractability is a rare indication for operative treatment of duodenal ulcer. Antisecretory medications and antibiotics targeting *H. pylori* have proved effective in healing duodenal ulcers and preventing recurrence. A small percentage of patients may present with nonhealing or recurrent ulcers despite maximal medical therapy. Patient noncompliance, malignancy, and Zollinger-Ellison syndrome should be excluded before performing surgery.

OPERATIVE APPROACH

A variety of factors influence the surgeon's choice of operation for duodenal ulcer. Important elements include patient age, comorbid conditions, hemodynamic status, previous duodenal ulcer, NSAID use, and adequacy of medical therapy. Choice of operation is also largely influenced by the surgeon's experience and personal preference. In general, nonresective ulcer operations have a lower morbidity and mortality rate but a higher ulcer recurrence rate when compared with resective procedures. In the setting of acute bleeding or perforation, there is an increasing trend among surgeons to forgo an acid-reducing operation in preference for damage control and *H. pylori* eradication. Recent reports indicate in this era of effective acid suppression and *H. pylori* treatment, a definitive ulcer surgery in the emergent setting may not be necessary. The impact of this practice on long-term ulcer recurrence remains to be seen.

Bleeding

Massive bleeding is usually the result of transmural ulceration along the posterior duodenal wall, causing erosion of the gastroduodenal artery. Emergent surgical intervention is required when bleeding is refractory to endoscopic therapy or in the presence of hemorrhagic shock. Preoperative resuscitation is essential. Once the patient is taken to the operative theater, a nasogastric tube and Foley catheter should be placed. An upper midline incision is used, extending from the xiphoid to just above the umbilicus. A Kocher maneuver is performed to mobilize the duodenum. The pylorus is identified by palpation and visualization of the pyloric vein. Two silk traction sutures are placed superior and inferior to the pyloric ring. A longitudinal pyloromyotomy is performed, extending approximately 3 cm on each side of the pylorus (Fig. 1). Upon opening of the duodenal bulb, digital pressure is applied over the ulcer base to temporize bleeding and allow resuscitation before suture control is obtained. Proper control of bleeding requires ligation of the gastroduodenal artery proximal and distal to the site of penetration. A third suture, a U stitch, is placed medially to control the transverse pancreatic branch (Fig. 2).

After bleeding has been controlled, we usually proceed with pyloroplasty and truncal vagotomy. The gastric mucosa may be biopsied for histologic analysis for *H. pylori*. The longitudinal pyloromyotomy is closed transversely in a Heineke–Mikulicz fashion with a single layer of 3-0 silk sutures (Fig. 3). Transverse closure reduces gastric outlet obstruction following vagotomy.

For acute duodenal ulcer bleeding, we usually proceed with truncal vagotomy. Exposure to the distal esophagus is provided by dividing the triangular ligament and the peritoneal lining overlying the gastroesophageal junction. The esophagus is gently mobilized and encircled with a Penrose drain. The anterior or left vagal trunk is usually located along the anterior midportion of the esophagus.

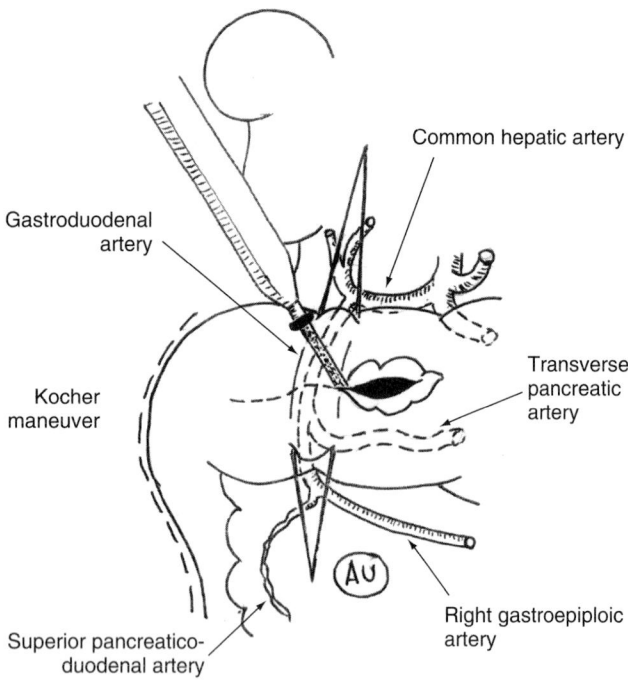

Figure 1 Longitudinal pyloromyotomy and relevant vasculature for bleeding duodenal ulcer.

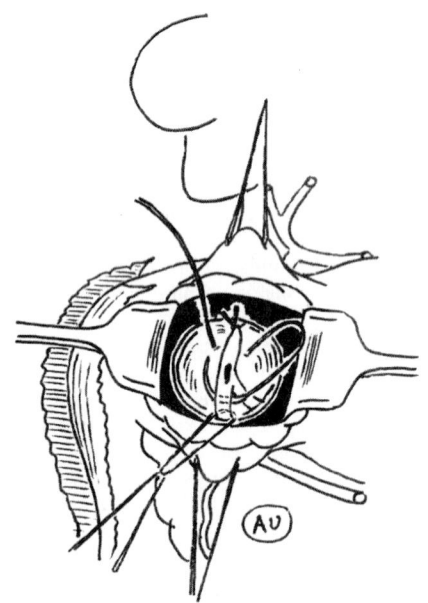

Figure 2 Three-point suture ligation of the gastroduodenal and transverse pancreatic arteries for bleeding duodenal ulcer.

The posterior or right vagal trunk is more variable in position and slightly larger in size. Complete vagotomy requires transection of the vagal trunks proximal to the hepatic and celiac branches. Clips are placed proximally and distally on the vagi, and a 2-cm segment of each nerve is transected. The esophagus should be skeletonized for 5 to 7 cm proximal to the gastroesophageal junction to ensure that all accessory vagal fibers are transected.

Truncal vagotomy may be deferred in unstable or moribund patients or in those who have not received previous medical therapy. Some surgeons report controlling acute ulcer bleeding through a lateral duodenotomy and replace vagotomy and pyloroplasty with *H. pylori* eradication and medical acid suppression.

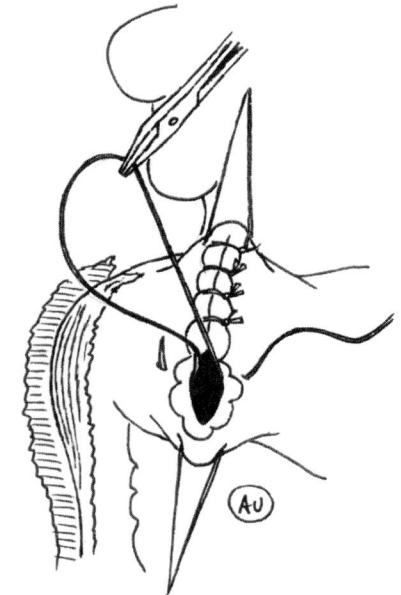

Figure 3 Heineke-Mikulicz pyloroplasty.

Truncal vagotomy and antrectomy is an alternative operation for bleeding duodenal ulcer and is the procedure of choice for chronic bleeding. Antrectomy refers to a 35% distal gastrectomy with complete resection of all gastrin-producing antral mucosa. Surgical landmarks for gastric resection include the third vein distal to the gastroesophageal junction along the lesser curvature and the point along the greater curvature at which the epiploic vessels are in nearest proximity to the gastric wall. Gastrointestinal continuity is restored with a gastroduodenostomy (Billroth I) or gastrojejunostomy (Billroth II). Vagotomy and antrectomy have a lower rate of ulcer recurrence but higher operative morbidity and mortality compared with vagotomy and pyloroplasty.

Perforation

Surgical options for perforated duodenal ulcer are simple patch closure with *H. pylori* eradication and patch closure with proximal gastric vagotomy. Simple patch closure alone should be performed in patients with hemodynamic instability, those with perforation of more than 24 hours' duration, and those whose perforation is clearly associated with NSAID use. Exposure to the duodenal perforation is provided by an upper midline incision. Primary closure of the perforation is usually accomplished with three sutures (Fig. 4). The tails of the sutures are subsequently used to anchor a vascularized omental patch. The abdomen is irrigated to reduce the risk of postoperative abscess formation. Patients should be tested for *H. pylori* with a breath test or serologic studies. *H. pylori* eradication is essential and will decrease ulcer recurrence.

Proximal gastric vagotomy should be performed in stable patients who have failed or are noncompliant with medical therapy. Exposure of the distal esophagus allows identification of the anterior and posterior vagal trunks. The distal 4 to 6 cm of esophagus is denervated by ligating branches of the major trunks. The criminal nerve of Grassi, arising from the posterior vagus to innervate the gastric cardia, must be identified and divided (Fig. 5). Neurovascular ligation is continued along the anterior aspect of the lesser curvature to a point approximately 4 cm proximal to the pylorus. The nerve of Laterjet, or crow's foot, is preserved to supply vagal innervation to the pyloric region (Fig. 6). Entering the lesser sac will provide excellent exposure for ligation of the posterior neurovascular bundles.

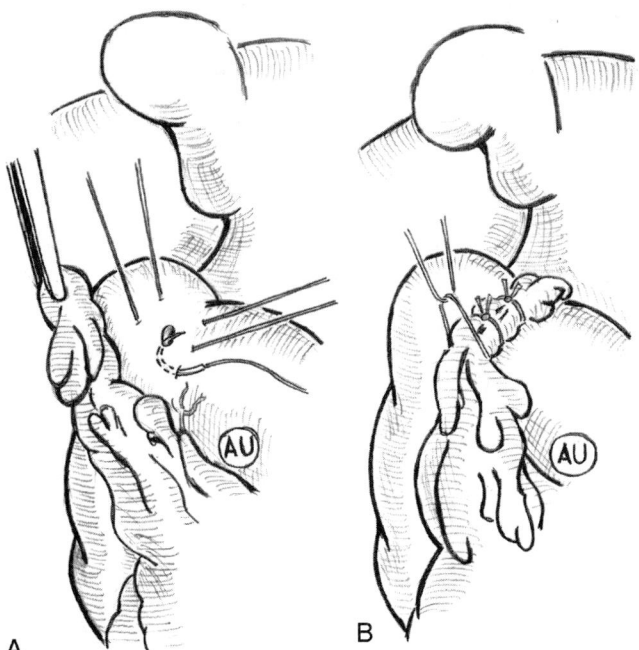

A   B

Figure 4   Omental patch closure of perforated duodenal ulcer.

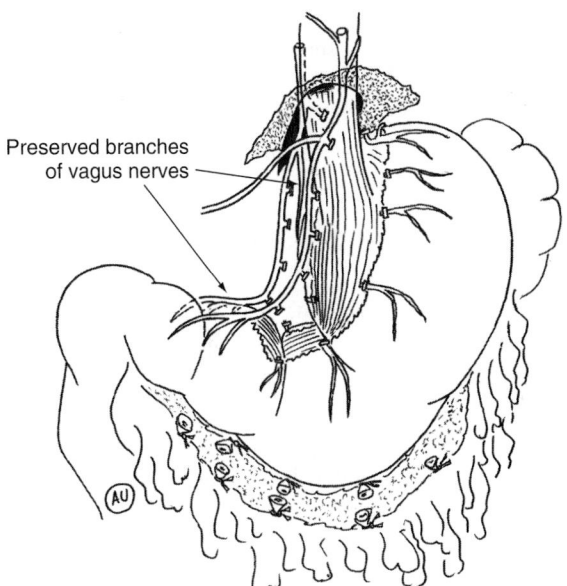

Figure 6   Proximal gastric vagotomy.

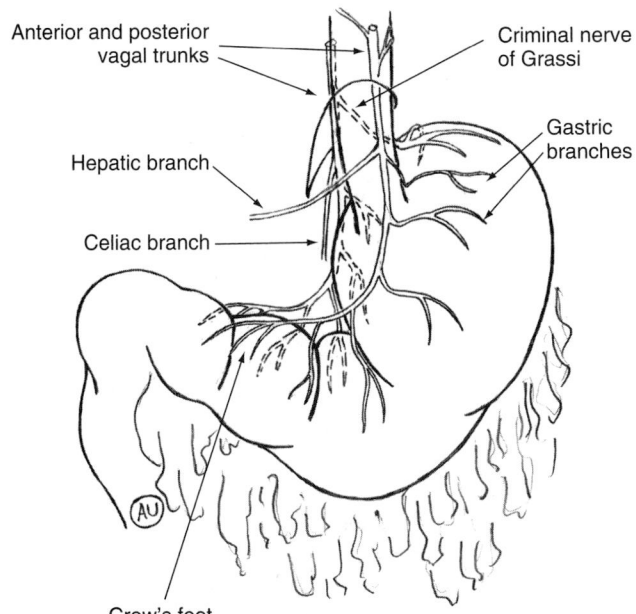

Figure 5   Anatomy of vagal nerves.

Obstruction

Although rarely performed, truncal vagotomy and antrectomy is our preferred operation for pyloric obstruction secondary to duodenal ulcer. It is important to assess the condition and mobility of the duodenum intraoperatively before proceeding with a definitive procedure. Severe pyloric inflammation may complicate efforts for reconstruction. If a tension-free anastomosis can be completed, we usually perform vagotomy and antrectomy with Billroth I reconstruction. Otherwise, a retrocolic Billroth II anastomosis is performed.

Noncompliance of the duodenal stump following antrectomy with Billroth II reconstruction can make duodenal closure extremely difficult and subject to disruption. Duodenal stump leak is a life-threatening complication, causing severe intra-abdominal sepsis. Diagnosis requires wide drainage and reclosure with a lateral tube duodenostomy.

Intractability

Operative intervention for the intractable duodenal ulcer has almost disappeared. Proximal gastric vagotomy is recommended in the few patients who have duodenal ulcer disease refractory to medical management. This procedure can be performed electively as previously described.

▍ COMPLICATIONS

Sound clinical judgment and precise surgical technique result in acceptably low perioperative morbidity and mortality. Complications of surgical therapy include ulcer recurrence, dumping syndrome, postvagotomy diarrhea, and gastroparesis. Ulcer recurrence is less than 2% with vagotomy and antrectomy, 5% with vagotomy and pyloroplasty, and 10% to 20% with proximal gastric vagotomy. Incomplete vagotomy, retained gastric antrum, or Zollinger-Ellison syndrome should be considered in patients with recurrent duodenal ulcer. The diagnosis of Zollinger-Ellison syndrome is confirmed by the presence of fasting hypergastrinemia while off proton pump inhibitors and a secretin stimulation test. An increase in serum gastrin of 200 pg/ml or greater strongly suggests the presence of a gastrinoma.

Dumping syndrome may occur after any form of vagotomy and is characterized by postprandial tachycardia, diaphoresis, abdominal pain, and diarrhea. These symptoms usually improve with time, dietary modification, or octreotide. Conversion to Roux-en-Y gastrojejunostomy may be required for persistent debilitating symptoms.

Postvagotomy diarrhea consists of watery stools occurring approximately 30 minutes to 1 hour after meals. As with dumping, symptoms generally improve with time. Octreotide and antimotility agents may be beneficial in some patients.

Gastroparesis is a common complication following antrectomy for preoperative gastric outlet obstruction. Initial management consists of prokinetic agents including Reglan and erythromycin. Persistent gastroparesis may warrant further operation.

LAPAROSCOPIC SURGERY

In recent years, there has been increasing enthusiasm among surgeons for the application of minimally invasive techniques to the management of duodenal ulcer disease. Standard ulcer operations, including truncal vagotomy, proximal gastric vagotomy, pyloroplasty, and antrectomy, have proved technically feasible with a laparoscopic approach. These procedures, however, should only be considered by those with advanced laparoscopic skills. Early results with this approach have been encouraging. Until data from long-term follow-up are available, the role of minimally invasive surgery for duodenal ulcer disease remains to be established.

Currently, laparoscopic surgery is most applicable for the treatment of perforated duodenal ulcer and intractability. For these procedures, the patient is placed in a modified lithotomy position, in slight reverse Trendelenburg, with the surgeon standing between the legs. Port placement is similar to that for other upper GI procedures. The perforated ulcer is closed with intracorporeal sutures and buttressed with an omental tongue, and the abdominal cavity is extensively irrigated. In selected patients, a definitive laparoscopic antiulcer procedure is performed. Proximal gastric vagotomy can be accomplished as previously described using the harmonic scalpel. An alternative and less time-consuming procedure is a posterior truncal vagotomy with anterior seromyotomy (Taylor procedure).

Laparoscopic repair of perforated duodenal ulcer has acceptable morbidity and mortality compared with open procedures. Several reports demonstrate decreased postoperative analgesia requirements, decreased incidence of wound infection, shorter hospital stays, and earlier return to work with minimally invasive techniques. Up to 20% of laparoscopic repairs require conversion to an open procedure. Preoperative risk factors for conversion include

Table 4: Risk Factors for Conversion of Laparoscopic to Open Repair of Perforated Duodenal Ulcer

Shock
Duration of symptoms >24 hours
Confounding medical condition
Age >70 years
Poor laparoscopic experience
ASA III–IV
Ulcers >6–10 mm in diameter
Ulcers with friable edges

presence of shock and duration of symptoms greater than 24 hours (Table 4). Long-term data for ulcer recurrence are currently being evaluated.

SUGGESTED READINGS

Dubois F: New surgical strategy for gastroduodenal ulcer: laparoscopic approach, *World J Surg* 24:270, 2000.

Jamieson GG: Current status of indications for surgery in peptic ulcer disease, *World J Surg* 24:256, 2000.

Lassen A, Hallas J, Schaffalitzky de Muckadell OB: Complicated and uncomplicated peptic ulcers in a Danish county 1993–2002: a population-based cohort study, *Am J Gastroenterol* 101:945, 2006.

Lunevicius R, Morkevicius M: Management strategies, early results, benefits, and risk factors of laparoscopic repair of perforated peptic ulcer, *World J Surg* 29:1299, 2005.

Millat B, Fingerhut A, Borie F: Surgical treatment of complicated duodenal ulcers: controlled trials, *World J Surg* 24:299, 2000.

Ng EK, et al: Eradication of *Helicobacter pylori* prevents recurrence of ulcer after simple closure of duodenal ulcer perforation: randomized controlled trial, *Ann Surg* 231:159, 2000.

Sarosi GA Jr, Jaiswal KR, Nwariaku FE, and others: Surgical therapy of peptic ulcers in the 21st century: more common than you think, *Am J Surg* 190:775, 2005.

Smith BR, Stabile BE: Emerging trends in peptic ulcer disease and damage control surgery in the *H. pylori* era, *Am J Surg* 71:797, 2005.

ZOLLINGER-ELLISON SYNDROME

Samuel E. Rice-Townsend, MD, and
Jeffrey A. Norton, MD

In 1955, at a meeting of the American Surgical Association, Drs. Robert Zollinger and Edwin Ellison first described a syndrome characterized by severe peptic ulcer disease in association with hypersecretion of gastric acid and non–beta islet cell tumors of the pancreas. We now understand that Zollinger-Ellison syndrome (ZES) is usually caused by a gastrin-secreting duodenal or pancreatic neuroendocrine tumor, or *gastrinoma,* more commonly found in the duodenum than the pancreas.

ZES is rare. It is the underlying cause of peptic ulcer disease in only 0.1 to 1.0% of cases, but it is responsible for closer to 2% of recurrent peptic ulcer disease. The syndrome occurs in a sporadic and familial

form. It is sporadic in 80% of cases and familial as part of the multiple endocrine neoplasia syndrome type 1 (MEN-1) 20% of the time (Table 1). Gastrinoma is the most common functional pancreatic neuroendocrine tumor in patients with MEN-1. Patients with ZES and MEN-1 are more likely to have multiple pancreatic or duodenal tumors than their counterparts with sporadic disease. Gastrinomas should be categorized as malignant. They have the potential to metastasize, and approximately one third of patients have evidence of lymph node, liver, or distant metastasis at the time of diagnosis.

DIAGNOSIS

Clinical Presentation

Clinical manifestations of ZES are mostly attributable to the hypersecretion of gastric acid. The most common symptoms are epigastric pain, heartburn, dysphagia, and diarrhea. Peptic ulceration is seen in 90% of patients with ZES. The proximal duodenum is the most common site of ulcers, but lesions in more unusual locations such as the distal duodenum and jejunum also occur. The ulcers associated with ZES recur much more frequently than sporadic ulcers and can

Table 1: Features of Multiple Endocrine Neoplasia Type 1 (MEN-1)

	MEN-1	Gene: MEN-1 (11q13) Pattern of Inheritance: AD
Location of Disease	Expression	Penetrance by Age 40
Parathyroid	Parathyroid adenoma	90
Pancreas/ Duodenum	Gastrinoma	40
	Insulinoma	10
	Glucogonoma, VIPoma, somatostatinoma	2
Anterior Pituitary	Prolactinoma	20
Other	Gastric enterochromaffin-like tumor	10
	Facial angiofibromas	85
	Collagenomas	70
	Lipomas	30

AD, autosomal dominant; *VIP*, vasoactive intestinal peptide.
Percentages from Brandi ML, Gagel RF, Angeli A, and others: J Clin Endocrinol Metab *86:5658, 2001.*

perforate; up to 10% of patients present initially with a perforated ulcer. Approximately 10% of patients have evidence of lower esophageal inflammation or even stricturing. Gastric acid hypersecretion can also cause a secretory diarrhea, which is seen in up to 40% of patients with ZES. Diarrhea is the sole presenting complaint in 20% of individuals. In advanced cases, patients may experience symptoms related to the size of the primary tumor itself or its metastases.

The diagnosis of ZES is commonly made several years after initial presentation. This is most likely due to a combination of factors. First, ZES is rare and may not initially be considered as a possible cause of symptoms. Second, hypergastrinemia can occur as a manifestation of a multitude of other diseases and conditions (Table 2). Certain cardinal signs demand a workup for ZES. These include ulcers located in the distal duodenum or jejunum, multiple or recurrent ulcers and ulcers associated with diarrhea. It is also important to consider ZES in any patient with peptic ulcer disease and primary hyperparathyroidism or nephrolithiasis or with a family history suggestive of MEN-1.

Diagnostic Testing

ZES is diagnosed by measuring a fasting serum level of gastrin and basal acid output (BAO). A secretin stimulation test is positive in approximately 90% of patients with ZES. Measurement of serum gastrin level is the initial test of choice for any patient suspected of having ZES. All patients with ZES have a serum gastrin level >100 pg/ml, with many patients having levels greater than 1000 pg/ml. Acid suppression therapy used to treat peptic ulcer disease also raises the serum gastrin level, and therefore patients should discontinue all proton pump inhibitors (PPIs) and H_2 antagonists 3 to 7 days before measurement of gastrin to ensure test accuracy. Moreover, a true elevated serum gastrin level is not specific for ZES and may be seen in a number of other conditions, including pernicious anemia, renal failure, and atrophic gastritis. To make the unequivocal diagnosis of ZES, BAO must also be measured and shown to be elevated (>15 mEq/hr or >5 mEq/hr if the patient has had prior acid reduction surgery). The combination of an elevated fasting level of gastrin and BAO is diagnostic of ZES.

Furthermore, the diagnosis of ZES can be confirmed using the secretin stimulation test. Patients with ZES have a paradoxical increase in serum level of gastrin in response to secretin. This test is particularly useful in equivocal cases in which the gastrin level is not markedly elevated and is helpful in differentiating gastrinomas from other causes of hypergastrinemia. It is performed by measuring basal serum gastrin, administering a 2 U/kg bolus of secretin intravenously, and then repeating serum gastrin levels at 2-, 5-, 10-, and 15-minute time points. To make the diagnosis of ZES, secretin stimulation must result in a >200 pg/ml increase in serum gastrin level. Recent results suggest that an increase of only 120 pg/ml is sufficient. This test is more than 93% sensitive for ZES.

Tumor Localization

Ideally, the precise location of the gastrinoma and any metastases should be determined preoperatively. This is accomplished using a combination of noninvasive imaging studies (Table 3). Approximately 80% of all gastrinomas are found within the *gastrinoma triangle,* an anatomic area that includes the first, second, and third portions of the duodenum and the head of the pancreas (Fig. 1). The primary tumor has, however, also been previously localized to extra-pancreatic, extra-intestinal sites in the body such as the ovary and the heart, making full-body imaging a requirement. Somatostatin receptor scintigraphy (SRS) is the imaging technique of choice for localizing both the primary and metastatic tumor. The radiolabeled somatostatin analog ^{111}In-pentetreotide has a high affinity for the type-2 somatostatin-receptor expressed by 80% of gastrinomas. This analogue binds to receptors on the surface of cells within the gastrinoma and thus reveals the location of the tumor (Fig. 2). With the ability to detect 80% of all gastrinomas and a specificity approaching 100%, SRS is better than all other imaging studies combined. Computed tomography (CT) can be helpful in conjunction with SRS to measure tumor size accurately and to determine its proximity to neighboring structures such as blood vessels (Fig. 3). CT also plays a crucial role in ZES/MEN-1 patients for whom only imageable tumors are resected. Although magnetic resonance imaging detects only approximately

Table 2: Other Conditions Associated with Hypergastrinemia

Pernicious anemia
Atrophic gastritis
Use of proton pump inhibitor
Renal insufficiency
Gastric outlet obstruction
G-cell hyperplasia
Retained gastric antrum

Table 3: Comparison of Studies to Localize Gastrinomas

Tumor Localization Study	Percent positive
Ultrasound	21
Computed tomography scan	38
Angiography	47
Any conventional imaging study	60
Secretin angio/PVS	82
Somatostatin receptor scintigraphy	84

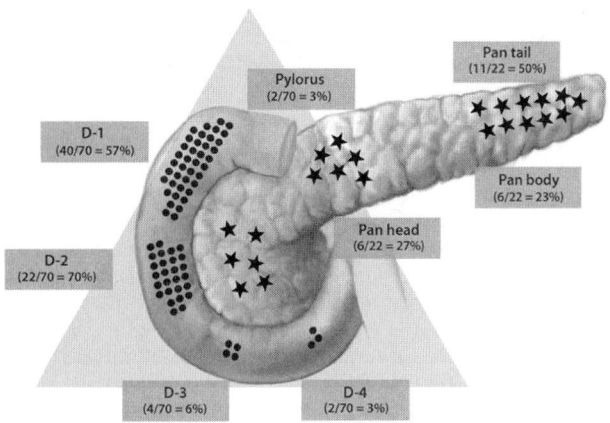

Figure 1 *Gastrinoma triangle* with probable locations of tumor. Note that duodenal gastrinomas are much more likely to be proximal than distal, whereas pancreatic gastrinomas are found uniformly throughout.

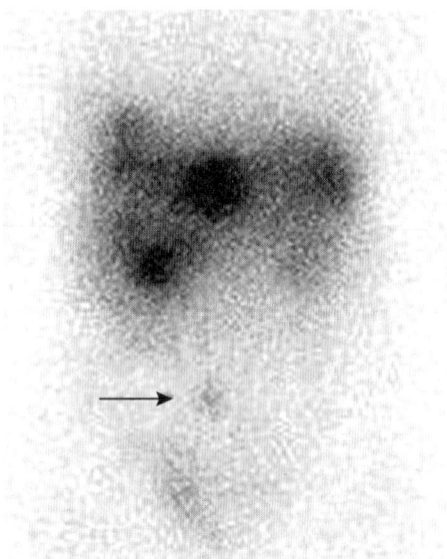

Figure 2 A positive Somatostatin receptor scintigraphy study demonstrating duodenal gastrinoma *(arrow)* and bilateral liver metastases.

25% of gastrinomas, this imaging modality may have utility in differentiating metastatic lesions from benign hemangiomas in the liver.

Unfortunately, noninvasive preoperative testing fails to detect tumor in up to 20% of patients with ZES. More invasive studies, including intraoperative studies, can be performed to help detect and localize disease in this subset of individuals. Provocative intra-arterial secretin testing can be used to localize gastrinomas to a particular region of pancreas. This test is performed by selectively injecting secretin into the superior mesenteric artery, the hepatic artery, or the splenic artery and then measuring serum gastrin levels in the hepatic vein seconds later. An increase of >50% in the serum gastrin level indicates the region of gastrinoma. In our experience, however, these occult gastrinomas localized by secretin angiogram are almost always in the gastrinoma triangle, making this study unnecessary. Careful exploration of the duodenum including duodenotomy is the critical maneuver in finding these tumors. Intraoperative ultrasound facilitates the localization and removal of pancreatic gastrinomas but is not useful in the visualization of duodenal gastrinomas.

TREATMENT

Before treatment is planned and instituted, MEN-1 must be ruled out in all patients with ZES. MEN-1 involves the pituitary, parathyroid and pancreas (see Table 1). The syndrome is identified by a careful family history and by measuring serum levels of calcium, intact parathyroid hormone, prolactin and pancreatic polypeptide, fasting glucose, and insulin. In instances in which MEN-1 may be present, the gene for MEN-1 should be sequenced to make an unequivocal diagnosis. The treatment for ZES in the context of MEN-1 is different, making it necessary to distinguish these cases from the sporadic cases.

Medical Management

Formerly, all patients with gastrinoma underwent total gastrectomy for relief of their symptoms, as was originally recommended by Zollinger and Ellison. With the advent of PPIs and H_2 receptor antagonists, patients' symptoms can now be effectively controlled medically (Fig. 4). PPIs are the medication of choice because H_2 receptor antagonists often require progressively higher doses and are associated with long-term failure. Omeprazole or lansoprazole are usually dosed at 20 to 40 mg twice daily. Dose adjustments should be made on the basis of BAO measurements because relief of symptoms is not a reliable indicator of effective acid control. Maintenance of BAO below 10 mEq/hr allows for healing of ulceration and prevents ulcer recurrence. In patients with reflux

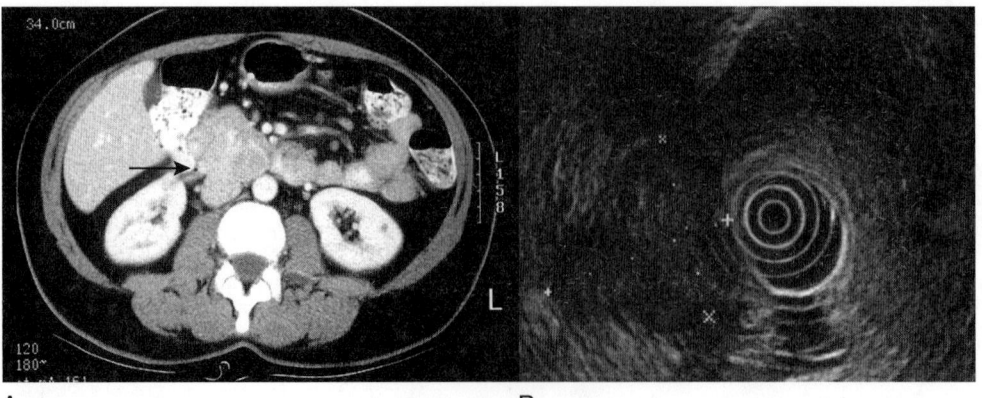

Figure 3 **(A)** Computed tomography showing duodenal gastrinoma in a patient with multiple endocrine neoplasia syndrome type 1. **(B)** Endoscopic ultrasound of the same tumor.

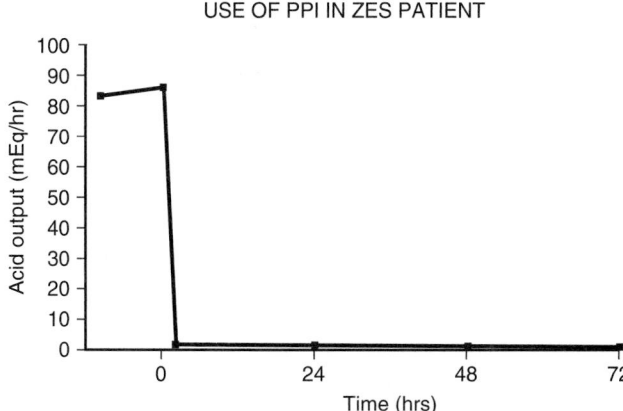

USE OF PPI IN ZES PATIENT

Figure 4 Use of proton pump inhibitors (PPIs) dramatically decreases the acid output and the associated symptoms. PPI was administered at time 0, and acid rapidly decreased. Acid output should be maintained less than 10 mEq/hour to control symptoms.

esophagitis secondary to ZES or prior ulcer surgery, BAO should be maintained below 5 mEq/hr.

Long-term medical management of ZES with acid suppression may have associated risks. Animal studies demonstrate an increased incidence of gastric malignancy. Additionally, some MEN-1 patients have developed diffuse malignant gastric carcinoid tumors after long-term acid-suppression therapy. Thus periodic gastric surveillance endoscopy should be performed on any patient treated with long-term PPI therapy for ZES.

Surgical Management

Since Zollinger and Ellison first described the syndrome, the focus of surgical therapy has shifted from treatment of the peptic ulcer disease for symptomatic relief to the more recent interest in removal of the tumor for potential cure and prolongation of survival. Although patients with ZES treated with PPIs need not undergo gastrectomy for symptomatic relief, the malignant potential of the tumor demands surgical intervention. The long-term survival of patients with ZES is primarily determined by the malignant nature of the tumor, with the most important determinant of survival being the presence or absence of hepatic metastases. Our recent comparison of ZES patients treated with surgery and those treated with medical management alone demonstrated that the

disease-related survival at 15 years is significantly higher in those individuals treated with surgery (Fig. 5). Moreover, routine surgical exploration has been shown to decrease the rate at which patients develop liver metastases, and 50% of patients with sporadic ZES enjoy long-term cure after surgical intervention. Thus it is recommended that all patients with sporadic ZES, even those without clearly imageable tumor, undergo surgical exploration for potential cure and prolongation of survival.

The intraoperative search for gastrinomas is performed using palpation, an extended Kocher maneuver (Fig. 6), complete mobilization of the pancreas, intraoperative ultrasonography, and duodenotomy. Gastrinomas located within the pancreatic head should be enucleated. A tumor within the tail of the pancreas may either be excised or resected, depending on the size and relationship to the pancreatic duct. Distal pancreatectomy-splenectomy is performed only if multiple pancreatic body or tail tumors (or both) are present that cannot be individually enucleated. If multiple pancreatic head tumors are identified, a proximal pancreaticoduodenectomy may be the surgical procedure of choice.

Duodenal tumors are often missed by preoperative and intraoperative localization studies. Duodenotomy has been shown to improve both the tumor detection rate and the cure rate of ZES. Incising the duodenal wall at the anterolateral surface of the second portion of the duodenum affords the opportunity to palpate the wall of the duodenum carefully between two fingers. Duodenal gastrinomas originate in the submucosa and cause dimpling of the mucosa. They are palpable as a firm nodule. The surgeon must be careful to avoid confusing the ampulla and the minor papilla on the medial wall of the duodenum with tumor. Once identified, tumors in the duodenal wall are completely excised, along with a small rim of normal duodenum (Fig. 7, A). Duodenal gastrinomas may be multiple in MEN-1 patients (Fig. 7, B). This technique allows for the excision of small duodenal gastrinomas that were previously undetectable. Since we began using the strategy of opening the duodenum, we have found and removed gastrinomas in every patient explored for ZES.

Lymph nodes can be the site of primary gastrinoma or of metastatic disease. Inspection and formal removal of the peripancreatic, periduodenal, and portohepatic lymph nodes are a routine part of surgical intervention in the management of ZES.

The role of proximal pancreaticoduodenectomy, or Whipple operation, in ZES is controversial. On the basis of studies demonstrating increased cure rates post-Whipple resection, some surgeons recommend that this procedure be routinely performed in a certain subset of patients with ZES. This includes patients with multiple duodenal or pancreatic head tumors, a large pancreatic head, or duodenal tumor that cannot be enucleated (see Fig. 3), multiple

Figure 5 Surgery improves disease-related survival in Zollinger-Ellison syndrome. Disease-related survival at 15 years is significantly improved by surgery (98% vs. 74%).

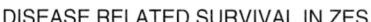

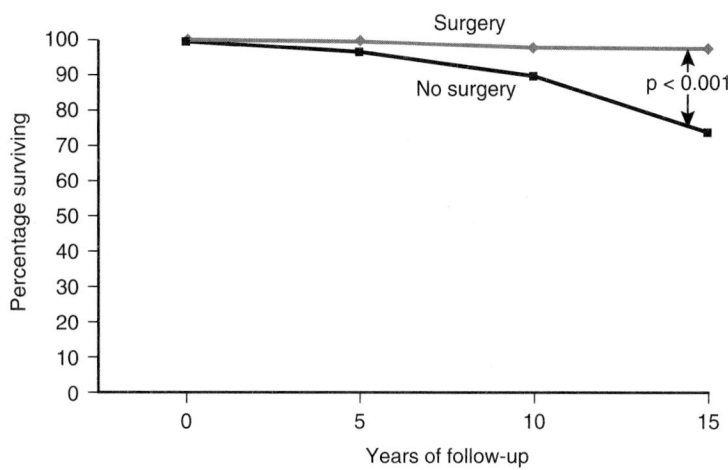

DISEASE RELATED SURVIVAL IN ZES

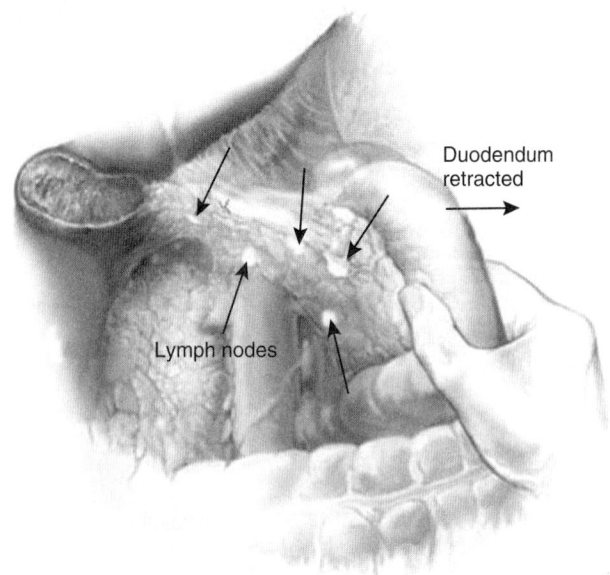

Duodendum retracted →

Lymph nodes

Figure 6   Kocher maneuver as part of the intraoperative search for gastrinomas. The duodenum is retracted to examine the structures on the underside of and beneath the pancreas. Lymph nodes to be examined are highlighted (*thin arrows*).

involved lymph nodes in the context of a duodenal or pancreatic head tumor, and patients not cured after standard removal of a duodenal or pancreatic head tumor regardless of lymph node status. Before this practice is generally accepted as the standard of care, there are important considerations that must be addressed. Patients with ZES currently enjoy a relatively long life expectancy. Although surgery significantly improves survival, the 15-year disease-related survival without surgery is still approximately 75%. The long-term complications of Whipple resection and their frequency must be studied and weighed against the true benefit afforded to these patients who are completely asymptomatic on medical therapy.

Surgical Treatment of Zollinger-Ellison Syndrome in Multiple Endocrine Neoplasia Syndrome Type I

Gastrinoma is the most common functional pancreatic neuroendocrine tumor in MEN-1. Approximately 50% of patients with MEN-1 develop gastrinoma by age 50. These tumors are more likely to be multiple than in sporadic cases, and surgery is less likely to result in cure. In patients with primary hyperparathyroidism (HPT) in addition to ZES, resection of parathyroid hyperplasia has been

shown to reduce significantly the end-organ effects of hypergastrinemia. Thus, MEN-1 patients with both ZES and primary HPT should undergo subtotal (three-and-a-half gland) parathyroidectomy before resection of the gastrinoma is considered.

Numerous studies have shown a strong correlation between primary tumor size and the development of liver metastases, which are the primary determinants of long-term survival. For this reason, it is generally agreed that the principal goal of surgery in MEN-1 patients should be to remove imageable gastrinomas (2–3 cm) in an attempt to prevent future liver metastases. An imageable tumor in the head of the pancreas should be enucleated if possible. When the imageable tumor is in the tail, a distal pancreatectomy is the preferred surgical procedure because it allows concomitant removal of other pancreatic neuroendocrine tumors that are usually present microscopically and on intraoperative ultrasound. A duodenotomy, as previously described, should be performed to identify and remove small gastrinomas in the wall of the duodenum. In MEN-1 patients, multiple duodenal gastrinomas are generally present, and a careful attempt to remove all duodenal neuroendocrine tumors should be made (see Fig. 7, *B*). Extensive sampling of the peripancreatic head lymph nodes should be carried out. If tumors in the pancreatic head are large or if there is extensive metastatic involvement to multiple lymph nodes, a Whipple operation should be considered.

Since the early 1990s, it has been generally agreed that the majority of gastrinomas in patients with ZES and MEN-1 are located in the duodenum. Despite our better understanding of the primary tumor location, the surgical cure rate of gastrinomas in the context of MEN-1 is disappointingly low without an aggressive Whipple resection. A Whipple resection may , however, have unacceptably high morbidity and mortality in patients who are known to have excellent 15-year survival outcomes with this less aggressive surgery. The operation is more extensive and makes repeat surgery technically more difficult. Moreover, if a patient develops liver metastases after a Whipple operation, liver embolization is no longer a treatment option because of the increased risk of ascending cholangitis and liver abscess. For MEN-1 patients, who have a higher incidence of disease recurrence following surgery, these are all notable considerations that must be taken into account when planning surgical intervention.

Treatment of Metastatic Disease

Although most gastrinomas have a lower malignant potential than carcinomas, there is a significant decrease in patient survival after a tumor has spread to the liver and an additional significant drop if metastases are multiple (Fig. 8). We now have long-term follow-up data indicating that tumors associated with sporadic ZES and ZES in MEN-1 metastasize with a similar frequency. Hepatic metastases can be dealt with medically or surgically. Medical therapy aimed at treating hepatic metastases includes interferon-α,

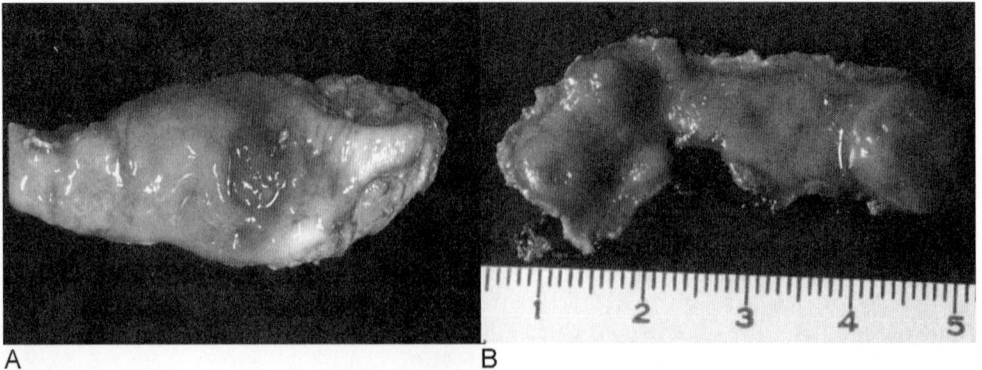

A   B

Figure 7   **(A)** Solitary duodenal gastrinoma in a sporadic patient vs. **(B)** Multiple duodenal gastrinomas in a multiple endocrine neoplasia syndrome type I patient. (*See color insert Figure 7.*)

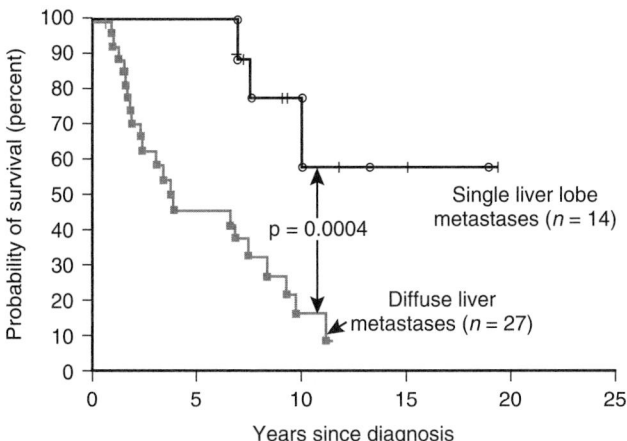

Figure 8 Liver metastases are the single most important factor affecting survival in patients with Zollinger-Ellison syndrome. Patients with single liver lobe metastasis *(open circles)* that have been removed surgically have a significantly better probability of survival at 10 years than those with diffuse bilobar liver metastases *(closed squares).*

chemotherapy, and hepatic artery embolization. Surgical resection of liver metastases may result in both outstanding relief of symptoms and long-term survival (see Fig. 8, single liver lobe metastases). Our current approach is to perform surgical resection of well-differentiated hepatic metastases in patients for whom it is estimated that 90% of the gross tumor in the liver can be effectively resected. We believe that tumors identified by SRS, which by definition express the somatostatin receptors on the cell surfaces, tend to be more highly differentiated. These tumors may be effectively controlled with somatostatin analogues postoperatively to inhibit growth. Long-acting somatostatin analogues cause gallstones, and thus a cholecystectomy should be performed at the time of the liver resection in these patients.

OUTCOMES

Surgery for ZES improves the disease-related survival at 15 years from 74% to 98% and offers the possibility of a complete cure. A cure after surgical treatment is defined as a normal fasting serum level of gastrin, negative secretin stimulation test, and no evidence of tumor on CT or SRS. The surgical cure rate in patients with sporadic ZES is 60% postoperatively, 40% at 5 years, and 34% at 10 years.

The recent routine use of duodenotomy in patients with sporadic gastrinoma has not only increased the detection of duodenal gastrinomas but has actually resulted in an improved cure rate for patients undergoing surgical treatment of ZES. Duodenotomy also decreases the death rate associated with gastrinoma, although it has no apparent effect on the development of liver metastases.

Gastrinomas of the duodenum and pancreas have a similar rate of metastases overall, but pancreatic gastrinomas are more likely to metastasize to the liver. Because the presence of liver metastases is the main determinant of survival, pancreatic gastrinomas are associated with a lower long-term survival compared with duodenal gastrinomas.

With less than a Whipple operation, the cure rate for patients with ZES in MEN-1 is low, at 0% to 10% and 25% per published reports. Fortunately, these patients have an excellent long-term survival without surgery. Even with metastatic disease, their 15-year survival is 52%. By resecting imageable tumors to prevent spread of the tumor to the liver, survival outcomes appear to be further improved.

SUGGESTED READINGS

Akerstrom G, Hessman O, Hellman P, and others: Pancreatic tumours as part of the MEN-1 syndrome, *Best Pract Res Clin Gastroenterol* 19:819, 2005.

Gibril F, Jensen RT: Advances in evaluation and management of gastrinoma in patients with Zollinger-Ellison syndrome, *Curr Gastroenterol Rep* 7:114, 2005.

Gibril F, Schumann M, Pace A, and others: Multiple endocrine neoplasia type 1 and Zollinger-Ellison syndrome: a prospective study of 107 cases and comparison with 1009 cases from the literature, *Medicine (Baltimore)* 83:43, 2004.

Gibril F, Venzon DJ, Ojeaburu JV, and others: Prospective study of the natural history of gastrinoma in patients with MEN1: definition of an aggressive and a nonaggressive form, *J Clin Endocrinol Metab* 86:5282, 2001.

Kloppel G, Anlauf M: Epidemiology, tumour biology and histopathological classification of neuroendocrine tumours of the gastrointestinal tract, *Best Pract Res Clin Gastroenterol* 19:507, 2005.

Norton JA: Surgical treatment and prognosis of gastrinoma, *Best Pract Res Clin Gastroenterol* 19:799, 2005.

Norton JA: Surgery and prognosis of duodenal gastrinoma as a duodenal neuroendocrine tumor, *Best Pract Res Clin Gastroenterol* 19:699, 2005.

Norton JA: Surgery for primary pancreatic neuroendocrine tumors, *J Gastrointest Surg* 10:327, 2006.

Norton JA, Alexander HR, Fraker DL, and others: Does the use of routine duodenotomy (DUODX) affect rate of cure, development of liver metastases, or survival in patients with Zollinger-Ellison syndrome? *Ann Surg* 239:617; discussion 626, 2004.

Norton JA, Fang TD, Jensen RT: Surgery for gastrinoma and insulinoma in multiple endocrine neoplasia type 1, *J Natl Compr Canc Netw* 4:148, 2006.

Norton JA, Jensen RT: Resolved and unresolved controversies in the surgical management of patients with Zollinger-Ellison syndrome, *Ann Surg* 240:757, 2004.

Oberg K, Eriksson B: Endocrine tumours of the pancreas, *Best Pract Res Clin Gastroenterol* 19:753, 2005.

POSTGASTRECTOMY SYNDROMES

Magesh Sundaram, MD, and David W. McFadden, MD

INTRODUCTION

The advent of effective pharmacotherapy for peptic ulcer disease and recognition and treatment of *Helicobacter pylori* have decreased the number of elective operations that require partial or total gastrectomy. The leading indications for gastric resection now include complications of ulcer disease, neoplasms, and bariatric surgery. We do not focus on the complications seen after bariatric surgery because these are covered elsewhere in this book but instead discuss the recognition and management of the classic postgastrectomy syndromes. Today's surgeon may be consulted to manage the patient with a remote history of an ulcer operation who presents with postgastrectomy syndromes; surgeons must also be cognizant to avoid the creation of postgastrectomy syndromes when performing gastric surgery. The surgeon must keep in mind that both anatomic and functional physiologic changes after gastric surgery lead to these syndromes. Remedial operations for the disorders of mechanical origin will often be effective, whereas operations

Table 1: Avoidance of Postgastrectomy Syndromes

A. Thorough preoperative evaluation—tests to consider before the gastric operation for benign disease:

   1. Esophagogastroduodenoscopy

   2. Upper gastrointestinal series

   3. Check for *Helicobacter pylori*

   4. Serum salicylate level

   5. Serum gastrin level

   6. Gastric emptying scan

   7. Duodenogastric reflux scan

   8. Gastrointestinal tract motility assessment

   9. Gastric analysis

B. Thoughtful operative planning: some issues to consider when planning a first gastric operation (especially in patients with nonmalignant disease):

   1. Consider highly selective vagotomy or selective vagotomy instead of truncal vagotomy

   2. Consider a potentially reversible operation instead of an irreversible operation (e.g., gastrojejunostomy instead of pyloroplasty; duodenal switch instead of subtotal gastrectomy with Roux-en-Y)

   3. Delayed gastric emptying may be made worse by vagotomy or gastrectomy

   4. Duodenogastric reflux may be made worse by pyloroplasty

   5. Global gastrointestinal tract dysmotility may be exacerbated by most gastric operations

   6. Why does the patient have an ulcer and why can it not be treated medically?

   7. In the *Helicobacter* proton pump inhibitor era, is a bigger operation better?

   8. Avoid gastric resection if the patient cannot afford to lose 10 pounds

should be reserved until medical and dietary conservative measures have failed for syndromes caused by altered physiologic function (Table 1).

DUMPING SYNDROME

One of the most common postgastrectomy syndromes is dumping syndrome. Although this disorder may be partially recognized in 25% to 50% of gastric surgery patients, only 5% will have a complete manifestation that is clinically relevant and requires the surgeon's attention. Postgastrectomy dumping syndrome presents in two distinct forms, early and late dumping; incidence is approximately 75% and 25%, respectively. The signs and symptoms of early dumping syndrome occur within 10 to 30 minutes after eating and comprise nausea, fullness, cramping abdominal pain, and diarrhea. Associated vasomotor symptoms include diaphoresis, weakness, dizziness, palpitations, and a need to lie down. The normal stomach averts too-rapid passage of solids and liquids into the small intestine. In the postgastrectomy state, rapid and direct passage of hyperosmolar chyme into the small intestine leads to osmolarity-based fluid shifts from the intravascular space to the bowel lumen. The resultant distension and increased peristalsis produces the typical bloating, cramping, and diarrhea. Associated intravascular volume depletion leads to the symptoms of dizziness, weakness,

tachycardia or palpitations. Neurohormonal gut peptides including enteroglucagon, serotonin, vasoactive intestinal peptide, motilin, and neurotensin have all been implicated as causative agents in early dumping syndrome.

Late dumping syndrome presents 2 to 3 hours after eating a meal with symptoms typical of hypoglycemia: weakness, diaphoresis, flushing, and dizziness. The pathophysiologic event in late dumping is the presentation and rapid absorption of a high carbohydrate load from the small intestine, with resultant hyperglycemia and a rapid systemic insulin response. Excessive insulin response, however, leads to systemic hypoglycemia within 2 to 3 hours after the meal, with symptomatic presentation of hyperinsulinemia.

The diagnosis of dumping syndrome must exclude other postgastrectomy syndromes such as delayed gastric emptying, afferent loop syndrome, distal obstruction, and recurrent–marginal ulceration. Radionuclide gastric emptying scan, upper endoscopy, and upper GI series may all be used; paying close attention to the presenting symptomatology, which should be reproducible, is also important.

Both forms of dumping syndrome should initially be treated with dietary and medical management. Dietary modification includes small, frequent meals with complex, not simple, carbohydrates and the addition of dietary fiber. Meals should be taken "dry," with liquids taken an hour or more after the meal. Beyond dietary modification, medical treatment of severe dumping syndrome consists of octreotide, the commercially available analogue of somatostatin. Octreotide, from 100 to 500 μg twice daily, slows gastric emptying, counters the pro-motility neural gut peptides, and inhibits insulin release. Side effects of octreotide therapy include steatorrhea, from pancreatic exocrine function inhibition; hyperglycemia or hypoglycemia; and cholelithiasis. Although up to 90% of patients experience symptomatic relief acutely with octreotide, long-term therapy is less clearly beneficial. Acarbose is a medical agent not available in the United States that competitively inhibits digestion of sugars but may also induce malabsorption.

Remedial operations for dumping syndrome should be reserved for symptomatic patients who have failed conservative measures and who have been observed over months by a multidisciplinary team of gastrointestinal (GI) specialists. Even in these cases, the surgeon should not rush to offer surgical therapy because the available surgical options may have variable results in individual patients. If a Billroth I or II gastrojejunostomy is present, conversion to a Roux-en-Y yields symptomatic relief in up to 85% to 90% of patients with dumping (Fig. 1). If the existing gastric remnant above the Billroth gastrojejunostomy is large, it should be pared down to avoid marginal ulceration or gastroparesis. Although patients with a pyloroplasty may be successfully managed with pyloric muscle repair or reconstruction, a more definitive operation for this subset would be the "duodenal switch" Roux-en-Y. Henley's interposition of an isoperistaltic jejunal loop between the stomach and the duodenum, although effective acutely, does not provide long-term symptomatic relief (Fig. 2). Placement of a 10-cm reversed jejunal segment between the stomach and the intestine has also been described but is rarely used because of the risk of mesenteric torsion and obstruction requiring reoperation (Fig. 3).

Minimizing the risk of dumping syndrome in the first gastric operation requires an examination of gastric emptying with radionuclide scan and endoscopy. Selective vagotomy procedures may be preferable to truncal vagotomy.

AFFERENT LIMB SYNDROME

Afferent limb syndrome occurs in patients with a Billroth II gastrojejunostomy in which the duodenal limb carrying the biliary and pancreatic juices to the stomach may become acutely or chronically obstructed. Factors that promote the development of afferent loop obstruction include an excessively long duodenal limb,

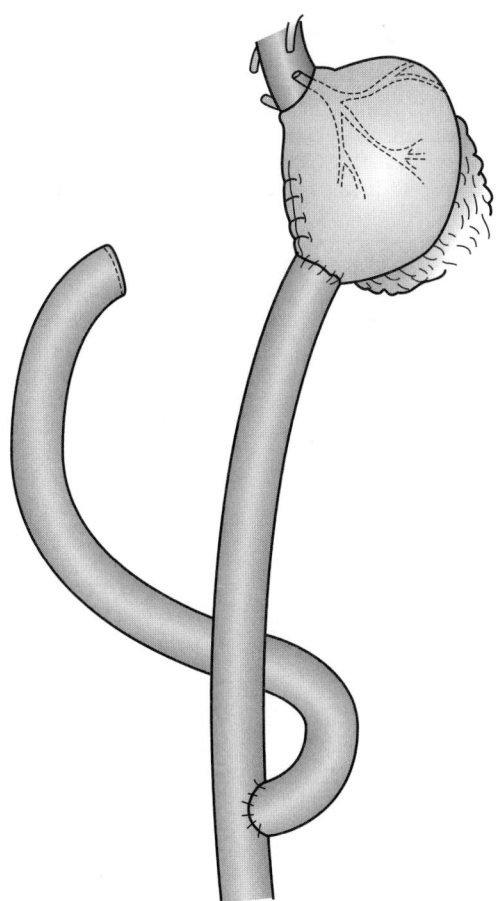

Figure 1 Conversion of a Billroth I and Billroth II gastrectomy to a Roux-en-Y anastomosis.   *From Cameron JL, editor: Current surgical therapy, ed 5, St. Louis, 1995, Mosby.*

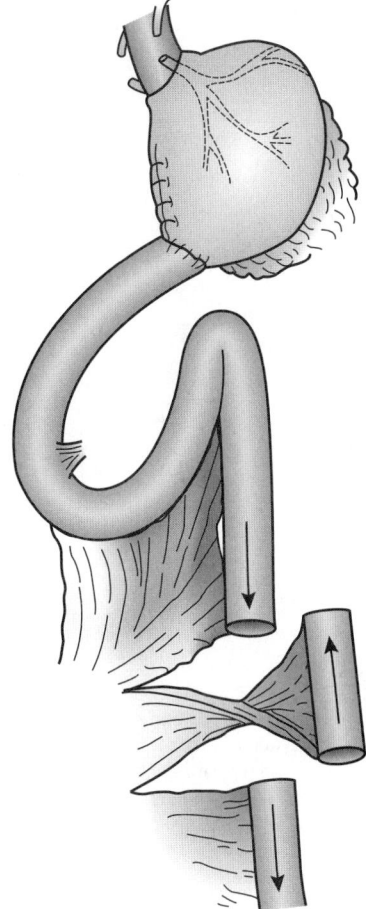

Figure 2 Interposition of a reversed 10-cm jejunal segment 100 cm beyond the ligament of Treitz may be useful for severe, intractable debilitating postvagotomy diarrhea.   *From Cameron JL, editor: Current surgical therapy, ed 5, St. Louis, 1995, Mosby.*

antecolic placement of the gastrojejunostomy, internal hernias or adhesions, anastomotic stricture or ulceration, or recurrence of carcinoma. Acute and chronic presentations of afferent limb syndrome exist.

Acute afferent loop obstruction manifests with fever, tachycardia, nonbilious vomiting, and severe epigastric pain. Bacterial overgrowth combined with the increasing intraluminal pressure from continued pancreaticobiliary secretion into the obstructed duodenum may rapidly lead to necrosis and septic shock. In the acute postoperative setting after gastrectomy operations, afferent loop obstruction is commonly the underlying etiology in duodenal stump blowout. Diagnosis of an acutely obstructed afferent limb is made with radiologic imaging (computed tomography [CT] or ultrasound) demonstrating a fluid-filled duodenal loop. Elevated liver function tests and amylase may be mistaken for pancreatitis or gallstone pathologies. Endoscopic entrance into and drainage of the nonischemic afferent limb may provide temporary relief of the acute obstruction and allow for correction of the patient in shock before surgical relief.

The chronic presentation of afferent limb syndrome is displayed in a stereotypical fashion. The postprandial patient presents with increasing epigastric pain that is dramatically relieved by explosive bilious vomiting. The vomitus does not contain foodstuff, which has passed into the efferent limb, and vomiting the contents of the obstructed duodenum relieves symptoms. These two symptoms are not seen with bile alkaline reflux gastritis, which is in the differential diagnosis (vide infra) for afferent limb syndrome in which the vomitus does contain food and does not relieve the epigastric pain. Other considerations in the differential diagnosis would

include recurrent/marginal ulceration, anastomotic stricture, and remnant carcinoma. Endoscopy can readily evaluate and exclude these other disorders.

The acute afferent limb syndrome is a classic example of a closed-loop obstruction of the GI tract and is a surgical emergency that, left untreated, carries mortality rates of 50%. In the acute setting, the afferent limb and duodenal stump must be examined for viability. If extensive necrosis is present, debridement and drainage are indicated, and pancreaticoduodenectomy is rarely necessary. The unstable patient with acceptable viability may be amenable to tube duodenostomy. Patients presenting with chronic afferent limb syndrome will gain excellent symptomatic relief with the remedial conversion of the Billroth II to a Roux-en-Y. Creation of a Braun enteroenterostomy between the afferent and efferent limbs is also effective.

To minimize the risk of afferent limb syndrome, the surgeon must create a retrocolic short-limbed gastrojejunostomy that lies horizontally, without vertical angulation and verify the patency of the afferent aspect of the completed gastrojejunstomy anastomosis. Early anastomotic stricture formation must be recognized and treated with endoscopic dilatation.

POSTVAGOTOMY DIARRHEA

Patients who have undergone truncal vagatomy may present in the early postoperative period with diarrhea. Clinically significant in

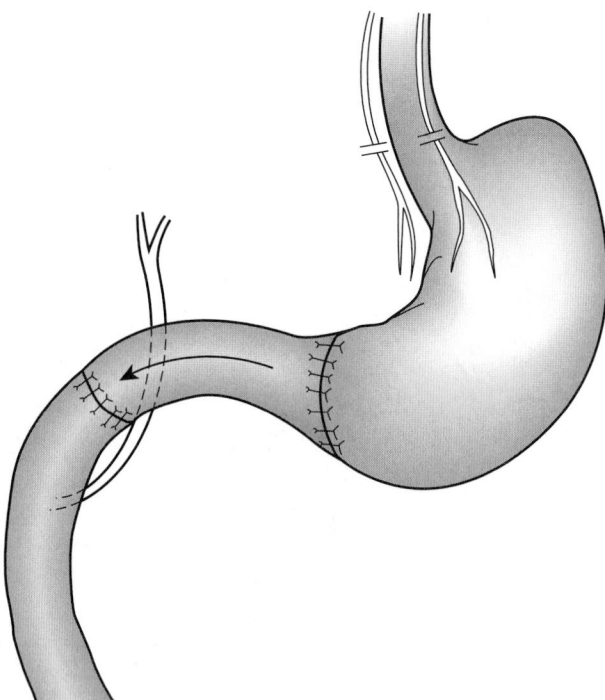

Figure 3   Henley jejunal interposition procedure was originally proposed for dumping syndrome, but it has been used more recently for bile reflux gastritis. The jejunal segment is placed in isoperistaltic fashion and should be 20 to 40 cm long.   *From Cameron JL editor: Current surgical therapy, ed 7, St. Louis, 2001, Mosby.*

approximately 5% of patients, it is persistent and considered chronic and debilitating in only 1% to 2%. Other possible etiologies that must be excluded include bacterial overgrowth, antibiotic-associated colitis, inflammatory bowel disease, malabsorption, and dumping. Steatorrhea and laxative abuse can be readily demonstrated and excluded.

The presumption that central nervous system control of gut motility and secretion is impaired by truncal vagotomy is intuitive; however, no direct evidence for this as a cause of persistent diarrhea has been demonstrated in the postvagotomy state. Mechanisms that have been proposed include rapid gastric emptying, loss of bile salts from the enterohepatic circulation, intestinal dysmotility, and bacterial overgrowth.

Remedial operations to reduce gastric emptying have not been successful in the treatment of postvagotomy diarrhea and may lead to a new set of problems, such as anastomotic stricture and obstruction. Medical management of postvagotomy diarrhea is similar to the management of dumping syndrome: small, dry meals and increased dietary fiber to increase intestinal transit time. When increased bile salt excretion is demonstrated, cholestyramine is beneficial in binding some of the lost bile acids. Unlike dumping syndrome, octreotide may worsen this disorder by decreasing pancreatic exocrine secretion and steatorrhea.

Only when all other causes of diarrhea have been excluded and the patient is debilitated by postvagotomy diarrhea is a remedial operation to decrease intestinal transit time offered. The recommended procedure is creation of a 10-cm reversed or antiperistaltic jejunal loop 100 cm distal to the ligament of Treitz. Benefits are seen in 50% to 70% of patients.

The surgeon must consider a selective vagotomy rather than a truncal vagotomy in the treatment of intractable ulcer disease to minimize the potential for postvagotomy diarrhea.

BILE ALKALINE REFLUX GASTRITIS

Destruction, bypass, or removal of the pylorus allows for the presentation of bile alkaline material from the duodenum into the stomach. Although all patients who have had gastrectomy procedures performed can be demonstrated to have bile reflux into the stomach on endoscopy, the majority are asymptomatic. Only 3% to 5% of patients will have symptomatic presentation of this disorder. The most common procedures these patients have had are Billroth II gastrojejunostomy, Billroth I gastroduodenostomy, and pyloroplasty. Nausea, epigastric pain, and burning are the typical symptoms, which may be exacerbated by eating, leading to food aversion and weight loss. Bilious vomiting with retained foodstuff does not relieve the epigastric pain, in contrast to the previously described symptoms of afferent limb syndrome. The differential diagnosis that must be entertained includes delayed gastric emptying or obstruction, small bowel obstruction, and recurrent ulcer. Endoscopy often reveals an inflamed, erythematous gastric mucosa with stagnant pools of bile in the dependent stomach. Hypochlorhydria or achlorhydria may be confirmed, and biopsy of the gastric mucosa demonstrates loss of parietal cells with intestinal changes of the gastric glands. The inciting event in both symptomatic and asymptomatic patients is the breakdown of the gastric mucosal barrier function from persistent exposure to the bile salts.

Hypergastrinemia from causes such as Zollinger-Ellison syndrome, retained antrum, or incomplete vagotomy should be excluded when hyperchlorhydria is identified on gastric analysis. Delayed gastric emptying should be excluded. Technetium scans with and without cholecystokinin will confirm continued bile reflux into the stomach, and provocative testing with bile salt ingestion may confirm the patient in whom remedial operations would be of benefit. Medical management of bile alkaline reflux gastritis includes sucralfate to promote gastric mucosal barrier defense, as well as pro-motility agents to improve gastric emptying.

Documented bile alkaline reflux gastritis is the most common postgastrectomy syndrome for which a remedial operation is clearly beneficial. Patients who have had a truncal vagotomy with pyloroplasty should be converted to a Roux-en-Y with an antrectomy to reduce the risk of ulcers. Patients who have had a prior Billroth I or II reconstruction should have remedial conversion to a Roux-en-Y with a 45- to 60-cm jejunal limb. Less attractive alternatives include the Henley jejunal loop interposition and the Braun enteroenterostomy. Although up to 85% of patients who receive a Roux-en-Y conversion have symptomatic relief, the resultant configuration carries the risks of marginal ulceration unless a vagotomy is added and malabsorption or obstruction if an excessively long limb is created. If some degree of gastroparesis is documented on preoperative evaluation, the patient may be at risk for Roux stasis syndrome, and therefore the remedial operation should include a near-total (90%–95%) gastrectomy above the Roux-en-Y.

GASTRIC STASIS AND ROUX STASIS SYNDROME

Gastroparesis and stasis in the Roux limb, or Roux stasis syndrome, are well-recognized postsurgical disorders. Early manifestation occurs in the immediate postoperative period and is marked by prolonged hospitalization, as well as patient and clinician frustration. This is often referred to as gastric atony or gastric ileus and is more pronounced in patients undergoing surgery for preexisting gastric outlet obstruction.

Patients who have had previous gastrectomy with Roux-en-Y may present with the chronic form of stasis in the gastric remnant or in the Roux limb, collectively called Roux stasis syndrome. Patients symptomatic of this disorder will exhibit great difficulty in gastric emptying, epigastric pain, vomiting, and weight loss. Bloating, early satiety, and intermittent vomiting of undigested food may also be seen as part of the presentation. Endoscopy and an upper GI series will demonstrate a dilated gastric remnant, dilatation of the Roux limb, or both. Stagnant food material and bezoars may be found in the stomach.

Other postgastrectomy disorders such as anastomotic stricture, adhesions or internal hernias, distal mechanical obstruction, recurrent ulcer, and remnant carcinoma must be excluded in establishing the diagnosis of gastroparesis or Roux stasis syndrome. In the acute postoperative phase, small bowel obstruction from adhesions and internal hernias must be ruled out. Neurohormonal imbalances caused by postoperative medications and diabetic gastroparesis must also be considered. Often a preexisting gastric dysmotility condition is made worse with the vagotomy or gastrectomy procedure. Diabetes, hypothyroidism, collagen vascular diseases, and neuropathies and myopathies must be considered before the first gastric operation on a patient.

Roux stasis syndrome has elements of both gastroparesis and decreased jejunal peristalsis, but the latter alone will not produce the clinical symptoms of this disorder. Diagnosis is made with confirmatory delayed gastric emptying scan combined with an upper GI series showing dilated stomach or Roux limb (or both) without evidence of kinking, obstruction, or anastomotic stricture. Manometry may be useful in establishing the impaired motility in these segments.

Early or postoperative gastroparesis should be managed with nasogastric decompression, correction of electrolyte and metabolic derangements, and nutritional support. Medications such as opiates, calcium channel blockers, and anticholinergics should be avoided. Pro-motility agents such as metoclopramide are more effective in stimulating a response in the gastroparesis setting than in the Roux stasis setting. Intravenous or oral erythromycin, used as a motilin receptor stimulant, also has some effect in improving gastric emptying in the postsurgical patient. We have had some success with urecholine in this setting.

If gastroparesis or Roux stasis syndrome is seen in the chronic setting and is refractory to medical management, remedial operations have limited success. If a vagotomy and pyloroplasty has been previously performed, gastroparesis can be treated with a distal hemigastrectomy and a Billroth I or II reconstruction. For gastroparesis in a patient with Billroth I or II anatomy, a near total gastrectomy with a Roux-en-Y esophagojejunostomy should be favored. Roux stasis syndrome is best treated with a total gastrectomy, resection of the dilated jejunal limb, and reconstruction with a Roux-en-Y esophagojejunostomy (Fig. 4). Clinical improvement in 75% to 80% of patients is seen with this extensive procedure.

RECURRENT ULCERATION

Greater understanding of vagal anatomy, more precise surgical technique, and addition of ulcer-treating medical pharmacotherapy have led to a decrease in ulcer recurrence rates after surgery for ulcer disease. The accepted rates of ulcer recurrence after vagotomy and pyloroplasty or highly selective vagotomy are approximately 10%, whereas the rate is 1% to 4% after vagotomy and antrectomy. Initial duodenal ulcer disease will typically recur in the stomach or the jejunum associated with Billroth reconstruction. When patients recur with a jejunal ulcer below the Billroth gastrojejunostomy, it is referred to as a "marginal ulcer."

Symptoms of recurrent ulcer include epigastric pain or burning that is exacerbated by eating and relieved with antacid use. Hemorrhagic ulcers will be seen in one third of patients, but perforation in the recurrent ulcer is much less common. Refractory pain and obstruction may also be associated with the recurrent ulcer.

Patients with ulcer recurrence after previous ulcer operations should be evaluated for retained antrum, incomplete vagotomy, Zollinger-Ellison syndrome, gastric cancer, and incompletely treated

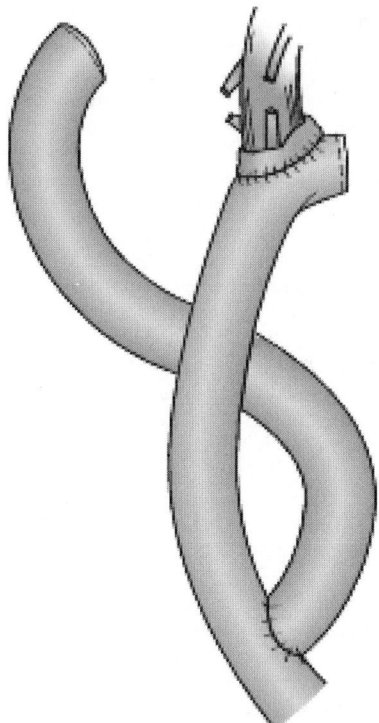

Figure 4 Near-total gastrectomy for Roux syndrome and postsurgical gastroparesis. *From Cameron JL editor: Current surgical therapy, ed 5, St. Louis, 1995, Mosby.*

H. pylori. More commonly, an inadequate ulcer operation was performed previously. Workup should include upper endoscopy, upper GI series, gastric emptying scan, and gastrin levels. If Zollinger-Ellison syndrome is suspected, a secretin challenge test is appropriate in which a gastrinoma is the only condition that will produce a paradoxical rise in gastrin after administration of secretin. Identification and resection of the gastrinoma is the appropriate treatment for recurrent ulcers in this setting.

Aggressive medical management with an *H. pylori* regimen, H_2 receptor, or proton pump antagonists should first be tried for a period of weeks to months before considering remedial surgery for recurrent ulcers. The complications of hemorrhage, obstruction, intractable pain, and perforation are, of course, indications for surgical attention. If an incomplete vagotomy is identified, a thoracoscopic truncal vagotomy or a highly selective vagotomy are recommended remedial operations. If a highly selective vagotomy were previously performed, a truncal vagotomy and antrectomy would be a corrective alternative. If retained antrum is documented by endoscopy, CT scan with oral contrast, or upper GI series, the residual antrum should be resected back to the first portion of the duodenum, as marked by the gastroduodenal artery and intraoperative frozen section analysis. Recurrent gastric ulcers should always be biopsied to exclude carcinoma and then reresected with a "generous" hemigastrectomy.

REMNANT CARCINOMA

The altered gastric milieu after a partial gastrectomy with a Billroth I or II reconstruction leads to development of hypochlorhydria or achlorhydria and intestinal metaplasia, potentially leading to dysplasia and carcinoma. Gastric stump, or remnant, carcinoma is a late consequence of ulcer surgery, occurring 15 to 20 years later. Patients who have undergone a Billroth II reconstruction after antrectomy appear to have up to a sixfold increased risk of remnant carcinoma. There is no indication of increased risk of cancer with a vagotomy and drainage procedures, however.

The typical presentation of this postgastrectomy disorder is in an elderly patient with remote history of an ulcer operation presenting with vague abdominal discomfort or pain, bloating, and weight loss. The symptom of early satiety is not associated with remnant carcinoma. However, these patients may have had chronic postgastrectomy symptoms, leading them to ignore any acceleration of their symptoms with the development of the carcinoma, and therefore to have an advanced stage of cancer at presentation.

Diagnosis must be confirmed with upper endoscopy with biopsies. The ulcerated, irregular-appearing anastomosis must be adequately biopsied in multiple places to confirm the suspicion of remnant carcinoma. Computed tomography scan of the abdomen is a useful staging modality for determining metastatic disease, as well as local resectability. Total gastrectomy with Roux-en-Y esophagojejunostomy is the treatment of choice.

NUTRITIONAL AND METABOLIC CONSIDERATIONS

The alteration or resection of the proximal GI tract can lead to chronic nutritional and metabolic changes in the postgastrectomy patient. The current explosion of gastric volume reduction procedures in bariatric surgery to produce capacity-based weight loss is well recognized. The patient who has undergone an ulcer-related operation can be expected to show some degree of weight loss after the procedure, but the effect is not persistent in terms of chronic weight loss. The degree of initial weight loss often parallels the magnitude of the initial operation. Gastric capacity, altered intake, and malabsorption are all factors in the associated weight loss.

Diversion of the food stream away from the duodenum, or resection of the duodenum or proximal jejunum, will affect the absorption of iron and calcium. An acidic environment promotes absorption of iron. Significant, long-term decrease in iron absorption will put these patients at risk for chronic anemia.

Partial or total gastrectomy may lead to significant reduction of the parietal cell mass, the main site of production of intrinsic factor. Enteric absorption of vitamin B12 can be impaired by the lack of intrinsic factor production in these patients. They should be monitored for signs of megaloblastic anemia. All patients who have had a total gastrectomy should receive lifelong monthly injections of vitamin B12 as supplementation.

Calcium absorption occurs primarily in the duodenum, which may be bypassed by creation of a gastrojejunostomy or Roux-en-Y. Patients may also experience gastroparesis or intestinal stasis, leading to bacterial overgrowth. Because bacterial overgrowth may interfere with fat absorption and vitamin D is a fat-soluble vitamin, these patients may have impaired vitamin D absorption in addition to the calcium losses. Therefore patients who have had surgical alteration of the proximal GI tract should be monitored for bone density loss and be supplemented appropriately with calcium and vitamin D.

Suggested Readings

Bouras EP, Scolapio JS: Gastric motility disorders: management that optimizes nutritional status, *J Clin Gastroenterol* 38:549–557, 2004.
Loeffel RJ: Prevalence of upper abdominal complaints in patients who have undergone partial gastrectomy, *Can J Gastroenterol* 14:681–684, 2000.
Scholmerich J: Postgastrectomy syndromes-diagnosis and management, *Best Pract Res Clin Gastroenterol* 18:917–933, 2004.
Uklea A: Dumping syndrome: pathophysiology and treatment, *Nutr Clin Pract* 20:517–525, 2005.

MALLORY-WEISS SYNDROME

Sean P. Harbison, MD, and Daniel T. Dempsey, MD

INTRODUCTION

Today Mallory-Weiss syndrome (MWS) is hardly a surgical disease. Rarely do patients with this interesting problem of upper gastrointestinal (GI) bleeding from linear mucosal tear(s) at the gastroesophageal junction require an operation. But it is important for the practicing surgeon to be familiar with this disorder. First, it accounts for 5% to 15% of patients admitted to hospital with upper GI bleeding. Second, MWS probably represents an even larger percentage of surgical consultations for upper GI bleeding because the typical arterial hemorrhage is sometimes frighteningly brisk and the patients quite ill. Finally, endoscopic (and certainly laparoscopic or open surgical) techniques of hemostasis are effective for control of hemorrhage in the small minority of patients who do not stop bleeding spontaneously.

It is likely that the earliest description of MWS was by Quincke, who in 1879 reported three cases of GI hemorrhage resulting from bleeding sites at the gastroesophageal junction. In 1929, G. Kenneth Mallory and Soma Weiss refined these earlier observations and

described the eponymous syndrome of upper GI hemorrhage arising from linear disruptions in the gastroesophageal mucosa in patients with antecedent alcohol-induced retching or vomiting. With the advent of flexible endoscopy in the 1970s, MWS (vomiting, hematemesis, and alcohol abuse) was recognized as a common cause of upper GI bleeding. Currently all acute linear mucosal lacerations or disruptions in the region of the gastroesophageal junction, whatever the cause, are referred to as Mallory-Weiss lesions. Although vomiting, retching associated with alcohol abuse remains a recognized cause of Mallory-Weiss mucosal tears, multiple causes other than alcoholism have been described. Although most of these causes are associated with vomiting, retching, or esophagogastric instrumentation, rarely no antecedent history or apparent cause of Mallory-Weiss lesions is discerned. Perhaps a more modern definition of the MWS would be vomiting or retching, upper GI bleeding, and typical linear mucosal tear(s) at the GE junction.

PATHOPHYSIOLOGY

Mallory-Weiss tears probably occur because of an abrupt increase in the gradient between intragastric and intrathoracic pressure, causing rapid and forceful distention of the region of the esophagogastric junction. Forceful vomiting results in spastic closure of the pylorus and retrograde propulsion of gastric contents with simultaneous relaxation of the lower esophageal sphincter and diaphragmatic hiatus. Rapid centrifugal dilatation of the GE junction results in linearly oriented mucosal tears. (Fig. 1, A and B) As noted, forceful vomiting or retching for any reason may produce

Study	N	% Male	Mean age	%EtOHism	%Cirrhosis	%Naus/Vom	Hematem (%)	% Active bleeding	%Assoc Sx (UGI)
Llach	63	63	51	36.5	12.6	29	82.5	73	
Sugawa	224	79.5	38	30.3		44		25	75
Luc	40	80	52(M) 73(F)	75			87.5		42
Huang	35	82		14	20	39	97	20	57
Park	34	97	52	50			91	19	31
Laine	44		43.5	47				25	

Figure 1   Clinical presentation summary, Mallory-Weiss syndrome.

Mallory-Weiss lesions. In addition to alcohol abuse, MWS has been associated with cardiopulmonary resuscitation, seizures, straining during childbirth or defecation, cancer chemotherapy, hyperemesis gravidarum, blunt abdominal trauma, transesophageal echocardiography, esophagogastroduodenoscopy, illicit drug ingestion, aspirin use, colonoscopy preparation with electrolyte–polyethylene glycol solution, ipecac treatment, general anesthesia, nasogastric intubation, food impaction, gastroenteritis and even primal scream therapy. It is notable that retrograde prolapse of the proximal stomach into the esophagus or the thorax during a spontaneous valsalva or vigorous coughing in patients with Mallory-Weiss tears has been documented. This phenomenon suggests that forceful prolapse of the gastric cardia into the thorax in a patient with a sliding hiatal hernia may actually physically tear the mucosa.

MWS should be considered in the differential diagnosis in most patients with acute upper GI hemorrhage. Large studies using flexible endoscopy have shown that MWS accounts for 5% to 15% of hospital cases with acute upper GI bleeding. The disorder is not uncommonly associated with alcohol abuse, particularly when there has been retching or emesis following an alcoholic binge. In one of the first descriptive studies of the endoscopic era, Knauer found that 58 of 528 consecutive patients endoscoped for upper GI bleeding had Mallory-Weiss lesions as the cause of bleeding. Associated upper GI lesions were common. Michel and colleagues found the classic triad of vomiting, hematemesis, and alcoholism in 30 of 40 patients with endoscopically proved MWS. Sliding hiatal hernia seemed to be an associated factor in both of these early studies. A male predominance (male:female ratio between 2:1 and 7:1) exists for Mallory-Weiss tears, even in abstemious populations. The mean age at diagnosis ranges from 40 to 60, but MWS has been described in the pediatric population.

Endoscopy reveals a single mucosal tear in 80% to 90% of cases, although multiple lacerations have been described; two tears have been noted in 8% to 15% of cases, and three tears or more have been noted in only 1% to 8% of cases. The most common location of the laceration(s) is along the lesser curvature of the stomach just distal to the esophagogastric junction (50% to 83%), whereas 10% to 23% of tears occur along the greater curvature under the diaphragm, and 4% to 18% occur posteriorly and 3% to 7% anteriorly (see Fig. 2). The higher frequency of tears in the area of the phrenoesophageal ligament along the lesser curvature at the esophagogastric junction seems to support the hypothesis of "burst" type pathophysiology; the phrenoesophageal ligament is the most fixed point of the gastroesophageal junction and is stressed maximally during forceful dilatation from vomiting. Mallory-Weiss tears are approximately 1 to 5 cm in length and generally occur just distal to the esophagogastric junction. The lacerations rarely involve the esophagus alone. After mucosal disruption, the rich submucosal blood supply in the region produces arterial bleeding. Hiatal hernia has been implicated as a risk factor in the development of Mallory-Weiss tears. It has been suggested that the presence of a hiatal hernia predisposes to the formation of a tear upon the application of a large pressure gradient. However, the presence of a hiatal hernia is found in only a minority of patients. It has been observed that those patients with hiatal hernia tend to have gastric cardia lesions, whereas patients without hiatal hernia tend to develop gastroesophageal junction lesions. Not surprisingly, the presence of portal hypertension has been associated with increased severity of bleeding and mortality rates

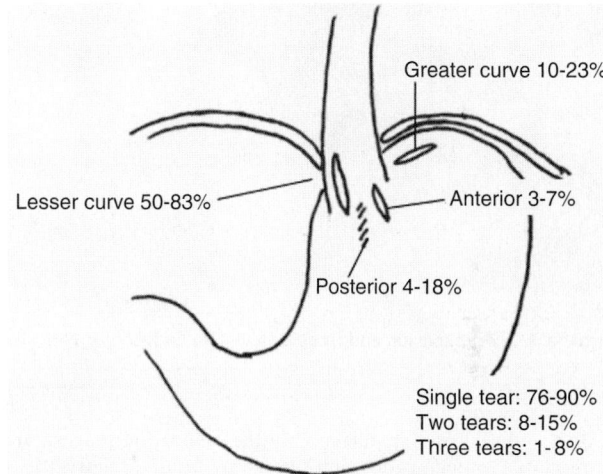

Figure 2   Distribution of Tear(s), Mallory-Weiss syndrome.

in patients with Mallory-Weiss hemorrhage. Sugawa noted that portal hypertension and cirrhosis were present in 6 of 8 individuals who died in a large series of 224 patients treated for MWS over a 10-year period. This unusually high mortality rate is probably due mostly to the underlying degree of functional liver impairment, but the role of portal hypertension in this hemorrhagic malady should not be trivialized.

DIAGNOSIS

MWS presents as hematemesis in approximately 90% of cases. The clinical triad of vomiting, retching, and subsequent hematemesis occurs in approximately half of patients, but 30% to 50% of patients have no history of vomiting. Melena may be the presenting symptom in up to 10% of patients. A third of patients with MWS give a history of aspirin or nonsteroidal anti-inflammatory drug use. Occasionally epigastric or back pain may be present, although bleeding from Mallory-Weiss tears is most often painless.

Although the presence of one or more predisposing risk factors in the patient history may move MWS to the top of the differential diagnosis, the definitive diagnosis is confirmed by flexible upper endoscopy. The use of contrast radiographic studies (i.e., barium swallow or upper GI series) for the diagnosis of MWS is not indicated and should only be entertained when perforation is considered (in which case a gastrograffin swallow or computed tomography scan should be the initial study). Although a history of vomiting and retching is frequently elicited in both MWS and Boerhaave's syndrome (discussed elsewhere in this volume), there is no evidence that these two diagnoses are pathophysiologically related nor that one problem predisposes or leads to the other. MWS rarely if ever perforates, and Boerhaave's syndrome rarely if ever bleeds significantly.

At endoscopy, Mallory-Weiss lesions appear as linear lacerations of the mucosa of the gastric cardia; the tear or tears may extend to the gastroesophageal junction or even into the distal esophagus (see

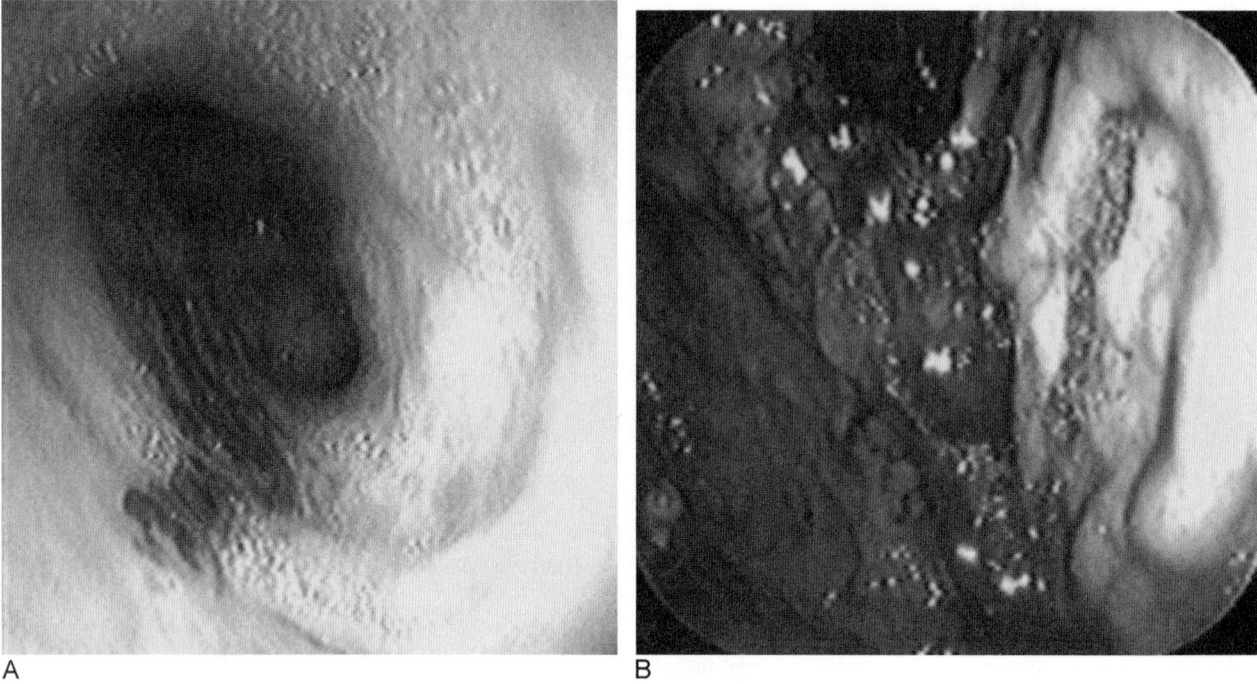

Figure 3 **(A)** Superior endoscopic view. **(B)** Endoscopic retroflexion view.

Fig. 3, *A* and *B*). Tears involving only the esophageal mucosa are uncommon. Optimal endoscopic visualization of Mallory-Weiss tears is accomplished by retroflexion of the scope to view the gastroesophageal junction (see Fig. 2, *B*). Additional possible sources of upper GI bleeding, including esophageal varices, gastritis, duodenitis, and peptic ulceration, are present in up to 80% of patients with MWS. It is therefore imperative to perform a complete esophagogastroduodenoscopy whenever possible.

One advantage of upper endoscopy as the primary diagnostic modality for Mallory-Weiss tears is the fact that a therapeutic hemostatic maneuver may be done simultaneously if indicated (see later discussion). Other useful but usually unnecessary diagnostic modalities for MWS include tagged red blood cell scanning and selective mesenteric arteriography. The latter may also be therapeutic because it allows for the option of selective angioembolization or infusion of vasoconstrictive agents (see later discussion).

MANAGEMENT

Most patients (up to 90%) with MWS will stop bleeding with resuscitation and observation only. The 10% to 20% of patients with shock, low hematocrit, high transfusion requirement, coagulopathy, liver disease, or endoscopic findings of active bleeding or visible vessel may need aggressive treatment of the bleeding and, rarely, may require operation. Patients with these risk factors have high mortality (10% to 20%) and require intensive care and prudent intervention (Fig. 4). In this cohort of patients with risk factors for poorer outcome, volume resuscitation with crystalloid should be instituted through large-bore peripheral intravenous access. Transfusion should be considered, and efforts to correct coagulopathy, if present, should be included as part of the initial resuscitation. Nasogastric tube placement and gastric lavage with warm (not cold) saline to clear the blood from the stomach allows for more accurate endoscopic assessment of active hemorrhage. Whether a Mallory-Weiss tear predisposes to perforation during instrumentation is unclear, but this theoretical possibility should be kept in mind. Any complaint of chest or abdominal pain should prompt an

upright chest x-ray before intubation or instrumentation of the upper GI tract; and, if the pain is severe, the diagnosis of MWS should be questioned and contrast radiography considered. Vital signs and urine output are usually sufficient to assess the adequacy of resuscitation. On the other hand, selected stable patients without risk factors may be managed in short-stay units or even on an outpatient basis. Healing of Mallory-Weiss tears has been observed endoscopically to occur within 48 hours from the initial

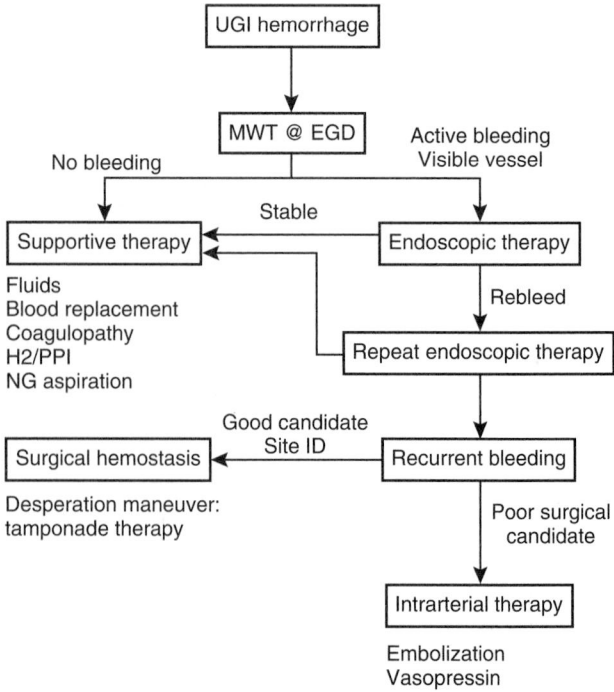

Figure 4 Suggested treatment algorithm, Mallory-Weiss syndrome.

presentation. Healing is probably enhanced by acid suppression, and proton pump inhibitors should be administered to all patients with MWS.

Endoscopic Therapy

Chung and colleagues evaluated 76 patients prospectively over 6 years and suggested that endoscopic treatment was unnecessary in Mallory-Weiss tears not bleeding at the time of endoscopy. As mentioned, selected stable patients without active bleeding may be managed with early discharge. In some series, up to 25% to 50% of patients have been found to have active hemorrhage at the time of initial endoscopy. Because this is one of the factors that defines the group at risk for complications or death, endoscopic hemostasis should be considered in these patients. Endoscopic therapy has largely supplanted angiography and surgery for the control of hemorrhage in patients with MWS. Four endoscopic methods for hemostasis have been used with high success rates: injection therapy, electrocoagulation, band ligation, and hemoclipping. The efficacy and benefits of each of these treatments are summarized in Figure 4.

Injection therapy is a well-established, effective, and safe treatment of Mallory-Weiss tears. Two broad groups of agents have been used to achieve hemostasis: vasoconstrictors (e.g., epinephrine) and sclerosants (e.g., polidocanol, ethanol). Combinations of vasoconstrictors and sclerosing agents have also been used safely. Epinephrine (1:10,000) is currently the most commonly used agent for injection therapy of Mallory-Weiss lesions. Some authors report effective hemostasis in 100% of patients treated by injection of epinephrine and polidocanol. Two to six milliliters of epinephrine (1:10,000) and 4 to 12 ml of 1% polidocanol were injected surrounding the base of Mallory-Weiss tears or visible vessels. Llach and colleagues randomized 63 patients with MWS to a control group (endoscopy and no injection therapy) or injection therapy with a combination of epinephrine and policocanol. Eight patients (26%) rebled in the control group versus only 2 (6%) in the treatment group ($p < .05$). There were no serious treatment-related complications in either group. Sclerotherapy is a particularly useful adjunct for high-risk patients who may have underlying cirrhosis, liver dysfunction and portal hypertension. Esophageal perforation is an oft-mentioned but unusual complication of sclerotherapy for MWS and occurs in less than 1% of patients. Most often Mallory-Weiss tears occur on the gastric side of the gastroesophageal junction and thus pose a low risk for full thickness ischemia and subsequent perforation after sclerotherapy. Epinephrine and ethanol have also been used for injection therapy, with success rates of greater than 90%. Failure of endoscopic injection therapy occurs only rarely and is most often related to active hemorrhage that limits visibility.

Endoscopic electrocoagulation has been shown to be safe and effective for the control of bleeding in MWS. In a randomized prospective control trial, coagulation therapy using an endoscopic multipolar or bipolar electrocoagulation cautery probe provided significantly greater hemostatic efficacy compared with sham therapy (100% vs. 13%) and significantly decreased transfusion requirements. Because of their wide availability, electrocoagulation and injection therapies are the most prevalent therapeutic interventions used to treat Mallory-Weiss hemorrhage.

Endoscopic hemoclipping and band ligation are two mechanical endoscopic techniques that have been applied successfully to control hemorrhage from Mallory-Weiss tears. Band ligation uses an endoscopic applicator that draws tissue into an overtube via suction. Deployment of one or more elastic bands around the tissue accomplishes hemostasis. Another mode of mechanical hemostasis employs one or more hemostatic clips placed via an endoscopic clip applier. Endoscopic band ligation has achieved high rates of hemostasis, as high as 100%, in its application to both nonvariceal and

variceal sources of upper GI hemorrhage. Hemoclip placement was introduced later and is less prevalent than band ligation but equally effective, safely arresting hemorrhage in up to 100% of subjects. Hemoclips have been used successfully for treatment of arterial bleeding secondary to peptic ulceration and Dieulafoy's lesions as well as Mallory-Weiss tears. Because of their successful use, endoscopic mechanical hemostasis has been suggested as effective therapy for patients who have portal hypertension and MWS. The literature also describes effective use of combination injection and mechanical therapy. In a prospective randomized study of hemoclipping versus epinephrine injection therapy, Huang found each modality to be equally efficacious and safe, resulting in a 100% rate of initial hemostasis.

Existing level 1 data suggest that endoscopic therapy is safe and effective as the primary diagnostic and therapeutic modality in the treatment of upper GI hemorrhage caused by MWS. Both injection and mechanical methods are equally effective, and often a combination is used. Most endoscopists currently use whichever modality is most readily available and most familiar.

Angiographic Therapy

Angiotherapy uses interventional radiologic techniques to deliver selectively either vasoconstrictors (e.g., vasopressin) or embolizing agents to the bleeding site. Both methods have been used with success in MWS; selective embolization of the left gastric artery and its branches and selective intra-arterial vasopressin infusion have achieved hemostasis in up to 94% of cases. Angiotherapy is generally thought to be riskier than endoscopic therapy. Catheter-related complications (bleeding, thrombosis, embolism) may occur, and local ischemia and infarction are rare but possible. Intra-arterial vasopressin is associated with a risk of myocardial infarction. These methods should therefore be reserved for patients who have failed endoscopic therapy or are a prohibitive surgical risk.

Direct tamponade of bleeding Mallory-Weiss tears with nasoenteric or oroenteric tubes such as the Sengstaken–Blakemore tube has been suggested as a method for achieving hemostasis, and this treatment has been used with success. However, the use of compression therapy increases the risk of aspiration and could theoretically convert a partial-thickness lesion into a full-thickness perforation. Balloon tamponade is also contraindicated in patients with hiatal hernia, which coexists not infrequently with the MWS. This treatment should therefore be considered only rarely, perhaps as a last resort in patients on mechanical ventilation who have failed other, more standard, therapies.

Surgical Therapy

Surgical intervention for MWS is rarely necessary in current clinical practice. During the pre-endoscopy era before the 1970s, surgical intervention approximated 50% for Mallory-Weiss hemorrhage. Recent published series report surgical intervention in less than 3% of cases. Today operation is considered for those few patients who are acceptable surgical risks and have failed endoscopic therapy. Patients deemed too great a surgical risk may be considered candidates for angiotherapy or, under dire circumstances, compression therapy. Classically, surgical control of bleeding from Mallory-Weiss tears is accomplished via a longitudinal proximal anterior gastrotomy to gain access and visualization of the gastroesophageal junction. Subserosal blood staining of the soft tissues at the gastroesophageal junction on initial exploration of the area has been observed as characteristic of Mallory-Weiss bleeding and may be useful as a guide to the location of the mucosal tear. Control of hemorrhage is achieved by oversewing the tear with absorbable sutures. Ligation of the ascending branch of the left gastric artery on the lesser curvature of the gastric cardia should be considered.

Study	N	Tx Modality	% Hemostasis	% Requiring Surgery	LOS (Days)	Rebleed Rate (%)	Blood Tx Units	Mortality
Llach	63	Endoscopic Inject + Sclero	100	0	3.4	3	0.5	0
Sugawa	224	Conservative (90%) Endoscopic (9%) Surgery (3%) Tamponade (1%)	100 45 100 50	7/224 (3%)		11/224 (4.9%)		8/224 (3.5%) Total pts
Luc Encompasses Pre-endoscopic data	40	Conservative (77.5%) Surgery (22.5%)	87 100	9/40 (22.5%)		0	8.6	7.5% Total pts
Huang	35	Endoscopic Clip placement Injection	100 100	0 0	8.2 4.5	2/35 (6%)	2.2 1.9	1/35 (3%)
Park	34	Endoscopic Band ligation Injection	100 94	0 0	5.0 4.2	0 0	4.8 3.4	0 0
Laine	44	Endoscopic Coagulation	90	0	4.4	0	2.4	0

Figure 5 Treatment outcomes summary, Mallory-Weiss syndrome.

Localization of the site of hemorrhage is often difficult or impaired by active hemorrhage. Good light, appropriate retractors, and suction are required. Placing laparotomy packs in the stomach and sequentially inspecting all of the gastric mucosa facilitates exposure and may help to locate the source of bleeding. Intraoperative endoscopy may also aid in location of an occult bleeding source. It is important for the surgeon to consider other possible esophagogastric bleeding sources if the Mallory-Weiss lesion cannot be located or appears trivial.

Combined laparoendoscopic techniques for locating and oversewing Mallory-Weiss tears have been described. Under endoscopic guidance, full-thickness absorbable sutures are laparoscopically placed at the gastroesophageal junction at the site of hemorrhage, and the ascending branch of the left gastric artery may be clipped or divided with the harmonic scalpel. An alternative laparoscopic technique would be to obtain pneumoperitoneum in the standard fashion, create two gastrotomies, and place the transabdominal laparoscopic trocars into the gastric lumen. Insufflation of the stomach is then established, and the Mallory-Weiss tear(s) can be suture ligated intragastrically under direct visualization. Whatever the surgical technique, care must be taken not to narrow or occlude the gastroesophageal junction. The need for surgical intervention in MWS currently identifies a patient at higher risk for complications and mortality because of the underlying severity of bleeding or comorbidities.

OUTCOMES

Mallory-Weiss syndrome is a common cause of upper GI hemorrhage, with a self-limited course in approximately 90% of cases. Spontaneous cessation of bleeding results from conservative, supportive therapy and suffices in most patients. Patients with active hemorrhage or an exposed visible vessel at initial endoscopy and an initial hematocrit of less than 30%, shock, underlying coagulopathy, or liver dysfunction are at increased risk for failure of conservative therapy and are predisposed to rebleeding and a more complicated hospital course. This subset of patients should be considered for therapeutic intervention. Endoscopy is the first-line diagnostic and therapeutic modality. Endoscopic injection of vasoconstrictors or sclerosants, electrocautery, and mechanical methods are all effective in achieving hemostasis in experienced hands

(Fig. 5). Rebleeding of Mallory-Weiss tears has been reported to occur in 0% to 5% of patients after initial endoscopic therapy. In almost all cases, rebleeding is successfully stopped using repeat endoscopic therapy. Other treatment modalities, including angiotherapy and surgical intervention, are required in less than 5% of cases. Overall risk of mortality from Mallory-Weiss syndrome is less than 5%.

SUGGESTED READINGS

Barkun A, Bardou M, Marshall JK: Nonvariceal Upper GI Bleeding Consensus Conference Group, Consensus recommendations for managing patients with nonvariceal upper gastrointestinal bleeding, *Ann Intern Med* 139:843, 2003.

Bataller R, Llach J, Salmeron JM, and others: Endoscopic sclerotherapy in upper gastrointestinal bleeding due to the Mallory-Weiss syndrome, *Am J Gastroenterol* 89:2147, 1994.

British Society of Gastroenterology Endoscopy Committee: Non-variceal upper gastrointestinal haemorrhage: guidelines, *Gut* 51(suppl 4):iv1, 2002.

Chung IK, Kim EJ, Hwang KY, and others: Evaluation of endoscopic hemostasis in upper gastrointestinal bleeding related to Mallory-Weiss syndrome, *Endoscopy* 34:474, 2002.

Ellenhorn JD, LaQuaglia MP, Geer RJ: Exposure of the mucosa of the gastroesophageal junction in patients with Mallory-Weiss tears, *Surg Gynecol Obstetr* 177:91, 1993.

Fisher RG, Schwartz JT, Graham DY: Angiotherapy with Mallory Weiss Tear, *AJR* 134:679, 1980.

Gawrieh S, Shaker R, Treatment of actively bleeding Mallory-Weiss syndrome: epinephrine injection or band ligation? *Curr Gastroenterol Rep* 7:175, 2005.

Huang SP, Wang HP, Lee YC, and others: Endoscopic hemoclip placement and epinephrine injection for Mallory-Weiss syndrome with active bleeding, *Gastrointest Endosc* 55:842, 2002.

Knauer CM: Mallory-Weiss syndrome, Characterization of 75 Mallory-Weiss lacerations in 528 patients with upper gastrointestinal hemorrhage, *Gastroenterology* 71:5, 1976.

Kortas DY, Haas LS, Simpson WG: Mallory Weiss tear predisposing factors and predictors of a complicated course, *Am J Gastroenterol* 96: 2863, 2001.

Laine L, Electrocoagulation in the treatment of active upper gi tract hemorrhage, *N Engl J Med* 316:1613, 1987.

Llach J, Elizalde JI, Guevara MC, and others: Endoscopic injection therapy in bleeding Mallory-Weiss syndrome: a randomized controlled trial, *Gastrointest Endosc* 54:679, 2001.

McNatt SS, McFadden DW: Mallory-Weiss syndrome. In Cameron JL, editor: *Current surgical therapy*, ed 8, Philadelphia, 2004, Elsevier.

Michel L, Serrano A, Malt RA: Mallory-Weiss syndrome, evolution of diagnostic and therapeutic patterns over two decades, *Ann Surg* 192:716, 1980.

Park CH, Min SW, Sohn YH and others: A prospective randomized trial of endoscopic Band Ligation vs epinephrine injection for actively bleeding Mallory Weiss syndrome, *Gastrointest Endosc* 60:22, 2004.

Sugawa C, Benishek D, Walt A: Mallory Weiss syndrome, a study of 224 patients, *Am J Surg* 145:30, 1983.

Yamaguchi Y, Yamato T, Katsumi N, and others: Endoscopic hemoclipping for upper GI bleeding due to Mallory-Weiss syndrome, *Gastrointest Endosc* 53:427, 2001.

MORBID OBESITY

Todd M. McCarty, MD, and Jeffery Lamont, MD

INTRODUCTION

Obesity is an increasing health care problem in the United States. Two thirds of the American population is considered overweight, defined as a body mass index (BMI) between 25 and 30 (BMI = wt [kg] / ht [m^2]). Approximately 30% of Americans aged 20 years and older are considered obese (BMI >30). More than 50 million Americans are obese and are at risk of or are experiencing obesity-related health problems. Obesity is associated with a variety of severe health problems, listed in Table 1. In 1998, it was estimated that 9.1% of all health care expenditures were overweight and obesity related, accounting for more than $96.2 billion of expense, in 2002 dollars. The key to improving or eliminating obesity-related illness and its expenses is weight loss. An innumerable number of exercise, pharmacologic, nutritional, and spiritual programs exist to promote weight loss, but all are plagued by the difficulty in sustaining weight loss in most individuals. The modern surgical approach to obesity is highly successful in allowing loss of at least 50% of excess body weight in 80% to 90% of individuals along with improvement of medical comorbid factors.

PATIENT SELECTION

The National Institutes of Health issued a consensus statement in 1991 regarding the effectiveness of bariatric surgical procedures in treating severe obesity. This was updated in 2004 by the American Society of Bariatric Surgery, which issued a review and recommendations of current surgical techniques. Appropriate candidates for bariatric surgery should be morbidly obese, that is, have a BMI ≥40 (Table 2). Patients with a BMI >35 are appropriate surgical candidates as long as obesity-related comorbidities exist. Extending bariatric surgery to patients with BMI <35 with severe comorbidities is the subject of clinical evaluation and is not routinely

Table 1: Health Consequences of Obesity (A Partial List)

Hypertension
Dyslipidemia (e.g., high total cholesterol or high levels of triglycerides)
Type 2 diabetes
Coronary heart disease
Stroke
Gallbladder disease
Osteoarthritis
Sleep apnea and respiratory problems
Some cancers (endometrial, breast, and colon)

Table 2: Patient Eligibility Requirements for Bariatric Surgery

BMI >40
BMI >35 with comorbid conditions
Failure to lose weight with nonsurgical methods
Medically compliant patient
No uncontrolled psychiatric or substance abuse problems
Medically able to undergo a surgical procedure

BMI, body mass index.

recommended at this time. Patients should have attempted weight reduction by nonsurgical means and failed in the past and should have realistic expectations regarding the utility and effectiveness of the surgical procedure. Noncompliant patients and patients with severe psychiatric illnesses or substance abuse are poor candidates for bariatric surgery. No strict age criteria exist; however, the benefits of long-term health improvements tend to wane in the elderly patient. Bariatric surgical procedures have been approved by Medicare as long as the provider meets certain performance criteria.

Most institutions providing bariatric surgical procedures stress the importance of a multidisciplinary approach. At Baylor University Medical Center, all patients are evaluated preoperatively by a nutritionist and a psychologist, as well as the surgeon, to ensure that patients' motivations and expectations of surgical weight loss are appropriate. All patients are required to attend an educational seminar regarding the various surgical procedures for morbid obesity, their expected morbidity, and their outcomes. Patients are counseled about the need for long-term follow-up, vitamin supplementation, and dietary compliance following the surgery. Patients are also encouraged to attend support group meetings or to discuss their medical care in a Web-based forum for assistance with various psychosocial issues regarding weight loss and weight loss surgery.

OPERATIVE PROCEDURES

Restrictive versus Malabsorptive Mechanism

Bariatric surgical procedures can be classified on the basis of their mechanism of action. Restrictive procedures involve the creation of a small gastric pouch causing a feeling of satiety for the patient. Examples are the vertical banded gastroplasty, the adjustable gastric banding, and the pouch created in the Roux-en-Y gastric bypass (RYGB). Malabsorptive procedures involve creating a long channel from the stomach or pouch before anastomosis with a biliopancreatic limb. This prevents nutrients from being absorbed effectively before mixing with bile and pancreatic juice. Examples of this mechanism are the RYGB and the biliopancreatic diversion or duodenal switch.

Roux-en-Y Gastric Bypass

Roux-en-Y gastric bypass is currently the gold standard for bariatric surgical procedures and is the most common bariatric procedure performed at Baylor University Medical Center. It is both restrictive and malabsorptive in its mechanism of action, allowing loss of 60% to 70% excess body weight at 2 years. The creation of a small gastric pouch is restrictive, in that it allows a patient to feel satiated after a small meal. The gastric pouch also bypasses the fundus of the stomach, where the hormonal stimulus for hunger, ghrelin, is elaborated. The malabsorptive component of RYGB is a long roux limb that is connected to the biliopancreatic limb 100 cm (BMI <50) or 150 cm (BMI ≥50) from the gastrojejunostomy. In addition, some patients experience "dumping syndrome," which is a feeling of panic, cramping abdominal pain, and diarrhea following "sugary" intake (e.g., soda). This is a strong reinforcement to the patient regarding appropriate dietary modifications following RYGB. RYGB is considered the gold standard because it has been shown in prospective trials to be superior to vertical banded gastroplasty and laparoscopic banding in terms of total weight loss and durability of weight loss.

At Baylor University Medical Center, RYGB is performed exclusively via the laparoscopic technique. The procedure described here has been modified over a series of more than 3500 procedures in the 6 years previous to this writing. The surgeon stands to the patient's right side and the assistant to the left, along with a camera operator and scrub nurse. Four 12-mm trocars are placed. The greater omentum is divided in the middle, and the ligament of Treitz (LT) is identified. Forty centimeters from the LT, the bowel is divided with a 60-mm white/vascular ENDO-GIA stapler (U.S. Surgical, Norwalk, CT). A 100 or 150-cm roux limb is measured and a side-to-side stapled anastomosis is created with the 60-mm stapler. All small-bowel anastomoses are created with white/vascular staple loads. A 5-mm trocar is placed just under the xiphoid process, through which a grasping instrument grasps the right pillar of the esophageal hiatus for retraction of the left hepatic lobe. We have found this to provide adequate exposure without the need for a separate retractor or assistant. The stomach is retracted and the position for the gastrojejunostomy is chosen near the lesser curve of the stomach. The pouch can be measured with an endoluminal balloon; however, with experience, a small 20- to 30-ml pouch can be accurately estimated. The vagal nerves are spared, and the lesser sac is entered bluntly. A longitudinal gastrotomy is performed, and the anvil of a 25-mm EEA stapler (U.S. Surgical) is placed endoluminally with an angled instrument. This is retrieved at the site of gastrojejunostomy with a small gastrotomy created with the post of a Harmonic Scalpel (Ethicon, Somerville, NJ). The greater curve gastrotomy is stapled closed. The stomach is transected with green loaded staples with Peristrip reinforcements (Synovis, St. Paul, MN). The gastrojejunostomy is then created with the EEA stapler in the antecolic position, and the open end of the jejunum is closed with a linear stapler. The anastomosis is reinforced with two absorbable sutures. The anastomosis is tested for leaks by instilling 50 ml of methylene blue containing saline via orogastric tube with distal limb occlusion. If a leak occurs, it is closed with suture and retested. With experience, the average time for this procedure is 45 minutes.

Several portions of the procedure and the subsequent care path have evolved that have helped to diminish the postoperative complication rates. The laparoscopic approach has the obvious value of preventing postoperative incisional hernia and promoting early ambulation while minimizing the need for intravenous narcotics. A change in the gastrojejunal anastomotic size from 21 to 25 mm has led to a decreased rate of stricture. The roux limb is considered antecolic based on the occurrence of transmesocolic internal hernias following excessive weight loss. Low–molecular-weight heparin was administered preoperatively but is now given following the procedure, which has diminished the problem of endoluminal anastomotic bleeding.

Postoperative care protocol includes observation in the postoperative recovery room for 4 hours while the patient receives a centrally acting alpha-2 adrenergic agonist (dexmedetomidine) for pain management. Patients are then transferred to a general care floor with patient-controlled analgesic pump with morphine sulfate and sequential progression from ice chips to low carbohydrate clear liquid diet on the first day. Patients do not undergo routine upper gastrointestinal (GI) series. Hospital discharge occurs when stability of clinical and laboratory parameters is achieved. Patients are seen in the clinic at 2 weeks, 6 weeks, 6 months, and then annually. In a consecutive series of 2000 patients at Baylor University Medical Center, 84% were discharged from the hospital within 23 hours of surgery. Readmission rate within 30 days was 1.7%.

Early postoperative complications (<30 days) in our experience included gastrojejunostomy stricture (0.8%), internal hernia (0.6%), gastrojejunal hematoma (0.2%), and gastrojejunostomy leak (0.2%). Late complications (>30 days) included internal hernia (2.5%), gastrojejunal stricture (1.3%), gastrogastric fistula (0.2%), and marginal ulcer (0.2%). Anastomotic strictures are effectively treated with endoscopic balloon dilatation along with proton pump inhibitors, should ulceration be a component. Gastrogastric fistula is usually managed conservatively along with endoscopic treatment (fibrin glue, closure with clips or sutures). An occasional patient with a gastrogastric fistula will require surgical revision. Mortality was 0.1% in this series. Long-term nutritional deficiencies are possible following RYBG, requiring patients to take supplemental calcium, vitamin B12, and a multivitamin containing iron for life.

Laparoscopic Adjustable Banding (Lap Band)

The Lap Band is a purely restrictive method of surgical weight loss. Its advantages are the avoidance of GI anastomoses and the fact that it is easily reversible. Introduced in the early 1990s, it gained wide acceptance in Europe. Currently one device has been approved for use by the U.S. Food and Drug Administration (Lap-Band; Inamed Health, Santa Barbara, CA). The band is placed via a laparoscopic approach around the cardia of the stomach, creating a small 15-ml pouch. The dissection proceeds from the base of the right crus, along the left crus to the angle of His (the pars flaccida approach); this has been shown to prevent band migration. The anterior wall of the stomach is sutured over the band to further prevent a "slipped" band. The Lap Band is then connected to a subcutaneous port but is not inflated on the day of surgery. This procedure is usually performed on an outpatient basis. Patients are followed in the clinic at 2 weeks, 4 weeks, 6 weeks, 6 months, and then annually. These patients often require frequent office visits for band fills to adjust the band appropriately.

Morbidity with Lap Band placement is reported at 5% with a mortality of 0.1%. Complications include "slipped" band, erosions and ulcerations, port pocket complications, and dysphagia. Patients are not required to take supplemental calcium or vitamin B12, but a multivitamin is recommended.

Vertical Banded Gastroplasty

Vertical banded gastroplasty (VBG) was first introduced in the 1970s and was widely used. It is a purely restrictive form of weight loss surgery. Although mostly performed open, it can now be performed laparoscopically. No gastric transaction or anastomoses are required. The procedure involves the creation of a stapled pouch from angle of His, parallel to the lesser curve of the stomach, with a volume of 15 to 25 ml. The outlet of the pouch is restricted by either a silicone or Marlex ring. The silicone ring is usually placed with a special notched stapler used to partition the stomach. The Marlex ring is usually placed around a defect in the stomach created by an EEA stapler. Regardless of the ring type, the outlet of the pouch is usually 0.75 to 1.25 cm in diameter.

Morbidity related to an open VBG includes the potential for wound infection and incisional hernia. Complications specific to VBG are staple line breakdown and fistula, diminishing the effectiveness of the procedure and gastric erosion of the band. Particulate food may obstruct the outlet and require endoscopic removal. Outlet obstruction following VBG usually requires surgical revision because the ring cannot be endoscopically dilated.

Biliopancreatic Diversion and Duodenal Switch

Both of these procedures are malabsorptive in mechanism. They are most often performed in the open setting but can be performed laparoscopically. At the extremes of weight (BMI >60), some surgeons recommend a two-staged procedure. Biliopancreatic diversion (BPD) was originally described in Italy and involves a partial gastrectomy, leaving a 150-ml pouch. This is drained by a roux limb, which is anastomosed to the biliopancreatic limb approximately 50 to 150 cm from the ileocecal valve. The duodenal switch (DS) is an American adaptation of the BPD that entails a tabularizing gastrectomy, preserving the pylorus. This pylorus is connected to a roux limb with downstream construction similar to the BPD.

Complications associated with BPD and DS include dumping syndrome in BPD and nutrient deficiencies in both procedures. Patients are given supplemental calcium, vitamin B, and multivitamins to prevent these complications and must consistently ingest adequate protein.

Outcomes

Weight loss following bariatric surgical procedures is typically 50% to 70% of total excess body weight (TEBW) by 2 years. RYGB is associated with 65% to 70% loss of excess body weight at 2 years. Results from the Lap Band include weight loss of 50% excess body weight at 2 years. Longer-term results are necessary to clarify the durability of the Lap Band over time. The expected weight loss following VBG is 55% to 60% TEBW, whereas BPD and DS are associated with 60% to 70% weight loss. Effective weight loss with any bariatric surgical procedure requires patient compliance with dietary modifications and is optimal when exercise is a component of the patient's lifestyle.

Emerging Technology

Several procedures are being investigated as new surgical options in the management of morbid obesity. Sleeve gastrectomy, resection of the lateral portion of the stomach (a component of DS), is gaining popularity and can be converted to DS or RYGB or inadequate weight loss. Gastric myoelectrical stimulation involves the laparoscopic placement of leads into the muscular layer of the stomach.

These leads are connected to a subcutaneous electronic pulse generator (Transcend IGS; Transneuronix, Mt. Arlington, NJ), which provides low-level gastric stimulation, causing a feeling of satiety. The advantage of this approach is to avoid the surgical and nutritional complications of other bariatric surgeries and the maintenance of normal anatomy.

Endoscopic approaches to obesity involve endosurgical restrictive procedures. These will involve endoluminal suturing and partitioning of the stomach, creating a gastric pouch or an endoscopic vertical banded gastroplasty type of construction. Such techniques are available clinically for the treatment of gastroesophageal reflux disease, but bariatric procedures are still the subject of research. Endoscopic suturing may be useful in revisional bariatric procedures, such as an enlarged pouch following a previous RYGB. A clinical trial investigating this procedure is planned. Endoscopically placed intragastric balloons with volumes of approximately 600 ml have been described for weight loss purposes. Its mechanism of action may be in part due to its influence on plasma ghrelin levels, as well as a restrictive mechanism. Its results have been modest.

QUALIFICATIONS FOR PERFORMANCE OF BARIATRIC SURGERY

The American Society of Bariatric Surgery lists several surgeon qualifications for the performance of bariatric surgical procedures. These include documented training in bariatric procedures, working in a multidisciplinary patient care environment, the ability to care for short- and long-term complications, and the mechanism to provide long-term follow-up. Procedure-specific qualifications also exist.

SUGGESTED READINGS

Buchwald H, Avidor Y, Braunwald E and others: Bariatric surgery: a systematic review and meta-analysis, *JAMA* 292(14):1724–1737, 2004.
McCarty TM, Arnold DT, Lamont JP and others: Optimizing outcomes in bariatric surgery: outpatient laparoscopic gastric bypass, *Ann Surg* 242(4):494–498, 2005.
McCarty TM: Can bariatric surgery be done as an outpatient procedure? *Adv Surg* 40:99–106, 2006.

GASTRIC ADENOCARCINOMA

Clifford S. Cho, MD, and Murray F. Brennan, MD

INTRODUCTION

Epidemiology and pathogenesis

Over the past century, mortality from gastric cancer has steadily declined. Once the most common source of cancer-related death in developed nations, it is currently the fourteenth most common oncologic cause of mortality in the United States. Nevertheless, gastric cancer remains a significant worldwide health problem, accounting for 880,000 new diagnoses and 650,000 deaths in 2000. Proximal gastric cancers are increasing in parallel with esophageal adenocarcinoma. Risk factors for gastric cancer include *Helicobacter pylori* infection, exposure

to potential carcinogens (including tobacco, salt, and nitrites), obesity, prior gastrectomy, pernicious anemia, and familial history of gastric cancer. Recently, inactivating mutations of the membrane glycoprotein E-cadherin have been linked to tumorigenesis, invasion, and metastasis. Levels of soluble E-cadherin appear to serve as an effective prognostic marker associated with adverse survival outcomes.

Pathology

Adenocarcinomas comprise approximately 90% of gastric tumors and are broadly categorized into two Lauren histotypes: the intestinal, or well-differentiated type, and the diffuse, or poorly differentiated type. The intestinal type arises from gastric mucosa and is associated with older patients and distal tumors. The diffuse type is believed to originate from the lamina propria of the stomach and grows in an infiltrative, submucosal pattern. Associated with younger patients and proximal tumors, the diffuse form also appears to be more strongly associated with early metastases. Corresponding to the increasing incidence of proximal gastric tumors, the incidence of diffuse type gastric cancer has been increasing in recent years. Early gastric cancers are a pathologic subtype confined within the gastric mucosa or submucosa and are being diagnosed with increasing frequency.

The most commonly adopted pathologic staging system in contemporary use is the updated American Joint Committee on Cancer/International Union Against Cancer (AJCC/UICC) system (Table 1). T status is defined by depth of gastric wall invasion: T1 lesions are invasive into the lamina propria or submucosa; T2a lesions invade into the muscularis propria and T2b lesions into the submucosa; T3 lesions penetrate the serosa and are therefore full-thickness lesions; T4 lesions are invasive into adjacent anatomic structures (e.g., peritoneum, colon). N status is now defined by the number of nodal metastases identified, with N1 disease defined by metastases present in 1 to 6 regional lymph nodes, N2 disease by metastases in 7 to 15 regional nodes, and N3 disease by metastases in more than 15 regional lymph nodes. A sufficient number of lymph nodes (≥ 15) must be removed and pathologically examined to permit accurate staging.

Table 1: American Joint Committee on Cancer/International Union Against Cancer (AJCC/UICC) Gastric Cancer Staging System

Tumor:	Tx	Primary tumor cannot be assessed		
	T0	No evidence of primary tumor		
	Tis	Carcinoma in situ: intraepithelial tumor without invasion of lamina propria		
	T1	Tumor invades lamina propria or submucosa		
	T2	Tumor invades muscularis propria or subserosa		
	T2a	Tumor invades muscularis propria		
	T2b	Tumor invades subserosa		
	T3	Tumor invades serosa (visceral peritoneum) without invasion of adjacent structures		
	T4	Tumor invades adjacent structures		
Nodes:	Nx	regional lymph nodes cannot be assessed		
	N0	No regional lymph node metastases		
	N1	Metastases in 1 to 6 regional lymph nodes		
	N2	Metastases in 7 to 15 regional lymph nodes		
	N3	Metastases in more than 15 regional lymph nodes		
Metastases:	Mx	Distant metastases cannot be assessed		
	M0	No distant metastases		
	M1	Distant metastases		
Stages:	0	Tis	N0	M0
	IA	T1	N0	M0
	IB	T1	N1	M0
		T2a/b	N0	M0
	II	T1	N2	M0
		T2a/b	N1	M0
		T3	N0	M0
	IIIA	T2a/b	N2	M0
		T3	N1	M0
		T4	N0	M0
	IIIB	T3	N2	M0
	IV	T4	N1-3	M0
		T1-3	N3	M0
		any T	any N	M1

Diagnosis and Staging

Because of the vague complex of symptoms (abdominal pain, dyspepsia) typically referable to early-stage gastric cancers, many cases of gastric adenocarcinoma in the United States present at an advanced stage. The most common physical examination finding is that of a palpable abdominal mass; classical physical examination findings of Sister Mary Joseph's periumbilical nodes, Blumer's shelf drop metastases into the prerectal peritoneal space, or Virchow's left supraclavicular lymph nodes are unusual and indicative of late-stage disease. The diagnostic modality of choice is endoscopy. Adjunctive use of endoscopic ultrasound (EUS) may permit identification of transmural (T3) involvement with approximately 80% accuracy or pathologically enlarged lymph nodes with approximately 50% accuracy. EUS may be used to direct clinical protocols of preoperative chemotherapy for patients with locally advanced lesions. The role of computed tomography (CT) is primarily for the detection of metastatic disease. Detection of metastases is enhanced with the use of diagnostic laparoscopy, which has demonstrated a yield of 20% to 30% in identifying patients with irresectable disease not previously appreciated on conventional cross-sectional imaging. Cytologic analysis of peritoneal washings obtained at the time of laparoscopy may also provide additional prognostic information for use in treatment selection. In a recent analysis of patients undergoing complete (R0) resection after diagnostic laparoscopy confirming no evidence of visible metastases, patients with negative peritoneal cytology demonstrated a median survival of 98.5 months compared with a median survival of 14.8 months among those with positive peritoneal cytology (Table 2).

SURGERY

Extent of Gastrectomy

Prospective randomized controlled trials have established that there is no difference in survival outcome between total and subtotal gastrectomy after R0 resection. Quality of life analyses demonstrate a favorable profile for patients treated with subtotal gastrectomy. Proximal subtotal gastrectomy has also demonstrated oncologic equivalence to total gastrectomy for proximal tumors. However, further analysis of morbidity and quality of life are necessary before advocating general adoption of this procedure. Because of the potential for submucosal spread, 6 cm has been suggested as a gross resection margin. The management of microscopically positive margins is an area of some controversy. Repeat resection to negative margins provides

Table 2: Median and 5-Year Overall Survival after R0 Resection Stratified by AJCC/UICC Stage

Stage	n	Median Overall Survival (months)	5-Year Overall Survival (%)
IA	333	Not reached	92
IB	299	Not reached	75%
II	374	54	49
IIIA	383	35	33
IIIB	179	18	13
IV	127	15	11

From the Memorial Sloan-Kettering Cancer Center database, July 1985 to December 2005.

a potential survival benefit for patients with microscopically positive margins (R1 resection), but only for those patients with N0 or N1 nodal status; the presence of N2 nodal disease appears to nullify any additional prognostic significance attributable to margin status.

Extent of Lymphadenectomy

Extent of lymphadenectomy remains controversial. Nodal stations historically have been defined according to their proximity to the stomach. D0 dissection refers to a (typically palliative) resection in which no effort is made to resect lymph nodes; D1 lymphadenectomy includes perigastric lymph node stations, and D2 lymphadenectomy incorporates lymph node stations along the main trunks of the celiac axis. Extended D2 lymphadenectomy has been championed by Japanese surgeons who have suggested significant improvements in overall survival with the adoption of extended D2 lymph node dissection. Several Western prospective randomized trials have examined the impact of extended D2 lymphadenectomy on outcome. The British Medical Research Council prospective randomized trial comparing D1 and D2 lymphadenectomy showed a significant increase in postoperative morbidity with no improvement in overall or recurrence-free survival. The Dutch Gastric Cancer Group prospective randomized trial of D1 versus D2 lymphadenectomy, which used an experienced Japanese surgeon as an instructor and intraoperative monitor to confirm adequacy of nodal dissection, also showed higher postoperative morbidity after D2 dissection with no improvement in survival. However, distal pancreatectomy and splenectomy were often incorporated into D2 dissection in both trials, and subgroup analyses have suggested that the performance of pancreatosplenectomy contributed significantly to the morbidity and possibly influenced the long-term mortality of patients undergoing extended lymphadenectomy. Subsequent nonrandomized single-center trials comparing D1 and D2 lymphadenectomy without pancreatosplenectomy have observed similar

morbidity and favorable survival among patients undergoing D2 dissection. Many centers staffed with experienced surgeons have documented the ability to perform D2 lymphadenectomy with operative morbidity rates no higher than those observed after limited D1 lymphadenectomy. An additional benefit of aggressive lymphadenectomy is in the accuracy of staging. A review of 1083 patients undergoing R0 resection at the Memorial Sloan-Kettering Cancer Center (MSKCC) demonstrated that the number, and not the location, of positive lymph nodes was of considerable prognostic importance. According to current AJCC guidelines, N1 disease is defined as positive nodal metastases in 1 to 6 regional lymph nodes, N2 disease is defined as 7 to 15 nodal metastases, and N3 as >15 nodal metastases; accurate nodal staging by examination of least 15 resected lymph nodes conferred a significant improvement in prognostication. Furthermore, resection of at least 15 lymph nodes resulted in significant incremental improvements for all stages. In all likelihood, this phenomenon is due to stage migration; the ability to classify patients more accurately by interrogating more lymph nodes decreases the likelihood that patients with occult nodal metastases are erroneously understaged.

Operative Technique

The conduct of gastrectomy with D2 lymphadenectomy commences with careful abdominal exploration to exclude the possibility of undiagnosed distant metastases. After resectability is confirmed, the avascular plane between the greater omentum and transverse colon is sharply incised (Fig. 1, A). The greater omentum is then dissected off of the colon, and the anterior sheath of the transverse mesocolon is removed along an avascular plane down to the level of the pancreas (Fig. 1, B). Classically, the pancreatic capsule is taken with the specimen, but this should be done selectively because proof of its oncological value is limited. The lateral attachments of the greater omentum are divided, as are the

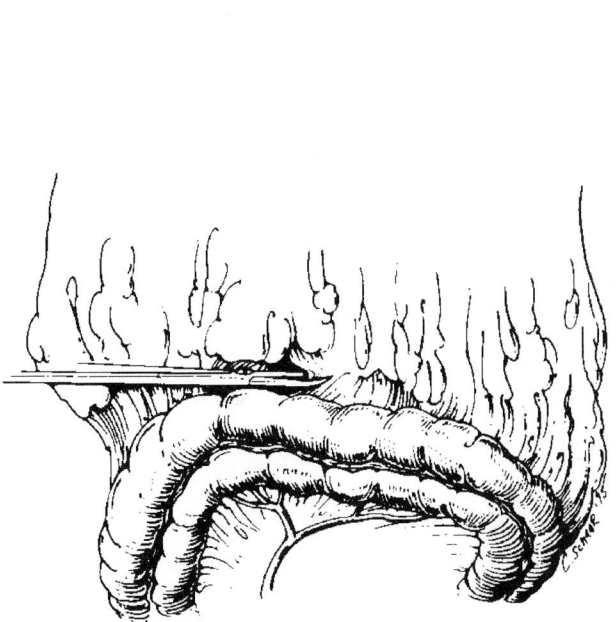

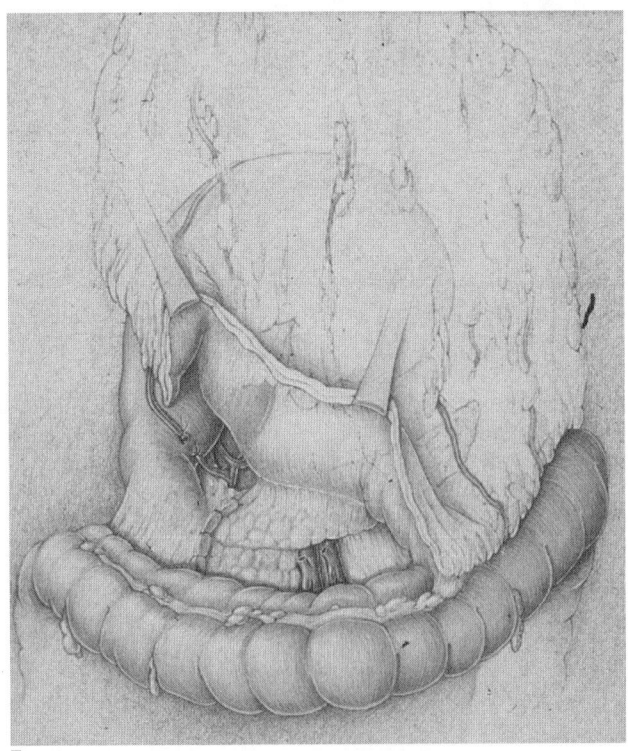

A   B

Figure 1 **(A)** The avascular plane between the greater omentum and transverse mesocolon is incised. **(B)** The greater omentum is dissected off of the colon along the avascular plane between the anterior and posterior sheaths of the transverse mesocolon. Dissection is carried down to the level of the pancreas.

(continued)

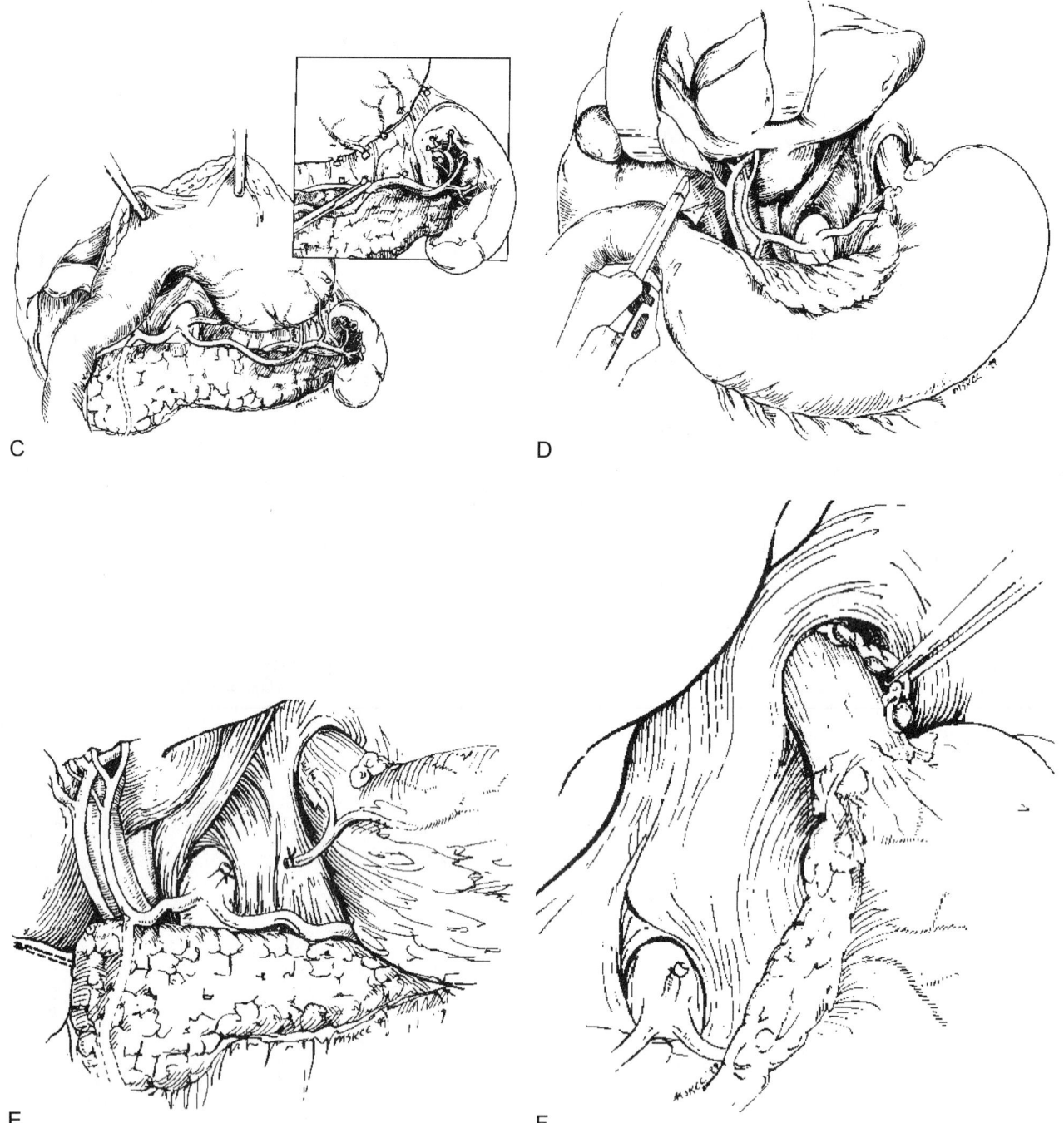

C

D

E

F

Figure 1 **Cont'd—(C)** The lateral attachments of the stomach and short gastric vessels are divided. Inset: The splenic artery is dissected along the superior border of the pancreas. Nodal tissue is dissected down to the level of splenic hilus. **(D)** The duodenum is identified and divided with the GIA linear stapler. **(E)** Nodal dissection proceeds from the porta hepatis toward the celiac axis along the superior border of the pancreas. The left gastric artery is divided at its origin. **(F)** Nodal dissection continues along the right diaphragmatic crus and esophageal hiatus. The left paracardial nodes are taken during total gastrectomy.

short gastric vessels (Fig. 1, C); the extent of dissection along the greater curvature of the stomach is dictated by the planned extent of gastric resection, that is, distal subtotal versus total gastrectomy. The duodenum is isolated and typically divided with the GIA stapling device (US Surgical, Norwalk, CT), with care taken to avoid a retained antral remnant (Fig. 1, D). Dissection is carried along the porta hepatis toward the celiac axis to incorporate all nodal tissue anterior to the portal vein with the resected specimen. Nodal tissue between the superior border of the pancreas and the common

hepatic artery is reflected toward the celiac axis. The left gastric artery is identified and divided at its origin from the celiac axis (Fig. 1, E), and all nodal tissue is swept off the right crus from the esophageal hiatus (Fig. 1, F). The proximal splenic artery is dissected along the superior border of the pancreas and nodal clearance proceeds toward the splenic hilum (see Fig. 1, C, inset). For distal subtotal gastrectomy, the proximal margin is divided with the GIA stapler; for total gastrectomy, the esophagus is encircled, controlled with a Satinsky clamp, and sharply transected.

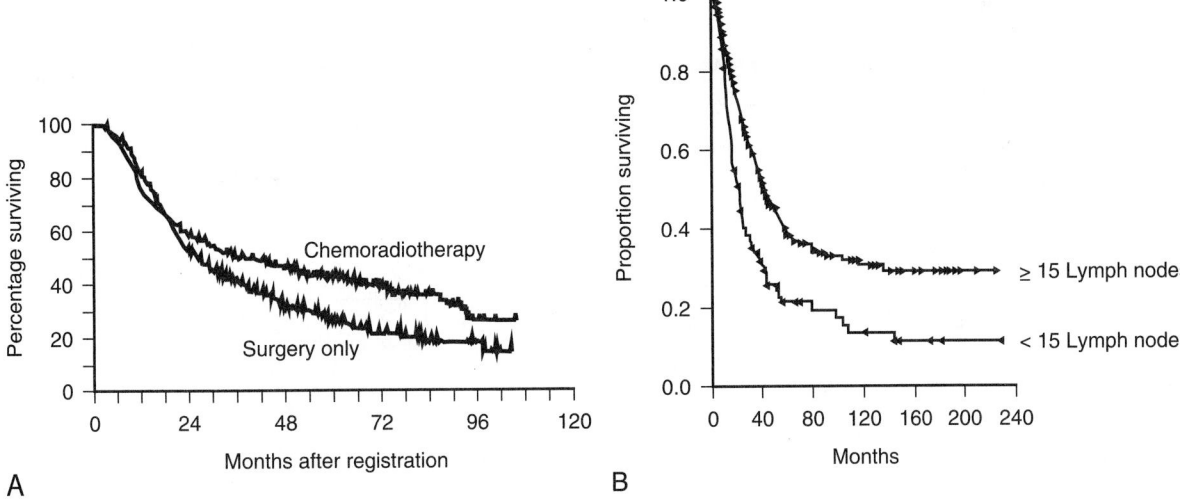

Figure 2 Comparison of Kaplan-Meier survival curves analyzing influence of adjuvant chemoradiation and extent of nodal dissection. **(A)** Overall survival of patients randomized to surgery alone (median survival = 27 months, *n* = 275) and surgery and chemoradiation (median survival = 36 months, *n* = 281) (*p* = .005). **(B)** Overall survival of patients with stage IIIA gastric cancer after R0 resection with fewer than 15 lymph nodes removed (median survival = 22 months, *n* = 116) or 15 or more lymph nodes removed (median survival = 42 months, *n* = 267) (*p* < .0001).   *Part A is from MacDonald JS, Smalley SR, and others: N Engl J Med 345:725, 2001. Part B data are from the MSKCC database, July 1985 to December 2005.*

Proximal margins are routinely submitted for frozen section confirmation of microscopic tumor clearance. Reconstruction is then performed, either with a Billroth II gastrojejunostomy or Roux-en-Y gastrojejunostomy after distal subtotal gastrectomy, or with a Roux-en-Y esophagojejunostomy after total gastrectomy. No convincing evidence exists to support the routine construction of a jejunal pouch after total gastrectomy.

COMBINED MODALITY THERAPY

Adjuvant Therapy

A recent analysis of 1172 patients undergoing R0 curative resection of gastric cancer at MSKCC identified a 42% incidence of recurrent disease after long-term follow-up. Fifty-four percent of recurrences included locoregional loci of disease, and 51% included distant loci. Seventy-nine percent of these recurrences were identified within 2 years of resection; the median time from recurrence to death was 6 months. The high likelihood of both local and distant recurrent disease exemplified by the results of this analysis has motivated interest in combined modality adjunctive therapies for resected gastric cancer. Numerous analyses and meta-analyses of adjuvant chemotherapy with or without radiation have failed to demonstrate consistently any significant impact on survival after curative resection. However, adjuvant chemoradiation has been suggested as the standard of care in the United States on the basis of the results of the Intergroup 0116 prospective randomized controlled trial comparing postoperative 5-fluorouracil and leucovorin and external beam radiation therapy versus observation. A significant improvement in overall and disease-free survival was observed among patients receiving adjuvant chemoradiation. This trial has been criticized for its flawed quality control of surgical therapy. Entry criteria included the recommendation that patients undergo D2 lymphadenectomy; analysis of resected specimens demonstrated that only 10% of patients had D2 lymphadenectomy, and 54% of patients had less than a D1 lymphadenectomy. It is unlikely that the incremental survival

benefit attributed to adjuvant chemoradiation in this trial would exceed that which would be expected simply as a result of more accurate staging after comprehensive lymphadenectomy of ≥15 lymph nodes (Fig. 2).

Neoadjuvant Therapy

Review of the Intergroup 0116 trial confirms that only 64% of patients assigned to receive postoperative chemoradiation were able to complete the prescribed therapy. The potential benefits of preoperative administration of chemotherapy (e.g., improved patient tolerance before surgical intervention, the ability to assess disease response in vivo, enhanced pharmacologic delivery of chemotherapeutic agents, potential tumor downstaging) have motivated a great deal of interest in neoadjuvant therapy for gastric cancer. The oncological benefit of neoadjuvant chemotherapy or chemoradiation remains controversial. Presented results of the recently completed MAGIC trial comparing preoperative and postoperative epirubicin, cisplatin, and 5-fluorouracil to surgical therapy alone suggest the presence of improved resectability and more durable overall and progression-free survival after perioperative chemotherapy. Of note, radiotherapy was not used in this study. Currently, parameters guiding appropriate patient selection for neoadjuvant therapy are not available. At MSKCC, a protocol for neoadjuvant chemotherapy is reserved for patients with radiographic and endoscopic evidence of at least T3 or N1 disease.

PROGNOSTICATION

The current AJCC staging system stratifies expected outcomes (Fig. 3), but the significant variability of survival that exists within stage groups results in suboptimal prognostication of individual patient outcomes. Relying on a large, single-institution database, a nomogram has been established that permits accurate prediction of individual outcomes for patients undergoing R0 resection of gastric adenocarcinoma (Fig. 4). This nomogram relies on multiple variables beyond those incorporated in the conventional AJCC

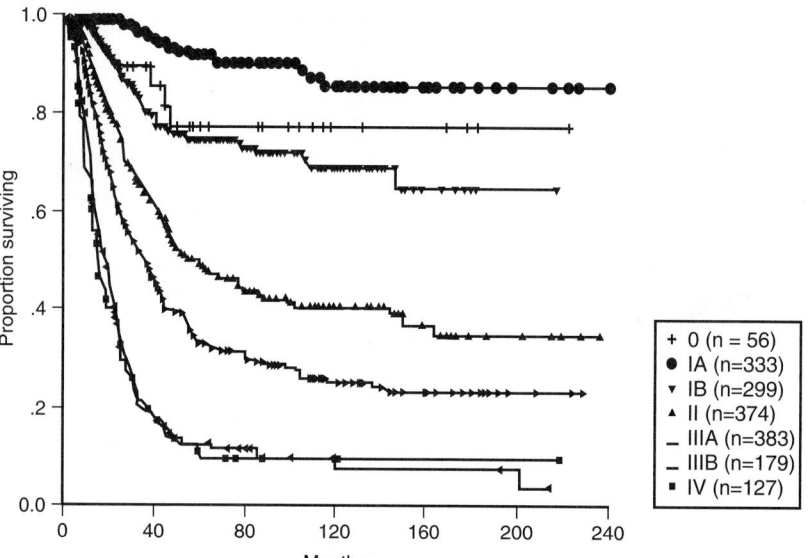

Figure 3 Kaplan-Meier survival curves after R0 resection stratified by American Joint Committee on Cancer/International Union Against Cancer (AJCC/UICC) stage. Note that stage 0 denotes in situ gastric cancer. *Data are from the Memorial Sloan-Kettering Cancer Center database, July 1985 to December 2005.*

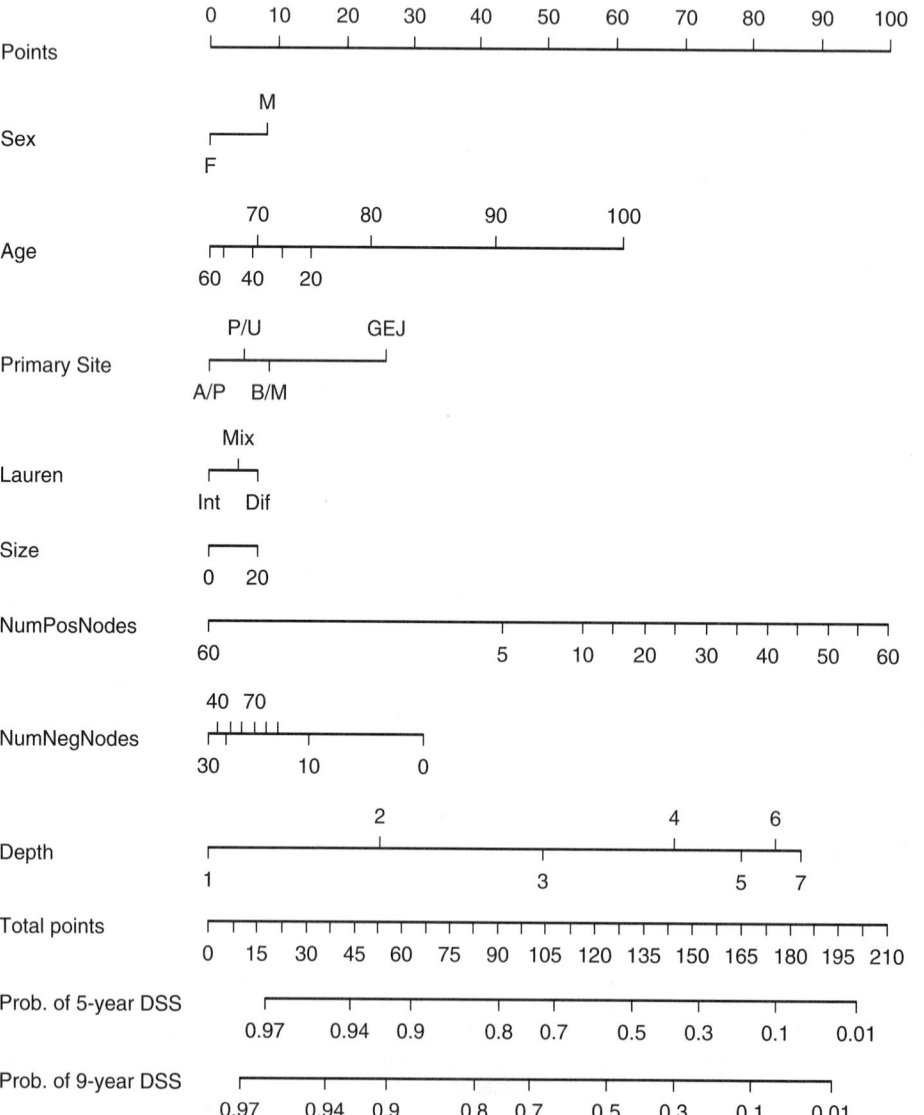

Figure 4 Gastric cancer postoperative nomogram for prediction of disease-specific survival after curative R0 resection. *From Kattan MW, Karpeh MS, Mazumdar M, and others: J Clin Oncol 21:3647, 2003.*

Tumor Size Node Status Metastasis (TNM) classification system (including patient gender, age, anatomic site, Lauren classification, nodal status, and tumor depth). This nomogram has since been validated at multiple institutions and may provide a means of patient prognostication or stratification for purposes of designing future clinical trials. The identification and adoption of additional prognostic variables (e.g., E-cadherin levels) may provide further optimization of nomogram predictive ability in the future.

PALLIATION

Because of the grim prognosis of patients with advanced gastric cancer and the inability to perform curative resection in approximately half of patients presenting with this disease, palliation is an important component of therapy. The role of surgical intervention in the palliation of patients with untreatable gastric adenocarcinoma is an area of considerable controversy. Gastrectomy for patients with advanced disease is associated with significant perioperative morbidity (54%) and mortality (6%). Although this is likely to be due to the deconditioned functional status of many patients with advanced gastric adenocarcinoma, palliative gastrectomy cannot be universally justified as a prophylactic measure. Longitudinal follow-up of patients whose planned gastrectomies were aborted because of the observation of previously undetected metastases at the time of diagnostic laparoscopy found that only 50% of such patients eventually required some form of therapeutic intervention for the onset of symptoms related to advancing tumors (e.g., hemorrhage, obstruction), and only 12% ultimately required some form of operative intervention; the majority of patients with irresectable gastric cancer never develop complications that would necessitate palliative gastrectomy.

SUMMARY

Epidemiologic analysis suggests a demonstrable trend toward more proximal and aggressive variants of gastric adenocarcinoma. For the subset of patients with resectable disease, surgical intervention remains the cornerstone of potentially curative therapy. R0 resection optimizes outcome; extended lymphadenectomy maximizes staging and may provide limited survival benefit. Significant advancements have been achieved in our ability to prognosticate outcomes accurately after curative resection. Further analysis is necessary to delineate accurately the role and optimal delivery of adjunctive forms of therapy.

SUGGESTED READINGS

Cuschieri A, Weeden S, Fielding J, and others: Patient survival after D1 and D2 resections for gastric cancer: long-term results of the MRC randomized surgical trial. Surgical Co-operative Group, *Br J Cancer* 79:1522, 1999.

Bonenkamp JJ, Hermans J, Sasako M, and others: Extended lymph-node dissection for gastric cancer, *N Engl J Med* 340:908, 1999.

Karpeh MS, Leon L, Klimstra D, and others: Lymph node staging in gastric cancer: is location more important than number? An analysis of 1,038 patients, *Ann Surg* 232:362, 2000.

Kattan MW, Karpeh MS, Mazumdar MS, and others: Postoperative nomogram for disease-specific survival after an R0 resection of gastric carcinoma, *J Clin Oncol* 21:3647, 2003.

MacDonald JS, Smalley SR, Benedetti J, and others: Chemoradiotherapy after surgery compared with surgery alone for adenocarcinoma of the stomach or gastroesophageal junction, *N Engl J Med* 345:725, 2001.

GASTROINTESTINAL STROMAL TUMORS

David T. Efron, MD

In 2001, Joensuu and colleagues reported in the *New England Journal of Medicine* remarkable regression of a metastatic gastrointestinal stromal tumor (GIST) in response to oral treatment with the tyrosine kinase inhibitor imatinib. This proof of concept ushered in an exciting new era in the treatment of these tumors, not only providing an effective new chemotherapy for stromal tumors for which there previously was none but also serving as a paradigm for the notion of targeted molecular therapy. This advance notwithstanding, the management of GISTs remains ensconced in the surgical arena and presents a challenge to the gastrointestinal surgeon.

EPIDEMIOLOGY

Although stromal tumors are the most common gastrointestinal mesenchymal neoplasms, they are still uncommon, with an annual incidence in the United States of approximately 3000 to 6000 per year. They demonstrate a fairly equal distribution between men and women, although some studies suggest a slight male prevalence.

GISTs are most commonly identified in patients in the seventh decade of life, although they may arise at any age. Additionally, GISTs have been identified from sites throughout the alimentary tract; however, the stomach is the most frequent site of occurrence (45%–65%), followed by the small bowel (15%–25%), large bowel including the rectum (5%–10%), esophagus (5%–10%), and duodenum (3%–5%). Primary mesenchymal tumors can arise outside of the alimentary tract in locations such as the omentum, pancreas, and other retroperitoneal structures, as well as the gastrointestinal (GI) mesentery. Although most GISTs are sporadic, both an association with neurofibromatosis and familial KIT germline mutation have been reported.

HISTOPATHOLOGY

The histopathologic diagnosis and characterization of GISTs has had a unique evolution over several decades. Demonstrating characteristics of smooth muscle under light microscopy, these neoplasms were initially identified as leiomyomata when demonstrating benign features or leiomyosarcomata when malignancy was identified. As pathologists' diagnostic strategies improved, this characterization came into question. Subsequent examination under electron microscopy suggested some cellular features consistent with neural elements, bringing into question whether smooth muscle was the true cell of origin. In an attempt to characterize these tumors more accurately, batteries of immunohistochemical markers were used to help differentiate the various potential subtypes of these tumors from true smooth muscle or neural neoplasms. These include S100 (neural elements), desmin (intermediate filaments of muscle), actin (alpha smooth muscle actin), vimentin (mesenchymal tissue), and CD 34 (vascular–endothelial markers). Cellular proliferation markers include Ki-67 and proliferating cell nuclear antigen (PCNA). Of the immunohistochemical markers, the most important remains CD 117 or KIT. Although the other immunohistochemical markers are variably expressed in GISTs, KIT expression is identified on up to 95% of GISTs and thus plays a central role in the diagnosis of these tumors.

KIT, a transmembrane growth factor receptor with tyrosine kinase activity, is normally inactive. When bound, KIT activates cascades including MAP kinase, STAT5, RAS, JAK2, and PI3 kinase leading to cellular proliferation, adhesion, and differentiation.

The c-KIT proto-oncogene found on chromosome 4q11-q12 controls KIT expression.

Constituative activation of the KIT receptor has been shown to occur as a result of several mutations in the c-KIT proto-oncogene, thus providing a continual stimulus for proliferation. This "gain of function" behavior likely plays a significant role in the biological behavior of GISTs. Platelet-derived growth factor receptor–alpha is another tyrosine kinase receptor for which alterations in activity may play a role in GIST tumorgenesis and behavior. This may be especially important in patients whose GIST does not express KIT.

Although KIT is expressed by nearly all GISTs, a multifaceted approach to the identification of these tumors is still of value. For the small percentage of patients who demonstrate a KIT-negative specimen, expanded immunohistochemistry, electron microscopy, and even tumor genotyping are beneficial. One cell that fits all of these characteristics is the interstitial cell of Cajal. Identified as the intestinal pacemaker cell, it has both smooth muscle and neural elements and expresses CD 117, thus making it an excellent candidate as the progenitor of these neoplasms.

Unlike other GI malignancies, the behavior of GISTs is at times difficult to predict on pathology. The surest indicator of malignancy is the identification of metastatic disease (before or during operative intervention) or invasion of adjacent organs (seen at the time of operation); however, all stromal tumors may potentially display malignant behavior. A number of characteristics have shown some ability to predict how GISTs will behave, including size, mitotic rate, DNA ploidy, cellular proliferation markers, telomerase activity, and suppressor gene hypermethylation.

The two most important remain size and mitotic rate. Small tumors with diameters less than 2 cm and less than 5 mitoses per high-powered field generally exhibit benign behavior. Conversely, tumors with diameter greater than 10 cm and demonstrating greater than 10 mitoses per high-power field consistently behave as malignant lesions. Those tumors of intermediate size or moderate mitotic activity pose a greater challenge to predict behavior accurately. Although each serves as an independent predictor of prognosis, neither small size nor low mitotic rate confirm benign behavior.

A 2001 Consensus Conference on GISTs established criteria to delineate the graded risk of malignant behavior on the basis of size and mitotic rate (Table 1). Prediction of prognosis and follow-up is determined accordingly. Metastatic spread is almost never via the lymphatic system. Invasion of adjacent organs, metastasis to the liver, and to extra-abdominal sites such as the lungs are the most common sites for metastatic disease.

PRESENTATION

The most common presenting symptoms of GISTs are GI bleeding, abdominal discomfort, and abdominal mass. These all likely result from the fact that GISTs are typically fast-growing neoplasms that often outgrow their blood supply. As a result, they frequently develop a necrotic center. When this fistulizes to the enteric lumen, GI bleeding ensues that at times can be quite profuse. Alternatively, some GISTs may grow to considerable size before causing symptoms related to displacement of neighboring structures, such as bloating, early satiety, or palpable mass. As with other tumors that arise in certain locations, GISTs may also present with site-specific symptoms

Table 1: Proposed Approach for Defining Risk of Aggressive Behavior in Gastrointestinal Stromal Tumors

	Size*	Mitotic Count†
Very low risk	<2 cm	<5 per 50 HPF
Low risk	2–5 cm	<5 per 50 HPF
Intermediate risk	<5 cm	6–10 per 50 HPF
	5–10 cm	<5 per 50 HPF
High risk	>5 cm	>5 per 50 HPF
	>10 cm	Any mitotic rate
	Any size	>10 per 50 HPF

HPF = high power fields.
*Size represents the single largest dimension. Admittedly this may vary somewhat before and after fixation and between observers. There is a general but poorly defined sense that perhaps the size threshold for aggressive behavior should be 1–2 cm less in the small bowel than elsewhere.
†Ideally mitotic count should be standardized according to surface area examined (based on size of high power fields), but there are no agreed definitions in this regard. Despite inevitable subjectivity in recognition of mitoses and variability in the area of high power fields, such mitotic counts still prove useful.

including dysphagia (esophageal or gastroesophageal junction), obstruction (small bowel), obstructive jaundice (duodenal), or palpable rectal mass (rectal).

GISTs are commonly identified incidentally in the workup of other lesions or at laparotomy for other pathology. These are frequently of smaller size, and prognosis depends largely on the patient's primary pathology.

DIAGNOSIS

GISTs are most frequently diagnosed in the workup of symptoms not specific to these masses. As a result, and depending on their location, they may be identified as masses on endoscopic evaluation (esophagogastroduodenoscopy and colonoscopy), contrast radiography (upper GI/small-bowel follow through or enema) or two-dimensional imaging (computed tomography [CT] scan or magnetic resonance imaging [MRI]). Endoscopic visualization often demonstrates evidence of an extrinsic mass impinging on the gastric lumen without a discrete mucosal lesion. Endoscopic biopsy in this case usually will show normal mucosa. Ulceration of the mass into the gastric lumen may also be seen. Similarly contrast radiography will likely suggest a mass causing smooth extrinsic compression of the bowel lumen. The most useful radiologic study for the diagnosis of GISTs is the CT scan. Not only does this demonstrate size and anatomic location of the mass, it may also demonstrate features suggestive of stromal tumors (well vascularized, necrotic center, heterogeneous appearance) and may provide evidence of metastatic disease at workup. Unfortunately neither CT nor MRI can accurately predict whether the tumor has grown into adjacent structures.

Fluorodeoxyglucose positron emission tomography ([18]FDG-PET) has been shown to be sensitive in identifying metabolic activity within these tumors; however, it is not specific and is likely most useful at present in identifying metastatic disease or metabolic activity in tumors undergoing molecular therapy.

The radiographic appearance of these lesions strongly indicates resection, and histopathologic diagnosis is made subsequently. Transcutaneous biopsy carries with it the risk of rupture of the pseudocapsule and dissemination of disease; it is contraindicated in the workup of nonmetastatic GISTs. Transcutaneous biopsy, however, is helpful in patients with known metastatic disease because it confirms a tissue diagnosis and guides potential tyrosine kinase therapy.

TREATMENT—PRIMARY TUMORS

Molecular therapy options notwithstanding, surgery remains the treatment of choice for primary nonmetastatic stromal tumors and represents the only chance for cure. On gross inspection, GISTs are characterized as well-circumscribed masses. They are usually irregular in shape, encased by a pseudocapsule that defines the margin of the tumor (Fig. 1). The tumor is often saprophytic in nature

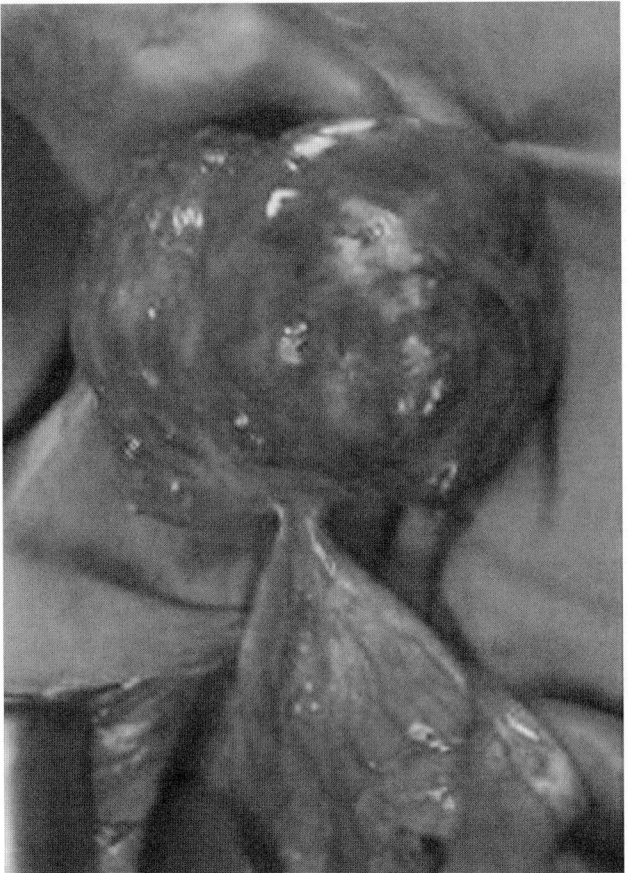

Figure 1 Typical gastric stromal tumor with a discrete stalk and clearly evident pseudocapsule. This tumor is well treated with wedge resection of the gastric wall. *From Efron DT, Lillemoe KD: Adv Surg 39:193, 2005.*

with regard to blood supply (likely secondary to rapidity of growth), and these vessels must be carefully ligated as the pseudocapsule is cleared from the surrounding structures. These tumors must be manipulated carefully because they are frequently delicate and are at significant risk of rupture, resulting in immediate intraperitoneal tumor seeding.

GISTs are often attached to the wall of the GI tract by a small stalk, thus wedge resection or limited segmental resection suffices in many cases (Fig. 1). Margins along the bowel wall must be clear of disease (2–3 cm are usually adequate), but wide margins of resection have shown no benefit. Because these tumors rarely demonstrate lymphatic spread, routine lymphatic dissection is not warranted. Not uncommonly GISTs will invade adjacent structures, necessitating en bloc resection (Fig. 2). Because it is impossible to predict radiographically which tumors will have done this, the surgeon must be prepared to perform an extensive resection. Determination of resection margin may be difficult in tumors that invade surrounding structures or the retroperitoneum.

With the exception of the aforementioned common principles, the operation of choice obviously depends on the origin of the tumor. Gastric GISTs may be treated with simple wedge resection or may require partial or total gastrectomy. Small- and large-bowel GISTs are most frequently well managed by segmental resection. Periampullary lesions may require pancreaticoduodenectomy. Laparoscopic resection has been accomplished in a number of reported cases and series, although appropriate selection is vital given the friable nature of the pseudocapsule and the potential for rupture with manipulation.

RECURRENCE, FOLLOW-UP, AND SURVIVAL

The recurrence rate of GISTs is 20% to 50% despite successful complete surgical resection. Recurrence is usually early within the first 2 years postoperatively, and therefore early close follow-up and postoperative surveillance are warranted. The National Comprehensive Cancer Network guidelines recommend abdominal and pelvic CT scanning every 3 to 6 months for the first 5 years postresection. Late recurrence, although reported, is uncommon. Local, intra-abdominal recurrence is the most likely site, followed by metastatic spread to the liver. Distant spread of disease beyond the abdominal cavity to the bone or lungs is less common and represents late disease.

In the era before imatinib, overall 5-year survival ranged from 30% to 65%. Primary predictors remain size and mitotic rate, although factors such as complete resection, violation of the pseudocapsule (during resection), and site of origin have also been shown to be contributory. Given the impact that tyrosine kinase

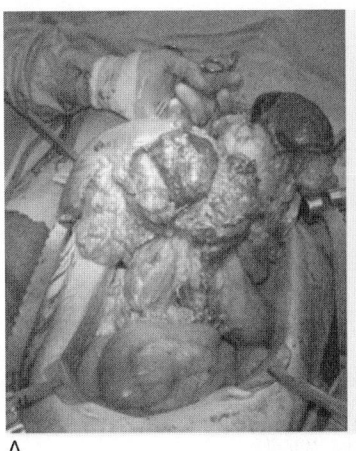
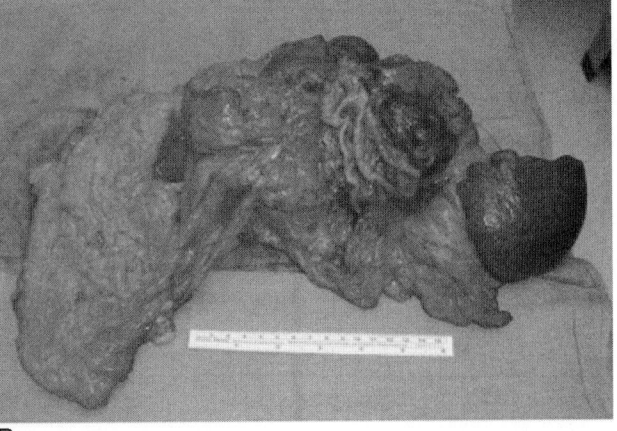

A   B

Figure 2 **(A)** Large gastric stromal tumor invading multiple structures in the left upper quadrant necessitating en bloc resection (excised specimen seen in **B**). *From Efron DT, Lillemoe KD: Adv Surg 39:193, 2005.*

inhibition therapy has had on the treatment of GISTs, the overall prediction of survival is likely to be revised.

[18]FDG-PET appears to be of increasing value in monitoring the progress of patients with metastatic or recurrent GISTs, especially in patients undergoing treatment with tyrosine kinase inhibitors. Changes in metabolic activity precede those seen on conventional CT imaging and thus may allow for earlier decision making with regard to therapeutic strategies. More recent experience with combined [18]FDG-PET and CT imaging also holds further promise because metabolic and precise anatomic imaging are combined.

TREATMENT—METASTATIC AND RECURRENT DISEASE

Figure 3 outlines the basic treatment scheme for GISTs. GISTs historically have been refractory to conventional chemotherapy and radiotherapy. These modalities have largely been replaced by tyrosine kinase inhibitor strategies. For patients with evidence of metastatic disease on initial presentation, imatinib is initiated as a first-line therapy. Imatinib is taken orally and is well tolerated, with primary side effects reported to be fatigue, diarrhea, nausea, rash, abdominal pain, skeletal muscle cramps, and periorbital edema. Optimal dosing of imatinib is not yet well established. Although it is increasingly clear that doses above 400 mg per day carry little

extra benefit, higher doses (800 mg/day) may be used with success for patients with GISTs refractory to lower dosing.

At present in this setting, lifetime therapy is indicated. A small percentage of patients will be resistant to imatinib and demonstrate progression of disease on therapy; as many as 50% of patients may develop resistance to imatinib after several years of therapy, most likely the result of additional KIT mutation. For these patients, alternative tyrosine kinase inhibitors such as SU11248 and AMG706 have shown promise and are under investigation.

Imatinib therapy will often hold in check the progression of disease and will occasionally shrink the tumor, although complete response is rare. Maximal response is usually identified within the first 6 months of initiation of imatinib therapy. For patients with metastatic disease at presentation, surgical resection of primary and metastatic disease is subsequently indicated if excision of gross disease is possible with acceptable morbidity because this likely reduces the chance of developing resistance to tyrosine kinase therapy. There is no proven benefit to cytoreductive surgery in the absence of complete resection.

In addition to resection of recurrent local disease, aggressive management of hepatic disease appears to impart a survival benefit for patients with discrete disease. As with other metastatic liver lesions, options include anatomic and nonanatomic liver resection, ultrasound-guided radiofrequency ablation, and hepatic artery embolization. It is unclear exactly how tyrosine kinase therapy will alter this approach.

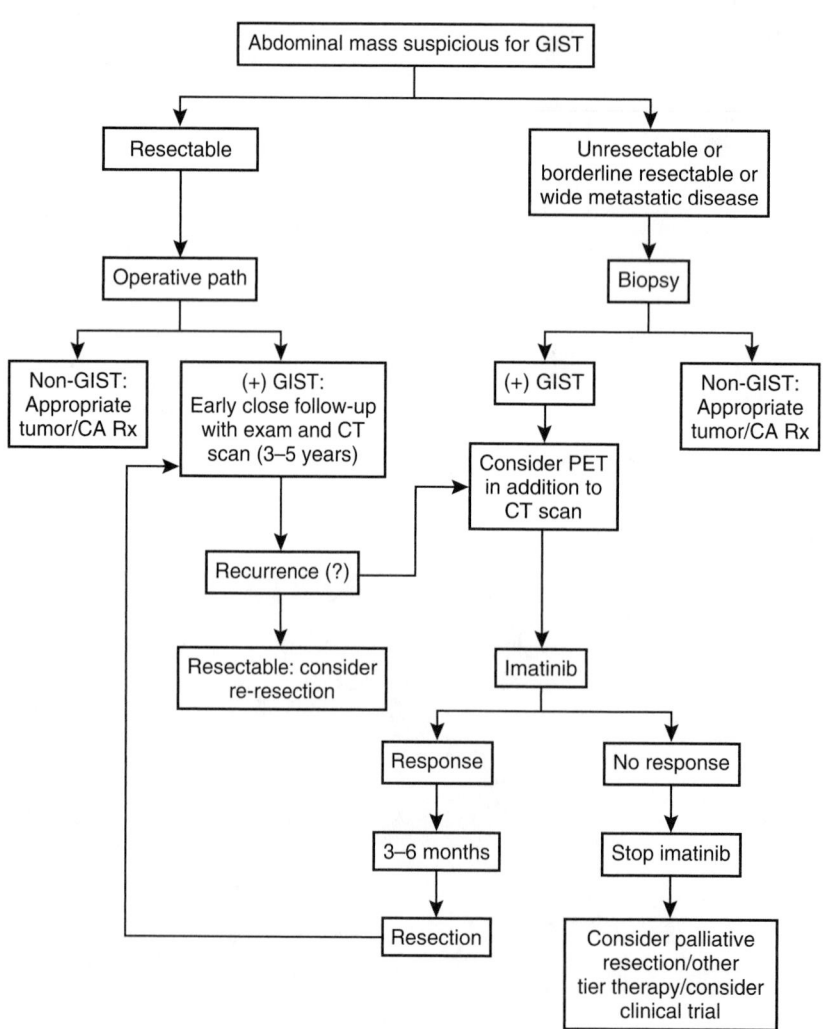

Figure 3 Simple proposed decision tree for the management of gastrointestinal stromal tumor *(GIST). CT,* computed tomography; *PET,* positron emission tomography. *From Efron DT, Lillemoe KD: Adv Surg 39:193, 2005.*

Given the high recurrence rate despite complete surgical resection, several ongoing studies are assessing the routine use of imatinib following complete resection of intermediate-risk and high-risk GISTs. For patients with technically unresectable primary disease, a certain small percentage of patients will shrink tumor mass and convert to potential candidates for surgical extirpation. Appropriate neo-adjuvant application of imatinib therapy is also under study.

SUGGESTED READINGS

Joensuu H, Roberts PJ, Sarlomo-Rikala M, and others: Effect of the tyrosine kinase inhibitor STI571 in a patient with a metastatic gastrointestinal stromal tumor, *N Engl J Med* 344:1052, 2001.

Fletcher CD, Berman JJ, Corless C and others: Diagnosis of gastrointestinal stromal tumors: a consensus approach. *Int J Surg Pathol* 10:81, 2002.

Efron DT, Lillemoe KD: The current management of gastrointestinal stromal tumors, *Adv Surg* 39:193, 2005.

Schnadig ID, Blanke CD: Gastrointestinal stromal tumors: imatinib and beyond, *Curr Treat Options Oncol* 7:427, 2006.

Gold JS, Dematteo RP: Combined surgical and molecular therapy: the gastrointestinal stromal tumor model, *Ann Surg* 244:176, 2006.

National Comprehensive Cancer Network: Sarcoma guidelines, http://www.nccn.org/. Accessed 2006.

SMALL BOWEL

SMALL BOWEL OBSTRUCTION

Kurtis A. Campbell, MD

Despite ever-increasing medical and surgical advances, small bowel obstruction remains a common problem. Postoperative adhesions are the cause of approximately three fourths of all these obstructive events, a change historically from the early 20th century, when hernias were the primary etiology. It is interesting to note that the advent of laparoscopic surgery has not had a significant impact on this incidence. Nearly one third of these obstructions attributable to adhesions will likely occur in the first year after laparotomy, with two thirds of those arising in the early postoperative period. Now the second most common cause, hernias are followed by obstruction caused by tumor, with the most common being metastatic colorectal cancer. Although interesting from a pathogenetic viewpoint, intussusception (Fig. 1), bezoar, gallstone ileus, Crohn's disease, and volvulus are all uncommon causes of small bowel obstruction.

Approximately 50% of patients with small bowel obstruction attributable to adhesion require surgery, and this percentage is higher when other causes of obstruction are also included. Landercasper and colleagues (1993) reported that the risk of recurrent obstruction in the subsequent 10 years was 42% for patients with small bowel obstruction, 29% for those treated with surgery, and 53% for those treated nonoperatively. Whether a patient can be managed nonoperatively is a judgment that is based on a number of factors, including probable etiology, previous surgery, incomplete versus complete obstruction, first occurrence versus recurrent, patient condition, and imaging study results. Inappropriate delay can be devastating, and most series report a significantly increased mortality in the setting of strangulation and resultant ischemia, some higher than 33%.

INITIAL EVALUATION

The aims of the initial evaluation of these patients should be to assess the degree of metabolic derangement and volume depletion and to determine the possible need for and timing of surgery. The accurate diagnosis and management of small bowel obstruction begins with a good history and physical examination. Typical symptoms include nausea, vomiting, distention, crampy abdominal pain that is classically periumbilical, and decreased or absent flatus and bowel movement. All of these will vary depending on the location of obstruction (proximal vs. distal), the time between onset and presentation, and the degree of obstruction (incomplete vs. complete). Physical examination should focus on both systemic signs and those specific to the abdomen. Laboratory studies help to assess physiologic status and may provide supporting evidence of the presence or absence of ischemia.

Diagnostic imaging should begin with plain films of the abdomen (supine and erect) and an upright chest radiograph. The latter is important to evaluate for pneumoperitoneum and for aspiration in the patient who has been vomiting. In those patients requiring further diagnostic imaging, computed tomography (CT) scan has supplanted the small bowel series as the study of choice. Sensitivity and specificity have been shown to approach 100% in prospective trials. Not only can the scan evaluate for degree of obstruction, it can potentially identify the transition point, a mass lesion as the cause of obstruction or intussusception (Fig. 2), or a hernia with obstruction (Fig. 3). Moreover, CT scan is sensitive for strangulation and the pneumoperitoneum indicative of perforation. It is a particularly important study in the patient with a history of malignancy to differentiate the potential etiologies of recurrent disease or adhesion and in the patient who has early postoperative obstruction to exclude ischemia, abscess, or other morbidity as an underlying cause (Fig. 4). Some have argued that repeat CT scan is a preferred serial imaging study over plain films in the patient who is undergoing nonoperative management because the scan can readily detect early signs of bowel ischemia, including wall thickening, free peritoneal fluid, or pneumatosis intestinalis.

Small bowel series should be reserved for those patients undergoing nonoperative management who remain without signs of strangulation but in whom the obstruction fails to resolve. Enteroclysis, whereby the proximal small bowel is intubated under fluoroscopic guidance and then instilled with air (or a plug of cellulose) and contrast, should be used even more selectively. These studies are sensitive and specific, with contrast in the cecum by 24 hours highly predictive of eventual spontaneous resolution (see Abbas and colleagues, 2005). There are no good data, however, to support the therapeutic use of water-soluble contrast to alleviate partial small bowel obstruction. This contrast medium represents a substantial intraluminal osmotic load and can significantly worsen metabolic derangement in the acute patient.

The use of ultrasound should not be overlooked in the patient with small bowel obstruction. Suri and colleagues (1999), as well as other authors, have shown ultrasound to be more sensitive and specific than plain radiographs in the diagnosis of small bowel obstruction. It may be particularly useful in the pregnant patient or as a bedside test in the critically ill.

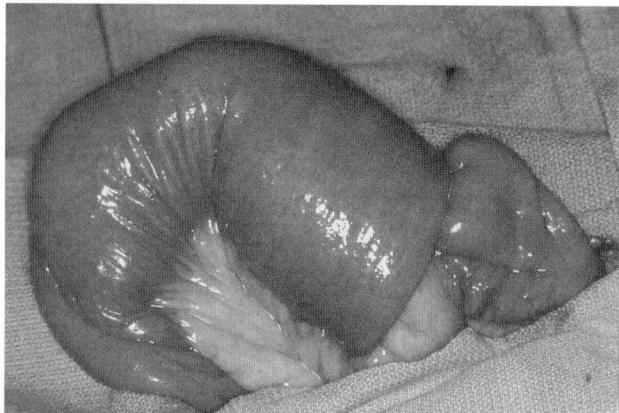

Figure 1   Small bowel intussusception.

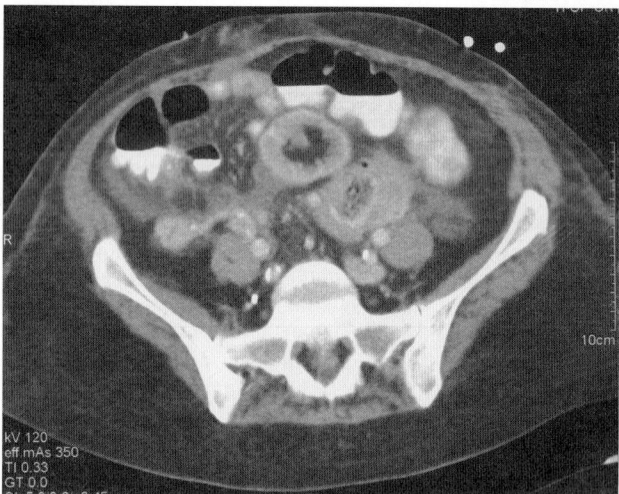

Figure 2   Computed tomography scan of small bowel intussusception with typical target sign.

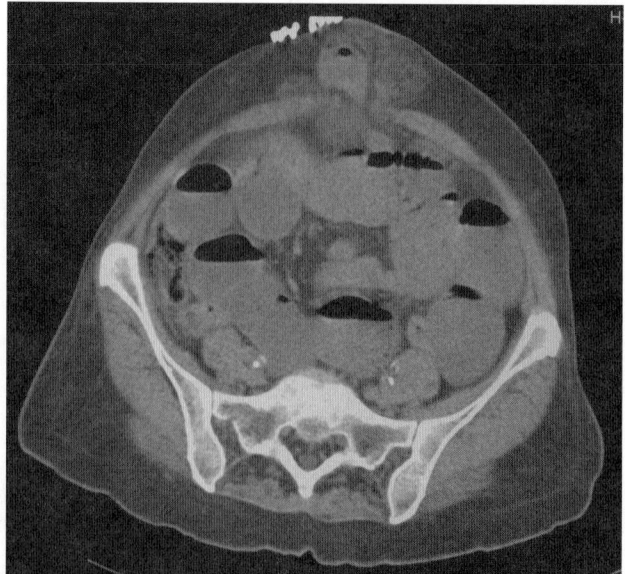

Figure 3   Computed tomography scan of complete small bowel obstruction due to incisional hernia.

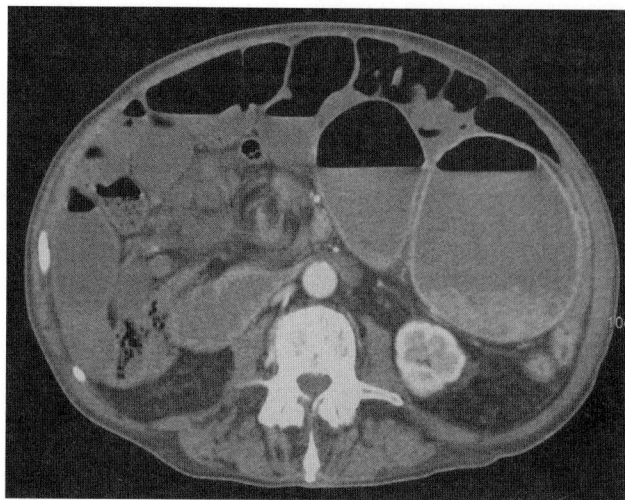

Figure 4   Computed tomography scan of small bowel volvulus with notable mesenteric torsion.

Small bowel obstruction should be differentiated from nonobstructive motility disorders such as paralytic ileus or pseudo-obstruction. Paralytic ileus likely occurs to some extent after nearly all open abdominal procedures. Either disorder can be caused by other major surgery, trauma, intestinal ischemia, peritonitis, or electrolyte derangement. These patients can develop the same symptoms as obstruction but should be distinguishable by history and appropriate radiographic imaging.

NONOPERATIVE MANAGEMENT

Appropriate nonoperative (or preoperative) management of the patient with small bowel obstruction begins with aggressive resuscitation of fluid and electrolyte disorders. A prolonged course before presentation with significant nausea and vomiting will result in a hypochloremic, hypokalemic metabolic alkalosis with paradoxical aciduria. Appropriate intravenous access, close monitoring of urinary output with a Foley catheter, and hemodynamic and electrolyte reassessment are all essential.

The instrument of gastrointestinal decompression has long been a subject of study and debate but has become less so in recent years. A standard-length nasogastric tube should be used to decompress the stomach. This provides patient comfort, prevents further gas and fluid accumulation proximally, and allows for the serial assessment of antegrade fluid movement (character and volume). These tubes only lessen the risk of aspiration if they are attended to because they render both the lower and upper esophageal sphincters incompetent. The use of long intestinal tubes (Miller-Abbot, Baker, Cantor) are theoretically advantageous but have been shown in several prospective trials not to increase the incidence of spontaneous small bowel obstruction and in fact may delay operative intervention.

The use of narcotic pain medicine remains controversial in the patient who is undergoing serial examination and attempted nonoperative management. Certainly special consideration should be given to the patient who may already be receiving narcotics: a postoperative patient, the chronic pain patient, trauma patients, and a patient with known intra-abdominal malignancy. One could argue that if the patient requires opiate medication for adequate analgesia from symptoms of small bowel obstruction, perhaps he or she belongs in the operating room. In addition, Sarr and colleagues (1983), as well as other authors, have shown that constant abdominal pain could not be used to predict accurately the presence of strangulation and that experienced clinicians are wrong more than 50% of the time in predicting the presence of gangrenous bowel.

Certain patient groups are more likely to be successfully managed nonoperatively. The most obvious would be the patient with a low-grade incomplete small bowel obstruction. These patients with less pain, less distention, and improving imaging studies can be slowly challenged with a diet as they continue to progress. This group may well benefit from a small bowel series or enteroclysis if there is not continued resolution after a period of several days or if they fail with diet challenge.

Another group that benefits from a course of nonoperative management is patients with early postoperative obstruction following an abdominal operation. Pickleman and Lee (1989) have shown that approximately 90% of these patients resolve without surgery. This group of patients and those with low-grade incomplete obstruction may be best managed with total parenteral nutrition while they undergo gut rest, nasogastric decompression, and intravenous hydration to avoid the sequelae of prolonged negative nitrogen balance.

Patients with recurrent small bowel obstruction also warrant an attempt at nonoperative management, particularly in the setting of multiple previous operations or in those who have a history of successful treatment without surgery. This group also benefits from the adjunctive treatment of parenteral nutrition, especially if treatment requires an extended nonoperative course. This is acceptable in the patient who remains clinically stable and shows no evidence of a worsened intra-abdominal process.

Typically, the obstructed patient with Crohn's disease presents with an incomplete obstruction. In this setting, particularly if the presentation represents the index symptomatic event for a specific site of obstruction or stricture, these patients should be managed conservatively. In addition to the standard nonoperative measures and total parenteral nutrition, this course may be benefited by steroids or other immunosuppressive therapy. Even during surgery, the use of these medications has been reported not to increase perioperative complications in this patient population.

Small bowel obstruction related to trauma is most likely to occur in children. Incomplete or complete obstruction by intramural hematoma is most likely to involve the duodenum. Nonoperative management is appropriate in the patient who does not present with or develop peritonitis. Fibrosis may have occurred if symptoms persists beyond 2 weeks, so in this subset, surgery should be considered. Drainage of only the hematoma is usually sufficient; however, these patients can also develop delayed fibrosis and recurrent obstruction.

OPERATIVE MANAGEMENT

More than half of all patients admitted to the hospital with small bowel obstruction will require surgery. This is particularly true in certain groups, especially those with complete small bowel obstruction or patients with high-grade incomplete small bowel obstruction, the former subset being less than 20% likely to be managed nonoperatively. Certainly those patients who present with significant abdominal pain and signs of ongoing inflammation, with fever, increased heart rate, and leukocytosis should be prepared for the operating room without delay. Surgery should also be strongly considered for patients who are clinically stable but who do not respond promptly within 12 to 24 hours to appropriate nonoperative management.

Those patients who present with small bowel obstruction and no previous history of abdominal surgery almost certainly warrant operative management. In these patients, adhesions are much less likely, but incarcerated hernia, tumor, or the index presentation of previously undiagnosed Crohn's disease should be considered. Goals of the operation should include correction of the obstruction and appropriate management of the underlying etiology.

Those patients with a history of intra-abdominal malignancy require special consideration. Especially in the setting of known recurrent disease, these patients are not infrequently relegated to nonoperative therapy. In fact, two thirds of these patients will have a surgically correctable small bowel obstruction, usually either from an adhesion or a resectable portion of their malignant disease. The remaining third will likely have carcinomatosis, and unless this clinical diagnosis can be made with preoperative imaging, these patients likely warrant operative management. Butler and colleagues (1991) have shown that these obstructions are more likely due to recurrent disease when they occur earlier after the initial surgery for malignancy, and adhesions become the more likely cause at a later time period (21 vs. 61 months). This is no doubt due to the prolonged survival of the latter group.

Adult intussusception (see Figs. 1 and 2) is much less common than in the pediatric population. In the child, these are nearly always ileocolic, and surgery is reserved for those patients who cannot be successfully managed with radiographic reduction or in those who manifest perforation. In the adult, there is usually a distinct pathologic lead point that is malignant in 50% of patients. Thus the adult with intussusception typically requires operative management.

Those patients with recurrent small bowel obstruction who fail a prolonged course of nonoperative management or who deteriorate will require surgery. These patients frequently have a history of multiple abdominal operations and can represent challenging problems. The incision orientation can be debated, but most surgeons would advocate a long midline incision with careful entry into the peritoneal cavity, preferably in a previously unopened portion. These patients frequently do not have a well-defined focus of obstruction and require careful adhesiolysis from the ligament of Treitz to the ileocecal valve. In this group, Weigelt and colleagues (1980), as well as other authors, have advocated the use of a long intestinal tube placed through a Stamm gastrostomy and manually progressed to the terminal ileum. This tube plication effectively forces the small bowel to develop a gentle serpentine course throughout its length. Although the patient can be advanced to a liquid diet around the tube, it is recommended that it remain in place for approximately 3 weeks.

Patients with intraluminal obstruction almost always require surgery. The two most common obstructions of this rare etiology are bezoars and gallstone ileus, the latter representing 1% to 2% of all small bowel obstructions. Gallstone ileus patients will typically present with radiographically depicted gallstones that are unusually located, pneumobilia from the biliary enteric fistula, and small bowel obstruction. Operative management includes enterotomy and stone removal or small bowel resection for severely impacted stones, palpation of the remainder of the gastrointestinal tract for other stones, cholecystectomy, and surgical management of the enteric side of the fistula. The fistula can also occur from the distal common bile duct to the duodenum, and thus the biliary side may also need to be managed with a Roux-en-Y choledochojejunostomy.

Occasionally, a patient with early postoperative small bowel obstruction will not respond to nonoperative management. In these patients, the timing of the necessary surgery is a critical decision. If, on the basis of clinical course, the patient does not require reoperation within the first 10 days, then it is likely best to wait until he or she has reached 4 weeks postoperative unless the clinical picture will not allow it. During the 10- to 30-day postoperative period, adhesions, like other inflammatory tissue during this period of healing, are vascular, cohesive, and thickened.

SPECIAL TECHNICAL CONSIDERATIONS

When the operation has progressed to achieve correction of the obstruction, careful and complete assessment of bowel viability must take place. Many times the bowel will be clearly pink, and this determination is easily made with subjective criteria. On occasion, however, this may prove more difficult, and in fact some subjective signs, such as motility, can be misleading. In these instances, patience and warmth should be used liberally. The peritoneal cavity should be copiously irrigated with warm saline; presumably the patient has been kept warm with extremity forced air warming blankets. The wound should then be covered to prevent further heat and fluid loss, and up to 10 minutes should be allowed to pass. If, after this time, bowel viability remains questionable, two standard adjuncts, Doppler and fluorescein, should be used. Bulkley and colleagues (1981) have shown intravenous fluorescein (1000 mg) and Woods lamp illumination to be more accurate than standard Doppler or subjective assessment of intestinal ischemia. In some centers laser Doppler flowmetry is available. If, after these maneuvers, nonviability remains unclear and if an overwhelming length of small bowel might be lost, then many would advocate returning to the operating room 24 hours later for a final assessment. Some have suggested performing that repeat operation laparoscopically with port placement at the time of the initial closure. Certainly if the length of bowel in question is limited, much of this effort is likely better spent in resecting that segment expeditiously.

Many surgeons suggest that luminal decompression is an important step to enhance blood flow to the distended, edematous, and previously obstructed bowel wall and to facilitate closure of the abdomen. Classically performed by milking content retrogradely toward the nasogastric tube, this maneuver can cause small bowel wall trauma or result in aspiration if not performed with the cooperation of the anesthesia team and thus must be done with considerable caution. Alternatively, accomplishing this through the enterotomy of an anastomosis must be achieved without spillage of intestinal content into the peritoneal cavity.

LAPAROSCOPY

Indications for laparoscopy in the management of patients with small bowel obstruction continue to increase. There are no clear contraindications, but it is reasonable to suggest that laparoscopic surgery is relatively contraindicated in the patient with massive small bowel distention, those with multiple previous laparotomies, the patient with early postoperative obstruction, or in the setting of obvious perforation and peritonitis.

The initial trocar placement should be accomplished using an open technique, with subsequent placements performed under direct vision. The use of atraumatic grasping instruments, liberal use of table positioning with the aid of the anesthesia team, and examination of the bowel in retrograde fashion beginning at the ileocecal valve are all steps that enhance success, which has been reported to be as high as 60% to 80%. Retrospective data suggest that the laparoscopic approach to small bowel obstruction may result in shorter hospital stays and earlier return of bowel function.

ADHESION PREVENTION

Attempts to prevent small bowel obstruction have concentrated mainly on the prevention or control of adhesion formation. Early techniques consisted of suturing or plicating the bowel during surgery for obstruction into conformations or anatomic patterns to prevent future obstruction. The tube or stitchless plication has been advocated by some but is not widely used.

A number of chemical agents have been tried to prevent postoperative adhesions. These have included nonsteroidal anti-inflammatory drug solutions, steroid solutions, lubricants, chemotherapeutic agents, fibrinolytic compounds, and dextran. Most have resulted in an increased incidence of postoperative intra-abdominal infection complications.

Bioresorbable barrier membrane technology currently shows the greatest promise in adhesion prevention. Two are currently available: Intercede (oxygenated regenerated cellulose; Ethicon, Somerville, NJ) and Seprafilm (sodium hyaluronate–based carboxymethylcellulose; Genzyme, Cambridge, MA). Although somewhat cumbersome and difficult to handle, these membranes have been shown experimentally and clinically to prevent adhesions to intra-abdominal surfaces on which they are placed. They are particularly useful in the setting of an anticipated or probable reoperation, making reentry into the peritoneal cavity technically easier. Neither material, however, has been shown to decrease the incidence of postoperative small bowel obstruction secondary to adhesions. Indeed, some experimental data suggest that the use of these membranes results in an increased incidence of intra-abdominal infection complications. Nonetheless, they represent an important step in the ongoing effort to reduce the incidence of small bowel obstruction.

SUGGESTED READINGS

Abbas S, Bissett I, Parry B: Oral water soluble contrast for the management of adhesive small bowel obstruction, *Cochrane Database Syst Rev* CD004651, 2005.

Bulkley GB, Zuidema GD, Hamilton SR, and others: Intraoperative determination of small intestinal viability following ischemic injury: a prospective, controlled trial of two adjuvant methods (Doppler and fluorescein) compared with standard clinical judgment, *Ann Surg* 193:628, 1981.

Butler JA, Cameron BL, Morrow M, and others: Small bowel obstruction in patients with a prior history of cancer, *Am J Surg* 162:624, 1991.

Landercasper J, Cogbill TH, Merry WH, and others: Long-term outcome after hospitalization for small-bowel obstruction, *Arch Surg* 128:765, 1993.

Pickleman J, Lee RM: The management of patients with suspected early postoperative small bowel obstruction, *Ann Surg* 210:216, 1989.

Sarr MG, Bulkley GB, Zuidema GD: Preoperative recognition of intestinal strangulation obstruction: prospective evaluation of diagnostic capability, *Am J Surg* 145:176, 1983.

Strickland P, Lourie DJ, Suddleson EA, and others: Is laparoscopy safe and effective for treatment of acute small bowel obstruction? *Surg Endosc* 13:695, 1999.

Suri S, Gupta S, Sudhakar PJ, and others: Comparative evaluation of plain films, ultrasound and CT in the diagnosis of intestinal obstruction, *Acta Radiol* 40:422, 1999.

Weigelt JA, Snyder WH, Norman JL: Complications and results of 160 Baker tube plications, *Am J Surg* 140:810, 1980.

POSTOPERATIVE ILEUS

Andreas M. Kaiser, MD, and Robert W. Beart, Jr., MD

Postoperative ileus is an expected motility disorder of the intestinal tract that develops in the course of an operation and general anesthesia. Abdominal operations are undoubtedly the most frequent triggers, but other types of operations and anesthesia or sedation may result in various degrees of intestinal motor dysfunction. Even general anesthesia or sedation alone is generally anticipated to result in some degree of intestinal paralysis. For this reason, elective procedures require several hours of fasting before anesthesia and a postoperative delay of oral intake for a few hours.

Most commonly, the suppression of coordinated propulsions is temporary and self-limited. Definitions of the duration of this "normal" depression vary in the literature but most often do not exceed 72 to 96 hours. From a practical standpoint, it is generally recommended to distinguish two forms of postoperative gastrointestinal dysfunction: (1) recovery of upper gastrointestinal (GI) function (small bowel, stomach), which should occur within 24 to 48 hours, and (2) recovery of lower GI function (colon), which may take up to 2 to 4 days. Prolonged postoperative ileus, however, is a dysmotility persisting beyond this expected time frame and represents a significant problem in the management of surgical patients. Because of the inability to resume or advance an oral diet as planned, postoperative ileus is a common reason for delayed discharge and extended length of hospital stay, resulting in tremendous cumulative health costs.

CLINICAL PRESENTATION

The symptoms of postoperative ileus depend on the anatomic level of the dysmotility and may be subtle in the beginning. Delayed recovery of the upper GI function includes a lack of appetite, inability to tolerate or advance oral intake, epigastric fullness or pressure, heartburn, and burping. As the pathologic condition progresses, nausea and vomiting occur. In case a nasogastric tube is already in place and verified to be in correct position, persistent high output is a reliable indicator of nonresolved postoperative ileus. Delayed recovery of lower GI function often presents as increasing abdominal distention, diffuse rather than colicky discomfort, and lack of passage of flatus or stool. Nausea and vomiting are relatively late symptoms of lower GI dysfunction. It is not an uncommon clinical scenario that the upper GI function initially recovers in a timely manner, allowing temporarily for some oral intake, but the patient subsequently experiences a setback secondary to the delayed recovery of lower GI function.

Systemic effects of prolonged postoperative ileus include loss and third spacing of fluids, electrolyte and acid–base abnormalities, tachycardia, and, later, hypotension. Malnutrition may result from ileus that persists beyond 5 days. It is important to rule out differential diagnoses and potential surgery-related complications such as anastomotic leaks, mechanical bowel obstruction (e.g., kinking, volvulus, internal hernia, adhesions), persistent ischemia, interloop abscess, aspiration, and so on. Fever and rising white blood cell counts should therefore be subject to concern and trigger appropriate evaluations.

PATHOGENESIS

The exact pathogenesis for postoperative ileus remains unclear and subject to both research and ongoing speculations, but the clinical

Table 1: Triggers of Postoperative Ileus

Category	Examples
Surgery, trauma	Laparotomy
Retroperitoneal/ mediastinal pathology	Hematoma, infection
Metabolic disorders	Hyponatremia, hypokalemia, hypomagnesemia, uremia, diabetic coma
Endocrine disorders	Adrenal insufficiency, diabetes, hypothyroidism
Drugs	Anesthesia, exogenous/endogenous opiates, psychotropics, anticholinergics
Spine	Vertebral and spinal cord injury
Infection	Peritonitis, sepsis, systemic inflammatory response syndrome
Cardiopulmonary failure	Right ventricular failure, low cardiac output, hypoxia
Vascular	Underperfusion, portal hypertension, portal vein thrombosis

picture appears to be the common final pathway of several unrelated pathologic conditions. Among these are both intrinsic and extrinsic factors (see Table 1), which may either coexist or be present at different times. The normal motility and propulsion of the intestines depends on intact morphology and function of the longitudinal and circular muscle fibers, as well as a proper autonomic nerve function (enteric nervous system). Complex interactions between autonomic–enteric and central nervous system functions, as well as local messenger substances in response to fasting or feeding, are responsible for the coordinated cyclic smooth muscle activity and the pace of the migrating motor complex. Any condition that interferes with this relatively labile equilibrium may activate central nervous system reflex pathways and the sympathetic system, resulting in a disorganized irregular electrical activity, and triggers a paralysis of a particular bowel segment. Similarly, a focal morphological alteration of the bowel secondary to injury, disease, or inflammation may directly interrupt or even reverse the antegrade propagation of coordinated contractions or the inflammatory cascade may result in a release of active mediators (e.g., nitric oxide) and proinflammatory cytokines that inhibit the intestinal motility.

PREVENTION

The underlying disease process necessitating an operation in a patient is an independent parameter, which as such cannot be affected. Particularly in case of a disease complication with a nonelective presentation, aggressive and timely management is of utmost importance to minimize the overall duration of the intestinal and peritoneal exposure to these negative impacts. For example, a rapid intervention for a perforated viscus will not only limit the risk of uncontrolled sepsis but also intercept the diffuse inflammatory damage of the bowels. Elective procedures may allow for optimization of the patient's underlying general condition and nutritional status (serum albumin) before the surgery is performed.

In view of the multifactorial pathogenesis and the fact that the need for surgery and anesthesia cannot be obviated, a multimodal approach is necessary to avoid prolonged postoperative ileus. Several intraoperative and postoperative strategies have to be considered to avoid and minimize risk factors and promote a timely return of gastrointestinal function.

Surgeon- and Surgery-Related Factors

Intraoperative management and tissue handling are among the most important parameters that the surgeon can directly influence. Relevant factors include the duration of the surgery and exposure of the bowels to room air and lower-than-body temperature, the extent and density of lysed intraperitoneal adhesions present from previous surgeries, and the extent to which the bowels have to be mechanically manipulated, exteriorized, and potentially devascularized. Intraoperative blood loss has been found to correlate with the incidence of postoperative ileus but rather may reflect the difficulty of a particular procedure than a true cause. A careful balance has to be found between minimizing operative time and the risk of causing inadvertent tissue damage by rushing through a procedure.

In lieu of the conventional approach with an open laparotomy, many abdominal surgeries can be performed laparoscopically or can be laparoscopically assisted. The laparoscopic approach offers several advantages and is generally considered to be less traumatic, but may significantly prolong the duration of the procedure. Even though not all studies have shown a relevant superiority of the laparoscopic approach, an increasing body of evidence indicates that, in experienced hands, intestinal function is less affected and shows a more rapid return to normal. The reasons for this difference are still being explored by experimental data and seem only in part to be the result of decreased postoperative pain and pain medication. Most notably, however, the physiologic and moist environment and the temperature within the peritoneal cavity are preserved throughout the procedure, large-surface bowel manipulations are avoided, and formation of adhesions is reduced. Furthermore, the primarily limited maneuvering space and visibility tend to deteriorate rapidly if there is relevant bleeding into the operative field. The surgical technique during laparoscopy has therefore evolved and follows more carefully the anatomic avascular planes. This minimizes blood loss and in itself may reduce surgical trauma to the intestines.

Pain Management

Anesthesia and the postoperative pain management are among the most relevant contributing factors to postoperative bowel dysmotility. Administration of exogenous opiates or endogenous opiate pathways exerts an inhibitory effect on smooth muscle contractility. Whenever possible, pain management therefore should also rely on nonopiate drugs. In particular, nonsteroidal anti-inflammatory drugs (NSAIDs) are of importance because they not only decrease opiate consumption but may also play a role in resolving the ileus by inhibiting the prostaglandin-mediated inflammation and depression of smooth muscle contractility.

With the presence in the body of three types of opiate receptors with different functions and anatomic distributions, this intestinal inhibitory effect is mostly mediated by μ_2 receptors. Although opiate antagonists such as naloxone successfully reverse the intestinal dysmotility, they also block the pain control. Research efforts have therefore focused on drugs that could be used to treat intestinal motility disorders selectively. Alvimopan and methylnaltrexone are two novel, peripherally acting, competitive μ-opioid receptor antagonists that do not cross the blood–brain barrier. Both substances are currently being evaluated for their potential in preventing and treating postoperative ileus. Although some shortening of the postoperative ileus and hospital stay has been observed, the final word on its clinical significance and best dosage is still out.

Epidural Anesthesia

Epidural anesthesia, preferably at a thoracic level, has been shown to provide excellent postoperative pain control while avoiding the inhibitory side effects of patient-controlled intravenous opiate administration. This results in a pharmacologic sympathectomy that in theory promotes intestinal motility. In addition to local anesthetics, low doses of epidural opiates enhance the analgesic effect without having a negative impact on respiratory and intestinal depression. However, controlled trials have provided conflicting data on the actual benefit of epidural anesthesia on resolving postoperative ileus.

Fast-Track Postoperative Management

Enteral feeding has fundamental benefits such as prevention of intestinal mucosal atrophy or acalculous cholecystitis. Furthermore, it is the most important stimulus of intestinal motor activity. Traditional postoperative pathways, with routine placement of a nasogastric tube and bowel rest until passage of flatus or stool, promote rather than prevent intestinal inactivity. Newer fast-track protocols avoid routine nasogastric tubes but recommend forced early ambulation and nutrition, often in combination with opiate-sparing pain management (e.g., with epidural anesthesia). If, on postoperative day 1, the patient does not complain of nausea or vomiting, clear liquids are started and the diet advanced as tolerated. Supportive means may include use of chewing gums, even though recent prospective randomized trials raised doubts about its effectiveness. In any case, this aggressive management approach has resulted in significantly faster reconvalescence with a reduction of the postoperative bowel recovery time and the length of stay, even though an estimated 15% of patients will suffer a setback and may require readmission to the hospital.

TREATMENT

Depending on the nature of the disease, the surgical procedure, and the point at which the prolonged postoperative ileus becomes manifest, its management may vary. The diagnosis is generally a clinical one, but additional diagnostic tests may be appropriate and include blood work and abdominal x-rays or a computed tomography scan to rule out a localized problem and confirm the diffuse bowel distention without transition point. Residual free air from the laparotomy should be absorbed within 7 to 10 days and has to be distinguished from new and pathologic extraluminal air pockets. Contrast studies are rarely necessary unless an anastomotic leak must be ruled out.

Immediate management steps consist of correction of any electrolyte and acid–base imbalances, fluid resuscitation, and placement of a nasogastric tube for decompression and prevention of repeated vomiting and to reduce the risk of aspiration. Underlying pathologic conditions (e.g., cardiopulmonary function, renal function, diabetes, adrenal insufficiency, hypothyroidism) require appropriate attention. The duration of this management is determined by serial assessment of clinical parameters to include the output from the nasogastric tube, the evolution of the abdominal distention, and the onset of passage of flatus or stool. In case the ileus persists for more than 5 days or malnutrition preexists, parenteral nutrition should be initiated and maintained until adequate caloric intake by enteral route is ensured. In case of an exceptionally long duration of intestinal dysfunction, replacement of the nasogastric tube by a percutaneous endoscopic gastrostomy (PEG) tube may be considered for reasons of patient comfort.

Evidence of a surgical complication may require abdominal re-exploration, but the window of opportunity is generally limited to the first 7 to 10 days. Although formation of relevant new adhesions may be a factor for the clinical picture of prolonged postoperative ileus, reintervention for lysis of these adhesions is rarely of any benefit because the adhesions re-form quickly. Furthermore, it can be anticipated that the density of fresh postoperative adhesions within the peritoneal cavity will be most extensive in the period 2 to 4 weeks after the surgery and occasionally amounts to a "hostile abdomen." After a peak, a steady decline of the adhesion density can generally be observed, but there is wide interindividual variability. Efforts to decrease the extent and impact of postoperative adhesions have been numerous, but so far success has been limited. Even the more promising tools (e.g., sodium hyaluronate–based bioresorbable polysaccharide membranes) that were found to result in a statistically significant reduction of adhesions have not provided any advantage with regard to preventing postoperative ileus.

Although most cases of prolonged postoperative ileus will eventually resolve within 5 to 7 days, it is recommended to reassess the patient's overall management and medications to eliminate potentially aggravating factors as previously discussed. Efforts to reduce opiate-based pain control and instead use NSAIDs (e.g., by rectal route) might offer an alternative with less negative impact. Metoclopramide or selective serotonin 5-HT3 receptor antagonists (e.g., odansetron) may be useful to suppress borderline nausea but do not otherwise contribute to the resolution of postoperative ileus. The use of prokinetic, that is, motility-promoting agents to accelerate gastric emptying and colonic transit time, is tempting, but the clinical success is often disappointing. Erythromycin could not be confirmed to have any benefit. Cisapride, one of the few successful prokinetic agents, was taken off the market because of rare life-threatening cardiac arrhythmias. Neostigmine, an inhibitor of the acetylcholinesterase, results in increased parasympathetic activity and may help to restimulate the intestinal and colonic motility, but its use is somewhat limited by side effects of bradycardia and abdominal cramping. Serotonin 5-HT4 receptor antagonists such as tegaserod have primarily been explored for their beneficial role in irritable bowel syndrome and functional constipation or gastroparesis. These motility-enhancing drugs may offer new options in the treatment and prevention of prolonged postoperative ileus but will first have to be investigated to that extent.

SUMMARY

Postoperative ileus remains a significant problem that results in significant morbidity and tremendous health care cost. The current management primarily focuses on a multimodal preventive approach that includes less traumatic surgeries, opiate-sparing pain control, and fast-track recovery protocols. The treatment includes nasogastric tubes on demand rather than by routine and in the future may increasingly rely on motility-promoting drugs.

SUGGESTED READINGS

Kehlet H, Williamson R, Buchler MW, and others: A survey of perceptions and attitudes among European surgeons towards the clinical impact and management of postoperative ileus, *Colorectal Dis* 7:245, 2005.

Luckey A, Livingston E, Tache Y: Mechanisms and treatment of postoperative ileus, *Arch Surg* 138:206, 2003.

Mattei P, Rombeau JL: Review of the pathophysiology and management of postoperative ileus, *World J Surg* 30:1382, 2006.

Person B, Wexner SD: The management of postoperative ileus, *Curr Probl Surg* 43:6, 2006.

Roberts DJ, Banh HL, Hall RI: Use of novel prokinetic agents to facilitate return of gastrointestinal motility in adult critically ill patients, *Curr Opin Crit Care* 12:295, 2006.

CROHN'S DISEASE OF THE SMALL BOWEL

Yoav Mintz, MD, and Mark A. Talamini, MD

INTRODUCTION

Crohn's disease is a transmural inflammatory process that can affect any location along the gut but most commonly affects the distal small bowel. Its etiology is unknown, it is slightly more common in women than men, and its peak incidence is in the third decade of life. Approximately 40% of patients with newly diagnosed Crohn's disease have ileocolic disease, 30% have disease limited to the small bowel, and 30% have disease involving only the colon or anorectum.

Surgical treatment for Crohn's is not curative. The primary goals of treatment are alleviating symptoms and improving patients' quality of life. Crohn's patients are best treated today using a multidisciplinary team approach. Centers treating Crohn's disease within the category of inflammatory bowel disease (IBD) use the collaboration of experts in each medical field involved in IBD (i.e., gastroenterologists, surgeons, radiologists, and nutritionists). Both medical and surgical treatments are continuously evolving, and those treating Crohn's disease should stay up to date on the new drugs and on the surgical and invasive radiology options available. This team approach is especially beneficial in Crohn's disease because this disease is still not fully understood, and extensive research is performed continuously. This chapter focuses on surgical management of Crohn's disease of the small bowel, but surgeons should be familiar with the medical management offered to ensure that their patients have received the most up-to-date medical treatment.

MEDICAL MANAGEMENT

Most patients with Crohn's disease will seek medical help through their primary care physician or gastroenterologist. The initial treatment will always be medical unless a severe complication has occurred. Medical management is targeted either to induce remission of an acute flare or to maintain remission. Drugs commonly used to treat the disease are listed in Table 1.

Table 1: Common Drugs used for Medical Therapy in Crohn's Disease

Mild Active Disease	Induction of Remission	Maintenance of Remission
5-ASA	Corticosteroids	Azathioprin
	Infliximab	6-mercaptopurine
		Methotrexate
		Infliximab

According to the World Congress of Gastroenterology (1998), Crohn's disease can be simply classified into three patterns of disease behavior: stricturing, perforating, and inflammatory. The stricturing pattern is characterized by the development of fibrosis and stenosis of segments of bowel, causing partial or complete bowel obstructions. Typically patients will go through cycles of inflammation and repair that will, over time, increase the thickness of the bowel wall and cause intestinal obstruction. Medical therapy will initially resolve the inflammation and relieve the mechanical obstruction. Repeated episodes will eventually cause stenosis and strictures that are no longer treatable by medicines, and patients will be referred for surgery. The perforating pattern is characterized by the development of an intra-abdominal abscess or fistula. This entity is best treated with a combined medical and surgical approach. Abscesses can be drained by means of invasive radiology, and not all fistulae are necessarily an indication for surgery. The inflammatory pattern is characterized by the absence of strictures or fistulae and tends to be more diffusely distributed through the length of the bowel. This entity is usually treated medically, with surgery being reserved for refractory cases.

Treatment of Active Inflammatory Crohn's Disease

Mild disease is usually treated with aminosalicylates, which are anti-inflammatory drugs. These include the 5-aminosalicylate (5-ASA) derivatives. As a class, these drugs are not always effective. In an acute episode or Crohn's flare, the goal of treatment is to induce remission. The gold standard therapy for induction of remission is still corticosteroids. Up to 70% of patients will respond to this treatment within a week. Having achieved remission, the next goal is sustaining the remission. For this, corticosteroids should not be the drug of choice because of their well-known side effects and the complications of long-term use. Budesonide, a synthetic glucocorticoid, is often used to induce remission because of its reduced systemic absorption. Although this drug is less likely to cause severe side effects, its reduced systemic absorption still can cause adrenal suppression. Before surgery, a careful history should be taken regarding corticosteroid therapy to decide whether the patient requires perioperative coverage of steroids because of long-term adrenal suppression.

Infliximab is a monoclonal antibody directed against tumor necrosis factor alpha (TNF-α), a cytokine that plays an important role in the development of inflammatory reactions. It was introduced in 1998 and has revolutionized the treatment of Crohn's disease. It is indicated for the treatment of moderately to severely active Crohn's disease resistant to conventional therapy. Up to 70% of patients respond to induction therapy within 1 to 2 weeks with a single infusion. This drug is expensive, however, and associated with an increased risk of serious opportunistic infections such as tuberculosis, listeriosis, and aspergillosis. Furthermore, infusion reactions occur in 3% to 17% of the patients and are associated with the formation of antibodies to infliximab. For this reason, the concomitant use of immunosuppressants with infliximab is recommended.

Natalizumab is a humanized monoclonal antibody against α_4 integrin that inhibits leukocyte adhesion and migration into inflamed tissue. It was initially believed that treatment with this drug induced clinical remission and improved the quality of life of patients with Crohn's disease. However, a recent prospective controlled double-blind study showed that induction therapy with natalizumab resulted in only a small, nonsignificant improvement in response and remission rates. Patients who did respond had significantly increased rates of sustained response and remission if natalizumab was continued at 4-week intervals. The benefit of this drug remains to be determined and weighed against the risk of serious adverse events, including progressive multifocal leukoencephalopathy.

Following the successful treatment of an acute flare, the goal of medical therapy becomes maintaining remission. Although corticosteroids can achieve long-term remission, the serious side effects of long-term systemic administration make their use problematic. The two most common steroid-sparing alternative drugs used for maintenance of remission are azathioprine (AZA) and 6-mercaptopurine (6-MP). These immunosuppressive agents act by inhibiting DNA synthesis, thereby suppressing cytotoxic T-cell and natural killer cell function. Both are effective for induction and maintenance of remission, but both have a long latency period (3 to 6 months) and therefore are usually used only for maintenance therapy. The treatment should start while response is induced with other methods. Close observation is warranted while treating patients with AZA and 6-MP because of their serious potential side effects. Bone marrow suppression, hepatotoxicity, and pancreatitis may occur, and weekly blood count monitoring is necessary during initial treatment. Methotrexate (MTX) is a second-line immunosuppressant used for the treatment of Crohn's disease. Similarly to AZA and 6-MP, it has a slow onset of action (1 to 3 months). Hepatotoxicity is the major concern when using MTX, which has a higher risk for liver damage in patients with increased risk for hepatotoxicity (chronic alcohol consumption, obesity, hyperglycemia, chronic viral hepatitis).

Infliximab has a rapid onset of action and therefore can be used for the treatment of induction, as well as for maintenance of remission. Up to 53% of patients remain in remission when treated at weekly intervals. The duration of efficacy of this drug is of approximately 8 to 12 weeks.

Treatment of Active Perforating Crohn's Disease

This pattern of disease includes the occurrence of intra-abdominal abscesses and fistulae. When an abscess is present, control of sepsis is the first aim of treatment. This can usually be accomplished by antibiotic therapy combined with image-guided or (rarely in this era) surgical drainage. After the sepsis has been resolved, a secondary evaluation of the patient and the disease is undertaken, and the disease is treated according to the patients' clinical status and nutritional condition. Most often, a period of medical management allows the inflammation to subside sufficiently to provide for a safer surgical approach.

Fistula management in Crohn's disease is challenging because a fistula is usually a reflection of active inflammation. The correct approach depends greatly on the type and location of the fistula. There are three main types of fistulae: enterocutaneous, enteroenteral, and enterovesical fistulae.

Enterocutaneous fistulae occur in approximately 4% of patients with Crohn's disease. They are a result of either a direct extension of a sinus tract from the diseased bowel through the abdominal wall or a percutaneous drainage of an intra-abdominal abscess with continuing drainage from the diseased bowel through the abscess cavity to the skin. An enterocutaneous fistula is not an absolute indication for surgery. The treatment is individualized according to the clinical status of the patient and the output of the fistula. These fistulae usually do not have such a high output as to cause fluid and electrolyte imbalances, but their presence may still be suggestive of severe underlined disease. If the patient's clinical status is satisfactory, nonoperative management can be initiated using a combination of antibiotic therapy together with nutritional support and medical treatment. Infliximab has a 61% to 69% response rate for closure of Crohn's-related fistulae. Fifty-three percent of patients remain in remission with continuous therapy. Even if unsuccessful, the time spent pursuing nonoperative treatment allows the tissue inflammation to subside. Enteroenteral fistulae used to be considered an indication for surgery. In 1982, Cameron and colleagues studied the natural history of enteroenteral fistulae and demonstrated a comparable outcome between surgical therapy and initial medical therapy in terms of morbidity and mortality. These fistulae are usually asymptomatic and are not by themselves considered an indication for surgery. Surgery is indicated, however, if these fistulae are associated with an acute exacerbation refractory to medical therapy, an abdominal mass, bleeding, or malnutrition.

Patients with enterovesical fistulae may present with any combination of the following symptoms: recurrent urinary tract infections (88%), pneumaturia (88%), fecaluria (38%), or hematuria (63%). These fistulae should, in general, be treated surgically because of the continuing insult to the kidneys from chronic urinary tract infection.

SURGICAL MANAGEMENT

The objectives of surgical treatment in Crohn's disease are to treat complications, relieve symptoms, and maximize quality of life. Unfortunately, most patients afflicted with Crohn's disease severe enough to require chronic medical attention will at one time or another require surgical intervention. The most common surgical procedure performed is small bowel resection. This is effective at relieving symptoms, improving quality of life, and reducing the need for powerful medications. However, the loss of small bowel length may eventually lead to problems related to vitamin absorption, fluid management, and nutrient absorption. Therefore small bowel resection, if necessary, should always be limited to the minimal length necessary to resolve the acute complication. If adequate, stricturoplasty may be performed rather than bowel resection for resolving obstructive symptoms.

Indications for Operation

Surgery is indicated for complications of Crohn's disease. The most common such complications are listed in Table 2. Failure of medical management could be defined as the failure of medical therapy to relieve the symptoms of the disease or the recurrence of symptoms following an attempt to withdraw induction therapy following remission. In these situations, the inflammatory process might not be amenable to medical treatment, or an additional unrecognized complication may exist. Intestinal obstruction occurs either in an acute flare or as a chronic partial obstruction that may evolve into a complete obstruction. An obstruction resulting from an acute inflammatory process can usually be treated medically. Surgery is an option for unresolved symptoms in patients already at maximal medical therapy. Chronic partial obstruction, however, is usually a result of a stricturing pattern of disease where the bowel wall is thickened, causing a narrow fixed and unpliable lumen. In these situations, the inflammatory process is not the cause of obstruction. The obstruction is caused by extensive scarring and fibrosis in the segment of bowel. Surgery is therefore the only option for treatment.

Enteroenteral fistula is not an indication for surgery by itself, but it may reflect the presence of severe disease. Surgery is usually indicated for enterocutaneous, enterovaginal, and enterovesical fistulae. The first two, however, can initially have a trial of medical closure before surgery. Enterovesical fistulae are always an indication for surgery because of the repeated bouts of injury to the kidneys during recurrent urinary tract infections.

Table 2: Indications for Operation in Crohn's Disease

Failure of medical management	Hemorrhage
Intestinal obstruction	Perforation
Enteric fistula	Growth retardation
Inflammatory mass/abscess	

An intra-abdominal abscess occurs when a diseased segment of bowel perforates through the entire bowel wall into the peritoneal cavity. This is usually a gradual process, and therefore the escaping bowel contents are usually enclosed by surrounding bowel loops and omentum. An abscess will not respond to medical treatment and requires drainage. If possible, the abscess should be drained using an image-guided percutaneous approach as the initial treatment. After sepsis is resolved and nutritional status improved, a definitive surgical treatment can be planned.

Gastrointestinal bleeding occurs more frequently when the colon is involved in the disease. Hemorrhage from the small bowel is infrequent and usually indolent. It may cause severe anemia requiring blood transfusions, and surgery is therefore indicated. Free perforation in Crohn's disease is rare because of the slow nature of the inflammatory process. However, it can occur in heavily medicated immunosuppressed patients because the therapy can impair the natural processes that should contain bowel contents and create an abscess. In these situations, the initial clinical appearance of the patient may be misleading, and peritonitis may be masked by high-dose steroid treatment. This is a good reason to obtain a computed tomography (CT) image for patients presenting acutely with Crohn's disease.

Growth retardation occurs in 15% to 40% of children with Crohn's disease. Corticosteroid treatment is not the only cause for retardation of growth because it is observed in patients treated with steroid-sparing drugs as well. It is believed that the disease itself is the main reason for the growth retardation. It may be that specific nutritional therapy may prevent loss of height in this patient population. These issues make surgical intervention more favorable in prepubertal children with refractory disease that does not respond to nutritional therapy.

Preoperative Evaluation and Preparation

Before an elective operation for Crohn's disease, a patient's gastrointestinal tract must be studied thoroughly. Several imaging modalities are available, and a reliable "map" of the current disease state is achieved by the integration of information from multiple studies. A contrast radiographic study (small bowel series) is the most directly visual study for acquiring information about the overall bowel length, the location of the disease, the presence of fistulae, and the nature of existing strictures. A CT scan is beneficial to provide information regarding bowel-wall thickening (especially if performed with water contrast), mesentery thickening, and retroperitoneal disease. Colonoscopy is important to determine whether the large bowel is involved in the disease. This is particularly important because it is more difficult to evaluate Crohn's disease of the colon intraoperatively by observing its external appearance. Video capsule endoscopy is an emerging technology for visualizing the small bowel mucosa in its entire length. Several reports have demonstrated the capsule's ability to diagnosis subtle Crohn's disease in suspected cases undetected by conventional imaging modalities. The diagnosis is achieved through the demonstration of mucosal alterations along the small intestine. The clinical significance of these findings is not yet entirely clear because these lesions have also been demonstrated in asymptomatic volunteers.

The patient's nutritional status should be evaluated before surgery. In patients with significant malnutrition, steps should be taken to rectify this before surgery; these steps include the initiation of intravenous parenteral nutrition if necessary. This may require home nutritional support until weight loss is at least reversed. Tube feeding or oral supplementation with nonsolid food may be an option in patients without significant obstruction symptoms.

A standard bowel preparation should be performed preoperatively unless the patient has a long-term, high-grade obstruction. In these cases a prolonged period of clear liquid diet only in combination with oral antibiotics just before surgery will likely suffice. Recent evidence that bowel preparation is not necessary for elective non-IBD colon surgery is unlikely to apply to the specific situation of Crohn's disease. All patients are given prophylactic intravenous antibiotics just before surgery. Fluid and electrolyte imbalances and any existing anemia should also be corrected before surgery. If a diversion is possible, a stoma site should be marked preoperatively.

Operative Management

Small Bowel Resection

The most common operation performed for Crohn's disease is small bowel resection. Careful judgment should be employed before resecting bowel because of the nature of this recurrent disease and the possible need for repeated operations. In general, it is helpful to follow the guidelines listed in Table 3. Before resection it is important to determine the length of healthy bowel. Patients with multiple segments of diseased bowel or who have had multiple operations for Crohn's complications are at risk for short bowel syndrome if the operation is not carefully planned. If possible, only that diseased bowel causing the acute complication should be resected. All other nonobstructing segments of diseased bowel do not necessarily require resection. If additional asymptomatic strictures are discovered at surgery, the surgeon should consider performing stricturoplasty rather than resection. In an attempt to salvage as much intestinal length as possible, resection margins should be minimal and limited to achieve macroscopically normal bowel. Recurrence rates do not increase when microscopic Crohn's disease is present at the resected margins. The incidence of immediate postoperative complications (leak with fistula or abscess; obstruction) also is not increased. Therefore extensive resection margins are unnecessary.

Recurrent operations for Crohn's disease complications may warrant strategies different from resection and stricturoplasty. Generally one should avoid bypassing a diseased segment of bowel because of the risk of hemorrhage, perforation, and future malignancy in the nonfunctional loop of bowel. However, in extreme situations, such as patients with extensive dense adhesions and prior bowel resections unsuitable for further resections, or duodenal Crohn's disease, a bypass may be the only option.

Resection of Crohn's-diseased bowel segments can be difficult. The mesentery is often markedly thickened and shortened. Division and ligation of blood vessels in this setting should be performed gradually and meticulously. To avoid bleeding, take small bites of the mesentery, use 2-0 ties, and slide the knots in conjunction with the clamp release so that the suture does not saw through the vessels. Another option for division of the mesentery is the Ligasure device (ValleyLab, Boulder, CO). When used properly, this device effectively seals and divides even difficult mesentery.

Table 3: Guidelines for Operative Management

Determine length of healthy bowel

Resect only the segment causing complication

Determine whether resection or stricturoplasty is more appropriate

Resection to grossly negative margins

Bypass only if the duodenum is involved, if resection is technically impossible, or in short bowel syndrome

If there is a high risk for complications, protect the anastomosis with diversion

Following resection, an intestinal anastomosis could be performed using either a standard stapling or a hand-sewn technique. When dealing with edematous or dilated bowel, a hand-sewn technique allows for better adjustment of the two segments of bowel. In cases of severe sepsis, poor nutritional status, diffuse peritonitis, or high-dose steroid treatment, protection of the anastomosis with a diverting ileostomy may be advisable.

Crohn's-Related Fistula

Surgical treatment of Crohn's-related fistula disease can be both a technical and a judgment challenge. The fistula site is usually enveloped by several bowel loops involved in the inflammatory process. Depending on the degree of inflammation, identifying and isolating the diseased bowel loop driving the fistula without injuring the surrounding innocent bowel can be difficult. Preoperative evaluation, particularly in terms of radiologic studies, can save time and effort in the operating room. After the origin and the target organ of the fistula have been traced and isolated, the fistula is divided, and the diseased bowel loop is resected. The target, innocent organ is only secondarily involved and usually does not require resection because of the Crohn's disease. It may, however, be so badly damaged by the fistula and inflammation that repair is not possible, and resection is necessary. In cases of enterovesical fistula, division of the fistula is followed by primary repair of the bladder defect. Care should be taken not to injure the trigon area while suturing. Fortunately, these fistulae are usually located on the anterior peritoneal surface away from the trigon. Preoperatively placed ureteral catheters can be helpful to identify the ureters within the inflammatory mass. In cases of enterocutaneous fistula, detachment of the fistula tract from the abdominal wall along with resection of the diseased bowel suffices.

Stricturoplasty

Stricturoplasty may be appropriate for any Crohn's patient undergoing surgery for obstructive symptoms. It is a surgical technique applied for preservation of bowel length. It is particularly important in patients who have already had bowel resections and for whom yet another surgical procedure is needed for obstructive symptoms. With this technique, the obstruction is released without loss of any bowel absorptive surface. Leaving the diseased bowel in place does, however, expose the patient to a potential malignant degeneration from the remaining Crohn's disease. Although the risk for malignancy is remote, it is meaningful, and during the stricturoplasty, a biopsy from the most diseased bowel mucosa should always be taken in case there is any unexpected dysplasia in the specimen.

A short stricturoplasty is performed in a standard fashion similar to Heinneke–Mikulicz pyloroplasty. A longitudinal incision is performed along the antimesenteric side of the stricture, and the bowel is closed in a transverse fashion. A single layer of 3-0 silk stitches is usually sufficient. It is our practice to mark the stricturoplasty site with a metal clip to distinguish this area when future imaging studies are performed. In case of a long strictured segment, the Finney-type stricturoplasty can be useful. In this procedure, the enteroenterostomy is performed after the affected bowel is folded onto itself in a U shape. In case of a particularly long stricture, a side-to-side isoperistaltic stricturoplasty, developed by Michelassi, could be performed. The bowel is divided transversely at the midstricture, both strictured areas are opened, and the antimesenteric faces of bowel are sewn one to the other in an isoperistaltic antimesenteric manner.

Minimally Invasive Surgery for Crohn's Disease

Traditionally patients with complications of Crohn's disease who require surgical treatment are operated via laparotomy. The need to palpate the entire bowel to delineate the extent and severity of the disease, together with the division of thickened mesentery that demands special attention, dictated the surgical approach. In the late 1990s, however, it became apparent that selected patients might benefit from a minimally invasive surgery (MIS) approach. The length of hospital stay, the postoperative morbidity rate, and the median overall costs during the first 3 postoperative months have been shown to be significantly lower in patients operated by an MIS approach. Furthermore, a laparoscopic approach enables quicker initiation of steroid treatment if necessary and reduces the adhesion formation to allow a safer and quicker access to the abdomen for recurrent disease. The indications for surgery should not differ between open and laparoscopic approach. An additional indication for laparoscopy is for diagnostic purposes. Patients with suspected Crohn's disease but with extensive negative workup can benefit from a diagnostic laparoscopy, and this should be recognized as an excellent diagnostic tool.

Not all patients with Crohn's disease are good candidates for MIS, and careful selection before surgery is mandatory to ensure successful results. Contraindications for MIS in Crohn's disease include patients with a known "frozen" abdomen, and emergent operations (i.e., active bleeding, peritonitis, complete small bowel obstruction). General contraindications for laparoscopy apply as well (uncorrected coagulopathy, hemodynamic instability, severe heart failure, severe chronic obstructive pulmonary disease, and so forth).

Surgical Technique

Following the preoperative evaluation and preparation of the patient, the procedure begins with achievement of pneumoperitoneum. Either a Veress needle or Hassan techniques are used. A 30-degree laparoscope is inserted, and initial evaluation of the abdomen is performed. On the basis of initial findings, two more 5-mm trocars are usually placed at the midline, one just above the symphysis pubis and the other in the upper abdomen. Using these ports, the entire bowel can be evaluated. In cases of small bowel resection, the affected part of the bowel is identified and grasped by one of the instruments. A 4- to 5-cm periumbilical or suprapubic (Pfannenstiel) incision is performed, and the diseased bowel is delivered through this incision onto the abdominal wall. The actual bowel resection and anastomosis including the mesenteric vessel division is performed on the abdominal wall. The drawback of performing the mesenteric vessel ligation through a small incision is the risk of tearing the vessels in their intra-abdominal portion because of extensive tension on the mesentery. Therefore division of the mesentery and bowel can be performed laparoscopically in cases of short and thickened mesentery. In these circumstances, the use of ultrasonic scissors or Ligasure device is imperative.

In case of terminal ileitis requiring an ileocolic resection, an additional trocar may be needed but should not be placed in potential ileostomy sites unless one is planned. The cecum and ascending colon are mobilized laparoscopically until the bowel and mesentery freely reach the abdominal wall. Resection and anastomosis are performed in the same fashion as described earlier. If a diversion is necessary, it is performed laparoscopically by delivering the bowel through the premarked ostomy site.

The most common reason for conversion from laparoscopic to open technique is the presence of dense adhesions, which prevents safe dissection between tissues (47% of cases). Neither the presence of a prior abdominal operation nor the number of abdominal operations serves as a predictor to conversion. Other reasons for conversion include extensive inflammation, size of inflammatory mass, and the inability to safely dissect a fistula from the involved healthy organ.

SPECIAL SITUATIONS

Crohn's Disease During Pregnancy

Patients with inactive Crohn's disease are as fertile as the general population. Thus approximately 25% of women with a diagnosis of this disease will conceive. Maintaining adequate disease control is crucial for both maternal and fetal health. Active Crohn's disease during pregnancy has been shown to increase the incidence of fetal loss, stillbirths, preterm delivery, low birth weight, and developmental defects. In general, these problems are due to the disease itself rather than to Crohn's medications used during pregnancy. Therefore it is advisable to work toward clinical remission before attempting conception. The indications for surgery in pregnant Crohn's disease women are the same as for nonpregnant patients. However, the diagnosis is usually much more difficult. Standard radiologic imaging such as small bowel series, barium enemas, and CT scans carry with them radiation risk to the fetus. Endoscopy, ultrasound, and magnetic resonance imaging are helpful in the diagnosis of abscesses and free perforations in these situations. There are only a few case reports of surgery in Crohn's disease during pregnancy. In a severely ill pregnant Crohn's patient, continued illness has a greater risk to the fetus and mother than surgery. The goals of surgical intervention are to resolve the acute problem and achieve full-term delivery. In the instance of a potentially difficult anastomosis, a temporary ileostomy may be preferable to reduce the risk of postoperative complications.

Unexpected Intraoperative Diagnosis of Crohn's Disease

A diagnosis of Crohn's disease could be made intraoperatively in patients undergoing emergent abdominal operations. Patients with perforations or abscesses caused by Crohn's disease are treated in the same manner as described earlier. In the setting of operation for suspected appendicitis or small bowel obstruction, however, it is not always necessary to go forward with surgical resection in the acute setting. Patients who have not been diagnosed with Crohn's disease before the surgery and have not yet had medical treatment for the disease may be better managed by making the diagnosis in the operating room, followed by medical treatment after the operation. The decision should be made according to the extent of the disease, the nature of the disease (acute inflammation or stricture), the patient's age, and overall clinical status. In case of suspected appendicitis, an appendectomy should be considered only if the disease is distant from the terminal ileum and the cecum is not involved. Performing an appendectomy on involved bowel could result in a leak or fistula. However, an appendectomy in young patients would rule out the diagnosis of appendicitis in future right lower quadrant pain and tenderness.

SUGGESTED READINGS

Broe PJ, Bayless TM, Cameron JL: Crohn's disease: are enteroenteral fistulae an indication for surgery? *Surgery* 91:249, 1982.

Domenech E. Inflammatory bowel disease: current therapeutic options, *Digestion* 73(suppl 1):67, 2006.

Fazio VW, Marchetti F, Church M, and others: Effect of resection margins on the recurrence of Crohn's disease in the small bowel. A randomized controlled trial, *Ann Surg* 224:563, 1996.

Milsom JW: Laparoscopic surgery in the treatment of Crohn's disease, *Surg Clin North Am* 85:25, vii, 2005.

Schmidt CM, Talamini MA, Kaufman HS, and others: Laparoscopic surgery for Crohn's disease: reasons for conversion, *Ann Surg* 233:733, 2001.

Talamini MA, Broe PJ, Cameron JL: Urinary fistulae in Crohn's disease, *Surg Gynecol Obstet* 154:553, 1982.

STRICTUREPLASTY IN CROHN'S DISEASE

Robert R. Cima, MD, and John H. Pemberton, MD

Crohn's disease (CD) is one of the major categories of nonspecific inflammatory bowel disease; ulcerative colitis (UC) is the other. Unlike UC, which is limited to the rectum and colon, CD affects any location along the intestine. Although CD predominantly affects the small bowel, it frequently involves the colon, rectum, and perianal region. Sometimes these areas may be involved simultaneously or at separate times during the course of the disease. Unlike UC, in which the intestinal manifestations of the disease are cured with removal of the rectum and colon, surgery for CD is directed at relieving symptoms and should not be considered curative but rather an adjunct to maximal medical therapy. Surgery should be considered only after careful consultation with the patient and with a gastroenterologist experienced in the medical management of the patient's disease.

The symptoms of CD are related to the transmural inflammation of the bowel wall that characterizes the disease. When this inflammatory process is allowed to progress to abscess formation, enteroenteral or enterocutaneous fistula, perforation, and strictures often occur. Stricture formation most commonly becomes symptomatic when it occurs in the small bowel. The primary surgical treatment of symptomatic CD is resection of the involved bowel with either restoration of intestinal continuity or a stoma. Unfortunately, a high percentage of CD patients coming to surgery after maximal medical management must have reoperation to manage recurrence of their disease. In these patients, repeated bowel resection may lead to problems related to decreased length of the small bowel, including vitamin and nutrient malabsorption and volume depletion. Strictureplasty is a useful surgical technique that relieves the obstructive symptoms caused by small bowel strictures while preserving intestinal length and thus, it is hoped, avoiding the complications of repeated small bowel resection. Table 1 lists indications, and Table 2, contraindications for strictureplasty in Crohn's disease.

Table 1: Indications for Strictureplasty

A single obstructing fibrotic small bowel stricture

Diffuse involvement of the small bowel with strictures

Any stricture in the setting of previous small bowel resections or known short bowel syndrome

Table 2: Contraindications to Strictureplasty

Free or contained perforation of the bowel associated with the stricture

Multiple strictures in a short segment in a patient who has not had prior small bowel resections or in a patient with sufficient small bowel length

Strictures that are close to an area of proposed resection

Any stricture with pathologic evidence of dysplasia or malignancy

Strictureplasty was first performed in patients with a technique used in the treatment of tubercular strictures of the small bowel. Lee and Papaioannou first reported strictureplasties for the treatment of Crohn's strictures in 1982. Strictureplasty gained broader acceptance after a number of groups reported that there was no difference in recurrence of Crohn's in patients who had resections limited to only the areas of grossly involved disease as opposed to those who had wide margins showing no microscopic evidence of disease. These findings, together with the well-known complications of extensive bowel resection, have led to a philosophy of minimizing the amount of small bowel resection in patients with CD. Strictureplasty took this precept even further, leaving diseased bowel in situ but surgically redesigning the involved segment to allow free passage of bowel contents.

PATIENT SELECTION

It is now accepted that CD patients may manifest different presentations of the disease. Although any Crohn's patient undergoing surgery for obstructive disease symptoms might be a candidate for a strictureplasty, those patients who will most benefit are those who develop recurrent strictures. The etiology of bowel stricturing is most likely related to repeated episodes of inflammation, resolution, and remodeling of the bowel wall, leading to replacement of the normally pliable tissue with a thickened, nonpliable bowel wall segment that eventually narrows the lumen. This results in obstructive symptoms. The time course of this process varies and may be modified by medication such as steroids, immunomodulators, or biological therapies such as infliximab. However, over time the involved segment of bowel becomes less responsive to increasingly aggressive medical management. Eventually surgical intervention becomes necessary.

Strictureplasty may be performed in the ileum, jejunum, duodenum, and even the colon. The nature of the stricture and the amount of the remaining bowel are key factors in determining whether a strictureplasty is appropriate. Strictureplasty is not an option in the setting of bowel perforation or extensive inflammatory phlegmon in the involved segment of bowel. Strictureplasty has less of a role in severely thickened bowel or in an extremely long strictured segment.

PREOPERATIVE EVALUATION AND PREPARATION

A number of issues must be considered before recommending elective surgery in a patient with Crohn's disease. Patients should have received optimal medical treatment for their disease. Furthermore, any septic focus should be controlled with antibiotics, percutaneous drainage, or both. Equally important is an evaluation of nutritional state. Patients who are nutritionally compromised should undergo nutritional repletion either by a liquid enteral diet or intravenous hyperalimentation to reverse their catabolic state before surgery. Although nutritional repletion may not eliminate the need for surgery, it has been shown to reduce postoperative complications.

A key for optimal surgical outcome is clearly defining the scope and nature of the patient's past and current disease activity. Obtaining a thorough history of prior operations and operative reports is helpful to determine the patient's anatomy. Colonoscopy should be performed to determine whether there is any colonic disease that might require surgical treatment. Furthermore, any colonic stricture must undergo biopsies to rule out the possibility of malignancy. Although colonic strictureplasty may be considered if there is a real need to preserve colonic length, the risk of an occult malignancy in a colonic stricture is relatively high, and resection should be the standard treatment.

Most important in preoperative planning is defining small bowel disease activity. Traditionally, a small bowel series is used to map the distribution of disease activity. This study provides information on the number and length of strictures, the presence of any unsuspected enteroenteral fistulae, contained perforations, and an estimate of small bowel length. New technology, computed tomographic (CT) enterography using a high-resolution scanner, provides images that substitute for a small bowel series. This study also provides additional information that a small bowel study may miss, such as an occult abscess or evidence of disease distal to a high-grade obstruction. A final important planning step is to discuss the possible need for a temporary or permanent stoma. Stoma sites should be marked on the patient's abdomen even if there is only a small chance that a stoma will be needed because unexpected intraoperative findings may change the scope of the operation and necessitate a stoma. Proper placement of a stoma is important for successful long-term function.

SURGICAL STRATEGY

Strictureplasty should be considered an option in any patient with CD who presents with obstructive symptoms. The goal is to prevent significant bowel loss related to resection. In patients requiring multiple operations, the surgeon must be concerned about loss of bowel length, which may result in short bowel syndrome. The length of bowel necessary for support by oral nutrition varies from patient to patient, but in general, at least 100 to 125 cm of small bowel is considered necessary to avoid supplemental intravenous alimentation or hydration. Some patients who have lived with chronically obstructed bowel may be able to tolerate shorter lengths of remaining bowel because of physiologic adaptation of the bowel. Another important consideration when evaluating a patient with stricturing Crohn's disease is the possibility of an occult malignancy. It is recommended that any stricture being prepared for strictureplasty should have frozen section analysis during the operation to rule out dysplasia or malignancy. This is particularly important in patients in whom a previous bypass procedure has been performed.

OPERATIVE TECHNIQUE

On initial exploration of the abdomen, all evidence of disease should be carefully noted and obvious strictures marked. Each area of involved bowel should be examined for any other pathology that might preclude a strictureplasty, such as a fistula or localized abscess. The length of bowel remaining in situ must be assessed. If the patient has adequate bowel length and the strictures are close to each other, it might be safer to perform a single resection and anastomosis rather than multiple strictureplasties. However, if residual bowel length is a concern, strictureplasties are indicated. It is also important at the end of the operation to document the remaining length of small bowel by actual measurement.

The technique used for a strictureplasty depends on the length of the stricture. For strictures less than 4 to 5 cm in length, the procedure is similar to the Heineke–Mikulicz pyloroplasty performed for pyloric stenosis. This strictureplasty (Fig. 1) is performed by first placing two 3–0 sutures, either nonabsorbable or absorbable, on the side of the bowel at the midportion of the stricture to act as stay sutures after the bowel is opened along the antimesenteric edge. The surgeon accesses the bowel by making an antimesenteric longitudinal incision with electrocautery. This incision divides the stricture and should be carried out at an equal distance proximally and distally into normal, thin-walled,

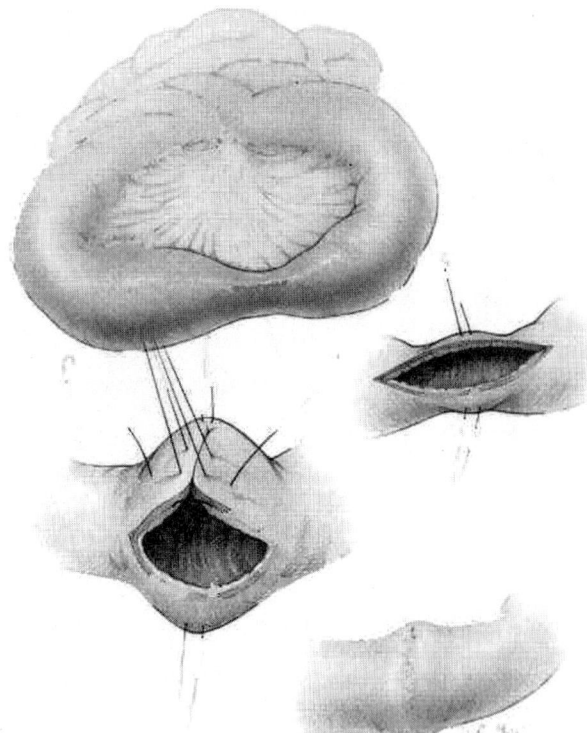

Figure 1 A Heineke–Mikulicz strictureplasty on an isolated stricture. In this drawing, a single-layer everting technique is performed to close the longitudinal enterotomy transversely, reconstituting an unobstructed lumen.

nondiseased bowel. For ease of closure, it is essential that the longitudinal incision stays truly on the antimesenteric border.

It is important to obtain excellent hemostasis because bleeding from a strictureplasty site is one of the most common and troubling postoperative complications. Then mucosal biopsies of the stricture for frozen section analysis are obtained to rule out the presence of dysplasia or malignancy. This is especially important if an ulcer is noted. The stay sutures are pulled perpendicular to the long axis of the bowel (see Fig. 1). Then the enterotomy is closed in two layers, although many authors have described single-layer closures.

This transverse closure is ideal for short strictures but not for longer areas. Fazio and others have widely proposed marking strictureplasty sites with a single metal clip on the adjacent mesentery so that these areas can be identified when future small bowel studies are performed if the patient becomes symptomatic again. However, in the era of CT enterography, this practice is probably unnecessary.

As noted previously, it is important to identify all the strictures along the bowel. However, visual and tactile external evaluation of the bowel may not identify all small bowel strictures. A number of techniques have been described to evaluate intraoperatively the internal diameter of the small bowel lumen. In essence, these techniques all rely on the introduction of a device, most commonly a balloon-tipped catheter, into the bowel that can be passed along its length to assess whether there are any obstructions to easy passage. The best way of introducing the balloon is through the enterotomy made for the first strictureplasty. We use a long jejunal Baker tube with an inflatable balloon at the distal end. The tube is passed to the end of the small bowel manually, and then the balloon is inflated with 12 to 15 ml of saline, to approximately 1.5 cm in diameter. Any point along the length of the small bowel where easy passage of the balloon is hindered is marked, and a strictureplasty is performed. Several devices, including rigid balls, have been

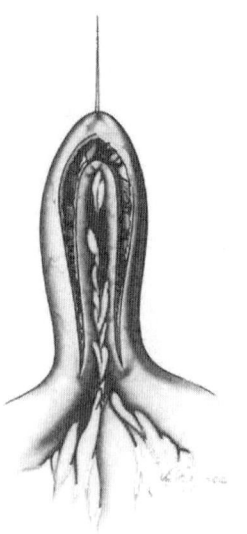
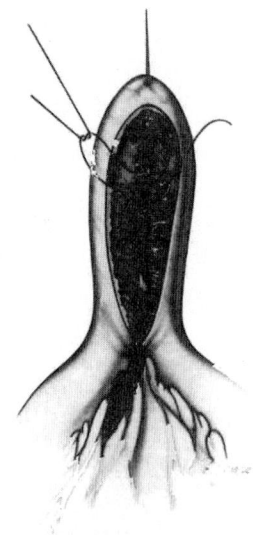
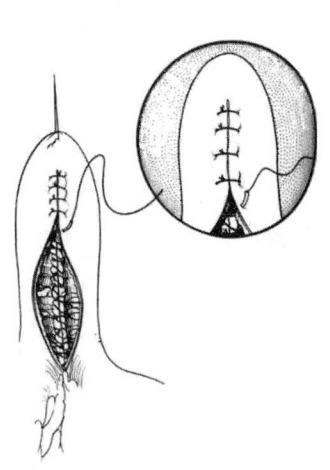

Figure 2 A Finney strictureplasty can be used for the treatment of a long stricture. The enteroenterostomy is performed after the stricture is divided along the antimesenteric border, and the involved bowel is folded onto itself in a U shape. The cut edges of the bowel on the interior of the U are sutured together as the back wall of the anastomosis, and the outer edges are sutured together as the front wall.

described but really confer no real advantage over the more readily available jejunal tube with a balloon.

Although there is no defined upper limit of strictureplasties that can be performed safely, each strictureplasty site represents a potential site for a leak, which can be a catastrophic complication in a patient with Crohn's disease. Therefore the decision to perform multiple strictureplasties instead of a single resection must be weighed carefully.

Other unusual configurations for strictureplasty may be useful and are designed to be used for longer strictures (>4–5 cm) or for multiple strictures in a short segment of bowel. The Finney strictureplasty (named after the Finney pyloroplasty) resembles a side-to-side anastomosis (Fig. 2). This strictureplasty may be useful in a patient with a long stricture or for a segment with multiple short strictures closely grouped together with intervening dilated short segments of bowel. The bowel is folded at the stricture, with the normal proximal and distal bowel brought alongside one another.

If a hand-sewn technique is used, there are two options. First, if the strictured area is mildly stenotic and the bowel is of reasonable quality, the entire stricture may be opened along the antimesenteric border, and a hand-sewn, essentially side-to-side anastomosis may be performed along the length of the enterotomy. Second, if the stricture is too tight or the bowel is not suitable for suturing, then a true side-to-side anastomosis between the proximal and distal normal bowel can be performed, leaving the strictured segment in place as a short bypassed segment. Similarly, if a stapling device is used, a side-to-side anastomosis can be fashioned between the normal proximal and distal bowel, leaving the strictured segment in continuity. The concern with this type of strictureplasty is that it results in a bypassed segment. Although the segment is short, there are concerns about possible complications, including bacterial overgrowth and malignant degeneration.

In patients with two strictures in close proximity, the bowel is entered on the antimesenteric border, and both strictures are divided, as is the normal intervening segment. The resulting long enterotomy is closed transversely (Fig. 3).

When the bowel is markedly dilated proximal to a short stricture, the size discrepancy between the proximal and distal normal bowel often precludes a Heineke-Mikulicz strictureplasty. In these instances, a Moskel-Walske-Neumayer strictureplasty is performed (Fig. 4). This strictureplasty is essentially a Y-to-V advancement flap closure of the stricture. The stricture is opened along the antimesenteric border as a Y-shaped enterotomy, with the Y portion in the dilated bowel just proximal to the stricture. The strictured

segment is then pulled apart, and the antimesenteric segment of the proximal bowel is advanced into the strictured area and closed in a transverse fashion, with one side of the closure being normal bowel along the entire length and the other being the two strictured bowel edges.

Michelassi has developed a unique procedure for dealing with the most difficult type of stricture, long (>20 cm) or a series of strictures in close proximity. In these highly unusual patients, a long segment of bowel that would result in a prohibitively extensive resection can be retained as a side-to-side isoperistaltic stricture-plasty (Fig. 5). In this technique, the bowel is completely divided transversely at the middle of the strictured segment. Unlike other strictureplasties, the mesentery is divided perpendicular to the long axis of the bowel to permit the two segments of bowel to be over-lapped and positioned side-to-side along the entire length of the divided segments. Both strictured segments are opened along the antimeseneteric border, and the antimesenteric faces of bowel are sewn one to the other in an isoperistaltic fashion. This technique has the advantage of not leaving bypassed bowel segments. Because a small number of patients require this type of strictureplasty, reports of long-term functional results are limited.

Some authors have advocated colonic strictureplasty, but such an operation has limited appeal because the colon is not essential for nutrient absorption and an isolated colonic stricture could harbor an occult malignancy. However, there may be patients in whom preservation of colonic mucosal surface area in the setting of an existing short bowel is important for water and electrolyte homeostasis. In this rare circumstance, an isolated colonic strictureplasty may be performed after the stricture has been extensively biopsied to ensure that there is no evidence of dysplasia or malignancy.

RESULTS

Nearly all series of strictureplasties are single institutional reports. Dietz and colleagues have reported the safety and long-term efficacy of strictureplasty in 314 patients with obstructing small bowel Crohn's disease. They reviewed 1124 strictureplasties performed in 314 patients. The overall morbidity was 18%, and septic complications occurred in 5%. Crohn's disease recurred in 34% of patients with a median follow-up of 7.5 years. The only significant predictor of recurrence was earlier age at the time of the index strictureplasty. These data were predominantly collected before the routine use of immunomodulators and biological therapies such as infliximab in the treatment of Crohn's disease. Similar findings were reported

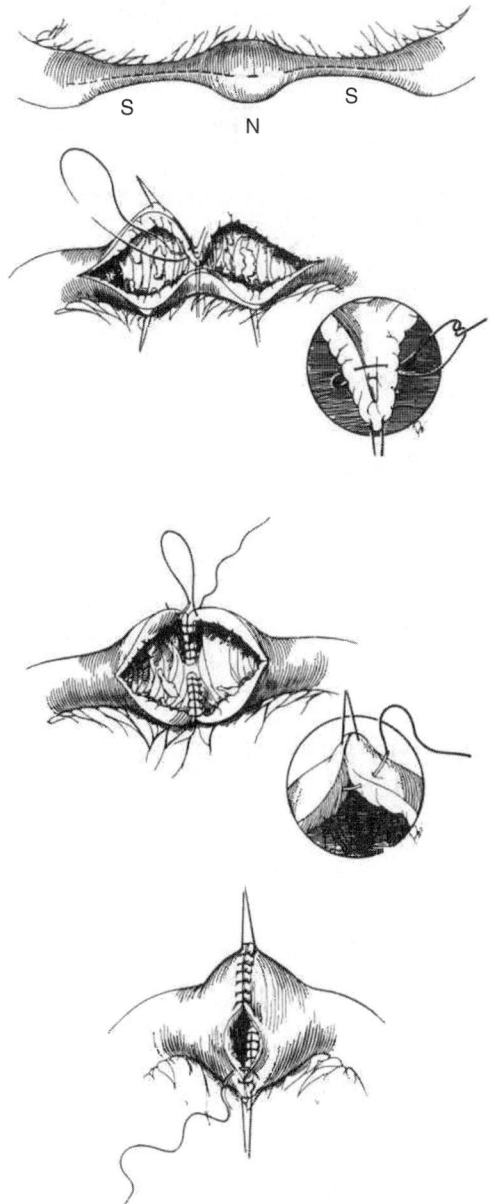

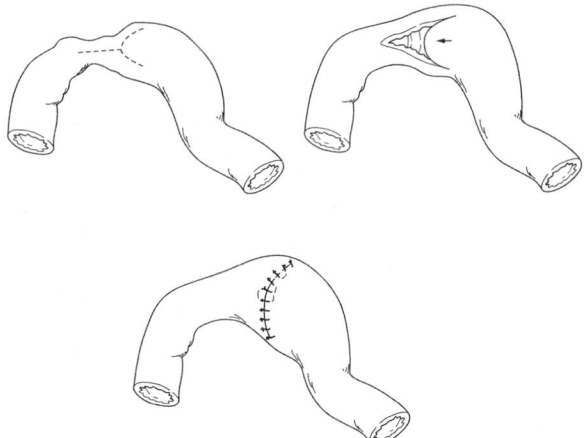

Figure 4 The Moskel-Walske-Neumayer strictureplasty is used when there is a significant size difference between the proximal and distal bowel segments adjacent to a short stricture. Instead of a longitudinal incision, a Y-shaped enterotomy is performed, and then the enterotomy is closed in a transverse fashion. *From Tichansky D, Cagir B, Yoo E, and others: Dis Colon Rectum 43:911-919, 2000.*

Figure 3 A modified Heineke–Mikulicz strictureplasty can be used for two short-segment strictures that are close to one another with a normal or dilated segment of bowel between them.

by Fearnhead and colleagues, who performed 479 strictureplasties in 100 patients.

An interesting meta-analysis of the available literature was performed by Tichansky and colleagues, who analyzed 1825 strictureplasties performed in 506 patients, as reported in 15 articles. They found that 90% of all strictures treated with strictureplasties were less than 10 cm in length. The Heineke–Mikulicz technique was used in 85%, and 13% were treated with a Finney strictureplasty. Forty-four percent of all procedures included a concurrent bowel resection.

Overall the literature supports the safety and efficacy of strictureplasty in the treatment of obstructing small bowel Crohn's disease, with nearly all studies reporting acceptable operative morbidity and recurrence rates, comparable to traditional resectional surgery. There are too few data to make recommendations regarding the use of this technique for colonic strictures.

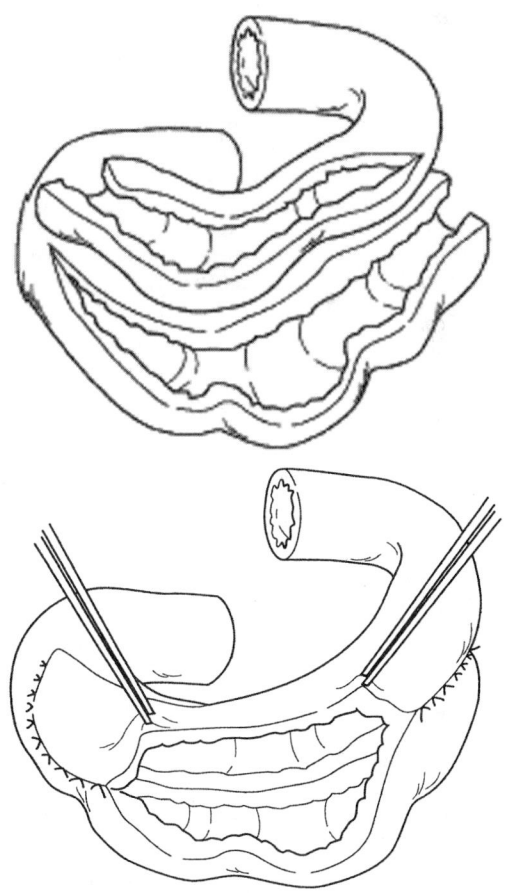

Figure 5 Side-to-side isoperistaltic strictureplasty is used for a long segment of involved bowel that would require resection because of multiple consecutive strictures. The involved bowel is divided in the midportion of the segment and a minimal portion of mesentery to allow the two segments to be slid over one another and laid side to side in an isoperistaltic fashion. An enteroenterostomy is performed, with the two cut edges closest to one another being closed as a back wall and the others being closed as the front wall. *From Tichansky D, Cagir B, Yoo E, and others: Dis Colon Rectum 43:911-919, 2000.*

SUMMARY

The primary role of strictureplasty is to preserve small bowel length in patients who have severe diffuse medically refractory disease or in patients who have recurrent disease. The goal is to preserve bowel length without constructing long bypass segments. In situations in which the integrity of the strictureplasty is in question or a long bypass segment will be constructed, the patient is best served by the surgeon's performing a resection rather than risk the associated complications of leaks from multiple strictureplasties or of bacterial overgrowth and bowel dysfunction caused by a bypassed segment. When strictureplasty is used appropriately, it is an important and useful operation for patients with complex Crohn's disease.

SUGGESTED READINGS

Dietz DW, Laureti S, Strong SA, and others: Safety and longterm efficacy of strictureplasty in 314 patients with obstructing small bowel Crohn's disease, *J Am Coll Surg* 192:330, 2001.
Fearnhead NS, Chowdhury R, Box B, and others: Long-term follow-up of strictureplasty for Crohn's disease, *Br J Surg* 93:475, 2006.
Lee EC, Papaionnou N: Minimal surgery for chronic obstruction inpatients with extensive or universal Crohn's disease, *Ann R Coll Surg Engl* 64:229, 1982.
Michelassi F: Side-to-side isoperistaltic strictureplasty for multiple Crohn's strictures, *Dis Colon Rectum* 39:344, 1996.
Roy P, Kumar D: Strictureplasty, *Br J Surg* 91:1428, 2004.
Wolff BG: Factors determining recurrence following surgery for Crohn's disease, *World J Surg* 22:364, 1998.

SMALL BOWEL TUMORS

Vitaliy Y. Poylin, MD, and Josef E. Fischer, MD

INTRODUCTION

Tumors of the small bowel are rarely encountered in general practice. Although the small bowel accounts for more than 90% of the mucosal surface of the gastrointestinal (GI) tract, these tumors represent only 1.0 to 1.5% of all GI neoplasms.

Factors thought to explain this disparity include the presence of high levels of secretory immunoglobulins (IgA), rapid transit time, presence of pancreatic enzymes, and low bacterial loads. Small bowel tumors have shown a slight predominance in African Americans, but this is not well established. There is a clear association with inflammatory bowel disease and a slight increase in the incidence of these tumors over the past 30 years, although no clear explanation has yet been proposed.

Most tumors of the small intestine are benign (Table 1) and show minimal or no clinical symptoms, whereas malignant tumors are more likely to be symptomatic, leading to their eventual diagnosis. Unfortunately, these lesions often are not discovered until they have metastasized to distant sites. An estimated 30% of patients with malignant neoplasms of small bowel have metastatic disease at the time of presentation. In operations for otherwise unexplained enteritis, small bowel adenocarcinoma is not recognized up to 50% of the time. The rarity of small bowel tumors, coupled with delayed presentation and nonspecific symptoms, complicates their diagnosis and treatment.

CLINICAL PRESENTATION

The presenting signs and symptoms of small bowel tumors are nonspecific and often poorly defined (Table 2). Benign masses are most often asymptomatic and discovered during radiological studies, surgery, or autopsy. When symptomatic, benign tumors present as intussusception, obstruction of the small bowel, intermittent abdominal pain, nausea, and vomiting. Intermittent gastrointestinal bleeding occurs in approximately 10% of cases and is more common with hemangiomas and spindle cell tumors. Weight loss is the most common symptom of malignant tumors. A large proportion of patients are significantly malnourished by the time they present to the surgeon. Abdominal pain is described as crampy, generalized, and intermittent. Although symptoms of obstruction may be the initial presentation, this likely marks advanced stage in the disease process, given the liquid consistency of small bowel contents. Along with obstruction, bleeding may also be an initial presenting symptom of malignant tumors. Perforations from small bowel tumors are rare and are more likely to be due to metastatic disease. Jaundice is also uncommon, with the exception of periampullary masses, and usually represents a poor prognosis, with likely liver metastases.

Table 1: Incidence of Small Bowel Tumors (Operative Series)

Type	Frequency (%)
Benign	30–40
GIST (benign or leiomyoma)	30–40
Adenoma	20–30
Lipoma	15
Hemangioma	10
Other	15
Malignant	60–70
Adenocarcinoma	30–50
Carcinoid	20–30
Lymphoma	15
GIST (malignant)	10–20

GIST, gastrointestinal stromal tumor.

Table 2: Clinical Presentation of Small Bowel Tumors

Occurrence: Benign Tumors		Occurrence: Malignant Tumors	
Symptom	**%**	**Symptom**	**%**
Asymptomatic	>50	Weight loss	>90
Pain	20–30	Abdominal pain	80
Obstruction	20	Obstruction	15–35
Bleeding	10	Abdominal mass	15
		Bleeding	10
		Perforation	10
		Jaundice	1–2

Modified from Ashley SW, Wells SA, Jr: Semin Oncol 15:116, 1988.

DIAGNOSIS

Many diagnostic modalities are available to aid in the discovery of suspected small bowel neoplasms. It is essential to communicate a suspected diagnosis to the radiologist to improve chance of diagnosis. Plain films may readily demonstrate an obstructive pattern or evidence of perforation, but they remain nonspecific and are generally not helpful. Upper GI (UGI) and small bowel follow through (SBFT) studies have been traditionally used to diagnose small bowel neoplasms. These studies are easy to perform, readily available, well tolerated, and cost effective but are limited by sensitivities of approximately 50% each.

Computerized tomography (CT) is gaining an increased role in the diagnosis of this disease. With the significantly improved quality of axial CT scans in recent years, the sensitivity of this modality has reached 57% to 65%. It is particularly useful in identifying proximal jejunal tumors. In addition to localizing the mass, a CT scan can be helpful in identifying extraluminal extension of the disease, the degree of wall invasion and surrounding tissue involvement, and lymphatic and intra-abdominal spread. In some instances, CT may also aid in histologic diagnosis for masses with a certain radiological appearance. Magnetic resonance imaging (MRI) is generally not used because it is more costly and does not provide information beyond that obtained by CT. Enteroclysis, a more difficult study to perform, involves advancement of an orointestinal or nasointestinal tube into the small bowel, with subsequent performance of a single or double contrast study. Sensitivity of enteroclysis for small bowel tumors can approximate 90%.

In recent years, there has been an increased use of oral endoscopic capsules, offering yet another diagnostic modality. Appealing because of its ability to visualize distal jejunal and ileal lesions that could otherwise only be visualized during surgery, this technique also has many potential drawbacks: difficulty of tumor localization, limited mucosal evaluation secondary to obscured views (because of small bowel contents), and inability to reexamine areas of potential pathology. The usefulness of this method and its sensitivity in comparison with other methods has yet to be determined.

Gastroduodenoscopy and small bowel enteroscopy are useful in identifying duodenal and proximal jejunal tumors (Fig. 1). They also provide an opportunity for tissue diagnosis with biopsy. They are, however, limited by their inability to access distal pathology.

In cases with GI bleeding with rates of at least 0.1 to 1.0 ml/min, angiography and 99Tc red-cell scintigraphy may be useful. These modalities are usually employed following negative upper and lower endoscopies. Although sensitivity may approach 80%, careful patient selection is necessary to achieve these high diagnostic rates.

BENIGN TUMORS

Adenoma

Adenomas comprise the second largest group of benign tumors (after GI stromal tumors [GISTs]) and may be associated with familial syndromes, such as familial adenomatous polyposis and Gardner's syndrome. There are three types of adenomas in the small bowel: tubular, villous, and Brunner gland. Tubular adenomas are often pedunculated and have low malignant potential. Villous adenomas have a much higher rate of malignant conversion, especially when their size increases beyond 2 cm. Brunner gland adenomas arise from hyperplastic exocrine glands in the proximal duodenum. These tumors are generally asymptomatic and have no malignant potential.

Because most adenomas are found in the duodenum, they can often be diagnosed and managed by EGD (esophagogastroduodenoscopy). Endoscopic excision alone is generally appropriate for tubular and Bruner gland adenomas. In contrast, endoscopic therapy is only appropriate with villous adenomas if complete excision can be safely accomplished, and transduodenal resection and local excision should be considered. If clear margins cannot be achieved or an invasive component is identified, pancreatoduodenal resection should be performed. Adenomas found more distally in the small bowel may become leading points for intussusception or a source of bleeding, necessitating their removal by simple segmental resection.

Lipoma

Lipoma is rarely found in the small intestine, most commonly occurring in the duodenum and jejunum (Fig. 2). Presenting symptoms include bleeding (can be occult or brisk), an intussusception, or

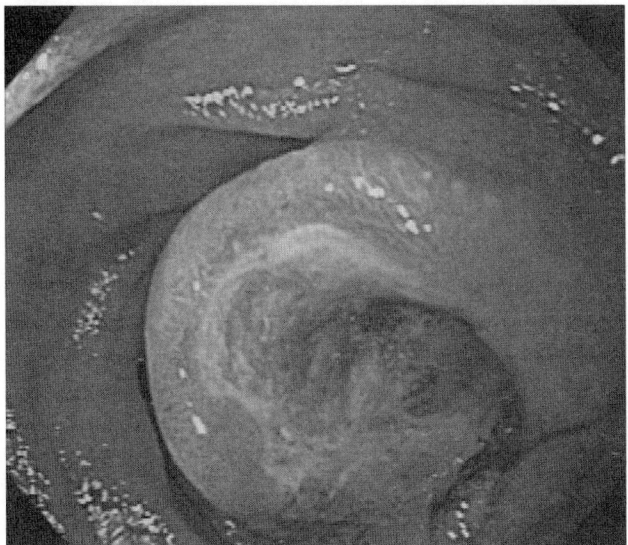

Figure 1 Endoscopic picture of gastrointestinal stromal tumors in the proximal jejunum.

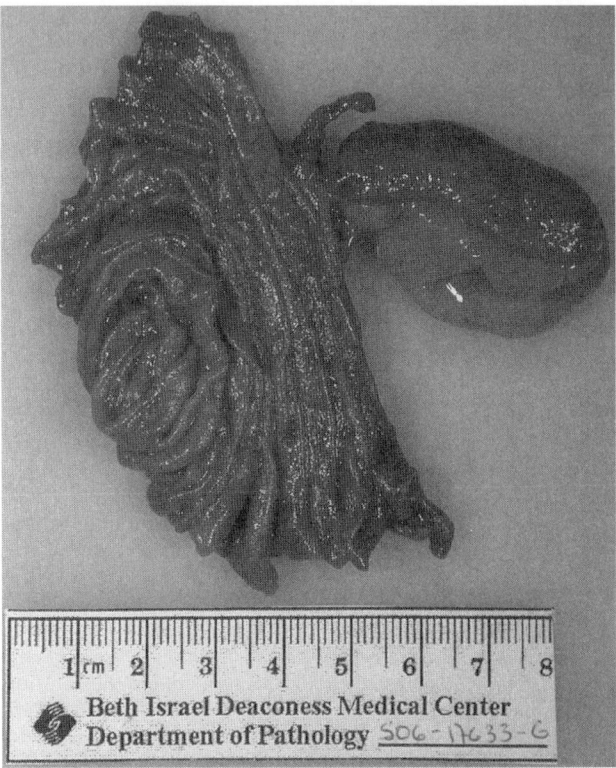

Figure 2 Gross picture of lipoma of the jejunum.

obstruction. Lipomas can usually be identified by CT scan because of their high fat content. Treatment is required only for symptomatic lesions, and this can be done by either endoscopic or segmental resection.

Hemangioma

Hemangiomas are another uncommon small bowel tumor. They may be single or multiple and may involve the entire GI tract as seen in Osler-Weber-Rendu disease. Diagnosis can be established by endoscopy or bleeding studies. Treatment by segmental resection or endoscopy is similar to that for lipomas but necessary only if the tumor is symptomatic.

Hamartoma

Seen almost exclusively in Peutz-Jeghers syndrome, this tumor is an autosomal-dominant disorder characterized by mucocutaneous melanotic pigmentation and multiple gastrointestinal polyps. Polyps have the potential to cause obstruction or intussusception. If resection is necessary, it should be limited to the area of active disease. These patients have an increased risk of adenocarcinoma and should be monitored closely.

MALIGNANT TUMORS

Carcinoid

Carcinoid tumors arise from enterochromatic-type Kulchitsky cells. Because of the distribution of these cells, carcinoid most often originates in the terminal ileum and appendix. Proximal ileal and jejunal locations are less likely, with nearly 80% of the tumors found within 2 feet of the ileocecal valve.

Primary tumors are usually singular, small (<2 cm), submucosal, and yellow-orange in color, although in some cases, multicentric disease can be found. Because of the slow development of carcinoid, many are found incidentally during surgery or autopsy. Similar to other small bowel tumors, symptomatic carcinoid presentation is vague, and metastatic disease is common at the time of initial presentation. Carcinoid tumors usually present with obstruction; bleeding or perforation are rare. It is thought that because of local effects of serotonin and growth factors, mesenteric fibrosis and desmoplastic reactions develop. As these progress, the mesentery will commonly constrict, pulling the tumor closer to the retroperitoneum. This kinking and fibrosis are often found at operation to be the cause of the obstruction.

Carcinoid syndrome is a rare manifestation of this disease, found in only 10% of the patients, and is caused by high levels of serotonin and other amines. Symptoms include diarrhea and flushing (lasting seconds to minutes) and, less commonly, bronchospasm, hypotension, tachycardia, coma, and death. Serotonin is readily cleared from portal circulation by the liver, thus carcinoid syndrome occurs only with liver or extramesenteric metastasis, when serotonin and other substances can be absorbed into systemic circulation by bypassing the liver. Natural progression of carcinoid syndrome includes eventual fibrosis of the pulmonic valve, leading to right-sided heart failure.

Although carcinoid tumors can be diagnosed by measuring levels of serotonin in the urine, relatively high levels are necessary for detection. CT scanning can efficiently demonstrate location, retroperitoneal extension, and mesenteric metastasis. Mesenteric mass with radiating densities is considered pathognomonic for carcinoid tumor. An octreotide scan can detect carcinoid tumor with more then 90% sensitivity and should be used as part of

metastatic workup in these patients. A positron emission tomography scan with labeled serotonin is also sensitive and is gaining popularity for diagnosis and follow-up.

Management of a carcinoid tumor depends on the location and size of the mass. Small duodenal tumors can be managed by enucleation, but larger masses require pancreatoduodenectomy. Tumors of the ileum and jejunum should be treated by en bloc resection if possible. Removal of lymphatic metastases has been shown to slow progression of the disease and lessen the number of future abdominal complications. Care should be taken to inspect the full length of the bowel to look for multicentric disease. Liver metastases should be removed by resection or ablation to lessen the chances of the patient's developing carcinoid syndrome. Surgeons should be aware that manipulation and general anesthesia may cause life-threatening carcinoid crisis, and intravenous somatostatin should be on hand for immediate administration.

Adjuvant therapy is generally not useful for carcinoid because these tumors show only a 20% to 30% response to chemotherapy and no response to radiation therapy. Octreotide can be used for palliation in severe cases and has been shown to decrease symptoms in nearly 30% of patients for more than 2 years. The overall 5-year survival rate is 60%, with an increase to nearly 100% for small tumors. Even in the presence of metastatic disease, median survival exceeds 15 years for patients with resectable lesions. Survival of patients with resectable liver metastasis is approximately 50% and decreases to less than 42% if metastases are nonresectable. During prolonged medical therapy, mesenteric fibrosis may progress, with an increased chance of vascular and intestinal entrapment. Early operation has been linked to better outcomes.

Adenocarcinoma

Adenocarcinoma accounts for 30% to 50% of malignant small bowel tumors, occurring more frequently in the duodenum than in the distal small bowel. The most important risk factor for development of adenocarcinoma is the presence of Crohn's disease. The incidence of Crohn's carcinoma seems to be 25 to 100 times more than the expected chance of carcinoma in enteritis and has different demographic distribution from that of spontaneous adenocarcinoma. One of the most common sites of occurrences of adenocarcinoma complicating Crohn's disease is following bypass. Initially Ginsberg and Garlock, two New York City surgeons active in the early surgical therapies of regional enteritis, carried out ileoceacectomy, but the mortality was excessive. Bypass was then used heavily, leaving the areas of acute inflammation and sepsis in place. After a latency period of 15 to 20 years, a number of those patients presented with adenocarcinoma. These patients are no longer appearing because in the late 1950s and early 1960s resection and end-to-end or end-to-side anastomosis became standard, and bypass essentially disappeared. Other risk factors include familial adenomatous polyposis, celiac sprue, cystic fibrosis, and a family history of hereditary nonpolyposis colorectal cancer.

The most common presenting symptoms include abdominal pain, weight loss, feelings of fullness and signs of obstruction. Diagnosis of adenocarcinoma depends on the location. EGD with biopsy is a common modality used for duodenal masses, whereas enteroclysis and other contrast studies can be employed for distal locations. On contrast studies, adenocarcinoma appears as an annular or apple core lesion with ulceration. CT scanning is also useful to assess location and resectability.

Surgical resection is the centerpiece of adenocarcinoma management. Periampular disease should be treated with a Whipple procedure. It is interesting to note that patients who undergo pancreatoduodenectomy are more likely to be disease free than patients with more distal disease who undergo resection. This phenomenon is most likely due to the earlier detection of duodenal masses, as well as the lymphadenectomy associated with Whipple procedures.

Distal duodenal and ileal and jejunal adenocarcinoma should be managed by en bloc resection with wide margins. A wide wedge of the mesentery should be taken because of the high incidence of local nodal metastasis. Before resection, extensive exploration should be performed to rule out serosal and liver metastasis. However, with the exception of extensive disease, local lymph node invasion is not a contraindication for surgery. In fact, removal of these nodes has been shown to decrease the rate of local recurrence and improve quality of life by decreasing the rate of future episodes of obstructions and bleeding. For distal ileal locations, right colectomy should be performed in conjunction with small bowel resection because it affords more effective node dissection.

Successful removal of the tumor and lymph node involvement are the biggest predictors of long-term survival. If lymph node invasion is present, 5-year survival for jejunal and ileal disease decreases from 70% to 80% to 10% to 15%. Tumor location also affects long-term prognosis, as mentioned earlier, with duodenal disease having better outcomes. Unfortunately, less than 50% of the small bowel adenocarcinomas are contained and nearly 25% present as stage IV disease. The value of chemoradiotherapy is not well defined. Most oncologists recommend adjuvant therapy, although benefits are not clear.

Lymphoma

The third most common type of malignant small bowel neoplasm, lymphoma accounts for 15% of patients with small bowel tumors. This disease usually appears in the fifth and sixth decade of life, with a slight male predominance. Most of these tumors are non–Hodgkin's B-cell lymphomas with intermediate or high-grade features arising from small bowel–associated lymphoid tissue and are more likely to come from the ileum than jejunum. Patients with malabsorptive syndromes or immunocompromised states have a greater chance of lymphoma development. These categories include Crohn's disease, celiac sprue, AIDS, systemic lupus erythematosus, and transplant recipients.

Small bowel lymphoma usually presents with some combination of abdominal pain, fatigue, fever, malaise, and weight loss. Generalized lymphadenopathy is common, and a palpable abdominal mass can be identified in 18% to 30% of patients. One fourth of patients present with obstruction, intussusception, or hemorrhage. Mediterranean lymphoma, a variant most commonly found in underdeveloped countries, presents with diarrhea, steatorrhea, and colicky pain.

The diagnosis of lymphoma can be made using contrast studies, which commonly reveal thickened mucosa, or CT scan, showing thickened bowel wall, enlarged nodes, and often a mass.

Resection of the affected small bowel and its adjacent mesentery is the first-line therapy, and there is significantly improved survival if complete resection can be achieved. Debulking is considered beneficial as long as nutritional absorption is not compromised. During operation, thorough exploration should be performed for staging purposes.

Chemotherapy, although commonly offered, does not show clear survival benefits. Radiation therapy is beneficial; however, it is associated with multiple complications. Overall prognosis is poor and depends on the disease stage. Five-year survival is 20% to 40% for localized disease and less than 1 year for disseminated disease.

Gastrointestinal Stromal Tumors

Gastrointestinal stromal tumors (GISTs) represent 10% to 20% of small bowel malignancies. GISTs are thought to originate from the intestinal cell of Cajal, intestinal pacemaker cells, or a common

progenitor of the two. Both cells have similar histochemical and immunochemical appearance, and both express the transmembrane tyrosine receptor CD117 (KIT). Staining with monoclonal antibody for expression of KIT has become the gold standard for GIST identification. GIST attracts widespread attention because the principal genetic defect responsible has been identified to be a gain-of-function mutation in the c-kit proto-oncogene. In some cases, platelet derived growth factor–a (PDGF-a) has been found responsible. A specific molecular inhibitor of both factors, imatinib mesalet (Gleevec [Novartis Pharmaceuticals, East Hanover, NJ]) has been developed.

GISTs distribute evenly throughout the small bowel. These tumors arise from the submucosa and can be recognized by their smooth appearance (Fig. 3). As a result of their slow growth rates, the tumors often remain asymptomatic for long periods of life. Patients usually present with abdominal pain, weight loss, and obstruction caused by external compression. The tumors tend to be vascular, and as they become larger, central necrosis and bleeding can develop. Nearly 50% of people have an abdominal mass by the time of presentation. These tumors often have a "dumbbell" configuration, with small intraluminal component and a large extraluminal component.

CT scan is useful for both diagnosis and metastatic workup, and a large round mass with central necrosis can usually be identified. SBFT may show external compression from the smooth mass and occasionally a contrast-filled cavity secondary to necrosis (Fig. 4). The rendering of central necrosis may contribute to presentation of these tumors with rapture. The vascular nature of GIST is a factor in presentation that can mimic ruptured aortic abdominal aneurysm and sudden abdominal pain and hypotension. The ruptured tumor is likely malignant and accompanied by peritoneal carcinomatosis.

Despite the fact that complete resection can be achieved in 85% of patients, GISTs have a high rate of recurrence and metastatic potential. In fact, 5-year disease-free survival is only 50%. The introduction of Gleevec has reshaped the treatment approach for GIST. This medication has minimal toxicity and primary response rates of nearly 60%. Surgery is still the treatment of choice for primary nonmetastatic disease, and segmental resection with tumor-free margins is usually sufficient. These tumors metastasize hematogenously, and extensive local resection is not indicated. Locally advanced and metastatic disease carried a dismal prognosis in the pre-Gleevec era, with no significant benefits of surgical resection. Today new indications for surgery have emerged in these groups. Patients who initially have a global response to Gleevec

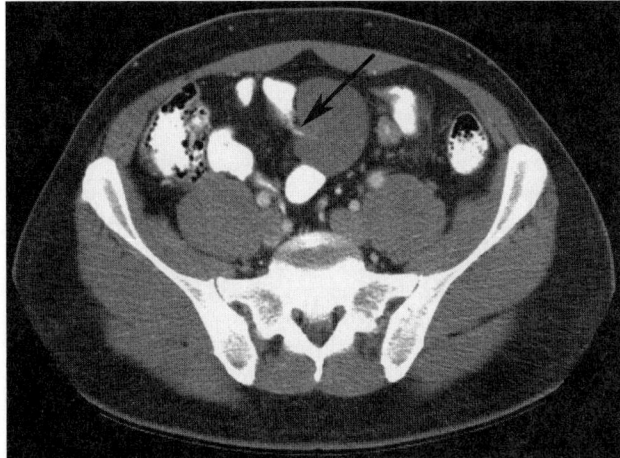

Figure 3 Computerized tomogram of a patient with small bowel gastrointestinal stromal tumors. Communication with the bowel lumen often seen in these tumors (*arrow*).

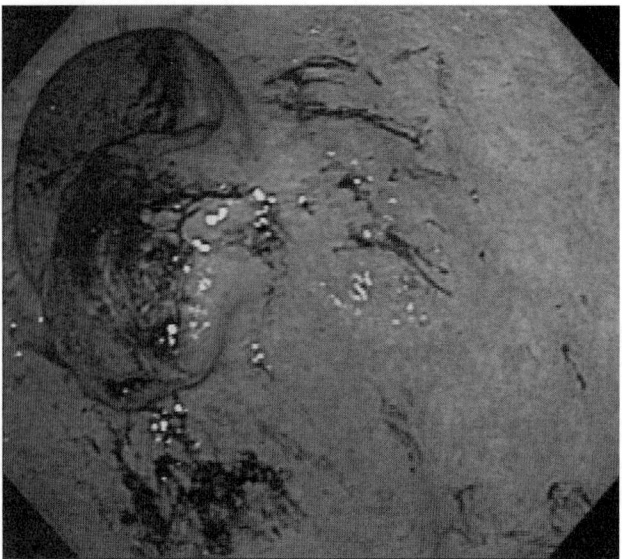

Figure 4 Endoscopic picture of gastrointestinal stromal tumors in the stomach with typical smooth surface and often-seen pedunculated appearance.

Table 3: Malignant Risk for Gastrointestinal Stromal Tumors

Risk	Size (cm)*	Mitotic Count (/50 HPF†)
Very low	<2	<5
Low	2–5	<5
Intermediate	<5	6–10
		<5
High	>5	>5
	>10	Any mitotic count
	Any size	>10

Modified from Fletcher CD, Berman JJ, Corless C, and others: Hum Pathol 33:459, 2002.
*Size is the single largest dimension.
†Mitotic count per 50 high-power fields.

Metastatic Disease

Metastases to the small bowel are most common type of all tumors found in the small bowel. Abdominal pain, weight loss, nausea, vomiting and bleeding are the most common presenting symptoms. Primary sites include colorectal cancer (most common), melanoma, pancreatic, ovarian, and lung carcinoma. Resection should be performed only for palliative purposes.

SUGGESTED READINGS

Akerstrom GP, Hellman P, Hessman O, and others: Management of midgut carcinoids, *J Surg Oncol* 89161, 2005.
Ashley SW, Wells SA Jr. Tumors of the small intestine, *Semin Oncol* 15:116, 1988.
Naef M, Buhlmann M, Baer HU: Small bowel tumors: diagnosis, therapy and prognostic factors, *Langenbecks Arch Surg* 384:176, 1999.
Neuhaus SJ, Clark MA, Hayes AJ, and others: Surgery for gastrointestinal stromal tumour in the post-imatinib era, *ANZ J Surg* 75:165, 2005.
Stahl D, Tyler G, Fischer JE: Inflammatory bowel disease—relationship to carcinoma, *Curr Probl Cancer* 5:1, 1981.

but later develop resistance or have stable disease while still on treatment seem to benefit from resection of the primary site. It is important to note that these indications have not yet been confirmed in long-term studies. Recurrent disease or recurrent disease after surgery is now treated primarily with imatinib and subsequently appears to offer only minimal benefit. Another approach currently under investigation is the use of Gleevec as a neoadjuvant agent and possibly in patients with complete resection. Although histopathologic distinction between benign and malignant GIST can be made on the basis of tumor size, site, and mitotic rate, many people doubt whether these tumors are ever really benign (Table 3).

DIVERTICULOSIS OF THE SMALL BOWEL

Douglas Bernstein, MD, Frederic E. Eckhauser, MD, and Martin A. Makary, MD, MPH

Diverticulosis of the small bowel is an uncommon condition that is clinically significant because of the potential gravity of its complications. The overall prevalence of small bowel diverticulosis is reported to be between 0.3% and 4.5% by autopsy series and is approximately 1% on the basis of small bowel contrast studies performed for unrelated reasons. Less than 4% of all small bowel diverticula cause symptoms. However, complications such as malabsorption, obstruction, hemorrhage, inflammation, and perforation are well documented in the literature.

There are two types of small bowel diverticula. These include false diverticula that arise in the duodenum and jejunoileum and true diverticula that arise in the distal ileum (Meckel's diverticulum). Duodenal and jejunoileal diverticula are acquired defects of the intestinal wall. They occur on the mesenteric aspect of the bowel at the points where nutrient blood vessels penetrate through the intestinal wall. Mucosa and submucosa herniate through these weak points, forming thin-walled diverticula that lack a muscular layer and lie embedded between the leaves of the mesentery. By comparison, a Meckel's diverticulum is a "true" diverticulum. As such, it is a congenital anomaly and contains all layers of the normal intestinal wall. Meckel's diverticula are located on the antimesenteric portion of the bowel. The symptoms, diagnostic evaluation, and surgical treatment of these diverticula vary considerably.

DUODENAL DIVERTICULA

Pathogenesis and Diagnosis

A duodenal diverticulum is most often diagnosed as a solitary extraluminal protrusion that occurs during or after the fifth decade of life. These diverticula account for 45% of all small bowel diverticula. Although less than 1% require treatment, surgery for duodenal diverticula is associated with significant morbidity and mortality.

Duodenal diverticula are characteristically located within 2 cm of the ampulla of Vater. Defects in the muscularis propria caused by penetration of the pancreatic and biliary ducts predispose to the development of "perivaterian" or "juxtaampullary" pulsion (false) diverticula. Proximity to the ampulla may cause sphincter dysfunction. Patients most commonly present with symptoms of biliary or pancreatic duct obstruction, including cholangitis, jaundice, or pancreatitis. Other less common presenting symptoms include inflammation, perforation, and hemorrhage. Duodenal diverticulitis may also present as epigastric pain radiating to the back or right shoulder and is often accompanied by nausea, vomiting, fever, and leukocytosis. It is frequently confused with peptic ulcer disease or other etiologies of pancreaticobiliary obstruction. Perforation most commonly occurs in the retroperitoneum adjacent to the second portion of the duodenum. Significant gastrointestinal bleeding may present as hematemesis, melena, or even hematochezia and requires surgical treatment.

The diagnostic modalities of choice to diagnose a duodenal diverticulum include esophagogastroduodenoscopy (EGD) or endoscopic retrograde cholangiopancreatography (ERCP). Both techniques provide direct visualization of the diverticulum, demonstrate its anatomic relationship to the ampulla, and facilitate transendoscopic intervention when indicated. Other useful diagnostic adjuncts include contrast radiography with small bowel follow-through and computerized tomography with both oral and intravenous contrast.

Treatment

The operative treatment of duodenal diverticula may be difficult. Endoscopic interventions, which primarily include sphincterotomy and stent placement, have been used successfully but carry a risk of iatrogenic perforation and retroperitonitis. If endoscopic interventions fail to relieve symptoms, surgery may be necessary. The surgical approach is fairly standard. An extensive Kocher maneuver is performed to mobilize and expose the duodenum. The next step is to clarify the anatomic relationship between the diverticulum and contiguous biliary or pancreatic ductal structures. The ampulla of Vater and any accessory pancreatic or biliary ducts should be positively identified. A metal probe or soft rubber catheter should be placed within the ampulla and accessory ducts for the duration of the operation. Retrograde access to the bile duct can be obtained using a transampullary approach. More complicated cases often require antegrade placement of a transampullary catheter via the cystic duct or a through small choledochotomy incision. The antegrade approach may be more useful in cases in which the presence of common bile duct calculi already dictates formal exploration of the common bile duct.

After the ampulla and any anatomic irregularities have been identified, simple diverticulectomy and primary closure may suffice, especially if no ducts are involved and there is no evidence of retroperitoneal contamination. To avoid developing a stricture of the duodenum, a tension-free, two-layer transverse or oblique closure should be performed. Inversion and simple oversewing of the diverticulum are no longer recommended.

For a wide-based diverticulum, there are two options. These include diverticulectomy, with placement of a jejunal serosal patch to close the defect, or segmental resection with end-to-end anastomosis. The latter is especially useful for duodenal diverticula that arise distal to the ampulla of Vater. If the ampulla is located within or directly adjacent to a diverticulum, surgery can be technically challenging and is potentially associated with significant morbidity. In such cases, a Roux-en-Y biliary bypass should be considered. This approach preserves sphincter function, diverts the enteric stream from the duodenum, and facilitates safe repair of the duodenal defect caused by the presence of the diverticulum.

The enteric stream can be diverted to treat perforations associated with significant retroperitoneal contamination. This reduces the incidence of high-output duodenal fistulae. Surgical options include an antrectomy with Billroth II gastrojejunal anastomosis or duodenal exclusion with simultaneous placement of gastrostomy and jejunostomy tubes for decompression and enteral feeding, respectively. It should be emphasized that few cases of perforation will require such extensive intervention; most are amenable to drainage alone.

All patients requiring surgery for duodenal diverticula should undergo cholecystectomy. This helps to prevent biliary stasis and calculus formation and avoids future diagnostic dilemmas. Duodenal diverticula that are discovered incidentally at laparotomy or following routine contrast studies rarely merit surgical intervention.

INTRALUMINAL DIVERTICULA

Although most duodenal diverticula are extraluminal in location, intraluminal or "windsock" diverticula are occasionally encountered in clinical practice. These are large, congenital saccular lesions originating from the second portion of the duodenum. Such diverticula may extend as far as the fourth portion of the duodenum. Small bowel obstruction is the most common complication of an intraluminal diverticulum arising in duodenum. The majority of such cases are associated with other anatomic abnormalities, including congenital biliary cysts, annular pancreas, malrotation, superior mesenteric artery compression syndrome, omphalocele, and various cardiac and urogenital abnormalities. A windsock diverticulum is best diagnosed with a barium contrast examination of the duodenum. A symptomatic windsock diverticulum is usually treated by primary excision.

JEJUNOILEAL DIVERTICULA

Pathogenesis and Diagnosis

Diverticula of the jejunum and ileum comprise 25% of all small bowel diverticula but are most likely of all small bowel diverticula to become symptomatic. Jejunoileal diverticula are commonly seen as multiple lesions. The incidence is highest in the jejunum and decreases more distally in the small intestine: 80% occur in the jejunum, 15% occur in the ileum, and 5% along the length of the entire small intestine. Patients who present with symptomatic diverticula are generally older than 50 years of age.

The pathogenesis of jejunoileal diverticula is related to myoneural abnormalities that originate in the myenteric plexus. Manometric studies have demonstrated dysmotility of the migrating motor complexes. This leads to spastic contractions of the bowel wall that create excessive and prolonged intraluminal pressures. This so-called jejunal dyskinesia is thought to play an integral role in the formation of jejunoileal diverticula.

Jejunal dyskinesia also contributes to the primary symptoms of small intestinal diverticula. Approximately 3.5% to 12% of patients show signs of chronic malabsorption caused by stasis and bacterial overgrowth within the diverticula. Clinical symptoms may include abdominal pain, steatorrhea, hypoproteinemia, megaloblastic anemia, and neuropathy. Inflammation, perforation, mechanical obstruction, and hemorrhage each occur in approximately 2% to 4% of patients with jejunoileal diverticula. Jejunoileal diverticula tend to occur on the mesenteric side of the bowel. Consequently, perforation may cause localized peritonitis that is walled off by the adjacent mesentery. Clinical manifestations of inflammation or perforation may be indistinguishable from acute appendicitis, and the diagnosis can often be made only by laparoscopy or laparotomy.

The preferred study for establishing the diagnosis of jejunoileal diverticula is an enteroclysis or dedicated small bowel contrast study. Computerized tomography or conventional contrast radiography of the gastrointestinal tract may be useful, but an enteroclysis is more likely to provide a definitive diagnosis. Clinical evidence of anemia, abdominal pain, and radiographic evidence of dilated small bowel loops, suggests the diagnosis of jejunoileal diverticulosis. There is no role for traditional endoscopy, but capsule endoscopy may place an increasing role in the future. An arteriogram or a tagged red blood cell scan may provide useful information in patients with evidence of occult or frank gastrointestinal hemorrhage.

Treatment

Uncomplicated jejunoileal diverticulitis can be treated conservatively, but laparoscopy or laparotomy is warranted for serious complications such as refractory inflammation, perforation, mechanical obstruction, or hemorrhage. To avoid complications such as intra-abdominal sepsis, anastomotic failure, and fistula formation, segmental resection is generally the preferred approach.

Malabsorption from bacterial overgrowth should first be treated medically. First-line therapy typically consists of metronidazole, with or without tetracycline, and aggressive vitamin supplementation. In the 25% of patients for whom medical therapy fails, segmental resection is recommended. Surgical excision should not be considered in an asymptomatic patient with jejunoileal diverticula that are discovered incidentally. In general, there is no role for prophylactic resection.

MECKEL'S DIVERTICULA

Pathogenesis and Diagnosis

Meckel's diverticula are true diverticula that contain all layers of the normal bowel wall. They constitute the most common congenital abnormality of the small bowel and comprise 25% of all small bowel diverticula.

During the fifth week of fetal gestation, the vitelline (omphalomesenteric) duct is obliterated. Failure of the duct to obliterate may lead to the formation of an ileo-umbilical fistula, a vitelline duct cyst, or, most commonly, a Meckel's diverticulum. A Meckel's diverticulum typically is located on the antimesenteric border of the ileum. Its blood supply arises from an anomalous branch (persistent right vitelline artery) of the superior mesenteric artery. Half of Meckel's diverticula contain heterotopic mucosa, of which gastric (75%) and pancreatic mucosa (15%) occur most commonly.

The "Rule of Two" classically describes the major clinical features of a Meckel's diverticulum. This anomaly is present in 2% of the population, is approximately 2 inches in length, occurs within 2 feet of the ileocecal valve, and may contain two types of heterotopic mucosa. Most patients develop symptoms within the first 2 years of life.

In children, lower gastrointestinal bleeding is the most common clinical manifestation of a Meckel's diverticulum. In fact, these anomalies are the most common cause of lower gastrointestinal bleeding in pediatric patients. Bleeding may present as melena or hematochezia. The cause is usually an ulcer that develops on the bowel wall opposite the diverticulum, in response to acid secretion from the heterotopic mucosa.

In the adult population, small bowel obstruction is the most common clinical manifestation and occurs in 45% of symptomatic patients. Obstruction may be secondary to an intussusception, a volvulus, or incarceration of the diverticulum within a Littre's hernia.

Diverticulitis occurs in 25% of patients and may be indistinguishable from acute appendicitis. The cause of inflammation is usually a fecalith or peptic acid exposure leading to ulceration. Hemorrhage occurs in 20% of patients, is generally painless, and results from ulceration of the bowel wall opposite the diverticulum. Neoplasms are rare.

The diagnosis of a Meckel's diverticulum can be made by contrast radiography or a radionuclide scan that uses ^{99m}Tc-pertechnetate. Because the radioisotope is taken up selectively by gastric mucosa, a positive scan occurs only in patients with a diverticulum that contains ectopic gastric mucosa. The scan is therefore most useful in cases of ulceration associated with gastrointestinal bleeding. The sensitivity of a Meckel's scan is approximately 85%, but the diagnostic yield can be improved by pretreating the patient with glucagon or pentagastrin. Selective arteriography may be useful to diagnose the site of bleeding if the rate of blood loss exceeds 0.5 ml/minute. The most useful arteriographic finding is a nonbranching end artery in the lower right abdomen that contains a cluster of small tortuous vessels at its distal end.

Despite the use of enteroclysis, radionuclide scintigraphy, and selective arteriography, most bleeding Meckel's diverticula are diagnosed at the time of exploratory surgery. Some authors have even suggested that radionuclide scintigraphy adds unnecessary time and expense to the evaluation and recommend exploratory laparoscopy as the first-line diagnostic and therapeutic modality.

Treatment

The surgical approach to a Meckel's diverticulum is determined primarily by the patient's clinical presentation. Small bowel obstruction should be treated as quickly as possible but only after the patient has been stabilized. In general, wedge excision of the diverticulum with a two-layer closure of the bowel wall is sufficient. Resection using a surgical stapler is also acceptable.

In patients with evidence of significant inflammation, hemorrhage, or a wide-based diverticulum, segmental resection with end-to-end anastomosis is generally the preferred approach. Patients who present with hemorrhage should always be treated with segmental resection rather than diverticulectomy because the bleeding ulcer is commonly on the wall opposite the diverticulum. The resected bowel should be opened to ensure that the ulcer has been completely excised. Any patient who requires surgery for a symptomatic Meckel's diverticulum should also undergo appendectomy to avoid future diagnostic dilemmas.

It is widely agreed that a Meckel's diverticulum that is discovered in a young child, whether symptomatic or discovered incidentally, should be removed. In contrast, there is considerable controversy as to whether an incidental Meckel's diverticulum should be resected in an adult. A review of the literature suggests that most surgeons do not recommend resection for an incidental Meckel's diverticulum in a patient 18 years or older. Relative indications for incidental diverticulectomy include the presence of palpable heterotopic tissue, signs of prior diverticulitis, and the presence of a mesodiverticular band. The nature of the symptoms and the pathology that led to the surgery, as well obstacles to future laparotomy such as abdominal radiation or adhesions, are also relative indications for resection of an asymptomatic diverticulum.

SUGGESTED READINGS

El-Haddawi F, Civil ID: Acquired jejuno-ileal diverticular disease: a diagnostic and management challenge, *ANZ J Surg* 73:584, 2003.

Gross SA, Katz S: Small bowel diverticulosis: an overlooked entity, *Curr Treat Options Gastroenterol* 6:3, 2003.

Kouraklis G, Mantas D, Glivanou A, and others: Diverticular disease of the small bowel: report of 27 cases, *Int Surg* 86:235, 2001.

Lempinen M, Salmela K, Kemppainen E: Jejunal diverticulosis: a potentially dangerous entity, *Scand J Gastroenterol* 9:905, 2004.

MESENTERIC VASCULAR DISEASE OF THE SMALL BOWEL

Jason F. Hall, MD, and Charles M. Ferguson, MD

INTRODUCTION

The vasculature of the abdominal viscera consists of three major vascular pedicles that are joined at several levels by collateral arcades. Although ischemic insults to this system are rare, they are often catastrophic unless promptly recognized and appropriately treated. Even with timely diagnosis, the mortality and morbidity associated with this diagnosis is high. Most series have reported mortalities as high as 60% to 70%. As the population ages, the incidence of mesenteric ischemia is increasing. The clinician must have a high degree of suspicion in persons presenting with abdominal pain without impressive physical findings. Once mesenteric ischemia is suspected, a diagnostic test is necessary to confirm the diagnosis.

Mesenteric ischemia is classically divided into acute and chronic. Acute mesenteric ischemia can be also further subdivided into four distinct mechanisms. These presentations include embolic, thrombotic, nonocclusive, and venous thrombosis. Chronic mesenteric ischemia is typically the result of long-standing, atherosclerotic, flow-limiting lesion.

ACUTE MESENTERIC ISCHEMIA

Clinical Presentation

The differing pathophysiologic processes responsible for acute mesenteric ischemia can result in varied clinical presentations. The classical description of a patient with an embolus to the mesenteric vessels is one of severe and constant abdominal pain that is not accompanied by physical findings of the same magnitude. Patients commonly have associated nausea, vomiting, and diarrhea. The diagnosis should certainly be suspected in any patient with atrial fibrillation, mural thrombus following myocardial infarction, cardiac valvular lesions, or risk factors for cholesterol embolization.

Patients with thrombosis of a mesenteric vessel typically describe prodomal symptoms that are consistent with a preexisting history of chronic mesenteric ischemia. These include postprandial pain, weight loss, nausea, and sitophobia. Nonocclusive mesenteric ischemia occurs in patients with widespread vasoconstriction. This condition is most commonly identified in critically ill patients with cardiogenic or septic shock and is often worsened by the patient's need for systemic vasopressors to maintain cerebral perfusion. Patients with mesenteric venous thrombosis often present much later in their clinical course and complain of diffuse abdominal pain that may be associated with nausea, anorexia, and diarrhea. These symptoms are typically insidious in onset and commonly occur over the course of weeks. Unfortunately, the mild nature of the symptoms makes diagnosis extremely difficult, such that most patients are not diagnosed until infarction and peritonitis are present.

The common endpoint of all these processes is bowel ischemia and necrosis. Should transmural necrosis occur, patients present with the typical constellation of findings, including fever, pain, septic shock, and peritonitis.

Diagnosis

As with any abdominal complaint, the history and physical examination are essential in developing suspicion of this diagnosis, but there are no basic radiological or laboratory tests that are diagnostic of mesenteric ischemia. As expected, many patients will have leukocytosis, and some will have elevated liver function tests. A more ominous sign is the development of lactic acidosis. Plain abdominal films may demonstrate thumbprinting of the small bowel, reflecting an edematous intestinal wall. This finding seldom spares the patient a more complex diagnostic procedure.

Computed tomographic angiography (CTA) and magnetic resonance angiography (MRA) are commonly used to establish the diagnosis of mesenteric ischemia. Helical, multidetector, multislice CTA is particularly useful because it can delineate the vascular anatomy in three dimensions. In addition, it can lend information about the condition of the small bowel and act as convenient screening tool for other abdominal conditions masquerading as ischemia. Findings of pneumatosis, small bowel wall thickening, portal venous gas, or obstruction of the mesenteric vessels are all suggestive of mesenteric ischemia. Recent prospective cohort trials assessing the efficacy of CTA have identified a 96% sensitivity and 94% specificity for diagnosing acute mesenteric ischemia. CT tends to be the initial test of choice when mesenteric ischemia is suspected in our institution.

Magnetic resonance angiography has undergone great advances over the past several years. Clinicians are now able to obtain high-resolution imaging of the mesenteric vessels in several three-dimensional views. MRAs are typically performed with gadolinium, which is significantly less nephrotoxic than contrast agents used for CTAs. This is often a consideration in elderly patients with tenuous renal function. Both MRA and CT scan are excellent for imaging ostial lesions but are less sensitive in imaging the distal branches of the celiac and superior mesenteric axes. Although MRA is widely available, the overall reliability of the technique is sometimes questionable. In addition, in our institution it is impractical to transport critically ill patients to the MRI suite.

Mesenteric angiography still remains the gold standard for establishing the diagnosis of mesenteric ischemia because it provides detailed imaging of both the proximal and distal mesenteric vasculature. The images are thought to be superior to those obtained by noninvasive means. Embolic disease typically presents as an obstruction just distal to the middle colic branch of the superior mesenteric artery (SMA). Thrombotic disease typically involves the ostia of the celiac or superior mesenteric artery resulting from long-standing atherosclerotic disease. Mesenteric angiography is not only diagnostic but can also be therapeutic in cases of nonocclusive ischemia because papaverine can be infused. There is growing experience with embolectomy using catheter-based techniques, and patients with chronic stenoses can often be treated with angioplasty and stenting.

Management

The management of acute mesenteric ischemia is slightly varied depending on its etiology. All patients are aggressively resuscitated with isotonic fluids, and all laboratory abnormalities are corrected. Because most patients are elderly and ill, they require placement of invasive hemodynamic monitors. Patients with peritonitis certainly mandate immediate exploration. It is helpful to prepare the thighs in case saphenous vein is required for patch angioplasty.

Patients with embolic disease typically present with sparing of the proximal jejunum and distal large bowel because the embolus is usually located just distal to the middle colic artery. The abdomen should be explored through a generous midline incision, and no bowel resections should be performed before vascular inflow is addressed. The SMA is exposed by retracting the transverse mesocolon cephalad and eviscerating the bowel to the patient's right side (Fig. 1). The ligament of Treitz is divided, and the SMA exposed. It is often necessary to fully mobilize the left renal vein to gain adequate control of the SMA (Fig. 2). Small jejunal branches limit exposure of the origin of the SMA but should be preserved to maintain flow to the distal duodenum and proximal jejunum. After proximal and distal control is achieved, systemic heparin is administered. A transverse arteriotomy and embolectomy are performed using a 4 F Fogarty catheter (Fig. 3). This is best performed with loupe magnification. The catheter is passed distally 15 to 20 cm and gently withdrawn, taking care not to injure the intima. Proximal inflow is ensured, and the vessel is flushed with heparinized saline solution before closure of the arteriotomy. If embolectomy is not fruitful, the diagnosis is generally thrombosis, and the surgeon must be prepared to perform a bypass procedure. The arteriotomy is closed with interrupted proline sutures. If there is any question of luminal narrowing, patch angioplasty techniques should be performed using either saphenous vein or polytetrafluoroethylene (PTFE) patch.

Patients with acute thrombosis of the SMA present with no sparing of the proximal jejunum because their lesions are typically ostial. If this diagnosis is suspected, the surgeon should be prepared to perform a retrograde bypass. The SMA is exposed as previously described. A vertical arteriotomy is performed because an endarterectomy is sometimes necessary. Bypass grafts are most commonly constructed with greater saphenous vein, although synthetic materials also have been used with success. The distal anastomosis is usually constructed first in an effort to avoid kinking after the small

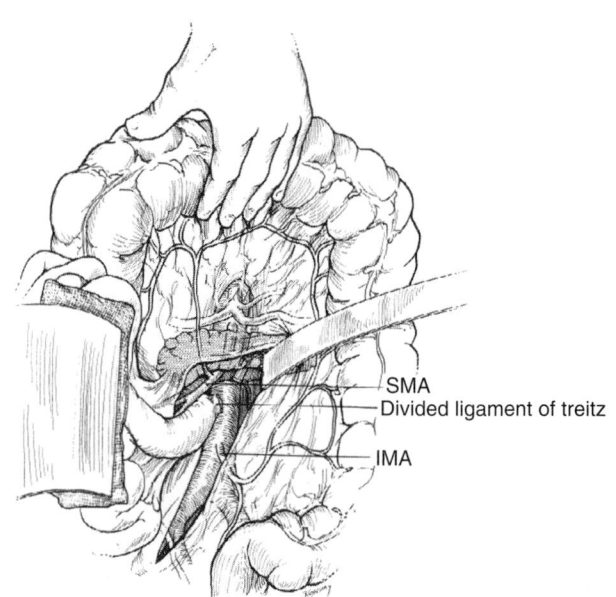

Figure 2 The ligament of Treitz is divided over to expose the superior mesenteric artery at the base of the small bowel mesentery. *From Kazmers A: Ann Vasc Surg 12:191, 1998.*

bowel is laid in position. The proximal anastomosis can be constructed on the infrarenal aorta or on the iliac vessels. (Fig. 6) After revascularization, there must be communication between the surgical and anesthesia teams because reperfusion can lead to sudden physiologic and metabolic derangements, including hypotension, hyperkalemia, and profound acidosis. Several authors have

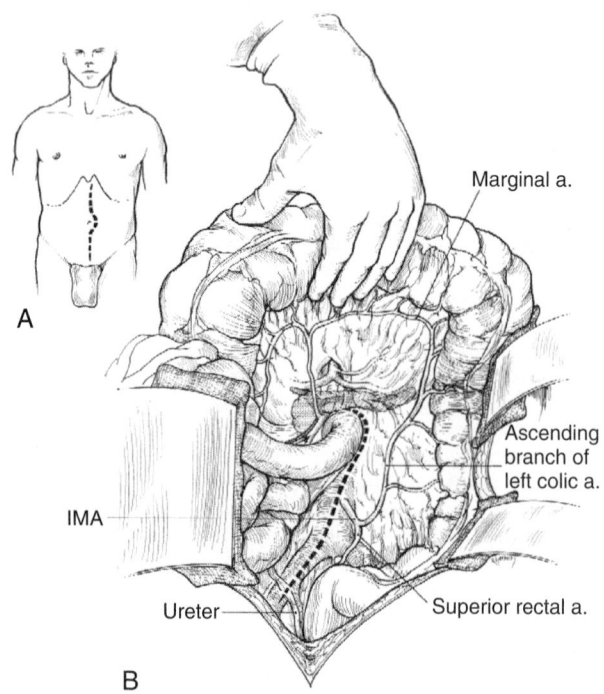

Figure 1 **(A)** A midline incision is carried from xiphoid to pubis. **(B)** SMA is exposed by reflecting the transverse colon superiorly and moving the small bowel to the patient's right side. The retroperitoneum is divided. *From Kazmers A: Ann Vasc Surg 12:190, 1998.*

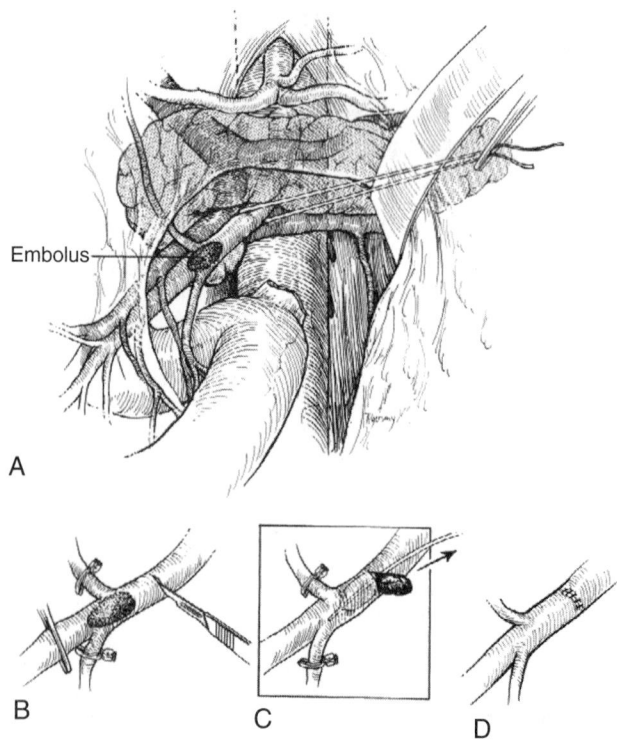

Figure 3 **(A)** Exposure of superior mesenteric artery by reflection of Ligament of Treitz. **(B)** A transverse arteriotomy is performed transversely, proximal to the middle colic branch of the superior mesenteric artery. **(C)** Embolectomy is performed with a 4-F embolectomy catheter. **(D)** Artery is closed with interrupted praline suture. *From Kazmers A: Ann Vasc Surg 12:192, 1998.*

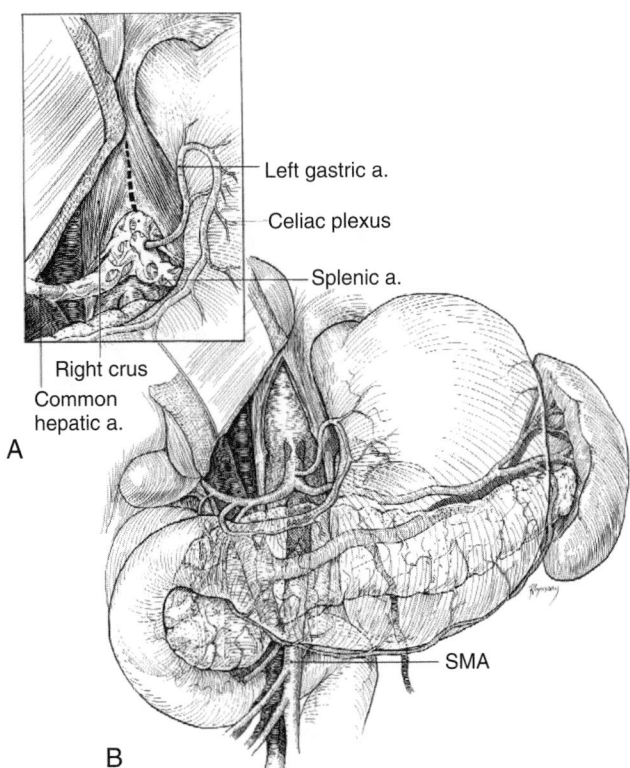

Left gastric a.

Celiac plexus

Splenic a.

Right crus

Common hepatic a.

A

SMA

B

Figure 4 Retrograde mesenteric bypass can be constructed from the infrarenal aorta or from the right **(A)** or left **(B)** iliac artery. *From Kazmers A: Ann Vasc Surg 12:305, 1998.*

recommended the use of postrevascularization papaverine infusions, but this approach is certainly not universal.

Bowel viability must be assessed 20 to 30 minutes following revascularization. The small bowel should be assessed using peristalsis, color, and palpable arterial pulsations as primary markers of bowel viability. Portable Doppler probes are commonly used to examine the antimesenteric aspect of the bowel for pulsations. Finally, intravenous fluorescein can be administered and the bowel examined for fluorescence after several minutes using a Wood's lamp, a technique of particular value to the colorblind surgeon. Any frankly necrotic bowel segments should be resected, but bowel resection should be conservative because marginal-appearing bowel may improve over the course of hours. It is at this point that the decision to perform a second-look laparotomy is generally determined. Although this stance in management has been advocated for several years, its efficacy is equivocal.

Although surgical revascularization remains the main treatment for acute mesenteric ischemia, several case reports and small series report the use of angiographic techniques for the treatment of acute mesenteric ischemia. Most of these reports have used streptokinase, urokinase, or recombinant tissue plasminogen activator. Although the majority of the ventures were successful, their small numbers make it unlikely that most centers will have any significant experience with these techniques, thus making their applicability limited. We currently consider this an investigational approach.

Nonocclusive mesenteric ischemia is typically diagnosed with contrast angiography or at exploration for peritonitis when areas of ischemic or infracted bowel are found with normal arterial pulsations. There is no surgical treatment of this problem except for resection of frankly necrotic small bowel. Several reports have demonstrated a benefit to the infusion of papaverine. This approach has decreased mortality rates in comparison with historical controls.

Mesenteric venous thrombosis (MVT) is often associated with other intra-abdominal disorders. The diagnosis is typically established with CT scan demonstrating delayed or lack of passage into the portal vein. Treatment of MVT consists of systemic anticoagulation and search for an underlying clotting disorder. Should frank peritonitis develop, patients must undergo exploratory laparotomy and resection of any infarcted bowel. The length of anticoagulation has not been formally determined, but most patients are placed on warfarin (Coumadin) for 3 to 6 months. As with acute myocardial infarction, thrombolytic techniques have been proposed by infusing thrombolytic agents into the SMA, internal jugular, or portal vein. This experience consists of mainly case reports and, although results are encouraging, there is no clear-cut evidence of its effectiveness. We tend to use thrombolytic therapy at our institution in patients with MVT and no signs of bowel infarction. Although there are reports of portal embolectomy for MVT (both operative and percutaneous), the results are unimpressive, and we have no experience with these techniques.

CHRONIC MESENTERIC ISCHEMIA

Clinical Presentation

Patients with chronic mesenteric ischemia present with symptoms that have usually developed over a prolonged period of time. Their complaints are characterized by weight loss, intestinal angina, and sitophobia. Most patients will have a concomitant history of peripheral vascular disease or heart disease. Although patients with chronic mesenteric ischemia typically are not critically ill, this condition can be quite debilitating. The goal of therapy therefore is not only to improve the vascular inflow before the onset of thrombotic acute mesenteric ischemia but also to improve the patient's ability to eat.

Diagnosis

The range of possible investigations does not differ greatly from those available to diagnose acute mesenteric ischemia. Abdominal CTA and MRA are useful in diagnosis. Contrast arteriogram remains the standard imaging study for the complete assessment of the abdominal vasculature. Duplex ultrasonography is often used to detect the degree of stenosis of the splanchnic vessels. It is highly specific for the detection of stenoses (92%–100%) but has a lower sensitivity (70%–89%). Because of the extensive collateralization of the mesenteric vasculature, there is no absolute correlation of degree of stenosis and degree of chronic mesenteric ischemia. Ultimately, the diagnosis of chronic mesenteric ischemia is a clinical one, and no one radiological study is diagnostic absent of clinical symptoms.

Management

Once the diagnosis of CMI is established, revascularization of the bowel is indicated. Traditionally, this is accomplished with open surgical bypass to the superior mesenteric artery, celiac artery, or both. Advances in endovascular techniques now allow lesions to be addressed percutaneously. The modern surgeon must be aware of both techniques and their potential applicability to diverse situations.

Surgical bypass techniques have been demonstrated to provide symptomatic relief in 96% of patients. Surgical bypass can be accomplished in several ways. Some authors advocate revascularization of both the celiac and superior mesenteric axes. Proponents invoke long-term data suggesting superior graft patency and survival. Another potential advantage of this approach is redundant circulation should one graft thrombose. The patient is most often approached through a midline incision. This technique can be accomplished by constructing a sequential vein graft from the aorta to the SMA and then to the celiac or hepatic artery. Alternatively, a bifurcated PTFE graft can be anastomosed to the aorta and then to each axis separately. Single-vessel revascularization (usually the SMA) is another viable option. Most recent data reflect a high patency rate (79%) at 9 years for bypasses to the SMA alone. Single-vessel revascularization can be a midline or retroperitoneal incision.

The second choice that must be made when preparing a mesenteric bypass is the site of origination of the graft. Grafts are considered antegrade if they are located above the celiac axis. They are considered retrograde if they are located on the infrarenal aorta or iliac vessels. Antegrade bypasses are advantageous because the graft conformation tends to be straighter and avoids kinking. However, clamping a calcified supraceliac aorta can lead to distal embolization, placing renal function at risk. To perform an antegrade bypass, the surgeon exposes the aorta by dividing the gastrohepatic ligament and exposing the anterior aspect of the aorta above the celiac axis (Figs. 5 and 6). The exposure of the infrarenal aorta or iliac vessels is technically easier and familiar to most surgeons. Fashioning of the retrograde bypass is key because there is a high risk of kinking. (Fig. 4)

Lastly, one must decide whether to use prosthetic materials or saphenous vein as bypass graft. Several studies have demonstrated no clear advantage to either type of graft. Prosthetic grafts tend to be less prone to kinking; however, there is a slightly higher risk of infection. The converse is true of saphenous vein grafts.

Endovascular techniques have grown in popularity as experience with catheter-based interventions has increased. These techniques have been especially helpful in patients with high preoperative risk. Patients are typically accessed through transfemoral techniques. Digital subtraction angiography of the abdominal aorta and

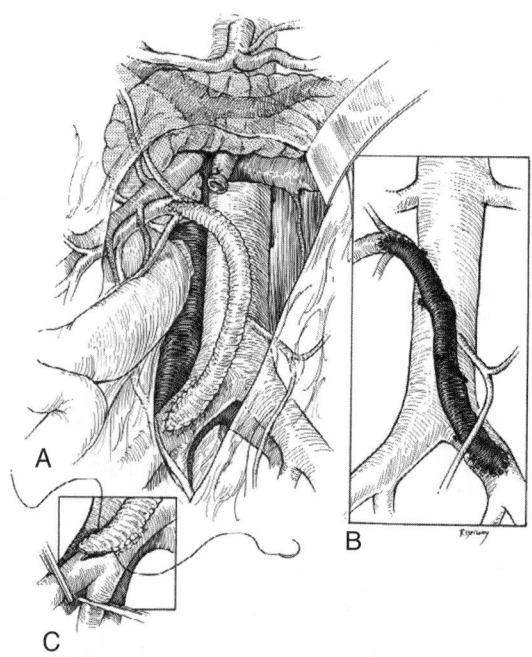

Figure 6 **(A)** An end-to-side aorto-common hepatic artery anastomosis is constructed. The aorta-superior mesenteric artery (SMA) limb is commonly passed behind the common hepatic artery. This is then tunneled behind the pancreas. **(B)** Alternatively, the aorta-SMA bypass limb can be passed in front of the common hepatic artery. *From Kazmers A: Ann Vasc Surg 12:305, 1998.*

selective catheterization of the affected vessels is performed. Lesions in the mesenteric vessels are usually treated with angioplasty first. Indications to stent a vessel include a residual narrowing greater than 30%, dissection, or a clinically significant pressure gradient. Steinmetz and colleagues reported a series of 19 patients undergoing endovascular treatment of chronic mesenteric ischemia as a first choice. Of the 16 patients seen in follow-up at 3 months, 15 had cessation of chronic abdominal pain. Over a mean follow-up of 31 months, the authors observed three cases of symptomatic restenosis. Other authors have quoted a survival of 76% and clinical success rate of 83% over 5 years of long-term follow-up. Although these results do not approach those of surgical revascularization, they demonstrate that percutaneous techniques can be useful in the appropriate clinical setting.

CONCLUSION

Acute and chronic mesenteric ischemia present uncommon challenges in diagnosis and operative treatment. Patients with acute mesenteric ischemia should be diagnosed early and treated aggressively. Patients should be evaluated with abdominal CT scan and angiography if necessary. Embolectomy and surgical bypass are the mainstays of therapy. Nonocclusive ischemia can be diagnosed with angiography and, if possible, treated with intra-arterial or intravenous papaverine. Mesenteric venous thrombosis is treated with anticoagulation, with bowel resection as necessary.

Chronic mesenteric ischemia is typically diagnosed using techniques similar to those used to diagnose acute mesenteric ischemia. Demonstration of stenosis with intestinal angina and weight loss is highly diagnostic. For suitable surgical candidates, surgical revascularization is the mainstay of therapy. Angioplasty and stenting have been shown by some groups to have decreased morbidity and mortality, although their long-term outcomes do not approach those of open surgery.

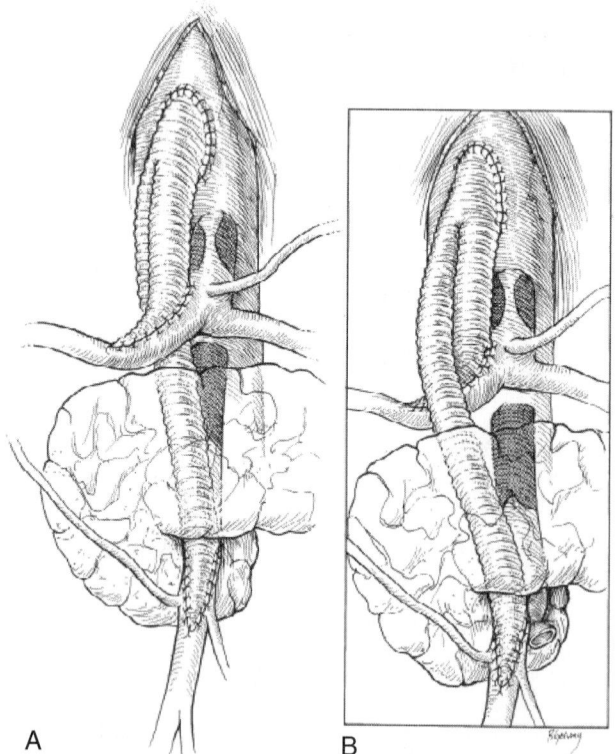

Figure 5 **(A)** The gastrohepatic ligament has been divided, and the right crus has been exposed. **(B)** Division of the right crus with retraction of the esophagus to the left exposes the distal thoracic aorta. *From Kazmers A: Ann Vasc Surg 12:302, 1998.*

Suggested Readings

AGA technical review on intestinal ischemia, *Gastroenterology* 188:954, 2000.

Boley SJ: Initial results from an aggressive approach to acute mesenteric ischemia, *Surgery* 82:848, 1977.

Bowersox JC, Zwolak RM, Walsh DB, and others: Duplex ultrasonography in the diagnosis of celiac and mesenteric artery occlusive disease, *J Vasc Surgery* 14:780, 1991.

Kazmers A: Operative management of acute mesenteric ischemia, *Ann Vasc Surg* 12:187, 1998.

Kazmers A: Operative management of acute mesenteric ischemia, *Ann Vasc Surg* 12:192, 299, 302, 305, 1998.

Kihara TK, Blebea J, Anderson KM, and others: Risk factors and outcomes following revascularization for chronic mesenteric ischemia, *Ann Vasc Surg* 13:37, 1999.

Kirkpatrick ID; Biphasic CT with mesenteric CT angiography in the evaluation of acute mesenteric ischemia: initial experience, *Radiology* 229:91, 2003.

Matsumoto AH, Angle JF, Spinosa DJ, and others: Percutaneous transluminal angioplasty and stenting in the treatment of chronic mesenteric ischemia: results and long term follow up, *J Am Coll Sur* 194(suppl 1): S22, 2002.

Moneta GL, Yeager RA, Dalman R, and others: Duplex ultrasound criteria for the diagnosis of splanchnic artery stenosis or occlusion, *J Vascular Surg* 14:511, 1991.

Park WM Cherry KJ Jr, Chua HK: Current results of open revascularization for chronic mesenteric ischemia: a standard for comparison, *J Vasc Surg* 35:853, 2002.

Rivitz SM, Geller SC, Hahn C, and others: Treatment of acute mesenteric venous thrombosis with transjugular intramesenteric urokinase transfusion, *J Vasc Interv Radiol* 6:219, 1995.

Simo G, Echenagusia AJ, Camunez F, and others: Superior mesenteric arterial embolism: local fibrinolytic treatment with urokinase, *Radiology* 20:775, 1997.

Steinmetz E, Tatou E, Flavier-Blavoux C, and others: Endovascular treatment as first choice in chronic intestinal ischemia, *Ann Vasc Surg* 16:693, 2002.

Turegano Fuentes F, Simo Muerza G, Echenagusia Belda A, and others: Successful intraarterial fragmentation and urokinase therapy in superior mesenteric artery embolism, *Surgery* 117:712, 1995.

Ward D: Improved outcome by identification of high-risk nonocclusive mesenteric ischemia, aggressive reexploration, and delayed anastomosis, *Am J Surg* 170:5777, 1995.

Yankes JR: Percutaneous transhepatic recanalization and thrombolysis of the superior mesenteric vein, *Am J Roentgenol* 151:289, 1988.

ENTEROCUTANEOUS FISTULA

Edmund S. Kassis, MD,
and Martin A. Makary, MD, MPH

The management of an enterocutaneous fistula (ECF) continues to be a challenging problem, even for the most experienced surgeon. Enterocutaneous fistulae are frequently complicated by associated abscesses, sepsis, electrolyte derangements, dehydration, and malnutrition. Despite advances in antimicrobial and nutritional therapy, the overall mortality in patients with ECF remains high, ranging from 10% to 20% depending on coexisting conditions.

■ ETIOLOGY

The vast majority of enterocutaneous fistulae occur as a complication of an abdominal operation, usually involving a bowel anastomosis, repair of an enterotomy, or unrecognized bowel injury. There are several risk factors for the development of ECF, most of which are related to tissue integrity and healing (Table 1).

Table 1: Differential Diagnosis for an Enterocutaneous Fistula

Anastomotic leak
Unrecognized enterotomy
Fascial suture through bowel
Ischemic bowel segment
Erosion into bowel by suction drains or mesh
Perforated viscous (e.g., peptic ulcer or colonic diverticula)
Local inflammation (e.g., Crohn's disease)

A technical error in creating a bowel anastomosis in the setting of a malnourished patient is the most notorious setting for an ECF. Anastomoses are more likely to leak in the context of malnutrition because of compromised tissue integrity. Hypoalbuminemia is one marker of nutritional status, and a serum albumin level less than 3.0 is a known risk factor for the development of an ECF. Local inflammation resulting from an abscess or enteric spillage is another major cause of anastomotic breakdowns. Accordingly, emergency abdominal procedures and contaminated operations are well-described risk factors for the formation of an ECF. For example, patients who present with a colonic perforation involving significant enteric spillage and a local inflammatory response are often best managed by creating an ostomy, deferring a bowel anastomosis to a second-stage operation after the infection has cleared and the inflammation resolved.

Another risk factor for the formation of an ECF is a history of steroid administration. Steroids can be a major contributing factor leading to bowel perforation and poor tissue healing, given the effect that steroids can have on decreasing bowel integrity and the response to injury. In cancer patients, radiation and chemotherapy are known to be associated with an increased risk for ECF. Such factors are predisposing causes of decreased tissue integrity, a problem that can lead to bowel perforation with the onset of a stress, such as a bowel obstruction. In some instances, an ECF can be the first manifestation of a gastrointestinal (GI) perforation secondary to a distal obstruction. Inflammatory bowel disease, diverticulitis, and invasive malignancies are also known to be conditions at risk for ECF.

Finally, ECF can be common among trauma patients with an open abdomen being managed with local wound care. In the surgical management of critically ill trauma patients, surgeons may choose to leave the abdomen open to avoid the risk of postoperative abdominal compartment syndrome or because the fascia simply will not approximate. These patients are often managed with a dressing placed directly on exposed bowel, a scenario at high risk for the development of an ECF. When dealing with exposed bowel, we recommend using a plastic nonadherent dressing for short-term management and gauze lubricated with Vaseline or other lubricant on the bowel to protect it from the mechanical debridement after a few days. An ECF commonly occurs when dressings on exposed bowel are peeled off during routine dressing changes. Vacuum dressings have been used on bowel directly with good results; however, low suction settings and such nondebriding dressings should be used to protect the bowel whenever possible. Rates of ECF with exposed bowel can be as high as 50%, and thus special precautions, with dressing changes and early closure of the abdomen or skin grafting, are warranted to reduce this risk.

DIAGNOSIS

The classic presentation of an ECF begins with a local wound infection following abdominal surgery. After the wound is opened, drainage is noted from the base of the wound immediately or 1 to 2 days later. The appearance or odor of enteric contents is diagnostic of an ECF. The fascia often separate to some degree. In fact, leakage of enteric contents is a common cause of dehiscence and evisceration; this should be considered in any patient with a wound infection, fascial separation, or drainage from a wound. The other common setting in which an ECF presents, as discussed earlier, is during a dressing change in a patient with an open abdomen. Enteric drainage is often visualized at a single location in the wound, and this is diagnostic. When such drainage is unrecognized and persistent, it may result in wound nonhealing.

An upper GI contrast study or computed tomography (CT) scan can often demonstrate an ECF. Alternatively, contrast can also be injected into a chronic fistula tract to locate where the communication exists along the alimentary tract, although this is ideally performed after a fistula tract has formed. Proximal GI fistulae are more prone to electrolyte abnormalities, fluid losses, and malnutrition because water and nutrients are not absorbed distally. Distal GI fistulae can sometimes have no fluid or electrolyte sequelae because they may function as a well-developed distal ileostomy or colostomy.

TREATMENT GOALS

Early recognition is critical to prevent severe and life-threatening metabolic, septic, and nutritional complications of ECF. Interventions should focus on resuscitation, correction of electrolyte abnormalities, control of sepsis, nutritional support, and skin care.

Resuscitation and Correction of Electrolyte Disturbances

The typical patient suffering from an ECF has had a slow postoperative recovery, often involving a prolonged ileus, fever, and wound complications. Third-space fluid losses can be profound, resulting in hypovolemia and shock. Prompt resuscitation with isotonic crystalloid solution and correction of electrolyte disturbances are the crucial first steps in the management of these patients.

Control of Sepsis

Uncontrolled sepsis is the major cause of mortality in patients with ECF. Early recognition and drainage of an abdominal abscess can be lifesaving. Although broad-spectrum antibiotics are the first step in management, treatment of the underlying cause is the overriding principle of treating sepsis. Image-guided drainage can preclude the need for early surgical intervention, which carries a high perioperative mortality. Early surgical intervention should be considered only in septic patients with uncontrolled leakage of enteric contents into the abdomen or associated abscesses that are not amenable to percutaneous drainage. Thus the initial questions in the management of an ECF are the following:

Is the patient septic?
Can the sepsis be treated with percutaneous drainage of an inciting fluid collection?

If the patient is not septic, an attempt at nonoperative management of the ECF should be attempted. A study by Reber and colleagues demonstrated that after the initial sepsis is controlled, 90% of ECFs close spontaneously within 1 month. Not only can patience on the part of the surgeon eliminate the need for future surgery but if the ECF persists, time will allow for a fistula tract to mature.

If the patient is septic (or becomes septic during conservative management) and percutaneous drainage of a fluid collection is not warranted or cannot be performed, then surgical exploration may be necessary to control the leakage of enteric contents as the underlying source of the patient's sepsis. This can be accomplished by resection of the leaking segment, internal or wide external drainage (or both) with large surgical drains, or conversion of the leakage site to an ostomy.

Definitive Care

The overall spontaneous closure rate of an ECF is 10% to 40% with conservative management alone. The use of tissue glues, somatostatin, infliximab (anti-tumor necrosis factor antibody), or a combination of these for the treatment ECF has yielded scant success in small studies and case reports, but these studies lack adequately powered control groups to permit any meaningful recommendations to use them. An ECF that persists 4 to 8 weeks after the resolution of sepsis and nutritional deficits is unlikely to close spontaneously, especially when the output is high (>500 ml/24 hours). These patients should be considered for a definitive operation to resect the fistula tract and the involved segment of bowel electively. Factors associated with failure of an ECF to close spontaneously include high output, malnutrition, and a distal bowel obstruction (Table 2).

We typically wait 3 to 6 months to perform an elective operation for a persistent ECF. To achieve the optimal chance of success at the time of surgical exploration, the fistula should be anatomically delineated. Preoperative imaging modalities such as a fistulogram and a CT scan are used to identify the location of the enterotomy, the presence of distal obstruction, and intestinal continuity. At the time of operation, the bowel is mobilized, and the fistulae and involved segment of bowel are resected. A primary anastomosis should be performed in the elective setting. Because the dissection can be complex and extensive, given a recent history of inflammation, the bowel should be carefully inspected to identify and repair inadvertent enterotomies or serosal tears.

Nutritional Support

Patients with an ECF are often malnourished, especially when the fistula is proximal and has a high output. Several reports have demonstrated a reduction in the complications of high-output ECF with aggressive and early nutritional support. Furthermore,

Table 2: Factors Inhibiting Spontaneous Closure of an Enterocutaneous Fistula

| High fistula output (>500 ml/24 hours) |
| Short fistula tract |
| Abscess |
| Distal bowel obstruction |
| Foreign body |
| Malignancy |
| Radiation |
| Steroids |
| Chronic epithelialization |

the rate of spontaneous closure of an ECF is enhanced dramatically with improved nutrition.

Patients with an ECF are often severely catabolic, with depletions in lean body mass, acute phase proteins, albumin, and prealbumin. In the early phase of treatment, restoration of nutritional stores is essential. In profoundly malnourished patients, protein and caloric requirements may be as high as 1.5 to 2 g/kg/day and 40 kcal/kg/day, respectively. It must be remembered that this support cannot overcome continued catabolism. Therefore control of sepsis, when present, is always the first priority.

Enteral versus Parenteral Nutrition

There is increasing evidence that enteral feeding is associated with maintenance of mucosal integrity and improved immunologic host defenses. In addition, enteral nutrition is associated with fewer septic complications. The beneficial effect of enteral nutrition may be realized even if only 10% to 20% of nutritional requirements are administered. These reasons, coupled with cost considerations, appear to make enteral nutrition the desired means of nutritional support. However, patients with a proximal ECF, prolonged ileus, bowel obstruction, or short bowel syndrome may not tolerate enteral nutrition. Furthermore, patients who are profoundly malnourished may not have nutritional requirements met by enteral nutrition and require parenteral support. Finally, enteral feeding may prolong closure of an ECF if feeding causes the fistula output to increase significantly. When the output is high or when uncontrolled enteric leakage into the abdomen is causing sepsis, we make the patient NPO (no oral food intake) and use parenteral nutrition. The practice of promoting healing and closure with enteric feeding should be individualized on the basis of the fistula output and the overall health and nutritional status of the patient.

Skin Care

An ECF from a visible enterotomy involving a segment of exposed bowel is rarely amenable to primary surgical closure. Control of the enteric drainage out of the wound should be the goal. Skin grafting over the remaining area of the wound is one strategy used to control enteric drainage within a large wound. A subsequent operation to close the abdomen is performed several months later and can be combined with a definitive fistula tract and bowel resection. Hernia repairs involving prosthetic mesh may require a separate operation if there is significant enteric contamination associated with the bowel resection.

SUGGESTED READINGS

Chamberlain RS, Kaufman HL, Danforth DN: Enterocutaneous fistula in cancer patients: etiology, management, outcome, and impact on further treatment. *Am Surg* 64:1204, 1998.
Jernigan TW, Fabian TC, Croce MA: Staged management of giant abdominal wall defects: acute and long-term results. *Ann Surg* 238:349, 2003.
Lynch AC, Delaney CP, Senagore AJ: Clinical outcome and factors predictive of recurrence after enterocutaneous fistula surgery. *Ann Surg* 240:825, 2004.

MANAGEMENT OF SHORT BOWEL SYNDROME

Jon S. Thompson, MD

Short bowel syndrome (SBS) is characterized by malabsorption and malnutrition, which generally occur when less than 180 cm of functional intestine remains in adults. The severity of the clinical features of SBS depends on several factors, including not only the extent of resection but also the site of resection, the underlying intestinal disease, the presence or absence of the ileocecal valve, the functional status of the remaining digestive organs, and the adaptive capacity of the intestinal remnant. Three fourths of these instances result from massive intestinal resection and 25% from multiple sequential resections of the small intestine. Approximately two thirds of patients who develop SBS survive from that hospitalization, and a similar percent are alive 1 year later. Patients' long-term outcome is primarily determined by their age and underlying disease. However, a number of deaths are caused by complications directly related to the management of SBS.

The pathophysiologic changes that occur in SBS relate to the loss of intestinal absorptive surface and more rapid intestinal transit. Malabsorption of nutrients results in malnutrition and weight loss, diarrhea and steatorrhea, vitamin deficiency, and electrolyte imbalance. Other specific complications include an increased incidence of nephrolithiasis from hyperoxaluria, cholelithiasis secondary to altered bile salt and bilirubin metabolism, and gastric hypersecretion. Bacterial overgrowth can also occur secondary to mechanical obstruction or primary motor abnormalities. In patients dependent primarily on parenteral nutrition (PN), liver disease has been an increasingly important factor in mortality. Functional and structural adaptation of the remaining intestine occurs after massive intestinal resection, resulting in improved absorption of nutrients and a decrease in diarrhea within the first few months after resection. The degree of adaptation that occurs depends on the extent and site of resection, the provision of enteral nutrients, and the response to gastrointestinal hormones and other regulatory polypeptides.

Early management of the patient with SBS is that of the critically ill surgical patient having recently undergone intestinal resection and other concomitant procedures. Thus controlling sepsis, maintaining fluid and electrolyte balance, and initiating nutritional support are important in the early management of these patients. Beyond this phase, the primary goals of management of SBS are to maintain adequate nutritional status, maximize the absorptive capacity of the remaining intestine, and prevent the development of complications related to both the underlying pathophysiology and the nutritional therapy itself. Surgical approaches have become increasingly important and generally include preserving the intestinal remnant, maximizing or improving the function of the intestinal remnant, and augmenting intestinal length via transplantation.

THERAPEUTIC GOALS

Maintain Nutritional Status

The most important therapeutic objective in the management of SBS is to maintain the patient's nutritional status. By necessity this is achieved primarily by parenteral nutrition (PN) support in the early postoperative period (Table 1). This therapy includes not

Table 1: Nutritional Support for Short Bowel Syndrome

Parenteral nutrition usually required early
Transition parenteral nutrition to enteral feeding
Optimize diet
Maximize intestinal absorption
Long-term parenteral nutrition for permanent intestinal failure

Table 2: Dietary Recommendations for Short Bowel Syndrome

Colon in Continuity	No Colon in Continuity
Carbohydrate	
50%–60% of caloric intake	40%–50% of caloric intake
Complex carbohydrates	Complex carbohydrates
Fat	
20%–30% of caloric intake	30%–40% of caloric intake
Ensure adequate essential fats	Ensure adequate essential fats
MCT/LCT	LCT
Protein	
20%–30% of caloric intake	20%–30% of caloric intake
High biologic value	High biologic value
Fiber	
5–10 gm soluble fiber/day for	5–10 gm soluble fiber/day for
Net secretors	Net secretors
Oxalate: Restrict	No restriction
Fluids	
ORS and/or hypotonic	ORS

LCT, long-chain triglycerides; MCT, medium-chain triglycerides; ORS, oral rehydration solution.

only provision of energy substrates and protein but also fluid, electrolytes, minerals, vitamins, and micronutrients. Fluid and electrolyte losses from the gastrointestinal tract may be great during the early postoperative period. Most patients require approximately 35 kcal/kg/day and 1.0 to 1.5 g/protein/kg/day with appropriate additives.

Enteral nutrition support can be started early after operation when the ileus has resolved. With time, an increasing amount of nutrients will be absorbed via the enteral route; this is important for maximizing intestinal adaptation and for preventing complications related to PN. As their conditions improve and intestinal adaptation occurs, many patients are able to absorb the necessary nutrients entirely via the enteral route. Intestinal remnant length has important prognostic implications in this regard. Patients with more than 180 cm small intestine remaining generally require no PN, those with more than 90 cm small intestine and particularly with colon will generally require PN for less than 1 year, and those with less than 60 cm small intestine will likely require permanent PN.

During the transition from parenteral to enteral nutrition support, the primary objectives are to maintain a stable body weight and prevent large fluctuations in fluid balance. Metabolic monitoring is necessary to detect and correct any metabolic abnormalities and micronutrient deficiency. Because it is not clear whether parenteral nutrients suppress appetite, PN should be gradually decreased only as enteral intake increases. A marked increase in gastrointestinal fluid loss is a sign that further increases in enteral feeding will not be tolerated. As parenteral requirements diminish, intermittent PN can be instituted, reducing hours of therapy during the day and eventually alternating days.

Maximize Enteral Nutrient Absorption

Dietary management for an individual patient with SBS is determined by a variety of factors, including intestinal remnant length and location, any underlying intestinal disease, and the status of the remaining digestive organs. The existence of a stoma is also an important consideration because diarrhea and perianal complications may markedly diminish oral intake. Thus patients with stomas may be more likely to take a greater percentage of their calories enterally. Patients with SBS, in fact, may develop hyperphagia to overcome their inefficient absorption. Continuous rather than intermittent enteral feeding may permit greater absorption of nutrients in patients with remnants less than 90 cm. Separating solid and liquid meals may aid absorption of solids.

The optimal diet for patients with SBS is determined primarily by whether the colon is in continuity (Table 2). Initially a high-carbohydrate, high-protein diet is appropriate to maximize absorption. Provision of nutrients in their simplest form so that digestion does not become an important part of the absorptive process is one strategic approach. Simple sugars and dipeptides and tripeptides are rapidly absorbed from the intestinal tract. However, partially hydrolyzed diets appear to be just as effective and are less expensive. Fat absorption requires more digestion unless the fat is supplied in the form of medium-chain triglycerides. Stool fat

increases markedly, however, with remnants less than 60 cm. The ability to absorb these nutrients does improve with time, thus the diet should be continually modified. Other problems, such as lactase deficiency, may also be present. Hypo-osmolar diets are started initially to minimize gastrointestinal fluid losses. More complex diets can be ingested later. Because jejunal mucosa is relatively permeable, isotonic feedings are particularly important with jejunal remnants. Ingestion of a glucose–electrolyte oral rehydration solution with a sodium concentration of at least 90 mmol/L optimizes water and sodium absorption in the proximal jejunum and prevents secretion into the lumen. Pectin may improve absorption by prolonging transit time and serving as a source of short chain fatty acids. The role of specific nutrients (e.g., glutamine) and growth factors such as growth hormone and glucagon-like peptide 2 (GLP-2) in improving nutrient absorption is currently being evaluated.

Another important aspect of the dietary management is to provide a diet that will maximize the intestinal adaptive response. Provision of fat, particularly long chain triglycerides, and dietary fiber may be particularly important in this regard. Glutamine may also be trophic to the gut. Although these nutrients may act directly to stimulate intestinal adaptation, the meal may also stimulate intestinal adaptation via endocrine or paracrine effects. Growth factors (e.g., growth hormone and GLP-2) may also stimulate intestinal adaptation and are currently under investigation in the clinical setting.

Minimizing gastrointestinal secretion and controlling diarrhea are also important goals for maximizing absorption (Table 3). The addition of dietary fiber is useful in patients who are net fluid secretors. Several agents are useful for improving absorption via their antisecretory and antimotility effects, including narcotics such as codeine and diphenoxylate and atropine (Lomotil) and the peripherally acting narcotic loperamide. Somatostatin and its long-acting analogue octreotide improve diarrhea by increasing small intestinal transit time, reducing salt and water excretion, as well as gastric hypersecretion. However, they may not be effective long term and have potentially deleterious effects, including steatorrhea, inhibition of intestinal adaptation, and increased incidence of cholelithiasis. Thus octreotide should not be used routinely for the management of chronic diarrhea. Both H_2 receptor antagonists

Table 3: Medical Treatment of Short Bowel Syndrome

Slow transit
Loperamide, Lomotil, narcotics
Reduce gastrointestinal secretion
H₂ receptor antagonists
Proton pump inhibitors
Octreotide*
Clonidine*
Treat bacterial overgrowth
Antibiotics
Probiotics
Prokinetics
Pharmacologic treatment
Growth hormone
Glutamine

*Off-label use.

and proton pump inhibitors have been shown to be effective in controlling gastric hypersecretion. Recent studies suggest that the alpha 2-adrenergic receptor agonist clonidine may also reduce fluid loss in those patients. Cholestyramine may also be beneficial when the diarrhea is related to the cathartic effect of unabsorbed bile salts in the colon. Bile acid malabsorption is difficult to detect, and thus cholestyramine should be tried on patients with ileal resections of less than 100 cm.

Pharmacologic therapy for SBS is a rapidly expanding area of investigation. A variety of growth factors and other substances have been identified that promote intestinal growth or enhance absorptive function. Although a number of agents with these effects have been studied experimentally, only a few drugs are being used clinically. Growth hormone has trophic and pro-absorptive effects on the gut, as well as other metabolic effects. Glutamine is the preferred enterocyte fuel. There are several unresolved issues related to timing, dose, duration of therapy, and route of delivery for these agents.

Initial efforts in this area were led by Wilmore and Byrne. They initiated a protocol that included a high-carbohydrate, low-fat diet, glutamine, and high-dose growth hormone (GH). In an initial unblinded, uncontrolled study, there was improved fluid and electrolyte absorption and nutrient absorption with weight gain in SBS patients. Subsequent studies by these investigators demonstrated that 60% of patients were weaned off PN, and 30% reduced PN requirements. This 4-week intensive regimen led to apparent benefit at 1-year follow-up. However, it was unclear which of these components was actually responsible for improved absorption. More recently, a randomized, placebo-controlled, double-blind clinical trial was undertaken comparing GH + diet, GH + glutamine + diet, and glutamine + diet. GH + glutamine + diet and GH + diet permitted more PN weaning than glutamine + diet, but only GH + glutamine + diet maintained the effect at 3 months. This suggests that GH and glutamine may have beneficial effects. However, growth hormone alone has not had a consistent beneficial effect in other randomized, blinded, placebo-controlled crossover studies. Both are available for clinical use.

Currently GLP-2 appears to be another agent that has promise for promoting intestinal absorption and adaptation. In an open-label study, Jeppesen reported improved absorption in eight SBS patients receiving exogenous GLP-2. A long-acting analogue is now available. This drug is still investigational, and an international multicenter trial is currently under way in SBS patients.

Table 4: Restoration of Intestinal Continuity

Advantages
Absorptive capacity increased
Energy from short-chain fatty acids
Intestinal stoma avoided
Infectious complications reduced
Transit time prolonged
Disadvantages
Bile acid diarrhea
Dietary restrictions
Perianal complications
Risk of nephrolithiasis

Epidermal growth factor (EGF) stimulates intestinal adaptation and is pro-absorptive in experimental studies. A recent clinical trial in pediatric SBS patients of enteral recombinant EGF found increased carbohydrate absorption and tolerance to enteral feeds. However, ongoing administration was required for sustained improvement. This agent remains investigational.

An important clinical issue is whether to establish intestinal continuity in patients who have a colonic remnant. There are both advantages and disadvantages to restoring continuity (Table 4). The colon may in fact improve intestinal absorption by increasing the absorptive surface area, deriving energy from short-chain fatty acids and prolonging transit time, particularly if the ileocecal valve is intact. It also improves quality of life by avoiding a stoma. However, the response of the colon to luminal contents is somewhat unpredictable. Bile acids may in fact cause a secretory diarrhea. Perianal problems can be disabling and decrease the patient's oral intake. Oxalate is absorbed primarily in the colon, and patients are thus at increased risk for the formation of calcium oxalate stones. We found that only 20% of patients who initially had a stoma formed ultimately had continuity restored with a satisfactory outcome. This decision should be considered on an individual basis, depending on the length of the intestinal remnant, the status of the ileocecal valve and colon, and the patient's overall condition. Generally, at least 90 cm of small intestine are required to prevent severe diarrhea and perianal complications.

Prevent Complications

Metabolic complications are common in SBS patients (Table 5). Patients are at risk for dehydration and renal dysfunction. Hypocalcemia is a common problem related to poor absorption and binding by intraluminal fat. Maintaining adequate levels of calcium, magnesium, and vitamin D supplementation are important to minimize bone disease. Hyperglycemia and hypoglycemia are frequent complications of patients receiving a large amount of their calories parenterally. Both metabolic acidosis and alkalosis can occur.

Table 5: Complications in Short Bowel Syndrome

Therapy related	Physiologic
• Metabolic	• Bacterial overgrowth
• Nutritional	• Cholelithiasis
• Infectious	• Nephrolithiasis
• Liver disease	• Gastric hypersecretion

A specific problem is D-lactic acidosis, which results from bacterial fermentation of unabsorbed nutrients, particularly simple sugars.

Specific nutrient deficiencies need to be prevented and monitored closely. These include iron and vitamin deficiencies, as well as micronutrients, such as selenium, zinc, and copper. Because fat is poorly absorbed, fatty acid deficiency can also occur. Serum free fatty acid levels and triene-to-tetraene ratios may need to be monitored periodically to determine the need for supplementation and response to treatment. In general, the enteral intake must greatly exceed the absorptive needs to ensure that these needs are being met.

Catheter-related sepsis is an important problem that often necessitates rehospitalization and replacement of catheters. Attention to technique and meticulous patient education are important to prevent this complication. Catheter thrombosis is another frequent problem. In patients who require total parenteral nutrition permanently, this may become an important factor in the patient's survival because vascular access may not be achievable indefinitely.

PN-induced liver disease is another potential long-term problem (Table 6). This appears to be a multifactorial process that is often reversible but may lead to severe steatosis, cholestasis, and eventually cirrhosis. It occurs more frequently in children and accounts for one third of deaths of patients on long-term PN. It can be minimized by providing as large a portion of the calories as possible enterally, avoiding overfeeding, using mixed fuels (< 30% fat), and preventing specific nutrient deficiencies. Treating bacterial growth and preventing recurrent sepsis are also important. Ursodeoxycholic acid administration may also be beneficial.

Bacterial overgrowth may result from impaired motility or stasis caused by obstructive lesions. Depending on the bacterial species present, secretory diarrhea may also occur. Bacterial overgrowth requires a high degree of suspicion for diagnosis. This complication should be suspected when a patient's absorptive capacity and stool habits change acutely. This may result from a mechanical obstruction or a blind loop, which can be relieved by operation. However, it is often a primary motor abnormality, which requires intermittent therapy with antibiotics. Colonization of the lumen with probiotics is another potential therapy.

Cholelithiasis occurs in 30% to 40% of SBS patients. Long-term PN causes both altered hepatic bile metabolism and gallbladder stasis. Biliary sludge forms within a few weeks of initiating PN if there is no enteral intake but rapidly disappears when enteral nutrition is resumed. Patients receiving PN are at risk for both cholelithiasis and hepatocellular dysfunction and thus require careful clinical evaluation. Intestinal mucosal disease and resection, particularly of the ileum, cause bile acid malabsorption, leading to lithogenic bile and the formation of cholesterol stones. The risk for cholelithiasis is significantly increased if less than 120 cm of intestine remains after resection, the terminal ileum has been resected, and PN is required. The incidence of cholelithiasis can by minimized by providing nutrients enterally whenever possible. Patients totally dependent on PN may be treated with intermittent cholecystokinin (CCK) injections to prevent stasis and formation of sludge. Administration of intravenous lipids also stimulates gallbladder emptying. Cholelithiasis is more likely to be complicated in patients with SBS and requires more extensive surgical treatment. Prophylactic cholecystectomy should be considered when laparotomy is being undertaken for other reasons.

Table 6: Prevention of Liver Disease

- Maximize enteral feeding
- Avoid overfeeding
- Use mixed fuels (<30% fat)
- Prevent nutrient deficiencies
- Treat overgrowth and sepsis

Nephrolithiasis, primarily calcium oxalate stones, also occurs with some frequency. Oxalate is normally bound to calcium in the intestinal lumen and is not absorbed. Decreased availability of calcium secondary to reduced intake or binding by intraluminal fat leaves free oxalate in the lumen. Thus the oxalate is absorbed in the colon and forms calcium oxalate in the urine. Nephrolithiasis is unusual in patients with intestinal resection and jejunostomy but occurs in one fourth of such patients with an intact colon within 2 years of resection. Nephrolithiasis can be prevented by maintaining a diet low in oxalate, minimizing intraluminal fat, supplementing calcium orally, and maintaining a high urinary volume. Cholestyramine, which binds oxalic acid in the colon, is another potential treatment.

Gastric hypersecretion is a potential problem in patients with SBS. Massive intestinal resection can cause gastric hypersecretion as a result of parietal cell hyperplasia and hypergastrinemia. This phenomenon is usually transient, lasting several months, and presumably involves loss of an inhibitor from the resected intestine. The associated hyperacidity exacerbates malabsorption and diarrhea. About one fourth of patients undergoing massive resection develop peptic ulcer disease. Treatment of gastric acid secretion may improve absorption but also prevents peptic ulcer disease. Control of acid secretion by H_2 receptor antagonists or proton pump inhibitors should be initiated in the perioperative period after resection and maintained until the increased acid production resolves. A few patients eventually require surgical intervention, but gastric resection should be avoided when possible.

SURGICAL STRATEGIES

Preserve Intestinal Remnant

Abdominal reoperation is required in approximately 50% of patients with SBS after their discharge from the hospital. Intestinal problems are the most frequent indication. An important goal in any reoperation in patients with SBS is to preserve the intestinal remnant length. Resection can often be avoided by using intestinal tapering to improve the function of dilated segments, employing stricturoplasty for benign strictures, and using serosal patching for certain strictures and chronic perforations. Resection should be limited in extent when it cannot be avoided. Depending on the previous operations performed, patients will occasionally have intestinal segments that can be recruited into continuity at the time of reoperation. This should always be given careful consideration. It is always important to document the length of intestine remaining during any operation on a patient with SBS.

Surgical Therapy for the Short Bowel Syndrome

There are several goals of surgical therapy for the short bowel syndrome (Fig. 1). One has been to slow intestinal transit by the construction of artificial valves, reversing intestinal segments, interposing colonic segments into the small intestine, and other innovative approaches such as intestinal pacing. Another goal has been to improve the function of existing intestine. For example, stenotic segments cause partial obstruction, which could lead to malabsorption. This can be managed by relieving the obstruction, often with a simple approach such as a stricturoplasty. Furthermore, dilatated dysfunctional segments aggravate malabsorption. These can be treated by tapering enteroplasty. For patients with particularly short remnants, increasing intestinal surface area is the best option for improving nutrient absorption. Intestinal lengthening procedures combine tapering with lengthening and are applicable in some patients. However, intestinal transplantation may be the final solution to this problem.

Figure 1 Surgical procedures for improvement of intestinal function in short bowel syndrome. *Reproduced from Thompson JS , Langnas AN, Pinch LW, and others: Ann Surg 222:600, 1995.*

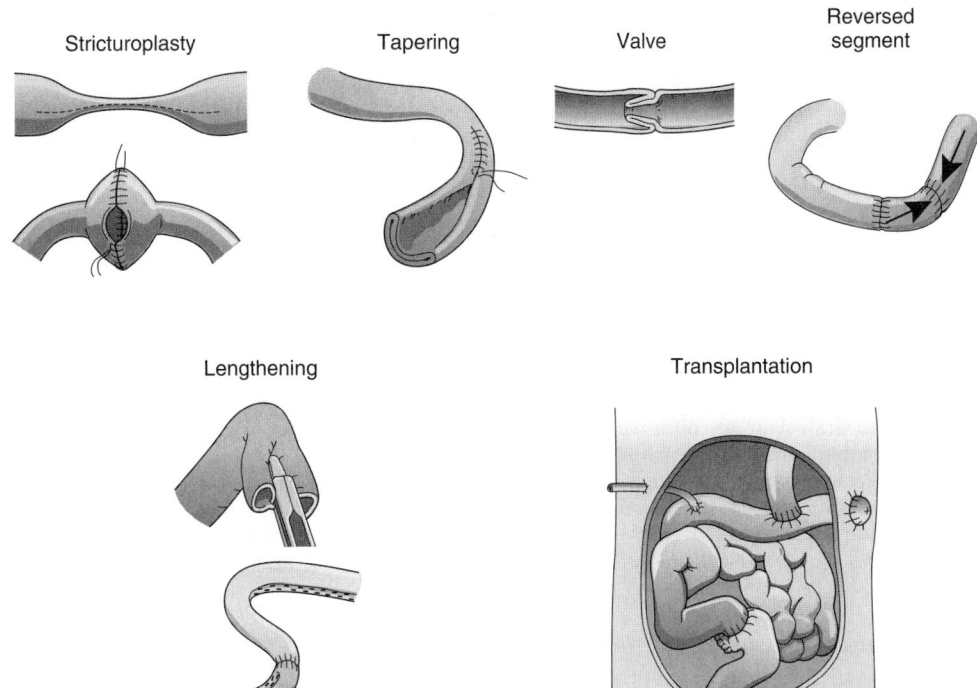

The surgical approach to the patient with SBS depends on several factors. The nature of nutritional support is obviously the primary determinant as to whether operation should be considered. In our experience, half of patients with SBS are able to sustain themselves on enteral nutrition alone. Operation should be considered cautiously and generally performed in these patients only if they demonstrate worsening malabsorption, are at risk for requiring PN, or have other symptoms related to malabsorption. Almost half of patients who are stable on long-term PN are candidates for operation, with the goal in this group being primarily to get the patient off PN. Patients who develop significant complication while dependent on PN have more compelling reasons to undergo operation. Most of these patients should undergo intestinal transplantation because many will die. Although liver disease is certainly the most frequent indication for transplantation, difficult vascular access and recurrent sepsis are also considerations. Patient age and underlying disease are also important factors. Children are much more likely to adapt to enteral nutrition but are also more likely to be candidates for operative treatment. In our experience, adult patients with mesenteric vascular disease and children with necrotizing enterocolitis undergo operation less frequently.

The choice of operation for SBS is influenced by intestinal remnant length, intestinal function, and the caliber of the intestinal remnant (Fig. 2). These factors allow identification of several patient groups that might be treated by specific surgical procedures.

Figure 2 Surgical management of short bowel syndrome. *Reproduced from Thompson JS, Langnas AN, Pinch LW, and others: Ann Surg 222:600, 1995.*

SURGICAL MANAGEMENT OF THE SHORT BOWEL SYNDROME

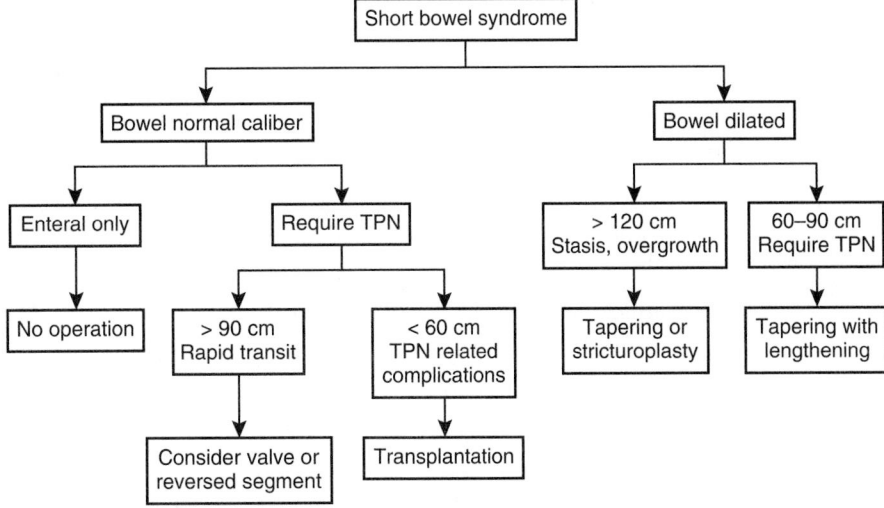

Adequate Remnant Length with Dilated Bowel

Adult patients with intestinal remnants greater than 120 cm are likely to be sustained on enteral nutrition alone, particularly if the ileocolonic junction is intact. However, these patients may develop dilatated bowel secondary to obstruction, often at the site of a previous anastomosis. A useful approach to these patients is to relieve the intestinal obstruction, often with a stricturoplasty, although other procedures may be necessary. Children with remnants greater than 60 cm usually are sustained on enteral nutrition alone. Dilatation of the intestinal remnant occurs more frequently in children and appears to have a different pathophysiologic basis. This may be a variant of intestinal pseudo-obstruction. Only one fourth of children with a significantly dilatated bowel have mechanical obstruction, but they routinely have bacterial overgrowth. Thus for children, a tapering enteroplasty is often the appropriate therapy and also deals with any obstructive component present. This can be accomplished either by excising the redundant bowel along the antimesenteric border or simply imbricating it; the latter is our preferred approach. Motility is generally slow to return. Recurrent dilatation is a concern, given the underlying pathophysiology, and we have found it necessary to reoperate on a few of our patients for this problem.

Moderate Remnant Length with Rapid Transit

A challenging group of patients are those who have shorter remnant (90–120 cm in adults) and signs of rapid transit. Slowing the rapid intestinal transit may permit these patients to be supported by enteral means alone. There are several possible approaches to this problem. Creation of various artificial valves to replace the ileocecal valve has been attempted. We have generally performed the valve procedure by creating a sphincter similar to that used in the continent ileostomy procedure but of shorter length (2 cm). We have had a favorable result in one adult and one child with this valve. Outcomes have not been uniformly successful in the few other reports, however. Reversing 10- to 15-cm intestinal segments has also been used in SBS. Longer segments are more likely to be associated with chronic obstruction, whereas the shorter segments have less influence on intestinal transit and function. More than 40 patients have been reported in the literature, and although documentation is usually not extensive, clinical improvement has often been reported. Some concerns have been raised about long-term function with the procedure. Both isoperistaltic and antiperistaltic colon interposition have been attempted. Although it appears that transit time may be prolonged because of the intrinsic differences in motility between the colon and small intestine, actual benefit has been difficult to show in a few anecdotal reports. Intestinal pacing has also been attempted on the basis of laboratory studies suggesting that it may be possible to pace the small intestine with electrodes in a retrograde fashion. However, attempts to do this clinically have proved unsuccessful.

Patients with Short Remnant and Dilatated Bowel

Patients with short remnant length (<90 cm in adults and <30 cm in children) and dilatated intestinal segments represent a more difficult problem. Even though the dilatated segment could be tapered, this still does not result in enough functional bowel to avoid PN. In this situation, we and others have found intestinal lengthening to be the optimal treatment. There are currently two techniques. Intestinal tapering and lengthening via the Bianchi procedure (Fig. 1) involves dissection along the mesenteric edge of the bowel to allocate terminal blood vessels to either side of the bowel wall. Longitudinal transection of the bowel is then performed, usually with a stapling device that creates two parallel limbs of a smaller caliber. These can then be anastomosed to lengthen the intestinal remnant. More than 100 cases have been reported, mostly in children. Segments have been lengthened up to 55 cm, and overall improved

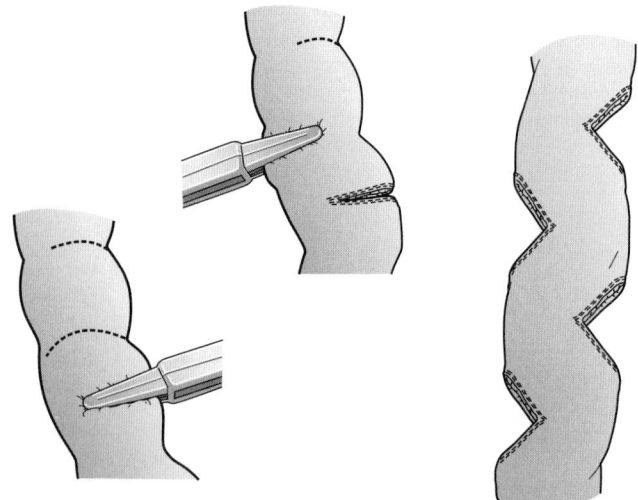

Figure 3 Serial transverse enteroplasty procedure (STEP). *Reproduced from Thompson JS: Surgery 135:465, 2004.*

nutrition resulted in approximately 90% of patients. Complications have been reported in 20% of procedures, which not surprisingly include ischemia, and anastomotic leaks. Recurrent dilatation has been a concern. However, follow-up for as long as 10 years suggests that this procedure has long-term benefit.

More recently, an alternative method of lengthening, termed *serial transverse enteroplasty procedure* (STEP), has been introduced (Fig. 3). This involves serial transverse applications of a linear stapler from opposite directions, dividing the bowel from either the mesenteric and antimesenteric sides or transversely. The length of the transverse division is determined by the intestinal diameter. This procedure avoids the difficult dissection along the mesenteric border of the Bianchi procedure and the end-to-end anastomosis. The bowel may have to be more dilatated to use this technique. It is more feasible in challenging areas such as near the ligament of Treitz. Our initial experience with this technique has been favorable.

One of the limitations of the intestinal lengthening procedures is that they can be applied only to a fairly select group of patients who have both a short intestinal remnant and an intestinal diameter greater than 3 to 4 cm. To improve the applicability of this technique, surgeons have used sequential operations employing first a procedure such as inserting an artificial valve, to produce intestinal dilatation, and then performing the lengthening at a later time.

Short Remnant Length and Parenteral-Nutrition-Related Complications

Patients with short intestinal remnants (<60 cm in adults and <30 cm in children) who develop complications related to PN represent a challenging group. For these patients, intestinal transplantation is the ideal solution. Patients with liver failure and SBS have been candidates for combined liver and small intestine transplantation. The patients who have reversible liver dysfunction or who have adequate liver function but other complications such as difficult vascular access and recurrent infection are candidates for solitary intestinal transplantation. More recently, isolated liver transplantation has been advocated for patients with irreversible liver failure and SBS that can be rehabilitated. The significant mortality rate among patients developing PN-induced complications justifies what continues to be a formidable operative approach.

More than 1000 intestinal transplantations have been performed worldwide in humans since the early 1990s. These have included primarily isolated small intestinal grafts (40%) and combined liver and small intestinal grafts (40%), with fewer, more extensive cluster grafts (20%). The majority of the transplant recipients are children.

Although the morbidity and mortality rates remain significant, 80% of patients who survive the procedure long term have been able to discontinue PN and return to more normal function. Reported patient survival has been 80% at 1 year and 50% at 3 years. Currently liver and small intestine transplantation has a survival similar to hepatic and cardiac transplants. Isolated intestinal transplants are comparable in outcome to kidney and pancreas.

It is hoped that with greater experience and improved results, this therapy can be extended to other patients with SBS. The more successful recent outcome has been related, in part, to the use of the new immunosuppressive agent, tacrolimus. However, other innovative approaches to modifying the immune response may lead to further improvement. The ethical and technical aspects of using living related donors for intestinal transplantation are currently being considered. Of all of the surgical approaches, intestinal transplantation has the greatest potential for treating these patients, both in terms of the number of patients who would benefit and the functional improvement derived. Transplantation is clearly appropriate for individuals with anticipated survival of less than 12 months related to PN-induced complications. A more aggressive approach to the use of intestinal transplantation, particularly solitary transplantation, is justified in patients with signs of early liver dysfunction and other severe complications of nutritional therapy.

MULTIDISCIPLINARY APPROACH

Comprehensive care of intestinal failure patients requires a multidisciplinary approach. A physician leader with expertise in gastrointestinal disease should coordinate the efforts. Gastrointestinal surgical expertise in both adult and pediatric patients is required, and the presence of a transplant surgeon broadens the therapeutic options. Administrative support to coordinate the process and database is essential. A nurse coordinator is indispensable in day-to-day management. A nutritionist is essential. Psychologists and social workers are important for addressing psychosocial issues. This multidisciplinary effort should optimize patient outcome.

SUGGESTED READINGS

Grant D, Abu-Elmagd K, Reyes J, and others: 2003 Report of the Intestine Transplant Registry, *Ann Surg* 241:607, 2005.
Buchman AL, Scolapio J, Fryer J: AGA technical review on short bowel syndrome and intestinal transplantation, *Gastroenterology* 124:1111, 2003.
Dibaise J, Young RJ, Vanderhoof JA, and others: Intestinal rehabilitation and the short bowel syndrome, *Am J Gastr* 99:1823, 2004.
Jeppesen PB: The use of hormonal growth factors in the treatment of patients with short bowel syndrome, *Drugs* 66:581, 2006.
Thompson JS: Surgical rehabilitation of intestine in short bowel syndrome, *Surgery* 135:465, 2004.

SMALL BOWEL CARCINOID TUMORS

Lindsey N. Jackson, MD, and B. Mark Evers, MD

S mall bowel carcinoid tumors are rare neuroendocrine neoplasms with a predilection for the alimentary tract. Originally described by Lubarsch in 1888 and later named *Karzinoide* by Oberndorfer in 1907 to describe their relatively indolent nature, carcinoid tumors are morphologically and biochemically diverse, with site of origin dictating behavior. Carcinoid tumors can synthesize a variety of bioactive substances, including serotonin, chromogranin, histamine, tachykinins, prostaglandins, and intestinal hormones. Up to 64% of carcinoid tumors are localized to the midgut, with a majority found within 2 to 3 feet from the ileocecal valve.

Carcinoid tumors comprise approximately 20% to 30% of small bowel tumors. Small bowel carcinoid tumors are derived from enterochromaffin cells (Kulchitsky cells) in the crypts of Lieberkühn, and, in contrast to carcinoids arising in other organs, they generally produce serotonin as their principal product. Thus tumors in this location most commonly produce the classic carcinoid syndrome. Small bowel carcinoids are multicentric in approximately one fourth of cases, with multiple primary small bowel carcinoids present in approximately 30% of patients with primary ileal tumors. They are associated with a synchronous noncarcinoid malignancy, most commonly colonic adenocarcinoma, in 10% to 20% of patients and are associated with multiple endocrine neoplasia type I in approximately 10% of cases.

Small bowel carcinoid tumors are usually small, firm submucosal nodules on gross examination (Fig. 1); the cut surface is typically yellow in color. Their indolent nature and submucosal location generally lead to a significant delay in presentation, with metastases often present at the time of diagnosis. A prominent characteristic of small bowel carcinoids is their ability to elicit an intense desmoplastic reaction that may lead to mesenteric fibrosis, intestinal kinking, and partial or intermittent bowel obstruction (Fig. 2). Microscopically, the tumors are composed of sheets of small, round, well-differentiated neuroendocrine cells and can be identified by silver impregnation staining. There is no defined classification system for these tumors, and prognosis is dependent on location, size, presence of metastasis, and functional status.

CLINICAL PRESENTATION

Carcinoid Tumors

Carcinoid tumors have protean clinical manifestations that depend largely on the bioactive substances produced. The majority of tumors are diagnosed at the time of emergency surgery, performed without knowledge of the diagnosis; bowel obstruction is a

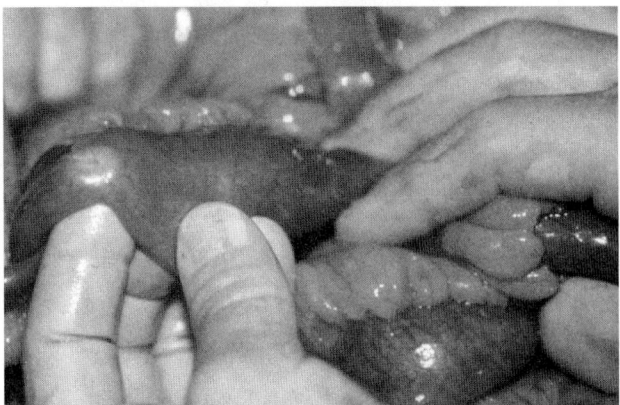

Figure I Midgut carcinoid in terminal ileum. *From Åkerström G, Hellman P, Hessman O, and others: Best Pract Res Clin Gastroenterol 19:5, 717, 2005.*

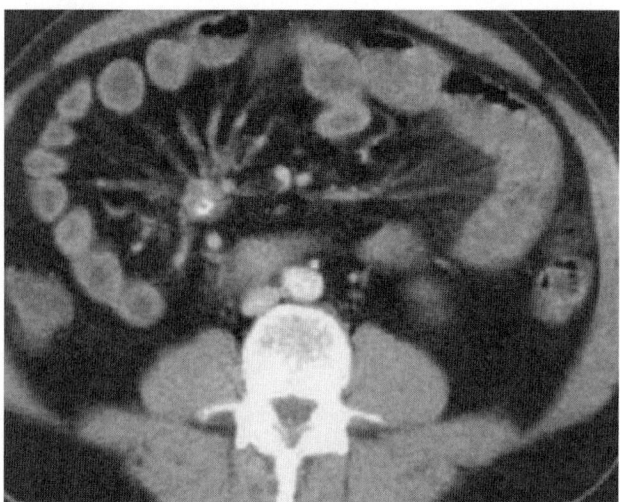

Figure 2   Abdominal computed tomography scan illustrating carcinoid-associated mesenteric fibrosis.   *From Lal A, Chen HL: Curr Opin Oncol 18:1, 9, 2006.*

common presentation. In the absence of carcinoid syndrome, the most common symptom is vague abdominal pain, which may be due to intestinal obstruction, mass effect, intussusception, adhesions, or hypermotility. Diarrhea may also occur as a result of partial bowel obstruction rather than the secretory diarrhea associated with carcinoid syndrome. A rare but emergent presentation is intestinal ischemia secondary to venous thrombosis associated with mesenteric shortening and kinking, a result of the intense fibrotic desmoplastic reaction associated with these tumors.

Carcinoid Syndrome

The classic carcinoid syndrome occurs in approximately 20% of patients with midgut carcinoid tumors and typically includes vasomotor, cardiac, and gastrointestinal manifestations. Secreted products of small intestinal tumors drain into the porta hepatis, resulting in first-pass metabolism by the liver; therefore the syndrome occurs only in the presence of retroperitoneal tumor invasion or hepatic metastasis. Symptoms include diarrhea, cutaneous flushing, and abdominal cramping and occur secondary to the elaboration of a variety of systemic humoral factors, including serotonin, histamine, dopamine, vasoactive intestinal peptide, 5-hydroxytryptophan, and prostaglandins. Flushing of the face, neck, and upper chest may be either short lived or violaceous flushing of longer duration. Asthmatic episodes may occur in temporal association with flushing symptoms. Carcinoid syndrome–associated diarrhea is episodic, explosive, and watery and is the only symptom clearly linked to excessive serotonin levels. Hepatomegaly may be present and is often related to tumor burden. As many as two thirds of patients with carcinoid syndrome develop carcinoid heart disease, the hallmark of which is idiopathic fibrous endocardial thickening of the right heart resulting in tricuspid or pulmonic valve stenosis or regurgitation, leading to heart failure and the possible need for valve replacement (Fig. 3). Pellagra (dermatitis, dementia, diarrhea) may be present, reflecting a diversion of dietary tryptophan to tumor hormone production, with a resultant decrease in nicotinic acid pools.

▆ DIAGNOSIS

In 30% to 50% of cases, the carcinoid tumor is diagnosed unexpectedly at the time of emergency surgery performed for bowel obstruction, intussusception, or other abdominal pathology. For patients who present with a history consistent with carcinoid

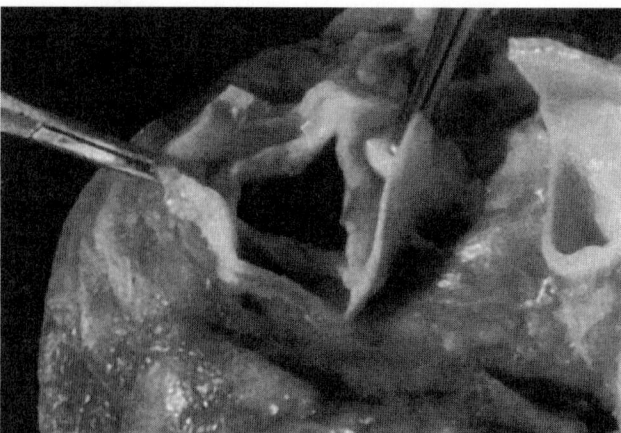

Figure 3   Fibrotic pulmonary valve from a patient with carcinoid heart disease.   *Courtesy James R. Stone, MD, PhD, Department of Pathology, Brigham and Women's Hospital, Boston.* (**See** *color insert Figure 8.*)

syndrome or with small bowel tumor or liver metastases discovered incidentally on radiographic studies, specific testing is warranted.

Biochemical Diagnosis

The cornerstone of the biochemical diagnosis is measurement of 24-hour urinary 5-hyroxyindoleactic acid (5-HIAA), the primary serotonin metabolite, which is 75% sensitive for detecting primary tumors in the absence of metastatic disease and 100% sensitive and specific for detecting metastatic disease. The best screening plasma evaluation is the measurement of chromogranin A, which is elevated in more than 80% of patients with carcinoid tumors. Measurements of serotonin, neurotensin, or neurokinin A are other diagnostic possibilities, although less sensitive.

Radiographic Studies

The most appropriate initial radiographic study is an abdominal computed tomography (CT) scan, which may identify a primary tumor, mesenteric thickening and shortening, hepatic involvement, and lymph node metastasis. Barium radiographic studies may reveal filling defects resulting from bowel thickening and fibrosis (Fig. 4). Angiography and ultrasound may be useful to define the extent of mesenteric or hepatic involvement. Endoscopically accessible lesions may be further investigated with endoscopic ultrasound imaging to delineate invasion and local nodal involvement. Positron emission tomography (PET) is another alternative, although results are often equivocal compared with other diagnostic modalities. Radiolabeled somatostatin analogue scintigraphy with ^{111}In-labeled pentetreotide or octreotide, which capitalizes on somatostatin receptor expression by a majority of these tumors, is currently the staging technique of choice, localizing both primary and metastatic tumors with a sensitivity approaching 90%. An added benefit of scintigraphy is that one dose of ^{111}In-labeled pentetreotide administered preoperatively can aid in diagnosis and preoperative planning, provide intraoperative localization of the radiolabeled probe, and evaluate for residual disease postoperatively.

▆ TREATMENT

Although surgery remains the most effective treatment for carcinoid tumors, the approach is often multidisciplinary, incorporating novel biologic therapies, especially in cases of advanced disease.

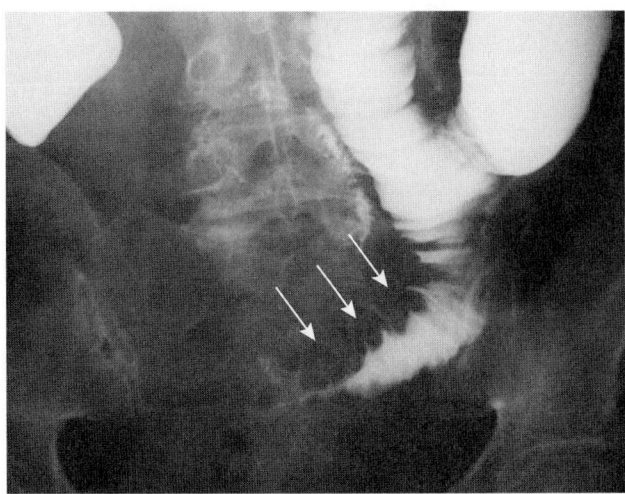

Figure 4 Obstructing carcinoid of the proximal ileum. Small bowel follow-through study shows lumen narrowing, tethering, and fixation attributable to the tumor's growing into the mesentery. *From Gore RM, Berlin JW, Mehta UK, and others: Best Pract Res Clin Gastroenterol 19:2, 245, 2005.*

Preoperative Considerations

Caution is warranted in the preoperative management of patients with carcinoid tumors because anesthesia and operative stress may precipitate a carcinoid crisis characterized by bronchospasm, hypotension, tachycardia, flushing, and arrhythmias in up to 11% of patients. Although patients with carcinoid syndrome are at greatest risk of developing this complication, any patient undergoing resection of a carcinoid tumor may be affected. Thus the perioperative management of patients undergoing carcinoid resection should include preoperative administration of the somatostatin analogue octreotide, either subcutaneously or intravenously, which significantly decreases the risk of carcinoid crisis. Carcinoid crisis, if it develops intraoperatively, is treated with an intravenous bolus of 50 to 100 μg octreotide, followed by a continuous infusion at 50 μg per hour. Intravenous antihistamine and hydrocortisone may also be of some benefit; albuterol is helpful if bronchospasm develops.

Surgery

Surgical resection remains the cornerstone of carcinoid treatment, with primary tumor location, size, and the presence or absence of metastatic disease dictating operative management. Surgery can be categorized as adequate resection with curative intent, resection of regional or distant metastatic disease with cytoreductive intent, or resection of disease for symptom palliation only. Intraoperative localization can be accomplished using a variety of techniques, including intraoperative ultrasound imaging, endoscopy, endoscopic tattooing, or palpation. Additionally, preoperative administration of radiolabeled somatostatin analogues and operative detection with a gamma-detecting probe can be used to identify primary tumors, metastatic disease, and lymph node involvement. The location of the primary tumor, after identified, and the presence or absence of metastatic disease determine the operative approach.

Isolated duodenal carcinoid tumors are rare and are frequently identified during routine upper endoscopy. Lesions are most commonly localized to the first or second part of the duodenum (>90%), and treatment is based on the size of the lesion. Up to 89% of duodenal carcinoids are smaller than 2 cm at diagnosis, with 85% localized to the mucosa or submucosa. Endoscopic resection or local excision is employed for tumors smaller than 1 cm; approximately 25% of duodenal carcinoids are resected with this approach. Transduodenal excision or segmental resection should

be considered for lesions between 1 and 2 cm. Larger lesions (>2 cm) require segmental resection, and, if they are in the second portion of the duodenum, pancreaticoduodenectomy may be indicated. A thorough exploration of the abdomen should be conducted to rule out multicentric lesions.

Carcinoid tumors of the jejunum and ileum are generally diagnosed operatively because the clinical presentation is most commonly small bowel obstruction; they are more infrequently discovered incidentally at the time of operation for other pathology. Because carcinoid tumors are common small intestinal neoplasms, a high index of suspicion of a carcinoid tumor should exist if a small intestinal mass or mesenteric fibrosis is present. In the unusual case of early disease and primary tumor less than 1 cm in size, segmental resection and careful inspection of the entire bowel and mesentery should be performed. However, the typical finding at laparotomy is a small primary tumor with extensive mesenteric metastases and fibrosis (Fig. 5). Tumors most commonly arise in the distal ileum, and tumors in this location carry a greater risk of multicentricity and metastasis; size is a less reliable predictor of malignant potential for tumors in this site. Primary tumors, after they are identified, and mesenteric metastases, if present and

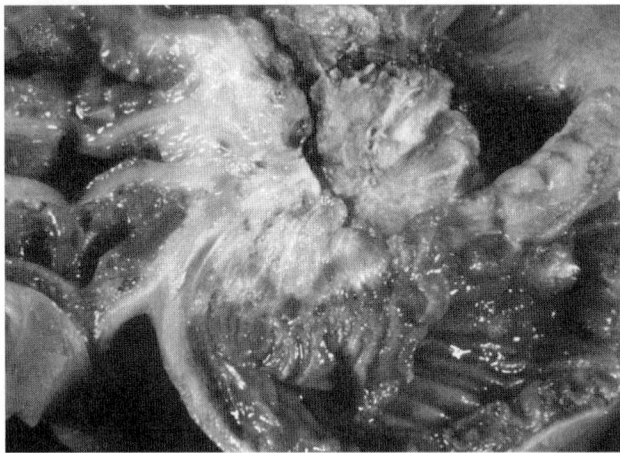

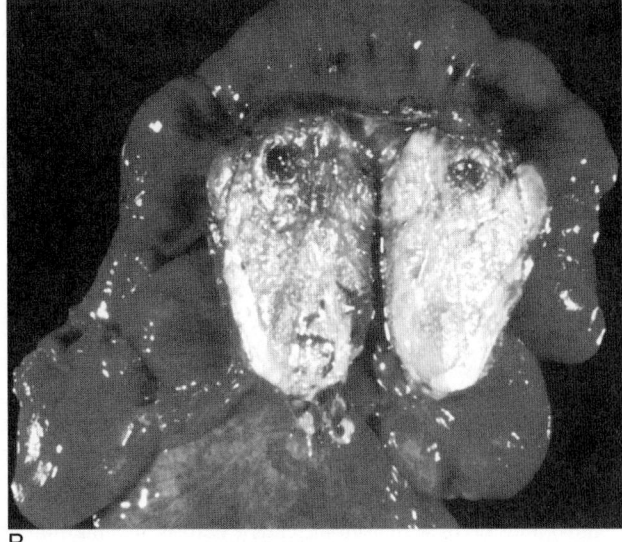

Figure 5 Gross pathologic characteristics of a small bowel carcinoid tumor. **(A)** Carcinoid tumor of the distal ileum with an intense desmoplastic reaction and fibrosis of the bowel wall. **(B)** Mesenteric metastases from a carcinoid tumor of the small bowel. *From Evers BM, Townsend CM Jr, Thompson JC, in Schwartz SI, editor: Principles of surgery, New York, 1999, McGraw-Hill, p. 1217. (See color insert Figure 9.)*

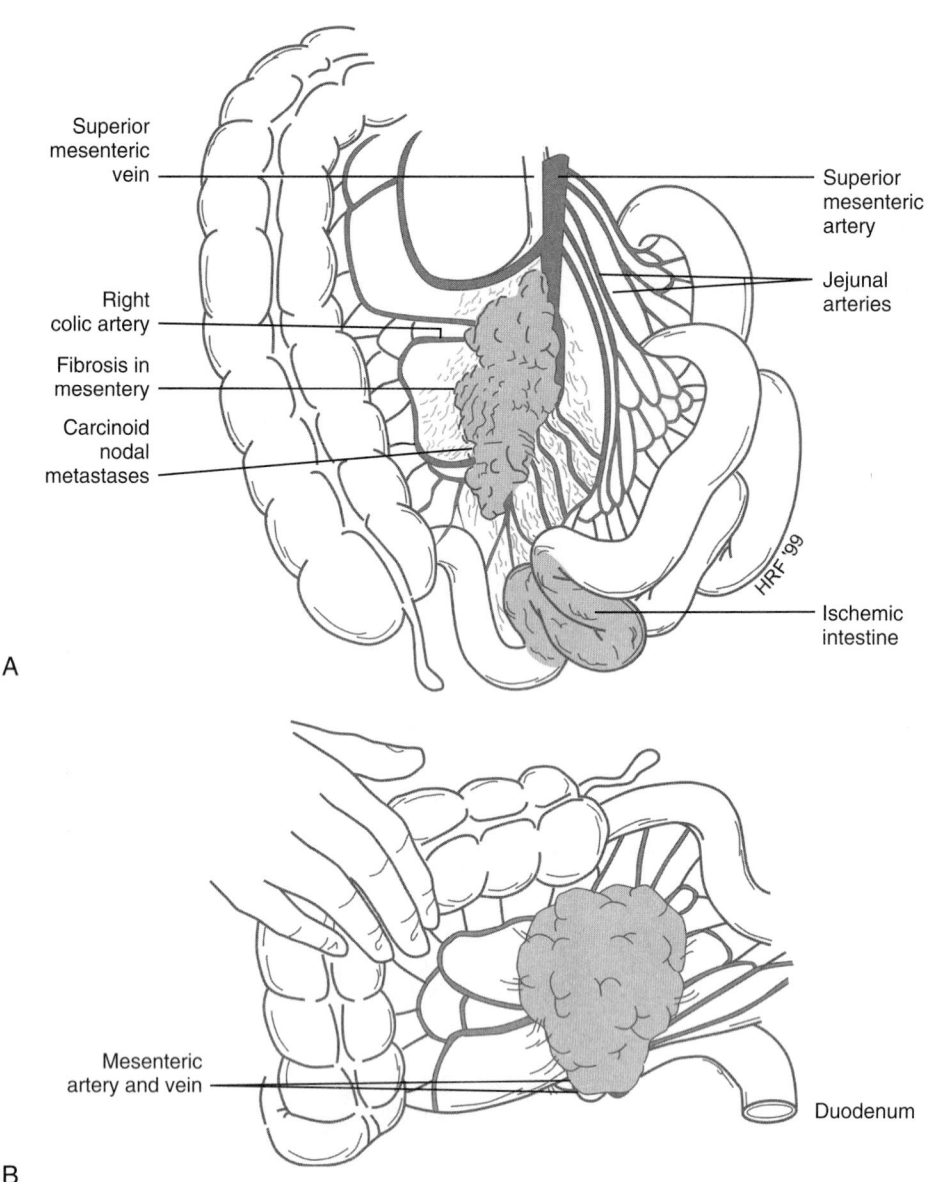

A

B

Figure 6 Resection of carcinoid primary tumor and mesenteric metastasis. **(A)** Mesenteric tumor may extensively involve the mesenteric root. **(B)** Mobilization of the cecum, terminal ileum, and mesenteric root by separation of retroperitoneal attachments allows the tumor to be lifted, approached from a posterior angle, and separated from the duodenum and main mesenteric vessels, with preservation of intestinal vascular supply and intestinal length. *From Åkerström G, Hellman P, Hessman O, and others: Best Pract Res Clin Gastroenterol 19:5, 717, 2005.*

limited, should be treated by wedge resection; care should be taken to clear any lymph node metastases that may be present by careful dissection around the mesenteric artery.

Advanced Disease

Advanced carcinoids may appear inoperable when fibrosis and gross metastases encase the major mesenteric vessels; however, aggressive dissection and debulking, even if total resection is not possible, has demonstrated a significant survival advantage. In one series, resection of the primary tumor with extensive debulking resulted in a doubling of median survival (from 69 months to 139 months). In cases of significant mesenteric fibrosis, mobilization of the right colon and small intestinal mesentery to the level of the lower pancreatic border with division of fibrotic posterior adhesions should be carefully undertaken so that the extent of disease can be more clearly assessed. The superior mesenteric artery and vein should be identified and followed dorsally in the elevated mesenteric root, and vessels should be further exposed by division of the right colon mesentery along the right colic or ileocolic artery, with medial extension of the incision to expose the mesenteric root.

Arteries and veins should be dissected free from surrounding tumor (Fig. 6). Vascular collaterals and arcades should be preserved, and intestinal resection should be reserved until dissection of the mesenteric tumor is complete in an effort to determine bowel viability. Intestinal resection should be as limited as possible to avoid sequelae associated with short bowel syndrome.

Liver Metastases

Approximately half of patients with carcinoid tumors have liver metastases at the time of diagnosis (Fig. 7). Radical resection is the treatment of choice for unilobar disease, leading to an increase in median survival from 48 months to 216 months in one study; however, most hepatic metastases are diffuse at presentation. Dearterialization is an option for disseminated metastases. Because the blood supply of liver metastases is predominantly arterial, whereas hepatic parenchyma obtains 75% to 80% of its blood supply from the portal vein, embolization of arterial blood flow will cause preferential ischemia of the metastases with relative sparing of hepatic tissue. After portal vein patency has been ensured, dearterialization can be accomplished via ligation, embolization, or

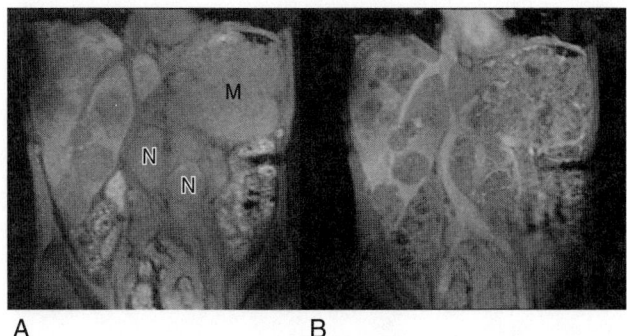

A   B

Figure 7 Large metastatic mesenteric carcinoid. **(A)** Gradient-recalled echo T1-weighted noncontrast magnetic resonance image demonstrates a large left upper quadrant mass *(M)* with multiple lymph node *(N)* and hepatic metastases. **(B)** Following intravenous injection of contrast medium, enhancement of the tumor and metastases is evident following gadolinium administration. *From Gore RM, Berlin JW, Mehta UK, and others: Best Pract Res Clin Gastroenterol 19:2, 245, 2005.*

chemoembolization. If chemoembolization is employed, simultaneous infusion of octreotide may cause intratumoral slowing of blood flow, improving the efficiency of chemoembolization. According to one series, dearterialization by embolization or chemoembolization leads to tumor regression in approximately 65% of patients; when combined with sequential chemotherapy, approximately 78% of tumors regress. Alternatively, cryosurgery or thermal ablation using radiofrequency may be used. In one small study of five patients undergoing cryosurgery, four of the five experienced symptomatic relief for more than 3 months; 6-month survival was 80%, and 1-year survival was 60%. The largest study of radiofrequency ablation combined the data accrued for the treatment of liver metastases from midgut carcinoid ($n = 23$) with those from other neuroendocrine tumors ($n = 19$), for a total of 198 tumors in 42 patients; successful ablation was reported in more than 90% of cases, but survival data for patients with midgut carcinoid were not available. There are currently no prospective randomized trials examining the advantages of these treatment modalities. Lastly, liver transplantation may be considered for patients with extensive liver tumor burden and hepatic failure. Recent meta-analysis has demonstrated a 50% 1-year survival and 24% 5-year disease-free survival for patients undergoing liver transplantation, but further analysis is needed. An algorithm for the treatment of advanced stage carcinoid is presented in Figure 8.

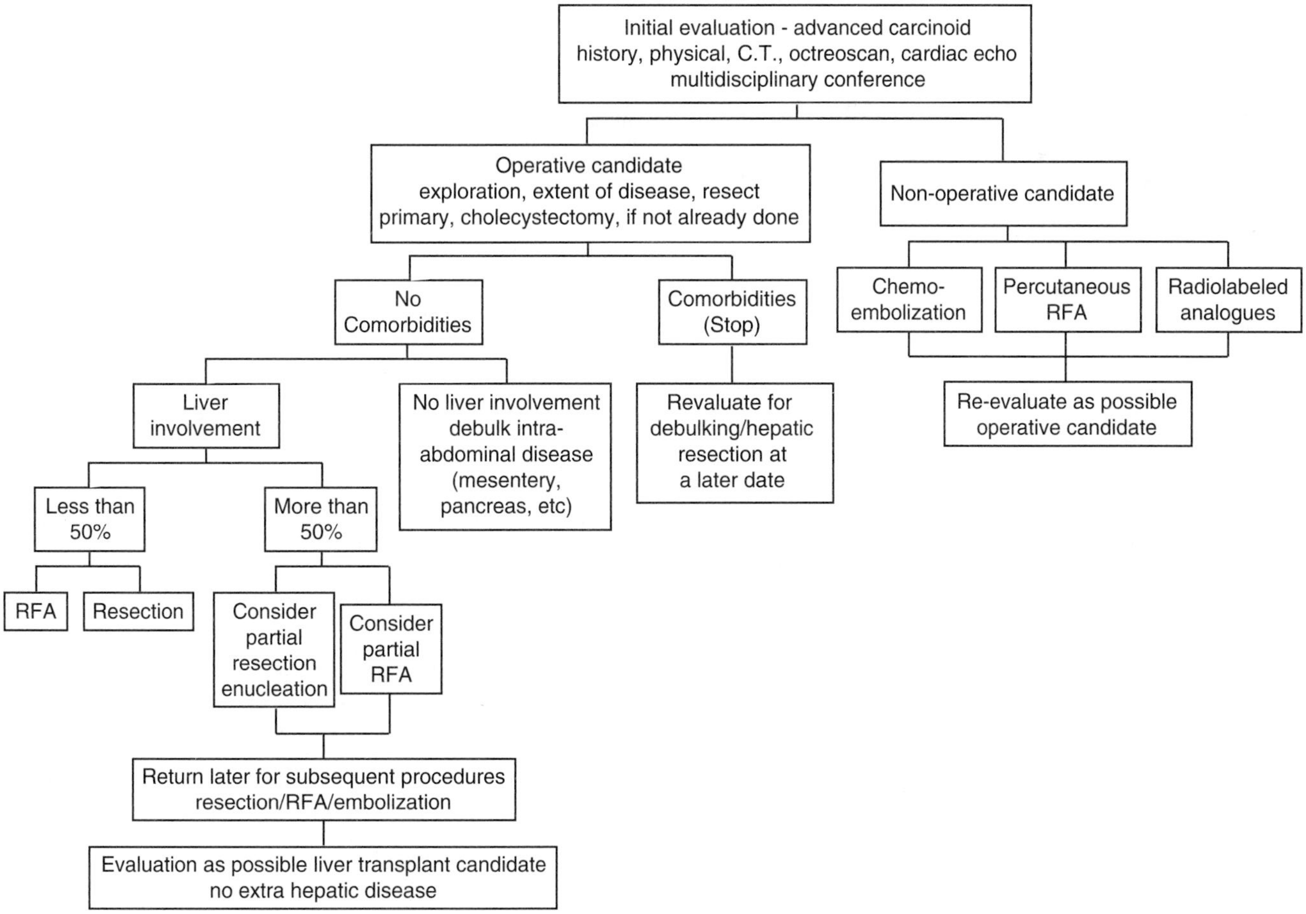

Figure 8 Suggested algorithm for surgical strategy with advanced stage carcinoid. *From Boudreaux JP, Putty B, Frey DJ, and others: Ann Surg 241:6, 839, 2005.*

Medical Therapy

Treatment with somatostatin analogues, including octreotide and lanreotide, has proved to be the foundation of the management of advanced carcinoid disease by palliating symptoms of carcinoid syndrome and reducing pain associated with residual tumor burden. These analogues may have the added benefit of slowing tumor growth and angiogenesis. A side effect of treatment with somatostatin analogues is biliary sludge and cholelithiasis, thus cholecystectomy may be indicated during laparotomy if treatment with these medications is used for residual disease. Interferon-α (IFN-α) similarly palliates symptoms of carcinoid syndrome, reduces hormone secretion, and may inhibit tumor growth and angiogenesis. Chemotherapeutic agents such as streptozocin, doxorubicin, 5-fluorouracil (FU), and cyclophosphamide have been used in the treatment of small intestinal carcinoids but are of questionable benefit, given the low proliferation rate of these tumors and the incidence of side effects.

PROGNOSIS

According to the Surveillance, Epidemiology, and End Results (SEER) database (1973–1999), the 5-year survival rate is 59.9% for localized small intestinal carcinoid tumors, 72.8% for regional disease, and 32.9% for distant disease; the overall 5-year survival is 60.5%. Liver metastasis was thought to be the largest contributor to mortality in these patients; however, bowel obstruction or ischemia (or both) has proved to be the cause of death in a majority of patients. This has led to a more aggressive surgical approach in the management of advanced disease. Debulking, treatment with somatostatin analogues, and extensive lymphadenectomy have been shown to double life expectancy in these patients. Patients should be closely followed after resection; measurement of serum chromogranin A is the most sensitive predictor of recurrence.

SUGGESTED READINGS

Åkerström G, Hellman P, Hessman O and others: Management of midgut carcinoids, *J Surg Oncol* 89:161, 2005.

Boudreaux JP, Putty B, Frey DJ, and others: Surgical treatment of advanced-stage carcinoid tumors: lessons learned, *Ann Surg* 241:839; discussion 45, 2005.

de Vries H, Verschueren RC, Willemse PH, and others: Diagnostic, surgical and medical aspect of the midgut carcinoids, *Cancer Treat Rev* 28:11, 2002.

Evers BM, Parekh D, Townsend CM Jr., and others: Somatostatin and analogues in the treatment of cancer. A review, *Ann Surg* 213:190, 1991.

Evers BM: Small intestine. In Townsend CM Jr., editor: *Sabiston's textbook of surgery: The biological basis of modern surgical practice*, ed. 17, Philadelphia, 2004, Elsevier Saunders, p. 1323.

Modlin IM, Kidd M, Latich I, and others: Current status of gastrointestinal carcinoids, *Gastroenterology* 128:1717, 2005.

Moertel CG, Sauer WG, Dockerty MB, and others: Life history of the carcinoid tumor of the small intestine, *Cancer* 14:901, 1961.

Oberndorfer S: Karzinoide tumoren des dunndarms, *Frankf Z Pathol.* 1:426, 1907.

Thompson GB, van Heerden JA, Martin JK Jr., and others: Carcinoid tumors of the gastrointestinal tract: presentation, management, and prognosis, *Surgery* 98:1054, 1985.

Woodside KJ, Townsend CM Jr, and Evers BM: Current management of gastrointestinal carcinoid tumors, *J Gastrointest Surg* 8:742, 2004.

MOTILITY DISORDERS OF THE STOMACH AND SMALL BOWEL

Corey W. Iqbal, MD, Michael S. Kasparek, MD, and Michael G. Sarr, MD

The surgeon most commonly encounters motility disorders of the gastrointestinal (GI) tract under two circumstances—postoperatively as the gut recovers from anesthesia or as a consequence of planned (or unplanned) functional or directed denervations. Primary motility disorders are less commonly the realm of the surgeon, but because they may masquerade as GI obstructions, one requires a working knowledge of their presentation and management. This chapter addresses motility disorders of the stomach and small bowel.

MOTILITY DISORDERS OF THE STOMACH

Gastric dysmotility manifests one of two ways: rapid transit (dumping, postvagotomy diarrhea) or delayed transit (gastroparesis). These disorders encompass a broad spectrum of etiologies, most of which can be managed successfully medically and rarely necessitate operative intervention. Symptomatology can span from mild or even asymptomatic disease to debilitating disease leading to weight loss and malnutrition. Surgeons should be familiar with the potential etiologies and management of these disorders because many are sequelae from operative procedures (e.g., vagotomy, gastrectomy); moreover, refractory disease may warrant surgical evaluation and possibly operative therapy in selected patients.

Dumping and Postvagotomy Diarrhea

Rapid transit disorders are exclusively a consequence of previous gastric or perigastric operative procedures—most commonly after a vagotomy with a gastric drainage procedure or gastrectomy—the key, however, is the vagotomy. Rapid transit disorders can be subdivided into *dumping syndrome* and *postvagotomy diarrhea*. The pathophysiology of both involves ablation of vagally mediated receptive relaxation, the physiologic process that allows for accommodation by the stomach after ingestion of a meal, that is, the stomach "relaxes" to accept the volume of the meal with minimal change in intragastric pressure. In the absence of receptive relaxation, the stomach fails to relax, and intragastric pressure increases. Because emptying of liquids is controlled largely by pressure in the proximal stomach, this increased intraluminal pressure leads to a rapid emptying of liquids. The resultant rapid gastric emptying is further exacerbated by the presence of a drainage procedure (pyloroplasty, gastroenterostomy), which impedes outflow resistance to gastric contents.

Dumping is characterized clinically by nausea, abdominal pain, diaphoresis, and palpitations 15 to 30 minutes after a meal, often followed by diarrhea 30 to 60 minutes later. In addition to the loss of receptive relaxation and outflow resistance of the stomach, dumping syndrome is associated with release of vasoactive substances from the gut mucosa in response to entry of hyperosmolar, carbohydrate-rich meals including neurotensin, vasoactive intestinal peptide, pancreatic polypeptide, motilin, peptide YY, and enteroglucagon, which stimulate GI secretions and motility; it is the release of these vasoactive substances that causes the symptomatology. Up to 25% of patients undergoing gastric resection with a vagotomy and drainage procedure will develop some clinical symptoms of dumping syndrome.

In contrast to the more common, early dumping syndrome, late dumping occurs approximately 2 hours postprandial associated with symptoms of hypoglycemia. Fortunately, this problem is much less common than early dumping, occurring in only 2% of patients. After ingestion of a meal, the overzealous release of enteroglucagon causes hyperglycemia, which then triggers an exaggerated release of insulin and subsequent hypoglycemia. Patients eat to restore their blood glucose levels, and a vicious cycle is initiated. More than 80% of patients, however, improve with time and dietary modification. Refractory cases should be managed with a trial of subcutaneous octreotide, which is effective in approximately 50% of patients.

The diagnosis of dumping can usually be made from a thorough history. Radionuclide scintigraphy can confirm rapid gastric emptying but is rarely, if ever, necessary. Dumping can usually be managed via dietary modification, specifically by eliminating carbohydrate-rich foods. Failure to improve with dietary changes warrants pharmacologic intervention. Octreotide may resolve explosive diarrhea, as well as inhibit release of GI neuropeptides; however, it is not without side effects, including cholestasis and gallstone formation, the painful injections required, and its high cost.

Because clinically relevant dumping almost always resolves in the first year postoperatively, operative intervention should be delayed and considered only in patients with refractory disease persisting for more than 1 year who have truly intractable symptoms resulting in weight loss and malnutrition. Several options exist for correction of dumping syndrome, although none is foolproof. Pyloric reconstruction (after previous pyloroplasty) to create greater resistance to gastric outflow or conversion of a Billroth II to a Billroth I–type reconstruction to reestablish duodenal drainage may be used, but with acknowledged limited success. Use of a 10-cm interposition, antiperistaltic segment of jejunum taken 100 cm distal to the ligament of Treitz, although initially promising, has not yielded satisfactory results. Conversion of a Billroth II to a Roux-en-Y gastrojejunostomy is probably the most appropriate procedure for refractory dumping syndrome because the Roux anatomy tends to slow gastric emptying.

Postvagotomy diarrhea can be difficult to distinguish from dumping syndrome. Nonetheless, it is an important distinction because the two vary in terms of their pathophysiology, treatment, and prognosis. Similar to dumping, postvagotomy diarrhea is attributed in part to loss of receptive relaxation, as well as other effects on small bowel motility, resulting in a markedly increased transit and bile acid malabsorption; the bile acid malabsorption leads to a decrease in water absorption in the colon and subsequent diarrhea. Unlike dumping, postvagotomy diarrhea is not related to a drainage procedure, nor is it related to hyperosmolality or other foodstuffs. Symptoms are similar to dumping; however, they occur 30 to 60 minutes postprandial. These symptoms are usually not severe enough to lead to malnutrition.

The mainstay of treatment of these rapid emptying disorders is dietary modification, primarily by avoiding carbohydrate-dense foods and with bulk-forming agents such as fiber supplements. If diarrhea persists, pharmacologic agents such as octreotide or bile acid resins (or both) may be used to target bile acid malabsorption; opiates can be tried to slow transit for symptomatic relief. Refractory postvagotomy diarrhea is rare and may initiate a Roux-en-Y conversion or an interposition segment of antiperistaltic jejunum; however, the surgeon must emphasize to the patient that results are not good. Many experts believe that postvagotomy diarrhea is untreatable.

Delayed Gastric Emptying

Slow gastric transit time is referred to globally as *delayed gastric emptying* (DGE) or gastroparesis. Recently, more specific etiologies of slow gastric transit include impaired fundic relaxation, antral hypomotility, antral dilatation, dyssynchronous antroduodenal coordination, pylorospasm, visceral hypersensitivity, and gastric dysrhythmias. These states are characterized by early satiety, nausea, vomiting, regurgitation, fullness, and bloating. The symptoms may range from mild to severe and can be confused with dyspepsia or reflux symptoms. In contrast to dumping syndrome, liquids are better tolerated. The pathophysiology of DGE can be broken into two categories: primary and secondary causes.

Primary causes for DGE cover a broad range of etiologies, most commonly diabetic gastroparesis and idiopathic gastroparesis, but other disorders associated with neuropathy can lead to DGE as well. Connective tissue disorders such as scleroderma; infiltrating diseases such as amyloidosis; abuse of medications including opiates, anticholinergics, and other psychotropics; hypothyroidism; and idiosyncratic reactions to ill-defined viral infection can contribute to gastroparesis, the latter most commonly in young women.

Secondary DGE is a postoperative consequence of vagotomy that results in an atonic, nondistensible stomach/gastric remnant caused by a loss of receptive relaxation or by denervation of the antrum and pylorus. Some element of DGE occurs in approximately 30% of patients undergoing vagotomy (with or without a gastric resection and drainage procedure). Other operative procedures, such as fundoplication, esophagectomy, gastric bypass, Whipple procedure, and cardiac or pulmonary operations may be associated with DGE, in some instances believed secondary to vagal injury or vagal dysfunction (e.g., fundoplication). Postoperatively, there are two forms of DGE—early postoperative DGE and late DGE, the latter possibly better termed *gastroparesis*. The former presents immediately postoperatively. The cause of this postoperative gastric "ileus" is not well understood, but it usually resolves within 6 weeks. Well-known causes that should be excluded are intra-abdominal sepsis or anastomotic leak, such as after a pancreatectomy at the site of pancreaticoenterostomy.

Gastroparesis occurs to some extent in up to 30% of patients undergoing Roux-en-Y reconstructions of GI continuity, the so-called Roux stasis syndrome. This condition can be difficult to manage medically, especially with severe symptoms, and on occasion it may require a near-total gastrectomy, which is effective, however, in only approximately 50% to 70% of patients. Some authors have suggested the use of an "uncut" Roux limb to avoid transection of the jejunum, which disrupts aborally propagated electrical pacemaker signals from the duodenum.

The most important concept in the workup of these patients is to exclude mechanical obstruction in the pylorus, gastroenterostomy, or small bowel, best achieved with endoscopy or contrast radiographs. Probably the most important symptom is the vomiting of food ingested the day before; in the absence of mechanical obstruction, this symptom is virtually pathognomonic of gastroparesis. Gastric emptying can be "confirmed" by several direct and indirect studies. Nuclear scintigraphy (gastric emptying study) is the most widely used tool, but radiopaque markers, such as barium pellets, real-time ultrasonography, magnetic resonance imaging, epigastric electrical impedance, manometry, use of a barostat, and carbon breath tests, although more specialized, can be used as well. Endoscopy will exclude anastomotic stricture and may also show retained food. The astute clinician will not be fooled into the diagnosis of "bile reflux gastritis" simply by the presence of bile in the stomach; gastroparesis allows accumulation of refluxed enteric content (bile) in the noncontractile stomach.

First-line therapy for these patients is dietary modification with small, more frequent, low-fat meals. Because liquids are better tolerated, liquid caloric supplements can be used as well. Prokinetic agents can be tried if diet alone does not control the patient's symptoms; however, such prokinetics as erythromycin, metoclopramide, and domperidone (which is not currently available in the United States) are usually ineffective; cisapride has been removed from the market (and did not work well); and tegasarod, a 5-HT4 agonist, although promising, is still under investigation. More recently, gastric pacemaking has been introduced as a treatment modality; however, its efficacy in decreasing vomiting is possibly worthwhile, but its efficacy in speeding gastric emptying has not been demonstrated as of yet. Patients unable to maintain adequate caloric intake should be supported aggressively with enteral feedings through an enterostomy tube or, if unable to tolerate enteral nutrition, by parenteral nutrition.

In the setting of weight loss and failure to maintain nutrition by oral intake, operative intervention may be entertained. The procedure of choice is a near-total gastrectomy to eliminate the noncompliant, noncontractile stomach. This aggressive procedure can be curative in 50% to 66% of patients; however, up to 25% may still require enteral support, and up to 25% may require parenteral support.

PRIMARY MOTILITY DISORDERS OF THE SMALL BOWEL

Most motility disorders of the small bowel manifest as slow transit and intestinal distention. Such a scenario mimics mechanical small bowel obstruction. Suspicion of and subsequent differentiation of mechanical from functional "obstruction" is important because treatment varies markedly.

Chronic Intestinal Pseudo-obstruction

Chronic intestinal pseudo-obstruction (CIP), a rare progressive disorder that can affect the entire GI tract, usually presents with clinical and radiologic signs of intestinal obstruction but in the absence of any mechanical obstruction. Familial and sporadic forms occur in children, as well as in adults, and manifest as visceral myopathies, neuropathies, or so-called intermediate histologic changes of the neuromuscular architecture of the intestine. In children, CIP may be associated with developmental abnormalities of the urinary tract, pyloric stenosis, intestinal atresia, and abnormalities of intestinal rotation, suggesting an as yet undefined genomic abnormality. In adults, CIP can be sporadic or familial, but it is often secondary to various systemic disorders, a characteristic that can affect the management and outcome of these patients (e.g., connective tissue diseases, amyloidosis, diabetic neuropathy, progressive systemic sclerosis, hypothyroidism, paraneoplastic syndromes, drugs with anticholinergic properties, Chagas's disease, and radiation enteritis). A form of CIP can also complicate certain neuromuscular diseases, such as Duchenne muscular dystrophy, Parkinson's disease, myotonic dystrophy, and mitochondrial myopathies.

Clinically these patients present with abdominal pain and distension, nausea, vomiting, and altered bowel movements, but they can also have dysphagia and gastroesophageal reflux with esophageal involvement, postprandial bloating, early satiety with gastric involvement, and constipation with colonic involvement. Patients with bacterial overgrowth secondary to the delayed small bowel transit may have diarrhea.

Physical examination often reveals a distended abdomen, with a tympanic percussion and "obstructive" or absent bowel sounds. Because the history and physical examination are not definitive, radiologic studies are required and usually obtained with an initial suspicion of mechanical small bowel obstruction. A plain radiograph commonly demonstrates dilatated bowel at varying regions but cannot exclude reliably a mechanical obstruction. An upper GI contrast series or computed tomography (CT) may show delayed but still present passage of oral contrast through the entire small intestine (all of which is dilatated) and into the colon, thereby excluding a relevant mechanical obstruction. If necessary, patency of the colon can be demonstrated on a retrograde contrast study. When the diagnosis is suspected but still unconfirmed, manometric studies may allow further differentiation of the functional obstruction of CIP from a mechanical obstruction with some reliability.

When an underlying mechanical obstruction cannot be excluded and there are no previous pathognomonic signs of CIP, these patients often undergo exploratory celiotomies, which reveal dilated small bowel but without a site of mechanical obstruction. Further operative intervention should be avoided whenever possible, because these patients are susceptible to developing adhesive mechanical obstruction in the future. Nevertheless, if a mechanical obstruction cannot be excluded or if the patient's condition deteriorates, an exploration should be performed. If possible, a laparoscopic approach is best, because should no point of obstruction be found, postoperative adhesion formation should be minimal, thereby preventing future adhesion problems with differentiation of adhesive from functional obstruction during episodes of symptomatologic exacerbation.

When the diagnosis is secure, the management of CIP is primarily supportive. Inability to ingest sufficient oral nutrition to maintain health usually precipitates the use of parenteral nutrition because enteral nutrition is not a viable option with their dysfunctional gut. Parenteral nutrition is also associated with the risk of liver failure, especially in children. The only curative approach for these malnourished children and adults with CIP is small bowel or multivisceral transplantation, the results of which have improved exponentially since 2000. Therefore patients with CIP on long-term parenteral nutrition should be referred to a transplant center for future consideration for small intestinal transplantation (Fig. 1, Table 1).

Bacterial overgrowth can be treated with alternating courses of oral antibiotics (ciprofloxacin, metronidazole, or doxycycline) to minimize diarrhea. Medical stimulation of GI motility is of questionable efficacy, but octreotide, erythromycin, and metoclopramide may be of benefit in some patients. Cisapride was helpful in some patients with CIP but is no longer available routinely in the United States.

In the patient with refractory symptoms, operative palliation may have a role. Rare patients have localized disease amenable to segmental resection or bypass; on occasion, the dysfunctional bowel involves only the duodenum, and some temporary benefit may be realized by a tailoring duodenoplasty. Temporary "venting" enterostomies can provide considerable symptomatic relief from abdominal distention. Enteral feeding tubes can occasionally be inserted distal to the functionally obstructed bowel; however, such ostensibly "localized" disease is unusual, and the CIP usually follows a relentless, progressive course to involve more and more of the gut. In the diffuse form of CIP, extended resections are not beneficial.

SECONDARY MOTILITY DISORDERS OF THE SMALL BOWEL

Ileus

The most common form of small bowel dysmotility seen by surgeons is postoperative ileus, which can develop after intra-abdominal operations and even after nonabdominal surgery. Normally, the usual patterns of small bowel motility are disrupted early postoperatively after an intra-abdominal operation. This "physiologic,"

Figure 1 Algorithm for the treatment of chronic intestinal pseudo-obstruction.

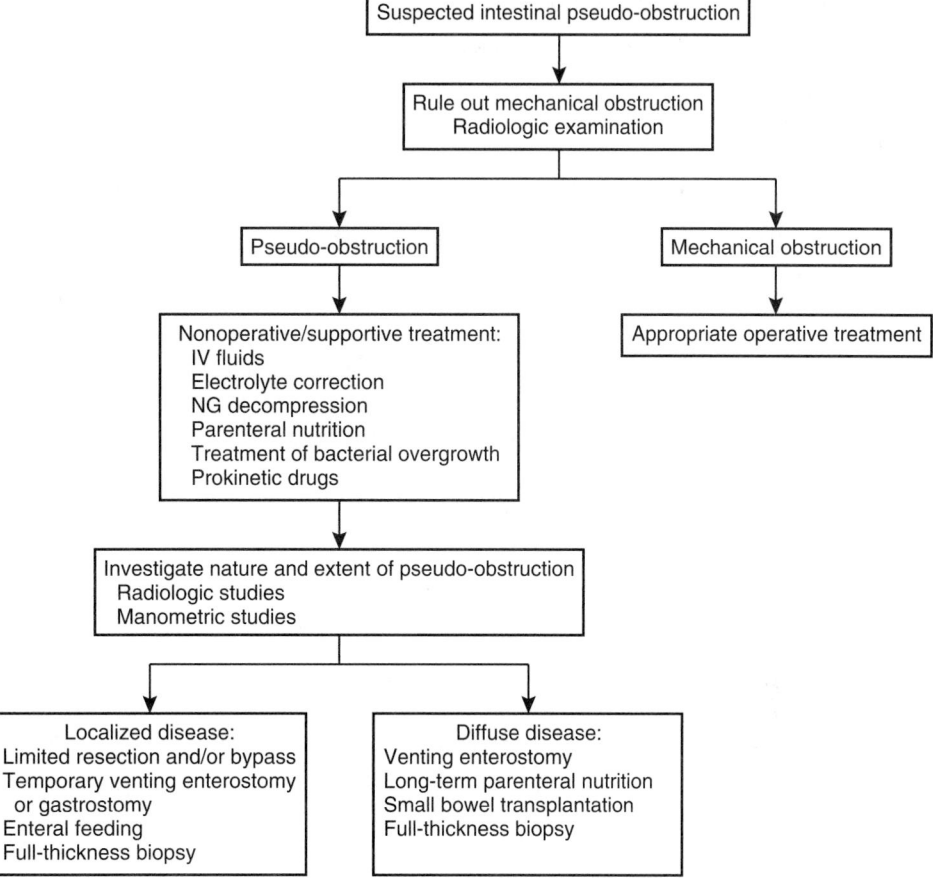

Table 1: Criteria for Operative Treatment in Patients with Presumed Chronic Intestinal Pseudo-Obstruction

1. Failure of nonoperative, supportive management
   Severe, symptomatic distention (venting, enterostomy)
   Persistent vomiting (gastrostomy)
2. Complications (perforation, ischemia, etc.)
3. Localized pseudo-obstruction (resection, bypass)
4. Enteral nutritional support (when possible)

postoperative ileus appears to be a short-lived, neurally mediated reflex response to the operative trauma that may be exacerbated by drugs used during anesthesia coupled with narcotic forms of postoperative analgesia. Physiologic ileus of the small bowel should not last more than a day (the postoperative ileus of the large intestine, in contrast, usually persists for 3–5 days). A more prolonged ileus, often called *adynamic ileus,* may be related to "overactivity" of the sympathetic innervation to the gut related to systemic stress, intra-abdominal sepsis, or retroperitoneal processes (neoplasms, operations, etc.), generalized electrolyte abnormalities, or by a prolonged inflammatory response associated with the release of inhibitory neurotransmitters within the gut wall, leading to a prolonged dysmotility. This form of adynamic ileus is also associated with a colonic ileus and distention.

Although these forms of ileus usually resolve spontaneously, certain measures may accelerate the recovery of motility and gut function and shorten the hospital stay. Postoperative ileus appears less likely after laparoscopic surgical techniques. The use of epidural preemptive analgesia—preferably with local anesthetics—may shorten postoperative ileus, although this topic remains controversial.

Management of postoperative ileus is primarily supportive. Aggressive attempts to correct electrolyte disturbances, treat intra-abdominal infections, and provide nutritional support represent the mainstays of active therapy. If recurrent vomiting occurs, a nasogastric tube should be considered. Erythromycin and metoclopramide are more effective for the treatment of gastric disorders. Neostigmine, an acetylcholinesterase inhibitor, has proved effective in selected patients, but patients with a history of myocardial infarction, arrhythmia, asthma, or concurrent use of beta-blockers should be monitored for parasympathetic side effects. Depending on the underlying cause, nonoperative management is usually successful.

An entity that mimics postoperative ileus but may require reoperation is *early postoperative small bowel obstruction* (EPSBO). This entity is a true mechanical small bowel obstruction, but because it manifests in the early postoperative period, it may be overlooked as such and assumed to be the functional obstruction of postoperative ileus. As with any mechanical obstruction, strangulation obstruction is a possibility, and thus EPSBO must at least be considered even in the postoperative period. Unlike postoperative ileus, which manifests immediately after operation, EPSBO often has a window of return of gut function (as expected) followed by loss of gut function. In most patients, these obstructions are secondary to development of adhesions and often resolve with observation, but other causes, such as acute internal herniation, intussusception, and port-site herniation after laparoscopy, must be considered and usually require surgical treatment. EPSBO also occurs in patients with peritoneal carcinosis or a frozen abdomen and after excessive adhesiolysis.

Table 2: Management of Postoperative Ileus and EPSBO

Early Postoperative Ileus (Postoperative day 3–5)

Perioperative: Consider laparoscopic surgery and/or epidural anesthesia; avoid fluid overload
Postoperative: Correct fluid and electrolyte imbalance; avoid nasogastric tube; minimize use of opioids; early enteral nutrition and ambulation; oral laxatives

Prolonged Postoperative Ileus (Beyond Postoperative day 5)

Rule out underlying causes (infection, intra-abdominal abscess)
Correct fluid and electrolyte imbalance; consider nasogastric tube and parenteral nutrition when recurrent vomiting occurs; minimize use of opioids; stimulation of GI motility (e.g., neostigmine)

EPSBO (Intestinal Obstruction After Initial Return of Bowel Function)

Rule out underlying cause (herniation, strangulation, intussusception, inflammation, trocar-site herniation)
Conservative but close observational treatment when no reoperation is indicated:
- Correct fluid and electrolyte imbalance; consider nasogastric tube and parenteral nutrition when recurrent vomiting occurs; minimize use of opioids; stimulation of GI motility (e.g., neostigmine, Gastrografin)
- Consider reoperation if GI transit cannot be restored within 2 weeks
- Prolonged conservative treatment can be justified in "hostile abdomen" (after excessive adhesiolysis, frozen abdomen, radiation enteritis, peritoneal carcinosis)

EPSBO, early postoperative small bowel obstruction; *GI,* gastrointestinal.

Diagnosis of EPSBO can be difficult. Plain abdominal radiographs in EPSBO often demonstrate dilatated, air-filled loops of small bowel, but an important distinction is the more distal collapsed loops of small bowel and no distention of the colon. Functional studies, such as an upper GI contrast study or the Gastrografin challenge test, can help to detect mechanical obstruction. Abdominal CT with water-soluble oral contrast is best to detect internal herniations or extra-luminal pathologies; in addition, fluid collections or abscesses can be recognized and treated by CT-guided drainage.

Two forms of EPSBO deserve mention. Trocar-site herniations represent a special entity of EPSBO. In patients after laparoscopy, the sudden development of a small bowel obstruction should precipitate consideration of and evaluation for a port-site herniation by ultrasonography or CT; the presence of this diagnosis requires immediate reoperation (Table 2). The second form of notable EPSBO is the difficult–to–diagnose internal hernias that can occur after laparoscopic bariatric procedures (Roux-en-Y gastric bypass and duodenal switch with biliopancreatic diversion). Overlooking these internal, often strangulating hernias can lead to catastrophic outcomes.

SUGGESTED READINGS

Behrns KE, Sarr MG: Diagnosis and management of gastric emptying disorders. In Cameron JL, editor: *Advances in surgery,* Vol. 27, Chicago, 1994, Mosby-Year Book, p. 233.

Bond GJ, Reyes JD: Intestinal transplantation for total/near-total aganglionosis and intestinal pseudo-obstruction, *Sem Pediatr Surg* 13:286, 2004.

Forstner-Barthell AW, Murr MM, Nitecki S, and others: Near-total completion gastrectomy for severe postvagotomy gastric stasis: analysis of early- and long-term results in 62 patients, *J Gastrointest Surg* 3:15, 1999.

Kelly KA, Sarr MG, Hinder RA: Disorders of gastrointestinal motility and emptying after gastric surgery. In Kelly KA, Sarr MG, Hinder RA, editors: *Mayo Clinic gastrointestinal surgery,* Philadelphia, 2004, WB Saunders, p. 127.

Murr MM, Sarr MG, Camilleri M: The surgeon's role in the treatment of chronic intestinal pseudoobstruction, *Am J Gastroenterol* 90:2147, 1995.

Sajja SBS, Schein M: Early postoperative small bowel obstruction, *Br J Surg* 91:683, 2004.

Smith DS, Williams CS, Ferris CD: Diagnosis and treatment of chronic gastroparesis and chronic intestinal pseudo-obstruction, *Gastroenterol Clin N Am* 32:619, 2003.

LARGE BOWEL

VIRTUAL COLONOSCOPY

Karen M. Horton, MD, and Elliot K. Fishman, MD

INTRODUCTION

Colon cancer is the third most common cancer in the United States and accounts for approximately 56,000 deaths per year. Despite a variety of colon cancer screening tests available today, participation remains low. Virtual colonoscopy is a relatively new and novel way to screen for colon polyps and cancers. The technique was first described in 1995. Early attempts at virtual colonoscopy were limited by both computed tomography (CT) scanner technology and limited software resources. However, since the mid-1990s, there have been significant advancements in CT scanner technology, including the introduction of multi-detector row CT, which allows fast high-resolution imaging. These new scanners, in combination with sophisticated three-dimensional (3D) software packages, now make virtual colonoscopy more accurate, affordable, and user friendly. This chapter describes the current status of virtual colonoscopy for colon cancer screening.

TECHNIQUE

Colon Preparation

To perform a high-quality virtual colonoscopy, colon cleansing is necessary. A variety of colon-cleansing preparations are available. These include magnesium citrate, phospho-soda, and polyethylene glycol solutions. In our practice, we routinely use phospho-soda preparations. We find that this does a good job of cleansing the colon and leaves little residual fluid. However, elderly patients or patients with renal or cardiac issues cannot take phospho-soda, and therefore we use polyethylene glycol for these patients. Recently there have been reports of phosphate-induced nephropathy in patients with no history of cardiac or renal issues. Therefore many institutions have switched to polyethylene glycol. This is an excellent bowel preparation, although it leaves a moderate amount of fluid, and this can be a challenge when performing virtual colonoscopy. Whatever colon preparation is chosen, it is important to begin the preparation the day before the study to ensure complete colonic cleansing.

In addition to the colon cleansing, to perform high-quality virtual colonoscopy, stool tagging is also necessary. Stool tagging is a method by which residual stool in the colon is "tagged" with a high-density contrast agent so that it can be easily identified on CT (Fig. 1). If stool tagging is not used, it is often difficult or impossible to distinguish small stool particles from polyps. Stool tagging consists of both solid and liquid stool tagging. Solid stool tagging is accomplished with diluted barium agents, which are consumed during the colonic preparation the day before the study. These barium agents combine with any residual solid stool. Therefore, during the study, if there is adherent stool, it will appear white on the CT scan. In addition to the solid stool tagging, iodinated oral contrast is also administrated the day before the CT colonoscopy. This is a liquid water-soluble iodine-based contrast agent that increases the density of any residual fluid. Therefore if there is residual fluid, it will also appear high density on the CT and can be easily identified. If liquid stool tagging is not used, residual fluid can hide small polyps.

Because of the complexity of the bowel preparation and stool tagging procedure at our institution, we prepare a bowel prep and tagging kit, which is mailed to the patient along with instructions before the study. This avoids confusion and helps achieve high-quality preparation.

Colonic Distention

In addition to the bowel cleansing and stool tagging, is important to distend the colon adequately. Although somewhat controversial in the literature, at our institution, we routinely administer 1 mg of glucagon 10 minutes before the study. This helps to relax the colon and, in our opinion, results in better colonic distention and improved patient tolerance.

When the patient is on the CT table, a small tube is inserted into the rectum. To distend the rectum, there are two options; room air versus carbon dioxide. If room air is used, a small handheld balloon pump inflates the colon. However, most busy practices doing virtual colonoscopy use carbon dioxide. The advantage of carbon dioxide is that it is well tolerated by patients and is absorbed. Therefore most patients feel comfortable within a half hour of the study. Carbon dioxide is administered through an electronic insufflator. The insufflator inflates the colon to a preset pressure. During the examination, if the patient loses some air, the pump will automatically reinflate. When using room air, approximately 1 to 2 L of air is necessary. With carbon dioxide, it is usually between 3 and 4 L of air.

Colon insufflation is started in the left lateral decubitus position. After adequate insufflation, the patient lies supine for the first scan. The exam is performed in both the supine and prone positions. This ensures adequate distention of all segments of the colon (Fig. 2). Also, if there is residual fluid or stool, it will shift when the patient changes positions (Fig. 3).

Computed Tomography Scan Protocol

For high-quality virtual colonoscopy, thin-slice collimation is necessary. We use our 64-slice multidetector row scanner. This

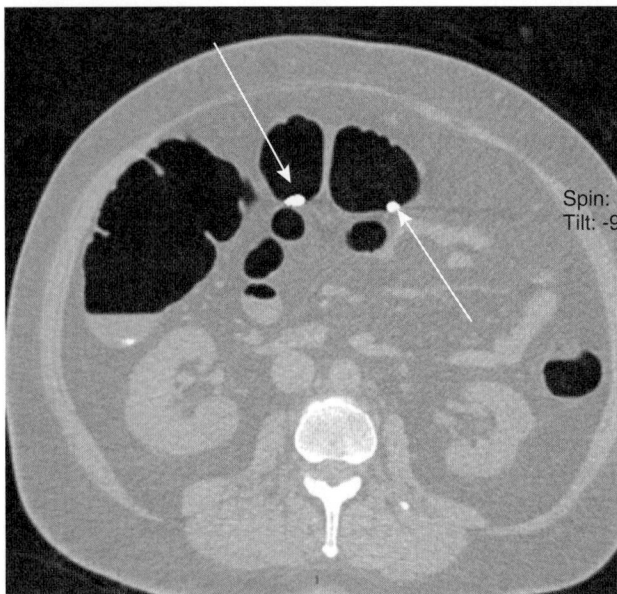

Figure 1 Axial image from virtual colonoscopy study shows air distention of the colon. The patient ingested a stool-tagging agent during the bowel cleansing. Two high-density foci are seen with in the transverse colon *(arrows)*. The stool-tagging agent is a dilute barium solution that mixes with residual stool. Therefore residual stool appears white on the computed tomography scan, allowing easy identification.

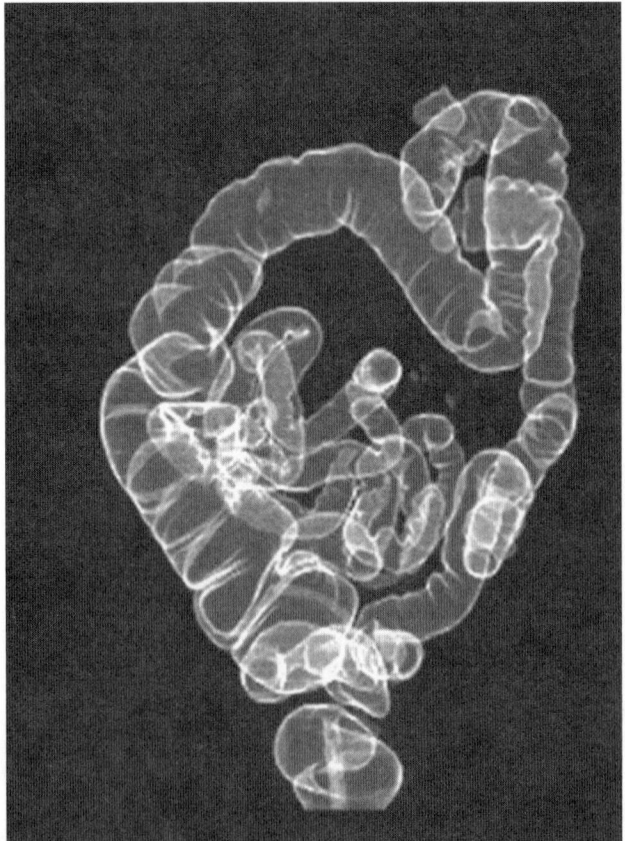

Figure 2 Global coronal view of the air-distended colon. This is a computed tomography examination in which the air-filled colon is accentuated. It resembles a double contrast barium enema. This view is useful in assessing adequate distention of the colon. The colon must be completely distended to detect polyps.

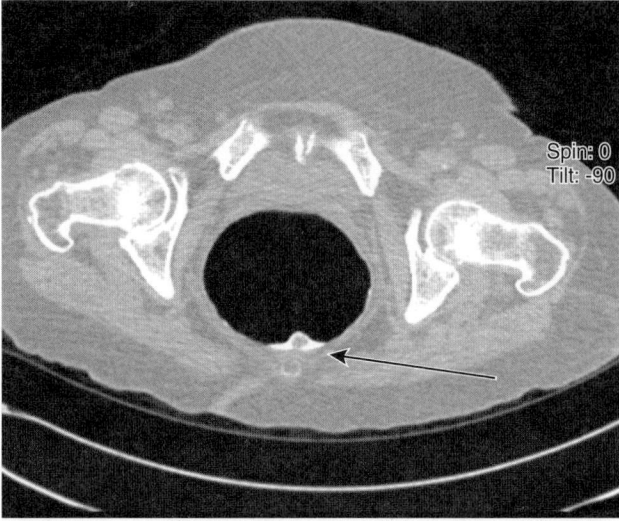

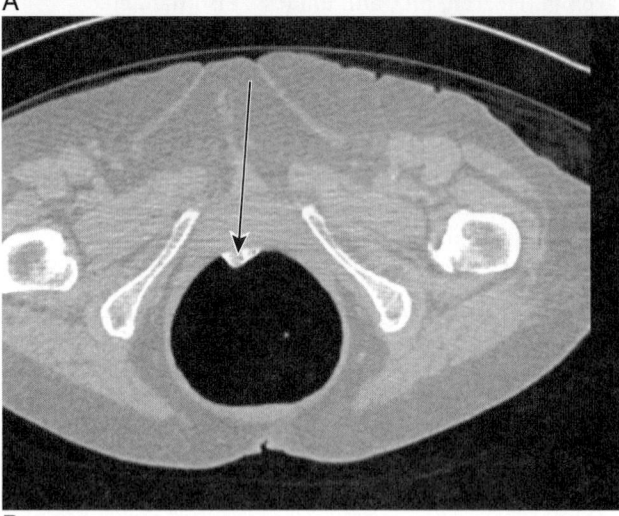

Figure 3 Axial images from virtual colonoscopy in the supine **(A)** and prone **(B)** positions. Minimal residual stool and tagging agent is identified in the rectum on both prone and supine images *(arrow)*. Note that the position of the residual stool changes between the prone and supine view, indicating that it is mobile. This confirms that this is indeed residual stool rather than a polyp, which would not change in position with patient movement.

allows submillimeter collimation. The 64.0 × 0.6–mm collimator setting is used to create 1-mm slices, which are reconstructed every 0.8 mm. This results in isotropic imaging. This means that high resolution is maintained in all imaging plains. Therefore the axial, coronal, and sagittal imaging and the 3D imaging will be of extremely high resolution. This is crucial to detect small polyps.

Radiation dose can be minimized because there is high contrast between the soft-tissue polyps and the air-filled colon. For routine studies, we therefore use mAs of 50, kVp of 120. This results in an estimated total radiation dose of 6.9 mGy. This is an acceptable dose that is typically similar to a barium enema. To put this in perspective, the background radiation dose from the environment in a year's time is 3 mGy.

With a 64-slice multidetector scanner, the average breath hold is 8 to 10 seconds. Even elderly patients can tolerate this procedure easily.

INTREPRETATION

Interpretation of virtual colonoscopy studies requires special software and dedicated training. There are two interpretation strategies. Some radiologists concentrate primarily on a two-dimensional (2D) review. This means spending the majority of their time reviewing the axial images of the colon, using lung windows to visual the small polyps. Radiologists typically scroll through the images starting at the rectum and continuing to the cecum and then scroll down to the rectum again. This is done on both the prone and supine data sets. Multiplanar reconstructions can be used for problem solving. In addition, the endoluminal fly-through views, which simulate the view at conventional colonoscopy, are used primarily as problem-solving tools. Other radiologists rely primarily on the endoluminal fly-through views and use the axial images and multiplanar reconstructions for problem solving (Fig. 4). This method is referred to as a primary 2D read with 3D problem solving. Both interpretation strategies are somewhat time-consuming initially. However, with experience, most examinations can be reviewed within 10 to 15 minutes. Regardless of the interpretation method used, it is essential that both the prone and supine data sets be reviewed.

Polyps appear as filling defects within the air-filled colon (Figs. 5 and 6). The presence of the stool tagging helps to distinguish stool from true polyps (see Figs. 1 and 4). Considering what we know about polyp size and malignancy, it is essential that polyps greater than 5 mm (especially those ≥1 cm) be detected with high sensitivity and specificity. Virtual colonoscopy has limited sensitivity and specificity for lesions smaller than 5 mm. However, because polyps of less than 5 mm are almost never malignant, the detection of these small lesions is not crucial, especially if the patient will be screened at regular 5- to 10-year intervals.

Flat lesions can be a challenge on both the 2D and 3D imaging but are also somewhat difficult at conventional colonoscopy. However, with experience, these lesions also can be detected. Radiologists attempt to confirm the presence of a polyp on both the prone and supine images, increasing reader confidence. Computer-aided detection software is now available that can help to detect polyps.

In addition to a comprehensive examination of the colon, the virtual colonoscopy exam requires careful review of the extracolonic structures. The published literature reports that significant extracolonic findings are seen in approximately 10% of patients undergoing virtual colonoscopy, including aneurysms, lung nodules, gallstones, renal cell cancers, and other abnormalities.

HOW GOOD IS IT?

Most of the literature on the virtual colonoscopy was published in the 1990s using high-risk patients with either family history of colon cancer or polyposis syndromes. Also, single detector and early multidetector CT scanners were used, and these could acquire only 3- to 5-mm slices. Therefore when reviewing the old literature, one must consider the limitations of both the software and hardware of that time. However, even early published studies were somewhat promising, especially in high-risk patients.

Today the question remains, can virtual colonoscopy be used as a screening study in asymptomatic patients? There are two large published studies regarding asymptomatic screening. The largest study to date was published by Pickhardt in 2003. This trial included more than 1200 asymptomatic patients at average risk for colon cancer. In the study, patients underwent CT colonoscopy and conventional colonoscopy on the same day. Both studies were blinded. The CT results were excellent, with a sensitivity and specificity of greater than 90% for lesions larger than 8 mm. In fact, the CT scan detected more polyps than the conventional colonoscopy. This study gained widespread attention for virtual colonoscopy. However, a few months later, a study was published in the *Journal of the American Medical Association* (*JAMA*), including another asymptomatic patient population, this time of 600 subjects. The results of this study were dismal. The CT scan detected fewer than 50% of the 1-cm polyps. One difficulty with this study was that it involved older data sets and inexperienced radiologists. In the *JAMA* study, the radiologists had only minimal experience interpreting virtual colonoscopy scans before joining the study.

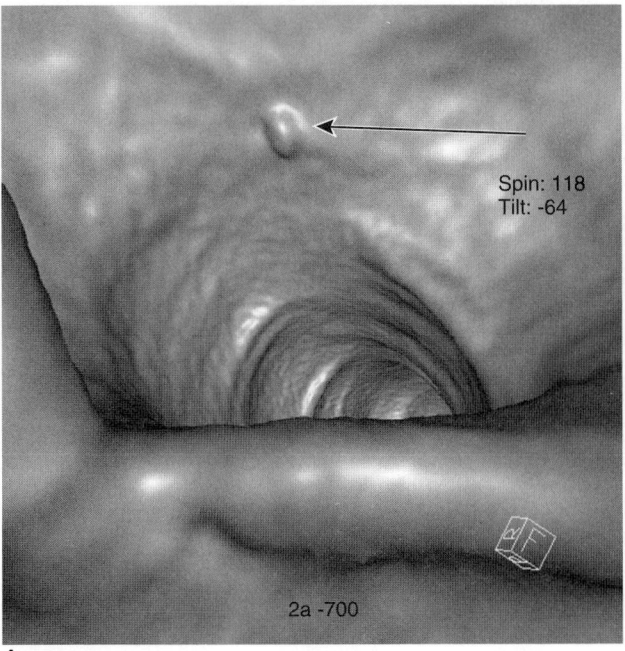

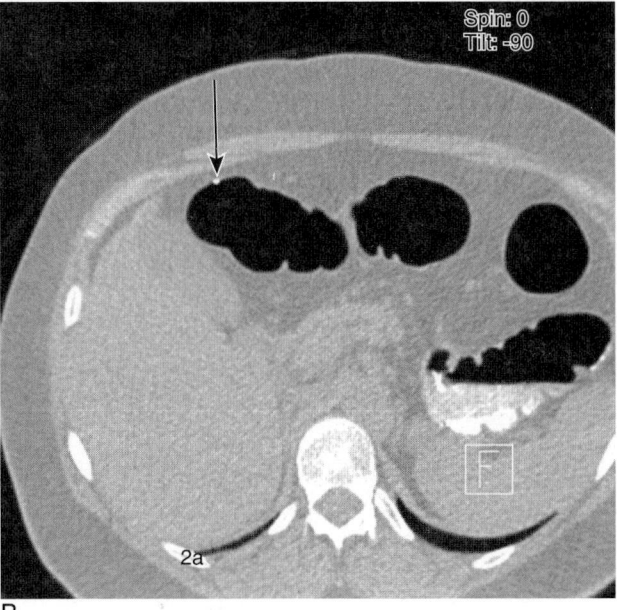

A   B

Figure 4 **(A)** Endoluminal view demonstrating a small polypoid lesion in the colon. When lesions are detected on the three-dimensional (3D) endoluminal views, they must be correlated with the axial or multiplaner reconstruction. **(B)** The small polypoid defect detected on the endoluminal views appears to be a small high-density stool particle on the axial images. This is an example of how the radiologist must correlate the 3D images with the conventional CT scan. (*See color insert Figure 10.*)

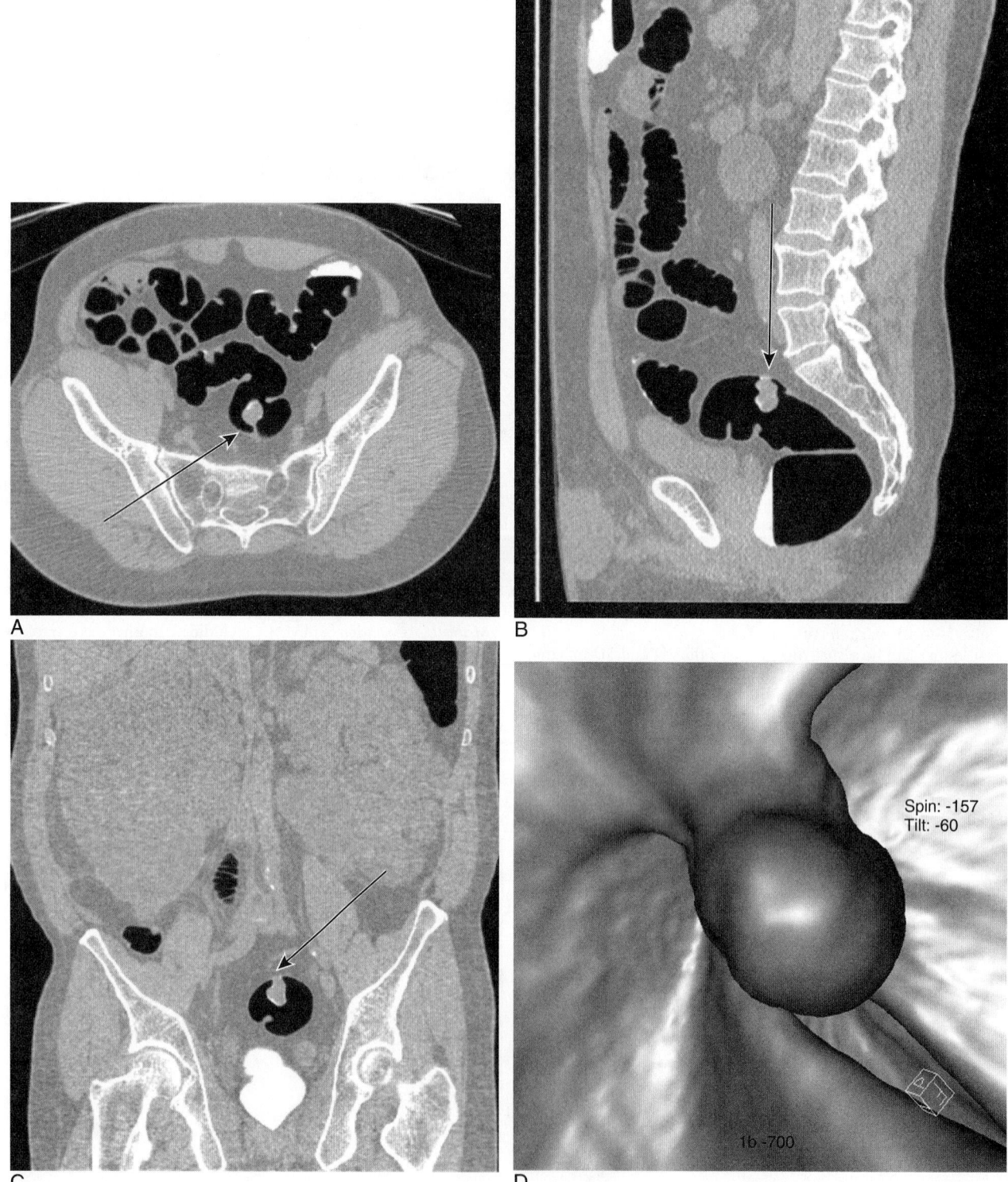

Figure 5 A villous adenoma (2.5 cm) in the rectum. This is easily identified on the axial images **(A)**, sagittal images **(B)**, coronal images **(C)**, and the three-dimensional endoluminal view **(D)**. (*See color insert Figure 11.*)

It is clear from the review of the literature that it is easy to obtain poor results using virtual colonoscopy. However, some promising studies show that with careful attention to colonic preparation and scanning technique and with experienced readers, it is possible to obtain excellent results. The largest study in an asymptomatic patient is ongoing. This is the ACRIN (American College of Radiology Imaging Network) study. It will involve more than 2300 asymptomatic patients who will undergo both CT colonoscopy and conventional colonoscopy on the same day. Fifteen institutions are involved, and all the radiologists were

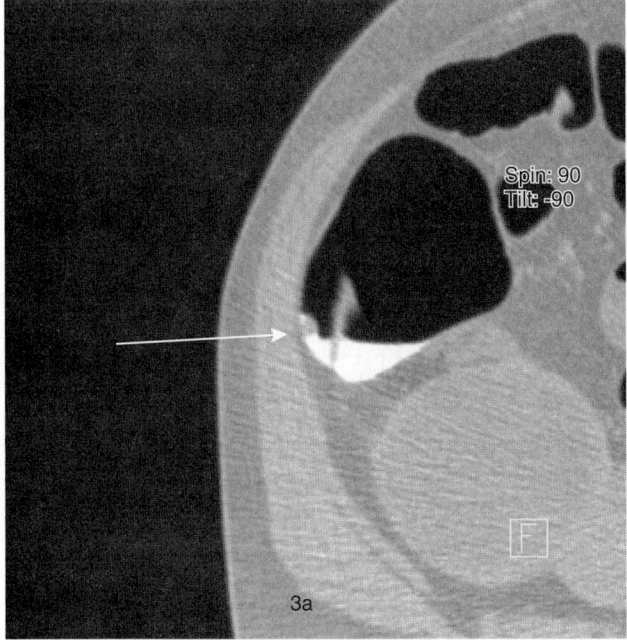

A

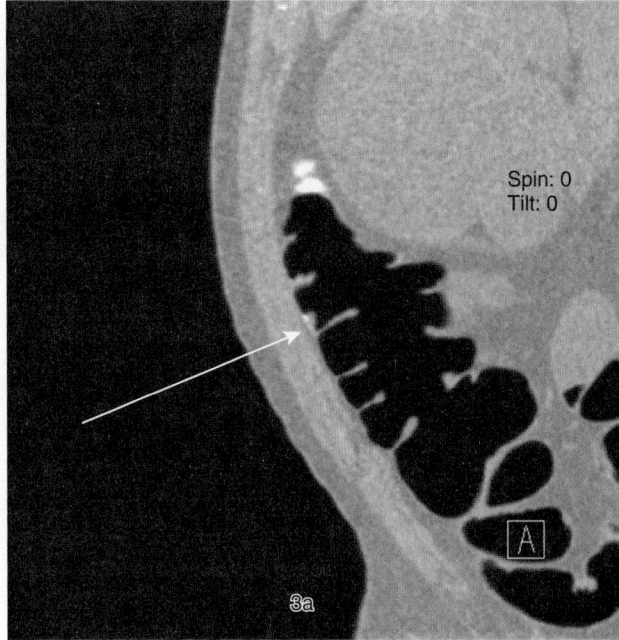

B

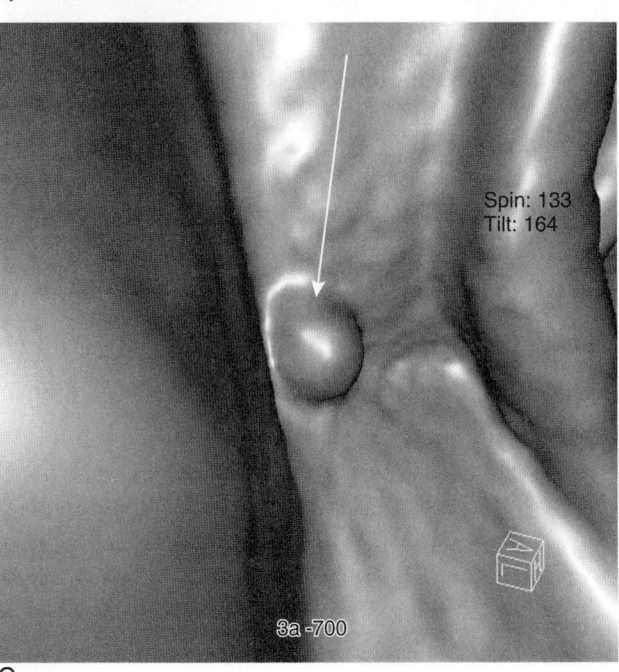

C

Figure 6 Polyp of 8 mm in the ascending colon. Small polyps can be a challenge during virtual colonoscopy but with careful review can be detected reliably. This small polyp is seen in the ascending colon on the axial images **(A)**, coronal images **(B)**, and the three-dimensional endoluminal view **(C)**. (*See color insert Figure 12*.)

specifically trained and had to pass a proficiency test before joining the trial. The results of this study will be available in approximately 2 years and will help to determine the future of virtual colonoscopy.

LIMITATIONS

There are some limitations to using CT for colon cancer screening. First, obviously, is the radiation issue. There is no way to perform the study without exposing the patient to radiation. This is always a concern in an asymptomatic population. However, as described earlier, there are methods to reduce the radiation to an acceptable level, especially for a study performed every 5 to 10 years.

Second, residual stool can be a limitation. Residual stool can mask or simulate polyps. However, as described earlier, the use of the fecal solid and liquid tagging agents greatly reduces this difficulty. Also, it is worth the effort to review the preparation instruction with the patients ahead of time and to answer any questions that may arise. Well-informed patients tend to have better preparation.

The third limitation is the cost. At this time, most insurance carriers will not pay for a true screening virtual colonoscopy.

Charges vary from $500 to $1500 across the country. It is likely that more insurance companies will start to cover this procedure after the results of the ACRIN screening trial have been published. It is clear that if virtual colonoscopy is going to be viable screening study, insurance companies must cover it and the cost must be reasonable.

Some insurance companies will pay for virtual colonoscopy in the setting of a recent failed colonoscopy. Also, select carriers will pay for virtual colonoscopy in patients in whom conventional colonoscopy is high risk, such as elderly patients or patients on anticoagulant therapy. It offers an alternative to a barium enema in these patient populations.

Another limitation of virtual colonoscopy is the current lack of sufficient radiologist training. Virtual colonoscopy is a relatively new study with a novel method of interpretation. Radiologists are not trained in virtual colonoscopy during their residency. Therefore dedicated training of residents, fellows, and practicing radiologists is necessary. This may require the use of known data sets or even perhaps specialized certification in this technique.

CURRENT UTILIZATION

At our institution, we routinely do virtual colonoscopy in patients after failed colonoscopy and in high-risk frail patients or those on anticoagulation. Also, we have found virtual colonoscopy to be useful in visualizing the colon proximal to an obstructing mass or stricture. We also perform screening virtual colonoscopy in a variety of patients, but as mentioned earlier, insurance companies typically do not reimburse these studies at this time.

FUTURE DIRECTIONS

Computer-aided diagnosis software (CAD) is currently available from most manufacturers and has the potential to aid in review of these large data sets. CAD will not likely replace radiologist interpretation but may act as a "second look," much as it does for mammography. Another potential innovation will be improved subtraction software, which is designed to subtract any residual tagged stool from the colon, thereby allowing a faster review of the study data set.

CONCLUSION

Virtual colonoscopy is a promising technique, and it is hoped that it will encourage more people to be screened for colon polyps and cancer. The technique involves colonic cleansing, stool tagging, and air distention of the colon. A relatively low-dose CT scan is performed in both prone and supine positions. Dedicated imaging software and adequate radiologist training are necessary for accurate interpretation. Large screening studies are being performed in an asymptomatic population at this time, and the results of these are anxiously awaited to determine the fate of virtual colonoscopy.

SUGGESTED READINGS

Cotton PB, Durkalski VL, Pineau BC, and others: Computed tomographic colonography (virtual colonoscopy): a multicenter comparison with standard colonoscopy for detection of colorectal neoplasia, *JAMA* 291:1713, 2004.

Pickhardt PJ: Virtual colonoscopy: issues related to primary screening, *Eur Radiolo* 15(suppl 4):D133, 2005.

Pickhardt PJ, Choi JR, Hwang I, and others: Computed tomographic virtual colonoscopy to screen for colorectal neoplasia in asymptomatic adults, *N Engl J Med* 349:191, 2003.

Taylor SA, Halligan S, Burling D, and others: Computer-assisted reader software versus expert reviewers for polyp detection on CT colonography, *AJR Am J Roentgenol* 186:696, 2006.

Yee J: Screening CT colonography, *Semin Ultrasound CT MR* 24:12, 2003.

DIVERTICULAR DISEASE OF THE COLON

Matthew R. Dixon, MD, and Judith L. Trudel, MD, MSc, MHPE

The term *diverticular disease* refers to a spectrum of clinical presentations associated with the presence of diverticulae, or outpouchings on the colon. Diverticulosis is defined as the presence of these outpouchings, usually occurring at the site where blood vessels penetrate the bowel wall. Diverticulitis refers to the presence of inflammation or infection around a colonic diverticulum.

The incidence of diverticulosis increases with age; in Westernized countries, it is estimated be present in approximately 30% of people at age 60 and 60% of people older than age 80. The presence of diverticulae is not necessarily associated with symptoms or clinical disease. Most patients are diagnosed incidentally at the time of screening colonoscopy, barium enema, or computed tomography (CT) scan for unrelated symptoms. Diverticulae most often arise in the sigmoid colon but may be seen in all colonic segments.

The vast majority of patients with diverticulosis are asymptomatic. When symptomatic, 10% to 30% may eventually develop a complication warranting surgical intervention. Overall, approximately 1% of all patients with diverticular disease require surgical intervention. Surgical treatment for diverticular disease may be indicated in selected cases of massive diverticular bleeding and in selected cases of diverticulitis.

EVOLVING CONTROVERSIES IN THE SURGICAL MANAGEMENT OF DIVERTICULAR DISEASE

The surgical management of diverticular disease continues to be a "hot topic" in modern surgery. In the early 1980s, much of the debate centered on the necessity and short- and long-term safety of the three-stage approach for perforated diverticulitis. We now recognize that primary resection is usually safe and feasible at the time of initial operation in almost all cases. In the late 1980s, the introduction of image-guided percutaneous catheter drainage (PCD) of diverticular abscesses revolutionized our acute management strategy, allowing for interval colonic resection with primary anastomosis in most cases. The most recent controversies revolve around the indications for surgery in cases of uncomplicated and complicated diverticulitis (Table 1). There is a trend toward nonsurgical conservative management in many presentations of diverticular disease. Although surgical treatment of diverticular disease remains indicated in selected cases, the controversial issues are addressed in the appropriate sections throughout this chapter.

Table 1: Diverticulitis: Indications for Surgery

Strictly Indicated by Available Literature	Available Literature Conflicting	Previous Indications no Longer Well Supported by Available Data
Diffuse peritonitis	Following successful percutaneous drainage of abscess	Uncomplicated first episode, even in patients aged <50
Free perforation	Uncomplicated; second and third episodes	
Obstruction		
Stricture		
Fistula		
Immunocompromised patients		
≥4 uncomplicated episodes		

DIVERTICULAR BLEEDING

Approximately 50% of massive lower gastrointestinal (LGI) bleeding is caused by diverticular disease. Bleeding is a feature of diverticulosis; it is rarely, if ever, seen with diverticulitis. Massive painless LGI bleeding results from the erosion of enlarged diverticulae into neighboring blood vessels (vasa recta). It stops spontaneously in more than 70% of cases, thus avoiding the need for surgical intervention. Surgery may be indicated in acute cases in which bleeding does not cease spontaneously, in acute cases of failure to control massive LGI bleeding, or in cases of recurrent massive LGI bleeding originating from diverticular disease.

The investigation and management of massive LGI bleeding is not the focus of this chapter. Ideally, the exact source of bleeding should be identified preoperatively, and resection should be limited to the involved segment. If the source of bleeding is not known, blind subtotal colectomy with ileorectal anastomosis is recommended because lesser segmental resections are associated with a 30% rebleeding rate.

UNCOMPLICATED DIVERTICULITIS

Diverticulitis refers to the presence of inflammation or infection around a colonic diverticulum. The trigger for inflammation or infection remains unknown. It is believed that microperforation at the site of a single diverticulum initiates the cascade of events leading to clinical diverticulitis. *Uncomplicated diverticulitis* is defined as diverticulitis in the absence of any complications, namely, abscess, free perforation, fistulization, or stenosis.

Clinical Diagnosis and Evaluation

Patients with uncomplicated diverticulitis typically present with abdominal pain, fever, and elevation of their white blood cell (WBC) count. Pain from diverticulitis classically localizes to the left lower quadrant, but in cases of sigmoid redundancy, abdominal pain may manifest in adjacent quadrants wherever sigmoid colon is present. Patterns of disease presentation may differ according to ethnicity: in patients of Asian or African descent, right-sided diverticulae are more prevalent, and therefore right-sided symptoms occur with more frequency.

Patients with milder forms of diverticulitis are often managed as outpatients by primary care physicians. The diagnosis of acute uncomplicated diverticulitis can be made purely on clinical grounds; CT scan is not mandatory to confirm the diagnosis of acute uncomplicated diverticulitis in a patient with left lower quadrant pain, low-grade fever, an elevated WBC count, and tenderness or a mass in the left lower quadrant. However, surgeons must be aware of the possibility that antibiotics may have been given for an episode of presumed diverticulitis without the diagnosis being firmly established. When planning elective surgery for patients with presumed recurrent episodes of diverticulitis, it is essential to review all available evidence (including CT scans) to make sure the clinical and radiologic findings support the diagnosis. Keep in mind that pain caused by colonic spasm or irritable bowel syndrome is usually self-limited and that CT scan findings will likely be negative; a "response to empirical antibiotic therapy" does not constitute indirect evidence that diverticulitis was the original diagnosis.

Most patients presenting to an emergency department undergo CT scanning before surgical consultation. CT scan is useful to (1) rule out complicated diverticulitis in patients with severe clinical findings on presentation, (2) diagnose diverticulitis in patients with atypical symptoms such as right-sided abdominal pain (Fig. 1), (3) reevaluate patients who do not improve or resolve after 48 hours of treatment, and (4) plan future management.

Management

The mainstay of treatment for uncomplicated diverticulitis is bowel rest and antibiotic therapy. Medical management of acute uncomplicated diverticulitis results in complete resolution without recurrence in at least 70% of cases.

Depending on the severity of the disease, some patients may be managed on an outpatient basis, with diet restricted to clear liquids and oral antibiotics. The most frequent aerobic bacteria involved in diverticulitis are *Escherichia coli*, *Proteus*, *Klebsiella*, and *Enterococcus*; the most frequent anaerobic bacterium is *Bacteroides fragilis*.

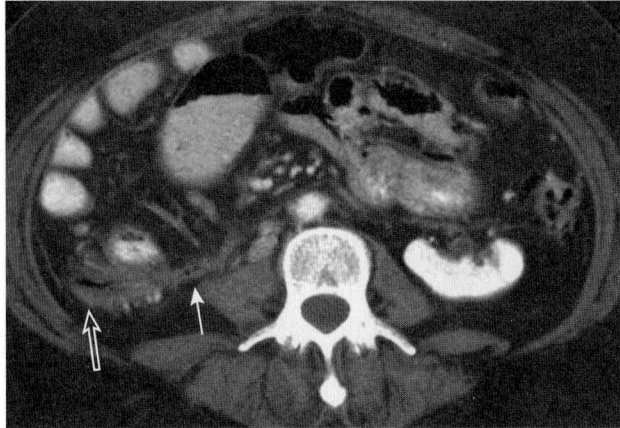

Figure 1 Computed tomography scan of a patient with right lower quadrant abscess *(open arrow)* secondary to perforated sigmoid diverticulitis. The closed arrow shows the normal appearing appendix. *From Am J Roentgenol* © 2005 American Roentgen Ray Society.

Broad-spectrum antibiotics providing both aerobic and anaerobic coverage (e.g., combination of ciprofloxacin and metronidazole) should be used. Clinical improvement must be assessed by serial abdominal exams, serial WBC, and close monitoring of the patient's temperature. Patients demonstrating clinical improvement may progress to a full liquid diet and then to a soft diet. Patients with more severe disease at the onset, outpatients who fail to improve, and outpatients who show signs of clinical deterioration should be admitted to the hospital and provided intravenous resuscitation and antibiotics. The use of a single antibiotic (e.g., cefotetan) may be adequate as long as broad-spectrum aerobic/anaerobic coverage is provided. Close monitoring as described earlier is mandatory. Patients with reassuring clinical signs may be discharged after a brief hospital stay after their pain has resolved and they demonstrate that they can tolerate a soft diet and bowel function has resumed. Patients who fail to improve within 48 hours or who deteriorate clinically should undergo a CT scan and surgical evaluation.

After the acute episode has resolved, colonoscopy to exclude underlying malignancy is recommended. Elective colonoscopy should be performed on an outpatient basis at a time interval that allows for optimal resolution of the diverticular inflammation. Many surgeons choose to wait 6 to 8 weeks because of the underlying concern that microperforations could be aggravated by colonic insufflation. Additionally, sigmoid spasm often persists for several weeks after an acute episode of diverticulitis, making the examination painful for the patient and difficult for the endoscopist. If disturbing features such as weight loss, significant changes in bowel habits, microcytic anemia, or a strong family history of colorectal cancer make the likelihood of malignancy much higher, it may be reasonable to modify this approach to expedite the diagnosis and treatment of an underlying malignancy.

ROLE OF ELECTIVE SURGERY IN ACUTE UNCOMPLICATED DIVERTICULITIS

Surgery is not indicated after a single episode of uncomplicated diverticulitis, irrespective of patient age. Age alone should not be used as an indication for operation after a first episode of diverticulitis. Current practice guidelines recommend that surgery should be offered to patients after two documented episodes of uncomplicated diverticulitis. Factors influencing recommendation to an individual patient include patient's fitness for surgery, number and severity of attacks, rapidity and completeness of response to medical therapy, and persistence of residual symptoms after completion of treatment.

These recommendations regarding the timing of surgery for uncomplicated diverticulitis are in evolution. Recent studies suggest that surgery should probably be reserved for patients with more recurrent episodes of uncomplicated diverticulitis (Table 1).

The rationale behind this recommendation is based on data from several recently published studies. First, a minority of patients with uncomplicated diverticulitis experience a recurrence or require eventual surgical intervention. A large retrospective cohort study of more than 3000 patients (mean follow-up 8 years) showed that only 13% of 2366 patients managed nonoperatively during their initial episode and who declined subsequent elective resection eventually had recurrence; all of the recurrences were safely managed nonoperatively (see Broderick-Villa and others 2005). Second, reserving colectomy for patients with several episodes of diverticulitis may provide a more optimal risk-to-benefit ratio for patients with diverticulitis. Salem and colleagues (2004) published a decision analysis showing that performing colectomy after the fourth rather than the second episode of diverticulitis resulted in fewer deaths, fewer colostomies, and significant cost savings, irrespective of patients' age. Third, counseling patients that a preemptive elective

colectomy is necessary to avoid the possibility of an emergent stoma for a future complicated episode may not be accurate. Somesakar and colleagues (2002) and Chapman and colleagues (2005) looked at patients presenting with perforated diverticulitis and found that the majority presenting with life-threatening diverticular disease had not had antecedent diverticular events.

As mentioned earlier, age alone should not be used as an indication for operation after a first episode of diverticulitis. Younger patients (<50) were previously thought to have more virulent disease with initial and future episodes. A growing body of evidence suggests that this may not be the case. Although younger patients may have a higher chance of developing recurrent episodes and eventually needing surgery, elective surgery for uncomplicated diverticulitis in young patients should follow the guidelines for patients of any age.

There are notable exceptions in which an aggressive early surgical approach is indicated. Evidence suggests that immunocompromised patients have a much higher incidence of free perforation, even with uncomplicated episodes. Transplant patients and other chronically immunocompromised patients such as patients with AIDS should be offered surgery after their first documented episode of diverticulitis.

PRINCIPLES OF SURGICAL RESECTION FOR UNCOMPLICATED DIVERTICULITIS

The goal is to remove the diseased diverticular segment and resect the remaining distal sigmoid colon down to the rectum. The anastomosis must be in the rectum. Any sigmoid colon between the area of disease and the rectum is considered to be a part of the "high-pressure zone" of the sigmoid colon. Failure to resect the distal sigmoid, even in absence of grossly visible diverticular disease, is the primary cause of recurrent sigmoid diverticulitis after surgery.

The diseased area is characterized by the presence of hypertrophied muscular layers. Therefore the proximal margin of resection should be in an area where the wall of the colon appears normal on palpation and inspection. It is not necessary to resect all of the diverticulae-bearing colon proximally. An open or laparoscopic approach may be used, depending on surgeon preference. It should be noted that although usually technically feasible, the decision to proceed laparoscopically should depend on the comfort and laparoscopic expertise of the surgeon, because the dissection required to resect a severely diseased sigmoid colon can pose significant challenges. Regardless of surgical approach, ureteral stents may be helpful to aid in identifying ureters during the dissection. Table 3 summarizes the principles for surgical resection of both uncomplicated and complicated diverticulitis.

COMPLICATED DIVERTICULITIS

Complicated diverticulitis is defined as diverticulitis associated with abscess formation, free perforation, fistula formation, or stenosis.

Contained Perforation: Pericolic and Pelvic Abscesses (Hinchey Stages I and II)

Table 2 provides the clinical staging for perforated diverticulitis. Although microperforation is considered a sine qua non condition for all types of diverticulitis, pericolic and pelvic abscesses are due to a contained colonic macroperforation. Diverticulitis-associated abscesses are usually diagnosed by CT scan. Our ability to manage abscesses by image-guided percutaneous catheter drainage (PCD) has revolutionized the management of this problem. Before PCD,

Table 2: Clinical Staging of Perforated Diverticulitis

	Hinchey Staging (1978)	Hughes/Cuthbertson/ Carden Staging (1963)
Stage I	Pericolic or intramesenteric abscess	Local peritonitis
Stage II	Walled-off pelvic abscess	Local pericolic or pelvic abscess
Stage III	Generalized purulent peritonitis caused by rupture of an abscess into general abdominal cavity	Generalized peritonitis caused by ruptured pericolic or pelvic abscess
Stage IV	Generalized fecal peritonitis caused by free perforation	General peritonitis caused by free perforation of the colon

presence of an abscess almost always mandated a staged surgical intervention with initial surgical drainage and colostomy, followed by interval resection. Successful PCD of diverticulitis-associated abscesses now allows for interval colonic resection with primary anastomosis in most cases.

It is not always necessary to drain all abscesses immediately. For pericolic and intramesenteric abscesses, initial management with intravenous antibiotics and close observation may be appropriate, reserving PCD for patients who fail to improve rapidly from a clinical standpoint. The threshold for PCD should remain low. Drains may be removed after clinical symptoms improve and drain output is minimal or ceases. After successful nonoperative management, patients may undergo elective colonoscopy in 6 to 8 weeks and receive counsel regarding surgical options.

The necessity of elective interval resection following successful PCD of abscesses is currently questioned. Classically, the finding of a diverticulitis-associated abscess was considered a "complication of the complication" (diverticulosis is the disease, diverticulitis is a complication of the disease, and abscess is a complication of the complication) that mandated elective interval colectomy. Conflicting data continue to fuel the controversy. Whereas data of Broderick-Villa and others (2005) support long-term nonoperative management even in patients with abscesses, several smaller case series suggest that patients with a history of abscess have a higher chance of recurrence. Additional data are needed to identify patients at high risk for recurrence following successful PCD of a diverticular abscess to provide appropriate surgical counseling.

When performed electively, surgery should follow the principles of surgical resection outlined for cases of uncomplicated diverticulitis. If semiurgent or urgent surgery is mandated by failure of nonoperative management, the principles of surgical resection should follow the outline given under surgical management of free perforation.

Free Perforation: Purulent and Fecal Peritonitis (Hinchey Stages III and IV)

Hemodynamic instability is frequent in this group of patients, with shock, diffuse generalized peritonitis on examination, and free air on imaging studies. Aggressive fluid resuscitation and intravenous broad-spectrum antibiotics should begin immediately and continue throughout the postoperative period. Fluid requirements may be considerable as a consequence of widespread peritoneal inflammation. Early intensive care unit monitoring with the addition of a central venous catheter to assist in resuscitation should be strongly considered.

Urgent operative management is the treatment of choice for patients with perforated diverticulitis. Primary resection should be performed at the time of the initial operation; this is safe and feasible in almost all cases (see Chandra, 2004). Clinical staging alone (see Table 2) cannot be used to dictate operative management. Factors influencing the decision include (1) overall patient stability, (2) the degree and type of peritonitis (purulent or fecal peritonitis), and (3) the condition of the colon, particularly if primary anastomosis is contemplated. The safest option when treating patients with severe sepsis and generalized purulent or fecal peritonitis is limited resection with colostomy and closure of the distal rectum (Hartmann's procedure) or mucus fistula. Mucus fistula maturation is not necessary; the bowel can be stapled and secured above fascia but below skin at the lower end of the incision, obviating the need for two appliances.

Principles of Surgical Resection for Perforated Diverticulitis

It may be helpful to begin by mobilizing the bowel proximal to the point of inflammation, identifying the ureter and working distally after dividing the proximal sigmoid colon. Ureteral stents may be helpful to aid in identifying ureters during the dissection. Ideally the goal of resection remains to remove the diseased diverticular segment and any distal sigmoid colon. The distal margin of resection should be in the proximal rectum. The only two exceptions to this rule are (1) if the patient is too unstable to undergo an extensive procedure, in which case only the perforated segment is excised and the remaining sigmoid resection and anastomosis are performed at a later date; and (2) if the surgeon chooses to bring out a mucus fistula and the length of the distal sigmoid is necessary to reach the abdominal wall. In each of these cases, the patient should be informed, and the operative report should clearly document that resection of the residual sigmoid colon will be needed at the time of future surgery, particularly if laparoscopic reversal is considered.

Although it is crucial for the distal margin to be in proximal rectum, excessive rectal mobilization (particularly in the presacral space) should be avoided because it makes future reversal of a colostomy more technically difficult. In some cases of extensive fecal or purulent soiling, it may be prudent to resect only the perforated segment, thus minimizing contamination of pristine planes for future surgery.

The decision to perform a primary anastomosis and whether to protect it with a diverting ileostomy again hinges on overall patient

Table 3: Principles of Resection for Diverticulitis (Uncomplicated and Complicated)

- Perform primary resection even when operating urgently for complicated diverticulitis
- Proximal resection margin should be in normal colon without palpable hypertrophy of muscularis layer
- Distal resection margin must be in proximal rectum, where tenia coli coalesce
- It is not necessary to resect all diverticulae-bearing proximal colon
- Perform oncologic operation (en bloc resection, high vascular ligation) if cancer has not been excluded preoperatively by endoscopy
- Preoperative ureteral stent placement may aid in identifying ureters for both open and laparoscopic cases
- If complete resection of distal sigmoid was not done at the time of initial operation, document in the operative note and tell the patient

stability, the degree and type of peritonitis, and the condition of the colon. Hemodynamically stable patients with purulent peritonitis may be treated with primary anastomosis and a diverting loop ileostomy. The condition of the bowel is critical: the bowel ends should be healthy, noninflamed, and well vascularized. Splenic flexure mobilization may be necessary to achieve a tension-free anastomosis, but is not mandatory in all cases. Although the use of mechanical bowel preparation to ensure anastomotic healing has recently been questioned in elective colon resections, these data cannot be extrapolated to critically ill patients with severe peritonitis. Intraoperative colonic lavage allows for optimal preparation with minimal complications in selected patients; care must be taken to also irrigate the rectum distal to the anastomosis.

Fecal diversion with a loop ileostomy facilitates subsequent takedown to restore intestinal continuity. Selected patients with a contained perforation that has been completely resected, leaving only normal tissues, may be candidates for a primary anastamosis without diversion, but this option should be reserved for the rare patient with these most reassuring clinical features.

Diverticular Fistula Formation

Diverticular fistulae arise when the inflamed colon erodes into adjacent organs, thus causing a fistulous connection. The most common fistulae are colovesical fistulae. Patients present with pneumaturia and fecaluria. The finding of air within the bladder on CT is considered pathognomonic. Women who have had hysterectomies may present with a colovaginal fistula, manifested by recurrent vaginal infections or passage of flatus and stool per vagina. Less commonly, diverticulitis may cause fistulae to the ureter, the prostate, the fallopian tubes or the uterus. Preoperative endoscopy is recommended in order to exclude cancer, because this would affect surgical approach.

At the time of surgery, blunt dissection should be used to separate the diseased colon from the affected organ. Standard sigmoid resection with resection with primary anastomosis to the proximal rectum can then be performed. After colonic resection, the "end" organ heals spontaneously; partial resection or closure of the bladder or vagina is not necessary. Foley catheter drainage of the bladder may be used for approximately 1 week; complete bladder healing should be confirmed by cystogram before removal of the catheter. More complex fistulae involving the prostate or the ureter may best be treated in conjunction with a urologist or gynecologist.

If cancer cannot be excluded preoperatively, an oncologic en bloc resection should be performed. Blunt dissection is discouraged because it could potentially violate resection planes. The resected specimen should immediately be opened by the pathologist to confirm mucosal integrity.

Diverticular Stenosis and Obstruction

Repeated episodes of diverticulitis may result in stenosis of the inflamed segment. Patients may or may not report a classic history of prior diverticulitis episodes. Although patients may complain of constipation or a change in bowel habits, stenosis may also be discovered incidentally during barium enema or routine screening colonoscopy. Inability to pass the colonoscope through a stenotic segment is an indication for surgical resection because preoperative exclusion of malignancy is impossible. Elective resection should follow oncologic resection principles.

In the event of acute large bowel obstruction secondary to diverticular stenosis, surgery is indicated. Resection with primary anastomosis, with or without proximal diversion, may be performed safely in these conditions, as long as the bowel ends are suitable for anastomosis. On-table colonic irrigation may be helpful. Bridge intraluminal stenting of benign diverticular strictures is associated with more complications than stenting of cancers and has limited usefulness, given the availability of surgical resection.

Suggested Readings

Broderick-Villa G, Bruchette RJ, Collins JC, and others: Hospitalization for acute diverticulitis does not mandate routine elective colectomy, *Arch Surg* 140:576, 2005.

Chandra V, Nelson H, Larsen DR, and others: Impact of primary resection on the outcome of patients with perforated diverticulitis, *Arch Surg* 139:1221, 2004.

Chapman J, Davies M, Wolff B, and others: Complicated diverticulitis: is it time to rethink the rules? *Ann Surg* 242:576, 2005.

Hinchey EJ, Schaal PGH, Richards GK: Treatment of perforated diverticular disease of the colon, *Adv Surg* 12:85, 1978.

Further Reading

Hughes ESR, Cuthbertson AM, Carden ABC: The surgical management of acute diverticulitis, *Med J Aust* 1:780, 1963.

Salem L, Veenstra DL, Sullivan SD, and others: The timing of elective colectomy in diverticulitis: a decision analysis, *J Am Coll Surg* 199:904, 2004.

Somasekar K, Foster ME, Haray PN: The natural history diverticular disease: is there a role for elective colectomy? *J R Coll Surg Ed* 47:481, 2002.

Chronic Ulcerative Colitis

Anna Serur, MD, Frank J. Caliendo, MD,
Luz P. Angel, MD, and John A. Procaccino, MD

Chronic ulcerative colitis (UC) is a diffuse inflammatory bowel disease of unknown etiology affecting the mucosa of the colon and rectum. Speculations regarding the cause of this disease include genetic predisposition, autoimmunity, viral or bacterial etiologies, and environmental factors, but no specific cause has been identified. Ulcerative colitis is limited to the mucosa and submucosa of colorectum. The rectum is always involved, and the disease progresses continuously from that point proximally.

The usual presentation of UC includes bloody diarrhea, increased frequency of bowel movements, and abdominal pain. The course of the disease is variable, ranging from mild to severe. Medical therapy is indicated as first-line therapy, producing remission in the vast majority of patients (Table 1). However, it is estimated that approximately 30% of patients will require surgical management. Historically, surgery was offered only late in the course of the disease, and the premorbid state of these patients led to unfavorable outcomes. Today, operations are performed earlier, with concomitant excellent results. Patients are also at risk for developing extracolonic manifestations of UC, such as pyoderma gangrenosum, erythema nodosum, ankylosing spondylitis, and sclerosing cholangitis.

Table 1: Medical Therapy for Ulcerative Colitis

Symptomatic Agents	Steroids
Antidiarrheals	Oral corticosteroids
Antispasmodic	IV corticosteroids
Cholesteramine	IV ACTH
	Topical steroids
Sulfasalazine Compounds	**Immunomodulators**
Oral sulfasalazine	6-MP
Topical sulfasalazine	Cyclosporine
Oral 5-ASA & analogues	Infliximab
Topical 5-ASA & 4-ASA	
	Antibiotics
	Metronidazole
	Fluoroquinolones
	Miscellaneous

IV, Intravenous; *ACTH,* adenocorticotropic hormone.

INDICATIONS FOR OPERATION

Surgical indications can be categorized as either emergent or elective (Table 2). Indications for emergency surgery include ongoing hemorrhage, development of toxic megacolon, and free perforation. Indications for elective operation are failure to respond to maximal medical therapy, inability to cope with side effects of medications used to control disease, development of dysplasia or carcinoma, and growth retardation.

Massive lower gastrointestinal hemorrhage is rare in ulcerative colitis but occasionally develops. Uncontrolled bleeding requires prompt intervention after appropriate stabilization. Patients with toxic megacolon usually present with signs of sepsis, such as tachycardia, tachypnea, fever, acidosis, and leukocytosis. Dilatation of the transverse colon (8-cm diameter) on a flat plate of the abdomen is diagnostic (Fig. 1). This condition requires urgent admission to the intensive care unit, maximal medical therapy with broad-spectrum intravenous antibiotics, aggressive fluid and electrolyte replacement, and serial abdominal x-rays. The therapeutic benefit of steroids in this scenario is controversial, but patients who were previously on steroids would require stress doses of corticosteroids. If the patient's condition deteriorates or does not improve in 24 to 72 hours, urgent colectomy is indicated. Toxic megacolon or the progression of severe disease may lead to colon perforation. These patients usually present with overt peritonitis; however, if their disease is being treated with high-dose steroids, one may not elicit peritoneal signs on examination. Radiologic evidence of free air is a clear-cut indication for emergent operation.

Table 2: Indications for Surgery in Ulcerative Colitis

Urgent Surgery	Elective Surgery
Ongoing hemorrhage	Failure of medical therapy
Toxic megacolon	Intolerable side effects of medical therapy
Colonic perforation	Development of dysplasia
Fulminant ulcerative colitis	Carcinoma
	Colonic stricture
	Growth retardation in children

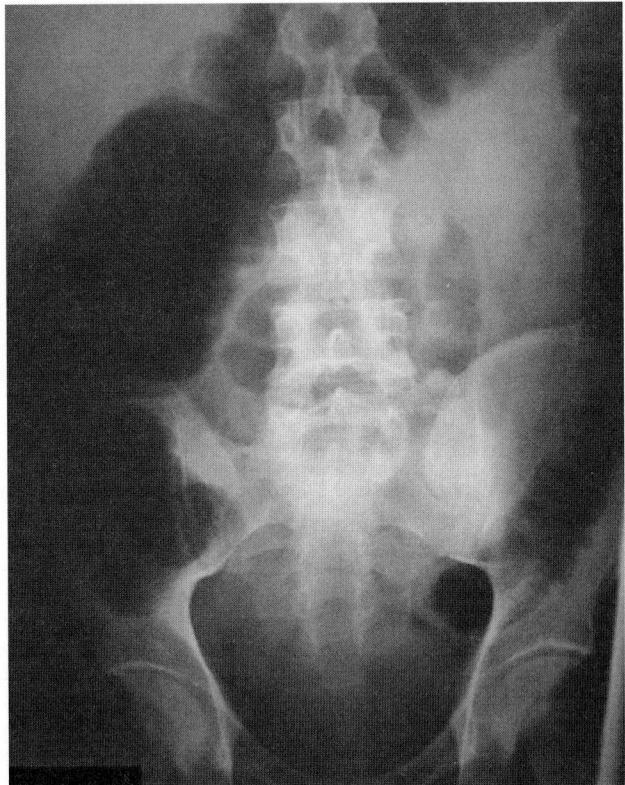

Figure 1   Toxic megacolon.

The most common indication for elective surgery is intractability of symptoms despite maximal medical therapy. Medications used to treat UC can themselves be associated with intolerable side effects, thereby requiring surgery. Long-standing UC puts a patient at a significantly increased risk for developing carcinoma of the colorectum. Thus patients who have had UC for 10 years or more should have an annual screening colonoscopy, with multiple random biopsies taken. Colonoscopies should not be performed during an acute flare to make a more accurate histologic assessment. If dysplasia is found, surgery is indicated. Development of a stricture in a patient with UC is considered malignant unless proven otherwise. Growth retardation occurs in some young patients and is a reason for elective surgical intervention. Extraintestinal manifestations of UC usually parallel the activity of colonic disease and are rarely an indication for surgery. It should be noted that sclerosing cholangitis is unaffected by colectomy, where as the other symptoms usually resolve after colectomy.

SELECTION OF OPERATIVE PROCEDURE

The operative procedure selected must be matched to the patient and, most importantly, to the indications for surgery (Table 3). In the urgent setting, when surgery is performed for toxic megacolon, bleeding, or perforation, the operative procedure of choice is subtotal colectomy with end ileostomy. Ongoing bleeding from a retained rectal stump has been reported in approximately 12% of patients but usually resolves spontaneously without further intervention.

The gold standard for elective colectomy for UC is panproctocolectomy and continent reconstruction with ileoanal J-pouch. The absolute contraindications to this operation include Crohn's disease (because of high recurrence rate found in the ileum used for

Table 3: Surgical Alternatives for Ulcerative Colitis

Emergency Operation	Elective Operation
Blowhole colostomy, loop ileostomy	Panproctocolectomy with permanent end ileostomy
Subtotal colectomy with end ileostomy	Subtotal colectomy with ileorectal anastomosis
Panproctocolectomy with permanent end ileostomy	Proctocolectomy with continent ileostomy (Kock pouch)
	Panproctocolectomy with ileal pouch-anal anastomosis with or without diverting ileostomy

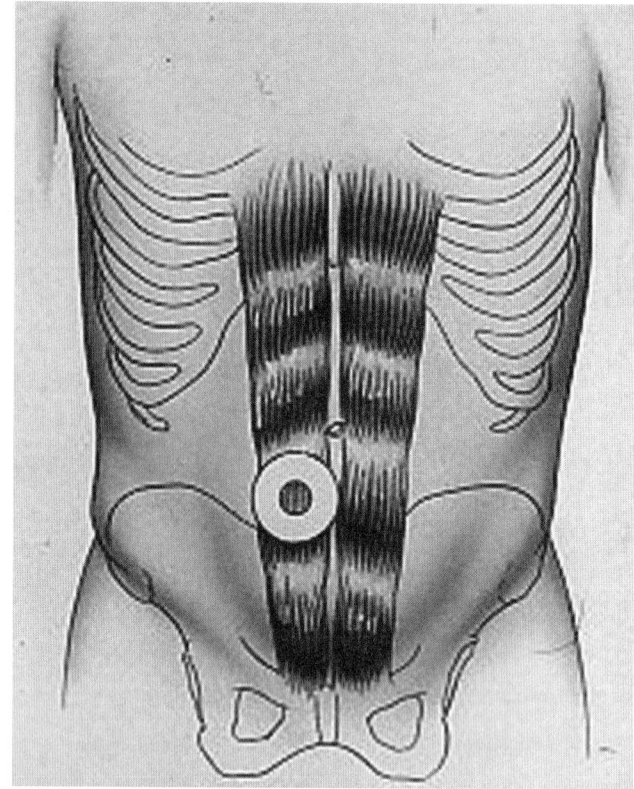

Stoma marking

Figure 2 Ostomy siting.

reconstruction), history of previous extensive small bowel surgery, perianal disease, sphincter trauma or dysfunction, and advanced carcinoma of the rectum. Advanced age is a relative contraindication because of the poor sphincter function that is a natural consequence of aging. We rarely offer this operation to patients older than 65 years of age without anal manometric studies to document adequate sphincter function. A survey from the Mayo Clinic evaluated 1386 patients who underwent ileal J-pouch-anal anastomosis; the median age was 32 years, only 16% were older than 45 years of age, and none were older than 65 years. Functional outcomes were much worse in patients who were older than 45 years at the time of the operation.

Patients who cannot have continent reconstruction should have a panproctocolectomy and a permanent end ileostomy. This is the safest operation, is 100% curative, and permits patients to have a virtually normal life. The Kock continent ileostomy is now rarely used and is reserved for patients who underwent a proctocolectomy with sphincter removal who now desire to avoid a permanent external appliance. It is associated with a high rate of complications, occasionally requiring an emergent reoperation.

Ileorectal anastomosis is another option that can be considered in a highly selective group of patients—namely, those with minor rectal disease or so-called "rectal sparing" (in these patients, a diagnosis of Crohn's disease should be seriously entertained and investigated), those who have contraindications to an ostomy such as ascites and portal hypertension, and those who absolutely refuse an ostomy but cannot undergo a restorative procedure. A number of these patients will require a proctectomy at a later time, either for intractable symptoms or development of carcinoma.

TECHNICAL CONSIDERATIONS

Subtotal Colectomy and Ileostomy

Even in the emergency setting, a site for the ostomy should be selected preoperatively with the patient in the upright sitting position. The ostomy should be sited at the apex of the infraumbilical fat mound and brought out through the rectus abdominus muscle (Fig. 2). A generous midline incision is made, affording exposure to the splenic flexure. Occasionally, a very dilated colon, especially in toxic megacolon, can create technical challenges. Colonic decompression may decrease operative time and minimize complications. Colonic decompression is performed by placing a purse-string suture in the area of dilated colon and using a 14-gauge angiocatheter to decompress the colon. On removal of the angiocatheter, the purse string is tied to prevent contamination. If free perforation is encountered, it can be closed expeditiously with suture or a staple device. Colectomy is performed in the

standard fashion. It is unnecessary to perform high ligation of the mesenteric vessels. All small bowel is preserved by selecting the proximal margin of resection just proximal to the ileocecal valve. Ideally, the ileocecal vessels are preserved so the blood supply to the subsequent pelvic pouch is preserved.

Selection of the distal margin and management of the rectosigmoid stump are significant considerations. Carrying the distal margin of resection as far as possible during the initial emergency surgery is not only unnecessary for the recuperation from the toxic state but will complicate subsequent surgery. As long as the entire abdominal colon is removed, eliminating the majority of the toxic source, patients do well. The distal margin is selected at a location that will allow the rectosigmoid stump to be brought up above the fascial level in the inferior aspect of the midline wound. The stump is closed with a TA stapler (US Surgical, Norwalk, CT), and the staple line is brought out above the fascia but below the skin. The serosa is tacked in position to the fascia with absorbable 3–0 sutures. In approximately one third of patients, the staple line will break down and a controlled fistula will develop, as opposed to pelvic sepsis if the stump were to remain in the peritoneal cavity. Ongoing rectal bleeding is rare. If it occurs, it can easily be controlled by dilute saline/epinephrine enemas and other local means. A final advantage of the longer rectal stump is that it facilitates the subsequent reoperation. The longer stump makes for easy identification of the remaining rectosigmoid and allows the rectal dissection to be performed in virgin planes, decreasing the difficulty and incidence of autonomic nerve injury.

Proctocolectomy and Ileostomy

Once considered the gold standard, proctocolectomy with end ileostomy still affords excellent results. This operation is performed in one stage, is curative, and is associated with the lowest complication rates. The disadvantage is that it leaves the patient with a permanent ileostomy and thus an altered body image.

Again, it is imperative to mark correctly the future stoma site. A midline vertical incision is made to provide access to the flexures and the pelvis. The colon is resected in a standard fashion, without high ligation of vessels unless surgery is performed for malignancy. Exposure is facilitated by the use of self-retaining retractors.

After the superior hemorrhoidal vessels are ligated above the sacral promontory, traction on the rectum toward the pubis allows exposure of the presacral space. This plane is identified by encountering the areolar tissue between the fascia propria of the rectum and the more dense presacral fascia. Appropriate exposure is achieved by the use of a St. Mark's pelvic retractor. If this plane is maintained, the sympathetic autonomic nerves that reside behind the presacral fascia will not be damaged. Complete posterior mobilization to the level of the levator complex should be accomplished before lateral dissection. Lateral dissection is accomplished by applying traction on the rectal specimen with one hand and traction on the ipsilateral pelvic sidewall with the pelvic retractor. As the lateral stalks are encountered and taken, the dissection plane should be close to the fascia propria of the rectum to avoid damage to the parasympathetic nerves. Finally, anterior rectal mobilization is carried out by applying posterior traction on the rectum toward the sacrum and using the pelvic retractor to elevate the prostate (in males) or vagina (in females). In males, the rectal side of Denonvillier's fascia is incised. In the female, the rectovaginal plane is entered, exposing the longitudinal muscle fibers of the rectum and avoiding entrance into the profuse vascular plexus on the posterior aspect of the vagina and vagina itself.

After circumferential complete rectal mobilization is accomplished from above, attention is directed to the perineum to complete the procedure. If surgery is not performed for cancer, an intersphincteric dissection is performed to keep the perineal wound as small as possible (Fig. 3). After an anal purse-string suture is placed, an intersphincteric plane is palpated and developed by injection of saline/epinephrine solution (1:250,000). An intersphincteric incision is made, and Allis clamps are placed on the internal sphincter to act as traction devices. This plane is continued cephalad until the perirectal plane developed from above is encountered. This then detaches the rectal specimen from the pelvic floor attachments. The rectum is delivered into the perineal wound through the posterior pelvic floor defect. The intersphincteric

technique leaves a smaller perineal wound that closes easily primarily and has a lower rate of wound complications and nonhealing.

Great care must be taken to construct the stoma because it is permanent. The ileostomy should be brought out through the rectus abdominus muscle in the previously marked site. To have the ostomy upright and everted after its construction, occasionally the ileocolic vessel has to be sacrificed, and the ostomy maintained on the arterial arcade of the terminal ileum. Sutures to mature the ostomy should not be brought out through the skin but rather in a subcuticular fashion to avoid implanting potentially viable ileal mucosal cells around the ostomy. This can potentially create a moisture problem and a long-term problem with pouching the ileostomy.

Colectomy and Ileorectal Anastomosis

Colectomy and ileorectal anastomosis for ulcerative colitis is rarely performed. This operation is offered only when the rectal disease is relatively minor and the patient is off local therapy. The distal margin of resection is at approximately the 13- to 15-cm level or at the level of the sacral promontory. Transecting the rectum at this level obviates the need for deep pelvic dissection and avoids possible autonomic nerve damage. The anastomosis is performed either with an endorectal circular stapler or manually, hand-sewing the anastomosis in a single layer with 3–0 absorbable sutures. We prefer to use a larger diameter stapler, at least 28 mm, to avoid an anastomotic stricture. If the terminal ileum does not admit this diameter, a hand-sewn anastomosis is performed.

Proctocolectomy and Continent Kock Ileostomy

This procedure was first described by Professor Nils Kock of Sweden in 1963, and it eliminated the need for a permanent external appliance. Many modifications have occurred since that time. Because of the high rate of complications, this procedure is rarely performed. It involves the formation of a low-pressure reservoir with synchronous construction of a continent nipple valve.

A total of 60 cm of terminal ileum is needed to construct the pouch with the valve. Three 15-cm limbs are constructed similar to the letter S. The three limbs are sutured together, and an enterotomy is made along the long axis of the pouch approximately 1 cm away from the staple line. This S-pouch construction allows less tension on the suture line overlying the nipple valve and allows the afferent limb to enter the pouch at its base rather than the apex, so there is less chance of obstruction. Approximately 15 cm of terminal ileum is needed for the pouch outlet (5 cm) and nipple valve construction (10 cm). The nipple valve is constructed by using Babcock clamps to intussuscept the 10-cm segment of ileum leading out of the pouch. The intussusception is then maintained by several firings of the TA stapler, taking care to place two rows of staples on either side of the mesentery, thus preserving the blood supply to the valve. The anterior wall of the reservoir is then closed, and the outlet of the Kock pouch is secured to the abdominal wall flush to the skin. This ileostomy can be placed lower down on the abdominal wall than a conventional ileostomy and intubated for evacuation as needed (Fig. 4).

Most complications of the Kock continent ileostomy are related to the nipple valve. Some studies quote a 30% to 50% rate of nipple valve slippage. This leads to inability to intubate the pouch and incontinence of the valve. This problem leads to a high reoperative rate. A number of modifications have been proposed, including rotating the valve, excising mesenteric fat to decrease mesenteric bulk, using a mesenteric sling of either fascia or Mersilene, stapling the valve to the pouch wall, and encircling the valve with a loop of small bowel. All of these measures have been helpful but have failed to eliminate the problem of valve slippage.

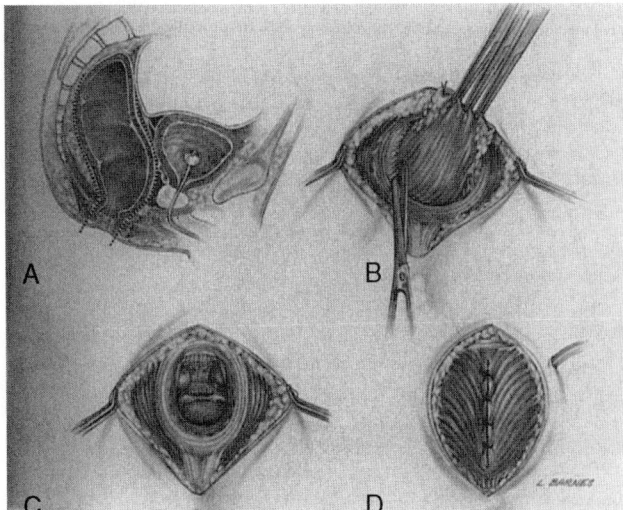

Figure 3 Intersphincteric proctectomy. **(A)** Outline of the resection. **(B)** Dissection of the intersphincteric plane. **(C)** Specimen removed. Levators and external sphincter. **(D)** Closure of the levators and external sphincter.

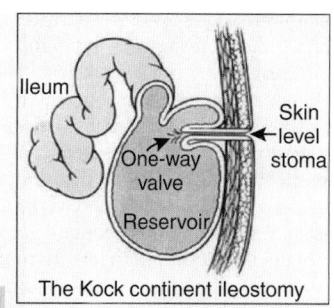

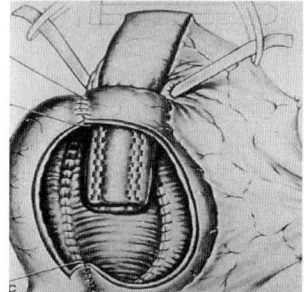

Figure 4 Kock ileostomy.

Continent Reconstruction with Ileal-Pouch-Anal Anastomosis

The pouch procedure, or "ileoanal pull-through," was first described by Sir Alan Parks in the *British Journal of Surgery* in 1980. Since its initial description, many technical modifications have been made, allowing the procedure to be performed safely with excellent success rates and good functional outcomes. Some controversies still exist regarding certain technical aspects of the procedure. The patient is placed in a modified dorsolithotomy Trendelenburg position with the left arm tucked. The abdominal colectomy and proctectomy are performed as described for panproctocolectomy. The ileum is transected just at the ileocecal valve region, and the rectal excision is completed down to the level of the levator complex from above. At this point, the rectum can be transected if a rectal mucosectomy is to be performed, or a stapling device, TA-30 (US Surgical, Norwalk, CT), can be used to close off the anorectal cuff if a double-staple technique is to be used (Fig. 5).

One of the most significant controversies involves the decision to perform distal rectal mucosectomy. Advocates of mucosectomy believe that all rectal mucosa should be removed to preclude the possibility of rectal strip colitis and future development of malignancy. Those who advocate the stapling technique believe that functional results are superior when stripping is not performed. It is technically easier to perform, less time consuming, and more readily fitted to the anatomically deep, narrow pelvis. It is our practice to perform the stapling technique routinely and to perform mucosectomy only when the operation is being done for familial polyposis or for dysplasia or frank carcinoma. It must be stressed that even when mucosectomy is performed, the mucosa may regenerate or remain as intramuscular islands. One of the pitfalls of the stapling technique is leaving too long of a rectal stump. One means of preventing this problem is to have an assistant perform a rigid proctosigmoidoscopy after the completion of the abdominal rectal mobilization. After the dentate line is identified, the scope is advanced 2 cm, and a marking suture is placed from above. The stapler is applied at this mark, and the specimen is removed.

The mucosectomy is performed using the Lone Star anal self-retaining retractor (Lone Star Medical Products, Stafford, TX) to evert the anus. Saline/epinephrine solution (1:250,000) is injected submucosally. Mucosectomy can be performed either with a scissor technique or with electrocautery, removing an intact cuff of distal

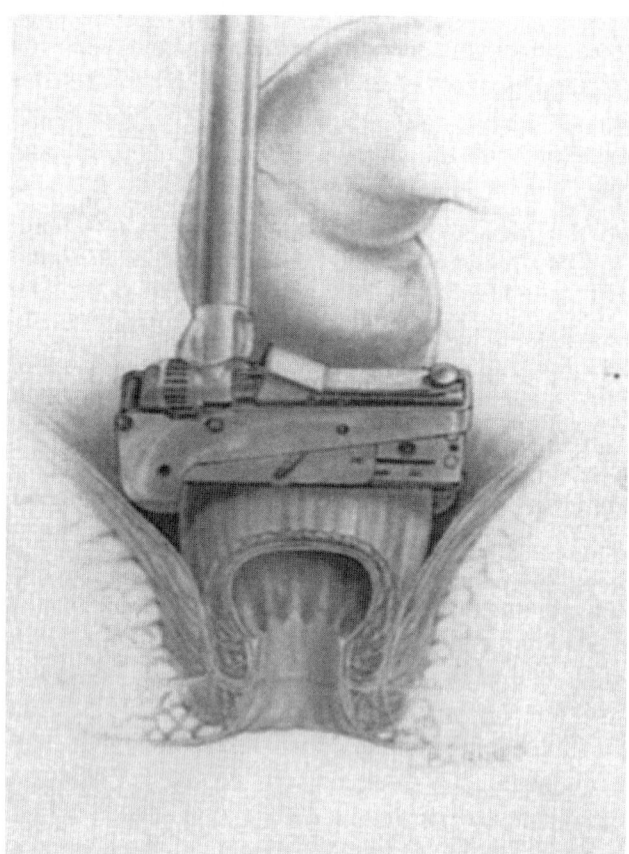

Figure 5 Linear stapling of the distal rectum.

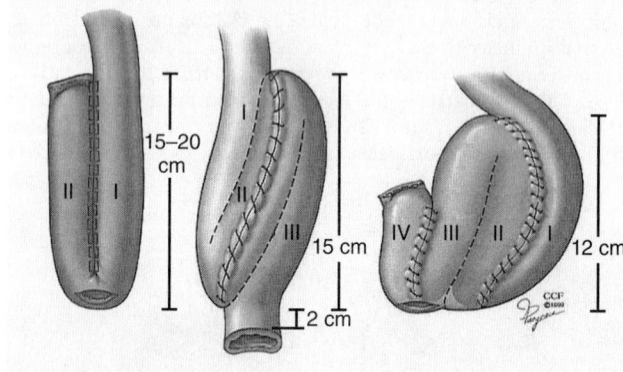

Figure 6 Different pouch configurations.

rectal mucosa from the dentate line to the top of the remaining rectal muscular cuff.

After the distal margin is prepared, attention should be shifted to pouch construction. Parks' initial description was of a three-limb S-pouch. In 1980, Utsunomiya described the two-limb J-pouch, and Nichols outlined the construction of the four-limb W-pouch (Fig. 6). Cohen and McLeod found that regardless of pouch construction, no functional difference existed after 6 months. Thus, because of technical ease of construction and elimination of any efferent limb that can lead to obstructed defecation, we routinely perform a J-pouch. After closing off the terminal ileum with a linear stapler, two 18- to 20-cm limbs of the terminal ileum are measured and folded back on themselves. An apical enterotomy is made, and a GIA 75 stapling device (US Surgical, Norwalk, CT) is fired sequentially to construct the pouch (Fig. 7).

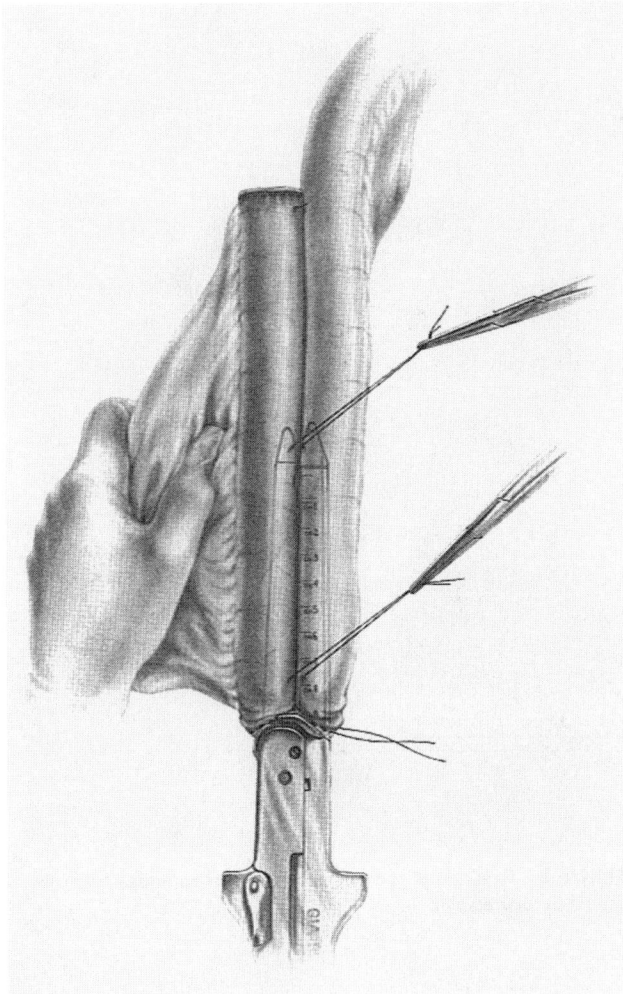

Figure 7 Construction of the J-pouch using the linear stapling device.

The anvil of a circular stapler is then placed in the apical enterotomy, and a purse-string suture is placed to secure it. The circular stapler is then passed transanally, and the anastomosis is created (Fig. 8). Great care must be taken to ensure that no surrounding tissue or adjacent structures are incorporated (i.e., vagina or prostate). After inspection of the tissue donuts, it is our practice to fill the pelvis with saline and test for leak by insufflating air through a rigid proctoscope. The anastomosis is also visually inspected. If the mucosectomy technique is used, following pouch construction a single-layer, hand-sewn anastomosis is performed with 2–0 absorbable full-thickness sutures through the pouch to the anal sphincter at the level of the dentate line.

In an attempt to accomplish a tension-free anastomosis, the maximal length of the ileal mesentery can be achieved by mobilizing the superior mesenteric artery up to its origin over the duodenum and the pancreas (Fig. 9). Also, transverse incisions in the peritoneum overlying the superior mesenteric artery (SMA) can be created every 2 to 3 cm to achieve an additional few centimeters in length (Fig. 10). As long as the pouch apex extends a few centimeters below the pubic symphysis, adequate tension-free anastomosis can be performed.

Another area of debate is the use of the diverting loop ileostomy. The use of the temporary ileostomy is based on the individual patient and the given operation. The patient who undergoes an elective operation who is well nourished, is not anemic, is not taking high-dose steroids, and has a technically good pouch construction may not require a diversion. If a diverting ileostomy is used,

a pouchogram is performed in approximately 6 to 8 weeks. When this confirms an intact pouch, the ileostomy is closed.

LAPAROSCOPIC MANAGEMENT OF ULCERATIVE COLITIS

The laparoscopic approach to patients with UC is slowly gaining acceptance as surgeons become more comfortable performing complex operations with the use of the laparoscope. All studies regarding laparoscopic colon surgery thus far have been favorable. They have demonstrated more rapid return of bowel function and reduced length of stay. Laparoscopic colon surgery has been shown to be safe and "less disfiguring."

Electively, a laparoscopic panproctocolectomy and continent reconstruction with an ileoanal J-pouch can be performed. This can be approached by "pure" laparoscopic means or by a hand-assisted method.

We use a hand-assisted method in our practice. A Pfannensteil incision is made 0.5 cm less that the operator's glove size, 1 cm above the symphysis pubis, through which a hand-assist device is inserted. A 10-mm port is placed in the supraumbilical area for a 30-degree 10-mm camera. Two 5-mm ports are placed on either side of the umbilicus lateral to the rectus muscles (Fig. 11). With the use of the Gelport (Applied Medical, Rancho Santa Margarita, CA), instruments can actually be placed through the device itself, thereby decreasing the total number of trocars required. The colon is mobilized in a lateral- to-medial fashion, similar to open technique. Some surgeons prefer to use medial-to-lateral approach. The mesentery is taken laparoscopically with the use of a ligasure device (ValleyLab, Boulder, CO). The terminal ileum is then carefully transected with a laparoscopic stapler, and the entire abdominal colon is drawn out through the suprapubic site. The lower pelvic dissection, creation of J-pouch, and ileal pouch to anal anastomosis are then performed through the Pfannensteil incision in the same fashion as in open surgery.

SURGICAL COMPLICATIONS

Surgery for UC is generally safe, with a mortality rate of less than 1% even when performed in the emergency setting. As with other surgery, complications include wound infection, thromboembolic events, and pulmonary complications. There are also complications specific to rectal surgery. In males, autonomic nerve damage caused by proctectomy can result in bladder dysfunction and erectile dysfunction such as retrograde ejaculation and impotence. With meticulous attention to detail during the perineal dissection, the incidence can be kept as low as 1% to 2%. In females, infertility can result from pelvic adhesions, but most patients can conceive normally and deliver vaginally.

Small bowel obstruction (SBO) can develop in approximately 20% of patients who have undergone abdominal surgery. The incidence of adhesions can be reduced by the application of hyalurinidase bioresorbable membrane, Seprafilm (Genzyme, Cambridge, MA). Conservative management with intravenous hydration, nasogastric decompression, and bowel rest are often sufficient for the resolution of the SBO.

Complications related specifically to ileal pelvic pouch reconstruction are subdivided into early and late. Early complications involve pelvic sepsis caused by an anastomotic leak either from the ileoanal anastomosis or from the pouch itself. It occurs in approximately 8% to 10% of patients. This can lead to peripouch pelvic abscess formation, which, if not treated expeditiously, can lead to loss of pouch compliance and poor functional outcome. Most anastomotic leaks are treated successfully with drainage and antibiotics. If patients fail conservative management, the pouch is taken down and reconstructed or converted to a permanent ileostomy.

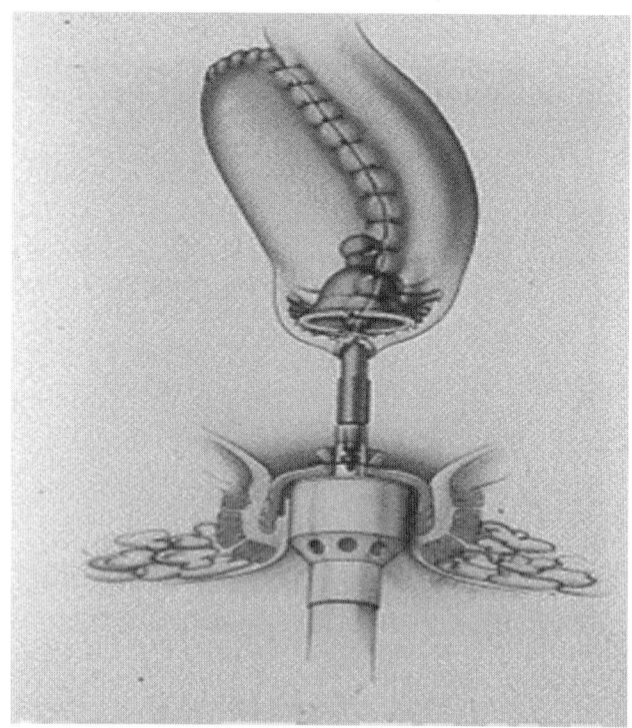

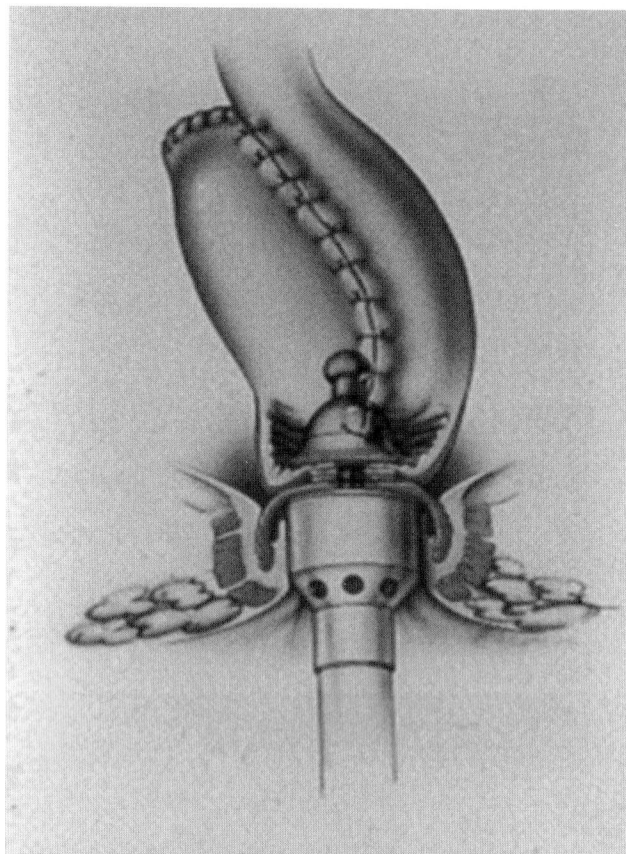

Figure 8 Creation of the ileal-pouch anal anastomosis with the use of circular stapler.

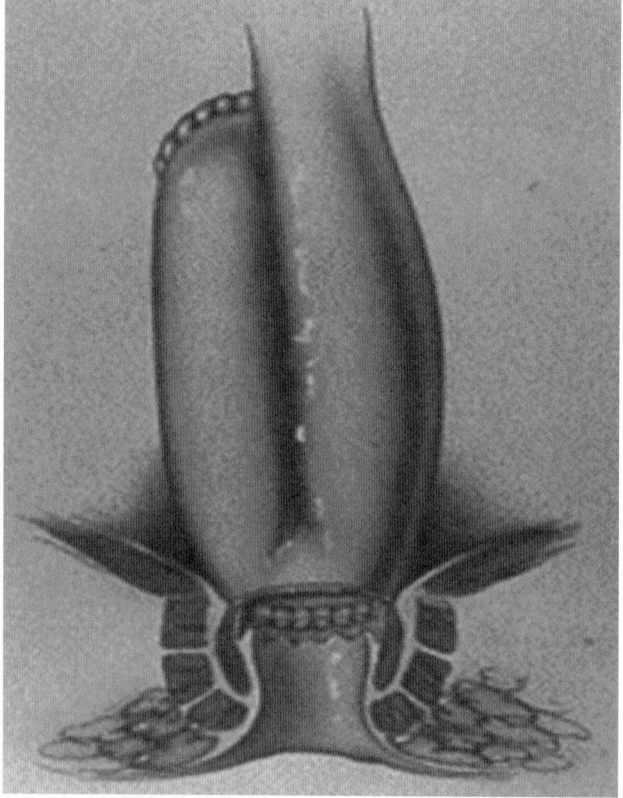

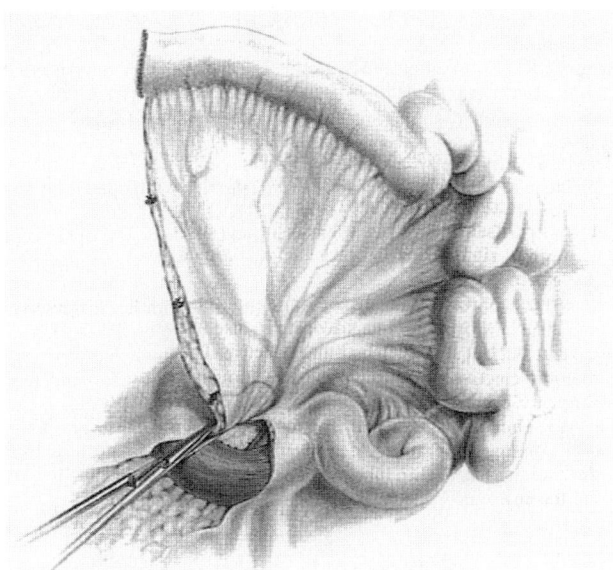

Figure 9 Superior mesenteric artery mobilization up to its origin over the duodenum and the pancreas.

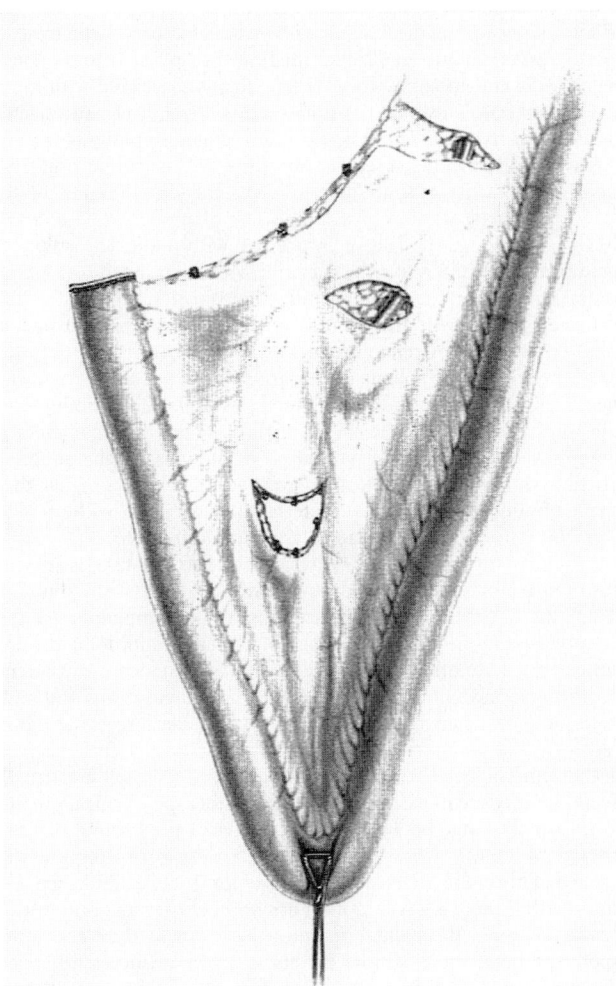

Figure 10 Incisions in the small bowel mesentery can provide further length.

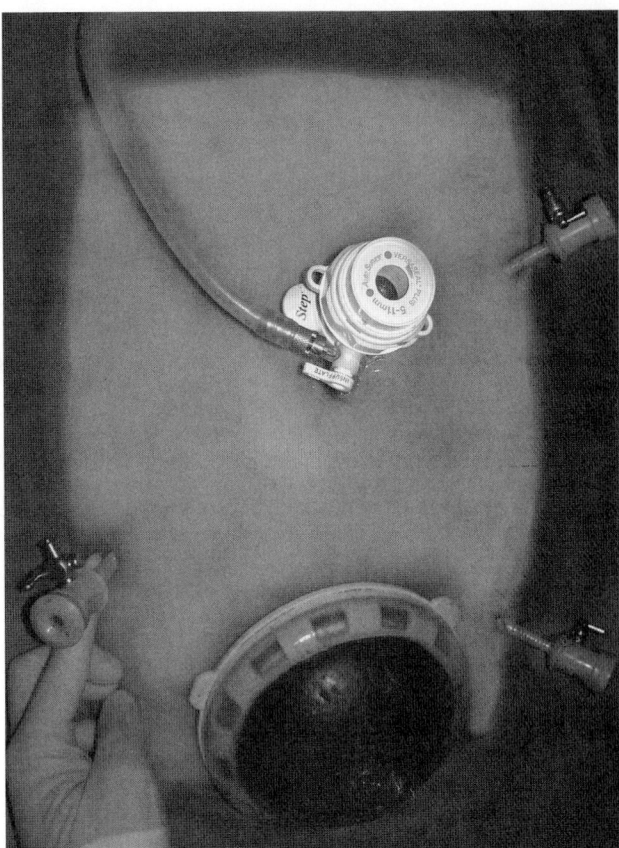

Figure 11 Port placement in laparoscopic-assisted total proctocolectomy.

The most common late complication after pelvic pouch surgery is pouchitis occurring in 25% to 30% of patients. Pouchitis is a nonspecific inflammation of the pouch mucosa, possibly related to stagnation of anaerobic bacteria in the pouch or to an immune mediated entity (it is rarely seen in pouches constructed for familial adenomatous polyposis [FAP]). Patients usually present with malaise, frequent watery stools, new onset rectal bleeding, and incontinence that is worse at night. The diagnosis is confirmed with pouchoscopy and responds quickly to a course of metronidazole or ciprofloxacin for 10 or 14 days. Probiotics and nonsteroidal enemas have been used with some limited success. If pouchitis becomes refractory, a diagnosis of Crohn's disease should be ruled out.

Patients who have undergone stapled restorative proctocolectomy should have an annual pouchoscopy and biopsy of the pelvic pouch and retained 1 to 2 cm of anal canal to screen for the development of dysplasia.

RESULTS

Most patients who undergo any surgical procedure for UC do extremely well, reporting great improvement in the quality of life. Although most patients adapt well to their procedure, patients who have undergone ileal pouch-anal surgery seem to have fewer restrictions on their physical activities and lifestyle.

Patients who have undergone pelvic pouch surgery report four to seven semiformed, toothpaste-consistency bowel movements daily. The neorectum is compliant and allows deferral of defecation. Urgency and incontinence are rare, occurring more frequently at night and more often in older patients, perhaps because of the decreased anal resting and squeeze pressures. Moreover, there is no deterioration of function with time. Ileal-pouch-anal anastomosis has become the standard procedure for patients requiring surgery for UC. The long-term results are excellent, with more than 97% of patients keeping their pouch with excellent functional outcomes and an extremely high quality of life.

In our practice, of 140 patients who underwent total proctocolectomy with ileal J-pouch-anal anastomosis, 99% of patients had good to excellent functional outcomes. Indications for surgery included FAP (n = 3) and UC (n = 137), with the mean age of patients being 35 years, ranging from 6 to 63 years. In our series, there were 6 anastomotic leaks (4.2%), 2 pouch-vaginal fistulae (1.4%), and 3 small bowel obstructions (2.1%) requiring reoperations. Only one pouch had to be excised in a patient who was later diagnosed with Crohn's disease. Pouchitis occurred in 40 patients (14.3%) and was managed conservatively with probiotics, antibiotics, and altered diet.

SUGGESTED READINGS

Coffey JC, Winter DC, Neary P, and others: Quality of life after ileal pouch-anal anastomosis: an evaluation of diet and other factors using the Cleveland Global Quality of Life Instrument, *Dis Colon Rectum* 45:30, 2002.

Corman ML: *Colon and rectal surgery*, ed 5, Philadelphia, 2005, JB Lippincott.

Lovegrove RE, Constantinides VA, Heriot AG and others: A comparison of hand-sewn versus stapled ileal pouch anal anastomosis (IPAA) following proctocolectomy: a meta-analysis of 4183 patients, *Ann Surg* 244(1):18, 2006.

Marcello PW, Milson JW, Wong SK and others: Laparoscopic restorative proctocolectomy: case-matched comparative study with open restorative proctocolectomy, *Dis Colon Rectum* 43(5):604, 2000.

McNevin MS, Bax T, MacFarlane M and others: Outcomes of a laparoscopic approach for total abdominal colectomy and proctocolectomy, *Am J Surg* 191(5):673, 2006.

Parks AG, Nicholls RJ, Belliveau P: Proctocolectomy with ileoanal reservoir and anal anastomosis, *Br J Surg* 67:533, 1980.

Procaccino JA: Tough topics in inflammatory bowel disease: management of ulcerative proctosigmoiditis, post graduate course in colon and rectal surgery, *ACS Clin Congress Manual 30*, 1998.

Reilly WT, Pemberton JH, Wolff BG and others: Randomized prospective trial comparing ileal pouch-anal anastomosis performed by excising the anal mucosa to ileal pouch-anal anastomosis performed by preserving the anal mucosa, *Ann Surg* 225:666, 1997.

CROHN'S COLITIS

Susan Galandiuk, MD

Crohn's disease (CD) has been steadily increasing in frequency since its initial clinical report by Dr. Burril Crohn and colleagues in the *Journal of the American Medical Association* in 1932. Its frequency currently is estimated to be 10 to 15 per 100,000. There are currently a wide variety of medical treatments, and CD affecting the colon is, for the most part, a medically treated disorder. Indications for surgery have changed and evolved over time. As medical therapy has improved, the surgical options have broadened and expanded. There are different issues to take into account, such as colon cancer risk, as well as issues with respect to fertility and pregnancy in women. Unlike ulcerative colitis (UC), in which the predominant symptom is bloody diarrhea, CD is more frequently associated with abdominal pain. Symptoms of both disorders can, however, be identical. Regardless of disease site, with CD it is important to examine both the macroscopic and microscopic pattern of inflammation with respect to the presence of skip areas. This is a characteristic manifestation of disease wherein normal areas are interspersed between diseased areas, both microscopically and macroscopically. Macroscopically, this applies with respect to continuity of colonic inflammation from the dentate line. It is important to remember that granulomas, although pathognomonic for CD, are present only in approximately 35% of cases. Microscopically, the presence of lymphoid aggregates without an overlying ulcer can be indicative of the presence of CD. In 10% of patients affected with inflammatory bowel disease affecting the colon, one is unable to definitively categorize patients as having either CD or UC. These patients are categorized as having indeterminate colitis. Correct pathologic diagnosis is important, because the type of surgery performed for a presumed diagnosis of CD as compared with a diagnosis of Crohn's colitis differs, as will be discussed later. In approximately 40% of patients, there is a disparity in diagnosis between general and specialist pathologists. This can make it particularly challenging for treating clinicians to accurately identify whether patients have CD or UC.

MEDICAL THERAPY

Medical therapy plays a vital part in the treatment of patients with Crohn's colitis before and after surgery. Knowledge of the benefits and limitations of medical therapy is essential to the surgeon treating patients with colonic CD. Initial medical therapy of Crohn's colitis begins with anti-inflammatory therapy that is associated with minimal side effects. This includes sulfasalazine (Azulfidine) and related medications. Because Azulfidine is not tolerated in patients with an allergy to sulfa products, separation of the sulfa-pyridine ring from the 5-amino-salisylic acid moiety led to the development of the 5-ASA products, which are the mainstay of modern CD and UC therapy (Table 1). If disease is present within the left colon or rectum, topical release products can provide high local 5-ASA concentrations. These products include suppositories, administered at bedtime, which treat the rectum and lower sigmoid as well as small-volume 5-ASA retention enemas. Enemas treat the left colon up to the level of the splenic flexure if administered at bedtime with the patient recumbent in the left lateral position. These products are safe and have minimal side effects. If they are not effective, medical therapy is escalated to the next level. Antibiotics can be added at any time during therapy. Most patients with CD have a higher than average number of luminal bacteria than patients without CD. Ciprofloxacin and metronidazole are commonly used. Metronidazole in tablet form frequently causes nausea; metallic taste is another common complaint. When administered in capsule form at a dose of 375 mg 3 times per day after meals, these complaints are frequently absent. In a large number of patients, antibiotic therapy alone or added to other therapy will result in dramatic improvement. If symptoms have not improved with 5-ASA medications and antibiotics, the next step is usually steroid therapy. Because of the significant side effects of steroids, including weight gain, aseptic necrosis of the femoral head, and cataract formation, steroids are usually given in high dose in what is termed "pulse therapy." Typical starting doses usually range between 40 and 60 mg of prednisone per day, tapered by 10 mg every 2 weeks until a dosage of 10 mg/day is reached. This is then halved to 5 mg/day for 2 weeks, and then discontinued. If there is a resumption of symptoms at any point during steroid weaning, the patient resumes the previous dose and again tapers, perhaps more slowly. If this is again unsuccessful, pulse therapy is tried. If this is not successful several times, an attempt is made to wean the patient off steroids using another medication for long-term maintenance. The most common choices would be

Table 1: Common Anti-inflammatory and Antimetabolite Medications Used for Crohn's Colitis

Drug Class	Drug	Brand Name	Unit Dose	Dose & Interval	Side-Effects	Drug Distribution
Anti-inflammatory	Sulfasalazine	Azulfidine	500 mg	2 by mouth qid	Mylagia Pancreatitis Oligospermia	Colon
	5-ASA oral	Pentasa	500 mg	2 by mouth qid	Interstitial nephritis Intolerance	Stomach, small bowel, colon
		Asacol	400 mg	2 by mouth tid		Terminal ileum, colon
		Dipentum	250 mg	2 by mouth bid		Colon
		Colazal	750 mg	3 by mouth tid		Colon
	5-ASA topical	Canasa	1000 mg	Suppositories at bedtime		Rectum
		Rowasa	4 g	Retention enema at bedtime		Rectum, sigmoid, left colon to Splenic flexure
Anti metabolite	Azathioprine	Imuran	2 mg/kg body weight	Every day, with serial CBC and LFT	Leukopenia Pancreatitis Nausea Lymphoma	Systemic
	6-Mercaptopurine	Purinethol	1.5 mg/kg body weight			

bid, Twice daily; *CBC,* complete blood count; *LFT,* liver function test; *qid,* 4 times/day; *tid,* 3 times/day.

antimetabolites (Table 1), including azathioprine or 6-mercaptopurine. Although approximately 5% of patients experience side effects, many of these are managed or minimized with serial blood work monitoring. The occurrence of serious side effects can be predicted with some reliability by testing for the type of genetic variant of the enzyme that a patient has that is responsible for drug metabolism. Patients who have a variant of the enzyme that does not metabolize this drug will predictably have serious side effects. This assay is commercially available and predicts which patients will have significant toxicity and in whom these drugs should not be used. These are, however, maintenance medications and, unlike steroids that work immediately and that can be used in flares, once they are started, typically take 4 to 6 months for their effects to become apparent. For this reason, after they are begun, it will take some time until patients can be weaned off the steroids.

Antitumor necrosis factor (anti-TNF) drugs have taken an increasing role in both the acute and maintenance treatments of CD, and especially in the treatment of Crohn's colitis. Currently, infliximab (Remicade; Centocor, Horsham, PA) and adalimumab (Humira; Abbott Laboratories, Abbott Park, IL) are the only anti-TNF agents that the Food and Drug Administration has approved for Crohn's disease. Etanercept is a drug that targets TNF that is approved for other indications. Remicade is a chimeric monoclonal anti-TNF alpha-antibody that contains both murine and human components. It is given intravenously over 2 hours, most commonly at a dose of 5 mg/kg body weight, and is used both in the acute and maintenance therapies of CD. Typically it is administered as a 3-dose induction treatment, with a dose at weeks 1, 2, and 6, and as maintenance treatment every 8 weeks. Adalimumab is administered subcutaneously every 2 weeks with a starting dose of 160 mg, then 80 mg, then 40 mg/dose maintenance. Common side effects of therapy include allergic reactions and reactivation of tuberculosis or histoplasmosis in patients who have had these disorders previously.

CLASSIFICATION OF CROHN'S DISEASE

There have been attempts to categorize the behavior of CD by many, including perhaps the most common classification scheme, the

Vienna classification of CD, which classifies CD based on three characteristics, that is, the behavior of disease; age of diagnosis (before or after age 40); and disease location with respect to upper GI, small bowel, ileocolic or colon. Recently, this has been modified in the Montreal classification (Table 2). It is thought that patients can display more than one pattern of behavior. As early as the 1950s, Marshak and Wolf suggested that, over time, CD progressed from an inflammatory type of disease to a more fibrotic form. It is logical to assume that medications that reduce edema and inflammation, such as steroids, would treat an inflammatory, edematous type of disease well, and that, as disease progresses toward a more fibrotic stage associated with significant fibrosis, this would respond less

Table 2: Montreal Classification of Crohn's Disease*

Age of Diagnosis of Crohn's Disease	Location of Crohn's Disease	Crohn's Disease Behavior
A1: 16 years old or younger	**L1:** Ileal	**B1:** Nonstricturing, nonpenetrating
A2: Age 17–40	**L2:** Colonic	**B2:** Stricturing
A3: >age 40	**L3:** Ileocolonic	**B3:** Penetrating
	L4: Isolated upper gastrointestinal disease†	**p:** Perineal disease modifier added to B1-B3 with concomitant perineal disease

A, Age of diagnosis; *L,* location of Crohn's disease; *B,* Crohn's disease behavior.

*Modified from Satsangi J, Silverberg MS, Vermeire S, Colombel J-F: Gut 55:749–753, 2006.

†L4 can be added as a modifier to L1-L3 when concomitant upper gastrointestinal disease is present.

well to medical therapy. Patients with significant obstruction caused by fibrotic Crohn's strictures typically have associated symptoms, including abdominal pain, increased abdominal distention, postprandial nausea, and vomiting. Many patients who have this pattern of disease progress to a perforating type of CD. There can be so much pressure on luminal Crohn's ulcers proximal to the obstruction that these in turn will actually perforate and lead to intra-abdominal abscess formation, which in turn will perforate into an adjacent structure, becoming a fistula to that structure. This can be manifest as an enteroenteric fistula, enterocolic fistula, enterovesical fistula, and so forth. Because of the proximity of the terminal ileum and the sigmoid colon, the most common colonic fistula by far is the ileosigmoid fistula.

The three behavior patterns of CD, that is, inflammatory, fibrostenosing, and penetrating, can therefore easily be interrelated and occur in the same individual over time.

INDICATIONS FOR SURGERY IN PATIENTS WITH CROHN'S COLITIS

Surgery for CD is indicated in several scenarios, and the philosophy of surgery for CD is based on the fact that one cannot cure CD by surgery as one can cancer and that it can recur. Therefore the aim has been to be "conservative," that is, treat the specific problem and do not excise more bowel than is necessary. This approach has long been applied with respect to the small bowel, but only recently with respect to the colon. General indications for surgery for CD include (1) obstruction, (2) intra-abdominal abscess not amenable to drainage guided by computed tomography (CT), (3) symptomatic fistulae, (4) the treatment or prevention of colorectal cancer or dysplasia, (5) failure to grow and develop normally in children, (6) side effects of medical therapy, and (7) failure of medical therapy to control symptoms of disease.

Obstruction

Obstruction is a common indication for surgery in small bowel and ileocolic CD but can also be an indication for surgery in patients with colonic CD. This condition can be due to a segmental colonic stricture that requires resection or to an anal canal/rectal stricture that requires either proctectomy and/or diversion. (Figs. 1 and 2).

Intra-Abdominal Abscess

Intra-abdominal abscess formation formerly was a universal indication for surgery. However, with the advent of CT-assisted drainage techniques, many intra-abdominal abscesses can now be treated without surgery and then with either more aggressive medical therapy or surgery, instituted at an elective time after the major sepsis has resolved and provided that there is no associated obstruction. As is the case with any other septic event, if an abscess is drained at the time of surgery, primary anastomosis should not be attempted because of the high risk of anastomotic leakage. In this scenario, rather than performing an end stoma and separate mucous fistula, one can perform the back row of the anastomosis between the proximal and distal limbs of bowel and exteriorize this segment as a loop stoma. In this manner, after the patient has sufficiently recovered postoperatively, 8 to 12 weeks later, this can often be closed without a formal relaparotomy.

Symptomatic Fistulae

It was formerly thought that all patients with enteroenteric fistulae required surgery; however, this is no longer the case. Many patients

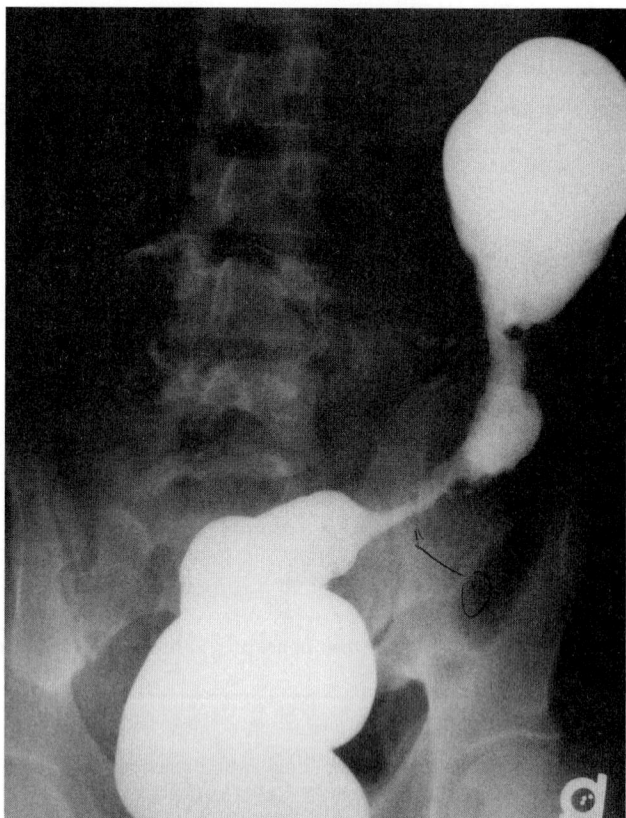

Figure 1 Radiographic contrast study showing sigmoid colon stricture secondary to Crohn's disease. This stricture caused symptoms of severe abdominal pain and diarrhea and was refractory to medical therapy. (*See color insert Figure 13.*)

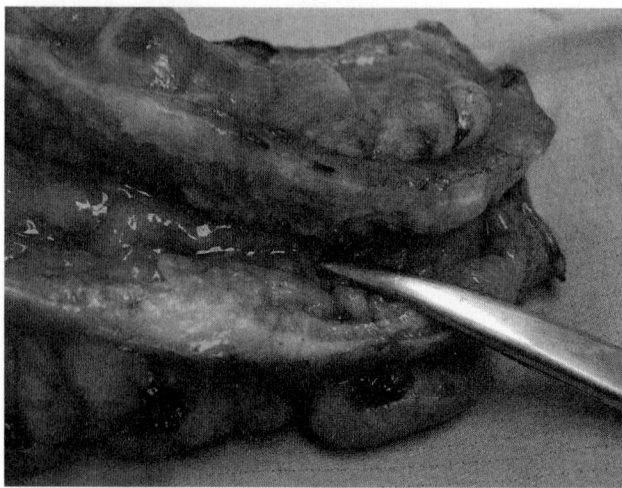

Figure 2 Sigmoid colon stricture with associated fistula indicated at tip of Mayo scissors. This stricture also was refractory to steroid and antimetabolite therapy and required segmental sigmoid resection. (*See color insert Figure 14.*)

with complex enteroenteric fistulae are relatively asymptomatic. However, patients with enterovesical fistulae who require chronic antibiotic suppression to avoid urinary tract infection, those with symptomatic enterovaginal fistulae draining large amounts of stool uncontrollably through the vagina, and patients with high-volume enterocutaneous fistulae all will require surgical correction (Fig. 3).

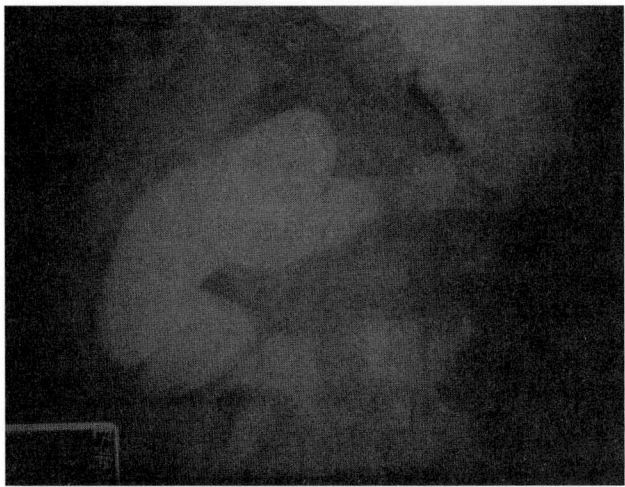

Figure 3 Gastrografin enema demonstrating large enterovesical fistula in patient with Crohn's colitis. This patient developed recurrent urinary tract infections despite continued antibiotic suppression, had severe associated bladder spasm, and required surgical resection and repair. (*See color insert Figure 15.*)

Colorectal Cancer and Dysplasia

Colorectal cancers that form in patients with inflammatory bowel disease generally affect patients at a younger age than in patients with sporadic colorectal cancer. Those patients who have a family history of colorectal cancer are at an even greater risk. Those patients who have colonic involvement of CD also are at a higher risk. The colorectal cancer risk is generally thought to be threefold that of the general population. Both CD and UC are considered to be high-risk groups with respect to colorectal cancer and should correspondingly undergo colonoscopy more frequently. There is indication from several large Canadian studies that chronic use of 5-ASA medications may indeed lower colorectal cancer risk.

Failure of Children to Grow

Failure of children to grow normally is an indication for surgery in CD patients and is extremely important. Failure to recognize this in a timely fashion can result in failure of a child to develop long-bone growth normally. Long-bone growth is assessed both by monitoring linear growth using nomograms and by assessing insulin-like growth factor 1 level and bone densitometry for age-specific bone development. If these are abnormal, strong consideration should be given to placing the child on growth hormone therapy in addition to changing the therapy for the patient's inflammatory bowel disease, be it with surgery or a change in medical therapy.

Side Effects of Medical Therapy

Patients who have significant side effects of medical therapy may frequently be candidates for surgery. Such side effects of medical therapy are numerous, as discussed earlier.

Failure of Medical Therapy to Control Symptoms

Failure of medical therapy to control symptoms is perhaps one of the most frequent indications for surgery, despite the growing armamentarium of medical options available to patients. One of the most serious and life-threatening indications for surgery with respect to failure of medical therapy is *toxic megacolon*. This term

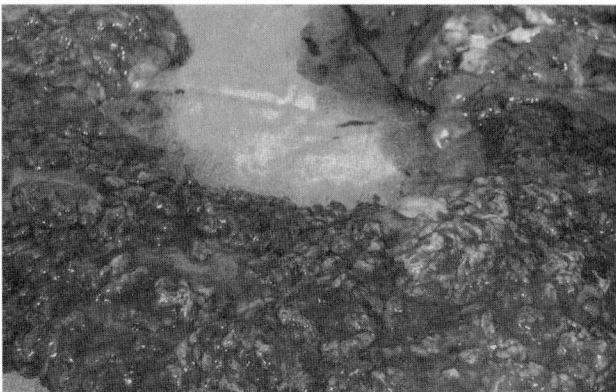

Figure 4 Endoluminal appearance of a colectomy specimen shortly after resection in a patient with toxic megacolon. Note the almost "autolytic" appearance of the colon, which was close to perforation. (*See color insert Figure 16.*)

is used to describe an entity that can occur with any kind of colitis, whether it is due to inflammatory bowel disease or colitis resulting from an infectious etiology. This is present when three or more of the following criteria are present: white blood cell count >12,500; tachycardia >100; a serum albumin <3 g/dl; a body temperature >38.5 degrees; and/or the diameter of a transverse colon on an abdominal film >5 cm. This typically means that the colitis has become so severe that there is actually resulting endotoxemia, with real danger of colonic perforation. In this circumstance, urgent surgery is required (Fig. 4).

Severe Perianal Disease

Patients with colonic Crohn's disease may also require surgery because of the coexistence of severe perianal CD (Fig. 5). This seems to occur more commonly in patients with Crohn's colitis.

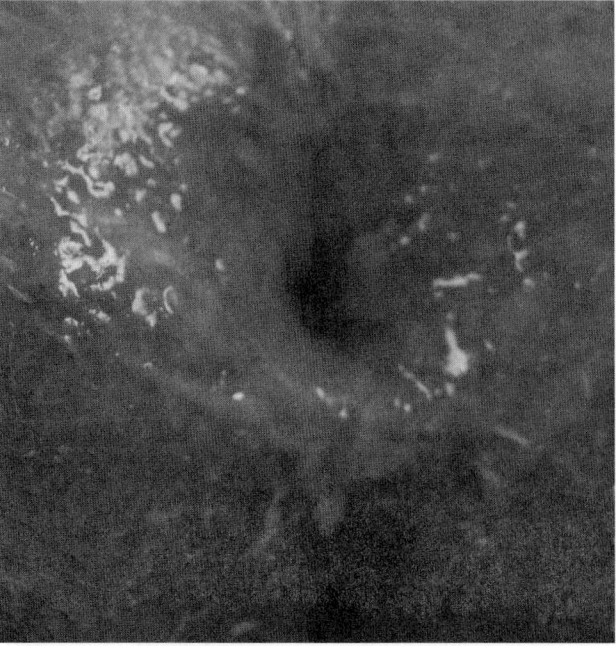

Figure 5 Severe perianal Crohn's disease stricture resulting in severe diarrhea, perianal excoriation, and small fistula right posteriolaterally. Note purulent discharge from anal canal. (*See color insert Figure 17.*)

Colonic Crohn's disease requires surgery in nearly equal frequency for severe perianal disease, disease-causing fistulae and abscesses, failure of medical therapy, and failure to thrive.

CHANGING SURGICAL TRENDS AND THE ROLE OF RECTAL COMPLIANCE

Surgery for CD of the colon and rectum has undergone a shift toward more conservative resection since the early 1990s. Before then, most patients with colonic CD were treated largely with total proctocolectomy and end ileostomy or, if they had relative rectal sparing, were offered subtotal colectomy and ileorectal anastomosis. Total proctocolectomy and ileostomy is still the operation associated with the lowest risk of recurrence of CD, estimated to range from 15% to 25% at 10 years in the absence of small bowel disease. Today, with the advent of more effective medical therapy to control colonic CD along with the recognition of the important water-absorbing role of the colon, more "colon conserving" surgery with segmental resection is being performed for segmental colonic CD. However, it must be realized and made clear to patients that this type of surgery is associated with a higher recurrence rate than proctocolectomy and ileostomy. In the young, compliant patient, however, this may lead to many years of delay or even avoidance of ileostomy. Here, the same criteria as with small bowel Crohn's surgery apply, that is, resecting and anastomosing into palpably normal bowel, resecting fibrotic stenosed segments, and diverting in the presence of gross purulence. The decision to avoid permanent diversion is made largely clinically on the basis of visual endoscopic inspection of the rectum, insufflation of air, and a documentation of patient symptoms. If the rectum is not pliable and does not distend on insufflation of air, whether on rigid proctoscopy or flexible endoscopy, this indicates that there has been significant transmural Crohn's proctitis and that the rectum has lost its reservoir function. These individuals do not do well functionally. They have incredible urgency and poor functional results, which are recorded by their symptoms. Usually, if this is explained to them, they will concede and accept diversion. If on the other hand, the rectum is pliable and distensible on insufflation of air, patients generally do well from the point of view of bowel function.

Every year, many patients with Crohn's disease of the colon inadvertently undergo colectomy and ileal pouch anal anastomosis under the presumed diagnosis of UC. Many of these patients do well, provided they do not have a history of perianal disease. Some have worse functional results than patients with UC and require more antidiarrheals. Some patients, however, develop Crohn's disease of the small bowel in the ileal pouch that cannot be controlled by medical therapy and that requires surgical resection of the ileal J-pouch and end ileostomy. Ileal j-pouch anal anastomosis should not knowingly be performed in a patient with Crohn's disease because of the danger of Crohn's disease developing in the pouch and the associated loss of large segments of small bowel should surgery be required. Table 3 lists the different types of procedures that are performed for patients with CD affecting the colon, both without and with perianal CD.

SURGERY FOR PERIANAL CROHN'S DISEASE

Perianal Crohn's disease can occur alone or together with Crohn's disease in other gastrointestinal locations. It frequently occurs in conjunction with Crohn's colitis and may therefore need to be addressed in conjunction with that illness. It may cause the patient relatively few symptoms or may be the source of almost disabling symptoms, as in the case of some high-output rectovaginal fistulae or painful cleft perineum, which occurs commonly in adolescents

Table 3: Operations Performed for Crohn's Colitis with and without Perianal Crohn's Disease

Operations for Colonic Disease	Operations for Perianal Crohn's Disease
Total proctocolectomy and end ileostomy	Fistulotomy for low fistulae
Subtotal colectomy and ileorectal anastomosis	Seton insertion or advancement flap repair for high fistulae
Segmental colectomy	Abscess drainage
Temporary proximal diverting ileostomy	Anal canal dilatation for anal canal Crohn's disease strictures
Colectomy and ileal J-pouch anal anastomosis*	Temporary or permanent fecal diversion

*Often inadvertently performed with a presumed preoperative diagnosis of ulcerative colitis.

and young adults. By and large, perianal Crohn's disease should first be treated medically and be treated surgically only if there are abscesses, symptomatic fistulae, or unacceptable function. Fistulae are a reflection of active distal rectal disease. It is paramount to do a digital exam to exclude the presence of an anal canal Crohn's disease stricture as an additional distal obstruction and factor contributing to persistence of the fistula. In the presence of a distal stricture, *no* medical therapy can be effective. In this scenario, there are three options: (1) regular dilatation of the stricture by the physician or (2) by the patient, or (3) permanent diversion, with or without proctectomy. If a patient is plagued by recurrent abscesses, placement of a *seton* is indicated. This is any type of device that is inserted into a fistula tract to facilitate drainage and that is designed to prevent the external fistula opening from closing and a recurrent abscess from forming at that site. I favor the use of large vessel loops that can easily be led through fistula tracts. They are washable and do not cause fecal material to adhere. Others prefer using 2–0 silk suture or other materials. These setons can be left in place for months or years, provide for drainage, and avoid the pain associated with abscess formation (Fig. 6). Since one cannot

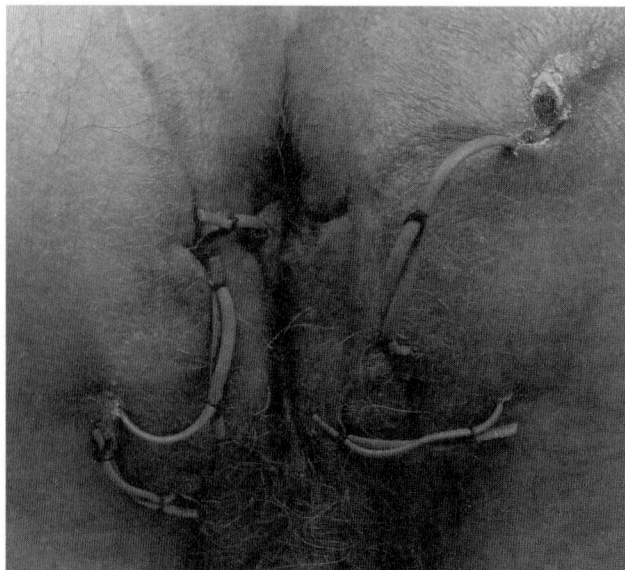

Figure 6 Perianal Crohn's disease resulting in recurrent abscesses and fistulae. The patient underwent placement of multiple setons. Here, blue vessel loops were used for this purpose to prevent abscesses from forming and to provide for continued drainage of the fistula tracts. (*See color insert Figure 18.*)

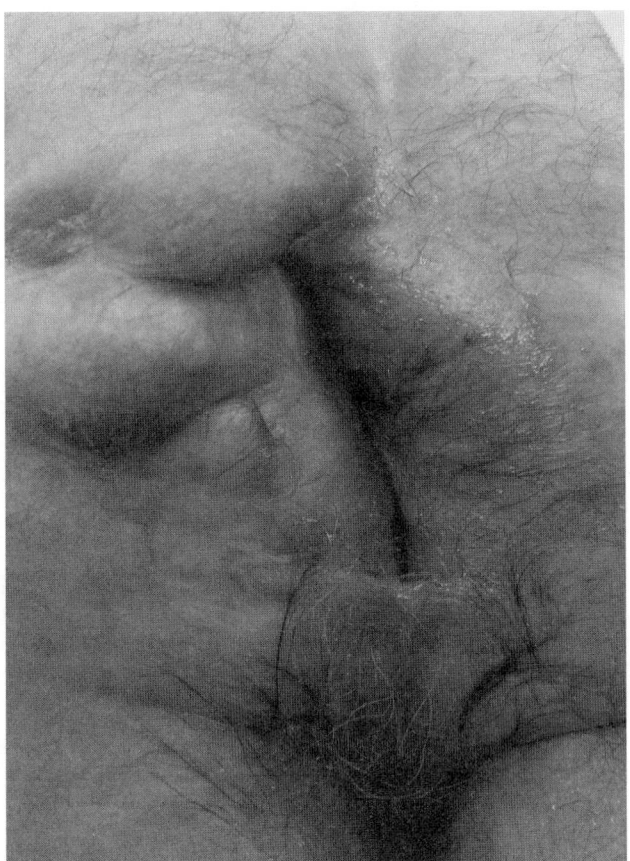

Figure 7 Severe deformity of the anal canal in a patient who has undergone multiple and extensive prior fistulotomies and abscess drainage procedures that have resulted in incontinence. (*See color insert Figure 19.*)

forecast the activity of Crohn's' disease in the future or the need for subsequent abdominal resective surgery, one wishes to minimize and even avoid surgery on the anal canal that divides or injures the anal sphincter, such as fistulotomy or fistulectomy. Unwise fistulotomies and abscess drainage procedures can lead to significant anal canal deformity and fecal incontinence (Fig. 7). The repair of rectovaginal fistula in patients with Crohn's disease is difficult. In the presence of active distal rectal Crohn's disease, even with diversion, rectal advancement flap repair techniques even in expert hands have often been unsuccessful.

CONCLUSION

Surgery for Crohn's colitis must be individualized for each patient. Generally, surgery is performed for complications of the disease. The goal of surgery is to be conservative and remove as little colon as possible, choosing margins of resections on the basis of palpably normal bowel. Diversion is used selectively in cases of abscess and frank purulence. Advances in medical therapy have led to a wider choice of options in surgical therapy for patients with Crohn's colitis, permitting some patients to avoid permanent diversion.

SUGGESTED READINGS

Farmer M, Petras RE, Hunt LE, and others: The importance of diagnostic accuracy in colonic inflammatory bowel disease, *Am J Gastroenterol* 95(11):3184–3188, 2000.

Galandiuk S, Kimberling J, Al-Mishlab TG, Stromberg AJ: Perianal Crohn disease: predictors of need for permanent diversion, *Ann Surg* 241:796–802, 2005.

Marshak RH, Wolf BS: Chronic ulcerative granulomatous jejunitis and ileo-jejunitis, *AJR Am J Roentgenol* 70:93, 1953.

Morpurgo E, Petras R, Kimberling J, and others: Characterization and clinical behavior of Crohn's disease initially presenting predominantly as colitis, *Dis Colon Rectum* 46:918, 2003.

Satsangi J, Silverberg MS, Vermeire S, Colombel J-F: The Montreal classification of inflammatory bowel disease: controversies, consensus, and implications, *Gut* 55:749–753, 2006.

Sonoda T, Hull T, Piedmonte MR, and others: Outcomes of primary repair of anorectal and rectovaginal fistulae using the endorectal advancement flap, *Dis Colon Rectum* 45:1622, 2002.

ISCHEMIC COLITIS

C. Neal Ellis, MD

Ischemic colitis is the most common form of intestinal ischemia. The clinical spectrum can range from transient, self-limited ischemia to acute fulminant transmural injury with bowel necrosis. Classically, ischemic colitis is suspected in elderly, critically ill patients with multiple comorbid conditions who present with abdominal pain, bloody diarrhea, and fever. With the increased use of computerized tomography and endoscopy to evaluate abdominal pain, ischemic colitis is frequently being diagnosed in "atypical" situations. In fact, 10% to 20% of patients are younger than 40 years of age and only half of the patients will have bleeding or diarrhea. The diverse causes, listed in Table 1, and the variable clinical presentations make the diagnosis and management of ischemic colitis a challenge.

CLINICAL PRESENTATION

Clinical findings and symptoms depend on the extent of the vascular injury. Most patients present with nongangrenous ischemia characterized by the acute onset of mild, crampy abdominal pain localized to the area of ischemic colon. The pain is usually associated with an urge to defecate. During the first 24 hours, there is commonly passage of blood, either bright red or maroon, which may be associated with diarrhea. Blood loss is generally minimal, without hemodynamic compromise or the need for transfusion. Profuse bleeding should prompt investigation for another source. Some individuals develop an ileus with anorexia, nausea, and abdominal distention.

Findings on physical examination may range from mild tenderness over the involved colon in early or limited ischemia to peritonitis from severe ischemia, with transmural necrosis of the bowel. Given the vascular anatomy of the colon, the areas most prone to ischemic damage are the "watershed" areas where the superior mesenteric, inferior mesenteric, and iliac arteries meet, such as the splenic flexure and sigmoid colon.

Table 1: Etiologies of Ischemic Colitis

Systemic shock (hypovolemic, septic, neurogenic)

    Cardiogenic (cardiac failure, dysrhythmias, coronary artery bypass surgery)

Vascular

    Major artery occlusion (aortic dissection, thrombotic, embolic)

    Surgical (aneurysmectomy, colectomy)

    Small artery occlusion (diabetes, atherosclerosis)

        Vasculitis (systemic lupus erythematosus, polyarteritis nodosa, thromboangiitis obliterans, rheumatoid, sickle cell disease, Takayasu arteritis, Wegner granulomatosis)

    Venous thrombosis

        Inflammatory (appendicitis, diverticulitis, pancreatitis)

        Hypercoagulable states

            Malignancy

            Factor deficiency (protein C, protein S, antithrombin III, Van Leiden, paroxysmal nocturnal hemoglobinuria, anticardiolipin syndrome, protein C resistance)

Colonic obstruction/dilatation

    Mechanical (neoplasm, impaction, volvulus, intussusception, stricture, hernia)

    Pseudo-obstruction (Ogilvie syndrome, toxic megacolon, colonoscopy)

Medications (see Table 2)

Other (airplane flights, marathon running)

Basic laboratory studies are normal in most patients with self-limiting ischemic colitis. Severe ischemia with infarction of a segment of the colon may lead to a leukocytosis or a metabolic acidosis. Although laboratory markers of ischemia, such as elevated serum lactate, lactate dehydrogenase, or alkaline phosphatase may be present, these findings are uncommon in mild ischemia and not present in severe ischemia until late in the clinical course.

RADIOLOGY

Findings on plain abdominal radiographs are generally nonspecific in mild to moderate ischemia, but these studies are important to exclude other conditions, such as intestinal obstruction or perforation. Although not commonly obtained, barium enema has been reported to show the suggestive findings of "thumbprinting," longitudinal ulcers, sacculation, or transverse ridging in up to 75% of patients with ischemic colitis. Computerized tomography (CT) is more frequently used for the evaluation of abdominal pain and may show circumferential wall thickening in up to 89% of patients with ischemic colitis. Other findings suggestive of severe ischemia include pneumatosis coli and gas within the portal vein.

Abdominal ultrasonography and mesenteric angiography have also been used in the evaluation of ischemic colitis. Ultrasonography has been reported to detect colonic abnormalities in up to 90% of patients with ischemic colitis. Ultrasound with color Doppler can detect patency of mesenteric veins and absent or diminished flow in ischemic bowel wall in 80% of patients. Most ischemic colitis is the result of nonocclusive or venous disease rather than arterial insufficiency, thereby limiting the role of visceral angiography. Patients with known predisposing factors such as a cardiac thrombus, hypercoagulable conditions, or evidence of arterial insufficiency on CT may benefit from angiography and possible treatment with thrombolytics or vasodilators.

ENDOSCOPY

Although invasive, colonoscopy has become the gold standard for the diagnosis of ischemic colitis because of its greater sensitivity for detecting mucosal changes and the ability to obtain biopsy specimens if needed. Colonoscopy is usually preferable to flexible sigmoidoscopy in most circumstances because the area of ischemia will be proximal to the splenic flexure in 30% to 40% of patients. This is particularly important because ischemia of the right colon has been reported to have a worse prognosis. In general, to minimize the risk of perforation, the colonoscope should not be passed beyond the affected area, and overinflation of the bowel should be avoided. In early stages of ischemia, petechial hemorrhages interspersed with areas of pale edematous mucosa will be found during endoscopy. This may progress to segmental erythema with or without ulcerations. A single longitudinal inflamed or ulcerated strip of colon, the "single stripe sign," may be present in limited ischemia. More severe ischemia results in dusky, gray or black mucosa with or without pseudopolyps or pseudomembranes. Chronic ischemia may result in a colonic stricture, decreased haustrations, and mucosal granularity.

There are no endoscopic findings specific to ischemic colitis, and therefore the complete clinical picture must be considered. Colitis related to other etiologies should be considered. In particular, inflammatory bowel disease, infectious colitis, and drug-associated colitis should be excluded. Endoscopic findings that favor ischemic colitis over inflammatory bowel disease include segmental area of injury, abrupt transition between normal and affected mucosa, and rectal sparing. Examination of the stool for ova and parasites, enteric pathogens, and *Clostridium difficile* toxin can help to evaluate for these etiologies. Patients may be reluctant to admit to misuse of some of the drugs listed in Table 2, but with nonjudgmental questioning and education stressing the importance of identifying the etiology, most patients will provide the necessary information.

On histologic examination of biopsy specimens, mucosal edema with distorted crypts, mucosal and submucosal hemorrhage, inflammation, intravascular thrombi, and necrosis can be seen with ischemic colitis. Less crypt damage and more inflammation will be seen in biopsies from patients with inflammatory bowel disease. The presence of a hyalinized, hemorrhagic lamina propria and full-thickness mucosal necrosis may help to differentiate ischemic colitis with pseudomembranes from *C. difficile* colitis.

TREATMENT

The management of ischemic colitis is determined by the degree of ischemia (Fig. 1). The challenge is that there are no means reliably to distinguish self-limiting ischemia from ischemia that results

Table 2: Medications That May Cause Colonic Ischemia

Digitalis

Estrogens (oral contraceptives)

Antihypertensives (diuretics, calcium channel blockers)

Vasopressors (ephedrine, pseudoephedrine, phenylephrine hydrochloride (Neo-Synephrine), phenylephrine, vasopressin, norepinephrine, epinephrine)

Cocaine

Nonsteroidal anti-inflammatory agents

Amphetamines (methamphetamine)

Psychotropic drugs

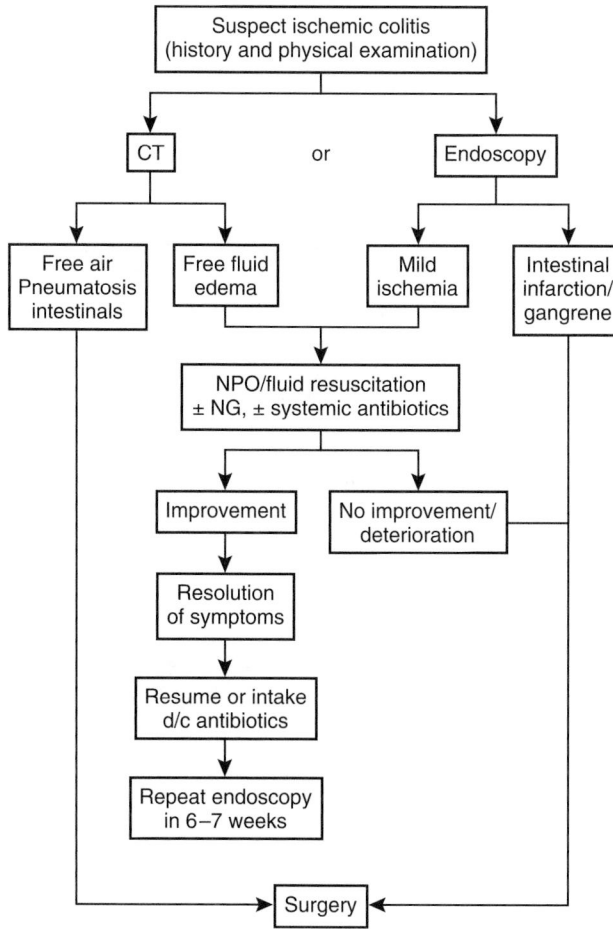

Figure 1 Management of ischemic colitis.

Emergent Surgery

Despite appropriate nonoperative therapy, in 20% of patients, colonic ischemia will progress. Worsening abdominal pain or peritonitis, as well as increasing leukocytosis and fever, are indications for emergent surgical intervention. Intraoperatively, the decision about what to resect is based on the assessment of the viability of the involved bowel. Methods that can be used to assess viability in questionable areas include intravenous infusion of fluorescein dye with use of the Woods lamp and the presence of a Doppler signal in the antimesenteric border. Palpation of a pulse in the mesentery has been described but is unreliable to determine viability because thrombosis of the microvasculature may have occurred, with infarction of the bowel despite flow being present in the larger mesenteric vessels. In situations in which there are large segments of involved bowel with questionable viability, a planned second-look procedure may avoid unnecessary resection of bowel that appears questionable initially but will recover. Whether planned or not, continued clinical deterioration with a worsening metabolic acidosis or a nonviable stoma are indications for reexploration.

In general, resection is reserved for areas of transmural ischemia or infarction. Although ischemia limited to the mucosa is not an indication for resection, it is a contraindication for primary anastomosis. Most commonly, either the bowel ends after resection are left in the abdomen if a second-look procedure is planned or a stoma with Hartmann pouch is created. Although these stomas are thought to be temporary, 30% to 40% of patients will not have bowel continuity restored, and thus creation of a well-placed and functioning stoma is important. In the unusual circumstance of ischemia confined to the right colon, a primary anastomosis can be considered if both the ileum and transverse colon appear well vascularized and the patient's overall condition allows.

Elective Surgery

Occasionally, the damage from limited ischemia may not heal completely despite resolution of the acute event resulting in chronic segmental colitis. This condition is characterized by persistent diarrhea, protein loss, bleeding, or stricture formation with obstructive symptoms. Patients with mild symptoms may be followed by periodic endoscopy to document lack of progression to more advanced stages. Elective resection of the involved colonic segment should be considered if there is bleeding, diarrhea, or enteral protein loss that persists for more than 2 weeks because these patients are at an increased risk of bowel perforation. Elective resection should also be considered if a stricture develops with significant obstructive symptoms or if the stricture prevents appropriate screening of the proximal colon for neoplasms. In these circumstances, resection of the involved segment is sufficient, and most of these patients will be candidates for primary anastomosis.

in bowel necrosis and infarction. Careful monitoring for persistent for worsening abdominal pain, leukocytosis, fever, and peritonitis are used to guide therapy.

Nonoperative Management

A trial of nonoperative therapy is indicated for the majority of patients with ischemic colitis. This consists of identification and correction of any of the possible etiologies of ischemic colitis (listed in Table 1), bowel rest to decrease colonic oxygen requirements, and intravenous fluids to improve perfusion. Optimization of cardiac function and oxygenation is essential. In critically ill patients with other comorbidities and an uncertain hemodynamic status, pulmonary artery catheterization may be helpful to assess fluid status and cardiac function. Although there is a lack of prospective clinical data, empiric broad-spectrum antibiotic administration has been advocated and is frequently used to minimize bacterial translocation and sepsis. Any medications that the patient is receiving with the potential to cause intestinal ischemia (Table 2) should be discontinued if possible. In patients with an associated ileus, nasogastric tube decompression may be beneficial. Bowel stimulants and cathartics should be avoided because they may, rarely, induce colonic perforation.

In 60% to 80% of patients, acute colonic ischemia will resolve within 24 to 48 hours with nonoperative therapy. However, the endoscopic and radiologic abnormalities may persist for up to 2 weeks after an episode of limited ischemia. With ischemia that results in colonic ulceration, it may take up to 6 months for complete resolution of the endoscopic findings.

Outcomes

The prognosis for patients with ischemic colitis is dependent on their overall medical condition, the degree of the ischemia, and the identification of a reversible cause. Patients with mild self-limited ischemia related to a correctable cause or medication have an excellent prognosis, with complete resolution of the symptoms in 24 to 48 hours and little risk of recurrence. Patients with chronic segmental colitis also have an excellent prognosis after elective resection of the involved segment. If the etiology of the ischemia cannot be corrected, as in cases of congestive heart failure, the prognosis is much worse, with the possibility of continued ischemia and progressive damage to the colon. The worse outcomes are seen in patients who undergo an emergency resection for infarcted bowel in which mortality rates are reported to be 50% overall and as high as 80% if there is perforation.

SELECTED READING

Biaxauli J, Kiran RP, Delaney CP: Investigation and management of ischemic colitis, *Cleve Clin J Med* 70:920, 2003.

Brandt LJ, Boley SJ: AGA technical review on intestinal ischemia, *Gastroenterology* 118:954, 2000.

Green BT, Tendler DA: Ischemic colitis: a clinical review, *South Med J* 98:217, 2005.

Medina C, Vilaseca J, Videla S, and others: Outcome of patients with ischemic colitic: review of 53 cases, *Dis Colon Rectum* 47:180, 2004.

Sreenarasimhaiah J: Diagnosis and management of ischemic colitis, *Curr Gastroenterol Rep* 7:421, 2005.

CLOSTRIDIUM DIFFICILE COLITIS

Karen E. Deveney, MD

The association between antibiotic use and the entity called pseudomembranous colitis was first noted in the early 1950s, but the clear link between clindamycin and pseudomembranous colitis dates to the work of Tedesco and others in 1974. *Clostridium difficile* was identified as the offending organism shortly thereafter, and it was soon recognized that the colitis is mediated through a bacterial toxin. Over the past 25 years, *C. difficile* colitis has emerged as a significant cause of morbidity and death in patients who have been exposed to antibiotics. Although clindamycin was the first antibiotic described as causing *C. difficile* colitis, cephalosporins became the most common antibiotic class precipitating *C. difficile* infection in the 1990s, at least in part because of their widespread use. More recently, fluoroquinolones have been recognized to cause *C. difficile* infection more frequently than any other class of antibiotics. Although *C. difficile* was initially acquired in the hospital, the indiscriminate use of antibiotics has resulted in the appearance of *C. difficile* as a community-acquired infection as well, presenting in patients who have never been hospitalized. It has also increasingly appeared in immunocompromised patients, some of whom have no documented history of antibiotic use. With the progressive increase in illness severity of hospitalized patients, it is not surprising that *C. difficile* colitis has become a significant cause of morbidity and death in transplant patients, patients receiving chemotherapy for cancer, dialysis patients, and other immunocompromised individuals.

PATHOPHYSIOLOGY

The pathophysiology of *C. difficile* colitis involves the destruction of the normal bacterial flora in the colon, usually by antibiotic use, followed by colonization with the gram-positive anaerobic bacillus *C. difficile* and the release of toxins that attack the colonic mucosa and create inflammation and cell death. The dead cells form a gelatinous surface or pseudomembrane, hence the name pseudomembraneous colitis. Although the exact mechanism of action of toxins A and B is not clearly delineated, it has been demonstrated that the toxins bind to membrane receptors and distort the cell, creating cell rupture and stimulating the elaboration of cytokines. The factors influencing the severity of the colitis include both the virulence of the organism and the resistance of the host. Phage typing in specific institutions and regions has shown that some strains of *C. difficile* are associated with more severe forms of colitis than others.

A virulent strain may produce an epidemic of severe cases of colitis in a hospital or community before running its course. A heightened vigilance is thus warranted when a cluster of severe cases occurs. Evidence also exists that patients who are most susceptible to the toxic effects of *C. difficile* have a lack of immunoglobulin A or G antibody to toxin A in the colonic lumen. The presence of immunoglobulin G antibody appears to block the binding of toxin A to the intestinal receptor and may prohibit or attenuate the effects of *C. difficile* in that host. This finding raises the possibility that immunization against *C. difficile* toxins may provide a potential preventive mechanism in the future.

C. difficile forms heat-resistant spores that can persist in the environment for months or years. Hospitals and nursing homes are particularly prime sites for survival of *C. difficile*, an organism that can frequently be cultured from equipment, floors, and furniture in these institutions. Health care personnel can also spread the infection on their hands or on stethoscopes. Careful epidemiologic studies have documented spread from patient to patient in nursing units. *C. difficile* infection is therefore largely preventable if careful attention is paid to good infection control practices such as handwashing, cleansing of equipment, and use of disposables whenever possible.

PRESENTATION

The mildest forms of *C. difficile* infection include the asymptomatic carrier state and simple colitis, a diarrheal illness without pseudomembranes visible on endoscopic examination. These patients are not severely ill; the former requires no treatment at all, and the latter responds readily to oral metronidazole. Pseudomembranous colitis represents a further progression in the severity of the disease. Although these patients have significant diarrhea, they are not toxic. As long as they are not nauseated and are able to eat, oral metronidazole is effective and adequate therapy.

The most treacherous form of *C. difficile* colitis is that of fulminant colitis, characterized by a constellation of systemic symptoms and signs in addition to diarrhea: fever, hypotension, abdominal pain, nausea, abdominal distention, and leukocytosis. The fever and leukocytosis are often striking and severe.

Not only is the incidence of *C. difficile* colitis increasing with time, so also is the percentage of cases presenting with serious, fulminant colitis and requiring fluid resuscitation, aggressive parenteral antibiotic treatment, and even colectomy. The factors responsible for the increased incidence and severity of *C. difficile* colitis include the overuse of antibiotics, inattention to preventive measures, and increased acuity of hospitalized patients.

DIAGNOSIS AND MANAGEMENT

The diagnosis of *C. difficile* infection should be considered in any patient with recent antibiotic treatment who presents with diarrhea. If the patient is not severely ill, treatment can wait until the stool test for *C. difficile* toxin is positive. If the patient is still taking the

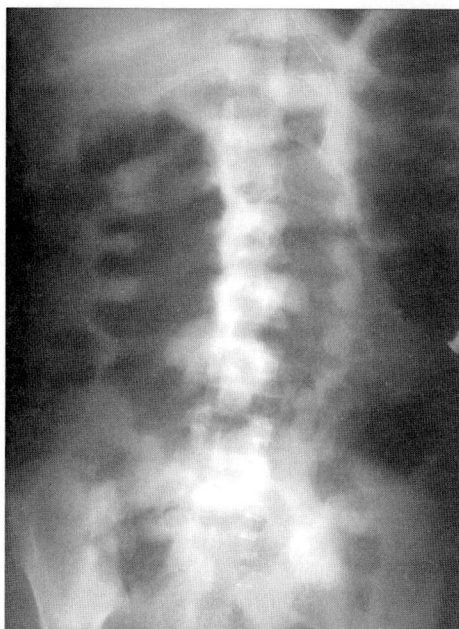

Figure 1 Abdominal films in patients with *Clostridium difficile* colitis may show a thickened colonic wall with "thumbprinting."

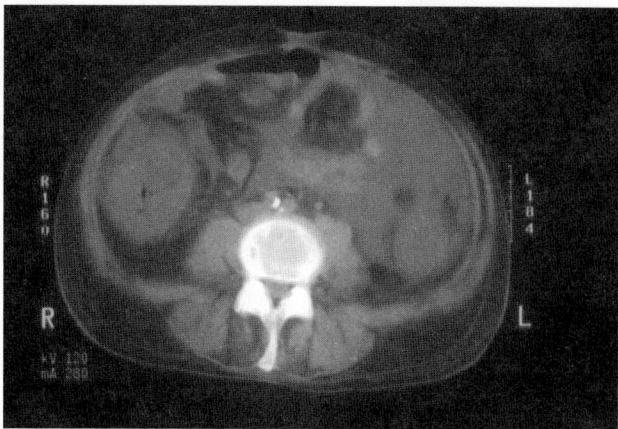

Figure 2 Computerized tomographic scan of the abdomen frequently shows a markedly thickened colon in patients with fulminant *Clostridium difficile* colitis.

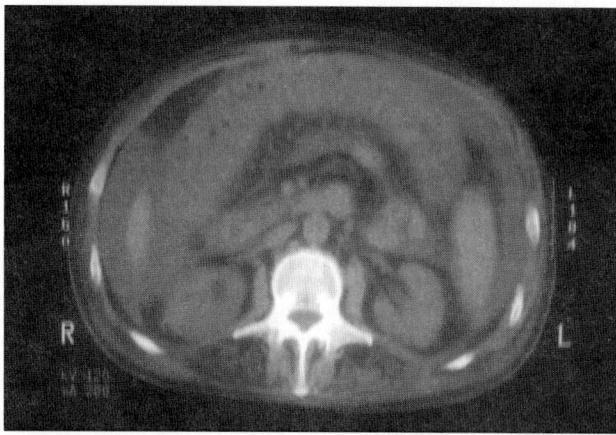

Figure 3 This image of the same patient as Figure 2 shows marked edema of the transverse colon.

offending antibiotic, it should be stopped, if possible. When the stool toxin test is shown to be positive, specific treatment for *C. difficile* is begun. Both oral vancomycin (125–500 mg four times daily) and metronidazole (500 mg four times daily) are adequate treatment, although metronidazole is the first line of therapy because of its low cost and the rapid response to treatment that is usually seen. One week's therapy is usually sufficient. Most people with simple diarrhea caused by *C. difficile colitis* can be treated as outpatients.

If the patient presents with not only diarrhea but also with tachycardia, fever, and leukocytosis, admission to the intensive care unit is warranted because the disease can rapidly worsen. Stool for *C. difficile* toxin should be sent to the laboratory immediately if the infection is suspected to be the cause of the patient's symptoms. If the patient is sufficiently toxic to be hypotensive, tachycardic, and hemodynamically unstable, treatment should be initiated before waiting for results of the *C. difficile* stool toxin study. Abdominal films (Fig. 1) will often show a thickened colonic wall with thumbprinting, but the most revealing study is an abdominal computed tomography (CT) scan, which will show a markedly thickened colonic wall (Figs. 2 and 3). Although oral metronidazole or vancomycin is preferred therapy for milder forms of *C. difficile* infection, this treatment is inadequate in patients with fulminant disease. When patients are unable to eat because they have an ileus, intravenous metronidazole is the treatment of choice and should be given in a dose of 500 mg every 6 hours. For the treatment of *C. difficile* colitis, vancomycin is effective only in the oral form. Although vancomycin has been delivered transrectally as treatment for *C. difficile* colitis, this method is anecdotal and without adequate evidence to support it.

Occasionally patients with fulminant colitis will have such a severe ileus that they do not have diarrhea. Although it is unusual, individuals can also develop fulminant *C. difficile* colitis without known previous antibiotic treatment. Because unexplained fever, tachycardia, leukocytosis, and abdominal distention and tenderness almost invariably prompt evaluation with a CT scan of the abdomen, adequate information to suspect *C. difficile* colitis is almost always promptly available. Immediate treatment with intravenous metronidazole is imperative. If confirmation is desired, a limited unprepped flexible sigmoidoscopy will reveal pseudomembranes, which are uniformly present when disease is this severe. The clinical presentation and CT scan are usually sufficient, however, to launch both general and specific treatment.

Patients with fulminant colitis will require vigorous fluid resuscitation in the intensive care unit and close monitoring of their clinical condition, including vital signs, hourly urine output, renal function tests, and white blood cell count.

The decision to perform a colectomy on a patient with severe *C. difficile* colitis is a matter of surgical judgment rather than a specific complex of symptoms and findings.

Problems in defining the exact indications for and timing of surgery include the small numbers of operated patients in most series, the lack of an accurate definition of the patient's illness severity, the uncontrolled retrospective nature of all of the published studies, wide variation in the patients' comorbidities, and even interobserver variation in assessment of the patients' overall condition and prognosis. Whether to perform a colectomy and at what point to do so with the best chance of a favorable outcome requires mature judgment that considers patients' underlying illnesses and their likely outcomes, the degree of compromise of vital organ function, whether metronidazole and fluid resuscitation appear to have improved the patient's condition, and the views of patients or their families about how aggressive treatment should be. When fulminant colitis is present and has not stabilized after a few hours of aggressive therapy, it is unlikely to do so, and surgery is most likely warranted unless the patient's condition is otherwise sufficiently poor that meaningful survival is unlikely. Waiting so long to decide on operation that multisystem organ failure has occurred

Table 1: *Clostridium Difficile* Colitis

Author	Year	N	Mortality (%)	Operation Required (%)	Surgical Mortality (%)
Lipsett	1994	3300	?	0.39	38
Prendergast	1994	201	8	1?	100?
Jobe	1995	201	3.4	5	30
Morris	2002	157	15.3	7.6	25
Dallal	2002	2334	13.5	1.9	57

will result in poor survival rates from surgery for *C. difficile* colitis, as several studies with high mortality rates (5%–100%) have shown. Operating too soon, however, will produce positive survival statistics while unnecessarily sacrificing a few colons that might not need to have been removed. Once full-blown, severe colitis has commenced, effective treatment with antibiotics and supportive measures alone are doubtful. The earliest sign of compromise of an organ system such as kidneys, heart, or lungs (systemic inflammatory response syndrome/acute respiratory distress syndrome) should prompt consideration of colectomy. Any chance for patient survival is compromised by delay.

The appropriate operation to perform in the patient with fulminant *C. difficile* colitis is an abdominal colectomy with ileostomy and preservation of a short rectal stump at the peritoneal reflection. Partial colectomy is associated with a significantly increased mortality compared with abdominal colectomy. One series showed a mortality of 67% with partial colectomy compared with 15% for total abdominal colectomy.

Findings at surgery are an edematous colon and friable tissues. Although it is clearly unnecessary to perform a high ligation of the mesenteric vessels to control the disease, the colectomy may be performed more efficiently if the named mesenteric vessels are ligated and divided before they branch. The rectum should be divided with a 4.5-mm stapling device at or just below the peritoneal reflection to minimize the degree of affected tissue remaining. In this severely ill population, proctectomy is ill advised, as is the laparoscopic approach. The simplest and quickest operation that can be done will best serve the patient. If the patient survives operation, intestinal continuity can later be restored by ileoproctostomy or, in a few patients with concomitant ulcerative colitis, a completion proctectomy and ileoanal pouch. In the survivor of the initial insult, good functional long-term results are possible.

Over the past 15 years the hospital population has become sicker, with more comorbid conditions and greater immune compromise. The overall mortality rate among patients diagnosed with *C. difficile* colitis has increased fivefold (Table 1). Early recognition of the disease and prompt treatment, along with early operation when the disease is clearly progressing, have been proposed to decrease this high mortality rate.

At one institution, evaluation of hospitalized patients treated for *C. difficile* infection during two time periods (1984–1994 and 1994–2000) showed an increased incidence and an increased need for surgery in an increasingly ill and immunocompromised patient population in the most recent time period (Table 2). In the early study, 20% of the patients were immunocompromised compared with 33% more recently. Operation was required in 7.6% of the patients compared with 5% in the earlier time period. Surgical mortality was statistically the same in both groups. Because the

Table 2: Evolution of a Disease in One Institution

	1984–1994 (%)	1994–2000 (%)
Mortality	3.4	15.3
Operation performed	5.0	7.6
Surgical mortality	30.0	25.0
Immunocompromised patients	20.0	33.0

patient population currently developing *C. difficile* colitis is an increasingly ill one with immunosuppression and multiple comorbidities, it remains to be seen whether earlier surgery can decrease the high mortality rates seen in some surgical series that exceed 50%. Of note, the studies with the highest mortality list indications for surgery such as hypotension requiring vasopressors despite adequate volume resuscitation or evidence of organ failure. In these studies, colectomy was likely performed too late. Studies in which abdominal colectomy and ileostomy is performed as soon as it is clear that medical therapy is not reversing the condition but pulmonary and renal function are still preserved show lower morality rates of 25% to 30%. The most successful outcomes are seen when there is little delay from the onset of symptoms to beginning medical treatment and early colectomy is performed if response to therapy is not seen promptly.

ACKNOWLEDGMENT

Portions of this chapter were presented by the author at the American College of Surgeons Postgraduate Course, October 12, 2004.

SUGGESTED READINGS

Dallal RM, Harbrecht BG, Boujoukas AJ, and others: Fulminant *Clostridium difficile*: an underappreciated and increasing cause of death and complications, *Ann Surg* 235:363, 2002.

Jobe BA, Grasley A, Deveney KE, and others: *Clostridium difficile* colitis: An increasing hospital-acquired illness, *Am J Surg* 169:480, 1995.

Lipsett PA, Samantaray DK, Tam ML, and others: Pseudomembranous colitis: A surgical disease? *Surgery* 116:491, 1994.

Morris AM, Jobe BA, Stoney M, and others: *Clostridium difficile* colitis: an increasingly aggressive iatrogenic disease? *Arch Surg* 137:1096, 2002.

Prendergast TM, Marini CP, D'Angelo AJ, and others: Surgical patients with pseudomembranous colitis: Factors affecting prognosis, *Surgery* 116:768, 1994.

LARGE BOWEL OBSTRUCTION

Bruce G. Wolff, MD, and Anne-Marie Boller, MD, MA

INTRODUCTION

Large bowel obstruction may present as a manifestation of an acute process or as the culmination of a progressive, chronic disease state. Obstruction of the large bowel may occur in all age groups, with distinctly differing etiologies. When obstruction presents emergently, surgical intervention is associated with a higher morbidity and mortality. Management options are widely divergent; prudent evaluation and an expedient diagnosis are paramount in patients presenting with obstructive symptoms.

ETIOLOGY

Causes of large bowel obstruction may result from mechanical or adynamic causes (Table 1). The most common etiology for mechanical obstruction in adults is colorectal carcinoma (90%), followed by volvulus (5%) and diverticular disease (3%). Additional mechanical causes include inflammatory bowel disease, anastomotic strictures following a surgical resection, and colonic ischemia. Mechanical obstruction also results from congenital causes, including Hirschsprung's disease, imperforate anus, meconium ileus, and microcolon. Adynamic obstruction, or pseudo-obstruction, is another cause of large bowel obstruction.

CLINICAL PRESENTATION

A careful history and physical examination are the initial steps in the evaluation and diagnosis of large bowel obstruction. The patient's age, comorbidities, and presenting symptoms will influence the focus of the subsequent diagnostic workup. Young patients and newborns present with Hirschsprung's disease and imperforate anus as the underlying etiology of their disease, whereas obstruction in the elderly more frequently reveals an underlying carcinoma or diverticular disease. The patient's medications should be extensively

Table 1: Causes of Large Bowel Obstruction

Mechanical Causes
Carcinoma—colon and rectum, extracolonic
Volvulus—sigmoid and cecal
Diverticulitis
Inflammatory bowel manifestations
Anastomotic stricture
Intussusception
Adynamic Causes
Colonic pseudo-obstruction
Colonic dysmotility
Congenital Causes
Hirschsprung's disease
Imperforate anus

reviewed. History of previous polyps, cancer, or surgery should be documented.

Symptoms of large bowel obstruction include abdominal pain, obstipation, abdominal distention, nausea, and vomiting. Patient history should elucidate the timing of symptoms and rapidity of the onset. Acute onset of symptoms and abdominal distention may be the first manifestations of sigmoid volvulus, whereas obstruction secondary to carcinoma may manifest with an insidious change in bowel habits and abdominal distention.

Physical examination may reveal signs that further clarify the diagnosis of large bowel obstruction. A complete physical examination should always proceed with a thorough abdominal evaluation, noting any signs of peritonitis, tympany, or masses. Hernias must be ruled out and a mandatory digital rectal examination performed to exclude the presence of a fecal or neoplastic mass. Fever and tachycardia accompany perforation, inflammation, and diverticulitis, whereas the presence of hematochezia alerts the examiner to the potential for cancer, ischemia, or inflammatory mucosal injury. Feculent breath may accompany large bowel obstruction.

DIAGNOSIS

Radiographic evaluation should proceed with the goal of differentiating mechanical obstruction from pseudo-obstruction, localizing the site of obstruction and potentially establishing its cause. Plain radiographic abdominal films may demonstrate colonic distention and can be diagnostic. The "bent inner tube" appearance (Fig. 1) is a classic sign of sigmoid volvulus. An abdominal series, including flat and decubitus views and an upright chest radiograph, may demonstrate air-fluid levels, pneumoperitoneum, and decompressed bowel distal to the obstruction. Cecal dilatation

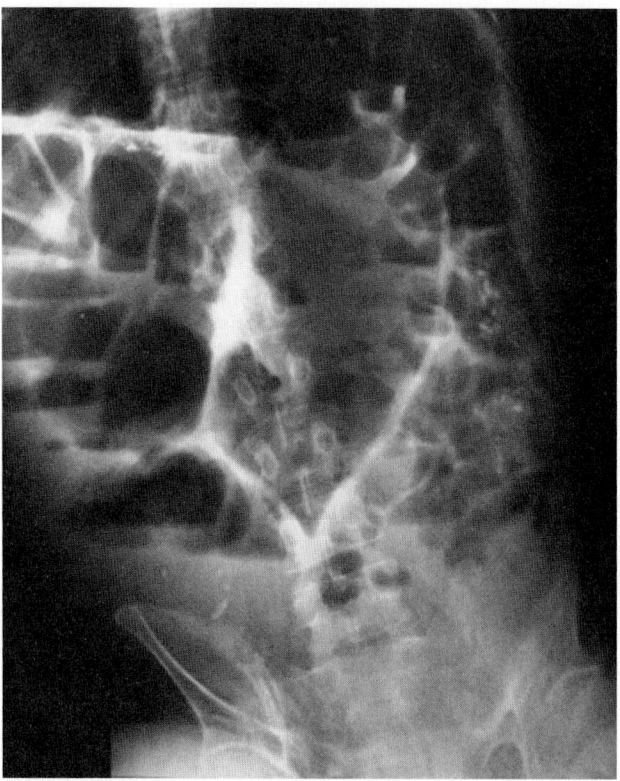

Figure 1 Abdominal film of a sigmoid volvulus. *From Frizelle FA, Wolff BG: Adv Surg 29:131, 1996.*

greater than 12 cm may be established on a plain abdominal film and indicates an increased risk for perforation because of the associated increase in luminal pressure, reflected by Laplace's law.

Diagnostic evaluation should proceed to a water-soluble contrast enema, avoiding barium when a perforation is suspected. A contrast enema may be therapeutic when the underlying etiology is fecal impaction and diagnostic in differentiating pseudo-obstruction from mechanical obstruction. After exclusion of a mechanical obstruction by contrast enema, pseudo-obstruction may be treated successfully with subsequent colonoscopic decompression and conservative management. In the case of sigmoid volvulus, the classic "bird's beak" may be apparent after contrast enema and may also be therapeutically managed with a colonoscopy. Mechanical obstruction is often readily apparent after an enema, and the water-soluble contrast assists in clearing the colon distal to the obstruction of débride. A classic "apple-core" narrowing may be present on contrast enema evaluation, supporting a diagnosis of an obstructing carcinoma.

A computed tomography (CT) scan may complement the radiographic evaluation of obstructing carcinomas by assessing lymph node involvement, metastases, and the stage of the disease. For diverticular disease, a CT scan may further define the extent of pericolonic inflammation and the dimensions of the abscess cavity and determine the ability of the team to address the cavity percutaneously. Identification of a "transition zone," marking the transition from proximally dilated colon to distally compressed bowel, is often difficult to assess on a CT scan.

PREOPERATIVE MANAGEMENT

Patients with bowel obstruction frequently present with dehydration as a culmination of the loss of edema and interstitial fluid caused by the luminal obstruction, combined with the loss of fluid and electrolytes resulting from recurrent emesis. Intravenous resuscitation should be immediately initiated with crystalloid and electrolyte replacement. Preoperative preparation of the patient should include the insertion of a nasogastric tube if the patient suffers from ongoing emesis, with careful attention to precautions against aspiration during intubation.

Laboratory analysis should evaluate the hemoglobin level, electrolytes, creatinine, and a coagulation panel. Efforts should proceed until laboratory and clinical parameters (urine output) reflect adequate resuscitation. Signs and symptoms of perforation mandate immediate operative intervention, but in their absence, a bowel preparation and careful resuscitation further prepare the patient for surgery. Timely administration and subsequent discontinuation of perioperative antibiotics should be initiated. All preoperative informed consent should include discussion of the potential need for a stoma operation.

SURGICAL MANAGEMENT

Carcinoma

Obstruction of the large bowel is most commonly associated with malignancy in the adult patient. Left-sided bowel obstructions occur more frequently than right-sided obstructions. Operative management after appropriate resuscitation is dependent on the location of the lesion and the intra-abdominal findings on laparotomy.

Right-sided obstruction should be resected with primary anastomosis, following decompression of the dilated, proximal bowel. A right hemicolectomy may be performed, even in the absence of a bowel preparation, and fecal diversion is rarely warranted.

Left-sided lesions may be amenable to a number of surgical interventions. Surgical decisions regarding resection are dependent

on the urgency of the clinical situation, patient variables, and the intra-abdominal environment. Patients presenting with a left-sided obstruction and signs of perforation or sepsis should be taken to the operating room immediately. After a complete evaluation of the bowel, the obstructed segment should be surgically resected by the most expeditious and safe means, respecting oncologic principles when appropriate. Two-stage procedures may be necessary in the emergent setting.

In patients who present without signs or symptoms of perforation, resuscitation and bowel preparation should be initiated. On completion of these maneuvers, the patient may proceed to the operating suite for resection of the obstructing bowel segment. Primary anastomosis may be completed, with subtotal colectomy or a segmental resection, provided the bowel is viable and the anastomosis is free of tension. Advantages of one-stage procedures include shorter hospital stay, reduced morbidity and mortality rates, and avoidance of a stoma and subsequent operative procedures.

The SCOTIA (subtotal colectomy versus on-table irrigation and anastomosis) Study Group conducted a prospective randomized trial in patients with malignant left-sided large bowel obstruction. They compared two one-stage procedures, subtotal colectomy and segmental resection with on-table lavage. Mortality and complication rates did not significantly differ when comparing subtotal colectomy with segmental resection following an on-table lavage. At 4 months follow-up, the subtotal colectomy patients had significantly more frequent bowel movements than their counterparts in the segmental resection group. Patients who have simultaneous cecal perforation or synchronous cancer lesions are appropriately addressed with a subtotal colectomy. Two-stage procedures may be considered for unstable patients, inexperienced surgical teams, and immunocompromised patients. It should also be remembered that approximately 30% of patients receiving a diverting ostomy at the time of their initial operation for an obstruction fail to return for subsequent closure and restoration of intestinal continuity.

Hemodynamically unstable patients with large bowel obstruction, who are poor operative candidates at presentation, may benefit from a cecostomy tube. The tube may be placed in the radiology suite or the operating room. A midline incision exposes the cecum, which is then elevated into the field. The tube may be placed through the appendicial stump or through the anterior teniae more distal from the ileocecal valve. Placing the tube through the appendix places an unusual torsion on the cecum, and, if possible, the anterior tenia is the better choice. After a purse-string suture is placed, an enterotomy is created and a Foley catheter, Malecot or pediatric feeding tube is placed into the ascending colon (Figs. 2 and 3). The tube should be run through a few folds of omentum, interposed between the colon and the abdominal wall, to facilitate quick, spontaneous closure when the tube is removed. The cecostomy tube is thus placed with minimal risk and provides proximal decompression of dilated large bowel and a means for distal bowel preparation for those patients who may benefit from a delayed, elective resection.

Volvulus

Management of large bowel volvulus is dependent on the location of its occurrence. The sigmoid colon is the most common location for obstruction related to a volvulus (Fig. 4). Sigmoid volvulus may be treated with endoscopic reduction. The flexible endoscope is inserted to the level of the obstruction with minimal insufflation. Any evidence of ischemia or mucosal insult should be noted. At the point of obstruction, the operator insufflates and attempts to induce uncoiling of the affected bowel. If this procedure is successful, a rectal tube should be inserted and left in place for up to 72 hours.

Failure of conservative endoscopic management or any evidence of compromised bowel or perforation necessitates surgical

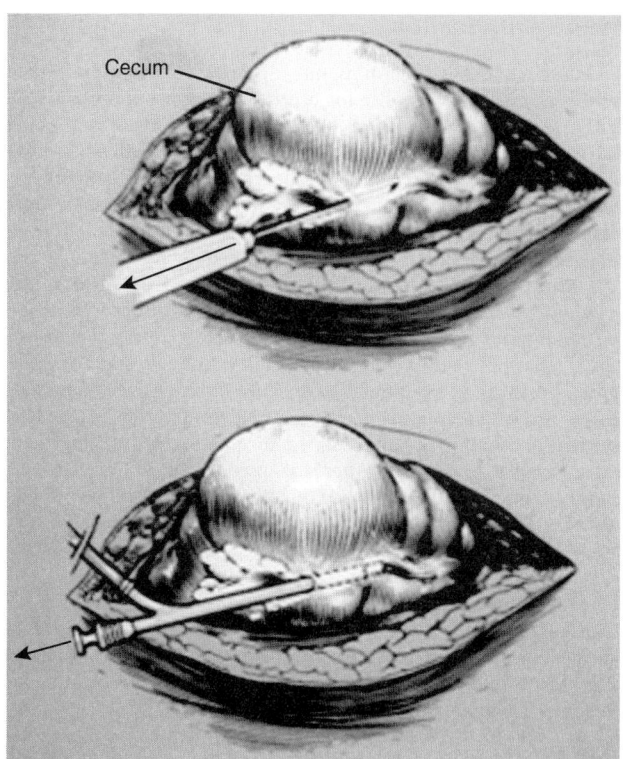

Figure 2 Tube cecostomy: aspiration with needle and trocar. *From Wolff BG: Volvulus of the colon. In Cameron JL: Current surgical therapy, ed 7, Philadelphia, 1989, Elsevier Mosby.*

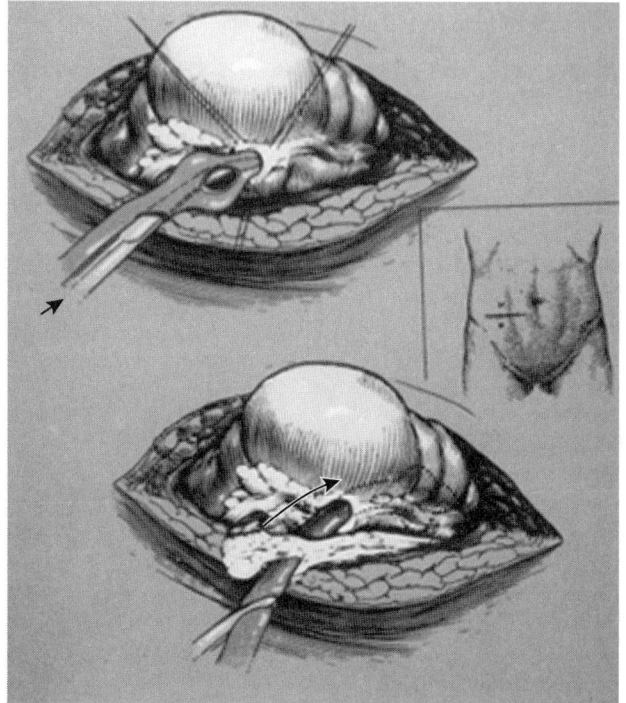

Figure 3 Method of tube cecostomy showing incision and tube site. *From Wolff BG: Volvulus of the colon. In Cameron JL: Current surgical therapy, ed 7, Philadelphia, 1989, Elsevier Mosby.*

COLONIC VOLVULUS
Olmsted County, 1960–1980

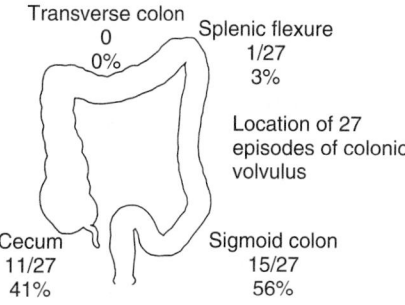

Figure 4 Distribution in 27 cases of colonic volvulus in Olmsted County, Minnesota, over a 20-year period. *From Wolff BG: Volvulus of the colon. In Cameron JL: Current surgical therapy, ed 7, Philadelphia, 1989, Elsevier Mosby.*

intervention. The affected segment is addressed with a sigmoid colectomy and primary anastomosis, providing the bowel is viable. Laparoscopic resection is considered an appropriate venue for the resection of sigmoid volvulus in experienced surgical hands. Simple decompression and sigmoidopexy to the abdominal wall is associated with high recurrence rates and should be performed only in patients unsuitable for segmental resection.

The cecum is the second most common location for an obstruction related to a volvulus. Unlike a sigmoid volvulus, cecal volvulus is rarely corrected endoscopically. Recurrence rates with endoscopic reduction are unacceptably high, and the danger of perforation with endoscopic insufflation precludes this procedure in almost all cases. The cecum may present with a complete clockwise rotation and volvulus or a bascule. A bascule occurs when the cecum is incompletely fixed to the abdominal wall, allowing it to fold onto itself and create an obstruction. Surgical management for either volvulus or bascule may include right hemicolectomy or cecopexy. Resection of the cecum with primary ileocolic anastomosis is sufficient to prevent significant recurrence and should be performed in the setting on nonviable colon. Cecopexy to the lateral abdominal sidewall is associated with a recurrence rate of 30% in some cases. When cecopexy and tube cecostomy (Figs. 2 and 3) are performed together, colonic decompression and cecal fixation are simultaneously accomplished, with recurrence rates that are significantly improved over cecopexy alone.

Diverticular Disease

Diverticular disease is the third most common cause of large bowel obstruction. Frequently presenting with left lower abdominal pain, tachycardia, and leukocytosis, patients may have radiologic findings consistent with a diverticular abscess, inflammation, or perforation. All patients should be adequately resuscitated and started on broad-spectrum antibiotics. Lesions amenable to a percutaneous approach should be addressed with CT or ultrasound-guided drainage of the associated abscess. The majority of patients will recover with this conservative management. The debate continues regarding the correct timing of surgical intervention for known diverticular disease. Despite presenting with an obstruction, most patients will continue to be considered for an elective, one-stage resection following their second attack of diverticulitis.

Diverticular patients who present with signs and symptoms of sepsis, have a significant lesion that is not amenable to percutaneous drainage, or have fecal contamination should undergo immediate laparotomy. The affected diverticular segment should be resected back to healthy-appearing bowel, and a Hartmann's pouch and end colostomy created. After a sufficient period of time, allowing for the resolution of the intra-abdominal inflammation, the patient may return for a second surgery in which the colostomy may be taken down and a primary anastomosis completed.

Intussusception

Intussusception is a rare form of mechanical large bowel obstruction in the adult that involves the telescoping of a segment of bowel into an adjacent, distal segment. Intussusception is the underlying etiology for 1% to 5% of adult large bowel obstructions. Less than 5% of all intussusception cases occur in the adult population, and 95% occur in the pediatric population. Pediatric patients usually have an ileocolic intussusception of benign origin, and more than 90% of cases can be successfully reduced with an air contrast enema. In the adult population, the intussusception is usually the product of a lead point lesion. Lead point lesions may be carcinomas, Meckel's diverticulum, colonic diverticulum, or polyps. In adults, intussusception must not be addressed with radiologic decompression alone because of the potential for underlying malignancy. At laparotomy or laparoscopy, the entire bowel should be evaluated, looking for any suspicious pathology. The intussusception should be milked out from the intussusceptum in a distal to proximal direction, without pulling on the bowel. After it is reduced, the involved area should be meticulously inspected and examined for the underlying cause of the intussusception. Affected bowel should be resected using appropriate oncologic techniques when cancer is the cause of obstruction. Primary anastomosis is acceptable in the setting of viable, healthy bowel.

Fecal Impaction

Fecal impaction can cause a mechanical obstruction in the distal colon. This etiology is often associated with diet, medications, and patient institutionalization. Digital decompression and subsequent enemas are frequently sufficient to relieve the obstruction. Following decompression, a heightened awareness to medications and bowel habits is required, especially in the nursing home setting.

Pseudo-Obstruction

Colonic pseudo-obstruction is an adynamic condition in which there is no mechanical cause for obstruction. Patients present with signs and symptoms of bowel obstruction and a plain radiograph that reveals massive distention of the large bowel. Patients are frequently elderly or institutionalized, bedridden, and on psychogenic medications including anticholinergics; further, they often have comorbidities including Parkinson's disease, multiple sclerosis, or paraplegia. Initial management should include resuscitation and a CT scan to rule out any mechanical etiology for the obstruction. Colonoscopy may be initiated and often results in decompression and resolution of the problem. If colonoscopy is unsuccessful, neostigmine has been proved–effective in this setting. Neostigmine reestablishes coordinated peristalsis of the bowel through its cholinergic agonist effects. Neostigmine may cause bradycardia, and this medical intervention should be administered in a monitored setting, with readily available atropine. After the pseudo-obstruction resolves, careful attention should be turned to patients' medication profile and daily bowel habits and a bowel regime should be implemented.

CONCLUSION

Advances in perioperative and intraoperative techniques have, in recent years, allowed for more and safer one-stage procedures for patients with acute large bowel obstruction.

SUGGESTED READINGS

Benacci J, Wolff BG: Cecostomy: therapeutic indications and results, *Dis Colon Rectum* 38:530, 1995.
Frizelle FA, Wolff BG: Colonic volvulus, *Adv Surg* 29:131, 1996.
Gordon PH, Nivatvongs S: *Principles and practices of surgery for the colon, rectum, and anus*, ed 2, St Louis, 1999, Quality Medical.
Keighley MRB, William N: *The anus, rectum and colon*, ed 2, London, 1999, Saunders.
SCOTIA Study Group: Single-stage treatment for malignant left-sided colonic obstruction: a prospective randomized clinical trial comparing subtotal colectomy with segmental resection following intraoperative irrigation, *Br J Surg* 82:1622, 1995.
Wolff BG: Volvulus of the colon. In Cameron JL: *Current surgical therapy*, ed 7, Philadelphia, 130, 1989, Elsevier Mosby.

ACUTE COLONIC PSEUDO-OBSTRUCTION (OLGILVIE'S SYNDROME)

Amy L. Halverson, MD

Acute colonic pseudo-obstruction is the clinical presentation of colonic distention in the absence of a mechanical obstruction. This condition is thought to result from an imbalance in the autonomic nervous system. Physiologic stress acting via direct innervation or through inflammatory mediators may stimulate sympathetic innervation and suppress parasympathetic innervation, resulting in an inhibitory effect on colonic motility. Multiple pharmacologic and metabolic factors can also alter the normal function of the colon. Acute colonic pseudo-obstruction may occur following surgery. It may also be seen after extensive burn injury, trauma, neurologic injury, sepsis, and in individuals with a malignancy (Table 1). Less commonly, it is seen in

Table 1: Predisposing Conditions Associated with Acute Colonic Pseudo-Obstruction

Surgery (laparotomy, orthopedic, cesarean section, thoracic, cardiovascular, renal transplantation)
Trauma (fractures, burns)
Infection (pneumonia, sepsis)
Cardiac (myocardial infarction, heart failure)
Neurological (Parkinson's disease, spinal cord injury, multiple sclerosis, Alzheimer's disease)
Cancer
Metabolic (hypokalemia, hyponatremia)

individuals without any identifiable contributing factors. Of the various medications that may contribute to acute colonic pseudo-obstruction (Table 2), opiate analgesics are the most frequently implicated.

Presenting signs and symptoms include abdominal distention, abdominal pain, constipation, or diarrhea. Abdominal radiographic images typically show marked colonic dilatation (Fig. 1). Colonic pseudo-obstruction is a diagnosis of exclusion and should be made only after ruling out other causes of distention, such as a mechanical obstruction or toxic megacolon resulting from acute colitis. A water-soluble contrast enema is useful to evaluate for a mechanical obstruction and may have the therapeutic advantage of evacuating contents from the colon. Limited proctoscopy may be performed to assess for colitis or a distal obstruction.

Table 2: Medications Associated with Acute Colonic Pseudo-obstruction

Narcotic analgesics
Anticholinergics (Atrovent, Spiriva)
Tricyclic antidepressants (imipramine, amitriptyline, nortriptyline)
Phenothiazines (chloromazine, trifuroperazine, thioridazine)
Antiparkinson drugs (levodopa, selequiline, amantadine)
Calcium channel blocking agents
Clonidine

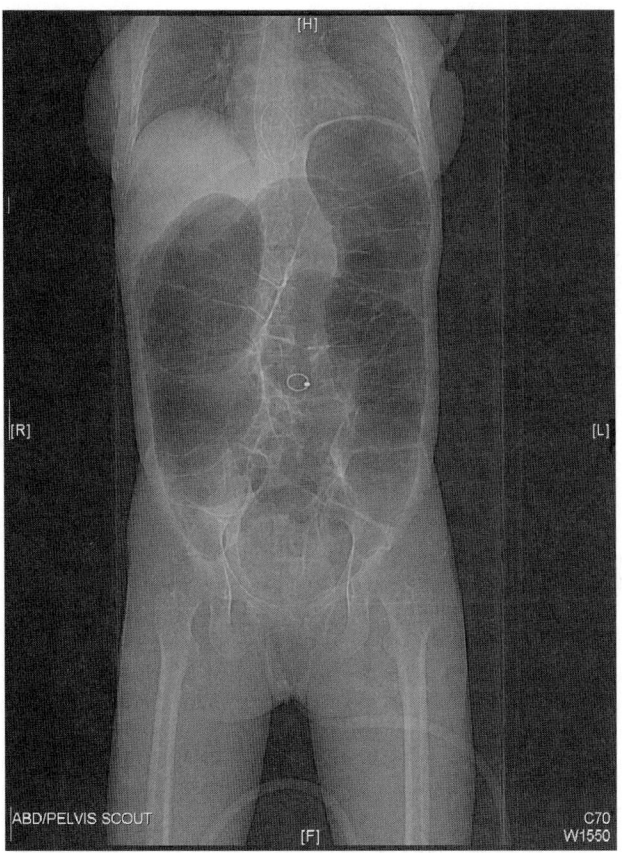

Figure 1 Abdominal radiograph showing marked colonic dilatation.

TREATMENT

Identifying and correcting any contributing factor is the first step in treating the pseudo-obstruction. Narcotic medications should be decreased or discontinued if possible. Electrolyte abnormalities should be corrected. Other commonly used elements of conservative treatment include discontinuation of oral intake, nasogastric decompression, and the placement of a rectal tube. Colonic dilatation resolves in approximately 80% of individuals within 48 hours with supportive treatment alone (Table 3).

Pharmacologic Treatment

Neostigmine, a reversible acetylcholinersterase inhibitor, potentiates the action of acetylcholine on the muscarinic parasympathetic receptors in the colon, resulting in increased colonic motility. Neostigmine is 90% effective in treating colonic pseudo-obstruction. A single dose of 2 mg is administered intravenously over 3 to 5 minutes. Improvement in colonic distention usually occurs within several minutes of neostigmine administration. The duration of action of neostigmine is approximately 1 to 2 hours. The effect may be prolonged in individuals with renal insufficiency. The parasympathomimetic action of neostigmine may cause bradycardia; therefore the administration should be performed with the patient supine and with continuous cardiac monitoring. Atropine (1 mg) should be available at the bedside to treat symptomatic bradycardia (Table 4). Other side effects of neostigmine include abdominal cramping, excessive salivation, nausea, and syncope. Patients should be monitored for approximately 30 minutes following neostigmine administration. Neostigmine should not be used if there is suspicion of colonic ischemia or perforation. Other contraindications include pregnancy, severe active bronchospasm, cardiac arrhythmias, and renal failure. Recurrent colonic dilatation following initial successful decompression with neostigmine has been reported to occur in 10% to 40% of individuals. A second dose of neostigmine may be administered to patients who do not respond or who have recurrent colonic distention following the first dose.

Colonoscopy

Several series have reported success rates between 60% and 84% for colonoscopic decompression of colonic pseudo-obstruction. Colonoscopy is indicated for individuals with persistent colonic dilatation after 24 to 28 hours of supportive care who have failed

Table 3: Supportive Therapy for Acute Colonic Pseudo-obstruction

Correct fluid and electrolyte abnormalities
No oral intake, nasogastric decompression
Rectal tube to gravity drainage
Limit offending medications

Table 4: Administration of Neostigmine

Neostigmine, 2 mg, intravenous infusion over 3–5 minutes
Atropine 1 mg available at the bedside
Continuous electrocardiographic monitoring and clinical assessment for 30 min
Patient supine, on bedpan

treatment with neostigmine or who have contraindications to its use. It should not be performed if peritonitis or perforation is suspected. Oral bowel preparation should not be administered before colonoscopy. Colonoscopy for pseudo-obstruction is technically challenging and should be performed with minimal additional insufflation. Success rates have been reported to be better when the cecum or ascending colon is reached compared with procedures that do not reach hepatic flexure. Prolonged efforts to reach the cecum in this setting are not prudent. A decompression tube may be placed at the time of colonoscopy. This is accomplished by advancing a guidewire through the scope and passing the tube over the guidewire. Fluoroscopy may be helpful to facilitate advancement of the guidewire and decompression tube. If colonoscopic decompression is performed without tube placement, approximately 30% of patients require repeat colonoscopy.

Percutaneous Tube Cecostomy

Percutaneous cecostomy has been used as an alternative to laparotomy for individuals who fail treatment with neostigmine and colonoscopic decompression. These techniques should not be used in individuals with peritonitis or suspected colonic ischemia. The placement of a percutaneous cecostomy tube has been described using both radiographic and endoscopic techniques. The radiographic technique involves percutaneous placement of an 8- to 12-F catheter using a Seldinger or trocar puncture technique with radiographic confirmation of correct placement of the tube in the cecum.

The described technique for endoscopic placement is similar to that used for percutaneous endoscopic gastrostomy. The standard, commercially available percutaneous endoscopic gastronomy kits with a 20-F tube may be used. The one substitution for these kits is that a standard colonoscopic polypectomy snare is used instead of the shorter snare provided with the kit. The site for the tube cecostomy is determined by transillumination and endoscopically observed indentation in response to pressure exerted with a finger on the abdominal wall. After successful placement, the cecostomy tube is placed to low intermittent suction or gravity drainage and flushed intermittently. Reported complications after tube cecostomy include pressure necrosis from the external bumper, the development of hypertrophic granulation tissue, cellulitis of the abdominal wall, leakage around the catheter, and bleeding at the insertion site.

Surgery

When nonoperative measures fail to relieve colonic distention, surgical intervention is indicated. If the patient develops signs or symptoms of ischemic bowel, exploratory laparotomy should be performed promptly. The procedure performed is dependent on the presence of ischemia or necrosis on the bowel. If there is no ischemia in the bowel wall, a tube cecostomy or blowhole cecostomy may be created. Either procedure may be performed under local anesthesia through a small right lower quadrant incision. If colonic necrosis or perforation is present, segmental colonic resection with end ileostomy and mucous fistula should be performed. Surgery for acute colonic pseudo-obstruction is associated with a high mortality—in some reports as high as 50%. The high surgical morbidity and mortality is most often due to the comorbidities commonly seen in these patients.

PROGNOSIS

Colonic distention may recur following neostigmine administration or colonoscopic decompression. The daily oral administration of polyethylene glycol electrolyte solution may be helpful to increase the sustained response rate after initial therapeutic intervention.

Persistent colonic distention may lead to ischemia and perforation in the cecum. Overall mortality for acute colonic pseudo-obstruction is 15%, increasing to 36% in patients who progress to colonic ischemia and perforation. Predictors of perforation include advanced age, increased cecal diameter, and delayed colonic decompression. In a review of 400 cases, Vanek and colleagues found the frequency of cecal perforation to be 23% in individuals with a cecal diameter greater than 14 cm measured on plain abdominal films, compared with a 7% rate of perforation with cecal diameter between 12 and 14 cm and no perforation in individuals with a cecal diameter of less than 12 cm. Delay in successful treatment is also an important predictor of outcome. Cecal perforation and mortality is rare in individuals successfully treated within 2 days. When colonic decompression is delayed beyond 6 days, the mortality rate may increase to more than 70%.

SUMMARY

Acute colonic pseudo-obstruction is a functional disorder of the colon diagnosed by the presence of signs and symptoms of acute colonic obstruction in the absence of a mechanical obstruction. In most patients, symptoms resolve within 24 to 72 hours with conservative management, including the identification and correction of predisposing factors. If symptoms progress or do not improve with conservative measures, intravenous neostigmine may be administered. Failure of neostigmine may be followed by colonoscopic decompression. Given the efficacy and safety of neostigmine, early administration within 24 hours of diagnosing acute colonic pseudo-obstruction is reasonable. There have been no clinical trials directly comparing the efficacy of neostigmine and colonoscopy. Surgery is reserved for cases in which other measures have failed or when patients have worsening abdominal pain, fever, leukocytosis, or other indicators of colonic ischemia or perforation.

SUGGESTED READINGS

Jetmore AB, Timmcke AE, Gathright JB Jr, and others: Ogilvie's syndrome: colonoscopic decompression and analysis of predisposing factors, *Dis Colon Rectum* 35:1135, 1992.

Ponec RJ, Saunders MD, Kimmey MB: Neostigmine for the treatment of acute colonic pseudo-obstruction, *N Engl J Med* 341:137, 1999.

Saunders MD, Kimmey MB: Systematic review: acute colonic pseudo-obstruction, *Aliment Pharmacol Ther* 22:917, 2005.

Vanek VW, Al-Salti M: Acute pseudo-obstruction of the colon (Ogilvie's syndrome), *Dis Colon Rectum* 29:203, 1986.

Colonic Volvulus

David A. McClusky III, MD, and Aaron S. Fink, MD

Colonic volvulus occurs when a portion of large bowel and its associated mesentery folds around a fixed point, causing strangulation of vascular structures, a closed intestinal loop, or both. For a volvulus to occur, a segment of excessively mobile bowel rotates around a fixed and tapered fulcrum within the mesentery or along the bowel wall. Anatomic factors that predispose patients to volvulus formation include an elongated colon and mesocolon; incomplete fixation of the colon's peritoneum to the abdominal wall; mesenteric foreshortening resulting from congenital bands or adhesion formation; disruption of the supporting gastrocolic, lineocolic, phrenocolic, and renocolic ligaments; or mass effect. The most common sites of colonic torsion include the sigmoid colon (~60%) and the terminal ileum and cecum (~40%). Volvulus of the transverse colon and splenic flexure are rare occurrences. Although the overwhelming majority of incidents are isolated to one area, synchronous and metachronous torsion have also been reported.

Colonic volvulus is the third most common cause of large-bowel obstruction in the United States, accounting for approximately 5% of all intestinal obstructions. Although information regarding the true incidence is scant, a report from Olmsted County, Minnesota, noted that the condition occurred in 3 of every 100,000 patients annually; in New York, 1 in 10,000 hospital admissions were attributed to volvulus. Studies in Africa, Eastern Europe, India, and Iran note a higher incidence, with 30% to 75% of all intestinal obstructions attributed to colonic volvulus. Theories regarding these geographic differences include the higher altitude in some of these regions, as well as the tendency to consume a predominantly high-fiber, high-residue diet. As dietary habits change in some areas of the world (e.g., the former Soviet Union), the incidence of volvulus appears to decrease, approaching that seen in Western Europe and the United States.

Volvulus of the colon is the leading cause of strangulated large bowel obstruction, with 50% to 80% mortality rates in cases involving intestinal ischemia. Because mortality rates are significantly lower in cases without ischemic change (0%–7%), early diagnosis and treatment are of primary concern.

SIGMOID VOLVULUS

Sigmoid volvulus, the most common type, is associated with an overall mortality ranging from 7% to 20%. In the United States, sigmoid volvulus occurs most commonly in men, African Americans, the elderly, and institutionalized patients. In the latter groups, chronic constipation and the frequent use of laxatives or enemas are believed to cause chronic distention with resultant elongation and redundancy of the sigmoid and mesosigmoid; the latter changes predispose the bowel to twisting. High-fiber and high-residue diets produce a fecal load that similarly elongates the colon, possibly explaining the higher incidence of volvulus in geographic regions where such diets are widespread. Other risk factors include pregnancy (the gravid uterus pushes the sigmoid up and over its mesentery); air travel; pelvic malignancy; megacolon (e.g., inflammatory bowel disease, Chaga's disease); Parkinson's; lead poisoning; and vitamin B deficiency. Sigmoid volvulus has also been observed after colonoscopy and laparoscopic cholecystectomy.

In cases of sigmoid volvulus, the freely mobile sigmoid rotates axially around the inferior mesenteric vessels between the fixed

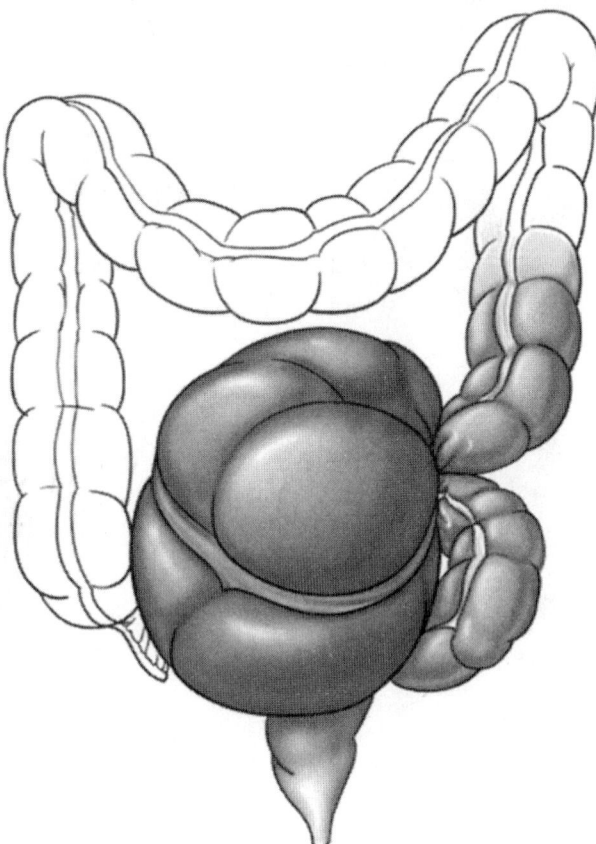

Figure 1 Torsion of a sigmoid volvulus leads to obstruction and ischemia.

proximal and distal colon; obstruction occurs after a 180-degree torsion (Fig. 1). Although torsion can occur in either a clockwise or counterclockwise direction, the counterclockwise direction is more common. The colon can also twist around the bowel wall itself as the forces of axial mesenteric torsion pull the bowel wall against its posterior point of peritoneal fixation. This less common form of torsion completely obstructs the bowel lumen, given the resultant closed loop.

In cases of simple obstruction, the sigmoid colon can tolerate a higher intraluminal pressure because of its muscular wall and small diameter. Eventually, peristalsis moves gas and liquid into a trapped loop, leading to venous occlusion, increasing distention, and finally arterial occlusion. A less common but more acute form of obstruction can also occur if the torsion is severe enough to occlude the inferior mesenteric vessels from the outset.

If gangrene is not present, patients present with the rapid onset of colicky abdominal pain, abdominal distention, and obstipation. Although not universal, the presence of vomiting portends a poorer prognosis if it presents before or concomitant to these associated symptoms. Physical examination often reveals a distended tympanitic abdomen, normal or high-pitched bowel sounds, and minimal tenderness. Forty percent of the time, plain abdominal films may reveal a markedly dilated colon loop projecting to the right upper quadrant with its resultant "omega loop" or "bent inner tube" sign (Fig. 2). On computed tomography (CT) scan, a "whirl" sign may be present if the axial cuts transect the site of volvulus perpendicularly. This appearance is created as the afferent and efferent loops lead to a central segment of twisted bowel and mesentery. Additional CT findings may include a radial or U-shaped

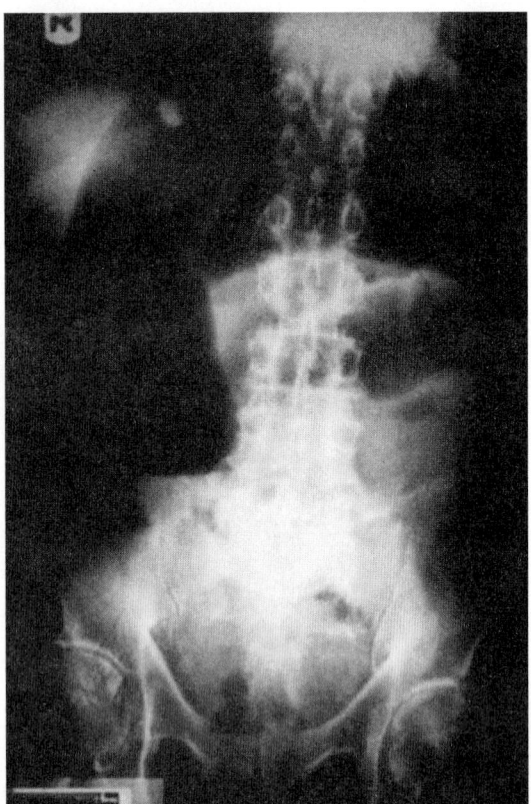

Figure 2 Radiologic examination reveals a dilated loop of intestine pointing toward the right upper quadrant, suggestive of sigmoid volvulus.

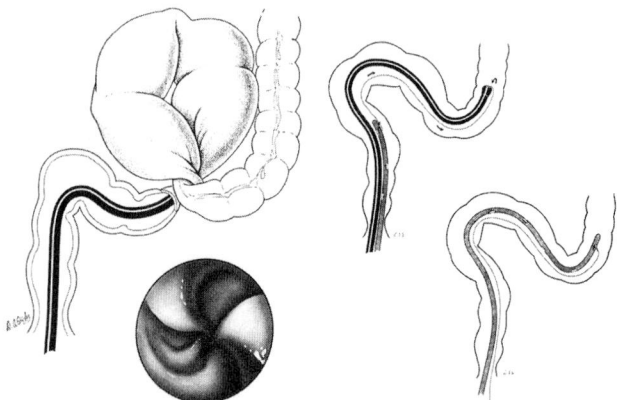

Figure 3 Schematic demonstrating endoscopic decompression of a sigmoid volvulus.

configuration of distended bowel loops, with a triangular tapering of the collapsed bowel at the site of torsion, thrombosis of the mesenteric vessels, or fat attenuation around the site of torsion. Additional testing, including a barium enema, is usually not indicated. If obtained, the classic "bird's beak" deformity (a barium or Gastrografin column ending sharply at the point of torsion) is a specific diagnostic indicator.

We initially evaluate all patients for the signs and symptoms of gangrenous bowel. An urgent laparotomy is mandated if suspicion for ischemia is high (e.g., elevated body temperature, leukocytosis, peritoneal signs, free abdominal air, significant acidosis, or early sepsis). If obvious gangrene is found, detorsion is avoided and resection of the involved segment with end colostomy and Hartmann's pouch is recommended. In more severe cases, a second-look laparotomy may be necessary. If the bowel appears viable at laparotomy, a 180-degree clockwise detorsion is performed. The bowel is then warmed and observed for pink coloration, peristalsis, and palpable arterial pulsations. If viability remains uncertain, the bowel can be examined with a Doppler probe or a Woods lamp following intravenous fluorescein administration. If the bowel is viable, resection with primary anastomosis is then performed except in elderly patients with multiple comorbidities.

If signs or symptoms of bowel ischemia are absent, we proceed to either rigid or flexible proctosigmoidoscopy. Both measures provide a safe means by which to examine the bowel mucosa, as well as to decompress the dilated loop (Fig. 3). The patient is placed in a lateral decubitus position, and the endoscope is passed until the volvulus is encountered, usually 15 to 20 cm from the anal verge. The scope is then carefully advanced through the narrowed area, often resulting in a rapid decompression of liquid stool and gas. Undue pressure must be avoided to avoid perforation; the procedure should be aborted if there is any resistance. Excess air and liquid are suctioned from the colonic lumen, after which a soft

25- to 32-F rectal tube is inserted into the dilated lumen, maintaining decompression for 48 to 72 hours. In cases in which endoscopic detorsion is unsuccessful, a barium enema may achieve detorsion in approximately 5% of patients; this intervention must be avoided if there is concern for colonic ischemia or perforation.

Recurrence of sigmoid volvulus after endoscopic detorsion ranges from 30% to 90%; in addition, morbidity and mortality increase with each successive detorsion. For this reason, after decompression, many patients undergo colonic lavage as plans are made for elective sigmoid resection during the same admission. The mortality of elective resection is low (1%–5%), with an equally low recurrence rate (~5%). We perform both open and laparoscopic resections because the two methods have been shown to be equally safe and effective. Currently, the choice of technique and conduct of the procedure depends on patient and surgeon preference.

When operative risk is prohibitive, some surgeons have attempted percutaneous endoscopic transcolonic tube placement during a second endoscopic procedure. The long-term efficacy of such measures remains unknown. Given our limited experience with this technique, we prefer to monitor these patients with frequent follow-up visits and offer additional endoscopic detorsion if necessary.

CECAL VOLVULUS

In the 1940s, cadaver studies demonstrated that the cecum fails to fuse to the retroperitoneum in nearly 25% of the population. This lack of fixation creates a significantly mobile ileocecal region that can form two types of volvulus: a clockwise axial torsion around the ileocolic vascular pedicle (90%; Fig. 4) or an inferior to superior cecal fold volvulus ("cecal bascule") forming a closed-loop obstruction (10%). Despite this high rate of inadequate fixation, cecal volvulus accounts for only 1% of all large bowel obstructions. This observation suggests that additional factors, including adhesive disease (acquired or congenital), pregnancy, malignancy, trauma, or conditions leading to cecal distention (distal large bowel obstruction, megacolon, positive pressure ventilation) must be present for such torsion to occur.

As with sigmoid volvulus, patients with cecal volvulus can present with either acute or chronic symptoms, although the former situation is much more common. Patients present acutely with nausea, vomiting, abdominal distention, and crampy pain. Physical examination reveals a distended, tympanic abdomen with minimal tenderness.

Although plain radiography is diagnostic in 25% to 40% of cases, cecal volvulus is often confused with sigmoid volvulus because the distended cecum can appear in either the right or left abdomen (Fig. 5). Radiologic findings generally suggest small bowel obstruction, with loops of distended, fluid-filled small bowel to the right of the distended colon. The classic "coffee-bean" or "comma" sign (a distended cecum with a single fluid level and haustral creases pointing toward the left upper quadrant) may be seen. Occasionally, the ileocecal valve can be visualized because of the gaseous distention of the cecum. As in sigmoid volvulus, the "whirl sign" (spiraled loops of cecum and terminal ileum twisted around the ileocolic mesentery) may be seen on CT scan. Although not necessary, contrast studies will reveal a tapered lumen culminating in a pointed blockage within the right lower quadrant.

Because endoscopic decompression is rarely successful (5%), treatment usually requires laparotomy. We remain interested in preoperative endoscopic decompression, however, because the detorsed bowel wall is thicker and less edematous and therefore more amendable to operative intervention.

As with sigmoid volvulus, the primary consideration is colonic viability. Thus if gangrenous bowel is identified, detorsion is avoided and right hemicolectomy is performed. Although ileostomy and mucous fistula creation together represent traditional management, primary anastomosis of ileum to transverse colon is equally safe in hemodynamically stable patients. Primary anastomosis should be avoided in patients with hemodynamic instability, peritoneal contamination, colonic perforation, or a markedly dilatated transverse colon.

In those with a viable right colon, detorsion alone is associated with a high recurrence rate (20%–40%), demanding additional measures. In our experience, both cecopexy and resection with primary anastomosis are equally safe and offer similar recurrence rates (5%–15%). We perform cecopexy in hemodynamically stable patients without significant distention and unequivocally viable bowel. We take care to fix the taenia of the cecum and entire right colon to the lateral abdominal wall using nonabsorbable suture. Although we do not routinely use a peritoneal flap, others have described this maneuver as a means of preventing recurrence. We reserve resection for those situations in which the bowel is of marginal viability or its wall has become atrophic or edematous, complicating placement of adequate seromuscular stitches. We use both open and laparoscopic access to accomplish these procedures, depending on patient and surgeon preference. We do not use cecostomy tubes because of their high rate of leakage (40%), infection, fistula formation, or cecal necrosis.

TRANSVERSE COLON VOLVULUS

Volvulus of the transverse colon is unusual, representing only 4% of all cases of colonic volvulus. It is more common in middle-aged women, especially those who have had prior abdominal surgery. Congenital factors include a mobile right colon, long transverse mesocolon, or hepatodiaphragmatic interposition of the colon (Chilaiditi syndrome). The clinical presentation is similar to that of any colonic obstruction. The radiographic appearance resembles that of cecal volvulus, with a single, markedly dilatated colon loop in the upper or middle abdomen; in contrast to cecal volvulus, however, two air-fluid levels are generally observed in transverse colon volvulus. The diagnosis is rarely made preoperatively because of this condition's infrequent occurrence.

Management is similar to that of cecal volvulus. After reduction, nonviable bowel is resected with creation of a colostomy and mucous fistula. If viable, either colopexy or resection is acceptable. We generally perform a resection because the excessively redundant colonic loop often precludes identification of an appropriate point for fixation.

SPLENIC FLEXURE VOLVULUS

This rare form of colonic volvulus occurs when the splenic flexure's normal fixation (phrenocolic, gastrocolic, and splenocolic ligaments) is disrupted. Although the condition has been reported following congenital band formation or left upper abdominal trauma, most

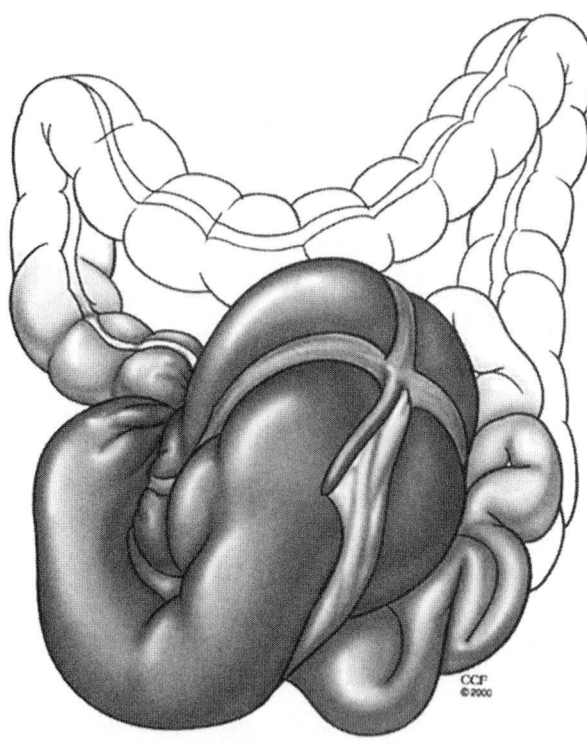

Figure 4 Schematic demonstrating the origin of a cecal volvulus.

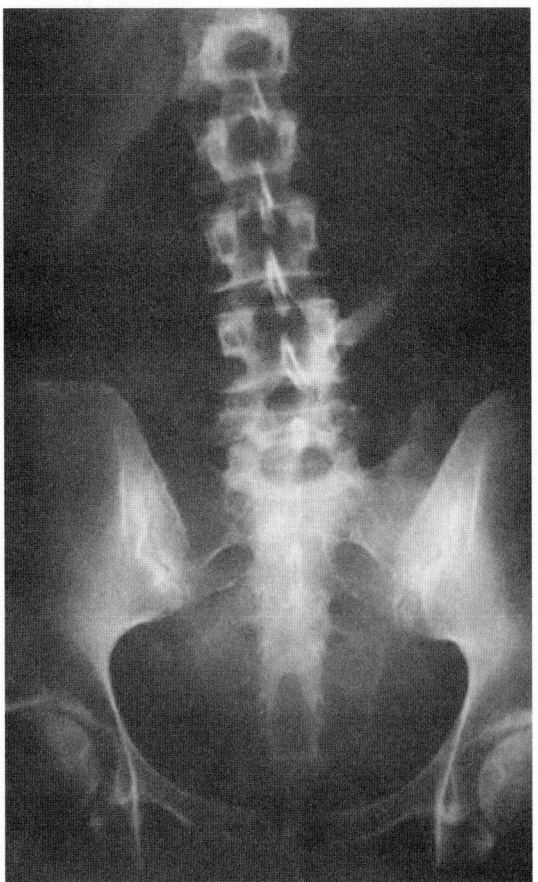

Figure 5 The dilated intestinal loop pointing to the left upper quadrant on this radiologic exam was caused by a cecal volvulus.

cases are seen in patients with previous abdominal surgery. Patients generally present with pain, obstipation, and distention. Although nonoperative reduction has been described, surgical treatment with resection or colopexy is generally performed to reduce the risk of recurrence. Because of the rarity of this condition, limited data exist to support any one therapy.

Suggested Readings

Ballantyne GH: Review of sigmoid volvulus: history and results of treatment, *Dis Colon Rectum* 25:494, 1982.

Ballantyne GH, Brandner MD, Beart RW Jr, and others: Volvulus of the colon. Incidence and mortality, *Ann Surg* 202:83, 1985.

Grossman EM, Longo WE, Stratton MD, and others: Sigmoid volvulus in Departments of Veterans Affairs Medical Centers, *Dis Colon Rectum* 43:414, 2002.

Haskin PH, Teplick SK, Teplick JG, and others: Volvulus of the cecum and right colon, *JAMA* 245:2433, 1981.

Madiba TE, Thomson SR: The management of cecal volvulus, *Dis Colon Rectum* 45:264, 2002.

Matsumoto S, Mori H, Okino Y, and others: Computed tomographic imaging of abdominal volvulus: pictorial essay, *Gastrointest Radiol* 55:297, 2004.

Renzulli P, Maurer CA, Netzer P, and others: Preoperative colonscopic derotation is beneficial in acute colonic volvulus, *Dig Surg* 19:223, 2003.

Tejler G, Joborn H: Volvulus of the cecum. Report of 26 cases and review of the literature, *Dis Colon Rectum* 31:445, 1988.

RECTAL PROLAPSE AND OBSTRUCTED DEFECATION

Susan L. Gearhart, MD

Disorders of defecation continue to be challenging medical problems and remain a poorly understood clinical entity. The disorders of defecation discussed in this chapter include rectal prolapse and obstructed defecation. There are three types of rectal prolapse: full-thickness rectal prolapse (procidentia), mucosal prolapse, and internal intussusception. Obstructed defecation, also know as nonrelaxing puborectalis, is the attempt to defecate against a closed anal canal passageway and is a component of the pathophysiology of rectal prolapse. Rectal prolapse is commonly found in female patients, with a female-to-male ratio that approaches 6:1 in adults. Whereas the incidence of rectal prolapse increases with increasing age in females, males have an equal incidence per decade throughout adult life. Longitudinal radiographic studies have demonstrated that the development of prolapse is a gradual process that begins as internal rectal intussusception and progresses to frank prolapse. The current theory of why rectal prolapse occurs relates to disorders of defecation that lead to excessive straining. Overtime, this will weaken the supportive structures of the pelvic floor and sphincter complex, allowing for herniation of bowel, bladder, or uterus through the pelvic outlet.

Frequently the symptom of rectal prolapse is a manifestation of the more common disorder known as pelvic organ prolapse. In fact, 1 of 10 women will require surgery for pelvic organ prolapse by age 80 years. Table 1 lists other findings of pelvic organ prolapse commonly seen in patients with symptomatic rectal prolapse. Anatomic findings commonly associated with procidentia include a deep cul-de-sac or pouch of Douglas, a redundant sigmoid colon, atonic levator ani muscles, laxity of the rectal support structures, and external anal sphincter weakness.

PRESENTATION AND ASSOCIATED FINDINGS

The presentation of rectal prolapse is rectum protruding from the anus. The rectum may spontaneously reduce or require manual reduction. On rare occasions, the rectum may incarcerate, requiring a laparotomy to reduce it to its normal location. Other related symptoms include rectal bleeding from irritation of the mucosa, tenesmus, and incomplete evacuation. It is important to differentiate full-thickness prolapse from mucosal prolapse, which is associated with hemorrhoids. Full-thickness rectal prolapse is the circumferential, full-thickness protrusion of the rectal wall through the anal orifice. Mucosal prolapse is the result of breakdown or laxity of the connective tissue between the submucosa and muscular portion of the anal canal, resulting in a protrusion of only the rectal mucosa through the anal orifice. Symptoms associated with mucosal prolapse are often the same as those associated with full-thickness prolapse. During physical examination, the classical distinction between full-thickness rectal prolapse and mucosal prolapse is the presence of circumferential folds seen in full-thickness rectal prolapse and radial folds with mucosal prolapse.

The functional defecatory disorders commonly found with all types of rectal prolapse are listed in Table 2. Chronic constipation and fecal incontinence are the most common symptoms. The association of constipation with rectal prolapse is evident in the increased incidence of this disorder among individuals with colonic inertia and obstructed defecation secondary to nonrelaxing puborectalis. Obstructed defecation often develops from the functional defecatory disorder of nonrelaxing puborectalis. Other causes of obstructed defecation include the presence of a rectocele or enterocele. Defecation occurs through a coordinated effort involving relaxation of the anal sphincter complex as well as the puborectalis muscle. The puborectalis muscle acts like a sling to create an angle between the rectum and the anal canal. Relaxation of this sling obliterates the angle, providing a direct passage of stool from the rectum through the anal canal. Paradoxical puborectalis muscle contraction during defecation maintains or exaggerates the anorectal angle, resulting in a functional resistance to defecation. This coordinated contraction can also be lost with the presence of a large enterocele or rectocele. An enterocele or rectocele results from a laxity within the rectovaginal septum, which allows either the posterior wall of the rectum or bowel from the peritoneal cavity to herniate within the pouch of Douglas.

Table 1: Other Related Pelvic Floor Findings Associated with Rectal Prolapse

Associated Finding	Incidence (%)
Perineal descent	67
Vaginal prolapse	57
Enterocele	47
Rectocele	44
Cystocele	33

Table 2: Defecatory Dysfunction Associated with Rectal Prolapse

Functional Problem	Incidence (%)
Fecal incontinence	50–75
Chronic constipation	30–67
Obstructed defecation	33
Solitary rectal ulcer	12
Colonic inertia	10

Fecal incontinence occurs in the majority of patients with all types of rectal prolapse, and the incidence increases with age and duration of the prolapse. It is thought that fecal incontinence is the result of a combination of an increase in intrarectal pressure as a result of the prolapse, as well as stretch injury to the pudendal nerves. The increase in the intrarectal pressure minimizes the normal pressure difference that exists between the rectum and the anal canal, resulting in incontinence. Stretch injury to the pudendal nerves that innervate the anal sphincter complex occurs as a result of excessive straining and recurrent prolapse of the pelvic floor. Fortunately, correction of the prolapse improves symptoms of fecal incontinence in nearly 80% of patients.

EVALUATION

All patients presenting with rectal prolapse should undergo a complete history and physical examination. Associated symptoms of pelvic organ prolapse should be ascertained. An emphasis should be placed on risk factors for anesthesia, because this information may affect the surgeon's choice of procedure. Patients who are a high operative risk may benefit from a less invasive procedure to fix the prolapse. The physical examination should include careful evaluation of the perineum and prolapsed rectum. With the patient in lithotomy position, the perineum should be inspected in the relaxed position, as well as during straining. During straining, the prolapsed rectum can often be seen, as can an enterocele or rectocele protruding into the posterior vaginal wall. If the prolapse is not easily demonstrated, the use of an enema may help. A digital rectal examination performed during straining can often demonstrate the lack of fixation of the rectum posteriorly and the presence of internal intussusception. If a laxity exists within the rectovaginal septum, a rectocele may be present.

Additional investigations in patients with rectal prolapse and obstructed defecation should include a colonoscopy or barium enema. Both tests provide an evaluation of the colonic mucosa for a lead point causing intussusception or other abnormalities, such as diverticular disease or solitary rectal ulcer, which may influence the type of procedure performed. Because these patients can manifest with several associated pelvic floor abnormalities, an assessment of pelvic floor anatomy and physiology is required. Depending on associated symptoms, tests may include cinedefecography, pelvic floor dynamic magnetic resonance imaging (MRI), anorectal manometry, endorectal ultrasound, electromyography (EMG), and colon transit studies.

Cinedefecography and dynamic pelvic floor MRI are both useful tests to evaluate the pelvic floor in patients with obstructed defecation and rectal prolapse. Cinedefecography is a test performed by the instillation of contrast into the rectum, vagina, and bladder and allowing the patient to evacuate the contents in the normal sitting position while real-time images are obtained. Cinedefecography can detect occult intussusception and rectal prolapse with a sensitivity of 100% and a specificity of 93%. Other abnormalities

that may be detected include paradoxical puborectalis contraction and pelvic floor weakness such as rectocele, enterocele, and cystocele. In contrast, dynamic pelvic floor MRI is performed with the installation of contrast into the rectum and vagina; however, the patient must be kept in the supine position. The patient is asked to bear down to the point of defecation while images are obtained. This test will identify a pelvic floor hernia.

Anorectal manometry and endorectal ultrasound are performed when there are symptoms of fecal incontinence associated with rectal prolapse. Often this may be useful for evaluation of occult sphincter defects, especially in older parous women. Patients with lower resting and maximal squeeze pressures are less likely to recover sphincter control following rectal prolapse repair. EMG studies have been used to identify patients with paradoxical puborectalis contraction (nonrelaxing puborectalis). This study can be performed with surface or needle EMG within the anorectal muscle. Surface EMGs tend to be less sensitive in identifying incomplete pelvic floor relaxation, and needle EMGs are not well tolerated by the patient. In addition, the balloon expulsion test can be performed at the same time anorectal manometry is performed. The balloon catheter used during this procedure is inflated with 50 to 100 ml of water, and the patient is asked to expel the balloon. Patients without obstructed defecation should easily expel the balloon.

Patients with long-standing constipation who have rectal prolapse should undergo colonic transit studies. This study uses 24 radiopaque markers that are ingested by the patient. Sequential daily plain abdominal films are performed to demonstrate the movement of stool throughout the colon. Patients with total colonic inertia will retain at least 80% of the markers equally distributed throughout the colon at 5 days. Patients with obstructed defecation will have markers concentrated near the rectosigmoid junction. Failure to recognize and treat a dysfunctional colon or obstructed defecation may result in continued straining and ultimately recurrent prolapse.

MANAGEMENT OPTIONS

The goal of treatment is the restoration of normal anatomy and correction of any associated physiologic disorder. Successful treatment results in long-lasting symptom relief and is accomplished best by nonoperative and operative techniques.

Nonoperative Management

Nonoperative therapy should be initiated in all patients with disorders of defecation. Initial treatment should include high-fiber therapy. This is best accomplished with fiber supplements so that a total of 30 g of fiber are consumed per day. Biofeedback is the mainstay therapy for obstructed defecation secondary to paradoxical puborectalis contraction and internal intussusception. Biofeedback training is aimed at suppressing the inappropriate contraction of the pelvic floor during defecation. This may result in a reduction in the time spent straining at defecation and prevent recurrence of prolapse.

Operative Management

Operative repair is indicated for full-thickness prolapse, mucosal prolapse, symptomatic enterocele, and rectocele. Operative repair has a limited role in internal intussusception and no role in nonrelaxing puborectalis. Several types of repair for full-thickness rectal prolapse exist; the indication for each type and recurrence rates are listed in Table 3. Other parameters used to compare outcomes among procedures include persistent or new symptoms of

Table 3: Indications and Recurrence Rates for Perineal versus Abdominal Procedures for Full-Thickness Rectal Prolapse

Procedure	Indication	No. of studies	Recurrence (%)
Anal encirclement	Bedridden, high surgical risk	8	0–60
Delorme	Bedridden, high surgical risk	8	5–21
Perineal rectosigmoidectomy	High surgical risk	11	0–44
Ripstein rectopexy	Prolapse without constipation, fecal incontinence	12	0–13
Wells rectopexy	Prolapse without constipation, fecal incontinence	6	2–10
Suture rectopexy	Prolapse without constipation, fecal incontinence	7	0–5
Resection rectopexy	Prolapse withconstipation, no fecal incontinence	4	0–6
Anterior resection	Prolapse associated with severe solitary rectal ulcer syndrome	3	4–9

Modified from Farouk R, Duthie GS: Eur J Surg 164(5):323, 1998.

constipation or fecal incontinence. In general, the literature supports the use of abdominal procedures rather than perineal procedures for rectal prolapse because of the associated decrease in recurrence rates. The goal of the abdominal approach, whether laparoscopic or open, is mobilization and posterior fixation of the rectum to the presacral fascia. The goal of the perineal procedure is partial or complete removal of the prolapsed rectum through the perineum with minimal operative risk to the patient. Therefore if a patient's physical condition does not allow for an abdominal procedure, then a perineal procedure is warranted.

Operative Indications

Rectal Prolapse without Constipation

Up to 50% of patients who present with rectal prolapse do not have a long-standing history of constipation. Historically, patients who underwent a rectopexy alone for rectal prolapse without constipation had an increased rate of postoperative defecatory dysfunction. For this reason, rectopexy and resection was recommended. However, after careful evaluation of the pelvic anatomy, it has been demonstrated that during mobilization of the lateral attachments of the rectum, several nerves important in rectal function can be injured. Recently, several studies have demonstrated that a rectopexy can be successfully performed alone if the lateral attachments of the rectum are preserved, preventing denervation of the rectum. It is therefore recommended that in patients without constipation, rectopexy be performed alone through an abdominal approach, with minimal chance of recurrence.

Rectal Prolapse with Constipation

Patients with long-standing constipation who do not have a colonic motility disorder on a Sitzmark study should undergo a resection rectopexy (Frykman and Goldberg procedure). If a colonic motility disorder is identified, further studies beyond the scope of this chapter should be performed to evaluate for gastric or small bowel dysmotility. If isolated colonic dysmotility is present, the patient may be offered a subtotal colectomy with ileorectal anastomosis and rectopexy.

Rectal Prolapse with Fecal Incontinence

Up to 70% of patients may complain of some degree of fecal incontinence. This is primarily due to an increase in intrarectal pressure. With ongoing straining and prolapse, pudendal nerve injury may occur, leading to worsening incontinence. In the presence of severe incontinence, I favor a rectopexy alone because the combination of a resection and rectopexy may make the symptoms of incontinence worse. In general, a combined approach for sphincter muscle repair

at the time of rectopexy is avoided because symptomatic incontinence improves in most patients.

Mucosal Prolapse

The surgical management of mucosal prolapse is best described by the treatment of hemorrhoids. The goal or repair for mucosal prolapse is to resuspend the mucosa within the anal canal. This can be accomplished with a conventional hemorrhoidectomy or stapled hemorrhoidectomy.

Enterocele and Rectocele

Rarely does an enterocele occur without evidence of complete pelvic organ prolapse. In general an enterocele can be repaired easily while a repair for rectal prolapse is performed. Symptomatic rectoceles commonly occur without evidence of complete pelvic organ prolapse. A rectocele less than 2 cm in size is generally treated with nonoperative management.

Operative Techniques

For all abdominal and perineal procedures including rectopexy without resection, all patients should undergo mechanical bowel preparation. Appropriate preoperative antibiotic coverage and antithrombotic therapy should be given. A decision regarding the use of a laparoscopic or an open procedure is made on the basis of the patient's previous surgical history, weight, and known contraindications to laparoscopic surgery.

Laparoscopic Approach

During the laparoscopic approach, the patient is placed in lithotomy and Trendelenburg positions throughout most of the procedure. Initially, a pnuemoperitoneum is achieved by using either the Hassan technique or with the Visiport with a standard insufflation pressure of 12 mm Hg. Four trocars are used (three 12-mm and one 5-mm port). A 12-mm port is placed in the supraumbilical region for insertion of the camera. Two trocars are placed on the right side, with one placed in the right midquadrant and one in the right lower quadrant, avoiding the inferior epigastric vessels. An additional trocar is placed in the left lower quadrant to assist in retracting the left colon and in performing an intracorporeal anastamosis. Alternatively, one trocar is placed in the suprapubic position, which will aid in tacking mesh to the presacral fascia if a Wells procedure is performed (discussed subsequently).

The sigmoid colon and the rectum are mobilized to free the retroperitoneal structures, including the left ureter and the hypogastric nerves. The space between the fascia propria of the rectum and the presacral fascia is opened down to the levator muscles. Care must be taken to avoid mobilization of the lateral attachments of the rectum, which includes the middle hemorrhoidal artery. Preservation of these lateral attachments prevents injury to the innervation of the rectum and preserves rectal function. The anterior reflection of peritoneum within the pouch of Douglas in female patients should always be opened to help minimize this space and prevent enterocele formation. If a sigmoid resection is planned, the resected bowel can be removed by enlarging the midline camera port or through a left lower quadrant incision. The sigmoid colon is removed, and either an intracorpeal or extracorporeal anastomosis is performed. The lateral attachments of the rectum are then secured to the presacral fascia/periosteum with nonabsorbable sutures (Fig. 1).

The addition of mesh to laparoscopic rectopexy is known as the Wells procedure. The mesh is introduced into the abdomen through one of the 12-mm ports. This mesh is then placed posterior to the rectum along the presacral fascia beginning at the sacral promontory. The mesh is secured by laparoscopic tacker (Origin Medsystems, Cupertino, CA). The lateral edges of the mesh are then secured to the lateral attachments of the rectum. Some proponents of this procedure cut the mesh into a T shape to allow for more ease in securing the mesh to the lateral attachments of the rectum. The Wells procedure is a modification of an earlier procedure known as the Ripstein rectopexy (see the subsequent discussion on the open abdominal approach).

Open Abdominal Approach

As in most procedures for pelvic organ prolapse, the patient is placed in the lithotomy position. For the open abdominal approach, I favor a Pfannenstiel incision. Although several authors favor a lower midline, I find that because the surgeon does not need to mobilize the splenic flexure, a Pfannenstiel incision works well and patients like the cosmetic benefits. A Balfour retractor can be used to retract the edges of the wound, and a bladder extension and a retracting extension can be placed to assist in retracting the small bowel from the pelvis. Dissection begins along the peritoneal reflection on each side of the rectosigmoid approximately 5 cm proximal to the pelvic brim. At this point, the left ureter

should be identified and protected. If a resection is to be carried out, the redundant bowel is isolated. The splenic flexure is not mobilized because this provides additional fixation to the colon. I prefer to perform the pelvic mobilization before dividing the bowel. With anterior retraction on the rectosigmoid, the presacral space can be entered. Care must be taken to preserve the lateral sympathetic and parasympathetic pelvic nerves. The dissection is taken posteriorly to the coccyx. The lateral dissection should not be taken down past the middle hemorrhoidal vessels because this may lead to rectal denervation and worsening obstructive defecation. The anterior dissection of the rectum is performed to allow for further mobilization and for closure of a deep pouch of Douglas.

After mobilization is complete, the bowel is resected and the redundant sigmoid colon is removed. The bowel is anastomosed without tension. Thereafter the rectopexy can be performed. A suture rectopexy is performed by tacking the lateral preserved attachments of the rectum to the presacral fascia at the level of S2 or S3. Four or six sutures can be used and placed from distal to proximal. If alternative material is to be used in this procedure, Teflon, Gortex, or Marlex mesh is usually used to secure the rectum. The mesh is secured to the sacrum, and this mesh is wrapped around the rectum, anchoring it to the muscularis propria and leaving a 1-cm separation on the anterior wall of the rectum to prevent luminal narrowing.

Perineal Approach

The perineal approaches used to repair rectal prolapse in patients at high operative risk include the perineal rectosigmoidectomy (Altmeier procedure) and the Delorme procedure. The patient can be positioned in the lithotomy or prone-jackknife position. The perineal rectosigmoidectomy is performed with the rectum fully prolapsed. Anal retracting sutures or the Lone Star retractor (Lone Star Medical Products, Stafford, TX) can be used to assist with exposure. A circumferential full-thickness incision is made 1 cm (hand sewn) to 3 cm (stapled anastomosis) above the dentate line (Fig. 2, *A* and *B*). It is important to maintain rotation of the rectum, and this can be facilitated by grasping the anterior rectum with a Babcock clamp. The anterior wall of the hernia sac is identified and opened, allowing the rectum to be circumferentially freed from the hernia sac. After the rectum is

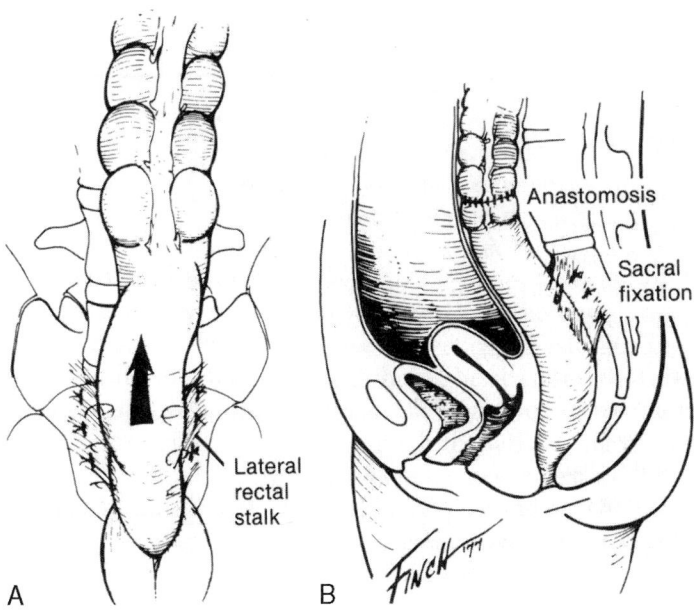

Figure I Anterior **(A)** and sagittal **(B)** views of fixation of the lateral ligaments of the rectum to the presacral fascia and periosteum of the sacrum. *From Gordon PH. In Gordon PH, Nivatvonys S, editors: Principles and practice of surgery for the colon, rectum and anus, ed 2, St. Louis, 1999, Quality Medical Publishing.*

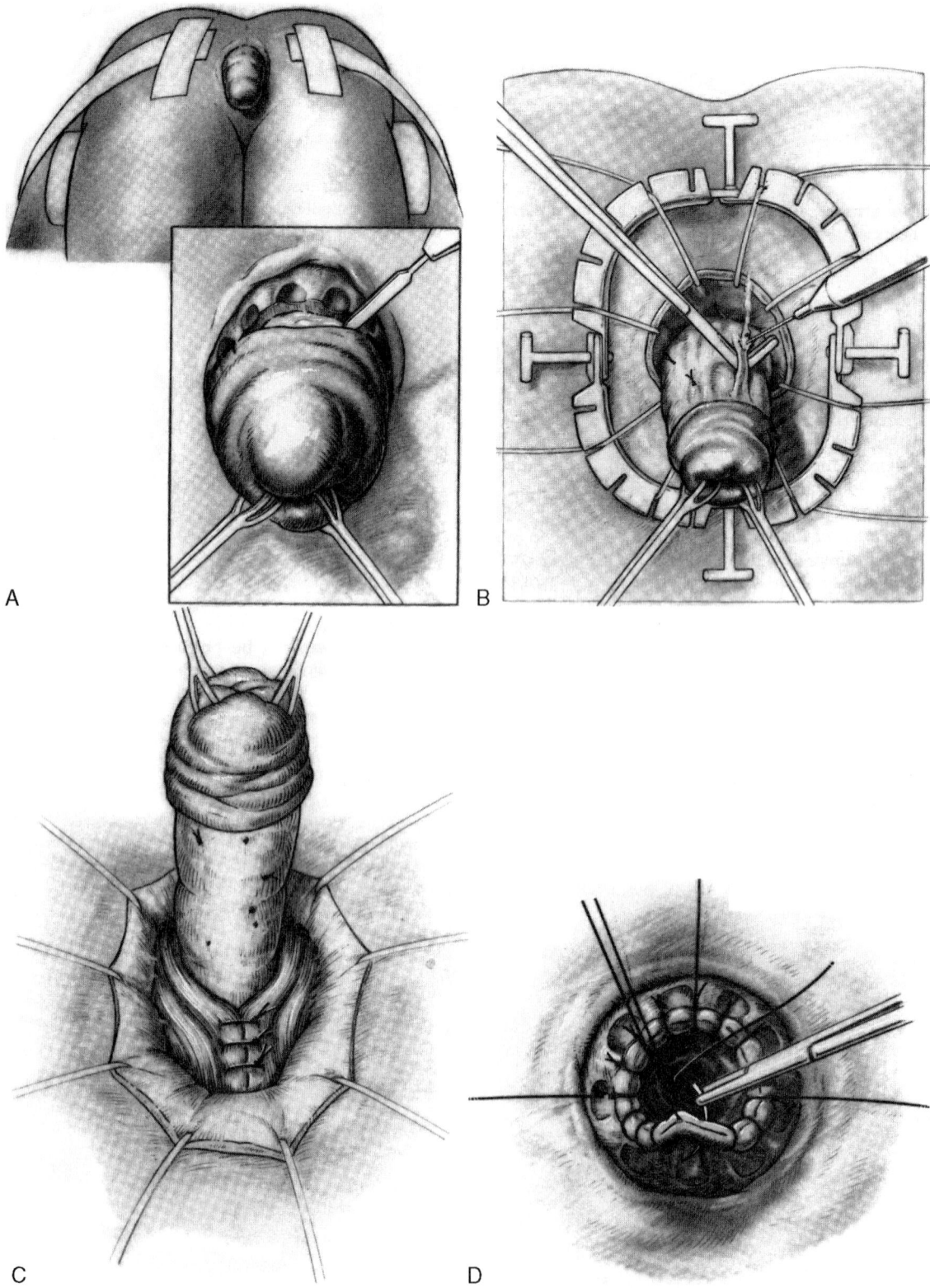

Figure 2 Perineal rectosigmoidectomy for full-thickness rectal prolapse. **(A)** The rectal mucosa is incised, and the hernia sac is entered. Two Babcock clamps are used to maintain the orientation of the rectum. **(B)** The mesorectum is divided. A Lone Star retractor facilitates exposure. **(C)** Plication of the herniated levator ani muscles. **(D)** A hand-sewn anastomosis is performed between the rectal remnant and the distal colon. *From Williams JG, Madoff RD. In Fielding LP, Goldberg SM, editors: Rob & Smith's operative surgery, surgery of the colon, rectum and anus, ed 5, Oxford, 1992, Butterworth-Heinemann.*

mobilized, the mesenteric attachments are freed by careful division with ligation of major vessels. This maneuver additionally frees the rectum. Any laxity in the levator muscles should then be repaired with plication to create a snug fit. After the correct bowel orientation is confirmed, the redundant bowel is transected. A hand-sewn anastomosis can be performed, reapproximating the proximal and distal ends (Fig. 2, *C* and *D*) Alternatively a stapled anastomosis can be performed with the use of end-end circular stapler.

Delorme Procedure

The Delorme procedure is a best described as a sleeve resection of only rectal mucosa that is removed from the prolapsed rectum. This is facilitated by infiltrating the submucosa with lidocaine and epinephrine (1:100,000). The denuded rectal muscular wall is plicated in four quadrants like an accordion, and the remaining mucosal rings are reapproximated. It is recommended that an absorbable suture such as 2–0 Vicryl be used (Fig. 3). Further sutures may be needed to complete the mucosal anastomosis.

Rectocele Repair

It is my preference to repair this defect through a perineal transvaginal approach in a combined procedure with the urogynecologist. A longitudinal incision is made in the posterior vaginal wall, together with a transverse incision at the introitus. The rectovaginal septum is entered and mobilized laterally. If sufficient later support fiber within the septum can be identified, these are drawn together and reapproximated. Alternatively, either fascia lata or allogenic graft may be used. It is best to avoid the use of mesh in this area because the risks of erosion and dysparunia are high.

CONCLUSION

The problems of rectal prolapse and obstructed defecation remain challenging for the surgeon. Key aspects of the care of these patients include careful preoperative evaluation for identification of any associated abnormalities that may lead to early failure, the use of combined operative and nonoperative strategies, and patient education. These patients often require a multidisciplinary approach.

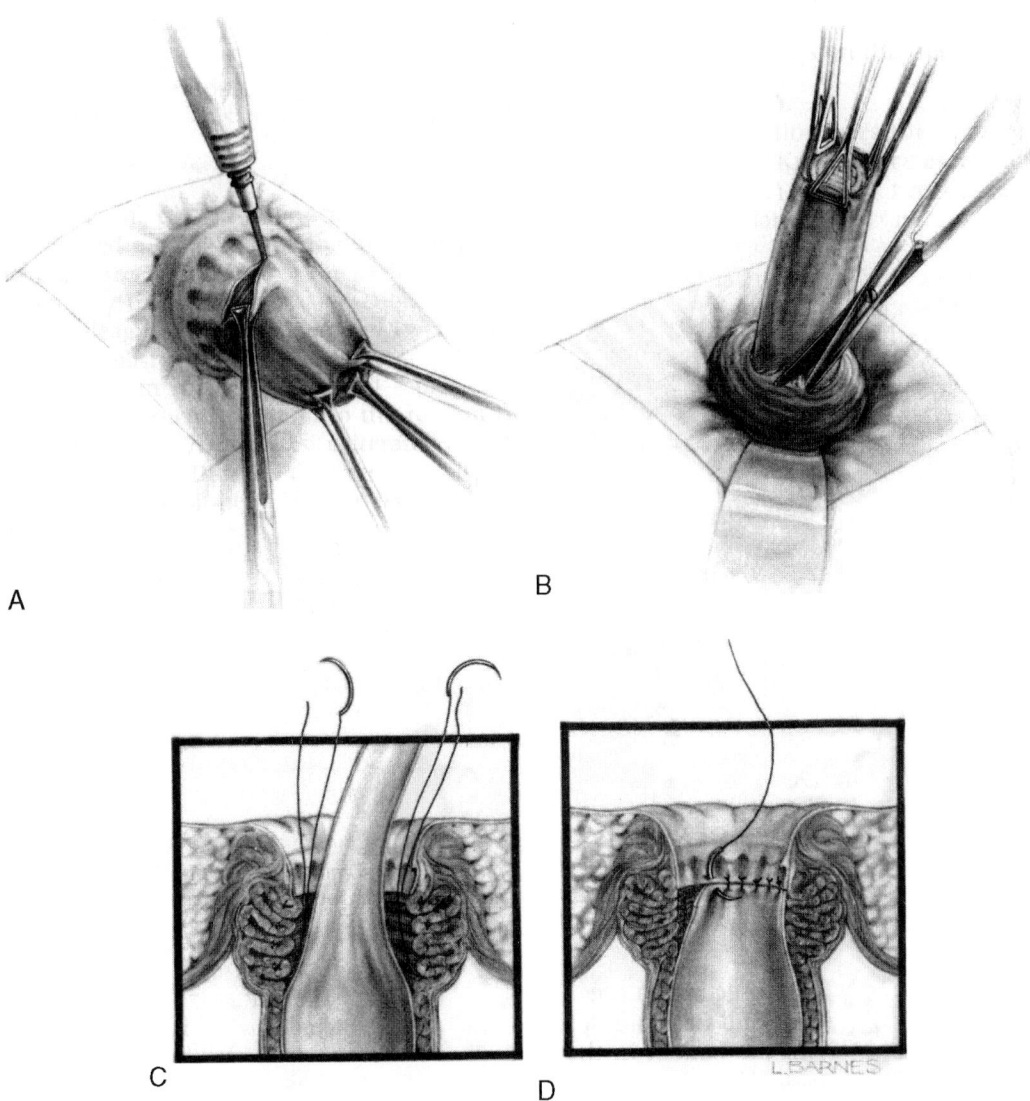

A

B

C

D

Figure 3 The Delorme procedure for full-thickness rectal prolapse. **(A)** After injecting the submucosa with a dilute lidocaine and epinephrine solution, the rectal mucosa is circumferentially incised above the dentate line. **(B)** Mucosal stripping is performed to the furthest extent. **(C)** The remaining muscular wall of the rectum is plicated to the intact muscular portion of the anal canal. **(D)** The mucosal edges are reapproximated. *From Corman ML. In Corman ML, editor: Colon and rectal surgery, ed 4, Philadelphia, 1998, Lippincott Williams & Wilkins.*

Although there are various approaches for these disorders, the best is that which is tailored to the specific patient.

SUGGESTED READINGS

Andromanakos N, Skandalakis P, Troupis T, and others: Constipation of anorectal outlet obstruction: pathophysiology, evaluation, and management, *J Gastroenterol Hepatol* 21:638, 2006.

Bruch H, Herold A, Schiedeck T, and others: Laparoscopic surgery for rectal prolapse and outlet obstruction, *Dis Colon Rectum* 42:1189, 1999.
Larulf R, Madoff R, Goldberg S: Rectal prolapse, *Curr Probl Surg* 38:757, 2000.
Madbouly K, Sheir K, Elsobky E, and others: Clinically based management of rectal prolapse, *Surg Endoscopy* 17:99, 2003.
Scaglia M, Fasth S, Hallgren T, and others: Abdominal rectopexy for rectal prolapse, Influence of surgical technique on functional outcome, *Dis Colon Rectum* 37:805, 1994.

SOLITARY RECTAL ULCER SYNDROME

Janice F. Rafferty, MD

Solitary rectal ulcer (SRU) is the physical manifestation of a syndrome that includes severe defecatory dysfunction. Although the clinicopathologic features of solitary rectal ulcer syndrome (SRUS) are well described, the varied endoscopic findings associated with SRUS, along with its infrequency in the general population, can make it a diagnostic dilemma. The majority of patients are under 50 years of age, and thus the condition is often mistaken for inflammatory bowel disease or rectal adenocarcinoma. It is most likely an underdiagnosed condition in the pediatric population. Delayed and incorrect diagnosis is common. Ultimately the diagnosis arises when the thoughtful clinician has a high index of suspicion and combines a thorough exploration of the patient's elimination pattern with radiographic findings and biopsy results. Making the correct diagnosis is critical to devising the appropriate treatment strategy for this benign disease process.

ETIOLOGY

The common denominator in SRUS is rectal dysfunction, but patients will rarely offer this information to the clinician voluntarily. Rectal dysfunction, and the consequent poor toileting habits of those affected, results in a marked microscopic abnormality of a portion of the rectal wall. Excessive straining to defecate creates high intra-abdominal pressure, forcing the rectal mucosa through the contracting muscles of the pelvic floor and into the anal canal, which in theory causes congestion, edema, and ulceration. Repeated digitation and even an enema tip can cause rectal ulceration. Chronic insult of the rectal mucosa can lead to hypertrophy and polypoid change.

CLINICAL FINDINGS

When pressed, patients consistently describe passage of bloody mucus with bowel movements, the need to strain, a sense of incomplete evacuation, frequent attempts to stool, and tenesmus. Some have incontinence. Thorough and explicit questioning will reveal a history of prolonged sitting on the toilet, excessive straining, digitation or splinting to evacuate stool, and multiple trips to the toilet every day to attempt to evacuate. Rarely is significant hemorrhage seen, but up to 2.8% of massive lower gastrointestinal bleeding is due to SRUS.

Examination should be performed with the patient in a prone jackknife position so that the examiner can evaluate perineal contour; a flattened perineum is consistent with loss of muscular and ligamentous perineal support and pelvic descent and suggests a generalized pelvic floor abnormality. Digital rectal exam may show an anal sphincter with high tone and nodularity and firmness of a segment of the distal rectal wall. Mucosal changes are most commonly located on the anterior rectal wall. Proctoscopic exam should be done even if flexible endoscopy was performed; this allows accurate localization and repeat large biopsies to confirm the diagnosis. Hyperemic mucosa with shallow ulceration will be seen in the distal rectum, often on the anterior rectal wall, on average 4.7 cm $\pm$ 1.5 cm from the dentate line. Polypoid change surrounds the ulcer in up to one third of patients, and multiple ulcers are seen in 30%. Even circumferential stenosis of the rectum has been caused by SRUS. The terms "solitary" and "ulcer" associated with this syndrome are therefore imprecise. An important examination technique is to observe patients while they are straining on the commode. This will reveal full-thickness prolapse that, if present, will influence treatment strategy.

DIAGNOSTIC TESTS

Biopsies are the best diagnostic test and are often read as consistent with prolapse, similar to stress-related mucosal injury. The most common misdiagnosis is inflammatory bowel disease, specifically Crohn's disease. There should be no evidence of adenomatous change. Up to 38% of patients with SRUS have histologic changes that mimic sessile serrated polyps, which are epithelial proliferative lesions. In a small percentage of cases, serrated polyps have focal loss of hMLH1 gene expression, which may translate to an increased propensity for neoplastic change. Therefore these rectal ulcers should be closely followed with proctoscopy and biopsy. Thickened muscularis propria is seen in SRUS but not in complete rectal prolapse. It is critical that histologic changes consistent with SRUS are differentiated from malignancy and endometriosis because submucosal infiltrating adenocarcinoma and endometriosis are occasionally misidentified as SRUS.

Defecography is the most informative test after biopsy and is abnormal in 75% of those with SRUS. Findings most often are internal intussusception, pelvic floor descent, and delayed or incomplete rectal evacuation. These are an important finding on defecography because the vast majority of patients with delayed rectal emptying have poor relief of symptoms with surgery.

Several other tests are complementary but not wholly necessary. Balloon expulsion testing will show that more than half of patients cannot pass a small water-filled balloon while sitting on the toilet because of nonrelaxing puborectalis. Colonic transit study should be obtained to rule out colonic inertia as a component of defecatory dysfunction. Transrectal ultrasound shows marked thickening of the internal sphincter and muscularis propria. Barium enema demonstrates the ulceration, nodularity, and occasionally a stricture. Pelvic floor testing is usually not helpful but will demonstrate reduced compliance of the fibrotic rectal wall if studied.

THERAPY

Nonsurgical

Treatment of SRUS is aimed at restoration of normal habits of defecation. Behavior modification is critical. The addition of insoluble dietary fiber, fluid, and occasionally laxatives is helpful. Physical therapy aimed at normalization of pelvic floor relaxation and contraction is useful. Biofeedback has been studied; it often leads to improvement of symptoms, whether or not the ulcer is healed. Biofeedback is more successful if the patient demonstrates anismus or evidence of nonrelaxing puborectalis. Mucosal blood flow is seen to improve after biofeedback and correlates with ulcer healing and symptom resolution. Positive effects degenerate over time in some patients. Psychiatric evaluation for occult obsessive disorders may prove necessary.

Many topical therapies have been tried, with limited success. Topical steroids and anti-inflammatory compounds, sucralfate enemas, and fibrin glue have all been described with minimal gain. Argon plasma coagulation may represent a therapeutic approach for bleeding SRUS.

Surgical

Surgery should be reserved for highly select cases with severe refractory symptoms, such as bleeding that requires transfusion, obstructing stricture, and complete rectal prolapse. The surgeon must keep in mind that even with correction of the anatomic defect, patients rarely change toileting habits without intense behavioral therapy, so symptoms may persist or recur. Surgical success is achieved in 50% to 79% of patients when SRUS is found in the presence of complete rectal prolapse but is much less effective when no prolapse is found. Preoperative delayed or incomplete rectal evacuation, tenesmus, and digitation correlate with poor outcome after surgery. Open or laparoscopic mesh rectopexy can be successful when used for the treatment of complete rectal prolapse with SRUS, leading to ulcer healing and long-term improvement in symptoms and quality of life. If rectopexy is combined with sigmoid resection, the anastomosis should lie at the top of the rectum where the taenia splay out to avoid decreased rectal capacity and anastomotic complications. Local excision of the ulcer may be necessary if the diagnosis is not firm following superficial biopsies; transanal endoscopic microsurgery for ulcer excision has been used in a small number of cases. Other operative management strategies include mucosectomy with or without plication of the muscular wall (Delorme procedure) and colostomy. Salvage colostomy is performed in up to 30% of patients who are treated for SRUS with an operation.

OUTCOMES

While short-term surgical results in select patients are favorable, reports on long-term outcome are few, and usually disappointing. Complete "cure" of SRUS is uncommon, and complete mucosal healing cannot be expected. A realistic goal with combination therapy is minimization of symptoms.

SUGGESTED READINGS

Bishop PR, Nowicki MJ: Nonsurgical therapy for solitary rectal ulcer syndrome, *Curr Treat Options Gastroenterol* 5:215, 2002.

Chiang JM, Changchien CR, Chen JR: Solitary rectal ulcer syndrome: an endoscopic and histological presentation and literature review, *Int J Colorectal Dis* 21:348, 2006.

Choi HJ, Shin EJ, Hwang YH, and others: Clinical presentation and surgical outcome in patients with solitary rectal ulcer syndrome, *Surg Innov* 12:307, 2005.

Felt-Bersma RJ, Cuesta MA: Rectal prolapse, rectal intussusception, rectocele, and solitary rectal ulcer syndrome, *Gastroenterol Clin North Am* 30:199, 2001.

Halligan S, Nicholls RJ, Bartram CI: Proctographic changes after rectopexy for solitary rectal ulcer syndrome and preoperative predictive factors for a successful outcome, *Br J Surg* 82:314, 1995.

Malouf AJ, Vaizey CJ, Kamm MA: Results of behavioral treatment (biofeedback) for solitary rectal ulcer syndrome, *Dis Colon Rectum* 44:72, 2001.

Martin de Carpi J, Vilar P, Varea V: Solitary rectal ulcer syndrome in childhood: a rare, benign, and probably misdiagnosed cause of rectal bleeding. Report of three cases, *Dis Colon Rectum* 50:534, 2007.

Rao SS, Ozturk R, De Ocampo S, Stessman M: Pathophysiology and role of biofeedback therapy in solitary rectal ulcer syndrome, *Am J Gastroenterol* 101:613, 2006.

Sitzler PJ, Kamm MA, Nicholls RJ, McKee RF: Long-term clinical outcome of surgery for solitary rectal ulcer syndrome, *Br J Surg* 85:1246, 1998.

Stoppino V, Cuomo R, Tonti P, and others: Argon plasma coagulation of hemorrhagic solitary rectal ulcer syndrome, *J Clin Gastroenterol* 37:392, 2003.

Tweedie DJ, Varma JS: Long-term outcome of laparoscopic mesh rectopexy for solitary rectal ulcer syndrome, *Colorectal Dis* 7:151, 2005.

RADIATION INJURY TO THE SMALL AND LARGE BOWEL

Najjia N. Mahmoud, MD, and Robert D. Fry, MD

Radiation therapy is an important component of the multidisciplinary treatment of a variety of pelvic malignancies, including those of gynecologic, urologic, and rectal origin. The benefit of radiation therapy for certain pelvic tumors has been conclusively demonstrated, but its exact role continues to evolve. A quarter of a century ago, it was generally thought that radiation provided no benefit for patients afflicted with rectal cancer because such cancers were resistant to radiation. However, experience has shown that rectal cancer is only moderately resistant to this modality and that higher doses of radiation often result in a dramatic therapeutic response. Unfortunately, the higher levels of radiation required to obtain this response approach the levels that can be tolerated by the normal organ and may exceed the levels tolerated by adjacent organs. For example, the moderately high dose of radiation (5040 cGy) commonly used to treat rectal cancer would cause severe organ damage if delivered directly to the small intestine.

Furthermore, the effects of radiation on various pelvic cancers have been shown to be augmented by intravenous chemotherapy delivered in conjunction with the radiation. This radiation-sensitizing effect unfortunately also extends to normal tissue. The combination of chemotherapy and radiation directed at advanced cancers has often (although not invariably) resulted in a marked regression, or downstaging, of the tumor. Some authors have reported highly selected cases of rectal cancer being eradicated with chemotherapy and radiation as the only treatment modalities.

Unfortunately the relatively high levels of radiation required to achieve a therapeutic response often result in collateral damage to the primary and adjacent organs. Radiation injury to the small intestine can cause diarrhea, malabsorption, stricture, obstruction, hemorrhage, perforation, and fistulization. Of the 100,000 patients annually receiving radiation therapy for pelvic malignancies, it is estimated that 70% will develop acute enteritis, and 5% to 15% of those patients will sustain chronic symptoms. As many as half of the patients in this latter group require surgical intervention.

PATHOGENESIS OF RADIATION DAMAGE

Radiation causes apoptosis and cell death by nonspecifically targeting cellular DNA, cytoplasmic proteins, and membrane-bound lipids. Tissues such as bone marrow and gastrointestinal epithelial cells have high mitotic indices and are particularly prone to damage. Radiation toxicity can be either acute or chronic. Acute symptoms may occur almost immediately after initiation of treatment and include nausea, diarrhea, cramping, tenesmus, and bleeding. Symptoms may occur almost immediately after initiation of treatment. Microscopically, distortion of the crypt-villus architecture is caused by shortening of the fili of the brush border. Hyperemia, edema, and mucosal ulceration correlate with patient complaints. The symptoms of chronic radiation injury are caused by transmural damage that evolves weeks to years after the completion of radiotherapy. The underlying pathophysiology is an obliterative endarteritis resulting in ischemia and fibrosis. Pale, stiff, noncompliant intestine is the clinical hallmark of this disease.

RISK FACTORS

Radiation toxicity is not entirely predictable, with some patients affected more severely than others. Risk factors for significant injury, both acute and chronic, have been broadly defined. Most reviews and case series have found higher risk of injury with administration after radical hysterectomy or other pelvic operations, thin body habitus, and vaginal brachytherapy. Some have found an association with advanced age. The strongest correlation with injury is dose—as the total dose and dose fractionation increases, the risk of damage does as well. At doses of 45 Gy, chronic radiation injury is observed in 5% of patients; at 65 Gy, 50% sustain chronic damage. Most current therapeutic regimens are within this dosage range. The size of the field of radiation is important as well. Those patients requiring extended fields (proximal to the sacral promontory or inclusive of the inguinal nodes, for example) are more prone to enteric damage (Table 1).

Table 1: Radiation Therapy Oncology Group/ European Organization for Research and Treatment of Cancer Chronic Radiation Morbidity for Small or Large Intestine

Grade	Criteria
1	Mild diarrhea, mild cramping, bowel movement <5 times daily, slight rectal bleeding
2	Moderate diarrhea and colic, bowel movement >5 times daily, intermittent rectal bleeding
3	Obstruction or bleeding requiring surgery
4	Necrosis, perforation, fistula
5	Death directly related to radiation last effects

RADIATION ENTERITIS

The treatment of acute radiation enteritis rarely involves operative intervention. Nausea, diarrhea, tenesmus, and bleeding are usually palliated with hydration, antiemetics, antidiarrheals, anti-inflammatory suppositories, and, if necessary, by decreasing the radiation dose fractionation or temporarily interrupting treatment.

Chronic radiation damage can result in diarrhea, malabsorption, lower gastrointestinal bleeding, obstruction (from strictures or adhesions), and fistulization between loops of bowel, or between bowel and adjacent visceral structures or the skin (Fig. 1). Rarely, enteroaortic or enteroiliac fistulae have been described. As many as half of patients affected by chronic changes require surgical treatment. Because perioperative morbidity and mortality are high (30%–50% and 5%–15%, respectively), operative procedures are usually reserved for the most refractory of symptoms, particularly obstruction, perforation, fistulae, and hemorrhage. Those with milder symptoms are preferably managed with antimotility agents, low-fiber diets, and optimal nutrition.

Surgery

Radiation enteritis is one of the most challenging conditions in surgery. Radiation injury may involve any portion of the small intestine, but the terminal ileum is most frequently affected. The cecum and sigmoid colon are the most commonly affected large bowel structures because of their low-lying position. The operative findings often include dense, inflammatory adhesions; unsuspected fistulae and strictures; and brittle, friable tissues. Patients with these complex problems benefit by having surgeons with specific experience in the management of such issues with backup from a high-volume intensive care unit and a good postoperative surgical nutrition support team.

Diagnosis is usually directed by the patient's symptoms. A thorough preoperative evaluation typically includes a small bowel contrast study, a barium enema, and a colonoscopy. Capsule endoscopy is generally avoided when near-obstructing lesions are suspected because of the risk of complete obstruction by the capsule itself. A nutritional preoperative assessment includes calculation of body

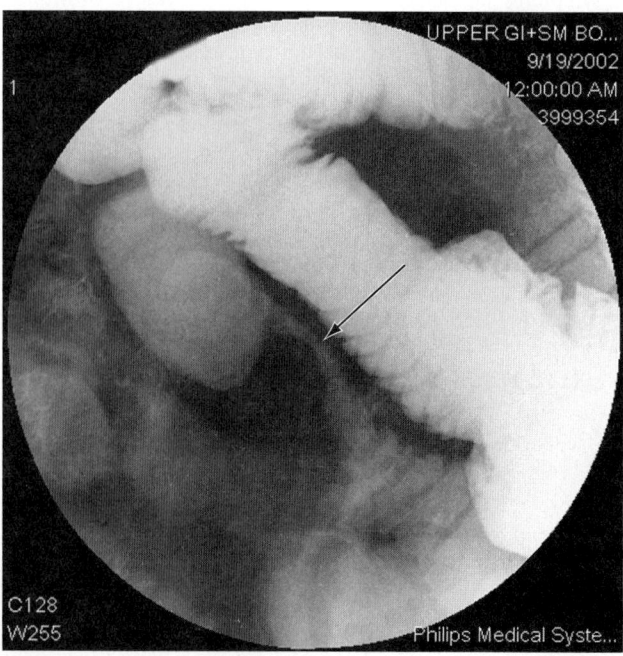

Figure 1   Radiation stricture of the terminal ileum.

Table 2: Surgery for Radiation Enteritis

Ensure adequate nutritional status preoperatively, using total parenteral nutrition if necessary

Consider ureteral stents

Limit lysis of adhesions

Resect and anastomose if possible

Bypass for extensive distal disease and bowel fixed deep in the pelvis

Attempt to use disease-free bowel for the anastomosis for resection or bypass (the transverse colon is often a good target)

The use of stricturoplasty has been limited and should not be used if resection is feasible

Total exclusion is a good option for fistulae in the setting of severe disease or involvement of the irradiated bladder

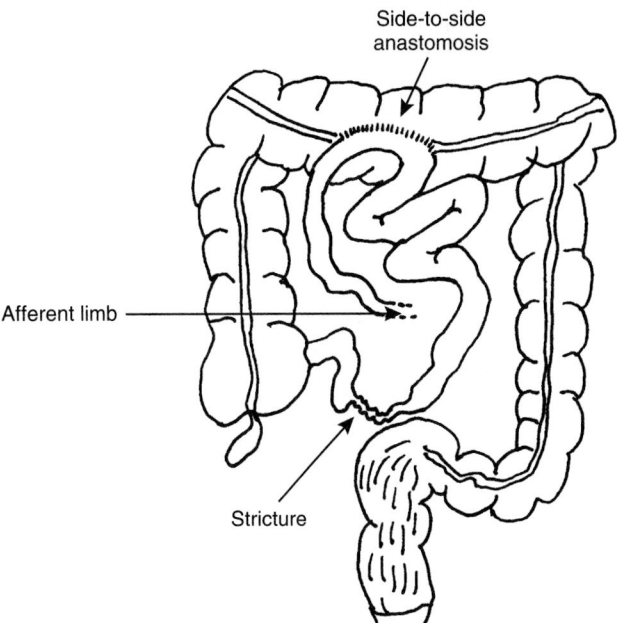

Figure 2 Side-to-side small bowel–transverse colon anastomosis bypassing a strictured segment of terminal ileum. *Adapted from Cameron JL:* Current surgical therapy, *ed 8, Philadelphia, 2004, Elsevier Mosby.*

mass index and measurement of markers of nutritional status such as prealbumin. Most surgeons advocate preoperative total parenteral nutrition (TPN) or oral nutritional supplementation in patients with significant indicators of malnutrition.

In general, operations for small bowel complications typically involve resection and reanastomosis, whereas those for colonic damage entail proximal diversion or resection with temporary diversion. Meticulous dissection and lysis of dense, inflammatory, nonobstructing adhesions to access the area of concern are usually required. Sharp dissection with careful attention to avoid unintended enterotomies is mandatory. Careful inspection and immediate repair of enterotomies and large areas of deserosalization help to prevent the dreaded consequence of postoperative abdominal sepsis and fistula formation. Resection of strictured, fistulized, or ulcerated bowel is currently advocated. Surgeons with experience often emphasize the importance of using nonirradiated intestine for at least one component of any anastomosis, if at all possible. Although there is scant evidence to support this method, it is a practice based on good surgical technique and represents a logical approach (Table 2).

In the past, bypass of obstructed segments was widely practiced. Although the indications for bypass are the same as for resection (primarily obstruction and fistulization), the practice was advocated because of its simplicity and lower risk of harm to adjacent structures (Fig. 2). This technique fails to eradicate diseased tissues, however, and does little to eliminate the risk of bleeding, perforation, abscess formation, and bacterial overgrowth (blind loop syndrome). Additionally, a low but real risk of cancer in the bypassed loop exists, increasing with time. Improvement in stapling devices, suture material, critical care, and nutrition, as well as a better understanding of the nature of the disease itself, has resulted in decreased use of bypass procedures for radiation injuries. Even so, bypass may yet be useful in the ill patient with dense pelvic adhesions and a readily identifiable afferent and efferent loop in whom extensive dissection may be more injurious than helpful. Proximal diversion (loop colostomy) may be definitive treatment for patients with extensive rectal disease for whom proctectomy may confer unacceptable risk. Interposing healthy tissue between suture lines in irradiated bowel or bladder is advocated as a way of reducing the likelihood of fistulization between anastomoses. Omentum usually serves this purpose.

Because the reoperation rate for chronic radiation injury is high (40%), short bowel syndrome is a significant concern when planning any operation for radiation enteritis. Stricturoplasty for short-segment radiation strictures in TPN-dependent patients or those at risk for TPN dependency has been described as an alternative to resection. Both Heineke-Mikulicz and Finney reconstruction are potential methods to preserve small bowel. Although it has

worked well for patients in limited case series with no anastomotic leaks reported, stricturoplasty is advocated only in patients with diffuse enteritis who have few other options available.

Surgery for radiation enteritis must be individualized. Good preoperative patient assessment, sharp dissection, careful tissue handling, quick recognition and repair of enterotomies, and the use of interposing healthy tissue when possible may help to reduce the risk of complications.

Surgical Outcomes

Long-term outcome and life expectancy in patients operated on for complications of chronic radiation enteritis are not well documented. A French surgical cooperative group published the most recent (2001) review of treatment and outcomes from 109 patients operated on for radiation-related complications from 1984 to 1994. Regimbeau and colleagues retrospectively analyzed patient risk factors, distribution of disease, recurrence rates, complications, and survival. Patients undergoing bypass ($n = 42$) were compared with those resected ($n = 65$). The overwhelming indication for surgery was intestinal obstruction from strictures or adhesions (82%). Thirty percent of patients experienced postoperative morbidity, with anastomotic leak occurring in 11 patients, 5 of whom had undergone bypass surgery. Overall operative mortality was 5%, whereas the mortality associated with leak was 18%. Operative morbidity did not correlate with the type of surgical management but was influenced by the urgency of the operation. Emergent procedures resulted in postoperative morbidity of greater than 40%. The reoperation rate was 50% in the bypass group and 34% in the resection group. At the end of the follow-up period, 55% of patients required a stoma. Overall survival in patients without evidence of recurrent cancer ($n = 91$) was 85%, 79%, and 69% at 1, 3, and 5 years, respectively. Patients with bypass had a 5-year survival rate of 51%, whereas those resected had a 71% survival rate in the same period of time. Resecting affected bowel, when possible, is advisable; it appears to reduce the rate of reoperation and is associated with increased survival.

Whether performing resection or bypass, avoidance of anastomotic leak remains a major technical concern. Anastomotic leak rates as high as 37% have been described, but most reported rates are below 10%. Inclusion of nonirradiated bowel in the anastomosis is often advised. The proximal transverse colon is infrequently affected by radiation, thus is often used as the distal end of an anastomosis. Regimbeau and colleagues did not find any difference between the complication rate of small bowel–transverse colon and small bowel–small bowel anastomoses in their cooperative review, but others have. One surgeon noted a leak rate of 50% before 1977, after which he changed his practice, creating only small bowel–transverse colon anastomoses, resulting in a decrease in leak rate to 7% with no other major changes in technique.

RADIATION PROCTITIS

The rectum is the most frequently affected gastrointestinal site of radiation injury. Although the rectum is more resistant to radiation damage than small bowel or colon, its fixed position and close proximity to treated organs make it vulnerable. Damage to the rectum is described as acute or chronic proctitis. It is dose-dependent and associated exclusively with radiation for pelvic malignancies. Acute rectal radiation toxicity affects 50% to 70% of patients receiving radiation and is manifested by cramps, minor bleeding, mucus discharge, tenesmus, and diarrhea. The rectum appears edematous and beefy red, with occasional superficial ulceration or mucosal sloughing. Almost all these cases are self-limited and resolve when treatment ends. It is important to avoid aggressive surgical treatment in patients with acute proctitis. Deep biopsies of mucosa or excision of hemorrhoids in such circumstances provides little benefit and carries significant risk of bleeding, fistula formation, and nonhealing wounds.

Chronic radiation proctitis appears months to years following treatment, with median onset at approximately 1 year. Symptoms are similar to those of acute proctitis, but the rectum is pale and noncompliant, with telangiectasias visible. Strictures and fistulae to adjacent organs may be present. Chronic proctitis may bleed heavily at times, requiring hospitalization and blood transfusion. The estimated incidence of chronic radiation proctitis is unknown, but conservative estimates indicate that approximately 3% of patients are affected after prostate radiation by any method. Although radiation proctitis can be associated with any pelvic malignancy, it is believed to occur most frequently following treatment for prostate cancer.

Treatment and Outcomes

Supportive management of acute radiation proctitis consists of hydration, antidiarrheals, and, in more troublesome cases, steroid or 5-aminosalicylate enemas. Rarely does any significant bleeding occur, and there is no role for operative intervention.

The treatment of chronic radiation proctitis is divided into topical treatments and ablative techniques. Rectal and oral steroid preparations, sucralfate, nonsteroidal anti-inflammatory drugs, and short-chain fatty acid enemas have been used, but none have been shown to be superior to ablative methods and few have compared favorably with placebo. Little evidence supports their routine use. Ablative techniques include topical formalin application, laser, and argon beam coagulation (ABC). Ease of use and efficacy have made formalin application and ABC the most commonly used methods.

Topical formalin is believed to cause a chemical cauterization of the friable mucosal neovessels responsible for bleeding associated with radiation proctitis. Topical formalin in concentrations of 4% is instilled into the rectum directly through a rigid proctoscope by syringe or via soaked gauze pads or long cotton-tipped applicators. The formalin is allowed to remain in contact with mucosa for 2 to 3 minutes and is then evacuated by suction or removal of the applicator. A slight blanching of the mucosa is often visible. The procedure can usually be performed in the office, with no sedation and no bowel preparation other than an enema. The perianal skin is subject to burn and irritation by the formalin and must be carefully protected during application and removal of the chemical.

Complications are rare, with perianal pain and irritation most commonly reported, although anal ulceration and worsening of preexisting rectal strictures have been infrequently observed. Most patients require repetitive applications, usually performed on a weekly or biweekly basis until significant diminution of bleeding occurs. Short-term success rates from small retrospective studies reveal satisfactory control of bleeding in 59% to 100% of patients. Successful responders show minimal relapse at 1 year. No prospective studies of this treatment have been conducted. Quality of life, long-term efficacy, and complication rates are unknown.

Laser therapies include both argon and neodymium:yttrium-aluminum-garnet (Nd:YAG) systems. Because of the equipment expense, need for protective precautions, and risk of bowel perforation, most endoscopists have abandoned these options for endoscopic ABC. The technique involves application of bipolar diathermy current using inert argon gas as a conducting medium. The beam produces an arc of cautery that produces a superficial burn over a large area of affected mucosa. Pooled blood creates a barrier between the arc and the mucosa, however, rendering it ineffective in patients with bleeding at the time of treatment. Patients should have a complete bowel prep before treatment to optimize visualization of the mucosa. Complications are uncommon, but perforation, ulceration, and bleeding have been reported.

As with formalin therapy, repeat ABC treatment is usually required. Two to four applications result in a significant decrease in blood loss in two thirds of patients, with significantly less recurrence and anemia compared with medical therapy. Durability of response appears to be similar to formalin therapy in the short and mid-term (6 months to 1 year).

Fistulae

Radiation-induced rectovaginal and rectourethral fistulae are the most severe consequence of radiation therapy and represent exceedingly difficult management problems. Rectovaginal fistulae may result from technical mistakes such as incorporation of the posterior vaginal cuff in the staple line during low anterior resection following neoadjuvant chemoradiation for rectal cancer. The problem may also occur when anterior rectal tumors involute following radiation therapy, creating a defect in the septum in the area formerly occupied by the tumor. Most patients with rectourethral fistulae have a history of rectal or urethral stricture requiring intervention, rectal biopsy, rectal argon beam therapy, or transurethral prostate resection after radiation.

Diagnosis and localization is usually made by proctoscopy. Contrast studies (barium or Gastrografin enema) may be useful in some cases, and pelvic computed tomography scan or magnetic resonance imaging is required to rule out recurrence or associated abscess. Recurrent malignancy must be ruled out, and small biopsies of the area are often warranted before definitive therapy.

Radiation-induced fistulae will not heal by primary intention. The goals of surgery are to close the fistula, preserve sphincter function if possible, and minimize morbidity and healing time (Table 3). Healthy, nonirradiated tissue must be interposed between the rectum and the vagina or urethra, and temporary urinary or fecal diversion is required (Fig. 3). Permanent diversion with a proximal diverting colostomy or a suprapubic tube is definitive therapy in those with comorbidities precluding surgery. Preoperative considerations for reconstruction include absence of recurrent malignancy, minimal inflammation and fibrosis, and normal

Table 3: Surgical Principles for Rectovaginal/Rectourethral Fistula Repair

1. Fistulae will not heal by secondary intention, even with diversion
2. Malignancy must be ruled out preoperatively
3. Healthy, nonirradiated tissues should be incorporated into the repair (local or free flap)
4. Temporary intestinal diversion is usually necessary

Table 4: Surgical Options for Rectovaginal/Rectourethral Fistulae*

Local Procedures	Abdominal Approaches
Gracilis flap	Rectus flap
Sartorius flap	Resection with colonic J-pouch
Martius flap (labial bulbocavernosus)	Resection with straight colorectal/coloanal anastomosis[†]
Medial fasciocutaneous thigh flap	

*Temporary diverting ostomy is advisable in all cases.
[†]Omental interposition flap should be used between the anastomosis and the radiated rectum or urethra, if possible.

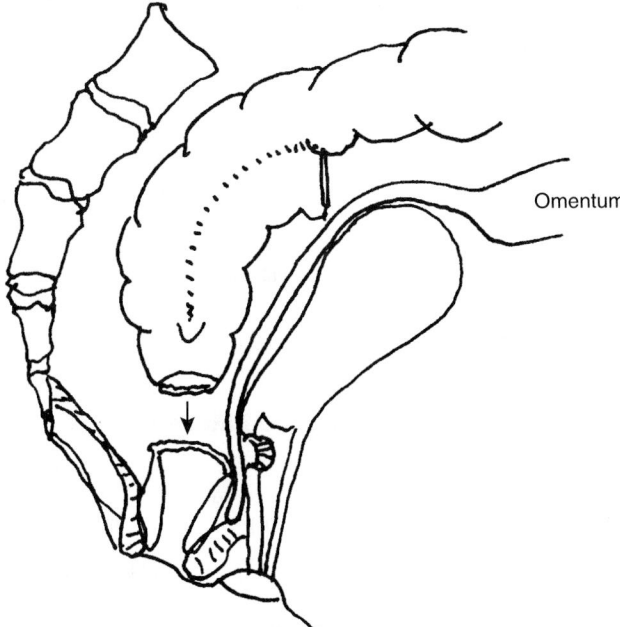

Omentum

Figure 3 Abdominal approach to a midlevel rectovaginal fistula demonstrating the use of a colon J-pouch. The coloanal anastomosis is below the level of the posterior vaginal defect, which is left open to granulate closed. This may also be done with a straight anastomosis. The omental flap is an important additional buttress between the vagina and colon, serving to separate the strictures and reduce the probability of recurrent fistulazation. *Adapted from Cameron JL:* Current surgical therapy, *ed 8, Philadelphia, 2004, Elsevier Mosby.*

continence. Options for surgical reconstruction depend on where the fistula is located. Low and mid-rectovaginal and rectourethral fistulae may be amenable to perineal approaches using local flaps. High fistulae, however, are almost always better treated by excising the affected rectum via an abdominal approach and advancing nonirradiated colon to an anastomosis below the fistula site. Using a buccal mucosa free flap is a described method for reconstructing a large urethral defect. Other options for both rectourethral and rectovaginal fistulae include gracilis and rectus pedicle flaps, as well as omental interposition following rectal resection (Table 4).

Surgical Strategies for Prevention of Radiation Enteritis

The introduction of three-dimensional conformal radiation therapy and intensity modulated radiation therapy has been the most significant advance in reducing radiation morbidity. Improved technology has resulted in more specific radiation delivery in doses that are better tolerated. Multiple radiation angles and fields reduce the dose to any one surrounding organ while maximizing impact at the target. Postoperative radiotherapy may be indicated for patients following major extirpative abdominal procedures for gynecologic, prostate, or rectal malignancies. Pelvic surgery increases the probability of radiation enteritis or proctitis by causing adhesions that fix loops of bowel in place and subjecting them to repeated episodes of irradiation. It may also open up extraperitoneal spaces from which bowel was previously excluded by the pelvic peritoneum. Surgically excluding bowel from the pelvis in cases requiring adjuvant radiation is a well-described strategy for prevention of radiation injury. However, no prospective data documenting a superior approach or long-term efficacy exist. The approach may be tailored to the patient's anatomy. The simplest technique is to simply fill the pelvis with the retroverted uterus, if available. Closing redundant retroperitoneal tissue over the pelvic inlet just below the sacral promontory, carefully avoiding the ureters is an alternative, if possible. The best-described and most commonly used techniques involve creation of an omental sling sewn to the retroperitoneum. Careful suture placement is required to prevent damage or occlusion of ureters. All described techniques involve suturing omentum to the ascending and descending colon and retroperitoneum above the level of the sacral promontory, using the omental tissue itself as a sling or hammock encasing the small bowel and excluding it from the pelvis. In the absence of native tissue, an absorbable mesh sling such as Vicryl can be used to close off the pelvic inlet by suturing a single layer to the parietal peritoneum circumferentially from the level of the umbilicus to the sacral promontory. Complications can include small bowel obstruction from herniation through gaps in the mesh and obstruction from adhesions. Securing the mesh or omentum with a running suture may reduce this risk.

SUGGESTED READINGS

Denton AS, Andreyev HJN, Forbes A, and others: Systematic review for non-surgical interventions for the management of late radiation proctitis, *Br J Cancer* 87:134, 2002.

Regimbeau JM, Panis Yves, and others: Operative and long term results after surgery for chronic radiation enteritis, *Am J Surg* 182:237, 2001.

Tagkalidis PP, Tjandra JJ: Chronic radiation proctitis, *ANZ J Surg* 71:230, 2001.

Waddell BE, Rodriquez-Bigas MA, Lee RJ, and others: Prevention of chronic radiation enteritis, *J Am Coll Surg* 189:611, 1999.

SURGERY OF THE POLYPOSIS SYNDROMES

James M. Church, MD

INTRODUCTION

Hereditary colorectal cancer syndromes are rare, accounting for less than 5% of all colorectal cancers. However, although these syndromes are rare, the patients and families affected by them present unique challenges to their caregivers. Issues of screening, diagnosis, timing and nature of surgery, and follow-up apply to several organs and require specialized knowledge and experience. Hereditary colorectal cancer syndromes can be conveniently considered as those associated with polyposis and those without polyposis. The "flagship" of hereditary colorectal cancer polyposis syndromes is familial adenomatous polyposis (FAP), which is most common and on which many of the principles of treatment of other syndromes are based. Other polyposis syndromes include *MYH* associated polyposis (MAP), hyperplastic polyposis (HPP), and the hamartomatous polyposes (Peutz-Jehger's syndrome [PJS]), juvenile polyposis (JPS), and *PTEN* hamartoma tumor syndrome (PHTS). The hereditary nonpolyposis colorectal cancer syndromes are Lynch syndrome and family cancer syndrome X. The purpose of this chapter is to review the surgical treatment of the hereditary colorectal polyposis syndrome and to provide the current surgical strategies for managing affected patients.

OVERVIEW OF CARE

Care of patients with hereditary colorectal cancer is best provided in a multidisciplinary setting in which counseling, gastroenterology, and surgery appointments can be coordinated and schedules made that are appropriate for each family and each patient. Experience, expertise, and interest are important components of a unit that will face complex decision making and that must understand the intricacies of making a genetic diagnosis. There are relatively few centers with the necessary level of interest, experience, and expertise, but those that exist are open to requests for consultation, so that the individual health care provider need not face the challenges of hereditary colorectal polyposis alone.

FAMILIAL ADENOMATOUS POLYPOSIS

Familial adenomatous polyposis (FAP) is an autosomal dominantly inherited syndrome of colorectal cancer predisposition caused by a germline mutation of *APC*. *APC* is a key "gateway" tumor suppressor gene in the Wnt/wingless pathway, by which cell growth is inhibited or enhanced. *APC* has several other functions in the cell, including cell-cell adhesion (via e-cadherin), chromosomal segregation, microtubule assembly, cell cycle regulation, and apoptosis (programmed cell death). Sporadic *APC* mutations or loss of heterozygosity are involved in a high proportion of sporadic colorectal cancers, underlining the importance of the protein in tumor suppression.

Mutations in *APC* usually cause a truncated protein by creating a "stop" codon that halts protein transcription. The clinical effect of a mutation seems to depend in part on its location in the gene,

reflective of a "genotype-phenotype association" that is at times important in determining surgical strategy. Mutations at the beginning of the gene (exons 3 and 4) almost always cause an attenuated form of polyposis, with fewer than 100 adenomas and a cancer risk that is delayed at least 2 decades compared with classic FAP. Mutations at the other end of the gene (the 3′ end of exon 15) are also associated with attenuated polyposis but confer a high risk of desmoid disease. Severe polyposis (>1000 adenomas) is found with the "hot-spot" mutation in codon 1309, and with other mutations close by, in exon 15G. Although this genotype suggests that early radical surgery is indicated, this is usually obvious from the clinical presentation. There does not seem to be a particular genotype that favors the upper gastrointestinal manifestations of FAP (fundic gland polyps and duodenal adenomas). However, other important genotype-phenotype associations involve Gardner's syndrome (the combination of polyposis and osteomas, epidermoid cysts, extra teeth, and desmoids, found with mutations in codons 1220–1440), and congenital hypertrophy of the retinal pigmented epithelium (CHRPE) (codons 840–1220). Although genotype-phenotype correlations are helpful in managing patients, they are not exact. There can be significant intrafamilial variation in expression of the same mutation, suggesting that modifying genes or factors are operating.

Cancer Risk in Familial Adenomatous Polyposis

Almost all patients carrying a germline *APC* mutation will develop colorectal cancer, with the median age at diagnosis approximately 39 years. This risk is most obvious in patients who are diagnosed by symptoms in which the incidence of colorectal cancer at diagnosis is greater than 60%. When patients are asymptomatic, the incidence of cancer at presentation drops significantly. Colorectal cancer is rare in teenage FAP patients, allowing surgery to be delayed until physical and social maturity is reached.

Extracolonic cancers in FAP may occur in several organs. The duodenum is most commonly affected, with cancers of the stomach, thyroid (papillary carcinoma usually in women), liver (hepatoblastoma in children), bile ducts, adrenal, and brain also seen.

Aims of Colorectal Surgery in Familial Adenomatous Polyposis

Surgery cannot cure disease caused by an inherited mutation. The primary aim of colorectal surgery in FAP is to prevent death from colorectal cancer. Because this involves removal of all or almost all of the large intestine, the functional outcomes of surgery and their effects on quality of life are important. This is especially so in young, often asymptomatic patients who are at a critical time in their social, academic, and physical development. To take such young, carefree men and women and create symptoms of fecal seepage, stool frequency, incontinence, and anal irritation is not desirable. Decisions about the timing and type of prophylactic colorectal surgery in a patient with FAP are therefore critical.

Timing of Surgery

In general, symptomatic patients who are discovered to have FAP undergo their surgery without undue delay. Their risk of cancer is high, and colonoscopy can identify suspicious-looking lesions. An accurate examination of the rectum to exclude cancer is essential because neoadjuvant chemoradiation should be used liberally here to prevent the need for postoperative radiation, which may cause irreparable and permanent damage to an ileal pouch. In patients in whom an accurate rectal examination is not possible in the office, examination under anesthesia is recommended.

Asymptomatic patients diagnosed by genetic or endoscopic screening do not always require quick surgery. A full colonoscopy allows assessment of the severity of the polyposis (see Table 1), and if the polyposis is mild or attenuated, surgery may be deferred. If surgery is deferred indefinitely, colonoscopy should be done at least yearly to guard against progression of the polyposis and the appearance of cancer. The ideal time for prophylactic colectomy is in the late teens and early 20s. At this time, there is usually physical and emotional maturity, and with laparoscopic technique the downtime associated with surgery is short. Bowel function in the young shows a greater capacity to adapt to colectomy or proctocolectomy and pouch, although even a temporary ileostomy can be distressing to teenagers or young adults.

Recently there has been a trend to try to delay surgery in patients at high risk of developing desmoid tumors. Because 80% of mesenteric desmoids follow abdominal surgery, and there is no predictably effective treatment other than adriamycin-based

chemotherapy, the rationale is that by delaying surgery, the development of desmoids may be delayed. This approach is reasonable because the risk of desmoids is inversely related to the severity of polyposis. However, its effectiveness has not been measured objectively.

TYPE OF SURGERY

When the decision to perform colon surgery for FAP has been made, the type of surgery must be chosen. There are three main options: colectomy and ileorectal anastomosis (IRA), proctocolectomy and ileal-anal pouch anastomosis (IPAA), and proctocolectomy and ileostomy. Each of these choices has its advantages and disadvantages, listed in Table 2. Table 3 shows the breakdown of primary prophylactic colorectal surgery performed for FAP at the Cleveland Clinic over 50 years from 1950. The effect of the advent of the ileal-anal pouch can be seen.

Colectomy and Ileorectal Anastomosis

Colectomy and IRA has been used for treatment of FAP since 1919. It removes the risk of colonic cancer while preserving reasonable bowel function and per anal defecation. The advent and spread of laparoscopic techniques in colon surgery has made this a relatively trauma-free procedure, and it is the operation of choice for patients with attenuated and mild polyposis, as defined in Table 1. Points of technique are as follows.

1. In a slim woman, it may be possible to perform the colectomy and IRA through a Pfannenstiel incision without laparoscopic equipment. A preoperative erect abdominal x-ray (KUB) will usually show the position of the flexures and give an indication

Table 1: Severity of Colorectal Polyposis

Severity	Number of Polyps
Oligopolyposis	3–100
Attenuated FAP	<100
Mild FAP	100–1000
Classical FAP	>1000
Profuse FAP	"Carpeting"

FAP, Familial adenomatous polyposis.

Table 2: The Surgical Options in Familial Adenomatous Polyposis

	Ileorectal Anastomosis	Ileal Pouch-Anal Anastomosis, Hand sewn	Ileal Pouch-Anal Anastomosis, Stapled	Proctocolectomy and Ileostomy
Advantages	Simple surgery No stoma Good function No impact on ability to conceive No threat to pelvic nerves	Removes almost all colorectal mucosa	Removes almost all colorectal mucosa Function good	Removes all the colorectal mucosa Lowest rate of complication No anal symptoms
Disadvantages	Risk of rectal cancer	Function unpredictable Complex surgery Highest rate of complications Decrease in ability of a woman to conceive Possibility of damaging pelvic nerves Temporary stoma Risk of anastomotic and pouch neoplasia	Complex surgery Temporary stoma Risk of anastomotic, ATZ and pouch neoplasia Decrease in ability of a woman to conceive Possibility of damaging pelvic nerves	Permanent ileostomy Risk of damage to pelvic nerves
Indications	<20 rectal adenomas <1000 colorectal adenomas	>20 rectal adenomas >1000 colorectal adenomas, or colorectal cancer Adenomas in ATZ	>20 rectal adenomas >1000 colorectal adenomas, or colorectal cancer ATZ clear	Ultra low rectal cancer Inability to have pouch because of inadequate mesenteric length (often desmoids) or poor sphincter function

ATZ, Anal transition zone.

Table 3: Colorectal Surgery for Familial Adenomatous Polyposis at the Cleveland Clinic, Cleveland: 1950–2000

	Pre-Pouch Era, 1950 to 1982	Pouch Era, 1983 to 2000
Ileorectal anastomosis	69	168
Ileal-anal pouch anastomosis	0	139
TPC, ileostomy	5	9
Total	74	306

TPC, Total protocolectomy.

whether this nonlaparoscopic, minimally invasive technique is possible.

2. Remove the entire colon. For ease of postoperative surveillance, there should not be a rectosigmoid angle. This means taking the resection into the rectum, as indicated by confluence of the tenia. This usually leaves a 15-cm rectum. Leaving less than 10 cm is likely to have an adverse impact on bowel function. For older patients, over age 60 years, who usually have attenuated polyposis, leaving some sigmoid colon is reasonable to prevent disabling diarrhea. The downside to this is the need to pass the sigmoidoscope around the rectosigmoid for postoperative surveillance.
3. Use oncologic technique. Occasionally an unsuspected cancer is present in the colon or rectum. Therefore the surgeon takes the omentum with the specimen, divides the mesenteric vessels high up, and opens the specimen before it leaves the operating room.
4. An ileorectal anastomosis can be tricky because the terminal ileum and upper rectum have different diameters and wall thicknesses. Although there are multiple technical options for the anastomosis, an end-to-end, hand-sewn anastomosis is safe.
5. Laparoscopic mobilization of the colon minimizes the length of incisions, an important consideration in young, active patients. It may reduce the risk of desmoid disease.
6. The mesenteric defect at the ileorectal anastomosis is closed, or there may be herniation of a loop of small intestine through it.
7. If there are a few large rectal polyps, it is advisable to remove these ahead of the IRA so that cancer can be excluded. Small polyps need not be treated because there is a 60% chance that these will regress spontaneously postoperatively.
8. The specimen is opened in the operating room and palpated for areas of hardness that may signal cancer. If there are suspicious areas, the surgeon ensures that the resection was as radical as is possible.

Postoperatively the course is usually smooth, especially if the surgery has been minimally invasive and the patient is young. If the pathology report shows no cancer and the preoperative proctoscopy did not show any worrisome lesions, the first surveillance proctoscopy can be in a year.

Total Proctocolectomy and Ileorectal Anastomosis

Publicized by Sir Alan Parks in the late 1970s, the technique of total proctocolectomy and ileorectal anastomosis (IRA) has evolved over the ensuing 27 years. From an S-pouch with a long mucosectomy and a long cuff of rectal muscle to a J-pouch and a stapled anastomosis just above the dentate line, the surgery has become safer and quicker and has a better functional outcome. Controversy still exists, however, regarding the place of mucosectomy and hand-sewn IPAA and the use of a temporary ileostomy for fecal diversion while the pouch heals. It is again important to remember that FAP

is not cured by surgery and that the surgery is tailored to the severity of the disease in any particular patient. Thus when the anal transition zone (ATZ) is clear of polyps, a stapled IPAA is reasonable. When the ATZ is involved by adenomas, it should be stripped out. Either way, yearly surveillance is necessary because there are reports of cancer in the area of the ATZ after each technique for IPAA. Although mucosectomy reduces the rate of ATZ neoplasia, it does not eliminate it, so yearly surveillance must continue. The issue of a one-stage versus two-stage IPAA is more difficult to decide. In favor of a one-stage pouch is the fact that patients are generally asymptomatic, especially compared with patients who have active colitis. Furthermore, they are on no immunosuppressive medications and, apart from the polyps, have a healthy bowel. They should have a low risk of a leaking anastomosis or pouch. On the other hand, pouch leaks can occur even in patients with FAP, and in a young, relatively asymptomatic person, they can be disastrous. It is also apparent that when a newly constructed IPPA is not diverted, postoperative ileus is often prolonged, and even when the ileus resolves, bowel function is suboptimal. This is then an individualized decision made after weighing the pros and cons for each patient.

An IPAA is not made entirely with minimally invasive techniques. After mobilization of the colon, a Pfannenstiel incision is used to allow construction of the pouch. This leads to the potential problem of making a right lower quadrant ileostomy and then closing the Pfannenstiel incision. The closure may disturb the alignment of the layers in the abdominal wall and cause some obstructive "shuttering" of the ileostomy. Other points of techniques are as follows.

1. An oncologic technique is used. Occasionally an unsuspected cancer is present in the colon or rectum. Therefore the surgeon takes the mesenteric vessels high up and opens the specimen before it leaves the operating room.
2. It is important to determine how easily the apex of the ileum will reach the anus before the rectum is removed. In obese men, there may be a significant amount of tension on the mesentery, and leaving a small amount of rectum is reasonable if there are no concerning polyps in this area. Mucosectomy should not be performed unless the surgeon is fairly certain that the pouch will reach to the dentate line.
3. Other techniques to reduce tension on the pouch mesentery include making a series of transverse incisions in the peritoneum over the superior mesenteric artery, constructing an S-pouch instead of a J-pouch and ensuring that mobilization of the mesentery is complete up to the pancreas. The length of a J-pouch is determined by its lead point being the apex of the superior mesenteric artery.
4. The surgeon ensures that the pouch mesentery is straight.
5. When a stapled anastomosis is performed, guide the stapler cartridge through the anus with a hand supporting the rectal stump from within the pelvis. This prevents inadvertent perforation of the transverse staple line by the cartridge.
6. If the upper anus is stapled off approximately 2 cm above the dentate line with a 30-mm transverse stapler, and a 33-mm circular stapler is used for the anastomosis, 1 cm more of anus will be removed in the donut, and the entire transverse staple line may be excised. This gives a "single" staple anastomosis within 1 cm of the dentate line, which is perfect.
7. The anastomosis is tested by insufflating air through a rigid proctoscope with the pelvis full of saline.
8. If there is a leak in a patient in whom there is some tension at the anastomosis, it is better to drain the pelvis from above, place a 30-F Foley catheter in the pouch, and perform an ileostomy. Attempts at transanal repair of the leak are usually unsuccessful and may tear the pouch. In a patient with FAP with healthy tissues, the leak will often heal spontaneously.
9. The ileostomy should be as close to the pouch as possible.

Total Proctocolectomy and Ileostomy

The now largely historic options of total proctocolectomy and end ileostomy, or continent ileostomy, still have some advantages to offer patients. Both procedures guarantee complete excision of the colorectal mucosa, something that IRA and IPAA cannot. Both procedures avoid anal incontinence and seepage, and the end ileostomy offers a minimal chance of further intestinal surgery. The great disadvantage of the continent ileostomy is its potential for complications that require pouch revision, but well-motivated patients are sometimes prepared to undergo multiple revisions to keep their continent ileostomy. Continent ileostomy is an option that should be considered only when an experienced surgeon is available to perform the surgery and its follow-up.

RECTAL CANCER AFTER ILEORECTAL ANASTOMOSIS

The literature is full of reports of relatively high rates of rectal cancer after an IRA, reaching up to 42% at 30 years of follow-up. However, interpretation of this literature must take into account the limited surgical options for patients with FAP operated before IPAA had been described. In pre-pouch days, patients with severe polyposis usually underwent IRA because the only alternative was an end ileostomy. Now such patients have an IPAA as their primary procedure. Therefore reports of cancer in IRAs performed before the pouch era are irrelevant to a consideration of IRA now, when only patients with mild or attenuated polyposis are offered that option.

THE EFFECT OF DESMOIDS ON SURGERY

Desmoid disease is found in 31% of patients with FAP and consists of fibromatous plaques or tumors that usually develop intra-abdominally, where they cause puckering and scarring of adjacent tissues. The most common location is in the small bowel mesentery, often at the root. Mesenteric desmoid disease interferes with mobilization of the small intestine and, when found during pouch surgery, may prevent a pouch from being made or from reaching the bottom of the pelvis. If a pouch will reach, desmoid disease may make the creation of an ileostomy impossible. Most often desmoid disease develops after the primary prophylactic surgery, causing bowel obstruction or intestinal fistulae.

Not all FAP patients have an equal risk of desmoid disease. Desmoids are part of Gardner's syndrome and occur with increasing frequency as the germline mutation is found more often at $3'$ of codon 1220. Women develop desmoids more frequently than men, and most desmoids develop within 5 years of an abdominal surgery. Patients who are found, by virtue of their genotype or phenotype, to be at risk for desmoid disease should be counseled that the proposed surgery may not be possible or that the surgical strategy may have to be changed if desmoids are found. Thus a proposed IPAA may become an IRA or an end ileostomy if desmoid disease is found.

FUNCTIONAL RESULTS AND QUALITY OF LIFE

There is no doubt that an ileorectal anastomosis offers an excellent quality of life. Ileorectal anastomosis in which the rectum is preserved results in an acceptable number of stools per day (average four) with minimal urgency and incontinence. Young patients do especially well because they are able to adapt to the change in their physiology almost seamlessly. However, as patients with an IRA age, they are at risk of developing urgency and incontinence. In elderly patients, particularly when there has been scarring resulting from multiple polyp coagulations, the rectum loses its compliance and the sphincters begin to lose some of their strength. The main difference between a rectum and an ileal pouch is that the rectum has effective peristalsis: it can propel stool outward and therefore create urgency. By contrast an ileal pouch has no effective peristalsis and must empty by gravity or increased abdominal pressure brought about by straining. Thus incomplete evacuation is a common problem in pouch patients, leading to frequent defecation and seepage. Patients with an IPAA should be advised to keep their stool somewhat liquid and to take enough time on the toilet to allow efficient emptying of their pouch. A recent meta-analysis of 12 studies comparing IRA and IPAA in 1002 patients showed that bowel frequency, nocturnal defecation, and use of pads were all more frequent in the IPAA group. Predictably IPAA patients had less urgency (as discussed earlier). There was no difference between IRA and IPAA in the incidence of bowel obstruction, postoperative hemorrhage, anastomotic leak, and wound infection.

CONTROL OF NEOPLASIA

Although neoplasia often occurs in the rectum after an IRA, recent studies have shown that it also may occur in the ileal pouch, the ATZ, and even in an ileostomy because the combination of the *APC* mutation and stasis of stool brings about the genetic sequence that has its culmination in an adenoma. The time to postsurgical neoplasia varies according to the organ; for the rectum, it is often 3 to 4 years. For the ileal pouch, it is 5 years and more; for the ATZ it is 3 years or more, and for the ileostomy, it is 15 to 20 years. Therefore continued surveillance is necessary.

FLEXIBLE ENDOSCOPY

The rectum, ATZ, and pouch are best examined using a flexible sigmoidoscope. In patients with a narrowed IPAA, a pediatric scope may be necessary. Two enemas are given as a preparation, and additional enemas may be required if the preparation is inadequate. No compromise in the adequacy of the preparation is allowable because advanced polyps and cancers can be flat and are easily covered by stool. The examination must be as comfortable and discrete as possible so that a high level of compliance with further examinations is encouraged. The bowel is inspected carefully, and polyps greater than 5 mm are snared. Polyps less than 5 mm, unless they are ulcerated or suspicious in other respects, can be left alone. The ATZ is carefully inspected on withdrawal, and if adenomatous epithelium is seen, an examination under anaesthesia is necessary to treat it. Air is aspirated as completely as possible before the scope is removed.

Steadily increasing numbers and size of adenomas are evidence of increasing instability of the rectal and pouch mucosa. Vogel and Church published a score incorporating the number, size, and histology of the polyps, analogous to the Spigelman staging system for duodenal adenomas, which may help in deciding when proctectomy is necessary. In patients with an IRA, proctectomy must be considered in the light of the patient's comorbidity, age, body shape, and preferences. Chemoprevention is an alternative to proctectomy, and both celecoxib and sulindac are effective in minimizing the number of adenomas. Careful examinations must continue, however, because cases of cancer have been described in patients whose polyps were apparently abrogated by sulindac. Chemoprevention seems most appropriate in the ileal pouch because pouch removal leads to a permanent stoma.

TRANSANAL EXCISION

In some patients with a stapled IPAA, the ATZ becomes covered by adenomas. In this case, the residual ATZ must be stripped out completely and the pouch advanced to the dentate line. The less residual anorectal mucosa there is, the easier the procedure. If there is 4 cm or more of residual ATZ and rectal mucosa, abdominal pouch mobilization and a repeat IPAA accomplished hand sewn is the preferred treatment. Certainly 3 cm or less of ATZ can readily be stripped out from below by a transanal approach. A smart strategy is to perform the procedure in two stages, working on half the circumference at each stage and allowing healing between stages. In this way, the tendency to create a stenosis at the anastomosis is avoided.

PROCTECTOMY AND SECONDARY TOTAL PROCTOCOLECTOMY AND ILEORECTAL ANASTOMOSIS

If rectal polyposis develops in a patient with an IRA, if a large villous lesion is seen, or if a lesion with severe dysplasia or invasive cancer is found, proctectomy is indicated. Reoperative surgery in patients with FAP can be difficult because of the intense adhesions that some patients generate or the inflammatory adhesions caused by chronic rectal cautery. Furthermore, desmoid disease may make the rectal excision challenging and the creation of an IPAA impossible. Patients must be informed of the possibility of ending up with a permanent ileostomy. The principles of reoperative surgery are as follows.

1. Where planes are obliterated, work close to the organ being dissected.
2. Ureteric stents should be used to allow easier identification of the ureters.
3. The pelvis is entered behind the superior rectal artery and dissected posteriorly in the plane between the fascia propria of the rectum and the presacral fascia.
4. Before performing a mucosectomy, the surgeon estimates the potential reach of a J-pouch.
5. The surgeon should remain close to the low rectum anteriorly to avoid entering the vagina or damaging the nervii erigentes.
6. The terminal ileum above an IRA is often considerably dilated. This does not mean that the pouch can be shorter because the dilatation confers no benefit in terms of pouch function.

SURGERY FOR DESMOID TUMORS AND THEIR COMPLICATIONS

Desmoid disease presents a wide variety of clinical situations, ranging from white plaques or sheets on the mesentery that pucker the bowel and may cause an obstruction to huge intra-abdominal tumors that can cause fistulae, hemorrhage, or free perforation. The primary treatment of intra-abdominal desmoid tumors in FAP is medical, using a variety of drugs that include nonsteroidal anti-inflammatory agents such as celecoxib and sulindac, estrogen-blocking drugs such as tamoxifen and raloxifen, and chemotherapeutic drugs such as vinblastine, methotrexate, and adriamycin. Surgery for intra-abdominal desmoids is a remedy of last resort, because the tumor infiltrates the root of the small bowel mesentery and welds it to the retroperitoneum. Complete excision is rarely possible and is achieved at the cost of resection of large amounts of small intestine. Even then, the risk of recurrence of the desmoid tumor is high. Typically complications of the desmoid, such as obstruction

Table 4: A Staging System for Intra-Abdominal Desmoid Tumors

Stage I	Asymptomatic disease that is not growing and <10 cm in maximum diameter
Stage II	Minimally symptomatic disease that is not growing or >10 cm maximum diameter
Stage III	Symptomatic disease, slowly growing, or obstructive complications
Stage IV	Symptomatic disease, rapidly growing, or severe complications (e.g., fistula)

From Church J, Berk T, Boman BM, and others: Dis Colon Rectum 48:1528, 2005; used with permission.

and fistula, can be dealt with by bypass or proximal diversion. The surgical strategy is to mobilize bowel above and below the area of involvement with the desmoid and then assess how much bowel is at risk, how much normal bowel is present away from the desmoid, and the likely functional sequelae of bypass or diversion. The worst situation occurs when an attempt is made to excise the desmoid or liberate involved bowel, and holes are made in the small bowel that cannot be effectively repaired or diverted. The surgeon is committed to resection, which may be a difficult, bloody procedure. It is better to back out before this happens. Treatment of intra-abdominal desmoids can be guided by a desmoid staging system, shown in Table 4.

Abdominal wall tumors present a different situation. These tumors are more readily excised, and the recurrence rate is low. These tumors, if growing, should undergo early surgery because the larger they are, the larger the abdominal wall defect that must be corrected. They are excised with a 1-cm margin, and the defect is filled with synthetic material such as Gortex. Postoperatively, prophylactic sulindac (150 mg twice daily) may help to prevent or delay recurrence.

SURGERY FOR UPPER GASTROINTESTINAL TRACT POLYPS

Duodenal/periampullary cancer is the second most common malignancy in FAP and the third most common cause of death. The combination of bile, adenomatous mucosa, and a mutated *APC* seems to promote neoplasia. Adenomas cluster around the duodenal papilla, and 50% of normal-appearing papillae have adenomatous mucosa. More than 90% of FAP patients develop duodenal adenomas, but fewer than 10% ever develop cancer. All patients are entered into a program of surveillance using esophagogastroduodenoscopy at regular intervals, with the time between scopes being determined by the Spigelman severity score for duodenal polyposis. This score is presented in Table 5. A recent study by Groves and colleagues showed that the risk of cancer was 0 in

Table 5: The Spigelman Staging System* for Upper Gastrointestinal Manifestations of Familial Adenomatous Polyposis

Points	1	2	3
Number of polyps	1–4	5–20	>20
Size of polyps (mm)	1–4	5–10	>10
Histology	Tubular	Tubulovillous	Villous
Dysplasia	Mild	Moderate	Severe

*Spigelman stage I, score 1–4; stage II, score 5–6; stage III, score 7–8; stage IV, score 9–12.

patients with Spigelman stage I neoplasia in the duodenum, 2% with score II, 2% with stage III, and 36% with stage IV. Patients with a score of IV are clearly at high risk of developing duodenal cancer and should be offered a pancreas-preserving duodenectomy. Patients with biopsy-proved cancer that is resectable should undergo a pancreatico-duodenectomy. Mackey and colleagues recently reported a series of 21 patients undergoing pancreas-preserving duodenal resection for advanced duodenal neoplasia. There were no deaths, a complication rate of 38%, and a low recurrence rate (9.5% at 6.5 years follow-up).

OTHER POLYPOSES

MYH-Associated Polyposis

MYH-associated polyposis is a recessively inherited syndrome of colorectal adenomatous polyposis and cancer that is due to inheriting biallelic mutation in *MYH*. *MYH* is a gene involved in the base-excision repair pathway that repairs oxidative damage to the DNA. Defective oxidative repair predisposes to G-C to A-T transversions in the DNA, causing mutations and, in particular, mutations in *APC*. These secondary *APC* mutations cause a syndrome of mild and attenuated polyposis, with 2 or 3 to more than 700 synchronous colorectal adenomas, colorectal cancer, and possibly upper gastrointestinal polyps as well.

Patients with MAP typically have oligo (<100) polyposis and a weak family history of colorectal cancer. Genetic testing for *MYH* mutations is reasonable in patients with more than 10 synchronous adenomas and either a weak or an absent family history of colorectal cancer. In practical terms, if the adenomas can be controlled endoscopically, this is a satisfactory alternative, although it means frequent colonoscopies and polypectomies. If the adenoma burden clearly cannot be dealt with or controlled endoscopically, then colectomy is needed. The definition of a "colonoscopically controllable" polyp burden is likely to vary according to the expertise and patience of the endoscopists. The technique of colectomy is similar to that for colectomy and ileorectal anastomosis in FAP.

Hyperplastic Polyposis

Hyperplastic polyposis is uncommon but carries a high risk of colorectal cancer. It is defined as at least 30 hyperplastic polyps scattered around the colon and rectum, or at least 5 hyperplastic polyps proximal to the sigmoid colon of which at least 2 are greater than 10 mm in size, or any number of hyperplastic polyps in a patient with a first-degree relative who has hyperplastic polyposis. Hyperplastic polyposis predisposes to colorectal cancer by the methylator phenotype in which excess methylation throughout the DNA causes inactivation of a number of tumor suppressor genes. Histologically the CIMP (CpG island methylator phenotype) produces serrated polyps, including serrated adenomas and mixed hyperplastic/adenomatous polyps. Ultimately the patients develop a CIMP cancer. Review of the literature of hyperplastic polyposis shows a rate of associated colorectal cancer of approximately 50%, with cancers occurring at presentation or after diagnosis while patients are on surveillance. Therefore colectomy and IRA is a reasonable option in patients with an unstable colorectal epithelium as evidenced by recurrent polyps despite frequent colonoscopies.

Hamartomatous Polyposes

There are three major syndromes of hamartomatous polyposis, with varying risks of colorectal cancer. These are summarized in Table 6.

Peutz-Jegher Syndrome

The Peutz-Jegher syndrome (PJS) is due to autosomal dominant inheritance of a mutation in *STK11*. It is characterized by hamartomatous polyps that occur mostly in the small intestine but also the colon, stomach, and duodenum. Peutz-Jeghers hamartomas are distinguished from juvenile polyps by the presence of smooth muscle bundles in the submucosa that give the polyps a "branching tree" appearance. Polyps in PJS can displace the underlying epithelium and appear as a pseudo-carcinomatous invasion of the muscularis mucosa.

PJS is defined as the presence of Peutz-Jegher polyps and at least two of the following: a positive family history, hyperpigmentation of the lips and buccal mucosa, and small bowel polyposis.

Patients with PJS often present in the first or second decade of life with bowel obstruction resulting from intussusception of a small bowel polyp. Often, surgery is needed to resect the intussuscepting polyp. At this time, a thorough search of the entire gastrointestinal tract for other polyps is made, and all lesions are removed or cauterized. This "clean sweep" approach results in fewer repeat laparotomies than treating only the symptomatic lesions. Recently surveillance of these patients has become easier with capsule endoscopy replacing push endoscopy of the small bowel. Esophagogastroduodenoscopy, capsule endoscopy and colonoscopy are indicated every 3 to 4 years, depending on the finding of the most recent examinations.

As shown in Table 6, patients with PJS are at high risk of a range of extracolonic cancers. Screening for these tumors is an important part of management of these patients.

Table 6: Summary of the Hereditary Hamartomatous Polyposes

Syndrome	Genes	Location of Polyps	Extracolonic Cancers	Risk of Colorectal Cancer	Surgery
Peutz-Jehgers syndrome	STK11	Stomach, small bowel, colorectum	Pancreas, lung, breast, ovary, testis, esophagus, endometrium	84x	Treat complications, such as intussusception with small bowel obstruction; "clean sweep"
Juvenile polyposis	SMAD4, BMPRIA	Stomach, small bowel, colon	Nil	9% to 50%	Colectomy and IRA vs. IPAA
PHTS	PTEN	Colon	Thyroid, breast, endometrium	No increased risk	Colectomy and IRA if there are "dangerous" polyps

IPAA, Ieal-anal pouch anastomosis; *IRA,* ileorectal anastomosis.

Juvenile Polyposis

Juvenile polyposis is an autosomal dominantly inherited syndrome featuring the presence of multiple juvenile polyps. Juvenile polyps are traditional hamartomas (without the mucosal smooth muscle of the Peutz-Jehger's polyp). These polyps are found predominantly in the colon and are the most common type of polyp found in children. Juvenile polyposis is defined as follows:

1. more than five juvenile polyps of the large intestine, or
2. multiple juvenile polyps throughout the GI tract, or
3. any number of juvenile polyps *and* a family history of juvenile polyps.

The number of polyps in a patient with juvenile polyposis can vary from 5 or 6 to hundreds. When juvenile polyps are profuse, patients are symptomatic with bloody diarrhea, mucus discharge, and protein-losing enteropathy. The risk of colorectal cancer is significantly enhanced in these patients, and if colectomy is not performed for symptoms, it is recommended as a prophylaxis against cancer. There is a high rate of recurrence of juvenile polyps in the rectum after IRA, requiring proctectomy. Polyps also recur in an ileal pouch, although they disappear with sulindac therapy. In mild cases, surgery may not be necessary, and patients can be followed by regular colonoscopies. The genotype has some influence on the phenotype.

Phosphatase and Tensin Homologue Tumor Hamartoma Syndrome

The PTEN tumor hamartoma syndrome is a term that includes a number of rare polyposes, such as Cowden's syndrome, Bannayan-Ruvalcaba-Riley syndrome, and proteus syndrome. These syndromes feature a variety of craniofacial, soft tissue, and musculoskeletal abnormalities, but patients can also develop colorectal polyps of a variety of histologic types. There may be adenomas, fibromas, ganglioneuromas, lipomas, hamartomas (juvenile), and hyperplastic polyps. As shown in Table 6, there is no overall increased risk of colorectal cancer, although some patients may be at risk by virtue of their particular polyp burden. Some of these patients may need a colectomy and IRA.

Suggested Readings

Aziz O, Athanasiou T, Fazio VW, and others: Meta-analysis of observational studies of ileorectal versus ileal pouch-anal anastomosis for familial adenomatous polyposis, *Br J Surg* 93:407, 2006.

Bertario L, Russo A, Sala P, and others: Hereditary Colorectal Tumours Registry. Genotype and phenotype factors as determinants of desmoid tumors in patients with familial adenomatous polyposis, *Int J Cancer* 95:102, 2001.

Bjork JA, Akerbrant HI, Iselius LE, and others: Risk factors for rectal cancer morbidity and mortality in patients with familial adenomatous polyposis after colectomy and ileorectal anastomosis, *Dis Colon Rectum* 43:1719, 2000.

Bulow S: Results of national registration of familial adenomatous polyposis, *Gut* 52:742, 2003.

Chan AO, Issa JP, Morris JS, and others: Concordant CpG island methylation in hyperplastic polyposis, *Am J Pathol* 160:529, 2002.

Church J: Anatomy of a gene, *Semin Colorectal Surg* 1995.

Church JM: Other polyposis syndromes, *Sem Colon Rectal Surg* 6:61, 1995.

Church J: Ileoanal pouch neoplasia in familial adenomatous polyposis: an underestimated threat, *Dis Colon Rectum* 48:1708, 2005.

Church J, Berk T, Boman BM, and others: Staging intra-abdominal desmoid tumors in familial adenomatous polyposis: a search for a uniform approach to a troubling disease, *Dis Colon Rectum* 48:1528, 2005.

Church J, Burke C, McGannon E, and others: Risk of rectal cancer in patients after colectomy and ileorectal anastomosis for familial adenomatous polyposis: a function of available surgical options, *Dis Colon Rectum* 46:1175, 2003.

Church JM, Fazio VW, Lavery IC, and others: Quality of life after prophylactic colectomy and ileorectal anastomosis in patients with familial adenomatous polyposis, *Dis Colon Rectum* 39:1404, 1996.

Church J, Kiringoda R, LaGuardia L: Inherited colorectal cancer registries in the United States, *Dis Colon Rectum* 47:674, 2004.

Church JM, McGannon E, Burke C, and others: Teenagers with familial adenomatous polyposis: what is their risk for colorectal cancer? *Dis Colon Rectum* 45:887, 2002.

Church JM, McGannon E, Hull-Boiner, and others: Gastroduodenal polyps in patients with familial adenomatous polyposis, *Dis Colon Rectum* 35:1170, 1992.

De Cosse JJ, Bulow S, Neale K, and others: Rectal cancer risk in patients treated for familial adenomatous polyposis, The Leeds Castle Polyposis Group, *Br J Surg* 79:1372, 1992.

Dunlop MG: British Society for Gastroenterology; Association of Coloproctology for Great Britain and Ireland. Guidance on gastrointestinal surveillance for hereditary non-polyposis colorectal cancer, familial adenomatous polyposis, juvenile polyposis, and Peutz-Jeghers syndrome, *Gut* 51(suppl 5):V21, 2002.

Eng C: PTEN: one gene, many syndromes, *Hum Mutat* 22:183, 2003.

Fearnhead NS, Britton MP, Bodmer WF: The ABC of APC, *Hum Mol Genet* 10:721, 2001.

Giardiello FM, Brensinger JD, Tersmette AC, and others: Very high risk of cancer in familial Peutz-Jeghers syndrome, *Gastroenterology* 119:1447, 2000.

Groves CJ, Saunders B, Spigelman A, and others: Duodenal cancer in patients with familial adenomatous polyposis (FAP): results of a 10 year prospective study, *Gut* 50:636, 2002.

Hartley JE, Church JM, Gupta S, and others: Significance of incidental desmoids identified during surgery for familial adenomatous polyposis, *Dis Colon Rectum* 47:334, 2003.

Hernegger GS, Moore HG, Guillem JG: Attenuated familial adenomatous polyposis: an evolving and poorly understood entity, *Dis Colon Rectum* 45:127, 2002.

Higuchi T, Jass J: My approach to serrated polyps of the colorectum, *J Clin Pathol* 57:682, 2004.

Hyman NH, Anderson P, Blasyk H: Hyperplastic polyposis and the risk of colorectal cancer, *Dis Colon Rectum* 47:2101, 2004.

Jones S, Emmerson P, Maynard J, and others: Biallelic germline mutations in MYH predispose to multiple colorectal adenoma and somatic G:C–>T:A mutations, *Hum Mol Genet* 11:2961, 2002.

Latchford AR, Sturt NJH, Neale K, and others: A 10-year review of surgery for desmoid disease associated with familial adenomatous polyposis, *Br J Surg* 93:1258, 2006.

Mackey R, Walsh RM, Chung R, and others: Pancreas-sparing duodenectomy is effective management for familial adenomatous polyposis, *J Gastrointest Surg* 9:1088, 2005.

Nessar G, Fazio VW, Tekkis P, and others: Long-term outcome and quality of life after continent ileostomy, *Dis Colon Rectum* 49:336, 2006.

Oncel M, Church JM, Remzi FH, and others: Colonic surgery in patients with juvenile polyposis syndrome: a case series, *Dis Colon Rectum* 48:49, 2005.

Oncel M, Remzi FH, Church JM, and others: Benefits of "clean sweep" in Peutz-Jeghers patients, *Colorectal Dis* 6:332, 2004.

Penna C, Tiret E, Parc R., and others: Operation and abdominal desmoid tumors in familial adenomatous polyposis, *Surg Gynecol Obstet* 177:263, 1993.

Remzi FH, Church JM, Bast J, and others: Mucosectomy vs. stapled ileal pouch-anal anastomosis in patients with familial adenomatous polyposis: functional outcome and neoplasia control, *Dis Colon Rectum* 44:1590, 2001.

Remzi FH, Fazio VW, Gorgun E: The outcome after restorative proctocolectomy with or without defunctioning ileostomy, *Dis Colon Rectum* 49:470, 2006.

Sarre RG, Jagelman DG, Beck GJ, and others: Colectomy with ileorectal anastomosis for familial adenomatous polyposis: the risk of rectal cancer, *Surgery* 101:20, 1987.

Sayed MG, Ahmed AF, Ringold JR, and others: Germline SMAD4 or BMPR1A mutations and phenotype of juvenile polyposis, *Ann Surg Oncol* 9:901, 2002.

Soares J, Lopes L, Vilas Boas G, and others: Wireless capsule endoscopy for evaluation of phenotypic expression of small-bowel polyps in patients with Peutz-Jeghers syndrome and in symptomatic first-degree relatives, *Endoscopy* 36:1060, 2004.

Vogel J, Church J: Post-operative endoscopic surveillance of rectal pouch following total abdominal colectomy with IRA and total proctocolectomy with IPAA in FAP and HNPCC. In Wilcox CM, editor: *Techniques in gastrointestinal endoscopy*, New York, 2006, Elsevier.

Vogel J, Church JM, LaGuardia L: Minimally invasive pouch surgery predisposes to desmoid tumor formation in patients with familial adenomatous polyposis, *Dis Colon Rectum* 48:662, 2005.

Wang L, Baudhuin LM, Boardman LA, and others: MYH mutations in patients with attenuated and classic polyposis and with young-onset colorectal cancer without polyps, *Gastroenterology* 127:9, 2004.

Wu JS, Paul P, McGannon EA, and others: APC genotype, polyp number, and surgical options in familial adenomatous polyposis, *Ann Surg* 227:57, 1998.

COLON CANCER

Michael A. Choti, MD

Large bowel cancer is the fourth most common malignancy in the United States, with more than 148,000 new cases in 2006, ranking behind lung, breast, and prostate cancer. With 55,170 estimated deaths, it is second to lung cancer as the leading cause of cancer-related deaths. These tumors can be further divided by the anatomic location of the tumor into colon and rectal cancer. Colon cancers are those that arise in the portion of the large bowel that is within the peritoneal cavity, from the cecum to the peritoneal reflection where the large bowel becomes the rectum. The distinction from rectal cancer, although seemingly somewhat arbitrary, is important for several reasons. Clinical presentation, the operative management, and the type of adjuvant therapy offered differ between colon and rectal cancer. Of all large bowel cancer, the colonic site makes up approximately 70%. Like rectal cancer, colon cancer management requires a multidisciplinary team approach to optimize detection, treatment, and subsequent surveillance.

SCREENING AND PRESENTATION

Colon cancer screening has been shown to reduce cancer-related mortality. The success of screening programs is one of the reasons cited for the decline in mortality rates from colorectal cancers since the late 1980s. The goal of screening is to detect early-stage cancer and premalignant adenomatous polyps. A variety of screening methods exist, including colonoscopy, flexible sigmoidoscopy, barium enema, and fecal occult blood testing (FOBT). More recently, computed tomographic colography or virtual colonoscopy is gaining acceptance in selected circumstances.

In individuals at average risk, screening is generally recommended to begin at age 50. Recommended screening options include colonoscopy every 5 to 10 years, flexible sigmoidoscopy every 5 years, annual FOBT, or a combination of these. Despite these recommendations, less than half of average-risk Americans comply with these guidelines, considerably fewer than of the number who comply with guidelines for other diseases, including breast and prostate cancer screening. Persons at higher risk should be screened earlier and more frequently. Specifically, individuals with a first-degree relative who has colorectal cancer or adenomatous polyps should have colonoscopy beginning at age 40 or 10 years younger than their youngest affected relative. Patients who have had a previous polyp or cancer removed should have repeat colonoscopy every 3 years. Patients at risk for hereditary syndromes such as familial adenomatous polyposis or hereditary nonpolyposis colon cancer should be screened frequently, receive genetic counseling and testing, and consider prophylactic colectomy in some cases.

The most common presenting symptoms are blood per rectum, anemia, change in bowel habits, or change in stool character. In contrast to rectal cancer, colon cancer rarely presents with anal pain, tenesmus, or incontinence. The location of the tumor within the colon often dictates the type of symptoms experienced. Right-sided tumors tend to present with anemia or related constitutional symptoms of anemia. Obstruction from right-sided tumors is more common when located near the ileocecal valve. Left-sided tumors are more likely to present with obstruction, largely because of the narrow bowel caliber, circumferential growth pattern, and firmer stool consistency. Evident blood in the stool and a change in stool caliber are also more commonly seen with distal colon cancer.

DIAGNOSIS

After cancer is suspected through either screening or symptoms, it is imperative that a thorough evaluation be performed. A complete history and physical examination is necessary to assess comorbid conditions before treatment. A detailed family history is important to determine the possibility of a familial or hereditary syndrome. Physical examination is most often unremarkable but can help to determine the presence of advanced disease through findings such as hepatomegaly, adenopathy, or an abdominal mass. A complete colonoscopy should be performed, if possible, before definitive therapy to confirm the histologic diagnosis and to rule out synchronous polyps or cancers. In addition, colonoscopic tattooing of the index lesion is important when the tumor is small or has been endoscopically excised to facilitate localization of these lesions at the time of operation.

In addition to routine laboratory blood studies, a preoperative serum carcinoembryonic antigen (CEA) measurement can be useful in both prognosis and postoperative surveillance. An elevated preoperative CEA is more likely associated with advanced disease and is an independent predictor of poor outcome. While a preoperative CEA level is advocated as a guide to postoperative management, it is important to realize that a normal preoperative CEA should not influence the utility of CEA for postoperative surveillance. Patients with normal levels at presentation, when the disease is clinically localized, often develop CEA elevation with recurrence. Liver function tests can also be useful as a preoperative indicator of metastatic liver disease.

The role of radiographic studies before surgical therapy is controversial. Preoperative computed tomography (CT) of the abdomen can detect evidence of locally advanced or metastatic disease. Approximately 20% of patients have metastatic disease at the time of presentation, and preoperative identification may result in different initial management. Preoperative CT can help identify patients with advanced disease in which treatment is clearly palliative and thereby obviate or help to limit the extent of surgery and minimize morbidity. Conversely, the identification of resectable and potentially curable liver metastases before the initial colonic resection can allow for the planning of a combined surgical approach or a more careful intraoperative assessment of the liver with intraoperative ultrasonography. Others argue that the extent of disease can often be assessed during surgery, and the surgical plan should account for multiple possibilities. Many surgeons, however, do obtain an abdominal CT to gain as much information as possible before surgery, particularly in those with locally advanced disease or if CEA is elevated.

Positron emission tomography (PET) or PET-CT is being used with increasing frequency for staging patients with various malignancies. PET has been found to be useful in patients with advanced colorectal cancer, primarily to assess chemotherapy response or to stage patients before resection of liver metastases. Current evidence on cost-effectiveness does not support its routine use in staging patients with primary colon cancer. Perhaps as PET becomes less costly, we may be seeing increased utilization for primary colon cancer staging.

STAGING

Historically, various staging systems have been used in colorectal cancer, contributing to some confusion. Currently, these previous staging systems have largely been supplanted by the TNM (*T*, primary tumor; *N*, regional lymph nodes; *M*, distant metastasis) staging system. This system was developed by the American Joint Committee on Cancer in cooperation with the TNM Committee of the International Union Against Cancer and is currently accepted as the universal staging system for colorectal cancer. In the sixth edition, modifications have been added incorporating more detailed stratification of stages II and III that more accurately reflect prognosis (Table 1).

SURGICAL MANAGEMENT

The management of colon cancer depends on the stage at presentation. In patients with localized and potentially curable disease, surgical resection is generally the primary and initial therapy, followed by adjuvant chemotherapy in some cases. When patients present with advanced incurable disease, chemotherapy is often the first line of therapy, and palliative resection is reserved for cases of locally symptomatic disease.

Colon Resection

The goals of surgical therapy with curative intent are to achieve complete removal of the primary cancer with adequate tumor-free

Table 1: TNM Classification for Colorectal Cancer Staging

Stage 0	Tis, N0, M0
Stage I	T1, N0, M0
	T2, N0, M0
Stage IIA	T3, N0, M0
Stage IIB	T4, N0, M0
Stage IIIA	T1, N1, M0
	T2, N1, M0
Stage IIIB	T3, N1, M0
	T4, N1, M0
Stage IIIC	Any T, N2, M0
Stage IV	Any T, Any N, M1

Primary tumor (**T**): *Tis*, Carcinoma in situ: intraepithelial or invasion of the lamina propria; *T0*, no evidence of primary tumor; *T1*, tumor invades submucosa; *T2*, tumor invades muscularis propria; *T3*, tumor invades through the muscularis propria into the subserosa or into nonperitonealized pericolic or perirectal tissues; *T4*, tumor directly invades other organs or structures and/or perforates visceral peritoneum. Regional lymph nodes (**N**): *N0*, no regional lymph node metastasis; *N1*, metastasis in 1 to 3 regional lymph nodes; *N2*, metastasis in four or more regional lymph nodes.
Distant metastasis (**M**): *M0*, no distant metastasis; *M1*: distant metastasis.
From the American Joint Committee on Cancer TNM staging system, ed 6.

margins, an anatomically complete lymphadenectomy of the surrounding lymph nodes, and en bloc resection of any involved adjacent organs. Between 80% and 90% of patients are appropriate candidates at presentation for an attempt at curative resection. The extent of colonic resection is determined by the vascular pedicles to achieve an adequate regional lymphadenectomy. This often requires resection of a larger segment of bowel beyond that necessary simply to obtain negative margins. The pericolic and intermediate draining lymph nodes are removed as part of a curative resection. Regional nodes are located along the course of the major vessels supplying the colon, along the vascular arcades of the marginal artery and adjacent to the colon along the mesocolic border. Resection of intermediate and pericolic nodes requires ligation and division of the main vascular trunks to the affected colon segment. In tumors located between vascular pedicles (e.g., hepatic or splenic flexure), extended colectomy is performed to remove nodes along both associated vascular pedicles. More extensive colonic resections, including subtotal or total colectomy, are typically reserved for those patients with multiple tumors or in cases in which a prophylactic component is being performed for those at risk for metachronous disease.

All operations with curative intent must include a through exploration of the abdominal cavity for evidence of metastatic disease. Peritoneal surfaces, omentum, and para-aortic nodes should be grossly assessed. Particular attention should be directed to the liver, the most common site for metastatic disease. Visualization and careful manual palpation of the liver should be conducted, including the periportal nodal region. Intraoperative ultrasound (IOUS) can be used in some cases to assess the liver more carefully. In cases in which liver metastases are known to be present on the basis of preoperative imaging, IOUS should be considered to assess potential resectability of the hepatic metastases.

Tumors of the cecum and ascending colon are typically managed with a right hemicolectomy. This involves resection of the terminal ileum, cecum, and ascending colon including the hepatic flexure. High ligation of the ileocolic and right colic vessels provides for an adequate lymphadenectomy. Tumors of the transverse colon are often managed with a transverse colectomy, including the middle colic and lymphatics. Left hemicolectomy is performed for tumors arising in the descending colon and includes ligation of the left colic artery. The splenic flexure is mobilized and the transverse colon is anastomosed to the proximal rectum. For sigmoid cancers, either a left hemicolectomy or a sigmoid colectomy can be performed. When performing the bowel anastomosis, various methods can be used, including hand-sewn or stapling techniques.

Laparoscopic Colectomy

The widespread application of laparoscopic approaches to common general surgical operations has changed abdominal surgery. This technology has also been applied to resections of the colon. Compared with other commonly performed laparoscopic procedures such as cholecystectomy, laparoscopic colon resection is technically more challenging because of necessary mobilization and the anastomosis that must be performed. Concerns about this approach include difficulty localizing small lesions because of the lack of the ability to palpate the colon. Preoperative colonoscopic tattooing of the lesion, as well as the ability to perform intraoperative colonoscopy, can help find such small lesions.

Early experience with this technique raised concerns about the oncologic adequacy of the laparoscopic approach. More recent studies, including randomized trials comparing the two approaches, have shown comparable outcomes. The advantages of the laparoscopic approach over open surgery, however, are less evident than with other laparoscopic operations. Laparoscopic colon resections tend to take longer to perform, require more expensive operative equipment, and still require an incision for removing the specimen and performing the anastomosis. Studies to date have shown some reduction in length of hospital stay and pain medication requirements. These findings, as well as the increasing adoption of hand-assisted techniques, have supported expansion of laparoscopic colectomy for large bowel cancer.

Importance of Adequate Lymph Node Assessment

The number of lymph nodes examined influences the accuracy of staging and the prognosis. In addition, the principal current indication for the recommendation of postoperative adjuvant chemotherapy is the involvement of any regional lymph nodes. Therefore complete and accurate pathologic lymph node staging documentation is crucial in the management of patients with colon cancer. The National Comprehensive Cancer Network (NCCN) recommends that no fewer than 12 nodes be microscopically examined to determine the nodal status accurately. Examination of fewer nodes is associated with the risk of understaging patients and with inaccurate survival prognostication. This is particularly true for "assumed" stage II colorectal cancers in patients who may inappropriately be deprived potentially beneficial chemotherapy. Several series have shown that stage II cancers with limited number of nodes examined (fewer than 8–12 nodes, depending on the series) have a significantly worse prognosis than those with higher nodes assessed (Fig. 1). Similarly, total nodal count has also been shown to affect the staging and survival of stage III patients.

Both surgical technique and thoroughness of the pathologic evaluation contribute to variation in the number of nodes contained in a specimen. The pathologist should use extreme diligence in the dissection of colectomy specimen. If fewer than 12 nodes are found despite a thorough search, the use of additional techniques, such as fat clearing, is encouraged.

One method used to facilitate special nodal assessment is to identify the node or nodes most likely to be involved. This technique, called sentinel lymph node mapping, is commonly used for lymph node staging of breast cancer and melanoma. Some investigators have studied its role in colorectal cancer as well. When this technique performed, vital dye or fluorescein is typically injected into the colon tumor during surgery, and the nodes are assessed minutes later. It can be carried out either in vivo or ex vivo immediately following resection. Although it may be helpful in identifying small pericolic nodes that could be overlooked otherwise, the value of upstaging colorectal cancer by detecting micrometastases remains to be validated. Moreover, unlike the cases of breast and skin cancer, mapping of the sentinel nodes for colorectal cancer does not change the surgical procedure significantly or obviate the need for complete lymphadenectomy.

Management of Obstructing or Perforated Colon Cancer

The management of obstructing or perforated colon cancer presents unique considerations. When patients present with urgent evidence of obstruction without the opportunity to prepare the bowel, they must be expediently resuscitated and undergo immediate surgical exploration. If the obstruction is due to a proximal lesion near the ileocecal valve, a right hemicolectomy with primary anastomosis may be performed safely in most cases, even with an unprepared colon. More distal obstructions are problematic because the proximal colon is dilatated and typically full of stool. After the involved segment of colon is resected, on-table lavage can be performed. This involves mobilization of the colon, attachment of large-bore sterile tubing to drain the effluent, and instillation of a large volume of warm saline through a catheter placed through an appendicostomy or the terminal ileum. The distal segment of bowel can be washed out from below. This technique can allow for a primary anastomosis in some cases, provided the bowel is relatively nondilatated and healthy appearing.

Perforations at the tumor site can present either as locally contained abscesses or as free perforation with peritonitis. In addition, obstructing tumors can result in colonic perforation, typically proximal to the tumor or at the cecum. In the case of contained perforations, abscesses can be drained percutaneously with subsequent investigations and elective surgical management. Free perforation with peritonitis is a surgical emergency that necessitates rapid resuscitation and operation. In the setting of gross fecal contamination, resection of the tumor and perforation are performed when possible with a proximal colostomy or ileostomy (Hartman procedure). In some cases, a primary anastomosis can be performed with a protecting proximal ostomy. An unprotected anastomosis without diversion is ill advised in these unstable patients.

Adjuvant Therapy

Despite apparently curative resections, many colorectal cancer patients develop recurrence of their disease. Among lymph node–positive patients, 30% to 70% develop recurrence and eventually die from recurrent disease. The goal of adjuvant therapy is to provide additional treatment to those patients most likely to experience recurrence while avoiding overtreatment in those with only a modest chance of benefit. Current standard recommendations are that all medically appropriate patients who are node positive (stage III disease) receive adjuvant chemotherapy. There is also a trend toward treating some stage II patients, particularly those with other poor prognostic features. These features include poorly differentiated histology, vascular or lymphatic invasion, bowel obstruction, T4 tumor, or fewer than 12 lymph nodes evaluated.

The choice of adjuvant chemotherapy can vary, depending on patient performance status and comorbid conditions. All chemotherapeutic regimens are fluoropyrimadine based, including 5-fluorouracil (5FU) and leucovorin (LV) or oral capecitabine. Recent randomized studies, including the MOSAIC trial, have demonstrated improved survival of infusion 5FU-LV with oxaliplatin (FOLFOX) over 5FU-LV alone in patients for postoperative adjuvant therapy for colon cancer. Ongoing randomized trials are examining whether the addition of biologic therapies such as cetuximab or

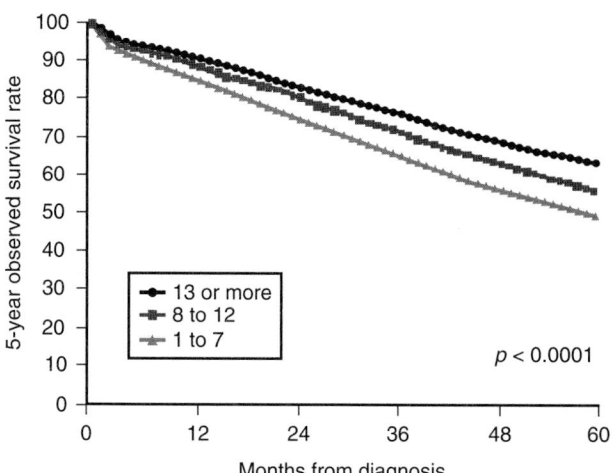

Figure 1 Kaplan-Meier 5-year survival curves of surgically resected T3N0 colon cancers by the number of regional lymph nodes pathologically examined. *From Swanson and others: Ann Surg Oncol 10:65, 2003.*

bevacizumab improve outcomes. Other trials are incorporating molecular risk stratification to select those who may derive benefit from postoperative adjuvant therapy. Unlike with rectal cancer, adjuvant radiation therapy for colon cancer is rarely indicated.

FOLLOW-UP

Following patients after treatment for colon cancer serves several functions. First, surveillance attempts to identify recurrent disease at a time when it is potentially resectable for cure. Second, following patients with colonoscopy can identify metachronous polyps or cancers at an early stage. A balance must be struck between accomplishing these goals and providing care that has minimal morbidity and is cost-effective. On the basis of available data, guidelines for follow-up have been developed, including by the NCCN. Patients with T2 or greater tumors should be followed with history and physical examination and a CEA level every 3 months for the first 2 years after treatment and then every 6 months for the next 3 years. If rising CEA is identified, further testing should be performed, including imaging studies and colonoscopy. CT scan is the most frequently used imaging modality. If negative with a continuing rise of the CEA, PET imaging should be considered. In addition, PET can be useful in cases in which resection of metastatic disease is being considered to rule out more extensive disease. In cases in which the primary tumor is of early stage (Tis, T1) or in which the patient may not be a candidate for aggressive treatment of recurrent disease, follow-up testing can be more limited.

Colonoscopy should be performed at 1 year postoperatively or within 6 months if a complete colonoscopy was not possible preoperatively because of obstruction or perforation. If the postoperative colonoscopy is free of polyps, repeat surveillance every 3 years is generally recommended. In patients in whom adenomas are found or if a hereditary syndrome is present, annual colonoscopy should be considered.

Suggested Readings

Benson AB, Choti MA, Cohen AM, and others: NCCN practice guidelines for colorectal cancer, *Oncology* 14:203, 2000.

Bertagnolli M, Miedema B, Redston M, and others: Sentinel node staging of resectable colon cancer: results of a multicenter study, *Ann Surg* 240:624; discussion 628, 2004.

Clinical Outcomes of Surgical Therapy Study Group: A comparison of laparoscopically assisted and open colectomy for colon cancer, *N Engl J Med* 13;350:2050, 2004.

Saha S, Seghal R, Patel M, and others: A multicenter trial of sentinel lymph node mapping in colorectal cancer: prognostic implications for nodal staging and recurrence, *Am J Surg* 191:305, 2006.

Swanson RS, Compton CC, Stewart AK, and others: The prognosis of T3N0 colon cancer is dependent on the number of lymph nodes examined, *Ann Surg Oncol* 10:65, 2003.

Wee CC, McCarthy EP, Phillips RS: Factors associated with colon cancer screening: the role of patient factors and physician counseling, *Prev Med* 41:23, 2005.

Rectal Cancer

Nita Ahuja, MD

Treatment for rectal cancer has improved in recent years with increased rates of sphincter salvage and improvements in local recurrence rates with total mesorectal excision and modern chemoradiation regimens. The continuing evolution of chemotherapy drugs in colorectal cancer and the integration of biologic markers in the near future make it crucial for the treating surgeon to integrate multimodality therapy within a team approach in the treatment of rectal cancer patients.

INCIDENCE

In 2006, the American Cancer Society estimated that there would be 148,610 new cases of colorectal cancer, with 41,930 cases of rectal cancer. Colorectal cancer remains a leading cause of cancer death with an estimated 55,170 deaths in 2006, making it the second leading cause of cancer death in men and the third leading cause of cancer death in women. However, incidence rates of colorectal cancers declined 1.8% per year from 1998 to 2002 because of improved screening and polyp removal. In addition, mortality rates from colorectal cancer have also declined since the mid-1990s, at an average of 1.8% per year because of decreasing incidence and improvements in survival.

RISK FACTORS

The greatest risk factor for colorectal cancer is age. The median age at diagnosis for colorectal cancer was 71 years on the basis of Surveillance, Epidemiology, and End Results (SEER) incidence rates for 2002 to 2003. Only 4.4% of colorectal cancers were diagnosed in patients aged less than 45 years, whereas 67% of colorectal cancers were diagnosed in patients over age 65.

Colorectal cancer is thought to occur in a stepwise fashion from adenoma to carcinoma, as described by Fearon and Vogelstein, with accumulation of genetic and epigenetic changes that transform the normal mucosa to adenomas and then to invasive carcinoma. Certain inherited genetic syndromes such as familial adenomatous polyposis (FAP) and hereditary nonpolyposis colorectal cancer (HNPCC) are associated with a high incidence of colorectal cancer, but these conditions account for less than 5% of all colorectal cancers. Patients with FAP (and its variants Gardner syndrome, Turcot syndrome, and attenuated adenomatous polyposis coli) have an inherited germline mutation in the so-called gatekeeper gene *APC* (adenomatous polyposis coli), which is autosomal-dominant. Patients with FAP develop hundreds to thousands of adenomas during early childhood and cancers by age 45. The attenuated form of *FAP* (AFAP) has a similar risk of colorectal cancer but results in fewer adenomas and an older age at diagnosis. Patients with FAP should undergo a prophylactic proctocolectomy with ileoanal anastomosis in their late teens or early 20s. HNPCC, also known as Lynch syndrome, is more common than FAP, and patients with this disorder have an inherited, autosomal-dominant mutation in the mismatch repair genes. These patients often have right-sided colon cancers with a younger mean age at diagnosis of 48 years, and have higher incidence of synchronous and metachronous lesions, but may have better survival compared with age-matched sporadic colorectal cancers. HNPCC patients also have an increased risk of endometrial and gastric cancers. These patients can be diagnosed on the basis of the clinical Amsterdam criteria. In addition, another 15% of sporadic colorectal cancers acquire defects in their mismatch repair pathway via methylation of the *MLH1* gene, the so-called microsatellite-instability-high colorectal cancers and display mutations in the *BRAF* gene and hypermethylation of multiple tumor-suppressor genes. These patients have right-sided colon cancers and appear to display an alternative pathway of colorectal carcinogenesis linked to serrated adenomas and hyperplastic polyposis syndrome.

Patients with a personal or family history of colorectal cancer or polyps are at a threefold to sixfold increased risk of colorectal cancer. Patients with inflammatory bowel disease also have an elevated risk of colorectal cancer dependent on the extent and duration of disease. The cumulative risk of colon cancer in patients with ulcerative colitis is 8% at 20 years and 18% at 30 years. This is in contrast to the average individual whose lifetime incidence of colorectal cancer is 6%. The risk of cancer is also elevated in patients with long-standing Crohn's colitis or ileitis to a similar extent. Colorectal cancer in patients with inflammatory bowel disease is often subtle and multifocal, with few mucosal aberrations. Malignancy more often occurs in the region affected by the disease the longest, the rectosigmoid region in ulcerative colitis and the proximal colon in Crohn's disease. Colorectal cancer in patients with inflammatory bowel disease is frequently preceded by the development of dysplasia in flat mucosa and occasionally surrounding a polypoid lesion or mass.

Multiple other predisposing factors have been implicated in colorectal cancer in large epidemiologic studies; these include dietary factors such as consumption of red meat, caffeine intake, and folate levels and lifestyle factors such as obesity, alcohol consumption, and cigarette smoking. Several studies have suggested that regular use of anti-inflammatory drugs, such as aspirin and use of 3-hydroxy-3-methylglutaryl coenzyme A (HMG-CoA) reductase inhibitors (statins) may reduce colorectal cancer risk. However, these drugs are not currently recommended for prevention.

PREOPERATIVE STAGING AND WORKUP

Most patients present to the surgeon with a diagnosis of rectal cancer. However, elements of the history, physical examination, and preoperative staging are helpful to assess patient's overall physical condition, need for neoadjuvant therapy, and need for local excision versus radical resection. In the history, it is important to inquire about preoperative sphincter and sexual function, especially as sphincter-salvage procedures are being considered. In addition, the presence of predisposing conditions such as HNPCC or inflammatory bowel disease may affect the extent of planned surgical treatment. The presence of symptoms such as pelvic pain can indicate to the surgeon potential sacral involvement, and the presence of obstipation or constipation can indicate a bulky obstructing lesion.

The digital rectal examination and rigid proctoscopy are essential to determine clinical staging and the need for neoadjuvant therapy and for planning surgical therapy. If the rectal lesion is palpable on digital rectal examination, it should be documented whether the tumor is anterior or posterior and mobile or fixed to surrounding structures. Ulceration, size of the tumor, and extent of circumferential involvement of the bowel wall by the tumor are additional features on physical exam that will influence surgical decision making. Finally, relationship of the tumor to the sphincter mechanism is important, rather than the distance of the rectal cancer from the anal verge because the anal verge is a nonreproducible landmark with significant interindividual variation (Fig. 1). Rigid proctoscopy can accurately assess the proximal and distal levels of the cancer and the relation to the sphincter muscles and to the vagina or prostate. In addition, the diagnosis of invasive cancer can be confirmed by biopsy, if not already performed. A complete evaluation of the colon, preferably with a colonoscopy, is essential because 3% to 5% of patients have synchronous proximal carcinoma. However, patients with synchronous cancers have the same prognosis as a patient with a solitary cancer when the highest stage of disease is compared. In patients who are unable to undergo a complete colonoscopy secondary to a near-obstructing lesion, virtual colonoscopy (see Fig. 2) or double-contrast barium enema are potential alternatives to evaluate the proximal colon.

Figure I Anatomy of the rectum.

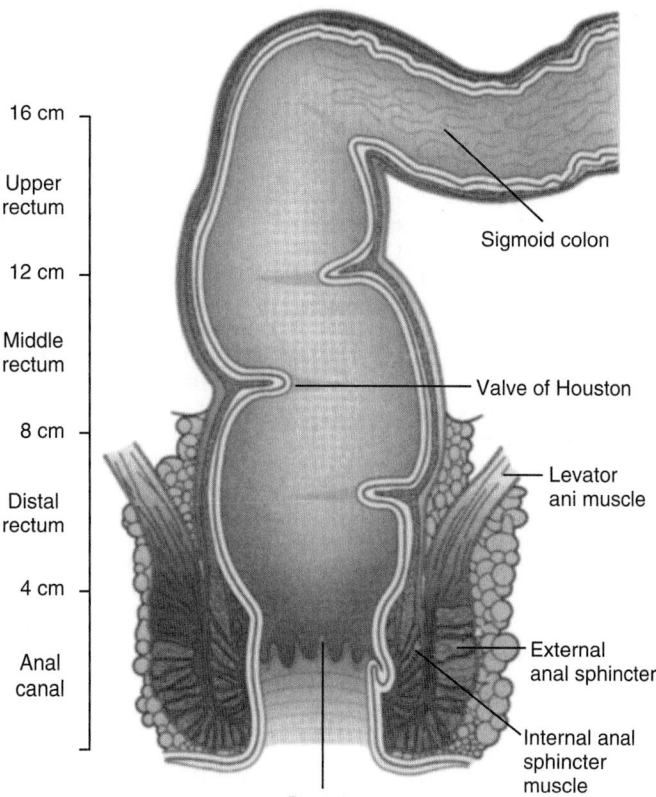

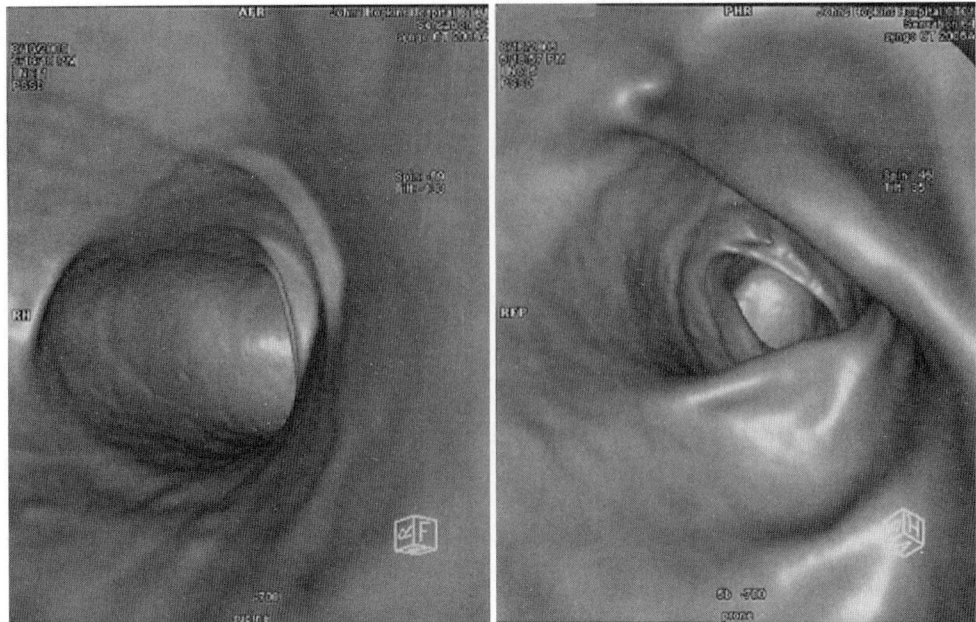

Figure 2 Images from virtual colonoscopy of the normal proximal colon of a patient with an obstructing rectal cancer.

All patients should have basic laboratory studies, such as a complete blood count and electrolytes. Other tests, such as electrocardiogram and stress test, can be performed selectively to assess patient's condition. A baseline carcinoembryonic antigen (CEA) level should be obtained in all patients, according to guidelines issued by the National Comprehensive Cancer Network. Patients with high preoperative CEA levels (>5 ng/ml) may have a worse prognosis compared with stage-matched patients. CEA levels can be used to follow up response to neoadjuvant therapy. In addition, an elevated preoperative CEA level that does not normalize following surgery may imply the presence of persistent disease. However, CEA levels are most useful in identifying recurrent disease during surveillance. All patients should undergo a chest x-ray to exclude pulmonary metastases. In additional, computerized tomography (CT) scans of the abdomen and pelvis are helpful for evaluating distant metastases and tumor-related complications (such as obstruction, perforation, fistula formation) and may be helpful to evaluate regional tumor extension and regional lymphatic metastases. The sensitivity of CT scans for detecting distant metastasis is higher (75%–87%) than for detecting nodal involvement (45%–73%) or the depth of transmural invasion (approximately 50%).

Endorectal ultrasound (ERUS), on the other hand, is superior to CT scan for locoregional staging. ERUS is an office-based procedure that should be performed preoperatively on all patients with rectal cancer. Figure 3 shows a schematic view of the layers seen on ERUS, and Figure 4 shows examples of rectal cancers. The ERUS generates images that demonstrate the depth of invasion of rectal cancer (T stage) as well as nodal involvement (N stage). The accuracy of ERUS for correctly predicting tumor stage ranges from 80% to 95%, compared with 65% to 75% for CT and 75% to 85% for magnetic resonance imaging (MRI). However, the accuracy of ERUS for predicting nodal status (approximately 70%–75%) is similar to that of CT (55%–65%) and MRI (60%–65%). The accuracy for nodal involvement requires that nodes be larger than 5 mm. In addition, ERUS allows the possibility of performing fine needle aspiration (FNA) biopsy, which may improve the accuracy of nodal staging. A modified ERUS-guided staging system has been proposed, as shown in Table 1. However, there is considerable

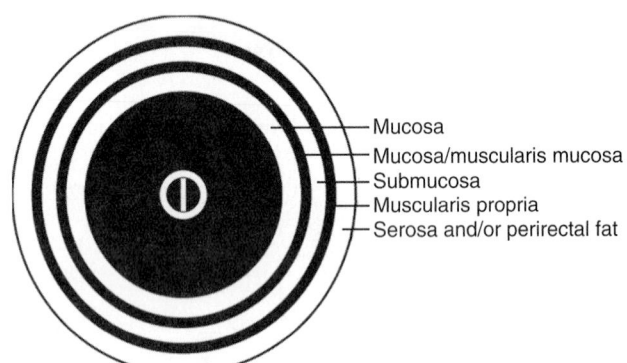

Figure 3 Schematic drawing of the layers seen in endorectal ultrasound.

interobserver variability, a significant learning curve associated with performing ERUS, and limitations in staging patients with near-obstructing cancers and downstaged cancers after chemoradiation therapy. Another potential concern with the use of ERUS is the potential for overstaging patients with early-stage disease (i.e., T1/2 N0) for neoadjuvant strategies. The ability of ERUS for locoregional staging may have been overestimated in the literature because of publication bias based on a recent study of more than 4000 patients. ERUS had an overall accuracy of 85% and 75% for T-staging and N-staging, respectively, in this study.

MRI with endorectal coil and phased-array MRI are additional newer modalities useful for locoregional staging of rectal cancers. Unlike ERUS, MRI is less dependent on operator and technique and may allow study of stenotic tumors. In addition, MRI can help in assessing the likelihood of a tumor-free resection margin by visualizing tumor involvement of the mesorectal fascia and surrounding organs in up to 100% of patients (see Fig. 5) and help to stratify patients for neoadjuvant therapy. MRI, like ERUS, is limited in restaging patients treated with preoperative

Figure 4 Endorectal ultrasound demonstrates a uT3 rectal cancer on the left and an enlarged lymph node on the right.

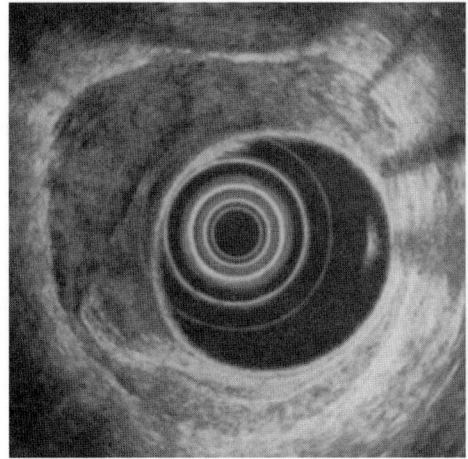
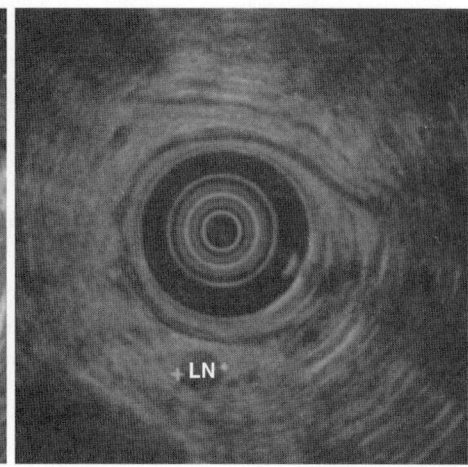

Table 1: Endorectal Ultrasound (ERUS) Staging of Rectal Cancers

T stage	Ultrasound Findings
uT1	Confined to the mucosa and submucosa
uT2	Invading into but not through the muscularis propria
uT3	Invading into the perirectal fat
uT4	Invading into an adjacent organ
uN0	No lymph node enlargement present
uN1	Lymph node enlargement present

chemoradiation because it cannot differentiate treatment-induced fibrosis from viable tumors.

Positron emission tomography (PET) combined with CT scan is an emerging modality. The role of PET scan in initial staging of rectal cancers is unclear at present, limited by data size. However, PET/CT may have a role in managing local recurrence and imaging of metastatic disease as well as monitoring response to therapy.

STAGING

The original staging of rectal cancer was based on the Duke's classification in the 1930s, which was then modified by Astler-Coller in the 1950s to classify rectal tumors according to a predicted 5-year survival. Currently, the TNM (*T*, primary tumor; *N*, regional lymph nodes; *M*, distant metastasis) system as proposed by the American Joint Commission on Cancer (AJCC) is commonly used based on the TNM staging (see Tables 2 and 3). The most recent 2002 version of AJCC TNM staging divides stage III disease into prognostically distinct A, B, and C categories depending on depth of the primary tumor and number of involved nodes. In addition, the new edition considers smooth metastatic nodules in the perirectal fat to be lymph node metastases, but irregularly contoured metastatic nodules in the peritumoral fat are considered vascular invasion and are classified in the T category as either a V1 (microscopic vascular invasion) or V2 (macroscopic vascular invasion). In addition, the importance of clearing the radial margin during surgery

is highlighted, as is the importance of removing an adequate number of lymph nodes during surgical resections. In general, 12 lymph nodes should be harvested during surgery in patients who have not received neoadjuvant therapy to adequately stage the patient

The College of Independent Pathologists recently published a consensus statement on independent prognostic factors in colorectal cancer that have been shown to have category I evidence including tumor thickness (T stage) and nodal involvement (N stage), presence of residual disease, lymphovascular invasion, and preoperative elevation of serum CEA antigen. Factors with category IIA evidence included tumor grade, radial margin status (for resection specimens with nonperitonealized surfaces), and residual tumor in the resection specimen following neoadjuvant therapy. Histologic grade, biologic features such as microsatellite instability, and chromosome 18q loss are considered, at present, to have category IIB evidence as prognostic factors.

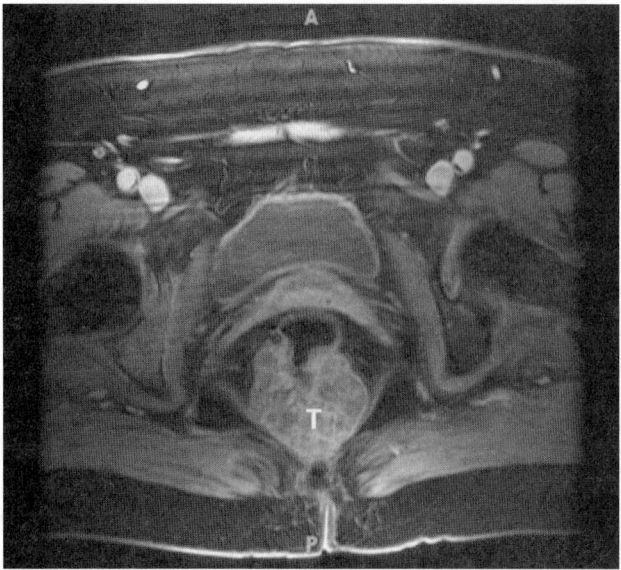

Figure 5 Magnetic resonance imaging demonstrates a rectal cancer that abuts the levators muscles, right more than left. Posteriorly the tumor extended into the presacral space to the coccyx but did not involve the coccyx.

Table 2: Current Staging System Based on TNM Classification

Primary Tumor (T)

T_X	Primary tumor cannot be assessed
T0	No evidence of primary tumor
Tis	Carcinoma in situ: intraepithelial or invasion of lamina propria
T1	Tumor invades into the submucosa
T2	Tumor invades into the muscularis propria
T3	Tumor invades through the muscularis propria into the subserosa or into nonperitonealized pericolic or perirectal tissues
T4	Tumor directly invades other organs or structures, and/or perforates visceral peritoneum

Regional Lymph Nodes (N)

NX	Regional lymph nodes cannot be assessed
N0	No regional lymph node metastasis
N1	Metastasis into 1 to 3 regional lymph nodes
N2	Metastasis into 4 or more regional lymph nodes

Distant Metastasis (M)

MX	Distant metastasis cannot be assessed
M0	No distant metastases
M1	Distant metastases present

Stage	TNM	Dukes*	MAC*
0	Tis N0 M0	—	—
I	T1 N0 M0	A	A
	T2 N0 M0	A	B1
IIA	T3 N0 M0	B	B2
IIB	T4 N0 M0	B	B3
IIIA	T1-T2 N1 M0	C	C1
IIIB	T3-T4 N1 M0	C	C2/C3
IIIC	Any T N2 M0	C	C1/C2/C3
IV	Any T Any N M1	—	D

*Modified from American Joint Committee on Cancer, AJCC Cancer Staging Manual, ed 6, 2002.). Used with the permission of the American Joint Committee on Cancer (AJCC), Chicago, Illinois. The original source for this material is the AJCC Cancer Staging Manual, Sixth Edition (2002) published by Springer-New Youk, www.springeronline.com.

Table 3: Stage at Presentation for Rectal Cancer

TNM Stage	Percentage of patients
Stage 1	34
Stage 2	25
Stage 3	26
Stage 4	15

From Jessup JM, Stewart AK, Menck HR: SO Cancer 83:2408, 1998.

In rectal cancer, the clinical staging is based on the integration of history and physical examination, biopsy results, and the results of the various imaging modalities, including ERUS, CT, MRI, and PET scan. However, definitive pathologic staging is carried out after surgical resection.

NEOADJUVANT THERAPY

Neoadjuvant therapy, including preoperative radiation therapy and chemoradiotherapy, is increasingly used in the management of distal rectal cancers for sphincter-salvage and converts a distal rectal cancer, which requires an abdominoperineal resection (APR), to a sphincter-saving low-anterior resection (LAR). In addition, neoadjuvant therapy is used for large, locally invasive or node-positive (T3 or T4, and/or N1) rectal cancer instead of postoperative radiation therapy, followed by total mesorectal excision (TME). In 1990, the National Institutes of Health Consensus Conference recommended postoperative chemoradiation for patients with transmural and/or nodal positive cancer (stage II/III). However, most centers currently have shifted to a neoadjuvant paradigm for treatment of locally advanced rectal cancer because of downstaging associated with improved tumor resectability, higher sphincter-salvage rates, and lower toxicity with neoadjuvant chemoradiation. In addition, complete pathologic responses can be seen in 10% to 25% of patients, and these patients may have improved overall and disease-free survival on the basis of results from single-institution series. There have been multiple large trials on the utility of preoperative radiation therapy, some of which are now summarized.

The Swedish Rectal Cancer Trial randomized 1168 patients to receive short-course radiation therapy (25 Gy in five fractions over 1 week) followed by surgery compared with surgery alone. Patients in the radiation arm had improvement in both local control (89% vs. 73%) and overall survival (58% vs. 48%). However, patients in the irradiated arm had a twofold to fourfold higher rate of hospital admissions for gastrointestinal issues (bowel obstruction, abdominal pain) at 10-year follow-up.

The Medical Research Council/National Cancer Institute of Canada trial, presented at the American Society of Clinical Oncology meeting in 2006, randomly assigned 1350 stage 1 to III rectal cancer patients to preoperative radiation therapy similar to the Swedish trial, but postoperative chemotherapy was offered to all patients with positive circumferential margins and/or positive nodes. Preoperative radiation therapy showed a benefit in local control (5% vs. 11% local recurrence) and in disease-free survival (80% vs. 75%) but not in overall survival (81% vs. 79%) at a median follow-up of 3 years.

The Dutch trial randomized 1861 patients to either TME or preoperative high-dose radiation followed by TME and showed no survival benefit for preoperative radiation but showed improvement in 5-year local recurrence rates (11.4% vs. 5.8%).

The available data, including meta-analyses, show that preoperative radiation therapy is associated with better local control. However, the Swedish approach of high-dose, short-course preoperative radiation therapy is generally not used in the United States because of potential of increased surgical morbidity and to integrate preoperative chemotherapy with radiation. The trials highlighting use of preoperative chemoradiation are now summarized.

The recently published European Organization for Research and Treatment of Cancer (EORTC) 22921 trial randomized T3 or T4 rectal cancers into four arms of preoperative radiation therapy or chemoradiation and the potential addition of postoperative chemotherapy to both the preoperative arms. The 5-year overall survival was similar (65.2%) in all groups. However, the addition of chemotherapy preoperatively or postoperatively resulted in improved local control.

The German Rectal Cancer Group compared preoperative and postoperative chemoradiation in treatment of stage II or III rectal cancers. There was no difference in overall survival in the two groups, but there was a significant reduction in local recurrence (6% vs. 13%) and treatment toxicity in the preoperative group.

Surgical resection is usually performed 6 to 8 weeks after completion of neoadjuvant therapy to allow maximal response to neoadjuvant therapy and to allow patients to recover. Some investigators have recently suggested that patients who have significant or complete response to neoadjuvant therapies be treated by transanal excision or observation alone. However, at present, preoperative staging modalities such as ERUS, MRI, or fluorodeoxyglucose (FDG)-PET scanning are unable to distinguish between treatment-related fibrosis and residual tumor and thus do not allow us to select the patients who have had complete pathologic response. Moreover, 1.8% to 16% of patients who have a complete pathologic response in their primary tumor still have lymph node involvement. At present, all patients should continue with definitive surgical therapy after neoadjuvant therapy unless they are enrolled in a clinical trial.

■ SURGICAL THERAPY

Patients with early-stage, distal rectal cancers limited to the submucosa (T1N0M0) without high-risk features can be treated by local excision with curative intent. Local excision techniques include transanal, transsphincteric, and transcoccygeal (Kraske resection) techniques. Transsphincteric and transcoccygeal resections are associated with a high rate of complications, including fecal fistulae and incontinence, and have been abandoned. Local palliative procedures including fulguration and radiation are options for patients who are medically unfit or unwilling to undergo major surgery. High T1 rectal tumors not amenable to a transanal approach and rectal tumors that have invaded the muscularis propria (T2N0M0) are treated with radical rectal surgery in medically fit patients. Patients with locally advanced disease (T3/T4 and/or N1) are generally treated first with preoperative chemoradiation followed by radical resection. In patients with resectable metastatic disease, a variety of factors, including patient comorbidities, resectability of metastases, and patient symptoms, must be considered in planning timing of chemotherapy and surgery. In patients with unresectable metastatic disease, surgical resection of the primary rectal lesion can be performed for palliative purposes in selected circumstances. Careful preoperative staging with the modalities discussed earlier, including surgical biopsy and ERUS, is important in stratifying patients appropriately.

Local Transanal Excision

The goal of local excision procedures is to perform a full-thickness resection of the primary rectal cancer with a 1-cm margin. Transanal excision can be performed in highly selected T1 rectal cancers with minimal morbidity and excellent functional outcomes. Patient selection is based on preoperative staging and on the probability of harboring nodal metastases, which increases with the depth of tumor invasion. Transanal local excision does not remove the lymph node-bearing tissue (i.e., the mesorectum), and optimal patient selection is needed to identify patients who have a low risk of nodal metastases. The risk of nodal metastases is estimated at 0% to 12% for T1 tumors; 12% to 28% for T2 tumors, and 36% to 79% for T3 cancers. Other features that have been associated with an increased risk of lymph node metastases include poor differentiation, lymphovascular invasion, and size greater than 3 cm. The Haggitt criteria also describe levels of invasiveness in pedunculated lesions. Cancers are deemed to be Haggitt level 1 to 4, depending on invasion into the head, neck, stalk, or base of the polyp. The incidence of lymph node metastasis has been correlated with the Haggitt level in a number of studies and ranges from 1% in Haggitt level 1 to 15% to 25% in Haggitt level 4.

However, in recent studies even T1 rectal cancers have shown a high rate of local recurrence with long-term follow-up at 10 years, with rates averaging 10% to 25% and survival rates ranging from 70% to 85%. The risk of local recurrence for T2 cancers is much higher, ranging from 25% to 62% with local excision alone. The addition of modern chemotherapy and radiation regimens may allow resection of T2 rectal cancers in selected patients. The American College of Surgeons Oncology Group has initiated a phase 2 trial (Z6041) with aggressive neoadjuvant chemoradiation (capecitabine and oxaliplatin plus radiation) followed by local excision for uT2N0 rectal cancers, and this trial may clarify indications for local excision in T2 cancers.

The generally accepted criteria for transanal excision are shown in Table 4. All patients undergoing transanal excision should be counseled preoperatively that if the local transanal excision reveals unfavorable features or higher-stage lesion (i.e., T2 or greater) or if the lesion is in an area that does not permit re-excision to clear margins, the patient must proceed with radical surgery with a TME, which may necessitate an LAR or an APR.

On the basis of selected small series, there is a potential role for salvage surgery in patients who develop a local recurrence after transanal excision, with 5-year disease-free survival ranging from 50% to 88%. Patients who undergo local excision should be followed carefully and for a long period of time because local recurrences are being seen at 5 years or more after local excision. The role of adjuvant radiation and chemotherapy in these patients is unclear.

Technique of Transanal Excision

The patient is placed in the lithotomy position for posterior tumors or the prone jackknife position for anterior tumors, and a rolled towel is placed under the sacrum to elevate and project the pelvis forward. In addition, the buttocks are spread wide apart and secured with tape. The surgery is usually performed under general anesthesia, although spinal or local anesthesia with sedation may be used in patients with extensive comorbidities. The lesion should be within reach of the anal canal and below the peritoneal reflection. The upper limit of resection is usually 6 to 8 cm from the dentate line. Posterior masses generally are technically easier than anterior masses. A full mechanical bowel preparation is recommended preoperatively to improve visualization and limit postoperative impaction.

A self-retaining retractor such as the Lone Star retractor (Lone Star Medical Products, Stafford, TX) or Gelpi retractors may be used to efface the anus. In addition, a handheld bivalve retractor, a Ferguson-Hill retractor, or a Fansler operating anoscope may be used to provide exposure of the lesion. Deep retractors such as narrow Deaver retractors are also helpful for exposing more proximal cancers.

The procedure is begun by performing a circumferential anal block with a local anesthetic with epinephrine. This aids in hemostasis and also to relax the sphincter. It is also helpful to place a traction suture 2 cm distal to the lesion to help facilitate its prolapse into the operating field. The electrocautery (or laparoscopic

Table 4: Criteria for Transanal Excision of Rectal Cancers

T1N0M0 lesions

- Should be within 8 to 10 cm of the anal verge
- Less than 4 cm wide
- Involve less than one third the circumference of the rectum
- No lymphatic or vascular invasion, no perineural invasion
- Well differentiated or moderately differentiated

instruments) is used to mark a 1-cm margin circumferentially, and the rectal wall is incised full thickness down to perirectal fat. Orientation of the specimen must be maintained at all times. The specimen must be removed in one piece, and after the tumor is removed, it is inspected to confirm that adequate margins have been obtained. The specimen is pinned to a board and marked for orientation before histologic examination. The proper orientation of the tumor is essential because any positive margin requires further assessment. The defect in the rectum is closed with simple or vertical mattress interrupted absorbable sutures. Alternatively, the defect in the rectal wall may be closed as the dissection proceeds, and each suture can be used for traction to keep the lesion in view. The operative site is irrigated with sterile water to minimize the risk that viable tumor cells will be left in the rectal wall. If the rectal wall defect is extraperitoneal, it may be left open to heal secondarily; however, we prefer to close all rectal wounds primarily. After the defect is closed, the surgeon should perform proctoscopy to ensure that the rectal lumen has not been compromised. Patients can begin clear fluids on recovery from anesthesia and be discharged on a normal diet the following day. Postoperative complications are minor, ranging from bleeding, urinary retention, and local infection.

Transanal Endoscopic Microsurgery

Transanal endoscopic microsurgery (TEM) is an option for local excision of rectal cancers in the upper and middle rectum that would not be accessible by transanal technique. It is a relatively new technique, first described by Buess in 1983. The advantage of TEM is that it allows precise excision of tumors while maintaining a constant view of the margin. TEM uses a specialized long operating 40-mm endoscope to allow for full-thickness rectal resection with intraluminal closure of the defect. The TEM instrumentation includes a binocular operating microscope with video projection and long proctoscope and operating surgical instruments. The procedure begins with insufflation of CO_2 into the rectum via a 4-cm operating rectoscope, and endoscopic instruments are then inserted and used under magnification to perform the local resection. The tumor is removed using bipolar electrocautery, which is mounted on a multifunction instrument with cutting and coagulating diathermy and suction and irrigation devices. The TEM scope allows access to tumors located up to 10 cm anteriorly, 15 cm laterally, and 18 cm posteriorly. Lesions selected for TEM include benign lesions and selected low-risk T1 rectal cancers as discussed earlier. Distal rectal lesions often are not amenable to TEM because there is difficulty in maintaining an adequate seal around the scope.

During TEM, if the peritoneal cavity is entered, conversion to an open procedure is required. Patients may also experience a short-term decrease in anorectal function. The principles of resection are the same as for transanal endoanal excision, and if adverse tumor features are found on the pathology, the patient must undergo more radical resection.

Radical Resection

Several principles must be addressed during all radical surgery for rectal cancers and include the principles of TME, importance of circumferential and distal resection margins, and autonomic nerve preservation.

The importance of the circumferential margin in rectal cancer surgery has been highlighted only recently. The circumferential margin is assessed by serial slicing and evaluation of multiple coronal sections of the tumor and mesorectum. Circumferential margins less than 2 mm may be associated with higher local recurrence, distant metastases, and death; all efforts should be made to obtain a negative circumferential margin, including en bloc resection of adjacent structures.

Traditionally, distal margins of 2 to 5 cm were considered standard in surgery for rectal cancers. Recent studies have shown that distal margins less than 2 cm are not associated with higher local recurrence or reduced survival. In fact, a distal margin of as small as 1 cm may be adequate to allow sphincter preservation in patients who receive chemoradiation therapy. Distal spread greater than 1 cm beyond the mucosal edge of the rectal cancer is seen in only 10% of cases, which are poorly differentiated and have node-positive lesions. Thus patients should get a 2-cm distal resection margin when feasible, although acceptable oncologic results may be attained with distal margins of at least 1 cm, especially in patients who have received neoadjuvant chemoradiation therapy.

TOTAL MESORECTAL EXCISION

TME was described in 1982 by Heald and colleagues and is now considered the gold standard for surgical treatment of middle and lower third rectal cancers. The basic principle of TME consists of excising the tumor en bloc with its blood and lymphatic supply (i.e., the mesorectum). This principle is based on the original observations of Moynihan in 1908 regarding potential pathways for lymphatic spread and also on the hypothesis of Heald that the mesorectum represents embryological advantages, conferring protection against tumor dissemination until the terminal stages. The TME concept is based on the premise that locoregional recurrence in rectal cancer results from incomplete clearance of the rectal mesentery, including its blood supply and lymphatic drainage (Figs. 6 and 7). Thus TME dissection in conjunction with

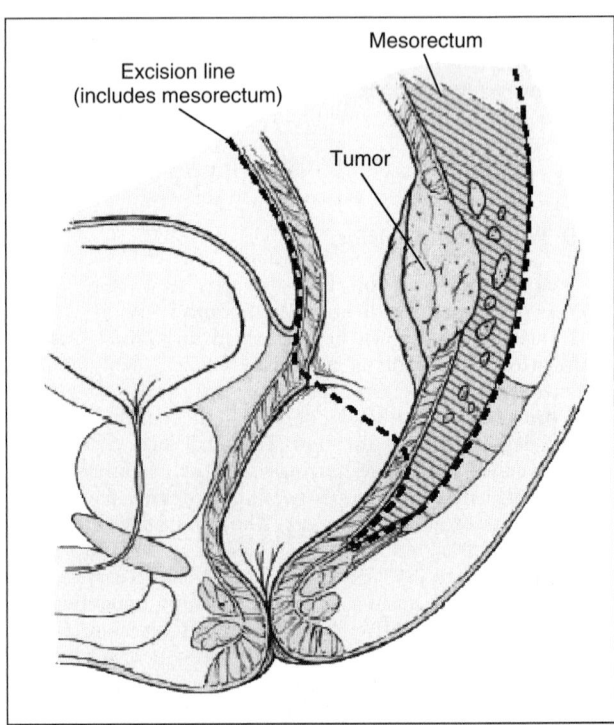

Figure 6 Total mesorectal excision, with the dashed lines indicating the extent of procedure. *From Nelson H, Sargent DJ: N Engl J Med 345:690.*

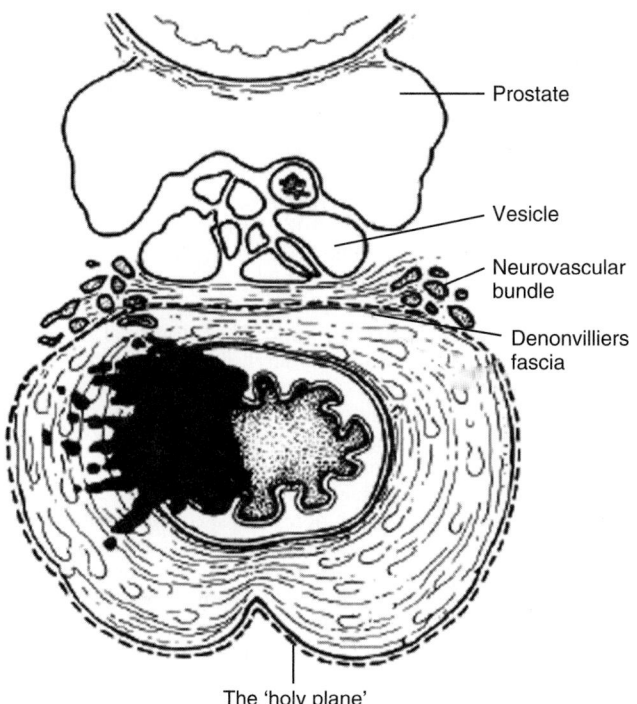

Prostate

Vesicle

Neurovascular
bundle

Denonvilliers
fascia

The 'holy plane'

Figure 7 The "holy plane" of total mesorectal excision in relation to anterior anatomy in a male patient. *From Heald RJ, Moran BJ: Sem Surg Oncol 15:66, 1998.*

either LAR or APR requires en bloc removal of the entire mesorectum, including the mesorectal distal to the tumor, which contains the draining lymph nodes of the rectum as an intact unit. The initial report by Heald and colleagues documented a 0% 2-year local recurrence rate, without the benefit of adjuvant radiotherapy in their initial series of 100 cases and 8% at 10 years among patients who had curative resection.

TME dissection occurs in the areolar plane between the visceral fascia that envelops the rectum and mesorectum and the parietal fascia that envelops the pelvic wall structures (Fig. 6). The procedure facilitates obtaining a negative circumferential and distal margin and lowers the local recurrence rates. Local recurrence rates approximate 6.5% from multiple published series (Table 5). This is in contrast to local recurrence rates of 14% to 40% in series before the advent of TME dissection. TME also allows preservation of the function of autonomic nerves and reduces the likelihood of postoperative genitourinary dysfunction, such as impotence, retrograde ejaculation, and urinary incontinence. However, TME dissection may be associated with an increase in the rate of anastomotic leak.

AUTONOMIC NERVE PRESERVATION

The hypogastric nerve arises from the ventral nerve roots of T12 to L3 and supplies sympathetic nerve innervation. The hypogastric nerve may be associated with the visceral fascia of the mesorectum. Injury to the hypogastric plexus results in increased bladder tone, impaired ejaculation, and dyspareunia in women. The parasympathetic innervation (nervi erigentes) arises from the S2 to S4 ventral nerve roots and is found on the pelvic sidewall. Injury to these nerves can lead to erectile dysfunction, voiding issues, and impaired vaginal lubrication. During TME, sharp meticulous dissection facilitates identification and preservation of the autonomic nerves.

SPHINCTER-SALVAGE PROCEDURES

In most patients, the decision to perform a sphincter-saving operation or an APR has already been made. However, in distal rectal cancers, this decision may not be made until the rectum has been fully mobilized and the distal margin assessed.

All radical resections for rectal cancer use the same technique for mobilizing the rectum and achieving proximal, lateral, and radial margin clearance. Anterior resections are classified as high, low, or extended low, depending on the extent of rectal mobilization and resection and on the level of the anastomosis. Sphincter preservation is usually possible in patients for rectal cancers located greater than 1 cm above the uppermost portion of the anorectal ring, in patients who have acceptable preoperative anorectal function and those who have reasonable pelvic anatomy. However, in a patient with preexisting anorectal dysfunction, a colostomy may often provide better quality of life than persistent postoperative perineal morbidity. In general, sphincter-preserving operations are more likely to occur in a thin patient with a wide pelvis compared with an obese patient with a narrow pelvis.

The possibility of a permanent or temporary diverting stoma should be discussed at length with the patient. Patients should be seen by an enterostomal therapist for counseling and for marking the abdominal wall for either a colostomy or ileostomy (or both).

Patients should receive an intravenous antibiotic before induction of anesthesia. An epidural catheter is often placed for postoperative analgesia. A Foley catheter is placed. In selected patients with a large bulky rectal tumor or in reoperative procedures, ureteral stents may be placed to facilitate intraoperative identification of the ureters. The patient is placed in the modified lithotomy position with the legs in stirrups using Allen or Yellow Fin–style stirrups, with the hips minimally flexed and abducted, knees flexed, and the feet flat in the stirrups. The surgeon should confirm that there is no pressure on the peroneal nerve or bony prominences. In addition, the buttocks should be positioned at the edge of the

Table 5: Long-term Outcomes with TME from Selected Series

Study (yr)	No. of Patients	Follow-up (months)	Study Design	Local Recurrence (%)
Heald (1998)	519	99	Retrospective	8.0 at 10 years
Enker (1995)	246	72	Retrospective	7.3
Zaheer (1998)	514	60	Retrospective	5.7
Havenga (1999)	1411	60	Retrospective	7.6
Martling (2000)	381	24	Prospective with historical controls	6.0
Kapiteijn (2001)	1748	24	Randomized control trial	8.2
				2.4 with preoperative XRT
Wibe (2002)	686	14–60	Retrospective	7.0

XRT, Radiation therapy.

table on a roll that elevates them, allowing access to the anus. The positioning in stirrups is invaluable in allowing an assistant to be positioned between the legs to help with retraction of the bladder and vagina. In addition, it allows access to the anus for placement of a circular stapler for sphincter-restorative procedures. Finally, the surgeon can use this position in mobilizing the splenic flexure. All patients should also have compression stockings with pneumatic compression devices with heparin, unless contraindicated. After the patient is under anesthesia, a digital rectal examination and rigid proctoscopy is performed to empty the rectum and reassess the rectal cancer. The involvement of the sphincter is assessed, and the distal edge of the tumor is noted. In addition, a rectal washout is performed using a large Foley catheter with a 30-ml balloon inflated, and washout of the rectum is performed with normal saline mixed with diluted povidone-iodine solution.

A low midline incision is made, avoiding any potential ostomy sites extending inferiorly to the pubis. The operating surgeon should be positioned on the patient's left side. Self-retaining retractors, such as the Bookwalter, are placed, and an abdominal exploration is performed to evaluate for presence of metastatic disease. The small bowel is then packed away.

Step1: Mobilization of the colon. The sigmoid and left colon are mobilized by incising the white line of Toldt up to the splenic flexure while retracting the rectosigmoid to the right. The left ureter and gonadal vessels are identified using sharp and blunt dissection, and the sigmoid mesentery is separated from the retroperitoneum. The right ureter is usually easier to find in its typical location as it crosses the iliac artery. The mobilization of the splenic flexure is continued and extended proximally to the left transverse colon. This process may be facilitated by the surgeon's moving between the legs to increase the exposure of the splenic attachments, which should be taken with sharp meticulous dissection. Injury to the spleen can occur at this point from traction being applied to the omentum rather than to the spleen itself.

Step 2: Ligation of inferior mesenteric artery (IMA). The surgeon now continues mobilization of the rectosigmoid anteriorly and to the left to identify the base of the inferior mesenteric artery and vein. After the IMA is identified, it is helpful to define an avascular plane on either side of the base of the artery. Ligation of the IMA can then be performed after confirming that there is adequate collateral blood flow through the marginal artery of Drummond. A high ligation of the IMA is performed approximately 1 cm from its origin from the aorta to preserve the para-aortic sympathetic plexus. The right and left ureter should have been identified before ligating the IMA. High ligation of the IMA is preferred because it ensures adequate reach of the proximal colon without tension when performing the anastomosis. After this, we usually divide the sigmoid–descending colon junction with a linear stapler. The mesentery to the sigmoid–descending colon is scored, and then the marginal arcades are clamped, divided, and ligated. If a pouch is planned, the surgeon must ensure that the proximal end of the colon reaches beyond the pubis symphysis without tension.

Step 3: TME with autonomic nerve preservation. The TME dissection is continued by exposing the avascular plane posterior to the rectum and anterior to the sacral promontory (see Fig. 8, A). This is facilitated by retracting the rectosigmoid anteriorly and inferiorly. Sharp dissection under direct visualization should be performed to separate the shiny posterior surface of the mesorectum from the sacrum. The patient may also be placed in Trendelenburg position. The hypogastric nerves should be identified at the sacral promontory as they descend into the presacral space. These nerves must be preserved posteriorly to maintain postoperative genitourinary function. Both ureters should be identified and retracted laterally. The presacral fascia is incised down to the retrosacral or Waldeyer's fascia, a thickened band attaching the rectum to the endopelvic fascia at the S4 level. After the Waldeyer's fascia is incised, the dissection then continues beyond the coccyx, and attention is paid to the anterior curve of the coccyx to avoid

injury to the presacral veins. A lighted St. Mark's retractor facilitates this dissection.

The posterior dissection is performed as far as possible and then the lateral dissection is begun. The surgeon must identify the nervi erigentes on the lateral pelvic sidewalls or "stalks" and preserve them (Fig. 8, B). The lateral dissection is again facilitated by having the assistant stand between the legs and by using the St. Mark's retractor to retract the lateral sidewall while the surgeon retracts the rectum and mesorectum medially. Adequate tension is essential during this lateral dissection to stay within the "holy plane" as defined by Heald (Fig. 7). The middle rectal artery can generally be cauterized, although if it is present as a large vessel, it should be ligated during the lateral dissection. The integrity of the endopelvic fascia should be maintained at all times during the dissection. The lateral dissection ends at the levator muscles, which form the inferior boundary of the pelvic cavity.

The anterior dissection is then begun. This dissection is often the most difficult because the planes of dissection are less discrete and the mesorectum is thin. Placing the patient in reverse Trendelenburg position may facilitate this dissection. The dissection is continued by incising the cul-de-sac and incising Denovilliers' fascia. The dissection is performed in a plane parallel to Denovilliers' fascia between the rectum and the posterior wall of the seminal vesicles (in men) (Fig. 7) or vagina (in women) (Fig. 8, C and D). The assistant can again use the lip of the St. Mark's retractor to elevate these structures anteriorly while the surgeon retracts posteriorly. Dissection is continued to the levator ani muscles, indicating that the entire mesorectum has been mobilized. Involvement of any of the structures in the pelvis, such as bladder, ovary, prostate, or sacrum, by contiguous involvement from the tumor requires en bloc removal of these organs. In patients with a narrow pelvis, the anterior dissection can be facilitated by having the assistant between the patient's legs apply cephalad pressure to the anus to elevate the levator ani and distal rectum toward the surgeon.

Step 4: Margin assessment and anastomosis. After the TME is complete, the point of transaction is chosen distal to the tumor. Recent studies have shown that a 2-cm margin is adequate for an oncologic resection. The level of transection can be confirmed by digital examination or rigid sigmoidoscopy. However, if an adequate distal margin cannot be attained, the surgeon must proceed with an APR. In addition to the distal margin, clearance of the circumferential margin is important, as discussed earlier, and may require resection of en bloc structures. After the point of transection is decided, electrocautery is used to dissect the mesorectal fat until the rectum is cleared circumferentially. The bowel is clamped with a noncrushing clamp distal to the tumor to perform another rectal washout. A transverse anastomosis (TA) stapler is then placed distal to the clamp. The stapler is fired and the rectum divided sharply and handed off the field, leaving a closed rectal stump for anastomosis. The size of the TA stapler used (30, 45, or 60 mm) depends on the depth and diameter of the pelvis.

The surgeon should inspect the resected specimen to determine the distal and radial margin and the integrity of the mesorectal dissection. The specimen should be oriented for the pathologist, and frozen sections of the margins can be obtained. If the margins are inadequate, the surgical plan must be altered to improve clearance of the margin and reduce the risk of local recurrence.

After the specimen is removed, the pelvis should be irrigated with normal saline and hemostasis should be ensured. Posterior bleeding may be seen secondary to injury to the sacral veins and is usually controlled by direct pressure.

Although there are many choices of anastomosis, the end-to-end is the traditional method. Most surgeons use the double-stapled end-to-end anastomosis, although a hand-sewn anastomosis can be performed (Fig. 8, E). The operating field is isolated with towels in preparation of manipulation of the proximal colon. The proximal end of the colon is prepared by clearing off the residual fat, and then the staple line is excised. Sizers are used to select a

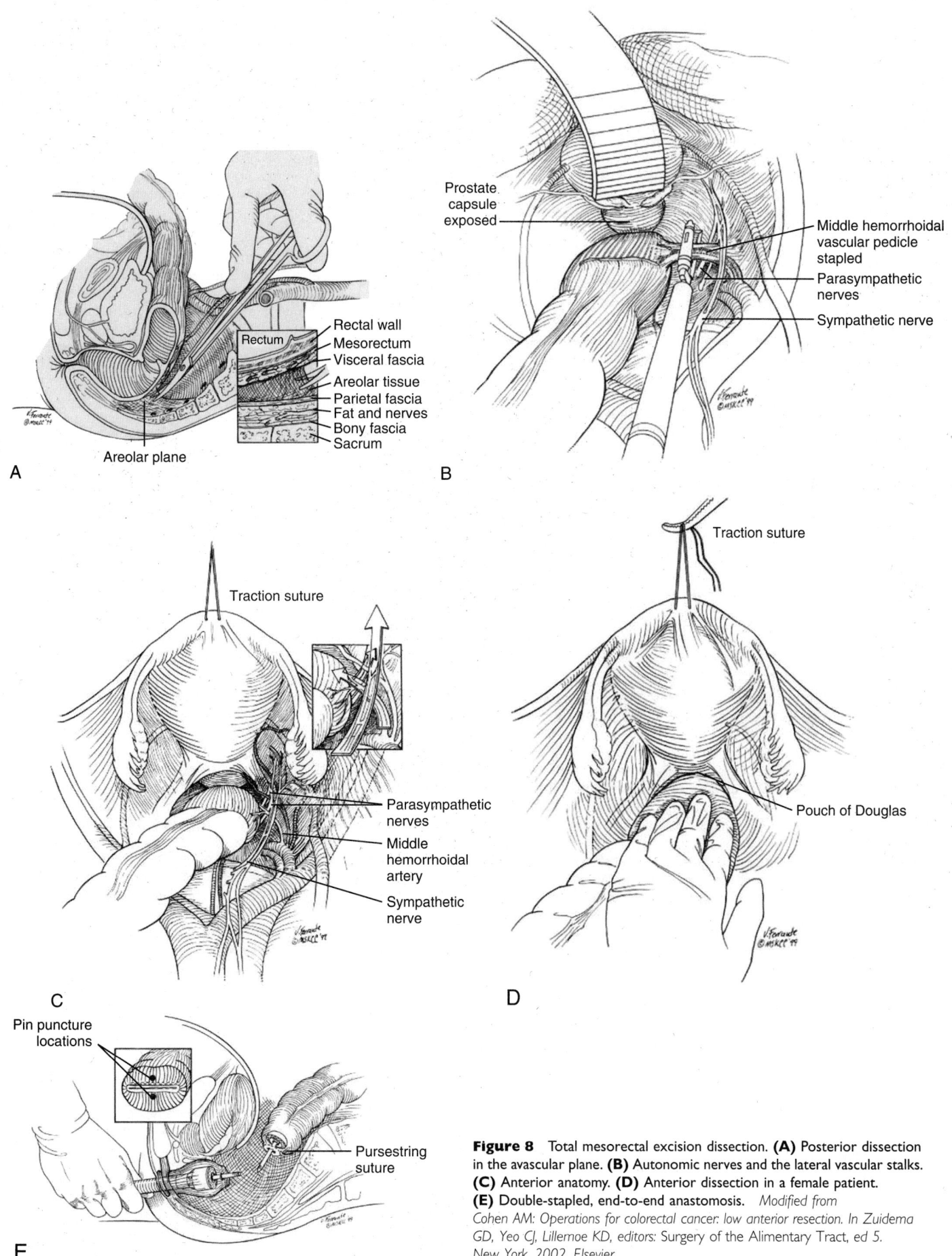

A

Rectal wall
Mesorectum
Visceral fascia
Areolar tissue
Parietal fascia
Fat and nerves
Bony fascia
Sacrum

Rectum

Areolar plane

B

Prostate capsule exposed

Middle hemorrhoidal vascular pedicle stapled

Parasympathetic nerves

Sympathetic nerve

C

Traction suture

Parasympathetic nerves

Middle hemorrhoidal artery

Sympathetic nerve

D

Traction suture

Pouch of Douglas

E

Pin puncture locations

Pursestring suture

Figure 8 Total mesorectal excision dissection. **(A)** Posterior dissection in the avascular plane. **(B)** Autonomic nerves and the lateral vascular stalks. **(C)** Anterior anatomy. **(D)** Anterior dissection in a female patient. **(E)** Double-stapled, end-to-end anastomosis. *Modified from Cohen AM: Operations for colorectal cancer: low anterior resection. In Zuidema GD, Yeo CJ, Lillemoe KD, editors: Surgery of the Alimentary Tract, ed 5. New York, 2002, Elsevier.*

staple diameter. A purse-string suture of 2–0 or 3–0 polypropylene is placed using full-thickness bites at 2-mm intervals. The anvil of the appropriately sized circular stapler is inserted and the purse-string suture is tied around the shaft. The circular stapler, without the anvil but with a trocar attachment, is inserted into the anus and advanced proximally to the apex of the closed rectal stump. The trocar is introduced through or adjacent to the staple line. The anvil and stapler are joined. At this point, the colon is inspected to ensure that no adjacent tissue is entrapped and the mesentery of the bowel is not twisted. The stapler is fired, opened slightly, and then removed. This is the second stapling line in the double staple technique. The stapler is then inspected on a separate table to see that the tissue from the proximal and distal bowel is intact in two rings (i.e., "the doughnuts").

The integrity of the anastomosis is confirmed by insufflating air into the rectum with a proctoscope while the anastomosis is under water and the surgeon inspects for air leaks. The proximal bowel should be clamped during this test. In addition, the proctoscope allows direct visualization of the anastomosis to look for bleeding.

In patients with a low coloanal anastomosis and those who have received neoadjuvant chemoradiation, we routinely perform a diverting loop ileostomy at a site marked preoperatively. The ileostomy can usually be reversed within 12 weeks of surgery. The ileostomy is created by making a 2-cm diameter skin opening. The dissection is then carried down to the anterior rectus sheath. The fascial sheath is opened in a cruciate fashion with muscle splitting and then the posterior peritoneum is opened. The ileum is brought through the opening. It is important to identify the proximal and distal ends, and often a marking suture is placed on the proximal end. The ileostomy is matured at the end following fascial and skin closure of the midline incision and placement of sterile dressing. The ileum is then incised transversely 1 cm above the skin on the distal limb of the loop. The cut edges of the ileum are then sewn to the skin with interrupted absorbable sutures, and the proximal limb can then be everted. A diverting stoma does not protect against anastomotic leakage or prevent anastomotic complications, but it does diminish the morbidity resulting from leakage and reduce the likelihood of an emergency operation. The loop ileostomy is also easier to close than a diverting colostomy. Stoma formation is performed with a plastic ileostomy rod to prevent retraction during the initial postoperative period, and the rod is removed on postoperative day 5. A presacral sump drain is also placed and brought out through the skin opposite to the ileostomy.

A hand-sewn end-to-end colorectal anastomosis can be performed, if desired, in one or two layers with interrupted sutures. The sutures are all placed first, and then we "parachute" the proximal colon to the rectal cuff as the sutures are tied down. The knots are generally placed on the inside to invert the mucosa. Alternatively, a hand-sewn anastomosis can be performed transanally.

Coloanal Anastomosis

Patients with particularly low anastomoses often have poor functional outcomes with straight coloanal or low colorectal anastomoses, reporting urgency, frequency, seepage, and incontinence.

Colonic J-Pouch

A colonic J-pouch is considered for low anastomoses less than 5 cm from the dentate line. The J-pouch was first described in 1986 to increase colonic reservoir and improve quality of life following coloanal anastomosis. The EORTC conducted a randomized, prospective trial comparing the quality of life after a straight coloanal anastomosis with a J-pouch coloanal anastomosis and showed improved functional outcome and quality of life after J-pouch anastomosis. The improvement seen with the J-pouch is most apparent in the first year following surgery. There is no advantage to the J-pouch in patients whose anastomoses are more proximal than

8 cm from the dentate line. The splenic flexure must have been mobilized to provide adequate bowel length. The distal descending colon is folded into a J configuration, with the efferent limb of the J-pouch being 5 to 6 cm. The linear stapler is inserted through a colotomy on the antimesenteric side of the inferior-most aspect of the J-pouch, then closed and fired. Multiple firings of the stapler may be needed. The staple line is checked for bleeding, and then the anvil of the circular stapler is placed using a purse-string suture. Further steps in the anastomosis are as described earlier. We routinely use a diverting loop ileostomy for patients with a J-pouch.

Transverse Coloplasty

A colonic J-pouch is not possible in approximately 25% of patients because of a narrow pelvis or inadequate reach of the proximal colon. In these patients, a transverse coloplasty, which was first described in 1997, is a suitable alternative. A recent randomized trial demonstrated comparable functional results between transverse coloplasty and J-pouch coloanal reconstruction. A longitudinal colotomy is initiated on the antimesenteric border at a point 5 cm from the cut end of the descending colon and extended proximally for 8 to 10 cm. The colotomy is then closed transversely, similar to a Heineke-Mikulicz pyloroplasty with absorbable suture. An end-to-end anastomosis is then performed with the circular stapler in the usual manner, and a diverting ileostomy is made. However, the coloplasty has been thought to be associated with a higher leak rate, ranging from 7% to 16% compared with J-pouch reconstruction, and is reserved only for patients not amenable to a J-pouch reconstruction. The functional advantages of both coloplasty and colonic J-pouches are best seen in the first 2 years after operation, including improvements in symptoms of urgency, frequency, nocturnal stooling, and continence.

Abdominoperineal Resection

Ernest Miles described the first APR operation in 1908. Currently, patients who are not amenable to sphincter salvage undergo APR resection, which involves the en bloc resection of the rectosigmoid, the rectum with the mesorectum, and the anus along with its surrounding mesentery and perianal soft tissues. There is increasing utilization of restorative procedures after radical surgery for rectal cancer, but on the basis of SEER registry data, APR is still performed in 30% to 55% of patients in the United States.

The abdominal portion of the operation is performed in a manner similar to the sphincter-salvage approach described earlier with a total mesorectal excision. In patients in whom an APR is planned preoperatively, the anus should be closed circumferentially with a heavy, purse-string suture before starting the surgery to prevent stool contamination during the procedure. The total mesorectal excision should be carried down to the levator muscles inferiorly. After the rectum is fully mobilized, the surgeon stands between the legs to perform the perineal excision. A two-team approach may also be used to expedite the surgery.

The perineal dissection is accomplished by making an elliptical incision around the anus. The elliptical incision should extend from the perineal body anteriorly to the coccyx posteriorly. Dissection is continued with electrocautery through the ischiorectal fat. A self-retaining retractor is useful to facilitate deep dissection. We prefer to use the Lone Star retractor, which has adjustable, flexible hooks that can be placed circumferentially to evert the tissues out. The dissection is carried outside of the external sphincters toward the coccyx. The anococcygeal ligament is palpated posteriorly and incised, creating an opening between the left and right levator muscles. At this point, it is helpful for the perineal surgeon to insert an index finger into the pelvis to guide the division of the posterolateral soft tissue with electrocautery, by hooking the index finger under the levator muscles laterally on each side. A vessel-sealing device, such as the LigaSure (Valleylab,

Boulder, CO), is useful during the deeper dissection. The anterior dissection should be done last. A narrow Deaver or appendectomy retractor may be used to improve the retraction during the deeper dissection. When the perineal opening is wide enough, the proximal end of the specimen is passed from the abdominal portion through the perineum in the opening between the coccyx and the anus. The everted specimen is then used to help provide traction to develop the anterior dissection plane. In male patients, the anterior dissection requires careful attention to avoid injury to the urethra or the prostatic capsule, which may result in excessive bleeding. As the dissection proceeds, it is helpful to palpate the Foley catheter during anterior dissection to remain in the right plane. In female patients, a bulky anterior lesion may necessitate a posterior wall vaginectomy to ensure a negative margin.

After the specimen is freed circumferentially, it is inspected and sent for pathologic evaluation. The pelvis is irrigated, and hemostasis is achieved. The perineal incision is then closed in several layers with absorbable sutures to minimize the risk of perineal wound infection. A drain should be placed in this space below the peritoneal reflection and be brought out either transabdominally or through the perineum. We prefer also to mobilize and place an omental pedicle in the pelvis to keep the small bowel out of the pelvis and decrease the risk of subsequent pelvic adhesions, as well as to facilitate healing.

The end colostomy is created in a site marked preoperatively by the enterostomal therapist. The colostomy site opening is created, similar to the loop ileostomy described earlier, in the left lower quadrant. The mobilized colon is passed through this site, but it is not matured until the abdominal incision is closed and a dry sterile dressing has been applied. The colon is secured to the peritoneal cavity circumferentially as it exits the abdomen. The colostomy is generally matured using an eversion technique and secured to the skin with interrupted 3–0 absorbable sutures.

The mortality rate from radical rectal surgery is approximately 2%, with the majority of deaths related to cardiopulmonary complications. The overall risk of anastomotic leak after rectal surgery is approximately 5% but can increase in patients who have a low coloanal anastomosis, those who are immunosuppressed, and those who have undergone neoadjuvant chemoradiation therapy. The risk of autonomic nerve dysfunction has declined from between 60% and 85% to less than 15% in most current series with TME dissection.

Laparoscopic Approaches

There are no prospective, randomized trials on laparoscopic resection of rectal cancers. Thus definitive recommendations cannot be made. However, small, nonrandomized studies show that laparoscopic-assisted TME is feasible when performed by experienced laparoscopic surgeons. Oncologic outcomes appear comparable to open approaches, and the laparoscopic approach may provide decreased short-term morbidity, including less pain, less postoperative ileus, and shorter length of stay.

ADJUVANT THERAPY

The reported 5-year survival rates for rectal cancer shown by Jessup and colleagues using the National Cancer Data Base are shown in Fig. 9. Adjuvant therapy in rectal cancer is given both to improve locoregional control and to lower the risk of systemic disease. Multiple studies have documented the benefit of radiation therapy to reduce the risk of local recurrence, as discussed in the section on neoadjuvant therapy. The risk of local recurrence in the modern era of TME is significantly lower than the historical range of 30% to 60%, ranging from 3.5% to 13%. The addition of radiation therapy to TME lowers the risk of local recurrence further, as

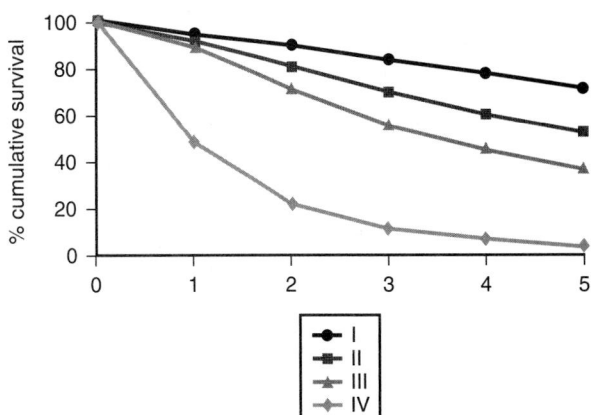

Figure 9 Survival patterns in rectal cancer. *From Jessup JM, Stewart AK, Menck HR: Cancer 83:2408, 1998.*

demonstrated in the Dutch trial (from 8.2% to 2.4%). Furthermore, radiation appears to have improved benefit, if given in the preoperative setting, based on the data from the German trial in which the local recurrence was reduced in the arm given preoperative chemoradiation (6% vs. 13%).

No trial to date has conclusively shown that adjuvant chemotherapy improves survival in patients who have undergone neoadjuvant chemoradiation. However, the NCCN guidelines and our protocol are to give 5-FU-based chemotherapy to all patients who received neoadjuvant chemoradiation. Most chemotherapy regimens contain infusional 5-FU and may include other drugs such as oxaliplatin or irinotecan.

SURVEILLANCE

The risk of second primary colorectal cancer is 1.5% at 5 years in patients with resected stage II and III disease. In addition, 40% to 50% of patients will experience a recurrence after curative resection. The risk of recurrence is highest in the first 2 years; 75% to 80% of recurrences are seen in the first 2 years and 90% within the first 4 years. We follow patients with a history and physical examination every 3 months for the first 2 years, then every 6 months for 3 years, and then annually. Serum CEA level is also monitored at similar intervals. A colonoscopy is performed at 1 year after the initial surgery and then every 3 to 5 years if the patient remains polyp free. We also perform a CT scan of the chest, abdomen, and pelvis at 1 year.

RECURRENT AND METASTATIC DISEASE

Patients who recur after local resection can be managed with salvage surgery if they have local disease only. These patients should then undergo radical surgery along with adjuvant chemotherapy and radiation therapy. In several small series, these patients have a 50% to 88% 5-year disease-free survival. Weiser and colleagues described 49 patients who underwent salvage surgery after local excision of rectal cancer. Of these patients, 55% required an extended pelvic dissection with en bloc resection of adjacent pelvic organs, and 58% had recurrence or died of disease within 33 months; 5-year disease-specific survival was 53%. Patients who experience recurrence with widely metastatic disease after local excision of rectal cancer should be managed in the context of a multidisciplinary team, although some of these patients may benefit from palliative surgery. Resection of isolated metastatic disease in the liver or lung (or both) has been shown to have long-term survival benefit in multiple studies and is discussed elsewhere.

In the current era of rectal surgery with TME, the local recurrence rates after radical surgery are 3% to 5%. Approximately 7% to 20% of these patients with local recurrences can undergo repeat resection with a repeat LAR, APR, or pelvic exenteration. An anastomotic recurrence after a high anterior resection may be treated with a repeat LAR or may require an APR. Local recurrences after an APR are usually not amenable to surgery and often require an exenteration or sacrectomy (or both). Patients considered for repeat resection should be chosen carefully after extensive staging to rule out systemic metastatic disease, with modalities such as CT, MRI, and FDG-PET/CT scans used to perform an operation with curative intent. These patients should also receive multimodality therapy to maximize the survival benefit. In patients with widespread systemic metastases and local symptomatic recurrence, a palliative procedure may be performed using local techniques such as excision, fulguration, endorectal stents, or chemoradiation.

SUGGESTED READINGS

Bosset J, Collette L, Calais G, and others for EORTC Radiotherapy Group Trial 22921: Chemotherapy with preoperative radiotherapy in rectal cancer, *New Engl J Med* 355:1114, 2006.

Heald RJ, Moran BJ: Embryology and anatomy of the rectum, *Sem Surg Oncol* 15:66, 1998.

National Comprehensive Cancer Network. Rectal cancer (NCCN Practice Guidelines in Oncology), http://www.nccn.org/professionals/physician_gls/PDF/rectal.pdf.

Paty PB, Nash GM, Baron P, and others: Long-term results of local excision for rectal cancer, *Ann Surg* 236:522, 2002.

Stipa F, Chessin DB, Shia J, and others: A pathologic complete response of rectal cancer to preoperative combined-modality therapy results in improved oncological outcome compared with those who achieve no downstaging on the basis of preoperative endorectal ultrasonography, *Ann Surg Oncol* 13:1047, 2006.

Weiser MR, Landmann RG, Wong WD, and others: Surgical salvage of recurrent rectal cancer after transanal excision, *Dis Colon Rectum* 48:1169, 2005.

THE USE OF ^{18}F-FLUORODEOXYGLUCOSE POSITRON EMISSION TOMOGRAPHY IN THE MANAGEMENT OF COLORECTAL CANCER

Tobias Leibold, MD, Ignacio A. Echenique and José G. Guillem, MD, MPH

^{18}F-Fluorodeoxyglucose positron emission tomography (^{18}F-FDG-PET) imaging has been successfully used in the diagnosis, staging, and treatment monitoring for a number of cancers, including ovarian, breast, lung, and colorectal. The ability of ^{18}F-FDG-PET to visualize metabolic activity distinguishes it from morphologic imaging modalities such as computerized tomography (CT) and magnetic resonance imaging (MRI). ^{18}F-FDG-PET provides an opportunity for enhanced differentiation between benign and malignant neoplasms, as well as differentiation between treatment effects, fibrosis, and viable tumor.

This chapter discusses indications for ^{18}F-FDG-PET during the diagnosis, treatment, and follow-up of colorectal cancer.

BASIC THEORY: ^{18}F-FLUORODEOXYGLUCOSE POSITRON EMISSION TOMOGRAPHY

^{18}F-FDG is a glucose analogue that carries a positron-emitting isotope (^{18}F). According to the Warburg effect, ^{18}F-FDG is preferentially taken up by metabolically active cells with upregulated cell surface glucose transporters and increased rate of glycolysis. ^{18}F-FDG decays by positron emission, and after traveling up to a few millimeters, the positron collides with an electron to produce a pair of annihilation photons. These photons are emitted in opposite directions and, after being detected by the PET scanner, can be localized to their source to construct a whole body image. Images can be displayed in a coronal, sagittal, and transverse manner. Normal PET scans demonstrate physiologic ^{18}F-FDG uptake in the brain, heart, colon, bladder, stomach, kidney, spleen, liver, and bone marrow. Because of the distance a positron travels before annihilation and other physical factors including the size of the detector system, the resolution of PET images is currently limited in lesions below 1 cm. Similarly, because of a wide variation in tumor metabolic activity, the sensitivity of ^{18}F-FDG-PET for detecting primary and recurrent mucinous cancer is generally lower than that reported for nonmucinous adenocarcinomas.

SCREENING AND STAGING OF COLORECTAL CANCER

It has been demonstrated that ^{18}F-FDG-PET can detect both malignant and premalignant colorectal lesions. However, the sensitivity is dependent on the size and the grade of dysplasia. For example, it has been reported that ^{18}F-FDG-PET detects 100% of colorectal cancers 2 cm or larger but only 17% of cancers smaller than 2 cm, including premalignant adenomas. It has also been shown that the sensitivity of ^{18}F-FDG-PET increases with the grade of dysplasia, from approximately 33% for adenomas with low-grade dysplasia to 89% for carcinomas. Furthermore, false-positive findings are not insignificant, mostly because of inflammation from diverticulitis or segmental colitis. Given the expense of ^{18}F-FDG-PET and its limited accuracy for detecting small lesions, it does not qualify as a colorectal cancer screening modality in its present form.

In terms of staging, the requirements for colon cancer differ from those for rectal cancer. For colon cancer, identification of distant metastatic disease is more important than T- and N-staging because the extent of mesenteric resection of the primary colon cancer is not influenced by T and N stage. However, the presence of distant metastatic disease in an otherwise asymptomatic colon cancer patient may justify upfront systemic chemotherapy rather than an initial resection of the primary colon cancer. For rectal cancer, accurate T- and N-staging is essential to determine whether neoadjuvant therapy is required and whether a sphincter-preserving surgical procedure can be performed. However, because ^{18}F-FDG-PET is not able to differentiate between the layers of the bowel wall, it is therefore unable to define level of invasion (T-level). Similarly, the sensitivity and specificity of ^{18}F-FDG-PET for detecting regional lymph node involvement range between 22% and 29% and 88% and 96%, respectively. This limitation is due to resolution of PET scanners and signal overlap with the primary tumor. Given the higher sensitivity of magnetic resonance imaging (MRI) and endorectal ultrasound (EUS), ^{18}F-FDG-PET in its present form does not appear to provide any further reliable information on regional lymph node staging in patients with rectal cancer. Therefore the potential role of ^{18}F-FDG-PET in the initial staging of colorectal cancer is the detection of distant disease. Although there are conflicting reports, ^{18}F-FDG-PET appears to be superior to CT and MRI in detecting distant metastases of colorectal cancer. In fact, ^{18}F-FDG-PET can identify colorectal liver metastases with up to 95% sensitivity.

In summary, although ^{18}F-FDG-PET may not have a role in screening for colorectal cancer, it seems to be the most accurate imaging modality for detecting distant metastatic disease in patients with colon and rectal cancer and has the potential to alter treatment decisions.

ASSESSMENT OF RESPONSE TO NEOADJUVANT THERAPY IN RECTAL CANCER

Because a number of studies have demonstrated improved local control following neoadjuvant therapy, preoperative radiation- or radiochemotherapy has evolved into the preferred treatment paradigm for patients with locally advanced rectal cancer. It has been reported that with preoperative radiochemotherapy, downstaging of rectal cancer can be achieved in up to 75% of cases. Accurately identifying patients with a great response to neoadjuvant therapy may direct treatment toward sphincter-preserving surgery or less aggressive surgical approaches. However, CT, MRI, and EUS appear unable to assess response because they cannot accurately differentiate scar, fibrosis, and viable tumor. Although the sensitivity of ^{18}F-FDG-PET may be reduced after recent chemotherapy, a study from Memorial Sloan-Kettering Cancer Center (MSKCC) demonstrated that ^{18}F-FDG-PET detected 100% of patients with response to neoadjuvant therapy and accurately estimated the extent of pathologic response in 60% of patients. Furthermore, the results indicated that ^{18}F-FDG-PET assessment of response to neoadjuvant therapy may predict long-term outcome in patients with locally advanced rectal cancer. Of particular interest is the potential for differentiation between responders and nonresponders early during the course of their neoadjuvant treatment. At this stage, treatment alterations, including a change to alternative chemotherapeutic agents or abandonment of ineffective neoadjuvant therapy to save resources and minimize the delay to definitive surgery, could further improve the outcome in patients with locally advanced rectal cancer. In ovarian and breast cancer, a number of studies have reliably predicted response to treatment as early as after the first cycle of neoadjuvant treatment.

In summary, because it has been suggested that in patients with a great response to neoadjuvant therapy local surgical approaches could be an alternative to radical surgery, assessment of response by ^{18}F-FDG-PET may have the potential to identify these patients preoperatively. Metabolic changes occur earlier than measurable tumor shrinkage, and thus only functional imaging modalities such as ^{18}F-FDG-PET can provide an early assessment of response to therapy.

FOLLOW-UP AND MANAGEMENT OF RECURRENT COLORECTAL CANCER

Because 20% to 60% of patients with colorectal cancer experience recurrence following an initially curative resection, follow-up of these patients is important to detect recurrences in an asymptomatic and potentially curative stage. Therefore imaging modalities are routinely used in various follow-up programs. However, their beneficial effect on reresection rates and overall survival has yet to be fully defined. In this setting, there are actually three scenarios in which ^{18}F-FDG-PET can be helpful. First, if used routinely, ^{18}F-FDG-PET may detect and localize unsuspected locally recurrent and distant metastatic colorectal lesions. Second, ^{18}F-FDG-PET may help differentiate among scar, fibrosis, and viable tumor in cases in which recurrent colorectal cancer is suspected or other imaging modalities show no evidence of disease despite an elevated carcinoembryonic antigen (CEA). Third, ^{18}F-FDG-PET may help to determine resectability in patients with diagnosed recurrent colorectal cancer at high risk for unresectable disease.

The use of ^{18}F-FDG-PET in the routine follow-up of curatively resected colorectal cancer patients has rarely been studied because the direct costs of ^{18}F-FDG-PET are still high and the cost effectiveness of follow-up programs in colorectal cancer is already questionable. However, because many intensive follow-up programs include CT as a routine imaging modality, with further improvements and reductions in cost it is likely that ^{18}F-FDG-PET could be used in combination with CT, such as PET-CT, to obtain simultaneous functional and anatomic information.

To discuss the role of ^{18}F-FDG-PET in patients with suspected recurrent colorectal cancer, it is necessary to differentiate between hepatic metastases and locally recurrent disease. As mentioned earlier, conventional imaging modalities such as CT and MRI have limited ability to distinguish scar from viable tumor, especially in patients with rectal cancer following preoperative radiochemotherapy in which anatomic changes resulting from inflammation and scarification are common. In our experience, as well as that of others, ^{18}F-FDG-PET turned out to be an accurate imaging modality, with a sensitivity of 84% and a specificity of 88% in detecting local pelvic recurrence in patients with rectal cancer following preoperative radiochemotherapy. In terms of detecting intrahepatic disease, it seems that ^{18}F-FDG-PET is equal to CT or MRI, but it has been reported that for the detection of recurrent intrahepatic tumors after liver resection, ^{18}F-FDG-PET has clear advantages.

Because it has been demonstrated that 70% of patients with asymptomatic recurrent colorectal disease present with elevated plasma CEA concentrations, serial CEA measurements are widely used in the follow-up of colorectal cancer patients. However, imaging studies often do not show any evidence of recurrent disease despite increasing CEA levels. Therefore it has been reported that ^{18}F-FDG-PET is a valuable tool in patients with a rising CEA and can detect recurrent disease with a positive predictive value of 89% and a negative predictive value of 100% in patients in whom conventional imaging techniques show no evidence for recurrent local or distant disease.

In summary, the optimal use of ^{18}F-FDG-PET in the routine follow-up and management of patients with recurrent colorectal cancer remains to be defined. It is unlikely that ^{18}F-FDG-PET qualifies for a routine follow-up imaging modality in its present form. For recurrent colorectal cancer, ^{18}F-FDG-PET shows promise and may currently be used to (1) verify nonspecific findings detected on conventional imaging modalities, (2) evaluate an unexplained CEA elevation, and (3) identify occult unresectable disease preoperatively.

PREDICTING RESECTABILITY

Several studies have also examined the role of ^{18}F-FDG-PET on selection of patients for resection of hepatic colorectal metastases and local recurrences. It has been reported that ^{18}F-FDG-PET as a whole-body imaging technique is the most accurate imaging modality for detecting extrahepatic disease and that it can predict the patients who are most likely to benefit from a second surgical procedure (Figs. 1 and 2). In fact, a study from MSKCC examined the role of ^{18}F-FDG-PET in predicting resectability in a group of 40 patients being considered for resection of hepatic colorectal metastases but at high risk for unresectable disease by clinical criteria. In 23% of cases, ^{18}F-FDG-PET identified unresectable disease and avoided unwarranted liver resection. However, ^{18}F-FDG-PET influenced the clinical management in 40% of cases either by avoiding unnecessary liver resection or by guiding surgery in patients in whom resectable extrahepatic disease was detected.

^{18}F-FLUORODEOXYGLUCOSE POSITRON EMISSION TOMOGRAPHY/ COMPUTED TOMOGRAPHY

In the last few years, several studies have examined the accuracy of combined PET/CT scanners in staging and restaging rectal cancer under the hypothesis that simultaneously obtained metabolic activity and anatomic changes improve diagnostic accuracy for tumor staging and restaging compared with separately acquired PET or CT. In a study of 51 patients with suspected recurrent colorectal cancer, PET/CT demonstrated a significantly higher accuracy of staging than PET alone (88% vs. 71%). A recently published study evaluated the efficacy of combined PET/CT in the evaluation of primary colorectal cancer. PET/CT altered management in 24% of patients with primary colorectal cancer presenting with elevated CEA levels (>10 ng/ml) or equivocal findings on CT scans.

It appears that PET/CT is significantly more accurate than PET or CT alone for staging and restaging colorectal cancer. However, adequately powered randomized trials are required to confirm these results, as well as the impact of PET/CT on assessment of tumor response.

SUMMARY

^{18}F-FDG-PET is a valuable tool in the management of several malignancies, including colorectal cancer. Although its role in the screening for and the initial local staging of colorectal cancer may be limited, in patients with suspected distant disease ^{18}F-FDG-PET can help to determine operability. In terms of rectal cancer response to neoadjuvant therapy, ^{18}F-FDG-PET has clear advantages compared with other imaging modalities and may be able to predict response early during the course of treatment. The use of ^{18}F-FDG-PET during follow-up of colorectal cancer patients has yet to be defined. However, for patients with suspected recurrent disease, ^{18}F-FDG-PET can be used to determine unresectable disease and therefore identify patients unlikely to benefit from an exploratory laparotomy. It is anticipated that the fusion of PET and CT will further improve the accuracy of ^{18}F-FDG-PET. However, this requires further study.

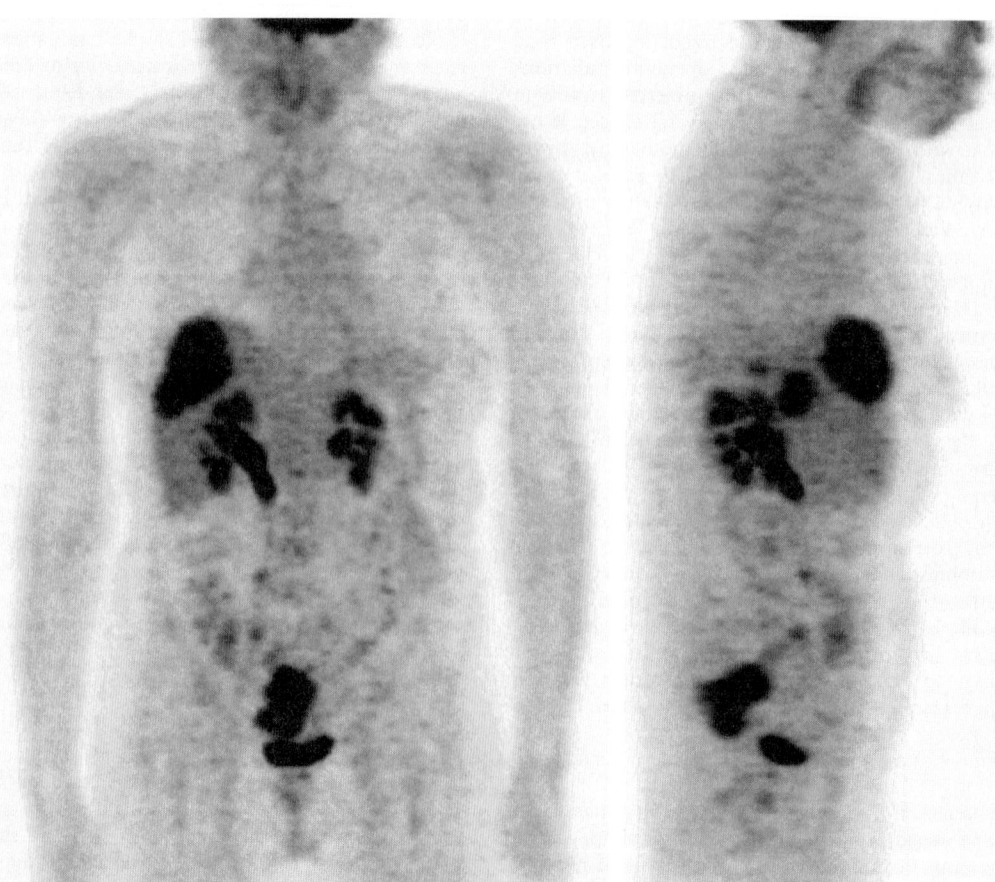

Figure 1 ^{18}F-FDG-PET showing a large rectal mass with FDG uptake in liver segments 7 and 8 consistent with metastatic rectal cancer. *^{18}F-FDG-PET*, ^{18}F-Fluorodeoxyglucose positron emission tomography.

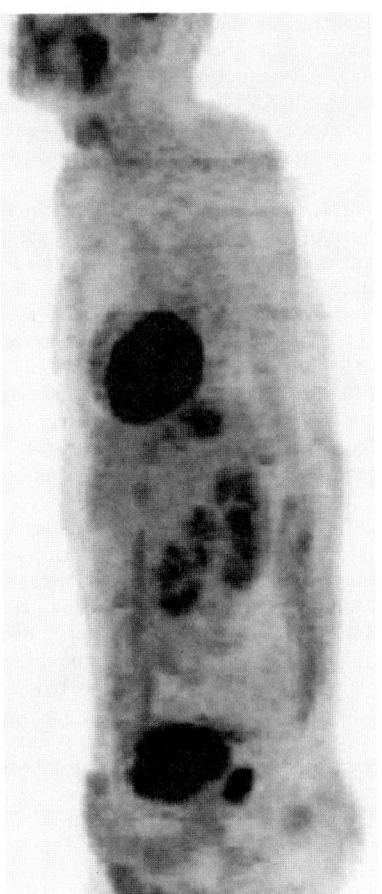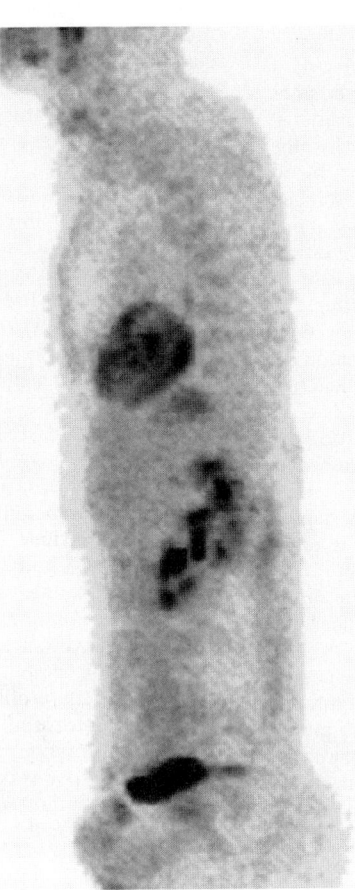

Figure 2 ^{18}F-FDG-PET before and after preoperative combined modality therapy showing a complete metabolic response of the primary rectal tumor without evidence of distant disease. *^{18}F-FDG-PET*, ^{18}F-Fluorodeoxyglucose positron emission tomography.

SUGGESTED READINGS

Chessin DB, Kiran RP, Akhurst T, and others: The emerging role of 18F-fluorodeoxyglucose positron emission tomography in the management of primary and recurrent rectal cancer, *J Am Coll Surg* 201:948, 2005.

Guillem JG, Moore HG, Akhurst T, and others: Sequential preoperative fluorodeoxyglucose-positron emission tomography assessment of response to preoperative chemoradiation: a means for determining long-term outcomes of rectal cancer, *J Am Coll Surg* 199:1, 2004.

Guillem JG, Puig-La Calle J Jr, Akhurst T, and others: Prospective assessment of primary rectal cancer response to preoperative radiation and chemotherapy using 18-fluorodeoxyglucose positron emission tomography, *Dis Colon Rectum* 43:18, 2000.

Libutti SK, Alexander HR Jr, Choyke P, and others: A prospective study of 2-[18F] fluoro-2-deoxy-D-glucose/positron emission tomography scan, 99mTc-labeled arcitumomab (CEA-scan), and blind second-look laparotomy for detecting colon cancer recurrence in patients with increasing carcinoembryonic antigen levels, *Ann Surg Oncol* 8:779, 2001.

Moore HG, Akhurst T, Larson SM, and others: A case-controlled study of 18-fluorodeoxyglucose positron emission tomography in the detection of pelvic recurrence in previously irradiated rectal cancer patients, *J Am Coll Surg* 197:22, 2003.

ADJUVANT TREATMENT FOR COLORECTAL CANCER

Jeff Infante, MD, and Wells Messersmith, MD

OVERVIEW

Colorectal cancer (CRC) is the second-leading cause of cancer mortality in the United States. In 2005, it was estimated that there were 145,290 new cases of cancer of the colon and rectum in the United States and an associated 54,200 deaths from this disease. Almost 40% of patients with newly diagnosed colorectal carcinoma have locoregional spread of the disease at diagnosis, and 19% have distant metastasis.

Surgical resection remains the foundation of a curative approach in both colon and rectal cancer. Failure after potentially curative resection is believed to be due to the presence of micrometastatic disease that was not removed during the operation. Chemotherapy and radiation therapy, either in the adjuvant (postoperative) or neoadjuvant (preoperative) setting, have been shown to decrease the risk of recurrence and increase survival. In the adjuvant setting, many patients must be treated to save one life. Therefore rational therapeutic choices must offer a better chance at cure yet should not be associated with excessive morbidity and mortality because many patients would be cured with surgery alone.

STAGING

Formal colorectal cancer staging is essential to establish the risk of recurrence and to ensure that the goals of care are curative rather than palliative, as in the advanced disease setting. The National Comprehensive Cancer Network (NCCN) recommends that the preoperative workup include a colonoscopy, complete blood counts, comprehensive electrolyte panel, carcinoembryonic antigen (CEA) serum level, computed tomography (CT) scan of the abdomen and pelvis, chest radiograph, and a pathologic review. Positron emission tomography (PET) is not routinely indicated but is often used if there are suspicious findings on the CT scan suggesting disease outside the colon. In general, the preoperative workup in rectal cancer is similar to that of colon cancer, with the optional addition of a pelvic magnetic resonance imaging (MRI) or endoscopic ultrasound to help better define the depth of invasion and lymph node spread. In rectal cancer, there is increasing evidence supporting the early use of PET/CT scans to provide additional staging information. Accurate preoperative staging is critical because rectal cancer therapy is often neoadjuvant as opposed to adjuvant. The staging information from a posttreatment pathologic specimen is often limited and less accurate.

The true pathologic stage is defined after the appropriate surgical procedure. Upon its introduction in 1987 by the American Joint Committee on Cancer, the TNM (T, primary tumor; N, regional lymph nodes; M, distant metastasis) staging system has largely replaced the Duke's and other older staging systems for colorectal cancer. The 5-year survival rates for both colon and rectal cancer are stage dependent. For patients with stage I disease, surgery alone is the treatment of choice because the 5-year survival is greater than 90%. As discussed in this chapter, the more extensive the disease and the more aggressive the biology, the greater the benefit of the adjuvant therapy.

ADJUVANT THERAPY FOR COLON CANCER

5-Fluorouracil-Based Regimens

The antifolate 5-fluorouracil (5-FU) has been the cornerstone of chemotherapy for CRC since the 1960s. A metabolite of 5-FU, fluorodeoxyuridine monophosphate (FdUMP), inhibits thymidylate synthase (TS) and thus interferes with DNA synthesis. 5-FU is also incorporated into RNA, which disrupts protein synthesis. Studies

did not show a survival advantage for adjuvant 5-FU until it was combined with a biomodulator. Leucovorin (folinic acid), levamisole (an antihelminthic agent), and methotrexate were all explored as modulators of 5-FU. Leucovorin (LV) has been accepted as the standard biomodulator and increases cytotoxicity by stabilizing the FdUMP/TS complex and increasing the intracellular pool of reduced folate.

Multiple prospective trials have shown the clinical benefit of postoperative 5FU in combination of either leucovorin or levamisole (Table 1). Shorter courses of 6 to 8 months of adjuvant 5FU/LV were equivalent to 12 months of therapy. The National Surgical Adjuvant Breast and Bowel Project C-03 trial showed that 6 months of 5FU and LV each given weekly at 500 mg/m^2 for 6 of 8 weeks (Roswell Park Regimen) were superior to combination therapy with methyl 1-[2-chloroethyl-3-(4methyl-cyclohexyl)] (CCNU), vincristine, and 5FU. The incremental increases in disease-free survival (DFS) from 64% to 73% and in overall survival (OS) from 77% to 84% were proportionally similar to other randomized trials with 5FU and LV.

There are numerous 5-FU dosing schedules. In the adjuvant setting, these include bolus daily for 5 days every 4 weeks, the so-called Mayo Clinic regimen; weekly for 6 of every 8 weeks, or Roswell Park regimen; and infusional schedules. Unlike the metastatic setting, continuous infusion 5-FU (CIFU) has not shown superiority over bolus-type adjuvant regimens. There was no difference in DFS or OS, but there was a suggestion that it may have an improved toxicity profile.

The convenience of oral therapy and the prospect of avoiding long-term intravenous access complications, such as thrombosis and infection, have stimulated the development of oral fluoropyrimidines. Capecitabine is a fluoropyrimidine carbamate that is converted to 5-FU in a three-step enzymatic cascade. Preclinical studies have shown that capecitabine exhibits selectivity for neoplastic cells because the final enzymatic conversion involves thymidine phosphorylase, which is preferentially expressed in tumor as opposed to normal tissues. Twice-daily oral administration simulates continuous infusion of 5-FU without the costs and inconvenience of a pump.

The X-ACT trial showed that capecitabine was at least equivalent to bolus 5-FU in the adjuvant setting. This noninferiority trial randomized 1987 patients with resected stage III colon cancer to 6 months of adjuvant capecitabine 1250 mg/m^2 twice day for 2 weeks of a 3-week schedule or to bolus 5-FU 425 mg/m^2 and LV 20 mg/m^2 daily days 1 through 5 of a 28-day cycle (Mayo Regimen). The 3-year DFS was 64.2% in the capecitabine arm compared with 60.6% in the bolus 5-FU arm. With a hazard

Table 1: Selected Trials of Adjuvant Chemotherapy for Colon Cancer

TRIAL	Description	N	3-year DFS	p Value
NSABP C-03	Intravenous 5-FU (Roswell Park Regimen) vs. methyl CCNU, vincristine, and 5-FU	1081 patients with Duke's B/C colon cancer	73% vs. 64%	.004
X-ACT	Capecitabine 1250 mg/m^2 orally twice daily vs. bolus intravenous 5-FU (Mayo Regimen)	1987 patients with resected stage III colon cancer (noninferiority trial)	64.2% vs. 60.6%	<.001*
MOSAIC	FOLFOX-4 vs. infusional 5-FU/LV	2246 patients with stage II/III colon cancer	78.2% vs. 72.9%	.002
NSABP C-07	FLOX vs. bolus weekly 5-FU/LV	2407 patients with stage II/III colon cancer	76.5% vs. 71.6%	<0.004

DFS, Disease-free survival; 5-FU, 5-fluorouracil; FLOX, bolus weekly 5-FU/LV with biweekly oxaliplatin; FOLFOX-4, oxaliplatin, folinic acid, and 5-fluorouracil combination; LV, leucovorin; methyl CCNU, 1-[2-chloroethyl-3-(4methyl-cyclohexyl)].
*Equivalence trial.

ratio of 0.87 and a $p < .001$, this study met its primary endpoint of equivalent DFS. The side effect profiles are slightly different, with capecitabine having an increased risk for hand-foot syndrome but markedly improved reductions in neutropenia and stomatitis seen in the bolus regimen. It remains unknown whether capecitabine is equivalent to infusional schedules of 5-FU when added to oxaliplatin and bevacizumab, pending the results of the AVANT trial.

Oxaliplatin-Based Regimens

Oxaliplatin is a third-generation platinum compound that cross-links DNA and induces apoptosis. Oxaliplatin has properties that are distinct from other platinum compounds such as cisplatin and carboplatin. The preclinical models showed both activity in cisplatin-resistant CRC cell lines and synergism when combined with 5-FU. Oxaliplatin causes little nephrotoxicity, ototoxicity, and alopecia but shares bone–marrow-suppressive properties and has its own sensory neuropathy that is typically reversible, cumulative, and exacerbated by exposure to cold.

Oxaliplatin was quickly moved to the adjuvant setting after initial studies showed its efficacy in the second-line metastatic setting. The MOSAIC trial randomized 2246 stage II (node negative) and stage III patients to receive either oxaliplatin, folinic acid and 5-FU (FOLFOX-4) combination or infusional 5-FU/LV. The infusional 5-FU was given every 2 weeks on a 28-day cycle as LV 200 mg/m^2 over 2 hours followed by bolus 5-FU 400 mg/m^2, and then a 22-hour infusion of 5-FU at 600 mg/m^2 on days 1 and 2. FOLFOX-4 included the same regimen of 5-FU/LV with the addition of oxaliplatin at 85 mg/m^2 over 2 hours every 2 weeks of a 28-day cycle. The probability of being free of disease at 3 years was 78.2% in the FOLFOX-4 arm compared with 72.9% in the infusional 5-FU/LV arm. Subgroup analysis revealed that stage III patients derived more benefit as evidenced by DFS (72% receiving FOLFOX-4 treatment vs 65% receiving 5-FU/LV, $p = .0002$) than stage II patients (87% receiving FOLFOX-4 vs. 84% receiving 5-FU/LV, $p = $ ns). Oxaliplatin regimens are still restricted by its dose-limiting toxicity of neuropathy, which seriously affected 12% of patients during trial, but the percentage of patients affected drops to 0.5% after 18 months. Although follow-up has not been long enough to see a statistically significant improvement in OS, a recent update showed the persistent improvement in DFS. Moreover, 3-year DFS has been shown to be well correlated with overall survival across multiple colorectal trials.

The benefit of oxaliplatin does not appear to be dependent on the schedule of 5-FU/LV. NSABP C-07 randomized 2407 patients with stage II/III colon cancer to bolus weekly 5-FU/LV (Roswell Park) or to FLOX (the same 5-FU/LV regimen with biweekly oxaliplatin). The improvement in the hazard ratios and DFS was similar to that seen in the MOSAIC trial. The probability of being alive and free of disease at 3 years was 76.5% in the oxaliplatin arm compared with 71.6% in the control arm. Although the efficacy of FLOX looks similar to the infusional 5-FU used in the MOSAIC trial, it does appear to be slightly more toxic, with increased diarrhea and dehydration. Final results are awaited.

Irinotecan-Based Regimens

Irinotecan (also called cpt-11) is a camptothecin derivative that inhibits topoisomerase I by stabilizing DNA breaks that arise in DNA uncoiling for transcription and replication. Two randomized controlled trials showed improved survival in patients receiving irinotecan along with 5-FU/LV, compared with 5-FU/LV alone, as first-line therapy in metastatic disease. Despite the proven benefit in advanced disease, preliminary results from three large trials do not support the use of irinotecan in the adjuvant setting. CALGB

C89803 compared a bolus version of irinotecan with 5-FU/LV (IFL) with 5-FU/LV alone and found increase in grade III–IV toxicities (neutropenia, neutropenic fever, and death on treatment) without an improvement in DFS. PETACC-3 and Accord02/FFCD9802 compared the addition of irinotecan with infusional 5-FU and also found increased toxicities in the experimental arm with no improvement in DFS in patients with stage III colon cancer (without post hoc statistical analysis). On the basis of early data from these trials, irinotecan-based regimens cannot be recommended in the adjuvant setting.

Irinotecan is hydrolyzed in the liver to its active metabolite, SN-38, which in turn is glucuronidated to an inactive form by uridine diphosphate glucuronosyltransferase isoform 1A1 (UGT1A1). The adverse events associated with irinotecan, including diarrhea, bone marrow suppression, and nausea or vomiting, have been shown in retrospective studies to correlate with polymorphisms of UGT1A1. A diagnostic test has been approved by the U.S. Food and Drug Administration (FDA), and several current trials include adjustment of irinotecan dosages on the basis of genetic profiles (pharmacogenomics) of these metabolic enzymes.

Current Trials and Future Directions

The two most recent FDA-approved therapies in metastatic colon cancer are "targeted," "biologic" agents rather than standard cytotoxic drugs. Both agents are monoclonal antibodies. Bevacizumab targets the vascular endothelial growth factor (VEGF) pathway and cetuximab is directed against the epidermal growth factor receptor (EGFR) pathway.

Bevacizumab (rhuMAb VegF; Avastin [Genentech, South San Francisco, CA]) is a humanized recombinant monoclonal antibody directed against VEGF. By binding ligand and preventing signaling of the VEGF receptor, bevacizumab is thought to interfere with the recruitment and growth of tumor-feeding blood vessels. Two phase-III trials have shown an improvement in both DFS and OS after the addition of bevacizumab to 5-FU based regimens combined with either oxaliplatin or irinotecan in the metastatic setting. Side effects seen in these trials thought to be due to the addition of bevacizumab included reversible hypertension and proteinuria, as well as rare serious side effects (albeit not statistically significant) such as gastrointestinal perforation, wound dehiscence, bleeding, and clotting. NSABP C-08 and MOSAIC-2 are two prospectively randomized trials designed to determine whether bevacizumab improves survival over FOLFOX-4 in the adjuvant setting.

Cetuximab (Erbitux [ImClone Systems, New York, NY, and Bristol-Myers Squibb, New York, NY]) is a monoclonal antibody directed against EGFR, which is involved in multiple growth signaling pathways. Cetuximab received FDA approval for treatment of irinotecan-resistant metastatic disease in 2004. In irinotecan-refractory disease, a 22% response rate was reached in patients treated with cetuximab/irinotecan compared with an 11% response rate with cetuximab as a single agent in a randomized phase II trial. The side effects of cetuximab are relatively mild, with an acneiform rash over the face, chest, and back occurring in most patients. Allergic reactions also occur (unlike bevacizumab, cetuximab is not fully humanized). The U.S. Intergroup N0147 trial is comparing FOLFOX-4 with and without cetuximab in the adjuvant setting for stage III colon cancer.

Role of Molecular Profiling

The role of molecular biomarkers to prognosticate as well as predict response to adjuvant therapy continues to evolve. This is an important clinical need because the majority of patients with stage II and III colon cancer are cured with surgery alone. Patients with tumors who have defects in their mismatch repair genes have a significantly better prognosis than their microsatellite-stable counterparts; however, there is a suggestion that they are less responsive to adjuvant 5–FU-based therapy. Loss of heterozygosity at chromosome 18q in microsatellite stable tumors has been shown to predict for a worse prognosis for stage III colon cancers following adjuvant therapy. In addition to using markers of neoplastic genetic alterations to help predict outcome, there is strong push to develop molecular predictors of efficacy and toxicity of chemotherapy on the basis of individual genotypes. Currently the evidence does not support the use of these markers to predict who will benefit from adjuvant therapy.

Role of Adjuvant Therapy after Hepatic Resection

Adjuvant chemotherapy is commonly recommended following resection of hepatic colorectal metastasis despite the fact that minimal data support its use. There are many unknowns, including the timing of resection, optimal drug combination, schedule, and duration of therapy. Because the presence of hepatic metastasis confers stage IV (advanced) status, either FOLFOX-4 or folinic acid, 5-FU, and irinotecan (FOLFIRI) for 4 to 6 months is often used. A targeted biologic agent may be considered despite the lack of data supporting use in stage II/III disease. Because of the risk of wound complications and other issues, it is recommended that bevacizumab be discontinued 8 weeks before or after major surgical procedures. If possible, enrollment in a clinical trial is recommended.

ADJUVANT THERAPY FOR RECTAL CANCER

As in colon cancer, surgical resection remains the cornerstone of the curative approach. However, unlike colon cancer, there is a significant tendency for local failure after potentially curative resection. Improvements in the initial surgical procedure by performing a total mesorectal excision (TME) have reduced but not eliminated the risk of local recurrence. Salvage surgical procedures are technically difficult and often unsuccessful. The morbidity associated with local recurrence can be a clinical nightmare for both the patient and the treating physician. Therefore the major difference in the adjuvant treatment paradigm for rectal as compared with colon cancer is the addition of radiation therapy to address the risk of local failure.

Role of Adjuvant Chemotherapy and Radiation

Studies in the 1980s and early 1990s solidified the superiority of postoperative chemoradiation over surgery alone and surgery followed by radiation without chemotherapy. Chemoradiation reduced the risk of local failure, distant failure, and the risk of death. In both studies, chemoradiation involved the use of semustine (methyl-CCNU) in addition to 5-FU. Semustine carries a small but real risk of acute myeloid leukemia and is no longer used in adjuvant regimens for rectal cancer. The North American intergroup trial confirmed the lack of additional benefit of semustine in addition to 5-FU and has established the role of continuous infusion 5-FU with radiation. Comparing continuous infusion 5-FU (225 mg/m^2 per day for 5 weeks) to bolus 5-FU (500 mg/m^2 days 1–3 and days 36–39) at 4 years, the time to relapse was improved from 53% to 63%, and survival was improved from 60% to 70%. Unlike colon cancer, biomodulation with leucovorin or levamisole has not increased the efficacy of 5-FU in rectal cancer. Intergroup study 0144 completed accrual in 2000 and is designed to determine

whether continued systemic therapy with infusional 5-FU improves survival over just using it during radiation. In general, adjuvant therapy is recommended for any tumor that is T3 or greater in size or is node positive.

Role of Neoadjuvant Chemotherapy and Radiation

The neoadjuvant approach is particularly attractive in rectal cancer because downstaging may increase ease and rates of respectability, allow potential sphincter preservation, and increase compliance by avoiding long postoperative recoveries. The Swedish Rectal Cancer Trial was the first to show that a short-term regimen of high-dose preoperative radiotherapy (25 Gy in five fractions 1 week before resection) decreased the rate of local recurrence and improved survival compared with surgery alone .

The German phase III EORTC 22921 study was the first study to complete accrual in comparing neoadjuvant therapy with combined 5-FU/radiation to postoperative adjuvant 5-FU/radiation (Fig. 1). Patients with tumor extending through the muscle wall or with positive nodes were randomized to preoperative or postoperative chemoradiation. In both arms, the radiation (5040 GY in 28 fractions) was combined with 5-FU (1000 mg/m^2 over 120 hours during the first and fifth week). All patients received additional systemic 5-FU for 4 months. The study failed to see an improvement in overall survival, but preoperative therapy was associated with an improved rate of local control (6% failure at 5 years compared with 13%), reduced acute and chronic toxicity, increased compliance, and an increased rate of sphincter preservation in patients with low-lying tumors. Interestingly, posttreatment pathology results proved to be highly prognostic. Patients whose posttreatment tumors showed marked regression or negative nodes had improved DFS.

Posttreatment Surveillance

The majority of patients with colorectal cancer undergo surgery with curative intent following diagnosis. Unfortunately, 30% to 50% of these patients will relapse and eventually die of their disease. Unlike most other solid tumors, salvage resection of solitary or oligometastases to the liver and lungs may result in either long-term DFS or possible cure. The best approach to surveillance remains controversial. The NCCN recommendations are similar to American Society of Clinical Oncology guidelines (Table 2): history and physical every 3 months for 2 years and then every 6 months for years 3 to 5, CEA every 3 months for 2 years and then every 6 months for years 3 to 5, and a colonoscopy within 1 year following resection (within 6 months if the patient presented with obstruction and a complete preoperative colonoscopy could not be performed) and then every 1 to 3 years on the basis of the findings. Chest, abdominal, and pelvic CT scans may be considered annually for patients at high risk of recurrence, including those with poorly differentiated histologic grade and perineural or venous invasion. If the patient is postmetastectomy for synchronous liver disease, the recommendation for CT scans may be increased to every 3 to 6 months. PET scans are not recommended during regular surveillance; however, some evidence supports their use in the situation of a rising CEA without CT evidence of disease.

Current Recommendations

The magnitude of benefit from adjuvant therapy appears to be proportional to the risk of relapse on the basis of pathologic stage. For stage III (node-positive) patients, the evidence supports the use of adjuvant chemotherapy for 6 months following resection.

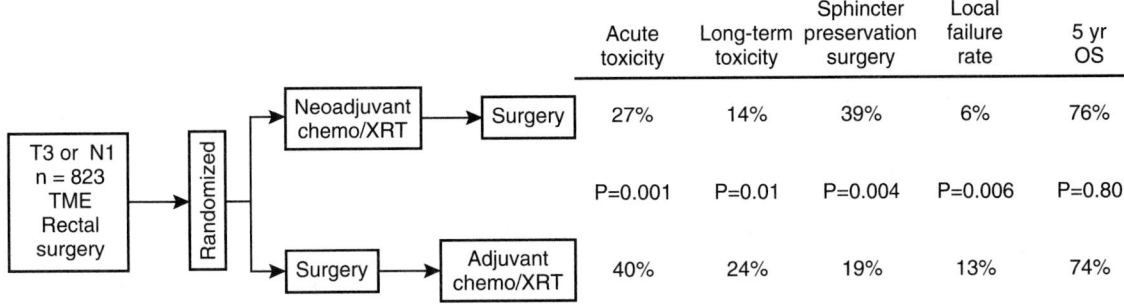

		Acute toxicity	Long-term toxicity	Sphincter preservation surgery	Local failure rate	5 yr OS
Neoadjuvant chemo/XRT → Surgery		27%	14%	39%	6%	76%
		P=0.001	P=0.01	P=0.004	P=0.006	P=0.80
Surgery → Adjuvant chemo/XRT		40%	24%	19%	13%	74%

Chemoradiation consisted of:
- 5040 cGY in 180 cGy fractions
- 5-FU 1000 mg/m²/day over 120 hours during week 1 and week 5
- All subjects received adjuvant 5-FU × 4 months

Figure I Neoadjuvant versus adjuvant chemoradiation for rectal cancer.

Table 2: Summary of the National Comprehensive Cancer Network Practice Guidelines for Surveillance after Surgery and Adjuvant Therapy for Colorectal Cancer

History and Physical Examination	Every 3 Months for 2 Years and Then Every 6 Months for a Total of 5 Years
CEA	Every 3 months for 2 years and then every 6 months for 5 years for lesions ≥T2
Colonoscopy	Perform in 1 year. If abnormal, repeat in 1 year. If no polyps found, repeat every 2–3 years. If a preoperative colonoscopy could not be performed because of obstruction, must be done in 3–6 months. For patients with rectal cancer who did not receive pelvic radiation, alternatives may include a flexible sigmoidoscopy every 6 months for 5 years.
CT scans	May be considered annually for people at high risk of recurrence as defined by poorly differentiated histologic grade and tumors with perineural or venous invasion. If the patient is postmetastectomy for synchronous liver disease, the recommendation for CT scans may be increased to every 3–6 months.

CEA, Carcinoembryonic antigen; *CT,* computed tomography.

FOLFOX-4, capecitabine, or intravenous 5-FU/LV are all reasonable alternatives. FOLFOX-4 has the most convincing efficacy data but is associated with increased toxicities compared with 5-FU/LV alone. Irinotecan-based regimens cannot be recommended in the adjuvant setting. For stage II (node-negative) patients, the absolute benefit appears to be real but much smaller. The current trials were not powered to see a difference in this subgroup, so the role of adjuvant treatment for stage II patients is controversial. Following the NCCN practice guidelines, FOLFOX-4 or 5-FU is often considered if the pathology displays high-risk features such as poor differentiation, lymphatic or vascular invasion, bowel obstruction, inadequate staging (<12 lymph nodes removed), perforation, or direct extension into other organs. For stage II patients with no high-risk features, observation is often recommended, but enrollment in a clinical trial is preferred.

The evidence also suggests that the elderly receive the same benefit from adjuvant chemotherapy as do younger patients. A pooled analysis of three randomized clinical trials suggested that efficacy of adjuvant 5-FU-based chemotherapy was maintained in the elderly (defined as 70 years of age or older) and that toxicity was similar to younger patients except for leukopenia in one study. Currently molecular markers are not recommended to dictate treatment options until further data are available.

Although no survival benefit was achieved with preoperative compared with postoperative chemoradiotherapy, we suggest that preoperative chemoradiotherapy is the preferred treatment for patients with locally advanced rectal cancer, given that it is associated with a superior overall compliance rate, an improved rate of local control, reduced toxicity, and an increased rate of sphincter preservation in patients with low-lying tumors.

SUGGESTED READINGS

Andre T, Boni C, Mounedji-Boudiaf L, and others: Oxaliplatin, fluorouracil, and leucovorin as adjuvant treatment for colon cancer, *N Engl J Med* 350:2343, 2004.

Benson AB III, Schrag D, Somerfield MR, and others: American Society of Clinical Oncology Recommendations on Adjuvant Chemotherapy for Stage II Colon Cancer, *J Clin Oncol* 22:3408, 2004.

Boice JD, Greene MH, Killen JY, and others: Leukemia after adjuvant chemotherapy with semustine (methyl-CCNU)-evidence of a dose-response effect, *N Engl J Med* 314:119, 1996.

Cunningham D, Humblet Y, Siena S, and others: Cetuximab monotherapy and cetuximab plus irinotecan in irinotecan-refractory metastatic colorectal cancer, *N Engl J Med* 351:337, 2004.

de Gramont A, Figer A, Seymour M, and others: Leucovorin and fluorouracil with or without oxaliplatin as first-line treatment in advanced colorectal cancer, *J Clin Oncol* 18:2938, 2000.

de Gramont A, Boni C, Navarro M, and others: Oxaliplatin/5FU/LV in the adjuvant treatment of stage II and stage III colon cancer: efficacy results with a median follow-up of 4 years, *J Clin Oncol* [meeting abstracts] 23 (suppl 16):3501, 2005.

Desch CE, Benson AB III, Somerfield MR, and others: Colorectal cancer surveillance: 2005 Update of an American Society of Clinical Oncology Practice Guideline, *J Clin Oncol* 23:8512, 2005.

Douillard JY, Cunningham D, Roth AD, and others: Irinotecan combined with fluorouracil compared with fluorouracil alone as first-line treatment for metastatic colorectal cancer: a multicentre randomised trial, *Lancet* 355:1041, 2000.

Ellis LM, Curley SA, Grothey A: Surgical resection after downsizing of colorectal liver metastasis in the era of bevacizumab, *J Clin Oncol* 23:4853, 2005.

Francini G, Petrioli R, Lorenzini L, and others: Folinic acid and 5-fluorouracil as adjuvant chemotherapy in colon cancer, *Gastroenterology* 106:899, 1994.

Gastrointestinal Tumor Study Group: Prolongation of the disease-free interval in surgically treated rectal carcinoma, *N Engl J Med* 312:1465, 1985.

Gearhart SL, Frassica D, Rosen R, and others: Improved staging with pretreatment positron emission tomography/computed tomography in low rectal cancer, *Ann Surg Oncol* 13:397, 2006.

Giantonio BJ, Catalano NJ, Meropol PJ, and others: High-dose bevacizumab improves survival when combined with FOLFOX4 in previously treated advanced colorectal cancer: results from the Eastern Cooperative Oncology Group (ECOG) study E3200, *J Clin Oncol* [meeting abstracts] 23 (suppl 16):2, 2005.

Havenga K, Enker WE, Norstein J, and others: Improved survival and local control after total mesorectal excision or D3 lymphadenectomy in the treatment of primary rectal cancer: an international analysis of 1411 patients, *Eur J Surg Oncol* 25:368, 1999.

Hurwitz H, Fehrenbacher L, Novotny W, and others: Bevacizumab plus irinotecan, fluorouracil, and leucovorin for metastatic colorectal cancer, *N Engl J Med* 350:2335, 2004.

International Multicentre Pooled Analysis of Colon Cancer Trials (IMPACT) investigators: Efficacy of adjuvant fluorouracil and folinic acid in colon cancer, *Lancet* 345:939, 1995.

Jeffery GM, Hickey BE, Hider P: Follow-up strategies for patients treated for non-metastatic colorectal cancer, *Cochrane Database Syst Rev* CD002200, 2002.

Jemal A, Murray T, Ward E, and others: Cancer statistics, 2005, *CA Cancer J Clin* 55:10, 2005.

Jessup JM, Stewart A, Greene FL, and others: Adjuvant chemotherapy for stage III colon cancer: implications of race/ethnicity, age, and differentiation, *JAMA* 294:2703, 2005.

Kawato Y, Aonuma M, Hirota Y, and others: Intracellular roles of SN-38, a metabolite of the camptothecin derivative CPT-11, in the antitumor effect of CPT-11, *Cancer Res* 51:4187, 1991.

Krook JE, Moertel CG, Gunderson LL, and others: Effective surgical adjuvant therapy for high-risk rectal carcinoma, *N Engl J Med* 324:709, 1991.

McLeod HL, Watters JW: Irinotecan pharmacogenetics: is it time to intervene, *J Clin Oncol* 22:1356, 2004.

Meyerhardt JA, Mayer RJ: Systemic therapy for colorectal cancer, *N Engl J Med* 352:476, 2005.

Miwa M, Ura M, Nishida M, and others: Design of a novel oral fluoropyrimidine carbamate, capecitabine, which generates 5-fluorouracil selectively in tumours by enzymes concentrated in human liver and cancer tissue, *Eur J Cancer* 34:1274, 1998.

Moertel CG, Fleming TR, Macdonald JS, and others: Intergroup study of fluorouracil plus levamisole as adjuvant therapy for stage II/Duke's B2 colon cancer, *J Clin Oncol* 13:2936, 1995.

Moertel CG, Fleming TR, Macdonald JS, and others: Levamisole and fluorouracil for adjuvant therapy of resected colon carcinoma, *N Engl J Med* 322:352, 1990.

National Comprehensive Cancer Network: *Clinical practice guidelines* (website), http://www.nccn.org. Accessed April 30, 2006.

O'Connell JB, Maggard MA, Ko CY: Colon cancer survival rates with the new American Joint Committee on Cancer Sixth Edition Staging, *J Natl Cancer Inst* 96:1420, 2004.

O'Connell MJ, Mailliard JA, Kahn MJ, and others: Controlled trial of fluorouracil and low-dose leucovorin given for 6 months as postoperative adjuvant therapy for colon cancer, *J Clin Oncol* 15:246, 1997.

O'Connell MJ, Martenson JA, Wieand HS, and others: Improving adjuvant therapy for rectal cancer by combining protracted-infusion fluorouracil with radiation therapy after curative surgery, *N Engl J Med* 331:502, 1994.

O'Connell MJ, Laurie JA, Kahn M, and others: Prospectively randomized trial of postoperative adjuvant chemotherapy in patients with high-risk colon cancer, *J Clin Oncol* 16:295, 1998.

Parker SL, Tong T, Bolden S, and others: Cancer statistics, 1997, *CA Cancer J Clin* 47:5, 1997.

Pinedo HM, Peters GF: Fluorouracil: biochemistry and pharmacology, *J Clin Oncol* 6:1653, 1988.

Popat S, Hubner R, Houlston RS, Systematic review of microsatellite instability and colorectal cancer prognosis, *J Clin Oncol* 23:609, 2005.

Poplin EA, Benedetti JK, Estes NC, and others: Phase III Southwest Oncology Group 9415/Intergroup 0153 randomized trial of fluorouracil, leucovorin, and levamisole versus fluorouracil continuous infusion and levamisole for adjuvant treatment of stage III and high-risk stage II colon cancer, *J Clin Oncol* 23:1819, 2005.

Raymond E, Buquet-Fagot C, Djelloul S, and others: Antitumor activity of oxaliplatin in combination with 5-fluorouracil and the thymidylate synthase inhibitor AG337 in human colon, breast and ovarian cancers, *Anticancer Drugs* 8:876, 1997.

Ribic CM, Sargent DJ, Moore MJ, and others: Tumor microsatellite-instability status as a predictor of benefit from fluorouracil-based adjuvant chemotherapy for colon cancer, *N Engl J Med* 349:247, 2003.

Saltz LB, Cox JV, Blanke C, and others: Irinotecan plus fluorouracil and leucovorin for metastatic colorectal cancer, *N Engl J Med* 343:905, 2000.

Saltz LB, Niedzwiecki D, Hollis D, and others: Irinotecan plus fluorouracil/leucovorin (IFL) versus fluorouracil/leucovorin alone (FL) in stage III colon cancer (intergroup trial CALGB C89803), *J Clin Oncol* [meeting abstracts] 22(suppl 14):3500, 2004.

Sargent DJ, Goldberg RM, Jacobson SD, and others: A pooled analysis of adjuvant chemotherapy for resected colon cancer in elderly patients, *N Engl J Med* 345:1091, 2001.

Sargent DJ, Wieand HS, Haller DG, and others: Disease-free survival versus overall survival as a primary end point for adjuvant colon cancer studies: individual patient data from 20,898 patients on 18 randomized trials, *J Clin Oncol* 23:8664, 2005.

Sauer R, Becker H, Hohenberger W, and others, for the German Rectal Cancer Study Group: Preoperative versus postoperative chemoradiotherapy for rectal cancer, *N Engl J Med* 351:1731-1740, 2004.

Swedish Rectal Cancer, Trial, Improved survival with preoperative radiotherapy in resectable rectal cancer, *N Engl J Med* 336:980, 1997.

Tepper JE, O'Connell M, Niedzwiecki D, and others: Adjuvant therapy in rectal cancer: analysis of stage, sex, and local control-final report of Intergroup 0114, *J Clin Oncol* 20:1744, 2002.

Twelves C, Wong A, Nowacki MP, and others: Capecitabine as adjuvant treatment for stage III colon cancer, *N Engl J Med* 352:2696, 2005.

van Cutsem E, Labianca R, Hossfeld D, and others: Randomized phase III trial comparing infused irinotecan/5-fluorouracil (5-FU)/folinic acid (IF) versus 5-FU/FA (F) in stage III colon cancer patients (pts), (PETACC 3), *J Clin Oncol* [meeting abstracts] 23(suppl 16):LBA8, 2005.

Watanabe T, Wu TT, Catalano PJ, and others: Molecular predictors of survival after adjuvant chemotherapy for colon cancer, *N Engl J Med* 344:1196, 2001.

Wolmark N, Wieand S, Kuebler JP, and others: A phase III trial comparing FULV to FULV + oxaliplatin in stage II or III carcinoma of the colon: results of NSABP Protocol C-07, *J Clin Oncol* [meeting abstracts], 23 (16_suppl):LBA3500, 2005.

Wolmark N, Rockette H, Fisher B, and others: The benefit of leucovorin-modulated fluorouracil as postoperative adjuvant therapy for primary colon cancer: results from National Surgical Adjuvant Breast and Bowel Project protocol C-03, *J Clin Oncol* 11:1879, 1993.

Ychou M, Rauol JL, Douillard JY, and others: A phase III randomized trial of LV5FU2+CPT-11 vs. LV5FU2 alone in adjuvant high risk colon cancer (FNCLCC Accord02/FFCD9802), *J Clin Oncol* [meeting abstracts] 23 (suppl 15):3502, 2005.

Zaniboni A: Adjuvant chemotherapy in colorectal cancer with high-dose leucovorin and fluorouracil: impact on disease-free survival and overall survival, *J Clin Oncol* 15:2432, 1997.

Useful Websites

For Clinical Calculators
http://www.mayoclinic.com/calcs/colon
www.adjuvantonline.com
For Patient Handouts
http://www.plwc.org

Tumors of the Anal Region

Jennifer M. Ayscue, MD, and Lee E. Smith, MD

Tumors of the anal region are uncommon. It was estimated that approximately 4660 new cases of anal cancer would be diagnosed in 2006. Most cases are in non-Hispanic whites, and women outnumber men in those cases not associated with the human immunodeficiency virus (HIV). In HIV-positive patients, men are diagnosed more frequently than women and at a younger age. In addition, there is an increased risk of anal cancer in young men who have sex with men, regardless of HIV status. Women have more anal canal cancers, whereas men more often have distal anal tumors. Overall, 75% of anal cancers are located in the anal canal, and the remaining 25% are anal margin tumors.

Significant risk factors for anal region tumors include infection with human papillomavirus (HPV), anal intercourse, smoking, lowered immunity, HIV infection, and p53 mutation. HPV infection is a major cause of anal cancer, especially types 16, 18, 31, 33, and 35. HPV-6 and HPV-11 are associated with benign genital condylomata, whereas types 16 and 18 are associated with in situ and invasive lesions. Unfortunately, therapy for HIV has not been shown to decrease risk for anal tumors. Screening for anal tumors includes inspection and digital examination of the anus and rectum and bilateral palpation for inguinal lymphadenopathy. Anal PAP smear and high-resolution anoscopy is sometimes used for high-risk patients.

The wide range of benign, premalignant, and malignant tumors of the anal region reflects its variation in anatomy and histology. Anatomically, there are two regions: the first is the anal canal, extending from the puborectalis muscle proximally, down to the anal margin, which begins at the junction between the internal and external anal sphincters (anal verge); second is the perianal skin, extending out for approximately 5 cm. Histologically there are three regions of the anal canal. The columnar mucosa is above the dentate line. At the dentate line, there is a zone of transitional mucosa with cuboidal, columnar, squamous, and transitional epithelial cells. Below the dentate line lies nonkeratinizing squamous cell epithelium, which merges with the hair-bearing epidermis at the anal verge (Fig. 1).

Most anal canal tumors are epidermoid, and these are further classified as squamous cell cancers, basaloid tumors, or mucoepidermoid tumors. These cancers behave similarly. Basaloid tumors originate from the anal transition zone, and the cells resemble those of basal cell cancers of the skin, although the anal basaloid cancer may metastasize.

Tumors above the dentate line drain via the inferior mesenteric nodal system and internal pudendal, hypogastric, and obturator nodes of the internal iliac system. Below the dentate line, drainage is to the superficial inguinal nodes and, less commonly, to the femoral and external iliac nodes.

PRECURSORS OF INVASIVE MALIGNANT NEOPLASMS

Anal Canal Precursors

Condyloma are the physical manifestations of HPV infection in the form of anal warts. The presence of condyloma is common but not necessary for malignant transformation of the distal anal canal.

Anal intraepithelial neoplasia (AIN) is a term that describes dysplastic changes of the epithelium of the anal canal. AIN I changes are limited to the lower third of the epithelium. AIN II involves changes of the lower two thirds of the epithelium, and AIN III represents full-thickness changes. These neoplastic changes are usually seen in the background of HPV infection, especially type 16. AIN is more prevalent in the immunosuppressed population and may be found in as many as half of these patients. It is uncertain as to whether AIN progresses to anal cancer, but it has been suggested that AIN III portends a higher risk of developing cancer than AIN I or II. Therefore it is important to examine these patients regularly with

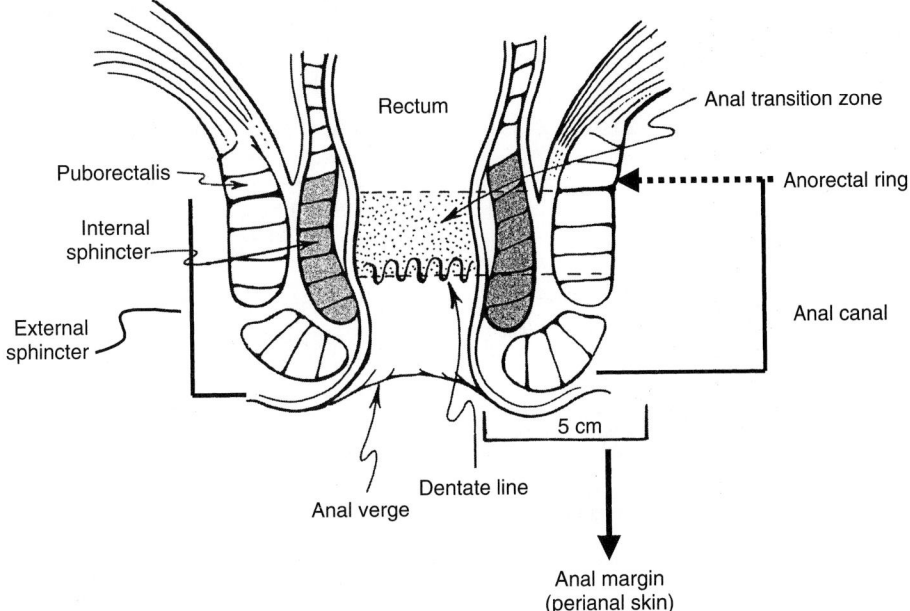

Figure 1   Anatomy of the anorectal region.   *From Sternberg JA, Gemlo BT: Current surgical therapy, ed 7, St Louis, 2001, Mosby.*

anoscopy, proctoscopy, and possibly high-resolution anoscopy. Any suspicious lesions should be biopsied. AIN I or II lesions may be followed closely or excised, depending on the extent of the lesions and patient immunologic status because wound healing may be an issue. AIN III lesions merit stronger consideration for surgical therapy, again taking into account extent of disease and patient immune status. Surgical therapy may include wide local excision with closure by primary or secondary intention or skin grafts or flaps.

Adenomas of the anal canal are found above the dentate line. Pedunculated polyps may be snared, but sessile polyps are better treated with full-thickness excision with a 1-cm margin, superficial to the internal sphincter. Because of possible recurrence, follow-up with frequent anal examination is necessary.

Anal Margin Precursors

Dysplasia of the anal margin is divided into low grade and high grade. High-grade dysplasia/carcinoma in situ of the perianal skin is termed Bowen's disease and is considered by many to be synonymous with AIN III. It is associated with HPV types 16 and 18. Symptoms are perianal itching and skin irritation and sometimes visible plaques. Diagnosis is obtained with biopsy in which characteristic vacuolated cells with hyperchromatic nuclei are seen. Bowen's disease is usually indolent and progresses to cancer in less than 5% of patients. Therapy consists of either perianal mapping biopsies with wide local excision or excision of only grossly evident lesions.

Paget's disease of the perianal skin is an adenocarcinoma in situ similar to that seen in the breast or axilla and is rare. Patients present with symptoms of pruritus ani as well as signs of a scaly, erythematous rash. Biopsy with slide preparation using periodic acid–Schiff (PAS) stain is diagnostic. Because there is a 50% to 70% association for an underlying lower gastrointestinal malignancy, screening examinations should be performed. The most commonly associated malignancies are apocrine or eccrine carcinomas, rectal adenocarcinoma, and anal carcinoma. Paget's is slow to mature but may become invasive in up to 40% of untreated patients. Treatment consists of wide local excision guided by mapping biopsies or frozen section. Wounds may be left open or primarily closed if the area is small. Larger wounds require skin graft or a flap procedure. If invasion is identified in the specimen, abdominoperineal resection and possibly chemoradiation are indicated. Long-term follow-up of these patients to exclude recurrence of Paget's or development of underlying malignancy is mandatory.

■ INVASIVE NEOPLASMS

Anal Canal Malignancies

Squamous cell carcinoma (SCC) comprises approximately 80% of anal canal cancers. Others included in the World Health Organization classification of carcinoma of the anal canal include adenocarcinoma (rectal type, of anal glands, and within anorectal fistula), mucinous adenocarcinoma, small cell carcinoma, and undifferentiated carcinoma. Other anal canal tumors include melanoma, gastrointestinal stromal tumors, lymphoma, and neuroendocrine tumors. Common symptoms of SCC include anal bleeding, pain, mucous discharge, fecal incontinence, and the feeling of a mass in the anus. Careful examination of the anus reveals a mass or villiform lesion that may harbor the cancer. Notation as to the size and position of the tumor, the extent of any lateral invasion, and whether the mass is fixed to the prostate, vagina, or bony pelvis is important to clinical staging. Palpation of perirectal and bilateral inguinal lymph nodes should also be performed. Biopsy of the anal mass and any enlarged lymph nodes

is necessary. Colonoscopy is not a substitute for an anal examination but is performed to exclude other lesions of the colon. Further workup may include anal ultrasound, computed tomography (CT), or magnetic resonance imaging (MRI) imaging of the abdomen, pelvis, and chest or radiography of the chest. HIV testing is appropriate.

Tumors of the anal canal are staged differently from the anal margin (Table 1, *A* and *B*). Melanoma, carcinoid tumors, and sarcomas are excluded from this staging system. As many as one third of anal SCCs have lymph node metastases at the

Table 1A: TNM Classification for Tumors of the Anal Canal

Primary Tumor (T)

TX	Primary tumor cannot be assessed
T0	No evidence of primary tumor
Tis	Carcinoma in situ
T1	Tumor ≤2 cm in greatest dimension
T2	Tumor >2 cm but ≤5 cm in greatest dimension
T3	Tumor >5 cm in greatest dimension
T4	Tumor of any size invading adjacent organ(s) (e.g., vagina, urethra, bladder; direct invasion of the rectal wall, perirectal skin, subcutaneous tissue, or the sphincter muscle is not classified as T4)

Regional Lymph Nodes (N)

NX	Regional lymph nodes cannot be assessed
N0	No regional lymph node metastasis
N1	Metastasis in perirectal lymph nodes(s)
N2	Metastasis in unilateral internal iliac and/or inguinal lymph nodes(s)
N3	Metastasis in perirectal and inguinal lymph nodes; and/or bilateral internal iliac; and/or inguinal lymph nodes

Distant Metastasis (M)

MX	Distant metastasis cannot be assessed
M0	No distant metastasis
M1	Distant metastasis

Table 1B: TNM Grouping by Stage for Tumors of the Anal Canal

Stage Grouping			
Stage 0	Tis	N0	M0
Stage I	T1	N0	M0
Stage II	T2	N0	M0
	T3	N0	M0
Stage IIIA	T1	N1	M0
	T2	N1	M0
	T3	N1	M0
	T4	N0	M0
Stage IIIB	T4	N1	M0
	Any T	N2	M0
	Any T	N3	M0
Stage IV	Any T	Any N	M1

T, Primary tumor; *N*, regional lymph nodes; *M*, distant metastasis.

time of diagnosis, and approximately 50% have local spread into the anal sphincter or surrounding soft tissues. Metastases, most commonly to the liver and lungs, are present in 5% to 10% at diagnosis and may ultimately appear in 10% to 30% after treatment.

SCC of the anal canal was historically treated by abdominoperineal resection (APR) with or without a groin dissection, but this was associated with a high morbidity and an overall survival of only 40% to 70%. However, in 1974, when Dr. Norman Nigro first noted that specimens he resected after preoperative chemoradiation contained no tumor, he developed a protocol to study patients using this modality. Patients were given radiation with concurrent 5-fluorouracil (5-FU) and mitomycin C (MMC). He and other investigators subsequently confirmed the efficacy of this regimen in more than 500 patients in mostly nonrandomized series with 5-year survival rates of 65% to 85% with minimal sphincter loss or need for a colostomy. Because of the high toxicity profile for MMC, recent studies using cisplatin in place of MMC have shown promising results, with complete response rates of 70% to 95% and less toxicity. Currently, most patients receive a modified version of the Nigro protocol as standard first-line therapy. Between 65% and 80% of patients maintain anal function after combined-modality treatment, but colostomies may be necessary in 2% to 10% of patients because of incontinence, stenosis, or pain. Patients who have incontinence of stool or a malignant fistula at the time of diagnosis should undergo APR with either preoperative or postoperative chemoradiation.

Follow-up of treated patients should include digital rectal exam with proctoscopy and nodal exam every 2 months in the first year, once every 3 months in the second year, once every 6 months years 3 to 5, and yearly thereafter. A CT of the chest, abdomen, and pelvis is recommended after 6 months to a year and then as indicated. If there is suspicious or recurrent disease, the patient's stage should be reevaluated by CT of the chest, abdomen, and pelvis, MRI of the pelvis (or both), and perhaps by fluorodeoxyglucose positron emission tomography scan. Tumors 2 cm or smaller are cured with initial therapy in 80% of cases, whereas those 5 cm or larger are cured in fewer than 50% of cases. Median time to regression of tumor is 12 weeks from the start of therapy, although it can take up to 36 weeks. Most recurrences occur within 2 years of treatment. Routine biopsies of the site or regressing tumor are not necessary. Persistent or recurrent local disease may be treated with additional chemoradiotherapy if the maximal dose has not been reached. Otherwise, abdominoperineal resection followed by chemotherapy with cisplatin with or without 5-FU is a good choice. A 5-year survival rate of approximately 50% may be expected. Radical inguinal node dissection may be beneficial for persistent or recurrent lymphatic metastases if maximal doses of radiation have been given. Distant metastatic disease is generally managed with palliative intent and generally consists of chemotherapy with cisplatin and/or 5-FU. Resection of solitary or small numbers of liver or lung metastases may be considered in lower-risk patients if the primary disease is controlled.

Adenocarcinoma of the anal ducts or glands are purported to behave more like low rectal adenocarcinomas than anal epidermoid carcinomas. We recommend an APR with neoadjuvant chemoradiotherapy using a 5-FU/leucovorin-based regimen. Five-year survival rates (60%) and recurrence rates (20%–50%) are poorer with these low-lying lesions compared with mid- and upper-rectal lesions when matched stage for stage.

Melanoma of the anal canal is rare but deadly, with a 5-year survival rate as low as 6% to 25%. It is the third most common site for melanoma after cutaneous and ocular. Melanocytes may be present anywhere in the anal canal, may give rise to pigmented or nonpigmented lesions, or may look like a thrombosed hemorrhoid. From 30% to 70% are amelanotic, which may lead to delay in diagnosis. Up to 60% of patients have metastatic disease at the time of diagnosis and most recurrences are systemic. Patients who have demonstrated long-term survival have had tumors less than 2 mm deep at time of excision. Because these tumors are not responsive to chemotherapy or radiation and have such a poor survival rate, wide local excision or APR is generally recommended. Although the few reported long-term survivors had an APR, most patients die of the disease regardless of extent of resection. Therefore, APR may only be beneficial for local palliation.

Gastrointestinal stromal tumors of the anal canal include rhabdomyosarcoma, leiomyosarcoma, fibrosarcoma, and liposarcoma and are treated similarly. Malignancy is determined by size of the lesion and number of mitoses per high-power field. Wide local excision is necessary and may require APR if the anal sphincter is involved by the tumor. Chemotherapy may be used for aggressive or metastatic disease.

Anorectal lymphoma is most commonly seen in patients with HIV or other types of immunocompromised patients. Commonly, a palpable mass demonstrates high-grade B-cell lymphoma when biopsied. Workup includes CT scans and bone marrow biopsy. Therapy involves chemoradiotherapy, although patients with systemic symptoms generally do poorly.

Small cell or neuroendocrine tumors are rare in the anal region. They appear as high-grade neoplasms that are highly infiltrative and exhibit early metastases mainly to liver and lungs. Localized disease is treated with surgery with or without radiation therapy, whereas metastatic disease is treated with the chemotherapy regimen used to treat small cell lung cancer, cisplatin, and etoposide.

Anal Margin Malignancies

The majority of anal margin tumors are keratinizing SCCs. They are similar to SSCs found elsewhere on the body and so are staged and treated similarly (Table 2, *A* and *B*). SCCs of the anal margin are slow growing and spread mainly to inguinal lymph nodes. Treatment of well-differentiated T1 lesions consists of wide local excision or chemoradiotherapy. More advanced tumors are

Table 2A: TNM classification for Tumors of the Anal Margin

Primary Tumor (T)	
TX	Primary tumor cannot be assessed
T0	No evidence of primary tumor
Tis	Carcinoma in situ
T1	Tumor <2 cm, superficial, or exophytic
T2	Tumor 2–5 cm or with minimal dermal invasion
T3	Tumor >5 cm or with deep dermal invasion
T4	Tumor extension into muscle or bone

Regional Lymph Nodes (N)	
Nx	Regional lymph nodes cannot be assessed
N0	No regional lymph node metastasis
N1	Perirectal nodes
N2	Unilateral internal iliac and/or inguinal nodes
N3	Perirectal and inguinal nodes or bilateral internal iliac or inguinal nodes

Distant Metastasis (M)	
M0	No distant metastasis
M1	Distant metastasis

T, Primary tumor, *N,* regional lymph nodes; *M,* distant metastasis.

Table 2B: TNM Grouping by Stage for Tumors of the Anal Region

Stage Grouping			
Stage 0	Tis	N0	M0
Stage I	T1	N0	M0
Stage II	T2	N0	M0
	T3	N0	M0
Stage IIIA	T1	N1	M0
	T2	N1	M0
	T3	N1	M0
	T4	N1	M0
Stage IIIB	T4	N1	M0
	Any T	N2	M0
	Any T	N3	M0
Stage IV	Any T	Any N	M1

T, Primary tumor; *N*, regional lymph nodes; *M*, distant metastasis.

treated with local and inguinal radiation therapy and chemotherapy. Treatment failures may benefit from wide local excision or APR and inguinal lymph node dissection for positive nodes. The 5-year cancer-specific survival ranges from 70% to 90% with local control rates of 65% to 85%.

Verrucous tumors, also known as Buschke-Lowenstein tumors or giant condyloma, may emanate from the anal canal or margin. They are exophytic, warty, gray-white, soft to firm masses and are locally invasive, but rarely metastasize. Verrucous tumors resemble condyloma microscopically and are treated by wide excision, which may require an APR if the sphincter complex is significantly involved. Skin reconstruction is often necessary. Radiation therapy is not currently recommended for these patients.

Basal cell carcinomas of the anal margin are rare and similar to those found elsewhere on the body. Wide local excision is the treatment of choice, and re-excision is performed for this commonly recurring tumor. Five-year disease-free survival is near 100%.

Kaposi's sarcoma rarely occurs on the perianal skin. It is composed primarily of spindle cells and small blood vessels. Kaposi's sarcoma is radiosensitive, although the brown pigmentation may remain permanently. Chemotherapy is reserved for generalized disease.

SUGGESTED READINGS

Billingsley K, Stern LE, Lowy AM, and others: Uncommon anal neoplasms, *Surg Oncol Clin North Am* 13:375, 2004.

Clark MA, Hartley A, Geh GI: Cancer of the anal canal, *Lancet Oncol* 5:149, 2004.

Malik U, Mohiuddin M: Cancer of the anal canal, In Abeloff MD, Armitage JO, Niederhuber JE, and others, editors: *Clinical oncology*, ed 3, Philadelphia, 2004, Churchill Livingstone.

Rousseau D, Jr, Petrelli NJ, Kahlenberg MS: Overview of anal cancer for the surgeon, *Surg Oncol Clin North Am* 3:249, 2004.

Shank B, Enver W, Flam M, and others: Neoplasms of the anus, In Bast R, Kufe D, Pollack R, editors: *Cancer medicine*, Ontario, 2003, BC Decker.

Skibber J, Rodriguez-Bigas MA, Gordon PH: Surgical considerations in anal cancer, *Surg Oncology Clinics North Am* 13:321, 2004.

Strauss R, Procaccino J, Moffa M, and others: Bowen's disease and Paget's disease. In Fazio V, Church J, Delancy C, and others, editors: *Current therapy in colon and rectal surgery*, ed 2, Philadelphia, 2005, Mosby.

COLORECTAL POLYPS

Anthony J. Senagore, MD, MS, MBA

INTRODUCTION

A colorectal polyp is an intraluminal mass lesion arising from the mucosa of the colon and rectum. Although a number of other lesions can present as luminal masses but are covered by normal mucosa, such as lipomas, carcinoid tumors, and leiomyomas, they should not be referred to as polyps. These lesions are outside the scope of a discussion regarding colonic polyps and are not discussed further in this chapter.

The molecular alterations that lead to the development of colorectal polyps have become increasingly understood. This improved correlation between histology and genotype has provided an alteration in recommendations related to treatment and risk reduction of cancer. Colonic polyps may also be a component of a variety of acquired or familial syndromes, many of which are potentially malignant conditions. These polyposis syndromes are described in more detail in another chapter of this text but are reviewed briefly here.

The management of colorectal polyps is related primarily to the risk of malignancy, and this indirect evidence has resulted in a significant increase in the use of screening colonoscopy. Larger polyps may also prompt treatment as a result of hemorrhage, obstruction, or intussusception. Endoscopic evaluation of polyps frequently allows complete excision of the lesion but at the least allows for histologic confirmation of the polyp type. Flexible endoscopy has proved to be a safe and highly effective means of treating colorectal polyps.

HISTOPATHOLOGY OF POLYPS

Hyperplastic Polyps

The relationship between hyperplastic polyps and colon cancer is controversial; however, the risk appears to be only slightly increased. Hyperplastic polyps contain an increased number of glandular cells with decreased cytoplasmic mucus but lack nuclear hyperchromatism, stratification, or atypia. These types of polyps are not considered neoplastic and generally do not confer a higher risk of colorectal cancer, especially small polyps located in the rectum. Factors associated with an increased risk for malignancy with hyperplastic polyps include large polyp size (>1 cm diameter); right colon lesions; a mixed adenoma/hyperplastic histology; more than 20 hyperplastic colonic polyps; familial hyperplastic polyposis; and a family history of colorectal cancer. Serrated adenomas represent a type a polyp previously classified as hyperplastic; however, these lesions appear to have an increased risk factor for colon cancer, as are typical adenomas. These serrated polyps tend to be larger, right-sided, and associated with BRAF genetic mutations and DNA methylation.

Hamartomas

A third histologic category of colorectal polyps is hamartomas. These types of polyps occur most commonly in association with one of three autosomal-dominant familial syndromes: Peutz-Jeghers syndrome, juvenile polyposis, and Cowden syndrome. Historically these syndromes have been considered benign; however, it is now clear that these lesions have malignant potential, and patients with these syndromes should undergo regular colonoscopic surveillance.

Peutz-Jeghers syndrome results from a mutation of the *STK11* gene and is associated with a typical phenotype that includes perioral-pigmented spots and multiple hamartomatous small bowel polyps. The polyps in this syndrome may be complicated by intussusception, bleeding, and obstruction early in life. After the third decade of life, there is a 2% to 13% risk for gastrointestinal (GI) cancer.

Juvenile polyposis is diagnosed when a young patient has 10 or more hamartomatous GI polyps. Lesions frequently occur in the colon but may develop anywhere within the GI tract. The initial symptom is often bleeding resulting from auto-amputation of the polyp. The mutations in this syndrome occur in the *SMAD4/DPC4* and *PTEN* genes. Colon cancer affects up to 50% of persons with juvenile polyposis and may occur in the fourth decade of life.

A final syndrome of juvenile and other hamartomatous polyps within the colon and throughout the gastrointestinal tract is Cowden syndrome. It results from a mutation of the *PTEN* gene. Colorectal cancer is not an established major risk in this syndrome, and no specific surveillance is recommended.

Adenomas

Approximately 10% to 25% of average-risk asymptomatic patients over age 50 have an adenomatous polyp. These lesions are characterized by histologic architecture that may be tubular (65%–85%), tubulovillous (10%–25%), or villous (5%–10%). Advanced lesions are defined by size greater than 1 cm, percentage of villous architecture, severe dysplasia, and carcinoma. Identification of a distal adenoma on flexible sigmoidoscopy should prompt a complete colonoscopy because of the approximately 2%–6% risk of proximal adenomatous lesions. Conversely, a small hyperplastic polyp is not an indication for colonoscopy in itself. The causal relationship between adenomas and colorectal cancer has been called the adenoma-carcinoma sequence. This relationship is supported by the following data: (1) almost all colon cancer arises within an adenoma, as evidenced by residual polyp in many colon cancers, (2) an approximately 30% incidence of synchronous adenomas in colon cancer resection specimens, (3) an increased risk of colon cancer with larger and increasing numbers of adenomatous polyps, (4) the high incidence of colorectal cancer in patients with familial adenomatous polyposis, and (6) the 4% risk after 5 years and 14% after 10 years in unresected polyps.

The development of colorectal polyps and subsequent cancer is believed to be the result of a cascade of sequentially accumulated genetic mutations. These mutations are a combination of loss of function and gain in function defects. Mismatch repair genes are directly tied to the hereditary nonpolyposis cancer syndrome; however, they are also involved in 15% of sporadic colon cancers. Similarly, the APC mutation is the causal mutation in familial polyposis; however, the defect can be seen in more than 80% of sporadic colon cancers and appears to be an early mutation leading to sporadic adenomatous polyps. Although 50% to 80% of benign polyps harbor the APC mutation, the transition to malignancy requires additional mutations. The loss of the deleted in colon cancer (DCC) gene appears to play a key role in the transition to a more advanced adenoma because of dysfunction of a neural cell adhesion molecule receptor and alterations in apoptosis. Another commonly altered gene is *p53*, which normally allows for arrest of the cell cycle to provide sufficient time for either DNA repair or apoptosis if the damage is too severe. A mutation of the *p53* gene appears a key component in the transition from advanced adenoma and carcinoma. The *K-ras* gene is involved in signal transduction from the cell membrane to the nucleus and gain of function mutation leads to increased replication and the development of the exophytic growth of adenomas. This mutation can be found in more than 50% of colon cancers.

COLONOSCOPIC POLYPECTOMY

Polypectomy has proven to be an effective means of colorectal cancer prevention because it allows for the identification of the mucosal lesions and subsequently removal with forceps or snares. Most endoscopists recommend removal of lesions greater than 5 mm using hot biopsy polypectomy and use of the snare for larger lesions. Snare excision offers a larger specimen and histopathologic evaluation of the stalk (or base) to allow better definition of the level of superficial malignancy. Large lesions may be removed using a piecemeal excisional technique, which will allow for sequential excision of the entire lesion. In some cases, these larger sessile lesions may be better treated with injection of saline in the submucosal plane to separate the lesion from the muscularis propria and to allow safer removal of the lesion with electrocautery. Contraindications to colonoscopy polypectomy include anticoagulation, bleeding diathesis, obvious invasive malignancy, or acute colitis.

With modern techniques, complications with colonoscopic polypectomy are uncommon and usually mild. The most common serious complication is bleeding, which occurs in 1.4% of polypectomies and usually starts 7 days after the procedure. Perforation occurs in up to 0.3% of patients, and postpolypectomy serosal burns—manifest by abdominal pain, fever, and leukocytosis—develop in 0.3% of patients. The majority of patients who present with free air identified after polypectomy may be observed and treated with intravenous antibiotics. However, the patients should be carefully followed as inpatients for any signs of clinical deterioration, worsening physical examination findings, or signs of infection, which would indicate laparotomy. An alternative approach is early laparoscopic identification of the perforation and primary repair, unless there is significant fecal soiling, peritonitis, or identification of malignancy on evaluation of the polypectomy specimen.

Surveillance strategy after polypectomy should be based on the risk of patients as defined by the index colonoscopic polypectomy. Increased risk is defined as follows: (1) three or more adenomas removed, (2) high-grade dysplasia, (3) villous features, or (4) an adenoma greater than or equal to 1 cm in size. Lower risk is defined by one or two small (<1 cm) tubular adenomas with no high-grade dysplasia. High-risk patients should have a repeat colonoscopy at 3 years, and low-risk patients may safely defer colonoscopy for 5 to 10 years. Patients with hyperplastic polyps may defer for the same 10-year follow-up recommended for average-risk people (see Fig. 1).

APPROACH TO THE MALIGNANT POLYP

As mentioned earlier, the key to high-quality polypectomy is complete excision, which should include the entire stalk to its base at the submucosa of the adjacent bowel surface. This will allow optimal histologic evaluation of the margins. The risk of malignancy in polyps ranges from 2% to 10%, and the risk increases with size (40% at 2 cm) and high-risk histology, which includes dysplasia and villous architecture. However, if the polyp is deemed benign and completely excised, then there is no need for resection. The term "carcinoma in situ" should be abandoned because it leads

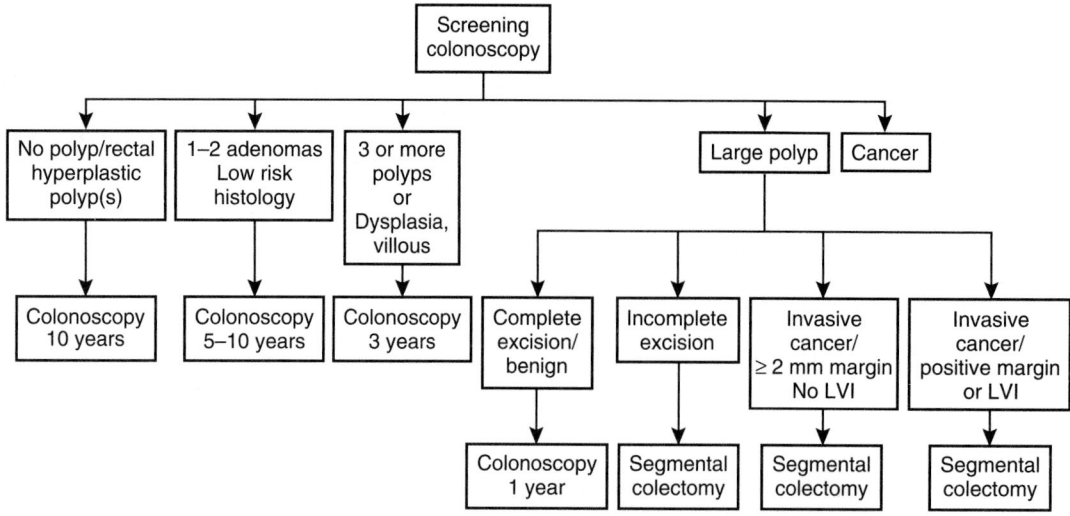

Figure I Algorithm for outcomes with screening colonoscopy. *LVI,* Lymphovascular invasion.

to confusion in the management decisions. Criteria for safe observation of the patient with a malignant polyp include complete excision, a resection margin of 2 mm, and absence of vascular or lymphatic invasion. Alternatively, incompletely resected polyps, positive margins, or evidence of vascular or lymphatic invasion should undergo an oncologic segmental resection. Recent data confirm that more than 20% of patients with colonoscopically unresectable lesions harbor invasive cancer in the polyp. This population is increasingly being managed with a laparoscopic oncologic segmental resection.

SUGGESTED READINGS

Hassan C, Zullo A, Risio M, and others: Histologic risk factors and clinical outcome in colorectal malignant polyp: a pooled-data analysis, *Gastroenterology* 98:371, 1990.

Levine JS, Ahnen DJ: Clinical practice. Adenomatous polyps of the colon, *N Engl J Med* 355:2551, 2006.

O'Brien MJ, Winawer SJ, Zauber AG, and others: The National Polyp Study. Patient and polyp characteristics associated with high-grade dysplasia in colorectal adenomas, *Gastroenterology* 109:1801, 1995.

Pokala N, Delaney CP, Kiran RP, and others: Outcome of laparoscopic colectomy for polyps not suitable for endoscopic resection, *Dis Colon Rectum* 47:1789; discussion 1796, 2004.

Seitz U, Bohnacker S, Seewald S, and others: Is endoscopic polypectomy an adequate therapy for malignant colorectal adenomas? Presentation of 1149 patients and review of the literature, *Dis Colon Rectum* 48:1588, 2005.

Volk EE, Goldblum JR, Petras RE, and others: Management and outcome of patients with invasive carcinoma arising in colorectal polyps, *Gastroenterology* 109:1801, 1995.

Winawer SJ, Zauber AG, Fletcher RH, and others: Guidelines for colonoscopy surveillance after polypectomy: a consensus update by the US Multi-Society Task Force on Colorectal Cancer and the American Cancer Society, *CA Cancer J Clin* 56:143; quiz 184, 2006.

MANAGEMENT OF PERITONEAL SURFACE MALIGNANCY: THE SURGEON'S ROLE

Jesus Esquivel, MD, and Paul H. Sugarbaker, MD

INTRODUCTION

The earliest success with the surgical management of metastatic disease was complete resection of locally recurrent colon and rectal cancer. Next the resection of liver metastases from the same disease was shown to be of benefit in a selected group of patients. Extension of the concept of complete surgical eradication of metastatic disease to bring about long-term survival to patients with peritoneal surface malignancy has recently been reported from several institutions. Appendix cancer is the paradigm for successful treatment of peritoneal carcinomatosis.

PRINCIPLES OF MANAGEMENT

The successful treatment of peritoneal surface malignancy requires a combined approach that uses peritonectomy procedures and perioperative intraperitoneal chemotherapy. To balance the risks and benefits, knowledgeable patient selection is mandatory. Both visceral and parietal peritonectomy are necessary for complete cytoreduction, which is essential for treatment to result in long-term survival. Between one and six peritonectomy procedures may be required. Their use depends on the distribution and extent of invasion of the malignancy disseminated within the peritoneal space. The question of when to pursue cytoreduction and when to accept palliative debulking as the proper treatment may present a difficult surgical problem.

Changes in the surgeon's use of chemotherapy in patients with peritoneal carcinomatosis, peritoneal sarcomatosis, and peritoneal mesothelioma have occurred and caused favorable results of treatment. A change in route of drug administration has occurred. Chemotherapy is given intraperitoneally or by combined intraperitoneal and intravenous routes. A change in timing has also occurred in that chemotherapy begins in the operating room and may be continued for the first 5 postoperative days. Third, a change in selection criteria for treatment of abdominal and pelvic malignancy has occurred. With the nonaggressive peritoneal surface malignancies as an exception, the lesion size of peritoneal implants is of crucial importance. Only patients with small intraperitoneal tumor nodules that have a limited distribution within the abdomen and pelvis are likely to show prolonged benefit.

Complete cytoreductive surgery is necessary before the intraperitoneal chemotherapy instillation, and this is unlikely for advanced sarcomatosis or carcinomatosis. However, as much as is possible, normal peritoneum is not resected; only parietal or visceral surfaces visibly involved by cancer are removed. Aggressive treatment strategies for an advanced and invasive intraperitoneal malignancy will not produce long-term benefits and are often the cause of excessive morbidity or mortality. Treatments to prevent the occurrence or eradicate established seeding must be initiated as early as is possible in the natural history of these diseases to achieve the greatest benefits. In some patients, the cytoreduction and intraperitoneal chemotherapy should be considered with the management of the primary cancer.

PERITONECTOMY PROCEDURES

Construction of the Surgical Field to Provide Simultaneous Exposure of the Abdomen and Pelvis

A self-retaining retractor is positioned so that continuous retraction of all parts of the abdominal incision occurs (Fig. 1). The retraction system must be securely anchored to the operating table to provide for continuous unencumbered visualization of the large operative field. The electrosurgical dissection is with a ball tip that allows contouring of the plane of dissection. The electrosurgery is used on pure cut at high voltage for dissection. When small bleeding points are encountered, high-voltage electrocoagulation is used. Frequent irrigation of the operative field with a saline solution cools the tissues irrigates away blood or blood

products that may accumulate and increases the conduction of the electrosurgical current.

Parietal Peritoneal Stripping from the Anterior Abdominal Wall

A single entry into the peritoneal cavity in the upper portion of the incision allows the surgeon to assess the requirement for a complete parietal peritonectomy. If cancer nodules are palpated on the parietal peritoneum, a decision for a complete dissection is made. Except for the small defect in the peritoneum required for this peritoneal exploration, the remainder of the peritoneum is left intact.

After dissecting generously the peritoneum on the right and left sides of the bladder, the apex of the bladder is localized and placed on strong traction using a Babcock clamp. The peritoneum with the underlying fatty tissues is stripped away from the surface of the bladder.

The self-retaining retraction system is steadily advanced more deeply into the abdominal cavity (Fig. 2). This optimizes the broad traction at the point of dissection of the peritoneum and its underlying tissues. It is most adherent directly overlying the transversus muscle. In some instances, blunt dissection from inferior to superior aspects of the abdominal wall facilitates clearing in this area. As the dissection proceeds to the peritoneum overlying the paracolic sulcus (line of Toldt), it becomes more rapid because of the loose connections of the peritoneum to the underlying fatty tissue at this anatomic site.

Peritoneal Stripping from Beneath the Hemidiaphragms

To begin peritonectomy of the left and right upper quadrants, the peritoneum is progressively stripped off the posterior rectus sheath. Strong traction combined with ball-tip electrosurgical dissection allows separation of peritoneal surface tumor from all normal tissue, including the diaphragmatic muscle, the adrenal glands, and the superior half of perirenal fat. The dissection between diaphragm muscle and its peritoneal covering must be performed with electro-evaporative surgery, not by blunt dissection. Numerous blood vessels between the diaphragm muscle and its peritoneal surface must be electrocoagulated before their transection, or unnecessary bleeding will occur as the divided blood vessel retracts into the muscle of the diaphragm. The stripping of the tumor from the undersurface of the diaphragm continues until the bare area of

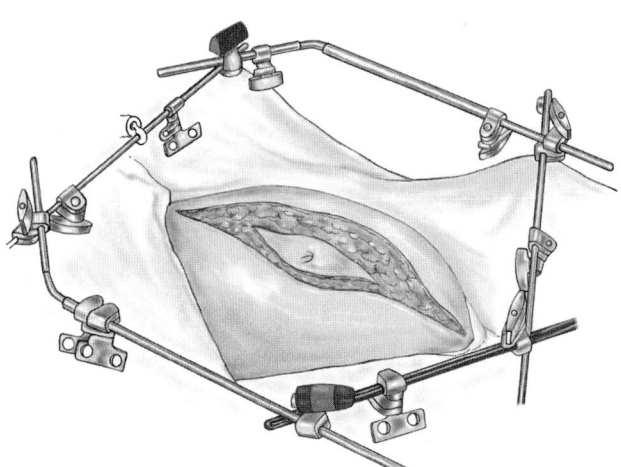

Figure 1 Self-retaining retractor and elliptical incision.

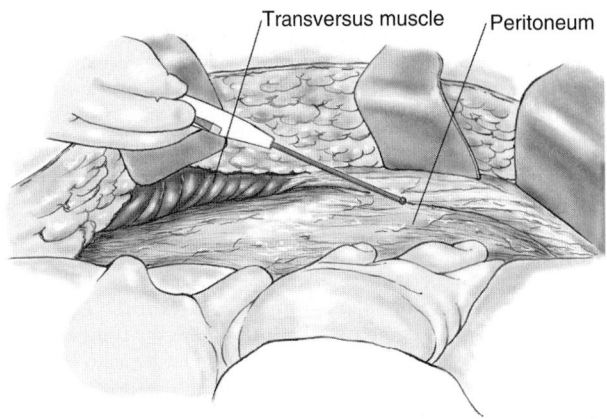

Figure 2 Parietal peritoneal dissection to the paracolic sulcus and beyond.

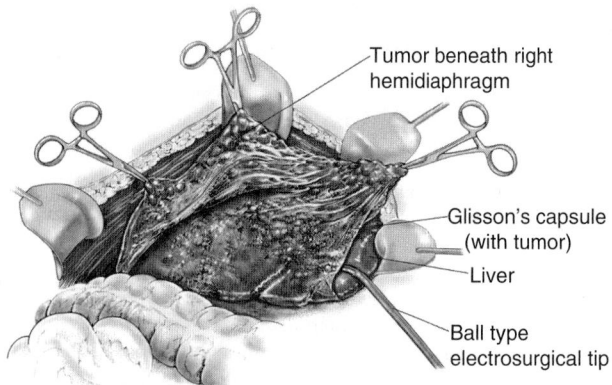

Figure 3 Peritoneal stripping from beneath the right hemidiaphragm and electroevaporation of tumor from the surface of the liver.

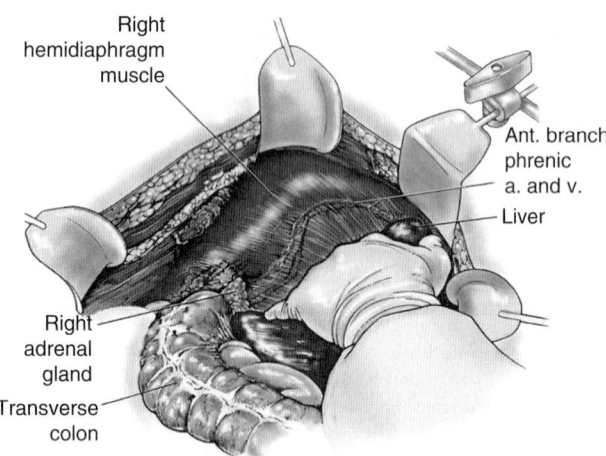

Figure 4 Completed right subphrenic peritonectomy.

the liver is encountered. At that point, tumor on the superior surface of the liver is electroevaporated until the liver surface is cleared. With ball-tipped electrosurgical dissection, a thick layer of tumor may be lifted off the dome of the liver by removing Glisson's capsule (Fig. 3). The dissection continues laterally on the right to encounter the perirenal fat covering the right kidney. The right adrenal gland is also visualized and carefully avoided as the tumor is stripped from the right subhepatic space. Care is taken not to traumatize the vena cava or to disrupt the caudate lobe veins that pass between the vena cava and segment 1 of the liver.

With strong upward traction on the right costal margin by the self-retaining retractor and medial displacement of the right liver, one can visualize the completed right subphrenic peritonectomy (Fig. 4).

Greater Omentectomy and Splenectomy

To remove a large volume of tumor from the midabdomen, a greater omentectomy-splenectomy is performed. The greater omentum is elevated and then separated from the transverse colon using electrosurgery. This dissection continues beneath the peritoneum that covers the transverse mesocolon to expose the inferior edge of the pancreas. The gastroepiploic vessels on the greater curvature of the stomach are clamped, ligated, and divided. The short gastric vessels are also transected. The mound of tumor that covers the spleen is identified. With traction on the spleen, the

peritoneum anterior to the pancreas involved by tumor is stripped from the gland using electrosurgery. This freely exposes the splenic artery and vein at the tail of the pancreas. These vessels are ligated in continuity and proximally suture ligated. The surgeon must avoid the main left gastric artery and its branches and the left gastric vein to preserve the sole remaining vascular supply to the stomach.

Cholecystectomy with Stripping of the Hepatoduodenal Ligament

The gallbladder is removed in routine fashion from its fundus toward the cystic artery and cystic duct. Blunt dissection of the base of the gallbladder away from the common duct and right hepatic artery distinguishes these structures from the surrounding tumor and fatty tissue. These structures are ligated and divided.

The triangular ligament of the left lobe of the liver was resected in performing the left subphrenic peritonectomy. This completed, the left lateral segment of the liver is retracted left to right to expose the hepatogastric ligament in its entirety. A circumferential release of this ligament from the fissure between liver segments 2, 3, and 1 and from the arcade of right gastric artery to left gastric artery along the lesser curvature of the stomach is required. After electrosurgically dividing the peritoneum on the lesser curvature of the stomach, digital dissection with extreme pressure from the surgeon's thumb and index finger separates lesser omental fat and tumor from the vascular arcade. As much of the anterior vagus nerve is spared as is possible. The tumor and fatty tissue surrounding the right and left gastric arteries are split away from the vascular arcade. In this manner, the specimen is centralized over the major branches of the left gastric artery. With strong traction on the specimen, the lesser omentum is released from the left gastric artery and vein (Fig. 5).

Stripping of the Floor of the Omental Bursa

A Dever retractor or the assistant's fingertips beneath the left caudate lobe are positioned to expose the entire floor of the omental bursa. Electroevaporation of tumor from the caudate process of the left caudate lobe of the liver may be necessary to achieve this exposure. Ball-tip electrosurgery is used cautiously to divide the peritoneal reflection of liver onto the left side of the subhepatic

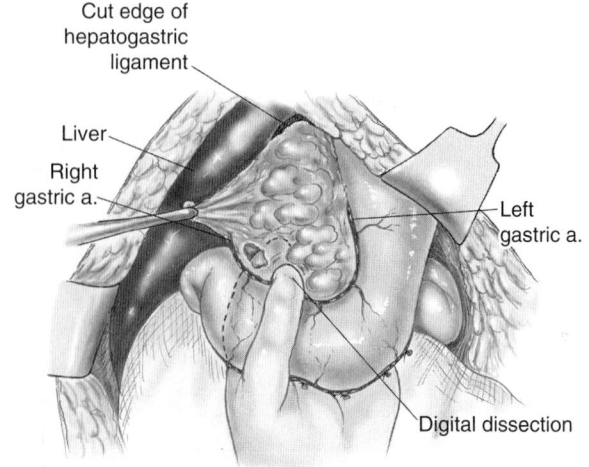

Figure 5 Circumferential resection of the hepatogastric ligament and lesser omentum by digital dissection.

vena cava. After the peritoneum is divided, Russian forceps assist in a blunt stripping of the peritoneum from the superior recess of the omental bursa, from the crus of the right hemidiaphragm and from beneath the portal vein. Electroevaporation of tumor from the shelf of liver parenchyma beneath the portal vein and joining right and left aspects of the caudate lobe may be required. Care is taken while stripping the floor of the omental bursa to remain superficial to the right phrenic artery.

Resection of Rectosigmoid Colon, Uterus, and Cul-de-Sac of Douglas

To begin rectosigmoid colon resection, a linear stapler is used to divide the sigmoid colon just above the limits of the pelvic tumor; this is usually at the junction of sigmoid and descending colon. The vascular supply of the distal portion of the bowel is traced back to its origin on the aorta. The inferior mesenteric artery and vein are ligated, suture ligated, and divided. This allows one to pack all the viscera, including the proximal descending colon, into the upper abdomen.

Ball-tipped electrosurgery is used to dissect at the limits of the pelvic peritonectomy (Fig. 6). The surgeon works in a centripetal fashion. Extraperitoneal ligation of the uterine arteries is performed just above the ureter and close to the base of the bladder. In women, the bladder is moved gently off the cervix, and the vagina is entered. The vaginal cuff anterior and posterior to the cervix is transected using ball-tipped electrosurgery, and the rectovaginal septum is entered. Ball-tipped electrosurgery is used to divide the perirectal fat beneath the peritoneal reflection. This ensures that all tumors that occupy the cul-de-sac are removed intact with the specimen. The rectal musculature is skeletonized using ball-tipped electrosurgery. Preservation of the lower half of the rectum will allow for a larger stool reservoir and diminish frequent bowel movements. A roticulator stapler (Autosuture, Norwalk, CT) is used to close off the rectal stump, and the rectum is sharply divided above the stapler.

CURRENT METHODOLOGY FOR DELIVERY OF HEATED INTRAOPERATIVE INTRAPERITONEAL CHEMOTHERAPY

In the operating room, heated intraoperative intraperitoneal chemotherapy is used. Heat is part of the optimizing process and is used to bring as much dose intensity to the abdominal and pelvic surfaces as is possible. Hyperthermia with intraperitoneal chemotherapy has several advantages. First, heat by itself has more toxicity for cancerous tissue than for normal tissue. This predominant effect on cancer increases as the vascularity of the malignancy decreases. Second, hyperthermia increases the penetration of chemotherapy into tissues. As tissues soften in response to heat, the elevated interstitial pressure of a tumor mass may decrease and allow improved drug penetration. Third, and probably most important, heat increases the cytotoxicity of selected chemotherapy agents. This synergism occurs only at the interface of heat and body tissue at the peritoneal surface.

After the cancer resection is complete, the Tenckhoff catheter and closed suction drains are placed through the abdominal wall and made watertight with a purse-string suture at the skin. Temperature probes are secured to the skin edge. The skin edges are secured to the self-retaining retractor with a long-running no. 2 monofilament suture. A plastic sheet is incorporated into these sutures to create a covering for the abdominal cavity. A slit in the plastic cover is made to allow the surgeon's double-gloved hand access to the abdomen and pelvis (Fig. 7). During the 90 minutes of perfusion, all the anatomic structures within the peritoneal cavity are uniformly exposed to heat and chemotherapy. The surgeon gently but continuously manipulates all viscera to keep adherence of peritoneal surfaces to a minimum. Roller pumps force the chemotherapy solution into the abdomen through the Tenckhoff catheter and pull it out through the drains. A heat exchanger keeps the fluid being infused at 44° to 46°C so that the intraperitoneal fluid is maintained at 42° to 43°C. The smoke evacuator is used to pull air from beneath the plastic cover through activated charcoal, preventing contamination (by chemotherapy aerosols) of air in the operating room.

After the intraoperative perfusion is complete, the abdomen is suctioned dry of fluid. The abdomen is then reopened, retractors repositioned, and reconstructive surgery is performed. It should be reemphasized that no suture lines are constructed until after the chemotherapy perfusion is complete. One exception to this rule is closure of the vaginal cuff to prevent leakage of intraperitoneal chemotherapy solution.

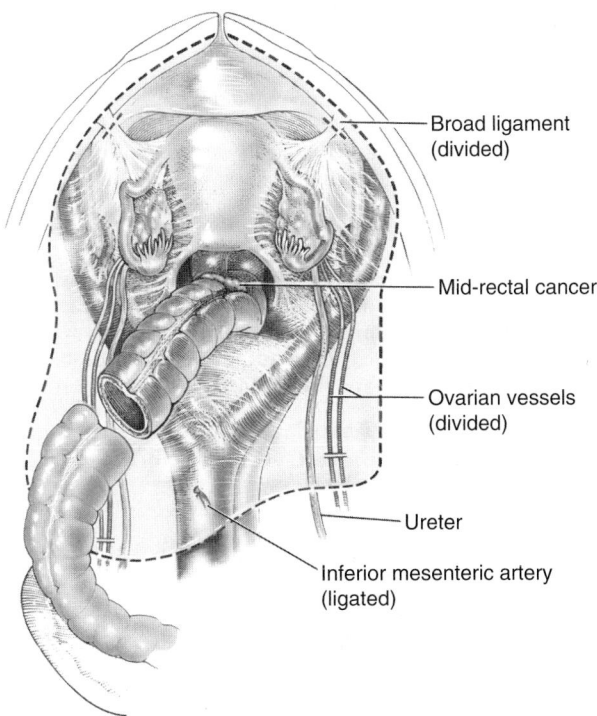

Broad ligament (divided)

Mid-rectal cancer

Ovarian vessels (divided)

Ureter

Inferior mesenteric artery (ligated)

Figure 6 Limits of the complete pelvic peritonectomy.

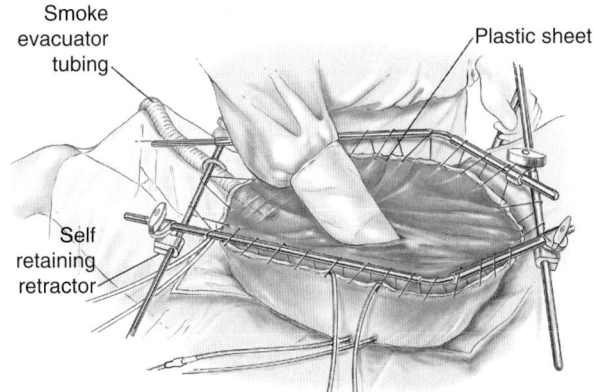

Smoke evacuator tubing

Plastic sheet

Self retaining retractor

Figure 7 Coliseum technique for heated intraoperative intraperitoneal chemotherapy. Surgical manipulation of the abdominal contents after complete resection of cancer ensures uniform distribution of heat and chemotherapy.

CLINICAL RESULTS OF TREATMENT

Appendix Cancer and Pseudomyxoma Peritonei

The paradigm for treatment of peritoneal carcinomatosis is appendiceal malignancy. The experience with nearly 800 patients treated over a 25-year time span is available. The survival of all patients is approximately 50% at 20 years.

Appendiceal Malignancy as a Paradigm

The appendiceal malignancies are characterized by unique clinical features that facilitate the successful treatment documented with this tumor. Spread from appendiceal tumors usually occurs in the absence of lymph node and liver metastases because small tumors early in the natural history of the disease will cause appendix obstruction and appendix perforation. This results in a release of tumor cells into the free peritoneal cavity. The seeding of the abdomen occurs in almost every patient before lymph node metastasis or liver metastasis has occurred. Second, there is a wide spectrum of invasion that these tumors exhibit. The ones that are minimally invasive can be totally resected using peritonectomy procedures to achieve a clear margin. Third, the majority of these tumors are mucinous. The texture of the implants allows greater penetration by chemotherapy than is possible with solid tumors. Finally, the malignancy disseminates so that all of its components are within the regional chemotherapy field. If the intraperitoneal chemotherapy is successful in eradicating the residual tumor on peritoneal surfaces, the patient will be a long-term survivor. Survival was significantly correlated with the completeness of cytoreduction (Fig. 8).

Colon Cancer Peritoneal Carcinomatosis

To date, approximately 200 patients have been treated who have peritoneal carcinomatosis from colon cancer. The Peritoneal Carcinomatosis Index provided a score valuable in selecting patients for treatment (Fig. 9). In patients who had a complete cytoreduction, there was marked improvement in survival; patients with residual disease show the expected short survival associated with peritoneal carcinomatosis from colon cancer (Fig. 10). These data suggest an early aggressive approach to peritoneal surface spread of adenocarcinoma of the colon in selected patients.

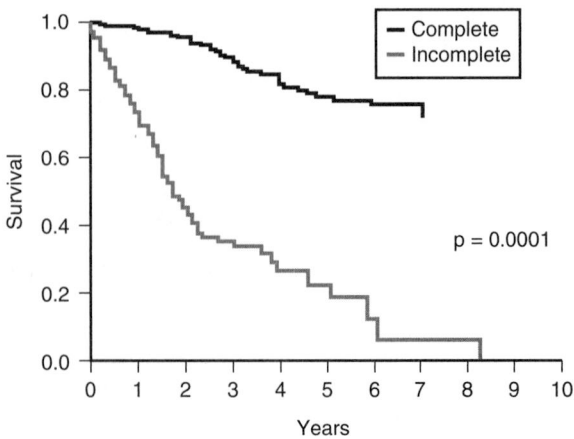

Figure 8 Survival of appendiceal malignancy with established peritoneal surface disease by completeness of cytoreduction.

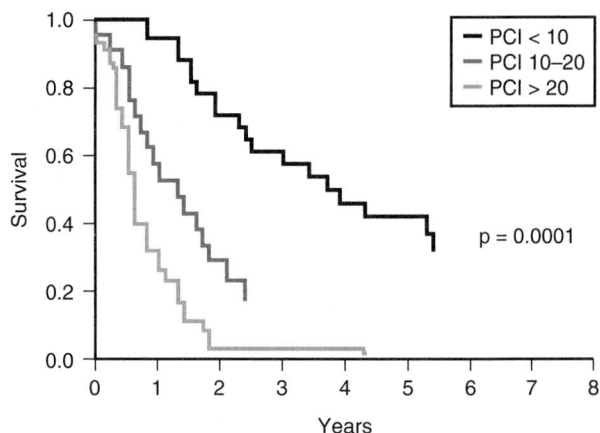

Figure 9 Survival of patients with peritoneal carcinomatosis from colon cancer by extent of peritoneal surface malignancy. Peritoneal Cancer Index *(PCI)* is a composite score of lesion size 0 to 3 in abdominopelvic regions 0 to 12.

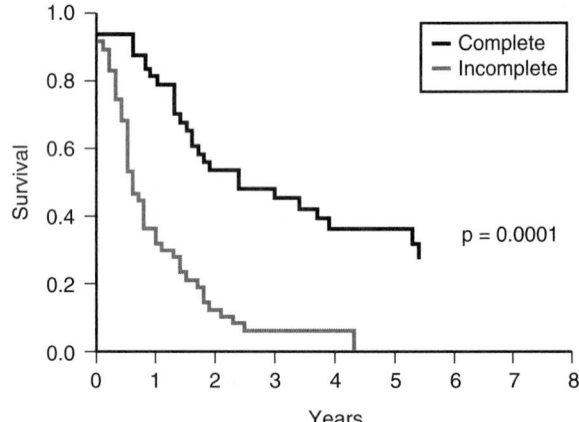

Figure 10 Survival of patients with peritoneal carcinomatosis from colon cancer by completeness of cytoreduction.

Selection Criteria

Proper patient selection is paramount to maximize benefits and minimize costs and morbidity in this group of patients. A list of clinical and radiologic features associated with an increased chance of having a complete cytoreduction is summarized in Table 1.

Morbidity and Mortality of Phase II Studies

The morbidity and mortality of 200 consecutive patients who had cytoreductive surgery and heated intraoperative intraperitoneal chemotherapy for peritoneal carcinomatosis has been reported. In these patients, there were three treatment-related deaths (1.8%). Peripancreatitis (7.1%) and fistulae (4.7%) were the most common

Table 1: Variables Associated with Increased Chances of a Complete Cytoreduction

ECOG performance status 2 or less
No evidence of extra-abdominal disease
Up to three small, resectable liver metastases
No evidence of biliary obstruction
No evidence of ureteral obstruction
No evidence of intestinal obstruction at more than one site
No evidence of bulky tumor at the hepatogastric ligament
Peritoneal Cancer Index of 20 or less

ECOG, Eastern Cooperative Oncology Group.

major complications. There were 25.3% of patients with grade III or IV complications.

Following these treatments, the patient is maintained on parenteral feeding for 2 to 3 weeks. Approximately 20% of patients, especially those who have had extensive prior surgery or who have a short bowel, will require parenteral feeding for several weeks after leaving the hospital.

SUGGESTED READINGS

Esquivel J, Sugarbaker PH: Elective surgery in recurrent colon cancer with peritoneal seeding: when to and when not to proceed [editorial], *Cancer Ther* 1:321, 1998.

Stephens AD, Alderman R, Chang D, and others: Morbidity and mortality of 200 treatments with cytoreductive surgery and hyperthermic intraoperative intraperitoneal chemotherapy using the Coliseum technique, *Ann Surg Oncol* 6:790, 1999.

Sugarbaker PH: Peritonectomy procedures, *Ann Surg* 221:29, 1995.

Sugarbaker PH, Yu W, Yonemura Y: Gastrectomy, peritonectomy and perioperative intraperitoneal chemotherapy: the evolution of treatment strategies for advanced gastric cancer, *Semin Surg Oncol* 21:233, 2003.

Vermess M, Doppman JL, Sugarbaker PH, and others: Computed tomography of the liver and spleen with intravenous lipoid contrast material: review of 60 examinations, *AJM Am J Roentgenol* 138:1063, 1982.

SURGICAL MANAGEMENT OF CONSTIPATION

Charles M. Friel, MD, and Ann C. Lowry, MD

Constipation is a common complaint accounting for frequent visits to primary care physicians. There are multiple causes of constipation, ranging from poor dietary habits to systemic medical conditions such as hypothyroidism. Simple measures such as increasing fiber and fluid intake, increasing exercise, and osmotic laxatives resolve the symptoms in the overwhelming majority of patients. Symptoms in patients with medical causes for their constipation can be well managed after the primary disease is controlled. However, a small subset of patients with chronic constipation require evaluation for possible surgical intervention. Even in busy referral practices, the number of patients who require surgery for constipation should be limited. Therefore to ensure optimal surgical results, proper patient selection is critical.

■ HISTORY AND PHYSICAL

A thorough history helps to identify patients with constipation who may benefit from surgery. The provider must have a clear understanding of what the patient means by "constipation." A common misconception is that a healthy person should have one formed stool daily. Constipation is defined as having fewer than three bowel movements per week. While many patients are concerned about the frequency of their bowel movements, others experience difficulty with defecation. Patients describe straining and a feeling of incomplete evacuation. Some patients require digital manipulation, whereas others apply perineal or transvaginal pressure for successful defecation. This type of symptom is better categorized as obstructive defecation. Although both decreased frequency and straining can be described as "constipation," distinguishing issues of frequency from obstructive defecation can be helpful because the treatment options may be different.

The duration of the problem is also a critical parameter. Most surgically correctable forms of constipation or obstructive defecation are longstanding; many patients have had problems their entire life. A recent change in stool pattern is more indicative of a new structural problem, systemic illness, or medication side effect. In addition to duration, associated symptoms should be identified. Patients with severe pain with defecation may have an anal fissure, and the associated "constipation" may be secondary to apprehension. Fecal soiling, generally associated with fecal incontinence, may be due to overflow and helps to diagnose patients with fecal impaction or, in children, encopresis. A history of multiparity and associated urinary symptoms or pelvic organ prolapse suggests more diffuse pelvic floor dysfunction. All of these parameters help the physician to make a definitive diagnosis and direct therapy.

Although the physical examination is often unremarkable, it remains an important part of the evaluation. Patients with poor colonic transit, such as slow transit colonic inertia or Hirschsprung's disease, often have abdominal distention, and in some cases a stool-filled colon can be palpated. Close inspection of the anorectal and perineal region is also important. With the patient in the left lateral decubitus position, he or she should be asked to strain. A clinically significant rectocele may be readily visualized because it bulges into the vaginal introitus in women and can be confirmed on digital rectal exam. Rectal prolapse, which is usually evident by history, may also be visualized. Under normal conditions, movement of the perineum should be limited, even during straining. The perineal descent syndrome is diagnosed when the perineum bulges and descends several centimeters below the ischial tuberosities.

A digital rectal examination should then be performed. Fecal impaction and low-lying rectal cancer are readily apparent. By applying anterior pressure with the examining finger, a rectocele can be visualized as the weakened rectal vaginal septum is displaced into the vaginal introitus (Fig. 1). Finally, the

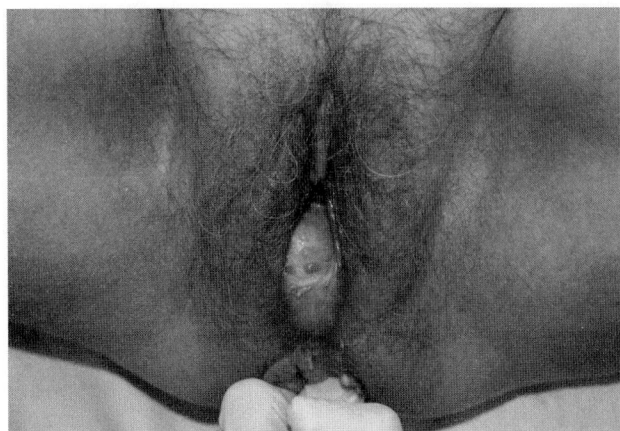

Figure 1 Rectocele demonstrated on physical examination with anterior pressure on digital rectal exam. (*See color insert Figure 20.*)

puborectalis muscle should be palpated. This is best accomplished by hooking the examining finger posteriorly over the coccyx. With the finger in the anal canal, the patient should be asked to perform the valsalva maneuver as if trying to move his or her bowels. Under normal conditions, there should be relaxation of the anal canal, which can often be appreciated as the anal sphincter relaxes and the anal canal opens slightly. Anismus, or nonrelaxation of the puborectalis muscle, should be considered if there is paradoxical puborectalis contraction when the patient strains.

TESTING

Patients referred for surgical management of constipation often require further testing. Anorectal manometry uses pressure transducers to measure anal canal pressure while the patient is resting, squeezing, and straining. With straining, the anal sphincter should relax, resulting in decreased pressure within the anal canal. If the pressure increases with straining, anismus is confirmed. High resting pressures are more consistent with hypertrophy of the internal sphincter muscle.

In addition to measuring anal pressures, anal manometry can be used to measure the presence or absence of the rectoanal inhibitory reflex. Rectal distention normally results in reflex relaxation of the anal sphincter and is referred to as the rectoanal inhibitory reflex. The presence of a rectoanal inhibitory reflex excludes the diagnosis of Hirschsprung's disease, whereas the absence of this reflex suggests the possibility of this disease.

Sponge electromyogram (EMG) can be used to measure the activity of the puborectalis muscle with the patient resting, straining, and squeezing. Under normal conditions, the measured electrical activity decreases when a patient strains and the puborectalis muscle relaxes. Increased electrical activity during straining indicates paradoxical contraction of the puborectalis muscle and confirms anismus.

The balloon expulsion test helps to diagnose obstructed defecation. An approximately 50-ml balloon is placed within the rectum and inflated. The patient is then asked to evacuate the balloon; evacuation is readily accomplished in patients with normal pelvic floor function. However, evacuation is difficult or impossible in patients with anismus.

Radiographic examination is also helpful in the evaluation of patients with chronic constipation. A stool-filled colon on a simple abdominal film will help to support a patient's assertion of infrequent bowel movements (Fig. 2). A barium enema can be given to identify any structural abnormalities, such as colon cancer or a diverticular stricture. Colonic transit time can be measured by having the patient ingest a capsule containing multiple radiopaque markers. Daily abdominal x-rays are then obtained. Normal subjects will pass 80% of the markers by day 5 and 100% by day 7. Retained markers that are evenly distributed throughout the colon indicate a colonic motility disorder. Markers that are clumped in the rectosigmoid region suggest that the primary problem is obstructed defecation and not transit.

An excellent functional examination is defecography, a dynamic test performed under fluoroscopic guidance. A barium paste is instilled in the rectum, and the patient is asked to evacuate the paste while being fluoroscopically evaluated. The entire procedure is videotaped, which provides an excellent visualization of the defecatory process for that patient. In a patient with normal defecation, the anorectal angle opens readily and the paste is easily evacuated. Anismus is diagnosed in patients who tighten or fail to relax the anal rectal angle and cannot evacuate the barium. Anatomic abnormalities such as rectoceles, enteroceles, sigmoidoceles, and intussusceptions may also be visualized.

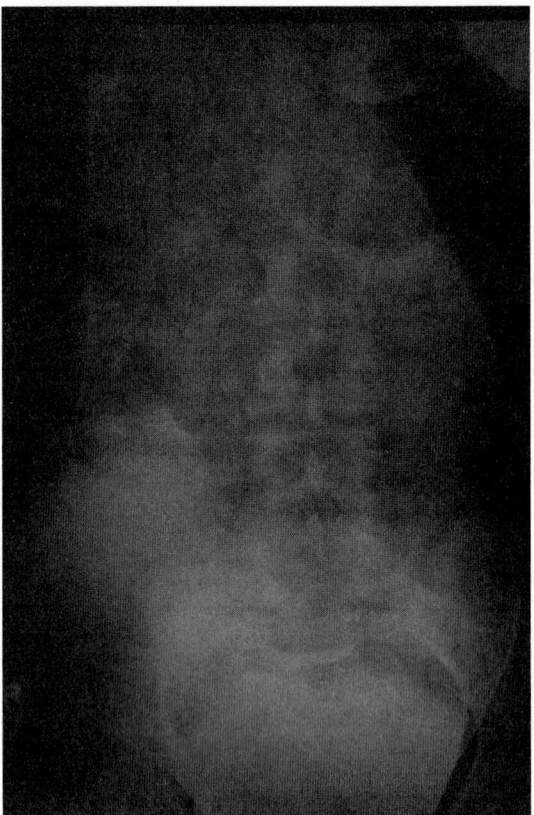

Figure 2 Abdominal x-ray showing massive stool-filled colon in a patient with chronic constipation.

SPECIFIC DISORDERS

Perineal Descent Syndrome

Perineal descent syndrome is diagnosed when there is significant downward descent of the perineum when the patient strains. Although corrective procedures have been described, most surgeons feel this condition is not surgically correctable. Therefore patients with perineal descent syndrome should be referred for biofeedback.

Anismus

Anismus (nonrelaxation of the puborectalis muscle, paradoxical contraction of the puborectalis muscle, pelvic floor dyssynergia) is diagnosed by a combination of the history, physical exam, defecography, sponge EMG, and anorectal manometry. Patients should be referred for biofeedback to help retrain the pelvic musculature. Although the majority of patients learn to relax their pelvic floor muscles appropriately, not all experience relief of their symptoms. Currently there is no good surgical solution for anismus.

Slow Transit Colonic Inertia

Slow transit colonic inertia can be surgically corrected, but careful patient selection is critical to success. Typical patients are adult women who have had a long history of chronic constipation that is unresponsive to high-fiber diets and over-the-counter laxatives. Associated symptoms often include bloating, straining, and abdominal pain. Before surgery is offered, it is imperative that all patients have a full and complete evaluation. All patients should have either a colonoscopy or a barium enema to rule out any structural abnormalities. Hypothyroidism and hypercalcemia must be excluded. Patients must have documented colonic dysmotility by an abnormal colonic transit study. A small bowel follow through should be obtained to ensure that the patient does not have a generalized motility disorder, which is unlikely to improve with surgery. Finally, defecography should be normal, without evidence of anismus or other pelvic floor abnormalities.

If a motility disorder isolated to the colon is confirmed by these studies, a total abdominal colectomy with an ileorectal anastomosis may be beneficial. This procedure can be done either open or laparoscopically. Controversy still exists regarding whether the anastomosis must be performed to the true rectum or to the distal sigmoid colon. Leaving large amounts of abdominal colon is likely to result in surgical failure. However, an anastomosis made too low in the rectum can lead to chronic diarrhea, which can be equally disabling, especially if associated with incontinence.

Some patients with slow transit also have anismus on defecography. Under these circumstances, colectomy alone is unlikely to improve their quality of life. These patients should be referred for biofeedback as their initial treatment. If after biofeedback their evacuation improves but frequency remains an issue, colectomy may be cautiously considered.

Before surgery, proper counseling is important. Patients must understand that an abdominal colectomy is major surgery with the possibility of significant complications, including anastomotic leak, diarrhea, incontinence, and small bowel obstruction. Therefore surgery should be considered only for patients with disabling symptoms. Furthermore, although most patients focus on the need to have a bowel movement, there is often a multitude of associated complaints, such as abdominal pain. Although total abdominal colectomy almost always improves the frequency of defecation, many of these other symptoms may persist. Some studies suggest that surgery for colonic inertia, although successful at increasing the frequency of bowel movements, does not necessarily improve the overall quality of life. To maximize patient satisfaction, these expectations must be clearly delineated before surgery (Table 1).

Adult Hirschsprung's Disease

Hirschsprung's disease is generally considered a pediatric disorder. The diagnosis is first suggested by failure of the newborn to pass meconium and is ultimately confirmed by full-thickness rectal biopsies demonstrating the lack of ganglion cells within the myenteric plexus. There are a host of procedures, all of which are variations on coloanal pull-through procedures, to treat this problem in pediatric patients. For a full discussion of the pediatric population, the reader is referred to a textbook on pediatric surgery.

On occasion, some patients with Hirschsprung's disease are not diagnosed until adulthood. Generally these patients present having had a lifelong struggle with constipation. Mental retardation and, more specifically, Down syndrome, may complicate and delay the diagnosis. Because the aganglionic segment is often short in this setting, this disease is also referred to as short segment Hirschsprung's disease. As in the pediatric population, a dilatated, stool-filled colon is common. If the diagnosis is suspected, anal manometry is an easy and effective screening test. If the rectoanal inhibitory reflex is present, the diagnosis of Hirschsprung's disease can be excluded. However, if the reflex is absent, full-thickness rectal biopsies are necessary to confirm the diagnosis.

The agangiolonic segment of Hirschsprung's disease is typically less extensive when diagnosed in adulthood. Therefore it is possible to consider less complex therapy. Although most children require some sort of coloanal pull-through operation, an alternative surgical approach for short segment disease is a rectal myectomy. This procedure is performed via a transanal approach with the patient in the lithotomy position. A transverse incision is placed posteriorly in the dentate line and a submucosal-mucosal flap approximately 1 cm in width is raised, exposing the circular muscle of the internal sphincter and the distal rectal wall. A strip of muscle is then excised as high as can be reached via this approach. Ideally, the dissection should extend to a level where the ganglion cells are present. The submucosal-mucosal flap is then reapproximated to the dentate line, completing the procedure. Although this operation is uncommon, there are reports of success, despite leaving a portion of distal rectum without ganglion cells. Because this operation is performed transanally, the potential for serious complications is low. Therefore this approach may be the best initial treatment.

If symptoms persist after a rectal myomectomy, a more extensive procedure should be considered. In this situation, the treatment principles of adult Hirschsprung's disease are similar to the pediatric population. Because the normal proximal colon may become dilatated, a temporary loop colostomy may be necessary to allow the colon to decompress to its normal diameter. Subsequently the distal diseased segment is resected, and a distal

Table 1: Results of Surgery for Slow Transit Colonic Inertia

Author	Year	Number of Patients	Bowel Movements/Day	Persistent Abdominal Pain (%)	Satisfaction (%)
Preston	1984	21	3.0	50	63
Yoshioka	1989	40	3.0	39	58
Piccirillo	1995	54	3.7	10	94
Lubowski	1996	52	4.0	52	90
Pluta	1996	24	2.6	17	92
Platell	1996	96	5.0	55	82
Bernini	1998	90	2.8	44	78
Mollen	2001	21	2.8	81	76
Webster	2001	55	3.0	19	89
Fitzharris	2003	75	*	41	93
Knowles[†‡]	1999	—	2.9	41	39–100

*Ninety-five percent of patients had an increase in bowel frequency.
[†‡]Review and summary of the literature.

anastomosis performed. Most of the pediatric procedures use a variation of coloanal techniques, hoping to limit the pelvic dissection and therefore some of the potential complications, such as impotence. However, those techniques are somewhat unfamiliar to surgeons caring for adults, whereas a low anterior resection with a low-stapled coloanal anastomosis is commonly performed. Therefore the best operation in the adult population is a low anterior resection with a stapled coloanal anastomosis. Care must be taken to carry the dissection to just above the anorectal ring. If this is not possible, a mucosectomy with a hand-sewn coloanal anastomosis can be performed. Although there is a risk of sexual dysfunction from the pelvic dissection, experience from surgery for ulcerative colitis would suggest that this risk is minimal in young patients.

Rectoceles

Patients with rectoceles commonly present with difficult evacuation. Frequently patients describe applying perineal or transvaginal pressure to move their bowels successfully. Clinically significant rectoceles can generally be diagnosed with a thorough history and physical examination. Patients note a bulging at the vaginal introitus. Urinary and sexual symptoms should be explored because a rectocele is often associated with other pelvic pathology.

On physical examination, the rectal vaginal septum can be seen bulging into the vaginal introitus with straining. Digital rectal and pelvic examinations should be done to distinguish a rectocele from a cystocele or vaginal vault prolapse. Defecography confirms the presence of a rectocele (Fig. 3). Large rectoceles may not empty on defecography without perineal or transvaginal pressure. Such an observation confirms the clinical significance of a large rectocele and assures the surgeon and patient that surgery is likely to provide relief. Small rectoceles (<2 cm in size) that empty easily on defecography are unlikely to be the source of symptoms and generally do not require surgery.

Rectoceles can be repaired via a transanal, perineal, or transvaginal approach. Because most rectoceles are actually repaired by gynecologists, a transvaginal approach is most common. With the patient in the lithotomy position, a transverse incision is made in the vaginal mucosal just proximal to the introitus. A mucosal-

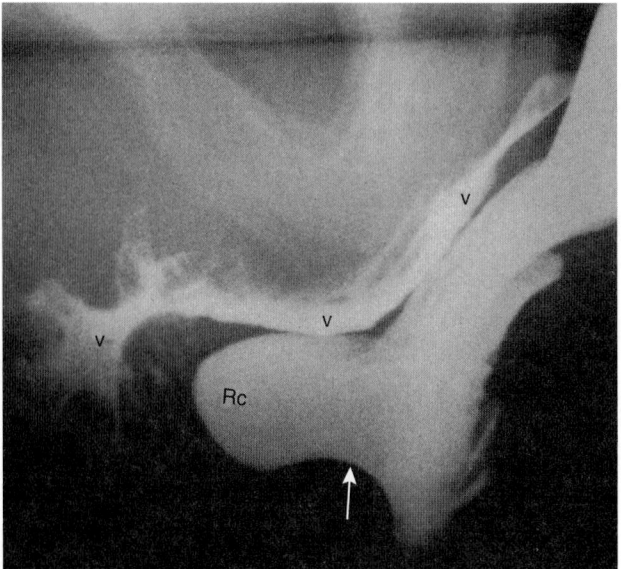

Figure 3 Defecography showing large rectocele. *Rc*, Rectocele; *V*, vagina.

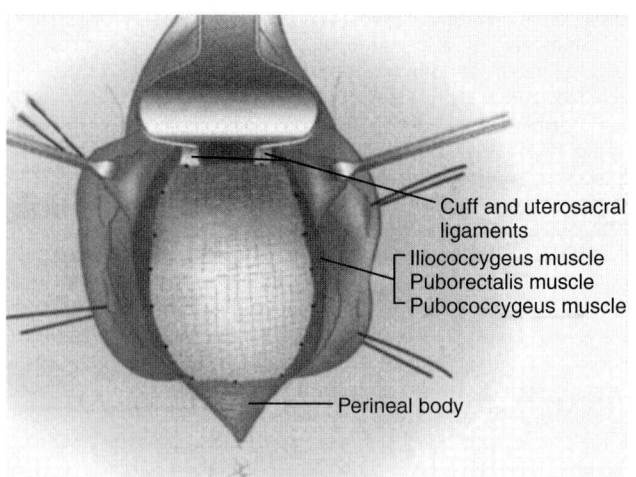

Figure 4 Rectocele repair using an implant to reinforce rectal vaginal septum.

submucosal flap is raised, thus exposing the weakened rectal vaginal septum. Care must be taken to avoid rectal injury to prevent the dreaded complication of a rectovaginal fistula. The dissection should continue to the apex of the vagina. The rectal vaginal septum and levator muscles are then reinforced using a series of imbricating stitches. Finally, the mucosal-submucosal flap is then reapproximated, completing the procedure.

A recently popularized alternative is referred to as the site-specific repair. In this repair, a perineal incision is made just at the vaginal introitus. The vaginal wall is separated from the rectovaginal septum. Defects are typically paravaginal, central, or transverse. If a specific defect can be identified in the rectovaginal septum, it is repaired. If the entire septum is lax, it can be reinforced with materials such as cadaveric fascia lata, porcine dermal xenografts, or synthetic mesh (Fig. 4).

More recently several reports have described using stapled transrectal rectal resection (STARR) to treat rectoceles and intussusceptions associated with obstructive defecation. Two firings of a circular stapler are used to resect sequentially the anterior rectal wall and subsequently the posterior rectal wall, thus eliminating redundant tissue. Early reports seem promising, but further study is clearly indicated. A multicenter clinical trial is currently recruiting patients to answer some of these unresolved questions.

Finally, in women who are elderly, frail, or unwilling to have surgery, a pessary should be considered. Pessaries placed within the vagina can provide much needed pelvic support. In addition to rectoceles, pessaries are also used to treat uterine prolapse and cystoceles. A number of types are available, and women need to be individually fitted to account for anatomic differences.

It is important to recognize that most of the surgical repairs for a rectocele stress the same fundamental principles; the weakened rectal vaginal septum is exposed and then reinforced. The debate focuses on how to access this dissection (e.g., transvaginal, transanal, transperineal) and how to reinforce the septum (e.g., direct repair, mesh). It is not surprising, therefore, that published reports have similar success rates (Table 2). The exception, however, is the STARR procedure. This procedure, which involves a full-thickness resection of the anterior and posterior rectal wall, deviates from the more traditional procedures. The early reports seem promising, with few anatomic recurrences and high rates of symptomatic improvement. Nevertheless, long-term results are still required before it can be widely advocated. Detractors of this approach note the potential for serious complications, including pelvic sepsis, rectovaginal fistula, bleeding, and incontinence. Unfortunately, these complications are also well described with the more traditional surgical approaches.

Table 2: Results of Surgery for Rectocele Repairs

Author	Year	Number of Patients	Type of Repair	Mesh	Recurrent Rectocele (%)	Improvement of Constipation (%)	Follow-up (months)
Van Laarhoven	1999	15	Transperineal	Both	60	87	27.0
Van Laarhoven	1999	7	Transanal	No	14	43	27.0
Nieminen	2004	15	Transvaginal	No	7	93	12.0
Nieminen	2004	14	Transanal	No	40	73	12.0
Boccasanta*	2004	90	STARR	No	0	81	16.0
Thornton	2005	40	Transanal	No	NS	55	20.0
Thornton	2005	40	Laparoscopic	No	NS	28	76.0
Abramov	2005	124	Site-specific	No	44	20	12.2
Abramov	2005	183	Transvaginal	No	18	18	12.4
Altman	2006	23	Transvaginal	Yes	41	30	38.0

An author listed consecutively represents comparative approaches described in a single study. *NS,* Not stated.
*Combination of rectocele and internal intussusception.

Interpreting the literature on rectocele repairs can be difficult because there are few randomized, prospective studies comparing the various techniques. Furthermore, the selection criteria and definitions of success are often different. Length of follow-up is another critical parameter because many reports in the literature highlight short-term success that may decline with long-term follow-up. The mere observation that there are a multitude of approaches suggests that there is no clear advantage of one technique over another. No matter the approach, many women do have sustained symptomatic improvement and are satisfied with the surgical result. However, these successes are by no means universal. Ironically, some women experience symptomatic relief despite an anatomic recurrence of the rectocele (Table 2).

Enteroceles and Sigmoidoceles

Enteroceles and sigmoidoceles may impede defecation and may cause pelvic discomfort. Women complain of perineal pressure with straining. Often it is difficult to diagnose these abnormalities and to determine their clinical significance. On physical examination, the perineum should be carefully examined with straining. In addition, the patient should be asked to strain while the surgeon performs a digital rectal exam. If the surgeon feels a bulging in the anterior cul-de-sac, an enterocele or sigmoidocele may be present. Either diagnosis can be confirmed by defecography, which may show a separation of the rectum and vagina with straining. This observation is greatly facilitated by having contrast material in both the small intestine and the vagina in addition to the usual barium paste in the rectum. If an enterocele or sigmoidocele impairs rectal emptying on defecography, it is reasonable to conclude that it may contribute to the patient's symptoms.

Surgery is appropriate if an enterocele or sigmoidocele is thought to be clinically significant. However, patients should be carefully counseled that surgical results are varied and that surgery may not relieve all their symptoms. When using the transabdominal approach, the general principle is to obliterate the deep anterior cul-de-sac through which the small bowel or redundant sigmoid colon may bulge. If vaginal vault prolapse is also present, both issues may be addressed with a sacrocolpopexy. If there is concomitant rectal prolapse, posterior rectal mobilization with rectopexy is the primary procedure, which generally elevates the anterior cul-de-sac and contributes to repair of the enterocele. Additionally, successive stitches can be placed between the peritoneum of the anterior rectal wall to the peritoneum of the posterior bladder and vagina, thus obliterating the space of the anterior cul-

de-sac. A significantly redundant sigmoid colon may also require simultaneous resection.

Stomas

Although certainly not the initial treatment, creation of a colostomy or ileostomy may be appropriate for patients with severe and disabling constipation or pelvic floor dysfunction. Stomas are appropriate only after an extensive evaluation and trials of all conservative approaches. Patients can usually be adequately managed with a combination of biofeedback, dietary manipulations, and osmotic laxatives. However, in some patients, these interventions are unsuccessful, and the constipation continues to be disabling. At this point, a discussion regarding stoma creation is appropriate. In patients who clearly have isolated anismus, the creation of an end colostomy should be effective. However, in patients who might have simultaneous slow transit colonic inertia, an ileostomy may be more appropriate. Both can easily be accomplished through laparoscopic or open techniques. Before the creation of a stoma, extensive counseling is necessary.

Patients with spinal cord injuries may also be best served with the creation of a well-functioning colostomy. A bowel management program for patients with paraplegia and quadriplegia can be intensive, often requiring daily enemas and manual disimpaction. Frequently the bowel program cannot be achieved by the patient alone and requires the assistance of another person. Bowel management may be simplified by the creation of a colostomy. Furthermore, many of these patients, especially those with paraplegia, can manage the colostomy alone, thus increasing their independence. Even in patients who cannot handle their own colostomy, management is often easier for the caregivers. An extensive discussion among the patient, the caregivers, and the patient's physicians is necessary before the creation of a stoma. However, more commonly, patients with spinal cord injuries struggle with defecation for years, unaware that there may be an excellent surgical alternative.

■ SUMMARY

Constipation is a common medical problem. The overwhelming majority of patients who experience constipation never require surgery. However, in a select subset of patients, both functional and structural problems can be identified that may be appropriately treated with surgery. Careful evaluation is critical to identify those few patients who may respond. Frequently there are associated pelvic floor abnormalities that should be simultaneously evaluated and repaired. Even after careful evaluation, extensive preoperative counseling is necessary to define patient and surgeon expectations; realistic expectations may help to maximize patient satisfaction.

Suggested Readings

Altman D, Zetterström J, López A, and others: Functional and anatomic outcome after transvaginal rectocele repair using collagen mesh: a prospective study, *Dis Colon Rectum* 48:1233; discussion 1241; author reply 1242, 2005.

Boccasanta P, Venturi M, Stuto A, and others: Stapled transanal rectal resection for outlet obstruction: a prospective, multicenter trial, *Dis Colon Rectum* 47:1285; discussion 1296, 2004.

FitzHarris GP, Garcia-Aguilar J, Parker SC, and others: Quality of life after subtotal colectomy for slow-transit constipation: both quality and quantity count, *Dis Colon Rectum* 46:433, 2003.

Knowles CH, Scott M, Lunniss PJ: Outcome of colectomy for slow transit constipation, *Ann Surg* 230:627, 1999.

Preoperative Bowel Preparation

David A. Margolin, MD, and Charles B. Whitlow, MD

The rationale for preoperative mechanical and antibiotic bowel preparation is to decrease the bacterial count in the colon, with the ultimate goal of decreasing surgical site infections (SSI) and the anastomotic leak rate. Additional benefits of mechanical preparation may include improved bowel handling and facilitation of intraoperative endoscopy. Surgical tradition and medicolegal concerns also contribute to current preoperative bowel preparation practices. The aim of this chapter is to reinforce the need for appropriate preoperative antibiotic coverage and, on the basis of current literature, challenge the dogma of mechanical bowel preparation despite its pervasive use.

ANTIBIOTIC PROPHYLAXIS

The use of antibiotic prophylaxis in elective colon surgery is mandatory. Oral antibiotics reduce intraluminal and mucosal bacterial counts, and parenteral antibiotics reduce systemic bacterial counts at the tissue level. Current practice is to use either one or both of these routes of antibiotic administration. No matter the route of delivery, it is important to choose antibiotics with an appropriate spectrum: those that cover both aerobic bacteria (e.g., *Escherichia coli*) and anaerobic organisms (e.g., *Bacteroides* spp.). Aside from the appropriate choice of antibiotics, the timing and duration of therapy is key.

In 1972, Nichols and Condon introduced an oral antibiotic regimen consisting of 1 g neomycin and 1 g erythromycin base. This regimen is rapidly and highly bacteriocidal against colonic pathogens, has limited systemic absorption, and has low systemic and local toxicity. Using this regimen combined with mechanical bowel preparation, they were able to decrease the wound infection rate from 35% to 9%. In a 2003 survey by Zmora and colleagues, 75% of colorectal surgeons reported using oral antibiotic prophylaxis. Interestingly, 71% of those using oral antibiotics questioned their usefulness, and 11% thought them to be of no value. Because of the common gastrointestinal side effects associated with erythromycin, many surgeons have replaced it with 500 mg of metronidazole with equal efficacy. Regardless of the antibiotic regimen chosen, the dosing interval is crucial. Antibiotics should be administered 19, 18, and 9 hours before the scheduled start of surgery.

An enormous variety of intravenous antibiotic regimens have been used to decrease infectious complications in colonic surgery. Common to all effective regimens is broad-spectrum coverage of typical colonic flora. At present, most surgeons prescribe either a second- or third-generation cephalosporin or a fluoroquinolone plus metronidazole. Unfortunately, two of the most widely used second-generation cephalosporins are no longer available. Cefotetan is no longer manufactured, and currently there is a national shortage of cefoxitin. Ampicillin-sulbactam has filled this void.

In addition to the particular antibiotics used, the timing and duration of therapy play a prominent role in decreasing infectious complications. Intravenous antibiotics should be administered within 60 minutes of skin incision to ensure adequate drug tissue levels. However, studies have demonstrated that administration of parenteral antibiotics on induction have also achieved sufficient tissue levels. Despite this, our practice is to administer intravenous antibiotics in the preoperative holding area immediately before transport to ensure that the drugs are indeed given and that there is an appropriate interval to obtain satisfactory tissue levels.

With regard to duration of antimicrobial therapy, a single dose of an appropriate antibiotic given before surgery is adequate. Studies have shown no benefit of multidose compared with single-dose therapy in reducing SSI. However, this single-dose recommendation does not include redosing antibiotics for procedures that exceed the half-life of the antibiotic. Postoperative antibiotic administration increases the risk of drug-resistant bacteria and antibiotic-associated complications.

Although there is no controversy regarding the need for antibiotics, there is controversy over the route of administration. Numerous trials have shown no single regimen to be superior in reducing SSI when using combined oral and intravenous antibiotics compared with oral or intravenous antibiotics alone. In three surveys of colorectal surgeons between 1990 and 1997, approximately 84% of respondents used a combination of oral and intravenous antibiotics for prophylaxis.

Our current practice is to use only intravenous antibiotics. Because of the reasons previously stated, this is a single dose of either 3 g of ampicillin-sulbactam or 500 mg ciprofloxacin and 500 mg metronidazole. We believe this a rational approach given (1) the lack of demonstrated benefit of the combination oral and intravenous antibiotics, (2) the lack of demonstrated benefit and potential deleterious effects of multiple doses of intravenous antibiotics, (3) the gastrointestinal side effects of the oral antibiotics, and (4) perceived problems of patient compliance with oral antibiotics.

MECHANICAL BOWEL PREPARATION

Since 1887, when Halsted described intestinal anastomosis, the idea of mechanically preparing the bowel has become accepted surgical practice. In the previously mentioned surveys, 100% of surgeons used some form of mechanical preparation. There are two oral preparations routinely used today, polyethylene glycol (PEG) and sodium phosphate (NaP).

PEG is an inert, osmotically active polymer that is mixed with an electrolyte solution, resulting in an isosomotic preparation that acts to lavage stool from the colon lumen. The electrolyte content combined with the osmotic activity of PEG prevents net absorption or excretion of water and electrolytes. Typically, 4 L of PEG is ingested over 2 to 3 hours. This produces good to excellent cleansing in most patients without causing significant fluid or electrolyte derangements. These issues are of particular importance in elderly patients or those with renal insufficiency or congestive heart failure. Nausea, vomiting, and patient compliance are obstacles to achieving adequate results in some patients. This has been addressed by the addition of flavor additives and a reduced volume preparation in which patients take four bisacodyl tablets and half the normal volume of PEG. Some surgeons also routinely prescribe metoclopramide to hasten gastric emptying or an antiemetic such as promethazine.

NaP is a hypersomolar oral saline laxative. Unlike PEG, smaller volumes of NaP can produce adequate bowel cleansing with better patient compliance. Patients are instructed to consume 45 ml of sodium phosphate diluted in clear liquids (15 ml NaP in 240 ml) in two doses separated by 10 hours. The timing of this should be such that the patient is not kept awake evacuating the entire night before the procedure. Sodium phosphate tablets are also available and are equally efficacious. Four tablets with 8 oz of clear liquid are taken every 15 minutes for a total of 28 tablets. In May 2006, the Federal Drug Administration issued a warning regarding oral NaP for bowel preparations in elderly patients, those with underlying kidney disease or dehydration, or those taking medication that affect renal perfusion (diuretics, angiotensin converting enzyme inhibitors, angiotensin receptor blockers, and nonsteroidal anti-inflammatory drugs). These patients are at increased risk for developing acute renal failure because of the relatively large phosphate load, fluid shifts, and decreased intravascular volume associated with NaP preparations. However, both the avoidance of this complication and improved efficacy can be achieved by appropriate patient selection and consumption of large volumes (2 to 3 L) of clear liquids as part of this preparation.

Even with its widespread use, the role of mechanical bowel prep in elective colon and rectal surgery has been called into question. With modern antibiotics and good surgical technique, does mechanical bowel preparation decrease the infectious complications of wound infection and intra-abdominal abscess, as well as the anastomotic leak rate? Six randomized controlled trials since 1992, including more than 1500 patients, have demonstrated no difference in infectious complications or leak rates between patients who were prepared or not prepared. A meta-analysis published by the Cochrane Library, updated in 2004, also showed no difference in these parameters. Despite this information, our current practice is a full mechanical preparation with PEG in most instances. Because the potential for change in practice patterns and surgical doctrine is enormous, we await the results of an appropriately powered randomized controlled trial to clarify the issue of mechanical preparation in elective colon surgery.

UNUSUAL CIRCUMSTANCES

Patients with partial large bowel obstruction provide a challenging scenario. Because they are unable to tolerate large volumes, PEG is not indicated. It has been our practice in patients with minimal retention of water-soluble contrast on postevacuation radiographs to attempt a "slow preparation." It is paramount that the patient be well hydrated and his or her electrolytes corrected before initiation of this preparation. In addition, vigilance and a low threshold to abort the preparation or operate is required. Fifteen milliliters of NaP is given, and the patient is monitored and examined before subsequent doses given at 4-hour intervals. After 12 hours, the dose may be increased to 30 ml if previous doses have been tolerated. Emesis or abdominal pain are indications to cease this preparation and consider operative intervention.

Before ileostomy or colostomy closure, patients often have large amounts of inspissated mucous in the defunctionalized segment. This can make passage of a circular stapler difficult and interfere with the anastomosis. Because this segment cannot be prepared orally, we irrigate with saline through a large urinary catheter placed via the anus and then suction any residual mucus under direct vision with a rigid proctoscope.

SUGGESTED READINGS

Bucher P, Gervaz P, Soravia C, and others: Randomized clinical trial of mechanical bowel preparation versus no preparation before elective left-sided colorectal surgery, *Br J Surg* 92:409, 2005.

Clarke JS, Condon RE, Bartlett JG: Preoperative oral antibiotics reduce septic complications of colon operations: results of prospective, randomized, double-blind clinical study, *Ann Surg* 186:251, 1977.

Geunaga K, Atallah AN, Castro AA, and others: Mechanical bowel preparation for elective colorectal surgery (Cochrane Review), *The Cochrane Library*, Issue 1, Oxford, 2006, Update Software.

Nichols RL, Choe EU, Wheldon CB: Mechanical and antibacterial bowel preparation in colon and rectal surgery, *Chemotherapy* 5(suppl 1):115, 2005.

Zmora O, Wexner SD, Hajjar L, and others: Trends in preparation for colorectal surgery: survey of the members of the American Society of Colon and Rectal Surgeons, *Am Surg* 69:150, 2003.

ACUTE APPENDICITIS

Genevieve B. Melton, MD, and Mark D. Duncan, MD

Inflammation of the appendix, including subsequent clinical sequelae of abscess and perforation, was first described in 1886 by Reginald Fitz. Today acute appendicitis is the most common surgical emergency of the abdomen, with more than 250,000 appendectomies performed annually in the United States. Although the diagnosis of appendicitis in a young man with acute abdominal pain localized to the right lower quadrant can be clear-cut, the clinical diagnosis may be less straightforward in women of childbearing age and at the extremes of age. In these patients, appendicitis can still be a challenging clinical entity to diagnose in a timely, accurate, and cost-effective manner. Important considerations for surgeons and areas of debate include investigative radiology tests such as computed tomography (CT) and ultrasonography and the use of laparoscopy as a diagnostic and therapeutic approach. As with other etiologies of the acute abdomen, early, accurate recognition of patients requiring urgent operative repair should be the overriding principle in the workup and treatment of patients with suspected appendicitis. Delayed diagnosis in the treatment of acute appendicitis is associated with higher rates of perforation, with resultant increased morbidity and mortality.

PRESENTATION OF ILLNESS

Appendicitis is most frequently a disease of young and healthy individuals. The location, timing, and character of pain and associated symptoms are key factors to elicit in understanding the presentation of disease. The classic presentation is an individual with cramping, intermittent abdominal pain, usually beginning in the periumbilical or epigastric region and that subsequently migrates to the right lower quadrant. As the course of appendicitis progresses, pain progresses from intermittent and cramping to constant and sharp in nature. If the appendix does not lie in an anterior or pelvic position, the diagnosis of appendicitis may be more difficult, leading to potential delay. In particular, a retrocecal appendix may not cause local signs of peritonitis. The timing of nausea can also help to distinguish appendicitis, in which nausea follows the pain, from gastroenteritis, in which nausea typically precedes pain. Most patients present with anorexia. A low-grade fever is often present in uncomplicated appendicitis. High fevers are atypical for simple appendicitis and may be a sign of perforation, appendiceal abscess, or another disease process. Other clinical entities to be considered in the differential diagnosis include urinary tract infection, renal calculi, gastroenteritis, gynecologic diagnoses such as ruptured ovarian cyst or pelvic inflammatory disease, cholecystitis, diverticulitis, or small bowel obstruction.

PATHOPHYSIOLOGY

The exact pathophysiology of acute appendicitis is not entirely clear, but the prevailing theory is that appendiceal luminal obstruction is the key mechanism. In children, lymphoid hyperplasia, often in the setting of infection or dehydration, is thought to be the most common etiology of obstruction. In the adult population, fecaliths, as well as rare scarring or tumor, are the main causes of obstruction leading to acute appendicitis. Obstruction causes distention of the lumen of the appendix, yielding increased intramural and intraluminal pressures. This leads to lymphatic and vascular compromise with ischemia and then necrosis of the appendix with associated bacterial overgrowth. In the first 24 hours, the great majority of patients have inflammation and possibly necrosis, with perforation uncommon. Approximately two thirds of patients with perforated appendicitis have had symptoms for more than 48 hours. Early in appendicitis, the most common bacteria are aerobic organisms. In contrast, late appendicitis is associated with mixed infections. Common organisms associated with late appendicitis are *Escherichia coli*, *Streptococcus* species, *Proteus*, *Bacteroides fragilis*, and *Pseudomonas* species.

DIAGNOSIS

History and Physical

Initial features in the history are typically nonspecific, including indigestion, change in bowel habits, and malaise. Following this, patients most typically experience visceral-type pain in the periumbilical or sometimes epigastric region that is characteristically intermittent, poorly localized, and often not terribly severe. Nausea and vomiting, which can occur, usually follow the onset of pain. Similarly, fever may be present and usually occurs following the onset of pain. The presence of high fever (>39.4°C) may be a sign of a perforated appendix. Early stages of appendicitis may not elicit tenderness on physical examination. Signs of localized inflammation or peritonitis occur as the disease progresses. Patients with an appendix in the anterior position typically have tenderness in the right lower quadrant near McBurney's point (two thirds of the distance from the umbilicus to the anterior superior iliac crest), often associated with peritoneal signs. In contrast, patients with a retrocecal appendix often have less

Table 1: Maneuvers on Physical Examination in Patients with Suspected Appendicitis

Maneuver	Description
Rovsing's sign	Palpation of the left lower quadrant eliciting pain in the right lower quadrant
Obturator sign	Pain with internal rotation of the hip (pelvic appendix)
Iliopsoas sign	Extension of the right hip eliciting pain in the right hip (retrocecal appendix)

impressive tenderness. Tenderness in patients with a pelvic appendix is often below McBurney's point. These patients often have symptoms of dysuria, urinary frequency, diarrhea, or tenesmus. Several classical maneuvers on physical examination to aid in the diagnosis of appendicitis have been described (Table 1).

Laboratory Examination

Laboratory tests are not a primary diagnostic modality in appendicitis, although they are helpful in ruling out other conditions and assessing metabolic derangements from dehydration and other electrolyte abnormalities. The white blood cell count in patients with simple appendicitis is typically mildly elevated, but it may be normal in 30% of cases. More than 95% of patients, however, have a left shift in their differential. Urinalysis is useful for ruling out a urinary tract infection or a stone in the urinary tract. Sterile pyuria or hematuria is observed in approximately a third of patients with appendicitis because of secondary inflammation onto the bladder and ureter. In sexually active or menstruating women, a urinary beta-human chorionic gonadotropin is mandatory to rule out pregnancy, including possible ectopic pregnancy. One may also obtain cervical cultures if pelvic inflammatory disease is suspected.

Imaging Studies

In general, a patient with a history and physical examination strongly suggestive of appendicitis should undergo prompt appendectomy without further imaging studies. In cases in which the presentation of appendicitis is not typical and the diagnosis is unclear, radiographic studies are key clinical tools. Abdominal x-rays in patients with appendicitis may demonstrate a fecalith, loss of the psoas shadow, deformity of the outline of the cecum, or a "sentinel loop" of small bowel in the right lower quadrant. However, plain films need not be routinely performed in patients with appendicitis because these findings are often subtle and not sensitive or specific for appendicitis. The two most widely used radiologic modalities for the diagnosis of appendicitis are ultrasonography and CT. The strengths and weaknesses of each modality were recently analyzed in a systematic review by Terasawa and colleagues. The authors demonstrated that CT had an overall sensitivity of 0.94 (confidence interval [CI]: 0.91–0.95) and specificity of 0.95 (CI: 0.93–0.96), whereas ultrasonography had an overall sensitivity of 0.86 (CI: 0.83–0.88) and a specificity of 0.81 (CI: 0.78–0.84) with a positive likelihood ratio 5.8 (CI: 3.5–9.5).

Findings strongly suggestive of acute appendicitis on standard abdominal CT scan include (1) a thick wall (>2 mm), often with "targeting" (concentric thickening of the inflamed appendix wall); (2) increased diameter of the appendix (>7 mm); (3) an appendicolith (seen in ~25%); (4) a phlegmon or abscess; or (5) free fluid. Stranding of the adjacent fatty tissues in the right lower quadrant is usually seen (Fig. 1). Air in the appendix or a contrast-filled appendiceal lumen without other abnormalities on CT virtually

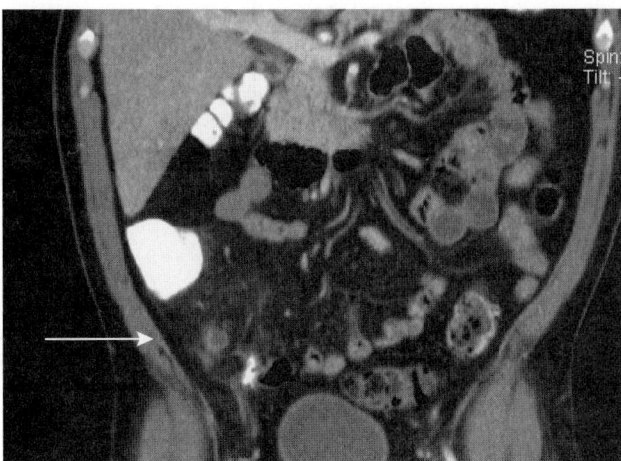

Figure 1 Computed tomography scan, coronal view, demonstrating acute appendicitis with increased diameter of the appendix and right lower quadrant stranding.

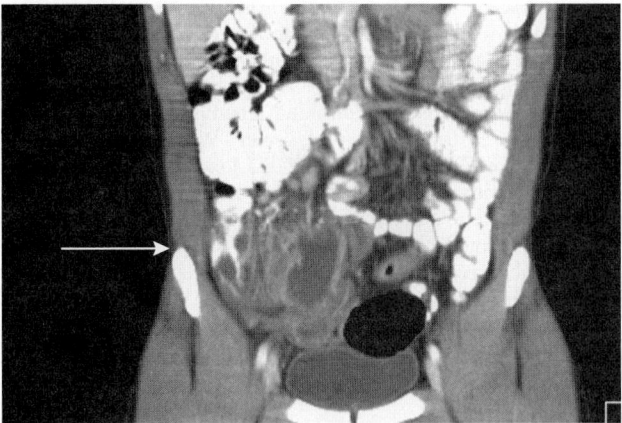

Figure 2 Computed tomography scan, coronal view, demonstrating periappendiceal abscess.

eliminate appendicitis as a diagnosis. However, appendicitis is not excluded if the appendix is not visualized on CT scan. If patients present early in their course, only minimal inflammatory changes may be seen. Computed tomography is also useful in diagnosing an appendiceal abscess (Fig. 2) and can guide percutaneous drainage of the abscess. Some have advocated the use of CT with rectal contrast alone and the use of thin cuts through the right iliac fossa, so-called appendiceal CT. In contrast to complete abdominal CT, which takes up to 2 hours with standard oral preparation to perform, appendiceal CT can be performed within 15 minutes. The main disadvantage of this technique is that it may not reveal pathology in other portions of the abdomen. Therefore workup of patients must continue if the study is negative. The choice of which study is superior remains an area of debate. Practically the type of CT performed can often depend on institutional preference and experience.

Ultrasonography can be particularly useful for examining pelvic pathology in women, especially with the technique of endovaginal ultrasound. Findings on ultrasonography suggestive of appendicitis include a thickened wall (>2 mm), increased appendiceal diameter (>6 mm), or free fluid. Whereas CT is performed with a low variability protocol and can often be interpreted by the surgeon, ultrasound is highly operator-dependent and may require a radiologist to interpret. Ultrasound can also be difficult to perform well in obese patients and in patients with a large amount of bowel gas overlying the appendix.

MANAGEMENT OF APPENDICITIS

General Management Issues

In all cases of suspected appendicitis, patients should have fluid and electrolyte balances corrected, and appropriate antibiotics should be administered. Andersen and colleagues recently examined antibiotic use for suspected appendicitis with a systematic review. The authors included 45 studies with 9576 patients and compared antibiotic treatment versus placebo in patients with suspected appendicitis (both uncomplicated and perforated) undergoing appendectomy. Use of antibiotics was found to be superior to placebo with respect to wound infection, intra-abdominal abscess, and length of stay with no apparent difference according to the method (open or laparoscopic) of appendectomy. If nonperforated appendicitis is suspected, surgery is indicated using either traditional open or a laparoscopic approach. Because of the acute nature of the condition, patients with acute appendicitis are frequently cared for by the on-call surgeon. The choice of procedure is dictated primarily by the experience of the treating surgeon, which may vary significantly even within an institution. Laparoscopic appendectomy is rapidly becoming the more common approach. Following surgery for nonperforated appendicitis, most patients are discharged within 24 to 48 hours. General requirements for discharge include being afebrile for 12 to 24 hours and tolerance of a diet. Patients are started on clear liquid following surgery and advanced as tolerated to an unrestricted diet. It is our practice to continue antibiotics for up to 24 hours after surgery in patients with nonperforated appendicitis; there is evidence only that perioperative antibiotics are beneficial, and no firm guidelines are available for exact antibiotic timing with current clinical evidence.

Perforation or rupture of the appendix may be suspected preoperatively or may not be confirmed until the time of surgery. In either case, prompt appendectomy is suitable. In most cases, appendectomy can be performed in standard laparoscopic or open fashion. Rarely, if necrosis is extensive and tissue quality is poor, an ileocecectomy may be required. Antibiotic coverage in patients following appendectomy for perforated appendicitis should involve 5 to 10 days of broad-spectrum antibiotics. Typical regimens include single therapy with piperacillin/tazobactam or triple therapy with ampicillin, gentamicin, and metronidazole. Patients may also have a postoperative ileus, and their diet should be advanced only as bowel function clinically returns. These patients are at risk for postoperative abscess, and a high clinical suspicion for abscess is warranted in those with fevers or ileus persisting beyond 3 to 5 days following appendectomy for perforated appendicitis.

In the case of periappendiceal abscess, the management algorithm is less straightforward and should be tailored to the individual patient. Treatment options include immediate appendectomy or percutaneous drainage, typically with interval appendectomy. Patients who have a well-delineated appendiceal abscess respond best to initial percutaneous drainage with CT guidance. The goal of percutaneous drainage is to allow inflammation to subside. This may alleviate the potential need for extended bowel resection and can help to stabilize an otherwise ill patient. These patients require an extended course of broad-spectrum antibiotics. In patients undergoing initial percutaneous drain placement, it is our practice to follow this in 6 to 8 weeks with an interval appendectomy, with the rationale that these patients are at risk for recurrent inflammation. Recent studies have challenged this notion, citing low rates of subsequent appendectomy in patients followed nonoperatively after CT-guided drainage of appendiceal abscess. Further evaluation of this strategy is required before it can be clearly advocated. Older patients should be considered for a colonoscopy or barium enema after resolution of the acute abscess to rule out colonic pathology (e.g., diverticular disease or malignancy) as the etiology for periappendiceal abscess before surgical intervention, or particularly if no surgery is planned.

Laparoscopic Versus Open Approach

Surgical options include both open and laparoscopic approaches. Although laparoscopic appendectomy may require longer operative time and greater hospital costs, it has also been associated with less postoperative pain and possibly shorter lengths of hospital stay. Laparoscopic surgery may be especially helpful in the treatment of patients with a less certain diagnosis. A systematic Cochrane review recently examined the diagnostic and therapeutic differences between the two approaches. The review included 54 studies, of which 45 compared laparoscopic appendectomy to open appendectomy in adults. Most consistently, laparoscopic appendectomy was associated with a decreased wound infection rate (approximately half the risk) and increased intra-abdominal abscess rate (approximately twice the risk). The review also suggest the following: reduction in hospital stay by 1.1 days in patients with laparoscopic approach, return to normal activity and work 6 and 3 days earlier with laparoscopic appendectomy, longer duration of surgery by 12 minutes with laparoscopy, decreased pain by an average of 9 points of 100 on a visual analogue scale, and increased hospital costs with laparoscopic appendectomy. The benefit of diagnostic laparoscopy was most evident in fertile women, in whom the rate of negative appendectomy with no final diagnosis was decreased. From these reports, most advocate laparoscopy if the clinician's index of suspicion is moderate to high, but several other items remain in the differential diagnosis. In particular, women may benefit from a laparoscopic approach, which may reveal other pelvic pathology, because they are more likely to have a negative appendectomy. The laparoscopic approach can also be helpful in obese patients in whom exposure with the standard open approach may require a larger incision.

Open Surgical Approach

The traditional open surgical approach involves an incision approximately 4 cm long centered over McBurney's point, lateral to the rectus sheath. It cannot be overemphasized that by staying lateral to the rectus sheath, anatomic clarity is easily achieved. This incision can be oblique along skin folds or transverse, which is more easily extended for increased exposure. The dissection is carried through the subcutaneous tissues to the external oblique fascia, which is then sharply incised. The muscle-splitting technique is then used to bluntly separate the external oblique fibers, followed by the internal oblique and transversus abdominis muscle fibers. The peritoneum is carefully entered. This layer-by-layer anatomic exercise is one of the joys of general surgery. On entry to the peritoneal cavity, turbid or murky fluid may be encountered; we do not advocate culture of peritoneal fluid because the results so rarely affect clinical management. To locate the appendix, a finger is swept lateral to medial in the right paracolic gutter. If the appendix is not found with this maneuver, the teniae coli can be followed to the base of the cecum, where the appendix originates. After it is located, adhesions can be freed from the appendix (and any surrounding structures), and it can be delivered through the incision with care to avoid tearing and possible spilling enteric contents. The mesoappendix is divided between Rienhoff clamps and tied off using 3–0 suture. The appendix is then ligated at its base with 2–0 absorbable suture, clamped distal to this, and sharply excised. The appendiceal stump is cauterized to prevent mucocele formation. If the appendiceal stump appears weak or necrotic, a purse-string suture or Z-stitch may be placed in the cecum to invert the base into the cecum. The surgical bed should be thoroughly irrigated with saline.

Closure of the incision is performed in layers with 3–0 and 2–0 absorbable suture on the peritoneum and internal oblique fascia. Irrigation is performed between each layer. The external oblique fascia is closed with a running 0 or 1 monofilament absorbable suture and may be infused with local anesthetic to improve analgesia. The skin is closed with 4–0 absorbable suture or surgical staples. Primary closure is the general rule for nonperforated appendicitis because wound infection is less likely. In the case of perforated appendicitis, skin closure options include primary closure as described earlier, loose partial closure, delayed primary closure, or secondary closure. If there is heavy fecal contamination, secondary closure is our general practice; loose partial closure with gauze packing between sutures is suitable for most other cases of perforated appendicitis.

Laparoscopic Surgical Approach

The laparoscopic approach for appendectomy can be performed using a variety of techniques. Decompression of the stomach and bladder is performed using a nasogastric or orogastric tube and a Foley catheter. Port placement is somewhat discretionary, with the general principle being triangulation to allow adequate visualization and exposure. We use the Hassan technique to directly place an umbilical 10-mm port for the camera. Two other ports are then placed under direct visualization: a single 12-mm port placed in the left abdomen inferior to the umbilical port and a single 5-mm port placed in the suprapubic region along the midline. After the appendix is identified, it is grasped at its tip and retracted anteriorly. This maneuver exposes the mesoappendix, which can then be divided using ligaclips, endostapler with vascular cartridge, LigaSure (Valleylab, Boulder, CO), or harmonic scalpel. The appendix is further cleared of any adhesions, and attention is then focused on division of the appendix from the cecum. We routinely have used the laparoscopic GIA stapler for the division of the appendix. Care must be taken to fire the device across healthy, unaffected tissue, which may include a portion of the cecum. The divided appendix is delivered through the 12-mm port site using an EndoCatch bag (US Surgical, Norwalk, CT) to avoid wound contamination. Irrigation is routinely employed. If there is an obvious abscess cavity, the abscess should be evacuated thoroughly and a drain placed. This is uncommon because even ruptured appendicitis rarely requires a drain.

Negative Appendectomy

In a number of series, up to 20% of patients with suspected appendicitis are found intraoperatively to have a normal appendix. If a normal appendix is encountered intraoperatively, it is important to address other possible etiologies and to remove the normal appendix to avoid possible confusion about future abdominal pain. Removal of the appendix is especially important if the procedure is performed using a standard open right lower quadrant incision. Other causes to look for explicitly in the operating room include terminal ileitis, Meckel's diverticulitis, mesenteric adenitis, cholecystitis, colonic diverticulitis, and pathology of the uterus, ovary, or fallopian tube. There may be rare patients with a low suspicion for acute appendicitis for whom it is important to rule it out definitively, in which case diagnostic laparoscopy without planned appendectomy if the appendix is normal may be an appropriate choice.

SPECIAL CONSIDERATIONS

Children

Age is one of the predominant factors in the consideration of acute appendicitis. Children with acute appendicitis often have associated diarrhea and may not have symptoms of anorexia. Despite reluctance on the part of some practitioners to expose children to radiation, CT has been demonstrated to be highly accurate in the diagnosis of appendicitis and can be helpful in those with an atypical presentation. In neonates and infants, the differential diagnoses include midgut volvulus, pyloric stenosis, Meckel's diverticulitis, and intussusception.

Elderly

Although diverticulitis and colonic neoplasms are more common in the elderly and can present similarly to appendicitis, appendicitis in the elderly is not uncommon; the estimated incidence in patients older than 65 years of age is approximately 1 in 2000. Elderly patients often may not be able to give a detailed history, and the acute abdomen may present with few or minimal subtle signs. CT is particularly helpful in this setting. Again, if a normal appendix is found intraoperatively, other causes of symptoms, including perforated colon cancer or diverticulitis of the cecum or sigmoid colon, should be sought.

Pregnancy

The most common general surgery emergency in pregnancy is acute appendicitis. The incidence of acute appendicitis is estimated at 0.1% of all deliveries, and it occurs with equal frequency during all three trimesters. The pregnant patient with suspected appendicitis can be difficult to diagnose. As the uterus enlarges, the appendix is pushed more cephalad, making the location of tenderness typically in the right upper quadrant or right flank. Ultrasound may be helpful in making the diagnosis and is preferred in early pregnancy to avoid the possible teratogenic effects of ionizing radiation. Late in pregnancy, when the effects of ionizing radiation are fewer, CT can be particularly helpful. The diagnosis and treatment of appendicitis in a timely manner is especially important in pregnancy because of the potential devastating effects on the fetus. Whereas nonperforated appendicitis carries a fetal mortality rate of less than 5%, perforated appendicitis is associated with a fetal mortality rate of more than 20%. Although appendicitis occurs equally during all trimesters of pregnancy, perforated appendicitis occurs most frequently in the third trimester, when clinical presentation and diagnosis can be particular challenging, again underscoring the importance of early recognition and management.

Immunocompromised Patients

Immunocompromised states include organ transplantation, immunosuppressive therapy for autoimmune or neoplastic pathology, and AIDS. These patients may show only mild tenderness on examination and have other items that should be considered in their differential diagnosis, including mycobacterial infection, cytomegalovirus, and fungal infections. In addition, enterocolitis is an important cause of abdominal pain and fever in patients with neutropenia, which can occur secondary to chemotherapy. CT is an important tool for the diagnostic workup of these patients, which can be particularly challenging. Although it is important to be clinically cautious in immunocompromised patients, it is also essential not to delay operative treatment in patients in whom there is a strong suspicion of appendicitis.

SUGGESTED READINGS

Andersen BR, Kallehave FL, Andersen HK: Antibiotics versus placebo for prevention of postoperative infection after appendectomy, *Cochrane Database of Systematic Review*, Oct 18(4):CD001546, 2004.

Fitz RH: Perforating inflammation of the vermiform appendix with special reference to its early diagnosis and treatment, *Am J Med Sci* 92:321, 1886.

Flum DR, Koepsell T: The clinical and economic correlates of misdiagnosed appendicitis: nationwide analysis, *Arch Surg* 137:799, 2002.

Paulson EK, Kalady MF, Pappas TN: Suspected appendicitis, *N Engl J Med* 348:236, 2003.

Sauerland S, Lefering R, Neugebauer EA: Laparoscopic versus open surgery for suspected appendicitis, *Cochrane Database of Systematic Review*, Oct 18(4):CD001546, 2004.

Terasawa T, Blackmore CC, Bent S: Systemic review: computed tomography and ultrasonography to detect acute appendicitis in adults and adolescents, *Ann Intern Med* 141(7):537, 2004.

HEMORRHOIDS

Sharon G. Gregorcyk, MD, and Philip J. Huber, Jr., MD

Hemorrhoids are a common problem and are one of the oldest ailments known to mankind. Although the majority of patients with anal complaints blame their problems on hemorrhoids, only approximately a third of these symptoms actually result from hemorrhoids. Other conditions causing anal complaints include pruritus ani, anal fissure, fistula-in-ano, abscess, and condyloma acuminata. Often a patient has hemorrhoids that are actually asymptomatic, but they have one of these other conditions causing symptoms that they erroneously attribute to their hemorrhoids. Surgeons who treat hemorrhoids should be familiar with these other conditions so that they can properly treat the patient.

ETIOLOGY AND CLASSIFICATION

Hemorrhoids are related to fibrovascular cushions that are a normal part of the anal canal anatomy. These cushions are thought to contribute to fecal continence by engorging and closing off the anal canal when one coughs, sneezes, or strains as with lifting. Typically there are three fibrovascular cushions, and they are located in the left lateral, right posterior, and right anterior anal canal (Fig. 1). Accessory hemorrhoidal complexes can often be found to vary the presentation.

Hemorrhoids occur when these normal fibrovascular cushions remain engorged or enlarged. It is believed that this enlargement results from chronic straining such as with constipation, diarrhea, or prolonged attempts at defecation. Over time with straining, the fibrovascular cushions lose their attachment to the underlying anorectal wall. This can then lead to bulging or prolapse of the tissue. With internal hemorrhoids, the overlying mucosa can become thin and friable, leading to bleeding from the underlying arteriovenous plexus.

Classically hemorrhoids are categorized as internal hemorrhoids, which are located above the dentate line, and external hemorrhoids, which are located below the dentate line. A combination of internal and external hemorrhoids also exists (Fig. 1). Internal hemorrhoids are further classified into four categories:

Grade I—bleeding without prolapse
Grade II—prolapse that spontaneously reduces
Grade III—prolapse that has to be manually reduced
Grade IV—irreducible, incarcerated prolapse

The classification of internal hemorrhoids is thus determined by the history and not necessarily by the physical exam.

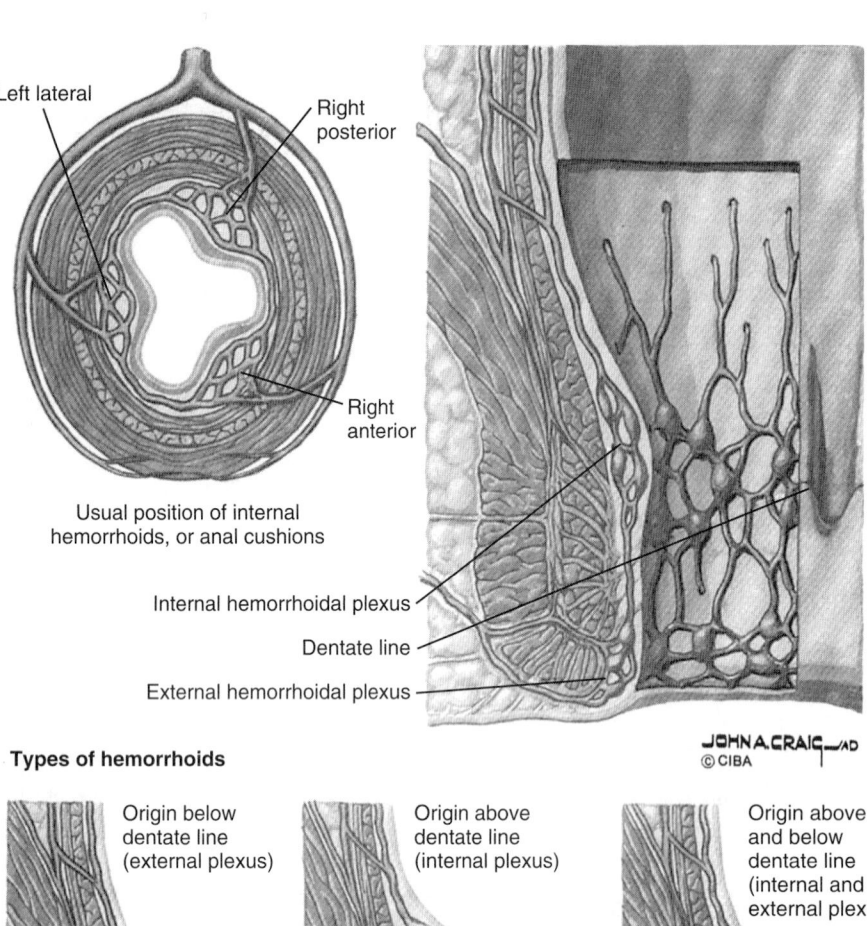

JOHN A. CRAIG—AD
©CIBA

Figure 1 Positions and types of hemorrhoids.

Left lateral

Right posterior

Right anterior

Usual position of internal hemorrhoids, or anal cushions

Internal hemorrhoidal plexus

Dentate line

External hemorrhoidal plexus

Types of hemorrhoids

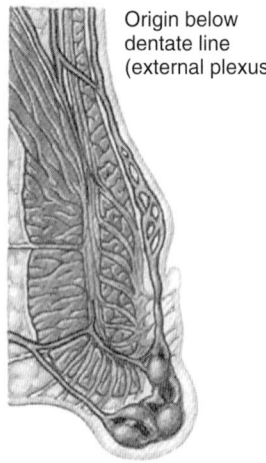

Origin below dentate line (external plexus)

External hemorrhoid

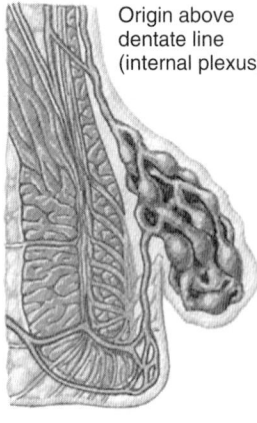

Origin above dentate line (internal plexus)

Internal hemorrhoid

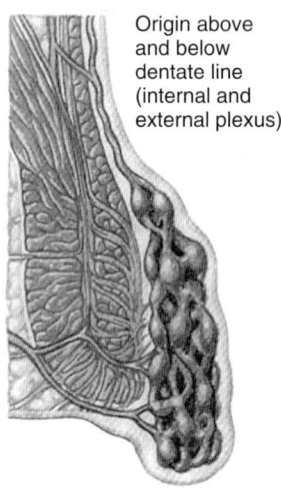

Origin above and below dentate line (internal and external plexus)

Mixed hemorrhoid

SYMPTOMS

Symptoms caused by hemorrhoids include bleeding, prolapse, swelling, and, rarely, pain. The bleeding that occurs with hemorrhoids is bright red because it is arterial in nature. It may be seen when the patient wipes after a bowel movement or may actually drip into the toilet bowl. Some patients will report bleeding without a bowel movement, but this is much less common. One must be cautious about attributing all anorectal bleeding to internal hemorrhoids. Proximal pathology such as proctitis or a tumor may be the source of the bleeding, and in most cases endoscopy is indicated to rule out a more proximal source. If the bleeding is atypical for hemorrhoids—for example, it is mixed in with stool or is not bright red, endoscopy is mandatory. Even young patients can have alternative pathology. Tragically the diagnosis of some rectal cancers has been significantly delayed in both young and old

patients because of a physician's finding hemorrhoids on examination and erroneously attributing the patient's symptoms to them.

Pain in the anal region is routinely blamed on hemorrhoids, although it is rarely the cause. Pain fibers are not present proximal to the dentate line, so simple internal hemorrhoids do not hurt. With fourth-degree internal hemorrhoids, the inability to reduce the hemorrhoids is uncomfortable. Subsequent swelling, irritation from mucous, and inflammation of the surrounding external tissue in these cases can be painful. If strangulation ensues, the patient will have extreme pain, bleeding, and possibly even signs of systemic illness.

External hemorrhoids may present simply as redundant skin in the anal region. Some patients complain of swelling of this external tissue, especially at the end of the day. This swelling can cause some discomfort but is not usually described as pain. Significant pain can occur with external hemorrhoids when they become acutely thrombosed.

TREATMENT OF HEMORRHOIDS

There are a wide variety of treatments for hemorrhoids. Choosing the appropriate therapy must take many factors into account: type of symptoms, severity and quality of those symptoms, duration of symptoms, and the patient's preference. Completely asymptomatic hemorrhoids require no treatment other than educating the patient to prevent future problems.

Thrombosed external hemorrhoids are unique in their management and are addressed separately here. The pain associated with thrombosed external hemorrhoids is at its height in the first 48 to 72 hours. If a patient presents during this time period with severe pain that is not improving, excision of the external hemorrhoid is recommended to speed relief of symptoms. This typically can be performed in the office setting with local anesthetic but may sometimes require the operating room. Thrombectomy alone is not recommended because of the risk of rethrombosis. If the patient presents with pain that is already improving, no surgical intervention is recommended because the thrombosis is resolving on its own and a surgical wound could cause as much or more trouble. However, if the patient continues to experience recurring thrombosed external hemorrhoids at the same location, elective excision is indicated.

Treatment options in general for hemorrhoids can be classified into three categories: medical therapy, office procedures, and operative therapy. With hemorrhoids that are simple and not significantly symptomatic, medical therapy and office-based procedures are typically chosen as the treatment options. More symptomatic hemorrhoids, including grades III and IV internal hemorrhoids, are routinely better treated with operative therapy.

Medical Therapy

The aim of medical therapy is to correct the cause of that individual's hemorrhoids. Thus efforts are placed at avoiding straining from constipation, diarrhea, or prolonged efforts at defecation. This requires primarily dietary and lifestyle modifications. Decreasing straining with stools by increasing fiber consumption and water intake is the main medical treatment for symptomatic hemorrhoids. A fiber supplement such as psyllium is useful to accomplish this goal. Fiber therapy may also help those patients with diarrhea by adding bulk to the stool, resulting in more formed stools with a decrease in frequency.

Topical steroids and other over-the-counter ointments and creams have no proven efficacy in treating hemorrhoids, although they may give the patient temporary comfort. Micronized, purified flavonoids derived from citrus fruit have been shown in studies to relieve bleeding from grades I and II hemorrhoids, but the long-term benefits are not known. We do not routinely recommend the use of flavonoids and instead instruct our patients on fiber, increased water intake, and cessation of the habit of reading on the toilet. These recommendations alone are effective in managing most grade I and some grade II symptomatic hemorrhoids.

Office Procedures

A number of office-based procedures are available to control hemorrhoid symptoms. Office-based practices typically define minimal maneuvers that are relatively less painful than an operation and do not require anesthetic for patient tolerance. Office procedures include rubber-band ligation, sclerotherapy, infrared coagulation, bipolar coagulation, and direct current electrotherapy, all of which are performed through a fenestrated anoscope. All of these techniques attempt to decrease the vascularity of the internal hemorrhoid and increase its fixation to the anorectal wall. Thus they are aimed at treating the symptoms of bleeding and prolapse. Patients best suited for office-based procedures are those with grades I or II hemorrhoids and select grade III hemorrhoids.

Rubber-Band Ligation

Rubber-band ligation is by far the most frequently practiced technique in office-based procedures and is frequently performed in the operating room as well. It is the most effective of the office procedures. The technique uses an instrument that delivers one or two circular rubber rings around an internal hemorrhoid at the base to constrict the blood supply and create a zone of necrosis and reactive ulceration (Fig. 2). The tissue subsequently sloughs, and the base fixes to the sphincter. Placement of the bands is critical so as not to incorporate the dentate line in the target. Crimping or pulling the dentate line can result in significant pain. Multiple devices are marketed for band ligation, and instruments that use suction within the bander device to pull the column into the drum permit "one-handed" delivery, which is advantageous.

Rubber-band ligation is not painless, and patients can be fairly uncomfortable even when placement appears perfect. A single hemorrhoid or multiple hemorrhoids may be treated per session. Discomfort increases with the number of hemorrhoids treated in a session, and most surgeons do not advocate banding three columns in one setting. If only one hemorrhoid is banded at the first encounter, it can give the patient an introduction to the treatment. At a repeat visit, more columns can be treated at one time because the patient is experienced. Band retention usually lasts for 2 to 10 days. The rubber promotes the inflammatory response that leads to tissue fixation at the ulcer. Repeat banding is best performed after a 4-week interval to allow the inflammatory response to subside.

Pertinent to rubber-band ligation is a satisfactory target. Although this technique is touted for any and all sizes of hemorrhoids, it is not easy or even a good idea if the column is too small or too snug on the sphincter. Similarly, the hemorrhoid can be too large to fit into the device.

Rubber-band ligation is performed without anesthetic, and it is usually well tolerated. The patient can feel the "lump" that accrues with band application, and there is typically a dull ache or sensation of the need to have a bowel movement. Nonsteroid anti-inflammatory drug therapy is usually sufficient for pain control. Discomfort can last for days but is generally 24 to 48 hours. Severe pain is unusual and worrisome. Pelvic sepsis syndrome has been reported and can be fatal. The exact pathophysiology of this syndrome is not known. The triad of symptoms for this sepsis syndrome is severe pain, urinary retention, and fever. Patients developing any of these symptoms after band ligation must be evaluated for pelvic sepsis syndrome and should be warned at the time of ligation. Fortunately, this is a rare complication.

Other complications of rubber-band ligation include local abscess and bleeding. In a Veteran's Administration study of more than 250 band applications, there were two abscesses and two bleeding events. Both bleeding events occurred in patients on warfarin; the risk of bleeding with warfarin is well recognized—and a relative contraindication to band ligation. Other series confirm complication rates between 0.5% and 8.0%. Minor complications of band slippage, external hemorrhoid thrombosis, and minor bleeding from the ulcer occur in less than 5% of patients. Patients who are immunocompromised are at increased risk with band ligation. It is probably best to select another method of office-based procedure to control symptomatic hemorrhoids in this population.

Rubber-band ligation is a durable procedure. Control of symptoms is typically good. Recurrent symptoms can occur over time, but years of successful control of symptoms is likely. Less than 10% of patients have persistent symptoms that require surgery.

Sclerotherapy

Sclerotherapy for internal hemorrhoids has been a reliable, if less durable, form of hemorrhoidal control dating back to the 1860s. This method is usually reserved for patients with small internal hemorrhoids or those who cannot tolerate other methods.

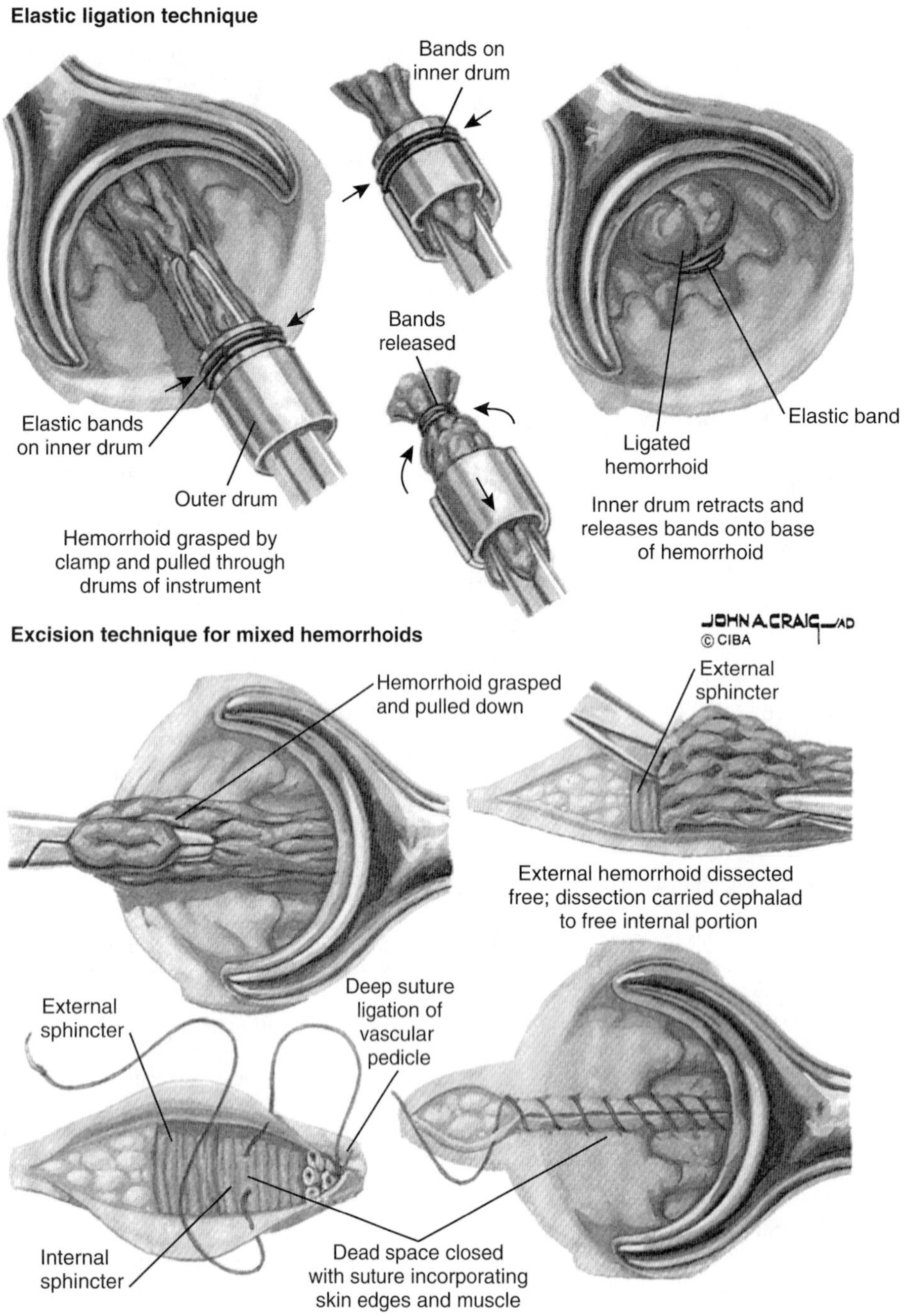

Elastic ligation technique

Figure 2 Elastic ligation and excision.

Bands on
inner drum

Elastic bands
on inner drum

Outer drum

Hemorrhoid grasped by
clamp and pulled through
drums of instrument

Bands
released

Elastic band

Ligated
hemorrhoid

Inner drum retracts and
releases bands onto base
of hemorrhoid

Excision technique for mixed hemorrhoids

JOHN A. CRAIG AD
© CIBA

Hemorrhoid grasped
and pulled down

External
sphincter

External hemorrhoid dissected
free; dissection carried cephalad
to free internal portion

External
sphincter

Deep suture
ligation of
vascular
pedicle

Internal
sphincter

Dead space closed
with suture incorporating
skin edges and muscle

There are two types of sclerotherapy techniques, each incorporating its own sclerosing solution. Oil-based (usually cottonseed) injections are performed with an 18-gauge spinal needle targeted into the submucosa at the cephalad portion of the hemorrhoid complex (Fig. 3). One to two milliliters is ample to sclerose a hemorrhoid. Larger amounts may result in pain. The second technique involves use of an aqueous solution formerly called Sotradecol, now Ethamolin (QOL Medical, Kirkland, WA), which is also used in esophageal and cutaneous varices. This solution is injected through a 25-gauge spinal needle directly into the internal hemorrhoid column through a single site but moving the needle carefully to spread 2 ml of solution. When the needle is removed, a cotton pledget is left over the site, and the anoscope is withdrawn, leaving pressure at the site for 30 seconds. Both of the techniques shrink the hemorrhoid effectively. One or two columns can be treated at a single visit. The procedure is usually well tolerated. Patients may

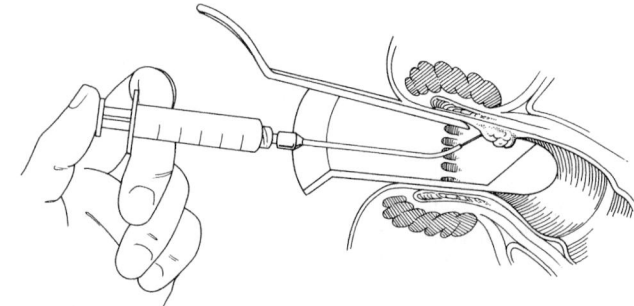

Figure 3 Sclerotherapy.

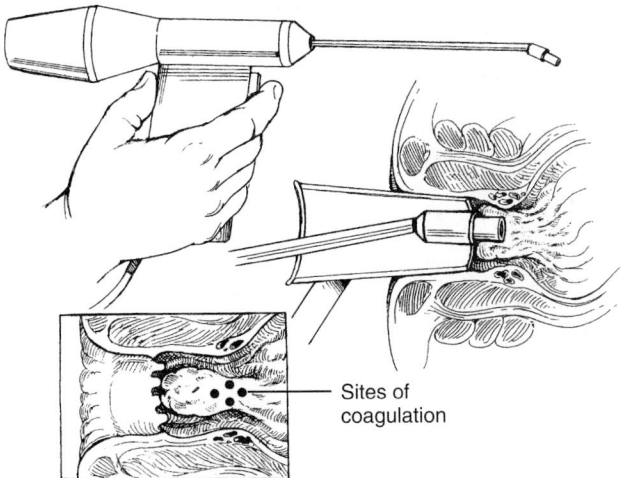

Figure 4 Infrared photocoagulation.

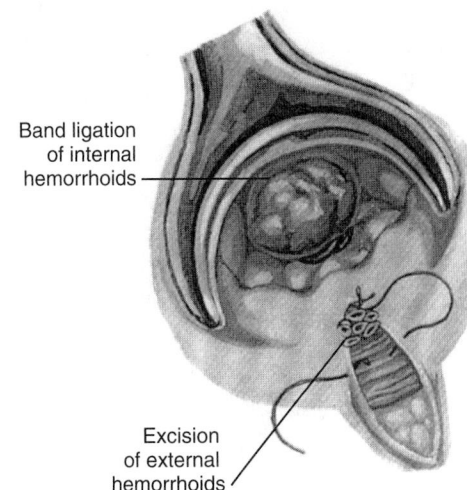

Figure 5 Combination of procedures.

experience a "burning" sensation. Solution should be kept in the submucosa and not injected into the sphincter. Sepsis is a possible sequela, and urinary retention has been reported. Control of hemorrhoid symptoms is typically good, but this is the least durable technique over time.

Infrared Coagulation, Bipolar Coagulation, and Direct Current Electrotherapy

Energy in various forms can be applied to the internal hemorrhoids to coagulate the tissue, resulting in eventual tissue sloughing and ulceration. This increases fixation to the anal musculature. Infrared coagulation, bipolar coagulation, and direct current therapy are all variations that work. Through a slotted anoscope, the energy is applied at the apex of the internal hemorrhoids at the top of the anal canal.

Infrared coagulation is the most popular of these three techniques and uses infrared radiation from a tungsten-halogen lamp. The energy is delivered by a probe that is placed in direct contact with the tissue at the apex of the hemorrhoids. Each hemorrhoid is coagulated at three to four sites, with the energy being delivered at a recommended 1.5-second pulse (Fig. 4). Multiple hemorrhoids can be treated at one visit. Studies show that infrared coagulation is less painful than rubber-band ligation, but significantly more sessions are required for effective treatment. Although infrared coagulation is not effective in treating substantial prolapsing tissue, it has a 67% to 96% success rate in treating bleeding from grades I and II hemorrhoids.

Bipolar coagulation is applied with a probe to the apex of the hemorrhoids in 1-second pulses of 20 watts. It usually takes less than 30 seconds to achieve the desired coagulation of the underlying tissue, compared with applications of up to 14 minutes using direct current electrotherapy. This time difference is responsible for the lack of popularity of the use of direct current. Both techniques have good success rates in controlling bleeding, but neither is useful for significant prolapse. The complication rate of these techniques is approximately 10% and includes complications such as bleeding and pain.

Operative Therapy

Surgical hemorrhoidectomy with excision of internal and external hemorrhoids is the most effective treatment for hemorrhoids, but it is also the most painful and has the highest complication rate. For some patients, it is the absolute best option. Other patients do not require extensive surgery, and their operative therapy can be tailored to be less invasive and, in turn, less painful. Suture ligation, excision,

and even stapled hemorrhoidopexy may be performed alone or in various combinations (Fig. 5). The key is to tailor the patient's surgery to his or her individual pathology, symptoms, and needs.

Although some patients acquiesce to surgery only after they have failed less invasive treatment, others have hemorrhoidal disease so severe that initial operative intervention is warranted. These patients also tend to respond better to surgery than patients with lesser symptoms, tolerating the pain better. Patients with grade IV hemorrhoids obviously fit into this category. Also patients with large grade III or large, swollen external hemorrhoids may select for operative therapy. Another indication for surgery may simply be patient preference. Some patients shun the nonoperative approaches because of the time involved with return appointments and treatments or the presumed nuisance.

Most of the procedures can be performed under a local anesthetic with sedation. Other anesthesia options include spinal and general anesthesia. Preoperative antibiotics are not necessary except for those comorbid conditions that require prophylaxis. We prefer the prone jackknife position with or without a Wilson frame. The buttocks are taped apart for exposure. Regardless of anesthesia used, a local anesthetic is infiltrated both for pain control and for assistance with hemostasis. For the stapled hemorrhoidopexy, the application of local anesthetic is described separately. For all excisional techniques, the authors use a 1:1 mixture of 1% lidocaine with epinephrine and 0.25% bupivicaine with epinephrine. If the patient has a spinal or general anesthetic, the lidocaine is omitted. It is our preference to first inject proximally within the anal canal, infiltrating submucosally, as well as into the intersphincteric space. A perianal block is then completed by injecting in four quadrants around the anus—bilateral, anterior, and posterior—infiltrating both deep and superficially. A total of approximately 30 ml of local anesthetic is used for the procedure.

During an emergent hemorrhoidectomy for incarcerated, gangrenous hemorrhoids, the injection of local anesthetic with epinephrine into the edematous tissue is of great benefit in reducing the edema. The anesthetic is massaged into the tissue, and often the hemorrhoids can then be reduced (Fig. 6). This reduction in the amount of edema allows for better definition of the hemorrhoids so that normal skin is spared in excising the hemorrhoidal tissue.

With the vascular nature of hemorrhoids, coagulopathic patients are at much greater risk, and anticoagulants such as warfarin should be stopped. Preferably the patient should be off aspirin as well. Caution is also advised in the severely immunocompromised patient. A nonhealing, infected anal wound would in most cases be worse than any hemorrhoid symptoms. Because this is a well-vascularized area, healing is not routinely a problem.

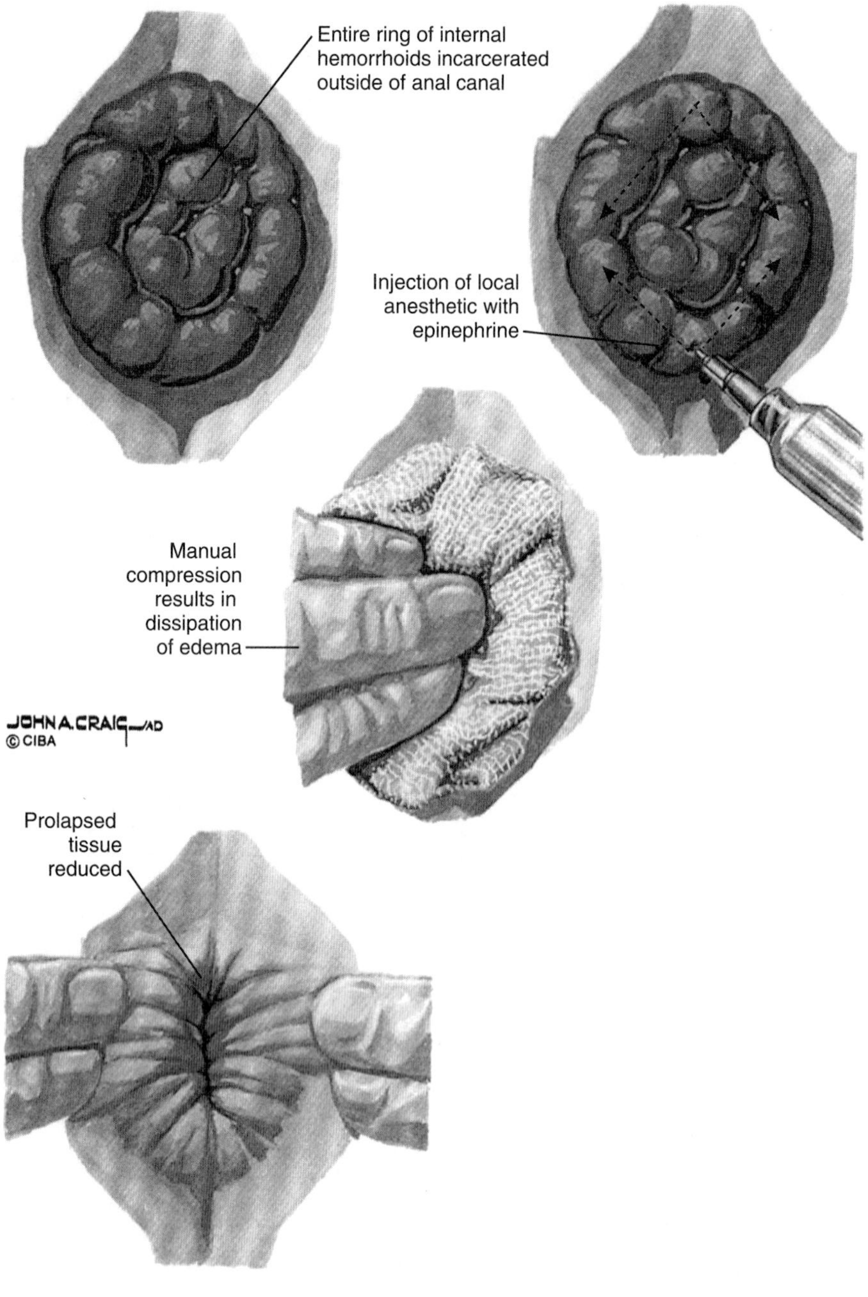

Entire ring of internal
hemorrhoids incarcerated
outside of anal canal

Figure 6 Reduction of
incarcerated hemorrhoids.

Injection of local
anesthetic with
epinephrine

Manual
compression
results in
dissipation
of edema

JOHN A. CRAIG—AD
©CIBA

Prolapsed
tissue
reduced

Surgical Hemorrhoidectomy

The most common excisional hemorrhoidectomy technique in the United States is known as the Ferguson hemorrhoidectomy, named after the Ferguson Clinic in Grand Rapids, Michigan, where it was in frequent use. It is also commonly referred to as the closed hemorrhoidectomy. After the local anesthetic has been infiltrated, a medium Hill-Ferguson retractor is inserted to expose the anal canal. The hemorrhoid complex is grasped with a hemostat for retraction, and a 3–0 Vicryl suture is placed in a figure-eight fashion just proximal to the apex of the internal hemorrhoid and tied to ligate the vascular pedicle. This suture is left in place to be used in closing the wound after excision. A 15-blade scalpel is used to make an elliptical incision around the internal and external hemorrhoidal complex, with the incision tapering in at the anoderm to limit the amount of anoderm excised and prevent long-term anal stenosis. The hemorrhoidal tissue is then dissected off of the underlying sphincter

muscles with scissors or scalpel (Fig. 2). Electrocautery may also be used but may not provide good visualization of the plane between the hemorrhoidal tissue and the sphincter muscle. The correct plane is essential to avoid injury to the sphincter. The hemorrhoid is then amputated distal to the suture ligation, and the wound is closed with a running stitch extending out to the anoderm. Small bites are taken in the underlying muscle to tack the mucosa down and to prevent a space for fluid to collect. The mucosa is mobile, and great care must be taken to avoid pulling it out to the anal verge and creating an ectropion. One to three hemorrhoids may be excised in this manner. Energy sources such as laser, LigaSure (Valleylab, Boulder, CO), and Harmonic scalpel (Johnson & Johnson Gateway, Piscataway, NJ) have been used, with none having a clear advantage over another or over sharp excision.

The Milligan-Morgan hemorrhoidectomy, also known as the open hemorrhoidectomy, is performed similarly to the Ferguson technique with regard to excision. The mucosal defect is then closed, but the anoderm is left open. This wound heals secondarily over 4 to 8 weeks. The closed and open techniques have been compared with one another with no significant difference being found in pain or complications. Both techniques carry the risk of bleeding (2%–4%), urinary retention (2%–32%), infection (0.5%–5.5%), stenosis (0%–6%), and incontinence (2%–12%). The complication rates are less with surgeons experienced in anal surgery.

Regardless of the technique used, postoperative pain remains a problem. Although some advocate routine internal sphincterotomy to assist with pain control, randomized studies do not support its effectiveness and actually show an increase in incontinence rates. Therefore sphincterotomy should only be performed if indicated by the presence of an anal fissure. We routinely use narcotics and scheduled ketorolac when possible for postoperative pain control. Scheduled diazepam as a muscle relaxant can be selectively added. Avoidance of constipation postoperatively is important, and stool softeners and mild laxatives are recommended as needed. Caution against diarrhea must also be exercised.

Amputative Hemorrhoidectomy

Amputative hemorrhoidectomy is an excisional technique that deserves special mention. Walter Whitehead is credited with the initial description of an "amputative" hemorrhoidectomy technique, which addressed complete excision of internal hemorrhoids and subcutaneous excision of external hemorrhoids with anal skin advancement flaps into the anal canal to reestablish the mucocutaneous junction (dentate line). This procedure, which requires a thorough knowledge of the anatomy of the anal canal and skilled surgical technique, is satisfactory for removal of complex hemorrhoids. It preserves the anoderm, which is then used to cover the sphincter, combining a functional outcome with good cosmetic results. Regrettably, subsequent attempts to duplicate this procedure were incorrectly performed with pull-out of mucosa to the anal verge (ectropion), circumferential scar stricture, and a resulting wet stenotic outlet, ironically termed "Whitehead deformity."

Correct application of the Whitehead technique can propose a successful outcome for a patient with the worst kind of presentation, that is, fourth-degree hemorrhoids, incarcerated circumstances, or severe prolapsing internal hemorrhoids with circumferential swollen external hemorrhoids. Stricture is a definite risk, but is not often encountered in experienced hands—less than 3% in our personal series. The cosmetic result is typically excellent with a smooth anal outlet and no tags. Because of the complications from inappropriate technique, the Whitehead hemorrhoidectomy is performed by few surgeons in the United States.

Stapled Hemorrhoidopexy

The circular stapled hemorrhoidopexy has been the most recent addition to hemorrhoid surgical management. Dr. Antonio Longo from Italy described the first large experience with division of the hemorrhoid blood supply with simultaneous excision of redundant anorectal mucosa and fixing of the tissue into the upper anal canal to correct prolapse of the hemorrhoid complexes. Credited with causing less pain, the procedure does not involve any incision of tissue at or below the dentate line.

Adequate training with proctoring is strongly advised or enforced, because improper use risks devastating complications such as rectovaginal fistula, substantial hemorrhage, retroperitoneal sepsis, and rectal perforation. The technique uses a modified 33-mm circular stapler called the "PPH" (*procedure for prolapsing hemorrhoids*), made by Ethicon (Ethicon Endo-Surgery [J&J], Cincinnati, OH).

An operating anoscope is inserted and sutured in place to the skin. A 2–0 Prolene purse-string suture is placed submucosally above the apices of the internal hemorrhoids, approximately 4 cm proximal to the dentate line (Fig. 7). This purse-string must be carefully positioned, staying at the same level circumferentially with bites being placed superficially and avoiding any large gaps between stitches. The opened circular stapler is inserted, and the purse-string is tied down onto the shaft. The suture is used to pull the tissue into the jaws of the stapler. A counter-stitch may be placed opposite to the starting site of the purse-string before inserting the stapler to balance the pull of tissue into the stapler. The stapler is closed. In female patients, before firing the device, the surgeon inserts a finger into the vagina to ensure that the vaginal septum has not been included. After the stapler is fired and removed, the staple line is inspected for bleeders and defects. Meticulous attention to hemostasis is essential, and all bleeders should be oversewn. The application of bupivicaine with epinephrine should be postponed until after hemostasis is achieved.

With recent long-term follow-ups, this technique appears to provide durability similar to that of conventional surgical extirpation. Multiple studies comparing stapled hemorrhoidopexy to excisional hemorrhoidectomy show decreased postoperative pain and quicker return to normal activity in the stapled group. The complication rates were equivalent. A study comparing stapled hemorrhoidopexy to rubber-band ligation revealed more pain in the stapled group but a higher success rate. Distinct advantages of stapled hemorrhoidopexy over banding are that it represents a single procedure for internal hemorrhoids and that larger hemorrhoids can be addressed. Selection of patients for this procedure is paramount, with the optimal target group being patients with large prolapsing internal hemorrhoids. Adding procedures to the

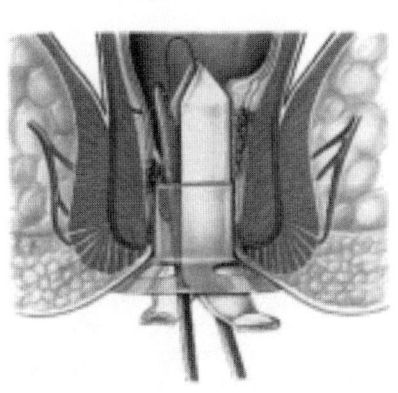
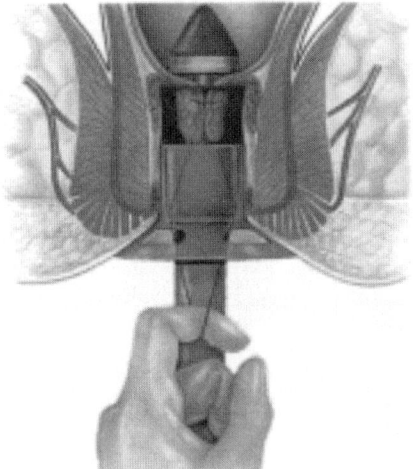
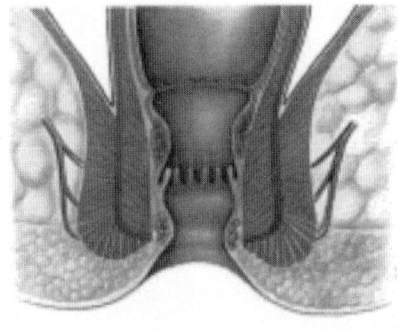

Figure 7 Stapled hemorrhoidectomy.

hemorrhoidopexy, such as tag excision, invites additional complications and pain. Although hemorrhoidopexy has been suggested to cause regression of external hemorrhoids, published and personal data are not as enthusiastic.

Suggested Readings

Arbman G, Krook H, Haapaniemi S: Closed vs open hemorrhoidectomy—is there any difference? *Dis Colon Rectum* 43:31, 2000.

MacRae HM, McLeaod RS: Comparison of hemorrhoidal treatment modalities. *Dis Colon Rectum* 38:687, 1995.

Salvaiti EP: Nonoperative management of hemorrhoids, *Dis Colon Rectum* 42:989, 1999.

Senagore AJ, Singer M, Abcarian H, and others: A prospective, randomized, controlled trial comparing stapled hemorrhoidopexy and Ferguson hemorrhoidectomy: perioperative and one-year results, *Dis Colon Rectum* 47:1824, 2004.

Standards Practice Task Force of the American Society of Colon and Rectal Surgeons: Practice parameters for the management of hemorrhoids (revised), *Dis Colon Rectum* 48:189, 2005.

Anal Fissures

Meagan Costedio, MD, and Peter A. Cataldo, MD

SIGNS AND SYMPTOMS

An anal fissure is a painful linear ulcer of the squamous epithelium usually extending from just above the dentate line to the anal verge. The ulcer lies in the posterior midline of the anal canal in 90% of cases (Fig. 1) but can also occur in the anterior midline. Anterior fissures are more commonly found in female patients.

This disorder is common and can affect patients at any age. Symptoms of anal fissure are characteristic and often diagnostic of the disease. The majority of patients describe the onset as a sharp, tearing pain that is initiated by the passage of stool, persists for hours, and is often associated with bright red rectal bleeding. At times patients associate constipation or, less commonly, severe diarrhea with the onset of symptoms. Patients may also complain of pruritus, swelling, or discharge, but these symptoms are less common. In the office, visual inspection while gently opening the anus often identifies the fissure. The anal region is often exquisitely tender, and a digital rectal examination may not be possible secondary to discomfort.

Fissures can be divided into primary and secondary types. Primary fissures can be found in the midline and are instigated by mechanical trauma, whereas secondary fissures are less classic in presentation and occur as a result of a predisposing illness. Primary fissures can be further divided into acute and chronic subtypes. Acute fissures are tears in the anoderm that bleed easily with minimal granulation tissue and have been present for less than 6 weeks. Approximately 20% of these patients do not heal after 6 weeks

despite conservative management and progress to chronic fissures. These lesions are characterized by visible internal sphincter fibers at the base of the fissure, indurated skin edges, an edematous fibrous skin tag (sentinel pile), or a hypertrophied anal papilla (Fig. 1). Chronic anal fissures require a more aggressive treatment regimen, with the aim of decreasing the mean anal resting pressure (MARP).

Secondary fissures are commonly off midline, painless, multiple, and refractory to medical and surgical therapies. Important predisposing conditions include local or systemic malignancy, Crohn's disease, tuberculosis, syphilis, trauma, and acquired immunodeficiency syndrome (AIDS). It is important to recognize secondary fissures and undertake further investigation into their underlying cause because treatment of the primary disease is necessary to achieve healing.

PATHOGENESIS

The pathogenesis of anal fissures is currently unknown. The initial epithelial disruption is thought to be a result of mechanical trauma, for example, constipation, diarrhea, or surgery. Eighty percent of the time, this epithelial process heals with conservative management, but if persistent, the tear will lead to resultant internal anal sphincter spasm and hypertonia. The current theory regarding chronic fissures is that this series of events results in constriction in the blood flow to the anoderm through the hypertonic sphincter and relative ischemia, which leads to impaired healing. Cadaveric studies have shown fewer blood vessels in the posterior anal canal compared with the rest of the anorectal region, and this observation may help to explain why fissures most often occur posteriorly. Data indicate that some patients with chronic anal fissures have raised MARPs greater than 80 to 100 mm Hg. As this pressure approaches arteriolar pressures, blood flow is decreased, leading to impaired wound healing. These data all lend support to the theory that chronic anal fissures are actually ischemic ulcers.

MANAGEMENT

Medical

The majority of primary acute anal fissures heal with conservative medical management consisting of constipation prevention, anal hygiene, and symptom control. The use of increased fluids and fiber supplementation in conjunction with stool softeners, sitz baths, and topical anesthetics results in healing in up to 50% of chronic fissures, which is higher than in untreated patients, although not significantly. Despite the fact that these treatments do not show a statistically significant improvement in healing compared with placebo, they have no side effects, are reasonably inexpensive, and may also aid in symptom amelioration.

Topical nitric oxide donors are used to treat chronic anal fissures and have been proved to reduce resting anal pressure, as well as to

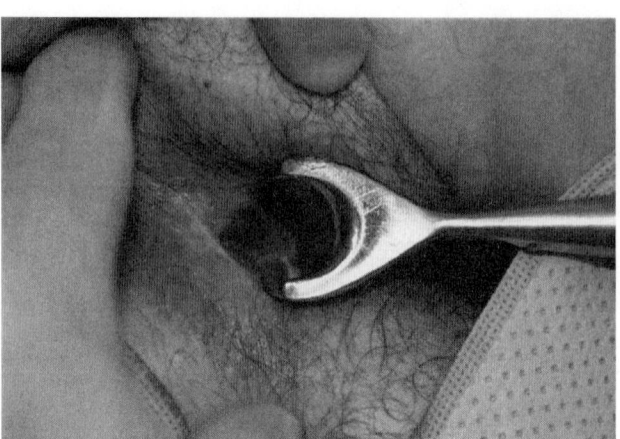

Figure 1 Chronic posterior anal fissure. (*See color insert Figure 21.*)

increase anoderm blood flow. Studies have shown a large variation in efficacy of topical nitrate therapy from 30% to 88%. Overall the data show that nitroglycerin is marginally better than placebo in healing chronic anal fissures. Although some studies demonstrate improved initial healing rates, they have also shown high recurrence rates. The chief side effect of nitrates is headache, with an incidence of 20% to 30%. The current recommendation for dosing is 1 to 1.5 g of 0.2% nitroglycerin cream applied three times daily to the anal margin for 8 weeks.

Calcium channel blockers (CCBs) decrease the internal sphincter tone and vasodilate the anodermal blood vessels in a similar manner to nitrates. Topical CCBs are associated with healing rates of 65% to 95% in chronic fissures, which are significantly better than placebo or oral CCBs. Topical CCBs are minimally absorbed, resulting in decreased systemic side effects. The most common side effect is perianal dermatitis, which responds to cessation of treatment. No randomized controlled studies of CCBs versus nitrate preparations have been performed, but there is evidence that healing rates are similar, and side effects of CCBs are more tolerable than those of nitroglycerin. CCBs may soon prove to be an adequate replacement for nitroglycerin ointments. The current recommendation for CCB dosing is 1 to 1.5 g of 0.2% nifedipine ointment to the perianal area twice a day.

Botulinum toxin A (Botox; Allergan, Irvine, CA) decreases resting anal pressure, leading to its use in the treatment of chronic anal fissure. The mechanism for the decrease in the anal canal tone is not clearly understood, because the internal sphincter, which is composed of smooth muscle, should be minimally affected by botulinum toxin. This decrease in pressure occurs within a few hours of injection, relieves pain quickly, and lasts for up to 3 months.

The data in the botulinum toxin literature are inconsistent, much like the other medical modalities presented above. Healing rates range from 43% to 88%, but these include differing dosing and injection regimens. Overall, botulinum toxin demonstrates similar efficacy and recurrence rates to the topical medications, but is clearly inferior to surgery. A key benefit of botulinum toxin compared with topical treatment is a one-time injection at an office visit and decreased concern with patient compliance. The main complication of Botox includes a low incidence of incontinence to stool and flatus. This is always temporary and often improves before the end of the 3-month period of action. There are also reports of perianal thrombosis, which can cause exquisite pain. Botox is the primary form of botulinum toxin A that is currently used, and dosing has been studied extensively. It appears that higher doses work better to a plateau dose of 30 units. Currently guidelines suggest that injections of approximately 15 units of Botox into the right and 15 units into the left lateral internal sphincter have the greatest effect (see Fig. 2).

Botulinum toxin is particularly appealing to patients who present with concerns about continence. A single study suggests that Botox administration in addition to fissure debridement in the operating room allows better accuracy of injection and improves healing. This small study demonstrates a 90% healing rate, but these patients were not followed for recurrence. We agree that this is a reasonable alternative to Botox alone and may produce healing rates superior to those of medical therapies in those concerned about potential incontinence caused by lateral internal sphincterotomy.

Current studies are considering other medical therapies for chronic anal fissure. These new agents include alpha-1 adrenoreceptor antagonists, cholinergic agonists, and phosphodiesterase inhibitors. All of these medications show promise in decreasing MARP but have not been evaluated in prospective randomized trials.

Surgery

Anal dilatation was used in the early treatment of anal fissure. This technique was abandoned secondary to high incontinence rates,

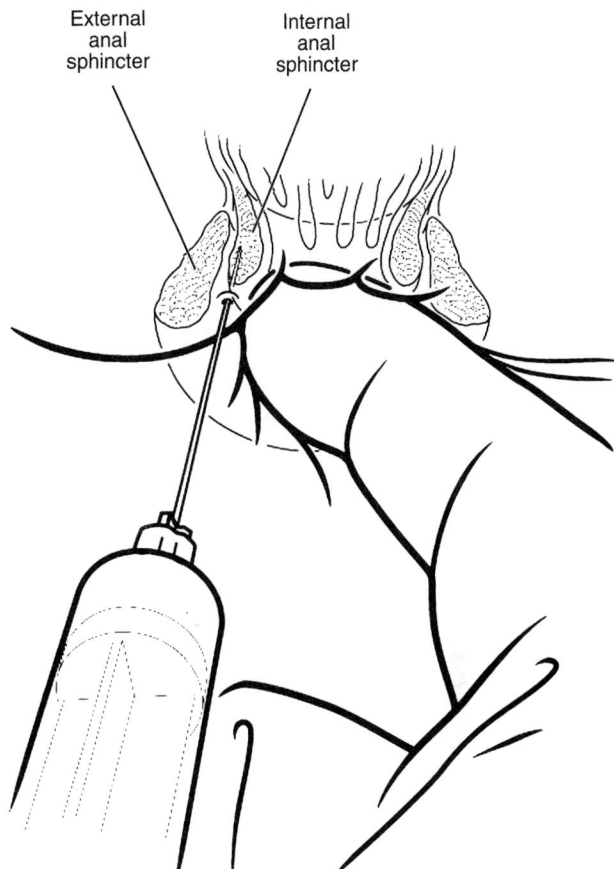

Figure 2 The internal anal sphincter is palpated and identified with the nondominant hand facilitating Botox injection directly into the muscle.

most likely related to inconsistency in dilatation. The more controlled lateral internal sphincterectomy (LIS) has now become the treatment of choice for management of chronic anal fissures. Healing rates are consistently at or above 95%, and recurrence rates are as low at 3%. The most significant complication associated with LIS is incontinence, which is reported to be between 0% and 36% to flatus, between 1% and 21% to liquid stool, and between 0% and 5% to solid stool. Other rare complications include bleeding, urinary retention, pain, and abscess. Overall less than 7% of patients experience long-term problems.

LIS is designed to cut a portion of the internal anal sphincter and can be performed through an open incision or via a closed technique. The procedure can be performed under local anesthesia with a pudendal nerve block, regional anesthesia, or general anesthesia. The patient is placed in the prone jackknife, lithotomy, or Symes position. A 1-cm incision is made, preferably in the left lateral aspect of the anal verge (see Fig. 3) because posterior incisions can leave keyhole deformities and have been associated with wetness and soiling. It is important to ensure the incision is in the perianal skin and not in the anal canal because incisions in the anal canal heal poorly. The internal sphincter is then grasped with an Allis clamp and is divided only to the proximal extent of the fissure in a limited technique. Currently, a limited internal sphincterotomy is advocated because of lower rates of postoperative incontinence and similar healing rates compared with traditional sphincterotomy. In theory, the high-pressure zone associated with a chronic fissure extends only to the proximal extent of the fissure. Therefore the sphincterotomy should not extend beyond this point.

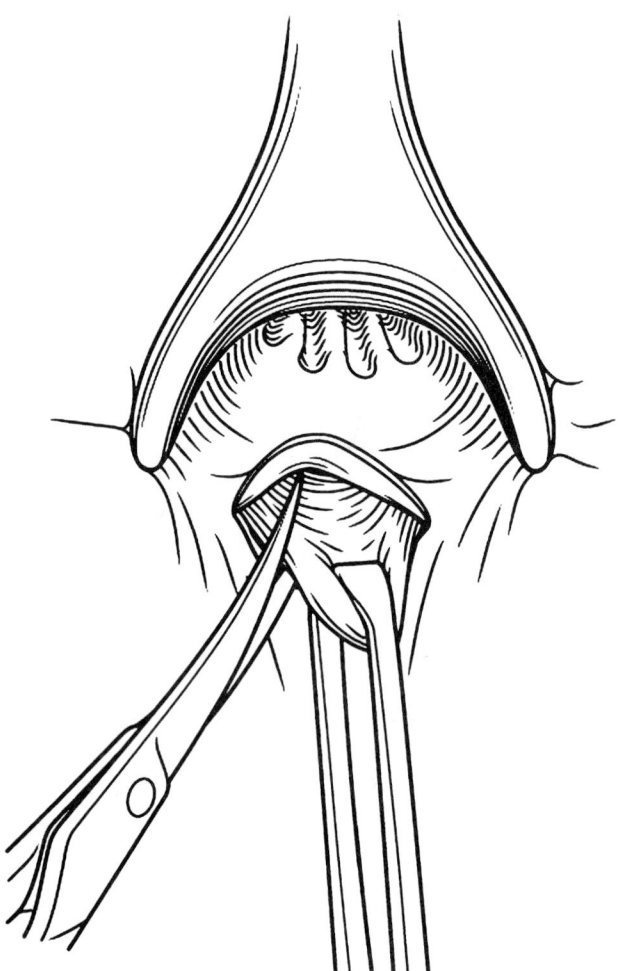

Figure 3 The internal sphincter is grasped with an Allis clamp, pulled partially through the wound, and transected for 4 to 5 mm.

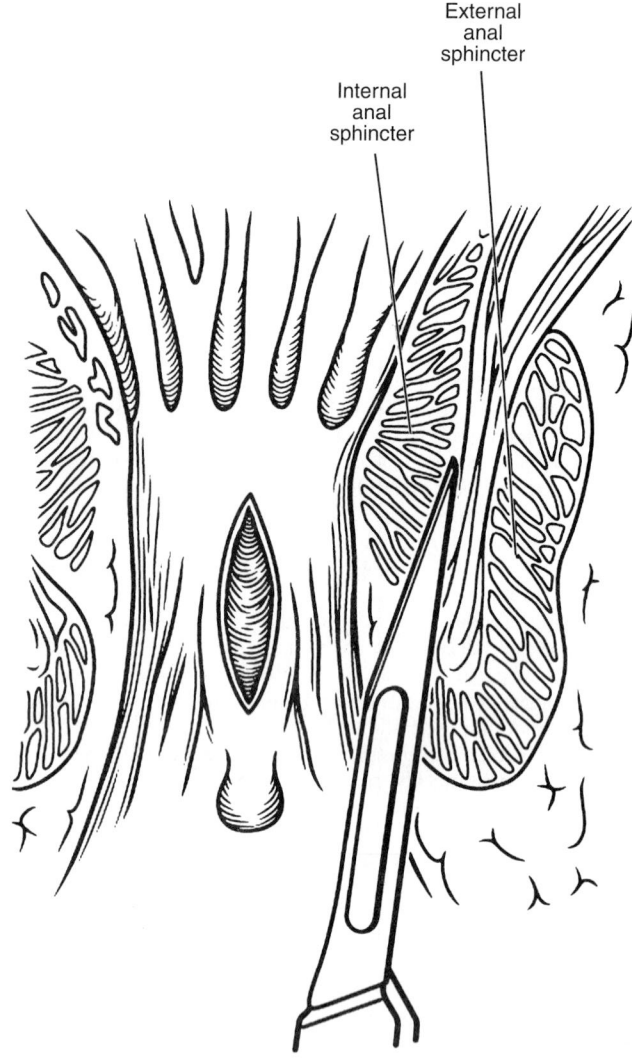

Figure 4 For closed sphincterotomy, a no. 11 blade is inserted into the intersphincteric groove, and the distal 4 to 5 mm of the internal sphincter are transected. A finger within the anal canal is used to judge the extent of the transection and to avoid mucosal injury.

In addition, external sphincter injury should be avoided in an effort to decrease the risk of incontinence. The incision is left open or closed depending on surgeon preference.

The closed technique is performed using a bivalve speculum to tighten the sphincters so the intersphincteric groove can be identified. The sphincterotomy is made through a stab incision distal to the intersphincteric groove (see Fig. 4). The open and closed techniques demonstrate similar healing and recurrence rates.

Anal advancement flap is a technique that is not as well studied as LIS but may be useful in patients with chronic fissures and low MARPs. This technique entails advancing a vascularized flap of perianal skin adjacent to the fissure. There are various techniques, including Y-to-V advancement flaps, house flaps, and island flaps. All achieve the same goal—closing the fissure defect with normal, well-vascularized skin while preventing tension. A Y-V anoplasty is performed as follows: first, the fissure bed is debrided. This will serve as the stem of the Y. Distal to this, a triangular segment of skin is mobilized and elevated off the subcutaneous fat. The flap is then advanced to cover the defect created by the fissure, thus changing the Y configuration to a V. This technique has not been studied in prospective randomized trials but has produced adequate healing rates in small retrospective reviews. This technique should be performed by a specialist, but it is an important option for an appropriate patient with continence concerns. The main complication is dehiscence of the flap, with few reports of incontinence.

Patients who present with prior alterations in continence, low resting pressures, or recurrence after prior sphincterotomy should be treated with special consideration. These patients are more likely to develop incontinence with a typical LIS. All of these patients should have preoperative manometry and possibly ultrasonography. If the pressures are high, a repeat or initial sphincterotomy can be performed on the opposing side. Patients with chronic fissures and low resting anal tone may be candidates for other medical therapies or an advancement flap procedure to preserve continence.

SUMMARY

There are multiple options available for the management of chronic anal fissures. First-line treatment includes fluids, fiber, stool softeners, and sitz baths. Nitrates, calcium channel blockers, and Botox all demonstrate similar healing rates; all are superior to placebo and inferior to LIS, but nitrates have more systemic side effects. The choice to use each should be based on cost, patient compliance, patient lifestyle, and side effects. LIS, open or closed, is the gold standard treatment, with superior healing and lower recurrence rates compared with other treatments available, with the rare undesirable side effect of incontinence. All patients with noncharacteristic anal fissures or those refractory to therapy should be examined further for primary pathology. Patients with altered continence or low MARPs should be treated cautiously and offered more extensive medical therapy, perhaps in combination with fissurectomy or advancement flap to avoid incontinence.

SUGGESTED READINGS

Fazio VW CJ, Delaney, CP: *Current therapy in colon and rectal surgery,* Philadelphia, 2005, Elsevier Mosby.

Gordon PH, Nivatvongs S: *Principles and practice of surgery for the colon, rectum, and anus,* ed 2, St. Louis, 1999, Quality Medical.

Orsay C, Rakinic J, Perry WB, and others: Practice parameters for the management of anal fissures (revised), *Dis Colon Rectum* 47:2003, 2004.

Schoetz D: Anal fissure and stenosis, *Sem Colon Rectal Surg* 8:1, 1997.

ANORECTAL ABSCESS AND FISTULA

Sean C. Glasgow, MD, and David W. Dietz, MD

Anorectal abscess and fistula are common, age-old afflictions in humans, with the earliest known descriptions of the diseases and their treatment outlined in the Egyptian Chester Beatty papyrus circa 1550 BC. A simplified approach to pelvic sepsis designates the abscess as the acute manifestation of infection, with the fistula representing the chronic stage of the same disease. However, both abscess and fistula can occur independently of the other. Adequate initial treatment helps to minimize subsequent complex fistula formation and facilitates additional surgical therapy. Although anorectal abscesses are common, their exact incidence in the general population is unknown. Approximately 40% of patients with abscesses eventually develop a fistula-in-ano. Successful treatment of these disorders with minimal morbidity requires knowledge of the anatomic spaces surrounding the anorectum and the various potential clinical presentations, application of traditional surgical principles, and employment of specific techniques tailored for each patient.

ANORECTAL ABSCESS

Several large series have demonstrated that the peak incidence of anorectal abscess occurs during the third decade of life, although they may occur at any age. Incidence increases in the spring and summer months and in warm climates. There is a slight male predominance. Although predisposing factors include diabetes mellitus, Crohn's disease, and human immunodeficiency virus (HIV) infection or other causes of immunosuppression, the majority of anorectal abscess occur in otherwise healthy individuals. A thorough understanding of the pelvic anatomy (including the potential perianal and perirectal spaces) is central to the treatment of anorectal abscesses. Inadequate initial treatment of an abscess can result in systemic sepsis and places the patient at an increased risk for a subsequent anorectal fistula with ongoing local sepsis and possible sphincter damage. Although the vast majority of abscesses are of cryptoglandular origin, one should also keep in mind a differential diagnosis that includes hidradenitis suppurativa, deep pilonidal abscess, anal tuberculosis or actinomycosis, and malignancy of the anal verge or anal canal.

Etiology

According to the widely accepted cryptoglandular theory, anorectal abscesses are believed to arise from one of the 10 to 15 anal crypts (of Morgagni) that are located circumferentially at the dentate line. These crypts empty the anal glands that facilitate defecation by lubricating stool and are positioned in the plane between the internal and external anal sphincters. Septic foci originating within these cryptoglandular structures may then propagate along paths of least resistance, dissecting between, through, or above the sphincter complex. Cultures generally demonstrate enteric bacteria, with a mix of gram-negatives and anaerobes. As previously mentioned, immunosuppressive and gastrointestinal inflammatory conditions predispose to the formation of anorectal abscesses. Other less common causes are listed in Table 1.

Anatomy and Classification

Anorectal abscesses are typically classified according to anatomic location; such classification is useful not only for descriptive purposes but also for determining treatment and prognosis. Abscesses may occur in the perianal, ischiorectal (or ischioanal), intersphincteric, postanal, submucosal, or supralevator spaces. Perianal abscesses are the most common, occurring in the space that surrounds the anus and becomes continuous with the fat of the buttocks. This space is caudal and lateral to the sphincter muscles. The ischiorectal (or ischioanal) space is lateral to the anal canal; it is bounded superiorly by the levators, inferiorly by the transverse perineal septum, medially by the external sphincter, and laterally by the ischial tuberosity. As the name implies, intersphincteric abscesses occur between the internal and external sphincters in a lateral or anterior position. Submucosal abscesses are superficial to the internal sphincter and above the dentate

Table 1: Etiology of Anorectal Abscess

Cryptoglandular
Iatrogenic
Perineal trauma
Anal or low rectal cancer
Postoperative anastomotic leak
Radiation injury
Inflammatory bowel disease
Acquired immunodeficiency syndrome
Invasive fungal infection
Hidradenitis suppurativa
Diverticulitis
Intra-abdominal infection
Anal fissure
Osteomyelitis

line. Finally, the supralevator space lies cephalad to the levator ani musculature. An abscess in this location may arise from the upward extension of an intersphincteric abscess or the downward extension of an intra-abdominal process such a diverticulitis or tubo-ovarian abscess.

Particular mention should be made regarding the postanal space, which is bounded by the levators superiorly and the external sphincter inferiorly. The postanal space communicates with the lateral ischiorectal fossae, and postanal infection frequently spreads in a lateral direction to involve these spaces. Failure to recognize the so-called horseshoe abscess at the time of surgical drainage can lead to ongoing infection and subsequent systemic illness, with possible sphincter destruction. Additionally, lateral abscesses typically communicate with the rectum in the posterior midline via the postanal space; this concept is discussed further later in the chapter.

Presentation and Diagnosis

Perianal Abscess

Perianal abscesses are the most common subtype of anorectal abscess, accounting for 40% to 45% of cases. Patients complain of severe perianal pain of short duration that occurs independent of defecation, persists throughout the day, and may be relieved with warm baths. Pain is aggravated with sitting or straining. They may also note fever and localized swelling. Patients should be queried about prior abscesses, prior anorectal surgery, any history of immunocompromise or recurring infections in other locations, and symptoms suggestive of inflammatory bowel disease.

Examination reveals a tender, erythematous bulge adjacent to the anal verge, with varying degrees of fluctuance, induration, and overlying cellulitis. In patients with perianal abscesses, the fullness should not extend above the dentate line, and the presence of rectal fullness would suggest a different diagnosis. Bimanual examination in women is important to rule out involvement of the rectovaginal septum. Spontaneous drainage to the perianal skin commonly occurs.

Ischiorectal (Ischioanal) Abscess

Given the relatively large potential space composed of ischiorectal fat and loose areolar tissue, abscesses in this location may attain large size and present with diffuse gluteal swelling. Because the abscess may be asymptomatic initially, patients often present at a later stage with extensive fat and soft tissue necrosis. Extension of the infection across the postanal space results in bilateral ischiorectal abscesses ("horseshoe abscess"). Less commonly, bilateral communication can occur across the anterior deep anal space.

Intersphincteric Abscess

Intersphincteric abscesses are relatively rare, comprising between 2% and 5% of anorectal abscesses in most series. In addition, they can be difficult to diagnose because findings on physical examination are less pronounced. Patients may complain of dull, constant anal aching. External findings are generally lacking. Digital rectal exam produces exquisite tenderness at the site of the abscess; localized swelling may also be appreciated at or above the dentate line. Intersphincteric abscesses are most commonly associated with anorectal fistulae and are the most likely abscess to recur.

Postanal Abscess

Barring lateral extension into the ischiorectal fossa (e.g., a horseshoe abscess), infection contained in this location between the levators superiorly and the external sphincter inferiorly may be difficult to diagnosis. Patients present with either a dull ache or sharp posterior anal pain. Discomfort may preclude a thorough anal examination, and patient symptoms often are similar to those of posterior anal fissures. Examination under anesthesia should be performed in any patient with severe postanal pain to exclude an abscess because undiagnosed pelvic sepsis in the postanal or intersphincteric spaces can result in severe functional morbidity.

Submucosal Abscess

Patients with submucosal abscesses may complain only of a dull perirectal ache or fullness and often lack external signs of infection. Findings on examination include a tender swelling cephalad to the dentate line.

Supralevator Abscess

Supralevator abscesses comprise between 2.5% and 9% of all anorectal abscesses. They arise either from cephalad progression of an intersphincteric source to a position above the puborectalis, or more commonly, caudal extension of an intra-abdominal source such as diverticulitis or pelvic inflammatory disease. Similar to intersphincteric abscesses, they can be difficult to diagnose solely on the basis of symptoms, with patients typically complaining only of dull rectal aching. Systemic symptoms such as fever and shaking chills may be observed. Cross-sectional tomographic imaging with either computed tomography (CT) or magnetic resonance (MRI) aids in diagnosing the supralevator abscess and provides further information regarding possible intra-abdominal etiologies.

Treatment

The definitive treatment of an anorectal abscess is incision and drainage. Depending on the location of the abscess and patient tolerance, this can often be accomplished at the bedside or in the clinic under local anesthesia. However, one must bear in mind that the relative tissue acidity surrounding an abscess reduces the effectiveness of injectable local anesthetics, making drainage under either regional or general anesthesia a reasonable alternative. Examination under anesthesia also may suggest the etiology of the fistula, as discussed later. Key tenets of abscess drainage include complete disruption of loculations with either a hemostat or the surgeon's finger, drainage of any collections adjacent to the primary abscess, and some method to prevent premature closure of the skin over the abscess cavity. Any patient with an associated mass or ulcerated lesion or a history of recurrent perianal abscesses or fistulae should undergo surgical biopsy of the tract to exclude the diagnoses of inflammatory bowel disease or malignancy. Commonly required surgical instruments are depicted in Fig. 1.

A common technique for drainage of a perianal abscess consists of a cruciate incision made over either the point of maximal prominence or to include any site of spontaneous drainage. Excision of the dermis at the corners of the incision can prevent premature skin closure. Gauze packing of most anorectal abscesses is impractical because of their locations. An alternative method drains the abscess by a small stab incision with subsequent placement of a 10-F to 16-F mushroom catheter in the abscess cavity to permit drainage. This technique, initially described by Beck and associates in 1988, limits the size of the wound and may be better tolerated by patients. The catheter usually remains in place without the discomfort of an anchoring stitch and can be removed in the clinic 5 to 10 days later, although it can be left in place for several months if necessary. Regardless of method used, the

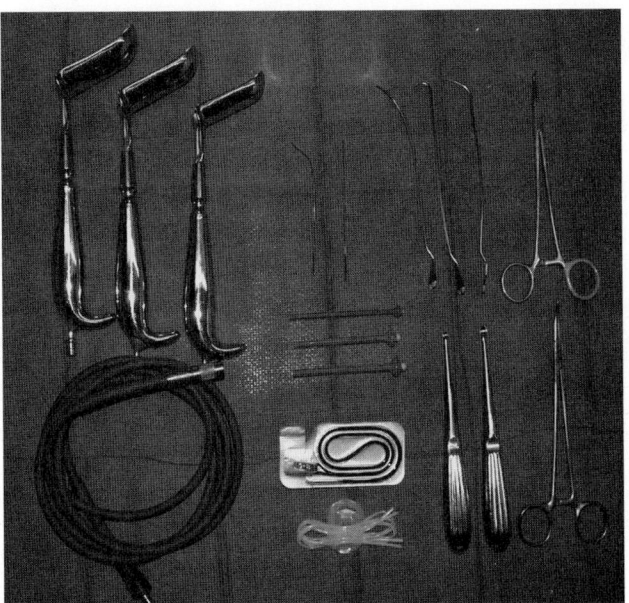

Figure 1 Useful instruments for the surgical treatment of anorectal abscesses and fistulae include lighted Hill-Ferguson retractors, fistula and lacrimal duct probes, curettes, fine-tipped thin tonsil and right-angle clamps, Silastic setons, mushroom catheters (10 to 16 F), and a syringe and angiocath for peroxide or methylene blue injection.

incision should be made as close to the anal verge as feasible to limit the length of any resulting fistula.

The role of primary fistulotomy at the time of anorectal abscess drainage is debatable. In an early large series from Cook County Hospital, Read and Abcarian reported that patients who underwent fistulotomy concurrent with drainage had half the abscess recurrence rate of those who did not during a 3-year follow-up. Conversely, Vasilevsky and Gordon found that only 37% of patients undergoing isolated abscess drainage developed a subsequent symptomatic fistula-in-ano. Schouten and van Vroonhoven confirmed these results in a prospective randomized controlled trial comparing drainage with concurrent fistulotomy against drainage alone; 41% of patients in the drainage-only arm experienced recurrent or persistent abscesses. Notably, they also found that disturbances of anal function were higher in the drainage-plus-fistulotomy group. Therefore there appears to be little role for primary fistulotomy because approximately 60% of patients with anorectal abscesses do not develop subsequent clinically apparent fistulae, and primary fistulotomy may unnecessarily impair continence. In addition, exploration for possible fistulae during the acute inflammatory stage may produce false tracts. If an obvious anorectal fistula is present at the time of abscess drainage, it is our practice to pass a noncutting Silastic (Dow Corning, Midland, MI) seton through the tract to facilitate thorough drainage of the abscess and prevent recurrence until definitive treatment of the fistula is performed.

Ischiorectal abscesses are managed similarly to perianal abscesses. When present, a horseshoe abscess can be drained by incisions over both ischiorectal fossae; a Penrose drain can be placed through both incisions to allow adequate evacuation of the postanal space. In men, fistulotomy (consisting of division of the internal sphincter) can be performed to treat isolated postanal abscesses. However, division of the sphincter muscle in women should not be undertaken at the time of abscess drainage.

Unroofing the overlying mucosa then dividing the internal sphincter as necessary treats submucosal and intersphincteric

abscesses. Hemostasis is achieved by oversewing the mucosal edges. Alternatively, intersphincteric abscesses can be drained by inserting a small mushroom catheter into the abscess cavity via a stab incision overlying the intersphincteric groove.

Treatment of a supralevator abscess first requires identification of its site of origin (e.g., pelvic infection vs. perianal). Abscesses arising from cephalad spread from the ischiorectal fossae or an intersphincteric source are treated with wide drainage into the rectum. CT-guided drainage catheters may be needed to adequately evacuate the supralevator space, particularly if accumulation is due to an extension from an abdominal source such as diverticulitis. Rarely, fecal diversion via colostomy is required to control pelvic sepsis, especially in patients with inflammatory bowel disease.

Postoperative Care

Patients generally only require a single dose of intravenous antibiotics covering gram-negative and anaerobic bacteria at the time of abscess drainage. However, certain patient populations should be treated with prolonged parenteral antibiotics, most notably if there is extensive cellulitis surrounding the drained abscess cavity (Table 2). Most patients can be discharged to home immediately following incision and drainage. Bulking agents can ease the pain of bowel movements and reduce constipation. Warm sitz baths are taken several times per day. Excessive administration of intravenous fluids, older age, severe pelvic disease, and male gender are all risk factors for urinary retention; Foley catheters are used on an as-needed basis.

Outcomes

Approximately 10% of patients develop a recurrent anorectal abscess following drainage. Retrospective studies have reported recurrence rates up to 68% in patients deemed "inadequately treated" at the time of initial diagnosis, emphasizing the importance of completely disrupting loculations, debriding any frankly necrotic tissue, and providing a durable means for drainage. As previously mentioned, approximately 40% of patients develop subsequent symptomatic anorectal fistulae, although many more likely have occult fistulae. Anorectal abscesses are the first manifestation of disease in 5% to 36% of Crohn's disease patients, and more than half with perianal disease develop recurrent abscesses despite maximal treatment. For this reason, a history of recurrent anorectal abscesses should prompt proctoscopy with rectal mucosal biopsies.

Table 2: Indications for Parenteral Antibiotics in Anorectal Abscess

Prosthetic cardiac valve
Mitral valve prolapse
Extensive periabscess cellulitis
Necrotizing infections
Systemic sepsis
Immunocompromised states
Diabetes mellitus
Acquired immunodeficiency syndrome
Bone marrow transplant recipient
Active chemotherapy
Prolonged corticosteroid use

FISTULA-IN-ANO

Surgical intervention for fistula-in-ano is highly effective and can yield tremendous relief for patients afflicted with this common malady. Fistulae typically arise from a localized infection of the anal glands and present clinically following abscess drainage, although inflammatory bowel disease, traumatic injury, and certain bacterial and fungal infections also may be causative. The natural history of fistula-in-ano is not well described; however, a sizable percentage may undergo spontaneous resolution without surgical intervention. Symptomatic anorectal fistulae can cause soiling, anal pruritus, recurrent pelvic sepsis, and general chronic discomfort. Because of the potential for an iatrogenic temporary or permanent alteration in fecal continence, asymptomatic fistulae should be left untreated unless there is serious concern for recurrent anorectal abscess or there is suspicion of underlying maliganancy. Treatment of the complex fistula-in-ano requires a detailed knowledge of the anatomy of the sphincter mechanism, as well as familiarity with new and evolving techniques.

Anatomy and Classification

An anorectal fistula is an abnormal communication between the anal canal or rectum and the perianal skin. These epithelialized tracts are typically the direct consequence of anorectal abscesses, and although an abscess may drain in any direction, approximately two thirds of anorectal fistulae follow an intersphincteric path. Initially proposed in 1976, Parks's classification schema for anorectal fistulae still serves today as a useful and functional system for not only delineating anatomy but also determining treatment (Fig. 2). A key tenet of managing the anorectal fistula is Goodsall's rule, which states that external fistulous openings anterior to a transverse line through the anus will open radially into the anal canal in a direct line at the dentate, whereas fistulae with perianal skin openings posterior to this line will follow a more circumferential route and originate in the posterior midline (Fig. 3). Accordingly, a posterior fistula typically is longer and follows a more tortuous course. Fistulae may also be defined as either simple or complex. In general, complex fistulae are those other than submucosal, intersphincteric, or low transsphincteric fistulae and those arising in patients with inflammatory bowel disease or prior sphincter injury. Patients with complex fistulae are at increased risk for both recurrence and treatment-related incontinence.

Principles of Treatment

Ensure Resolution of Perianal Sepsis

With the possible exception of submucosal fistulae, definitive fistulotomy should be deferred until the initiating abscess has

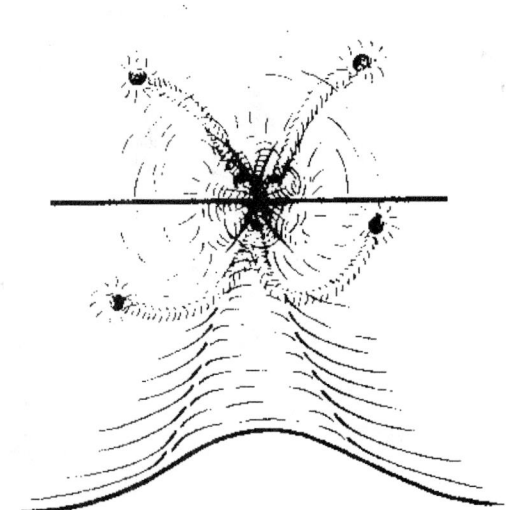

Figure 3 Goodsall's rule. *From Atlas of colorectal surgery, New York, 1996, Churchill Livingstone.*

been fully drained and there is no suggestion of ongoing localized infection (purulent drainage, cellulitis). Most anorectal abscesses are successfully treated with a single drainage procedure, followed by fistulotomy 4 to 6 weeks later if a fistula persists. However, patients with Crohn's disease, a history of recurrent fistulae or abscesses, or immunosuppressive disorders may require multiple reexaminations under anesthesia to ensure adequate resolution of perianal infection. In patients with complex fistulae, it is a sound strategy to employ draining Silastic setons placed loosely through the fistula to prepare the tract for definitive treatment.

Define the Anatomy

Determination of the course and type of anorectal fistula is best accomplished by an examination under anesthesia. Gentle passage of a lacrimal probe through the external opening is usually successful at delineating the internal communication. Retraction of the secondary opening at the skin with an Allis clamp can straighten the fistula and aid passage of the probe. Care must be taken to avoid creating false passages into the rectum, which might turn an otherwise simple fistula into a markedly more complex situation. If gentle probing fails to reveal the primary opening, dilute methylene blue or hydrogen peroxide can be injected through the external opening. When the fistulous tract cannot be delineated on examination, either MRI or transrectal ultrasound (TRUS) may prove useful. Trials from St. Mark's Hospital initially reported that high-resolution MRI using an endorectal coil successfully identified the internal opening in up to 80% of patients with fistulae. A subsequent comparison trial by West and colleagues demonstrated good concordance among MRI, hydrogen peroxide–enhanced TRUS, and findings at surgery with regard to fistula type, presence of secondary tracts, and the location of the primary opening. Thus MRI and TRUS should be regarded as complementary diagnostic tests to operative examination in patients with occult internal openings.

Determine Risk of Incontinence

Before fistulotomy, all patients should be informed of the risk of fecal incontinence because most surgical treatments require division of some portion of the internal sphincter musculature. Data

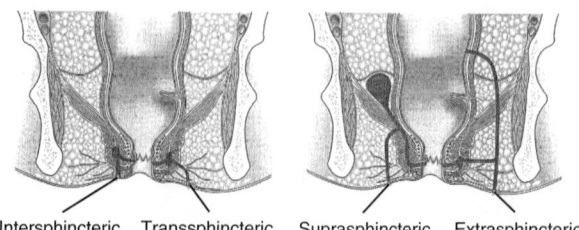

Intersphincteric Transsphincteric   Suprasphincteric Extrasphincteric

Figure 2 Parks's classification of anorectal fistulae.

from the University of Minnesota indicate that up to 45% of patients undergoing fistulotomy report some postoperative change in their continence. Risk factors predictive of incontinence include female gender, a high (extrasphincteric) fistula, and a history of prior fistula surgery. Incontinence also increases linearly with the amount of external sphincter divided during fistulotomy. Anteriorly located fistulae are particularly problematic in women because of their thinner perineal body. Other factors influencing the treatment decision include any history of sphincteric injury (such as episiotomy) and preexisting bowel dysfunction or inflammatory bowel disease that predispose to diarrhea. Identification of a patient at an increased risk for incontinence may bias initial attempts at treatment toward the various sphincter-sparing options described later.

Surgical Options

The choice of definitive treatment for an anorectal fistula is dictated by its type, position, patient comorbidities, and surgeon preference (Table 3). Options include fistulotomy, cutting seton, anorectal mucosal advancement flaps, fibrin glue injection, or use of a collagen plug. Most fistula surgery can be performed on an outpatient basis. Patients take nothing by mouth after midnight prior to surgery, and an enema is administered the morning of surgery to empty the rectal vault. Either general or regional anesthesia can be combined with a bilateral perianal block using a 1:1 mixture of 1% lidocaine and 0.5% bupivicaine. Our practice is to position the patient on the basis of the location of the anorectal pathology. Lesions involving the anterior anal canal are usually approached with the patient in the prone jackknife position, whereas lesions in the posterior anal canal are best visualized in lithotomy. Postoperatively, patients are prescribed adequate narcotic analgesics and continue twice daily sitz baths and bulking agents.

Fistulotomy

Surgical fistulotomy remains the mainstay for treating submucosal and low intersphincteric fistulae. After passage of a probe through the tract and out the internal opening, the anorectal mucosa is divided using electrocautery, followed by division of the internal sphincter down to the probe. The lining of the tract is then curetted and irrigated to remove any granulation tissue. Hemostasis is obtained either with cautery or by running 3–0 chromic sutures along the mucosal edges; this also serves to marsupialize the tract and may help prevent premature closure and diminish the risk of fistula recurrence.

Care must be taken in performing a fistulotomy under certain circumstances. Whereas men generally tolerate division of the entire internal sphincter without changes in fecal continence, women may suffer incontinence after only a small portion of the muscle is divided. Additionally, fistulotomies performed in the anterior position in women are particularly hazardous, especially in the context of prior episiotomy. In these cases, we favor either an anal mucosal advancement flap or collagen plug repair as a means of preserving the remaining sphincter musculature. Alternatively, a partial fistulotomy (e.g., Parks's fistulotomy) can be performed, with the remaining sphincter encircled with a noncutting seton; resolution using this method is approximately 70% at 8 weeks.

Cutting Seton

Cutting setons are most useful for transsphincteric fistulae, when there is concern of injury to the external anal sphincter. The theory behind the use of a cutting seton is to slowly divide a portion of the external sphincter while allowing scar formation to prevent the circumferential retraction (and possible functional compromise) that occurs with acute surgical transection. The cutting seton, typically an 0 silk suture, is tied to the proximal end of the probe and pulled through the transsphincteric fistula. The perianal skin and the internal sphincter are divided using electrocautery; then the seton is tightly secured against the underlying muscle. The seton is tightened during follow-up clinic visits every 2 weeks to slowly cut through the remaining muscle. Cutting setons can be uncomfortable and may require several months for complete treatment; this technique generally has been replaced with newer methods.

Advancement Flap

Anorectal mucosal advancement flaps are best employed for anterior transsphincteric fistulae in women or fistulae in patients with preexisting impaired sphincter function. The primary principle is exclusion of the internal opening from the fecal stream. A thick, broad-based, U-shaped flap is elevated, beginning at the internal opening of the fistula and continuing for 4 to 5 cm cephalad. The flap consists of mucosa, submucosa, and fibers of the internal sphincter muscle. The flap should be mobilized enough so that a tension-free suture line will result, but care must be taken to keep the base of the flap as wide as possible to avoid ischemia. After the flap has been elevated, the fistula tract through the sphincter should be curetted and then closed with 2–0 Vicryl suture. After hemostasis has been ensured, the flap is brought down over this repair and sutured to the distal anal canal mucosa with interrupted 3–0 chromic sutures. A small mushroom catheter can be placed into the external opening to provide counter drainage. Patients are typically kept nothing-per-mouth for 48 hours to prevent bowel movements and are continued on intravenous antibiotics.

Fibrin Glue Injection

Fibrin glue injection has gained in popularity over the last 10 years because of its low risk-to-benefit ratio. It has advantages over fistulotomy in that there is no risk for incontinence following the procedure, and unsuccessful treatment of the fistula does not preclude further surgical options. It also is fairly simple to perform. Fibrin glue should only be used in linear, nonbranching fistulae without evidence of persistent infection. After both openings of the fistula are delineated, the tract is lightly debrided by passing a knotted silk suture or gauze sponge. The fistula is irrigated with saline or dilute hydrogen peroxide. An angiocatheter then is passed via the external opening into the fistula, and a total of 5 ml of a commercially available combination of fibrinogen and thrombin (Tisseel; Baxter, Deerfield, IL) is injected. After a large bead of fibrin glue is created at the internal opening, the catheter is slowly withdrawn while the tract is completely filled. Gluing is terminated at the external opening by creating a second large bead to complete a "dumbbell" configuration.

Table 3: Surgical Treatment by Type of Anorectal Fistula

Subcutaneous	Fistulotomy
Intersphincteric	
Low	Fistulotomy
High	Advancement flap, fibrin glue or collagen plug
Transsphincteric	Advancement flap, fibrin glue or collagen plug
Suprasphincteric	Advancement flap, fibrin glue or collagen plug
Extrasphincteric	Address the pelvic or intra-abdominal source

We routinely secure the fibrin matrix using a single absorbable suture through the internal opening. Patients are discharged the same day with instructions to avoid straining, coughing, or tub bathing for 1 week to prevent extrusion of the fibrin glue plug from the fistula.

Collagen Plug

With initial results first reported in 2004 at the American Society of Colon and Rectal Surgery annual meeting, the collagen plug is a novel treatment for high intersphincteric, transsphincteric, and suprasphincteric fistulae that would almost certainly lead to incontinence if treated by fistulotomy. The early experience with this technique used self-fashioned conical plugs composed of lyophilized porcine intestinal submucosa. The plug creates a collagen scaffold for tissue ingrowth while excluding the internal opening from the fecal stream. Preformed tapered plugs with a 6-mm maximal diameter are now commercially available (Surgisis AFP; Cook Surgical, West Lafayette, IN). The plug is prepared by tying a suture to the tail (narrow end). Care must be taken to avoid enlarging the fistula; for this reason, we do not routinely irrigate or curette the tract itself. After passage of a probe through the tract, the tied suture and plug are pulled through the internal opening until the tapered plug is snug in the fistula. The excess plug within the rectal lumen is trimmed flush with the mucosa, then secured using a 2–0 Vicryl stitch at the internal opening (Fig. 4). Excess length at the skin opening also is trimmed.

Outcomes

Direct comparison of results for the various treatments for anorectal fistula is difficult because of the heterogeneity of the disease and multitude of therapeutic options (Table 4). Generally, techniques involving the direct division of internal or external sphincter muscles produce the highest healing rates. Unfortunately, they also have the highest risk of fecal incontinence, with up to 45% of patients reporting altered continence following fistulotomy and cutting seton deployment. The remaining techniques virtually eliminate the risk of causing incontinence, but the fistula healing rate is inferior to that achieved with simple fistulotomy. Variable success rates (40%–60%) are reported for mucosal advancement flaps, with breakdown or infection of the flap a not uncommon occurrence even in the hands of experienced colorectal surgeons. Cintron and colleagues conducted the largest

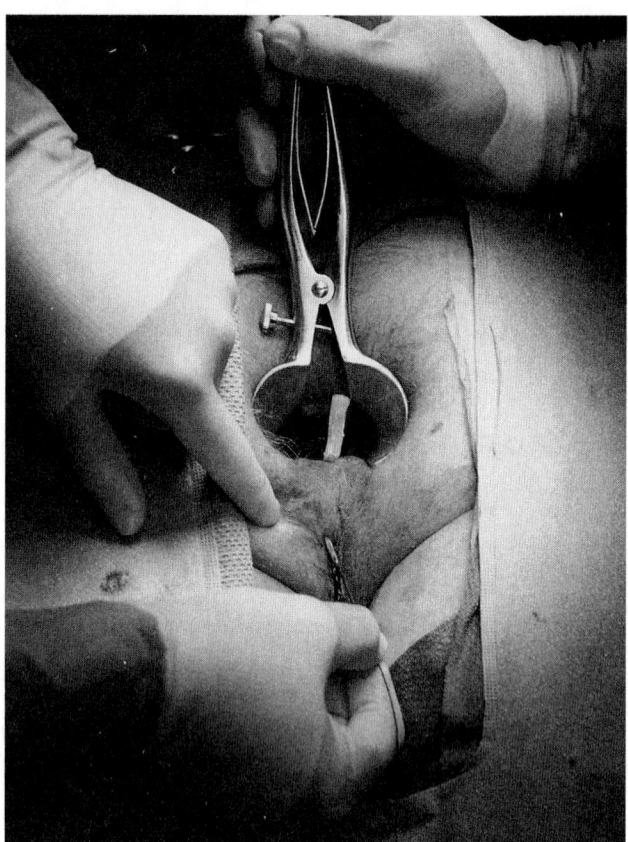

Figure 4 Positioning of a collagen plug in a simple anterior anal fistula.

series examining the use of fibrin glue injection. They reported an overall success rate of 66%, with recurrence varying according to the complexity of the fistula. Others have found that although skin healing is present in a majority of patients at 2 weeks, only 14% remain healed at 16 months. Our own long-term results using fibrin glue showed an overall healing rate of only 31% at a median of 23 months follow-up. Additionally, repeat treatment was successful in only 12%. Preliminary reports of the collagen plug technique are

Table 4: Outcomes for Various Fistula Treatments

Author	Method	No. Patients	Follow-Up	Recurrence (%)	Altered Continence (%)
Hamalainen & Sainio (1997)	Cutting seton	35	NR	6	51
Dziki & Bartos (1998)	Cutting seton	32	NR	0	19
Hyman (1999)	Advancement flap	33	NR	19	0
Schouten, Zimmerman, & Briel (1999)	Advancement flap	44	NR	25	38
Cintron and others (2000)	Fibrin glue	79	12 months	39	NR
Lindsey and others (2002)	Fibrin glue	19	14 months	37	0
Loungnarath and others (2004)	Fibrin glue	39	23 months	69	0
Singer and others (2005)	Fibrin glue	75	27 months	67	0
Johnson, Gaw, & Armstrong (2006)	Collagen plug	15	3 months	13	NR

NR, Data not reported.

favorable, with Johnson and colleagues reporting an 87% success rate at a mean follow-up of 13 weeks versus only 40% for patients treated with fibrin glue. Although median time to failure was only 4 weeks, whether the collagen plug provides a durable cure is unknown because data regarding long-term outcomes are lacking.

Fistula-in-Ano and Crohn's Disease

Between 20% and 56% of Crohn's patients develop perineal disease, with a majority having either anorectal abscesses or fistulae. Although the scope of this chapter precludes a full discussion of this difficult topic, a few key management points should be noted. Patients with Crohn's disease are at increased risk for developing perianal carcinomas, and the presence of mucinous discharge from a fistula tract or persistent induration in a nonsuppurative area should prompt a biopsy. Fistulization occurs through the low rectal mucosa, generally producing higher and more complex tracts. After active infection has been drained (often with multiple loose setons left in place for weeks), a trial of nonoperative therapy may be attempted, consisting of oral ciprofloxacin with metronidazole and immunosuppressives such as azathioprine or 6-mercaptopurine. The ACCENT II study examined infliximab (Remicade; Centocor, Malvern, PA) infusions for patients with perianal Crohn's fistulae and found a 69% initial response rate. However, 42% of initial responders developed recurrences at 1 year despite maintenance infliximab therapy. Overall, symptomatic relief is reported in up to 90% of patients treated nonoperatively; however, relapse is common upon cessation of medication. Patients with multiple complex tracts (e.g., "watering-can perineum," Fig. 5) may benefit from fecal diversion by a loop ileostomy; although this does not alter the natural course of the disease, it will likely improve symptoms. Refractory perineal disease eventually requires proctectomy with permanent fecal diversion.

SUGGESTED READINGS

Cintron JR, Park JJ, Orsay CP, and others: Repair of fistulae-in-ano using fibrin adhesive: long-term follow-up, *Dis Colon Rectum* 43:944, 2000.

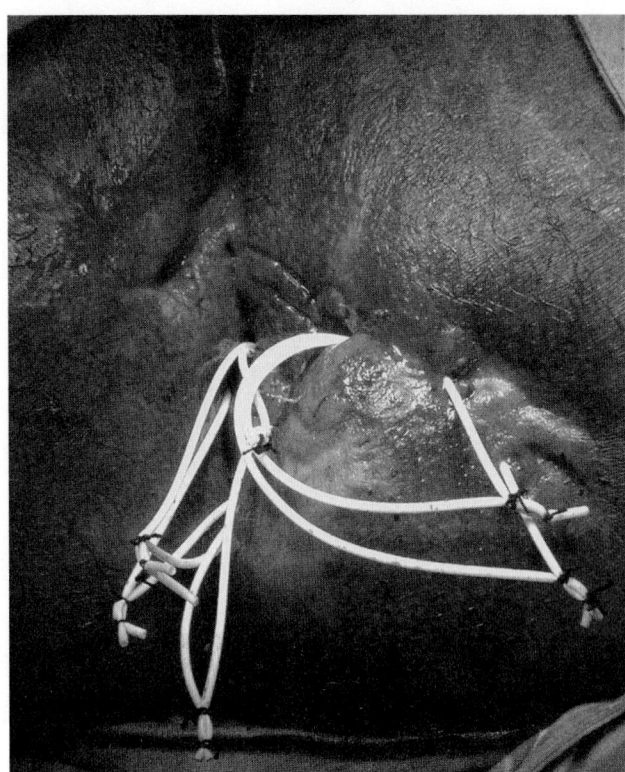

Figure 5 Multiple complex anorectal fistulae resulting from Crohn's disease.

Johnson EK, Gaw JU, Armstrong DN: Efficacy of anal fistula plug vs. fibrin glue in closure of anorectal fistulae, *Dis Colon Rectum* 49:371, 2006.
Loungnarath R, Dietz DW, Mutch MG, and others: Fibrin glue treatment of complex anal fistulae has low success rate, *Dis Colon Rectum* 47:432, 2004.
Pemberton JH: Anorectal sepsis. In Keighley MRB, Pemberton JH, Fazio VW, and others, editors, *Atlas of colorectal surgery*, New York, 1996, Churchill Livingstone.

ANORECTAL STRICTURE

John G. Carson, MD, and Michael J. Stamos, MD

INTRODUCTION

Anal stenosis refers to a nonspecific narrowing of the anal canal, whereas anal stricture is the result of the replacement of normal pliable anal canal and anoderm with scarring, tumor, or inflammation. Anorectal stricture refers to a narrowing in the anal canal as bordered by the anal verge at the caudal end and the pelvic floor at the cranial end. Anorectal stricture is most commonly caused by postoperative scarring, although the potential etiologies are numerous. Table 1 lists the more common causes of anorectal strictures.

ETIOLOGY

Anal stricture is most often iatrogenic but may be secondary to such diverse entities as hemorrhoidectomy, excision of low rectal tumors, resection of perianal skin lesions, trauma, inflammatory bowel disease, sexually transmitted diseases, chronic diarrhea, local radiation

therapy, and scarring after manual anal dilatation. A classic example is found as a complication after a Whitehead hemorrhoidectomy, now rarely performed. In this procedure, hemorrhoids are excised by a circumferential incision to remove all hemorrhoid tissue. A mucosal defect (ectropion) may result, often associated with an anorectal stricture that is commonly referred to as a Whitehead deformity. In one somewhat older series of 212 patients, anal stenosis was the result of hemorrhoid surgery in 87.7% of the cases, and

Table 1: Causes of Anorectal Stricture

Previous Surgery	Miscellaneous	Neoplasia
Fistulae	Sphincter hypertrophy	Bowen's disease
Hemorrhoids	Inflammatory bowel disease	Paget's disease
Fissures	Laxative abuse	Verrucous carcinoma
	Trauma	Squamous cell carcinoma
	Tuberculosis	Giant condyloma acuminata
	Sexually transmitted diseases	

Table 2: Classification of Anorectal Stricture

Based on Severity	Based on Level of Stenosis
Mild: tight anal canal can be examined by a well-lubricated finger or a medium Hill-Ferguson retractor	Low: distal anal canal at least 0.5 cm below the dentate line
Moderate: forceful dilatation is required to insert either the index finger or a medium Hill-Ferguson retractor	Middle: 0.5 cm proximal to 0.5 cm distal to the dentate line
Severe: neither the little finger nor the small Hill-Ferguson retractor can be inserted without forceful dilatation	High: proximal to 0.5 cm above the dentate line

current "open" hemorrhoidectomy procedures will result in postoperative anal stenosis up to 5% of the time, although most resolve with conservative therapy. Stapled hemorrhoidectomy or hemorrhoidopexy results in anal or rectal stenosis in approximately 3% of cases, the majority of which resolve without specific therapy.

DIAGNOSIS

Common patient complaints include difficulty with defecation, diminishing stool caliber, incomplete rectal emptying (clustering of bowel movements), and occasionally tenesmus. Sufferers have frequently resorted to laxatives, enemas, and suppositories to achieve short-term relief. Such symptomatic treatment may often worsen the situation and allow a stenosis to progress to a stricture resulting from the lack of chronic dilatation achieved with proper stool bulk. Physical examination findings are typically notable for the physician's being unable to perform an adequate digital examination. Findings often demonstrate a conical narrowing of the anal canal. Examination often must be performed under anesthesia to arrive at a definite diagnosis and treatment plan. A symptomatic anorectal stricture warrants treatment, with the type of treatment dependent on the severity, the exact location, and the comorbid features of the patient. Any history of predisposing factors, such as previous anorectal surgery, laxative abuse, sexually transmitted disease, and inflammatory bowel disease should be obtained. Additionally, any element of anal incontinence should be noted and graded by severity.

Anal stricture should be classified to degree of severity as well as location and length or extent of the anal canal. Classification allows more accurate comparison of treatment outcomes and selection of appropriate therapy.

Table 2 describes a useful classification of anorectal strictures, with severity ranging from mild to severe and location based on relationship of the stricture to the dentate line. The location may include more than one level for long strictures.

TREATMENT

Medical Treatment

Conservative treatment has often included trials of laxatives, suppositories, and enemas. These methods may temporarily relieve symptoms but often worsen the situation and do not treat the narrowed canal. Fiber and bulk agents are more appropriate because they act to chronically dilatation the canal. Bulk agents may also be helpful to maintain an adequate lumen in the posttreatment period if surgical correction or dilatation is necessary.

Anal dilatation may be used with mixed results. Except for mild cases, typically the initial dilatation is performed with the patient under anesthesia, followed by self-digitation or dilatator use at home. This may be an effective treatment for mild to moderate strictures. In addition, this may have a role in patients who are less than optimal operative candidates, such as elderly or infirm patients, those with Crohn's disease, or those with prior pelvic radiation. Dilatation may also be useful following operative repair of a stricture (e.g., anoplasty), if results are not ideal. In this situation, dilatation would not be used until 6 to 8 weeks or longer following operation. Some studies have found dilatation to be responsible for incontinence, however, leading to another problem; thus avoiding dilatation that is too forceful is key. Other complications of manual dilatation under anesthesia include hematoma formation in the sphincter, which could result in fibrosis and progressive stenosis.

Surgical Treatment

Many operative procedures for correction of anal stricture have been described. The various forms range from excision of eschar and stricturotomy/sphincterotomy to anoplasty with cutaneous advancement flap.

Excision of Eschar and Stricturotomy/Strictureplasty

For a patient with a mild to moderate degree of short-length stricture, the fibrous tissue may be incised or excised. The resultant defect may be closed transversely to avoid recurrence (strictureplasty). For narrow "weblike" strictures resulting from ileoanal or coloanal anastomosis, multiple stricturotomies in all four "quadrants" with dilatation can be an effective means of management. Additionally, although not truly a stricture, a "functional" anal stenosis often complicates an anal fissure and may be treated with topical therapy, injections of Botox (Allergan, Irvine, CA), or a classic lateral sphincterotomy.

Advancement Flaps

Many types of anoplasty have been described. All share the common theory of excision of scar tissue with movement of normal local tissue into a surgically created defect to prevent restricturing. The success of the flap depends on the basic theory of flap transfer: tension-free advancement with preservation of maximal flap blood supply. The flaps that we describe here are as follows: Martin's flap anoplasty, Y-V, V-Y, house, diamond, U-flaps, and C-plasty and S-plasty flaps. The Lone Star retractor (Lone Star Medical Products, Stafford, TX) has been instrumental in facilitating essentially all of the operative approaches with minimization of anal dilatation and thus subsequent defecation disturbances.

Martin's flap anoplasty

Mucosal advancement flap or Martin's flap anoplasty is particularly useful for high strictures. An oval-shaped defect results from a longitudinal incision with or without excision of the scar. An internal sphincterotomy may be performed if functional stenosis is also present, although this increases the risk of continence disturbance. The anal mucosa above the defect is elevated, advanced, and then sutured at the distal edge of the defect with absorbable sutures. An ectropion may result if the flap is advanced too far and sutured to the anal verge. Success rates of 70% to 80% can be expected with good patient selection. This flap may be combined with a house or other cutaneous flap for long strictures (see Fig. 1).

Y-V flap

This option also begins with an elliptical longitudinal incision/excision of the strictured area. This is the base of the Y. Next a flap of perianal skin is raised, forming the open tip of the Y. The flap is then advanced cranially into the surgical defect and secured with absorbable sutures to result in a V-shaped closure (see Fig. 2).

V-Y, house, diamond, and U-flaps

The V-Y, house, diamond, and U-flaps are based on the anoderm or perianal skin located distal to the strictured area. The flap shape

Figure 1 Mucosal (Martin's) advancement flap: longitudinal incision is made over the strictured area in anal canal. Proximal rectal and anal mucosa are then undermined through transverse incision starting at the proximal end of a previously made longitudinal incision. The flap is then sutured to the distal edge of internal anal sphincter, leaving open the most distal aspect of the wound. *From Liberman H, Thorson AG: Am J Surg 179:325, 2000, with permission from Excerpta Medica, Inc.*

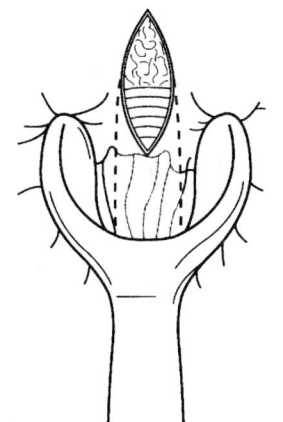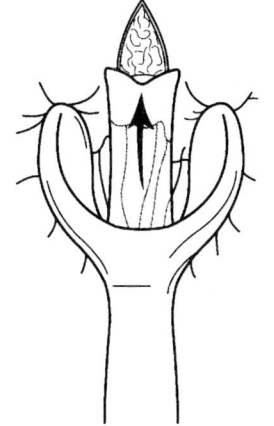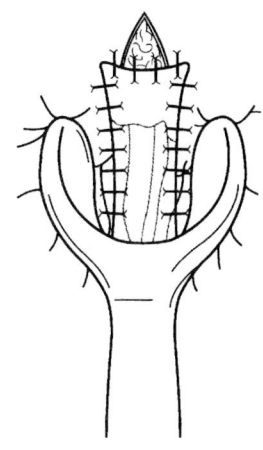

Figure 2 Y-V flap: an initial relaxing incision is made overlying the area of the stricture. This corresponds to the vertical limb of the Y. Distally, diagonal limbs of the Y are created in the perianal area, and the resultant flap, in the shape of a V, is sutured to the apex of the relaxed wound. *From Liberman H, Thorson AG: Am J Surg 179:325, 2000, with permission from Excerpta Medica, Inc.*

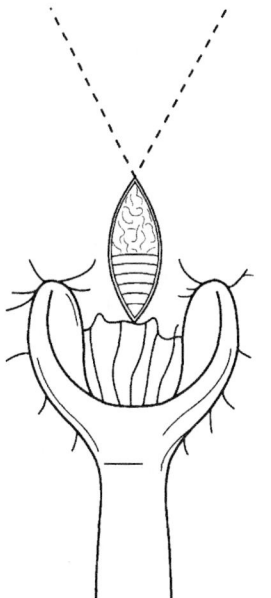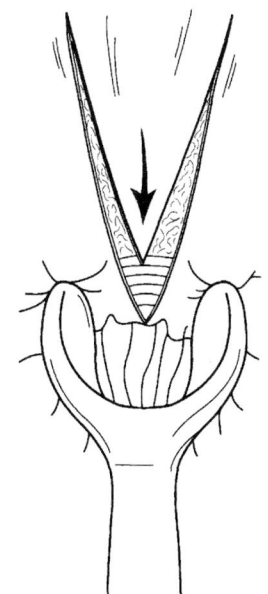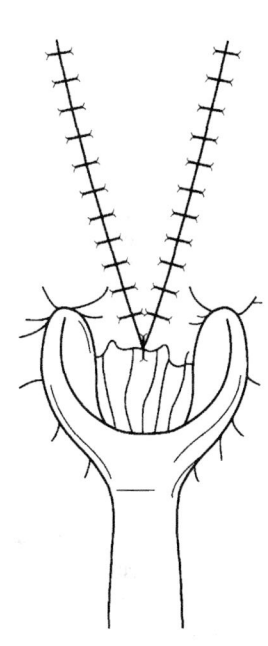

and dimensions vary; however, the techniques and principles are the same. The house, diamond, and U-flaps allow for more tissue to be transferred into the stenosed canal than the V-Y or Y-V flaps and theoretically are thought to provide a better repair, particularly for longer and higher strictures. The house flap in particular provides greater coverage of the anal canal. The strictured area is incised, and the scar is excised. The flap is then marked out, and the edges are incised; then the entire flap is advanced based on its subcutaneous blood supply. The incisions around the flap must be through the skin down to the underlying fat or muscle to ensure easy advancement. Absorbable sutures are used to secure the flap in place. The donor site is most often closed primarily, although if necessary, grafted tissue may be used or the defect may be allowed to heal by secondary intention. These flaps may be performed bilaterally for more severe strictures and combined with mucosal advancement flaps for longer strictures (see Fig. 3).

C and S rotation flaps

Extensive recurrent strictures may be repaired with S-plasty and C-plasty flaps. S-flaps were described by Ferguson for the treatment of extensive anal stenosis associated with Whitehead deformity. These flaps require larger incisions and are therefore less frequently used. They may be particularly useful following failure of more conservative advancement flaps. Once the flaps are made, they are then rotated into place and secured with absorbable sutures. The donor site is closed primarily (Fig. 4).

Postoperative Care

Most flaps are performed as an inpatient procedure, with a 1-night stay primarily for pain control. Preoperative mechanical bowel preparation is typically used, and parenteral antibiotics are recommended; however, postoperative antibiotics are not used. Patients should be placed on a high-fiber diet and encouraged to increase fluid consumption; 30 ml mineral oil daily for the first 2 to 3 days will facilitate the first bowel movement without excessive trauma or pain. Ketoralac and other narcotic-sparing pain medications are used to avoid postoperative constipation. Local wound care with brief sitz baths is used after the first 72 hours, and showers are taken for hygiene and comfort. Topical anesthetic may be used for the first 2 weeks. Patients should follow up in 14 to 21 days.

Results

A list of common complications of surgical repair may be found in Table 3, although the most common significant problems are failure with restricture and fecal incontinence. Most procedures may be performed with good results (success rates of 70% to 80% can be expected) and few complications. Minor incontinence fortunately is usually temporary (see subsequent discussion). Most complications may be treated with conservative management, depending on the severity.

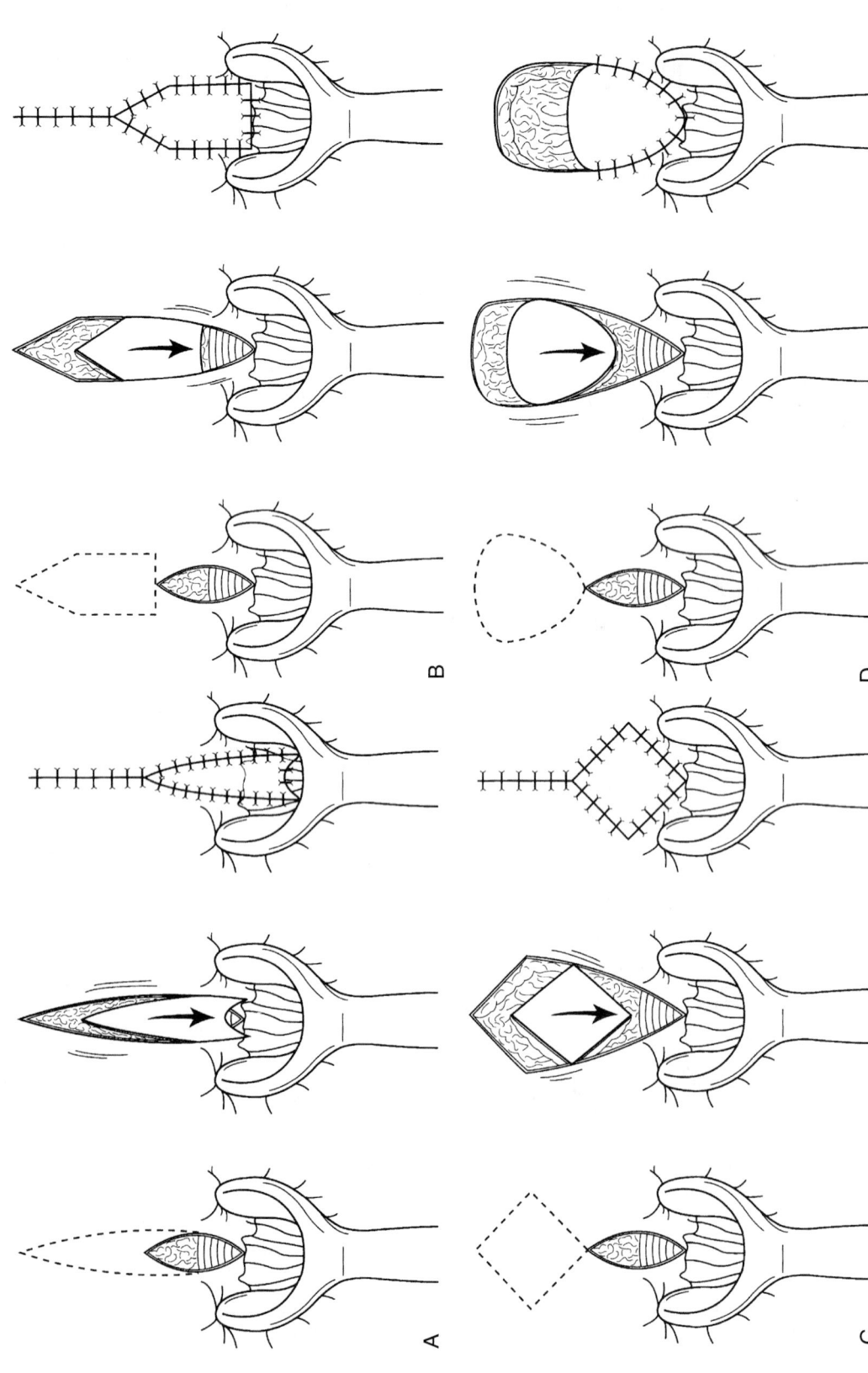

Figure 3 **(A)** V-Y flap: after a longitudinal incision is made over the strictured area, a V-shaped incision is made in perianal skin, with the wide area of the V oriented proximally into the anal canal. The resultant island of tissue is advanced into the anal canal and sutured in place. The donor site is then closed, leaving the inverted Y configuration of final suture lines. **(B)** House flap: after an incision is made overlying the strictured area, a transverse incision is made at each end of the initial incision and the edges undermined, allowing the wound to assume a rectangular shape. The flap is then configured in perianal skin in the shape of a house. The base is oriented proximally and the roof distally. Walls of the house are of the same length as the initial incision made in the anal canal. The width of the flap is designed to accommodate the width of the rectangular wound. The island of tissue is mobilized into a defect in the anal canal and sutured in place with 2–0 absorbable sutures. The roof of the house allows the donor site to be primarily closed with 3–0 absorbable sutures. **(C)** Diamond flap: This method follows the same principles as a V-Y flap. The difference is that a diamond-shaped island of tissue is advanced into the anal canal. After adequate mobilization of the island flap, it is sutured in place in the anal canal. **(D)** U-flap: an incision used to mobilize tissue to cover the strictured area has the shape of a broad U. After adequate mobilization of the island flap, it is sutured in place in the anal canal. *From Liberman H, Thorson AG: Am J Surg 179:325, 2000, with permission from Excerpta Medica, Inc.*

Figure 4 Rotational S-plasty: Areas of scar tissue within the anal canal are excised. A full-thickness flap in the shape of an S is configured in the perianal area. After adequate mobilization is achieved, the flap is rotated to cover the resulting defect in the anal canal. *From Liberman H, Thorson AG: Am J Surg 179:325, 2000, with permission from Excerpta Medica, Inc.*

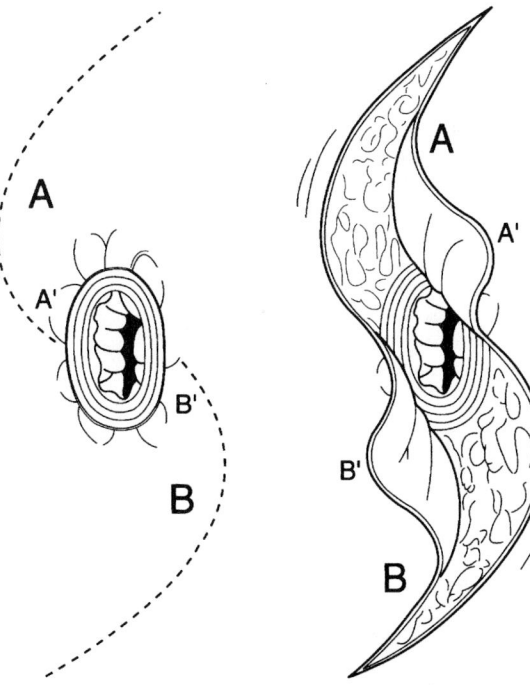

Table 3: Complications of Surgical Repair of Anorectal Stricture

Flap necrosis	Hematoma	Hypertrophic scar
Suture line disruption	Ectropion	Ischemic contracture
Restenosis	Abscess	Fecal incontinence
Urinary tract infection	Chronic pain	Fistula

Special Considerations

Patients with inflammatory bowel disease are at higher risk of failure and must be made aware of this. In the presence of active inflammatory bowel disease, the repair should be delayed to first achieve optimal medical management. In an immunocompromised patient, such as an HIV-positive patient with an acceptable CD-4 count and a low viral load, anoplasty may still be an acceptable option; however, a transplant patient may be best treated in a more conservative fashion (e.g., dilatation or diversion). Diabetes and smoking lead synergistically to treatment failure. Operative treatment should be held until glucose is controlled and smoking cessation achieved. Patients with history of prior radiation to either the perineum or pelvis are at the highest risk for failure. Adequate counseling must be made available with alternative treatment options.

Sphincter Function and Continence

Before operative repair, many patients have some soilage resulting from imperfect anal closure from local scar tissue. These symptoms are resolved after surgery in many patients, although this is difficult if not impossible to predict. If a sphincter is nonfunctional or poorly functional before surgery, it will most likely be so after repair. Current recommendations do not include anal manometry or anal ultrasound before repair; in fact these are often impossible or unreliable because of the local anatomy. Most incontinence that will improve will do so within 4 to 6 weeks after repair. Incontinence that persists beyond this time should be evaluated and treated if possible.

SUGGESTED READINGS

Ferguson J: Repair of "Whitehead deformity" of the anus, *Surg Gynecol Obstet* 108:115, 1959.
Khubchandani IT: Anal stenosis, *Surg Clin North Am* 741353, 1994.
MacDonald A, Smith A, McNeill AD, and others: Manual dilatation of the anus, *Br J Surg* 79:1381, 1992.
Milsom JW, Mazier WP: Classification and management of postsurgical anal stenosis, *Surg GynecolObstet* 163:60, 1986.
Trevisani G, Hyman N: Surgical options for anal stenosis, *Sem Colon Rectal Surg* 8:46, 1997.

PRURITUS ANI

Christopher Kenyon, MD, and Anthony
R. MacLean, MD

INTRODUCTION

Pruritus ani refers to itching and burning of the perianal skin. These symptoms can be troublesome and embarrassing for the patient, and they are often refractory to initial attempts at treatment. The diagnosis and management of this condition can also be challenging for the physician. Patients may present with perianal pruritus for which there is no identifiable etiology (idiopathic pruritus ani) or with pruritus that is secondary to another primary colorectal or perianal disease, dermatologic condition, or infectious etiology. This chapter reviews the causes of anal pruritus and the approach to managing the patient with pruritus ani.

PREVALENCE AND ETIOLOGY OF THE CONDITION

Pruritus ani is a relatively common disorder that typically affects individuals between the ages of 30 and 70. It is estimated that 1% to 5% of the population are afflicted with this condition, and males are more commonly affected than females, with a ratio of 4:1. The prevalence of anal pruritus in the population is likely higher than that seen in clinical practice. Many individuals do not seek medical attention for this symptom complex, nor for many other conditions involving the anorectum, because of concerns related to social embarrassment. A telephone survey by Nelson and Abcarian of a random sample of the general population between the ages of 50 and 65 demonstrated that 20% of individuals had ongoing symptoms attributable to anorectal disorders and that the majority of these individuals had not sought medical attention.

Pruritus ani may be localized to a defined area, or it may be widespread in the perianal region. Symptom onset is typically gradual. Often the burning sensation is worse at night or in warm, moist climates. This is an unpleasant and troubling sensation that often leads to scratching or self-medication with over-the-counter topical preparations. Unfortunately, scratching and the use of these ointments may actually exacerbate the problem and result in excoriation of the perianal skin.

Pruritus ani is frequently classified into two groups: primary or idiopathic pruritus ani and secondary pruritus ani. Secondary causes include fistula-in-ano, anal fissures, hemorrhoids, rectal prolapse, fecal incontinence, and colorectal and anal neoplasia. It is important to point out that the itching sensation is typically more severe, persistent, and of shorter duration in individuals presenting with anorectal malignancy. Pruritus ani may also be secondary to dermatologic conditions including contact dermatitis, psoriasis, and lichen sclerosis or occur in conjunction with various bacterial, viral, and parasitic infections.

Most authors feel that pruritus ani is most commonly idiopathic and not due to an underlying anorectal condition. However, Daniel and colleagues challenged this notion when they identified a cohort of patients with pruritus ani and followed them for 2 years, attempting to identify how frequently anal pruritus was associated with anorectal malignancy. In their study, 25% of patients had primary, or idiopathic pruritis ani, whereas 75% had a concomitant anorectal cause for their symptoms. Of these patients, 20% suffered from hemorrhoids and 12% had an anal fissure. Rectal cancer was present in 11% of these individuals, anal cancer was found in 6%, adenomatous polyps were noted in 4%, and colon cancer was found in 2%.

PATIENT EVALUATION

The evaluation of a patient with pruritus ani should start with a careful history and physical examination. Patients should be questioned about abdominal pain, altered bowel habits, and rectal bleeding. Rectal bleeding or symptoms suggestive of a change in bowel habit should be appropriately investigated. Recommended investigations include colonoscopy or barium enema, particularly for individuals older than age 40 or with a family or personal history of colorectal cancer. The history should also focus on potential causes of the symptoms, including dietary factors such as coffee consumption, alcohol consumption, and use of tobacco and medications, as well as systemic causes including diabetes mellitus, liver disease, and blood dyscrasias such as aplastic anemia and leukemia (Table 1). A careful physical examination should include visual inspection of the perianal skin, as well as a digital rectal examination, anoscopy, and sigmoidoscopy. Any suspicious lesions should be biopsied. This can usually be accomplished with a simple punch biopsy of the involved skin. Acute pruritus ani often presents with a symmetric area of erythema around the anal opening, whereas chronic pruritus ani is often associated with areas of pale macerated skin, edema, and radial thickening. Pruritus can be further classified using the Washington Hospital criteria as follows: stage I consists of skin that is red and inflamed; stage II consists of white, lichenified skin; and stage III involves lichenified skin coincident with coarse ridges of skin and ulceration.

Table 1: Etiology of Idiopathic Anal Pruritus

Local Irritants

Fecal
Poor hygiene
Diet (coffee, tea, cola, chocolate, citrus fruits, spicy foods, tomatoes, beer, dairy products)
Drugs (mineral oil, docusate)

Moisture

Obesity
Heat
Athletic activity
Snug underwear

Miscellaneous

Excessive wiping with toilet paper
Soaps
Perfumes
Topical medications/"-caine" anesthetics
Witch hazel
Drugs (colchicines, quinidine, tetracycline, erythromycin)

TREATMENT

Idiopathic Pruritus Ani

Idiopathic or primary pruritus ani is a challenging and frustrating problem for both the patient and the clinician. Patients frequently have long-standing symptoms and have used a variety of prescription and over-the-counter treatments. The exact inciting agent in these cases has not been well defined, but various irritants have been implicated. Fecal soilage has been implicated as a causative agent in many patients. Feces contain endopeptidases of bacterial origin, as well as other potential allergens and bacteria. These enzymes are capable of causing irritation and pruritus. As such, any condition resulting in fecal soiling of the perianal region may be a potential cause of pruritus ani. This includes fistula-in-ano, fecal incontinence, chronic diarrhea, and poor anal hygiene.

Certain medications are known to cause pruritus ani. Among the most common agents associated with the condition are colchicine, quinidine, tetracycline, and erythromycin. Other agents that result in loosening of stool or diarrhea may cause or exacerbate a pruritic response. This includes stool-softening agents such as mineral oil and docusate. In addition, any agent that induces a histamine release has the potential to cause anal pruritus.

Some foods have been implicated in pruritus ani. Frequently associated foods include coffee, cola, tea, chocolate, spicy foods, citrus foods, and others. It is unclear how these foods may result in perianal irritation, but there are a few proposed mechanisms. Caffeinated products may contribute to perianal irritation by acting in a fashion similar to the way they are believed to act in exacerbations of gastroesophageal reflux disorder; that is, they may cause transient, inappropriate relaxation of the internal anal sphincter. Other irritants such as spicy foods, citrus foods, and tomatoes may alter the pH of stool, resulting in local perianal irritation.

A patient deemed to have idiopathic pruritus ani can be difficult to manage clinically. However, the majority should respond to conservative measures and reassurance about the benign nature of their

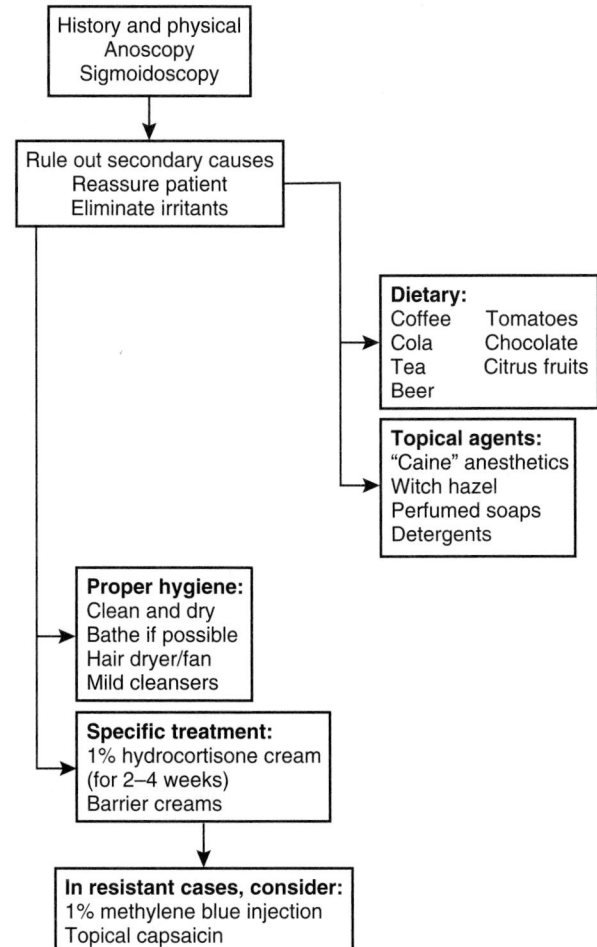

Figure 1 Treatment algorithm for pruritus.

medications may offer some relief of symptoms when applied at bedtime and may prevent nocturnal itching and scratching.

A minority of patients do not respond to conservative measures. For these individuals, a variety of therapies have been attempted. Local irradiation and perianal skin excision are among the more radical procedures that have been described, and in general should be avoided. Local methylene blue injection for these patients has been described. A recent report documented the experience of 30 patients undergoing treatment with a 1% local injection of methylene blue. In this small study, 24 patients (80%) described relief of their symptoms. Originally described in the 1960s, the therapy is thought to destroy dermal nerve endings in the perianal skin, thereby offering relief. The most frequent side effect was a sensation of numbness that resolved over a period of a few weeks. Another small study showed similar benefit; however, the patients all had persistent perianal numbness.

Topical capsaicin has also shown some benefit in patients with intractable pruritus ani. Capsaicin is a natural alkaloid derived from plants of the Solanaceae family. It is a commonly used and safe anti-itch medication. The exact mechanism of action is unknown, but capsaicin is thought to have a depressant effect on the synthesis, release, and storage of substance P. Substance P is a neuropeptide that mediates the pain and itching sensations from the periphery to the central nervous system. A clinical trial demonstrated benefit in 31 of 44 patients. Patients applied a thin layer of a capsaicin cream three times a day. Four patients left the study because of a burning sensation upon application of the cream. However, there were no other major side effects attributed to capsaicin therapy. Twenty-nine patients were applying capsaicin once daily and described themselves as symptom free at a mean follow-up time of 8 months.

Secondary Pruritus Ani

Infectious Causes

Pruritus ani may occur secondarily to certain infectious conditions (Table 2). Bacteria, viruses, and parasites are all capable of inciting a pruritic reaction. Erythrasma is a cutaneous bacterial infection caused by the organism *Corynebacterium minutissimum*. This commonly presents with mild brownish-red scaling lesions in the inguinal folds and perianal skin. A Woods lamp will demonstrate an intense coral-red fluorescence of the lesion. Other common perianal bacterial infections are caused by beta-hemolytic streptococci groups A, B, and G. This is a superficial skin infection with an eczema-like appearance. Hidradenitis suppuritiva, caused by gram-positive organisms, can also lead to cellulitis and itching. Antibiotics may improve the course of all of these conditions; hidradenitis may require surgical excision, however.

Viral infections such as herpes simplex and human papillomavirus can lead to pruritus ani. In particular, condylomata acuminate can cause functional changes of the anal sphincter, leading to minor fecal leakage and subsequent itching. Herpes simplex is characterized by small, painful vesicles during an eruption and can be treated with oral acyclovir. Condylomata are treated with topical podophylline, topical 5-fluorouracil, cryotherapy, or surgical excision or fulguration.

The most common parasitic infection resulting in pruritus ani is that caused by *Enterobius vermicularis*, or pinworms. The hallmark of pinworm infection is nocturnal pruritus. The diagnosis can be made by microscopic evaluation of cellophane tape applied to the perianal region. Treatment consists of mebendazole for both the affected individual and all family members.

Dermatologic Causes

The most common dermatologic causes of pruritus ani are contact dermatitis, lichen sclerosus et atrophicus, and psoriasis

problem. Conservative strategies should begin by eliminating possible irritating factors, both dietary and pharmaceutical—that is, topical or systemic medications. Dietary modification should include removing possible irritants from the diet, although there is no good evidence that this is effective. Foods such as milk that may promote loose stools should also be removed from the diet of susceptible patients. A high-fiber diet should be encouraged because this may promote bulking of the stool and reduce fecal leakage and soiling. Appropriate perianal hygiene should be instituted. The goal of hygienic therapy should be to keep the perianal skin clean and dry, to remove any fecal debris, and to avoid injuring the skin by excessive wiping. Harsh cleansing agents or soaps should be avoided. Patients may find it helpful to bathe after defecation if possible. Other strategies may include the use of medicated wipes or premoistened tissues. Drying the area with a fan or hair dryer can be helpful, although somewhat difficult to accomplish. Patients should avoid vigorous rubbing because this may damage the skin and promote breakdown of the epidermis. A small randomized trial comparing the use of topical steroids to a mild cleansing agent demonstrated that maintaining good hygiene relieved the symptoms of patients with idiopathic pruritus ani as effectively as a topical steroid (Fig. 1).

Further conservative strategies for patients with idiopathic pruritus ani include the use of a 1% topical steroid cream. This can be applied twice daily to relieve symptoms and promote healing. Prolonged use of topical steroids may cause thinning and atrophy of the skin; therefore they should be used over a limited time span. Topical anti-itch

Table 2: Etiology of Secondary Pruritus Ani

Colorectal and Anal Causes

Hemorrhoids

Fistula-in-ano

Anal fissure

Hidradenitis suppurativa

Pilonidal sinus

Perianal Crohn's disease

Anal neoplasms

Anal canal cancer

Anal margin cancer

Paget's disease

Bowen's disease

Rectal neoplasms

Rectal adenoma

Rectal cancer

Rectal prolapse

Fecal incontinence

Chronic diarrhea

Dermatologic Causes

Contact dermatitis

Lichen sclerosis

Psoriasis

Radiation dermatitis

Other

Infectious Causes

Bacterial

Erythrasma (*Corynebacterium minutissimum*)

Staphylococcus aureus

Streptococci groups A, B, and G

Gonococcus

Chlamydia

Syphilis

Viral

Herpes virus

Human papillomavirus

Mulloscum contagiosum

Parasitic

Pinworms (*Enterobius vermicularis*)

Scabies

Fungal

Candida

Systemic Causes

Diabetes mellitus

Liver disease, jaundice

Leukemia

Aplastic anemia

Lymphoma

(see Table 2). Psoriasis does not commonly affect the perianal region, but when it does, it occurs in the pattern of so-called reverse psoriasis. The rash is scaly and asymmetric. Treatment should be undertaken in consultation with a dermatologist.

Contact or allergic dermatitis may be due to a number of possible irritants. It may be associated with mild soaps, deodorant sprays, perfumes, or alcohols contained in feminine hygiene products. More commonly it is associated with repeated exposure to topical medications, including the local anesthetics of the "caine" group, antibiotics, or antihistamines contained in many of the topical preparations used to treat itching and hemorrhoidal-type symptoms. Contact with allergens such as "poison oak" and "poison ivy" may also cause pruritus ani. In persistent cases, a search for possible offending agents should be made, patch tests considered, and any potential inciting agents avoided.

Lichen sclerosis is a condition thought to be caused by cell-mediated autoimmunity that progresses from an intensely itchy erythematous reaction into a thickened, indurated, slightly raised macular reaction. It most commonly affects perimenopausal women and is associated with involvement of the vulva and vagina in 60% of female patients. Dermatologic consultation should be sought in these cases also.

Anorectal Causes

Anal fissures, fistulae, hemorrhoids, and neoplasms can all result in pruritus ani (see Table 2). The itching sensation is often worse during and immediately after defecation. Fistulae cause pruritus because of the chronic irritation resulting from fluid draining from the external opening. Prolapsed hemorrhoids may also lead to a chronic drainage of mucus at the level of the perianal skin, resulting in irritation of the region. Additionally, prolapsing internal and external hemorrhoids may impair good hygiene, resulting in chronic irritation secondary to feces left in the folds of the perianal skin. Rectal prolapse may similarly result in a moist perianal environment, resulting in irritation and pruritus ani. Other conditions resulting in leakage of stool, such as fecal incontinence or chronic diarrhea, expose the perianal skin to the damaging products of stool, which may result in anal pruritus. Correction of the underlying anorectal condition should improve the irritation of the perianal region and resolve the itching.

In summary, pruritus ani is a common condition that can often be successfully diagnosed and treated with a careful and thorough approach. Treatment consists of identifying and addressing the cause, minimizing further injury of the perianal skin, and maintaining close follow-up with the patient to ensure healing and relief of symptoms.

Suggested Readings

Daniel GL, Longo WE, Vernava AM: Pruritus ani. Causes and concerns, *Dis Colon Rectum* 37:670, 1994.

Lysy J, Sistiery-Ittah, Israelit Y, and others: Topical capsaicin-a novel and effective treatment for idiopathic intractable pruritus ani: a randomized, placebo controlled, crossover study, *Gut* 53:1323, 2003.

Mentes BB, Akin M, Leventoglu S, and others: Intradermal methylene blue injection for the treatment of intractable idiopathic pruritus ani: results of 30 cases, *Tech Coloproctol* 8:11, 2004.

Nelson RL, Abcarian H, Davis FG, and others: Prevalence of benign anorectal disease in a randomly selected population, *Dis Colon Rectum* 38:341, 1995.

Oztas MO, Oztas P, Onder ML: Idiopathic perianal pruritus: washing compared with topical corticosteroids, *Postgrad Med Journal* 80:295, 2004.

FECAL INCONTINENCE

Madeleine Poirier, MD and Herand Abcarian, MD

INTRODUCTION

Fecal incontinence (FI) is a disabling disease with severe psychosocial implications. In general, it is defined as the involuntary passage of liquid, solid stool, or flatus. The impact on the quality of life for patients suffering from FI is significant and can lead to work absenteeism, depression, and social isolation. The true prevalence and incidence of FI is difficult to ascertain because of the embarrassment and social stigma leading to underreporting by affected patients. In the general population within the United States, FI is an important burden, and its prevalence has been estimated to be between 2% and 18%. In the elderly population, reports have observed prevalence as high as 60%. Because the U.S. population is aging, FI represents a rising public health concern.

ETIOLOGY

Basic understanding of pelvic floor anatomy is essential to appreciate the etiology and treatment of FI. Sphincter function, rectal sensation, adequate capacity and compliance, colonic transit time, stool consistency, and cognitive and neurologic function are all factors that influence continence. The sphincter mechanisms are the internal sphincter (IAS), the external anal sphincter (EAS), and the puborectalis muscle (PR). The IAS, an involuntary muscle, is the continuation of the smooth muscle of the rectum. It accounts for 80% of the resting pressure of the anal canal and is innervated by the autonomic nervous system (parasympathetic and sympathetic fibers). The rectoanal inhibitory reflect (RAIR) is defined as relaxation of the IAS secondary to rectal distention. The EAS is a voluntary muscle and is responsible for the squeeze pressure in maintaining continence. It is innervated by the pudendal nerve (S2, S3, and S4). The U-shaped PR muscle surrounds the rectum and is also innervated by the pudendal nerve. It maintains the rectoanal angle, which widens during defecation.

The IAS and EAS can be torn or divided during vaginal delivery, trauma, or anorectal surgery, leading to sphincter defect and possible fecal incontinence. The stretch of the pudendal nerve during delivery may lead to malfunction of the PR and EAS. The PR muscle may also form a more obtuse angle than normal in neurologic conditions such as spinal cord injury, thus leading to FI.

Compliance of the rectum is also important, and conditions that overdistend the rectum (fecal impaction) or decrease compliance (e.g., radiation therapy, chronic inflammation) combined with abnormal stool consistency may lead to FI. Table 1 summarizes the main etiologies of FI.

EVALUATION

History and Physical Examination

The first step in the evaluation of FI is a thorough history focused on symptomatology and quality of life. The distinction among seepage, poor hygiene, and FI can be easily made by

Table 1: Etiology of Incontinence

Postsurgical
Anorectal surgery
Sphincter saving operation
Obstetric Injury
Trauma (impalement, etc.)
Sphincter impairment
Procidentia
Imperforated anus
Radiation injury
Rectal cancer
Neurogenic
Trauma
Spinal cord injuries
Multiple sclerosis
Aging
Dementia
Diabetes
Miscellaneous
Fecal impaction
Chronic anorectal inflammation
Colitis/proctitis
Laxative abuse
Psychotropic drugs
Large prolapsing hemorrhoids
Idiopathic

obtaining a complete history. Consistency of the stool, aggravating factors, and diet are useful determinants of the patient's symptoms. The severity of the FI can also be easily obtained with the use of one of the validated incontinence scoring indices such as FISI (Fecal Incontinence Severity Index), the Wexner or Cleveland Clinic scoring system. These provide an objective assessment of the patient's incontinence. Validated quality-of-life questionnaires are also available for objective evaluation; the two most commonly used are the FIQL (Fecal Incontinence Quality of Life Questionnaire) and the SF-36. Neither of these questionnaires is perfect or universally applicable but, when used consistently by the same physician, they can be useful for assessment of FI.

Patient medical and surgical history such as previous anorectal surgery, trauma, obstetric injury (episiotomy, vaginal tears), and medical conditions such as diabetes, inflammatory bowel disease, dementia, and neurologic conditions may help to determine the contributing factors to FI.

Complete anorectal examination is mandatory in the evaluation of FI. Evaluation begins with the perianal skin, where signs of erythema, moisture, fecal soilage, previous scars, presence of cloaca, anal deformity (e.g., keyhole, Whitehead deformity, anal stenosis), fistula or mass can be assessed. Digital rectal examination is then performed to evaluate the presence of anal sphincter defect, stricture of the anal canal, or anal/rectal mass and to assess anal sphincteric resting and squeeze pressures, as well as the presence of rectal procidentia, rectocele, or mucosal prolapse.

Physiology Testing, Imaging, and Endoscopy

Anorectal physiology testing is a common adjunct in the evaluation algorithm of FI and can help to determine treatment. Anorectal manometry provides information about resting and squeeze pressure of the anal sphincter and helps to identify sphincter dysfunction in anatomically normal or abnormal sphincters. Pudendal nerve terminal motor latency study (PNTML) evaluates pudendal neuropathy, but its value might be less important as a diagnostic tool than in predicting therapeutic outcomes.

Endoanal ultrasound is the most useful imaging study in the evaluation of FI. Its accuracy has been repetitively validated in the literature. It provides a reliable means of identification of sphincter defects and should be used in all women with FI and previous vaginal deliveries. New reports on the use of magnetic resonance imaging with an endoanal coil for anal sphincter evaluation are appearing in the literature, but no studies have demonstrated a clear advantage over endoanal ultrasound. Defecography and flexible endoscopy (sigmoidoscopy and colonoscopy) can be used in selected patients on the basis of the history compatible with obstructed defecation and risk factors for malignancy.

TREATMENT

Nonsurgical

Dietary Manipulation and Pharmacology

First-line therapy in the management of mild FI is conservative and includes dietary manipulation. Patients are instructed to increase their dietary fiber to 30 g per day. This if often better accomplished with the help of fiber supplements. Avoidance of specific foods has been shown to improve mild symptoms of FI; the most common culprits include caffeine, chocolate, citrus fruits, spicy foods, and beer. Identification of allergy or intolerance to lactose or gluten and other malabsorption disorders should also be considered and treated accordingly. Some patients may benefit from regular consultations with a registered dietitian or nutritionist.

Opiate derivatives are the mainstay of the pharmacologic management of FI; these are antidiarrheal medications that can be taken orally, such as codeine, loperamide and diphenoxylate HCL, and tincture of opium. These all act via opiate receptors to slow down peristalsis, increase colonic transit time, and increase water reabsorption. Some studies have shown that loperamide may also increase anal pressure. Anticholinergics help slow colonic transit.

Regularly scheduled saline or tap-water enema may also help to maintain continence by emptying the rectum, and polyethylene glycol or lactulose can be used to treat constipation and fecal impaction, thus preventing overflow incontinence.

Biofeedback

The treatment of FI with biofeedback has been reported extensively in the literature. Initial studies observed an overall efficacy of biofeedback ranging from 50% to 90%, but most of these studies did not have a control group. A Cochrane review of the subject showed the paucity of eligible studies for comparison (only five) and concluded that the small number of studies and the weakness of their methodological and statistical analysis did not allow an adequate analysis of the efficacy of biofeedback in the management of FI. Norton and colleagues conducted a prospective randomized study comparing four treatment groups. No difference was found among any of the groups. Moreover, when the groups were stratified for evidence of obstetric injury (i.e., IAS or EAS defect), it did not correlate with the outcome. Other studies such as the one performed by Mahony and colleagues evaluated the success of biofeedback in the treatment of postobstetric injury FI. In this study, 96% of women had ultrasound evidence of EAS defect, and biofeedback showed significant improvement in incontinence as well as improvement in quality of life. However, a few studies have suggested that education alone may be sufficient to improve FI and quality of life and that biofeedback may be only as good as the enthusiasm of the therapist delivering the therapy. There has been concern about the possible time-related decay in the long-term benefit of biofeedback therapy. Although there is a paucity of data on this subject, a recent nonrandomized study has shown a sustained improvement in FI with biofeedback therapy alone. Biofeedback therapy for the treatment of FI is safe and in selected patients proves to be effective.

SURGICAL PROCEDURES

Sphincteroplasty

In patients in whom preoperative evaluation demonstrates a sphincter defect, surgical repair is the preferred treatment. The main indications include sphincter defect secondary to obstetric injury, trauma, or iatrogenic injury secondary to anorectal surgery. Our preferred method of sphincter repair (i.e., overlapping sphincteroplasty) includes a full preoperative mechanical bowel preparation, a single dose of perioperative antibiotic, and insertion of a Foley catheter. The operation is performed with the patient in the prone jackknife position under regional or general anesthesia. A dilute solution of lidocaine 0.5% with epinephrine (1:200,000) is injected subcutaneously along the length of the incision to assist with hemostasis. A "smiling" incision is made in the perineum and is extended laterally and cephalad. Skin and anodermal flaps are raised inferiorly and superiorly and retracted to provide optimal exposure. The rectovaginal septum is separated until the puborectalis muscle is palpated. The cut ends of the EAS are then identified and mobilized sufficiently to allow for a 2-cm overlap without tension. The IAS is identified, mobilized, and repaired in a vertical fashion with 2 to 3 interrupted absorbable sutures. An anterior levatorplasty is then performed by approximating the PR muscles in the midline with interrupted absorbable sutures. This recreates the perineal body by interposing a layer of muscle between the rectum and vagina. This is especially useful when a rectovaginal fistula is seen in association with sphincter injury. Overlapping sphincteroplasty is then performed. The EAS muscle overlap is created in a "vest over plants" fashion using absorbable mattress sutures, utilizing the scarred ends of the EAS. If the cut ends of the muscle are too far apart, simple reapproximation of the muscle can be performed with mattress sutures. Hemostasis is ensured to avoid hematoma formation and subsequent infection. The skin can be closed horizontally or vertically depending on the tension of the skin edges. Vertical mattress stitches of 3–0 absorbable material are used and the center part of the incision is left open to allow drainage. No drain is used (Fig. 1)

Patients are usually kept overnight for pain control and then sent home 24 to 48 hours after surgery with a strict bowel regimen of stool softeners, fiber supplements, and warm showers. Sitting should be avoided for 5 to 7 days. Complications from sphincteroplasty are uncommon but include bleeding, urinary retention, and infection.

Although the overlapping technique is most commonly used, no clear benefit is reported in the literature between overlapping versus approximation technique of sphincteroplasty. Continence after

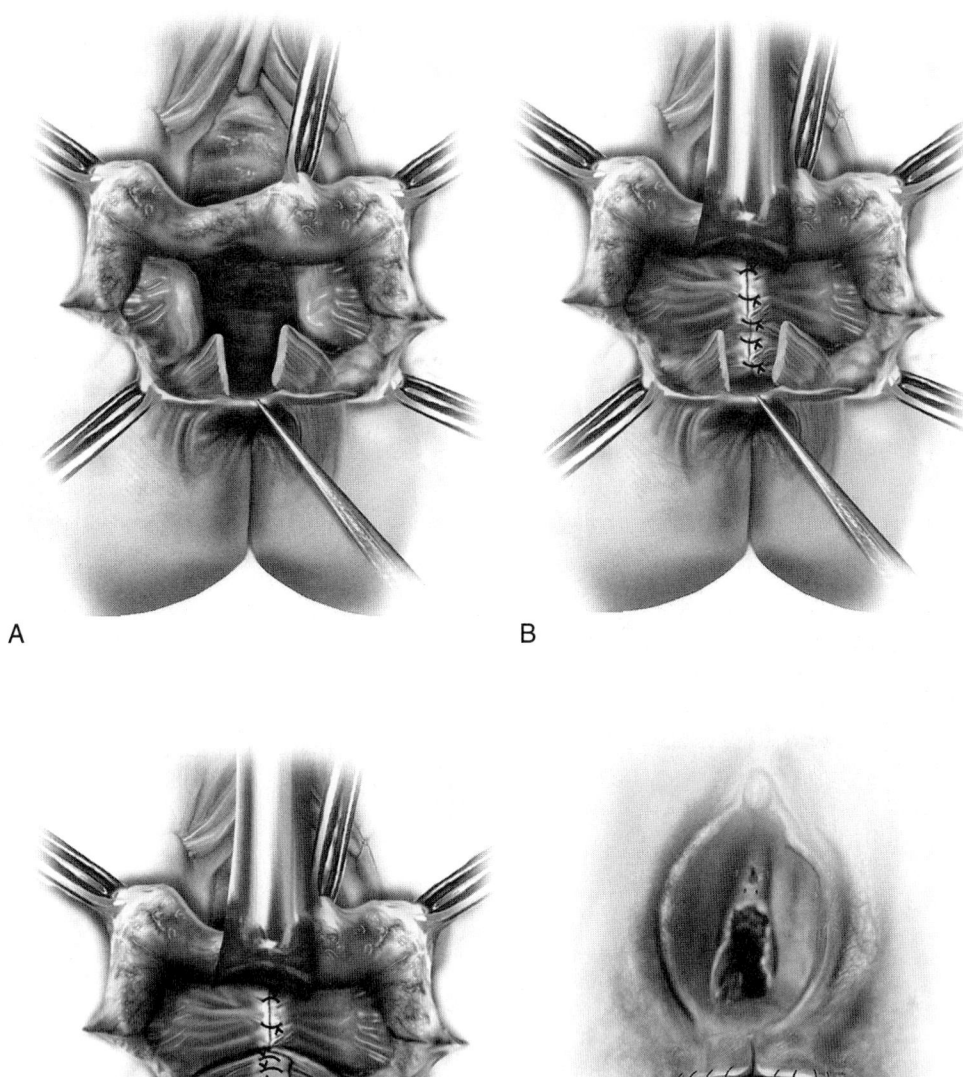

A

B

C

D

Figure 1 Sphincteroplasty. **(A)** The rectovaginal septum is dissected. **(B)** The puborectalis muscles are approximated in the midline. **(C)** The external sphincter is repaired in a vest over pants (overlapping) technique external sphincter repair. **(D)** The skin is partially closed to ensure drainage.

sphincteroplasty is excellent at short-term follow-up. Most studies demonstrate improved functional outcome of approximately 80% at 12 months. Most recently, a growing body of evidence demonstrated that the success of the procedure may deteriorate with time, and only half of patients remain satisfied with the procedure at 3 to 5 years follow-up.

Endoanal ultrasound can be performed in patients who complain of no improvement or recurrent symptoms postoperatively. If the repair is disrupted, patients may undergo a repeat sphincteroplasty; otherwise biofeedback therapy or sacral nerve stimulation are possible alternatives.

Muscle Transfer Procedures

Gracilis transposition was originally introduced by Pickrell in 1952. This was in reality a "living Thiersch" procedure, and the patients opened and closed the anal canal by abduction and adduction of the thigh. In 1986, the operation was modified to stimulated (dynamic) graciloplasty to include an implanted stimulator in the abdominal wall. The procedure involves harvest of the gracilis muscle from the thigh, using its distal end to encircle the anus and create a neosphincter. The stimulator, via chronic contraction, converts type II (fast-twitch muscle fibers) to type I (slow-twitch

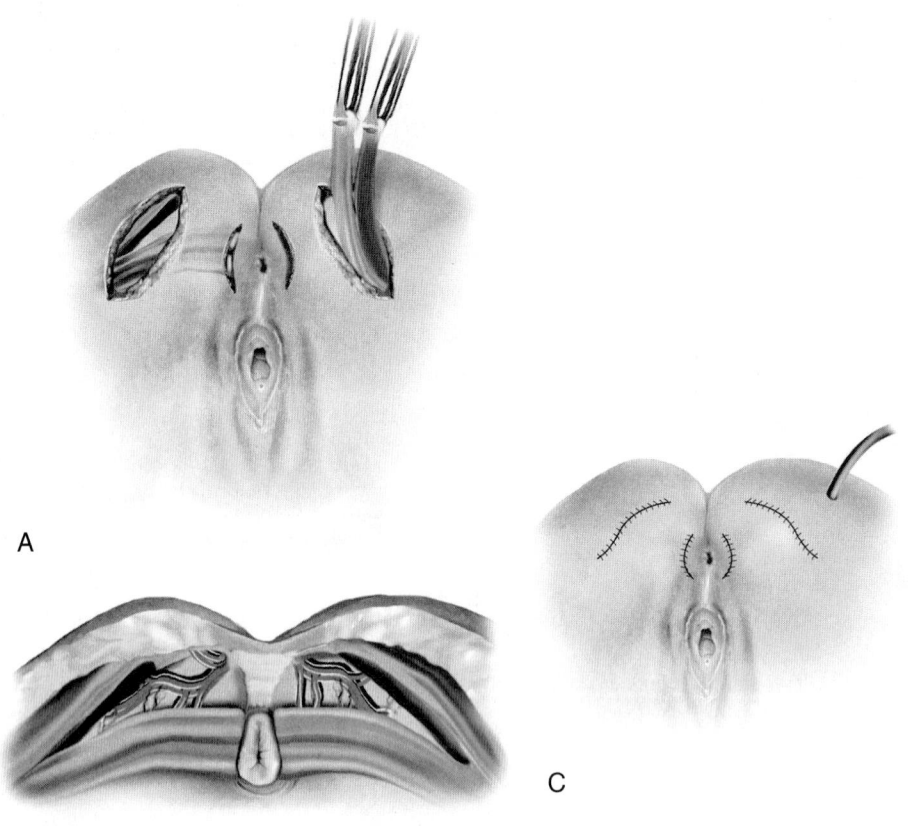

A

B

C

Figure 2   Gluteus maximus transfer. **(A)** Detached gluteus maximus muscle is bifurcated, rotated inferiorly, and then tunneled subcutaneously to encircle the anus. The ends of each of the bifurcated limbs from the same side are sutured together to form two opposing voluntary muscle slings. **(B)** Overview of the completed operation. Note the location of the neurovascular bundles *(arrow)*. When the body of the gluteus maximus muscle contracts, the anal canal is pulled posteriorly. **(C)** Suction drains are placed subcutaneously to evacuate the dead space created by the skin flaps in the postoperative period.   *From Pearl RK, Prasad ML, Nelson RL, and others:* Dis Colon and Rectum *34(6):478, 1991.*

muscle fibers), which are most resistant to fatigue. Long-term success of stimulated graciloplasty as measured by improvement in continence and quality of life, is seen in approximately 60% of patients. The morbidity of this procedure is significant, with infection being the most common complication and cause of failure. Some studies have demonstrated rates of complication as high as 74%. This procedure is still used in Europe and Canada but is no longer available in the United States.

Gluteus Maximus Transfer

Most patients contract their gluteus when asked to tighten their anal sphincters. This has led some surgeons to detach a section of the gluteus maximus from the coccyx and split the segment into two longitudinal strips. A subcutaneous tunnel is then constructed around the anal canal, and the strips of muscle on each side are inserted into this space anterior and posterior to the anal canal and then sutured to the strips from the opposite side, essentially surrounding the anal canal with gluteal muscle strips. The incisions are irrigated with antibiotic solution and closed. The operation may be performed under covering colostomy. Devesa and his colleagues reported improvement in continence in 67% of 20 patients with total incontinence (Fig. 2).

Novel Procedures

Sacral Nerve Stimulation

Sacral nerve stimulation (SNS) was initially used for the treatment of urinary incontinence but has been used for the treatment of FI

since 1995, and its popularity is rising as more data become available. SNS is indicated in patients suffering from FI with either normal or minimally damaged anal sphincters or patients with failed surgical repair. The exact mechanism(s) of action are unclear, but hypotheses are as follows: (1) effect is via efferent motor neuron leading to muscle contraction with stimulation and (2) effect is via regulation of rectal sensitivity and contractility via the sacral nerves. The procedure is performed in three stages. The first consists of identification of the sacral nerve roots, which optimally lead to contraction of the anal sphincter and pelvic floor muscles (S2–S4). This is performed in the operating room under general anesthesia. The second stage consists of a trial, between 1 and 2 weeks, of a temporary stimulator. If the patient's symptoms of FI improve, a permanent electrode and generator are implanted in the abdominal wall or buttock in the third stage (Fig. 3).

Results of SNS have been encouraging. Initial clinical studies reported an overall success rate of 80% with modest-sized cohorts. More recently, a multicenter study has confirmed these results. Although long-term data are lacking, the results of this low-morbidity procedure are encouraging. The most common complications of this procedure are the dislodgement of the electrodes and infection.

Artificial Bowel Sphincter

Patients who have failed medical or surgical therapy (or both) and those who are not candidates for sphincteroplasty, such as patients with extensive sphincter disruption from trauma, may be good candidates for the artificial bowel sphincter (ABS). The Acticon Neosphincter (American Medical Systems, Minnetonka, MN) is a completely implantable device. The ABS consists of three parts: the fluid-filled occlusive perianal cuff, a control pump, and a

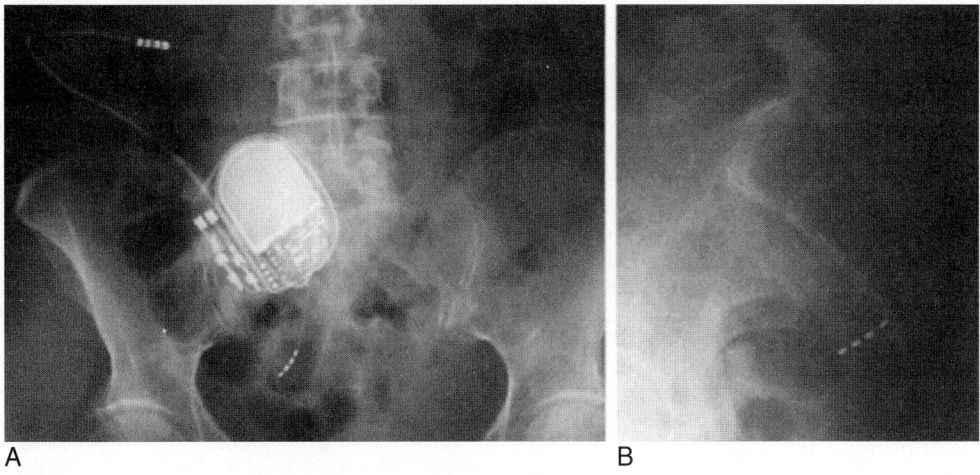

Figure 3 Sacral nerve stimulation. Anteroposterior and lateral x-ray demonstrating the permanent electrode on S3 and the impulse generator. *From Matzel KE, Kamm MA, Stösser M, and others: Lancet 363:1270, 2004.*

Figure 4 Functioning of the artificial bowel sphincter (ABS) **(A)** anal occlusion. Pressure is equilibrated throughout the system, ensuring pressurization of the cuff and thus automatic closure of the anal canal at a predetermined pressure level approximately equal to that of the pressure-regulating balloon selected for implantation. **(B)** Anal opening, controlled by the patient. The pressure equilibrium in the system is interrupted by the active transfer (manipulation of the control pump) of the fluid from the cuff to the pressure-regulating balloon. **(C)** Progressive anal closure (arrows indicate the direction of fluid transfers within the system after defecation). *Courtesy Paul-Antoine Lehr, MD, University Hospital of Nantes, Nantes, France.*

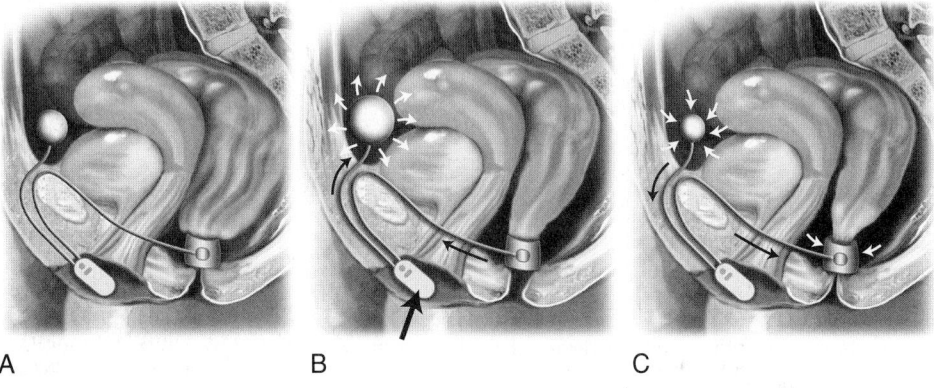

pressure-regulating balloon. The three parts are connected via kink-resistant tubing.

The function of the ABS is semiautomatic. Resting anal pressure is maintained by the occlusive perianal cuff via transmission of the pressure gradient from the pressure-regulated balloon located in the abdomen. Patients initiate defecation by applying 5 to 15 squeezes on the control pump, leading to transfer of fluid from the pressure-regulated balloon and allowing anal opening. Passive transfer of fluid from the pressure-regulated balloon to the cuff subsequently occurs within 5 to 8 minutes after anal opening and restores the resting anal pressure.

ABS is implanted under full mechanical bowel preparation, pre-operative skin care (2 povidone-iodine showers), single-dose peri-operative antibiotics, and with the patient in dorsal lithotomy position. A transverse perianal incision is made, and a tunnel is bluntly created around the anal canal. The ABS device is then prepared on a sterile back table while the length of the occlusive cuff is chosen with a sizer. A Pfannenstiel incision is made, and an extraperitoneal pocket is prepared underneath the rectus muscle. The perianal cuff is placed first, and a tunnel is created to reach the extraperitoneal pocket and place the pressure-regulated balloon. The abdominal incision is closed, and the control pump is placed in the scrotum or labium majora. All tubing is connected, and all skin incisions closed. The pump is deactivated and emptied at the end of the procedure for 8 weeks to allow for healing. The patient is then readmitted for 1 day for ABS activation. Teaching of the device use is provided at the same time (Fig. 4).

A multicenter cohort study of 112 patients demonstrated 85% successful outcome in patients who retained their ABS, whereas 51 patients (45%) and 41 patients (37%) required surgery for either revision or explantation. More recently (2003), the University of Minnesota published its experience with ABS; two groups of patients were identified, those receiving ABS between 1989 and 1992 ($n = 10$) and those who received the ABS between 1995 and 2001 ($n = 37$). The latter group had an overall success of 49%, and those patients who retained their ABS in that group had 100% successful outcome. The rates of revision and infection in that group were 37% and 34% respectively. The most common complication after ABS implantation remains infection, which often leads to revision or explantation.

Secca

Patients with fecal incontinence who fail medical therapy and who are not surgical candidates are targeted by this minimally invasive approach. The Secca procedure delivers circumferential temperature-controlled radiofrequency (RF) energy to the anal sphincters. The procedure can be performed on an outpatient basis with conscious sedation and pudendal nerve block. The patient is placed in the left lateral decubitus, prone jackknife, or lithotomy position. The Secca device is then inserted inside the anal canal, and RF energy is delivered circumferentially in a 4-quadrant approach starting just distal to the dentate line and moving in 1-cm increments proximally in the anal canal. The data available on the Secca procedure are limited. Takahashi and others reported the initial pilot study of Secca in 10 patients with improvement in Cleveland Clinic Florida Fecal Incontinence scores. The results were sustained at 2-year follow-up. A multicenter double-blind study comparing Secca to placebo has recently been completed, but results are not yet available (Fig. 5).

Malone Antegrade Continent Enema

Patients with congenital anorectal anomalies who failed previous repair and patients with neurologic disorders are the optimal candidates for this procedure. Patients undergo full mechanical bowel preparation. Through a right lower quadrant transverse incision, the appendix is identified and its patency verified. The appendix is divided at its base and rotated 180 degrees. A myotomy is created at the antimesenteric tenia of the cecum, and an appendicocecal anastomosis is performed and tunneled under the previously created myotomy. A small incision is created at the base of the umbilicus, the base of the appendix is spatulated, and appendicoumbilical anastomosis carried out with interrupted fine sutures. A pediatric feeding tube is kept in place for 2 to 3 weeks as a stent, after which a contrast study is performed to exclude anastomotic leak. Patients are then taught to irrigate through their umbilical appendicostomy to cleanse the colon and prevent FI (Fig. 6).

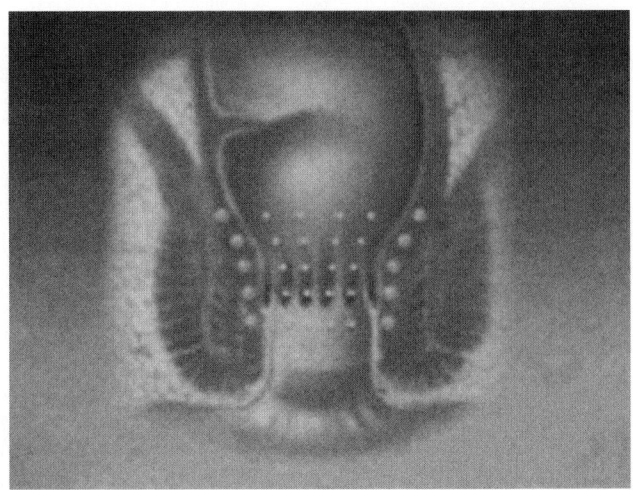

Figure 5 Secca procedure. Thermal lesions are delivered in a stepwise manner to all quadrants of the anal canal, beginning just distal to the dentate line and progressing proximally. *From Takahashi T, Garcia-Osogobio S, Valdovinos MA, and others: Dis Colon Rectum 46:711.* (See color insert Figure 22.)

The results of the Malone antegrade continent enema (MACE) in the treatment of FI are limited to case series in the pediatric literature with short follow-up. In our series of MACE procedures, 5 of 18 patients had a MACE for fecal FI and 4 of 5 (80%) had successful outcome at follow-up.

Thiersch Procedure

In patients whose incontinence is related to recurrent rectal procidentia, anal encirclement may be used as a last resort to keep the rectal protrusion reduced permanently. This operation can be performed under local anesthesia and conscious sedation. A 3-cm-deep circumanal tunnel is created, and 1.5-cm-wide nonabsorbable mesh (such as 4-ply polypropylene) is inserted into the tunnel at

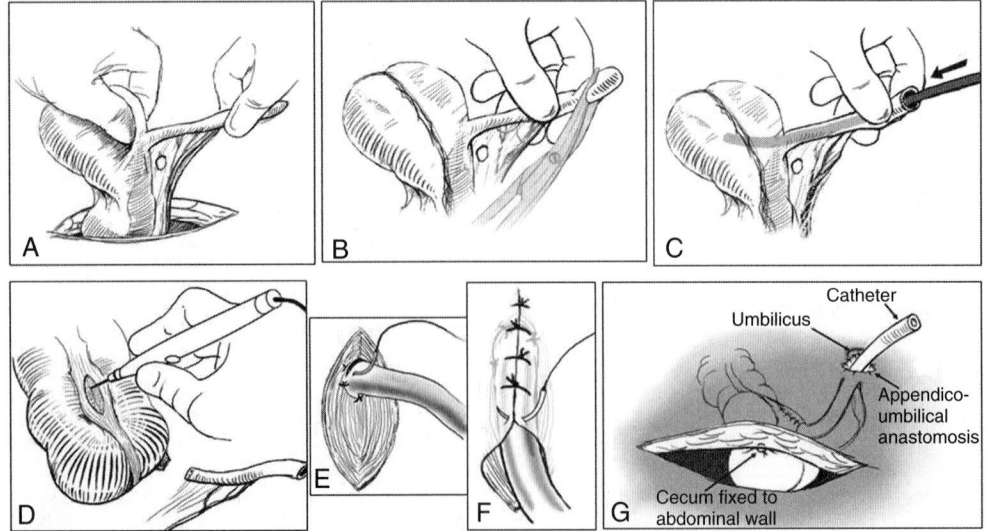

Figure 6 Schematic representation of Malone antegrade continent enema (MACE) technique at our institution. **(A)** Isolation of appendix and of appendiceal artery. **(B)** Preparation of appendiceal cannulation by excision of appendiceal tip. **(C)** Cannulation of appendix to ensure patency. **(D)** Myotomy of cecum over tenia coli after transection of appendix performed. **(E)** After 180-degree rotation of the appendix, an appendicocecostomy anastomosis is performed with interrupted suture. **(F)** Tunneling of the appendix with muscular and serosal layer of cecum. **(G)** Final result demonstrating the appendix brought through umbilicus as an appendicoumbilical stoma and the cecum being fixed to anterior abdominal wall. *From Dis Colon Rectum, in press.*

the level of the deep EAS. The mesh is tightened and sutured to itself, leaving the anal canal open around a no. 16 Hegar dilator. Complications include infection, fecal impaction, and, rarely, erosion of mesh into the anorectal lumen.

Colostomy

For patients with perianal trauma, those who have failed or cannot afford ABS, or those with severe radiation therapy injury leading to disabling FI and poor quality of life, a stoma may be the only solution left to restore functional outcome. Colostomy should be placed as distal as possible to avoid large mucous leaks.

CONCLUSION

FI is a disabling condition affecting a significant portion of the population. The rising age of the population is likely to be associated with an increase in the prevalence of FI. In the treatment of FI, a complete history to establish the etiology of fecal incontinence is the main step that guides appropriate therapy. Overlapping sphincteroplasty remains the first-line treatment of sphincter defect. However, in view of its questionable long-term success, newer and less invasive procedures such as SNS are gaining popularity. At present, the indications for these novel procedures often overlap, and as more data become available, clinicians will be better able to determine individualized treatments on the basis of appropriate patient selection.

SUGGESTED READINGS

Bharucha AE: Outcome measures for fecal incontinence: anorectal structure and function, *Gastroenterology* 126(suppl 1):S90, 2004.
Madoff RD: Surgical treatment options for fecal incontinence, *Gastroenterology* 126(suppl 1):S48, 2004.
Rockwood TH, Church JM, Fleshman JW, and others: Patient and surgeon ranking of the severity of symptoms associated with fecal incontinence, *Dis Colon Rectum* 42:1525, 1999.

RECTOVAGINAL FISTULA

N. Anh Tran, MD, and Alan G. Thorson, MD

INTRODUCTION

Although not a life-threatening disease, a rectovaginal fistula can produce symptoms that are traumatic to the patient, affecting aspects of intimacy, social function, and wellbeing. Because this condition is of a particularly sensitive nature, care of the patient should address all of these aspects, as well as the anatomic problem.

ETIOLOGIES

The majority of rectovaginal fistulae are a result of obstetric trauma. Those especially at risk are women who have sustained a forceps delivery, episiotomy, or third- or fourth-degree laceration. Approximately 5% of vaginal deliveries are associated with such lacerations; 1% to 2% of those sustaining injury will develop a rectovaginal fistula. Thus the risk of rectovaginal fistula following vaginal delivery is roughly 1 per 1000 deliveries.

The second most common cause is inflammatory bowel disease. Rectovaginal fistulae associated with Crohn's disease can be exceptionally difficult to treat. Other causes include radiation; penetrating trauma; diverticulitis (particularly if the patient has had a previous hysterectomy); foreign bodies (long-standing pessaries); cancer; and any previous pelvic, perineal or rectal surgery (especially vaginal hysterectomy and low anterior resection) (Table 1).

CLINICAL MANIFESTATIONS

Patients with a rectovaginal fistula generally describe gas or stool passing through the vagina. They may have a foul-smelling drainage or give a history of fecal incontinence, often not realizing that the leakage of stool is actually exiting the vagina rather than the anus.

Physical examination should start with inspection of the perineum. Any scars from a previous episiotomy or anorectal surgery should be noted. Patients with associated incontinence may have a patulous anus. Sphincter tone should be assessed. The perineal body can be particularly thin, especially in those who have sustained obstetric trauma. Digital examination may reveal induration at the site of the fistula. Bimanual examination of the rectovaginal septum also may be helpful. Anoscopy or a vaginal speculum examination may reveal granulation tissue marking the fistula site.

If a fistula cannot be identified but the patient's history is consistent with one, other methods of diagnosis include the methylene blue tampon test and the vagina "bubble" test. The methylene blue test involves placing a tampon in the vagina and then giving the patient a methylene blue enema. If the tampon stains blue, this confirms the presence of a fistula. The "bubble" test entails positioning the patient in lithotomy position, filling the vagina with water, and performing rigid proctoscopy with insufflation. The vagina is then inspected for any bubbles to confirm the diagnosis of a fistula.

OTHER STUDIES

Pelvic floor laboratory studies are crucial to determine the presence of a sphincter injury (which could alter surgical management) or pudendal neuropathy (which may affect an otherwise successful

Table 1: Etiologies of Rectovaginal Fistula

Trauma	Obstetric (forceps delivery, episiotomy, third- and fourth-degree laceration)
	Foreign body (pessaries)
	Accidental/nonaccidental (sexual abuse)
Postsurgical	Anorectal (fistulotomy)
	Vaginal (hysterectomy, rectocele repair)
	Abdominal (hysterectomy, low anterior resection, pouch procedure)
Infection	Cryptoglandular abscess, diverticulitis, tuberculosis
Inflammatory bowel disease	Crohn's disease
Neoplasm	Anal, rectal, vaginal, leukemia
Radiation	External beam, brachytherapy

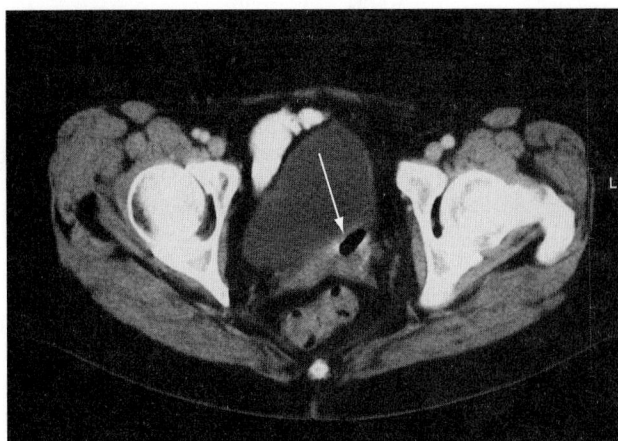

Figure 1   The arrow points to air in the vagina on this computed tomography scan of a rectovaginal fistula.

repair). Such studies are essential to the workup of any patient who has a prior history of birth trauma or has symptoms of incontinence. These studies generally consist of anorectal manometry, transanal ultrasound, and pudendal nerve terminal motor latencies.

Although not helpful in diagnosing low rectovaginal fistulae, imaging studies such as computed tomography (CT) scan or barium enema may visualize higher fistula tracts. CT scans should be performed with intravenous and rectal contrast. Even if the tract is not directly visualized, air or contrast within the vagina may suggest the presence of a fistula (Fig. 1).

CLASSIFICATION OF RECTOVAGINAL FISTULA

Rectovaginal fistulae are commonly classified according to location, complexity, or size but may be most appropriately classified by etiology. Low fistulae are usually simple and caused by obstetric trauma. High fistulae often require a more invasive repair, frequently necessitating an abdominal approach. These fistulae originate from diverticulitis, radiation, or previous pelvic surgery.

PREOPERATIVE PREPARATION

If the fistula is the result of a traumatic vaginal delivery and appears immediately postpartum, it is preferable to wait at least 3 months before performing any local repair. This allows for the inflammation to resolve and for fibrosis to develop. The presence of fibrosis is helpful in supporting sutures should the patient require sphincter repair. Also, the waiting period may permit the fistula to heal completely without intervention. In the interim, symptoms can be improved with stool bulking or mild constipation with loperamide or other antidiarrheals.

The importance of adequate drainage before repair cannot be overemphasized. Any associated abscesses should be drained and a noncutting, Silastic (Dow Corning, Midland, MI) seton placed if necessary. Even anatomically excellent repairs can be marred by wound dehiscence caused by ongoing infection.

The type of preoperative preparation usually depends on the particular procedure that is planned for the repair. For simple advancement flaps, a Fleet enema on the morning of the procedure is usually adequate. For more involved repairs such as an overlapping sphincteroplasty, a full mechanical bowel prep is preferred. This usually gives the patient at least 2 days before her first bowel movement, allowing additional healing time without the nuisance of fecal stream.

SURGICAL MANAGEMENT

Transanal Procedures

Transanal procedures have the advantage of repairing the fistula from the high-pressure side of the rectovaginal septum. Exposure is not equivalent to a transvaginal approach but is almost always adequate. Transanal repairs are ideal for low rectovaginal fistulae and can be combined with fecal diversion for fistulae of complicated etiology.

Endorectal Advancement Flap

This technique is the mainstay for uncomplicated, low rectovaginal fistulae (Fig. 2). It can usually be performed in the outpatient setting. The prone position allows for good exposure of the fistula on the anterior wall. Both the anus and vagina should be prepped. A Fansler operative anoscope also aids in exposure. As with much of anorectal surgery, a good headlight is invaluable. After identification of the fistula site, a trapezoid flap is outlined, orienting the base cephalad and the apex caudad. A curvilinear incision has also been described. The base should be at least twice as wide as the apex, with the apex encompassing the fistula site. The flap (containing mucosa, submucosa, and the circular layer of muscle) is elevated with electrocautery. Some prefer injection of an epinephrine solution prior to flap elevation, believing that this aids the dissection. Saline can be used as well but does not provide the benefit of hemostasis. Placing a finger within the vagina to lead dissection and avoid "buttonholing" can also be helpful.

After the fistula is exposed, it can either be cored out completely or simply curetted, removing all granulation tissue. An interrupted, absorbable suture is used to close the remaining defect in the muscular layer. The internal opening is excised from the flap, and the flap is mobilized sufficiently to close the wound without tension. The wound is then closed with interrupted, 3–0 absorbable suture, tacking the corners down first to assist in placement of the remaining stitches. It is not necessary to close the vaginal opening as long as the high-pressure zone of the rectum has been treated. Postoperative care includes a high-fiber diet, sitz baths, and a tap-water enema on the third postoperative day if there has not yet been a bowel movement. Prevention of impaction is imperative to avoid disruption of the suture line.

Fistulotomy

Because fistulotomy would divide the sphincters in an area that is already particularly susceptible to injury, one should undertake this alternative with extreme caution. To best preserve sphincter function, we recommend a staged fistulotomy with placement of an abrading suture for a minimum of 8 weeks to allow for fibrosis and then removal of the seton via division of the remaining muscle fibers. This technique should be limited to the superficial fistula to avoid alterations in continence status. It is rarely used.

Fibrin Glue

Fibrin glue presents a minimally invasive manner with which to treat rectovaginal fistulae. Because it preserves sphincter function, it would seem to be an attractive alternative to sphincter-dividing techniques such as fistulotomy. However, this technique cannot be recommended as a good alternative because results have not proved reliable in the treatment of rectovaginal fistulae. Most surgeons who use fibrin glue recommend that the fistula be adequately drained. A Silastic, noncutting seton may be placed for a number of weeks before injection of fibrin glue. After adequate drainage, the seton is removed, and the tract is curetted. Fibrin glue is packaged such that the two ingredients (fibrinogen and thrombin) are combined via a Y-connecter. The blunt needle is placed through the external (vaginal) opening and, ideally, would

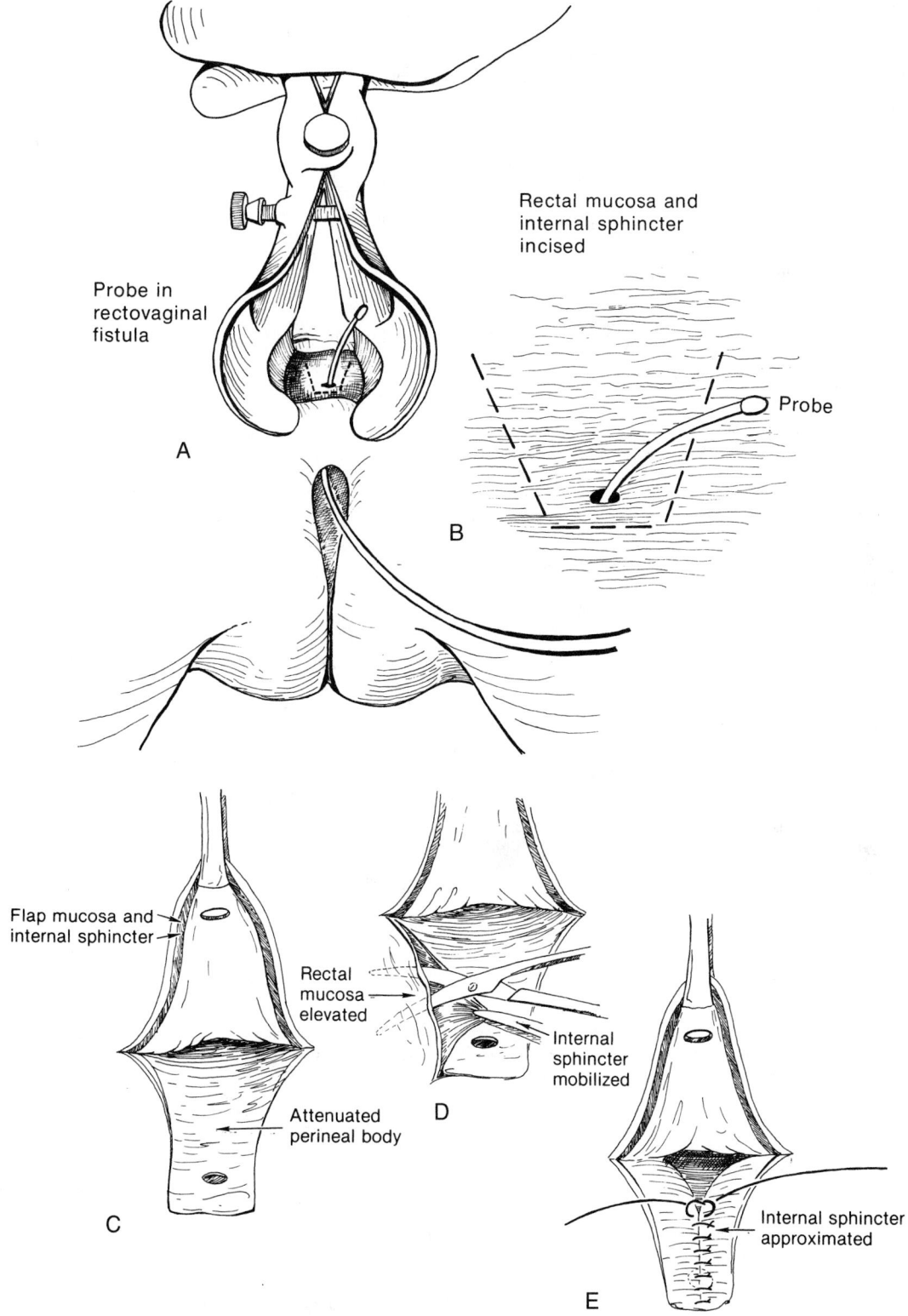

Probe in rectovaginal fistula

Rectal mucosa and internal sphincter incised

Probe

A

B

Flap mucosa and internal sphincter

Rectal mucosa elevated

Internal sphincter mobilized

Attenuated perineal body

Internal sphincter approximated

C

D

E

Figure 2 **(A)** The fistula is confirmed with passage of a fistula probe. **(B)** A flap is outlined with the base two times the width of the apex. **(C)** The flap of mucosa, submucosa, and internal sphincter is raised from apex to base, which should extend at least 4 cm proximal to the fistula. **(D)** The internal sphincter is mobilized laterally on both sides. **(E)** The mobilized internal sphincter is closed over the vaginal fistula opening with 2–0 polyglycolic acid sutures. *From Goldberg SM, Gordon PH, Nivatongs S: Essentials of anorectal surgery, Philadelphia, 1980, JB Lippincott, Fig. 25.5, pp 326-327.*

(continued)

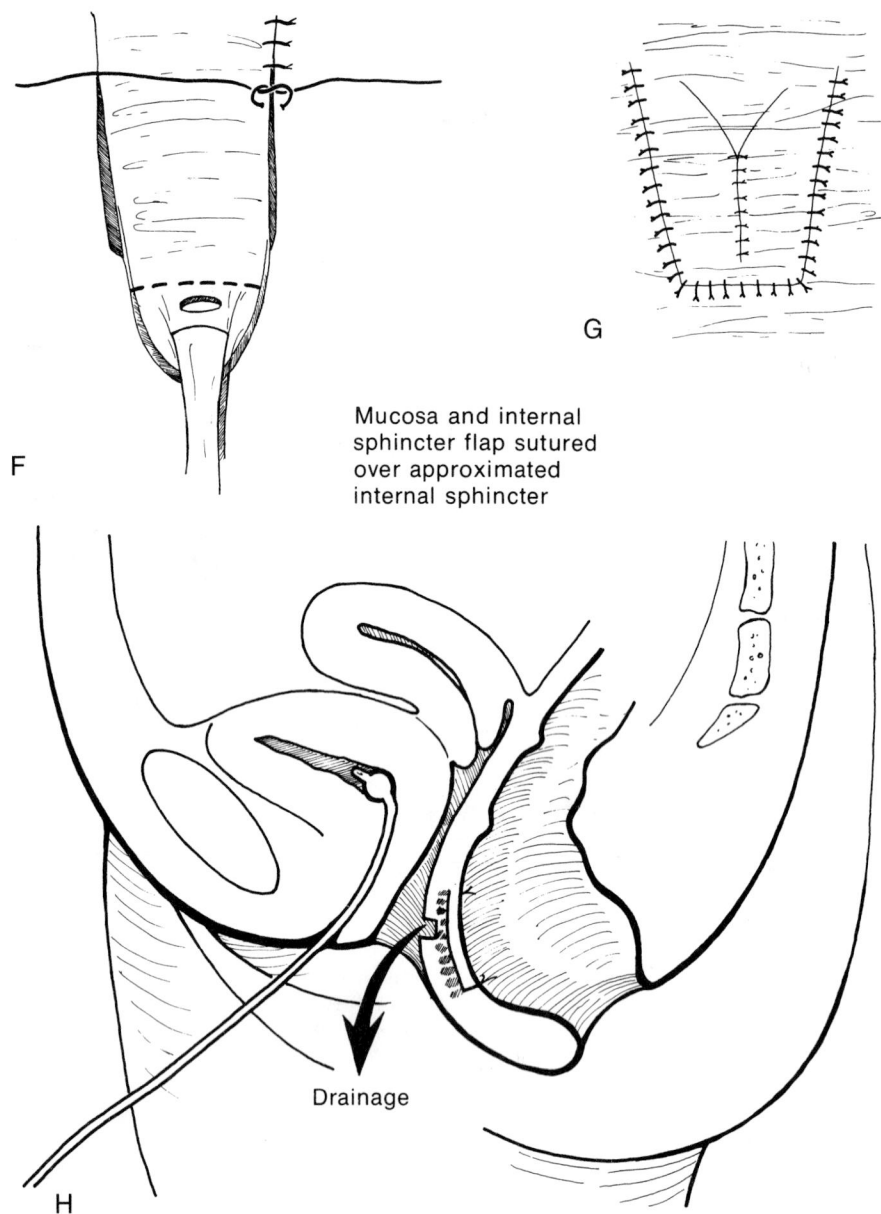

Mucosa and internal
sphincter flap sutured
over approximated
internal sphincter

Drainage

Figure 2 Cont'd—**(F)** Excess flap to include the rectal fistula opening is excised. **(G)** The flap is sutured in place using 3–0 polyglycolic acid sutures. **(H)** The vaginal side is left open for drainage. *From Goldberg SM, Gordon PH, Nivatongs S: Essentials of anorectal surgery, Philadelphia, 1980, JB Lippincott, Fig. 25.5, pp 326-327.*

be seen coming out of the internal (rectal) opening. As it is withdrawn, one injects the glue at a steady pace, ensuring that it fills the entire fistula tract. If the compound is allowed to sit within the blunt needle for any period of time, it will clot, and a new needle will have to be used. Some authors advocate closing the internal or the external openings (or both) with a figure-of-eight suture. Limited data are available because studies usually involve small numbers. It has been suggested that low success rates with fibrin glue are secondary to the fact that most rectovaginal fistulae have a short tract.

Bioprosthetic Plug

The bioprosthetic plug is composed of a rolled sheet of bioabsorbable xenograft, made of porcine intestinal submucosa

(Surgisis AFP; Cook Biotech, West Lafayette, IN). It is tapered on one end to facilitate insertion. As with fibrin glue, it is important to ensure adequate drainage before placing the fibrin plug. Although early reports described curettage of the tract, more recent reports have discouraged any disruption of the tract. With or without curettage, a probe is placed into the tract from the external opening to the internal opening. A suture placed on the tapered end of the plug is secured to the probe and the plug pulled into the tract. The larger end is thus lodged at the internal opening. The excess is trimmed, and the plug is secured in place with a figure-of-eight suture while mucosa is closed over the plug. The external opening is usually left open, and excess plug trimmed at this level. The plug presents the same problem seen with fibrin glue in that rectovaginal fistulae generally have short tracts, making failure more likely.

Transperineal Procedures

Transperineal repairs involve an incision across the perineal body. This allows for excellent exposure of the rectovaginal septum but also requires careful dissection of both rectal and vaginal mucosa. It is important to avoid buttonholing either of these because doing so may compromise the repair. Transperineal procedures have the benefit of interpositioning well-vascularized tissue (usually muscle) between the rectum and vagina and thereby increasing the odds of a successful repair. We prefer the prone position for these repairs.

Overlapping Sphincteroplasty

This alternative is ideal for the patient with a concomitant sphincter injury. The technique of overlapping sphincteroplasty is discussed elsewhere in this text. In regard to rectovaginal fistulae, the addition of this procedure to an advancement flap greatly increases success rates.

Layered Closure

This technique reconstructs the initial injury of a third-degree or fourth-degree laceration with excision of the fistula by dividing through the perineal body. The perineum is then repaired in layers by sequentially closing the rectal mucosa, rectal muscular wall, the vaginal muscular wall, and then the vaginal mucosa. Each layer must be sufficiently mobilized with careful dissection to ensure a proper tension-free closure. The drawback to this technique is the mandatory division of the anal sphincters. Because of the considerable risk of incontinence, this repair should not be used unless the patient already has an appreciable sphincter defect. Such a defect can be demonstrated on transanal ultrasound with the fibers of the external sphincter splaying anteriorly.

Repair with Interposition

The most well known of these procedures is the Martius graft, which involves transposition of the bulbocavernosus muscle with its labial fat pad. This is tunneled to lie between the rectum and the vagina at the site of the fistula after it has been excised. Other tissues that have been used for such interposition include the gracilis, sartorius, and gluteus maximus muscles. The use of Surgisis mesh has also been described. These repairs have the added benefit of introducing a well-vascularized pedicle, which can be particularly helpful in radiation-induced fistulae.

Transvaginal Procedures

Transvaginal approaches do not have the advantage of expressly treating the high-pressure zone of the rectum. Advancement flaps through the vagina are approached in a similar manner to endorectal flaps. An effort should be made to close the rectal opening separately.

Abdominal Procedures

High rectovaginal fistulae are usually a complication of low anterior resection, hysterectomy, or diverticulitis (these actually being colovaginal fistulae). These are best treated by an abdominal procedure. In the case of diverticulitis, sigmoid resection down to the decussation of the teniae with simple closure of the vaginal defect should be sufficient. Interposition with an omental tongue may improve success rates. Fistulae resulting from complications of low anterior resection or hysterectomy can be treated with simple closure with

interposition of an omental flap or reresection. Reoperation in this setting is notoriously difficult, and consideration should be given to whether the patient's symptoms warrant embarking on such a difficult procedure. In the especially infirm and frail, one might contemplate end colostomy alone.

OUTCOMES

Rectovaginal fistulae are notoriously difficult to treat, but interpreting the data of previous studies can be even more challenging. Most studies encompass all anorectal fistulae, with rectovaginal fistulae being one tiny subcategory. Thus the numbers are usually small and the techniques used varied, making it problematic to draw substantial conclusions.

Although endorectal advancement flaps have been the most studied, results are varied. Sonoda and colleagues reported success in only 16 of their 37 patients who underwent advancement flaps, giving a morbid 43% success rate. Mizrahi and colleagues fared a bit better, with a success rate of 56%. Tsang and colleagues compared advancement flaps with sphincteroplasty, finding a distinct advantage to sphincteroplasty if, of course, a sphincter defect exists (success rates were 41% vs. 80%). Lowry and colleagues studied 81 patients with simple rectovaginal fistulae. They all underwent advancement flap, with 25 undergoing concomitant sphincteroplasty, and the overall success rate was 83%. Kodner and colleagues reported an overall success rate of 84% in a population of 107 patients.

Complications include wound dehiscence, wound infection, recurrence, and incontinence. For sphincteroplasties, wound dehiscence has been reported at 8.5% and wound infection 5.7%. Recurrence can be affected by a number of factors. The most notorious are Crohn's disease and previous radiation, which are discussed separately in the following section. Previous repairs also adversely affect recurrence rates. Lowry's study with advancement flaps revealed that success rates incrementally decreased with the number of previous repairs (see Table 2). This disturbing finding has been duplicated in other studies. Such data highlight the importance of a secure, well-executed (technically sound) first repair. If a first repair fails, all subsequent repairs are dogged with skewed tissue planes and extensive scarring. It cannot be overemphasized that if a surgeon is unfamiliar in treating rectovaginal fistulae, he or she should promptly refer to a subspecialist.

Reporting of incontinence as a complication of rectovaginal fistula repairs can be an exceptionally thorny issue. As would be expected, incontinence rates are higher with sphincter-dividing procedures such as fistulotomy and layered closure. As reported by Tsang and colleagues, incontinence rates after flap repair remained constant. In the same study, as expected, incontinence rates improved by 44% with sphincteroplasty.

Table 2: Success Rates and Number of Previous Repairs

No. Previous Repairs	Success Rate (%)
0	88
1	85
2	55

From Lowry AC, Thorson AG, Rothenberger DA, and others: *Dis Colon Rectum* 31:676, 1988.

SPECIAL CONSIDERATIONS

Radiation-induced fistulae and fistulae secondary to Crohn's disease warrant special consideration. Increased used of radiation for pelvic cancers either preoperatively or postoperatively has made this complication especially pertinent. Those particularly at risk have usually received doses exceeding 5000 cGy. The possibility of recurrent cancer must be thoroughly evaluated before any treatment of the fistula. If there is no recurrent cancer, rigid proctoscopy should be performed to evaluate the extent of radiation damage to the rectum. If the rectum is noncompliant or if the mucosa is especially friable, then simple flap advancement is likely to fail. If a local repair is to be attempted, one should consider buttressing the repair with muscle (both the sartorius and gracilis have been described) to increase vascularization to the area and diverting the fecal stream with a colostomy or diverting loop ileostomy. If local repair is not an option, one could consider abdominal resection or diverting colostomy alone.

Crohn's disease should be suspected in any patient who has undergone multiple failed attempts to treat a rectovaginal fistula. These fistulae are particularly difficult to treat, and repairs are prone to failure. Medical therapy should be optimized before any efforts at repair. When contemplating repair, one should first determine whether the rectum is actively inflamed. If so and if there is existing infection, a noncutting Silastic seton should be placed for drainage. If proctitis is present but there is no active infection, fibrin glue can be attempted, but it is associated with high recurrence rates. In the patient who does not have proctitis, an advancement flap can be considered. The Cleveland Clinic group has reported a 50% success rate with advancement flaps in anorectal and rectovaginal fistulae in Crohn's patients, with patients on higher dose steroids trending toward a higher failure rate. A rectal sleeve advancement flap as described by Berman has been used with some success for complicated perianal Crohn's disease. This involves elevating a circumferential flap to be advanced down after excision of diseased tissue. Some have postulated that local repair in combination with fecal diversion could increase success. In the face of severe proctitis and perianal disease, total proctocolectomy with end ileostomy remains an option of last resort.

SUGGESTED READINGS

Lowry AC, Thorson AG, Rothenberger DA, and others: Repair of simple rectovaginal fistula. Influence of repairs, *Dis Colon Rectum* 31:676, 1988.
Saclarides TJ: Rectovaginal fistula, *Surg Clin North Am* 82:1261, 2002.
Sonoda T, Hull T, Piedmonte MR, and others: Outcomes of primary repair of anorectal and rectovaginal fistulae using the endorectal advancement flap, *Dis Colon Rectum* 45:1622, 2002.

CONDYLOMA ACUMINATA

Katherine Facklis, MD, and Phillip Fleshner, MD

Condyloma acuminata is one of the most common problems a surgeon sees, and the incidence is increasing at an alarming rate. The disease is caused by human papillomavirus (HPV), a double-stranded DNA virus that invades the basal layer of the skin. Over the characteristic 6-week inoculation time, the virus replicates in the nucleus, and the cells migrate upward through the various layers of the squamous and transitional epithelium. As a result, this condition is difficult to eliminate. The rationale for treatment includes eradication of exophytic, pruritic growth and impedance of the virus' vertical and horizontal transmission. Although this disease can occur in heterosexual men and women, it is most common in male homosexuals, and it can be associated with other sexually transmitted diseases. One retrospective review of 677 patients with human immunodeficiency virus (HIV) showed that 119 (19%) had anal condyloma.

PRESENTATION

Condyloma have a characteristic appearance of small, discrete, elevated, pink to gray, velvety growths in the anal canal, perianal skin, and urogenital region. They rarely extend to the rectum but are confined to the squamous epithelium and anal transitional zone. Treatment of the external component will fail if the patient has internal warts. Anoscopy is an essential part of the examination. It is important to look and feel for any other growth over the entire perineum so that disease in this area can also be treated. Female patients should undergo gynecologic evaluation, in particular vaginal speculum examinations and Pap smears. HIV testing is a good idea in all condyloma patients.

THERAPY

Current treatment options include topical therapies such as podophyllin and podofilox, bichloroacetic and trichloroacetic acids, cryotherapy, 5-fluorouracil (5-FU), and imiquimod (Aldara; 3M Pharmaceuticals, St. Paul, MN). Other options include interferon (IFN), vaccines, and surgery. The Standards Task Force of the American Society of Colon and Rectal Surgeons has developed recommendations for treating anal condyloma. If the lesions are limited to the perianal skin, topical medications, local destruction, and immunotherapy can be useful treatments. Patients with extensive perianal or anal canal condyloma usually require more aggressive treatment. Pretreatment strategies should focus on finding associated sexually transmitted diseases such as HIV, examining sexual partners, and performing Pap smears.

Topical Therapies

Podophyllin and Podofilox

Podophyllin is a cytotoxic chemical that can be used externally only. It cannot be used in pregnant women or women of childbearing age because it is teratogenic. It is irritating, and the area should be cleansed 6 to 8 hours after application. This method usually requires multiple treatments. Optimal results are seen with either a 10% or 25% concentration. Studies have shown only 22% of patients to be free of warts after 3 months of therapy. Large doses of the chemical can cause hepatic, renal, gastrointestinal, and neurologic problems. Podophyllin can cause severe necrosis, scarring, and fistulae. Podofilox (0.5%) is a standardized compound unlike podophyllin, and it also has fewer associated complications. It eliminates growth of HPV-infected cells by disrupting the G2 phase of the cell cycle. The medication, which can be applied by patients, is used twice a day for 3 consecutive days followed by 4 days without treatment each week for 4 weeks. Cure rates with this treatment are only 20% to 50%. Many surgeons believe it may be most useful as prophylaxis against recurrence.

Chloroacetic Acid

Chloroacetic acids denature cellular proteins and are powerful keratolytic agents and cauterants. This treatment is applied directly to internal and external anal warts and can be repeated every 1 to 2 weeks. An applicator is used, and for internal lesions cotton is then wiped over the area before allowing the anal canal to collapse on itself. Local tissue sloughing does occur, but the chemical is less painful than podophyllin and can treat a larger volume of warts in one application. Systemic absorption is not a problem. The cure rates are reported to be only in the 20% to 40% range.

Cryotherapy

Cryotherapy is indicated for patients with few heavily keratinized warts. Multiple treatments are well tolerated and do not require anesthesia; however, this therapy has been of limited use in the anal canal. Criticism regarding excessive postprocedural discomfort has limited the utility of this approach. The standard procedure includes application of the cryotherapy probe or cotton-tipped applicator to the lesion for 30 to 120 seconds. The technique requires careful control of the depth and width of the wound. Local tissue reaction is common. Reported cure rates are between 30% and 50%.

5-Fluouracil

5-FU is a pyrimidine antagonist that disrupts the S-phase of the cell cycle. The 5% cream is applied twice a day for 2 weeks. Less than 10% systemic absorption occurs. Topical 5-FU may be most helpful as a postoperative adjunct in especially resistant cases, or it can be used as nonoperative therapy. Postoperative treatment can be initiated within 4 weeks and consists of weekly applications of 5% cream for 6 to 8 weeks. Local irritation is common. The cure rates range from 40% to 60%. Its use is contraindicated in pregnancy.

In 1988, Krebs followed postoperative patients who received adjuvant 5-FU and found a lower recurrence rate (decreased from 38% to 13%). In 1990, Reid found an increased cure rate, from 15% to 50%. Theses authors concurred that therapy with 5-FU should be started early after surgery to lower recurrent disease significantly.

Immunomodulators

Other innovative treatments have also been introduced. Some have found more clinical use than others. Aldara 5% cream (imiquimod 250 mg) is applied every other night and rinsed off in the morning. It is used until the lesions clear or for a maximum of 4 months. The cream stimulates the immune system by an unknown mechanism. One report noted cure rates of 40%. The recurrence rate is 11%. Side effects include erythema, burning pain, and itching. It can be used preoperatively for large lesions or postoperatively to prevent recurrence. An intra-anal formula/indication

is in development. Isotretinoin is a vitamin A derivative with antiproliferative activities on various epithelial tissues. One trial reported 75% cure rates. Topical thiotepa and intralesional bleomycin have also been used to treat condyloma with varying results. Cidofovir gel (topical 1% HPMPC (S)-1-(3-hydroxy-2-phosphonyl methoxy propyl cytosine in Beeler base) is an acyclic nucleoside phosphonate analogue with broad antiviral activity. It was found to treat effectively three immunocompromised patients with severe relapsing infections caused by HPV. Another study evaluated cidofovir in 49 HIV-positive patients with condyloma acuminata. No systemic toxicity was observed. There was a 65% response rate (complete or partial response greater than 50% decrease in size). Reversible application site reactions were observed in 40% of patients. Its main therapeutic value is to supplement electrosurgery when there is recurrence. There are no long-term randomized studies available, and its expense prohibits widespread use.

Interferon

Human leukocyte IFN disrupts viral replication and release, improves T-cell and macrophage activity, and protects uninfected cells. The major side effect is a flulike syndrome seen in up to 50% of patients. Theoretically, IFN can be used via three routes: systemic, topical, and intralesional. Of the three, intralesional IFN has the best results and fewest side effects and is the only indication approved by the U.S. Food and Drug Administration (FDA). Injection of 1 million International Units under each lesion two times per week for 3 to 8 weeks has produced cure rates approaching 60%. The maximal dose per session is 2.5 million International Units. The use of local anesthesia is usually necessary. Eron and colleagues conducted a randomized, controlled study in which 257 patients had intralesional injections of IFN. Significant reductions in condyloma volume were seen. Our own group performed a prospective randomized controlled study in which one group of patients underwent surgical excision and fulguration followed by injection of 500,000 International Units of IFN-alfa-n3 into each of the four quadrants of the anal canal. The control group had four saline injections after the same procedure. A statistically significant difference in the 12% recurrence was noted in the IFN group versus the 39% rate seen in the control subjects. More recent randomized, controlled trials have shown no benefit of IFN over less costly regimens. Systemic IFN and topical IFN have also not been effective.

Molecular hybridization studies revealed HPV DNA sequences in adjacent tissue after CO_2 laser removal, and these patients had an increased recurrence rate. Of 20 patients, 11 (55%) had negative margins and only a 9% recurrence rate. Positive margins were noted in 9 of the 20 patients (45%), and 67% of these patients had recurrences. This study demonstrated that HPV is often present in clinically and histologically normal cutaneous epithelium adjacent to condyloma and strongly suggests that its presence is related to the development of new lesions. These findings may help to solidify the role for IFN, particularly after surgical excision. The surgical ablation of warts may expose virus particles and virus-infected keratinocytes to immune and inflammatory cells in the epidermis and upper dermis with a weak specific-nonspecific immune response. IFN, an immunostimulant, may augment this response. In addition, IFN may limit the local spread of HPV through its antiviral and antiproliferative action.

Immunotherapy

Abcarian and Sharon introduced the concept of immunotherapy. Autogenous vaccine was prepared from homogenized condyloma tissue (5 g). The vaccine (0.5 ml) was given subcutaneously in the deltoid weekly over 6 consecutive weeks. Vaccines were frozen between injections. Of 200 patients over an 8-year study period, 84% had excellent results, 11% had fair results, and no improvement was observed in 5% of patients. No adverse reactions or complications were reported. Half of the 5% of patients with poor results were actually cured after their second course of immunotherapy. Long-term results were good.

Usman found a 44% cure rate 6 weeks after immunotherapy; 1 year later, none of these patients' symptoms had recurred. Eftaiha and colleagues also studied immunotherapy for treatment of anal condyloma and found that 94% of patients responded. Wiltz and colleagues studied patients who had surgery followed by vaccination and compared these results with those reported for other modalities. They found this therapy to be superior to any other medical or surgical treatment. Current FDA regulations prohibit shipping of vaccines across a state line, so the vaccine must be prepared locally. More recent data have shown less efficacy with this treatment. Additionally, a new HPV vaccine is now available. It will be interesting to speculate whether use of this vaccine will aid in primary prevention and also whether it can help in prophylaxis after surgical treatment.

Surgery

Surgery is consistently the best treatment approach for initial therapy and recurrent disease. The cure rates are approximately 60% to 90%. There are three techniques: scissor excision, laser therapy, and excision and fulguration. It is important to avoid wide tissue destruction, remove fumes, and send tissue for biopsy. Viral DNA typing has no proven benefit in diagnosis or management.

Scissor excision can be performed after submucosal or subcutaneous injections of 0.5% or 1.0% lidocaine or 0.25% to 0.5% bupivacaine with epinephrine. The injection allows for elevation of the tissue and maximal preservation of normal skin and mucosa.

Laser therapy for anal condyloma has no proven benefits over excision and fulguration, which is the gold standard technique. Billingham and Lewis performed a controlled study on 38 patients. The left half of the anus was treated with CO_2 laser, the other half with classical surgical excision. The authors reported more pain and earlier recurrence in the laser-treated group. In addition, this treatment is more expensive and requires special training, and vaporization of the viral particles can expose the surgeon and others in the operating suite to the virus. Another randomized study by Duus and others found no significant difference in the rate of recurrence, scar formation, postoperative pain, or time to healing between laser and conventional surgical techniques.

Excision and fulguration with electrocautery is the optimal therapy for anal condyloma. Application of the needle-tip electrode causes the viral particle to explode. The tissue is then wiped with a dry gauze sponge or with a curette. The burn should not be deep into the dermis or fat. Patients experience significant postoperative pain and can develop anal strictures. Patients are then seen every few weeks for the first few months to treat any recurrent lesions as soon as they present. Recurrence rates range from 10% to 25%. Yet another comparative study showed electrodessication to be superior to cryotherapy, which, in turn, was superior to podophyllin therapy. Patients should be informed of the recurrent nature of this problem and that treatment and close follow-up may be longer than anticipated. Suppressive therapy with 5-FU or imiquimod (Aldara; 3M Pharmaceuticals, St. Paul, MN) should be considered. In addition, HIV-positive patients should have aggressive antiviral therapy. Daily cleansing with soap and water and sitz baths are helpful in the postoperative period.

TREATMENT APPROACH

The treatment approach to anal condyloma should first begin with anoscopy. If disease is limited to the perianal region, initial therapy can consist of podofilox (Condylox; Watson Pharmaceuticals, Corona, CA), podophyllin, bichloroacetic or trichloroacetic acids, or liquid nitrogen. In these patients, we favor imiquimod (Aldara) supplemented with bichloroacetic acid in the office. Recurrent disease can be treated with surgery and imiquimod. For patients with anal canal disease, initial treatment is surgery and imiquimod; recurrence is also treated with surgery, and with imiquimod or 5-FU postoperatively. Patients must be followed closely for recurrence: monthly for the first 3 months then every 2 to 3 months until they are free of disease for 1 year. Of these patients, 10% to 75% have recurrent disease. Bichloroacetic acid can be applied in the office and supplemented with imiquimod use at home. HIV-positive patients who are otherwise doing well can tolerate aggressive treatment as well as patients who are HIV negative.

The most common subtypes of HPV are 6 and 11. Subtypes 16,18, and possibly 31, 33, and 35 have been associated with malignant transformation. HPVs express E6 protein, which complexes with the p53 tumor-suppressor protein and therefore diminishes p53-related regulatory mechanisms. HIV may help to potentiate this process. HPV-16 DNA was seen in 56% of anal squamous cell carcinomas (SCCs), and HPV 18 DNA was seen in 5% of anal SCCs. HPV-16 DNA that was detected in anal cancer had predominantly integrated into the host-cell DNA. This state is distinct from the vegetative episomal state that viral DNA usually has in premalignant cells.

In clinically normal HIV-positive men, HPV can have an abnormal histologic appearance. The entity anal intraepithelial neoplasia (AIN) has been found in routine anal scrapings in HIV-positive patients and appears to be related to the level of immunosuppression rather than to the specific subtype of HPV. Two small reports failed to show progression from AIN to SCC. Its prevalence and true malignant potential are uncertain; however, 40% of cases recur after treatment, and AIN is commonly seen in the adjacent mucosa of patients with anal SCC. Patients found to have AIN should be followed every 3 months, and a biopsy should be performed if suspicious areas are present.

HIV-positive patients and patients with AIN are special cases. Anal cartography (anal mapping) is slowly becoming available in certain practices. This involves high-resolution anoscopy and directed ablation. Anal Pap smears are also being performed more readily. It is important to speak to the pathologist to ensure of the availability and diagnostic acumen for reading this information. Studies are currently underway to formulate a protocol for patients with condyloma and possibly AIN.

Goldstone and Ufford studied male homosexuals with benign anal disorders and found that their incidence of AIN or SCC was 44% despite a lack of visible condyloma. Cytologic examination was recommended, and biopsies were performed on any further abnormalities. HIV-positive patients had a higher prevalence of AIN and SCC (71% vs. 46%) over HIV-negative patients. The area most often affected by AIN and SCC was the squamocolumnar junction. Another study by Youk and colleagues found HPV-16 DNA present in 21 of 21 anal epidermoid carcinomas. All controls were negative for HPV DNA. In addition, in that specific population, the common sequence variation of the E7 gene in the anal cancer patients was also identified in female patients with cervical cancer.

Karamanoukian and colleagues conducted a retrospective chart review and found 20 patients with HIV and HPV with circumferential anal dysplasia who were followed over 2 years. Only one patient progressed to invasive carcinoma and had the additional risk factor of a previous flame burn. These authors' preliminary findings suggest that physical examination alone could be safely used to follow HIV patients with squamous dysplasia.

Metcalf and Dean attempted to identify risk factors that might promote progression to dysplasia in patients with anal condyloma.

Through a retrospective chart review of 103 male patients, they concluded that homosexual or bisexual orientation, disease above the dentate line, and immunosuppression significantly increased the risk of dysplasia. The increased risk in these patients was believed to necessitate close observation and possible biopsy in all patients.

GIANT CONDYLOMA ACUMINATA

Giant condyloma acuminata is a variant of anal condyloma that invades deeply into adjacent tissue and has a high rate of recurrence (66%) and malignant transformation (56%). No metastases have been identified. Creasman and colleagues hypothesized that this lesion lies along the spectrum from anal condyloma to SCC. In addition, Chu and colleagues found that one third of these patients with malignant behavior had associated fistulae. Wide local resection to negative 1-cm margins is the treatment of choice. Flaps or skin grafts may be necessary. If the sphincter is involved, abdominoperineal resection (APR) should be performed. These lesions can recur in up to 50% of patients if treated with surgery alone. Vaccine therapy was evaluated by Abcarian in 1976 and Eftaiha in 1982 and was found to be effective alternative therapy for recurrent condyloma and giant condyloma acuminata. Chemoradiation combined with surgery may improve the cure rate. In one case report in which the lesion was too large to treat with wide excision, intravenous 5-FU, mitomycin C, and extended-field radiation (45 cGy) with follow-up abdominoperineal resection were used. In fact, at APR, no residual tumor was found. Chu and colleagues confirmed this finding in a patient with a recurrent, inoperable lesion that was treated with radiotherapy and pelvic perfusions of 5-FU and cisplatin followed by radical surgery. Although superior results have been seen with radical surgery over chemoradiotherapy or local excision (or both), preoperative chemoradiotherapy followed by radical surgery seems to be an effective treatment option worthy of further investigation.

SUGGESTED READINGS

Beck DE, Jazo RG, Zajac RA: Surgical management of anal condylomata in the HIV-positive patient, *Dis Colon Rectum* 33:180, 1990.

Beck DE, Wexner SD: *Fundamentals of anorectal surgery*, ed 2, Philadelphia, 1998, WB Saunders.

Bonnez W, Elswick RK, Bailey-Farchione A, and others: Efficacy and safety of 0.5% podofilox solution in the treatment and suppression of anogenital warts, *Am J Med* 96:420, 1994.

Cardamakis EK, Kotoulas IG, Dimopoulos DP, and others: Comparative study of systemic interferon alfa-2a with oral isotretinoin and oral isotretinoin alone in the treatment of recurrent condyloma acuminata, *Arch Gynecol Obstet* 258:35, 1996.

Corman ML: *Colon and rectal surgery*, ed 5, Philadelphia, 2005, Lippincott Williams & Wilkins.

Cowsert LM, Fox MC, Zon G, and others: In vitro evaluation of phosphothionate oligonucleotides targeted to the E2 mRNA of papillomavirus: potential treatment for genital warts, *Antimicrob Agents Chemother* 37:171, 1993.

Dodi G, Infantino A, Moretti R, and others: Cryotherapy of anorectal warts and condylomata, *Cryobiology* 19:287, 1982.

Douglas J, and others: A phase I/II study of cidofovir topical gel for refractory condyloma acuminatum in patients with HIV infection, Poster presented at the 4th Conference on Retroviruses and Opportunistic Infections, Washington, DC, January 22-26, 1997.

Eron LJ, Judson F, Tucker S, and others: Interferon therapy for condyloma acuminata, *N Engl J Med* 315:1059, 1986.

Fleshner PR, Freilich MI: Adjuvant interferon for anal condyloma, *Dis Colon Rectum* 37:1255, 1994.

Megyeri K, Au WC, Rosztoczy I, and others: Stimulation of interferon and cytokine gene expression by imiquimod and stimulation by Sendai virus utilize similar signal transduction pathways, *Mol Cell Biol* 15:2207, 1995.

Snoeck R, Van Ranst M, Andrei G, and others: Treatment of anogenital papilloma virus infections with an acyclic nucleoside phosphonate analogue, *N Engl J Med* 333:943, 1995.

MODERN MANAGEMENT OF PILONIDAL DISEASE

Jan Rakinic, MD

ETIOLOGY

Pilonidal disease is a relatively common problem, with an incidence of approximately 0.7% in young adults. Men are afflicted 2 to 4 times as frequently as women. Pilonidal disease is commonly accepted to be an acquired condition, with embedded hairs in the tissues of the intergluteal cleft as the genesis of the problem. Observations supporting the acquired theory include the occurrence of pilonidal sinus in unusual locations such as the umbilicus, axilla, interdigital clefts, and healed amputation stumps; recurrence after adequate excision; and higher incidence in hirsute persons.

DIAGNOSIS

Pilonidal disease may present as an acute abscess, a simple pilonidal cyst, or a complicated or recurrent sinus. Local cellulitis alone may be conservatively managed with antibiotics directed at skin flora. Anecdotally, it is thought that many of these patients will eventually present with an abscess or mature sinus; however, there are no long-term observational data confirming this.

A painful fluctuant mass in the sacrococcygeal area is the most common initial presentation. Minor cellulitis may also be observed, with few local signs aside from tenderness. With either of these presentations, primary midline openings or pits may be seen in the gluteal cleft approximately 5 cm cephalad to the anus; at times these pits can be obscured by local edema. Chronic sinus tracts become lined with squamous epithelium and extend for a variable distance, almost always in a cephalad direction. There may be branching tracts, and loose hairs may be seen protruding from the midline pits. Secondary openings, often the location of spontaneous abscess drainage, are notable for the presence of granulation tissue and seropurulent discharge.

Although few sinus tracts run in a caudad direction, these may be difficult to distinguish from fistula-in-ano or hidradenitis. Careful examination will reveal one or more midline pits in the intergluteal cleft. Differential diagnosis also includes skin furuncle, syphilitic or tubercular granuloma, osteomyelitis with draining sinuses, and actinomycosis, which can be indistinguishable from pilonidal sinus.

MICROBIOLOGY AND ANTIBIOTIC USE

Pilonidal abscesses are polymicrobial with anaerobes predominating, especially *Bacteroides* species and anaerobic cocci. In contrast, preoperative cultures of chronic pilonidal sinuses contain more aerobes. A study comparing intravenous preoperative cefoxitin to no antibiotic before pilonidal sinus excision and primary closure showed no difference in wound complications, healing within 4 weeks, or recurrence, with 6 to 30 months of follow-up. Another study concluded that preoperative clindamycin conferred no advantage with respect to wound healing. Administration of perioperative antibiotics at primary pilonidal sinus excision is therefore not supported by medical literature; however, antibiotics may be considered in selected situations such as the diabetic or otherwise immunologically vulnerable patient, or in recurrent disease with cellulitis or compromised tissues.

PILONIDAL ABSCESS

Abscesses usually present cephalad and lateral to the infected sinus. Drainage can almost always be accomplished under local anesthetic in the office or emergency department. The incision should be made off the midline because wounds in the intergluteal cleft tend to heal poorly and slowly. If present, hair in the cavity should be removed and the wound curetted. Postoperatively, the wound is cleansed daily in the shower. An area of 2 to 3 cm surrounding the wound should be maintained hair-free for 3 months following healing. This will cure pilonidal disease in 60% to 70% of patients. However, it can be difficult for a young adult to follow this course of therapy for reasons of body habitus, extreme hirsutism, or lack of commitment to the treatment plan. Laser depilation of the buttocks and gluteal cleft has been used in patients with multiple recurrent episodes, resulting in durable long-term healing. It is unlikely that this modality would be used in the setting of straightforward pilonidal disease.

MANAGEMENT OF PILONIDAL SINUS

Statement of the Issue

Pilonidal disease is reported to be the cause of countless hours of time lost from employment and school; often it is the treatment for pilonidal disease that is the culprit. Wide excision of the sinus, leaving a large wound in the gluteal cleft, requires daily dressing changes for 6 to 8 weeks, with resultant loss of productivity in the afflicted young adult population. The surgical literature contains an array of surgical approaches for pilonidal sinus management. As in any disease with a spectrum of possibilities for presentation, treatment must be tailored to the extent of disease. Although there have been advocates of conservative management of pilonidal sinus since the mid-1960s, limited surgical therapy appears to be gaining more attention in the last 5 years.

Management Options for Uncomplicated Pilonidal Sinus

Wide Excision

All sinus tracts are excised along with a 5-mm rim of normal tissue down to the sacrococcygeal fascia, producing a large wound. This may be primarily closed, with more rapid healing; however, recurrence is as high as 40%. When the wound is left open to granulate, complete healing takes an average of 2 months, requiring frequent dressing changes, with an attendant loss of work and school time, as well as costs incurred for frequent wound care. Wide excision offers no advantage over marsupialization (discussed later) for simple sinuses and should be avoided.

Marsupialization

With this approach the sinus tracts are opened in the midline and debris curetted. The fibrous tissue of the sinus is not excised but sutured to the wound edges to produce a smaller, shallower wound compared with wide excision. Daily wound cleansing and dressing changes are still required. Healing usually occurs within 6 weeks. Recurrence is reported as low as 10%. This approach has the advantage of simplicity but the drawback of prolonged dressing changes.

Nonexcisional Management

Excision of the midline pits with cleansing of hair and debris from the sinus cavity was described in 1965 by Lord and Millar, who used a thin bottle brush to cleanse the sinus, which was not excised. Bascom described a lateral incision for entry and curettage of the cavity (Fig. 1), which is not excised; however, the midline pits are excised. His long-term results were published in 1983. Both approaches require long-term removal of local hair for best results.

Phenol Injection

Phenol instillation into the sinus has enjoyed some popularity in Europe but has not been widely used in the United States. One to two milliliters of 80% phenol is injected into the sinus, taking great care to protect the normal skin. The intense inflammation destroys the epithelial lining and removes embedded hairs. There is considerable postoperative pain, requiring inpatient pain management for 24 to 48 hours. Removal of surrounding hair is considered essential. This treatment can be repeated at 4- to 6-week intervals as necessary. Median time to healing is 1 to 2 months, with a reported approximate cure rate of 70%.

Sinus Excision

The acquired theory of pilonidal disease describes an inflammatory process confined to the subcutaneous tissues, and excision of involved tissue alone should be sufficient treatment. As such, the approach of sinus excision has become more widely used. The goal is complete sinus excision without unnecessary removal of any normal tissue, unlike the classic wide excision. Sinus excision can be performed with a midline approach (Fig. 2, A), often leaving

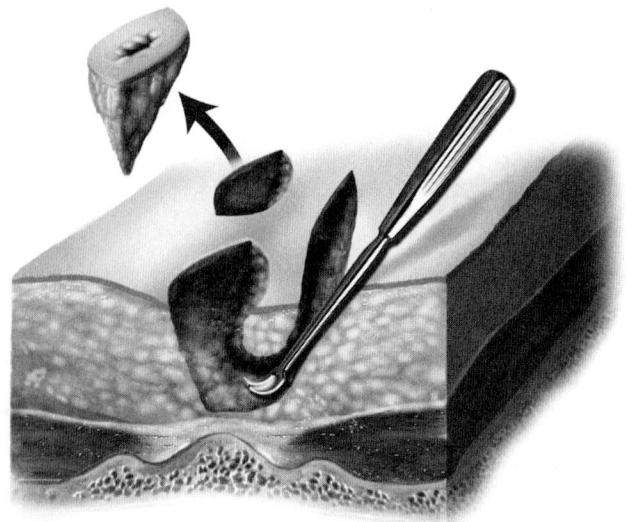

Figure 1 The incision is made lateral to the pilonidal sinus cavity, and the cavity is curetted. Pits are excised separately or en bloc. *Adapted from Nivatvongs S: Pilonidal disease. In Gordon P, Nivatvongs S, editors: Principles and practice of surgery for the colon, rectum, and anus, St. Louis, 1992, Quality Medical.*

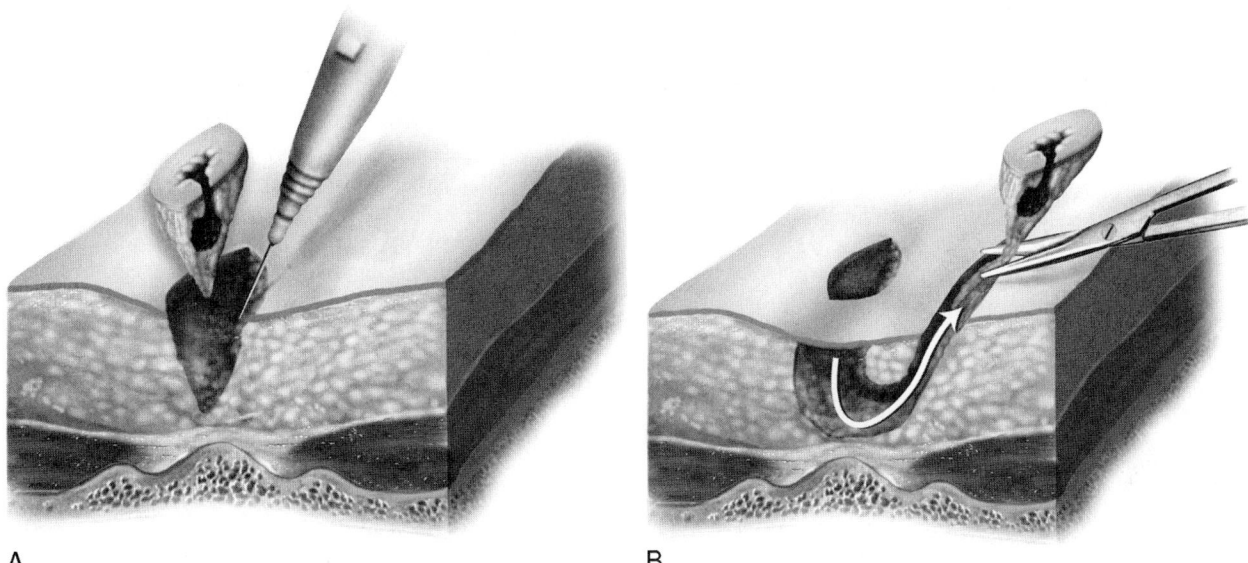

A   B

Figure 2 **(A)** Sinus removal with a midline approach. The sinus and midline pit(s) are excised through a midline incision that encompasses the pit(s). **(B)** Sinus removal through a lateral approach. A rice-grain-sized incision around each pit allows the midline pit(s) to be removed en bloc with the underlying sinus. The specimen is extracted through the lateral incision.

the wound open to heal secondarily or through a lateral incision with en bloc excision of the sinus and the connected midline pits (Fig. 2, *B*). After en bloc excision of the sinus and midline pits through the lateral incision, the lateral skin incision is closed, leaving the small sites of the excised midline pits to heal secondarily. This lateral approach is my technique of choice for uncomplicated pilonidal sinus and can also be used in selected recurrences.

Sinus excision techniques provide shorter operative time and less time off work compared with marsupialization and wide local excision techniques, and are usually performed as outpatient surgery. Rates of complication and recurrence are at least equivalent.

Topics of Debate

Incision Off Midline

Many surgeons have observed poor healing with incisions in the gluteal cleft. Postulated causes include poorer blood supply; depth of the cleft; the nature of a moist, bacteria-rich area; and unavoidable motion caused by ambulation. The location of pilonidal sinus has made complete avoidance of the midline difficult. There has been considerable enthusiasm for placing the primary incision for pilonidal sinus excision laterally (see Fig. 2, *B*); however, this is less likely to be possible with a large or complex sinus unless a flap closure is used (see subsequent section).

Flap Closure for Primary Pilonidal Sinus

Procedures that rotate or advance adjacent tissue for closure of the midline wound have traditionally been reserved for use in complex, recurrent pilonidal sinuses. However, several groups have been using such flap closure in the treatment of primary pilonidal sinus with good results. A number of flap designs have been described or adapted for this application, including the sliding Karydakis flap, Bascom's cleft closure, and various flaps that rearrange local tissue. Most avoid a suture line in the midline gluteal cleft. However, wound separation or infection, with potential flap loss, can be a serious complication and must be considered before using flap closure for management of primary pilonidal sinus.

Karydakis Flap

Karydakis popularized an advancing flap method, which he advocates for use in primary pilonidal sinus management. An eccentrically placed elliptical incision is made, encompassing the sinus and all midline pits (Fig. 3). After adequate sinus excision, a thick flap *(inset)* is mobilized to allow advancement to the other side for closure, avoiding a wound in the midline and making the superior part of the gluteal cleft flatter. A closed suction drain is generally used. In a series of 1687 patients, 8.5% developed hematoma or infection. Of 671 patients followed for 7 months to 6 years, nine (1.3%) experienced recurrence.

Cleft closure

Cleft closure as described by Bascom has similarities. Here the line of contact of the buttocks is marked, and the buttocks are taped apart (Fig. 4). A triangular section of skin surrounding the unhealed wound (inset) is excised, with its apex above and lateral to the cleft apex. All granulation and hair are debrided from the cavity; no mobilization of fat or muscle is performed. The skin flap is raised out to the previously marked line and, with the tapes released, positioned to overlap the contralateral wound edge. Any excess skin is removed from the flap. Subcutaneous tissues and skin are closed over a suction drain. The gluteal cleft is now obliterated. This procedure can be performed on an outpatient basis. Recurrence is reported as low as 4%. This procedure cannot be used when previous wide excision has left significant tissue tension in the area.

Local flaps

Z-plasty flattens the superior part of the gluteal cleft and provides horizontal length. After sinus excision (Fig. 5), limbs of the Z are marked at a 30-degree angle to the long axis of the wound. Flaps of skin and subcutaneous fat are raised and transposed, and the skin is closed.

The *rhomboid flap* has a broad, well-vascularized pedicle that is unlikely to necrose. The procedure begins with excision of the sinus and all midline pits using a rhombic incision (Fig. 6). The flap, consisting of skin and fat to the level of gluteal fascia, is outlined as shown and rotated into place, flattening the gluteal cleft.

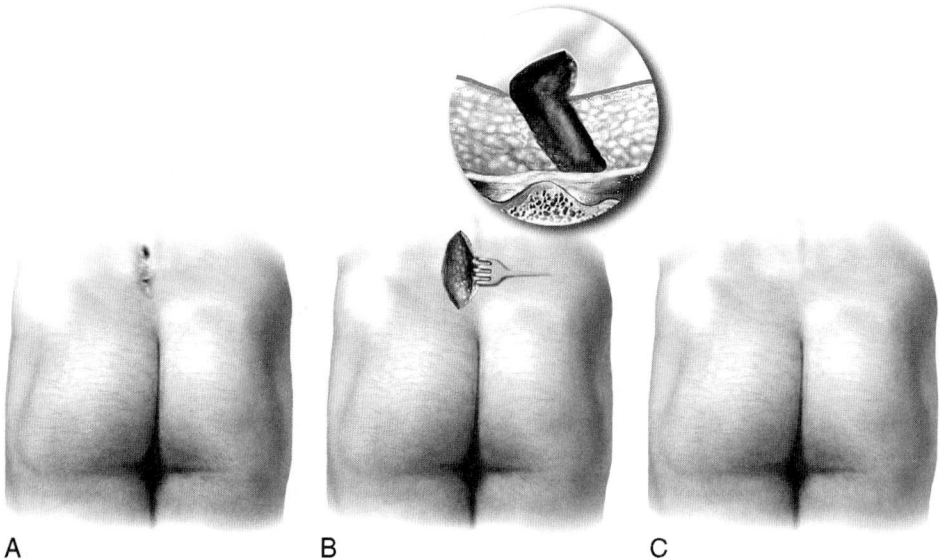

Figure 3 Karydakis sliding flap. **(A)** The sinus is excised to the sacrococcygeal fascia, with the incision made off the midline (Inset). **(B)** A full-thickness flap is raised on one side. **(C)** The flap is slid to opposite side and wound closed, remaining off the midline. *Adapted from Nivatvongs S: Pilonidal disease. In Gordon P, Nivatvongs S, editors: Principles and practice of surgery for the colon, rectum, and anus. St. Louis, 1992, Quality Medical.*

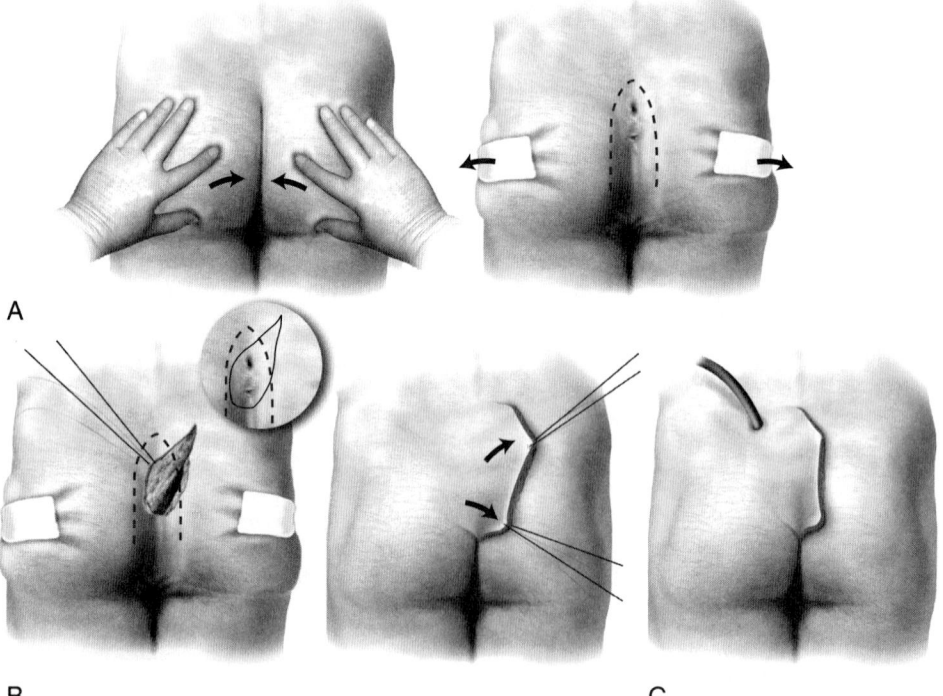

Figure 4 Cleft closure. **(A)** Lines of buttock contact are marked, and the buttocks are then taped apart. **(B)** The unhealed wound is excised in a triangular shape off the midline. The skin flap is raised out to the previously marked line on the side where less skin was removed, then tapes are released. The skin flap is positioned and excess skin trimmed. **(C)** A closed suction drain is placed in subcutaneous tissue before skin closure. *Adapted from Nivatvongs S: Pilonidal disease. In Gordon P, Nivatvongs S, editors: Principles and practice of surgery for the colon, rectum, and anus. St. Louis, 1992, Quality Medical.*

The flap is secured, and the donor site is closed primarily. Use of closed-suction drains is usual, although the necessity for a drain is being reexamined.

V-Y advancement flaps can be used unilaterally or bilaterally, depending on the wound size (Fig. 7). A unilateral flap can cover a defect diameter of 8 to 10 cm. Here the flap is composed of skin, fat, and gluteal fascia; the medial aspect of the flap can be used to eliminate dead space in a deep wound. At completion of the procedure, the gluteal cleft is eliminated. Final placement of a suture line in the midline may be considered a drawback of this procedure. Drains are commonly used, perhaps because this procedure is usually performed in the setting of complex recurrent pilonidal sinus in a multiply operated field.

RECURRENT PILONIDAL SINUS DISEASE

Rates of recurrence vary widely (0%–40%) among published series (see Table 1). Causes are poorly understood; some have suggested that recurrence represents unsuccessful initial control of the disease, with conditions that contributed to the first sinus still present. Others consider wound infection to be the inciting cause of recurrence. A Norwegian group reported on 197 patients treated with sinus excision and primary closure. All received perioperative antibiotics. Wounds failed to heal primarily in 49%. Infection occurred in 34%. Recurrence was 15%. Cox regression analysis showed that a wound complication was an independent predictor

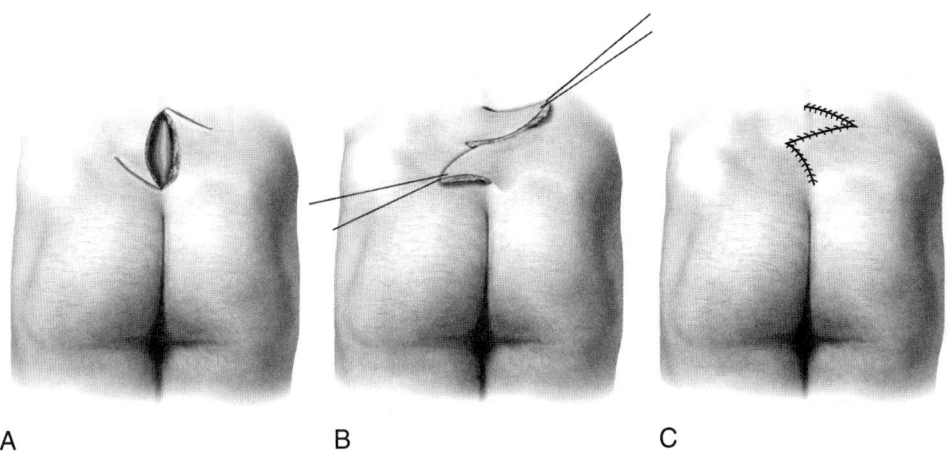

Figure 5 Z-plasty closure after midline excision. **(A)** After sinus excision, limbs of the Z are marked at a 30-degree angle to the long axis of the wound. **(B)** Full-thickness flaps are raised and transposed. **(C)** The wound is closed. *Adapted from Nivatvongs S: Pilonidal disease. In Gordon P, Nivatvongs S, editors: Principles and practice of surgery for the colon, rectum, and anus, St. Louis, 1992, Quality Medical.*

Table 1: Comparison of Treatment Methods for Pilonidal Disease

Method	IP or OP Treatment	Dressing Changes Required	Weeks to Healing (Average)	Recurrence (%)
Abscess drainage/Shaving	OP	Yes	3–4	25–40
Phenol injection	IP	No	4–8	30
Conservative Excision	OP	No	3	16
Marsupialization	OP	Yes	6	8
Wide local excision only	OP	Yes	8	Up to 38
Wide local excision, primary closure	OP	No	4–8	Up to 38
Excision, advancement flap	IP	No	3–4	6–20
Karydakis advancement flap	IP	No	3	1.3
Bascom cleft closure	OP	No	3	3.3

IP, Inpatient; *OP,* outpatient.

of recurrence. Antibiotic treatment was not a significant predictor of recurrence.

Recurrent pilonidal sinuses can be treated in the same way as the initial sinus. However, if there is a third or fourth recurrence, a different approach should be considered. The choice of approach depends on the extent of disease. No primary closure or flap should be performed if there is any cellulitis or infection. Control of sepsis is an important first step. This includes adequate abscess drainage, avoiding too small incisions.

The choice of definitive procedure depends on the anticipated wound size after adequate excision of all involved tissue. If the wound is shallow with a diameter of 10 to 15 cm, and the surrounding tissue has sufficient laxity, primary closure may be possible. Any of the flaps described earlier can also be used in this instance, depending on available local tissue. Disease excision followed by skin grafting remains an option that is sometimes overlooked. This requires a longer hospital stay, produces an additional

(donor site) wound and scar, and may be cosmetically less acceptable to patients.

Larger, deeper wounds require more tissue to fill the space, and preoperative planning is essential. The gluteus maximus fasciocutaneous or musculocutaneous flap (Fig. 8) may be considered in this setting. After excision of all involved tissue, the flap is raised, consisting of skin, subcutaneous fat, gluteus maximus fascia, and sometimes muscle. The flap is rotated into place, filling the dead space with bulky, well-vascularized tissue. Large defects can be managed easily. The gluteal cleft is flattened, and there is no midline suture line. However, the procedure is longer and requires a significant hospital stay, and there is commensurately higher morbidity should the flap fail.

Seroma and hematoma are the most common complications of all these flaps. Although the issue of drain necessity has not been decided, many surgeons continue to use small closed suction drains to avoid seroma and hematoma. No study has shown complications

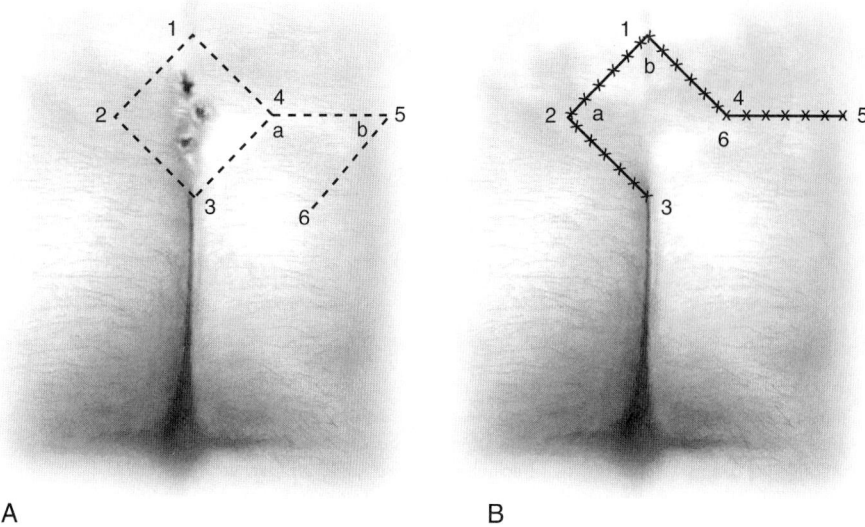

A

B

Figure 6 Rhomboid flap. The pilonidal sinus is excised in a diamond shape. **(A)** Rhombic flap is incised as shown, including skin and subcutaneous tissue. **(B)** The flap is rotated into place and secured. The donor site is closed primarily. *Adapted from Nivatvongs S: Pilonidal disease. In Gordon P, Nivatvongs S, editors: Principles and practice of surgery for the colon, rectum, and anus, St. Louis, 1992, Quality Medical.*

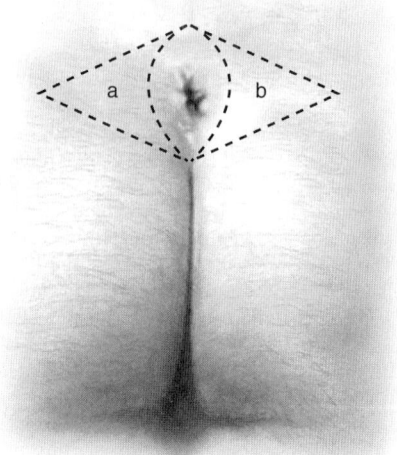

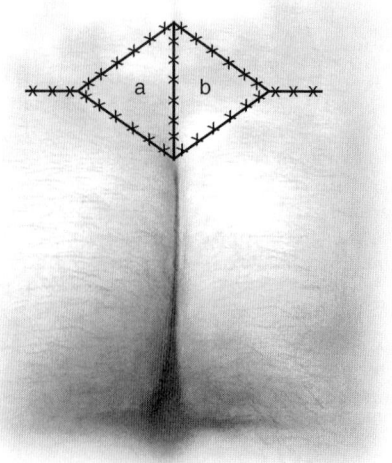

A

Figure 7 V-Y advancement flaps. This can be performed unilaterally **(A)** or bilaterally **(B)**, depending on the defect size after sinus excision. Donor sites are closed primarily. *Adapted from Nivatvongs S: Pilonidal disease. In Gordon P, Nivatvongs S, editors: Principles and practice of surgery for the colon, rectum, and anus, St. Louis, 1992, Quality Medical.*

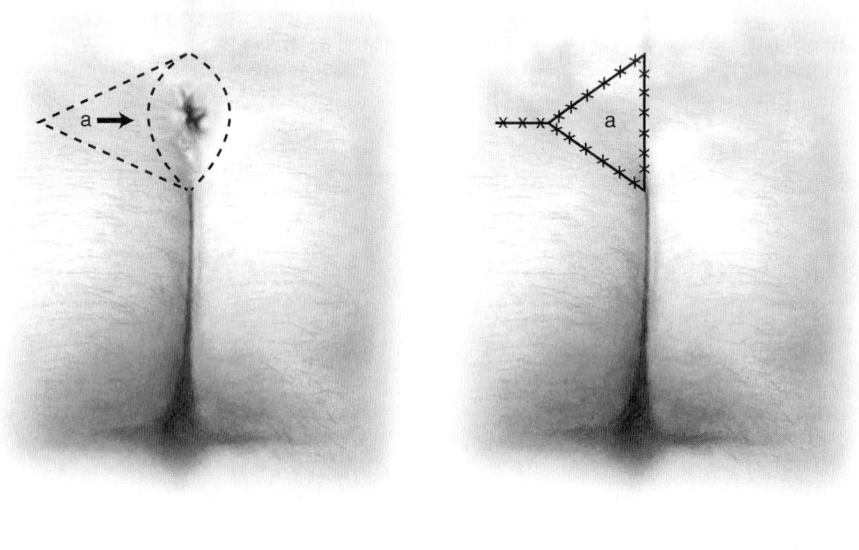

B

Figure 8 Gluteus maximus rotational flap. After sinus excision, the flap is rotated into place as shown.

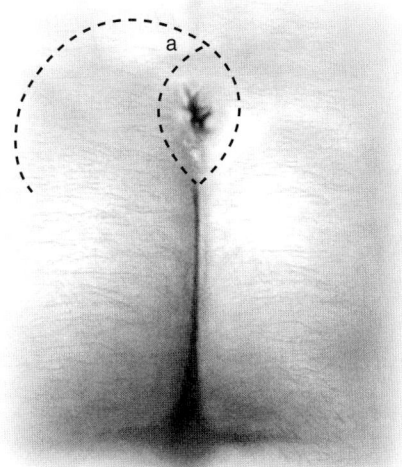
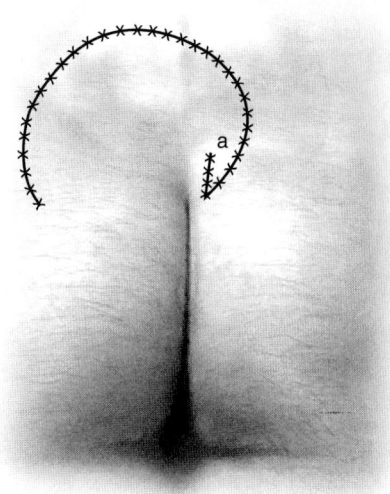

associated with drain use, although some report a longer hospital stay associated with it.

ADJUNCTS TO SURGICAL EXCISION

Fibrin glue has recently been used as an adjunct to surgical therapy of pilonidal sinus. Fibrin glue is injected into the wound cavity following excision with or without primary closure or pit excision with sinus curettage. Patient satisfaction and healing in these small studies was good; recurrence was 0% to 17% with follow-up of 10 to 23 months. The reported series are observational. No prospective study has been reported.

Vacuum-assisted closure (VAC) has produced good results in many types of complicated wounds and has recently been used in wounds of complex pilonidal disease. The VAC system has been used both as a primary wound treatment after excision of large complex pilonidal sinuses and also over split-thickness skin grafts for a period of 4 days postoperatively. The VAC was well tolerated and produced wound closure sooner than traditional open wound management. Although the reported series are small, all have found a shorter hospital stay, a diminished need for further surgical intervention, and improved cosmetic result superior to that after traditional dressing changes. The cost for this therapy will probably limit its use to complex or recurrent cases. Data from a prospective study would be welcome.

CARCINOMA IN PILONIDAL SINUS

Carcinoma arising in pilonidal sinus is rare. Most are well-differentiated squamous cell cancers. Lesions appear as friable ulcers with fungating, rapidly growing margins. Treatment is wide excision with reconstruction by grafting or flap closure. Recurrence rates approach 50%; 5-year survival is 51%. Any palpable inguinal nodes should be biopsied; if positive for tumor (as are 14% at the time of diagnosis), the prognosis is particularly poor. Adjunct radiotherapy decreases recurrence. Any benefit from chemotherapy has yet to be shown.

SUMMARY

Treatment of pilonidal sinus has often caused postoperative disability disproportionate to the severity of the original problem. The goal of therapy should be limiting recurrence while minimizing patient morbidity and inconvenience. Limited resection of pilonidal sinus has gained popularity over wider excision, with the advantages of outpatient performance, smaller wound, fewer dressing changes (none if the wound is closed primarily), and acceptable rates of morbidity and recurrence. Similarly, flap closure after primary pilonidal sinus excision is gaining wider acceptance, with reasonable rates of morbidity and recurrence.

Extensive recurrent pilonidal sinus and the unhealed wound remain difficult management issues. Flap closure of these larger wounds is almost always necessary. At times, local advancement or rotational flaps may not be feasible because of local tissue loss, and more extensive flap techniques, including the gluteus maximus fasciocutaneous or musculocutaneous flap, may be required. These complex flaps require a prolonged inpatient stay, as well as more intensive nursing and wound care, and potential flap loss bears commensurately more serious implications. Newer techniques of wound management, including vacuum-assisted closure, should prove to be advantageous when dealing with the complex pilonidal wound.

SUGGESTED READINGS

Akca T, Colak T, Ustunsoy B, and others: Randomized clinical trial comparing primary closure with the Limberg flap in the treatment of primary sacrococcygeal pilonidal disease, *Br J Surg* 92:1081, 2005.

Chaudhry V, Hyser MJ, Gracias DH, and others: Colonoscopy: the initial test for acute lower gastrointestinal bleeding, *Am Surg* 64:723, 1998.

Oncel M, Kurt N, Kement M, and others: Excision and marsupialization versus sinus excision for the treatment of limited chronic pilonidal disease: a prospective, randomized trial, *Tech Coloproctol* 6:165, 2002.

Petersen S, Koch R, Stelzner S, and others: Primary closure techniques in chronic pilonidal sinus: a survey of the results of different surgical approaches, *Dis Colon Rectum* 45:1458, 2002.

Sondenaa K, Diab R, Nesvik I, and others: Influence of failure of primary wound healing on subsequent recurrence of pilonidal sinus. Combined prospective study and randomized controlled trial, *Eur J Surg* 168:614, 2002.

APPROACH TO LOWER GASTROINTESTINAL BLEEDING

Charles E. Lucas, MD, Anna M. Ledgerwood, MD, and Choichi Sugawa, MD

DEFINITION

Lower gastrointestinal bleeding (LGIB) is defined as bleeding that arises distal to the ligament of Treitz. The most common cause of hematochezia, however, is upper gastrointestinal bleeding (UGIB). Melena indicates UGIB. Consequently, the initial evaluation of hematochezia in stable patients should include nasogastric aspiration to show a bilious return followed by esophagogastroduodenoscopy (EGD); severe rebleeding from a postpyloric peptic ulcer may occur in patients with bilious nasogastric aspirate. This rules out UGIB, thereby allowing a more systematic approach to LGIB.

LGIB can be categorized as minor, major, or massive. Diverticular disease is the most common cause of LGIB, although the incidence of the many causes of LGIB is variable (Table 1). Minor LGIB is likely due to hemorrhoids, inflammatory bowel disease (IBD), nonspecific infectious colitis, arteriovenous malformations (AVMs), colon polyps, or colon cancers. Patients with minor LGIB have stable vital signs and are often worked up as outpatients. Patients with major or massive LGIB, however, require hospital evaluation and treatment. Major LGIB causes a change of vital signs, an altered level of consciousness, or the need to transfuse two or more units of blood for continued bleeding. Massive LGIF requires 10 or more blood transfusions to restore or maintain vital signs. This overview focuses on major and massive LGIB.

Table 1: LGIB in an Urban Emergency Center

Source of Bleeding	Percent
Colonic diverticula	32.7
Hemorrhoids	27.1
Cancer	8.1
Inflammatory bowel disease	6.7
Angiodysplasia	5.3
Polyps	4.9
Ischemic colitis	4.5
Rectal ulcer	2.4
Post polypectomy	0.6
Miscellaneous	7.7

Sources of lower gastrointestingal bleeding *(LGIB)* in 695 patients examined by one endoscopist at an urban medical center.

ETIOLOGY OF MAJOR AND MASSIVE LOWER GASTROINTESTINAL BLEEDING

The most common defined cause of major or massive LGIB is colonic diverticulosis (Table 1; Fig. 1). AVMs of the cecum and ascending colon may also cause severe hemorrhage. Another important source of major/massive LGIB is of undefined origin; this category ranges from 14% to 30% depending on the criteria used to define bleeding of diverticular origin. Less common causes of major/massive LGIB include diffuse mucosal ischemia (Fig. 2, *A*), sometimes after aortic graft replacement, diffuse ischemia from mesenteric occlusive disease, stercoulceration of the rectum, colitis of various etiologies, and colon cancers. LGIB may also be influenced by medications; nonsteroidal anti-inflammatory drugs (NSAIDS) increase the incidence of bleeding from colonic diverticula or may also cause focal bleeding from small bowel or colon ulcers (Fig. 2, *B*). LGIB more commonly occurs in the elderly patient, especially when significant comorbidities exist. Major/massive LGIB in the child is likely arising from a Meckel's

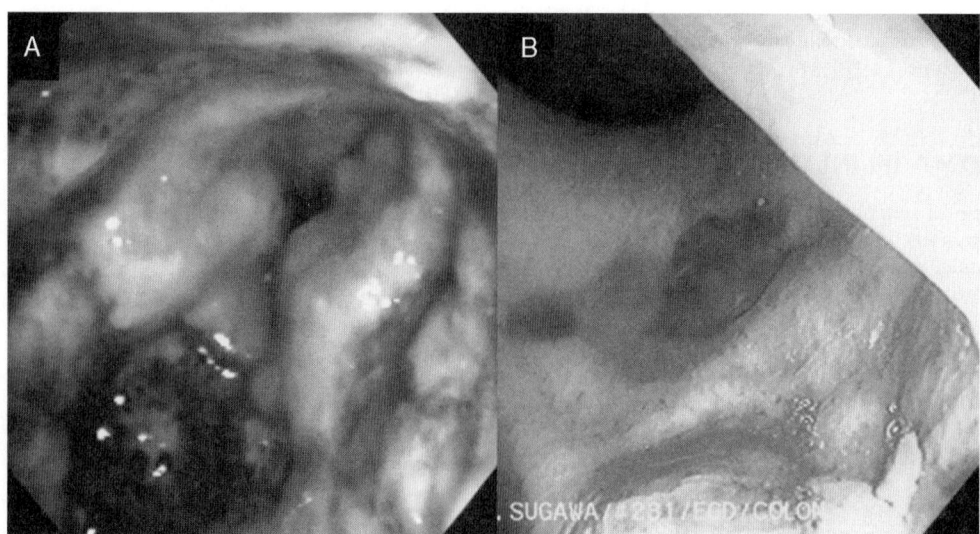

Figure 1 **(A)** Bleeding ischemic colitis. **(B)** Bleeding rectal ulcer.

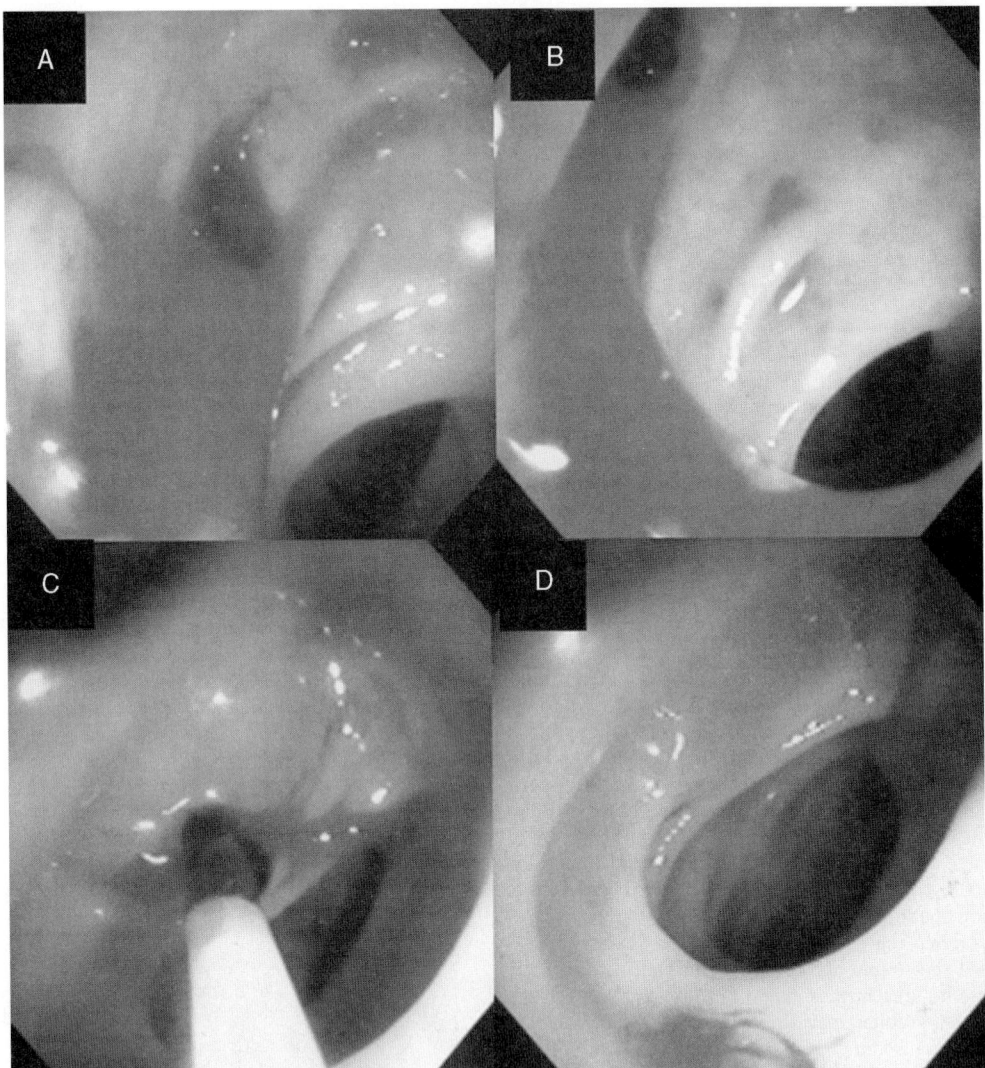

Figure 2 (**A** and **B**) Active bleeding from a colonic diverticulum. (**C**) Endoscopic injection of 10 ml 1:10,000 epinephrine in saline. (**D**) No further bleeding after successful injection.

diverticulum. Patients taking warfarin, heparins (fractionated or unfractionated), or inhibitors of platelet aggregation have an increased propensity for bleeding from any source. Reversal of the coagulopathy by the administration of plasma and, if necessary, platelets is an essential part of the initial resuscitation. Ongoing monitoring of coagulation is vital.

CLINICAL APPROACH

Initial therapy should be directed toward appropriate resuscitation with crystalloid solution and blood, supplemented by fresh frozen plasma (FFP), platelets, or both, as needed. Most patients with coagulopathy and major/massive LGIB can be successfully treated by reversing the coagulopathy without operative intervention.

EMERGENCY EXPLORATORY LAPAROTOMY FOR LOWER GASTROINTESTINAL BLEEDING OF UNKNOWN ORIGIN

After a UGIB source has been ruled out, the patient who remains severely hypotensive and too precarious for colonoscopy despite

aggressive resuscitation and reversal of coagulopathy is best transported to the operative suite for exploratory laparotomy; adjunctive therapy may include intraoperative colonoscopy and, in rare instances, enteroscopy. This is an undesirable setting for the surgeon who may perform a "blind" total abdominal colectomy (TAC) with ileoproctomy or ileostomy when the LGIB is later found not to be of colonic origin.

When exploration in this unstable patient reveals a colon full of blood and no blood in the small intestine, the safest and most expeditious procedure is TAC with ileoproctostomy; when the patient's condition precludes a primary anastomosis, the procedure should be an end ileostomy and a Hartman pouch. Although some surgeons prefer routinely to perform an ileostomy with Hartmann pouch after emergency TAC because the bowel has not been prepped, the rapid bleeding serves as a purge so that the colon is clean. This is a safe anastomosis. The fact that these procedures are performed blindly because the bleeding site has not been seen preoperatively highlights the risk of exploratory laparotomy for major/massive LGIB because of refractory shock. This "blind" TAC, however, will remove the source of bleeding from the two common causes of major/massive LGIB—namely, diffuse diverticulosis and colonic AVMs. Although colonic diverticula in most patients are confined to the left colon, the subgroup of patients with major/massive LGIB from diverticula have pandiverticulosis and usually (60%) are bleeding from the right colon; likewise, most bleeding from colonic AVMs is right sided.

When blood is seen in the small intestine during emergency laparotomy in the unstable patient, a source of bleeding can sometimes be identified by palpation of a mass, visualization of abnormal vessels on the mesentery border, or isolated small bowel diverticula. When multiple small bowel diverticula are present and there is significant blood within the small bowel, surgical devascularization of the diverticula on the mesentery border followed by inversion with seromuscular sutures may be successful.

URGENT NONOPERATIVE EVALUATION OF LOWER GASTROINTESTINAL BLEEDING SOURCE

Fortunately, most patients respond to resuscitation. The decision tree is then based on whether the patient has continued bleeding but is stable or the bleeding has stopped. Stable patients with continued bleeding are candidates for colonoscopy, a tagged red blood cell (RBC) bleeding scan, or mesenteric angiography. Colonoscopy after an antegrade colon preparation with a purge procedure is the diagnostic procedure of choice for its accuracy (53% to 97%) in lesion localization and its therapeutic capability. Simultaneous endoscopic therapies include polypectomy, thermotherapy for AVMs, epinephrine injection for bleeding diverticulosis, and combination injection and thermotherapy for bleeding ulcers, including postpolypectomy ulcers. The bleeding scans are performed with the intravenous infusion of technetium-labeled RBCs; the test will be positive when the bleeding is occurring at greater than 0.1 ml/minute. The positive scans do not identify the exact point of bleeding, however, and in our experience have been of little help in the decision-making process. Mesenteric angiography identifies the specific branch that is bleeding and thereby better directs the surgeon toward the source of bleeding during laparotomy; the bleeding rate must be greater than 0.5 ml/minute for this test to be positive. The angiographer may stop bleeding by the infusion of vasopressin, autologous clots, small particles of Gelfoam (Pfizer, New York, NY), or coils. Although complications such as bowel ischemia or rebleeding may occur following angiographic therapy, the temporary cessation of bleeding facilitates a more thorough evaluation and a more deliberate approach to operative intervention. Unfortunately, many radiologists will not perform angiography with potential angiographic intervention unless there has been a prior RBC scan that shows active bleeding.

When blood is seen endoscopically in the colon without a specific source of active bleeding, examination of the terminal ileum may show blood passing from a more proximal location; the source of bleeding in this setting is presumed to be the small bowel. When colonoscopy identifies blood coming from the small bowel, a more deliberate evaluation should be performed. This would include endoscopic assessment of the distal ileum, angiography if bleeding persists, or push enteroscopy of the proximal small bowel in the stable patient. Contrarily, when the effluent from the terminal ileum contains no blood, the colon is presumed to be the site of active bleeding. This presumption is really a "best guess."

NONEMERGENT OPERATION FOR LOWER GASTROINTESTINAL BLEEDING

The decision to operate for continued bleeding is based on the amount of bleeding and the history of previous bleeds. When continued bleeding requires four or more blood transfusions in the absence of a coagulopathy, urgent operative intervention

during the same hospitalization is associated with a better long-term outcome; this magnitude of bleeding predicts rebleeding without operation. Likewise, rebleeding while in hospital predicts later rebleeding if an operation is not performed. This "urgent" operation performed during the same hospitalization should be designed to remove all of the sites of potential bleeding even when hemorrhage, on this occasion, arises from a known site of the colon. We have performed right colectomy for a massive LGIB proven by angiography to be from right-sided AVMs or diverticular disease only to have recurrent LGIB from left colon diverticula (Fig. 3). Thus right colectomy with careful preservation of the terminal ileum is excellent for AVMs or diverticular bleeding in the absence of left-sided diverticular disease; TAC is best for patients with pandiverticulosis even though the site of bleeding is right sided. One of the often-reported complications of TAC is incapacitating diarrhea, especially in the elderly. This complication can be reduced or eliminated by dividing the distal ileum as it enters the cecum; this requires a few extra minutes to take down the fatty hood over the distal 3 inches of terminal ileum. Preserving this ileum segment eliminates incapacitating diarrhea in most patients. Although diverticula may extend distally to the level of true rectum, the distal colonic transaction is made at the proximal portion of the rectosigmoid colon, thus making the primary anastomosis technically easier in this high-risk patient. Rebleeding from the distal 2 or 3 cm of the rectosigmoid colon is rare, and we have never seen it. We prefer an end-to-end hand-sewn anastomosis to maximize preservation of every millimeter of absorptive ileal mucosa; the difference in circumference between the smaller ileum and the wider rectosigmoid colon is dealt with by incising the ileum along the antimesenteric border.

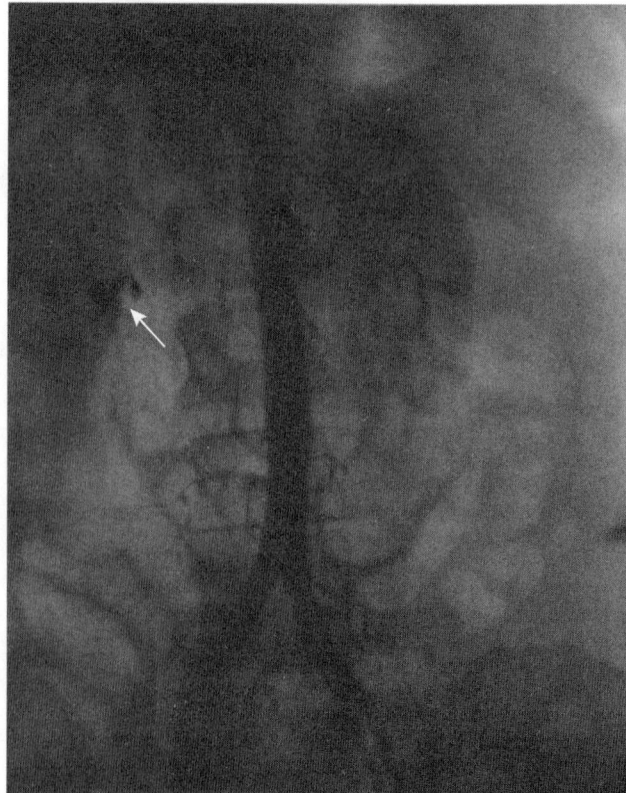

Figure 3 This 56-year-old patient, treated by right hemicolectomy for massive bleeding (24 RBC transfusions/10 hours) from a bleeding right-sided diverticulum shown here required left colectomy 21 months later for massive bleeding (14 transfusions) from a left-sided diverticulum.

DIAGNOSTIC ASSESSMENT AFTER BLEEDING CEASES

Most LGIB stops regardless of etiology. After bleeding stops, the most informative examination is colonoscopy. This permits the endoscopic treatment of vascular ectasia even when not actively bleeding and defines the extent of diverticular disease (Fig. 4). Because bleeding has ceased, no blood is seen at the ileal orifice even if the LGIB originated from the small bowel. When the indications for operative intervention are met, this conundrum may result in a TAC for right-sided vascular ectasia and pandiverticulosis even though the source of bleeding is the small intestine. When the colonoscopy is entirely normal, LGIB is presumed to be of small bowel origin. Push enteroscopy in the stable patient allows visualization of the distal duodenum and proximal 3 to 5 feet of jejunum. Colonoscopy, in an attempt to identify cryptic bleeding, can be extended to assess the distal 25 cm of ileum. Lesions that can be identified and sometimes treated by these techniques include vascular ectasis, polyps, and acute ulcers. Even when the site of bleeding cannot be controlled endoscopically, identification of the source of bleeding helps to direct the successful surgical approach. When the push enteroscopy of the proximal jejunum and the colonoscopy with examination of the distal ileum are negative, the LGIB is presumed to arise from the midportion of the small intestine. This can be assessed by means of angiography in patients with AVMs or by means of an air contrast small bowel follow through in patients with polyps. The identification of either will allow for a successful operative intervention with resection of the segment of arteriovenous malformation or small bowel polyp. When all studies, including the upper endoscopy, push enteroscopy, colonoscopy with distal ileoscopy, mesenteric angiography, and air contrast small bowel follow through, are negative the bleeding is likely to be coming from the midportion of the small bowel. Capsule endoscopy may help to identify the cause of obscure LGIB. Patients who meet the indications for operative intervention can often be successfully treated by laparotomy and specifically looking for a source of bleeding coming from that portion of the small bowel that could not be visualized by the push enteroscopy or colonoscopy with terminal ileoscopy. Often the source of LGIB is apparent.

OPERATIVE INTERVENTION FOR RECURRENT LOWER GASTROINTESTINAL BLEEDING

The vast majority of patients can be successfully managed without operation for the first episode of severe LGIB. When the number of transfusions required during this first episode exceeds four, the likelihood for rebleeding after discharge is significantly increased. A decision must therefore be made as to whether the patient should undergo prophylactic operation to prevent rebleeding or simply be observed, knowing that rebleeding is a significant risk. This decision must take into account comorbidities, which are common in patients with major/massive LGIB. Because both vascular ectasia and pandiverticulosis are diseases of aging, one expects that there will be significant comorbidities including hypertension, diffuse vascular disease, cerebral vascular disease, diabetes melitis, and obesity. Patients with these comorbidities are at risk for either having an operation on the first admission to prevent rebleeding or being

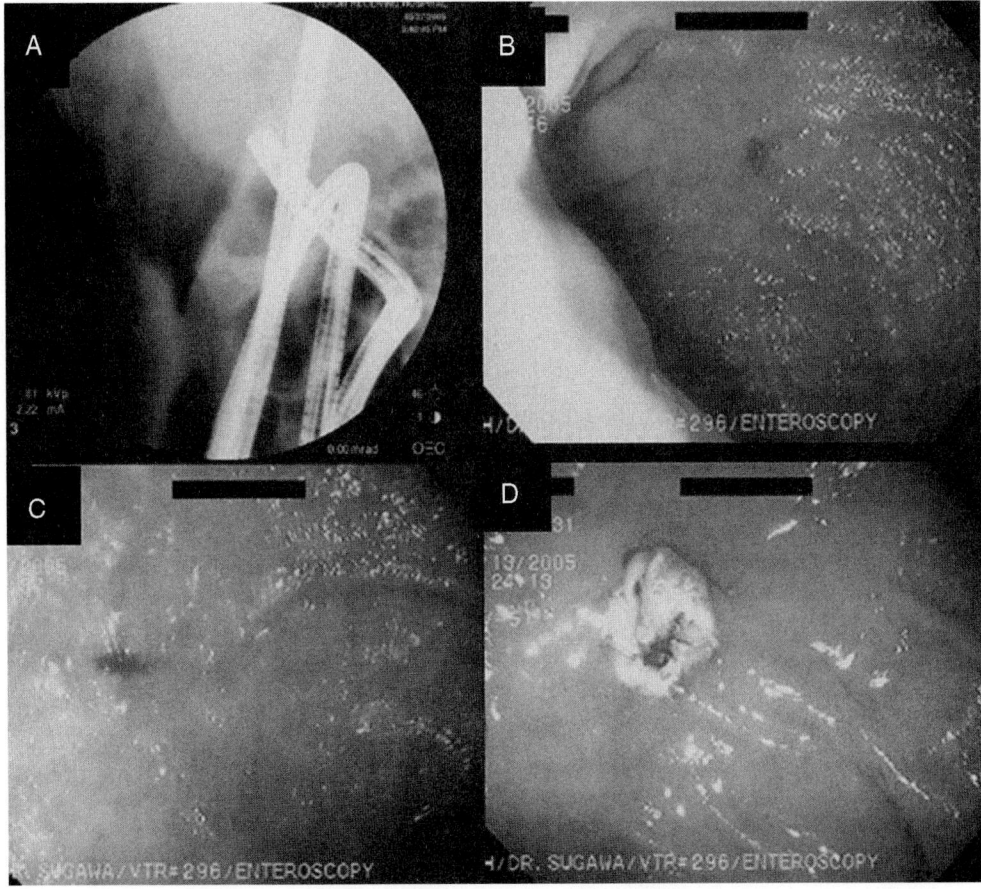

Figure 4 Enteroscopy (**A**) showing nonbleeding vascular ectasia in the jejunum (**B** and **C**) treated by thermal therapy with heater probe (**D**).

observed nonoperatively knowing that a severe recurrent episode of bleeding will aggravate the multiple comorbidities. Recognizing this dilemma, we favor operative intervention on the first hospitalization in patients who require more than six blood transfusions in the absence of a coagulopathy.

When patients requiring fewer than four blood transfusions are successfully treated nonoperatively, there is still a significant risk for rebleeding. This risk is enhanced in patients who are placed back on warfarin (Coumadin; Bristol-Myers Squibb, New York, NY) therapy for such things as atrial fibrillation or prior cerebral vascular attacks. Balancing the risks of Coumadin with the risks of coronary artery ischemia while off Coumadin is an important consideration. Often the risk of anticoagulation in these patients is greater than the risk of coronary artery thrombosis or carotid artery thrombosis. When rebleeding occurs in the patient who has been discontinued from anticoagulant therapy and requires additional blood replacement for maintenance of vital signs, operative intervention is indicated. This decision must, however, reflect comorbidities and the relative risk of operative intervention.

Many years ago, Robert Burns, the poet laureate of Scotland wrote, "the best laid plans of mice and men oft go awry." This is nicely demonstrated in a patient whom we treated some years ago. An elderly woman presented with massive LGIB requiring 11 blood transfusions. Upper endoscopy was normal; lower endoscopy showed pandiverticulosis, colonic blood with no active bleeding, and no blood at the terminal ileum. TAC was performed, and she recovered uneventfully. Three serious rebleeding episodes occurred over the next 18 months. Multiple studies including push enteroscopy and air contrast small bowel series showed multiple small bowel diverticula. No bleeding site was seen on endoscopy or on angiography. After the third recurrent hemorrhage, she underwent laparotomy with devascularization and inversion of approximately 50 of the largest diverticula. Over the next 3 years, she had multiple rebleeding episodes of unknown origin. Fortunately, during one recurrent hemorrhage, an active bleeding diverticulum was seen in the proximal jejunum. Laparotomy and resection of this diverticulum was curative. She lived many more years. This sequence of events predictably occurs in a small number of patients with severe LGIB when bleeding is presumed to arise from pandiverticulosis but the actual site of bleeding is not visualized. Fortunately, the "best guess" decision at the time of operative intervention is usually successful.

SUGGESTED READINGS

Chaudhry V, Hyser MJ, Gracias DH, and others: Colonoscopy: the initial test for acute lower gastrointestinal bleeding, *Am Surg* 64:723, 1998.

Farner R, Lichliter W, Kuhn J, and others: Total colectomy versus limited colonic resection for acute lower gastrointestinal bleeding, *Am J Surg* 178:587, 1999.

Lin S, Rockey DC: Obscure gastrointestinal bleeding, *Gastroenterol Clin N Am* 47:136, 2005.

Miller M Jr, Smith TP: Angiographic diagnosis and endovascular management of non-variceal gastrointestinal hemorrhage, *Gastroenterol Clin N Am* 34:735, 2005.

Newhall SG, Lucas CE, Ledgerwood AM: Diagnostic and therapeutic approach to colonic bleeding, *Am Surg* 47:136, 1981.

Stollman NH, Raskin JB: Diverticular disease of the colon, *J Clin Gastroenterol* 29:241, 1999.

NEWER TECHNIQUES IN LIVER SURGERY

Rebecca Taylor, MD, and Yuman Fong, MD

INTRODUCTION

It is only in the past 20 years that hepatic surgery has been safe enough to be practiced widely. Improvements in patient selection, preoperative preparation, intraoperative technique, and the use of combined modality treatments have resulted in safer surgeries and improved oncologic outcomes. These advances have enabled surgeons to adopt a more aggressive surgical approach to malignant lesions in the liver and have expanded the indications for curative surgical resections for primary hepatocellular carcinoma (HCC) and hepatic metastases.

PREOPERATIVE PREPARATION

Assessment of Hepatic Reserve

Postresection hepatic failure is a devastating complication. When the remaining liver remnant is too small, immediate hepatic failure leads to multisystem organ failure and death, whereas a marginal remnant results in the cycle of complications, prolonged stay in the intensive care unit, and progressive liver failure over weeks, resulting in eventual death.

The future liver remnant (FLR) can be estimated by a number of methods. In general, resection of the right lobe, including segment IV, removes 85% of the liver volume, and it is in these situations that postoperative hepatic reserve may be in jeopardy. For a more precise estimate of the FLR, three-dimensional computed tomography (CT) volumetry is useful. The FLR can be expressed as a percentage of the total liver volume as measured on the preoperative CT or as estimated on the basis of patient size and body surface area. The latter method is called *the standardized FLR measurement*, and a correlation between this value and operative outcome has been established.

As a general rule, hepatic resection can be undertaken in patients with normal hepatic parenchyma when vascular inflow-outflow and biliary drainage can be preserved in two adjacent liver segments with remnant volume of at least 20% of the total estimated liver volume. When the liver parenchyma is compromised by chronic liver disease, high-dose chemotherapy, or severe fibrosis,

a remnant volume of more than 40% is advisable. However, if the specimen is extensively involved with tumor replacing the normal parenchyma, compensatory hypertrophy of the uninvolved side has usually already occurred, and the risk of hepatic insufficiency is negligible.

Although a number of other functional tests have been developed and evaluated, the most notable being indocyanine green retention, none has gained widespread use. A simple and reliable measure of hepatic function in patients with cirrhosis is the Child–Pugh classification. In general, only patients with a Child-Pugh score of less than 7 are candidates for liver resection, and patients with a serum bilirubin more than twice normal or clinically or radiologically detected ascites should also be excluded.

Preoperative Portal Vein Embolization

When an adequate FLR is the only obstacle to a curative hepatic resection, portal vein embolization (PVE) may be used. This procedure, performed several weeks before the scheduled hepatic resection, redirects the portal blood flow toward the hepatic segments that will remain after the resection. The basis of this technique is the ability of the normally quiescent liver to respond to hypoxic or surgical insults with a rapid and massive proliferation of hepatocytes, resulting in the recovery of functional liver mass within 2 weeks (Fig. 1). The clinical rationale for using preoperative PVE is primarily to increase the functional mass of the FLR and therefore reduce the risk of postresection metabolic changes and liver failure. In addition, it is thought to minimize the effects of the abrupt elevation of portal pressure in the FLR that occur during a hepatectomy and can lead to hepatocellular damage in the FLR. The peak hepatocyte replication occurs at 3 to 4 days in the normal liver; the rates of regeneration are slower in the cirrhotic liver, with an overall reduced capacity to respond to the stimulus.

PVE is generally performed in the interventional radiology suite. Every branch of the portal tree to be resected should be occluded to minimize the development of portoportal collaterals that will limit regeneration. A number of embolic agents have been used, including absolute alcohol, fibrin glue with iodized oil, and polyvinyl alcohol, with no significant differences in the rate of hypertrophy or final volume but varying rates of portal vein recanalization.

There is minimal inflammation and no hepatic distortion seen following PVE, and the procedure is generally well tolerated. Patients may experience vague right upper quadrant pain, nausea and vomiting, and a low-grade fever. Complications are mainly technical and include bleeding such as subcapsular hematoma; hemoperitoneum; and hemobilia, arteriovenous fistula, and portal vein thrombosis. However, transient liver failure may occur. Clinically, overt portal hypertension is the only absolute contraindication to PVE, but relative contraindications include tumor

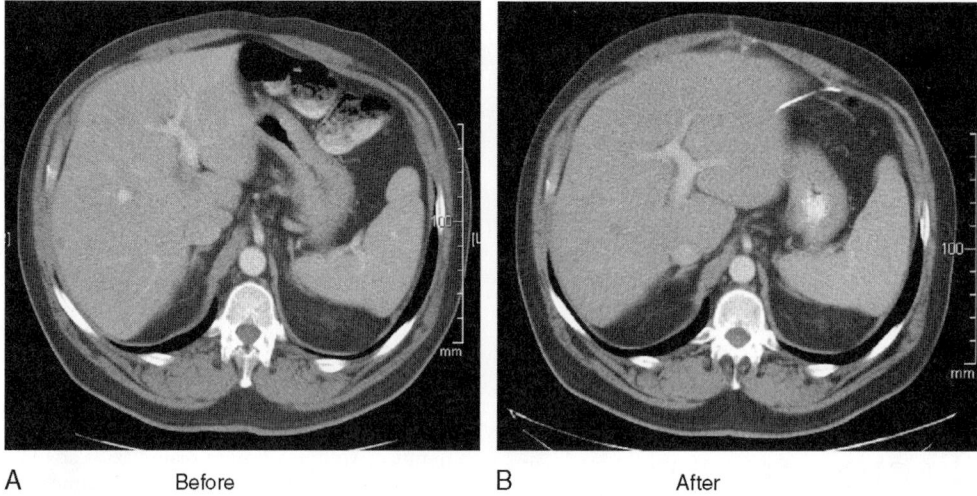

A   Before   B   After

Figure 1 Computed tomography scan of the liver before **(A)** and after **(B)** portal vein embolization to increase the future liver remnant.

invasion of the portal vein or occlusion resulting in portal flow already being diverted, biliary tree obstruction (drainage is recommended), mild portal hypertension, renal failure, and uncorrected coagulopathy.

The outcomes in patients with chronic liver disease undergoing preoperative PVE and resection are better in comparison with resection alone. The incidence of postoperative complications, liver failure, and death are reduced in this population with the use of PVE, and therefore the overall rate of survival is significantly better. In persons with no underlying liver disease, PVE significantly increases the volume of the FLR, reduces the incidence of postoperative complications and length of stay, and increases the number of patients eligible for curative resection. Recurrence in the liver after PVE and resection is also more often amenable to further treatment.

Assessment of Resectability

Resectability can be assessed in many patients using preoperative imaging. Tumors that are situated within the liver parenchyma at a distance from major vascular structures with no lesions detected outside the planned area of resection are clearly resectable. Tumors that are multiple and bilateral with little parenchymal sparing are, obviously, unresectable. In contrast, tumors that are closely applied to or even invading the major hilar structures or the inferior vena cava (IVC) are difficult to evaluate with preoperative imaging alone, and surgeons should be cautious about declaring these tumors unresectable before exploration and hepatic mobilization. Slow-growing tumors with smooth margins that compress surrounding structures (pushing tumors) are nearly always resectable, whereas tumors with irregular margins are more likely to be invasive. Even IVC and portal vein involvement are no longer absolute contraindications because techniques such as major vascular reconstruction have been perfected, and other techniques such as ex vivo resection have been developed.

In the setting of colorectal cancer metastases, bilobar metastases were previously considered a contraindication for a curative resection. Increasingly, the use of multimodal therapy using chemotherapy, PVE, and ablative techniques combined with a staged resection has extended the indications for curative surgery. The use of neoadjuvant chemotherapy in unresectable patients may render up to 40% of patients eligible for resection. If the FLR is marginal, PVE may be used. If a single lesion remains outside the area of resection,

then ablative techniques, such as radiofrequency ablation, can be used. Alternatively, a two-staged resection may be planned. In the first stage, the liver segments with the highest number of tumors are removed, followed by chemotherapy to suppress tumor growth while the hepatic remnant hypertrophies. After the FLR has achieved an adequate volume, the second surgery is undertaken to remove the remaining tumors. Approximately one third of patients with bilobar tumors can undergo this type of procedure, but among these patients the 3-year survival rate is 35%. The use of neoadjuvant chemotherapy has been associated with severe steatohepatitis, particularly in obese patients, and hepatic fibrosis, making resection more technically challenging.

Preoperative Hepatic Arterial Embolization

Vascular tumors that derive most of their blood supply from the hepatic artery, such as primary HCC and secondary neuroendocrine tumors, are most likely to respond to embolization. The indications for embolization are preoperative and palliative. The rationale for preoperative transcatheter arterial chemoembolization (TACE) in HCC is that it will induce tumor necrosis and therefore limit the spillage and vascular dissemination of viable tumor cells during resection, particularly in larger tumors with capsular invasion and vessel involvement. A number of studies have demonstrated a significant reduction in extrahepatic and diffuse intrahepatic tumor recurrence with an improved disease-free survival. The practice is controversial, however, because other studies were unable to show any differences in long-term survival and because preoperative TACE may make liver resection more difficult owing to the development of inflammation of the porta and perihepatic adhesions. In patients with metastatic neuroendocrine tumors to the liver, preoperative embolization is used to reduce the vascularity and volume of a single metastasis before resection. Palliative hepatic bland and chemoembolization are also used for both tumor types.

INTRAOPERATIVE ASSESSMENT

Anesthetic Technique

The possibility of significant intraoperative hemorrhage should be considered, and therefore intraoperative monitoring with a central

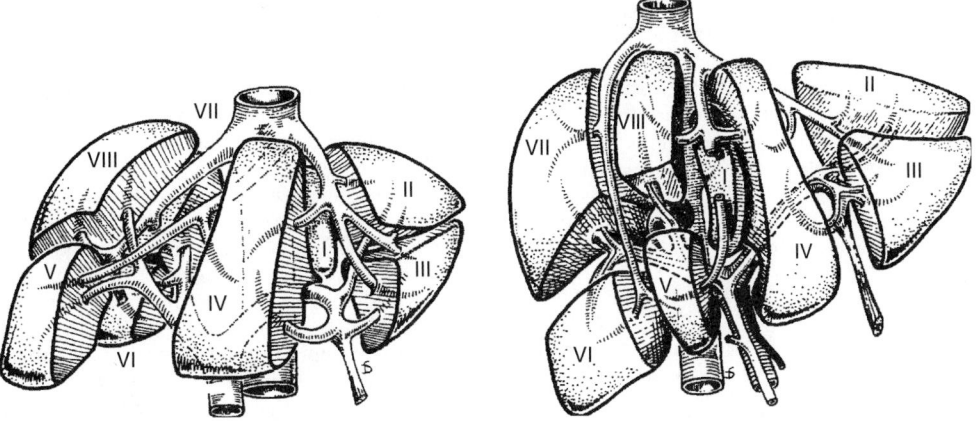

Figure 2 Functional division of the liver into segments according to Couinaud's nomenclature. *From Schulick R: Newer techniques in liver surgery. In Cameron JL, editor: Current Surgical Therapy, ed 7, Philadelphia, 2001, Elsevier Mosby, p. 328.*

venous catheter and adequate intravenous access and facilities for rapid transfusion should be established. Maintaining the central venous pressure less than 5 mm Hg limits IVC distention and thereby minimizes venous bleeding during parenchymal transection. This requires intraoperative fluid restriction and acceptance of a marginal urine output (25 ml/hr). The patient should be kept in 15 degrees of the Trendelenburg position to improve cardiac preload and to prevent air embolism. After the resection is complete, the intravascular volume can be immediately re-expanded. When feasible, healthy patients are encouraged to donate 2 units of autologous blood before surgery.

Surgical Technique

Hepatic Anatomy

Hepatic resections require a precise understanding of surgical anatomy of the liver, the portal triads and hepatic veins that supply and drain each independent segment (Fig. 2). The liver is divided by Cantlie's line, which runs from the gallbladder bed anteriorly to the suprahepatic IVC posteriorly and marks the path of the middle hepatic vein. The three hepatic veins (right, middle, and left) divide the liver into four sectors (left lateral, left medial, right anterior, and right posterior), and these are further subdivided into segments by the transverse plane, along which lie the right and left portal veins. These eight segments, defined by Couinaud, have their own vascular inflow, outflow, and biliary drainage. The right hepatic vein separates the right anterior sector (segments V and VIII) from the right posterior sector (segments VI and VII). In the left lobe of the liver, the umbilical fissure separates the left lateral sector (segments II and III) from the left medial sector (segment IV). The caudate lobe is segment I which derives portal structures from the right and left side and has venous drainage directly into the IVC.

The portal structures outside of the liver are not surrounded by a fibrous sheath and can be dissected separately. The right portal vein and hepatic duct follow a short extrahepatic course before entering the liver and dividing into the anterior and posterior sectoral branches. The left hepatic duct follows a longer and more horizontal course at the base segment IV before entering the umbilical fissure and sending branches to segments II and III and "feedback branches" to segment IV. Within the liver, the portal structures are enveloped in a fibrous sheath, which is an extension of Glisson's capsule. This distinguishes them from the thin-walled hepatic veins, both visually and on ultrasound scan.

Incision and Exposure

Although the incision used depends on the type of resection to be undertaken, adequate exposure is imperative (Fig. 3). The lower chest should always be exposed in case a median sternotomy or thoracoabdominal incision is necessary to gain access to the suprahepatic IVC. An extended right subcostal incision provides excellent exposure for both right and left hepatectomy and has been associated with a lower hernia rate than the Mercedes incision (bilateral subcostal incision with vertical midline extension). After the abdomen is opened, a complete exploratory laparotomy should be performed, with attention to evaluating lymph nodes along the

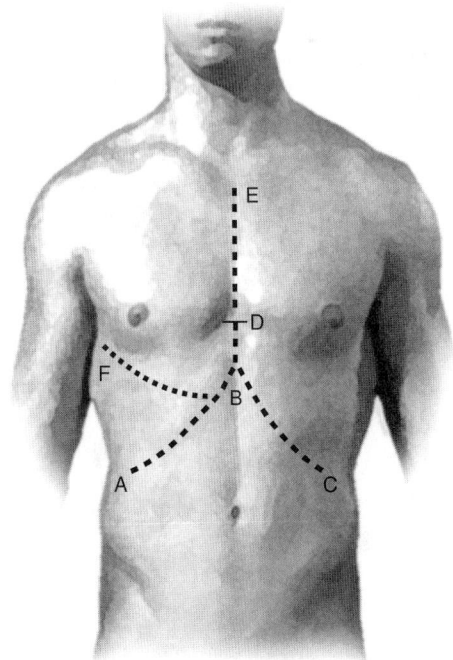

Figure 3 The incisions used for partial hepatectomy. *(A, B, C, D)* "Rooftop" incision with vertical extension. *(D, E)* Median sternotomy. *(F)* Right thoracic extension. *From Blumgart LH: Liver resection for benign disease and for liver and biliary tumors. In Blumgart LH and Fong Y, editors: Surgery of the liver and biliary tract, ed 3, Edinburgh, 2000, Churchill Livingstone, p. 1653.*

hepatic artery and celiac axis and palpating the liver with two hands to detect previously undetected additional metastases. The ligamentum teres and the falciform ligament are divided up to the suprahepatic IVC posteriorly. To mobilize the right lobe of the liver, the right triangular ligament is incised to expose the bare area. The liver can then be rotated to the left, and the venocaval ligament is divided with an ENDO-GIA stapler (US Surgical, Norwalk, CT) or scissors, exposing the retrohepatic IVC. The left lobe of the liver is mobilized by division of the left triangular ligament at its apex on the far left, exposing the bare area, left hepatic vein, and upper IVC.

Vascular Inflow and Outflow Control

Intraoperative blood loss is a primary determinant of perioperative outcome. Vascular occlusion techniques selectively reduce the blood flow to the liver before parenchymal transection. Typically, vascular inflow is controlled first, followed by vascular outflow, and both can be managed either inside or outside of the liver. Preoperative assessment of the hepatic vascular anatomy, such as a high-quality triphasic CT scan, is necessary to define the anatomic relationship of the tumor to the major hepatic blood vessels.

Vascular inflow control can be obtained by extrahepatic dissection of the porta hepatis or intrahepatic pedicle ligation. Extrahepatic dissection increases the risk of biliary injury, especially on the right side, where anatomic variations of the major sectoral ducts are common. For this reason, many surgeons reserve this approach for tumors that are close to the hilum and for which pedicle ligation might compromise tumor clearance. Intrahepatic pedicle ligation can be performed before or during parenchymal transection. The pedicles are easily and directly accessed through small hepatotomies made at specific locations on the inferior surface of the liver (Fig. 4, A and B), and this technique has been greatly facilitated by the use of ENDO-GIA vascular staplers. Pedicle ligation results in segmental hepatic ischemia and the characteristic demarcation demonstrating the plane for parenchymal transection. For a detailed description of the use of staplers for vascular control and

for the placement of hepatotomies for segmental portal pedicle ligation, the reader is referred to Fong and Blumgart (1997).

Vascular outflow control further reduces bleeding during parenchymal transection. It is obtained by isolation and ligation of one of the three main hepatic veins. Despite their short course, these veins can usually be isolated extrahepatically near their junction with the IVC. Once again, vascular staplers may be helpful. In tumors located near the hepatic vein trunks and IVC, this technique facilitates tumor clearance and reduces the risk of major hemorrhage.

Total liver inflow occlusion may be achieved by applying a tourniquet to the hepatoduodenal ligament (Pringle maneuver, Fig. 5). Although it is effective at reducing blood loss, even after selective inflow ligation has been performed, it may also induce ischemia and portal hypertension. A noncirrhotic liver can tolerate total inflow occlusion for 60 minutes or more, but in patients with liver dysfunction, that time may be significantly shorter. Applying the Pringle maneuver for 10 minutes at a time, followed by reperfusion, may protect the liver from subsequent prolonged ischemia, a technique called *ischemic preconditioning*. This technique of intermittent clamping, compared with continuous clamping, improves overall parenchymal tolerance with no increase in operative blood loss. Total vascular exclusion includes total inflow occlusion and control of the infrahepatic and suprahepatic IVC. This technique can be associated with significant hemodynamic instability and unique complications, such as spontaneous splenic rupture.

Parenchymal Transection

Parenchymal division should be performed along anatomic planes to minimize blood loss. The parenchyma should be opened completely from anterior to posterior because this avoids working in a hole and prevents blood from pooling and obscuring the area of transection. A number of techniques can be used; none has been shown to have a clear advantage. The crushing technique uses a Kelly clamp to open the hepatic parenchyma, bluntly exposing the vessels and biliary radicals that can be clipped or tied. Vascular staplers, such as the

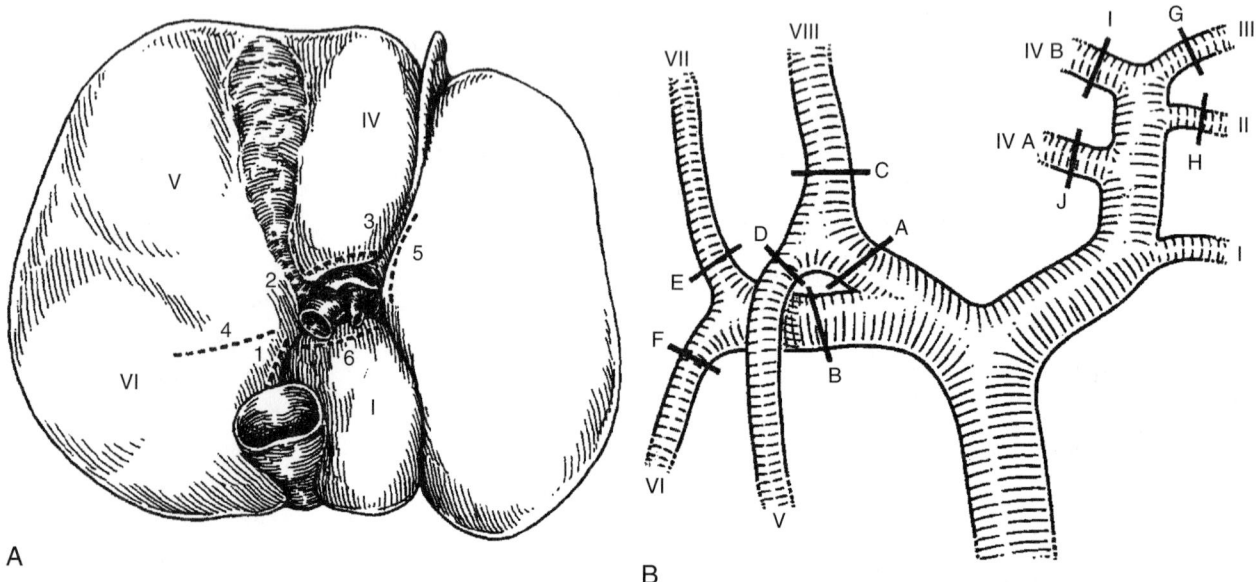

Figure 4 **(A)** Sites for hepatectomy in portal pedicle isolation. The undersurface face of the liver is illustrated. Dotted lines indicate sites for hepatectomy. Incision at 3 allows lowering of the hilar plate. Incisions at 1 and 2 allow control of the right main pedicle. Incisions at 1 and 4 allow control of the right posterior pedicle. Incisions at 2 and 4 allow control of the right anterior pedicle. Incisions at 3 and 5 allow control of the left pedicle. **(B)** Distribution of pedicles and points of control (A–J) for segmental resections. Note that control of the anterior **(A)** or posterior **(B)** sectoral pedicles allows anterior or posterior right sectorectomy. Control of pedicles at points A, I, and J allows central hepatectomy. *Part A: From Schulick R: Newer techniques in liver surgery. In Cameron JL, editor: Current Surgical Therapy, ed 7, Philadelphia, 2001, Elsevier Mosby, p. 331. Part B: From Blumgart LH: Liver resection for benign disease and for liver and biliary tumors. In Blumgart LH and Fong Y, editors: Surgery of the liver and biliary tract, ed 3, Edinburgh, 2000, Churchill Livingstone, p. 1683.*

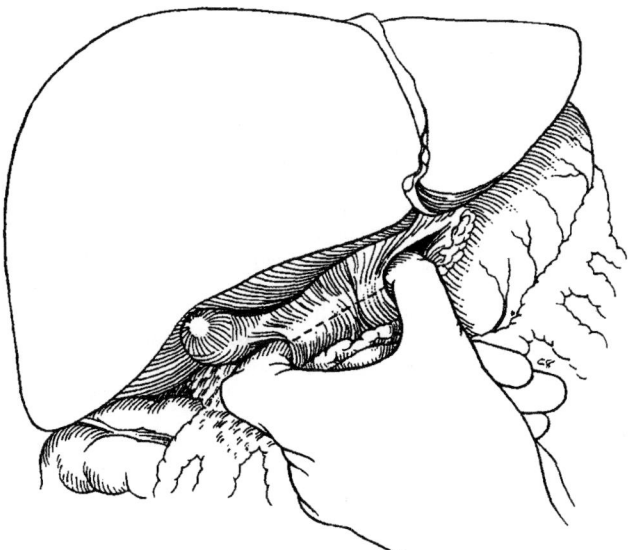

Figure 5 Pringle maneuver. Access to the porta hepatis is achieved by inserting an index finger into the foramen of Winslow and the thumb through the defect created in the gastrohepatic ligament. For total inflow occlusion, a traumatic vascular clamp or Silastic (Dow Corning, Midland, MI) loop can be placed and tightened. *From Schulick R: Newer techniques in liver surgery. In Cameron JL, editor: Current Surgical Therapy, ed 7, Philadelphia, 2001, Elsevier Mosby, p. 330.*

slim-linear ENDO-GIA, are useful in dividing major vessels and pedicles within the liver. Hemostasis of the cut surface of the liver can be obtained with argon beam coagulation or a hemostatic compound, such as Avitene (Davol, Cranston, RI). When the liver is fibrotic from cirrhosis or chemotherapy, the organ fractures more easily, resulting in bleeding. In these cases, newer instruments such as the ultrasonic dissector or water jet dissector may be preferable. In addition, vascular staplers are useful in dividing major vessels and pedicles within the liver. Recently developed dissecting and sealing devices use radiofrequency ablation (RFA) energy to precoagulate the parenchyma before transection, resulting in the occlusion of small vessels and bile ducts. These devices are designed be hemostatic without the need for inflow occlusion.

A tumor-free surgical margin within the hepatic parenchyma is essential because patients with histologically positive margins do as poorly as patients with resectable liver metastases not removed. Adjuvants to improve outcomes in close or positive margins have been used, including edge cryotherapy or RFA with TissueLink (TissueLink Medical, Dover, NH).

Hepatectomy and Hepatic Lobectomy

There are essentially five types of major hepatic resection as defined by Couinaud (Table 1). In a right hepatectomy, complete mobilization along the IVC before parenchymal transection is a basic maneuver. However, when right-sided tumors are extremely large or are invading the diaphragm, mobilization may be difficult. In these cases, an anterior approach, with parenchymal transection from the anterior surface down to the IVC, reduces tumor dissemination resulting from manipulation and avoids compression of the remnant liver. This technique is facilitated by the hanging liver maneuver, which involves exposure and blunt dissection of the suprahepatic IVC (between the right and middle hepatic veins) and the infrahepatic IVC (posterior to the caudate and to the left of the right hepatic vein). Blind dissection continues along the anterior surface of the IVC until a tape can be passed along its length and pulled upward (Fig. 6), effectively elevating the liver away from the anterior surface of the IVC. This maneuver provides

Table 1: The Five Types of Major Hepatic Resection as Defined by Couinaud

Hepatic Resection	Segments
Right hepatic lobectomy (Right hepatectomy)	V, VI, VII, VIII
Left hepatic lobectomy (Left hepatectomy)	II, III, IV
Extended right lobectomy (Right trisegmentectomy)	IV, V, VI, VII, VII, sometimes I
Extended left lobectomy (Left trisegmentectomy)	II, III, IV, V, VIII, sometimes I
Left lateral segmentectomy	II and II

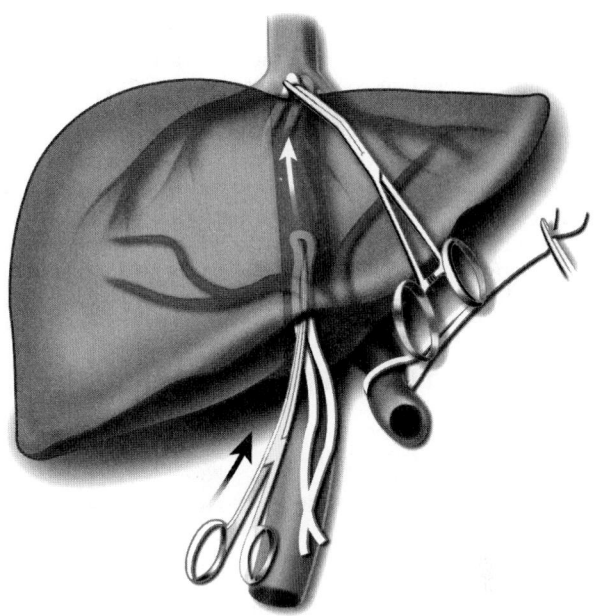

Figure 6 Hanging maneuver time is realized after lifting the liver with a tape. This prepares a better and safer parenchymal transection without mobilization of the right liver. *From Belghiti J, Guevara OA, Noun R, and others: J Am Coll Surg 193(1):109–111, 2001.*

excellent exposure to the transection surface in the deep parenchyma and protection of the anterior surface of the IVC; and, when rotated to the left, the tape defines the plane of transection along the left side of the middle hepatic vein.

Segmental Hepatic Resections

A detailed understanding of the segmental anatomy of the liver and significant advances in imaging technology have led to parenchymal-sparing hepatic resections. Segmentectomies have the advantage of preserving functional liver parenchyma and therefore minimizing physiologic impact compared with classic major liver resection, while respecting the anatomic boundaries between individual segments, unlike nonanatomic wedge resection. Each segment is supplied by its own portal pedicle and is separated by relatively avascular planes, making hepatic parenchymal transection technically easier. Moreover, most tumors grow within a segment or spread along portal pedicles, thereby respecting the anatomic boundaries between segments and providing an oncologic rationale for performing segmental resection. This concept is illustrated by the higher margin–positive rate (16% vs. 2%) and inferior survival following nonanatomic wedge resection compared with segmentectomy. Segmental resections are also particularly useful for patients with HCC, bilobar metastases, or those undergoing repeat hepatic resections because they provide parenchymal sparing.

MINIMALLY INVASIVE HEPATIC RESECTION

Although laparoscopy is routinely used for marsupialization of hepatic cysts, wedge resections of benign lesions and small tumors, and staging in the setting of colorectal metastases, it has only recently been used to perform hepatic resections. In comparative studies with open liver surgery, operative time was longer with laparoscopy, but mean hospital stay was shorter, whereas blood loss, morbidity, and mortality were similar. The location of the lesions is critical in determining the feasibility of laparoscopic resection. Lesions located along the free edge of the liver (segments II and VI), as well as the left lateral segment, are technically most suited to laparoscopic resection, as are smaller lesions (<5 cm). In most series, the conversion rate is approximately 10% to 20%, and failure to control bleeding is the most important reason. The ultrasonic scalpel is a useful tool during laparoscopic parenchymal transection because it coagulates blood vessels and biliary radicals up to 3 mm in diameter with minimal thermal energy spread and no plume production. Tumor recurrence does not appear to be increased by the laparoscopic approach, and disease-free survival appears to be equivalent for both HCC and colorectal cancer metastases.

ALTERNATIVE LIVER THERAPIES

Radiofrequency Ablation

Although surgery is still considered the preferred treatment for primary and metastatic hepatic malignancies, RFA is emerging as the primary modality for tumor ablation in lesions not amenable to surgical resection. The technique involves the transfer of electric energy to induce thermal injury within the tissue. An alternating current in the radiofrequency range is applied to the tissue via an electrode. Because the tissue has a relatively high electrical resistance, the alternating electric field results in ionic friction. This generates heat that desiccates the surrounding tissue, leading to coagulation necrosis. The minimum temperature threshold is approximately 50°C, with an optimal temperature of 80° to 100°C. Temperatures above 110°C result in charring, which increases the resistance around the electrode, thereby reducing the transfer of thermal energy. The zone of thermal ablation is based on the size and shape of the electrode used, and strategies involving novel probe designs, such as internally cooled and multi-tined expandable electrodes, have been developed to maximize the zone of ablation. A 5-cm sphere of thermal ablation is approximately the limit for a single electrode, and this can be used to treat a tumor no larger than 3 cm in its longest dimension to ensure that a 1-cm margin around the entire tumor is obtained. Larger tumors can be treated by the use of multiple overlapping applications. Large vessels such as the hepatic veins act as heat sinks by removing the thermal energy in the blood. This effectively protects the vessel wall from thermal injury but may also limit the ablation efficacy in these tumors. Unfortunately, these are often the tumors that are not amenable to surgical resection.

The indications for RFA continue to evolve, but as a general principle, the patient should not be a candidate for hepatic resection and successful treatment of the hepatic tumor should improve the patient's prognosis. Patients may be inoperable because of poor general health or cirrhosis or unresectable because of tumor location or distribution. In addition, RFA may be used as an adjuvant modality at the time of hepatic resection to treat tumors that are not amenable to surgical resection or as an alternative to repeated resection in patients with a hepatic recurrence after resection. A limited life expectancy (<6 months), severe cirrhosis, or portal vein thrombosis are considered contraindications to RFA. As the number of lesions increases, the potential for complications increases and the theoretical benefit decreases; therefore many centers prefer to treat patients who have four or fewer lesions.

Prospective studies of colorectal metastases comparing surgical resection, surgical resection plus RFA, and RFA alone demonstrate that overall and recurrence-free survival is superior with surgery (4-year survival of 65% for surgery vs. 36% for combined and 22% for RFA alone), but all groups had better survival than patients treated with chemotherapy alone. This suggests that patients who can undergo local treatment of isolated hepatic tumors with RFA improves survival. In patients with HCC and cirrhosis who were not candidates for surgery, RFA used as the primary therapy resulted in a 5-year survival of 48% with a recurrence rate of 81% for new tumors and 10% for local tumor progression. Major complications occur in approximately 6% after RFA and include hepatic abscess, bile leak, intrahepatic hematoma or hemoperitoneum, pneumothorax and pleural effusion, intestinal perforation (percutaneous technique only), hepatic failure, and death. The results with RFA and indications for its use will continue to expand as our experience and understanding of this technique evolve.

Microwave Ablation

Microwave coagulation causes molecular vibration of dipoles, such as water, producing frictional heat and thermal coagulation, similar to RFA. The coagulative necrosis produced around the microwave needle is rapid, resulting in the formation of a tissue coagulum that prevents further dissipation of heat into the tissue, limiting the area of necrosis. The microwave needle must therefore be advanced 5 to 10 mm through the tumor and surrounding tissue, or multiple needles are required. Studies with microwave coagulation have demonstrated efficacy with both HCC and colorectal metastases with a low local recurrence rate (<10%), but survival appears to be inferior to hepatic resection. The results with RFA and microwave coagulation and indications for their use will continue to expand as our experience and understanding of these techniques evolve.

SUGGESTED READINGS

Fong Y, Blumgart LH: Useful stapling techniques in liver surgery, *J Am Coll Surg* 185:93, 1997.

FURTHER READINGS

Abdalla EK, Barnett CC, Doherty D, and others: Extended hepatectomy in patients with hepatobiliary malignancies with and without preoperative portal vein embolization, *Arch Surg* 137:675, 2002.

Adam R, Avisar E, Ariche A, and others: Five-year survival following hepatic resection after neoadjuvant therapy for nonresectable colorectal, *Ann Surg Oncol* 8:347, 2001.

Blumgart LH, Fong Y, editors: *Surgery of the liver and biliary tract*, ed 3, Edinburgh, 2000, Churchill Livingstone.

Launois B, Jamieson GG: The importance of Glisson's capsule and its sheaths in the intrahepatic approach to resection of the liver, *Surg Gynecol Obstet* 174:7, 1992.

HEPATIC ABSCESS

Conrad H. Simpfendorfer, MD, and J. Michael Henderson, MD

Hepatic abscess is an uncommon disease that continues to present a challenge in diagnosis and treatment. Changing patient populations have resulted in a different profile of hepatic abscess in larger referral hospitals: immunocompromised patients and patients having various invasive ablative procedures for liver tumors are a new emerging population at risk for liver abscesses. Hepatic abscesses are separated into three major categories according to their causative microorganisms: (1) pyogenic, which are typically polymicrobial, are caused by aerobe and anaerobic bacteria; (2) amebic, which are due to *Entamoeba histolytica*; and (3) fungal, which are usually caused by *Candida* species. The overwhelming majority of liver abscess cases in the United States are pyogenic, accounting for approximately 80%. Amebic and fungal abscesses each represent approximately 10% of hepatic abscess cases.

Over the past half-century, the morbidity and mortality rates of hepatic abscess have declined considerably. Advancements in radiologic technology, improved antimicrobial agents, and improved treatment algorithms and techniques have contributed to greater success in management of hepatic abscess.

PYOGENIC LIVER ABSCESS

Epidemiology

In 1938, Oschner and DeBakey described 47 patients with pyogenic liver abscess and gave a review of the world literature. They reported an incidence of 8 per 100,000 hospital admissions. Patients were typically in their 20s or 30s, and the pyogenic liver abscess was largely attributed to pyelophlebitis from complicated appendicitis. Today pyogenic liver abscess is by far the most common form of liver abscess in the United States, with a reported incidence ranging from 8 to 22 cases per 100,000 hospital admissions. A slight increase has been noted since 1970, with current reports placing the incidence at 10 to 15 cases per 100,000 admissions. The increase may be attributed to improved detection and a rising incidence in the treatment of benign and malignant biliary tract disease. Along with a slight increase in the incidence of pyogenic liver abscess, a profound change in epidemiology has emerged since Oschner and DeBakey's classic publication. Since the introduction of effective antibiotics, the average patient with pyogenic liver abscess is now typically between 50 and 60 years of age, and the cause of the abscess is often of biliary tract origin.

Pathogenesis

The liver is normally a sterile organ that is typically able to clear portal venous bacterial loads on a regular basis. A liver abscess occurs when both a bacterial source and a route for inoculation exist and the initial inflammatory response fails to clear the infection from the liver. The potential routes for hepatic invasion are the (1) biliary tree, (2) portal vein, (3) hepatic artery, (4) direct extension, and (5) trauma. Although these routes of infection provide a pathway for identifying a potential source of infection, cryptogenic abscesses are still common and predominate in many series.

Ascending suppurative cholangitis is now the most common identifiable cause of pyogenic abscess. Biliary obstruction from benign or malignant disease results in bile stasis, bacterial colonization, infection, and ascension into the liver. In the Western world, biliary obstruction from hepatobiliary malignancy is becoming a more predominant factor in pyogenic abscess, whereas in Asia, recurrent pyogenic cholangitis from intrahepatic stones is still a common cause. Other causes include Caroli's disease, invasion of the biliary tree by *Ascaris lumbricoides*, or previous biliary-enteric anastomosis.

Pyelophlebitis from any infectious disorder of the gastrointestinal tract may result in pyogenic abscess. Appendicitis, diverticulitis, pancreatitis, omphalitis, inflammatory bowel disease, pelvic inflammatory disease, or postoperative infection can result in ascending portal vein infection and liver abscess.

Generalized septicemia or bacteremia can spread to the liver via the hepatic artery. This can occur with endocarditis, line sepsis, pneumonia, osteomyelitis, or even dental infection. Frequently, patients with severe sepsis are found to have multiple microabscesses at autopsy.

Direct extension can occur from gastric or duodenal perforation, suppurative cholecystitis, or contact with subphrenic or perinephric abscesses. Trauma, either penetrating or blunt, may result in hematoma and devitalized liver tissue that is susceptible to infection. Penetrating injuries allow for the direct inoculation of external bacteria, whereas additional organ injuries may provide secondary sources of bacterial infection.

Iatrogenic causes, including hepatic arterial embolization, hepatic arterial chemoembolization, radiofrequency ablation, ethanol injection, and cryotherapy for liver lesions have all been associated with liver abscess. The incidence of liver abscess formation after radiofrequency ablation ranges from 1.7% to 5.8%, and for transcatheter arterial chemoembolization (TACE) the incidence is reported to be between 0% and 2.7%. The major determining factor for liver abscess formation following either radiofrequency ablation or chemoembololization is prior bilioenteric anastomosis. In a study by Kim and colleagues, the risk of hepatic abscess complication in patients who had undergone Whipple procedure was more than 800 times greater than patients without bilioenteric anastomosis.

Hepatic abscess is a rare complication after orthotopic liver transplantation and is frequently associated with hepatic artery thrombosis. Tachopoulou and colleagues reported an incidence of 4.8 patients per 1000 transplant patient-years. Liver aspirates grew gram-positive aerobic bacteria in 50% of isolates and gram-negative aerobic bacteria in 30% of isolates, and anaerobes or yeast were found in 10% of isolates each. The mortality rate for liver transplant patients who developed hepatic abscess was 42% compared with 28% for all liver transplant patients.

Microbiology

With the various routes of infection, microorganisms recovered from pyogenic liver abscess generally reflect the underlying pathologic process and include aerobic and anaerobic organisms (Table 1). *Escherichia coli* and *Klebsiella pneumonia* are the most common aerobic organisms cultured and reflect the increased incidence of biliary tract source. Other commonly encountered aerobes include Enterococci and viridans streptococci, found primarily in polymicrobial abscesses. Whereas *Staphylococcus aureus* tends to be more commonly associated with monomicrobial abscesses, *Bacteroides* species is the most common anaerobic organism, followed by *Fusobacterium* and anaerobic streptococci. Anaerobic and mixed cultures of bacteria favor a colonic or appendiceal source. The increasing use of prompt empiric wide-spectrum antimicrobial therapy occasionally results in sterile abscess aspirates.

Table 1: Pyogenic Liver Abscess Microbiology

	Gram-negative Aerobes	Gram-positive Aerobes	Anaerobes
Common (≥10%)	*Escherichia coli* *Klebsiella*	*Staphylococcus aureus* *Enterococcus* spp. Viridans streptococci	*Bacteroides* spp.
Uncommon (1%–10%)	Pseudomonas *Proteus* Enterobacter *Citrobacter* Serratia	β-hemolytic streptococci	*Fusobacterium* Anaerobic streptococci *Clostridium* *Lactobacilli*

Diagnosis

Clinical Presentation

The classic triad of fever, jaundice, and right upper quadrant tenderness is found in only 10% of patients at presentation. Patients typically present with fever, chills, and abdominal pain, along with a variable array of nonspecific constitutional symptoms, including malaise, fatigue, anorexia, and weight loss. Systemic symptoms may be minimal in immunosuppressed patients. On physical examination, approximately half of patients have right upper quadrant tenderness or hepatomegally. Jaundice is seen in less than half and is commonly seen in patients with underlying biliary tract disease. Leukocytosis and anemia are present in the majority of patients, and abnormal liver function test results are common, with alkaline phosphatase being elevated in most patients. Blood cultures are positive in approximately half of patients.

Imaging

Radiographic imaging studies are essential in establishing the diagnosis of hepatic abscess. Abnormalities on plain x-ray of the abdomen and chest can be seen in 50% of patients. The findings are generally nonspecific and reflect signs of subdiaphragmatic pathology (e.g., elevated hemidiaphragm, right lower lobe atelectasis), and they provide little help in making the diagnosis. Ultrasound and computer tomography (CT) scan have the proven benefit of excellent sensitivity in visualizing the liver abscess and providing image-guided diagnosis and therapy.

Ultrasound is highly sensitive (80%–95%), noninvasive, and better at visualizing the biliary tree than CT scan, which makes it the ideal study for initial screening for hepatic abscess. Contrast-enhanced CT scan has a higher sensitivity (95%–100%) and the improved capability to demonstrate smaller and multiple abscesses. CT scan also has the added benefit of demonstrating any underlying primary pathology that may exist in the abdomen or pelvis. Ultrasound and CT scan also have the added benefit of providing image-guided percutaneous aspiration or drainage of the liver abscess (Fig. 1).

Magnetic resonance imaging (MRI) of the liver is another extremely sensitive technique for visualizing hepatic lesions but is less accessible, more costly, and not ideal for interventional procedures. Neither ultrasound, CT, nor MRI can readily differentiate pyogenic from amebic liver abscess.

Therapy

Treatment of pyogenic liver abscess involves not only therapy for the abscess but also identification and treatment of the underlying

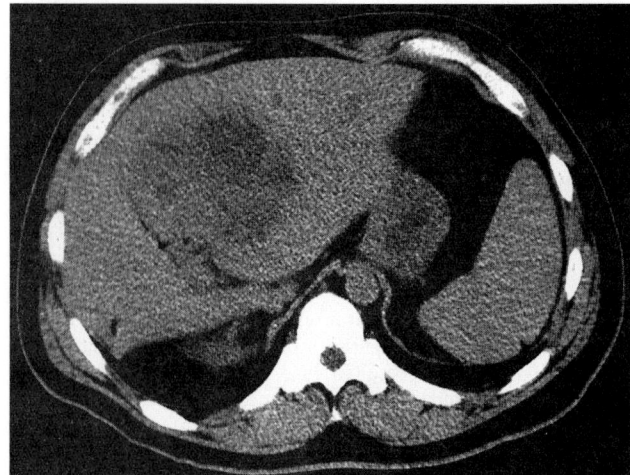

Figure 1 Computed tomography scan demonstrating hypodense abscess in left hepatic lobe. The patient has a history of Roux-en-Y hepatojejunostomy for common bile duct excision.

cause of the liver abscess. Pyogenic liver abscess is traditionally treated with the administration of antibiotics and drainage of purulent collections. Prompt administration of empiric antibiotic therapy and early diagnostic imaging with ultrasound and CT scan should be obtained whenever pyogenic liver abscess is suspected. Percutaneous aspiration or drainage should be performed if no intraabdominal disease requiring surgical intervention is identified. If a primary disorder is identified that requires operative treatment, surgical drainage of the liver abscess is performed in conjunction with the treatment of the underlying disease.

Antibiotics

Empiric antibiotic therapy should be initiated early, and treatment should be directed toward the suspected origin of infection. Blood specimens for culture and amebic serology should be obtained before administration of antibiotics when possible. Therapy should not be delayed for cultures from the abscess. Initial therapy includes broad-spectrum antibiotics that target aerobes and anaerobes. Combination regimens, including an aminoglycoside, metronidazole, and either ampicillin or vancomycin or a third-generation cephalosporin and metronidazole have traditionally been used as initial therapy. Metronidazole is used to empirically treat both anaerobes (especially *Bacteroides fragilis*) and *Entamoeba histolytica*. Single broad-spectrum agents such as ticarcillin-clavulanate, imapenem-cilastin, or piperacillin-tazobactam provide alternate therapy. The treatment should be tailored according to the final isolated organism and its antibiotic susceptibility profile. Typically pyogenic liver abscess is treated with 2 to 3 weeks of parenteral antibiotics, followed by 4 to 6 weeks of oral antibiotics.

Drainage

Although successful treatment of pyogenic liver abscess with antibiotics alone has been reported, the practice has been limited to selected patients, with mixed results. Antibiotic therapy without drainage should be considered only in those patients with small liver abscesses not amenable to drainage or in those for whom drainage presents an unacceptable risk. Antibiotic therapy along with aspiration or drainage of the abscess remains the standard of care.

Percutaneous Drainage

First introduced in 1953, percutaneous drainage of pyogenic liver abscesses did not gain widespread acceptance until the 1980s with

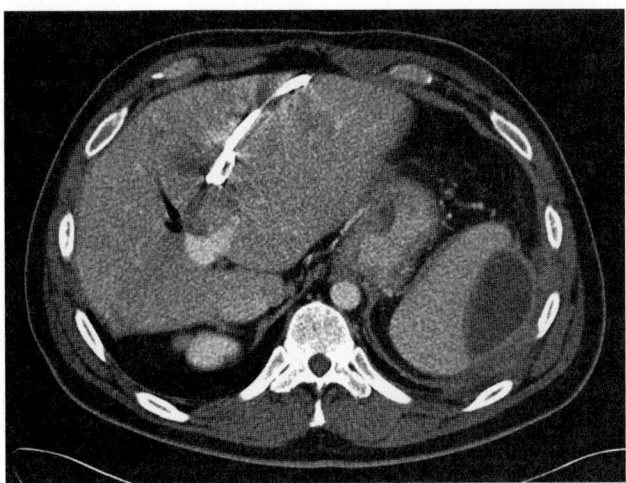

Figure 2 Computed–tomography-guided percutaneous drainage of left lobe pyogenic liver abscess. A drainage catheter is seen in good position, with marked decrease in size of the hepatic abscess.

the development and refinement of image-guided techniques. Ultrasound and CT scan provide excellent visualization of hepatic abscesses for percutaneous aspiration or placement of drainage catheters (Fig. 2). Aspiration alone is useful to obtain culture material during initial diagnosis or potentially as drainage of a small abscess in a healthy patient who is not responding to antibiotics alone. CT-guided percutaneous drainage of pyogenic liver abscess is performed using variable-sized catheters introduced over guidewires and tract dilators. Most abscesses, including those with loculations, can be successfully drained under CT guidance. Catheters may be upsized for better drainage, and loculations may be disrupted using aggressive percutaneous techniques. The catheter is usually placed to gravity bag or bulb suction and removed when the patient is no longer sick and the daily drainage from the abscess is scant. Occasionally repeated CT-guided aspiration or drainage of residual abscess is necessary for patients who fail to improve with initial percutaneous drainage and antibiotics. Thomas and colleagues reported a significant risk (26%) of postprocedure sepsis after percutaneous catheter drainage of hepatic abscess. Patients should therefore be carefully monitored after the procedure for any signs or symptoms of sepsis.

The role of percutaneous drainage in the patient with abscess related to an ablated liver tumor is questionable. If extensive necrosis has occurred, it may be necessary to drain frank pus, but the balance of risks must consider how far this may further disseminate tumor. Antibiotic therapy alone may be a better course.

Surgical Drainage

Open operative drainage of pyogenic liver abscess is reserved for patients who require surgery for concurrent gastrointestinal disease process that led to the formation of the abscess and for patients who are not candidates for or have failed percutaneous drainage. Before the introduction of antibiotics, Oschner and DeBakey advocated the extraperitoneal approach to liver abscess drainage to avoid contamination of the pleural or peritoneal cavities. The position of the abscess determined the location of extraperitoneal approach. Anterior abscesses are approached through a subcostal incision, and posterior abscesses are accessed through the bed of the 12th rib using a posterior retroperitoneal incision. Abscesses located high on the dome of the liver have been drained through transpleural approaches, resulting in a shorter drainage route. These approaches can still be used for patients with solitary liver abscess of known cause that has been treated adequately.

With the introduction of antibiotics and the improvements in surgical techniques, the transperitoneal approach for drainage of liver abscess has become the current standard. Many advantages are offered by this approach, including exposure and visualization of the entire liver, selection of an optimal drainage site, localization and treatment of multiple smaller abscesses with intraoperative ultrasound, exploration of the entire abdomen for a source of primary infection, and, finally, performance of intraoperative cholangiogram and common duct exploration if indicated.

Complete examination of the abdomen is performed before drainage of the liver abscess. The likelihood of missing an abdominal source of infection is significantly reduced with a high-quality contrast CT scan. After the entire abdomen has been explored and the primary focus of infection managed appropriately, liver palpation is performed carefully. Results of preoperative CT or ultrasound help to guide localization of liver abscesses. Smaller and deeper abscesses that are not obvious by palpation can be localized by intraoperative ultrasound. After the abscess has been identified, needle aspiration is performed, and the fluid is collected for aerobic and anaerobic cultures and Gram stain and examined for amebae. The peritoneal cavity is then protected by laparotomy pads, and adequate suction is made available. The abscess cavity is then drained dependently using blunt finger dissection. Multiloculated cavities are carefully opened, avoiding any increased hemorrhage. A biopsy of the abscess wall is obtained to rule out the presence of amebic trophozoites and to evaluate for the possibility of a necrotic, infected tumor. A second biopsy of normal-appearing liver should be obtained to rule out the presence of microscopic liver abscesses, which would require a longer course of intravenous antibiotics. Closed suction drains with or without Penrose drains are placed into the abscess cavity and adjacent perihepatic spaces and brought out through separate stab incisions. The drains may be used for irrigation and postoperative contrast studies to assess the size of the abscess cavity.

Debridement of necrotic liver tissue is occasionally necessary to control infection. Rarely, liver resection is required for multiple intrahepatic abscesses, infected liver malignancy, hepatolithiasis, or intrahepatic biliary stricture.

Drainage of pyogenic liver abscess through laparoscopic techniques has been reported in select patients. This approach allows the surgeon to drain the abscess and explore the entire abdomen with decreased patient morbidity. Laparoscopic ultrasound may be used to localize small abscess that are not readily visualized.

Results

Pyogenic liver abscess is almost uniformly fatal if left untreated. Since the introduction of broad-spectrum antibiotics and improvements in image-guided drainage, the mortality from pyogenic liver abscess has decreased dramatically. Currently, mortality rates are reported to be between 10% and 20%. An increased relative risk for mortality has been shown with biliary origin, presence of disseminated intravascular coagulopathy, multiple abscesses, an acute physiologic assessment and chronic health evaluation II (APACHE II) score of 10 or higher, and abnormal laboratory results of hemoglobin, alkaline phosphatase, aspartate transaminase, blood urea nitrogen, creatinine, albumin, prothrombin time, and blood culture.

The success rate of percutaneous catheter drainage with antibiotic therapy has been reported to be between 69% and 90% over the past 20 years. Simple aspiration with antibiotic therapy has reported success rates between 58% and 88%, although more than half of these patients require additional aspiration or drainage. No randomized prospective comparison has been made between open surgical drainage and percutaneous drainage or between percutaneous drainage and simple aspiration.

AMEBIC LIVER ABSCESS

Amebic liver abscess is the most common extraintestinal manifestation of the parasitic protozoan *E. histolytica*. The parasite has long been known to cause amebic dysentery, particularly in tropical climates and areas of unsanitary living conditions. The first North American case of amebic liver abscess was described by Sir William Osler in 1890 after amebae were discovered in both the stool and abscess fluid of a patient from Panama.

In the 1930s, a drastic reduction in mortality was demonstrated with the combination of therapeutic aspiration and amebicidal therapy. Until this time, both amebic and pyogenic liver abscesses were treated with open surgical drainage. Further advancement in management came with the introduction of serologic tests, improved radiologic imaging, and newer amebicidal agents.

Epidemiology

Amebiasis is a widespread parasitic disease affecting both developing and developed countries. The disease is most prevalent in tropical and underdeveloped countries where public health, sanitation, and personal hygiene are suboptimal. Mexico, India, East and South Africa, and areas of Central and South America have the highest endemic activity of *E. histolytica*. In 1995, the World Health Organization estimated that between 40 and 50 million people worldwide develop amebic colitis or amebic liver abscess, resulting in 40,000 to 100,000 deaths each year. The overall incidence of amebiasis is low in the United States, although increased travel to endemic areas, immigration, and a growth in the homosexual population may result in an increased incidence.

The typical patient diagnosed with amebic liver abscess in the United States is a young Hispanic male between 20 and 40 years of age who has a history of travel to an endemic area or emigration from Mexico or Southeast Asia. Amebic liver abscess is much more common in men, with a male preponderance in a ratio of 10:1 (male-to-female). The reason for this remains unclear, although it has been suggested that heavy alcohol consumption may play a significant role. Other associated risk factors common in patients with amebic liver abscess include impaired immunity, malnutrition, pregnancy, steroid use, and chronic infections such as tuberculosis or syphilis.

Pathogenesis

Humans are the principal host, and amebiasis occurs after ingestion of *E. histolytica* cysts through a fecal-oral route. The main source of infection is cyst-passing chronic patients or asymptomatic carriers who transmit the cysts through water and vegetables contaminated with feces, food contaminated by fertilizers or hands of infected food handlers, or by direct transmission. The cysts are ingested and pass unaffected through the stomach into the intestine, where excystation and liberation of the trophozoite form of the parasite occurs in the small intestine. In most patients, amebiasis results in asymptomatic colonization of the gastrointestinal tract, but some patients may develop invasive disease of the colon. Invasion by *E. histolytica* requires adherence of the trophozoites to the lumen of the bowel, cytolytic and proteolytic effects on the host tissue, and resistance to host defenses by the parasite. Lesions on the colon are typically described as being flask-shaped, with ulceration extending through the mucosa and muscularis mucosa into the submucosa. It is proposed that amebic liver abscess occurs when *E. histolytica* invades mesenteric venules and lymphatics and travels to hepatic venules by way of the portal vein. The trophozoites aggregate in the liver parenchyma where, through a process of acute inflammation, granuloma formation, and progressive tissue necrosis (hence the name *histolytica*), an amebic liver abscess is formed. The contents of the amebic abscess, which has been classically described as "anchovy paste," are acellular, proteinaceous debris and blood, surrounded by an outer rim of *Entamoebae* invading healthy hepatic tissue.

Diagnosis

Clinical Presentation

The presenting symptoms, signs, and radiologic features of amebic liver abscess are similar to those of pyogenic liver abscess and make the distinction between the two difficult. Given the differing epidemiology and pathogenesis of the disease, it is important to obtain a careful patient history, including emigration from or travel to an endemic area. As previously mentioned, 90% of cases involve young men, and in the United States the patient commonly has an Asian or Mexican background or has recently traveled to Central America. The majority of patients present with symptoms that develop over a few days to weeks. Typical symptoms include fever, chills, anorexia, right upper quadrant pain and tenderness, and hepatomegaly. Between 10% and 30% of patients have gastrointestinal symptoms that may include nausea, vomiting, abdominal cramping or distention, diarrhea, or constipation. Patients with amebic liver abscess rarely have concurrent dysentery, and most will not have detectable parasites in their stool.

Fever, hepatomegaly, and right upper quadrant tenderness are the most frequent findings on physical examination. Jaundice, septic shock, and a palpable mass are seen more commonly with pyogenic liver abscess and rarely with amebic liver abscess. Other physical findings may be discovered in patients with advanced amebic abscess and rupture into cavities adjacent to the liver. Intra-abdominal rupture may result in peritonitis, intrapericardial rupture may result in cardiac tamponade and failure, and pleural rupture may result in pleuritis and decreased breath sounds. Although less than 1% of patients develop brain infection from *E. histolytica*, a careful neurologic examination and mental status evaluation should be performed.

Laboratory data may reveal a mild to moderate leukocytosis, anemia, and nonspecific elevation of liver function tests. Eosinophilia is rarely seen in patients with amebic liver abscess. The overall incidence of liver function test abnormalities is similar to that seen with pyogenic liver abscess, although serum albumin, direct bilirubin, lactic dehydrogenase, and aspartate aminotransferase are more frequently abnormal in pyogenic liver abscess.

Because most patients do not have detectable parasites in their stool, serologic testing for antibodies to *E. histolytica* has become the critical test for diagnosing amebic liver abscess. Serologic tests include enzyme immunoassay (EIA), enzyme-linked immunosorbent assay (ELISA), indirect hemagglutinin assay (IHA), indirect immunofluorescent antibody (IFA), latex agglutination (LA), agar gel diffusion (AGD), and counter-immunoelectrophoresis (CIE). EIA is used most widely because it is a more simple, rapid, stable, and inexpensive test to perform. EIA has a reported sensitivity of 99% and specificity greater than 90%. Because the serologic assays detect specific antibodies to amebic antigens, a limitation of the test is that a positive titer may represent a previous infection rather than a current illness, and it may remain positive for up to 20 years (Table 2).

Imaging for amebic liver abscess is similar to that used for evaluation of pyogenic abscesses. Ultrasound, CT, and MRI are excellent at detecting and characterizing hepatic abscesses but are incapable of differentiating an amebic abscess from a pyogenic liver

Table 2: Comparison of Pyogenic and Amebic Abscess: Clinical Features

Clinical Features	Pyogenic Abscess	Amebic Abscess
Age (mean)	>50	20–40
Male:female	1:1	>10:1
Abscess number	≥1 in 50%	1 in ≥80% of chronic cases and 50% of acute cases
Travel/emigration history	No	Yes
Diabetes mellitus	Common	Uncommon
Alcohol abuse	Common	Common
Jaundice	Common	Uncommon
Pruritus	Common	Uncommon
Elevated bilirubin	Common	Uncommon
Elevated aspartate transaminase	Common	Uncommon
Elevated alkaline phosphatase	Common	Common
Positive blood culture	Yes	No
Positive amebic serology	No	Yes

abscess. A ^{99m}Tc nuclear hepatic scan is able to differentiate between a "cold" amebic liver abscess and a "hot" pyogenic abscess because of the presence of active leukocytes in the pyogenic abscess.

If clinical suspicion for amebic liver abscess is sufficiently elevated, then performing a diagnostic aspiration is usually unnecessary. Simple diagnostic aspiration may be used to rule out pyogenic liver abscess but should not delay initiation of amebicidal therapy if amebic abscess is suspected.

Therapy

Uncomplicated amebic liver abscess is generally treated with amebicidal drugs alone. Select patients may benefit from additional therapeutic options, including simple aspiration, percutaneous drainage, and open surgical drainage.

Antimicrobials

Metronidazole has been used for more than 30 years for the treatment of amebiasis and currently remains as the drug of choice for treating amebic liver abscess. Both systemic and intestinal amebiasis are effectively treated with metronidazole. Most patients have rapid clinical improvement in 72 hours, and more than 90% are cured with metronidazole, 750 mg orally three times a day for 10 days. Chloroquine may be substituted or added to the metronidazole therapy if patients do not tolerate metronidazole or fail to respond to metronidazole within 5 days. All patients who have been treated for amebic liver abscess should have additional treatment with a luminal agent such as iodoquinol, paromycin, or diloxanide furoate to eradicate the asymptomatic colonization state. A 10% relapse of infection has been reported in patients who fail to use a luminal agent.

Drainage

Because the majority of patients respond to amebicidal agents alone, the need for simple aspiration, percutaneous drainage, or open surgical drainage is rarely necessary. Some experts suggest that simple aspiration should be considered in patients with (1) abscesses greater than 5 cm in size because of the increased risk of rupture, (2) abscesses located in the left hepatic lobe because of the higher frequency of peritoneal leak or rupture into the pericardium and higher mortality, (3) failure to respond to drug therapy, and (4) suspicion that the abscess may be pyogenic or secondarily infected with bacteria.

Percutaneous drainage is seldom used for amebic liver abscess because of the success of amebicidal therapy with or without simple aspiration and the fear of bacterial superinfection. Similarly, open surgical drainage of amebic liver abscess is rarely performed and is reserved for patients with complications from rupture, failure to respond to medical therapy, and inadequate aspiration.

Results

Currently the majority of patients with amebic liver abscess show a rapid clinical response and high curative rates with timely amebicidal therapy. The mortality rates of patients with amebic liver abscess are reported to be from 0% to 18%. Higher mortality rates are seen in patients with delayed diagnosis, secondary bacterial infection, or complications (e.g., rupture into peritoneal, pericardial, or pleural cavity). The overall incidence of rupture ranges from 3% to 17%. Independent risk factors associated with poorer outcomes include elevated bilirubin (serum bilirubin level >3.5 mg/dl), encephalopathy, hypoalbuminemia (serum albumin level <2 g/dl), a high volume abscess cavity (volume >500 ml), and multiple abscesses.

Radiologic resolution of the amebic liver abscess does not coincide with the rapid clinical improvements seen with amebicidal therapy. Complete radiologic resolution of the liver abscess is seen on average in 3 to 9 months, with a range of 3 to 131 months. In some patients, CT scan continues to show abscess-related changes for more than 10 years. It is therefore unnecessary to have follow-up imaging studies in patients who have clinical resolution of signs and symptoms after treatment for amebic liver abscess.

FUNGAL LIVER ABSCESS

Fungal liver abscesses are being recognized with increased frequency and currently account for approximately 10% of hepatic abscesses. *Candida albicans* and other *Candida* species are found in approximately 80% of cases. *Aspergillus, Cryptococcus,* and mixed infections make up the remaining fungal pathogens. Fungal liver abscesses are usually multiple and usually occur in immunocompromised patients. Patients with leukemia receiving chemotherapy and patients with human immunodeficiency virus (HIV) infection typically have monomicrobial fungal infections, whereas patients with biliary malignancy and indwelling stents and frequent courses of antibiotics tend to develop polymicrobial fungal and bacterial abscesses.

Treatment

Fungal liver abscesses are treated with systemic antifungal therapy and drainage of the abscess cavity or cavities by simple aspiration, percutaneous drainage, or open surgical drainage. Amphotericin B is the first-line drug of choice for systemic antifungal therapy because of its broad fungal efficacy. Patients with mixed fungal and bacterial abscesses should also be started on the appropriate systemic antibiotic for the isolated bacteria.

Table 3: Comparison of Hepatic Abscess: Diagnosis and Treatment

Liver Abscess	Diagnosis	Treatment
Pyogenic	Clinical suspicion US or CT ± aspiration	Systemic antibiotics Drainage of abscess
Amebic	Clinical suspicion US or CT Positive amebic serology	Amebicidal therapy (e.g., metronidazole) Lumenal agent Drainage of complicated abscess
Fungal	Immunocompromised patient US or CT ± aspiration	Systemic antifungal (e.g., Amphotericin B) Drainage of abscess Systemic antibiotics for mixed abscess

CT, Computed tomography; *US,* ultrasound.

Voriconazole or Caspofungin may be used to treat patients who are not responding to Amphotericin B or who have aggressive infections caused by other fungal species (Table 3).

Results

Most patients with fungal liver abscess develop mixed fungal and bacterial abscesses, and only a few develop pure fungal abscesses. The overall mortality rate is approximately 50%. Mortality is significantly increased in patients who do not receive antifungal therapy early or before the development of fungemia. The type of drainage procedure does not affect the patient's survival.

SUGGESTED READINGS

Huang CJ, Pitt HA, Lipsett PA, and others: Pyogenic hepatic abscess: changing trends over 42 years, *Ann Surg* 223:600, 1996.
Johannsen EC, Sifri CD, Madoff LC: Pyogenic liver abscess, *Infect Dis Clin North Am* 14:547, 2000.
Hughes MA, Petri WA JR: Amebic liver abscess, *Infect Dis Clin North Am* 14:565, 2000.
Lipsett PA, Huang CJ, Lillemoe KD, and others: Fungal hepatic abscess: characterization and management, *J Gastrointest Surg* 1:78, 1997.
Pitt HA: Surgical management of hepatic abscess, *World J Surg* 14:498, 1990.

CYSTIC DISEASE OF THE LIVER

Reid B. Adams, MD, and Todd W. Bauer, MD

Nonparasitic cystic masses in the liver have an estimated prevalence of 5%. They are frequent incidental findings on abdominal imaging studies and during operative exploration or intraoperative hepatic ultrasonography. As a result, cystic liver masses and other incidentally discovered liver masses have become a common reason for referral to the general surgeon.

Hepatic cystic lesions are discovered throughout the age spectrum. In general, the lesions discussed here are more common in adults and women; this is particularly true in series reporting symptomatic patients. Although the vast majority of hepatic cystic lesions are benign, the differential diagnosis can include a number of entities including malignancies (Table 1). Pyogenic or parasitic cystic lesions are not discussed here but are reviewed elsewhere in this book.

As outlined in the following sections, cystic lesions pose several dilemmas to the practicing surgeon. The first is making a definitive diagnosis of the nature of the cystic lesion. The second is determining whether the patient's symptoms are related to the cystic lesion. The third is deciding whether and when to institute therapy for the lesion in question. Finally, a number of treatment options are available, resulting in the fourth issue, which is deciding the appropriate therapy for the patient.

PRESENTATION

The majority of hepatic cystic lesions are asymptomatic, discovered as incidental findings during radiographic studies. In a general

Table 1: Nonparasitic Cystic Lesions of the Liver

Simple cysts
Neoplastic cysts
Cystadenoma
Cystadenocarcinoma
Adult polycystic liver disease (APLD)
Associated with autosomal-dominant polycystic kidney disease (ADPKD)
Autosomal-dominant APLD not associated with ADPKD
Traumatic cysts
Perihepatic pseudocysts from acute pancreatitis
Other neoplasms
Metastatic mucinous adenocarcinomas
Cystic degeneration of primary or metastatic malignancies

surgeon's practice, the presentation of these cystic lesions will fall into several broad clinical scenarios:

A cystic liver mass is discovered in an asymptomatic patient.

A cystic liver mass occurs in a patient with a history of malignancy.

A cystic liver mass is discovered during evaluation for upper abdominal symptoms.

Asymptomatic Patient with an Incidental Liver Mass

The most common presentation of hepatic cysts is incidental discovery during evaluation for unrelated symptoms or for another disease in a patient with no history of malignancy or chronic liver disease. Because hepatic cysts are common, they are frequently found during ultrasonography (US) or computed tomography (CT) performed for unrelated reasons. After hemangiomata, hepatic cysts are the most common incidentally discovered lesions in the liver. Found in this context, "asymptomatic" refers to a patient undergoing imaging for some reason other than symptoms that could be attributed to the cystic lesion. The important issue in these patients is making a definitive diagnosis regarding the nature of this unsuspected cystic lesion.

Liver Mass in Patients with Malignancy

In a patient with a current or past history of malignancy, discovery of a cystic liver lesion on screening radiographic studies raises concern for metastatic disease. Because cystic lesions are common, the likelihood that one will be coexistent in this patient population is significant. Consequently, this poses a diagnostic challenge. As noted earlier, the critical issue in this patient population is definitively distinguishing a benign cystic lesion from a metastatic lesion.

Liver Mass Discovered during Evaluation for Upper Abdominal Symptoms

Symptoms referable to the upper abdomen often lead to diagnostic imaging. Because hepatic cystic lesions are common findings on imaging, the coexistence of symptoms and a cystic lesion is not unusual. In the majority of these patients, the cystic lesion does not adequately account for their symptoms. It is therefore imperative in these patients to search for other pathology that could account for their symptoms. In this group, the clinical challenge is determining causality between the cystic lesion and the patient's symptoms.

Clinical Manifestations of Hepatic Cystic Lesions

Symptomatic cystic lesions can present in a variety of ways (Table 2). The most common symptoms are abdominal pain or discomfort. Generally, these symptoms are vague, poorly localized, and reported as either intermittent or constant. Typically the pain is dull or low grade, with more intense pain or incapacitating symptoms being the exception. Less commonly, pain is reported in the flank, back, or shoulder. Symptoms related to mass effect appear to be the next most common. This group of patients describes abdominal fullness, bloating, the sensation of a mass, early satiety, nausea, or vomiting. Although complications in simple cysts are rare, the most common is intracystic hemorrhage. These patients can present with sudden, severe pain and a rapid increase in the size of the cyst. In some, the symptoms are mild or absent. Spontaneous rupture, infection, biliary compression with obstructive jaundice, and torsion have been reported, but these are exceedingly rare complications of cystic lesions.

Table 2: Clinical Presentations of Symptomatic Cystic Lesions

Common	Rare
Abdominal pain or discomfort	Fever or sweats
Abdominal fullness or distension	Back, flank, or shoulder pain
Early satiety, nausea, vomiting	Obstructive jaundice

A physiological explanation for the clinical symptoms associated with hepatic cystic lesions has been elusive. The most easily understood symptoms are those related to stretching of Glisson's capsule. Capsular stretching could account for the poorly localized pain, discomfort, and fullness associated with cystic lesions but clearly could explain symptoms only in those cysts abutting the capsule and distending it. More acute or intense pain may result from rapid distension of the capsule or inflammation associated with intracystic hemorrhage or infection. Likewise, symptoms of fullness, nausea, vomiting, or a palpable mass can readily be understood when a large cyst compresses an adjacent organ. However, when cystic lesions are confined within the hepatic parenchyma and do not affect the liver capsule, the understanding and assignment of symptoms to these lesions is much more problematic. The manner by which these intrahepatic cystic lesions cause symptoms (if there are any) remains unclear, especially because similarly placed intrahepatic malignancies or intrahepatic vascular thromboses are generally asymptomatic. This is an important consideration as one decides whether treatment is merited for this group of patients.

DIAGNOSIS

The diagnosis of hepatic cystic lesions is made by noninvasive radiographic studies. Incidental discovery of cystic lesions most often occurs during abdominal US or CT. The differential diagnosis for a cystic lesion is shown in Table 1. From a practical standpoint, the vast majority of these lesions are simple cysts. Generally, US or CT is diagnostic for these lesions.

Complex cysts pose a diagnostic challenge; these could represent a simple cyst with hemorrhage or infection, or a neoplastic cyst such as cystadenoma or cystadenocarcinoma. If the patient has had a prior hepatic procedure or a history of trauma, the cyst may be traumatic. Finally, in patients with a malignancy, the lesion could represent a cystic metastasis, such as a mucinous colon adenocarcinoma or cystic degeneration of a metastatic deposit. Additional imaging or diagnostic studies may be required to define the diagnosis.

If the diagnosis is equivocal, additional diagnostic imaging, primarily magnetic resonance imaging (MRI), is indicated. Laboratory studies in general are not helpful to define the diagnosis. The exception is laboratory studies of aspirated cyst fluid. Finally, the role for invasive studies is limited, except when cyst fluid chemistries or cytology are necessary.

Ultrasonography

Typical sonographic features allow an accurate diagnosis of cystic lesions by US in the majority of cases. Characteristic findings of a simple cyst include a well-circumscribed lesion; thin, almost imperceptible walls; a homogeneous anechoic pattern; and posterior acoustic enhancement (Fig. 1, *A*). These findings are diagnostic of a simple cyst. If the cyst fluid has echoic material or the patient presents in a fashion suggestive of intracystic hemorrhage, the US may be diagnostic. Clots within the cyst are echogenic and usually mobile, changing position within the cyst on repositioning of the patient. Cystic lesions with septations, debris, mural nodules, or projections or with a thick wall are indicative of a complex cyst (Fig. 1, *B*), typically a neoplastic cyst rather than a simple cyst. If the patient has a history of malignancy and develops a new cyst on serial imaging or has a cyst with atypical features, the concern for a metastatic lesion is increased. In these circumstances, additional evaluation is warranted.

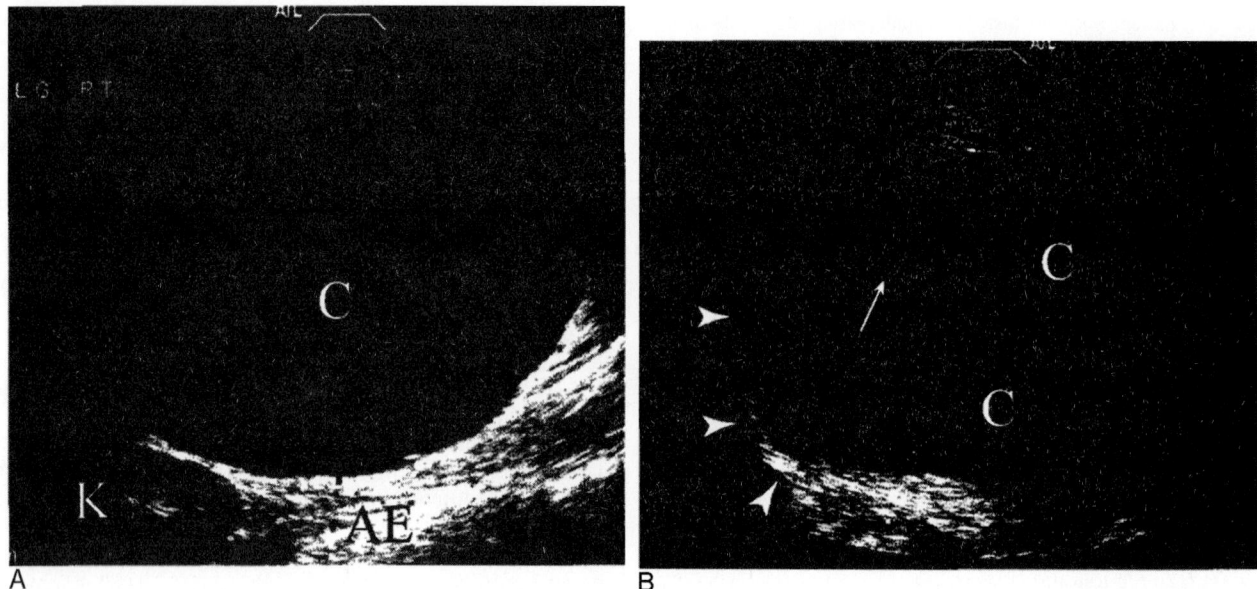

Figure 1 Ultrasound features of liver cysts. **(A)** Simple cysts *(C)* have anechoic fluid, a thin imperceptible wall, and posterior acoustic enhancement *(AE)*. No internal features are present. *K,* right kidney. **(B)** Complex cysts have echogenic material within them, including internal septa *(white arrow)*, debris, and mural nodules or projections. These cysts *(C)* are multilocular. A thick, irregular wall *(white arrowheads)* is frequently seen in complex cysts.

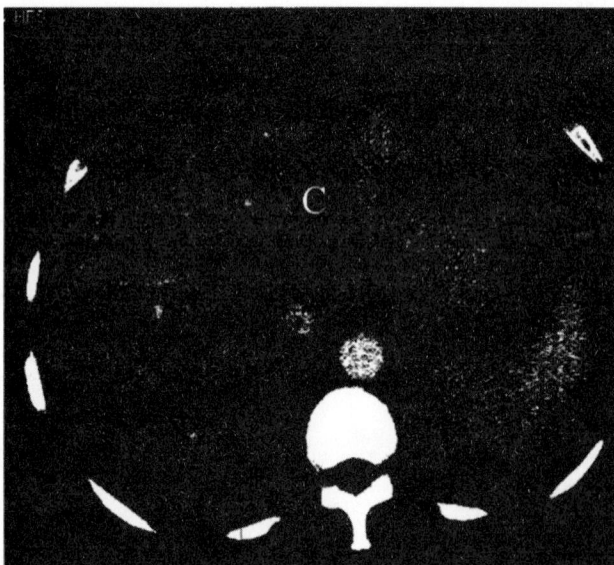

Figure 2 Computed tomography features of a simple cyst *(C)* are similar to those demonstrated on ultrasonography. Fluid density is similar to water. No internal debris, projections, or nodules are seen, and the walls are thin and imperceptible.

Computed Tomography

Hepatic cystic lesions are often incidental findings during CT. The typical features on a contrast-enhanced CT are similar to those found on US. Simple cysts typically have a well-defined, thin, almost imperceptible wall on CT (Fig. 2). The lesion is filled with a homogeneous, hypoattenuated fluid with Houndsfield units similar to water. Complex cysts have features similar to those seen on

US and MRI. The fluid within a complex cyst may have Houndsfield units denser than water; additionally, it may contain debris, fluid-fluid levels, or septations within the cyst. An advantage of CT over US is the ability to detect enhancement of the cyst wall. Enhancement of the cyst wall or within a mural nodule or papillary projection is concerning for a neoplastic process. However, many of these lesions are noted on general abdominal screening CT scans, and the study may not be diagnostic. Often, this is the case when the scanning times have not been optimized with the contrast bolus or when a noncontrasted scan has been performed. Small lesions (<2 cm) also fall into this category because they often are not well characterized on CT. If a small or any other lesion is suspected to be cystic, it can be well characterized by US, which is typically diagnostic in this setting. When US or CT is diagnostic for simple cysts, additional studies and follow-up are not required in the asymptomatic patient. When they are not diagnostic or when a complex lesion requires further characterization, our preference is to proceed directly to MRI.

Magnetic Resonance Imaging

MRI has become the imaging study of choice at many institutions for focal liver lesions. Compared with CT, MRI is superior for lesion detection and particularly for characterization. MRI is particularly useful in defining lesions smaller than 2 cm, a feature not shared by CT. The accuracy of MRI for diagnosing cystic lesions is high. Simple cysts have characteristic MRI features, including a well-defined, thin, imperceptible wall, and fluid signal intensity that is low on T1-weighted images and high on T2-weighted images (similar to cerebrospinal fluid). Simple cysts have no wall enhancement, nodules, or projections and no internal signals (Fig. 3, *A*). When MRI features confirm the diagnosis of a simple cyst, additional studies and follow-up are not required in the asymptomatic patient. An advantage of MRI over US and CT is the ability to characterize the fluid. Fluid signal characteristics different from water suggest hemorrhagic products, proteinous/mucinous fluid, or the

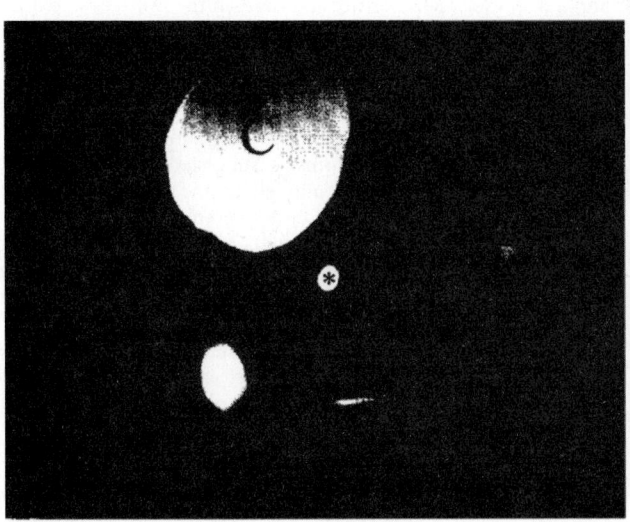 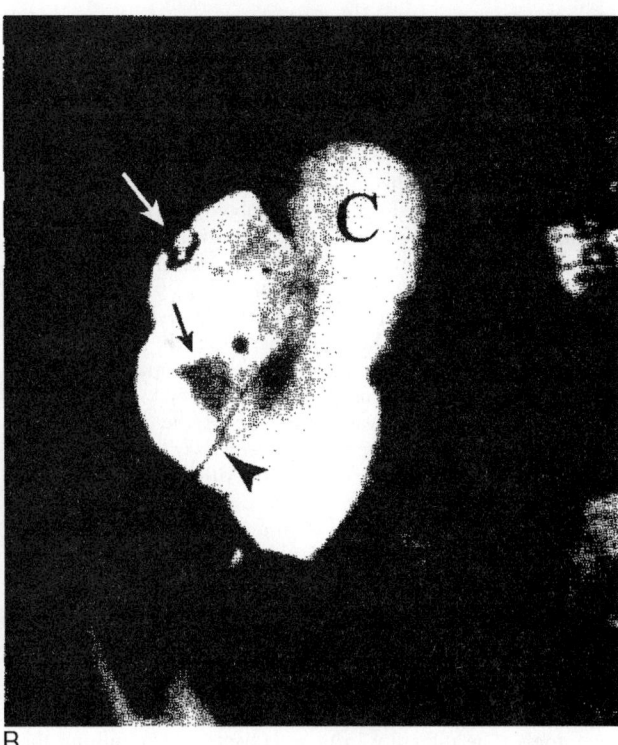

Figure 3 Magnetic resonance features of liver cysts. **(A)** Simple cysts *(C and asterisk)* are bright on T2-weighted sequences. The morphological features are similar to those seen on ultrasonography and CT. Simple cysts do no have wall enhancement on intravenous contrast-enhanced sequences. **(B)** Complex cysts *(C)* have fluid with a density different from water, and the fluid densities can differ within the same cyst. Complex cysts are multilocular with mural nodules, papillary projections, internal debris, and septations frequently present *(arrows and arrowhead)*.

presence of subtle mural nodules/projections. Similar to CT, an enhancing cyst wall or solid element is concerning for a neoplastic process (Fig. 3, *B*).

Nearly all initially undefined, incidentally discovered liver masses can be accurately characterized by the imaging studies described, particularly if the mass is cystic. Occasionally, however, diagnostic uncertainty persists regarding the nature of the cystic lesion. In these instances, percutaneous fluid aspiration and analysis can be helpful. Fluid appearance, the presence of mucin, chemical analysis (CEA, CA19-9, bilirubin), and cytology may be helpful in distinguishing cystic lesions from one another.

Cyst Fluid Analysis

Simple cysts frequently have thin, straw-colored fluid on aspiration. Cytological analysis demonstrates acellular fluid and the absence of mucin. Analysis of CEA, CA19-9, and total bilirubin is negative or normal. Uncommonly, several simple cysts are clustered, giving the imaging appearance of a complex cyst with septations. Fluid analysis can help differentiate this situation from a true complex cyst such as a neoplastic cyst.

Some simple cysts have bilious-appearing fluid. If the bilirubin is elevated in the fluid, the treatment options differ from those for simple cysts. Thin, darker fluid may be encountered in some cysts; if the bilirubin and tumor markers are normal and no hemorrhagic products are present, these cysts can be treated similarly to simple cysts. Evidence of blood or blood products in the fluid aspirate also affects therapy options.

Analysis of cyst fluid tumor markers is helpful to distinguish cyst types. Neoplastic cyst fluid has an elevated CA19-9, distinguishing it from a simple cyst. Recent evidence demonstrates a high sensitivity in this situation. Likewise, CEA is routinely elevated in neoplastic cysts but not by simple cysts. Together these markers have high sensitivity and specificity for distinguishing simple from neoplastic cysts. Whether a negative (normal) tumor marker level completely excludes a neoplastic cyst when the imaging is suggestive of one is unclear. No evidence exists to suggest that these tumor markers can distinguish cystadenoma from cystadenocarcinoma.

Cytological analysis of complex cysts may be helpful but is more commonly nondiagnostic. These specimens often have few cells to examine. Although those cells present may demonstrate cellular atypia, the cellular changes or amount of diagnostic material are often insufficient to allow a definitive diagnosis. Again, when the findings are positive, cytology is helpful. A negative cytology is nondiagnostic. Regardless of the cytology, the finding of mucin in the aspirate is suggestive of a neoplastic cyst.

DIAGNOSTIC FEATURES AND THERAPY OF SPECIFIC CYSTIC LESIONS

The treatment of hepatic cystic lesions depends on the cyst type and the presence of symptoms. Patients with asymptomatic benign hepatic cysts do not require intervention. When symptoms are present and referable to the cyst, a number of potential interventions are available, depending on the nature of the cyst. Neoplastic cysts have specific characteristics that must be recognized because they require therapy even in the absence of symptoms.

Simple Cysts

Simple cysts are by far the most common cystic lesions of the liver. They are lined by a single layer of cuboidal or low columnar epithelium and do not have malignant potential. These cysts can occur throughout all segments of the liver. Communication with the biliary tract is unusual. Approximately half of patients have a single cyst, whereas the remaining patients have two or more. A small number of patients have innumerable cysts; this is distinguished from adult polycystic disease, an entity in which more than 50% of the hepatic parenchyma is involved with cysts.

Simple hepatic cysts are asymptomatic in the vast majority (>90%) of patients; most are found incidentally by imaging or during operation. Imaging by US, CT, or MRI is diagnostic; the simplest and most cost-effective study is US (Figs. 1, *A*, 2, and 3, *A*). Under these circumstances, no additional evaluation or therapy is necessary (Table 3).

Probably the most difficult decision regarding simple cysts, after confirming the diagnosis, is deciding whether treatment is warranted (Table 4). Treatment is considered for a narrow range of specific indications: (1) significant symptoms in the absence of other potential etiologies, (2) intracystic hemorrhage, or (3) diagnostic uncertainty. The most common reason to consider treatment is for symptoms. The difficulty in these patients is determining the relationship between the symptoms and the cyst. Only when other potential etiologies such as gastroduodenal, biliary, pancreatic, renal, pulmonary, and musculoskeletal sources have been eliminated is active treatment considered. The most straightforward

Table 3: Features Typical of Simple Hepatic Cysts and Neoplastic Cysts

Simple	Neoplastic
Unilocular	Multilocular, septated
Thin, sharp, imperceptible wall	Thick, irregular wall
No mural nodules or projections	Mural nodules, projections present
Thin, watery, straw-colored fluid	Thick, green/brown fluid
No mucin present	Mucinous material in fluid
Normal CEA and CA19-9 in cyst fluid	Elevated CEA or CA19-9 in fluid

Table 4: Indications for Therapy—Simple Hepatic Cysts

Treatment Indicated

Severe, intractable symptoms

Absence of another etiology for symptoms

Intracystic hemorrhage

Diagnostic uncertainty

Treatment Not Indicated

Size of cyst alone

Vague symptoms with unclear association with cyst

Prophylaxis to prevent bleeding, rupture, or injury

group to reconcile includes patients with large cysts causing mass effect symptoms. The decision to treat these patients actively is more clear-cut than the other scenarios. In cases in which a patient has a large cyst stretching the liver capsule and abdominal complaints without another source for their symptoms, treatment also should be considered. More difficult is deciding treatment in those patients with abdominal complaints without an identifiable source and a liver cyst that does not impinge on the liver capsule. In this group, strong consideration should be given for a period of waiting before treatment in initiated. For patients with vague symptoms and a deeper cyst or a small capsular cyst of uncertain symptoms, an alternative approach is a diagnostic aspiration. If cyst aspiration relieves the patient's symptoms, a role for the cyst as the source of the symptoms is suggested. In the absence of relief, surgical intervention is unlikely to improve their symptoms. How often improvement after cyst aspiration is related to a placebo effect is unknown. Thus the decision to treat a cyst on the basis of the symptoms of abdominal pain, discomfort, or vague complaints should be considered only after eliminating another etiology as the source for the symptoms and probably only after a period of observation to ensure that the symptoms are persistent and troubling. Only when this approach fails and the patient continues to have significant symptoms should active treatment of the cyst be considered.

Hemorrhage into a cyst may result in symptoms or an incidentally discovered complex-appearing lesion. Imaging, particularly MRI, is useful to determine whether the lesion is a hemorrhagic cyst. Likewise, fluid aspiration demonstrating old blood products may confirm the diagnosis. Identifying hemorrhagic cysts is important because this finding affects the treatment options.

Diagnostic uncertainty, although unusual, can occur with simple cysts. This situation occurs when several simple cysts are adjacent to one another. The shared walls give the appearance of a complex, septated cyst. In the absence of symptoms and any mural nodules or enhancing walls, fluid aspiration may be helpful. A cytologically bland cyst with normal CEA, CA19-9, or both is consistent with a simple cyst(s). Another unusual situation occurs when a portal triad or hepatic vein traverses a simple cyst, again giving the appearance of a complex cyst. Ultrasonography with flow studies mapping the portal or hepatic vein can distinguish this entity from a neoplastic cyst. Again, fluid analysis in this unusual situation may be helpful.

In the past, growth of a cyst was used as an indication for treatment by some authors. Although larger cysts are more often associated with symptoms, no direct correlation between change in size and symptoms or complications is apparent from published studies. Thus treatment is not indicated simply because a cyst is present, on the basis of size alone, or for prophylaxis to prevent bleeding, rupture, or injury.

Treatment of Simple Cysts

Treatment options for simple hepatic cysts depend on their characteristics (Table 5). Percutaneous aspiration is a simple form of treatment that may provide temporary relief of symptoms. It is associated with recurrence in nearly 100% of cases. Repeated aspirations can result in cyst infection. Except in cases of diagnostic aspiration for fluid characterization or to assess relief of symptoms, simple aspiration is not indicated for definitive therapy. Cyst aspiration followed by injection of a sclerosing agent (ethanol, minocycline hydrochloride, or tetracycline hydrochloride) is effective in relieving symptoms in approximately 80% to 90% of patients. For patients with recurrence following sclerosis, a repeat procedure can be effective. Sclerosing agents destroy the lining epithelium, preventing further fluid secretion, and

Table 5: Therapeutic Options for Hepatic Cystic Lesions

Simple Hepatic Cysts

Percutaneous aspiration and sclerosis (medically unfit patient or declines surgery)

Cyst wall resection and epithelial ablation

Laparoscopic (treatment of choice)

Open–lesions located superiorly or posteriorly, adjacent to the diaphragm

Enucleation—deep cysts with little involvement of the liver capsule

Simple Hepatic Cysts with a Biliary Communication

Cyst wall resection and epithelial ablation, suture ligation of biliary communication

Laparoscopic (treatment of choice)

Open–lesions located superiorly or posteriorly, adjacent to the diaphragm

Enucleation–deep cysts with little involvement of the liver capsule

Simple Hepatic Cysts with Intracystic Hemorrhage

Percutaneous aspiration and sclerosis

Enucleation

Neoplastic Cysts

Enucleation (treatment of choice for cystadenoma)

Resection–known or likely malignant lesions (cystadenocarcinoma)

Adult Polycystic Liver Disease

Type I	Cyst wall resection with or without partial hepatectomy
Type II	Cyst wall resection with or without partial hepatectomy (anterior dominant cysts)
Type III	Partial hepatectomy (two adjacent segments must be spared) Liver transplantation

therefore reaccumulation, into the cyst. If the cyst fluid is bilious, sclerosis is contraindicated because a biliary communication is present and sclerosis may injure the biliary tract. Sclerotherapy is generally reserved for patients at high operative risk or who decline operative intervention.

Patients with symptomatic, simple cysts who are operative candidates should proceed with operative management because this approach has the lowest (<5%–10%) recurrence rate. The simplest form of therapy is resection of the exposed cyst wall as it protrudes from the surface of the liver. Transection of the cyst wall is performed at the interface between the cyst and the hepatic parenchyma. Terms such as *fenestration, unroofing,* or *marsupialization* all describe a similar operative technique. Removing a portion of the cyst allows drainage into the peritoneal cavity and access to its interior. Ablation of any remaining cyst wall lining by fulguration will minimize recurrences and the risk of ascites. The resected cyst wall should be submitted for frozen and permanent pathological examination to rule out a neoplastic cyst. Cyst resection can be accomplished by an open or laparoscopic approach. Currently, a laparoscopic approach is favored because ample evidence demonstrates treatment results equivalent to that of an open approach, coupled with the advantages of a laparoscopic approach. The conversion rate is low, and the postoperative stay, symptoms, and complications are comparable to laparoscopic cholecystectomy. If the cyst wall is consistent with a neoplastic cyst, conversion to enucleation of the cyst is appropriate and recommended.

Simple cysts with bilious fluid are treated similarly. Cyst wall resection allows access to the cyst interior. Careful inspection for the communicating biliary duct is required, followed by suture closure of this site to prevent bile peritonitis. Cyst lining fulguration, not including the biliary leak site, completes the treatment.

Simple cysts with hemorrhage require a different approach. Cyst aspiration with sclerosis or cyst resection by enucleation are appropriate strategies in this situation. Cyst wall resection and epithelial ablation are not recommended in these patients because a repeat bleeding episode from the cyst wall carries the risk of intraperitoneal hemorrhage.

Simple cysts rarely require techniques such as enucleation or hepatic resection. Cyst enterostomy is not indicated for these patients. The one instance when enucleation may be indicated, other than that described earlier, is the cyst with a small area of capsular involvement. These cysts can be difficult to open adequately, resulting in poor drainage and inadequate cyst lining ablation. Enucleation may be a better option for patients with deeper cysts with a minimal surface component. The other indication for enucleation or resection is the recurrence of a cyst following treatment. Recurrence may result from misdiagnosis of a neoplastic cyst. Otherwise, the more invasive options should be reserved for special circumstances.

Neoplastic Cysts

In comparison with simple cysts, neoplastic cysts are rare. Most are cystadenomas, a benign cystic neoplasm with purported malignant potential. Cystadenomas are slow-growing tumors lined with mucin-secreting cuboidal or columnar epithelium. Two types of cystadenomas are recognized: those that are associated with a mesenchymal stroma and those that are not. Those with stroma are surrounded by a thick, cellular layer that resembles ovarian stroma. Cystadenomas with mesenchymal stroma are seen exclusively in women. Currently, the clinicopathologic course of both types appears similar. Malignant transformation of the epithelium in cystadenomas is thought to lead to the even more rare cystadenocarcinoma. Neoplastic cysts are typically solitary lesions in the liver that can occur within any segment.

Unlike simple cysts, most neoplastic cysts present as symptomatic lesions. Abdominal pain, bloating, nausea, and vomiting are common presentations. Occasionally they may present with biliary obstruction from local compression. They occur more frequently in women, usually in patients older than 40 years of age. The mean age of patients with cystadenocarcinomas is 10 years greater than that of patients with cystadenomas.

Imaging by US, CT, or MRI provides the initial clues regarding the nature of these lesions (Table 3 and Figs. 1, *B,* and 3, *B*). Neoplastic cysts are complex cystic lesions with internal septations, debris, fluid density greater than water, mural abnormalities, or a combination of these. Evidence to support the suspicion of a cystic neoplasm includes a thickened, irregular wall with mural nodules or papillary projections. Wall enhancement is characteristic of neoplastic cysts. Although rare, the presence of invasion from the cyst wall into the surrounding hepatic parenchyma should elicit concern for a cystadenocarcinoma. Nearly all neoplastic cysts are multilocular or septated, but there have been reports of unilocular neoplastic cysts. Other than their unilocular appearance, they typically have the other features suggestive of a neoplastic cyst.

If diagnostic uncertainty persists, fluid aspiration for analysis can be helpful. The fluid may be straw colored and thin but most often is darker (green-brown), thicker, bloody, or mucinous. Cytology is useful if characteristic mucin-secreting epithelium or malignant cells are identified. In the absence of diagnostic cells, mucin present in the fluid is indicative of a neoplastic cyst. The absence of these characteristics does not rule out a neoplastic cyst. Elevated CEA or CA19-9 in the cyst fluid is highly suggestive of a neoplastic cyst. If a large solid component is present, biopsy of this area is more likely to be diagnostic than cytology of the fluid alone. However, in the presence of these imaging findings, biopsy is unlikely to change the treatment recommendations and should be avoided if resection is appropriate, regardless of the biopsy findings.

Treatment of Neoplastic Cysts

Neoplastic cysts should be treated by complete resection. Cyst wall excision is not appropriate because of the high rate of recurrence and the risk of malignancy. Generally, resection by enucleation is appropriate and sufficient treatment for cystadenoma. The associated risks are low, and enucleation preserves hepatic parenchyma; when performed appropriately, it is associated with no risk of recurrence. In the presence of imaging that is concerning for malignant features, local liver invasion, or a biopsy demonstrating malignancy, a formal hepatic resection to achieve negative margins is the appropriate choice.

Recently, some authors have suggested that the presence of intestinal metaplasia or atypia in the resected (sampled) cystadenoma wall be used as an indication for complete cyst resection. In those patients without metaplasia or atypia, they recommend cyst wall resection with thermal ablation of the remaining epithelium. For patients with metaplasia or atypia, complete resection is recommended. The rationale for this strategy is predicated on intestinal metaplasia or atypia being a precursor for malignancy. However, the primary literature on which this argument is based recommends complete resection of all cystadenomas, even in the absence of intestinal metaplasia or atypia. This is based on 30% of patients in their series having a cystadenocarcinoma with benign epithelium without intestinal metaplasia within the tumor. These authors also advocate complete resection because the cyst walls can be heterogeneous, which potentially leads to a sampling error for partially resected cysts. Finally, there are numerous reports in the literature regarding the inaccuracy of frozen section biopsies, including false-positive and false-negative findings. Therefore on the basis of our current understanding of these lesions, the safest strategy is complete resection of neoplastic cysts. Whether partial excision and epithelial ablation for cystadenomas is appropriate remains uncertain and therefore cannot be recommended as the standard approach at present.

Adult Polycystic Liver Disease

Adult polycystic liver disease (APLD) is the most frequent extrarenal manifestation of autosomal dominant polycystic kidney disease (ADPKD). Another autosomal dominant form of APLD is not associated with ADPKD. This form is associated with cysts in other organs, with the kidneys being the most common extrahepatic site. Hepatic cysts associated with ADPKD develop later in life than the renal cysts. They are more common in women. The cysts are lined with simple biliary epithelium without communication with the biliary tract.

Most patients with APLD are asymptomatic and do not require treatment. When symptoms develop, they usually result from the mass effect of the accompanying hepatomegaly. Other common complications are infection or hemorrhage into a cyst(s). Complications of rupture, portal hypertension, vena cava compression, malignant transformation, and hepatic insufficiency are rare.

Because symptoms are generally related to mass effect from hepatomegaly, most therapies are designed to reduce cyst or liver size, although the optimal management of APLD remains unresolved. Three forms of APLD have been described, and this classification is helpful in guiding therapy. Type I APLD is associated with large (10 cm), relatively fewer superficial cysts within the liver. There are relatively generous areas of spared normal parenchyma. Type II patients have multiple medium-sized cysts (5–7 cm) diffusely scattered throughout the liver with relative sparing of normal parenchyma. Type III cysts are small- to medium-sized cysts (<5 cm) diffusely scattered throughout the parenchyma with little identifiable normal hepatic parenchyma. Screening for cerebral aneurysms should be performed in these patients, especially those considering surgical therapy because they are present in 10% of this patient population.

Aspiration and sclerotherapy is useful in APLD in relatively few cases. Cyst wall resection is preferred for multiple cysts and can be effective for type I APLD. A laparoscopic approach, if feasible, is optimal for these patients. The superficial cyst wall(s) is resected, followed by excision of the internal septa (common walls) between the deeper cysts. Use of laparoscopic US is essential to guide the cyst wall resection, thereby avoiding major vascular and biliary structures, which are frequently draped around and between the multiple cysts. Despite adequate cyst wall resection, the stiff architecture of livers with APLD may not allow adequate hepatic volume reduction. In these cases, a combination of cyst wall resection and hepatic resection may be required at laparotomy. Resection should include the most polycystic segments of the liver to preserve hepatic function. Resection is contraindicated unless two or more contiguous hepatic segments are left behind and are relatively spared from the APLD. Resection is hazardous and difficult because of the distortion of the normal anatomic planes resulting from the cystic changes.

A few patients with anteriorly located type II APLD can be approached laparoscopically. More diffuse involvement requires an open approach to fenestration, with or without resection following the above guidelines.

Type III patients are problematic because they have few options. In general, if two adjacent segments can be spared, resection and cyst wall excision can be considered. If no adjacent segments are spared, liver transplantation is an option.

Miscellaneous Cystic Lesions

Traumatic Cysts

These are rare lesions noted in the context of prior hepatic trauma or invasive procedures. They may result from resorbing hematoma or a contained bile leak (biloma). Consequently, they lack an epithelial lining. The imaging appearance is similarly to simple cysts, except that a fluid-fluid level may be present if blood products are present in the cyst. The majority are incidental findings and do not require treatment. The rare symptomatic lesions (usually from mass effect) are treated similarly to simple hepatic cysts. The one caveat is treatment of bilomas. After opening the cyst, a search for an ongoing bile leak should be conducted. A leak should be suture ligated to prevent recurrence and bile peritonitis.

Hepatic Pseudocysts

Also rare, hepatic pseudocysts can develop during an episode of acute pancreatitis. These cysts have no epithelial lining. They are thought to occur as a result of fluid dissection into the hepatoduodenal ligament and the leaves of the gastrohepatic ligament. No therapy is necessary because these typically disappear following resolution of the pancreatitis.

Cystic Malignancies

Some adenocarcinomas have a high component of mucinous cells, such as mucinous colon cancer. In these tumors, disease metastatic to the liver can appear as cystic lesions. Likewise, some neuroendocrine carcinomas, sarcomas, and other malignancies metastatic to the liver can develop as cystic-appearing lesions, often resulting from central necrosis. Therefore in the context of a history of malignancy, cystic lesions should be viewed with suspicion. In general, US or other imaging can distinguish between the thin-walled, water-density-filled simple cyst and a cystic metastatic lesion. If diagnostic uncertainty exists, fine needle aspiration for cytology and fluid analysis may be helpful. If the diagnosis remains elusive and the patient is a candidate for resection of hepatic metastatic disease, treatment planning should proceed as if these were metastatic lesions and not simple cysts—in other words, by a formal hepatic resection.

TECHNICAL CONSIDERATIONS IN TREATING HEPATIC CYSTIC LESIONS

Percutaneous Chemical Sclerosis

This technique should be limited to the treatment of simple cysts or simple cysts with evidence of intracystic hemorrhage. It is not appropriate for neoplastic cysts. The procedure is typically performed on an outpatient basis under conscious sedation. Simple needle placement in the cyst or placement of a small indwelling catheter can be used to aspirate 25% to 30% of the fluid. The course of the needle or catheter should traverse as much normal liver as feasible en route to the cyst puncture site. This decreases the risk of leaking cyst fluid or sclerosant. If the fluid is bilious, no sclerosing agent should be instilled. In the absence of bile, water-soluble contrast is instilled into the cyst to exclude biliary communication with the cyst. If absent, a volume of absolute ethanol, minocycline, or tetracycline equivalent to the amount of fluid aspirated should be instilled into the cyst. The patient is rolled side to side and front to back, resting approximately 10 minutes in each position to allow sufficient contact time of the sclerosing agent with the cyst wall. The cyst is then aspirated completely. If the patient redevelops symptoms and a cyst, the process can be repeated.

Cyst Wall Resection (Fenestration, Unroofing, Marsupialization)

The principles for open or laparoscopic cyst wall resection are similar. A laparoscopic approach is preferred in most cases except as indicated. Understanding the preoperative imaging is critical to understanding the location of the major portal pedicles that are typically draped around the interior or posterior walls of these cysts (Fig. 4). Preoperative imaging can be supplemented by intraoperative US. Trocar placement depends on the cyst location. Most cysts requiring treatment have some component of the cyst wall adjacent to the surface of the liver. To begin, the cyst is punctured at its thinnest point, and the fluid is aspirated. If bile is present, the feeding duct must be located and ligated following cyst wall resection. The cyst wall is excised at its junction with the hepatic parenchyma (Fig. 5). This can be accomplished with a variety of tools. Simple cautery excision (hook or scissors) is not the best choice because larger vessels and biliary radicals can be present at this interface. Better choices include the ultrasonic coagulating shears or similar devices or linear endoscopic staplers. Occasionally, bile leaks or bleeding will require suture ligatures. After the cyst wall is excised, it is

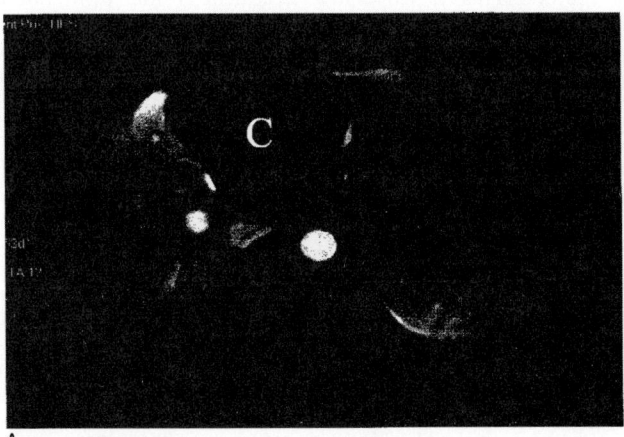
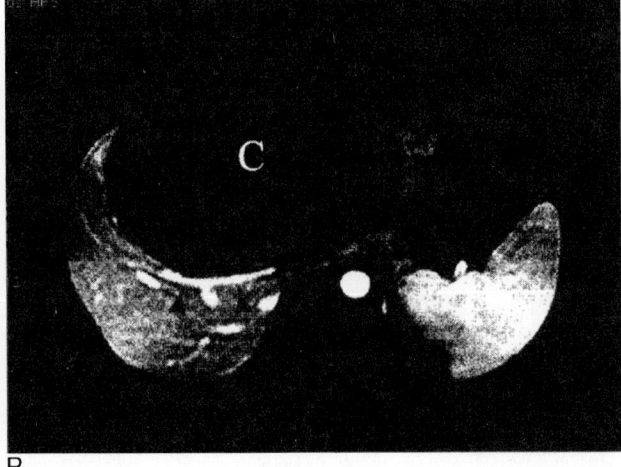

A   B

Figure 4 **(A)** Simple cyst *(C)* with the middle hepatic vein *(black arrow)* adjacent to the right wall of the cyst. The left hepatic vein *(black arrowhead)* is draped around the left side of the cyst. **(B)** A complex cyst *(C)* with internal septations. The right portal vein *(black arrowheads)* is splayed out along the posterior wall of the cyst.

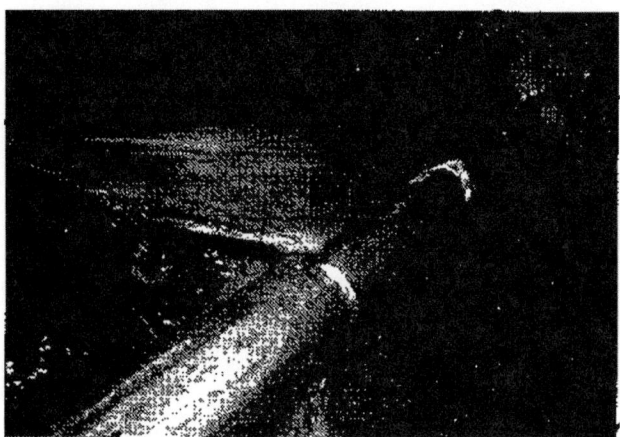

Figure 5   Excision of a simple cyst wall with the linear endoscopic stapler. The transection plane is the interface between the exposed cyst wall and the hepatic parenchyma.

sent to the pathology lab for frozen section to ensure the absence of a neoplastic cyst. If bile was present, the cyst interior should be inspected and the bile leak suture ligated. If this repair is near a major pedicle, performing an intraoperative cholangiogram is prudent. In the absence of a bile leak or following ligation of one, the cyst lining should be fulgurated. Our preference is to use the argon beam coagulator. If this is being performed laparoscopically, adequate venting of the peritoneal cavity by opening the other ports is mandatory to prevent excessive intra-abdominal pressure. Some authors advocate omental packing of the cyst cavity to prevent recurrence. The utility of packing has not been rigorously studied, and the benefit is unclear. Several authors do not advocate cyst-lining ablation. Others recommend ablation if less than 50% of the cyst wall was excised. Our preference is to ablate the lining in all cases unless most of the cyst wall has been excised. Ablation is simple, effective, and has little downside. Following uncomplicated cyst wall resection, most patients can be discharged the same day.

A limitation to the laparoscopic approach is a cyst located in the superior liver (segments VII and VIII) or posteriorly. An open approach is better for cysts in these positions to allow full excision of the cyst wall, which can be difficult laparoscopically. In addition, higher rates of recurrence have been reported following laparoscopic treatment of cysts in these locations. Adherence to the diaphragm with reaccumulation of cyst fluid has been postulated as the cause in these patients. This problem can be minimized by ablating the cyst lining, but this is also difficult laparoscopically. Consequently, an open approach is indicated for these patients.

Cystectomy (Enucleation)

Most neoplastic cysts or those recurrent following other treatments can be excised by enucleation. This technique is similar to the one used for hemangiomata. Enucleation is favored over hepatic resection because it is associated with minimal blood loss and fewer complications while preserving hepatic parenchyma. It is feasible because of the pseudocapsule that surrounds the cyst, resulting from compression of the adjacent normal hepatic parenchyma. Few or no vessels or bile ducts cross this space between the pseudocapsule and the cyst. Consequently, little blood loss results, and postoperative bile leaks are reduced or

eliminated. However, the vasculobiliary pedicle can be closely associated with the cyst wall, and care must be taken to avoid injury during enucleation (Fig. 4). Selective use of the Pringle maneuver when working near the major pedicles can minimize blood loss. Dissection within the plane of the pseudocapsule allows separation of the cyst from the liver parenchyma. To accomplish enucleation, Glisson's capsule is incised, and dissection is performed to find the plane of the pseudocapsule. Typically, this can be achieved using blunt dissection; however, the dissection can be facilitated with an ultrasonic dissector or hydrodissector. When it is within the plane, the cyst can be elevated out of the pseudocapsule, and the few crossing vessels within this space are ligated as they are encountered. The enucleation is relatively straightforward when in the appropriate plane. However, this dissection can be tedious and difficult when elevating the cyst wall off of a major pedicle. If elevation off of a pedicle cannot be safely achieved, an alternative is to leave the cyst wall in place as it drapes over the pedicle. The remnant cyst wall can be ablated with the argon beam coagulator, but care must be exercised to avoid injury to the underlying bile duct.

Alternatively, anatomic or nonanatomic resections can be used for excision if these can be completed in an easier and safer manner than enucleation. Standard resection techniques are used in these cases. Currently, there is no indication for cyst enterostomy.

SUMMARY

Simple hepatic cysts are common benign mass-occupying lesions in the liver. The vast majority are asymptomatic and do not require any therapy or continued follow-up. One of the primary issues regarding a cystic lesion is distinguishing it from the much more rare neoplastic cyst. This distinction is important because neoplastic cysts have malignant potential and require excision for treatment. In nearly all cases, noninvasive imaging can reliably distinguish between these two entities. Overall, US and MRI are the most useful tests. When left untreated, simple hepatic cysts typically do not become symptomatic, develop complications, or increase significantly in size. When therapy is contemplated for a presumed symptomatic lesion, care must be exercised to ensure that the symptoms are not attributable to another cause because this is the case in many patients. Furthermore, a period of observation or a diagnostic aspiration can be useful to determine whether symptoms are indeed resulting from the cyst. Finally, if operative treatment is offered, it should be tailored to the type of lesion. Simple hepatic cysts can be treated by cyst wall excision, whereas neoplastic cysts require enucleation or resection. These can often be performed laparoscopically and with minimal blood loss, little need for transfusion, and with negligible morbidity and mortality. Overall, however, there are few indications for operative therapy for simple hepatic cysts.

SUGGESTED READINGS

Arnold HL, Harrison SA: New advances in evaluation and management of patients with polycystic liver disease, *Am J Gastroenterol* 100(11):2569, 2005.

Devaney K, Goodman ZD, Ishak KG: Hepatobiliary cystadenoma and cystadenocarcinoma. A light microscopic and immunohistochemical study of 70 patients, *Am J Surg Pathol* 18:1078, 1994.

Dixon E, Sutherland FR, Mitchell P, and others: Cystadenomas of the liver: a spectrum of disease, *Can J Surg* 44:371, 2001.

Gigot JF, Jadoul P, Que F, and others: Adult polycystic liver disease: is fenestration the most adequate operation for long-term management? *Ann Surg* 225:286, 1997.

Gigot JF, Legrand M, Hubens G, and others: Laparoscopic treatment of non-parasitic liver cysts: adequate selection of patients and surgical technique, *World J Surg* 20:556, 1996.

Hansman MF, Ryan JA Jr, Holmes JH, and others: Management and long-term follow-up of hepatic cysts, *Am J Surg* 181:404, 2001.

Koffron A, Rao S, Ferrario M, and others: Intrahepatic biliary cystadenoma: role of cyst fluid analysis and surgical management in the laparoscopic era, *Surgery* 136:926, 2004.

Lewis WD, Jenkins RL, Rossi RL, and others: Surgical treatment of biliary cystadenoma. A report of 15 cases, *Arch Surg* 123:563, 1988.

Martin IJ, McKinley AJ, Currie EJ, and others: Tailoring the management of nonparasitic liver cysts, *Ann Surg* 228:167, 1998.

Montorsi M, Torzilli G, Fumagalli U, and others: Percutaneous alcohol sclerotherapy of simple hepatic cysts. Results from a multicentre survey in Italy, *HPB Surg* 8:89, 1994.

Thomas KT, Welch D, Trueblood A, and others: Effective treatment of biliary cystadenoma, *Ann Surg* 241:769; discussion 773, 2005.

Vogt DP, Henderson JM, Chmielewski E: Cystadenoma and cystadenocarcinoma of the liver: a single center experience, *J Am Coll Surg* 200:727, 2005.

ECHINOCOCCAL DISEASE OF THE LIVER

Timothy M. Pawlik, MD, MPH

INTRODUCTION

Echinococcus is a flat tapeworm characterized by a scolex with four suckers and a double row of 30 to 36 hooklets. The life cycle of *Echinococcus* alternates been carnivores and herbivores, with dogs being the definitive host. In general, tapeworm eggs are passed in the feces of infected dogs, which then in turn contaminate herbage that is subsequently eaten by intermediate hosts such as sheep or cattle. Once consumed, the ova hatch in the small intestine, penetrate the intestinal wall, and enter the portal system to reach the liver, lung, and other distant sites. Human infestation occurs with consumption of contaminated vegetables or through contact with infected animals or soil. Although echinococcosis is fairly uncommon in North America, it is endemic in Mediterranean countries, the Middle and Far East, and South America. However, the combination of travel and immigration has made echinococcus a worldwide disease.

Although there are four documented species, *E. granulosus* and *E. multilocularis* are most commonly associated with hydatid disease in humans. Infection with either species can result in hydatid disease anywhere in the body, with the liver being the most frequently involved organ (55%–80%) followed by the lung (10%–40%). Hepatic *E. multilocularis* is characterized by macroscopic appearance of an infiltrating mass composed of multiple small cysts. This alveolar form of hydatid disease lacks a limiting membrane, and the liver parenchyma near the mass is often atrophic with capsular retraction. In contrast, *E. granulosus* is more often characterized by a single cyst, with or without daughter cysts. In fact, up to 80% of patients present with a solitary cyst in a single organ. This chapter focuses on *E. granulosus* because it is the most common form of hydatid disease.

PATHOLOGY

In the liver, *E. granulosus* forms cysts that are constituted by an external acellular layer and an inner cellular germinal layer that produces the brood capsules containing protoscolicies, hydatid sand, or daughter cysts. The outer acellular layer is usually 2 to 5 mm thick and is composed of fibroblasts that produce a capsule of fibrous connective tissue called the *pericyst*. The pericyst is calcified in approximately half of patients. The inner germinal layer, in contrast, is where the actual echinococcal scoleces develop and where daughter cysts develop and then float freely in the cyst fluid. A small cyst might contain hundreds of protoscolicies, whereas a large cyst can contain tens of thousands of protoscolicies. In contrast, mature cysts may become inactive and further calcify.

PRESENTATION

The symptoms associated with hepatic *E. granulosus* can vary considerably. Hepatic hydatid cysts tend to grow slowly, displacing normal hepatic parenchyma and adjacent organs rather than infiltrating them. Because of this, patients can remain asymptomatic for prolonged periods of time. Typical signs and symptoms are usually nonspecific and may include abdominal pain, palpable abdominal mass, fever, fatigue, nausea, jaundice, and biliary cholangitis from rupture into the bile duct. Patients with exceptionally large cysts may also present with signs of vena cava compression or portal hypertension. Although uncommon, hydatid cyst rupture can result in a more dramatic clinical presentation characterized by anaphylaxis and shock.

Because of the paucity of pathonomonic signs and symptoms, the diagnosis of uncomplicated echinococcal infection is frequently made on the basis of clinical suspicion and epidemiologic data. In patients suspected of harboring echinococcus, serology may be helpful. Although eosinophilia is present in 20% to 25% of infected patients, it is only suggestive. In contrast, specific enzyme-linked immunosorbent assay (ELISA) and hydatid antigen immunobinding assays yield a sensitivity and specificity up to 95% and 90%, respectively. The accuracy of these serologic assays varies, however, with the location of the hydatid cyst (highest for hepatic cysts) and the patient's age. As such, serologic assays should be used mostly to confirm infection suspected on imaging studies.

IMAGING

Traditionally, ultrasound has been favored as the first-line diagnostic imaging tool. Ultrasound is inexpensive, noninvasive, and readily available. In addition, the specificity of ultrasound to rule out hepatic hydatid cystic disease has been reported to be as high as 90%. For these reasons, there has been extensive experience using ultrasound to characterize hepatic echinococcal disease. On ultrasound, hydatid cysts classically appear as thick-walled cysts that often have calcifications. Several investigators have proposed an ultrasonographic classification of hydatid disease. The ultrasound classification described by Gharbi is probably the most widely accepted (Table 1). However, more recently the World Health Organization (WHO) Working Group on Echinococcosis has proposed a standardized classification of cystic hydatid disease (Table 2). Ultrasonographic classification staging systems are not only diagnostically important but also clinically relevant because therapy is often stage based.

Cross-sectional imaging with computed tomography (CT) and magnetic resonance imaging (MRI) complements information obtained on ultrasound. CT and MRI can provide additional

Table 1: Gharbi's Classification of Cystic Hydatid Disease

Type	Ultrasound Features
I	Pure fluid collection
II	Fluid collection with split wall/detached membrane
III	Fluid collection with multiple septa/daughter cysts
IV	Heterogeneous hyperechoic cyst contents
V	Cyst with reflecting thick ± calcified wall

Adapted from Gharbi HA, Hassine W, Brauner MW, and others: Radiology 139:459, 1981.

Table 2: World Health Organization Classification of Cystic Hydatid Disease

Type	Ultrasound Features
CL	Unilocular lesion with no cyst wall visible
CE1	Unilocular lesion with cyst wall visible, hydatid sand, "snowflake" sign
CE2	Multivesicular lesion, multiseptated, honeycomb sign, daughter cysts visible
CE3	Unilocular lesion, detached laminated membrane inside cyst, "water lily" sign
CE4	Heterogeneous hypoechoic or hyperechoic lesion, no daughter cysts, degenerative contents
CE5	Thick calcified lesion, calcification partial to complete, cone-shaped shadow

Adapted from WHO Informal Working Group: Acta Tropica 85:253, 2003.

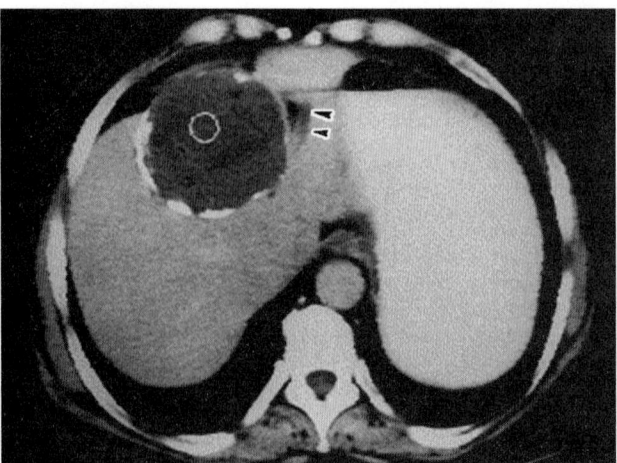

Figure 1 Computed tomography scan showing a 7.8-cm hepatic enchinococcal cyst with calcification of the pericyst and a CT density of 23.4 HU, causing mass effect with pericystic biliary dilatation *(arrowheads)*. *From Haddad MC, Al-Awar G, Huwaijah SH, and others: J Clin Imag 25:403, 2001. Used with permission.*

structural details and show more precisely the location and depth of the cyst within the liver (Fig. 1). The presence of daughter cysts and exogenous cysts can also be more clearly seen on CT and MRI. As such, ultrasound should be used in combination with either CT or MRI in the diagnostic workup of patients suspected of having hepatic echinococcal disease.

Endoscopic retrograde cholangiopancreatography (ERCP) may also provide valuable information. Communication of the hydatid cyst with the biliary tract may occur in up to 25% of patients. ERCP is clearly indicated when the patient presents with a complication such as cholangitis or jaundice. Its routine use in asymptomatic, uncomplicated hydatid liver disease is, however, more controversial. Some centers advocate routine use of ERCP to define the bile duct anatomy and to visualize subclinical connections between the cyst and the biliary system before surgery.

TREATMENT

Once hydatid disease is diagnosed, treatment should be initiated so that secondary complications can be prevented. The principle of hydatid disease treatment should center on eliminating the *Echinococcus*, preventing recurrence, and minimizing patient morbidity. Current treatment options include medical therapy, percutaneous management, or surgery. The ultrasound classification, location, size, number, and presence of associated complications help to dictate the therapeutic approach.

Medical Therapy

Chemotherapy with benzimidazole compounds (mebendazole and albendazole) is the medical treatment of choice. Chemotherapy is routinely administered before percutaneous or surgical management. Mebendazole is poorly absorbed in the intestine, and the mebendazole fluorinated analogue does not penetrate the cyst. In contrast, albendazole has significantly better intestinal absorption and undergoes a rapid first-pass metabolism in the liver. As such, albendazole has better tissue distribution and higher cyst fluid concentrations. Therefore albendazole is the drug of choice for medical therapy. The indicated dosage of albendazole is 10 to 15 mg/kg/day postprandially in two divided doses. More recently, praziquantel, a synthetic isoquinoline-pyrazine derivative, has been used in combination with albendazole. This combination may be more effective than albendazole monotherapy.

Despite the activity of these drugs toward *Echinococcus*, they should be considered parasitostatic and not parasiticidal because most patients develop recurrent disease following cessation of medical treatment. In fact, with medical treatment alone, only 30% of patients can expect clinical and radiographic resolution. Medical treatment therefore should be used primarily in conjunction with percutaneous drainage or surgery. According to the WHO guidelines, preoperative administration should begin between 1 and 4 days before surgery for albendazole and 3 months before surgery for mebendazole.

Percutaneous Aspiration, Injection, and Reaspiration

In the early 1980s, several reports of accidental percutaneous punctures of hepatic hydatid cysts were reported with no associated complications. Combined with the recent availability of chemotherapeutic agents with significant activity against *Echinococcus*, several investigators subsequently have begun to use transhepatic percutaneous drainage to manage hydatid cysts. With this technique, the hydatid cyst is percutaneously aspirated under ultrasonographic or CT guidance, followed by injection of a protoscolicidal agent and finally reaspiration of the cyst contents. Percutaneous aspiration, injection, and reaspiration (PAIR) can be performed using a single-needle puncture for both univesicular and mutlivesicular cysts. Patients undergoing PAIR typically receive oral benzimidazole therapy for 1 week before and 28 days after the procedure. Different scolicidal agents can be used during PAIR; however, 20% sodium chloride is most commonly used. Hypertonic saline has a high density and attenuation on CT imaging, which allows for evaluation of proper contact of the scolicidal agent with the cyst wall. In general, 95% ethanol is avoided, particularly if a communication between the cyst and the biliary system is suspected. Studies have shown that there is immediate detachment of the inner germinal layer from the pericyst after injection of the scolicidal agent. Following PAIR, the cyst fluid can be assessed to confirm the success of the procedure and the viability of any remaining protoscolices. PAIR is usually well tolerated. Complications include infection and leakage during the drainage, which can result in fever or, uncommonly, signs of anaphylaxis. Cyst decompression can also result in cyst-biliary communications, which can usually be managed by ERCP.

PAIR is indicated in patients with hepatic disease who refuse surgery, have multiple cysts, or who relapse after surgery. PAIR is contraindicated to treat cysts that are inaccessible to puncture or in those cysts that do not have a sufficient layer of hepatic tissue to allow transhepatic puncture.

Surgery

Surgical options for hepatic hydatid disease range from conservative procedures, such as simple cyst drainage and partial cystectomy, with or without omentoplasty, to radical procedures, such as total pericystectomy, partial hepatectomy, or hemihepatectomy. The conservative techniques focus on sparing hepatic tissue and removing the parasite while leaving part or most of the pericyst in situ. In contrast, more radical procedures remove the entire pericyst, with or without entering the cyst itself. Whether the surgeon should routinely use a conservative versus radical approach to hepatic hydatid disease is somewhat controversial but largely should be based on the size, site, and type of the cyst, as well as the surgeon's expertise.

Many surgeons use simple drainage and partial cystectomy, which is perhaps best suited to cysts on the periphery of the liver. Before entering the cyst, packing of the operative field with scolicidal agent-soaked gauzes is necessary to minimize the risk of peritoneal soilage and contamination. The cyst contents are then inactivated by aspirating the cyst using a closed system, followed by infusion of the scolicidal agent into the empty cavity (Fig. 2, A). If the cyst fluid is bile stained or connection with the bile ducts had previously been identified on ERCP, intracavitary scolicidal agents should be avoided. After evacuating the cyst contents and the scolicidal agent, the cyst should be unroofed, and part of the cyst wall removed so that the cavity can be fully explored. Any remaining debris should be cleared (Fig. 2, B). The cyst cavity should then be filled with an omental pedicle (Fig. 2, C).

Total pericystectomy can be performed with either an open or closed technique. In the open technique, the cyst is opened and the material removed, and a scolicidal agent is infused. When opening the cyst cavity, the surgeon must be certain not to spill the cyst contents. The pericyst wall is removed using sharp electrocautery or dissector (Fig. 3). Open pericystectomy is recommended when the cyst wall is thin and rupture is possible. With the closed technique, a plane is identified outside the pericyst,

and an en block pericsystectomy is performed without manipulating the contents of the cyst. During the removal of the pericyst, blood vessels and biliary structures are controlled with clips or sutures. Intraoperative ultrasonography (IOUS) may be useful to determine the relationship of the cyst to vascular and biliary structures within the liver parenchyma. The advantages of closed pericystectomy include leaving no residual adventia, eliminating scolicidal agents, and reducing the risk of biliary fistula. However, the closed technique is more technically demanding because hepatic parenchymal transection is required. In general, pericystectomy, as with simple cyst drainage and partial cystectomy, is best performed on cysts that are accessible along the periphery of the liver.

Laparoscopic treatment of liver echinococcosis has been increasingly proposed as an alternative therapeutic option. The laparoscopic approach can involve simple drainage, partial cystectomy, or even total pericystectomy. Proponents of the laparoscopic approach note that the technique allows the cavity of the cyst to be examined in more detail. Additional benefits are a shorter hospital stay and reduction of wound complications. A major disadvantage of laparoscopy, however, is the inability to prevent cavity content spillage under the high pneumoperitoneum intraabdominal pressures. Thus the puncture of the hydatid cyst without spillage of the cyst contents can be difficult during laparascopy. Several investigators have suggested various techniques to help minimize the potential risk of cyst leak. One technique involves fixing the cyst in the abdominal wall with a special umbrella trocar and suction with a specific suction device. Other investigators suggest that the patient be placed in Trendelenburg position and that the right subdiaphragmatic suprahepatic space be filled with an antiscolecoidal agent. Although there are no randomized trials comparing laparoscopic versus open surgery for hepatic hydatid disease, reported postoperative morbidity and mortality has generally been comparable. It is important to note, however, that patient selection is critical. The principles of laparoscopic surgery for hepatic hydatid disease should remain the same as with the open surgical technique. With this in mind, centrally located cysts are not amenable to either laparoscopic or open simple drainage or partial or total pericystectomy.

In general, liver resection is indicated when other, more conservative surgical therapies have failed or are contraindicated (e.g., deep-seated, centrally located cysts). Hepatic resection is also indicated for large hydatid cysts that have destroyed one or more liver segments or if the cyst is near major vascular or biliary structures. A formal hepatic resection should be undertaken only if complete excision of the cysts can be achieved. Unlike E. granulosa, which almost always presents as a single cyst, E. multilocularis can result in a more complicated disease process known as alveolar echinococcosis. In this variation of the disease, multiple cysts can form throughout the liver, leading to fulminant liver failure from biliary sclerosis, Budd-Chiari syndrome, or sclerosing cholangitis. Although this clinical scenario is rare, orthotopic liver transplantation may be the only potentially curative therapy.

Management of possible biliary communication within the hydatid cyst requires attention, regardless of the type of surgical procedure performed. As noted, preoperative ERCP can be helpful to identify biliary-cyst communications. However, exploration for biliary-cyst communication is mandatory in every patient. Patients with large cysts involving numerous hepatic segments or patients with a history of cholangitis should especially be suspected of harboring a biliary-cyst communication. Bile-stained cyst fluid is another clue that a communication exists. Once identified, communications smaller than 5 mm usually can be sutured. In contrast, biliary communications larger than 5 mm may be more difficult to manage. If simple drainage or partial cystectomy is planned, common duct exploration is mandatory with choledochoscopy. T-tube drainage can be used

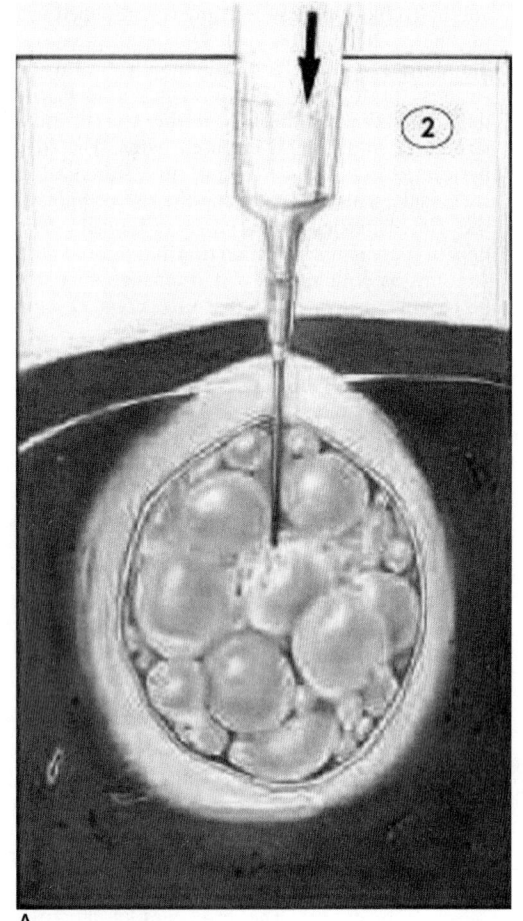

A

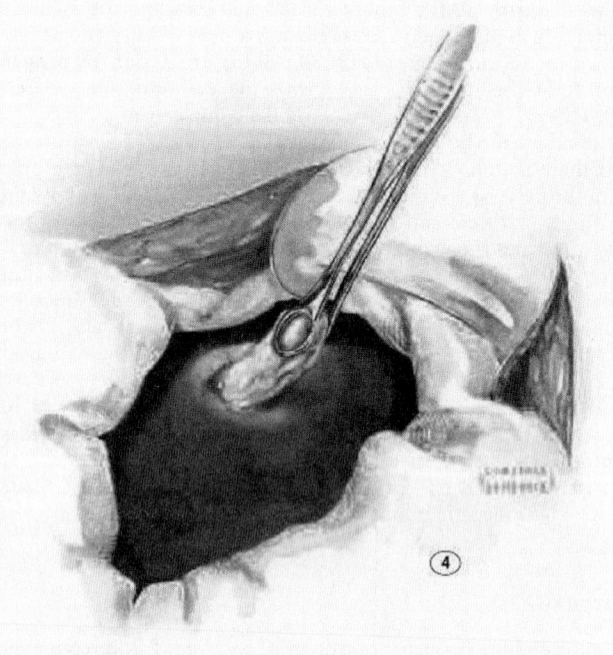

B

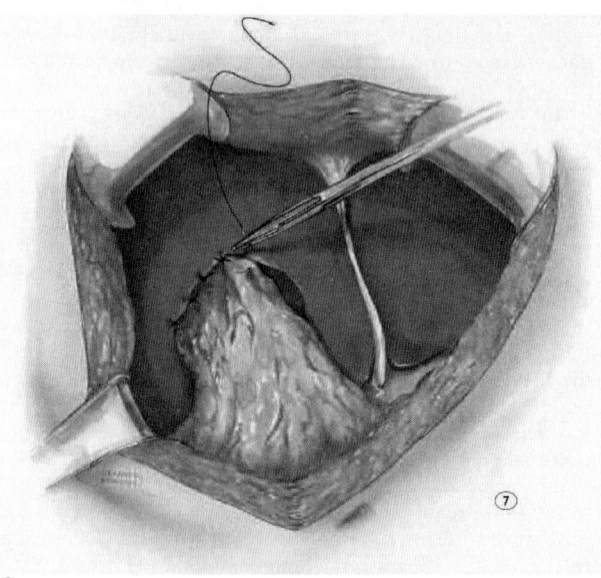

C

Figure 2 Open cysts drainage and evacuation. The cyst contents are inactivated by aspirating the cyst using a closed-system followed by infusion of the scolicidal agent into the empty cavity **(A).** The cyst is then unroofed and part of the cyst wall removed so that debris can be cleared **(B).** Finally, the cyst cavity is filled with an omental pedicle **(C).** *From Cameron JL, Sandone C: Atlas of surgery: gallbladder and biliary tract, the liver, portasystemic shunts, the pancreas, Hamilton, ON, Canada, 1990, BC Decker. Used with permission.*

to secure and decompress closure of a large duct. Internal drainage with a Roux-en-Y intracystic hepaticojejunostomy may also sometimes be necessary for large cysts in which large ducts have been disrupted. Another approach to deal with bile duct disruption is to convert to a formal hepatic resection, thereby

eliminating the need for bile duct exploration, repair, and T-tube drainage.

There is no formal consensus regarding the routine use of chemotherapy following surgery. WHO recommends postoperative use of scolicidal agents for 1 month (albendazole) or 3 months

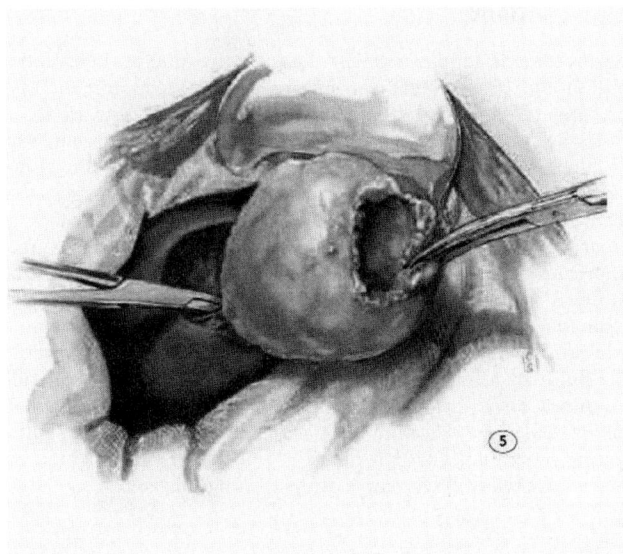

Figure 3 Pericystectomy can be performed with removal of the calcified pericyst either using sharp electrocautery or a dissector. *From Cameron JL, Sandone C: Atlas of surgery: gallbladder and biliary tract, the liver, portasystemic shunts, the pancreas, Hamilton, ON, Canada, 1990, BC Decker. Used with permission.*

(mebendazole) if there has been spillage of protoscolices at the time of surgery. Postoperative medical treatment is not indicated when there is no cyst spillage and the cyst has been completely removed.

CHOOSING A THERAPEUTIC STRATEGY

In general, the therapeutic approach to patients with hepatic ecchinococcal disease can be stratified according to the classification of the cystic hydatid disease. Patients with WHO classification CL, CE1, and CE3 cysts can frequently be treated with scolicidal chemotherapy. PAIR, however, is frequently required because chemotherapy alone often does not produce degenerative changes. Patients with CL, CE1, and CE3 cysts require surgery only if chemotherapy and PAIR fail. In contrast, CE2 hydatid cysts are much less responsive to chemotherapy and therefore should initially be managed by PAIR or surgery, depending on the drainability of the cyst contents, the number of daughter cysts, and the location of the cyst within the liver. Although PAIR may be possible for treatment of CE2 cysts when the number of daughter cysts is low, surgery is often necessary when there are numerous daughter cysts. Surgery is the treatment of choice for type CE4 and CE5 cysts, unless the cyst is completely calcified and inactive.

OUTCOME FOLLOWING TREATMENT OF HEPATIC HYDATID DISEASE

With advances in perioperative care and intraoperative techniques, the morbidity and mortality associated with the surgical treatment of hepatic hydatid disease has decreased dramatically. Shock secondary to protoscolice spillage should be a rare occurrence when the appropriate preoperative chemotherapy and intraoperative techniques have been used. For uncomplicated hydatid disease, morbidity and mortality have been reported to be in the range of 20% and 1%, respectively; in contrast, patients with complicated disease have a higher reported morbidity and mortality, in the range of 30% to 50% and 5%, respectively.

Overall, the long-term results of PAIR and surgery for hepatic hydatid cysts are excellent. Most series report recurrence rates less than 10%. However, because of the risk for reinfestation, every patient requires long-term follow-up with both serologic studies and radiographic imaging.

SUGGESTED READINGS

Alonso Casado O, Moreno González E, Loinaz Segurola C, and others: Results of 22 years of experience in radical surgical treatment of hepatic hydatid cysts, *Hepatogastroenterology* 48:235, 2001.

Balik AA, Basoglu M, Celebi F, and others: Surgical treatment of hydatid disease of the liver: review of 304 cases, *Arch Surgery* 134:166, 1999.

Gil-Grande LA, Rodriguez-Caabeiro F, Prieto JG, and others: Randomized controlled trial of efficacy of albendazole in intra-abdominal hydatid disease, *Lancet* 342:1269, 1993.

Khuroo JG, Wani NA, Javid G, and others: Percutaneous drainage compared with surgery for hepatic hydatid cysts, *N Engl J Med* 337:581, 1997.

World Health Organization.: Guidelines for the treatment of CE, *Bulletin of the WHO* 74:231, 1996.

BENIGN LIVER LESIONS

Jane M. Liaw, MD, and William C. Chapman, MD

Benign hepatic lesions are common, with an estimated incidence of 7% to 9%, and in one autopsy series, up to 20% of the population. They are discovered with increasing frequency with the advancement and widespread use of radiographic imaging studies, often incidentally. They may occur in the presence or absence of liver disease. Surgical intervention is not usually indicated because most of these lesions are asymptomatic with a benign natural history. However, a few of these tumors carry risk for clinical complications or malignant transformation or have overlapping radiographic features with malignant tumors, posing unique diagnostic and therapeutic challenges.

Important issues for consideration in the surgical evaluation of a liver mass include symptoms or the risk of symptoms and the magnitude of a possible surgical resection versus the need for long-term, possibly lifelong clinical follow-up. The single most important issue is diagnostic certainty. In this area, radiographic imaging studies are critical. Taken together with clinical presentation, most lesions can be accurately identified by characteristic imaging findings without the need for biopsy. Once lesions are identified, surgeons should understand the natural history of each entity, which heavily influences management strategies and the need for surgical intervention.

CYSTIC TUMORS

Hepatic cystic lesions are a common finding, usually discovered incidentally during workup for unrelated issues. Simple cysts have a reported prevalence of 5% in the United States. Other hepatic cystic tumors include cystadenomas, cystadenocarcinomas, hydatid cysts, and abscesses.

SIMPLE CYSTS

Pathogenesis

Simple cysts are usually congenital, a result of abnormal embryonal development of intrahepatic biliary ducts. These ducts fail to connect to their extrahepatic counterparts, forming intraparenchymal cysts. Simple cysts are solitary more than 50% of the time and asymptomatic more than 90% of the time. Size can range up to 20 cm, although most are less than 5 cm. Histologically, they consist of a single layer of cuboidal or columnar epithelium, with minimal surrounding fibrous stroma. The cyst almost always contains a clear, straw-colored serous fluid without bile.

Presentation

Simple cysts are usually found incidentally in female patients older than age 40. Cysts of less than 8 cm are almost always asymptomatic. Any symptoms are usually related to mass effect, causing pain in the right upper quadrant and occasionally early satiety. Rarely, intracystic hemorrhage and infection may develop. Ultrasound (US) is usually sufficient for diagnosis. On computed tomography (CT) and magnetic resonance imaging (MRI), cysts have a thin wall without enhancement and a fluid-filled appearance (Fig. 1). There are no internal features or septations.

Management

Asymptomatic simple cysts less than 8 cm require no intervention but should be observed. For smaller (<5 cm) symptomatic cysts or patients who are poor operative candidates, the cysts are sometimes aspirated and given injection with a sclerosing agent, such as ethanol or minocycline. However, chemical sclerosis results in a higher rate of recurrence and infection, especially for larger cysts. Thus patients with symptomatic cysts (>5 cm) should undergo laparoscopic or open cyst unroofing. A laparoscopic versus open approach is guided by the location of the cyst (i.e., readily accessible location of cyst wall on the liver surface). Typical straw-colored or clear fluid in an otherwise simple-appearing cyst does not require additional analysis (cytology, tumor markers, etc.). However, if the fluid has a bilious hue, the inner cyst wall should be carefully examined for a ductal communication, and if present, this should be ligated. Biliary communications are exceedingly rare in the setting of simple cysts that have not undergone manipulation but may occur following attempts at cyst aspiration.

Technical Tips

When simple cysts are unroofed, a wide opening should be created along an area where the cyst is thin walled with minimal overlying hepatic parenchyma. This approach minimizes the risk of cyst closure and recurrence and allows any continued fluid production by the cyst wall to drain freely into the abdominal cavity for resorption.

COMPLEX CYSTS

Multiple Cysts

If multiple simple cysts are seen, consider polycystic liver disease. This is an inherited condition (autosomal dominant), often found in association with renal cysts. US, CT, and MR imaging are all valuable diagnostic tools (Fig. 2). Although polycystic renal disease often leads to progressive renal insufficiency and end-stage renal failure, the majority of patients with polycystic liver disease remain asymptomatic with preserved liver function and do not require surgical intervention. Advanced disease often presents with chronic abdominal pain and tenderness in the right upper quadrant. Rarely, the polycystic liver can become massive in size and occupy a large majority of the abdominal cavity. Aggressive cyst unroofing and

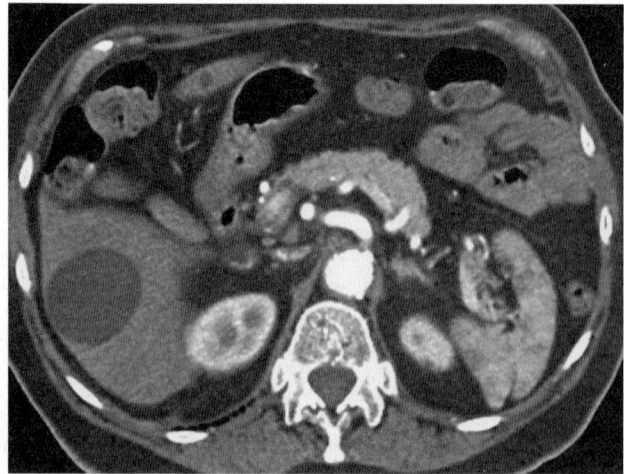

Figure 1 Simple cyst. Contrast-enhanced computed tomography scan demonstrating a simple cyst in right posterior liver (segment VI). Note fluid-filled structure with a thin, nonenhancing wall and absence of internal septations.

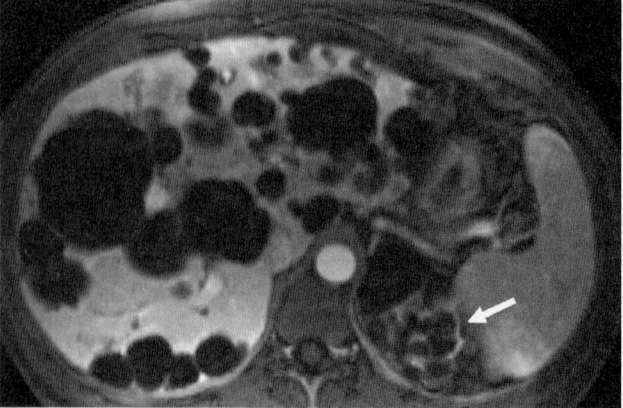

Figure 2 Magnetic resonance image in a patient with polycystic liver disease. There are multiple cysts of varying size scattered throughout the entire liver substance. Also note the multiple cysts involving the upper pole of the left kidney (arrow) in this patient with combined liver and kidney polycystic disease.

fenestration along with limited hepatic resection can provide relief of symptoms and reduce liver cyst volume, but relief is usually only transient because disease progression and cyst recurrence is the norm. Although kidney transplantation is commonly considered for renal failure associated with polycystic kidney disease, this is not the case for polycystic liver disease. Liver transplantation is rarely considered and usually only with significant end-stage liver symptoms such as portal hypertension or hepatic failure.

Cystadenomas

Biliary cystadenomas are uncommon, slow-growing complex cysts measuring up to 20 cm in size. They are benign but have malignant potential to transform into cystadenocarcinoma and thus should be surgically removed whenever recognized. The incidence is 50 to 1000 times less common than simple cysts, usually occurring in women older than age 40. Histologically, cystadenomas are multilocular lined by a single layer of cuboidal or columnar epithelium surrounded by thickened stroma. The diagnosis is made by the presence of mesenchymal tissue.

Presentation

Abdominal pain or discomfort, loss of appetite, nausea, and abdominal fullness are the presenting symptoms of cystadenoma. Jaundice may be present if the tumor compresses the biliary tree or if fistulization into biliary ducts occurs, allowing mucinous material to obstruct the biliary tree. On clinical examination, a large, hepatic mass may be palpated.

Radiologically, internal septations are almost always seen in cystadenomas on contrast-enhanced CT or MRI (Fig. 3). Cystadenomas have irregular borders and a thick stromal layer, and calcifications and mural nodules can occasionally be seen in the walls. MRI appearance varies, depending on the protein content of the fluid and the presence or absence of an intracystic soft-tissue component.

Technical Tips

It is the cyst wall and lining that carry the malignant potential for degeneration. Thus cyst wall enucleation (complete removal of epithelium) is indicated for the cystadenoma without malignancy. There is a high rate of recurrence and persistent malignant risk if only cyst unroofing is performed. If, during surgery, the diagnosis is uncertain, enucleation can be performed empirically or frozen sections may be sent for pathologic evaluation. If cystadenocarcinoma is found or strongly suspected, standard hepatic resection should be considered to ensure a margin-negative resection.

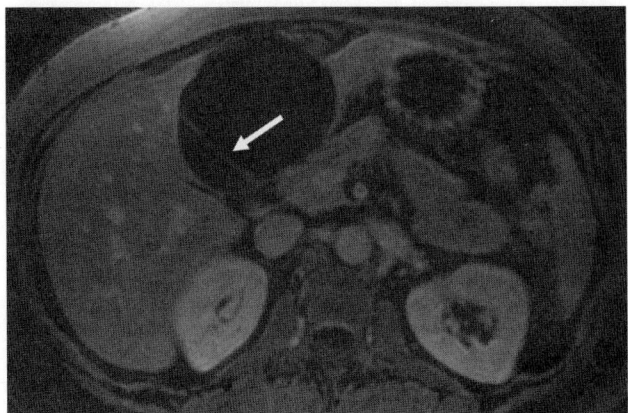

Figure 3   Biliary cystadenoma. Portal venous phase gadolinium-enhanced T1-weighted magnetic resonance image shows cystic mass in the porta hepatis containing a single septation with enhancement of the capsule and septa *(arrow)*.

Hydatid Cysts

Hydatid or echinococcal cysts should be considered in patients from endemic areas of the world with findings of complex hepatic cysts. These include the southwestern United States, Scotland, and many parts of Europe. These cysts are caused by the intestinal *Echinococcus* spp. tapeworm that infects dogs. Humans, sheep, pigs, and cattle are intermediary hosts infected by ingestion of paracystic eggs via direct contact with an infected animal or ingestion of contaminated food or water. Each cyst represents the larval form of the parasite and can be found in the liver, lungs, brain, and kidneys.

Presentation

Most patients are asymptomatic, but some may present with abdominal pain, fever, or hepatomegaly. Anaphylactic shock may follow cyst rupture into the peritoneal cavity. On US and CT, hydatid cysts have thick walls that are often calcified and contain debris. Intracystic septations are often present. Peripheral daughter cysts may be seen in mature cysts. MRI clearly demonstrates fine features of hydatid cysts, although diagnosis can be confirmed by serologic tests. Eosinophilia is often seen on routine complete blood count, typical of parasitic disease.

Management

Complete cyst enucleation can offer surgical cure, provided all cysts are removed and there are no extrahepatic sites of disease. Great care should be taken to keep the cyst intact because spillage of cyst contents may cause anaphylaxis. Although laparoscopic and open cyst drainage and unroofing have previously been reported as treatment modalities, we do not recommend these procedures because of the high risk of anaphylaxis (4%) and recurrence (9%). Antiparasitic drugs such as mebendazole and albendazole are useful adjuvant therapies and are usually started before surgical intervention.

Technical Tips

A right subcostal incision with midline extension or extension bilaterally generally provides adequate exposure to hydatid cysts in any location. Midline laparotomy is the approach of choice in patients with cysts in the left lobe, abdominal hydatidosis, or ruptured cysts. The area surrounding the cyst should be carefully packed with a layer of saline-soaked gauze, followed by laparotomy pads soaked with a protoscolicidal agent, such as 20% hypertonic saline, 0.5% cetrimide and 0.05% chlorhexidine, or 10% povidone-iodine. Intraoperative US may be useful for cyst identification. Manipulation of the liver and cyst area should be minimized to avoid iatrogenic rupture. Suction should be on hand in such a case. Again, complete removal of the cyst, any daughter cysts, and the pericyst layer is emphasized to prevent recurrence.

▉ SOLID TUMORS

Solid benign liver masses usually fall into one of the following categories: hemangiomas, focal nodular hyperplasia (FNH), hepatic adenoma, and miscellaneous.

Hemangiomas

Pathogenesis

Hemangiomas are the most common benign live tumor, with an estimated 3% incidence. These tumors arise from the endothelial lining of blood vessels as vascular ectasias and have been associated with high estrogen states including puberty, pregnancy, oral contraceptive use, and androgen treatment. Estrogen receptors have been found in some tumors, suggesting the role of hormones in pathogenesis and perhaps accounting for the prevalence of the tumor in women versus men.

Autopsy series report prevalances from 0.5% to as high as 20.0%. The female-to-male ratio is between 5:1 and 6:1. Hemangioma is usually found between the ages of 30 and 70 years, with a mean age of 45. It is common in children as well, accounting for 12% of all childhood hepatic tumors, although the natural history of hemangiomas in children is unlike that of adults and is regarded as a separate entity.

In infants and children, unlike adults, multiple hepatic hemangiomas may be accompanied by multiple cutaneous hemangiomas. Infantile hemangioma may present with hepatomegaly congestive heart failure resulting from significant shunting, whereas even large lesions are almost always asymptomatic in adults. Patients refractory to inotropics and diuretics may be treated with hepatic arterial embolization or direct surgical ligation. However, collateral vessels often develop rapidly following intervention. Rarely, pediatric hemangioma may present with jaundice, disseminated intravascular coagulation, or hemorrhagic shock from intraperitoneal rupture, requiring hepatic resection. Pediatric hepatic hemangiomas that are asymptomatic often regress after the first year of life and do not require intervention.

In adults, hepatic hemangiomas are also called *cavernous* hemangiomas. Tumors larger than 5 cm are historically called *giant* hemangiomas, although the term is not associated with greater potential for symptoms or complications. They are usually found subcapsular in the region of the right lobe, with sizes ranging from 1 to 20 cm. Grossly, the tumor is well circumscribed, compressible, and dark colored, owing to its blood-filled spaces. Microscopically, it consists of multiple, large vascular channels lined by a single layer of endothelial cells supported by collagenous walls. The hepatic artery supplies these tumors.

Presentation

The most common scenario is that of an incidentally discovered tumor found during ultrasonographic examination of the abdomen for unrelated reasons. Most tumors are less than 5 cm and asymptomatic. Symptoms are usually related to size or location, with tumors larger than 5 cm causing nonspecific abdominal pain. Peripherally located tumors may cause pain as a result of phlebitic irritation. Rarely, lesions may undergo spontaneous rupture, causing intermittent pain, although this risk is less than 1%.

Kasabach–Merritt syndrome is a rare syndrome characterized by thrombocytopenia and disseminated intravascular coagulopathy (DIC) in association with giant hemangiomas. Surgical and dental procedures often activate the consumptive cascade, and patients present with abdominal pain and bleeding within their hemangiomas. Interferon-alfa has been used in the management of this syndrome.

Radiographic Appearance

Hemangiomas have characteristic appearances on CT and MRI modalities. Radiographic imaging alone is usually sufficient for diagnosis, and patients rarely require additional studies. Noncontrast CT examination reveals well-defined, hypodense masses that may have calcifications and areas of fibrosis and central scarring.

Contrast-enhanced CT with delayed venous examination will demonstrate peripheral nodular enhancement and progressive centripetal fill-in (Fig. 4). This pattern is pathognomonic for hemangioma, and no further workup is required. Large areas of contrast pooling at the edges of the tumor are also characteristic on contrast-enhanced CT imaging.

On gadolinium-enhanced MRI, hemangiomas are hypointense on T1-weighted images and hyperintense on T2-weighted images. Tumors are isointense compared with cerebral spinal fluid and the gallbladder. Lesions of less than 2 cm will often appear hyperintense on both arterial and venous portal phases and may not show typical rapid contrast washout because of their small size. These should not be confused with hypervascular malignancies. If the diagnosis is in question, a Tc99-labeled red blood cell scan can be performed to make a definitive diagnosis.

Management

Hemangiomas almost never require surgical resection after the diagnosis is secure because most lesions are asymptomatic, and risk of spontaneous rupture is extremely small. For symptomatic lesions, simple enucleation is recommended because it preserves the maximal amount of functional liver. If significant bleeding is expected because of tumor location, an anatomic approach may be taken. Alternatively, hepatic resection and laparoscopic resection may be considered, depending on tumor location. In rare cases, transplantation has been reported for technically unresectable giant hemangiomata.

Technical Tips

Extrahepatic vascular control can be obtained by ligation of the right or left hepatic artery, depending on the location of the lesion. Gentle finger dissection in the plane between normal liver

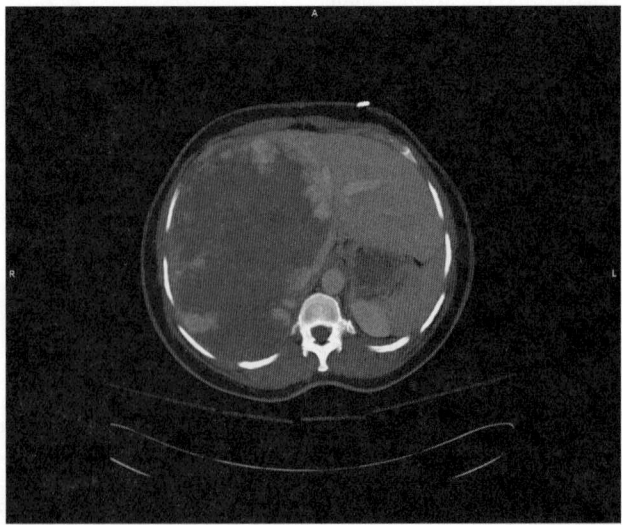
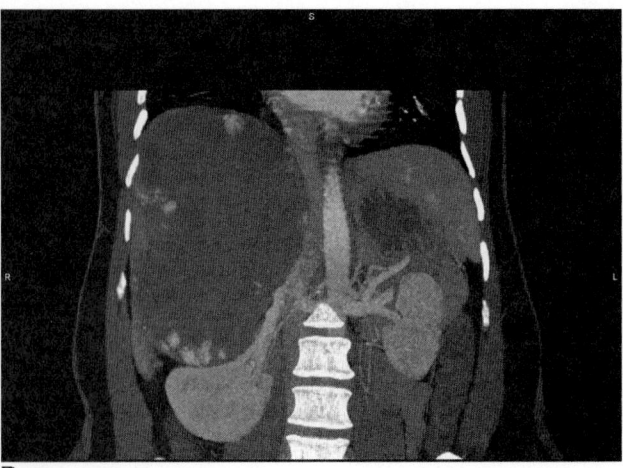

A   B

Figure 4 Giant cavernous hemangioma. **(A)** Contrast-enhanced axial computed tomography image demonstrates peripheral nodular enhancement with progressive centripetal fill-in. **(B)** Coronal image demonstrates inferior and medial displacement of right kidney and vena cava, respectively.

parenchyma and compressed tissue bordering the hemangioma can be used to shell out the tumor, ligating any vessels or bile ducts encountered. Blood loss is generally minimal because this plane is relatively avascular. Liver function is also mostly unaffected, even with removal of large hemangiomata. The raw surface of the remaining cavity can be coagulated using argon beam, and an omentoplasty may be used to cover the exposed surface.

Focal Nodular Hyperplasia

Pathogenesis

Focal nodular hyperplasia (FNH) is the second most common benign solid hepatic tumor (behind hemangioma), comprising 8% of all primary hepatic tumors. Prevalence of FNH is estimated to be 3% of the general population, predominantly in women in their third to fifth decades. The female-to-male ratio is between 6:1 and 8:1. Although a causal relationship has not been definitively shown, FNH is associated with oral contraceptive use, accelerating the growth of already existing tumors. It does not cause the formation of new lesions. FNH is considered a nonneoplastic, hyperplastic response to a congenital vascular malformation, rather than a hamartoma or response to ischemia, as previously thought. Most tumors are solitary, although they can be multifocal. Grossly, it is a well-circumscribed, nonencapsulated globular and lobulated tumor. Microscopically, FNH consists of benign-appearing hepatocytes with cords of fibrous septae radiating from a central scar, which comprises biliary structures of hepatocellular origin. This central scar can often be visualized on imaging studies. It consists of biliary ductules, cholangiolar proliferation with surrounding inflammation, and malformed arteries and capillaries. Portal veins are notably absent.

Presentation

Most patients present with an asymptomatic, solitary tumor of less than 5 cm near the hepatic surface. Only 10% of patients have clinical symptoms, such as epigastric or right upper quadrant pain. Most patients have normal liver function tests. Spontaneous rupture leading to hemorrhage is rare. To date, no cases of malignant degeneration have ever been described. Because of its benign clinical course, the distinction between FNH and other hypervascular hepatic tumors is critical.

Imaging

Presence of a central scar is the most characteristic feature of FNH on radiographic studies (Fig. 5). Other lesions may demonstrate a central scar similar to that of FNH. These include fibrolamellar variant of hepatocellular carcinoma, and hypervascular tumors such as hepatic adenoma and some metastases.

On US, FNH appears as a well-demarcated homogenous lesion. If the central scar can be seen, it is visualized as a hyperechoic band.

On noncontrast CT examination, FNHs are well defined, marginated, and hypodense or isodense. On contrast-enhanced multiphasic CT imaging, lesions are usually homogenous and isoattenuating to liver parenchyma before contrast injection. Lesions are bright, hypervascular with hypodense central scarring on arterial phase examination. If present, radiating hypodense fibrous bands and septa that arise from the scar are characteristic findings. FNH may be hypodense but often returns to isoattenuation on portal venous phases.

Ten-minute-delayed images often demonstrate increased contrast uptake in the scar and septa compared with surrounding liver parenchyma because of late opacification of the fibrotic components. Dilatated feeding arteries penetrating the central scar and draining veins at the tumor surface maybe observed in large FNH.

On T1-weighted MRI imaging, FNH is homogenous and slightly hypointense relative to the surrounding liver. On T2-weighted imaging, FNH is slightly hyperintense. It can also appear isointense on T1- and T2-weighted imaging.

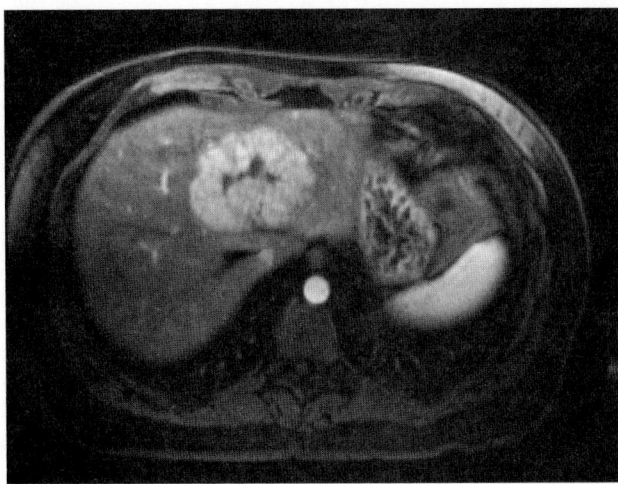

Figure 5 Focal nodular hyperplasia *(FNH)*. Arterial phase gadolinium-enhanced magnetic resonance image demonstrates hypervascular appearance of FNH with characteristic central scar.

Nuclear medicine imaging can sometimes be helpful to distinguish FNH from hepatic adenoma because sulfa-colloid is taken up by Kupffer cells (present in FNH), which are usually absent in adenoma. However, on scintigraphy with ^{99m}Tc-sulfur-colloid, FNH can have variable findings. If sulfa-colloid uptake is either the same as or increased compared with background liver, then this weighs against hepatic adenoma. When there is decreased uptake with this modality, it is not possible to rule out either tumor type.

On angiography, FNH displays a characteristic spoke-wheel pattern.

Management

Treatment strategy is heavily influenced by the certainty of diagnosis. In asymptomatic patients with a clear diagnosis, no further treatment is necessary, and the patient may be observed. In equivocal cases in which all imaging modalities fail to establish a firm diagnosis, biopsy is warranted for histologic examination. If possible, this should be performed laparoscopically. Surgical resection is usually indicated for patients with significant symptoms such as pain or when there is diagnostic uncertainty. Rarely, when resection is not possible in a patient with significant symptoms, transarterial embolization has been used as a treatment alternative. In patients with FNH and high estrogen state resulting from use of oral contraceptives, it is controversial whether to recommend that these be discontinued or that pregnancy be avoided. During pregnancy and postpartum state, patients should be observed and monitored with frequent US examinations. Postmenopausal women with FNH should be changed from oral estrogen treatment to transdermal delivery to decrease first-pass hepatic metabolism.

Hepatic Adenoma

Hepatic adenoma (HA) is a rare hepatic tumor that occurs predominantly in women aged 20 to 40 years, with a female-to-male ratio of at least 4:1 and reportedly as high as 11:1. It has a strong association with oral contraceptive use, with an incidence of 3 to 4 in 100,000 oral contraceptive users versus 1 in 100,000 nonusers. It occurs more frequently in long-term, high-dose estrogen use, and its withdrawal may induce tumor regression. It is also seen in androgen steroid therapy and anabolic steroid use, increasing the number, size, and incidence of HA in these patients. HA is also associated with diabetes mellitus and glycogen storage diseases, with 50% prevalence in type I (von Gierke's disease) and 25% in type III glycogen storage disease.

On gross inspection, HAs are mostly solitary (70%–80%), well circumscribed, round, and unencapsulated. A pseudocapsule is often present. Lesions are usually yellow-tan in color, with sizes of 5 to 15 cm in diameter, although tumors as large as 30 cm have been reported. Intratumoral fat, necrosis, and hemorrhage are often observed. Large subcapsular vessels are also common.

Histologically, hepatic adenomas are hypervascular tumors characterized by the benign proliferation of bile-producing hepatocytes, but no bile ducts can be seen, a key characteristic of HA. Cells are organized in plates separated by dilated sinusoids perfused by feeding arteries. Hepatocytes may contain fat and glycogen and occasional calcifications.

Presentation

Most patients present with a small, asymptomatic lesion. Multiple tumors are found in 10% to 30%, and more than 10 are designated liver adenomatosis. Larger HA tumors (>5 cm) can be associated with right upper-quadrant pain, fullness, or discomfort. Because of its hypervascular nature and lack of a capsule, HA carries a moderate to high risk of spontaneous rupture, associated with increasing size (>5 cm). When rupture occurs, it is intratumoral in one third of cases and intraperitoneal in two thirds of cases.

Rare cases of malignant degeneration have also been reported in patients with large or multiple tumors.

Hepatic adenomatosis is defined as the presence of more than 10 adenomas and is considered its own distinct disease entity. It has been reported in the absence of oral contraceptive and has a male-to-female ratio of 1:1. Histologically and on radiographic imaging, adenomatosis is similar to hepatic adenoma. Adenomatosis tends to be diffuse and has a higher risk of rupture and malignant transformation. Patients often present with abdominal pain, hepatomegaly, and impaired liver function. Because of its diffuse nature, complete resection often is not possible. Alternatively, hepatic artery embolization and radiofrequency ablation can be used in combination with resection. Occasionally, transplantation is required for definitive treatment.

Imaging

Hepatic adenomas appear variable and nonspecific on US examination, depending on tumor characteristics. Simple adenomas appear hypoechoic, whereas hemorrhagic or necrotic tumors have a mixed echoic pattern. Adenomas with fat components appear hyperechoic. Almost all lesions appear hypervascular.

On CT, adenomas often appear heterogeneous because of their mixed components of fat, hemorrhage, and necrosis (Fig. 6). On portal venous examination or delayed images, they may appear isodense. HAs are contrast enhancing because of their rich vascular supply and often show peripheral enhancement with centripetal progression, indicating the presence of large subcapsular feeding vessels and early draining veins.

On MRI, adenomas also appear heterogeneous, although often hyperintense on both T1- and T2-weighted images. Early contrast enhancement is often seen.

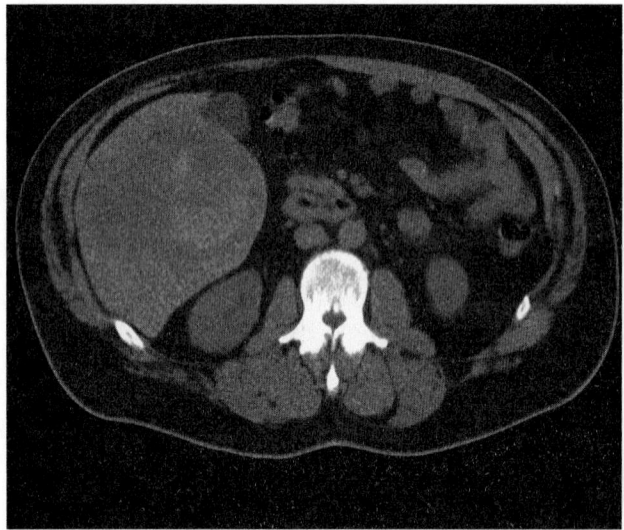

A

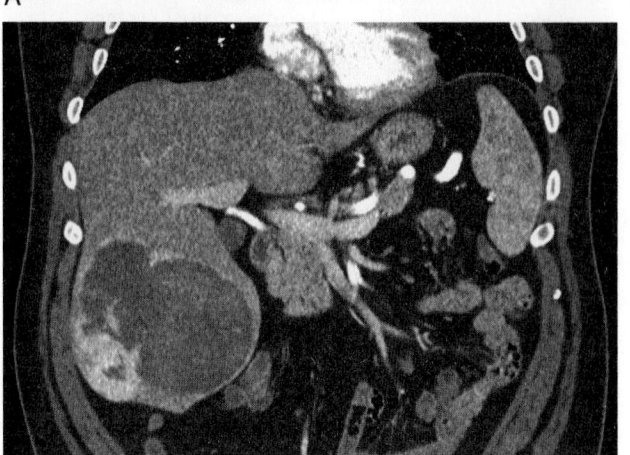

C

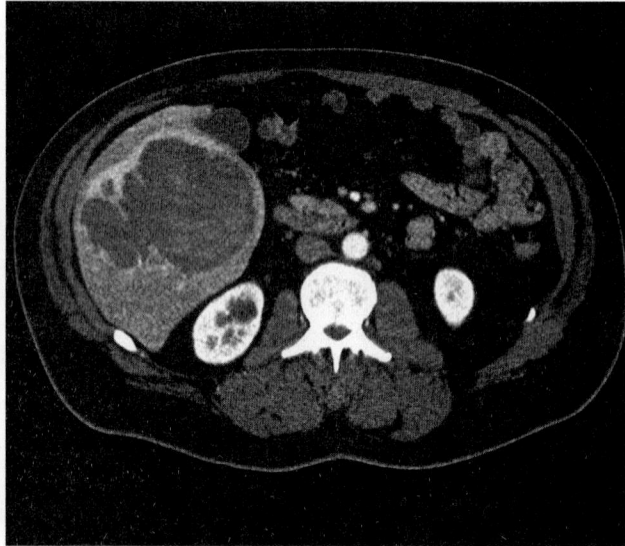

B

Figure 6 Hepatic adenoma with intratumoral rupture. **(A)** Non-contrast-enhanced computed tomography *(CT)* demonstrating a mixed echogenic pattern of ruptured hepatic adenoma. Note hyperintense signal suggestive of recent hemorrhage. **(B)** Contrast-enhanced CT showing peripheral enhancement of adenoma with mixed signal in areas of hemorrhage. **(C)** Coronal reconstruction of contrast-enhanced CT showing pedunculated appearance of adenoma involving segments V and VI.

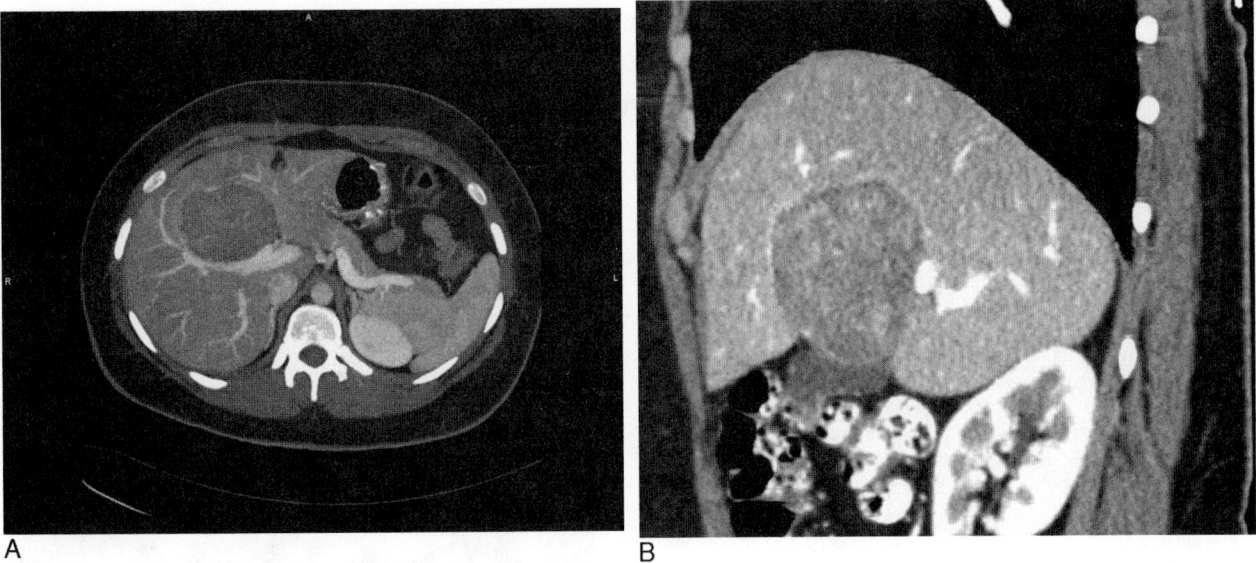

Figure 7 Large central hepatic adenoma. **(A)** Contrast-enhanced computed tomography demonstrating a 7-cm centrally located hepatic adenoma that was associated with right upper quadrant abdominal pain. **(B)** Sagittal image of tumor showing central location of adenoma and proximity to hilar structures. Following resection by central enucleation, the patient had uneventful recovery and has remained asymptomatic for 2.5 years of follow-up.

Management

Hepatic adenomas should generally be resected because of risk of spontaneous rupture, malignant transformation, and difficulty distinguishing these lesions from well-differentiated hepatocellular carcinoma (Fig. 7). However, in small, asymptomatic HA (<4–5 cm), discontinuation of estrogen and follow-up with scheduled imaging and serial alfa-fetoprotein measurements can also be considered. Surgical treatment options range from enucleation, resection, hepatic artery embolization, and transplantation. Enucleation is an effective treatment modality, and surgeons should aim for a 1- to 2-cm margin. Anatomic resection is also satisfactory. For tumors with active hemorrhage, hepatic artery embolization should be undertaken as acute treatment. After a period of recovery, the patient may be taken back for formal resection.

Suggested Readings

Al-Mukhaizeem KA, Rosenberg A, Sherker AH: Nodular regenerative hyperplasia of the liver: an under-recognized cause of portal hypertension in hematological disorders, *Am J Hematol* 75:225, 2004.

Besim H, Karayalcin K, Hamamci O, and others: Scolicidal agents in hydatid cyst surgery, *HPB Surg* 10:347, 1998.

Blumgart LH, Belghiti J, Jarnagin WR, and others, editors: *Surgery of the liver, biliary tract and pancreas* ed 4, Philadelphia, 2006, WB Saunders.

Buetow L, Pantongrag-Brown L, Buck JL, and others: Focal nodular hyperplasia: CT findings with emphasis on multiphasic helical CT in 78 patients, *Radiology* 219:61, 2001.

Chiche L, Dao T, Salame E, and others: Liver adenomatosis; reappraisal, diagnosis, and surgical management: eight new cases and review of the literature, *Ann Surg* 231:74, 2000.

Choi BY, Nguyen MH: The diagnosis and management of benign hepatic tumors, *J Clin Gastroenterol* 39:401, 2005.

Descottes B, Glineur D, Lachachi F, and others: Laparoscopic liver resection of benign liver tumors, *Surg Endosc* 17:23, 2003.

Dimick JB, Cowan JA Jr, Upchurg GR Jr: Hepatic resection in the United States: indications, outcomes, and hospital procedural volumes from a nationally representative database, *Arch Surg* 138:185, 2003.

Fulcher AS, Sterling RK: Hepatic neoplasms: computed tomography and magnetic resonance features, *J Clin Gastroenterol* 34:463, 2002.

Gibbs JF, Litwin AM, Kahlenberg MS: Contemporary management of benign liver tumors, *Surg Clin N Am* 84:463, 2004.

Grazioli L, Federle MP, Brancatelli G, and others: Hepatic adenomas: imaging and pathologic findings, *Radiographics* 21:877, 2001.

Herman P, Costa ML, Machado MA, and others: Management of hepatic hemangiomas: a 14-year experience, *J Gastrointest Surg* 9:853, 2005.

Horton KM, Bluemke DA, Hruban RH, and others: CT and MR Imaging of benign hepatic and biliary tumors, *Radiographics* 19:431, 1999.

Hussain SM, Zondervan PE, IJzermans JN, and others: Benign versus malignant hepatic nodules: MR imaging findings with pathologic correlation, *Radiographics* 22:1023, 2002.

Isozaki T, Numata K, Kiba T, and others: Differential diagnosis of hepatic tumors by using contrast enhancement patterns at US, *Radiology* 229:798, 2003.

Kammula US, Buell JF, Labow DM, and others: Surgical management of benign tumors of the liver, *Int J Gastrointest Cancer* 30:141, 2001.

Karavias DD, Tsamandas AC, Payatakes AH, and others: Simple (non-parasitic) liver cysts: clinical presentation and outcome, *Hepatogastroenterology* 47:1439, 2000.

Kayaalp C: Hydatid cyst of the liver. In Blumgart LH, Belghiti J, Jarnagin WR, editors: *Surgery of the liver, biliary tract and pancreas*, ed 4, Philadelphia, 2006, WB Saunders.

Kehagias D, Moulopoulos L, Antoniou A, and others: Focal nodular hyperplasia: imaging findings, *Eur Radiol* 11:202, 2001.

Kim J, Ahmad SA, Lowy AM, and others: An algorithm for the accurate identification of benign liver lesions, *Am J Surg* 187:274, 2004.

Mathieu D, Kobeiter H, Maison P, and others: Oral contraceptive use and focal nodular hyperplasia of the liver, *Gastroenterology* 118:560, 2000.

Mortele KJ, Ros PR: Cystic focal liver lesions in the adult: differential CT and MR imaging features, *Radiographics* 21:895, 2001.

Quaglia MA: Hepatic tumors in childhood, In Blumgart LH, Belghiti J, Jarnagin WR, editors: *Surgery of the liver, biliary tract and pancreas*, ed 4, Philadelphia, 2006, WB Saunders.

Seven R, Berber E, Mercan S, and others: Laparoscopic treatment of hepatic hydatid cysts, *Surgery* 128:36, 2000.

Tepetes K, Selby R, Webb M, and others: Orthotopic liver transplantation for benign hepatic neoplasms, *Arch Surg* 130:153, 1995.

Terkivata T, de Wilt JH, de Man RA, and others: Indications and long-term outcome of treatment for benign hepatic tumors: a critical appraisal, *Arch Surg* 136:1033, 2001.

Wanless IR: Benign liver tumors, *Clin Liver Dis* 6:513, 2002.

Yoon SS, Charny CK, Fong Y, and others: Diagnosis, management and outcomes of 115 patients with hepatic hemangioma, *J Am Coll Surg* 180:135, 2003.

LIVER HEMANGIOMA

Steven C. Cunningham, MD, and Robert C. Moesinger, MD

INTRODUCTION

Hepatic hemangiomata are congenital vascular malformations. As such, they enlarge by ectasia rather than neoplastic growth. Consistent with this nonneoplastic process, there are no known reports of malignant degeneration of liver hemangiomata. Grossly, these lesions are dark reddish-blue in color, spongy in texture, and well circumscribed with a pseudocapsule composed of adjacent compressed hepatic parenchyma and fibrous tissue. Histologic analysis reveals a matrix of endothelium-lined, blood-filled spaces with fibrous septae.

With an incidence in the general population of up to 7%, hemangiomata are the most common benign liver tumors. Consequently, they are often discovered incidentally during abdominal imaging or operative exploration for other pathology. There are reports of recurrence and enlargement in women who are pregnant or receiving hormone-replacement therapy, but a causal relationship to estrogen has never been proven. The most common age at diagnosis is in the fourth and fifth decades, with a female predominance of approximately 4:1. Multiple hemangiomata occur in a single patient in 20% to 50% of cases, depending on the series.

As described in detail in the following sections, a four-tiered approach to liver hemangiomata can be considered:

1. Given the presence of a mass in the liver, a definitive diagnosis of hemangioma must be made.
2. Given a firm diagnosis of hemangioma in a symptomatic patient, the surgeon must determine whether the hemangioma is indeed the cause of the symptoms.
3. The surgeon and patient must decide whether the symptoms are specific and severe enough to warrant operation.
4. The surgeon must determine the optimal surgical approach and procedure, for example, open versus laparoscopic and enucleation versus anatomic liver resection.

MAKING THE DIAGNOSIS

The diagnosis of liver hemangioma is usually made radiographically. The differential diagnosis of liver masses includes benign and malignant hepatic lesions: hepatic parenchymal lesions, for example, focal nodular hyperplasia, adenoma, regenerative nodule, and hepatocellular carcinoma; biliary parenchymal lesions, for example, biliary cyst, adenoma, and cholangiocarcinoma; mesenchymal lesions, for example, hemangioma, angiomyolipoma, and angiosarcoma; and finally, nonhepatobiliary metastatic lesions (which in North America are more common than primary hepatic malignancies), for example, colorectal carcinoma and other metastatic lesions, particularly of the gastrointestinal tract. Ultrasound (US), computed tomography (CT), and magnetic resonance imaging (MRI) are each individually capable of accurate diagnosis of liver hemangioma, but more than one may be used for confirmation when uncertainty exists.

The sonographic appearance of liver hemangioma is shown in Figure 1. Characteristically, the lesion is echogenic, well circumscribed, and homogeneous. Posterior acoustic enhancement is often seen, and

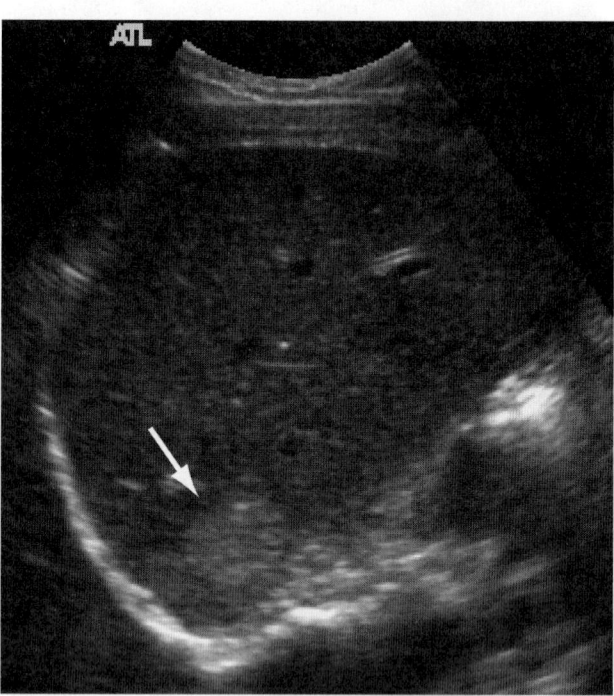

Figure 1 Characteristic transabdominal ultrasound appearance of a liver hemangioma. Arrow points to hemangioma with typical features: hyperechoic, well circumscribed, and homogeneous. *Courtesy Dr. W. Brandt, Department of Radiology, University of Virginia Health System.*

posterior shadowing is generally absent. Some lesions may appear isoechoic or hypoechoic with a hyperechoic rim. A patient with these typical findings and without evidence of malignancy or chronic liver disease requires no further diagnostic maneuvers or follow-up. If, however, the ultrasonic appearance is atypical, for example, a heterogeneous echo pattern, then additional investigations are warranted.

The CT appearance of liver hemangiomata is also characteristic (Fig. 2) and is an appropriate next step if US findings are inconclusive. Without intravenous contrast, hemangiomata are hypodense relative to the liver and well circumscribed. Following intravenous contrast administration, the arterial phase demonstrates peripheral nodular enhancement, which is followed by centripetal filling that becomes homogeneous on delayed images. Small (<2 cm) and large (>5 cm) hemangiomata may lack this pattern, the small lesions because the peripheral nodular pattern is missed and the large lesions because thrombosis or fibrosis may prevent complete opacificaton. Similar to US, CT is sufficient for establishing the diagnosis when the radiographic findings are typical.

When the diagnosis is still in question after US and CT, then MRI may be useful and is, in fact, the first-line imaging modality at some institutions. Although more cumbersome and expensive than US or CT, MRI is accurate (sensitivity and specificity approaching 100%) and particularly useful in characterizing lesions smaller than 2 cm. A typical MRI appearance is low intensity on T1-weighted images, high intensity on T2-weighted images, and, similar to CT, peripheral nodular enhancement after contrast administration (Fig. 3).

If the diagnosis is still in question after MRI or if MRI is not available, then single photon emission computed tomography (SPECT) with technetium-labeled red blood cells may be used. This modality has similar sensitivity and specificity to MRI for hemangioma if the lesion is greater than 3 cm and close to the liver surface.

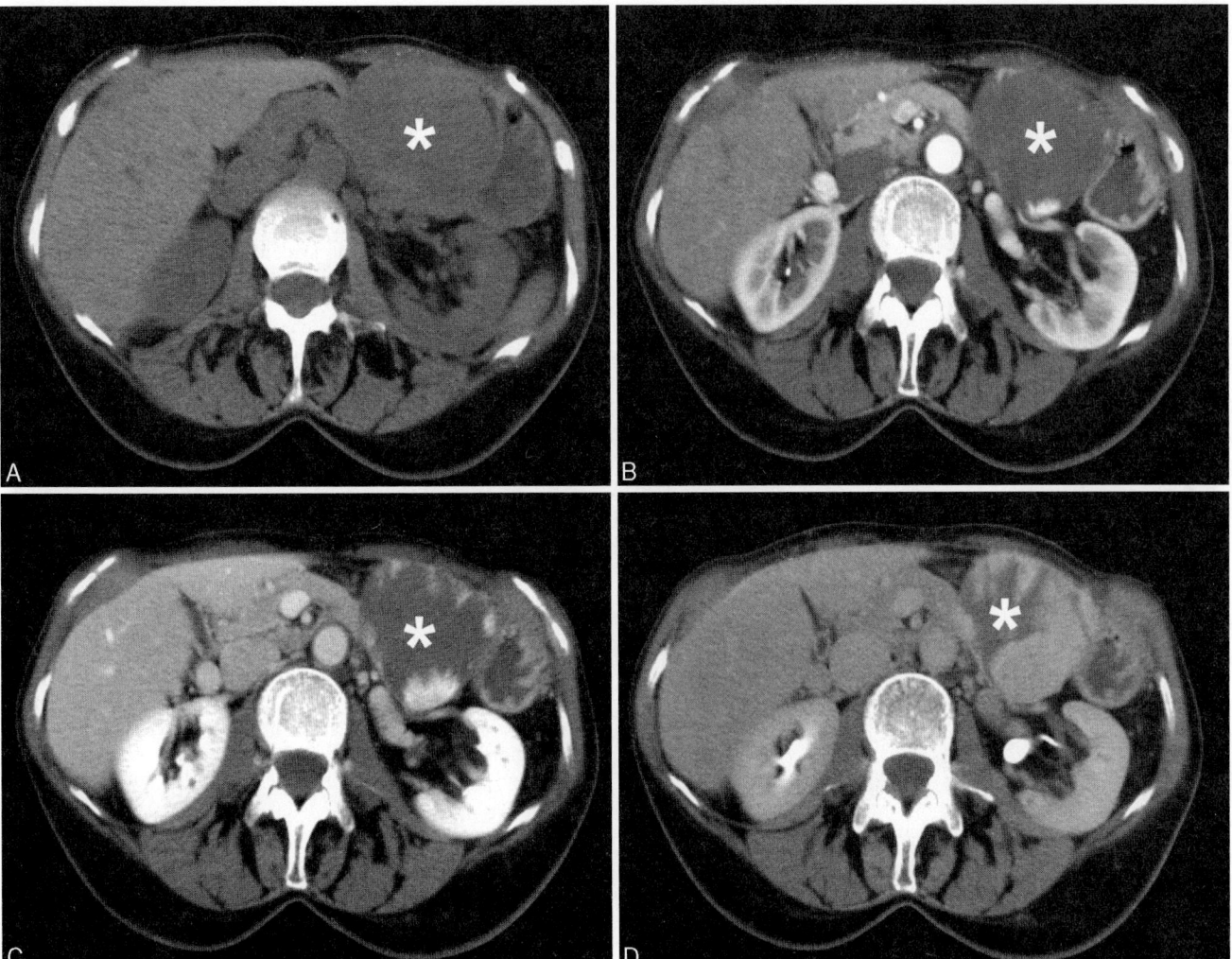

Figure 2 Characteristic computed tomography appearance of a liver hemangioma. Asterisk indicates the center of the hemangioma. **(A)** Well-defined, hypodense mass before intravenous contrast. **(B and C)** Peripheral, nodular enhancement early following administration of contrast. **(D)** Centripetal filling of the hemangioma by contrast on later images. *Courtesy Dr. S. Gay, Department of Radiology, University of Virginia Health System.*

Because liver hemangiomata are nonneoplastic and metabolically quiescent, they are not detected by positron emission tomography. If noninvasive imaging fails to secure the diagnosis, then hepatic angiography or percutaneous biopsy remain diagnostic options. Angiography may demonstrate dilatated and ectatic contrast-filled spaces with retention of contrast on the venous phase. The safety and efficacy of percutaneous fine needle or core biopsy in the diagnosis of liver hemangioma continue to be debated in the literature. Fortunately, the increasing accuracy of other modalities is largely rendering this debate moot.

Although a variety of tumor markers may be measured in patients with liver masses, none is specific or sensitive for liver hemangioma. In fact, the presence of an elevated tumor marker in a patient thought to have a liver hemangioma should cause a reevaluation of the diagnosis.

DETERMINING RELATIONSHIP OF DIAGNOSIS TO SYMPTOMS

The vast majority of liver hemangiomata present at autopsy or not at all. Because the incidence is so high, however, patients with known liver hemangiomata comprise a sizeable group. These are typically patients whose hemangiomata were detected as incidental findings. The vast majority of these patients are managed nonoperatively.

The more challenging patients are those who present with symptoms with evaluation that leads to a diagnosis of liver hemangioma. Unfortunately, symptoms typical of liver hemangioma, for example, pain, discomfort, fullness, and distention of the abdomen; pain in the back, flank, or shoulder; and nausea and vomiting are also entirely nonspecific. Therefore to determine confidently that the presenting symptoms are caused by the hemangioma, other common causes must be ruled out, including esophageal, gastroduodenal, biliary, pancreatic, renal, pulmonary, cardiac, and musculoskeletal causes. At least 50% of patients with a possible symptomatic liver hemangioma have another cause of their symptoms, and approximately 75% of the remaining patients have spontaneous resolution of symptoms.

Larger tumors are more likely to be symptomatic, and it is known that peripheral lesions stretching the liver capsule may cause well-localized somatic pain. It is more difficult to reconcile similar symptoms with a deep lesion not stretching the liver capsule, and in these cases well-localized somatic pain should not be attributed to a deep hemangioma. However, given that the parenchyma and the vessels within the parenchyma are innervated with nociceptive afferent

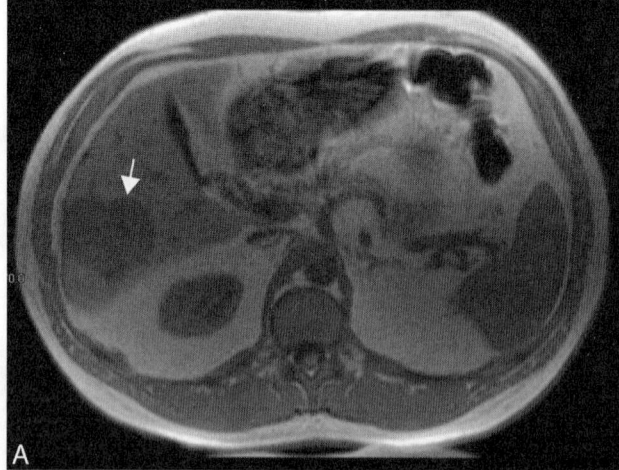

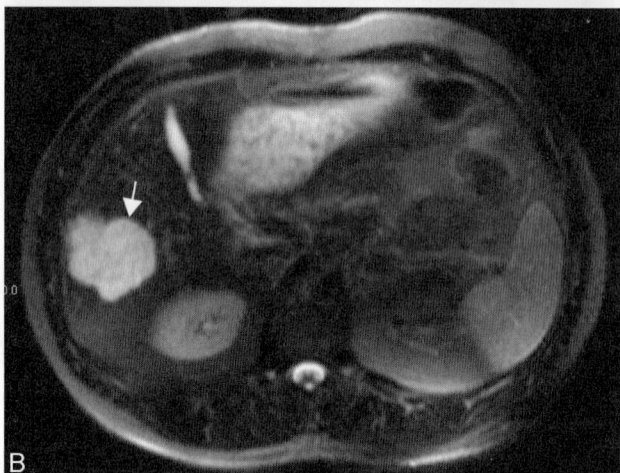

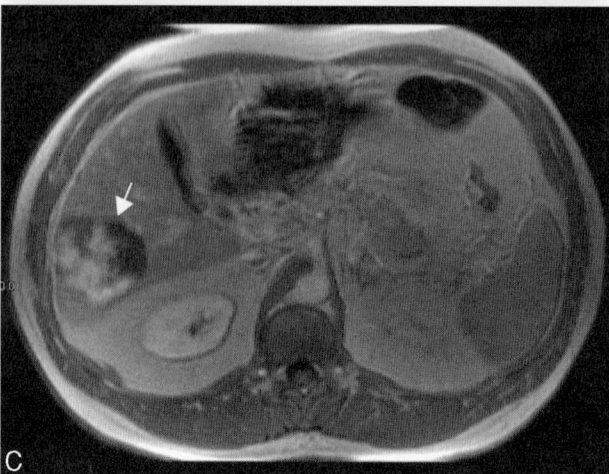

Figure 3 Characteristic transabdominal magnetic resonance image appearance of a liver hemangioma. Arrow points to hemangioma with typical features. **(A)** Well-defined lesion with low signal intensity on T1-weighting. **(B)** High signal intensity on T2-weighting. **(C)** Peripheral, nodular enhancement after gadolinium contrast administration. *Courtesy Dr. E. DeLange, Department of Radiology, University of Virginia Health System.*

fibers and that these tumors enlarge by ectatic dilatation and stretching of vessels, even deep lesions may be a source of pain despite being remote from the liver capsule. This pain, however, would not typically be somatic but rather visceral; poorly localized; and, as with other foregut structures, referred to the central epigastrium.

INDICATIONS FOR OPERATION

There are three main indications for operation: severe symptoms caused by the hemangioma, diagnostic uncertainty, and intraperitoneal hemorrhage. The most common is severe symptoms. Having determined that the hemangioma is causing symptoms, the surgeon and the patient must decide whether the symptoms are severe enough to warrant operation. This difficult decision is complicated by the knowledge that some patients—up to 36% in one large series—may have persistent symptoms after surgical treatment, even when the symptoms were attributed with certainty to the hemangioma. When patients with pain and a liver hemangioma are treated with analgesics and observation, the majority experience significant resolution of symptoms, suggesting that for symptoms to be an indication for operation, they need be not only severe but also persistent and refractory to nonoperative management.

Diagnostic uncertainty is an important indication for operation if all other noninvasive and invasive diagnostic attempts have been unsuccessful, particularly in a patient with historical or current evidence of malignancy. This may be accomplished by laparotomy or laparoscopy. In many cases, the diagnosis can be made by visual appearance alone, but intraoperative biopsy may be necessary.

Spontaneous rupture of a liver hemangioma is a rare event, but a patient presenting with hypotension and sudden severe abdominal pain and who is found to have intraperitoneal hemorrhage and a liver lesion does require emergent intervention. In most cases, however, the best option is to resuscitate the patient, embolize the tumor, and then reevaluate for elective resection. Prophylactic resection solely to prevent rupture is not indicated for enlarging hemangiomata because no correlation between size changes and symptoms or complications is evident from longitudinal studies.

SURGICAL APPROACH AND PROCEDURE

Liver hemangiomata may be approached either via laparoscopy or laparotomy. Most relevant procedures, including tumor removal and biopsy, have been performed and reported using the laparoscopic approach. Lesions especially amenable to laparoscopic approach are those that are small, superficial, and in Couinaud segments II and III. Worldwide, several hundred laparoscopic liver resections and enucleations of benign liver tumors in all segments except I and VII have been reported.

Removal of a liver hemangioma may be performed by enucleation, nonanatomic liver resection or anatomic liver resection. In experienced hands, resections may be performed with negligible mortality and low morbidity. Compared with liver resection, enucleation is preferred because it is associated with lower morbidity and preservation of hepatic parenchyma. These advantages are due to the presence of the pseudocapsule, which contains few vessels and few, if any, bile ducts. Some authors recommend temporary inflow occlusion for many enucleations, and this decision can be made on a case-by-case basis. In any case, enucleation is begun by incising Glisson's capsule and dissecting into the plane of the pseudocapsule, guided by intraoperative US as needed. The ultrasonic dissector, the hydrodissector, or blunt dissection may then be used to separate the hemangioma from the surrounding liver parenchyma along the plane of the pseudocapsule. The advantage of inflow occlusion is the resultant decompression of the hemangioma that facilitates dissection. Crossing vessels are ligated as encountered. After the mass is enucleated, inflow is restored and hemostasis is imposed on cut surfaces using manual compression, standard electrocautery, argon beam cautery, or sutures.

Resection of liver hemangiomata may be performed anatomically or nonanatomically (Fig. 4). The ease of either type of resection and the attendant morbidity depend primarily on the

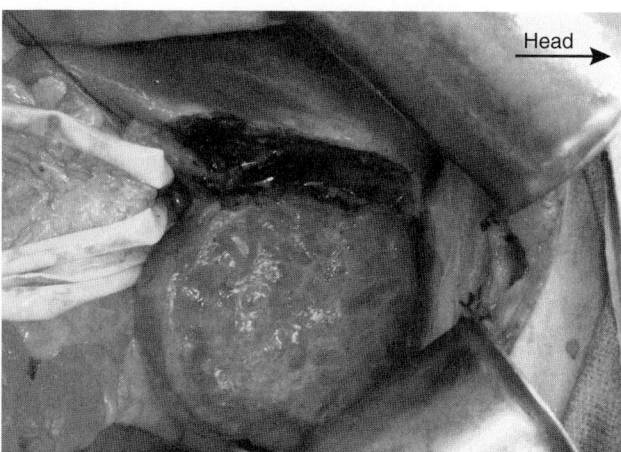

Figure 4 Intraoperative photograph. The patient's head is to the right. A large hemangioma in segments II, III, and IV is being enucleated. *Courtesy Richard Schulick, MD, Department of Surgery, Johns Hopkins Hospital.* **(See color Insert Figure 23.)**

tumor's location and size. Hemangiomata that are small, superficial, pedunculated, or in segments II or III are most easily removed, often by nonanatomic resection. However, resection of lesions that are large or deep within the liver can be associated with significant morbidity. In any case, standard operative principles of liver resection apply here as to other liver resections. Choice of abdominal incision, suction devices, intraoperative imaging, and method of dividing hepatic parenchyma are determined on an individual basis, depending on tumor characteristics and surgeon preference. Because these lesions are composed almost entirely of ectatic blood vessels, inflow occlusion results in substantial decompression, which facilitates tumor manipulation. Orthotopic liver transplantation and ex vivo resection with reimplantation of the liver also have been used to treat technically unresectable, large hemangiomata, but these are rather extraordinary undertakings.

NONOPERATIVE TREATMENT

Alternatives to tumor removal include selective hepatic embolization and local irradiation. The use of corticosteroids is of historical interest only. In some patients who cannot or do not wish to undergo tumor removal, alternative treatments may result in relief of symptoms. However, long-term, high-quality data supporting their use are lacking.

SPECIAL CIRCUMSTANCES

In the past, patients with liver hemangioma have been advised not to become pregnant lest the tumor enlarge or rupture. However, there is currently insufficient evidence to support such a recommendation. In fact, the overall risk of rupture is extremely small, and there are reports of women with giant hemangiomata carrying pregnancies to full term without complications.

Pediatric liver hemangioma is in many respects a different disease. It occurs predominantly in infants younger than 6 months old, with no gender predominance. Unlike the adult tumors, the pediatric hemangioma is more often characterized by a period of rapid growth followed by involution, multicentricity, and involvement of other organs, for example, skin, lung, and bone. Finally, the likelihood of some malignancies, especially hemangioendothelioma, is greater in children than in adults.

Some unusual complications deserve special mention. Budd–Chiari syndrome has been reported to occur secondary to caval compression and has at times been treated with transplantation. Kasabach–Merritt syndrome is characterized by a consumptive coagulopathy, thrombocytopenia, microangiopathic hemolytic anemia, and resultant ecchymoses and purpura. The association of this disorder with liver hemangioma has been reported but is rare. Finally, inflammatory hemangioma or hemangioma with systemic inflammatory response has been rarely described. These patients have hemangioma, usually large, and systemic symptoms including fever, night sweats, and malaise. Biochemical evidence of systemic inflammation can include elevated erythrocyte sedimentation rates, anemia, thrombocytosis, elevated fibrinogen, and normal liver function tests. Necrosis within the hemangioma has been proposed as an etiology. In these cases, resection has provided relief of symptoms.

SUMMARY

The most common primary tumor of the liver, hemangioma poses several challenges to the surgeon: making the diagnosis, establishing its relation or lack thereof to symptoms, determining indications for operation, and choosing the correct procedure. Diagnosis may be made on the basis of characteristic US, CT, or MRI findings, with uncommon need for other modalities. After diagnosis, the asymptomatic hemangioma requires no further treatment or follow-up, regardless of size or change thereof. Symptomatic patients may benefit from analgesics and supportive care and often experience resolution of symptoms. Severe, refractory symptoms are the most common indication for treatment. Although nonresective therapies have been reported, tumor removal, optimally via enucleation, is safe and effective at treating severe, refractory symptoms.

Suggested Readings

Borzellino G, Ruzzenente A, Minicozzi A-M, and others: Laparoscopic hepatic resection, *Surg Endosc* 20:787, 2006.

Herman P, Costa ML, Machado MA, and others: Management of hepatic hemangiomas: a 14-year experience, *J Gastrointest Surg* 9:853, 2005.

Özden I, Emre A, Alper A, and others: Long-term results of surgery for liver hemangiomas, *Arch Surg* 135:978, 2000.

Terkivatan T, de Wilt JH, de Man RA, and others: Indications and long-term outcome of treatment for benign hepatic tumors, *Arch Surg* 136:1033, 2001.

Yoon SS, Charny CK, Fong Y, and others: Diagnosis, management, and outcomes of 115 patients with hepatic hemangioma, *J Am Coll Surg* 197:392, 2003.

MALIGNANT LIVER TUMORS

Keith D. Gray, MD, Dario Ribero, MD, and
Jean-Nicolas Vauthey, MD

Because the surgical management of liver metastases is discussed in separate chapters, herein we focus on hepatocellular carcinoma (HCC), the fibrolamellar variant of HCC and intrahepatic cholangiocarcinoma (I-CCA). HCC is the most common primary liver cancer worldwide, affecting more than 600,000 people annually. Although less prevalent in the United States, the incidence is steadily increasing as a result of the spread of hepatitis C virus infection, and more than 16,000 patients are expected to die from HCC in 2007. In the majority of patients, HCC develops in a background of hepatitis B- and C-induced fibrosis or cirrhosis.

Because primary medical therapy has not offered durable results, surgical resection offers the only prospect for cure in patients with HCC, with 5-year survival rates ranging from 20% to 60%. Although the majority of patients with primary liver cancer are not surgical candidates because of the burden of hepatic tumor, the presence of extrahepatic spread, or the extent of underlying liver disease, liver resections are increasingly performed because of better perioperative care and improved imaging and surgical techniques. In selected patients with small HCCs and impaired liver function, orthotopic liver transplantation (OLT) represents the only surgical option. However, given the shortage of organs and restricted indications for OLT, liver resection is widely considered the mainstay of curative therapy in patients with preserved hepatic reserve.

PREOPERATIVE ASSESSMENT

As with any surgical procedure for neoplasm, optimal outcomes after hepatic resection are contingent on identifying appropriate candidates. The assessment of tumor extent is the essential step for determining resectability and the appropriate type of surgical resection. Along with tumor staging, meticulous preoperative evaluation of general medical fitness, underlying liver function, and size of the anticipated future liver remnant (FLR) is also critical to ensure suitable patient selection. Patient age alone should not be considered a contraindication for resection. However, in elderly patients, comorbid illnesses are prevalent and hidden medical diseases are not uncommon. Recently it has been reported that the presence of comorbidities was one of two independent factors predictive of postoperative mortality after extended hepatectomy. In general, patients with American Society of Anesthesiology (ASA) scores greater than 1 represent a population at greater risk for postoperative complications and death. The surgical risk becomes unacceptably high in patients with congestive heart failure, severe chronic obstructive pulmonary disease, and chronic renal failure.

At the University of Texas M.D. Anderson Cancer Center, each patient is first staged with a triple-phase helical computed tomography (CT) of the thorax and the abdomen. The enhancement patterns during the various phases of contrast circulation in the liver are used to characterize hepatic lesions. Hypervascular tumors, such as HCC or metastatic neuroendocrine tumors, are hyperdense during the early arterial phase, whereas hypovascular tumors, such as I-CCA and metastatic adenocarcinoma, are detected during the portal phase.

Magnetic resonance imaging (MRI) may be advantageous when contrast agents are contraindicated, better lesion characterization is necessary, or the anatomic relationship between tumor and major vascular or biliary structures requires further delineation. Because MRI is unreliable in detecting extrahepatic disease in the chest and peritoneum, its role as a primary imaging modality is limited, especially in patients with I-CCA who often present with advanced disease as a result of peritoneal seeding.

Evaluation of Tumor Extent

Because mortality rates after partial hepatectomy have fallen to near zero in recent years, many centers worldwide have expanded resection eligibility criteria to include tumors once considered unresectable: large HCCs, multinodular HCCs, and HCCs with portal vein or hepatic vein involvement. Concurrently, the surgical treatment of intrahepatic recurrence has become more frequent.

In Western countries, because of the lack of an effective HCC screening program, up to 50% of HCC is diagnosed at an advanced stage, with tumor diameters sometimes exceeding 10 cm. Despite the technical problems with liver mobilization and hepatic vein access and control encountered with large tumors, liver resection for large HCCs has been shown to be safe and effective. In a recent study, we reported 30-day mortality and 5-year survival rates of 5% and 27%, respectively, in 300 patients who underwent partial hepatectomy for HCCs larger than 10 cm. Because cadaveric OLT and radiofrequency ablation (RFA) are not indicated, surgical resection remains the option for cure of large HCCs.

Multinodular HCCs (more than 3 nodules or more than 1 nodule exceeding 3 cm in diameter) have been considered in some centers unsuitable for resection. However, an analysis of outcomes after resection in 380 patients with multinodular HCC showed a mortality rate of 2.4% and a 5-year survival rate of 39%. Surgical resection for these patients often requires major resection because of substantial tumor volume. Hence, when liver function permits and clearance of all tumor nodules is possible, en bloc extended hepatectomy, multiple bilobar resections, or hepatectomy plus effective local ablative therapy for treatment of contralateral nodules should be considered for patients with bilobar HCC.

HCCs with major portal or hepatic vein involvement represent a technical and oncologic challenge. Although these tumors are aggressive and often multifocal, hepatic resection for such tumors seems to be justified. We recently showed a survival benefit in 102 patients undergoing hepatic resection for HCC with major portal vein branch or hepatic vein involvement, with a 23% 5-year survival rate in those without cirrhosis. Another series from the Eastern countries recently reported a median survival of 3.4 years and 5-year survival of 42% in 23 patients with portal vein involvement, treated with partial hepatectomy.

Intrahepatic tumor recurrence (de novo HCC or intrahepatic metastases) represents the most common cause of treatment failure after curative liver resection, with a cumulative 5-year recurrence rate of 70% to 100%. Recurrence in the liver remnant occurs as a result of vascular invasion leading to microsatellite tumors within the liver ("early recurrence"), or second primaries associated with field effect from hepatitis and cirrhosis ("late recurrence"). From 10% to 31% of the patients can be treated with a second hepatectomy. Repeat hepatic resection has been proven to be a safe and worthwhile procedure, with mortality and 5-year survival rates of 0% to 8% and 50% to 69%, respectively.

Evaluation of Hepatic Function

In the Western countries, the Child-Pugh score has been used traditionally to estimate hepatic functional reserve. Usually only patients with Child-Pugh A are considered good candidates for hepatectomy, whereas death rates in patients with Child-Pugh C approach 50%. However, the Child-Pugh classification is a crude measurement and is prone to underestimate the surgical risk associated with undiagnosed or latent portal hypertension. Portal hypertension is present if the portal venous pressure is greater than 10 mm Hg and puts a cirrhotic patient undergoing liver resection at risk of major postoperative complications, such as variceal bleeding, endotoxemia, and hepatic decompensation. Thus clinical or radiologic evidence of portal hypertension, including splenomegaly, abdominal collaterals, thrombocytopenia (platelets $< 100,000/mm^3$), and esophagogastric varices are relative contraindications for resection. Additionally, as elevated liver function tests may infer active hepatitis, we consider patients with an abnormal bilirubin level (>1 mg/dL), an elevated aspartate aminotransferase level (>100 IU/L), or alanine aminotransferase level at least twice normal to be poor candidates for major hepatic resection.

Several hepatobiliary units, mostly in Eastern countries, have used more sophisticated quantitative liver function tests, such as indocyanine green (ICG) clearance, galactose elimination capacity, and aminopyrine clearance to predict the risk of postoperative liver failure. The most widely used and validated metabolic assessment is the ICG clearance test. Patient selection by ICG clearance test has significantly reduced the mortality rate in some centers to zero. In patients with cirrhosis, an ICG retention rate at 15 minutes (ICGR15) of ≤10% is considered the upper limit for safe resection of four or more segments of the liver because above this limit mortality rates rise threefold.

Evaluation of Future Liver Remnant Volume

Although useful for limited hepatic resections, ICG clearance and other hepatic reserve tests only estimate overall hepatic function but do not evaluate the functional reserve of the remnant liver necessary after major resection. Therefore in patients selected for major hepatectomies, attention has also focused on the future liver remnant (FLR) volume. Three-dimensional CT volumetry provides a thorough method for preoperatively measuring the FLR and is acquired by outlining hepatic segmental contours and calculating the volumes from surface measurement from each slice. Although direct measurement of the total liver volume (TLV) is feasible by CT volumetry, it has been suggested not to be relevant for surgical planning. A more accurate method uses the estimated TLV, which is calculated using a formula that relies on the linear correlation between TLV and body surface area (BSA): $TLV (cm^3) = -794.41 + 1,267.28 \times BSA (m^2)$. The ratio of the CT measured FLR volume to calculated TLV is defined as the "standardized FLR."

Using the standardized FLR measurement, a correlation between the anticipated liver remnant and operative outcome has been established. In 48 patients without chronic liver disease undergoing extended hepatectomy with and without preoperative portal vein embolization (PVE), we demonstrated significantly increased postoperative complication rates in patients with FLR volume less than 20% of the estimated TLV. Using a different BSA-based standardized method of remnant liver calculation in patients with chronic liver disease, Shirabe and colleagues reported that all deaths from liver failure after hepatectomy occurred in patients with an FLR volume less than 300 ml/m² (Fig. 1). Small liver remnant size has been associated with increases in portal pressure and flow, endothelial, and Kupffer cell injury and release of proinflammatory cytokines. Collectively these factors result in hepatocellular injury and impaired regeneration. Surrogate measures of the overall postoperative course (hospital stay) and intensive care unit stay also appear to be increased as liver remnant size decreases. Thus a small FLR seems strongly correlated with an increase in the morbidity and mortality of hepatic resection. In general, an FLR of 20% appears to be the minimum safe volume necessary following extended

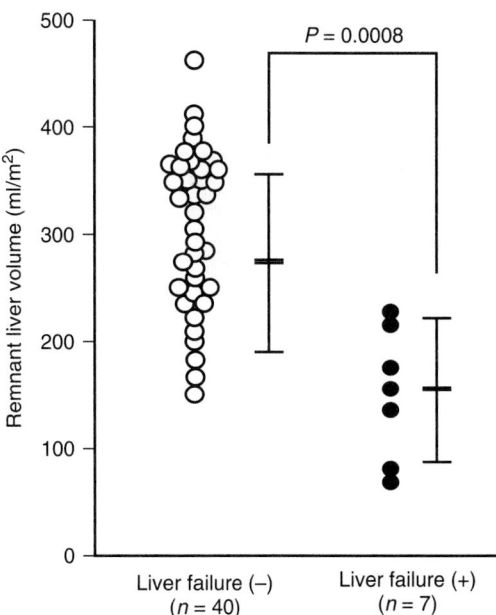

Figure 1 Small liver volume correlates with poor outcomes in patients with chronic liver disease. In this study, all deaths from liver failure occurred in patients with standardized liver remnants less than 300 ml/m² (mean 163 = 63 ml/m²). *From Shirabe K, Shimanda M, Gion T, and others: J Am Coll Surg 188:304, 1999. Used with permission.*

hepatic resection in patients with normal underlying liver and 40% in patients with chronic liver disease.

When the FLR is inadequate, portal vein embolizatoin (PVE) can be safely used to prime hypertrophy of the FLR and offer potentially curative hepatectomy to a subset of patients not previously considered optimal surgical candidates (Fig. 2). Under fluoroscopic guidance, PVE usually involves percutaneous cannulation of the ipsilateral portal vein and embolization of the entire portal vein tree to be resected using microparticles and microcoils (Fig. 3). The resultant redirection of portal flow to the FLR increases both volume and function of the nonembolized segments, as indicated by increased biliary excretion, increased technetium-99m-galactosyl human serum albumin uptake and improvement in postoperative liver function tests. Additionally, in patients with chronic liver disease, the appropriate use of PVE significantly decreases the number and severity of complications, the incidence of postoperative hepatic insufficiency, and death following major hepatic resection. The magnitude and rate of volume increase after PVE are less in patients with chronic liver disease compared with those with normal underlying liver. The combination of transarterial chemoembolization (TACE) of the tumor followed by PVE within 2 weeks may optimize the outcome of some patients with HCC and cirrhosis requiring major resection.

SURGICAL TECHNIQUES

Anatomic Resection

HCC has a high propensity to invade the portal and hepatic veins; thus the spread of HCC is essentially through the bloodstream—first via the portal vein to cause intrahepatic metastasis and later to extrahepatic organs such as the lungs, bone, and adrenal glands. On this basis, the standard surgical approach is an anatomic resection, which involves systematic removal of a hepatic segment confined by tumor-bearing portal tributaries that might contain portal metastases or daughter micronodules. Ultrasonography has

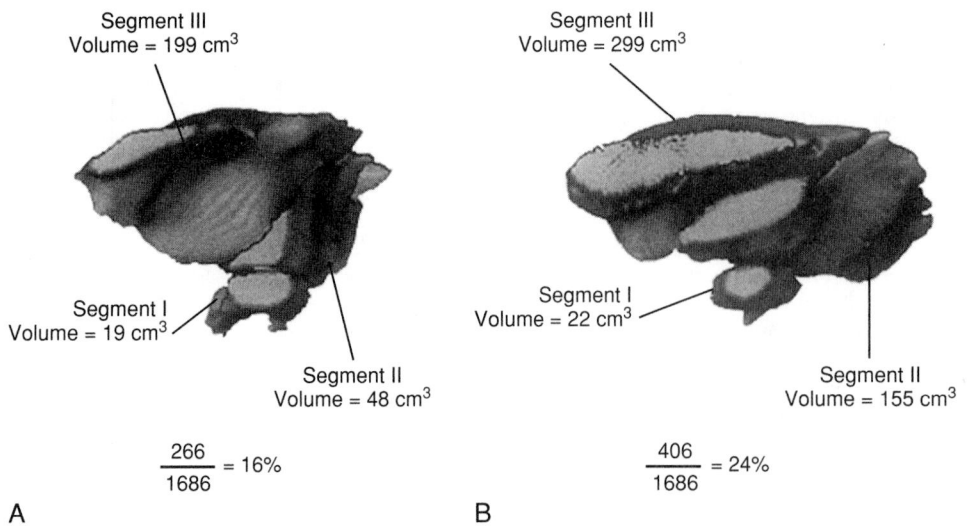

Segment III
Volume = 199 cm^3

Segment I
Volume = 19 cm^3

Segment II
Volume = 48 cm^3

Segment III
Volume = 299 cm^3

Segment I
Volume = 22 cm^3

Segment II
Volume = 155 cm^3

$$\frac{266}{1686} = 16\%$$

$$\frac{406}{1686} = 24\%$$

A

B

Figure 2 Hypertrophy of the future liver remnant (FLR) after portal vein embolization as determined by three-dimensional reconstruction of computed tomographic images. **(A)** Preembolization reconstruction with calculated volumes. **(B)** Postembolization reconstruction with calculated volumes showing resultant hypertrophy of the FLR. *From Vauthey JN, Chaoui A, Do KA, and others: Surgery 127:512, 2000. Used with permission.*

contributed significantly to the development of segment-oriented anatomic resection. Intraoperative ultrasound (IOUS) detects new lesions in up to 30% of cases, although only approximately 25% of these lesions turn out to be malignant.

The differential diagnosis (regenerative nodules, dysplastic nodules, or early HCCs) of such new lesions may be difficult, and intraoperative biopsy seems to be inadequate to solve this problem because of the lack of specific features.

Resection of Large Right-Lobe Tumors

Surgical resection of a large right-lobe tumor presents a challenging situation. With the conventional technique for hepatectomy, mobilization of the right lobe from the retroperitoneum and anterior surface of the inferior vena cava (IVC) may be difficult because of the tumor volume and adhesion to the diaphragm. To avoid these problems, the anterior approach can be used. After hilar control of the vascular inflow is achieved, the parenchyma is transected from the anterior surface of the liver down to the anterior surface of the IVC, without prior mobilization of the right lobe. After control of all venous tributaries to the IVC is achieved, including the right hepatic vein, the right lobe is detached from the diaphragm. In patients with large right-lobe HCCs, the anterior approach resulted in less intraoperative blood loss, lower transfusion requirements, a lower in-hospital death rate, and significantly better overall and disease-free survival compared with the conventional approach.

Because it may be difficult to control bleeding in the deeper parenchymal plane using this method, a technique of hanging the liver over an umbilical tape passed between the anterior surface of the IVC and the liver parenchyma ("liver-hanging maneuver") has been proposed. After dissection of the space between the right and middle hepatic veins and the anterior plane of the IVC, a vascular clamp is gently pushed cranially from below to blindly complete the dissection of the middle plane along the IVC. When the clamp appears between the right and middle hepatic veins, the tape is seized and passed around the hepatic parenchyma. The parenchymal dissection is facilitated by upward traction on the tape, allowing the surgeon to follow a direct plane and facilitating exposure and hemostasis of the posterior parenchymal plane in front of the IVC.

Prevention and Control of Bleeding

Many studies have shown that intraoperative blood loss and transfusion requirements are independent predictors of major morbidity and death from surgery. The Pringle maneuver (e.g., portal triad clamping) is effective in reducing blood loss at the time of hepatic transection. In patients with chronic liver disease, intermittent Pringle maneuver—that is, 15 minutes of inflow occlusion followed by 5 minutes of liver revascularization—has been demonstrated to be safer than continuous inflow occlusion and should be considered the technique of choice. However, the Pringle maneuver does not prevent back-bleeding from the hepatic veins. A direct association

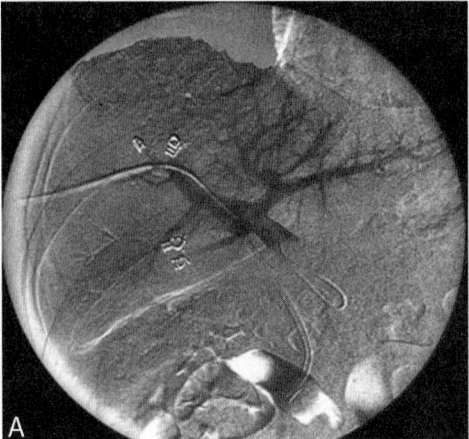
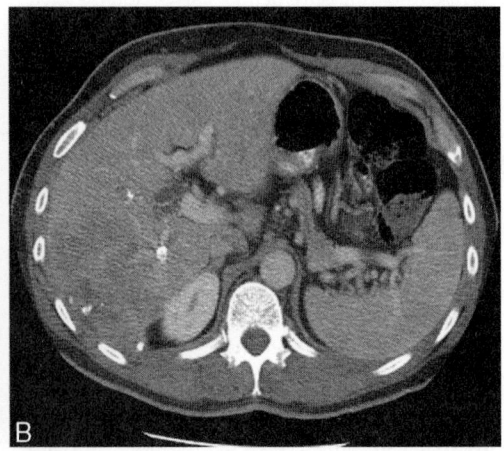

Figure 3   Transhepatic ipsilateral right portal vein embolization. Postprocedural portogram **(A)** and computed tomography scan show coils occluding the anterior and posterior branches of the right portal vein **(B)**. *From Ribero D, Abdalla EK, Thomas MB, and others: Expert Rev Anticancer Ther 6:567, 2006. Used with permission.*

has been demonstrated between mean caval pressure and blood loss. As hepatic vein pressure directly reflects the caval pressure, we maintain a low central venous pressure (<5 mm Hg) with minimal acceptable urine output (0.5 mg/kg/hr) in patients, until the parenchymal transection is completed.

Several parenchymal dissection techniques have been developed to minimize blood loss and expedite hepatic resection. Advances in instrumentation, such as development of the ultrasonic aspirator, jet cutter, argon beam coagulator, and saline-linked cautery, have all been purported to improve surgical technique. We recently combined saline-linked cautery with ultrasonic dissection, which allows a clear delineation of the vascular and biliary anatomy within the transection plane. This resulted in a significant decrease in total operative time and blood loss. The use of saline-linked cautery to coagulate small vessels minimized the need for suture control of intraparenchymal vessels and permitted rapid transection of the liver. This is of utmost importance because a faster parenchymal phase may reduce the time of the Pringle maneuver and thus may reduce ischemic injury of the liver (Fig. 4).

STAGING AND OUTCOMES AFTER RESECTION

Several studies from Asia, Europe, and North America have reported divergent outcomes and predictors of survival after resection in patients with HCC, resulting in a number of classification systems. Most of these staging systems (the Okuda staging system, the Cancer of the Liver Italian Program [CLIP] score, the Japan Integrated Staging [JIS] score, and the Barcelona Clinic Liver Cancer [BCLC] scoring classification) are "clinical" staging systems based on clinicoradiographic features, rather than pathologic findings, making them more applicable for patients with advanced disease.

Pathologic staging systems such as the American Joint Committee on Cancer (AJCC)/International Union Against Cancer (UICC) have been used traditionally for accurate prognostic assessment after resection. The AJCC/UICC staging system uses a tumor-node-metastasis (TNM) classification scheme to predict

survival after resection. Recently the International Cooperative Study Group for HCC reviewed the data from 557 patients who had undergone resection of HCC in centers in the United States, Europe, and Asia. Using multivariate analysis, microvascular invasion, invasion of a main portal or hepatic vein branch, severe fibrosis/cirrhosis, tumor number, and tumor size greater than 5 cm were found to be independent predictors of survival. On the basis of these data, a simplified AJCC/UICC TNM staging system was proposed, grouping three T-stage subgroups of patients with similar survival after stratification according to the prognostic factors. Vascular invasion was the major predictor of outcome after resection. Interestingly, in patients with a single tumor without vascular invasion, tumor size had no effect on survival irrespective of how tumor size was dichotomized (i.e., 2, 3, 4, 5, or 10 cm), whereas tumor size (>5 cm) had a significant effect on survival in patients with multiple tumors. This revised staging system was subsequently adopted in the new sixth edition of the AJCC/UICC TNM staging manual (Table 1).

Another important feature in the report from the International Cooperative Study Group was the recognition of the impact of the underling liver function on survival. The investigators found that the presence of severe fibrosis/cirrhosis was significantly associated with a worse 5-year survival, regardless of T-stage classification (Table 2). The strong effect of fibrosis/cirrhosis on survival may provide an explanation for the absence of overall survival differences among centers in the United States, Europe, and Japan, despite the difference in tumor stage at presentation. Therefore the AJCC/UICC incorporated into the new TNM (T = primary tumor; N = regional lymph nodes; M = distant metastasis) system the provision of a separate reporting of fibrosis in every resected case of HCC using the fibrosis classification proposed by Ishak (Ishak 0–2 represents no or minimal fibrosis, Ishak 3–4 incomplete bridging fibrosis, and Ishak 5–6 complete fibrosis and nodules). Patients with severe fibrosis/cirrhosis (Ishak score of 5–6) are staged as F1, whereas those patients with no or moderate fibrosis (Ishak score 0–4) are staged as F0. Although the impact of fibrosis/cirrhosis in the nontumorous liver on recurrence and long-term survival after resection of HCC is controversial, several recent studies have documented an association

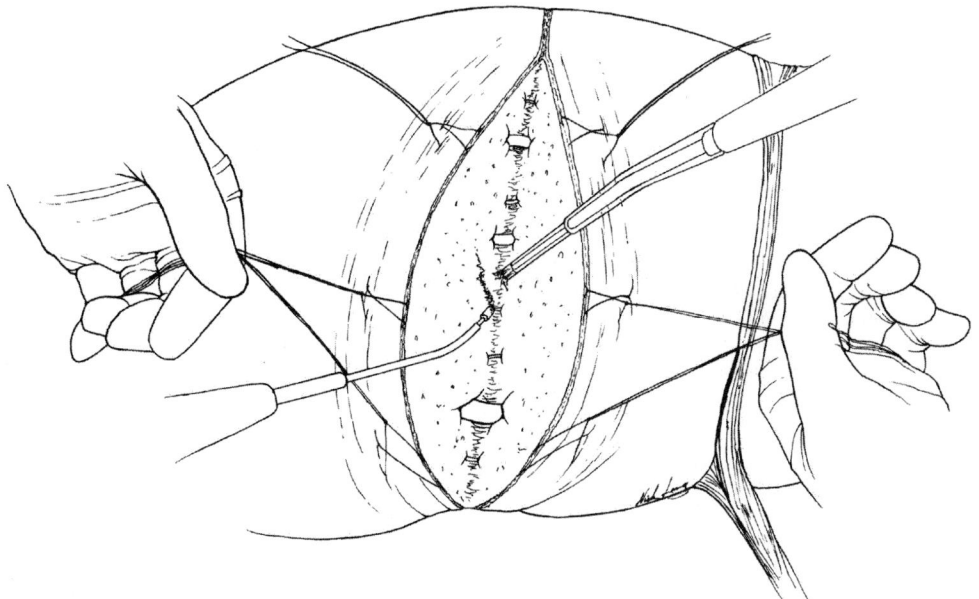

Secondary surgeon

Primary surgeon

Figure 4 Two-surgeon technique for hepatic parenchymal transection. Using the ultrasonic dissection device, the primary surgeon directs the dissection from the patient's left side. Simultaneously, the secondary surgeon operates the saline-linked cautery device from the patient's right side. Traction on 4-0 polypropylene stay sutures is used to expose the deepening transection plane. *From Aloia TA, Zorzi D, Abdalla EK, and others: Ann Surg 242:172, 2005. Used with permission.*

Table 1: American Joint Committee on Cancer/International Union Against Cancer 6th Edition Tumor-Node-Metastasis, Histologic Grade, and Fibrosis Scheme for Hepatocellular Carcinoma

Primary Tumor (T)

T1	Solitary tumor without vascular invasion
T2	Solitary tumor with vascular invasion or multiple tumors none more than 5 cm
T3	Multiple tumors more than 5 cm *or* tumor involving a major branch of the portal or hepatic vein(s)
T4	Tumor(s) with direct invasion of adjacent organs other than the gallbladder or with perforation of visceral peritoneum

Regional Lymph Nodes (N)

N0	No regional lymph node metastasis
N1	Regional lymph node metastasis

Distant Metastasis (M)

M0	No distant metastasis
M1	Distant metastasis

Stage Grouping

Stage I	T1	N0	M0
Stage II	T2	N0	M0
Stage IIIA	T3	N0	M0
Stage IIIB	T4	N0	M0
Stage IIIC	Any T	N1	M0
Stage IV	Any T	Any N	M1

Histologic Grade (G)

G1	Well differentiated
G2	Moderately differentiated
G3	Poorly differentiated
G4	Undifferentiated

Fibrosis Score (F)

F0	Fibrosis score 0–4 (no fibrosis to moderate fibrosis)
F1	Fibrosis score 5–6 (severe fibrosis to cirrhosis)

Adapted from Liver (including intrahepatic bile ducts). In Greene FL, Page DL, Fleming ID, and others, editors: American Joint Committee on Cancer Staging Manual, ed. 6. New York, 2002, Springer-Verlag, 131.

Table 2: Presence of Fibrosis Leads to Worse Prognosis for Each T Category

Group	Fibrosis	5-Year Survival (%)	p Value
T1-Solitary without vascular invasion	F0	64	.01
	F1	49	
T2-Solitary with vascular invasion or multiple tumors ≤5 cm	F0	46	.01
	F1	30	
T3-Major vascular invasion or multiple tumors >5 cm	F0	17	.005
	F1	9	

F0, fibrosis grade 0–4; F1, fibrosis grade 5–6, according to Ishak K, Baptista A, Bianchi L, and others: *J Hepatol* 22:696, 1995.
Adapted from Vauthey JN, Lauwers GY: J Hepatol 38:237, 2003.

describe the technique of PEI in 1986. Under ultrasonographic guidance, a 95% ethanol solution is injected percutaneously into the tumor, which generally must be less than 4 cm in diameter. Early reports indicated that tumors treated with PEI were reduced in size and that 48% of patients did not develop new local tumors at follow-up. Although the 5-year survival was 28%, which was significantly better than the control group, 66% of patients had tumor recurrence at distant sites. Subsequently, PEI was compared with resection in patients with HCC of less than 4 cm in diameter, and survival was found to be equivalent in both treatment groups, even though patients treated with PEI had worse underlying liver function. Most studies report an overall survival rate of 90% at 1 year and 45% to 75% at 3 years for PEI. The best results are obtained in solitary lesions less than 4 cm in diameter, especially when the tumor is well differentiated.

Although the majority of studies have not shown improved survival with the use of TACE as primary therapy for HCC, most studies do report significant response rates. Although response rates are between 24% and 55%, less than 20% of patients have a greater than 50% size reduction in their tumor mass after TACE. In a study of 185 patients with HCC who were not amenable to surgery, patients with small tumors (<4 cm) derived the most benefit from TACE, whereas poor response and significant side effects were seen in patients with large tumors, suggesting that TACE treatment offers little benefit in advanced HCC. Two recent randomized studies have shown an improvement in survival after TACE in selected patients. In each of these studies, the patients were stringently selected on the basis of age, extent of underlying liver disease (only Child A or B patients were eligible), lack of portal hypertension, and absence of extrahepatic spread. In the study by Lo and colleagues, chemoembolization resulted in a marked tumor response, and the actuarial survival was significantly better than in the control group (3 years, 26% vs. 3%; $p = 0.002$). Similarly, Llovet and colleagues reported a 36% improvement in 2-year survival after chemoembolization.

Another treatment aimed at local control in patients who are not candidates for traditional resection has been RFA. RFA is a localized thermal treatment technique that produces tumor destruction by heating tumor tissue to temperatures over 50°C, causing cytodestruction by denaturation of intracellular proteins, as well as dissolution and melting of the phospholipids membranes. Our group found that RFA produces effective local control of disease and can be performed safely with minimal complications. Although local tumor recurrence at the RFA site was only 3.6%, new liver tumors or extrahepatic metastasis developed in 45.5% of patients. Thus although local tumor control may be achieved to some measure with RFA, the high propensity for the disease to recur systemically emphasizes the need for additional systemic agents to aid in the control of distant disease.

between cirrhosis and recurrence. In a study of 145 patients who survived more than 5 years after resection of HCC, we have reported that recurrence rates were 31% in those patients with fibrosis/cirrhosis (Ishak 3–6) compared with only 7% in patients with no fibrosis or cirrhosis.

ABLATION THERAPY

Several ablative strategies have been developed to achieve local tumor control in patients with limited disease who are not suitable candidates for hepatic resection or OLT. These methods include percutaneous ethanol injection (PEI), transcatheter arterial chemotherapy (TACE), and RFA. Livraghi and colleagues were the first to

FIBROLAMELLAR VARIANT OF HCC

Fibrolamellar carcinoma (FLHCC) is a distinct clinical variant of HCC, usually occurring within the second and third decades of life with no gender predominance. The incidence of FLHCC has been reported in 6% to 23% of Western patients with HCC. Pathologically, FLHCC typically consists of well-circumscribed, large solitary lesions with a central scar arising in a noncirrhotic liver. In addition, viral hepatitis is uncommon and serum alpha-fetoprotein levels are usually within normal limits. CT and MRI often demonstrate a heterogeneous mass with a central scar that is similar to those seen in cases of focal nodular hyperplasia (FNH). Central calcifications within the mass help to distinguish FLHCC from FNH, but this is not specific. Existing data indicate a resectability rate of approximately 95% and improved survival after resection for patients with FLHCC compared with HCC patients. Moreover, survival times are longer in patients with recurrences of FLHCC than in patients with recurrence of classic HCC. Number of lesions and the presence of nodal disease represent significant predictors of survival after resection. The rate of lymph node metastasis is quite high in FLHCC, raising the question of en bloc lymphadenectomy at the time of the primary surgery. To date, no data have been reported to answer this question adequately.

Controversy exists as to whether resection or OLT for FLHCC provides superior survival. A review of the literature on transplantation for HCC showed that OLT is not appropriate for FLHCC without cirrhosis. A phase II trial conducted at our institution suggests a potential neoadjuvant role for continuous infusion of fluorouracil and subcutaneous interferon alfa-2b. In patients with advanced FLHCC there was a 62.5% response rate as compared to a 14% response rate in patients with HCC.

INTRAHEPATIC CHOLANGIOCARCINOMA

I-CCA is the second most common primary hepatic tumor and arises from the malignant transformation of the epithelial cells that line the bile ducts within the liver. Primary sclerosing cholangitis is the main risk factor in Western countries, and there also appears to be an association between I-CCA and cirrhosis. Three macroscopic types of I-CCA have been described: mass-forming, periductal infiltrating-type, and intraductal growth-type. Patients with mass-forming I-CCA (MFCC) do worse than patients with periductal infiltrating or intraductal I-CCA following resection. This may be in part due to a propensity for MFCC to have vascular invasion and lymph node metastasis. MFCC has the propensity to extend along the biliary tree in some patients, translating into significantly shorter survival.

Surgical resection offers the only chance for cure, with 5-year survival rates of 13% to 44%. Clinicopathologic factors that adversely affect survival are large tumors, vascular invasion, nodal involvement, bile duct involvement, multiple nodules, and margin status. Although lymph node involvement is common in IHCC, the extent of lymphadenectomy during resection has not been proven to affect survival.

OLT for I-CCA has resulted in largely disappointing outcomes and should not be considered except as part of specifically designed clinical trials.

SUGGESTED READINGS

Abdalla EK, Barnett CC, Doherty D, and others: Extended hepatectomy in patients with hepatobiliary malignancies with and without preoperative portal vein embolization, *Arch Surg* 137:675, 2002.

Aloia TA, Zorzi D, Abdalla EK, and others: Two-surgeon technique for hepatic parenchymal transection of the noncirrhotic liver using saline-linked cautery and ultrasonic dissection, *Ann Surg* 242:172, 2005.

Bilimoria MM, Lauwers GY, Doherty DA, and others: Underlying liver disease, not tumor factors, predicts long-term survival after resection of hepatocellular carcinoma, *Arch Surg* 136:528, 2001.

Curley SA, Izzo F, Ellis LM, and others: Radiofrequency ablation of hepatocellular cancer in 110 patients with cirrhosis, *Ann Surg* 232:381, 2000.

Esnaola NF, Mirza ND, Lauwers GY, and others: Comparison of clinicopathologic characteristics and outcomes after resection in patients with hepatocellular carcinoma treated in the United States, France, and Japan, *Ann Surg* 238:711, 2003.

Pawlik TM, Poon RT, Abdalla EK, and others: Critical appraisal of the clinical and pathologic predictors of survival after resection of large hepatocellular carcinoma, *Arch Surg* 140:450, 2005.

Vauthey JN, Lauwers GY, Esnaola NF, and others: Simplified staging for hepatocellular carcinoma, *J Clin Oncol* 20:1527, 2002.

HEPATIC MALIGNANCY: RESECTION VERSUS TRANSPLANTATION

Eric T. Castaldo, MD, and C. Wright Pinson, MD, MBA

INTRODUCTION

Of the many options available, hepatic resection and transplantation are two of the most effective methods of treating hepatic malignancy. Treatment of these tumors should be multidisciplinary, and multiple methods may be used over time in a given patient. Understanding these options, the pathology of various tumors; tumor stage, size, number and location; patient's underlying condition; and resources available are keys to selecting the optimal treatment choice for each patient.

The most common primary hepatic malignancy in the world is hepatocellular carcinoma (HCC). HCC is particularly prevalent in Asia and Africa. Approximately 80% of all cases of HCC arise in the setting of cirrhosis, and conversely 5% of cirrhotic patients develop HCC. Chronic infection with hepatitis B virus increases the likelihood of developing HCC eightfold. Chronic infection with hepatitis C virus (HCV) makes patients four times as likely to develop HCC. Food contamination with aflatoxin has been implicated in the development of HCC in Asia.

Cholangiocarcinoma (CCA) accounts for less than 2% of all human malignancies and 10% of hepatobiliary malignancies, representing the second most common hepatobiliary malignancy worldwide. CCA is a difficult disease to treat because patients often present late in their course when options are limited. Although CCA develops anywhere in the biliary tree, the most common site is at the biliary confluence.

Neuroendocrine tumors (NET) including carcinoid tumors are less common, often indolent tumors primarily arising in the gastrointestinal tract but occasionally in the liver. These tumors have been known to metastasize to the liver in up to 90% of patients. With a large enough tumor burden and excessive hormonal release, they can become symptomatic. Although cure is a rare outcome of surgical treatment, relief of symptoms from bulky liver metastasis and prolongation of life are attainable goals. Hepatic resection and transplantation should also be considered with hepatoblastoma and epithelioid hemangioendothelioma.

The organization of this chapter on resection and transplantation of hepatic tumors focuses on patient screening and evaluation, staging, and surgical management of the tumors just described. Other alternative techniques for the treatment of hepatic malignancy, such as chemoembolization, alcohol injection, chemotherapy, and thermoablation, are not discussed.

POPULATION SCREENING

Because the vast majority of patients in the United States with HCC have underlying cirrhosis, surveillance of these at-risk patients is important in identifying HCC at its earliest stages, when it is more amenable to curative therapies. The most common laboratory evaluation to screen at-risk patients is the serum alpha-fetoprotein (AFP). Serum AFP is elevated in 60% to 80% of patients with HCC. Levels of AFP greater than 400 ng/ml are highly suggestive of HCC (however, AFP levels can be this high in patients with HCV cirrhosis who do not have HCC). Using ultrasound in combination with AFP for screening raises the sensitivity and specificity of detecting patients with HCC. Ultrasound can detect between 60% and 80% of lesions as small as 1 cm and more than 95% of lesions 3 cm or greater, although this is dependent on the experience of the operator. Although there are no current specific screening protocols, most clinicians recommend screening of patients with cirrhosis at 3- to 6-month intervals.

The majority of cases of CCA are sporadic; however, many develop in patients with primary sclerosing cholangitis (PSC). Reports vary between 10% and 35% on the incidence of CCA in patients with PSC. The risk of developing CCA after a diagnosis of PSC is approximately 1.5% per year. Patients with PSC should be screened with the serum tumor markers carbohydrate antigen 19-9 (CA19-9) and carcinogenic embryonic antigen (CEA). If the Ramage score [CA19-9 + (CEA × 40)] is greater than 400, this is 90% specific for cholangiocarcinoma. The progression of symptoms of patients with PSC, such as increasing jaundice, pruritis, pain, liver enzymes, and cholangitis, is the hallmark of the development of CCA and should prompt an endoscopic retrograde cholangiopancreatography (ERCP).

PATIENT EVALUATION

The evaluation of a patient with a hepatic tumor should begin first with identification of any underlying liver disease. A directed history and physical examination should be performed to assess for the severity of liver disease and the presence of portal hypertension through evidence such as past hospitalizations for gastrointestinal hemorrhage, caput medusa, ascites, jaundice, gynecomastia, and musculoskeletal wasting. Full hepatitis profiles should be obtained to ascertain the cause of disease. Routine laboratory studies should be performed to determine the severity of hepatitis and whether coagulopathy is present, as well as to assess for the presence of the hepatorenal syndrome. Additional laboratory studies such as CA19-9, CEA, and 5-hydroxyindoleacetic acid (5-HIAA) should also be obtained, depending on the suspected diagnosis of the tumor.

The predominant cause of death following hepatic resection in patients with cirrhosis is liver failure. Thus the determination of hepatic reserve is important. This is assessed using the Child-Pugh classification (Table 1). Patients with Child-Pugh A cirrhosis can undergo resection with reported perioperative mortality rates between 0% and 5%. In general, Child-Pugh A patients can be

Table 1: Child-Pugh Classification of Cirrhosis

Parameter	1 Point	2 Points	3 Points
Albumin (g/dl)	>3.5	2.8–3.5	<2.8
Bilirubin (mg/dl)	<2	2–3	>3
INR	<1.7	1.7–2.3	>2.3
Ascites	None	Slight	Moderate
Encephalopathy	None	1–2	3–4

Child-Pugh classification is calculated by summing the points per parameter to arrive at a total between 5 and 15. *INR,* international normalized ratio. Grade A = 5–6, grade B = 7–9, Grade C = 10–15.

considered for resection of up to 50% of liver parenchyma. Perioperative mortality rates are greater for Child-Pugh B patients, approximately 10% to 15%; therefore only limited resection of these patients is possible—up to 25% of liver parenchyma. Perioperative mortality in Child-Pugh C cirrhosis exceeds 25% and is therefore a contraindication to resection. These patients are potential candidates for transplantation only.

Furthermore, an assessment of the functional hepatic capacity can be performed to help determine ability to tolerate resection. For example, the indocyanine green (ICG) clearance test is one of the best-known tests to predict the risk of postoperative liver failure. The amount of ICG remaining in the bloodstream of a patient with a normal liver 15 minutes after its injection should be less than 10%. A two-segment resection is likely to be tolerated if 15% to 20% of the dye remains at 15 minutes. A value of 21% to 30% is suggestive that a single segment or wedge resection is tolerable. A value of 40% or greater indicates that postoperative liver failure will likely occur even with a minimal resection.

In addition, the Model for End Stage Liver Disease (MELD) score is calculated to assess the severity of liver and kidney disease and is used to prioritize patients for transplantation and to predict preoperative and postoperative mortality. The MELD score ranges from 6 (less ill) to 40 (gravely ill) and is calculated from the following three laboratory measurements: serum creatinine, bilirubin, and international normalized ratio.

If transplantation is considered, further evaluation required includes a full psychosocial evaluation and the identification of a sufficient patient social support system. Patients who smoke are required to abstain for at least 3 months. Patients with a past history of alcohol use are required to abstain from alcohol ingestion for at least 6 months and go through a rehabilitation program. Consultations with specialists in hepatology, hematology, infectious disease, psychiatry, ophthalmology, and dentistry are performed. Full hepatitis and human immunodeficiency virus profiles and appropriate vaccinations must also be performed.

IMAGING

Computed tomography (CT) and magnetic resonance imaging (MRI) are the major modalities available for imaging. A triphasic CT scan is one in which hepatic imaging is performed before contrast and in both the arterial and venous phases. It is helpful to determine the anatomy of the tumor(s) and the proximity to major hepatic venous structures, as well as extension or gross invasion into the hepatic or portal veins. Additionally, certain tumors such as HCC, which derives its blood flow through the hepatic arteries, can be seen more readily during the arterial phase. CT is also used to estimate the future liver remnant (FLR) volume. This is an estimate of the remaining liver after resection and can be predictive of postoperative liver failure if the FLR is less than 40% of the whole liver. MRI is equally as good as triphasic CT to determine the relationships between tumor and the surrounding hepatic vasculature and is a good alternative in patients with allergies to intravenous contrast or in whom contrast nephropathy is a concern. Ultrasound imaging can be helpful to assess intrahepatic and portal vascular blood flow. Hepatic arteriography has been largely replaced by CT arteriography and MR arteriography to determine relationships of major vessels to tumors. More recently, three-dimensional image analysis techniques have become available. Initially applied to living-donor liver transplantation (LDLT), these techniques for estimating liver volumes, perfusion territory, and detailed intrahepatic anatomy have now been applied to liver resection. Three-dimensional modeling of patient anatomy closely resembles the actual pathologic findings found intraoperatively. ^{18}F-fluorodeoxyglucose positron emission tomography ([18]FDG-PET) has also been used in evaluating patients with HCC. It has limited use because the sensitivity for the detection of HCC is approximately 64%. It is helpful in patients who do accumulate FDG in demonstrating regional or distant metastases. PET with ^{11}C-acetate has been shown to be useful in the detection of HCC, with a sensitivity approaching 90%. Several studies have found [18]FDG-PET useful for both detecting and staging CCA. In a recent series, the sensitivity of [18]FDG-PET was 85% for detection of primary CCA of nodular morphology with a mass greater than 1 cm. It also allowed detection of unsuspected distant metastases and led to changes in surgical management in up to 30% of patients.

Imaging with three radiopharmaceuticals can be particularly useful when evaluating patients with metastatic NET: the radiolabeled somatostatin analogue (^{111}In-octreotide) scan, the norepinephrine analogue radio labeled meta-iodobenzylguanidine (MIBG) scan, and PET using FDG. These studies take advantage of selective uptake and concentration of the radionuclide carrier molecules by NET cells. These nuclear medicine studies have helped to (1) differentiate benign from malignant lesions; (2) differentiate postsurgical scar from recurrent tumor; (3) monitor treatment response; and (4) help to stage patients by identifying extrahepatic disease. They also are often used when tumor markers are rising in the absence of an identifiable source or further evaluation of equivocal lesions.

INVASIVE EVALUATION

Percutaneous liver biopsy of potentially resectable tumors is not often indicated for fear of seeding the biopsy track, especially in the case of HCC, in which the decision to operate is made on the basis of noninvasive clinical and radiographic criteria and does not require a tissue diagnosis. Biopsy is more valuable to determine whether cirrhosis is present in the unaffected portion of the liver. If a tissue diagnosis is required, as may be the case in CCA, ERCP with brushings can be performed safely. Laparoscopy with intraoperative ultrasound is another safe, effective method of obtaining biopsies and further assessing tumor extent that can help with the operative decision making. Some series have demonstrated that up to 22% of patients with HCC who undergo laparoscopy are deemed unresectable and therefore avoid laparotomy. Another series demonstrated that patients with indeterminate staging of HCC on the basis of radiographic studies were upstaged from their initial staging in 66% of cases.

TREATMENT

Hepatocellular Carcinoma

Surgical resection for noncirrhotic patients with HCC is a mainstay of therapy. Resectability is determined by the absence of distant metastatic disease and the anatomic relationship of the tumor to major hepatic vasculature. Intraoperative ultrasound is an excellent tool to determine these relationships and should be used when planning the feasibility of hepatic resection. Resections should be carried out with standard oncologic principles, including adequate surgical margins (1 cm) and with enough hepatic remnant to avoid postoperative liver failure. Preoperative portal venous embolization aids in the resection of large hepatic tumors by promoting

Table 2: AJCC/UICC TNM Classification of Hepatocellular Carcinoma, 6th edition (2002)

T1	Single tumor without vascular invasion
T2	Single tumor with vascular invasion or multiple tumors, none >5 cm
T3	Multiple tumors, any >5 cm, or tumors involving major branch of portal or hepatic veins
T4	Tumors with direct invasion of adjacent organs other than the gallbladder, or perforation of visceral peritoneum
N1	Regional lymph node metastasis
M1	Distant metastasis

Stage	Tumor	Node	Metastasis
I	T1	N0	M0
II	T2	N0	M0
IIIa	T3	N0	M0
IIIb	T4	N0	M0
IIIc	Any T	N1	M0
IV	Any T	Any N	M1

AJCC, American Joint Committee on Cancer; *M,* distant metastasis; *N,* regional lymph nodes; *T,* primary tumor; *UICC,* International Union Against Cancer.

hypertrophy of the future remnant. The pathologic staging according to the Tumor Node Metastasis system is presented in Table 2. It takes into account tumor size and its relation to surrounding vasculature, local regional metastasis, and distant metastasis. Although it is an excellent stratification scheme for determining prognosis after liver resection, it fails to stratify patients in accordance with their underlying liver disease, a major consideration in the surgical management of these tumors. Reports on survival following resection for HCC are variable and highly dependent on patient selection. Numerous series have analyzed independent predictors of survival. For example, one study from Japan demonstrated that 5-year survival in patients undergoing resection for tumors less than 2 cm had improved survival (66%) over patients undergoing resection for tumors 2 to 5 cm (52%) who, in turn, had improved survival over patients with tumors larger than 5 cm (37%). These figures are similar to a study from the United States in which patients with tumors larger than 5 cm demonstrated worse survival (32%) than those with tumors under 5 cm (43%). Both macroscopic and microscopic vascular invasion have been shown to affect negatively survival following resection. However, microscopic vascular invasion is not identified until after resection and does not influence the decision to operate. The number of nodules present is another independent predictor of survival. Several studies have demonstrated that 5-year survival is significantly worse in patients undergoing resection for multiple foci of HCC compared with single foci HCC. Additionally, outcomes are improved for multicentric HCC (maximum of three foci) with transplantation, and thus resection is relatively contraindicated in these patients. The results of resection for HCC for selected series are presented in Table 3.

The use of liver transplantation in the treatment of HCC has evolved significantly over the past few decades. In the 1980s, poor long-term survival (below 40%) was observed as patients with large tumors, macrovascular invasion, and extrahepatic spread were permitted to receive transplants, the accepted criteria of the time. In the 1990s, Bismuth and Mazzaferro established the Milan criteria for hepatic transplantation. They demonstrated that patients with a single tumor smaller than 5 cm or two or three tumors smaller than 3 cm undergoing transplantation had comparable long-term survival

Table 3: Results of Survival After Hepatic Resection for Hepatocellular Carcinoma in Selected Series

Author	Year	N	1-Year Survival (%)	3-Year Survival (%)	5-Year Survival (%)
Franco	1990	72	68	51	NR
Nagasue	1993	229	80	51	23
Llovet	1999	77	85	62	51
Zhou	2001	1000 (<5 cm)	91	77	65
		1366 (>5 cm)	76	48	37
Ercolani	2003	224	83	63	43
Shimozawa	2004	135	95	73	55

NR, Not reported.

(70%) to patients who were HCC free at the time of transplantation. These criteria are now universally accepted and are considered the standard for the listing of patients for transplantation. Recently some centers have been extending these criteria experimentally.

Before 2002, patients were placed on the liver transplant waiting list and received no priority associated with malignant disease. As a result, some patients with HCC experienced disease progression and were no longer suitable candidates for transplantation when a suitable liver was allocated. In 2002, the United Network for Organ Sharing began using the MELD system and as a matter of policy allocated additional points to patients with HCC in an effort to increase their competitiveness for a suitable organ. This was to ensure that these patients could be transplanted in a timely fashion (3 to 6 months) and limit disease progression while on the waiting list. This resulted in a substantial increase in the number of patients transplanted for HCC. Strategies that have been employed to manage tumors and prevent tumor progression for patients while they are on the transplant waiting list have been percutaneous radiofrequency ablation, transcatheter arterial chemoembolization, and percutaneous ethanol injection. These techniques are widely used and contribute to temporary local control of tumors. LDLT has become an attractive alternative to cadaveric transplantation because of the shortage of donor livers. Graft sizes from partial livers are smaller than a cadaveric graft. Because of the MELD exemptions, cirrhotic patients with HCC typically have more hepatic reserve than their cirrhotic counterparts without HCC listed for transplantation. Thus patients with HCC are able to tolerate smaller graft sizes. It is an area of debate as to whether patients undergoing LDLT should be held to the same strict criteria (Milan criteria) because of the potential unlimited resource of living donors. Prospective studies are necessary to determine whether expanding the criteria is efficacious.

The results of hepatic transplantation for HCC are equal or better than resection. A large series from Japan showed 1-, 3-, 5-, and 10-year survival rates of 85%, 64%, 45%, and 21%, respectively. When using the Milan criteria, the 3-year survival rate has been reported to be similar, between 74% and 84%. Results from selected series for transplantation for HCC are shown in Table 4.

In summary, treatment options for patients with HCC rely on a number of variables, and selection for therapeutic modality should be based on the number and sizes of tumors, underlying hepatic function, and the general condition of the patient. The best candidates for surgical resection for HCC are patients without cirrhosis and patients with Child-Pugh class A cirrhosis with a single tumor less than 5 cm in diameter in an anatomically favorable position, no evidence of macrovascular invasion, and the absence of the clinical stigmata of portal hypertension. Patients with Child-Pugh's class C cirrhosis should be considered for transplantation or one of the other methods of tumor control should they not be candidates for transplantation. A summary for treatment options can be seen in Table 5.

Fibrolamellar Carcinoma

Fibrolamellar carcinoma (FLC) is a histological variant of HCC that is distinct in its epidemiology and prognosis. FLC typically develops in younger patients (aged 20–40 years) without underlying liver disease. FLC is typically large and has the appearance of a central scar on CT scan. Because of the lack of underlying hepatic disease, these tumors are often more amenable to resection and are associated with improved survival over patients with typical HCC. Published series have reported a 5-year survival in resectable patients as high as 63%. Transplantation should also be considered in patients with FLC without evidence of distant metastatic disease who are unresectable.

Cholangiocarcinoma

The 1-year survival for patients with untreated CCA is approximately 25%. Survival can be improved with grossly complete surgical resection, which usually must be extensive and often includes partial hepatectomy. Unfortunately, CCA often presents (50%-90% of patients) with advanced American Joint Committee on Cancer stage III and IV and locoregional spread, making this complete resection difficult or impossible.

For isolated intrahepatic lesions in patients with good liver function, the appropriate liver resection is indicated. For extrahepatic lesions (Bismuth type I and II anatomic lesions), patients with good liver function are candidates for resection of the extrahepatic bile duct and bifurcation, including the caudate lobe behind the porta hepatis together with a periportal lymph node dissection, followed by reconstruction of the biliary system. Type III anatomic lesions require both a hemihepatectomy and extrahepatic bile duct resection. Patients with poor or declining liver function should not be considered for resection. Surgical mortality and morbidity

Table 4: Survival Following Liver Transplantation for Hepatocellular Carcinoma in Selected Series

Author	Year	N	1-Year Survival (%)	3-Year Survival (%)	5-Year Survival (%)
Mazzaferro	1996	48	90	84	NR
Hemming	2001	112	78	63	57
Roayaie	2002	43	90	58	44
Zavaglia	2005	155	84	75	72

NR, Not reported.

Table 5: Summary of Treatment Options for Hepatocellular Carcinoma

		Tumor Extent				
Operative Risk	Liver Function	Metastasis	Number	Volume	Size	Treatment
Good	Normal	No	Limited (≤4)	≤¾		Resection up to trisegmentectomy
Good	Child A or MELD <9	No	Limited	≤½		Resection up to lobectomy
Good	Child B or MELD 9–10	No	Limited	≤¼		Resection up to segmentectomy
Good	Normal, Child A or B	No	Limited		<3 cm	Resection, RFA, PEI, or cryosurgery
Good	Normal, Child A or B	No	Limited		<4 cm	Resection, PEI, or cryosurgery
Good	Normal, Child A or B	No	Limited		<6 cm	Resection or cryosurgery
Good	Child A or B	No	Multiple	Extensive		Chemoembolization or PEI
Fair, Poor	Child B or C or MELD >11	No	1 3		≤ 5 cm or ≤ 3 cm	Transplantation
Good	Child A or B	Yes	Any	Any	Any	Systemic chemotherapy or clinical trial
Poor	Child C	Yes	Any	Any	Any	Supportive care

Together, patient performance, liver function as assessed by Child-Pugh classification or Model for End-Stage Liver Disease *(MELD)*, and the extent of tumor influence the choice of treatment (last column). *PEI,* Percutaneous ethanol injection; *RFA,* radioablation.

following resection for CCA average approximately 10% and 30%, respectively. The 1-, 3-, and 5-year survival is variable but averages 70%, 35%, and 25%, respectively (see Table 6).

In the infancy of transplantation, CCA was an acceptable diagnosis for transplantation, given the limited survival following resection. In those series, which did not emphasize highly selected early-stage disease and neoadjuvant or adjuvant radiation and chemotherapy, the average 1-, 3-, and 5-year survivals were 43%, 30%, and 10%, respectively. Given the few long-term survivors, the high rate of early recurrence, the mortality and morbidity associated with transplantation, and the limited number of hepatic grafts, transplantation for the majority of patients with CCA ceased. In recent years, however, some investigators have challenged this dearth by developing new strategies for transplantation of patients with early-stage CCA (Table 7). Emphasizing neoadjuvant radiation and chemosensitization in operatively confirmed stage I or II hilar CCA has led to promising results. Patients undergoing transplantation using these protocols have demonstrated improved survival, up to 92% at 1 year, 82% at 3 years, and 82% at 5 years. Additionally, 1-, 3-, and 5-year recurrence rates were also improved at 0%, 5%, and 12%, respectively. In conclusion, although patients with CCA should undergo resection if possible, under strict research protocols at select centers, for patients with early stage CCA with anatomically unresectable (Bismuth type IV) lesions, hepatic transplantation is an acceptable therapy.

Neuroendocrine Tumors Including Carcinoid Tumors

Variable 5-year survival for untreated liver metastasis from NET has been reported, generally at 30% to 40%. Carcinoid tumors have a more favorable prognosis, but for those diagnosed with liver metastasis, 5-year survival is estimated at approximately 30% to 50%. Because these tumors characteristically are relatively slow growing and treatment response rates are different from a comparable tumor load of other types of metastasis, these patients deserve careful and thoughtful consideration of aggressive medical and surgical therapy. For example, functional hormonal blockade often provides significantly improved quality of life. Furthermore, tumor debulking or ablation can produce improved quality and length of life by decreasing the levels of circulating hormones produced by the tumor and resulting symptoms, improving other organ dysfunction such as heart failure, and improving gastrointestinal function and nutrition.

It is commonplace for liver metastases of NET to be bilobar, and patients with NET typically have a miliary pattern of disease and often present with distant disease. Therefore only approximately 10% to 20% of patients are candidates for resection, and even then total resection is not often accomplished. Nonetheless, this cytoreductive approach reduces clinical symptoms and improves the likely response of adjunct medical therapy. For NET this is reasonable because of slow tumor kinetics, the liver representing a great portion of the total tumor burden, the nodular displacing rather than invading growth pattern in the liver, and the efficacy of hormonal blockade. In general, palliative resection of hepatic metastases is believed to be a worthwhile endeavor if 80% to 90% of the gross hepatic tumor mass can be successfully resected and the surgical risk is low. Symptomatic improvement can be expected in the majority of these patients, and the duration of the clinical response is felt to be inversely proportional to the amount of residual tumor following resection.

Good candidates for operation are patients with 80% to 90% resectable tumors who are unresponsive to medical management, without extrahepatic dissemination, and with good overall function. Elevated venous pressures associated with carcinoid heart

Table 6: Survival Following Resection for Cholangiocarcinoma in Selected Series

Author	Year	N	1-Year Survival (%)	3-Year Survival (%)	5-Year Survival (%)
Pinson	1988	25	84	44	35
Madariaga	1998	62	73	40	21
Lillemoe	2000	109	68	30	11
Nishio	2005	301	80	35	22

Table 7: Survival Following Transplantation for Cholangiocarcinoma in Select Series

Author	Year	N	1-Year Survival (%)	3-Year Survival (%)	5-Year Survival (%)
O'Grady	1988	26	34	8	5
Shimoda	2001	25	71	35	NR
Sudan	2002	11	55	45	45
Rea	2005	38	92	82	82

N, Number; *NR*, not reported.

disease represent a contraindication to liver resection. Tumors can be enucleated or resected. Although there are no data from a randomized controlled prospective trial that clearly show improved survival after hepatic resection for NET, nonrandomized studies show improved 5-year survival. Resection of both the primary tumor and all gross metastatic disease is reported to provide 5-year survival of 70% to 85%, with a mortality and morbidity similar to resections for other indications. Even with palliative resection, 5-year survival is greater than 67%, which is better than other treatments or no treatment. Although liver transplantation theoretically might be efficacious for patients with NET because of their indolent course and especially so with isolated liver disease, in practice results have been mixed. The reported 5-year survival has ranged from 36% to 47% overall and up to 70% for carcinoid tumors. Recurrence-free 5-year survival has been less than 25%. Less than 1% of all liver transplantation has been performed for NET, and this indication is controversial, given the donor-liver shortage. Suggested current indications for transplantation include age younger than 50 years, primary tumor completely resected, absence of extrahepatic disease proven over a 6-month period, and excessive hormonal symptoms refractory to medical therapy.

Other Uncommon Liver Tumors

The main treatment for hepatoblastoma, the most common childhood hepatic malignancy, is cisplatin-based chemotherapy followed by surgical resection. Approximately 60% of patients are unresectable at the time of diagnosis. When followed by resection, 5- to 10-year disease-free survival of 80% has been demonstrated. Liver transplantation has been used for patients with hepatoblastoma who are unresectable after initial chemotherapy, have an incomplete resection, recur after resection, or develop liver failure secondary to chemotherapy. The long-term survival has been excellent, with published reports exceeding 80%. These results have led hepatoblastoma to become a widely accepted indication for liver transplantation.

Hepatic epithelioid hemangioendothelioma is a rare, multifocal tumor arising from the vascular endothelium. They are unusual tumors with unknown malignant potential that lie somewhere between benign hemangiomas and malignant angiosarcomas. The multifocal nature of the disease can often make these tumors difficult to resect and have made liver transplantation an attractive option. Although small, some series have demonstrated 5-year survival rates as high as 71%.

SUGGESTED READINGS

Bismuth H, Chiche L, Adam R, and others: Liver resection versus transplantation for hepatocellular carcinoma in cirrhosis, *Ann Surg* 218:145, 1993.

Fong Y, Sun RL, Jarnagin W, and others: An analysis of 412 cases of hepatocellular carcinoma at a Western center, *Ann Surg* 229:790, 1999.

Llovet JM, Schwartz M, Mazzaferro V: Resection and liver transplantation for hepatocellular carcinoma, *Semin Liver Dis* 25:181, 2005.

Mazzaferro V, Regalia E, Doci R, and others: Liver transplantation for the treatment of hepatocellular carcinomas in patients with cirrhosis, *N Engl J Med* 334:693, 1996.

Rea DJ, Heimbach JK, Rosen CB, and others: Liver transplant with neoadjuvant chemoradiation is more effective than resection for hilar cholangiocarcinoma, *Ann Surg* 242:451, 2005.

SURGERY FOR COLORECTAL LIVER METASTASES

Ronald P. DeMatteo, MD

INTRODUCTION

Partial hepatectomy remains the mainstay of therapy for select patients with liver metastases from colorectal cancer. Surgery has historically achieved a 5-year survival of approximately 40% and a cure rate of approximately 20%. Liver surgery is now routinely performed with less than 5% mortality because of advances in radiologic imaging, low central venous pressure anesthesia, and surgical techniques. Because of dramatic progress in systemic chemotherapy during the past 5 years, the median survival for patients with metastatic colorectal cancer treated medically is almost 2 years at present. Consequently, the results of partial hepatectomy will improve further. The preoperative considerations, operative principles, specific liver resections, and results for partial hepatectomy in patients with metastatic colorectal cancer are summarized in this chapter.

PREOPERATIVE CONSIDERATIONS

Evaluation

Several factors must be considered in evaluating a patient for partial hepatectomy: general medical condition of the patient, presence of extrahepatic disease, and features of the intrahepatic cancer. First, the patient must be healthy enough to tolerate the physiologic stress of liver surgery. A cardiology consultation is generally obtained in patients with significant comorbidities or those older than 65 years old. With careful selection, we have found that elderly patients have similar perioperative morbidity and mortality rates as younger patients. To survey for extrahepatic disease, we generally perform a computed tomography (CT) scan of the abdomen and pelvis, with oral and intravenous contrast, and a chest x-ray or CT scan of the chest. ^{18}F-fluoro-deoxyglucose positron emission tomography (^{18}FDG-PET) scans are also frequently obtained, but false negatives may occur after chemotherapy has been initiated. Magnetic resonance imaging (MRI) or ultrasound is sometimes useful to characterize a small liver lesion that may be a cyst. Ultrasound might also detect small liver tumors that are not seen on cross-sectional imaging. A recent (within 6 months) colonoscopy is usually necessary to screen for a second colorectal primary or an anastomotic recurrence. We have found that select patients who also have lung metastases benefit from liver and lung resection. Hepatectomy is generally contraindicated in patients with portal lymph node involvement or peritoneal disease, although this is being reevaluated because of the availability of more effective chemotherapy regimens.

The third consideration in performing a liver resection for metastatic colorectal cancer is the intrahepatic location of the disease with respect to major vascular and biliary structures and the distribution of tumors. The metastases must be completely removable, and even patients with more than four tumors appear to benefit from surgery. Up to 85% of a normal liver can be removed. The surgeon should strive for a 1-cm margin of normal tissue whenever possible.

Unresectable Disease

Unfortunately, most patients with colorectal metastases are not candidates for resection because of the extent of intrahepatic disease and the inability to preserve an adequate remnant of functional liver. It is rare for a solitary tumor to be unresectable, unless it involves the portal bifurcation or the confluence of the hepatic veins. A variety of approaches can enable surgery in patients considered to have unresectable disease by conventional criteria. In patients in whom the remnant is judged to be inadequate (<20% of functional liver) and thus the risk of postoperative hepatic insufficiency is high, preoperative portal vein embolization can be performed. This may be the case for a small, deeply placed tumor that requires a large sacrifice of parenchyma (e.g., extended resection plus caudate resection). In patients with steatosis, which is now commonly seen after prolonged chemotherapy, the necessary liver remnant size may be larger (i.e., >20% of functional liver). Portal vein embolization is performed ipsilateral to the intended resection to stimulate contralateral liver regeneration and increase the size of the intended liver remnant. However, whether portal vein embolization alters perioperative mortality in patients with either a normal or steatotic liver is unclear, although it probably reduces morbidity.

Another approach to the patient with unresectable disease isolated to the liver is to use preoperative chemotherapy to reduce the size and number of tumors. Chemotherapy can be delivered intravenously or via a surgically placed hepatic artery infusion pump. Both methods achieve response rates greater than 60% to 70%. The chance of converting a patient to have resectable disease appears to be between 15% and 30%. However, with prolonged use of drugs such as oxaliplatin and CPT-11, it is now typical for many patients to develop fatty livers, increasing the perioperative morbidity of partial hepatectomy. Bevacizumab (Avastin; Genentech, South San Francisco, CA) is now commonly used in multiagent chemotherapy. Because bevacizumab has been associated with both bleeding disorders and hypercoagulability, patients should not undergo surgery for at least 6 weeks after the last dose. For other chemotherapeutic agents, a wait of at least 2 weeks is advisable.

The remaining option for patients with unresectable disease is to perform either a combination of resection and ablation or staged hepatectomies. Resection plus intraoperative ablation is an acceptable approach, particularly if the ablated tumor is small (<3 cm). It is clear that radiofrequency ablation (RFA) or cryotherapy of large tumors (>3 cm) is associated with a high rate of local recurrence. RFA should be performed with overlapping applications to include a 1-cm rim of normal tissue whenever possible. Staged hepatectomies are occasionally indicated. The liver regeneration that occurs after the first hepatectomy allows for safer removal of the residual contralateral disease.

Timing of Hepatectomy

The optimal timing of liver resection in patients with a primary colorectal tumor and synchronous liver metastases is not well defined. If the patient has obstructive or bleeding symptoms, the primary tumor is usually resected first, and then systemic chemotherapy is administered to treat the liver disease; hepatectomy is subsequently considered. In the absence of symptoms from the primary, chemotherapy is generally the first line of therapy in patients with multiple, small liver tumors or those with substantial (>50% liver involvement) liver disease before surgery is considered. It is preferable to perform staged procedures if both the colorectal and liver resections are large (e.g., extended hepatectomy and low anterior resection); otherwise simultaneous resections are possible.

In patients with metachronous liver metastases, it is not clear whether chemotherapy or hepatectomy should be performed first. The rationale to perform chemotherapy first is that the response to the specific chemotherapy regimen can be assessed. As with most tumors, it appears that patients with disease responsive to chemotherapy fare better after surgery.

OPERATIVE PRINCIPLES

Hepatic surgery depends on a complete understanding of liver anatomy and comprises (1) liver mobilization and exposure, (2) vascular inflow and outflow control, and (3) biliary and parenchymal transection.

Anatomy

It is vital that the surgeon appreciates the three-dimensional anatomy of the liver and its vascular and biliary components (Fig. 1). The right and left liver are separated by Cantlie's line,

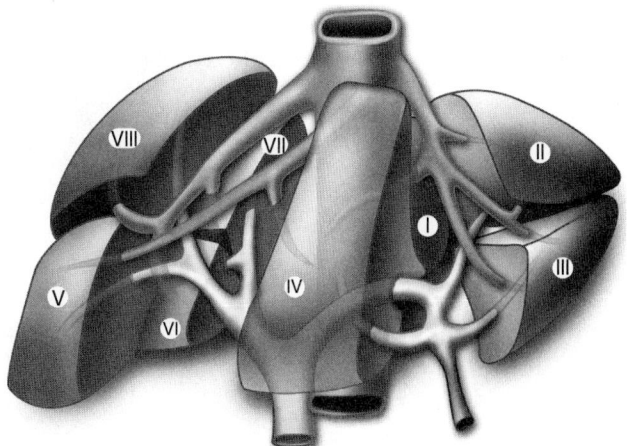

Figure 1 Segmental anatomy of the liver. The portal pedicles and the hepatic veins divide the liver into eight autonomous segments. *Reprinted from Blumgart LH: Liver resection for benign disease and for liver and biliary tumors. In Blumgart LH, Fong Y, editors: Surgery of the liver and biliary tract, ed 3, p 1643, Philadelphia, 2000, Churchill Livingstone. Used by permission of the publisher.*

an imaginary line that marks the plane between the gallbladder bed and the suprahepatic inferior vena cava (IVC). The eight segments of the liver are defined by the major hepatic veins and the portal inflow. Each segment is autonomous, with independent vascular supply, venous drainage, and biliary drainage. Consequently, any individual segment can be removed without disturbing the function of the remaining segments. The right liver is made up of an anterior section (segments 5 and 8) and a posterior section (segments 6 and 7). The falciform ligament and umbilical fissure separate the left lateral section (segments 2 and 3) from the medial section (segment 4) of the left liver. The caudate lobe (segment 1) is situated between the IVC and the portal vein caudally and the IVC and the middle and left hepatic vein trunks cephalad. The gastrohepatic omentum passes between the left portion of the caudate lobe and segments 2 and 3 to insert into the ligamentum venosum.

Within the liver, the portal structures (portal vein, hepatic artery, and bile duct) are contained in a common fibrous sheath that is readily distinguished from the thin walls of the hepatic vein branches. Outside the liver, the portal structures run separately. The right portal vein and right hepatic bile duct have a much shorter extrahepatic portion than the left portal vein and left hepatic duct, which are positioned horizontally at the base of segment 4. The main right portal structures branch into the right anterior and posterior pedicles to supply their respective sections. The left portal structures enter at the base of the umbilical fissure and then give rise to the segments 2 and 3 pedicles and "feedback" branches to segment 4 (Fig. 2). The main hepatic veins have a short extrahepatic course before they enter the IVC. The right hepatic vein runs between the right anterior and posterior sections (Fig. 3). The middle hepatic vein lies in Cantlie's line. The left hepatic vein separates segments 2 and 3 and typically joins the middle hepatic vein before entering the IVC. There are usually several small venules that drain directly into the retrohepatic IVC from the caudate and posterior right liver.

Liver Mobilization and Exposure

As with most operations, proper exposure is critical to safe and accurate liver surgery. The patient is positioned supine with both arms extended. The most commonly used incision is a right

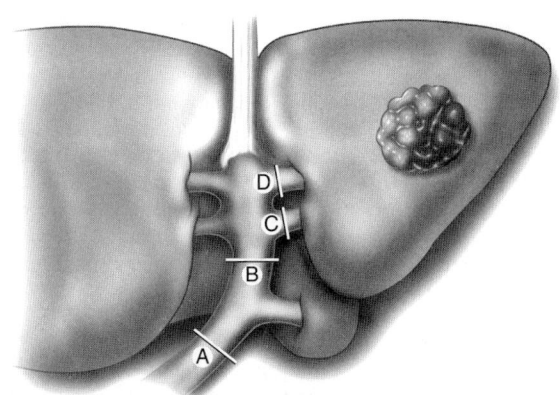

Figure 2 Anatomy of the umbilical fissure. The left liver and caudate lobe are devascularized by division of the left portal vein at position A. To preserve the caudate during a left hepatectomy, the left portal vein is divided at B. The segment 2 (C) and 3 (D) pedicles are shown, as well as the segment 4 "feedback" branches. *Reprinted from Blumgart LH: Liver resection for benign disease and for liver and biliary tumors. In Blumgart LH, Fong Y, editors: Surgery of the liver and biliary tract, ed 3, p 1643, Philadelphia, 2000, Churchill Livingstone. Used by permission of the publisher.*

subcostal incision with xiphoid extension. A midline incision can be used for a thin patient or for a left-sided resection. A right thoracoabdominal incision is generally required only when there is a massive right-sided tumor and the hepatic veins cannot be approached safely. A crossbar retractor is used to elevate the costal margins. The right liver is mobilized by dividing the peritoneal attachments between segment 6 and the retroperitoneum. The right triangular ligament that attaches the diaphragm to the right liver is divided to reveal the bare area of the liver and the right side of the suprahepatic IVC. The falciform ligament is followed cephalad to expose the anterior aspect of the suprahepatic IVC. The right liver is rotated to the left and upward to facilitate the retrohepatic caval dissection. Small draining veins are divided between clips starting from below and progressing cephalad (Fig. 3). The fibrous IVC ligament that conceals the lateral aspect

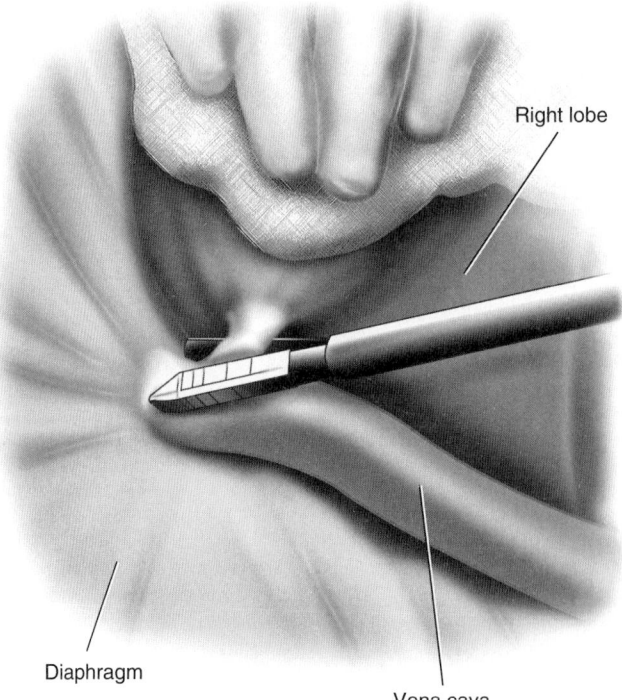

Right lobe

Diaphragm

Vena cava

Figure 3 Division of the right hepatic vein using an endovascular stapler. After the venules that drain directly into the vena cava have been divided, the right hepatic vein is isolated, the liver is rotated toward the left, and an endo-GIA vascular stapler is used to divide the vein. *Reprinted from Fong Y, Blumgart LH: J Am Coll Surg 185:97, 1997. Used by permission of Elsevier Science, Inc.*

of the right hepatic vein and IVC is transected (often using an endovascular stapler) to complete the mobilization of the right liver (Fig. 3). The left lateral section is mobilized by dividing the left triangular ligament from its lateral edge to the lateral margin of the left hepatic vein. Complete mobilization of the left liver requires division of the posterior caudate veins that drain directly into the IVC.

If tumor attachment to the diaphragm is encountered during liver mobilization, an en bloc diaphragm resection should be performed, even though true invasion by a colorectal liver metastasis is rarely present. After the relevant portion of liver is mobilized, bimanual palpation and intraoperative ultrasound are used to assess the extent of intrahepatic disease and identify any additional tumors.

Vascular Inflow and Outflow Control

Minimizing blood loss is critical to the success of liver surgery. Precise vascular control of the hepatic inflow and outflow vessels reduces bleeding during parenchymal transection and can be used to demarcate the anatomic boundaries of the liver. Hepatic inflow can be controlled by either (1) traditional dissection of the extrahepatic branches of the hepatic artery and portal vein before parenchymal transection or (2) pedicle ligation. Pedicle ligation involves dividing the portal pedicles within the liver before or during parenchymal transection. Via small hepatotomies, the pedicles can be rapidly isolated (Fig. 4). Alternatively, the pedicles can be located during parenchymal transection. After it is isolated, a pedicle can be quickly divided with a TA or GIA vascular stapler. Pedicle ligation is particularly advantageous if there has been previous right upper quadrant surgery, which may make hilar dissection hazardous.

The intrahepatic pedicle ligation approach is preferred for right-sided resections whenever possible. With this method, hilar dissection is avoided, and thus the risk of left bile duct injury is minimized. Right main pedicle ligation can be performed rapidly after the gallbladder is removed, caudal retrohepatic veins are divided, and the hilar plate is lowered to protect the left hepatic duct. Under Pringle control, a vertical hepatotomy is made in the gallbladder fossa and extended to the left just anterior to the

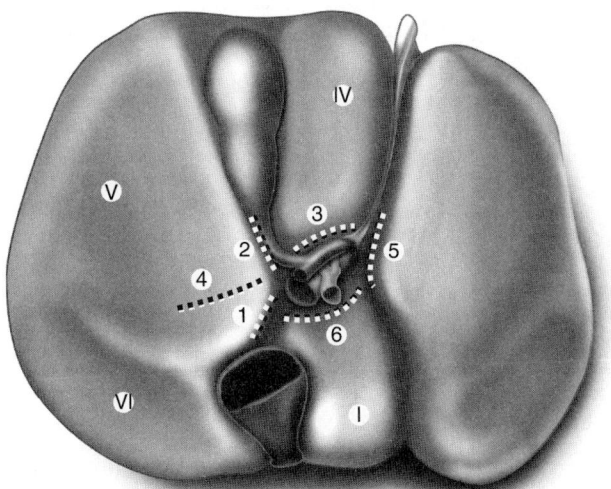

Figure 4 Location of hepatotomies for portal pedicle ligation. The undersurface of the liver is shown. The main right portal pedicle is isolated via hepatotomies 1 and 2, the right anterior pedicle via 2 and 4, the right posterior via 1 and 4, and the left portal pedicle via 3 and 5. *Reprinted from Fong Y, Blumgart LH: J Am Coll Surg 185:97, 1997. Used by permission of Elsevier Science, Inc.*

hilar plate. After a cruciate incision is made in the caudate process with cautery, a finger or clamp is passed into the liver to join the two hepatotomies and thereby encircle the right portal pedicle. Minor bleeding from middle hepatic vein branches may occur. The other method to isolate the intrahepatic right main pedicle is to divide the liver parenchyma first to expose the pedicle broadly. The right anterior and posterior sectional pedicles can also be selectively isolated with appropriate hepatotomies. The right posterior pedicle may be isolated with hepatotomies anterior to the fissure of Ganz and in the caudate process (Fig. 4). The right anterior pedicle may be isolated through incisions in the gallbladder fossa and anterior to the fissure of Ganz (Fig. 4). Liver demarcation after pedicle clamping is useful to confirm isolation of the correct pedicle and to guide the plane of parenchymal transection. The other approach to locate the right anterior or posterior sectional pedicle is to dissect starting from the right main pedicle.

The principal contraindication to a pedicle ligation maneuver is proximity of a tumor to the liver hilus because the oncologic margin may then be compromised; in this case, extrahepatic dissection with individual ligation of the portal vein and hepatic artery branches is preferred. This traditional technique takes longer and risks injury to the bile duct or vasculature, especially in the presence of anatomic variants. Even when extrahepatic dissection of the vascular inflow is performed, the right bile duct is generally divided within the liver to avoid biliary injury in the porta hepatis. For left-sided liver resections, extrahepatic dissection is usually performed instead of a pedicle approach.

Major bleeding during hepatectomy usually originates from the hepatic veins or IVC. Tumors located near the hepatic vein trunks or invading the IVC are particularly dangerous. Despite their short extrahepatic course, the three main hepatic veins can usually be isolated outside the liver. Early hepatic vein control decreases venous oozing during parenchymal transection and facilitates tumor clearance. Vascular staplers have greatly facilitated the process of dividing hepatic veins, especially in deep or obese patients when the use of vascular clamps is cumbersome. Although hepatic vein control can be safely obtained within the liver for tumors that are distant from the hepatic vein trunks, extrahepatic control of the relevant hepatic vein is preferable before parenchymal transection.

The right hepatic vein trunk is located by dividing the falciform ligament upward and to the right of the suprahepatic IVC. The trunk is readily identified at the notch it makes in the superior border of the liver. The vein is dissected, and the angle between the middle and right hepatic veins is cleared. The right liver is then mobilized, and the retrohepatic venules and IVC ligament are divided. The right hepatic vein is then encircled from above or below.

The left hepatic vein trunk is isolated after mobilization of the left lateral section of the liver, which is retracted to the right so that the ligamentum venosum can be divided cephalad. This exposes the angle between the posterior aspect of the left hepatic vein outside of the liver and the anterior surface of the IVC. It may be necessary to drop the top of the caudate off the IVC for better exposure. A tunnel is developed posterior to the left and middle hepatic veins, and a clamp is inserted from the left to emerge anterior to the IVC between the middle and right hepatic veins. The left and middle hepatic veins are divided at their common trunk or individually with vascular clamps or a stapler.

Biliary and Parenchymal Transection

Biliary injury during hepatectomy may occur when a tumor is near the hilus or an unrecognized anatomic variant is present. The hilar plate should be lowered routinely to allow the left hepatic duct to fall away from the base of segment 4. The bile duct is typically divided within the liver during right-sided liver resections, even when extrahepatic division of the artery and portal vein is performed. In contrast, the left bile duct may be divided safely outside the liver because of its extrahepatic length.

Parenchymal transection is performed along anatomic planes whenever possible to reduce blood loss. There are now numerous techniques to divide the liver parenchyma physically. A crushing technique using a Kelly clamp is simple and reliable. The use of vascular staplers to divide the parenchyma is less precise and should be avoided near a tumor to prevent compromising the surgical margin. In the presence of liver fibrosis, ultrasonic, thermal, or pressurized water dissection is used to reduce bleeding. Liver stitches are placed on either side of the intended line of transection to retract the liver open. Intrahepatic vessels and bile ducts are clipped or ligated. The Pringle maneuver is applied for 5- to 10-minute intervals during parenchymal division. Prolonged portal occlusion is avoided in steatotic livers. Most resections require less than 20 total minutes of Pringle occlusion. Low central venous pressure anesthesia is critical to minimize blood loss during liver transection. In the past, preoperative volume loading with crystalloid, albumin, blood, or fresh frozen plasma was used to blunt the anticipated blood loss. This approach actually exacerbated venous bleeding during mobilization and parenchymal division. Nowadays, central venous pressure is kept below 5 mm Hg by minimizing intravenous fluids, refraining from intraoperative blood transfusion unless there is significant (>25% of blood volume) hemorrhage, and accepting a urine output of 25 ml/hr. Intravenous nitroglycerin or nitroprusside is necessary rarely to lower the central venous pressure. Hemostasis of the liver edge is obtained with an argon beam coagulator, Avitene (Davol, Cranston, RI), Surgicel (Johnson & Johnson, New Brunswick, NJ), or suture ligation. Volume is restored after hemostasis is achieved. Abdominal drains generally are placed only if biliary reconstruction is performed.

SPECIFIC LIVER RESECTIONS

The common hepatic resections (Table 1) are described here. Specialty textbooks should be consulted for other types of resections, such as segmentectomy. Whenever possible, anatomic resection should be chosen over wedge resection. The main reason for this is that a segmental resection generally has a greater chance of achieving a negative margin of resection. Anatomic resection in colorectal cancer results in positive margins in only 2% of patients, compared with 16% for wedge resections at our institution. Furthermore, wedge resection of deep tumors is often associated with more bleeding because the hepatic vein branches that are typically located at the base of the tumor may not be sufficiently exposed to control them well. Wedge hepatectomy is usually performed only for small (<2 cm), superficial tumors for which wide margins can be readily achieved.

Table 1: Standardized Terminology of Hepatic Resections

Terminology	Segments
Right hepatectomy	5, 6, 7, 8
Right anterior sectionectomy	5, 8
Right posterior sectionectomy	6, 7
Left hepatectomy	2, 3, 4
Left lateral sectionectomy	2, 3
Left medial sectionectomy	4

From the Terminology Committee of the International Hepato-Pancreato-Biliary Association (www.IHPBA.org).

Staging laparoscopy is performed in high-risk patients (i.e., those with a risk score as defined below of greater than 2) or to evaluate specific abnormalities identified on preoperative imaging, such as a potential portal lymph node metastasis or peritoneal disease. Laparoscopic hepatectomy, with or without hand assistance, is evolving but is used mostly for minor hepatic resections of the left lateral section or superficial lesions. Intermittent Pringle control is used and the parenchyma is divided with a harmonic scalpel and vascular stapling. Hemostasis is obtained with a laparoscopic argon beam coagulator. Because laparoscopic resections tend to be wedge or atypical resections, care must be taken to achieve adequate tumor clearance. Improvements in laparoscopic instruments should promote the use of laparoscopic hepatectomy.

Right Hepatectomy

Right hepatectomy is the removal of segments 5, 6, 7, and 8. The right liver is mobilized, and the retrohepatic venules are divided to expose the right hepatic vein. A pedicle ligation approach is preferred to control the inflow. Generally, the gallbladder is removed, and the liver is split in the midline under Pringle control to expose the right main pedicle. Clamping the pedicle and the subsequent demarcation of the liver confirms correct identification of the pedicle. Extrahepatic dissection is performed when the tumor is close to the hilus. In this approach, the right hepatic artery is transected close to the liver, and its proximal stump is retracted to the left to expose the portal vein. A small caudate branch that arises from the posterolateral aspect of the right portal vein is divided, and the vein is then encircled. The vein is divided between clamps or with a vascular stapler. After the hilar plate is lowered, the right bile duct is usually divided within the liver during parenchymal transection to avoid injury to the left hepatic duct.

After the inflow is divided by the pedicle or extrahepatic approach, the right hepatic vein trunk is divided with a stapler. If it is necessary to divide the middle hepatic vein, this can usually be performed within the liver. Right liver mobilization is sometimes not possible, especially for large tumors at the dome of the liver. In these instances, an anterior approach is necessary. The liver is split, and the retrohepatic venules and the right hepatic vein are controlled within the liver.

Extended Right Hepatectomy

An extended right hepatectomy (also known as *right trisegmentectomy*) is a right hepatectomy plus removal of segment 4. There are two main differences from a right hepatectomy. First, the line of transection is more to the left. For tumors near the umbilical fissure, a formal dissection within the fissure may be necessary to obtain tumor clearance. For tumors at a distance from the umbilical fissure, the segment 4 feedback vessels can be divided within the liver parenchyma at a slight distance from the umbilical fissure. The plane of transection may be modified to preserve segment 4a or 4b, depending on the location of the tumors. The second major difference is that the middle hepatic vein must always be divided. This is generally performed within the liver unless a tumor lies near the middle hepatic vein trunk, in which case the vein is isolated just as it enters the liver. Because the middle and left hepatic veins usually join together before draining into the IVC, care must be taken not to injure the left hepatic vein if the proximal middle hepatic vein is divided.

Left Hepatectomy

Left hepatectomy is the resection of segments 2, 3, and 4. After the left liver is mobilized, the ligamentum teres is elevated, and the hilar plate is lowered. Extrahepatic dissection is performed to control the inflow at the base of the umbilical fissure. The left hepatic artery is located at the left edge of the porta hepatis. If an accessory or replaced left hepatic artery arising from the left gastric artery is present in the gastrohepatic ligament, it is divided. The left portal vein is then dissected and divided at the base of the umbilical fissure, above the origin of the caudate branches. The liver demarcates along the principal plane. Outflow control can be obtained within the liver or, if the tumor is close to the proximal left or middle hepatic vein, outside the liver. The left bile duct is divided outside the liver. It has a long extrahepatic course and is located just cephalad and behind the left portal vein. Parenchymal transection is performed in the principal plane starting in the gallbladder fossa and proceeding posteriorly. The dissection is carried to the left and becomes horizontal just above the hilar plate and the ligamentum venosum, thus separating the left liver from the anterior surface of the caudate.

Extended Left Hepatectomy

Extended left hepatectomy (also known as *left trisegmentectomy*) is a left hepatectomy plus removal of the anterior section of the right liver (segments 5 and 8). The procedure can be difficult to perform. The greatest risk is to the remaining posterior sector bile duct. The presence of a large inferior right hepatic vein allows sacrifice of the main right hepatic vein if necessary. It is essential to develop the proper plane of parenchymal transection. The plane begins several centimeters to the right of the gallbladder fossa and is parallel and just anterior to the right hepatic vein. Ideally, control of the right anterior sectoral pedicle is obtained to demarcate the horizontal plane of transection. This can be performed by following the main right portal pedicle into the liver or by finding the anterior sectoral pedicle deeper within the liver substance via splitting the liver.

Left Lateral Sectionectomy

The left lateral section (segments 2 and 3) is mobilized by dividing the left triangular ligament. If there is a bridge of liver tissue connecting segments 3 and 4, it is divided with cautery. If a tumor is near the umbilical fissure, then the segment 2 and 3 pedicles must be isolated and controlled separately within the umbilical fissure. For more laterally placed tumors, the liver is split from anterior to posterior, just to the left of the ligamentum teres and the falciform ligament. The inflow vessels and bile ducts are divided within the liver. The left hepatic vein is easily taken within the liver or, if a tumor is near the left hepatic vein trunk, it is taken outside the liver.

Other Procedures

The detailed procedures for other hepatic resections can be obtained from review articles or specialty textbooks cited at the end of the chapter. Isolated resection of segment 1 (caudate lobe) is performed either alone or in combination with hemihepatectomy. In either case, resection of the caudate is technically demanding because of its intimate relationship to the portal vein, IVC, and

hepatic veins. Segment 4 resection is relatively straightforward. Parenchymal transection begins at the inferior edge of the liver, and stay sutures are used to lift the segment upwards. The inflow and outflow are taken within the liver. In right posterior sectionectomy (segments 6 and 7), the right posterior portal pedicle is isolated using pedicle ligation. Pedicle clamping demarcates the liver section and guides the plane of transection. The right hepatic vein is isolated outside the liver and may have to be sacrificed, depending on the location of the disease. Central hepatectomy (segments 4, 5, and 8) is a combination of right anterior sectionectomy and segment 4 resection. The right anterior sectional pedicle is isolated by pedicle ligation or by tracing the right portal pedicle into the liver. The pedicle is clamped to reveal the right border of the resection. The left portion of segment 4 is divided near the umbilical fissure. Parenchymal transection is performed along the anterior border of the right hepatic vein and the left aspect of segment 4 until the two planes meet cephalad, where the middle hepatic vein is divided.

When tumors are poorly situated next to a contralateral main hepatic bile duct, it is sometimes necessary to perform a concomitant bile duct resection to obtain tumor clearance. Reconstruction is generally performed with a Roux-en-Y limb of jejunum. The use of an hepatic arterial infusion pump that is inserted at the time of hepatectomy has declined with the improved efficacy of systemic therapy. It is clear that regional arterial therapy does decrease intrahepatic recurrence, but the effect on overall survival is uncertain.

RESULTS

In 1001 patients with colorectal liver metastases who underwent hepatectomy at our institution, the perioperative mortality rate was 2.8%, median survival was 42 months, and 5-year actuarial survival was 37%. On multivariate analysis, there were five preoperative factors that predicted poor outcome: more than one tumor, tumor size greater than 5 cm, serum carcinoembryonic antigen (CEA) level greater than 200 ng/ml, positive nodal status of the primary colorectal tumor, and disease-free interval less than 1 year between the time of the colorectal primary and the liver metastases. Five-year survival depended on the preoperative "clinical risk score;" it was 44% in the presence of one risk factor, whereas it was 33% and 22% for those with three or all factors, respectively. A positive microscopic resection margin and extrahepatic disease also predicted poor survival. Further improvements in outcome after hepatectomy for colorectal metastases depend on the development of more effective systemic therapies to eradicate residual microscopic disease.

SUGGESTED READINGS

Bismuth H, Houssin D, Castaing D: Major and minor segmentectomies "reglees" in liver surgery, *World J Surg* 6:10, 1982.

Blumgart LH, Belghiti J, Buchler MW, DeMatteo RP, and others, editors: *Surgery of the liver and biliary tract* ed 4, St Louis, 2007, Elsevier.

Fong Y, Fortner J, Sun RL, and others: Clinical score for predicting recurrence after hepatic resection for metastatic colorectal cancer: analysis of 1001 consecutive cases, *Ann Surg* 230:309, 1999.

Liau K, Blumgart LH, DeMatteo RP: Segment-oriented approach to liver resection, *Surg Clin NA* 84:543, 2004.

COLORECTAL CANCER METASTATIC TO THE LIVER: RADIOFREQUENCY ABLATION

Anton J. Bilchik, MD, PhD

Surgical treatment is the gold standard for patients with liver metastases or primary liver tumors. Cure rates of 30% to 50% can follow the resection of liver metastases from colorectal cancer. Unfortunately, resection is possible in only approximately 20% of patients; most hepatic malignancies are surgically inaccessible or associated with a large tumor burden or inadequate hepatic reserve. Patients with unresectable disease may be candidates for systemic therapy, local ablative techniques (percutaneous ethanol injection, microwave tumor coagulation, interstitial laser photocoagulation, cryosurgical ablation, or radiofrequency ablation), or hepatic-directed therapy (hepatic artery ligation, chemoembolization, hepatic artery perfusion).

Cryosurgery freezes malignant tissues with liquid nitrogen and can destroy unresectable liver tumors while sparing normal tissue. Although a median survival of 26 to 30 months has been reported for patients treated with cryosurgery alone or in combination with hepatic resection, recurrence is common. Moreover, although cryosurgery can improve overall survival, it is associated with a relatively high rate of complications, including coagulopathy, hemorrhage, pleural effusion, parenchymal cracking, bile duct injury, and acute renal failure. Also, its instrumentation is cumbersome and expensive.

Unlike cryosurgical ablation, radiofrequency ablation (RFA) uses relatively inexpensive instrumentation and can be performed in the operating room via celiotomy or laparoscopy or in the radiology suite via a percutaneous approach. The application of high-frequency alternating current within tissue results in frictional heating of the tissue surrounding the electrode (Fig. 1). With a target temperature of greater than 90°C, larger zones of coagulative necrosis can occur. RFA has largely replaced cryosurgery for the treatment of unresectable metastases and can be used with other modes of liver-directed therapy such as resection and hepatic artery perfusion or in conjunction with systemic therapy for other sites of metastatic disease.

INDICATIONS AND PREOPERATIVE ASSESSMENT

Patients who present with primary or metastatic liver tumors should be evaluated for curative resection. Those whose performance status or disease location/distribution prohibits resection may be candidates for RFA. RFA has been used mainly for unresectable hepatocellular carcinoma or metastatic disease confined to the liver. Some patients have resectable disease but limited hepatic reserve; for example, a patient with hepatic recurrence after previous hepatectomy may not have sufficient hepatic reserve for additional resection. In other patients with bilobar disease, resection of larger lesions and RFA of smaller lesions can completely eradicate tumor while maintaining hepatic reserve. Finally, in patients who have multiple comorbid factors and are at high risk for general anesthesia, a less invasive approach such as percutaneous RFA may be preferable.

Because tumors may be deemed unresectable on the basis of size, number, location, or doubling time, the preoperative workup must include imaging to look for other sites of disease, prior response to other therapies, and the nature of the disease. Before RFA, all patients should undergo computed tomography (CT), magnetic resonance imaging (MRI), FDG-positron emission tomography (PET), or a combination of these modalities. Baseline hepatic function should be assessed through laboratory indicators of synthetic function and Child-Pugh classification of liver dysfunction. A thorough history and physical examination are essential to determine patient performance and treatment history.

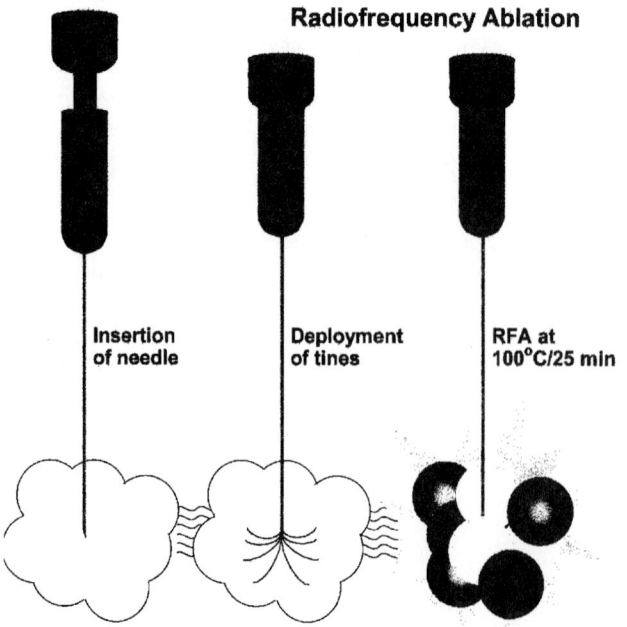

Radiofrequency Ablation

Insertion of needle

Deployment of tines

RFA at 100°C/25 min

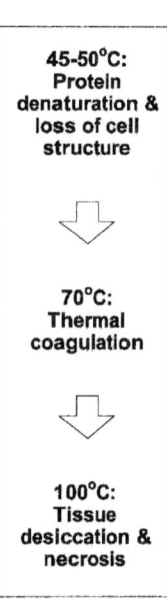

45-50°C: Protein denaturation & loss of cell structure

70°C: Thermal coagulation

100°C: Tissue desiccation & necrosis

Figure 1 A high-frequency alternating current heats the tissue surrounding the electrode. Current-induced ionic vibration leads to protein denaturation, thermal coagulation, and ultimately cell death. *From Bilchik AJ, Wood TF, Allegra DP: Oncologist 6:24, 2001. Reprinted with permission.*

TECHNICAL CONSIDERATIONS

RFA can be performed by celiotomy (open), laparoscopy, or a percutaneous approach. The choice of technique depends on the patient's condition, the number and location of liver tumors, and the skill of the physician performing the ablation. Each approach offers certain advantages and disadvantages that must be weighed to determine the best approach for the individual patient. In general, percutaneous RFA should be reserved for patients too ill to undergo laparoscopy/laparotomy and for patients who have undergone multiple prior laparotomies.

Open or Laparoscopic Radiofrequency Ablation

RFA via celiotomy (open RFA) or via laparoscopy is performed with ultrasound guidance in the operating room while the patient is under general anesthesia. An operative approach via laparoscopy or laparotomy allows detection of extrahepatic disease missed by preprocedure imaging. The ability to use intraoperative ultrasound during celiotomy or laparoscopy is also the most accurate method for the detection of small hepatic lesions. Approximately 12% of patients undergoing laparoscopy before RFA have extrahepatic disease and therefore will not be candidates for potentially curative procedures.

If the procedure is performed through a laparoscope, two ports are placed in the right upper quadrant because most patients have undergone a midline laparotomy (Table 1). A limited takedown of adhesions is performed. The liver is mobilized by taking down the falciform and triangular ligaments. A 30-degree angled laparoscope can be used to explore all parietal and visceral peritoneal surfaces, the lesser sac, omentum, and viscera. If extrahepatic disease is found, RFA should not be performed and systemic treatment should be considered.

At laparotomy or laparoscopy, a flexible 7.5-MHz intraoperative ultrasonography (IOUS) probe is used to evaluate all eight sections of the liver and determine the proximity of liver lesions to major vascular and biliary structures. The exact location of hepatic metastases affects the technical approach for RFA. The porta hepatis is examined, and enlarged lymph nodes are biopsied.

Resectable tumors should be resected; if a decision is made to proceed with RFA, the probe should be placed parallel to the IOUS probe. This is similar to the technique used for biopsy of breast lesions. Adjacent viscera is protected by blunt retraction. Ultrasonography is used to guide the probe into the lesion, and the ablation is monitored by real-time ultrasonographic imaging of an expanding hyperechogenic zone. Ultrasonography cannot reliably distinguish between ablated and normal tissue, and thus ablation should begin

Table 1: Steps for Laparoscopic Radiofrequency Ablation

1. Place two ports in upper abdomen.
2. Take down adhesions.
3. Explore peritoneal cavity.
4. Mobilize liver and protect adjacent viscera.
5. Evaluate porta hepatis and biopsy portal nodes if necessary.
6. Examine eight segments using flexible 7.5-mHz intraoperative ultrasound probe.
7. Place radiofrequency ablation probe parallel to ultrasound probe.
8. Ablate periphery of lesion.
9. Overlap ablations for larger lesions.
10. Cauterize probe track to minimize bleeding.

at the most posterior portion of the tumor. The probe then can be withdrawn in approximately 2-cm increments to create sequential overlapping zones of ablated tissue. Depending on the maximal ablation size achievable by the probe, multiple overlapping ablations may be necessary to destroy a tumor and produce a surrounding rim of necrosis. This can be technically challenging. If target temperatures are not reached, as may be the case for lesions near major vascular structures (heat-sink), the tines are withdrawn slightly or rotated approximately 45 degrees to increase the temperature in the region of ablation. Each ablation should include a 1-cm margin of normal parenchyma to ensure complete tumor destruction and reduce the risk of local recurrence.

After ablation, the probe track is cauterized as the RFA probe is withdrawn to prevent hemorrhage and tumor seeding. Patients are typically observed in the hospital overnight.

Percutaneous Radiofrequency Ablation

Percutaneous RFA is performed in the radiology suite by an experienced interventional radiologist; the procedure is guided by ultrasonography or CT while the patient is under local anesthesia and conscious sedation. Only an experienced interventional radiologist, in conjunction with a multidisciplinary team, should decide which tumors are safe and appropriate to ablate via this route.

Percutaneous ablation can damage structures unrelated to the ablation target. Diaphragmatic injuries are not uncommon because of poor diaphragmatic visualization. Transdiaphragmatic probe insertion can thus occur, even in CT-guided attempts to place the probe into high hepatic lesions. Misidentification and nonidentification of structures can also cause visceral injuries, such as bowel and ureteral complications. To avoid injury to adjacent structures, lesions approached percutaneously must therefore not be located close to visceral organs or biliary structures. Furthermore, the lesion size and location must be within the capacity of the percutaneous approach.

Because it is minimally invasive and has no cumulative toxicity, percutaneous RFA may be considered for hepatic recurrences (Fig. 2). Although repeat hepatic resection is associated with improved survival, a second surgery may be associated with a high morbidity because of inadequate hepatic reserve.

MONITORING AND FOLLOW-UP

The adequacy of ablation is typically monitored by CT or magnetic resonance imaging (MRI). The treatment area should encompass the tumor and at least a 1-cm rim of normal tissue. A CT scan is obtained 1 week after the procedure (baseline), at 3-month intervals during the first year, and every 6 months thereafter. The baseline image obtained with contrast enhancement reveals a hypovascular ablated field with a rim of hypervascular inflammatory tissue. The rim enhancement area should disappear over several months as inflammation resolves. Comparing preoperative imaging with postoperative imaging is important to determine the adequacy of treatment, and serial imaging is essential for early detection of recurrence. Recurrences appear as irregular nonenhancing areas on contrast CT. Postoperative PET scans are also useful to evaluate recurrence.

RESULTS

Laparoscopic and Laparotomy Radiofrequency Ablation

At the John Wayne Cancer Institute, combined laparoscopy and laparoscopic intraoperative ultrasound findings changed the

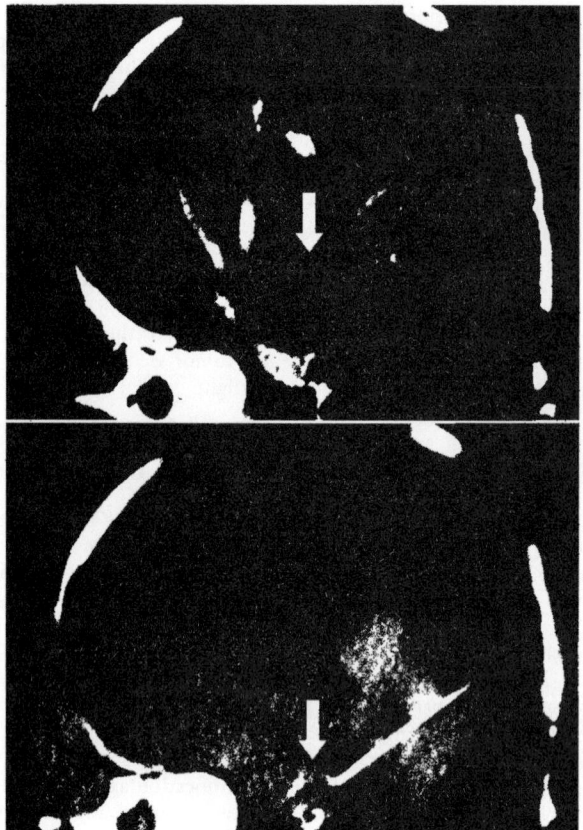

Figure 2 RFA site recurrences appear as a rim of increased contrast uptake around an ablation scar *(arrow, top panel).* Recurrences can be successfully ablated by a percutaneous approach *(arrow, bottom panel). From Wood TF, Rose DM, Chung M, and others: Ann Surg Oncol 7:593, 2000. Reprinted with permission.*

operative management in 32% of the patients. Laparoscopy detected more lesions in 11 of 50 patients, and laparoscopic intraoperative ultrasound detected more lesions in 18 of 50 patients. Most of the additional tumors were less than 1 cm in diameter and located on or near the surface of the liver. However, two patients had intraparenchymal lesions 1 to 2 cm in diameter that were missed by preoperative imaging. All additionally discovered hepatic tumors were ablated successfully. Laparoscopic RFA was also effective in 11 (41%) patients who had undergone prior laparotomies, specifically colectomy ($n = 7$), small bowel operations ($n = 3$), or cryosurgery ($n = 1$).

Although the local tumor recurrence rate at the RFA site was only 4.7% at a mean follow-up of 14 months, 16 (59%) patients experienced progression of disease in the liver and at other sites. This high rate of disease progression supports the value of a minimally invasive approach for unresectable hepatic tumors in this group of patients with a short expected survival. All patients tolerated the procedure extremely well, were discharged home in 1 day, and were able to perform most activities of daily living within 1 week.

The celiotomy approach, which requires inpatient admission, is the most invasive but also the most versatile. During open procedures, large and multiple tumors may be safely treated, and concurrent procedures such as resection and placement of a hepatic artery infusion pump can be performed. Both laparoscopy and laparotomy therefore provide better staging and may result in fewer complications because of the ability to protect vital structures.

Percutaneous Radiofrequency Ablation

Because percutaneous RFA is the least invasive technique and can be performed as an outpatient procedure or during a 23-hour stay, most published studies of RFA have used a percutaneous approach. Reported rates of local recurrence, complications, and survival are acceptable but require validation by follow-up data and prospective randomization. Percutaneous RFA relies on accurate preoperative location of hepatic tumors, which may fail to detect tumors smaller than 1 cm in diameter. Recent studies suggest that it is responsible for the largest number of documented complications, as well as the highest rates of recurrence. RFA under CT scan or transabdominal ultrasound guidance precludes the use of intraoperative ultrasound, and this may account for the higher local recurrence rate.

At the John Wayne Cancer Institute, 34 patients have undergone percutaneous RFA for 167 tumor recurrences. Twenty-six patients were treated twice, four were treated three times, three were treated four times, and one was treated eight times. The local recurrence rate was 19.8%, and the morbidity was 23.5% compared with 12% and 10% in patients undergoing single ablations. The median hospital stay was only 1 day. Multivariate analysis identified tumor size as the only significant predictor of recurrence. Because the number of ablations may be directly related to the risk of incomplete cytoreduction and subsequent tumor recurrence, it is not surprising that local recurrence and morbidity were higher in the serially ablated population. However, the nearly identical distribution of disease status for patients who underwent single versus serial ablations is intriguing and merits continued follow-up.

COMPLICATIONS

Reported morbidity and mortality rates associated with RFA can be difficult to interpret, in part because technical approaches vary. Some investigators combine RFA with other treatments such as liver resection; the addition of a second procedure may inflate the complication rate. Ablation of multiple tumors also increases the risk of complications such as bleeding or bile leak. Early studies often used multiple sequential RFAs for treatment of a single hepatic tumor because the monopolar electrode gave a smaller thermal ablation field than the current cluster electrodes. The multiple ablations required to destroy larger tumors increased the potential for complications.

Unfortunately, the reporting of morbidities is also not standardized. Some authors regard low-grade fevers, transient liver function test elevations, small pleural effusions, and right upper quadrant pain as minor complications, whereas others believe these are expected events that should not be reported. As expected, studies undertaken at institutions with skilled interventionalists or surgeons report fewer complications. Variations in patient selection and disease type also confound interpretation of results. For example, comorbid factors for patients with hepatocellular carcinoma are different from those for patients with colorectal metastases. The preprocedural state may influence the outcome of RFA.

Direct complications of RFA include biloma, biliary fistula, ascites, hepatic insufficiency, arteriovenous fistula, symptomatic pleural effusion, abscess, pain, hemorrhage, hydropneumothorax, pneumothorax, and thermal injury to surrounding structures. Burns related to grounding pads have also been reported; these can be avoided by proper positioning of the pads, by using a larger number of pads for longer ablations, and by carefully following the manufacturer's directions. Other potential complications are those related to an operative procedure, such as myocardial infarction, cardiac arrhythmias, and pneumonia.

At the John Wayne Cancer Institute, complications of RFA have mostly been related to infection (30%) and biliary injury (14%). Although no specific risk factors for infectious complications have yet been identified, we rigorously screen preoperatively for potential pulmonary, gastrointestinal, and indwelling catheter-related sources that may seed the RFA coagulum. The reported rate of biliary injuries is approximately 20%, in part because RFA is often the only treatment option for patients with peribiliary tumors. To ablate

Figure 3 After right hepatic lobectomy for colorectal metastasis *(upper left panel),* this patient developed an unresectable central hepatic metastasis that was approached percutaneously *(lower left panel).* After RFA, the hepatic and portal veins remained patent *(upper right panel).* However, the postprocedure course was complicated by a bile duct stricture and subsequent hepatic abscess, which were successfully managed by percutaneous drainage of the abscess and endoscopic placement of a biliary stent *(lower right panel).* From Wood TF, Rose DM, Chung M, and others: Ann Surg Oncol 7:593, 2000. Reprinted with permission.

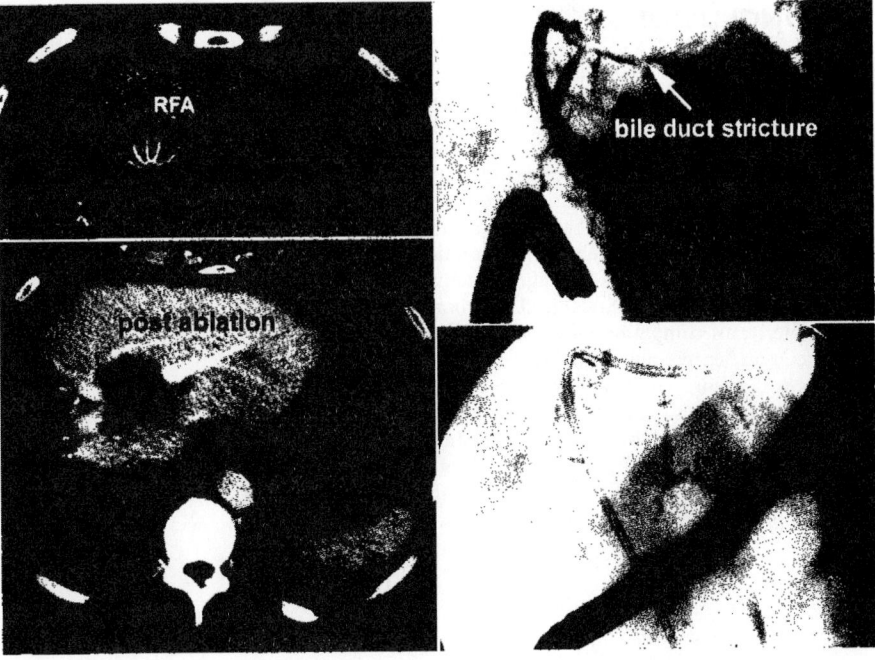

these tumors with less chance of biliary injury, we stent the biliary system via endoscopic retrograde pancreatography before RFA (Fig. 3). We have performed this procedure in 10 patients to date with no postablation injury. The stents are removed 4 to 6 weeks after the procedure.

RESPONSE RATES

Local recurrence rates after RFA are difficult to interpret across studies. Some authors report recurrences after complete ablation as determined by early postoperative CT or MRI images, whereas others do not confirm complete response by postoperative imaging and report recurrences based on follow-up imaging. Some investigators also report recurrence rates within the whole liver rather than at the site of ablation. The length of follow-up also affects the recurrence rate. Response rates vary from 48% to 98% across studies, in part because of differences in the size of treated lesions. Larger lesions typically require overlapping ablations. Areas of treated tumor may obscure ultrasound imaging of untreated tumor, resulting in higher treatment failures and recurrences.

The approach to RFA also influences response rates. One study reported that 6 of 76 patients who underwent percutaneous RFA had an incomplete response, whereas all 34 patients who underwent laparoscopic or open RFA had a complete response. This difference might be explained by better hepatic imaging with intraoperative ultrasonography during laparoscopy or celiotomy than with transabdominal ultrasonography during percutaneous RFA. Another possibility is that intraoperative probe positioning may be more accurate than percutaneous placement of the probe.

Tumor location adjacent to large vessels also influences response rates. Blood flow from large vessels will create a heat-sink effect that cools surrounding tissue and increases the temperature necessary for complete ablation. Large vessels are resistant to high temperatures that can damage surrounding tissue. Vascular inflow occlusion reportedly can increase the area of ablation in patients undergoing RFA of tumors larger than 35 mm or near large blood vessels. A Pringle maneuver therefore might improve the efficacy of ablation when tumors are near major blood vessels.

In general, the rate of recurrence increases with the size of the hepatic tumor and with the presence of tumor vascular invasion or hepatic dysfunction (or both). Data from the John Wayne Cancer Institute indicate that tumor size significantly influenced local recurrence of metastatic disease, independent of RFA technique. No study has shown that differences in technique influence the rate of recurrence after a complete response. Most studies also report local recurrence rates using first-generation RFA probes. Advances in probe technology and intraoperative imaging will probably decrease these rates. Indeed, we recently demonstrated that local recurrence rates after use of probes introduced between 2001 and 2004 were significantly lower than recurrence rates after use of older probes. Technologic advances such as the delivery of microwave current now allow destruction of lesions as large as 7 cm with a single ablation; higher temperatures reduce ablation time.

There are few reports of survival rates following RFA. Differences in patient selection, follow-up time, tumor type, and RFA approach make studies difficult to compare. The 3-year survival following RFA for colorectal cancer ranges from 37% to 46%. A retrospective analysis reported survival data for a 9-year series of patients treated with RFA alone or with resection. Many patients had extensive disease that had progressed on chemotherapy. At a mean follow-up of 33 months, the overall survival for patients with ablated colorectal liver metastases was 29.7 months. Of 521 tumors treated, 24% recurred. The incidence of local recurrence was significantly higher when tumor size exceeded 3 cm (28% vs. 17.8%; $p < .04$). Moreover, patients who had undergone RFA alone had a higher rate of recurrence than those treated with a combination of resection and RFA.

One retrospective study of 358 patients with colorectal liver metastases compared resection, RFA plus resection, RFA alone, and laparotomy with biopsy. RFA was used for cure when complete resection was not possible. All patient-related and tumor-related factors known to influence outcome were similar among the groups. The rate of recurrence was 84% after RFA alone, 63% after RFA plus resection, and 52% after resection alone. Local recurrence (in the area treated) was more common after RFA plus resection (9%) than RFA alone (5%) or resection alone (2%). The 3-year rate of overall survival was 73% after resection, 43% after RFA plus resection, and 37% after RFA alone. Patients who underwent RFA had a survival advantage over patients who underwent biopsy with or without chemotherapy.

CONCLUSIONS

Resection remains the first choice for patients with disease confined to the liver, in part because recent data demonstrate higher local recurrence rates after RFA than after resection. However, RFA is a useful adjunct to resection, and it may be a successful alternative to resection when extensive disease and limited hepatic reserve, bilobar disease, or medical conditions would preclude laparotomy. Recent data suggest that RFA may confer a survival advantage over chemotherapy alone, and a randomized multicenter phase III trial is evaluating the potential advantage of adding RFA to oxaliplatin-based chemotherapy. Outcome data from this trial and large multicenter trials comparing RFA and resection will help to establish a comprehensive algorithm for multimodal management of patients with colorectal hepatic metastases. In the meantime, RFA technology continues to evolve with the introduction of new probes that increase the field of ablation and simplify the technique. Microwave ablation has been introduced as a rapid method of delivering high temperatures to a large area of the liver, possibly reducing local recurrence rates.

SUGGESTED READINGS

Abdalla EK, Vauthey J-N, Ellis LM, and others: Recurrence and outcomes following hepatic resection, radiofrequency ablation, and combined resection/ablation for colorectal liver metastases, *Ann Surg* 239:818, 2004.

Ahmad A, Chen SL, Kavanagh MA, and others: Radiofrequency ablation of hepatic metastases from colorectal cancer: are newer generation probes better? *Am Surg* 72:875, 2006.

Amersi FF, McElrath-Garza A, Ahmad A, and others: Long-term survival after radiofrequency ablation of complex unresectable liver tumors, *Arch Surg* 141:581, 2006.

Bleicher RJ, Allegra DP, Nora DT, and others: Radiofrequency ablation in 447 complex unresectable liver tumors: lessons learned, *Ann Surg Oncol* 10:52, 2003.

Fahy BN, Jarnagin WR: Evolving techniques in the treatment of liver colorectal metastases: role of laparoscopy, radiofrequency ablation, microwave coagulation, hepatic arterial chemotherapy, indications and contraindications for resection, role of transplantation, and timing of chemotherapy, *Surg Clin North Am* 86:1005, 2006.

Livraghi T, Solbiati L, Meloni MF, and others: Treatment of focal liver tumors with percutaneous radio-frequency ablation: complications encountered in a multicenter study, *Radiology* 226:441, 2003.

Vivarelli M, Guglielmi A, Ruzzenente A, and others: Surgical resection versus percutaneous radiofrequency ablation in the treatment of hepatocellular carcinoma on cirrhotic liver, *Ann Surg* 240:102, 2004.

FACTORS AFFECTING MORBIDITY AND MORTALITY AFTER LIVER RESECTION

Nestor F. Esnaola, MD, MPH, and Steven A. Curley, MD

Expansion of the indications for resection in patients with primary and metastatic hepatic malignancies has led to a dramatic increase in the number of liver resections performed in recent years. Since the mid-1970s, the perioperative mortality rate of hepatectomy has decreased from as high as 20% before 1980, to less than 5% in recent series from high-volume centers. Several factors are likely responsible for the improvement in outcomes during this period, including improved patient selection, novel anesthetic techniques, better understanding of the functional anatomy of the liver, advances in surgical technique, and improvements in postoperative care.

PREOPERATIVE FACTORS

Age and Comorbidity

As with any major surgery, it is important to assess fully the general medical fitness of patients when selecting candidates for hepatic resection. Although hepatobiliary malignancies are particularly prevalent during the sixth to eighth decades of life, advanced age is often perceived as a rough proxy for occult comorbid illness and considered to be a relative contraindication to hepatectomy.

Recent large series using multivariate analyses, however, suggest that age alone has a marginal impact on perioperative outcomes when controlling for other patient-, liver-, and surgery-related factors. In contrast, the presence of active comorbidities has been shown to increase the risk of postoperative complications. In fact, an American Society of Anesthesiologists (ASA) risk score greater than 1 (denoting "a patient with mild systemic disease") was recently shown to double the rate of complications and increase the risk of death after hepatectomy by a factor of 10. More specifically, preoperative cardiovascular disease has been identified as an independent predictor of morbidity after resection, highlighting the importance of careful cardiovascular risk assessment and proactive management of cardiovascular disease prior to surgery. A careful pulmonary evaluation is also mandatory in patients with a history of heavy tobacco use, asthma, or chronic obstructive pulmonary disease, particularly because pulmonary complications, such as pneumonia and respiratory failure, have been reported to occur in up to 20% of patients. Although diabetes has been linked to abnormalities in liver metabolism and immune function, its impact on postoperative outcomes is debatable. Although some investigators have noted an increased association between diabetes and perioperative complications, recent studies suggest that this association is in fact mediated by the presence of secondary hepatic parenchymal abnormalities, such as steatosis, rather than by the disease itself.

Underlying Hepatic Function

A significant proportion of patients with primary and metastatic liver tumors present with underlying, preexisting liver disease. The function of the noncancerous liver must also be taken into account when selecting among various treatments because it can have a profound effect on both perioperative and long-term outcomes. The reported overall mortality rate of liver resection varies from less than 1% in patients with normal underlying parenchyma to 5% in patients with diseased livers, even at major hepatobiliary centers. In general, elective surgery is contraindicated in patients with evidence of active alcoholic or viral hepatitis and elevated transaminase levels indicative of ongoing, active hepatocyte damage. The risk of death in these patients has been reported to range from 9.5% to 55%, and surgery must be postponed until the transaminitis has resolved.

A significant percentage of patients referred for hepatic resection also have evidence of nonalcoholic fatty liver disease, which can have a significant negative impact on perioperative outcomes. The mildest form, steatosis, is characterized by accumulation of fat in the liver and is estimated to occur in 6% to 11% of the general population. In Western countries, steatosis is present in approximately 25% of liver donors and 20% of patients who present for liver resection. Pathologically, it is characterized by the percentage of hepatocytes with fat inclusions on hematoxylin and eosin staining and is usually quantified as "mild" (< 30%), "moderate" (30% to 60%), or "severe" (> 60%). In animal models, steatosis is associated with decreased adenosine triphosphate (ATP) production, impaired sinusoidal flow, and Kupffer cell dysfunction. In addition, fatty hepatocytes appear to be less tolerant of ischemic insults and have impaired ability to regenerate. In human subjects, steatosis has been linked to obesity, long-standing diabetes, and preoperative chemotherapy, and it has been associated with increased rates of postoperative infection and complications after liver resection (Fig. 1). In a recent study, moderate to severe steatosis was associated with a threefold increased risk of postoperative complication, even when controlling for age, comorbidity, and extent of resection. Although steatosis can result in soft, friable livers that can make parenchymal transection more difficult, the same study failed to show an association between degree of steatosis and blood loss, need for transfusion, operative time, or postoperative mortality.

Steatohepatitis, a more severe form of nonalcoholic fatty liver disease, is characterized by lobular inflammation and hepatocyte degeneration, which can eventually lead to parenchymal fibrosis and cirrhosis. It is rarely observed in the setting of obesity alone and is therefore thought to be mediated by a "second hit," which leads to lipid peroxidation and release of reactive oxygen species or endotoxemia. Steatohepatitis is associated with impaired hepatocyte proliferation because of alterations of the nuclear factor (NF)-kappa B pathway, which is involved in the priming phase of liver regeneration. Steatohepatitis has been observed after long-term total parenteral nutrition or jejunoileal bypass surgery and has been increasingly observed in patients with hepatic colorectal metastases treated with neoadjuvant chemotherapy. A recent study noted a fivefold increase in steatohepatitis at the time of hepatectomy in patients pretreated with irinotecan-based, but not oxaliplatin-based, therapy. Of note, patients with steatohepatitis had a markedly increased risk of 90-day mortality and death rate from postoperative liver failure compared with patients without steatohepatitis

(14.7% vs. 1.6%, and 5.8% vs. 0.6%, respectively). Neoadjuvant chemotherapy is increasingly being used in patients with hepatic colorectal metastases to reduce tumor size and increase the pool of resectable patients. Given the potential risks of chemotherapy-induced steatosis and steatohepatitis after hepatectomy, the use of neoadjuvant therapy in patients with resectable disease at presentation should be considered carefully.

The addition of bevacizumab, a monoclonal antibody to vascular endothelial growth factor A (VEGF-A), has been shown to improve response rates with neoadjuvant chemotherapy even further. A recent analysis of pooled data from two randomized trials revealed an increased risk of postoperative wound complications (13% vs. 3.4%) in patients with metastatic colorectal cancer who underwent surgery while on bevacizumab therapy. Given the fact that VEGF plays a central role in liver regeneration after hepatectomy and that hepatic steatosis has been shown to impair angiogenesis in animal models, concerns have been raised regarding the safety of combined bevacizumab and combined chemotherapy in the neoadjuvant setting. Bevacizumab has a relatively long half-life of approximately 20 days, and there is no reliable way to measure free circulating VEGF levels. Most experts currently suggest waiting at least 6 to 8 weeks after the last dose of bevacizumab before performing hepatectomy, although there are no preclinical or clinical data to support this recommendation.

Cholestasis is a major risk factor for poor outcome after liver surgery, even in noncirrhotics, and postoperative mortality rates approaching 20% have been reported. Cholestasis in the absence of obvious biliary obstruction can be a manifestation of serious, underlying hepatocellular dysfunction and can progress to hepatic failure and death if the cause cannot be readily identified and the process reversed. Obstructive jaundice, on the other hand, usually represents a potential reversible situation, and patients who are candidates for hepatectomy should be referred for immediate biliary decompression. After the biliary tree has been drained and serum bilirubin levels have returned to near normal (≤3 mg/dl), resection can be performed. Failure of laboratory studies to normalize after biliary drainage should be interpreted as a sign of ongoing hepatic insufficiency and is a contraindication to resection. A recent Japanese study estimated the safe and permissible limits of hepatectomy in patients with obstructive jaundice to be 48.7% and 71.6%, respectively. Preoperative portal vein embolization (see Residual Liver Volume later in the chapter) increased the safe limit of hepatectomy to 67.4%. Resections beyond the reported permissible limit, however, were associated with irreversible hyperbilirubinemia (>14.4 mg/dl) and liver failure.

Parenchymal fibrosis and cirrhosis resulting from chronic liver disease are associated with an increased risk of morbidity and mortality after hepatic resection. The wide range of reported mortality rates in "cirrhotic" patients speaks to the degree of heterogeneity within this group and highlights the need to grade the degree of fibrosis in the noncancerous liver to stratify patients better. In one study, the risk of death after hepatectomy was 0% in patients with grade 0 to 3 fibrosis (i.e., no fibrosis to portal inflammation with bridging fibrosis), compared with 32% in patients with grade 4 fibrosis (i.e., frank cirrhosis). Cirrhotic patients are commonly stratified using a combination of clinical, laboratory, and radiologic criteria. Most Western centers initially classify patients using the Child-Turcotte-Pugh (CTP) score (Table 1), which was specifically created and modified to stratify patients with cirrhosis with respect to perioperative risk. The CTP score is simple to use, serves as a rough measure of the synthetic and detoxifying capacity of the underlying liver, and has significant prognostic value in the postoperative setting. In patients undergoing major abdominal surgery, perioperative mortality rates of 10%, 30%, and 80% have been reported in class A, B, and C cirrhotics, respectively. Therefore only patients who are CTP class A are generally considered for major hepatic resections, whereas class B patients may be occasionally considered for minor resections of superficial tumors. A recent

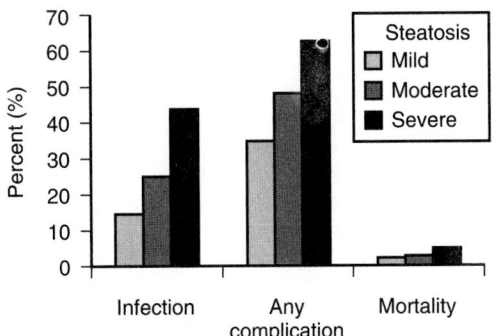

Figure 1 Association between hepatic steatosis and postoperative outcomes following elective hepatic resection. There is a direct relationship between increasing degrees of steatosis and rates of postoperative infection (p < .01) and overall complications (p < .01). There is also a trend toward increased mortality, although it is not statistically significant (p = .29). *Data from Kooby DA, Fong Y, Suriawinata A, and others: J Gastrointest Surg 7:1034, 2003.*

Table 1: Child-Turcotte-Pugh (CTP) Score to Assess Severity of Cirrhosis

Parameter	Points		
	1	2	3
Total bilirubin (mg/dl)	<2	2–3	>3
Serum albumin (g/dl)	>3.5	2.8–3.5	<2.8
International Normalized Ratio	<1.7	1.71–2.20	>2.20
Ascites	None	Suppressed with medication	Refractory
Hepatic encephalopathy	None	Grade I–II	Grade III–IV (or refractory)

Most authors place patients with 5 or 6 points in class A, 7 to 9 points in class B, and 10 to 15 points in class C.

study from the Mayo Clinic suggests that use of the Model for End-Stage Liver Disease (MELD) score in class A cirrhotics, a composite of the international normalized ratio, serum total bilirubin, and serum creatinine, may help to further stratify these patients before surgery. The postoperative mortality in class A patients with a MELD score of 8 or less was 0%, compared with 26% in patients with a MELD score of 9 or greater. MELD score was an independent predictor of mortality risk after resection, along with the ASA classification and clinical tumor symptoms.

Several tests have been developed that quantitatively measure the ability of the liver to extract, transform, and metabolize certain target substances. The most commonly used test is the indocyanine green (ICG) clearance test, which provides an indirect measure of hepatic blood flow. A multivariate analysis by a group in Hong Kong revealed that out of the various liver function tests, ICG clearance was the single best predictor of postoperative mortality after major resection for hepatocellular carcinoma. In patients with cirrhosis, an ICG retention at 15 minutes of less than 14% after an intravenous injection of 0.5 mg/kg is considered the safety limit for major resection (i.e., ≥3 segments). Despite its potential to identify "marginal" patients who might otherwise go on to resection, the ICG clearance is rarely used or is unavailable at most Western centers.

Portal hypertension is associated with an increased risk of serious bleeding and postoperative liver failure after hepatectomy. In class A cirrhotic patients, thrombocytopenia, grade II or III esophageal varices, splenomegaly, or ascites are signs of potentially significant portal hypertension and are widely considered to be contraindications to surgery. A more quantitative way to detect portal hypertension involves cannulating the femoral vein and advancing a balloon catheter to the main right hepatic vein under fluoroscopic guidance. By wedging the balloon at this site and occluding the vein, the hepatic venous pressure gradient (HVPG) can be measured. Although invasive, measurement of the HVPG can help to further stratify class A cirrhotics before major resection. In a study by the Barcelona group, unresolved hepatic decompensation occurred in 11 of 15 patients with an HVPG 10 mm Hg or greater, compared to 0 of 14 patients with a preoperative HVPG less than 10 mm Hg.

Residual Liver Volume

Before proceeding with hepatectomy, it is imperative to determine whether the volume of the liver that will remain after resection,

the future liver remnant (FLR), will be sufficient to sustain adequate hepatic function postoperatively. Direct measurement of the future liver remnant can be reliably and reproducibly performed using computed tomography (CT). The volume of the expected FLR is initially measured directly using three-dimensional, CT-volumetric analysis. The total liver volume (TLV) is then estimated using a formula relating TLV to body surface area (BSA): $TLV = -794.41 + 1267.28 \times BSA$ (m^2). The ratio of the FLR to the TLV is then calculated and expressed as a ratio. In patients with normal hepatic parenchyma, an FLR greater than 20% is generally recommended to minimize the risk of major postoperative complications, including postoperative liver failure. In patients with abnormal hepatic parenchyma (i.e., patients treated with neoadjuvant chemotherapy with steatosis or cirrhotics), an FLR greater than 30% is generally recommended. A recent study revealed that although only 10% of patients scheduled to undergo right hepatic hepatectomy had an FLR 20% or less, approximately 75% of patients scheduled to undergo extended right hepatectomy had an FLR 20% or less. The risk of postoperative complications approached 50% in patients with a preoperative FLR 20% or less, compared with approximately 10% in patients with a preoperative FLR above 20%. Therefore it is important to assess the FLR in patients who may require extended hepatectomy, particularly if they are suspected or known to have abnormal liver parenchyma.

In patients with an inadequate preoperative FLR, portal vein embolization (PVE) of the segments to be resected can be used to induce hypertrophy of the FLR and allow safe hepatic resection. PVE arose from the observation that tumor invasion of the portal vein results in ipsilateral lobe atrophy and contralateral lobe hypertrophy. PVE was initially used to induce lobar hypertrophy before surgery in patients with hepatocellular carcinoma and was later used to allow extended hepatic resections in patients with an inadequate FLR. PVE is performed via a percutaneous, transhepatic technique, and an ipsilateral approach to the relevant portal vein branches is used to avoid damage to the contralateral vasculature. Embolization is usually performed using polyvinyl alcohol and metal coils, and side effects include transient fever and pain. More serious complications are rare, and no deaths have been reported. On average, PVE can increase the FLR by 8% to 27%, and approximately 58% to 100% of patients go on to resection. In a recent study of patients with hepatic colorectal metastases treated with extended hepatic resection, the 5-year survival rate of patients pretreated with PVE was 40%, which compared favorably with a similar group of patients who did not require preoperative PVE. At our centers, we often consider preoperative PVE in patients with "normal" livers and an FLR 20% or less who require extended resection, as well as patients with steatosis or chronic liver disease with an FLR 30% or less who require major resection.

Complex Hepatectomy

A significant proportion of patients with primary biliary malignancies and hepatic colorectal metastases may require "complex hepatectomy," or performance of another major intra-abdominal procedure in addition to the primary hepatic resection at the time of presentation. This can include portal vein or caval resection, biliary resection and reconstruction, or other organ resection, such as colectomy or proctectomy. In a large series of patients with no underlying liver disease undergoing elective hepatectomy, the performance of an extrahepatic procedure was associated with a perioperative mortality rate of 5.8% (compared with 0.4% in patients treated with hepatectomy alone). Complex hepatectomy was an independent predictor of death in patients with malignancy, with a relative risk of 7.49. In a more recent series, complex hepatectomy was associated with increased blood loss, morbidity rate, and length of hospital stay. In patients who underwent major hepatic resections (three or more segments), complex hepatectomy was associated with a twofold increase in postoperative mortality rate (6.7% vs. 3%). Although complex hepatectomy often cannot be avoided in patients with biliary malignancies, careful consideration should be given to staged procedures in patients with asymptomatic, synchronous colorectal primaries, particularly if major resection or proctectomy is contemplated.

Suggested Preoperative Algorithm

Figures 2 and 3 outline our algorithms for assessing preoperative hepatic function and reserve in patients with presumably normal livers and patients with chronic liver disease. In asymptomatic, otherwise healthy patients, a thorough history and physical focusing on risk factors (e.g., previous transfusions, tattoos, alcohol use, intravenous drug use) and subtle symptoms or signs of occult, underlying liver disease is required. Screening liver function tests may also be useful, particularly in patients with hepatocellular carcinoma in whom the tumor may represent the first manifestation of chronic liver disease. In patients with abnormal serum liver function tests or evidence of significant steatosis on imaging studies, a liver biopsy can provide important diagnostic information and identify patients who might benefit from preoperative portal vein embolization. Patients with known chronic liver disease are initially stratified using CTP score. Class A patients are further stratified using MELD score or by measuring the HVPG, if available. In patients with grade 4 fibrosis and an FLR of 30% or less, preoperative PVE should be strongly considered.

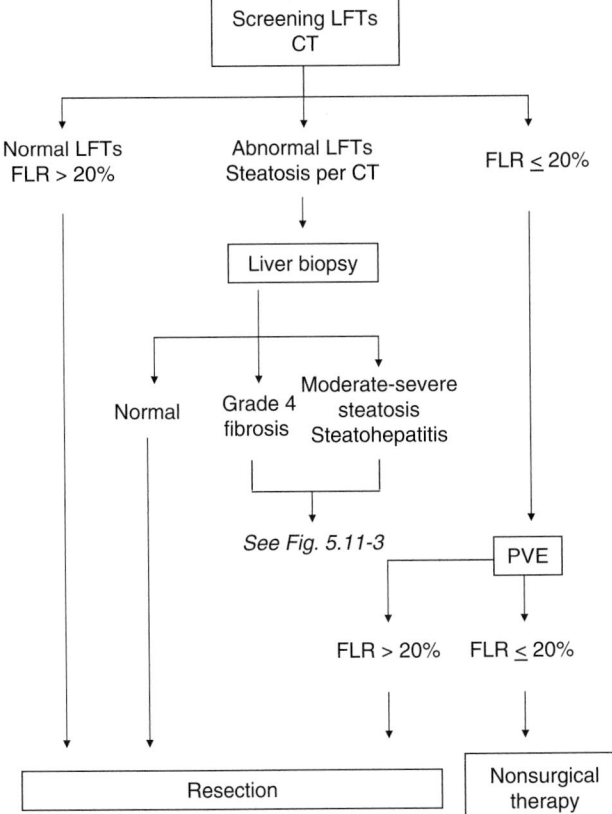

Figure 2 Suggested algorithm for assessment of hepatic reserve in patients with normal liver parenchyma. LFTs include serum bilirubin, alanine aminotransferase, aspartate aminotransferase, alkaline phosphatase, prothrombin time, and albumin levels. *CT,* Computed tomography; *FLR,* future liver remnant; *LFTs,* liver function tests; *PVE,* portal vein embolization.

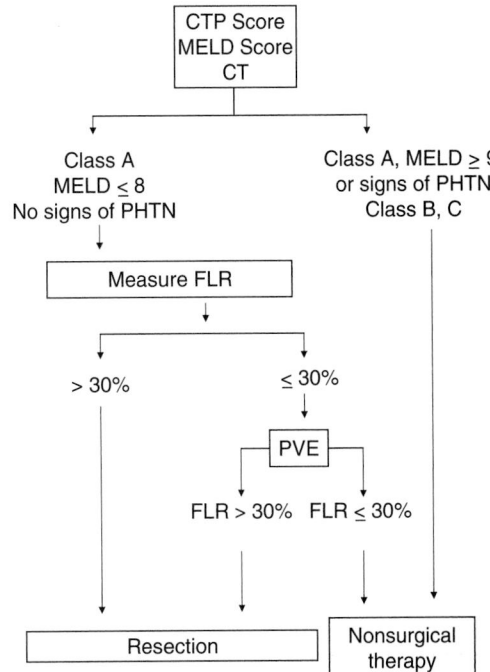

Figure 3 Suggested algorithm for assessment of hepatic reserve in patients with abnormal liver parenchyma. *CT,* Computed tomography; *CTP,* Child-Turcotte-Pugh; *FLR,* future liver remnant; *MELD,* Model for End-Stage Liver Disease; *PHTN,* portal hypertension; *PVE,* portal vein embolization.

INTRAOPERATIVE FACTORS

A thorough knowledge of the internal, functional anatomy of the liver is central to the safe conduct of hepatectomy. Serious hemorrhage is a major concern during resection and remains a major determinant of postoperative morbidity and mortality. Life-threatening hemorrhage is rare and is usually caused by damage to the hepatic veins near their junction with the vena cava during mobilization of the liver. In the vast majority of cases, oozing from the raw surface of the liver and from small branches of the portal and hepatic veins during parenchymal transection accounts for most of the blood loss. In response, several anesthetic and surgical techniques have been developed to minimize intraoperative blood loss and transfusion requirements during hepatectomy. These techniques have been rapidly incorporated into common practice since the mid-1990s and are likely responsible for the improvement in perioperative outcomes observed during this time.

Anesthetic Considerations

Thoracic epidural anesthesia is usually recommended for hepatectomy. It minimizes the amount of general anesthesia required during the case and allows for optimal postoperative analgesia with rapid recovery of pulmonary mechanics, gastrointestinal function, and ambulation. Use of a local anesthetic-opioid mixture in the epidural infusion also minimizes the use of narcotics during the immediate postoperative period, when liver metabolism may be compromised.

Maintenance of low central venous pressure (LCVP) while obtaining vascular control and during parenchymal transection is critical and has been shown to minimize blood loss and mortality after hepatectomy. After induction, patients are usually placed in the Trendelenburg position at 15 degrees, and intravenous fluids are reduced to a rate of 1 ml/kg/hour. General anesthesia is usually maintained using a combination of isoflurane (which provides vasodilation with minimal myocardial depression), muscle relaxants, and narcotics such as fentanyl or morphine, which minimize hypotension and potentiate vasodilation. Intravenous fluid boluses are given to keep urine output at approximately 25 to 30 ml/hour while keeping CVP between 0 and 5 mm Hg. After parenchymal transection and hemostasis is complete, euvolemia is restored using a combination of crystalloid and colloid solutions. During parenchymal transection, LCVP minimizes blood loss from intraparenchymal hepatic vein branches and enhances visibility, allowing for the identification and ligation of small hepatic vein and biliary branches and potentially minimizing the risk of postoperative bleeding and bile leaks. In a recent series of 496 LCVP-assisted major liver resections, the perioperative mortality rate was 3.8%, the median blood loss was 645 ml, and a mean of 0.9 ± 1.8 units of blood were transfused. These figures compared favorably with other contemporary series in which the reported blood loss ranged from 1000 to 1325 ml and patients received an average of 1.4 to 8.0 units of blood. Despite the use of relative hypovolemia, only 3% of patients experienced a clinically significant, persistent rise in serum creatinine, compared with 13% of patients previously resected without LCVP by the same group.

Vascular Control

After LCVP has been established, it is imperative to obtain vascular control before parenchymal transection, particularly if major resection is planned. This can range from simple portal triad clamping (PTC), also called the *Pringle maneuver*, to complete hepatic vascular exclusion (HVE), which involves PTC with clamping of the infrahepatic vena cava and suprahepatic vena cava above the hepatic veins. Although HVE is the safer option in patients with large, central tumors abutting the hepatic vein confluence, it requires mobilization of the entire retrohepatic vena cava, which adds significant complexity and risk to the case. In a recent prospective, randomized study comparing PTC versus HVE in noncirrhotic patients undergoing major hepatectomies, 14% of patients experienced unpredictable, hemodynamic instability during HVE despite the use of previous blood volume expansion and trial clamping. Although intraoperative blood loss and postoperative transaminase levels (indicative of hepatocellular injuring resulting from warm ischemia during clamping) were the same, there was a trend toward more pulmonary complications and intra-abdominal fluid collections in the HVE group, as well increased length of hospital stay.

Any clamping method is associated with a certain degree of warm ischemia and potential injury to the liver parenchyma, particularly in the setting of steatosis or chronic liver disease. Intermittent inflow occlusion avoids long periods of prolonged ischemia but is associated with ischemia-reperfusion injury in experimental models. A recent prospective, randomized trial compared intermittent PTC (consisting of alternating periods of clamping for 15 minutes and unclamping for 5 minutes) with continuous PTC during 86 LVCP-assisted liver resections. Although intraoperative blood loss was higher in the intermittent PTC group (530 ml vs. 280 ml), postoperative bilirubin and transaminase levels were higher in the continuous PTC group, particularly in patients with steatosis or chronic liver disease. Of note, two deaths and four episodes of major liver decompensation occurred in patients with diseased livers, all of whom underwent continuous PTC. It is postulated that intermittent PTC exposes liver cells to a sublethal stress that triggers defense mechanisms, such as the induction of heat shock proteins, which in turn protect cells from subsequent sublethal stress of the same type.

Parenchymal Transection Techniques

After LCVP has been established and vascular control has been obtained, the surgeon can proceed with ligation of the relevant vascular structures and parenchymal transection. Inflow control can be achieved extrahepatically (i.e., by dissecting out the relevant portal structures at the hepatic hilum) or intrahepatically (i.e., by creating strategic hepatotomies and identifying the portal sheaths within the liver parenchyma, as described by Launois and Jamieson). More recently, our group has described an ultrasound-guided technique of major hepatic resection using transparenchymal application of vascular staplers. After the gallbladder has been removed and the relevant lobe has been completely mobilized, an intraoperative ultrasound is performed to identify the right or left portal triads in relation to the middle hepatic vein. Depending on whether right or left hepatic hepatectomy is planned, the liver capsule is then scored along the medial aspect of the gallbladder fossa or the hilar plate, and a long clamp is advanced through the parenchyma anterior to the portal triad but posterior to the middle hepatic vein. A linear vascular stapler is then passed through this tract and used to divide the portal vein, hepatic artery, and hepatic duct with a single application. During right hepatic hepatectomy, outflow control is usually achieved extrahepatically by dividing the right hepatic vein below the hepatic vein confluence using a reticulating, endoscopic linear vascular stapler. After inflow and outflow control is achieved, parenchymal transection is performed with or without PTC, as needed. This technique was recently used in a series of 346 patients treated at the University of Texas M.D. Anderson Cancer Center. The average blood loss for all patients was 396 ml, with a mean warm ischemia (PTC) time of only 13.7 minutes and mean total operative time of 140.7 minutes. The morbidity and 90-day mortality rates were 29.5% and 1.4%, respectively. Although this technique is not appropriate in patients with centrally located tumors encroaching on the portal bifurcation, it is safe and minimizes blood loss, warm ischemia time, and operative time compared with recently published reports of patients resected using other techniques.

After vascular inflow and outflow control has been successfully achieved, a clear line of demarcation will usually appear along the projected plane of transection. Several techniques have been described to transect the liver parenchyma, including blunt dissection (using finger fracture or crushing clamp), ultrasonic aspiration (cavitational ultrasonic surgical aspirator), and water-jet dissection. In general, blunt dissection with a crushing clamp is preferred over finger facture because it allows better visualization and ligation of small venous and biliary branches. The choice of transection technique largely remains a matter of surgeon preference.

Prevention of Bile Leaks

Several techniques have been proposed to help identify bile leaks intraoperatively or minimize biliary complications postoperatively. Transcystic duct injection of saline or methylene blue has been described to help detect and ligate leaking bile ductules along the cut surface of the liver after parenchymal transection. A prospective, randomized trial using transcystic duct injection of normal saline alone showed an intraoperative bile leak rate of 41% in the test group but no difference in the rate of postoperative bile leakage between groups. Transcystic duct injection of a dilute methylene blue solution reduced the rate of postoperative bile leakage from 7.3% to 2.3% in a series of 304 of 616 consecutive hepatectomies. The majority of the bile leaks detected were either at the bile duct stump or the raw surface of the liver. Of note, 10% of patients who had a leaking site identified and ligated continued to leak postoperatively, highlighting the need for meticulous surgical technique. Finally, the routine use of closed-suction drains is associated with an increased risk of infected fluid collections postoperatively and is therefore reserved for high-risk cases involving biliary anastomoses or complex, extended resections.

POSTOPERATIVE FACTORS

Hypophosphatemia

Postoperative hypophosphatemia is a common problem after major hepatic resection and is usually observed between the second and fifth postoperative days. A significant proportion of patients can develop profound hypophosphatemia (<1.0 mg/dl), which has been associated with an increased risk of major postoperative complications (80% vs. 28%) and prolonged length of stay. The degree of postoperative hypophosphatemia after hepatectomy generally exceeds that observed after other major abdominal procedures and appears to be exacerbated by the use of aluminum-containing antacids, warm ischemia time, and extent of resection. Although the pathophysiology underlying posthepatectomy hypophosphatemia has not been fully defined, it is generally attributed to increased consumption of ATP by the regenerating liver. A recent study, however, noted evidence of inappropriate, transient renal wastage of phosphate during the same postoperative period, suggesting that hypophosphatemia may in part be mediated by the kidneys. Irrespective of its cause, frequent monitoring of serum phosphate levels is imperative after hepatectomy, particularly because replacement has been shown to have a protective effect.

Management of Biliary Complications

The rate of postoperative biliary complications in series published since the mid-1990s has ranged from 6% to 12%. Intra-abdominal abscesses secondary to bile leaks are the second leading cause of morbidity after pulmonary complications and have been associated with rates of intra-abdominal sepsis and mortality approaching 50%. Biliary complications after elective hepatectomy should ideally be managed aggressively but nonoperatively because reoperation is associated with a mortality rate of almost 40%. Although the location of bile leakage ultimately cannot be determined in a significant proportion of patients, common locations include the hepatic duct stump, bilioenteric anastomoses, and the raw surface of the liver. Bilomas are initially managed with CT-guided, percutaneous drains, and culture results are used to guide antibiotic therapy. Endoscopic retrograde cholangiopancreatography has been used to manage benign leaks with a success rate of 90% and is the preferred method to decompress the biliary system and facilitate closure of leaks. Although most leaks will close with nonoperative management, patience is necessary because drains may be required for several months.

Postoperative Liver Failure

Careful patient selection and improvements in surgical technique have resulted in a dramatic drop in the rate of postoperative liver failure. Postoperative liver failure is generally classified as either nonregenerative or cholestatic. Nonregenerative liver failure can

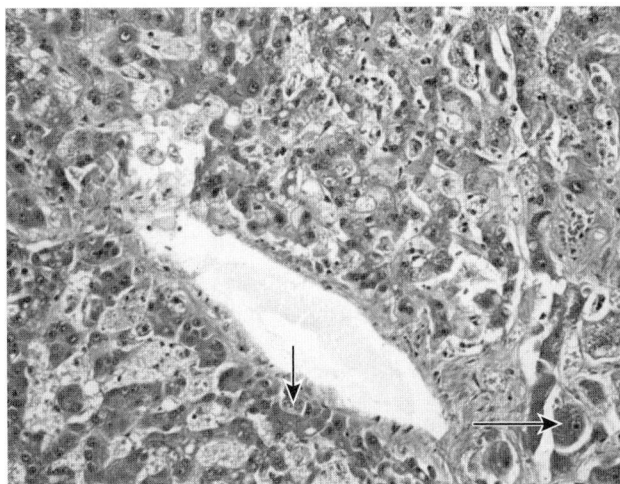

Figure 4 Example of cholestatic postoperative liver failure. Note presence of bile plugs, fibrosis in Disse's space, and hepatocyte regeneration.

be seen in the setting of ischemia or excessive hepatectomy with an inadequate FLR. It is characterized by increased apoptosis, decreased hepatocyte regeneration, and a rapid rise in serum liver function tests postoperatively. Cholestatic liver failure, on the other hand, is characterized by the presence of bile plugs, fibrosis in Disse's space, and hepatocyte regeneration (Fig. 4). The total serum bilirubin level rises more slowly in cholestatic liver failure and is generally considered irreversible after it reaches levels above 15 mg/dl. Cholestatic liver failure has been observed after excessive hepatectomy with an inadequate FLR but can also be triggered by postoperative infection. Therefore it is important to identify and aggressively treat potential sources of infection, such as pneumonia, cholangitis, or intra-abdominal abscesses in patients with persistently elevated or rising serum bilirubin levels after hepatectomy.

SUGGESTED READINGS

Jarnagin WR, Gonen M, Fong Y, and others: Improvement in perioperative outcome after hepatic resection: analysis of 1,803 consecutive cases over the past decade, *Ann Surg* 236:397; discussion 406, 2002.

Kooby DA, Fong Y, Suriawinata A, and others: Impact of steatosis on perioperative outcome following hepatic resection, *J Gastrointest Surg* 7:1034, 2003.

Lam CM, Lo CM, Liu CL, and others: Biliary complications during liver resection, *World J Surg* 25:1273, 2001.

Melendez JA, Arslan V, Fischer ME, and others: Perioperative outcomes of major hepatic resections under low central venous pressure anesthesia: blood loss, blood transfusion, and the risk of postoperative renal dysfunction, *J Am Coll Surg* 187:620, 1998.

Smith DL, Arens JF, Barnett CC Jr., and others: A prospective evaluation of ultrasound-directed transparenchymal vascular control with linear cutting staplers in major hepatic resections, *Am J Surg* 190:23, 2005.

Teh SH, Christein J, Donohue J, and others: Hepatic resection of hepatocellular carcinoma in patients with cirrhosis: Model of End-Stage Liver Disease (MELD) score predicts perioperative mortality, *J Gastrointest Surg* 9:1207; discussion 1215, 2005.

Vauthey JN, Pawlik TM, Ribero D, and others: Chemotherapy regimen predicts steatohepatitis and an increase in 90-day mortality after surgery for hepatic colorectal metastases, *J Clin Oncol* 24:2065, 2006.

PORTAL HYPERTENSION

PORTAL HYPERTENSION: THE ROLE OF SHUNTING PROCEDURES

Layton F. Rikkers, MD

During much of the latter half of the 20th century, surgical portosystemic shunts served as the mainstay of definitive therapy for patients with variceal bleeding. However, many developments since the mid-1970s have greatly narrowed the focus of shunt surgery in the management of patients with this life-threatening complication of portal hypertension. Endoscopic treatment, pharmacotherapy, liver transplantation, and, most recently, the transjugular intrahepatic portosystemic shunt (TIPS) all have a role in the treatment of these complex patients. As a result, fewer portosystemic shunt operations are being performed. In fact, most major medical centers could count on one hand the number of such operations performed annually in recent years. Because so few of these procedures are being performed, there is a lack of adequately trained surgeons to provide this service in the future. Because of the narrow indications and the lack of trained personnel to perform shunt surgery, the existence of these once commonly performed operations is threatened. The purpose of this chapter is to put portosystemic shunt operations in perspective as one of many therapeutic options for patients who bleed from esophagogastric varices. The surgical techniques for constructing a nonselective shunt (end-to-side portacaval shunt) and a selective shunt (distal splenorenal shunt) will also be described.

TYPES OF PORTOSYSTEMIC SHUNTS

All portasystemic shunts can be placed into one of three categories: (1) nonselective shunts that eliminate hepatic portal perfusion, (2) selective shunts that decompress esophageal and gastric varices but have the potential to maintain portal perfusion of the liver, and (3) partial shunts that incompletely decompress the entire portal venous system and also have the potential to preserve some portal flow to the liver.

Nonselective Shunts

There are two basic types of nonselective shunts (Fig. 1): (1) the end-to-side portacaval shunt, which directly diverts all portal flow to the inferior vena cava and (2) side-to-side portosystemic shunts, which leave the portal vein intact and decompress the liver, as well as the entire portal venous system.

The end-to-side portacaval shunt (Eck fistula) was the first shunt introduced into clinical practice and the first to be compared with other methods of managing variceal bleeding. Because portal blood contains hepatotrophic hormones and intestinally absorbed cerebral toxins, complete diversion of portal flow into the systemic circulation can result in accelerated hepatic failure and the development of portosystemic encephalopathy (PSE) in many patients. When the end-to-side portacaval shunt was compared with conventional medical management of the time in the 1970s, it was shown to be much more effective in preventing recurrent bleeding. However, most likely because of diversion of portal flow away from the liver, up to 40% of patients developed postoperative encephalopathy. Additionally, and surprisingly at the time, there was little survival advantage to the nonselective end-to-side portacaval shunt over medical management because of an accelerated onset of hepatic failure. These disappointing results stimulated the development of other types of shunting procedures.

Side-to-side portosystemic shunts were developed with the objective of preserving hepatic portal perfusion in addition to decompressing varices. However, it soon became apparent that these operations also completely divert portal flow away from the liver and convert the portal vein into an outflow track for hepatic arterial perfusion as well. The fact that these operations effectively decompress the liver, as well as the splanchnic venous circulation, make them effective in resolving medically intractable ascites and in preventing recurrent variceal bleeding. However, the resultant complete diversion of portal flow again results in a high frequency of postshunt encephalopathy and an acceleration of hepatic failure similar to that observed following the end-to-side portacaval shunt.

A variation on the theme of the side-to-side portosystemic shunt is the interposition graft shunt, usually made of synthetic material. These grafts can be placed in the portacaval, mesocaval, mesorenal, and splenorenal positions, all with the same effect of decompressing both the liver and the portal venous system as long as the grafts are 14 mm in diameter or greater. These shunts are hemodynamically indistinguishable from the side-to-side portacaval shunt but have the additional disadvantage of a high late occlusion rate secondary to thrombus forming in the synthetic graft. The likelihood of shunt failure can be lessened by using autogenous vein (internal jugular) rather than a synthetic graft.

The final variety of nonselective shunt is the conventional splenorenal shunt, which consists of splenectomy and anastomosis of the proximal end of the splenic vein to the left renal vein. Although early investigations of this procedure suggested that it more effectively preserved hepatic portal perfusion than any of the other nonselective shunts, further assessment showed that this was most likely due to a higher thrombosis rate of this shunt because the smaller diameter proximal splenic vein was used in

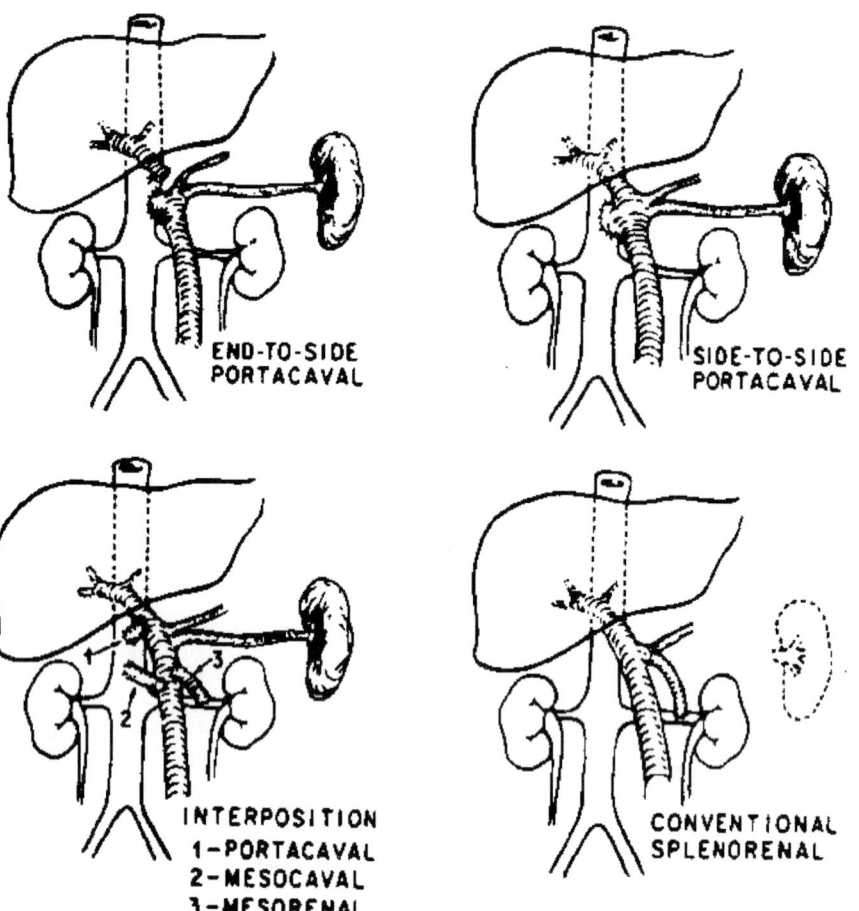

END-TO-SIDE
PORTACAVAL

SIDE-TO-SIDE
PORTACAVAL

INTERPOSITION
1-PORTACAVAL
2-MESOCAVAL
3-MESORENAL

CONVENTIONAL
SPLENORENAL

Figure 1 Nonselective shunts completely divert portal blood flow away from the liver. The side-to-side varieties decompress the liver, as well as the splanchnic viscera, and are effective in treating ascites and preventing variceal bleeding.

the anastomosis. Because splenectomy is a component of the conventional splenorenal shunt procedure, it has been used when severe hypersplenism complicates the portal hypertensive state, an uncommon occurrence.

Currently, indications for nonselective shunts are few. Because the TIPS procedure also serves as a side-to-side nonselective shunt but can be achieved without an open operation, it has generally replaced the various types of nonselective shunts. One of these operations may rarely be indicated in patients with both medically intractable ascites and recurrent variceal bleeding after TIPS failure. They may also be occasionally used in the desperate emergency setting when TIPS technology is not available. Another uncommon indication for a side-to-side shunt is the subacute Budd-Chiari syndrome before the onset of cirrhosis. After cirrhosis has developed, liver transplantation is a preferable option.

The end-to-side portacaval shunt is performed through a right subcostal incision. The right costal margin and the liver are retracted superiorly, and the peritoneum along the lateral edge of the hepatoduodenal ligament is incised, identifying the common bile duct. The bile duct is retracted medially, and the underlying portal vein is dissected from its bifurcation proximally down to its disappearance beneath the head of the pancreas (Fig. 2, *A*). The inferior vena cava is then identified in the retroperitoneum and freed over a sufficient length from the caudate lobe inferiorly so that a partially occluding vascular clamp can be applied. The portal vein is then ligated just distal to its bifurcation. After the portal vein is clamped as it enters the hepatoduodenal ligament from beneath the pancreas, it is divided and brought in a gentle arc to the inferior vena cava, where an end-to-side anastomosis is constructed after a small button of inferior vena cava is excised (Fig. 2, *B* and *C*). Two continuous sutures of 4-0 or 5-0

polypropylene are generally used. The same exposure is used for a side-to-side portacaval shunt, but the portal vein is not ligated. After a partially occluding clamp is placed on the inferior vena cava, the portal vein is occluded proximally and distally with either vascular clamps or Rommel tourniquets, and the anastomosis is constructed.

Selective shunts

The only selective shunt presently in use is the distal splenorenal shunt, conceived by Dr. W. Dean Warren in the late 1960s (Fig. 3). The objectives of this procedure are both effective variceal decompression and preservation of hepatic portal perfusion. Several studies have shown that these objectives are often achieved, at least in the short term. Over time, and especially in alcoholic cirrhotic patients, collaterals can develop through the pancreas that eventually divert portal flow away from the liver and to the shunt.

Several controlled trials have compared the selective distal splenorenal shunt with a variety of nonselective shunts. All of these studies have shown no difference in survival in the mainly alcoholic cirrhotic patients enrolled but a lower incidence of postshunt encephalopathy after the selective shunt in most of the trials. Other investigations have compared the distal splenorenal shunt with endoscopic therapy, and all of these have shown better prevention of recurrent variceal bleeding in the shunt groups. However, in most of the trials, no difference in survival has been apparent. Because of its lower frequency of postshunt encephalopathy, the distal splenorenal shunt is the most commonly used portosystemic shunting procedure in most areas of the world. Its use is generally confined to patients with preserved hepatic functional reserve

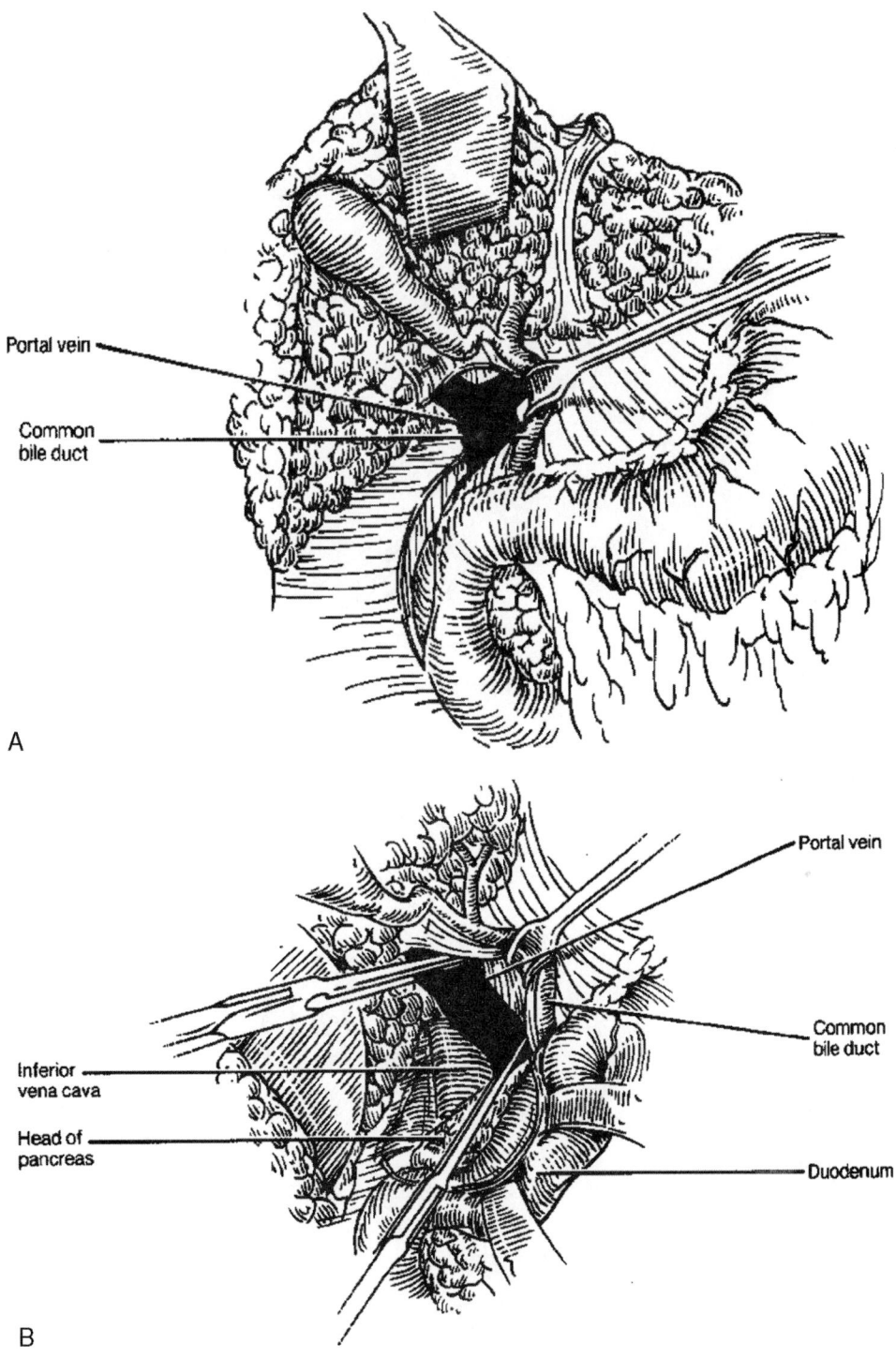

A

B

Figure 2 Construction of an end-to-side portacaval shunt. **(A)** The portal vein is dissected from its bifurcation down to the pancreas by incising the peritoneum over the lateral hepatoduodenal ligament and retracting the common bile duct medially. **(B)** The portal vein can then be ligated slightly distal to its bifurcation and a vascular clamp placed across it just before it disappears beneath the head of the pancreas.

(continued)

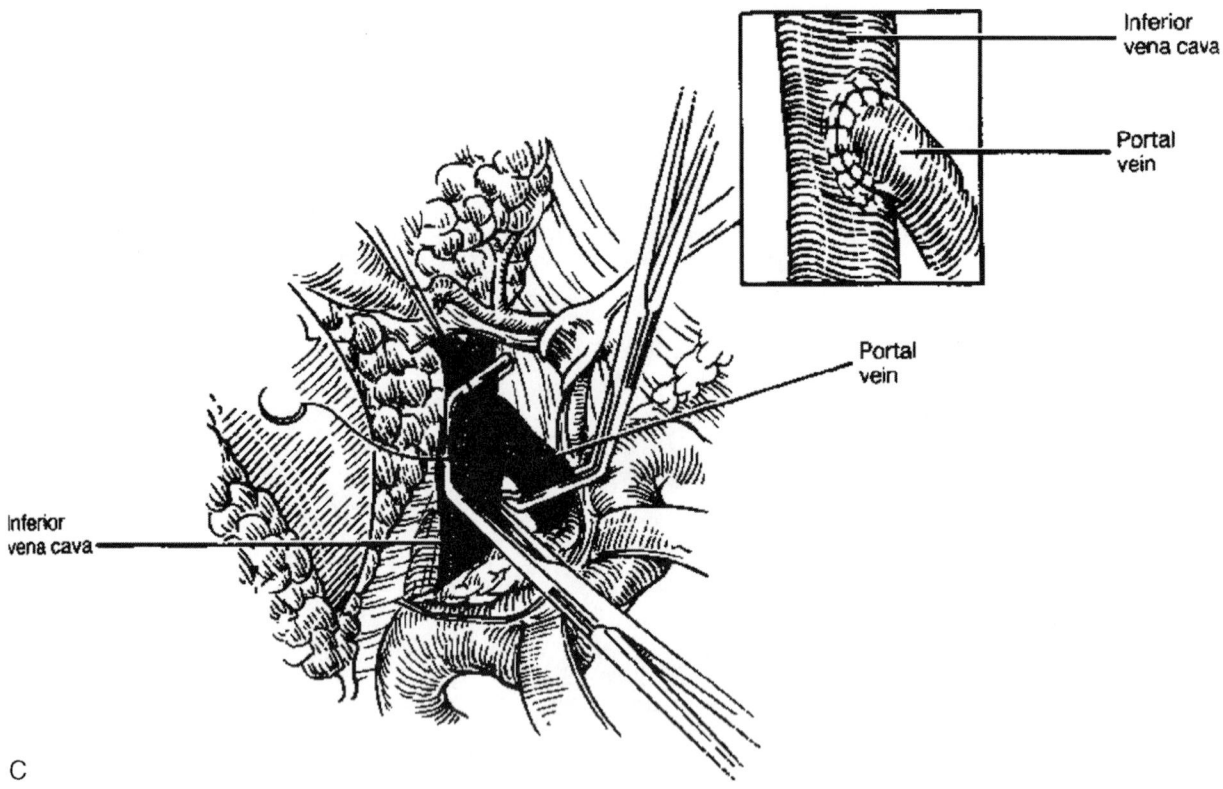

Inferior
vena cava

Portal
vein

Portal
vein

Inferior
vena cava

C

Figure 2 **Cont'd—(C)** The inferior vena cava is dissected from the caudate lobe inferiorly and a partially occluding clamp is placed across it. A small button of inferior vena cava is excised, the portal vein is brought down to it in a gentle arc, and an end-to-side anastomosis is constructed.

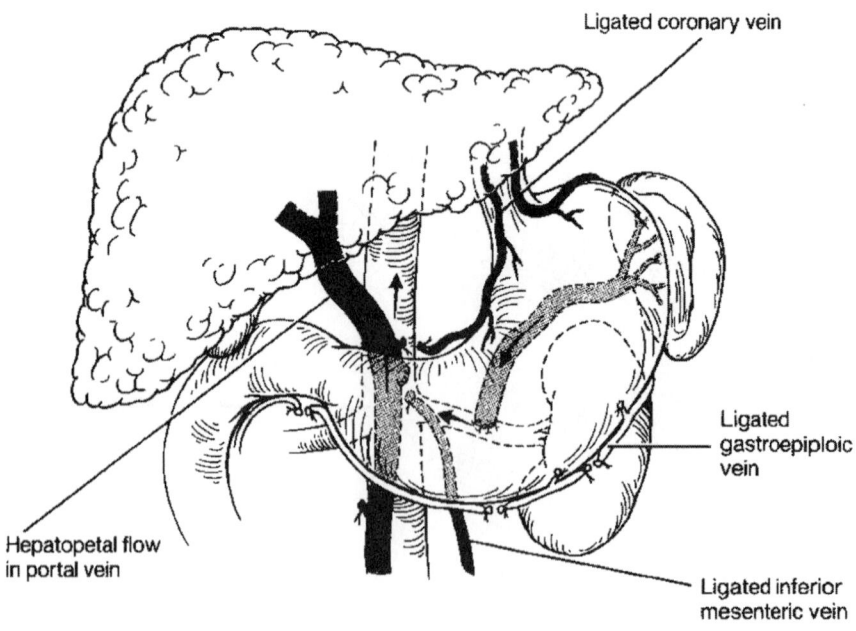

Ligated coronary vein

Ligated
gastroepiploic
vein

Hepatopetal flow
in portal vein

Ligated inferior
mesenteric vein

Figure 3 The selective distal splenorenal shunt effectively decompresses esophageal and gastric varices and also has the potential to maintain hepatic portal perfusion.

(Child-Pugh classes A and B) and to the elective setting. When applied in this population, operative mortality rates are generally less than 5%, the frequency of recurrent variceal bleeding is less than 10%, postshunt encephalopathy is unusual, and 5-year survival rates are in the range of 50% to 60%.

The presence of medically intractable ascites is a contraindication to the distal splenorenal shunt. Because one objective of the operation is to maintain mesenteric venous hypertension and retroperitoneal lymphatics are interrupted during the dissection of the left renal vein, this procedure tends to aggravate rather than relieve ascites. A relative contraindication is a splenic vein diameter less than 7 mm because the frequency of shunt thrombosis is considerably higher when such a small-diameter vein is used in shunt construction.

A multi-institutional study recently compared the distal splenorenal shunt with TIPS in patients with Child-Pugh class A or B cirrhosis. Surprisingly, there was no significant difference in recurrent variceal bleeding between the groups (distal splenorenal shunt, 5%; TIPS, 10%), but this represents the lowest rebleeding rate ever reported for the TIPS procedure, likely because of the close follow-up of the patients in this trial with duplex ultrasound and angiography, allowing reintervention when TIPS stenosis or occlusion developed. The major difference between groups in this investigation was a much higher reintervention rate in the TIPS patients (80%) than in the distal splenorenal shunt arm. The conclusion of this trial is that both TIPS and the distal splenorenal shunt are efficacious in good-risk patients who require portal decompression after failing endoscopic or pharmacologic therapy (or both). The advantage of TIPS is that it does not require an open operation, and the advantage of the distal splenorenal shunt is that it is a more durable procedure that does not require multiple reinterventions to maintain shunt patency. Many more TIPS procedures than distal splenorenal shunts are being performed throughout the United States, and this trend is likely to continue. As a result, the distal splenorenal shunt will likely have a narrow window in any algorithm for the management of variceal bleeding. It is currently most commonly performed in patients who fail TIPS and in those with normal livers and portal vein thrombosis who rebleed despite pharmacotherapy and endoscopic treatment. However, as demonstrated in the recently completed trial of TIPS versus the distal splenorenal shunt, it is also an excellent choice for good-risk cirrhotic patients who fail pharmacologic and endoscopic therapy and who will not require a liver transplant for several years, if ever.

The distal splenorenal shunt is a technically challenging operation that can be mastered by most surgeons who are well versed in the principles of vascular surgery. It is performed through an extended left subcostal incision. The gastrocolic ligament is taken down to the first short gastric vein, and the inferior border of the body and tail of the pancreas is mobilized (Fig. 4, A). The splenic vein is identified and meticulously dissected from the pancreas by ligating and dividing multiple small pancreatic branches (Fig. 4, B). After mobilizing 4 to 6 cm of the splenic vein, it is brought down in a gentle arc and anastomosed end-to-side to the left renal vein, which can be found in the retroperitoneum posterior to the splenic vein (Fig. 4, C). Patency can generally be assured if kinking and torsion of the splenic vein are avoided and the vein diameter is greater than 7 mm. Ligation of the coronary vein, gastroepiploic vein, and any other collaterals connecting the decompressed gastrosplenic and hypertensive superior mesenteric venous networks is an essential component of the operation if hepatic portal perfusion is to be preserved.

Partial Shunts

The objectives of the partial shunt are similar to those of the distal splenorenal shunt. Although incompletely decompressing the entire portal venous system, partial shunts also have the potential to preserve some hepatic portal perfusion while lowering portal pressure below that required for variceal bleeding (12 mm Hg). The only commonly applied partial shunt is the small-diameter interposition portacaval shunt, which uses a polytetrafluoroethylene graft as originally described by Sarfeh. In addition to placing the shunt, the coronary vein and other collateral vessels are ligated as in the distal splenorenal shunt procedure. A number of studies have shown that when the prosthetic graft is 10 mm or less in diameter, hepatic portal perfusion is preserved in most patients, at least during the early postoperative period. A single prospective randomized trial that enrolled a small number of patients showed a lower frequency of encephalopathy after the small-diameter

interposition portacaval shunt (8 mm) than following the larger diameter shunt (16 mm). However, because synthetic material is used in this procedure, a concern is that long-term shunt thrombosis rates will be higher than have been observed with the distal splenorenal shunt operation. Possibly for this reason, only a limited number of institutions have used the partial shunt approach in the management of variceal bleeding.

TREATMENT OF ACUTE VARICEAL BLEEDING

Because many patients with acute variceal hemorrhage have decompensated hepatic function, emergency treatment of their bleeding should be nonoperative whenever feasible. Endoscopic treatment (preferably variceal ligation) and pharmacotherapy (intravenous octreotide infusion) effectively control bleeding in more than 85% of patients. When these treatment modalities fail in the acute setting, TIPS rather than an operative shunt is the means by which portal decompression is achieved in most institutions. When TIPS is not indicated or the expertise is not available, an emergency portosystemic shunt operation, most commonly an end-to-side portacaval shunt or an interposition shunt, can be lifesaving. However, surgeons with the expertise to perform these operations when they are indicated are available in only a limited number of medical institutions throughout the United States.

If the emergency situation does mandate an operative shunt procedure, it is best to anticipate it and perform it early in the patient's course before extensive blood transfusions have been given and hepatic decompensation has developed. Patients with gastric variceal bleeding are more likely to require an emergency shunt operation because they tend to bleed more aggressively than patients with esophageal variceal bleeding and because endoscopic therapy is considerably less effective for gastric varices.

PROPHYLACTIC THERAPY OF VARICES

Prophylactic therapy of varices is treatment administered before development of an initial variceal hemorrhage. However, because only one third of patients with varices eventually bleed, many individuals undergoing prophylactic therapy are treated unnecessarily. In recent years, risk factors for an initial bleeding episode have been identified and include large size of varices, red color signs on the varices, and high variceal pressure. Trials in which only patients at high risk for bleeding are included have shown a substantial reduction in the initial bleeding episode when pharmacotherapy with nonselective beta blockade or endoscopic variceal ligation are used. There is little evidence that portal decompression either by means of TIPS or a shunt operation is beneficial in patients who have not previously bled from their varices.

PREVENTION OF RECURRENT VARICEAL BLEEDING

After a patient has bled from varices, the likelihood of recurrent bleeding at some time in the future exceeds 70%. This is the setting in which surgical portal decompression, although infrequently used in the present era, has been found to be most beneficial. Figure 5 is an algorithm for prevention of recurrent variceal hemorrhage. Patients who are present or future candidates for liver transplantation (abstinent alcoholic cirrhotics and patients with nonalcoholic cirrhosis) are managed somewhat differently than those individuals who will never be liver transplant candidates (active alcoholics, the elderly, and those with

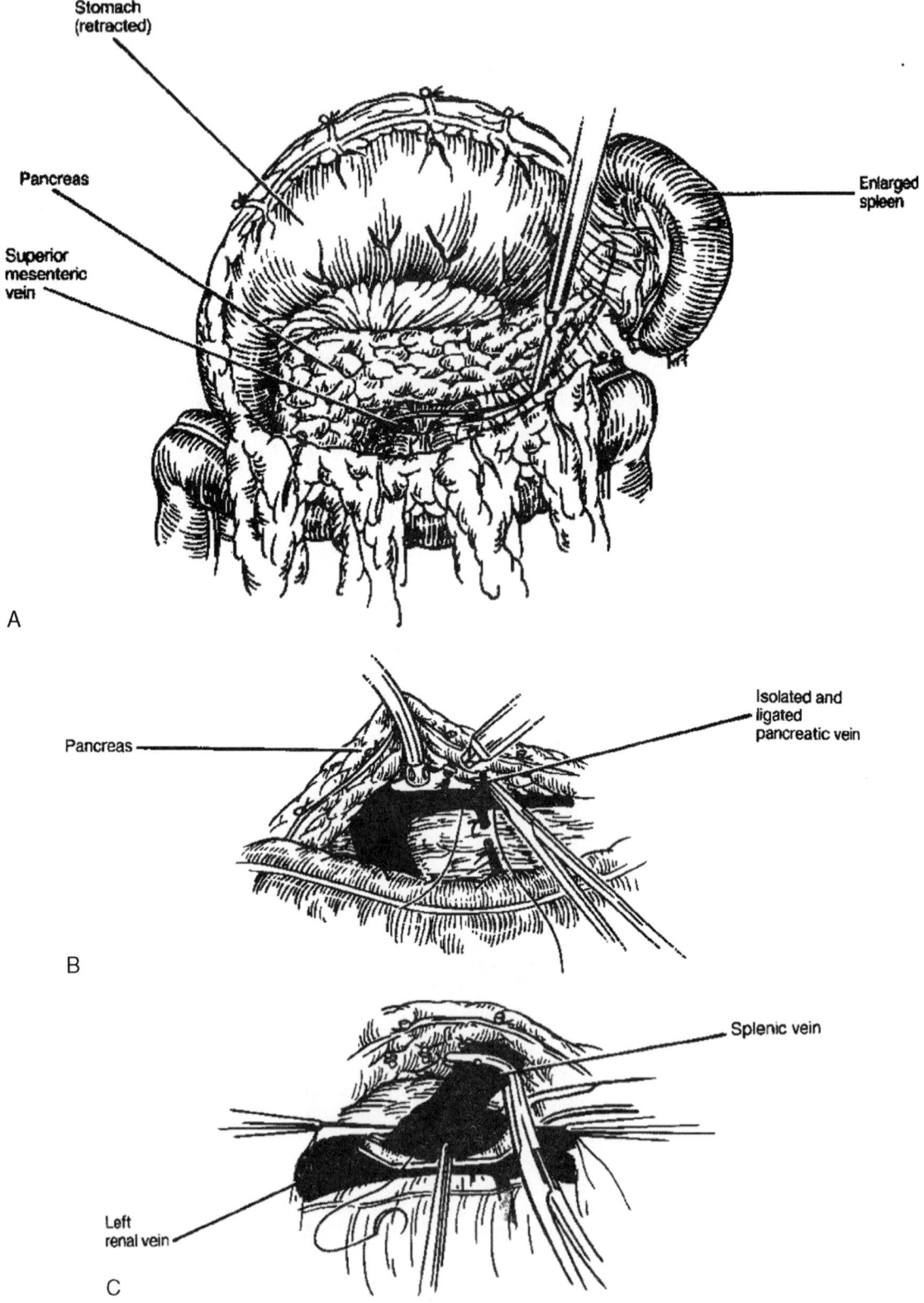

Figure 4 Construction of a distal splenorenal shunt. **(A)** After an extended left subcostal incision is made, the gastrocolic ligament is taken down from the pylorus up to the first short gastric vessels and dissection is begun along the inferior border of the pancreas. **(B)** The splenic vein is dissected from the body and tail of the pancreas by ligating and dividing multiple small pancreatic branches. **(C)** After a 4- to 6-cm length of splenic vein is dissected, it is ligated at its junction with the portal vein and divided. The left renal vein is identified in the retroperitoneum. After a partially occluding clamp is placed on the renal vein, a small button of vein is removed; the splenic vein is brought down in a gentle arc and an end-to-side anastomosis is constructed.

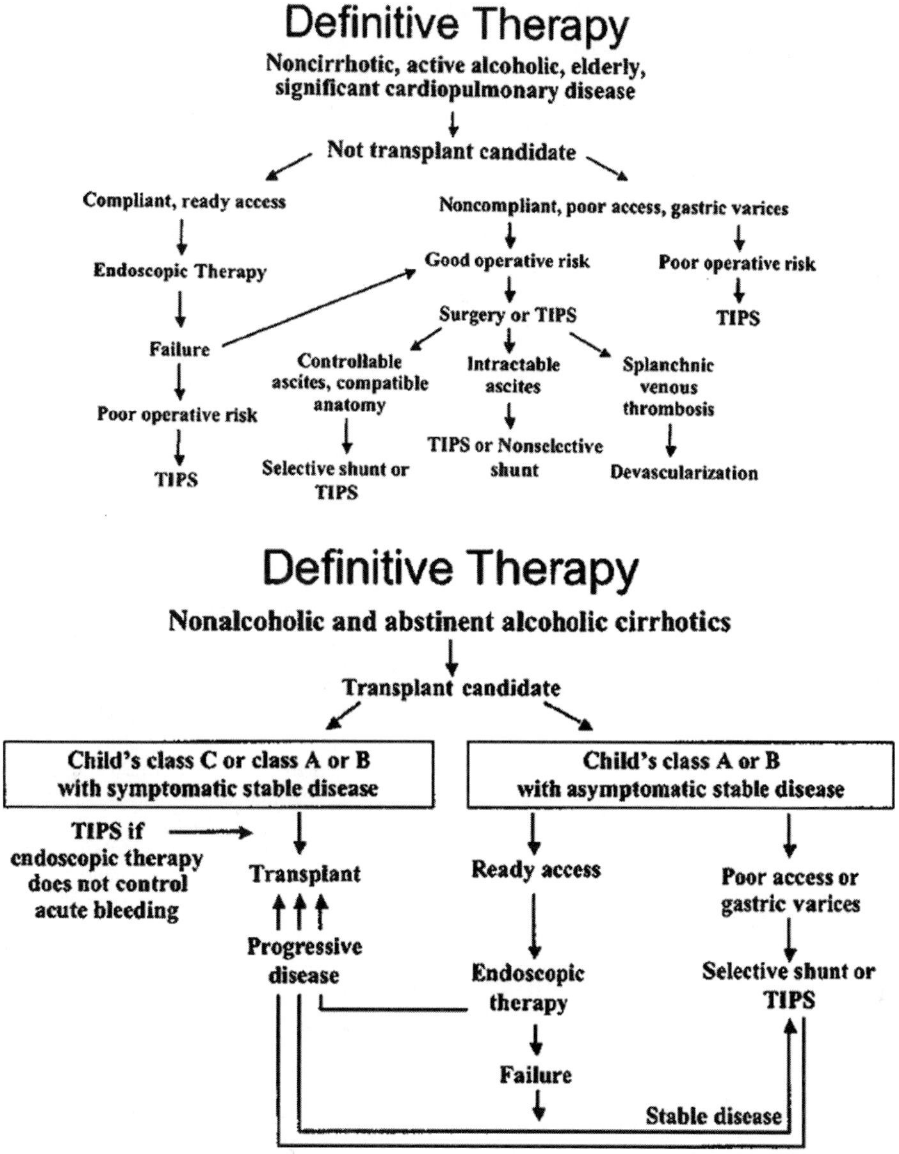

Definitive Therapy

Noncirrhotic, active alcoholic, elderly, significant cardiopulmonary disease

Not transplant candidate

Compliant, ready access → Endoscopic Therapy → Failure → Poor operative risk → TIPS

Noncompliant, poor access, gastric varices

Good operative risk → Surgery or TIPS

Poor operative risk → TIPS

Controllable ascites, compatible anatomy → Selective shunt or TIPS

Intractable ascites → TIPS or Nonselective shunt

Splanchnic venous thrombosis → Devascularization

Definitive Therapy

Nonalcoholic and abstinent alcoholic cirrhotics

Transplant candidate

Child's class C or class A or B with symptomatic stable disease

TIPS if endoscopic therapy does not control acute bleeding → Transplant ← Progressive disease

Child's class A or B with asymptomatic stable disease

Ready access → Endoscopic therapy → Failure

Poor access or gastric varices → Selective shunt or TIPS

Stable disease

Figure 5 Algorithm for definitive management of variceal bleeding in patients who are present or future transplant candidates and those who are unlikely to ever undergo liver transplantation.

limited physiologic reserve). Those individuals who are immediate transplantation candidates (limited hepatic functional reserve or poor quality of life secondary to their liver disease) should be managed with a TIPS procedure as a short-term bridge to transplantation if pharmacotherapy or endoscopic treatment fail to control their bleeding. They are given transplants as soon as possible. Patients with preserved hepatic functional reserve (Child-Pugh class A and B+) may not require liver transplantation for several years, and some may never require such treatment. These individuals require portal decompression when pharmacotherapy and endoscopic treatment fail to control bleeding. Either a TIPS or a distal splenorenal shunt is a reasonable alternative for these patients. The advantage of the TIPS is that it is nonoperative; a major disadvantage is that it requires multiple reinterventions in most patients to maintain patency. The advantage of the distal splenorenal shunt is that it is more durable than TIPS and seldom requires reintervention. Another theoretic advantage of the distal splenorenal shunt is that it has the potential of preserving hepatic portal perfusion. However, in the recent multi-institutional trial of TIPS versus the distal splenorenal shunt, these

procedures were equally efficacious with respect to preventing recurrent variceal bleeding and in the development of postshunt encephalopathy.

Those who are not currently and likely will never be transplant candidates are also initially managed with endoscopic or pharmacologic therapy (or both). When this treatment fails, as it is likely to in approximately one third of patients, some form of portal decompression is indicated. Patients who are poor operative risks should receive TIPS, and those who are good operative risks can be considered for either TIPS or an operative shunt. A selective distal splenorenal shunt is preferred for those individuals with compatible anatomy and manageable ascites. Patients with both variceal bleeding and medically intractable ascites should undergo a TIPS procedure and receive an operative nonselective shunt if the TIPS fails. Finally, there is a small cohort of patients with portal hypertension and bleeding varices who cannot undergo portal venous decompression because of diffuse splanchnic venous thrombosis. Many of these patients have normal liver function and a hypercoagulable state (e.g., myeloproliferative disorder, protein C or S deficiency, antithrombin III deficiency). Such patients are more likely to bleed from gastric varices than esophageal varices. When their bleeding cannot be controlled nonoperatively, they become candidates for extensive esophageal and gastric devascularization combined with splenectomy (modified Sugiura procedure). This operation has often been described to include esophageal transection with an EEA stapler, but in my experience, this is generally not necessary because gastric varices usually predominate. Additionally, esophageal varices can generally be controlled by endoscopic means when they are present or if they develop in the future.

SUGGESTED READINGS

D'Amico G, Pagliaro L, Bosch J: The treatment of portal hypertension: a meta-analytic review, *Hepatology* 22:332, 1995.
Henderson JM, Boyer TS, Kutner MH, and others: Distal splenorenal shunt versus transjugular intrahepatic portal systemic shunt for variceal bleeding: a randomized trial, *Gastroenterology* 130:1643, 2006.
Rikkers LF: The changing spectrum of treatment for variceal bleeding, *Ann Surg* 228:536, 1998.
Wright AS, Rikkers LF: Current management of portal hypertension, *J Gastrointest Surg* 9:992, 2005.

TRANSJUGULAR INTRAHEPATIC PORTOSYSTEMIC SHUNTS (TIPS)

Ashkan A. Malayeri, MD, Gregory Czuczman, BS, and Aravind Arepally, MD

INTRODUCTION

Portal hypertension is a common manifestation of cirrhosis and is responsible for the majority of morbidity and mortality from liver disease. It has been estimated that 5.5 million Americans have cirrhosis. The majority of these patients develop life-threatening complications of cirrhosis such as varices, ascites, and eventual liver failure.

Because of the medical complexity of patients with portal hypertension, the management of these cases requires a multidisciplinary approach. Although there are multiple medical, surgical, and endoscopic options available in treating portal hypertension, transjugular intrahepatic portosystemic shunts (TIPS) offers the only minimally invasive alternative to provide relief for the myriad symptoms related to portal hypertension. This procedure is relatively new, but it has been effectively implemented into clinical practice and is now available at most institutions. This chapter focuses on (1) current indications, (2) patient selection strategies, (3) technique of performing the procedure, and (4) procedure-related complications.

INDICATIONS

Because of refinement of techniques and equipment, TIPS has seen tremendous success and exponential growth. With this experience, indications and contraindications for both emergent and elective TIPS are now well described and established.

Variceal Bleeding

When portosystemic gradients reach levels greater than 12 mmHg, patients are at risk for the development of variceal bleeding. In clinical practice, variceal bleeding is seen in three distinct situations: a primary variceal bleed, refractory variceal bleeding, and recurrent variceal bleeds. Currently first-line therapy for primary variceal bleed is endoscopic band ligation or sclerotherapy combined with pharmacologic therapies such as nitroglycerin, somatostatin, and octreotide. Invasive procedures, such as TIPS and surgical shunts, should not be used as first-line therapy in patients with a primary variceal bleed or variceal bleeding that has been successfully controlled.

However, in patients with a primary variceal bleed, the risk of rebleeding is 50% and can be severely life threatening. Therefore in patients with rebleeding that cannot be controlled with endoscopic management (refractory variceal bleeding) or who continue to rebleed (recurrent variceal bleeding), TIPS is an excellent option for portal decompression. Results of meta-analytic studies have shown TIPS to be effective in 90% of patients in these situations. Furthermore, whether the source of bleeding is gastric or esophageal varices, TIPS is equally effective in controlling bleeding from both sites. Occasionally in patients with massive variceal bleeding, adjunctive embolization may be necessary to perform to control bleeding acutely and stabilize the patient.

Ascites

Ascites is said to be refractory to medical treatment when it is unresponsive to sodium restriction and the use of high doses of diuretics or when the patient is intolerant of diuretic therapy. This clinical picture is associated with a poor prognosis; approximately 50% of patients die within 12 months. A number of approaches have been taken in the management of patients with refractory ascites, including peritoneovenous shunts, repeated large-volume paracentesis (LVP), and TIPS. Peritoneovenous shunts have been abandoned, except in unusual circumstances, because of a lack of efficacy and the high rate of complication. Compared with LVP, patients who undergo TIPS procedure show improvement in their ascites without the need for paracentesis. Currently there is no significant difference in survival after TIPS and LVP, but recent studies have been disputing this notion. Finally, it is important to note that encephalopathy can occur more frequently in the TIPS groups compared with the LVP groups.

Refractory Hepatic Hydrothorax

Refractory hepatic hydrothorax is another complication of portal hypertension and is the result of fluid leak from the abdominal cavity through small defects in the diaphragm. In a series of small studies, the effect of TIPS on patients with recurrent hepatic hydrothorax has been relatively uniform, with either resolution of the hepatic hydrothorax or a decrease in the need for thoracentesis. Because the therapeutic alternatives in these patients are limited, TIPS is an important tool for the management of this complication of ascites. Overall survival in these patients is poor, and the impact of TIPS on the survival has not been determined. TIPS is effective in the control of hepatic hydrothorax, but it should be used only in patients whose effusion cannot be controlled by diuretics and sodium restriction.

Hepatorenal Syndrome

Hepatorenal syndrome (HRS) is a dreaded complication of cirrhosis and is associated with a poor prognosis. In type 1 HRS, renal failure occurs rapidly (over a 2-week period) and has the worst prognosis; in type 2 HRS, the renal failure develops more slowly with better prognosis. In a small series, the use of TIPS has been associated with improvements in renal function in these patients. However, performing TIPS in this patient population is difficult because of changes in fluid volumes and contrast load. Therefore further investigations with other pharmacologic therapies such as terlipressin and other vasoactive compounds are necessary before their role in the treatment of HRS is determined. TIPS is thus currently not recommended for the treatment of HRS, especially type 1 HRS, until the publication of more controlled trials.

Budd-Chiari Syndrome

Budd-Chiari syndrome (BCS) can occur from hepatic vein stenosis/occlusion or obstruction of the inferior vena cava. The most common presentation is subacute liver disease complicated by portal hypertension with ascites and varying degrees of liver failure. As a result of hepatic congestion, severe liver injury can occur. In the past, patients often were treated for symptoms and with anticoagulation therapy; in severe cases, surgical shunts were used. Although experience with BCS and TIPS is limited, current studies indicate that some patients may respond well to this procedure. Studies have demonstrated that patients with chronic and subacute disease may have relief of symptoms with improvement of liver function and a good intermediate (2 to 4 years) survival. However, patients with acute BCS seem to have poor survival rates. Whether this is related to progression of disease or sequelae of TIPS is not well known, and therefore further investigations are necessary. The decision to create a TIPS in a patient with Budd-Chiari syndrome should be made on the basis of the severity of disease; only patients with moderate disease appear to be reasonable candidates for a TIPS, whereas those with severe disease or acute hepatic failure may be best managed by liver transplantation.

Veno-occlusive Disease

Veno-occlusive disease (sinusoidal obstruction syndrome) is seen most commonly following hematopoietic stem cell transplantation. In patients with the severe form of the disease, ascites is common as a result of the development of portal hypertension. In these series, TIPS improved ascites and lowered levels of liver enzymes but did not affect serum bilirubin levels. Most of the patients died despite the creation of the TIPS; therefore the use of this modality to treat sinusoidal obstruction syndrome is not recommended.

Hepatopulmonary Syndrome

Hepatopulmonary syndrome is a complication of cirrhosis in which shunts develop in the lungs, leading to the development of hypoxia. A small study has shown that TIPS has a role in improving oxygenation and, to some extent, decreasing intrapulmonary shunt. With the current knowledge base, however, the use of TIPS to treat all hepatopulmonary syndrome patients cannot be recommended.

Portal Gastropathy

Portal hypertensive gastropathy (PHG) is usually an endoscopic diagnosis and is limited only to patients with portal hypertension. Gastric antral vascular ectasia is similar to PHG but can be seen in a variety of disorders, including cirrhosis. Therefore in patients with suspected PHG, differentiation from gastric antral vascular ectasia should be made by endoscopy before any therapy is initiated. The use of TIPS in the management of portal hypertensive gastropathy should be limited to those who have recurrent bleeding despite the use of beta-blockers. In a series of small studies, TIPS was shown to reduce the risk of bleeding and improve portal hypertensive gastropathy appearance on endoscopy. In contrast, bleeding from gastric antral vascular ectasia in patients with cirrhosis remains unaffected by TIPS and therefore it should not be used to control bleeding from this source in patients with cirrhosis.

LIVER TRANSPLANTATION

Patients who are candidates for liver transplantation may also benefit from TIPS procedure. Clinical presentation of these patients consists mainly of refractory bleeding from varices or refractory ascites associated with cirrhosis. TIPS is especially useful for short-term management of patients before liver transplantation because it does not interrupt the normal anatomic structure of the liver and portal system Moreover, lower portal pressure can make liver transplantation technically easier. However, TIPS cannot be recommended for preoperative portal decompression solely to facilitate liver transplantation. In patients who are candidates for liver transplantation, TIPS should be placed entirely intrahepatically. Inappropriate extension of the stent complicates the hepatectomy, and bare wires may be hazardous to the surgeon during the operation.

CONTRAINDICATIONS

Absolute contraindications to TIPS are polycystic liver disease, congestive heart failure, severe tricuspid regurgitation, and pulmonary hypertension (Table 1). Relative contraindications are mostly related to anatomic problems that can complicate the creation of the TIPS; these include portal vein thrombosis, hepatic vein obstruction, large hepatoma, hypervascular liver tumors, and encephalopathy. Because TIPS can be performed in these situations, the difficulty of this procedure and risk assessment should be balanced against the clinical necessity. Clinical situations with relative contraindications that justify TIPS placement include patients with refractory variceal bleeding or ascites with hepatoma or recanalization of occluded portal veins. Patients with Budd-Chiari syndrome and progressive liver failure in whom there are no patent hepatic veins are also candidates for TIPS placement.

Table 1: Contraindications to Transjugular Intrahepatic Portosystemic Shunts

Absolute Contraindications	Relative Contraindications
Severe hepatic encephalopathy	Hepatic vein thrombosis
Congestive heart failure	Severe coagulopathy
Severe pulmonary hypertension	Central hepatoma
Multiple hepatic cysts	Thrombocytopenia $<20,000/cm^3$
Active infection	Moderate pulmonary hypertension
	Portal vein thrombosis

PATIENT SELECTION

During the early experience with TIPS, most procedures were performed without adherence to strict selection criteria and resulted in poor outcomes. Before any intervention, a thorough evaluation and multidisciplinary consideration is mandatory. Careful clinical workup must identify evidence of cardiovascular, pulmonary, or renal disease. Mental status, quality of life, and ability to comply with follow-up must also be addressed. Laboratory evaluation of renal and liver function, as well as platelet count and clotting times, are necessary. Imaging studies should evaluate the patency of hepatic vasculature and identify any liver lesions.

In recent years many clinical variables were found to be associated with a poor outcome after TIPS placement, including high bilirubin, prolonged prothrombin time, high creatinine, encephalopathy, sepsis, the use of balloon tamponade for bleeding control, need for mechanical ventilation, use of vasoactive drugs for hemodynamic support, high number of sclerotherapy sessions, and emergency TIPS placement. Incorporation of several of these variables into prognostic scoring systems has been useful in patient selection and shared decision making.

Prognostic aids are not a substitute for clinical judgment but can help to identify patients at high risk for this procedure. A variety of scoring systems are available for stratifying patients on the basis of severity of liver disease. These include (1) Child-Pugh scores, (2) Model for End-Stage Liver Disease (MELD Score), and (3) Acute Physiology and Chronic Health Evaluation (APACHE) score. Use of a staging system will optimize patient selection by eliminating high-risk procedures, allowing for more valid comparisons among studies, and providing more accurate survival prediction for patients and their families.

It may be ideal first to distinguish patients who require an elective TIPS procedure from those needing emergency TIPS, which has a much higher mortality rate. For patients considered for elective TIPS procedures, both MELD and Child-Pugh scores have performed similarly in predicting survival and identifying patients likely to have a poor outcome. The MELD score is preferred by many, however, because the Child-Pugh score uses the subjective measurements of ascites and encephalopathy and imposes a ceiling effect on bilirubin levels, theoretically having less power in delineating advanced liver failure. Although stark cutoffs do not exist, favorable results are usually seen in patients with a MELD score of 17 or less, with excellent survival in those with MELD scores of 10 or below. Patients with MELD scores over 24 are at high risk for early mortality and should not undergo elective TIPS.

For patients considered for emergency TIPS, which has an early mortality of up to 50%, the Child-Pugh and APACHE II systems have proven useful in identifying patients at high risk. Patients with an APACHE II score over 18 and Child-Pugh class C cirrhosis have a dismal prognosis, with a 93.3% early mortality rate shown in one study. The Prognostic Index, however, is the only model to date that is based solely on emergently placed TIPS. Although not externally validated, the authors have found prospectively that scores above 18.52 have yielded a 100% 6-week mortality (42% of total deaths), making it difficult to recommend TIPS for high-risk patients in this category.

These prognostic tools are only one piece of the equation but are helpful in identifying patients at high risk and guiding decision making between patients and their physicians. Ideally, TIPS placement in any patient meeting minimal transplant criteria should be viewed as a bridge to transplantation.

TECHNIQUE FOR TIPS

Because TIPS is one of the most invasive percutaneous procedures performed at most institutions, only individuals with proper training and experience should perform it. On all patients a history is taken, and physical examination is performed to assess the physical status; standard laboratory data, which includes coagulation profile, liver function tests, and white blood cell count and platelet count, are essential. On the basis of these results, a MELD score is calculated before the procedure to assess the potential impact of this procedure on outcome. Using this score not only provides guidelines to the physician but can help to explain the potential severity of this procedure to patients and family while consent is obtained.

Before the procedure, dedicated imaging targeting the portal vein is mandatory. Magnetic resonance angiography (MRA) or computed tomographic angiography (CTA) are both adequate and can assess the location and patency of the portal vein. Doppler ultrasound can provide physiologic information but does not convey the full three-dimensional anatomic relationship of the portal vein to the hepatic veins, inferior vena cava, and other vital structures that is often necessary to perform this procedure. Finally, all patients require coverage with broad-spectrum antibiotics, and the procedure is performed with full conscious sedation. In extremely sick patients with variceal bleeding, the use of general anesthesia is mandatory to protect the airway from aspiration.

Accessing the Hepatic Veins

Because of the close proximity of the right hepatic vein to the portal vein, the right hepatic vein is used in the majority of TIPS procedures (Fig. 1). Under fluoroscopy, access into the right jugular vein is obtained with sonographic guidance, followed by the placement of an 11-F sheath (St. Jude Medical, St. Paul, MN). Using a 7-F MPA-1-guiding catheter (Cordis, Miami Lakes, FL), the right hepatic vein is cannulated with a Benson guidewire (Cook, Bloomington, IN). As the severity of cirrhosis increases, cannulating the hepatic veins can become more difficult. This difficulty is often related to a small, shrunken liver surrounded by ascites that is displaced centrally. In addition, the angle of the hepatic vein near the inferior vena cava increases with cirrhosis, and this can further hinder the cannulation of hepatic veins. When these situations occur, other catheters with sharper angulations may have to be used. If catheter selection is inadequate, either the middle or left hepatic veins can be used.

Carbon Dioxide Portography

The next step is to visualize the portal vein to facilitate transhepatic punctures (Fig. 1). Using the right hepatic vein, the surgeon removes the guiding catheter and exchanges it for a Berman wedge catheter (Arrow International, Reading, PA). Carbon dioxide (CO_2) has several advantages as a contrast agent: (1) it is readily available in most hospitals, (2) it is rapidly reabsorbed with blood, and (3) it can diffuse across liver parenchyma to opacify the portal vein. With the Berman wedge catheter inflated, CO_2 is injected rapidly using an AngioFlush III fluid management system (AngioDynamics, Queensbury, NY) and a 60-ml syringe. Image acquisition should be at six frames per second to capture the rapid distribution of the gas into the portal vein. Using both a frontal and lateral view, the surgeon should be able to readily identify the portal vein. After identification of the portal vein, simultaneous wedged pressures of the liver and right atrium should be performed to determine corrected sinusoidal pressures. Significantly elevated right atrial pressures should immediately preclude any TIPS procedure until a full cardiac evaluation is performed.

Portal Vein Cannulation

Currently, two needle systems are routinely used for transhepatic punctures of the portal vein (Figs. 2 and 3): Rosch-Uchida Liver

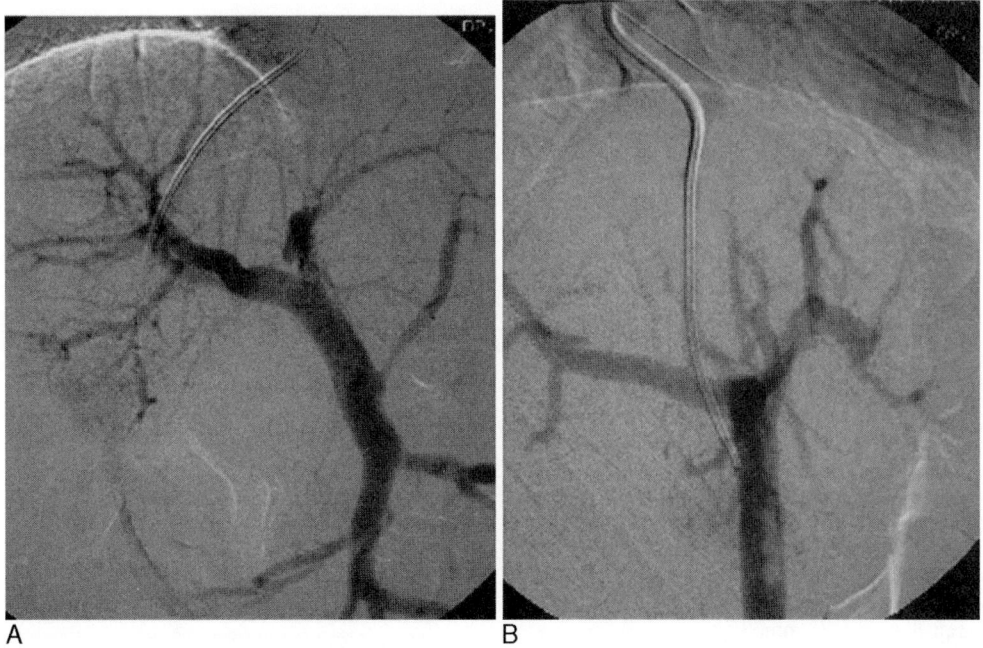

Figure 1 Frontal **(A)** and lateral **(B)** views: gaseous CO_2 is injected through a wedge catheter placed in the right hepatic vein to opacify the portal vein.

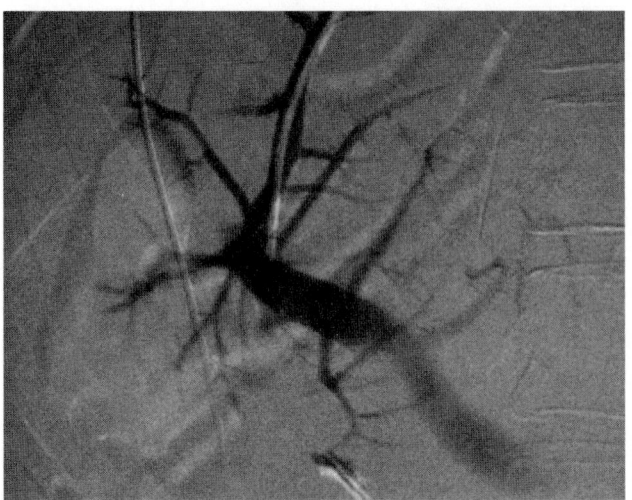

Figure 2 Transhepatic puncture of the portal vein using a Colapinto needle. Contrast is injected through the needle to opacify the portal vein.

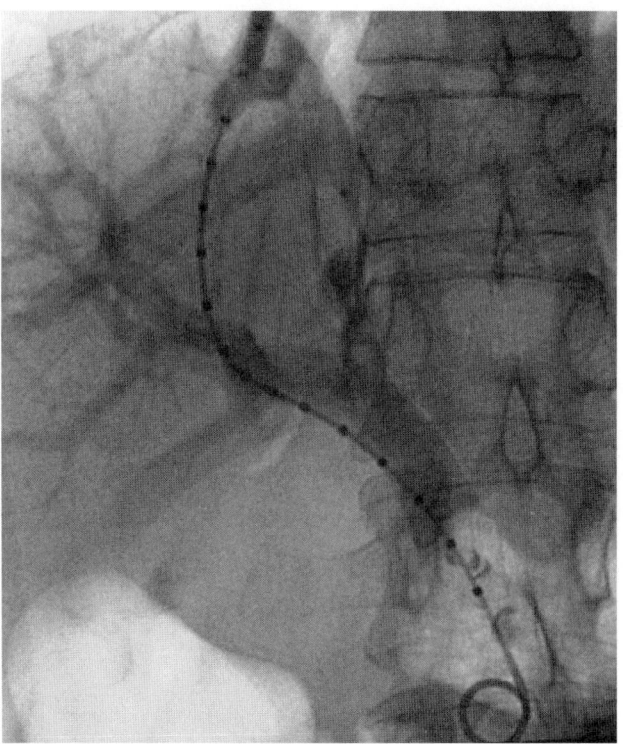

Figure 3 Pigtail catheter is advanced into the portal vein to obtain contrast portogram and direct portal pressures.

Access Set (Cook Medical, Bloomington, IN) or Colapinto needle (Cook Medical, Bloomington, IN). The Rosch-Uchida set is a smaller-caliber needle system that can minimize the trauma of transhepatic punctures; however, it can be inadequate with advanced cirrhosis because of the rigidity of the liver. In these situations, the Colapinto needle may be a better option.

After identification of the portal vein, the Berman wedge is exchanged for either the Rosch-Uchida or Colapinto needle set. Using the CO_2 portogram for guidance, the surgeon slowly performs needle advancement through the liver and in the general direction of the portal vein. After a needle pass, the surgeon gently withdraws the needle while aspirating with a 20-ml syringe. Often, multiple passes are required before the portal vein is accessed. Entry into the portal vein is demonstrated by an immediate return of venous blood into the syringe and subsequent confirmation with

contrast injection through the needle. The ideal entry point into the portal vein should be the main right portal vein trunk.

After portal vein entry has been confirmed, a Benson guidewire is advanced through the needle system and into the portal vein. Subsequently, the needle system is removed and exchanged for a pigtail catheter that is advanced into either the splenic or superior mesenteric vein (Fig. 3). Simultaneous pressures between the portal and right atrium should be obtained, followed by a formal contrast portogram to delineate the entire portomesenteric venous circulation.

Stent Placement

Before placement of a stent, the pigtail catheter is removed and exchanged for an angioplasty balloon to dilatate the transhepatic tract (Fig. 4). Although there are multiple stents available for TIPS, most surgeons primarily favor stent grafts (VIATORR, W.L. Gore, Flagstaff, AZ) because of their improved shunt patency.

The VIATORR stent graft is composed of a flexible self-expanding nitinol stent with a layer of tetrafluoroethylene (ePTFE). The stent-graft has a 2-cm-long unlined portal vein segment to maintain portal perfusion and a graft-lined segment (4 to 8 cm long) that is deployed within the intrahepatic tract and the hepatic vein from the portal ostium to the inferior vena cava (IVC). A circumferential radiopaque gold band identifies the junction between the two segments, and another radiopaque gold marker is incorporated into trailing edge of the device. The entire stent graft is constrained beneath a low-profile plastic introducer sleeve, which facilitates insertion of the leading end of the device through the hemostatic valve. Three stent graft diameters (8 mm, 10 mm, and 12 mm) are currently available.

For stent-graft insertion, the entire sheath system must be advanced 3 cm into the portal vein. The VIATORR device is introduced and advanced until the leading edge is at the tip of the sheath and the entire uncovered stent segment lies within the portal vein. With the delivery catheter held fixed in this position, withdrawal of the introducer sheath deploys the leading 2 cm of bare stent. The delivery catheter and the sheath are then pulled back until the junctional radiopaque marker is placed at the portal entry site. The introducer sheath is then fully retracted over the delivery

system to expose the entire stent graft. The covered portion is then deployed in the tract and hepatic vein by pulling the constraining PTFE tape. The stent graft is subsequently dilatated to its nominal diameter with balloon, followed by pressure measurements and portal venography. Embolization of varices can be performed through the TIPS, especially in cases where dilatation of the stent to 12 mm does not reduce the portosystemic gradient to less than 12 mmHg or 20% below the baseline. Technical success in performing this procedure is greater than 95%, and clinical success in managing the symptoms of portal hypertension is seen in more than 90% of patients.

COMPLICATIONS

Complications related to TIPS can be classified as acute and chronic (Table 2). Technical success from a TIPS procedure has been seen in more than 90% of patients. Acute complications related to the procedure include intraperitoneal hemorrhage from capsular perfora-

Table 2: Complications of Transjugular Intrahepatic Portosystemic Shunts

Complications	Frequency (%)
Shunt occlusion/stenosis	10–15
Encephalopathy	10–45
Malposition of stents	10–20
Transscapular perforation	1–2
Hemobilia	<5
Sepsis	210

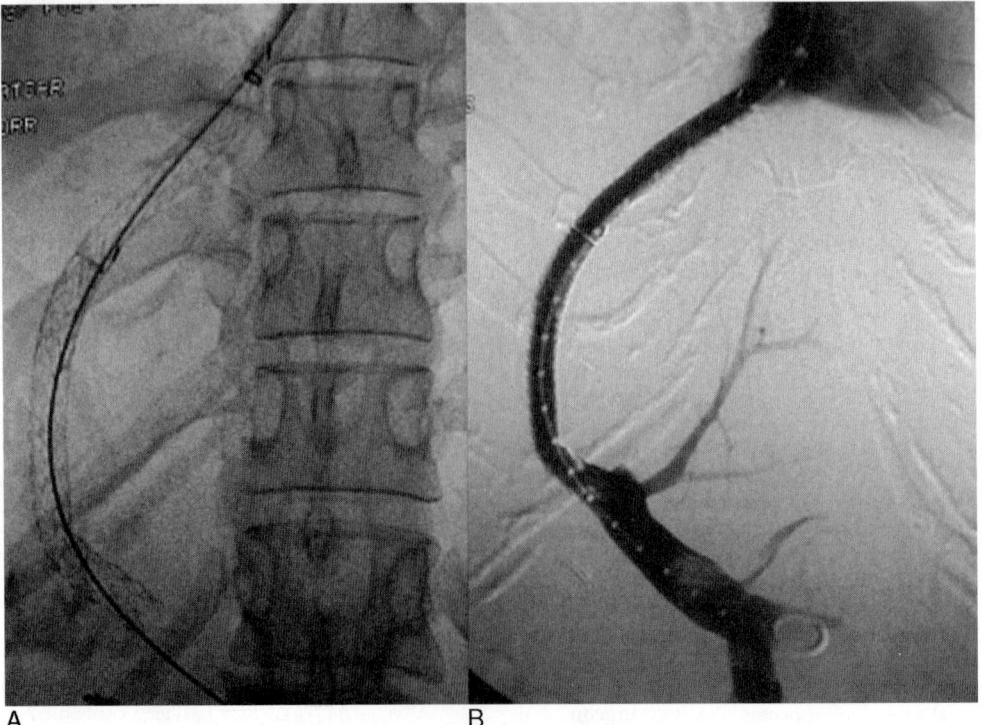

A   B

Figure 4 A self-expanding covered nitinol stent (Viabahn; W.L.Gore, Flagstaff, AZ) is deployed from the portal vein to the hepatic vein to create the transjugular intrahepatic portosystemic shunts shunt. **(B)** Portogram demonstrates the flow from the portal vein through the stent and to the right atrium. Some perfusion to the liver is maintained.

tion, hemobilia, and acute cardiopulmonary collapse from right heart failure. The frequencies of these complications are low and are usually managed with expectant monitoring. The most severe acute complication is acute or worsening hepatic failure after the procedure. This is often related to poor hepatic reserve and advanced liver disease (Child-Pugh class C). Although these high-risk patients should be screened before a TIPS procedure, unexpected hepatic failure may require emergent liver transplantation for salvage.

The two major long-term complications that have limited the efficacy of TIPS are hepatic encephalopathy and shunt dysfunction. Hepatic encephalopathy is often the result of poor portal perfusion because of significant shunting through the TIPS stent. Most often this is seen in patients with severe advanced liver disease and tends to occur within the first month. Reports from multiple studies have been variable but, in general, 15% to 40% of post-TIPS patients have some form of encephalopathy (mild to severe). Factors associated with encephalopathy include nonalcoholic liver disease, female sex, and prior history of encephalopathy. Most of these situations can be successfully managed with lactulose, protein restrictions, and elimination of any potential precipitating factors. In patients who do not respond, then the addition of neomycin or metronidazole should be considered. Finally, in patients who are refractory to any medical therapy and worsening encephalopathy, the TIPS shunt can be closed with novel percutaneous techniques.

TIPS dysfunction is defined as either occlusion of the TIPS shunt or stenosis resulting in loss of portal decompression and return of clinical symptomatology. Occlusions, although infrequent, occur within 24 hours and are usually a result of communication to the biliary system, hypercoagulable state or inadequate stent coverage of the TIPS tract. Unlike occlusion, stenosis occurs in a delayed manner and is the result of pseudointimal hyperplasia. Symptoms tend to occur when there is a 50% stenosis or an elevation of the portosystemic gradient greater than 12 mm Hg. Although there are no clear, definable guidelines for monitoring of TIPS stent, most interventionists use Doppler ultrasound for surveillance. However, sonographic studies can be imprecise and should not be the sole criteria in patients at high risk for stenosis or with clinical symptoms. An abnormal Doppler ultrasound performed with an experienced sonographer can be predictive of a stenosis. A normal study does not completely exclude a TIPS stenosis, however, especially in a patient with recurrent symptoms. In these situations, the only way to evaluate the patient is to access the shunt for formal venography.

■ CONCLUSION

Since the introduction of TIPS in 1990, it has become one of the main therapeutic options in the management of patients with portal hypertension. With incorporation of rapidly developing stent technologies and enhancement of patient selections, this procedure will continue to provide a minimally invasive safe option in patients with portal hypertension.

SUGGESTED READINGS

Angermayr B, Cejna M, Karnel F, and others: Child-Pugh versus MELD score in predicting survival in patients undergoing transjugular intrahepatic portosystemic shunt, *Gut* 52(6):879, 2003.

Bañares R, Casado M, Rodríguez-Láiz JM, and others: Urgent transjugular intrahepatic portosystemic shunt for control of acute variceal bleeding, *Am J Gastroenterol* 93(1):75, 1998.

Boyer TD, Haskal ZJ: American Association for the Study of Liver Diseases Practice Guidelines: the role of transjugular intrahepatic portosystemic shunt creation in the management of portal hypertension, *J Vasc Interv Radiol* 16(5):615, 2005.

Boyer TD, Haskal ZJ: The role of transjugular intrahepatic portosystemic shunt in the management of portal hypertension, *Hepatology* 41(2):386, 2005.

Brensing KA, Raab P, Textor J, and others: Prospective evaluation of a clinical score for 60-day mortality after transjugular intrahepatic portosystemic stent-shunt: Bonn TIPSS early mortality analysis, *Eur J Gastroenterol Hepatol* 14(7):723, 2002.

Encarnacion CE, Palmaz JC, Rivera FJ, and others: Transjugular intrahepatic portosystemic shunt placement for variceal bleeding: predictors of mortality, *J Vasc Interv Radiol* 6(5):687, 1995.

Ferral H, Gamboa P, Postoak DW, and others: Survival after elective transjugular intrahepatic portosystemic shunt creation: prediction with model for end-stage liver disease score, *Radiology* 231(1):231, 2004.

Ferral H, Patel NH: Selection criteria for patients undergoing transjugular intrahepatic portosystemic shunt procedures: current status, *J Vasc Interv Radiol* 16(4):449, 2005.

Forman LM, Lucey MR: Predicting the prognosis of chronic liver disease: an evolution from child to MELD. Mayo end-stage liver disease, *Hepatology* 33(2):473, 2001.

Molmenti EP, Segev DL, Arepally A, and others: The utility of TIPS in the management of Budd-Chiari syndrome, *Ann Surg* 241(6):978; discussion 982, 2005.

Montgomery A, Ferral H, Vasan R, Postoak DW: MELD score as a predictor of early death in patients undergoing elective transjugular intrahepatic portosystemic shunt (TIPS) procedures, *Cardiovasc Intervent Radiol* 28(3):307, 2005.

Patch D, Nikolopoulou V, McCormick A, and others: Factors related to early mortality after transjugular intrahepatic portosystemic shunt for failed endoscopic therapy in acute variceal bleeding, *J Hepatol* 28(3):454, 1998.

Rosado B, Kamath PS: Transjugular intrahepatic portosystemic shunts: an update, *Liver Transpl* 9(3):207, 2003.

Rubin RA, Haskal ZJ, O'Brien CB, and others: Transjugular intrahepatic portosystemic shunting: decreased survival for patients with high APACHE II scores, *Am J Gastroenterol* 90(4):556, 1995.

Salerno F, Merli M, Cazzaniga M, and others: MELD score is better than Child-Pugh score in predicting 3-month survival of patients undergoing transjugular intrahepatic portosystemic shunt, *J Hepatol* 36(4):494, 2002.

Portal Hypertension: Role of Liver Transplantation

Andrew M. Cameron, MD, PhD, Jonathan R. Hiatt, MD, and Ronald W. Busuttil, MD, PhD

Normal pressure in the portal vein varies between 3 and 7 mm Hg. In response to a variety of causes, most commonly cirrhosis from viral hepatitis or alcohol use, these pressures may become elevated. Lower-resistance venous collaterals then develop that may rupture and result in clinically significant upper gastrointestinal bleeding. Other sequelae of portal hypertension include ascites, hepatic encephalopathy, peripheral edema, and splenomegaly with thrombocytopenia from platelet sequestration (Table 1).

Orthotopic liver transplantation (OLT) is the optimal treatment for portal hypertension because it both decompresses the varices and corrects the underlying cause. While the patient is awaiting OLT, or in rare cases when OLT is not necessary, various treatment modalities to manage the sequelae of portal hypertension are available. Management algorithms are directed to symptomatic treatment or prevention of gastroesophageal variceal bleeding, ascites formation, and hepatic encephalopathy with the understanding that OLT represents the eventual final pathway for durable resolution of portal hypertension via treatment of its underlying cause. Ironically, the Model for End Stage Liver Disease (MELD) system in current use for liver transplant allocation is based on only three laboratory values: serum creatinine, total bilirubin, and international normalized ratio, none of which is directly related to a patient's degree of clinical disability from the sequelae of portal hypertension. The historical evolution of the understanding and management of portal hypertension is shown in Table 2.

This chapter considers the use of OLT for specific complications of portal hypertension. We also discuss technical issues related to transplantation in the setting of severe portal hypertension, as well as management of portal hypertension after OLT.

VARICEAL BLEEDING: MANAGEMENT ALGORITHM AND ROLE OF LIVER TRANSPLANTATION

Variceal bleeding is a major complication of advanced portal hypertension, with substantial morbidity and mortality. Although portal hypertension resulting from end-stage liver disease is a cardinal indication for liver replacement, isolated variceal bleeding can be managed successfully without liver transplantation. Also, some patients experience bleeding early in the course of transplant candidacy or at a time when a donor organ is not immediately available.

Mortality from bleeding esophageal or gastric varices is correlated linearly with hepatic function, measured by Child-Pugh grading; mortality for the index bleed is 5%, 18%, and 68% in grades A, B, and C patients, respectively. More than half of patients with esophagogastric varices never experience bleeding. These patients are managed with beta-blockers, which reduce portal pressure by constriction of the splanchnic vasculature and reduction of cardiac output. The use of prophylactic interventions has been debated. Although prophylactic surgical shunts have no role, endoscopic

therapies may be of benefit in reducing the risk of bleeding with grade 4 varices but lack a clear effect on mortality. Some centers use hepatic portal venous pressure for measurement of response to beta-blockade and other interventions.

Patients with acute variceal bleeding require emergent resuscitation, medical management, endoscopic diagnosis, and directed therapy. The algorithm for management of these patients is summarized in Figure 1. Patients are admitted to the intensive care unit (ICU) for resuscitation, monitoring, and procedures. Endotracheal intubation is often necessary for airway protection, especially during endoscopy. Large-bore venous access is secured, usually in a central vein. Clotting defects are corrected with transfusion of fresh frozen plasma and platelets. Ascites and infection with bacterial or fungal organisms should be identified and treated because these may complicate and exacerbate bleeding. Although a variety of vasoactive and other medications are available for control of variceal hemorrhage, the current regimen uses octreotide and pantoprazole. Octreotide is a synthetic analogue of somatostatin, a splanchnic constrictor and inhibitor of glucagon and other vasodilatory peptides. Pantoprazole suppresses gastric acid secretion by inhibition

Table 1: Portal Hypertension Overview

Definition	Portal Venous Pressure Exceeding the Normal Value of 3–7 mmHg, Typically Rising to 20–30 mmHg
Etiology	*Prehepatic*
	Portal vein thrombosis, splenic vein thrombosis
	Intrahepatic
	Presinusoidal
	Schistosomiasis, primary biliary cirrhosis, sarcoidosis
	Sinusoidal
	Cirrhosis (viral hepatitis, alcohol, etc.)
	Postsinusoidal
	Alcohol-induced central hyaline sclerosis
	Posthepatic
	Budd-Chiari, veno-occlusive disease, right heart failure
Collaterals	From: left gastric vein, short gastric veins
	To: intercostal, diaphragmatic, and esophageal veins
	Collateral: gastroesophageal Varices
	From: superior hemorrhoidal vein
	To: middle and inferior hemorrhoidal veins
	Collateral: hemorrhoids
	From: left portal vein via falciform ligament
	To: umbilicus and abdominal wall veins
	Collateral: caput Medusa
	From: liver via lienorenal ligament
	To: left renal vein
	Collateral: retroperitoneal veins
Clinical Sequelae	Gastroesophageal varices
	Ascites
	Hepatic encephalopathy
	Splenomegaly with thrombocytopenia

Table 2: Historical Timeline of Surgery for Portal Hypertension

1877	Nicolai Eck creates portacaval shunts in dogs to treat portal hypertension following portal vein ligation
1893	Ivan Pavlov studies physiology of portacaval shunt, describes "meat intoxication syndrome" (Nobel Prize in Medicine, 1894)
1906	Alexis Carrel publishes vascular technique of portacaval anastomosis (Nobel Prize in Medicine, 1912)
1945	A. O. Whipple reports portacaval shunts in humans
1963	Thomas Starzl reports first orthotopic liver transplantation in humans
1967	Warren and Zeppa describe series of distal splenorenal shunts
1979	Endoscopic gastroesophageal variceal therapy reported by Terblanche
1982	Colapinto reports transjugular intrahepatic portosystemic shunting in humans
1983	National Institutes of Health consensus conference on use of liver transplantation for treatment of end-stage liver disease

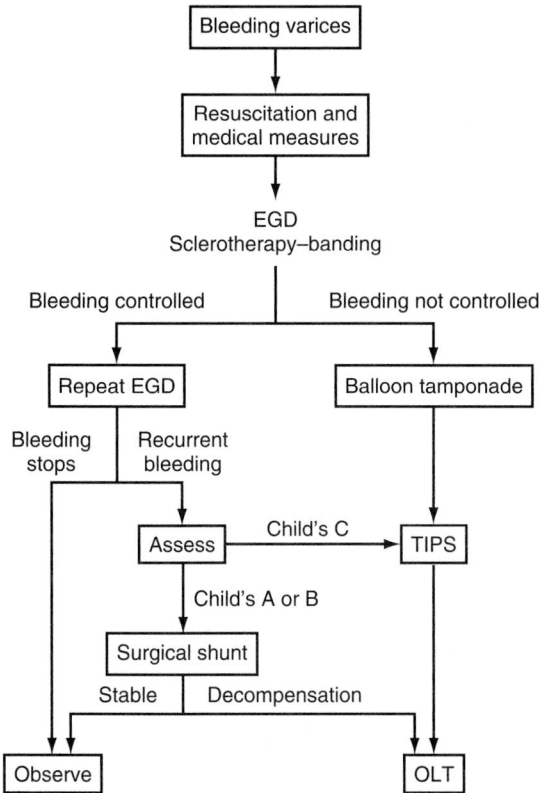

Figure 1 Management of acutely bleeding gastroesophageal varices. *EGD*, Esophagogastroduodenoscopy; *OLT*, orthotopic liver transplantation; *TIPS*, transjugular intrahepatic portosystemic shunt.

of the hydrogen-potassium adenosine tri-phosphate pump in the gastric parietal cell.

Endoscopic Diagnosis and Therapy

Emergent esophagogastroduodenoscopy (EGD) identifies the presence of varices and excludes other bleeding sources such as portal gastropathy, gastritis, or ulcer. Bleeding varices in the esophagus or esophagogastric junction are treated with injection sclerotherapy or variceal band ligation. The latter is more difficult to perform but has lower morbidity than sclerotherapy, which may be complicated by aspiration pneumonia or esophageal ulceration. In capable hands, bleeding is controlled by endoscopic measures in more than 90% of patients. With bleeding controlled, patients are observed closely, and repeat EGD is performed within the first week after the initial session. Bleeding that is uncontrolled by endoscopic measures represents a major challenge. Initial control is attempted with balloon tamponade using a Sengstaken-Blakemore tube. The next intervention is usually transjugular intrahepatic portosystemic shunting (TIPS). Liver transplantation is a therapeutic option for recalcitrant episodic bleeding, provided that the patient can be stabilized hemodynamically and an organ becomes available.

Bleeding may recur in patients whose bleeding was controlled initially by medical and endoscopic measures. In Child-Pugh class A or B cirrhosis with good liver function, a surgical shunt is performed. Various options are discussed next, but in general terms, the choice of shunt is determined by the portal anatomy and the likelihood and timing of liver transplantation.

Portosystemic Shunts

Shunts constructed between portal and systemic circulations are either selective or nonselective types. The latter (portacaval, mesocaval, TIPS) reduce portal pressure and have the advantages of ease of construction and durability but share the problems of encephalopathy and worsening liver function. Selective shunts, of which distal splenorenal is the most common, provide selective decompression of the portal-azygos system, and thus of the gastroesophageal varices, while preserving nutrient inflow to the liver via the greater splanchnic circulation (superior mesenteric and portal veins). The use of the distal splenorenal shunt is limited by its decreased efficacy in the acutely bleeding patient and its propensity to cause ascites. Additionally, there is an eventual loss of selectivity by gradual enlargement of pancreatic collaterals.

TIPS has become the first-line therapy for portal hypertension after immediate endoscopic control, despite few controlled studies confirming its benefit. The procedure is performed by interventional radiologists using fluoroscopic and sonographic guidance while the patient is under sedation and local anesthesia. A needle is passed from the middle hepatic vein into a portal vein branch, followed by guidewire passage through the needle and into the main portal vein. Next, portal pressure is measured; the tract is dilatated with a balloon; portography is performed; and an expandable stent is inserted, sometimes followed by a second stent if necessary to reduce the portal pressure gradient below 12 mm Hg. As with any nonselective shunt, hepatic encephalopathy may occur, as may liver failure from diversion of portal flow. The major complications of TIPS include shunt stenosis (33% to 66%); hepatic encephalopathy (15% to 30%); technical failure (5% to 10%); and portal or splenic vein thrombosis, worsening liver function, and chronic hemolysis (< 5% each).

Distal splenorenal shunt (DSRS) and nonselective shunts have been compared in many trials over the past quarter century. The prevailing conclusions from these reports are that rates of survival and recurrent bleeding are similar, but incidence of postoperative encephalopathy is lower with DSRS. Survival after DSRS in Child-Pugh grade A or B is better than that for patients with more severely compromised liver function. Another group of studies comparing DSRS with sclerotherapy has generally supported the concept of sclerotherapy for acute bleeding and DSRS for elective surgical correction of chronic or recurrent bleeding.

Orloff has been a consistent advocate of emergency side-to-side portacaval shunting for acutely bleeding esophageal varices. In a report of 400 patients, rates of 15-year survival and of recurrent encephalopathy were 57% and 8%, respectively, for the 220 patients treated after 1978. An earlier report described excellent results even with advanced disease: 5-year survival in 64% and postoperative encephalopathy in 18% of 94 Child-Pugh class C patients.

The mesocaval shunt, or H-graft, has been advocated as a bridge to liver transplantation because it is relatively easy to construct, avoids any dissection in the porta hepatis, and can be simply ligated at time of transplantation. A randomized prospective comparison of H-graft with small-diameter side-to-side portacaval shunt in good-risk patients found less encephalopathy and better preservation of liver function with the H-graft compared with a direct side-to-side portacaval shunt without prosthetic.

Portal vein thrombosis is an important cause of extrahepatic portal hypertension, particularly in children. Using an inferior mesenteric or internal jugular venous conduit, the Rex procedure reconnects the mesenteric system to the portal system at the Rex recessus, a bridge of liver tissue between segments 3 and 4. In the first U.S. series of Rex shunts, Bambini described the procedure as superior to DSRS for reasons including restoration of portal flow, normalization of portal venous pressure, and splenic decompression, with relief of secondary thrombocytopenia and leukopenia.

Splenectomy remains an option of last resort when no appropriate-caliber vessels remain patent for shunting. Thrombocytopenia and upper gastrointestinal (GI) bleeding may improve, especially in cases of sinistral (left-sided) portal hypertension, as it does with splenic vein thrombosis. Pediatric patients will require penicillin prophylaxis thereafter, as well as vigilance regarding postsplenectomy sepsis.

As shown in Figure 1, in the management of portal hypertensive gastroesophageal variceal bleeding, OLT has a role in patients with recalcitrant bleeding and underlying parenchymal failure and for those who have received shunts or medical management and in whom liver function is steadily worsening. When a liver is allocated to these patients via the MELD system, OLT will correct both the complications of portal hypertension and the underlying cause.

ASCITES AND HEPATIC ENCEPHALOPATHY: MANAGEMENT ALGORITHMS AND ROLE OF LIVER TRANSPLANTATION

Ascites

Ascites, or hepatic lymph, represents intraperitoneal accumulation of transudative fluid. The pathophysiology of ascites formation is poorly understood but probably is a function of low intravascular colloidal pressure and sodium retention in the setting of portal hypertension.

The evaluation of a patient with ascites includes abdominal paracentesis to exclude infection or spontaneous bacterial peritonitis (SBP). Fluid is sent for cell count with differential and bacterial culture with sensitivities. SBP is considered present when abdominal fluid contains more than 250 polymorphonuclear leukocytes per milliliter. The most common organisms include *Escherichia coli*, *Klebsiella*, and *pneumococcus*. Patients are treated with intravenous cefotaxime for 5 days at a dose of 2 g every 8 hours.

Ascites formation is managed first by fluid restriction (1500 ml/day), diuretics, and sodium restriction (2 g/day). This regimen controls ascites in 95% of patients. Diuretic dosages may be increased to include furosemide (80 mg) and spironolactone (200 mg) orally twice per day.

Ascites that is refractory to these measures is treated with serial large-volume paracenteses. TIPS has been shown in controlled trials to be inferior to medical management for ascites. LeVeen or Denver peritoneovenous shunts have been shown in controlled trials to decrease hospitalizations and diuretic doses, but poor long-term patency, excessive complications, and lack of demonstrable survival

advantage over medical therapy have largely led to their abandonment.

As with other sequelae of portal hypertension, refractory ascites ultimately may be controlled only by OLT, which serves to decompress elevated portal pressures and replace the underlying cirrhotic liver. Although the presence of ascites was part of the United Network for Organ Sharing allocation scoring system used until 2002, it does not figure into calculation of the MELD score. Patients with significant ascites and a low MELD score therefore require careful medical management as they await OLT.

Hepatic Encephalopathy

Hepatic encephalopathy (HE) describes the spectrum of reversible neuropsychiatric abnormalities seen in patients with liver dysfunction after exclusion of unrelated neurologic or metabolic abnormalities. HE is manifested clinically as increased fatigue, disturbance in sleep patterns, and asterixis and may progress to somnolence and eventual coma. Computed tomography, magnetic resonance imaging, and lumbar puncture tests are within normal limits in patients with HE, whereas serum ammonia levels will be elevated in 90% of patients. Ammonia is produced by enterocytes from glutamine and by colonic bacterial catabolism of nitrogenous sources such as ingested protein and secreted urea. A functioning liver clears portal vein ammonia, converting it to urea or glutamine and thereby preventing its entry into the systemic circulation.

Patients with HE often require transfer to an ICU, with intubation if the patient has become unarousable or unable to participate in care. Precipitating events that cause worsening HE must be considered in treatment strategies. Such events include infection (such as SBP), bleeding from varices or another source, electrolyte abnormalities (especially low potassium), drugs (benzodiazepines or other sedatives), and dehydration. In these cases the underlying cause of the decompensation must be addressed along with the resultant HE and any subsequent complications.

Strategies used to prevent worsening HE include a low protein diet (<40 g/day) and lactulose (30 ml orally or by nasogastric tube every 4 hours) titrated to five or six bowel movements per day or 1 L of diarrhea. Lactulose in HE is presumed to exert its effect by acidification of ammonia to the unabsorbable ammonium form in the intestine. Neomycin (3 g orally every six hours) can also be used for HE and acts by decreasing anaerobic bacterial growth in the intestines, with a resultant decrease in ammonia production.

Occasional patients will present with cirrhosis and resultant portal hypertension manifested almost exclusively by HE. In some cases, their HE may prove refractory to aggressive medical management and requires hospitalization until OLT, which represents the only hope for return to clinical normalcy. Current liver allocation policies using the MELD formula put such patients at a severe disadvantage and require aggressive advocacy by their physicians to seek an exception in MELD status for early OLT.

ORTHOTOPIC LIVER TRANSPLANTATION: TECHNICAL ISSUES RELATED TO PORTAL HYPERTENSION

Orthotopic Liver Transplantation with Portal Vein Thrombus and Orthotopic Liver Transplantation after Surgical Shunts or Transjugular Intrahepatic Portosystemic Shunting

Recipient hepatectomy in OLT can be made considerably more difficult by the presence of severe portal hypertension and varices. In such cases, total venovenous bypass may prove invaluable

(Fig. 2). Other technical challenges related to portal hypertension include OLT in the presence of portal vein thrombosis (PVT) and OLT after surgical portosystemic shunt or TIPS.

The presence and extent of PVT should be determined before transplantation whenever possible. Organ selection, the necessity for donor venous conduit, and intraoperative blood loss may all be affected. Extensive thrombosis of the portomesenteric system is rare and, if diagnosed preoperatively, will prevent futile attempts at PV thrombectomy. Alternatively, if proximal dissection proximally to the superior mesenteric-splenic vein junction behind the neck of the pancreas reveals a soft, patent portal vein, then thrombectomy with Fogarty catheters may be attempted.

Thromboendvenectomy is required in cases of more extensive thrombus. This can be followed by use of a Fogarty catheter or insertion of a PV bypass cannula, but the PV may be fragile at this point and prone to tearing. With chronic thrombotic occlusion extending below the superior mesenteric vein-splenic vein (SMV-SV) confluence, a donor venous conduit is used to construct a jump graft from patent recipient SMV to donor PV, as first described by Shaw.

Outcomes in recipients with PVT have improved in recent reports. At the University of California at Los Angeles (UCLA), a review of 1423 patients undergoing OLT revealed PVT in 70 patients (4.9%). The first 35 patients with PVT had a 66% survival (vs. 82% in a control patient group), whereas the latter 35 had an 82% survival at 1 year, compared with 85% in control subjects. Although mortality rates for OLT with or without PVT are now similar, greater morbidity with PVT has been demonstrated in several studies, including higher incidence of renal failure, transfusion requirements, and delayed graft function.

In cases in which patients have received prior surgical shunts, the portal vein may become shrunken and sclerotic, and pretransplant imaging is critical, that is, shunt patency may obviate the need for intraoperative portal venovenous bypass. However, it is our experience at UCLA that these cases can be technically demanding and that venovenous bypass (Fig. 2) remains a critical adjunct. Specifically, direct portacaval shunts require extensive hilar dissection, making subsequent OLT more difficult, and should be avoided in transplant candidates. These shunts require dismantling during OLT, with portal vein and inferior vena cava (IVC) control above and below the shunt before explantation. Subsequent sharp dissection with IVC repair and portal anastomosis can be difficult and may require portal venous extension with a donor iliac vein. OLT after mesocaval shunt is not as difficult; this shunt can serve to decompress portal hypertension during transplant and should be ligated after graft reperfusion. DSRS usually disturbs portal dissection only slightly and usually does not require ligation. Jenkins compared patients with (n = 81) and without (n = 247) DSRS before liver transplantation and found no differences in operative time, blood loss, and early mortality. Portal vein thrombosis occurred in five DSRS patients. The interval between DSRS and liver transplantation was more than 5 years, demonstrating the utility of the shunt procedure as a temporizing measure.

The number of patients coming to OLT after surgical shunt has declined over time with increasing use of TIPS. OLT in patients with prior TIPS can be difficult in cases of stent migration or placement

Figure 2 Venovenous bypass, allowing decompression of the splanchnic and systemic venous beds during orthotopic liver transplantation. *From Starzl TE, Demetris AJ: Curr Probl Surg 27:187, 1990.*

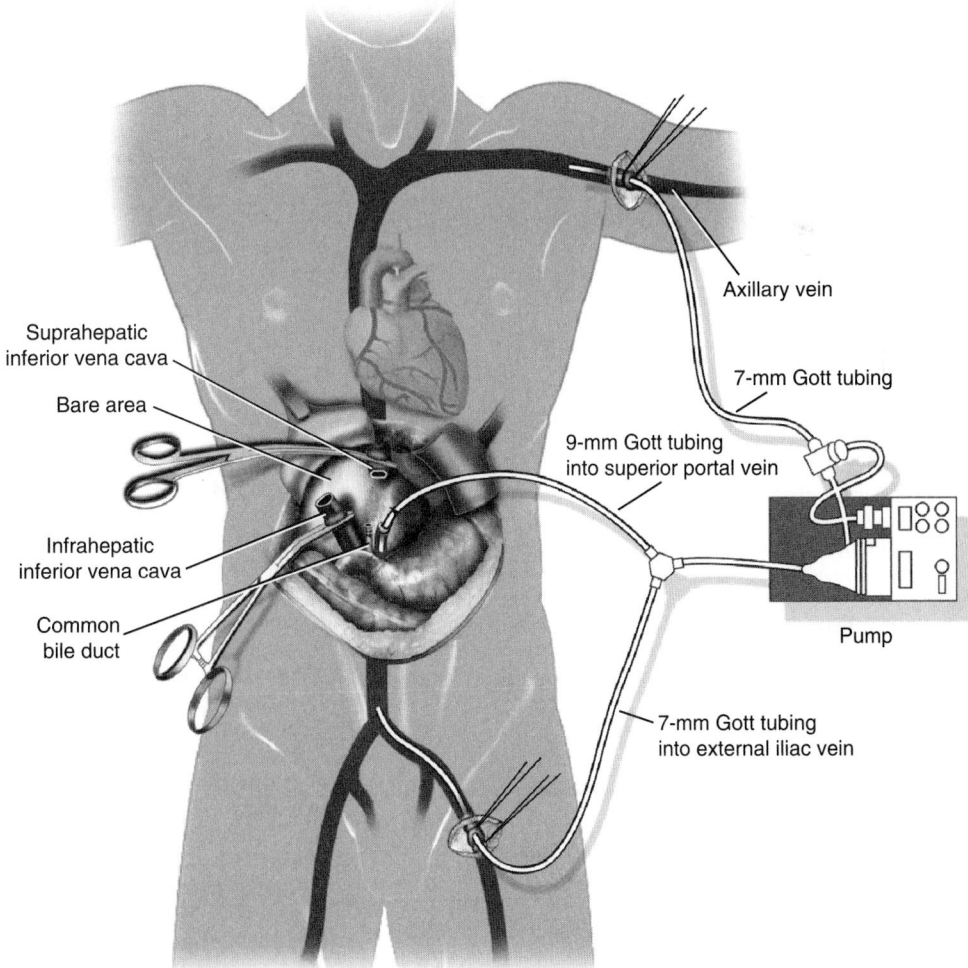

Suprahepatic inferior vena cava

Bare area

Infrahepatic inferior vena cava

Common bile duct

Axillary vein

7-mm Gott tubing

9-mm Gott tubing into superior portal vein

Pump

7-mm Gott tubing into external iliac vein

outside the liver, either in the suprahepatic IVC or extrahepatic portal vein. The latter case requires clamping below the stent, portal vein transection across the stent, and careful extraction of the remaining portion of the stent. In cases of IVC placement, TIPS extraction is again recommended. Rarely this requires performance of the suprahepatic IVC anastomosis in the pericardial space, open cardiotomy for removal, or incorporation of the stent-containing vessel wall into the anastomosis. Consenza performed a study of liver transplantation post-TIPS and found that TIPS did not affect operative time or transfusion requirements; portal vein thrombosis occurred in one patient and required thrombectomy at the time of transplantation.

Role of Living-Donor Liver Transplantation for Patients with Portal Hypertension

Adult-to-adult right hepatic lobe living donor liver transplantation (LDLT) has been developed over the past 15 years in response to donor scarcity and now is used for approximately 5% of all OLTs performed in the United States, or approximately 350 cases per year. Use of LDLT decreased over recent years with careful evaluation of advantages and disadvantages for donor and recipient. Right-lobe grafts are generally one third smaller than whole deceased-donor livers, and these partial grafts may represent a disadvantage to recipients with severe portal hypertension or others who are more critically ill.

Small-for-size syndrome (SFSS) occurs after hepatic resection or OLT with a small cadaveric graft or right-lobe LDLT, when reduced liver mass is insufficient to maintain normal function. The syndrome is characterized by postoperative liver dysfunction with prolonged cholestasis, coagulopathy, portal hypertension, and ascites, if severe. These features can persist for several weeks and may resolve, but half of OLT recipients with SFSS die of sepsis within 4 to 6 weeks. Recipient portal hypertension is thought to play an important pathophysiologic role. A graft weight to recipient body weight ratio (GRBWR) of greater than or equal to 0.8% gives graft and patient survivals greater than 90% in well-compensated patients. Heaton and coworkers have recommended a GRBWR of greater than or equal to 1.5% in patients with severe portal hypertension.

Inadequate functional liver mass, excessive portal perfusion, and exposure to gut-derived endotoxin contribute to morbidity after OLT in SFSS. Portal hypertension causes direct and indirect graft injury via hemodynamic interactions between portal vein and hepatic artery flow. SFSS grafts with a lower GRBWR show higher measured PV blood flow and correspondingly impaired hepatic artery (HA) flow. Moreover, there is a higher incidence of hepatic artery thrombosis (HAT) in SFSS grafts.

Ito performed a prospective trial measuring portal venous pressure in 79 cases of LDLT. Recipients of SFS grafts had significantly higher PVP, significantly worse survival, and higher incidence of bacteremia, cholestasis, prolonged PT, and ascites. Operative interventions reported to ameliorate SFSS include retention of donor middle hepatic vein with a right-lobe graft; recipient splenic artery ligation with or without splenectomy; and other measures, including graded portocaval shunt, portal vein band, or portomesenteric disconnection.

PORTAL HYPERTENSION AFTER ORTHOTOPIC LIVER TRANSPLANTATION

Portal Vein Thrombosis after Transplantation

In most cases of OLT with a graft of appropriate size, portal venous pressure should be decompressed effectively through the new low-resistance liver. In cases with persistence or recurrence of sequelae of portal hypertension, including ascites or variceal bleeding, technical complications such as PV thrombosis must be considered. Although recent series document PV patency following OLT at 95% to 100%, some centers continue to use preventive strategies, including prophylactic intravenous dextran and aspirin and color flow Doppler ultrasonography on the first postoperative day.

Early post-OLT PVT presents as liver failure, ascites, or GI bleeding, with high mortality. Immediate operative thrombectomy may salvage some grafts, but other patients require retransplantation. Percutaneous interventional methods including thrombolysis and stenting have been used, as well as systemic anticoagulation for patients in whom the 2- to 4-week postoperative timing makes reoperation ill advised. Late PVT generally presents with preserved liver function and can be managed with anticoagulation. In these patients, the sequelae of portal hypertension can be expected to recur, and consideration should be given to construction of a DSRS.

In the absence of vascular problems, recurrent sequelae may be unrelated to portal hypertension. Hepatic encephalopathy may take days to resolve after OLT, but long-term HE does not occur with good graft function. Other causes of mental status change, including cerebrovascular accident and drug toxicity (especially steroid effects and calcineurin inhibitor neurotoxicity), must be considered.

Gastroesophageal variceal bleeding after OLT also is rare. Varices persist after OLT but are decompressed when hepatic vessels are patent. Upper endoscopy should be performed for diagnosis and treatment, with consideration given to other causes of bleeding such as gastritis, peptic ulcer, or perioperative Mallory-Weiss tear. The last has been seen occasionally with our recent routine use of intraoperative transesophageal probes at UCLA.

Ascites after Orthotopic Liver Transplantation

Persistent ascites can occur after OLT and in most cases is seen with good graft function and in the absence of any technical problems. In these cases, ascites tends to resolve within 2 to 4 weeks of transplant. In a small subset of patients, ascites persist for longer periods. Investigators at the University of Pennsylvania found prolonged persistent ascites to be associated with hepatitis C virus (HCV) infection, significant ascites before OLT, and prolonged donor graft cold ischemia time. These patients are managed with fluid restriction, diuretic therapy, and even graft TIPS in extreme cases.

PORTAL HYPERTENSION IN CHILDREN: ROLE OF ORTHOTOPIC LIVER TRANSPLANTATION

Portal hypertension in children is less common than in adults, but the process of collateral formation is similar with resultant varices, ascites, and hypersplenism. As in adults, classification is according to etiologic site (Table 1). Prehepatic PV obstruction represents the most frequent cause of portal hypertension in children. PV obstruction is most commonly due to thrombosis or atresia, with neonatal omphalitis or venous catheterization as possible precipitating events. Congenital cardiac, vascular, and biliary anomalies may occur with PV obstruction, but most commonly the liver itself is normal.

Intrahepatic portal hypertension is associated with a variable degree of parenchymal dysfunction and is most commonly due to congenital hepatic fibrosis (CHF) or cirrhosis. CHF is an autosomal recessive disease including biliary dysplasia, renal abnormalities, portal hypertension, and minimal hepatic insufficiency. Cirrhosis, in contrast, is most commonly due to biliary atresia, cystic fibrosis, or alpha-1-antitrypsin deficiency disease.

Posthepatic portal hypertension from a suprahepatic obstruction (Budd-Chiari syndrome; BCS) is rare in children. The underlying etiology is seldom found but may be due to tumor, trauma, webbed IVC, sickle cell disease, or systemic lupus. Hypercoaguable defects that produce BCS in adults are rarely seen in children.

Treatment of portal hypertension in children is similar to that for adults. The risk of hemorrhage and the evolution of parenchymal liver dysfunction influence therapeutic management decisions. Algorithms (Fig. 1) again begin with endoscopic banding, followed by TIPS or surgical shunts if vessel size permits, and ultimately by OLT.

The risk of post-OLT PVT in children is between 1% and 15%, with a higher incidence seen in children smaller than 10 kg, in those with biliary atresia (BA), and in recipients of split liver grafts. The higher rate in BA is perhaps due to smaller patients, previous Kasai procedures, or atretic portal veins. Outcomes after PVT are so poor that preventive strategies with immediate postoperative use of heparin and dextran and transition to aspirin are used at UCLA and elsewhere.

SUMMARY

Portal hypertension may arise from a variety of causes but for U.S. adults is most commonly due to HCV or alcoholic cirrhosis. Therapy, surgical or otherwise, is directed at the sequelae of portal hypertension, including gastroesophageal varices, ascites, hepatic encephalopathy, and hypersplenism. In most cases, OLT is the optimal treatment because it decompresses portal pressures and treats the underlying cause of their elevation. Patients with parenchymal decompensation accompanying portal hypertension tolerate other operations poorly. Timing of OLT is restricted by limited organ availability and the current distribution system based on the MELD formula, which does not consider the clinical parameters directly related to portal hypertension. While a patient is awaiting OLT, the sequelae of portal hypertension are managed by a multimodality approach including lifestyle, medical, endoscopic, and surgical interventions. These interventions and portal hypertension itself may make eventual OLT more difficult, but this procedure alone represents the best opportunity for durable cure.

SUGGESTED READINGS

Botha JF, Campos BD, Grant WJ, and others: Portosystemic shunts in children: a 15-year experience, *J Am Coll Surg* 199:179, 2004.

Geevarghese SK, Hiatt JR, Busuttil RW: Management of portal hypertensive hemorrhage in the era of liver transplantation, In Busuttil RW, Klintmalm GB, editors: *Transplantation of the liver,* ed 2, Philadelphia, 2006, Elsevier Saunders.

Ito T, Kiuchi T, Yamomoto H, and others: Changes in portal venous pressure (PVP) in the early phase after living donor liver transplantation: pathogenesis and clinical implications, *Transplantation* 75:1313, 2003.

Knechtle SJ: Portal hypertension from Eck's fistula to TIPS, *Ann Surg* 238: S49, 2003.

Seu P, Shackleton CR, Shaked A, and others: Improved results of liver transplantation in patients with portal vein thrombosis, *Arch Surg* 131:840, 1996.

Stewart CA, Wertheim J, Olthoff K, and others: Ascites after liver transplantation—a mystery, *Liver Transpl* 10:654, 2004.

ENDOSCOPIC THERAPY FOR ESOPHAGEAL VARICEAL HEMORRHAGE

Priscilla Magno, MD, and Anthony N. Kalloo, MD

Esophageal variceal hemorrhage is a potentially life-threatening complication of portal hypertension. One third of cirrhotic patients with documented esophageal varices bleed within 2 years from the time of diagnosis. The mortality rate from the first upper gastrointestinal hemorrhage is 20% to 35% despite aggressive management and is 30% with subsequent bleeding episodes. Risk factors for variceal bleeding include advanced cirrhosis (Child-Pugh class B and C), large varices, proximal extension of varices, high portal pressure (hepatic venous wedge pressure gradient ≥12 mmHg), continued ingestion of alcohol, and hepatocellular carcinoma.

The initial management of an acute gastrointestinal hemorrhage is adequate resuscitation of the patient with replacement of intravenous fluid, blood, and clotting factors as needed. Uncooperative or combative patients and those presenting with massive hematemesis might benefit from endotracheal intubation for airway protection and controlled ventilation. Gastric lavage using a large-bore orogastric tube (32 F or greater) is useful to assess the amount of ongoing bleeding while clearing the stomach for better endoscopic viewing. After the patient has become hemodynamically stable, endoscopic evaluation of the upper gastrointestinal tract is the next step, even in patients with known previous esophageal variceal bleeding. It is important to establish the cause of bleeding because up to 25% of patients with known esophageal varices may also bleed from gastritis, portal gastropathy, and peptic ulcer disease. Indications for endoscopic therapy following diagnosis of esophageal varices include visualization of active bleeding from a varix, signs of recent bleeding from a varix (e.g., adherent blood clot), and large varices with no other explanation for bleeding.

Medical management of bleeding esophageal varices is initiated after the source of bleeding is documented to be variceal. Medical therapy consists of vasoactive drugs that lower portal pressure and the pressure in the collateral circulation by vasoconstriction of the splanchnic circulation. Two natural peptides, somatostatin and vasopressin, and their analogues octreotide and terlipressin improve the efficacy of endoscopic therapy in achieving initial control of both acute variceal bleeding and 5-day hemostasis. Vasopressin, a potent nonselective vasoconstrictor, was the first vasoactive agent used in the control of acute variceal bleeding. It must be administered at an intensive care unit through a central intravenous line at a rate of 0.1–1.0 unit/minute. Sublingual nitroglycerine is used in combination with vasopressin to reduce some of the associated adverse effects of vasopressin, such as myocardial ischemia and arterial hypertension, seen in approximately 25% of patients. The vasopressin analogue terlipressin has fewer side effects but is currently unavailable in the United States. Somatostatin and its longer acting analogue octreotide produce a selective splanchnic vasoconstriction and consistently decrease the azygous blood flow, a measure of variceal blood flow. These drugs can be administered even before endoscopy if the cause of hemorrhage is suspected to be variceal. An initial intravenous bolus dose (somatostatin, 250 µg; octreotide, 50 g) is followed by a continuous infusion (somatostatin 250 µg/hour; octreotide, 50 to 100 µg/hour) for 3 to 5 days after endoscopic treatment only if a portal hypertensive source of bleeding is documented.

The selective splanchnic vasoconstrictive action and reduced risk of systemic side effects favor the use of octreotide or somatostatin over vasopressin. In addition, the administration of broad-spectrum antibiotics (fluoroquinolones) for 5 to 7 days reduces the risk of complications from variceal bleeding (bacterial peritonitis, pneumonia, renal failure) in cirrhotic patients.

ENDOSCOPIC SCLEROTHERAPY

Since the mid-1930s, the endoscopic treatment of esophageal varices has been endoscopic injection sclerotherapy (EIS). Sclerotherapy is designed to control bleeding by thrombosing the veins or thickening of the mucosa overlying the veins. This technique, which is performed using a flexible upper endoscope, requires only a sclerotherapy needle and a sclerosing agent. The sclerosing agent is usually injected intravariceally but can be injected paravariceally (submucosa adjacent to a varix) or both. Depending on the size of the varix, 1 to 5 ml of sclerosing agent is injected into each column beginning at the gastroesophageal junction, proceeding in circumferential fashion into all columns. If a discrete site of bleeding is identified on the varix, the sclerosant injection is directed below the site of bleeding. Injections in the proximal and midesophagus are avoided because the sclerosant may escape into the azygous vein and then into the pulmonary circulation. Sodium morrhuate (5% solution), sodium tetradecyl sulfate (1%–3% solution), and ethanolamine oleate (5% solution) are the most commonly used sclerosant agents. There is a large variation in the actual type and the volume of sclerosing agent used, site of injection, and volume of agent used per session. Trials comparing various techniques or types of solution show no significant advantage of one method or agent. Irrespective of the agent or technique used, endoscopic sclerotherapy is effective in the initial control of hemorrhage in approximately 80% to 90% of patients.

After the initial sclerotherapy has been performed, subsequent sessions are scheduled to completely obliterate the varices in the distal esophagus and prevent rebleeding. Three to five weekly sessions of sclerotherapy appear to offer the best results in most patients. Esophageal ulcerations are present in almost 100% of all sclerotherapy cases if endoscopy is performed early enough after a sclerotherapy session. Sclerotherapy should not be performed if ulcerations are present because of an increased risk of esophageal perforation. A 1-week interval between sessions is sufficient to allow recovery from the previous sclerotherapy session. There is no benefit to performing endoscopic sclerotherapy in patients with known esophageal varices who have not had a history of bleeding.

Endoscopic sclerotherapy is associated with significant complications in up to 40% of patients. Injection site ulceration occurs in up to 100% of patients and is associated with recurrent bleeding in 2% to 13% of cases. This probably should not be considered a complication but an expected consequence of sclerotherapy. Esophageal strictures develop in 10% to 20% of patients, and most of these respond to bougienage. Also, chest pain, fevers, and respiratory complications have all been attributed to endoscopic sclerotherapy. Prophylactic antibiotics are recommended to prevent bacteremia and associated peritonitis after sclerotherapy. Acid suppressants and liquid sucralfate (1 g orally four times daily) have been suggested to be useful in reducing esophageal complications of sclerotherapy.

ENDOSCOPIC VARICEAL LIGATION

Endoscopic ligation of esophageal varices was first described by Stiegmann and colleagues in 1986. This technique employs the use of small elastic bands that are endoscopically placed over a suctioned varix. The obvious advantage of this technique is that it avoids the complications of injecting a sclerosing agent into the varix—namely, deep ulcerations, abscess formation, stricture

formation, and pulmonary complications. The advantages of endoscopic ligation for bleeding esophageal varices have been substantiated by several prospective studies. Although endoscopic sclerotherapy and endoscopic ligation are equally effective in both controlling of active bleeding and eradicating varices, endoscopic ligation has shown lower rates of complications, including rebleeding and mortality, and the need of fewer sessions to achieve variceal eradication.

The technique of variceal ligation essentially consists of deploying a tight elastic "O" band over a varix. These bands are stretched and preloaded onto a cylinder attached to the tip of an end-viewing endoscope. The varix is suctioned into the banding device and ensnared by a firing mechanism that deploys the band at the base of the varix (Fig. 1, A-C). The strangulated varix is dislodged from the banding device, undergoing necrosis and sloughing off the thrombosed varix and band approximately 1 week later. The introduction of multishot band devices allows the placement of 6 to 8 bands at a time and avoids the use of overtubes and their related complications. The new transparent cylinders have improved the reduced visibility caused by the banding device fitted at the tip of the scope. Ligation of esophageal varices is started at the gastroesophageal junction and continued cephalad. Bands can be placed directly on the site of active bleeding or both distal and proximal to the rent in the varix. Band ligation sessions are usually repeated at 1- to 2-week intervals until varices are obliterated; this is achieved in 90% of patients after 2 to 4 sessions. The recurrence of esophageal varices is more frequent in variceal banding ligation (30% to 48%) compared with sclerotherapy (8% to 30%). The difference in recurrence is based on the fact that band ligation obliterates varices on the mucosa and submucosa of the esophageal wall, excluding periesophageal and perforating veins, which are the determinant factors for recurrence.

Combined techniques of both esophageal variceal ligation with sclerotherapy have been suggested to improve variceal recurrence. In the synchronous combination, variceal ligation is performed first, followed by sclerotherapy into the stagnant varix above the ligation in the hope that the sclerosing agent will be trapped by the banded varix and thereby prevent the systemic complications of sclerotherapy. Recent meta-analysis demonstrated that the combination therapy provides no additional benefit over endoscopic variceal ligation and was associated with a higher complication rate and number of sessions. In the sequential therapy, variceal ligation is repeated

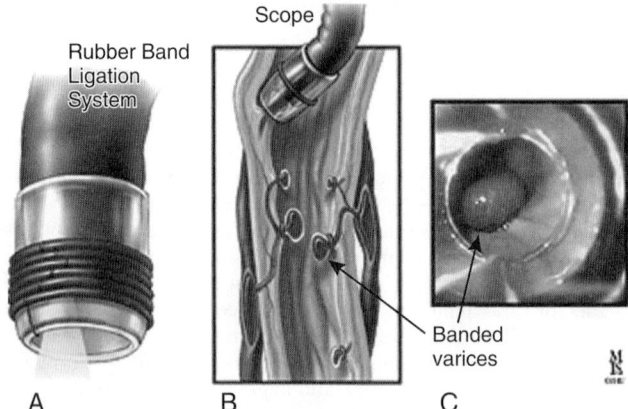

Figure I Endoscopic band ligation. **(A)** The multishot band device has 6 to 8 "O" elastic bands stretched and preloaded onto a transparent cylinder attached to the tip of an end-viewing endoscope. **(B)** The varix is suctioned into the banding device and ensnared by a firing mechanism that deploys the band at the base of the varix. **(C)** The strangulated varix is dislodged from the banding device, undergoing necrosis and sloughing of the thrombosed varix and band approximately 1 week later. *Used with permission from www.hopkins-gi.org.* **(See color insert Figure 24.)**

until the varices are reduced in size, followed by weekly small-volume sclerotherapy until complete eradication. One study has shown that the staged approach therapy required an equal number or more endoscopic sessions for variceal eradication but lower rates of rebleeding, variceal recurrence, and mortality than therapy with variceal ligation alone. Other investigators have found no difference in their studies. On the basis of current data, the initial bleeding control of variceal ligation only is comparable to any combination therapy. However, combination therapy may reduce the risk of variceal recurrence and rebleeding at a higher complication rate.

A new ligation device using a nylon snare has been recently introduced for achieving hemostasis and variceal eradication. The technique consists of using a small Endoloop (Ethicon Endosurgery, Somerville, NJ) snare that is closed onto the varix and then detached from the delivery system. A transparent ligation endcap cylinder with a rim on the inside is fitted onto the tip of the endoscope. The detachable Endoloop snare is inserted through a plastic sleeve introducer into the working channel of the endoscope. When the Endoloop emerges from the distal end of the channel, the head of the Endoloop opens and engages the distal rim of the endcap. The varix is suctioned into the transparent endcap, and the detachable Endoloop is positioned around it and tightened at the base of the aspirated varix. The suction is released, and the Endoloop is detached from the sleeve introducer. Additional ligations can be performed by reloading detachable Endoloops while the endoscope remains in the esophagus. The current design of the Endoloop snare and transparent endcap allows ligation of esophageal varices with the advantage of an improved visualization, tighter application, and an unlimited number of ligations at a time. A recent prospective nonrandomized study showed that the Endoloop device is as effective as band ligation for control of acute variceal bleeding, but no significant differences were found between these techniques with respect to rate of variceal eradication, the total number of treatment sessions required for variceal eradication, or the frequency of variceal recurrence. However, the Endoloop technique requires the assistance of skilled personnel and a longer procedure time than the preloaded multiple banding devices. Larger, randomized, controlled studies are necessary to validate the results of this small, nonrandomized, and underpowered study.

SUGGESTED READINGS

Kriege JEJ, Shaw JM, Bornman PC: The evolving role of endoscopic treatment for bleeding esophageal varices, *World J Surg* 29:966, 2005.

Lane L, Cook D: Endoscopic ligation compared with sclerotherapy for treatment of esophageal variceal bleeding: a meta-analysis, *Ann Int Med* 123:280, 1995.

Naga MI, Okasha HH, Gomaa MS, and others: Detachable Endoloop vs. elastic band ligation for bleeding esophageal varices, *Gastrointest Endosc* 59:804, 2004.

Saeed ZA: Endoscopic therapy of bleeding esophageal varices: ligation is still the best, *Gastroenterology* 110:635, 1996.

Stiegmann GV, Goff JS, Michaletz-Onody PA, and others: Endoscopic sclerotherapy as compared with endoscopic ligation for bleeding esophageal varices, *N Engl J Med* 326:1527, 1992.

Westaby D, Hayes PC, Gimson AE, and others: Controlled clinical trial of injection sclerotherapy for active variceal bleeding, *Hepatology* 9:274, 1989.

REFRACTORY ASCITES

Kevin A. Moreman, MD, and H. Franklin Herlong, MD

Although accumulation of fluid in the abdomen can result from many disorders, in more than 75% of patients with ascites, cirrhosis is the cause. Over a 10-year period, approximately 50% of patients with cirrhosis eventually develop ascites. The development of ascites carries an ominous prognosis, with a 2-year mortality greater than 50%. In patients with cirrhosis, sinusoidal hypertension is an essential element in the formation of ascites. This hypothesis is supported by the fact that postsinusoidal hypertension caused by disorders such as Budd-Chiari syndrome leads to a rapid accumulation of ascites, whereas a portal vein thrombosis causes marked splanchnic hypertension but rarely results in ascites. Increased renal retention of sodium caused by a complex combination of neurohumoral factors contributes to an expansion of the plasma volume that exacerbates hepatic lymph formation. When the production of hepatic lymph exceeds the capacity of the lymphatic system to return it to the systemic circulation, ascites accumulates.

DIAGNOSIS

A diagnostic paracentesis should be performed in all patients with new onset of ascites. Twenty milliliters of fluid is removed under sterile technique. Ten milliliters of fluid are inoculated into bacterial culture bottles at the bedside to maximize the yield of cultures in patients with peritonitis. Cell count with differential is performed on a 5-ml heparinized specimen, and another 5 ml of fluid is sent for total protein and albumin measurements. A simultaneous blood sample is sent for serum albumin concentration. Using these results, a serum-ascites albumin concentration gradient (SAAG) can be calculated by subtracting the ascites albumin concentration from the serum concentration (SAAG = serum albumin − ascites albumin).

The sinusoidal pressure threshold necessary for the formation of ascites is 12 mmHg. A SAAG of 1.1 g/dl correlates with sinusoidal pressure of 12 mmHg. Consequently, finding an SAAG greater than or equal to 1.1 g/dL indicates that the patient has sinusoidal hypertension that is likely the cause of the ascites. Although cirrhosis accounts for the vast majority of cases of sinusoidal hypertension, an elevation in sinusoidal pressure can also result from occlusion of the hepatic veins (Budd-Chiari syndrome), congestive heart failure, or constrictive pericarditis. In patients with congestion of the liver, the hepatic sinusoidal fenestrations remain intact. Hence the ascites fluid in outflow obstruction contains a high concentration of protein. In cirrhosis, the hepatic endothelium becomes capillarized by sinusoidal fibrosis, decreasing the permeability of protein. Consequently, in cirrhosis the SAAG is greater than or equal to 1.1, but the total protein is less than 2.5 g/dl. When ascites is caused by disorders of the peritoneum (peritoneal carcinomatosis, tuberculous peritonitis, pancreatic ascites, etc.), the sinusoidal pressure is normal, and the SAAG is less than 1.1 g/dl. However, the peritoneal surface has increased permeability with the exudation of protein into the ascites. Therefore using a combination of the SAAG and ascetic total fluid concentrations, most cases of ascites can be accurately characterized. Once the correct diagnosis is made, appropriate therapy can begin (see Tables 1 and 2).

TREATMENT OF ASCITES CAUSED BY CIRRHOSIS

The International Ascites Club established three grades of ascites on the basis of severity. Grade 1 ascites is detectable only by radiographic imaging with an ultrasound or computed tomography (CT) scan. Grade 2 ascites causes moderated symmetrical distention of the abdomen on clinical examination. Grade 3 causes exhibit abdominal distention, often with additional symptoms such as respiratory compromise, anorexia, and significant discomfort. This classification is useful in assigning treatment regimens. The medical treatment of ascites consists of a combination of dietary salt restriction and diuretics. In general, patients are initially started on a 2 g (88 mmol)/day sodium diet. Although more stringent dietary sodium restriction might lead to more rapid resolution of ascites, it is virtually impossible for most patients to adhere to such a diet on an ambulatory basis. In addition, these diets often are so unpalatable that the decrease in food intake can impair nutrition. Consultation with an experienced nutritionist can often improve compliance.

Patients with grade 1 ascites often can be treated with dietary salt restriction alone. Reducing salt intake should be sufficient to induce negative sodium balance and reduce the accumulation of ascitic fluid. Patients with grade 2 or 3 ascites require the addition of diuretic therapy to dietary salt restriction. In cirrhosis, hyperaldosteronism results in avid distal sodium reabsorption. Consequently, spironolactone, an aldosterone antagonist, is the most effective diuretic in the treatment of cirrhotic ascites. However, because of hyperkalemia and a prolonged half-life, this drug is rarely used as a single agent. The initial regimen consists of 100 mg of spironolactone plus 40 mg of furosemide given in the morning. If this combination fails to induce a significant diuresis within 3 to 5 days, both doses are increased, maintaining a 100 mg/40 mg ratio. The goal of therapy is to mobilize 0.5 kg of fluid per day in patients with no edema. A more aggressive diuresis can result in intravascular volume depletion with azotemia and worsening encephalopathy. A more vigorous diuresis (up to 1.0 kg per day) is permissible in patients who also have peripheral edema.

Patients with grade 3 ascites may require an initial large-volume paracentesis in addition to medical therapy. This is a safe procedure that can be performed on an outpatient basis and is more effective than diuretics in rapid removal of ascitic fluid. A paracentesis should generally be performed in the left lower quadrant, where the abdominal wall is thinner. A standard 18-gauge plastic catheter is inserted into the peritoneal cavity under local anesthesia. Inserting the distal end of the tubing into evacuated bottles hastens fluid removal. Specially modified needles with blunt tips and multiple side holes are available and eliminate the kinking commonly encountered with plastic catheters. Using a Z-track lessens the likelihood of a postparacentesis leak. When more than 5 L of ascitic fluid is removed, patients should receive 8 gm/L of fluid removed of albumin during the procedure to reduce the likelihood of postparacentesis hypotension and azotemia.

REFRACTORY ASCITES

In most patients with cirrhosis and ascites, medical therapy is effective in controlling fluid accumulation. However, approximately 10% to 15% of patients are refractory to medical therapy. Failure to respond to medical therapy carries an ominous prognosis; 50% of patients die within 1 year. In 2003, the International Ascites Club revised its criteria for refractory ascites to include the following two groups. In one group, designated "diuretic-resistant ascites," fluid accumulation cannot be prevented or controlled because of a lack of response to medical therapy. In the other group, designated

Table 2: Diagnosis, Treatment, and Prophylaxis of SBP and Variants

Diagnosis	Ascitic Fluid Cell Count	Culture Results
SBP		Positive
CNNA	>250 PMNs	Negative
MNNB	<250 PMNs	Positive (single organism)
Polymicrobial bacterascites	<250 PMNs	Positive (multiple organisms)

Treatment of SBP

- Treatment with cefotaxime 2 g IV every 8 hours for 5 to 7 days
- Administer albumin 1.5 g/kg body weight IV within 6 hours of diagnosis and another 1.0 g/kg on day 3 of hospitalization.

Treatment of CNNA

- Exclude tuberculous peritonitis or malignant ascites.
- Same as SBP

Treatment of MNNB

- No treatment unless fever, abdominal pain, or change in mental status

Treatment of Polymicrobial Infection

- Search for perforation or acute abdomen.
- Treatment is based on culture results and sensitivities.

Prophylaxis for Prevention of SBP

- Patients with one or more prior episodes of SBP should be treated with norfloxacin 400 mg daily or Bactrim DS daily.
- Some patients with an ascitic protein of <1.0 g should also receive prophylactic antibiotics.
- Patients with gastrointestinal hemorrhage should also receive prophylaxis with norfloxacin 400 mg by mouth twice daily for 7 days.

CNNA, Culture-negative neutrocytic ascites; *IV,* intravenous administration; *MNNB,* monomicrobial nonneutrocytic bacterascites; *SBP,* spontaneous bacterial peritonitis.

Table 1: Diagnostic Interpretation of SAAG and Total Protein in Ascitic Fluid

SAAG >1.1 g/dl Total Protein <2.5 g/dl	SAAG >1.1 g/dl Total Protein > 2.5 g/dl	SAAG <1.1 g/dl Total Protein >2.5 g/dl
Cirrhosis	Congestive heart failure	Tuberculosis
	Constrictive pericarditis	Malignancy
	Bacterial peritonitis	Pancreatitis
	Budd-Chiari syndrome (early)	

SAAG, Serum albumin-ascites albumin.

"diuretic intractable ascites," treatment with diuretics leads to unacceptable complications, including hepatic encephalopathy, renal impairment, hyponatremia, and hyperkalemia.

Before concluding that a patient has refractory ascites, it is important to identify and eliminate any complicating factors such as infection or the use of agents that reduce urinary sodium excretion. Nonsteroidal anti-inflammatory agents can significantly reduce urinary sodium excretion and inhibit diuresis. Simply discontinuing these agents may make patients responsive to medical therapy. It is also important to ensure compliance with dietary sodium restriction. Measuring 24-hour urinary sodium excretion can be helpful. If the patient is excreting more than 78 mEq of sodium in 24 hours or requires large-volume paracentesis more than every 2 weeks, then the patient is consuming more than 2000 mg of sodium daily. If the patient excretes less than 10 mEq of sodium daily while on sodium restrictions and maximal diuretic therapy, then the patient truly has refractory ascites.

Most patients with refractory ascites have hyponatremia, but few are symptomatic. Fluid restriction should be imposed only if the serum sodium is less than 125 mEq/L. Restricting fluid intake has no effect on ascites mobilization itself. The use of aquaretic agents that promote free water clearance has not been approved in the United States. Rapid correction of hyponatremia with hypertonic saline should be avoided.

LARGE-VOLUME PARACENTESIS

Patients with refractory ascites are treated initially with large-volume paracentesis (LVP). As previously described, this procedure can be safely performed on an outpatient basis. There is no proven benefit to correcting thrombocytopenia or a coagulopathy before performing the procedure. Routine culture of the fluid is not necessary because the prevalence of occult spontaneous bacterial peritonitis in asymptomatic outpatients is low. In some patients undergoing LVP (>5 L), activation of the renin-angiotensin system leads to vascular compromise with azotemia and hyponatremia. Often referred to as *postparacentesis circulatory dysfunction,* these complications can be reduced by infusing albumin during or shortly after the paracentesis is completed. If more than 5 L are removed, 8 g of albumin per liter of fluid removed should be given. LVP is safe and effective in eliminating ascites but does not prevent recurrence.

TRANSJUGULAR INTRAHEPATIC PORTOSYSTEMIC SHUNTS

Transjugular intrahepatic portosystemic shunt (TIPS) placement reduces sinusoidal hypertension and lessens ascites formation. This side-to-side shunt is placed by interventional radiologists through the right internal jugular vein under local anesthesia. A low-resistance channel is created between the intrahepatic portion of the portal vein and the hepatic veins by use of an expandable metal stent. The use of polytetrafluoroethylene-covered stents improves patency compared with uncovered, bare stents. TIPS should be considered in patients requiring more than 3 LVPs per month or in those who are intolerant to LVP because of complications. Successful TIPS placement results in improved renal function, sodium excretion, and general well-being. Contraindications to TIPS placement include congestive heart failure, biliary obstruction, sepsis, multiple hepatic cysts, pulmonary hypertension, international normalized ratio (INR) greater than 5, grade 3 or 4 encephalopathy, Child-Pugh score greater than 12, or age older than 75 years. Relative contraindications include hepatocellular carcinoma, hepatic vein occlusion, portal vein thrombosis, and platelets under 20,000.

The major complication of TIPS placement is hepatic encephalopathy, which occurs in approximately 25% of patients. Most patients who develop encephalopathy after TIPS placement respond to protein restriction and lactulose, but approximately 10% of patients develop refractory encephalopathy that is associated with a high mortality. Predictors of post-TIPS encephalopathy include pre-TIPS encephalopathy, age older than 69 years, and advanced liver disease. Shunt malfunction is common and may require additional procedures. Thrombosis after insertion occurs in approximately 10% of patients. Stenosis is seen in up to 75% of patients within 6 to 12 months. Ascites frequently reappears in these patients, requiring some form of revision to reestablish patency.

Successful placement of a TIPS results in improved renal function, sodium excretion, and general well-being. Meta-analyses of controlled trials comparing TIPS with LVP show that TIPS was superior in ascites control but did not improve overall and transplant-free survival and caused higher rates of encephalopathy. There was no difference in rates of liver failure, variceal hemorrhage, acute renal failure, hospitalization, or improvement in quality of life. One study showed that patients undergoing TIPS had significant improvement in their nutritional statuses. A multicenter trial studying quality of life showed similar results between LVP and TIPS. One study showed that TIPS was more expensive than LVP with albumin.

HEPATIC HYDROTHORAX

A variant of refractory ascites, hepatic hydrothorax, develops in approximately 10% of patients with cirrhosis. Hydrothorax results from the transmigration of ascitic fluid into the pleural space through pores in the diaphragm. Hepatic hydrothorax rarely responds to medical therapy and often requires TIPS placement as an alternative to repeated thoracentesis. Chest tube placement should never be attempted in patients with hepatic hydrothorax because this procedure is associated with a marked increase in mortality. In addition, pleurodesis is rarely effective.

OBSOLETE THERAPIES

Peritoneovenous shunts drain ascitic fluid from the peritoneum into the internal jugular vein through a subcutaneous tube. This therapy is associated with multiple complications, including disseminated intravascular coagulation, infection, variceal bleeding, and small bowel obstruction. Because of the high complication rate and no convincing survival benefit, this procedure should be considered only in patients with refractory ascites who are not candidates for LVP or TIPS. Side-to-side surgical shunts reduce sinusoidal hypertension and prevent ascites formation; however, poor long-term patency, excessive complications, and no improvement in mortality make this approach obsolete.

LIVER TRANSPLANTATION

The only definitive treatment for patients with refractory ascites is hepatic transplantation. Ideally patients should be considered for this therapy before they develop refractory ascites. Because the waiting time for transplantation often exceeds 1 year, the possibility of living donor should be explored in appropriate patients with refractory ascites.

SPONTANEOUS BACTERIAL PERITONITIS

When patients with cirrhosis develop refractory ascites, they are susceptible to bacterial infection of the ascitic fluid (spontaneous bacterial peritonitis [SBP]). Patients with advanced liver disease as measured by the Child-Pugh classification are at increased risk for this complication. Decreased opsonization of bacteria by the host immune response also promotes infection. Consequently, ascitic fluid with a low total protein and complement concentration may become infected more easily. Because clinically significant gastrointestinal bleeding is also a risk factor for SBP, prophylactic antibiotics should be administered promptly to any patient with ascites who has a gastrointestinal hemorrhage. A presumptive diagnosis of SBP is made when more than 250 polymorphonuclear leukocytes/mm³ are detected in ascitic fluid. Patients with neutrocytic ascites in whom ascitic fluid cultures grow no organisms have a similar prognosis as those with positive cultures and should be treated with a similar regimen. Cirrhotic patients with SBP are also at increased risk for renal insufficiency. Prompt administration of albumin when the diagnosis is made can reduce the likelihood of subsequent renal failure. Therefore 1.5 g/kg body weight of intravenous albumin is given within 6 hours of SBP detection and 1.0 g/kg on day 3.

Several regimens have proved efficacious in the treatment of SBP. Cefotaxime 2 g every 8 hours for 5 to 7 days is the most common antibiotic choice used for SBP treatment. Because of the risk of recurrent SBP after the first episode, patients should receive prophylaxis with 400 mg norfloxacin or 1 tablet of sulfamethoxazole and trimethoprim (Bactrim DS; AR Scientific, Philadelphia, PA) daily indefinitely. Some also advocate prophylaxis for those patients whose ascitic fluid contains less than 1 g of protein.

Suggested Readings

Boyer TD, Haskal ZJ: The role of transjugular intrahepatic portosystemic shunt in the management of portal hypertension, *Hepatology* 41:386, 2005.

Cardenas A, Gines P: Management of refractory ascites, *Clin Gastroenterol Hepatol* 3:1187, 2005.

Cardenas A, Gines P: Management of complications of cirrhosis in patients awaiting liver transplantation, *J Hepatol* 42:S124, 2005.

Hillebrand DJ, Runyon BA, Yasmineh WG, and others: Ascitic fluid adenosine deaminase insensitivity in detecting tuberculous peritonitis in the United States, *Hepatology* 24:1408, 1996.

Moore KP, Wong F, Gines P, and others: The management of ascites in cirrhosis: report on the Consensus Conference of the International Ascites Club, *Hepatology* 38:258, 2003.

Runyon BA: Ascites and spontaneous bacterial peritonitis, In Feldman M, Friedman LS, Sleisenger MH, editors: *Sleisenger and Fordtran's gastrointestinal and liver disease*, ed 7, Philadelphia, 2002, Saunders.

Runyon BA: Refractory ascites, *Semin Liver Disease* 13:343, 1993.

Hepatic Encephalopathy

Mack C. Mitchell, Jr., MD

Hepatic or portosystemic encephalopathy is a complex spectrum of reversible neuropsychiatric alterations that develop in patients with advanced chronic liver disease or in those with acute liver failure from any cause. Hepatic encephalopathy is a form of metabolic encephalopathy that is characterized by altered mental status, ranging from mild cognitive impairment to coma. In general, the signs and symptoms of hepatic encephalopathy are not specific to liver failure and therefore do not distinguish a hepatic etiology from other causes of metabolic encephalopathy. For that reason, some additional evidence of impaired liver function is necessary before the diagnosis of hepatic encephalopathy can be confirmed.

Symptoms of hepatic encephalopathy include impaired cognitive function, changes in personality, loss of the normal diurnal sleep cycle, confusion, repetitive behaviors, and ultimately a decline in the level of consciousness. The most characteristic physical finding in hepatic encephalopathy is asterixis, which is commonly seen in all forms of metabolic encephalopathy. Asterixis is a flapping tremor of the hands and arms that is most prominent when the arms are outstretched with extension of the wrists. In addition to confusion and a decline in level of consciousness, hyperactivity of the deep tendon reflexes, and rarely decerebrate posturing may occur. Focal neurologic findings may be present transiently in patients with hepatic encephalopathy, particularly in the more advanced stages, but these findings should always prompt a search for structural abnormalities within the central nervous system (CNS).

In most instances, hepatic encephalopathy occurs intermittently in patients with underlying liver disease, although in some patients with advanced stages of cirrhosis, the symptoms may be more persistent. To reflect these different situations and permit more precisely defined study, a classification of hepatic encephalopathy was proposed by a working group at the World Congress of Gastroenterology meeting in 1998. This classification scheme proposed defining three separate conditions: episodic (spontaneous or precipitated) encephalopathy, persistent encephalopathy, and minimal hepatic encephalopathy. The latter condition describes subtle changes in personality and behavior associated with cognitive impairment that may be apparent only with sensitive psychometric testing. However, patients with minimal hepatic encephalopathy may lack the judgment required to operate motor vehicles safely or to make complex decisions as a consequence of these changes. Another aspect of the classification scheme separates hepatic encephalopathy associated with acute liver failure from that occurring in patients with advanced chronic liver disease or the condition that results from portosystemic bypass shunts in patients without underlying liver disease (Table 1). The clinical stages of encephalopathy are generally agreed on and are detailed in Table 2. These stages are important in guiding therapy for hepatic encephalopathy. In the more advanced stages, careful attention must be given to supportive care, including protection of the airway. As discussed later, these aspects of care are essential in patients with acute liver failure in whom increased intracranial pressure may cause similar changes in level of consciousness.

PATHOGENESIS OF HEPATIC ENCEPHALOPATHY

Although many studies of the pathogenesis of hepatic encephalopathy have been conducted both in humans and in animal models, the exact etiology of the clinical syndrome is not known precisely. It is likely that many potentially neurotoxic substances accumulate as a result of impaired hepatic metabolism in patients with hepatic encephalopathy. Among these, ammonia is the one toxin that is consistently believed to play a pathogenic role in the altered level of consciousness in patients with hepatic encephalopathy. The evidence for a central role for ammonia is based on observations that

Table 1: Classification of Hepatic Encephalopathy

Encephalopathy associated with acute liver failure

Encephalopathy associated with portal-systemic shunts without liver disease

Encephalopathy associated with cirrhosis and portal hypertension

    Episodic

      Precipitated

      Spontaneous

      Recurrent

    Persistent

      Mild

      Severe

      Treatment dependent

    Minimal

Based on classification from Ferenci P, Lockwood A, Mullen K, and others: Hepatology 35:716, 2002.

Table 2: Clinical Stages of Hepatic Encephalopathy

Stage	Cognitive Function	Neurologic Signs
Minimal	No overt impairment	Changes detectable on psychometric testing
Stage 1	Sleep disturbance, inattention, personality changes	Tremor, poor fine-motor coordination
Stage 2	Drowsiness, disorientation to time, lethargy, poor computations	Asterixis, slurred speech, hypoactive reflexes
Stage 3	Poorly arousable, disorientation to place, amnesia,	Hyperactive reflexes, clonus, muscular rigidity
Stage 4	Coma, not arousable	Decerebrate posturing, no response to stimuli, loss of brainstem reflexes

patients with urea cycle defects in whom high levels of ammonia accumulate develop a condition that is similar to that seen in hepatic encephalopathy. Furthermore, ammonia will cause coma when administered to animals. Although the serum ammonia is often elevated in patients with hepatic encephalopathy, the exact level does not correlate well with the extent of impairment in cognitive function or the level of consciousness. Furthermore, ammonia can be elevated in other conditions, including urinary tract infections with urea splitting organisms, ureterosigmoidostomy, parenteral nutrition, inborn errors of metabolism (urea cycle defects), and following administration of some chemotherapeutic agents.

The gastrointestinal (GI) tract is the primary source of ammonia. Excessive ammonia is formed by bacterial degradation of nitrogenous compounds such as protein ingested as food or blood during GI bleeding. Ammonia is usually cleared with high efficiency during first pass of the portal blood through the liver in healthy individuals, but in patients with impaired liver function a significant amount reaches the systemic circulation, where it readily crosses the blood-brain barrier and alters function of the CNS. Recognition of the role of protein and bacteria in formation of ammonia has led to the development of much of the current therapy for hepatic encephalopathy.

Clinical conditions that result in excessive production of ammonia in the gut include GI bleeding, excessive ingestion of protein (particularly red meat), and constipation. Hypovolemia, dehydration, and metabolic alkalosis favor formation of the nonionized form of ammonia and may result in increased reabsorption of ammonia or increased renal production of ammonia. These conditions often precipitate episodes of hepatic encephalopathy. In addition, uremia and hypokalemia may also precipitate encephalopathy. Excessive use of diuretics is a major factor that causes hypokalemia, metabolic alkalosis, dehydration, and uremia.

In addition to ammonia, there is evidence that alterations in CNS neurotransmitters contribute to the pathogenesis of hepatic encephalopathy. Evidence also suggests that endogenous benzodiazepines or other gamma-aminobutyric acid-reactive substances may be involved, either through activation of peripheral benzodiazepine receptors or by creating imbalance between neuroexcitatory and neuroinhibitory pathways in the brain. In that regard, norepinephrine and glutamate may also be important contributors to the syndrome of hepatic encephalopathy. The involvement of neurotransmitters of the inhibitory type explains the clinical observation that sedatives, particularly benzodiazepines and barbiturates, often precipitate episodes of hepatic encephalopathy.

THERAPY FOR HEPATIC ENCEPHALOPATHY

Therapy for hepatic encephalopathy is dictated by the clinical situation in which encephalopathy develops and whether it develops spontaneously or in response to a precipitating factor. As noted earlier, several factors are frequently associated with episodes of hepatic encephalopathy in patients with otherwise compensated cirrhosis. These are listed in Table 3. Of these, azotemia (often attributable to diuretics), sedatives, infection, and GI bleeding account for the majority of episodes. The initial approach to the patient with suspected encephalopathy should focus on determining whether one of these factors might be involved.

Initial Approach to the Patient

The diagnosis of hepatic encephalopathy is based primarily on characteristic clinical manifestations occurring in a setting such as chronic liver disease or fulminant hepatic failure. Serum ammonia should be measured because elevation is supporting evidence of the diagnosis. Although arterial levels are more accurate, a venous sample is usually sufficient, but it is best to have the sample analyzed soon after collection. Serum electrolytes, blood urea nitrogen, and creatinine should be measured to look for evidence of hypokalemia, metabolic alkalosis, and uremia, all of which are known to precipitate

Table 3: Precipitating Factors in Hepatic Encephalopathy

Gastrointestinal bleeding

Sedative use

Hypovolemia

Uremia

Hypokalemia

Metabolic alkalosis

Excessive dietary protein

Infection

Constipation

hepatic encephalopathy. Complete blood counts and Hemoccult (Beckman Coulter, Fullerton, CA) testing of the stool are necessary to exclude GI bleeding and infection. In patients with ascites, diagnostic paracentesis should be performed to exclude spontaneous bacterial peritonitis, a site of infection that often lacks specific manifestations. The absence of fever or a white blood count (WBC) within the normal range does not exclude infection in patients with cirrhosis. WBC is usually less than 5000 in patients with portal hypertension; thus WBC of 10,000 should prompt concern, even though it is within the normal range for the laboratory. A computed tomography scan of the head is necessary to exclude other causes of altered mental status, particularly when there are focal neurologic defects. Although the electroencephalogram (EEG) may show characteristic triphasic delta waves, an abnormal EEG adds little except in instances where there is doubt regarding the diagnosis.

Specific Therapy to Decrease Toxins within the Gut

Ammonia and other potential toxins originate in the gut in patients with hepatic encephalopathy. Reducing the amount of nitrogen within the GI tract will ultimately reduce the amount available for bacterial production of ammonia. Although reducing dietary protein may improve encephalopathy, this measure can be counterproductive by contributing to malnutrition, particularly if the degree of protein restriction is severe (40 g) or if it is continued over a prolonged time. In patients who are comatose, dietary protein can be restricted completely for up to 48 hours or until improvement is noticed. Prolonged periods of protein restriction should be avoided in most patients. Studies of nutrition in patients with severe alcoholic hepatitis have demonstrated that high protein/high calorie diets improve rather than worsen spontaneous hepatic encephalopathy, probably through improving overall liver function. In patients with advanced cirrhosis who have frequent episodes of spontaneous encephalopathy, restricting protein to 60 to 70 g daily maintains adequate nutrition. Avoiding red meat and eating a higher proportion of vegetable-derived protein may be beneficial.

Lactulose and lacitol are nonabsorbable disaccharides that produce a high osmotic load in the GI tract after catabolism to short-chain fatty acids by gut bacteria. They act primarily as laxatives but may also lower the pH in the lumen, which in theory should decrease absorption of ammonia from the colon. Both are relatively well tolerated and lack serious toxicity. However, many patients complain of bloating and gassiness when they are ingested chronically. For long-term use, lactulose should be given in amounts sufficient to produce two to three soft but not watery bowel movements each day. This amount is usually 30 ml (20 g) twice daily. It can also be administered orally or by nasogastric tube in larger amounts to patients who require hospitalization for acute episodes of hepatic encephalopathy. In my experience, lactulose is more effective in improving hepatic encephalopathy in patients with GI bleeding than in those with spontaneous encephalopathy or that precipitated by other factors such as infection or azotemia, probably because it acts as a cathartic to eliminate blood from the GI tract. In certain situations such as constipation and GI bleeding, cleansing enemas or enemas containing lactulose can be used. This approach can be considered when it is not possible to administer these compounds orally.

A systematic review of the use of oral disaccharides in treating hepatic encephalopathy concluded that there was marginal benefit in improving hepatic encephalopathy, but when only high-quality trials were considered, there was no benefit. The authors of this Cochrane review also concluded that antibiotics were more effective and that oral disaccharides such as lactulose should not be used as a reference comparator in future studies.

Nonetheless, the safety and clinical experience with lactulose is considerable and therefore justifies continued use in some situations. However, the marginal efficacy in clinical trials suggests that its use should be tempered whenever problems such as uncontrollable diarrhea result.

Specific Therapy to Decrease Gut Bacteria

Poorly absorbed antibiotics such as neomycin were among the first drugs used to treat hepatic encephalopathy. Unfortunately, a small amount of neomycin is absorbed and may cause ototoxicity and nephrotoxicity after prolonged use, particularly in patients with underlying renal insufficiency. Because many patients with advanced cirrhosis also have renal impairment, neomycin is not generally an acceptable alternative to lactulose owing to safety concerns.

Metronidazole has also been used to decrease gut bacteria and therefore the production of ammonia. Few controlled trials of this medication are available, but anecdotal evidence suggests that it may be helpful in some patients.

Rifaximin is a poorly absorbed broad-spectrum antibiotic with activity against both gram-negative rods and gram-positive cocci, including *Enterococcus*. There is some activity against *Bacteroides*. A number of controlled trials have demonstrated that rifaximin given 400 mg 3/day is equivalent or superior to nonabsorbable disaccharides. A meta-analysis also confirmed greater improvement with this agent compared with disaccharides. Rifaximin has also been used for treatment of traveler's diarrhea and is approved by the Food and Drug Administration (FDA) for this indication but not for treatment of hepatic encephalopathy. However, on the basis of results from clinical trials, it may be approved soon. Because it is poorly absorbed and has few side effects, it can potentially be administered over a longer period of time in patients with chronic encephalopathy after transjugular intrahepatic portosystemic shunts or surgical shunts.

Other Therapy for Hepatic Encephalopathy

Benzodiazepines are known to precipitate episodes of hepatic encephalopathy in patients with advanced liver disease. This observation led to a hypothesis that alterations in the benzodiazepine receptor or endogenous benzodiazepine-like compounds might play a role in the pathogenesis of hepatic encephalopathy. The benzodiazepine receptor antagonist flumazenil has been tried with some success in patients with encephalopathy. Several small controlled trials have suggested possible benefit, and a systematic review confirmed more rapid improvement on flumazenil. However, flumazenil is not approved by the FDA for treatment of encephalopathy. It must be given intravenously and has a relatively short half-life, which limits its overall utility. The role of flumazenil in treatment of encephalopathy remains unclear, pending further randomized trials that determine longer-term outcome.

Approach to Patients with Hepatic Encephalopathy and Fulminant Hepatic Failure

The pathogenesis of hepatic encephalopathy in patients with fulminant hepatic failure likely differs from those with established portal systemic shunting. In particular, these patients are at risk for developing increased intracranial pressure from cerebral edema. The risk of edema is 25% to 35% in patients with grade III encephalopathy and up to 75% in those with grade IV coma. Management of patients with fulminant hepatic failure should ideally be carried out using a highly specialized approach that is usually available only in liver transplant centers. A retrospective comparison of treatment of early stages of hepatic encephalopathy with lactulose or no specific therapy did not show benefit in terms of overall outcome or improvement in encephalopathy. In

Table 4: Management of Hepatic Encephalopathy

Careful search and treatment of precipitating factors

   Gastrointestinal hemorrhage

   Electrolyte disturbances, particularly hypokalemia and
   metabolic alkalosis

   Hypovolemia (especially diuretic induced)

   Sedative use, particularly benzodiazepines and barbiturates

   Infection

   Uremia

Specific therapy for stage 0–II encephalopathy

   Lactulose 30 ml PO II–III times daily to produce 2–3 soft stools
   daily

   Rifaximin 400 mg PO three times daily

Specific therapy for stage III–IV encephalopathy

   Restrict dietary protein for 48 hours

   Lactulose as above

   Cleansing enemas for constipation or gastrointestinal bleeding

Fulminant hepatic failure

   Transfer to center with liver transplantation

   Search for precipitating factors as above

   No specific therapy for stages I–II

   Elevate head of bed to 30 degrees

   Mannitol infusion for evidence of increased intracranial pressure

   Consider hypertonic saline, hyperventilation if no response to
   mannitol

PO, Administered orally.

patients with more advanced stages of encephalopathy, careful monitoring of hemodynamic parameters is desirable. The head of the bed should be elevated to 30 degrees, and care should be undertaken to avoid Valsalva-like movements that could contribute to increase in intracranial pressure (ICP). The use of ICP-monitoring devices remains controversial, mostly because of the high rate of complications observed when the critical care team lacks experience with these devices or when patients have severe coagulopathy. Mannitol is used to induce osmotic diuresis in patients with decerebrate posturing or other evidence of increased ICP, although its prophylactic use is not recommended.

Hyperventilation, hypertonic sodium chloride infusion, and moderate hypothermia have all been used with limited success in treating increased ICP. There is no benefit to administration of corticosteroids.

Summary

Unfortunately there is little proof from randomized controlled trials to suggest that most specific therapy for hepatic encephalopathy is beneficial. Because many episodes of hepatic encephalopathy are precipitated by medications such as diuretics and sedatives, it is imperative that these agents be discontinued or used only with caution and with careful monitoring in patients with encephalopathy. Patients with GI bleeding probably improve more rapidly when given lactulose because of the cathartic effects. Protein restriction may be helpful for a short period of time, but for chronic treatment, only mild restriction is warranted to avoid adverse effects of malnutrition. The ultimate role of poorly absorbed antibiotics such as rifaximin has not yet been firmly established. An overall approach to therapy in patients with hepatic encephalopathy is summarized in Table 4. Fortunately, in most clinical situations, hepatic encephalopathy improves in parallel with the underlying liver disease.

Suggested Readings

Als-Nielsen B, Gluud LL, Gluud C: Benzodiazepine receptor antagonists for hepatic encephalopathy, *Cochrane Database Syst Rev* 2:CS002798, 2004.

Als-Nielsen B, Gluud LL, Gluud C: Non-absorbable disaccharides for hepatic encephalopathy: systematic review of randomized trials, *BMJ*; doi: 10.1136/bmj.38048.506134.EE [Epub March 30, 2004].

Cordoba J, Lopez-Hellin J, Planas M, and others: Normal protein diet for episodic hepatic encephalopathy: results of a randomized study, *J Hepatol* 41:38, 2004.

Ferenci P, Lockwood A, Mullen K: Hepatic encephalopathy—definition, nomenclature, diagnosis, and quantification: final report of the working party at the 11th World Congress of Gastroenterology, *Hepatology* 35:716, 2002.

Liu Q, Duan ZP, Ha DK, and others: Symbiotic modulation of gut flora: effect on minimal hepatic encephalopathy in patients with cirrhosis, *Hepatology* 39(5):1441, 2004.

Mas A, Rodes J, Sunyer L, and others: Comparison of rifaximin and lactitol in the treatment of acute hepatic encephalopathy: results of a randomized, double-blind, double-dummy controlled clinical trial, *J Hepatol* 38(1):51, 2003.

Shawcross D, Jalan R, and others: Dispelling myths in the treatment of hepatic encephalopathy, *Lancet* 365:431, 2005.

Budd-Chiari Syndrome

Andrew S. Klein, MD, MBA, and Steven Colquhoun, MD

INTRODUCTION

Hepatic venous outflow obstruction results in a rare form of portal hypertension called Budd-Chiari syndrome (BCS). Occlusion of the suprahepatic inferior vena cava, hepatic veins, or both secondary to intravenous membranous webs is a common cause of hepatic venous outflow obstruction in Asian populations. However, this is an unusual entity in Western countries, in which BCS is most commonly attributable to thrombosis of the major hepatic veins. This distinction has important therapeutic consequences because the intravascular webs responsible for the "Eastern" form of BCS are often amenable to mechanical disruption and obliteration by surgical or interventional radiological techniques. These same techniques are of little value in the management of the "Western" form of BCS, characterized by hepatic venous thrombosis.

In most cases of hepatic vein occlusion, a prothrombotic state can be identified as a predisposing factor. Polycythemia rubra vera is the most common of these conditions, which also include paroxysmal nocturnal hemoglobinuria; essential thrombocytosis; deficiencies in protein C, protein S, or antithrombin III; antiphospholipid antibody syndrome; and factor V Leiden mutation. Hypercoagulability related to oral contraceptive use or the postpartum state has also been implicated in the development of BCS. The etiology of

BCS must be considered when planning therapeutic options. Patients with paroxysmal nocturnal hemoglobinuria, for example, suffer from disseminated clotting, and prognosis is considered so poor with surgery that some would consider this disease a relative contraindication to liver transplantation (LT) or construction of a surgical shunt. Associated nonhematologic pathologies identified at the time of presentation should also be taken into consideration when determining the best treatment for BCS. These include but are not limited to the presence of cirrhosis, previous attempts at decompressive surgery, the presence of hepatocellular carcinoma, and coexistent viral hepatic infection. Pathophysiologically, BCS results in liver congestion, elevated sinusoidal pressure, erythrocyte extravasation into the hepatic parenchyma, and tissue hypoxia. The caudate lobe of the liver drains directly into the vena cava via multiple short veins that are usually spared in BCS. As a result, compensatory hypertrophy and hyperplasia in the unobstructed caudate lobe lead to the common finding of caudate lobe enlargement.

CLINICAL PRESENTATION AND DIAGNOSIS

Most BCS patients (~90%) present subacutely with ascites, abdominal pain, and tender hepatomegaly. The dominant clinical feature is the development of ascites in an otherwise healthy person without preexisting liver disease or recognized risk factors for a liver disorder. Liver function is generally preserved, and liver function tests are normal or minimally deranged. A small fraction of BCS patients (<5%) develop fulminant hepatic failure with massive hepatocyte necrosis, rapidly progressive encephalopathy, and profound coagulopathy. In an equally small number of patients, hepatic vein occlusion is initially silent clinically, and BCS is identified only when an evaluation, including vascular imaging, is performed in a patient with cryptogenic cirrhosis.

The diagnosis of BCS is established radiologically. Duplex ultrasonography is often the initial study and, in the hands of an experienced operator, can be an accurate test. Magnetic resonance imaging and magnetic resonance angiography (MRI and MRA), as well as rapid-sequence helical computed tomography (CT), can now provide highly detailed images that can be reconstructed in three dimensions. Despite the technological advances in MRI and CT, the inferior vena cavagram and hepatic venogram remain the diagnostic gold standard for BCS. Venography has the singular advantage of allowing the radiologist to measure venous pressures in the infrahepatic and suprahepatic vena cava, as well as in the right atrium. These measurements often factor heavily in the ultimate choice of therapy. Finally, a liver biopsy should be obtained from both hepatic lobes because the hepatic venous thrombosis may not have completely obstructed the right, middle, and left hepatic veins. The degree of necrosis, fibrosis, and cirrhosis identified histologically will influence treatment strategy.

TREATMENT

The primary goal of treatment for patients with BCS is reduction of hepatic congestion and associated sequelae such as significant ascites. A secondary but essential goal is the prevention of recurrence. Initial management of BCS focuses on control of the underlying disease; reduction of ascites with salt restriction, diuretics, and paracentesis; and anticoagulation. Thrombolysis has been reported to be effective in rare cases, but delivery of the thrombolytic agent "upstream" from the clotted hepatic veins is difficult or, in many cases, impossible. Anticoagulation should be viewed as a means to prevent clot progression or recurrent venous thrombosis, but it will not reverse established disease. Despite sporadic reports of successful treatment of BCS with anticoagulation and thrombolytic

therapy alone, most patients described in these studies have relatively short periods of follow-up. Extrapolation of results from such studies to recommendations that medical therapy by itself is appropriate for long-term management is not warranted at this time.

The natural history of unrelieved hepatic venous outflow obstruction is generally progressive liver failure with fibrotic and cirrhotic changes histologically. Cameron and colleagues have demonstrated progressive hepatocyte atrophy and impaired cellular regeneration in the setting of persistent sinusoidal congestion. In a study reported by McCarthy and colleagues, 12 of 14 patients with the BCS who were managed nonsurgically died within 6 months of diagnosis. An exception to this poor prognosis may be realized by the subset of patients determined to have incomplete hepatic venous obstruction.

SURGICAL AND RADIOLOGICAL MANAGEMENT

Selection of Therapy

A proposed algorithm for the treatment of BCS is shown in Figure 1. For the small fraction of patients who present with fulminant hepatic failure secondary to BCS, LT is the only curative option. However, transjugular portal systemic shunting (TIPS) has been shown in some cases to stabilize critically ill BCS patients while they are awaiting allocation of an acceptable hepatic allograft for transplantation. In patients who develop hepatic venous thrombosis secondary to metabolic defects localized to the liver (e.g., antithrombin III deficiency or protein C deficiency), LT offers the singular benefit of being curative. The treatment options for patients with chronic hepatic venous outflow obstruction who have histologic evidence of cirrhosis are also limited to total hepatectomy and liver replacement. The realization that cirrhotic patients will do poorly with nontransplant treatment strategies emphasizes the importance of obtaining bilobar liver biopsies in patients with BCS.

The treatment dilemmas are most problematic in the approximately 90% of all BCS patients who present subacutely and have potentially reversible liver injury. Before the application of LT became available to patients with BCS, surgical therapy focused on decompression of the obstructed liver by the conversion of the portal vein from an inflow vessel to an outflow tract. This was accomplished by construction of a nonselective mesenteric-systemic or portal-systemic shunt. Slakey and others have demonstrated excellent survival (75%–94% at 5 years) with such shunts, although it is well recognized that hemodynamic and anatomic factors may limit the options for shunt selection. The caudate lobe often hypertrophies in response to the dysfunctional state of the remaining part of the liver. This can result in external compression of the inferior vena cava (IVC) and subsequent partial or complete caval obstruction (Fig. 2). Significant obstruction, defined as a pressure gradient between the infrahepatic IVC and the right atrium exceeding 20 mmHg, is felt by many to be a contraindication to standard mesocaval or portocaval shunts because these forms of bypass will not effectively decompress the liver when the systemic venous reservoir is under high pressure. Shunt thrombosis is likely under these circumstances, and even if the shunt remains patent, sinusoidal hypertension will persist. A novel solution for BCS patients with caval obstruction proposed by Cameron and colleagues was to create a direct connection between the superior mesenteric vein and the right atrium. The initial experience with mesoatrial shunts at Johns Hopkins Hospital was encouraging, with 5-year patient survival of 68%. However, the primary patency rate of the mesoatrial shunt was determined to be only 46%. With more durable treatment alternatives now available, the current indications for a mesoatrial shunt are rare. One alternative solution takes advantage of developments in endovascular therapy wherein the caval obstruction is eliminated by first deploying an expanding metallic stent to dilatate a partially obstructed IVC (Fig. 3) and then

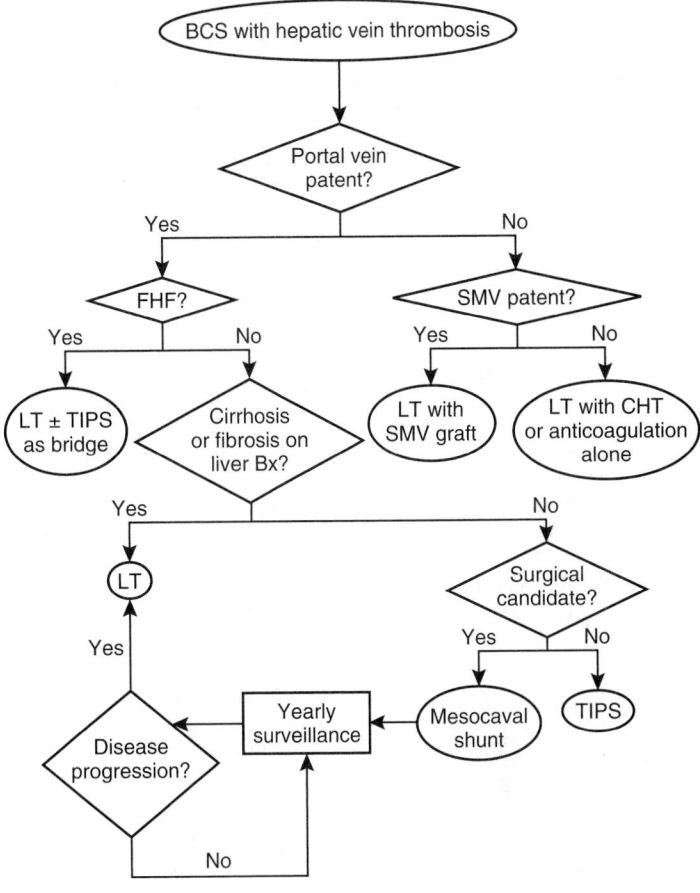

Figure 1 Treatment algorithm for patients with the Budd-Chiari syndrome. *Bx,* Biopsy; *CHT,* caval hemitransposition; *FHF,* fulminant hepatic failure; *LT,* liver transplant; *SMV,* superior mesenteric vein; *TIPS,* transjugular portalsystemic shunting.

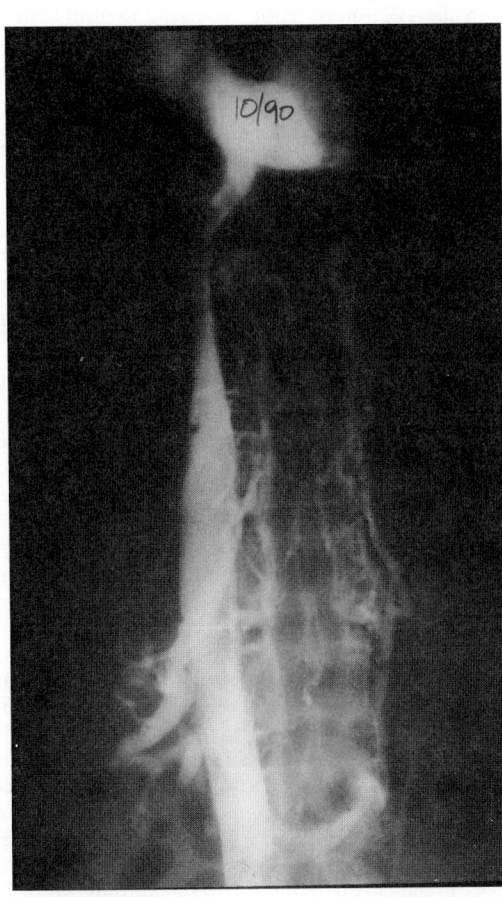

Figure 2 Partial occlusion of the inferior vena cava secondary to caudate lobe hypertrophy.

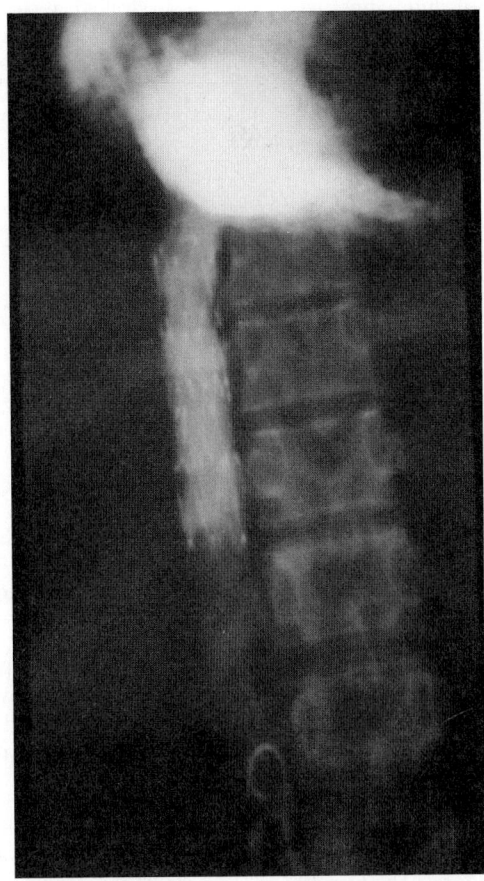

Figure 3 Successful endovascular stenting of externally compressed inferior vena cava.

constructing a standard mesenteric-systemic surgical shunt (e.g., a mesocaval shunt). Although effective in the short term, in some cases the indwelling caval stents have been shown to migrate above the diaphragm, even into the right atrium. This event can have dramatic consequences if an LT is indicated in the future, as discussed subsequently.

In the absence of vena caval obstruction, the selection of which shunt procedure is best has been a controversial topic. Orloff has had excellent results with the side-to-side portocaval shunt. However, this success has not been replicated elsewhere and may speak to the particular expertise or patient population present in a single institution. We and others have noted significant anatomic barriers to performing a portacaval shunt for patients with BCS. Notably, the presence of caudate lobe enlargement often renders a side-to-side portocaval shunt technically difficult unless a caudate lobe resection is performed before the side-to-side portocaval shunt is constructed. It is the bias of a growing number of surgeons that shunts requiring dissection or anastomosis (or both) of the portal vein itself are indicated in a dwindling number of situations. Because portacaval shunts must be disconnected at the time of LT, requiring extensive dissection of the porta hepatis, they have the disadvantage of potentially complicating subsequent LT. Several studies have documented increased blood loss, prolonged operating time, and prolonged postoperative hospital stays in LT recipients who had a previous portacaval shunt. Alternatively, mesocaval shunts are performed remotely from the porta hepatis, which is then not a reoperative field at the time of LT. At the conclusion of the LT, the mesocaval shunt is divided and oversewn or stapled. The mesocaval shunt may actually simplify the LT procedure by providing portal and systemic venous decompression during intraoperative venovenous bypass via a single femoral vein cannula. In a series from Pittsburgh, a preexisting mesocaval shunt appeared to confer a survival advantage to liver transplant recipients. The 5-year posttransplant survival was 35% for patients with a previously placed end-to-side portacaval shunt, 50% for patients with a side-to-side portacaval shunt, and 95% for patients with a mesocaval shunt. The survival for nonshunted patients was 65%.

Mesocaval Shunt for Budd-Chiari Syndrome: Technical Considerations

It is our preference to perform a mesocaval shunt C-shunt for BCS patients with potentially reversible hepatic injury who have no significant IVC obstruction (Fig. 4). This procedure can be performed rapidly; leaves the porta hepatis unscathed; and, in the event of a subsequent LT, can be easily ligated. With the patient prepped and draped in the supine position, a bilateral subcostal or an upper midline incision can be performed. We prefer the subcostal incision because it provides superior exposure and is the same approach that will be taken should an LT be required in the future. Although we have not observed this complication in BCS patients, the performance of a midline incision followed soon thereafter by a subcostal incision has been associated with tissue necrosis of the devascularized abdominal wall. A thorough exploration of the abdomen is performed, and the liver is characteristically noted to be swollen and firm, with a purplish discoloration. The small bowel is packed inferiorly with moist laparotomy pads. The transverse colon is reflected superiorly, and the middle colic vein is often an excellent landmark for identification of the superior mesenteric vein (SMV), located at the base of the transverse mesocolon to the right of the superior mesenteric artery. An oblique incision in the retroperitoneum is made to expose the SMV, which is then dissected from the first major bifurcation inferiorly to the neck of the pancreas superiorly. It is not necessary to mobilize the SMV circumferentially out of its retroperitoneal bed, but sufficient anterior and lateral

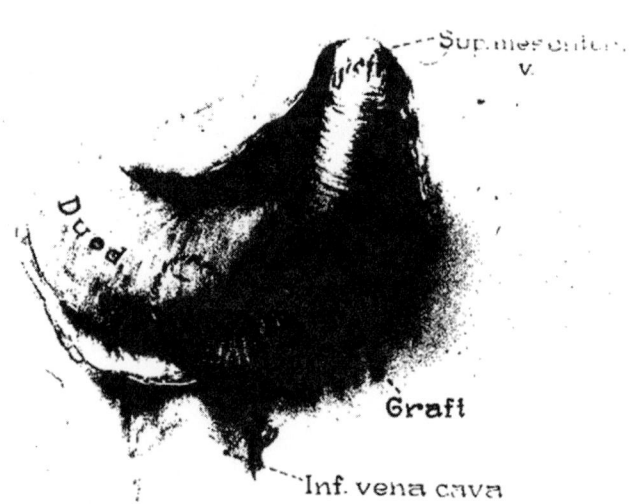

Figure 4 Mesocaval "C" shunt.

dissection is required to allow the placement of a side-biting vascular clamp. Small SMV branches may be ligated with fine monofilament suture ligatures and divided. Generally 4 to 5 cm of SMV must be exposed.

Attention is then turned to exposure of the infrarenal IVC. The duodenum is mobilized to the right with a generous Kocher maneuver. The anterior and lateral surfaces of the IVC are dissected, and to clear 5 to 6 cm of IVC, it is usually necessary to ligate and divide the gonadal vein. A Satinsky-type vascular clamp is applied to the IVC, an anterior venotomy is made, and a small ellipse of the anterior caval wall is excised. Fine monofilament stay sutures are placed in the IVC walls to keep the vessel splayed open while the anastomosis is performed. Low-porosity woven Dacron grafts or Gortex grafts 14 to 16 mm in diameter work well for these procedures. The ideal graft prosthesis is stiff enough to resist external compression from surrounding viscera but flexible enough to assume a gently curved shape without kinking. The graft is sewn end to side to the IVC with 4-0 nonabsorbable monofilament suture. The graft is then navigated around the third portion of the duodenum in a C-shaped curve. A small, side-biting clamp is applied to the SMV, which, it must be noted, in BCS patients—unlike patients with longstanding portal hypertension—is often thin walled and quite fragile. A venotomy is made in the SMV, and a single stay suture is placed in the left lateral SMV wall. An end-to-side anastomosis to the graft is performed with 5-0 nonabsorbable monofilament suture, beginning with a mattress suture at the inferior corner of the anastomosis and proceeding along the right lateral wall from inside the vessel to the superior corner stitch previously placed but not tied until the right wall of the anastomosis is completed. It is crucial that the assistant coapt the synthetic graft to the SMV while the first few stitches are placed in the anastomosis to prevent undue tension and subsequent tearing of the SMV, which could be catastrophic. The left side of the anastomosis is sewn from the outside; and before tying the running suture, caval and mesenteric vein clamps are released to flush air and clots from the lumen of the prosthesis. Another caveat is to avoid taking deep bites of the SMV wall that will "flatten" the anastomosis. Although deep bites would seemingly decrease the likelihood that the fragile SMV would tear, this technique produces a functional occlusion of flow from the SMV into the graft and increases the likelihood of shunt thrombosis.

It is occasionally necessary to use the suprarenal IVC as a target vessel (e.g., in patients with infrarenal IVC thrombosis or indwelling IVC filters). In this case, the dissection of the IVC must be carried superiorly to the inferior border of the liver to prevent tearing of the IVC or pericaval hepatic tissue when the vascular clamp is applied. For a suprarenal mesocaval shunt, the approach to the SMV is also slightly different. In this case, the dissection of the retroperitoneal tissue along the third portion of the duodenum is continued to expose the lateral border of the SMV, which is the first major vascular structure encountered. The orientation of the prosthetic graft for a suprarenal mesocaval shunt is in a more transverse plane around the second portion of the duodenum.

In many instances, surgical options may be limited simply because local surgical expertise is lacking. With increased availability of and enthusiasm for TIPS, the requisite institutional expertise with surgically constructed portal systemic shunts is, in many cases, absent. Even in training programs with access to a high volume of patients with portal hypertension, experience with portal venous decompression surgery is diminishing. Between 1995 and 1999, the surgical chief residents at the Johns Hopkins Hospital finished their training with a combined experience of four portal-systemic decompression procedures.

The Role of Transjugular Portal Systemic Shunting and Endovascular Interventions

Insertion of a TIPS stent has been shown to be an effective means to decompress the splanchnic circulation in patients with BCS. In his series of 11 patients with BCS who were treated with TIPS, Molmenti demonstrated that mean portal pressure was reduced by 43% and the portal vein/right atrium pressure gradient was reduced 73%. Although hemodynamic and physiologic improvement can be demonstrated with TIPS, occlusion is a common complication, occurring in 50% of patients in one of the larger clinical series. This limitation suggests that TIPS may be particularly useful as a temporizing measure but by many accounts lacks the durability of other therapies. TIPS may be best viewed as a bridge to transplantation rather than a destination therapy.

However, from a practical standpoint, the radiologic expertise required for successful TIPS stent insertion is far more likely to be present than is the local availability of a surgeon with the skills and experience necessary for construction of a mesenteric-systemic shunt. Additionally, it has been asserted that TIPS is more "compatible" with liver transplant surgery, should it be required, than are traditional surgical procedures. Nonetheless, misplacement or migration of TIPS stents is not uncommon, and such misadventures can have dire consequences at the time of a subsequent liver transplant. One BCS patient in our series, who underwent seven TIPS revisions following the placement of her first, developed hepatic venous outflow obstruction caused by the multiple TIPS stents. The metallic stents that extended from the patient's right atrium to the confluence of her superior mesenteric vein and splenic vein were densely incorporated into her heart and her splanchnic vasculature. This was a case in which the treatment created a problem that was more difficult to overcome than the original disease. The technical demands of the LT itself were further complicated in this case by the necessity following liver transplantation to place suprahepatic inferior vena caval stents to alleviate hepatic venous outflow obstruction in the new hepatic allograft caused by remnants of the TIPS stents. Others have quantified the potential penalty imposed on patients who receive TIPS before LT. In the series from Duke University, 33% of cases had misplacement of the stent inferiorly into the main portal vein, and blood transfusion requirements at the time of LT in the TIPS recipients were more than two times greater than those required for LT patients who did not have a previous TIPS. Although the Duke study was not limited to BCS patients, in the largest clinical series to date evaluating BCS patients who underwent LT, Mentha and colleagues determined that pre-LT TIPS was directly related to decreased patient survival.

Liver Transplantation

The first LT for the BCS was performed in 1974. Over the next 15 years, 1- and 3-year posttransplant patient survival rates for BCS (~70% and 45%, respectively) were determined to be inferior to what was observed for adult liver recipients in general. The improved success reported in more recent series (3-year survival rates of 69%–95%) has been attributed to (1) a decreased interval between the onset of symptoms and initiation of therapy, (2) early institution of anticoagulant or antithrombotic therapy (or both) posttransplantation, and (3) a commitment to lifelong anticoagulation for patients with a definable hypercoagulable state. The largest clinical series of patients with BCS treated by LT is derived from data reported by Mentha and colleagues, who surveyed the European Liver Transplantation Registry between 1988 and 1999. The researchers identified 295 patients transplanted for BCS; complete follow-up data were obtained for 248 patients. The actuarial survival was 75.6%, 71.4%, and 68% at 1, 5, and 10 years posttransplant, respectively. Late mortality was low in this study; only 9 patients died after 1 year. However, 27 patients (11%) developed some form of venous thrombosis despite anticoagulation therapy. Six of these patients had recurrent hepatic venous thrombosis. Most series, however, have suggested that early initiation of anticoagulation therapy has markedly reduced the incidence of recurrent BCS following LT. We would advocate lifelong anticoagulation following LT for patients with BCS, even in the absence of an identifiable hypercoagulable state. This strategy is not without penalty. The series from Cambridge reported a 44% incidence of nonfatal hemorrhage when a policy of early posttransplant anticoagulation was instituted, and the European multicenter clinical series identified 27 patients (11%) who had sustained a clinically significant hemorrhage that was related to anticoagulation. Nonetheless, there is general agreement that complications secondary to bleeding are generally more amenable to treatment than are complications secondary to thrombosis.

LT poses specific technical challenges for patients with BCS. The obstructed liver is generally enlarged, firm, and difficult to mobilize during the hepatectomy. A diffuse fibrotic reaction in the retroperitoneum, perhaps related to the hepatic vein thrombotic process, increases the difficulty of identifying, mobilizing, and controlling the IVC. Because the caudate lobe is enlarged and the hepatic veins orifices are occluded, the "piggyback" technique of LT may be particularly tricky. Control of the vena cava may actually require incision of the diaphragm and isolation of the vena cava within the pericardial sac.

Not infrequently, BCS patients with hypercoagulable conditions present with thrombosis of other large vessels in their splanchnic circulation. Portal vein occlusion presents a particularly difficult problem because a plan for restoring portal venous inflow to the transplanted liver must be devised before proceeding with LT. If the portal vein is occluded but the SMV is patent, pretransplant transhepatic cannulation of the portal vein with thrombolysis and venoplasty has been shown to be successful in a small number of patients. Alternatively, donor iliac vein can be used as a conduit from the recipient's SMV to the allograft portal vein. In cases in which both the portal vein and SMV are occluded, Tzakis and colleagues have performed LT with caval hemitransposition whereby the allograft portal vein is sewn end-to-side to the recipient's IVC. The IVC superior to this anastomosis is partially or totally ligated to preferentially direct systemic venous blood through the allograft portal vein. Patients treated with caval hemitransposition have persistent portal hypertension, as well as functional caval obstruction posttransplantation. Not surprisingly, morbidity and mortality are high in such patients, who arguably are best treated with anticoagulation alone with the hope that they will develop collateral splanchnic venous drainage and symptomatic improvement over time.

Despite the successful construction of mesenteric-systemic surgical shunts or the placement of TIPS stents, persistent liver injury with histologic progression to fibrosis and cirrhosis has been documented in some patients. Shunt patency does not necessarily ensure complete decompression of the congested hepatic sinusoids. For this reason, lifelong follow-up and tracking of hepatic function is indicated in BCS patients treated with surgical shunts or TIPS. As noted earlier, the impact of radiologic therapies for BCS following a subsequent LT cannot be neglected. It should be emphasized that intravascular stents (either a TIPS stent placed to decompress directly the hypertensive splanchnic circulation or a transcaval stent placed in a partially occluded IVC to improve the efficiency of a surgically placed mesocaval shunt) become densely incorporated into their resident blood vessels. Should these stents migrate into the main portal vein, the suprahepatic IVC, or the right atrium, significant technical difficulties may be encountered during isolation of the hepatic vasculature and subsequent explantation of the liver.

CONCLUSION

There is little controversy that LT offers the most effective therapy for the minority of individuals with either fulminant hepatic failure or the chronic cirrhotic form of BCS. However, most BCS patients present with acute or subacute manifestations of hepatic venous outflow obstruction. If long-term benefit were the sole benchmark by which treatment was selected for these patients, who represent the majority of BCS patients, there is general agreement that as a group, they will do best if given transplants. Unfortunately, from a practical standpoint, clinical outcomes alone cannot be used to determine whether LT is advisable for patients with BCS. A more restricted use of LT is mandated by (1) the widening gap between the number of patients who require LT and the static pool of donated organs, (2) the unpredictable availability of donor organs, (3) the need for and consequences of lifelong immunosuppression, and (4) the dramatically higher cost of transplant versus nontransplant therapies.

SUGGESTED READINGS

Attwell A, Ludkowski M, Nash R, and others: Treatment of Budd-Chiari syndrome in a liver transplant unit, the role of transjugular intrahepatic porto-systemic shunt and liver transplantation, *Aliment Pharmacol Ther* 20(8):867, 2004.

Brems JJ, Hiatt JR, Klein AS, and others: Effect of a prior portasystemic shunt on subsequent liver transplantation, *Ann Surg* 209:52, 1989.

Mentha G, Giostra E, Majno P, and others: Liver transplantation for Budd-Chiari syndrome: a European study on 248 patients from 51 centres, *J Hepatol* 44:520, 2006.

Molmenti EP, Segev DL, Arepally A, and others: The utility of TIPS in the management of Budd-Chiari Syndrome, *Ann Surg* 241:978, 2005.

Narayanan Menon KV, Shah V, Kamath PS: The Budd-Chiari Syndrome, *N Engl J Med* 350:578, 2004.

Slakey D, Klein AS, Venbrux AC, and others: Budd-Chiari syndrome: current management options, *Ann Surg* 233:522, 2001.

Srinivasan P, Rela M, Prachalias M, and others: Liver transplantation for the Budd-Chiari syndrome, *Transplantation* 73:973, 2002.

Venbrux AC, Mitchell SE, Savader SJ, and others: Long-term results with the use of metallic stents in the IVC for treatment of Budd-Chiari syndrome, *JVIR* 5:411, 1994.

GALLBLADDER AND BILIARY TREE

ASYMPTOMATIC (SILENT) GALLSTONES

Robert A. Garwood, MD, and John B. Hanks, MD

INTRODUCTION

Gallstone disease is one of the leading indications for surgery in the United States today, with approximately 500,000 cholecystectomies being performed every year. As much as 10% to 20% of the population will develop gallstones at some stage of life, and the incidence increases with age. The advent of laparoscopic cholecystectomy has done much to facilitate the management of this condition as symptoms or complications arise. However, when gallstones are found incidentally and are asymptomatic, management decisions have not been so clear-cut and controversy exists in the surgical literature.

EXPECTANT MANAGEMENT VERSUS PROPHYLATIC CHOLECYSTECTOMY

Natural history of "silent" gallstones does not appear to justify treatment with prophylactic cholecystectomy. Nearly 80% of patients remain asymptomatic throughout their lives, with only 1% to 4% progressing to symptoms or developing complications from gallstones annually. Only 10% of those found to have asymptomatic gallstones develop symptoms within the first 5 years after diagnosis, increasing only to 20% at 20 years. This was first demonstrated by Gracie and Ransohoff in their landmark study of 123 patients followed prospectively over a 15-year period. They showed that 10% of patients progressed to symptomatic disease at 5 years, 15% by 10 years, and 18% by 15 years. Overall, patients developed symptoms or serious complications, such as acute cholecystitis, at a rate of 1% to 2% per year, with most patients developing symptoms within 5 years. Critics of the study cited its homogenous population of primarily young white male patients. However, other investigators have shown similar results with more diverse patient populations. McSherry and colleagues studied 135 patients with asymptomatic gallstones and diverse ethnicity and gender. With a 58-month follow-up, 10% developed symptoms and only 7% required cholecystectomy at annual rates of 2.2% and 1.5%, respectively. Friedman and colleagues, in their review of the literature, looked at an ethnically diverse patient population as well. They showed that 3% to 4% of patients developed biliary symptoms in the first 10 years. Of these, nearly all patients who developed a complication had experienced previous symptoms; only 1% to 3% of patients with mild symptoms and 6% to 8% with severe symptoms progressed to have a complication.

Several investigators have attempted to identify local or patient factors that are predictive of gallstone disease progression. Generally most studies have not shown gallstone size or nature, gallbladder wall thickness, or gallbladder contractility to be significant predictors of progression to symptoms or complications. A few studies have demonstrated that patients with gallstones greater than 2.5 cm have higher rates of acute cholecystitis and a higher risk for developing gallbladder cancer. In addition, higher rates of gallbladder cancer have also been identified in patients with porcelain gallbladder and gallbladder polyps greater than 10 mm in diameter. Patient factors such as age, sex, or comorbidities such as diabetes have also been generally nonpredictive for progression to symptoms or complications. Two exceptions include the morbidly obese after bariatric surgery (30% develop gallstones) and patient status postcolectomy (20% will develop symptoms within 5 years).

Despite the relatively low risk of progression to symptomatic disease and complications, some proponents of prophylactic cholecystectomy have proposed early operation. It may be that the introduction of laparoscopic cholecystectomy, with its low morbidity and nearly zero mortality rates, might alter the risk-to-benefit ratio in favor of prophylactic cholecystectomy. Given the low risk of elective laparoscopic cholecystectomy, Patino and colleagues, in their review of the literature, proposed criteria for patients with a "high" risk for developing complications of asymptomatic gallstones who would benefit from prophylactic cholecystectomy (Table 1). However, although mean operative times and length of hospital stay are longer for laparoscopic cholecystectomy in the context of acute cholecystitis, the conversion rates (7.3% vs. 7.6%) and morbidity rates (8.7% vs. 9.6%) have not been shown to be significantly different. Furthermore, a follow-up study by Ransohoff comparing expectant management versus prophylactic cholecystectomy showed that patients undergoing prophylactic cholecystectomy had decreased survival. Using a decision analysis, they demonstrated that a 50-year-old and 30-year-old man, respectively, would lose 18 days and 4 days of life by undergoing a prophylactic cholecystectomy. A cost-effective analysis did not demonstrate a substantial difference between patients with silent gallstones who underwent an immediate cholecystectomy compared with those for whom an approach of watchful waiting was taken.

Overall, except for a few special situations, the natural history of asymptomatic gallstones appears to be that benign and expectant management is the recommended course of action.

SPECIAL CASES

Diabetes

In the past, management of diabetic patients with asymptomatic gallstones emphasized early cholecystectomy. The argument for

Table 1: Proposed Criteria for Prophylactic Cholecystectomy

Life expectancy >20 years
Calculi >2 cm in diameter
Calculi <3 mm and patent cystic duct
Radiopaque calculi
Gallbladder polyps
Nonfunctioning or calcified gallbladder
Women <60 years of age
Patients in areas with high prevalence of gallbladder cancer

prophylactic cholecystectomy was based on the assumption that these patients had diabetic autonomic neuropathy that masked the pain and signs associated with acute cholecystitis, and thus they presented with advanced disease and had more complications. Hickman and colleagues demonstrated that diabetic patients in general were subject to more infectious complications that contributed to mortality. Furthermore, when comparing diabetic with nondiabetic patients, Landau and colleagues found diabetics to have higher rates of infected bile, gangrene, gallbladder perforation, and surgical mortality in the setting of acute cholecystitis (21% vs. 9%).

More recent evidence demonstrates that a natural history of asymptomatic gallstones in diabetic patients has a lower risk of major complications than previously thought. The prevalence of gallstones in diabetic compared with nondiabetic patients (14.4% vs. 12.5%) is not significantly different, and the overall percentage of non-insulin-dependent diabetics who initially presented with symptoms or complications of gallstone disease is only 14.9% and 4.2%, respectively.

Furthermore, mortality and morbidity rates following surgery are not significantly different. Postoperation morbidity is primarily due to older age and concurrent cardiovascular and renal disease. Ransohoff and colleagues showed that age-adjusted risk for death increased by a factor of 2.2 for diabetic compared with nondiabetic patients; however, mortality was most significant for the age group older than 75 years. Thus prophylactic cholecystectomy did not appear justified.

Transplantation

The prevalence of cholelithiasis in transplant patients appears to range from 30% to 40%. Prophylactic cholecystectomy may well be warranted in prospective transplant patients. The high incidence of gallstones in this patient population has been attributed to cyclosporine. However, the type of organ transplantation is an important factor, and the incidence of gallstones and rates of complications varies among the organs transplanted. In a recent decision analysis by Kao and colleagues, prophylactic posttransplantation cholecystectomy resulted in less mortality than pretransplantation cholecystectomy and expectant management in heart transplant patients (5:1000 vs. 80:1000 vs. 40:1000 deaths, respectively) compared with renal/pancreas transplant patients where expectant management was found to be a safer course of management than prophylactic cholecystectomy (2:1000 vs. 5:1000 deaths, respectively).

Prophylactic cholecystectomy is not recommended in patients undergoing renal transplantation. Greenstein and colleagues followed renal transplant patients for 4 years and found only a 7% incidence of gallstones and 3% incidence of sludge. Of these patients, 87% remained asymptomatic, with only 7% patients developing acute cholecystitis and requiring subsequent uncomplicated laparoscopic cholecystectomy. Others have supported this evidence and have shown that the presence of gallstone disease does not negatively affect graft survival.

On the contrary, heart transplant patients have been shown to have higher rates of gallstone formation and gallstone-related complications. Peterseim and colleagues showed a 42% incidence of silent gallstones, with 58% of these cases developing symptoms within 2 years of heart transplant. Others have reported significantly increased mortality associated with the development of symptoms and complications and the need for emergent cholecystectomy in this group of patients. The Mayo Clinic reported that 36% of 178 heart-lung transplant patients had abnormal gallbladder ultrasound results, with 50% requiring intervention secondary to gallstone-related complications. The operative mortality rate was 29%. Milas and colleagues also showed a 30% incidence of gallstones, with nearly 50% of these patients going on to cholecystectomy secondary to symptomatic disease. However, they did not report any postoperative deaths in their study. This group concluded that screening ultrasound, followed by prophylactic laparoscopic cholecystectomy if stones are present, is prudent, given the high incidence of gallstones and the subsequent risk of progressing to symptomatic disease.

Hemoglobinopathies

Patients with hemoglobinopathies are at a significantly increased risk for developing pigmented stones. Gallstones have been reported in up to 70% of sickle cell patients, up to 85% of hereditary spherocytosis patients, and up to 24% of thalassemia patients. In sickle cell patients, complications from asymptomatic gallstones have been reported to be as high as 50% within 3 to 5 years of diagnosis. This has been attributed largely to the diagnostic challenge associated with symptomatic cholelithiasis versus abdominal sickling crisis.

Historically, the primary argument for expectant management in these patients was the significant morbidity and mortality associated with open operation. The advent of laparoscopic cholecystectomy, along with improvements in and understanding of the importance of preoperative hydration and transfusion, improved anesthetic technique, and postoperative care, have lowered the operative risk for these patients (especially sickle cell patients). Currently, elective laparoscopic cholecystectomy can be safely performed with minimal perioperative mortality and morbidity. Prophylactic cholecystectomy in these patients avoids future diagnostic confusion, as well as the mortality and morbidity risk associated with emergency surgery. Furthermore, cholecystectomy can and should be performed at time of splenectomy, whether open or laparoscopic.

Pappas and colleagues reported on 12 patients who underwent splenectomy without concomitant cholecystectomy for hemolytic diseases despite presence of silent gallstones. Two patients required surgery secondary to symptoms or complications within 2 to 3 weeks of splenectomy; the remaining 10 required surgery within the next 7.5 years. Thus current recommendations include prophylactic cholecystectomy if gallstones are present or concomitant cholecystectomy if splenectomy is planned.

Cirrhosis

Several studies have shown no significant differences in progression to symptoms from silent gallstones in cirrhotic patients compared with noncirrhotic patients. Castaing and colleagues reviewed gallstone disease in cirrhotic patients and found that 17% had gallstones, with 14% of these patients going on to have symptoms or complications requiring cholecystectomy. There was one postoperative death and one postoperative complication secondary to variceal bleeding. Sleeman and colleagues, in their review of 25 Child-Pugh class A and B cirrhotic patients who underwent laparoscopic cholecystectomy, reported the procedure to be feasible and safe in cirrhotic patients. Despite a 32% morbidity rate (wound hematoma, pneumonia, and ascites), they reported zero postoperative deaths and a mean length of stay of 1.7 days.

Although the natural history of asymptomatic gallstones in cirrhotic patients does not significantly differ from the general population, there are certain important specific risks to consider. Cirrhotic patients do develop more severe symptoms from acute cholecystitis. When severe symptoms occur, they may well be associated with increased morbidity and mortality. Furthermore, laparoscopic cholecystectomy, although safe and feasible, is more technically challenging in the context of cirrhosis and portal hypertension. The risk of hemorrhage from portal hypertension in the periumbilical area can affect trocar site placement. Varices in the perigastric and porta hepatis affect dissection. Therefore anatomic consideration and natural history of the clinical situation suggest that a course of expectant management is recommended in the cirrhotic patient.

Altered Nutrition

Total Parental Nutrition

A well-documented relationship exists between prolonged total parental nutrition (TPN) administration and the formation of gallstones. This has been shown to be secondary to multiple factors, such as gallbladder stasis and changed composition of bile. There may be nearly a 35% incidence of gallstone formation in these patients, among whom a larger than expected percentage progresses to symptomatic disease. Roslyn and colleagues reported a retrospective review of patients who underwent cholecystectomy for TPN-induced gallbladder disease. Of the 35 patients included in the study, 40% required emergent cholecystectomy, with an overall operative morbidity of 54% and mortality of 11%. The authors concluded that those on long-term TPN should have ultrasound surveillance and elective cholecystectomy when gallstones are detected.

Bariatrics

Rapid weight loss by any means markedly increases the incidence of gallstone formation from the 10% to 20% range in the general population to the 30% to 40% range in weight-reduction patients without previously documented gallstones. Pharmacologic prophylaxis with ursodiol has been shown to be an effective treatment in decreasing gallstone formation as long as the patient is compliant. Several studies have shown ursodiol compliance to be in the 64% to 85% range. In a review of 289 patients who underwent laparoscopic gastric bypass, Villegas and colleagues showed that when patients without documented gallstones at the time of surgery were treated with ursodiol and followed at 6 months with ultrasound examination, only 39 (22%) of 151 patients developed gallstones and 12 (8%) developed sludge. Eleven of these patients went on to cholecystectomy secondary to symptoms or complications from their gallstones. The authors recommended concomitant cholecystectomy when gallstones were documented preoperatively or intraoperatively. They further reported that doing so increased the technical difficulty of the case, often required placement of additional port sites, increased operative times by 20 to 49 minutes, and doubled the length of hospital stay from 2.5 to 4.5 days. There was no apparent effect on serious postoperative complications or mortality. Therefore they concluded that concomitant cholecystectomy at the time of laparoscopic gastric bypass was both feasible and safe. Given the available evidence, it seems reasonable to remove the gallbladder when gallstones are documented either preoperatively or intraoperatively and to treat patients undergoing bariatric surgery without documented gallstones with ursodiol.

INCIDENTAL CHOLECYSTECTOMY

The management of cholelithiasis found incidentally during an abdominal or alimentary tract procedure is controversial. Although concomitant cholecystectomy definitively removes the risk of gallbladder disease and its complications, it has the potential to increase patient morbidity and mortality. However, numerous authors have found concomitant cholecystectomy to be a safe and efficacious procedure. In a review of colorectal surgery patients, the Mayo Clinic found a 15% rate of symptomatic cholelithiasis over a 6-year period in patients with incidental cholelithiasis. They determined that the probability of requiring future cholecystectomy in this patient population was 12% at 2 years and 22% at 5 years. Saade and colleagues also looked at patients undergoing colorectal, gastric, and gynecological procedures over 4-year period. In the 109 patients studied, 78 (72%) had incidental cholecystectomy, with only 2 postoperative complications. Thirty-one patients (28%) had their gallbladders left in situ, with 12 remaining asymptomatic and 13 developing symptoms. Seven of these patients went on to open cholecystectomy 2 to 11 weeks later. Thompson and colleagues followed 56 patients found to have incidental gallstones at time of celiotomy; 33 underwent incidental cholecystectomy, with only 1 (3%) complication. Twenty-three patients had their gallbladders left in situ, with 16 of these developing complications, including 11 with acute cholecystitis, within 6 months. Fifteen (65%) of these patients subsequently underwent open cholecystectomy, with 6 patients (40%) requiring common bile duct exploration. McSherry and colleagues reviewed 137 patients undergoing incidental cholecystectomy for a variety of intra-abdominal procedures. Only three patients in this cohort had postoperative complications directly attributable to cholecystectomy. This is particularly true if the patient is older than 70 years of age. In a review of 4072 patients aged older than 70 years with cholelithiasis, Watemberg and colleagues showed increases in mortality, morbidity, and length of hospital stay for patients in whom incidental cholecystectomy was not performed. These increases were attributed to increased pulmonary complications, sepsis, and multiple organ failure. Therefore concomitant cholecystectomy is appropriate during abdominal or alimentary tract surgery in patients older than 70 years of age.

Management of incidental cholelithiasis during a vascular surgery procedure has been even more controversial because of the frequent use of prosthetic graft material. Concomitant cholecystectomy increases the risk for potential graft infection from bile spillage. However, despite this risk of potential contamination, several authors have reported data showing cholecystectomy to be feasible during vascular surgery. Ochsner and colleagues were among the first to show that concomitant cholecystectomy was safe during open abdominal aortic aneurysmectomies (AAAs). Fifty-one of 931 patients in their series underwent cholecystectomy at the time of AAA repair with no increase in mortality or morbidity. Ouriel and colleagues reported similar results in 42 of 845 patients found to have gallstones at the time of AAA repair. In the 18 patients who had simultaneous cholecystectomy during AAA repair, only one graft infection occurred, and this in a patient whose retroperitoneum was not closed before cholecystectomy. Furthermore, of the 11 patients who had aneurysmectomy without cholecystectomy, 9 developed acute cholecystitis within 3 years, with 1 death from biliary sepsis. Sonpal and colleagues reviewed 113 patients undergoing a major abdominal vascular procedure with prosthetic graft, of whom 7 had an incidental cholecystectomy. There were no complications, including graft infection, attributed to cholecystectomy, and the authors concluded that incidental cholecystectomy was safe following closure of retroperitoneum over the graft. Thus incidental cholecystectomy is supported during AAA repair provided that the graft is covered with peritoneum before proceeding with cholecystectomy.

SUMMARY

The finding of asymptomatic gallstones leads to a clinical decision challenge. The risk of a procedure must be balanced against the morbidity of progression to acute cholecystitis. Expectant management can take advantage of increased technology such as ultrasound and pharmacologic management (e.g., ursodiol) but requires patient compliance, as well as the physician's understanding of any underlying clinical disease (i.e., cirrhosis) that on its own can be associated with increased complications. The advent of laparoscopy has allowed the surgeon to use a technique with reduced morbidity. Finally, intraoperative concomitant cholecystectomy should be directed by the clinical circumstance—largely technical—and the best judgment of the operating surgeon.

Suggested Readings

Castaing D, Houssin D, Lemoine J, and others: Surgical management of gallstones in cirrhotic patients, *Am J Surg* 146:310, 1983.

Friedman G: Natural history of asymptomatic and symptomatic gallstones, *Am J Surg* 165:399, 1993.

Greenstein SM, Katz S, Sun S, and others: Prevalence of asymptomatic cholelithiasis and risk of acute cholecystitis after kidney transplantation, *Transplantation* 63:1030, 1997.

Juhasz ES, Wolff BG, Meagher AP, and others: Incidental cholecystectomy during colorectal surgery, *Ann Surg* 219:467, 1994.

Kao LS, Flowers C, Flum DR: Prophylactic cholecystectomy in transplant patients: a decision analysis, *J Gastrointest Surg* 9:965, 2005.

Milas M, Ricketts RR, Amerson JR, and others: Management of biliary tract stones in heart transplant patients, *Ann Surg* 223:747, 1996.

McSherry CK, Glenn F: Biliary tract surgery concomitant with other intraabdominal operations, *Ann Surg* 193:169, 1981.

Pappas C, Galanakis S, Moussatos G, and others: Experience of splenectomy and cholecystectomy in children with chronic haemolytic anaemia, *J Pediatr Surg* 24:543, 1989.

Patino JF, Quintero GA: Asymptomatic cholelithiasis revisited, *World J Surg* 22:1119, 1998.

Peterseim D, Pappas TN, Meyers CH, and others: Management of biliary complications after heart transplant, *J Heart Lung Transplant* 14:623, 1995.

Ransohoff DF, Gracie WA, Wolfensen LB, and others: Prophylactic cholecystectomy or expectant management for silent gallstones, *Ann Intern Med* 99:199, 1983.

Roslyn JJ, Pitt HA, Mann L, and others: Parenteral nutrition–induced gallbladder disease: a reason for early cholecystectomy, *Am J Surg* 148:58, 1984.

Sleeman D, Namias N, Levi D, and others: Laparoscopic cholecystectomy in cirrhotic patients, *J Am Coll Surg* 187:400, 1998.

Sonpal IM, Schreiber H, Byramjee AM, and others: The rational for incidental cholecystectomy during major abdominal vascular surgery, *Am Surg* 57:579, 1991.

Thompson JS, Philben VJ, Hodgson PE: Operative management of incidental cholelithiasis, *Am J Surg* 148:821, 1984.

Villegas L, Schneider B, Provost D, and others: Is routine cholecystectomy required during laparoscopic gastric bypass? *Obes Surg* 14:206, 2004.

Acute Cholecystitis

Harry Zemon, MD, and Todd A. Ponsky, MD

The gallbladder needs to be removed not because it contains stones but because it forms them.

Dr. Carl Langenbuch, who performed the first cholecystectomy on July 15, 1882.

INTRODUCTION

Since Langenbuch described the first cholecystectomy, this operation remains one of the most common operations performed by general surgeons. The technique for the operation has changed significantly over the past century with the advent of laparoscopy, but the general concept of the procedure, indications, and controversies remain.

PATHOPHYSIOLOGY

Acute cholecystitis (AC) is inflammation of the gallbladder that is usually caused by an obstruction of the cystic duct, most often by gallstones or biliary sludge. The mucosa of the obstructed gallbladder continues to secrete mucous, and the gallbladder becomes distended, resulting in venous congestion and eventual impediment of arterial inflow and ischemia. The inflammation can be sterile, but positive bacterial cultures of the bile or gallbladder are found in 50% to 75% of cases. Acute acalculous cholecystitis (AAC) occurs secondary to ischemia of the gallbladder wall and subsequent to chemical damage from bile stasis and increased lithogenicity of bile. AAC is often found in hospitalized acutely ill patients after trauma or burns. AAC also occurs frequently in patients who have experienced global ischemia, such as after cardiac surgery or those surviving cardiac arrest.

EPIDEMIOLOGY

Cholelithiasis is present in approximately 10% of adults. Only 30% of patients with asymptomatic cholelithiasis will go on to require a cholecystectomy at some point in their life. Thus incidental finding of cholelithiasis does not warrant removal of the gallbladder. The true incidence of AC is unknown. Estrogen production directly influences the production of gallstones. Therefore, patients who are female, overweight, or of childbearing age (younger than age 50) are at higher risk for cholelithiasis. Women in this age group are three times more likely to develop gallstones than men.

CLINICAL PRESENTATION

Most patients with AC will present with a constellation of symptoms and signs including right upper quadrant pain, nausea, vomiting, and fever. Patients frequently report a several-month history of symptoms of abdominal pain after a fatty meal that resolves over time. Some patients may report right shoulder pain, which results from deferred pain caused by diaphragmatic irritation.

DIAGNOSIS AND WORKUP

Patients with AC typically will have a low-grade fever, mild tachycardia, and right upper quadrant tenderness on physical examination. Some patients may have local or diffuse peritoneal signs. Patients often demonstrate inspiratory arrest with deep right upper quadrant palpation; this is known as Murphy's sign. Typically these patients have mild leukocytosis. A high leukocytosis may indicate a gangrenous or perforated gallbladder or the presence of another process such as pancreatitis, cholangitis, or even pneumonia. AC itself should not cause jaundice. If jaundice is present, one should consider obstruction of the common bile duct (CBD) as a diagnosis. AC can lead to jaundice in the rare case of Mirrizi's syndrome, in which external compression of the CBD occurs from a large cystic duct stone.

Abdominal ultrasound of the right upper quadrant remains the initial study of choice despite multiple peer-reviewed studies showing a sensitivity of only 60% to 70%. A computed tomography

(CT) scan is often performed to evaluate complications of cholecystitis but not as the initial study. Demonstration of gallbladder wall thickening, pericholecystic fluid, gallstones, or a combination of these are highly suggestive of AC. In cases of symptoms consistent with AC but negative on ultrasound, we perform a hepatobiliary iminodiacetic acid (DISIDA) scan (Figs. 1 and 2). This test, although more expensive than ultrasound, is approximately 90% to 97% sensitive. Some centers use the DISIDA scan as the primary study to diagnose AC.

One must differentiate the symptoms of biliary colic from AC. Patients with biliary colic are usually nontender, have resolving pain, and have no fever or leukocytosis. Patients with biliary colic will require surgery, but this should be scheduled on an elective basis.

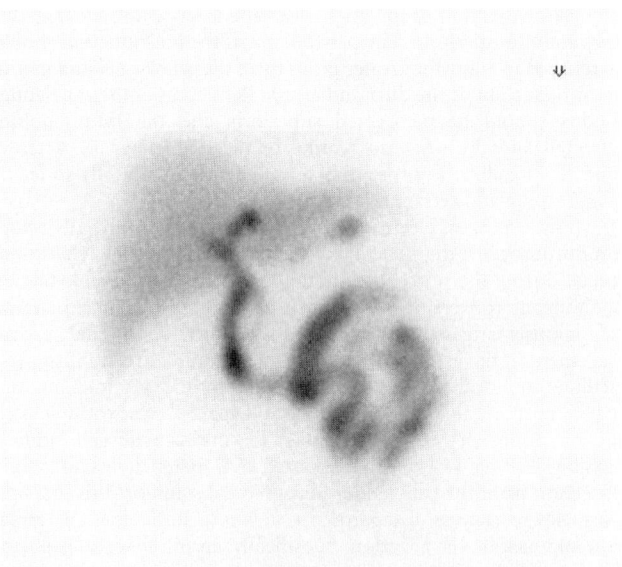

Figure 1   Technetium 99 hepatobiliary iminodiacetic acid (DISIDA) scan consistent with acute cholecystitis showing nonfilling of the gallbladder and transit of tracer into the duodenum.

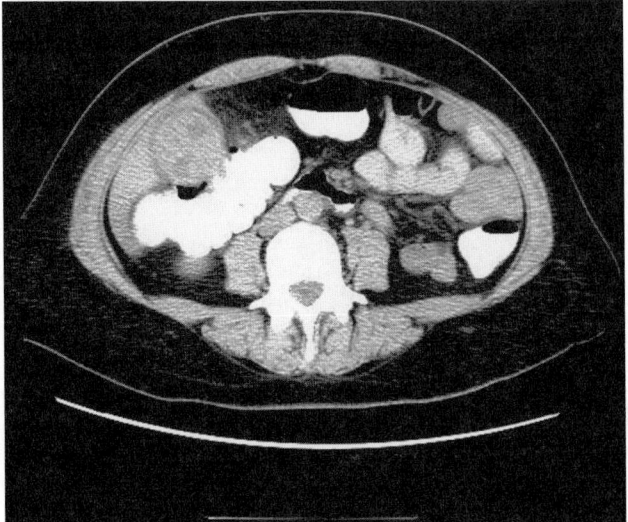

Figure 2   Computed tomography scan showing a thickened gallbladder wall, cholelithiasis, and pericholecystic fluid consistent with acute cholecystitis.

PREOPERATIVE CONSIDERATIONS

Antibiotics

The most commonly associated organisms of septic cholecystitis are *Escherichia coli, Klebsiella, Enterobacter, Enterococcus, Streptococcus, Bacteroides,* and *Clostridium.* Antibiotic therapy should be broad spectrum and directed at these organisms, such as a second-generation cephalosporin or fluoroquinalone. In a study from Greece, Dervisoglou and colleagues demonstrated a significant reduction in surgical-site infection by using ampicillin-sulbactam, which covers *Enterococcus.* Antibiotic therapy should be initiated on diagnosis of AC and discontinued after removal of the gallbladder. Extension of therapy to 5 to 7 days is warranted for those with emphysema or gangrene of the gallbladder, with empyema, or with continued signs of infections.

Early versus Delayed Surgery

Until recently, many surgeons believed that early surgery for acute cholecystitis, whether performed laparoscopically or open, carried higher risk for complications, increased operative times, and caused higher conversion rates. Many surgeons advocated a cool-down period in which patients were given 1 week of antibiotics and surgery was delayed for 6 to 10 weeks. Recently, however, this strategy of delayed surgery has been debated. The controversy surrounding timing of surgery for acute cholecystitis has been studied extensively. The benefits of early surgery, defined as 1 to 7 days from the onset of symptoms, have been substantiated by multiple randomized control trials (RCT). A meta-analysis of 10 RCTs by Shikata and colleagues comparing early versus delayed laparoscopic surgery shows that early surgery does not increase morbidity or mortality, nor does it increase conversion rates. Lau and colleagues, in a meta-analysis of 4 RCTs, also showed that early surgery for acute cholecystitis decreased total length of stay and reduced emergent readmission rates.

At our institution, most surgeons operate on patients with AC within the first 24 to 48 hours. Delaying surgery allows progression of the inflammatory process, which in turn can lead to induration, abscess, and necrosis of the gallbladder. Elderly, cirrhotic, diabetic, and immunocompromised patients are at higher risk for rapid progression to perforation and gangrene.

Comorbidities

Before proceeding with a cholecystectomy, the overall condition of the patient must be considered. For most patients, laparoscopic cholecystectomy is the next appropriate step after confirming the diagnosis of AC. In certain circumstances, however, immediate laparoscopic cholecystectomy may not be the safest course of action. In patients with significant hemodynamic instability, severe cardiomyopathy, active myocardial infarction, or any other comorbidity that makes surgery prohibitively unsafe, a percutaneous cholecystostomy tube should be placed. This can be performed at the bedside in the intensive care unit or, more typically, by interventional radiology.

Pregnancy

The management of the pregnant patient with AC also warrants special consideration. Laparoscopy during the first trimester is thought to affect organogenesis, possibly secondary to the vascular changes caused by carbon dioxide pneumoperitoneum. Open cholecystectomy has a 12% fetal loss rate in the first trimester. Surgery during the third trimester has a reported 30% to 40% rate of preterm labor and is a technically difficult operation laparoscopically because of the size of the uterus. Surgery is safest during the second trimester and carries the lowest incidence of preterm labor and fetal demise. If a pregnant patient in either the first or third trimester of pregnancy presents with mild AC that improves with intravenous antibiotics over 24 hours, it is most prudent to perform an interval cholecystectomy in either the second trimester or postpartum. However, given that any intra-abdominal infection may lead to fetal demise or preterm labor, a patient with severe AC should be managed with immediate cholecystectomy. The Society for American Gastrointestinal Endoscopic Surgeons recommends postponing surgery until the second trimester, insufflating the abdomen using the open Hassan technique and only to a pressure of 8 to 12 mm Hg. It is also recommended to perform fetal monitoring during the case. The use of intraoperative cholangiogram, prophylactic tocolytics, and fetal monitoring is variable among published practices.

OPERATIVE CONSIDERATIONS

Laparoscopic versus Open

The increased popularity of laparoscopy has dramatically increased the skill level and experience of graduating surgical residents. As such, most cases of acute cholecystitis are started laparoscopically and converted to open as needed. Absolute contraindications to laparoscopy are inability to tolerate the effects of general anesthesia and pneumoperitoneum or the presence of a coagulopathy. The decision to start with an open cholecystectomy is usually secondary to the patients' comorbidities and number of prior abdominal surgeries. Previous abdominal surgery is not a contraindication to laparoscopy at our institution. In cases of concern for umbilical adhesions, one can gain access via the open Hassan technique or at an alternate site such as the epigastric or right upper quadrant port sites. Ultimately, each case is judged individually on the basis of the surgeon's skill level and experience.

Anatomy

Fifteen to twenty percent of patients will have anomalous anatomy. As such, a thorough and complete knowledge of the normal and anomalous biliary and vascular anatomy is paramount to performing this operation. The most relevant cystic duct anomaly is a short cystic duct. In this circumstance, the right hepatic or CBD may be mistaken for the cystic duct and lead to transection (Figs. 3 and 4). Similarly, a short cystic artery may lead to inadvertent transection of the right hepatic artery. Ten to fifteen percent of patients have a replaced right hepatic artery with its origin from the superior mesenteric artery. This replaced right hepatic artery courses through the triangle of Calot, in closer proximity to the cystic duct, making it more vulnerable to injury during the dissection.

Lap Technique

The principles of a cholecystectomy are well established and focus on avoiding injury to the CBD. Standard laparoscopic techniques help avoid damage to surrounding structures. A basic tenet of this procedure is the identification of the infundibular-cystic duct (ICD) junction. Safe dissection of the cystic duct and artery must occur at this level and not inferiorly. The peritoneum at the ICD junction should be released to allow for greater mobility of the gallbladder and meticulous dissection of the duct and artery. Retraction of the gallbladder fundus should be performed superiorly and the infundibulum retracted laterally to avoid tenting of the CBD (Fig. 5). A tense, fluid-filled gallbladder should be drained laparoscopically to facilitate grasping and retraction of the gallbladder.

Minimization of electrocautery or other energy source dissectors minimizes occult thermal injury to surrounding bowel. Gallstones spilled during the procedure should be retrieved if possible but do not warrant conversion to an open procedure. Bile spilled should be copiously irrigated to avoid a nidus for intra-abdominal abscess. Placement of the gallbladder into an endoscopic extraction bag may facilitate removal of the gallbladder from the peritoneum and reduce port-site infection and stone spillage. Some advocate closed suction drains in Morrison's pouch for intrahepatic gallbladders, possibly leading to extensive exposed liver parenchyma following dissection from the gallbladder fossa. No data support this practice. Obstacles to successful laparoscopy relate to difficulties in retraction and lack of visualization. Specifically, an intrahepatic gallbladder or a gallbladder with a necrotic, friable wall may prevent proper retraction and safe dissection in the triangle of Calot. Bleeding and severe inflammation may prevent proper visualization of the cystic artery and duct. Dissection should not be attempted until the ideal exposure is obtained in any of these situations.

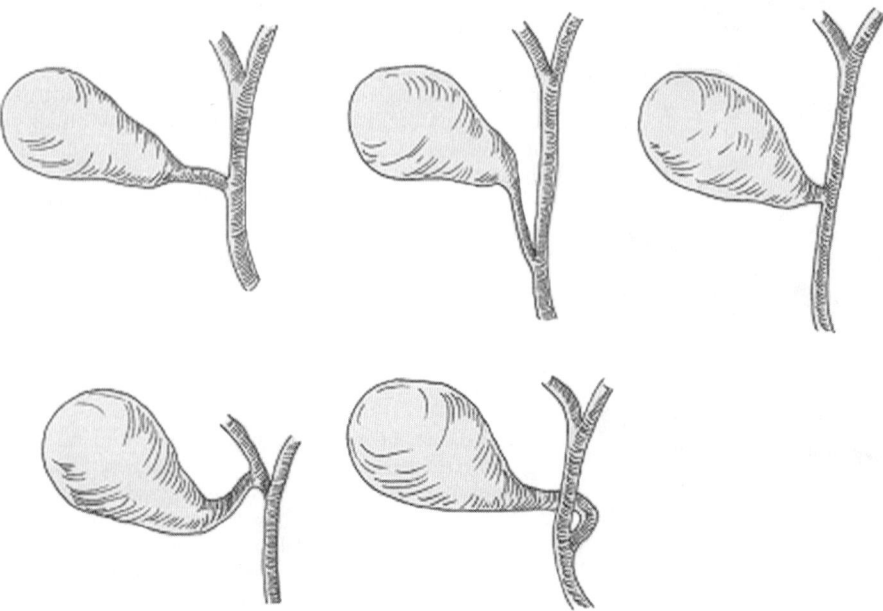

Figure 3 Variations of cystic duct anatomy.

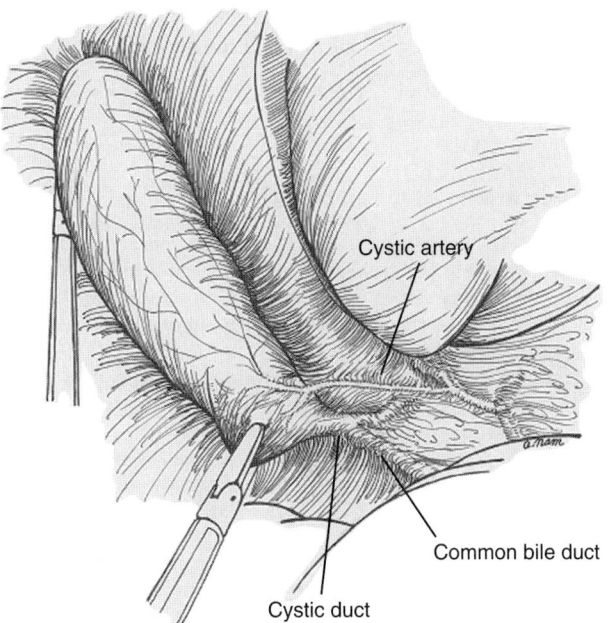

Figure 4 The common bile duct can be mistaken for the cystic duct if the latter is short, as shown here.

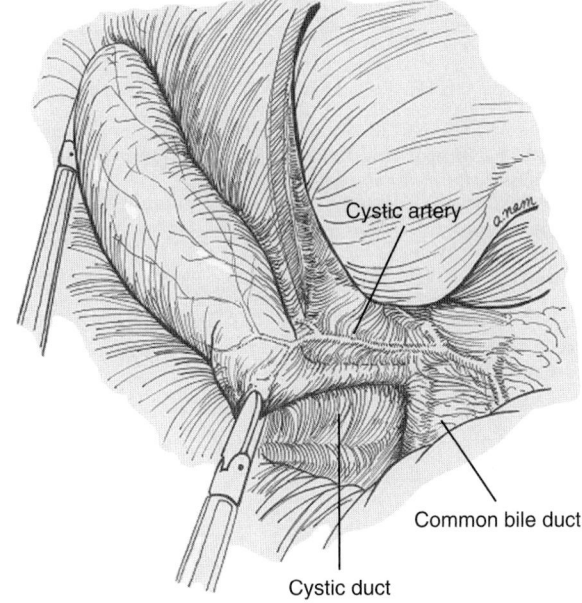

Figure 5 Proper retraction of the gallbladder.

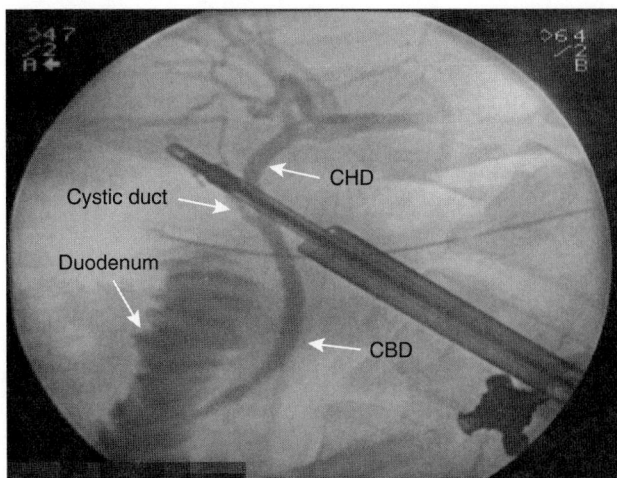

Figure 6 Normal intraoperative cholangiogram. *CBD*, Common bile duct; *CHD*, common hepatic duct.

Intraoperative Cholangiogram

Routine use of intraoperative cholangiogram (IOC) is controversial. Most surgeons advocate for selective approach to IOC when CBD stones are clinically suspected preoperatively or when the anatomy appears unclear intraoperatively.

Proponents of the selective approach argue that routine IOC unnecessarily adds time and expense to the operation because the vast majority of CBD stones are detected and treated preoperatively with endoscopic retrograde cholangiopancreatography (ERCP). They also contend that normal preoperative bilirubin translates to clinically insignificant stones that will pass spontaneously with no sequelae. Selective proponents also argue that the clinical impact and significance of occult retained stones are overstated. A review of the literature by Metcalfe and colleagues that included 5179 laparoscopic cholecystectomies performed without IOC and without preoperative indication of common bile duct stones demonstrated that only 0.6% developed symptoms from residual stones postoperatively. This study also showed no statistically significant difference in the rate of CBD transection during laparoscopic cholecystectomy with (0.02%) and without (0.09%) IOC.

Proponents for routine IOC argue for the importance of experience in both cystic duct cannulation and fluoroscopy interpretation (Fig. 6). In addition, proponents argue that IOC can exclude the presence of undiagnosed CBD stones that are found in 6% to 10% of elective cases with cholecystitis even with a normal preoperative bilirubin level. Undiagnosed retained stones in the CBD may pass on their own but can lead to back pressure on the cystic duct stump before they pass and possibly dislodge the cystic duct clips. If the stones do not pass, they may lead to obstructive jaundice and cholangitis, warranting a second procedure such as an ERCP or CBD exploration. In addition, IOC can help to identify aberrant anatomy and bile duct injury, allowing for decreased morbidity with early primary repair. In the academic training setting, IOC is used routinely to facilitate surgical resident education.

Intraoperative laparoscopic ultrasound for the detection of CBD stones is an alternative approach that is gaining popularity. In the hands of an experienced surgeon, laparoscopic ultrasound has been shown to safely detect CBD stones and identify biliary anatomy. As experience with ultrasound cholangiography increases, it may obviate the need for the more invasive intraoperative fluoroscopic cholangiograms.

Conversion from Laparoscopic to Open Cholecystectomy

Although laparotomy is associated with greater morbidity and prolonged hospital stays, conversion to open cholecystectomy is not a complication nor should it be considered a failure. Conversion to open cholecystectomy may provide improved visualization if the relevant anatomy is not discernible laparoscopically or if injury to a vital structure occurs. Rates of conversion reported in the literature are cited between 0% and 20%. The most common reasons cited for opening are uncertainty of anatomy, poor visualization, and injury to surrounding structures. Surgeon experience plays a role in the rate of conversion. In a Turkish study, Kama and colleagues found conversion rates to be 10% in the initial 100 patients and 4.1% in the subsequent 900. Independent risk factors for conversion include male gender, history of biliary disease, delay greater than 48 hours to surgery, white blood cell count greater than 18, obesity, and high American Society of Anesthesiologists classification.

Open Cholecystectomy

Open cholecystectomy is performed via a midline or subcostal incision. The hepatoduodenal ligament is palpated to familiarize the position of the common bile duct and to palpate for ductal stones. The cystic duct and artery are dissected and encircled with a silk tie but not ligated. The "dome down" approach is accomplished by placing a clamp on the fundus of the gallbladder and retracting inferiorly to expose the junction of the fundus and the edge of the liver. The peritoneum is incised along the border of the liver, releasing the gallbladder from its intrahepatic attachments. As the infundibulum-cystic duct junction is encountered, dissection of the lateral peritoneal attachment should occur along the medial side. After complete release of the gallbladder, lateral retraction exposes the final attachments, that is, the cystic duct and artery. Proximal and distal ligation of the artery and duct can now safely occur. Standard two-layer fascial closure is performed for the subcostal incision, and one-layer closure is performed for the midline approach.

Bailout Maneuvers

Even the most experienced surgeon will likely encounter a gallbladder that cannot be safely removed in its entirety. Long-standing inflammation and sclerosis around the porta hepatis and retroperitoneum prevents mobility and elevation of the biliary tree, in turn creating poor visualization of the biliary anatomy and hepatic vessels. There are several options at this point. The least invasive is a cholecystostomy tube and placement of closed-suction drainage tubes. Alternatively, partial removal of the gallbladder with ligation and suture closure of the infundibulum is a reasonable alternative to dissecting a cystic duct in a hostile cemented portal region. The remaining mucosal surface of the infundibulum is cauterized to prevent a mucocele. Similarly, a necrotic friable gallbladder without a tissue plain of the posterior wall can be left in situ rather than

attempting removal and potentially causing bleeding or injury to surrounding structures. In all of these instances, we recommend placement of a closed-suction drainage tube in the subhepatic space.

Complications of Cholecystitis

Progressive acute cholecystitis can lead to gangrene, empyema, and eventual rupture of the gallbladder wall. Spillage of infected bile can lead to peritonitis, sepsis, and death. Chronic cholecystitis can result in fistula formation with the duodenum or stomach, and this in turn can lead to gallstone ileus.

Minor complications of cholecystectomy are bleeding, wound infection, hernia, hematoma, and abscess from stone or bile spillage. Minor and clinically asymptomatic bile leaks are common after cholecystectomy. These leaks are usually caused by the division of small cholecystohepatic ducts, and the majority of these resolve without intervention or sequelae. Cystic duct leak is a rare complication that occurs in less than 1% of laparoscopic cholecystectomies. Diagnosis is often made by ERCP, sonogram, DISIDA, or CT. ERCP with ductal decompression by sphincterotomy and stent placement is the management of choice; however, it can also be managed by percutaneous drainage, laparoscopy, or laparotomy. Major complications such as bile duct injury occur in between 0.2% and 1.4% of cases. Open and laparoscopic operations have essentially equal rates of bile duct injuries, but the recent trend is toward fewer injuries with laparoscopy. This is most likely related to the fact that only the most difficult cases are converted to the open procedure.

Suggested Readings

Bhattacharya D, Ammori BJ: Contemporary minimally invasive approaches to the management of acute cholecystitis: a review and appraisal, *Surg Laparosc Endosc Percutan Tech* 15:1, 2005.
Flum DR, Koepsell T, Heagerty P, and others: Common bile duct injury during laparoscopic cholecystectomy and the use of intraoperative cholangiography, *Arch Surg* 136:1287, 2001.
Gurusamy KS, Samraj K: Early versus delayed laparoscopic cholecystectomy for acute cholecystitis, *Cochrane Database of Syst Rev* 2006, 4.
Shikata S, Noguchi Y, Fukui T: Early versus delayed cholecystectomy for acute cholecystitis: a meta-analysis of randomized controlled trials, *Surg Today* 35:553, 2005.

MANAGEMENT OF COMMON DUCT STONES

Brent D. Matthews, MD, and Steven M. Strasberg, MD

INTRODUCTION

Choledocholithiasis is present in 5% to 10% of patients who require surgery for symptomatic cholelithiasis. Common duct exploration and endoscopic retrograde cholangiography (ERC) are the two techniques available for stone removal. The classical surgical approach was open common duct exploration, which is rarely performed today; instead, bile duct exploration is performed

laparoscopically in most cases. Laparoscopic bile duct exploration may be performed via the cystic duct or through a choledochotomy. Although the techniques are highly successful, it seems that they are not widely practiced by U.S. surgeons today. This chapter describes the two laparoscopic techniques for duct exploration. A summary of the vanishing technique of open exploration is also given at the end of the chapter.

LAPAROSCOPIC MANAGEMENT OF COMMON BILE DUCT STONES

A single-stage laparoscopic procedure is the preferred treatment for choledocholithiasis in the presence of symptomatic cholelithiasis in many centers. The single-stage approach has been shown to be more economical and safer than laparoscopic cholecystectomy combined with postoperative ERC and endoscopic sphincterotomy. Postoperative ERC has a failure rate of 4% to 10%, and patients are at risk of requiring reoperation for open common bile duct exploration (CBDE). A randomized trial of laparoscopic CBDE versus postoperative ERC with or without sphincterotomy (S) in an intention-to-treat model reported that, by the end of treatment, duct clearance was 100% in the laparoscopic group compared with 93% in the postoperative ERC group; duration of treatment was a median of 90 minutes (range: 25–310) in the laparoscopic group compared with 105 minutes (range: 60–255) in the postoperative ERC group; and hospitalization was a median of 1 day (range: 1–26) in the laparoscopic group versus 3.5 days (range: 1–11) in the postoperative ERC ± S groups.

Although outcome data support the use of laparoscopic CBDE, a recent survey of practicing general surgeons in rural areas of the United States indicated that 45% perform laparoscopic CBDE, but only 21% practiced it as their preferred approach. Reasons given for not performing laparoscopic exploration were time constraints, lack of equipment, inadequate endoscopic backup, and insufficient laparoscopic technical capabilities. In fact, there appears to be a striking difference between the rapid and widespread adoption of laparoscopic cholecystectomy and the slow and localized use of laparoscopic bile duct exploration. Laparoscopic CBDE should be adopted and used by surgeons able to perform this advanced laparoscopic technique in the management algorithm for choledocholithiasis.

LAPAROSCOPIC TRANSCYSTIC EXPLORATION

Access and Flushing

Laparoscopic transcystic exploration is the preferred technique of most surgeons performing laparoscopic CBDE. It is highly effective when applied appropriately, and it avoids the more technically difficult exploration via choledochotomy. Common bile duct stones are verified before exploration, usually by percutaneous intraoperative cystic duct cholangiography. A 5-mm grasper is left attached to the gallbladder during cholangiography and serves as a ruler to measure stone and ductal diameters seen on the radiographs. Surgeons facile in sonography may also use this technique. Laparoscopic transcystic CBDE is performed through the cystic ductotomy used for cholangiography. A transcystic approach is favored when the following conditions are present: common bile duct is less than 6 mm in diameter, stones are located distal to the cystic duct–common bile duct junction, the cystic duct is greater than 4 mm in diameter, and fewer than 6 to 8 stones are present in the common bile duct. Common duct exploration of any type other than flushing through the cystic duct should be avoided if the common bile duct is 3 mm or less in diameter because injury to the bile duct is more likely. If stones less than 2 mm in diameter are present in any sized duct, forceful irrigation with saline after relaxation of the sphincter of Oddi by intravenous administration of 1 to 2 mg of glucagon will often flush stones into the duodenum. To facilitate this technique, the ampulla may be dilated under pressure monitoring after placement of a balloon-dilating catheter (4 to 6 mm) over a guidewire (0.028 to 0.035 inches) under fluoroscopic guidance. Repeat forceful irrigation of saline can subsequently be attempted. If simple flushing fails to clear stones of 3 mm or less, the surgeon should consider allowing them to pass on their own unless there is a history of gallstone pancreatitis.

Stone Extraction under Fluoroscopy

Transcystic fluoroscopic placement of a helical stone basket and stone extraction may be attempted primarily after unsuccessful attempts to flush the stones into the duodenum. Guidewire (modified Seldinger technique) and fluoroscopic guidance of the helical stone basket minimizes the potential complications of common bile

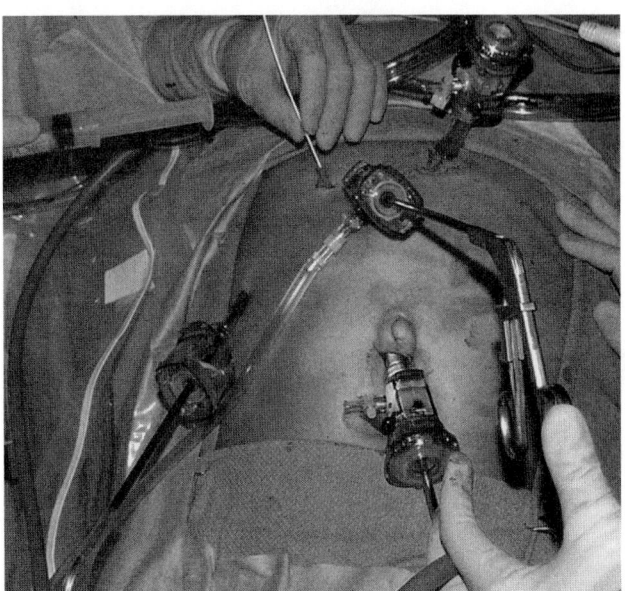

Figure 1 Manipulation of a biliary balloon-tipped catheter through a 14-gauge angiocatheter placed in the right upper quadrant for cholangiography.

duct perforation or impaction of the basket in the ampulla. The guidewires, biliary balloon-tipped catheters, and helical stone baskets can be manipulated through a 14-gauge angiocatheter initially placed in the right upper quadrant for cholangiography (Fig. 1). Use of the 14-gauge angiocatheter allows the operating surgeon and assistant to use all of the trocars placed for laparoscopic cholecystectomy and thus enhances the ability to retract the liver or manipulate the gallbladder.

Choledochoscopic Examination and Stone Extraction

Laparoscopic transcystic flexible biliary endoscopy is performed when the cystic duct is greater than or dilatable to 8 mm in diameter. Choledochoscopes from 3 to 10 F in diameter are available for transcystic exploration. We prefer a 3- to 5-mm instrument. The cystic ductotomy can be dilatated by balloon or mechanically with sequentially placed ureteral bougies to 8 mm in diameter or to a diameter no larger than the internal diameter of the common bile duct. Novel, peel-away 14-F catheters have been used to maintain access to the biliary system as an overtube during choledochoscopy. The peel-away catheter is inserted via the cystic duct over a guidewire after serial dilatation of the duct. The choledochoscope is introduced through the midclavicular 5-mm trocar and into the cystic ductotomy. Continuous saline infusion distends the common bile and common hepatic ducts and allows for manipulation and extraction of the stones. A video switcher for simultaneous monitor display of the laparoscopic and choledochoscopic images simplifies the procedure by eliminating the need for a second video monitor. The choledochoscope is manipulated with atraumatic grasping forceps, and the stones are removed using a helical stone basket passed through the working channel of the choledochoscope (Fig. 2, *A* and *B*). On occasion, the scope may be used to push stones through the ampulla of Vater into the duodenum. After stone extraction is completed, the ampulla is identified and the choledochoscope can usually be passed into the duodenum. The choledochoscope is advanced into the duodenum if possible. The opening into the duodenum appears as a dark slit. The scope is slowly pulled back. All four walls of the duct should be visible for the entire length of the passage. Failure to see all four walls may be due to deflection of the scope by

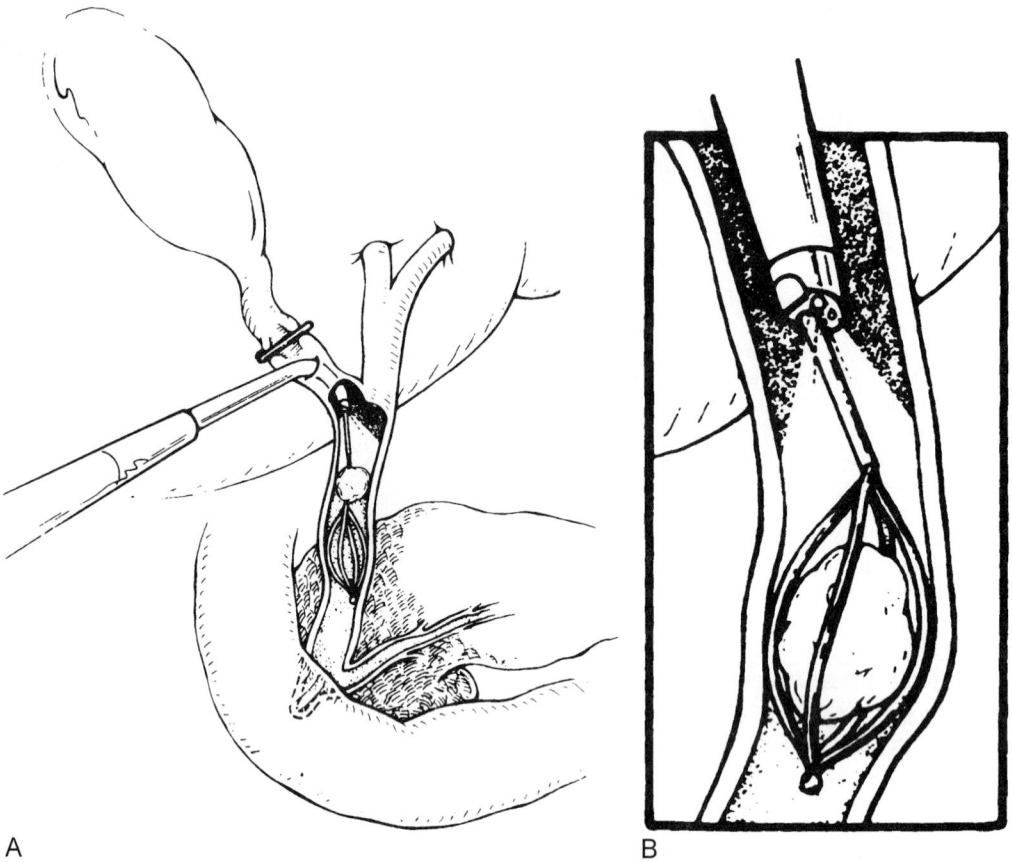

A   B

Figure 2 **(A)** Laparoscopic transcystic choledochoscopy is performed with the passage of a helical basket through the working channel of the choledochoscope. **(B)** A common bile duct stone is ensnared and extracted. *From Soper N. In Cameron JL, editor: Current surgical therapy, ed 7, Philadelphia, CV Mosby, 2001.*

a stone. If possible, the scope is then passed into the upper ducts. The common hepatic duct and the right and left ducts and their tributaries are explored as far as duct size will allow. Access to the common hepatic duct or more proximal ductal system is usually limited with a transcystic approach, and laparoscopic choledochotomy is typically required when stones are present in these locations.

Direct visualization of stones greatly improves the efficiency and speed of stone removal. Clearance of common bile duct stones is confirmed by a completion cholangiogram. Failure of dye to enter the duodenum is not unusual because of sphincter spasm after exploration and is not an indication for reexploration. A transcystic externalized biliary catheter (C-tube) or internalized biliary catheter (endobiliary stent) may be placed on completion of the procedure but is not mandatory unless the surgeon is concerned about the possibility of retained stones or debris or about ampullary stenosis resulting from edema. The catheters decompress the common bile duct in the immediate postoperative period and can be removed 10 to 21 days after insertion. The cystic duct is secured with clips or ligated with an Endoloop (Ethicon Endosurgery, Cincinnati, OH) or intracorporeal suture. The Endoloop or an intracorporeal-placed suture may be more secure than clips after vigorous manipulation of the cystic duct and is therefore the preferred method.

Results

The success rate of laparoscopic transcystic common bile duct stone exploration is 71% to 98%, and morbidity rates range from 0% to 14%. Cystic duct stump leaks, bile duct perforation, and pancreatitis are potential complications of a transcystic approach, and retained stones occur in 2% to 5% of patients. Failure of the transcystic approach may be due to inability to cannulate or dilate the cystic duct

or to extract large or multiple stones through the cystic duct. Treatment options include laparoscopic choledochotomy, open CBDE, or postoperative ERC with or without sphincterotomy. Recent studies indicate that laparoscopic transcystic exploration is more time efficient, is associated with decreased length of postoperative hospitalization, has less perioperative morbidity than laparoscopic choledochotomy, and is more cost effective than postoperative ERC. Maximal efficiency occurs when the equipment necessary for laparoscopic transcystic CBDE is readily available on specially organized instrument trays or carts (Fig. 3). Recent series have reported an increase of only 10 to 15 minutes in operative times for the addition of transcystic CBDE compared with laparoscopic cholecystectomy with intraoperative cholangiogram alone when performed in a structured operating room environment.

LAPAROSCOPIC CHOLEDOCHOTOMY

Indications

The decision to perform laparoscopic CBDE via a choledochotomy is influenced by multiple factors, including cystic duct and common bile duct anatomy; number, size, and location of common bile duct stones; inflammatory changes within the triangle of Calot; technical expertise; and availability of skilled biliary endoscopy for postoperative endoscopic retrograde cholangiography. Laparoscopic choledochotomy is an option after failure of transcystic techniques. For instance, if the cystic duct diameter is less than 4 mm or the cystic duct is tortuous and cannot be traversed with a guidewire, biliary balloon-tipped catheter, or retrieval basket or it cannot be

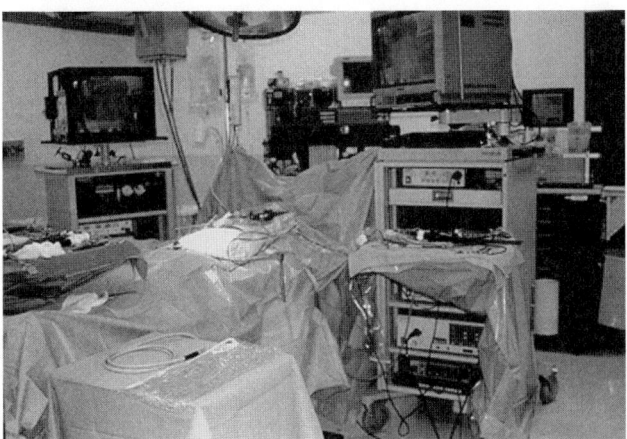

Figure 3 The equipment necessary for laparoscopic transcystic common bile duct exploration is readily available on specially organized instrument trays or carts to maximize efficiency. *From Petelin JB, Pruett CS. In: Cameron JL, editor,* Current surgical therapy *ed 8, Philadelphia, Elsevier Mosby, 2004.*

dilated to intubate a 5- to 10-F-diameter choledochoscope, then laparoscopic choledochotomy is preferred. Also choledochotomy is preferred when common bile duct stones are greater than 6 to 8 mm in diameter or proximal to the cystic duct–common bile duct junction because the success of laparoscopic transcystic exploration is low under these circumstances. Severe inflammation in the triangle of Calot may actually necessitate open CBDE, provided that the inflammation does not extend over the region of the common bile duct. Less conventional techniques (e.g., laparoscopic transcystic placement of a C-tube or internalized endobiliary stent and intraoperative or postoperative ERC± S, or laparoscopic transcystic balloon dilatation of the sphincter of Oddi and antegrade sphincterotomy) are appropriate if surgical or endoscopic procedural expertise is available in these techniques. Laparoscopic antegrade sphincterotomy requires antegrade (transcystic or via choledochotomy) introduction of an endoscopic sphincterotome through the ampulla and visualization via a side-viewing duodenoscope with subsequent sphincterotomy. This approach has been reported from only a few specialized centers. Laparoscopic choledochotomy requires expertise in intracorporeal suturing to close the choledochotomy primarily or over a T-tube, and this should be factored into the decision to perform a CBDE laparoscopically.

Technique

Laparoscopic choledochotomy is performed by making a longitudinal 1.0- to 1.5-cm incision with scissors on the anterior surface of the common bile duct at the level of the cystic duct–common bile duct junction. Placement of stay sutures on either side of the choledochotomy as routinely performed during open CBDE to maintain anterior traction on the common bile duct is optional and often not necessary. A 3-F or 4-F balloon-tipped catheter can be placed into the ductotomy to flush loose stones or debris. Subsequently it may be inflated and used to sweep the duct. However, laparoscopic exploration with a flexible choledochoscopy is usually the preferred technique for stone clearance. The flexible choledochoscope is introduced through the 5-mm midclavicular, right upper quadrant trocar and placed into the choledochotomy. The technique is similar to that described previously for transcystic choledochoscopy. The choledochotomy may be closed primarily or over a T-tube, C-tube, or internalized biliary catheter (antegrade stenting). Primary closure or closure over a C-tube or internalized biliary catheter is performed by intracorporeal suturing techniques with 4–0 monofilament or multifilament

absorbable suture in an interrupted fashion. Choledochoscopic or cholangiographic confirmation of a patent common bile duct before suture of the common bile duct is critical to avoid postoperative bile duct leaks if the choledochotomy is closed primarily without stenting. Access for ductal imaging is lost after primary closure or closure over an internalized biliary catheter, although the latter allows for continued decompression of the bile duct. The biliary catheter can be removed after 10 to 21 days or an appropriately designated time by snaring the internalized transampullary portion of the catheter in the duodenum using a flexible endoscope. Laparoscopic placement of a T-tube is comparable to an open technique. A 10- to 14-F T-tube is prepared and placed in the common bile duct. The ductotomy is closed by intracorporeal suturing techniques with 4–0 monofilament or multifilament absorbable suture in an interrupted fashion. After the security of the T-tube closure is confirmed by saline infusion, a completion cholangiogram is performed by externalizing the T-tube through one of the upper abdominal trocars and infusing water-soluble contrast during real-time fluoroscopy. After the completion of the laparoscopic cholecystectomy, the T-tube is externalized through the 5-mm midclavicular trocar site and sutured to the skin.

Results

The success rate of laparoscopic choledochotomy for common bile duct stone extraction is 85% to 97%, and morbidity rates range from 3% to 16%, with a slightly higher complication rate reported in several longitudinal, nonrandomized, and retrospective series for choledochotomy closure over a T-tube. Recent studies have indicated that laparoscopic CBDE and primary choledochotomy closure are safe, time-efficient, associated with a decreased length of postoperative hospitalization, and as cost effective as closure over a T-tube. Primary closure avoids potential complications of T-tube placement such as bile duct leak with inadvertent T-tube dislodgement, cholangitis, pancreatitis, or unintended suturing of the T-tube to the common bile duct. Bile duct leaks and subhepatic bilomas or abscesses have been reported after primary closure. Common bile duct strictures after laparoscopic choledochotomy with primary closure or closure over a T-tube have been reported infrequently with follow-up reported over 36 to 43 months.

OPEN COMMON BILE DUCT EXPLORATION

Open CBDE for extraction of gallstones, once a common procedure, is rarely performed today. Its chief indication is failure of other techniques. Laparoscopic and endoscopic techniques fail uncommonly, especially when referring doctors take advantage of expertise available in specialized centers for difficult cases. Some of the principles of open CBDE are still of use to those performing laparoscopic CBDE.

Chief among these are the following:

- Avoid CBDE when the common bile duct is less than 5 mm in diameter, and do not explore a bile duct that is 3 mm in diameter or less. The risk of injury to the bile duct rises with decreasing diameter. Stones smaller than 3 mm in diameter usually pass spontaneously and pose little risk unless the patient has previously had acute pancreatitis. In cases of gallstone pancreatitis, stones identified by cholangiography should be removed endoscopically when the duct is particularly small. This is a rare event. In case of a small bile duct, a transcystic approach may be attempted as described in the section on transcystic laparoscopic approaches. The indication for doing so is rare.
- Avoid forceful manipulation of instruments in the bile duct. The latter may result in false passages into the bowel or

retroperitoneum with consequent fistula or abscess and later stricture of the bile duct.
- An operative cholangiogram should be performed before ductal exploration to delineate the position and number of stones and to provide a roadmap to ductal anatomy. CBDE should always be completed by examination of the duct using choledochoscopy or cholangiography (preferably both).

The procedure is performed through a right subcostal or upper midline incision. An extensive Kocher maneuver is performed so that the retroduodenal and intrapancreatic bile duct can be palpated for stones. Exploration of the bile duct is often easier from the left side of the table. The common bile duct is identified by incising the overlying peritoneum and by following the cystic duct to its union with the common duct. Normally the structure is a green color, and small blood vessels are visible on its surface. The size of the common duct and the midplane of the duct are noted. After placing two stay sutures in the common duct, the duct is incised with a number 15 blade longitudinally at the level of the cystic duct entry. The incision should initially be made slightly to the left of the longitudinal midplane of what appears to be the common bile duct. This avoids opening into the septum of a fused cystic–common hepatic duct in the case of parallel insertion of the cystic duct that is present in about 20% of patients. Once the duct is opened, the side walls should be palpated with an instrument such as a Potts scissors placed into the duct to identify the center line (midplane) of the duct. The duct is then opened to approximately 1.5 cm. Obvious stones are extracted. Stones palpated in the duct may be milked up (or down) until they appear in the choledochotomy and can be extracted. Next the duct is explored with Randall stone forceps. The path of the duct is learned by allowing the closed forceps to find its way up and down the duct. The forceps is then reinserted in an open position and closed to grasp stones. One should be aware that when exploring upward, the confluence of ducts may be grasped and mistakenly thought to be a stone. Once a stone is grasped, it should be gently removed. Excessive force should not be used. Flexible spoons or scoops are also useful devices for removing stones. The bile duct should be irrigated using a catheter (Fig. 4) or directly with a bulb syringe, the tip of which has been wedged into the duct. Flushing the duct in this manner expands it around the stones and is particularly useful for intrahepatic stones. The choledochoscope may be used at open surgery to remove stones, as described in the laparoscopic section of this chapter. The biliary Fogarty catheter may be used as well, although we find it much less efficient than the traditional methods just described.

Ampullary patency can be proved by various means. One common technique is to use a metal sound such as a Bakes dilator. A small-diameter sound should be used, and the ampulla should not be dilatated with graduated sounds. Holding the sound between only the thumb and index finger avoids use of force. The presence of the sound in the duodenum is detected by the "steel sign," that is, seeing the tip of the sound through the duodenal wall. We prefer to prove patency using a biliary Fogarty catheter, which is flexible and tends to go into the duodenum easily when there is no obstruction. When there is free passage of the catheter for 20 cm into the bile duct without resistance, the balloon may be inflated and pulled back to identify the position of the sphincter of Oddi. When there is doubt, the surgeon should palpate the catheter in the duodenum before inflation.

Choledochoscopy is always performed using a flexible or rigid scope. At open surgery, stay sutures are crossed to retain saline, which is flushed into the duct under pressure.

When stones are identified, they may be removed using the techniques described earlier or using baskets passed via the scope as previously described.

Impacted stones represent a special case. Fortunately, they are rare and are usually diagnosed preoperatively. Severely impacted

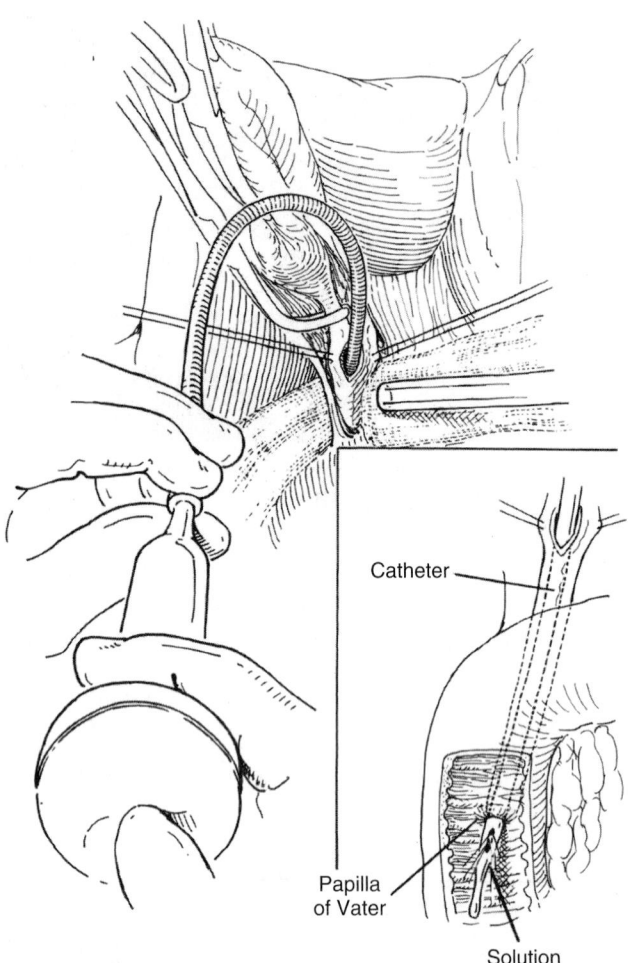

Figure 4 Flushing the common bile duct with normal saline through a 10-F red rubber catheter. *From Zollinger RM Jr, Zollinger RM: Atlas of surgical operations, ed 7, New York, 1993, McGraw-Hill.*

stones remain one of the uncommon indications for open exploration after other approaches fail. The safest and most effective way to deal with these stones is by electrohydraulic lithotripsy via the choledochoscope. This technique breaks the stones into small pieces, which then can be extracted. Laser energy has been used to do the same but is more expensive and has hazards not associated with the mechanical lithotripter. Electrohydraulic lithotripsy must always be performed under direct vision, and the active tip should be immediately adjacent to the stone. In the past, impacted stones at the lower end of the bile duct have been extracted by duodenotomy and sphincteroplasty. This is almost never required and should be performed only by surgeons who have experience in the technique. Pictures are sometimes shown in texts of incising the sphincter over a sound. This is an ideal method, but in the case of a truly impacted stone, a sound cannot be passed into the duodenum, and the incision must be made onto the impacted stone. If an impacted stone cannot be removed and experience in lithotripsy or sphincterotomy is lacking, then a T-tube should be placed and the operation terminated so that the patient may be referred for treatment of the stone. Removal can almost always be achieved by endoscopic or percutaneous means in specialized centers. This is preferable to duodenotomy and sphincteroplasty, in our opinion, because currently few surgeons have experience in this procedure.

After choledochoscopy is completed, a T-tube is sewn into place (Fig. 5). A 14-F (4.7 mm) or larger tube should be used.

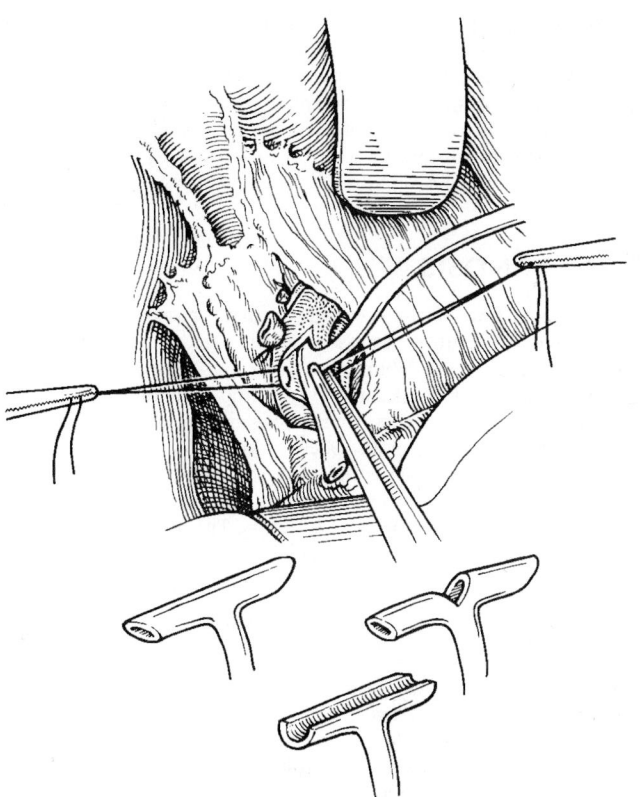

Figure 5 A T-tube is inserted in the common bile duct, and the choledochotomy incision is closed over it with fine Vicryl sutures. *From Zollinger RM Jr, Zollinger RM: Atlas of surgical operations, ed 7, New York, 1993, McGraw-Hill.*

Stones may be extracted through tube tracks of this size in the postoperative period if they are discovered on postoperative T-tube cholangiography. The limbs of the tube should be approximately 1 cm in length. A long limb passing into the duodenum may cause pancreatitis. Fashioning a small opening in the cross-limb just opposite to the union with the long limb allows the tube to bend for easier insertion and later extraction. The tube should fit loosely in the duct; if it is snug, it should be replaced with a smaller-sized tube. The tube should be moved down the duct so that the choledochotomy is sutured from above downward. This prevents the tube from pulling on the suture line when it is extracted. The duct is closed with fine absorbable suture (e.g., 3–0 chromic), taking bites 1 to 2 mm in depth and approximately 2 mm apart using running or interrupted technique. The last bites are alongside the exiting long limb of the T-tube to obtain a watertight seal. The T-tube is flushed with saline. We do this by inserting a 5-F infant feeding tube down the T-tube because this seems to best rid the tube and duct of air bubbles. A cholangiogram is obtained. Often dye will not enter the duodenum after the sphincter of Oddi has been instrumented. This should not be considered a reason for reexploration if the choledochoscopy has been adequate.

SUGGESTED READINGS

Fitzgibbons RJ, Gardner GC: Laparoscopic surgery and the common bile duct, *World J Surg* 25:1317, 2001.
Hungness ES, Soper NJ: Management of common bile duct stones, *J Gastrointest Surg* 10:612, 2006.
Lyass S, Phillips EH: Laparoscopic transcystic common bile duct exploration, *Surg Endosc* 20:S441, 2006.
Rhoads M, Sussman L: Randomized trial of laparoscopic exploration of common bile duct versus postoperative endoscopic retrograde cholangiography for common bile duct stones, *Lancet* 351:159, 1998.
Riciardi R, Islam S, Canete JJ, and others: Effectiveness and long-term results of laparoscopic common bile duct exploration, *Surg Endosc* 17:19, 2002.
Thompson MH, Tranter SE: All-comers policy for laparoscopic exploration of the common bile duct, *Br J Surg* 89:1608, 2002.

ACUTE CHOLANGITIS

**Siong-Seng Liau, MBChB Ed, MRCS Ed, and
Edward E. Whang, MD**

Acute cholangitis is an infectious syndrome affecting the biliary tract, for which biliary stasis and obstruction are prominent risk factors. The spectrum of clinical severity can range from mild to potentially life-threatening disease accompanied by septic shock and multiorgan dysfunction. Because of the propensity for rapid deterioration among patients with untreated acute cholangitis, expeditious diagnosis and therapy are essential.

EPIDEMIOLOGY AND RISK FACTORS

The median age of patients diagnosed with acute cholangitis is reported to range from 50 to 60 years, and incidence increases with age. The most important risk factors are biliary stasis or obstruction for which the most prevalent etiology is choledocholithiasis. In much of the world, secondary choledocholithiasis (caused by stones originating in the gallbladder) predominates; in Southeast Asia, however, where Oriental cholangiohepatitis is endemic, primary choledocholithiasis is an important cause of cholangitis. Other benign and malignant etiologies of biliary obstruction are listed in Table 1 and are discussed in greater detail elsewhere in this textbook.

An increasingly prevalent risk factor is iatrogenic biliary tract manipulation (Table 1), which in some centers, particularly those with active liver transplantation programs, is associated with up to 50% of cases of acute cholangitis. Specific risk factors in this context include endoscopic and percutaneous instrumentation of the biliary tract, indwelling biliary stents, anastomotic (biliobiliary or bilioenteric) strictures, and ischemic strictures of the biliary tract.

PATHOGENESIS

Mechanisms postulated to help maintain the normal sterility of the biliary tract include (1) an intact sphincter of Oddi that prevents reflux of duodenal contents into the common bile duct, (2) unimpeded efflux of bile from the common bile duct, (3) the presence of

Table 1: Etiologies of Acute Cholangitis

Noniatrogenic

Benign conditions
  Choledocholithiasis
    Primary
    Secondary
  Pancreatitis (chronic/acute), including pancreatic pseudocyst
  Papillary stenosis
  Mirizzi's syndrome
  Choledochal cysts (type V, Caroli's disease)
  Primary sclerosing cholangitis
Malignancies
  Pancreatic cancer
  Cholangiocarcinoma
  Porta hepatis tumor/metastasis

Iatrogenic

Obstructed biliary endoprosthesis
Iatrogenic biliary stricture
  Direct surgical trauma
  Ischemia-induced stricture
Anastomotic stricture (biliobiliary/bilioenteric anastomosis)

immunoglobulin A (IgA) in bile, and (4) the bacteriostatic properties of bile salts. When one or more of these defenses is breached or if a foreign body is present in the biliary tract where it can serve as a nidus for infection, cholangitis may ensue.

Most cases are thought to arise from direct ascent of bacteria from the duodenum into the common bile duct; hematogenous seeding of the biliary tract is likely to play only a minor role. Bacterial proliferation within the biliary tract, together with its entry into the systemic circulation via lymphatic and venous channels, results in the infectious manifestations of acute cholangitis. Increased pressure within the biliary tract, as occurs with biliary obstruction, promotes these processes.

Cultures of bile, intraductal stones, or indwelling stents from patients with acute cholangitis indicate a polymicrobial infection in most patients, with bowel flora being the most common isolates. The most commonly identified gram-negative bacteria are *Escherichia coli* (25% to 50% of cases), *Klebsiella* species (15% to 20% of cases), and *Enterobacter* species (5% to 10% of cases). The most commonly isolated gram-positive bacteria are *Enterococcus* species (10% to 20% of cases). The contribution of anaerobes such as *Bacteroides* and *Clostridium* species to the pathogenesis of acute cholangitis is controversial; however, they are not uncommonly cultured in specimens obtained from elderly patients and those who have undergone biliary tract instrumentation.

Although bacteria are responsible for the great majority of cases of acute cholangitis, other pathogens, such as helminths, fungi, and viruses (e.g., cytomegalovirus and Epstein-Barr virus) can cause this syndrome. These organisms should be considered in the appropriate clinical setting (e.g., in areas where parasitic infections are endemic and among immunocompromised individuals).

CLINICAL PRESENTATION

In 1877, Jean Charcot described the hallmarks of acute cholangitis: fever, jaundice, and right upper quadrant abdominal pain. Note that all three features of this eponymous triad are present in only

50% to 75% of patients with acute cholangitis. Fever is the most common symptom (present in 90% of cases), with jaundice and abdominal pain being less prevalent (present in 60% and 70% of cases, respectively). Reynold's pentad (described by Reynold and Dargon in 1959) denotes the presence of mental status derangements and hypotension, in addition to features of Charcot's triad, and is suggestive of severe disease and systemic sepsis.

DIAGNOSIS

Acute cholangitis is a clinical diagnosis that is based on the presence of the clinical features discussed earlier, together with supportive findings revealed by laboratory tests and radiographic studies. Because acute cholangitis can present without abdominal pain, particularly in elderly patients, absence of pain (or any of the individual symptoms and signs discussed earlier) does not rule out this diagnosis. Acute cholangitis therefore should also be considered in patients presenting with sepsis but without abdominal pain or tenderness who have appropriate risk factors. The differential diagnosis includes other conditions associated with right upper quadrant abdominal pain, jaundice, or fever, including cholecystitis, liver abscesses, and hepatitis.

Laboratory test findings typically associated with acute cholangitis include leukocytosis with neutrophilia and liver function test abnormalities suggestive of cholestasis (e.g., increased serum alkaline phosphatase, gamma-glutamyl transpeptidase, and conjugated bilirubin concentrations). Increased serum aminotransferase concentrations can occur with acute liver injury resulting from cholangitis-induced hepatic microabscess formation. Serum amylase concentration is elevated in up to 30% of patients with acute cholangitis. Blood cultures should be performed in all patients suspected of having cholangitis. In addition, cultures of bile aspirated from percutaneous biliary catheters or obtained during endoscopic retrograde cholangiopancreatography (ERCP) and of any indwelling biliary prostheses that are removed should be obtained. Although treatment should be initiated before culture results become available, they can be used in directing specific antibiotic therapy.

Imaging studies have the following roles in patients with suspected acute cholangitis: (1) they can confirm the presence of dilated bile ducts (a finding present in most cases of acute cholangitis), (2) they may reveal the specific etiology responsible for biliary obstruction (e.g., choledocholithiasis), (3) they can exclude other conditions in the differential diagnosis (e.g., acute cholecystitis), and (4) they can be used to guide therapeutic interventions (e.g., biliary drainage or removal of an obstructed biliary stent).

Transabdominal ultrasonography is the best initial imaging study in most patients with suspected acute cholangitis. It is noninvasive, rapid, cost-effective, and highly sensitive in the detection of biliary tract dilation. However, note that the absence of biliary tract dilation does not rule out acute cholangitis, especially if the ultrasound is obtained soon after acute onset of biliary obstruction, before the bile ducts have had time to dilate. Remember also that transabdominal ultrasonography is associated with relatively low sensitivity in the detection of choledocholithiasis.

In most patients with acute cholangitis, ultrasonography should be followed by endoscopic ERCP because it allows for both direct cholangiography and therapeutic intervention. Unavailability or failure of ERCP should prompt percutaneous transhepatic cholangiography (PTC). Patients with indwelling biliary catheters (e.g., T-tubes or U-tubes) can undergo cholangiography with contrast instilled into these tubes, if they are externally accessible. The therapeutic roles of ERCP and PTC are discussed subsequently.

Computed tomography (CT) scanning can reveal biliary tract dilatation and allows for global assessment intra-abdominal pathology, but it has poor sensitivity in the detection of intraductal stones. Magnetic resonance cholangiopancreatography (MRCP) has greater sensitivity for choledocholithiasis than CT scanning but is less widely available, and the prolonged duration of MRCP examinations limits their application in unstable patients. Endoscopic ultrasonography (EUS) is another imaging option with good sensitivity for choledocholithiasis. Because CT, MRCP, and EUS do not offer therapeutic capability, ERCP should not be delayed to obtain these imaging studies unless diagnostic uncertainty or relative contraindications to ERCP exist.

THERAPY

Therapy for acute cholangitis consists of three main components: (1) resuscitation, (2) antibiotics, and (3) biliary drainage (Fig. 1).

Resuscitation with administration of intravenous fluids and correction of electrolyte abnormalities should be initiated without delay. Given that urgent interventional or surgical procedures are likely to be required, attention should be directed to identifying and correcting coagulopathies that may exist (e.g., those resulting from vitamin K deficiency or sepsis-induced thrombocytopenia). Vigilant monitoring to ensure adequacy of resuscitation and early recognition of clinical deterioration (e.g., shock or mental status abnormalities) is essential. High-risk patients with significant comorbidities are best monitored in a dedicated intensive care unit, where invasive monitoring and inotropic support can be instituted.

Empiric broad-spectrum antibiotic administration should commence when the diagnosis of acute cholangitis is considered. Empiric therapy should be effective against both gram-negative and gram-positive bacteria (especially *Enterococcus*) and ideally should include antibiotics capable of achieving high concentrations within bile, even in the presence of biliary obstruction.

Our first-line regimen for the empiric therapy of acute cholangitis is the combination of a fluoroquinolone (e.g., levofloxacin) with metronidazole. We use metronidazole in this setting despite the low frequency with which anaerobes are isolated from bile cultures because (1) standard culture techniques underestimate the true prevalence of anaerobic infections, (2) anaerobes are prevalent in cultures of bile obtained from some patient groups (e.g., those with prior biliary instrumentation), and (3) metronidazole has a favorable safety profile.

Other antibiotics appropriate for empiric therapy include the combination of ampicillin and gentamicin, carbapenems (e.g., imipenem and meropenem), extended-spectrum penicillins (e.g., piperacillin), and penicillin/beta-lactamase inhibitor combinations (e.g., piperacillin-tazobactam, ampicillin-sulbactam, ticarcillin-clavulanate). Given the substantial risk of aminoglycoside-induced nephrotoxicity, we prefer to avoid gentamicin-based regimens unless specific reasons for their administration exist. Second- and third-generation cephalosporins, although providing excellent activity against gram-negative bacteria, provide poor coverage against *Enterococcus* species and are therefore not recommended.

With resuscitation and empiric antibiotic therapy, up to 85% of patients with acute cholangitis improve, even in the absence of interventional therapy. When culture results become available, antibiotics should be tailored to sensitivity findings. The duration of antibiotic therapy should be based on clinical response; for patients documented to have bacteremia, antibiotic courses lasting 1 to 2 weeks are recommended.

Patients who improve with resuscitation and antibiotics alone should undergo elective biliary drainage. However, the 15% to 20% of patients who fail to respond within 12 to 24 hours after initiation of conservative therapy should undergo emergent biliary decompression. Specific indications for emergent biliary drainage include persistent abdominal pain or hypotension, high fevers (>39°C), and mental status derangements.

In most cases, ERCP is the first-line modality for establishing biliary drainage, with PTC reserved for patients in whom ERCP fails or is unavailable. Patients with external biliary drains should have these drains placed to gravity drainage as soon as the diagnosis

of acute cholangitis is considered. Emergent surgical biliary decompression for acute cholangitis is largely of historical interest only; because of high associated mortality rates, its application should be limited to those rare cases in which neither ERCP nor PTC can be accomplished.

ERCP is effective in establishing biliary drainage in 90% to 98% of cases. In procedures performed for acute cholangitis, bile should be aspirated from the common bile duct to decompress it before injection of contrast for cholangiography. Occlusive cholangiography performed before ductal decompression, particularly in cases of suppurative cholangitis, can induce bacteremia, sepsis, and rapid decompensation. For patients in whom endoscopic sphincterotomy is contraindicated, such as those with persistent coagulopathy, temporizing biliary drainage can be achieved by placement of a nasobiliary drain or an internal biliary stent without sphincterotomy. More definitive therapy (e.g., endoscopic sphincterotomy and removal of intraductal stones followed by cholecystectomy) can then be accomplished electively, after these patients have stabilized. Other therapeutic applications facilitated by ERCP in patients with acute cholangitis include replacement of obstructed biliary stents and stenting or dilatation (or both) of benign biliary strictures.

If ERCP fails in establishing biliary drainage or if it is unavailable or contraindicated, then PTC with placement of an external biliary drain should be performed. PTC is reported to be successful in establishing biliary drainage in 90% of patients with biliary

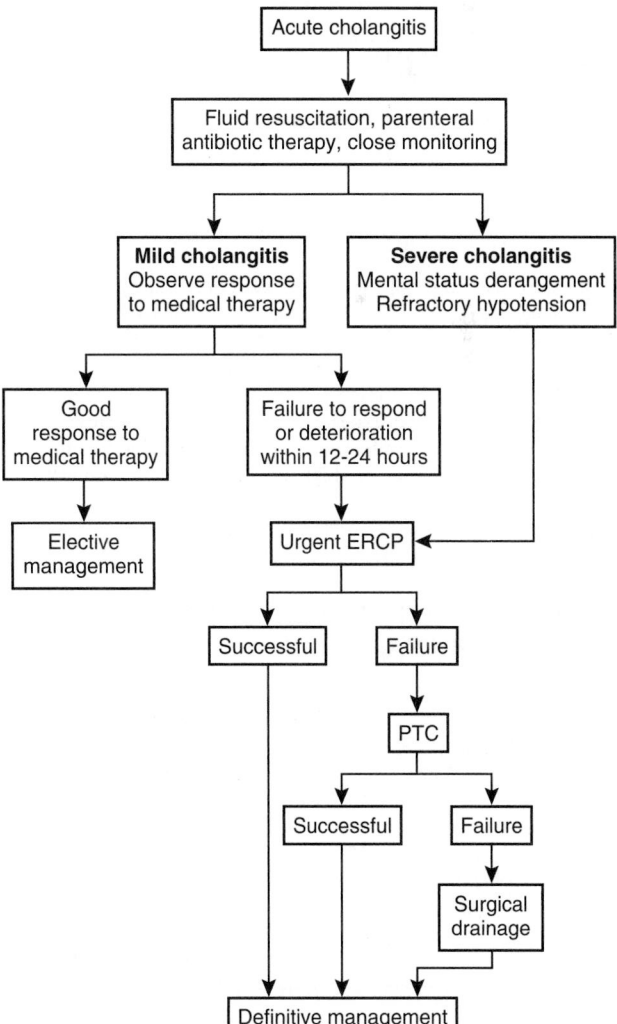

Figure 1 Clinical algorithm for management of patients with acute cholangitis.

obstruction; however, it is associated with high morbidity rates (up to 80% in some series). Serious complications of PTC include intraperitoneal hemorrhage, hemobilia, and bile peritonitis. Specific circumstances in which PTC may be required include intrahepatic biliary obstruction resulting from hepatolithiasis, proximal biliary obstruction caused by a hilar cholangiocarcinoma, and a papilla that is not endoscopically accessible (e.g., patients with a periampullary diverticulum or who have undergone an operation involving Roux-en-Y reconstruction). Percutaneous cholecystostomy is a technically easier alternative to PTC; however, the efficacy of this procedure in acute cholangitis is dependent on cystic duct patency, and the obstructing lesion must be located distal to the cystic duct–common duct junction.

Because of the high efficacy rates associated with ERCP and PTC, surgical biliary decompression in the acute setting should be applied only if these nonoperative procedures fail to achieve biliary drainage or are unavailable. Historical series suggest that emergency surgery in unstable patients with acute cholangitis is associated with perioperative mortality rates as high as 40%. If surgery is required, it should be limited to choledochotomy and biliary decompression with placement of a large-diameter (at least 16 F) T-tube. More extensive procedures such as formal common bile duct exploration, transduodenal sphincteroplasty, and biliary-enteric bypass are inappropriate in unstable patients.

Following biliary decompression and resolution of sepsis, patients should undergo definitive therapy, if indicated, on an elective basis. In this context, surgery plays an important role in the definitive management of conditions such as choledocholithiasis/cholelithiasis and benign and malignant biliary strictures. These procedures are discussed in further detail elsewhere in this textbook.

Suggested Readings

Lai EC, Tam PC, Paterson IA, and others: Emergency surgery for severe acute cholangitis. The high-risk patients, *Ann Surg* 211:55, 1990.
Millonig G, Buratti T, Graziadei ID, and others: Bactobilia after liver transplantation: frequency and antibiotic susceptibility, *Liver Transpl* 12:747, 2006.
Poon RT, Liu CL, Lo CM, and others: Management of gallstone cholangitis in the era of laparoscopic cholecystectomy, *Arch Surg* 136:11, 2001.

BENIGN BILIARY STRICTURES

**Marshall S. Baker, MD, MBA, and
Keith D. Lillemoe, MD**

Benign strictures of the biliary system are among the most challenging clinical problems faced by the general surgeon. Mismanagement of these entities frequently ends in potentially life-threatening complications, including cholangitis, cirrhosis, and portal hypertension. In contrast, appropriate technique and timing of intervention at centers experienced in hepatobiliary surgery have been shown to yield excellent and durable functional results. This chapter briefly reviews the etiology and classification of biliary injuries and strictures and describes an approach to the effective diagnosis and management of the most common strictures.

IATROGENIC BILE DUCT INJURY AND STRICTURE

Benign strictures are the end result of either inflammatory processes such as pancreatitis, biliary calculi and infection, or traumatic injury. Currently, the most common cause of bile duct strictures is iatrogenic biliary injury occurring during laparoscopic cholecystectomy. Multiple early reviews of large Medicare and private databases have demonstrated that the ascension of laparoscopic cholecystectomy during the decade of the 1990s was associated with a threefold to tenfold increase in the incidence of bile duct injury relative to that seen in the era of open cholecystectomy. Although the most recent comprehensive reviews of the National Inpatient Sample database suggests a late decrease in the rate at which operative repairs are required to manage biliary injury, the absolute number of bile duct injuries remains high despite improved clinical training, an increase in our collective laparoscopic experience, and heightened awareness.

The impact of biliary injuries is substantial. A retrospective review of the Medicare National Claims database demonstrated a statistical increase in long-term mortality for Medicare recipients suffering biliary injury following laparoscopic cholecystectomy compared with those without injury following laparoscopic cholecystectomy (adjusted hazard ratio of 2.8 at 3 years postoperative). Similarly, smaller prospective single-institution studies have demonstrated a substantial effect on the quality of life of patients suffering biliary injury and estimated the financial cost for the management of patients with biliary injury to be in excess of $50,000 per event.

Mechanisms of Bile Duct Injury

Iatrogenic injury during laparoscopic cholecystectomy is usually the result of a misidentification of the biliary anatomy by the operating surgeon. In the classic laparoscopic injury, excessive cephalad retraction of the gallbladder fundus or insufficient lateral retraction on the infundibulum aligns the cystic duct and the common bile duct. The common bile duct is then mistakenly perceived to be the cystic duct and is clipped and divided (Fig. 1). Technical issues—including the use of an end-viewing laparoscope that distorts the perspective of the operator, the excessive use of thermal cautery, and the tenting of the common bile duct by excessive lateral retraction on the infundibulum—and local environmental factors—including inflammation in the triangle of Calot (as during acute cholecystitis) and aberrant biliary anatomy (isolated right segmental hepatic duct arising from the common bile duct)—have also been implicated as factors conferring risk of biliary injury during laparoscopic cholecystectomy.

Preventing Iatrogenic Injury

Injury avoidance is always clearly preferable to managing a complication postoperatively. Much has been written about strategies to avoid biliary injuries during laparoscopic cholecystectomy. In the mid-1990s, Soper and Strasberg introduced the concept of the "critical view of safety" whereby the fundus of the gallbladder is retracted superiorly, the infundibulum is retracted laterally, and careful effort is made essentially to clear the triangle of Calot of all fat and fibrous tissue. This technique effectively lays bare the triangle and leaves only two potential structures connected to the lower end of the gallbladder: the cystic artery and cystic duct. Both

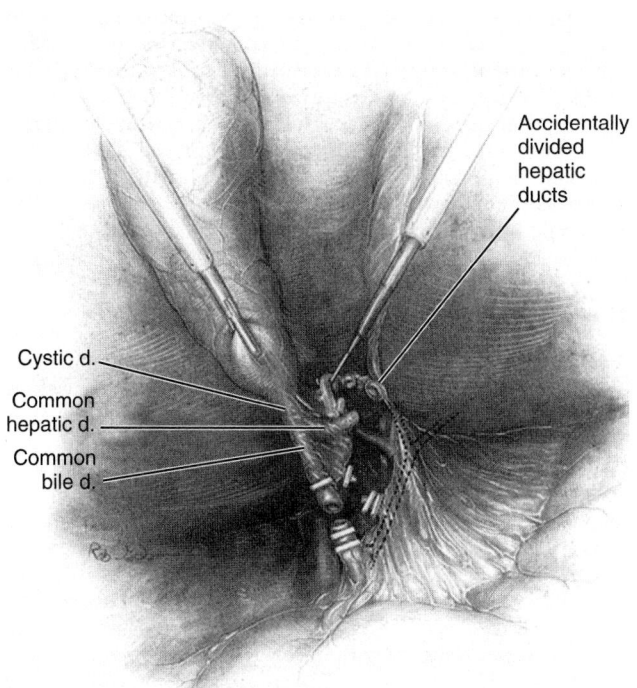

Figure 1 Classic injury during laparoscopic cholecystectomy. The common bile duct is mistaken for the cystic duct, and a length of the common duct is excised. *From Branum G, Schmitt C, Baillie J, and others: Ann Surg 217:532, 1993.*

of these may then be safely ligated. Most authors now identify this effort to dissect meticulously the triangle of Calot as the single most effective means of preventing iatrogenic biliary injury. Intraoperative cholangiography has also been identified as a strategy for avoiding biliary injury during laparoscopic cholecystectomy and has been extensively studied both retrospectively and prospectively. One recent large retrospective review of the Medicare database, adjusted for patient comorbidity and physician experience with cholangiography, found a 1.7-fold relative decrease in the rate of biliary injury when intraoperative cholangiography was used during laparoscopic cholecystectomy. However, results of the evaluation of cholangiography as an instrument of prevention are generally mixed, with some studies suggesting improved rates of injury, others demonstrating a lesser degree of injury, and others demonstrating no difference in either rates or degree of biliary injury when routine or elective cholangiography is compared with not using intraoperative cholangiography.

Classification of Injury

A number of classification schemes for benign biliary strictures have been described. The most widely used was developed in the era of the open cholecystectomy by Bismuth and defined the type of stricture based on the anatomic location with respect to the hepatic bifurcation. Strasberg and Soper subsequently modified the original Bismuth classification, attempting to better characterize patterns of injury seen following laparoscopic cholecystectomy (Fig. 2).

Clinical Presentation

Large series reviews have demonstrated that less than one third of iatrogenic injuries are detected at the time of the cholecystectomy.

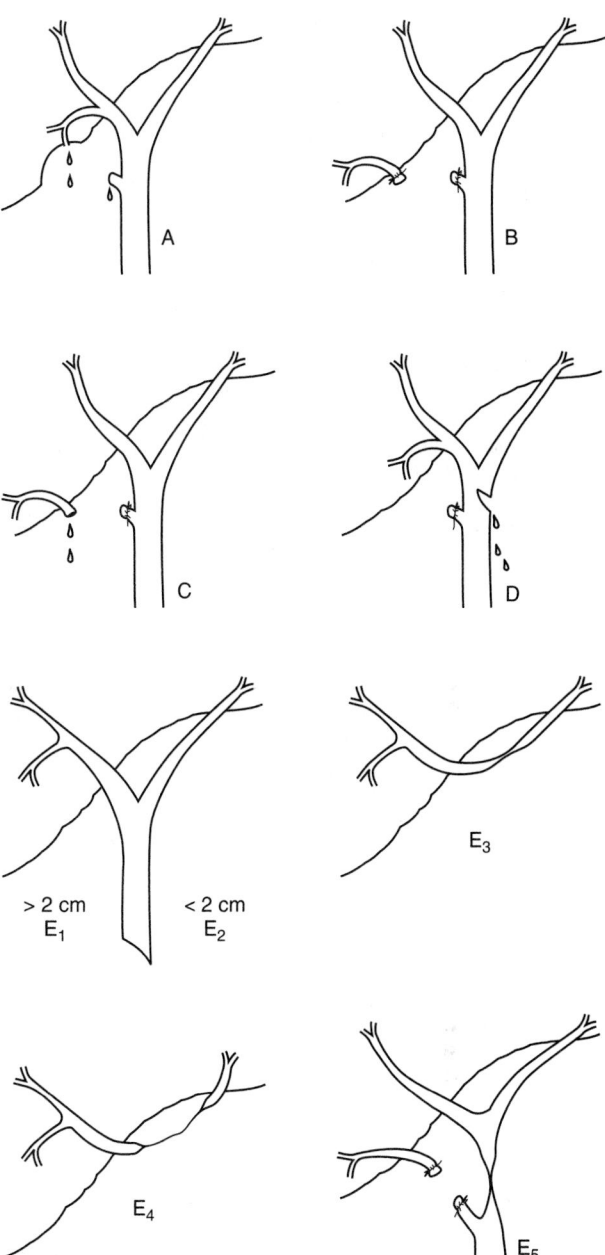

Figure 2 Strasberg-Soper classification of laparoscopic injuries to the biliary system. Type A injuries are leaks from the cystic duct or ducts at the hepatic resection bed (ducts of Luschka). Types B and C involve injuries to aberrant right hepatic ducts. Type E injuries are chronic strictures resulting from occult laparoscopic biliary injuries and are subclassified in a way similar to the original Bismuth scheme for benign biliary stricture.

Keys to intraoperative recognition of the injury include the finding of a persistent leak of bile from the liver or the soft tissue adjacent to the portahepatis or the finding of a "second" ductal structure during the completion of the cholecystectomy. The majority of bile duct injuries are detected postoperatively. Most commonly, the hepatic duct has been transected and incompletely clipped, resulting in bile leakage into the peritoneal cavity. Patients then present with increasing abdominal pain, distention, nausea, and emesis. Patients in whom the bile duct has been completely clipped present with pain and obstructive jaundice or, less commonly, pain and fever indicative of cholangitis. Such an atypical course from the routine recovery for a laparoscopic cholecystectomy should always prompt an evaluation for possible biliary injury.

Repair of the Immediately Recognized Injury

For cases in which an injury is recognized at the time of the cholecystectomy, prompt cholangiography is imperative. Intraoperative cholangiography confirms and better defines the injury, and the results of the cholangiogram will dictate further surgical management. If a segmental or accessory duct less than 3 mm in diameter has been injured and cholangiography demonstrates a segmental or subsegmental drainage by the injured ductal system, simple ligation of the injured duct will be adequate treatment. If the injured duct is 4 mm in diameter or greater or the cholangiogram demonstrates sectoral or lobar drainage, the injured duct is likely to have drained multiple hepatic segments or the entire right hepatic lobe. These injuries warrant operative repair, and laparotomy is indicated. The nature of that repair is dictated by the length of separation between opposed residual and viable ends of the injured duct. If the injured segment of the bile duct is short (<1 cm) and the two viable ends can be opposed without tension, an end-to-end anastomosis may be performed. A generous Kocher maneuver effectively mobilizes the duodenum out of the retroperitoneum and should be used to alleviate tension at the repair. For proximal injuries near the hepatic duct bifurcation or if the injured segment of the bile duct is longer than 1 cm, an end-to-end primary biliary anastomosis results in excessive tension and should be avoided. Under these circumstances, the distal bile duct should be oversewn and the proximal bile duct should be debrided of injured tissue and anastomosed to a Roux-en-Y jejunal limb in an end-to-side fashion.

A major objective of any reconstruction is the prevention of continued bile leak, which can be an ongoing source of infection and further morbidity. To this end, we recommend external transanastomotic biliary drainage for all immediate repairs. In the case of a primary end-to-end repair, this drainage may take the form of a T-tube placed through a separate choledochotomy above or below the anastomosis. In the case of the end-to-side Roux reconstruction, a transhepatic stent should be placed. In both cases, a closed suction drain is also placed behind the completed anastomosis so that any potential postoperative leak is well controlled.

Initial Management Following Delayed Recognition in the Postoperative Period

The initial management of a patient who presents in a delayed fashion following an injury during laparoscopic cholecystectomy depends on the nature of the injury and the mode and timing of presentation. In patients presenting early following cholecystectomy, the most common mode of presentation is a bile leak. In this situation, the result of reconstruction is almost always better if the definitive repair is made well after the leak and consequent intraabdominal inflammation and sepsis are controlled with percutaneous biliary drainage. If early laparotomy is performed in such cases, in the face of continued uncontrolled bile leak, the marked inflammation obscures the field and makes identification of the decompressed biliary system difficult, especially in the hands of the inexperienced biliary surgeon. Biliary reconstruction under these circumstances is technically difficult and frequently ends in long-term failure in the form of recurrent leak or biliary stricture. To avoid this, every attempt should be made to define the biliary anatomy using percutaneous cholangiography and to drain and control the bile leak with percutaneous biliary stents and percutaneous drains. The repair is ideally made 6 to 8 weeks after adequate control of the leak has been attained.

In patients who present with biliary stricture weeks to months after cholecystectomy, cholangiography is again essential to define the exact anatomy of the biliary system and the location of the stricture and to allow planning of the definitive repair. In patients with a stricture and symptoms of cholangitis, biliary decompression should be performed and is usually best accomplished with transhepatic percutaneous catheter placement. Parenteral antibiotics should be tailored to biliary cultures and continued until sepsis is controlled. In patients without evidence of cholangitis, preoperative biliary decompression has no demonstrable impact on outcome and should be avoided.

Definitive Management of Bile Duct Stricture

The method of choice for treating a bile duct transection or stricture continues to be the subject of some debate. There have been many recent advances in endoscopic and interventional techniques and in the accessibility of these technologies. Multiple interventional approaches are now readily available for patients who have biliary-enteric continuity, including transhepatic dilatation and stenting, as well as endoscopic balloon dilatation with and without stenting. The best results of nonoperative management are those achieved through endoscopic techniques. Several reports demonstrate successful alleviation of stricture in all treated patients with no evidence of recurrence at follow-up of almost 4 years. These series use aggressive stenting protocols requiring multiple repeated dilatations and stent changes. The average patient requires four stent placements and is treated for 12 months before there is complete resolution of clinical symptoms and radiologic evidence of the stricture. Unfortunately, in the era of laparoscopic cholecystectomy, most biliary injuries involve a complete transection of the bile duct or a complex stenosis that is not amenable to precutaneous or endoscopic therapy.

The goal of operative management of a bile duct stricture is the establishment of bile flow into the proximal gastrointestinal tract in a manner that prevents sludge, stone formation, cholangitis, restricture, and cirrhosis. A number of alternative strategies are available for surgical repair. Invariably there is loss of bile duct length as a result of fibrosis associated with the injury, and simple excision of a bile duct stricture with end-to-end ductal anastomosis or repair is rarely technically feasible. Typically some version of a biliary-enteric anastomosis is required. Several principles generally guide successful biliary-enteric reconstruction: (1) exposure of healthy proximal bile duct that provides drainage of the entire liver, (2) preparation of a suitable section of intestine that can be brought to the area of the stricture without tension, and (3) creation of a biliary-enteric anastomosis that approximates biliary to enteric mucosa. In almost all cases, these principles mandate that a hepaticojejunostomy constructed to a Roux-en-Y limb of jejunum be used.

The exact details of the reconstruction thus vary depending on the particular anatomic features of the stricture. For strictures in which there is a length of greater than 2 cm of healthy common hepatic duct preserved (Bismuth I), a simple end-to-side biliary-enteric anastomosis will suffice. For strictures in which a length of less than 2 cm of healthy hepatic duct is preserved (Bismuth II) or that involve the bifurcation of the hepatic duct but in which the right and left duct communicate (Bismuth III), it may be necessary to lower the hilar plate and extend the dochotomy along a short length of the right or left hepatic duct to allow a common biliary-enteric anastomosis. Strictures that completely separate the right and left systems (Bismuth IV and V) require separate right and left biliary-enteric anastomoses. In rare instances, suitable duct length outside the hepatic parenchyma cannot be obtained. These cases necessitate isolation of the intrahepatic biliary system. Intraoperative ultrasound is essential in these efforts. The segment II duct can be located and isolated as it courses superficially on the inferior posterior surface of segment II. The parenchyma is incised over the duct, and the duct is opened along its length for 2 cm. A side-to-side biliary-enteric anastomosis to a Roux limb is then created. Similarly, the segment 3 duct can be isolated on the medial anterior surface of segment 3 just lateral to the insertion of the falciform ligament. This duct is usually located deep within the liver parenchyma, and a wedge of liver parenchyma must be removed to complete the exposure of the duct.

The use of transanastomotic biliary stents is believed by many to be important in obtaining good long-term results following biliary-enteric reconstruction for biliary strictures. In most cases, the stents are placed preoperatively by interventional radiology to control the bile leak or cholangitis. At the time of exploration for definitive repair, the stents can facilitate the identification and dissection of the proximal biliary tree. The interventional stents are replaced at the time of the surgical repair with larger, soft silastic stents that serve to control bile flow in the event of an anastomotic leak and provide access for cholangiography and that may prevent stenosis reformation.

In the operative technique for biliary reconstruction with transanastomotic stents, the bile duct proximal to the injury is carefully dissected circumferentially in a cephalad direction for a distance not to exceed 5 mm. Excessive dissection should be avoided to prevent vascular compromise to this segment of the duct. The duct is opened, and the preoperative biliary catheter(s) identified. A radiologic guidewire is placed into these catheters. A series of progressively larger Coude catheters may then be passed over the guidewires to dilatate the biliary system, and appropriate large, soft silastic stents are then placed over the guidewires. The stents are 12 to 22 F in size and have multiple sideholes present along 40% of their length (Fig. 3). The sideholes are left to reside within the intrahepatic biliary tree and the portion of the Roux-en-Y jejunal limb used for the biliary anastomosis. The end of the stent without the sideholes exits through the hepatic parenchyma and is brought out through a stab wound in the upper anterior abdominal wall. After the stents have been placed, a Roux-en-Y limb is prepared and the anastomosis completed as an end-to-side hepaticojejunostomy. The anastomosis is usually achieved with interrupted 4–0 or 5–0 absorbable suture. Closed suction drains are placed behind the anastomosis. Postoperatively, the silastic stents are left to gravity drainage for 3 to 4 days. A postoperative cholangiogram is then performed, and, if that study is satisfactory, the stents are internalized and the diet advanced (Fig. 4). The length of time that the stents are left in place is variable and determined by the nature of the injury, the patient's clinical course, and follow-up cholangiography.

Long-Term Results of Surgical Reconstruction

The perioperative outcomes of surgical repair for biliary injuries following laparoscopic surgery were recently reported for a series of 200 patients undergoing management at the Johns Hopkins Hospital. In that series, the rate of perioperative complications was 43%. The most common complications were wound infections (8%), cholangitis (5.7%), and intra-abdominal abscess (2.9%). The postoperative mortality rate was 1.7%. Early postoperative cholangiography revealed an anastomotic leak in 4.6% and extravasation at the liver dome-stent site in 10.3% of patients. None of the patients required reexploration postoperatively. Postoperative radiologic intervention, including percutaneous abscess drainage, was required in nine patients (5.1%), and stent replacement was required in four patients (2.3%).

Several series have described excellent long-term results in patients who have undergone repair of established stricture during the era of open cholecystectomy, with long-term patency rates at

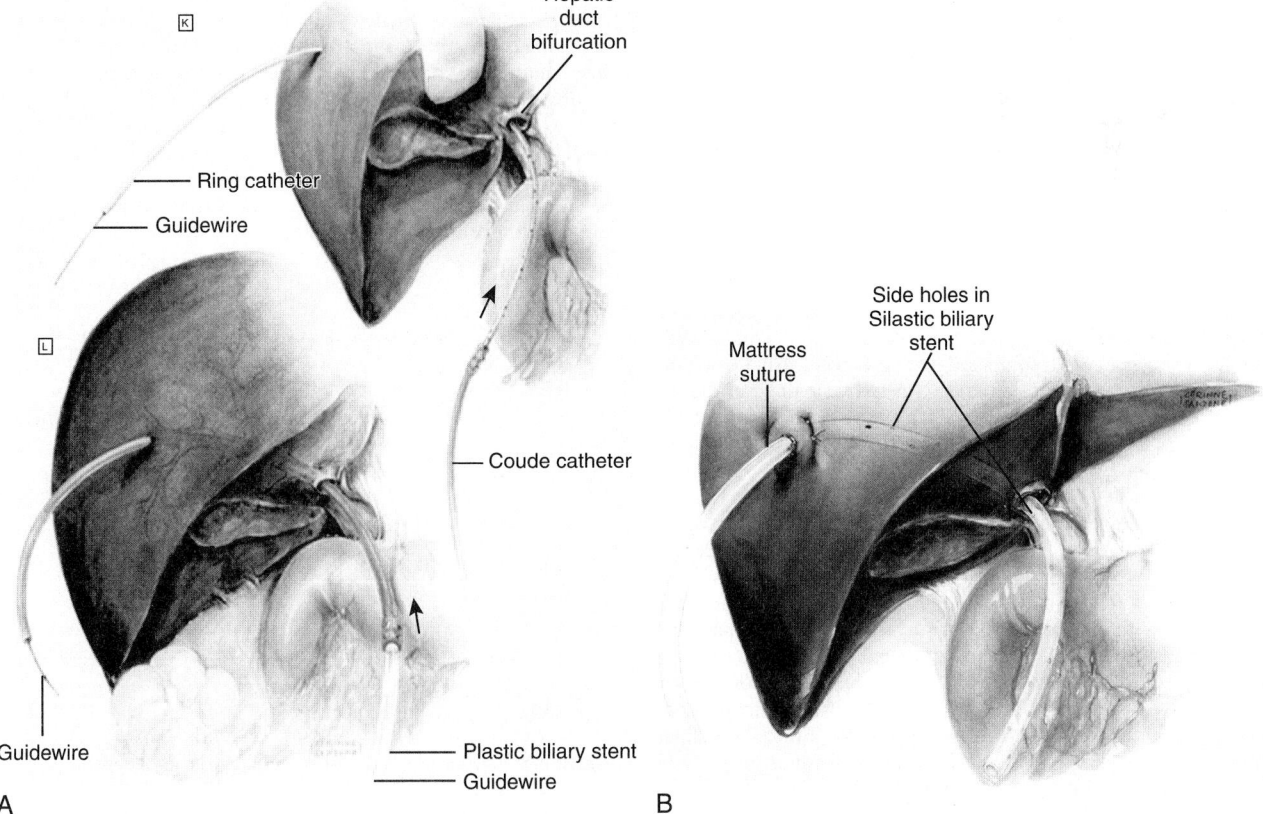

Figure 3 Preoperatively placed biliary stents are exchanged for soft silastic catheters that exit through the surface of the liver and the transected hepatic ducts. A surgical anastomosis is then constructed between the transected hepatic duct and a Roux Limb of the jejunum around the silastic stent.

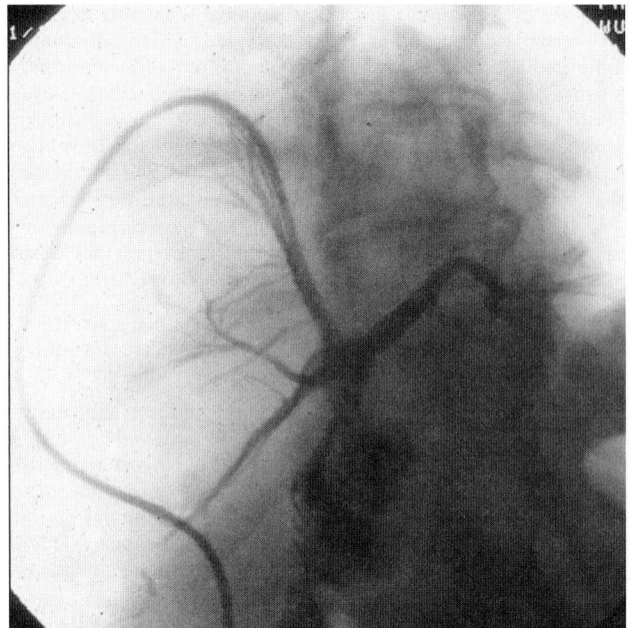

Figure 4 Postoperative cholangiogram demonstrating position of the transhepatic biliary stent in the right biliary system with free flow of contrast into the Roux limb and the left biliary system with no evidence of contrast extravasation.

70% to 90%. A number of smaller retrospective studies were reported in the 1990s with excellent short-term results following surgical reconstruction for iatrogenic biliary injury following laparoscopic cholecystectomy. The long-term results of reconstruction for these injuries remained to be determined, however, and multiple authors raised the question of whether the results after reconstruction in the era of open cholecystectomy can be translated to reconstructions following laparoscopic injury. These authors cite the complex nature of many of the injuries and the frequent association with significant inflammation and fibrosis secondary to sustained, unrecognized bile leak as potential variables that might confound the long-term success of the surgical reconstruction.

Stewart and Way have attempted to better delineate variables associated with successful reconstruction following biliary injuries during the era of laparoscopic cholecystectomy. In their report of the records of 85 patients who underwent 112 such biliary repairs, 64 repairs performed by the primary surgeon or a surgeon of comparable experience were compared with 46 reconstructions performed by biliary surgeons at tertiary referral centers. Four factors were found to determine the success or failure of the treatment in this series: (1) the performance of preoperative cholangiography, (2) the choice of repair, (3) the details of the operative repair, and (4) the experience of the surgeon performing the repair. Ninety-six percent of the procedures in which cholangiograms were not obtained before surgery were unsuccessful. Sixty-nine percent of the procedures for which cholangiographic data were incomplete were not successful. In contrast, when the cholangiographic data were complete, the initial repair was successful in 84% of patients. With regard to the type of repair performed: hepaticojejunostomy was more commonly associated with acceptable outcome than primary end-to-end repair. For each case in which a primary end-to-end repair was used to reconstruct a transected duct, the repair failed. In contrast, 63% of Roux-en-Y hepaticojejunostomies were successful. With regard to surgeon experience, initial repair by the original laparoscopic surgeon was successful in only 17% of patients, and in no case was a second or third repair by the primary surgeon successful. In contrast, patients whose first repair was by a biliary surgeon demonstrated a 94% success rate.

The largest prospective series examining outcome following surgery for stricture following laparoscopic cholecystectomy is a report of Lillemoe's experience at the Johns Hopkins Hospital during the decade of the 1990s. In that experience, a total of 156 patients underwent surgical repair of benign stricture following either laparoscopic or open cholecystectomy or other procedure during the decade of the 1990s. Sixty patients had undergone a previous attempt at repair. Eight patients had undergone more than one previous attempt at repair. The mean follow-up in this series was 57.5 months. One hundred forty-two patients had completed treatment and were available for evaluation. Of those, only 13 patients (9.2%) failed following surgical reconstruction. The success rate associated with the surgical repair for biliary injury incurred during laparoscopic cholecystectomy was in excess of 94% and was significantly better than the results for repair of strictures following other operations or trauma (Fig. 5). Each of those that failed underwent either surgical revision or balloon dilatation. Only three patients continued to require long-term biliary stents to prevent symptoms of biliary obstruction, cholangitis, or both. Therefore of the 142 patients who completed therapy, including subsequent interventional procedures, a successful outcome without stents was ultimately achieved in 139 (98%).

Effect of Surgical Repair on Quality of Life

Several studies have examined the question of quality of life following surgical repair of bile duct injury. Most demonstrate complete return of the individual to functional health. One recent comparison was made of the patients from the Johns Hopkins series who had undergone successful surgical reconstruction of a bile duct injury to age-matched healthy control subjects and to age-matched individuals who had undergone recent uncomplicated laparoscopic cholecystectomy. In that study, the authors sent a standardized quality-of-life assessment to the patients who had had a surgical reconstruction and to the age-matched control subjects. The findings demonstrate that the patients having successful bile duct reconstruction were not statistically different from control subjects in the assessment of their quality of life in physical and social functional domains, but that they scored less well in the psychological domains of the assessment tool. The presence of a lawsuit related to the injury appeared to be a significant factor negatively influencing quality of life in all domains.

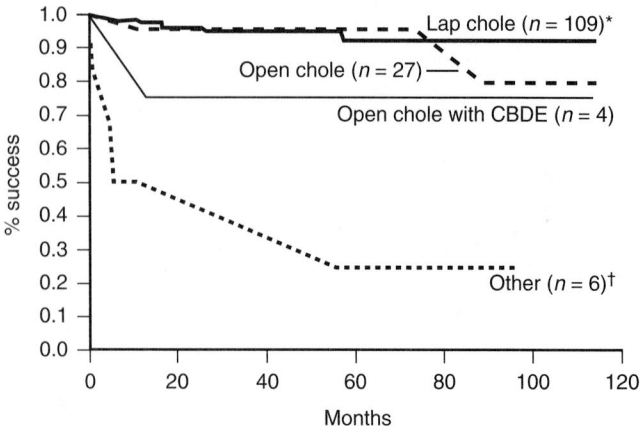

Figure 5 Actuarial success of surgical repair in patients with postoperative bile duct injury or stricture following various operations. *CBDE,* Common bile duct exploration; *Lap chole,* laparoscopic cholecystectomy; *open chole,* open cholecystectomy; *other,* other abdominal operation or trauma. *From Lillemoe KD, Melton GB, Cameron JL, and others: Ann Surg 232:430, 2000.*

NONIATROGENIC BILIARY STRICTURES

Chronic Pancreatitis

Chronic pancreatitis is an uncommon cause of biliary strictures. In these cases, fibrosis of the pancreatic parenchyma results in distal bile duct obstruction. These strictures classically involve the entire intrapancreatic segment of the common bile duct and are associated with dilatation of the entire biliary tree. In most cases, the cause of the chronic pancreatitis is alcohol abuse. The clinical presentation of the patients with biliary strictures secondary to chronic pancreatitis is variable. Some patients have no symptoms, and the diagnosis of biliary stricture is suggested by abnormal liver function tests. The serum alkaline phosphatase appears to be the most sensitive laboratory finding and is elevated in more than 80% of patients. The definitive evaluation of patients with a stricture caused by chronic pancreatitis is cholangiography. Endoscopic retrograde cholangiopancreatography and magnetic resonance cholangiopancreatography both have the advantage of also demonstrating pancreatic ductal anatomy and can thus help to determine surgical strategy for managing the chronic pancreatitis. A long, smooth, gradual tapering of the bile duct on cholangiography is an appearance most compatible with a benign stricture resulting from chronic pancreatitis. Provided that periampullary malignancy can be ruled out by clinical course or imaging studies, biliary bypass by either choledochoduodenostomy or choledochojejunostomy is indicated. Many surgeons prefer choledochoduodenostomy because it does not divert bile from the duodenum and leaves the jejunum intact for any associated procedures required for decompression of the pancreatic duct. In patients in whom malignancy cannot be excluded or in patients with significant chronic pain thought secondary to proximal pancreatic duct disease, pancreaticoduodenectomy is an effective procedure, providing both pain relief and permanent biliary diversion.

Cholelithiasis and Bile Duct Stricture

Biliary strictures caused by cholelithiasis are usually associated with a narrowing at the level of the common hepatic duct caused by stones impacted in the neck of the gallbladder. This narrowing is the result of either simple compression from a large stone in the cystic duct lying adjacent to the common hepatic duct or from chronic inflammation that extends from the neck of the gallbladder to the bile duct. Biliary obstruction by either means is known as *Mirizzi's syndrome* and is a relative contraindication to laparoscopic cholecystectomy because dissection in the triangle of Calot is made treacherous by local inflammation. In cases of duct compression associated with acute inflammation, the common hepatic duct almost always returns to normal after the offending stone has been removed by open cholecystectomy. In patients with chronic stricture or when a large fistula has developed between the gallbladder and the bile duct, reconstruction in the form of a Roux-en-Y hepaticojejunostomy may be necessary. In these cases, preoperative placement of a percutaneous transhepatic catheter facilitates the dissection and biliary reconstruction.

SUGGESTED READINGS

Dolan JP, Diggs BS, Sheppard BC, and others: Ten-year trend in the national volume of bile duct injuries requiring operative repair, *Surg Endosc* 19:967, 2005.

Flum DR, Cheadle A, Prela C, and others: Bile duct injury during cholecystectomy and survival in medicare beneficiaries, *JAMA* 290:2168, 2003.

Lillemoe KD, Melton GB, Cameron JL, and others: Postoperative bile duct strictures: management and outcome in the 1990s, *Ann Surg* 232:430, 2000.

Melton GB, Lillemoe KD, Cameron JL, and others: Major bile duct injuries associated with laparoscopic cholecystectomy: effect of surgical repair on quality of life, *Ann Surg* 255:888, 2002.

Sicklick JK, Camp MS, Lillemoe KD, and others: Surgical management of bile duct injuries sustained during laparoscopic cholecystectomy: perioperative results in 200 patients, *Ann Surg* 241:786, 2005.

Stewart L, Way LW: Bile duct injuries during laparoscopic cholecystectomy, *Arch Surg* 130:1223, 1995.

Strasberg SM, Hertl M, Soper NJ: An analysis of the problem of biliary injury during laparoscopic cholecystectomy, *J Am Coll Surg* 180:101, 1995.

COMPLICATIONS OF LAPAROSCOPIC CHOLECYSTECTOMY

Aaron Eckhauser, MD, and Kenneth W. Sharp, MD

Laparoscopic cholecystectomy has become the gold standard of treatment for patients with symptomatic gallstone disease. Numerous studies have shown the efficacy and safety of this procedure, as well as advantages such as reduced hospital stay, earlier recovery, fewer intra-abdominal adhesions, and a better cosmetic outcome compared with the open approach. A subset of patients cannot undergo laparoscopic cholecystectomy, and conversion to open surgery may be required because of technical difficulties or complications in as many as 5% of elective cholecystectomies for chronic cholecystitis and up to 30% of cholecystectomies performed for acute cholecystitis. Following cholecystectomy, the vast majority of patients experience resolution of their abdominal symptoms; however, a few either find their symptoms unchanged, complain of new upper gastrointestinal (GI) tract symptoms or have complications directly related to the surgical procedure. Complications following cholecystectomy can be defined as either early (within 1 year) or late (more than 1 year). We focus here on early postoperative complications.

EARLY POSTCHOLECYSTECTOMY PROBLEMS

Laparoscopic and open cholecystectomy has low complication rates (0.5%–5.0%). Most patients have an uncomplicated course following laparoscopic cholecystectomy and are discharged home within 24 hours of admission. Most patients recover rapidly and return to normal activity within 7 to 10 days postoperatively.

The most common complications following laparoscopic cholecystectomy include minor wound infections at the port sites and intraoperative bleeding. The incidence of wound infection is 0.4 to 1.1%. These are generally easily managed by opening the infected wound and administering oral antibiotics. Wound infections that progress to necrotizing infections are exceedingly rare following laparoscopic cholecystectomy.

The incidence of significant bleeding during laparoscopic cholecystectomy is less than 1% and accounts for many conversions to laparotomy. Bleeding typically results from trocar or Veress needle injury, liver laceration, or bleeding from the gallbladder fossa and

Table 1: Early Postcholecystectomy Complications

Spilled stones
Retained common duct stone
Bile duct leak
Bile duct injury
Bowel injury
Incidental gallbladder cancer

injury to the cystic artery or portal vessels. Trocar or Veress needle injuries occur in 0.1 to 0.25% of all laparoscopic procedures but account for a significant morbidity and mortality. The risk of this injury can be decreased by using an open technique to access the peritoneum. Early recognition of hypotension and bleeding is essential for prompt and successful management. Injury to an abdominal wall vessel such as the epigastric artery or vein can be reduced if trocar placement is lateral to the rectus sheath and transillumination is used to guide insertion. These injuries can be treated with full-wall thickness sutures or wound exploration and direct vessel ligation. Liver lacerations generally occur as a result of excess traction on the gallbladder or blind placement of instruments. These injuries can be reduced by avoiding excessive traction on the gallbladder, avoiding the falciform ligament when inserting the epigastric trocar, and using meticulous dissection in the plane between the gallbladder and liver. Bleeding from the cystic artery can usually be controlled with suction, irrigation, and cautery or clips, but conversion to an open procedure should not be delayed excessively. Radiographs of patients with injuries to the bile duct and subsequent strictures often show an unusually large number of clips in the hilum of the liver; thus blind placement of clips in a field obscured by blood is not safe and should be avoided. Injuries to the hepatic arteries or portal vein are heralded by massive bleeding, and visualization of the injury is virtually impossible without conversion to laparotomy.

The more serious early postcholecystectomy complications are listed in Table 1. The incidence of spilled gallstones is 3% to 33%; retained common bile duct stones, 0.7% to 1.5%; bile leak, 0.4% to 1.1%; bile duct injury, 0.25% to 0.6%; bowel injury, 0.2% to 0.6%; and incidental gallbladder cancer, up to 0.35%.

EVALUATION AND MANAGEMENT OF ACUTE POSTOPERATIVE PROBLEMS

The majority of patients who undergo laparoscopic cholecystectomy are discharged within 24 hours of operation. However, for those patients in the early postoperative period who have unresolved or persistent abdominal complaints (e.g., pain, anorexia, nausea, vomiting, and jaundice) or evidence of infection (e.g., fever and chills), a complete and timely evaluation of the patient must be undertaken to rule out an operative complication.

A focused history and physical exam should include onset, duration, localization, and severity of pain and any associated symptoms such as nausea, vomiting, fever, or chills. Laboratory evaluation should include a complete blood count, liver function tests, amylase, and lipase. Chest and abdominal x-rays may be performed, but the findings are often confusing and inconclusive. Atelectasis, pleural effusions, and small amounts of free air may be seen on postoperative radiographs, but large amounts of free air should heighten suspicion for a visceral injury.

Multiple noninvasive imaging tests can be used to evaluate the patient with persistent pain, fever, or nausea following laparoscopic cholecystectomy. Ultrasound is a quick and specific test to evaluate the presence of retained fluid collections in the abdomen and

around the liver. Computerized tomography (CT) is useful in identifying fluid collections and can facilitate percutaneous drainage procedures. Magnetic resonance cholangiopancreatography (MRCP) also provides excellent noninterventional imaging of the biliary tract, retained stones, the pancreas, and fluid collections. Magnetic resonance imaging is not used as commonly as CT to facilitate percutaneous procedures. Hepatobiliary imaging (technetium-99 m iminodiacetic acid [HIDA scan]) assesses hepatocellular function, flow of bile into the duodenum, and collections of extrabiliary radionuclide. HIDA scans can determine whether fluid collections originate from the biliary system and whether there is an active leak and may illustrate the rate of leakage. They do not precisely define the biliary tree anatomy, and further imaging is required if leaks are seen. For example, a leak from a duodenal injury may not be distinguished from a bile duct leak on HIDA imaging.

If qualified gastroenterologists or radiologists are available, endoscopic retrograde cholangiopancreatography (ERCP) and percutaneous transhepatic cholangiography (PTC) provide alternative invasive means of diagnosis and treatment. ERCP can be used to define biliary anatomy, evaluate biliary fistulae, and perform therapeutic interventions such as draining the bile duct in the case of a cystic duct stump leak, extracting retained common bile duct stones, and stenting or dilatating strictures. PTC can clearly define biliary anatomy and facilitate drainage of the biliary tree and stent placement. PTC and stent placement have several benefits: they allow local control of the biliary fistula; can be used as a landmark during surgery to identify the transected ducts, which are usually retracted into the hilum; and can aid postoperative control of biliary leaks.

Finally, if sophisticated facilities are not available for management of suspected leaks, retained stones, or injuries, referral to a tertiary center for evaluation and management should be emphasized. Surgical reexploration to assess and manage complications without sophisticated preoperative evaluation is a difficult operation and should be performed only in unusual situations.

Successful management of patients with biliary injuries following laparoscopic cholecystectomy includes (1) completely defining the nature of the injury, which may require cholangiography from above (a percutaneous transhepatic approach) and below (an endoscopic approach); (2) percutaneously draining the biliary system; (3) treating sepsis and periportal inflammation with antibiotics and drainage of collections; and (4) appropriate timing of expert, definitive repair.

Intra-abdominal fluid collections in the early postoperative period may be secondary to bile, blood, or enteric contents secondary to unrecognized bowel injury. We discuss the specific management of these injuries later in the chapter. It should be emphasized that postoperative fluid collections are common but rarely clinically significant. The majority of patients undergoing laparoscopic cholecystectomy have some postoperative intra-abdominal fluid found on a CT scan if they are scanned early in the postoperative period, yet less than 1% of all laparoscopic cholecystectomies are complicated by a clinically detectable leak.

Most clinically significant postoperative fluid collections are the result of bile duct injury or cystic duct stump leakage and require prompt attention. Morbidity and mortality rates in patients with undrained bile collections are high. Most patients with bile collections do not initially present with peritonitis, but with pain, fever, malaise, jaundice, or abnormal liver function tests. Prompt drainage of intra-abdominal bile is crucial to prevent severe complications such as sepsis and multiorgan failure. After intra-abdominal fluid has been detected, it should be percutaneously drained and cultured to guide appropriate antibiotic choice. Following drainage of a bile collection, the potential for immediate serious illness is reduced, and the injury can then be fully investigated with operative treatment executed in a more controlled and elective manner. The specific timing of scans, percutaneous drainage, and cholangiography can be tailored to the severity of each patient's illness: the more acutely ill the patient, the more acutely drainage must be accomplished.

SPILLED STONES

Perforation of the gallbladder with loss of bile and gallstones during laparoscopic cholecystectomy is relatively common, occurring in up to 30% of cholecystectomies. There is concern that retained intraperitoneal gallstones can cause abscess formation, inflammation, fibrosis, adhesions, cutaneous sinuses, and fistulae. The incidence of complications related to retained stones is reported in 0.08% to 0.3% of patients. Retained stones or fragments may not lead to complications if the bile is sterile, the fragments are small, and no other complications occur; they encyst in a fibrous capsule. Management recommendations for the optimal treatment of spilled stones range from conversion to full laparotomy and retrieval of all stones to copious irrigation and meticulous laparoscopic removal of all visible stones and fragments with careful postoperative observation.

Spilled stones in the presence of infected bile can lead to an inflammatory reaction and abscess formation. These usually occur early in the postoperative course but can present several years later with pain, fever, and intra-abdominal abscess on CT scan. Infectious complications are more common in the elderly and immunologically impaired, in whom infected bile is more common than in younger patients, who are more likely to have sterile bile present with their gallstones.

Abdominal wall abscesses resulting from retained stones at the port site are treated with local drainage and evacuation of all stones. Intra-abdominal abscesses resulting from retained stones after laparoscopic cholecystectomy can be drained percutaneously. Recurrence of intra-abdominal abscesses should heighten suspicion to the presence of a retained stone or foreign body. Treatment with percutaneous drainage is not likely to succeed if all the stones in an abscess cavity are not retrieved. Gallstones have also been found at distant sites, including hernia sacs, urine, and sputum.

All patients should be informed that stones were spilled into the abdominal cavity and that a potential for long-term complications exists. Early recognition of the complications of spilled intraperitoneal stones is critical for the safe diagnosis and treatment of symptomatic patients.

Retained Common Bile Duct Stones

The incidence of retained common bile duct stones following laparoscopic cholecystectomy is approximately 1.1% to 3.3% and is discussed in other chapters. The vast majority of retained common duct stones can be managed nonoperatively with endoscopic sphincterotomy and stone extraction. Some patients require operative treatment, including those with multiple or large stones and those patients with prior surgical therapy (e.g., Roux-en-Y gastric bypass or gastric resection with Billroth II anastomosis) that prevents endoscopic access to the ampulla.

Identification and Classification of Biliary Injury and Leak

Iatrogenic biliary tract injuries during cholecystectomy usually result in significant morbidity and require further intervention. Injuries include bile duct leaks, strictures, transection, or ligation. Significant postoperative bile leaks occur in up to 1% of patients following laparoscopic cholecystectomy.

Biliary injuries can be classified as described by Strasberg (Fig. 1). Strasberg type A injuries include leaks from the cystic

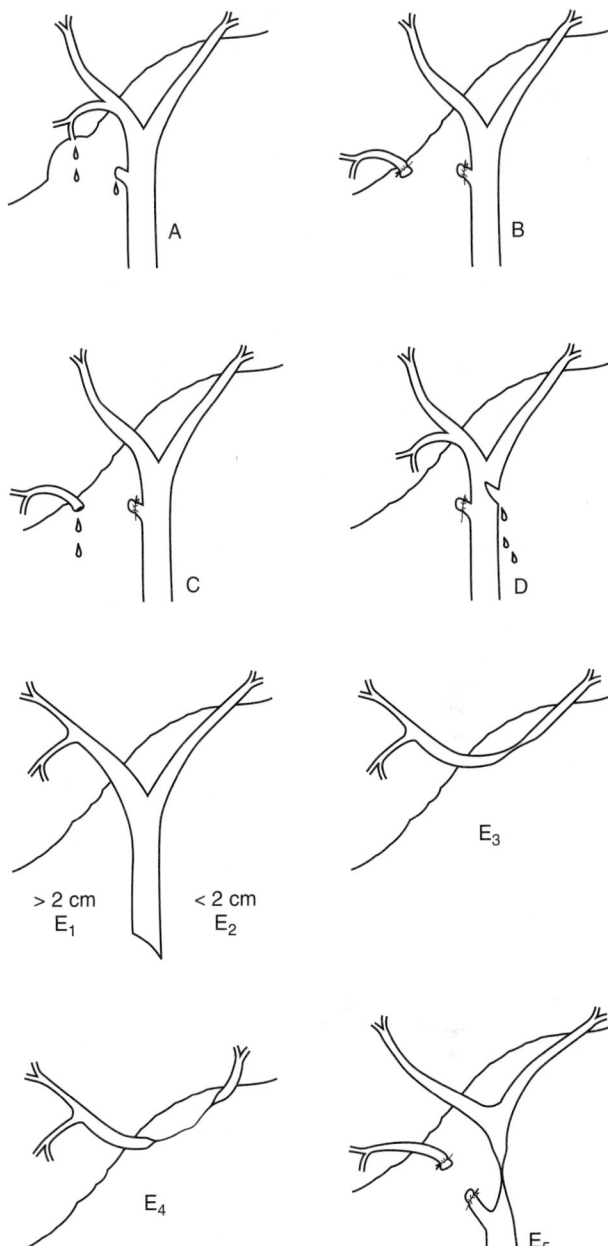

Figure 1 Strasberg classification of laparoscopic injuries to the biliary tract. Injuries of types A to E are illustrated. Type E injuries are subdivided according to the Bismuth classification. Type A injuries are cystic duct leaks or leaks from small ducts in the liver bed. Type B and C injuries almost always involve aberrant right hepatic ducts. Type D injuries are lateral injuries to major bile ducts. The notations >2 cm and <2 cm in type E1 and type E2 indicate the length of common hepatic duct remaining. *From Strasberg SM, Soper NJ: Benign biliary stricture. In Cameron JL, editor: Current surgical therapy, ed 8, Philadelphia, 2004, Elsevier Mosby.*

duct stump or minor ducts on the liver bed with intact intrahepatic and extrahepatic ducts. Leakage from the cystic duct occurs secondary to clip failure (improperly applied or crossed clips or inadequate occlusion of the entire width of the cystic duct) or a burst phenomenon in the presence of retained common duct stones; it may also be seen when the clips are applied too tightly and local ischemia leads to necrosis of the cystic duct stump. Patients with this type of injury present with symptoms related to the presence of intraperitoneal bile—namely, abdominal pain, anorexia, ileus, nausea, or bile peritonitis with sepsis. This injury may be recognized on HIDA scan as contrast extravasation from the bile duct but with radiocontrast also entering the duodenum via the common duct (with the caveat that a lateral bile duct injury may look the same). MRCP may identify this injury but does not offer an option for therapeutic intervention. Generally ERCP or PTC clearly identify this injury as contrast extravasation adjacent to cystic duct clips and provide an avenue for therapy.

Type B injuries occlude a portion of the biliary tree and may occur when the cystic duct drains into the right hepatic duct rather than the common duct. The right hepatic duct, or an aberrant right hepatic duct, is then mistaken for the cystic duct and is ligated or divided. Patients with type B injuries may remain asymptomatic as the obstructed lobe or segment atrophies and the remaining liver hypertrophies. Alternatively, they may present with pain or cholangitis in the occluded area. If the entire right or left hepatic duct is divided and occluded with clips, the patient will have abnormal liver tests for a long period but may not suffer any functional consequence if the remaining liver is normal.

A type C injury is a leak from a duct not in continuity with the common duct and is also known as a sectoral duct injury without occlusion of the injured duct, so that bile leakage into the peritoneal cavity occurs. Patients become symptomatic secondary to the presence of a peritoneal bile collection, presenting with pain, nausea, peritoneal irritation, and signs of sepsis. However, because the portion of the biliary tree draining into the peritoneum is not in communication with the common duct, distal stenting for this type of injury is ineffective. These injuries may not be evident on ERCP if the distal clips are intact and there is no extravasation from the hepatic ducts. PTC may also fail to demonstrate this injury if the contralateral intrahepatic duct is entered and dye shows only the proximal left and right hepatic ducts draining into the common hepatic duct. Radiographically these injuries are usually defined after percutaneous drainage of a bile collection, followed by establishment of a biliary fistula and subsequent contrast injection of the fistula.

The type D injury is a lateral injury to any extrahepatic duct, and, like many injuries, may be caused by cautery, scissors, or improper placement of clips. This injury may have several manifestations depending on whether the injury is a laceration, cautery burn, or partial clip obstruction. Partial lacerations from scissors or cautery injury present early with bile peritonitis. However, a cautery burn may present later as a stricture if there is not full thickness injury to the duct. Partial clip applications across the common hepatic or bile duct may present early with peritonitis if there is necrosis of the duct in that area, but more commonly they present later with a bilary stricture. Identification of these injuries depends on the presentation; patients with symptoms of bile collection are found after percutaneous drainage and ERCP/PTC; patients with bilary obstruction present with abnormal liver tests, jaundice, or late sepsis from cholangitis.

A type E injury is an excision or complete occlusion of the common hepatic or common bile duct that totally disrupts biliary-enteric communication. Type E injuries most commonly present with early sepsis and peritonitis if there is bile leaking from the duct injury or can present later with jaundice or cholangitis if the duct is totally occluded by clips or ligatures.

MANAGEMENT OF CYSTIC DUCT STUMP LEAK

Cystic duct leaks are usually treated with endoscopic transampullary stenting to decrease endobiliary pressure in addition to percutaneous drainage of localized bile collections. Endoscopic sphincterotomy may be necessary in some cases to facilitate stent placement but may fail when used alone (without stenting). Success with

nonoperative management of an isolated cystic duct stump leak approaches 90%. Some patients require laparoscopy and peritoneal lavage to remove large bile collections—especially if the bile has not localized to the perihepatic space and is located in multiple abdominal quadrants. Open surgical drainage or closure of cystic duct leaks is rarely necessary; surgical closure with clips or ligatures may be hazardous in an edematous and friable surgical field. If retained common duct stones are present in the face of a cystic duct leak, they must be removed to facilitate closure of the fistula. This is generally accomplished with an endoscopic sphincterotomy and stone extraction.

MANAGEMENT OF BILIARY INJURY

Endoscopy provides an effective diagnostic and therapeutic option for treatment of biliary leaks following laparoscopic cholecystectomy. An increasing number of reports now support the early use of ERCP to diagnose and better define the nature of the biliary injury and also to facilitate treatment, whether endoscopic or surgical. In a large retrospective study, Kaffes and colleagues found that the optimal treatment for simple bile duct leaks (especially cystic duct stump leaks) is placement of a straight plastic stent, at least 7 F, to eliminate the transpapillary biliary-duodenal pressure gradient. The stents can be removed after 4 weeks without follow-up cholangiogram unless there is a known or probable stricture. However, when the bilioenteric system is in discontinuity (as in types B, C, and E injuries), then ERCP is of less therapeutic benefit, and further imaging and intervention is required.

Recognition of a bile duct injury during cholecystectomy requires either direct repair with a stent or restoration of bilioenteric flow via a Roux-en-Y hepaticojejunostomy. Primary repair of a severed common bile duct is uncommon but may be feasible in selected cases where the ends of the bile duct are healthy, are free of cautery or crush injury, and have adequate blood supply (no injury to the hepatic artery or the 3 o'clock and 9 o'clock arterial supply of the bile duct). If there has been excision of a significant portion of the bile duct, primary repair over a T-tube may result in excessive tension and a later leak or stricture.

Type B biliary injuries may or may not require operative repair. If the injury involves a minor sectoral branch of the right hepatic duct, the patient may show elevated liver tests as the involved segment atrophies, but little long-term consequence will be noted unless infection occurs. Infection of a minor obstructed segment may be manageable with antibiotics alone or percutaneous drainage. Abscess formation is uncommon, and rarely are resection or debridement necessary. If the injury obstructs the main right hepatic duct or two or more subsegmental branches, then operative drainage with a Roux-en-Y hepaticojejunostomy will likely be necessary. Left hepatic duct injuries are less common than accessory right branches, but the same principles apply to management.

Type C injuries present earlier and with more sepsis and inflammatory changes than type B injuries because there is ongoing leakage of bile from the injured duct(s). However, if the injury is to a small sectoral right branch, simple percutaneous drainage will likely suffice with subsequent delineation of the exact duct injury pattern. If it is a minor duct transection, then fibrosis, sclerosis of the duct, and atrophy of the subsegment will occur over time. When a major right ductal injury is detected, operative repair is necessary with a Roux-en-Y hepaticojejunostomy.

Type D injuries, as mentioned earlier, present early with septic issues or later with obstruction. Early type D injuries (leak from cutting or cautery injuries) require drainage of biliary collections and delineation of the site and size of the leak. Repair will be best accomplished in a stable, nonseptic patient with good preoperative delineation of the anatomy. Preoperative placement of a PTC drain facilitates biliary drainage, and the catheter may be palpated in a thickened, scarred porta hepatis, thereby facilitating operative dissection. Tangential injuries are best treated with Roux-en-Y drainage procedures because primary repair is virtually impossible. Injuries that almost transect the bile duct are best treated by complete division and closure of the distal duct with hepaticojejunostomy proximally. Late-presenting Type D injuries are almost always treated with a Roux-en-Y hepaticojejunostomy as the most common treatment of a biliary stricture.

Type E injuries present early and again are best treated with establishment of drainage, delineation of the biliary anatomy, and repair after sepsis and inflammatory changes have subsided. Because these injuries involve transection of the duct, virtually all will require a Roux-en-Y hepaticojejunostomy. If the injury involves the bifurcation of the hepatic duct, repair will be difficult and may require two or more hepatic duct anastomoses.

The timing of biliary injury repair is controversial. There are clearly indications for early repair, for example, early recognition of a bile duct transection (especially intraoperative detection). Delayed repair is indicated in the unstable patient with overwhelming sepsis (although urgent operative intervention is necessary to establish good drainage if percutaneous routes are not available or if they fail). Lillemoe and colleagues reported the largest single-center experience with biliary tract injuries resulting from laparoscopic cholecystectomy. Their primary goal during the initial management is control of the bile leak and ongoing sepsis. This was uniformly accomplished in this series with PTC and external drainage. Bilioenteric reconstruction during acute inflammation and peritonitis is a difficult surgical procedure, and delayed repair several weeks after resolution of sepsis is more likely to be successful. Timing of operation (early, intermediate, and delayed, as indicated by clinical presentation), presenting symptoms, and prior attempt at repair had no influence on perioperative complications and length of stay. Ninety-eight percent of these injuries were repaired using a Roux-en-Y hepaticojejunostomy, with an excellent perioperative mortality and leak rate of 2.7% and 4.6%, respectively. When faced with a bilary injury, the surgeon must consider several factors in planning repairs: local availability of experienced radiologists for cholangiography and other percutaneous interventions; gastroenterologists with expertise in bilary tract manipulations; critical care facilities for critically ill patients; and, finally, the surgeon's own experience with difficult operations on the biliary tree in less than ideal conditions. These considerations and others such as medicolegal concerns may favor transfer of the patient to a tertiary center with a larger experience in managing these complications.

Early repair results in significant cost savings, decreased morbidity and mortality, and a shorter hospital stay with decreased outpatient visits. Early repair in experienced hands may also minimize hepatic damage and avoid cirrhotic parenchymal transformation. Delayed repair can be made technically more difficult by hilar plate retraction, retraction of anastomotic structures, and rotation of the hepatic pedicle.

▌ BOWEL INJURY

Bowel injury with perforation resulting from laparoscopic surgery is rare and occurs only in approximately 1.3 in 1000 patients. The small bowel (especially the duodenum) is the most frequently injured organ, followed by the colon and stomach. These injuries occur with trocar insertion (direct laceration); tearing or cutting injuries (sharp instruments or shearing of tissues during dissection of adhesions or adherent bowel); and thermal injuries (direct burns or arcing injuries). The majority of bowel injuries go unnoticed at the time of injury, with thermal injuries generally presenting later than nonthermal injuries. Electrocautery accounts for approximately 50% of injuries, followed by injury during Veress needle or trocar insertion.

All bowel injuries recognized at the time of operation should be repaired primarily. Laparoscopic repair of injury or enterotomy is safe and effective, but many operators convert to an open procedure if they are not completely sure of the extent of the injury or the security of the repair. Bowel injuries missed during cholecystectomy likely present early with abdominal pain, nausea, fever, and distention. Because small bowel contents are not as irritating to the peritoneum as gastric acid is (as in a perforated duodenal ulcer), these patients may not have classical signs such as a rigid, boardlike abdomen and absent bowel sounds. Typically, cautery injuries present several days later when the injury progresses to bowel wall necrosis and spillage of enteric contents. As discussed previously, patients presenting days after a laparoscopic cholecystectomy with fever, abdominal pain, nausea, and distention are suspected to have a biliary injury, and a CT scan will show intra-abdominal fluid; an HIDA scan may not show extravasation, however. Oral contrast administered for the CT may or may not show extravasation, and the absence of extravasation should not be taken as a gold standard for the absence of bowel injury. Aspiration under CT or ultrasound guidance may be necessary, and it should clarify that the fluid is enteric and alert the surgeon to the need for exploration.

Incidental Gallbladder Cancer

Unsuspected gallbladder cancer is rare, affecting less than 0.5% of patients with gallstones. Most of these are early-stage lesions detected by pathology as opposed to intraoperative detection, and there is controversy with regard to optimal treatment in patients with an incidental finding of gallbladder cancer. There is substantial concern about performing laparoscopic cholecystectomy for cancer because of the inability to attain adequate resection margins and the possibility of port site recurrence and peritoneal seeding of tumor.

Most patients found to have an unsuspected gallbladder cancer have early-stage lesions; advanced cancers will have visible extension into the liver, as well as metastases or peritoneal implants, and laparoscopic attempts at resection will likely be abandoned. Varshney and colleagues reported that simple cholecystectomy is adequate for T1a lesions (tumor invades lamina propria), with few patients progressing to develop port-site metastases or locoregional occurrence. Patients with T1b tumors (tumor invades muscular layer) may be cured by cholecystectomy, but there is controversial evidence to support port-site, liver-bed, and regional lymphadenectomy in a second radical operation. T2 tumors (tumor invades the perimuscular connective tissue but does not extend beyond the serosa or into the liver) require a second radical operation in patients considered fit for a curative resection. Few T3 and T4 tumors (perforates the serosa and extends into periportal structures and adjacent organs) can be cured, but a radical second operation may prolong survival and may serve a palliative purpose. These patients are often best served by referral to a specialist if the surgeon is not experienced in radical resection of the porta hepatis structures.

Patients who have laparoscopic cholecystectomy and are found to have incidental gallbladder cancer may develop port-site recurrences in up to 30% of cases. These recurrences are not dependent on direct tumor handling or extraction through the port site. Early peritoneal dissemination of tumor cells is a specific concern associated with laparoscopy.

▌ SUMMARY

Patients with symptomatic gallstone disease are well treated with a laparoscopic cholecystectomy but should be preoperatively counseled concerning the risk of perioperative complications because it is not the totally innocuous procedure that many patients believe. Although laparoscopic cholecystectomy is generally safe in the vast majority of cases, postcholecystectomy complications remain a significant source of concern for surgeons and warrant detailed laboratory and radiographic evaluation rather than assumption of a benign postoperative course.

SUGGESTED READINGS

Cohen J, Sharp K: Complications of laparoscopic cholecystectomy. In *Laparoscopic surgery of the abdomen:* New York, 2004, Springer-Verlag.

Deziel DJ: Complication of cholecystectomy: incidence, clinical manifestations, and diagnosis, *Surg Clin North Am* 74:809, 1994.

Kaffes AJ, Hourigan L, De Luca N, and others: Impact of endoscopic intervention in 100 patients with suspected postcholecystectomy leak, *Gastrointest Endosc* 61:269, 2005.

Lee CM, Stewart L, Way LW: Postcholecystectomy abdominal bile collections, *Arch Surg* 135:538, 2000.

Lee VS, Chari RS, Cucchiaro G, and others: Complications of laparoscopic cholecystectomy, *Am J Surg* 165:527, 1993.

Murr M, Gigot JF, Nagorney DM, and others: Long-term results of biliary reconstruction after laparoscopic bile duct injuries, *Arch Surg* 134:604, 1999.

Sicklick J, Camp M, Lillemoe K, and others: Surgical management of bile duct injuries sustained during laparoscopic cholecystectomy: perioperative results in 200 patients, *Ann Surg* 241:786, 2005.

Tumer AR, Yuksek YN, Yasti AC, and others: Dropped gallstones during laparoscopic cholecystectomy: the consequences, *World J Surg* 29:437, 2005.

Varshney S, Buttirini G, Gupta R: Incidental carcinoma of the gallbladder, *Eur J Surg Oncol* 28:4, 2002.

CYSTIC DISORDERS OF THE BILE DUCTS

Jayme E. Locke, MD, and Pamela A. Lipsett, MD

The average general surgeon will rarely encounter a biliary cyst. Although typically considered a disease of childhood, presenting with the triad of a right upper quadrant mass, jaundice, and abdominal pain, today an equal number of patients are first recognized in adulthood. Despite its rarity, biliary cystic disease is clinically important because it is associated with recurrent cholangitis, biliary stricture, choledocholithiasis, recurrent acute pancreatitis, and malignancy. Patients who present in adulthood often have symptoms or signs of gallbladder or pancreatic disease, and thus surgeons who operate in the abdomen must be familiar with this problem. In this chapter, the epidemiology, classification, etiology, diagnosis, management, and outcome of patients with biliary cysts are discussed.

EPIDEMIOLOGY

Cystic disorders of the biliary tree are seen across the world and across a spectrum of patient ages. Aside from biliary atresia, it is the most common congenital abnormality of the biliary tree and the most common cause of cholestatic jaundice in infancy, especially in Asia. The disease appears to be most common in Asian countries, with an estimated incidence of 1 in 13,000 compared with a worldwide incidence of 1 in 2 million live births. Biliary cysts are four times more common in women compared with men. Approximately 60% of patients are diagnosed with biliary cystic disease during their first decade of life, and 20% are diagnosed as adults.

CLASSIFICATION

Cystic dilatation of the bile duct, also known as *choledochal cyst disease,* occurs in many locations along the biliary tree and has been classified into several types. Today these malformations are most often classified according to the Todani modification of the Alonso-Lej classification (Fig. 1 and Table 1). The incidence of various types of choledochal cysts depends on the patient's country of origin and age of diagnosis. Traditionally the classic type and most common (50% to 80%) choledochal cyst is type I

disease: (1) cystic, (2) saccular, or (3) fusiform (Fig. 2) dilatation of the extrahepatic biliary tree. Type II cysts are simple diverticula of the extrahepatic biliary tree and account for 2% to 3% of all cysts. Recently a rare combination of type I cystic dilatation and a type II diverticulum was reported in four children. A type III cyst, also known as *choledochocele,* is a cystic dilatation of the intraduodenal portion of the extrahepatic biliary tree and is a distinct entity from peri-Vaterian duodenal diverticula. The true incidence of these cysts is unknown because they are likely underreported when diagnosed at endoscopic retrograde cholangiopancreatography (ERCP). Multiple dilatations of the intrahepatic and extrahepatic biliary tree are known as type IV cysts. Type IVA cysts are the second most common (30% to 40%) type of cysts seen in adults and may be quite difficult to treat. Caroli's disease, or a type V cyst, is confined to the intrahepatic portion of the biliary tree. This disease can be associated with periportal fibrosis and cirrhosis and may be confined to the left hepatic lobe, or it may be bilobar.

ETIOLOGY

The pathogenesis of biliary cysts is unknown, although most believe it is related to congenital factors, such as malunion of the pancreaticobiliary duct junction. Additional explanations of the etiology of biliary cysts include the following: (1) reflux of pancreatic juice into the biliary tree secondary to a long anomalous pancreaticobiliary channel; (2) an in utero accident; or (3) an acquired defect. None of these explanations is entirely satisfactory or accounts for the predilection of the disease for women or those of Asian descent. The increased identification of adults with this disease may reflect improved diagnostic modalities and suggests an acquired component to the disease.

DIAGNOSIS

The age of presentation and diagnosis of choledochal cyst disease, ranging from antenatal to neonatal to adulthood, depends in large part on the patient's country of origin. For example, in some countries, such as Japan, the disease is still most commonly seen in young childhood, whereas in the United States, an increasing number of patients present for diagnosis and treatment in adulthood. As previously noted, a choledochal cyst is most classically associated with the triad of jaundice, right upper quadrant pain, and an abdominal mass. However, this triad is present in less than 15% of all patients and is most commonly seen in children. Although a mass may be palpable as often as one third of the time in neonates and infants, this is uncommon in adults, presumably because of development of abdominal wall musculature. Table 2 demonstrates common presenting signs and symptoms seen in our series.

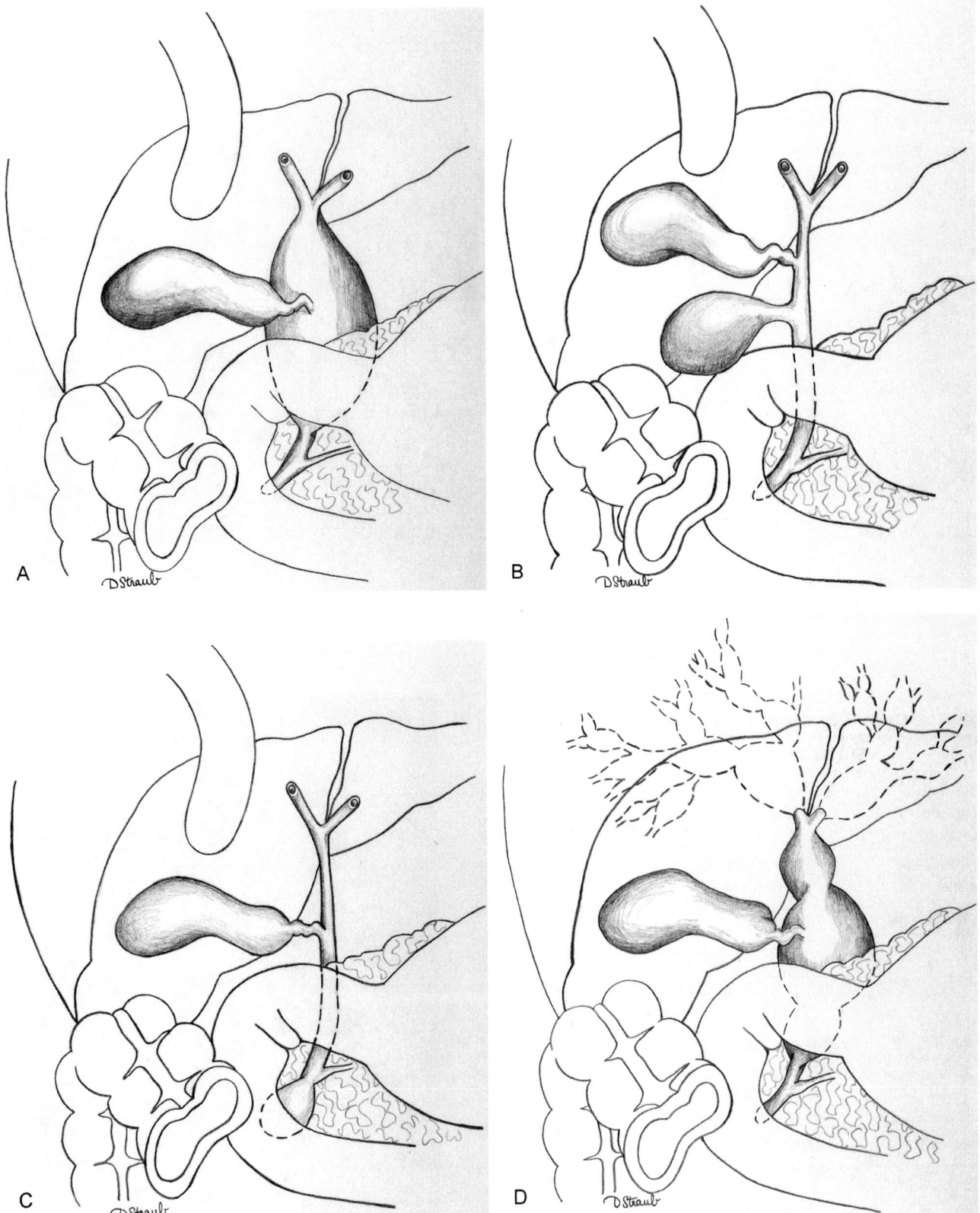

Figure 1 Classification of biliary cysts. **(A)** Type I. **(B)** Type II. **(C)** Type III. **(D)** Type IVA.

(continued)

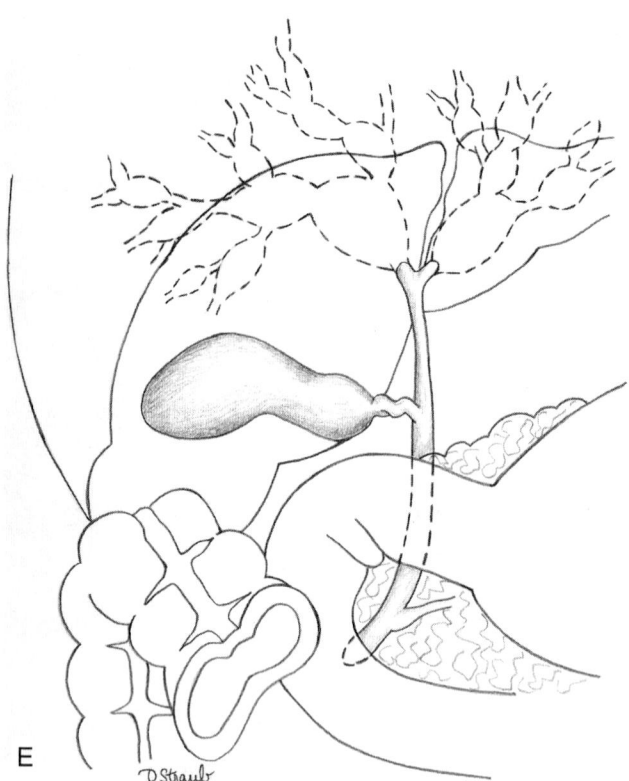

E

Figure I Cont'd—**(E)** Type V.
*From Lipsett PA, Pitt HA, Colombani PM,
and others: Ann Surg 220:644, 1994.*

Table I: Cyst Type Alonso-Lej/Todani Modification

Type	Description	% of All Cysts
Type I (choledochal cyst)	Cystic, fusiform saccular extrahepatic biliary dilatation	50%–80%
Mixed type I and II	Fusiform dilatation of the extrahepatic biliary tree in combination with a separate diverticulum, midportion of the common bile duct, with cystic duct entering in the right of the diverticulum	1%
Type II	Extrahepatic biliary diverticulum	2%–3%
Type III (choledochocele)	Dilatation of extrahepatic intraduodenal biliary tree	<10%
Type IVA	Intrahepatic and extrahepatic saccular/ cystic dilatation	30%–40%
B	Multiple extrahepatic cysts	<5%
Type V (Caroli's disease)	Intrahepatic biliary cyst	<10%

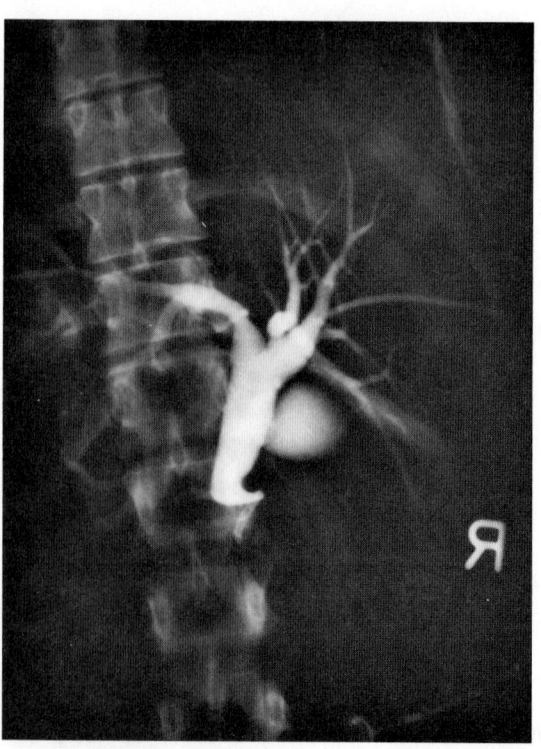

Figure 2 Percutaneous cholangiogram of a type I choledochal cyst. A fusiform pattern is easily seen.

Table 2: Common Presenting Signs and Symptoms of a Choledochal Cyst

Symptom	Children (n = 24) n (%)	Adults (n = 84) n (%)
Abdominal mass	9 (82)	4 (13)*
Abdominal pain	4 (36)	27 (87)*
Jaundice	7 (64)	13 (42)
Fever	2 (18)	8 (26)
Nausea/vomiting	2 (18)	9 (29)
Pancreatitis	0 (0)	7 (23)†
Prior cholecystectomy	0 (0)	16 (52)*

*$p < .01$ vs. children, chi square test.
†$p = .06$ vs. children, chi square test.
From Lipsett PA, Pitt HA, Colombani PM, and others: Ann Surg 220:644, 1994.

Adults are typically diagnosed with cystic dilatation of their bile ducts during workup for presumed cholecystitis or pancreatitis. Many adults present with jaundice, and, as a result, abnormal liver function tests are often seen. Liver function tests generally reflect a pattern of mechanical obstruction, with elevations in bilirubin, alkaline phosphatase, and gamma glutamyl transferase being most common. The transaminases (alanine and aspartate aminotransferases [SGOT/SGPT]) can be elevated to a lesser degree. Serum amylase may be elevated in patients presenting with acute abdominal pain and signs and symptoms of clinical pancreatitis.

Given recent advances in the diagnosis of antenatal choledochal cysts (type I), the differentiation between type I disease and biliary atresia is possible. Biopsy results can demonstrate the advanced liver disease associated with biliary atresia compared with the mild changes of early type I disease, identifying the need for earlier operation in the case of biliary atresia. Neonates, children, and young adults who present with jaundice and abdominal pain should be evaluated using abdominal ultrasound because this is the most cost-effective method. In this patient population, biliary cysts are high on the list of differential diagnoses. In an older patient, however, a computerized tomographic (CT) scan may provide additional information because the list of differential diagnoses is more expansive. A CT scan is easily read by surgeons and defines well the anatomy of the hepatobiliary and pancreatic regions in a jaundiced patient. Magnetic resonance cholangiopancreatography (MRCP) is increasingly used when available and frequently demonstrates the abnormal biliary anatomy, including an abnormal pancreaticobiliary union with a long common channel. Other methods of imaging the region, which are almost of historic use, have been employed, particularly nuclear scans. These tests provide little incremental information and are not frequently used today.

Precise definition of the biliary anatomy is necessary via cholangiography, which can be accomplished noninvasively via MRCP or invasively via ERCP or percutaneous transhepatic cholangiography (PTC). In adults, we prefer PTC and the placement of transhepatic stents, especially in patients with a type IV cyst, in whom resection of the bifurcation may be necessary and long-term stenting required. Because long common channels are often present and to avoid the development of periprocedural pancreatitis, placement of the stent through the ampulla should not be performed at the time of PTC. Similarly, during ERCP, care to avoid the pancreatic duct is important. ERCP may not define the most proximal biliary anatomy, which is often abnormal; in part this is why we prefer the transhepatic approach.

MANAGEMENT

Patients with bile duct cysts are at an increased risk of malignancy, whether in the bile duct, (cholangiocarcinoma), the gallbladder, or both. The cause of this increased risk for the development of cancer is unknown, but transformation to cancer on average occurs at least a decade earlier than the age of a typical cholangiocarcinoma, and advanced disease at the time of diagnosis is not uncommon. Possible reasons for the increased risk of cancer include bile stasis, superinfection, repeated episodes of inflammation, conversion of a bile salt to a carcinogenic substance by chronic infections, or some unknown factor related to the development of the congenital cyst.

Scattered reports suggest that percutaneous drainage of cysts should be used. This should be a rare management strategy aimed only at temporizing and stabilizing a patient in septic shock or some other abdominal catastrophe until appropriate resection can be performed. In addition, cyst bypass should not be used because of the increased risk of the development of cancer as just described. All patients with biliary cysts of type I, II, or IV should have the cyst excised. Although the mucosa of the cysts should be removed, in many patients the mucosa is replaced with fibrosis, and complete excision of the cyst is recommended.

OPERATIVE TECHNIQUE

Type I: Choledochal Cyst

The patient is explored through a midline incision, beginning with a search for possible malignancy. If the gallbladder has not been previously removed, it should be dissected free from the hepatic bed at this time (Fig. 3). The duodenum is freed from its attachments by a Kocher maneuver. The dissection may be approached from either a cephalad or caudad position. The common bile duct is encircled at its proximal extent, usually at or just below the bifurcation of the hepatic ducts. The distal-most portion of the cystic dilatation is identified and encircled as it enters the pancreas, and the retroduodenal portion of the common bile duct is separated from surrounding tissues (Fig. 4). The duct is then transected at the intrapancreatic portion with extreme care taken not to injure the pancreatic duct (Fig. 5). If dilatation of the bile duct is still present at the distal-most margin (duodenal), the mucosa must be stripped before closure. By elevating the cyst anteriorly (facilitated by the bile stent), the cyst is then dissected proximally, off the portal vein

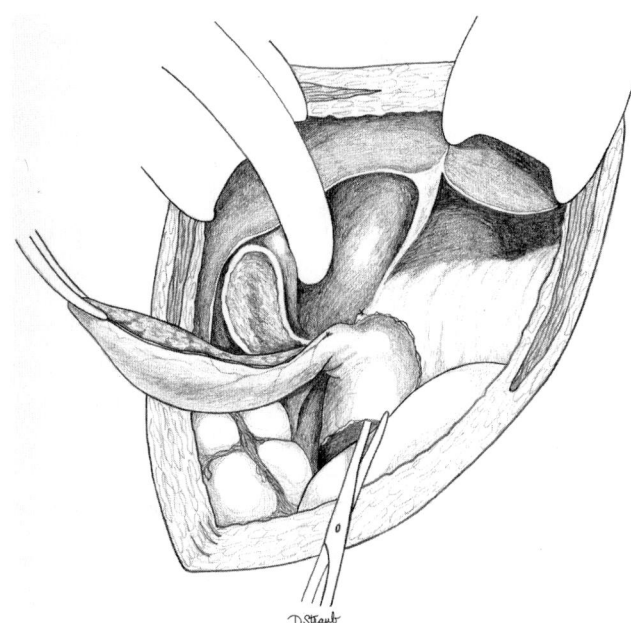

Figure 3 Dissection of the gallbladder from the hepatic bed.

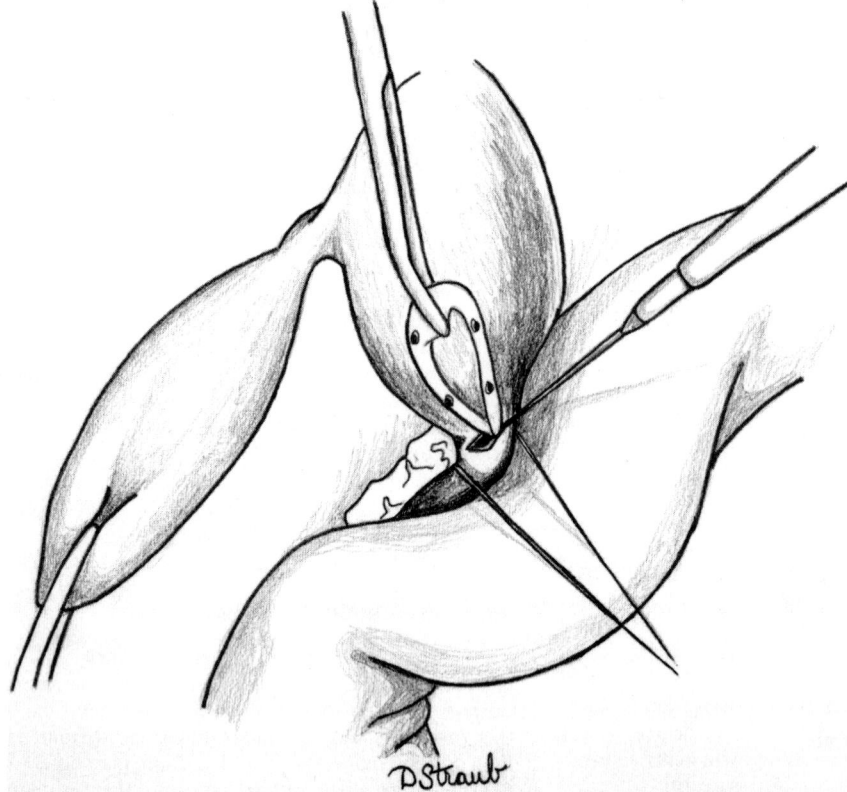

Figure 4 Transection of the distal choledochal cyst.

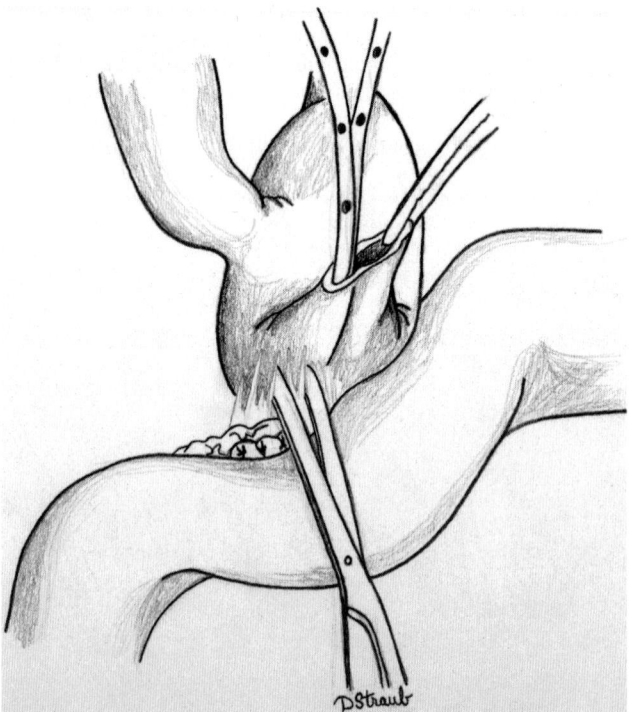

Figure 5 Distal dissection of the choledochal cyst as it enters the pancreas.

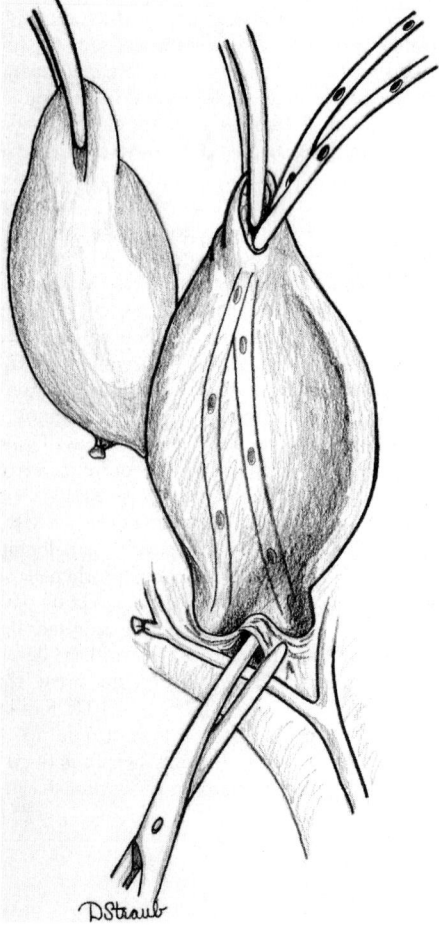

Figure 6 Proximal dissection of the cyst using the bile stent for anterior reflection.

(Fig. 6). Care must be taken to identify aberrant or variant biliary or vascular anatomy. Hemostasis must be meticulous. The cyst is usually transected just below the hepatic bifurcation. However, the hepatic bile ducts must be carefully examined for the presence of strictures, and a separate left and right hepatic duct anastomosis must be performed if strictures are present. Otherwise, a standard 45-cm Roux-en-Y loop is used for an end-side hepaticojejunostomy. The anastomosis is constructed with a single layer of absorbable

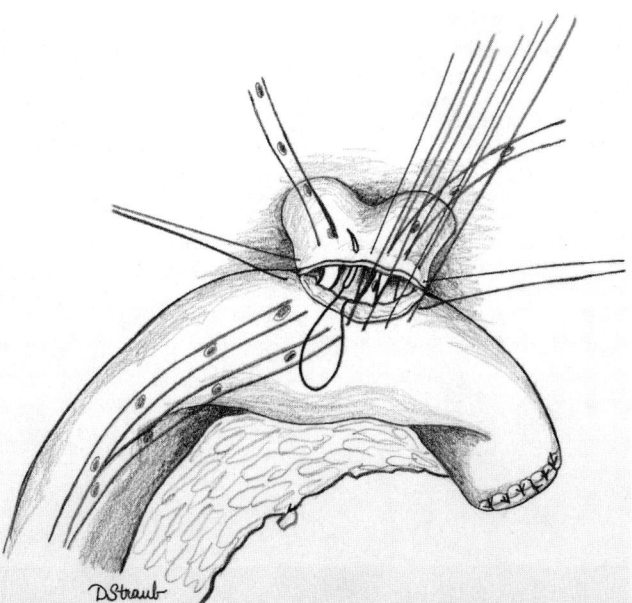

Figure 7 Construction of the Roux-en-Y anastomosis, anterior layer.

suture (Fig. 7). If a bile stent is present, the stent is placed into the jejunum after the posterior suture line is completed and the anterior suture line stitches placed and tied. In a patient with type IV cyst, placement of a Houston loop may be helpful. This loop is complexed to the abdominal wall and marked along its course with metallic clips to facilitate identification of the limb for future percutaneous access to the biliary tree. This is helpful because patients with type IV cysts are prone to recurrent hepatic stones. If the surgeon has advanced laparoscopic surgical skills, a type I choledochal cyst may be excised laparoscopically.

Occasionally, the inflammatory process surrounding the cyst is extensive, making excision seemingly hazardous. Because malignancy is always a concern, the cyst should be opened and the lining of the cysts excised. If this is technically difficult, the layers may be more easily separated by injection of saline into the wall of the cyst. A hepaticojejunostomy is then constructed as described earlier, leaving the cyst wall in place. However, as much as possible of the cyst wall should be removed. As a point of emphasis, leaving the cyst wall or any major part of it in place should be uncommon. Patients with a previous cystenterostomy can be approached in a similar fashion if the cyst cannot be excised. However, cancer may be present in this patient population, and frozen section may be necessary to rule out the presence of malignancy.

Type II: Bile Duct Cysts

Type II bile duct cysts are rare. They are easily treated with simple cyst excision. The defect in the wall of the common bile duct should be closed in a transverse rather than a longitudinal fashion. This requires mobilization of the bile duct to prevent tension and minimize the possibility of narrowing the lumen of the common bile duct.

Type III: Bile Duct Cysts—the Choledochocele

The risk of cancer in a type III cyst is not clear and may be lower than in other types of cysts. Accordingly, the absolute requirement for excision is less. In symptomatic patients, the cyst is approached from a lateral duodenostomy in the second portion of the duodenum. The pancreatic and bile ducts must be individually identified and are best intubated with a small silastic or feeding tube. The cyst is then excised. The mucosa of the bile duct and pancreatic duct is individually sutured to the duodenal mucosa using interrupted sutures. If necessary, sphincteroplasty may be performed. The duodenostomy is closed transversely.

Type IV: Bile Duct Cysts

In patients with a type IVA cyst, extrahepatic biliary resection, as with the type I cyst, is recommended. The entire involved portion of the extrahepatic biliary tree should be resected when possible. Usually, individual reconstruction of the left, right, and any accessory ducts is necessary. A hepaticojejunostomy is constructed as described earlier. Because these patients have the greatest likelihood of recurrent cholangitis, stricture formation, and hepatolithiasis, a Houston loop may be helpful. In all cases, marking the limb with metallic clips can assist in the future nonoperative management of complications. Large-bore silastic stents are best left in place in these patients to facilitate management of these problems.

Type V: Bile Duct Cysts

Caroli's disease is often confined to a single hepatic lobe, typically the left side. If cholangitis is present and the disease is confined to a single lobe, hepatic resection may be indicated. If a large cyst is present within a single inaccessible hepatic segment, the cyst can be unroofed to a Roux-en-Y limb. In some cases in which the intrahepatic disease has resulted in extensive fibrosis, liver transplantation may be a reasonable and effective choice.

PROGNOSIS

After a biliary cyst is recognized and diagnosed, management is usually straightforward in experienced hands. Patients who present with complications such as cholangitis or pancreatitis should be initially managed symptomatically until definitive surgical therapy is possible. In the perioperative period, the typical surgical problems can occur, but anastomotic leak is uncommon. Pancreatitis is a possible complication secondary to aggressive manipulation of the distal end of the cyst, involving the long common channel.

Late complications of cholangitis and anastomotic stricture are seen in as many as 25% to 35% of patients and can also include the development of both intrahepatic and bile duct stones. These complications appear to be greatest in type IV cysts and should be approached and treated aggressively. Occasionally, percutaneous dilatation of a biliary stricture may be helpful. Choledochoscopy can be used to extract stones directly and may also be used to survey for the development of malignancy.

Although technically challenging, patients with a history of biliary cystic disease that was previously bypassed should be offered the option of resection. However, patients with a history of either resection or bypass remain at a 20-fold increased risk for the development of malignancy. The risk of malignancy is less, but not eliminated, with resection, presumably because of field defects and exposure to carcinogens. Patients with a history of bile duct cyst excision should have lifelong follow-up.

Earlier identification of this disease has been seen with increased frequency and is likely to continue with evolving and improved, less invasive means of diagnosis. Future trends in the management of this disease may include more resections being performed with minimally invasive approaches, such as combined endoscopic and laparoscopic techniques.

SUGGESTED READINGS

De Vries JS, de Vries S, Aronson DC, and others: Choledochal cysts: age of presentation, symptoms, and late complications related to Todani's classification, *J Ped Surg* 37:1568, 2002.

Kaneyama K, Yamataka A, Kobayashi H, and others: Mixed type I and II choledochal cyst: a new clinical subtype? *Pediatr Surg Int* 21:911, 2005.

Lipsett PA, Locke JE: Biliary cystic disease, *Curr Treat Options Gastroenterol* 9:107, 2006.

Lipsett PA, Pitt HA: Surgical treatment of choledochal cysts, *J Hepatobiliary Pancreat Surg* 10:352, 2003.

Lipsett PA, Pitt HA, Colombani PM, and others: Choledochal cyst disease: a changing pattern of presentation, *Ann Surg* 220:644, 1994.

Plata-Munoz JJ, Mercado MA, and others: Complete resection of choledochal cyst with Roux-en-Y derivation vs. cystenterostomy as standard treatment of cystic disease of the biliary tract in the adult patient, *Hepatogastroenterology* 52:13, 2005.

Shi LB, Peng SY, Meng XK, and others: Diagnosis and treatment of congenital choledochal cyst: 20 years' experience in China, *World J Gastroenterol* 7:732, 2001.

Shimotakahara A, Yamataka A, Yanai T, and others: Roux-en-Y hepaticojejunostomy or hepaticoduodenostomy for biliary reconstruction during the surgical treatment of choledochal cyst: which is better? *Pediatr Surg Int* 21:5, 2005.

Soreide K, Korner H, Havnen J, and others: Bile duct cysts in adults, *Br J Surg* 91:1538, 2004.

Watanabe Y, Toki A, Todani T: Bile duct cancer developed after cyst excision for choledochal cyst, *J Hepatobiliary Pancreat Surg* 63:207, 1999.

Wiseman K, Buczkowski AK, Chung SW, and others: Epidemiology, presentation, diagnosis, and outcomes of choledochal cysts in adults in an urban environment, *Am J Surg* 189:527, 2005.

GALLSTONE ILEUS

Sam G. Pappas, MD, and Steven A. Ahrendt, MD

PATHOGENESIS

Gallstone ileus is mechanical obstruction of the gastrointestinal tract secondary to an impacted gallstone. This process starts with the impaction of a large gallstone within the gallbladder. Ischemia and pressure necrosis of the gallbladder wall lead to inflammatory adhesion of the gallbladder to adjacent viscera (duodenum, gastric antrum, transverse colon) and eventually to erosion of the gallstone into the adjacent structure with formation of a cholecystoduodenal, cholecystogastric, or cholecystocolonic fistula.

Larger gallstones (>2.5 cm) subsequently impact in the intestinal tract, producing signs and symptoms of small bowel obstruction. Most commonly, obstruction occurs in the narrower-caliber terminal ileum. Large gallstones passing through a cholecystocolonic fistula typically become impacted in the sigmoid colon. Impaction of a large gallstone in the duodenal bulb or pyloric channel leads to gastric outlet obstruction (Bouveret's syndrome). Occasionally gallstones produce intermittent symptoms (tumbling obstruction) as they pass distally in the gastrointestinal tract. The majority of stones smaller than 2 cm will not produce intestinal obstruction.

CLINICAL PRESENTATION

Gallstone ileus usually produces signs and symptoms consistent with acute small bowel obstruction. Most patients are female, and more than 50% have an antecedent history of biliary tract disease. The presence of comorbidities may delay the diagnosis of gallstone ileus in the elderly, and many patients present with symptoms of more than 4 days' duration. Patients may also note intermittent relief in their symptoms during the course of their illness. The intermittent symptoms result from the tumbling nature of the obstructing stone, causing intermittent obstruction followed by relief as the stone travels farther down the bowel until it again obstructs the bowel lumen.

DIAGNOSTIC IMAGING

Prompt diagnosis and appropriate therapy are critical to lowering the high morbidity and mortality of gallstone ileus in an elderly patient

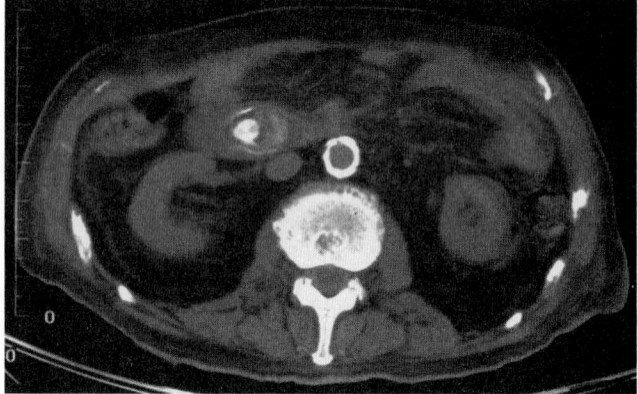

Figure 1 Computerized tomogram of a large calcified gallstone in the third portion of the duodenum. *Computed tomography scan courtesy Dr. Elin Angeid-Bachman, Department of Radiology, Medical College of Georgia, Augusta, Georgia.*

population. Abdominal plain films are usually the first radiologic study obtained in patients with signs and symptoms of small bowel obstruction. Classic findings (Rigler's triad) of gallstone ileus on plain abdominal films include pneumobilia, small bowel air-fluid levels compatible with obstruction, and an ectopic gallstone. However, these findings are present in only a minority of patients (30% to 35%) with gallstone ileus, and the sensitivity of abdominal plain films in making the diagnosis of gallstone ileus ranges from 40% to 70%.

Abdominal computed tomography (CT) has been used increasingly in the diagnosis and management of small bowel obstruction and is useful in the diagnosis of gallstone ileus. Features of gallstone ileus present on CT include an abnormal gallbladder containing air, an air-fluid level, or oral contrast; an ectopic gallstone; and dilatated small bowel consistent with obstruction (Fig. 1). Gallstone calcification is easier to detect by CT than plain films (25%) and has been reported in up to 100% of patients with large gallstones causing gallstone ileus. Oral contrast and intravenous contrast enhancement of the small intestinal wall may obscure calcified gallstones. Overall, CT has 93% sensitivity, 100% specificity, and 99% accuracy in diagnosing gallstone ileus.

MANAGEMENT

The appropriate management of gallstone ileus is operative relief of the intestinal obstruction with or without cholecystectomy and repair of the biliary intestinal fistula. Spontaneous relief is rare in patients with signs and symptoms of obstruction, and immediate operative intervention is warranted. Nausea, vomiting, and abdominal pain have usually been present for several days, and therefore preoperative correction of electrolyte abnormalities and fluid deficits and placement of a nasogastric tube are necessary.

Exploratory laparotomy with enterolithotomy remains the standard management strategy for patients with gallstone ileus. Every effort should be made to optimize the patient's status before surgical exploration because this disease primarily occurs in elderly patients with many preexisting comorbidities. We prefer a midline laparotomy to ensure adequate visualization of the entire bowel, with special attention to assessing the viability of the affected segment and the presence of additional intraluminal gallstones. After the entire bowel has been visualized, the stone is milked back to an unaffected segment of proximal bowel and delivered through a longitudinal enterotomy. Care is taken to avoid contamination of the peritoneal cavity, and the bowel is closed transversely in a standard two-layer closure. Small bowel resection should be reserved only for instances in which there is full-thickness ischemic necrosis at the impaction site because this approach may be associated with higher anastomotic leak rates. Primary anastomosis is usually feasible, although proximal enterostomy may occasionally be necessary, determined on the basis of surgeon judgment, intestinal viability, patient condition, and degree of contamination.

Considerable debate remains as to the preference of a one-stage versus a two-stage approach to managing the intestinal obstruction and definitive closure of the cholecystenteric fistula. The two-stage approach to managing these patients offers immediate operative relief of the obstruction with management of the fistula at a later date, when the patient's condition is optimal and the acute inflammatory process surrounding the biliary enteric fistula has resolved. Most patients tolerate this approach with reasonable morbidity and low mortality. The likelihood that the cholecystenteric fistula will cause a significant problem is low, and the spontaneous closure rate favors observation. We favor this approach in patients with significant comorbidities, lower performance status, intraoperative hemodynamic instability, or greater degrees of inflammation. In the largest review to date, Reisner and Cohen found a higher mortality rate associated with the one-stage approach compared with patients who underwent enterolithotomy alone.

The one-stage approach offers relief of the obstructing stone and prevention of future complications related to the presence of the bilioenteric fistula. In low-risk, stable patients, the one-stage strategy may be the preferred approach. Cholecystectomy and closure of the biliary enteric fistula should be undertaken only when the inflammatory process involving the gallbladder, duodenum, and extrahepatic bile duct is limited in extent. Most authors cite improved preoperative and postoperative care as reasons to support definitive management of both the obstructing stone and the presence of a cholecystenteric fistula.

Recent advances with minimally invasive techniques have led to increasing interest in managing these patients laparoscopically. Several authors have reported their experiences with laparoscopic-assisted enterolithotomy and have found success with this approach. A few technical aspects to this approach are worth mentioning. Access to the abdominal cavity for insufflation should be obtained using an optical trocar or under direct vision because

the bowel is often distended proximally and is at risk for injury if blind access is attempted. Conventional port access is obtained to facilitate exposure of the terminal ileum. The bowel is carefully manipulated using blunt graspers, and visualization of the entire bowel should be attempted. After the obstructing stone is discovered, the ileum is secured distally to the obstructing stone and grasped with an atraumatic grasper. The port site is enlarged, and the obstructed bowel segment is delivered through the wound. A longitudinal enterotomy is made to deliver the obstructed segment and is closed transversely to minimize narrowing the affected segment of bowel.

A recent report of successful management of proximal gallstone ileus with endoscopic approaches raises the possibility that not all patients require laparotomy. Bouveret's syndrome is a unique instance in which endoscopic therapies may be ideally suited to relieve the intestinal obstruction. Simple stone extraction and endoluminal stone ablative therapies for impacted stones have both produced acceptable outcomes. We consider this combined approach the preferred method of treatment. However, any signs of bowel compromise or decompensation warrant laparotomy.

OUTCOME

Outcome largely depends on the patient's preoperative status. Full recovery and resumption of normal bowel activity can be expected in most patients managed operatively. The incidence of postoperative infectious wound complications appears to be high (32% in one series), and consideration of delayed primary closure should be given if contamination is a problem. This risk also underscores the importance of judicious use of perioperative broad-spectrum antibiotics. Operative mortality may be higher in patients undergoing a one-stage approach, and the decision to perform both enterolithotomy and closure of the biliary-enteric fistula should not be taken lightly. In the largest review to date, Reisner and colleagues reported a higher operative mortality for a one-stage procedure compared with enterolithotomy alone (17% vs. 12%).

SUMMARY

Gallstone ileus remains a common cause of intestinal obstruction in the elderly population with significant comorbidities. Contrast-enhanced CT scanning is the preferred method of diagnosis. Once the condition is recognized, prompt surgical intervention remains the mainstay of therapy. Surgical approaches include open or laparoscopic enterolithotomy in most cases. Controversy remains as to whether to perform a one-stage versus a two-stage repair.

SUGGESTED READINGS

Kirchmayr W, Mühlmann G, Zitt M, and others: Gallstone ileus: rare and still controversial, *ANZ J Surg* 75:234, 2005.
Reisner RM, Cohen JR: Gallstone ileus: a review of 1001 reported cases, *Am Surg* 60:441, 1994.
Yu CY, Linn CC, Shyu RY, and others: Value of CT in the diagnosis and management of gallstone ileus, *World J Gastroenterol* 11:2142, 2005.

PRIMARY SCLEROSING CHOLANGITIS

Nicholas J. Zyromski, MD, and Henry A. Pitt, MD

Primary sclerosing cholangitis (PSC) is a poorly understood disease characterized by inflammatory strictures affecting both intrahepatic and extrahepatic bile ducts. The clinical course of PSC, although variable, is generally progressive, ultimately leading to cholestasis, hepatic cirrhosis, and death from liver failure. Cholangiocarcinoma develops in approximately 10% to 20% of patients with PSC and is the second leading cause of death in this patient population. No medical therapy has proved to be effective in delaying progression of disease or prolonging overall or transplant-free survival. A wide variety of percutaneous, endoscopic, and surgical approaches have been applied to patients with dominant strictures with little evidence to support the superiority of any one modality. Liver transplantation has emerged as the treatment of choice after hepatic cirrhosis develops.

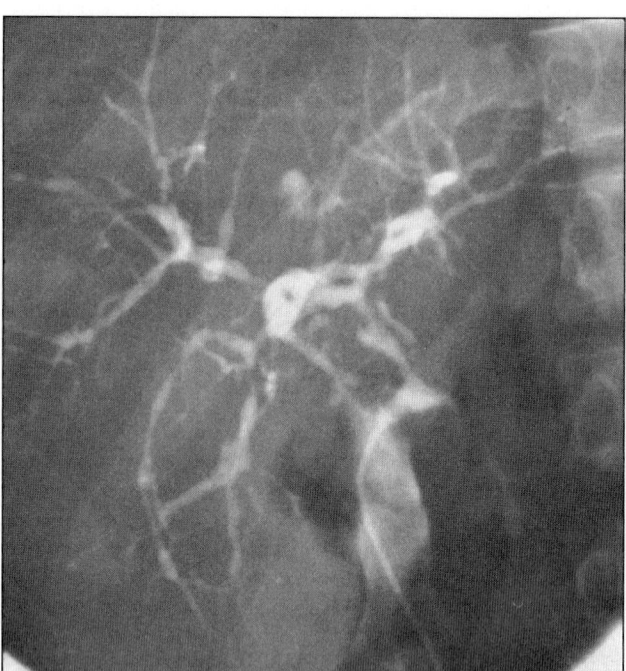

Figure 1 Endoscopic retrograde cholangiopancreatography demonstrating multiple intrahepatic and extrahepatic bile duct strictures characteristic of primary sclerosing cholangitis.

NATURAL HISTORY

Approximately two thirds of patients with PSC are male, with an average age of 42 at the time of diagnosis. The prevalence of PSC in the United States is approximately 6 per 100,000. Large population series have shown that the median survival from time of diagnosis to death or liver transplantation ranges from 12 to 18 years. The Mayo Model is a mathematical construct incorporating serum bilirubin, degree of hepatic fibrosis, presence of splenomegaly, and age. This model is widely used to predict survival and the optimal timing of liver transplantation. About 75% of patients have involvement of both intrahepatic and extrahepatic bile ducts, with 15% having only intrahepatic involvement and 10% having only extrahepatic involvement. The hepatic duct bifurcation is commonly involved in patients with extrahepatic ductal disease.

Approximately 70% of patients with PSC also have inflammatory bowel disease (IBD), most commonly ulcerative colitis. In contrast, only 10% of patients with inflammatory bowel disease develop PSC. Other autoimmune diseases associated less commonly with PSC include thyroiditis, ankylosing spondylitis, and celiac disease. PSC has been associated with a moderately increased risk for pancreatitis, pancreatic adenocarcinoma, and colorectal carcinoma. The association with cholangiocarcinoma is discussed in more detail later in the chapter.

DIAGNOSIS

The presentation of patients with PSC is widely variable. Many patients present with typical biliary symptoms of right upper quadrant pain, pruritus, and fatigue. Some patients are completely asymptomatic and diagnosed on the basis of abnormal liver function tests (e.g., the IBD patient screened for liver disease). Patients with small duct (intrahepatic) disease may present with end-stage liver disease and hepatic failure, and those with isolated extrahepatic strictures may have jaundice as the first clinical sign.

Endoscopic retrograde cholangiography (ERC) has historically been the gold standard for diagnosis of PSC and accurately demonstrates the intrahepatic and extrahepatic biliary tree more than 95%

of the time (Fig. 1). Disadvantages of ERC include the invasive nature of the test and potential for complications, including cholangitis, perforation of the biliary tree, pancreatitis, and hemorrhage. Recent advances in magnetic resonance technology have led to increased use of magnetic resonance cholangiography (MRC) in the diagnosis of PSC; indeed this test has supplanted ERC for screening purposes in many centers. MRC affords visualization of intrahepatic bile ducts proximal to high-grade strictures and, additionally, images the rest of the abdomen. The disadvantage of MRC is that it is a purely diagnostic test. Percutaneous transhepatic cholangiography in PSC is technically challenging even for an experienced interventional radiologist; however, this test is useful in select cases.

After the diagnosis of PSC has been secured, liver biopsy should be performed to document the degree of hepatic fibrosis. The possibility of lobar atrophy/hypertrophy should be considered when performing a liver biopsy in these patients. Additionally, colonoscopy is indicated in patients without the diagnosis of IBD to exclude this diagnosis.

CHOLANGIOCARCINOMA IN PRIMARY SCLEROSING CHOLANGITIS

Development of cholangiocarcinoma (CCA) is the most dreaded complication of PSC. The diagnosis of CCA is notoriously difficult in the face of multiple intrahepatic and extrahepatic bile duct strictures, and outcomes are uniformly poor. Cholangiocarcinoma is the second leading cause of death in most series of PSC. Population surveys and series of surgical resection have shown an incidence of CCA ranging from 8% to 18% (Table 1). Even the lower end of this range, however, represents an increased risk of up to 160 times that of the general population. Unsuspected ("incidental") cholangiocarcinoma is found in 3% to 9% of explanted livers at the time of transplantation for PSC despite aggressive preoperative screening protocols.

Table 1: Incidence of Cholangiocarcinoma in Select Series of Primary Sclerosing Cholangitis

First Author	Year	Study Type	N	CCA, n (%)
Tischendorf JJ	2006	Population	273	36 (13)
Burak K	2004	Population	161	11 (7)
Ponsioen CY	2002	Population	174	18 (10)
Boberg KM	2002	Population	394	48 (12)
Broome U	1996	Population	305	24 (8)
Solano E	2000	Transplant	111	3 (3)
Liden H	2000	Transplant	47	4 (9)
Graziadei IW	1999	Transplant	150	6 (4)
Goss JA	1997	Transplant	127	10 (8)
Ahrendt SA	1999	Surgical	139	25 (18)

CCA, Cholangiocarcinoma.

Cholangiocarcinoma is observed more frequently in the setting of IBD and in women; however, no correlation exists between development of hepatic cirrhosis and duration of PSC. Approximately half of patients developing CCA are diagnosed within 1 year of presentation with PSC, and many are diagnosed concurrently. Development of CCA may be suspected in the patient with sudden onset of jaundice, weight loss, and increasing abdominal pain; however, these symptoms are all nonspecific and may simply be related to progression of a benign stricture. Tissue histology is the gold standard for making the diagnosis of CCA; however, the sensitivity of biliary brushings and biopsy obtained at the time of ERC is less than 40%. Serum levels of the tumor marker carbohydrate antigen (CA)19–9 are usually elevated in patients with CCA. Although CA19–9 is relatively specific, it suffers from poor sensitivity and may be spuriously elevated (giving a false positive) in the setting of jaundice.

Computed tomography and MRC are becoming more sophisticated; however, their accuracy in diagnosing CCA remains less than 70%. The role of positron emission tomography in diagnosis of biliary malignancy has recently been evaluated; unfortunately, sensitivity and specificity are poor. Digital image analysis (DIA) and fluorescence in situ hybridization (FISH) are advanced cytologic techniques that have recently been applied to the diagnosis of CCA in PSC. Both tests attempt to define malignant cells by identification of chromosomal abnormalities (which are present in approximately 80% of biliary malignancies). Early studies with limited numbers of patients have been promising in the differentiation of benign from malignant strictures; however, the routine application of these tests is not yet universal.

Complete surgical resection offers the best prognosis for those patients developing CCA in the face of PSC. Patients with recurrent dominant strictures or those with cellular atypia or dysplasia on cytologic brushing or biopsy should therefore undergo operative exploration rather than repeated attempts at endoscopic diagnosis. Transplantation for CCA should be performed only under a strict protocol with neoadjuvant therapy.

MEDICAL THERAPY

On the basis of the putative underlying causes of PSC (i.e., autoimmunity, proinflammatory cytokines, infection, bile acid transporter/ion channel abnormalities), numerous agents have been tested in controlled clinical trials (Table 2). However, no medical therapy has been shown to slow the progression of disease, prolong survival, or improve outcomes in patients with PSC. The hydrophilic bile acid ursodeoxycholic acid (UDCA) is one of the most widely studied agents. Data from a large prospective, randomized trial of low dose

Table 2: Select Medications Studied in Treatment of Primary Sclerosing Cholangitis and Their Mechanism of Action

Agent	Mechanism of Action
Ursodeoxycholic acid (UDCA)	Hydrophilic bile acid
Prednisone	Corticosteroid
Budesonide	Corticosteroid
Colchicine	Mitotic inhibitor
Tacrolimus (FK 506)	Immunosuppressant
Methotrexate	Immunosuppressant
Mycophenolate Mofetil	Immunosuppressant
Perfinidone	Antifibrotic
Metronidazole	Antibiotic
Minocycline	Antibiotic
Etanercept	TNF-α inhibitor
Pentoxifylline	TNF-α inhibitor
Docosahexanoic acid	CFTR function

CFTR, Cystic fibrosis transmembrane conductance receptor; *TNF-α,* tumor necrosis factor-alpha.

(12–15 mg/kg daily) of UDCA demonstrated improvements in serum liver chemistry values but failed to show improvement in liver histology or transplant-free survival. Subsequent prospective studies using increased doses of UDCA have similarly failed to show beneficial effect on symptoms, serum liver chemistry values, quality of life, or transplant-free survival. Administration of both topical and systemic glucocorticoids also has been studied prospectively; to date, no evidence suggests that these medications improve any objective measure of outcome in PSC. Additionally, glucocorticoid administration may actually be dangerous because it carries an increased risk of infection and may mask symptoms of biliary infection. Current research is focused on targeted therapy with antifibrotic agents, agents that inhibit tumor necrosis factor (TNF), and inhibitors of toxic bile formation.

ENDOSCOPIC THERAPY

Beginning in the late 1980s and early 1990s, percutaneous transhepatic stenting and endoscopic dilatation with or without stenting began to be used to treat dominant strictures in PSC. The choice of a nonsurgical approach (i.e., percutaneous versus endoscopic) has depended largely on institutional expertise; however, with improvements in endoscopic techniques and technology, the majority of tertiary centers treating patients with PSC currently favor endoscopic over percutaneous approaches. Routine placement of endoscopic stents has fallen out of favor because the incidence of stent occlusion and cholangitis is significant, and prospective studies have failed to show their benefit. A clinical response can be demonstrated in up to 80% of patients after endoscopic balloon dilatation; however, to date, no prospective trial has demonstrated benefit in outcome or compared this modality directly to surgical resection of dominant extrahepatic stricture. Complications of endoscopic therapy arise in approximately 10% of patients and include bleeding, perforation, pancreatitis, and cholangitis. The majority of these complications resolve with medical management.

A representative series of patients with PSC and a dominant stricture treated endoscopically was recently reported from Indiana University. In this large series, 63 patients were treated endoscopically over a 6-year time period, with a median follow-up of 34 months. Sixty-one patients underwent balloon dilatation a mean of 2.3 ($\pm$ 2.0 SD) times. Fifty-three percent of patients had a temporary biliary stent placed. Seven patients died (five from liver failure, two from cholangiocarcinoma), and eight underwent liver transplantation. Cholangiocarcinoma was diagnosed in five patients (8%) in this series. Overall 1-, 3-, and 5-year survival was 97%, 87%, and 83%, respectively. These survival rates were significantly improved compared with survival predicted by the Mayo Risk Score (92%, 77%, and 65%, respectively). The authors appropriately concluded that these results should be viewed with caution because they provide only indirect evidence that endoscopic stenting improves survival in patients with PSC and dominant strictures. A persistent concern with prolonged endoscopic therapy is the delay in diagnosis of CCA.

SURGICAL RESECTION

In select patients with dominant extrahepatic strictures and no hepatic cirrhosis, resection of the extrahepatic biliary tree and reconstruction with a Roux-en-Y limb of jejunum and transhepatic

biliary stenting provides durable relief of jaundice, confirms or excludes the diagnosis of CCA, and delays the progression of hepatic cirrhosis and need for liver transplantation.

Ahrendt and colleagues at Johns Hopkins compared outcomes of 146 patients with PSC managed by surgical resection, percutaneous or endoscopic balloon dilatation with or without stenting, medical therapy alone, and transplantation. In noncirrhotic patients, overall 5-year survival (85% vs. 59%) and transplant-free survival (82% vs. 46%) were significantly longer in the resection group versus those managed with endoscopic or percutaneous balloon dilatation (Fig. 2, A and B). Importantly, CCA developed in 6% of the endoscopically treated group and none of the resected patients with long-term follow-up (>5 years). Patients with hepatic cirrhosis had longer survival after transplantation than after resection or endoscopic management.

In up to 80% of patients with dominant strictures, the hepatic duct bifurcation is involved; percutaneous stents are therefore placed preoperatively into both the right and left hepatic ducts. This maneuver greatly facilitates dissection of the hepatic bifurcation and provides stenting for the reconstructive hepaticojejunostomies. Transhepatic stents are virtually all colonized with bacteria; thus perioperative antibiotics are tailored to cover specific bacteria cultured from the bile and continued postoperatively until the patient remains afebrile for 24 hours to treat the mild cholangitis that occurs with intraoperative stent manipulation and cholangiography. High-quality computed tomography with intravascular contrast allows preoperative assessment of variant hepatic arterial anatomy, as well as the presence of atrophy/hypertrophy.

The general operative approach to resection of the extrahepatic biliary tree with Roux-en- Y cholangiojejunostomy over transhepatic stents is illustrated in Figure 3, A and B. An upper midline incision provides excellent exposure of the hepatic bifurcation and allows optimal positioning of the transhepatic stents on the abdominal wall. Careful abdominal exploration is undertaken, and suspicious lymph nodes are biopsied for frozen section. Intraoperative ultrasonography is routinely applied; suspicious intrahepatic nodules are likewise biopsied. The hepatic flexure of the colon is mobilized, and a Kocher maneuver is performed.

Cholecystectomy is performed if the gallbladder is in situ, and the common bile duct is divided close to the pancreas to remove

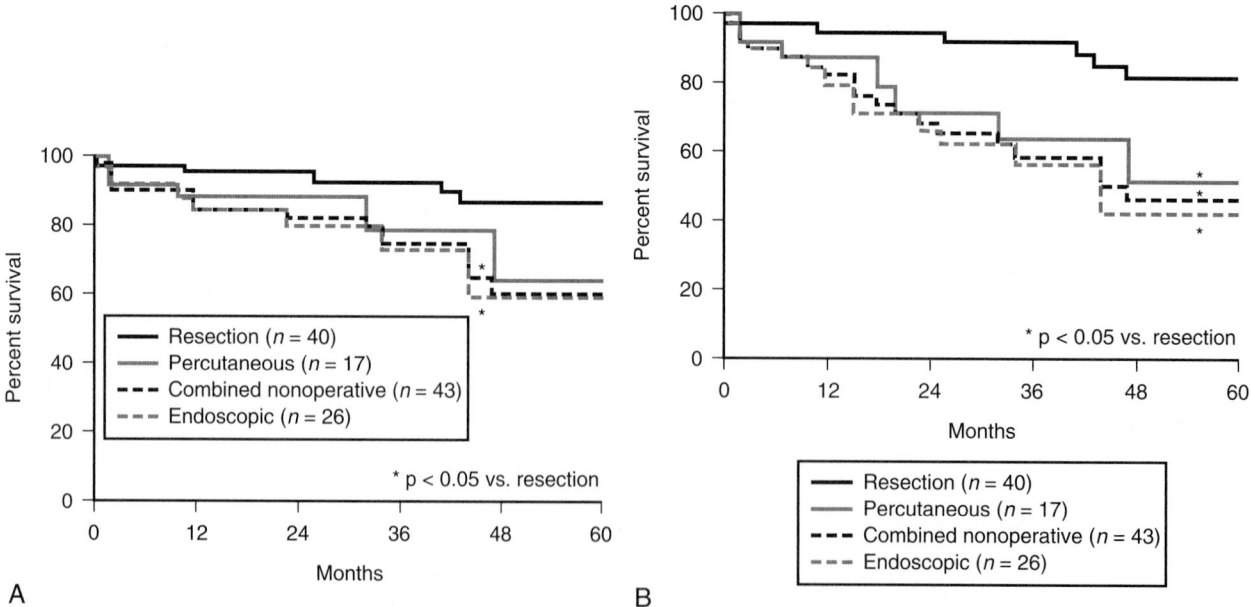

Figure 2 Overall (**A**) and transplant-free (**B**) survival curves for noncirrhotic patients undergoing resection, percutaneous, and endoscopic treatment of dominant extrahepatic biliary strictures in primary sclerosing cholangitis. *From Ahrendt SA: Ann Surg 227:419, 1998.*

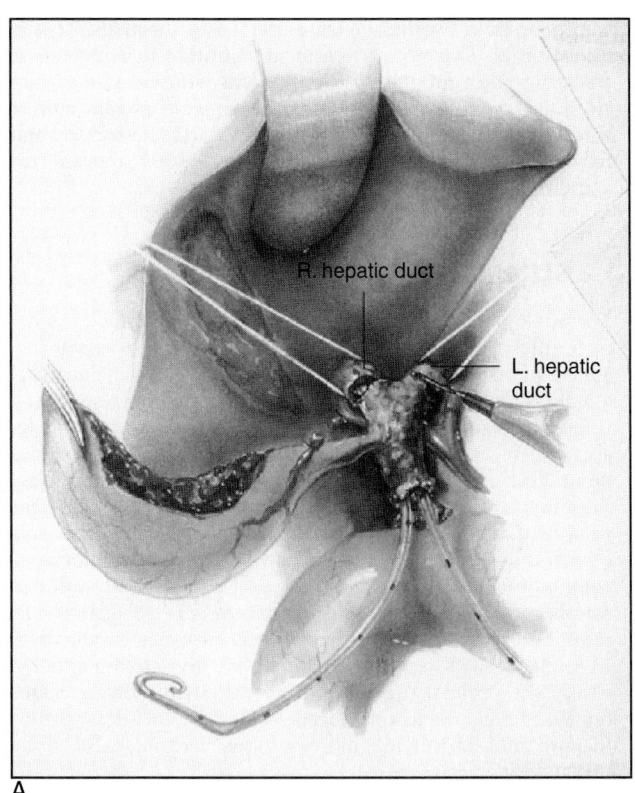
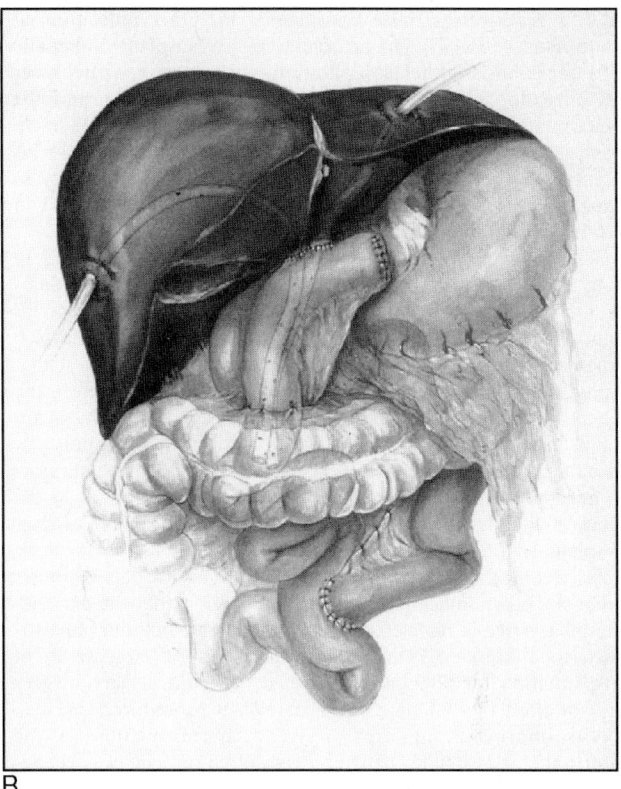

Figure 3 **(A)** The extrahepatic bile duct and hepatic duct bifurcation are removed. **(B)** Completed retrocolic Roux-en-Y cholangiojejunostomies with transhepatic stents. *From Cameron JL: Atlas of surgery, vol 1, Philadelphia, 1990, BC Decker, Inc., with permission.*

as much biliary epithelium as possible. The distal common bile duct at the edge of the pancreas is oversewn, and dissection continues proximally, lifting the bile duct off of the portal vein. The usual course of the right hepatic artery is to pass posterior to the common hepatic duct; such anatomy should be anticipated at this point of the dissection. The right and left main hepatic ducts are divided proximal to the bifurcation, and frozen sections are obtained of all margins to confirm the absence of malignancy. The preoperative transhepatic stents are exchanged for large Silastic catheters. A Roux limb of jejunum is brought through the transverse mesocolon to the right of the middle colic vessels, and cholangiojejunostomies are created around the Silastic catheters. Chromic sutures are placed at the exit site of the stents from the liver to minimize bile leakage.

Completion cholangiography is performed in the operating room to ensure optimal stent positioning and to exclude anastomotic leak. The Silastic stents are brought through the abdominal wall in a subcostal position away from the midline incision. Incorporation of a gentle curve is important to avoid kinking of the stent and to facilitate subsequent radiologic stent changes. Closed-suction drains are placed behind the cholangiojejunostomies and at the site of stent exit from the liver. Overall morbidity after extrahepatic biliary resection with Roux-en-Y biliary anastomosis is approximately 30% to 40%, and perioperative mortality is less than 3%. Specific complications include cholangitis, hemobilia, and bile leak; almost all are amenable to nonoperative management.

LIVER TRANSPLANTATION:

Liver transplantation is the optimal treatment modality for PSC after cirrhosis has developed. Approximately 5% of all liver transplants in the United States are performed for end-stage liver disease

secondary to PSC. Survival of patients after liver transplant for PSC is generally good; several large series have documented 5-year patient and graft survival of approximately 80% to 85% and 70% to 75%, respectively. These outcomes are modestly better than those of liver transplantation performed for other indications (Fig. 4). Patients transplanted for PSC have a somewhat higher retransplant

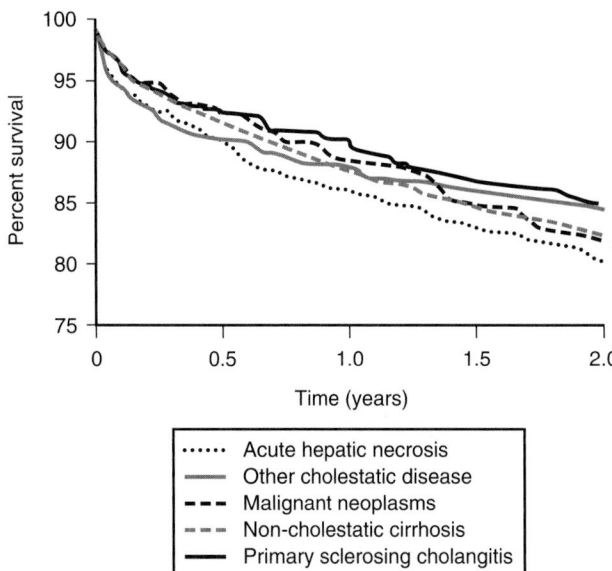

Figure 4 Survival curves for liver transplantation performed for primary sclerosing cholangitis versus other indications. *From LaRusso NF, Schneider BL, Black D: Hepatology 44:756, 2006.*

rate at 2 years versus those transplanted for other indications—9.6% versus 4.9%. The major cause for retransplant is hepatic artery thrombosis. Other complications include somewhat higher rates of acute cellular and chronic ductopenic rejection and the development of biliary strictures. Recurrent PSC may occur in up to one third of patients undergoing liver transplant, although this percentage is difficult to define precisely because of variability in diagnostic criteria and follow-up. Whether recurrence of PSC in the transplanted liver directly affects outcome is unclear.

Despite aggressive surveillance, unsuspected CCA is found in 3% to 9% of explanted livers of patients undergoing transplantation for PSC, again highlighting the difficulty in establishing this diagnosis preoperatively. Interestingly, data from both the Mayo Clinic and the University of California at Los Angeles suggest that finding a small (<1 cm) unsuspected CCA does not affect the long-term survival of these patients. Patients from these same series with a known diagnosis of CCA preoperatively had significantly worse outcomes. Outside of an investigational protocol using rigorous neoadjuvant chemoradiotherapy, the presence of CCA in the setting of PSC is generally considered a contraindication to liver transplantation.

The technical conduct of liver transplantation for PSC is similar to that for other indications, with the exception that the extrahepatic biliary tree is resected and the donor graft bile duct anastomosed to a Roux-en-Y limb of jejunum. Several large series of transplantation for PSC have confirmed that prior biliary surgery does not affect the outcome of the transplant procedure.

With improved long-term survival after transplantation, the importance of associated IBD and risk of colon cancer is recognized. Among patients with IBD, the risk of developing colonic malignancy is approximately 15% 5 years after liver transplantation. Aggressive screening protocols with colonoscopy are therefore warranted in this population. UDCA may decrease the risk of colon cancer in PSC patients with IBD and is commonly administered, although little evidence exists to support this treatment.

Outcomes of hepatic transplantation for PSC are improved if the transplant is performed before the development of cirrhosis. Therefore an unanswered question is whether patients with PSC should undergo early or late transplantation. The overall goals of early transplantation are to reduce the risk of CCA, improve survival, and reduce the overall cost of medical therapy. Because most CCAs are diagnosed within 1 year of diagnosis of PSC, early transplantation would play a small (4%) role in prevention and would not improve survival over 5 years. Additionally, early transplantation would increase the costs of medical care by 2 to 3 times. Therefore a treatment algorithm that includes early transplantation for the 10% of patients with established cirrhosis, biliary surgery for patients with dominant extrahepatic strictures (10%) or suspicion of CCA (10%), and late transplantation for low- and moderate-risk patients (70%) appears to be warranted.

SUMMARY

The etiology and pathogenesis of PSC are poorly understood, and no medical therapy has been shown to be effective in slowing the course of the disease. Endoscopic retrograde cholangiopancreatography is the gold standard for diagnosis. Magnetic resonance cholangiopancreatography techniques have improved, and this test is also widely used for diagnosis and surveillance. Cholangiocarcinoma develops in 8% to 18% of patients with PSC; however, the diagnosis of malignancy is notoriously difficult to differentiate from that of benign stricture. Endoscopic therapy with balloon dilatation is commonly applied; however, the risk of cholangiocarcinoma must be appreciated. For select patients with a dominant extrahepatic stricture (10%) or concern for malignancy (10%), resection of the extrahepatic biliary tree provides durable therapy. In patients with established cirrhosis, liver transplantation is clearly the optimal therapy. Current research efforts are focused on elucidating the etiopathogenesis of PSC, developing medical therapy, and identifying more sensitive techniques to diagnose malignancy.

SUGGESTED READINGS

Ahrendt SA, Pitt HA, Kalloo AN, and others: Primary sclerosing cholangitis: resect, dilate, or transplant? *Ann Surg* 227:412, 1998.

Ahrendt SA, Pitt HA, Nakeeb A, and others: Diagnosis and management of cholangiocarcinoma in primary sclerosing cholangitis, *J Gastrointest Surg* 3:357, 1999.

Baluyut AR, Sherman S, Lehman GA, and others: Impact of endoscopic therapy on the survival of patients with primary sclerosing cholangitis, *Gastrointest Endosc* 53:308, 2001.

Cameron JL, Pitt HA, Zinner MJ, and others: Resection of hepatic duct bifurcation and transhepatic stenting for sclerosing cholangitis, *Ann Surg* 207:614, 1988.

Graziadei IW, Weisner RH, Marotta PJ, and others: Long-term results of patients undergoing liver transplantation for primary sclerosing cholangitis, *Hepatology* 30:1121, 1999.

BILE DUCT CANCER

Steven C. Cunningham, MD, and Richard D. Schulick, MD

INTRODUCTION

Of the approximately 7500 annual new cases of cancer of the biliary system in the United States, approximately 5000 are bile duct cancers (cholangiocarcinomas), the remainder being cancers of the gallbladder. From the 1970s to the 2000s, the worldwide ratio of extrahepatic to intrahepatic cholangiocarcinoma has shifted from 1:2 to 1:1, together comprising 3% of all malignancies. Risk for the development of bile duct cancer is most strongly and relevantly associated with sclerosing cholangitis (8% to 20% lifetime risk) and choledochal cysts (3% to 28% lifetime risk). Asian descent and male gender confer a twofold and 1.5-fold increased risk, respectively.

Macroscopically, intrahepatic bile duct cancer has been classified on the basis of patterns of growth, including mass-forming, periductal infiltrating, and intraductal, whereas extrahepatic bile duct cancer may be sclerosing, nodular, or papillary. Microscopically, cholangiocarcinoma is most commonly a tubular adenocarcinoma, but papillary adenocarcinoma, signet-cell carcinoma, mucoepidermoid carcinoma, and other histological variants of cholangiocarcinoma may be uncommonly observed.

Various classification systems have been described, often broadly separating those arising within the liver from those arising without and subdividing the latter group into proximal, middle, and distal subgroups. At Johns Hopkins, we have favored the simpler—and

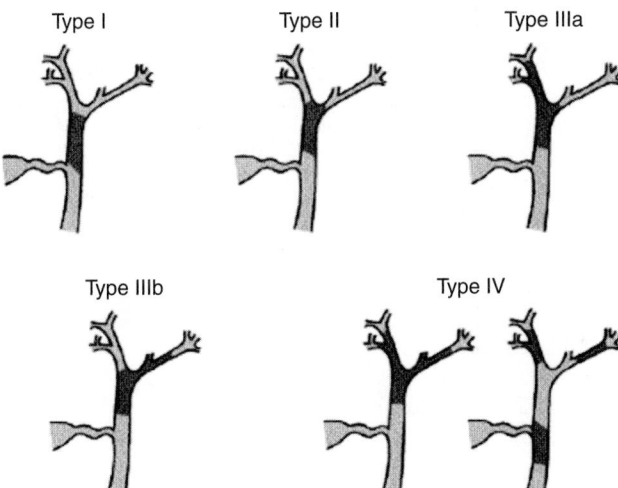

Figure 1 Classification of (peri)hilar cholangiocarcinoma according to the Bismuth-Corlette system. *From Lazaridis KN, Gores GJ: Gastroenterology 128:1655.*

clinically and surgically relevant—three-tiered classification system comprising intrahepatic, perihilar, and distal groups. Perihilar tumors may be further classified according to the Bismuth-Corlette system (Fig. 1).

DIAGNOSIS

Intrahepatic, perihilar, and distal bile duct cancers may each produce a unique set of symptoms, although overlap is common (Table 1). Intrahepatic lesions are significantly more likely to produce pain initially than perihilar or distal lesions and are typically associated with other nonspecific symptoms such as anorexia, weight loss, night sweats, malaise, and fatigue. Perihilar and distal lesions, by contrast, are significantly more likely than intrahepatic lesions to present with stigmata of biliary obstruction, especially jaundice, and commonly present with weight loss. Alkaline phosphatase and tumor markers (such as CEA and carbohydrate antigen 19–9) may be elevated in cases of bile duct cancer arising from any of the three locations but lack sensitivity and specificity.

Table 1: Signs and Symptoms of Cholangiocarcinoma

	Intrahepatic	Perihilar	Distal
Abdominal pain	XX*	X	X
Anorexia	X	X	X
Weight loss	X	XX	XX
Pruritis	X	X	X
Jaundice	—†	XXX	XXX
Distended palpable GB	—	—	X
Abnormal AP/GGT	X	X	X

From Nakeeb A, Pitt HA, Sohn TA, and others: Ann Surg 224:463, 1996.
AP, Alkaline phosphatase; *GB*, gallbladder; *GGT*, gamma glutamyl transpeptidase.
*Number of Xs indicates approximate relative likelihood of finding indicated signs or symptoms.
†$p < .05$

Several imaging modalities are available to assess resectability. The choice of imaging modalities depends in part on the anatomic structures of most interest. The general trend has been toward less invasive modalities of imaging. Although the bile ducts can be best visualized by endoscopic retrograde cholangiopancreatography (ERCP) or percutaneous transhepatic cholangiography (PTC), magnetic resonance cholangiopancreatography (MRCP) gives nearly equivalent imaging information and is noninvasive. Patients are often referred to our institution after placement of an endostent and cholangiography. If better delineation of the biliary tree is required, an MRCP is often helpful. If these modalities are insufficient to demonstrate the anatomy of the biliary tree, we occasionally have the patient undergo PTC. Major vascular involvement can be ascertained by multidetector computed tomography (CT); with three-dimensional reconstructions (3-D CT); by magnetic resonance angiography (MRA); or, historically, by traditional angiography. The liver parenchyma, as well as distant sites of metastasis, can also be studied using either CT or magnetic resonance imaging.

The differential diagnosis for cholangiocarcinoma includes benign biliary strictures as may result from diseases such as primary sclerosing cholangitis (PSC), choledocholithiasis, and Mirizzi's syndrome. The diagnosis of cholangiocarcinoma superimposed on PSC is especially challenging because there may not be a dominant biliary stricture. Nonbiliary malignancies, such as primary and metastatic liver cancers, and nonbiliary periampullary cancers are also in the differential diagnosis. If nonoperative management is pursued, percutaneous or endoscopic biopsy should be performed to establish the diagnosis. Otherwise, biopsy is not required.

STAGING

The American Joint Committee on Cancer staging system for cholangiocarcinoma does not adequately account for resectability. For this reason, Jarnagin and colleagues have recently proposed the Blumgart staging system (Table 2), which incorporates local tumor extent. In this system, tumors are classified according to three factors: bile duct involvement (according to the Bismuth-Corlette system, Fig. 1), portal vein invasion, and hepatic lobar atrophy. Using this system, Jarnagin and colleagues were able to predict resectability, metastasis, and survival in 219 patients.

PREOPERATIVE PREPARATION

Because of the potential for significant morbidity and mortality associated with cholangiocarcinoma resection, all patients considered for resection should receive preoperative treatment for correctable medical comorbidities, such as malnutrition, coagulopathy, and treatable cardiac, pulmonary, and renal disease.

The use of preoperative stenting is no longer routine and indeed may increase the rate of infectious complications. Nevertheless, biliary stenting is used in select cases. Potential advantages include decompressing an obstructed biliary tree (in patients with a bilirubin >15 mg/dl, to allow hepatic function to improve) and providing patients suffering from malnutrition, biliary sepsis, or other medical problems time to recover before an elective resection.

Because resection offers the only hope for a cure, all potentially resectable patients should be considered for operation unless prohibitive contraindications are present. Patient-related contraindications include severe medical comorbidities, especially major cardiopulmonary disease and cirrhosis. Blumgart and colleagues have proposed local tumor-related criteria for unresectability (Table 3). Tumor-related contraindications include involvement of bilateral secondary ducts or unilateral ducts with

Table 2: Staging of Cholangiocarcinoma

Staging System	Stage	Tumor	Node	Metastasis
AJCC TNM intrahepatic	I	T1	N0	M0
	II	T2	N0	M0
	IIIA	T3	N0	M0
	IIIB	T4	N0	M0
	IIIC	Any T	N1	M0
	IV	Any T	Any N	M1
		T1, solitary tumor without vascular invasion; T2, solitary tumor with vascular invasion or multiple <5 cm; T3, multiple >5 cm or major vascular involvement; T4, direct invasion of adjacent organ (not gallbladder) or perforation of visceral peritoneum; N1, regional LN metastases; M1, distant metastases.		
AJCC TNM extrahepatic	0	Tis	N0	M0
	IA	T1	N0	M0
	IB	T2	N0	M0
	IIA	T3	N0	M0
	IIB	T1 to T3	N1	M0
	III	T4	Any N	M0
	IV	Any T	Any N	M1
		Tis, carcinoma in situ; T1, confined to bile duct; T2, beyond bile duct; T3, invades liver, gallbladder, pancreas, or unilateral HA or PV; T4, invades other adjacent organs or main HA or PV; N1, regional LN metastasis; M1, distant metastasis		
Blumgart T-stage criteria perihilar		**Criteria**		
	T1	Tumor involving biliary confluence ± unilateral extension to second-order biliary radicles		
	T2	Tumor involving biliary confluence ± unilateral extension to second-order biliary radicles *and* ipsilateral portal vein involvement ± ipsilateral hepatic lobar atrophy		
	T3	Tumor involving biliary confluence + bilateral extension to second-order biliary radicles; or unilateral extension to second-order biliary radicles with contralateral portal vine involvement; or unilateral extension to second-order biliary radicles with contralateral hepatic lobar atrophy; or main or bilateral portal venous involvement		

Modified from AJCC Staging, 6th edition and Jarnagin et al, Ann Surg 234:507.
AJCC, American Joint Committee on Cancer; HA, hepatic artery; LN, lymph node; PV, portal vein; TNM staging system, T, primary tumor; N, regional lymph nodes; M, distant metastasis.

Table 3: Local Tumor-Related Criteria for Unresectability

1. Hepatic duct involvement up to secondary biliary radicals bilaterally

2. Encasement or occlusion of the main portal vein proximal to its bifurcation*

3. Atrophy of one hepatic lobe with contralateral encasement of portal vein branch

4. Atrophy of one hepatic lobe with contralateral involvement of secondary biliary radicals

5. Unilateral tumor extension to secondary biliary radicles with contralateral vein branch encasement or occlusion

*Relative criterion. Portal vein resection and reconstruction may be possible.
Modified from Jarnigan WR, Fong Y, DeMatteo RP, and others: Ann Surg 234:507, 2001.

contralateral vein branch compromise, encasement or occlusion of the main portal vein, and hepatic lobe atrophy with contralateral compromise of the secondary duct or portal vein branches.

RESECTION

Intrahepatic Resection

Intrahepatic cholangiocarcinomas are resected by standard hepatectomy techniques. Lesions are considered resectable if localized and if 25% or more of normal liver remnant can be maintained with adequate hepatic portal and arterial inflow, hepatic venous outflow, and biliary enteric drainage. For extensive lesions, consideration should be given to preoperative embolization of the involved side to increase the size of the future liver remnant.

Intrahepatic cholangiocarcinomas can be resected using anatomic and nonanatomic (large wedge resection) techniques.

Generally, smaller and more peripheral lesions can be resected with nonanatomic techniques. Larger lesions usually require formal anatomic resection such as right and left hepatectomy, right and left extended hepatectomy, left lateral sectionectomy, right posterior sectionectomy, and so on, which can be accomplished through an extended right subcostal incision. The first portion of the operation is devoted to confirming the absence of metastatic disease. For right and left hepatectomy or extended hepatectomy, the appropriate portion of the liver is mobilized by dividing the corresponding triangular ligament to expose the associated bare area of the liver. If present, the gallbladder is removed. Intraoperative ultrasound is used to survey the anatomy and to search for metastatic disease.

The right or left hepatic artery and portal vein can be controlled in the hilum of the liver. The corresponding right or left bile duct can also be divided in the hilum. Control of hepatic venous outflow can then be obtained by dividing the right or left hepatic vein. Alternatively, the hepatic vein can be divided later, intraparenchymally toward the end of the resection, but this may predispose to greater hepatic venous backbleeding. Intermittent Pringle maneuver of the proper hepatic artery and main portal vein can be used to decrease further bleeding from the remnant side. The parenchyma is then transected with any of a multitude of techniques, ranging from simple finger-fracture and Kelly clamp–fracture techniques to devices using ultrasonic, stapling, tissue-sealing, and water-jet technologies. Small vessels and ducts are controlled with clips, and larger ones are tied or stapled.

Perihilar Resection

Perihilar cholangiocarcinomas are often technically challenging because of the close proximity of vital structures in the porta hepatis. Resectability criteria were discussed earlier in the chapter. Consideration should be given to preoperative portal vein embolization of the portion of the liver that is to be resected to stimulate growth of the future liver remnant. Unlike cases of intrahepatic cholangiocarcinoma, in cases of perihilar tumors, the extrahepatic biliary tree and bile duct bifurcation are removed, extensive hilar lymphadenectomy is performed, and the biliaryenteric tract is reconstructed.

An extended right subcostal incision is favorable for dissection of the liver hilus. After metastatic disease is excluded, the gallbladder, if present, is separated from the gallbladder fossa, and the common bile duct is divided just cephalad to the pancreas. A frozen section is performed to confirm a negative margin. If this margin is positive, the disease cannot be resected without addition of pancreaticoduodenectomy. The extrahepatic biliary tree is then dissected, removing the perihilar lymphatic tissue en bloc, skeletonizing the hepatic artery and portal vein and exposing their bifurcations. Typically, the left hilar plate can be dissected to expose the left bile duct (Fig. 2). This left bile duct can then be divided near the umbilical fissure, and a frozen section can be performed to confirm a negative margin. If this margin is negative, then an extended right hepatectomy can be performed to resect the tumor. If this margin is positive, an attempt to dissect the right bile duct should be made to try to reach a negative margin on the main right bile duct or in the right posterior bile duct, in which case a left or extended left hepatectomy can be performed. The principles for performing the hepatectomy are as described previously for intrahepatic cholangiocarcinomas.

Reconstruction is typically performed using a Roux-en-Y limb of jejunum to the remnant bile duct(s). Most centers advocate liberal use of hepatectomy to gain a negative margin rather than simple excision of the bifurcation and extrahepatic biliary tree. Several authors have demonstrated a correlation between the rate of hepatectomy and the rate of margin-negative resection. Many centers also advocate routine resection of segment 1 because the

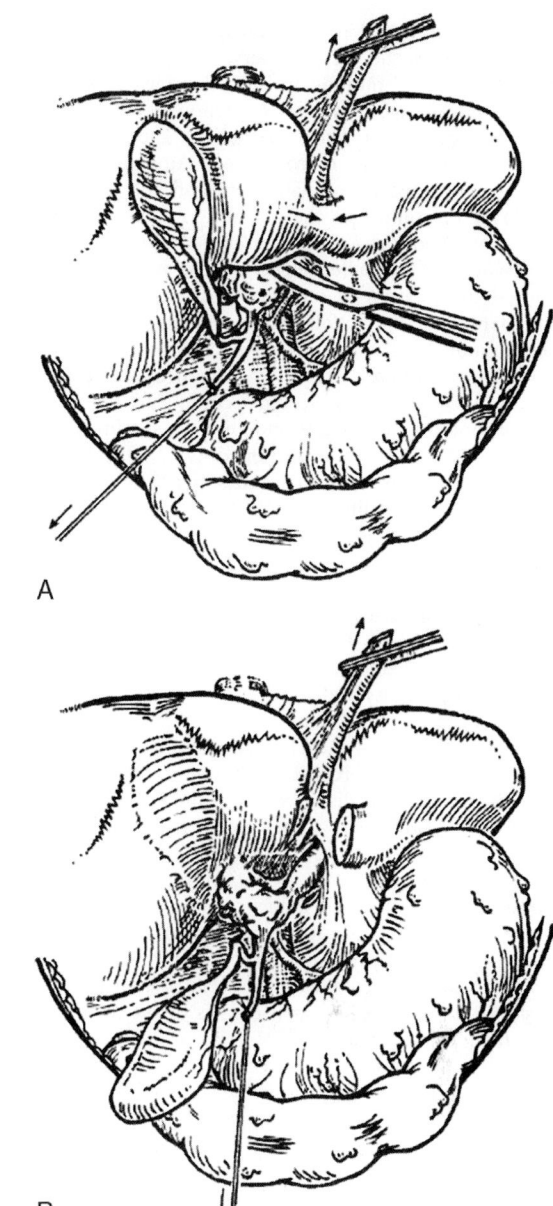

Figure 2   Dissection of the hilus of the liver. **(A)** With firm upward traction on the ligamentum teres, dissection at the base of the quadrate lobe (*scissors*) lowers the hilar plate. **(B)** The bridge of tissue between segments 3 and 4b (*arrows* in part A) is divided, further exposing the hilar structures.   *From Blumgart LH, Fong Y, editors: Surgery of the liver and biliary tract, Philadelphia, 2003, WB Saunders.*

caudate often has one or more bile ducts joining the main biliary tree within 1 cm of the bifurcation. Some have advocated the routine resection of the portal venous bifurcation and anastomosis of the main and left portal vein, citing improved clearance of tumor (because the venous bifurcation is often situated adjacent and posterior to the main tumor) and avoidance of dissecting the hilus with potentially resultant tumor dissemination.

Distal Cholangiocarcinoma Resection

Distal cholangiocarcinoma is resected with a pancreaticoduodenectomy. The main criteria for resectability include the absence of metastatic disease and lack of involvement of the portal and superior mesenteric veins, the hepatic artery, and the superior mesenteric artery. An upper midline incision provides good exposure for pancreaticoduodenectomy. This operation is well described in numerous publications. In brief, the patient is explored and the lack of metastatic disease is confirmed. An extensive Kocher maneuver is performed to evaluate the lesion and to palpate the relationship of the tumor to the portal and superior mesenteric veins and the superior mesenteric artery. At this point, a plane can often be dissected dorsal to the neck of the pancreas and ventral to the portal and superior mesenteric veins, proceeding caudad to cephalad. If present, the gallbladder is mobilized from the liver, and the common hepatic duct is divided above the insertion of the cystic duct or where required to obtain a negative margin, which should be confirmed by frozen section. Next the gastroduodenal artery should be divided to mobilize the specimen from the hepatic artery. The plane of dissection dorsal to the neck of the pancreas and ventral to the portal and superior mesenteric veins can be completed proceeding cephalad to caudad. The duodenum is divided 2 to 3 cm distal to the pylorus for a pylorus-preserving pancreaticoduodenectomy. Alternatively, an antrectomy can be included for a classic pancreaticoduodenectomy. The neck of the pancreas is then transected. The jejunum is divided 15 to 20 cm distal to the ligament of Treitz, and the proximal jejunum and fourth portion of the duodenum are then mobilized by dividing the ligament and the associated vessels in the mesentery of the mobilized small intestines. The proximal jejunum and fourth portion of the duodenum are then flipped dorsal to the root of the mesentery. The uncinate process of the pancreas and associated lymphatic tissues are then dissected off of the portal and superior mesenteric veins and superior mesenteric artery to remove the specimen.

Multiple options for reconstruction are available. A well-accepted sequence is to perform a duct-to-mucosa (or invaginated), end-to-side pancreaticojejunostomy and an end-to-side hepaticojejunostomy to the remnant jejunal limb brought through a defect in the right transverse mesocolon. Gastrointestinal continuity may be reestablished with an antecolic anastomosis of the duodenum (or stomach) to a downstream loop of jejunum. The jejunal limb placed through the mesocolon is secured to prevent herniation, and the defect at the ligament of Treitz is closed. Closed-suction drains are often placed, although some groups prefer not to use them.

OTHER TREATMENT MODALITIES

The use of adjuvant therapy is not well established. Several small trials of adjuvant chemotherapy have been reported, but these demonstrated only low partial-response rates and no major survival benefit. Some small studies have provided evidence of a modest improvement in survival after treatment of cholangiocarcinoma with external beam radiation treatment. Other studies have evaluated the role of liver transplantation in the treatment of cholangiocarcinoma, with varied success. In the absence of high-quality, more definitive evidence, chemoradiation adjuvant therapy and liver transplantation should be considered investigational.

PALLIATION

Palliative treatment of cholangiocarcinoma is an important subject because many patients will not be resectable. The primary aim of palliative treatment is to provide biliary drainage with long-term symptomatic relief. Endoscopic placement of biliary stents has low complication rates and high rates of symptomatic

relief for patients with biliary obstruction caused by unresectable tumors, especially those tumors within easy endoscopic reach. Their effectiveness, however, can be limited by frequent obstruction and the need for replacement. Self-expanding metallic biliary stents have improved patency compared with plastic stents but are more difficult to change when they do obstruct. Percutaneous biliary drainage is an acceptable alternative, especially when endoscopic expertise is not available, has failed, or is inappropriate for accessing multiple, isolated pockets that are infected or obstructed within the intrahepatic biliary tree. Revision of these percutaneous drains is relatively straightforward, and they can be kept internalized for physiologic excretion into the small intestine. Operative biliary-enteric bypass usually provides durable palliation of obstructive jaundice and is commonly performed after a patient has been explored and found to be unresectable; however, because of increased mortality and morbidity, it is usually not the first choice in patients who are deemed clearly to have unresectable disease as determined by imaging studies.

OUTCOMES

Cholangiocarcinoma resectability rates are reported to range from 30% to 50%. In our series of 564 operations, 430 (76%) underwent resection and 134 (24%) underwent palliation. The proportion of patients undergoing resection was far greater for distal lesions (96%) than for perihilar lesions (61%) or intrahepatic lesions (66%).

Complication rates after operation of cholangiocarcinoma range from 10% to 60%, depending in part on the location of the tumor. Resection of intrahepatic tumors is associated with lower rates of complications, whereas perihilar resections are generally associated with the highest rates. Operative mortality rates range in the literature from 0% to 15% and, as with complication rates, are highest for perihilar resections (Table 4). In our series, the overall complication rate was 35% and the operative mortality rate was 4%.

Survival following resection of cholangiocarcinoma depends on several factors, especially margin status, lymph node status, size, and differentiation. Stage may or may not correlate with survival, depending on the series and the staging system employed. In our series, margin status was the most robust predictor of outcome following resection of cholangiocarcinoma. When only R0 patients are analyzed, lymph node status is the only one of these factors that remains a significant predictor of survival. Because of the importance of margin status on survival, a more aggressive operation to achieve negative margins is warranted. In high-volume centers, this approach is associated with acceptable morbidity and mortality rates. In our series, twice as many hilar resections are currently performed with concomitant liver resection to achieve negative margins, compared with our early experience, consistent with the internationally observed correlation between the rate of hepatectomy and the rate of margin-negative resection.

Long-term survival rates for cholangiocarcinoma depend on tumor location and are highest for intrahepatic cancers and lowest for perihilar cancers (Table 4). In our series, the 5-year survivals for R0-resected intrahepatic, perihilar, and distal tumors were 63%, 30%, and 27%, respectively. Palliated patients have a median survival of less than 12 months.

CONCLUSIONS

Cholangiocarcinoma represents a spectrum of disease, and mortality from this disease remains high. Resection at an early stage remains the only chance for long-term survival.

Table 4: Review of the Literature

Author, Location, Year	Resected (N)	Liver Rx (%)	5-year Survival, R0	5-year Survival, All	Mortality (%)
Intrahepatic					
Pichlmayr, Germany, 1995	32	100	NR	17%	6
Jan, Taiwan, 1996	41	100	44%	27%	0
Casavilla, Pittsburgh, 1997	34	100	NR	31%	7
Lieser, Rochester, 1998	32	100	45%	NR	NR
Madariaga, Pittsburgh, 1998	34	100	51%	35%	6
Valverde, France, 1999	30	100	NR	22%	3
Inoue, Japan, 2000	52	100	55%	36%	2
Weber, New York, 2001	33	100	NR****	31%	3
DeOliveira, Baltimore, 2006	34	100	63%	40%	2
Perihilar					
Suigura, Japan, 1994	83	100	33%	20%	8
Su, China, 1996	49	50	34%	15	10
Nagino, Japan, 1998	138	90	26%	NR	10
Miyazaki, Japan, 1998	76	86	40%	26%	15
Madariaga, Pittsburgh, 1998	28	100	25%	9%	14
Kosuge, Japan, 1999	65	80	52%	35%	9
Neuhaus, Germany, 1999	95***	85	37%	22%	6
Jarnagin, New York, 2001	80	78	30%	NR	10
Kondo, Japan, 2004	40	78	NR**	NR	0
Rea, Rochester, 2004	46	100	30%	26%	9
Nishio, Japan, 2005	301	95	27%	22%	8
Dianant, Netherlands, 2006	99	38	33%	27%	15
Wahab, Egypt, 2006	73	100	NR	13%	11
DeOliveira, Baltimore, 2006	173	20	30%	10%	5
Distal					
Bortolasi, Rochester, 2000	15	0	NR	20%	0
Yoshida, Japan, 2002	27	0	44%	37%	4
DeOliveira, Baltimore, 2006	229	0	27%	23%	3

Modified from DeOliveira ML, Cunningham SC, Cameron JL, and others: Ann Surg 245:755, 2007.
NR, *Not reported.*
**3-Year survival was 44%.
***Included 15 hepatectomies with liver transplantation.
****3-Year survival was 62%.

Margin-negative resection is one of the most reliable predictors of survival. Further improvements in survival will be possible only if the disease can be diagnosed earlier and effective adjuvant or neoadjuvant therapy can be developed.

SUGGESTED READINGS

DeOliveira ML, Cunningham SC, Cameron JL, and others: Cholangiocarcinoma: 31-Year experience with 564 patients at a single institution, *Ann Surg* 245:755, 2007.

Jarnigan WR, Fong Y, DeMatteo RP, and others: Staging, resectability, and outcome in 225 patients with hilar cholangiocarcinoma, *Ann Surg* 234:507, 2001.

Lazaridis KN, Gores GJ: Cholangiocarcinoma, *Gastroenterology* 128:1655, 2005.

Nakeeb A, Pitt HA, Sohn TA, and others: Cholangiocarcinoma: a spectrum of intrahepatic, perihilar and distal tumors, *Ann Surg* 224:463, 1996.

Shaib Y, El-Serag HB: The epidemiology of cholangiocarcinoma, *Semin Liver Dis* 24:115, 2004.

Singhal D, van Gulik TM, Gouma DJL: Palliative management of hilar cholangiocarcinoma, *Surg Oncol* 13:59, 2005.

GALLBLADDER CANCER

Daniela P. Ladner, MD, and Sherry M. Wren, MD

INCIDENCE AND EPIDEMIOLOGY

Gallbladder cancer is rare in most Western countries and is associated with a poor prognosis even with modern surgical care. Although the majority of patients still present with advanced, unresectable disease, a small but increasing number of early-stage cases are found incidentally either during or after cholecystectomy that are potentially curable. Unfortunately, the overall 5-year survival remains a dismal 0% to 12%. It is the most common cancer of the biliary tract and the fifth most common malignancy of the gastrointestinal tract. In the United States in 2006, there were an estimated 8500 new cases and 3260 deaths from this cancer.

Worldwide the incidence of gallbladder cancer parallels the incidence of cholelithiasis. This may explain the higher incidence of gallbladder carcinoma in women because cholelithiasis and cholecystitis are more common in females. Populations that have prevalence for gallstones show a higher incidence. Thus women in Delhi, India, have the highest worldwide incidence, 21.5 per 100,000; by comparison, in the diverse U.S. population, the overall incidence of gallbladder cancer is 2.5 per 100,000, but it is significantly higher in the cholelithogenic Native American and Hispanic populations, and there is a 50% greater incidence of gallbladder cancer in Caucasians compared with African Americans. The frequency increases with age and usually presents between the sixth and seventh decades.

The strong association of gallbladder cancer with cholelithiasis (65% to 90%) raises the question of whether gallstones cause or predispose to cancer. Clearly the risk of cancer is actually minimal because the prevalence of people with gallstones in the United States is greater than 25 million individuals, but only 1% to 2% of patients who undergo a laparoscopic cholecystectomy for symptomatic cholelithiasis are diagnosed with gallbladder cancer. Gallstone size directly increases the relative risk of developing gallbladder cancer. Individuals with stones less than 3 cm have a relative risk of developing cancer of 2.5 compared with those having stones greater than 3 cm, which has a relative risk of 10. Currently there is no consensus that patients with large stones should be referred for prophylactic cholecystectomy.

Additional risk factors for development of cancer include adenomatous polyps, calcification of the gallbladder wall ("porcelain gallbladder"), and anomalous pancreaticobiliary duct junctions. In the last National Institutes of Health Consensus Guideline of Gallstones and Laparoscopic Cholecystectomy (1992), only porcelain gallbladder was considered an indication for prophylactic cholecystectomy because of the reported risk of cancer in up to 25% of patients with calcified gallbladder walls. Even this association has been questioned in recent studies that conclude that the risk of cancer in porcelain gallbladders has been significantly overestimated.

PATHOLOGY

Carcinoma of the gallbladder is believed to progress slowly from dysplasia through carcinoma in situ to invasive carcinoma over 15 years. More than 90% of patients have histological changes in the mucosa consistent with dysplasia and carcinoma in situ found adjacent to the gallbladder cancer. Chronic inflammation from stones or other processes is postulated to be the inciting event in the dysplasia to carcinoma pathway. The vast majority (80% to 95%) of gallbladder cancers are adenocarcinomas of papillary, tubular, mucinous, or signet-cell type. There is a small incidence of other pathologies including anaplastic carcinomas (7%), squamous cell carcinomas (1% to 6%), or adenosquamous cell carcinomas (1% to 4%). Other rare cancers include small-cell carcinomas, carcinoid, sarcoma, melanoma, and lymphomas.

One of the most interesting aspects of gallbladder cancer is its ability to spread both regionally and distant via four routes. First, cancer can have direct invasion through the gallbladder wall into the liver or other adjacent organs such as the colon or duodenum. High-risk hepatic areas for local extension are segments 4b and 5. This route is common because the majority of gallbladder cancers originate in the gallbladder fundus (60%). Tumors that start or extend to the gallbladder infundibulum can locally invade the cystic duct, common bile duct, and vascular structures in the hepatoduodenal ligament. The second route is dissemination via lymphatics. In the normal gallbladder, lymphatic channels run just beneath the muscle layer of the gallbladder wall. Tumors that invade deeper than the muscle layer are prone to lymphatic spread, which accounts for the large percentage of lymph node involvement in T2–T4 disease (Fig. 1). The third route is via hematogenous dissemination. The sites most involved by this path are the lung (>30%) and brain. Therefore it is critical to rule out pulmonary metastases in the evaluation of patients with T2 or greater disease.

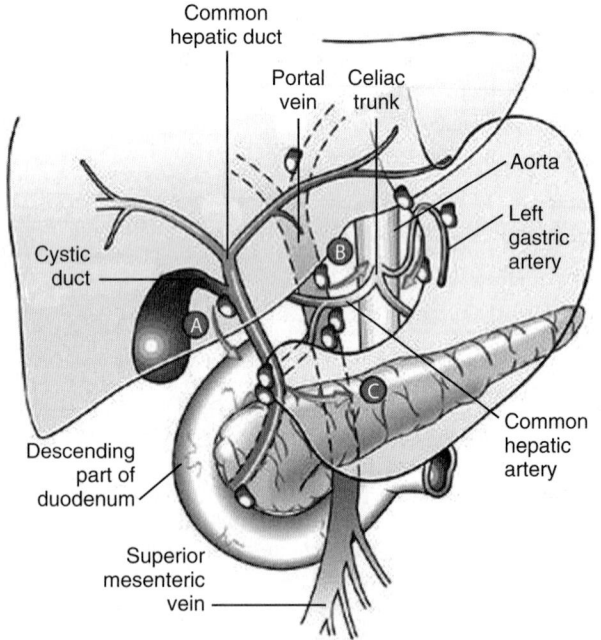

Figure 1 Patterns of lymphatic drainage from the gallbladder. **(A)** The main pathway of lymphatic drainage, and thus lymph node metastasis from gallbladder cancer, is to the cholecystoretropancreatic nodes. This pathway drains from the gallbladder to nodes along the cystic duct and common bile duct and then to nodes posterior to the duodenum and pancreatic head. **(B)** The cholecystoceliac pathway courses from the gallbladder through the gastrohepatic ligament to celiac nodes. **(C)** The third lymphatic drainage route is the cholecystomesenteric pathway, coursing from the gallbladder posterior to the pancreas to aortocaval lymph nodes. *From Keefe DMK, Frei E, Holland JF, and others: Holland-Frei cancer medicine, ed 6, Hamilton, Ontario, Canada, 2003, BC Decker Inc., fig. 102–1.*

Finally, the cancer can spread directly via the peritoneum. Gallbladder cancer has the ability to seed the peritoneum, surgical wounds, and laparoscopic port sites. Therefore advanced disease should be approached with a diagnostic laparoscopy before attempting laparotomy.

■ STAGING

The most recent (6th) edition of the American Joint Commission on Cancer Staging Manual (Table 1) attempted to clarify the staging protocol into potentially resectable lesions (stages 0, I, IIA, and IIB) versus probably unresectable lesions (stages III and IV). The sixth edition is different from the fifth edition (Table 2) in three key areas. First, T4 disease, which was previously defined on the basis of depth of tumor invasion into the liver or invasion

Table 1: UICC/AJCC TNM Classification (6th edition), 2002

T: Primary Tumors

Tx	Primary tumor cannot be assessed
T0	No evidence of primary tumor
Tis	Carcinoma in situ
T1	Tumor invades lamina propria or muscle layer
T1a	Tumor invades lamina propria
T1b	Tumor invades muscle layer
T2	Tumor invades perimuscular connective tissue, no extension beyond serosa or into liver
T3	Tumor perforates serosa (visceral peritoneum) or directly invades the liver and/or one other adjacent organ or structure, e.g., stomach, duodenum, colon, pancreas, omentum, extrahepatic bile ducts
T4	Tumor invades main portal vein or hepatic artery, or invades two or more extrahepatic organs or structures

N: Regional Lymph Nodes*

NX	Regional lymph nodes cannot be assessed
N0	No regional lymph-node metastasis
N1	Regional lymph-node metastasis

M: Distant Metastasis

MX	Distant metastasis cannot be assessed
M0	No distant metastasis
M1	Distant metastasis

Staging

Stage O	Tis	N0	M0
Stage IA	T1	N0	M0
Stage IB	T2	N0	M0
Stage IIA	T3	N0	M0
Stage IIB	T1, T2, T3	N1	M0
Stage III	T4	Any N	M0
Stage IV	Any T	Any N	M1

AJCC, American Joint Committee on Cancer; *UICC,* International Union Against Cancer.
*Cystic duct node and pericholedochal, hilar, peripancreatic (head only), periduodenal, periportal, celiac, and superior mesenteric nodes.

Table 2: UICC/AJCC TNM Classification (5th edition) 1997

T: Primary Tumors

Tx	Primary tumor cannot be assessed
T0	No evidence of primary tumor
Tis	Carcinoma in situ
T1	Tumor invades lamina propria or muscle layer
T1a	Tumor invades lamina propria
T1b	Tumor invades muscle layer
T2	Tumor invades perimuscular connective tissue, no extension beyond serosa or into liver
T3	Tumor invades/perforates the serosa and/or directly invades another organ, e.g., stomach, duodenum, colon, pancreas, omentum, extrahepatic bile ducts
T4	Tumor extends more than 2 cm into the liver and/or 2 or more adjacent organs

N: Regional Lymph Nodes*

NX	Regional lymph nodes cannot be assessed
N0	No regional lymph-node metastasis
N1	Metastases in cystic duct or pericholedochal and/or hilar lymph nodes
N2	Metastases in peripancreatic, periduodenal, periportal, celiac, and/or mesenteric lymph nodes

M: Distant Metastasis

MX	Distant metastasis cannot be assessed
M0	No distant metastasis
M1	Distant metastasis, lymph node involvement, beyond N2

Staging

Stage O	Tis	N0	M0
Stage I	T1	N0	M0
Stage II			
Stage III	T2	N0	M0
	T3	N0	M0
Stage IVA	T1, T2, T3	N1	M0
Stage IVB	T4	N0, N1	M0
	Any T	Any N1	M0, M1

AJCC, American Joint Committee on Cancer; *UICC,* International Union Against Cancer.
*Cystic duct node and pericholedochal, hilar, peripancreatic (head only), periduodenal, and periportal.

of adjacent organs, is now defined as invasion into extrahepatic organs or vascular involvement of the hepatic artery or portal vein. The second difference is that whereas earlier editions subdivided lymph node staging into N1–N3, the current manual categorizes lymph node involvement as only N0 or N1 disease. The final difference is in the overall stage groupings. In the new edition stage IV disease must have metastases; this was not true in the older edition, in which stage IV disease had to have only a T4 lesion or N2 involvement. It is critical when reviewing data to know which protocol was used for staging because the majority of data have been reported using the fifth or earlier editions, and clinical reports of survivorship in stage IV cases can be misleading if the reader assumes that this means metastatic disease.

CLINICAL PRESENTATION AND WORKUP

Gallbladder cancer can present either as an incidental finding postcholecystectomy, symptomatically with pain or jaundice, or when a mass is found on diagnostic imaging. When found incidentally at the time of surgery or by pathologic examination of a resected specimen, the diagnosis is often a surprise to both the patient and surgeon. Fortunately the majority of patients found to have unsuspected carcinoma on pathologic review have T1a mucosal lesions. The likelihood of metastases in these cases is low because the cancer has not accessed the lymphatic channels within the gallbladder wall. Simple cholecystectomy is the acceptable treatment as long as all margins, especially the cystic duct margin, are free of tumor. The 5-year survival rate for these patients is 85% to 100%. Incidental finding after laparoscopic cholecystectomy represents a new and sometimes difficult problem in the treatment of gallbladder cancer. New problems such as peritoneal seeding from spillage of gallbladder contents and direct seeding of trocar sites have become clinically recognized; these may have been exacerbated by not using a specimen bag to extract the gallbladder. Patients subsequently may present with stage IV disease with extensive peritoneal seeding even though their primary cancer was small. Recognition of this problem has prompted most surgeons to use extraction bags and to adopt a liberal policy of converting to an open procedure if there is any question of a cancer.

Of the patients who do not present with gallbladder cancer after routine cholecystectomy, most patients present with symptoms of pain (75%) or jaundice (45%). Nausea, vomiting, anorexia, and weight loss may also be present. The initial imaging study of a patient with gallbladder symptoms is often an ultrasound; the diagnostic accuracy of this examination is greater than 80% for gallstones but only 50% for gallbladder cancer. Although high-resolution ultrasonography can demonstrate bile duct obstruction, porta hepatis lymphadenopathy, direct liver extension of tumor, or even hepatic metastases, it is operator dependent.

Patients with suspicion for a gallbladder cancer should have either computerized tomography (CT) or magnetic resonance imaging (MRI); both are superior to ultrasound for delineating the extent of disease and local invasion. Imaging should also include the chest because this is a common site of distant disease. Both CT and MRI can demonstrate invasion of tumor into the hepatoduodenal ligament or adjacent liver, lymph node involvement, and encasement of the portal vein or hepatic artery. The extent of adjacent liver involvement is particularly important in planning the extent of liver resection. The finding of para-aortic or peripancreatic nodal disease beyond the head of the pancreas on imaging precludes curative resection. Recently positron emission tomography (PET) has proved to be the most sensitive modality for determining distant metastasis and can reduce nonproductive surgical explorations for unresectable disease. Magnetic resonance cholangiopancreaticography also can provide detailed information of possible bile duct involvement. In patients presenting with biliary obstructive symptoms, endoscopic retrograde cholangiography may be helpful in staging the disease, obtaining a tissue diagnosis, and alleviating the obstruction by placing a stent. Long strictures of the common hepatic duct are suggestive of advanced disease. In patients with advanced disease, for whom nonsurgical treatment is planned, fine needle aspiration cytology (FNAC) guided by ultrasound or CT is a highly sensitive tool to diagnose gallbladder cancer with a sensitivity greater than 88%.

Laboratory studies are generally nonspecific in gallbladder cancer. Serum alkaline phosphatase, alanine aminotransferase, and aspartate aminotransferase levels may be elevated, especially in the presence of advanced hepatic invasion or metastasis. Limited data are available concerning tumor markers and genetic changes occurring in gallbladder cancer. Carcinoembryonic antigen and carbohydrate antigen 19–9 levels have been shown to be elevated in gallbladder cancer in 18% and 30%, respectively. K-ras mutations and p53 tumor suppressor genes are reported in 39% to 59% and 35% to 92%, respectively. Evidence to mandate adoption of these markers into the preoperative workup is insufficient at this time.

SURGICAL PROCEDURES AND OUTCOMES

Surgery is the only potentially curative treatment for gallbladder cancer. Regrettably, most patients present with advanced disease, and curative resection is feasible in only 10% to 30% of patients. The overall 5-year survival of gallbladder cancer in collected reviews remains less than 5%. A more aggressive surgical approach to advanced regional disease has shown promise in improving survival in this patient population.

Treatment is based primarily on the T-stage of the tumor. Factors such as age, nutritional status, and cardiopulmonary and hepatic function must also be considered in choosing the appropriate treatment approach. Contraindications for surgical resection include liver metastases, malignant ascites, peritoneal metastases, distant disease, extensive involvement of hepatoduodenal ligament, encasement or occlusion of major vessels, and poor performance status. Studies also indicate that para-aortic lymph node involvement has an equal survival rate as gallbladder cancer with distant metastasis and therefore should be a contraindication to operation.

Early Lesions: Tis and T1a

For patients with early Tis or T1a stage cancers (invasion limited to the lamina propria), simple cholecystectomy is the treatment of choice. These patients have minimal chance of lymph node involvement. Cure rates with simple cholecystectomy are 85% to 100% as long as negative margins are obtained. If the cystic duct margin is involved, reexploration should be undertaken and common bile duct excision with biliary reconstruction should be performed. Laparoscopic and open cholecystectomies have shown equal survival rates and local control rates. However, it is our opinion that if a patient has suspected gallbladder cancer or a high-risk polypoid lesion, the laparoscopic approach should not be performed. This is because of the increased risk of peritoneal spread and seeding if there is spillage of gallbladder contents, as well as the possibility of trocar site tumor implantation, especially if specimen bags are not used or if they break.

T1b and T2 Tumors

In contrast to Tis and T1a tumors, T1b tumors (invasion of the muscle layer) have a 15% rate of lymph node metastasis, and in T2 tumors, regional lymph node metastasis are found in 40% to 80% of cases. Invasion of the perimuscular connective tissue of the gallbladder increases the chance of extension into the adjacent hepatic parenchyma. A simple cholecystectomy is not appropriate treatment for these tumors because the resection plane is subserosal and can leave cancer cells in the serosa that can extend into the liver.

Extended resection or radical cholecystectomy (Fig. 2) is associated with a much better overall survival rate for these lesions over simple cholecystectomy alone (19% to 40% vs. 61% to 100% for T2 lesions). As long as preoperative and intraoperative staging shows no obvious metastases or unresectable local disease, the gallbladder, gallbladder fossa, a minimum of 2 cm of hepatic parenchymal margin, and lymphadenectomy are performed. Lymphadenectomy consists of dissection of the lymph node beds in the

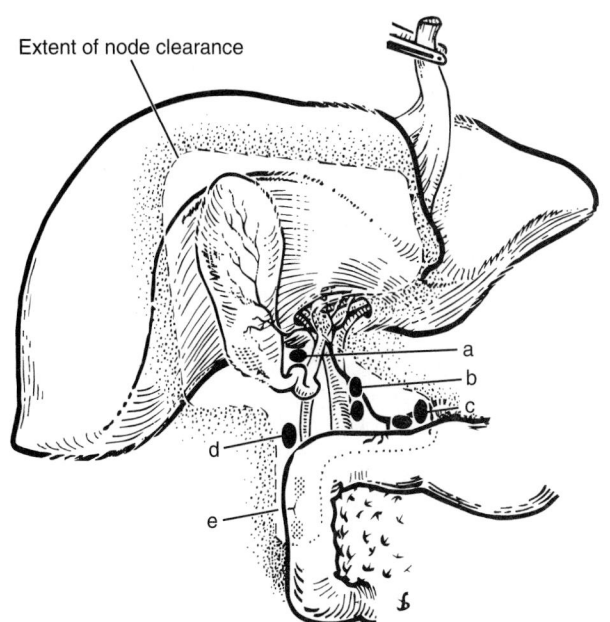

Extent of node clearance

a
b
c
d
e
f

Figure 2 Diagrammatic representation of the extent of lymph node dissection in an extended or radical cholecystectomy. *From Blumgart LH, Fong Y: Surgery of the liver and biliary tract, ed 3, Philadelphia, 2000, WB Saunders, fig. 53.8.*

porta hepatis, gastroduodenal ligament, gastrohepatic ligament, and a Kocher maneuver with removal of the lymph nodes along the posterior duodenum; some surgeons include nodes behind the pancreatic head. More extensive lymph node dissection has been performed in Japan, including removal of the lymph nodes along the vena cava and aorta. Present data do not suggest any survival benefit among patients undergoing this more aggressive approach. Most surgeons believe that to perform a porta hepatis dissection adequately, it is often necessary to resect the extrahepatic bile duct and undertake a biliary reconstruction, but this is not always necessary. Extrahepatic bile duct resection should be performed in patients who present with obstructive jaundice resulting from invasion of tumor and for tumors located in the neck of the gallbladder or in the cystic duct. It is unclear whether extrahepatic bile duct resection is of any benefit to patients who are not jaundiced preoperatively except to allow for a better lymphadenectomy. Extended cholecystectomy can be performed with minimal morbidity and a 1% mortality rate.

T3 and T4 Tumors

Patients with locally advanced T3 and T4 cancers may benefit from resection if there is no evidence of distant or peritoneal disease and a resection is technically feasible. There is no survival benefit if the tumor is not completely resected; therefore debulking operations play no role in this disease. Diagnostic laparoscopy should be strongly considered before exploratory laparotomy in locally advanced T3 or T4 tumors to identify patients with peritoneal seeding of the cancer and avoid unnecessary laparotomy. If the tumor locally invades the colon, duodenum, or liver, complete local resection, if possible, is indicated and can improve survival if negative margins can be obtained.

Recent reports demonstrate a 25% to 44% 5-year survival rate with radical surgery. The extent of hepatic resection is determined by the local invasion of liver. Lesions that have minimal extension into the liver can usually be approached with simple wedge or segment 4b and 5 resection. As the lesion size increases or vascular

structures are affected, more extensive resections are required. It does not appear that anatomic-based resections have any survival benefit over plain wedge resection, but often to obtain R0 resection in T4 tumors, larger liver resections are necessary. These can range from segment 4 and 5 removal; removal of segments 4, 5, 8; and right trisegmentectomy (segments 4, 5, 6, 7, and 8). Right hepatectomy without segment IV excision is generally not advisable because more than one third of advanced tumors involve the left lobe. In addition to hepatic excision, resection of adjacent organs such as colon, duodenum, or stomach may be necessary. Multivariate analysis of multiple recent reports support an aggressive surgical approach with extended liver resection to achieve R0 resection and improve overall survival in T4 tumors with no distant metastasis. Older data using AJCC 5th edition designation of stages III and IV (not M1 disease) have shown a survival benefit for patients in whom a complete resection can be achieved. In these reports, the 5-year survival after extensive resection was 35% to 55% for stage III and 17% to 33% for stage IV disease. The most important factor for survival is resection of the tumor with negative margins, preferably greater than 2 cm.

The ability to perform liver resection with far less morbidity and mortality than in the past is a factor in the improvement of survival from gallbladder cancer over the past decade. Intraoperative ultrasonography and preoperative imaging have improved operative staging and delineation of disease extent. Newer operative techniques using parenchymal division tools shorten operative time and blood loss and thereby reduce morbidity and mortality associated with liver resection. Mortality rates for major hepatectomies are 0% to 5% in the current literature.

There has been some move in Japanese centers to perform more radical operations such as pancreaticoduodenectomy in addition to liver resection in locally advanced gallbladder cancers. This combined operation has a reported in-hospital mortality of 15% and a morbidity of 54%. Given the present data, there is no proof of survival benefit for this aggressive approach in the treatment of gallbladder cancer, especially given the exponential increase of mortality and morbidity.

Gallbladder Polyps

The prevalence of gallbladder polyps in healthy patients ranges from 3% to 10% on ultrasound. Cholesterol polyps make up the vast majority of these lesions (46% to 70%). Other histologies include inflammatory, hyperplastic, adenoma (6%), and polyps with malignant changes (8%). Ultrasound is the most effective diagnostic method for detecting polyps. When large lesions (>1 cm) are found on ultrasound, CT should be performed to assess for possible gallbladder cancer. Most gallbladder polyps are small and benign and do not change in size over time. However, polyp size greater than 10 mm, broad-based sessile lesions, and age older than 50 years have been shown to be most predictive of malignancy. We suggest that laparoscopic cholecystectomy should be performed for these patients only when the suspicion for malignancy is low. If on the basis of these factors there is preoperative suspicion for gallbladder cancer, a simple open cholecystectomy with intraoperative frozen section should be performed. In patients with small polypoid lesions, ultrasound follow-up should be performed every 6 months and followed for 2 years to ensure a stable lesion.

Incidental Finding of Gallbladder Cancer

Incidental finding of malignancy after laparoscopic cholecystectomy occurs in 1% to 2% of laparoscopic cholecystectomies and represents a relatively new and challenging problem in the treatment of gallbladder cancer. With the advent of laparoscopic cholecystectomies in the late 1980s, new problems such as peritoneal seeding from spillage of gallbladder contents and direct seeding of trocar sites became clinically recognized. This may have been exacerbated by surgeons not using a specimen bag to extract the gallbladder. Fortunately, the majority of patients found to have carcinoma on pathologic review have T1a mucosal lesions. On the basis of multiple retrospective reviews, survival after laparoscopic cholecystectomy and incidental finding of gallbladder cancer for Tis and T1a, no further resection is necessary if the cystic duct margins are free of tumor. The 5-year survival rate for these patients is 85% to 100%.

During routine cholecystectomy, suspicion of cancer should be entertained if the procedure is more difficult or unusual than expected. Conversion to an open operation to prevent spillage and seeding should be considered. If a suspicious lesion is identified, a frozen section can be performed to confirm the diagnosis and to assess the depth of tumor invasion. If the diagnosis of T2 or greater gallbladder cancer is confirmed, the surgeon can proceed to an open radical cholecystectomy accordingly. Another choice is to perform simple cholecystectomy, closure, and image-guided staging, and then refer the patient to a local hepatobiliary expert. Long-term survival is the same if the extended cholecystectomy is performed at the initial operation or during a later operation.

Tragically, patients have presented with stage IV disease with extensive peritoneal seeding or port site disease even though their primary cancer was small or undetected after routine cholecystectomy. Port site seeding after laparoscopic cholecystectomy with presentation as advanced disease has been reported in 5% to 20% of cases. Recognition of this problem has prompted surgeons to use extraction bags and to adopt a liberal policy of converting to an open procedure if there is any question of a cancer because perforation and spillage has been reported to lead to a high rate (40%) of port site recurrence.

Patients who are found to have T1b or greater lesions on pathologic review of the gallbladder should be offered a resection to further treat their cancer. In the Memorial Sloan Kettering series, there was a significant survival difference in patients who underwent re-resection in cases of T2 cancers compared with those who did not (61% vs. 19%). Before resection, staging with imaging and possible laparoscopy should be performed to rule out distant disease or peritoneal spread. Some authors also advocate resection of port sites at time of resection, but this remains controversial.

UNRESECTABLE OR METASTATIC DISEASE: PALLIATIVE MANAGEMENT

Patients who present with locally unresectable or metastatic disease have an overall dismal prognosis, often with a survival of less than 1 year. Unfortunately, there is no effective adjuvant treatment for gallbladder cancers. The majority of patients require palliation for pain, jaundice, and possibly intestinal obstruction. Minimal morbidity is of great importance for any palliative procedures, considering that median survival in this group may be only 2 to 4 months. If unresectable disease is encountered during an exploratory laparotomy, jaundice and obstruction can be treated with choledochojejunostomy and gastrojejunostomy. Biliary obstruction can also be successfully treated with endoscopic or percutaneous drainage. In general, operative exploration should be avoided because median survival is already poor; endoscopic stent placement for biliary or intestinal obstructions can offer these patients symptom relief without the need for postsurgical recovery.

Chemotherapy and radiotherapy have been largely unsuccessful in treating this disease. Modest results have been reported with 5-fluorouracil (5-FU)-, gemcitabine-, or capecitabine-based single-agent and multiagent regimens. Response rates are low, but occasional disease stabilization can be achieved for a few months. Patients can also be referred for enrollment in a clinical trial or offered 5FU- or gemcitabine-based chemotherapy or best supportive care.

ADJUVANT TREATMENT AND SURVEILLANCE

At present, there are limited clinical trial data to support adjuvant treatment postresection because no prospective randomized trials have been performed. There are reports of small trials reaching different conclusions either in support of or against the use of adjuvant treatment. In the National Comprehensive Cancer Network guidelines, 5FU- or gemcitabine-based chemotherapy with radiation should be considered except in T1 or N0 patients. Clearly good clinical trials to answer this important question should be undertaken to guide management. Patients who have had complete resection may be offered imaging every 6 months to identify possible recurrences; this should be an individualized discussion with each patient. Recurrent disease often occurs locally in the liver and presents with jaundice. Patients may also present with peritoneal disease or distant disease. Supportive care or palliative chemotherapy can be given at that time.

CONCLUSION

Gallbladder cancer can be a treatable disease with good results even when presenting with more advanced local T stage or N1 disease. Recent literature supports the role of aggressive resection in patients with T1b or greater disease. Recognition of the mechanisms of disease spread have allowed for better preoperative staging and selection of operative candidates. The sixth edition of the AJCC staging manual clarified the staging protocol to help the clinician identify potentially resectable patients. Suspicious lesions should be approached with open surgical, not laparoscopic, techniques to avoid potential intraperitoneal spread of disease. However, laparoscopy is an important tool in the preoperative assessment of cases to undergo re-resection or in advanced cases to eliminate the presence of peritoneal seeds. Clinical trials are necessary to address a role of adjuvant treatment in this cancer. Overall the survival rate for patients presenting with advanced T stage disease is much better than it was 20 years ago. The role of radical surgery in locally advanced disease offers some chance for cure and certainly offers patients more hope than palliation alone.

Suggested Readings

Dixon E, Vollmer CM Jr, Sahajpal A, and others: An aggressive surgical approach leads to improved survival in patients with gallbladder cancer: a 12-year study at a North American Center, *Ann Surg* 241:385, 2005.

Lee KF, Wong J, Li JC, and others: Polypoid lesions of the gallbladder, *Am J Surg* 188:186, 2004.

Misra S, Chaturvedi A, Misra NC: Gallbladder cancer, *Curr Treat Options Gastroenterol* 9:95, 2006.

Wistuba II, Gazdar AF: Gallbladder cancer: lessons from a rare tumour, *Nat Rev Cancer* 4:695, 2004.

ANTIBIOTIC SELECTION IN BILIARY SURGERY

Donald E. Fry, MD

Disease of the gallbladder remains a common focus of attention for surgeons. Cholelithiasis results in surgical cholecystectomy, either by laparoscopic or a traditional open approach, for approximately 500,000 patients per year in the United States. Numerous other biliary tract procedures are performed by surgeons, gastroenterologists, and interventional radiologists because of biliary obstruction or for diagnosis of clinical conditions in which disease of the biliary tract is suspected. Significant colonization or active infection is commonly encountered in the course of these many interventions in the biliary tree, and infection as a complication from any of the many mechanical interventions is a continued source of concern. Thus antibiotics are commonly used for prevention of infection or for the treatment of clinical infection that is already present within the gallbladder and the bile ducts. Appropriate antibiotic use requires a complete understanding of the pathogenesis, microbiology, prevention, and treatment of these patients.

PATHOPHYSIOLOGY AND MICROBIOLOGY

In the absence of disease within the biliary tract, human bile does not have bacteria that can be cultured. Recovery of bacteria in the bile increases in probability either when calculi are present as a surface for microbial adherence or when obstruction to bile flow is present.

The mechanism by which bacteria gain access to the biliary tract remains poorly defined. Retrograde reflux of bacteria from the duodenum via the ampulla of Vater is an attractive hypothesis. However, microbial colonization of the proximal duodenum in patients with normal gastric acid production is quantitatively low. The valve function of the sphincter of Oddi and the normal antegrade flow of bile similarly minimize those bacteria present in the duodenum from gaining access to the biliary tract lumen. The increased incidence of positive bacterial cultures with acute cholecystitis and with distal biliary tract obstruction makes retrograde colonization unlikely. A second and more likely hypothesis is that microbes gain access to the bile via lymphatic or portal vein transport from the intestinal tract. The normal microbial filtration mechanism of the liver may result in proximal access of microbes into bile, and these colonists assume clinical significance only with the presence of calculi or with obstruction to normal flow. It is likely that transient, low-inocula microbial colonization occurs in all people and that normal flow of bile prevents invasive infection.

Infection within the gallbladder or within the duct system itself occurs when the microbe adheres to the mucosal surface, multiplies, and invades the wall of the biliary tree. Microbial invasion occurs because of high concentrations of microbes or because of injury to the mucosal surface that impairs the normal barrier and allows the pathogen a convenient location for adherence and growth. Obstruction increases the contact time that bacteria have with the biliary mucosa, and this may also neutralize benefits of immunoglobulin A antibody, which ordinarily would retard microbial adherence to mucosal cells. Invasion of bacteria provokes activation of the human inflammatory response, which then yields the characteristic signs and symptoms of biliary tract infection. Repeated activation and resolution of the inflammatory process yield collagen deposition in the wall of the gallbladder and the bile ducts. This leads to the severe scarring and distorted anatomy that is identified in the surgical management of many patients with chronic and recurrent biliary tract disease.

The most common bacteria that colonize human bile are aerobic enteric organisms. *Escherichia coli* is most common and is likewise the most common pathogen that is cultured from active biliary tract infection. *Klebsiella pneumoniae* is the next most common organism. *Enterococcus* species are cultured from bile but are much less commonly seen as pathogens in active infection, except in older and immunosuppressed patients. These three species are the most common aerobic bacteria to be cultured from the entire human gastrointestinal tract, but not from the duodenum. *Pseudomonas* species and *Enterobacter* species have traditionally been uncommon in bile but are seen in patients from nursing homes or among those who have had recent antibiotic therapy that has changed the enteric colonization of the patient.

Anaerobic species are much less frequently seen in bile. *Clostridium* species and *Bacteroides fragilis,* the two most commonly identified anaerobes in the human colon, are occasionally cultured from bile and are uncommonly cultured from clinical biliary tract infections. Anaerobes in bile are identified most commonly in the elderly population. The organisms that predominate in bile are representative of the entire gut and give additional credibility to the visceral lymph or venous drainage to the liver from the intestinal tract being the likely source for these bacteria.

PREVENTIVE ANTIBIOTICS

Preventive antibiotics are commonly used in patients who are undergoing cholecystectomy, even with laparoscopic cholecystectomy, although the data for benefit are not conclusive. With complex open biliary operations that involve resection of stricture or neoplasm with an enteric anastomosis of the common duct into the intestinal tract, preventive antibiotics should be used.

Table 1 identifies the common risk factors that are associated with patients having bactibilia and who represent the candidate group that should receive perioperative preventive antibiotics with biliary surgery. Because some of these variables may not be identified until the actual time of the procedure (e.g., the presence of common duct stones), a single preoperative dose of a safe and appropriate drug is commonly used by many surgeons for all cholecystectomy patients and seems warranted.

The principles for the administration of preventive antibiotics are those promulgated by the National Surgical Infection Prevention program. First, the antibiotic should be administered within

Table 1: Risk Factors Associated with Bactibilia and Patient Groups in Which Preventive Antibiotics Are Most Likely of Benefit

- Age >70 years
- Clinical jaundice
- Choledocholithiasis
- Acute cholecystitis
- Operation within 1 month of resolved acute cholecystitis
- Previous biliary tract surgery
- Chills or fever within 1 week of surgery
- Emergent biliary surgery

60 minutes of the surgical incision. It is a fundamental tenet of preventive antibiotic use that the antibiotic must be present in the tissues at the time of intraoperative contamination. Antibiotic can be started too early and be eliminated by the time the procedure and contamination actually occur, and drug given after the operation has begun or following completion of the procedure has no benefit.

Second, the antibiotic should have activity against the pathogens likely to be encountered during the procedure. In biliary surgery, this ordinarily includes coverage for *E. coli* and *K. pneumoniae* as the most likely biliary colonists. Enterococcal coverage with the preventive antibiotic choice has not been documented to be of value. This is likely because of the minimal virulence of this bacterium. Coverage for *Staphylococcus aureus* is generally desirable to cover for potential cutaneous contamination. Cefazolin has been the antibiotic most consistently chosen for this indication. For penicillin-allergic patients, a quinolone is a reasonable choice, although there are few data and no approved indication for it.

Third, the antibiotic should be discontinued after the procedure is completed. Most surgeons do not redose the antibiotic postoperatively unless there has been gross contamination (e.g., gallbladder leakage during removal) during the procedure. Even in conditions of gross contamination, there is no evidence that postoperative doses of the drug afford protection from surgical site infection. The increasing frequency and severity of *C. difficile* enterocolitis that is associated with antibiotic use is a strong argument against the continuation of preventive antibiotics into the postoperative period for biliary surgery patients.

Percutaneous and endoscopic manipulations for diagnostic and therapeutic indications have become common. There are no prospective data to direct decisively preventive antibiotic use in these patients because the postprocedural infectious events (not including technical errors from duct perforation) are low in frequency (<1%). Because obstruction or severe ductal disease is usually present in these patients, it can be safely assumed that colonization of the bile is present, and the administration of a single dose of a preventive antibiotic (e.g., cefazolin 1 g) immediately before the procedure is prudent. Again, continuation of the antibiotic because a stent or catheter remains in the biliary tree after the procedure is of no benefit to the patient.

Should antibiotics be continued or reinstituted in the laparoscopic cholecystectomy patient with a postoperative bile leak? This remains a difficult question. Drainage of the leak is obviously important and provides an opportunity to obtain cultures of the bile. If the patient has either positive cultures or a clinical response to the leak including fever, leukocytosis, or other symptoms of infection, then antibiotics should be used to cover either the culture-proved organism or the *E. coli* or *K. pneumoniae* that is likely to be present.

BILIARY TRACT INFECTION

Infection in the biliary tract may occur within the gallbladder itself or it may arise within the biliary ductal system that drains the liver. Although the bacteria are in the bile and the bile is commonly cultured to define the pathogen, the infection represents invasion of the tissues and is not an event within the aqueous medium of the bile itself. Antibiotic treatment depends on effective penetration of the drug into the infected tissues. Penetration of the antibiotic into the bile, as is commonly studied in pharmacokinetic studies, is not a requirement of the drug for effective treatment.

Acute Cholecystitis

Acute cholecystitis is the most common infection in the biliary tract. The clinical diagnosis is made in patients with acute onset of right upper quadrant abdominal pain, nausea, perhaps vomiting, and low-grade fever. Jaundice may or may not be present. Right upper quadrant tenderness with a positive Murphy's sign and rebound are usually seen. A palpable mass may be present. Ultrasound of the right upper quadrant usually establishes the diagnosis. Hepatobiliary iminodiacetic acid scan may be necessary in difficult diagnoses.

The principal treatment is cholecystectomy, and antibiotics are adjunctive treatment. Cholecystectomy is performed promptly unless the patient has medical conditions (e.g., uncontrolled diabetes) that require management before operation. For routine cholecystectomy, culture of the bile is not necessary; in clinical studies in which bile has been routinely cultured in patients with acute cholecystitis, as many as 50% do not grow any bacteria. Acute cholecystitis is sterile inflammation resulting from obstruction of the cystic duct in many patients. The presumption is that either *E. coli* or *K. pneumoniae* is the pathogen, and antibiotic therapy is addressed to these organisms. Cefazolin 1 to 2 g every 8 hours is appropriate. Piperacillin/tazobactam is commonly used at 3.375 mg every 6 hours, although the anaerobic coverage is unnecessary. Either quinolones or aminoglycoside choices also provide coverage for the target organisms. A spectrum of antibiotic therapy that is broader than cefazolin, or cefuroxime, is justified if the patient has been in a nursing home, has had a recent hospitalization, or has recently had a course of systemic antibiotics that could affect normal colonization.

The tendency is to extend antibiotic therapy too long for these patients. Cholecystectomy removes the patient's disease. The clinical syndrome of pain, fever, and leukocytosis quickly defervesce following definitive surgical care, and in most uncomplicated cases, the antibiotics can be discontinued within 24 hours of the operation. Early discontinuation of antibiotics may even be achieved with a "spill" of bile from the acutely inflamed gallbladder during cholecystectomy. Extending antibiotic therapy under these circumstances of notable intraoperative contamination may be appropriate, and clinical criteria should be used to discontinue the antibiotics.

Empyema of the Gallbladder

Empyema of the gallbladder can occur as a complication of acute cholecystitis, or it may complicate chronic gallbladder disease. In the acute infection scenario, patients present with severe clinical infection, appearing more toxic than typical cholecystitis patients. White blood cell counts tend to be higher, and clinical jaundice with elevated liver enzymes (e.g., aspartate aminotransferase, alanine aminotransferase) is more common than in conventional acute cholecystitis. In many respects, patients appear similar to those with ascending cholangitis.

At operation, the gallbladder is severely inflamed; disruption of the gallbladder is not uncommon. Indeed, it is the identification of frank pus rather than bile that establishes the diagnosis. Cultures are usually performed with the identification of pus. The bacteriology is typical of those organisms seen with acute cholecystitis.

Cholecystectomy is again the definitive treatment in that it represents complete removal of the infected structure. Antibiotic choices for the likely gram-negative rods are defined in Table 2. The pyogenic character of the infection is clinical evidence to implicate potential anaerobic participation and provides ample justification to add anaerobic coverage. Thus initial antibiotic therapy with cefazolin and metronidazole or piperacillin/tazobactam is appropriate until culture and sensitivity data are available. Because surgical therapy is usually effective, antibiotics for many patients can be discontinued within 2 to 3 days on the basis of clinical response. Severe contamination of the subhepatic space during cholecystectomy or from spontaneous perforation of the gallbladder with extraluminal pus at the time of operation commonly results in longer courses of therapy. Postoperative subhepatic abscess can be a complication following

Table 2: Possible Antibiotic Choices for *Escherichia coli* and *Klebsiella pneumoniae* in Patients with Active Biliary Tract Infection

Antibiotic Choice	Dose	Comment
Cefazolin	1–2 g Q 8 hr	Continues to be the choice in patients with mild-to-moderate infections
Cefuroxime	1–2 g Q 8 hr	Has a similar spectrum to cefazolin
Ampicillin/sulbactam	1.5–3 g Q 6 hr	Has a 20% to 30% pattern of *E. coli* resistance in some areas
Piperacillin/tazobactam	3.375 g Q 6 hr	Excellent gram-negative activity; good coverage of *Bacteroides fragilis* if necessary
Imipenem	1 g Q 12 hr	Broad coverage; not necessary in routine cases
Meropenem	1 g Q 12 hr	An equivalent choice to imipenem
Ertapenem	1 g Q 24 hrs.	Excellent gram-negative coverage but limited activity against *Pseudomonas* sp.
Aztreonam	1 g Q 12 hr	Good gram-negative coverage but no gram-positive or anaerobic spectrum
Fluoroquinolones	Variable	Limited data in this type of infection, but an appropriate gram-negative spectrum
Aminoglycosides	Variable	Use only for organisms that are resistant to other choices

Q, Every.

cholecystectomy for empyema of the gallbladder. Patients not having a prompt response to cholecystectomy should be evaluated for abdominal abscess with a computed tomography (CT) scan at 5 to 7 days following the procedure, and appropriate selection of antibiotics should be made.

Occasionally empyema of the gallbladder is seen as a complication of chronic cholecystitis and is an unanticipated finding with routine cholecystectomy. It tends to be seen in older patients and in patients with long-standing symptoms from cholelithiasis. Culture of the pus is important because older patients have more reasons (prior antibiotic therapy being most notable) to have some unusual bacteria in the gallbladder pus. Given that this is an incidental finding, treatment with antibiotics in the postoperative period should be dictated by the patient's clinical course. In this setting, antibiotics can usually be discontinued within 24 to 48 hours of the procedure. Cefazolin with or without metronidazole or piperacillin/tazobactam are dependable choices until the culture evidence is available.

Gangrenous/Ischemic Cholecystitis

Necrosis of the gallbladder wall is from the loss of tissue perfusion. Intraluminal pressure from severe acute cholecystitis may exceed the tissue perfusion pressure. Splanchnic arterial disease, inadequate cardiac output, systemic sepsis from another source, or hypovolemia can lead to gallbladder ischemia and so-called acalculous cholecystitis. Clinical findings are more subtle, and this presentation happens in hospitalized patients for other reasons. Perforation of the necrotic gallbladder wall is a common event and severely complicates patient management.

At cholecystectomy, patients can be subdivided into those with and without perforation of the gallbladder. Gangrenous cholecystitis without perforation is treated much like acute cholecystitis. Cholecystectomy has eradicated the source of the disease, and the usual antibiotic choices are used and discontinued on the basis of the postoperative clinical response of the patient.

Gallbladder perforation may be seen in the old and in the young. Ischemic cholecystitis with perforation in hospitalized patients requires more thought about antibiotic choices. Hospital-based, nosocomial pathogens are now a consideration and require that cultures and sensitivity data be obtained. Resistant *Enterobacter* species, *Pseudomonas aeruginosa,* and methicillin-resistant *S. aureus* are considerations. Broader-spectrum coverage with imipenem or meropenem are choices until culture results allow refinement of the antibiotic regimen. Therapy for

methicillin-resistant *S. aureus* should ordinarily be reserved until culture and sensitivity documentation is present. Because perforation from ischemic cholecystitis commonly occurs in conjunction with other illnesses, these patients require longer courses of therapy. By 7 days, consideration for discontinuation is appropriate, and patients with continued evidence of infection require an abdominal CT scan for the evaluation of abdominal abscess. Abscesses that are subsequently drained require culture confirmation of the pathogen because these infections become yet higher risks for hospital-based, resistant pathogens.

Ascending Cholangitis

Ascending cholangitis occurs with obstruction in the common or hepatic ducts, proliferation of bacteria proximal to the obstruction, and invasion of the microbe into the ductal tissues and hepatic parenchyma. The obstruction may be due to neoplasm of the pancreas or the biliary ducts, chronic pancreatitis, benign biliary stricture, or stricture related to prior biliary surgery. Ascending cholangitis presents with fulminate clinical sepsis of fever, leukocytosis, rapidly evolving jaundice, systemic toxemia, and even septic shock. Treatment is to drain the biliary tree mechanically, usually by operation but occasionally by minimally invasive methods. Antibiotic therapy target *E. coli* and *K. pneumoniae* if the infection presents as a community-based infection. Culture and sensitivity data are especially important if the patient has been in a nursing home, is currently or recently hospitalized, or has had antecedent antibiotic therapy. Under these circumstances, then, a carbapenem should be considered for resistant gram-negative rods. Methicillin-resistant *S. aureus* is a consideration, and vancomycin, linezolid, or daptomycin are choices after cultures have documented the pathogen. In the patient with chronic biliary obstruction that has been treated with repeated percutaneous and endoscopic manipulations, literally any bacterial pathogen and even *Candida* species are potential pathogens. Good sensitivity data are essential for a correct antimicrobial selection under these circumstances.

ACQUIRED IMMUNODEFICIENCY SYNDROME–ASSOCIATED CHOLANGIOPATHY

An unusual infection unique to patients with acquired-immunodeficiency syndrome (AIDS) is AIDS-associated cholangiopathy. These infections are a sclerosing cholangitis thought to be the direct invasion of the biliary ducts by an array of unusual opportunistic pathogens. The disease is characterized by right upper quadrant pain, elevated alkaline phosphatase, and characteristic changes on endoscopic retrograde cholangiopancreatography in a patient with established AIDS. Pathogens associated with this infection are cytomegalovirus, as well as the protozoan pathogens of *Cryptosporidium* species and *Microsporidia*. *Giardia* species, *Cyclospora cayetanensis*, *Isospora* species, and atypical mycobacteria are also pathogens. Antimicrobial therapy specific to these pathogens, especially the protozoans, has been ineffective. Current antimicrobial treatment is with highly active antiretroviral therapy to improve the patient's underlying immunosuppression from AIDS.

SUGGESTED READINGS

Chetlin SH, Elliott DW: Biliary bacteremia, *Arch Surg* 102:303, 1971.

Chetlin SH, Elliott DW: Preoperative antibiotics in biliary surgery, *Arch Surg* 107:319, 1973.

Fry DE, Cox RA, Harbrecht PJ: Empyema of the gallbladder: a complication in the natural history of acute cholecystitis, *Am J Surg* 141:366, 1981.

Fry DE, Cox RA, Harbrecht PJ: Gangrene of the gallbladder: a complication of acute cholecystitis, *South Med J* 74:666, 1981.

Lillemoe KD: Surgical treatment of biliary tract infections, *Am Surg* 66:138, 2000.

Thompson JE Jr, Bennion RS, Doty JE, and others: Predictive factors for bactibilia in acute cholecystitis, *Arch Surg* 125:261, 2000.

TRANSHEPATIC INTERVENTIONS FOR OBSTRUCTIVE JAUNDICE

Eleni Liapi, MD, Christos S. Georgiades, MD, and Jean-Francois Geschwind, MD

Obstructive jaundice is a challenging clinical problem and can be the primary presentation for a variety of pathologies both malignant and benign. Almost 90% of patients who present with painless jaundice have an underlying malignancy as the cause, with benign disease accounting for the remaining 10% to 20% (Table 1). Of the malignant causes of obstructive jaundice, the majority are due to pancreatic cancer (in the United States, 30,000 cases annually) and cholangiocarcinoma (5000 U.S. cases annually). Percutaneous biliary interventions have significantly increased in number and scope, offering diagnostic, therapeutic, and surgical adjunctive options that were previously unavailable.

Table 1: Causes of Obstructive Jaundice

Malignant (80%–90%)	Benign (10%–20%)
Cholangiocarcinoma	Choledocholithiasis
Pancreatic cancer	Pancreatitis
Gallbladder cancer	Primary sclerosis cholangitis
Hepatocellular carcinoma	Iatrogenic injury
Metastatic disease	Cholangitis
Radiation	
Ischemia	
Cystic disease	
Cystic fibrosis	

The vast majority of patients (90%) presenting with obstructive jaundice have a malignant obstruction of the biliary tree. Cholangiocarcinoma and pancreatic cancer account for most of the malignant causes by far. Of those with cholangiocarcinoma, 70% will have involvement of the biliary confluence at presentation, that is, Klatskin tumor, and therefore require bilateral biliary drainage. A minority of patients (usually younger patients) are obstructed secondary to stones or (increasing in frequency) as a result of iatrogenic injury. The latter is due to more frequent use of laparoscopic biliary procedures and an increasingly obese population.

The armamentarium of interventional radiology includes percutaneous transhepatic cholangiogram (PTC) and percutaneous biliary drain (PBD), among others. Indications for biliary interventions include diagnosis, staging, decompression for obstruction, diversion for leak, biopsy, and treatment for benign and malignant disease. These and their relative contraindications are summarized in Table 2.

Whether malignant or benign, the pathophysiology and anatomy of the obstructive lesion have critical ramifications for treatment,

Table 2: Types of Percutaneous Biliary Interventions and Relative Contraindications

Percutaneous Biliary Interventions	Contraindications (Relative)
Diagnostic or staging cholangiogram	Hypercoagulability Polycystic liver disease Severe ascites Diffuse tumor infiltration
Monitor treatment response (i.e., PSC, or s/p Whipple, or transplant)	
Decompression of obstructed system	
Endobiliary biopsy	
Cholangioplasty for benign stricture	
Catheter drainage	
Endostent placement	
Choledochoscopy	
Endobiliary lithotripsy	

PSC, Primary sclerosing cholangitis; *s/p,* status post.

Diagnostic percutaneous transhepatic cholangiogram (PTC) can provide invaluable information with regard to cause of obstruction and treatment planning. It can further provide information regarding the response to treatment, as when the patient is chemically treated for PSC. Furthermore, PTC provides a conduit for a variety of available interventions such as biopsy, cholangioplasty, and biliary stone management. The contraindications to percutaneous liver interventions are listed in the second column. These are relative and should not preclude the patient from a required intervention. Hypercoagulability can be reversed at least temporarily, and ascites can be drained. Polycystic liver disease used to be an absolute contraindication. However, more and more biliary interventions are performed in such patients with acceptable risk of complications. Diffuse tumor infiltration is a relative contraindication mainly because of limited life expectancy of the patient and a slightly higher risk of bleeding, but if clinically necessary it can be performed with acceptable risk profile.

prognosis, and patient outcome. Expertise in using these interventional tools and participation in interdisciplinary patient care by the interventional radiologist can offer substantial benefits to the patient and surgical team and can affect the outcome of any treatment. Additionally, because of the advanced skills and experience required of both the interventional radiologist and surgeon, the rarity of related cases, and the impact of such techniques on patient outcome, biliary pathology is most optimally addressed in a few specialized centers. This chapter provides an overview of the types of percutaneous biliary procedures available and describes those situations for which they are indicated and how they can help nonsurgical, presurgical, and postsurgical patients.

PERCUTANEOUS BILIARY INTERVENTIONS FOR OBSTRUCTIVE JAUNDICE

Percutaneous Transhepatic Cholangiogram

PTC was one of the first interventional procedures to be described in the radiologic literature and is the cornerstone for the development of all other percutaneous biliary interventions. Its objective is to opacify the biliary tree and thus to demonstrate the level and cause of obstruction. Interestingly, the technique has changed little since the 1970s, when the biliary Seldinger technique was introduced. Current advances in computed tomography (CT) and magnetic resonance imaging (MRI) have decreased the need for invasive imaging of the biliary tree with PTC. This technique is currently used mostly as a preliminary diagnostic step before PBD and stenting or when results from other noninvasive studies are incomplete or equivocal.

The patient is first placed in the supine position on the angiography table, followed by sterile preparation and draping.

A local anesthetic (2% lidocaine) is administered at the skin puncture site, and conscious sedation is administered for pain control (intravenous midazolam and fentanyl). General anesthesia may be needed in selected but rare cases.

Most PTCs are performed from the right midaxillary approach, although a subxiphoid (left biliary access) approach is occasionally needed. Traditionally, the right lobe is the preferred puncture site for PBD, mainly because right-sided access keeps the operator's hands out of the beam and achieves drainage of a larger volume of liver when there is obstruction at the liver hilum. However, left biliary drainage is not technically difficult, especially under ultrasound guidance, which may reduce the amount of radiation to the patient and operator. In addition, left biliary catheters are usually more comfortable for patients than those placed on the right side, primarily because they do not traverse the intercostal space. Some patients (i.e., those with a cholangiocarcinoma involving the hilum and central right and left hepatic ducts) may require bilateral access.

Figure 1 showcases the step-by-step procedure for a PTC. A diagnostic-quality PTC shows the level and degree of stenosis or obstruction, opacifies all the contiguous biliary tree, and provides information on the health of the biliary epithelium.

The technical success rate for PTC approaches 100% in patients with biliary dilatation and has been reported to be as high as 90% in patients with nondilatated systems. Significant frequent findings on cholangiography include biliary obstruction resulting from congenital abnormality, stone, tumor, focal stricture, or diffuse sclerosing cholangitis and bile leak resulting from tumor, trauma, and breakdown of a surgical anastomosis. Current screening methods are effective in differentiating surgical from medical biliary disease, and therefore a normal PTC study is rarely seen.

A large study of almost 3600 patients established the overall major complication rate of fine needle PTC to be 3%. Complications included death (0.14%); hemorrhage (0.28%); sepsis (1.8%); intraperitoneal bile leak (1%); and rare instances of pneumothorax,

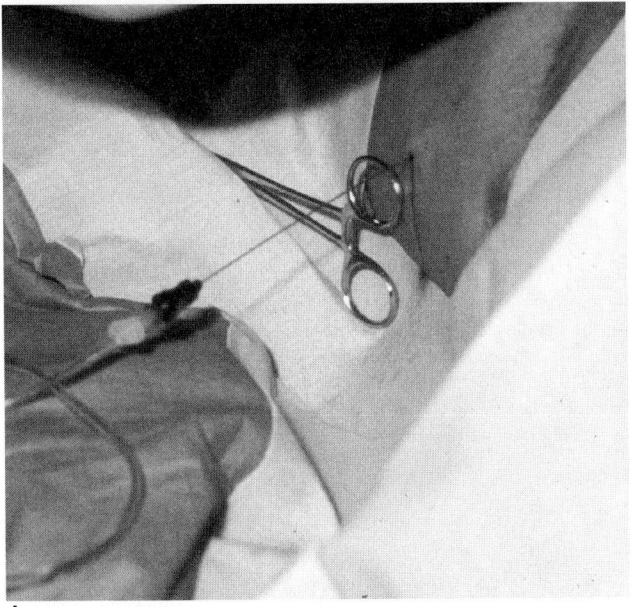
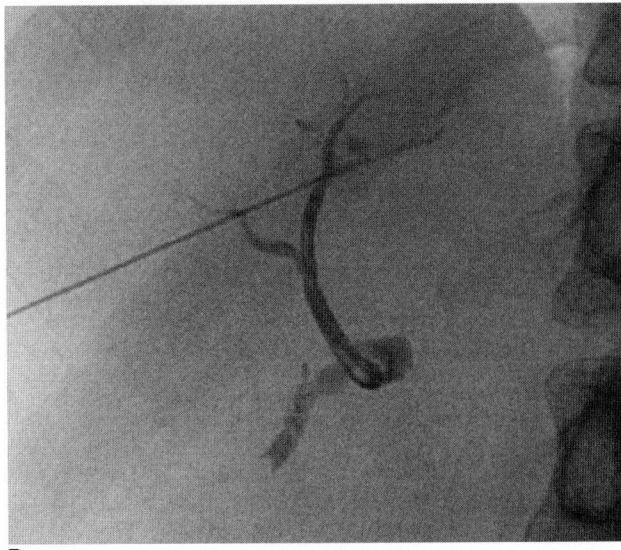

A   B

Figure 1 Step-by-step placement of right percutaneous biliary drain. After proper preparation and local anesthesia at the midaxillary line below the diaphragm *(A)*, a 22-g needle is used to opacify a dilatated biliary system *(B)*. Multiple random passes may be necessary, especially in a nondilatated system. After the system is opacified, a second needle is used to access a peripheral duct .

(continued)

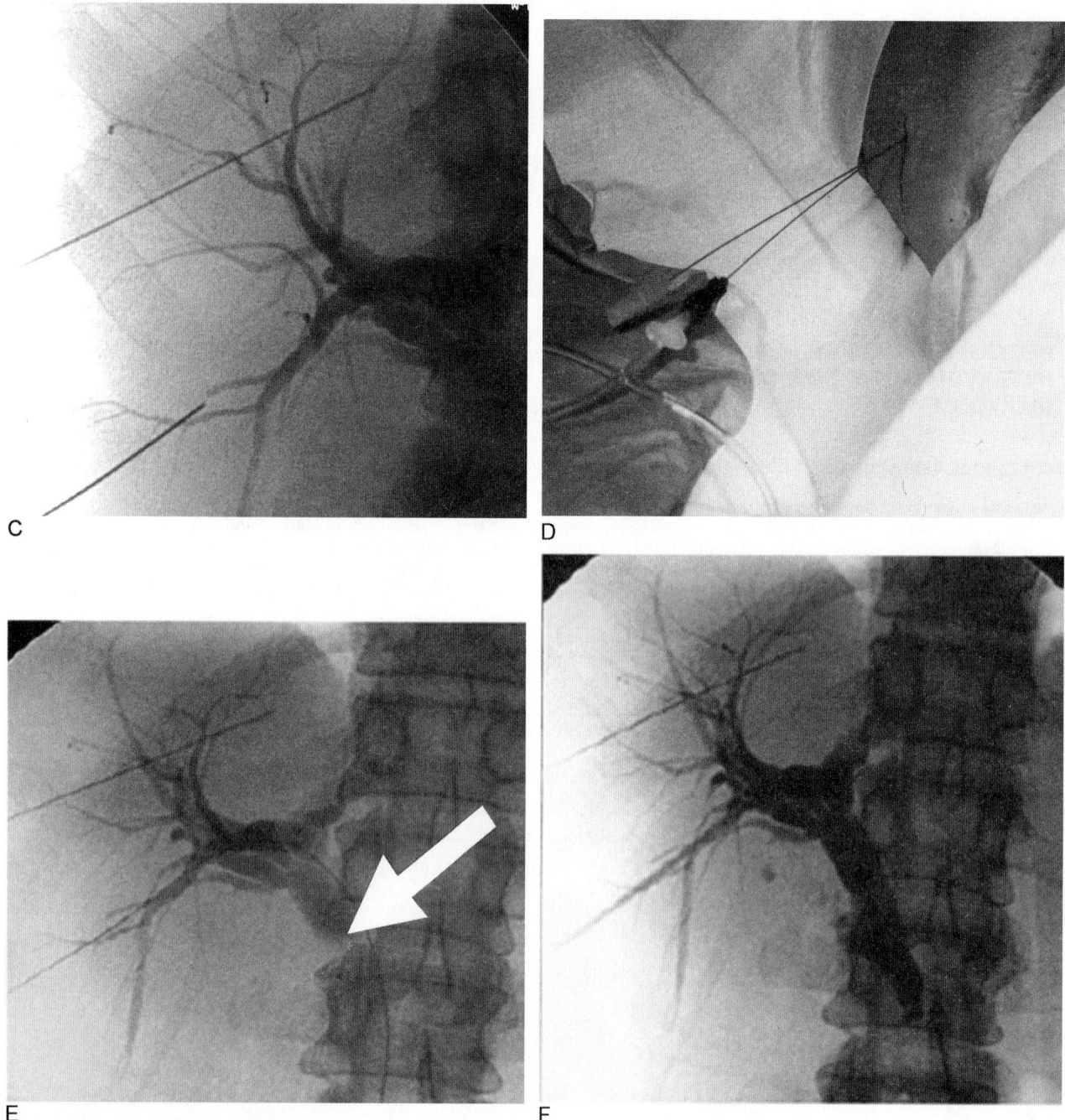

Figure 1 Cont'd—Multiple random passes may be necessary, especially in a nondilatated system. After the system is opacified, a second needle is used to access a peripheral duct *(C and D)*. A wire is advanced via the needle into the biliary system or into the duodenum if possible *(E)*. A sheath is placed over the wire after the needle has been removed *(F)* to provide secure access. A glide wire–catheter combination is then used to cross the obstruction into the small bowel *(G)*. The wire is exchanged for a stiffer one and a biliary catheter is finally advanced over it into the duodenum *(H)*. In this case, the obstructive lesion is a pancreatic cancer occluding the distal common bile duct *(arrow)*. The final cholangiogram *(H)* shows both the left and right biliary systems that have already decompressed.

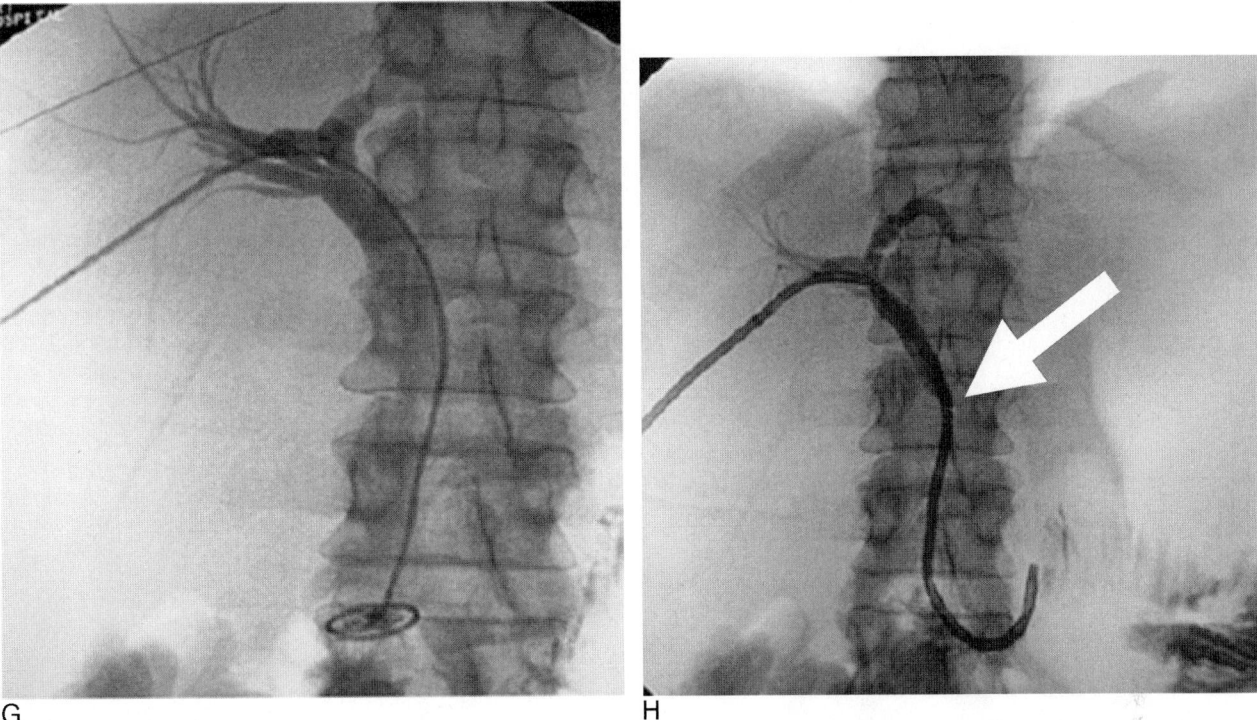

Figure 1 Cont'd—*(G)* The wire is exchanged for a stiffer one and a biliary catheter is finally advanced over it into the duodenum *(H)*. In this case, the obstructive lesion is a pancreatic cancer occluding the distal common bile duct *(arrow)*. The final cholangiogram *(H)* shows both the left and right biliary systems that have already decompressed.

hemothorax, contrast reaction, arteriovenous fistula, and vasovagal reaction. Risks of complication and death were higher for patients with malignant disease than for those with benign biliary disease. Complications following PTC (and catheter placement) are listed in Table 3. Figure 2 showcases a variety of obstructive biliary pathology seen on PTC.

Percutaneous Transhepatic Biliary Drainage

After delineating the biliary anatomy and identifying the pattern and level of obstruction with PTC, PBD is performed. Whereas for nondilatated biliary systems the most challenging aspect is actually obtaining biliary access, for an obstructed, dilatated system the difficulty is in crossing the lesion. This is usually achieved with a glide wire–catheter combination, following which a drain catheter is placed. PBD can be external or external-internal. When an external biliary drainage is placed, the tip of the catheter lies above the obstructing lesion. This occurs when the obstructing lesion cannot be crossed and thus the only route for bile drainage is external, through the PBD catheter. The catheter is connected to a gravity drainage bag and is secured to the skin to prevent inadvertent removal. In most cases, initial access, even though adequate for PTC, is inappropriate for placing a biliary catheter. If this is the case, a second, peripheral puncture of a horizontal duct is necessary (see Figure 1). In the external–internal drainage, a percutaneous catheter crosses the stricture so that the catheter's sideholes are placed above and below the obstructing lesion. This allows drainage of bile into the duodenum while correcting or maintaining fluid and electrolyte balance that may result from prolonged external biliary drainage. Eventually the external tube can be capped or completely internalized. There is little question that internal drainage is preferred over external; however, in few cases, internalization is not technically possible, and the patient is left with an external drain. Another difficult scenario may be encountered when a stricture is

too tight to be traversed. In such cases, an external catheter is initially inserted and, after a few days of external drainage, a channel through the stricture usually appears following resolution of tissue edema; this can be negotiated by the radiologist at a second session. Some

Table 3: Complications after Percutaneous Transhepatic Cholangiography and Catheter Placement

Complication	PTC	PBD	Risk Factor
Hemobilia	0.28%	8%	Central access
Biliary sepsis	1.8%	2.5%	Marked dilatation
Bile leak	1%	3%	Large bore access
Death	0.14%	1.7%	–
Biloma/abscess	–	0.5%	Improper drainage
Pneumo-, hemo-, bilothorax	rare	0.5%	High access
Vasovagal, contrast reaction	rare	Rare	–

PBD, Percutaneous biliary drainage; *PTC,* percutaneous transhepatic cholangiography.

PTC is a safe procedure with few clinically significant complications. Even those such as hemobilia are easily addressed with tube upsize in case of venous hemobilia (majority) and embolization in case of arterial hemobilia. The most common preventable complication is violation of the pleural space resulting in pneumo-, hemo- or bilothorax. If this occurs, a new lower access is required with removal of the original access needle/catheter. Because of more access attempts and larger caliber, the complication rate for PBD is slightly higher than that of PTC, albeit still low.

patients are managed for long periods of time with internal–external catheters, and this type of biliary drainage is associated with bile leaks, infection, patient discomfort, and psychological problems.

Successful cannulation of a dilatated biliary system is reported to be as high as 100% and on average 70% for a nondilatated system. Successful internalization is reported in more than 90% of all successful cannulations. Biliary tract complications can be divided into major and minor categories. The minor group includes leakage of bile, pain, mild venous hemobilia, biloma formation, fever and chills, and transient hyperamylasemia with or without clinical symptoms of pancreatitis. Major complications include sepsis (2.5%), significant venous hemobilia, arterial hemobilia, local infection (abscess, peritonitis, cholecystitis, pancreatitis) (0.5%), hemothorax or bilothorax (0.5%), and death. Complications are listed in Table 3.

Percutaneous Endobiliary Stenting

Endobiliary stents are short, metallic, supported mesh stents that span the biliary obstructive lesion only and enable internal drainage of bile across the lesion, thus circumventing the need for external catheters. Endobiliary stents are either bare metallic or polytetrafluoroethylene (PTFE) covered (Figure 3).

The initial steps of deploying a stent are similar to those of placing a biliary drain tube. An initial cholangiogram is performed to calculate the length of the stricture and the diameter of the duct. The stricture can be predilatated with a balloon, which facilitates easier passage of the stent that is oversized to the native diameter of the biliary duct. An 8- or 10-mm diameter stent should be selected regardless of common bile duct (CBD) diameter. Additionally, the length of the stent should be at least

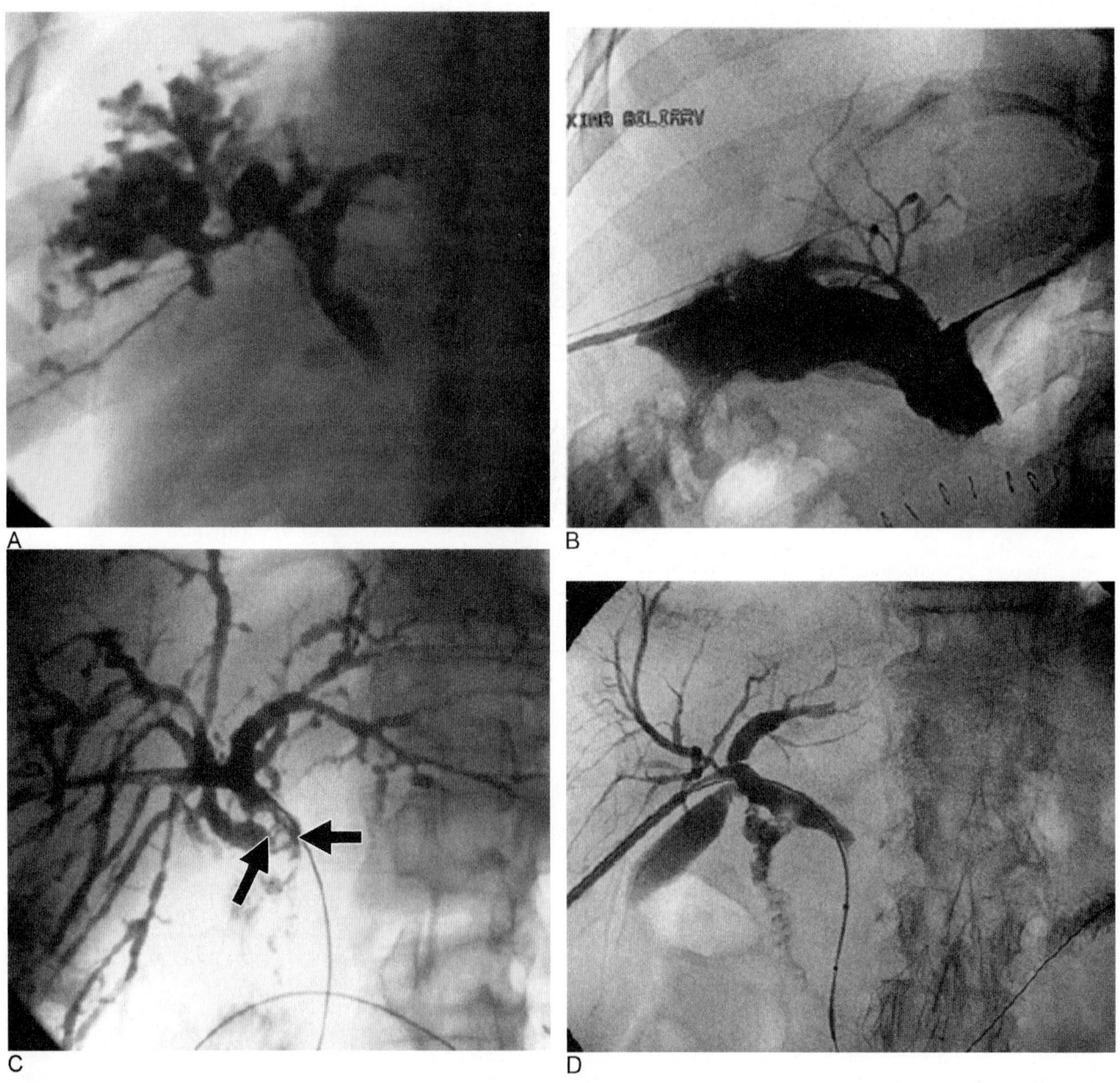

Figure 2 Spectrum of findings on percutaneous transhepatic cholangiogram. Intrahepatic cystic biliary dilatation indicative of Carolli's disease (A); large subhepatic contrast leak from a nondilatated biliary system caused by laparoscopic–cholecystectomy-related common bile duct injury (B); bile stone seen as a filling defect (arrows) in bile duct after Whipple's resection (C); distal common bile duct obstruction caused by pancreatic cancer (D); benign hepatojejunostomy anastomotic stricture after Whipple's resection.

patients are managed for long periods of time with internal–external catheters, and this type of biliary drainage is associated with bile leaks, infection, patient discomfort, and psychological problems.

Successful cannulation of a dilatated biliary system is reported to be as high as 100% and on average 70% for a nondilatated system. Successful internalization is reported in more than 90% of all successful cannulations. Biliary tract complications can be divided into major and minor categories. The minor group includes leakage of bile, pain, mild venous hemobilia, biloma formation, fever and chills, and transient hyperamylasemia with or without clinical symptoms of pancreatitis. Major complications include sepsis (2.5%), significant venous hemobilia, arterial hemobilia, local infection (abscess, peritonitis, cholecystitis, pancreatitis) (0.5%), hemothorax or bilothorax (0.5%), and death. Complications are listed in Table 3.

Percutaneous Endobiliary Stenting

Endobiliary stents are short, metallic, supported mesh stents that span the biliary obstructive lesion only and enable internal drainage of bile across the lesion, thus circumventing the need for external catheters. Endobiliary stents are either bare metallic or polytetrafluoroethylene (PTFE) covered (Figure 3).

The initial steps of deploying a stent are similar to those of placing a biliary drain tube. An initial cholangiogram is performed to calculate the length of the stricture and the diameter of the duct. The stricture can be predilatated with a balloon, which facilitates easier passage of the stent that is oversized to the native diameter of the biliary duct. An 8- or 10-mm diameter stent should be selected regardless of common bile duct (CBD) diameter. Additionally, the length of the stent should be at least

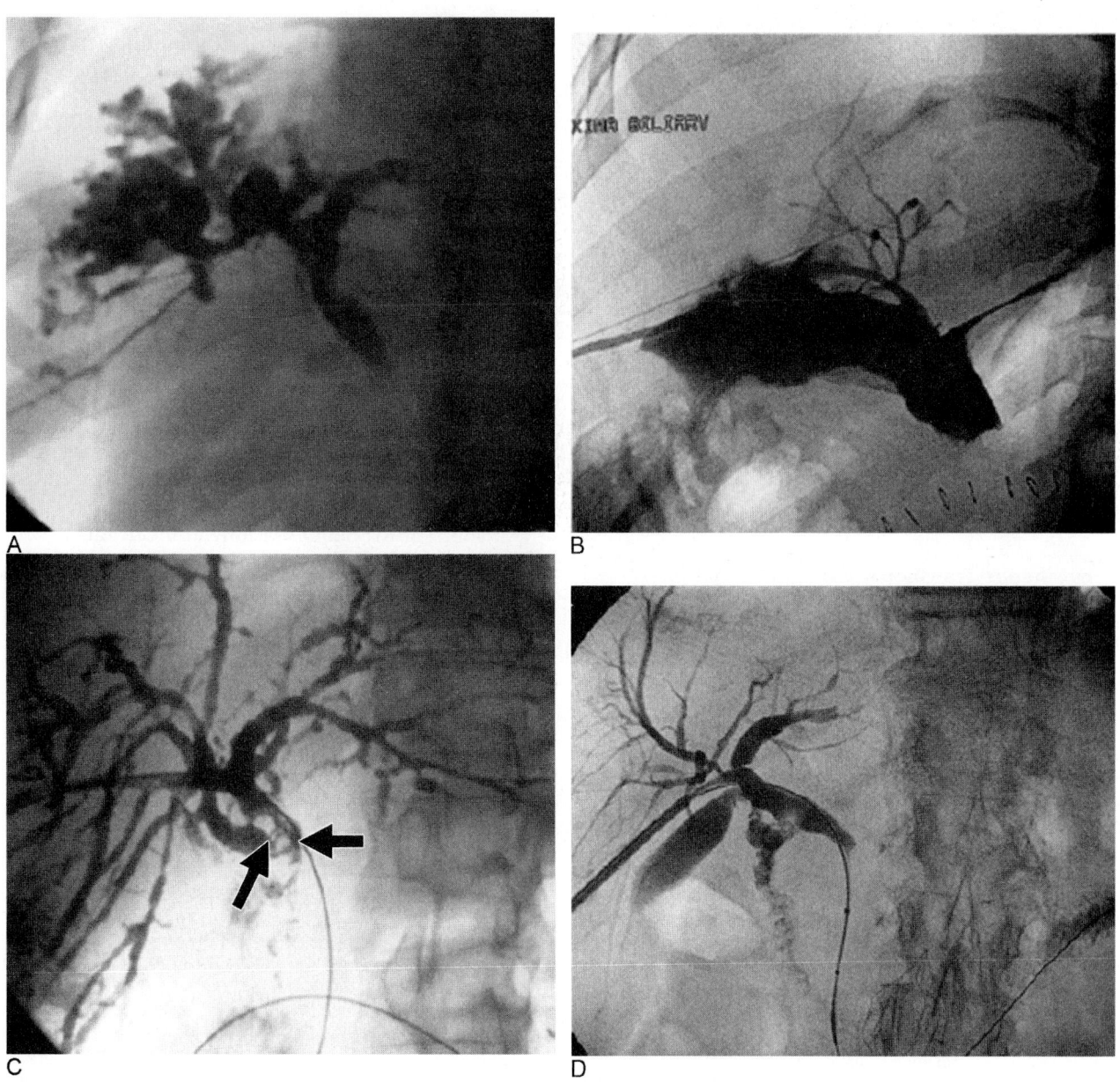

Figure 2   Spectrum of findings on percutaneous transhepatic cholangiogram. Intrahepatic cystic biliary dilatation indicative of Carolli's disease *(A)*; large subhepatic contrast leak from a nondilatated biliary system caused by laparoscopic–cholecystectomy-related common bile duct injury *(B)*; bile stone seen as a filling defect *(arrows)* in bile duct after Whipple's resection *(C)*; distal common bile duct obstruction caused by pancreatic cancer *(D)*; benign hepatojejunostomy anastomotic stricture after Whipple's resection.

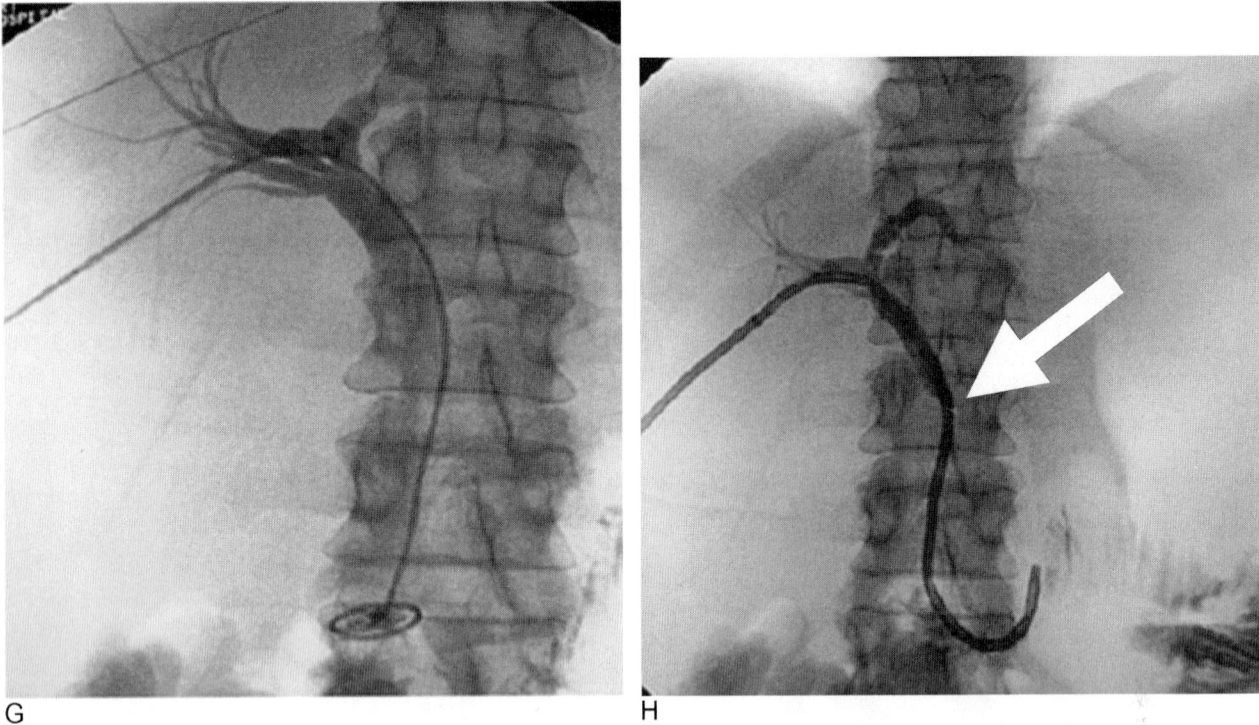

G   H

Figure 1 Cont'd—*(G)* The wire is exchanged for a stiffer one and a biliary catheter is finally advanced over it into the duodenum *(H)*. In this case, the obstructive lesion is a pancreatic cancer occluding the distal common bile duct *(arrow)*. The final cholangiogram *(H)* shows both the left and right biliary systems that have already decompressed.

hemothorax, contrast reaction, arteriovenous fistula, and vasovagal reaction. Risks of complication and death were higher for patients with malignant disease than for those with benign biliary disease. Complications following PTC (and catheter placement) are listed in Table 3. Figure 2 showcases a variety of obstructive biliary pathology seen on PTC.

Percutaneous Transhepatic Biliary Drainage

After delineating the biliary anatomy and identifying the pattern and level of obstruction with PTC, PBD is performed. Whereas for nondilatated biliary systems the most challenging aspect is actually obtaining biliary access, for an obstructed, dilatated system the difficulty is in crossing the lesion. This is usually achieved with a glide wire–catheter combination, following which a drain catheter is placed. PBD can be external or external-internal. When an external biliary drainage is placed, the tip of the catheter lies above the obstructing lesion. This occurs when the obstructing lesion cannot be crossed and thus the only route for bile drainage is external, through the PBD catheter. The catheter is connected to a gravity drainage bag and is secured to the skin to prevent inadvertent removal. In most cases, initial access, even though adequate for PTC, is inappropriate for placing a biliary catheter. If this is the case, a second, peripheral puncture of a horizontal duct is necessary (see Figure 1). In the external–internal drainage, a percutaneous catheter crosses the stricture so that the catheter's sideholes are placed above and below the obstructing lesion. This allows drainage of bile into the duodenum while correcting or maintaining fluid and electrolyte balance that may result from prolonged external biliary drainage. Eventually the external tube can be capped or completely internalized. There is little question that internal drainage is preferred over external; however, in few cases, internalization is not technically possible, and the patient is left with an external drain. Another difficult scenario may be encountered when a stricture is

too tight to be traversed. In such cases, an external catheter is initially inserted and, after a few days of external drainage, a channel through the stricture usually appears following resolution of tissue edema; this can be negotiated by the radiologist at a second session. Some

Table 3: Complications after Percutaneous Transhepatic Cholangiography and Catheter Placement

Complication	PTC	PBD	Risk Factor
Hemobilia	0.28%	8%	Central access
Biliary sepsis	1.8%	2.5%	Marked dilatation
Bile leak	1%	3%	Large bore access
Death	0.14%	1.7%	–
Biloma/abscess	–	0.5%	Improper drainage
Pneumo-, hemo-, bilothorax	rare	0.5%	High access
Vasovagal, contrast reaction	rare	Rare	–

PBD, Percutaneous biliary drainage; *PTC,* percutaneous transhepatic cholangiography.

PTC is a safe procedure with few clinically significant complications. Even those such as hemobilia are easily addressed with tube upsize in case of venous hemobilia (majority) and embolization in case of arterial hemobilia. The most common preventable complication is violation of the pleural space resulting in pneumo-, hemo- or bilothorax. If this occurs, a new lower access is required with removal of the original access needle/catheter. Because of more access attempts and larger caliber, the complication rate for PBD is slightly higher than that of PTC, albeit still low.

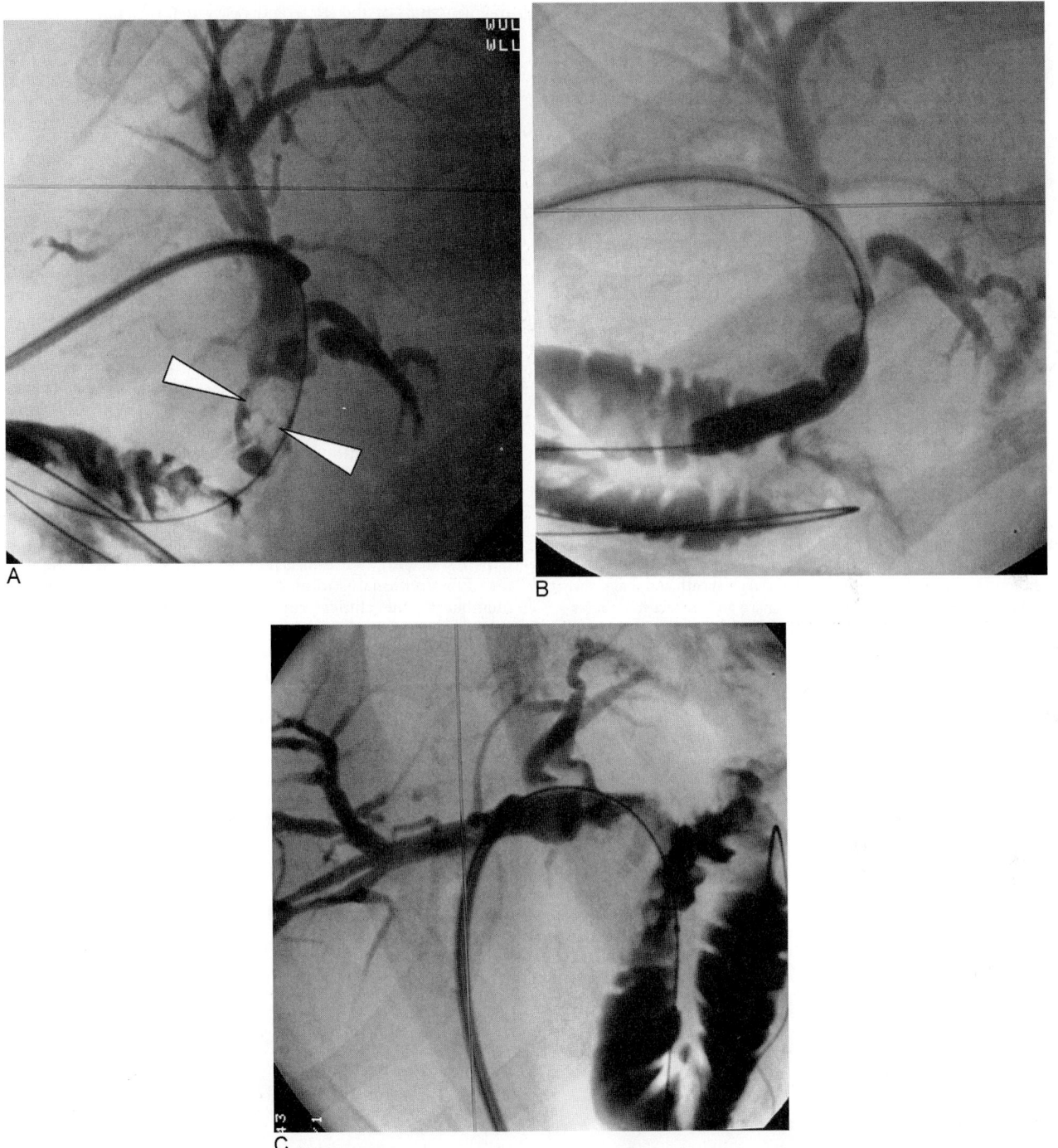

Figure 8 Percutaneous transhepatic cholangiogram (PTC) showing extraction of a common bile duct stone causing obstructive jaundice. Initial PTC reveals a large stone *(arrows)* appearing as a filling defect in the distal common bile duct in a patient after Whipple's surgery *(A)*. Balloon plasty of the hepatojejunostomy (HJ) and balloon extraction are performed *(B)*. In this maneuver the balloon is inflated above the stone and used to push the stone into the small bowel via the HJ. A follow-up PTC shows no residual stone and restoration of the flow of contrast into the small bowel *(C)*.

hepatojejunostomy (HJ). The latter, along with any condition that results in slow bile clearance or partial obstruction, can predispose to stone formation. Management of such patients is many times more difficult, especially for those who have undergone an HJ because the endoscopic route is no longer an option. Bile stones

can be managed by a variety of ways from a minimally invasive percutaneous approach. If the size of the stones is amenable, they can be simply "pushed" through the ampulla or HJ with an inflated balloon (Figure 8). Occasionally the ampulla or the HJ has to be pre-plastied with the balloon to allow for stone passage.

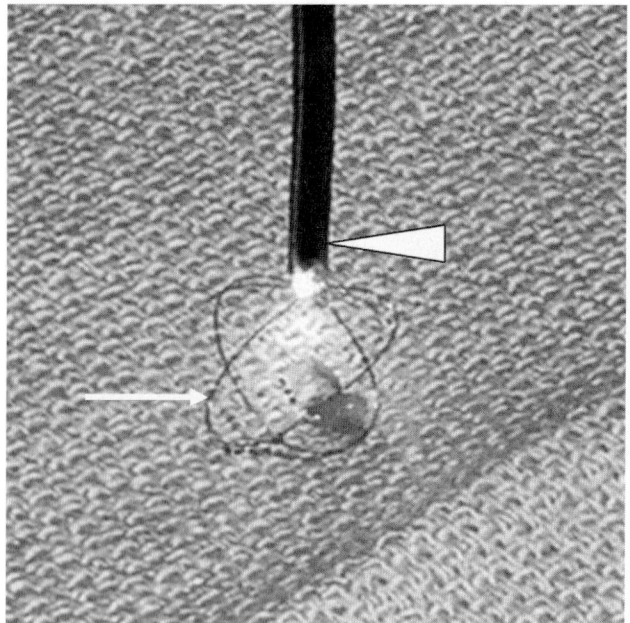

Figure 9 Basket retrieval of biliary stones is another option for the management of obstructive jaundice caused by choledocholithiasis. The basket *(arrow)* is placed into the bile ducts via a sheath and under direct choledochoscopy *(arrowhead)* is used to snare and extract the stones.

Alternatively, a stone "basket" can be used to retrieve the stones under either direct cholangioscopy or fluoroscopic guidance (Figure 9). Many times the stones are too large for either extraction option. If this is the case, the use of laser lithotripsy can facilitate fragmentation of the stone and easier removal. Biliary lithotripsy is performed under direct percutaneous cholangioscopic visualization with simultaneous fluoroscopic confirmation. After the stone is pulverized into smaller fragments, the fragments can be pushed into the small bowel. Figure 10 shows the use of biliary lithotripsy in a patient with massive bile stone rendered stone free after lithotripsy.

DISCUSSION

Obstructive jaundice presents a difficult clinical problem from both diagnostic workup and treatment points of view. Even though cross-sectional imaging (CT, MRI) can easily reveal the extent and distribution of biliary ductal dilatation, many times it fails to show the cause of obstruction. Percutaneous cholangiogram can characterize biliary lesions and help to diagnose a variety of benign and malignant states. Additionally, percutaneous biliary access offers the choice of a number of treatment interventions, including drainage of an obstructed biliary tree, placement of biliary endostent, biliary balloon plasty, endobiliary biopsy, embolization of bile leak, cholangioscopy, and stone extraction. These procedures require refined skills and experience and can be invaluable to surgeons and patients dealing with biliary pathology. Beyond these skills, the interventional radiologist must become a contributing member to the clinical care of these patients and coordinate this care with the rest of the interdisciplinary team. Whatever the cause and degree, obstructive jaundice can always be resolved with proper percutaneous interventions. In benign disease (strictures, stones, bile leak), percutaneous techniques can offer definitive treatment, whereas in malignant disease they can be an important adjuvant to surgical or medical treatment planning.

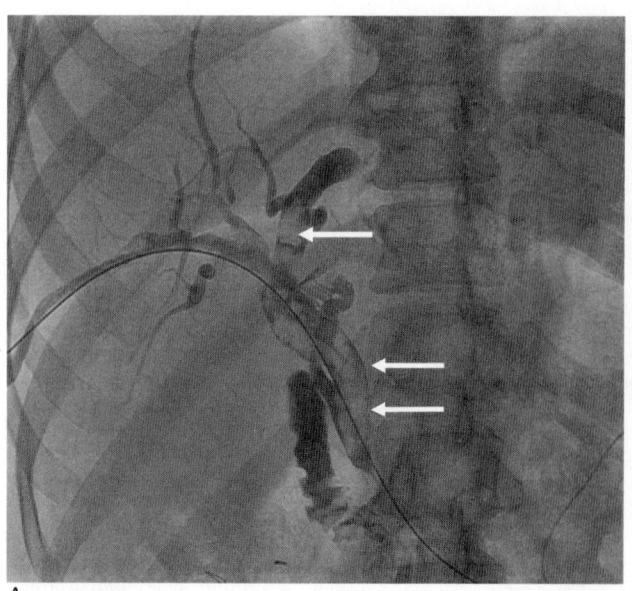

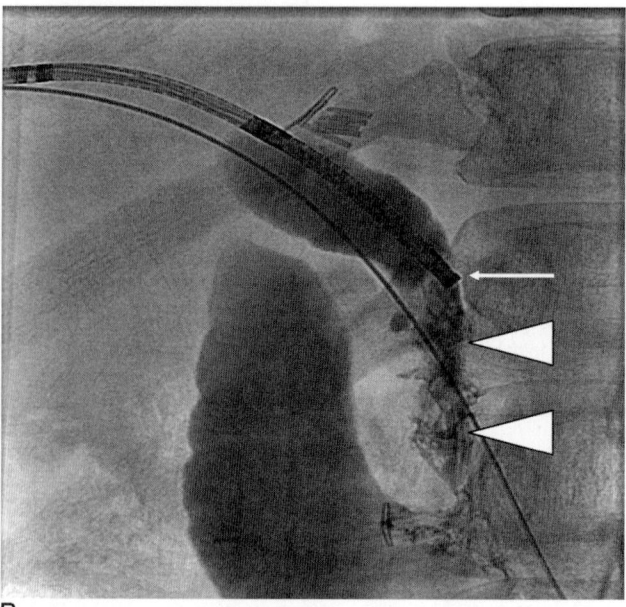

A   B

Figure 10 Percutaneous treatment of large biliary stones causing obstructive jaundice. A diagnostic cholangiogram shows large filling defects in the right, left, and common bile ducts of a patient *(A)*. The stones were too large to extract in whole. Under direct choledochoscopic *(arrow)* and fluoroscopic visualization the stones were broken by use of lithotripsy *(B)*.

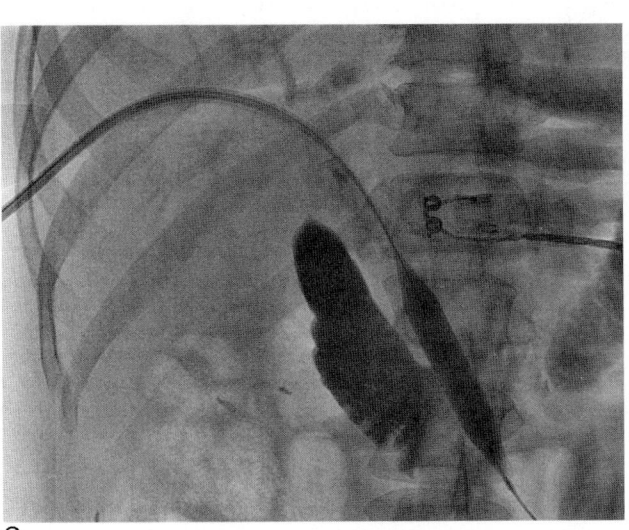
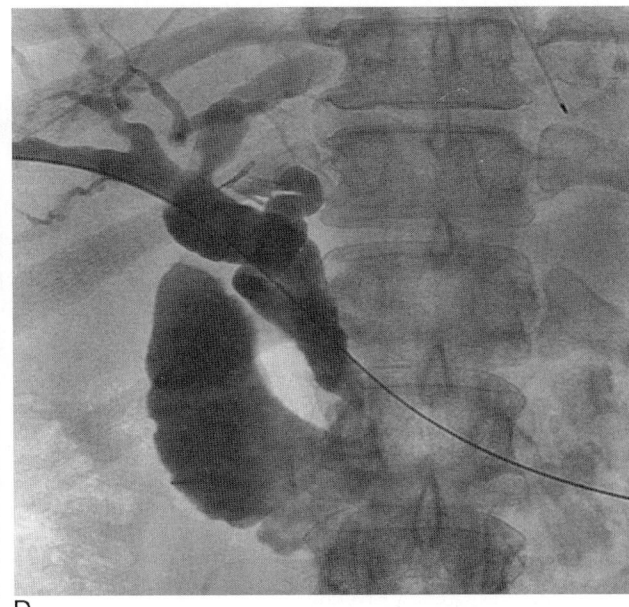

C

D

Figures 10 Cont'd—The tiny stone fragments *(arrowheads)* are visualized in the common bile duct. Then a balloon is used to push the fragments into the small bowel and clear the bile ducts *(C)*. Postprocedure cholangiogram shows complete resolution of cholelithiasis *(D)*.

SUGGESTED READINGS

Bezzi M, Zolovkins A, Cantisani V, and others: New ePTFE/FEP-covered stent in the palliative treatment of malignant biliary obstruction, *J Vasc Interv Radiol* 13:581, 2002.

Funaki B, Zaleski GX, Straus CA, and others: Percutaneous biliary drainage in patients with nondilated intrahepatic bile ducts, *AJR Am J Roentgenol* 173:1541, 1999.

L'Hermine C, Ernst O, Delemazure O, and others: Arterial complications of percutaneous transhepatic biliary drainage, *Cardiovasc Intervent Radiol* 19:160, 1996.

Pinol V, Castells A, Bordas JM, and others: Percutaneous self-expanding metal stents versus endoscopic polyethylene endoprostheses for treating malignant biliary obstruction: Randomized clinical trial, *Radiology* 225:27, 2002.

Savader SJ, Prescott CA, Lund GB, and others: Intraductal biliary biopsy: Comparison of three techniques, *J Vasc Interv Radiol* 7:743, 1996.

OBSTRUCTIVE JAUNDICE: ENDOSCOPIC THERAPY

David F. Hutcheon, MD

Endoscopic retrograde cholangiopancreatography (ERCP) is an integral part of the management of obstructive jaundice. It is a low-risk procedure that allows clear definition of the cause of obstructive jaundice, as well as therapy, in the same endoscopic session. With the advent of more sophisticated imaging studies, particularly magnetic resonance cholangiopancreatography (MRCP), ERCP is seldom used for diagnosis alone but continues to be a mainstay of therapy for obstructive jaundice.

Patients with obstructive jaundice present with symptoms of dark urine; jaundice; possibly abdominal pain; and, in the case of cholangitis, fever. Laboratory studies usually show an elevation in direct bilirubin. Alkaline phosphatase is usually elevated in excess of transaminases in cases of subacute or chronic jaundice, whereas transaminases frequently exceed alkaline phosphatase elevation in cases of acute biliary obstruction, such as choledocholithiasis.

The causes of obstructive jaundice are listed in Table 1. In the United States, choledocholithiasis and pancreatic carcinoma are the most common causes.

Imaging studies are extremely helpful in the preoperative diagnosis of obstructive jaundice. Studies usually indicate biliary ductal dilation proximal to the point of obstruction. Ultrasound is readily available and frequently the initial imaging method. Sensitivity for detection of biliary ductal dilation varies from 55% to 91%. Ultrasound is not sensitive for visualization of common bile duct (CBD) stones. Computed tomography scans accurately identify ductal dilation and masses, particularly of the pancreas.

MRCP and endoscopic ultrasound are comparable to ERCP, which is at present the gold standard, in providing images that delineate ductal dilation, as well as stones and strictures. All studies may miss small stones.

Endoscopic ultrasound can be performed in the same session as ERCP, providing information as to whether ERCP is necessary in cases of choledocholithiasis in which the stone may have passed or be retained.

The technique of ERCP has been well described. The patient is kept non per os, and in most cases antibiotics are administered intravenously before the procedure. Sedation with a combination of meperidine or fentanyl and diazepam (Valium; Roche Pharmaceuticals, Nutley, NJ) or midazolam has been traditional in the past. Recently, deeper sedation with propofol administered by an anesthesiologist is frequently used. A side-viewing endoscope

Table 1: Causes of Obstructive Jaundice

Benign

- Choledocholithiasis
- Benign biliary strictures—postoperative, sclerosing cholangitis, papillary stenosis, chronic pancreatitis, sphincter of Oddi dysfunction
- Choledochal cyst
- Parasitic disease
- External compression caused by portal lymphadenopathy, Mirizzi's syndrome, pancreatic pseudocyst

Neoplastic

- Pancreatic carcinoma
- Cholangiocarcinoma
- Gallbladder carcinoma
- Periampullary carcinoma
- Islet cell carcinoma
- Metastatic or adjacent neoplasms

is introduced through the mouth and passed into the stomach. The pylorus is passed by visualizing the opening and, as it is approached, elevating the endoscope tip so that the pylorus is just lost to view inferiorly. With gentle pressure, the scope passes through the pylorus. The tip is then passed into the second portion of duodenum, and the scope is retracted to straighten the loop of scope in the stomach and advance the tip of the endoscope distally, closer to the papilla of Vater. The endoscope has an elevator that allows raising and lowering of a cannula or sphincterotome, which is passed under direct vision into the papillary opening and then into the pancreatic or bile duct (Fig. 1). A hydrophilic or JAG guidewire (Boston Scientific, Natick, MA) may be passed through the cannula or sphincterotome to aid with ductal cannulation and avoid excessive papillary trauma. After cannulation, dye is injected under fluoroscopy, and a cholangiogram or pancreatogram is obtained. From the cholangiogram, a diagnosis of the cause of jaundice is usually evident.

Sphincterotomy is a technique that allows enlargement of the papilla of Vater opening by incising a 1- to 2-cm segment of duodenal wall, which is shared by the distal CBD. Incision beyond or lateral to the shared wall causes duodenal perforation, and thus precision is necessary to orient the incision and control the extent of the incision. This is accomplished using a bow-shaped sphincterotome with a wire through which current is applied to allow controlled cutting and coagulation. The speed of the cut is a function of the amount of current and the amount of pressure from the wire against the tissue. A minimal amount of wire is usually introduced into the bile duct (usually approximately one third of the length), and pressure is gently applied using the elevator. After the incision is made, stones may be extracted, strictures dilatated, and stents placed (Fig. 2).

CHOLEDOCHOLITHISIS

Choledocholithiasis is found in 8% to 18% of patients with symptomatic gallstones. Distal CBD obstruction by stones may lead to jaundice, pancreatitis, cholangitis, or any combination of these. Although some series suggest an advantage for laparoscopic bile duct exploration over ERCP and laparoscopic cholecystectomy at the time of surgery, most centers treat choledocholithiasis and chololithiasis with ERCP, sphincterotomy, and stone extraction,

followed by laparoscopic cholecystectomy. ERCP is successful in clearing the biliary ducts of stones in more than 90% of cases.

Identifying the individuals with cholelithiasis who also have choledocholithiasis is a challenge. Patients with clinical jaundice or cholangitis or ultrasonic findings of biliary dilatation or CBD stones have a greater than 50% risk of choledocholithiasis and should usually undergo ERCP. Patients with a history of jaundice or pancreatitis, elevated bilirubin, and alkaline phosphatase levels or multiple small gallstones have a 10% to 50% risk of CBD stones. Patients without these findings have a less than 5% risk of choledocholithiasis. MRCP and endoscopic ultrasound are increasingly useful in sorting the patients who should undergo ERCP for presumed CBD stones.

In the past, elderly patients with gallstones and choledocholithiasis were frequently treated with ERCP and stone extraction alone, without cholecystectomy. Two recent studies suggest that 24% to 47% of patients so treated will have recurrent biliary symptoms. With the low morbidity and mortality of laparoscopic cholecystectomy, a more aggressive surgical approach in most patients seems warranted.

The technique of stone extraction relies on an adequate sphincterotomy. It is important to cut entirely through the sphincter muscle and up to the top of the papillary bulge for large stones. Stones can be extracted with balloon catheters, which inflate a balloon above the stone and remove it by pulling the catheter and stone through the sphincterotomy site. For larger stones, I prefer using a stone basket, which is placed above the stone, then brought down into the vicinity of the stone. Shaking the basket by moving the catheter slightly in and out helps to engage the stone. The stone then can be pulled through the sphincterotomy. Large cholesterol stones are usually faceted on cholangiogram and frequently fragment on extraction. Bilirubin stones are frequently round and usually do not fragment; firm traction or mechanical lithotripsy may be necessary. When multiple stones are present in the bile duct, it is important to initially extract the distal stones and work up the duct to avoid impacting multiple stones in the distal duct. If there is any question of adequate clearance of the duct, it is prudent to leave a stent or nasobiliary tube. The nasobiliary tube has the advantage of allowing ad lib cholangiograms and irrigation but the disadvantage of being easily dislodged. I prefer the placement of an Amsterdam stent, which acts to prevent stone impaction and bile duct occlusion. In critically ill or coagulopathic patients, choledocholithiasis can be treated temporarily with the placement of a 7- or 10-F Amsterdam stent without sphincterotomy or stone extraction. This relieves the CBD obstruction and allows resolution of the acute situation. This approach is not uncommon in critically ill patients with cholangitis and choledocholithiasis. The stent obviously must be removed at a later date when the patient is more stable. More definitive therapy, such as sphincterotomy and stone extraction, can be carried out at that time as well.

CHOLANGITIS

Cholangitis is a result of biliary bacterial contamination and increased pressure resulting from obstruction. It occurs most frequently in patients with choledocholithiasis or prior biliary manipulation. Charcot's triad of fever, right upper quadrant pain, and jaundice occurs in 50% to 75% of cases. The most common organisms are *Escherichia coli*, *Klebsiella*, *Enterobacter*, and *Enterococcus*. Anaerobes such as *Bacteroides* and *Clostridia* may be present. Antibiotic therapy with ampicillin and gentamicin, imipenem or meropenem, or levofloxacin is recommended, with metronidazole added in severely ill patients. Eighty percent of patients respond to antibiotic therapy and may undergo ERCP therapy on an elective basis. Twenty percent require urgent endoscopic intervention with sphincterotomy and stone removal or stent placement before more definitive therapy.

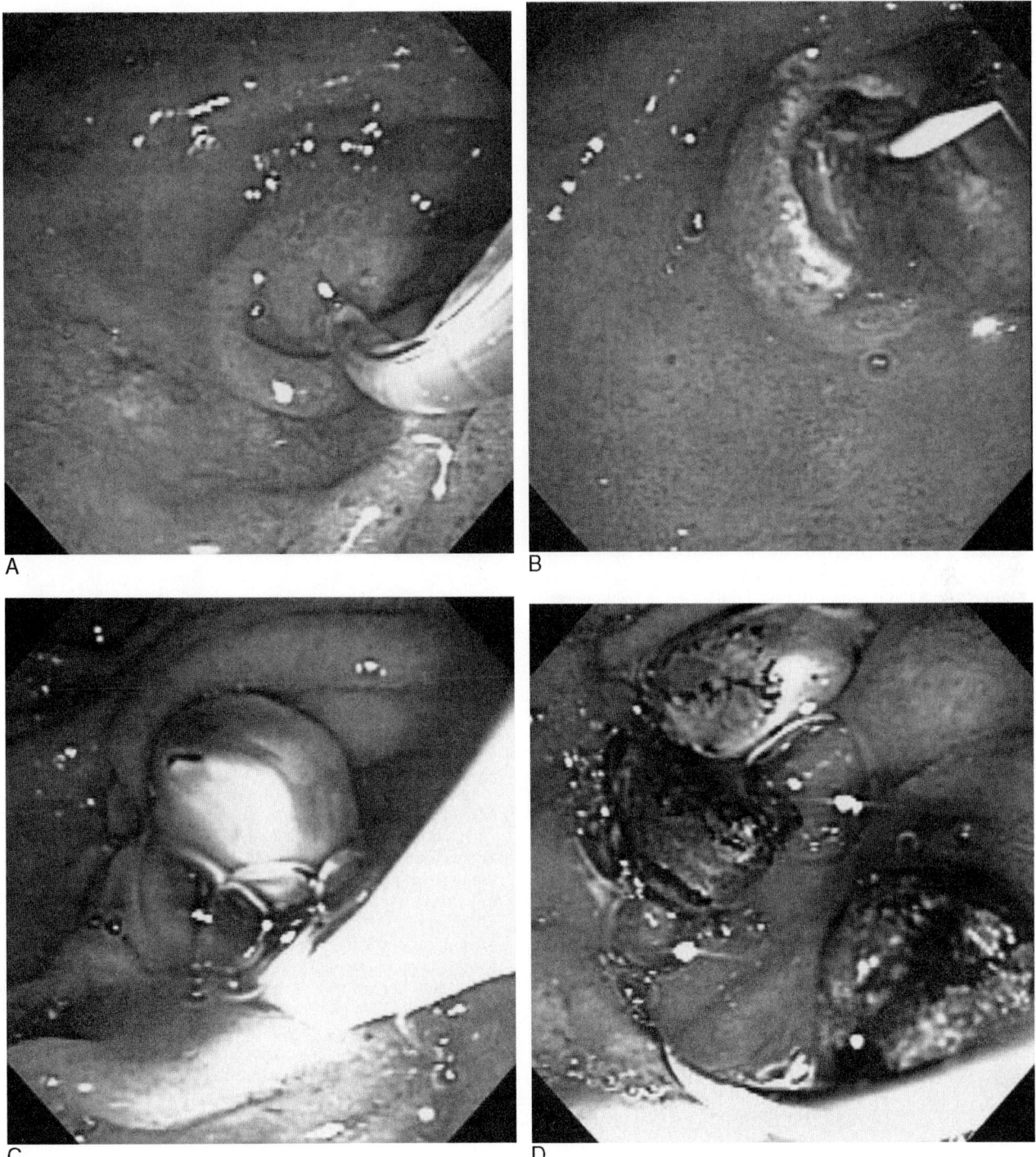

Figure 1 **(A)** Sphincterotome in normal papilla of Vater. **(B)** Papilla of Vater after sphincterotomy. **(C)** Stone being removed from papilla with balloon catheter. **(D)** Multiple stones in duodenum after extraction.

MALIGNANT BILIARY STRICTURES

Obstructive jaundice caused by malignant strictures is ideally treated with curative surgical resection. Biliary stenting is usually performed in unresectable patients or for biliary decompression before surgery. Tissue sampling from the stricture may be obtained through brush cytology in which a brush is passed into the bile duct and area of stricture and samples taken for cytology. Biliary brush cytology has a sensitivity of 35% to 70% and specificity greater than 90% in patients with malignant strictures. Small biopsy forceps may also

be passed into the bile duct and biopsies obtained. These yield sensitivities of 43% to 88%. In general, a positive cytology or biopsy is helpful, but a negative one does not rule out a malignant stricture.

Biliary stenting may be accomplished with either plastic or metal stents, both of which are highly efficacious in relieving obstruction. The advantages of metal stenting are larger luminal diameter and longer patency rates compared with plastic stents (Table 2). Plastic stents are readily removed and replaced, whereas metal stents are usually permanent and not removable because of tissue ingrowth into the interstices of the stent mesh. When metal stents occlude, a

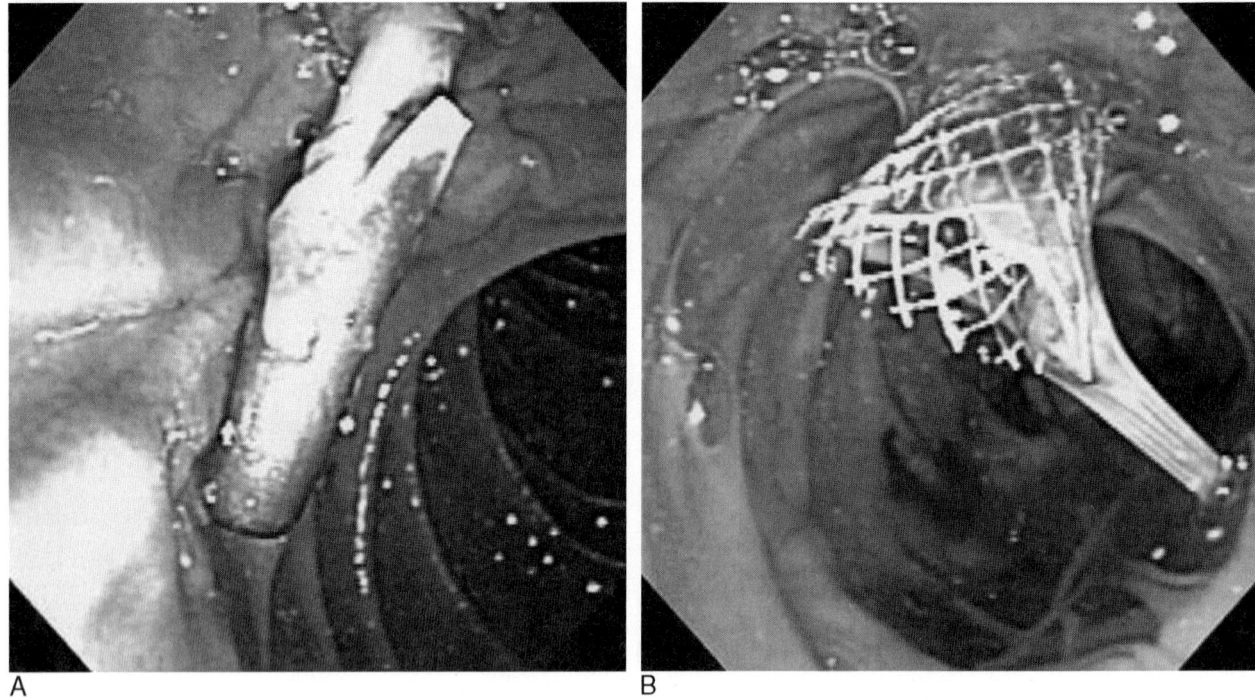

Figure 2 **(A)** Amsterdam 10-F plastic stent extending from papilla of Vater. **(B)** Biliary Wallstent extending from papilla of Vater with purulent drainage.

Table 2: Plastic versus Metal Stents for Malignant Biliary Obstruction

	Carr-Locke	Davids	Yoon
Successful placement			
Plastic stents	95%	95%	
Uncovered metal stents	98%	96%	
Mean time to obstruction			
Plastic stents	62 days	82 days	
Uncovered metal stents	111 days	273 days	319 days
Covered metal stents			398 days
Stents obstructing			
Plastic stents		54%	
Uncovered metal stents		33%	

second metal stent or plastic stent may be placed to alleviate obstruction. In general, plastic stents are replaced every 3 months.

Stenting may be performed with or without prior sphincterotomy. Sphincterotomy is frequently performed to allow ready access to the biliary tree. A hydrophilic or JAG guidewire is passed through a cannula, or a sphincterotome is passed through the area of stricture. It is usually not necessary to dilatate the stricture before stenting. If a plastic stent is being placed, a guide catheter is passed over the wire and into the right or left hepatic duct well above the stricture. The stent is then placed over the guide catheter and pushed into position with a pusher tube while an endoscopy technician maintains traction on the guide catheter to prevent advancement of the catheter. This is performed under fluoroscopic observation to maintain the guide catheter in position. When the stent is properly positioned, the guide catheter and wire are simultaneously withdrawn through the scope, with the pushing tube left in position against the position stent to prevent distal displacement of the stent. Bile drainage is usually evident through or around (or both) the stent after placement.

In placing metal stents, a guidewire is passed through the neoplastic stricture, as with plastic stents. The metal stent is then passed over the wire into position such that the proximal stent is 1 to 2 cm or more above the proximal extent of the stricture, and the distal portion extends 1 to 2 cm from the papilla. The stent is deployed in 1- to 2-cm increments under fluoroscopic guidance. It must usually be retracted toward the endoscope with each deployment because it tends to be pulled into the bile duct as the proximal portion of the stent deploys and expands. Both plastic and metal stents achieve successful biliary drainage in more than 90% of patients (Fig. 3).

In the past few years, plastic-coated metal stents have become available. These stents have a plastic coating on the interior that is designed to prevent ingrowth of tumor or hyperplastic tissue, which is a frequent cause of uncovered metal stent obstruction. Both ends of the stent have 0.5 cm of uncovered mesh to help anchor the stent. Advantages of the stent are a slightly longer patency than uncovered metal stents (Table 2) and the fact that they can be removed by placing a snare around the distal stent and pulling it out in the same manner as plastic stents are removed. Stent migration is more common with covered metal stents, and cholecystitis occurs in 3.5% to 3.8% of patients because of obstruction of the cystic duct.

Malignant strictures of the bifurcation such as Klatskin cholangiocarcinomas are more technically challenging and have lower success rates for endoscopic stenting than more distal malignant strictures. Transhepatic stenting is frequently preferred over endoscopic stenting. In patients with bilateral hepatic duct obstruction, unilateral stenting is as effective as bilateral stenting.

Periampullary neoplasms also present a challenge in that they are frequently friable and bleed with minor trauma. It is important

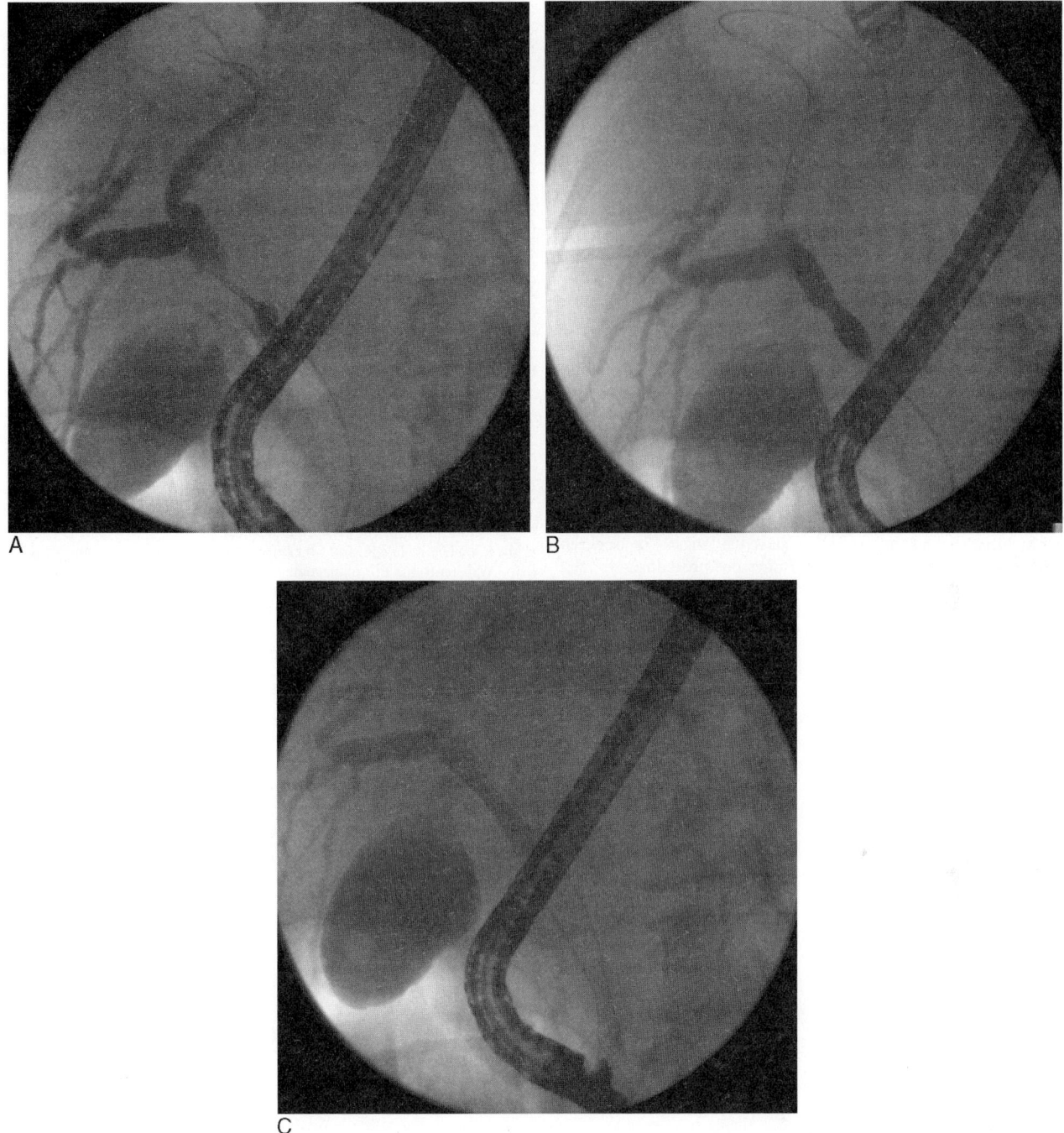

Figure 3 **(A)** Stricture in common hepatic duct. **(B)** Balloon dilatation of the stricture. **(C)** Wallstent in place through the common hepatic duct stricture.

to scrutinize the papilla to identify bile staining or other clue to the papillary orifice before attempted cannulation. Sphincterotomy alone can frequently relieve biliary obstruction in these patients if it can be extended above the neoplasm. If there is any doubt regarding adequate drainage, however, a stent should be placed.

BENIGN BILIARY STRICTURES

The most common causes of benign biliary strictures are ductal injury at prior biliary surgery, including liver transplantation, sclerosing cholangitis, and chronic pancreatitis. Benign strictures can be treated endoscopically by performing a biliary

sphincterotomy and balloon dilatation and placing 2 to 3 10-F stents through the area of stricture. Balloon dilatation is achieved by placing a sausage-shaped balloon at the tip of a catheter into the stricture and inflating the balloon under pressure. This is usually performed sequentially with any combination of balloons of 4, 6, 8 mm diameter. After dilatation, 2 to 3 stents are placed through the stricture to maintain patency and to prevent the scar tissue from retracting and restricturing. The stents are changed every 3 months for a period of at least 1 year. Success rates are variable. In one series of biliary strictures caused by chronic pancreatitis, the technique was successful in 59.1% of patients without pancreatic calcifications but in only 7.7% of patients with pancreatic calcification.

Table 3: Complications of Endoscopic Retrograde Pancreatography and Sphincterotomy

	Freeman (1996) %	Rabenstein (1999) %
Pancreatitis	5.4	4.7
Bleeding	2.0	2.0
Sepsis	1.5	1.4
Perforation	0.3	0.1

COMPLICATIONS OF ENDOSCOPIC RETROGRADE PANCREATOGRAPHY AND SPHINCTEROTOMY

Major complications of ERCP and sphincterotomy are listed in Table 3. The most common complication in most series is pancreatitis, followed by bleeding, cholangitis, and perforation. Risk factors for complications include difficulty with cannulation, precut sphincterotomy, sphincter of Oddi dysfunction, combined percutaneous-endoscopic procedures, and low case volumes by the endoscopist.

The risk of hemorrhage is increased in patients who are coagulopathic, bleed during the procedure, have cholangitis, or undergo anticoagulation therapy in less than 3 days postprocedure.

The risk of pancreatitis is increased in patients with pancreatic ductal injection, prior post-ERCP pancreatitis, young age, sphincter of Oddi dysfunction, normal bilirubin, and precut or pancreatic sphincterotomy. Stenting the pancreatic duct has been shown to decrease the risk or pancreatitis in high-risk individuals.

SUGGESTED READINGS

Baillie J, Paulson E, Vitellas K: Biliary imaging: a review, *Gastroenterology* 124:1686, 2003.

Carr-Locke D, Ball T, Connors P, and others: Multicenter randomized trial of Wallstent biliary endoprosthesis versus plastic stents [abstract], *Gastrointest Endosc* 39:310, 1993.

Davids P, Groen A, Raws E, and others: Randomised trial of self-expanding metal stents versus polyethylene stents for distal malignant biliary obstruction, *Lancet* 340:1488–1492, 1992.

Freeman ML, Nelson D, Sherman S, and others: Complications of endoscopic biliary sphincterotomy, *N Engl J Med* 335:909, 1996.

Freitas M, Bell R, Duffy A: Choledocholithiasis: evolving standards for diagnosis and management, *World J Gastroenterol* 12:3162, 2006.

Lau J, Leow C, Fung T, and others: Cholecystectomy or gallbladder in situ after endoscopic sphincterotomy and bile duct stone removal in Chinese patients, *Gastroenterology* 130:96, 2006.

Leung J, Rahim N: The role of covered self-expandable metallic stents in malignant biliary strictures, *Gastrointest Endosc* 63:1001, 2006.

Rabenstein T, Schneider H, Nicklas M, and others: Impact of skill and experience of the endoscopist on the outcome of endoscopic sphincterotomy techniques, *Gastrointest Endosc* 50:628, 1999.

Yoon W, Lee K, Lee K, and others: A comparison of covered and uncovered Wallstents for the management of distal malignant biliary obstruction, *Gastrointest Endosc* 63:9996, 2006.

THE PANCREAS

ACUTE PANCREATITIS

Zara Cooper, MD, MSc, and Stanley W. Ashley, MD

In the United States approximately 220,000 patients develop acute pancreatitis annually. In most, this is a benign and self-limited disease that resolves within 1 week with conservative management. However, as many as 20% develop severe acute pancreatitis, most often associated with pancreatic necrosis. Such disease is characterized by marked fluid sequestration, the systemic inflammatory response syndrome (SIRS), multiorgan dysfunction, and sometimes pancreatic infection and sepsis. In this group, mortality remains in the range of 10% to 15%.

Biliary disease and alcohol are responsible for most episodes of pancreatitis. A variety of other less frequent etiologies have been identified, and approximately 20% of cases remain idiopathic. Many of this latter group have biliary sludge or microlithiasis and, if they suffer a second episode, should undergo cholecystectomy. Likewise, patients with documented cholelithiasis and mild disease should undergo early cholecystectomy, preferably during the same hospitalization to prevent recurrence. For most of the other etiologies, recurrent episodes are prevented by eliminating the inciting agent when possible.

No matter the etiology, the inciting event leads to intra-acinar cell cleavage of trypsinogen to trypsin, with subsequent activation of other enzymes. The local inflammatory response in the pancreas is associated with the liberation of oxygen-derived free radicals and cytokines, including interleukin (IL)-1, IL-6, IL-8, tumor necrosis factor alpha (TNFα), and platelet-activating factor (PAF); these mediators play an important role in the transformation of a local inflammatory response to a systemic illness. Despite considerable experimental effort, it is still unclear why some patients develop only interstitial or edematous pancreatitis, whereas others progress to pancreatic necrosis. Likewise, our understanding of the pathogenesis of pancreatitis has had little impact on management to date. Trials with inhibitors of secretion, proteases, and even PAF have failed to demonstrate a benefit.

DIAGNOSIS AND STAGING

The early diagnosis and precise staging of disease severity are important goals in the initial evaluation and management. Not only must pancreatitis be differentiated from a myriad of other potential diagnoses, but patients should be stratified to identify those with severe disease and to guide appropriate therapy. The typical presentation includes low-grade fever, severe epigastric pain radiating to the back, abdominal tenderness, nausea, emesis, and leukocytosis. Diagnosis still largely depends on clinical suspicion and the presence of an elevated serum amylase and lipase. Amylase is less specific than lipase because elevation can be seen in a number of other settings, including perforated duodenal ulcer, small bowel obstruction, renal failure, and salivary disease. Lipase has a longer half-life and is 100% sensitive and specific when the cutoff for diagnosis is three times the upper limit of normal. Imaging studies may prove useful in equivocal cases.

Clinical judgment should guide the timing of such studies. Ultrasound may be appropriate to identify gallstones, particularly if elevations in the liver function tests raise concern for biliary obstruction and cholangitis. Endoscopic ultrasound (EUS) or magnetic resonance cholangiopancreatography (MRCP) are even more specific for obstructive disease. Early contrast-enhanced computed tomography (CT) is indicated if the diagnosis is in question but may fail to identify developing pancreatic necrosis until such areas are better demarcated, which may require 2 to 3 days after the initial clinical onset of symptoms. Although limited experimental evidence has suggested that intravenous contrast may exacerbate early pancreatic necrosis, clinical data to support this phenomenon are lacking. The sensitivity for identifying pancreatic necrosis, as opposed to interstitial or edematous pancreatitis, using contrast-enhanced CT scan approaches 100% after 4 days from presentation (Fig. 1). It is therefore reasonable to recommend an abdominal CT scan with oral and intravenous contrast in patients with clinical and biochemical features of acute pancreatitis who do not improve after several days of conservative management. Follow-up scans may be obtained with any signs of clinical deterioration.

After the diagnosis is established, it is important to identify patients with severe disease and institute aggressive therapy. To this end, the Ranson scoring system was developed (Table 1) and seems to be reasonably predictive of the subsequent course. A Ranson score of 3 or higher is generally associated with severe disease. A variety of attempts have been made to improve on this—the Glasgow and APACHE (Acute Physiology and Chronic Health Evaluation) II scores have been most commonly used and may have some minor advantages. The Balthazar score, based on the findings of CT scan, has been shown to be similarly accurate. Efforts have also been made to identify a single predictive marker. C-reactive protein (CRP) is perhaps the most reliable—a level greater than 150 mg/ml on the second day of symptoms predicts severe disease at least as well as the scoring systems using multiple criteria.

These tools are particularly useful for comparing patients in clinical trials. However, for the individual patient, clinical judgment, informed by an understanding of these scoring systems, is most important. The patient with signs of fluid sequestration (tachycardia, orthostatic hypotension, hemoconcentration, oliguria), confusion, hypoxemia, and hypocalcemia should receive aggressive resuscitation and monitoring, usually in an intensive-care setting. Age older than 55 years and morbid obesity are both

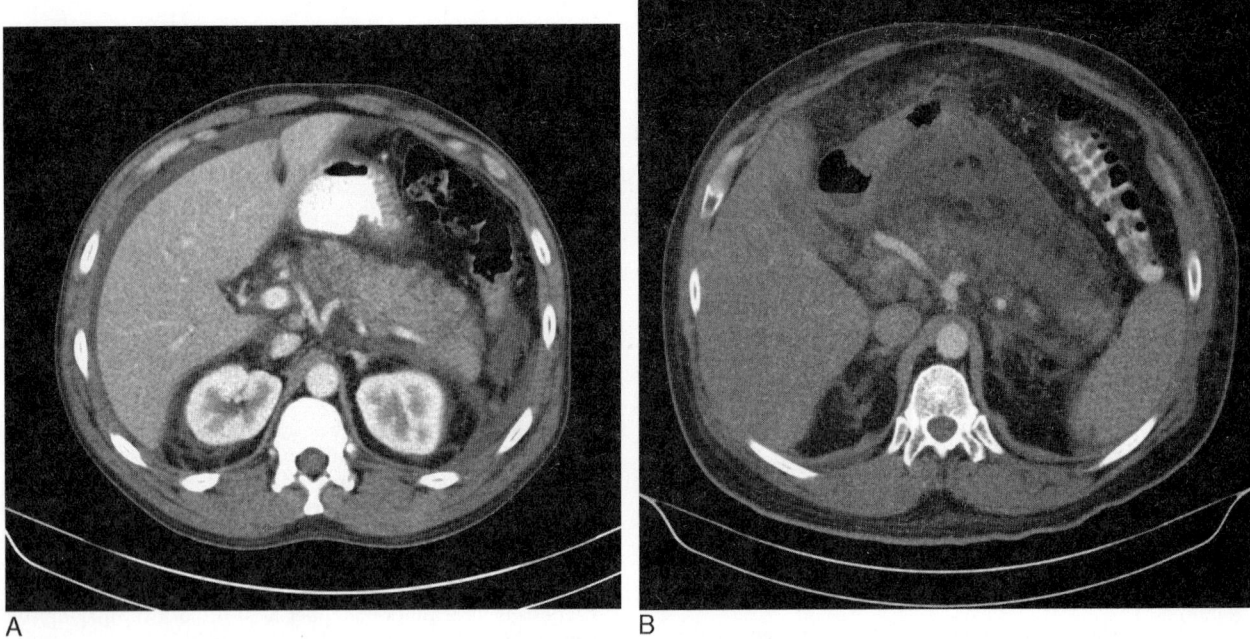

Figure 1 **(A)** Computed tomography *(CT)* of interstitial pancreatitis. Although there is diffuse swelling of the pancreas, it is uniformly enhanced after intravenous contrast. **(B)** CT of pancreatic necrosis. The diffusely swollen pancreas fails to enhance with intravenous contrast except in the extreme distal tail.

Table 1: Ranson's Score for Assessing the Severity of Acute Pancreatitis

On Admission	Within 48 Hours
Age >55 years	Drop in hematocrit >10%
WBC >16,000/mm^3	Fluid deficit >6 L
Serum glucose >200 mg/dl	Serum calcium <8/0 mg/dl
Serum LDH >350 mg/dl	Hypoxemia (pO$_2$ <60 mm Hg)
Serum AST >250 IU/L	Rise in BUN >50 mg/dl
	Albumin <3.2 g/dl

AST, Aspartate aminotransferase; *BUN,* blood urea nitrogen; *LDH,* lactate dehydrogenase, *WBC,* white blood cell count.

associated with a significant increase in morbidity and warrant more careful management, as well.

GENERAL MANAGEMENT

For the purposes of management, severe acute pancreatitis is conveniently divided into two clinical phases—an early vasoactive and a late septic phase. The vasoactive phase, typically during the first 2 weeks, is dominated by the consequences of SIRS, including massive fluid sequestration, respiratory failure, and renal insufficiency. The second phase of the disease is characterized by infection of pancreatic necrosis and subsequent sepsis. Both phases can result in multiorgan failure, the leading cause of death in acute pancreatitis, and management strategies are directed at preventing this complication.

Resuscitation and Supportive Measures

Aggressive fluid resuscitation is important to replenish extravascular or "third-space" fluid losses, which may be considerable.

Intravenous fluids at rates of greater than 250 ml per hour are often necessary to restore and maintain intravascular volume. This degree of fluid resuscitation is important to avoid systemic complications, particularly acute renal insufficiency, that may occur with hypovolemia. Furthermore, inadequate resuscitation has recently been shown to pose a significant risk for further pancreatic injury, particularly necrosis.

Close monitoring of respiratory, cardiovascular, and renal function is essential to detect and treat complications from the hypovolemia. Usually this means a Foley catheter for monitoring urinary output and continuous measurements of oxygen saturation. Patients with the most severe disease may also require continuous arterial and central venous or pulmonary artery pressure monitoring. Early intubation should be considered for patients with significant respiratory compromise.

Pain control is essential in these patients. Intravenous narcotics are often necessary; there is even some recent evidence suggesting that better pain control with an epidural catheter may improve outcomes. There is no evidence to support the routine use of a nasogastric tube to avoid pancreatic stimulation; however, paralytic ileus is not uncommon, and nasogastric tubes should be used in this circumstance to prevent emesis and aspiration pneumonia.

Nutrition

Limitation of enteral feeding to avoid stimulation of pancreatic exocrine secretion has traditionally been the norm. Recent data suggest that this is probably unnecessary. In mild pancreatitis, brief periods without oral intake may be appropriate, and a full diet is often tolerated after several days with resolution of the pain. More severe disease is associated with a hypercatabolic state and sometimes an ileus, which has led to the frequent use of parenteral nutrition in these patients. However, increasing evidence has suggested that enteral nutrition may be feasible, safe, and even desirable in severe pancreatitis. Several randomized trials have documented that enteral nutrition, when tolerated, has the advantage of avoiding the high cost of total parenteral nutrition (TPN), as well as catheter-related complications, particularly line sepsis; furthermore, the use of enteral nutrition, usually through a nasojejunal tube, may support intestinal mucosal integrity and avoid the alterations to intestinal barrier function and altered intestinal permeability associated with TPN. We believe that enteral nutrition should be used if tolerated; because of the risk of aspiration, we much prefer a jejunal route to nasogastric feeding.

Endoscopic Retrograde Cholangiopancreatography

The role of early ERCP in biliary pancreatitis remains controversial. Although there is proven benefit in patients with obstruction or cholangitis, its role in other patients with gallstone pancreatitis is less clear. Although two randomized trials demonstrated a significant reduction in morbidity with the routine use of ERCP, these studies included patients with known obstruction and cholangitis in the treated cohort. A more recent multicenter randomized study excluded patients with known biliary sepsis or obstruction and demonstrated increased complications and mortality in the ERCP group. At present, we believe that ERCP should reserved for those with clear evidence of biliary obstruction.

Prophylactic Antibiotics

Pancreatic infection is common with pancreatic necrosis, and the incidence of this increases with time, although it is unusual before the second week. Aerobic and anaerobic gastrointestinal flora are the primary organisms involved, and infections may be monomicrobial or polymicrobial. An association between pancreatic infection and mortality has been the rationale behind the widespread use of prophylactic systemic antibiotics in patients with pancreatic necrosis. Several animal studies have shown a benefit from early antibiotic administration, although this has not been as consistently demonstrated in humans.

Although several randomized trials have suggested reductions in the incidence of pancreatic infection with prophylactic antibiotics, recent attempts to address problems in the design of these studies have failed to demonstrate a reduction in either pancreatic infection or in mortality. The use of broad-spectrum antibiotics for this purpose is known to change the bacterial flora of pancreatic infection and has been demonstrated to encourage the development of antibiotic-resistant bacterial and fungal infections. Although many institutions still use routine prophylactic antibiotics, we have tried to minimize their use. The risk of superinfection is thought to be related to the length of treatment with prophylactic antibiotics, and, if they are administered, we limit their use to 7 to 10 days. An alternative approach is to administer fluconazole simultaneously.

▮ MANAGEMENT OF NECROSIS AND INFECTION

In most patients with severe disease, the initial CT scan is performed at a convenient time during the first week of hospitalization. Follow-up scans can then be obtained after any clinical deterioration. Accepted CT criteria for diagnosis of necrosis include either focal or diffuse well-marginated zones of nonenhanced pancreatic parenchyma greater than 3 cm or occupying more than 30% of the gland.

Recent series have suggested that even with documented pancreatic necrosis, a significant percentage of patients require no therapy other than the general measures outlined earlier. A relatively small group of patients may require operation for reasons other than

their pancreatic necrosis; for example, if another surgical emergency such as perforated viscus is suspected, surgery may be appropriate. In the remaining patients, there are only three indications for some form of intervention. The first, documented pancreatic infection, is undisputed. In contrast, operation in patients with severe sterile necrosis continues to be a subject of some controversy. Finally, delayed intervention for symptomatic organized necrosis is receiving increasing attention.

It has been generally accepted that infected pancreatic necrosis is an absolute indication for some form of drainage. With infection, mortality is virtually 100% without intervention, whereas recent series suggest that with appropriate therapy, it should approach that of those with sterile necrosis. Although some patients may have radiographic evidence of infection, emphysematous pancreatitis or extralumenal gas, CT-guided percutaneous fine-needle aspiration (FNA) is used to diagnose infection in the majority of patients. Although those with severe sterile necrosis alone, particularly with organ failure, may fail to improve clinically in the first 7 to 14 days, this is also the subset of patients in whom infection must be suspected. Unfortunately, both severe sterile necrosis and infected pancreatic necrosis may be associated with significant leukocytosis and fever, making a clinical distinction impossible. Aspiration of the necrotic pancreas or extrapancreatic fluid collections may be performed with minimal associated morbidity and, if negative, permit a nonoperative approach. Reported sensitivity and specificity for percutaneous aspiration are greater than 95%. Gram stains on the aspirate have been shown to be positive in the vast majority of cases later documented to have infection, permitting rapid decision making, although all samples should be sent for aerobic, anaerobic, and fungal culture. Studies employing repeated aspiration have established the natural history of infected necrosis. Although the interval from presentation with necrosis to infection is variable, the overall incidence increases up to 3 weeks. Repeat CT-guided aspirations are therefore recommended until clear clinical improvement is demonstrated.

As experience with FNA and conservative therapy has accumulated, clinicians have become increasingly comfortable with the concept of conservative, nonoperative management in the stable patient. Opponents of this strategy have continued to suggest that there are some patients with the most severe disease, on the basis of the severity of illness, extent of necrosis, or degree of organ failure, who might benefit from debridement regardless of the status of infection. Efforts have been made to establish criteria other than infection, such as extent of necrosis, that might identify patients who would benefit from debridement but have not been shown to be sufficiently specific to use as a basis for decision making. Although series advocating a more aggressive approach continue to be reported, most centers have adopted an increasingly conservative posture. However, there have been relatively few large studies analyzing the results of such an approach. The Bern group managed 86 patients prospectively using a strict conservative protocol and reported a mortality of 10% with just a single patient undergoing operation in the absence of documented infection. At Brigham and Women's Hospital, 99 consecutive patients with necrotizing pancreatitis were treated, with a mortality of 14%. In three, because of underlying medical problems, the decision was made initially not to intervene. Of the remaining 96 patients, 93 were managed with a conservative strategy, intervening only for documented infection; 3 had other indications for operation. In the 59 patients without infection who were managed conservatively, there were 7 deaths (11%) related to organ failure. In the 34 patients with infected necrosis, all underwent either surgery or percutaneous drainage, and 4 (12%) of this group died. These results suggest that conservative strategies can be applied successfully in most patients with this disease with reasonable outcomes. In addition, analyzing the patients who died, it was difficult to identify individuals who might benefit from a more aggressive strategy.

The conservative approach, operating only for documented infection, does produce a group of patients with sterile necrosis who suffer continuing pain, malaise, or inability to tolerate a diet. These patients have what we have defined as organized necrosis, which we suggest is a different pathologic process than acute necrosis, accompanied by maturation and demarcation of the inflammatory process. Nonrandomized series have demonstrated significantly better outcomes in patients undergoing late-versus-early debridement, and most surgeons would agree that operation is considerably facilitated by the demarcation that occurs. The exact indications and timing for surgery in this group deserve further study, although there is some indication that 4 weeks is an appropriate interval. Many of these patients may even undergo internal drainage into the stomach or a Roux-en-Y limb of jejunum.

Recent reports have also suggested that percutaneous approaches to debridement may be of benefit to some patients. Although the traditional teaching has been that pancreatic debris is too solid to be successfully managed with a percutaneously placed drain, the combination of larger catheters, placed through a Seldinger technique, with frequent irrigations has proved effective in some cases. Even when these patients ultimately require operation, such percutaneous approaches might delay the need for operative intervention until such time as the necrosis becomes better organized and demarcated, reducing the morbidity and mortality of operation. Although these data appear promising and suggest that such therapies might be applicable in a select group of patients, further study in a prospective series is necessary before such methods can be recommended as standard practice.

Pancreatic Debridement

Pancreatic necrosectomy or debridement should accomplish two primary goals: (1) the removal of all devitalized tissue and (2) the assurance of the postoperative removal of any products of ongoing inflammation that persist after debridement. Depending on the timing and indications for necrosectomy, these goals may be more or less difficult to accomplish. Late operation, after the necrosis has clearly demarcated, can usually be performed with considerable ease, and ongoing necrosis is seldom an issue. In contrast, when debridement is attempted early in the course of the pancreatitis, the extent is often limited by hemorrhage, and methods to control the ongoing necrosis are frequently necessary.

Although techniques of open debridement are fundamentally equal, postdebridement strategies differ considerably. Debridement may be combined with open packing, postoperative lavage, or closure with drains alone. Reported morbidity and mortality vary widely; comparisons among studies are difficult given a lack of standardization in disease severity and in criteria for operative management. The methods must be tailored to the individual patient, and each may have a role under specific circumstances.

Before surgical debridement, accurate preoperative imaging is essential. A high-quality CT scan with intravenous contrast is essential to identify areas of pancreatic or peripancreatic necrosis. Exploration of the pancreatic bed may be initiated via either a bilateral subcostal or midline incision. The lesser sac may be approached through either the gastrocolic ligament or the transverse mesocolon. Some have strongly advocated an approach to the lesser sac via the left side of the transverse mesocolon to avoid the dense inflammatory process that can obscure tissue planes between the stomach and transverse colon. The middle colic vessels present a potential anatomic barrier to the transmesocolic approach, although these vessels are often thrombosed in this setting. An additional advantage of the transmesocolic approach is that drains may be placed in a dependent position after debridement. Others have advocated an approach via the gastrocolic ligament for the primary reason that the inframesocolic space is typically uninvolved with peripancreatic inflammation and infection.

Pancreatic debridement is accomplished bluntly, primarily using finger dissection. The differentiation between necrotic and viable tissue, which is firm, is often best made by palpation. Necrotic debris should separate easily from the surrounding tissues, without extensive dissection. Debridement should therefore be limited to all clearly necrotic tissue that is easily separable from surrounding structures. Hemorrhage from inflamed retroperitoneal tissues is not uncommon; hemostasis may require packing of the cavity. Precise vascular control in an inflamed tissue field can prove difficult, if not impossible. If such is the case, hemostasis may require prolonged manual compression and possibly multiple sutures.

As the inflammatory mass is exposed during the course of the debridement, it may become necessary to extend the intra-abdominal dissection to expose fully all necrotic tissue. A complete search for and identification of all necrotic foci must be performed. For necrosis of the head of the pancreas, improved exposure may be achieved through either the right side of the mesocolon or an approach posterior to the second and third portions of the duodenum. Additional exposure may require mobilization of the hepatic and splenic flexures of the colon. Thorough exposure of all necrotic tissue may involve opening both paracolic gutters, the pararenal spaces, the retroperitoneum into the pelvis, or the gastrohepatic omentum.

Depending on the timing of operation, the debridement may be more or less complete. Early in the course of the disease, before the necrosum has completely demarcated, some borderline tissue may not be so easily removed, and ongoing necrosis may occur. The options for dealing with this include open packing, lavage, and simple closure over drains.

Open packing, or "marsupialization," accepts the need for recurrent pancreatic debridement and is usually mandated by diffuse hemorrhage, precluding further dissection. Laparotomy pads or other gauze are placed directly within the pancreatic bed, and some authors have recommended presoaking these packs in iodinated solutions. No attempt is made to close the fascia or skin, although occasionally a small number of extraperitoneal nylon stay sutures may be loosely tied to discourage evisceration. This results in an open communicating defect for planned reexplorations, which are performed in the operating room at 2- to 3-day intervals for additional debridement. After debridement has been achieved by open packing, the abdominal wound may either be left to heal entirely by secondary intention or undergo delayed primary closure.

Another approach is continuous postoperative high-volume lavage of the lesser sac. Beger has written extensively on this technique. Postoperative lavage is facilitated by the insertion of two to five large double-lumen tubes. After drain placement, the gastrocolic ligament may be sutured to form a closed compartment in the lesser sac. Continuous lavage is undertaken with hyperosmolar, potassium-free dialysate at approximately 2 L per hour, although irrigation with normal saline has also been used. Irrigation continues until the effluent is free of particulate matter. These drains are gradually downsized and eventually withdrawn.

When the initial debridement is considered complete, simple drainage with closed-suction drains may be adequate. The drains are subsequently removed as their output ceases, allowing the cavity to close.

No strict criteria have been proposed to select patients adequately for these various procedures, and the optimal method of drainage has not been examined in a prospective fashion. Reports of postoperative complications and mortality vary widely across series and probably are more a reflection of the indications and timing of operation than the procedure itself. To summarize, significant mortality is seen in all groups. Planned reoperation tends to be associated with a higher rate of gastrointestinal fistula. Closed drainage, in most series, is accompanied by a significant rate of reoperation. We continue to believe that each technique has its place. When early operation is mandated, open packing or lavage may be necessary to deal with the consequences of ongoing necrosis. If operation can be delayed, debridement with closed drainage and sometimes even internal drainage may be adequate.

In a series of 99 patients with pancreatic necrosis managed conservatively at the Brigham and Women's Hospital, operation was offered only for documented infection or for sterile pancreatic necrosis with persistent systemic illness. In this series, most patients were managed with closed drainage. The mean interval from presentation to surgery was 27 days. Of these patients, 31 (86%) were managed with debridement and closure over drains, 1 received postoperative irrigation, and 4 required open packing and planned reexploration. Nineteen patients (34%) developed complications, including 9% each with pancreatic or enteric fistulae and 15% with endocrine or exocrine insufficiency. Of patients managed with closure over drains, only 4 (13%) required reexploration because of persistent illness and presumed inadequate debridement.

Various endoscopic and minimally invasive techniques have recently been used to treat pancreatic necrosis. Endoscopic access through the posterior wall of the stomach, permitting serial irrigation and debridement, can be successful in the appropriate patient. Likewise, there have been numerous reports of retroperitoneal approaches using the laparoscope to explore and drain the peripancreatic area after dilatating a percutaneous drain tract. Such techniques can undoubtedly reduce the severity of the systemic inflammatory response and organ dysfunction associated with open pancreatic debridement. The primary risks of these procedures are an incomplete debridement of solid necrosum and inadequate drainage of the pancreatic bed. No randomized studies exist to compare these techniques with traditional open debridement. Furthermore, studies are difficult to compare given their small size, retrospective nature, and varying comorbidities and selection criteria. Most of these approaches require repeated debridement, usually under general anesthesia. Open surgical debridement remains the gold standard of treatment for surgical management of pancreatic necrosis. However, as management strategies become more nonoperative, it is likely that endoscopic and minimally invasive techniques will play an increasing role.

SUGGESTED READINGS

Ashley SW, Perez A, Pierce EA, and others: Necrotizing pancreatitis. Contemporary analysis of 99 consecutive cases, *Ann Surg* 234:572, 2001.

Ashley SW: Editorial. Operation for sterile pancreatic necrosis: an evolving strategy, *J Am Coll Surg* 181:363, 1995.

Baron TH, Morgan DE: Acute necrotizing pancreatitis, *N Engl J Med* 340:1412, 1999.

Buchler MW, Gloor B, Muller CA, and others: Acute necrotizing pancreatitis: treatment strategy according to the status of infection, *Ann Surg* 232:619, 2000.

Clancy TE, Benoit EP, Ashley SW: Current management of acute pancreatitis, *J Gastrointest Surg* 9:440, 2005.

MANAGEMENT OF GALLSTONE PANCREATITIS

Thomas J. Howard, MD

INTRODUCTION

Bile duct stones and sludge originating from the gallbladder are well-known causes of acute pancreatitis in 30% to 50% of patients, although the precise pathogenic mechanism is not entirely understood. Clinical evidence implicating the passage of small gallstones through the ampulla of Vater as a cause of acute pancreatitis is found in classic observational studies showing that gallstones are recovered from the stool in 85% of patients with acute biliary pancreatitis and in only 10% of patients with symptomatic cholelithiasis without pancreatitis. In patients with recurrent acute pancreatitis and biliary microlithiasis (cholesterol monohydrate or calcium bilirubinate crystals), therapy directed at alleviating the passage of microlithiasis through the ampulla of Vater (cholecystectomy, ursodeoxycholic acid, or endoscopic sphincterotomy [ES]) results in an 85% reduction in recurrent episodes of acute pancreatitis. Although the overall incidence of biliary pancreatitis in patients with documented gallstones is low, patients who have an episode of gallstone pancreatitis who do not have treatment directed at preventing recurrent passage of gallstones (cholecystectomy or ES) have a 90-day risk of recurrent pancreatitis, estimated to be approximately 50%. These data emphasize that the current management of gallstone pancreatitis uses both surgical (cholecystectomy) and endoscopic (ES) techniques to alleviate the source of gallstones or facilitate their passage through the sphincter of Oddi.

PATHOGENESIS

The pathogenesis of acute pancreatitis on a cellular level appears to be common to all etiologies of acute pancreatitis. After an initiating event (gallstone passage, alcohol consumption, drug toxicity), intracellular changes occur within the pancreatic acinar cells, resulting in inhibition of digestive enzyme secretion and colocalization of zymogen granules with lysosomal hydrolases, in turn leading to enzyme activation and acinar cell injury. This injury causes the elaboration of proinflammatory factors (including transcription factors nuclear factor kappa B; activator protein 1 [NF-κB, AP-1]; stress activated kinases, mitogen-activated protein kinase[MAPK], extracellular signal-regulated kinase[ERK]; interleukins [IL]-1, IL-6, IL-8; and other factors) that, in synergy with the patient's underlying genetic predisposition, result in pancreatic injury and a corresponding systemic inflammatory response syndrome (SIRS). This SIRS response can be mild and self-limiting or severe, producing circulatory changes within the pancreas, altered gut permeability, and end-organ damage predominantly manifest as acute respiratory distress syndrome or acute renal failure.

CLINICAL PICTURE

Patients with gallstone pancreatitis present with acute onset midepigastric abdominal pain that is sudden, abrupt and boring in character that can radiate to the back. The intensity of the pain increases over several hours and is commonly associated with nausea and vomiting. Physical findings in patients with acute pancreatitis are diffuse abdominal tenderness and, in some patients, rigidity and guarding that mimics an acute surgical abdomen. Patients with mild interstitial pancreatitis appear uncomfortable but not seriously ill, and their vital signs may be almost completely normal. In contrast, patients with severe acute pancreatitis appear ill and toxic, with tachycardia, tachypnea, and hypotension. Nausea and vomiting can be a prominent component in some patients and occasionally requires the insertion of a nasogastric tube for relief. As severe acute pancreatitis progresses (over the course of 6 to 12 hours), the abdomen becomes distended and typanitic from a paralytic ileus. Sequestration of fluid in the abdomen (ileus) and retroperitoneum (inflammation) produces severe dehydration (hypotension, tachycardia, dry mucous membranes, low urine output, and poor skin turgor). This physiologic state must be recognized promptly and treated aggressively with large-volume resuscitation to maintain organ perfusion and consequently minimize microcirculatory dysfunction, which can often lead to organ failure and an increased severity of pancreatitis. Large-volume resuscitation combined with increased capillary permeability in the lungs resulting from the SIRS requires supplemental oxygen and commonly mechanical ventilation to maintain adequate tissue oxygenation.

DIAGNOSIS

The diagnosis of gallstone pancreatitis is made on the basis of findings of acute pancreatitis in a patient with cholelithiasis or choledocholithiasis who lacks an alternative etiology such as alcohol use, hyperlipidemia, or exposure to drugs associated with acute pancreatitis. Given a patient with presumed gallstone pancreatitis, the diagnosis is supported by serum or urinary tests showing an elevated amylase or lipase level and confirmed by radiographic imaging studies showing gallstones or biliary microlithiasis and pancreatic inflammation.

An elevated serum amylase level (rises within 2 hours of disease onset, peaks within 48 hours) remains the best single test to make the diagnosis of acute pancreatitis. In patients with gallstone pancreatitis, a marked elevation (>1000 IU/L) is not unusual, although it should be emphasized that the extent of amylase elevation has no relation to the severity of acute pancreatitis. Because of an increased sensitivity and specificity for acute pancreatitis, lipase may actually be more valuable than amylase in making the diagnosis. In practical terms, most clinicians routinely obtain both tests. Hepatic transaminases, particularly alanine aminotransferase (ALT), are helpful to distinguish biliary pancreatitis from other causes of acute pancreatitis. Elevation of ALT greater than three times the upper limit of normal in the presence of acute pancreatitis has a 95% positive predictive value for gallstone pancreatitis. Unfortunately, only half the patients with gallstone pancreatitis show this level of ALT elevation, making the overall sensitivity of the test low.

Transabdominal ultrasound is the best initial test for establishing gallstones as the etiology of acute pancreatitis, with an overall accuracy rate of 70% to 80%. Although it carries a high sensitivity (>95%) for detection of gallstones in the gallbladder, it has a much lower sensitivity (40% to 60%) for choledocholithiasis. In selected situations, endoscopic ultrasound (EUS) has been a useful test to confirm choledocholithiasis because this modality has both a higher sensitivity (93%) and higher specificity (95%) than routine transabdominal ultrasound and can be particularly useful in the detection of biliary microlithiasis.

Thin-slice multidetector-row computed tomography (CT) with intravenous contrast is the most important radiographic test both to diagnose acute pancreatitis and to exclude other common intra-abdominal conditions that can mimic its clinical presentation, including perforated duodenal ulcer, internal hernia with closed-loop obstruction, or mesenteric infarction. The radiographic signs of acute pancreatitis using CT include a diffusely enlarged and hypoechoic gland with irregular contour (interstitial edema), peripancreatic stranding in the retroperitoneum, and mesenteric fat and extrapancreatic fluid collections involving the anterior pararenal space and lesser sac. In severe acute pancreatitis, failure of the pancreatic parenchyma to enhance during intravenous contrast administration suggests pancreatic necrosis. The CT abnormalities that occur in acute pancreatitis are virtually pathognomonic of the disease, with a reported specificity approaching 100%.

Magnetic resonance imaging (MRI) and magnetic resonance cholangiopancreatography (MRCP) are newer imaging techniques, and definition as to their exact role in patients with acute pancreatitis is evolving. One of the benefits of MRI compared with CT is that it does not require ionizing radiation or the administration of nephrotoxic intravenous contrast agents. Because of the MRCP component of the test, it is much more sensitive than CT in the diagnosis of both cholelithiasis and choledocholithiasis, and its multiplanar capabilities of imaging can be particularly helpful in diagnosing other uncommon etiologies of acute pancreatitis (i.e., intraductal papillary mucinous tumors or pancreas divisum). The disadvantages of using MRI in patients with acute pancreatitis are that it is currently more expensive and less widely available than CT; takes longer to perform (≈ 15 minutes); and, for optimal imaging, it requires patient participation that is often problematic in a sedated patient with abdominal pain and a severe acute illness.

THERAPY

Treatment of patients with gallstone pancreatitis is based on the disease severity of the underlying pancreatitis. Approximately 80% of patients have acute edematous pancreatitis that follows a mild, self-limited disease course and carries a low risk of complications or mortality. After resolution of the inflammatory process, the pancreas returns to its normal structure and function. Severe acute pancreatitis occurs in 20% of patients and is associated with organ failure (pulmonary, renal, hepatic) and local complications such as pancreatic necrosis, pancreatic abscess, or pseudocyst. These patients have a 30% to 50% morbidity rate and 10% to 30% mortality rate even with current state-of-the-art treatment. Furthermore, even after full recovery, most patients with severe acute pancreatitis and pancreatic necrosis have persistent structural (duct strictures) and functional damage (endocrine or exocrine insufficiency) to the pancreas.

Although it would be useful at the time of initial evaluation to be able to stratify patients with acute pancreatitis as to disease severity, there are currently no clinical assessment parameters, scoring systems, or radiographic imaging techniques that accurately prognosticate the clinical course with a high level of precision early in the disease process. It is for this reason that all patients with acute pancreatitis should be hospitalized for a period of observation (i.e., 48 to 72 hours) after the diagnosis is confirmed to assess fully the clinical course. Assay of C-reactive protein is the only easily available blood test in clinical practice that is a proved discriminator between mild and severe pancreatitis, using a cutoff level of 150 mg/ml at 48 hours after the onset of symptoms. Ranson's score is the most commonly used specific pancreatitis scoring system, combining 11 clinical data points (5 during the first 24 hours, and 6 during the next 24 hours), each of which is assigned a score of 1 point (Table 1). Scores of greater than or equal to 3 are considered consistent with severe pancreatitis. Mortality rates correlate with total score assigned: 0 to 2 points = less than 1% mortality; 3 to 4 points = 15% mortality; more than 6 points = 100% mortality. Limitations of the Ranson's score are that it evolves over a 48-hour period of time and is applicable only during the initial course of illness. The severity scoring system of the Acute Physiology and Chronic Health Evaluation (APACHE-II) has been validated in patients with acute pancreatitis and has been shown to have sensitivity and specificity similar to the other severity scoring systems, with total scores of 8 or more associated with severe pancreatitis. Unlike the Ranson's score, APACHE II scoring has additional value in that it can be used throughout the course of illness to monitor the clinical progress in individual patients. Unfortunately, this scoring system has failed to gain wider acceptance because it is cumbersome to calculate, relying on assigning a point value to 12 individual variable points, age points, and chronic health points that are added together to calculate the total score. The CT severity index (CTSI) is a scoring system based on imaging that uses contrast-enhanced multidetector-row CT scanning. This index combines the initial grading system with the presence and extent of pancreatic

Table 1: Comparison of the Clinical and Laboratory Data Used for Ranson's Criteria of Severity in Both Biliary and Nonbiliary Acute Pancreatitis

	Biliary Pancreatitis	Nonbiliary Pancreatitis
Admission		
Age	>70	>55
WBC (mm^3)	>18,000	>16,000
Serum glucose (mg/dl)	>220	>200
Serum LDH (U/L)	>400	>350
Serum AST (U/L)	>250	>250
Within 48 Hours		
Hematocrit fall (%)	>10	>10
BUN rise (mg/dl)	>2	>5
Serum calcium (mg/dl)	<8	<8
PaO$_2$ (mm Hg)	<60	<60
Base deficit (mEq/L)	>5	>4
Fluid sequestration (L)	>4	>6

Table 2: Grading System and Total Point Calculations for the Computed Tomography Severity Index (CTSI)

CT Grade	Points	Necrosis	Points	CTSI
A	0			
B	1	None	0	1
C	2	<30%	2	4
D	3	30%–50%	4	7
E	4	>50%	6	10

Definitions of CT grade: *A,* Normal pancreas; *B,* pancreatic enlargement; *C,* inflammation of pancreas and/or peripancreatic fat; *D,* single peripancreatic fluid collection; *E,* two or more fluid collections and/or retroperitoneal air.

necrosis (Table 2). Patients with grades A to E are assigned 0 to 4 points, to which are added 2, 4, or 6 points for up to 30%, up to 50%, or greater than 50% necrosis. The resulting severity scores correlate well with morbidity and mortality rates. Scores of 0 to 2 = 4% morbidity, 0 mortality; 3 to 6 = 35% morbidity, 6% mortality; and 7 to 10 = 92% morbidity, 17% mortality.

Mild Disease

Patients with mild acute pancreatitis from gallstones (Ranson's score <3, APACHE II <8, CTSI <2) require only supportive care. They are made NPO (nothing by mouth) and given intravenous fluids and electrolytes both to correct their calculated deficits and cover basal fluid requirements. Abdominal pain is controlled with narcotic analgesics, and antiemetics are provided. Patients are frequently reassessed for stability in vital signs, abdominal examination, and adequacy of urine output. Baseline white blood cell count, amylase level, and liver function tests (serum glutamic oxaloacetic transaminase, serum glutamic pyruvic transaminase, alkaline phosphatase, bilirubin) are repeated daily until both the patient's clinical course and laboratory values show a trend toward resolution of the acute inflammatory process.

As patients with mild pancreatitis improve clinically, oral intake can be resumed and advanced to a low-fat diet as tolerated. Often resolution of the hyperamylasemia lags behind the patient's clinical improvement. It is our practice to begin oral intake in patients who are clinically well (no fever, tachycardia) with few abdominal complaints who express an interest in food, even if their serum amylase values remain above the normal range. Persistent abdominal pain, fever, nausea, vomiting, or leukocytosis implies that the pancreatic inflammation has not settled to the point that oral intake can be resumed.

All patients with mild gallstone pancreatitis who are acceptable surgical candidates should undergo elective laparoscopic cholecystectomy with intraoperative biliary imaging (cholangiography or laparoscopic ultrasonography) after the acute inflammation has subsided and during their index hospitalization. Cholecystectomy is 97% effective in preventing recurrent episodes of gallstone pancreatitis and has a low procedure-related morbidity and mortality rate in this setting. Same-admission cholecystectomy prevents the high early recurrence rate (≈50%) of gallstone pancreatitis in patients discharged and scheduled for interval cholecystectomy. If intraoperative biliary imaging cannot be accomplished at the time of cholecystectomy, postoperative imaging is mandatory, using either MRCP or endoscopic ultrasound.

In severely debilitated patients with mild acute gallstone pancreatitis who are considered poor operative candidates for a laparoscopic cholecystectomy, prevention of recurrent gallstone pancreatitis can be accomplished using endoscopic sphincterotomy (ES), with a 94% to 97% success rate at 2 years' follow-up. This treatment, while leaving the gallbladder in situ, prevents recurrent pancreatitis by allowing free passage of stones, sludge, and debris through the ampulla of Vater. Although ES virtually eliminates the risk of recurrent pancreatitis, a significant drawback of this strategy is the high relative risk (20% to 40%) of biliary tract complications such as cholecystitis, jaundice, or cholangitis related to leaving a gallbladder with crystals, sludge, or stones in place. Given these limitations, ES is acceptable in highly selected situations as a temporizing measure or in poor-risk surgical patients to prevent recurrent gallstone pancreatitis.

Patients with gallstone pancreatitis who are found to have common bile duct stones at the time of laparoscopic or open cholecystectomy require stone removal. Transcystic or transcholedochal laparoscopic common bile duct exploration (CBDE), laparotomy with open common bile duct exploration and T-tube placement, endoscopic retrograde cholangiography (ERC) with or without ES, and percutaneous transhepatic cholangiography (PTC) with stone removal are all acceptable methods of clearing bile duct stones. The choice of one technique over the others is dictated by the particular circumstances surrounding the patient (clinical condition, biliary anatomy, hepatoduodenal inflammation, available bile duct access routes), the surgeon (expertise in advanced laparoscopic techniques), and the institution (fluoroscopic intraoperative imaging system, endoscopic expertise, interventional radiology expertise). Transcystic or transcholedochal laparoscopic CBDE has a reported success rate of 80% to 98% in experienced hands and is associated with a low procedure-related complication rate. At my own institution, access to a world-class gastrointestinal endoscopy group combined with my limited advanced laparoscopic skill set restricts me to an intraoperative attempt at laparoscopic transcystic CBDE and stone removal and, if this is technically difficult or unsuccessful, referral for ERC/ES. Other surgeons may favor laparoscopic CBDE, and in certain situations, conversion to an open laparotomy with common bile duct exploration and T-tube placement may be the best method to ensure clearance of common bile duct stones and prevention of recurrent bouts of pancreatitis or biliary sepsis.

Severe Disease

Patients with severe acute pancreatitis require aggressive, skilled critical care management to provide for adequate fluid resuscitation and support of organ function. The treatment of severe acute pancreatitis from gallstones differs from that of severe acute pancreatitis from other etiologies only in that the genesis of the pancreatic insult is biliary calculi, and their continued presence obstructing the ampullary orifice can increase the severity of acute pancreatitis.

Patients with severe gallstone pancreatitis (Ranson's >3, APACHE II >8, CTSI >2) who fail to improve substantially during the initial 24 hours of volume resuscitation and critical care management or those patients with initially mild prognostic signs who develop clinical deterioration should be considered for urgent ERC/ES to assess for ampullary obstruction. An elevated bilirubin level, severe and continuous epigastric pain, spiking fevers, or a bile-free gastric aspirate all imply persistent ampullary obstruction. Five randomized controlled clinical trials have addressed this issue. Despite significant differences in patient selection and timing of intervention in these trials, four were included in a recent meta-analysis attempting to pool results and obtain a firm consensus. In this analysis, an absolute risk reduction of 13% in complication rate and 4% in mortality rate were identified in favor of ERC/ES over conventional treatment. The most recent study, not included in the meta-analysis, shows that in patients with gallstone pancreatitis and ampullary obstruction, limiting the duration of obstruction to less than 48 hours using ERC/ES significantly decreases subsequent morbidity. Although relatively safe in the setting of severe acute pancreatitis, ERC/ES still carries a 5% to 10% failure rate to clear the common bile duct of stones and a 1% to 2% major morbidity rate of bleeding or perforation. Furthermore, the addition of pancreatography to ERC (i.e., ERCP) remains controversial in patients with severe acute pancreatitis and necrosis related to the possibility of infecting sterile pancreatic necrosis.

Cholangitis occurs in 3% to 14% of patients with acute gallstone pancreatitis. Fever (usually >38.5°C), right upper quadrant abdominal pain, and jaundice represent the classic Charcot's triad and mandate immediate intervention with fluid resuscitation, broad-spectrum antibiotic, and emergent ERC/ES with drainage of the biliary system. If ERC/ES are unavailable or unsuccessful, access to the biliary system can be achieved using either percutaneous transhepatic cholangiography (PTC) or laparoscopic or open cholecystectomy with intraoperative T-tube placement. If the pancreatitis is severe or the biliary sepsis profound, minimally invasive approaches (ERC/ES, PTC) are preferable over operative approaches that require a general anesthetic, assuming they can be carried out quickly and efficiently. When neither minimally invasive option is available, intraoperative T-tube placement using either a laparoscopic or open technique is the procedure of choice to decompress the obstructed biliary system effectively and resolve the biliary sepsis.

The main indication for surgery in patients with severe gallstone pancreatitis is sepsis resulting from infected pancreatic necrosis. Infection in pancreatic necrosis is documented by image-guided fine needle aspiration for Gram stain and culture. In patients with infected pancreatic necrosis and clinical sepsis, pancreatic debridement with external drainage combined with cholecystectomy with intraoperative cholangiography is the operation of choice. If choledocholithiasis is identified in this setting, the surgeon must make a decision on the basis of the patient's overall condition and the extent of necrosis and inflammation of the hepatoduodenal ligament as to whether an open CBDE with T-tube placement is advisable. This dissection can be particularly treacherous in the setting of infected pancreatic necrosis. Unfortunately, this same inflammation often obscures the duodenal landmarks, limiting the technical success of ERC/ES. In patients without cholangitis, successful management of the infected pancreatic necrosis leads to a resolution of duodenal edema, allowing for subsequent safe ERC/ES to address

the residual choledocholithiasis. In patients with cholangitis, placement of a simple T-tube to decompress the obstructed biliary system and allow postoperative access for subsequent percutaneous stone removal can be lifesaving. In certain situations, placement of a guidewire through the cystic duct and into the duodenum allows the endoscopist to have a vital landmark to identify the ampulla of Vater and facilitate cannulation of distal common bile duct, allowing endoscopic stone removal.

In patients with severe gallstone pancreatitis and sterile pancreatic necrosis, cholecystectomy should be delayed at least 3 weeks while supportive care is provided both to minimize the chance of secondarily infecting the pancreatic necrosis during instrumentation and to allow time for the acute inflammatory process in the hepatoduodenal ligament to subside. After this period of time, a laparoscopic approach to cholecystectomy is feasible, although it often requires more than the standard port placement to ensure adequate visualization of the anatomy. In patients with severe gallstone pancreatitis who have large peripancreatic fluid collections, the surgeon should wait at least 6 weeks after the initial event before considering cholecystectomy. The rationale for this timing is to allow for the maturation of peripancreatic fluid collections into mature pancreatic pseudocysts, which if persistent and symptomatic can be safely drained internally at the time of cholecystectomy.

PREGNANT PATIENTS

Gallstones and their complications are second only to appendectomy as the most common cause of nonobstetric surgery in pregnant patients. In mild gallstone pancreatitis, laparoscopic cholecystectomy is relatively safe in the second trimester, and biliary imaging can be achieved using laparoscopic ultrasound, endoscopic ultrasound, or MRI\MRCP. MRI, which uses no ionizing radiation, is not recommended during the first trimester, and use of contrast material is not recommended in pregnant patients. Fast MRI is useful in various obstetric settings and can provide more specific information with excellent tissue contrast and multiplanar views. Women in their first trimester of pregnancy should be managed conservatively until the second trimester, when an operation can be safely performed. Gallstone pancreatitis in the third trimester should be managed conservatively until after delivery, when treatment of these patients will mimic that of their nonpregnant counterparts.

Suggested Readings

Booerma D, Rauws EA, Keulemans YC, and others: Wait-and-see policy for laparoscopic cholecystectomy after endoscopic sphincterotomy for bile-duct stones: a randomized trial, *Lancet* 360:761, 2002.

Hungness ES, Soper NJ: Management of common bile duct stones, *J Gastrointest Surg* 10:612, 2006.

Nealon WH, Bawduniak J, Walser EM: Appropriate timing of cholecystectomy in patients who present with moderate to severe gallstone-associated acute pancreatitis with peripancreatic fluid collections, *Ann Surg* 239:741, 2004.

Sharma VK, Howden CW: Meta-analysis of randomized controlled trials of endoscopic retrograde cholangiography and endoscopic sphincterotomy for the treatment of acute biliary pancreatitis, *Am J Gastroenterol* 94:3211, 1999.

Toouli J, Brooke-Smith M, Bassi C, and others: Guidelines for the management of acute pancreatitis, *J Gastroenterol Hepatol* 17(suppl): S15, 2002.

Uhl W, Warshaw A, Imrie C, and others: IAP guidelines for the surgical management of acute pancreatitis, *Pancreatology* 2:565, 2002.

PANCREAS DIVISUM AND OTHER VARIANTS OF DOMINANT DORSAL DUCT ANATOMY

Andrew L. Warshaw, MD

Pancreas divisum, strictly defined, is an anatomic variant of pancreatic duct anatomy in which the dorsal and ventral ducts fail to fuse during embryogenesis. This necessitates that each duct must drain via its own separate orifice (the major papilla of Vater for the ventral duct of Wirsung, and the minor or accessory papilla for the dorsal duct of Santorini). Interest in the possible clinical significance of pancreas divisum has led to enlargement of the definition to include a group of anatomic variations, each of which necessitates drainage of a major fraction of pancreatic secretions via the accessory papilla. This cluster, characterized by the predominance of the dorsal duct, includes "partial" pancreas divisum in which the communicating link forms but is tiny and functionally inadequate and the ventral duct is completely absent. Although the appellation *pancreas divisum* is still in common usage, the term *dominant dorsal duct* is more inclusive (Fig. 1). A dominant dorsal duct occurs in more than 10% of Western populations.

The presumed basis of the pathophysiology is that the accessory papilla may be inadequate to serve as the outflow tract for up to 2 L/day of pancreatic secretions. The consequence is pathologically increased pressure in the pancreatic duct system that causes damage to the acinar tissues. The aim of logical therapy is thus to relieve the obstruction of the dorsal duct that otherwise could lead to pain, acute pancreatitis, and even fibrotic chronic pancreatitis.

CLINICAL PRESENTATION

Most people with dominant dorsal duct anatomy have no symptoms, and none may ever develop. Most instances are found incidentally during pancreatography, but pancreas divisum anatomy has been found to be significantly more common among patients who are investigated for unexplained pancreatitis than for biliary conditions. Pancreas divisum may actually be protective against gallstone-induced pancreatitis because the bile duct is separate from the principal pancreatic channel.

It is now widely accepted that dominant dorsal duct anatomic variants associated with accessory papilla stenosis can cause recurrent attacks of acute pancreatitis, proved by increases in serum amylase and lipase and by inflammatory changes. Most series are composed of a majority of women (3:1 over men), with an average age of 34 years at diagnosis. Whereas the dominant dorsal duct anatomy is congenital, it is unknown whether the accessory papilla stenosis is congenital or acquired. Reports of symptomatic pancreas divisum

Figure 1 Variants of pancreatic duct anatomy that allow for either ventral orifice drainage or obligate dorsal drainage via the accessory papilla (including pancreas divisum).

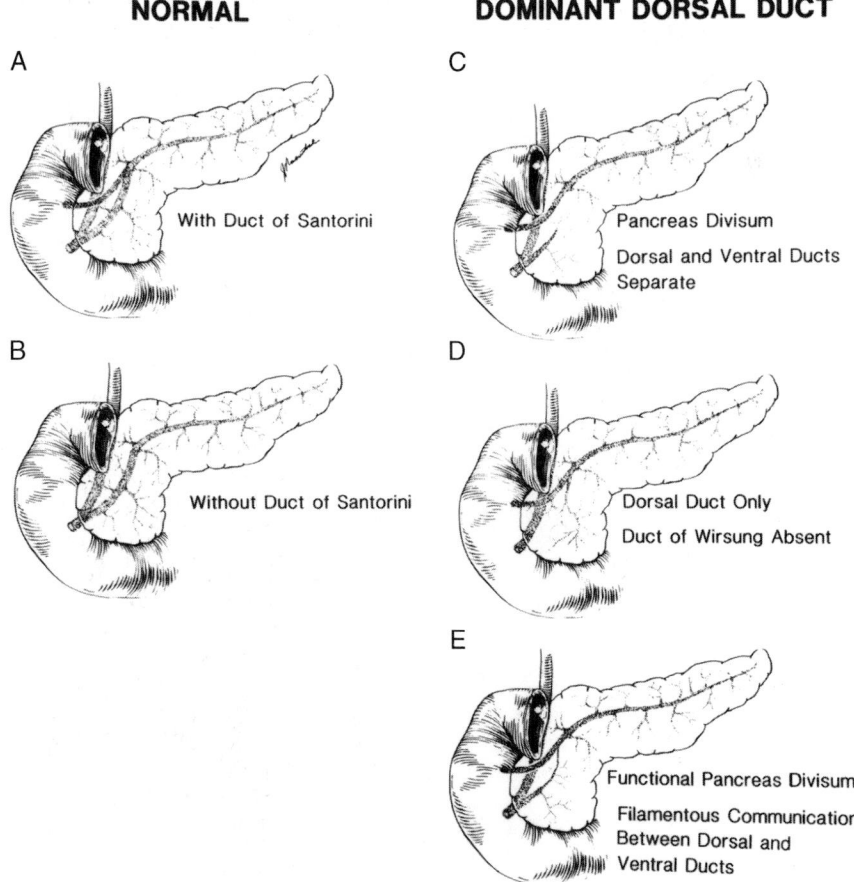

NORMAL

A   With Duct of Santorini

B   Without Duct of Santorini

DOMINANT DORSAL DUCT

C   Pancreas Divisum
Dorsal and Ventral Ducts Separate

D   Dorsal Duct Only
Duct of Wirsung Absent

E   Functional Pancreas Divisum
Filamentous Communication Between Dorsal and Ventral Ducts

in childhood are appearing, perhaps because of the greater awareness of the condition and better access to endoscopic retrograde cholangiopancreatography (ERCP) for children.

The association with established chronic pancreatitis is less clear or perhaps less frequent. Statistical analyses have not established a greater prevalence of pancreas divisum in patients with chronic pancreatitis, but there are striking and indisputable examples of severe acinar loss and fibrosis confined to the dorsal duct segment.

A syndrome of epigastric and back pain consistent with a pancreatic origin and without other demonstrable cause has also been attributed to pancreas divisum. The absence of objective correlates such as hyperamylasemia naturally engenders skepticism. The inability to exclude unrelated pathology, including psychopathology, has led to a much higher rate of treatment failure.

Longitudinal observations in these patients often indicate infrequent attacks of pancreatitis initially, perhaps only every year or two, but with increasing frequency with the passage of time. Similarly, pain may be sporadic at first but evolves to become daily and eventually continuous. Hyperamylasemia may be documented early but may cease to occur later, thus obscuring the objective diagnosis.

The attacks of pancreatitis in most patients tend to be mild. Pancreatic necrosis, pseudocysts, or other life-threatening complications have been rare. Similarly, progression to diabetes and exocrine insufficiency is unusual.

DIAGNOSIS

ERCP has been the means most commonly used to delineate the pancreatic duct system. Recently, the quality of magnetic resonance cholangiopancreatography (MRCP) has improved to the point that an accurate diagnosis of pancreas divisum or dominant dorsal duct without a ventral duct can be made by MRCP alone (Fig. 2).

Typically the ventral duct in pancreas divisum extends proximally only 2 to 4 cm from the major ampulla. It is formed from the confluence of fine, tapered secondary branches that service a part of the head and the uncinate process but do not extend to the midline (Fig. 3). This foreshortened ventral duct must not be confused with a ventral duct truncated by neoplasm (Fig. 4) or by stricture or obstruction acquired by scarring as a consequence of fibrosis in chronic pancreatitis or the necrotizing parenchymal destruction in acute pancreatitis. The morphology of this acquired ventral duct termination, called *false pancreas divisum,* is easily differentiated from the congenital anomaly in that the visualized portion of the main ventral duct is wider, may be longer, and terminates abruptly as a cutoff rather than tapering peripherally into its branch ducts.

Inability to locate a ventral duct at the major papilla by ERCP should raise the suspicion that there may not be a ventral duct—that the dorsal duct, emptying into the minor papilla, represents the entire pancreatic drainage system. Failure to appreciate this

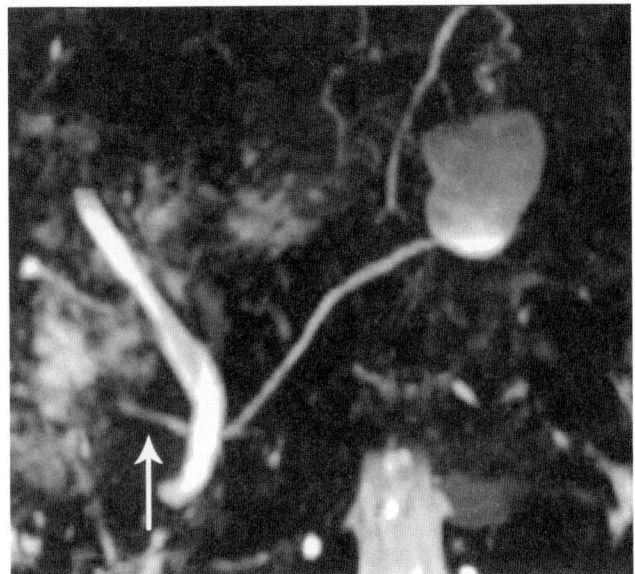

Figure 2 Magnetic resonance cholangiopancreatography demonstrating pancreatic duct anatomy of the classic pancreas divisum variation.

phenomenon has led to underestimation of the prevalence of dominant dorsal ducts and to potentially missed diagnoses. MRCP or cannulation of the dorsal duct via the accessory papilla is necessary to confirm the anatomy (Fig. 5) and to assess for chronic obstructive and inflammatory changes.

The dorsal duct, despite the typically small orifice of the accessory papilla, generally has a normal, nondilated appearance at pancreatography. Significant dilation has been exceptional, and true fibrotic chronic pancreatitis has been noted in only 3 of 200 pancreatograms in my series of symptomatic patients. Pancreatography is routinely performed in the fasting, unstimulated state, and dilatation may only occur episodically when the pancreas is actively secreting. Similarly, dilatation may occur after secretin stimulation, and this change may provide diagnostic and prognostic information.

Visual estimation of the presence or absence of accessory papilla stenosis by the endoscopist has been unreliable, as has been the difficulty or ease of cannulation. Manometry through this tiny channel has proved difficult and of poor predictive value in selecting patients for endoscopic or surgical treatment.

We described the use of ultrasonography during secretin stimulation to uncover functional papillary stenosis. The concept is based on an impeded egress of pancreatic secretions that may be

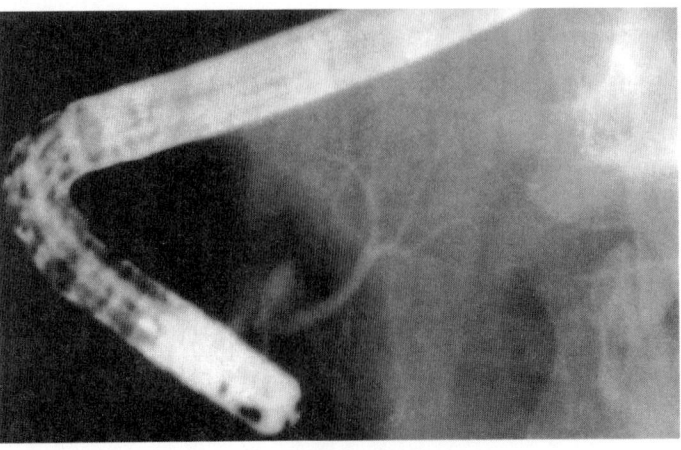

Figure 3 Endoscopic pancreatogram via the papilla of Vater. The pancreatic duct in the head of the gland is short and formed by the confluence of fine secondary branches.

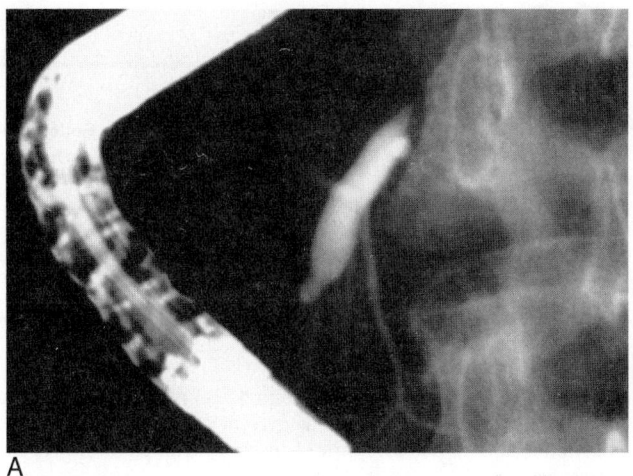
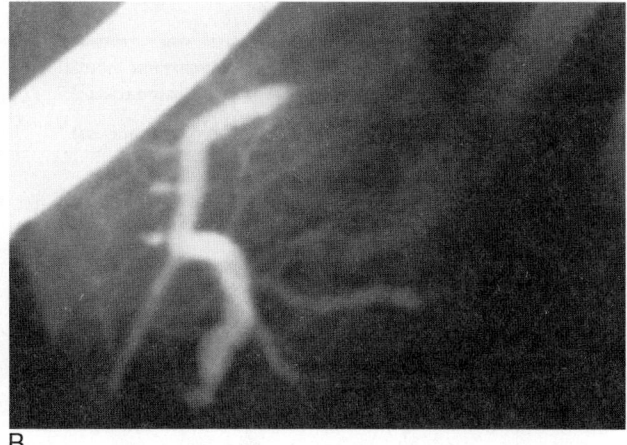

Figure 4 Pancreatograms illustrating "false pancreas divisum": **(A)** the duct abruptly terminates at a ductal adenocarcinoma. **(B)** The duct ends at the point of occlusive healing after necrotizing pancreatitis.

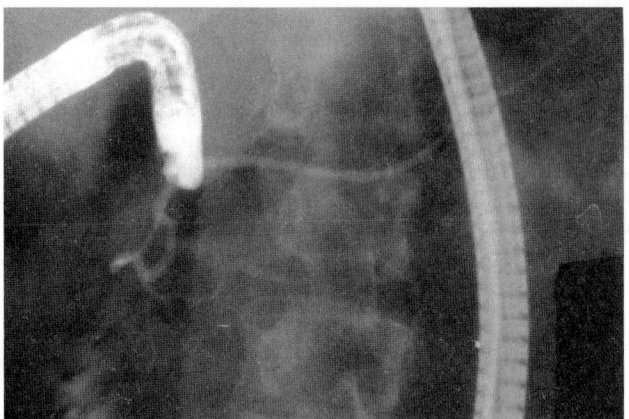

Figure 5 Endoscopic pancreatogram via the accessory papilla. The dorsal duct system serves the entire pancreas (absent ventral duct system).

inapparent at the typical baseline low-flow state but obvious during stimulated high flow. In my experience, prolonged dilatation of the pancreatic duct (for 20–30 minutes) occurs in accessory papilla stenosis, in contrast to the brief 1 to 3 minutes seen normally. Our studies indicate an 80% to 90% positive predictive value for successful amelioration of recurrent acute pancreatitis and, to a lesser extent, chronic pancreatic pain in patients with a positive ultrasound-secretin test (Table 1). More recently, endoscopic

Table 1: Chance of Beneficial Outcome after Accessory Papilla Sphincteroplasty

Ultrasound Secretin Test	Recurrent Acute Pancreatitis	Chronic Pain Only
Positive	90% (19/21)	94% (15/16)
Negative	64% (7/11)	21% (3/14)*

*$p < .0001$ versus positive test groups: $p < .05$ versus negative test with attacks.
From Warshaw AL, Simeone JF, Schapiro RH, and others: Am J Surg 159:59, 1990.

ultrasonography (EUS) and MRCP have also been used to monitor pancreatic duct size during secretin stimulation.

A therapeutic trial of dorsal duct stenting has been proposed to determine whether relief of the presumed ductal hypertension will relieve symptoms. If symptoms are frequent or continuous, a response may soon be apparent. If the pattern of the disease is one of occasional attacks, a much longer period of observation would be required, possibly confounded by placebo effect and risking stent-induced injury to the ducts.

THERAPY

Nonsurgical attempts to ameliorate symptoms have included (with no proved benefit) a low-fat diet, high-dose pancreatic enzymes, and long-acting somatostatin analogues. Chronic analgesics, particularly narcotics, should be used with caution. The only therapeutic strategy shown to be effective has been enlargement of the accessory papilla. It is noteworthy that either endoscopic or open surgical means have been used with comparable success, but in current practice, the endoscopic approach has supplanted surgical therapy in the great majority of new cases because the endoscopist, who sees the patient first, has the opportunity to determine the treatment plan.

ENDOSCOPIC THERAPY

Endoscopic approaches to the accessory papilla have evolved from balloon dilatation to long-term stenting, endoscopic sphincterotomy, and a combination of sphincterotomy and short-term stenting. The last is the currently accepted preference because the prior approaches induced too much pancreatitis and did not produce lasting benefit (sphincterotomy alone), induced irreversible stent-induced injury to the duct, and required frequent stent replacement for occlusion by debris. Nonetheless, a randomized (unblinded) trial of long-term stent therapy (Lans and colleagues) showed a 90% benefit attributed to stenting (>50% reduction in pain, reduced emergency department visits and hospitalizations) versus 11% among control subjects over a mean follow-up of more than 2 years.

Several investigators have reported successful use of a combination of sphincterotomy and short-term (2 weeks) stenting. Lehman and colleagues reported significant reduction in pain and hospital days per month in 13 of 17 (76%) patients with recurrent acute

Table 2: Outcomes of Accessory Papilla Sphincteroplasty for Dominant Dorsal Duct Syndromes (Pancreas Divisum)

	No. Patients	Recurrent Acute Pancreatitis No. (% success)	Chronic Pain only No. (% success)	Restenosis (%)	Mean Follow-up (Months)
Warshaw (1990)	88	43 (82)	45 (56)	7	53
Madura (1986)	30	11 (82)	19 (77)	—	31
Keith (1989)	21	13 (100)	8 (75)	5	53
Bradley (1996)	31	31 (84)	—	6	76

pancreatitis, 3 of 11 with chronic pancreatitis, and 6 of 23 with chronic pain. However, even with short-duration stenting, 50% had dorsal duct damage at the time of stent removal. Kozarek and colleagues reported good results in 11 of 15 (73%) patients with recurrent acute pancreatitis, 6 of 19 with chronic pancreatitis, and 1 of 5 with chronic pain; 20% of their patients had procedure or stent-related pancreatitis, and 12% had restenosis of the accessory papilla.

SURGICAL THERAPY

The operative approach to patients with dominant dorsal duct syndrome parallels that of endoscopic sphincterotomy and stenting but has the potential advantages of greater long-term patency and assured entry into the accessory papilla. The operation has been applied with success to symptomatic patients without changes of

chronic pancreatitis (Table 2). The practical reality of patient flow determines that most patients at present are referred to surgeons only after failure to accomplish endoscopic sphincterotomy or after restenosis.

Surgical enlargement of the accessory papilla is accomplished by sutured sphincteroplasty through a transverse duodenotomy (Fig. 6). The technique requires identification of the accessory papilla, which is located anterior and 2 to 3 cm proximal to the major papilla. The use of secretin stimulation may be helpful in visualizing the tiny papillary orifice. The orifice is cannulated with a fine probe and incised along its anterosuperior lip to eliminate the mucosal cap on the end of the duct, and the pancreatic and duodenal mucosae are approximated with fine, absorbable, synthetic sutures to control bleeding and to promote healing with minimal scar. A 5-F pediatric feeding catheter, left in the duct and brought out through the duodenum and abdominal wall, ensures unimpeded drainage during recovery and is removed in 2 to 3 weeks.

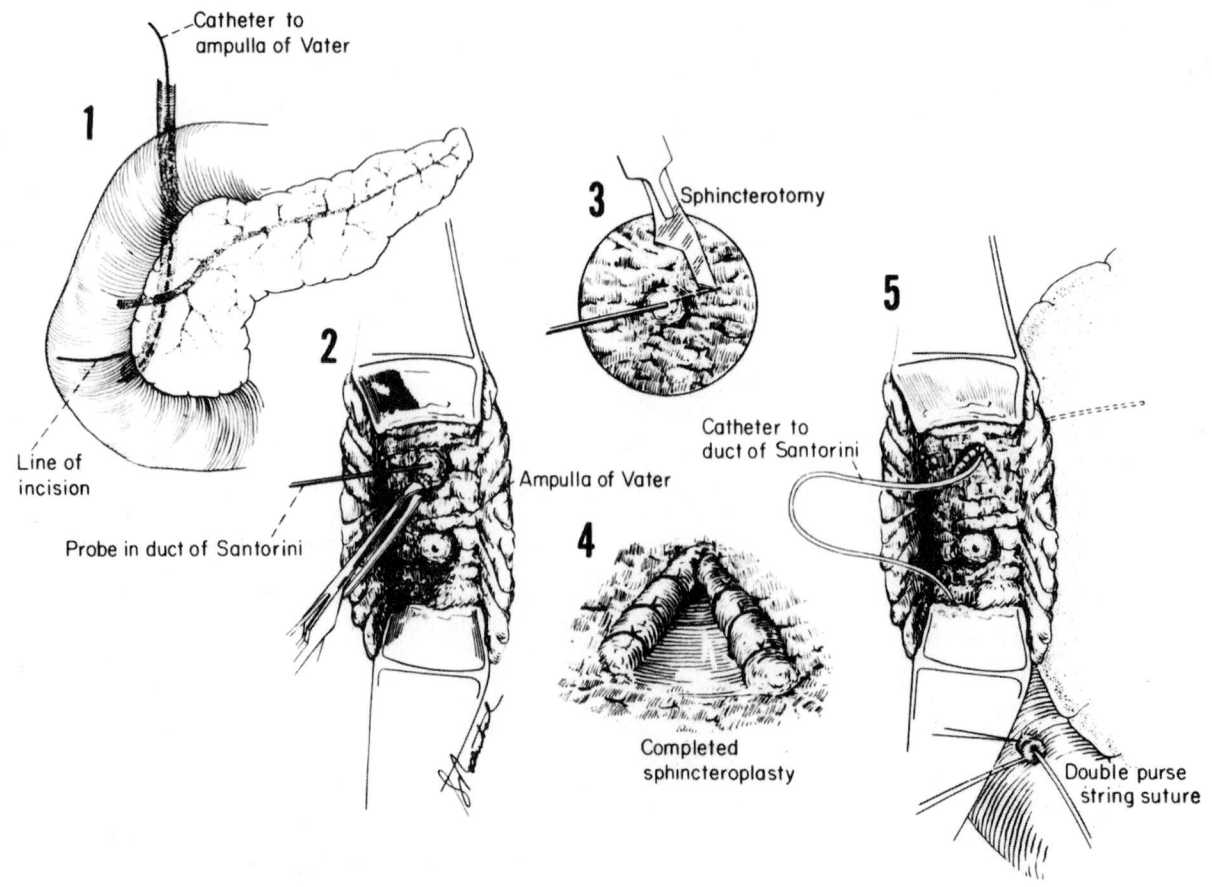

Figure 6 Technique of accessory papilla sphincteroplasty.

Our current experience of 170 patients mirrors our published long-term analysis of 88 patients treated by accessory papilla sphincteroplasty. At a mean follow-up of 53 months, 70% were significantly improved: 82% of those with documented recurrent acute pancreatitis and 92% of those with a positive ultrasound-secretin test (Table 1).

Mortality rates in published series have been less than 1%, and the complication rates approximately 4%. Endoscopic therapy or repeat sphincteroplasty for restenosis is efficacious less than half the time, and established fibrotic obstructive pancreatitis after sphincter therapy has failed may necessitate pancreaticoduodenectomy.

Accessory papilla sphincteroplasty is inappropriate and unsuccessful when there is morphologically established chronic fibrotic pancreatitis, calcification, or markedly dilatated ducts, with or without a "chain of lakes." Whether the chronic pancreatitis in such patients was caused by accessory papilla obstruction or is pathogenetically unrelated and coincidental is moot and of no importance to the choice of therapy. Chronic pancreatitis and its complications in patients with pancreas divisum are treated like those of any causation: side-to-side pancreaticojejunostomy (modified Puestow procedure) if the main duct is sufficiently dilatated; pancreaticoduodenectomy or duodenum-sparing pancreatic head resection if it is not.

As pancreas divisum becomes recognized and treated more frequently in childhood, the evolving principles of treatment appear to be the same as in adults.

Several cases of isolated ventral chronic pancreatitis in patients with pancreas divisum have been reported. The pathogenesis of this condition is not well understood, but successful relief of pain has been reported following either sphincteroplasty of the major papilla with pancreatolithotomy or pancreaticoduodenectomy.

SUGGESTED READINGS

Bradley EL, Stephan RN: Accessory duct sphincteroplasty is preferred for long-term prevention of recurrent acute pancreatitis in patients with pancreas divisum, *J Am Coll Surg* 183:65, 1996.

Catalano MF, Lahoti S, Alcocer E, and others: Dynamic imaging of the pancreas using real-time endoscopic ultrasonography with secretin stimulation, *Gastrointest Endosc* 48:580, 1998.

Keith RG, Shapero TF, Saibil FG, and others: Dorsal duct sphincterotomy is effective long-term treatment of acute pancreatitis associated with pancreas divisum, *Surgery* 106:660, 1989.

Kozarek RA, Ball TJ, Patterson DJ, and others: Endoscopic therapy in patients with pancreas divisum, *Dig Dis Sci* 40:1974, 1995.

Lans JL, Geenen JE, Johanson JF, and others: Endoscopic therapy in patients with pancreas divisum and acute pancreatitis: a prospective, randomized, controlled clinical trial, *Gastrointest Endosc* 38:430, 1992.

Lehman CA, Sherman S, Nisi R, and others: Pancreas divisum: results of minor papilla sphincterotomy, *Gastroinest Endosc* 39:1, 1993.

Madura JA: Pancreas divisum. Stenosis of the dorsally dominant pancreatic duct: a surgically correctable lesion, *Am J Surg* 151:742, 1986.

Neblett WW III, O'Neill JA Jr: Surgical management of recurrent pancreatitis in children with pancreas divisum, *Ann Surg* 231:899, 2000.

Warshaw AL, Cambria RP: False pancreas divisum: acquired pancreatic duct obstruction simulating the congenital anomaly, *Ann Surg* 200:595, 1984.

Warshaw AL, Simeone JF, Schapiro RH, and others: Evaluation and treatment of the dominant dorsal duct syndrome (pancreas divisum redefined), *Am J Surg* 159:59, 1990.

Warshaw AL, Simeone J, Schapiro RH, and others: Objective evaluation of ampullary stenosis with ultrasonography and pancreatic stimulation, *Am J Surg* 149:65, 1985.

PANCREATIC ABSCESS

Katherine A. Morgan, MD, and David B. Adams, MD

INTRODUCTION

The pancreatic abscess is a circumscribed collection of pus that appears adjacent to the pancreas in acute and chronic pancreatic injury. Management includes both operative debridement and drainage and image-guided percutaneous catheter drainage, depending on the degree of localized pancreatic and peripancreatic tissue destruction.

In most instances, a pancreatic abscess develops following the onset of acute necrotizing pancreatitis and disease severity is dependent on cytokine-mediated systemic injury and localized tissue destruction related to pancreatic enzyme activation. Abscess formation may occur in up to 70% of patients with severe acute pancreatitis with necrosis.

Acute pancreatitis is a protean disease characterized by inflammation and pancreatic enzyme activation with resultant local and systemic pathology of variable severity. Alcohol consumption and gallstone disease account for the vast majority of cases of acute pancreatitis in the United States. Most episodes of acute pancreatitis are self-limited, with minimal long-term morbidity and mortality. Approximately 15% to 20% of cases are severe, with associated systemic organ failure and local complications such as pancreatic pseudocyst, intra-abdominal or gastrointestinal hemorrhage, pancreatic or enteric fistulae, and pancreatic and peripancreatic necrosis. Optimal care depends on the support of a coordinated care system that offers the special expertise of surgeons, interventional radiologists, anesthesiologists, gastroenterologists, and critical care support services. Despite excellent care, patients with infected pancreatic necrosis may face mortality rates as high as 29%.

DEFINITIONS

The Atlanta classification system was established in 1992 to attempt to define various presentations of pancreatitis. *Necrotizing pancreatitis* was identified as pancreatitis with devitalized tissue. It was further classified as *noninfected pancreatic necrosis* and *infected pancreatic necrosis*. *Noninfected necrosis* implies that there is no documented infection of nonviable tissue. *Infected necrosis* refers to infection of the devitalized tissue, as documented by image-guided aspiration or by presumed infection, usually identified by extraluminal gas in the peripancreatic tissues on computed tomography (CT). *Pancreatic abscess* is defined as a collection of infected peripancreatic fluid in the absence of significant necrosis. The term used in this review, *infected pancreatic and peripancreatic fluid collections*, includes infected pancreatic necrosis (in which fluid is evident on CT scan), pancreatic abscess (a circumscribed collection of pus often adjacent to pancreatic necrosis), and infected pancreatic pseudocyst. Although the Atlanta classification is the most widely accepted clinically based classification system for acute pancreatitis, natural diseases operate in a continuum, so it is not always clear in acute patient management whether one is observing an infected pancreatic pseudocyst, a pancreatic abscess, or infected pancreatic necrosis. It is possible that there are overlapping or gray areas that are part of disease progression but that do not affect urgent patient-management decisions. As Bob Dylan said, "You don't need a weatherman to know which way the wind blows." What one does need to know is that infected pancreatic and peripancreatic fluid collections that lack substantial amounts of solid tissue necrosis can be safely managed with image-guided percutaneous catheter drainage. Infected fluid with substantial amounts of tissue necrosis requires operative drainage and debridement. When percutaneous catheter drainage fails, operative drainage is required. When operative drainage and debridement are complicated by recurrent abscess, percutaneous catheter drainage may be necessary and usually avoids reoperation.

INITIAL MANAGEMENT

An episode of acute pancreatitis is caused by an isolated insulting event that precipitates pancreatic enzyme activation and may lead to ductal disruption with local and systemic effects. In severe pancreatitis, the local effect is autodigestion with necrosis of pancreatic and peripancreatic tissues. The systemic effects are the result of the activation of the cytokine-mediated inflammatory cascade.

Systems for stratification of severity of illness have been used for acute pancreatitis (Ranson, Glasgow, Acute Physiology and Chronic Health Evaluation [APACHE] II) as outcome predictors. Rarely is there confusion in identifying patients with severe disease who require intensive care unit (ICU) resuscitation and monitoring. The inflammatory response with associated systemic capillary leak can be dramatic, with massive resuscitative fluid requirements. One does well to consider these patients as having a massive retroperitoneal burn. Monitoring for respiratory failure, with intubation and ventilatory support as needed, may be part of the initial care. Often cardiovascular monitoring with a pulmonary artery catheter and use of vasopressors and inotropes are necessary. Likewise, renal, hepatic, and immunologic failure can be swift and dramatic in these patients.

Substantial nutritional support is essential in these critically ill patients. Ileus is often present early in disease, but enteral alimentation is started as soon as the patient is able to tolerate it. Although there are many sources of infection of pancreatic necrosis, an important mechanism is translocation of organisms across the disrupted basement membrane of the gastrointestinal tract. Enteral feedings can help to maintain the integrity of the gut mucosal barrier. Ideally feedings are begun through a tube in the postpyloric position to minimize pancreatic stimulation, although the insult that incites the severe episode of pancreatitis is an isolated event, and reluctance for further pancreatic stimulation should not prohibit enteral feeding. Patients with severe pancreatitis and abscess frequently have gut dysfunction that necessitates use of total parental alimentation.

Empiric antibiotic therapy is initiated in patients with evidence of pancreatic necrosis on CT scan. A meta-analysis has shown a positive benefit for antibiotics in reducing mortality in severe pancreatitis, and many studies have shown diminished infectious complications. Imipenem, chosen for its gram-negative and anaerobic coverage and its excellent concentration into pancreatic tissue, is the antibiotic of choice. In those patients intolerant to carbapenems, a fluoroquinolone, also well concentrated into pancreatic tissue, is selected along with metronidazole. Because of recent trends of resistant gram-positive organisms in pancreatitis patients, vancomycin is frequently used. Fluconazole is added to antibiotic coverage when there is concern for yeast infection, particularly in patients who have received multiple broad-spectrum antibiotics and have continued high fever and signs of sepsis. In addition to gut translocation, infected central lines, the biliary system, and ascending duodenal infection via the pancreatic duct may be sources of pancreatic infection and should be considered in antibiotic selection.

ROLE OF COMPUTED TOMOGRAPHY SCAN

The diagnosis of severe acute pancreatitis is a clinical diagnosis made at the bedside by the patient's presentation and physiologic course. A diagnostic CT scan with oral and intravenous contrast is invaluable in a patient with organ failure, large resuscitative requirements, or an indeterminate diagnosis. Adequate hydration should be ensured in these patients, who are often hypovolemic before intravenous infusion of the radiographic contrast agent. In a normovolemic patient with minor renal insufficiency, renal protective measures such as acetylcysteine, bicarbonate, and hydration should be instituted before the study.

A CT scan with intravenous contrast can reveal areas of nonperfusion in the pancreas, suggestive of pancreatic necrosis. Early in the disease course, pancreatic edema and large amounts of peripancreatic fluid may result in overestimation of the degree of necrosis. As acute inflammation and edema resolve and fluid collections organize, CT provides more useful information in planning interventional strategies. CT scan may show extraluminal air in the retroperitoneum, indicative of infected pancreatic necrosis. However, conservative management of the patient without signs of sepsis may be successful even in the face of CT evidence of retroperitoneal gas. CT scan is valuable to assess local complications of pancreatitis that may alter management such as pseudocyst, fistula, or pseudoaneurysm.

In the patient with CT evidence of necrosis with fever, leukocytosis, or worsening organ failure, CT-guided aspiration of the pancreatic bed can confirm the diagnosis of infected necrosis. In the early course of severe acute pancreatitis, organ dysfunction from cytokine injury is a systemic problem that requires systemic therapy. Abscess and infection associated with pancreatic necrosis are unlikely to be the source of organ dysfunction, and thus CT aspiration of the pancreatic bed is unlikely to be of benefit early in the disease course. When pancreatic and peripancreatic fluid collections develop later in the course of disease in association with signs of sepsis, percutaneous catheter drainage of fluid collections has several benefits. First, it provides a source of culture material. Second, it may eradicate collections comprising tissue-destructive, enzyme-rich fluid. Third, it may ameliorate the septic course in patients with major medical comorbidity and high operative risk. Large volumes of infected, thick, necrotic tissue cannot be drained through a small catheter, but occasionally patients with infected, liquefied pancreatic necrosis avoid operative drainage and are salvaged with image-guided drainage.

OPERATIVE INDICATIONS

Management of pancreatic abscess cannot be separated from discussion of surgical management of acute pancreatitis. The International Association of Pancreatology has developed evidence-based guidelines on the surgical management of acute pancreatitis that are useful in patient management and form a basis for determining the quality of patient care delivery (Table 1).

Although patients with infected pancreatic necrosis require prompt debridement, expectant, nonoperative management for at least 4 weeks after onset of illness is optimal. This timing allows much of the evolution of the necrosis to mature and liquefy, making soft-finger debridement safer and protecting mesenteric vessels from operative injury. At 4 weeks, patients can usually undergo successful single-stage operative debridement. Expectant management of infected pancreatic necrosis has three risks: bleeding, perforation (with fistula formation), and obstruction. Enzymatic erosion of visceral vessels can cause bleeding from branches of the mesenteric and celiac axis. The splenic artery and the gastroduodenal artery are most commonly involved with this complication, but all retroperitoneal vessels are at risk. If the patient is hemodynamically stable and does not require emergent laparotomy, this complication is best managed with angiographic embolization. The enzyme-rich abscess fluid can erode into adjacent visceral organs, including stomach, duodenum, terminal bile duct, proximal jejunum, and colon. Fistulae are typically best managed conservatively, with assurance of appropriate drainage. The inflammatory

Table 1: International Association of Pancreatology Guidelines for the Surgical Management of Acute Pancreatitis

1. Mild acute pancreatitis is not an indication for pancreatic surgery.

2. The use of prophylactic broad-spectrum antibiotics reduces infection rates in computed tomography–proved necrotizing pancreatitis.

3. Fine needle aspiration for bacteriology should be performed to differentiate between sterile and infected pancreatic necrosis in patients with sepsis syndrome.

4. Infected pancreatic necrosis in patients with clinical signs and symptoms of sepsis is an indication for intervention including surgery and radiologic drainage.

5. Patients with sterile pancreatic necrosis should be managed conservatively and should undergo intervention only in selected cases.

6. Early surgery within 14 days after onset of the disease is not recommended in patients with necrotizing pancreatitis unless there are specific indications.

7. Surgical and other forms of interventional management should favor an organ-preserving approach, which involves debridement or necrosectomy combined with a postoperative management concept that maximizes postoperative evacuation of retroperitoneal debris and exudate.

8. Cholecystectomy should be performed to avoid recurrence of gallstone-associated acute pancreatitis.

9. In mild gallstone-associated acute pancreatitis, cholecystectomy should be performed as soon as the patient has recovered, ideally during the same hospital admission.

10. In severe gallstone-associated acute pancreatitis, cholecystectomy should be delayed until there is sufficient resolution of the inflammatory response and clinical recovery.

11. Endoscopic sphincterotomy is an alternative to cholecystectomy in those who are not fit to undergo surgery.

From Uhl W, Warshaw A, Imrie C, and others: IAP guidelines for the surgical management of acute pancreatitis, *Pancreatology* 2:565, 2002.

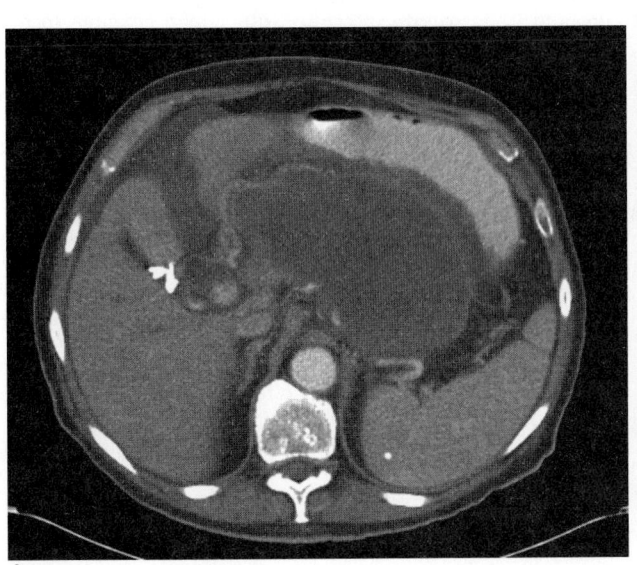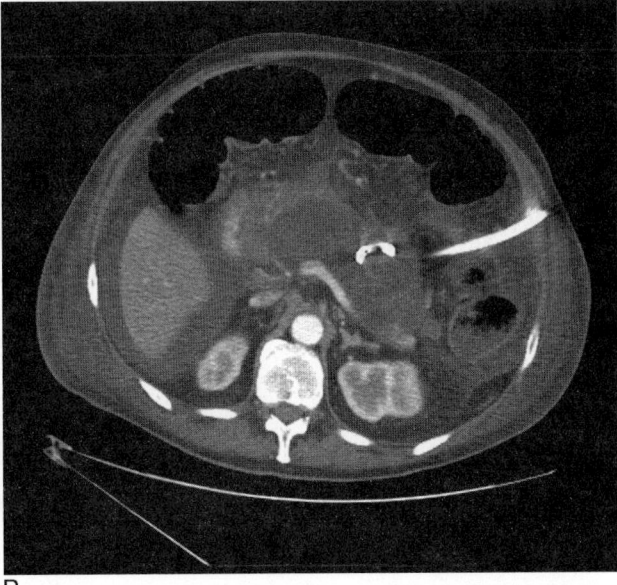

Figure 1   Pancreatic abscess in a patient with associated biliary obstruction **(A)** successfully managed with image-guided percutaneous catheter drainage **(B)**.

mass associated with a pancreatic abscess can also cause obstruction of the gastric outlet, the terminal bile duct, the proximal jejunum, or the transverse colon (Fig. 1). Obstruction can often be managed nonoperatively but at times may require external drainage, resection, or diversion of the involved structures.

PREOPERATIVE PREPARATION

Patient education is important in preoperative preparation for pancreatic abscess drainage and debridement. Patients and families should be aware that operation usually results in a systemic insult that puts the patient in a condition markedly worse than the

preoperative status. Worsening of the sepsis syndrome may put the patient in the ICU for weeks. It is not uncommon for patients to be readmitted several times to the ICU before convalescence. Many patients require hospital discharge to rehabilitation centers. It may be months to years to full recovery, but recovery can be complete and gratifying to patients, their families, and all involved in the patient's care.

TECHNIQUE

The goals of pancreatic debridement are fourfold. First, an extensive and gentle necrosectomy is undertaken. Second, the etiology of the pancreatitis is addressed, and cholecystectomy is performed if indicated and safe. When retroperitoneal inflammation extensively involves the porta hepatis and the hazards of cholecystectomy are great, gallbladder removal can de delayed. Third, the nutritional needs of the patient are addressed with enteral tube positioning. Fourth, closed-suction drainage of the exudative process and persistent pancreatic duct leak is established.

A midline incision permits easy access and exposure to the lesser sac. Abdominal reentry for subsequent operations is facilitated with a midline incision. The stomach and transverse colon are often intimately opposed from the inflammatory process, making access to the lesser sac through the gastrocolic ligament difficult. The avascular portion of the transverse mesocolon left of the middle colic vessels provides a safe window to enter the lesser sac and debride necrotic tissue in the left and right upper retroperitoneum and the lower left retroperitoneum and paracolic gutter (Fig. 2). The right lower retroperitoneum and paracolic gutter are entered through the mesocolon of the hepatic flexure when necrosis extends there. Persistent and gentle blunt finger dissection using the CT scan as a road map permits careful entry into all affected areas by hand and extraction of necrotic tissue with ringed forceps assistance as needed. A laparotomy pad can be positioned to provide gentle debridement of residual tissue after finger and forceps dissection. On occasion, a disconnected necrotic segment of pancreas is extracted in the debridement. Necrotic peripancreatic fat is most commonly the debridement target. Pulsatile saline lavage is used to complete the cavity debridement and irrigation. Bleeding that is encountered is usually from the granulation tissue in the walls of the cavity and can be managed with pressure or temporary packing. Mesenteric venous tributaries may bleed and are best managed with hemostatic metallic clips. Debridement in the region of the superior mesenteric vein and the portal vein should ensure that these structures are kept out of harm's way. Suture ligation of arterial hemorrhage may be necessary for hemostasis. In general, a pseudoaneurysm from a named vessel should be suspected from the preoperative CT and not encountered unexpectedly. If this does occur and attempts at hemostasis with suture ligation are impossible, one can pack the site of bleeding and transport the patient to the angiography department for embolization.

Jejunal feeding tubes are avoided in patients with severe necrosis and sepsis because associated jejunostomy tube complications

may be life threatening. Placement of a nasojejunal tube with intraoperative guidance into a postpyloric position is preferred. If the need for long-term feeding access becomes apparent in the postoperative period, endoscopic placement of a gastrojejunal feeding tube is undertaken.

Large, soft sump drains are placed into the lesser sac at the completion of the operation. They exit through separate sites and are used postoperatively for both drainage and irrigation. Drains are positioned at the transverse mesocolic window to avoid catheter trauma to the colon or stomach. Closed-suction drains may be placed within smaller cavities or recesses not well drained by the larger irrigating drains.

POSTOPERATIVE CARE

The sump drains are infused with saline irrigation at a rate of 50 ml/hr, and low constant suction is maintained through the sump port. Irrigation is continued until the drainage is clear, usually 5 to 7 days. When tube drainage diminishes to less than 50 ml per day, the tubes are withdrawn at a rate of 1 inch per day.

Postoperative fever or leukocytosis a week or more after surgery dictates CT scan evaluation. Between 10% and 20% of patients require an additional image-guided percutaneous drain. Reexploration for ongoing necrosis or undrainable pus is necessary in a minority of cases.

Enteric fistulae occur in approximately 10% of patients. Stomach, terminal bile duct, duodenum, proximal jejunum, and left transverse colon are all possible sites of fistula formation. Fistulae are initially managed expectantly with careful attention to nutritional support and image-guided drainage of associated fluid collections. Fistulae that do not resolve or that are associated with uncontrolled sepsis require operative management. Choice of external drainage, diversion, internal drainage, and resection depend on the condition of the patient and the status of the pancreatic disorder.

If there is a persistent pancreatic leak caused by ductal disruption, intravenous octreotide may facilitate patient management and accelerate fistula closure. When there is evidence of pancreatic ductal disruption, endoscopic retrograde cholangiopancreatography (ERCP) is undertaken to define the pancreatic ductal anatomy. Along with rendering a diagnosis, ERCP may be therapeutic. Transpapillary stent placement and sphincterotomy may facilitate fistula closure. Magnetic resonance cholangiopancreatography (MRCP) is rarely useful in identifying ductal disorders in the early postoperative setting because of pancreatic edema and peripancreatic fluid collections. If endoscopic management fails or if midbody pancreatic necrosis is identified, delayed operative intervention is undertaken. Patients with pancreatic necrosis and abscess frequently have ductal disruption at the pancreatic genu and are well managed in the long term with distal pancreatectomy and splenectomy.

IMAGE-GUIDED PERCUTANEOUS CATHETER DRAINAGE OF INFECTED PANCREATIC AND PERIPANCREATIC FLUID COLLECTIONS

Image-guided percutaneous catheter drainage of infected pancreatic and peripancreatic fluid collections is successful in well-selected patients. The acute pancreatic pseudocyst, characterized as an enzyme-rich collection of pancreatic fluid enveloped by a fibrous wall, may become secondarily infected. If the pseudocyst does not communicate with the pancreatic duct, percutaneous catheter drainage may lead to complete eradication of the infected pseudocyst. If duct communication exists, percutaneous catheter drainage

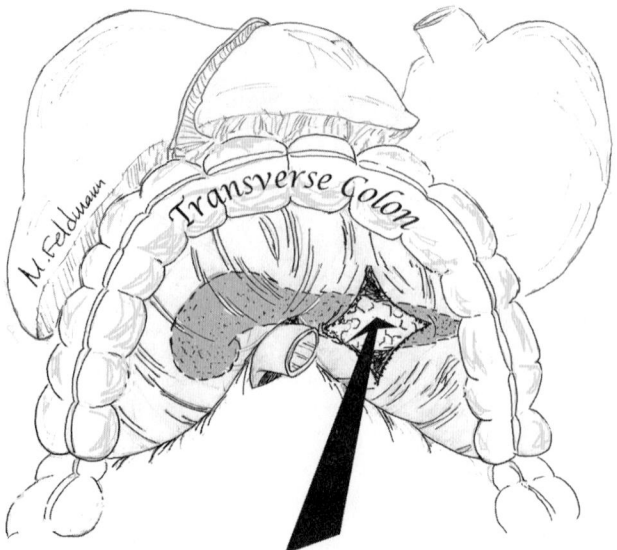

Figure 2 Transmesocolic approach for debridement and drainage of pancreatic necrosis and abscess.

may lead to resolution of the acute infection and allow elective management of the underlying ductal disorder with a pancreatic resection or drainage procedure. Similar to the infected pancreatic pseudocyst is the uncommon unilocular pancreatic abscess. Resolution of the uncomplicated pancreatic abscess can be expected with catheter drainage when it is easily accessible. Foreign bodies, solid necrotic tissue, and a persistent underlying pancreatic duct or gastrointestinal disruption are factors involved in abscesses that fail percutaneous drainage. More common than the simple pancreatic abscess is the abscess associated with infected pancreatic necrosis. A liquefied collection of pus and pancreatic secretions that develops later in the course of pancreatic necrosis may be successfully

managed with percutaneous catheter drainage in the absence of substantial amounts of solid necrotic tissue. Because it may be difficult to identify these patients on the basis of their clinical course and CT scan findings, percutaneous catheter drainage of pancreatic abscess that is unsuccessful should lead to early operative debridement and drainage (Fig. 3).

Percutaneous catheter drainage has been promoted as an effective temporizing measure in unstable patients with severe sepsis because it drains pus under pressure. Portal hypertension caused by prehepatic splanchnic venous occlusion is another situation in which percutaneous catheter drainage may be selected in a patient who otherwise would meet indications for operative drainage and

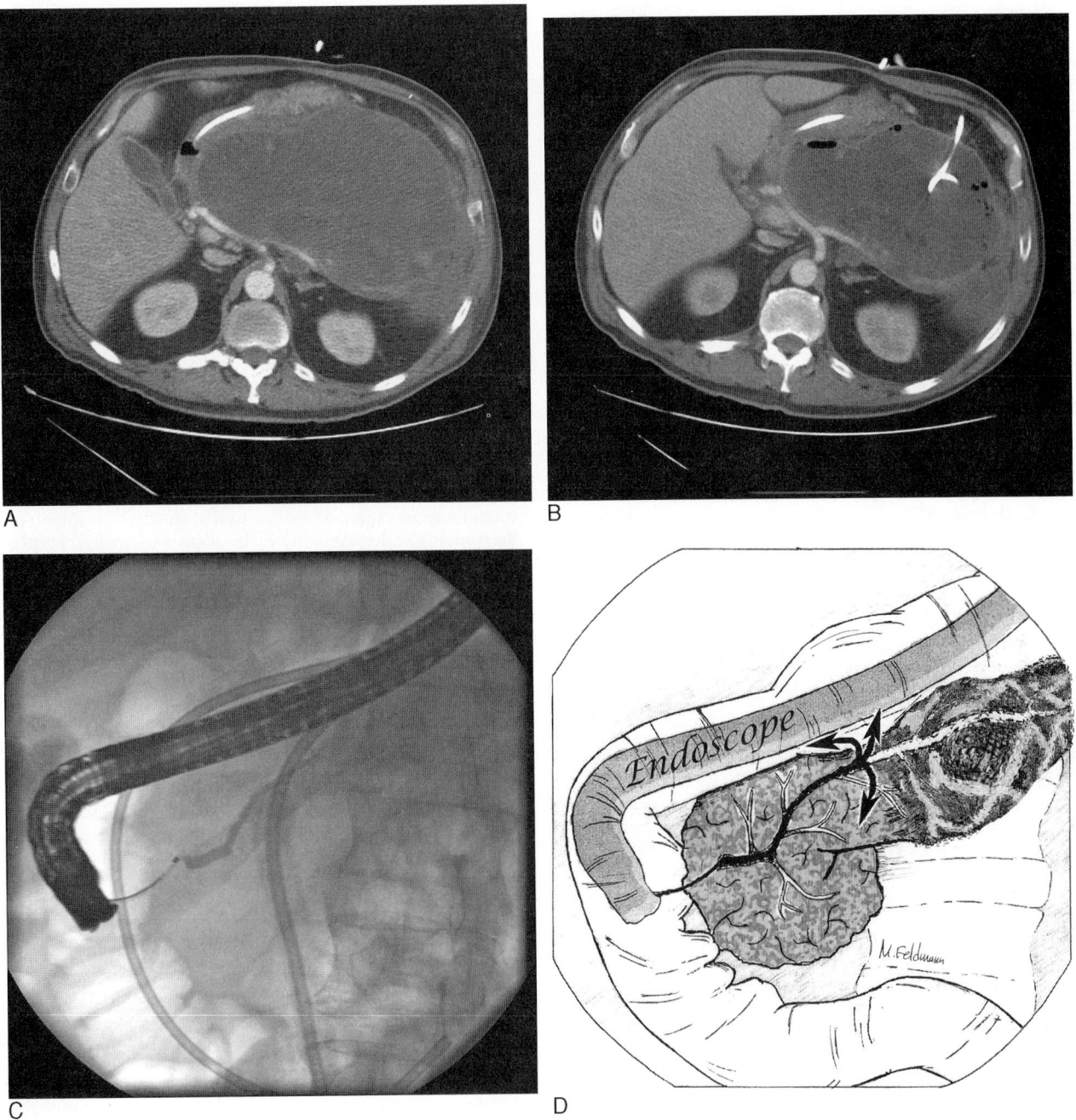

Figure 3 Pancreatic abscess and necrosis in a patient temporized with image-guided percutaneous drainage who required subsequent operative drainage and debridement. **(A)** Computed tomography *(CT)* scan shows a large pancreatic abscess and liquefied necrosis. **(B)** CT-guided percutaneous drain was placed into the peripancreatic fluid collection. **(C)** Endoscopic retrograde cholangiopancreatography demonstrates midbody ductal disruption in the same patient. **(D)** A line drawing that more clearly illustrates ductal leak and associated pancreatic tissue destruction.

debridement. Severe acute or chronic respiratory failure, severe cardiac dysfunction, and recent myocardial infarction are also conditions that would lead to consideration for percutaneous catheter drainage over operative drainage. Abscesses that develop after operations on the pancreas and in proximity to it show favorable outcomes with percutaneous catheter drainage.

When image-guided percutaneous catheter drainage is selected for management of pancreatic abscess, communication and collaboration with an experienced interventional radiologist are important. Initial placement of a single lumen 12- to 20-F pigtail catheter is undertaken under CT guidance with a Seldinger technique. Fluid Gram stain and culture are monitored to select specific antibiotic therapy. Drains are placed to a closed gravity system and are irrigated with sterile saline three times a day. Clinical signs of sepsis and weekly CT scans are used to assess the outcome. When sepsis and fluid collections do not resolve, catheter manipulations with larger catheters, sump catheters, and urokinase instillation have been used to improve catheter drainage. Multiple drains may be necessary for multilocular abscesses. The most common cause of failed percutaneous catheter drainage is inability to eradicate infected necrotic tissue. Necrotic peripancreatic tissue may not be readily apparent on CT scan.

Abscess eradication with percutaneous catheter drainage may be followed by the development of an external pancreatic fistula. Octreotide can be used to help optimize conditions for nonoperative closure. Persistent pancreatic fistulae are evaluated with sinogram and ERCP to define the underlying pancreatic ductal disorder and plan an appropriate operation.

ENDOSCOPIC AND LAPAROSCOPIC DIRECTED DRAINAGE OF INFECTED PANCREATIC AND PERIPANCREATIC FLUID COLLECTIONS

Endoscopic- and laparoscopic-assisted drainage of infected pancreatic necrosis, pancreatic abscess, and infected pancreatic pseudocysts has been reported from centers with advanced, specialized technical skills and long-standing experience in management of complicated pancreatitis. Most medical systems that manage these patients, however, have their most reliable experience with operative and image-guided drainage of infected pancreatic and peripancreatic fluid collections.

SUGGESTED READINGS

Adams DB, Harvey TS, Anderson MC: Percutaneous catheter drainage of infected pancreatic and peripancreatic fluid collections, *Arch Surg* 125:1554, 1990.
Baril NB, Ralls PW, Wren SM, and others: Does an infected peripancreatic fluid collection or abscess mandate operation? *Ann Surg* 231:361, 2000.
Mithofer K, Mueller PR, Warshaw AL: Interventional and surgical treatment of pancreatic abscess, *World J Surg* 21:162, 1997.
Rodriguez JR, Razo AO, Targarona J, and others: Debridement and closed packing for necrotizing pancreatitis: a 15 year experience, *Pancreas* 31:465, 2005.
Traverso LW, Kozarek RA: Pancreatic necrosectomy: definitions and technique, *J Gastrointest Surg* 94:36, 2005.

PANCREATIC PSEUDOCYSTS

Kevin E. Behrns, MD

Pancreatic pseudocysts result from excessive pressure within a pancreatic duct that ruptures and permits extravasation of enzyme-rich pancreatic fluid. In 1992, the International Symposium on Acute Pancreatitis formulated the following definition: "A pancreatic pseudocyst is a collection of pancreatic juice enclosed by wall of fibrous or granulation tissue which arises as a consequence of acute pancreatitis, trauma, or chronic pancreatitis." Because pancreatic fluid is encapsulated by fibrous tissue, a pseudocyst forms over several weeks as fibroblasts react to inflammation and lay down extracellular matrix proteins. Generally, a pseudocyst matures over 4 to 6 weeks, during which time the fibrous wall thickens and achieves near-maximal strength. In contradistinction, an acute fluid collection arises in the setting of acute pancreatitis and is characterized by a collection of nonenzymatic fluid that is a product of the acute inflammatory response but not the result of a disrupted pancreatic duct (Fig. 1). The difference between a pseudocyst and an acute fluid collection is crucial because an acute fluid collection invariably resolves spontaneously as the inflammatory process wanes. Therefore an acute fluid collection requires no treatment, whereas a pseudocyst may resolve, persist, or enlarge over time and cause complications.

ETIOLOGY AND PATHOGENESIS

Pancreatic pseudocysts develop in chronic pancreatitis (35%) more commonly than in acute pancreatitis (15%); however, many of the pseudocysts in chronic pancreatitis are small, cause no symptoms, and thus require no treatment. The pathogenesis of pseudocyst formation in acute and chronic pancreatitis differs significantly, and careful consideration of this critical distinction is important in determining treatment options. In acute pancreatitis, most often caused by gallstones or sporadic alcohol ingestion, the pancreas has not been previously injured. Consequently, the main pancreatic duct is often normal or has a single point of disruption that may heal well with minimal intervention. Chronic pancreatitis, however, is a unique disease in which repetitive alcohol use causes loss of acinar cells and deposition of collagen. This chronic, injurious process results in major changes in the architecture of the pancreas and, especially, the pancreatic duct, which may be strictured, dilatated, or obliterated. Therefore the treatment of a pseudocyst in the setting of chronic pancreatitis may differ significantly from that of a pseudocyst in acute pancreatitis.

In addition to distinguishing pancreatic pseudocysts in acute and chronic pancreatitis, pseudocysts must be differentiated from other cystic lesions of the pancreas, which constitute approximately 15% of all pancreatic cysts. Benign simple cysts are uncommon, but because of improved cross-sectional imaging, cystic neoplasms of the pancreas are identified with increasing frequency and must be discriminated from pseudocysts. Cystic neoplasms are not associated with a history of pancreatitis; may contain septa; have exuberant and calcium-containing wall growth; and have an epithelial lining that may undergo malignant transformation. Histologic assessment is mandatory when a pseudocyst cannot be confidently distinguished radiographically from a pancreatic cystic neoplasm.

Furthermore, pseudocysts may be associated with symptoms, whereas cystic neoplasms typically do not cause symptoms until they achieve a large size. However, nearly 25% of pseudocysts are less than 6 cm in size and cause few symptoms. Large pseudocysts may be associated with abdominal pain, nausea, vomiting, bloating, and other nonspecific symptoms. Moreover, pseudocysts cause complications that result in various clinical presentations.

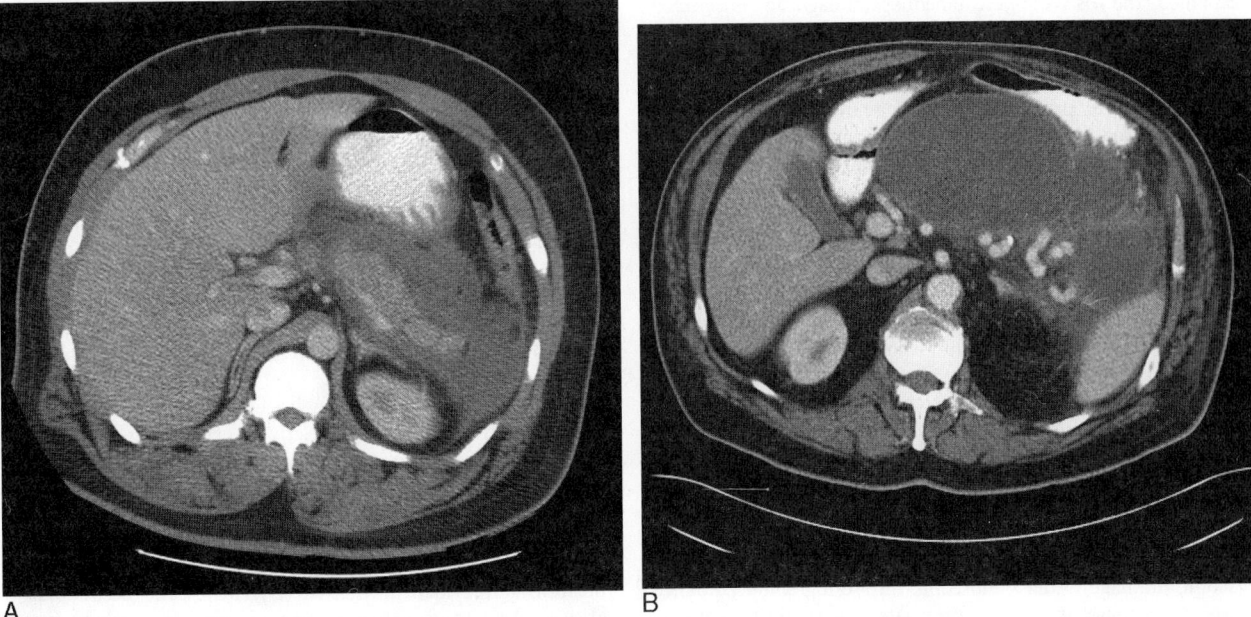

Figure 1   Computed tomography images of an acute fluid collection **(A)** and a pancreatic pseuodcyst **(B).** Note the well-developed fibrous wall of the pseudocyst in contrast to the indistinct border of the fluid collection.

As pseudocysts increase in size, gastroduodenal obstruction is manifest by early satiety, nausea, or vomiting, and biliary obstruction may result from a pseudocyst located in the head of the pancreas. Pseudocysts may also cause vascular compromise with thrombosis of the splenic, superior mesenteric, or portal veins that results in venous congestion and, rarely, in gastrointestinal bleeding. Pseudocyst erosion into an artery may cause bleeding, including hemosuccus pancreaticus, whereas erosion into the splenic hilum can lift off the capsule of the spleen and be associated with significant splenic hemorrhage. Finally, pseudocysts may become infected and require drainage to prevent sepsis or rupture freely into the peritoneal cavity and ultimately cause a pancreatic fistula.

DIAGNOSTIC EVALUATION

Since the mid-1980s, improved cross-sectional imaging has significantly enhanced the evaluation of cystic lesions of the pancreas. However, many pancreatic cystic lesions, especially those 2 to 3 cm in size, remain a diagnostic dilemma because of nonspecific features. Pseudocysts are typically discovered by either ultrasonography or computed tomography (CT) performed for abdominal symptoms. Refinements in imaging techniques, particularly thin-sliced, multidetector CT, permit detailed images that suggest unique cyst or pancreatic parenchymal features and allow accurate diagnosis. Differentiating pure cystic lesions from combined solid/cystic lesions is occasionally problematic, and magnetic resonance imaging (MRI) with T2-weighted sequences clearly demonstrates cystic, fluid-filled components of the lesion. MRI also has the distinct advantage of cholangiopancreatography that may demonstrate a cyst-pancreatic duct communication, which may be seen in pancreatic pseudocysts or intraductal papillary mucinous neoplasms. Endoscopic ultrasonography (EUS) has also enhanced visualization of pancreatic cysts. This technique provides a close, detailed view of cysts, and irregularity in the wall or fine septa within the cyst may be demonstrated. Furthermore, fine needle aspiration (FNA) of cyst fluid permits evaluation for cytology, tumor markers, mucin, and pancreatic enzymes. Generally, FNA of a pancreatic pseudocyst is acellular, has low tumor marker content such as carcinogenic embryonic antigen (CEA), carbohydrate

antigen (CA) 19–9, or CA 15–3; and contains no mucin but has a high amylase concentration. Finally, for small pancreatic cystic lesions, serial imaging can accurately detect incremental size increase, which may be an important factor in the treatment decision.

MANAGEMENT OPTIONS

Prior to the 1970s, treatment of pseudocysts was often empiric because of lack of natural history data. In 1979, however, Bradley and colleagues published the initial study examining the natural history of pancreatic pseudocysts and found that in 54 patients under serial observation, the risk of complications from an untreated pseudocyst increased after 7 weeks of observation. This risk (46%) was far higher than the risk of operation. Therefore for the next decade, pseudocysts that had not resolved by 6 weeks underwent operative therapy with a goal of enteric drainage. Outcomes from this period suggest that the overall mortality (7%) and morbidity rates (>40%) were relatively high. This protocol of management of pseudocysts persisted until the early 1990s, when two surgical studies suggested that the risk of complication from a pseudocyst was related to the size of the lesion. At this time, pseudocysts were readily identified and followed by CT, and Yeo and colleagues and Vitas and Sarr found that observation of asymptomatic pseudocysts less than 6 cm in size infrequently resulted in complications. In fact, in the Vitas and Sarr study, seven patients with pseudocysts greater than 10 cm were managed by observation. Thereafter an expectant approach to the management of asymptomatic, small pseudocysts was prevalent.

The period of minimal intervention, however, was relatively brief because of the introduction of percutaneous drainage of pseudocysts and acute fluid collections. This procedure was performed on numerous patients with little regard to adherence to a strict definition of a pseudocyst versus an acute fluid collection and little recognition that the pathophysiology of pseudocyst formation in acute and chronic pancreatitits differed. Thus many patients underwent percutaneous drainage of pseudocysts, and predictably the outcome was variable; more than 30% of patients subsequently required operative therapy. With the realization that poor results accompanied the use of percutaneous drainage in unselected patients and the more frequent use of cross-sectional imaging, medical and surgical pancreatologists have based treatment on the etiology of pancreatitis, status of the pancreatic duct, pancreatic parenchyma, and the patient's comorbid conditions.

Recently, evaluation and management of pancreatic pseudocysts has begun with identification of the cause of pseudocysts—acute versus chronic pancreatitis and symptom assessment. Although large, asymptomatic pseudocysts may be managed with watchful waiting, the risks of insidious complications such as venous thrombosis have not been documented. In symptomatic patients with chronic pancreatitis, careful examination of the cause of the symptoms (infection, gastroduodenal or biliary obstruction, venous thrombosis, fistula, rupture) should be sought, and cross-sectional imaging with CT or MRI is necessary. Because patients with chronic pancreatitis often have pancreatic duct strictures, imaging of the pancreas is necessary. This may be accomplished with magnetic resonance cholangiopancreatography (MRCP) or endoscopic retrograde cholangiopancreatography (ERCP). With the information from these two studies, medical and surgical pancreatologists can cooperatively create a management plan. The management approach depends on pseudocyst location and duct status. Either endoscopic drainage under endoscopic ultrasonographic guidance or surgical drainage may be appropriate. Alternatively, surgical enteric drainage may be more appropriate for giant pancreatic pseudocysts or those pseudocysts not amenable to endoscopic drainage. Percutaneous drainage is rarely appropriate for pseudocysts resulting from chronic pancreatitis.

Nealon and Walser recently demonstrated the importance of ERCP to define pancreatic ductal anatomy. They identified seven categories of ductal anatomy and determined the results of treatment on the basis of pancreatography. Patients with duct strictures, duct-cyst communication, and duct cutoff fared poorly with percutaneous drainage, and they suggested that these patients are more appropriately treated with surgical intervention. Because ERCP is invasive, however, recent studies have examined the role of MRCP and found that sensitivity of MRCP is poor, but specificity and overall accuracy are greater than 90%. Appropriate management of pseudocysts may be based on MRCP findings when these are taken in the context of CT or sonographic findings of the pancreatic parenchyma. MRCP, however, does not delineate well pancreatic duct side branch changes, and interpretation in a heavily calcified gland may be difficult.

In the past decade, endoscopic management of pseudocysts has become a primary mode of treatment. Two basic endoscopic approaches may be considered: (1) endoscopic transmural drainage and (2) transpapillary drainage. Transmural drainage is indicated when the pseudocyst deforms the gastric or duodenal wall that can be punctured easily. This method depends on the Seldinger technique of dilatating a track between the pseudocyst and alimentary tract lumen. Endoscopic ultrasonography, which can detect wall thickness, presence of varices, and the amount of pseudocyst debris, is helpful to predict the efficacy of endoscopic transmural drainage. Transpapillary drainage may be indicated in moderate-sized pseudocysts with a duct-cyst communication. Extensive necrosis or intracystic debris are relative contraindications for these methods.

For decades, surgical internal drainage of PP has led to the best long-term results. Recently, however, endoscopic drainage has produced equivalent results for straightforward pseudocysts. Therefore surgeons often treat the most complex pseudocyst that is associated with pancreatic duct changes in chronic pancreatitis. These include giant pseudocysts, multiple pseudocysts, and pseudocysts accompanied by multiple pancreatic duct abnormalities including strictures, stones, and duct cutoffs. Traditional enteric methods including cystgastrostomy, cystduodenostomy, and Roux-en-Y cystjejunostomy remain appropriate, but other options include lateral pancreaticojejunostomy; duodenal-sparing pancreatic head resection with pseudocyst incorporation with or without accompanying pancreatic duct drainage; and, infrequently, pancreatic resection. Recent surgical approaches consider not only pseudocyst drainage but also definitive treatment of chronic pancreatic pain. Internal drainage has long-standing good results, but patients with chronic duct changes can experience recurrent pseudocysts. In these patients with chronic disease, a more definitive duct procedure is attractive in those who have maintained abstinence from alcohol. Recent evidence suggests that lateral pancreaticojejunostomy alone (without PP drainage) is adequate surgical management for patients with chronic pancreatic pseudocysts. European clinical trials have shown good pain relief results with duodenal-sparing pancreatic head resections, but these operations have not been widely adopted.

Symptomatic patients with large pseudocysts who are treated appropriately should expect relatively expeditious relief of symptoms with excellent long-term outcomes. Patients with symptoms who have acute pancreatitis complicated by pseudocysts and associated with a normal pancreatic duct have good outcomes with endoscopic treatment by transpapillary drainage (cyst-duct communication identified) or transmural drainage (cyst-duct communication not evident). Alternatively, pancreatic pseudocysts that arise in the setting of chronic pancreatitis characterized by parenchymal and duct changes respond best to surgical drainage by cystenteric anastomosis, pancreatojejunostomy, or duodenal-sparing head resection. At least 85% of patients treated by these methods should achieve good long-term results in the absence of alcohol consumption. Percutaneous drainage is the treatment of choice for infected pancreatic pseudocysts that contain air, are associated with sepsis, and do not have extensive accompanying pancreatic necrosis.

PSEUDOCYSTS REQUIRING SPECIAL CONSIDERATION

Not infrequently, giant (>15 cm) pancreatic pseudocysts or pseudocysts complicated by splenic parenchymal involvement are encountered. Giant pseudocysts are treated best with Roux-en-Y cystjejunostomy that is placed in the most dependent location of the pseudocyst. This management provides adequate drainage with decreased likelihood of undrained portions of the cyst and subsequent sepsis. Furthermore, pseudocysts located in the pancreatic tail may cause splenic compromise by enzymes that dissect along the splenic hilum and cause digestion of the parenchyma. Disruption of the spleen may be accompanied by massive, life-threatening hemorrhage that requires emergent distal pancreatectomy and splenectomy. Typically, these pseudocysts result from chronic pancreatitis with pancreatic duct cutoffs, and therefore pancreatic resection must encompass the parenchyma containing the obliterated duct to avoid a pancreatic stump fistula. Blood loss in these challenging operations can be decreased by preoperative splenic artery embolization.

MANAGEMENT SCHEME

Because of the multiple options available for the treatment of pseudocysts, confusion regarding the best treatment option abounds. A proposed management scheme is shown in Figure 2. First, pseudocysts less than 6 cm in size rarely cause symptoms and typically can be managed with observation using serial cross-sectional imaging. Symptomatic pseudocysts require careful evaluation to determine the underlying cause of pancreatic inflammation. Pseudocysts arising in acute pancreatitis and not associated with extensive pancreatic

Figure 2 Management algorithm that may serve as a guideline for the treatment of pancreatic pseudocysts.

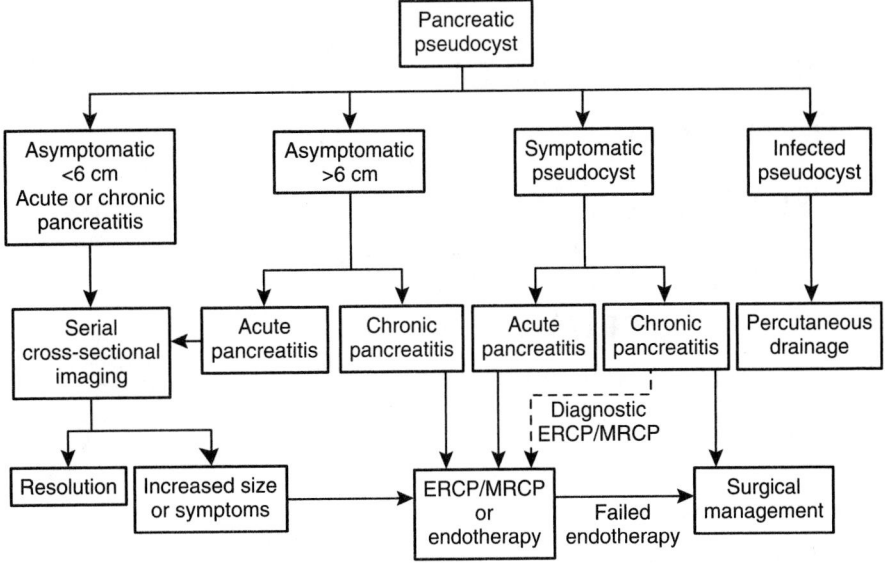

necrosis may be treated by endoscopic approaches. Alternatively, pseudocysts associated with significant pancreatic necrosis or those associated with chronic pancreatitis and duct changes should be managed by cystenteric drainage, pancreatojejunostomy, or pancreatic resection. Patients who have pseudocysts greater than 6 cm in size but who are asymptomatic present a challenging management dilemma for which no reliable evidence exists to guide treatment. In these patients with acute pancreatitis, serial imaging may demonstrate decreasing pseudocyst size over time, and close observation is reasonable. Patients with chronic pancreatitis are infrequently completely asymptomatic, however, and therefore treatment is often required.

SUMMARY

Recent management of pancreatic pseudocysts rests on differentiating acute from chronic pancreatitis and the associated duct abnormalities. Endoscopic methods are a primary treatment for pseudocysts, and newer operative procedures are good alternatives for the treatment of chronic pancreatitis associated with pseudocysts. Application of the appropriate treatment in symptomatic patients results in excellent long-term outcomes.

S U G G E S T E D   R E A D I N G S

Baillie J: Pancreatic pseudocysts (part I), *Gastrointest Endosc* 59:873, 2004.

Baillie J: Pancreatic pseudocysts (part II), *Gastrointest Endosc* 60:105, 2004.

Bradley E: A clinically based classification system for acute pancreatitis, *Arch Surg* 128:586, 1993.

Bradley E, Clements J, Gonzalez A: The natural history of pancreatic pseudocysts: a unified concept of management, *Am J Surg* 137:135, 1979.

Cahen D, Rauws E, Fockens P, and others: Endoscopic drainage of pancreatic pseudocysts: long-term outcome and procedural factors associated with safe and successful treatment, *Endoscopy* 37:977, 2005.

Heider R, Meyer A, Galanko J, and others: Percutaneous drainage of pancreatic pseudocysts is associated with a higher failure rate than surgical treatment in unselected patients, *Ann Surg* 229:781, 1999.

Morton JM, Brown A, Galanko JA, and others: A national comparison of surgical versus percutaneous drainage of pancreatic pseudocysts: 1997–2001, *J Gastrointest Surg* 9:15, 2005.

Nealon W, Walser E: Main pancreatic ductal anatomy can direct choice of modality for treating pancreatic pseudocysts (surgery versus percutaneous drainage), *Ann Surg* 235:751, 2002.

Vitas G, Sarr M: Selected management of pancreatic pseudocysts: operative versus expectant treatment, *Surgery* 111:123, 1992.

Yeo C, Bastidas J, Lynch-Nyhan A, and others: The natural history of pancreatic pseudocysts documented by computed tomography, *Surg Gyn Obstet* 170:411, 1990.

PANCREATIC DUCTAL DISRUPTIONS LEADING TO PANCREATIC FISTULA, PANCREATIC ASCITES, OR PLEURAL EFFUSION

L. William Traverso, MD, Mehran Fotoohi, MD, and Richard A. Kozarek, MD

DEFINITIONS

Pancreatic ductal disruption—A loss of ductal integrity anywhere in the pancreatic ductal system (i.e., a major pancreatic duct or a tertiary ductule) demonstrated by pancreatography (endoscopic retrograde cholangiopancreatography [ERCP]) or a sinogram through a percutaneous drain that reveals a pancreatic duct.

Pancreatic fistula—Passage of pancreatic juice through a pancreatic ductal disruption that exits the pancreatic parenchyma. This fistula can reside totally within the capsule of the pancreas and therefore can be minimal and self-healing. Alternatively, the fistula can breach the capsule of the pancreas, resulting in pancreatic juice entering the retroperitoneal or peritoneal cavities.

Pancreatic fluid collection—An accumulation of pancreatic juice (enzyme-rich fluid) in the peripancreatic area to include the adjacent retroperitoneal or peritoneal cavities (Fig. 1, *A*).

Pancreatic pseudocyst—A long-standing peripancreatic or intrapancreatic fluid collection that develops a significant wall (usually determined by imaging studies) (Fig. 1, *B*).

Pancreatic necrosis—Implies a permanent condition that will occur when a portion of the pancreas loses its blood supply. Unfortunately, the term *necrosis* is used interchangeably with *nonenhancement* of the gland during contrast-enhanced computed tomography (CT) (Fig. 1, *C*). It is "irreversible," yet many cases of "necrosis" will, after recovery, culminate in a patient with a normal pancreas on CT and ERCP. The confusion resides in overinterpreting the contrast-enhanced CT. Realize that CT nonenhancement could also be severe inflammation or a fluid collection. Necrosis might be present, but only time will tell.

Pancreatic pleural effusion—A collection of enzyme-rich pancreatic juice that collects in the pleural cavity on either side of the chest (Fig. 2). This collection originates from a pancreatic ductal disruption "fistulizing" into the retroperitoneum. The collection is not walled off in the extracapsular peripancreatic space but rather communicates through pleuroperitoneal foramina into the right or left pleural cavity. The location of the ductal disruption in the pancreatic ductal system determines whether the right or left pleural cavity is the site of collection (i.e., a ductal disruption dorsally over the portal vein might accumulate in the right chest, whereas a disruption dorsally from the pancreatic tail might accumulate in the left chest). The presence of a right or left pleural effusion is a clue to the site of the ductal disruption from within the pancreas.

Pancreatic ascites—A collection of pancreatic juice from a pancreatic ductal disruption that communicates into the peritoneal cavity, usually from the lesser sac (Fig. 3). This uncommon type of pancreatic fluid collection is not walled off to form a peripancreatic fluid collection or a pseudocyst and is fairly well tolerated by the patient unless the

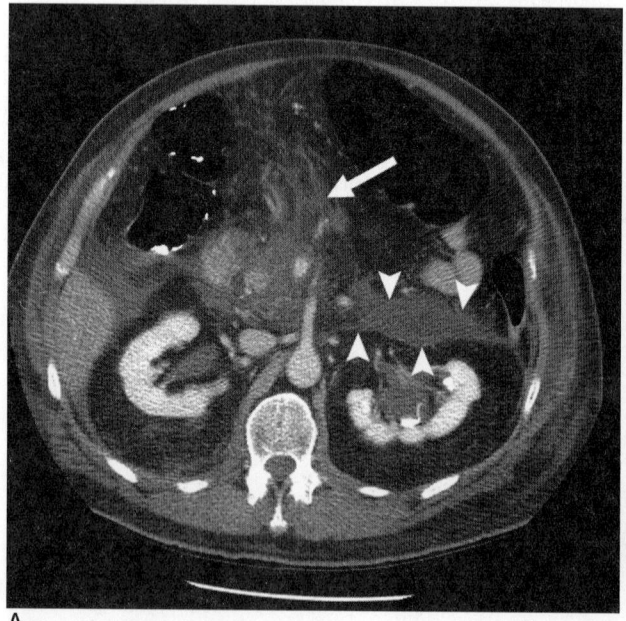
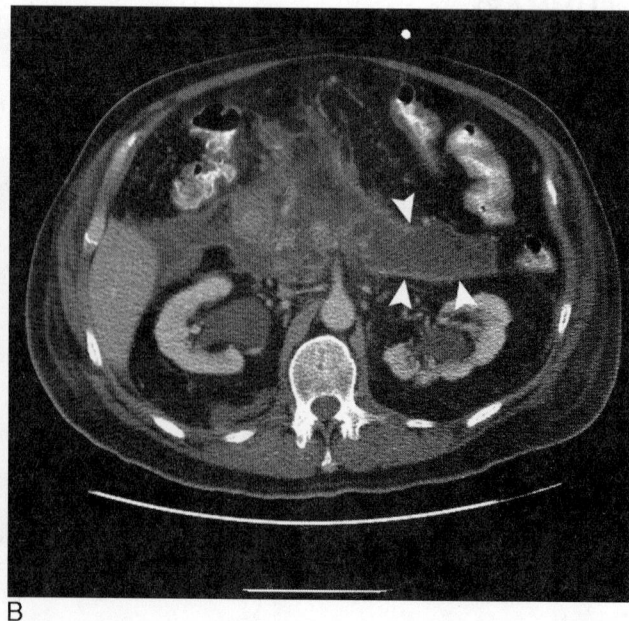

A   B

Figure 1   A 64-year-old male patient presenting with acute pancreatitis with nausea and abdominal pain. **(A)** The computed tomography *(CT)* image shows peripancreatic fluid *(arrowheads)*, later proved to be amylase rich. There are extensive inflammatory changes at the root of the mesentery *(arrow)*. **(B)** Follow-up CT scan 20 days later reveals evolution of the peripancreatic fluid with development of an enhancing wall *(white arrowheads)*, suggesting maturation of the collection.

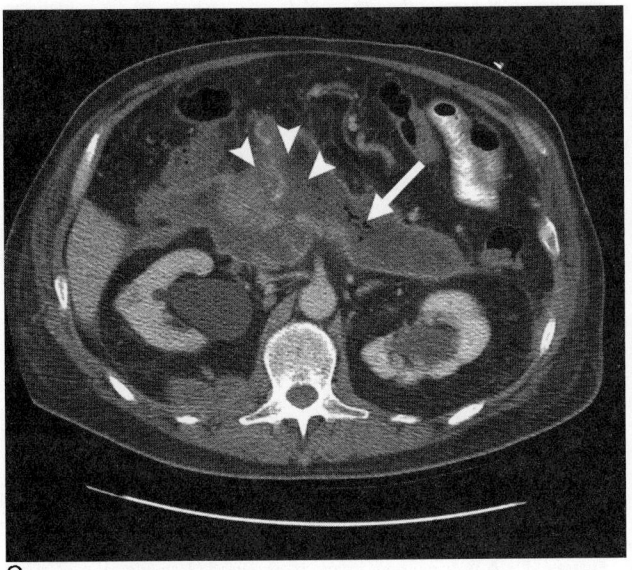

C

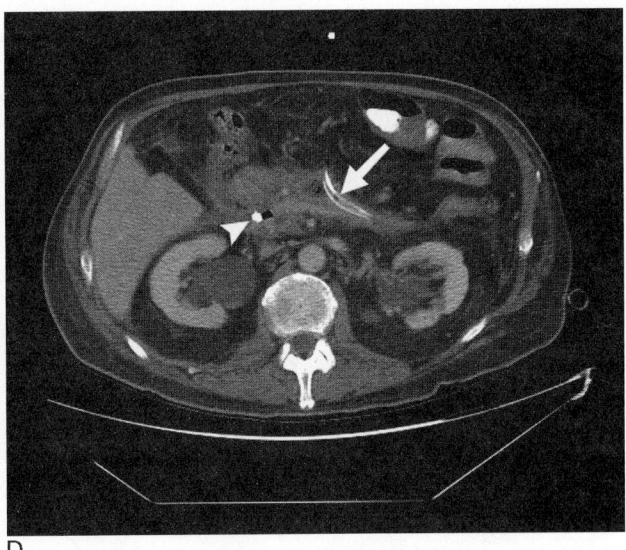

D

Figure 1 Cont'd—**(C)** Fourteen days later, another CT scan shows small pockets of gas within the collection *(arrow)* and development of surrounding infected peripancreatic nonenhancement, suggesting necrosis *(arrowheads)*. **(D)** After aggressive drainage of abdominal fluid collections with large-bore catheters up to 28 F *(white arrow)*, follow-up CT scan reveals near-complete resolution of the collection. Note the bile duct has a stent in place *(arrowhead)*.

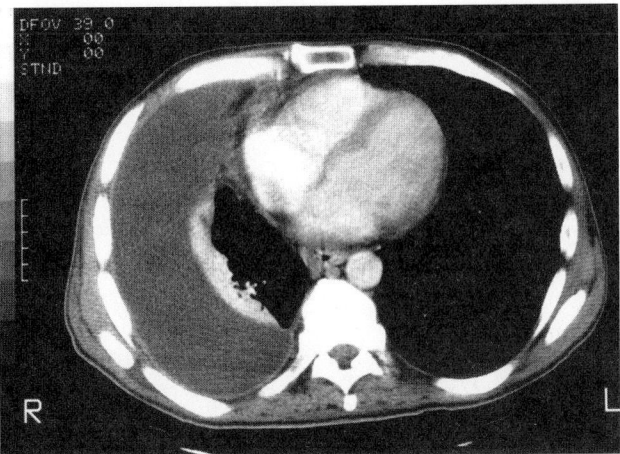

Figure 2 A right-sided amylase-rich pleural effusion is shown by computed tomography scan in a man with a dorsal-duct disruption at the genu of the pancreatic duct over the portal vein. The route to the right pleural cavity was through the retroperitoneum over the portal vein by way of the hepatoduodenal ligament through the pleuroperitoneal foramina of the diaphragm. *From Cameron JL, editor: Current surgical therapy, ed 6, Philadelphia, 1998, Mosby Yearbook, 510.*

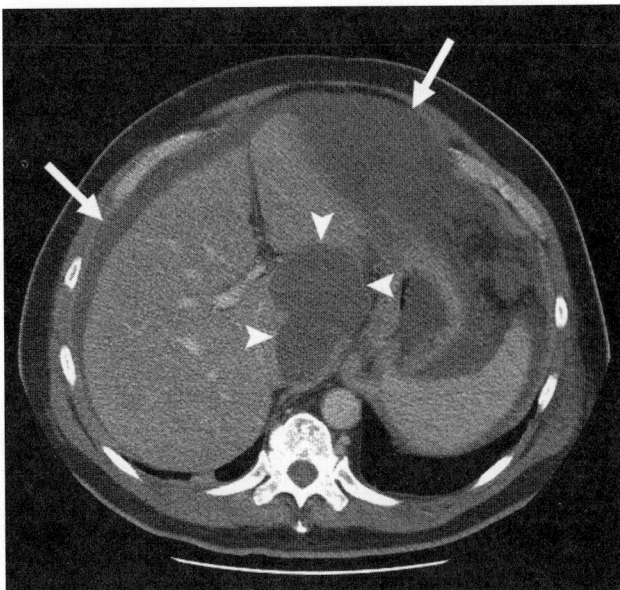

Figure 3 An abdominal computed tomography scan reveals pancreatic ascites around liver *(arrows)* and spleen. The patient was shown to have a downstream-duct disruption and disconnected gland in the area of the body of the pancreas. Pancreatic fluid leaked into the lesser sac *(arrowheads)* and then freely into the peritoneal cavity *(arrows)*.

proenzymes in the ascites become activated or the ascites becomes infected. Approximately half the cases have a concomitant pseudocyst present, suggesting that the etiology of the ascites might have been a leaking pseudocyst.

SITE OF PANCREATIC DUCTAL DISRUPTIONS

Our institutional approach to pancreatitis involves delineating pancreatic ductal anatomy if any patient develops persistent symptoms of pancreatitis. Approximately 90% of patients developing acute

pancreatitis present with a self-limiting course of abdominal pain and hyperamylasemia that resolves within 1 week. When clinical symptoms persist longer than a week, then most likely a complication of pancreatitis is developing. In the majority of our cases, this means a pancreatic ductal disruption will soon be demonstrable. Therefore when a patient reaches this clinical stage of persistent pancreatitis for longer than a week beyond the onset of symptoms, we find it useful to term this condition as *complicated pancreatitis*.

The majority of these patients undergo an ERCP, and two thirds are found to have a ductal disruption. The sites and frequency of disruption are depicted in Fig. 4. The presence of a ductal disruption is a predictor of outcomes. Therefore it is important to determine the presence and location of a disruption to treat patients promptly. The treatment has one goal: to halt the egress of pancreatic juice with its accompanying peripancreatic necrosis and complications. The end stage of a neglected peripancreatic fluid collection (whether it is a pseudocyst, ascites, or pleural effusion) includes infected necrosis, fistulization into a hollow organ, or ruptured pseudoaneurysm. These are demonstrated respectively in Figure. 1, *C*, and Figures 5 and 6.

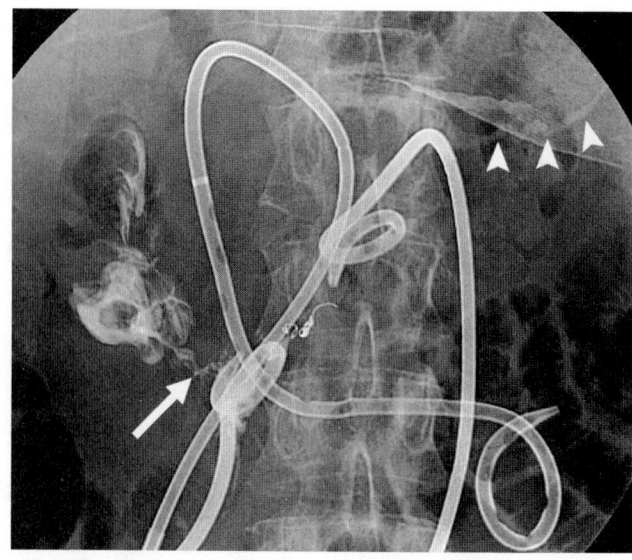

Figure 5 A fluoroscopic image is obtained after injection of contrast into left and right drainage catheters in a patient with pancreatitis whose disease was complicated by development of multiple peripancreatic fluid collections. The right inferior cavity has decompressed into the hepatic flexure of the colon *(arrow)*. Note the catheter in the superior left cavity opacifies a disrupted pancreatic duct at the neck of the pancreas. The duct in the body and tail fills with contrast *(arrowheads)*. The catheter in the center of this figure is a percutaneous transhepatic bile duct tube that passes through the ampulla to reside in the proximal jejunum.

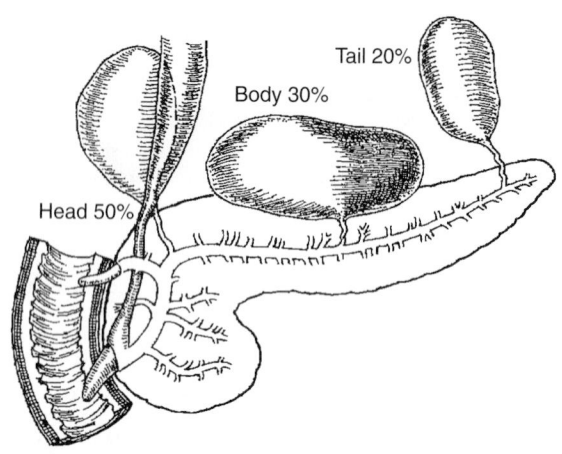

Figure 4 The site and frequency of pancreatic ductal disruptions in our institution are depicted in this line drawing. *From Cameron JL, editor:* Current surgical therapy, *ed 6, Philadelphia, 1998, Mosby Yearbook, 510.*

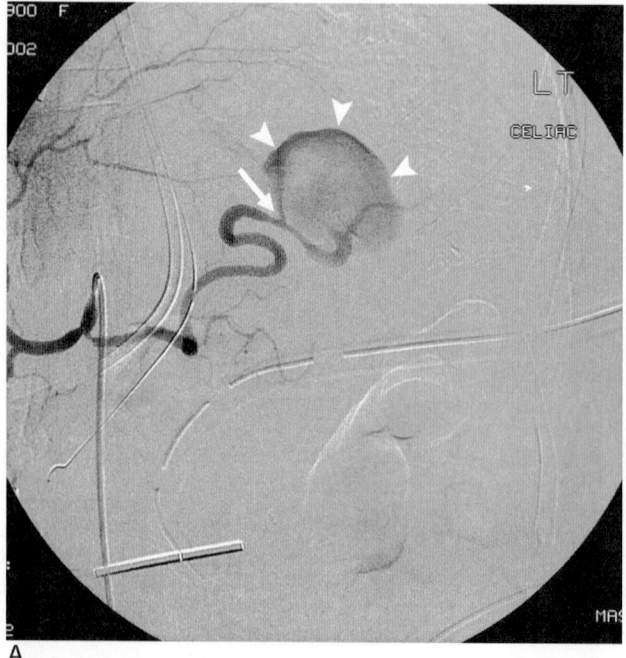

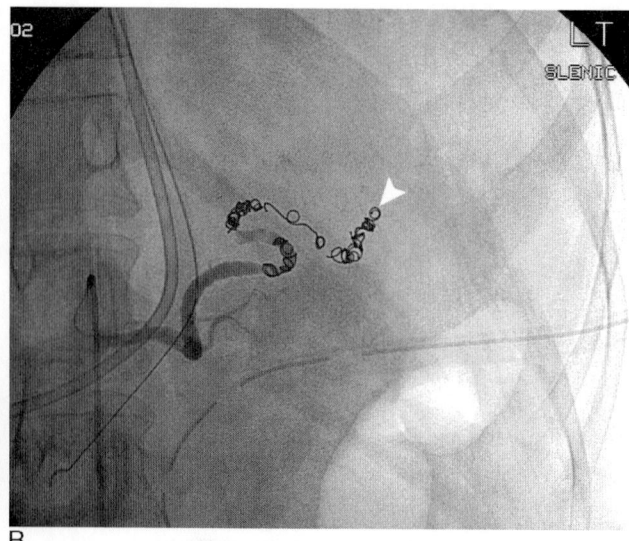

A   B

Figure 6 Digital subtraction arteriogram in a 46-year-old female patient with necrotizing pancreatitis and multiple drainage catheters who presented with severe bleeding through drainage catheters with cardiopulmonary arrest. **(A)** Emergent celiac arteriogram reveals extravasation of contrast from the midportion of the splenic artery into one of the drained cavities *(arrowheads)* through a pseudoaneurysm *(arrow)*. **(B)** Selective splenic arteriogram after successful occlusion of the artery with Gelfoam (Pfizer, New York, NY) and multiple coils *(one is marked with an arrowhead)* shows no flow within the artery and no extravasation.

RATIONALE FOR THERAPY

Management of peripancreatic fluid collections is based on the principle that all symptomatic patients should undergo "surgical drainage." By describing the management of pancreatic fluid collections, such as pleural effusion or pancreatic ascites, we hope to illustrate the common denominator in the management of symptomatic pancreatic fluid collections—drainage. By definition, an amylase-rich fluid collection can be derived only through the presence of a pancreatic-duct disruption. If a symptomatic pancreatic fluid collection is undrained, the following complications are possible: (1) peripancreatic necrosis with or without infection, (2) erosion into a blood vessel or a hollow viscus, or (3) communication with the free peritoneal cavity, mediastinum, or pleural cavities. Our premise is that most of the cases of severe pancreatitis seen in our institution are not related to parenchymal pancreatitis but rather to focal pancreatitis with pancreatic ductal disruption and some form of peripancreatic fluid collection. Our bias is not to wait for infection or necrosis but to halt the process. If patients with pancreatitis are not improving by 1 week after the onset of symptoms, assessments to find the ductal disruption must begin. The disruption must be decompressed from within and externally drained at its source. Logically this interrupts the process that could culminate in extension to even more severe peripancreatitis. In summary, the assessment involves delineating the ductal and parenchymal anatomy to determine the presence and location of ductal disruption with or without demonstrable fluid collection.

The assessment process begins with a dynamic bolus CT scan. The scan provides immediate information regarding the presence of pancreatic fluid collections, as well as their size and location. As mentioned earlier, the location of pancreatic fluid collections on CT scan are a clue to the location of duct disruptions. Pleural effusions are related to pancreatic juice leaking from a duct disruption and then penetrating the pancreatic capsule into the retroperitoneal space. When undrained, the dissecting fluid can enter the left pleural cavity from a disruption in the pancreatic tail or body and communicate into the left chest through pleuroperitoneal foramina. The juice can enter the right pleural cavity from a disruption in the region of the genu of the pancreatic duct, dorsally over the pancreatic head but ventral to the portal vein. This space is a channel to the thorax because the pancreatic juice can pass behind the hepatoduodenal ligament, through the pleuroperitoneal foramina, and into the right chest.

Pancreatic ascites accumulates from a major pancreatic ductal disruption anywhere in the ventral pancreas inside the lesser sac. The reason the pancreatic juice is not walled off and penetrates freely into the peritoneal cavity is unknown. Pancreatic fluid collections can also accumulate in the retroperitoneum by dorsal rupture through the pancreatic capsule from the tail to collect over the left renal space or from the dorsal head in the pancreaticoduodenal groove to collect over the right pararenal space. Pancreatic juice collections in these areas have difficulty traveling elsewhere, and they will form the classic pseudocyst. The inflammatory process ultimately results in a thickened wall. More common, however, is the lesser sac fluid collections that form a pseudocyst rather than pancreatic ascites.

The mature pseudocyst is uncommonly seen in our experience unless the patient has been referred after a prolonged hospital course. This observation results from our bias: all *symptomatic* fluid collections in our institution are drained with minimally invasive methods before a thickened wall develops. A rapid approach to decompress fluid collections may also explain the relative absence of peripancreatic necrosis in patients cared for at our institution (unless patients are transferred after delayed diagnosis and treatment).

MANAGEMENT OF PANCREATIC FLUID COLLECTIONS

Initial Therapy

In the presence of persistent fever, tachycardia, ileus, leukocytosis, and hyperamylasemia, a plethora of objective studies is not required to decide that a patient with symptomatic pancreatitis is not improving after the initial onset of the disease. Most likely, intensive resuscitation with intravenous fluids and antibiotics has already avoided pulmonary and renal complications. After this stage has been reached, an abdominal CT scan will indicate most accurately the presence of pancreatic fluid collections, as well as their size and location. It is at this time that an ERCP is considered at our medical center. Because pancreatography defines the pancreatic ductal anatomy, it is also possible to direct treatment simultaneously with endoscopic techniques. We do not believe that we introduce infection by ERCP if, and only if, the fluid collection (previously localized by CT) is drained during or immediately after this "assessment ERCP." Performing an ERCP without the capability of drainage is contraindicated. In contrast to clinical infection, however, the fluid collection cavity is often colonized by gut bacteria following drainage by percutaneous, endoscopic, or even open surgical techniques. However, if drainage by any route is successful, colonization does not lead to infection or sepsis.

When a disruption results in a pleural effusion or pancreatic ascites, classic medical therapy relies on the inhibition of pancreatic secretions by feeding clear liquids or the use of total parenteral nutrition. Other attempts at decreasing secretions have included oral pancreatic enzymes, diuretics, atropine, or somatostatin analogues. Somatostatin analogues can accelerate fistula healing or improve the success of medical therapy in a subset of patients (approximately half). Serosal apposition by repeated paracentesis or thoracentesis (occasionally an indwelling chest tube) has been recommended.

Endoscopic Drainage

In contrast to these approaches, our group has documented that endoscopic placement of transpapillary endoprostheses can decompress the pancreatic ductal system, relieve downstream obstruction, preclude the need for surgery, or convert an urgent need for surgery into an elective situation.

Pancreatic Effusions

Suppose a major pancreatic ductal disruption is present in the head of the pancreas (Fig. 7). This dorsal disruption results in an amylase-rich pleural effusion in the right pleural cavity (Fig. 2). An ERCP undertaken after antibiotic coverage both delineates the pancreatic ductal disruption and is used to place a 5- to 10-F transampullary pancreatic stent across the area of the pancreatic ductal disruption. Less commonly, in patients with an end-pancreatic fistula, the prosthesis is placed through the disruption and directly into the fluid collection. This procedure should not be undertaken if there is significant debris within the fluid collection because small-caliber stents may occlude, with resulting iatrogenic infectious complications. During the immediate poststenting period in our example patient, the pleural effusion was noted to decrease and the patient's symptoms improved. A subsequent follow-up ERCP is performed within 6 weeks. The transpapillary stent may or may not need to be exchanged. If the pancreatic ductal disruption has not healed at the time of follow-up ERCP, head resection may be required to ameliorate the problem. During the decompression period, neither somatostatin nor total parenteral nutrition is used, and the patient resumes a regular diet. Elective resectional therapy occurs at a time

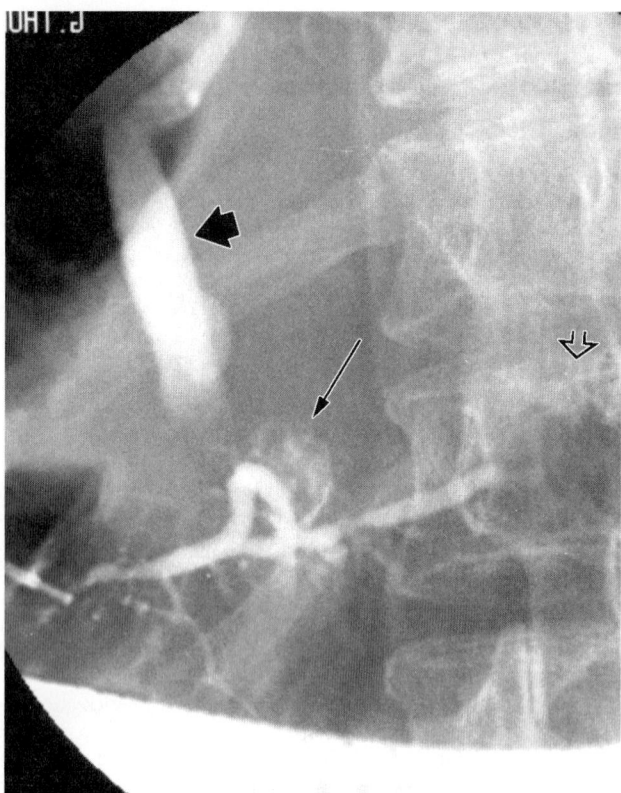

Figure 7   In a patient with pancreatic ascites and pancreas divisum, the dorsal pancreatic duct in the pancreatic head is leaking in two locations. The first is shown as contrast leaked through a disruption into the lesser sac *(thin closed arrow)*. The second is from the upstream pancreatic duct that is obstructed over the vertebral bodies. A faint collection of contrast in the lesser sac is marked with an open arrow. These disruptions accounted for the pancreatic ascites. Just before the pancreatic duct injection through the minor ampulla, the common bile duct *(large closed arrow)* had been filled from the major ampulla. After transminor papilla stenting, the ascites resolved, but pain continued, and the downstream disruption did not seal. An uncomplicated pancreatoduodenectomy resolved these problems when the inflammation was at a minimum.   *From Cameron JL, editor: Current surgical therapy, ed 6, Philadelphia, 1998, Mosby Yearbook, 510.*

when the patient is not sick, and the mortality and morbidity are minimal. In contrast, if the patient does not symptomatically improve after pancreatic duct stenting, percutaneous drainage is performed into the right chest to drain that fluid collection. Immediate surgical intervention is seldom required. If there is a concomitant lesser sac fluid collection, then a transgastric or transduodenal endoscopically placed double-pigtail stent into the fluid collection can ameliorate the fluid collection and allow the surgeon to proceed with elective resection (if necessary) at a future date. Because the lesser sac collection is from a ventral disruption of the pancreatic ductal system, it usually does not coincide with a pleural collection that originates from a dorsal disruption into a retropancreatic fluid collection.

Ductal disruptions in the head are frequently at the genu of the pancreatic duct in one of two directions—dorsally over the portal vein or ventrally into the lesser sac and toward the duodenum. In this latter instance, transduodenal endoscopic-drainage pigtail catheters may have to be used for a right-sided lesser sac collection. The process usually does not allow the pancreatic ductal rupture to seal, and a resection is required. Remarkably, a few main pancreatic ductal disruptions in the head heal and do not require surgery.

Pancreatic Ascites

Endotherapy depends on bypassing downstream obstruction that may be the cause of an upstream duct disruption. To decompress the isolated ductal system, a transpapillary stent is inserted to bypass the leak or concomitant ductal stenosis. The ascites is drained under ultrasound control. Usually the ascites has not reformed, and these previously recalcitrant pancreatic ascites patients are discharged within 1 week of stenting. A low-fat diet is begun after 12 hours, and almost all patients resolve their ascites without complication. The stent is removed after approximately 4 weeks. Long-term follow-up (3 years) has shown these cases of pancreatic ascites do not recur.

Surgical Management

The presence of a pancreatic duct disruption during acute pancreatitis is a predictor of outcomes in that mortality, length of stay, and the need for surgery are significantly higher if a disruption is present. The need for subsequent surgery such as debridement, a duct-drainage procedure, or resection is also increasingly necessary if ductal disruptions are present. The need for surgery in patients with pancreatic ascites or pancreatic enzyme-rich pleural fluid collections is not an issue. Minimally invasive maneuvers focused on isolating ductal disruption with drainage catheters allow the ascites and pleural effusions to resolve. Remaining for the surgeon to solve is the inability of the pancreatic ductal disruption itself to heal despite all of the previously discussed minimally invasive drainage procedures.

Keep in mind the caveat that after interventional radiologic and endoscopic treatments, the surgeon is seldom faced with the need to treat a pseudocyst with a pseudocystogastrostomy or other enteric drainage. The surgical challenge is not to focus on the ascites, pleural effusion, or pseudocyst. Rather the patient's problem stems from a persistent fistula that is usually managed by percutaneous drainage. An endoscopic pancreatic duct stent may or may not be in place. A persistent pancreatic fistula from the gland is usually observed in one of two clinical situations. First, there might be downstream ductal obstruction that cannot be decompressed, and the path of least resistance is through the external drainage catheter. The second possibility is the disconnected duct syndrome, in which the gland has been permanently separated at the pancreatic neck (because of necrosis of the pancreatic neck or body) from the downstream pancreatic parenchyma from the upstream disconnected segment. Therefore the result of this necrosis and loss of pancreatic parenchyma is an end-pancreatic fistula (Fig. 8).

To minimize surgical morbidity and mortality, the surgeon should first be patient for a number of weeks. An extended drainage time is used for peripancreatic fluid collections through percutaneous, transenteric, or transpapillary catheters. This allows the surrounding inflammatory process to subside as much as possible. The patient will benefit with the better outcomes of elective surgery. The goal of surgical treatment is termination of the chronic fistula, prevention of further pancreatitis, and parenchymal preservation. After 2 to 3 months, either the fistula will heal or surgical treatment is required.

A thorough knowledge of the ductal anatomy of each residual pancreatic segment is required to decide on the proper surgical treatment. These treatments include resection or enteric drainage. Head resection is required for downstream obstruction in the pancreatic head and upstream duct disruption that is also in the head of the gland (Fig. 7). The disconnected gland syndrome requires surgical treatment if it is associated with a persistent pancreatic fistula from the upstream segment. Resection of the upstream disconnected segment may be the best option, but if all of the pancreatic body and tail are present, an enteric drainage of that segment may be the surgeon's choice, provided that the remaining duct in the head and tail is normal. However, a distal pancreatectomy is usually used for most disruptions in the pancreatic body and for all tail disruptions. These

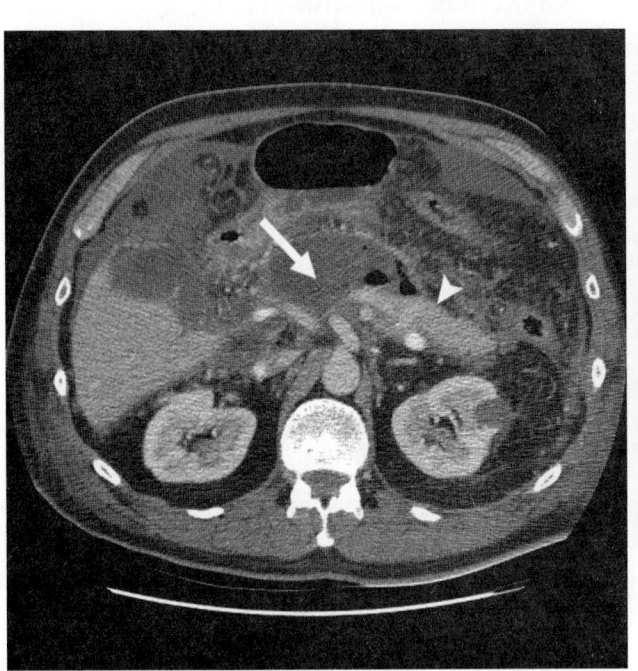
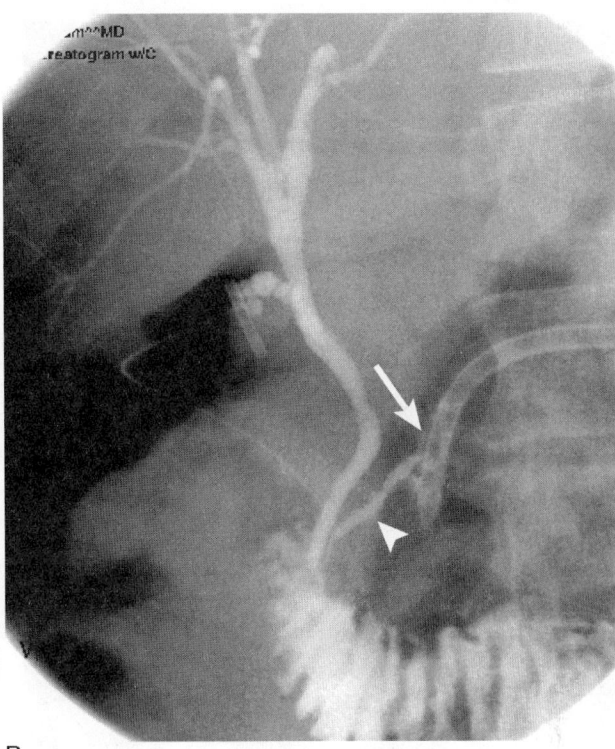

A   B

Figure 8 **(A)** Necrosis in the region of the pancreatic neck *(arrow)* resulted in disconnection of the head from the body of the pancreas shown in this computed tomography scan. Note the enhancing body and tail of the pancreas *(arrowhead)*. **(B)** An intraoperative cholangiogram through the cystic duct during necrosectomy showed free reflux of contrast up into the main pancreatic duct *(arrowhead)* and then into the cavity of necrosis where the pancreatic neck had been *(arrow)*. Overlying the latter is a percutaneous drain from the left anterior renal route that had been used in the preoperative period to allow for nonemergent necrosectomy after the inflammatory process had improved. Note the contrast filling the drain.

operations on the left side of the pancreas can be difficult because of surrounding postinflammatory scarring or if there is left-sided portal hypertension resulting from splenic vein occlusion.

SUGGESTED READINGS

Kozarek RA, Jiranek G, Traverso LW: Endoscopic treatment of pancreatic ascites, *Am J Surg* 168:223–228, 1994.

Lau ST, Simchuk EJ, Kozarek RA, and others: A pancreatic duct leak should be sought to direct treatment in patients with acute pancreatitis, *Am J Surg* 181:411, 2001.

Simchuk EJ, Traverso LW, Nukui Y, and others: Computed tomography severity index is a predictor of outcomes for severe pancreatitis, *Am J Surg* 179:352, 2000.

Werner J, Feuerbach S, Uhl W, and others: Management of acute pancreatitis: from surgery to interventional intensive care, *Gut* 54:426-436, 2005.

CHRONIC PANCREATITIS

James K. Fullerton, MD, and Gary C. Vitale, MD

Chronic pancreatitis is an ongoing inflammatory process characterized by irreversible destruction of the pancreas parenchyma and ductal architecture. This can lead to chronic abdominal pain, pancreatic exocrine insufficiency, and diabetes mellitus. The most common risk factor is alcohol use; 70% of patients with chronic pancreatitis have a history of alcohol abuse. Other, less common causes include hyperlipidemia, pancreas divisum, medications, traumatic strictures, hypercalcemia, cystic fibrosis, and genetic factors. Approximately 30% of patients have an unclear etiology and are given the diagnosis of idiopathic chronic pancreatitis.

Diagnosis is based on the clinical presentation and imaging studies. Patients present with epigastric pain that radiates to the back, as well as nausea, vomiting, and weight loss. In more advanced stages, patients can develop diabetes, malabsorption with streatorrhea, and biliary obstruction. Computed tomography (CT) is the most useful imaging technique for evaluating the parenchymal changes of the pancreas. CT can identify an inflammatory mass, pseudocyst, calcifications, and duct dilatation and can differentiate a malignant mass (Fig. 1). Endoscopic retrograde cholangiopancreatography (ERCP) is invaluable for evaluating the pancreatic duct and for conducting endoscopic therapeutic treatment. ERCP can demonstrate pancreatic duct dilatation and identify treatable pancreatic and biliary duct strictures (Fig. 2). Magnetic resonance imaging cholangiopancreatography (MRCP) can be useful when the diagnosis is unclear and when ERCP is unsuccessful in evaluating the pancreatic duct. Endoscopic ultrasonography (EUS) is also highly sensitive and specific for diagnosing chronic pancreatitis. EUS is helpful when the diagnosis is unclear, for evaluating cystic or solid lesions, and when biopsy is necessary.

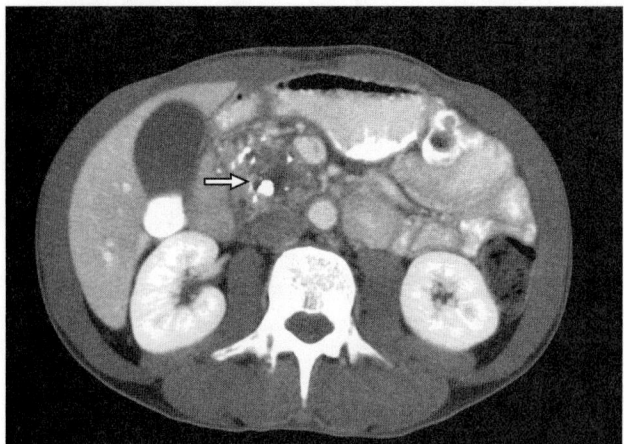

Figure 1 Computed tomography scan demonstrating changes of chronic pancreatitis. Note the calcifications within the pancreatic head *(arrow)*.

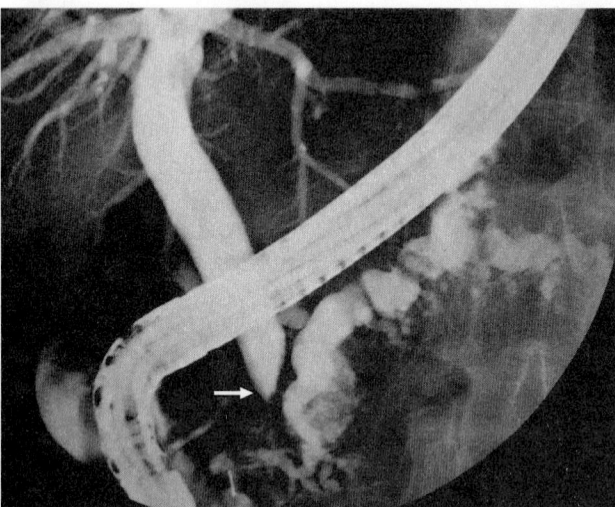

Figure 2 Endoscopic retrograde cholangiopancreatography demonstrating changes of chronic pancreatitis. Note the smooth, tapered distal bile duct stricture *(arrow)*, downstream pancreatic duct stricture with upstream dilatation, intrapancreatic duct stones, and secondary pancreatic duct branching.

Medical treatment should begin by eliminating potential etiologic agents and beginning a graduated pain medication regimen. Other important medical treatment modalities include maintaining a low-fat diet and pancreatic enzyme supplementation. When patients continue to have persistent abdominal pain, endocrine and exocrine dysfunction, and frequent hospitalizations, more invasive treatment modalities should be initiated. Interventional therapeutic endoscopy and surgery are beneficial for treating the debilitating pain and associated complications secondary to chronic pancreatitis.

The etiology of chronic pancreatitis pain is likely multifactorial. Proposed hypotheses include ductal and parenchymal hypertension, ischemia of the pancreatic parenchyma leading to a "compartment syndrome" of the pancreas, and peripancreatic perineural inflammation. This has led to the development of many endoscopic and surgical procedures in an attempt to reduce pain and treat the associated complications. It is important to remember that treatment must be individualized for each patient because no one procedure has been shown to be superior in the treatment of chronic pancreatitis.

ENDOSCOPIC TREATMENT FOR CHRONIC PANCREATITIS

The main treatment goal for interventional therapeutic endoscopy is relieving chronic pain via duct decompression. On the basis of surgical success of pancreatic duct drainage, endoscopic decompression of the pancreatic duct has become an important treatment option for physicians treating chronic pancreatitis. The indications for endoscopic therapy are listed in Table 1. After a treatable lesion is identified via ERCP, multiple endoscopic interventions can be used as initial lesion-directed treatment (Table 2). Endoscopic therapy offers the most minimally invasive treatment option, with lower morbidity and mortality than surgery. These procedures also do not preclude subsequent surgical intervention if symptoms persist.

Pancreatic duct stenting has gained acceptance as a first-line treatment in chronic pancreatitis for patients with a dominant pancreatic duct stricture and upstream dilatation. Pancreatic sphincterotomy is performed, and a guidewire is placed upstream to the stricture (Fig. 3). The stricture is then dilatated with a hydrostatic balloon catheter. Attempts can be made to remove pancreatic duct stones with retrieval wire baskets or balloons. Extracorporeal shock wave lithotripsy (ESWL) is occasionally necessary to fragment stones for removal. A polyethylene stent is placed to achieve ductal decompression by traversing the area of stricture (Fig. 4). Stent size ranges between 5 and 10 F, and lengths vary depending on stricture location.

Endoscopic management is also used to direct further treatments. Patients who receive pain relief with stenting are treated with stent exchanges and dilatations for 3 to 12 months. Patients who initially receive symptom relief from endoscopic ductal decompression but who continue to have recurrent symptoms after stent removal are more likely to respond to surgical drainage procedures. Patients who do not receive symptom relief are treated with surgical resection procedures, even if the pancreatic duct is dilatated.

Table 1: Indications for Therapeutic Endoscopy in Chronic Pancreatitis

Chronic pain unresponsive to medical therapy
Obstruction of the main pancreatic duct by stricture or stones
Pseudocyst resulting from downstream ductal obstruction and pancreatic duct leak
Distal common bile duct stricture

Table 2: Endoscopic Interventions for Chronic Pancreatitis

Obstruction of the main pancreatic duct
Pancreatic sphincterotomy
Pancreatic duct stricture dilatation
Pancreatic duct stone extraction
Pancreatic duct stent
Extracorporeal shock wave lithotripsy
Pseudocyst and pancreatic duct leak
Endoscopic cystgastrostomy
Endoscopic cystduodenostomy
Transpapillary stent
Common bile duct obstruction
Biliary sphincterotomy
Biliary duct dilatation and stenting

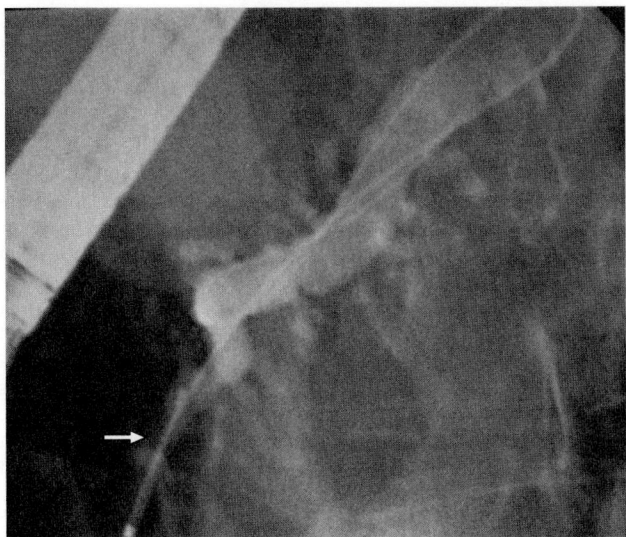

Figure 3 Endoscopic retrograde cholangiopancreatography demonstrating pancreatic duct stricture *(arrow)* with upstream dilatation. A guidewire is placed across the stricture.

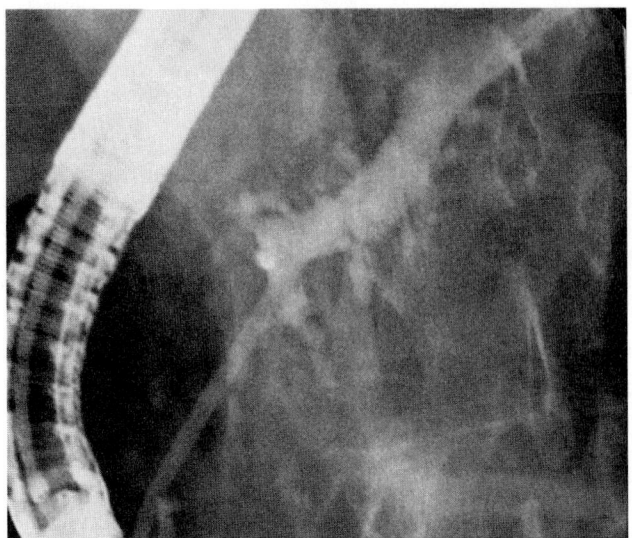

Figure 4 Pancreatic stent placement for duct decompression.

Studies demonstrate that approximately two thirds of patients have pain improvement after pancreatic duct stent placement. Patients also report an increased quality of life and decreased medication use. In a long-term follow-up study of more than 1000 patients, Rosch and colleagues demonstrated endoscopic treatment success in 65% of patients. Twenty-four percent of patients required surgery, and pancreatic function was not improved with stenting. At the University of Louisville, 89 patients were treated with pancreatic duct stenting over a 10-year period. Eighty-three percent of patients experienced a decreased pain level after pancreatic stenting. On a scale of 1 to 10, there was a decrease in pain level from 8.7 to 4.1 after stenting. Pain medication usage decreased in 47% of patients, 83% of patients considered their treatment successful, and 63% of patients had a documented decrease in narcotic use. Surgery was required in 12% of patients for persistent symptoms.

Complications of endoscopic treatment occur in approximately 15% of patients and are usually mild. The most common complications include mild pancreatitis, stent occlusion, migration of the stent, and duodenal erosions. Stent-induced pancreatic ductal changes in chronic pancreatitis patients are unlikely to have clinical relevance and are more likely to be seen in patients with normal pancreatic ducts. Endoscopic stenting is a safe and effective method for treating chronic pancreatitis secondary to strictures in the main pancreatic duct.

SURGICAL TREATMENT FOR CHRONIC PANCREATITIS

Surgery should be considered when patients have persistent symptoms despite aggressive nonsurgical management and anatomic changes consistent with chronic pancreatitis. Other indications for surgery include associated complications from pancreatitis and when pancreatic malignancy cannot be ruled out (Table 3). The goals of surgical treatment are to improve the patient's pain while preserving pancreatic function and to treat associated complications. Surgical procedures for the treatment of pain in chronic pancreatitis are listed in Table 4. The most appropriate surgical procedure depends on the extent of pancreatic parenchyma and duct disease, the response to endoscopic stenting, patient comorbidities, and the surgeon's experience.

Table 3: Indications for Surgery in Chronic Pancreatitis

Chronic abdominal pain unresponsive to nonsurgical therapies
Suspicion of pancreatic cancer
Persistent common bile duct obstruction unresponsive to endoscopic therapy
Duodenal obstruction
Splenic vein thrombosis with bleeding gastric varices
Symptomatic or enlarging pancreatic pseudocyst
Persistent pancreatic ascites or fistula

Table 4: Surgical Procedures for Treating Pain in Chronic Pancreatitis

Duct drainage procedures
Lateral Roux-en-Y pancreaticojejunostomy (Partington-Rochelle modification of Puestow-Gillesby procedure)
Combined resection-drainage procedures
Pancreaticoduodenectomy (Classic Whipple or pylorus-preserving)
Local resection of the head of the pancreas combined with longitudinal pancreaticojejunostomy (Frey procedure)
Duodenum-preserving pancreatic head resection (Beger procedure)
Resection procedures
Total pancreatectomy with or without islet cell autotransplantation
Distal pancreatectomy
Subtotal pancreatectomy
Neuroablative procedures
Thoracoscopic splanchnicectomy

Pancreatic Duct Drainage Procedures

Many surgical drainage procedures have been described in an attempt to reduce pancreatic duct pressure. In 1954, Duval described ductal drainage with a distal pancreatectomy, splenectomy, and an end-to-side distal Roux-en-Y pancreaticojejunostomy. This technique did not allow adequate drainage of the pancreatic duct in patients with the "chain of lakes," leading to the modification by Puestow and Gillespy in 1958. This included making a longitudinal incision in the pancreatic duct, distal pancreatectomy, splenectomy, and insertion of the pancreas into a loop of jejunum. This technique was modified by Partington and Rochelle in 1960. They described the now-standard side-to-side Roux-en-Y lateral pancreaticojejunostomy.

The lateral pancreaticojejunostomy preserves pancreatic parenchyma and avoids splenectomy while providing improved drainage of the pancreatic duct. It also eliminates the need to dissect the posterior pancreas off the portal vein and thus avoids a potential bleeding complication. A bilateral subcostal (chevron) incision is made and a thorough exploration is performed to rule out malignancy. Adhesions from the stomach to the anterior surface of the pancreas should be divided to expose the entire anterior surface of the pancreas. Palpation of the anterior surface of the pancreas usually identifies the soft-dilatated pancreatic duct. This is confirmed by aspirating the duct with a 22-gauge needle. If the pancreatic duct remains difficult to find, intraoperative ultrasound can be helpful. After the pancreatic duct is identified, electrocautery is used to cut down alongside the needle until the main pancreatic duct is entered. A right-angle clamp is then used to guide the process of opening the rest of the pancreatic duct. The duct should be opened as far as possible to allow maximal decompression of the duct. A Roux-en-Y jejunal limb is created and anastomosed to the pancreatic capsule alongside the opened pancreatic duct with an interrupted or continuous 3–0 nonabsorbable suture (Fig. 5).

Lateral pancreaticojejunostomy has demonstrated initial pain relief in 50% to 90% of patients. Some studies have shown up to a 50% decline in long-term pain relief, however. The morbidity ranges between 5% and 20%, with an early mortality rate of less than 1%. Lateral pancreaticojejunostomy is technically easier than the pancreatic resection procedures and has a lower morbidity and mortality rate. It is a good surgical option for patients who have initial pain relief with pancreatic duct stenting and a dilatated duct greater than 6 mm.

Combined Resection-Drainage Procedures

The pancreatic head can become inflamed and enlarged in patients with chronic pancreatitis and is often thought of as the "pacemaker of chronic pancreatitis." These patients do not respond well to pancreatic duct drainage procedures and are best served with a combined resective-drainage procedure for the treatment of pain.

Pancreaticoduodenectomy (Whipple or Pylorus-Preserving)

Pancreaticoduodenectomy is a good treatment option for patients who have an inflammatory mass in the head of the pancreas or a nondilatated pancreatic duct, or when there is no response from pancreatic duct stenting. It is also indicated when patients present with a distal bile duct stricture and a downstream pancreatic duct stricture from an inflammatory mass in the head. Surgical resection is also warranted when malignancy cannot be excluded. Pancreaticoduodenectomy removes the inflamed pancreatic head and provides adequate drainage of the pancreatic duct in most cases. It can be safely performed with an operative morbidity between 10% and 50% and mortality less than 2%. The most common complication of pancreaticoduodenectomy is delayed gastric emptying, seen in 20% of patients. Pancreatic fistula rates are low, between 5% and 10%. Long-term pain relief is demonstrated in 50% and 90% of patients.

The Whipple procedure and pylorus-preserving pancreaticoduodenectomy have demonstrated similar morbidity rates and pain relief in most studies, and either method is acceptable treatment for patients with chronic pancreatitis. Jimenez and colleagues compared pancreaticoduodenectomy with pylorus preservation or antrectomy in the treatment of chronic pancreatitis. There was a higher rate of delayed gastric emptying (33% vs. 12%) for the pylorus-preserving treated group. Postoperative enzyme supplementation and new-onset diabetes did not differ between groups. Pain relief was seen in 70% of patients having the standard Whipple and in 60% of the pylorus-preserving treated group. Traverso and Kozarek demonstrated pain relief in all patients undergoing pancreaticoduodenectomy, with 76% becoming pain free. The onset of diabetes was seen in 22% of patients and developed at least 1 year after surgery, suggesting continued disease in the pancreatic remnant.

Frey Procedure

In an attempt to reduce operative morbidity and endocrine and exocrine insufficiency, the Frey and Beger procedures were developed. The Frey procedure, first described in 1987, consists of a longitudinal pancreaticojejunostomy and "coring out" of the pancreatic head, leaving the duodenum and bile duct intact. Approximately 5 to 10 g of tissue is removed from the head of the pancreas. The ducts in the head of the pancreas are decompressed along with the main pancreatic duct out to the tail. Indications for the Frey procedure are similar to those of pancreaticoduodenectomy. It can be used in patients with a pancreatic duct size of 3 mm or greater. The main advantage of the Frey procedure is that it decompresses all of the ducts within the head of the pancreas and does not require dividing the pancreas above the portal vein, thus reducing the risk of bleeding. It can also treat an associated distal bile duct obstruction and decompress communicating pseudocysts.

The Frey procedure is begun in a similar manner as the lateral pancreaticojejunostomy. The main addition is in the "coring out" process of the pancreatic head. Hemostatic sutures are placed around the edge of the pancreatic head to help with hemostasis. Pancreatic tissue is removed from the anterior capsule and continuing downward to the level of the duct of Wirsung. Removing tissue deeper than the posterior aspect of the duct of Wirsung is not necessary. Approximately 5 mm of pancreatic tissue is left on the duodenum and to the right of the superior mesenteric vein to allow for the anastomosis. A Roux-en-Y limb of jejunum is then created to perform the longitudinal anastomosis to the pancreatic duct and cored-out head.

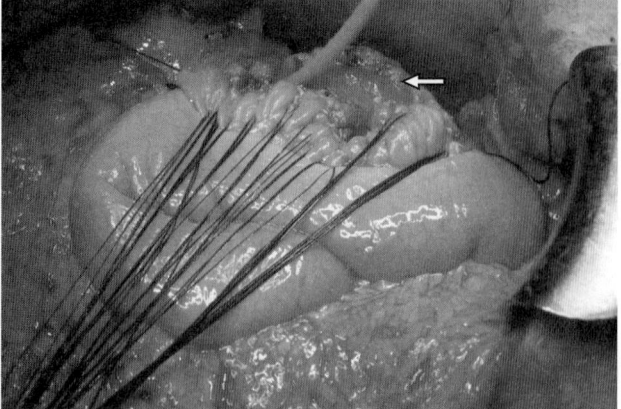

Figure 5   Lateral pancreaticojejunostomy demonstrating an anastomosis between the opened pancreatic duct (*arrow*) and Roux-en-Y limb of jejunum. (*See color insert Figure 25.*)

The Frey procedure offers pain relief in 75% to 90% of patients, with a morbidity of 15% and mortality less than 3%. Endocrine and exocrine insufficiency is low (5%–10%). A randomized prospective study by Izbicki and colleagues compared the Frey procedure with the pylorus-preserving pancreaticoduodenectomy. Both procedures had equal effectiveness in pain relief. Relief of symptoms was seen in 90% after the Frey procedure and 87% after the pylorus-preserving pancreaticoduodenectomy. Quality of life improved by 71% in the Frey procedure group and only 43% in the pylorus-preserving group. Morbidity was higher in the pylorus-preserving group (53.3%), including delayed gastric emptying in 30% of patients. The Frey procedure group had a complication rate of 19.4%. The advantages of the Frey procedure are that it drains the entire pancreatic duct, addresses disease within the pancreatic head, preserves pancreatic tissue, and avoids division of the pancreatic neck.

Beger Procedure

The duodenum-preserving pancreatic head resection was developed by Beger to remove the diseased pancreatic head while maintaining gastrointestinal continuity. The Beger procedure removes most of the pancreatic head by dividing the neck and leaving a rim of pancreas tissue between the common bile duct and duodenum. A Roux-en-Y jejunostomy is anastomosed to the remaining body and tail and to the small portion of pancreas adjacent to the duodenum. More pancreatic tissue is removed in the head of the pancreas than with the Frey procedure; however, there is the added difficulty of dissecting the pancreas off the underlying portal vein. Indications for this procedure are similar for the patients undergoing the pancreaticoduodenectomy and Frey procedure. The Beger and Frey procedures should not be performed when malignancy is suspected. The duodenal-preserving pancreatic head resection procedure offers excellent pain relief in approximately 70% to 95% of patients and a morbidity rate between 15% and 55%. In a long-term study by Beger, 91% of the patients were pain free up to 14 years after resection. The rate of hospital admissions for acute episodes of chronic pancreatitis dropped from 69% to 9% after surgery. Endocrine function was improved in 11% of patients, and 69% of patients were professionally rehabilitated.

A prospective randomized trial comparing the duodenal-preserving pancreatic head resection with the pylorus-preserving Whipple procedure demonstrated improved pain relief in the Beger procedure (75%) compared with the pylorus-preserving procedure (40%). The morbidity rates were similar between groups. Comparing long-term results of the Beger and Frey procedure in a randomized control trial, Izbicki and colleagues reported on 38 patients undergoing the Beger procedure and 36 patients undergoing the Frey procedure. The median follow-up was 104 months. There were no significant differences in the global quality of life, pain score, mortality, and exocrine/endocrine insufficiency between the two surgical groups. There was a high incidence of exocrine insufficiency in both groups (88% in the Beger group and 78% in the Frey group). Diabetes developed in more than 50% of patients in each treatment group. The development of pancreatic insufficiency and diabetes is likely related to further disease progression in the remaining pancreas and independent of the surgical procedure. Each of the combined resection-drainage procedures is effective in relieving pain in this difficult-to-treat patient group.

Pure Resection Procedures

Distal Pancreatectomy

Removing the distal portion of the pancreas can offer pain relief when the disease is confined to the tail. This is seen when there is a midduct stricture or pseudocyst in the body and tail of the pancreas. Preoperative evaluation with CT and ERCP is essential to rule out disease and strictures in the head of the pancreas. Removing the tail of the pancreas is relatively straightforward, and the spleen should be preserved when technically feasible. The spleen should be removed when preoperative imaging demonstrates splenic vein thrombosis or when there is significant inflammation surrounding the splenic vessels.

Results of distal pancreatectomy have been variable but can provide pain relief in 60% to 70% of patients. Hutchings and colleagues reported on 90 patients who had a distal pancreatectomy for chronic pancreatitis. Forty-eight (57%) patients had little or no pain on long-term follow-up. The morbidity rate was 28% for spleen-conserving procedures and 31% for those undergoing a splenectomy. The in-hospital mortality rate was 1%, and the late mortality rate was 10%. The diabetic risk was 46% over 2 years, and there was no change in exocrine function. Patients with pseudocyst disease or an inflammatory mass in the tail of the pancreas had the best outcome.

Total Pancreatectomy

Total pancreatectomy and subtotal pancreatectomy can offer similar pain relief compared with the other resective procedures. However, even when the entire pancreas is removed, 20% of patients continue to have chronic abdominal pain. Total pancreatectomy can also lead to significant endocrine and exocrine insufficiency. Thus this should not be the initial surgery, given the success rates of the previously described procedures. Total pancreatectomy may be warranted in patients who have continued debilitating pain, are already insulin-dependent diabetics, and have had previous resective surgery. Patient selection and education is essential to treating these difficult patients. There has been some success with autologous islet cell transplantation in patients undergoing total pancreatectomy, and this should be considered in young patients who fail previous treatment.

Neuroablative Procedures

Many procedures have been attempted to denervate the pancreas by disrupting the afferent pain nerves from the pancreas in hope of relieving chronic abdominal pain. Percutaneous and endoscopic celiac plexus blocks can offer initial pain relief in 50% of patients, but the effects are usually temporary. Bilateral thoracoscopic splanchnicectomy has recently been shown to offer a minimally invasive approach for pain control in chronic pancreatitis. General anesthesia is used, and the patient is placed in the prone position. Three 5-mm ports are used for each side: the scope port is placed 2 cm below the inferior angle of the scapula, and the two working ports are placed 2 cm superior and inferior to the scope port to produce triangulation. CO_2 insufflation to 8 mm Hg is used to help decompress the lung. Hook electrocautery is used to incise the pleura above the greater splanchnic nerve trunk. The greater, lesser, and least splanchnic nerves are identified and divided. Evaluation of the fatty tissue between the intercostal vessels is required to ensure division of any small nerve branches. Chest tubes are rarely necessary, and patients are discharged the following day.

In evaluating 20 patients undergoing bilateral thoracoscopic splanchnicectomy at the University of Louisville, 65% of patients had a decrease in pain level, and 53% demonstrated a decrease in pain medication use. Hospital admissions for pain decreased in 19 patients (95%).

Bilateral thoracoscopic splanchnicectomy is a minimally invasive procedure that can offer some pain relief with minimal morbidity and does not preclude other surgeries if necessary. It can be used after endoscopic treatment failure or after surgical failure before completion pancreatectomy is entertained. Treatment results for chronic pancreatitis are compared in Table 5. Our treatment algorithm for patients with chronic pancreatitis is demonstrated in Fig. 6.

Table 5: Treatment Results for Chronic Pancreatitis (%)

Procedure	Pain Relief	Morbidity	Early Mortality
Pancreatic duct stenting*	65–94	13–19	0–1
Lateral pancreaticojejunostomy†	65–86	6–21	0–1
Pancreaticoduodenectomy‡	40–100	20–53	0–2
Frey procedure§	75–90	8–22	0–3
Beger procedure[l]	75–95	8–29	0–1
Distal pancreatectomy¶	57–84	32–46	0–1
Thoracoscopic splanchnicectomy#	20–85	0–11	0

*Cremer 1991, Smits 1995, Rosch 2002, Vitale 2004.
†Prinz 1981, Adams 1994, Nealon 2001.
‡Buchler 1995, Martin 1996, Traverso 1997, Izbicki 1998, Jimenez 2000.
§Frey 1994, Izbicki 1998, Falconi 2006.
[l]Buchler 1995, Izbicki 1995, Buchler 1997, Beger 1999, Witzigmann 2003.
¶Schoenberg 1999, Hutchins 2002.
#Ihse 1999, Maher 2001, Howard 2002, Hammond 2004.

TREATMENT OF COMPLICATIONS FROM CHRONIC PANCREATITIS

Pancreatic Pseudocysts

Pancreatic pseudocysts may be seen in up to 40% of chronic pancreatitis cases. The pancreatic ductal rupture leading to the formation of these pseudocysts is usually associated with downstream duct obstruction. Most pseudocysts from chronic pancreatitis do not resolve spontaneously, unlike those seen with acute pancreatitis. It has been shown that asymptomatic pseudocysts can be followed, however. Treatment is pursued for symptomatic or enlarging pseudocysts or if there are associated complications (biliary or intestinal obstruction, infection, and bleeding).

Treatment options include percutaneous drainage, endoscopic drainage, surgical drainage, and resection. Endoscopic drainage has had an increasing role in the treatment of pseudocysts in recent years. Endoscopic drainage has a success rate of 65% to 90%, a complication rate ranging from 5% to 25%, and a recurrence rate of 5% to 20%. Pseudocysts can be drained through a transgastric, transduodenal, or transpapillary endoscopic route. Examination with CT and ERCP is essential to evaluate the pseudocyst location, size, and ductal anatomy before endoscopic drainage. It should be noted that 10% to 20% of pancreatic cystic

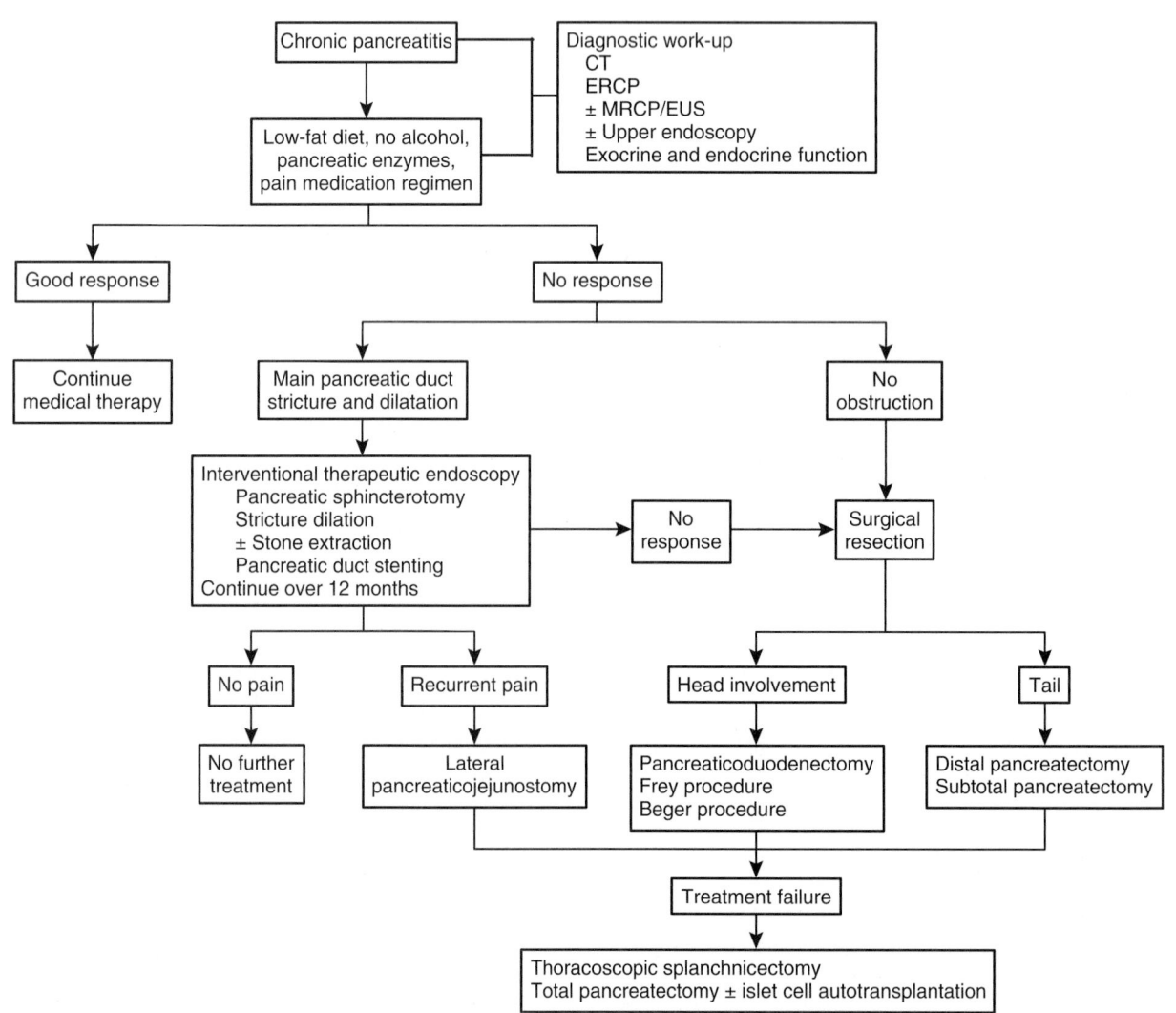

Figure 6 Treatment algorithm for chronic pancreatitis.

lesions are neoplastic, and patient selection is critical when endoscopic or percutaneous treatments are used. Caution should be exercised when there is no definite history of pancreatitis, the cyst wall is thick (>1 cm), and septations are noted on CT. When the diagnosis is uncertain, surgical drainage or resection should be performed.

Pseudocysts that communicate with the pancreatic duct on ERCP and are located in the head or body can be treated with transpapillary endoscopic drainage. This approach can also be used to treat a persistent pancreatic duct disruption causing ascites or fistula. Selective cannulation of the pancreatic duct is obtained, and pancreatic duct sphincterotomy is performed to allow improved drainage. A guidewire is passed through the pancreatic duct into the pseudocyst cavity, and stricture dilatation is performed if necessary. A pancreatic stent (5–10 F) is then placed into the cyst cavity. The stent is left in place for 8 weeks and replaced if necessary. Patients are followed with CT scans to ensure resolution of the cyst before removal of the stent.

If the pseudocyst does not communicate with the pancreatic duct on ERCP, transmural drainage is performed. Criteria for a transmural approach include visible bulging of the pseudocyst into the wall of the stomach or duodenum on endoscopy, less than 1 cm distance between the pseudocyst and stomach-duodenal lumen on CT scan, and the cyst wall must be mature (usually >4–6 weeks). The bulge of the pseudocyst is visualized with a side-viewing endoscope, and this position is maintained. A commercial cystotome or precut knife is used to puncture the cyst wall and enter the cavity (Fig. 7). Contrast is injected into the cyst cavity to ensure correct positioning, and a guidewire is passed into the cyst to maintain access to the cyst lumen. The opening is then enlarged with cautery using the cystotome or sphincterotome catheter to approximately 1 cm. The opening is balloon dilatated if necessary. One or more 10-F double pigtail stents are placed to maintain drainage (Fig. 8). These are usually removed in 2 months after resolution of the cyst is confirmed via CT scan.

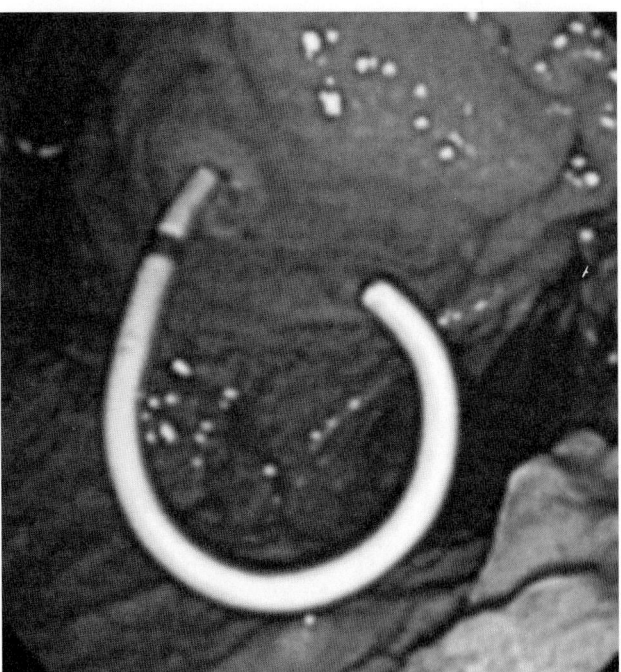

Figure 8   Endoscopic drainage of pancreatic pseudocyst. A 10-F pigtail stent is placed to maintain drainage of the pseudocyst. (*See color insert Figure 27.*)

The University of Louisville reported on a total of 36 endoscopic pseudocyst drainage procedures with a complete resolution in 83% of patients. Five patients required eventual surgery. The recurrence rate was 14%. There were no complications of bleeding; one patient developed pancreatitis that resolved in 1 week.

Surgical drainage of symptomatic pancreatic pseudocysts should be performed when endoscopic drainage is not feasible, when the pseudocyst recurs, or if there is a question of malignancy. Internal surgical drainage can be performed with a cystgastrostomy, cystduodenostomy, or cystjejunostomy, depending on the location of the cyst. Patients who have an associated dilatated pancreatic duct should also be treated with a lateral pancreaticojejunostomy. If the pseudocyst is located in the pancreatic tail, a distal pancreatectomy and splenectomy may be the best treatment option. Because of its high rate of persistent fistula formation, percutaneous drainage should be reserved for infected pseudocysts or when the patient is unsuitable for endoscopic or surgical drainage.

Distal Common Bile Duct Strictures

Distal common bile duct strictures can be seen in up to a third of patients with chronic pancreatitis. Periductal inflammation, fibrosis, and pseudocyst formation may cause progressive obstruction, leading to jaundice. The stricture on ERCP is usually seen as a long, smooth tapering of the distal bile duct. This appearance usually distinguishes it from a malignancy, but brushings of the stricture along with a CT scan should be obtained.

Intervention is indicated when patients develop jaundice, cholangitis, or biliary cirrhosis. In pain-free patients, a biliary enteric bypass, such as a Roux-en-Y choledochojejunostomy or choledochoduodenostomy, is a good treatment option. Patients with pain from pancreatic duct obstruction who are jaundiced can be treated with a combined resection-drainage procedure to deal with both obstructions.

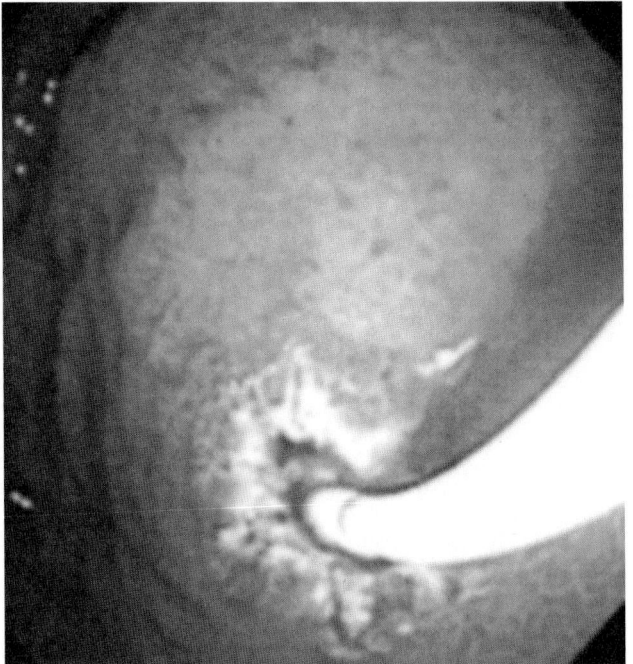

Figure 7   Endoscopic drainage of pancreatic pseudocyst. Cystotome is used to create the cystgastrostomy. (*See color insert Figure 26.*)

Endoscopic biliary stenting has recently been demonstrated to provide definitive treatment in patients with bile duct strictures caused by chronic pancreatitis. At the University of Louisville, 25 patients underwent endoscopic biliary stenting for jaundice and cholestasis secondary to chronic pancreatitis. Eighty percent of patients were treated successfully with no recurrence of the stricture at a mean follow-up of 32 months. Successful results require frequent dilatations, multiple simultaneous stents, and a duration of stenting usually of more than 12 months. Endoscopic stenting for biliary obstruction is a safe alternative to surgical drainage and should be considered for initial treatment because surgery can often be avoided.

SUGGESTED READINGS

Frey CF: The surgical management of chronic pancreatitis: the Frey procedure, *Adv Surg* 32:4185, 1999.

Izbicki JR, Bloechle C, Knoefel WT, and others: Surgical treatment of chronic pancreatitis and quality of life after operation, *Surg Clin North Am* 79:913, 1999.

Vitale GC, Cothron K, Vitale EA, and others: Role of pancreatic duct stenting in the treatment of chronic pancreatitis, *Surg Endosc* 18:1431, 2004.

Vitale GC, Lawhorn JC, Larson GM, and others: Endoscopic drainage of the pancreatic pseudocyst, *Surgery* 126:616, 1999.

Vitale GC, Reed DN, Nguyen CT, and others: Endoscopic treatment of distal bile duct stricture from chronic pancreatitis, *Surg Endosc* 14:227, 2000.

PERIAMPULLARY CANCER

O. Joe Hines, MD, and Howard A. Reber, MD

INTRODUCTION

The term *periampullary carcinoma* refers to cancers that arise from the pancreas, ampulla of Vater, bile duct, or duodenum. The most common of these tumors is a pancreatic adenocarcinoma, but because the clinical presentation, symptoms, and treatment of these lesions are often similar, they are appropriately discussed together. Nevertheless, as the management of periampullary tumors has evolved and more data and experience have accumulated, it has become apparent that some of these tumors have peculiar features that may justify somewhat different approaches. They certainly have vastly different survival statistics (e.g., pancreatic vs. ampullary cancer). Although preoperative imaging and tissue biopsy can help to determine the most likely diagnosis, the precise tumor type is often unknown preoperatively (e.g., pancreatic vs. cholangiocarcinoma), and a periampullary mass that appears to be a malignant neoplasm should be resected if assessment suggests this is feasible and it can be performed safely.

In the following discussion, we consider separately certain features of pancreatic, ampullary, biliary, and duodenal carcinomas. Because the most common of these neoplasms is a pancreatic cancer, most of the discussion is devoted to that topic. In addition, we include a detailed description of a pancreaticoduodenectomy, which generally is the operation appropriate for the management of all of these cancers.

PANCREATIC ADENOCARCINOMA

Pancreatic cancer is lethal, and in 2006 an estimated 33,730 Americans were diagnosed with this disease. This accounts for 2% of new cancer diagnoses. An estimated 32,300 Americans (16,090 men and 16,210 women) died during the same year, which makes this neoplasm the fourth leading cause of cancer death overall, and the cause of 6% (up from 5.5% the previous year) of cancer deaths in the United States. The most common form of pancreatic cancer is adenocarcinoma. Only approximately 23% of patients with cancer of the exocrine pancreas will be alive 1 year after their diagnosis; only approximately 4% will survive 5 years. Even for those people diagnosed with local disease who undergo surgical resection, the 5-year survival rate is only approximately 20%.

Patients with pancreatic cancer can present with a variety of symptoms, including weight loss, jaundice, abdominal or back pain, and, rarely, malabsorption. Approximately 20% of patients with pancreatic cancer will have had a new diagnosis of diabetes made within the previous 1 to 2 years. In fact, patients in their 50s with no risk factors for diabetes who present with a new diagnosis of diabetes should probably be screened for pancreatic cancer. Patients who present with back pain, which often is due to invasion of the retroperitoneal nerve plexuses by cancer, generally have advanced disease, which portends unresectability and a poor prognosis.

Evaluation

Initial evaluation of the patient should consist of a general assessment of the patient's condition and a complete medical history, including any history of chronic pancreatitis. In addition, a family history of pancreatic or breast cancer should be established. Recent estimates suggest that as many as 10% of pancreatic cancers have a familial genetic basis. The physical examination should focus on any evidence of metastatic disease, including palpation of the supraclavicular nodes and assessment of the liver. It is rare to be able to palpate the primary lesion by physical examination. Laboratory tests should include a complete blood count; liver function tests, including an albumin test to assess for nutritional status; and tests for tumor markers, including carbohydrate antigen 19–9 and carcinogenic embryonic antigen.

Although this initial evaluation is important to understand the full range of the patient's disease and to provide information about operative risk, the single most valuable study to stage patients with pancreatic cancer is the helical computerized tomographic (CT) scan performed as a pancreatic protocol scan (Fig. 1). Some physicians prefer a magnetic resonance imaging (MRI) to CT, and newer software and protocols for imaging the pancreas with MR may produce images that are as informative as those from a CT scan. The MRI scan also can be reconstructed to give an image of the pancreatic and bile ducts (magnetic resonance cholangiopancreatography) (Fig. 2). The pancreatic protocol CT requires that 2–3 mm collimation be performed through the pancreas itself during the administration of intravenous contrast and that separate scans for both the pancreas and the liver during the arterial and venous phases be performed. Appropriate software permits the creation of images that provide extraordinary detail of the tumor and its relationship to important adjacent structures. Nevertheless, for a variety of reasons, some patients still cannot be categorized with certainty into a "resectable" or "unresectable" group.

Both CT and MRI can provide three-dimensional (3D) reconstruction of the vascular structures surrounding the pancreatic lesion with excellent detail (Fig. 3). This has largely replaced the need for preoperative angiography for those who felt it was an important aspect of preoperative assessment. The images can be formatted to give a rotational image, allowing the surgeon to view the vasculature from several angles.

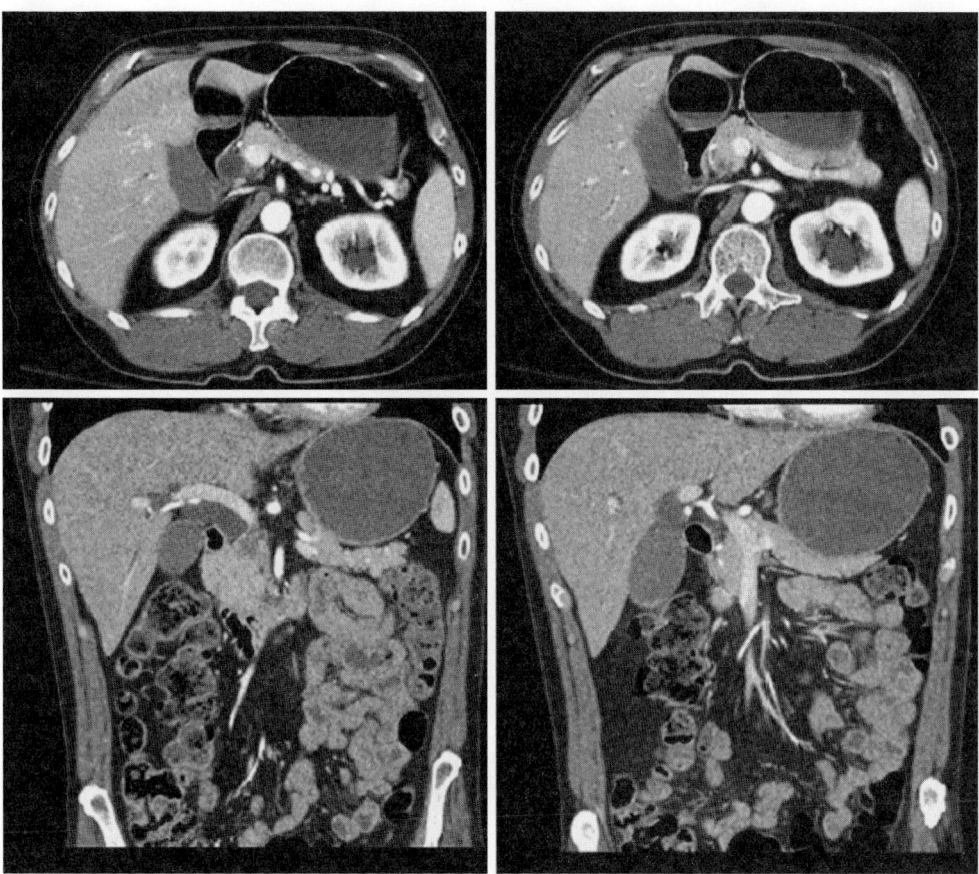

Figure 1 Pancreatic protocol helical computed tomography scan. The scan demonstrates extraordinary detail of a lesion in the uncinate and head of the pancreas. The coronal reconstruction demonstrates possible involvement of the portal vein by the lesion.

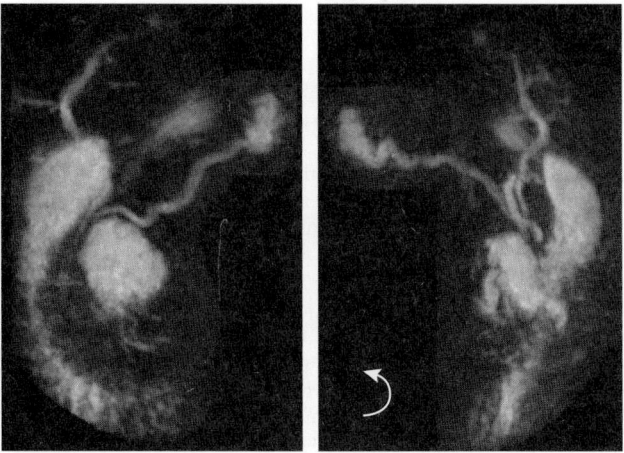

Figure 2 Magnetic resonance pancreaticocholangiography demonstrating a cystic lesion in both the head and tail of the pancreas. This image can be rotated, demonstrating the same from a posterior view.

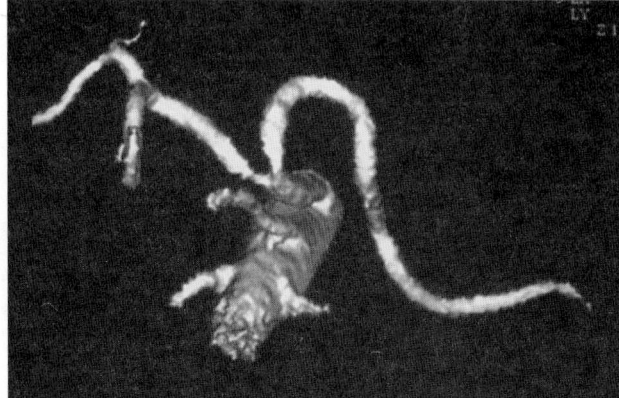

Figure 3 A three-dimensional reconstruction from a computed tomography scan of the aorta, celiac, superior mesenteric, and renal arteries. The common hepatic artery appears to have narrowing near its origin, which corresponds to involvement by a pancreatic cancer.

Patients with metastatic disease are not operative candidates. Locally advanced disease that includes involvement of the hepatic, celiac, or superior mesenteric arteries or involvement of the superior mesenteric or portal vein is generally felt to be unresectable by most pancreatic surgeons. However, a growing experience with patients who have superior mesenteric or portal vein involvement suggests that vein resection can be performed safely. Although the survival rate for these patients is similar to that of resected patients without vein involvement, no patients are cured. Patients with involved celiac or periaortic nodes (not normally resected as part of a pancreaticoduodenectomy) are considered unresectable. However, because enlarged lymph nodes identified on preoperative imaging studies may be either inflammatory or neoplastic, large nodes should not be a reason to deny a patient an operation and the chance for a resection.

The information provided by a pancreatic protocol CT allows for correct prediction of resectability approximately 85% of the time. Of the remaining 15% who are eventually found to be unresectable, approximately half have small liver or peritoneal metastases that are too small for the scan to have detected. The rest have extensive local disease, usually involving one or more of the major vessels already mentioned. In this latter group, there is usually a suggestion on the preoperative CT that the vessels may be involved, but some level of uncertainty persists, and the patient is explored to settle the issue. On the other hand, a loss of the normal fat plane between the superior mesenteric or portal vein and the tumor of more than 50% of the circumference of the vein likely represents true invasion and unresectability. These patients are generally not explored.

Endoscopic ultrasound (EUS) also has the potential to provide information about resectability, but the quality of the information is highly operator dependent. Generally we would not deny a patient the opportunity for resection solely on the basis of an EUS report that declared a lesion "unresectable" because of vascular involvement. In that case, we would require a CT scan that corroborated those findings. If the CT did not corroborate the findings, we would operate on the patient. EUS is a reliable way to establish a tissue diagnosis when required, although such diagnosis is not necessary preoperatively in most cases, and it should not be required routinely. It may be especially useful when suspicious celiac or periaortic lymph nodes are identified; fine needle aspiration of these may avoid surgery by confirming neoplastic involvement. The sensitivity of this approach is 85%, and specificity almost 100%.

Staging and Resectablity

The TNM (T = primary tumor; N = regional lymph nodes; M = distant metastasis) definitions and 6th edition of the American Joint Committee on Cancer (AJCC) staging for pancreatic cancer are shown in Table 1. Patients with stage 0, I, or II are generally considered resectable. Some surgeons will resect patients with stage III disease. Patients with tumor confined to the pancreas and lymph nodes that will be included in the resection and who have no vascular invasion are candidates for resection.

Chemoradiation

Neoadjuvant therapy for pancreatic cancer is not routinely performed, although theoretical reasons that support that approach have been articulated. We use it when the tumor appears to be locally invasive, raising a question about whether major vessels are involved that would preclude resection for cure. In approximately 10% of cases, downstaging occurs, which allows for resection. Adjuvant therapy is the standard of care, and most patients receive it. Debate continues about whether radiation in addition to chemotherapy is useful.

AMPULLARY CARCINOMA

Carcinoma of the ampulla of Vater is a rare tumor. The incidence has been estimated to be 6 per million persons per year. It is more likely to be resectable than other periampullary malignancies because these patients may present earlier with jaundice; the tumor also appears to be less aggressive than pancreatic or bile duct cancers. Patients commonly present with abdominal pain, jaundice, and weight loss. The resection rate is estimated to be approximately 80% of cases, which is much higher than for pancreatic cancer for which only approximately 15% to 20% of cases are resected. As with many of these periampullary cancers, the presence of lymph node metastasis, perineural invasion, and poor tumor differentiation negatively affect survival.

Table 1: The American Joint Committee on Cancer 6th Edition Staging System—Pancreatic Cancer

Primary Tumor (T)

T1	Tumor limited to the pancreas, ≤2 cm
T2	Tumor limited to the pancreas, >2 cm
T3	Tumor extends beyond the pancreas but without involvement of the celiac axis or the superior mesenteric artery
T4	Tumor involves the celiac axis or the superior mesenteric artery (unresectable primary tumor)

Regional Lymph Nodes (N)

N0	No regional lymph node metastasis
N1	Regional lymph node metastasis

Distant Metastasis (M)

M0	No distant metastasis
M1	Distant metastasis

Stage Grouping

0	Tis	N0	M0
Ia	T1	N0	M0
Ib	T2	N0	M0
IIa	T3	N0	M0
IIb	T1	N1	M0
	T2	N1	M0
	T3	N1	M0
III	T4	Any N	M0
IV	Any T	Any N	M1

Several reports have addressed the survival rate of patients with ampullary carcinoma, which is the highest of all of the periampullary cancers. The reported 5-year survival for ampullary cancers in the literature span a wide range varying from approximately 30% in some series up to 70% in others. A recent study from Seoul University reported 5-year cancer-specific survival of 59.8%. The Memorial Sloan-Kettering and University of California–Los Angeles (UCLA) Medical Center series have reported a 5-year cancer-specific survival of 46% and 67.7%, respectively.

Preoperative evaluation for lesions of the ampulla of Vater includes a high-quality CT scan and an EUS with biopsy or fine needle aspiration. As with pancreatic adenocarcinoma, ampullary cancer should be assessed for the presence of local invasion and distant disease, either of which may preclude resection. However, we occasionally resect patients with either ampullary or duodenal cancers who have liver metastases because palliation of either of these lesions is poor unless they have been removed (tumors left in situ tend to bleed, etc.). Of course the patient must be a good risk for major resection, and the extent of distant disease should be compatible with a significant survival. The AJCC staging system for ampullary carcinoma is shown in Table 2. Endoscopy and EUS allow biopsy of ampullary lesions to determine their true nature (i.e., whether they are benign adenomas or invasive neoplasms), as well as their depth of involvement into the duodenal wall. All patients with biopsy-proved cancers and those who appear to have lesions that penetrate the muscularis of the duodenum should have a pancreaticoduodenectomy. Patients who have what appear to be benign lesions can be managed with a local excision of the ampulla

Table 2: The American Joint Committee on Cancer 6th Edition Staging System—Ampulla of Vater Carcinoma

Primary Tumor (T)

T1	Tumor limited to ampulla of Vater or sphincter of Oddi
T2	Tumor invades duodenal wall
T3	Tumor invades pancreas
T4	Tumor invades peripancreatic soft tissues or other adjacent organs or structures

Regional Lymph Nodes (N)

N0	No regional lymph node metastasis
N1	Regional lymph node metastasis

Distant Metastasis (M)

M0	No distant metastasis
M1	Distant metastasis

Stage Grouping

0	Tis	N0	M0
Ia	T1	N0	M0
Ib	T2	N0	M0
IIa	T3	N0	M0
IIb	T1	N1	M0
	T2	N1	M0
	T3	N1	M0
III	T4	Any N	M0
IV	Any T	Any N	M1

of Vater. Occasionally this can be performed endoscopically. At the time of a surgical ampullectomy, a frozen section of the specimen should be performed; the diagnosis of cancer requires conversion to a pancreaticoduodenectomy. Although there are reports of local resection for patients with limited T1 carcinoma, we would not agree with that approach.

There are no trials indicating that chemotherapy or radiation improves survival from ampullary carcinoma, but resection clearly does (Table 3). Nevertheless, many of these patients receive adjuvant treatment.

CHOLANGIOCARCINOMA

These tumors are rare in the United States but more common in Asian countries and are often associated with a variety of chronic inflammatory conditions of the bile ducts (e.g., sclerosing cholangitis, parasitic infestations). Approximately 25% of bile duct cancers occur in the distal duct, and the symptoms are usually indistinguishable from pancreatic cancer. The diagnosis may be suspected if preoperative studies show an isolated bile duct stricture, with a normal pancreatic duct. Nevertheless, the diagnosis is usually not known until the pathologist examines the pancreaticoduodenectomy specimen. Prognosis is poor; the 5-year survival after resection is approximately 15%.

DUODENAL CARCINOMA

Adenocarcinoma of the duodenum is also a rare disease with a poorly defined natural history. Some evidence suggests that the incidence of duodenal polyps is rising. As with the relationship between colon cancer and colon polyps, duodenal cancers presumably originate from duodenal polyps. Duodenal carcinoma represents less than 0.5% of all gastrointestinal tract malignant neoplasms but accounts for up to 45% of small bowel cancers. Duodenal carcinomas can occur along the entire length of the duodenum. The disease is usually diagnosed at an advanced stage, and surgical resection is the only potentially curative treatment. Reported 5-year survival rates range up to 50%. Because of the small number of patients with this neoplasm, it has been difficult to determine the factors that influence survival. Controversial issues include the significance of the tumor stage and degree of differentiation, as well as the prognostic value of nodal status. Although a pancreaticoduodenectomy is indicated for these lesions, some data suggest that a segmental resection may be adequate for tumors that affect the most distal part of the fourth portion of the duodenum. Of course, these are not truly "periampullary" in location.

PANCREATICODUODENECTOMY

The Whipple resection can be performed as it was originally described, to include a partial gastrectomy (antrectomy) or as the pylorus-preserving modification. Most surgeons, including the UCLA group, prefer the pylorus-preserving operation. We reserve the standard Whipple resection for patients with larger tumors that appear to encroach on the proximal duodenum or gastric antrum. It is generally agreed that both operations are equivalent oncologically; we have not found that the incidence of complications, especially delayed gastric emptying ($\approx$15%), is higher when the pylorus is preserved. We are also not convinced that the long-term nutritional consequences are better for the patient with the pylorus-preserving technique, although this was the principle reason for its adoption.

Operative Technique

The operation is usually performed through a bilateral subcostal incision, but in thin patients, a midline incision also provides good

Table 3: Five-Year Observed Survival for Ampullary Cancers Comparing Recent Publications

Author	Institution	Year of Publication	Sample Size	5-Year Survival (%)
Howe JR and others	Memorial-Sloan Kettering, NY	1998	101	46
Duffy JP and others	UCLA Med Center, Los Angeles, CA	2003	55	67.7
Di Giorgio A and others	Catholic University School of Medicine, Rome, Italy	2005	64	64.6
Riall TS and others	Johns Hopkins Hospital, Baltimore, MD	2005	59	46[*†]
Brown KM and others	Loyola University Med. Ctr. Maywood, IL	2005	51	58
Kim RD and others	Toronto General Hospital, Canada	2006	43	51.4
Yoon Y and others	Seoul University, South Korea	2005	199	59.8

* Excludes perioperative deaths and patients lost to follow-up.
† Standard resection.

exposure. The following maneuvers are carried out, usually in this order: (1) assessment of the abdomen for metastatic disease; (2) mobilization of the duodenum and the head of the pancreas, with identification of the superior mesenteric vein; (3) mobilization of the stomach and proximal duodenum, with transection of the proximal duodenum (or stomach) as soon as the decision for resection has been made; (4) skeletonization of the structures of the porta; (5) cholecystectomy and division of the common bile duct; (6) mobilization and division of the proximal jejunum; (7) transection of the neck of the pancreas and division of the remaining attachments of the specimen to the superior mesenteric and portal veins and the superior mesenteric artery; and (8) reconstruction of gastrointestinal continuity.

Initial Assessment

After the abdomen has been entered, both lobes of the liver are inspected and palpated; all peritoneal surfaces are assessed for metastatic disease. The transverse colon is elevated, and its mesocolon, especially overlying the duodenum and head of the pancreas, is inspected. Occasionally the tumor will have grown through the mesocolon, where it can be seen and palpated as a firm nodularity. The area of the ligament of Treitz, the proximal jejunum, and the root of the small bowel mesentery are also inspected. A biopsy with frozen section should be taken of any suspicious lesion to rule out cancer. If none is found, any adhesions that may interfere with later exposure are lysed and a self-retaining retractor is placed.

Exposure, Mobilization, and Resection

The gallbladder and the right and left lobes of the liver are retracted cranially. We usually begin by performing an extensive Kocher maneuver to mobilize the duodenum and the head of the pancreas. The vena cava and the aorta are cleaned of soft tissue in the process, and the left renal vein is exposed, but we do not remove the soft tissue and nodes between the cava and aorta. Indeed, if the tumor is adherent to these structures or if the nodes are firm and appear to be involved by tumor, we confirm the presence of cancer by biopsy. Tumor involvement here is a contraindication to resection. As the duodenal mobilization proceeds distally, the hepatic flexure of the colon must be separated from it, and this begins to identify its mesocolon as a distinct structure. It is helpful at this point to retract the hepatic flexure and right colon caudally. Now the mobilization of the third and fourth portions of the duodenum continues until an opening is made in the peritoneum caudal to the duodenum and anterior to the aorta, to the left side of the peritoneal cavity (Fig. 4). This allows the surgeon to place a finger through to the area of the ligament of Treitz and proximal jejunum that will be approached later in the operation. This maneuver usually signals the end of the duodenal mobilization.

Inspection of the anterior aspect of the exposed pancreatic head reveals the avascular line of fusion between the mesocolon and the pancreas. The mesocolon should be separated from the head of the pancreas along this line and reflected medially to expose the superior mesenteric vein, which runs along the right lateral margin of this tissue. It is the superior mesenteric vein that limits the further medial separation of the transverse mesocolon from the neck of the pancreas and the retroperitoneal third part of the duodenum. The plane of dissection of the vein should be at the level of its adventitia. Several venous tributaries from the head of the pancreas run directly into the vein, and the larger ones should be ligated in continuity and divided at this point. The middle colic vein is usually preserved, but at either this point or later stage in the dissection the large gastroepiploic vein from the greater curve of the stomach should be divided close to where it enters the superior mesenteric vein. (The gastroepiploic vein may also join the middle colic vein

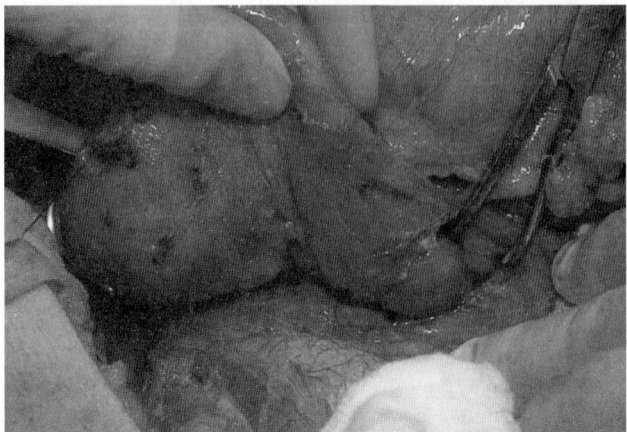

Figure 4 The mobilization of the third and fourth portion of the duodenum. The peritoneum (ligament of Treitz) is finally incised, signifying the completion of the mobilization. The clamp is seen under the ligament.

where the two run together for a short distance as the gastrocolic trunk, which then enters the superior mesenteric vein as a single vessel, discussed later) After the superior mesenteric vein has been cleaned of adherent tissue and the larger tributaries from the pancreas proximal to the middle colic vein have been divided (Fig. 5), we usually begin the dissection of the stomach and proximal duodenum. Separation of the neck of the pancreas from the vein is usually postponed until after that dissection has been performed.

The stomach is elevated and pulled cranially, and the gastrocolic omentum is entered, taking care to preserve the gastroepiploic arcade of vessels along the greater curve. Major vessels are ligated and divided, and an opening is created so that the avascular adhesions from the posterior surface of the stomach to the pancreas can be exposed and lysed. As one develops the dissection distally toward the pylorus, the avascular attachments of the transverse mesocolon to the gastrocolic omentum can be separated. Transillumination of the tissue allows for identification of the gastroepiploic vein, which should be ligated and divided before it enters the superior mesenteric vein or joins with the middle colic vein (discussed earlier). The gastroepiploic artery should also be ligated and divided. The dissection of the duodenum should continue at least 1 to 2 cm past the gastroduodenal artery, where it can be seen and felt on the surface of the pancreas. By this time, the dissection should have

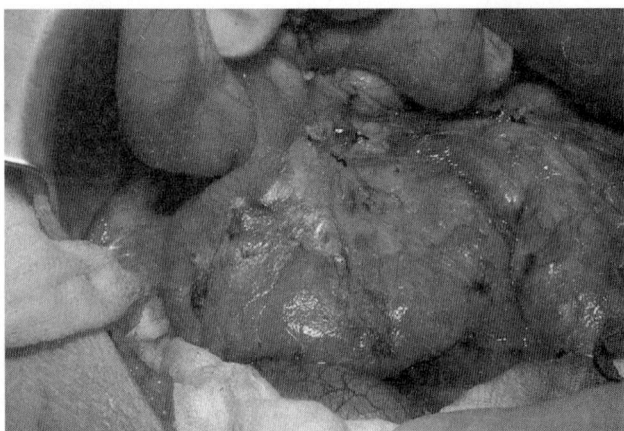

Figure 5 The superior mesenteric vein is exposed and visualized coming under the neck of the pancreas.

reached the same level and be in the same plane as the earlier dissection of the superior mesenteric vein and the neck of the pancreas where the vein disappears beneath it. Now we incise along the inferior margin of the pancreas for a distance of approximately 3 to 4 cm along the body of the gland. This allows one to deepen the dissection to the left of the neck of the gland and to reach the level where the later pancreaticojejunal anastomosis will take place. At this point, the dissection is usually through fatty areolar tissue, but occasionally a vessel is encountered that should be divided. By this time, it is often evident that the tumor is resectable (i.e., the tumor mass can be palpated and its position away from the superior mesenteric and portal veins can be confirmed). If this is the case, we then mobilize the lesser curve side of the distal stomach and proximal duodenum and divide the right gastric and duodenal vessels to a point opposite where the duodenum was mobilized and its surface cleaned on the greater curve side. This is performed a centimeter or so away from the duodenum to preserve collateral vessels to the gastroduodenal wall and in a fashion that avoids injury to the nerve of Latarjet. When the duodenum has been cleaned circumferentially, it is then transected with a stapler. More than 90% of our resections are performed as pylorus-preserving operations, but if a standard pancreaticoduodenectomy is to be performed, the duodenal dissection just described is not necessary and the stomach is transected at the level of the gastric antrum. Then the gastric staple line starting from the lesser curve side is buried using 3–0 seromuscular silk sutures, stopping approximately 4 to 5 cm from the greater curve margin. This will be the site of the eventual gastrojejunostomy (Hofmeister) during the later gastrointestinal reconstruction. In either case, the preserved stomach (and duodenum) is then retracted toward the left upper quadrant. This provides wide exposure of the hepatoduodenal ligament, which is dissected next. If it is still uncertain whether resection is possible after the duodenum has been cleaned circumferentially, we delay duodenal transection.

The hepatoduodenal ligament is dissected next. The soft tissue of the gastrohepatic ligament is opened in an avascular area to the left of the hepatic artery. The hepatic artery is then cleaned of its attached tissues, which contain fat, lymphatic channels, and lymph nodes, all of which will be removed. The right gastric and gastroduodenal arteries are divided close to their origins; a metal clip is also placed on the gastroduodenal artery stump. (Occasionally the right gastric artery is particularly large and well developed, which suggests that it should be preserved to maintain the blood supply of the distal stomach and duodenum.) This dissection is carried caudally to the superior border of the pancreas, which is also cleaned of adherent tissue. The lymph nodes that are typically found along the superior border of the neck of the pancreas, where the pancreatic transection will later occur, should be removed. This dissection should be sufficiently deep to expose both the splenic artery as it begins its course toward the spleen and the anterior surface of the portal vein. (If there were still a question of whether the tumor was adherent to the anterior surface of the portal vein, this can be resolved because the superior mesenteric vein below and the portal vein above are now exposed.) The anterior surface of the portal vein is now cleaned cranially along with the right and left hepatic arteries to the level at which the bile duct will be transected. The gallbladder is removed. We next transect the common hepatic duct. A right-angled dissecting clamp is inserted behind it, keeping close to its posterior surface, and a vessel loop is pulled through the opening. The duct is elevated so that a curved bulldog clamp can be applied to its proximal portion. The distal part is clamped with a tonsil clamp, and the duct is cut. If a stent had been placed preoperatively, it is removed at this time. The soft tissue and lymph nodes that are always present behind the bile duct are separated from it and allowed to remain in continuity with the specimen. Because this tissue is vascular, it must be ligated as it is separated piece by piece from the tissues that are to remain. Finally we pass a quarter-inch Penrose drain behind the neck of the pancreas and anterior

to the superior mesenteric/portal vein. This protects the vessels later when the neck of the pancreas is transected.

Next the ligament of Treitz and the proximal jejunum are exposed, requiring modification of the original exposure. While the surgeon stays anterior and medial to the inferior mesenteric vein at all times, the avascular peritoneal folds that are the ligament of Treitz are cut with electrocautery. Next the mesentery of the proximal jejunum is displayed, and the vascular arcades of the bowel are divided close to the bowel wall beginning approximately 4 to 6 inches from the ligament of Treitz. When a large enough opening has been created in the mesentery, a stapler is inserted through it and the jejunum is divided. With an Allis clamp providing tension on the proximal stapled end of the jejunum, the vessels in the mesentery are divided, progressing proximally until the retroperitoneal portion of the duodenum has been reached. We then pass the distal jejunum (which will eventually be anastomosed to the pancreas and bile duct) behind the small bowel mesentery, and the superior mesenteric artery and vein through the window in the peritoneum. The proximal duodenal-jejunal segment, which is part of the specimen, can also be delivered to the right side through the peritoneal opening at this time. Now retractors are repositioned for the final phase of the resection.

The neck of the pancreas is elevated from the underlying vein with the help of the Penrose drain. Hemostatic Prolene sutures (3–0) are placed through the pancreatic parenchyma at both the inferior and superior margin of the pancreas, on either side of the proposed line of transection (i.e., four sutures total), which usually overlies the vein. On the specimen side, the sutures can be placed to occlude most or all of the pancreatic parenchyma and the duct. On the side of the pancreas that will remain, the surgeon should try to avoid placing the superior margin suture in a way that might obstruct the pancreatic duct, which normally is situated closer to that margin and posterior in the gland. All of the sutures are tied tightly, but care should be taken to avoid tearing the pancreatic parenchyma. (If the pancreatic parenchyma is firm, these four sutures are not necessary.) Next the pancreatic parenchyma is divided with electrocautery; any bleeding from the cut surface is easily controlled with electrocautery.

The surgeon, who stands on the patient's left side, grasps the duodenum and head of the pancreas in the left hand and retracts it away from the portal vein (Fig. 6). The dissection begins at the cranial end of the specimen progressing distally, and the remaining attachments to the superior mesenteric and portal vein, the superior mesenteric artery, and the retroperitoneal tissues are ligated and divided.

The entire specimen is then sent to the pathology laboratory for frozen-section examination of the resection margins (duodenal, jejunal, pancreas, bile duct). If invasive cancer is seen in any of them, more tissue is resected until a negative margin is obtained.

RECONSTRUCTION

Pancreatic Anastomosis

An end-to-side pancreaticojejunostomy is performed first, usually by bringing the jejunum behind the superior mesenteric artery and vein, in a position similar to that occupied originally by the retroperitoneal duodenum. However, in patients with cancers arising in the third part of the duodenum, we prefer to bring the jejunum through a hole in the transverse mesocolon instead. This minimizes the potential for later obstruction of the jejunum if the cancer should recur in the retroperitoneum. The cut end of the pancreas is mobilized from the retroperitoneal tissues for a distance of 2 to 3 cm, and this may require division of a few venous tributaries to the splenic vein. The pancreatic duct is probed and its patency ensured past the point where the Prolene hemostatic suture had

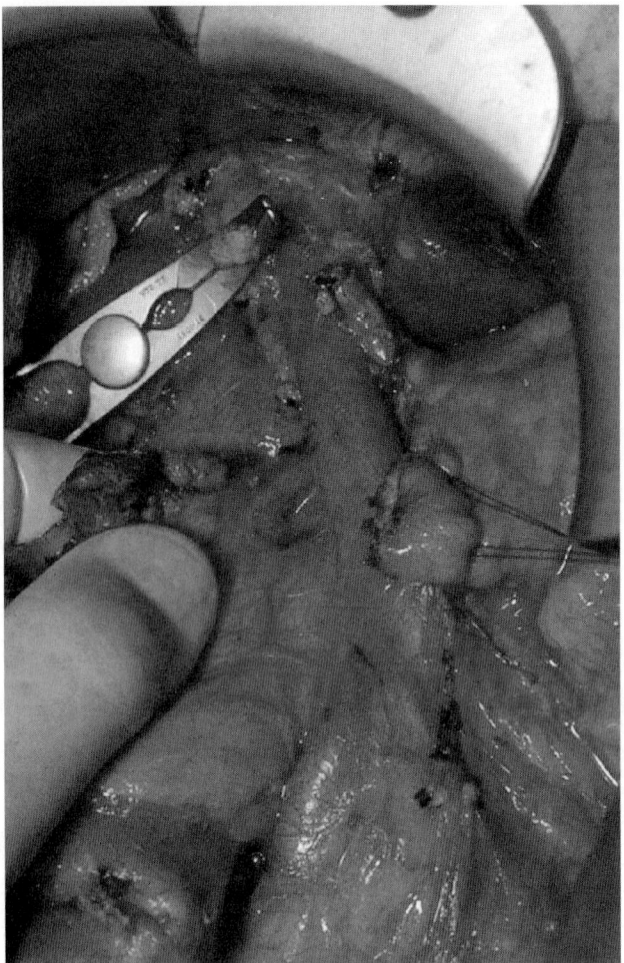

Figure 6   The final attachments of the pancreas are taken off the superior mesenteric/portal vein and superior mesenteric artery. The common duct is clamped with a bulldog clamp, and the cut edge of the distal pancreatic neck is seen with two Prolene sutures.

been placed earlier. Depending on the size of the duct, a 5- or 8-F pediatric feeding tube is inserted well into the duct so that it can be easily seen during the anastomosis. (We do not use a pancreatic duct stent, so this will be removed later.) The two-layer anastomosis is begun by placing a posterior row of three or four 3–0 horizontal silk mattress sutures from the pancreas to the bowel; after they are all placed, the sutures are tied as the first assistant brings the bowel to the pancreas to minimize the chances that the pancreatic parenchyma will tear. They are placed horizontally so that when they are tied, any pancreatic parenchymal vessels (which generally run transversely) are likely to be compressed; this minimizes bleeding from needle placement. The jejunum is then opened with electrocautery approximately 1 cm anterior to the line where the silk sutures have been tied. Two 3–0 Polydioxane (PDS) sutures are then placed at the posterosuperior margin of the anastomosis, the end of each is tied, and the short end is cut. Both of these sutures are placed from the mucosal side of the bowel and then through the pancreatic parenchyma approximately 1 cm back from the cut edge of the pancreas. The first suture is continued as the posterior row and should be placed through the lumen of the pancreatic duct as it passes near the duct and then through the full thickness of the bowel wall approximately 5 mm from the cut edge. This usually requires two or three sutures placed into the duct lumen in this fashion, even with the largest ducts (Fig. 7). This posterior-row suture is held after the inferior corner of the anastomosis is completed. Then

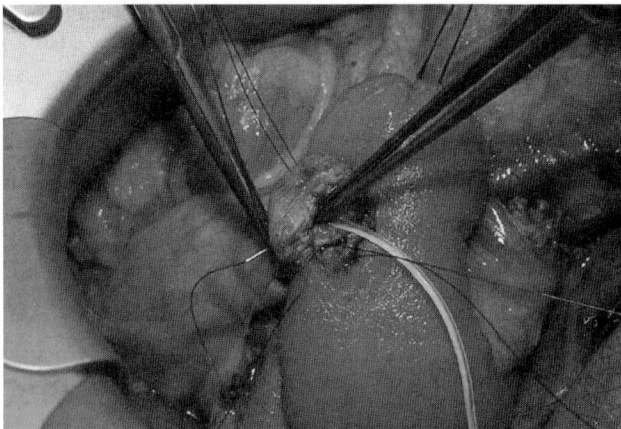

Figure 7   After an outer layer of 3–0 silk suture is placed, an inner layer of running 3–0 Polydioxane suture is used. The back layer of suture incorporates the pancreatic duct with two or three bites. The duct is seen cannulated with a pediatric feeding tube, which is removed before the completion of the anastomosis.

the second suture is brought from the inside of the bowel lumen, where it was tied, through the bowel wall so that the anterior row of sutures can be placed. Again, the sutures are placed through the lumen of the pancreatic duct before traversing the full thickness of the anterior bowel wall. The feeding tube helps to identify the duct lumen and aids in suture placement. When the sutures progress past the duct, the feeding tube should be removed. When the anterior row of sutures reaches the posterior one, the two PDS sutures are tied. The anastomosis is completed with the placement of the anterior row of 3–0 silk sutures in a fashion similar to the posterior row. This anastomosis results in the invagination of the cut end of the pancreas into the lumen of the bowel (Fig. 8).

Biliary Anastomosis

The hepaticojejunal anastomosis is performed next at a sufficient distance from the pancreas to avoid tension on the suture line, but not long enough to allow kinking of the bowel. The clamp is removed from the bile duct, a bile culture is taken, and hemostasis is obtained. A single-layer anastomosis using interrupted sutures of 4–0 or 5–0 PDS is performed. If the duct is smaller than 1 cm in diameter, a small T-tube is inserted through the wall of the bile duct proximal to the anastomosis. The distal limb of the T-tube lies in the jejunal limb. The tube is removed in the office 3 to 4 weeks later, usually without a prior cholangiogram.

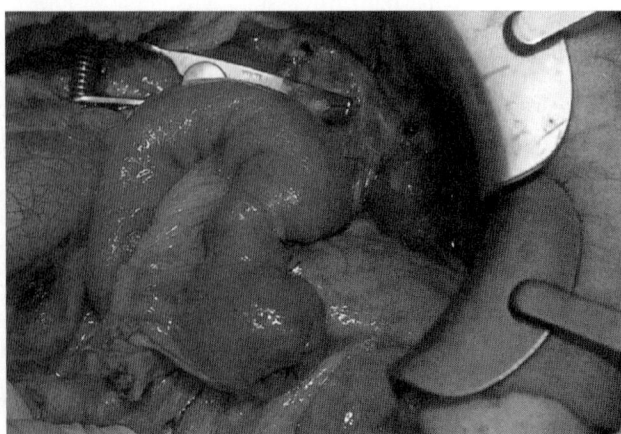

Figure 8   The completed pancreaticojejunostomy.

Duodenal Anastomosis

Finally, a retrocolic duodenojejunostomy is constructed approximately 30 cm distal to the choledochojejunostomy in a standard two-layer fashion. The duodenum (or proximal stomach, in the case of a standard Whipple resection) is usually brought through an opening in the transverse mesocolon, but sometimes an antecolic anastomosis is performed in obese individuals.

Two closed-suction drains (e.g., no.10 Jackson Pratt) are placed close to the pancreatic and hepatic duct anastomoses. The pancreatic drain is led though a hole in the transverse mesocolon, behind the stomach, and then between the pancreaticojejunostomy and the left lobe of the liver. The biliary drain is placed behind the hepaticojejunostomy. They are brought out of the abdomen separately on the right (hepatic duct anastomosis) and the left (pancreatic anastomosis) sides. After this, the abdomen is irrigated again, and it is closed in layers.

POSTOPERATIVE CARE

Patients do not routinely require time in the intensive care unit postoperatively. The nasogastric tube is removed on the morning of the first postoperative day, and the patient is encouraged to ambulate. A clear liquid diet is usually started on the fifth postoperative day, and most patients are able to advance to a regular diet over the next 24 to 48 hours. If there is no evidence of a biliary leak, the biliary drain is removed the day after the patient begins oral intake. The pancreatic drain is removed on the day of discharge as long as there is no pancreatic leak. Most patients are released from the hospital within 7 to 10 days of operation.

CONCLUSIONS

Periampullary cancers (pancreatic, bile duct, ampulla of Vater, duodenal) are lesions that often present with similar symptoms, require a similar preoperative assessment, and generally are best managed with the same operation—a pancreaticoduodenectomy. This procedure is now performed safely in major centers throughout the world, with operative mortality rates less than 5% and often less than 1%, although there is still significant morbidity. Despite the similarities among these cancers, their prognosis varies considerably, probably because of their underlying biological aggressiveness. Improvements in prognosis will likely result from earlier diagnosis and better chemotherapeutic approaches, rather than from changes in operative technique.

SUGGESTED READINGS

Allema JH, Reinders ME, van Gulik TM, and others: Results of pancreatico-duodenectomy for ampullary carcinoma and analysis of prognostic factors for survival, *Surgery* 117:247, 1995.

Alwmark A, Andersson A, Lasson A: Primary carcinoma of the duodenum, *Ann Surg* 191:13, 1980.

Barnes G Jr, Romero L, Hess KR, and others: Primary adenocarcinoma of the duodenum: management and survival in 67 patients, *Ann Surg Oncol* 1:73, 1994.

Brown KM, Tompkins AJ, Sherri Y, and others: Pancreaticoduodenectomy is curative in the majority of patients with node-negative ampullary cancer, *Arch Surg* 140:529, 2005.

Delcore R Jr, Connor CS, Thomas JH, and others: Significance of tumor spread in adenocarcinoma of the ampulla of Vater, *Am J Surg* 158:593, 1989.

Di Giorgio A, Alfieri S, Rotondi F, and others: Pancreatoduodenectomy for tumors of Vater's ampulla: report on 94 consecutive patients, *World J Surg* 29:513, 2005.

Duffy JP, Hines OJ, Liu JH, and others: Improved survival for adenocarcinoma of the ampulla of Vater: fifty-five consecutive resections, *Arch Surg* 138:941, 2003.

Hayes DH, Bolton JS, Willis GW, and others: Carcinoma of the ampulla of Vater, *Ann Surg* 206:572, 1987.

Hines OJ, Reber HA: Pancreatic surgery, *Curr Opin Gastroenterol* 21:568, 2005.

Hines OJ, Reber HA: Technique of pancreaticojejunostomy for the normal pancreas: reconstruction after pancreaticoduodenectomy, *J Hepatobiliary Pancreat Surg* 13:185, 2006.

Howe JR, Klimstra DS, Moccia RD, and others: Factors predictive of survival in ampullary carcinoma, *Ann Surg* 228:87, 1998.

Jemal A, Siegel R, Ward E, and others: Cancer statistics, 2006, *CA Cancer J Clin* 56:106, 2006.

Joesting DR, Beart RW Jr, van Heerden JA, and others: Improving survival in adenocarcinoma of the duodenum, *Am J Surg* 141:228, 1981.

Kim RD, Kundhal PS, McGilvray ID, and others: Predictors of failure after pancreaticoduodenectomy for ampullary carcinoma, *J Am Coll Surg* 202:112, 2006.

Lu DS, Reber HA, Krasny RM, and others: Local staging of pancreatic cancer: criteria for unresectability of major vessels as revealed by pancreatic-phase, thin-section helical CT, *AJR Am J Roentgenol* 168:1439, 1997.

Nakase A, Matsumoto Y, Uchida K, and others: Surgical treatment of cancer of the pancreas and the periampullary region: cumulative results in 57 institutions in Japan, *Ann Surg* 185:52, 1977.

Neoptolemos JP, Talbot IC, Carr-Locke DL, and others: Treatment and outcome in 52 consecutive cases of ampullary carcinoma, *Br J Surg* 74:957, 1987.

Riall TS, Cameron JL, Lillemoe KD, and others: Pancreaticoduodenectomy with or without distal gastrectomy and extended retroperitoneal lymphadenectomy for periampullary adenocarcinoma, *J Gastrointest Surg* 9:1191, 2005.

Rose DM, Hochwald SN, Klimstra DS, and others: Primary duodenal adenocarcinoma: a ten-year experience with 79 patients, *J Am Coll Surg* 183:89, 1996.

Ryder NM, Ko CY, Hines OJ, and others: Primary duodenal adenocarcinoma: a 40-year experience, *Arch Surg* 135:1070, 2000.

Scott-Coombes DM, Williamson RCN: Surgical treatment of primary duodenal carcinoma: a personal series, *Br J Surg* 81:1472, 1994.

Sohn TA, Lillemoe KD, Cameron JL, and others: Adenocarcinoma of the duodenum: factors influencing long-term survival, *J Gastrointest Surg* 2:79, 1998.

Talamini MA, Moesinger RC, Pitt HA, and others: Adenocarcinoma of the ampulla of Vater. A 28-year experience, *Ann Surg* 225:590, 1997.

Yoon YS, Kim SW, Park SJ, and others: Clinicopathologic analysis of early ampullary cancers with focus on the feasibility of ampullectomy, *Ann Surg* 242:92, 2005.

PALLIATIVE THERAPY FOR PANCREATIC CANCER

Theodore N. Pappas, MD, and Sebastian G. de la Fuente, MD

Pancreatic adenocarcinoma continues to be the fourth leading cause of cancer-related deaths in the United States, accounting for 6% of all cancers for both males and females. In 2006, the American Cancer Society estimated 33,730 new cases of pancreatic cancer, with approximately 32,300 deaths. Even with the advent of accurate diagnostic tools and potent chemoradiation therapies, the prevalence of pancreatic cancer and cancer-related mortality has remained steady through the years. At the time of diagnosis, the vast majority of patients will have locally advanced or metastatic disease not amenable to surgical resection. Even after resection, the 5-year survival rate is approximately 15% to 20% in patients having surgery in high-volume institutions.

Following standardized preoperative staging, tumor resectability may be decided intraoperatively. A tumor in the head of the pancreas is deemed unresectable if there is evidence of (1) celiac or superior mesenteric arterial vascular invasion or encasement; (2) hepatic metastases; (3) peritoneal metastases; (4) extra-abdominal metastases; (5) or metastases to lymph nodes outside of the resection area, for example, para-aortic, celiac, and so forth (Table 1). If vascular invasion is limited to the superior mesenteric or portal veins, surgeons familiar with the technique may attempt vascular reconstruction, although there is no level-I evidence that this will alter the prognosis.

In patients with unresectable disease at time of laparotomy or with prohibitive risks for resection, palliative intervention is performed. The goal of palliative therapy is to alleviate symptoms associated with biliary obstruction, duodenal obstruction, or tumor-related pain. Traditionally, surgical bypass was the preferred method of choice in patients considered unresectable; however, there is growing interest in less invasive approaches such as endoluminal stenting. Stents are associated with reduced rates of complications and mortality but higher incidence of recurrent obstruction compared with surgery (Table 2).

PRESENTATION AND DECISION-MAKING ALGORITHM

The initial evaluation of the patient presenting with suspected pancreatic cancer should include a detailed history and physical examination. The classic presentation of pancreatic cancer is obstructive

Table 1: Determinants of Pancreatic Cancer Unresectability

Vascular invasion*
Hepatic metastases
Peritoneal disease
Extra-abdominal metastases
Metastases to lymph nodes outside of the resection area

*If cancer has invaded into the portal or superior mesenteric vein, a potentially curative resection may be attempted. Curative resections with or without venous resection carry similar prognoses.

Table 2: Comparison between Endoscopic Stents and Surgery for Biliary Decompression

	Endoscopic Stents (n = 789)		Surgical Bypass (n = 180)	
	Range	Mean	Range	Mean
30-Day mortality	0–20	14	0–31	12
Hospital stay (days)	3–26	7	19–30	17
Success rate (%)	82–100	90	75–100	93
Early complications (%)	8–34	21	6–56	31
Late complications (%)	13–45	28	5–47	16

Modified from Watanpa P, Williamson RCN: Br J Surg 79:8, 1992.

jaundice. Jaundice results from obstruction of the intrapancreatic portion of the common bile duct and can be accompanied by pruritus, light stools, and dark urine. If left untreated, biliary obstruction can lead to severe pruritus and worsening hepatic function, exacerbating the patient's overall medical condition; therefore early decompression of the biliary system is usually recommended. Epigastric pain is also present in up to 80% of patients and is described as dull and radiating to the back. Weight loss can be significant and may be related to appetite loss, early satiety, diarrhea, and other factors. Duodenal obstruction is present in approximately 5% to 10% of patients with unresectable pancreatic cancer, although a higher number suffer from nausea and vomiting at presentation. Historical reports have shown that gastric outlet obstruction symptoms can be the first and only sign of advanced pancreatic cancer in up to 7% of patients. These symptoms have direct effects not only on quality of life but also on the patients' nutritional status. For this reason, optimizing gastric emptying is of crucial importance in this population. A small number of patients may also present with acute pancreatitis.

The diagnostic algorithm consists of routine laboratory tests, including liver function tests, amylase, lipase and serum tumor markers, and computed tomography (CT) with intravenous and oral contrast. Endoscopic ultrasonography (EUS) to obtain a biopsy is also part of the preoperative workup, especially if the patient is to undergo neoadjuvant therapy. Other imaging tests that facilitate preoperative staging include magnetic resonance imaging (MRI) and MR cholangiopancreatography (MRCP) if the CT scan is not definitive.

If the cancer has been classified as unresectable on the basis of preoperative imaging, biliary and duodenal drainage may be accomplished by either nonsurgical or surgical interventions with good results (Fig. 1). Historically, surgery has been associated with superior success rates in decompressing the bile system but higher postoperative early morbidity and mortality than endoluminal stents. By contrast, stents offer a less invasive alternative but appear to be associated with higher reocclusion rates and costs (Fig. 2; Table 2). For duodenal obstructions, gastrojejunostomy has been traditionally recommended; however, more recently the use of self-expandable metal enteric stents has been reported as an effective alternative to surgical therapy (Fig. 3).

PALLIATION OF PATIENTS FOUND TO BE UNRESECTABLE ON PREOPERATIVE WORKUP

Palliation of patients found to be unresectable on preoperative staging is generally nonsurgical. Surgery is limited for those who failed nonsurgical management or have significant complications from it. For biliary decompression, stents can be placed either

Figure 1   Decision-making algorithm for unresectable pancreatic cancer patients.* Many patients undergoing laparoscopy have stents placed ahead.

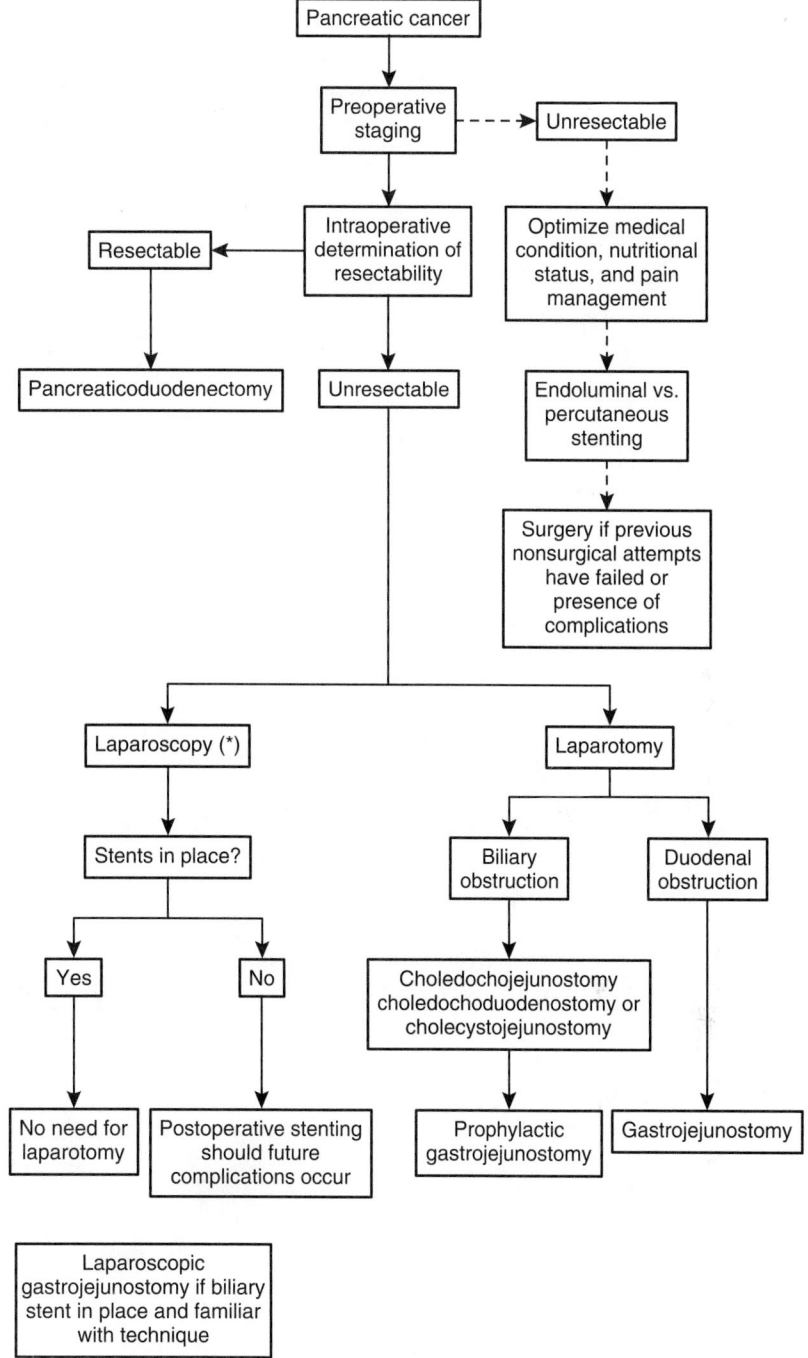

percutaneously or endoscopically, although the great majority are inserted across the obstruction at endoscopy. A prospective randomized trial has shown that endoscopic stenting has a significantly higher rate of jaundice relief (81% vs. 61%) and significantly lower 30-day mortality than percutaneous stent placement. Commercially available stents are constructed of either plastic or metal. Randomized prospective trials have found that relief of jaundice is equally successful with both types of stent; however, metal stents are associated with a lower relative risk of recurrent biliary occlusion (Table 3). This reduction in the risk of reocclusion with metal stents has resulted in fewer reinterventions but is not associated with increased survival. Studies have also shown that occlusion of plastic stents is related to bacterial colonization with biliary sludge deposition in the luminal surface of the stent and bilioduodenal

reflux. Newer metal stents with coating are being developed and less spacing between struts evaluated to reduce the risk of tumor ingrowth resulting in obstruction. Because of the elevated costs of self-expanding metal stents, cost-effective analysis has shown that these stents are justified if expected survival is more than 6 months.

For duodenal obstruction, endoscopic stenting has been shown to be as effective as gastrojejunostomy in terms of overall survival and has been associated in retrospective reports with shorter hospital stays and faster return to oral diet. A recent meta-analysis reviewed all patients published in the literature who underwent duodenal stenting for malignant gastric outlet obstruction. Of the total 606 patients identified, stent placement was successful in 97%. All of these patients were able to resume oral intake, with 87% taking soft solids or a full liquid diet and final resolution of symptoms occurring

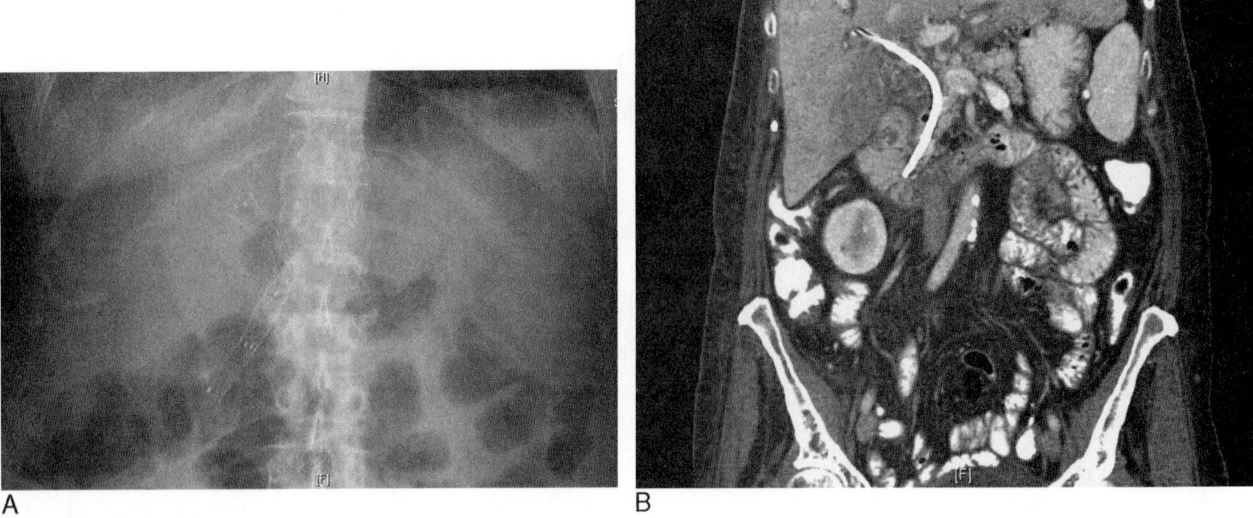

Figure 2 Abdominal plain x-ray **(A)** and computed tomography scan with coronal cuts **(B)** demonstrating self-expanding metal stent in the biliary system of a patient with unresectable pancreatic cancer.

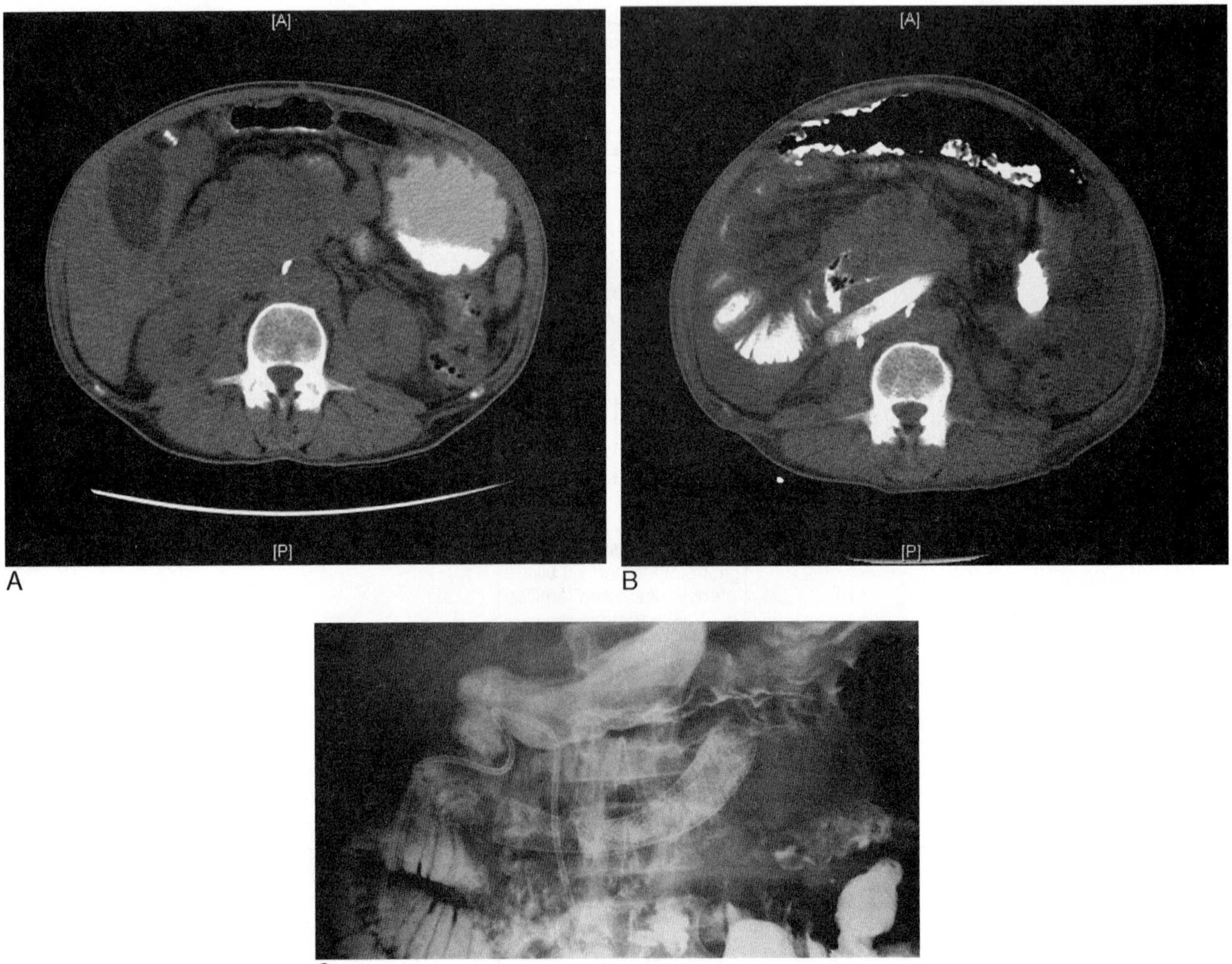

Figure 3 Abdominal computed tomography of patient with large pancreatic mass obstructing the second and third portions of the duodenum **(A)**. The patient underwent endoluminal stent placement with symptomatic relief **(B)**. Two endoluminal self-expanding metal stents were required to alleviate his symptoms **(C)**.

Table 3: Prospective Trials Comparing Recurrent Biliary Obstruction between Self-Expanding Metal Stents versus Plastic Stents

Review: Palliative biliary stents for obstructing pancreatic carcinoma
Comparison: 02 Metal versus Plastic Stent
Outcome: 08 Recurrent biliary obstruction prior to death/end of study

Study	Metal n/N	Plastic n/N	Relative Risk (Fixed) 95% CI	Weight (%)	Relative Risk (Fixed) 95% CI
Carr Locke 1993	11/88	10/78		10.8	1.00 [0.45, 2.22]
Davids 1992b	16/40	30/50		28.9	0.01 [0.38, 0.88]
Kaassis 2003	11/59	22/59		22.7	0.50 [0.27, 0.94]
Knyrim 1993	0/31	12/31		12.4	0.50 [0.21, 0.10]
Prat 1998a	0/34	24/33		25.2	0.24 [0.11, 0.52]
Total (95% Cl)	259	257		100.0	0.52 [0.39, 0.00]

Total events: 50 (Metal), 08 (Plastic)
Test for heterogeneity CHi-square = 8.92 df = 4 p = 0.141 I^2 = 42.2%
Test for overall effect z = 4.44 p<0.00001

0.1   0.2   0.5   1   2   5   10
Favors metal   Favors plastic

From Moss AC, Morris E, MacMathuna P: Palliative biliary stents for obstructing pancreatic carcinoma, *Cochrane Upper Gastrointestinal and Pancreatic Diseases Group Cochrane Database of Systematic Reviews*, 2006.

after a mean of 4 days. There were no documented procedure-related mortalities, but some of the complications noted were stent occlusion resulting from tumor ingrowth in 18%, stent migration in 5%, and bleeding and perforation in 1.2% of patients. Recently a small prospective randomized trial comparing laparoscopic gastrojejunostomy with endoscopic duodenal stent placement confirmed this, but the small number of patients enrolled in the study ($n = 27$) precludes drawing definitive conclusions.

PATIENTS FOUND TO BE UNRESECTABLE DURING LAPAROTOMY

Patients with pancreatic cancer that is unresectable at the time of the staging laparotomy (Table 1) undergo palliative surgical therapy. Biliary bypass can be accomplished by a hepatico-[choledocho]-jejunostomy, cholecystojejunostomy, or choledochoduodenostomy. Several studies in the late 1980s found that choledochojejunostomy is preferred over a cholecystojejunostomy because it offers less postoperative morbidity and mortality and facilitates biliary drainage. Choledochojejunostomy can be performed through a right subcostal or upper midline incision. If the gallbladder is present, a cholecystectomy is performed. The dilatated common bile duct (or common hepatic duct) is identified and exposed proximal to the obstruction. The enteric anastomosis can be made to either a simple jejunal loop or a Roux-en-Y limb (preferred). For side-to-side anastomoses, the bowel is anchored to the bile duct with stay sutures. A 2-cm longitudinal incision is created in the duct adjacent to the small bowel. Using absorbable sutures, the surgeon performs a single-layer anastomosis of enteric bowel wall to bile duct. A drain is left in place in proximity to the anastomosis because there is an expected leak rate of 5% or less with bilio-enteric anastomoses in general. If a stent was placed preoperatively, the abdomen should be irrigated with warm saline to decrease the incidence of wound infection or abdominal abscess because these infectious complications are more common when stents are in place. Alternatively, a choledochoduodenostomy can

be fashioned if there is no obvious invasion of cancer to the duodenum. DiFronzo and colleagues retrospectively reviewed a series of 71 consecutive patients who underwent choledochoduodenostomy for biopsy-proved unresectable pancreatic cancer. Patients experienced a rapid resolution of jaundice with a postoperative mortality of only 3%. There were no leaks or recurrent biliary obstruction in his series. Technically, a choledochoduodenostomy is a relatively straightforward procedure. After the common bile duct is identified, a 2-cm choledochotomy is made longitudinally, and the anastomosis to the duodenum is created with a single layer of interrupted absorbable sutures. Several retrospective studies have shown that a choledochoduodenostomy provides results similar to those of a hepaticojejunostomy (Table 4).

Duodenal obstruction relief is surgically achieved with a gastrojejunostomy. A gastrojejunostomy allows emptying of gastric contents into the jejunum distal to the enteric obstruction. The gastrojejunostomy can be constructed in an antecolic or a retrocolic manner, depending on the operating surgeon's familiarity with the technique. Previous concerns regarding the risk of anastomotic obstruction with retrocolic anastomoses because of the proximity of the tumor to the anastomosis have not been confirmed in randomized trials. To perform a retrocolic gastrojejunostomy, a segment of jejunum is located approximately 15 to 20 cm from the ligament of Treitz and is brought to the greater curvature of the stomach through a window made in the colonic mesentery. The segment of intestine is then tacked to its new location with two silk sutures, and a common enterotomy and gastrotomy are made with electrocautery. The anastomosis is created with staplers or a single-layer suture technique. The anastomosis is fixed to the colonic mesentery to prevent migration of the small bowel into the lesser sac. These patients should be started on H2-blockers or proton pump inhibitors after surgery to prevent marginal ulcer formation. A single-center randomized trial from Johns Hopkins University has demonstrated that a retrocolic anastomosis provides better emptying than an antecolic anastomosis. In contrast, Yilmaz and colleagues prospectively compared two types of gastric bypasses in patients undergoing biliary bypass for cancer of the pancreatic head who were not suitable for

Table 4: Comparative Analysis of Recurrent Biliary Obstruction following Choledochoduodenostomy, Choledochojejunostomy, or Cholecystojejunostomy in Patients with Unresectable Pancreatic Cancer

	No. Patients with Recurrent Biliary Obstruction/Total Patients (%)		
Author	Choledochoduodenostomy	Choledochojejunostomy	Cholecystojejunostomy
Aranha and others	0/8 (0%)	N/A	N/A
Singh and others	4/16 (25%)	8/60 (13%)	10/74 (13%)
Potts and others	1/61 (1.6%)	2/25 (8%)	6/32 (18%)
Welvaart and others	N/A	1/5 (20%)	4/25 (16%)
Huguier and others	83/1159 (7.1%)	39/611 (6.4%)	14/237 (5.9%)
Deziel and others	0/8 (0%)	5/39 (12.8%)	6/28 (21%)
DiFronzo and others	0/71 (0%)	N/A	N/A
Total	88/1323 (6.6%)	55/740 (7.4%)	40/396 (10.1%)

N/A, not available.
Modified from DiFronzo LA, Egrari S, O'Connell TX: Arch Surg 133:820, 1998.

curative resection but with no signs of duodenal obstruction. Twenty-two patients underwent an antecolic, isoperistaltic gastrojejunostomy, jejunojejunostomy, and hepaticojejunostomy, and the remaining 22 had an antecolic, antiperistaltic gastrojejunostomy. No difference was found in the incidence of postoperative complications, time to oral diet, relaparotomy rate, late upper gastrointestinal bleeding, mortality, duration of hospital stay, or survival. The antiperistaltic technique was associated with less delayed gastric emptying, but this was not significant. However, the small number of patients in this study makes a type II error possible. Human and animals studies have shown that interpolating a longer segment of jejunum in the anastomosis has no effect on the gastric emptying of either solids or liquids. In summary, retrocolic gastrojejunostomy may be superior to antecolic, but the difference is likely small.

The decision whether to perform a prophylactic gastrojejunostomy in patients found to be unresectable has been the subject of some debate. Because a significant number of patients will eventually develop gastric outlet obstruction at some point during their disease, a prophylactic gastrojejunostomy at the time of the biliary bypass despite the absence of preoperative obstructive symptoms is the routine care for most specialized surgeons. Lillimoe and colleagues were the first to demonstrate in a prospective randomized trial that performing a prophylactic gastrojejunostomy does not increase perioperative morbidity, mortality, or length of hospital stay. In their series, 194 patients with unresectable disease were randomized to receive either a prophylactic retrocolic gastrojejunostomy or no gastrojejunostomy. No postoperative deaths were seen in either group, and morbidity rates were indistinguishable. The postoperative length of stay in the gastrojejunostomy group was 8.5 ± 0.5 days and 8.0 ± 0.5 days for the no-gastrojejunostomy group. Furthermore, 19% of patients who did not undergo a gastrojejunostomy experienced late gastric outlet obstruction requiring therapeutic intervention. Van Heek and colleagues in a European prospective multicenter trial subsequently confirmed these data by randomizing patients to a hepaticojejunostomy and retrocolic gastrojejunostomy or a hepaticojejunostomy alone. Postoperative clinical symptoms of gastric outlet obstruction were found in 5.5% of patients with the double bypass, compared with 41.4% of those in the single-bypass group ($p = .001$). The authors did not find any difference in the quality of life between the groups; however, the double-bypass group had less need for reoperation (2.8% vs. 20.7%, $p = .04$). Because of the significance of these findings, the trial was stopped earlier than planned.

In summary, palliation at the time of open failed attempt at resection surgery should include a Roux-en-Y biliary bypass to the common duct (preferred) and a retrocolic gastrojejunostomy (preferred), which is recommended for clinical gastric outlet obstruction or prophylactically in patients with no obvious evidence of obstruction.

PALLIATIVE CARE FOR PATIENTS WITH UNRESECTABLE PANCREATIC CANCER AT STAGING LAPAROSCOPY

Since the mid 1990s, widespread accessibility to minimally invasive techniques has broadened the armamentarium of surgeons for the staging and treatment of pancreatic cancer. Laparoscopy has been found to prevent unnecessary laparotomies and enables detection of small, intra-abdominal lesions that are undetectable in preoperative radiographic examinations.

Controversy surrounds the management of patients who are found to have unresectable disease on staging laparoscopy. If the surgeon is familiar with the laparoscopic gastrojejunostomy technique and the patient has a biliary stent in place, laparoscopic duodenal bypass is appropriate because success rates in the hands of an experienced laparoscopic surgeon are similar to those of an open approach. On the contrary, some surgeons prefer not to perform a laparoscopic palliative procedure at the time of the staging laparoscopy and treat any potential biliary and duodenal obstructions with endoluminal stents. In a retrospective review of 155 consecutive patients with unresectable, histologically proved pancreatic adenocarcinoma undergoing surgery at Memorial Sloan-Kettering Cancer Center, Espat and colleagues analyzed the frequency of surgical bypasses performed prophylactically at the time of staging laparoscopy or afterward. In this series, 98% of patients did not require a subsequent open surgical procedure to treat biliary or duodenal obstruction. In those in whom a stent had not been placed preoperatively, endoscopic treatment was successfully achieved postoperatively. The authors concluded that surgical biliary bypass should be advocated only for patients with obstructive jaundice who failed endoscopic stent placement and that open gastroenterostomy should be reserved for patients who have confirmed duodenal obstruction.

Therefore if patients have adequate palliation preoperatively and are found to have unresectable pancreatic cancer at the time of laparoscopy, no further palliation is required at that time.

OUTCOMES OF NONOPERATIVE VERSUS SURGICAL BILIARY DRAINAGE

Overall, survival in patients with unresectable pancreatic cancer is approximately 5 to 6 months and is independent of the type of procedure performed. Comparative studies have been conducted to evaluate nonoperative biliary drainage versus surgical palliation for malignant obstructive jaundice (Table 2). Data from three prospective randomized trials comparing plastic stents with chole-cystojejunostomy or choledochoduodenostomy showed no difference in the relative risk for technical or therapeutic success between stenting and surgery. The incidence of all complications was lower in those receiving stenting. The 30-day mortality also showed a trend favoring stenting; however, this did not reach statistical significance. These studies showed no difference in survival or quality of life between groups; however, hospital stay was shorter for the patients who received stents. No randomized prospective study exists to date comparing metal stents with choledochojejunostomy or any other surgical technique.

TUMOR-RELATED PAIN

Pain control for patients with unresectable pancreatic cancer can be achieved with systemic therapy or neurolysis of the celiac plexus. Systemic therapy includes the use of nonsteroidal anti-inflammatory agents and opiates, which can be administered either orally, intravenously, or transdermally. The four most commonly used techniques for celiac block or neurolysis of the splanich nerves include operative injection at the time of laparotomy, thoracoscopic neurolysis, endoscopic ultrasonography–guided celiac injection, and percutaneous CT-guided injection.

CELIAC PLEXUS BLOCK

Eisenberg and colleagues conducted a meta-analysis to assess the efficacy and safety of neurolytic celiac plexus block for the treatment of cancer-related pain. The study included data of 24 retrospective and prospective papers with a total of 1145 patients. Short-term analgesic efficacy (1–14 days subsequent to the block) was reported in 89% of patients. Further analysis of 274 patients with successful results indicated that 59% experienced complete and 41% experienced partial early (2 weeks or sooner) pain relief. The longer-term outcome (up to 3 months or beyond) was reported in 273 patients; approximately 90% maintained partial or complete pain relief. Data from 53 patients in six studies indicated that 73% and 92% had partial to complete relief when death occurred within or beyond 3 months, respectively. With regard to side effects and complications associated with neurolytic celiac plexus block, most were transient, including local pain in 96% of patients, diarrhea in 44%, and hypotension in 38%. Serious neurologic complications, such as lower extremity weakness, paresthesia, epidural anesthesia, and lumbar puncture, occurred in 1% of patients. Nonneurologic adverse effects occurred in an additional 1% and included pneumothorax; shoulder, chest, and pleuritic pain; and hematuria. No mortality was reported related to the technique. It was concluded from this meta-analysis that neurolytic celiac plexus block has a long-lasting analgesic efficacy with common but transient adverse effects. Recently celiac block has been achieved laparoscopically in nine patients with unresectable disease with no immediate technical difficulties.

All of these techniques have been shown to be effective at relieving pain in patients with unresectable pancreatic cancer, although the best approach should be tailored to each patient on the basis of the degree of pain, limitation of daily activities, and life expectancy.

SPECIAL CONSIDERATIONS

Palliative Pancreaticoduodenectomy

A retrospective review of patients with nonmetastatic pancreatic cancer but positive surgical margins revealed that pancreaticoduodenectomy might offer survival benefits similar to those of biliary and gastric bypass. This finding has yet to be proven in randomized

prospective studies, however. Although the incidence of complications has decreased dramatically over the past 2 decades and the 30-day mortality is less than 5% in high-volume centers following pylorus-preserving pancreaticoduodenectomy, further research is warranted to determine the long-term outcomes and quality of life in patients undergoing resective procedures for margin-positive pancreatic cancers. Research is under way to determine the role of adjuvant chemoradiation in patients who underwent pancreaticoduodenectomy with positive surgical margins. At this time, pancreaticoduodenectomy with palliative intent is not recommended.

Palliative Chemoradiation

The benefits of palliative chemotherapy and radiation in unresectable pancreatic cancer are limited. Several chemotherapeutic regimens have been studied for these patients; unfortunately, objective responses have been disappointing. Frey and colleagues randomized 152 Veterans Administration patients with advanced pancreatic cancer to no treatment versus chemotherapy with 5-fluorouracil and lomustine without any observed benefit on survival. Forty-three patients were randomized by Palmer and colleagues to no therapy versus a combination of 5-fluorouracil, doxorubicin (Adriamycin; Pharmacia, Milan, Italy), and mitomycin. A survival benefit was noted for the chemotherapy-treated patients, but quality of life was not determined in this study. The single-agent gemcitabine has been used in patients with advanced pancreatic cancer after a superior clinical response was demonstrated in a randomized study comparing it with 5-fluorouracil. In this trial, 126 patients with advanced symptomatic pancreatic cancer were administered either gemcitabine at 1000 mg/m^2 weekly for 7 weeks followed by 1 week of rest, then weekly for 3 weeks every 4 weeks thereafter ($n = 63$), or 5-fluorouracil 600 mg/m^2 once weekly ($n = 63$). The outcome measured was clinical response, which was a composite of measurements of pain, Karnofsky performance status, weight, response rate, time to progressive disease, and survival. In this series, 23.8% of gemcitabine-treated versus 4.8% of 5-fluorouracil-treated patients experienced a clinical response ($p = .0022$). The median survival duration was also significantly increased in the group receiving gemcitabine (5.65 vs. 4.41 months, $p = .0025$). More recently, a randomized controlled multicenter phase III trial showed that a four-regimen therapy with cisplatin, epirubicin, fluorouracil, and gemcitabine might be of some benefit for patients with advanced disease.

The radiation options for patients with locally advanced pancreatic cancer include external beam radiation therapy with chemotherapy; intraoperative radiation therapy; and, more recently, external beam radiation therapy with novel chemotherapeutic and targeted agents. Although poorly documented in many studies, some reports have shown symptomatic relief using these techniques in up to 50% of patients. Studies in the 1980s have demonstrated that a combination of radiation (4000 or 6000 cGy) and chemotherapy is superior to either therapy alone; however, no studies to date have documented an objective survival increment with these therapies.

CONCLUSIONS AND OVERALL PROGNOSIS

The 5-year survival in patients with resectable pancreatic cancer who undergo pancreaticoduodenectomy is between 6% and 36% in high-volume, specialized centers. However, the overall prognosis in patients who are found to be unresectable at the time of laparotomy is grim. Unresectable patients who undergo palliative surgery are expected to have a 1-, 2-, and 4-year survival of approximately 25%, 9% and 6%, respectively.

Staging of pancreatic cancer is made preoperatively, but the final decision of whether a tumor is resectable is often made intraoperatively. Patients found to be unresectable at the initial workup should undergo palliative nonoperative therapy if possible. Endoscopic stenting of the bile duct and duodenum provides adequate palliation in most patients. If patients undergoing surgery for possible resection are found to have unresectable cancer, biliary and gastric bypass provide excellent palliation. Patients with endoscopic palliation who are found at staging laparoscopy to be unresectable usually do not require further palliation. The management of pain in patients with unresectable pancreatic cancer is crucial, and this can be achieved with a variety of oral medications and percutaneous techniques with good results. To date, there is no role for palliative pancreaticoduodenectomy. Palliative chemoradiation in patients with advanced pancreatic cancer is often used with modest results.

Suggested Readings

Burris HA 3rd, Moore MJ, Andersen J, and others: Improvements in survival and clinical benefit with gemcitabine as first-line therapy for patients with advanced pancreas cancer: a randomized trial, *J Clin Oncol* 15:2403, 1997.

Chekan EG, Clark L, Wu J, and others: Laparoscopic biliary and enteric bypass, *Semin Surg Oncol* 16:313, 1999.

DiFronzo LA, Egrari S, O'Connell TX: Choledochoduodenostomy for palliation in unresectable pancreatic cancer, *Arch Surg* 133:820, 1998.

Eisenberg E, Carr DB, Chalmers TC: Neurolytic celiac plexus block for treatment of cancer pain: a meta-analysis, *Anesth Analg* 80:290, 1995.

Espat NJ, Brennan MF, Conlon KC: Patients with laparoscopically staged unresectable pancreatic adenocarcinoma do not require subsequent surgical biliary or gastric bypass, *J Am Coll Surg* 188:649, 1999.

Lillemoe KD, Cameron JL, Hardacre JM, and others: Is prophylactic gastrojejunostomy indicated for unresectable periampullary cancer? A prospective randomized trial, *Ann Surg* 230:322, 1999.

Moss AC, Morris E, MacMathuna P: Palliative biliary stents for obstructing pancreatic carcinoma. Cochrane Upper Gastrointestinal and Pancreatic Diseases Group, *Cochrane Database Syst Rev* 3, 2006.

Van Heek NT, De Castro SM, van Eijck CH, and others: The need for a prophylactic gastrojejunostomy for unresectable periampullary cancer: a prospective randomized multicenter trial with special focus on assessment of quality of life, *Ann Surg* 238:894, 2003.

Watanpa P, Williamson RCN: Surgical palliation for pancreatic cancer: developments during the past two decades, *Br J Surg* 79:8–20, 1992.

Yilmaz S, Kirimlioglu V, Katz DA, and others: Randomized clinical trial of two bypass operations for unresectable cancer of the pancreatic head, *Eur J Surg* 167:770, 2001.

Neoadjuvant and Adjuvant Therapy of Pancreatic Cancer

Vincent J. Picozzi, MD, MMM

INTRODUCTION

Pancreatic cancer now represents the fourth most common cause of cancer death in the United States. More than 30,000 deaths per year occur in the United States from this disorder, and more than 200,000 people succumb annually to pancreatic cancer worldwide. Only 2% of patients with pancreas cancer survive 5 years, representing the poorest 5-year survival statistic for any major cancer. Given these statistics, pancreatic cancer may be the most underappreciated and understudied condition in all of oncology.

The situation for patients with resectable pancreatic cancer is little better than for the patient group as a whole. In general, the only patients with pancreatic cancer with potential for protracted survivals are those who are able to undergo complete resection of their cancers. Thus the pancreaticobiliary surgeon plays a critical role in the curative therapy of pancreatic cancer. However, management of pancreatic cancer is just as challenging from the perspective of the surgeon as it is from the perspectives of other oncology disciplines. In the United States, only approximately 15% of patients (≈4500 patients per year) with pancreatic cancer are able to undergo surgery with curative intent. Although the operative mortality for pancreaticoduodenectomy has declined substantially at large-volume centers over the past several decades, a significant fraction of patients still undergo surgery at low- and moderate-volume centers where operative mortalities remain greater than 10%. Furthermore, outcomes from pancreaticoduodenectomy as a sole modality for the treatment of resectable pancreatic cancers remain

Table 1: Results of Pancreaticoduodenectomy-Only Resected Pancreatic Cancer

Author	No. Patients	Median Survival (Months)	Overall Survival (5 Year)
GITSG	22	11	0
Bakkevold	31	11	8
EORTC	54	13	8
ESPAC-1	69	17	8

EORTC, European Organization for the Research and Treatment of Cancer; *ESPAC,* European Study Group for Pancreas Cancer; *GITSG,* Gastrointestinal Tumor Study Group.

surprisingly poor. Median survival after pancreaticoduodenectomy alone for such patients remains disappointingly low (on the order of only 1 year even in contemporary series), with long-term survivals of 10% or less (Table 1).

ADJUVANT THERAPY OF PANCREATIC CANCER

Why Are the Results So Poor?

Why are the results of surgery alone as a sole modality for the treatment of resectable pancreatic cancer so poor? First, virtually all (80%–90%) of such patients experience early systemic recurrence (median time to recurrence was 8 months in one series). This means that, although surgery may be necessary for the curative treatment of pancreatic cancer at this time, it is not sufficient for cure for most patients, even if successfully performed. Pancreatic cancer must be thought of as a systemic illness in all patients, even those resected. Increases in cure rates in the future will ultimately depend on systemic therapy.

Second, even with successful surgery, up to 50% of patients or more experience a local recurrence of their cancer in the peripancreatic bed (with local recurrence rates even higher in patients with microscopically positive margins at surgery). Thus local recurrence, as well as systemic recurrence, must be considered when adjuvant therapies for resected pancreatic cancer are developed. This implies a potential role for radiation therapy as adjuvant treatment for resected pancreas cancer, provided that systemic therapy is not compromised by the use of radiation therapy and additional reductions in local recurrence rates can be achieved with combined modality treatment over the use of systemic therapy only.

Finally, patient comorbidities and postoperative complications may affect the ability to give effective adjuvant therapy for resected pancreatic cancer. The average age of patients with pancreatic cancer is nearly 65 years; cardiovascular, gastrointestinal, and renal comorbidities are common in these patients. Also, in addition to perioperative mortality, postoperative complications (e.g., anastomotic leaks, altered gastric emptying, etc.) may further compromise the ability to deliver postoperative therapy; indeed, 20% to 30% of resected patients fail to receive any adjuvant therapy even at large and experienced centers.

Therefore effective adjuvant therapy for resected pancreas cancer must consider each of the following four factors: (1) systemic recurrence, (2) local recurrence, (3) therapeutic toxicity and patient comorbidity, and (4) patient and physician acceptance.

Given these considerations, why has it been so difficult to develop improved therapeutic outcomes for patients with resected pancreatic cancer? First, as noted, patient age and comorbidity conspire against the ability to deliver effective adjuvant therapy to such patients. Second, pancreatic cancer is difficult to diagnose, particularly at an early stage. As stated earlier, only 15% of patients present as candidates for curative resection, and many of them have already had symptoms for a number of months. Effective prevention and screening techniques for pancreatic cancer and simple systemic therapy for pancreatic cancer are not available.

Third, systemic therapy for pancreatic cancer has been much less effective than it is for other cancers. Even now, response rates of 30% to systemic therapy for patients with advanced disease are considered good, and overall survivals for patients with advanced disease have improved by only a few months over supportive care, results that are much poorer than those achieved for breast and colon cancers, for example. Also, the systemic therapies that have achieved the best response rates (mostly gemcitabine-based combinations) have yet to be applied to resected disease.

Fourth, many types of physicians (medical oncologists, radiation oncologists, gastrointestinal endoscopists, radiologists, pathologists, and others) are involved in the care of pancreatic cancer patients. It takes optimal multidisciplinary coordination to provide ideal care for such patients; few medical centers have the full array of physician interests, abilities, skills, and cooperation to provide such care. Coupled with this is the realization that most of these physician groups have little direct experience caring for pancreatic cancer patients who receive adjuvant therapy. For example, the average medical oncologist in the United States only sees one patient with resected pancreatic cancer every 2 or 3 years; as a result, the majority have never seen a long-term pancreatic cancer survivor.

This leads finally to perhaps the biggest obstacle to the care of the (resected) pancreatic cancer patient: pessimism. Physicians (particularly nonsurgical physicians) have little positive personal experience to energize them. Patients have no ready cohort of similar individuals with whom to share experiences and successes. Of course, all parties know the discouraging statistics on pancreatic cancer either from the medical literature or from the Internet. Thus many patients are doomed to failure from the start simply for lack of optimism and effort.

Key Historical Studies

Any analysis of adjuvant therapy for pancreatic cancer begins with the Gastrointestinal Tumor Study Group (GITSG) trial published in 1985 using postoperative radiation therapy and bolus 5-fluorouracil (FU)[1]. An initial prospective, randomized study compared pancreaticoduodenectomy only ($n = 22$ patients) with pancreaticoduodenectomy plus postoperative chemoradiation ($n = 21$ patients) in patients with resected (R0) pancreatic adenocarcinoma. In the chemoradiation arm of the trial, radiation therapy was administered as two 20-Gy fractions separated by a 2-week break (40 Gy total). Chemotherapy consisted of 5-FU (500 mg/m^2) given as an intravenous (IV) bolus on days 1 to 3 of each radiation course; patients were then given the same dose of 5-FU weekly for 2 years or until disease progression. With chemoradiation, there were significant improvements in both median (20 months vs. 11 months; $p = .05$) and 2-year (43% vs. 18%; $p = .05$) overall survival. Subsequently, an additional 30 patients were treated by the GITSG according to the experimental (chemoradiation) arm of the initial experience; results at 2 years were similar to those reported originally.

The results of the GITSG trial were regarded by many as definitive evidence in support of the role of 5-FU-based chemoradiation as adjuvant treatment for resected pancreatic cancer. However, a number of limitations of this study (only 43 patients randomized within 7 years, no pretreatment stratification, few [28%] node-positive patients, and no margin-positive patients, and approximately one quarter [24%] of patients treated more than 10 weeks after pancreaticoduodenectomy) led others to question the validity of the results. The results were duplicated but not surpassed in a variety of phase II experiences, principally in the United States, including some large patient experiences at premier institutions. One particularly important experience was reported by Sohn and colleagues from Johns Hopkins, in which, in a retrospective review of more than 350 patients, the 5-year actual survival of patients receiving 5-FU-based adjuvant chemoradiation was approximately 20% in contrast to less than 10% for those who did not receive adjuvant treatment As such, this approach to the adjuvant therapy of pancreatic cancer became a standard of care in the United States, and in much of the world, and exists as such even to this day.

Investigational Approaches

The questions remain, however, as to whether this is indeed the best addition to surgery for the curative treatment of pancreatic cancer and which approaches might offer superior outcomes. In this regard, four potential approaches exist: (1) neoadjuvant therapy (chemotherapy or chemoradiation), (2) adjuvant chemotherapy as a sole additional modality to surgery, (3) alternative (chemo)therapy to 5-FU before and after chemoradiation, (4) novel chemoradiation combinations.

Each of these approaches has been explored over the past decade and remains under active clinical investigation.

▊ NEOADJUVANT THERAPY

Neoadjuvant therapy has a variety of potential advantages, both theoretical and practical. First, remembering recurrence patterns after pancreaticoduodenectomy, neoadjuvant drug therapy provides immediate systemic therapy for a disease that is systemic at diagnosis and thus requires effective systemic treatment as soon as possible. Patients who receive adjuvant drug therapy in a "classic" fashion frequently fail to begin treatment for several months. Second, remembering the fraction of patients who fail to receive adjuvant drug therapy postoperatively because of postoperative complications, a greater percentage of patients may be able to receive effective systemic therapy if it is given neoadjuvantly rather than adjuvantly. Third, therapy given neoadjuvantly may be more effective than therapy given adjuvantly because of the nonimpaired perfusion of the tumor bed. Fourth, neoadjuvant therapy may improve the percentage of R0 resection rates, particularly important given that patients with R1 or R2 resections are virtually never cured of their disease and live on average only a matter of months. Finally, patients with rapidly progressive systemic disease may be more readily identified and thus spared the morbidity of pancreaticoduodenectomy. One set of investigators interested in this approach reported that patients who demonstrated disease progression after preoperative chemoradiation had a median life expectancy of only 7 months. Thus a variety of compelling reasons exist to explore the neoadjuvant approach to therapy.

Most clinical trials of neoadjuvant therapy for resected pancreatic cancer have used a combined modality approach. In an initial trial performed by the Eastern Cooperative Oncology Group (ECOG), 53 patients with potentially resectable pancreatic cancer received chemoradiation consisting of 50.4 Gy external beam radiation, continuous infusion 5-FU (1000 mg/m^2 given on days 2–5 and 29–32), and mitomycin C (10/mg^2 on day 2). The results of the study were disappointing; 51% of patients required hospitalization for toxicity, with two toxic deaths resulting from biliary sepsis; only 45% of patients ultimately underwent pancreaticoduodenectomy. Median survival of the patients able to complete all therapy successfully was only 16 months. Given the toxicity displayed by neoadjuvant chemoradiation, other investigators have used different neoadjuvant approaches, including the use of alternative systemic agents (including gemcitabine both as an individual agent and in combination with paclitaxel, and cisplatin) and shortening the course of chemoradiation (i.e., to 30 Gy). Although these approaches have reduced therapeutic toxicity (hospitalization rates typically 10% to 40%), no convincing gains have been made to date in terms of resection rates (typically 50% to 70%) or overall survival (typically 18 to 25 months for resected patients).

ADJUVANT CHEMOTHERAPY

Intellectual leadership in the use of adjuvant chemotherapy has largely come from Europe. The appeal of chemotherapy as a sole therapeutic modality is obvious. Given the frequency of systemic recurrence, the ability to use maximally effective systemic therapy (limited during radiation therapy) while avoiding the toxicities of combined modality treatment should provide maximum systemic benefit.

Two clinical trials in particular illustrate the importance of chemotherapy in the adjuvant therapy of pancreatic cancer. The first is the European Study Group for Pancreas Cancer (ESPAC)-1 trial. As published in 2004, the ESPAC-1 trial randomized 541 patients from 11 countries to receive one of four adjuvant therapies in a 2 by 2 factorial design. The four study arms were: (1) pancreaticoduodenectomy only, (2) chemoradiation using the GITSG regimen, (3) adjuvant chemotherapy consisting of IV bolus 5-FU (425 mg/m^2/day and folinic acid (20 mg/m^2/day) given on 5 consecutive days every 28 days for six cycles, and (4) both chemoradiation and postchemoradiation chemotherapy. Although interpretation of this trial is complicated, the authors demonstrated a statistically superior survival in patients who received adjuvant chemotherapy versus those who did not (20.1 vs. 15.5 months, $p = 0.009$). Conversely, patients who received chemoradiation had a slightly inferior survival to those who did not (15.9 vs. 17.9 months, $p = 0.05$). The survival in each of the four study arms was as follows: pancreaticoduodenectomy only, 16.9 months; chemoradiation alone, 13.9 months; chemotherapy alone, 21.6 months; and both chemoradiation and chemotherapy, 19.9 months. Although the trial is highly controversial with respect to its interpretations surrounding the (lack of) efficacy of chemoradiation, it does emphasize the importance of systemic chemotherapy in improving outcomes following surgery for resected pancreatic cancer.

This point is even more clearly emphasized by a second trial performed in Germany (CONKO-001 trial) that randomized patients

with resected pancreatic cancer to gemcitabine (1000 mg/m^2 IV bolus weekly, 3 times every 28 days for 6 cycles) to observation only. This trial, involving 368 patients, was first reported in 2005 and showed a clear advantage to gemcitabine adjuvant therapy over observation with respect to median disease-free survival (14.2 months vs. 7.5 months, $p = 0.0001$). At the time of its initial analysis, the trial had not (yet) shown an overall survival advantage for the gemcitabine arm; however, this may have been due to the interim nature of the analysis and the fact that many patients on the observation arm crossed over to single-agent gemcitabine after relapse.

ALTERNATIVE CHEMOTHERAPY BEFORE AND AFTER 5-FU-BASED CHEMORADIATION

A third way to enhance the efficacy of adjuvant treatment for resected pancreatic cancer is to change the systemic therapy administered before or after (or both) 5-FU-based chemoradiation. Given the difficulty of achieving adequate resection margins following pancreaticoduodenectomy, radiation therapy seems useful in several ways. First, it could reduce the incidence of positive margins following surgery. Second, it could reduce local recurrence rates when used in conjunction with surgery. Finally, it could reduce the significant morbidities that occur from local recurrence. Bolus 5-FU (as used in the GITSG trial) is now felt to have little or no activity in advanced pancreas cancer.

The Radiation Therapy Oncology Group 9704 trial, the first large-scale randomized clinical trial for the adjuvant therapy of pancreatic cancer successfully conducted in the United States, represents the foremost research effort directed at modifying chemotherapy before and after chemoradiation. In this trial, 442 eligible patients were given 50.4 Gy radiation therapy and continuous infusion 5-FU 250 mg/m^2/day throughout radiation. Patients were randomized between before and after continuous infusion 5-FU (250 mg/m^2/d for 3 weeks) and gemcitabine (1000 mg/m^2 IV bolus 3 of 4 weeks) given over 3 weeks before and 12 weeks subsequent to radiation. Patients with pancreatic head ($n = 380$) cancers, but not body or tail cancers, displayed statistically improved survival when gemcitabine rather than 5-FU was administered (median survival 18.8 months vs. 16.7 months, 3-year overall survival 31% vs. 21%, $p = .05$). Also of note was the incidence of grade III or higher toxicity in this trial (over 60% in the 5-FU arm, approximately 80% in the gemcitabine arm). Thus if 5-FU-based chemoradiation is used, gemcitabine appears to be the superior agent to use both before and after chemoradiation. Yet to be tested are other drug combinations (most particularly gemcitabine-based combinations) used in conjunction with 5-FU-based chemoradiation as adjuvant therapy for pancreatic cancer.

NOVEL CHEMORADIATION COMBINATIONS

If one believes in the efficacy of chemoradiation as demonstrated by the GITSG trial, then this efficacy might be enhanced by novel chemoradiation combinations that would improve both local and systemic anticancer effects. Efforts in this area can be divided into two groups, chemoradiation regimens that are gemcitabine based and those that are 5-FU based. With respect to the former, most studies have been performed on patients with locally advanced pancreas cancer. Experience to date has suggested that the use of gemcitabine with radiation therapy is doable, but associated with significant toxicity, especially hematologic and gastrointestinal toxicity (including bowel perforation).

Exemplary with respect to respectable patients is the most recent MD Anderson Cancer Center experience reported by

Table 2: Phase II Results Virginia Mason Protocol Compared with Other Major Clinical Trials

Author	No. Patients	Median Survival (Months)	Overall Survival (2 Year)	Overall Survival (5 Year)
GITSG	43	21	43	19
Johns Hopkins	366	21	39	16
EORTC	114	16	29	10
ESPAC-1	289	22	40	21
Virginia Mason	43	44	58	42

EORTC, European Organization for the Research and Treatment of Cancer; ESPAC, European Study Group for Pancreas Cancer; GITSG, Gastrointestinal Tumor Study Group.

Varadhachary and colleagues. They employed in 78 potentially resectable patients both the gemcitabine/cisplatin chemotherapy "doublet" (gemcitabine 750 mg/m^2 and cisplatin 30 mg/m^2 every 2 weeks for 4 cycles and 30 Gy radiation in 10 fractions together with gemcitabine 400 mg/^{2} IV bolus for 4 administrations, all given neoadjuvantly. Ninety-four percent of patients completed the therapy, and 66% underwent successful resection. Median survival of the study group was 21 months, similar to previous results.

With respect to novel 5-FU-based chemoradiation, the most promising approach to date has been reported from Virginia Mason Hospital using cisplatin and alpha-interferon in conjunction with infusional 5-FU during chemoradiation (the so-called Virginia Mason protocol). The logic behind this approach was to create a combination of drugs that were synergistic both with respect to radiosensitization and with respect to cytotoxicity. The specific regimen as it is now employed consists of 50.4 Gy of radiation given over 28 fractions days 1 to 38 (with reduced radiation field size to minimize toxicity) combined with 5-FU 175 mg/m^2 IV via continuous infusion IV days 1 to 38, cisplatin 30mg/m^2 given weekly (days 1, 8, 15, 22, 29, and 36), and alpha-interferon 3 by 10^6 million units every Monday, Wednesday, and Friday during treatment (17 treatments total, days 1–38). Two 6-week infusions of continuous infusion 5-FU at a dose of 200 mg/m^2 daily separated by a 2-week break (weeks 11 to 16 and 19 to 24) complete the therapy. The toxicity of this regimen proved to be significant (70% of patients required interruption in chemoradiation, and approximately 40% were hospitalized at some point during treatment for therapy-related toxicity). However, despite a patient population that was prognostically adverse on the basis of pathologic features (Table 2), the 5-year actual (not actuarial) overall survival for the initial patient group of 42 patients with head of pancreas lesions has remained more than 40%.

(NEO)ADJUVANT THERAPY OF PANCREATIC CANCER—LESSONS LEARNED AND FUTURE DIRECTIONS

On the basis of the foregoing experiences, the following general conclusions seem applicable to the (neo)adjuvant therapy of pancreatic cancer: (1) long-term survivorship with surgery only is poor. (2) Chemotherapy clearly appears to improve overall survivorship following surgery for pancreatic cancer and thus should be offered to all patients capable of receiving it as part of an adjuvant therapy program (CONKO-001 trial, ESPAC-1). (3) Both 5-FU and gemcitabine appear to have value in this regard; which single agent is superior is yet to be determined with certainty (RTOG 9704, ESPAC-3). (4) To what extent radiation therapy adds to the effectiveness of chemotherapy as adjuvant treatment for pancreatic cancer is not yet clear. (5) Neoadjuvant therapy for resectable pancreatic cancer, although attractive in theory, has yet to be proved beneficial and thus remains an area for clinical investigation and not standard practice. (6) Many therapeutic approaches to pancreatic cancer for advanced pancreatic cancer, including chemotherapeutic drug combinations, "targeted" therapies, and immunotherapy, are just beginning to receive wide-scale test as part of adjuvant therapy for pancreatic cancer. (7) Single-institution experience suggests it may be possible to achieve better overall survival statistics in the near future for the (neo)adjuvant treatment of pancreatic cancer (Virginia Mason experience). (8) Referral of patients with resectable pancreatic cancer to experienced, high-volume treatment centers may optimize patient outcomes in terms of both overall survival and toxicity avoidance.

Drawing from these lessons, a wide variety of clinical trials is currently under way or in development around the world to improved therapeutic outcomes for resected pancreatic cancer (Table 3). With respect to neoadjuvant therapy, additional

Table 3: Major Ongoing Clinical Trials Resected Pancreatic Cancer

Cooperative Group	Trial Type	# Patients	Protocol Schema
ESPAC-3	Phase III	990	gem × 6 cycles vs. 5-FU/leucovorin × 6 cycles
EORTC 40013	Phase II/Phase III	538	gem × 2 cycles → gem/XRT vs. gem × 4 cycles
ACOSOG Z05031	Multi-institutional Phase II	89	cisplatin/5-FU/alpha-interferon/XRT → 5-FU × 2 cycles
ECOG 2204	Randomized phase II	126	gem × 1 cycle plus XRT/capecitabine/ plus gem × 5 cycles with bevacizumab vs. cetuximab
JHMI J9988	Phase II	60	vaccine → 5-FU based chemoradiation → vaccine

ACOSOG, American College of Surgeons Oncology Group; ECOG, Eastern Cooperative Oncology Group; EORTC, European Organization for the Research and Treatment of Cancer; ESPAC, European Study Group for Pancreas Cancer; 5-FU, 5-fluorouracil; gem, gemcitabine; GITSG, Gastrointestinal Tumor Study Group; JHMI, Johns Hopkins Medical Institutions; XRT, x-ray therapy.

trials, using either the MD Anderson model of chemoradiation or chemotherapy alone in a fashion analogous to that used in the MAGIC (**M**edical Research Council **A**djunct **G**astric **I**nfusional **C**hemotherapy) trial performed in patients with localized gastroesophageal cancer. As in the MAGIC trial, the ESPAC-3 trial (which randomizes 5-FU/leucovorin as used in the ESPAC-1 trial against gemcitabine as used in the CONKO-1 trial) studies the use of chemotherapy as a sole therapeutic modality. This trial will soon be ready for analysis.

Multiple trials of interest involving chemoradiation are also ongoing. The European Organization for the Research and Treatment of Cancer (EORTC) is conducting a phase II/ III trial (EORTC 40013) comparing bolus gemcitabine (1000mg/m^2 weekly 3 times every 28 days) followed by weekly gemcitabine combined with radiation as adjuvant therapy versus bolus gemcitabine only. The American College of Surgeons Oncology Group has completed a phase II trial (ACOSOG Z05031) that will assess the reproducibility of the Virginia Mason experience in a multi-institutional setting. Other centers in the United States (Washington University in St. Louis; MD Anderson Cancer Center) and Europe (Heidelberg) are also exploring this approach.

Studies are also under way using radiation therapy in combination with capecitabine (a 5-FU pro-drug) and drugs targeted against growth factor receptors on the surface of cancer cells (so-called targeted therapies). ECOG is investigating in a randomized phase II study a chemoradiation combination of capecitabine and either bevacizumab or cetuximab; gemcitabine given with either bevacizumab and cetuximab before and after chemoradiation in a fashion analogous to that used in RTOG 9704. Finally, a novel approach to adjuvant therapy that involves vaccination with allogeneic tumor cells genetically modified to express costimulatory cytokines (in this case, sargramostin) is under investigation at Johns Hopkins. Initial results from this experience (JHMI J9988) have been encouraging, producing initial results similar to those seen in the Virginia Mason experience.

ROLE OF THE SURGEON

In conclusion, the pancreaticobiliary surgeon plays a pivotal role in the (neo)adjuvant therapy of pancreatic cancer that extends far beyond mere operative skill. First, the pancreaticobiliary surgeon must select with thought and accuracy those patients who are candidates for a treatment approach that, although potentially curative, is also exceedingly difficult both physically and emotionally. Second, because surgery alone has clearly been shown to be insufficient to maximize overall survival among resected

patients, the pancreaticobiliary surgeon must be aware of novel (neo) adjuvant therapeutic approaches to pancreatic cancer (such as the ones described in this chapter) and be willing to participate in clinical trials designed to test these approaches. Third, pancreaticobiliary surgeons must recognize their role as essential members of an entire team of physicians—including radiologists, pathologists, gastroenterologists, medical oncologists, and radiation oncologists—each of whose skills and cooperation are essential to optimizing patient outcomes. Fourth, the pancreaticobiliary surgeon must maintain a volume of surgical activity that enables superior surgical outcomes and minimizes morbidity and, if not, to refer to high-volume centers that specialize in the (neo)adjuvant treatment of resected pancreatic cancer. Finally, the pancreaticobiliary surgeon must pay assiduous attention to the postoperative recovery and rehabilitation of the resected patient, and especially to their nutritional, gastroenterologic, and psychologic recovery, so that the remaining treatment can be delivered with promptness and success.

If pancreaticobiliary surgeons can fulfill these roles, they will serve an indispensable purpose in contributing to the improved survival for patients with localized pancreatic cancer that seem certain to come in the near future.

SUGGESTED READINGS

Kalser MH, Ellenberg SS: Pancreatic cancer; adjuvant combined radiation and chemotherapy following curative resection, *Arch Surg* 120:899, 1985.

Neoptolemos JA, Stocken DD, Friess H, and others: A randomized trial of chemoradiotherapy and chemotherapy after resection of pancreatic cancer, *N Engl J Med* 350:1200, 2004.

Neuhaus P, Oettle H, Post S, and others: A randomized, prospective, multicenter phase III trial of adjuvant chemotherapy with gemcitabine vs. observation in patients with resected pancreas cancer, *Proc ASCO* 311s (abstract 4013), 2005.

Picozzi VJ, Traverso LW: The Virginia Mason approach to localized pancreatic cancer, *Surg Onc Clin North Am* 13:663, 2004.

Pisters PWT, Wolff RA, Janjan NA, and others: Preoperative paclitaxel and concurrent rapid-fractionation radiation for resectable pancreatic adenocarcinoma: toxicities, histologic response rates, and event-free outcome, *J Clin Oncol* 20:2537, 2002.

Regine WF, Winter KW, Abrams R, and others: RTOG 9704: a phase III study of adjuvant pre and post chemoradiation, 5-FU vs. gemcitabine for resected pancreatic adenocarcinoma, *Proc ASCO* 42:181s (abstract 4007), 2006.

Sohn TA, Yeo CJ, Cameron JL, and others: Resected adenocarcinoma of the pancreas—616 patients; results, outcomes, and prognostic indicators, *J Gastrointest Surg* 4:567, 2000.

UNUSUAL PANCREATIC TUMORS

Kacy Phillips, MD, Jason B. Fleming, MD, Eric P. Tamm, MD, and Douglas B. Evans, MD

INTRODUCTION

Patients may be referred to a surgeon for a mass in the pancreas after cross-sectional imaging has been obtained to investigate a gastrointestinal or abdominal complaint that may or may not be related to the pancreas. The pancreatic mass may appear cystic or solid or may have cystic and solid components. The widespread use of cross-sectional abdominal imaging has increased the number of patients with such incidental pancreatic lesions. The difficulty in confirming the diagnosis on the basis of imaging studies alone and the frequent complexity of obtaining a tissue diagnosis (because of the anatomic location of the pancreas) make incidental pancreatic lesions a diagnostic and treatment challenge for many physicians. This chapter provides a differential diagnosis for incidental and rare pancreatic lesions and reviews treatment recommendations on the basis of histologic diagnosis.

GENERAL APPROACH TO PATIENTS WITH A PANCREATIC MASS

High-quality imaging is necessary for the proper management of patients with a pancreatic mass. Following a complete history and physical examination, we use a multislice or multidetector computed tomography (MDCT) to image the pancreas. This allows visualization of the entire pancreas at peak contrast enhancement. The scanned data can then be processed and displayed in three-dimensional and multiplanar formats, allowing assessment of the relationship of the low-density tumor to important adjacent vascular structures: the celiac axis, superior mesenteric artery (SMA), and superior mesenteric-portal vein (SMPV) confluence. Patients with a clinical history suggesting pancreatic cancer (biliary obstruction, weight loss, abdominal discomfort and pain) who do not have a low-density mass identified by CT should undergo upper endoscopy and endoscopic ultrasound (EUS). EUS-guided fine needle aspiration (FNA) is the procedure of choice for obtaining the cytologic diagnosis of a pancreatic or periampullary neoplasm. However, FNA should be avoided if biopsy results would not influence the treatment plan. Appropriate uses of EUS-guided FNA biopsy include the following:

- patients with presumed resectable adenocarcinoma of the pancreas eligible for neoadjuvant protocol-based therapy,
- patients with locally advanced or metastatic tumors of the pancreas in whom a cytologic diagnosis is necessary for the delivery of systemic therapy or local-regional chemoradiation,
- patients who are suspected to have pancreatic metastases or large cell lymphoma, and
- patients with cystic neoplasms, especially those in whom non-operative management would be appropriate such as those with suspected small mucinous neoplasms, serous cystadenomas, or lymphoepithelial cysts.

INTRADUCTAL PAPILLARY MUCINOUS NEOPLASM

Intraductal papillary mucinous neoplasms (IPMNs) form an increasingly well-recognized yet rare category of pancreatic neoplasms. IPMNs are defined by the World Health Organization as papillary mucin-producing neoplasms arising in the main pancreatic duct or its major branches. Although the true incidence of IPMNs remains unknown, they are thought to represent approximately 1% of pancreatic neoplasms and up to one fourth of pancreatic cystic neoplasms. IPMNs are best known for their thick, mucin-rich fluid exuding from the ampulla as seen at the time of endoscopic retrograde cholangiopancreatography (ERCP). IPMNs are distinguished from mucinous cystic neoplasms by their direct communication with the main or branch pancreatic ducts (Fig. 1), their proximal location, male predominance, occurrence

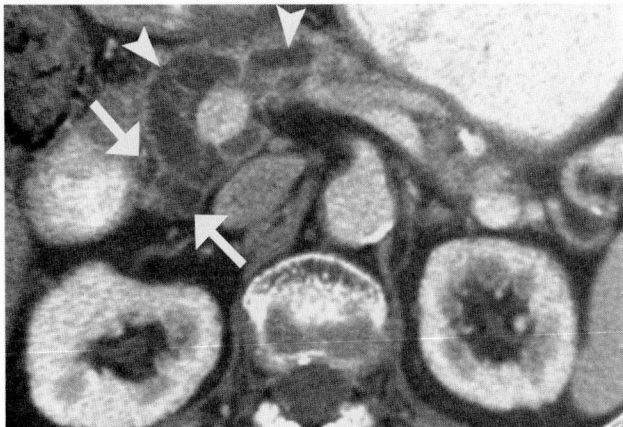

Figure I   Axial contrast-enhanced computed tomography of main duct type intraductal papillary mucinous neoplasms. The main pancreatic duct *(white arrowheads)* is dilatated with mucin. Multiple cystic lesions in the pancreatic side branches *(white arrows)* are also seen.

in older patients (usually in the seventh decade of life), and absence of ovarian-like stroma on histologic sections (found in mucinous cystic neoplasms). In contrast, mucinous cystic neoplasms (MCNs) occur as circumscribed unilocular or multilocular cysts at least partially encapsulated by fibrous tissue with no communication with the pancreatic ducts; they arise most often in the body or tail of the pancreas, have a female predominance, and usually occur in younger individuals (aged 40 to 50 years).

Important points to remember in the management of patients with suspected or proven IPMN include the following:

- Malignant (invasive) IPMN is more likely with proximal tumor location, main pancreatic duct involvement, and large tumor size.
- Low-level serum elevations of carbohydrate antigen (CA) 19–9 do not accurately distinguish invasive from noninvasive IPMN.
- IPMNs are often noninvasive (with or without dysplasia or carcinoma in situ), and therefore even a malignant diagnosis by FNA does not confirm invasive disease. For almost any primary tumor, the diagnosis of invasion can be made definitively only when tumor cells are seen infiltrating through the basement membrane into surrounding connective tissue. To appreciate this finding microscopically, histologic tissue sections are necessary and, in the case of IPMN, may require excision of the entire mass to find the focus of invasive disease necessary for this diagnosis. Despite this limitation, FNA is of value in the management of selected patients with suspected IPMN. For example, FNA biopsy results document the presence or absence of mucin when the radiographic characteristics of a cystic neoplasm are not typical for IPMN, and therefore the differential diagnosis may include other nonmucinous tumors. In contrast, in a good-risk patient in whom main duct IPMN is apparent on CT or endoscopy (mucin seen extruding from the ampulla), FNA biopsy is unlikely to provide additional information that would alter a recommendation for surgery.

The consensus statement from the International Association of Pancreatology for management of IPMNs and MCNs of the pancreas supports resection of all main-duct IPMNs (duct diameter >10 mm) and mixed-variant IPMNs in good-risk surgical candidates. In patients of advanced age or with significant medical comorbidities, it is important to remember that the risk for invasive cancer is low in patients with a main pancreatic duct diameter of less than 15 mm and no visible mural nodules (on CT or EUS); observation may be reasonable in such patients. Because the incidence of invasive cancer is lower in branch-duct IPMNs, a less aggressive surgical approach can be supported. Serial observation is appropriate for asymptomatic patients with branch-duct IPMNs less than 30 mm in size with a main duct of less than 10 mm and no visible mural nodules.

MUCINOUS CYSTIC NEOPLASM

Mucinous cystic neoplasms account for only 2% of pancreatic neoplasms but 30% of pancreatic cystic neoplasms. These usually present as a cystic mass located in the body or tail of the pancreas in women in their 40s or 50s. Although detailed natural history studies are not available, it is generally believed that MCNs increase in size and risk of malignancy over time. As is often seen in colon adenocarcinoma, MCNs are thought to have the potential to progress from cellular atypia to frank malignancy. The distal location of these lesions makes jaundice a rare symptom in affected patients, but many present with pain. The presence of any symptom is associated with an increased risk for malignancy. Imaging of an MCN with CT or magnetic resonance imaging (MRI) usually identifies a thick wall around the cyst that is not present with serous cystadenomas, and the identification of calcification within the wall also supports the

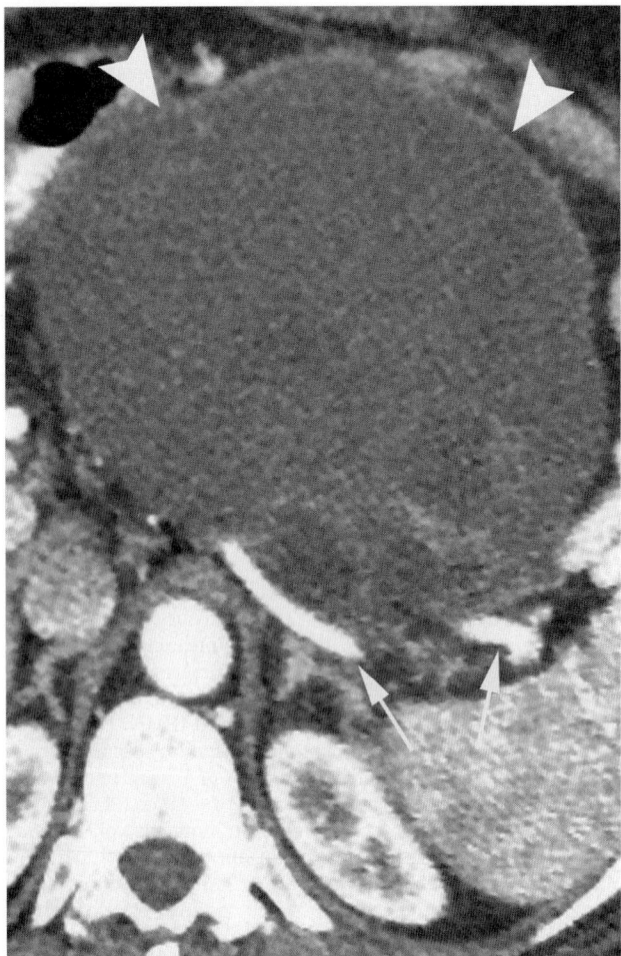

Figure 2 Axial contrast-enhanced computed tomography of a mucinous cystic neoplasm demonstrating a large cystic mass *(white arrowheads)* with internal septations compressing the splenic artery *(white arrows).*

diagnosis of an MCN. It should also be remembered that MCNs can present with a large, unilocular or a smaller, multilocular architecture (Fig. 2). Examination by ERCP or magnetic resonance cholangiopancreatography (MRCP) demonstrates that MCNs rarely communicate with the main pancreatic duct, which distinguishes MCN from IPMN. The thick cyst wall can appear similar to that seen with a pancreatic pseudocyst, and it is often necessary to distinguish MCNs from pancreatic pseudocysts by cross-sectional imaging in combination with EUS-guided FNA. Aspiration of the cyst contents identifies clear, thick, mucin-rich fluid within MCNs and thin, dark, opaque, nonmucinous fluid within pseudocysts. Biopsy is also necessary to confirm the presence of mucin when the differential diagnosis contains nonmucinous cysts. The presence of elevated levels of tumor markers, such as carcinogenic embryonic antigen (CEA), in the cyst fluid is usually a reliable method to differentiate MCNs from serous cystadenomas or pseudocysts. As is the case with IPMNs, FNA cannot reliably distinguish invasive from noninvasive MCNs, and the definitive diagnosis of an MCN requires tumor removal and the identification of a distinctive, ovarian-like stroma within the cyst wall on histologic sections.

The malignant potential of MCNs supports current recommendations that MCNs be resected in all suitable operative candidates. Distal pancreatectomy is usually the required operation because of the distal location of most MCNs. Frozen-section examination of the pancreas margin is recommended because a suspected MCN

could represent an IPMN with invasive disease at the margin. Laparoscopic pancreatectomy may be considered when the risk for invasive carcinoma is thought to be low, the cyst is small (<3 cm), and it has no visible evidence of mural nodules or calcification. The risk of recurrence following resection of MCNs without invasive carcinoma should be zero, unlike the situation with noninvasive IPMNs in which the remaining pancreas is at risk for the development of additional neoplasms. In contrast, patients who have undergone resection of malignant (invasive) MCNs have a significant risk of recurrence and should have a follow-up program similar to that for patients with typical pancreatic ductal adenocarcinoma.

SEROUS CYSTADENOMA

Serous cystadenomas are usually composed of multiple small cysts filled with serous fluid and account for 1% to 2% of all pancreatic neoplasms and one quarter of all cystic pancreatic tumors. Serous cystadenomas are distributed evenly throughout the pancreas and are often found incidentally on CT (Fig. 3) or ultrasound. When serous cystadenomas become symptomatic, it is usually because of large size (up 15 cm), and symptoms are caused by tumor impingement on adjacent viscera. For example, serous cystadenomas in the pancreatic head may cause gastric outlet obstruction or, rarely, may obstruct the bile duct. Serous cystadenomas typically have a

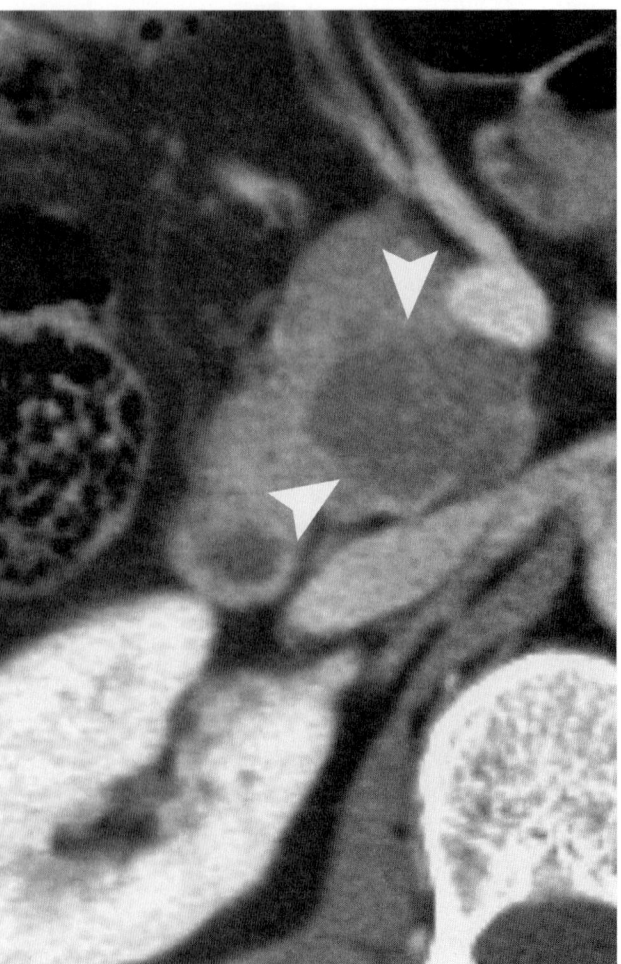

Figure 3 Axial contrast-enhanced computed tomography of a serous cystadenoma demonstrating a complex cystic lesion in the pancreatic head *(white arrowheads).* The lesion shows a "ground glass" appearance secondary to many tiny cysts.

female predominance, which is similar to MCNs, but these patients usually present later in life (the mean age at presentation is 61 years). Unlike MCNs, serous cystadenomas lack mucin and are generally believed to carry no risk for transformation to invasive cancer. On CT imaging, serous cystadenomas display a thin-walled capsule; this is unlike MCNs, which have a characteristically thick epithelial wall. Two additional distinct characteristic findings seen on CT images are the sunburst pattern of calcification with a central scar and honeycombing of the cyst by thin-walled septae. Similar to MCNs, serous cystadenomas do not communicate with the main pancreatic duct. The epithelial lining of these cysts can become denuded, making it difficult to distinguish these from pseudocysts or MCNs, and the diagnosis may necessitate using a periodic acid-Schiff (PAS) stain following biopsy or resection to identify the glycogen-positive clear cells characteristic of cystadenoma.

Serous cystadenomas are generally thought to be benign. A malignant variant of the benign serous cystadenoma may exist, termed *serous cystadenocarcinoma*, and a handful of such cases have been reported, although all are rather poorly documented. Pathological examination of the malignant variant is microscopically identical to serous cystadenomas, with only the presence of metastases to distinguish them as malignant. Therefore clinicians should consider serous cystadenomas to be benign cystic neoplasms of the pancreas. If the diagnosis is confirmed by either radiographic imaging (classic findings of sunburst calcification, central scar, and internal honeycomb appearance) or FNA biopsy (absence of mucin, low CEA level in the cyst fluid, positive PAS stain for glycogen), surgery is not indicated unless local symptoms are present or tumor size suggests that symptoms will develop. Clearly it is inappropriate to consider resection of a serous cystadenoma of small size in an asymptomatic patient of any age, or one of any size in an asymptomatic patient of advanced age or with significant medical comorbidities. After they are identified, cystadenomas can be expected to increase in size at a rate of approximately 0.6 cm per year; however, tumors larger than 4 cm at the time of discovery may increase up to 2 cm per year and are thus more likely to be associated with new or progressively worsening symptoms. On the basis of these observations, surgery has been recommended for reasonable surgical candidates with lesions 4 cm or larger.

Although the vast majority of serous cystadenomas have a microcystic pattern with cysts lined by simple, cuboidal cells, a macroscopic variant can occur. Macrocystic serous cystadenomas are also benign, but they can appear similar to MCNs on CT and EUS, possibly resulting in their surgical resection because of concern over a mucinous (premalignant) neoplasm. Macrocystic serous cystadenomas do not exhibit the typical honeycomb pattern or classic sunburst pattern of calcification within a central scar that is seen with microcystic adenomas on CT imaging. Also, they predominantly occur in women in the fifth decade, which is younger than patients with microcystic adenomas, who present in the seventh decade. Lastly, macrocystic serous cystadenomas, like MCNs, frequently appear as solitary cysts that do not communicate with the pancreatic ducts on cross-sectional imaging. Unlike MCNs, macrocystic serous cystadenomas have a relatively higher male-to-female ratio, a higher frequency of tumors occurring in the head of the pancreas, and smaller cyst size. Knowledge of these distinguishing clinical features in addition to FNA sampling for the presence of mucin should be used to differentiate these two forms of cystic neoplasms preoperatively.

LYMPHOEPITHELIAL CYST

Lymphoepithelial cysts (LECs) are rare (64 cases have been described in the literature since its first description in 1985) benign cystic lesions of uncertain origin that are predominately identified in men (a 4:1 male-to-female ratio) between the fifth and sixth decades of life. The majority of lymphoepithelial cysts are detected incidentally by abdominal ultrasound or CT images. Lymphoepithelial cysts

are often greater than 5 cm in size and may be located throughout the pancreas yet rarely cause symptoms such as abdominal pain or gastric outlet obstruction. On CT imaging, lymphoepithelial cysts are seen as low attenuation, multilocular (60%) or unilocular (40%) neoplasms with a thin, enhancing rim of fibrous tissue. Lymphoepithelial cysts are usually positioned just beneath the surface of the pancreas, and the cyst cavity is not contiguous with the main pancreatic duct. The cysts are filled with a dense material composed mainly of debris, keratin, and cholesterol crystals, and MRI can often detect the lipid component of these cysts. Additionally, the high keratin content of cyst fluid often produces a high signal on T1-weighted images and a low signal on T2-weighted images; this distinguishes lymphoepithelial cysts from other cystic neoplasms.

Histologic sections of lymphoepithelial cysts identify a thin wall of keratinized stratified squamous epithelium that is surrounded by mature lymphoid tissue with intervening germinal centers. The squamous epithelium is responsible for the keratin and debris within the cyst. Immunohistochemical examination of cells from this keratin layer stain positive for the presence of the CA19–9 antigen, and cyst fluid often contains high levels (in the malignant range) of tumor markers such as CEA and CA19–9 and variable levels of amylase. Reliance on these findings alone could lead to the resection of this benign lesion, and thus it is recommended that squamous cells, keratin debris, lymphocytes, and cholesterol crystals be searched for within the cyst contents following aspiration biopsy; their presence confirms the diagnosis of a lymphoepithelial cyst. Most lymphoepithelial cysts would be observed (and surgery avoided) if the diagnosis is secure and the patient asymptomatic. If the cyst is causing biliary or gastric outlet obstruction, there may be a role for intraoperative biopsy to guide the extent of resection. We prefer to avoid pancreaticoduodenectomy for a benign lesion such as this. In contrast to the intraoperative management of mucinous and serous lesions, internal drainage into a Roux-en-Y limb of jejunum is a reasonable option for large lymphoepithelial cysts that would otherwise involve a complex multiorgan resection.

LYMPHOPLASMACYTIC SCLEROSING PANCREATITIS

Lymphoplasmacytic sclerosing pancreatitis (LPSP), a recently recognized form of autoimmune pancreatitis, is a rare condition that clinically and radiographically mimics pancreatic adenocarcinoma. The presenting symptoms of patients with LPSP may include abdominal pain, jaundice, exocrine pancreatic insufficiency, and diabetes mellitus. Patients with LPSP usually have no history of alcohol abuse or gallbladder disease, but the patient or his or her family often has a history of other autoimmune diseases. CT images often show an enhancing and diffusely enlarged pancreas with no evidence of pancreatic duct dilatation and no surrounding edema or inflammation, as one would usually see with diffuse pancreatitis (Fig. 4). MRI confirms the enlargement but can also identify a low-density, capsulelike rim corresponding to inflamed pancreatic tissue. ERCP, if performed, usually identifies narrowing of the intrapancreatic common bile duct and narrowing or obliteration of the pancreatic duct at one or multiple sites.

LPSP is believed to be an autoimmune disease, but knowledge of the pathophysiology is incomplete. An important clinical observation was the identification of high serum concentrations of the immunoglobulin (IgG) subclass 4 fraction of gamma globulins within the serum of many of these patients. This has helped to define LPSP as unique from other diverse causes of chronic inflammation of the pancreas and biliary tree including pancreatic cancer, classic chronic pancreatitis, primary biliary cirrhosis, and primary sclerosing cholangitis. To improve the predictive value of the presence of serum IgG4, some investigators have combined serum IgG4 levels with measurement of other serum antibodies against pancreas-

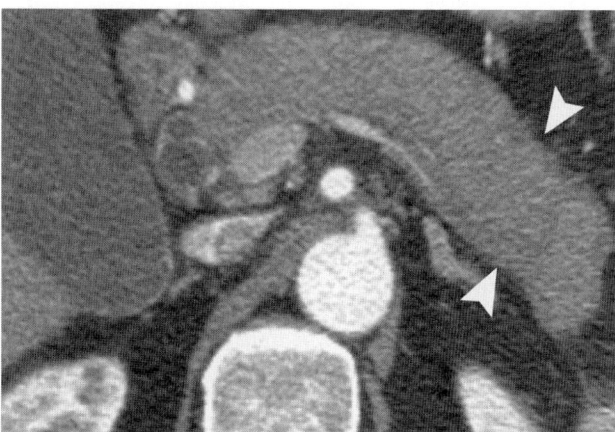

Figure 4 Axial contrast-enhanced computed tomography of lymphoplasmacytic sclerosing pancreatitis. The pancreas shows diffuse thickening throughout (*white arrowheads*).

specific antigens, such as anticarbonic anhydrase II. Combining these serum tests with a history of autoimmune disease greatly increases the likelihood of autoimmune pancreatitis in the appropriate clinical setting. Approximately 70% of specimens resected from patients with autoimmune pancreatitis have moderate to large numbers of IgG4-positive plasma cells in and around ducts, interlobular fibrous tissue, and peripancreatic fat. In contrast, only 11% to 12% of specimens from patients with chronic pancreatitis and ductal adenocarcinomas have this finding. Consequently, the presence of infiltrating lymphocytes within the stroma of the pancreas may help to identify these patients preoperatively. EUS-guided biopsy has been offered as a possible means to obtain tissue to identify IgG4-positive plasma cells and other lymphocytic infiltrates within the pancreas, but current reports in the literature do not suggest that it is a reliable method for decision making because only one third of biopsy specimens from patients with confirmed autoimmune pancreatitis exhibited lymphocyte infiltration into the stroma.

In an effort to establish standardized diagnostic criteria for autoimmune pancreatitis, the Japan Pancreas Society proposed use of the following data: (1) radiologic imaging demonstrating diffuse swelling of the pancreas and segmental or diffuse irregular narrowing of the main pancreatic duct, (2) laboratory data consisting of an elevated IgG or detection of autoantibodies, and (3) histopathologic evidence of lymphoplasmacytic infiltration and fibrosis. According to these recommendations, the diagnosis of autoimmune pancreatitis requires one of two scenarios: (1) all of the criteria are present or (2) criterion 1 is present in addition to either criterion 2 or criterion 3. Given the similarity in clinical presentation between LPSP and pancreatic adenocarcinoma, LPSP is a challenging diagnosis to make even in the proper clinical setting and with typical radiographic imaging findings.

After LPSP is diagnosed, the mainstay of treatment is systemic corticosteroids, particularly for patients with symptoms such as abdominal pain, jaundice, and steatorrhea. The recommended starting dose of glucocorticoid therapy is 30 to 40 mg of prednisone per day (or 0.6 to 0.8 mg/kg/day) until symptoms improve, followed by a steroid taper to 5 to 10 mg per day. If the patient has an intact pancreas (has not had surgical resection), a radiographic response to steroid therapy should be observed within 4 weeks. If no reduction in the pancreas enlargement is seen, the diagnosis of LPSP should be reconsidered. Because of the obstructive jaundice often seen with LPSP (resulting from stenosis of the intrapancreatic common bile duct), polyethylene stents are usually inserted into the bile duct in addition to the administration of oral steroids. The bile duct narrowing usually resolves within 2 to 3 months so that the biliary stent can be removed. The level of serum IgG4 and other autoantibodies should also decrease with steroid therapy. The long-term prognosis of LPSP treated with steroids is uncertain, and relapse is possible.

ACINAR CELL CARCINOMA

Acinar cell carcinoma (ACC) represents less than 2% of all pancreatic malignancies. The patients normally present in the fifth to seventh decades of life, with a male predominance of 2 to 1. Similar to more common pancreatic tumors, ACCs are usually found within the head of the pancreas, and thus the most common presenting sign or symptom is biliary obstruction. Additionally, patients often complain of abdominal pain and bloating because these tumors are usually large at diagnosis, ranging from 10 to 15 cm. On CT scan, an ACC appears as a sizable pancreatic mass with a well-defined enhancing capsule and internal calcifications. Significant central hypodensity is frequently present. On pathologic examination, ACCs appear grossly as soft and fleshy tumors with scattered areas of hemorrhage and necrosis. Histologically, the acinar cells undergo differentiation into clusters of cells around a small central lumina and often appear similar to pancreatic endocrine tumors. A pathologist can differentiate between ACC and neuroendocrine tumors by using immunohistochemistry staining patterns. Both react strongly for pancytokeratin, but only pancreatic endocrine tumor cells react with synaptophysin and chromogranin.

A unique feature of ACC is the ability to release lipase into the circulation; this is believed to cause systemic manifestations such as polyarthralgia, subcutaneous fat necrosis, and erythema nodosum-like rashes with peripheral eosinophilia. The skin nodules should not be mistaken for metastatic disease because this could result in inappropriate or delayed therapy. When elevated, the lipase levels do not appear to correlate with extent of disease or prognosis; however, the levels decrease in response to surgical resection of the ACC. It has recently been recognized that ACC can, in some cases, produce alpha-fetoprotein (AFP), which is detectable within the serum. Although AFP production does not predict the development of liver metastases, serum AFP levels are useful for diagnosis and as a marker for evaluating recurrent disease and therapeutic response.

ACCs have an aggressive biologic behavior, with overall survival rates only slightly better than pancreatic ductal carcinoma. In the most comprehensive series to date, 39 patients treated for ACC experienced a median survival of 19 months. The best results are obtained in those patients with tumors confined to the pancreas that can be resected with a negative margin (36-month median survival). More than half of the patients with ACC present with metastatic disease and are not candidates for surgery. Even if a complete resection can be achieved, approximately three quarters of these patients will develop metachronous recurrent disease. Most recurrences occur at distant sites, suggesting that local control can be achieved but that hematogenous metastases drive the poor prognosis. The aggressive natural history of ACC indicates that adjuvant systemic therapy might improve patient survival. Unfortunately, because of the rarity of this disease, limited data are available to recommend a specific treatment regimen. The drugs most commonly used have been 5-fluorouracil, streptozotocin, cisplatin, and doxorubicin. In the largest reported series describing the use of systemic therapy, 22 chemotherapy regimens were administered to 18 patients, and only 2 of 18 patients experienced a partial response to therapy. The combination of chemotherapy and radiotherapy may be beneficial, but clinical experience is limited.

SOLID-PSEUDOPAPILLARY TUMOR

Solid-pseudopapillary tumor (SPT) of the pancreas is the name recommended by the World Health Organization for a rare and generally benign pancreatic tumor that represents 1% to 2% of all

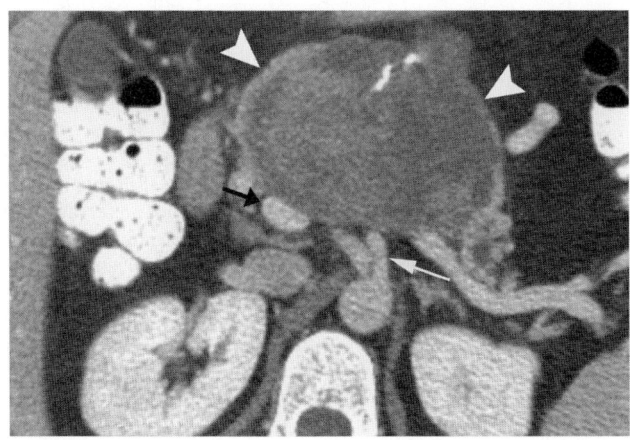

Figure 5 Axial contrast-enhanced computed tomography of a large pseudopapillary tumor arising in the body of the pancreas (*white arrowheads*). The tumor compresses the main portal vein (*black arrow*) superior to the splenoportal confluence and contacts the anterior walls of the splenic artery and the common hepatic artery (*white arrow*), which have separate origins from the aorta.

pancreatic neoplasms. Although 90% of these tumors are identified in women of childbearing age (mean age: 27 years), no association between SPT and reproductive hormone signaling has been established. For as yet unknown reasons, most cases involve African American and Asian women. Patients with SPTs often present incidentally or with symptoms secondary to the mass effect of a large tumor causing nausea, vomiting, and vague abdominal pain. Although SPTs are often large (8–10 cm on average) at presentation, they are generally indolent. Of the 450 previously reported patients with SPTs, metastatic disease occurred in 20 (≈4%). The most common site of distant disease is the liver, with lymph node and peritoneal metastases rarely seen. In most studies examining the clinical outcome of SPTs, no clinicopathologic factors predictive of prognosis have been identified.

CT examination demonstrates a well-encapsulated tumor with solid and cystic components that are not true cysts but necrotic tumor resulting from hemorrhagic degeneration (Fig. 5). The solid areas of the tumor are well circumscribed with a thick fibrous capsule, whereas the cystic portions are often calcified. Histologically, the tumor architecture consists of papillary configurations attached to a fibrovascular stalk. On high-power microscopy, tumor tissue is characterized by the presence of foamy macrophages, cholesterol granulomas, and necrotic tissue. Although the lineage of cellular differentiation that occurs in the formation of SPTs remains unclear, immunohistochemical staining displays a characteristic immunophenotype; vimentin protein is consistently expressed, and other markers of neuroendocrine or exocrine differentiation are absent. The diagnosis of SPT using FNA biopsy can be difficult, and in such cases the clinical presentation and radiographic findings usually aid in making the correct preoperative diagnosis.

Treatment of SPT is primarily surgical, and the goal of surgery is complete resection of the tumor with a negative margin; lymphadenectomy is probably not necessary. More than 95% of patients with SPT are cured with complete surgical resection, and the size of the lesion is not a predictor of unresectability. In fact, SPTs 20 to 30 cm in size have been successfully removed in several series. These tumors rarely invade contiguous structures, obstruct the bile duct, or occlude the superior mesenteric-portal vein confluence. However, vascular invasion can occasionally be seen, and reports have demonstrated long-term survival after resection of these tumors in continuity with the portal vein or hepatic artery. Metachronous recurrence of SPT after complete resection of local disease is rare but theoretically possible because these tumors are occasionally

malignant. Consequently, a follow-up regimen involving periodic (6- to 12-month intervals) cross-sectional imaging appears most reasonable. No clinicopathologic factors, including tumor size, vascular, lymphatic, or perineural invasion, have been used to predict recurrence or overall survival, primarily because of the rarity of malignant SPTs. Experience with adjuvant therapy is limited, and the treatment of metastatic disease is largely anecdotal; radiotherapy has been used infrequently.

PANCREATIC LYMPHOMA (NON-HODGKIN'S TYPE)

Non-Hodgkin's lymphoma arises in extranodal tissue in up to 40% of reported cases, although primary pancreatic lymphoma is exceedingly rare. The clinical presentation of patients with pancreatic lymphoma is often nonspecific, consisting of weight loss, nausea, vomiting, and abdominal pain. B-type lymphoma symptoms such as fever and night sweats may be present. CT images may suggest the diagnosis of pancreatic lymphoma by the presence of a bulky pancreatic mass with surrounding lymphadenopathy. CT evidence of a bulky pancreatic mass in the absence of weight loss, back pain, and extrahepatic biliary obstruction (normal serum bilirubin associated with an elevated lactate dehydrogenase) should cause one to consider lymphoma in the differential diagnosis.

EUS-guided FNA combined with expert cytopathology can usually establish the diagnosis of lymphoma. In a retrospective review from our institution, we evaluated the characteristics of 11 patients diagnosed with pancreatic lymphoma over a 15-year period. Five of six patients who underwent FNA biopsy had the diagnosis established correctly. However, 3 of the 11 patients underwent surgical resection for presumed pancreatic endocrine or exocrine carcinoma (followed by chemotherapy). Control of the disease was accomplished, but similar results may have been achieved with systemic chemotherapy alone. A report from The Johns Hopkins University has suggested that surgical resection may have a role in the treatment of early pancreatic lymphoma. These researchers reported three patients with early-stage pancreatic lymphoma who underwent pancreaticoduodenectomy for suspected periampullary adenocarcinoma and who were disease free at 5-year follow-up. This anecdotal experience suggests that pancreatic resection may be associated with a therapeutic benefit in an occasional patient found to have small-volume lymphoma who underwent initial operation because of the concern over a possible periampullary or pancreatic adenocarcinoma.

Systemic treatment of pancreatic lymphoma traditionally has involved cytotoxic chemotherapy. The most common chemotherapy regimens include cyclophosphamide, doxorubicin (Adriamycin; Pharmacia, Milan, Italy), vincristine, and prednisone (CHOP). Complete remission can be expected with multidrug chemotherapy in 60% to 80% of patients with early-stage non-Hodgkin's lymphoma. However, recurrence is more common in patients older than age 60. More recently, rituximab (a chimeric murine/human monoclonal antibody directed against the CD20 antigen found on lymphocytes) has been combined with CHOP, resulting in improved response rates and long-term survival for patients with diffuse, large B-cell lymphomas.

METASTASES TO THE PANCREAS (RENAL CELL CARCINOMA)

Metastases to the pancreas (pancreatic parenchyma) are rare. The most common primary cancer to metastasize to the pancreas is renal cell carcinoma. Other malignancies known to metastasize to the pancreas include melanoma, non–small-cell lung cancer, breast cancer, and colon cancer. However, a metastasis to a peripancreatic

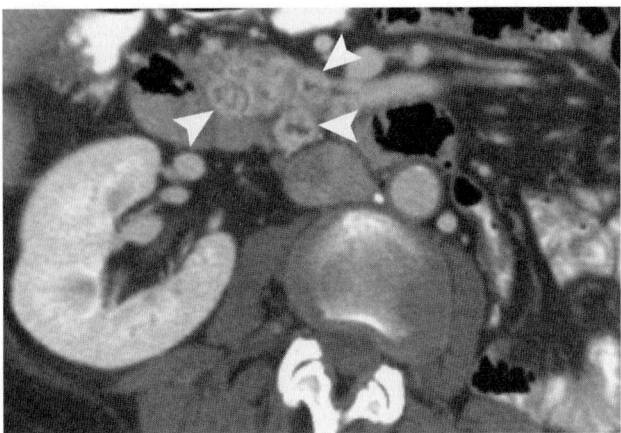

Figure 6 Axial contrast-enhanced computed tomography demonstrates multiple small hypervascular metastases *(white arrowheads)* in the pancreatic head resulting from renal cell carcinoma.

lymph node(s) is often incorrectly interpreted as a pancreatic metastasis; such is the case with most solid tumors other than renal cell carcinoma. In general, metastasis to the pancreas carries the same poor prognosis as metastasis to other visceral sites. As such, most patients with a pancreatic metastasis likely possess additional sites of disease, and a thorough staging evaluation should be performed on the basis of the cancer diagnosis. Renal cell carcinoma metastatic to the pancreas is unique in that there is often a long disease-free interval (often 10 years or more) from nephrectomy to the recognition of pancreatic metastases. In addition, patients with isolated renal cell metastases to the pancreas may experience a prolonged disease-free course postpancreatectomy.

Renal cell carcinoma is the most common malignancy producing metastases limited to the pancreas that are amenable to surgical resection. The tumors in these patients can be identified secondary to local symptoms from tumor growth such as jaundice or bleeding but are often found as part of routine follow-up imaging. As in other visceral sites, the metastatic tumors usually appear on CT as hypervascular spherical masses (Fig. 6) within the parenchyma of the pancreas (ductal adenocarcinomas appear hypovascular). Renal cell metastases can be confused with other hypervascular lesions of the pancreas such as neuroendocrine tumors or accessory splenic tissue. In patients with a history of renal cell cancer, the CT

findings are so characteristic that a biopsy is often unnecessary. However, a tissue diagnosis obtained by EUS-FNA is helpful if the diagnosis is uncertain or a nonoperative approach is planned.

Surgical treatment of renal cell carcinoma metastatic to the pancreas must be individualized, with an emphasis on the medical comorbidities of the operative candidate, the extent of disease, and the disease-free interval from nephrectomy. The goal should be adequate tumor resection with negative margins and preservation of some pancreatic mass when possible to prevent insulin-dependant diabetes mellitus. Surgical therapeutic options include pancreaticoduodenectomy; distal pancreatectomy; segmental resection; and, in some cases, total pancreatectomy; all interventions are based on the number and location of the metastases. Retrospective reviews suggest that resection of renal cell carcinoma metastases to the pancreas can greatly benefit a carefully selected group of patients.

SUGGESTED READINGS

Bouvet M, Staerkel GA, Spitz FR, and others: Primary pancreatic lymphoma, *Surgery* 123:382, 1998.

Capitanich P, Iovaldi ML, Medrano M, and others: Lymphoepithelial cysts of the pancreas: case report and review of the literature, *J Gastrointest Surg* 8:342, 2004.

Goh BK, Tan YM, Yap WM, and others: Pancreatic serous oligocystic adenomas: clinicopathologic features and a comparison with serous microcystic adenomas and mucinous cystic neoplasms, *World J Surg* 30:1553, 2006.

Hamano H, Kawa S, Horiuchi A, and others: High serum IgG4 concentrations in patients with sclerosing pancreatitis, *N Engl J Med* 344:732, 2001.

Holen KD, Klimstra DS, Hummer A, and others: Clinical characteristics and outcomes from an institutional series of acinar cell carcinoma of the pancreas and related tumors, *J Clin Oncol* 20:4673, 2002.

Martin RC, Klimstra DS, Brennan MF, and others: Solid-pseudopapillary tumor of the pancreas: a surgical enigma? *Ann Surg Oncol* 9:35, 2002.

Raut CP, Cleary KR, Staerkel GA, and others: Intraductal papillary mucinous neoplasms of the pancreas: effect of invasion and pancreatic margin status on recurrence and survival, *Ann Surg Oncol* 13:582, 2006.

Tanaka M, Chari S, Adsay V, and others: International consensus guidelines for management of intraductal papillary mucinous neoplasms and mucinous cystic neoplasms of the pancreas, *Pancreatology* 6:17, 2006.

Tseng JF, Warshaw AL, Sahani DV, and others: Serous cystadenoma of the pancreas: tumor growth rates and recommendations for treatment, *Ann Surg* 242:413, discussion 419, 2005.

Von Hoff DD, Evans DB, Hruban RH: *Pancreatic cancer*, Sudbury, MA, 2005, Jones and Bartlett.

INTRADUCTAL PAPILLARY MUCINOUS NEOPLASMS OF THE PANCREAS

Kenneth J. Woodside, MD, and Taylor S. Riall, MD

Intraductal papillary mucinous neoplasms (IPMNs) have recently been recognized as a distinct subset of pancreatic cystic neoplasms. The proportion of IPMNs relative to other pancreatic neoplasms has increased since the mid 1990s, with IPMNs now comprising approximately 20% of resected pancreatic neoplasms. This increase is likely due to a number of factors, including increased

recognition of the disease, improved pathologic criteria, improved cross-sectional imaging, and a true increase in IPMN incidence. In general, these lesions are thought to be more frequently benign than pancreatic ductal adenocarcinoma. However, malignant degeneration sequentially occurs as the lesions age, similar to the adenoma-carcinoma sequence in colorectal cancer. These lesions are best managed surgically, with oncologic resection to tumor-free margins.

PATHOLOGY

First described in 1982 by Ohashi and colleagues, IPMNs are cystic, intraductal, mucin-producing neoplasms that often demonstrate significant pancreatic ductal dilatation (Fig. 1). The majority of these lesions are located in the head, neck, or uncinate process (70%), but body or tail lesions are not uncommon. Diffuse involvement or multifocal involvement of the duct is also possible. Classification of IPMNs is based on the 1996 World Health Organization

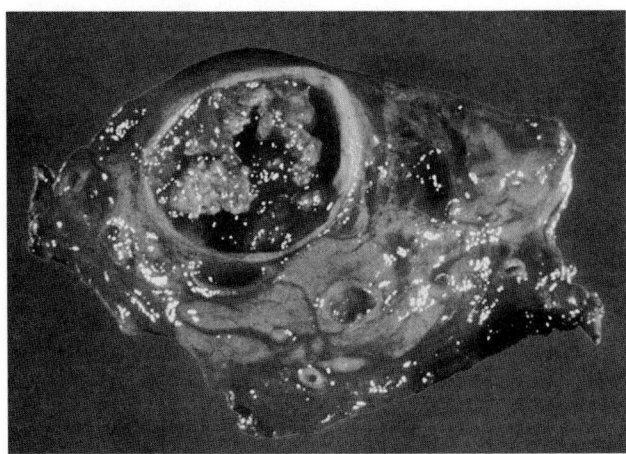

Figure 1 Gross photograph of a main duct intraductal papillary mucinous neoplasm demonstrating a cross section of the gland through the main pancreatic duct. The main pancreatic duct is massively dilatated with papillary fronds growing within the duct itself. (See *color insert Figure 28.*)

criteria. On histologic assessment, IPMNs demonstrate tall, columnar, mucin-containing epithelium, with or without papillary projections, which extensively involve the main pancreatic duct or major side branches. They lack the ovarian stroma characteristic of mucinous cystic neoplasms (MCN). IPMNs must be 1 cm or larger and grossly or radiographically identifiable, which helps to differentiate them from pancreatic intraepithelial neoplasia. Depending on whether the tumor is centered in the main pancreatic duct or major side branches, IPMN lesions are classified as main duct, branch duct, or combined variants, with approximately 50% of IPMNs presenting as branch-duct variants, whereas main-duct and combined variants each make up approximately one quarter of IPMNs. IPMNs are differentiated from MCNs by several features, shown in Table 1. It is critical to distinguish IPMNs from MCNs because the prognoses for long-term survival and recurrence are markedly different for each diagnosis.

Table 1: Comparison of Clinical Features of MCN and Branched-Duct IPMN

	MCN	IPMN
Age	Perimenopausal	Elderly
Sex (% female)	>95%	30%–50%
Location	Majority in the pancreatic body and tail	Majority in the pancreatic head
Calcification	Rare	No
Common thick capsule	Yes	No
Ovarian stroma	Present	Absent
Main pancreatic duct involvement	Rare	Yes but not always demonstrable
Main pancreatic duct	Normal or deviated	Normal (branch duct variant) or dilated (main duct or combined variant)

IPMN, Intraductal papillary mucinous neoplasms; *MCN*, mucinous cystic neoplasms.
Modified from Tanaka M, Kobayashi K, Mizumoto K, and others: J Gastroenterol 40:669, 2005. *Used with permission from Springer-Verlag.*

Sixty percent to seventy percent of IPMNs are noninvasive tumors, and 30% to 40% demonstrate invasive cancer on final pathology. Noninvasive subtypes based on histologic grade include IPMN adenoma, borderline IPMN, and IPMN with carcinoma in situ (CIS). Similar to the colorectal adenoma-carcinoma sequence, these noninvasive subtypes are thought to be stages in development toward invasive (malignant) IPMN or intraductal papillary mucinous carcinoma, with progression from benign to malignant disease estimated to occur over approximately 5 years. Pathologic tumor types of invasive cancers include tubular, colloid, mixed, and anaplastic variants, with colloid tumors having the best prognosis.

CLINICAL PRESENTATION

IPMNs typically present in the seventh decade of life, with a mean age of approximately 67 years at presentation. However, benign disease likely occurs earlier: mean age of presentation of patients with IPMN adenoma is 63 years, increasing to 67 years for those with borderline or CIS-containing IPMNs and 68 years for those with invasive carcinoma. Some studies have shown a slight male predominance. Gender and race distribution are similar for those with noninvasive and invasive disease.

Although a majority of patients have historically presented with symptoms, increased use of computed tomography (CT) in recent years has resulted in more frequent incidental detection of these lesions. As with most pancreatic neoplasms, typical symptoms are relatively nonspecific and include abdominal pain, weight loss, diarrhea, nausea, and vomiting (Table 2).

Table 2: Demographics and Presenting Symptoms of IPMNs

	Noninvasive IPMNs	Invasive IPMNs	*p* Value
N	84	52	
Demographics			
Mean age	63.2 ± 4.0 years (adenoma)	68.1± 1.5 years	.08*
	66.7 ± 1.6 years (borderline/CIS)	≈	
Gender	61% male	52% male	ns
Race	90% Caucasian	87% Caucasian	ns
Presenting Signs/Symptoms			
Obstructive jaundice	7%	33%	<.001
Abdominal pain	51%	54%	ns
Weight loss	20%	44%	.002
Nausea/vomiting	21%	2%	.002
Acute pancreatitis	13%	12%	ns
Gastrointestinal bleed	2%	4%	ns
Fever/chills	4%	0%	ns

CIS, Carcinoma in situ; *IPMN*, intraductal papillary mucinous neoplasms; *ns*, nonsignificant.
**p* value for adenoma vs. carcinoma.
From Sohn TA, Yeo CJ, Cameron JL, and others: Ann Surg 239:788, 2004. *Used with permission from Lippincott Williams & Wilkins.*

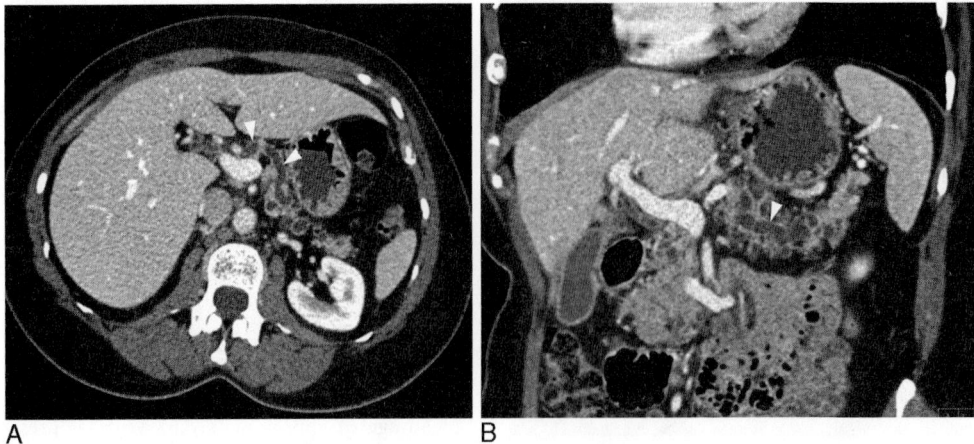

Figure 2 Three-dimensional computed tomography of a combined variant intraductal papillary mucinous neoplasm. **(A)** The axial image shows marked diffuse dilatation of the main pancreatic duct. **(B)** This reformatted coronal image on the same patient shows multiple cystic lesions communicating with the main pancreatic duct. These cystic lesions represent the branch duct involvement.

Patients may also present with obstructive jaundice or acute or recurring pancreatitis, suggesting more diagnostic specificity. Patients with invasive IPMN are more likely to present with obstructive jaundice, new-onset diabetes mellitus, and weight loss, whereas those with noninvasive disease are more likely to have nausea and vomiting.

DIAGNOSIS AND PREOPERATIVE MANAGEMENT

With the increased use of cross-sectional imaging, many of these lesions are already identified, either incidentally or as part of an abdominal pain workup, by the time the patient sees a surgeon. A thin-cut three-dimensional (3D) abdominal CT scan should assess for a cystic lesion and ductal dilatation (Fig. 2, *A* and *B*), as well as for signs of lymphadenopathy, organ invasion, or liver metastasis. In addition, a CT scan helps with assessment for resectability (e.g., superior mesenteric artery, superior mesenteric vein, portal vein, or inferior vena cava involvement) and operative planning. If additional detail is required, a magnetic resonance cholangiopancreatography (MRCP), which may reveal additional filling defects in the main or side branches of the pancreatic duct, can be obtained. Preoperative workup should also include a chest radiograph to assess for lung metastasis, liver function tests to assess for obstruction, amylase and lipase to assess for pancreatitis, and albumin to assess for malnutrition.

Endoscopic retrograde cholangiopancreatography (ERCP) can be used to identify the ductal lesion and communication with the main duct for branch variants, coupled with brushings or mucus sampling. The classical triad of ERCP findings includes a bulging ampulla, mucin extrusion from the ampulla (Fig. 3), and a dilatated duct. Mucus samples have high mucin and amylase levels and can have elevated carcinogenic embryonic antigen (CEA) levels. Carbohydrate antigen (CA) 19–9 levels are variable, and CA153 levels are low. In contrast, MCN typically demonstrates normal or low amylase and high CA15–3 levels. Similarly, if diagnosis is in doubt, an endoscopic ultrasound (EUS)-guided fine needle aspiration (FNA) can be obtained, providing both fluid and tissue, but this is often unnecessary in the presence of the findings just cited.

Preoperative differentiation of malignant versus benign IPMN is difficult. Liver metastases obviously indicate malignancy, as would any known distant metastatic lesion. Atypical cells on

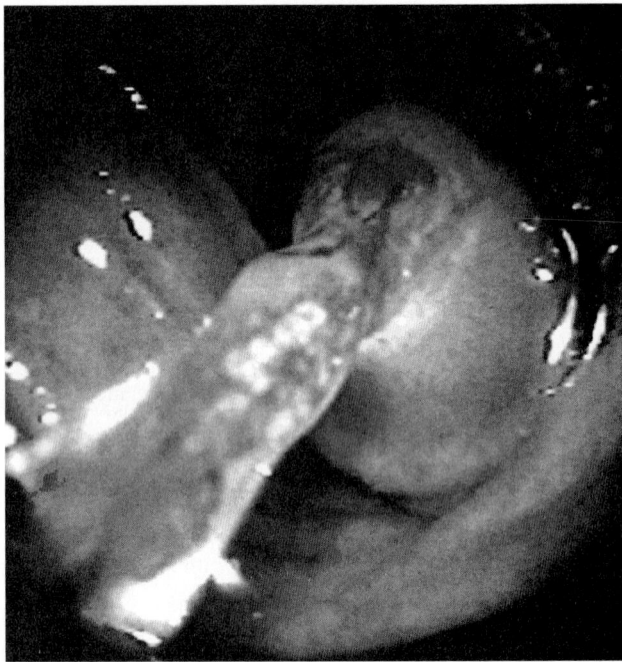

Figure 3 Patulous bulging ampulla with extruding mucin seen at endoscopy. *From Conlon KC: J Clin Oncol 23:4518, 2006. Used with permission from the American Society of Clinical Oncology.* **(See color insert Figure 29.)**

FNA are predictive of malignancy. Main-duct variant lesions are more likely to be malignant than branch-duct variants. Furthermore, marked main-duct dilatation ($\geq$12 mm), tumor size ($\geq$30 mm), and mural nodules in the duct are suggestive of malignancy, as are obstructive jaundice, new-onset diabetes, and elevated alkaline phosphatase levels. Because true determination of malignant potential is difficult and more benign lesions are likely to progress toward malignancy, a high index of suspicion must be maintained.

EXTRAPANCREATIC NEOPLASMS

Patients with IPMNs have a high incidence (24% to 39%) of metachronous extrapancreatic neoplasms and must be evaluated for other lesions for either concurrent or postoperative management. Gastric and colorectal adenocarcinomas have been most frequently reported, although lung, biliary, thyroid, and liquid tumors have been reported as well. Often, patients with IPMN are older, so it is difficult to determine whether this increased frequency is from advanced age or actually from the pathophysiology of IPMN. Abdominal lesions can often be handled concurrently, whereas those outside of the operative field or low in the intestinal tract may best be approached at a different time. In high-risk patients, the additional stress of the expanded operation may also alter the risk-to-benefit ratio of the operation enough to alter the operative plan.

MANAGEMENT

After the patient is nutritionally replete, operative intervention should proceed. When indicated, the operative approach for curative resection is based on location and characteristics of the lesion. However, the mass may not be well visualized on cross-sectional imaging, but the dilatated duct and mucin may be well demonstrated. All main duct lesions should be resected, as should branch duct lesions with main duct involvement, larger size (>3 cm), mural nodules, main duct dilatation (>6 mm), obstructive jaundice or pancreatitis, or other symptoms. Smaller (<3 cm), asymptomatic, branch duct variant lesions can be followed clinically with serial cross-sectional imaging in higher-risk patients because these lesions have a low likelihood of progressing to invasive disease (0% to 5%).

The type of resection is based on location of the tumor. For head, neck, or uncinate process tumors, a pylorus-preserving pancreaticoduodenectomy (Whipple procedure) is preferred, with a classic pancreaticoduodenectomy reserved for tumors with proximal duodenal or gastric invasion or involvement. A distal pancreatectomy should be performed for body or tail lesions. Smaller, well-localized pancreatic neck lesions without invasive cancer may be treated by a central pancreatectomy (Fig. 4), although lesions amicable to this type of resection are relatively rare.

IPMNs tend to grow longitudinally along the duct, rather than radially into the parenchyma, requiring stringent use of intraoperative frozen sections of the margin of resection, with particular attention paid to the duct itself. In addition, synchronous IPMN lesions are described that may require additional resection. In fact, the use of intraoperative pancreatoscopy with a choledochoscope may be indicated if preoperative imaging is less than adequate.

If the surgical margin is continually positive or multiple lesions are found throughout the duct, the surgeon must be prepared to perform a total pancreatectomy in patients who are an appropriate surgical risk. Because 15% of patients may require a total pancreatectomy, patients should provide consent for the possibility of this operation preoperatively as a contingency to its possible need. A recent international consensus meeting on IPMNs addressed the management of positive surgical margins at the time of resection. Although the authors acknowledged that the relative risk and biological significance of the varying grades of IPMNs cannot yet be fully understood, they made several recommendations on the basis of grade. For IPMN adenoma, no further resection is recommended. IPMNs with borderline atypia may require further resection if there are more papillary nodules, florid papilla formation, or other concerning findings. For IPMNs with CIS or invasive carcinoma, complete tumor resection is recommended. Total pancreatectomy is not routinely recommended for prevention of recurrence if disease in the unresected segment is not proved. In addition, for particularly poor-risk patients with limited life expectancy, a lesser procedure with close follow-up may be indicated because the disease is more indolent than pancreatic ductal adenocarcinoma.

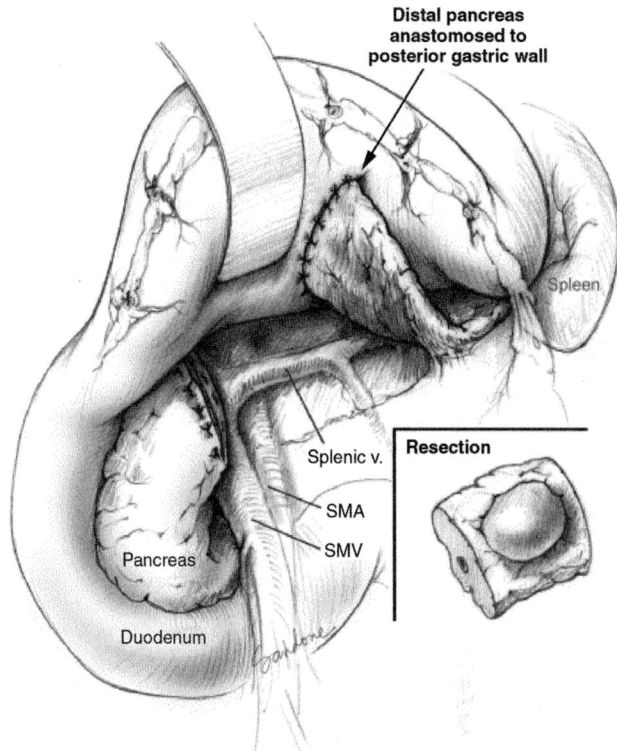

Figure 4 A view of the completed pancreaticogastrostomy *(PG)* and oversewn proximal pancreatic remnant. The inset depicts the specimen properly oriented and ready to be sent to the pathology laboratory for diagnosis and margin assessment. *From Efron DT, Lillemoe KD, Cameron JL, and others: J Gastrointest Surg 8:532, 2004; Used with permission from Elsevier Inc.*

POSTOPERATIVE MANAGEMENT

Initial perioperative management of IPMN patients is dependent on the particulars of their operation. Perioperative mortality ranges from 0% to 4%. However, for patients undergoing pancreaticoduodenectomy, the overall complication rate is 30% to 40%, with delayed gastric emptying (12% to 20%) and pancreatic fistula (10% to 15%) occurring most frequently. Intra-abdominal abscess (5% to 7%), wound infections (4% to 10%), and pneumonia (~2%) also occur with some frequency. Pancreaticobiliary complications occur, with bile leak occurring in less than 4% of patients, pancreatitis in less than 2% of patients, and cholangitis in less than 2% of patients. Pancreatic fistula formation for patients undergoing distal pancreatectomy is approximately 5%.

Those with new-onset postoperative diabetes mellitus should be treated with insulin rather than oral agents because this condition results from insulin insufficiency as a result of loss of pancreatic mass rather than from insulin resistance. Those patients requiring total pancreatectomy require both aggressive diabetic management, often by an endocrinologist, and pancreatic enzyme replacement. Pancreatic enzyme replacement must be appropriately timed before the meal and should be of an adequate amount to maintain the weight of the patient and prevent steatorrhea.

PROGNOSIS

In recent large studies, long-term actuarial survival for patients with noninvasive IPMN is 77% to 100% at 5 years. Of note, several deaths in the noninvasive group occurred as a result of disseminated adenocarcinoma in multiple series. For those with

IPMN adenoma, borderline IPMN, and IPMN with CIS, there are no significant differences in survival. For patients with IPMNs with invasive carcinoma, long-term actuarial survival was less promising but still better than that seen in patients with pancreatic ductal carcinoma. Five-year survival is 36% to 60% for these patients, with disseminated adenocarcinoma responsible for the majority of deaths in these patients. Although main-duct variant IPMN is perceived as having a worse outcome compared with branch-duct variant IPMN, recent larger studies have not supported this contention. For invasive IPMN, lymph node involvement, vascular invasion, and tubular variant type are consistently associated with decreased survival (Table 3). Patients with colloid carcinoma variant have a 5-year survival of 72% to 83%, whereas those patients with tubular variant have a 5-year survival of 24% to 50%. Patients with lymph node involvement have a 5-year survival of 0% to 30%, whereas patients with vascular invasion have the worst prognosis. Patients with residual invasive disease at the surgical margin have poor survival, with a 1-year survival rate of approximately 40% and a 5-year survival rate approaching zero. However, for patients with noninvasive IPMN, the surgical margin is less predictive of both survival and recurrence. Many patients with negative margins have recurrence, and many with positive margins never develop clinical recurrence.

IPMN recurrence may occur from residual disease, recurrent disease, or a synchronous lesion that was not detected at the first operation. For those with noninvasive IPMN, recurrence rates are 1% to 20%, whereas those with invasive IPMN demonstrate recurrence rates of 44% to 65%, with approximately 90% of recurrences occurring within 3 years of initial resection. Recurrences in patients with noninvasive disease can be either invasive or noninvasive and are independent of the margin status at the initial resection. Resection of noninvasive recurrences with completion pancreatectomy is associated with a good prognosis. An invasive recurrence has a significantly lower 5-year survival, with the majority of the recurrences unresectable on presentation.

FOLLOW-UP

Given the concern for recurrence following resection of both benign and malignant IPMNs, these patients must undergo careful postoperative surveillance. Abdominal CT scans or other cross-sectional imaging should be obtained at 6-month intervals for those patients with invasive disease. For those patients with noninvasive disease, the interval can be lengthened if there is no recurrence over several years. For recurrent disease, aggressive surgical intervention with completion pancreatectomy is usually indicated. In addition, given the concern for extrapancreatic neoplasms in patients with IPMNs, an aggressive lifelong screening regimen for other cancers must be employed, including interval endoscopy and chest radiographs.

For patients with unresected IPMNs, yearly cross-sectional imaging should be obtained if the lesion is less than 1 centimeter. For lesions of 1 to 2 cm, cross-sectional imaging should be obtained at 6- to 12-month intervals. For lesions of more than 2 cm, cross-sectional imaging should be obtained at 3- to 6-month intervals. The decision to proceed to operative resection should be based on symptoms, the overall operative risk, lesion growth, and cancer risk. Patients with branch-duct variants that are asymptomatic are at lower risk of invasive disease. If symptoms are present or the lesion develops main-duct involvement, larger size (>3 cm), mural nodules, main-duct dilatation (>6 mm), obstructive jaundice, or pancreatitis, resection is indicated.

Table 3: Association of Prognostic Factors with Outcome in Patients with Invasive IPMNs

Factor	N	5-Year Survival (%)	Log Rank (p Value)
Lymph node status			
Negative	20	73	
Positive	10	30	.02
Vascular invasion			
Absent	26	74	
Present	4	0	.009
Serum bilirubin			
Normal	19	67	
Elevated	11	38	.05
Percent invasive			
1%–49%	16	72	
50%–100%	14	44	.24
Size invasive			
–1 cm	17	56	
>1.0 cm	13	42	.56
Type of invasive tumor			
Colloid	13	72	
Tubular	17	50	.15

IPMN, Intraductal papillary mucinous neoplasms.
From D'Angelica M, Brennan MF, Suriawinata AA, and others: Ann Surg 239:400, 2004. *Used with permission from Lippincott Williams & Wilkins.*

Suggested Readings

Chari ST, Yadav D, Smyrk TC, and others: Study of recurrence after surgical resection of intraductal papillary mucinous neoplasm of the pancreas, *Gastroenterology* 123:1500, 2002.

Choi MG, Kim SW, Han SS, and others: High incidence of extrapancreatic neoplasm in patients with intraductal papillary mucinous neoplasms, *Arch Surg* 141:51, 2006.

D'Angelica M, Brennan MF, Suriawinata AA, and others: Intraductal papillary mucinous neoplasms of the pancreas: an analysis of clinicopathologic features and outcomes, *Ann Surg* 239:400, 2004.

Efron DT, Lillemoe KD, Cameron JL, and others: Central pancreatectomy with pancreaticogastrostomy for benign pancreatic pathology, *J Gastrointest Surg* 8:532, 2004.

Hruban RA, Takaori K, Klimstra DS, and others: An illustrated consensus on the classification of the pancreatic intraepithelial neoplasia and intraductal papillary mucinous neoplasms, *Am J Surg Pathol* 28:977, 2004.

Jang JY, Kim SW, Ahn YJ, and others: Multicenter analysis of clinicopathologic features of intraductal papillary mucinous tumor of the pancreas: is it possible to predict malignancy before surgery? *Ann Surg Oncol* 12:124, 2005.

Salvia R, Fernandez-del Castillo C, Bassi C, and others: Main-duct intraductal papillary mucinous neoplasms of the pancreas: clinical predictors of malignancy and long-term survival following resection, *Ann Surg* 239:678, 2004.

Sohn TA, Yeo CJ, Cameron JL, and others: Intraductal papillary mucinous neoplasms of the pancreas: an increasingly recognized clinicopathologic entity, *Ann Surg* 234:313, 2004.

Sohn TA, Yeo CJ, Cameron JL, and others: Intraductal papillary mucinous neoplasm of the pancreas: an updated experience, *Ann Surg* 239:788, 2004.

Tanaka M, Chari S, Adsay V, and others: International consensus guidelines for management of intraductal papillary mucinous neoplasms and mucinous cystic neoplasms of the pancreas, *Pancreatology* 6:17, 2006.

MANAGEMENT OF PANCREATIC ISLET CELL TUMORS EXCLUDING GASTRINOMA

Herbert Chen, MD, FACS

INTRODUCTION

Pancreatic islet cell tumors are rare neoplasms with an incidence of 1 per 100,000. There are approximately 2500 new cases of pancreatic islet cell tumors each year in the United States. Pancreatic islet cell tumors are can be functional (associated with a clinical syndrome related to hormones secreted by the tumor) or nonfunctional (the lack of symptoms or hormone production by the tumor). They can occur sporadically or in association with an inherited syndrome such as multiple endocrine neoplasia type 1 (MEN1) or Von Hippel-Lindau disease. The types of pancreatic islet cell tumors that are discussed in this chapter, as well as some of their characteristics, are shown in Table 1.

INSULINOMA

Diagnosis

Insulinomas are the most common type of pancreatic islet cell tumor. They occur more commonly in women in the fifth or sixth decade. These tumors secrete insulin or, less commonly, proinsulin, which leads to the clinical syndrome of hypoglycemic symptoms, low blood glucose (<40 mg/dl), and relief with administration of glucose, referred to as Whipple's triad. These symptoms are often exacerbated with fasting and relieved by food consumption. Patients have an elevated serum insulin or proinsulin level in the setting of a low or normal glucose level (ratio >0.3). A serum C-peptide level should be obtained (and >1.7 ng/ml in the case of insulinoma) to rule out exogenous insulin administration. Patients may occasionally be admitted to the hospital for diagnosis. During this time, patients must fast and serum insulin levels are monitored for up to 72 hours. Several provocative tests are used to clarify the diagnosis of insulinoma. The tolbutamide provocative test takes advantage of the propensity of tolbutamide to stimulate synthesis

and release of endogenous insulin. Patients with insulinoma have persistent hypoglycemia (<50 mg/dl) and elevated serum insulin levels for 2 to 3 hours after the test. In the glucagon-stimulation test, patients with insulinoma have a rapid rise in glucose and then develop severe hypoglycemia with persistent hyperinsulinism. This test is normal in patients with reactive hypoglycemia and detects insulinoma with a sensitivity of 72%. The final provocative test mentioned here is the calcium infusion test. Intravenous calcium causes a rise in insulin in patients with insulinoma within 2 hours of infusion. Normal patients have no significant change in insulin or glucose serum levels.

Imaging and Preoperative Preparation

The majority of insulinomas are small (<2 cm), solitary, benign (>90%) and uniformly distributed throughout the pancreas. Computed tomography (CT), transabdominal ultrasound, and magnetic resonance imaging (MRI) have sensitivity greater than 50% (Fig. 1). Unlike other pancreatic islet cell tumors, insulinomas are rarely detected with somatostatin (octreotide) radionucleotide scanning. Endoscopic ultrasound has reported sensitivities up to 80%. Arteriography with portal venous sampling has sensitivity in the 80% to 90% range but is an invasive procedure. The most

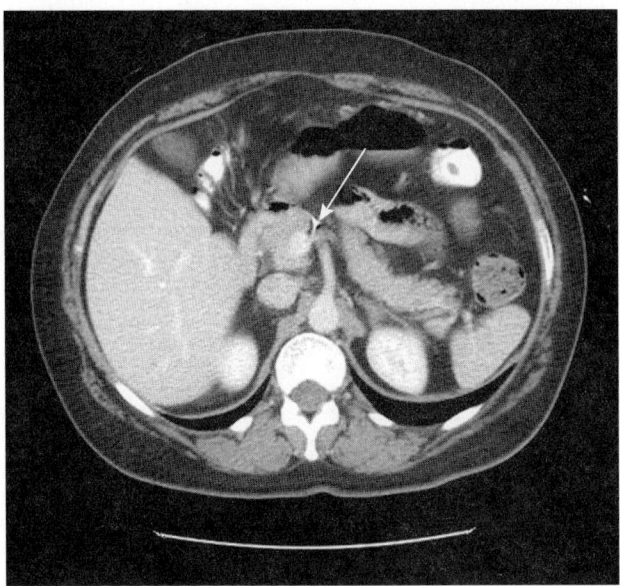

Figure 1 Abdominal computed tomography scan depicting a hypervascular lesion in the head of the pancreas (insulinoma).

Table 1: Summary of Pancreatic Islet Cell Tumor Types

Tumor	% Malignant	% Multicentric	% Outside Pancreas	5-Year Survival	% Associated with MEN-1
Insulinoma	10	5–10	<3	97	5
Gastrinoma	60–90	60–70	40	60–70	25
Glucagonoma	50–80	<5	<5	50–60	1–20
VIPoma	40–70	<5	<10	50	5
Somatostatinoma	75	<5	30–40	40	45–50
Nonfunctioning and PPoma	>60	<5	<5	30–50	20–40

PPoma, Pancreatic polypeptide-secreting tumor; *VIPoma*, vasoactive intestinal peptide-secreting tumor.
Modified from Mansour JC, Chen H: J Surg Res 120:139, 2004.

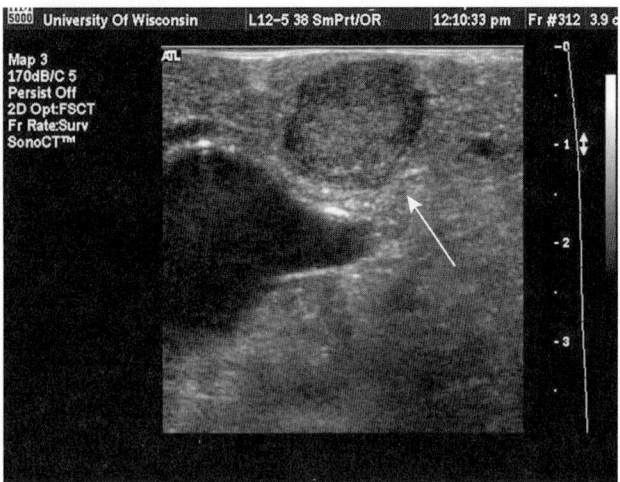

Figure 2 Intraoperative ultrasound confirms the insulinoma seen in Figure 1.

sensitive imaging technique is intraoperative ultrasound, which localizes more than 90% of insulinomas. Combined with palpation, almost 100% of insulinomas can be found with intraoperative ultrasound (Fig. 2).

Therefore after the biochemical diagnosis of insulinoma is made, we usually obtain a CT scan and, if it is negative, an endoscopic ultrasound. Localization is performed to determine whether laparoscopic resection is possible. Even if the lesion does not localize, we still proceed to the operating room and perform intraoperative palpation and ultrasound for localization. Preoperative control of hypoglycemia includes frequent meals (six times/day) and a reduction in strenuous exercise. Many authors recommend diazoxide (150–800 mg/day) preoperatively to control hypoglycemia. Diazoxide is a nondiuretic benzothiadiazine that acts on beta cells to decrease insulin secretion. In 50% of patients with insulinomas, diazoxide can control blood glucose at least temporarily.

GLUCAGONOMA

Diagnosis

Patients typically present in the fifth decade of life with an even gender distribution. Glucagonomas are rare tumors that cause the "4D syndrome": diabetes, dermatitis, deep vein thrombosis, and depression. Additional findings associated with glucagonoma include cheilitis, anemia, weight loss, hypoaminoacidemia, and other neuropsychiatric symptoms. Patients often present with elevated glucose and a characteristic rash called *necrolytic migratory erythema* seen on the face, lower abdomen, perineum, and lower extremities. Skin biopsy can occasionally confirm the diagnosis. The diagnosis of glucagonoma is made by a serum glucagon level of greater than 500 pg/ml.

Imaging and Preoperative Preparation

Because glucagonomas are rare and often go undiagnosed for many years, they tend to be large at the time of presentation (>5 cm) and metastatic (75%). Thus CT or MRI often detects the lesion. Octreotide scanning has a sensitivity exceeding 75%. Glucagonomas tend to be solitary and more commonly occur in the body and tail of the pancreas. Diabetes is present in 75% to 95% of patients with glucagonoma. The hyperglycemia is typically mild with a mean hemoglobin A1C of 9.8 controlled by diet, oral hypoglycemics, insulin, or a combination of these. Preoperatively these patients

require aggressive nutritional support in light of their prolonged catabolic state. This may include oral supplements, high protein diets, tube feedings, or total parenteral nutrition. Topical and oral zinc (200 mg twice a day) may help to improve symptoms from the rash. Up to 30% of patients with glucagonoma have deep venous thrombosis. In light of this unique association, heparin prophylaxis should be considered in these patients. Some have proposed the use of perioperative aspirin and dipyridamole as well.

VASOACTIVE INTESTINAL PEPTIDE-SECRETING TUMOR

Diagnosis

Vasoactive intestinal peptide-secreting tumors (VIPomas) are also extremely rare tumors that cause the "WDHA syndrome": watery (secretory) diarrhea, hypokalemia, and achlorhydria. WDHA syndrome has also been called pancreatic cholera or Verner-Morrison syndrome. Other symptoms include abdominal pain, flushing, muscle weakness, and weight loss and can often be mistaken for carcinoid syndrome. The diagnosis is made by a serum VIP level >200 pg/ml. These tumors occur with a frequency of 1 per 10,000,000 per year. They arise in the pancreas more than 90% of the time but have also been described in the colon, bronchus, adrenals, liver, and sympathetic ganglia. Adults typically present between ages 30 and 50 years.

Imaging and Preoperative Preparation

VIPomas are typically solitary and greater than 3 cm in diameter with 75% located in the tail of the pancreas. The majority of VIPomas can be localized with CT or MRI. Octreotide scanning is also highly sensitive. Sixty to eighty percent are metastatic at the time of diagnosis. The first course of action after VIPoma has been diagnosed is to correct aggressively the dehydration and metabolic derangements intrinsic to the syndrome. Octreotide can stop the diarrhea and allow for the correction of hypokalemia and other metabolic abnormalities in the majority of these patients.

SOMATOSTATINOMA

Diagnosis

Somatostatinomas are the rarest pancreatic islet cell tumor. These tumors are often discovered incidentally during evaluation or operation for an unrelated complaint or problem. The classic symptoms associated with these tumors are diabetes mellitus, caused by the inhibitory effects of somatostatin on insulin release; cholelithiasis, caused by decreased gallbladder contractility and cholecystokinin release; and steatorrhea, caused by the inhibition of pancreatic enzyme secretion, bicarbonate secretion, and intestinal absorption. Diabetes and gallstones occur with a frequency of 60% and 70%, respectively, in patients with these tumors. Patients with duodenal tumors may present with obstructive symptoms. An elevated somatostatin level (>10 ng/ml) confirms the diagnosis. The median age at diagnosis is 50 years, and gender distribution is equal.

Imaging and Preoperative Preparation

Most somatostatinomas are solitary. Up to 70% of these tumors are located in the pancreas. Even though somatostatin-secreting delta cells are diffusely located throughout the pancreas, two thirds of pancreatic somatostatinomas are located in the head of the pancreas. Most of the extrapancreatic tumors are located in the duodenum, ampulla, or remaining small bowel. Somatostatinomas often go undiagnosed for years and are therefore large (>5 cm) at the time of presentation. The majority of somatostatinomas are metastatic at presentation (75%) and can be localized with CT or MRI. Octreotide scanning is also highly sensitive.

PANCREATIC POLYPEPTIDE-SECRETING TUMOR

Diagnosis

The third most common type of islet cell tumor is a pancreatic polypeptide-secreting tumor (PPoma). The function of pancreatic polypeptide is not completely understood. Patients present with weight loss, jaundice, and abdominal pain. The diagnosis is confirmed by pancreatic polypeptide levels greater than 300 pg/ml. Because other pancreatic islet cell tumors may secrete pancreatic polypeptide, to be classified as a PPoma, more than 50% of the tumor must stain for pancreatic polypeptide by immunohistochemistry.

Imaging and Preoperative Preparation

PPomas tend to be large by the time of diagnosis and are usually seen in CT or MRI. Octreotide scanning is also sensitive for the detection of these tumors. Preoperative preparation involves control of serum glucose levels.

NONFUNCTIONAL ISLET CELL TUMORS

Diagnosis and Imaging

Nonfunctional islet cell tumors histologically resemble other pancreatic islet cell tumors but do not secrete biologically active substances that result in a detectable clinical syndrome. Most likely, they secrete low levels of hormones, biologically inactive hormones, or hormones that are currently unidentified. Most of these tumors, however, secrete chromogranin A, which can be detected in the serum and thus confirm the diagnosis. Most patients present with abdominal pain or other vague symptoms, prompting diagnostic studies. Almost all of nonfunctional islet cell tumors are diagnosed by CT or MRI because of the lack of symptomatology.

SURGICAL TREATMENT OF PANCREATIC ISLET CELL TUMORS

Figure 3 illustrates a proposed treatment algorithm for pancreatic islet cell tumor. After appropriate preoperative serum marker testing including chromogranin A levels, abdominal CT scan is performed. In patients with a negative CT or suspected metastatic disease, somatostatin receptor scintigraphy (octreotide scan; Fig. 4) should be used to define the extent of disease. Surgical resection remains the only curative therapy for patients with pancreatic islet cell tumors. In the absence of metastatic disease, operative exploration and curative resection should be considered for all patients with pancreatic islet cell tumors.

Open Approach

When performing an open surgery, I prefer a midline incision. After a careful evaluation for metastatic disease, including palpation and ultrasound of the liver and examination of the peritoneal surfaces and intra-abdominal organs, the duodenum is widely Kocherized. The lesser sac is entered through the gastrocolic ligament. The pancreas is then evaluated with palpation and intraoperative ultrasound. Any suspicious lesions can be biopsied with fine needle aspiration if necessary. If the primary lesion cannot be identified, intraoperative endoscopy with transillumination of the duodenum can be performed, especially in the case of a gastrinoma.

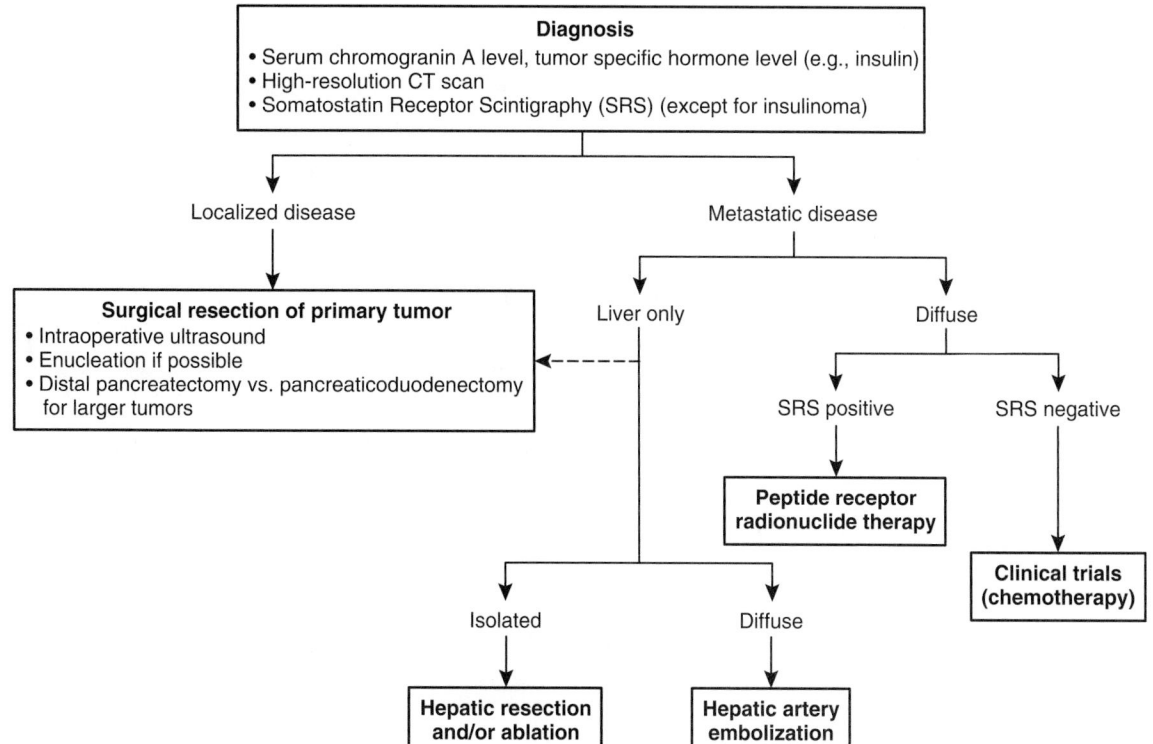

Figure 3 Algorithm for treatment of patients with pancreatic islet cell tumors. *Modified from Chen H: SSAT/AGA/ASGE State of the Art Conference on Pancreatic Neuroendocrine Tumors: consensus statement,* J Gastrointest Surg 10:321, 2006.

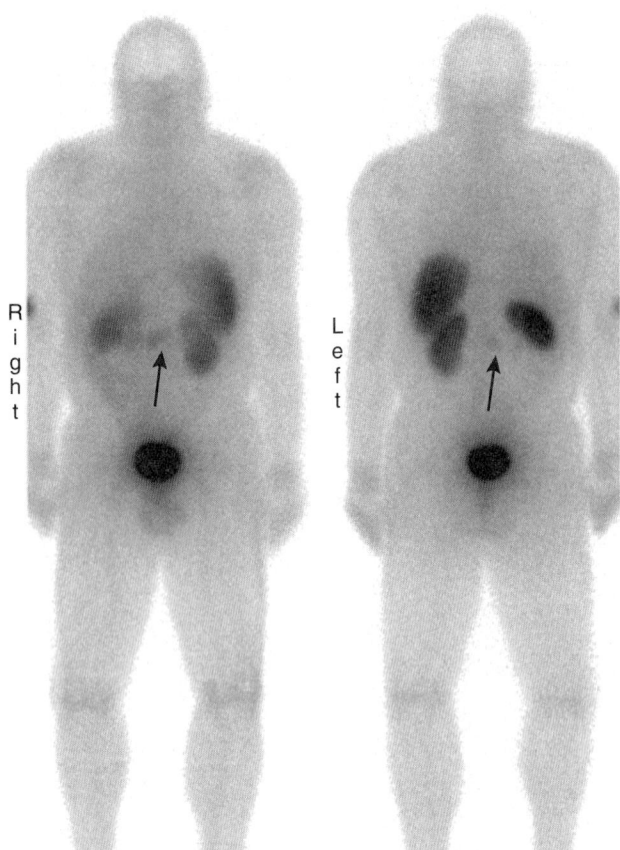

Figure 4 Somatostatin (octreotide) receptor scintigraphy is often helpful in localizing metastases. This patient presented with recurrent islet cell tumor in a lymph node *(arrow)*.

In the case of insulinomas, because the vast majority are benign and solitary, enucleation is the procedure of choice, when possible. Intraoperative ultrasound is critical to evaluating the relationship of the lesion to the pancreatic duct. With the other pancreatic islet cell tumors, a formal pancreatic resection is recommended, given that the chance for malignancy is much higher and that the diagnosis of benign versus malignant is often not possible in the absence of gross metastatic disease. For lesions in the tail of the pancreas, distal pancreatectomy (with or without splenic preservation) should be undertaken. Pancreatic islet cell tumors in the head of the pancreas require a Whipple procedure (pancreaticoduodenectomy).

Laparoscopic Approach

There is growing experience with laparoscopic pancreatic resections. Insulinomas in particular are the ideal lesion for a minimally invasive approach because they are solitary and often in the tail of the pancreas. A transabdominal exploration is carried out with a laparoscope, together with laparoscopic ultrasound. Similar to the open approach, ultrasound evaluation should include the liver and pancreas. The most common laparoscopic procedure for pancreatic islet cell tumors is distal pancreatectomy and splenectomy, although enucleation is also possible.

The technique of laparoscopic distal pancreatectomy has been nicely described by Nakeeb. The patient is positioned either supine in low lithotomy or a semilateral position with the left side up. Five ports are placed along the right subcostal margin. The pancreas is widely exposed by dividing the gastrocolic omentum from the pancreatic head to the splenic flexure of the colon. The splenocolic

ligament is then divided, and the colon reflected inferiorly. Initial dissection is directed medial to the pancreatic lesion in the tail. Sharp dissection is used to elevate the pancreatic body and identify the splenic vein posterior to the pancreas. Both the splenic vein and artery are looped. The pancreatic parenchyma is then divided with the harmonic scalpel or an endoscopic stapler, controlling the small pancreatic branches of the splenic vein and artery with the harmonic scalpel or small clips. Some surgeons advocate oversewing of the pancreas with a series of interrupted horizontal mattress sutures using an absorbable suture.

TREATMENT OF METASTATIC DISEASE

Most patients with pancreatic islet cell tumors (with the exception of insulinoma) present with metastatic disease (Fig. 5). Pancreatic islet cell tumors are one of a small number of tumors for which surgical debulking may confer some survival advantage. The treatment algorithm for metastatic disease is also shown in Figure 3. In addition, the often-crippling symptoms associated with many of these tumors may be eased by decreasing tumor load. In a series of patients with unresectable disease who underwent surgical debulking, 50% of patients reported an improvement in symptoms for a mean duration of 39 months. In the setting of liver-only metastatic disease, aggressive resection of the primary tumor with resection, or ablation of liver lesions (or a combination of these) should be considered.

Hepatic Resection

Aggressive resection of hepatic metastatic disease seems to be associated with improved overall survival. In recent series, the 5-year survival for patients treated with hepatic resection was 76%. We have demonstrated the benefits of aggressive hepatic resection for metastatic neuroendocrine tumors including pancreatic islet cell tumor. Complete resection of neuroendocrine hepatic metastases

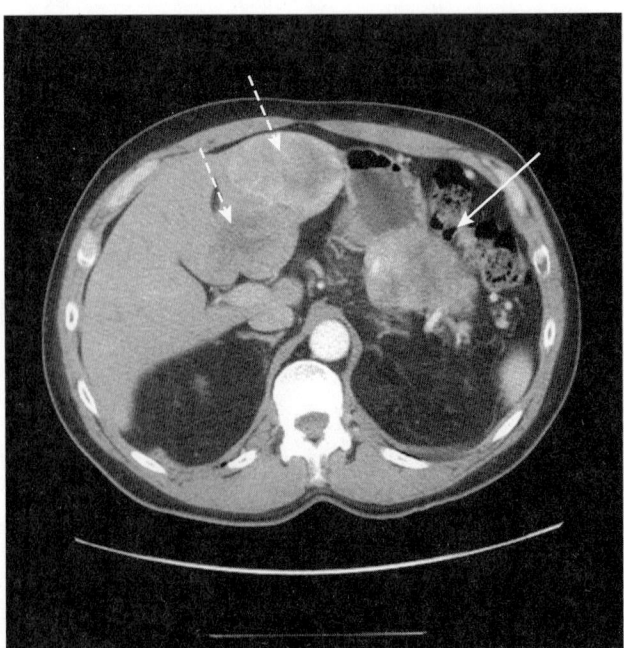

Figure 5 Computed tomography scan of a patient with metastatic islet cell tumors to the liver. *Solid arrow,* primary tumor in the tail of the pancreas. *Dotted arrow,* two liver metastases in the left lobe.

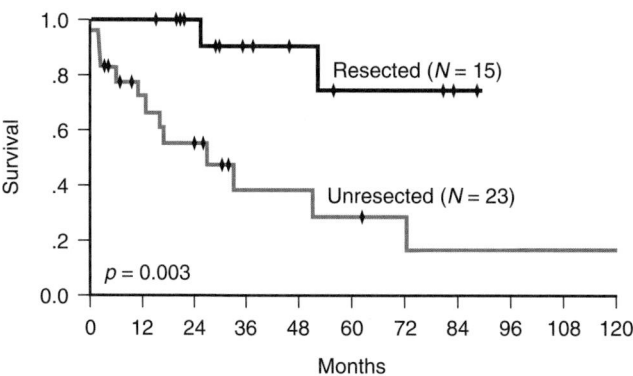

Figure 6 Effect of complete resection of pancreatic endocrine tumors on overall survival. *From Chen H, Hardacre JM, Uzar A, and others: JACS 187:88, 1998. Reprinted with permission.*

resulted in a prolonged 5-year survival compared with those patients incompletely resected (73% vs. 25%) (Fig. 6). I concur with most authors in my recommendation to consider hepatic resection if more than 90% of the tumor can be excised and less than 75% of the liver is involved.

Radiofrequency and Cryoablation

Radiofrequency ablation (RFA) and cryoablation have been shown to treat hepatic metastases from pancreatic islet cell tumors effectively in a number series. These ablation techniques are often used in combination with hepatic resection in patients with multiple, bilobar liver lesions. RFA can also be performed percutaneously in isolation as well.

Peptide Receptor Radionuclide Therapy (Radioactive Octreotide or MIBG)

Several reports of radiolabeled somatostatin analogues have been published. This technique involves the fusion of octreotide to a beta-emitting radionuclide resulting in ^{90}Yttrium-DOTA-labeled or ^{111}Indium-DTPA,D-Phe1. The side effects of this therapy are similar to those for more traditional radiation therapies and include nausea, vomiting, and renal toxicity. In addition, 34% of patients may develop lymphocytopenia. In a study of 38 patients with advanced neuroendocrine tumors treated with ^{111}Indium-DTPA-octreotide, 30% of patients demonstrated a reduction in tumor size. Another option is radioactive ^{131}I-methyliodobenzyl-guanidine scintigraphy (MIBG). ^{131}I-MIBG has been most commonly used in Europe and has been found in a series of 30 patients to have a 60% symptomatic response rate.

Hepatic Artery Embolization

Hepatic artery embolization (HAE) is predicated on the anatomic observation that most tumors within the hepatic parenchyma receive the bulk of their blood supply from the hepatic artery, whereas the portal vein supplies most of the normal hepatic parenchyma. Chemoembolization involves infusion of vaso-occlusive material into the hepatic artery to reduce blood supply to the tumor along with an infusion of high-dose chemotherapy. Coils, Gelfoam (Pfizer, New York, NY), polyvinyl alcohol, and iodinated oil have been used to embolize arteries with the addition of doxorubicin, cisplatin mitomycin C, streptozocin, and 5-fluorouracil. None of these combinations has produced significantly superior results. Contraindications to this procedure include tumor comprising more than 50% of the hepatic volume, bilirubin greater than 2.0, aspartate aminotransferase greater than 100, or portal vein thrombosis. Interpreting the studies on this topic is made difficult by the fact that most series are small with carcinoid and pancreatic islet cell tumors intermixed. Multiple studies have shown short-lived reductions in hormonal levels in more than 90% of patients. Unfortunately, these responses have lasted for little more than a year. Complication rates in these trials approach 20%, and mortality rates were 6%.

Chemotherapy

The presence of somatostatin receptors on many pancreatic islet cell tumors provides not only a useful tool for tumor localization but also a weapon to treat unresectable disease. Predictably, tumors such as gastrinomas, glucagonomas, VIPomas, nonfunctional tumors, and carcinoids with high-affinity somatostatin receptors are most amenable to this therapy. The development of lanreotide, an intramuscular version of octreotide with a much longer half-life and equal effectiveness, has simplified this therapy considerably. Treatment side effects with either medication include nausea, vomiting, abdominal pain, steatorrhea, diarrhea, and cholelithiasis. Symptomatic and biochemical responses occur in 60% to 90% of patients treated with somatostatin analogues. The median duration for this improvement is approximately 12 months until the tumors become refractory to the somatostatin analogue. The tumoricidal effects of somatostatin analogues are weak. Only 5% to 15% of patients have a documented reduction in tumor load, with stabilization of tumor progression in 35% to 80% of patients. High-dose somatostatin therapy for patients failing or developing resistance to standard somatostatin analogue therapy involves the administration of greater than 3000 μm per day. These patients have a symptomatic and biochemical response only 50% of the time, with only 11% of the tumors shrinking.

Unfortunately, the experience with multiple regimens of chemotherapy has been disappointing to date. Standard chemotherapy regimens are generally not useful in this disease, and new studies should incorporate novel mechanisms of action. Thus we highly encourage patients with metastatic pancreatic islet cell tumor to consider enrollment in ongoing clinical trials. However, several available strategies are currently being tested that may result in durable treatment for these patients. It is hoped that with the maturation of ongoing clinical trials and directed laboratory research, we will find a tolerable and effective treatment for patients with diffuse metastases from pancreatic islet cell tumors.

SUGGESTED READINGS

Chen H: SSAT/AGA/ASGE State of the Art Conference on Pancreatic Neuroendocrine Tumors: Consensus Statement, *J Gastrointest Surg* 10:321, 2006.
Chen H, Hardacre JM, Uzar A, and others: Isolated liver metastases from neuroendocrine tumors: does resection prolong survival? *J Am Coll Surg* 187:88, 1998.
Jensen RT: Pancreatic neuroendocrine tumors: overview of recent advances and diagnosis, *J Gastrointest Surg* 10:324, 2006.
Mansour JC, Chen H: Pancreatic endocrine tumors, *J Surg Res* 120:139, 2004.
Musunuru S, Chen H, Rajpal S, and others: Metastatic neuroendocrine hepatic tumors: resection improves survival, *Arch Surg* 141:1000, 2006.
Nakeeb A: The role of minimally invasive surgery for pancreatic pathology. In Cameron JL, editor: *Advances in surgery*, Philadelphia, 2004, Elsevier.

TRANSPLANTATION OF THE PANCREAS

Miguel Tan, MD, CM, MSc, and Joseph Keith Melancon, MD

INTRODUCTION

The first pancreas transplant was performed in December 1966 at the University of Minnesota by Drs. Richard Lillehei and William Kelly. Over the past 40 years, pancreas transplantation has evolved from an experimental procedure with a high failure rate to a commonly performed procedure with excellent long-term outcomes that rival those of other abdominal organ transplants. It is currently the standard for surgical management of diabetes. Unlike exogenous insulin therapy, pancreas transplantation allows for tight, physiologic control of blood glucose with a beneficial effect on secondary diabetic complications such as retinopathy, neuropathy, and nephropathy. Although insulin therapy remains the primary treatment for the vast majority of diabetics, for an expanding population of brittle diabetics, whole-organ pancreas transplant is the best option. Until isolated islet transplantation becomes a viable long-term alternative for maintaining euglycemia, the only reliable option for beta-cell replacement is whole-organ pancreas transplantation.

Despite its overall excellent outcomes, this operation remains a technically challenging endeavor. In addition to the recipient operation itself, procurement and meticulous technique in the backtable preparation of the pancreaticoduodenal graft are important to ensure good outcome. Unlike kidney or hepatic allograft, the pancreas is a relatively low-flow organ and is prone to thrombosis. Peripancreatic inflammation and edema are also poorly tolerated and can increase the risk of infection and graft failure.

A direct correlation exists between donor and recipient obesity and poor outcomes after transplantation. However, when donor and recipient selection is optimized and a technically successful operation performed, long-term tight glycemic control is possible with some evidence of stabilization and in some cases improvement of secondary complications of diabetes that, left unchecked, would ultimately lead to significant patient morbidity and mortality.

With the alarming increase of type 1 and type 2 diabetes mellitus worldwide, demand for beta-cell replacement therapy will continue to grow. Because islet transplantation and stem cell techniques remain in their infancy, the only reliable beta-cell replacement strategy is currently whole-organ pancreas transplantation.

INDICATIONS

Pancreas transplantation can achieve long-term, sustained euglycemia and can successfully abrogate hypoglycemic unawareness that can be life threatening in brittle diabetics. It remains the only reliable procedure for recapitulating native beta-cell function. Any nonobese diabetic with end-stage renal disease should be considered for a simultaneous kidney and pancreas transplantation. Even traditional critics of pancreas transplantation agree that both morbidity and mortality are deceased in this patient group after pancreas transplantation.

Pancreas transplantation alone (PTA) remains controversial, but momentum is currently swinging to favor both pancreas-after-kidney transplantation (PAK) and PTA. With modern immunosuppression and surgical technique, morbidity associated with these procedures is acceptably low with high patient satisfaction rates.

All brittle diabetics without significant surgical contraindications can be considered for pancreas transplantation. Patients should be thin (body mass index <30), relatively healthy (no severe cardiopulmonary disease), and not at the extremes of age (younger than 16 or older than 55).

TECHNICAL CONSIDERATIONS

In this section, we concentrate on key points and potential pitfalls in both the donor and recipient operations. All phases of pancreas transplantation, including procurement and bench work, are integral parts of obtaining good outcomes, and meticulous attention should be paid to proper execution of all phases.

Organ Procurement from a Deceased Donor

The goal of pancreas procurement from a deceased donor is to obtain an allograft that will have the best chance of euglycemic function in the recipient. Visualization of the graft by the procuring surgeon is one of the key determinants in making this judgment. Key characteristics to be noted are the degree of intraparenchymal fat and the texture of the organ. The pancreas should be soft without hard or firm areas suggestive of pancreatitis or scarring. The parenchyma should be salmon colored with minimal fatty infiltrate. Furthermore, edematous pancreases from overresuscitated donors should be considered carefully because this may predispose the allograft to subsequent graft pancreatitis.

Another consideration is the expected total ischemia time. This not an insignificant issue, especially with the number of organs that are now transported cross-country. Total ischemia times exceeding 20 hours are associated with an increase in graft thrombosis, anastomotic leaks, and wound infection and should be used with caution.

Organ procurement is often performed as a multivisceral procedure involving harvest of other organs by multiple surgical teams. (Detailed descriptions of this can be found in the Suggested Reading section of this chapter). Briefly, after appropriate exposure is obtained, the infrarenal and suprahepatic aorta are exposed and encircled with heavy umbilical tape. The superior mesenteric artery (SMA) is identified by mobilizing the small bowel cephalad until the left renal vein is encountered. The SMA can be palpated just superior to this structure and should be encircled with a vessel loop.

After the portal dissection is completed, the splenic artery should be encircled with a vessel loop. The lesser sac may be opened at this point to allow exposure of the pancreas. The duodenum is flushed with 250 ml of antibiotic/iodine solution via the nasogastric tube. Most of the pancreatic dissection may be carried out in a bloodless field once perfusion is initiated. When all surgical teams are ready, cold perfusion of the organs is initiated. After 1 L of perfusate is flushed through the aortic cannula, the vessel loops on the SMA and splenic artery are tightened to restrict further flow into the pancreas and prevent excessive perfusion and distention of the organ.

After the portal vein is divided, the pancreas is mobilized by grasping the spleen and sharply dividing the retroperitoneal attachments. The superior and inferior borders are mobilized sharply, carrying out the dissection toward the head of the pancreas. The inferior mesenteric vein (IMV) should be ligated during dissection of the inferior border. The spleen is left attached to the tail of the pancreas to act as a "handle" to minimize manipulation of the pancreas itself. The duodenum is divided just distal to the pylorus using a GIA stapling device (US Surgical, Norwalk, CT). The duodenum is subsequently divided distal to the pancreatic head with a second GIA stapler. At this point, the organ should be attached by the root of the small bowel mesentery, which can be divided with a third GIA reload. Finally, the SMA is divided close to its origin at the aorta.

Pancreas Bench Preparation

Meticulous bench work is essential to minimize postreperfusion hemorrhage. The spleen is removed by either ligating the individual vessels at the tail of the pancreas with 2–0 and 3–0 silk ties or dividing these vessels with a vascular GIA stapler and oversewing the staple line with 4–0 polypropylene. The superior and inferior borders of the allograft should be divested of excess fat using 3–0 silk ties because this redundant adipose tissue tends to necrose and may act as a nidus for abscess formation. Care should be taken not to injure the splenic vessels as they run along the border of the pancreas when removing the peripancreatic fat. The proximal duodenum is then imbricated with running 4–0 polypropylene suture to reinforce the staple line. This minimizes the risk of duodenal stump leak. The mesenteric staple line is oversewn with running 4–0 polypropylene suture as well. A ganglionectomy is performed by ligating the thick tissue around the SMA and splenic artery using 2–0 and 3–0 silk ties. Care should be taken when ligating tissue around the SMA on the side of the pancreatic head because injury to the inferior pancreaticoduodenal branch may occur.

Finally, arterial reconstruction of the SMA and splenic artery is completed by using a Y-graft consisting of iliac vessel procured from the donor (Fig. 1). For size matching and orientation purposes, the internal iliac artery branch of the Y-graft is usually anastomosed to the allograft splenic artery, and the external iliac branch is anastomosed to the SMA using running 7–0 polypropylene suture (Figs. 2 and 3).

The Recipient Operation: Pitfalls, Key Points, and Decision Making

Although a number of variants exist in implanting the pancreas allograft, including use of living donor allografts, segmental, and duct-injected grafts, fundamentally two aspects of pancreas implantation must be addressed: (1) vascular inflow and outflow and (2) exocrine drainage.

Inflow and outflow may be established by employing systemic vessels such as the iliac artery and vein or portal drainage, using a tributary of the portal vein for outflow. Portal drainage may be advantageous in that it mimics the normal physiologic route of blood draining from the native pancreas. It has been postulated that

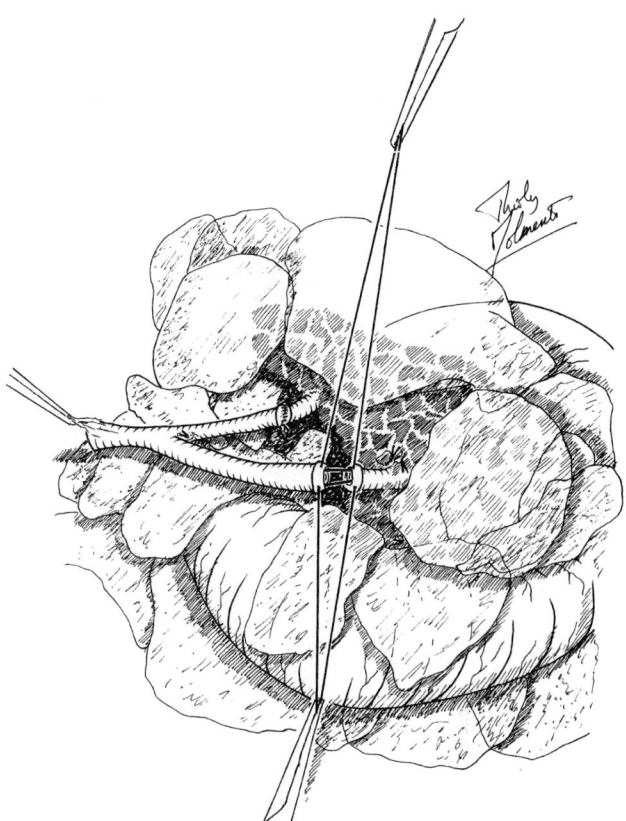

Figure 2 The internal iliac artery of the donor has been anastomosed to the splenic artery of the pancreas. The external iliac artery is being anastomosed to the superior mesenteric artery.

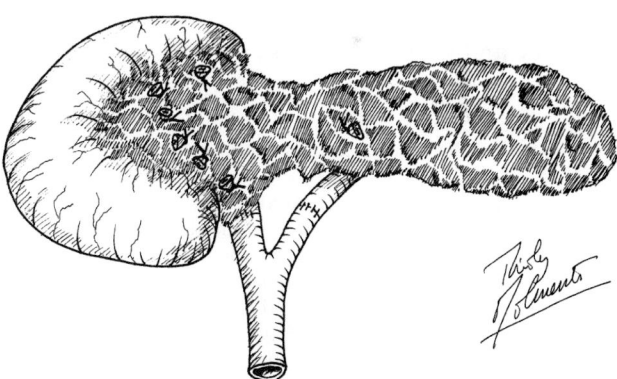

Figure 3 The pancreas allograft is ready for implantation. The arterial supply has been addressed. The spleen has been amputated, and the duodenum trimmed to an appropriate size.

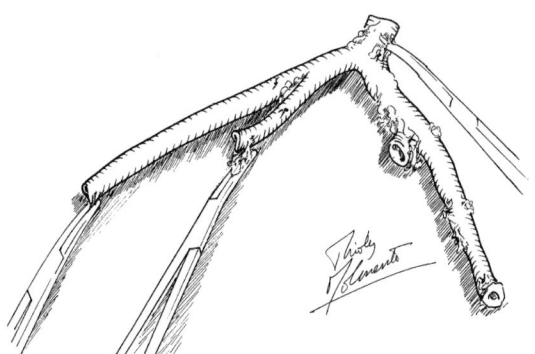

Figure 1 The iliac vessels of the donor are procured. The artery is subsequently used to create a single inflow tract to the superior mesenteric and splenic arteries of the pancreas graft.

this "first-pass" effect through the portal circulation may lead to decreased rejection rates and lack of hyperinsulinemia, which can occur with systemically drained allografts. However, its effect on overall graft survival is unclear.

Because of the low-flow nature of the pancreas allograft and other technical considerations, one must be cognizant of the risk of graft thrombosis using portal drainage. To achieve a good technical outcome with portal drainage, the portal vein of the allograft must be aligned along the longitudinal axis of the SMV in a manner such that the vein does not twist. It is not advisable to perform the venous anastomosis to the recipient SMV if the branch is too small or the overlying mesenteric fat is too thick because this increases the risk of venous thrombosis. Because of the orientation of the pancreatic head, it is generally not possible to perform a bladder anastomosis, committing one to enteric drainage, which can be problematic if the transplant duodenum appears less than ideally perfused after vascular continuity is reestablished. We reserve portal drainage for well-selected recipients, and it has been our practice to perform systemic vascular drainage in most recipients because many of our recipients are less than ideal.

The next consideration is exocrine drainage. Enteric drainage is performed when possible in simultaneous pancreas-kidney (SPK) transplants because this abrogates the postoperative complications associated with bladder drainage, including significant dehydration, electrolyte imbalances, and cystitis. However, in instances when the allograft duodenum does not appear to be well perfused or may be at increased risk for anastomotic leak, use of bladder drainage is warranted. If a small anastomotic leakage occurs in this situation, it can often be remedied with conservative maneuvers such as prolonged bladder catheterization. Conversely, loss of anastomotic integrity in an enterically drained allograft often leads to significant intra-abdominal infection or abscess, requiring reexploration and graft compromise.

In PTA and PAK transplants, we tend to favor bladder drainage because it allows for easy detection of graft rejection by monitoring urinary amylase levels. Unlike the SPK situation, in which pancreas rejection tends to be concordant with kidney rejection, one cannot use increasing creatinine as a marker for pancreas rejection in PTA and PAK transplants. After glucose metabolism is clinically impaired and the recipient presents with hyperglycemia, it is often difficult to salvage the graft. Serum amylase and lipase are not always reliable indicators because these markers may be elevated in conditions other than rejection. Urinary amylase provides early warning of graft dysfunction.

Overall, approximately 10% to 15% of bladder-drained recipients require enteric conversion after their transplant. This is particularly pronounced in male recipients, who tend to suffer more from dehydration and electrolyte disturbances.

Systemic and Enteric Drainage

An intra-abdominal approach is taken using a generous midline incision. The allograft is preferably placed in the right lower quadrant because the iliac vessels are easier to mobilize on this side. The common external and internal iliac arteries are mobilized and encircled with vessel loops. The external and common iliac veins are mobilized lateral to the artery, and any hypogastric branches are ligated and divided to allow for a tension-free anastomosis with the graft portal vein. In cases with a particularly short portal vein, an extension graft may be constructed from a piece of donor iliac vein. We routinely administer intravenous heparin before clamping the vascular structures. The portal vein is anastomosed in an end-to-side fashion to the recipient external iliac vein using running 6–0 polypropylene suture. The Y-graft is anastomosed to the recipient common iliac artery using running 5–0 polypropylene.

The head of the pancreas is oriented in a caudad position in the event that bladder drainage must be performed. After the graft is reperfused and adequate hemostasis is achieved, a loop of proximal jejunum is brought down to the graft duodenum in a tension-free manner, and a side-to-side enteroenterostomy is performed with an inner layer of running absorbable suture and an outer layer of nonabsorbable suture (Fig. 4). If a tension-free enteroenterostomy is not possible, a defunctionalized Roux-en-Y limb may be constructed.

Systemic and Bladder Drainage

The vascular anastomosis is carried out in the same fashion as described earlier. The cystoenterostomy may be performed using a

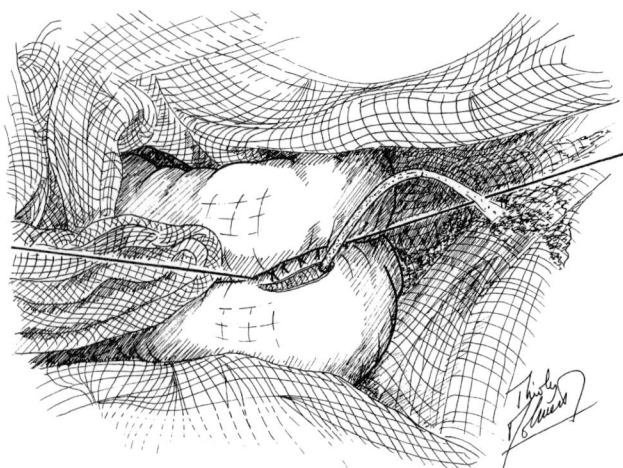

Figure 4 A two-layer anastomosis between the donor duodenum and recipient jejunum is constructed. Note the pancreatic and duodenal secretions emanating from the incised duodenal wall.

two-layer handsewn anastomosis similar to the enteroenterostomy described, or it may be performed using a 28-F end-to-end anastomosis (EEA) stapler. Using a stapled anastomosis requires creating a cystotomy in the anterior wall of the bladder to place the anvil of the EEA. The staple line should be inspected from within the bladder and reinforced with a running 4–0 absorbable suture for hemostasis. The anterior cystotomy is closed with two or three layers of absorbable 3–0 suture (Fig. 5).

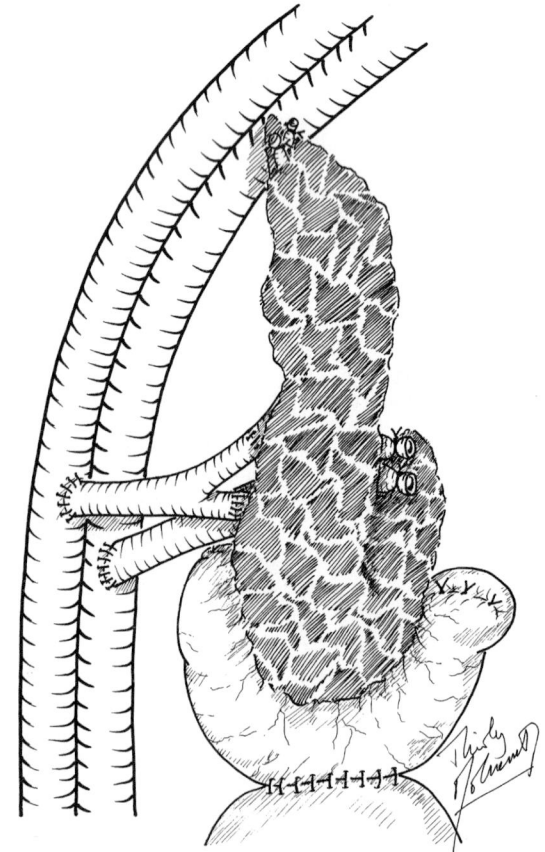

Figure 5 View of an implanted allograft with systemic venous output and bladder drainage of exocrine products.

Portal and Enteric Drainage

The transverse colon is reflected superiorly to expose the root of the small bowel mesentery. The peritoneal layer overlying the SMV and its tributaries is divided. The SMV is carefully mobilized for a length of 10 to 12 cm (Fig. 6). The iliac artery on the right is mobilized and encircled with vessel loops. After the decision has been made to proceed with the venous anastomosis on the basis of the size of the SMV, an adequate-sized tributary distal to the SMV is selected for the anastomosis (Fig. 7). We do not routinely perform the anastomosis directly to the proximal SMV or other large tributary because of the concern that, in the event of venous thrombosis, the clot may propagate into the portal system with

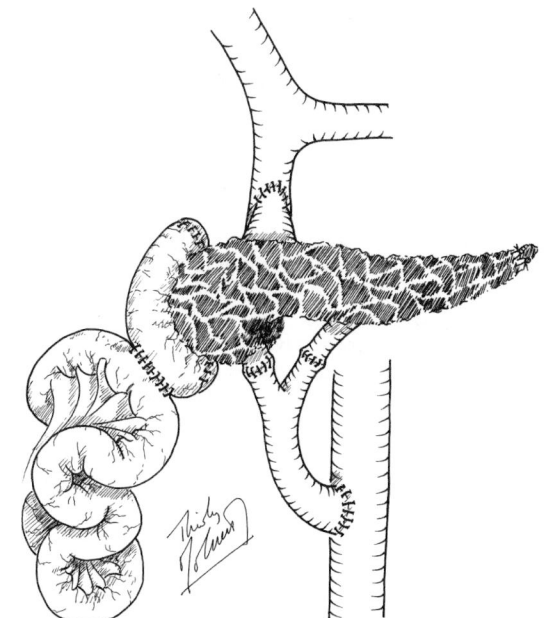

Figure 8 View of the implanted allograft with portal venous output and enteric drainage of exocrine products.

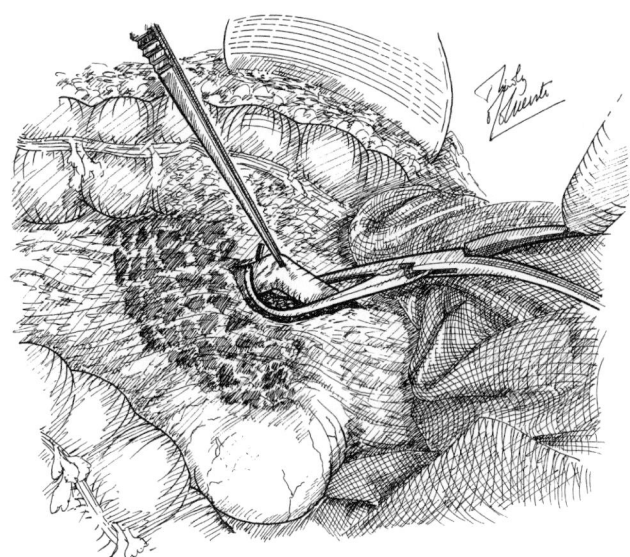

Figure 6 The superior mesenteric vein of the recipient is dissected free of surrounding tissues.

catastrophic results on visceral venous outflow. The arterial anastomosis is performed by passing the Y-graft with an arterial extension graft through the small bowel mesentery in the shortest line to the selected site on the iliac artery. An end-to-side anastomosis is then performed. The enteroenterostomy is handled in the same fashion as described earlier, taking note that to have proper alignment of the vascular anastomoses, the head of the pancreas is oriented in a cephalad direction (Fig. 8). Bladder drainage in this situation is usually not feasible.

POSTOPERATIVE MANAGEMENT

The postoperative management of pancreas transplant patients is challenging. Even before transplantation, these patients often suffer from vasculopathy, autonomic dysfunction, and gastrointestinal dysmotility, which remains after successful transplantation. Their wounds heal slowly, and the risks of infection and rejection increase.

Because of the increased risk of graft rejection compared with kidney or liver transplantation, we use induction immunosuppressive therapy, preferring polyclonal T-cell depleting agents (thymoglobulin) for the first few days postoperatively. We begin maintenance with triple-drug immunosuppression (tacrolimus, mycophenolate mofetil, and prednisone) immediately after the operation. Because of the risk of early pancreatitis, intravenous octreotide is administered for the first 4 postoperative days. To mitigate the risk of graft thrombosis, low-dose heparin is also infused (500 units/hour) for the first 4 days after transplantation. Patients then begin aspirin therapy at a dose of 81 mg daily for 1 year. All enterically drained grafts have nasogastric decompression until return of bowel function, and all urinary-bladder-drained grafts have indwelling bladder catheterization for 3 weeks postoperatively to decrease the likelihood of leakage.

In all bladder-drained grafts, urinary amylase production is monitored after the discontinuation of octreotide, carefully surveying for an acute decrease in amylase levels, which correlates well with acute rejection. In enterically drained grafts, renal function is monitored if performed as a concomitant transplant (SPK). A kidney biopsy is performed if there is any increase in

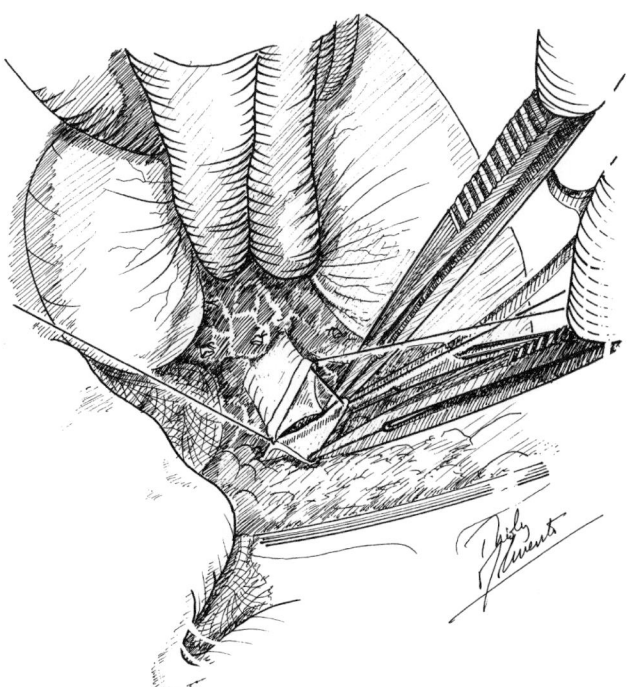

Figure 7 The donor portal vein is anastomosed in an end-to-side fashion to the recipient superior mesenteric vein.

serum creatinine; if not a concomitant transplant, a percutaneous pancreas biopsy is performed if there is a significant increase in serum amylase or lipase, looking for signs of acute rejection (i.e., lymphocytic ascinitis and isletitis).

OUTCOMES

Outcomes after pancreas transplantation have improved markedly since the mid 1990s and now rival those of other solid organ transplants. The 1-year graft survival after SPK transplantation is 85%, and the 3-year graft survival is 78%. The 1-year patient survival is 95%, and the 3-year patient survival is 90%. Although graft survival rates are approximately 5% less after solitary pancreas transplantation, patient survival is excellent, reflecting a younger, relatively healthy demographic in the solitary pancreas transplant recipient group.

COMPLICATIONS

A high index of suspicion is important when caring for pancreas transplant patients. One must be meticulous in the workup of even the most benign of symptoms. Constipation after pancreas transplantation can herald an intra-abdominal abscess or an acute rejection. Because the pancreas graft does not benefit from the copious intragraft perfusion of other vascularized transplants, fluid collections or infections can quickly compromise blood flow to the graft and cause thrombosis. Patients who complain of malaise or abdominal colic should be quickly admitted and surveyed for intra-abdominal infection. These patients can have surprisingly benign physical examinations, although they have significant intra-abdominal pathology.

Acute rejection is poorly tolerated in a pancreas transplant graft and when suspected must be quickly diagnosed and treated.

Hyperglycemia after transplantation has a poor prognosis and is a late occurrence after acute rejection. Acute rejection is usually treated with polyclonal antibody (thymoglobulin 6–8 mg/kg) because these rejections are usually steroid resistant.

CONCLUSIONS

Pancreas transplantation can successfully address the most distressing problems experienced by labile diabetics. Having good alpha- and beta-cell function allows these patients to avoid the comorbidities associated with the twin terrors of hypoglycemia and hyperglycemia. The morbidity and mortality associated with brittle diabetes is reduced, affording these patients longer, more productive lives. The future of islet replacement therapy may rest with alloislet transplantation or some other form of cell-replacement therapy, including stem cells or xenografts; however, at present and for the foreseeable future, pancreas transplantation remains the best option for labile diabetics.

Suggested Readings

Gruessner RWG, Sutherland DER, editors: *Transplantation of the pancreas,* London, 2004, Springer-Verlag.

Humar A, Kandaswamy R, Drangstveit MB, and others: Prolonged preservation increases surgical complications after pancreas transplants, *Surgery* 127:545, 2000.

Humar A, Matas AJ, Payne WD, editors: *Atlas of organ transplantation,* London, 2006, Springer-Verlag.

Tan M, Kandaswamy R, Sutherland DER, and others: Laparoscopic donor distal pancreatectomy for living donor pancreas and pancreas-kidney transplantation, *Am J Transplant* 5:1966, 2005.

Troppmann C, Gjertson DW, Cecka JM, and others: Impact of portal venous pancreas graft drainage on kidney graft outcome in simultaneous pancreas-kidney recipients reported to UNOS, *Am J Transplant* 4:544, 2004.

THE SPLEEN

SPLENECTOMY FOR HEMATOLOGIC DISORDERS

Molly L. Sebastian, MD, and Michael R. Marohn, DO

Splenectomy continues to find common therapeutic indications for hematologic disorders in which the spleen plays a pathologic role. The role of laparoscopy for splenectomy has continued to expand, aided both by new technologies and techniques.

Hematologic disorders can be categorized by a variety of criteria, including by the origin of the disorder: splenic origin, peripheral blood cell origin, bone marrow origin, or genetic origin. Indications for splenectomy for hematologic disorders can be for symptoms, an enlarged spleen, hematologic abnormality, or for diagnostic and staging information (Table 1). Indications can also be organized around the cell line abnormality: platelet disorders, red cell disorders, white cell disorders, and bone marrow disorders. We have organized this section around the underlying mechanism of the hematologic disorder: autoimmune and idiopathic disorders, cell membrane disorders, genetic disorders, disorders of white cell origin, and disorders of the bone marrow (Table 2). Therapeutic splenectomy rarely cures the underlying hematologic disease, but in many of these disorders, splenectomy can significantly ameliorate the pathologic effects of splenic sequestration and symptomatic splenomegaly, can correct the hematologic abnormality, and can aid in diagnosis and staging. Removal of the spleen can play an important role in reducing the morbidity of hematologic conditions.

INDICATIONS

Autoimmune and Idiopathic Disorders

Idiopathic Thrombocytopenic Purpura

Idiopathic thrombocytopenia purpura (ITP) is the most common indication for elective splenectomy in the United States. It is an acquired disorder characterized by splenic production of immunoglobulin (Ig) G that induces splenic sequestration and destruction of platelets. The hallmarks of this condition are low platelet levels, ecchymoses, purpura, petechiae, and abnormal bleeding (e.g., heavy vaginal bleeding, bleeding gums, gastrointestinal bleeding, hematuria, etc.). Intracranial bleeding, which can be lethal, affects 1% to 2% of these patients and may occur early in the course of the disease. ITP can occur in the presence of human immunodeficiency virus, acquired immunodeficiency syndrome, and systemic lupus erythematosus.

The management for childhood ITP is different from that for adults, particularly with regard to the role of splenectomy. Children tend to present acutely. The condition is often self-limited in children, with more than 70% of cases resolving spontaneously. Splenectomy for childhood ITP is rarely indicated, reserved for the rare case of severe, symptomatic thrombocytopenia of greater than 1 year's duration that is refractory to medical management (including corticosteroids and intravenous infusion of immunoglobulin [IVIG] therapy).

In adults, the thrombocytopenia associated with ITP is usually morbid and requires intervention. Women are affected more commonly than men. Bleeding is rarely intense and may be cyclical. The first-line therapy is medical. Initial therapy is oral steroid administration (1.0–1.5 mg/kg per day), with a response typically seen within 3 weeks. In severe cases, with platelet counts under 5000/mm^3, IVIG at 1.0 g/kg per day for 2 to 3 days is administered. Initial response rates to medical therapy are between 50% and 75%, but relapses are common, with permanent cure from medical therapy reaching 15% to 20%. Generally, splenectomy is indicated in adults with ITP if the patient does not improve after 8 weeks of steroid therapy or if the thrombocytopenia recurs after steroids are tapered or terminated. Intracranial hemorrhage is an indication for emergent IVIG and splenectomy.

The spleen is not enlarged in ITP, making laparoscopic splenectomy an attractive therapeutic option for these patients.

In the operating room, platelet transfusions are held until the splenic artery has been doubly ligated or clamped. Even for patients with particularly low platelet counts, platelet pack transfusion is held for intraoperative use to avoid platelet consumption within the spleen. Intraoperative platelet transfusion is held unless there is persistent bleeding after the spleen has been removed. Because the splenic tissue is the source for this disorder, a key component of operative strategy is a thorough inspection of the abdomen for accessory spleens. Accessory spleens are reported in up to 30% of patients with ITP. They are most commonly located in the gastrosplenic, gastrocolic, or lienorenal ligaments but can reside throughout the peritoneal cavity. Presence of an unresected accessory spleen can result in recurrence of ITP. In patients who have recurrent symptoms following splenectomy, a ^{99m}Tc-labeled red cell or ^{111}In-labeled platelet scan can be performed to identify the location of the accessory spleen and facilitate resection, with removal of the remnant accessory spleen typically associated with ITP cure.

Splenectomy results in surgical cure of 75% to 85% of patients with ITP. Even in the remaining 15% to 25% with persistent postsplenectomy thrombocytopenia, petechiae, ecchymosis, and significant bleeding are uncommon.

Table 1: General Indications for Splenectomy for Hematologic Disorders

Symptomatic splenomegaly
Hypersplenism
Hematologic abnormality, including disorders of platelets, red cells, white cells, or bone marrow origin
Diagnosis and staging

Table 2: Indications to Consider Splenectomy for Hematologic Disorders

Autoimmune and Idiopathic Disorders

Idiopathic thrombocytopenia purpura (ITP)
Thrombotic thrombocytopenic purpura (TTP)
Idiopathic autoimmune hemolytic anemia (AIHA)
Felty's syndrome (autoimmune neutropenia)
Sarcoidosis

Cell Membrane Disorders

Hereditary spherocytosis
Hereditary elliptocytosis
Hereditary pyropoikilocytosis
Hereditary hydrocytosis
Hereditary xerocytosis

Genetic Deficiencies

Thalassemia (Mediterranean anemia or Cooley's anemia)
Sickle cell anemia
Gaucher's disease
Pyruvate kinase deficiency
Glucose-6-phosphate dehydrogenase deficiency

Disorders of White Blood Cell Origin Causing Hypersplenism

Hodgkin's lymphoma
Non-Hodgkin's lymphoma
Chronic lymphocytic leukemia
Chronic myelogenous leukemia
Hairy cell leukemia

Disorders of the Bone Marrow

Myelofibrosis with myeloid metaplasia
Myeloproliferative disorders

Thrombotic Thrombocytopenic Purpura

Thrombotic thrombocytopenic purpura (TTP) is a rare and dangerous disorder in which the arterioles and capillaries have anomalous hyaline membranes that cause platelet aggregation and occlusion. There is minimal inflammation associated with this process, but it has a dramatic hematologic impact. The classic pentad of clinical signs of TTP is purpura, fever, microangiopathic hemolytic anemia, neurologic deficits, and renal dysfunction (hematuria or renal failure). In approximately 5% of cases, TTP first appears during pregnancy.

The recommended initial therapy for TTP is plasmaphoresis, often repeated until the process reverses. Unfortunately, TTP is characterized by rapid onset and progressions, often with a fatal outcome because of intracranial hemorrhage or renal failure. Mortality is greater than 60% for patients who do not respond to plasmapheresis. Platelet administration in TTP patients is typically avoided because their administration has been associated with clinical deterioration.

Splenectomy in TTP, coupled with high-dose steroids, can play a role for patients who relapse or who fail repeated plasma exchange transfusions. Unfortunately there is only a 40% cure rate with splenectomy for TTP.

Idiopathic Autoimmune Hemolytic Anemia

Idiopathic autoimmune hemolytic anemia (AIHA) is characterized by splenic autoantibody production. Red blood cells opsonized by these autoantibodies can either become sequestered in the spleen or undergo phagocytosis in the peripheral circulation. This disorder is more prevalent in female patients. AIHA can occur at any age, but most afflicted patients are older than 50 years of age.

Steroids are the first-line therapy (1.0–2.0 mg/kg per day of corticosteroids until hematocrit rises). Splenectomy is a second-line therapy for AIHA patients who fail steroid therapy. Splenomegaly is present in more than half of the cases, and thus the role of laparoscopic splenectomy is selective. Splenectomy is effective in correcting the anemia of AIHA in 80% of cases.

Felty's Syndrome (Autoimmune Neutropenia)

Felty's syndrome is an uncommon disorder that includes splenomegaly, neutropenia, and rheumatoid arthritis. Felty's syndrome patients can also have thrombocytopenia and anemia. All of these conditions leave patients vulnerable to aggressive infections.

They are initially treated with steroids. Splenectomy can be helpful in correcting the neutropenia that can hamper the patient's ability to fight infection. In some cases, the neutropenia persists despite splenectomy, but the neutrophil response to infectious agents is improved. Frequent need for transfusion (>1 per month), thrombocytopenia, and recurrent infections are also indications for splenectomy. Because splenomegaly is a hallmark of Felty's syndrome, the role of laparoscopic splenectomy should be selective.

Sarcoidosis

A hallmark of sarcoidosis is the formation of noncaseating granulomas. Approximately one quarter of patients with sarcoidosis have granulomatous involvement of the spleen, causing splenomegaly. Of these patients, 20% have hypersplenism, in which the enlarged spleen is hyperactive, resulting in thrombocytopenia. This low platelet count generally improves after splenectomy. These patients can also have anemia, neutropenia, and spontaneous splenic rupture. Because of the common splenomegaly and hypersplenism, the role of laparoscopic splenectomy for these patients is selective.

Cell Membrane Disorders

Hereditary Spherocytosis

Hereditary spherocytosis (HS) is the most common congenital anemia for which splenectomy is performed. In this autosomal-dominant disorder, a deficiency of spectrin is passed from one generation to the next (75% of patients with HS have a family history of the disorder). Lack of spectrin erythrocyte membrane protein leads to loss of red blood cell membrane surface area and causes the characteristic shape of HS red blood cells, called *spherocytes*. These abnormal red blood cells are less deformable and have increased osmotic fragility, and therefore they cannot easily pass through the splenic pulp and have increased tendency to be sequestered and destroyed within the spleen. Patients present with anemia, jaundice, and splenomegaly. The splenomegaly develops by the time the patient is 1 year old. By age 5, many patients with HS have pigmented gallstones. Pigmented gallstones are present in 30% to 60% of HS patients. The diagnosis of HS is made by analysis of a peripheral blood smear displaying the spherocytes. Although the spherocytes persist, these patients are cured of their anemia and jaundice with splenectomy. Removal of the gallbladder in the same procedure is warranted if the patient has developed gallstones. The surgeon should try to delay splenectomy until the patient is 4 years old if possible to reduce the risk of overwhelming postsplenectomy infection (OPSI). There are recent reports of partial splenectomy for HS without recurrence in 1 to 2 years of follow-up, but the long-term durability of this approach has yet to be established. With appropriate skill and correctly sized instruments, laparoscopic splenectomy combined with cholecystectomy, if indicated, is a good option for these patients.

Hereditary Elliptocytosis

Hereditary elliptocytosis is an uncommon condition affecting 1 in every 2000 people. It has a milder clinical course than HS, with the elliptical red blood cells more deformable and more robust than spherocytes. Patients are usually asymptomatic. Splenectomy is indicated only if the patient develops a severe anemia requiring transfusion more frequently than once a month. If splenectomy is required, as with HS it is curative of the anemia.

Hereditary Pyropoikilocytosis

A recessive variant of HS, hereditary pyropoikilocytosis is a rare disorder that results in distorted red blood cell membranes. The severity of the anemia is extremely variable. If the disorder is manifest in childhood, it is most likely to resolve spontaneously. If it does not resolve, the patient usually requires splenectomy to control the anemia, with an expectation of 100% resolution of the associated anemia, as with HS.

Hereditary Hydrocytosis

This condition is characterized by increased water content in the red blood cell membrane. These cells are more fragile than normal red blood cells (also more fragile than red cells in hereditary xerocytosis). As a result, this condition can lead to rapid destruction and sequestration of red cells by the spleen, causing hemolytic anemia. Splenectomy is curative for the anemia.

Hereditary Xerocytosis

Hereditary xerocytosis is characterized by decreased water content in the cell membrane. Patients with this rare condition are less likely to require splenectomy than patients with hereditary hydrocytosis.

Genetic Deficiencies

Thalassemia (Mediterranean Anemia or Cooley's Anemia)

Thalassemias are autosomal-dominant deficiencies in hemoglobin synthesis. The red blood cells have intracellular precipitation of excess globin chains. These intracellular precipitates lead to the premature destruction of red blood cells when they are filtered in the spleen. There are several subtypes, determined on the basis of which globin chain is defective (α, β, γ, or δ). The beta subtype is the most common thalassemia in the United States. Individuals who are homozygous (thalassemia major) have a more severe clinical presentation, whereas the heterozygous patients (thalassemia minor) can be asymptomatic. Clinical signs of thalassemia major include growth retardation, pallor, extremity ulcers, gallstones, enlargement of the head, and splenomegaly. Peripheral blood smear may show "target cells," which are nucleated red blood cells with relatively washed-out appearance of the cytoplasm.

Thalassemia major patients benefit from splenectomy if they require frequent transfusions (>1 per month), suffer from severe pain caused by splenic infarct, or have severe thrombocytopenia (<20,000 platelets/mm^3).

Sickle Cell Anemia

Sickle cell anemia is a hereditary hemolytic anemia caused by a single amino acid substitution on the beta chain of the hemoglobin molecule, which imbues the red blood cell with a tendency to sickle and stiffen in relatively hypoxic environments such as the red pulp of the spleen. The altered hemoglobin molecule is called *hemoglobin S* (Hb-S). Because the red cells are less flexible, they tend to cause infarcts in the microvasculature, felt to be the source of the severe pain commonly associated with "sickle cell crisis." Because of this process of repeated microvascular infarcts, patients who are homozygous for sickle cell anemia undergo autosplenectomy usually by the time they are 5 years old.

Although it is rare for sickle cell anemia patients to require splenectomy, splenic abscess or acute sequestration may be indications. Splenic abscess may complicate splenic infarct, making splenectomy of benefit. Splenectomy does not affect sickling, but elective splenectomy is a consideration following one major acute splenic sequestration crisis to avoid the 40% to 50% probability of subsequent acute sequestration crises, which can be associated with as high as 20% mortality rate. The incidence of acute sequestrations in patients with sickle cell disease is approximately 5%, with approximately 3% requiring splenectomy. Key perioperative management principles for sickle cell patients include adequate hydration and avoidance of hypothermia.

Gaucher's Disease

Gaucher's disease is a familial disorder in which abnormal storage of glycolipid cerebrosides into reticuloendothelial cells occurs. It is associated with splenomegaly and lymph node enlargement as a result.

Although splenectomy does not alter the course of a patient with Gaucher's disease, it is the procedure of choice if there are signs of hypersplenism (thrombocytopenia that may be associated with anemia and neutropenia). After splenectomy, the thrombocytopenia improves. Some authors have proposed performing a partial splenectomy for hypersplenism in Gaucher's disease to limit the hypersplenism while preserving some splenic function.

Pyruvate Kinase Deficiency

Pyruvate kinase deficiency can cause a profound anemia that can be improved with splenectomy, although in some cases postoperative thrombosis involving the portal or hepatic veins has been reported if the hemolysis does not resolve.

Glucose-6-Phosphate Dehydrogenase Deficiency

When patients lack glucose-6-phosphate dehydrogenase (G-6-PD) enzyme, they are at risk for developing a significant hemolytic anemia when taking certain medications. Splenectomy is rarely, if ever, indicated for the anemia associated with G-6-PD.

Hereditary High Red Phosphatidylcholine Anemia

Splenectomy is contraindicated in hereditary high red phosphatidylcholine anemia.

Disorders of White Blood Cell Origin

Hodgkin's Lymphoma

Staging laparotomy for Hodgkin's lymphoma is a procedure of historical interest. This invasive procedure involved liver biopsy, splenectomy, removal of any enlarged or abnormal lymph nodes, and sampling from the periaortic, mesenteric, and hepatoduodenal lymph nodes.

Current management of Hodgkin's disease incorporates adequate staging as assessed in the history and physical examination, combined with chest, abdomen, and pelvis computed tomography (CT) scan. Chemotherapy is the mainstay of treatment for this disease. Radiation therapy can be used in early stages (stage IA or IIA), with chemotherapy as the second-line therapy for nonresponders. Because these patients are nearly always treated with chemotherapy, there is no benefit to performing an invasive staging procedure that may delay their treatment.

Patients with Hodgkin's disease occasionally require splenectomy for symptomatic splenomegaly or for thrombocytopenia or leukopenia that interferes with their medical therapy.

Non-Hodgkin's Lymphoma

Non-Hodgkin's lymphoma is the most common kind of lymphoma. Splenectomy is reserved for non-Hodgkin's lymphoma patients who have significant symptoms from splenomegaly (secondary to lymphatic infiltration) or pancytopenia, with frequent transfusion requirements resulting from hypersplenism. In these cases, splenectomy can improve patients' symptoms.

Chronic Lymphocytic Leukemia

Chronic lymphocytic leukemia (CLL) is a low-grade neoplastic process characterized by accumulations of functionally incompetent B cells. In advanced stages of the disease, splenomegaly is common. Like patients with other neoplastic disorders, CLL patients can develop significant symptoms from the mass effect of the enlarged spleen (feelings of abdominal pressure, pain, and gastric compression). Secondary hypersplenism can develop in the enlarged spleen and cause anemia and thrombocytopenia.

Splenectomy improves the thrombocytopenia associated with CLL in 70% to 80% of patients and anemia in 60% to 70% of patients, with the benefit lasting more than a year. Patients in the advanced stages of CLL who have failed multiple courses of chemotherapy or who have a small spleen do not respond as well to splenectomy. Terminal patients have significantly increased operative morbidity and should not undergo routine splenectomy.

Chronic Myelogenous Leukemia

Ninety percent of patients with chronic myelogenous leukemia (CML) have the characteristic Philadelphia chromosome—a reciprocal translation between chromosomes 9 and 22.

Select patients in the advanced stages of the disease can benefit from splenectomy to relieve symptoms of splenomegaly or to reduce their need for frequent transfusions. Several studies have shown an objective benefit to these patients with relatively low morbidity of the operation.

Hairy Cell Leukemia

In "hairy cell" leukemia, a B cell with irregular cytoplasmic protrusions invades the bone marrow and the spleen. It is a low-grade leukemic disorder that typically affects men who are older than age 50.

Although splenectomy was a major component of the treatment algorithm in the past, it has been supplanted by chemotherapeutic agents—specifically, pentostatin and cladribine (purine nucleoside analogues), which yield a complete response rate in 80% to 90%

of patients, with longer duration than the effect from splenectomy. Splenectomy is reserved for palliation of splenomegaly in "hairy cell" leukemia patients who fail medical management.

Disorders Related to the Bone Marrow

Myelofibrosis with Myeloid Metaplasia

Myelofibrosis with myeloid metaplasia is a chronic myeloproliferative disorder in which immature myeloid precursor cells are released into the circulation and settle in the reticuloendothelial organs (particularly the spleen and liver). Splenomegaly develops when these cells initiate extramedullary hematopoiesis (i.e., marrow function outside of the bone marrow). Up to 75% of these patients develop massive splenic enlargement. Because of the presence of the large spleen and propensity for hematopoiesis, either thrombocytopenia or thrombocytosis can exist.

These patients often require splenectomy to alleviate the symptoms from the mechanical effect of their enormous spleen. Associated disorders can include esophagogastric varices resulting from portal hypertension (these varices resolve after splenectomy), thrombocytopenia, anemia, or pain caused by splenic infarcts. In the postoperative period, these patients are at high risk for developing thrombocytosis and portal vein thrombosis. A recent review of the Mayo Clinic's 30-year experience in splenectomy for this disorder suggested that platelet-lowering therapy may be helpful to reduce postoperative thrombotic complications. Platelet-lowering therapy in this study consisted of medical therapy with hydroxyurea, aspirin, or anagrelide, and platelet apheresis if the platelet count was higher than 1 million. Portal vein thrombosis can present as prolonged postoperative ileus, new-onset ascites, hepatic insufficiency, and vague abdominal discomfort. The treatment is intravenous heparin infusion with transition to warfarin for 6 months of therapy while collateralization occurs. An operative strategy proposed in the Mayo Clinic review to minimize the risk of postoperative portal vein thrombosis was ligating the splenic vein flush at its confluence with the superior mesenteric vein to maintain laminar flow in the area. This maneuver is often difficult to achieve because of dense adherence of the splenic vein to the posterior aspect of the pancreas.

Myeloproliferative Disorders

Myeloproliferative disorders represent a spectrum of panproliferative abnormalities manifest by abnormal proliferation within the bone marrow and hematopoietic elements including acute and chronic myeloid leukemia, chronic myelomonocytic leukemia, polycythemia vera, essential thrombocythemia, and myelofibrosis. Splenectomy does not cure the underlying disorder but may ameliorate symptoms if splenomegaly has developed. Splenectomy offers little benefit for essential thrombocythemia or polycythemia vera until myelofibrosis has developed.

PREOPERATIVE MANAGEMENT

For elective splenectomy, regardless of approach, vaccination against encapsulated organisms (*Haemophilus influenzae B*, polyvalent *Pneumococcus,* and *Meningococcus* vaccines) is generally recommended to occur 2 weeks before the procedure whenever possible.

Preoperative imaging of the spleen, with a CT scan or ultrasound of the abdomen showing the size of the spleen and its proximity to surrounding structures, can be helpful in planning operative strategy. CT imaging has advantages over ultrasound beyond splenic size determination, providing better delineation of the spleen, vascular relationships, and detection of accessory spleens. For massive splenomegaly, preoperative splenic artery embolization can be helpful to reduce intraoperative blood loss.

On the day of surgery, appropriate preoperative antibiotic should be infused within 30 minutes of skin incision. Patients who are at risk for adrenal insufficiency resulting from recent steroid use should receive stress dose steroids (usually 100 mg of intravenous hydrocortisone with rapid taper postoperatively). An oral gastric or nasogastric tube is placed to decompress the stomach. This step facilitates dissection of the short gastric vessels along the greater curvature of the stomach.

OPERATIVE STRATEGY

During open splenectomy, short gastric vessels are serially ligated; this may include suture ligation. During laparoscopic splenectomy, devices such as the LigaSure (ValleyLab, Boulder, CO) device, harmonic scalpel, or endoclips can be used when dividing the short gastric vessels. Many surgeons leave in a nasogastric tube postoperatively overnight to minimize the risk of gastric distention disrupting a short gastric vascular pedicle. At open surgery, the splenic pedicle can be divided with ligatures, typically with vessels individually isolated and suture ligated at open surgery and divided using a vascular GIA stapling device (US Surgical, Norwalk, CT). At laparoscopic surgery, the splenic pedicle is often divided using an EndoGIA (US Surgical, Norwalk, CT) stapling device with vascular staples.

Coagulopathy and portal hypertension are relative contraindications to splenectomy.

Several approaches are used to manage the splenic artery. Ligation can be achieved by entering the lesser sac and dissecting the artery free from the pancreas. The splenic artery should be doubly ligated whenever possible. In ITP, this step is performed before platelets are infused (unless significant thrombocytopenia and hemorrhage necessitate earlier use). Accomplishing this step early in the operation facilitates optimal timing for platelet transfusion and limits operative blood loss. An alternate approach to early control of the splenic artery in the lesser sac involves managing the splenic artery at the splenic hilum as outlined earlier.

The ligamentous attachments to the spleen should be divided under direct vision. After the spleen is mobilized, the splenic bed should be closely inspected for hemostasis and for accessory spleens. Bleeding along the diaphragmatic portion of the splenic

bed is the most common source identified at the time of reexploration. Careful inspection of the abdomen for the presence of accessory spleens is also important for good outcomes, particularly with splenectomy for hematologic disorders. The incidence of accessory spleens is reported to be as high as 30% among the general public.

Percutaneous drainage is not used for routine splenectomy but should be a consideration if a distal pancreatectomy was performed coincident to splenectomy because of the high rate of fistula formation.

LAPAROSCOPIC SPLENECTOMY

Advances in laparoscopic technology and techniques have expanded the role of laparoscopic splenectomy since its inception in 1991 by Delaitre and Maignien. Elective laparoscopic splenectomy is most commonly performed for hematologic disorders. Multiple series have shown a consistent trend for laparoscopic splenectomy, resulting in shorter length of hospital stay and lower morbidity, albeit operative times are longer for these procedures (Table 3).

Size matters for laparoscopic splenectomy. In ITP, the spleen is usually small, making this disorder ideally suited for a laparoscopic splenectomy. In general, the size of the spleen is the most important technical consideration when preparing for a laparoscopic approach. When measured in the craniocaudal axis on CT or ultrasound imaging, the spleen should be less than 20 to 25 cm in length for laparoscopy to be feasible. There are exceptions to this rule, but this measurement is the current general practice among experienced minimally invasive surgeons. Increasing availability of expertise with various hand-assisted surgery devices has expanded the size criteria for successful laparoscopic splenectomy. Kirkwood and colleagues recently reported their series of laparoscopic splenectomies for massive splenomegaly (>17 cm craniocaudal length), which showed a higher rate of conversion to an open procedure for massive splenomegaly but also an increasing role for use of a hand port in the cases that stayed with a laparoscopic approach in these patients.

Hand-assisted laparoscopic surgery (HALS) uses a combination of laparoscopic and "open" splenectomy techniques. HALS employs a device to enable intra-abdominal placement of a hand and

Table 3: Outcomes after Laparoscopic and Open Splenectomy

Study	OR Approach	N	Spleen Size (g)	Mean OR Time (min)	Reoperation for Bleeding (%)	Estimated Blood Loss (ml)	Length of Stay (days)	Morb. (%)	Mort. (%)
Kirkwood 2006	Lap	85	—	233	1	707	2–5	7	0
	Open	26	—	128	12	770	7–13	24	12
Puglisi 2006	Lap	379	1200	140	—	—	5.5	17.8	0.5
Brunt (meta-analysis) 2003	Lap	2119	—	180	—	—	3.6	15.5	0.6
	Open	821	—	114	—	—	7.2	26.6	1.1
Sweeney 2003	Lap	101	191–1295	138–190	—	307–1060	3.5–6.3	18	4
Donohue 2003	Lap	42	157	167	—	—	3.31	24	—
	Open	44	273	119	—	—	5.34	39	—
Heniford 2002	Lap	49	600–4750	171	—	114	2.3	6	0
Witzke 2000	Lap	197	289.7	145	—	161	2.7	8.4	0

Lap, Laproscopic; *Morb,* morbidity; *Mort,* mortality; *OR,* operative.

forearm through a small incision while maintaining pneumoperitoneum to facilitate palpation, dissection, retraction, or specimen removal. The length of the required hand port incision correlates mainly with breadth of surgeon's palm (approximates the surgeon's glove size, i.e., 6.5–8.0 cm). For a large spleen, it can help the surgeon to manipulate the organ with less trauma. Placement of the HALS device is important. There is a need for "stand-off" distance between the hand port and the target organ so that the surgeon's hand has working room and does not interfere with laparoscopic instruments or camera view. In splenectomy, the most common site is the upper midline.

Laparoscopic splenectomy is an excellent option for an expanding group of indications but requires an experienced laparoscopic team.

POSTOPERATIVE MANAGEMENT AND COMPLICATIONS

In all patients who have undergone splenectomy, vaccination is an important consideration. The ideal timing for vaccination (as discussed in Preoperative Management section) is 2 weeks before the operation. If this was not accomplished, the next best option is to vaccinate the patient just before discharge. Careful counseling of patients and communication with their primary care providers should also take place because these vaccinations must be repeated every 5 years.

In the immediate postoperative period, the patient should be monitored for bleeding and infection. Patients with fever and elevated white blood cell counts should be treated empirically with antibiotics and evaluated with CT scan looking for abscess. A rare but potentially lethal complication of splenectomy is OPSI, which is associated with up to 50% mortality. The typical scenario is a late postoperative patient who develops an upper respiratory infection that progresses rapidly to sepsis and multisystem organ failure. Although the lifetime risk of OPSI in the general population ranges from 1% to 4%, in patients who undergo splenectomy for hematologic disorders, particularly children younger than age 4 who have thalassemia or sickle cell disease, the incidence of OPSI is increased, reported to be as high as 12% to 15%. Infection is able to spread so aggressively because of the blunted immune response characterized by decreased levels of IgM and opsonins, clearance of encapsulated organisms, complement fixation, and filtration. The most common offending organisms implicated with OPSI are: *H. influenza, Pneumococcus, Meningococcus,* and *Escherichia coli.* OPSI risk management is best treated with prevention, but if suspected, early use of broad-spectrum antibiotics and supportive measures can be lifesaving for these vulnerable patients until the diagnosis of OPSI can be ruled out. Many surgeons provide antibiotic prophylaxis during the first 2 years following splenectomy for children whose indication is a hematologic disorder.

Postsplenectomy patients are at risk for thrombotic complications, particularly thrombosis in the remnant of the splenic vein. Thrombi can propagate to the mesenteric and portal venous systems. Such patients can present with ileus, abdominal pain, and ascites. Patients with myeloproliferative disorders are felt to be at

Table 4: Complications after Splenectomy

| Hemorrhage |
| Atelectasis |
| Pneumonia |
| Pleural effusion |
| Subphrenic abscess |
| Pancreatitis |
| Pancreatic fistula |
| Portal vein thrombosis |
| Overwhelming postsplenectomy infection |
| Persistence of hypersplenism (unresected accessory spleen) |

particularly increased risk of this complication and should be treated with prophylactic platelet-lowering medication.

Some data suggest that patients who undergo splenectomy have increased lifetime risk of malignancy, as well as accelerated atherosclerosis.

After successful splenectomy, a patient will have target cells (immature cells), Howell-Jolly bodies (nuclear remnants), Heinz bodies (denatured hemoglobin), and Papenheimer bodies (iron granules) on their peripheral blood smear. If these features are absent in the peripheral red blood cells, the patient may have an unresected accessory spleen. A patient with symptoms of hypersplenism despite splenectomy may have had a failed operation because of an undetected accessory spleen and may require reexploration. A technetium scan can be helpful to localize the residual splenic tissue. Selective embolization has been reported as an alternative to reoperation in these patients.

Surgical complications of laparoscopic splenectomy are similar to those for the open splenectomy, including pneumonia, left pleural effusions, atelectasis, and injury to adjacent organs (e.g., stomach, pancreas) (Table 4). Hemorrhage is a known source of complications with splenectomy; transfusion rates with splenectomy range from 3% to 5% for all indications. Laparoscopic splenectomy is associated with slightly higher bleeding problems, and open splenectomy is associated with higher incidence of pulmonary-related complications. Portal vein thrombosis is a risk and is particularly associated with myeloproliferative disorders.

SUGGESTED READINGS

Heniford BT, Park A, Walsh RM, and others: Laparoscopic splenectomy with normal-sized spleens versus splenomegaly: does size matter? *Am Surg* 67:854, 2001.

Mahon D, Rhodes M: Laparoscopic splenectomy: size matters, *Ann R Coll Surg Eng* 85:248, 2003.

Marohn MR, Steele K, Lawler LP: Minimally invasive surgical and image guided interventional approaches to the spleen. In Yeo C, editor: *Shackelford's surgery of the alimentary tract,* ed. 6, Philadelphia, 2007, WB Saunders, p. 1780.

Park A, Marcaccio M, Sternbach M, and others: Laparoscopic vs. open splenectomy, *Arch Surg* 134:1263, 1999.

CYSTS, TUMORS, AND ABSCESSES OF THE SPLEEN

Thomas McIntyre, MD, and Michael E. Zenilman, MD

Cysts, tumors, and abscesses of the spleen are entities that occur rarely but often require surgical treatment (Table 1).

CYSTS

Splenic cysts are classified as either primary (true) or secondary (false) on the basis of the presence of an epithelial lining of the lumen. False cysts are also referred to as *pseudocysts*.

Primary (True)

Primary cysts with an epithelial lining are either parasitic or non-parasitic. In the United States, approximately 5% of splenic cysts are parasitic. However, in geographic regions where hydatid disease is endemic, such as South America and parts of the Mediterranean region, most splenic cysts are parasitic.

Parasitic

Parasitic cysts occur after infection by the *Tinea echinococcus*. The most common organism is *Echinococcus granulosus*, which forms a unilocular cyst. Rare infections from *E. multilocularis* and *E. vogeli* form multiloculated cysts. These cysts are typically asymptomatic and are associated with manifestations of echinococcal disease elsewhere. The most common organ affected is the liver, followed by the spleen and lungs. A parasitic cyst should be suspected if the splenic cyst has wall calcifications and internal daughter cysts. Serologic testing for parasite antibodies should be performed to confirm diagnosis. In all cases, splenectomy is indicated to avoid the potential complications of rupture and bacterial superinfection. Splenectomy should be combined with medical management of echinococcal disease. Appropriate intraoperative precautions and surgical techniques should be used to minimize cyst rupture and intraperitoneal contamination.

Nonparasitic

Nonparasitic epithelial lined cysts account for 20% of all splenic cysts and can be congenital or neoplastic. Neoplastic splenic cysts are exceedingly rare. Congenital cysts are either epidermoid or dermoid and are usually detected in children or young adults. Epidermoid cysts account for 90% of all nonparasitic true cysts.

Symptomatic splenic cysts can cause left upper quadrant pain, early satiety, and postprandial nausea and vomiting. Of asymptomatic patients, half have a palpable mass on physical examination. Computed tomography (CT) scan typically shows a solitary cyst with occasional wall calcifications.

Secondary (False)—Pseudocysts

Secondary cysts or pseudocysts account for the vast majority of splenic cysts seen in the United States. The spleen is the most commonly injured organ following abdominal trauma, and most secondary cysts are posttraumatic in origin. They may also occur in association with a pancreatic pseudocyst after acute pancreatitis and splenic infarcts or infections. The diagnosis of splenic pseudocysts is increasingly common because of the widespread nonoperative management of splenic trauma and increased use of CT scanning as a diagnostic modality.

Treatment

Indications for treatment of splenic cysts are based on the patient's symptoms and cyst diameter (Fig. 1). Possible complications of an untreated cyst include spontaneous rupture with peritonitis or bleeding, abscess formation, hypersplenism, and portal hypertension. For asymptomatic cysts of less than 5 cm, conservative treatment is advocated because these cysts often resolve. If the cyst is greater than 5 cm or symptomatic, surgical intervention is recommended. Percutaneous drainage should be avoided because of the high incidence of recurrence and subsequent inflammatory reaction that ensues, rendering subsequent operations difficult.

Figure 1 Algorithm for treatment of splenic cysts. *Adapted from Hansen MB, Moller AC: Surg Laparosc Endosc Percutan Tech 14:316, 2004.*

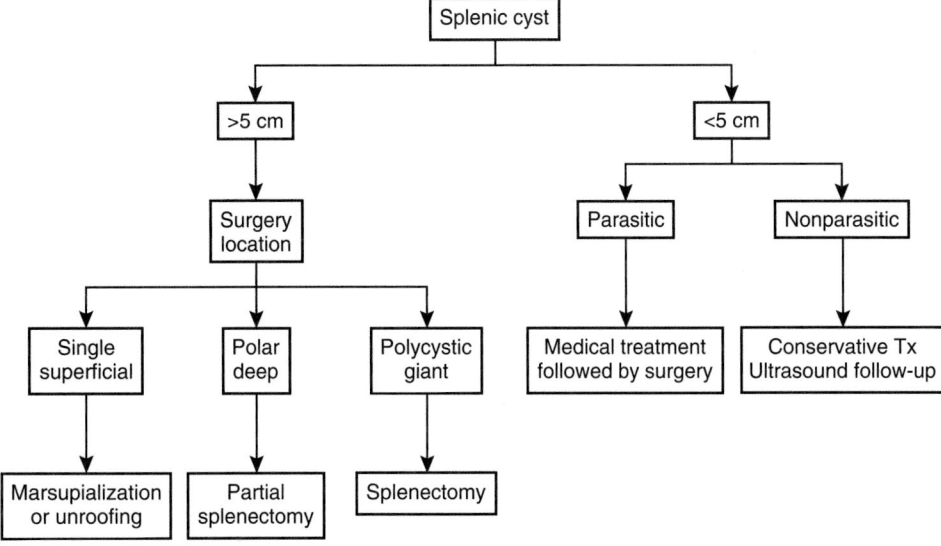

Table 1: Classification of Splenic Cysts, Tumors, and Abscesses

Cysts

Primary (True)
  Parasitic
  Nonparasitic
    Congenital
      Epidermoid
      Dermoid
    Neoplastic
Secondary (false)—pseudocysts

Tumors

Malignant
  Lymphoproliferative disease
    Non-Hodgkin's lymphoma
    Hodgkin's disease
    Hairy cell leukemia
    Chronic lymphocytic leukemia
  Myeloproliferative disease
    Chronic myelogenous leukemia
    Myelofibrosis
  Primary tumors
    Angiosarcoma
  Metastatic tumors
Benign
  Hemangiomas
  Hamartomas
  Lymphangiomas

Abscesses

Bacterial
Fungal

Surgical options include complete or partial splenectomy, unroofing of the cyst, and fenestration. All of these can be accomplished by open or minimally invasive techniques. A spleen-preserving, minimally invasive procedure is recommended, if possible. Splenic preservation is advocated because the spleen plays an important role in regulation of the circulating blood volume, hematopoesis, protection against infection, and malignancies.

Splenectomy

Complete splenectomy is recommended in polycystic cases and when cysts are inaccessible for fenestration or partial splenectomy. Splenectomy should be performed laparoscopically when possible. The laparoscopic procedure typically places the patient in the lateral position and uses four subcostal ports. The spleen is first mobilized from its attachments to the colon and retroperitoneum. The short gastric vessels can be clipped and divided or taken with a harmonic scalpel or LigaSure device (ValleyLab, Boulder, CO). The vascular pedicle can then be isolated and divided. The specimen is placed in a bag, morcellated, and removed from one of the subcostal port sites.

Partial Splenectomy

At least 25% of the splenic parenchyma should be preserved to ensure adequate postoperative splenic function. Partial splenectomy is recommended if the cyst cavity is deep within the splenic parenchyma. In general, splenic cysts respect the segmental blood supply of the spleen, making it possible to perform partial splenectomy without major blood loss. Control of splenic arterial inflow and complete splenic mobilization are first performed. Segmental vessels are ligated until a desired line of ischemic demarcation is achieved. Transection and hemostasis of the splenic parenchyma is undertaken within the cyanotic area using a variety of techniques: finger or scalpel fracture, electrocautery, clips, staplers, argon beam coagulation, sutures, or topical hemostatic agents. Polar lesions are more amenable to a laparoscopic approach.

Unroofing or Fenestration

These techniques are recommended for superficial and peripherally located cysts and can almost always be performed laparoscopically. The major problem with unroofing and fenestration is a slightly higher risk of recurrence. In most cases, however, the residual cysts are small and asymptomatic. To reduce the risk of reappearance, the surgeon should remove as much cyst wall as possible and fill the resulting parenchymal defect with omentum.

TUMORS

Malignant

Malignant tumors of the spleen can be grouped into these categories: lymphoproliferative diseases, myeloproliferative diseases, primary splenic (nonlymphoid) neoplasms, and metastatic lesions. In lymphoproliferative and myeloproliferative diseases, the spleen is rarely the primary site of malignancy and is usually secondarily involved.

Lymphoproliferative Disease

Non-Hodgkin's lymphoma (NHL) is the most common malignancy involving the spleen (Fig. 2). It is rarely the primary site of malignancy but is secondarily involved in up to 40% of all patients with NHL. After a diagnosis is made, multiagent chemotherapy with or without radiation is the primary mode of treatment. Splenectomy is reserved for patients who develop cytopenias or symptomatic splenomegaly. Splenectomy in these patients improves peripheral blood counts but has no effect on long-term survival.

Hodgkin's disease is a highly curable disease that progresses in a predictable fashion from one nodal group to another. Critical to effective treatment is accurate staging on the basis of the extent of disease. It is difficult to determine the presence of infradiaphragmatic disease in patients with clinical stage I or stage II supradiaphragmatic disease. Up to 35% of all stage I and stage II patients have occult splenic disease or upper abdominal nodal involvement. This was the rationale for staging laparotomies in the past. Because of the dramatic improvements in radiographic imaging and chemotherapeutic regimens, currently less than 5% of patients require staging laparotomy. An abdominal CT scan is currently the principal investigational tool for infradiaphragmatic disease, although staging laparotomy is still considered the most accurate technique to determine abdominal disease. Staging laparotomy should be performed only if results would change the final treatment regimen. The staging procedure can be safely performed laparoscopically and should include inspection of the peritoneum, splenectomy, wedge and core biopsies of the liver, and biopsies of the para-aortic, iliac, portal, and mesenteric lymph node basins.

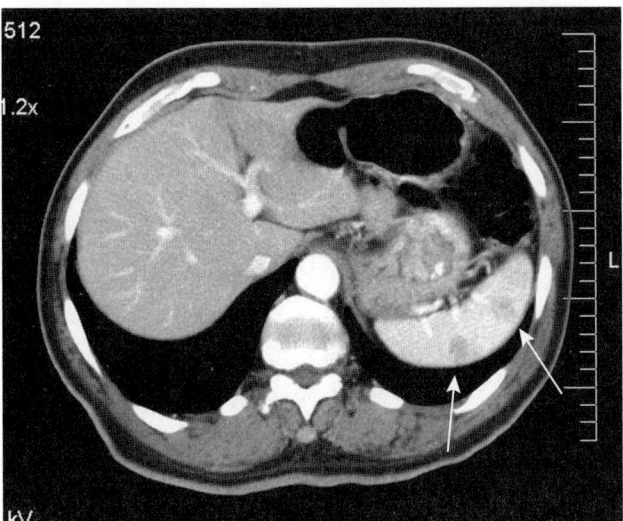

Figure 2 Abdominal computed tomography scan of a 72-year-old man with weight loss and weakness that shows multiple hypodense lesions in the spleen *(arrows)*. Splenectomy was performed and revealed non-Hodgkin's lymphoma.

Hairy cell leukemia is a lymphocytic leukemia that manifests as splenomegaly and pancytopenia. In patients with symptomatic hypersplenism, splenectomy is beneficial. It is associated with improved overall survival, likely because of the reduced risk of complications associated with pancytopenia.

Chronic lymphocytic leukemia is treated with splenectomy only in patients with symptomatic splenomegaly or cytopenias resulting from hypersplenism. There is no increase in survival; however, there is a substantial reduction in peripheral lymphocyte count and transfusion requirements.

Myeloproliferative Disease

Chronic myelogenous leukemia accounts for 30% of all adult leukemias. Splenectomy during the blastic or accelerated phase of the disease has been shown to improve quality of life and decrease transfusion requirements. Myelofibrosis is a rare disorder that is universally fatal, with mean survival of 5 years. Splenectomy has a palliative role in reducing transfusion requirements, improving quality of life.

Primary (Nonlymphoid) Neoplasms

Angiosarcoma is the most common nonlymphoid malignant tumor of the spleen. These tumors grow rapidly and metastasize early, and thus they carry a poor prognosis. Splenectomy is indicated but rarely curative. Other exceedingly rare malignancies include fibrosarcomas, leiomyosarcomas, plasmacytomas, malignant fibrous histiocytomas, and vascular tumors such as hemangiosarcomas and lymphangiosarcomas.

Metastatic Tumors

Metastatic involvement of the spleen from nonlymphoid malignancies is rare and usually a manifestation of disseminated disease. Splenic metastases are usually seen in association with widespread visceral metastases. The involvement of the spleen may be a function of the immunologic role of the spleen and its ability to eliminate microscopic metastatic disease. Cancers known to metastasize to

the spleen include breast, lung, melanoma, ovarian, endometrial, gastric, colonic, and prostate. Splenectomy is acceptable when a thorough workup reveals solitary splenic metastases and the primary tumor is controlled. Splenectomy can also be justified in conjunction with an abdominal debulking procedure for ovarian carcinoma.

Benign

The discovery of benign splenic tumors has become more common because of improvements in CT technology and its widespread use. They are usually found incidentally and are seldom symptomatic. Hemangiomas are the most common benign tumors of the spleen. They are typically associated with hemangiomas of other intra-abdominal organs, particularly the liver. The associated risks include rupture and hemorrhage. These tumors do not require treatment unless they become symptomatic as a result of splenomegaly or they produce a consumptive coagulopathy, thrombocytopenia, microangiopathic anemia, or disseminated intravascular coagulation.

Hamartomas of the spleen can be either cystic or solid. These lesions rarely become symptomatic because of their size, and splenectomy is reserved only as a necessary diagnostic maneuver.

Lymphangiomas are benign cystic tumors that are rare and occasionally lead to hypersplenism. They are commonly associated with lymphangiomas of the liver and lesions in other parts of the body including the lung, skin, and bone. Splenectomy is indicated only to alleviate symptoms or confirm a diagnosis. Other benign tumors of the spleen include lipomas, angiomyolipomas, leiomyomas, hemangioendotheliomas, and hemangiopericytomas.

Treatment

Splenectomy is accepted as the surgical procedure for nearly all tumors of the spleen that require treatment. Some small benign lesions may be amenable to partial splenectomy, but for malignant diseases, splenectomy is the rule. Several series comparing splenectomy for benign and malignant tumors have demonstrated that splenectomy can be safely performed laparoscopically for malignant disease with similar outcomes.

ABSCESSES

Splenic abscesses are rare. In untreated patients, mortality rates approach 100%; however, with appropriate treatment, mortality rates are reduced to nearly 14%. The majority of abscesses arise from hematogenous spread from a distant primary septic focus, such as bacterial endocarditis, intra-abdominal infections including pyelonephritis, and direct introduction of bacteria into the bloodstream from intravenous drug use. They may also arise as a secondary infection in a splenic hematoma after a noninfectious embolic event or trauma. Finally, direct penetration of the splenic parenchyma can also result from an adjacent intra-abdominal process. Because of the increased incidence of human immunodeficiency virus and more aggressive chemotherapy and immunosuppression for organ transplantation, immunodeficiency is becoming a more frequent risk factor.

Most patients present with fever, fatigue, abdominal pain, and leukocytosis. Only approximately half of patients will have positive blood cultures. CT scan is the diagnostic procedure of choice, showing a low-density lesion that does not enhance with intravenous (IV) contrast. The gram-positive aerobic organisms *Staphylococcus* and *Streptococcus* are the most common bacteria cultured. Gram-negative organisms such as *Salmonella* are also seen, as well as polymicrobial flora. Fungal organisms such as *Candida* and *Aspergillosis* represent approximately 8% of all cases and are more commonly found in immunosuppressed patients.

Treatment

Splenectomy is the definitive treatment for splenic abscesses. Treatment with IV antibiotics remains a cornerstone of treatment as well. Broad-spectrum antibiotics should be used after the diagnosis is made until the regimen can be tailored to specific culture data. Percutaneous aspiration can be used to direct antimicrobial therapy. Percutaneous drainage is increasing in popularity as a treatment option and is safe in carefully selected patients. Failure rates for percutaneous drainage range from 50% to 60%, and patients require lengthier hospital stays. It should be reserved for patients unable to tolerate surgery or as a temporizing measure for patients requiring stabilization. Despite the rarity of these lesions, several small series have demonstrated that splenectomy can be performed laparoscopically in this cohort of patients.

OVERWHELMING POSTSPLENECTOMY SEPSIS

Splenectomy increases a patient's risk for routine bacterial infection and, more important, for overwhelming systemic sepsis (OPSS), which is usually associated with gram-positive encapsulated organisms. The incidence of OPSS is highest in children—it has been reported to be as high as 4%—but adults are also considered high risk. The mortality rate of OPSS is approximately 50%. Vaccinations against *Streptococcus pneumoniae, Haemophilus influenzae,* and *Neisseria meningitis* should be given 2 weeks before surgery. If this is not possible, vaccination should be delayed until 2 weeks postoperatively. Given that the highest incidence of OPSS has been shown to be in the first year postsplenectomy, some advocate providing low-dose prophylactic penicillin to high-risk patients in the first year after operation.

SUGGESTED READINGS

Burch M, Misra M, Phillips E: Splenic malignancy: A minimally invasive approach, *Cancer J* 11:36, 2005.
Carbonell A, Kercher K, Matthews B, and others: Laparoscopic splenectomy for splenic abscess, *Surg Laparosc Enodosc Percutan Tech* 14:289, 2004.
Hansen M, Moller A: Splenic cysts, *Surg Laparosc Enodosc Percutan Tech* 14:316, 2004.
Heniford BT, Mathews B, Answini G: Laparoscopic splenectomy for malignant diseases, *Sem Laparosc Surg* 7:93, 2000.

SPLENIC SALVAGE PROCEDURES: THERAPEUTIC OPTIONS

Adil H. Haider, MD, MPH, and Edward E. Cornwell III, MD

Pursuit of organ preservation in patients with an injured spleen combines the appropriate selection of patients managed nonoperatively with the application of available technical modalities in patients requiring surgical intervention. The widespread acceptance of splenic salvage grows from concerns for the physiologic risk of the asplenic state, which includes possible susceptibility to nonfatal infections, as well as overwhelming postsplenectomy infection (OPSI), which is rare but lethal in adults. Some guidance regarding nonoperative management (NOM) of splenic trauma is obtained from evidence-based medicine guidelines generated by the Eastern Association for the Surgery of Trauma (EAST).

In describing two methods of splenic salvage, (1) NOM and (2) techniques in operative splenorrhaphy, it must be emphasized that some patients with splenic injury are best served by splenectomy. A patient's life should never be jeopardized to preserve the spleen.

NONOPERATIVE MANAGEMENT

Although selective nonoperative management of blunt splenic injuries in children has been accepted for decades, considerable evolution of thought has occurred regarding its efficacy in adults. Currently the proportion of patients with splenic injuries managed nonoperatively has grown to more than 70%, owing to improvements in computed tomography (CT) scanning technology and advancing techniques in angioembolization of the spleen. Development of the field has also been enhanced by the utility of the American Association for the Surgery of Trauma (AAST) Organ Injury Scale. The scale enables researchers and clinicians to make comparisons according to a standard approach, aiding in therapeutic and research decisions (Table 1).

Table 1: American Association for the Surgery of Trauma—Organ Injury Scale for the Spleen

Grade*	Injury Type	Description of Injury
I	Hematoma	Subcapsular, <10% surface area
II	Laceration	Capsular tear, <1 cm parenchymal depth
	Hematoma	Subcapsular, 10%–50% surface area; intraparenchymal, <5 cm in diameter
	Laceration	Capsular tear, 1–3 cm parenchymal depth that does not involve a trabecular vessel
III	Hematoma	Subcapsular, >50% surface area or expanding; ruptured subcapsular or parenchymal hematoma; intraparenchymal hematoma ≥5 cm or expanding
	Laceration	>3 cm parenchymal depth or involving trabecular vessels
IV	Laceration	Laceration involving segmental or hilar vessels producing major devascularization (>25% of spleen)
V	Laceration	Completely shattered spleen
	Vascular	Hilar vascular injury with devascularized spleen

*Advance one grade for multiple injuries up to grade III.
From Moore EE, Cogbill TH, Jurkovich GJ, and others: J Trauma 38;323, 1995.

Criteria for Patient Inclusion

Patients with blunt splenic injuries must meet the following criteria to be considered candidates for NOM (Table 2): (1) hemodynamic stability, (2) CT documentation and classification of the injury, (3) absence on CT scan of intra-abdominal (hollow viscus) or retroperitoneal (duodenum, pancreas, kidney) injuries mandating operative intervention, and (4) transfusion of fewer than 2 units of packed red blood cells (PRBCs). Restricting transfusions to fewer than 2 units of PRBCs is extremely important because, along with the known infectious risks associated with blood transfusions, compelling evidence now identifies blood product transfusion as an independent risk factor for complications in the injured patient. Other exclusion criteria for NOM are patients in whom coagulopathy cannot be reversed and those who must receive urgently anticoagulation therapy (e.g., a patient with an artificial heart valve or a trauma victim with blunt carotid injury requiring anticoagulation).

Particulars of Nonoperative Management

In 2003, the Eastern Association for the Surgery of Trauma (EAST) published practice management guidelines for patients with blunt liver or spleen injuries derived from the best available evidence. Their level-2 recommendations suggest that age, neurologic status, or associated injuries do not preclude NOM in a hemodynamically stable patient and that an abdominal CT scan is the most reliable method to assess the severity of organ injury. Level-3 evidence suggests that this initial CT scan be obtained with intravenous and oral contrast to enhance its ability to delineate associated injuries.

The optimal success rate with NOM is obtained when CT scanning is combined with careful serial clinical examinations. Patients should be observed in a setting in which serial physical examinations, vital sign readings, and hematocrit determinations can be performed, and there should be immediate operating availability in case of acute change in clinical examination. A suggested NOM scheme for blunt splenic injury is depicted in Figure 1.

Angioembolization of the Splenic Artery

Initially described in 1995, angiography and embolization of the splenic artery have become accepted adjuncts for NOM in patients with blunt splenic injury. Routine performance of an angiogram on all patients with splenic injury has been found to be unnecessary because few patients with grade I or grade II splenic injury require an interventional procedure. Earlier recommendations of performing splenic angiography on all patients with "contrast pooling" or a "contrast blush" on the initial CT scan have given way to greater emphasis on the grade of injury. Angiography of the splenic artery should be considered in patients with grade III and higher splenic injuries (Fig. 2) and in patients with frank splenic artery hemorrhage delineated on the initial CT scan.

Table 2: Criterion for Nonoperative Management of Blunt Splenic Injury

1. Hemodynamic stability
2. Documented computed tomography classification of injury
3. Absence of additional injuries requiring operative intervention
4. Transfusion of fewer than 2 units packed red blood cells

A multicenter study performed under the auspices of the Western Trauma Association (WTA) showed that grade of injury best predicts need for a vascular embolization procedure (placement of coils or Gelfoam [Pfizer, New York, NY]) and outcomes. In this study, with the adjunctive use of angioembolization procedures, more than 90% of patients with grade III splenic injuries and 80% of patients with grades IV and V splenic injuries were successfully managed without an operation. The study did not detect any differences between the types of embolization material used; nor was there a difference between coils versus Gelfoam in terms of success rates between main splenic artery embolization and super selective embolization techniques in which the more distal splenic artery segments were embolized. The study also determined that the main predictor of failure of angioembolization is the presence of an arteriovenous fistula on the initial CT scan. The researchers suggested that hemodynamically unstable patients and older patients (aged >55 years) had a higher likelihood of angioembolization failure.

Progression of Care

Studies are currently being performed to determine the optimal time a patient receiving nonoperative therapy should be kept NPO (nothing by mouth) and on bed rest and when they should be initiated on deep venous thromboembolism prophylaxis. Other questions under study are when such patients can be safely discharged home and resume normal activity and whether they require follow-up radiographic imaging for their splenic injury. In the meantime, surgical attitudes have been surveyed; a poll of EAST members published in 2005 revealed that approximately 50% of surgeons would recommend that a patient with a grade I or grade II splenic injury return to light normal activity at 2 weeks and that they would not order a routine follow-up CT scan for such patients. However, the same groups of surgeons responded that they would recommend a patient with a higher-grade injury wait at least 4 to 6 weeks before resuming normal activities and obtain a follow-up CT scan. The physicians surveyed seemed to be in agreement with level-3 guidelines from EAST that recommend obtaining a follow-up CT scan in patients with grade III or higher splenic injuries and in patients with high-risk occupations (e.g., athletes, construction workers) before granting them medical clearance for normal activity.

Success of Nonoperative Management

A multi-institutional trial sponsored by EAST and published in 2000 revealed a NOM success rate of 89% (1488 patients at 27 centers). In 2004, the AAST spleen study group reported a 96% success rate with NOM (300+ patients). In children the reported failure rate for NOM is less than 2%. The most common cause for failure of NOM is bleeding in the first 96 hours. If the patient becomes hemodynamically unstable, emergent splenectomy is indicated. If the patient remains stable, a repeat CT scan may be performed with intravenous contrast. On occasion, the initial CT may not reveal the true grade of splenic injury, or an injured vessel that was previously in spasm may have relaxed and start to hemorrhage. Patients with such findings may benefit from angioembolization. However, if the patient has required 2 or more units of blood or has undergone prior angioembolization, operative intervention is indicated. Other causes for NOM failure include late bleeding (before or after discharge), abscess formation, and splenic artery pseudoaneurysm.

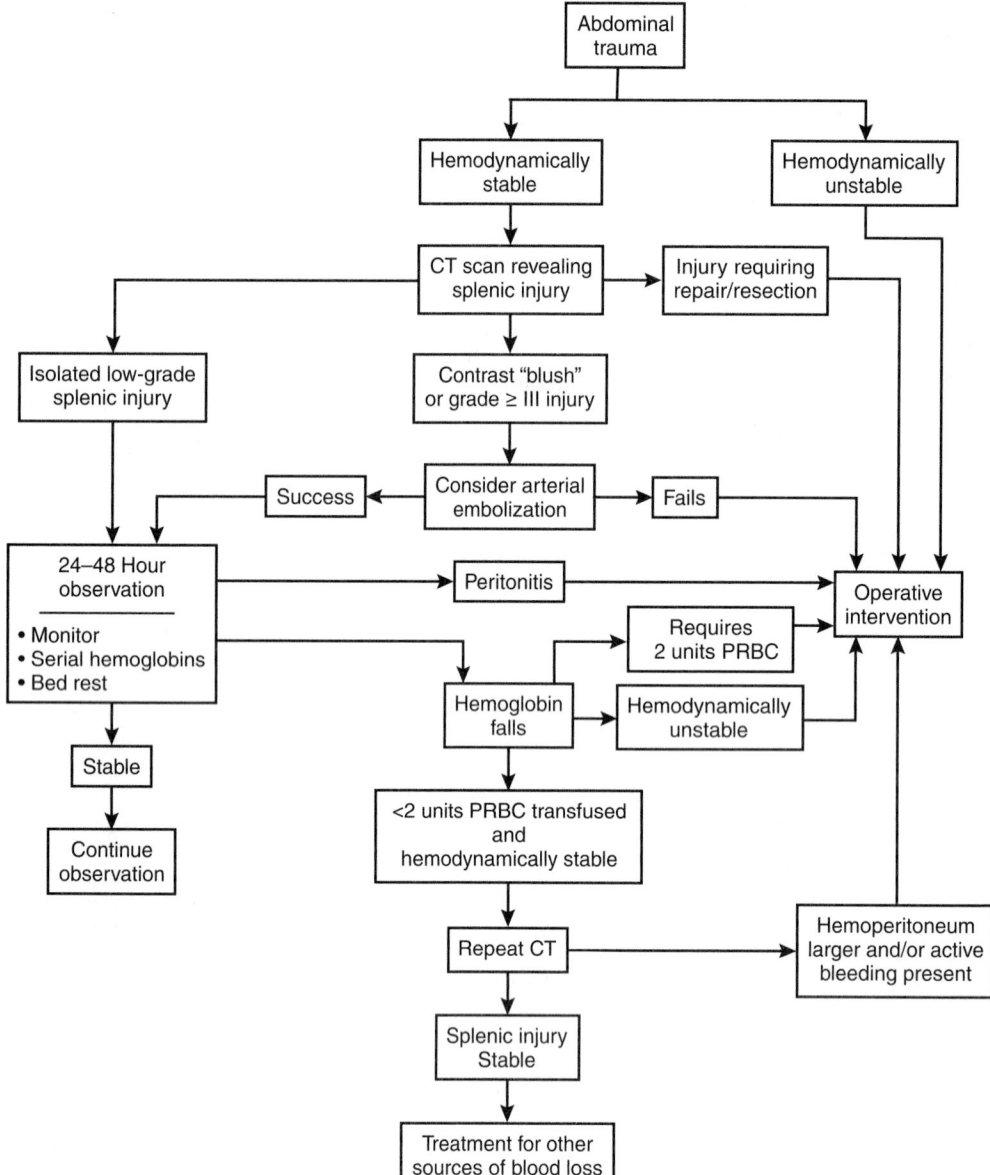

Figure 1 Algorithm for nonoperative management of blunt splenic injuries.

PRBC = packed red blood cells.

SPLENORRHAPHY

By the early 1980s, techniques of splenorrhaphy were fairly well standardized, including adequate exposure and splenic mobilization by division of avascular ligaments; facilitated organ repair, which was usually achieved with topical hemostatic agents; suture repair; partial splenectomy; or a combination of these. Three major adjuncts to operative splenic repair were introduced by the late 1980s: argon beam coagulation (ABC), fibrin glue, and polyglycolic mesh wrap.

The decision to save rather than remove an injured spleen requires consideration of the total complex of the patient's injuries. Splenic salvage should not be attempted in unstable patients undergoing damage-control surgery. Similarly, a patient with severe head injury requiring intracranial pressure monitoring or a wide mediastinum that must be worked up deserves expeditious splenectomy so

that other diagnostic and therapeutic maneuvers may be pursued. Likewise, a patient should not be subjected to multiple transfusions because of excessive surgical persistence at repairing a nonsalvageable spleen.

After the decision to attempt splenorrhaphy has been made, adequate exposure and mobilization are mandatory. Attempting to repair an incompletely mobilized spleen is a frustrating exercise in futility for both the surgeon and assistant. Division of avascular ligaments (lienophrenic, lienorenal, and lienocolic) is essential to mobilize the spleen medially out of its bed and up into the operative field close to the midline position of its embryological origin (Fig. 3). After the spleen has been mobilized, assessed, and debrided of frankly devitalized fragments, hemostasis may be achieved by a combination of topical hemostatic agents such as microfibrillar collagen (e.g., Avitene; Davol, Cranston, RI)), methylcellulose (e.g., Surgicel; Johnson & Johnson, New Brunswick, NJ) or mattress

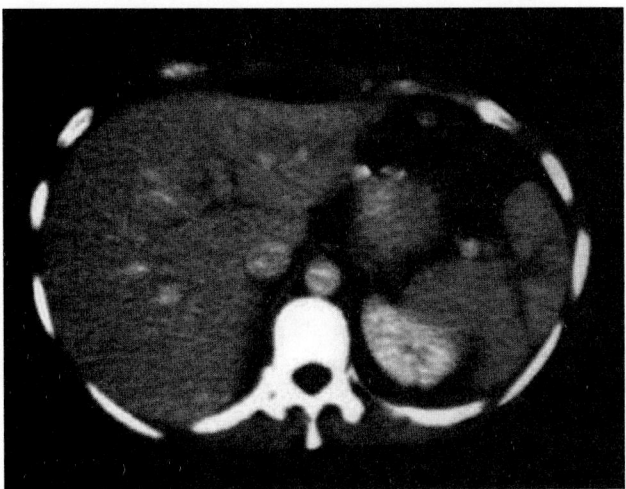

Figure 2 Computed tomography image depicting grade III splenic injury. *Photo credit: Eduardo Bastos, general surgeon, Marilia, Brazil; reproduced with permission from www.trauma.org.*

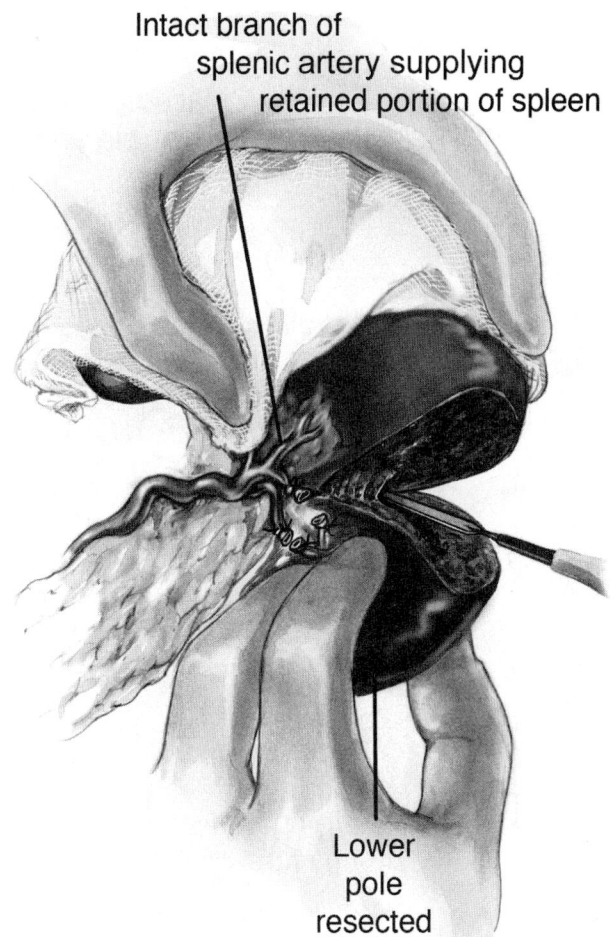

Figure 4 To achieve hemostasis, the splenic artery branch to the lower pole of the spleen is ligated. Subsequently, an anatomic resection of the lower pole of the spleen is performed. *From C. Sandone, Johns Hopkins School of Medicine, Baltimore, MD. Reproduced with permission.*

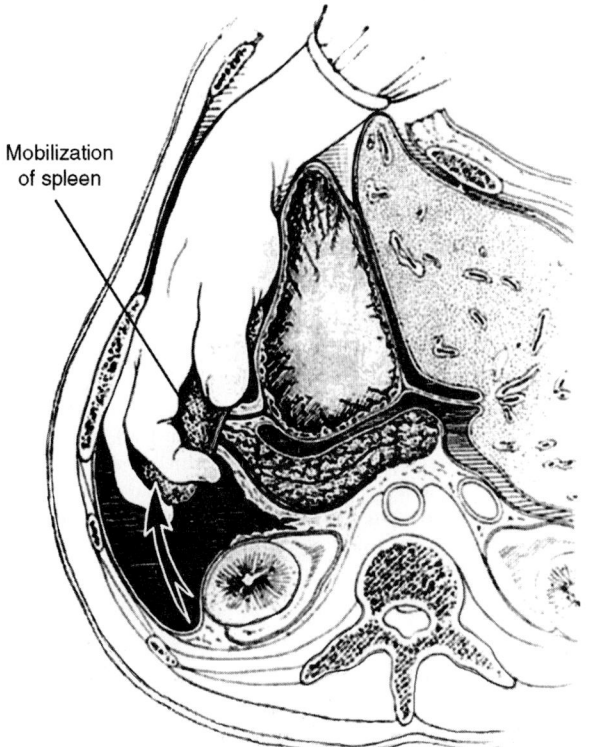

Figure 3 After division of avascular ligaments, the spleen can be mobilized medially, up into the operative field, close to the midline position. *From Trunkey DD: Spleen. In Blaisdell FW, Trunkey DD, editors: Trauma management, vol 1: abdominal trauma, New York, 1982, Thieme. Reproduced with permission.*

50% of the splenic parenchyma attached to an identifiable vessel is viable, partial splenectomy may be performed, and splenic immune function can be expected to be maintained. Early demarcation of the segment of the spleen to be removed with the electrocautery device facilitates exposing intrasplenic vessels for individual suture ligation, which should proceed meticulously. Occasionally, cross-clamping the splenic hilum may be temporarily required if manual compression does not produce adequate hemostasis. The resected margin of the spleen is then oversewn with mattress sutures with or without pledgets (Fig. 5). If necessary, a blunt liver needle may be used to place such mattress sutures.

Argon Beam Coagulator

ABC is an electrocoagulation system that should not be confused with the argon laser. No eyewear is required. The instrument achieves hemostasis by using inert gas as a medium to conduct radiofrequency energy (Fig. 6). The gas is emitted as a constant flow at room temperature from a hand piece and nozzle that blows away blood and debris to optimize visualization. The first

sutures (e.g., 3–0 Prolene; Ethicon, Piscataway, NJ) placed either directly or over Teflon pledgets.

Partial splenectomy may be selected when early ligation of a branch of the splenic artery to a segment of the spleen results in major progress toward hemostasis (Fig. 4). Provided that

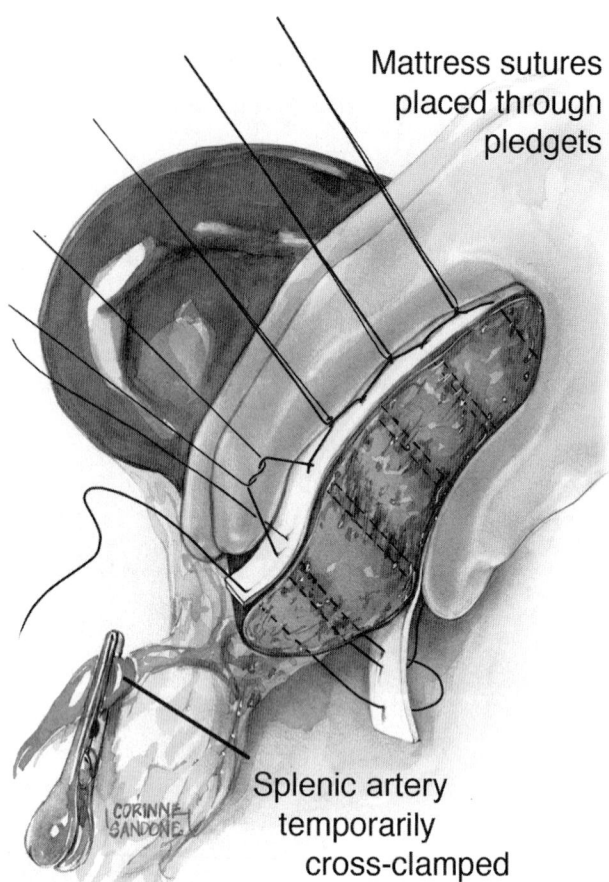

Mattress sutures
placed through
pledgets

Splenic artery
temporarily
cross-clamped

Figure 5 Manual compression and, if necessary, clamping of the splenic artery, provide necessary hemostasis required to oversew the margin of the retained spleen. Teflon pledgets are employed to prevent a suture from cutting through the otherwise friable tissue. *From C. Sandone, Johns Hopkins School of Medicine, Baltimore, MD. Reproduced with permission.*

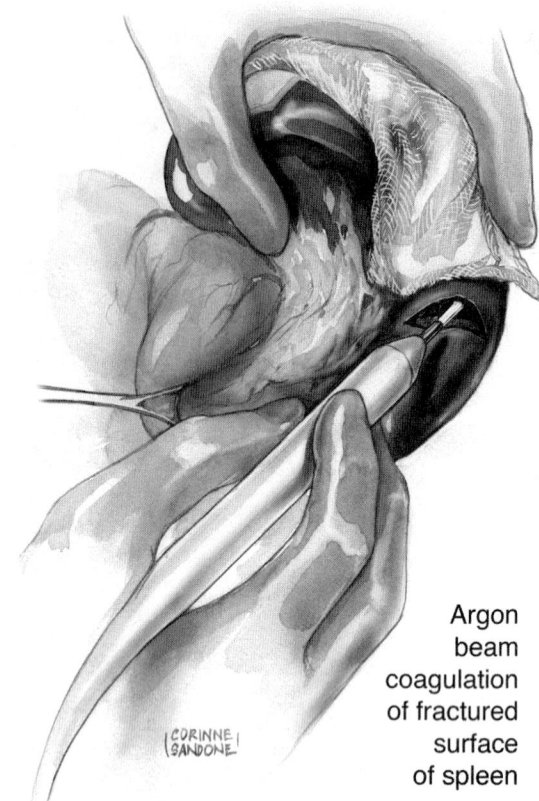

Argon
beam
coagulation
of fractured
surface
of spleen

Figure 6 Argon beam coagulator. *From C. Sandone, Johns Hopkins School of Medicine, Baltimore, MD. Reproduced with permission.*

large clinical series using the ABC for splenic salvage was published in 1991. This report concluded that most spleens with superficial lacerations are easily salvaged with standard topical maneuvers and that the ABC offers a technical advantage in patients with deep parenchymal injuries. In the ensuing decade, the ABC has achieved wide acceptance in the management of both spleen and other solid organ injuries.

Absorbable Mesh Wrap

Polyglycolic mesh wrap is another modality reported to be useful in splenic salvage. The injured spleen is passed through an enlarged hole in the mesh fashioned for this purpose. The mesh is then wrapped around the spleen and sutured to itself to provide tamponade (Figs. 7 and 8) Recent reports have also suggested incorporating methylcellulose into the mesh to help "bulk it up." In this technique, multiple layers of methylcellulose are placed directly onto the injured surfaces, after which the mesh is secured around the spleen, enhancing the tamponade effect. Previous concerns of possible mesh infection, especially in the setting of hollow viscus injury, have proved to be unfounded on the basis of large series of patients.

Fibrin Glue

Early impressive laboratory experience with fibrin glue, which consists of fibrinogen, dried thrombin, and calcium chloride, prompted its emergence in the clinical area. Commonly available fibrin sealants such as Tisseal (Immuno, Vienna, Austria) and Crosseal (Omrix Pharmaceuticals, Brussels, Belgium) may be applied directly to the injured surfaces of the spleen to achieve immediate hemostasis, especially on linear tears and cracks. Recent reports have demonstrated application of fibrin sealants to "glue together" massively injured spleens and then performance of mesh splenorrhaphy. Using this approach, grades IV and V injured spleens have been salvaged.

Laparoscopy

The role of minimally invasive surgery in isolated splenic injury appears to be limited. Hemodynamically unstable patients warrant a laparotomy, and most hemodynamically stable patients can undergo nonoperative management successfully. Laparoscopy may play a role in patients who undergo laparoscopic evaluation for traumatic left-side diaphragmatic hernia. If the patient has an associated splenic injury and is hemodynamically stable, a laparoscopic splenorrhaphy can be attempted.

■ RECOMMENDATIONS

Careful selection, CT scan imaging and serial clinical examinations are crucial to the successful nonoperative management

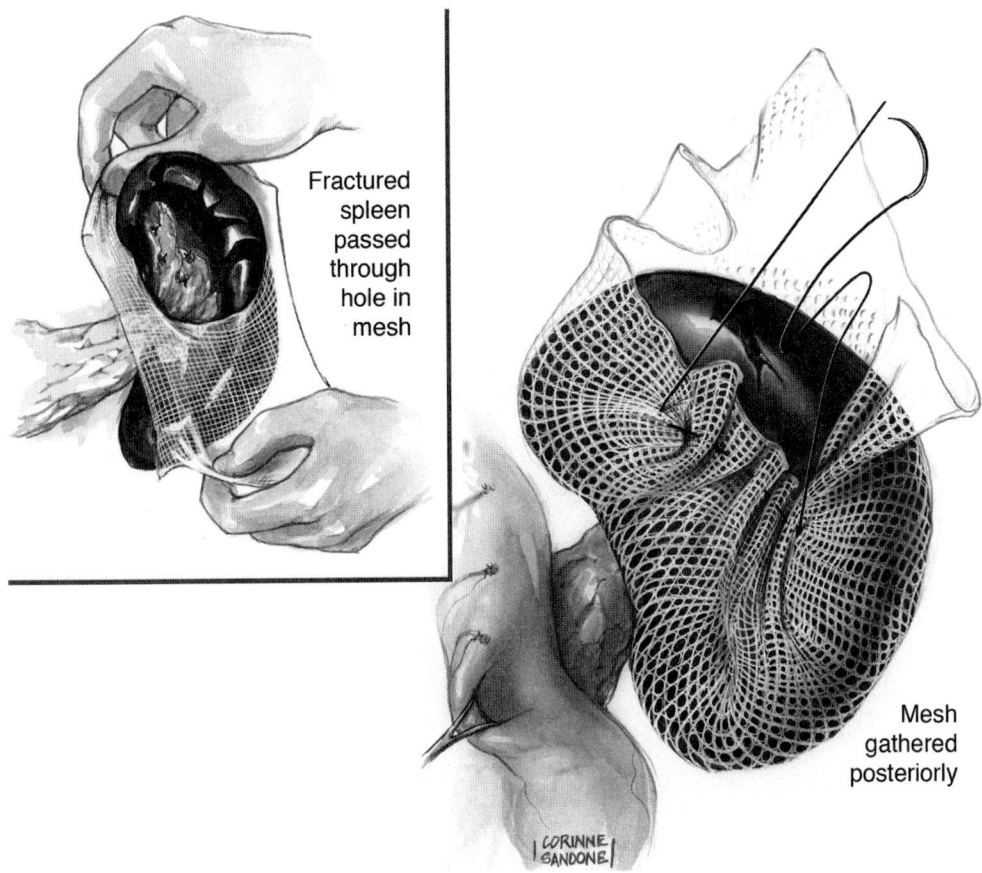

Figure 7 Mesh splenorrhaphy: injured spleen is passed through an enlarged hole in the mesh. The mesh is then wrapped around the spleen and sutured to itself. *From C. Sandone, Johns Hopkins School of Medicine, Baltimore, MD. Reproduced with permission.*

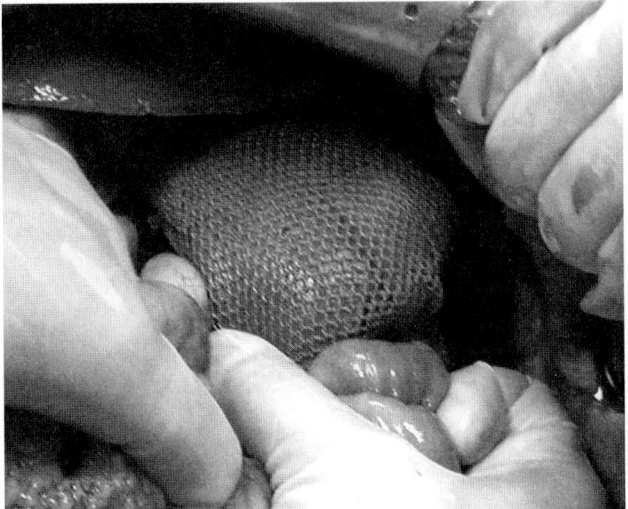

Figure 8 Mesh splenorrhaphy in situ with Surgicel placed directly over the injured portion of the spleen, before suturing to secure the mesh. *Photo Credit: Horacio A. Massotto, MD, Costa Rica. Reproduced with permission from www.trauma.org.* **(See color insert Figure 30.)**

of patients with blunt splenic injuries. Angioembolization has furthered our ability to salvage a patient's spleen without an operation. Patients requiring surgical intervention are best managed with adequate exposure and mobilization. ABC, fibrin glue, and absorbable mesh wrap appear to have advanced the art of splenic salvage beyond the level achieved by topical hemostatic agents, suturing, and partial splenectomy. With these technical considerations combined with careful selection of candidates for nonoperative management, we have evolved to a point at which most patients with splenic injuries can undergo successful splenic salvage.

SUGGESTED READINGS

Dunham CM, Cornwell EE, Militello P: The role of argon beam coagulator in splenic salvage, *Surg Gynecol Obstet* 173:179, 1991.

EAST Practice Management Guidelines Work Group. *Practice management guidelines for the non-operative management of blunt injury to the liver and spleen* (Web site), Eastern Association for the Surgery of Trauma, 2003. www.east.org/tpg/livspleen.pdf. Accessed on June 14, 2006.

Haan HM, for the Western Trauma Association Multi-Institutional Trials Committee: Splenic embolization revisited: a multicenter review, *J Trauma* 56:542, 2004.

Richardson JD: Changes in management of injuries to the liver and spleen, *J Am Coll Surg* 200:648, 2005.

HERNIA

GROIN HERNIA

Leena Khaitan, MD, and J. Barry McKernan, MD, PhD

INTRODUCTION

Repairs of hernias of the groin are among the most commonly performed procedures by the general surgeon today, with almost as many types of repairs as there are hernias. Hernias of the groin include those through the direct, indirect, femoral, and obturator spaces; all can be congenital or acquired. These hernias can be unilateral or bilateral and can be primary or recurrent. This anatomy is one of the most complex for a surgeon in training to master. Intricate knowledge of this anatomy allows the surgeon to repair the defects effectively using the best technique and materials available.

Diagnosis of hernias is primarily directed by patient history and physical examination. In describing their history, patients often report the presence of a bulge in the groin that is noted with an activity associated with and increase in intra-abdominal pressure (e.g., coughing, sneezing, jumping, lifting a heavy object). The bulge may be constant or may change in size over the course of time. The bulge and any associated discomfort are often greatest in the evening hours and least in the morning, after the patient has been supine for several hours. The physical examination should be performed with the patient in both supine and upright positions. The presence of a defect can sometimes be made more obvious by having the patient cough during the examination. Obturator hernias are extremely uncommon and difficult to diagnose on physical examination. They are not considered further in this chapter.

During the history and physical, the surgeon should consider several questions: (1) Is the hernia palpable or visible? (2) Is the hernia reducible or incarcerated? (3) Is there a contralateral hernia? (4) Has the hernia been repaired before, and if so, by which technique? (5) Is the testicular examination normal? (6) Is there an associated hydrocele?

INDICATIONS

Some surgeons may argue that the mere presence of a hernia warrants repair. Does this still stand true? In the past, the argument was that if the hernia is not repaired electively, the patient has the potential to present emergently with compromised viability of the bowel, requiring a much more invasive operation. Today recommended elective open and laparoscopic techniques use the placement of a mesh material to provide stronger repair and lower recurrence rates. The introduction of foreign material and the repair of the hernia itself can have potential adverse consequences with short- and long-term complications. Inguinodynia is one of the most challenging conditions to treat, and most often its etiology is iatrogenic. Therefore the indications for hernia repair have evolved such that the surgeon must have an educated discussion with the patient before repair. One must discuss the following questions: (1) Is the hernia symptomatic? (2) Is the hernia reducible? (3) How long has the hernia been present? After one has the answers to these questions, indications for repair include (1) relief of symptoms; (2) prevention of progression and further weakening of the abdominal wall; and (3) prevention of complications of acute incarceration and strangulation. Workman's compensation or employment issues must also be addressed.

TIMING OF THERAPY

A recent randomized controlled trial was performed in the United States to determine whether all groin hernias must be repaired. Indeed, for minimally symptomatic patients, observation is acceptable. Thus physicians can tell their patients that the chance of a having a complication resulting from an unrepaired hernia is extremely low. The patient should also realize, however, that of those who decide on observation, almost a quarter go on to repair within the next 2 years secondary to a progression of symptoms.

For those who choose elective repair, timing is dependent on patient and surgeon convenience. Most of these procedures are performed on an outpatient basis. The next discussion with the patient should focus on the type of hernia repair.

CONTRAINDICATIONS

For elective repair, contraindications are relatively few. Absolute contraindications to elective repair include pregnancy and active infection; after these conditions are resolved, repair can be considered. The presence of ascites may make repair difficult, and the indications for repair of hernias in these patients should be examined carefully. Such procedures in these patients have a higher likelihood of postoperative complications. Because of the many options available for repair and anesthesia, limitations to repair secondary to anesthesia intolerance are unusual.

ANESTHESIA

Hernia procedures can be performed under spinal, general, or local anesthesia with intravenous sedation (monitored anesthesia care [MAC]). The factors that determine choice of anesthesia include patient and surgeon preference, type of procedure performed (open or laparoscopic), hernia characteristics (recurrent, large, slider, bilateral), and the patient's ability to cooperate. For patients undergoing an open repair, MAC with local or spinal anesthetic can be used. For all patients undergoing a laparoscopic repair, general anesthesia is required to allow adequate relaxation of the abdominal wall and insufflation of the preperitoneal space. General anesthesia can also be used for patients with questionable airways and those unable to cooperate (e.g., because of dementia) or for more challenging cases. Even with general anesthesia, it is helpful to inject incision sites with a long-acting local anesthetic (0.25% Marcaine [bupivacaine hydrochloride]; Sanofi Winthrope Pharmaceuticals, New York, NY) to help the patient with analgesia during the postoperative recovery period.

HERNIA REPAIR OPTIONS

A multitude of hernia repairs have been described, and it has been said that the best hernia repair is the one that a surgeon knows how to do well. Hernia repairs can be categorized as follows.

- **Open**
  - Suture-based: Bassini, McVay, Shouldice, and so on
  - Mesh-based: "plug and patch," Lichtenstein, Gilbert, Stoppa, Kugel
- **Laparoscopic**
  - Total extraperitoneal (TEP): split mesh, rectangular mesh, preformed mesh
  - Transabdominal preperitoneal (TAPP)

The choice of technique is based on three factors: patient preference, surgeon expertise, and ability of the patient to tolerate anesthesia.

When patients present for a hernia repair, among their many concerns will be the size of the incision, the magnitude of postoperative pain, and the recovery time. Physicians can discuss not only their own experience but also the published data. In experienced hands, laparoscopic repair can offer advantages for all of these considerations, although the VA Cooperative study questions this assertion. Nevertheless, extensive published literature from experienced minimally invasive surgeons supports the benefits of laparoscopy, and we prefer a laparoscopic approach because of these benefits. We also believe it provides better repair for our patients. Particularly in young, active individuals, a laparoscopic approach restores one's normal lifestyle more quickly.

Other concerns for the surgeon include training, experience, type of hernia, and cost. Surgical training can be variable, and not all surgical residents are comfortable performing a laparoscopic repair of a primary unilateral hernia. The learning curve for the laparoscopic inguinal hernia repair has been reported to be anywhere from 1 to 50 cases. Surgeons who do not feel they have achieved proficiency in laparoscopic repair should offer patients the repair they are comfortable performing.

Many studies have evaluated costs of the various procedures, and although the laparoscopic procedure may be more expensive initially, the cost to society and the patient is reduced given decreased infection rates, reduced use of analgesia, and quicker return to work. For recurrent and bilateral hernias, laparoscopic repair has become the procedure of choice for most surgeons.

If one does choose the open approach, suture-based repairs have become almost extinct (except in a few specialized centers). Most repairs in adults should be performed with mesh in a tension-free fashion to achieve lower recurrence rates. Previous concerns of infection, extrusion, and other complications have not materialized. We have learned that different mesh materials act differently in different people. All meshes have some degree of contraction, and some will cause scarring to the degree that patients may feel they have a "plate" in their bodies. The objective is to place lightweight mesh but provide adequate scaffolding for collagen deposition so that patients will not know the mesh is there after the healing process is complete. Therefore macroporous mesh weaves are increasingly preferable. It remains unclear whether a hydrophilic or hydrophobic material allows the better ingrowth.

When laparoscopic repairs are compared with open, suture-based repairs, laparoscopic repair undoubtedly offers the advantages of quicker return to work and reduced pain. When laparoscopic repair is compared with open mesh repairs, many studies find the magnitude of difference to be much less. With the open, tension-free approach and the use of mesh, the incidence of pain and recurrence has improved. Nevertheless, we feel that the laparoscopic approach is better for most of our patients. Recent comparison studies have shown long-term groin pain to be as high as 20% with open repair and 1% or less with laparoscopic repair.

When considering whether to offer patients a laparoscopic or open procedure, one must also consider patients' ability to undergo anesthesia. If a patient cannot tolerate general anesthesia, we consider the open repair.

An open procedure may be considered in those patients who have had prior irradiation, especially if performed more than 2 years earlier, or a lower midline procedure that has been in the preperitoneal space (prostate surgery, bladder suspension procedures). For those patients, unless the surgeon has excellent experience, the preperitoneal space cannot be easily or adequately dissected to place the mesh appropriately, and a Lichtenstein may be preferred.

LAPAROSCOPIC HERNIA REPAIR OPTIONS

Laparoscopic repair can be performed by entering the peritoneal cavity (TAPP procedure) or by staying in the preperitoneal space (TEP procedure). Surgeons who prefer TEP state that it can be performed with several advantages: less dissection, less time, and avoidance of the peritoneal cavity. The disadvantages are that it is more costly and performed in a smaller space and that the intra-abdominal organs cannot be assessed. Those who are proponents of TAPP note the following advantages: better visualization of the abdominal anatomy, better for teaching the anatomy, and less expensive (no dissecting balloon). The disadvantages are the longer time and the difficulty in reperitonealizing the mesh, which increases the likelihood that the mesh may come in contact with bowel (see Table 1). We prefer the TEP approach.

Other considerations for laparoscopic hernia repair are the type of mesh to use and whether to fixate it. We prefer a rectangular piece of mesh. It can be either slit for the cord structures or placed without a slit. If a keyhole method is used, care must be taken to overlap the mesh well or place an additional piece of mesh over the slit. Preformed mesh options are also available. Of these, our preferred mesh materials are Prolene (Ethicon, Piscataway, NJ) and Parietex (Autosuture, Norwalk, CT); the latter has a flap that encircles the cord and then is affixed in place with Velcro (Velcro USA, Manchester, NH). Because it encircles the cord and is preformed, Parietex requires less fixation. If a large enough piece of mesh is used, fixation may be avoided. However, this usually means no keyhole and requires a much larger area of dissection.

TOTAL EXTRAPERITONEAL TECHNIQUE

Patients undergoing TEP are given general anesthesia; their arms are tucked, if possible, and a Foley catheter is placed (this step in optional; note that the bladder must be empty). Cases anticipated to be longer or more complex may be facilitated by the placement of a Foley catheter. The camera operator stands on the opposite side of the table from the surgeon. An infraumbilical incision is made, and blunt dissection exposes the anterior rectus sheath, which is then grasped just off of the midline with Kocher clamps. The fascia is then incised and S retractors are used to separate bluntly and elevate the rectus muscle from the posterior rectus sheath and peritoneum (Fig. 1). Stay sutures of 0 Vicryl

Table 1: Laparoscopic Inguinal Hernia Repair

Name	Features	Advantages	Disadvantages
Transabdominal preperitoneal (TAPP)	1. Preperitoneal space dissection via the familiar intra-abdominal laparoscopic view 2. Indirect sac easily reduced or transected 3. Large prosthesis placed in preperitoneal space 4. Peritoneum closed over prosthesis to prevent bowel adhesions	1. Diagnostic laparoscopy and in conjunction with other laparoscopic procedure 2. Prosthesis is covered by peritoneum (suture or staple) 3. Indirect hernias easier to repair than with TEP 4. 30-degree scope preferred 5. Preferred for both TAPP or TEP recurrences	1. Morbidity is increased because of potential intra-abdominal injuries 2. Potential for adhesive complications of bowel entrapment through a defect of reperitonealization
Total extraperitoneal (TEP)	1. Dissection of preperitoneal space begins at umbilicus, external to the intra-abdominal cavity (i.e., extraperitoneal) avoiding intra-abdominal adhesions 2. After the preperitoneal space in groin is developed, the mesh placement is similar to TAPP	1. Peritoneal cavity is never entered 2. Direct inguinal hernias easier to repair 3. 45-degree scope preferred 4. Easier to perform than TAPP with obese patients 5. Bilateral hernias are easier to operate than with TAPP 6. Shoulder pain often absent	1. Technically most difficult repair 2. Peritoneal breach is common, especially for difficult dissection (breaches should be closed to prevent bowel entrapment)

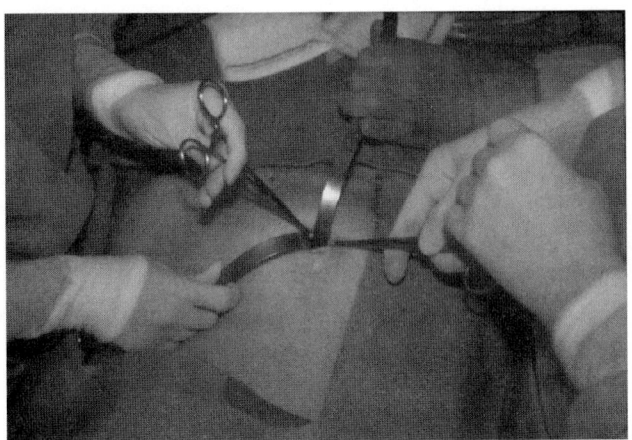

Figure 1 S retractors are used to separate bluntly and elevate the rectus muscle from the posterior rectus sheath and peritoneum.

(Ethicon, Somerville, NJ) are placed in the fascia to secure the Hasson trocar during the procedure and to aid facial closure at the conclusion of the procedure. The patient is then placed in the Trendelenberg position. An Origin PDB 1000 (Autosuture, Norwalk, CT) preperitoneal distention balloon is used to expand the preperitoneal space carefully under direct vision with a 0-degree telescope (Fig. 2, A). Initially, the balloon is inserted by elevating the rectus muscle and angling the tip of the balloon toward the pubis. The balloon is distended with the pump while the surgeon observes the rectus muscles anterior to the pubis and Cooper's ligament laterally. The distention is carried out just enough to allow placement of the other trocars. The balloon is not used to perform the entire dissection. If the balloon tip will not pass easily to the pubis, the Hasson canula is placed through the periumbilical; incise beneath the rectus muscle in the preperitoneal space; insufflation at 10 mm is initiated. The operating laparoscope with a blunt dissector through the operative port is inserted through the Hasson cannula, and dissection is carried out to the pubis and preperitoneal space (Figs. 2, B; 3, 4, and 5). If the preperitoneal space cannot be safely distended, the procedure can be converted to a TAPP.

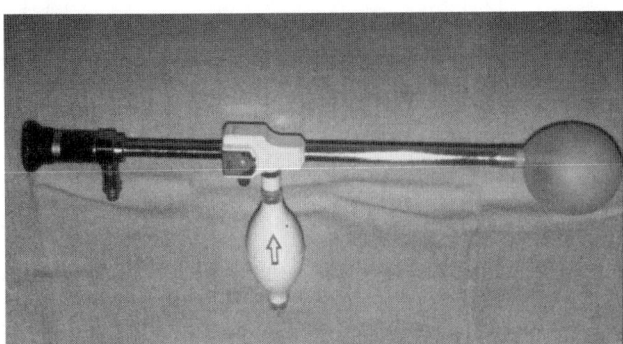

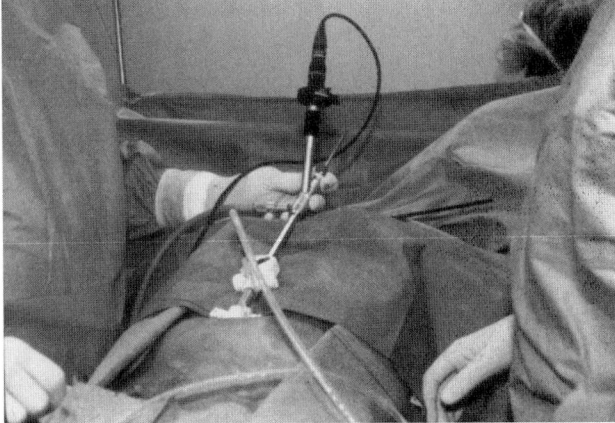

Figure 2 **(A)** The Origin PDB1000 preperitoneal distention balloon is used to carefully expand the preperitoneal space. **(B)** The operative laparoscope with a blunt dissector through the operator port is used to dissect the preperitoneal space under direct visualization.

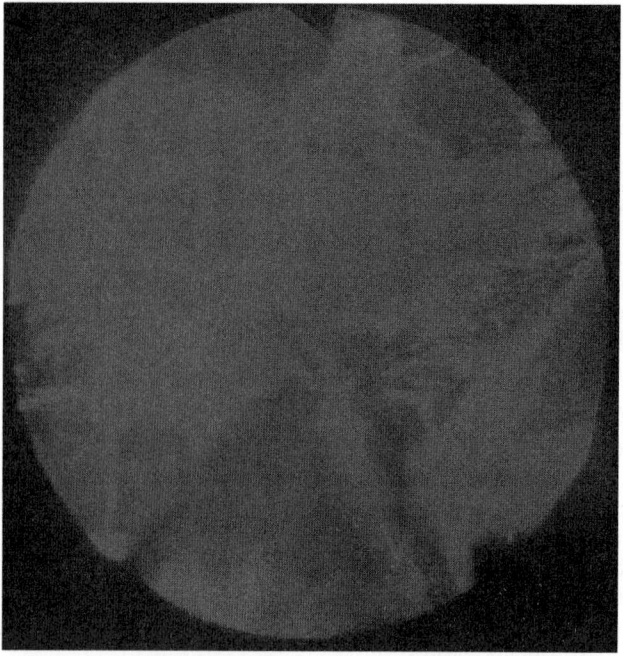

Figure 3   Visualization of the preperitoneal space with a blunt probe through an operative telescope.

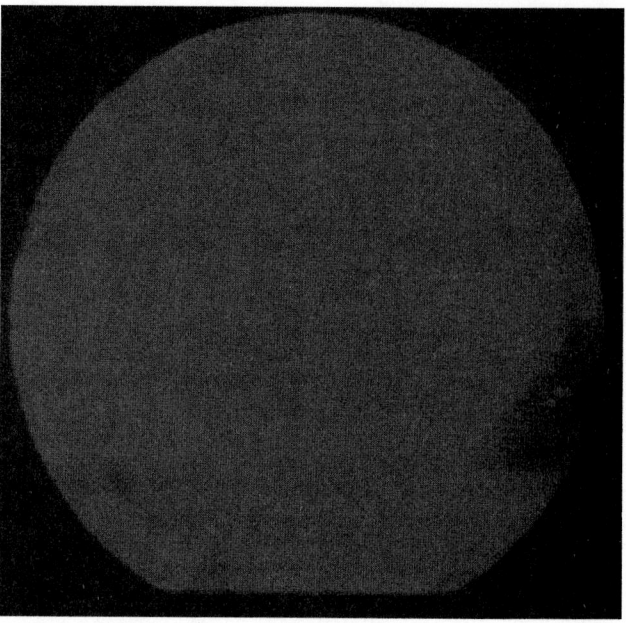

Figure 5   Completed tunnel dissection down to the symphysis pubis.

Hernia puncture sites

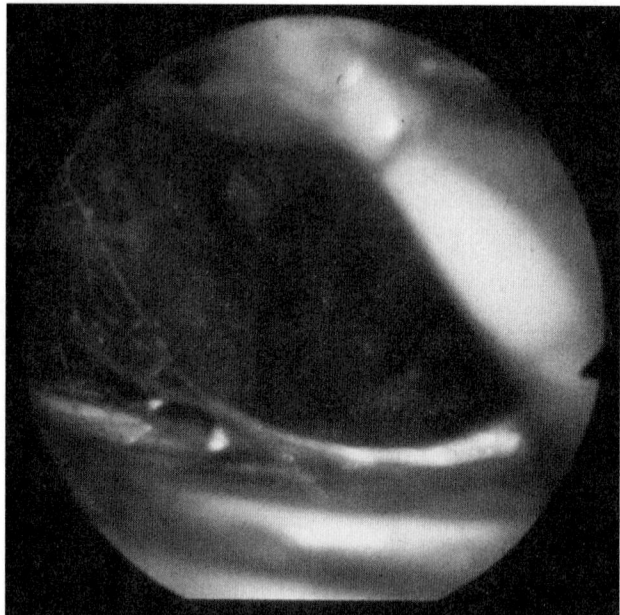

Figure 4   Resultant tunnel dissection for trocar placement.

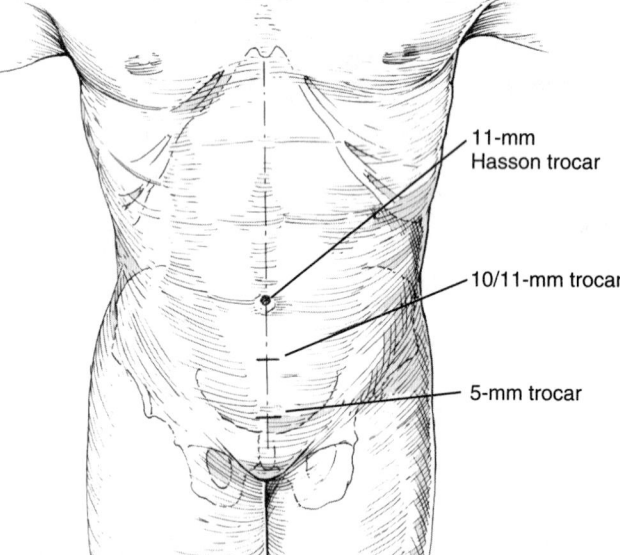

11-mm
Hasson trocar

10/11-mm trocar

5-mm trocar

Figure 6   A 5-mm cannula is placed approximately one finger breadth above the pubis, and the second, a 10/11 trocar, is placed midway between the 5-mm and Hasson canula in the midline.

The preperitoneal space is almost always insufflated and maintained with CO_2 to a pressure of 10 mm Hg (higher pressures may result in significant subcutaneous emphysema in lean patients). Additionally, two cannulas are placed in the midline under direct visualization; the first, a 5-mm cannula, is placed approximately one finger breadth above the pubis; the second, a 10/11 trocar, is placed midway between the 5-mm and Hasson cannulas in the midline (Fig. 6). Placement of the 10/11 trocar is associated with the greatest risk of invading the peritoneal cavity. To aid

in its placement, after the skin incision is made, a no. 11 blade is carefully inserted under direct visualization through the midline fascia into the preperitoneal space; a hemostat is then passed through this incision, and the fascia is widened to accept easily the bladed or shielded cannula.

The 0-degree telescope is now exchanged for a 45-degree telescope. A regular, blunt grasper is used in the left hand, and a suction irrigation device is placed in the right hand (most dissection is blunt and usually bloodless). Anatomical proficiency is critical

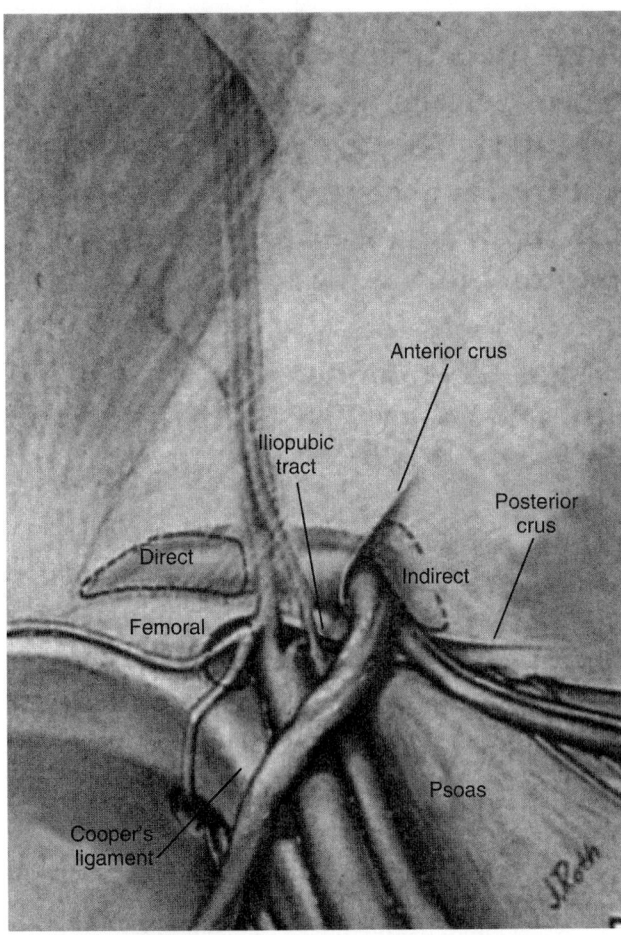

Figure 7 Anatomy of the right groin with direct, indirect, and femoral hernia areas outlined.

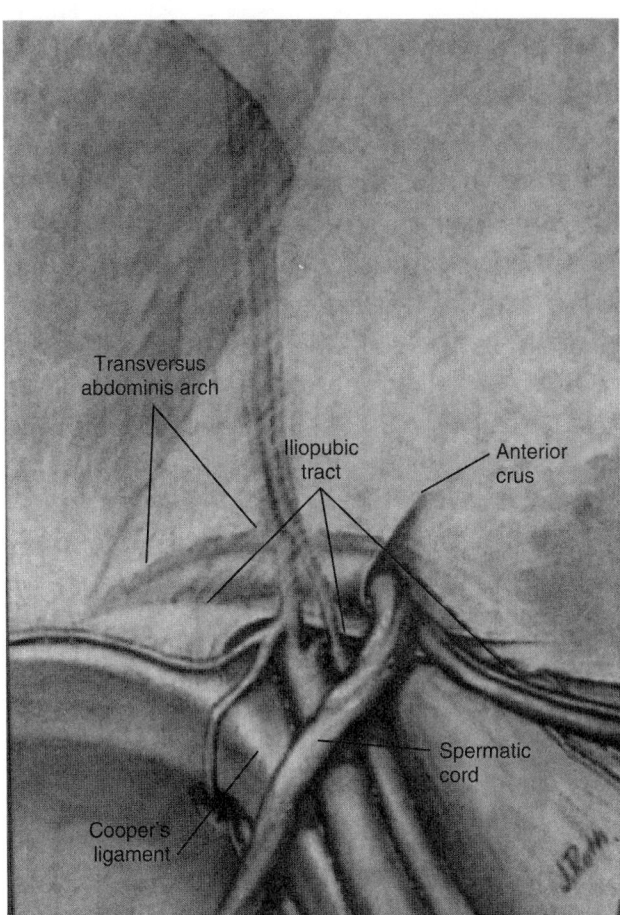

Figure 8 Anatomy of the right groin marking the iliopubic tract, cord structures, Cooper's ligament, and major groin vessels.

to the laparoscopic repair. (Figs. 7, 8, and 9) Dissection begins at the pubis and is carried laterally along Cooper's ligament to the iliac vein (Fig. 10). The inferior epigastric vessels are identified and in place anteriorly to prevent obscuration of the operative field. If injured, the inferior epigastric vessels are ligated or cauterized using bipolar cautery. Monopolar cautery is less effective than bipolar cautery. The area of the direct defect is now inspected, and any preperitoneal fat in this area is reduced (Fig. 11). The dissection is carried lateral to the inferior epigastric vessels to expose the spermatic cord inferiorly and anterior laterally to the iliopubic tract. This dissection is accomplished by using the instruments in a "chopsticks" fashion in the plane of the cord structures by hugging the rectus muscle anteriorly (Fig. 12). Any lipoma of the spermatic cord must be exposed and, if present, reduced because this may be mistaken or confused postoperatively for a retained indirect hernia. The indirect hernia sac is identified and reduced unless the sac extends below the external ring into the scrotum, in which case complete dissection is avoided. Instead, the sac is ligated proximally with suture, leaving the distal sac open. Particular attention is paid to hemostasis at this point of the procedure. In the event of a large, either chronically or acutely incarcerated hernia, it is sometimes helpful to place an optically dilating trocar into the peritoneal cavity to inspect for possible injury to the peritoneum during dissection or reduced bowel contents, to check the viability of reduced bowel, or to aid in the reduction of the hernia.

The hernia repair is completed using a 3 × 5–inch piece of Prolene polypropylene mesh. We have used this size at our center since 1990. However, this is the minimal size and requires sTAPPle fixation. A 1.75-inch cut is made vertically in the mesh 2 inches

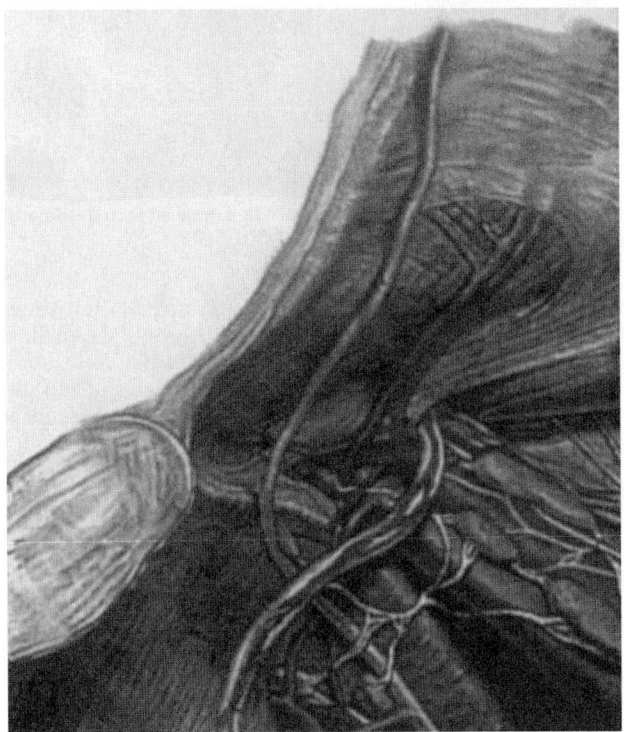

Figure 9 Although complex, all major components must be mastered for anatomic proficiency.

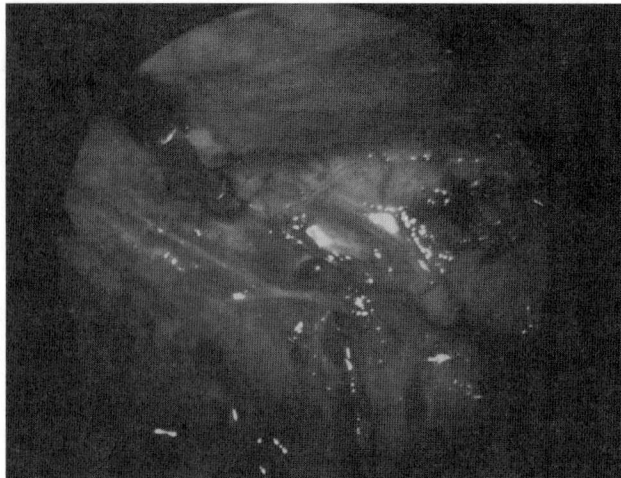

Figure 10   Dissection begins at the pubis and is carried laterally along Cooper's ligament to the iliac vein. (*See color insert Figure 31.*)

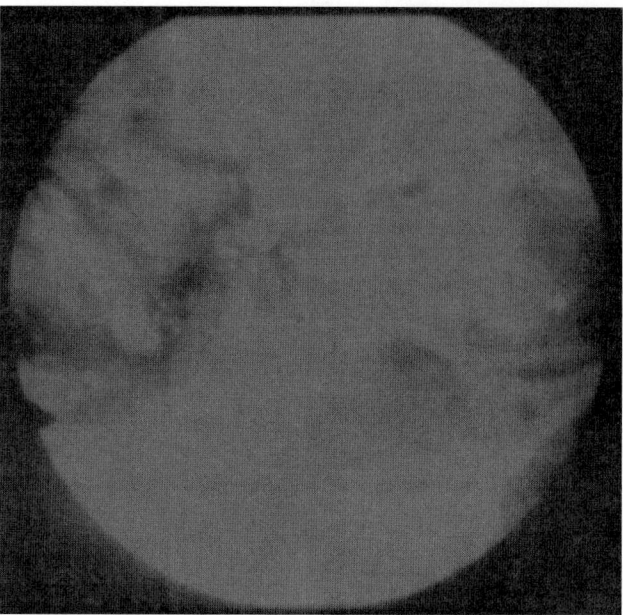

Figure 12   Complete peritoneal dissection exposes Cooper's ligament; cord structures; and, laterally, the iliopubic tract.

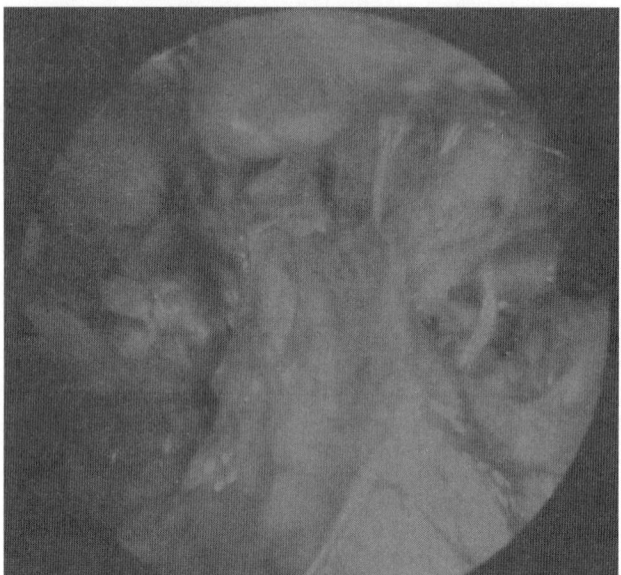

Figure 11   The area of the direct defect is now inspected, and any preperitoneal fat in this area is reduced.

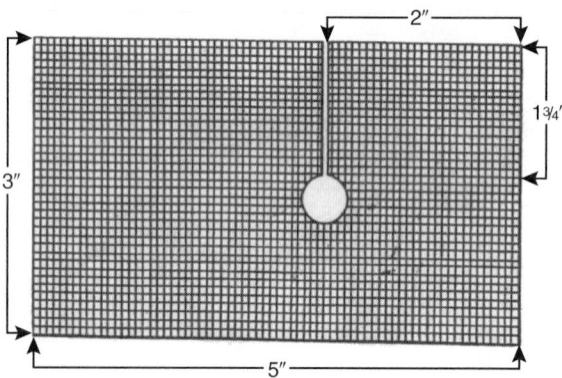

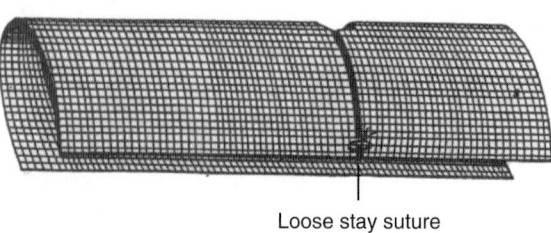

Loose stay suture

Figure 13   Using 3- × 5–inch piece of Prolene polypropylene mesh, a 1.75-inch cut is made vertically in the mesh 2 inches from the cephalad portion of the mesh, and a 1-cm hole is created for the cord structures to pass through. The mesh is folded, and a suture is placed for security, facilitating mesh placement.

from the cephalad portion of the mesh, and a 1-cm hole is created for the cord structures to pass through (Fig. 13). The mesh is folded, and a suture is placed for security, facilitating mesh placement. The vas deferens, spermatic artery, and vein are carefully dissected free from the lateral pelvic wall, enabling the mesh to be placed behind the cord structures (Fig. 14). The Prolene mesh is then inserted through the 10/11-mm cannula in proper orientation for easy positioning.

The surgeon must exercise considerable care, during dissection and severance of an indirect sac and in sTAPPle placement for securing the prosthetic mesh, not to compromise or injure the cord structures. The mesh is brought behind the cord structures and positioned to pass through the 1-cm hole in the mesh. The stay suture is cut, and the mesh is elevated into position (Fig. 15). Care is taken not to compromise the cord structures by deliberate placement of the first two keyhole sTAPPles. Two or three sTAPPles are then placed to close the keyhole (Fig. 16). STAPPles are no longer placed laterally, but if there is some surgical indication for lateral sTAPPles, they should be placed anterior to the iliopubic tract and

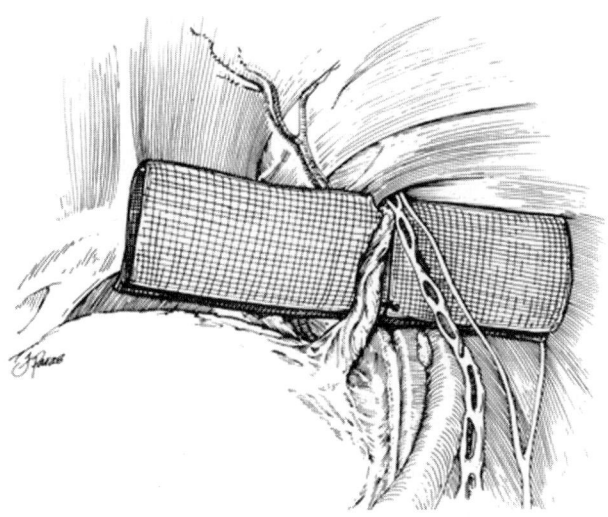

Figure 14 Folded mesh placed behind cord structures is shown.

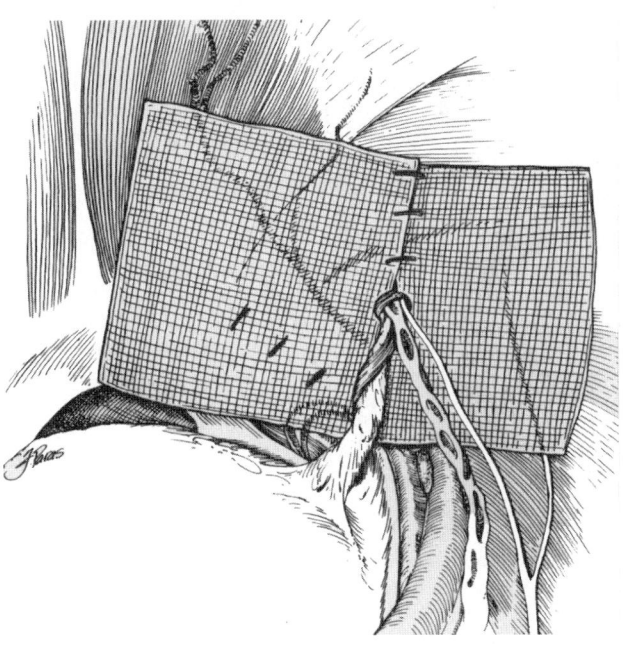

Figure 16 Placement of staples to close the keyhole and attachment to Cooper's ligament.

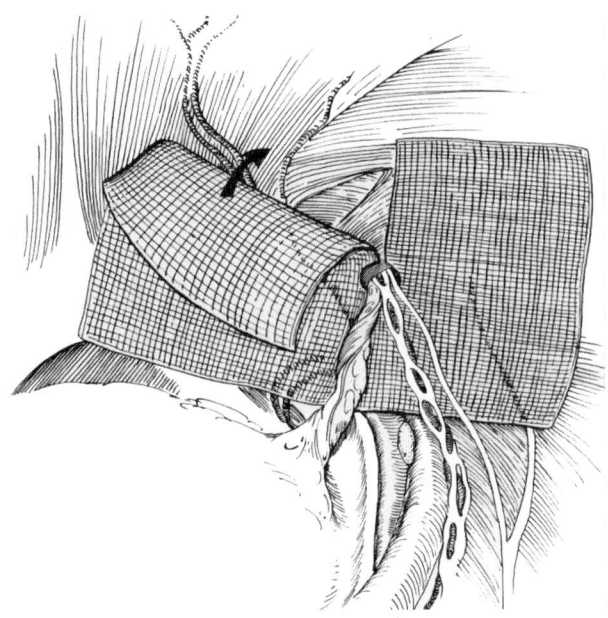

Figure 15 After the stay suture is cut, the mesh is elevated into position.

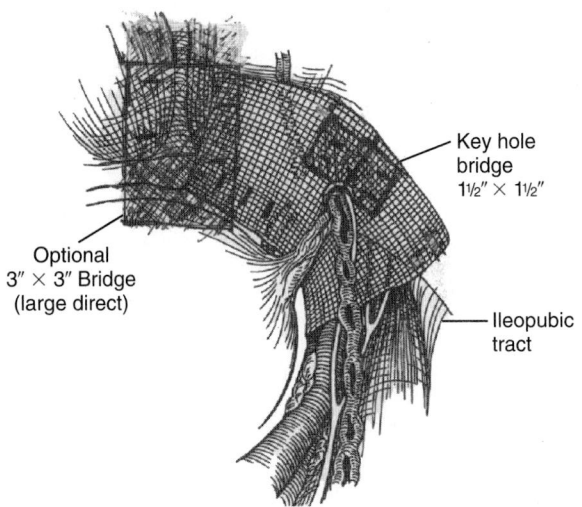

Figure 17 Bridge for the keyhole and an optional midline bridge for bilateral or large direct.

cord structures. The mesh is then tacked along Cooper's ligament and, optionally, anteriorly in the posterior aspects of the rectus muscle. STAPPles are not placed below the iliopubic tract, lateral to the internal ring. Except for the sTAPPles in Cooper's ligament, external counterpressure on the stapling device will help to ensure that sTAP-Ples are not placed such that nerve injury may occur. At this point, the keyhole is reinforced with a 1 × 1–inch piece of Prolene mesh that is referred to as a "bridge reinforcement" (Fig. 17) to prevent a recurrent indirect hernia (all 6 recurrences in the initial 1000 cases occurred through the keyhole that was not bridged). It is acceptable to perform the procedure without the use of the keyhole, but we find that the keyhole aids in proper positioning and orientation of the mesh.

In cases of a unilateral hernia, during the preoperative preparation of the patient, consent is obtained for bilateral herniorrhaphy. The opposite side is examined, and the occult hernia (occurs up to

50% of the time) is repaired if found. The two pieces of Prolene mesh are tacked together at the pubis. In cases of large bilateral direct hernia, an additional 3 × .75–inch piece of mesh is centered at the pubis and secured to the previously placed mesh (Fig. 17). This prevents protrusion of the mesh through a large direct defect. The mesh is also tacked around the opening in the facial defect in a large direct hernia to stabilize and prevent protrusion of the mesh.

Incarcerated hernias can present a difficult problem for the surgeon who is operating from the posterior approach. In dealing with an irreducible hernia, if the extraperitoneal dissection procedure fails, a transabdominal trocar is placed lateral and slightly above the periumbilical trocar the paramedian position opposite the incarcerated hernia. In 50% of these types of cases, contents of the sac can be reduced by use of an operative laparoscope with a grasper through the operative channel by manually pulling gently on the bowel. If this maneuver fails, the surgeon makes a 1-inch incision in the groin and dissects down to the external inguinal ring. The fibers of the external ring are carefully divided, and in most cases, this allows the hernia to be easily reduced. However, if this does not permit complete reduction, the surgeon must consider the possibility of adhesions in the hernia sac. In this case, the surgeon may open the sac via the previously made 1-inch groin incision; the adhesions are lysed and bowel or omentum reduced before proceeding to repair the hernia preperitoneally. If either of these methods does not permit reduction, the hernia must be approached anteriorly (to date we have not had such a case).

All trocar sites and areas of dissection are inspected for hemostasis, 30 ml of 0.25% Marcaine is injected via the side port of the blunt-tipped trocar, and the CO_2 is allowed to escape from the preperitoneal space. The fascia at both 10/11-mm trocar sites are closed with the 0 Vicryl sutures. Skin is closed with a subcuticular suture.

Key Points

In a preperitoneal hernia repair, knowledge of the anatomy is critical (Figs. 10.1-7, 10.1-8, and 10.1-9). The direct and indirect spaces are clearly delineated by their relation to the inferior epigastric vessels. Laterally, one must stay above the iliopubic tract when placing tacks to avoid catching any of the sensory nerves to the groin region. One way to avoid complication is to palpate the fixation device anterior to the iliac crest across the abdominal wall before placing any tacks.

For patients who have had prior preperitoneal procedures, a TAPP procedure should be considered. Also use TAPP when assessment of intraperitoneal organs is indicated (see Table 1) or to visualize intra-abdominal contents following a TEP via a paramedian incision with optical entry.

▌ CONCLUSIONS AND OPINIONS

Open, mesh-based repairs are clearly better than the suture-based tension repairs in terms of patient discomfort and recurrence.

The TEP and the open mesh repairs are reported to have similar or better results in terms of patient discomfort and hernia recurrence. However, operative time with TEP is often reduced, and as with all laparoscopic repairs, it also has the added advantage of allowing the surgeon to evaluate both sides. It has been reported that up to 50% of patients have bilateral hernias on laparoscopic visualization, yet clinically only one side was palpable. Thus both sides can be repaired with little additional operative time and without additional incisions.

With regard to prostheses, a new area of interest is low-weight meshes. More studies are being performed on available mesh materials. When considering a mesh material, assess its degree of contraction and ingrowth and the size of the hernia because these are the most important factors in the effectiveness of the mesh. Meshes

with high contraction rates lead to hernia recurrence if the mesh is cut small. Macroporous weaves provide excellent scaffolding for collagen deposition and remain compliant with the abdominal wall. However, if the hernia defect is large, more compliant meshes may protrude or prolapse through the defect. Fixation or large defect overlap aids the high flexibility of these meshes. By choosing the best mesh material, and more important the largest workable size, we maximize long-term function for our patients.

Laparoscopic repair is initially a more costly procedure to perform; however, the decreased procedure time, quicker recovery, and reduced long-term groin pain, along with the fact that fewer infections occur, easily make up for the operative cost. For recurrent or bilateral hernias, laparoscopic repair should be the procedure of choice. Recurrent inguinal hernias with posterior or anterior repairs are best treated laparoscopically (TEP or TAPP), not only to repair symptomatic recurrence but to evaluate the opposite side. Recurrent open posterior or laparoscopic repairs are usually more easily performed using the TAPP method.

The only case in which a suture-based open repair should be considered is in infants and in women of childbearing age. Women may wish to avoid mesh if they plan to become pregnant or in the presence of gross contamination.

In conclusion, both open and laparoscopic repairs are effective when performed appropriately by a skilled surgeon. Surgeons should select the repair method they feel most comfortable performing.

S U G G E S T E D R E A D I N G S

Andersson B, Hallen M, Leveau P, and others: Laparoscopic extraperitoneal inguinal hernia repair versus open mesh repair: a prospective randomized controlled trial, *Surgery* 133:464, 2003.

EU Hernia Trialists Collaboration: Repair of groin hernia with synthetic mesh: meta-analysis of randomized controlled trials, *Ann Surg* 235:322, 2002.

Fitzgibbons RJ Jr, Giobbie-Harder A, Gibbs JO, and others: Watchful waiting vs repair of inguinal hernia in minimally symptomatic men: a randomized clinical trial, *JAMA* 295:285, 2006.

Gonzalez R, Fugate K, McClusky D 3rd, and others: Relationship between tissue ingrowth and mesh contraction, *World J Surg* 29:1038, 2005.

Gonzalez R, Ramshaw BJ: Comparison of tissue integration between polyester and polypropylene prostheses in the preperitoneal space, *Am Surg* 69:471; discussion 476, 2003.

McKernan JB: Prosthetic inguinal hernia repair using a laparoscopic extraperitoneal approach, *Sem Lap Surg* 1:116, 1994.

Neumayer L, Giobbie-Harder A, Jonasson O, and others: Veterans affairs cooperative studies program 456 investigators. related articles, links open mesh versus laparoscopic mesh repair of inguinal hernia, *N Engl J Med* 350:1819–1827, 2004.

McKernan JB, Laws H: Laparoscopic repair of inguinal hernias using totally extraperitoneal prosthetic approach, *Surg Endosc* 7:26, 1993.

Winslow ER, Quasebarth M, Brunt LM: Perioperative outcomes and complications of open vs. laparoscopic extraperitoneal inguinal hernia repair in a mature surgical practice, *Surg Endosc* 18:221, 2004.

The Management of Recurrent Inguinal Hernia

Gregory J. Mancini, MD, and Bruce J. Ramshaw, MD

INTRODUCTION

Treatment of more than 750,000 inguinal hernias is performed annually in the United States, making it the most common operation performed by general surgeons. Various techniques have been developed and modified, each with the primary goal of minimizing hernia recurrence. The use of permanent mesh prosthetics and the development of laparoscopic techniques have each made a significant impact on hernia recurrence. They have also created new problems and questions for surgeons.

Numerous studies have been published comparing the various current hernia repair techniques. Although many are well designed and well intentioned, most are severely hindered by low follow-up numbers, short follow-up periods, and low surgeon experience (primarily in the technique of laparoscopic hernia repair). Large studies for inguinal hernia repair report recurrence rates ranging from less than 1% to more than 10%. Most would concede that this rate is two to three times higher in the general population. This means that nearly 40,000 inguinal hernia repairs are performed annually for hernia recurrence.

Recurrence in today's era of hernia surgery poses unique problems for the surgeon. Nearly 90% of primary adult hernia repairs have a prosthetic mesh implanted. This means that in addition to the anatomic distortion from the first repair and from the hernia recurrence, surgeons must contend with anatomic distortion caused by the chronic host-mesh inflammatory response.

The technical complexity of recurrent hernia surgery, the increased incidence of recurrences, and the higher rates of complications make patient counseling a critical component of the management of recurrent inguinal hernias.

MECHANISM OF HERNIA RECURRENCE

The mechanism of recurrence greatly depends on the type of prior hernia repair, the location and type of mesh prosthetic implant, and patient comorbidities. Patient selection and patient preparation before hernia repair are critically important to the success of a recurrent hernia repair.

Impact of Patient Characteristics

Several risk factors are potentially associated with higher rates of recurrence after hernia repair. These include diabetes mellitus, obesity, wound infection, immunosuppression, chronic obstructive pulmonary disease (COPD), and smoking.

Diabetes with poorly controlled blood glucose levels is associated with both impaired neutrophil function and decreased collagen synthesis by fibroblasts, resulting in higher infection rates and poor collagen deposition.

Heniford and colleagues have shown that obese patients have increased intra-abdominal pressures compared with nonobese patients, resulting in chronically elevated tension forces on the hernia repair.

Wound infections are known to produce proteases and collagenases that alter the extracellular matrix composition and delay wound healing.

Immunosuppression, whether intrinsic or iatrogenic, reduces macrophage function, fibroblast synthesis of collagen, and phenotypic expression of myofibroblasts responsible for wound contracture.

COPD with a chronic cough generates repeated high-pressure strain on a hernia repair. A cough or Valsalva can create intra-abdominal pressures exceeding 100 mm Hg.

On the basis of recent studies, smoking has the greatest association with hernia recurrence, with an odds ratio greater than two. It has been shown to inhibit fibroblast migration to the wound and to alter extracellular matrix composition, resulting in poor wound healing.

Impact of the Type of Initial Hernia Repair

The Shouldice repair, developed by Dr. Edward Shouldice in 1954, is a multilayered abdominal wall closure of the inguinal canal. The benefits of this technique are its ability to be performed under local anesthesia, low cost, and the avoidance of implanting a foreign body mesh prosthetic. Recurrence rates for hernias repaired at the Shouldice clinic are reported to be 1% to 2%. A recent European multicenter randomized clinical trial revealed a recurrence rate of 6.7% at 5 years. Ninety-five percent of recurrences were categorized as direct space defects. Beets and colleagues reported a 15% recurrence rate at a 14-year follow-up interval. The observations made in these and other studies validate the mechanism of recurrence in this repair. The technique requires the division of the transversalis fascia, which effectively disrupts the floor of the inguinal canal. Tissue tension is created by suture reapproximation of the attenuated layers of the abdominal wall. The inherently poor-quality tissue, constant intra-abdominal pressure forces, time, and patient comorbidities lead to weakening of the repair and eventual hernia recurrence.

A tension-free hernia repair is currently the most common technique used to treat inguinal hernia. The Lichtenstein repair and its variations, which include the plug-and-patch repair, account for nearly 75% of hernia repairs performed in the United States. Key principles of this repair include the complete reduction of the hernia sac and the implantation of a permanent mesh prosthetic as a tension-reducing bridge covering the fascial edges of hernia defect. Benefits of this technique include its ability to be performed under local anesthesia but at increased costs compared with the Shouldice repair because of the mesh. Additional benefits when compared with tissue repair techniques include lower recurrence rates, less postoperative pain, and quicker return to activities. The vast majority of synthetic material used in the tension-free repair is some type of heavyweight polypropylene mesh. Over the past decade, research regarding surgical mesh composition has revealed significant deficiencies in biocompatibility. Long thought to be inert, mesh prostheses have now been shown by mounting evidence to induce a chronic inflammatory reaction. This chronic foreign body reaction is likely responsible for both success in reducing hernia recurrence and failure related to the mechanism of recurrence, chronic pain, and tissue stiffness. Explant studies of mesh removed during hernia reoperations show significant macroscopic and microscopic changes in both the mesh and native tissue. Grossly, a chronic scar plate is observed including the mesh and local tissue. Contraction of the mesh up to more than 80% from the original size is likewise observed in some patients. Histologically, significant inflammatory cell infiltration is seen with mononucleated giant cells indicative of foreign body reaction. Additionally, altered ratios of type I/III collagen are observed, suggesting poor-quality scar formation.

The failure mechanism clinically observed in the tension-free repair is due to the contracted mesh pulling away from poor-quality native fascia, allowing hernia recurrence at the edges of the mesh. Interstitial hernia recurrences through defects in the transversals fascia, deep to the mesh, have also been observed.

The laparoscopic approach accounts for approximately 15% of inguinal hernia repairs in the United States. Numerous studies comparing various open techniques to laparoscopic techniques have been conducted. Instead of settling the debate about the optimal repair, these studies have intensified this discourse. Advocates for laparoscopic repair point out the shorter recovery time, reduced postoperative pain, and optimal mesh coverage of the myopectineal orifice. Contrarians point out the increased costs, long learning curve, and potential complications of the laparoscopic technique. Overall, recurrence rates for the laparoscopic approach range from less than 1% to more than 10% in most randomized clinical trials. Similar to the open repair, heavyweight polypropylene is the mesh most commonly used in laparoscopic inguinal hernia repair. This material in the preperitoneal space is subject to similar host-mesh inflammatory response as the anteriorly placed mesh. Significant differences between the two include the mesh size and vector forces experienced by the mesh. Mesh placed behind the abdominal wall musculature is pushed against the hernia defect by intra-abdominal forces. Mesh size recommended for the laparoscopic repair is at least 12 × 15 cm, compared with 3 × 8 cm for the open, tension-free repair. The different sizes and locations of the mesh for open, tension-free and laparoscopic inguinal hernia repair techniques clearly demonstrate that they are not similar repairs. The laparoscopic approach allows for a much wider coverage of the myopectineal orifice in a space completely behind (inside) the defect (Figs. 1, 2, and 3). A retrospective review of the laparoscopic hernia repair shows that the mechanism of recurrence is herniation around the edges of mesh or through a mesh slit, if the mesh is cut. Technical errors that contribute to recurrence are failure to dissect the hernia sac adequately off of the cord structures, inadequate fixation of the mesh over the entire myopectineal orifice, and inadequate mesh coverage because of small mesh implant size or secondary to chronic mesh contraction.

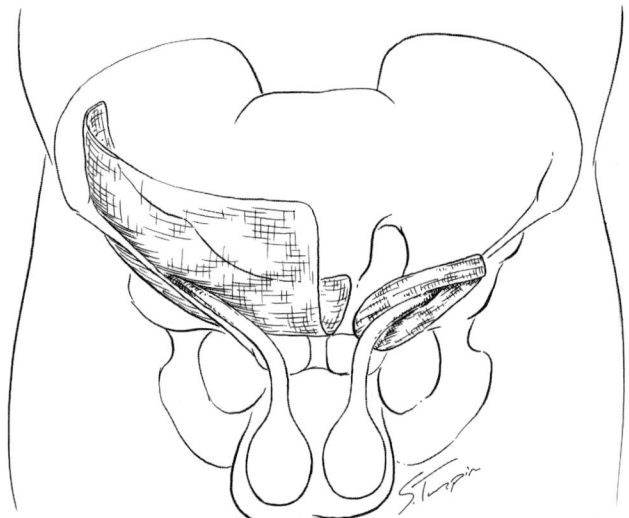

Figure 2 A transparent view of the lower abdomen showing typical mash placement for open, tension-free *(left)* and laparoscopic *(right)* inguinal hernia repairs.

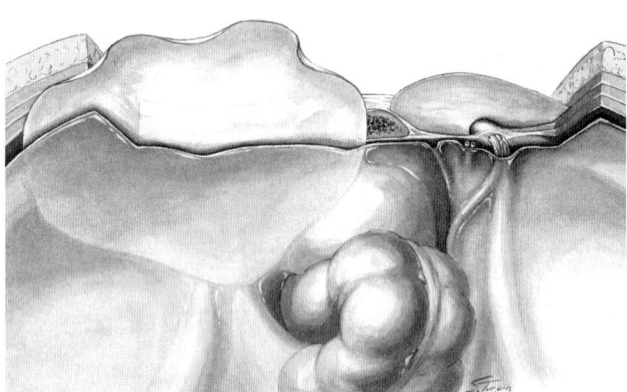

Figure 3 A posterior (internal) view of the lower abdomen showing typical mesh placement for an open, tension-free *(right)* and a laparoscopic *(left)* inguinal hernia repair.

INDICATIONS FOR RECURRENT HERNIA REPAIR

A key to success in the treatment of inguinal hernia complications is to separate patients with hernia recurrence from those with chronic groin pain. The two most common presentations of recurrent inguinal hernia are a recurrent groin bulge or groin pain. The primary goal for the surgeon is to decide whether the bulge or pain represents a true hernia recurrence or a new disease process. In the previously operated groin with a mesh implant, this clinical decision can be difficult. If the presence of a recurrent hernia cannot be discerned by physical examination, the use of radiography may be indicated. CT herniography has a sensitivity of 75% for detecting inguinal defects, but for recurrent hernias, this number is likely lower. Although not commonly used, ultrasound or x-ray herniography may dynamically show a hernia recurrence. If either physical examination or

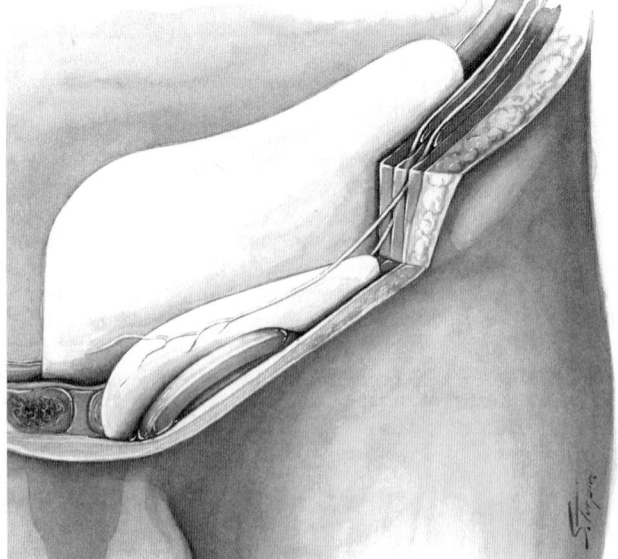

Figure 1 An anterior view of the left groin showing the typical size and location of meshes placed open (as in a Lichtenstein procedure) and laparoscopically.

radiographic study demonstrates hernia recurrence, hernia repair is indicated. However, if neither reveals a hernia, cautious reevaluation of treatment goals and options should be discussed with the patient. An attempt to improve patient symptoms with nonsurgical options, such as pain management or physical therapy, may be warranted. Alternative nonoperative interventions, such as trigger point injections or medications such as gabapentin or amitriptyline, can be helpful in chronic pain scenarios.

SURGICAL TECHNIQUES TO TREAT RECURRENT INGUINAL HERNIA

The surgical approach used to treat a recurrent inguinal hernia may depend on the type of prior hernia repair, the prosthetic implant used, and the symptoms presenting with the recurrence. In most cases, we feel a laparoscopic approach provides the best technique both to diagnose the mechanism of recurrence and to repair the recurrent hernia defect. When the prior hernia repair is a tissue repair or a tension-free repair with mesh placed anterior to the fascia, the preperitoneal space has not been violated. A total extraperitoneal preperitoneal (TEP) approach can be used in this setting with results approaching that of a primary TEP procedure. This approach avoids the previously operated anterior space with mesh and scarring and minimizes potential injury to the inguioinguinal and iliohypogastric nerves as well. It is especially important in reoperative hernia surgery to be aware of the course of the deep and more superficial nerves coursing through the groin (Figs. 4 and 5)

When a recurrence has developed after an open repair in which the preperitoneal space has been violated, such as with a Prolene Hernia System (Ethicon, Piscataway, NJ), a laparoscopic approach, or a Kugel repair (Bard, Murray Hill, NJ), the laparoscopic TEP approach may be difficult. During balloon dissection, the peritoneum may tear and not create the extraperitoneal workspace that is necessary. In this case, a transabdominal preperitoneal approach (TAPP) should be used. This allows the surgeon to complete the mobilization of the peritoneum from the cord structures and to identify the location of the recurrence. In addition to reducing the hernia sac, the surgeon can excise the old mesh, if necessary and if safety can be ensured. The type of new mesh should be chosen on the basis of the proximity to bowel structures. If the peritoneum can be adequately reapproximated and will cover the mesh completely, a lightweight polypropylene or polyester mesh

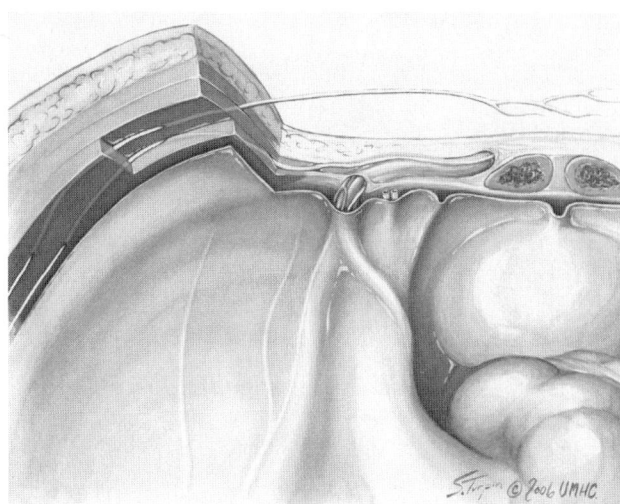

Figure 5 Posterior (interior) view of the left groin showing the nerves at risk during inguinal hernia repair.

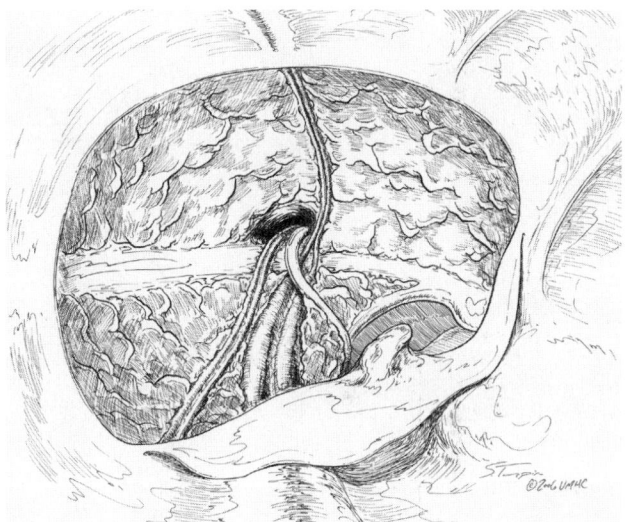

Figure 6 Exposure of the left groin from a transabdominal approach. The peritoneum has been incised, and the indirect hernia sac has been reduced.

may be placed in a standard TAPP fashion. More commonly, the peritoneum is adherent to mesh and tears during the dissection of the extraperitoneal space. In this setting, the mesh is fixed to the fascia, and the peritoneum is not closed (Figs. 6, 7, and 8). This procedure is a transabdominal preperitoneal approach without reperitonealization (TAPPWR), and a mesh designed for intraabdominal use should be employed.

Similarly, in the scenario of recurrence after either a TEP or TAPP hernia repair, we prefer the TAPPWR approach. Because the most common cause of recurrence is related to herniation around the mesh, the key to the recurrent repair is a wide dissection of the lower abdominal wall and groin region. Wide mobilization of the peritoneum is begun away from scar tissue and previous mesh, eventually working toward the area of the previous repair. After the hernia sac is reduced, a mesh designed for intra-abdominal use is placed. Spiral tack fixation is performed medially at the pubic tubercle and Cooper's ligament, laterally to the abdominal wall superior to the iliac crest and superiorly at the rectus muscle.

In a situation in which the surgeon is uncomfortable with the TEP or TAPP approaches, an open hernia repair may be performed.

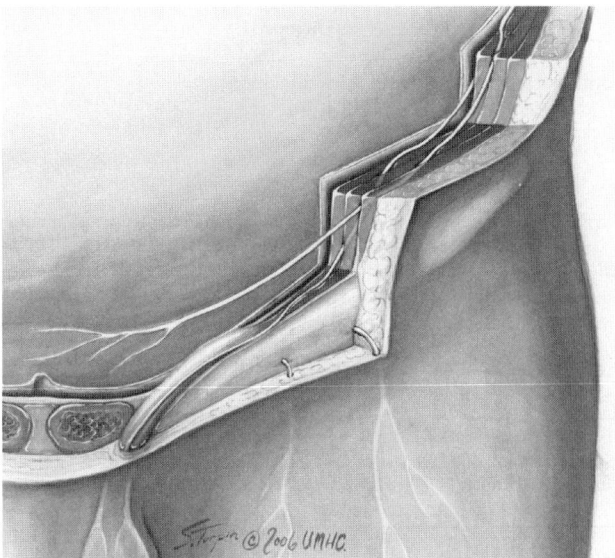

Figure 4 Anterior view of the left groin showing the nerves at risk during inguinal hernia repair.

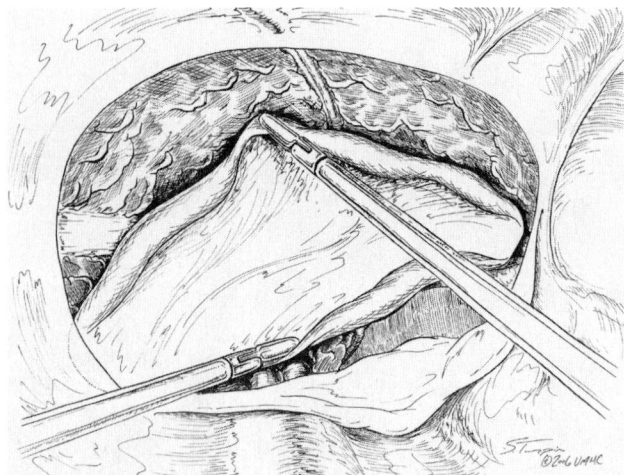

Figure 7 A mesh designed for intra-abdominal placement is introduced and positioned to cover the entire myopectineal orifice.

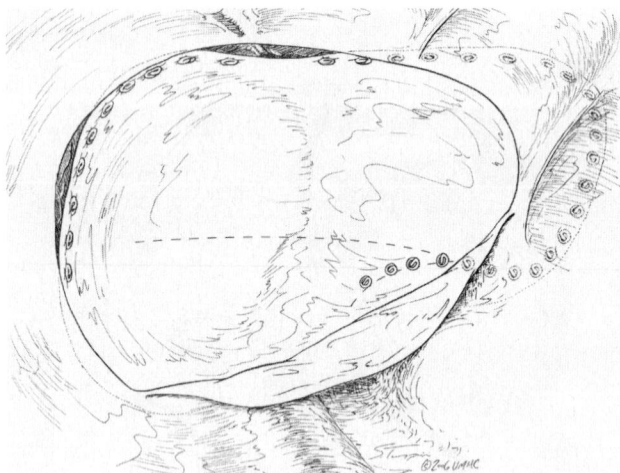

Figure 8 The mesh is fixed to the abdominal wall with a point fixation device or sutures (or both), and the peritoneum is left open.

This can be achieved under local, regional, or general anesthesia in accordance with the profile and preferences of the patient and surgeon. The benefit to the surgeon of a conscious patient is the ability to perform a Valsalva maneuver on command to demonstrate the location of a small hernia defect. Goals in the open approach are to identify and reduce the hernia sac, define the extent of the hernia defect, preserve cord structures of the groin, and repair the hernia defect with mesh in a tension-free manner. This may or may not require partial or whole mesh excision. The difficulty of this technique greatly depends on the complexity of the hernia defect and the inflammatory reaction to the previous mesh prosthesis. The patient should be counseled regarding the risks of postoperative pain or paresthesia, testicular atrophy, and hernia recurrence.

RESULTS OF TREATMENT

Few studies compare recurrence rates and patient outcomes after primary and recurrent hernia repairs. One such study is based on a Swedish hernia registry. This study reports 4.6% reoperation rate within 2 years of repair for recurrent hernia compared with 1.7% reoperation rate after primary repairs. Further review of the

literature shows that outcomes after repair of recurrent hernias are worse overall compared with those following primary repair. After the repair of a recurrent hernia, patients have higher complication rates, longer periods of convalescence, a greater incidence of chronic groin pain, and higher recurrence rates.

More studies comparing the various techniques for repairing recurrent hernias are necessary. No randomized controlled studies have compared open anterior with laparoscopic hernia repair for recurrent hernias. Feliu and colleagues reported a nonrandomized trial comparing an open preperitoneal and a laparoscopic TEP repair for recurrent hernias. This study reported statistically equivalent outcomes and recurrence rates for the two groups. Several studies purport the benefits of the laparoscopic TEP repair in the setting of a recurrence after an anterior repair, with complication and recurrence rates nearly equal to those of a primary repair. When the laparoscopic TEP approach is performed after a preperitoneal hernia repair has failed, the potential for complications related to scar tissue in the extraperitoneal space may be increased. When a laparoscopic TAPP approach is performed by experienced surgeons in the setting of recurrence, the outcomes and recurrence rates are favorable. Currently there are no consensus or treatment algorithms regarding the optimal approach to repairing recurrent inguinal hernias. Future studies in this area are greatly needed.

DISCUSSION

Recurrent inguinal hernias are a difficult problem to manage. Although improvements in hernia technique and prosthetic materials are thought to have reduced their incidence, hernia recurrence is a common problem that most general surgeons face in their practice. The technical complexity of recurrent hernia surgery, the increased incidence of recurrences, and the higher rates of complications make patient counseling a critical component to managing recurrent inguinal hernias. Our preference is to tailor our operative approach according to the patient's previous hernia repair history. For previous anterior repairs, with or without mesh, we prefer to perform a laparoscopic TEP hernia repair. If mesh has been placed in the preperitoneal or intra-abdominal location, we perform a laparoscopic TAPP or TAPPWR, depending on the condition of the peritoneum and the ability to cover the mesh implant. Mesh in the preperitoneal or intra-abdominal location may have to be partially or completely removed to allow for optimal tissue approximation for the new mesh.

ACKNOWLEDGMENTS

Administrative Assistant: Brandy Stockton
Medical Illustrator: Stacy Turpin

SUGGESTED READINGS

Barrat C, Surlin V, Bordea A, and others: Management of recurrent inguinal hernias: a prospective study of 163 cases, *Hernia* 7:125, 2003.
Feliu X, Torres G, Vinas X, and others: Preperitoneal repair for recurrent inguinal hernia: laparoscopic and open approach, *Hernia* 8:113, 2004.
Felix EL: A unified approach to recurrent laparoscopic hernia repairs, *Surg Endosc* 15:969, 2001.
Frankum CE, Ramshaw BJ, White J, and others: Laparoscopic repair of bilateral and recurrent hernias, *Am Surg* 65:839, 1999.
Ramshaw BJ, Abiad F, Voeller G, and others: Polyester (Parietex) mesh for total extraperitoneal laparoscopic inguinal hernia repair: initial experience in the United States, *Surg Endosc* 17:498, 2003.
Ramshaw BJ, Shuler FW, Jones HB, and others: Laparoscopic inguinal hernia repair: lessons learned after 1224 consecutive cases, *Surg Endosc* 15:50, 2001.
Ramshaw BJ, Tucker JG, Conner T, and others: A comparison of the approaches to laparoscopic herniorrhaphy, *Surg Endosc* 10:29, 1996.

Incisional, Epigastric, and Umbilical Hernias

Anthony P. Tufaro, DDS, MD, and Kurtis
A. Campbell, MD

Any evisceration of the abdominal contents through a fascial defect is defined as a hernia and can result in loss of abdominal domain and abdominal visceral disproportion. Three fascial defects—incisional, epigastric, and umbilical hernias—commonly seen are reviewed in this chapter. The underlying etiology can differ for each type, yet the exacerbating factors and the factors that predispose to their recurrences are common to all. Umbilical hernias are true congenital fascial defects that often present at birth and may not completely close; epigastric hernias are considered acquired because they rarely present at birth but often relate to the anatomy of the midline fascial decussations; and incisional hernias are secondary to a prior surgical procedure.

INCISIONAL HERNIA

An incisional hernia is an inclusive term for any abdominal wall defect in the site of prior surgical incisions or trocar and drain sites, all causing a fascial defect. The vast majority of these are ventral; less commonly, incisional hernias may be found in the flank or even lumbar area. The incidence of incisional hernia is 2% of patients following an open, clean, elective surgery, increasing to 20% in contaminated surgical procedures. A postoperative wound infection also correlates with a higher incidence of postoperative incisional hernia. Within 6 months of a surgery, 50% of hernias become evident, and the majority occur by 2 years. Exacerbating factors are obesity; chronic obstructive pulmonary disease (COPD) or respiratory insufficiency; prior wound infections; prostatism; chronic constipation; pregnancy; ascites; and any cause of chronically increased intra-abdominal pressure. The predisposing factors for a ventral hernia are identical to those for an incisional hernia and include obesity and other conditions that cause rectus diastasis and attenuation of the native fascia. As we approach epidemic proportions of obesity in Western society, the challenging problems of incisional and ventral hernias will also markedly increase.

Also contributing to incisional hernias are etiologies of poor wound healing, such as smoking; poorly controlled diabetes; steroid use; radiation; systemic immunosuppression; multiple parallel incisions in the fascia; or multiple prior surgeries causing areas of ischemia or poorly perfused abdominal wall. Likewise, genetic factors such as defective collagen synthesis or crosslinking abnormalities secondary to Marfan's or Ehler-Danlos's diseases can also cause defective fascial wound reparation.

The primary reasons for incisional hernias are (1) an abdominal wall closure under tension with shearing of sutures in the fascia, (2) postoperative seroma collection leading to a higher incidence of postoperative infection, and (3) frank infection from a contaminated emergent procedure or one involving fascitis and necrosis leading to frank tissue loss. Incisional hernias can vary from being small and barely detectable to involving the whole abdominal wall with almost the entirety of the abdominal contents eviscerating into the hernia sac. The exacerbating factors already mentioned lead to the expected and continued enlargement of the fascial defect over time. The large hernias are truly challenging management problems because their reduction back into the abdominal cavity can cause abdominovisceral disproportion and thus cardiovascular compromise with abdominal compartment syndrome or respiratory embarrassment resulting from compromised ventilation. The nontrivial recurrence rate for incisional hernia repairs is 20% to 46% because the reduction of a large hernia reestablishes significant abdominal domain that is directly correlated with increased abdominal pressure. This pressure is the precise reason for their occurrence in the first place, as well as for their recurrence.

Before any surgery, it is important to identify the status and topography of the patient's entire abdominal wall to plan for definitive abdominal wall reconstruction. Preoperatively, careful determination of the location and extent of the fascial defect, the viability and stability of neighboring soft tissue, and the medical stability of the patient are essential. It is necessary to map out all prior incisions and crossing incisions, ostomy sites, or areas healed by secondary intention. Imaging by computed tomography (CT) scan with oral contrast delineates the hernia entirely in more than 90% of cases and can sufficiently identify incarcerated viscera protruding into the fascial defect and hernia sac. CT also detects chronically incarcerated omentum versus bowel; it is not uncommon to detect incarcerated bladder in the lower abdominal defects. Imaging permits identification of the primary defect and some associated smaller defects, which may have been undetected clinically. The unappreciated smaller defects are often associated with a recurrence following a primary repair and are at risk of enlarging following repair of the larger defect.

Incisional hernias can run the gamut from a small, minor repair to one of the most complex and challenging management problems. Larger hernia defects are associated with higher recurrence rates; in fact, fascial defects of only 4 cm are associated with a threefold increase in recurrence. Thus direct closure has not represented the standard. Direct closure may occasionally be appropriate for small fascial defects with well-vascularized soft tissue and fascia but should be avoided in acutely infected wounds, prior radiation, in any setting with preexisting tissue loss, or of any moderate size. The long-standing guiding principle for standard fascial closure is that sutures are placed consistently 1 cm apart and 1 cm from the fascial edge. Any deviation from a meticulous technique of consistent suture placement increases the incidence of wound failure. Failure to recognize even minor fascial defects at the time of the initial repair, such as those created by a needle hole in the fascia during closure, can lead to recurrence when placed under tension during closure and subsequent function. Inception of the hernia can occur in the operating room even with improper anesthetic relaxation, which leads to sudden increased tension and a shearing of the sutures through the fascia. Thus the requirements essential for a standard repair include the following: (1) deep anesthetic relaxation in the repair of a moderate or large hernia size, (2) an extensive lysis of adhesions to separate normal viscera from hernia sac, and (3) a strategy for the loss of abdominal domain. This regaining of abdominal domain following the reduction of viscera into the abdominal cavity can cause postoperative critical care issues of compromised respiratory mechanics and cardiovascular compromise, as well as the potential for abdominal compartment syndrome (Fig. 1). The extent of the lysis of adhesions essential to reduce the viscera and define adequate fascial borders can stimulate extensive fluid-seeking behavior postoperatively that is in turn problematic and can contribute to an abdominal compartment syndrome if left unchecked.

The technique in abdominal wall reconstruction must incorporate an understanding of its complexity and versatility as a three-tiered structure, permitting pliability and dynamic changes in intra-abdominal pressures. The abdominal wall is a lattice of crossing musculature and has a unique anatomy in that most of the

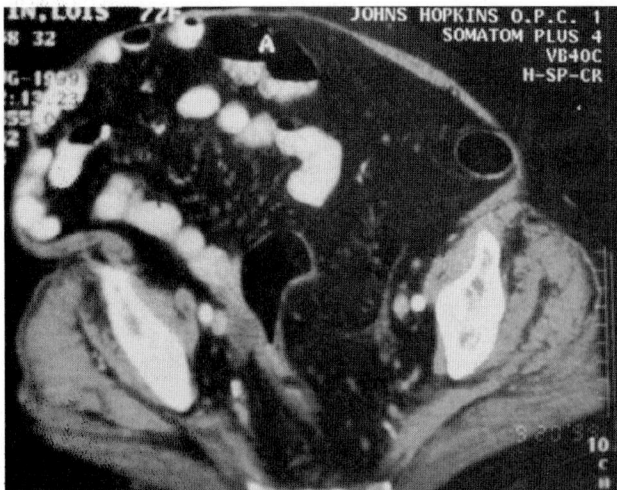

Figure 1 Computed tomography scan of a massive incisional hernia with marked loss of domain.

muscles insert only into an aponeurosis or tendon, as opposed to a bone or cartilage. The lateral musculature combines three sets of muscles at angles, which insert into broad central aponeuroses, which likewise insert into a midline tendon (the linea alba). The central aponeuroses encase the rectus abdominis muscles, which span from the ribs to the pubis inferiorly and insert into four tendinous transverse bands in the rectus muscle. Of note, nonmidline incisions, which do not run parallel to the nerves or vessels, can sever the blood and nervous supply to the abdominal wall, leading to muscular atrophy or areas of compromised perfusion.

TECHNIQUE

Over the past 6 years, we have developed a tension-free technique for the management of complicated incisional-ventral, flank, and lumbar hernias. We have applied our scheme in recurrent hernias, in the presence of infected and exposed prosthetic material. We have also applied it to patients with enterocutaneous fistulae and ostomies, which combine the complexity of large complicated hernias in the problematic setting of chronically infected skin. More than 340 patients have been treated in this fashion with a recurrence rate of approximately 1.8%. All of the recurrences have been in patients with ostomies, and all are parastomal recurrences.

There are three basic principles to this technique. First is *the separation of the lipocutaneous layer* from the patient's native fascia. This allows the entire area at risk in the abdominal wall to be visualized, from the xiphoid process to the pubic symphysis. Often other areas of fascial defects are found that would have subsequently led to a hernia. After the skin and subcutaneous fat, which is often scarred, are mobilized from the fascia, it is much easier to mobilize the myofascial layer toward the midline for closure without tension. By mobilizing the fat and skin, one is also able to resect the scarred and excess skin so that the closure can be approximated with healthy stable tissue.

The second principle is that we always obtain *a biologic closure* over the viscera. The separation of the lipocutaneous layer facilitates this in most cases by allowing primary fascial closure and establishing a normal visceral domain and abdominal contours. When there is still a defect in the fascial closure, rather than place undue tension on the fascial closure, we elect to use a bioprosthetic to separate viscera from our mesh onlay. This avoids the problem of bowel ingrowth into mesh. The use of sheets of impervious material is always fraught with problems, such as seroma and subsequent infection, and we avoid their use. Acellular dermis, our material of choice, allows for

tensionless closure, placement of mesh without the problem of bowel injury, and avoidance of seroma formation seen with impervious sheets of prosthetic material. Acellular dermis also has the potential for vascular ingrowth. The material is placed as an "inset" without undue tension (Fig. 2). It is measured and constructed to size and sutured with interrupted horizontal mattress sutures, using a permanent suture. In our experience, the bioprosthetic materials do not tolerate tension; they will become thin or attenuated, and they potentially fail if close attention is not paid to this point.

The use of mesh is the gold standard to reduce the rate of hernia recurrence for any sizeable hernia defect and has been shown to reduce long-term failure rates from 25% to 52% to 11% to 21%. Thus the third principle is *the fixation of a permanent mesh,* such as polypropylene, as a "quilted mesh onlay" (Fig. 3). The most important step is the fixation of the mesh to stable anatomic points. The first principle of lipocutaneous separation from fascia now allows access for the mesh to be fixed to the periosteum of ribs, anterior superior iliac spine, pubic symphysis, and the inguinal ligament. Careful evaluation of all failed attempts at prior repair reveals that the point of failure is often at the interface of prosthetic material with native tissue. By fixing the mesh to stable points outside the area at risk of

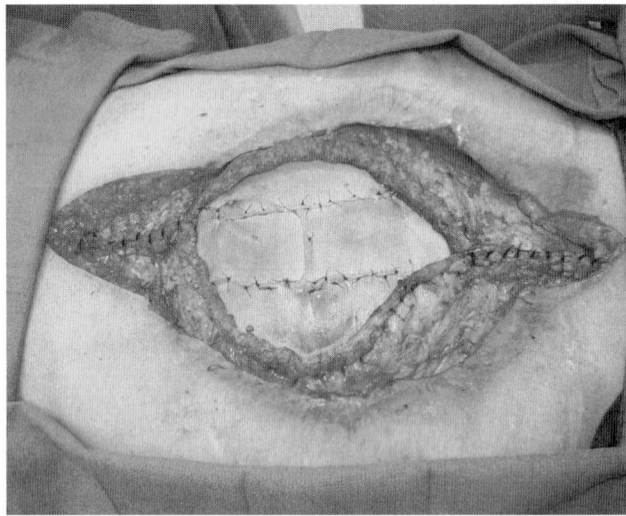

Figure 2 Acellular dermis used as inset for biologic closure over bowel.

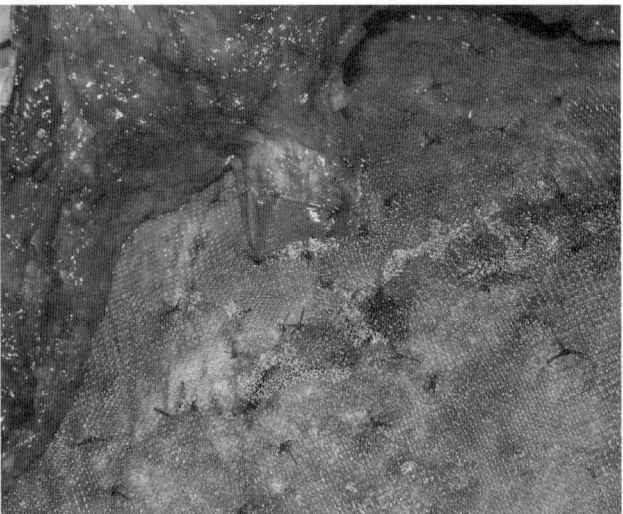

Figure 3 Quilted mesh onlay fitted around the ileal conduit with acellular dermis collar.

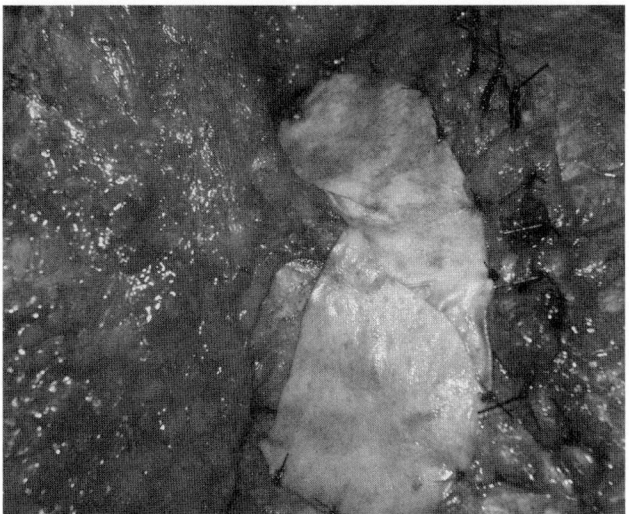

Figure 4 Acellular dermis fitted around an ileal conduit to protect the intestinal conduit and to reinforce the native fascia.

further hernias, we have reduced the recurrence rate to zero in our patients without ostomies. The mesh is "quilted" to the patients' abdominal wall. This technique eliminates the possibility of seroma formation under the mesh and thus of potential infection. By placing the mesh in intimate contact with the native tissue, the forces of the abdominal wall are transferred to the stable structures mentioned earlier. This "load transfer" takes the stress of the abdominal wall in function and distributes the stress to structures that will not fail.

The quilting process allows for soft-tissue ingrowth in just a few weeks, which then transforms the abdominal wall into a single stable construct. The entire wall has been evaluated from xiphoid process to pubic symphysis and covered with a strong material anchored to stable structures, leading to rapid ingrowth of tissue and a total reconstruction of the abdominal wall.

Wound-healing problems are seen in approximately 17% of our patients. The wide undermining can render the relatively hypovascular, subcutaneous fat ischemic, leading to eventual skin and fat necrosis and requiring debridement and local wound care. Preservation of one or two large lateral perforators prevents this problem and decreases wound-healing issues. Even in cases of wound or incisional breakdown, we have not seen frank infection of the mesh or the need to remove the large implant. In a small number of cases—fewer than 10—a small area of mesh that has not become fully incorporated and became exposed with wound breakdown is excised. This usually happens either in the midline, where the irregular contours can make close adaptation of mesh to the fascia difficult, or between widely spaced quilting sutures. Even with an open wound, vascularized soft tissue usually grows through the mesh with dressing changes or a vacuum-assisted closure device. This is because the material is quilted in place, and soft-tissue ingrowth is a rapid process.

This technique is used in the presence of ostomies by placing a collar of acellular dermis at the base of the stoma to separate it from the mesh and avoid possible erosion (Fig. 4). The technique used in the presence of ostomies has a slightly higher recurrence rate. The recurrences present as parastomal hernias and can be fixed with a parastomal approach without complication.

LAPAROSCOPY

Laparoscopic incisional hernia repair is increasingly used in the management of patients with incisional hernias. Laparoscopy permits an underlay technique with intraperitoneal placement of the prosthesis, and in principle this technique is similar, although one

layer deeper, to the open Stoppa repair, which is a retrorectus onlay. Following laparoscopic adhesiolysis, the prosthetic is placed intraperitoneally and sutured circumferentially to the full thickness of the abdominal wall. The advantages of laparoscopy include an ability to detect "Swiss cheese"–type defects, decreased length of hospital stay, and wound complication rates. Complication rates can occur in 5% to 15% of patients and include an inadvertent enterotomy, which precludes completion of the operation; seroma between the mesh and the hernia sac because the sac is left in situ; suture site pain secondary to nerve entrapment; and a wound infection. Recurrence rates are reported to be between 2% and 17%. A strong emphasis is on appropriate fixation of the prosthesis (expanded polytetrafluoroethylene [Teflon]) in laparoscopic hernia repair, with large, nonabsorbable sutures providing strong and reliable fixation of the prosthesis. Hernia tacks and staples are not sufficient as the primary source of attachment but are welcome to fill gaps between the sutures. The technique of a tension-free intraperitoneal placement of a prosthetic graft mandates broad anchorage of the mesh, such that there is an overlap of the hernia margin of 3 to 4 cm. Application of laparoscopy is not always a good option for challenging hernias and may not be feasible in all patients, such as in cases with extensive intra-abdominal adhesions or large recurrent hernias and patients with enterocutaneous fistulae and ostomies.

UMBILICAL HERNIAS

Congenital umbilical hernias are the most common abdominal wall defect in children, and surgical repair is delayed until after 2 to 4 years of age because of the high incidence of spontaneous closure. Soon after birth, the umbilical ring begins to contract, reinforced by the lateral umbilical ligaments (obliterated umbilical arteries), or the round ligament (umbilical vein), or urachus. The 10% of umbilical hernias detected in adults are presumed to be congenital and present three times more frequently in women. These are most often seen in multiparous women because of the significant contractile stress during parturition or in patients with chronically increased abdominal pressure such as those with ascites, prostatism, COPD, constipation, or obesity. The size of umbilical hernias can vary, and notably a large hernia with a narrow fascial neck has the potential for strangulation. Commonly the presentation is of chronically incarcerated omentum, but the herniation may represent bowel strangulation. Differential diagnosis of an umbilical mass also includes an omphalomesenteric duct, urachal cyst, or Sister Mary Joseph node. Operative indications include symptoms such as pain, nausea, signs of obstruction, disproportionate hernia size compared with fascial neck, skin discoloration or changes, and ascites. Symptoms, particularly those in a high-risk patient with multiple medical comorbidities such as hypertension, uncontrolled diabetes, and obesity, should be the indication for elective repair. Ignoring risk factors actually puts patients at a far greater risk when the hernia continues to enlarge or they present for emergent repair, which may lead to poor outcome and higher morbidity and mortality.

TECHNIQUE

Most umbilical hernias can be repaired electively in an outpatient setting using a variety of anesthetic techniques because they are typically relatively small and do not represent a large loss of domain. A curved infraumbilical incision can easily identify the defect at the base of the umbilical stalk, and direct dissection of the musculoaponeurotic edges around the hernia then facilitates reduction of the bowel. The principles are the same as those discussed for incisional hernias and include careful evaluation of the topography of the abdominal wall, clearance of the musculoaponeurotic edge of more than 2 cm in all directions, and avoidance of excess tension. Sutures should be carefully and consistently placed 1 cm apart and 1 cm across for equal distribution of pressure. Primary closure of the fascia is ideal and may require mobilization of the skin and subcutaneous tissue far enough on the fascia to reapproximate native fascia. Large defects may require alloplastic prosthetic or bioprosthetic material to reinforce the fascial closure and to enhance a tension-free closure. Component separation is not advised because relaxing incisions in the lateral anterior rectus sheaths do not relieve tension at the umbilicus as a result of the tendinous insertion into the rectus abdominis muscles at the umbilicus.

EPIGASTRIC HERNIA

Epigastric hernias typically are in the midline along the linea alba from the xiphoid down to the umbilicus and have a prevalence of 1% to 5% of the population; male patients present with this type of hernia three times more commonly than women. More than 20% of epigastric hernias are multiple. The linea alba is a decussation of fibers forming an aponeurosis between the rectus sheaths, and herniation can occur between attenuated aponeurotic fibers. Nearly all epigastric hernias occur when there is only a single decussation of aponeurotic fibers, as opposed to the typically redundant, multiple decussation of aponeurotic fibers. In fact, the linea alba is wider in the upper abdomen and thus may have more attenuated decussating fascial fibers, which leads to the higher incidence of epigastric hernias than those in the infraumbilical region, where the linea alba is narrower and more redundant. The etiology of epigastric hernias is partially congenital because of the underlying anatomic differences of midline decussation and partially acquired from stress on the linea alba —the majority occur in 20- to 50-year-old adults. Most epigastric hernias are small and in the midline, usually containing only preperitoneal fat. Body habitus or obesity may make the typically palpable mass in the midepigastrium indistinguishable from the surrounding fat and can often be recognized by the symptoms of exacerbation of pain on exertion and relief on reclining. Imaging by ultrasound or CT scan may be essential in more rotund or obese patients.

TECHNIQUE

Surgical therapy is indicated in all adult patients who are symptomatic or after a diagnosis is established. Methods for repairing an epigastric defect depend on the size of the defects. Conversion of epigastric fascial defects into one midline incision, which is then closed primarily, is recommended to incorporate the commonly associated multiple epigastric hernias or umbilical hernias into one repair. A midline vertical incision is made overlying the hernia, and the linea alba is exposed around the neck of the defect and extended in a vertical direction to identify other coexisting fascial defects. After the defect is identified, the preperitoneal fat or sac is reduced; rarely is there a hernia sac associated with a primary epigastric defect. After the hernia contents are reduced, digital exploration of the preperitoneal plane superiorly and inferiorly to identify occult fascial defects ensures the identification of other herniations, as well as an umbilical hernia. The fascial edges are cleared approximately 2 cm in all directions. Most repairs can be accomplished as a primary fascial repair but have a recurrence rate of 5% to 10%. If the defect is greater than 2 to 3 cm, reinforcement of the primary fascial repair with alloplastic material (polypropylene) or bioprosthetic materials such as acellular dermis sutured in place using interrupted nonabsorbable sutures adds strength to the fascial repair. Again the problem of identifying high-risk patients arises, and meticulous care to identify and avoid the reasons for recurrences is essential to avoid failure at the interface of the implant and native fascia.

SUGGESTED READINGS

Askar OM: Surgical anatomy of the aponeurotic expansions of the anterior abdominal wall, *Ann R Coll Surg Engl* 55:313, 1977.
Gilbert AI, Graham MF, Voigt WJ: Infected grafts on incisional hernioplasties, *Hernia* 1:77, 1997.
Heniford BT, Park A, Ramshaw BJ, and others: Laparoscopic ventral and incisional hernia repair in 407 patients, *J Am Coll Surg* 190:645, 2000.
LeBlanc K, Bellanger D: Laparoscopic repair of paraostomal hernias: early results, *J Am Coll Surg* 194:232, 2002.
Novitsky YW, Porter JR, Rucho ZC, and others: Open preperitoneal retrofascial mesh repair for multiply recurrent ventral incisional hernias, *J Am Coll Surg* 203:283, 2006.
Ramshaw B, Esartia P, Schwab J, and others: Comparison of laparoscopic and open ventral herniorrhaphy, *Am Surg* 65:827, 1999.
Read R: Metabolic factors contributing to herniation: a review, *Hernia* 2:51, 1998.
Steinwald PM, Mathes SJ: Management of the complex abdominal wall wound, *Adv Surg* 35:77, 2001.
Stoppa RE: The treatment of complicated groin and incisional hernias, *World J Surg* 13:545, 1989.
Sugarbaker P: Peritoneal approach to prosthetic mesh repair of paraostomy hernias, *Ann Surg* 201:344, 1985.
Velasco M, Garcia-Urena MA, Hidalgo M, and others: Current concepts on adult umbilical hernia, *Hernia* 3:233, 1999.

SPIGELIAN, LUMBAR, AND OBTURATOR HERNIATION

Thomas Rauth, MD, MPH, Michael Holzman, MD, MPH, and John Tarpley, MD

INTRODUCTION

"You see what you look for and you diagnose what you know." Every surgeon has heard this aphorism, or a variant of it, at some point during his or her training. It speaks to familiarity with clinical encounters and the knowledge of physical examination findings. Although applicable to routine physical diagnosis, it is most relevant when discussing rare clinical conditions. Appropriately it prefaces a review of the less common abdominal wall defects: the Spigelian, lumbar, and obturator hernias.

Few surgeons have significant clinical experience with these hernias, and some may go their entire careers without ever managing one. Although their sequelae can be life threatening, the prevalence of these hernias is low. Thus they are often overlooked during physical examination and not considered in the differential diagnosis for bowel obstruction or generalized peritonitis. However, the rarity with which they present does not obviate the need for their review; rather, it is the reason for it.

SPIGELIAN HERNIA

Spigelian hernia is the congenital or acquired protrusion of a peritoneal sac, organ, or properitoneal fat through the Spigelian

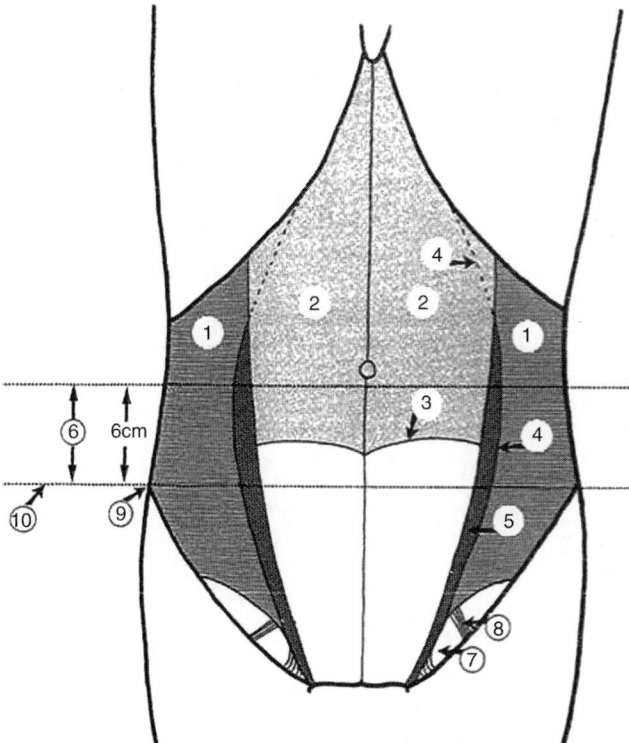

Figure 1 Diagrammatic representation of posterior view of the anterior abdominal wall. External oblique, internal oblique, and rectus abdominis muscles have been cut away. *1,* Transversus abdominis muscle; *2,* dorsal lamella of the rectus sheath; *3,* semicircular line (of Douglas); *4,* semilunar line (of Spigel); *5,* Spigelian aponeurosis; *6,* Spigelian hernia belt; *7,* Hesselbach's triangle; *8,* inferior epigastric vessels; *9,* anterior superior iliac spine; *10,* interspinal plane. *From Skandalakis PN, Zoras O, Skandalakis JE, and others: Am Surg 27:42, 2006. Used with permission.*

aponeuroses (Figs. 1, 2 and 3). Although it is the most common of the spontaneous lateral ventral hernias, it is found in only 1% to 2% of the population with hernia defects. Described by Josef T. Klinkosh in 1764, the Spigelian aponeuroses and its hernia defect are named after the anatomist who first described the semilunar line, Adriaan van der Spieghel (Flemish anatomist 1578–1625).

The Spigelian aponeurosis is the aponeurotic portion of the transverse abdominal muscle found between the semilunar line laterally and the lateral edge of the rectus muscle medially. The semilunar lines are two curved lines that mark the transition of the transversus abdominis from muscle to aponeurosis. The lines course from the costal margin of the ninth rib superiorly to the pubic spine inferiorly. Although herniation through the Spigelian aponeurosis can occur at all levels of the abdominal wall, it occurs most commonly below the level of the umbilicus. This region, termed the *Spigelian hernia belt,* is a 6-cm transverse band with the inferior border marked by a line connecting the anterior superior iliac spines. The Spigelian aponeurosis is widest in this region and weakest at the intersection of the arcuate and semilunar lines. Recall that the arcuate line, also known as the arcuate fold, semicircular line, or line of Douglas, marks the inferior border of the posterior rectus sheath. Above the arcuate line, the internal oblique aponeurosis splits to ensheath the rectus muscle. Here the anterior division of the rectus sheath is reinforced by the aponeurosis of the external oblique, whereas the posterior sheath is reinforced by the aponeuroses of the transversus abdominus and transversalis fascia. Below the arcuate line, the aponeuroses of the transversus abdominus and internal oblique condense to pass

anterior to the rectus muscle with the external oblique. In this region, the posterior belly of the rectus abdominus is bordered only by the transversalis fascia. It is the absence of the posterior rectus sheath that contributes to the relative weakness of the Spigelian aponeurosis below the arcuate line, and attenuation of its tendinous insertions into the rectus sheath leads to the fascial defect and herniation. Hernia defects found inferior and medial to the inferior epigastric vessels are more likely to be direct inguinal hernias through Hesselbach's triangle than the less commonly encountered "low Spigelian hernia."

Spigelian hernias most commonly present between the fourth and seventh decades of life but have been described in the pediatric population. Many of these patients have had previous abdominal operations or have chronic conditions leading to elevated intra-abdominal pressure (obesity, pulmonary disease, prostatic hypertrophy, multiple pregnancies). The presenting complaint is classically of abdominal pain and a palpable abdominal wall mass. As with other hernias, the physical examination is facilitated with the patient standing. Other times, the hernia may not violate the aponeurosis of the external oblique, making it difficult to appreciate in all but the leanest individuals. If Spigelian hernia is not included in the differential diagnosis of a patient who presents with bowel obstruction, diagnosis is frequently made at the time of abdominal exploration. The fascial defect is often small (1–2 cm in diameter) with a fibrous edge, making incarceration comparatively frequent. The hernia sac consists of attenuated transversalis fascia overlying properitoneal fat and the peritoneal sac. Although it may contain small bowel or omentum, large bowel, ovaries, testes, Meckel's diverticula, and the bladder have been reported within these hernias. Both ultrasound and computed tomography (CT) are useful in making the diagnosis of Spigelian hernia. Ultrasound evaluation has the advantages of being portable and able to generate real-time images with the patient upright to increase the rate of detection. In the patient with bowel obstruction and an unrevealing or equivocal physical examination, contrasted CT may reveal the diagnosis of Spigelian hernia. However, CT imaging may miss the hernia if it reduces spontaneously with the patient supine, or it may fail to detect a small fascial defect with simple axial imaging.

Repair of Spigelian hernias has traditionally been performed through an open approach. Herniorrhaphy should be performed in a tension-free manner either by direct aponeurotic approximation or by applying a prosthetic patch. A transverse incision is made over the abdominal wall mass or fascial defect identified on imaging studies. Dissection is carried through the aponeurosis of the external oblique until the hernia sac is identified. The attachments of properitoneal fat and attenuated transversalis fascia are dissected free from the fibrous edge of the defect in the Spigelian aponeurosis. If possible, the intact peritoneal sac should be reduced into the abdomen. If the peritoneal sac is redundant, violated, or cannot easily be mobilized from the fascial edges, it should be excised, and the hernia contents inspected and placed back into the abdominal cavity. When the hernia is incarcerated, extending the aponeurotic defect medially with electrosurgery or sharp dissection may facilitate reduction. In the setting of strangulation and visceral compromise, resection and anastomosis can be performed through the same incision after the defect is widened medially toward the rectus. Primary repair is performed by reapproximating the aponeurotic defect of the transversus abdominus and internal oblique using nonabsorbable interrupted sutures. The external oblique aponeurosis may be closed in a similar fashion, thus overlapping and buttressing the repair beneath. If herniorrhaphy cannot be performed in a tension-free manner, a prosthetic patch may be used. We favor an expanded polytetrafluoroethylene (ePTFE) composite mesh or other nonadhesive, nonabsorbable products (coated polyester) for intraperitoneal herniorrhaphy when the prosthesis is exposed to bowel. Polypropylene

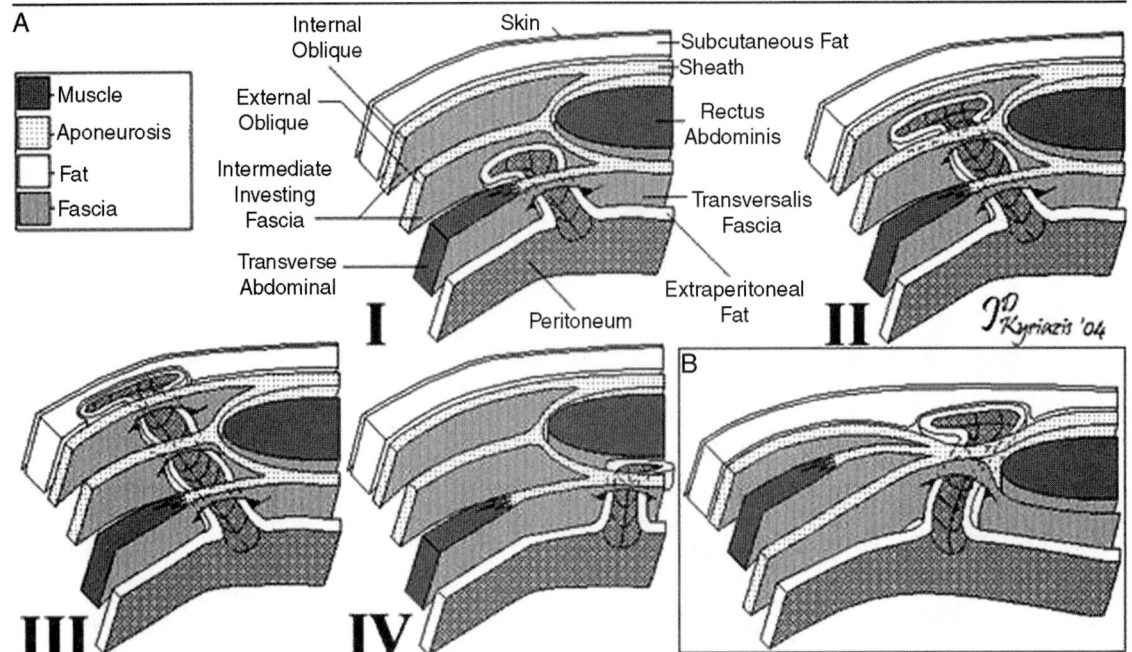

Figure 2 Three-dimensional schematic presentation of cross section of the abdominal wall in vicinity of the left border of the sheath of the rectus abdominis muscle, posterior view. Spigelian hernia sac is shown at various surgical levels: **(A)** above the semicircular line (of Douglas). *(I)* Superficial to the aponeurosis of the transverse abdominal muscle; *(II)* superficial to the aponeurosis of the internal oblique; *(III)* superficial to the aponeurosis of the internal oblique muscle; *(IV)* penetrating the posterior lamina of the rectus sheath. **(B)** Below the semicircular line (of Douglas). *From Skandalakis PN, Zoras O, Skandalakis JE, and others: Am Surg 27:42, 2006. Used with permission.*

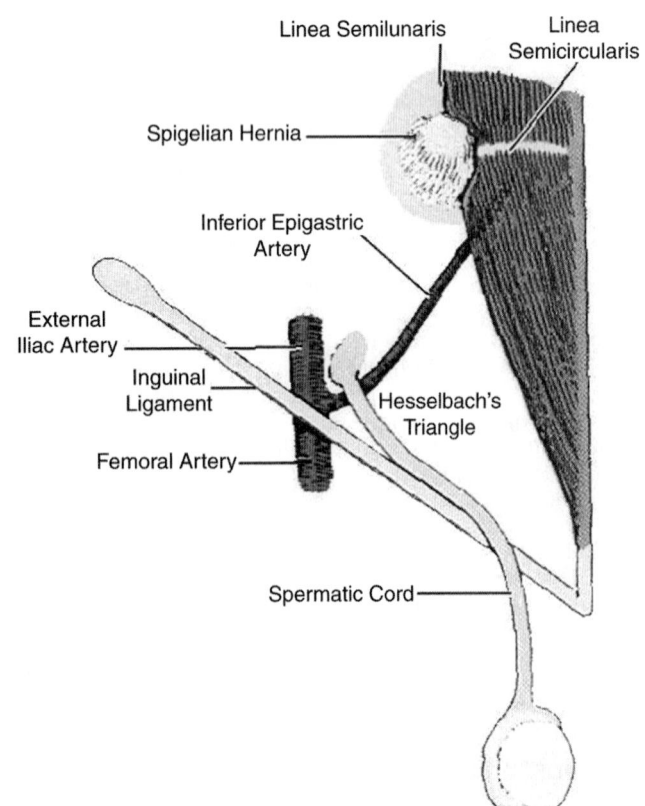

Figure 3 Schematic representation of relations of a Spigelian hernia to inguinal structures. *From Skandalakis PN, Zoras O, Skandalakis JE, and others: Am Surg 27:42, 2006. Used with permission.*

plugs and onlays may be used if the peritoneum is not violated. The use of a nonabsorbable prosthesis is contraindicated in the setting of a contaminated wound, and primary repair is indicated. For large hernia defects in a contaminated field, temporary or absorbable materials or even autogenous fascia lata may be used to provide a tension-free repair.

The laparoscopic approach to Spigelian herniorrhaphy is well described. For the surgeon skilled in advanced laparoscopy, the minimally invasive approach allows for the complete exploration of the peritoneal cavity when the diagnosis of hernia is uncertain at the time of operation, as well as for clear identification of the aponeurotic defect. We prefer the intraperitoneal approach over the properitoneal approach for laparoscopic repair of Spigelian hernias. Abdominal access is obtained through an umbilical port. Two additional working ports are placed under direct visualization such that the operative field is triangulated by these ports. As with open repair, an ePTFE mesh or composite product is the preferred prosthesis for intraperitoneal repair. Adhesiolysis is performed, and the contents of the hernia sac are carefully reduced. To account for contraction of the prosthesis, the mesh is sized so that there is at least a 4-cm overlap around the edge of the defect. Transabdominal suture fixation of the mesh is performed radially around the defect, and an intra-abdominal tacker is used to secure the edges of the mesh to prevent bowel incarceration. If strangulated bowel is encountered laparoscopically, resection can be performed extraperitoneally through a small midline incision or intraperitoneally for surgeons comfortable with laparoscopic resection and anastomosis. Herniorrhaphy can then be performed through a noncontaminated open approach or laparoscopically using one of the absorbable, bioprosthetic products or other temporary material, autogenous fascia lata, direct suture, or even leaving the hernia repair for another day. The reported recurrence rate for both open and laparoscopic repairs of Spigelian hernias is low.

LUMBAR HERNIA

Hernias of the posterior abdominal wall or lumbar hernias occur infrequently, with approximately 300 cases reported in the literature. Approximately 20% of lumbar hernias are considered congenital, occurring in infants and children with musculoskeletal defects of the posterior abdominal wall. The remaining 80% are termed *acquired* and may be classified as primary or secondary. Primary lumbar hernias comprise the majority and occur spontaneously as a result of chronically elevated intra-abdominal pressures, excessive weight loss, and age. Secondary lumbar hernias make up approximately 25% of all lumbar hernias and are the result of prior trauma, surgical intervention, or infection.

The area of the posterior abdominal wall defined by the twelfth rib superiorly, iliac crest inferiorly, erector spinae muscles medially, and external oblique muscle laterally is known as the *lumbar region*. Although several areas within this region are prone to weakness, the two most frequently cited are the superior lumbar triangle of Grynfeltt-Lesshaft and the inferior lumbar triangle of Petit (Fig. 4). The superior triangle is larger and more constant in shape than the inferior one. Its boundaries consist of the twelfth rib superiorly, the lateral edge of the quadratus lumborum medially, and the posterior free edge of the internal oblique muscle laterally. The latissimus dorsi makes up the roof of the triangle. Herniation occurs most commonly through the upper portion of the triangle at the inferior edge of the twelfth rib where the intercostal neurovascular bundle pierces the abdominal wall. The inferior triangle is smaller and less constant in shape and size. The iliac crest forms the base of the triangle. The medial border arises from the lateral free edge of latissimus dorsi and lateral border of the triangle from the posterior margin of the external oblique.

The natural history of these hernias is one of increasing size and symptomatology. They carry a 25% risk of incarceration and 8%

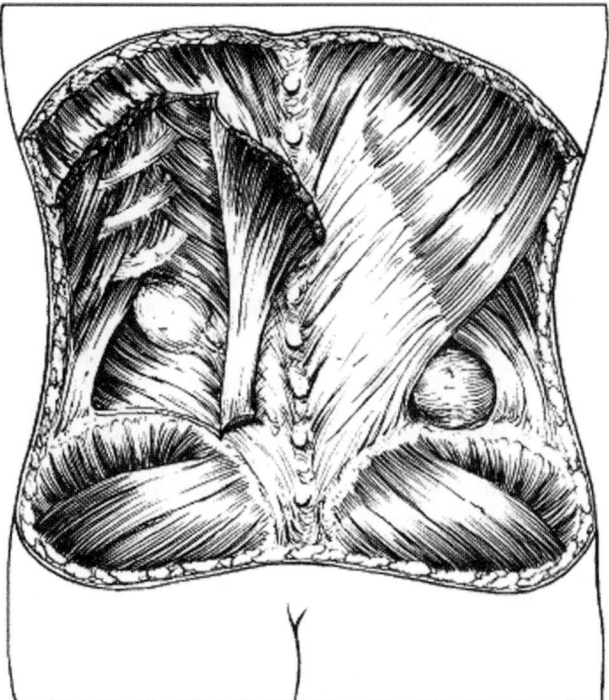

Figure 4 Anatomic relationships of lumbar or dorsal hernia. (Adapted from Netter.) On the left, lumbar or dorsal hernia into space of Grynfelt. On the right, hernia into Petit's triangle (inferior lumbar space). *From Doherty GM, Way LW: Current surgical diagnosis and treatment, ed 12, Norwalk, CT, 2006, Appleton and Lange, p. 776. Used with permission.*

risk of strangulation. Because lumbar hernias enlarge over time and become progressively more symptomatic and disfiguring, it is recommended that repair be performed at the time of diagnosis if the patient can tolerate general anesthesia. The typical presentation is a unilateral bulge in the flank first noted by the patient. Patients may describe a feeling of fullness in the region with radiation to the lower back and thigh. Many times an incision from a previous renal or adrenal operation is present in the area of concern. The hernia is more easily appreciated with the patient standing; coughing may generate an impulse over the flank.

The location of the hernia defect, absence of defining signs and symptoms, and the rarity with which it presents make the diagnosis of lumbar hernia difficult at times. Lumbar hernias may be confused with soft-tissue tumors and lipomas, panniculitis, hematoma, or abscess. In fact, most masses of the posterior abdominal wall do not prove to be lumbar hernias. Radiographic imaging can be helpful in both making the diagnosis and planning repair. A contrasted CT scan of the abdomen and pelvis helps to delineate the extent of the muscular defect, the contents of the hernia sac, and its relation to the structures of the abdomen and retroperitoneum.

Traditionally the repair of lumbar hernias has been performed through open techniques. Numerous methods for herniorrhaphy have been reported, including primary repair, open mesh repair, and the use of tissue transfer with aponeurotic flaps. With the patient in a semilateral or lateral position, the thigh is extended at the hip, the table is flexed, and the kidney rest elevated to increase the space between the twelfth rib and iliac crest to expose the lumbar region maximally. An oblique incision is made over the defect beginning posterosuperiorly and ending anteroinferiorly. After the hernia sac is identified, it should be carefully dissected from the surrounding tissues to reveal the borders of the musculofascial defect. Redundant hernia sac should be ligated and excised. A complete extraperitoneal repair can be performed, but the nature of the hernia, previous operations and the difficulty in securing the fascial edges of the defect usually make violating the peritoneal cavity unavoidable. Entering the sac reveals small and large bowel, the appendix, omentum, spleen, stomach, and ovaries. The mesocolon may be misidentified as properitoneal adipose tissue, and injury to the colonic blood supply can ensue.

With exploration and dissection complete, the bed is flattened and the kidney rest retracted to take the imposed tension out of the repair. Small defects may be repaired primarily using interrupted nonabsorbable sutures. For hernias of the superior triangle, the transversalis fascia may be approximated to the transversus abdominus muscle, lumbocostal ligament, and the periosteum of the twelfth rib for the first layer. Approximating the lateral free edge of the internal oblique to the quadratus lumborum or serratus posteroinferior buttresses the repair as a second layer. For hernias of the inferior triangle, the transversalis fascia may similarly be approximated to the transversus abdominus muscle as the deep layer. The second layer is fashioned by approximating the free edge of the external oblique to the fascia of the latissimus dorsi muscle.

For lumbar hernias that cannot be repaired primarily, the use of a mesh prosthesis or adjacent tissue transfer is required to achieve a satisfactory tension-free repair. Polypropylene, polyester, and ePTFE mesh products may be used in the intraperitoneal and properitoneal position as inlays or, more rarely, they may serve to reinforce a primary repair as an onlay. When placed against bowel, we favor either ePTFE or a composite product to limit the risk of significant adhesions. The mesh is sized so that there is at least a 4-cm overlap between mesh and fascial edge of the defect to accommodate contraction of the mesh and enlargement of the hernia. In the setting of a contaminated field, the use of autogenous tissue is indicated, providing reinforcement to the repair without the risk of a foreign body. Aponeurotic flaps from the gluteus maximus muscle may be used to reinforce or minimize tension in larger repairs of the inferior triangle, and free fascia lata grafts may facilitate the repair of moderate-sized defects in the superior triangle.

Both small intestinal submucosa and human acellular dermis are alternatives to autogenous tissue in the contaminated field and have been used with reported success in small case reports in the repair of hernias of the posterior abdominal wall.

It is becoming increasingly evident that the traditional open repair of lumbar hernias has several limitations. Limited fascial strength and opposing lines of tension in the muscle surrounding the defect make secure primary repair difficult. The implantation of mesh is a more desirable approach; however, it requires a large incision, and adequate visualization of the entire defect is often compromised. Using techniques borrowed from laparoscopic ventral hernia repair, the laparoscopic approach to lumbar herniorrhaphy facilitates visualization of the abdominal wall defect and allows for a secure, tension-free repair without the morbidity or postoperative pain of a large, open incision. Reports document shorter hospitalizations and fewer analgesic requirements with the laparoscopic approach. With the patient in the semilateral position, pneumoperitoneum is established through an umbilical port. Two additional working ports may be placed in the midline above and below the umbilicus. The hernia is gently reduced using blunt dissection, minimizing the use of electrocautery. With the fascial defect visualized, the mesh is sized to allow for at least 4 cm of overlap. We again favor ePTFE or a composite product for intraperitoneal herniorrhaphy. Transabdominal fixation of the mesh with nonabsorbable suture is achieved using a laparoscopic suture passed through 2-mm stab incisions. For hernias of the superior triangle, the suture is passed around the twelfth rib to anchor the mesh superiorly, taking care to avoid the pleural space. For hernias of the inferior triangle, the mesh may be anchored to the iliac crest. A 3-mm drill bit is used to create holes in the iliac crest 1 cm from the edge through which the suture may be passed and secured. A laparoscopic tacker helps to obliterate spaces left between sutures at the edge of the mesh. Transabdominal fixation sutures can lead to nerve entrapment. Severe pinpoint pain at a suture site in the postoperative period may require removal of the suture.

OBTURATOR HERNIA

Herniation through the obturator canal, the most common of the pelvic floor hernias, occurs infrequently, accounting for less than 0.1% of all hernias (Fig. 5). The obturator foramen is located in the anterolateral pelvis and is formed by the rami of the ischium and pubic bones. The largest foramen in the body, it is nearly completely obliterated by the obturator membrane, a fibrous, four-layer musculoaponeurotic sheath. The obturator canal is situated in the most cephalad portion of the foramen, with the superolateral wall of the canal being the pubic ramus. The canal is approximately 0.2 to 0.5 cm wide and courses obliquely from the pelvis for 2 to 3 cm, wherein reside the obturator nerve, artery, vein, and fat pad. The obturator nerve is the superior-most structure within the neurovascular bundle. On entering the thigh, the nerve divides into the anterior and posterior divisions, supplying sensory innervation to the upper thigh and motor innervation to the adductor group, obturator externus, gracilis, and pectineus. The obturator artery is a branch of the hypogastric artery, although variant vasculature is frequently encountered, with the artery originating from the external iliac or inferior epigastric arteries. Anomalous arterial and venous connections between the obturator and external iliac systems, collectively known as the *corona mortis,* are a potential source of life-threatening hemorrhage and must be considered at the time of operation.

Obturator hernias occur in thin, elderly women in their seventh or eighth decades six times more frequently than in any other age or gender category. It is believed that the wider female pelvis and relatively larger obturator foramen predispose this group to herniation. Ninety percent of cases present as bowel obstruction, and most will have not had previous abdominal or pelvic operations.

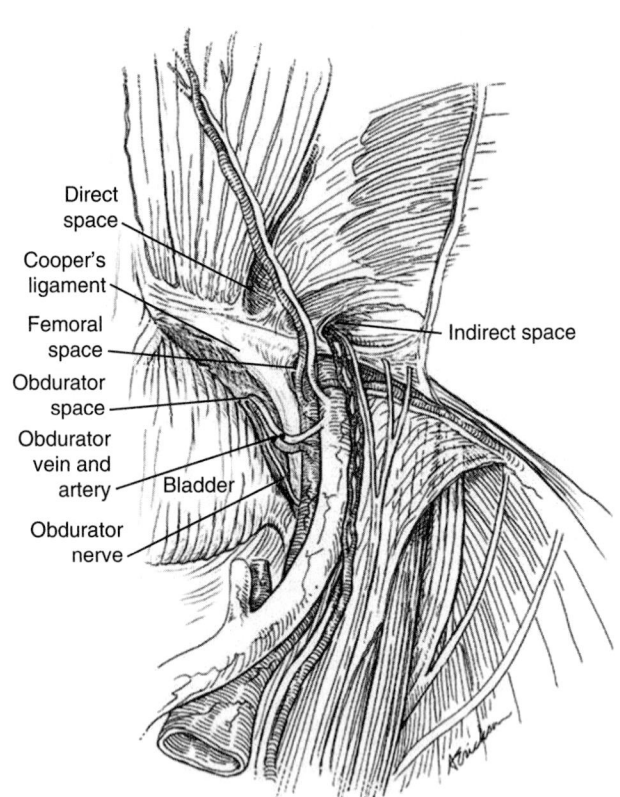

Figure 5 Anatomy of the preperitoneal space. *From Shapiro K, Patel S, Choy C, and others: Surg Endosc 18;954, 2004. Used with permission.*

Approximately 40% of patients present with the referred pain of the Howship-Romberg sign caused by compression of the anterior division of the obturator nerve against the pubic ramus by the hernia sac. It is characterized by hip and medial thigh pain that is exacerbated by extension and external rotation of the thigh. Physical examination rarely reveals the cause of generalized peritonitis or obstruction in patients with obturator hernia. A faint bruise may appear in the femoral triangle, evidence of the extravasation of bloodstained fluid from strangulated bowel. Sepsis of the thigh is rare. A careful vaginal examination may reveal a tender mass in the region of the obturator foramen, but rectal examination is often unremarkable. If the clinical situation permits, radiographic imaging, such as contrasted CT or ultrasonography, may reliably diagnose obturator hernia. CT is considered truly specific for the preoperative diagnosis of obturator hernia and can provide additional information regarding the level and degree of obstruction. Alternatively, ultrasound provides real-time imaging that can accurately assess bowel wall thickness, as well as peristalsis. The image quality of ultrasound is not dependent on intravenous contrast, a potential benefit when selecting the imaging modality for a frail, dehydrated, elderly woman with significant comorbidities. However, the diagnosis is usually made at the time of laparotomy for complete bowel obstruction.

The patient with an obturator hernia is treated operatively. Because the diagnosis is rarely made prior to exploration, the hernia is usually discovered after finding a loop of incarcerated ileum in the pelvis at the time of urgent laparotomy. Steep Trendelenburg facilitates the visualization of the obturator foramen. The incarcerated bowel may be reduced manually. If it cannot be reduced or if there is concern that any additional manipulation may cause further injury or contamination, the obturator membrane may be incised posteromedially over a clamp (parallel to the neurovascular bundle) to facilitate reduction. Bowel resection is performed as indicated and is required 50% of the time. The contralateral pelvic sidewall must be routinely explored to rule out underlying hernia of the opposite obturator canal. Similarly the femoral canal, Hesselbach's triangle, and the internal ring are inspected to rule out synchronous hernias.

If the patient remains hemodynamically stable following reduction of the hernia, herniorrhaphy may be performed. The sac is emptied and its contents inspected. The sac is then inverted or ligated and divided. The ligated stump may be fashioned to the obturator membrane to create a plug. The repair can be buttressed using peritoneum, an autogenous fascial flap, omentum, or a pedicle of uterine ligament. If gross contamination is present, primary tissue apposition will usually suffice. If this provides insufficient coverage of the defect, one of the acellular tissue matrices may be used to reinforce the repair. Alternatively, polypropylene or ePTFE mesh onlays may be used to cover the foramen in the absence of peritoneal sepsis and gross contamination. The mesh is fashioned to the anterior abdominal wall at Cooper's ligament, taking care to avoid compression of the obturator nerve. If polypropylene mesh is used, it must be placed in the properitoneal space or covered with peritoneum to prevent contact with bowel. It is postulated that the recurrence rate for hernias repaired with simple tissue apposition is less than 10%. However, because of the advanced age and comorbidities of the patient population with obturator hernia, the long-term recurrence rate is not known.

For the rare patient in whom an obturator hernia is diagnosed preoperatively in a hemodynamically normal patient without evidence of intestinal strangulation, several strategies exist for the properitoneal approach. The thigh, inguinal, and midline approaches all provide access to the properitoneal space for the open repair of an obturator hernia. However, visualization of the neurovascular structures is limited with these techniques. Alternatively, the laparoscopic properitoneal approach can provide excellent, bilateral visualization of the obturator canal and associated neurovascular structures, as well as the femoral canal, Hesselbach's triangle, and internal inguinal ring. With the bladder retracted medially, the properitoneal fat can be swept off of Cooper's ligament, and the obturator vessels can be seen coursing toward the foramen. Gentle retraction reduces the hernia. In this setting, a large piece of polypropylene mesh can be placed in the properitoneal space to obliterate the obturator foramen and cover the femoral canal, Hesselbach's triangle, and internal inguinal ring.

SUGGESTED READINGS

Arca MJ, Heniford BT, Pokorny R, and others: Laparoscopic repair of lumbar hernias, *J Am Coll Surg* 187:147, 1998.

Losanoff JE, Richman BW, Jones JW: Obturator hernia, *J Am Coll Surg* 194:657, 2002.

Fitzgibbons RJ Jr, Gerson AG, editors: *Nyhus and Condon's hernia*, ed 5, Philadelphia, 2002, Lippincott, Williams and Wilkins.

Skandalakis LJ, Androulakis J, Colborn GL, and others: Obturator hernia. Embryology, anatomy, and surgical applications, *Surg Clin North Am* 80:71, 2000.

Skandalakis PN, Zoras O, Skandalakis JE, and others: Spigelian hernia: surgical anatomy, embryology, and technique of repair, *Am Surg* 72:42, 2006.

ENDOCRINE GLANDS

ADRENOCORTICAL TUMORS

James A. Lee, MD, and Electron Kebebew, MD

INTRODUCTION

The adrenal glands are paired retroperitoneal organs located superior to the kidneys and lateral to the diaphragmatic crura. They are divided into a medullary portion that secretes catecholamines and a cortical portion that secretes steroid hormones. The cortex makes up 80% of the adrenal's volume and is further divided into the zona glomerulosa (which produces aldosterone) and the zona fasciculata and zona reticularis (which produce glucocorticoids and sex hormones). There are two main categories of tumors of the adrenal cortex that require surgical intervention: hyperfunctioning tumors (aldosteronomas, Cushing's syndrome, virilizing/feminizing syndrome) and nonfunctioning tumors that may be malignant (adrenocortical cancer and metastatic disease) (Fig. 1). The need for and approach to adrenalectomy are determined by a thorough history and physical examination, biochemical testing, and imaging studies to localize the adrenal tumor.

Since the mid 1990s, laparoscopic adrenalectomy has emerged as the best approach for treating most adrenal tumors. Several studies have demonstrated that patients have less pain, shorter recovery times, and fewer complications after laparoscopic adrenalectomy than after open adrenalectomy procedures. Adrenocortical cancer is a relative contraindication to laparoscopic adrenalectomy. However, as surgeons have gained experience with laparoscopic techniques, many have used laparoscopic adrenalectomy for localized adrenocortical cancer and metastasis and for large tumors suspicious for malignancy, and the short-term results have been similar to those for open adrenalectomy.

ALDOSTERONOMA

Primary hyperaldosteronism accounts for approximately 1% of all cases of hypertension and is typically refractory to medical therapy. The classic Conn's syndrome is characterized by hypertension, hypokalemia, and polyuria (Fig. 2). Patients may also present with muscle weakness, polydipsia, headaches, and fatigue. In addition to low potassium levels, electrolyte abnormalities may include hypernatremia and a hypochloremic metabolic alkalosis. The diagnosis is confirmed by a concomitant elevated plasma aldosterone concentration (PAC), low plasma renin activity (PRA), and a PAC:PRA ratio greater than 25 to 30. PRA is suppressed by feedback inhibition from excess aldosterone. If necessary, the diagnosis may be confirmed by the aldosterone suppression test, which demonstrates elevated urinary aldosterone levels (>12 µg per day) during saline infusion.

Excess aldosterone secretion is caused by a unilateral adrenocortical adenoma (aldosteronoma) in two thirds of patients and by bilateral hyperplasia (idiopathic hyperaldosteronism) in approximately one third. Only 1% of cases are caused by a unilateral hyperplasia. Five percent of cases are caused by angiotensin-II responsive adenomas, and less than 1% are caused by familial hyperaldosteronism type I (glucocorticoid-remediable hyperaldosteronism) and familial hyperaldosteronism type II. Rarely an adrenocortical carcinoma may secrete aldosterone along with other hormones. It is crucial to differentiate between an aldosteronoma and bilateral hyperplasia because the treatments differ radically. In comparison with patients with bilateral hyperplasia, patients with an aldosteronoma are often younger and have more severe hypertension, more profound hypokalemia (<3.0 mEq/L), and higher urinary and plasma aldosterone (>25 mg/dl) levels. ^{131}I-6 beta-iodomethyl-19-norcholesterol (NP-59) scans and postural stimulation tests are seldom necessary because of the increasing sensitivity of computed tomography (CT) scanning. CT scanning of the abdomen with thin cuts (3-5 mm) through the adrenal glands is the best way to distinguish aldosteronoma from bilateral hyperplasia. Most clinically significant aldosteronomas are hypodense, measure 0.5 to 2.0 cm, and are readily seen on CT scans. However, small tumors (<0.5 cm) and micronodular hyperplasia may be mistaken for bilateral hyperplasia. When a unilateral adrenal lesion is seen on CT scan, the diagnosis of aldosteronoma is confirmed.

If there is adrenal hypertrophy, bilateral nodules, or no lesions, selective venous catheterization for aldosterone sampling is warranted to lateralize the hyperfunctioning adrenal gland.

In selective venous catheterization, blood samples for cortisol and aldosterone are obtained from both adrenal veins and at various points along the inferior vena cava, either with or without adrenocorticotrophin hormone (ACTH) stimulation. The objectives of the procedure are to cannulate successfully both adrenal veins and to lateralize the tumor. Failure to cannulate the right adrenal vein is a common problem because it is typically a short branch that drains directly into the inferior vena cava. An adrenal vein-to-inferior vena cava cortisol ratio of at least 3:1 indicates that the adrenal vein has been successfully cannulated. Less than a 3:1 ratio indicates a failure to cannulate and therefore a failed procedure. Lateralization of an aldosteronoma or unilateral adrenal hyperplasia is confirmed if the adrenal vein aldosterone to cortisol ratio is at least five times higher on one side. If the ratios from one side to the other are similar, bilateral hyperplasia should be suspected and medical management with spironolactone started. Bilateral adrenalectomy is not indicated for bilateral hyperplasia.

The best treatment approach for an aldosteronoma or unilateral adrenal hyperplasia is laparoscopic adrenalectomy. Before surgery, patients usually begin taking spironolactone, a competitive inhibitor of aldosterone, to control hypertension and normalize their

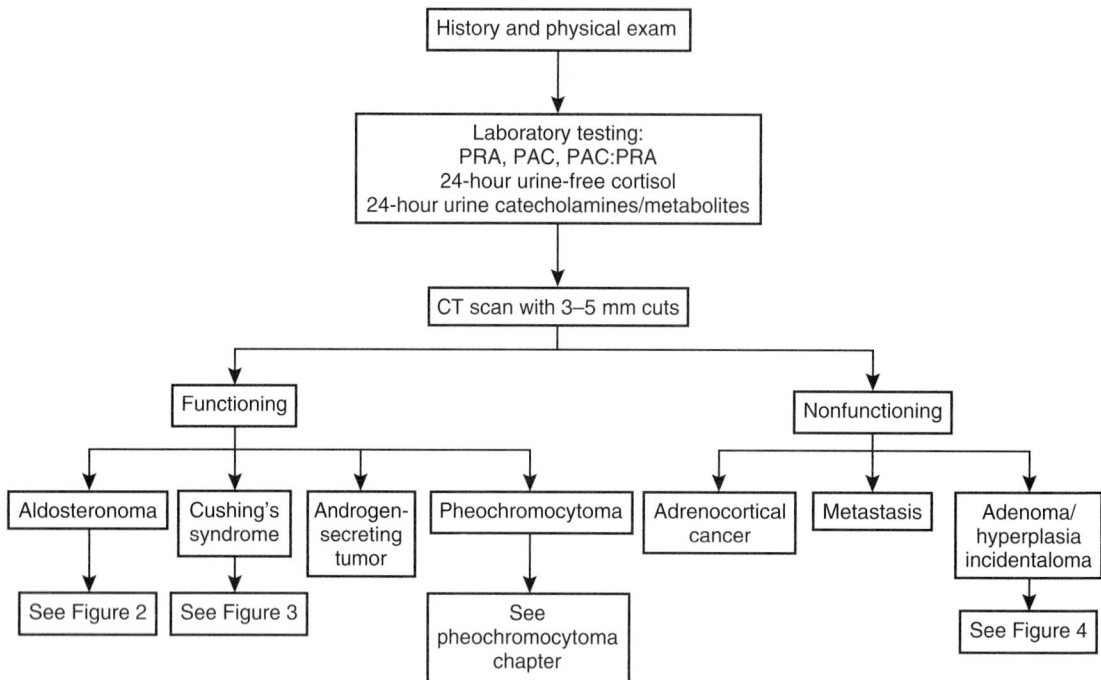

Figure 1 Overview of adrenal tumors.

potassium levels. Other antihypertensives and potassium supplements are added as needed. Adrenalectomy corrects hypokalemia almost immediately in more than 95% of patients. More than 75% of patients will have improvement, if not resolution, of hypertension within 1 month of their operation. Two thirds of responders will be off all antihypertensives, and one third will require fewer medications than they required preoperatively. Spironolactone treatment and potassium supplementation should be discontinued immediately after the operation. Recurrence is rare because almost all aldosteronomas are benign.

ADRENAL CUSHING'S SYNDROME

Cushing's syndrome is caused by glucocorticoid excess and is characterized by central obesity (90%), hypertension (85%), moon facies, easy bruisability, skin changes (purple striae, hirsutism, acne, plethora), weakness, depression, polyuria, and glucose intolerance or diabetes mellitus. Exogenous steroid use is the most common cause of Cushing's syndrome. The etiology of endogenous glucocorticoid hypersecretion can be divided into ACTH-dependent (secondary adrenal) and ACTH-independent (primary adrenal) causes. ACTH-dependent tumors overproduce ACTH, thereby stimulating excess glucocorticoid secretion from the adrenal cortex and resulting in bilateral adrenal hyperplasia. They comprise 80% of cases and are caused by pituitary adenomas/hyperplasia (also known as *Cushing's disease*) and ectopic ACTH-secreting tumors (small cell lung cancer, bronchial carcinoid tumors, thymomas, and pancreatic islet cell tumors). In contrast, ACTH-independent tumors (referred to as *adrenal Cushing's syndrome*) hypersecrete glucocorticoids directly and are caused by adrenocortical adenomas, adrenocortical carcinomas, or macronodular or micronodular hyperplasia.

The diagnostic workup for Cushing's syndrome involves first confirming the diagnosis and then differentiating between ACTH-dependent and independent tumors. The common finding in all patients with glucocorticoid hypersecretion is the loss of normal hypothalamic regulation of cortisol secretion. One of the first signs is the loss of diurnal variation of cortisol levels. An elevated

24-hour urinary-free cortisol is the most sensitive and specific test (95% and 98%, respectively) for making the diagnosis of Cushing's syndrome (Fig. 3). Irrespective of tumor type, all patients with Cushing's syndrome are unable to suppress cortisol levels after overnight low-dose dexamethasone suppression testing. In cases in which there is a high index of suspicion but a negative or equivocal 24-hour urinary-free cortisol test, a formal low-dose dexamethasone suppression test can be performed to exclude Cushing's syndrome.

After the diagnosis is confirmed, further biochemical testing determines the type of tumor involved. First, plasma ACTH levels differentiate between ACTH-dependent and ACTH-independent tumors. Low ACTH levels (<5 pg/ml) signify an ACTH-independent tumor because excess glucocorticoid suppresses pituitary release of ACTH. In contrast, an elevated ACTH level (>15 pg/ml) indicates lack of feedback inhibition and therefore an autonomous ACTH-producing tumor. A high-dose dexamethasone suppression test can further distinguish between a pituitary and ectopic cause. The ACTH level is suppressed by pituitary tumors but not by ectopic ACTH-producing tumors. Furthermore, an ACTH level greater than 500 pg/ml is typically associated with an ectopic ACTH-producing tumor. The corticotropin-releasing hormone (CRH) stimulation test can distinguish pituitary pathology from adrenal and ectopic ACTH tumor. When stimulated with CRH, pituitary lesions increase ACTH secretion by at least 35% above baseline, whereas the others do not.

After the diagnosis is made, CT, magnetic resonance imaging (MRI), or both are used for localizing the tumor and therapeutic planning. MRI with gadolinium contrast and thin cuts through the sellar region can verify the presence of a pituitary adenoma or hyperplasia in patients with suspected Cushing's disease. Pituitary tumors are either resected transsphenoidally or irradiated if the patient is a poor surgical candidate. For recurrent or persistent Cushing's disease, bilateral adrenalectomy can be curative. The search for ectopic ACTH-producing tumors begins with a CT of the chest and may proceed to an abdominal CT with thin cuts through the pancreas. In cases of adrenal Cushing's syndrome, an abdominal CT with thin cuts through the adrenal bed determines whether a unilateral adenoma or bilateral hyperplasia is present.

Figure 2 Aldosteronoma.

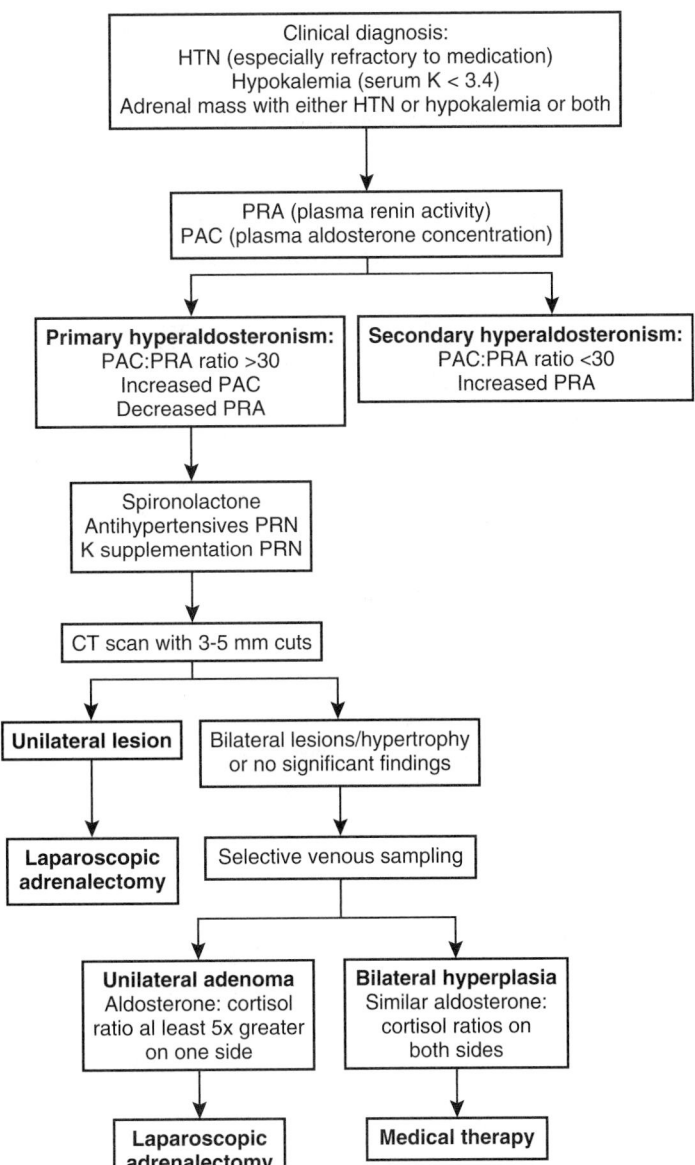

Clinical diagnosis:
HTN (especially refractory to medication)
Hypokalemia (serum K < 3.4)
Adrenal mass with either HTN or hypokalemia or both

↓

PRA (plasma renin activity)
PAC (plasma aldosterone concentration)

Primary hyperaldosteronism:
PAC:PRA ratio >30
Increased PAC
Decreased PRA

Secondary hyperaldosteronism:
PAC:PRA ratio <30
Increased PRA

Spironolactone
Antihypertensives PRN
K supplementation PRN

CT scan with 3-5 mm cuts

Unilateral lesion   Bilateral lesions/hypertrophy
or no significant findings

Laparoscopic adrenalectomy   Selective venous sampling

Unilateral adenoma
Aldosterone: cortisol
ratio al least 5x greater
on one side

Bilateral hyperplasia
Similar aldosterone:
cortisol ratios on
both sides

Laparoscopic adrenalectomy   **Medical therapy**

Patients with Cushing's syndrome should be given perioperative stress-dose steroids consisting of hydrocortisone 100 mg intravenously every 6 to 8 hours. The steroids are then tapered to an oral regimen in the postoperative period. Typically the contralateral adrenal gland is suppressed and may remain so for weeks to months after the operation. In addition, one dose of preoperative antibiotics should be given because patients with Cushing's syndrome are more prone to infections. Adrenal Cushing's syndrome is typically caused by unilateral adenomas, which are usually small and perfectly suited to laparoscopic adrenalectomy. However, adrenocortical cancers may also secrete cortisol. Known or suspected adrenocortical cancers should be removed using an open adrenalectomy approach to ensure complete resection. However, several groups have reported similar success rates with laparoscopic en bloc resections for localized adrenocortical cancers. Although rare, bilateral nodular hyperplasia can cause Cushing's syndrome. Patients with bilateral nodular hyperplasia should have bilateral laparoscopic adrenalectomy. These patients require lifetime glucocorticoid and mineralocorticoid (Florinef [Bristol-Myers Squibb, New York, NY] 0.1 mg/day) replacement.

VIRILIZING AND FEMINIZING TUMORS

Adrenal tumors secreting sex hormones are usually symptomatic but are rare. Because of their rarity, routine biochemical testing for sex steroid levels in patients with an adrenal incidentaloma should be considered only if there is clinical evidence of virilization or feminization. Unfortunately, more than 80% of these adrenocortical tumors are malignant. Almost all feminizing tumors and up to one half of virilizing tumors are adrenocortical cancers.

Women with hirsutism, irregular menses, and other virilizing signs may have a hypersecreting adrenal tumor, congenital adrenal hyperplasia, or cystic ovarian disease. Elevated levels of serum testosterone, serum dihydroepiandrostenedione, and 24-hour urine 7-hydroxysteroids and 17-ketosteroids establish the diagnosis of a virilizing tumor. The dexamethasone suppression test can differentiate between adrenal and ovarian causes. Serum androgens and 24-hour ketosteroids will be suppressed if produced by ovarian tumors but not when produced by adrenal tumors. Men with gynecomastia, impotence, loss of libido, or testicular atrophy may have a hypersecreting adrenal tumor or testicular tumor. Elevated

Overnight low-dose dexamethasone suppression test

May be used to confirm the diagnosis or in cases where the 24-hour urine-free cortisol level is equivocal but the diagnosis is strongly suspected from clinical parameters
1) Dexamethasone 1 mg PO at 11 PM
2) Check plasma cortisol at 8 AM
3) If cortisol is not suppressed below 5 mcg/dl, the patient has Cushing's syndrome

Overnight high dose dexamethasone suppression test

1) Check baseline plasma and 24 hour urine free cortisol
2) Dexamethasone 8 mg PO at 12 AM
3) Check AM plasma and 24 hour urine free cortisol
4) If plasma cortisol < 5 ng/dl and UFC decreases by 50%, then the patient has Cushing's syndrome (i.e., pituitary cause); otherwise, the patient has an adrenal or ectopic cause

Corticotropin-releasing hormone stimulation test

May be used to differentiate between pituitary and adrenal/ectopic Cushing's
1) CRH IV given
2) Check serum ACTH and cortisol Q 15 minutes
3) If serum ACTH increases > 35% above baseline, the patient has Cushing's syndrome (i.e., pituitary cause); otherwise, the patient has an adrenal or ectopic cause

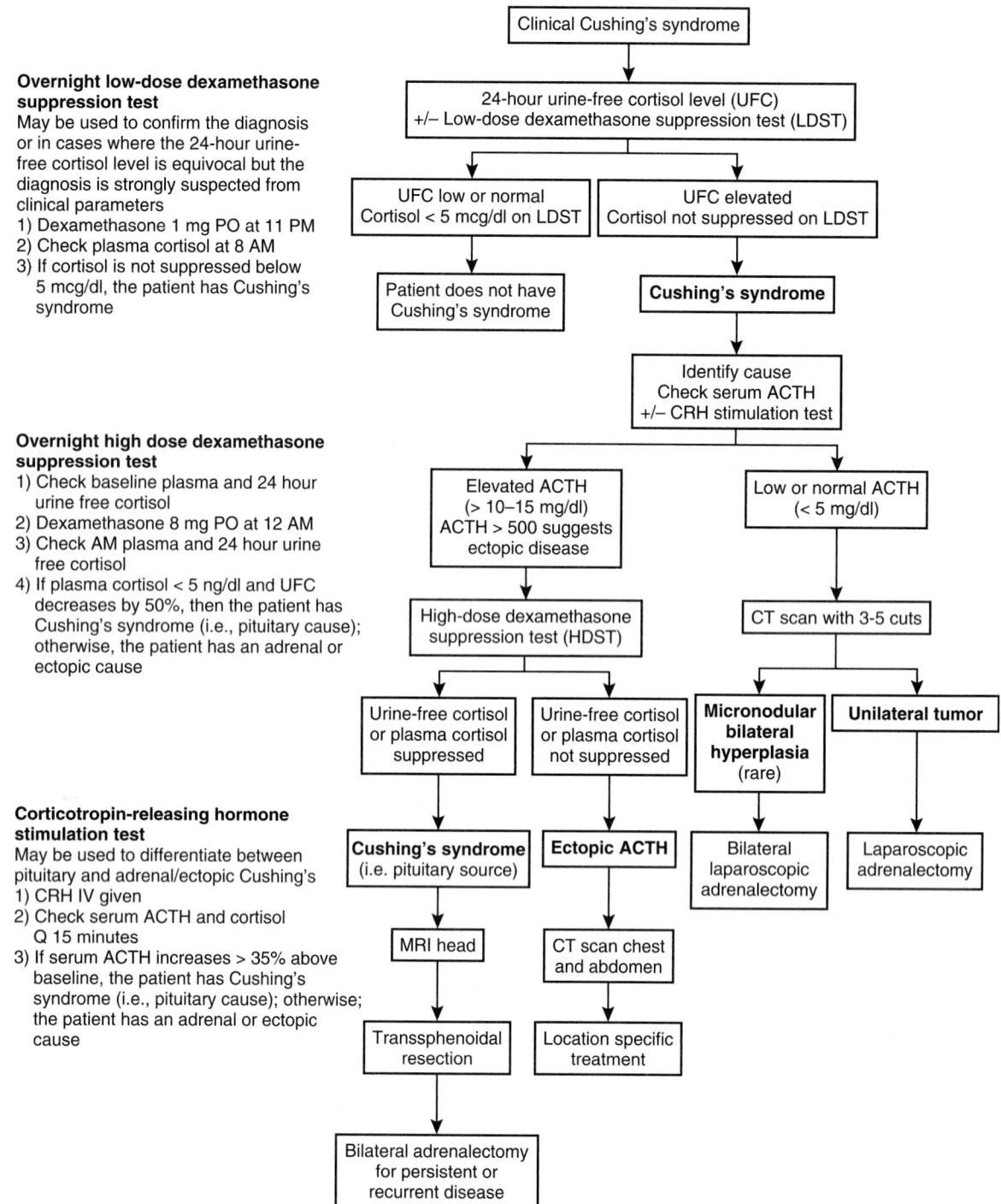

Figure 3 Cushing's syndrome.

serum estrogen and suppressed follicle stimulating hormone, luteinizing hormone, and gonadotropins confirm the diagnosis of a feminizing tumor.

A CT scan of the abdomen with thin cuts through the adrenal gland generally identifies the presence of an adrenal tumor. For small tumors with no malignant features on CT scan, a laparoscopic approach may be attempted as long as the surgeon has a low threshold for converting to a hand-assisted or open approach if features of a malignant tumor are found during the operation or if a complete resection with negative margins cannot be performed.

ADRENOCORTICAL CANCER

Adrenocortical cancer accounts for 1% of adrenal tumors and is a rare cancer, with an incidence of 1 person per million in the United States each year. The median age at diagnosis is 40 to 50 years, and there is a 1:1 female-to-male ratio. Sixty percent to 80% of adrenocortical cancers are functioning, with 30% secreting cortisol, 20% androgens, 10% estrogen, 35% mixed hormones, and 1% aldosterone. The remaining tumors are nonfunctioning and are usually diagnosed as a large symptomatic mass, although 1% to 5% present as incidentalomas. Typically adrenocortical cancers are large, and the diagnosis should be suspected in any adrenocortical mass greater than 6 cm. Although potentially curable with complete surgical resection, only two fifths of patients have disease confined to the adrenal gland at the time of diagnosis. One fifth of patients have regional disease, and two fifths have metastatic disease at diagnosis.

The surgeon should have a high index of suspicion for cancer when dealing with a functioning tumor secreting multiple hormones such as androgens or estrogen because they are more likely to be malignant. On CT scan, adrenocortical cancers tend to be heterogeneous with irregular borders and areas of hemorrhage or tumor necrosis. Several studies have demonstrated that a tumor having Hounsfield units greater than 20 is more likely to be malignant. Less than 5% of most adrenocortical cancers are 6 cm or less in size, and many investigators have reported an average tumor size of 12 to 16 cm. CT scans should also be carefully reviewed for signs of invasion into adjacent structures and organs, as well as for regional lymphadenopathy, metastases, and inferior vena cava thrombus. The most common sites for metastatic disease include the liver, lung, peritoneum, and bones. On MRI, gadolinium washes out of adenomas rapidly but persists in malignant tumors. MRI is also useful to confirm the extent of disease, as well to assess for invasion into the vasculature. Invasion into the inferior vena cava and the presence of tumor thrombus are considered regional disease, and resection with or without venovenous bypass is warranted.

Many studies show that complete en bloc resection of adrenocortical cancer and involved structures, including the periadrenal fat, is the only chance for cure. Most surgeons recommend open adrenalectomy as the safest operation for patients with suspected adrenocortical cancer. With complete resection, the 5-year survival for stage I and II tumors is 40% to 60% (Table 1). For stage III disease (any size but with local invasion into adjacent organs), the 5-year survival rate is 20% to 30%, even with complete resection. Only 10% of patients with stage IV disease (distant metastases, local organ invasion, or invasion up to local organs with positive nodes) survive beyond 1 year. Often palliation is the only reason to operate on patients with stage IV disease, especially if the tumor is functioning or the patient has local significant symptoms from the tumor. The risk of recurrence increases with stage of disease, with up to 85% of patients developing local recurrence or metastatic disease. Of recurrences, 68% occur locally and in lymph nodes. Of distant metastases, 71% occur in the lung, 42% in the liver, and 26% in the bone.

Table 1: TNM Staging for Adrenocortical Carcinoma

TNM	
T1	Tumor <5 cm, no invasion
T2	Tumor ≥5 cm, no invasion
T3	Any size with invasion up to, involving, adjacent organs
T4	Any size, invading adjacent organs
N0	No positive regional nodes
N1	Positive regional nodes
M0	No metastases
M1	Metastases
Stage	
I	T1 N0 M0
II	T2 N0 M0
III	T1 N1 M0, T2 N1 M0, T3 N0 M0
IV	TX NX M1, T3 N1, T4

T, Primary tumor; *N,* regional lymph nodes; *M,* distant metastasis.

Mitotane is the most common adjuvant therapy used in patients with residual, recurrent, or metastatic disease. A pesticide analogue, mitotane is a direct adrenolytic agent. Several series report disheartening low remission rates of 20% to 35%. However, mitotane is effective in palliating symptoms of functioning tumors, with 80% of patients demonstrating a decrease in cortisol hypersecretion. As with patients who undergo bilateral adrenalectomy, patients treated with mitotane must receive glucocorticoid and mineralocorticoid replacement. Several groups are studying mitotane combined with etoposide and cisplatin in prospective trials.

ADRENAL METASTASES

An adrenal mass should be suspected of being a metastasis in a patient with a history of cancer. In up to 30% to 75% of such cases, the mass is metastatic. Lung cancer (especially small cell), renal cell carcinoma, melanoma, gastrointestinal cancer, breast cancer, lymphoma, and hepatocellular carcinoma are the most common metastases to the adrenal gland. Discovering multiple synchronous metastases is more common than finding a single adrenal metastasis. Patients with multiple lesions have a poor prognosis and do not benefit from adrenal metastasectomy.

Patients with a solitary adrenal mass and symptoms suggestive of malignancy should have screening colonoscopy, mammography, and a chest x-ray to identify the primary tumor. Bilateral lesions, large tumors, irregular borders, local invasion, hemorrhage, and tumor necrosis are suggestive of malignant disease. Positron emission tomography scanning may be helpful to differentiate between metabolically active malignant disease and benign pathology and to identify other metastatic foci. To confirm the diagnosis, fine needle aspiration may be performed but only after a pheochromocytoma has been definitively ruled out. Inadvertent biopsy of a pheochromocytoma is potentially lethal.

Patients with solitary synchronous or metachronous adrenal metastases may benefit from adrenalectomy. Outcomes are particularly favorable when there has been a long disease-free interval between initial resection of the primary tumor and discovery of the adrenal metastasis. The same principles for resection of adrenocortical cancers (described earlier in this chapter) apply, and a complete en bloc resection must be performed. Fortunately, isolated adrenal metastases are often smaller and encapsulated within the adrenal gland. Several groups have shown that laparoscopic adrenalectomy results in treatment that is equally effective as open adrenalectomy. After adrenalectomy, the 5-year survival rate is 25%, with a mean survival ranging from 20 to 30 months, in contrast to 6 to 8 months in patients who do not undergo resection.

ADRENAL INCIDENTALOMA

Because the topic of adrenal incidentaloma is covered in more detail in another chapter, only a few overarching themes are presented here. Adrenal incidentalomas are defined as adrenal tumors discovered on diagnostic imaging for nonadrenal disorders. The prevalence of adrenal incidentalomas has increased as a result of the improved sensitivity and more widespread use of imaging techniques. The prevalence of incidentalomas is approximately 4% on abdominal imaging studies and increases as the age of the study cohort increases. The main criteria for resection of incidentalomas are hormonal hypersecretion and a risk of cancer (Fig. 4). Tumor size, imaging features, and a history of extra-adrenal malignancy are used to determine the risk that an adrenal incidentaloma is a malignant tumor. Most experts agree that a tumor 6 cm or greater in size should be resected because the risk that it is an adrenocortical cancer is estimated to be 35% to 98%. For tumors measuring 4 to less than 6 cm in greatest dimension, the malignant potential is low but not insignificant. Therefore there is no clear consensus on treatment of these tumors as outlined by the National

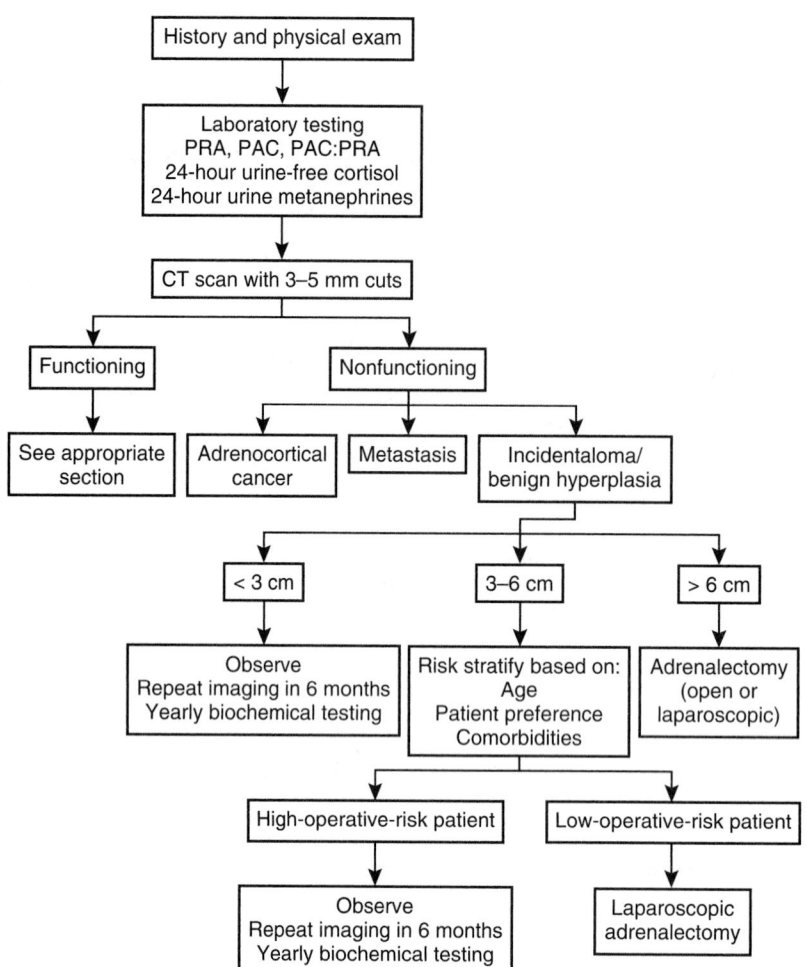

Figure 4 Incidentaloma.

Institutes of Health State of Science Conference. For such tumors, size, patient preference, age, and comorbidities should be considered when determining whether observation with follow-up imaging or adrenalectomy is indicated. Unless there is clear evidence of malignancy, these tumors may be resected laparoscopically. The surgeon can convert to an open or hand-assisted operation if malignant features are found intraoperatively, or a complete laparoscopic resection cannot be performed. Patients with tumors that are less than 4 cm in greatest dimension or of 4 to less than 6 cm and treated nonoperatively should undergo follow-up monitoring with repeat abdominal imaging every 6 months to a year and with yearly screening for cortisol and catecholamine hypersecretion for up to 5 years. Twenty-five percent of incidentalomas will grow, and 20% will hypersecrete over a 10-year follow-up period.

SURGICAL APPROACHES FOR ADRENALECTOMY

Laparoscopic adrenalectomy is the procedure of choice for most adrenocortical tumors that are localized and smaller than 6 cm. Tumors that are larger than 6 cm are more technically challenging to remove laparoscopically and are more likely to be malignant. An open adrenalectomy approach should be used for adrenocortical tumors that have extra-adrenal tumor extension or that are associated with regional lymphadenopathy (Fig. 5). An anterior (through a subcostal or midline incision), posterior, or thoracoabdominal approach may be used for an open adrenalectomy, and each has its advantages and disadvantages. An anterior approach using a

subcostal or midline incision is most commonly used but is associated with longer recovery time; higher risk of poor wound healing, especially in patients with Cushing's syndrome; and a higher risk of cardiopulmonary postoperative complications than the posterior retroperitoneal approach. The posterior retroperitoneal approach is best suited for small adrenal tumors (<6 cm) and in patients with intraperitoneal adhesions from a previous laparotomy or peritonitis. Although a thoracoabdominal approach is associated with significant morbidity, it may be necessary to perform an en bloc resection of a large, malignant, and locally invasive adrenal tumor.

Laparoscopic adrenalectomy may be performed using a lateral transabdominal, lateral, or posterior retroperitoneal approach. Patient outcome is similar among the three laparoscopic adrenalectomy approaches and better than open adrenalectomy. In some cases, it may be reasonable to perform a hand-assisted laparoscopic adrenalectomy, and these three approaches (laparoscopic, hand-assisted, and open) should be viewed as a continuum from least to most invasive approaches.

Technique of Laparoscopic Adrenalectomy (Lateral Abdominal Approach)

The lateral transabdominal laparoscopic approach for adrenalectomy is most commonly used. The patient is positioned in the lateral decubitus position so that gravity will help retract the viscera away from the field of dissection. The operating surgeon and assistant stand on the same side, facing the patient, with the assistant standing more cephalad. Depending on surgeon preference, three

Figure 5 Open adrenalectomy approaches. **(A)** Anterior approach via subcostal or midline incision. **(B)** Posterior approach through a hockey-stick incision. **(C)** A thoracoabdominal approach. *Adapted from Kebebew E, Duh Q-Y: Operative strategies of adrenalectomy. In Doherty GM, Skogsied B, editors: Surgical endocrinology, Philadelphia, 2000, Lippincott Williams & Wilkins.*

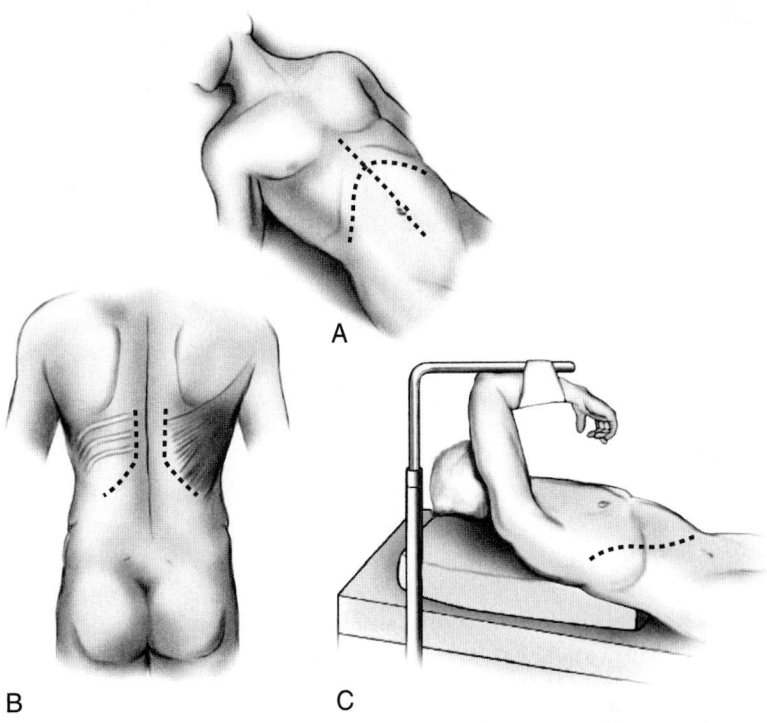

to four trocars are placed subcostally from the midclavicular to midaxillary line, approximately 2 to 3 cm apart. For a right adrenalectomy, we use four trocars. For a left adrenalectomy, we often use only three ports because the spleen is more readily retracted by gravity than the liver (Fig. 6).

The technique for laparoscopic adrenalectomy has four important steps (Table 2). The left adrenal gland lies posterior to the tail of the pancreas and spleen, whereas the right adrenal gland lies posterolateral to the inferior vena cava (Fig. 7). The first step is to expose the superior and medial borders of the adrenal

Figure 6 **(A)** Positioning for laparoscopic adrenalectomy using the lateral transabdominal approach. **(B)** Port placement for a right laparoscopic adrenalectomy. **(C)** Port placement for left laparoscopic adrenalectomy. *Used with permission from the Columbia On-line Curriculum Project.*

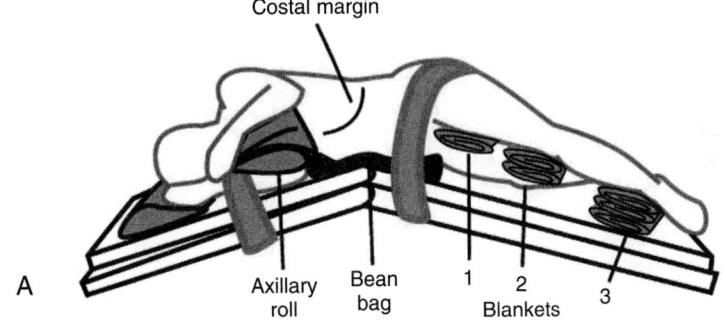

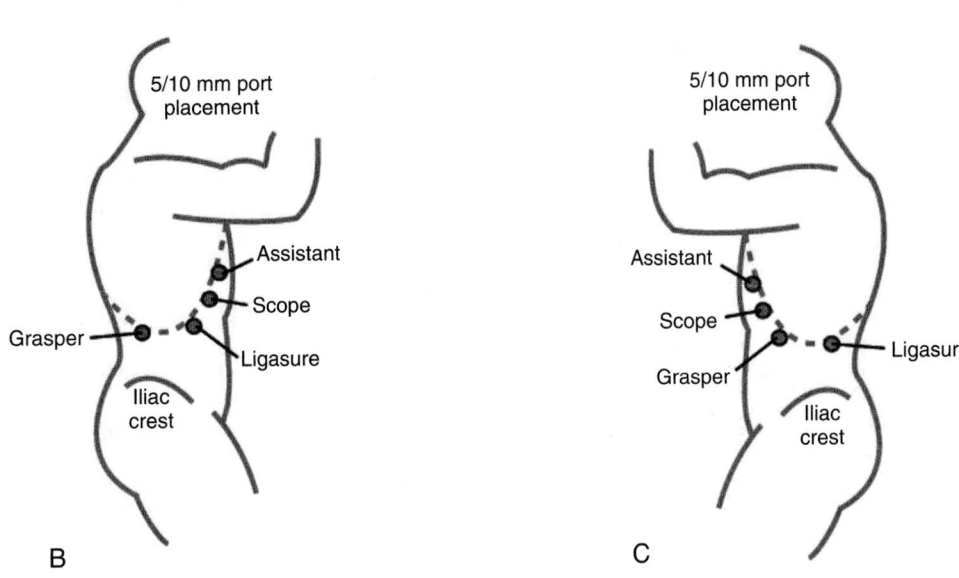

Table 2: Technique of Laparoscopic Adrenalectomy (Lateral Transabdominal Approach)

- Position: lateral decubitus
- Survey the abdomen for pathology
- Adrenalectomy technique in 4 steps
- **Step 1: Exposing the adrenal gland**
  - Incise the lateral attachments to allow medial rotation of either the spleen/pancreas or liver and dissect peritoneum free from the interface between the adrenal and either the spleen/pancreas or liver.
- **Step 2: Dissection of adrenal gland**
  - Starting with the most cephalad attachments to the diaphragm and moving toward the renal hilum, carefully dissect one layer at a time between the adrenal gland and either the spleen/pancreas or liver.
  - Retract the adrenal laterally and inferiorly as you progress.
  - Identify the adrenal vein.
- In a left adrenalectomy, the inferior phrenic vein usually joins the adrenal vein and the splenic vessels typically "point" to the adrenal vein.
- In a right adrenalectomy, the adrenal vein is short and usually comes directly off the posterior, medial surface of the IVC.
  - When cutting the vein, do NOT pass point because there is often a small artery that runs in close proximity that must be cauterized or ligated.
  - In 5%-10% of cases, there is more than one adrenal vein (accessory adrenal veins are more common on the right side).
- **Step 3: Mobilizing free the adrenal gland from the renal hilum**
  - Be careful not to ligate a superior pole vessel to the kidney because this may cause postoperative hypertension, and be sure to maintain your dissection plane right over the renal capsule.
- **Step 4: Completing the adrenalectomy**
  - Cut through the fat between the kidney and adrenal gland, hugging the kidney, using the LigaSure (Valley Lab, Boulder, CO), harmonic scalpel, or cautery.
  - Pushing the clamp on the top of the kidney will define the perfect plane,
  - Remove en block the retroperitoneal fat with the adrenal gland.

IVC, Inferior vena cava.

gland. In a right adrenalectomy, the triangular ligament of the liver is divided while the assistant provides gentle medial retraction with the fan retractor to expose the adrenal gland and inferior vena cava (Fig. 7, *A*). The dissection of the right adrenal gland is started below the liver edge to view directly the superior and medial border of the adrenal gland and continued clockwise, dividing the artery and main adrenal vein. Similarly, the first step for a left adrenalectomy is to incise the lateral attachments of the spleen so that the spleen and tail of the pancreas may be rotated medially to expose the adrenal gland (Fig. 7, *B*). Again, the dissection for the left adrenal gland begins by dividing the superior and superior-medial attachments below the diaphragm. The adrenal gland is dissected counterclockwise. This technique allows excellent visibility and clear identification of the adrenal vein and multiple adrenal arteries entering the medial portion of the gland. Freeing the superior pole in the beginning allows for inferolateral retraction of the adrenal gland.

The adrenal glands have an extensive subcapsular vascular plexus fed by multiple branches from the inferior phrenic artery (superior adrenal arteries), aorta (middle adrenal arteries), and renal artery (inferior adrenal arteries). Although the arterial supply is highly variable, the venous drainage is generally into a single adrenal vein. The right adrenal vein is short and drains directly into the posterolateral surface of the inferior vena cava. In rare cases, an aberrant right adrenal vein may drain into the right hepatic vein or renal vein. In contrast, the left adrenal vein drains into the left renal vein, typically after joining with the inferior phrenic vein. Multiple veins may be encountered in 5% to 10% of cases and are usually found draining the right adrenal gland. Although some authors advocate ligating the

adrenal vein as soon as possible, we wait until we encounter the vein in the course of the superior to medial dissection of the gland. The adrenal vein is then ligated with clips and divided. Large adrenal arteries and parasitic vessels are also clipped. The cautery, harmonic scalpel, or LigaSure (ValleyLab, Boulder, CO) are usually sufficient to divide normal caliber adrenal arteries.

The periadrenal tissue is then dissected layer by layer around the renal hilum to avoid injury to or ligation of the superior pole vessels to the kidney because this may lead to postoperative hypertension. The adrenal gland is then dissected free from the kidney and posterior abdominal wall, taking most of the apical perirenal and retroperitoneal fat with the specimen. Direct manipulation of the adrenal gland must be avoided to prevent tumor rupture because most adrenocortical tumors are easy to fracture. Instead, the periadrenal fat may be grasped with an atraumatic grasper. The adrenal specimen is placed into an impermeable specimen bag and fractured into smaller pieces with a ring forceps and extracted piecemeal.

SUMMARY

Adrenocortical tumors are a diverse family of neoplasms. The primary goals during workup are to determine whether an adrenocortical tumor is functioning and the risk of malignancy. Hypersecreting tumors and tumors suspicious for malignancy should be resected. Laparoscopic adrenalectomy is the best surgical approach except in cases of known adrenocortical cancer or when complete resection cannot be performed.

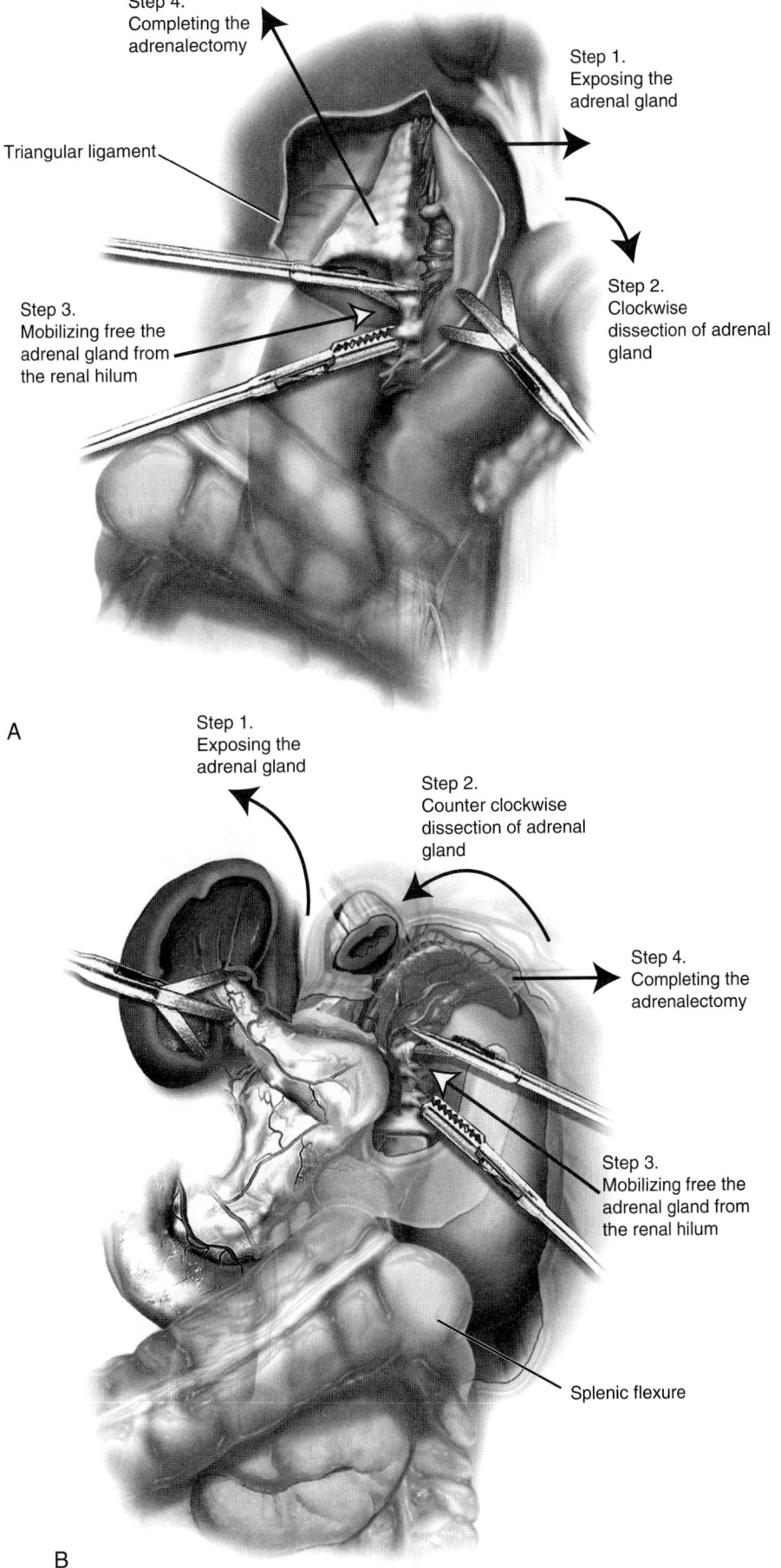

Figure 7 Technique and steps for laparoscopic adrenalectomy using a lateral transabdominal approach. **(A)** Right adrenalectomy. **(B)** Left adrenalectomy. *Adapted from Kebebew E, Duh Q-Y: Operative strategies of adrenalectomy. In Doherty GM, Skogsied B, editors: Surgical endocrinology, Philadelphia, 2000, Lippincott Williams & Wilkins.*

Suggested Readings

Al Fehaily M, Duh QY: Clinical manifestation of aldosteronoma, *Surg Clin North Am* 84:887, 2004.

Kebebew E Duh QY: Operative strategies of adrenalectomy. In: Doherty GM, Skogsied B, editors: *Surgical endocrinology.* Philadelphia, 2000, Lippincott Williams & Wilkins.

Kebebew E, Reiff E, Duh QY, and others: Extent of disease at presentation and outcome for adrenocortical carcinoma: have we made progress? *World J Surg* 30:872, 2006.

Kebebew E, Siperstein AE, Clark OH, and others: Results of laparoscopic adrenalectomy for suspected and unsuspected malignant adrenal neoplasms, *Arch Surg* 137:948, 2002.

Kebebew E, Siperstein AE, Duh QY: Laparoscopic adrenalectomy: the optimal surgical approach, *J Laparoendosc Adv Surg Tech* 11:409, 2001.

Sturgeon C, Kebebew E: Laparoscopic adrenalectomy for malignancy, *Surg Clin North Am* 84:755, 2004.

PHEOCHROMOCYTOMA

Geoffrey B. Thompson, MD, and Clive S. Grant, MD

Pheochromocytomas (and their extra-adrenal counterpart—paragangliomas) arise within chromaffin cells and sustentacular cells of the adrenal medulla and extra-adrenal paraganglia. The first successful adrenalectomies for pheochromocytoma were performed concomitantly in 1926 by Mayo in Rochester, Minnesota, and Roux in Switzerland. Pheochromocytoma has an incidence of approximately two to eight cases per million persons annually and is responsible for a curable form of hypertension in 0.1% to 1.0% of all hypertensive patients. Unfortunately, as many as 800 persons die annually in the United States from complications associated with an unsuspected pheochromocytoma. One third of sudden deaths occur during or shortly after operative procedures, delivery, or minor operations. Males and females are equally affected, and the peak age of presentation is seen in the fourth and fifth decades. Traditionally, pheochromocytoma has been referred to as the "10% tumor" with 10% being bilateral, 10% malignant, 10% extra-adrenal, 10% hereditary, and 10% arising in children.

With modern molecular analysis, as many as one fourth of the patients with apparently sporadic pheochromocytoma may be found to be carriers of mutations in the RET gene (associated with Multiple Endocrine Neoplasia type 2); the VHL gene associated with von Hippel–Lindau disease; and, rarely, neurofibromatosis type 1. Mutations of the genes coding for succinate dehydrogenase, subunit D or B, which encode mitochondrial enzymes involved in oxidative phosphorylation, have also been identified in association with familial paraganglioma syndromes and, rarely, pheochromocytomas.

Classically, pheochromocytomas secrete epinephrine, norepinephrine, or dopamine, but a cadre of other hormones have also been isolated from these tumors, including adrenocorticotropin, corticotropin releasing factor, neuron-specific enolase, interleukin 6, vasoactive intestinal peptide, neuropeptide Y, calcitonin, PTH-rP, and chromogranin A.

Malignancy appears to be more commonly associated with extra-adrenal sites and in women. The diagnosis of malignancy rests solely on the presence of invasion of locoregional structures or the presence of distant metastatic disease.

PRESENTATION AND DIAGNOSIS

The hallmark clinical presentation of pheochromocytoma is that of a hypertensive "spell." Nonfunctioning pheochromocytomas are uncommon, and when detected radiographically as an incidental finding, are often associated, albeit in retrospect, with some clinical manifestations. That having been said, approximately 10% of the benign sporadic pheochromocytomas seen at Mayo Clinic were initially classified as adrenal incidentalomas. The constellation of headache, sweating, palpitations, and paroxysmal hypertension combine to form the prototypical "spell." Sustained hypertension may be seen in approximately 50% of patients with pheochromocytoma. A number of factors may precipitate a spell, including vigorous physical exercise, defecation, ingestion of alcohol, and sexual intercourse. Spells associated with urination may indicate a paraganglioma of the urinary bladder.

In patients who are not pharmacologically blocked, severe and sometimes lethal paroxysms have occurred with invasive procedures, such as diagnostic percutaneous needle biopsies, angiography, delivery, general anesthesia, and surgical procedures. Less common symptoms include nausea, flushing, heat intolerance, anxiety, abdominal pain, and glucose intolerance. Patients often describe a feeling of "doom and gloom" and pounding headaches described as crippling. Patients can present in cardiogenic shock and multiorgan failure from an acute catecholamine-induced cardiomyopathy. A more chronic cardiomyopathy associated with pheochromocytoma, if recognized early, may be reversible with tumor excision.

DIAGNOSIS

Figure 1 provides a management algorithm for pheochromocytoma. When suspected, patients should undergo biochemical testing for 24-hour urinary excretion of total metanephrines and fractionated catecholamines. This combination, when normal, essentially rules out a pheochromocytoma. Less than 1% of sporadic pheochromocytomas and paragangliomas are missed by these screening tests. The measurement of plasma metanephrines and normetanephrines has high sensitivity and specificity for detecting pheochromocytomas but has a higher false-positive rate than that described for urinary studies. When there is a high index of suspicion, particularly in kindred members with known genetic mutations predisposing to chromaffin tumors and in children in whom 24-hour urine collection may be problematic, plasma studies become more valuable. With regard to the urinary studies, any laboratory value above the upper limit of normal for total metanephrines and any value twofold or greater above the normal for fractionated catecholamines is considered positive. A number of drugs can interfere with the measurement of urinary catecholamines and their metabolites, most notably tricyclic antidepressants.

Only pheochromocytomas and paragangliomas arising specifically in the organ of Zuckerkandl can metabolize norepinephrine to epinephrine via the PNMT enzyme. Other paragangliomas do not possess this enzyme and are unable to secrete epinephrine. This can be a valuable observation when trying to localize the site of origin. Provocative testing is obsolete and potentially dangerous and should not be used.

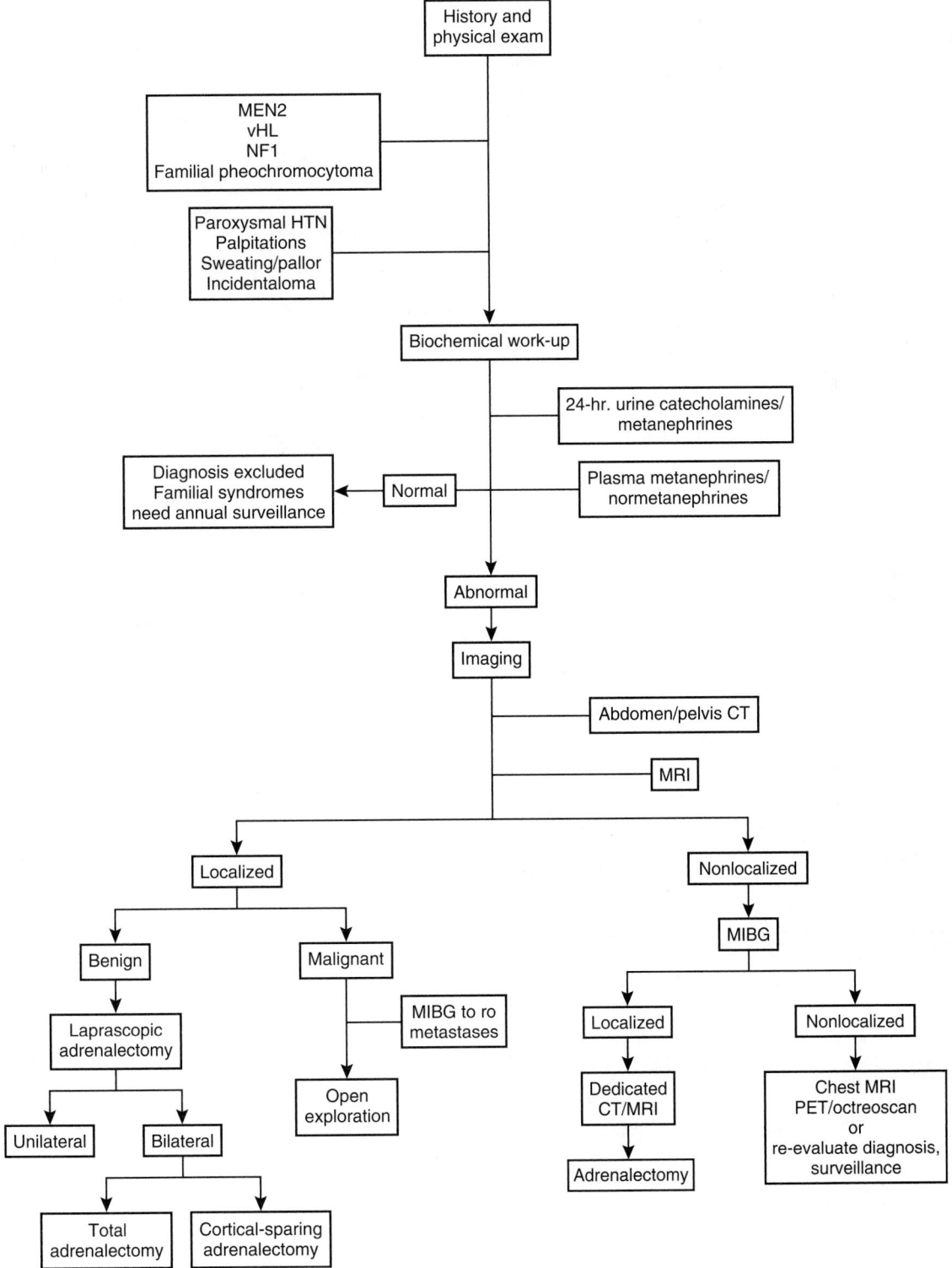

Figure 1 Management algorithm for pheochromocytoma.

■ LOCALIZATION

Computerized tomography (CT) (Fig. 2, with thin cuts through the adrenal glands) represents the best and most cost-effective imaging modality for localizing pheochromocytomas. The overall accuracy of CT scanning is greater than 90%. Although older reports cautioned against the use of intravenous contrast for fear of precipitating a hypertensive crisis, this is no longer a concern with the use of present-day contrast agents. In fact, the uptake of contrast by an adrenal mass is one of the radiographic phenotypes that raises the suspicion of a pheochromocytoma.

Magnetic resonance imaging (MRI) (Fig. 3, *A* and *B*) is also a useful imaging modality because pheochromocytomas and paragangliomas display high signal intensity on T2-weighted images and have high water density on chemical-shift MRI, thus providing both anatomic and physiologic evidence of a possible pheochromocytoma.

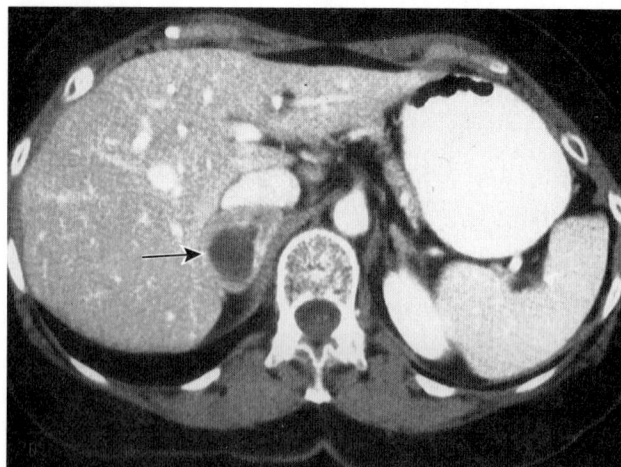

Figure 2 Computed tomography scan demonstrating right adrenal pheochromocytoma with classic cystic degeneration.

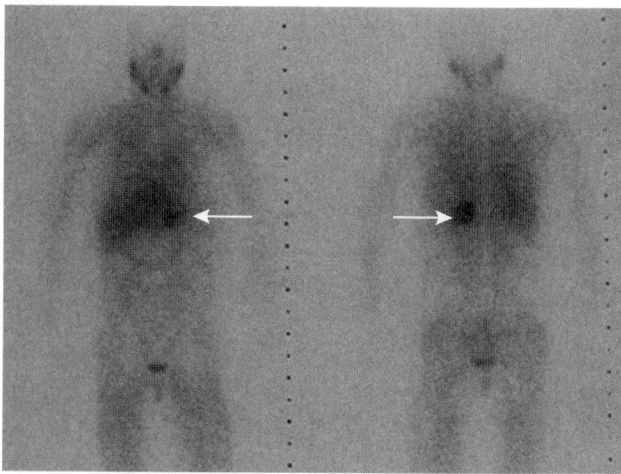

Figure 4 ^{123}I metaiodobenzylguanidine scan demonstrating a left-sided pheochromocytoma.

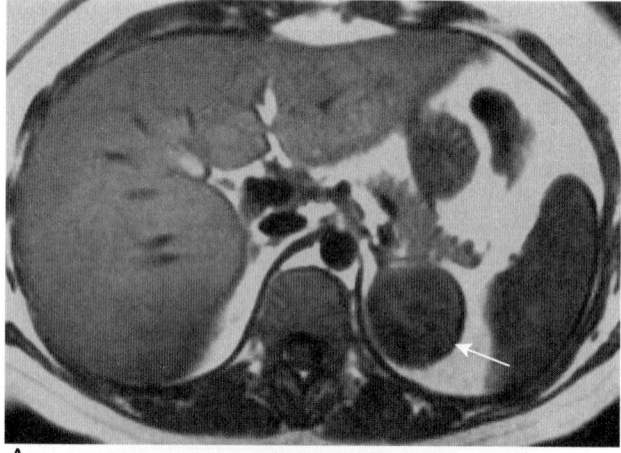

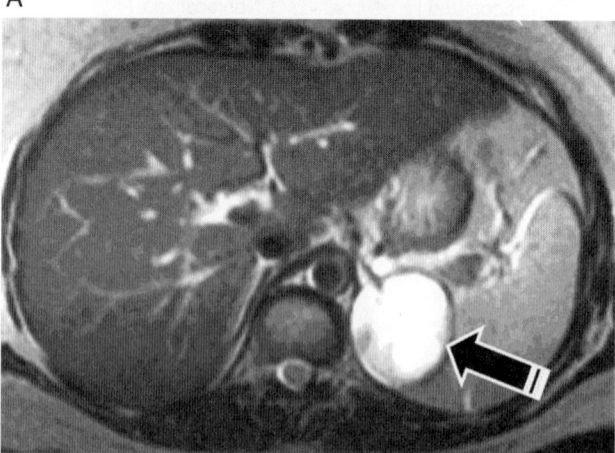

Figure 3 **(A)** Left-sided pheochromocytoma on T1-weighted magnetic resonance imaging (MRI) scan. **(B)** T2-weighted MRI demonstrating high signal intensity characteristic of a pheochromocytoma.

This is the imaging modality of choice in pregnant women, thus avoiding fetal exposure to ionizing radiation. It is also helpful in the presence of large tumors, both intra-adrenal and extra-adrenal, for identifying possible vascular invasion or tumor thrombus formation. It may also be better at detecting multiple tumors in patients with familial paraganglioma syndrome, in which tumors may arise anywhere from the base of the skull to the bladder.

Metaiodobenzylguanidine (MIBG) (Fig. 4) is an agent that is concentrated in adrenergic vesicles. Nuclear scintigraphy using either I^{123} MIBG or ^{131} MIBG has a reported sensitivity of 80% to 90%. It has been used at some centers as a primary imaging modality but is used more often to rule out synchronous lesions or metastatic disease. I^{123} MIBG has been reported to have higher sensitivity and specificity than I^{131} MIBG and also permits the addition of single photon emission computed tomography (SPECT) for improved localization. The isotopes are not readily available, and the protocol for its use is cumbersome, limiting its clinical utility. Somatostatin receptor scintigraphy (octreotide scanning) has also been shown to identify some chromaffin tumors. Positron emission tomography (PET) scanning can visualize some pheochromocytomas and paragangliomas not identified by MIBG scanning. A number of different PET isotopes are under investigation.

PERIOPERATIVE MANAGEMENT

After the biochemical diagnosis has been made, alpha-adrenergic blockade should begin immediately. We have had the most success using phenoxybenzamine, typically beginning at a dose of 20 to 30 mg daily in divided doses and working up to increasingly higher doses until the desired end point is reached. Orthostatic hypotension and nasal stuffiness are the desired end points. Patients are instructed to consume highly salted foods. Patients are encouraged to increase their fluid intake so as to expand their intravascular volume in response to the pharmacologic vasodilation. Over a period of 7 to 14 days, this renders the patient normotensive and euvolemic, thus minimizing the risks of wide blood pressure swings intraoperatively and profound hypotension after tumor removal. We generally add a beta-blocker 2 to 3 days before surgery if tachyarrhythmias are present. Beta-blockers should never be instituted before adequate alpha blockade because of the risk of unopposed alpha stimulation leading to possible severe hypertension, pulmonary edema, and congestive heart failure. A number of other pharmacologic agents have been used with variable degrees of success, including selective alpha-1-adrenergic blocking agents such as prazosin, doxazosin, or terazosin. Other agents include angiotensin-converting enzyme inhibitors and calcium channel blockers. For patients with severe clinical manifestations, especially with a history of cardiogenic shock, myocardial infarction, or recent stroke, we favor the use of Demser (Merck, Whitehouse Station, NJ), which is highly effective at depleting catecholamine stores. Others have also recommended the combined alpha-blocker and beta-blocker labetalol; however, less flexibility exists with the use of this fixed combination.

INTRAOPERATIVE MANAGEMENT

Appropriate pharmacologic agents must be available at the time of induction. As a minimum, a large-bore peripheral intravenous catheter, a radial arterial line, and a urinary catheter should be in place. In patients who have had a severe preoperative course or in whom underlying cardiac pathology is a concern, central venous access is obtained. Rarely is a Swan-Ganz catheter necessary. Sodium nitroprusside is a valuable pharmacologic agent used intraoperatively for rapid control of acute hypertension and can provide second-by-second blood pressure control. Other anesthesiologists prefer intermittent small doses of esmolol instead. Hypotension is managed with phenylephrine or ephedrine and volume expansion with crystalloid and blood as indicated. Rarely is lidocaine necessary for ventricular arrhythmias.

OPERATIVE TECHNIQUE

In the early years of adrenal surgery for pheochromocytoma, tumors were approached anteriorly through an upper midline or transverse epigastric incision. This approach provided excellent exposure so that the patient could be "dissected away" from the tumor, indicating the importance of a limited no-touch technique. This also provided the easiest access to the draining central vein, the early ligation of which was thought to be essential in terms of the intraoperative management and reduction of wide blood pressure swings. The open approach also permitted a thorough evaluation of the contralateral adrenal gland and the midline for possible associated paragangliomas in the days before the availability of advanced preoperative imaging techniques. The open anterior approach today is reserved for large pheochromocytomas (Fig. 5) and obviously malignant pheochromocytomas for which wide exposure is essential, especially if the need arises for en bloc resection of adjacent structures, vascular thrombectomy, or vascular resection and reconstruction.

Unlike other intra-abdominal operations, operations for paraganglioma or pheochromocytoma should begin with a limited exploration and an initial approach directed toward the tumor. This limits any periods of hemodynamic instability. Care should be taken to avoid excessive manipulation of the primary tumor. For tumors on the right side, the right lobe of the liver exposure is facilitated by the use of a third-arm mechanical retractor. The peritoneal attachments to the right lobe of the liver are divided, and the liver is mobilized to the patient's left, exposing the underlying vena cava and retroperitoneum. For larger tumors, the duodenum may require kocherization, along with mobilization of the hepatic flexure of the colon, but for smaller tumors, this is generally not necessary.

Dissection begins at the level of the right renal vein, along the lateral aspect of the vena cava. The vena cava is carefully dissected away from the tumor using a combination of Ligaclips (Ethicon, Somerville, NJ), and the ultrasonic dissector until the short right adrenal vein is reached more cephalad in a posterolateral position off the vena cava. This vein is isolated, doubly clipped, and divided. During this first part of the dissection, an arterial branch from the aorta may be encountered, which can either be clipped or divided using the ultrasonic dissector. After the central vein is divided, dissection is carried superiorly. Arterial branches from the phrenic artery and any additional venous branches encountered (<5% of cases) are divided. The inferior aspect of the gland is then mobilized, staying well away from the tumor capsule. The surgeon often encounters a major arterial branch coming from the renal artery, which can be divided at this point. Care must be taken to avoid injury to accessory renal arteries or polar vessels during this part of the dissection. After this last arterial branch is divided, there is usually little else tethering the tumor other than loose areolar attachments to the diaphragm, Gerota's fascia, and the kidney. After the primary tumor is out and the patient is stable, the surgeon can proceed with further inspection for lymphadenopathy, metastatic disease, and other chromaffin tumors when suspected. Drains are not used, and patients can often return to a regular hospital room, unless comorbidities or intraoperative complications warrant the need for intensive care monitoring. Bleeding and hypotension are the biggest concerns in the immediate postoperative period but are rarely problematic in a properly executed operation.

An open left adrenalectomy is performed either through the lesser sac or, preferably, via medial visceral rotation of the spleen, pancreas, and stomach, exposing the underlying adrenal and kidney. This is a particularly valuable approach for large or malignant tumors in this region. On this side, we often expose the superior aspect of the renal vein where it gives rise to the adrenal vein. The latter can be doubly clipped, proximally and distally, and divided. In addition, the inferior phrenic vein, draining into the adrenal vein, often requires division. We then mobilize the lateral aspect of the tumor away from the kidney, including some of Gerota's fascia, to be absolutely certain that capsular disruption is avoided. Working from above down and below up with the ultrasonic dissector, we sequentially take the inferior, medial, and superior arterial branches, thereby removing the tumor.

The inferior pole of the adrenal gland, on the left side, often extends down into the region of the renal hilum, and thus particular attention should be applied to avoid injury to the renal vasculature, including accessory polar vessels. Drains are not placed unless concerns arise regarding a possible pancreatic injury during its mobilization.

Regardless of the operative approach, care must be taken to avoid disruption of the tumor capsule, which can lead to tumor recurrence years later, even for benign pheochromocytomas. After this occurs, cure is often difficult, if not impossible, to achieve and may require repeated tumor debulking procedures.

Open-Flank Approach

The open-flank approach really plays no role in our modern-day operative armamentarium. Although it can provide excellent exposure for adrenalectomy, the long-term complications from flank incisions, including denervation, flank bulging, and hernia formation, negate its value over other available approaches today.

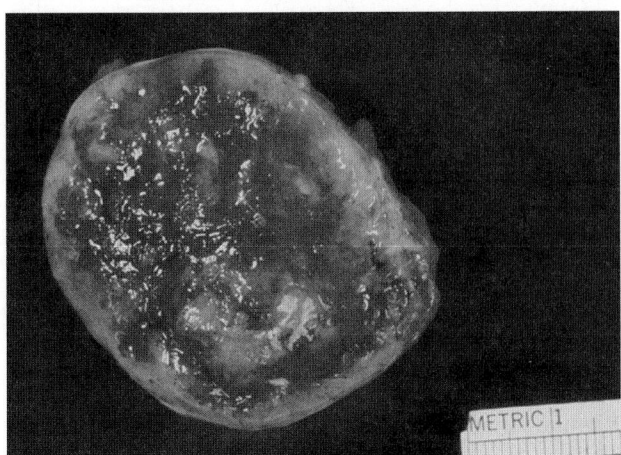

Figure 5   Large 8-cm pheochromocytoma.

Open Posterior Adrenalectomy

Because of limited exposure, concerns regarding optimal anesthetic management, and inability to explore for other possible sites of pheochromocytoma and paraganglioma, the open posterior approach was generally frowned on for many years. However, with improvements in anesthetic management and tumor localization, surgeons began to explore the possibility of removing well-localized small pheochromocytomas through a posterior approach because the open posterior adrenalectomy had shown benefits over the open anterior approach when used for other small functioning and nonfunctioning adrenal neoplasms. With excellent preoperative blockade and intraoperative anesthetic management, posterior adrenalectomies became more commonplace for pheochromocytomas because there was less associated ileus, atelectasis, pain, need for blood transfusions, and recuperative time. It was only with long-term follow-up studies that the drawbacks of open posterior adrenalectomy became apparent—namely, the muscle denervation, flank bulging, and dysesthesias that were reported in more than half of the patients undergoing open posterior adrenalectomy. The procedure still has a limited role when laparoscopic techniques are not possible because of extensive intra-abdominal adhesions, although some experts today have been able to carry out successful posterior retroperitoneoscopic adrenalectomies in these situations.

The open posterior approach is carried out with the patient placed prone on the operating table. After routine prepping and draping, a hockey-stick incision is made in the paravertebral region based on the twelfth rib. The incision is deepened down through the latissimus dorsi muscle and the posterior lamella of the lumbodorsal fascia. The sacrospinalis muscle is retracted, exposing the underlying twelfth rib, which is excised, taking care to avoid injury to the subcostal nerve. The anterior lamella of the lumbodorsal fascia is then incised, at which point Gerota's fascia becomes visible, along with the diaphragm and parietal pleura. The pleura is swept off of the diaphragm with a blunt dissector, and a small portion of the diaphragm is incised toward the spine. A mechanical retractor helps facilitate exposure. The adrenal gland is exposed and carefully mobilized and removed in a fashion similar to that described for the open approach. If the parietal pleura is breached, a small catheter is inserted into the pleural face through the opening, approximated by a purse-string suture. The air is evacuated, followed by removal of the tube and tightening of the purse-string suture. Rarely is a chest tube indicated postoperatively.

Lateral Transperitoneal Laparoscopic Adrenalectomy

This operation, popularized by Gagner in the early 1990s, has become the gold standard for most benign-appearing pheochromocytomas less than 8 cm in size. Concerns regarding increased hemodynamic instability as a result of the CO_2 insufflation have not been as much of an issue as was once thought and can be obviated by adequate preoperative preparation in most cases.

On the right side, the patient is positioned in a near-total lateral decubitus position with the right side up. After routine prepping and draping and CO_2 insufflation, four 10-mm trocars are placed along the right subcostal region, with the lateral-most port being in the midaxillary line. The operation is then performed as described in the open anterior approach, and the adrenal gland removed intact in an Endobag (Tyco Healthcare, Princeton, NJ). Care must be taken to avoid rupture of the Endobag during delivery because this may lead to a sudden catecholamine infusion via absorption through the peritoneal cavity, resulting in a hypertensive crisis.

On the left side, three or four ports are used in the lateral decubitus position; a fourth port for retraction of Gerota's fascia and the kidney in obese patients may be necessary. The adrenal gland is exposed after performing a medial visceral rotation and mobilized as in an open anterior operation.

POSTOPERATIVE MANAGEMENT

After routine laparoscopic adrenalectomy for pheochromocytoma, most patients are able to return to a regular room and resume a general diet within 12 to 24 hours. It is common for the patient's blood pressure to remain slightly below 100 systolic for the first 12 hours after surgery, until the preoperative doses of dibenzyline have been metabolized.

We hold all antihypertensive medications postoperatively unless the patient had been taking a beta-blocker chronically. Diet progression is rapid. Patients are often dismissed within 24 to 48 hours after surgery. Before dismissal, we routinely draw plasma metanephrines and normetanephrines to serve as a baseline for future reference. These may be slightly elevated shortly after surgery as a result of the stress response but can be repeated in a few weeks' time (or urinary studies performed) to confirm the success of the procedure.

All of the tumors are evaluated for DNA ploidy. Diploid tumors never behave in a malignant fashion. However, 30% of nondiploid tumors may behave so and may recur in the future. We generally recommend lifelong follow-up with yearly urinary studies because recurrences have been noted as far out as 30 years following operation.

PARAGANGLIOMAS

Paragangliomas can occur anywhere from the base of the skull to the bladder, including the inner ear. From a general surgeon's standpoint, most are intra-abdominal, either within the organ of Zuckerkandl, near the takeoff of the inferior mesenteric artery, or between the aorta and left renal vein. For most of these, vascular invasion is rare, but more than 40% of these tumors behave in a malignant fashion. Unlike pheochromocytomas that have a nice rim of cortex surrounding the actual tumor, paragangliomas oftentimes are adherent to surrounding structures. We therefore strongly recommend that all of these be removed in an open fashion to avoid tumor spillage. When they are large and invasive, concomitant resection of surrounding structures, including major vessels with vascular reconstruction, can be undertaken because this represents our best available form of therapy.

LESS COMMON SITUATIONS

Malignancy

The most common sites for metastases for pheochromocytomas and paragangliomas are bone, lung, liver, and retroperitoneal and mediastinal lymph nodes. Although there are isolated instances of prolonged survival, patients with distant metastases generally have 5-year survivals ranging from 30% to 45%. MIBG scanning can be particularly helpful in identifying sites of metastatic disease, but these are not always positive, and other tests such as PET scanning and octreotide scanning may demonstrate evidence of metastatic disease not seen by MIBG scanning or other conventional imaging. When metastases are surgically resectable, reoperation is worthwhile, but more often than not, palliation rather than cure is the rule. Bone pain can be effectively palliated with external beam radiation, and others have reported successful palliation with the use of therapeutic I^{131} MIBG. Combination chemotherapy using cyclophosphamide, vincristine, and dacarbazine has proved effective against some malignant pheochromocytomas, with response rates in the 60% to 70% range.

Resection of Pheochromocytoma in Pregnancy

Pheochromocytoma in pregnancy is extremely rare but carries with it a maternal mortality rate of 40% and a fetal death rate of more than 50%. When suspected, urinary catecholamines should be measured

because these do not fall outside the normal values during pregnancy. Because of the lack of ionizing radiation, MRI is the localization test of choice. Preoperative alpha blockade and then beta blockade are used as they are in the nonpregnant patient. What is best for the mother is best for the baby. Pheochromocytoma is a life-threatening tumor and must be treated. If the mother is beyond the 24th week, it is not unreasonable to attempt to bring the fetus to a safe gestation, using pharmacologic blockade, but this requires close monitoring. After the fetus is mature, a cesarean section is performed under a single anesthetic, followed immediately thereafter by tumor excision.

There have been case reports describing successful laparoscopic adrenalectomy during early pregnancy without morbidity or long-term consequences to the mother and fetus.

Multiple Endocrine Neoplasia Type 2 Syndrome

Pheochromocytomas occur in approximately 40% of patients with multiple endocrine neoplasia type 2 syndrome (MEN 2) syndrome. There is often antecedent adrenal medullary hyperplasia. The tumors can be multifocal and bilateral. In the past, we routinely performed bilateral adrenalectomy on these patients, but the risk of Addisonian crisis is not insignificant. In as many as half the patients, contralateral adrenalectomy has proved unnecessary, at least within the first 5 years of follow-up. With the advent of laparoscopic adrenalectomy, the trend now is to remove the affected side and observe the contralateral side until there is biochemical and radiographic evidence of disease. Some authors have proposed cortical-sparing partial adrenalectomies for MEN 2 patients, but given the presence of adrenal medullary hyperplasia, there are at least theoretical concerns regarding transecting such glands as opposed to removing them in their entirety.

OTHER ASSOCIATED CONDITIONS

Pheochromocytoma can develop in the setting of other neuroectodermal disorders, including type 1 von Recklinghausen's neurofibromatosis, von Hippel-Lindau (vHL) disease, Sturge-Weber syndrome, and tuberous sclerosis. The incidence of pheochromocytoma developing in patients with vHL varies from 10% to 20%, but some kindreds are more prone to pheochromocytomas than others. In some families, the only manifestation of vHL is isolated solitary pheochromocytomas. The tumors in vHL may be bilateral and extra-adrenal but are rarely malignant. Cortical-sparing adrenalectomies (open and laparoscopic) have been performed in selected vHL patients. Carney's syndrome includes the association of gastric epithelial leiomyosarcoma (GIST tumors), pulmonary chondromas, and extra-adrenal paragangliomas.

SUMMARY

Pheochromocytomas and their extra-adrenal counterparts may present as incidentalomas but more often than not are detected clinically by the presence of "spells." The diagnosis is confirmed with biochemical urinary testing for catecholamine excess and localized, most often, by conventional cross-sectional imaging (CT), supplemented by MRI, and nuclear scintigraphy. Preoperative pharmacologic blockade is essential for safe intraoperative and postoperative management of these patients. A number of surgical approaches are used to remove pheochromocytomas; laparoscopic adrenalectomy has become the most popular approach. It is both safe and effective when used for nonmalignant pheochromocytomas less than 8 cm in size when performed by experienced surgeons. It has the advantages of faster recuperation, shorter hospital stays, less pain, and better cosmesis. Lifelong follow-up is essential because even seemingly benign pheochromocytomas have recurred 30 years postoperatively. Other tumors may arise metachronously in previously unsuspected familial cases. Patients with familial syndromes associated with pheochromocytomas and paragangliomas are becoming increasingly recognized. Even solitary pheochromocytomas and paragangliomas may have a familial basis, more so than was once thought, based on our improved understanding of the molecular biology of these tumors.

SUGGESTED READINGS

Gagner M, Lacrois A, Bolté E: Laparoscopic adrenalectomy in Cushing's syndrome and pheochromocytoma, *N Engl J Med* 327:1033, 1992.

Grant CS: Pheochromocytoma. In: Clark OH, Duh Q-Y, Kebebew E, editors: *Textbook of endocrine surgery*, ed 2, Philadelphia, 2005, Elsevier Saunders, p. 621.

Inabnet W, Pitre J, Bernard D, Chapuis Y: Comparison of the hemodynamic parameters of open and laparoscopic adrenalectomy for pheochromocytoma, *World J Surg* 24:574, 2000.

Kudva YC, Young WF Jr, Thompson GB, and others: Adrenal incidentaloma: an important component of the clinical presentation spectrum of benign sporadic adrenal pheochromocytoma, *Endocrinologist* 9:77, 1999.

Sawka A, Jaeschke R, Singh R, and others: A comparison of biochemical tests for pheochromocytoma: measurement of fractionated plasma metanephrines compared with the combination of 24-hour urinary metanephrines and catecholamines, *J Clin Endocrinol Metab* 85:553, 2003.

Thompson GB, Grant CS, Schlinkert RT, and others: Laparoscopic versus open posterior adrenalectomy: a case-control study of 100 patients, *Surgery* 122:1132, 1997.

ADRENAL INCIDENTALOMA

L. Michael Brunt, MD, and Jeffrey F. Moley, MD

Adrenal incidentaloma is the most common adrenal lesion encountered by surgeons today because of the increased used of cross-sectional imaging in clinical practice. Incidentally discovered adrenal lesions are found in 1% to 5% of patients undergoing abdominal computed tomography (CT), most commonly for the evaluation of abdominal pain. Most adrenal incidentalomas are clinically silent and nonfunctioning and are rarely the source of the patient's pain. When faced with an adrenal incidentaloma, the surgeon should attempt to answer two questions: (1) Is the lesion hypersecreting adrenal hormones? and (2) Is it malignant or potentially malignant? If the answer is yes to either of these assessments, adrenalectomy may be indicated. Surgeons should therefore be familiar with the essential biochemical tests necessary to assess hormonal activity of an adrenal tumor and should understand the key imaging features associated with benign versus malignant lesions to select patients properly for adrenalectomy.

DIFFERENTIAL DIAGNOSIS

The differential diagnosis and frequency of various tumors presenting as adrenal incidentalomas is shown in Table 1. The most common lesions overall are nonfunctioning cortical adenomas, and the most common functioning tumors are subclinical

Table 1: Nature of Adrenal Incidentalomas Removed in 1303 Cases from Compiled Surgical Series*

Functioning Lesions	N (%)
Nonfunctioning adenoma	786 (60)
Pheochromocytoma	94 (7.2)
Subclinical Cushing's syndrome	86 (6.6)
Aldosteronoma	31 (2.4)
Nonfunctioning Lesions	
Adrenocortical cancer	112 (8.6)
Metastatic cancer	41 (3.1)
Myelolipoma	47 (3.6)
Other*	106 (8.1)

*Most commonly adrenal cysts and ganglioneuromas.
Derived from Brunt LM, Moley JF: The pituitary and adrenals. In Townsend CM, editor: Sabiston's biologic basis of modern surgical practice, ed 17, Philadelphia, 2004, WB Saunders, p. 1070.

cortisol-producing adenomas (subclinical Cushing's syndrome) and pheochromocytomas. Primary adrenal cortical cancers account for up to 9% of incidentalomas, and adrenal metastases most commonly occur in the setting of other metastatic disease. A variety of other nonfunctioning lesions, such as myeloliopmas, are detected as incidentalomas and should be considered in the differential diagnosis. Occasionally patients may have bilateral adrenal lesions detected as incidentalomas. The differential diagnosis in such cases includes bilateral pheochromocytomas, metastases, lymphoma, myelolipomas, and infection (e.g., tuberculosis). The key features of these various lesions that occur incidentally as opposed to symptomatic presentations are discussed in the following sections.

Nonfunctioning Cortical Adenomas

Nonfunctioning cortical adenomas account for 60% or more of incidentalomas in major series. These lesions are characterized radiographically by their homogeneity and low attenuation values on CT imaging as discussed further below. Most adenomas are less than 4 cm in size, but they may be up to 6 cm in diameter or occasionally even larger. Adrenalectomy is indicated for those larger than 4 cm or with imaging characteristics that are atypical for an adenoma.

Aldosteronoma

Aldosterone-producing adenoma (aldosteronoma) is the most common hypersecretory adrenal lesion, and in recent years, it has been recognized as occurring in up to 12% of hypertensive patients. However, aldosteronomas are not often discovered as incidentalomas because of their small size (1.0–1.5 cm or smaller). Hyperaldosteronism should be screened for in any patient with an incidentaloma who has hypertension or hypokalemia. Patients with adrenal incidentalomas who are normotensive and normokalemic do not require testing for this diagnosis.

Initial biochemical screening should consist of measurement of plasma aldosterone and plasma renin activity. A ratio of aldosterone to renin greater than 20 with a plasma aldosterone greater than 15 ng/dl is suggestive of the diagnosis and should lead to further testing. Measurement of a 24-hour urine collection for aldosterone, sodium, and potassium while on a high-salt diet or during saline loading is typically performed. A 24-hour urine aldosterone greater than 12 µg/dl is confirmatory of the diagnosis. Urinary potassium

is usually greater than 30 mEq per 24 hours. Because approximately 35% of patients with primary hyperaldosteronism have idiopathic hyperaldosteronism resulting from bilateral cortical hyperplasia, adrenal vein sampling for aldosterone and cortisol to determine whether the source of increased aldosterone production lateralizes to one adrenal is recommended for all patients with bilateral adrenal nodularity, normal adrenals, or a unilateral nodule under 1 cm.

Subclinical Cushing's Syndrome

Abnormalities in cortisol secretion without overt signs of Cushing's syndrome have been reported in up to 20% of patients with adrenal incidentalomas. In a review of more than 1400 patients with incidentalomas, 7.8% had subclinical Cushing's syndrome (SCS). A variety of biochemical abnormalities define SCS, including failure to suppress cortisol with dexamethasone, loss of diurnal variation in cortisol secretion, low or suppressed plasma adenocorticotropin hormone (ACTH), lack of ACTH response to corticotropin-releasing hormone, and elevated 24-hour urine-free cortisol. The latter, however, is often a late finding associated with emerging clinical signs. Patients with SCS have a higher incidence of hypertension, diabetes, and obesity compared with other patients with adrenal incidentalomas. In a recent review, hypertension was present in 76% of patients, diabetes in 30%, and obesity in 52%.

The natural history of SCS has not been extensively studied, but in one series the incidence of progression to overt Cushing's syndrome was 12.5% at 1 year. The diagnosis of SCS is generally established by demonstrating that plasma cortisol levels do not suppress after a low-dose dexamethasone test. In this test, 1 to 3 mg of dexamethasone is given at 11 P.M., and an 8 A.M. plasma cortisol is collected the next morning. Normal individuals should suppress to less than 3 µg/dl. Patients who fail to suppress should undergo further testing with plasma ACTH and 24-hour urine-free cortisol measurement.

Most endocrine surgeons recommend adrenalectomy for patients with SCS who are suitable candidates for surgery. Improvements in weight loss, hypertension, and blood glucose control have been observed in most reported series of patients treated surgically. Although supporting data are lacking, an increased risk of osteoporosis has also been hypothesized in SCS because of the potential for steroid-induced increased rate of bone turnover. Although this has not been clearly shown, the osteoporosis risk may be a further reason to consider adrenalectomy, especially in women.

Patients with biochemical evidence of SCS are at increased risk for adrenal insufficiency after adrenalectomy and therefore should be given supplemental glucocorticoids postoperatively. Similarly, all patients with adrenal incidentaloma who are undergoing adrenalectomy should be tested for this possibility preoperatively to prevent an acute adrenal crisis. Up to 12 months may be required for the pituitary-adrenal axis to recover normal function.

Pheochromocytoma

Pheochromocytoma is the second most common secretory tumor among series of adrenal incidentalomas. Overall approximately 5% of incidentalomas are found to be pheochromocytomas, and up to 10% of all pheochromocytomas may present originally as incidentalomas. These lesions are typically clinically silent except for the presence of hypertension, but spells of palpitations, headache, sweating, tremor, pallor, and anxiety are usually absent. Because of the potential for a life-threatening hypertensive crisis in patients undergoing adrenalectomy for unsuspected pheochromocytoma, all patients with adrenal incidentalomas should be evaluated for this possibility.

The diagnostic evaluation for pheochromocytoma consists of measurement of plasma- fractionated metanephrines or 24-hour urine measurement of catecholamines and metanephrines. Plasma-

fractionated metanephrine measurement is simpler to perform and is preferred in most institutions. However, false-positive results may occur, and further testing with urine catecholamines and metanephrines is recommended in equivocal cases.

Pheochromocytoma may be suspected on CT imaging by its heterogeneous appearance (Fig. 1; see imaging description later in the chapter). Pheochromocytomas also have a typically bright appearance on T2-weighted MRI sequences. Adrenalectomy is recommended for all patients with incidentally discovered pheochromocytomas. Patients should be prepared for surgery preoperatively with alpha-receptor blockade with phenoxybenzamine to prevent intraoperative hypertensive exacerbations. Beta blockade is reserved for patients with predominately epinephrine-secreting tumors or in the setting of persistent tachycardia after alpha blockade.

Adrenocortical Carcinoma

Adrenal cortical cancers are rare tumors with an incidence of approximately 1 in 1 to 1.5 million population. Most adrenal cancers are large at the time of presentation, with a mean tumor size greater than 10 cm in diameter. Although more than 90% of these tumors are larger than 6 cm, smaller adrenal cancers do occur; in one series, 16% of adrenal cancers were less than 5 cm in diameter. Approximately half of adrenal cancers are hypersecretory with clinical and biochemical features of either Cushing's syndrome, virilization, or mixed features.

The incidence of primary adrenocortical cancer in major series of adrenal incidentalomas has ranged from 1.2% to 22.0% with an average incidence of 8.6%. Only 4 (1.2%) nonfunctioning adrenal cancers were found in the Mayo Clinic series of 342 adrenal incidentalomas. In a national database study from Italy of 380 incidentalomas that were selected for adrenalectomy, 44 patients were proved to have primary adrenal carcinomas for an incidence of 12.4%. The probability that an incidentaloma is a primary adrenal cancer increases with increasing size of the lesion. Assessment of the risk of an adrenal incidentaloma for adrenal cancer is made not only on the basis of size but also on other imaging characteristics as discussed subsequently.

Adrenal Metastases

The adrenal gland is a relatively common site for metastasis, although this usually occurs in the setting of extra-adrenal metastatic disease.

As a result, few adrenal metastases are amenable to surgical resection (only 3% of surgically resected incidentalomas in the series in Table 1 were adrenal metastasis). Cancers that most commonly metastasize to or involve the adrenal gland include renal, lung, melanoma, breast, and lymphoma. Most adrenal metastases are greater than 3 cm in diameter and have imaging characteristics that are suspicious for malignancy, such as higher attenuation on CT and no loss of signal on MRI chemical shift imaging. Adrenalectomy is appropriate for the patient with a solitary adrenal metastasis. Positron emission tomography (PET) may be helpful to exclude extra-adrenal metastatic disease that may not be apparent on conventional cross sectional imaging. Fine needle aspiration (FNA) biopsy should be reserved primarily for the patient in whom a tissue diagnosis will alter therapy, but is not warranted if the lesion is amenable to resection and the patient is an appropriate surgical candidate.

Other Adrenal Lesions

A variety of other lesions may present as incidentalomas, including cysts, myelolipomas, and hemorrhage. These lesions can usually be distinguished by their imaging characteristics, and further workup may not be necessary. Myelolipomas are benign masses composed of fat and bone marrow elements and are one of the more common lesions to present as an incidentaloma. They can become large (up to 10–15 cm) and are characterized radiographically by the presence of macroscopic fat (Fig. 2). Myelolipomas do not have to be removed unless they are symptomatic, which is uncommon, or if they are enlarging.

DIAGNOSTIC EVALUATION

Evaluation of Hormonal Function

Our diagnostic algorithm for evaluating adrenal incidentalomas is outlined in Figure 3. For lesions that do not look like cysts or myelolipomas, the first step is to perform a biochemical evaluation to determine whether the lesion is hormonally active. All

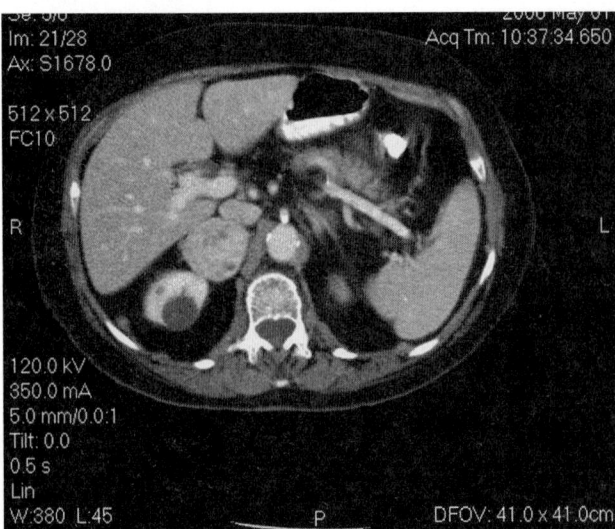

Figure 1 Computed tomography scan of a right adrenal pheochromocytoma. Note the heterogenous appearance and areas of calcification and hemorrhage.

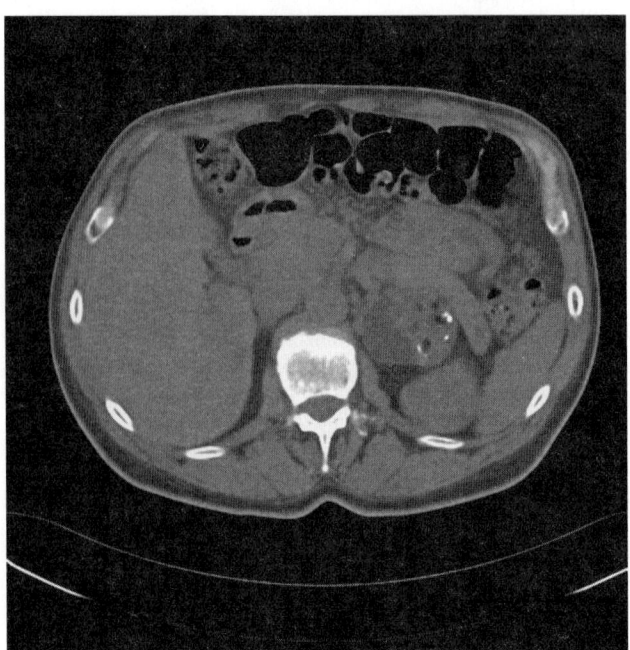

Figure 2 Computed tomography scan of left adrenal myelolipoma. The low attenuation areas within the lesion are due to macroscopic fat.

DIAGNOSTIC EVALUATION

```
                            ┌─────────────────────────┐
                            │  Adrenal incidentaloma  │
                            └─────────────────────────┘
                    ┌───────────────┴───────────────────┐
          ┌──────────────────────┐          ┌──────────────────────────┐
          │ Biochemical evaluation│          │ Radiographic assessment  │
          └──────────────────────┘          └──────────────────────────┘
```

| Plasma fractionated metanephrines or 24-hr urine catecholamines and metanephrines | Overnight Dexamethasone (DM) test (1 mg DM at 11 PM, 8 AM plasma cortisol) | PAC:PRA* (only if hypertensive and/or hypokalemic) | Imaging review (lesion size, attenuation, homogeneity) |

```
                                                          │
                                                ┌───────────────────┐
                                                │  MRI if CT is     │
                                                │  indeterminate    │
                                                └───────────────────┘
```

Figure 3 Diagnostic algorithm for adrenal incidentalomas.

patients should undergo screening for pheochromocytoma with measurement of either plasma-fractionated metanephrines or a 24-hour urine collection for catecholamines and metanephrines. Our preference, for reasons of simplicity, is to obtain plasma meta-nephrines as the initial screening test for pheochromocytoma and only to order a 24-hour urine test for catecholamines and metabolites if the plasma metanephrines are abnormal. Urinary vanillylmandelic acid has a higher incidence of false-positive results and is not usually measured. Screening for subclinical hypercortisolism should consist of an overnight dexamethasone test as described earlier. If the patient fails to suppress cortisol levels to less than 3 to 5 μg/dl with dexamethasone, further testing should be carried out with measurement of 24-hour urine cortisol and plasma ACTH levels. Screening for hyperaldosteronism with measurement of plasma aldosterone and renin levels is performed only if the patient has hypertension or is hypokalemic.

RADIOGRAPHIC ASSESSMENT

An important part of the initial evaluation is a careful review of all radiographic studies. Most patients have had their incidentaloma diagnosed with a CT scan, and the CT should be reviewed for lesion size, homogeneity, invasiveness, and attenuation values. Adenomas are typically smooth, homogenous, well-circumscribed lesions that are less than 6 cm in size. Because they contain abundant intracellular lipid, they are relatively low in attenuation on unenhanced CT scans (<10 Hounsfield units), which is lower attenuation than liver or kidney but higher than retroperitoneal fat (Fig. 4). However, some adenomas have higher attenuation values that may overlap with those seen in primary and metastatic adrenal malignancies. Furthermore, most CT scans in which the incidentaloma was identified were administered with intravenous contrast, so attenuation values may not be available. Adrenal cortical carcinomas are usually inhomogeneous in appearance, with areas of necrosis, hemorrhage, or calcification. They may also have irregular margins and evidence of local invasiveness or regional lymphadenopathy. Attenuation values are usually greater than 18 Hounsfield units. Pheochromocytomas appear as round or oval masses with smooth margins and are similar in density to liver on unenhanced scans. Larger pheochromocytomas often have inhomogeneous or cystic areas (Fig. 1). Because they are highly vascular, they enhance prominently with intravenous contrast.

MRI may be useful in further characterizing the nature of the adrenal mass if it is not clearly identified as an adenoma by CT criteria. On T2-weighted MRI, adenomas are typically low in signal, whereas pheochromocytomas and metastases are bright in appearance. Chemical shift imaging is an MRI sequence that makes use

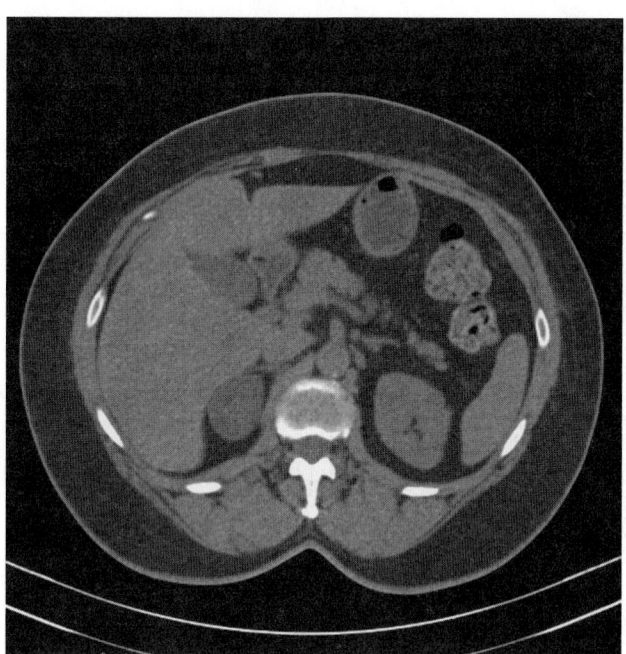

Figure 4 Unenhanced computed tomography scan of right adrenal adenoma. The lesion is smooth, homogeneous, and low in attenuation.

of the differential lipid versus water content of adrenal masses. With this technique, separate pulse signals are generated for protons in water versus fat. On in-phase MRI, the signal pulse is such that the protons in water and fat are "in phase" together, whereas in opposed-phase sequences, the signal from protons in fat is subtracted from those in water. As a result, benign lesions such as adenomas that have a mixture of fat and water density will have a loss of signal intensity on opposed-phase compared with in-phase sequences (Fig. 5). Malignant lesions and pheochromocytomas typically have little intracellular fat and as a result show no loss of signal intensity on opposed-phase imaging. In some series, the presence of a loss of signal on opposed-phase images has been highly specific for the diagnosis of an adenoma.

The role of PET imaging in the evaluation of adrenal incidentalomas has not been well defined and is not recommended except in the setting of patients with a known extra-adrenal malignancy. In such patients, PET imaging may be useful to search for extra-adrenal metastatic disease before recommending adrenalectomy for a potentially resectable metastasis.

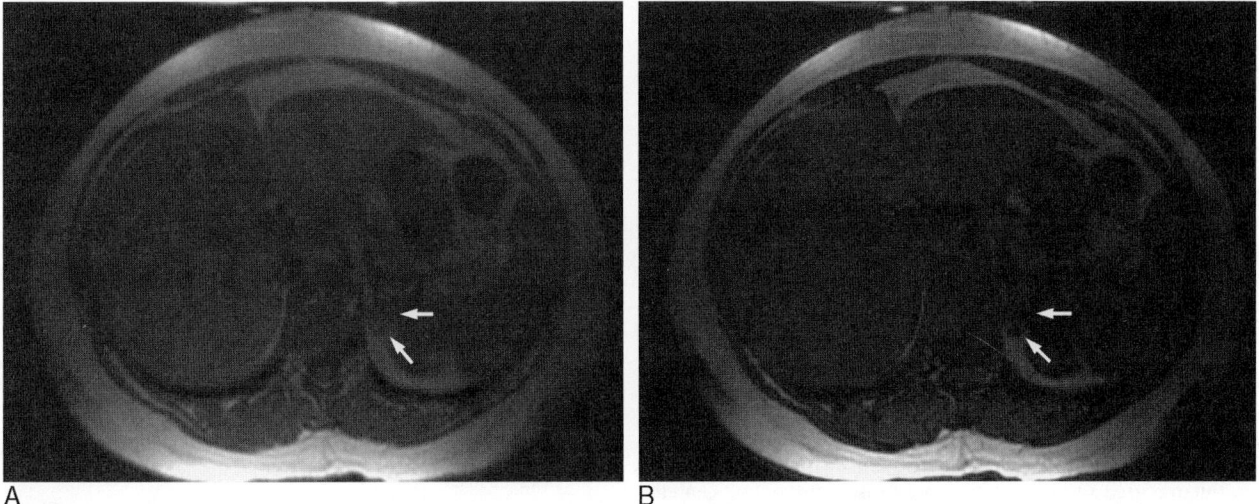

Figure 5 Chemical shift magnetic resonance imaging sequence of a left adrenal adenoma *(arrows).* **(A)** In-phase sequence; **(B)** opposed-phase sequence. Note the loss of signal intensity of the lesion on the opposed phase image.

TUMOR SIZE

The size of an adrenal incidentaloma is also an important variable in assessing the malignant potential of an adrenal lesion. Most adrenal cortical carcinomas are larger than 6 cm, but smaller primary adrenal cancers have been observed. Because survival is better for early (stage I and II) adrenal cancers, most endocrine surgeons recommend a 4-cm size threshold for removal of an incidentaloma. In the National Italian Study Group series of adrenal incidentalomas, a size cutoff of 4 cm for performing adrenalectomy resulted in a 90% sensitivity for detecting adrenal carcinoma, although 76% of lesions less than 4 cm were still benign. Adrenal metastases may also be large but are more likely to overlap with adenomas in terms of size than primary adrenal cancers. Therefore size is only one parameter that should be considered in weighing the risk of malignancy, and lesions with a concerning imaging phenotype should be removed regardless of size.

FINE NEEDLE ASPIRATION BIOPSY

FNA biopsy is rarely indicated in patients with adrenal incidentalomas. FNA biopsy is not usually capable of distinguishing benign from malignant primary adrenal tumors, and the decision regarding removal should instead be based on lesion size and imaging characteristics, as discussed earlier. Although metastatic lesions to the adrenal gland can usually be diagnosed by needle biopsy, a biopsy is indicated in this setting only if it will alter the therapeutic approach. For example, a biopsy should be unnecessary in a patient with a solitary adrenal lesion that is radiographically suspicious for a metastasis and appears resectable. Adrenal biopsy should never be undertaken unless a pheochromocytoma has been excluded biochemically because of the risk of precipitating a hypertensive crisis.

MANAGEMENT

The frequent detection of adrenal incidentalomas radiographically and the availability of a minimally invasive approach to adrenalectomy should not result in liberalization of the indications for adrenalectomy. Surgery should be reserved for incidentalomas that are secreting excess adrenal hormones and those that, on the basis of size and other imaging characteristics, have an increased likelihood of malignancy (Fig. 6). For all other lesions, observation is the most appropriate course. Evidence of excess hormone secretion may develop in up to 20% of patients who are followed and is more common in patients with lesions greater than 3 cm. The most likely condition to appear is subclinical Cushing's, and therefore repeat biochemical testing with an overnight dexamethasone test is appropriate at 1 year and annually for 3 to 4 years, after which time the risk plateaus.

Figure 6 Management algorithm of adrenal incidentaloma.

ADRENAL INCIDENTALOMA MANAGEMENT ALGORITHM

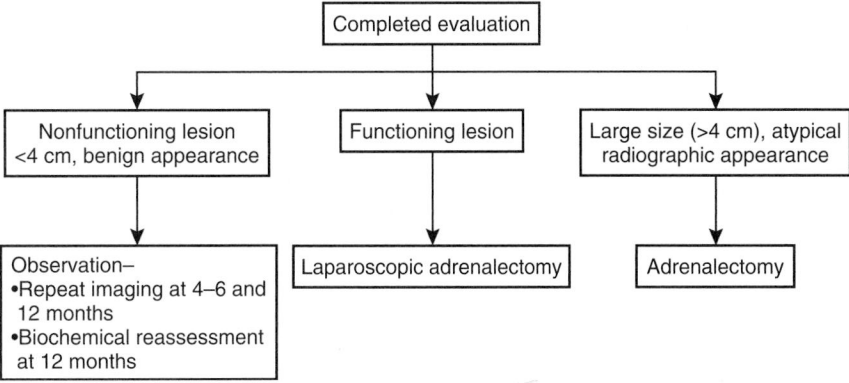

Repeat imaging is recommended within 4 to 6 months of detection of the incidentaloma and again at 1 year. Lesions that are stable in size and appearance over that time frame are not likely to change further and may not require further imaging or can be followed at longer intervals. In a study of 229 patients who were followed prospectively for a median of 25 months, an increase in incidentaloma size of 0.5 cm or larger was observed in 17 patients (7.4%) and enlargement of 1.0 cm or more occurred in 12 patients (5.2%).

Laparoscopic adrenalectomy is appropriate for most patients with incidentalomas that require removal. The only absolute contraindication to a laparoscopic approach is local invasion by the tumor. Large lesions greater than 6 cm are more difficult to remove laparoscopically and also pose a greater risk of adrenal malignancy. Local tumor recurrences have been reported after removal of unsuspected primary adrenal cancers by several groups, although local recurrence rates have been similar to those reported historically for open adrenalectomy. Preliminary data also suggest that the laparoscopic approach is safe for removal in selected patients with adrenal metastases, but reported series have all come from high-volume centers with substantial laparoscopic experience, and long-term follow-up studies are lacking. Therefore surgeons who attempt removal of large adrenal lesions or lesions with other imaging features suspicious for malignancy should be highly experienced in laparoscopic adrenalectomy techniques. Regardless of the nature of the lesion or the surgical approach, removal of an intact specimen with negative surgical margins should be the primary goal.

Patients with SCS should receive perioperative supplemental steroids and may require several weeks to months of replacement therapy before recovery of the pituitary-adrenal axis. Patients with biochemical suspicion of a pheochromocytoma should be prepared for surgery with phenoxybenzamine to prevent a hypertensive crisis intraoperatively. Most patients can be discharged within 1 day of laparoscopic adrenalectomy.

SUGGESTED READINGS

Brunt LM, Moley JF: Adrenal incidentalomas, *World J Surg* 25:905, 2001.

Bulow B, Jansson S, Juhlin C, and others: Adrenal incidentaloma follow-up results from a Swedish prospective study, *Eur J Endocrinol* 154:419, 2006.

Grumbach MM, Biller BMK, Braunstein GD, and others: NIH Conference: management of the clinically inapparent adrenal mass, *Ann Intern Med* 138:424, 2003.

Mansmann G, Lau J, Balk E, and others: The clinically inapparent adrenal mass: update in diagnosis and management, *Endocr Rev* 25:309, 2004.

Sippel RS, Chen H: Subclinical Cushing's syndrome in adrenal incidentalomas, *Surg Clin N Am* 84:875, 2004.

Young WF: Management approached to adrenal incidentalomas: a view from Rochester, Minnesota, *Endocrinol Metab Clin N Amer* 29:159, 2000.

MANAGEMENT OF THYROID NODULES

Elizabeth A. Mittendorf, MD, and Christopher R. McHenry, MD

A thyroid nodule is a discrete lesion within the thyroid gland. Such lesions are common in the United States, with a prevalence of 4% to 7% for palpable nodules. However, nonpalpable nodules discovered incidentally on ultrasound or at autopsy suggest an overall prevalence of 19% to 67%. With an estimated annual incidence rate of 0.1%, approximately 300,000 new nodules are identified yearly. Thyroid nodules are four times more common in women than in men, and the incidence increases with age, radiation exposure, and reduced iodine intake. The prevalence of nodular thyroid disease has been reported to be 15% in areas of iodine deficiency.

The majority of thyroid nodules are benign. Colloid nodules, cysts, and thyroiditis account for approximately 80%, and benign follicular and Hurthle cell adenomas account for 10% to 15% of all thyroid nodules. Only 5% of thyroid nodules are malignant. In 2008, an estimated 33,550 new cases of thyroid cancer are expected to occur in the United States, and approximately 1530 patients are expected to die from thyroid cancer. The challenge for a clinician is to distinguish patients with malignancy, who are treated surgically, from patients with benign disease, who are followed clinically. This is accomplished by a diagnostic approach that consists of routine fine needle aspiration biopsy (FNAB), a routine screening third-generation thyrotropin (thyroid-stimulating hormone [TSH]) level, and selective use of high-resolution ultrasound (US) and iodine-123 (I-123) thyroid scintigraphy. In this chapter, we review the diagnostic approach for evaluating a patient with a thyroid nodule, summarized in Figure 1.

CLINICAL EVALUATION

Nodules that are larger than 1 cm in size are considered clinically significant and require further evaluation. With increasing radiographic evaluation of the neck, including duplex scanning for carotid artery disease and magnetic resonance imaging (MRI) for cervical spine disease, more nodules less than 1 cm in size are being identified. A selective approach to the workup of these smaller nodules is advocated. Patients with a personal history of prior thyroid lobectomy for carcinoma, a family history of thyroid cancer, a history of head and neck irradiation, or a nodule with suspicious sonographic findings should undergo further evaluation regardless of nodule size.

Evaluation begins with a thorough history and physical examination. Pertinent historical features that should increase suspicion for malignancy include age younger than 20 or older than 60 years, male sex, a history of head and neck irradiation, or total body irradiation for bone marrow transplantation. The risk of malignancy is twofold higher in patients younger than 20 years. A history of familial medullary thyroid cancer (MTC), multiple endocrine neoplasia (MEN) type 2, familial papillary thyroid cancer (PTC), familial polyposis coli, Cowden's disease, and Gardner's syndrome also increases the concern that a nodule is malignant.

Patients should be questioned about recent onset of hoarseness, dysphagia, or dyspnea, as well as about the rate of growth of the nodule. These are all nonspecific but potentially worrisome findings. For example, hoarseness may be indicative of tumor invasion of the recurrent laryngeal nerve. Dysphagia may be the result of esophageal compression, and dyspnea may be indicative of tracheal compression from a large benign or malignant goiter. A slow but progressive increase in nodule size over the course of weeks to months is worrisome for malignancy, whereas a rapid increase in size should raise concern for an anaplastic carcinoma or a primary lymphoma. Patients should also be questioned about neck pain and symptomatology suggestive of hyperthyroidism or hypothyroidism. Neck pain may occur as a result of hemorrhage into a nodule or may be a manifestation of thyroiditis. Hyperthyroidism and

Figure I Algorithm for the evaluation of patients with a thyroid nodule. *TSH,* Thyroid stimulating hormone; *US,* ultrasound; *FNAB,* fine needle aspiration biopsy.

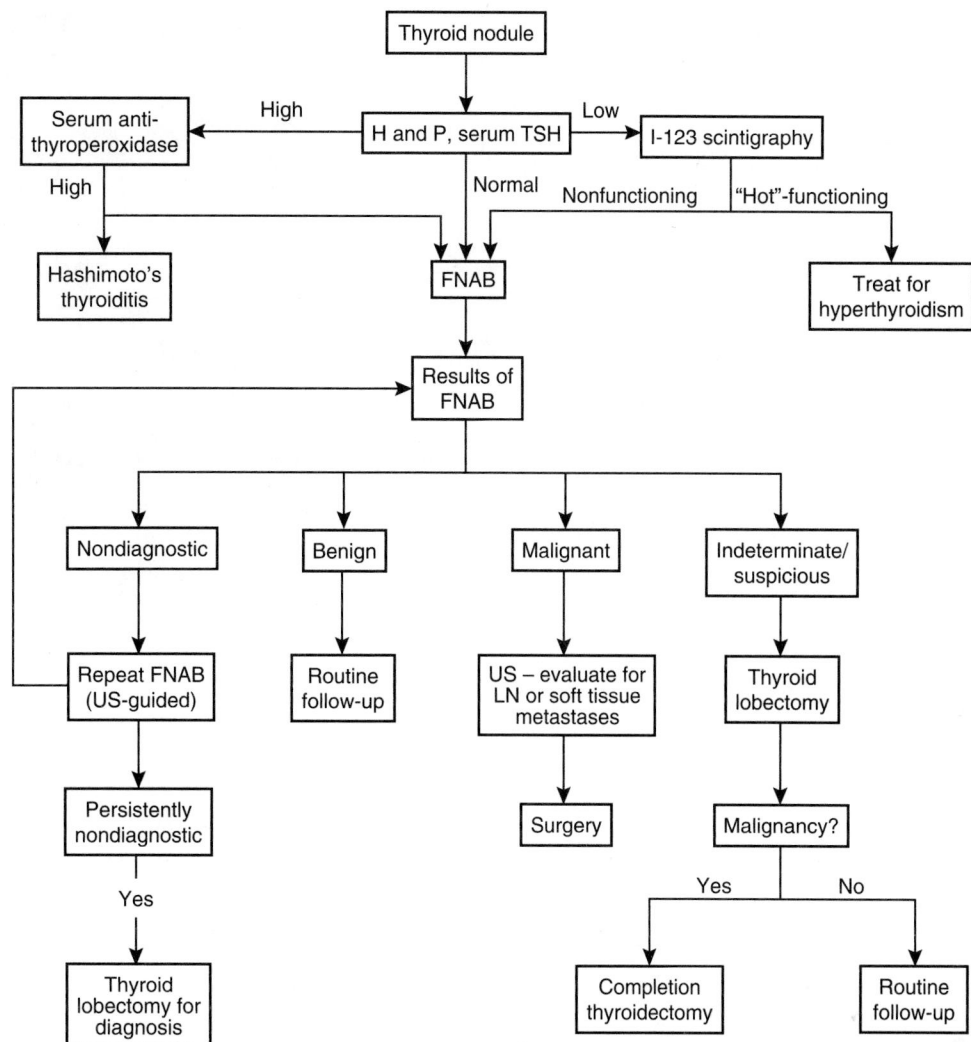

LABORATORY EVALUATION

The only laboratory test that must be performed routinely in the evaluation of a patient with a thyroid nodule is a third-generation TSH level. In the majority of patients, the TSH level will be normal, indicating that the patient is euthyroid. Approximately 10% of patients with a solitary nodule have a suppressed TSH level, which suggests a benign hyperfunctioning nodule. In these patients, a free thyroxine and a free triiodothyronine level should be measured. An I-123 thyroid scan is obtained to distinguish a hyperfunctioning ("hot") nodule (Fig. 2, *A*) from a hypofunctioning ("cold") nodule (Fig. 2, *B*) in a patient with Graves' disease. If the thyroid scan confirms a functioning nodule in the setting of a low TSH, no further diagnostic evaluation is necessary. The incidence of malignancy in patients with a hyperfunctioning nodule is less than 1%. The patient can be treated with a thyroid lobectomy or with radioiodine ablation. Patients with thyrotoxicosis and a hypofunctioning nodule should undergo FNAB.

In patients with a dominant thyroid nodule and an elevated serum TSH level, a free T4 and serum antithyroperoxidase antibody level should be obtained. An elevated serum antithyroperoxidase antibody level is indicative of Hashimoto's thyroiditis. In these patients, an FNAB is indicated to rule out malignancy, including lymphoma, which accounts for a minority of thyroid cancers but is known to be associated with Hashimoto's thyroiditis.

hypothyroidism are usually associated with benign disease. Patients with a solitary thyroid nodule and hyperthyroidism may have an autonomous functioning follicular adenoma or a hypofunctioning nodule with underlying Graves' disease. The majority of patients with thyroid carcinoma are asymptomatic and euthyroid.

Physical examination alone detects only 40% of nodules that are greater than 1.5 cm. This is related to a posterior or substernal location of a nodule, a patient's body habitus such as a short, thick neck; obesity or kyphosis; and clinician inexperience. If a nodule is identified on physical examination, particular attention should be paid to its size, shape, consistency, location, and mobility. The presence of tracheal displacement, cervical lymphadenopathy, and substernal extension of the nodule should also be assessed. Patients with a large nodule that extends substernally may have a Pemberton's sign. This refers to facial plethora, neck vein distention, and difficulty breathing from a narrowing of the thoracic inlet that occurs when patients elevate their arms above their head. Physical examination has a low sensitivity and specificity. However, the finding of a firm or hard nodule, fixation of the nodule to surrounding tissues, or ipsilateral cervical lymphadenopathy is suggestive of malignancy. A paralyzed vocal cord documented by laryngoscopy is also highly suggestive of carcinoma. Neck tenderness on palpation is usually a manifestation of thyroiditis.

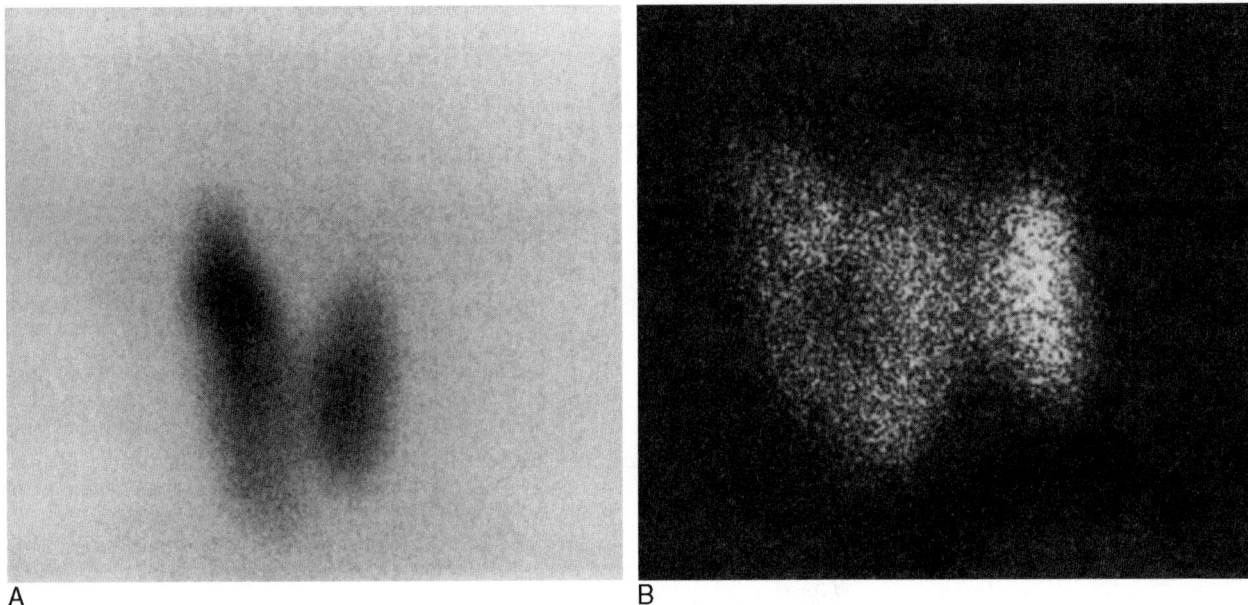

A   B

Figure 2 Results of Iodine-123 thyroid scan showing a hyperfunctioning ("hot") nodule **(A)** and a hypofunctioning ("cold") nodule **(B).** *From McHenry CR: Goiter and nontoxic benign thyroid conditions. In Bland KI, editor: The practice of general surgery, Philadelphia, 2002, WB Saunders, p. 1043. Reproduced with permission.*

In patients with a family history of MTC or MEN 2, a basal serum calcitonin level should be obtained. Baseline levels of calcitonin greater than 100 pg/ml are highly suggestive of MTC. In patients without a history of familial MTC, routine calcitonin testing is not recommended because large studies of nodular thyroid disease have reported a prevalence of MTC of less than 1.5%.

FINE NEEDLE ASPIRATION BIOPSY

FNAB is the diagnostic procedure of choice in the evaluation of thyroid nodules. Since it became widely adopted in the early 1990s, the routine use of FNAB has resulted in a reduction of unnecessary testing, fewer operations, and an increased cancer yield when thyroidectomy is recommended; furthermore, the percentage of patients undergoing thyroidectomy has declined by 25%, whereas the yield of carcinoma has increased by 50%.

FNAB can be performed as either a palpation-guided or US-guided procedure. If the patient has a palpable nodule, an FNAB is performed at the initial clinic visit before any other diagnostic study. To perform an FNAB, the patient is positioned supine with the neck extended. The nodule is then identified and stabilized between the clinician's two fingers. Biopsy is then performed using a 22-gauge, 1.5-inch needle attached to a 10-ml disposable syringe. The needle is moved vigorously up and down while continuous suction is applied to the plunger of the syringe to disrupt the follicular epithelium. Aspirated material in the hub of the needle is then smeared on a slide and either fixed with alcohol or allowed to air dry. It is then submitted for staining and cytologic evaluation. It should be emphasized that this technique provides a cytologic rather than histopathologic diagnosis because it cannot provide any information about capsular or vascular invasion. Patients tolerate this procedure well, and it has a low rate of complications.

The results of cytologic analysis of FNAB specimens are divided into four main categories: nondiagnostic, benign, indeterminate/suspicious for neoplasm, and malignant (Table 1). In the absence of cytologic findings consistent with malignancy, a biopsy is considered adequate only if it contains at least 6 groups of 10 or more well-preserved follicular epithelial cells on one or more slides. Specimens not fulfilling these criteria are categorized as

nondiagnostic. Nondiagnostic aspirates account for 10% to 20% of all FNAB results. Aspirates are more likely to be nondiagnostic if the nodule has a predominant cystic component or if the nodule is small or difficult to palpate. The reported incidence of malignancy is 5% to 10% in patients with a thyroid nodule and a nondiagnostic FNAB, and therefore a repeat FNAB should always be obtained. For patients with a nondiagnostic palpation-guided FNAB, a repeat FNAB can be obtained under ultrasound guidance. Using US guidance, an adequate specimen is obtained in 50% of patients with a previously nondiagnostic palpation-guided FNAB. In the majority of these patients, repeat FNAB confirmed a benign lesion and helped to avoid an unnecessary operation. If FNAB is persistently nondiagnostic, thyroid lobectomy is recommended with frozen section exam of the nodule.

Decreasing the rate of nondiagnostic aspirates is one of the purported benefits of US-guided FNAB. This is attributed to

Table 1: Fine Needle Aspiration Biopsy Cytologic Diagnoses

I. Nondiagnostic

II. Benign
   a. Colloid nodule
   b. Adenomatous hyperplasia
   c. Thyroiditis

III. Indeterminate or suspicious
   a. Consistent with a follicular neoplasm
   b. Consistent with a Hurthle cell neoplasm
   c. Suspicious for papillary carcinoma

IV. Malignant
   a. Papillary carcinoma
   b. Medullary carcinoma
   c. Anaplastic carcinoma
   d. Lymphoma
   e. Metastatic carcinoma

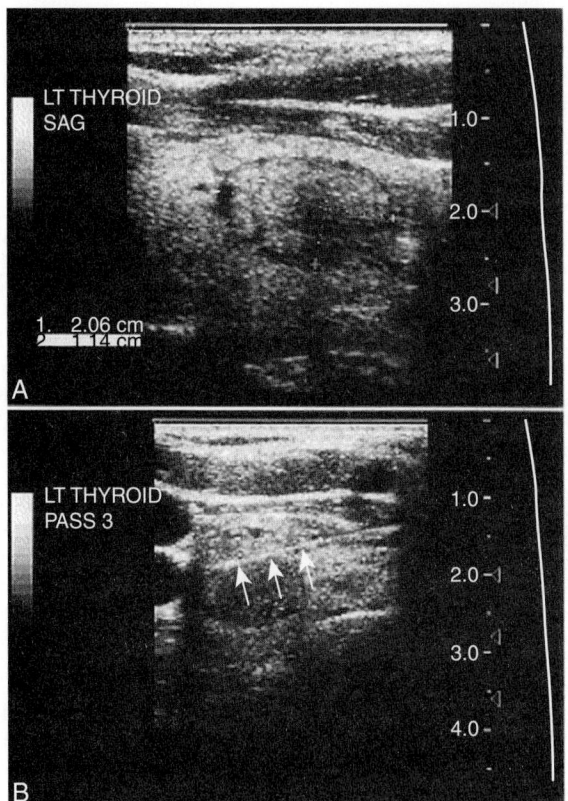

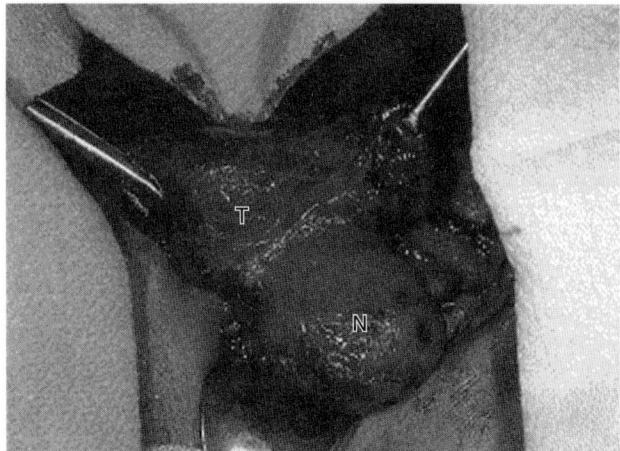

Figure 4 Intraoperative photograph of a lobe of the thyroid gland *(T)* elevated anteromedially with 3-cm nodule *(N)* arising from posterior surface that was not palpable on physical examination. *From Miteendorf EA, Tamarkin S, McHenry CR: Surgery 132:648, 2002. Reproduced with permission.*

Figure 3 Ultrasound examination of thyroid gland demonstrating a 1.1 × 2.1 cm nodule in sagittal plane **(A)** and the same nodule in a transverse plane **(B)** with needle *(arrow)* within the nodule. *From Mittendorf EA, Tamarkin S, McHenry CR: Surgery 132:648, 2002. Reproduced with permission.*

continuous visualization of the needle during insertion and sampling (Fig. 3). This may be most helpful when evaluating a complex nodule with cystic and solid components because the cyst fluid that is obtained is often acellular, and the residual solid component is often difficult to palpate. US guidance ensures that the biopsy needle is within the solid portion. Visualization provided by US is also important when sampling smaller nodules or those that are difficult to palpate. Several factors can contribute to a lesion being difficult to palpate, including nodule size and location and patient body habitus. Nodules arising from the posterior surface of the thyroid are frequently not palpable (Fig. 4). A nodule may be difficult to palpate in a patient with kyphosis, a short, thick muscular neck, or with extensive adipose tissue. In patients with a nonpalpable nodule identified incidentally by imaging obtained for an unrelated indication, US guidance is required for FNAB.

Approximately 70% of FNAB specimens are benign. Benign lesions include adenomatous or hyperplastic nodules, colloid nodules, simple cysts, and Hashimoto's thyroiditis. There is a known association between Hashimoto's thyroiditis and thyroid lymphoma. A repeat FNAB specimen should be obtained in patients with Hashimoto's thyroiditis for flow cytometry to evaluate for monoclonality to exclude the possibility of lymphoma. In addition, repeat FNAB in a patient with an initial benign cytologic diagnosis may be of value when the cytologic specimen contains abundant red blood cells that obscure the evaluation of the follicular cell nuclei, a nodule is greater than 4 cm because of an increased risk of a sampling error, a nodule is difficult to palpate raising concern for sampling error, or a nodule undergoes progressive enlargement. Patients with a benign FNAB are asked to return in 6

months, at which time they are evaluated for an increase in nodule size or development of compressive symptoms. If the patient is asymptomatic and there is no change in the nodule size, follow-up with history, physical examination, and a screening serum TSH level is recommended at yearly intervals. Yearly US evaluation can provide objective measure of nodule size when necessary. Thyroidectomy is recommended for a progressive increase in nodule size and development of compressive symptoms.

The false-negative rate for FNAB is 2% to 5%. The most commonly reported causes of false-negative FNAB results include sampling and cytodiagnostic errors. Sampling errors tend to occur with particularly small or large nodules, hemorrhagic nodules, or multinodular glands. Some authors have found that the false-negative rate is increased in patients with complex solid-cystic nodules. More often, complex nodules with a cystic and solid component are a cause for a nondiagnostic rather than false-negative FNAB.

The cytologic category that is referred to as indeterminate or suspicious for neoplasm accounts for approximately 15% to 20% of all FNAB results. These include specimens for which a definitive cytologic diagnosis cannot be made and those suspicious for follicular neoplasm, for Hurthle cell neoplasm, and for papillary carcinoma. FNAB specimens from follicular neoplasms are hypercellular with a monotony of cells and often present in a microfollicular arrangement with diminished or absent colloid. A Hurthle cell neoplasm is diagnosed when an aspirate consists of a predominance of Hurthle cells, usually with absent or scanty colloid and a paucity of other cells. It is the presence of capsular or vascular invasion that distinguishes a benign follicular or Hurthle cell adenoma from a follicular or Hurthle cell carcinoma. As a result, cytologic analysis of FNAB specimens cannot differentiate benign and malignant follicular or Hurthle cell lesions. The risk of malignancy is approximately 20% in nodules with an FNAB interpreted as a follicular or Hurthle cell neoplasm. At present, there are no clinical, imaging, or cytologic features accurate enough to determine which patients have a malignancy; therefore patients require thyroid lobectomy to make a definitive diagnosis. If the final pathology reveals a clinically significant carcinoma, completion thyroidectomy is performed. Alternatively, patients are counseled regarding the 20% risk of their lesion being malignant and may be offered total thyroidectomy as their initial surgical procedure. Such an approach eliminates the need for reoperative surgery should the final pathology reveal malignancy; however, it guarantees that the patient will require thyroid hormone replacement therapy.

FNAB specimens that have some, but not all, of the cytologic features for PTC in association with otherwise benign cytologic features are also classified as indeterminate. The risk of malignancy in a patient with an FNAB result interpreted as suspicious for PTC is approximately 40% to 50%. The best management strategy for these patients is to proceed with thyroid lobectomy and frozen section examination. If the frozen-section examination confirms the presence of PTC, a total thyroidectomy is completed.

FNAB is malignant in approximately 5% of patients with a dominant thyroid nodule. Because the false-positive rate for patients with a malignant FNAB is 1% to 2%, definitive therapy is recommended on the basis of the cytologic result alone. The malignancies that FNAB can reliably identify include papillary, medullary, and anaplastic thyroid cancer. FNAB may also be helpful in diagnosing metastatic cancer and lymphoma.

FNAB has a sensitivity of greater than 90% for diagnosing PTC, which accounts for 70% to 80% of all cases of thyroid malignancy. Cytologic criteria that are necessary to make a definitive diagnosis of PTC include large monolayer sheets of follicular epithelial cells with enlarged nuclei containing fine powdery chromatin, intranuclear cytoplasmic inclusions and nuclear grooves, and papillary structures with or without tall columnar cells. For patients with a thyroid nodule 1 cm or larger and an FNAB diagnosis of PTC, a total thyroidectomy is the preferred treatment. Some authorities recognize a group of low-risk patients who can be treated with thyroid lobectomy and isthmusectomy. A complete discussion regarding these recommendations is beyond the scope of this chapter.

Cytologic criteria necessary to make a diagnosis of MTC include an absence of colloid; the variable presence of amyloid (present in one third of cases); polygonal-, triangular-, or spindle-shaped cells; and eccentric, bipolar, and hyperchromatic nuclei. Calcitonin immunostaining is diagnostic. If the diagnosis of MTC is made, patients should undergo screening for MEN 2 with evaluation of the *RET* proto-oncogene. If MEN2 is diagnosed, the patient requires further evaluation for the presence of hyperparathyroidism or a pheochromocytoma. At minimum, patients with MTC should be treated with a total thyroidectomy and central compartment lymph node dissection.

Cytologic features indicative of anaplastic carcinoma include a highly cellular pattern with associated necrosis and marked pleomorphism. Nuclei can be giant or spindle shaped. Anaplastic carcinoma is usually suspected on the basis of clinical presentation, including a history of rapid nodule enlargement and a hard, fixed mass identified on physical examination.

ADJUNCTS TO FINE NEEDLE ASPIRATION BIOPSY

The indeterminate cytologic FNAB result is one of the limitations of FNAB in the evaluation of a thyroid nodule. In up to 20% of patients, FNAB cytology unfortunately cannot discriminate between benign and malignant thyroid nodules, and these patients require thyroid lobectomy for diagnosis. This has led to an interest in identifying molecular markers that can help to differentiate benign and malignant neoplasms preoperatively and improve the initial surgical decision-making process. Preliminary studies examining immunohistochemical markers such as galactin-3 and human bone marrow endothelial cell (HBME-1) have shown some promise. Mutations in the *BRAF* gene are common in human cancers, and several investigators have reported a transversion, activating mutation in 30% to 70% of PTCs. Importantly, this mutation has been reported to be specific for PTC and has not been identified in benign thyroid neoplasms. *BRAF* mutations therefore have the potential to serve as specific molecular markers for PTC. *BRAF* mutations can be easily and reliably demonstrated, and investigators have already used them to identify correctly 50% of PTCs.

Genes modulating angiogenesis have been evaluated in an attempt to identify differentially expressed genes that may help to distinguish benign from malignant thyroid neoplasms. Using a technique of complementary DNA (cDNA) array analysis confirmed by real-time quantitative polymerase chain reaction (RT-PCR), it has been shown that the combined use of angiopoietin 2 (ANGPT2)and the tissue inhibitor of metalloproteinase 1 (TIMP1) mRNA expression levels was able to distinguish malignant from benign thyroid neoplasms with a sensitivity of 90%, a specificity of 85%, a positive predictive value of 75%, and a negative predictive value of 94%. These diagnostic markers may help to improve the diagnostic accuracy of FNAB.

Genes regulating cell invasion have also been evaluated as potential diagnostic markers of malignancy. Using extracellular matrix and adhesion molecule cDNA array analysis comparing benign lesions to malignant lesions, six differentially expressed genes have been identified. Using RT-PCR, it has been documented that the mRNA expression in three of these genes is high in malignant lesions. Excluding cases of PTC that are usually accurately diagnosed by FNAB, the levels of ECM1 and TMPRSS4 mRNA expression were higher in follicular thyroid cancers and the follicular variant of PTC than in hyperplastic nodules and follicular adenomas. Subsequently, ECM1 and TMPRSS4 expression analysis has been shown to improve the diagnostic accuracy of FNAB in 92% of indeterminate or suspicious results. If the risk of malignancy of a thyroid nodule could be reliably predicted by measuring mRNA expression levels ECM1 and TMPRSS4, or any of the other molecular markers, it would significantly decrease the number of diagnostic thyroidectomies performed and the cost of evaluation and management of a patient with a thyroid nodule. Questions persist regarding the technical feasibility of cDNA analysis or RT-PCR on FNAB specimens. Further investigation is required to determine the clinical utility of these techniques.

DIAGNOSTIC IMAGING

High-Resolution Ultrasound

The increased use of US as an office-based adjunct to physical examination has resulted in recommendations from the American Thyroid Association and the American Association of Clinical Endocrinologists to use US in the initial evaluation of all patients with a thyroid nodule. Whether US examination is necessary for evaluation of all patients with nodular thyroid disease remains a subject of debate. US is indicated for evaluation of patients with nondiagnostic palpation-guided FNAB. In 50% of these patients, US facilitates obtaining a diagnostic aspirate. US is also useful in the evaluation of patients with nodules that are difficult to palpate because of the nodule size or location or the patient's body habitus. For patients referred with a nonpalpable nodule identified incidentally on imaging obtained for an unrelated indication, US is valuable to better characterize the nodule. Finally, a US examination is obtained preoperatively in patients with a thyroid nodule and a malignant FNAB to evaluate for abnormal lymph nodes in the central and lateral neck. Preoperative, high-quality US in these patients has been shown to detect lymph node or soft-tissue metastases in neck compartments believed to be uninvolved by PE in almost 40% of patients. Finding metastatic disease preoperatively alters the surgical procedure in these patients, facilitating complete resection of disease and helping to minimize local and regional recurrence.

Although certain sonographic features should raise suspicion for malignancy (Table 2), the presence or absence of these sonographic findings cannot reliably distinguish benign from malignant lesions. As a result, all patients with a nodule 1 cm or larger in size should be evaluated with FNAB. For lesions less than 1 cm in size however,

Table 2: Sonographic Features That Can Be Associated with Malignancy

Indistinct or irregular margins
Intranodular calcifications
Hypoechogenicity
A nodule that is taller than it is wide
Increased intranodular vascular markings
Suspicious lymph nodes

such sonographic findings may help to determine which nodules warrant FNAB versus observation (Table 2). Additional findings suggesting local invasion or the presence of lymph node metastases are worrisome for malignancy and warrant immediate FNAB, regardless of the nodule size. Sonographic findings suggestive of invasion include the extension of irregular hypoechoic lesions beyond the thyroid capsule or invasion of adjacent musculature.

Additional Imaging Modalities

Iodine-123 thyroid scintigraphy also has utility in selected patients with a thyroid nodule (Table 3). On the basis of the pattern of radionuclide uptake, nodules are classified as hyperfunctioning ("hot"), isofunctioning, or nonfunctioning ("cold"). Hyperfunctioning nodules almost never represent malignant lesions. Isofunctioning and hypofunctioning nodules have a reported 5% to 10% risk of malignancy. Because more than 80% of nodules are hypofunctioning and only 5% to 10% are malignant, the predictive value of thyroid scintigraphy for the presence of malignancy is low. Because of the low specificity of I-123 thyroid scintigraphy, its routine use in the evaluation of patients with nodular thyroid disease is not recommended.

I-123 thyroid scintigraphy is of value in patients with a solitary nodule and suppressed TSH to distinguish a functioning nodule, which has a less than 1% incidence of malignancy, from a hypofunctioning nodule in a patient with Graves' disease, which has an approximate 10% risk of malignancy. If a functioning nodule is confirmed, the patient requires no further evaluation and can be treated with a thyroid lobectomy or radioiodine. A hypofunctioning nodule in a patient with Graves' disease should be evaluated with FNAB, and a total thyroidectomy recommended for an FNAB that is malignant or suspicious for malignancy. I-123 thyroid scintigraphy is also indicated in patients with a thyroid nodule, a suppressed TSH level, and an FNAB that is consistent with a follicular neoplasm or persistently nondiagnostic. In these clinical scenarios, it is also important to distinguish a hyperfunctioning from a hypofunctioning nodule. Thyroidectomy is recommended when a hypofunctioning nodule is identified because of a 20% to 30% incidence of malignancy in patients with a follicular neoplasm and a 10% incidence of malignancy in patients with a persistently nondiagnostic FNAB. Other imaging modalities such as computed tomography (CT) or magnetic resonance imaging (MRI) cannot distinguish between benign and malignant nodules and are not

Table 3: Selected Indications for Iodine-123 Thyroid Scintigraphy in Patients with a Dominant Thyroid Nodule

Low TSH before performing FNAB
FNAB consistent with a follicular neoplasm and a low serum TSH level
Persistently nondiagnostic FNAB and a low serum TSH level

FNAB, Fine needle aspiration biopsy; *TSH,* thyroid stimulating hormone.

indicated in the initial evaluation of a thyroid nodule. CT or MRI are of value for assessment of nodule size, substernal extension, and nodule displacement or impingement on adjacent structures. CT is the modality of choice for assessment of tracheal diameter.

SPECIAL SITUATIONS

Multinodular Goiter

Patients with multiple nodules have the same risk of malignancy as patients with a solitary nodule. Therefore if FNAB is performed only on the largest nodule, a thyroid cancer may be missed. Patients with a multinodular goiter should therefore undergo US evaluation to identify all nodules greater than 1 cm. Those with suspicious sonographic characteristics (Table 2) such as the presence of microcalcifications, hypoechogenicity, and intranodular hypervascularity should be identified and preferentially biopsied. If no nodules have suspicious sonographic features, the likelihood of malignancy is low, and then it is reasonable to perform FNAB on only the largest nodules.

Patients presenting with a multinodular goiter and suppressed TSH level (i.e., toxic multinodular goiter) should have I-123 scintigraphy performed to confirm that there are no cold or hypofunctioning nodules. If a hypofunctioning nodule is identified, it should be evaluated by FNAB.

Cystic Thyroid Nodule

The term *cystic thyroid nodule* refers to any fluid-filled nodule. Cystic nodules account for approximately 15% to 37% of all nodules that are surgically excised. Most cystic thyroid nodules represent cystic degeneration of some underlying neoplasm or nonneoplastic nodule. Cystic nodules also include true or simple cysts, which are characterized by the presence of an epithelial lining, but they are rare.

The evaluation and management of a patient with a cystic thyroid nodule is the same as for a solid nodule with a few caveats. FNAB is performed, and the cystic component of the nodule is completely aspirated. FNAB is also performed on the residual solid component of the mass. The cyst fluid, as well as the cellular material in the hub of the biopsy needle, is submitted for cytologic evaluation. FNAB of cystic nodules has been associated with a greater frequency of nondiagnostic results related to a higher frequency of acellular aspirates. Repeat FNAB is recommended for all patients with recurrent cysts and an initially nondiagnostic FNAB. US-guided FNAB may be of value to ensure biopsy of the solid component of the cystic nodule. FNAB results in cyst resolution in approximately 15% of patients.

Thyroidectomy is recommended for all patients with a cystic thyroid nodule who have (1) a prior history of head and neck irradiation, (2) an abnormal FNAB, (3) a recurrent cyst with a persistent nondiagnostic FNAB, and (4) compressive symptoms unrelieved by evacuation of cyst fluid. A nondiagnostic FNAB should not be equated with benign disease. Patients with a thyroid nodule and a persistently nondiagnostic FNAB have previously been reported to have an 8% incidence of carcinoma.

Percutaneous injection of sclerosing agents such as tetracycline, ethanol, and OK-432 has been used for treatment of recurrent cystic thyroid nodules. Injection therapy should be used selectively for patients with a recurrent cystic thyroid nodule and a definitive benign cytologic diagnosis. It should not be used for patients with an abnormal or persistently nondiagnostic FNAB result because it does not deal with the possibility of an underlying malignancy.

Nodule in Patients with a History of Head and Neck Irradiation

Radiation exposure to the thyroid gland is a risk factor for the development of well-differentiated thyroid cancer, most commonly PTC. This exposure may be environmental or the result of prior radiation treatment to the head and neck region. The development of thyroid cancer usually occurs many years after the exposure occurs. Latency periods as long as 40 years following initial exposure to radiation are not unusual. In a patient with such a history who presents with a thyroid nodule, the risk of malignancy is approximately 40%. In these patients a thorough discussion regarding the risk of thyroid cancer is undertaken, and the therapeutic alternatives are reviewed. Patients are offered total thyroidectomy or further evaluation with FNAB. If the FNAB is diagnostic of malignancy, total thyroidectomy is recommended. If the FNAB is benign, the patient may be followed clinically. For patients with a history of head and neck irradiation and a nondiagnostic or indeterminate aspirate, a total thyroidectomy is recommended.

Thyroid Nodule in Pregnancy

There are data to suggest that pregnancy is associated with an increase in the size of a preexisting thyroid nodule or the appearance of new nodules. It is hypothesized that this may be due to a negative iodine balance that frequently occurs during pregnancy. A thyroid nodule identified in a pregnant patient should be managed in the same manner as in a nonpregnant woman except that the use of radioactive agents for either diagnosis or treatment should be avoided. Patients should have a serum TSH level measured. If the serum TSH is suppressed, further evaluation should be deferred until after the pregnancy, when an I-123 thyroid scan can be performed. For patients with a normal or high serum TSH, FNAB should be performed. If a cytologic diagnosis of malignancy is made, surgery is indicated; however, the timing of thyroidectomy remains debated. Thyroidectomy can be safely performed during the second trimester. Others recommend waiting until the postpartum period, on the basis of data that have demonstrated no difference in recurrence or survival rates between women with well-differentiated thyroid cancer operated on during or after pregnancy. A reasonable approach to the management of a malignant nodule identified early in the pregnancy is to follow it sonographically. If it increases significantly in size, thyroidectomy can be performed during the second trimester. If the nodule remains stable, surgery can be performed after delivery. For patients diagnosed later in their pregnancy, thyroidectomy in the postpartum period is appropriate. If the FNAB is interpreted as indeterminate or suspicious for malignancy, it is reasonable to follow the patient clinically in combination with US examination during the pregnancy. Pregnancy may cause a misleading diagnosis of follicular neoplasm because of a physiologic increase in follicular epithelium. Repeat FNAB and, if indicated, thyroidectomy, can be performed in the postpartum period.

SUGGESTED READINGS

Kebebew E, Peng M, Reiff E, and others: ECM1 and TMPRSS4 are diagnostic markers of malignant thyroid neoplasms and improve the accuracy of fine needle aspiration biopsy, *Ann Surg* 242:353, 2005.

Kouvaraki MA, Shapiro SE, Fornage BD, and others: Role of preoperative ultrasonography in the surgical management of patients with thyroid cancer, *Surgery* 134:946, 2003.

McHenry CR, Slusarczyk SJ, Askari AT, and others: Refined use of scintigraphy in the evaluation of nodular thyroid disease. *Surgery* 124:656, 1998.

McHenry CR, Slusarczyk SJ, Khiyami A: Recommendations for management of cystic thyroid disease, *Surgery* 126:1167, 1999.

Mittendorf EA, McHenry CR: Follow-up evaluation and clinical course of patients with benign nodular thyroid disease, *Am Surg* 65:653, 1999.

Mittendorf EA, Tamarkin SW, McHenry CR: The results of ultrasound-guided fine-needle aspiration biopsy for evaluation of nodular thyroid disease, *Surgery* 132:648, 2002.

Xing M, Vasko V, Tallini G, and others: BRAF T1796A transversion mutation in various thyroid neoplasms, *J Clin Endocrinol Metab* 89:1365, 2004.

NONTOXIC GOITER

Martha A. Zeiger, MD

The word *goiter* is derived from the French (*goitre*) and Latin (*guttur*), both meaning throat. A goiter is defined as an enlargement of the thyroid gland and is considered endemic when it involves more than 10% of the population. For the majority of the world population, the presence of a goiter is secondary to iodine deficiency. The disorder is especially found in high mountain regions that are far from the ocean, such as the Himalayas and the Andes. In these regions and in lowlands away from the ocean, thyroid enlargement is believed to be secondary to goitrogens found in food staples such as maize, bamboo shoots, and sweet potatoes. The prevention of goiter was first conceived and demonstrated in 1921 with the introduction of salt iodination in Switzerland and the United States. In developing countries where salt is not often used, iodination of vegetable oil serves as a substitute. A goiter can be nontoxic and multinodular; it can be due to Graves' disease, Hashimoto's thyroiditis, de Quervain's thyroiditis, or Riedel's thyroiditis. The focus of this chapter is nontoxic goiter and its evaluation and treatment.

The first reported thyroidectomy performed was in Paris in 1791 by Pierre-Joseph Desault. Until the twentieth century, most patients undergoing thyroidectomy succumbed to either bleeding or infection. Indeed, the perioperative mortality was as high as 40% in the middle of the nineteenth century. It was only with the introduction of antisepsis, hemostasis, and general anesthesia in the 1840s that thyroid surgery became safe. One of the first surgeons to use anesthesia, antisepsis, and good hemostasis was Theodore Kocher from Bern, Switzerland, and his pioneering efforts in thyroid surgery resulted in a Nobel Prize in 1909. In the United States, William S. Halsted continued the tradition of improving the surgical technique involved in thyroidectomy in the 1880s and even designed instruments for this operation. Charles Mayo, George Crile, and Frank Lahey all continued the trend of decreasing the mortality and morbidity associated with thyroid surgery, making their greatest impact on the surgical management of Graves' disease.

In the evaluation of a multinodular goiter, it is important to ascertain whether the patient has local symptoms, whether the goiter is toxic or nontoxic, whether any of the nodules harbor a cancer, the number and bilaterality of the nodules, and appropriate treatment options for each particular patient. In taking a history, it is important to elicit whether the patient experiences a cough, shortness of breath, stridor, or hoarseness; whether the patient has had episodes suggesting choking or aspiration, dysphagia, or pain; and finally, whether the patient has cosmetic concerns. In determining whether the patient has a toxic or nontoxic goiter, signs and symptoms of hyperthyroidism can be usually be determined by history and physical examination. However, the sine qua non for the differential diagnosis of hypothyroidism or hyperthyroidism is serum thyroid stimulating hormone (TSH). In the examination of a patient with a goiter, it is important to determine whether the goiter is confined to the neck or whether it has a substernal component (Figs. 1 and 2); whether tracheal deviation is present; the size and consistency of the goiter; and the mobility of the vocal cords by either indirect or direct laryngoscopy.

Physical examination often reveals whether the patient has bilateral nodules. However, should there be any question in this regard, ultrasound is particularly useful in determining how many nodules there are, whether the nodules are bilateral, or whether they have suspicious ultrasound characteristics because these factors may affect the surgical approach. Additional and useful imaging includes computed tomography (CT) scan of the neck and chest, especially if the goiter is substernal. One must also be cognizant of the rare intrathoracic or aberrant thyroid, a congenital abnormality in which the blood supply arises from intrathoracic vessels and the thoracic thyroid is separate from the cervical thyroid. For these rare cases, the surgeon may have to perform a

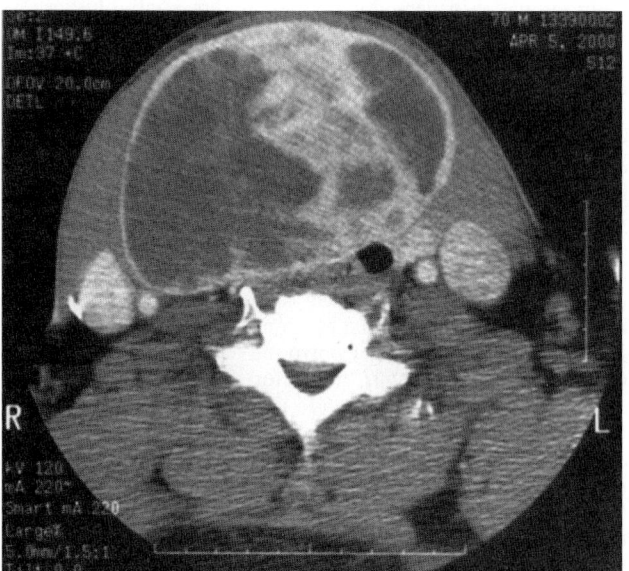

Figure 1 Massively enlarged goiter with marked tracheal deviation.

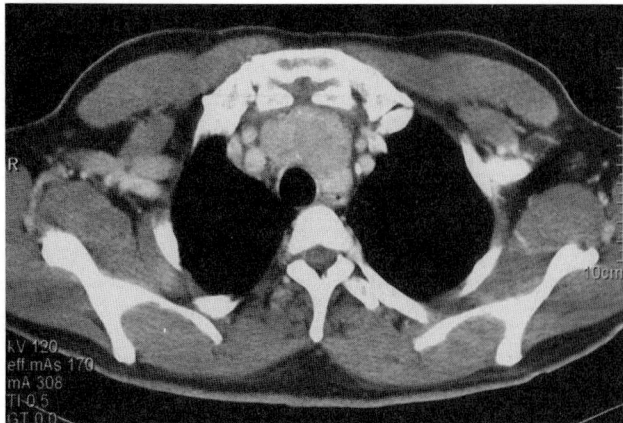

Figure 2 Goiter with a significant substernal component.

median sternotomy or a posterolateral thyroidectomy to gain access to the blood supply. Fine needle aspiration (FNA) in the evaluation of a multinodular goiter is important if the patient is to be managed medically or to determine whether the patient should have a thyroid lobectomy or total thyroidectomy. Any suspicious or malignant lesion should be addressed surgically. Tollin and others published a series of 61 patients with multinodular goiter and found 5% of nodules to be malignant on FNA, a percentage consistent with the overall rate of malignancy in solitary thyroid nodules.

What are treatment options for nontoxic thyroid goiter besides surgical resection? Some endocrinologists believe that thyroid hormone suppression may be indicated and useful. Others believe, especially in the high-risk patient, that radioiodine therapy is efficacious. Should the patient be symptomatic or should there be concern about a malignancy, surgery is generally recommended. Interestingly, a survey of the European Thyroid Association found 52% recommending thyroid hormone suppression, 67% radioiodine therapy, and 10% surgery, although they preferred the latter if the goiter was large or suspicious. Gharib and Mazzaferri summarized the literature from 1986 to 1996 that examined thyroxine suppression therapy for solitary and multinodular disease. They reported that only 10% to 20% of nodules actually respond to this treatment. Importantly, however, there is frequently a spontaneous decrease in the size of nodules. Furthermore, there is also no evidence that thyroxine therapy prevents the formation of new nodules. These authors therefore concluded that use of thyroxine-suppressive therapy should be discouraged. With regard to radioiodine therapy as a treatment option, Nygaard and others published their series of 69 patients treated with radioiodine, and of these, two thirds responded within 2 years with a 60% reduction in size. However, approximately 22% became hypothyroid, requiring thyroid hormone replacement. Less impressive were results from Le Moli and others, who reported on 50 patients, of whom three quarters responded but with only a 13% decrease in goiter volume; half required thyroid hormone replacement.

Should the patient require surgery, the standard surgical approach to thyroid operations generally suffices. The patient is placed in the semi–Fowler's position with the neck hyperextended, and a standard Kocher incision is performed. Superior and inferior platysmal flaps are created to thyroid cartilage and sternal notch, respectively. Rarely does the patient require a T-extension vertically to the sternal notch or an upper limited median sternotomy for a goiter that extends substernally. The strap muscles usually are divided longitudinally and reflected laterally. The strap muscles may also require division horizontally to deliver an especially large gland into the neck.

In general, most vessels can be ligated within the neck. A convenient and efficient technique includes hemoclipping the vessels on the specimen side and placing a tie on the patient side of the goiter. Other surgical techniques may include the use of a bipolar electrosealing device. For surgical closure the strap muscles are closed longitudinally with a running locking suture and closed transversely with interrupted figure of eight suture if they have been divided horizontally. The platysma is closed with interrupted suture, and the skin is closed with a subcuticular stitch. The patients are generally hospitalized overnight and are discharged on the following day after serum calcium has been checked. They are then begun on thyroid hormone replacement 3 to 4 days after surgery.

In summary, the majority of investigators and clinicians believe that surgery should be the first line of treatment for thyroid goiter if the patient is symptomatic, if there is a concern for malignancy, or for cosmetic reasons. If the patient is particularly high risk medically, radioiodine treatment can be considered. Following this, however, patients must be followed with regular serum TSH to be certain that they do not develop hypothyroidism.

SUGGESTED READINGS

Franko J, Kish KJ, Pezzi CM, and others: Safely increasing the efficiency of thyroidectomy using a new bipolar electrosealing device (Liga-Sure) versus conventional clamp-and-tie technique, *Am Surg* 72:132, 2006.

Gharib H, Mazzaferri EL: Thyroxine suppressive therapy in patients with nodular thyroid disease, *Ann Intern Med* 128:386, 2006.

Le Moli R, Wesche MF, Tiel-Van Buul MM, and others: Determinants of long-term outcome of radioiodine therapy of sporadic non-toxic goitre, *Clin Endocrinol (Oxf)* 50:783, 1999.

Nygaard B, Hegedus L, Gervil M, and others: Radioiodine treatment of multinodular non-toxic goitre, *BMJ* 307:828, 1993.

Tollin SR, Mery GM, Jelveh N, and others: The use of fine-needle aspiration biopsy under ultrasound guidance to assess the risk of malignancy in patients with a multinodular goiter, *Thyroid* 10:235, 2000.

THYROID CANCER

Rasa Zarnegar, MD, and Orlo H. Clark, MD

INTRODUCTION

Thyroid cancer is the most common endocrine malignancy, accounting for more than 95% of all endocrine cancers. In 2005, according to the American Cancer Society, there were 25,690 newly diagnosed cases, accounting for 1.5% of all new cancers and 1490 deaths. The Surveillance, Epidemiology, and End Results (SEER) program of the National Cancer Institute estimates the prevalence of thyroid cancer as 327,000 cases in the United States, which represents less than 0.1% of the population. Thyroid cancer is increasing faster than any other cancer in the United States at a rate of 4.3% per year. Although it is increasing in all ethnic groups, white males have shown the most rapid rise in new cases. The spectrum of thyroid cancer ranges from occult papillary thyroid carcinoma, which has a relatively benign course, to aggressive anaplastic thyroid carcinoma. Fortunately, more than 90% of all thyroid cancers are well differentiated, and individuals with these tumors have a good long-term prognosis.

The diagnosis, treatment, and follow-up for thyroid cancer is a rapidly evolving field as more sensitive imaging modalities such as ultrasound, fine needle aspiration (FNA), genetic testing, and serum markers begin to play roles. Several important techniques that have come to the forefront of diagnosis are ultrasound scanning of the neck preoperatively and postoperatively to evaluate and monitor the extent and persistence or recurrence of disease. Ultrasound-guided FNA of suspicious thyroid and neck nodules for diagnosis has increased the sensitivity of cancer detection. Serum markers, thyroglobulin (TG) for well-differentiated thyroid cancer, and calcitonin and carcinogenic embryonic antigen (CEA) for medullary thyroid cancer are also important and sensitive methods for detecting persistent or recurrent disease.

The extent of surgical treatment for thyroid cancer is a controversial topic. The goals of initial therapy for the management of thyroid cancer should include the following: (1) removal of primary tumor, disease that extends beyond the thyroid capsule, and involved cervical lymph nodes; (2) minimization of treatment- and disease-related morbidity; (3) accurate disease staging; (4) facilitation of postoperative treatment with radioiodine when appropriate; (5) accurate long-term surveillance; and (6) minimization of the risk of recurrent local and metastatic tumor. In this chapter, we highlight important steps in the diagnosis and treatment of thyroid cancer and address controversial issues.

CLINICAL PRESENTATION AND DIAGNOSIS

Most thyroid cancer patients present clinically with a palpable thyroid nodule. These are usually asymptomatic. In rare cases, patients present with hoarseness, pain, dysphagia, dyspnea, coughing, or choking spells. Pain associated with a malignant thyroid lesion should raise the suspicion for medullary thyroid carcinoma, anaplastic carcinoma, or lymphoma. Virtually all patients who present with cervical lymphadenopathy caused by metastatic tumor have an ipsilateral thyroid cancer, and in 20%, the primary thyroid cancer is nonpalpable.

Although clinically apparent thyroid cancer is relatively uncommon, clinically unapparent or occult thyroid cancer is common. We define an occult thyroid cancer as a lesion under 10 mm that is an unexpected and incidental finding during thyroidectomy or autopsy. The prevalence of occult thyroid cancer at autopsy in the United States averages 3.6%.

In evaluating patients for thyroid cancers, clinical history and physical examination remain the cornerstone of appropriate management. Pertinent historical factors predicting malignancy include a history of head and neck irradiation; total body irradiation for bone marrow transplantation; exposure to fallout from the explosion of the Chernobyl nuclear power plant in 1986, especially in children; a family history of thyroid cancer; and rapid growth or hoarseness. Children, men, and adults older than 60 years have an increased risk of malignancy. Personal and family history of other endocrine disorders, specifically hyperparathyroidism, pituitary adenomas, pancreatic islet cell tumors, adrenal tumors, and breast cancer increase the risk of thyroid cancer. A family history of papillary or medullary carcinoma (multiple endocrine neoplasia [MEN] syndromes), familial polyposis, Gardner's syndrome, and Cowden's syndrome are also risk factors for thyroid cancer.

With the discovery of a thyroid nodule, a physical examination focusing on the thyroid gland and adjacent cervical lymph nodes should be performed. Pertinent physical findings suggesting possible malignancy include a "gritty texture" of the thyroid nodule, cervical lymphadenopathy, vocal cord paralysis, and fixation of the nodule to surrounding tissue. Patients presenting with hoarseness or patients planned for reoperation should have a direct laryngoscopy before any surgical intervention to document the function of the vocal cords.

High-resolution thyroid ultrasonography has become an extension of the physical examination in the evaluation of thyroid disease. With a high-frequency transducer of 10 to 13 MHz, nodules as small as 2 mm can be detected in the thyroid. As technology improves, the haunting prospect that thyroid nodules could be imaged in more than half the population aged older than 50 years is becoming a clinical reality. Recent investigations have documented that three sonographic features were significant independent risk factors for malignancy: irregular margins, intranodular vascular pattern, and microcalcifications.

FNA biopsy (FNAB) is the most reliable and cost-efficient method for evaluating thyroid nodules. These should now routinely be performed under ultrasound guidance for small or difficult-to-palpate or complex nodules to reduce failure rates. Using ultrasound criteria, FNAB of the most suspicious nodules, not the largest nodules, has the highest predictive value for detecting malignancy. FNAB is not as accurate in radiation-induced thyroid cancer or in patients with a family history of thyroid cancer; these patients should undergo surgical resection if there is clinical suspicion of malignancy. An algorithm for the evaluation of thyroid nodules is shown in Figure 1.

Preoperatively, all patients should therefore undergo ultrasound examination of the thyroid gland and cervical lymph nodes, as well

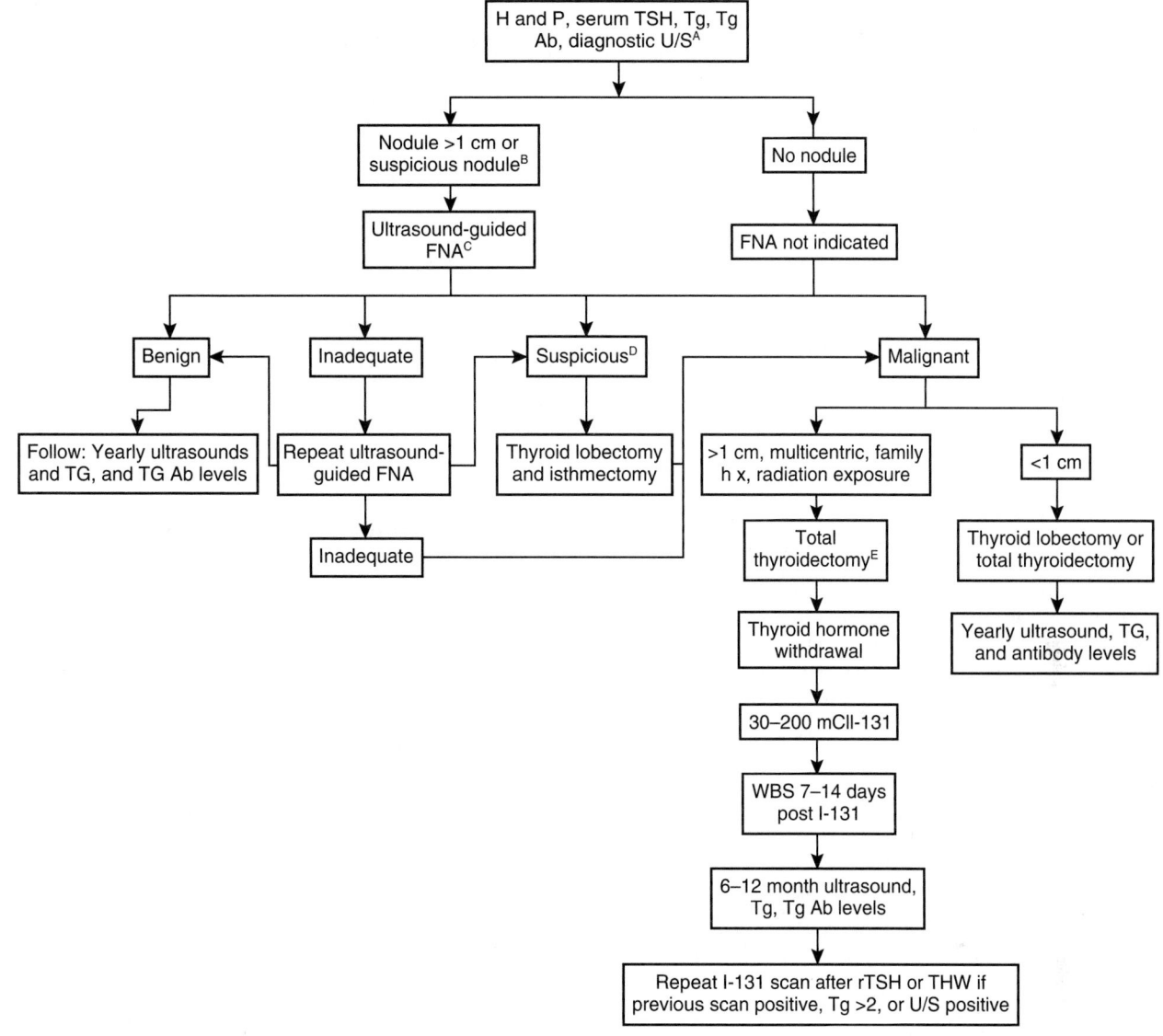

Figure 1 Algorithm for the evaluation and treatment of patients with one or more thyroid nodules. *(A)* Patients with family history of thyroid cancer or history of exposure to a low-dose therapeutic and who have a thyroid nodule have an approximately 40% risk of thyroid cancer, and thus a total or near total thyroidectomy is recommended. *(B)* A suspicious nodule has irregular borders, increased vascular flow, and microcalcifications. *(C)* For nodules suspicious for papillary thyroid cancer, repeat fine needle aspiration or frozen section may be helpful, but these procedures are not recommended for follicular and Hurthle cell neoplasms. *(D)* Total or near total thyroidectomy is recommended.

as thyroid function tests. When differentiated, thyroid cancer is suspected or proved on a serum thyroglobulin, and antithyroglobulin antibody levels and blood calcium levels should be obtained. In the case of medullary thyroid cancer, serum calcitonin, CEA, and calcium levels should be obtained. All patients with medullary thyroid cancer should also be tested for the RET proto-oncogene and evaluated for pheochromocytoma and hyperparathyroidism before surgery.

WELL-DIFFERENTIATED THYROID CARCINOMA

Papillary Thyroid Carcinoma

Papillary thyroid cancer is the most common endocrine malignancy and has accounted for approximately 80% of new cases of thyroid cancer in the United States. Papillary thyroid cancers, including

mixed papillary follicular thyroid cancer, follicular variant of thyroid cancer, and diffuse sclerosing papillary thyroid cancer, are associated with the best prognosis. It is somewhat surprising that patients with papillary thyroid cancer, especially young patients, do so well because most of these tumors are multifocal (<80%), and cervical lymph nodes are common, at least microscopically, in up to 80% of cases. Some patients have poorly differentiated papillary thyroid cancer, including tall-cell and columnar tumors, and these patients have a worse prognosis.

Papillary thyroid cancer is at least twice as common in women as men and has a peak age of presentation of 38 to 45 years. This tumor also accounts for 90% of radiation-induced thyroid cancer and is familial in 5% of patients.

Patients can be separated into low- and high-risk groups on the basis of patient age, grade of tumor, and extent and size of tumor (AGES); age, metastases, extent, and size (AMES); or metastasis, age, completeness of resection, local invasion, and tumor size (MACIS) (Table 1). Other classification systems include the TNM

Table 1: Classification of Low-versus High-Risk Patients Using the AGES System

Variable	Low Risk	High Risk
Age	Women <50 years Men <40 years	Women > 50 years Men > 40 years
Grade	Well differentiated	Poorly differentiated Fibrous struma Insular, mucoid, columnar, and tall-cell variant
Extent	Confined to the thyroid	Invasive to adjacent tissues or distant metastases
Size	Tumor with maximal diameter <4 cm	Tumor with maximal diameter >4 cm

AGES, Patient age and grade, extent, and size of tumor.

Table 2: AJCC Staging System for Papillary and Follicular Thyroid Carcinoma

Definition	
T1	Tumor diameter 2 cm or smaller
T2	Primary tumor diameter > 2 to 4 cm
T3	Primary tumor diameter > 4 cm limited to the thyroid or with minimal extrathyroidal extension
T4$_a$	Tumor of any size extending beyond the thyroid capsule to invade subcutaneous soft tissues, larynx, trachea, esophagus, or recurrent laryngeal nerve
T4$_b$	Tumor invades prevertebral fascia or encases carotid artery or mediastinal vessels
TX	Primary tumor size unknown, but without extrathyroidal invasion
N0	No metastatic nodes
N1$_a$	Metastases to level VI (pretracheal, paratracheal, and prelaryngeal/Delphian lymph nodes)
N1$_b$	Metastasis to unilateral, bilateral, contralateral cervical or superior mediastinal mode metastases
NX	Nodes not assessed at surgery
M0	No distant metastases
M1	Distant metastases
MX	Distant metastases not assessed

Stages	Patient Age < 45 Years	Patient Aged 45 Years or Older
Stage I	Any T, and N, M0	T1, N0, M0
Stage II	Any T, any N, M1	T2, N0, M0
Stage III		T3, N0, M0 T1, N1$_a$, M0 T2, N1$_a$, M0 T3, N1$_a$, M0
Stage IVA		T4$_a$, N0, M0 T4$_a$, N1$_a$, M0 T1, N1$_b$, M0 T2, N1$_b$, M0 T3, N1$_b$, M0 T4$_a$, N1$_b$, M0
Stage IVB		T4$_b$, Any N, M0
Stage IVC		Any T, Any N, M1

Used with permission of the American Joint Committee on Cancer (AJCC), Chicago, IL. The original source for this material is the *AJCC Cancer Staging Manual*, ed 6, New York, 2002, Springer-Verlag.
From *AJCC cancer staging manual, ed 6, New York, 2002, Springer Verlag*.

(Table 2), the European Organization for the Research and Treatment of Cancer (EORTC), and others. Unfortunately, all the classification systems are based on postoperative findings. These classifications help predict tumor behavior, however, because the risk of death from thyroid cancer in the low-risk group is approximately 5% versus the high-risk group at 40%. Fortunately, most patients (70%) are in the low-risk group. Other histological factors that predict the behavior of thyroid cancer include (1) ploidy of the tumor, (2) adenylate cyclase response to thyroid stimulating hormone (TSH), (3) radioiodine uptake, (4) a positive positron emission tomography scan, and (5) epidermal growth factor (EGF) receptor level and various gene profiles.

The extent of surgical resection for papillary thyroid cancer is controversial. We recommend a total or near total thyroidectomy (Fig. 2) and selective nodal resection when postoperative treatment with iodine-131 (I-131) is considered. Low-risk patients, who have papillary thyroid cancer of less than 1 cm, can be treated by thyroid lobectomy and isthmectomy; reoperation is generally not indicated unless the tumor is multifocal, associated with nodal metastases, or with local invasion. Total thyroidectomy has a complication rate of less than 2% when performed by surgeons experienced in this field and has been shown to be associated with fewer recurrences and improved survival. Surgeons who advocate lobectomy and isthmectomy for low-risk patients cite the recurrence rate of less than 5% in the thyroid bed, which can be cured surgically, and the increased risk of complications with more extensive operations. However, the distinct benefits of total thyroidectomy include (1) the thyroid tissue is removed so that postoperative radioiodine scanning and ablative therapy can be effective, (2) serum thyroglobulin levels are rendered more sensitive for detecting recurrent or persistent disease, (3) intrathyroidal cancer that is present in more than 50% of patients is removed, and (4) the small risk of a differentiated thyroid cancer becoming an undifferentiated cancer is decreased.

The role of lymph node dissection in papillary thyroid cancer and the prognostic importance of nodal metastases are also controversial. Micrometastasis to cervical lymph nodes is common in papillary thyroid cancer (80%). The indolent course of most of these metastases provides evidence that prophylactic cervical lymph node dissection is not warranted. Routine preoperative ultrasonography of the neck detects suspicious nodal disease. Therefore functional neck dissection and central neck dissection should generally be performed only in patients with clinical or sonographic evidence of lymph node involvement. Intraoperative enlarged lymph nodes in the central and lateral neck should be removed and submitted for frozen section. If positive, a formal lymph node dissection should be undertaken. Formal lymph node dissection is preferable to "berry picking" because it is associated with a lower incidence of subsequent recurrent disease. It also helps to minimize the need for repeat surgery for recurrent lymph node metastases, which can be difficult in a scarred operative field. Some expert surgeons routinely perform a central node dissection as part of the initial operation, irrespective of sonographic findings, to reduce the risk of recurrent disease in the central neck, leading to repeat surgery. We are concerned that such treatment may increase the frequency of hypoparathyroidism. Recurrence of papillary thyroid cancer can occur anytime during the patients' lifetime, thus lifelong surveillance is required. Unfortunately approximately one third of patients who develop recurrent thyroid cancer eventually die from it.

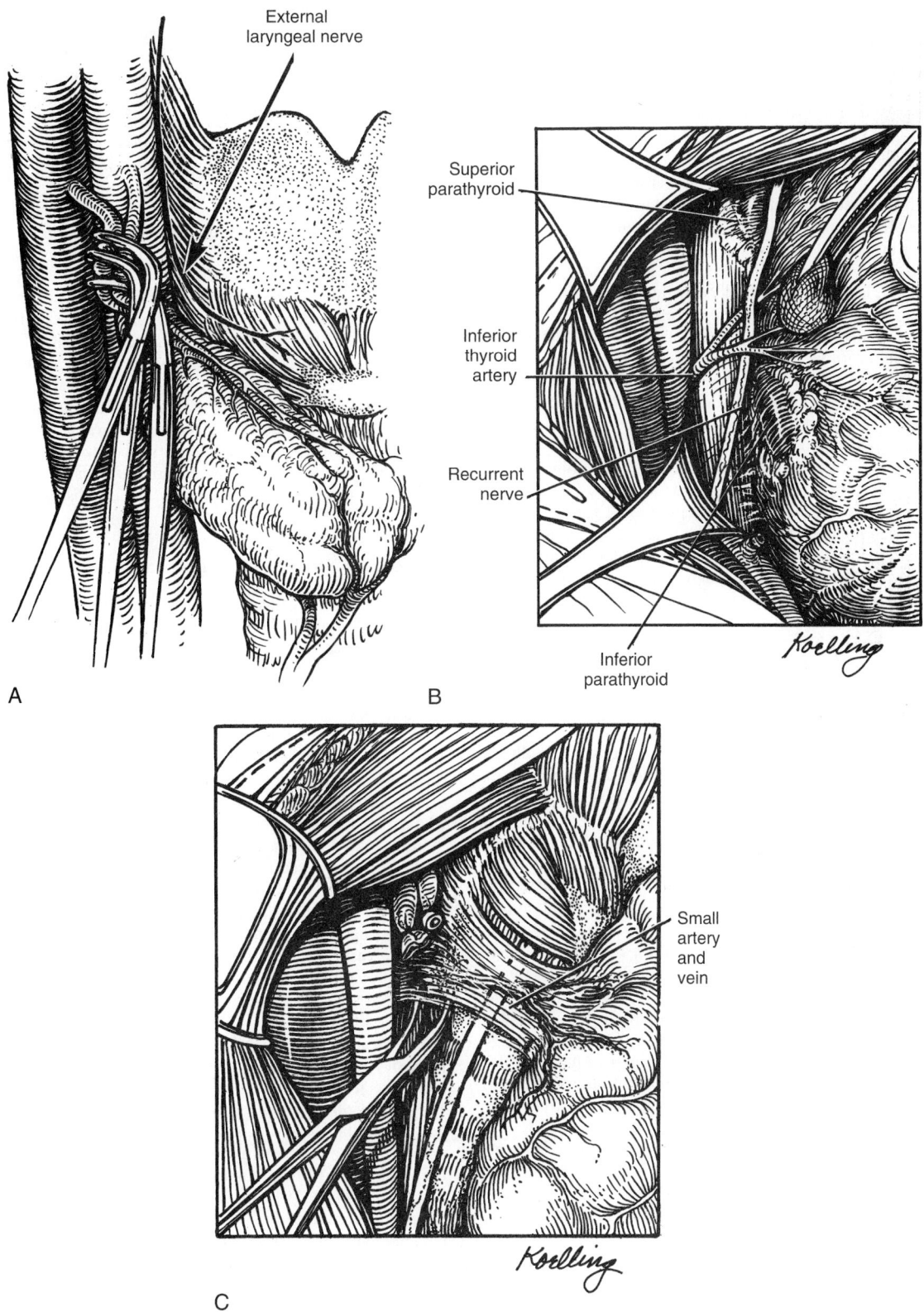

Figure 2 Thyroidectomy: **(A)** Superior pole, **(B)** the lateral dissection and the recurrent laryngeal nerve, and **(C)** the ligament of Berry. *From Clark OH: Endocrine surgery of the thyroid and parathyroid glands, St. Louis, 1985, Mosby.*

Follicular Thyroid Carcinoma

Follicular cancer accounts for approximately 10% of all thyroid malignancies. Although follicular thyroid cancer can occur in any age group, these patients are typically older than are patients with papillary thyroid cancer group, usually in the sixth decade of life. As with papillary thyroid cancer, the female-to-male ratio is between 2:1 and 5:1.

Follicular thyroid cancer usually presents as a slowly growing solitary thyroid nodule. Occasionally it also exhibits local symptoms. Rarely patients with follicular cancer present with symptoms of distant metastasis to the bone, lung, brain, and liver because these tumors, unlike papillary cancers, have a tendency to spread hematogenously. Less than 6% of follicular thyroid cancers metastasize to the cervical lymph nodes. Approximately 25% of patients have extrathyroidal invasion, and 10% to 33% have distant metastasis at the time of initial diagnosis.

The prognosis of follicular cancer is slightly worse than that for papillary cancer. Depending on the stage of the patient at presentation, overall survival ranges from 43% to 95% at 10 years. However, unlike patients with papillary thyroid cancers, those with follicular thyroid cancer who have not experienced recurrence within 12 years of their initial operation are usually cured. Therefore lifelong surveillance is not necessary. The important prognostic factors include the following: (1) presence of metastatic disease (2) older age (usually >40 years), (3) degree of invasion (microcapsular vs. angioinvasion with or without capsular and widely invasive), and (4) degree of tumor differentiation. The staging of follicular cancer is based on the TNM staging system of thyroid cancer (Table 2).

Without evidence of metastatic disease, it is difficult preoperatively to determine whether a patient with a solitary thyroid nodule has follicular cancer. These patients usually have undergone FNAB. However, FNAB is unable to distinguish benign from malignant follicular neoplasms because this technique evaluates cellular features. Approximately 20% of patients with FNAB consistent with follicular neoplasm have cancer. To distinguish benign from malignant follicular neoplasm, the whole specimen must be evaluated for vascular and capsular invasion.

Because the diagnosis of follicular cancer cannot be made on FNAB, the recommended initial operation is lobectomy and isthmectomy. Frozen sections are usually of limited utility in determination of malignancy. However, careful gross evaluation, attention to the clinical situation, and judicious use of frozen section analysis may make the need for total thyroidectomy apparent at the initial operation. If the tumor has evidence of vascular invasion or is widely invasive on final pathology, the patient should undergo a completion thyroidectomy. The clinical importance of capsular invasion is more controversial; some centers will and others will not perform a completion thyroidectomy if the patient has minimal capsular invasion. During the initial thyroid operation, usually thyroid lobectomy, the surgeon should not manipulate the contralateral lobe, thus leaving this an unviolated field and making the completion thyroidectomy easier and with less risk of complication. Lymph node dissection is rarely warranted because nodal metastases are uncommon.

Hurthle Cell Carcinoma

Hurthle cell cancer accounts for approximately 3% of all thyroid cancers. As with follicular cancer, it has a peak incidence in the fifth and sixth decades. The female-to-male ratios range from 2:1 to 10:1. Men with Hurthle cell neoplasms have a higher relative risk of malignancy. Previous radiation exposure has been correlated with an increase in bilateralism and multicentricity of Hurthle cell neoplasms, as well as an increased incidence of contralateral non–Hurthle cell malignant thyroid lesions. Radiation exposure, age, and familial Hurthle cell tumors are associated with an increased risk

of these neoplasms. The 10-year survival of Hurthle cell carcinoma is 70%. The cause-specific 20-year mortality for this carcinoma has been reported to range from 20% to 35%. Prognosis generally depends on extent of disease at the initial diagnosis and the extent of resection. The TNM staging system for thyroid cancer is used for classification of Hurthle cell carcinoma (Table 2).

Most patients with Hurthle cell neoplasms present with a solitary nodule. FNAB can reliably diagnose these neoplasms, but similar to follicular neoplasms, it cannot determine malignancy, which occurs in 35% of patients. Malignancy is determined by capsular or vascular invasion. In patients presenting with malignant lesions, 70% to 80% are confined to the gland, 10% to 20% have lymph node metastasis, and 15% have distant metastasis, most commonly to bone or lung.

Careful surgical exploration should always be undertaken to detect the presence of obvious malignant disease. In patients with obvious malignant disease or contralateral nodular disease, or in patients with a history of childhood head and neck radiation, a one-stage total thyroidectomy is the preferred approach. For the routine patient with a solitary nodule, surgical management should consist of lobectomy and isthmectomy. Frozen section is inherently unreliable in Hurthle cell neoplasm, similar to follicular neoplasm, and should be used judiciously. Lymph node dissection is indicated only for clinically or sonographically evident disease.

Medullary Thyroid Carcinoma

Medullary thyroid cancer (MTC) accounts for 7% of thyroid cancers and 15% of all thyroid cancer–related deaths. Approximately 75% of the cases are sporadic, and 25% are hereditary. These tumors originate from c cells or parafollicular cells and may be associated with c-cell hyperplasia. Because of the location of the parafollicular cells, these tumors are almost always located laterally at the junction of the upper two thirds of the thyroid gland at approximately the level of the cricoid cartilage. In the sporadic form, there is usually a single focus of malignancy and unilateral disease in 85% of cases, compared with the hereditary form, in which the disease is multifocal and bilateral in 90% of cases and there is c-cell hyperplasia.

MTC is associated with the RET proto-oncogene mutation. The hereditary forms of MTC are MEN 2A, MEN 2B, and familial MTC (FMTC). These causes of MTC all have point mutations in the RET proto-oncogene. A diagnosis of isolated FMTC is made when three or more cases are identified in a family without other associated endocrinopathies. Ten percent of patients with apparent sporadic MTC also have a de novo mutation in the RET proto-oncogene. Thus all patients with MTC should be RET proto-oncogene tested. Genetic testing and surgical treatment should begin no later than 5 years of age in MEN 2A and soon after birth in MEN 2B.

In the absence of a family history of MTC, no clues distinguish MTC from other thyroid pathology. The diagnosis is usually suspected on the basis of characteristic cytological features and the presence of immunostaining for calcitonin on FNAB specimen. Blood testing for calcitonin and CEA may also be informative. After the diagnosis of MTC is made, it is important to screen the patients for pheochromocytoma and hyperparathyroidism because 20% of patients have these associated conditions.

In the presence of a history of hereditary MTC, the workup is more extensive. MEN 2 and its characteristic clinical presentations are shown in Table 3. It is important to screen patients for these associated clinical syndromes. MEN 2A is the most common syndrome, accounting for two thirds of the patients with familial MTC. Pheochromocytoma and hyperparathyroidism are expressed in 42% and 35% of cases, respectively. MEN 2B is associated with pheochromocytoma in 50% and neural gangliomas in 100% of cases. Patients with MEN 2B also exhibit skeletal abnormalities (Marfanoid-like body habitus), poor dentition, mucosal neuromas, enlarged nerves, and megacolon.

Table 3: Multiple Endocrine Neoplasia 2 and Its Clinical Variants and Syndromes

Syndrome	Characteristic Features
MEN2A	MTC
	Adrenal medulla (pheochromocytoma)
	Parathyroid glands
FMTC	MTC
MEN2A with cutaneous lichenamyloidosis	MEN2A and a pruritic cutaneous lesion located over the upper back
MEN2A or FMTC with Hirschsprung's disease	MEN2A or FMTC with Hirschsprung's disease
MEN2B	MTC
	Adrenal medulla (pheochromocytoma)
	Intestinal and mucosal ganglioneuromatosis
	Characteristic habitus, marfanoid

Lymph node metastases are positive in 70% of patients with palpable disease. Moley and colleagues showed that with palpable unilateral MTC, 81% of patients had central node disease, 81% had ipsilateral cervical node disease, and 44% had contralateral cervical nodal disease. In patients with bilateral MTC, 78% had central node disease, 71% had ipsilateral cervical node disease, and 49% had contralateral cervical node disease.

Serum markers for calcitonin support the diagnosis and correlate with tumor bulk, nodal, and distant metastasis. A calcitonin level greater than 1000 pg/ml after total thyroidectomy with no evidence of recurrence in the neck invariably indicates the presence of distant metastases (usually micrometastases in the liver). Some surgeons perform a diagnostic laparoscopy during the original operation to document liver disease in these patients because the liver is the most common site of MTC metastases. MTC can also metastasize to the lung and bone. High CEA levels correlate with a poorer prognosis. Patients with flushing and diarrhea also have a worse prognosis, as do patients with MEN 2B.

Prevention or cure of MTC is by surgery, and success is mainly dependent on the initial stage of the disease and the adequacy of the initial operation. Therefore surgeries for MTC should be performed in RET-positive patients with familial disease before the age of possible malignant progression. Current studies support the need for total thyroidectomy before age 6. Skinner and colleagues showed that for RET-positive patients who are younger than age 6 and are ultrasound and calcitonin negative, a prophylactic central neck dissection is not necessary. Delay necessitates nodal resection and exposes these patients to an unacceptably high risk of metastatic MTC, which may preclude biochemical cure. The goal is to perform thyroidectomy before basal and stimulated calcitonin levels become elevated.

Surgical management for MTC depends on the presentation of the disease. Children with MEN 2B or RET codon mutations 883, 918, or 922 (or a combination of these) are classified as high risk and should have their thyroidectomy and central node dissection before 1 year of age or at diagnosis in those with an increased calcitonin. If metastases are identified, a more extensive node dissection may be appropriate. Children with MEN 2A and familial MTC without other endocrinopathies should have a total thyroidectomy and central node dissection by age 5. In sporadic MTC, a routine ipsilateral central and lateral functional lymph node dissection should be performed. Current recommendations on the treatment of occult MTC are reoperation and neck dissection with an elevated basal or stimulated pentagastrin, microcarcinomas >5 mm in diameter, or when it is difficult to ensure prolonged follow-up for the patient.

Central lymph node dissections increase the risk of recurrent laryngeal nerve injury and hypoparathyroidism. If the vascular supply to a parathyroid is disrupted, it should be autotransplanted into the sternocleidomastoid or, in patients with MEN 2A, into the nondominant forearm because the latter patients are more likely to develop graft-dependent hyperparathyroidism. If a patient with MEN 2A has associated hyperparathyroidism, the abnormal parathyroid gland(s) should be removed selectively. All normal parathyroid glands should be marked. Some of the abnormal parathyroid glands should be cryopreserved to decrease the risk of permanent hypoparathyroidism. If the parathyroid tumor is possibly the last parathyroid gland, it should be autotransplanted to the nondominant forearm. Approximately 95% of the autografts generally function adequately within 4 to 6 weeks.

In patients with recurrent MTC, a decision regarding reoperation must be made. Reoperations are usually palliative in that the blood calcitonin level rarely becomes undetectable. As a rule, more extensive initial operative therapy and a meticulous lymph node dissection of all compartments of the neck and perhaps the mediastinum are necessary for cure. MTC is not amenable to radioiodine therapy, and other adjuvant therapy is performed only in clinical trials. Several clinical trials are currently available for patients with MTC.

Several recent reports document that a faster calcitonin doubling time correlates with a poorer prognosis. When calcitonin-doubling times are less than 6 months, patients had a 10-year survival of 8% compared with 100% when the doubling time was longer than 2 years.

Anaplastic Thyroid Carcinoma

Fortunately anaplastic thyroid cancer (ATC) is a rare tumor, accounting for 1% to 2% of thyroid malignancies in the United States. Unlike well-differentiated thyroid cancer, ATC is invariably lethal and accounts for more than half of the deaths from thyroid cancer. Survival is measured in months. ATC occurs most commonly within well-differentiated thyroid cancer; this transformation occurs in approximately 1% of patients with differentiated cancers. ATC occurs most commonly in patients older than 60 years and usually presents as a rapidly expanding thyroid mass that is firm to hard and frequently fixed. The tumor may compress the trachea and infiltrate the skin, causing overlying necrosis. Lymph node enlargement is frequent (84%) and early. Local tumor extension can cause fixation of the larynx, esophagus, and carotid vessels. Patients can present with hoarseness because of vocal cord paralysis resulting from direct extension. Symptoms such as dysphagia, dysphonia, and dyspnea are common. Systemic metastases occur in 75% of patients, usually involving the lungs, bone, brain, and adrenal glands.

The diagnosis of ATC can be established by FNAB. The diagnosis of ATC must be differentiated from that of lymphoma and poorly differentiated medullary carcinoma, and appropriate immunophenotyping and other marker examinations may be required.

The standard form of treatment of thyroid cancer has been complete tumor removal, but in ATC, this maneuver is usually not curative because many patients present with distant metastases. Multimodality treatment seems to have slightly improved outcomes. The Swedish group from the Karolinska Medical Center indicated that multimodality treatment consisting of radiation, chemotherapy, and then surgery, followed by further radiation and chemotherapy, provides the best results, and we have used this approach. Besides tumor resection, tracheostomy may be indicated for advanced disease.

The outcomes of most trials using multimodal therapy indicate local control in 22% to 76% of patients. However, median survival ranges from 2.5 to 9 months, with 2-year survival of less than 20%. Factors favoring prolonged survival included younger age (<45 years), female, tumors smaller than 6 cm, disease confined to the neck, and complete resection. Unfortunately, the current treatments still have a limited role in the management of ATC because the majority of patients die within months of their diagnosis from local invasion or distant metastases.

Lymphoma

Primary lymphomas of the thyroid are rare, accounting for only 1% to 2% of thyroid malignancies and less than 2% of extranodal lymphomas. Most thyroid lymphomas are non–Hodgkin's B-cell lymphomas, although Hodgkin's disease of the thyroid has been described. Thyroid lymphomas are predominantly associated with Hashimoto's thyroiditis and may be histologically difficult to distinguish from this chronic lymphocytic disease. The relative risk of lymphoma in these patients is 70 to 80 times higher than general population control individuals.

Most patients present with a several-week history of a rapidly enlarging goiter and respiratory difficulty. Typically the patients are female in their seventh decade of life with a long-standing history of Hashimoto's thyroiditis. It is usually painless and often associated with hoarseness and dysphagia. Less commonly patients may present with tracheal compression. On physical examination, patients usually have a firm thyroid either unilateral or bilateral with possible fixation to adjacent structures. Lymphadenopathy is common.

Clinically primary lymphoma poses a diagnostic and therapeutic challenge because it can present in a fashion similar to ATC. As a result, it is essential to distinguish these two entities because they have different therapeutic and prognostic implications. FNAB has helped distinguish these two conditions preoperatively and has decreased the need for open biopsy. Up to 88% of thyroid lymphomas are diagnosed on FNA alone, although core needle biopsy or open surgical biopsy may be warranted. Staging for lymphoma is shown in Table 4.

Surgery plays a limited role in thyroid lymphoma unless the diagnosis is not established. Thyroid lymphomas have been shown to be both radiosensitive and chemosensitive; therefore most current recommendations are to treat these tumors with a combined modality therapy. Doxorubicin-based combination chemotherapy deceases the chance of distant metastasis. In B-cell lymphoma of mucosa-associated lymphoid tissue (MALT) of the thyroid, radiation alone has resulted in a 96% complete response, with only a 30% relapse rate.

Advanced stage of the tumor, size greater than 10 cm, mediastinal involvement, and the presence of dysphagia are poor prognostic factors. Most recurrences occur within the first 4 years. The overall survival for primary thyroid lymphoma is 50% to 70%, ranging from 80% in stage IE to less than 36% in stage IIE and IVE in 5 years.

Table 4: Staging for Thyroid Lymphoma

Stage IE	Localized disease within the thyroid
Stage IIE	Disease confined to thyroid and regional lymph nodes
Stage IIIE	Disease on both sides of diaphragm
Stage IVE	Disseminated disease

LONG-TERM FOLLOW-UP FOR PATIENTS WITH THYROID CANCER

Well-Differentiated Thyroid Cancer

Papillary thyroid cancer recurs or persists in approximately 25% of patients, and 80% of these recurrences are in the neck. Recurrence occurs most commonly in the first 2 years after thyroidectomy. In papillary thyroid cancer, however, recurrence can occur up to 45 years after surgery, whereas virtually all patients with follicular and Hurthle cell cancer recur before 12 years after surgery.

The current recommendations for postoperative follow-up of well-differentiated thyroid cancer, except for particularly low-risk patients, are thyroid remnant ablation and TSH suppression. Radioiodine ablation is recommended for patients with papillary thyroid cancers larger than 1.5 cm, multifocal tumors, and for those with lymph node metastases. Invasive follicular and Hurthle cell cancer also warrant radioiodine therapy. We routinely use 30 to 50 mCi of radioiodine in low-risk patients and 100 to 200 mCi of radioiodine in high-risk patients. The initial radioiodine treatment should be performed under hormone withdrawal 6 to 8 weeks postoperatively in an iodine-deficient patient. Patients should have a TSH; thyroglobulin; and, if pregnancy is a possibility, a pregnancy test before I-131 scanning and ablation therapy, as well as posttreatment imaging.

TSH is known to stimulate tumor growth, invasion, angiogenesis, and thyroglobulin secretion. Therefore patients are placed postoperatively on thyroid hormone at a dosage of approximately 1 mg/lb. In low-risk patients, we maintain the serum TSH level just below the lower limit of the normal range between 0.1 and 0.4 mU/ml. In high-risk patients, the dosage is adjusted to maintain a serum TSH level less than 0.1 mU/ml because this has been reported to improve tumor-free survival. Adverse effects of TSH suppression may include the known consequences of subclinical thyrotoxicosis, including exacerbation of angina, atrial fibrillation, and osteoporosis in postmenopausal women.

External beam radiation and chemotherapy have a limited role in the postoperative management of thyroid cancer patients. External beam radiation is used infrequently in the management of thyroid cancer except as a palliative treatment for locally advanced unresectable disease, positive tumor margins, or recurrent disease after re-resection. Chemotherapy has shown only minimal benefit in the treatment of well-differentiated thyroid cancer. New clinical trials have recently become available.

Follow-up is different for patients at low, intermediate, and high risk of having persistent or recurrent disease. Low-risk patients are defined as patients with no local or distant metastases; complete resection of tumor contained within the thyroid with no locoregional invasion; tumor without aggressive histology; and, if radioiodine was given, no uptake outside of the thyroid bed. Intermediate-risk patients have microscopic invasion of tumor into the perithyroidal soft tissue at initial surgery or tumor with aggressive histology or vascular invasion. High-risk patients have macroscopic tumor invasion, incomplete tumor resection, distant metastases, or radioiodine uptake outside the thyroid bed on the posttreatment scan after thyroid remnant ablation.

The absence of persistent disease in patients who have undergone at least a total thyroidectomy and thyroid remnant ablation comprises no clinical evidence of tumor, no imaging evidence of tumor, and undetectable serum thyroglobulin levels during TSH suppression and stimulation in the absence of interfering antibodies.

All patients with a history of well-differentiated thyroid cancer should have yearly cervical ultrasound scanning, as well as thyroglobulin and thyroglobulin antibody levels. Approximately 20% of patients who are clinically disease free with serum thyroglobulin levels less than 2 ng/ml during thyroid hormone suppression will have a thyroglobulin level greater than 5 ng/ml after recombinant human TSH (rhTSH) or thyroid hormone withdrawal. One third of this group will have persistent disease identified on imaging studies. Therefore a serum thyroglobulin level above 5 ng/ml after rhTSH stimulation is highly sensitive in identifying patients with persistent disease. Furthermore, the clinical significance of minimally detectable thyroglobulin levels is unclear, especially if only detected after TSH stimulation. Twenty-five percent of patients with thyroid cancer have antithyroglobulin antibodies, and follow-up with thyroglobulin will be insensitive. In this group, serial serum antithyroglobulin antibody measurements may serve as an imprecise surrogate marker to detect recurrence.

The current guidelines for the long-term follow-up of patients with well-differentiated thyroid cancer are shown in Figure 1. Accurate surveillance for possible recurrence and treatment in patients thought to be free of disease is a major goal of long-term follow-up.

Medullary Thyroid Cancer

Blood calcitonin monitoring is the most sensitive test to identify persistent recurrent tumor in patients with MTC. Patients may have locoregional or distant metastasis as their primary site of recurrence. Ultrasound of the neck by an experienced ultrasonographer is the most sensitive method for identifying residual disease. If the plasma calcitonin is not elevated, patients should continue to undergo basal and provocative testing annually for 5 years. Calcitonin levels in the normal range after total thyroidectomy suggest persistent disease. Calcitonin levels greater than 1000 pg/ml indicate distant metastasis. Chemotherapy plays a limited role in advanced surgically unamenable MTC in clinical trials. Radioiodine may play a role for destroying residual normal thyroid tissue and for patients with mixed tumors of follicular and parafollicular cell origin. Its role is still controversial, however. New clinical trials are currently available.

SURGICAL APPROACHES FOR THYROID CANCER

Thyroid Lobectomy and Isthmectomy: Total Thyroidectomy and Thyroid Lobectomy and Isthmectomy

Total thyroidectomy is the operation of choice for well-differentiated thyroid cancer. In minimally invasive (capsular invasive) follicular and occult papillary thyroid cancers, a more limited initial operation is a thyroid lobectomy and isthmectomy.

During a total thyroidectomy, the patient is placed in the supine position with the arms tucked and the neck extended. The patient is then positioned with the head up (at 30 degrees). After skin preparation, an incision is placed in a natural skin fold (Zeus line in men, Venus line in women). These lines are areas with the least tension, allowing for better scar healing. Ideally this line is one fingerbreadth below the cricoid cartilage, which centers it over the middle of the thyroid gland. After the skin incision is made, usually 3 to 5 cm, skin flaps are mobilized superiorly to the thyroid cartilage and inferiorly to the sternal notch. The median raphe is then opened along its vertical course, and the muscle plane between the sternohyoid and sternothyroid muscle is opened medial to lateral until the ansa cervicalis is identified laterally. The sternothyroid is then mobilized off the thyroid gland. It is important to start the dissection on the side of the primary tumor. After mobilization of the sternothyroid,

the carotid artery is identified laterally and retracted. The dissection is carried bluntly medial to the carotid artery superiorly to identify the superior pole vessels. These are taken close to the thyroid gland, after retracting the thyroid laterally and caudally, to avoid injury to the external laryngeal nerve. After mobilization of the superior pole, the dissection is continued laterally and inferiorly. During these steps, it is important to identify the recurrent laryngeal nerve and the parathyroid glands. The recurrent laryngeal nerve runs in the tracheoesophageal groove on the left and is deep to the inferior parathyroids and medial to the superior parathyroid gland before entering the cricothyroid membrane. On the right, the nerve has a slightly more oblique course, and in less than 1% of cases, it is nonrecurrent. Up to 20% of recurrent laryngeal nerves are branched. It is important to preserve all the parathyroids on their vascular pedicle and sweep them off the thyroid gland. If a parathyroid is compromised, it should be autotransplanted in the ipsilateral sternocleidomastoid unless otherwise indicated. When mobilizing the thyroid, it is important not to disrupt the tumor capsule to avoid spillage. Sterile water is helpful if the capsule is disrupted. After mobilization of the thyroid gland on the tumor-containing side, the contralateral thyroid lobe should be removed in similar fashion. When there is concern for injury to the nerve or parathyroids on the first side, a more limited dissection on the contralateral side should be performed. If performing a lobectomy and isthmectomy, the contralateral thyroid lobe should not be manipulated as previously mentioned. In all cases, a thorough search for a pyramidal lobe should be performed. After thyroidectomy and adequate hemostasis, the muscle layers should be closed separately and the platysma reapproximated before skin closure.

CENTRAL NECK DISSECTION

Central neck dissections are an important part of the initial operation in MTC and in patients with thyroid cancer of follicular thyroid cancer who have clinically suspicious nodes. It is important to remove all lymph tissue from the central compartment when performing this procedure. The central compartment is defined by the borders of the carotid arteries laterally, the cricoid cartilage superiorly, the clavicles caudally, and the trachea and esophagus medially. Meticulous dissection is required to remove all pretracheal and tracheoesophageal nodes without injuring the parathyroid glands or the recurrent and external laryngeal nerves. If the parathyroids are injured, they should be autotransplanted. If the nerve is injured, it should be repaired immediately with an 8–0 Prolene suture (Ethicon, Somerville, NJ).

Functional Neck Dissection

Functional neck dissection, also referred to as a modified radical neck dissection, involves removing level 2 through level 4 jugular lymph nodes (Fig. 3). The lateral border of dissection is the lateral border of the sternocleidomastoid. This procedure has a better cosmetic result than radical neck dissections, which are disfiguring because they involve resection of the sternocleidomastoid and the internal jugular. When performing a modified radical or functional neck dissection, it is important to identify and preserve the phrenic nerve, the thyrocervical trunk, the brachial plexus, the thoracic duct, and the spinal accessory nerve. We also preserve the cervical sensory nerves. Meticulous dissection is required for optimal outcomes with this procedure. Level 1 and level 5 are infrequently involved with metastatic nodes so that nodal resection of these areas is usually unnecessary.

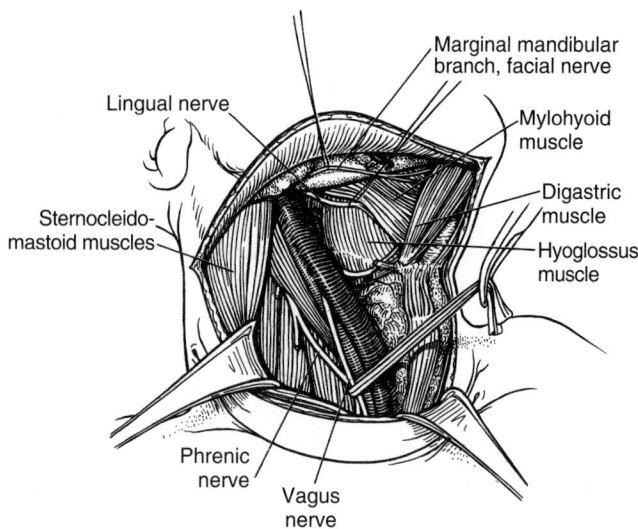

Figure 3 Lateral neck dissection.

Metastatic and Recurrent Disease

There is controversy on the management of recurrent cervical disease identified clinically on sonogram. At the University of California at San Francisco, we believe that reoperation is indicated in these patients and that it should focus on removal of suspicious lesions. Because reoperation in a scarred neck increases the rate of complications, the extent of the operation should be limited, and preoperative ultrasound guidance is helpful. We recommend preoperative needle localization for recurrent lymph nodes in the central neck. Some groups have advocated alcohol injection or radiofrequency ablation for the treatment of these recurrences; these techniques are experimental, however.

SUGGESTED READINGS

Cooper DS, Doherty GM, Haugen BR, and others: Management guidelines for patients with thyroid nodules and differentiated thyroid cancer, *Thyroid* 16:109, 2006.

Clark OH, editor: *Endocrine surgery of the thyroid and parathyroid glands,* St Louis, 1985, Mosby.

Clark OH, Duh QY, Kebebew E, editors: *Textbook of endocrine surgery,* ed 2, Philadelphia, 2006, Elsevier.

HYPERTHYROIDISM

Clive S. Grant, MD, and Geoffrey B. Thompson, MD

Hyperthyroidism has a prevalence of 2% in women and 0.2% in men; the term refers to thyroid gland hyperfunction. Hyperthyroidism can have many causes, and determining the cause is essential to formulate a rational treatment plan. Whereas thyrotoxicosis resulting from Graves' disease most commonly develops during the second to fourth decades of life, nodular goiter with hyperthyroidism evolves with increasing age and most commonly in geographic regions where dietary iodine is insufficient.

Medical options for definitive treatment of hyperthyroidism include antithyroid drugs and radioactive iodine administration. Surgical management of hyperthyroidism, which is generally highly safe and effective, is considered for the following conditions:

- Graves' disease,
- Toxic nodular goiter, either single or multiple nodules (Plummer's disease), and
- Amiodarone-induced thyrotoxicosis.

SYMPTOMS AND DIAGNOSIS

Patients with overt thyrotoxicosis may have symptoms of heat intolerance; palpitations; fatigue; weight loss; diaphoresis; muscle weakness; anxiety; insomnia; nervousness or restlessness; irritability; emotional lability; and, in women, irregular menses. Clinical findings may include tremor; tachycardia; goiter; lid lag; proptosis; periorbital edema; exophthalmos; chemosis; hyperreflexia; warm, moist skin; dermopathy; and pretibial edema.

In overt thyrotoxicosis, serum thyroid stimulating hormone (TSH) is decreased, and serum levels of free thyroxine (T4), free tri-iodothyronine (T3), or both are elevated. In subclinical hyperthyroidism, TSH levels are decreased, but T4 and T3 levels remain normal. Radioactive iodine uptake is elevated in Graves' disease and may be either elevated or normal in nodular goiter with hyperthyroidism. In contrast, the uptake is low or undetectable in thyroiditis or amiodarone-associated thyrotoxicosis. A thyroid scan may be helpful to distinguish Graves' disease (i.e., diffuse uptake) from toxic multinodular goiter (i.e., focal areas of increased uptake with intervening suppressed uptake). Additionally, elevated levels of thyroperoxidase (TPO) antibodies are characteristic of autoimmune thyroiditis (Hashimoto's disease). Table 1 provides a summary of disease states related to hyperthyroidism.

GRAVES' DISEASE

Graves' disease is an autoimmune systemic disorder, and hyperthyroidism is caused by thyroid receptor antibody (TRAB) binding to and stimulating the TSH receptor, resulting in excessive synthesis and secretion of thyroid hormone. The thyroid glands are usually diffusely and symmetrically enlarged and firm.

Antithyroid Drugs

Thioamides including propylthiouracil (PTU, given three times daily) and methimazole (once daily dose) decrease thyroid hormone synthesis and control hyperthyroidism in 90% of patients within several weeks. The intent is to induce remission, but despite continuous treatment over 12 to 18 months, relapse occurs after discontinuing the drug in 60% to 80% of patients. Minor side effects occur in 5%, and agranulocytosis occurs in 0.5%. In the United States, these drugs are seldom favored for definitive

Table 1: Summary of Hyperthyroid Disease States

Disease	Diagnostic Features	Preoperative Preparation	Operation
Graves' disease	↑ T4, T3, TSI, TPO ↓ TSH ↑ Symmetrical radioiodine uptake, scan Diffuse goiter Eye signs	Antithyroid drugs Beta-blockers Iodine drops	Bilateral near-total or total thyroidectomy
Unilateral toxic nodule	↑ T4, T3 ↓ TSH Single "hot" nodule on scan; remaining thyroid suppressed	None	Unilateral thyroid subtotal or total lobectomy
Multinodular goiter	↑ T4, T3 ↓ TSH Multiple "hot" nodules on scan; remaining thyroid suppressed	None	Bilateral near-total or total thyroidectomy (conservative)
Amiodarone-induced thyrotoxicosis	↑ T4, T3 ↓ TSH Taking amiodarone Minimal or no uptake on thyroid scan	Cardiac evaluation relative to the use of amiodarone	Bilateral near-total or total thyroidectomy
Autoimmune thyroiditis	↑ T4, T3, TPO ↓ TSH Minimal or no uptake on thyroid scan	None	Nonsurgical

T3, Free tri-iodothyronine; *T4*, free thyroxine; *TPO*, thyroperoxidase; *TSH*, thyroid stimulating hormone; *TSI*, thyroid stimulating immunoglobulin.

treatment but are commonly used for preoperative preparation or for temporary management of pregnant patients with Graves' disease.

Radioactive Iodine

Treatment with iodine-131 (I-131) is highly effective in Graves' disease, resulting in relief of hyperthyroidism in more than 90% of patients with a single dose. It is the treatment chosen for the vast majority of Graves' patients in the United States. These patients commonly, if not intentionally, become hypothyroid, which is usually easily managed with replacement T4. Side effects include neck pain from radiation thyroiditis, especially in larger goiters, sialadenitis and dry mouth, temporary worsening of thyrotoxicosis, and sometimes worsening of Graves' ophthalmopathy. Prophylactic simultaneous administration of glucocorticoids may ameliorate the neck pain and worsening eye signs. Return to euthyroidism is delayed for several weeks. Some patients have significant fear of any radioactivity, although the frequencies of major genetic or carcinogenic effects have not increased in more than 25 years of follow-up experience with adults. Conflicting studies, however, still exist. I-131 is contraindicated during pregnancy or in lactating mothers and has been used in relatively few children and adolescents because of the lack of data regarding long-term effects. Recurrence and need for more than a single dose of I-131 in young patients seems more prevalent.

Surgery

Bilateral near-total or total thyroidectomy is virtually 100% effective in permanently curing hyperthyroidism resulting from Graves' disease. It predictably results in the need for replacement T4 treatment, which is inexpensive and free of side effects at proper dosages and can be precisely managed with minimal blood testing. Thyroidectomy rapidly resolves hyperthyroidism and can be performed within 10 days of establishing the diagnosis, usually requiring only a single night of hospitalization. It is equally effective for all age groups, establishes definitive pathology for any accompanying suspicious nodules or thyroid cancer (5%), precludes any fear of radiation, and may be used safely during the second trimester of pregnancy and in lactating mothers. It is highly effective in young patients and is associated with improvement of eye signs in 85% of cases. Whether total thyroidectomy predictably improves the eye signs of Graves' disease remains an unresolved debate.

The risk of permanent recurrent laryngeal nerve damage ranges from 0% to 5%, and transient neurapraxia may occur in a similar number. Permanent hypoparathyroidism is thought to occur more frequently in Graves' disease than other bilateral thyroidectomy operations but should not exceed 1% to 4%. Careful identification and preservation of even a single, well-vascularized parathyroid gland is sufficient for eventual normal parathyroid function. Autotransplantation of excised parathyroid glands, minced into 1-mm fragments and placed in muscular pockets of the sternocleidomastoid muscle, should function within weeks to months in 95% of patients. Normal parathyroid function based solely on transplanted parathyroid tissue probably requires at least two parathyroid glands.

A few technical points that may be of help include (Fig. 1):

- After the thyroid gland has been mobilized and elevated out of its bed, the recurrent laryngeal nerve (RLN) can be detected beneath fat and other soft tissue by palpating it against the trachea, below the level of the thyroid gland.
- The vascular supply to both superior and inferior parathyroid glands enters from the anterior aspect. Therefore transecting soft tissue just barely anterior to these glands threatens devascularization.
- The superior parathyroid gland and the RLN can be visualized and saved by preserving a small remnant of thyroid tissue just anterior to the parathyroid gland and its blood supply and

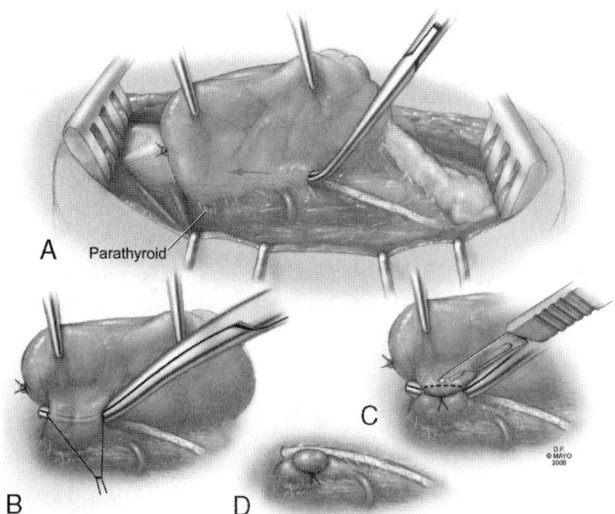

Figure 1 Method for preserving the superior parathyroid gland in near-total thyroidectomy. **(A)** An Adson right-angle clamp is advanced immediately adjacent and on top of the recurrent laryngeal nerve (areolar space along the recurrent laryngeal nerve [RLN] allows easy, nonforceful opening of this plane) until the tip of the clamp can be seen medial and superior to the remaining attached superior aspect of the thyroid lobe. **(B)** A tie is passed through the dissected opening, anterior to the RLN, which is confirmed through this maneuver to be safe from ligation or transaction. **(C)** After the ligature is tied with a small remnant of thyroid preserved anterior to the superior parathyroid gland (visible posterior to the small thyroid remnant), the bridge of thyroid tissue is transected with a scalpel, protecting the RLN with the clamp. **(D)** After the bridge is transected, the RLN is fully exposed, the tiny thyroid remnant retracts posteriorly with the protected superior parathyroid gland, and the remaining thyroid lobe can be easily and safely excised. *Copyright DF Mayo, 2006.*

developing the areolar space adjacent to the RLN as illustrated in Figure 1. The amount of thyroid tissue preserved is no more than 100 to 200 mg.

The surgical scar ranges up to 7 cm, depending on the patient's body habitus, and may represent the single most difficult obstacle to a surgical approach when initially consulting on a young female patient. However, the necessity of prolonged frequent daily antithyroid medication or the perceived specter of radioactive treatment often come to outweigh this issue.

Preoperative preparation is absolutely required. For most patients, antithyroid drugs (discussed earlier) are instituted for 3 to 6 weeks with a goal of nearly normalizing the T3 and T4. The addition of beta-blocking agents such as propranolol or atenolol rapidly controls the adrenergic side effects of excess T4 and T3 such as tachycardia, tremor, and diaphoresis. The administration of iodine in the form of super-saturated potassium iodide or Lugol's solution was often used as the sole means of preoperative preparation in the past. It rapidly but temporarily restores normal thyroid function and reduces thyroid gland vascularity.

TOXIC SINGLE ADENOMA

Toxic adenomas are single, benign, monoclonal thyroid tumors that autonomously oversecrete thyroid hormone. The nodule is usually 3 cm or larger, evolves through a course of subclinical to overt hyperthyroidism, and is virtually never malignant.

Antithyroid Drugs

Whereas hyperthyroidism can be controlled with antithyroid drugs (thioamides), remission does not occur, recurrence inevitably develops when the medication is discontinued, and lifelong treatment is unacceptable. Therefore these drugs are seldom if ever chosen as definitive treatment.

Radioactive Iodine

Radioactive iodine is effective with little risk to surrounding structures or of causing radiation-induced tumors. The nodules may shrink to some extent but rarely disappear. Euthyroidism is reestablished in at least 80% of patients with a single dose. However, variability in size of the nodule, uptake, and dose of radioiodine administered may lead to either recurrence or hypothyroidism. Pregnancy and lactation are contraindications to ^{I}I-131.

Surgery

Subtotal or total lobectomy to resect the hot nodule is virtually 100% effective in controlling hyperthyroidism. Most patients are restored to euthyroidism if the remaining thyroid gland is normal. The risk of RLN paralysis is 1% or less, hypoparathyroidism is essentially unknown, and other surgical complications are rare. The surgical scar, hospitalization, anesthesia, and cost are the principal deterrents to a surgical approach.

TOXIC MULTINODULAR GOITER (PLUMMER'S DISEASE)

First described by H.S. Plummer in 1913, this condition is unremitting; it often develops slowly and with more subtle symptoms than Graves' disease. A long phase of subclinical hyperthyroidism can precede the appearance of overt symptoms. Cardiac symptoms such as tachycardia, heart failure or arrhythmia, and atrial fibrillation are most frequent. In addition, unexplained, asymptomatic weight loss may occur in older patients with toxic multinodular goiter (MNG). Patients may also experience local pressure complications of large nodular goiters such as tracheal, esophageal, or jugular venous compression (Pemberton's sign: facial plethora, inspiratory stridor, and venous congestion when arms are raised above the head).

Antithyroid Drugs

For the same reasons as for single toxic adenoma, thioamides are virtually never used as definitive treatment, but rather as preoperative preparation.

Radioactive Iodine

Increasingly, I-131 has been advocated in the treatment of toxic MNG. Radioactive iodine (radioiodine) offers an attractive alternative to thyroidectomy in patients who present high operative risk. In addition, it is often used for smaller goiters without local pressure symptoms. Cardiac symptoms are more prevalent in radioiodine-treated patients. On average, resolution of hyperthyroidism with radioiodine takes 5 to 6 months, reduces the goiter size by approximately 40%, is associated with subsequent hypothyroidism in approximately 10% of cases, and 15% to 25% of patients may require a second dose. Complications are rare with the exception of radiation-related thyroiditis causing neck pain.

Surgery

The advantages of surgical treatment for MNG include prompt, permanent resolution of hyperthyroidism; removal of the goiter, resolving any associated compressive or cosmetic problems; and treatment of associated malignancy. With conservative, bilateral, near-total thyroidectomy, virtually all patients have their hyperthyroidism resolved within a month postoperatively. All are started on replacement T4 because surgically induced hypothyroidism is the desired operative goal.

Because of the size of MNG, the surgical risks are often higher than either bilateral thyroidectomy for cancer or Graves' disease. Bleeding and postoperative hematoma are more likely due to the markedly enlarged and plentiful thyroid vasculature. The RLNs may be more difficult to identify because of anatomic displacement by nodules or difficulty with exposure from the sheer size of the goiter. Equally difficult to identify may be the parathyroid glands in large MNG. For these reasons, a few technical hints may be of help:

- A larger incision is usually necessary to gain adequate exposure.
- Reverse Trendelenburg position reduces venous pressure and bleeding.
- Careful dissection and preservation of the sternohyoid strap muscles are valuable to protect the trachea at the time of closure. However, the sternothyroid muscles are often thin, splayed over the surface of the goiter, and may be sacrificed.
- Although the goiter may be large, the isthmus is often still narrow. Early transection of the isthmus with careful control of the paired inferior thyroid veins and control of the confluence of three veins along the superior border of the isthmus yields an exposed trachea, which serves as a useful landmark in later dissection.
- Early ligation of the superior thyroid artery along the anterior superior surface of the superior pole may be easier than expected because it is often elongated by the goiter extending substernally. This reduces the inevitable bothersome bleeding associated with mobilization and resection of the large nodular lobe.
- Blunt finger dissection on the surface of the thyroid lobe, carried posteriorly and inferiorly immediately under the strap muscles, facilitates mobilization of the inferior pole of the lobe out of its bed.
- As the lobe is mobilized, it is helpful to recall that no anatomic structure of importance crosses transversely across the carotid artery from the base of the neck to the thyroid cartilage (except the middle thyroid vein, which is sacrificed). To expose the carotid over this length facilitates further dissection, particularly identification of the RLN.
- With a large goiter elevated out of its bed, the trachea and esophagus are often rotated anteriorly, exposing the RLN to potential danger. With the lobe thus elevated, however, the nerve is usually taut and easily palpated. After the RLN is exposed and protected, resection may begin.
- The inferior parathyroid seems more variable in location because of the distortion caused by the large goiter. However, following the cervical extension of the thymus (and associated vein) to the inferior pole of the thyroid often leads to this parathyroid gland. Less variable is the deep, posterior position of the superior parathyroid gland. The inferior parathyroid gland is often excised, biopsied for identity confirmation, and autotransplanted into the sternocleidomastoid muscle, whereas the superior parathyroid gland can be more easily protected in situ.
- If the inferior parathyroid has been excised, there is nothing of importance to save anterior to the RLN, inferior to the lower pole of the thyroid, or around to the midline surface of the trachea; this soft tissue may be sacrificed.
- Lobectomy is undertaken by circumferential dissection facilitated by earlier isthmic transection.

AMIODARONE-ASSOCIATED THYROTOXICOSIS

Amiodarone is an iodine-rich (37% by molecular weight) class III antiarrhythmic agent that was initially introduced for refractory arrhythmias but has seen increasing usage because of its effectiveness. Even conventional doses of this drug result in large expansion of the iodine pool. Often amiodarone-associated thyrotoxicosis (AAT) occurs in patients with significant cardiac dysrhythmias who do not tolerate the cardiac effects of hyperthyroidism. Two forms have been described. Type I develops in patients with preexisting goiter, resulting in excessive hormone production from the marked iodine excess. Type II occurs without preexisting thyroid disease from a chemical-induced thyroiditis and resultant release of hormone. Type II is more common in the United States, occurring in 2% of patients treated with amiodarone. AAT is notoriously refractory to medical management, with low radioactive iodine uptake, thereby precluding use of I-131 for treatment. Discontinuation of amiodarone may help, but often this is a poor choice in patients with life-threatening arrhythmias. Additionally, the long half-life of the drug requires weeks to months for the hyperthyroidism to resolve.

Antithyroid Drugs

Although thioamides have been used with some success, inadequate results are the rule. Only if hyperthyroidism is mild and amiodarone can be discontinued do antithyroid drugs have the likelihood of prolonged success.

Radioactive Iodine

Because the iodine uptake is low in the usual type II AAT patients, radioiodine is not an option.

Surgery

Thyroidectomy offers many of the same benefits as have been discussed in previous sections: prompt and permanent control of hyperthyroidism, low risk of RLN damage or hypoparathyroidism, short hospitalization, and quick recovery. However, this group of patients is at the highest risk of all patients undergoing thyroidectomy; almost all of the risk is related to the severity of their cardiac disease. These patients often have severe cardiac failure, life-threatening arrhythmias, and ejection fractions of 10% to 30%. Despite their high operative risk, thyroidectomy is efficacious in treating AAT, and most patients ultimately recover well.

SUGGESTED READINGS

Houghton S, Farley D, Brennan M, and others: Surgical management of amiodarone-associated thyrotoxicosis: Mayo Clinic experience, *World J Surg* 28:1083, 2004.
Kang A, Grant C, Thompson G, van Heerden J: Current treatment of nodular goiter with hyperthyroidism (Plummer's disease): surgery versus radioiodine, *Surgery* 132:916, 2002.
O'Brien T, Gharib H, Suman V, and others: Treatment of toxic solitary thyroid nodules: surgery versus radioactive iodine, *Surgery* 112:1166, 1992.
Sherman J, Thompson G, Lteif A, and others: Surgical management of Graves' disease in childhood and adolescence: an institutional experience, *Surgery* 140:1056, 2006.
Stice R, Grant C, Gharib H, van Heerden J: The management of Graves' disease during pregnancy, *Surg Gynecol Obstetr* 158:157, 1984.

THYROIDITIS

James A. Stefater and Alan P. B. Dackiw, MD

Thyroiditis, or inflammation of the thyroid, is classified into three main subtypes: 1) chronic, 2) subacute, and 3) acute. A discussion of the three types—their etiology and pathogenesis, clinical presentation, differential diagnosis, and clinical management—is principally a medical concern. However, an understanding of the classification and disease progression of thyroiditis can serve as an important guide to the surgeon assessing and following a patient with thyroiditis. Furthermore, in some cases, surgery may be warranted. For these reasons, a discussion of thyroiditis is of relevance to the practicing surgeon.

CHRONIC THYROIDITIS

There are two types of chronic thyroiditis: Hashimoto's thyroiditis, the most common inflammatory disease of the thyroid, and Riedel's thyroiditis, a rare fibroinflammatory disorder.

Hashimoto's Thyroiditis

Hashimoto's thyroiditis is also called *chronic lymphocytic thyroiditis, chronic progressive thyroiditis, struma lymphomatosa,* and *autoimmune chronic lymphocytic thyroiditis.* Hashimoto's thyroiditis is an autoimmune disorder that, like almost all forms of thyroiditis, primarily affects women; up to 95% of cases of Hashimoto's disease occur in women. Several theories exist as to the mechanism of autoimmune initiation, but regardless of etiology, patients present with elevated levels of circulating antibodies to thyroglobulin, thyroid peroxidase, and thyrotropin receptor. Most likely, autoimmune initiation is a result of both genetic predisposition and environmental factors. A strong correlation has been observed between development of Hashimoto's and HLA-DR5. Additionally, a family history of autoimmune disorders has been shown to be a significant risk factor. A possible explanation for the increasing prevalence of Hashimoto's in the West may be the direct correlation between iodide intake and thyroid autoantibody levels. A viral component has been postulated but remains unsubstantiated.

Clinical Presentation

Hashimoto's is the most common cause of hypothyroidism in the United States. Twenty percent of patients present with hypothyroidism and 5% present with hyperthyroidism. Patients have a relatively small, firm gland that is usually symmetrical but can be irregular. Usually patients present asymptomatically, and the goiter is found during routine physical examination. Occasionally patients may report awareness of a painless anterior neck mass. The presence of distinct nodules in the gland may indicate a benign nodule, a thyroid lymphoma, or a papillary thyroid cancer.

Differential Diagnosis

Two important considerations include nontoxic multinodular goiter and thyroid lymphoma. The former is characterized by more distinct nodules in the gland, a euthyroid patient, and decreased circulating levels of the previously noted relevant antibodies. Thyroid lymphoma can be a serious complication of Hashimoto's,

and a fine needle aspiration (FNA) biopsy is recommended for any patient presenting with nodules or a rapidly increasing goiter.

Clinical Management

For patients with overt hypothyroidism, it is necessary to prescribe thyroid hormone replacement therapy with the intent of establishing normal thyroid stimulating hormone (TSH) levels. Hormone replacement therapy for patients with subclinical hypothyroidism (normal free thyroxine [T4], free tri-iodothyronine [T3], and antibody levels but elevated TSH) is more controversial. In a study that followed patients for 20 years, 55% of female patients eventually developed hypothyroidism, and the progression rate for men has been reported to be even higher. Therefore hormone therapy is generally recommended for women and indicated for males. In general, patients with TSH levels greater than 10 mU/L should receive therapy, and in all cases, long-term follow-up is necessary.

The Surgeon's Role

Papillary thyroid carcinomas may also occur in the setting of Hashimoto's thyroiditis. Surgery is indicated if malignancy is suspected from FNA biopsy. Additionally, thyroidectomy may be required in a patient with compressive symptoms from a large goiter or for cosmetic purposes. Surgical resection of a thyroiditis gland may be more technically challenging because of increased vascularity; the gland's firm, woody character; and dissection of the parathyroids off the gland itself.

Riedel's Thyroiditis

Riedel's thyroiditis is also called Riedel's struma or invasive fibrous thyroiditis. The etiology of Riedel's thyroiditis is unknown. Some researchers postulate an autoimmune etiology, which is indicated by the presence of thyroid antibodies in up to 67% of patients, patient susceptibility to other autoimmune disorders, occasional lymphoid infiltration, and a strong response in some patients to steroid therapy. Because the hallmark of Riedel's thyroiditis is the replacement of thyroid parenchyma with fibrous tissue, others have suggested an unknown fibrotic disorder.

Clinical Presentation

As with most types of thyroiditis, women are more susceptible to Reidel's thyroiditis (by a ratio of 3 to 1), especially women between the ages 30 and 60 years. Patients present with a painless, hard, "woody" thyroid gland that is fixed to the adjacent tissue. Over the course of months or years, patients experience symptomatic compression of the trachea, esophagus, or recurrent laryngeal nerves. Replacement of the thyroid and surrounding tissue with fibrous tissue can result in hypothyroidism (observed in one third of patients) and hypoparathyroidism (less common). In extreme cases, vocal cord paralysis may result.

Differential Diagnosis

Riedel's thyroiditis can be distinguished from Hashimoto's thyroiditis by serological profile, pathology, or the lack of a goiter (goiters are present in Hashimoto's and absent in Riedel's). Thyroid lymphoma and carcinoma can be difficult to distinguish, and therefore biopsy is recommended. Biopsy in this disease demonstrates a sparsely cellular aspirate with fibrosis, lymphocytes, and plasma cells.

Clinical Management

Medical therapy for symptomatic Riedel's thyroiditis may include high-dose systemic steroids, which have proved effective in some patients. Additionally, for unknown reasons, antiestrogen therapy with tamoxifen may be helpful. For patients remaining resolutely hypothyroid, thyroid hormone replacement therapy is indicated.

The Surgeon's Role

Symptoms of Riedel's are rarely alleviated with medical therapy alone. Isthmusectomy and resection have proved useful in relieving symptoms of compression. Also, because of the "rock-hard" nature of the thyroid gland, FNA biopsy may not be feasible, and open biopsy is required.

SUBACUTE THYROIDITIS

The two types of subacute thyroiditis are distinguished by the presence or absence of their most prominent symptom: pain. Painless thyroiditis has been divided into silent and postpartum forms depending on temporal occurrence. In the postpartum form, painless thyroiditis is fairly common with subsequent pregnancies. Painful thyroiditis is rare.

Painless Thyroiditis

Painless thyroiditis is also called lymphocytic thyroiditis with spontaneously resolving hyperthyroidism, subacute lymphocytic thyroiditis, painless lymphocytic thyroiditis, subacute nonsuppurative thyroiditis, atypical subacute thyroiditis, hyperthyroiditis, and silent thyroiditis. If painless thyroiditis occurs after pregnancy, it is designated specifically as postpartum thyroiditis. Painless thyroiditis is an autoimmune disorder. Patients typically have elevated thyroid peroxidase antibody levels and lymphocytic infiltration of the thyroid. Additionally, many patients with painless thyroiditis also present with other autoimmune disorders. A genetic predisposition has been proposed, and some patients possess HLA-DR3, -DR4, or -DR5 haplotypes. In postpartum thyroiditis, an autoimmune etiology is even more likely. Women who develop a postpartum thyroiditis have elevated thyroid peroxidase antibody titers in early pregnancy. Also, the risk of developing a postpartum thyroiditis is increased with subsequent pregnancies, and 50% of affected women have a positive family history for the disease.

Clinical Presentation

Painless thyroiditis affects women more than men, usually between the ages of 30 and 60 years. Depending on the study, between 2% and 21% of women are affected postpartum. The disease has a four-stage clinical course that is well characterized: (1) destruction-

induced thyrotoxicosis, (2) euthryoidism, (3) hypothyroidism, and (4) return to euthyroidism (Fig. 1). However, approximately 40% of patients follow the classical clinical course, with 30% presenting with thyrotoxicosis alone and 30% presenting only with hypothyroidism. Women diagnosed with postpartum thyroiditis usually show signs of thyrotoxicosis 2 weeks to several months after pregnancy, progress to the hypothyroid stage after 3 to 6 months and usually return to a clinical and biochemical euthyroid state after 1 year. Throughout the disease progression, there is a complete absence of pain and systemic conditions such as fever. The gland is usually firm and nontender with symmetrical, modest enlargement. Unfortunately, nearly one third of affected patients become permanently hypothyroid.

Differential Diagnosis

During the thyrotoxicosis stage, physicians should rule out Graves' disease. Usually with thyroiditis, the onset of hyperthyroidism is more abrupt. Relative to a patient with Graves' disease, patients presenting with thyroiditis have a lower serum T3 to T4 ratio, higher serum thyroglobulin levels preceding thyrotoxicosis, the presence of antithyroid peroxidase antibodies, and the absence of thyrotropin receptor antibodies. The clinical course closely resembles the other type of subacute thyroiditis, painful thyroiditis, and the two diseases can be distinguished simply by the presence or absence of pain.

Clinical Management

During the thyrotoxic stage, hyperthyroidism can be treated with beta-adrenergic-blocking drugs, but because of the transient nature of symptoms, many patients do not require therapy. The hypothyroid stage can be treated with standard hormone replacement therapy and is especially warranted in women wishing to become pregnant.

The Surgeon's Role

Thyroidectomy is rarely indicated and should be performed only on patients with severe, recurrent episodes of thyroiditis.

Painful Thyroiditis

Painful thyroiditis is also called de Quervain's disease, granulomatous thyroiditis, pseudogranulomatous thyroiditis, acute simple thyroiditis, noninfectious thyroiditis, and giant-cell thyroiditis. This condition is the most common cause of a painful thyroid gland. Painful thyroiditis has a viral etiology. Frequently, this type of

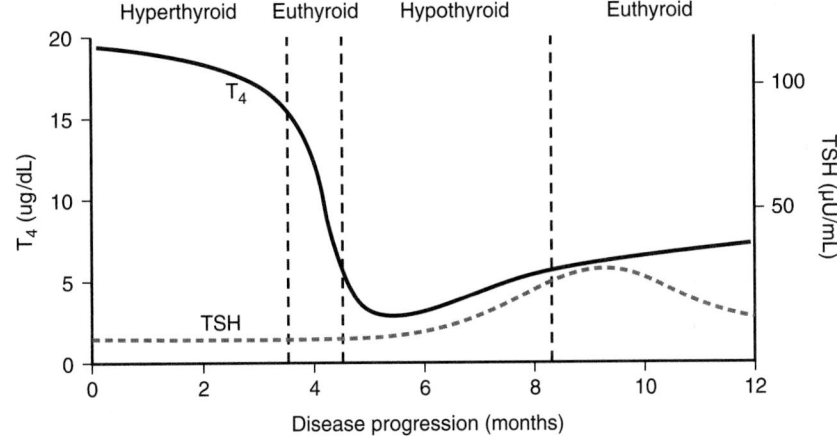

Figure I Schematic representation of the disease progression of subacute thyroiditis. Approximately 40% of patients follow this clinical course. The solid line represents T₄ levels; the small-dashed line represents TSH levels. *Adapted from Woolf PD: Thyroiditis. In: Falk SA, editor, Thyroid disease: Endocrinology, surgery, nuclear medicine, and radiotherapy, ed 2, 1997, Philadelphia, Lippincott-Raven, 393-410.*

thyroiditis is preceded by upper respiratory infection, appears to be self-limiting, and increases in prevalence seasonally. Patients with other viral infections have a greater risk of developing painful thyroiditis. Patients with the HLA-B35 haplotype are reported to have a genetic predisposition to this disease.

Clinical Presentation

Women between the ages of 30 and 40 years are at the greatest risk of contracting painful thyroiditis. Patients present with pain that can radiate toward the jaw and ear. This pain is often exacerbated by swallowing or neck movement. Patients occasionally present with high fever (up to 105 degrees), edema, and other flulike symptoms. The thyroid gland is enlarged, asymmetrical, exquisitely tender, and firm. The overlying skin may be erythematous and warm. The disease course is identical to painless thyroiditis, proceeding in four stages: thyrotoxicosis, euthyroid, hypothyroid, and return to euthyroid (Fig. 1). Patients usually return to a euthyroid state (90%), but some may be permanently hypothyroid.

Differential Diagnosis

If patients initially present with hyperthyroidism, Graves' disease should be ruled out. A painful form of Hashimoto's thyroiditis should also be considered and may be distinguished from painful thyroiditis by serology. Acute thyroiditis (discussed later) may be ruled out by measuring TSH levels or thyroxine levels (decreased and increased respectively for painful thyroiditis; normal for acute thyroiditis). Additionally, acute hemorrhage into a thyroid nodule or cyst may resemble painful thyroiditis but can be further distinguished by ultrasound.

Clinical Management

Because the disease course is usually self-limited, treatment is directed at symptom control alone and is specific for each phase of the disease. Similar to the treatment of painless thyroiditis, beta-blockade is indicated to treat the symptoms of hyperthyroidism. If severe thyrotoxicosis is present, rapid control of hyperthyroidism can be achieved using iopanoic acid (Telepaque; Amersham Health, Princeton, NJ), which inhibits the peripheral deiodination of T4. Note that antithyroid therapy is not indicated because thyroid hormone synthesis is not elevated. Also similar to the treatment of painless thyroiditis, symptoms of hypothyroidism can be alleviated with thyroid hormone replacement therapy. To treat the pain associated with this disease, nonsteroidal anti-inflammatory medications and salicylates are prescribed, but prednisone may also be used for severe pain at up to 40 mg/day.

The Surgeon's Role

Thyroidectomy is indicated only for patients with prolonged thyroiditis that proves unresponsive to conventional medical therapy.

ACUTE THYROIDITIS

Acute thyroiditis is also called *acute suppurative thyroiditis, infectious thyroiditis,* and *bacterial thyroiditis.* The disease is an uncommon thyroid condition and the only type of thyroiditis that affects women and men equally. The etiology of acute thyroiditis is almost always bacterial but can also be fungal, mycobacterial, or parasitic. In general, the thyroid is extremely resistant to bacterial infection because of its extensive blood and lymphatic supply, high iodide content, and fibrous capsule. When infections do occur, they are most commonly the result of direct spread from a persistent pyriform sinus fistula or thyroglossal duct cyst. Infections can also be initiated by the hematogenous or lymphatic routes and secondary to penetrating trauma of the thyroid. A wide variety of pathogens have been isolated from

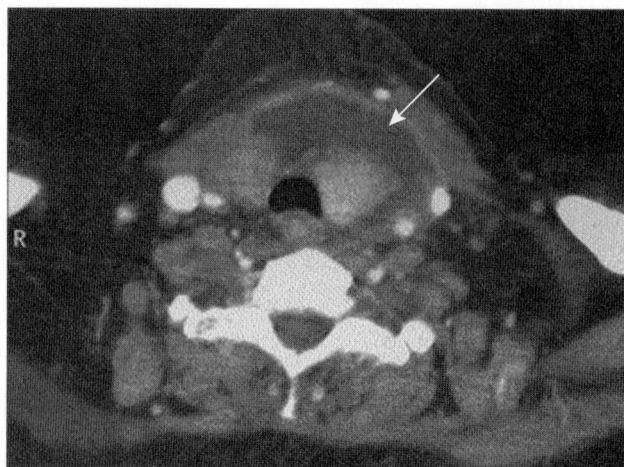

Figure 2 Computed tomography of the neck showing the abscess overlying the left lobe of the thyroid *(arrow).* *From Dunham B, Nicol TL, Ishii M, and others: Lancet, 368(9548):1742, 2006.*

infected tissue, but pediatric infections closely reflect the pharyngeal flora. *Staphylococcus* is responsible for one third of adult infections. The remaining portion consist of a number of gram-negative organisms, including *Brucella melitensis, Capnocytophaga ochracea, Eikenella corrodens, Haemophilus influenzae, Moraxella nonliquefaciens, Salmonella paratyphi,* and *Serratia marcescens.* Immunosuppression is also a risk factor for acute thyroiditis, making patients with acquired immunodeficiency syndrome particularly susceptible. Numerous patients with *Pneumocystis carinii* infection of the thyroid have been identified.

Clinical Presentation

In adults, two thirds of patients have a preexisting thyroid disorder, including simple goiter, nodular goiter, Hashimoto's thyroiditis, or thyroid cancer. Additionally, many patients present with an upper respiratory infection. As noted, children are particularly susceptible to acute thyroiditis. The majority of children present with a persistent left pyriform sinus fistula, and thus unilateral infection of the left lobe is most common (Fig. 2). Patients generally have severe neck pain that radiates down the neck and to the jaw. Additionally, localized warmth, tenderness, fever, dysphagia, and erythema are all common symptoms. Rarely some patients may develop transient vocal cord palsy.

Differential Diagnosis

The differential diagnosis for acute thyroiditis is complicated and extremely important. An 8.6% mortality rate has been reported for acute thyroiditis, with most of the deaths resulting from an incorrect diagnosis. Subacute painful thyroiditis can be ruled out because patients with acute thyroiditis have a normal 24-hour radioactive iodide uptake. Additionally, patients presenting with acute thyroiditis are usually euthyroid. Hashimoto's thyroiditis can be differentiated by serology. Thyroid carcinoma should be carefully considered. One study outlined several variables that help to distinguish acute thyroiditis from malignancy. The following variables increased a patient's risk of carcinoma: old age, dysphagia, right lobe involvement, larger lesions, anemia, and sterile thyroid aspirates. Other medical considerations include suppurative lymphadenitis, thyroglossal duct or branchial cleft cyst, Ludwig's angina, and dissecting retropharyngeal abscess. These conditions can be diagnosed with a careful analysis of clinical history, physical examination, diagnostic tests, and imaging.

Clinical Management

Treatment is essential and mainly consists of parenteral antibiotics and abscess drainage, when appropriate.

The Surgeon's Role

Drainage of abscesses may be achieved via aspiration, wide-bore needle, or open surgical drainage. Additionally, in order to prevent relapse, cases of acute thyroiditis caused by left pyriform sinus fistulas must be surgically addressed. Fistulectomy and complete resection of the sinus tract and the area of the thyroid where this tract terminates are therefore required.

SUMMARY: SURGICAL THERAPY

While treatment of thyroiditis is mainly a medical concern, the different types of thyroiditis all have an immediate or at least potential surgical role. In the treatment of all types of thyroiditis, FNA biopsy may be indicated to rule out malignancy. Additionally, Hashimoto's thyroiditis can result in symptoms of compression or cosmetic deformity that indicate thyroidectomy. Treatment of Reidel's thyroiditis may require surgery to relieve compression where isthmusectomy and limited resections are indicated or when open biopsy is necessary rather than FNA. The two types of subacute thyroiditis are usually treated medically, and surgery is used only in the rare instance in which the patient has prolonged, unresponsive thyroiditis. Finally, in the management of acute thyroiditis, surgical drainage may be required, and fistulectomy is indicated in most instances.

Table 1: Summary of the Clinical and Biochemical Characteristics of the Five Subtypes of Thyroiditis

Subtypes	Neck Pain	Goiter	TSH	T4	Anti-TG	Anti-TP	Anti-TR
Chronic Thyroiditis							
Hashimoto's	No	Yes	May be elevated	May be decreased	Present	Present	Present
Riedel's	No	No	May be decreased	May be decreased	Antibodies present in 67% of patients		
Subacute Thyroiditis							
Painless	No	Yes	Decreased*	Elevated*	Absent	Present	Variable
Painful	Yes	Variable	Decreased*	Elevated*	Absent	Absent	Absent
Acute Thyroiditis							
Acute	Yes	Yes	Normal	Normal	Absent	Absent	Absent

TSH, Thyroid-stimulating hormone; *T4*, thyroxine; *TG*, thyroglobulin; *TP*, thyroid peroxidase; *TR*, thyroid receptor.
*Levels at beginning of disease course (see Fig. 1).

Table 2: Summary of Patient Presentations and Appropriate Therapies

Subtypes	Etiology	Indications	Therapy
Chronic Thyroiditis			
Hashimoto's	Autoimmune	Hypothyroidism (20%) Hyperthyroidism (5%) Suspension of malignancy Compressive symptoms	Thyroid hormone replacement therapy Beta-blockers FNA biopsy, thyroidectomy, or lobectomy Total thyroidectomy
Riedel's	Unknown	Hypothyroidism (33%) Hypoparathyroidism (rare) Edema and fibrosis (up to 33%) Compressive symptoms (common)	Thyroid hormone replacement therapy Hormone replacement therapy High-dose systemic steroids, antiestrogen therapy Partial thyroidectomy, isthmusectomy
Subacute Thyroiditis			
Painless	Autoimmune	Hyperthyroidism (usually transient) Hypothyroidism	Beta-blockers Thyroid hormone replacement therapy
Painful	Viral	Hyperthyroidism (common) Hypothyroidism (25–50%) Pain (100%)	Beta-blockers, ipodate Thyroid hormone replacement therapy salicylates, prednisone
Acute Thyroiditis			
Acute	Bacterial fungal mycobacterial parasitic	Detection of infection Thyroid abscess Left pyriform sinus fistula Compressive symptoms	Parenteral antibiotics Drainage via aspiration, wide-bore needle or open surgical drainage Fistulectomy Thyroidectomy

FNA, Fine needle aspiration.

SUGGESTED READINGS

Baloch ZW, LiVolsi VA: Pathology of thyroid gland. In: LiVolsi VA, Asa SL, editors: *Endocrine pathology*, Philadelphia, 2002, Churchill Livingstone, 65–67.

Dunham B, Nicol TL, Ishii M, and others: Suppurative thyroiditis, *Lancet*, 368(9548):1742, 2006.

Farwell AP, Braverman LE: Inflammatory thyroid disorders, *Otolarygol Clin North Am* 29:541, 1996.

Woolf PD: Thyroiditis. In: Falk SA, editor, *Thyroid disease: Endocrinology, surgery, nuclear medicine, and radiotherapy*, ed 2, Philadelphia, 1997, Lippincott-Raven, 393–410.

PRIMARY HYPERPARATHYROIDISM

Sanziana Roman, MD, and Robert Udelsman, MD, MBA

The parathyroid glands were first discovered by Sir Richard Owen in 1852 while he was performing a postmortem examination of an Indian rhinoceros; they were reported in humans by Ivar Sandstrom, a Swedish medical student, in 1880. In 1915, a Viennese surgeon, Friedrich Schlagenhaufer, suggested that an enlarged parathyroid gland should be excised. This later ushered the treatment of primary hyperparathyroidism. Later, William S. Halsted had observed severe hypocalcemia after total thyroidectomy and demonstrated that parathyroid transplantation in dogs was lifesaving. He described the parathyroid blood supply and promoted gentle manipulation of normal parathyroid glands to avoid ischemic injury. The first parathyroidectomy was performed by Felix Mandl in Vienna in 1924 on Albert Gahne, a tram conductor. In the United States, the first parathyroidectomy was performed by I.Y. Olch in 1928 at the Barnes Hospital of Washington University in St. Louis. Solomon A. Berson and Rosalyn S. Yalow identified and measured parathyroid hormone (PTH) in serum in 1963 and were awarded the Nobel Prize.

INCIDENCE AND DIAGNOSIS

Primary hyperparathyroidism (PHPT) is defined as a disorder of inappropriate or excessive secretion of PTH by one or more of the parathyroid glands, leading to hypercalcemia. Patients have normal renal function. The prevalence of PHPT has been reported to be between 1 and 5 patients per 1000 persons, with a female-to-male ratio of 4:1. This increases up to 13 patients per 1000 persons after age 65.

PTH directly mediates osteoclast activity in conjunction with 1,25-dihydroxycholecalciferol, as well as various interleukins. Increased levels of PTH stimulate renal tubular reabsorption of filtered calcium. Hypercalcemia inhibits antidiuretic hormone, leading to relative nephrogenic diabetes insipidus. Symptoms of mild to moderate hypercalcemia may include increased thirst and urinary frequency, constipation, anorexia, nausea, muscle weakness, and neurocognitive deficits such as depression and spatial memory loss. Nephrolithiasis may result from compensatory renal hypercalciuria. Cardiac manifestations of moderate to severe hypercalcemia (serum calcium >12 mg/dl) or rapidly increasing serum calcium levels include decreased repolarization time associated with shortened QT interval, bradycardia, and first-degree atrioventricular (AV) block. Chronic PHPT can lead to bone loss, osteoporosis, and fractures. Hypertension and diabetes can also be worsened by PHPT.

In the United States, more than 40% of patients currently diagnosed with PHPT are considered minimally symptomatic or asymptomatic, often having the diagnosis made incidentally on routine blood laboratory examinations. The diagnosis of PHPT requires the findings of elevation or inappropriate levels of serum calcium and intact PTH (iPTH) levels, normal renal function, and normal or increased urinary calcium excretion. Benign familial hypocalciuric hypercalcemia (FHH) results in mildly elevated, asymptomatic serum calcium and iPTH levels and should be excluded by measuring the 24-hour urinary calcium/creatinine clearance. If this is less than 0.01, a diagnosis of FHH should be entertained. Patients with this autosomal-dominant condition do not benefit from parathyroidectomy.

Primary hyperparathyroidism is caused by a solitary parathyroid adenoma in 80% to 85% of patients. Multigland hyperplasia is responsible for PHPT in 15% to 20% of cases, whereas parathyroid carcinoma occurs in less than 1% of patients.

TREATMENT

Indications for Surgery

The most effective treatment and the only chance for cure of PHPT is surgical parathyroidectomy. Although the development of symptoms in PHPT, such as nephrolithiasis, pathologic bone fractures, severe hypercalcemia or crisis, and declining renal function, is a clear indication for surgical treatment, the debate for medical treatment and follow-up versus surgical referral in patients who are deemed asymptomatic or minimally symptomatic still remains. The 1991 National Institutes of Health (NIH) Consensus Meeting and the 2002 NIH Workshop on PHPT recommended criteria for surgical treatment in these patients (Table 1).

Medical Treatment

Asymptomatic patients with mild to moderate PHPT may be treated expectantly with interval follow-up and medications. Patients should avoid either dehydration or intake of excess calcium. Serum vitamin D levels should be monitored and restored, if necessary. Patients taking thiazide diuretics or lithium may have mild elevations of serum calcium and iPTH levels without pathologic PHPT.

Table 1: Guidelines for Surgical Intervention in Asymptomatic Patients with Primary Hyperparathyroidism, Based on the National Institutes of Health Workshop, 2002

- Age <50 years
- Ca ≥1 mg/dl above normal
- 24-hour urinary calcium >400 mg
- Creatinine clearance reduced by 30%
- Bone mineral density t score ≤2.5 any site
- Failure of medical management

These patients should have a biochemical reassessment after discontinuing these medications for a month before the diagnosis of PHPT can be made with certainty.

Oral bisphosphonates such as alendronate or risedronate may be beneficial against bone loss, but etidronate and clodronate have not shown long-term efficacy in PHPT. Raloxifene and salmon calcitonin by nasal spray or injection have not been evaluated for mild PHPT. Calcimimetic agents, which are calcium-sensing receptor agonists, such as cinacalcet, are often used in secondary HPT but are not approved for routine treatment of PHPT.

Patients who are not referred for surgical treatment should be monitored on a biannual basis with testing of serum levels of calcium, iPTH, creatinine, and urinary creatinine clearance. Further recommendations of the 2002 NIH workshop include measurements of yearly 24-hour urinary calcium excretion and bone mass density every 1 or 2 years. If stability is established over 3 to 4 years, the follow-up interval may be increased. Prospective studies of the clinical course of patients with mildly asymptomatic PHPT have shown that up to 30% of patients have evidence of disease progression, with worsening hypercalcemia, hypercalciuria, or bone density loss within 10 years of diagnosis.

Surgical Treatment

All patients with PHPT who are symptomatic, as well as asymptomatic patients included in the NIH criteria and patients who cannot have adequate medical follow-up, should be referred for parathyroidectomy. The traditional bilateral neck exploration for parathyroidectomy under general anesthesia has been the gold standard for decades, with cure rates of more than 95% when performed by experienced parathyroid surgeons. With the development of minimally invasive techniques, aided by advances in preoperative parathyroid imaging and the development of rapid PTH assays, the current surgical standards of parathyroidectomy are changing. The 2002 NIH Workshop recommends that all patients referred for surgical evaluation should have preoperative localization studies to determine the feasibility of minimally invasive parathyroidectomy (MIP) or unilateral exploration. MIP employing local or regional anesthesia on an outpatient basis has been shown to have cure rates equal to standard parathyroidectomy. MIP is also associated with a significant decrease in operating time and costs.

Preoperative Localization and Imaging Techniques

Noninvasive preoperative localization studies include [99m]technetium-sestamibi scintigraphy with or without single photon emission computed tomography (SPECT), ultrasonography, computed tomography (CT), magnetic resonance imaging (MRI), and thallium-201/technetium pertechnetate scanning. More recently, four-dimensional (4D) CT and positron emission tomography (PET)-CT studies also have been employed successfully for parathyroid localization. The single best study is sestamibi combined with SPECT. Sestamibi, a monovalent lipophilic cation, diffuses passively across cell membranes and concentrates in mitochondria. Hence it is preferentially concentrated in mitochondrial-rich adenomatous and hyperplastic parathyroid tissue because of increased blood supply, higher metabolic activity, and an absence of p-glycoprotein on the cell membrane. Sestamibi imaging can be performed preoperatively or within hours of the parathyroidectomy procedure for use of the intraoperative gamma probe for detection of the adenomatous parathyroid glands.

The sensitivity of sestamibi scanning is reported to be between 67% and 90%. This decreases in multiglandular disease or patients with secondary hyperparathyroidism. The addition of SPECT improves the accuracy of localization by allowing visualization of structures in an anterior-posterior plane. It is helpful in the detection of smaller, posteriorly placed parathyroid adenomas (Fig. 1). If unequivocal, this imaging technique can obviate additional studies, unless major coexisting thyroid pathology is suspected. False-positive sestamibi scan can occur because of the existence of other metabolically active tissues, such as occult cancer or hyperplastic thyroid tissue. Addition of a complementary imaging modality, such as ultrasound, can be helpful.

Ultrasound is noninvasive, relatively inexpensive, and useful in patients with concomitant thyroid disease or nodules. It is, however, operator dependent and limited to the neck area. It has a 48% to 74% true-positive rate (Fig. 2). When used in combination with sestamibi, the combined true-positive rate is 90%.

CT and MRI scans provide cross-sectional imaging and are useful for ectopic parathyroid glands in the mediastinum, retroesophageal space, carotid sheath, and other ectopic positions. Parathyroid adenomas appear intense on MRI T2-weighted images. These imaging modalities are often used as secondary studies, confirming an ectopically located parathyroid gland seen on sestamibi or in the reoperative setting.

Figure I Anterior-posterior projection of [99m]technetium-sestamibi scan showing retained uptake in a parathyroid adenoma. **(A)** Submandibular glands. **(B)** Increased uptake in a right-sided parathyroid adenoma. Addition of coronal single photon emission computed tomography (SPECT) image showing uptake in the parathyroid adenoma in the upper right gland (A, submandibular glands). **(C)** Lateral projection SPECT showing uptake to be posterior, thus making the diagnosis of a superior parathyroid gland adenoma. A, superimposed submandibular glands, B, posterior parathyroid adenoma.

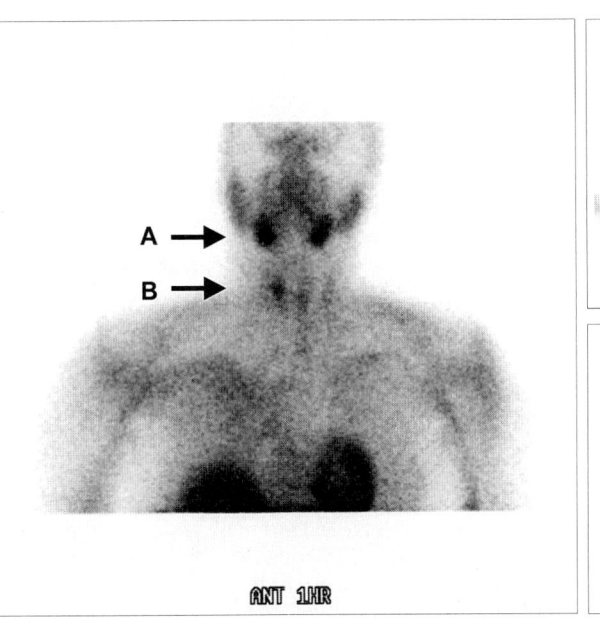

ANT 1HR

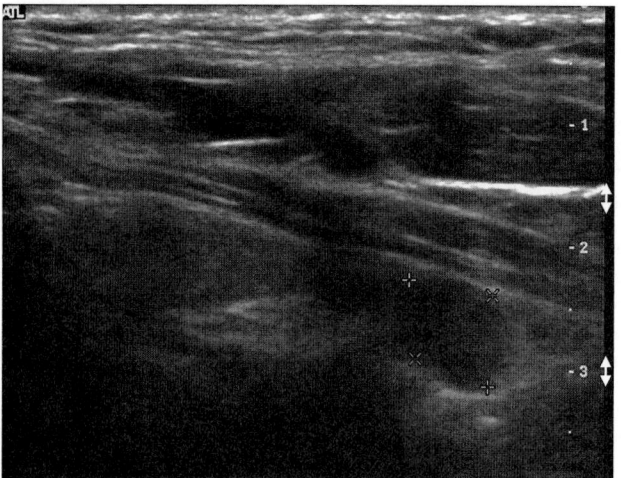

Figure 2 Ultrasound of an inferior parathyroid adenoma. The gland is enlarged, measuring more than 1 cm; hypoechoic; and well circumscribed.

Invasive imaging modalities are reserved for patients who require reoperations for failed initial parathyroidectomy, or for recurrent disease, and who have negative, discordant, or equivocal noninvasive localization studies. The most effective invasive study is the selective angiography with venous sampling of iPTH. This technique is particularly efficacious with the rapid iPTH assay in the angiography suite, allowing real-time guidance of PTH levels and anatomic correlation. Arterial phase studies of parathyroid adenomas have a characteristic blush because of their increased vascularity. The sensitivity of these invasive studies is 60%. Because of the requisite expertise and time of performing these invasive studies, experienced and dedicated centers are optimally suited for referral of reoperative patients.

Sestamibi scanning tends to have a lower sensitivity in the reoperative setting, but ultrasound can yield good results, especially by allowing fine needle aspiration of a suspicious nodule and employing the rapid PTH assay to analyze the aspirate. A 10-fold elevation of PTH levels in the aspirate compared with serum levels confirms parathyroid tissue.

Rapid Intraoperative Parathyroid Hormone Assay

The rapid intraoperative PTH assay (IOPTH) is a useful adjunct. It may be used to confirm adequate removal of hyperfunctioning parathyroid glands and to predict a curative procedure. It is based on the concept that removal of the hyperfunctioning parathyroid gland(s) will result in a rapid and significant decrease in the serum PTH levels. Failure of the serum PTH levels to decrease more than 50% of baseline strongly suggests the presence of residual hyperfunctioning PTH secreting glands.

Conventional Bilateral Neck Exploration

The conventional surgical approach for parathyroidectomy is bilateral exploration of the neck with visualization of all parathyroid glands before excision of the abnormal tissue. It is an established, safe operation with a cure rate of more than 95% and a low rate of complication. It has traditionally been performed without preoperative localization studies. It is usually performed under general anesthesia, and the patient is generally admitted to the hospital overnight for observation. After anesthesia is induced, the patient is placed in the semi-Fowler "sniffing position" for adequate exposure and

extension of the anterior neck. A 3- to 5-cm cervical Kocher incision is made and extended through the subcutaneous tissue and platysma muscle. A subplatysmal flap is developed up to the level of the thyroid cartilage, laterally to the sternocleidomastoid muscles and inferiorly to the sternal notch. After these flaps are developed, a self-retaining retractor can be placed to give appropriate exposure.

Because parathyroid adenomas statistically arise more commonly in the right lower parathyroid gland, we prefer to start the dissection on the right side of the neck.

The strap muscles are separated in the median raphe and dissected laterally off the thyroid capsule from the thyroid cartilage to the sternal notch. The middle thyroid veins are almost always preserved.

The recurrent laryngeal nerve and inferior thyroid artery are identified. The thyroid lobe is mobilized medially. The lower parathyroid gland is usually found in the thyrothymic tract, inferior to the thyroid lobe and anterior to the recurrent laryngeal nerve. This parathyroid gland may lie within the capsule of the lower thyroid pole. The superior parathyroid gland is usually within 1 cm of the recurrent laryngeal nerve as it enters the cricothyroid membrane, posterior to the superior pole of the thyroid. All parathyroid glands should be identified before excision of the abnormal gland(s). This is particularly important for patients with multigland disease who will undergo a subtotal parathyroidectomy, in which preferentially the most normal-appearing gland can be chosen to become the partial remnant. We do not recommend routine biopsy of normal parathyroid glands. If the intraoperative PTH assay is available, fine needle aspiration of an excised parathyroid gland can be used in conjunction with the IOPTH to confirm parathyroid tissue in lieu of frozen-section biopsy. In situ biopsy or aspiration of enlarged glands is generally not recommended because these techniques are associated with parathyromatosis.

Parathyroid glands are often located in a mirror image on the contralateral side, making bilateral exploration easier. Aberrant or ectopic parathyroid tissue has been noted in 15% to 20% of autopsy studies. The vast majority of aberrant hyperfunctioning parathyroid glands can be extirpated successfully through a standard neck exploration. Missing ectopic superior glands are searched for in the retropharyngeal, retroesophageal, posterior mediastinal, intrathyroidal, and the carotid sheath locations. Ectopic inferior glands are often found inside the inferior thyroid capsule or lower pole thyroid parenchyma, carotid sheath, or the thymus—anterior mediastinum. If a single gland is not found, ipsilateral ligation of the inferior thyroid artery can be considered to devascularize the missing parathyroid gland. Alternatively, a thyroid lobectomy can be performed on the ipsilateral site. Intraoperative ultrasound examination may be helpful if an intrathyroidal parathyroid gland is suspected. Intraoperative lateralization of the abnormal parathyroid tissue can be obtained by bilateral internal jugular vein sampling for IOPTH.

Up to 20% of patients have parathyroid glands extending into the mediastinum. Most of these can be extracted through the neck by performing a cervical thymectomy (Table 2). Transsternal mediastinal exploration is required in only 1% to 2% of cases. Subcarinal parathyroid adenomas may be accessed via either partial or complete median sternotomy, whereas posterior mediastinal parathyroid adenomas may require a thoracotomy, although successful resection of these adenomas using video-assisted thoracoscopic surgery is becoming more popular. These procedures are not generally performed at the same time as the primary neck exploration.

Minimally Invasive Parathyroidectomy and Unilateral Exploration

Because 85% of PHPT results from a single adenoma, directed surgery following accurate preoperative localization is becoming more frequent. Minimally invasive parathyroidectomy (MIP), minimal access parathyroidectomy, or unilateral explorations employ directed neck exploration under regional or local anesthesia in the

Table 2: Intraoperative Algorithm for Searching for a "Missing" Parathyroid Gland

Open and inspect the thyroid capsule; palpate the gland/intraoperative ultrasound.

⇩

Dissect the superior thymic/paratracheal tissue; complete a cervical thymectomy (for missing inferior parathyroid glands).

⇩

Mobilize the pharynx and esophagus to look in the parapharyngeal and retropharyngeal and esophageal spaces (for missing superior parathyroid glands).

⇩

Open the carotid sheath and expose the common carotid throughout its course in the neck; inspect for potential parathyroid glands.

⇩

Ligate the ipsilateral inferior thyroid artery and/or perform a thyroid lobectomy. Record location of all confirmed glands identified.

⇩

Terminate procedure; follow the patient for evidence of persistent hypercalcemia. Reimage the patient for evidence of ectopic parathyroid adenomas.

ambulatory setting. These procedures generally require positive preoperative localization. The procedure is usually performed under locoregional analgesia with monitored anesthesia care and sedation, with confirmation of adequacy of resection employing the IOPTH.

The superficial cervical block is often administered by the surgeon using 1% lidocaine with 1:100,000 epinephrine. The patient is positioned in the neck-extension, semi-Fowler ("sniffing") position and prepared; 10 ml of local anesthetic are administered deep to the posterior border of the ipsilateral sternocleidomastoid muscle, with additional lidocaine administered along the anterior border and the anterior neck as needed. Usually 18 to 25 ml of analgesic are used. Intravascular injections must be avoided. Bupivacaine is less desirable because of its long-acting deleterious effects if injected intravascularly. Anesthesia of the recurrent laryngeal nerve is a potential temporary side effect that may be dangerous if both nerves become anesthetized, leading to respiratory compromise. Sedation with fentanyl, midazolam, or both is used to minimize patient anxiety while allowing the patient to phonate.

The 2.5- to 4.0-cm Kocher incision is used for the vast majority of patients. A lateral incision along the sternocleidomastoid muscle can be employed in remedial cases. Measurement of IOPTH can be performed by placing an 18-gauge intravenous (IV) catheter in the arm of the patient and withdrawing 3 ml of blood per measurement. A baseline IOPTH is obtained before the procedure is started. Propofol can interfere with the PTH assay, and therefore it should be discontinued at least 5 minutes before PTH measurement. After the parathyroid adenoma is excised, IOPTH measurements are obtained every 5 minutes for up to 15 minutes, if necessary. A 50% decline in IOPTH from baseline within 10 minutes into the normal range denotes successful extirpation of the disease, and the procedure can be terminated. This percent decline has proven to be predictive of cure in 96% of cases. A fall of IOPTH less than 50% from baseline, plateauing of the level above the normal range, or rebound elevation of IOPTH levels signals the presence of residual multigland disease. In this setting, continued exploration of all

glands may become necessary. Bilateral neck exploration can be performed under regional anesthesia, with conversion to general anesthesia if the patient is uncomfortable.

The vast majority of patients having MIP are discharged on the day of surgery. Symptomatic hypocalcemia is less likely to occur in patients who have undergone MIP. Serum calcium and iPTH levels are measured within the first week of follow-up and at 6 months. Increased oral calcium supplementation of 1500 to 2000 mg per day and vitamin D repletion may be indicated for several months postoperatively after successful parathyroidectomy.

MIP has cure and complication rates similar to those achieved by conventional bilateral exploration (cure: 96% vs. 98%; complications: 3% vs. 1.5). MIP has shorter operating times (1 hour for MIP vs. 2.4 hours for the conventional operation) and significant reduction in hospital stays (0.24 days vs. 1.64 days), with more than $2000 savings per total charges per patient. Operative failures also decrease with the use of the IOPTH.

Radioguided Parathyroidectomy

Radioguided parathyroidectomy is another minimal access technique. It is an extension of the sestamibi localization study. Five milliequivalents of ^{99m}Tc-sestamibi is administered IV approximately 1 hour before neck exploration. Using similar anesthetic techniques, as described earlier and a handheld gamma probe, the area of highest radioactivity is found in the neck and a 2- to 3-cm incision is performed directly over this site. The parathyroid adenoma is dissected, employing the same principles described earlier. The parathyroid adenoma should have gamma counts of at least 20% greater than the thyroid background counts. Although this technique appears attractive, most endocrine surgery centers have not found it to be advantageous. IOPTH appears more useful than gamma probe counts to ensure the success of the operation.

TREATMENT OF HYPERCALCEMIC CRISIS

Patients with PHPT seldom present with symptoms and extremely high or rapidly increasing serum calcium levels. Urgent medical and surgical treatment is necessary in these patients, who present with severe dehydration, hypotension, altered mental status, and dysrhythmias. The initial management requires aggressive rehydration with normal saline at a rate of 300 ml/hr. This restores the intravascular volume contraction and promotes renal excretion of calcium. Fluid overload must be avoided. Loop diuretics can be used to reduce fluid overload and inhibit calcium resorption in the loop of Henle, thus promoting increased renal calcium excretion. Patients with renal failure should be dialyzed with low-calcium dialysate.

A variety of pharmacologic agents can be employed to lower serum calcium levels after rehydration. Glucocorticoids lower calcium by inhibiting the effects of vitamin D, increasing renal calcium excretion, and inhibiting osteoclast-activating factor. The initial dose of hydrocortisone is 200 to 400 mg IV per day for 3 to 5 days. Bisphosphonates inhibit osteoclast activity, thus preventing bone resorption induced by PTH. Pamidronate (90 mg IV) or zoledronic acid (4 mg IV initial treatment, 8 mg on retreatment) normalizes calcium levels in most patients.

Calcitonin acts quickly (within 24 to 48 hours) to lower serum calcium levels and is more effective when used in combination with glucocorticoids. It should not be used in patients with salmon allergies.

After patients with PHPT and hypercalcemic crisis are stabilized and serum calcium levels have been reduced to acceptable levels, preoperative localization studies should be obtained expeditiously in anticipation of an urgent parathyroidectomy.

POSTOPERATIVE MANAGEMENT

Patients who undergo conventional bilateral neck explorations may require an overnight hospital stay, whereas most patients who undergo MIP or unilateral explorations are treated as outpatients. Patients should be instructed about the symptoms of hypocalcemia (perioral and digital paresthesias) and instructed to take 1500 to 3000 mg of calcium supplementation per day. Calcium carbonate is most easily absorbed and tolerated. Mild postoperative hypocalcemia occurs in up to 25% of patients. Neck hematomas and recurrent laryngeal nerve injuries are rare (1% to 2%).

Calcium supplementation should be continued for approximately 3 months to avoid potential reactive secondary hyperparathyroidism of a chronic hypocalcemic state. A normal serum calcium and intact PTH level at 6 months postoperatively denotes cure. Persistent hyperparathyroidism is diagnosed if biochemical evidence of PHPT occurs within the initial 6-month postoperative period. It is due to a missed parathyroid adenoma or unrecognized multigland disease. Recurrent hyperparathyroidism results from the development of another parathyroid adenoma or hyperplasia after a 6-month period of normocalcemia. This may occur in up to 10% of patients long term.

SUGGESTED READINGS

Bilezikian JP, Potts JT Jr, Fuleihan EH, and others: Summary statement from a workshop on asymptomatic primary hyperparathyroidism: a perspective for the 21st century, *J Clin Endocrinol Metab* 87:5353, 2002.

Roman SA, Sosa JA, Mayes L, and others: Parathyroidectomy improves neurocognitive deficits in patients with primary hyperparathyroidism, *Surgery* 138:1121, 2005.

Sosa JA, Powe NR, Levine MA, and others: Cost implications of different surgical management strategies for primary hyperparathyroidism, *Surgery* 124:1028, 1998.

Udelsman R: Six hundred fifty-six consecutive explorations for primary hyperparathyroidism, *Ann Surg* 235:665, 2002.

Udelsman R, Aruny JE, Donovan PI, and others: Rapid parathyroid hormone analysis during venous localization, *Ann Surg* 237:714; discussion 719, 2003.

PERSISTENT OR RECURRENT HYPERPARATHYROIDISM

Elizabeth A. Mittendorf, MD, and Nancy D. Perrier, MD

Primary hyperparathyroidism (PHPT), an endocrinopathy involving calcium metabolism, is treated by parathyroidectomy.

Traditionally, parathyroidectomy has involved exploration of all four parathyroid glands. With the improvement of preoperative localization studies and the introduction of intraoperative adjuncts such as the rapid intraoperative parathyroid hormone (IOPTH) assay, minimally invasive parathyroidectomy (MIP) has increasingly become the surgical procedure of choice. Regardless of the operative approach, cure, defined as eucalcemia 6 months after parathyroidectomy, is achieved in more than 95% of patients with PHPT when the operation is performed by an experienced endocrine surgeon.

A patient who does not achieve or maintain eucalcemia in the 6 months following parathyroidectomy is considered to have persistent disease, which occurs in approximately 5% of patients. If a patient has an apparently successful operation but develops hypercalcemia in the setting of an inappropriately elevated parathyroid hormone (PTH) level more than 6 months following parathyroidectomy, the patient is considered to have recurrent disease. Recurrent disease is uncommon, occurring in less than 1.5% of patients in large series from experienced endocrine centers. In this chapter, we review the pathophysiology, evaluation, and treatment of patients with either persistent or recurrent hyperparathyroidism.

ANATOMY AND PATHOPHYSIOLOGY

The normal locations of the parathyroid glands are fairly consistent. Fig. 1 depicts the positions in which parathyroid glands are most often found. Superior glands are commonly located superior to the inferior thyroid artery and posterior to the recurrent laryngeal nerve. They are often juxtaposed to the posterior capsule of the thyroid parenchyma. In such locations, the gland may be

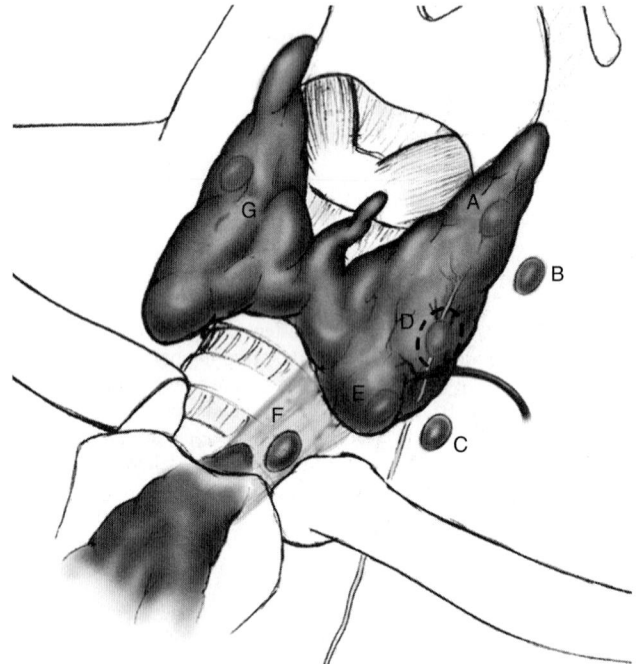

Figure 1 Parathyroid localization nomenclature. *(A)* Superior gland, in proximity of posterior surface of thyroid parenchyma. May be intracapsular or compressed. *(B)* Superior gland, fallen posteriorly into tracheoesophageal groove. May not contact the posterior surface of thyroid tissue. Found in the region of the craniocaudal confines of the thyroid lobe. *(C)* Superior gland, fallen posteriorly into tracheoesophageal groove. May not contact the posterior surface of thyroid tissue. Caudal-inferior to craniocaudal confines of thyroid lobe. *(D)* In the midregion of the posterior surface of the thyroid parenchyma. Could be superior or inferior gland because the nerve is not visible. Near junction of recurrent laryngeal nerve and inferior thyroidal artery. *(E)* Inferior gland in inferior region of thyroid parenchyma, which lies in anteroposterior plane of the thyroid, anterior to the trachea. *(F)* Inferior gland that has descended into thyrothymic ligament or superior thymus. May appear to be "ectopic" or in mediastinum. Anteroposterior view shows it anterior and near the trachea. *(G)* Intrathyroidal parathyroid (rare).

intimately attached to the undersurface of the thyroid within the thyroid capsule *(A)*. Some superior glands, especially heavy adenomatous glands, fall posteriorly in the tracheoesophageal groove. Such glands may not be in contact with the thyroid parenchyma *(B* and *C)*. Inferior glands usually lie near the inferior pole of the thyroid and are inferior to the inferior thyroid artery and medial and anterior to the recurrent laryngeal nerve *(E)*. Enlarged, heavy, inferior glands may fall anteriorly into the thyrothymic ligament *(F)*. Intrathyroidal parathyroid glands are rare but do occur *(G)*. Ectopic locations of parathyroid glands include within the carotid sheath, in the anterior mediastinum (nonthymic), and in a high cervical, undescended position. Supernumerary glands occur in 7% to 10% of the population.

Persistent hyperparathyroidism occurs when residual hyperfunctioning parathyroid tissue remains in the neck following parathyroidectomy. Failed initial neck explorations result from (1) failure to localize a parathyroid adenoma, (2) inadequate resection of multigland disease, or (3) implantation of cells from a fractured parathyroid adenoma (parathyromatosis). Failure to localize an adenoma can be due to a missed gland in the neck or a gland in the mediastinum that is out of reach of cervical dissection.

A review from the Mayo Clinic found that the majority of missed abnormal parathyroid glands were in usual anatomic locations. A small number were intrathyroidal or were found within the carotid sheath, anterior to the trachea, or in a retroesophageal location. When the Mayo Clinic group compared patients with persistent disease referred from outside institutions with their own first-time failures, they found that most referred patients had a missed single adenoma (82%); missed single adenomas accounted for only 15% of their first-time failures. Interestingly, all of the missed single adenomas from their institution were mediastinal glands, and the patients were subsequently cured following mediastinal exploration.

In a review of the University of California, San Francisco, experience with reoperative parathyroidectomy, investigators found that the previous operation in patients with persistent hyperparathyroidism was a bilateral approach with reported four-gland exploration in almost 90% of patients and a limited approach in only 10%. Interestingly, four parathyroid glands were actually identified in less than 25% of the patients in the bilateral approach group. The findings from these two experienced endocrine centers support a recommendation that initial exploration be performed by a surgeon with thorough knowledge of the anatomy and embryology of the cervical and mediastinal regions.

Inadequate excision of hyperplastic tissue in patients with multigland disease also results in persistent hyperparathyroidism. Multigland disease has historically accounted for 15% of cases of PHPT. In series reporting the results of MIP, multigland disease was found in 3% to 10% of cases. This frequency of multigland disease is based on early data that do not show an increased rate of persistent or recurrent disease in the MIP era. Longer follow-up is necessary to confirm this operative success rate. These findings, however, suggest that some of the glands removed at the time of four-gland exploration may not be hyperfunctioning despite the fact that they appear enlarged. With MIP, when an IOPTH assay is used, a 50% drop from baseline in the IOPTH value 5 to 10 minutes after resection suggests that all hyperfunctioning tissue has been removed, regardless of the number of glands resected and their gross appearance. This approach is dependent on a low false-positive rate for IOPTH assays. A false-positive IOPTH assay result would be a value that drops by more than 50% despite the fact that additional hyperfunctioning parathyroid tissue remains. Equivalent cure rates with standard four-gland exploration and MIP confirm that this functional, as opposed to anatomic, approach to parathyroidectomy is effective.

A final cause of persistent disease is parathyromatosis, which occurs when there is gross rupture of the tumor capsule during the initial operation. This can lead to implantation of adenomatous or hyperplastic parathyroid cells in surrounding soft tissue and muscle. This condition is difficult to cure by reoperation because of dense dissemination of parathyroid cells.

In contrast to persistent disease, in which residual hyperfunctioning parathyroid tissue remains in the neck following parathyroidectomy, recurrent hyperparathyroidism results from postoperative development of autonomous hypersecretion by presumed, previously normally functioning parathyroid glands. Fortunately, except in patients with familial hyperparathyroidism, recurrent disease is rare.

INDICATIONS FOR REOPERATION

When recommending initial parathyroidectomy, the majority of endocrine surgeons take into consideration criteria outlined by a National Institutes of Health consensus conference statement (Table 1). However, reoperative parathyroid surgery is technically more difficult and associated with greater rates of morbidity. In addition, patients frequently have greater anxiety because of the initial failure to cure their disease, the prospect of continued disease-related complications, or the possibility of an additional surgical procedure, with its increased cost and risk of complications. For these reasons, the indications for reoperation should be more stringent than those used for initial exploration. Reoperative parathyroidectomy should be performed in patients with ongoing nephrolithiasis, worsening renal function, worsening bone disease as evidenced by bone mineral density scores, associated neuromuscular or psychiatric symptoms, worrisome hypercalcemia, or a combination of these (Table 1). These indications may be modified if two or more concordant imaging studies localize an enlarged parathyroid adenoma.

Table 1: Indications for Initial versus Reoperative Parathyroidectomy

Indications for Initial Parathyroidectomy*	Indications for Reoperative Parathyroidectomy for Persistent or Recurrent Disease
Serum calcium level >1 mg/dl above the upper limit of normal	Ongoing nephrolithiasis
Age <50 years	Worsening renal function
Osteoporosis (T-score ≤2.5 at any site)	Worsening bone disease as evidenced by bone mineral density scores
Creatinine clearance decreased by >30%	Associated neuromuscular symptoms
24-Hour urinary calcium excretion >400 mg/day	Associated psychiatric symptoms
Typical bone, renal, gastrointestinal, or neuromuscular symptoms	Worrisome progressive hypercalcemia
History of life-threatening hypercalcemia	
Medical surveillance not desirable or not possible	

*Criteria outlined by a National Institutes of Health consensus conference statement.

PREOPERATIVE EVALUATION

History, Physical Examination, and Laboratory Evaluation

The evaluation and management of patients with persistent or recurrent hyperparathyroidism are complex. The initial step in the evaluation of these patients is to confirm the diagnosis. Serum calcium and intact PTH levels should be checked to ensure that both are inappropriately elevated. An elevated PTH level in the setting of a normal calcium level occurs postoperatively in up to 30% of patients who undergo parathyroidectomy and is not indicative of persistent disease. Several potential etiologies for this phenomenon have been described, including a secondary response to bone remineralization (i.e., hungry bone syndrome), low vitamin D levels, and impaired renal function. In the majority of these patients, the PTH level normalizes over time. Conversely, an elevated calcium level in the setting of an appropriately low PTH level suggests a misdiagnosis. In these patients, the possibility of a concomitant malignancy should be excluded. Additional laboratory evaluations that should be undertaken in all patients with concern for persistent or recurrent disease include measurements of serum vitamin D (25-hydroxy), magnesium, phosphorous, blood urea nitrogen, and creatinine. A 24-hour urinary calcium level should also be checked to evaluate for benign familial hypocalciuric hypercalcemia, a condition that does not require parathyroidectomy.

Evaluation of persistent or recurrent disease should also include a thorough medical history. One should inquire about a family history of endocrinopathies, including multiple endocrine neoplasia syndromes and familial PHPT. It may be helpful to ask about a family history of kidney stones, significant ulcer disease, thyroid cancer, and pancreatic or adrenal tumors, which may be common in families with hereditary disease that has not yet been diagnosed. The presence of a familial endocrinopathy syndrome suggests multigland disease. Male gender or young age at the time of diagnosis should also increase suspicion regarding the presence of multigland disease.

During the physical examination, particular attention should be paid to factors that may have caused previous imaging studies to be inaccurate and surgical exploration to be difficult, such as a large body mass index or the presence of a goiter or thyroid nodules. The location of the previous incision should be noted. Before undertaking reoperative parathyroidectomy in any patient, laryngoscopy should be performed to assess for possible vocal cord paralysis related to the previous operation.

Review of Previous Reports

Before performing reoperative surgery, the surgeon should obtain as much information regarding the initial surgical procedure as possible. Review of localization studies such as sestamibi scans or ultrasound examinations obtained before the initial parathyroidectomy may provide insights into what the findings at the time of initial surgery should have been. Discussion with the surgeon who performed the initial parathyroidectomy, if not the current surgeon, or review of an operative report detailing the procedure can determine whether the intraoperative findings correlated with the preoperative images. The operative report provides details regarding whether a four-gland exploration or MIP was performed, which parathyroid glands were identified, and which were removed. For glands identified in expected anatomic locations, note should be made of their described appearance and whether they were biopsied and confirmed to be parathyroid tissue. The operative report should also indicate the amount of time spent exploring the neck, which sites of potential ectopic glands were evaluated, and whether the thymus was delivered into the operative field and inspected or

removed. Factors that could complicate the identification of parathyroid glands such as coexisting thyroid pathology (e.g., Hashimoto's thyroiditis or a multinodular goiter) or the presence of benign enlarged lymph nodes should also be noted.

The pathology report from the initial surgery should also be meticulously reviewed. This report provides details regarding the size, weight, and cellularity of the pathologic tissue that was removed, as well as information about any normal tissue that was resected. Additional biopsies that were performed should be noted. The performance of multiple biopsies of tissue that proved to be thyroid nodules, lymph nodes, or benign fat suggests difficulty in identifying parathyroid tissue.

Preoperative Localization

For patients undergoing reoperative parathyroidectomy, a minimum of two concordant imaging studies is required. If preoperative localization is successful, the rate of cure with reoperative parathyroidectomy is greater than 90%. When preoperative localization is not successful, the cure rate drops to between 60% and 70%.

Multiple imaging modalities have been used including sestamibi scanning, ultrasonography (US), computed tomography (CT), and selective venous sampling (SVS). Studies have suggested that increasing numbers of concordant true-positive localization studies result in improved surgical cure rates. Common initial localization studies performed on patients with persistent or recurrent disease are ^{99m}technetium (^{99m}Tc)-sestamibi single photon emission computed tomography (SPECT)-CT and high-resolution, real-time neck US. Sestamibi scanning can visualize hyperfunctioning parathyroid glands and help to lateralize the hyperfunctioning glands to one side of the neck. When this test is ordered, it is important to request mediastinal views to evaluate for an ectopic gland in the mediastinum, as well as jaw views to evaluate for an undescended gland. Sestamibi is most valuable in identifying a hyperfunctioning adenoma that was not found during the initial surgical procedure. Sestamibi is not as valuable in evaluating patients with multigland disease.

High-resolution, real-time US must be performed by an experienced ultrasonographer. The performance and interpretation of a US study is aided by knowledge of the results of prior localization studies and intraoperative findings. US is able to provide good anatomic information, but it is unable to assess the hypersecretory status of any lesion identified. Fine needle aspiration biopsy for cytologic confirmation and PTH assay can be performed at the time of US evaluation. Studies have shown that US with cytologic and biochemical confirmation improves the accuracy of US alone in confirming parathyroid tissue from 65% to greater than 80% and the sensitivity from 75% to 90%. Often sestamibi and US provide concordant data; therefore the two studies are frequently adequate to localize an adenomatous gland before reoperation.

Four-dimensional CT (4D-CT) has recently been described for the preoperative evaluation of patients with parathyroid disease. This imaging modality is similar to CT angiography. In addition to generating detailed multiplanar images of the neck, 4D-CT visualizes differences in the perfusion characteristics of hyperfunctioning parathyroid glands (i.e., rapid uptake and quick washout) compared with normal parathyroid glands and other structures in the neck. The images generated by 4D-CT therefore provide both anatomic information and a correlate of function (perfusion) with a single modality. Early studies suggested that 4D-CT has higher sensitivity than sestamibi scanning and US in lateralizing hyperfunctioning parathyroid glands to one side of the neck. The greatest benefit of 4D-CT, however, is its ability to identify precisely the location of parathyroid tumors in the neck. Figure 2 shows a 4D-CT scan obtained in a patient with persistent hyperparathyroidism who had previously undergone four-gland exploration. The 4D-CT scan clearly demonstrates an abnormal parathyroid gland in

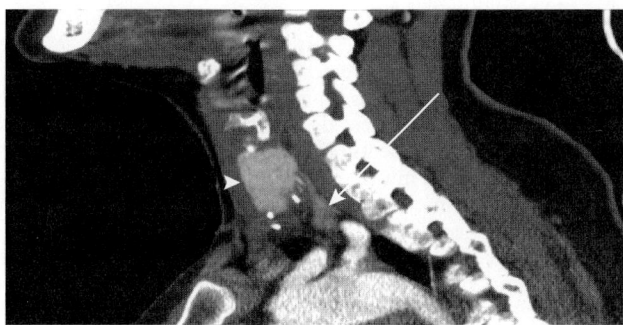

Figure 2 Four-dimensional computed tomography scans obtained on a patient with persistent hyperparathyroidism who had undergone prior four-gland exploration. An abnormal left superior parathyroid adenoma measuring 2 cm superoinferior by 7 mm anteroposterior was identified. The adenoma (arrow) is seen on its vascular pedicle in the tracheoesophageal groove well below the left lobe of the thyroid (arrowhead). The lesion showed vigorous enhancement with rapid washout, consistent with a parathyroid adenoma.

the left neck measuring 2 cm superoinferior by 7 mm anterior-posterior. The adenoma was interpreted as a superior gland that had fallen into the tracheoesophageal groove. It showed vigorous enhancement with rapid washout, findings consistent with a parathyroid adenoma. After this localization study was performed, the patient was taken to the operating room and the lesion was easily identified and removed during focused reexploration.

If noninvasive localization procedures provide discordant or indeterminate results, SVS should be considered. This technique requires catheterization of multiple veins in the neck and mediastinum, including the superior, middle, and inferior thyroid veins and the subclavian vein. Blood samples are obtained from these veins and assessed using a rapid PTH assay. The ability to obtain the results quickly allows the interventional radiologist performing the procedure to obtain additional samples from any site where subtle but potentially significant changes in PTH levels are detected. In addition, because parathyroid adenomas have increased vascularity, they have a characteristic blush on arteriograms, which can be performed selectively on the basis of venous regionalization. Studies looking at the accuracy of SVS of intact PTH levels in difficult cases of recurrent or persistent hyperparathyroidism have shown true-positive results in 75% of patients. False-positive rates are approximately 15%, and the results are indeterminate in approximately 5% of cases. Unfortunately, SVS is costly, time consuming, and difficult to perform. To achieve optimal results, the procedure must be performed by an experienced interventional radiologist.

REOPERATIVE PARATHYROIDECTOMY

Reoperative parathyroidectomy is more challenging than an initial exploration, with a lower cure rate (89% vs. >95%) and greater morbidity. Patients must therefore be counseled regarding the possibility of persistent disease and complications. The incidence of vocal cord paralysis is greater after reoperative parathyroidectomy, with a recurrent laryngeal nerve injury rate of approximately 4% depending on the extent of exploration during previous operation(s). In addition, there is a higher incidence of aparathyroidism resulting in hypocalcemia caused by devascularization of normal parathyroid glands during the neck dissection, particularly if patients had a prior four-gland exploration. This aparathyroidism may be permanent. Patients should be advised that such an outcome would require lifelong calcium and vitamin D supplementation.

If preoperative localization studies suggest that a directed approach is possible, this is preferred because it helps to reduce

operative morbidity by minimizing the dissection that must be performed in an already scarred neck where normal tissue planes are destroyed and identification of normal structures is challenging. In large series treating patients with persistent or recurrent hyperparathyroidism, directed parathyroidectomy was successfully performed in more than 70% on the basis of the preoperative localization tests in association with the previous operative and histologic findings.

Several strategies may be helpful when performing reoperative parathyroidectomy. One technique is to use a lateral approach between the infrahyoid muscles and sternocleidomastoid muscle; this approach may offer easier access, especially to superior glands that have fallen posteriorly. Whenever feasible, the recurrent laryngeal nerve should be identified because it provides a level of comfort to know where the nerve is when resecting presumed abnormal parathyroid tissue. When abnormal glands are identified, frozen-section evaluation should be performed to get histologic confirmation that hyperplastic parathyroid tissue has been removed. It is also possible to aspirate the resected tissue and send the aspirate for determination of PTH levels. To perform this aspiration, a 25-gauge needle is used on a 5-ml syringe. Approximately 1 ml of normal saline is drawn up into the syringe, after which the tissue is directly aspirated until a small flash is seen in the needle hub. The contents of the syringe are placed into a purple top ethylenediamine tetraacetic acid tub and sent for biochemical analysis. PTH values that exceed the maximal concentration of the assay (>1900 pg/dl) confirm that the tissue is of parathyroid origin. The additional intraoperative adjuncts described in the following section can be helpful when performing reoperative parathyroidectomy.

INTRAOPERATIVE ADJUNCTS

Intraoperative Parathyroid Hormone Assay

IOPTH assays provide objective evidence of the adequacy of resection. When good preoperative localization studies suggest a single adenoma, a focused exploration can be undertaken. Before resection of the suspected abnormal parathyroid tissue, blood is obtained from either the ipsilateral internal jugular vein or a peripheral vessel. Additional blood samples are obtained 5 and 10 minutes after excision. If a peripheral site is used, no intravenous fluid should be infused on the ipsilateral side because the infusant may dilute the specimen. An intraoperative decline in the PTH level of 50% or more from the baseline value, and preferably into the normal PTH range, confirms that the resected tissue was likely the cause of persistent disease. No further exploration is required in these cases; a decrease of 50% or more from the baseline PTH level has been shown to be a reliable predictor of a successful operation in patients with persistent or recurrent hyperparathyroidism, with sensitivity and positive predictive values greater than 90%. If a 50% drop in IOPTH level is not achieved, further exploration should be considered to look for multigland disease. If a directed approach was attempted, this may require conversion to a standard cervical exploration.

For patients in whom review of the outside operative notes, pathology reports, and preoperative localization studies suggest multigland disease, the surgery may begin as a four-gland exploration. IOPTH assays can still assist in confirming the adequacy of resection. Some authors have reported data suggesting that increasing the degree of decline in PTH level from 50% to 70% from baseline at 20 minutes after excision is more accurate in patients with multigland disease.

Intraoperative PTH is a useful adjunct that must be taken in context with good clinical judgment. For example, in a patient with a preoperative calcium level of 12.0 mg/dl and preoperative imaging that suggests a single adenoma, if a relatively small gland weighing only 150 mg is identified at the time of directed parathyroidectomy and IOPTH drops 51%, further exploration should be considered. In contrast, if a large, 3-g adenoma is found in the anticipated anatomic location and IOPTH drops only 35%, we would consider the possibility of a laboratory error, dilution of the sample if drawn peripherally, or other source of contamination. The IOPTH can be repeated. It is likely that the large adenoma is the source of persistent disease in this scenario, and further exploration is likely not warranted.

Intraoperative Ultrasound

Intraoperative US has been demonstrated to be effective in identifying intrathyroidal parathyroid adenomas. However, a limitation of this technique is differentiating an intrathyroidal parathyroid adenoma from a thyroid colloid nodule. In cases of reoperative parathyroidectomy, we use US to identify intrathyroidal lesions and to provide guidance for fine needle aspiration. The cytopathologist can then assist in differentiating between the two entities. After resection, we again use an IOPTH assay, with a 50% or greater drop confirming the adequacy of resection.

Nerve Monitoring

The routine use of intraoperative nerve monitoring remains debated. Nerve monitoring can aid in the identification of the recurrent laryngeal nerve in a densely scarred operative field. Its greatest benefit may be confirmation of nerve, after it is identified in scarred tissue, if identification is not certain. It may be particularly useful in facilitating identification of the nerve if the parathyroid gland to be excised is near the midposterior surface of the thyroid gland. The intricacies of this technique usually require that it be performed regularly to allow confidence in its use. Attention must be paid to multiple details such as equipment function, placement of the probe, probe accuracy and interpretation of results. If not part of routine care, it may be too cumbersome and misleading for occasional use.

Cryopreservation and Autotransplantation

In patients undergoing reoperative parathyroidectomy who have had multiple prior procedures with resection or manipulation and potential devascularization of multiple glands, parathyroid tissue should be cryopreserved. This tissue serves as an important "insurance policy" for the patient should the resected tissue be the only parathyroid tissue remaining. If aparathyroidism occurs and cryopreserved tissue is successfully autotransplanted, it can significantly affect the patient's quality of life. To cryopreserve, confirmed parathyroid tissue that is removed from the neck at the time of surgery is morcellated into 20- to 30-mm pieces. These pieces are placed in a sterile Petri dish with Tis-Sol solution. A freezing medium is then added, after which the mixture is transferred into two to three sterile vials and frozen at −80°C. In a recently reported series looking at the long-term functionality of parathyroid autografts, approximately 60% of delayed, cryopreserved parathyroid autografts were found to be functional. Of these, 40% enabled patients to achieve full parathyroid competency without any supplementation. A long duration of cryopreservation is a significant predictor of graft failure. We do not recommend transplantation greater than 24 months after freezing.

The success rate for fresh parathyroid autografts has been reported to exceed 80%. For this reason, in patients who have already had multiple glands removed, autotransplantation into the nondominant brachioradialis muscle at the time of reoperative parathyroidectomy is preferred. Resected parathyroid tissue is minced into 1-mm fragments. A 1- to 2-cm incision is made, after which a pocket in the muscle is created, and 10 to 20 of the parathyroid pieces are inserted. The pocket is closed and tagged with hemoclips or Prolene (Ethicon, Somerville, NJ) for future site identification if necessary. The forearm is used preferentially over the sternocleidomastoid muscle in the neck because the forearm is easier to reexplore if the patient were to have persistent or recurrent disease caused by the autotransplanted tissue. In addition, it is easier to identify PTH gradients with peripheral blood draws if the tissue is autotransplanted into the forearm.

Radioguided Parathyroidectomy

Radioguided parathyroidectomy is a technique that combines ^{99m}Tc injection and intraoperative gamma probe for parathyroid tissue localization. This combination technique has the greatest utility in the identification of a single adenoma; its utility is limited in patients with multigland disease or concomitant nodular thyroid disease.

On the morning of surgery, the patient receives 15 to 20 mCi of ^{99m}Tc. After a delay of 60 to 90 minutes, which allows for washout of the ^{99m}Tc from the thyroid gland, the patient proceeds to the operating room. The gamma probe can be used to identify the site with the highest count transcutaneously, thereby indicating the most appropriate location to make an incision for directed parathyroidectomy. The gamma probe can be used intraoperatively to direct the surgeon to the adenoma; it can reliably differentiate pathological parathyroid lesions from other structures in the neck, including lymph nodes and normal parathyroid glands. After the suspected abnormal tissue is resected, the gamma probe is used to obtain an ex vivo count to confirm retention of the radioisotope. An IOPTH assay is used to confirm the adequacy of resection.

Another adjunct, methylene blue injection, has been described for use in conjunction with radioguided parathyroidectomy. Methylene blue stains both normal and abnormal parathyroid glands, thereby facilitating their intraoperative identification. Methylene blue (7.5 mg/kg in 500 ml of 5% dextrose in water) is administered intravenously over 60 to 90 minutes, with the rate being adjusted to complete the infusion at the time of skin incision. Local effects, most commonly discomfort at the infusion site, are experienced by approximately 70% of patients. In less than 8% of patients, a more serious side effect such as local edema or thrombophlebitis occurs.

SUGGESTED READINGS

Cohen MS, Dilley WG, Wells SA, and others: Long-term functionality of cryopreserved parathyroid autografts: a 13-year prospective analysis, *Surgery* 138:1033, 2005.

Jones JJ, Brunaud L, Dowd CF, and others: Accuracy of selective venous sampling for intact parathyroid hormone in difficult patients with recurrent or persistent hyperparathyroidism, *Surgery* 132:944, 2002.

Sebag F, Shen W, Brunaud L, and others: Intraoperative parathyroid hormone assay and parathyroid reoperations, *Surgery* 134:1049, 2003.

Thompson GB, Grant CS, Perrier ND, and others: Reoperative parathyroid surgery in the era of sestamibi scanning and intraoperative parathyroid hormone monitoring, *Arch Surg* 134:699, 1999.

SECONDARY AND TERTIARY HYPERPARATHYROIDISM

Sanziana A. Roman, MD, and Julie Ann Sosa, MA, MD

HISTORY

The last major organ to be recognized in humans was the parathyroid glands, which were discovered in 1880 by a Swedish medical student, Ivar Sandstrom. In the early 1900s, Erdheim demonstrated that all four parathyroid glands were enlarged in osteomalacia and rickets. Albright first suggested a relationship between chronic renal disease and hyperparathyroidism in 1934; however, he suggested that bone disease seen in patients with renal failure resulted from acidosis rather than hyperparathyroidism. Castleman and Mallory described the pathologic finding of chief cell hyperplasia leading to marked parathyroid gland enlargement. In 1959, Stanbury and Lumb described three types of skeletal problems in renal failure: renal rickets, osteomalacia, and renal osteitis fibrosa. They also reported the first subtotal parathyroidectomy as definitive therapy. In 1971, Wilson reported a 7-year experience with surgically treated patients with severe secondary hyperparathyroidism (2PHPT) and renal failure, showing that subtotal parathyroidectomy is an effective means of preventing the progression of osteitis fibrosa.

PATHOPHYSIOLOGY

Most commonly 2PHPT occurs in patients with end-stage renal disease (ESRD), but it also compensates for the true hypocalcemia associated with some diseases of the gastrointestinal tract, bone, or other endocrine organs. A defect in mineral homeostasis leads to a compensatory increase in parathyroid gland function and size. The pathogenesis of 2PHPT in chronic renal failure has multiple contributing factors, such as possible genetic mutations, altered vitamin D (calcitriol) metabolism and resistance, an impaired calcemic response to parathyroid hormone (PTH), phosphate retention, and altered PTH metabolism. The pathways leading to 2PHPT have different predominating factors, depending on the severity of renal failure. Early in the disease, mutations in the calcium-sensing receptor (CaSR) and possible defects in calcitriol receptors lead to incipient 2PHPT. Subtle decreases in calcitriol levels, increasing serum phosphate levels, and the direct action of calcitriol and phosphate on the parathyroid glands further potentiate 2PHPT. In progressing renal failure, calcitriol deficiency becomes important and phosphate retention plays a major role in worsening 2PHPT. Changes in calcium set points, increasing skeletal resistance to PTH, and parathyroid gland hyperplasia contribute to the development of severe 2PHPT.

With prolonged compensatory stimulation, a hyperplastic gland occasionally develops autonomous function. This state is referred to as *tertiary hyperparathyroidism* (3PHPT). St. Goar was the first to recognize this entity in patients who underwent renal transplantation. Reversal of parathyroid hyperplasia should theoretically be expected after successful renal transplantation. Nevertheless, studies show that hypercalcemia can persist in the range of 8.5% to 53% of transplant recipients. Of these, less than 1% requires parathyroidectomy. In the transplant patient, there may be additional factors that can contribute to persistent 3PHPT, including use of steroids, cyclosporine, and thiazide diuretics, as well as glomerular filtration rate (GFR) alterations caused by tubular injury or rejection episodes.

MEDICAL THERAPY

Virtually all patients with chronic renal failure requiring hemodialysis (HD) have some degree of 2PHPT. Hyperphosphatemia, vitamin D deficiency, and resulting hypocalcemia traditionally have been treated by effective dialysis and correction of uremia, calcium supplementation, phosphate restriction, and the administration of phosphate binders and vitamin D derivatives. These treatments have moderate efficacy. One problem encountered can be attributed to hypercalcemia resulting from the administration of calcium salts as a phosphate binder and the calcemic action of vitamin D. Hypercalcemia and hyperphosphatemia (as measured by the calcium-phosphate product) can result in accelerated systemic calcifications. Non-calcium-containing phosphate binders (sevelamer hydrochloride and lanthanum) and vitamin D analogues that suppress PTH secretion with minimum calcemic action have been developed. These "noncalcemic" vitamin D derivatives include 19-nor-1-alpha, 25-dihydroxyvitamin D2 (paricalcitol), 1-alpha-hydroxyvitamin D2 (doxercalciferol), 22 oxa-calcitriol (maxacalcitol), and F6-calcitriol (falecalcitriol).

Recent developments have been made in the modulation of the CaSR using calcimimetic agents. Cinacalcet, a calcimimetic agent that acts as an allosteric activator of the CaSR, has proved to be an effective therapy for 2PHPT because it simultaneously reduces the concentrations of PTH, calcium, and phosphate in dialysis patients. It is absorbed rapidly from the gastrointestinal tract and reaches peak plasma levels within 2 to 3 hours after the oral administration of the drug, corresponding also to a plasma PTH concentration decrease of up to 60% to 70% after a single administration. The plasma PTH response is linearly dose dependent up to 200 mg cinacalcet every 24 hours. The pharmacokinetics of cinacalcet are not affected by dialysis.

Calcimimetic agents are now one of the primary therapeutic interventions for 2PHPT. The extent to which they improve clinical outcomes in the long run remains unclear. A recent analysis of Medicare parathyroidectomy rates between 1992 and 2002 in the United States showed an increasing number of surgical interventions between 1998 and 2002, despite the fact that this period overlapped with the development and dissemination of these new medical treatment alternatives for 2PHPT.

INDICATIONS FOR SURGERY

Failure of Medical Management

More than 300,000 people are undergoing therapy for ESRD in the United States. Virtually all of these patients eventually suffer from 2PHPT. The mortality rate for dialysis patients is approximately 20% per year. Associated diabetes, cardiovascular disease, decreased nutritional status, and certain demographic factors (i.e., older age, male gender) have been related to increased morbidity and mortality. A nationally representative database of more than 40,000 HD patients found that elevated serum phosphate levels greater than 5 mg/dl, hypercalcemia, and moderate 2PHPT (serum PTH levels >600 pg/ml) were associated with an increased relative risk of death, as well as increased risk of cardiovascular morbidity and fractures. Lower levels of serum PTH and normal levels of calcium and phosphate did not show increased risks. Hyperphosphatemia, hypercalcemia, and moderate-severe hyperparathyroidism despite adequate uremic control with dialysis and medical management are indications for surgical therapy (Table 1).

Table 1: Indications for Parathyroidectomy

Secondary Hyperparathyroidism	Tertiary Hyperparathyroidism (after Renal Transplantation)
Worsening disease with failure of appropriate medical management	Subacute severe hypercalcemia (Ca^{2+} >12.5 mg/dl)
• PTH >600 pg/ml	Persistent hypercalcemia 2 years after transplantation associated with
• $[Ca^{2+} \times PO_4^-]$>50	• Renal function decline without graft rejection
• Hypercalcemia	• Osteodystrophy
Renal osteodystrophy	• Pancreatitis
Calciphylaxis	• Nephrolithiasis
Uremic pruritus	
Persistent anemia	

PTH, Parathyroid hormone.

Renal Osteodystrophy

Renal osteodystrophy includes osteitis fibrosa, osteomalacia, and adynamic bone disease. Osteitis fibrosa is caused by high levels of PTH coupled with increased cytokines production and low calcitriol levels. It is associated with osteopenia, long-bone fractures, and decreased strength resulting from dystrophic bone formation. Renal osteomalacia is marked by accumulation of nonmineralized osteoid and is not responsive to administration of vitamin D (Fig. 1). It has been associated with aluminum toxicity. Adynamic bone disease is marked by hypocellular bone surfaces with little or no evidence of remodeling. This disease is common in patients with normal or low PTH and aluminum intoxication. These "normal" PTH levels cannot maintain normal rates of bone remodeling. This need for increased bone remodeling may actually be a stimulus for subsequent parathyroid oversecretion. Osteitis fibrosa is most often improved by parathyroidectomy.

Calciphylaxis

Calciphylaxis, also named calcific uremic arteriolopathy, is a rare, severe complication of 2PHPT characterized by calcification of the media of small-to-medium-sized arteries, resulting in ischemic damage in dermal and epidermal structures. The diagnosis of calciphylaxis is usually based on clinical findings of characteristic skin lesions and can be supported by microscopic examination of skin biopsy. The skin lesions appear as violaceous, painful areas, livedo reticularis, advancing to hard, tender erythematous plaques with central ulcerations, leading to stellate eschars (Fig. 2). Parathyroidectomy can be effective in slowing progression and allowing healing of the wounds with intensive local therapy. Parathyroidectomy is also the only effective treatment for patients with calciphylaxis in 3PHPT. Transplant-associated immunosuppression can worsen calciphylaxis. Sympathectomy aimed at relieving vasoconstriction in the periphery is not helpful in treating these ulcers.

Other Indications

Patients with uremic pruritus despite intensive HD can be ameliorated within days of parathyroidectomy. Anemia is a common finding in ESRD patients because of the deficiency of endogenous erythropoietin. PTH may directly inhibit renal and extrarenal production of erythropoietin. Improvements in anemia have been reported after parathyroidectomy in patients with 2PHPT.

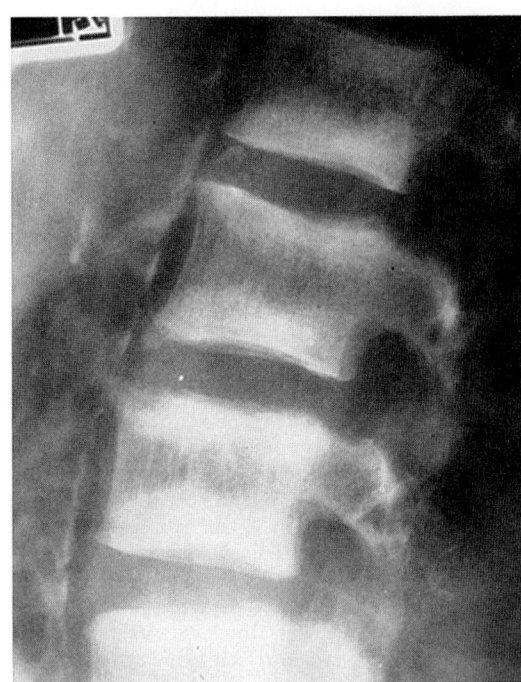

Figure 1 Lateral radiograph of the thoracic spine in a patient with end-stage renal disease showing bandlike regions of increased opacity at the superior and inferior margins of the vertebral bodies. This is typical of the "rugger jersey spine" sign.

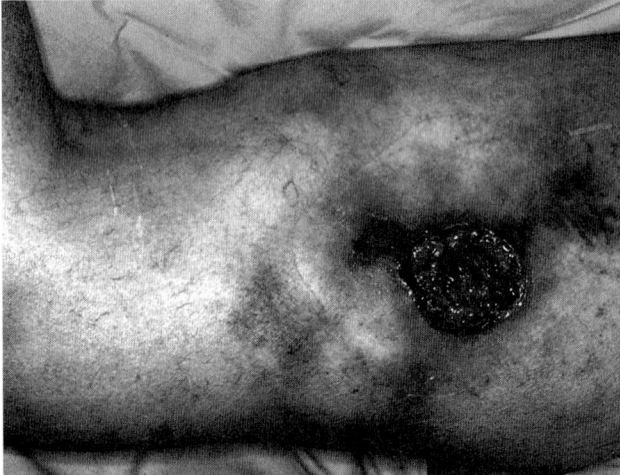

Figure 2 Eschar formation with central ulceration in a patient with end-stage renal disease and calciphylaxis.

Severe 2PHPT in Pretransplant Patients

Patients with serum levels of PTH greater than 600 pg/ml awaiting renal transplantation should have surgical correction of their 2PHPT before transplantation because postoperative hypercalcemia and 3PHPT can threaten the viability and longevity of the renal graft. Patients who are pretransplantation are best served by a subtotal parathyroidectomy (discussed later), with preservation of a well-vascularized, in situ parathyroid gland remnant to minimize the risk of permanent hypoparathyroidism.

PERIOPERATIVE CARE

Preoperative Management

Patients with 2PHPT are chronically ill and often have a number of comorbid conditions, including underlying cardiac disease, hypertension, and diabetes. It is essential that these patients are medically optimized before parathyroidectomy, and communication across treating physicians in Surgery, Anesthesiology, and Nephrology is particularly critical. In dialysis-dependent patients, electrolyte, volume, and coagulation abnormalities should be normalized, and coordination of parathyroidectomy with dialysis days is important. Uremic platelet dysfunction should be anticipated, and treatment with desmopressin acetate (DDAVP) or platelet transfusion can be used in severe cases of uncontrolled diffuse microvascular bleeding or thrombocytopenia.

Unlike primary hyperparathyroidism, which usually results from a single parathyroid adenoma, 2PHPT and 3PHPT result from hyperplasia of all parathyroid tissue. Because formal bilateral neck exploration is always indicated, preoperative imaging studies are generally unnecessary. If preoperative imaging has been performed and reveals a single focus of disease (i.e., enlarged parathyroid gland on ultrasound or intense focus of activity on nuclear medicine scan), a formal four-gland exploration is still necessary because the hyperplastic parathyroid glands frequently have different sizes and functional set points. In patients who previously have had parathyroidectomy and who have persistent or recurrent hyperparathyroidism, usually because of a supernumerary or heterotopic parathyroid gland, preoperative imaging is essential because it can focus exploration or even facilitate the performance of minimally invasive parathyroidectomy (MIP). In the reoperative setting, two corroborating studies are best. The favored method of parathyroid imaging is sestamibi with single photon emission computed tomography (SPECT). Because it can capture whole-body uptake of [99m]technetium-sestamibi, it is useful to identify the site of disease in patients who have undergone total parathyroidectomy with heterotopic autotransplantation. Additional imaging modalities include dedicated neck ultrasound, magnetic resonance imaging (MRI), computed tomography (CT), and angiography with selective venous sampling using the rapid PTH assay in the interventional radiology suite.

Postoperative Management

In the early postoperative setting after surgery for 2PHPT or 3PHPT, there is often symptomatic hypocalcemia. Symptoms of hypocalcemia include perioral numbness, paresthesias, and muscle cramps or carpopedal spasm. These symptoms can in turn provoke patient anxiety and hyperventilation, leading to worsening of the hypocalcemia. Severe hypocalcemia can lead to tetany and convulsions. It results from surgically induced hypoparathyroidism and from acute deposition of calcium into the bones ("hungry bone" syndrome). Preoperative elevation in serum alkaline phosphatase level can predict severity of this phenomenon.

All patients should be started on oral calcium supplementation in addition to oral calcitriol 0.5 to 4.0 g per day. Patients who have undergone total parathyroidectomy with autotransplantation experience more profound and prolonged hypocalcemia than patients after subtotal parathyroidectomy. Adequate intravenous access is essential preoperatively for frequent blood draws and for intravenous calcium administration in the postoperative setting. The administration of a calcium gluconate drip (10 g of calcium gluconate in a liter of normal saline started at 30 ml/hour and titrated appropriately for symptoms and serum calcium level) should be anticipated, particularly if the calcium level drops below 7.5 mg/dl. Simultaneously, patients on HD or peritoneal dialysis should be administered high-calcium dialysate during this period.

Oral calcium and calcitriol supplementation should be continued for at least 4 weeks or until serum calcium levels have stabilized.

SURGICAL TECHNIQUE

Parathyroidectomy for 2PHPT and 3PHPT is usually carried out under general anesthesia, although locoregional anesthesia with sedation can be used in select patients. Patients should be placed in the semi-Fowler position with the neck in extension and all appropriate pressure points padded. A 3- to 5-cm transverse cervical incision is made and extended through the subcutaneous tissue, and subplatysmal flaps are raised superiorly and inferiorly to the level of the thyroid cartilage and the sternal notch, respectively, and laterally to the sternocleidomastoid muscles. The strap muscles should be separated in the median raphe and dissected laterally off the thyroid capsule. The middle thyroid veins can be ligated and divided to allow full mobilization of the thyroid lobes anteromedially. Hemostasis is crucial at all times.

The recurrent laryngeal nerve and inferior thyroid artery should be identified. In most patients, the recurrent laryngeal nerve lies in the tracheoesophageal groove. The lower parathyroid gland is normally found in the thyrothymic tract, inferior to the thyroid lobe and anterior to the recurrent laryngeal nerve. The parathyroid gland may lie within the capsule of the lower thyroid pole. A common location for the superior parathyroid gland is within 1 cm of the recurrent laryngeal nerve as it pierces the cricothyroid membrane, posterior to the superior pole of the thyroid. All glands should be identified and their locations recorded before excision. This is particularly important for subtotal parathyroidectomy, for which the most normal-appearing gland can preferentially be chosen to become the partial remnant. Some surgeons recommend biopsy of each gland with frozen-section identification. The intraoperative rapid PTH assay is especially helpful when the surgeon has difficulty distinguishing among thyroid tissue, lymph nodes, or a parathyroid gland. Aspiration of parathyroid tissue with a 25-gauge needle with washing of the aspirate in 3 ml of 0.9% saline yields off-scale values, thereby securing the tissue diagnosis. Intraoperative needle aspiration has become a useful alternative to frozen section for parathyroid gland identification. This is preferentially performed ex vivo because in situ biopsy or aspiration of enlarged glands is potentially associated with parathyromatosis.

Parathyroid glands are often found in ectopic locations along their embryologic migration path. Aberrant parathyroid tissue has been noted in 15% to 20% of autopsy studies. The vast majority of patients who have aberrant parathyroid glands in the neck can be treated successfully through a standard neck exploration. Missing superior glands may be found in the retropharyngeal or retroesophageal planes, the posterior mediastinum, inside the upper or posterior thyroid capsule, and the carotid sheath. Inferior glands may be found inside the thyroid capsule or lower pole thyroid parenchyma, carotid sheath, and thymus/anterior mediastinum (Fig. 3). If a gland is not found, ipsilateral ligation of the inferior thyroid artery can be performed, which devascularizes the majority of parathyroid glands, or ipsilateral hemithyroidectomy can be considered. Up to 20% of patients have parathyroid glands in the superior mediastinum, but most of these can be extracted through the neck by performing a cervical thymectomy. Patients with 2PHPT and 3PHPT have a higher incidence of supernumerary glands because of the physiologic stimulation of growth of

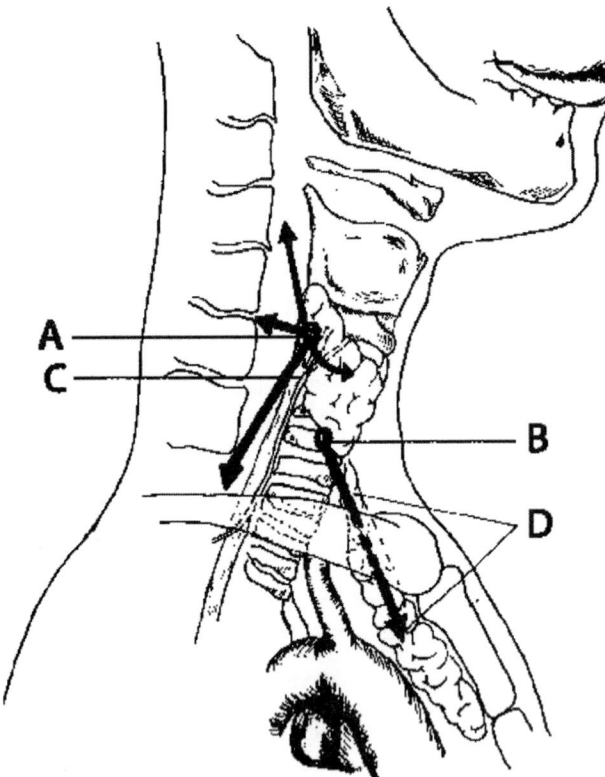

Figure 3   Possible anatomic locations of ectopic parathyroid glands. (A) Superior parathyroid gland; (B) inferior parathyroid gland; (C) recurrent laryngeal nerve; (D) thyrothymic tract and thymus.

parathyroid rests. Therefore cervical thymectomy should be standard at the time of parathyroidectomy. Direct mediastinal exploration is required in only 1% to 2% of cases.

Subtotal Parathyroidectomy versus Total Parathyroidectomy with Heterotopic Autotransplantation

After the first successful surgical intervention by Stanbury in 1960, subtotal parathyroidectomy became the standard operative strategy. In 1975, with the demonstration of parathyroid autograft function by PTH assay and forearm autotransplantation, total parathyroidectomy with heterotopic autotransplantation became popular. Total parathyroidectomy without autotransplantation has been described but is not widely in use. The debate over which procedure is better has been long-standing.

Both approaches require a thorough neck exploration through a cervical incision. When performing subtotal parathyroidectomy, it is advisable to choose the easiest accessible gland for the vascularized remnant. Most often this will be an inferior gland because of its more anterior location. If the remnant appears ischemic, a second gland should be chosen. Surgery consists of removal of three (or more if supernumerary glands are identified) glands in toto and 50% to 75% removal of one gland with preservation of a viable, histologically confirmed remnant weighing approximately 30 to 40 mg. Marking the remnant with a titanium clip enables hemostasis of the gland and later identification if necessary.

Use of the intraoperative, rapid PTH assay can help to ensure that adequate tissue has been resected. Results from this chemiluminescence immunometric assay are available within 12 to 15

minutes. Unlike primary HPT, for which rapid PTH measurements documenting a decrease in PTH of greater than 50% from baseline into the normal range predicts cure, for 2PHPT or 3PHPT, the absolute value of PTH measurement is most important in predicting long-term control of disease. The size of the parathyroid remnant can be tailored on the basis of the rapid PTH value, which optimally falls into the normal range or at least to less than 100 pg/ml.

There are several advantages to subtotal parathyroidectomy. A well-vascularized, orthotopic gland will regain function earlier and maintain it more easily than an autotransplanted gland, which requires neovascularization after transplantation. This might be particularly important in a noncompliant patient who is less likely to take calcium supplementation faithfully postoperatively. Choosing an accessible gland and marking it with a clip for potential identification makes reexploration easy without significant complications. Finally, avoiding an arm incision allows easier hemodialysis access later. The disadvantages are that a second neck surgery is necessary if hyperparathyroidism recurs, and the patient may develop hypoparathyroidism with significant hypocalcemia if the remnant is not well vascularized.

Total parathyroidectomy with autotransplantation removes all identified glands and uses an easily accessible area, most commonly the forearm or the sternocleidomastoid muscle, for the site of implantation. The gland to be transplanted is minced into 1-mm pieces, and 12 to 18 pieces are embedded in well-vascularized muscle and marked with a stitch or titanium clip. Neovascularization then occurs over several weeks. The principle advantages of this technique are that residual parathyroid function is easily followed and recurrences can be treated by partial resection under local anesthesia without the need for cervical reexploration. There are several disadvantages. More aggressive medical treatment is necessary postoperatively to maintain adequate serum calcium levels and avoid serious hypocalcemic complications. Autograft failure can lead to persistent hypoparathyroidism, which can be profound. Retrieval of all small grafts may be difficult at reoperation. Implantation into muscle may interfere with future HD access, and invasive growth of autografts into muscle and adjacent tissue requiring radical resection has been described.

Subtotal parathyroidectomy seems to be the preferred surgical approach. Overall recurrence of 2PHPT varies from 5% to 17%. Nodular proliferation in glands seems to predispose to recurrence more often than homogeneous gland hyperplasia. Cryopreservation of excised tissue is essential if total parathyroidectomy with autotransplantation is planned should the autograft prove to be nonfunctional. The resected parathyroid gland is minced into 1- to 2-mm fragments and kept on ice. The fragments are stored in sterile RPMI solution with 10% autologous serum and 10% dimethyl-sulfoxide and frozen to -80° C. They can be kept in liquid nitrogen in a tissue bank. Cryopreservation is not available at all centers.

A recent meta-analysis by Richards of 504 patients undergoing reoperative exploration for 2PHPT between 1983 and 2004 found that 36% of patients underwent subtotal parathyroidectomy, and 64% had total parathyroidectomy with autotransplantation. Overall, 83% of patients had recurrent 2PHPT and 17% had persistent disease resulting from missed in situ glands, supernumerary glands, or inadequate resections. In a small randomized trial by Rothmund comparing subtotal parathyroidectomy and total parathyroidectomy with autotransplantation, total thyroidectomy had somewhat lower long-term rates of 2PHPT recurrence. Overall, recurrence rates vary from 5% to 17% in the literature.

In 3PHPT, subtotal parathyroidectomy is the preferred surgical approach. Because patients with 3PHPT have normal renal function following successful renal transplantation, there is less chance of recurrence from parathyroid hyperplasia; therefore total parathyroidectomy with heterotopic autotransplantation is associated with an unnecessarily higher risk of hypoparathyroidism. Single adenoma excision often leads to failure.

SUMMARY

There have been significant advances in the medical management of 2PHPT; calcimimetic agents such as cinacalcet have reduced the need for early parathyroidectomy, although they may have increased the need for surgery for severe 3PHPT. Overall, subtotal parathyroidectomy remains the preferred approach for the surgical management of 2PHPT and 3PHPT, with the useful addition of the rapid PTH assay as a guide for extent of resection. Parathyroidectomy should be performed by experienced endocrine surgeons because operative volume has been shown to be a predictor of patient outcome.

SUGGESTED READINGS

Block GA, Klassen PS, Lazarus M, and others: Mineral metabolism, mortality, and morbidity in maintenance hemodialysis, *J Am Soc Nephrol* 15:2208, 2004.

Foley RN, Li S, Liu J, and others: The fall and rise of parathyroidectomy in U.S. hemodialysis patients, 1992–2002, *J Am Soc Nephrol* 16:210, 2005.

Goodman WG: Calcimimetics: a remedy for all problems of excess parathyroid hormone activity in chronic kidney disease? *Curr Opin Nephrol Hypertension* 14:355, 2005.

Richards ML, Wormuth J, Bingener J, and others: Parathyroidectomy in secondary hyperparathyroidism: Is there an optimal operative management, *Surgery* 139:174, 2006.

Sosa JA, Powe NR, Levine MA, and others: Thresholds for surgery and surgical outcomes for patients with primary hyperparathyroidism: a national survey of endocrine surgeons, *J Clin Endocrinol Metab* 83:2658, 1998.

THE ROLE OF STEREOTACTIC BREAST BIOPSY IN THE MANAGEMENT OF BREAST DISEASE

Monica Morrow, MD, and Kathryn Evers, MD

INTRODUCTION

Although screening mammography reduces breast cancer mortality, the majority of nonpalpable lesions that are detected in screening programs are benign. Surgical excisional biopsy after preoperative needle localization for diagnosis, although a proved safe and accurate procedure, can be the most expensive component of a mammography screening program. Stereotactic needle biopsy of nonpalpable lesions is an equally accurate and less expensive technique that avoids surgery for benign lesions and reliably identifies malignancies, facilitating the performance of definitive surgery with a single operative procedure. This chapter focuses on the techniques, indications for, and results of stereotactic biopsy.

TECHNIQUE

Equipment

In most cases, stereotactic biopsy is performed on a dedicated table with the patient in prone position. These units allow access to the breast from multiple positions, including access parallel to the compression plate. Add-on units that can be used with standard mammography equipment are also available. Older add-on units require the patient to be in the seated position, whereas the newer versions allow the biopsy to be performed in the lateral decubitus position. These devices are less expensive than the old models and do not require dedicated space. However, operator access to the breast is more limited, and the ability of the patient to see the needle increases the risks of both patient motion and vasovagal reactions. All types of stereotactic units require mammographic breast compression and a motionless, cooperative patient to ensure accurate lesion sampling.

Lesion Targeting

Stereotactic localization uses the principle of parallax to determine the lesion position in three-dimensional space. The x (horizontal) and y (vertical) coordinates of the lesion to be sampled are determined from the scout film. A stereotactic pair, consisting of two angled radiographic views, is acquired with the x-ray beam 15 degrees on either side of the center and is used to determine the precise depth (z coordinate) of the mammographic lesion. The physician targets the lesion by marking the lesion in each image of the stereotactic pair (Fig. 1). A computer algorithm uses simple geometric relations to calculate the depth (z axis) of the lesion on the basis of the geometric "shift" between the two views. The biopsy needle apparatus, supported by a stage attached to the equipment, is moved to the calculated x and y coordinates. The needle is then advanced to the calculated depth. A stereotactic pair of images is then performed (prefire pair), the biopsy gun is fired, and an additional set of images is obtained (postbiopsy pair). Digital imaging improves the accuracy of the procedure because the shortened procedure time makes it less likely that the patient will move. Generally the patient will be in compression for 20 to 40 minutes for this procedure.

Biopsy Needles

Most biopsies are performed using directional vacuum-assisted devices, although automated biopsy guns are still used by some practices. The vacuum-assisted devices have gained acceptance because of the speed with which the specimens can be obtained, the need to insert a needle only once, the larger size of the specimens, and the ability to obtain diagnostic samples even if targeting is not perfect. The major negative factor associated with the use of these devices is the increased cost compared with automated guns. In most instances, this is more than offset by the improved diagnostic ability of these devices. A vacuum is used to pull the sampled tissue into the cutting chamber of the probe. A rotating cutting needle is automatically advanced into this chamber. The specimen is then cut and withdrawn through the outer needle. The probe can be rotated through a full 360 degrees, or samples can be obtained in a specific quadrant.

Automated, spring-loaded biopsy guns use a double-action needle that consists of an inner trocar with a sample notch and an outer cutting cannula. The gun rapidly advances the needle into the breast, taking a core of tissue during its excursion. This must be removed from the needle after obtaining each specimen, requiring multiple needle insertions.

Standard probe sizes for the vacuum-assisted biopsy guns range from 8- to 11-gauge, whereas the automated biopsy guns are typically 14-gauge needles. The volume of tissue obtained using the vacuum devices is generally approximately twice as large as that retrieved using the automated guns.

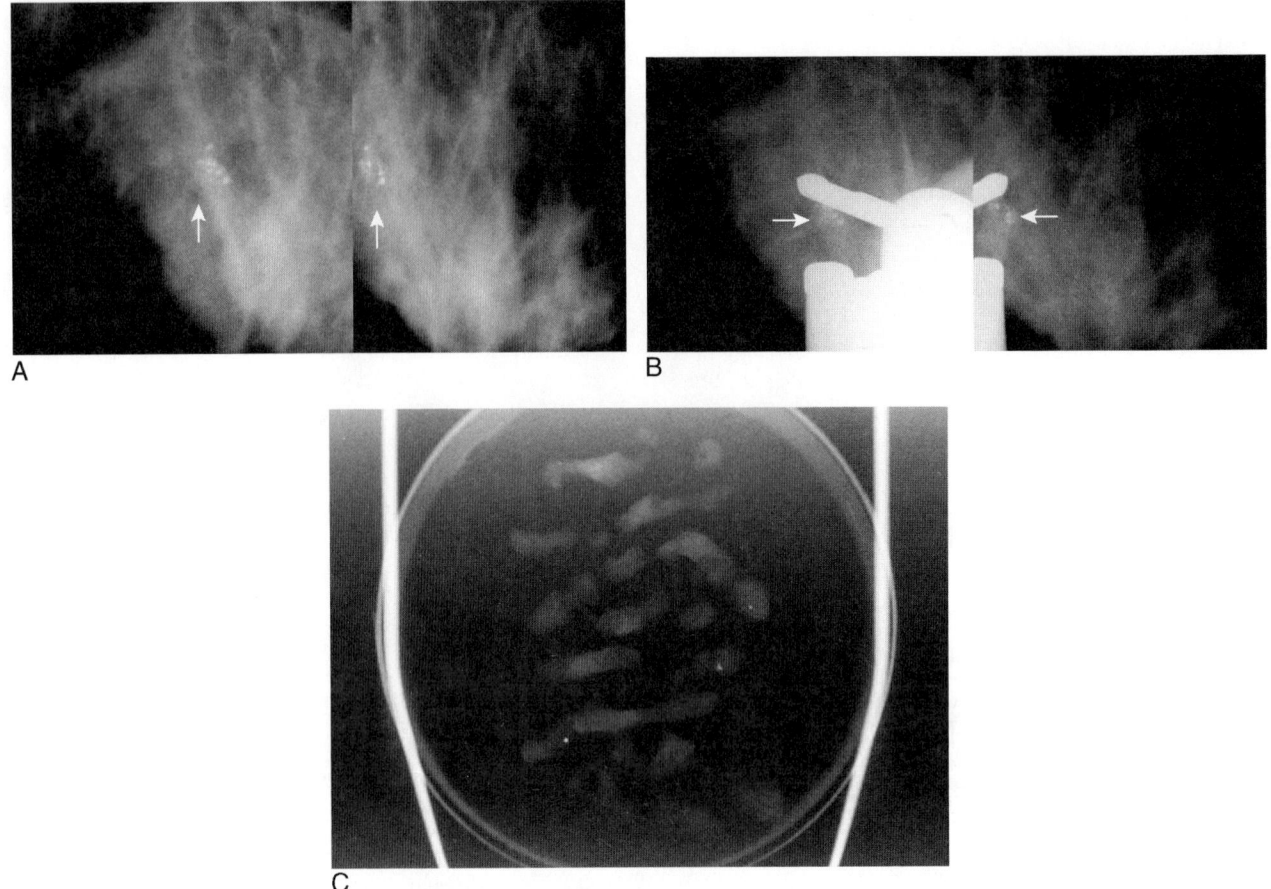

Figure 1   Stereotactic needle biopsy of a cluster of indeterminate calcifications. **(A)** Prebiopsy, stereotactic pair shows a cluster of indeterminate calcifications *(arrow)*. **(B)** Stereotactic pair obtained with the 9-gauge directional vacuum-assisted probe in place reveals the calcifications *(arrow)* immediately below the trough of the needle. **(C)** Core specimen radiograph demonstrates multiple calcifications to be present, confirming adequate sampling. Histology: Severely atypical ductal hyperplasia.

Core Specimen Handling

Histologic samples obtained with core biopsy needles are radiographed if the lesion contains microcalcifications, to ensure adequate sampling, and are then preserved in formalin for histologic evaluation. Multiple core biopsy samples are necessary to ensure accurate sampling of different areas of the lesion. In most cases, accurate lesion sampling can be achieved by obtaining four core samples for masses and 6 to 12 core samples for microcalcifications. The number of core samples required decreases as the size of the biopsy probe increases.

Patient Selection

Patient cooperation is key to successful lesion sampling because the patient must remain motionless for the duration of the procedure, often 20 to 40 minutes. Patients with severe coughing or anxiety may move too much to allow accurate targeting. Patients who are unable to lie prone because of abdominal or spinal problems may not be able to undergo stereotactic biopsy. Stereotactic tables have a patient weight limit (usually approximately 300 lbs, 135 kgs) that, if exceeded, can result in damage to the motorized table moving apparatus. In one study, 8% of cancellations of stereotactic biopsy were due to the patient's inability to tolerate the procedure.

It can be difficult to perform stereotactic biopsy of breast lesions that are superficial or near the nipple because of the inability to place the area in proper compression. Lesions that are near the chest wall may not be able to be targeted because it is difficult to image posterior tissue using the prone biopsy tables. Patients with thin breasts may not have enough tissue to allow for needle excursion. This can be overcome to some extent through the use of the "lateral arm." This apparatus is included with newer prone biopsy tables and allows the needle to be accurately placed into a lesion from a direction parallel to the plane of compression rather than perpendicular to it. With the use of the lateral arm, few lesions are inaccessible because of excessive compressibility. Lesions that are extremely superficial in the breast may not be accessible for stereotactic biopsy because there is insufficient tissue superficial to the lesion to permit effective action of the vacuum apparatus.

Ultrasound-guided biopsy is an alternative that should be considered for all lesions that can be visualized with this modality. Ultrasound guidance has the advantages of avoiding breast compression, making the procedure more comfortable for the patient, and of eliminating exposure to ionizing radiation. Also, lesions close to the chest wall, superficially placed in the breast, or near the nipple can be sampled using ultrasound guidance.

▮ INDICATIONS

Stereotactic biopsy should not replace a complete imaging workup. An imaging workup is essential to completely analyze the abnormality, assess the degree of suspicion, and exclude multiple lesions. A review of 89 cancelled stereotactic core needle biopsies reported the reasons for cancellation to be lack of a recognizable lesion in

Table 1: Contraindications to Stereotactic Core Biopsy

Patient unable to lie prone or cooperate
Patient weight >300 lbs.
Lesion location superficial or near nipple
Breasts too thin to allow needle excursion
Lesion suitable for short interval follow-up (Breast Imaging Reporting and Data System 3)

Table 2: Indications for Surgical Biopsy after Stereotactic Biopsy

Discordance between imaging findings and pathologic diagnosis
Atypical hyperplasia, ductal or lobular
Lobular carcinoma in situ
Papillary lesions
Phyllodes tumor
Radial scar

29%, reassessment of the lesion as benign in 19%, and benign cysts in 25%. This same study reported that a complete imaging workup, including ultrasound, would have avoided the delay in diagnosis and anxiety produced by scheduling (and canceling) a stereotactic biopsy in 48% of patients. Contraindications to stereotactic biopsy are summarized in Table 1.

LESION SELECTION

The American College of Radiology Breast Imaging Reporting and Data System (BI-RADS) has developed a lexicon for mammography in an effort to standardize mammographic reporting, reduce confusion in breast imaging interpretation, and facilitate outcome monitoring. The five final assessment BI-RADS categories are (1) negative, (2) benign finding, (3) probably benign finding, (4) suspicious abnormality, and (5) highly suggestive of malignancy. Lesions categorized as BI-RADS 3, probably benign, are usually managed by 6-month follow-up mammography, whereas lesions in categories 4 and 5 (i.e., suspicious or highly suggestive of malignancy) require histologic sampling and are candidates for stereotactic biopsy. Although some advocate needle biopsy of low-suspicion lesions to lower the anxiety of nervous women who do not wish to undergo follow-up, a study assessing patient stress reported the overall stress experienced by women who underwent core biopsy to be significantly greater than that reported in the group who were followed up with mammography.

Image-guided needle biopsy can decrease the number of operations performed and the time to definitive treatment in women with breast cancer. If the cancer diagnosis is made by preoperative core needle biopsy, definitive lesion removal and axillary surgery can be performed in a single operation. Morrow and colleagues compared prospectively the number of surgical procedures to completion of local therapy after core biopsy and surgical biopsy on the basis of lesion type, degree of suspicion, and type of local therapy for 1852 abnormalities in 1550 consecutive patients. The benefit of core biopsy in reducing the number of surgical procedures was seen for all types of mammographic abnormalities and in patients having mastectomy or axillary surgery. In patients having lumpectomy alone, surgical biopsy was as likely as core needle biopsy followed by lumpectomy to be the definitive surgical procedure. In a companion cost analysis study, core biopsy resulted in cost savings for all clinical scenarios.

Stereotactic biopsy is extremely useful in the evaluation of patients with multiple suspicious lesions to determine whether multicentric cancer, contraindicating breast-conserving surgery, is present. Making this determination nonsurgically preserves the skin envelope of the breast and facilitates skin-sparing mastectomy with immediate reconstruction.

ACCURACY RATE

The accuracy of image-guided core needle biopsy is comparable to surgical biopsy, and it is clear that experienced operators can obtain adequate samples the majority of the time. In a prospective study of 2403 image-guided breast biopsies performed using standardized protocols at 22 institutions, the overall sensitivity, specificity, and accuracy of the core biopsy was 0.91, 1.00, and 0.98 respectively. The accuracy in diagnosing masses (0.99) was found to be significantly greater than for diagnosing calcifications (0.96; $p < .001$). A recent meta-analysis comparing outcomes of vacuum-assisted biopsy and core biopsy using stereotactic guidance demonstrated a lower rate of nondiagnostic samples and a decrease in pathologic underestimation with the vacuum-assisted biopsy devices. In a study examining the influence of the number of specimens on diagnostic accuracy for 11-gauge vacuum-assisted biopsies, 12 specimens were found to optimize diagnostic accuracy, and increasing the specimen number did not improve diagnostic yield.

Correlation of the radiographic findings with the pathologic diagnosis is essential to avoid missed cancers. Concordance and adequate lesion sampling are easier to assess when the targeted lesion contains microcalcifications, and specimen radiography is standard practice to ensure adequate sampling of lesions containing calcifications. Discordant imaging and histopathologic results are an indication for repeat biopsy. In the meta-analysis, 23% of nondiagnostic specimens were found to be malignant. Inaccurate lesion targeting is the most common cause of nonconcordant samples. Partial concordance is encountered when the degree of carcinoma is underestimated. As many as 10% to 20% of patients diagnosed with ductal carcinoma in situ by 14-gauge core biopsy or vacuum-assisted stereotactic biopsy will have foci of invasion at surgery. Indications for surgical biopsy after core biopsy are listed in Table 2.

LESION REMOVAL

Lesion removal may occur inadvertently during core sampling of a small lesion. This occurrence is of no concern when the pathology is benign but has important practical implications when surgical excision is necessary because of a pathology report of atypia or malignancy. Mammographic changes such as air or hematoma from the core biopsy resolve completely in time, leaving no residual mark at the site of the biopsy. Placement of a small metallic clip at the biopsy site serves to identify the site for subsequent surgical excision even if the mammographic lesion has been completely removed. However, it is important to confirm that the clip is accurately placed at the biopsy site and for surgeons to be aware that as many as 57% of clips are placed more than 5.0 mm from the biopsy site, sometimes necessitating a larger surgical excision to ensure complete removal of the biopsy site.

PATHOLOGIC INDICATIONS FOR SURGICAL BIOPSY

Lack of concordance between the pathologic and imaging findings, as discussed earlier, is an indication for either repeat stereotactic biopsy if a targeting problem is identified or needle localization and surgical excision of the lesion. A number of pathologic diagnoses are also indications for surgical excision, and these are summarized in Table 2. Atypical hyperplasia, either ductal or lobular, is a marker of an increased risk of breast cancer when diagnosed by excisional biopsy. When atypical hyperplasia is encountered in core samples, surgical excision is indicated because it may coexist with adjacent intraductal or invasive carcinoma in as many as 18% to 50% of cases. Even with large vacuum biopsy devices, underestimation of disease remains a problem. The same rationale exists for biopsying lesions diagnosed as lobular carcinoma in situ by core biopsy. Core biopsy is not capable of differentiating benign from malignant papillary lesions or benign from malignant phyllodes tumors, nor can it distinguish between fragments of radial scar and well-differentiated carcinomas.

OTHER PATHOLOGY ISSUES

Needle biopsy techniques may displace intraductal carcinoma into adjacent breast parenchyma, resulting in a mistaken diagnosis of invasion in the surgical specimen. The presence of fragments of epithelium in artificial spaces accompanied by hemorrhage, inflammation, and granulation tissue should alert the pathologist to this diagnosis. Seeding of the needle track with invasive carcinoma may also occur as a result of core biopsy. This phenomenon was identified in 42% of patients when the interval from core biopsy to surgical excision was less than 15 days compared with 15% of patients who had definitive surgery more than 28 days after core biopsy ($p < .005$), indicating that these cells are not viable. It is not necessary to excise the core needle track as part of breast-conserving surgery.

COMPLICATIONS

Complications of needle biopsy are similar to those of needle localization procedures and may include bleeding, infection, and vasovagal reactions.

Using a 14-gauge needle, the estimated frequencies of hematoma and infection are each less than 2 in 1000. The complication rates with the 14-gauge vacuum-assisted biopsy are similar to that with 14-gauge automated biopsy guns. Bruising at the biopsy site and mild tenderness are expected symptoms and of no clinical concern. Permanent mammographic scarring or architectural distortion has not been observed as a result of needle core biopsies. Pneumothorax following ultrasound-guided core biopsy is possible but extremely rare.

SUMMARY

Imaging-guided percutaneous breast biopsy is the procedure of choice for the evaluation of most nonpalpable breast lesions. There are several advantages to percutaneous breast biopsy over open surgical biopsy. Percutaneous biopsy is fast, inexpensive, and avoids the scarring often associated with surgical biopsy. A benign concordant needle biopsy result avoids a surgical biopsy, thereby reducing the cost of screening. Although a small percentage of women who undergo percutaneous biopsy also require a surgical biopsy because of insufficient sampling, indeterminate results, or radiographic-histopathologic discordance, studies have shown a cost savings of 23% to 50% with the use of needle-core biopsy instead of surgery.

SUGGESTED READINGS

Diaz LK, Wiley EL, Venta LA: Are malignant cells displaced by large gauge biopsy of the breast? *Am J Radiol* 173:1303, 1999.
Fahrbach K, Sledge I, Cella C, and others: A comparison of the accuracy of two minimally invasive breast biopsy methods: A systematic literature review and metaanalysis, *Arch Gynecol Obstet* 274:63, 2006.
Fajardo LL, Pisano ED, Caudry DJ, and others: Stereotactic and sonographic large-core biopsy of nonpalpable breast lesions: results of the Radiologic Diagnostic Oncology Group V Study, *Acad Radiol* 11:293, 2004.
Golub RM, Bennett CL, Stinson T, and others: Cost minimization study of image-guided core biopsy versus surgical excisional biopsy for women with abnormal mammograms, *J Clin Oncol* 22:2430, 2004.
Morrow M, Venta L, Stinson T, and others: Prospective comparison of stereotactic core biopsy and surgical excision as diagnostic procedures for breast cancer patients, *Ann Surg* 233:537, 2001.

BENIGN BREAST DISEASE

Julie R. Lange, MD, ScM

INTRODUCTION

Surgeons are often called on to evaluate breast problems. Each breast complaint must be evaluated and resolved as an individual event, with goals of providing a diagnosis, providing reassurance if benign, and reinforcing a plan for ongoing breast cancer screening. This chapter reviews the appropriate evaluation of common breast problems, as well as the management of common benign breast disorders, and briefly reviews current screening recommendations.

EVALUATION OF COMMON PRESENTING COMPLAINTS

General Considerations

Evaluation of a breast problem begins with a history and physical examination. Evaluation is influenced by the patient's age, the physical findings, and the perceived level of breast cancer risk. Women younger than age 50 are likely to have a benign cause for a breast complaint. The chance that a breast complaint is caused by an underlying cancer increases with age, and a new or changing breast complaint in a woman past the age of menopause should be viewed with suspicion. Physical examination includes visual inspection for asymmetry and skin lesions such as rash, retraction, or erythema. Palpation should thoroughly cover all areas of both breasts and should include examination of the axillary and supraclavicular node basins.

Today almost every breast complaint requires breast imaging to characterize any physical abnormalities, to guide further evaluation, and to provide guidance for targeted biopsy if indicated. For most patients younger than 30 years, diagnostic ultrasound is the study of choice; mammography is seldom helpful because of the density of the breasts in young adulthood and because of the low likelihood of cancer in this population. Between 30 and 39 years, diagnostic mammography is indicated because some patients in this age range have reasonably interpretable mammograms, and even with dense breast tissue, it may be possible to see abnormal microcalcifications or other abnormalities. Targeted breast ultrasound is warranted as well. At age 40 and older, evaluation should include bilateral mammogram with diagnostic views of the areas of clinical concern, with targeted ultrasound as needed. In general, mammography and ultrasound are sufficient imaging for evaluation of most breast complaints; more costly imaging such as MRI should be reserved at this time for diagnostic problems that cannot be resolved by the above measures. When a biopsy is indicated, the procedure of choice today is usually a radiologic-guided core biopsy rather than a surgical biopsy.

Breast Mass

Breast mass remains the most common breast complaint and is generally accompanied by substantial patient anxiety because most women are well aware that a breast mass can be a presenting symptom of breast cancer. In the premenopausal years, most breast masses are ultimately found to be a cyst, fibrocystic changes, or a fibroadenoma, with relatively few cancers. Nonetheless, ruling out a cancer is the most important part of the evaluation of a breast mass. After menopause, a new breast mass should be assumed to be a cancer unless proven benign. The basic evaluation outlined earlier should allow the examiner to form an initial impression of whether the lesion is likely to be a cyst (fluid-filled on ultrasound), fibroadenoma (smoothly marginated solid mass in a premenopausal woman), or cancer (ill-defined or spiculated solid density). Today most solid masses are evaluated for definitive diagnosis by radiologic-guided core needle biopsy. If the lesion is seen well on ultrasound, ultrasound-guided core needle biopsy is the preferred technique.

Nipple Discharge

Nipple discharge is common and usually of benign etiology. Most women who have lactated can induce a small amount of discharge, usually from both nipples and multiple ducts; this type of induced discharge is a normal finding and requires no specific evaluation. True galactorrhea is uncommon and characterized by copious bilateral discharge in a nonlactating woman that is spontaneous and persistent, milky, and from multiple ducts. It has an underlying physiologic cause such as hyperprolactinemia related to pituitary tumor, hypothyroidism, or drug side effect and should be evaluated with prolactin and thyrotropin levels. Basic age-appropriate breast evaluation is warranted to rule out coexisting breast disorders. Patients with true galactorrhea should be referred to an endocrinologist for management.

Nipple discharge that requires surgical evaluation is spontaneous and recurrent, generally unilateral, and from a single duct. It may be sanguineous or serous. Testing for occult blood or cytology of nipple discharge are of little use because they are not definitive and do not yield sufficient evidence to obviate the need for a surgical biopsy. Evaluation begins with physical examination and with mammogram and ultrasound. If a specific, targetable suspicious lesion such as abnormal microcalcifications or solid mass is found, the lesion should undergo a core needle biopsy. If no suspicious lesion is found, an excisional biopsy of the offending duct is likely necessary to make a specific diagnosis and rule out cancer. A ductogram (galactogram) is often useful in preoperative planning to identify ductal filling defects. If a specific filling defect is seen, it may provide guidance in how the excisional biopsy is performed. Most causes of nipple discharge are benign, especially in younger women, and common causes are benign papilloma, duct ectasia, and fibrocystic changes. The risk of cancer in patients presenting with nipple discharge increases with age.

Breast Pain

Mastalgia is common throughout life, especially during the reproductive years; it is usually related to fibrocystic and hormonal changes and is seldom associated with a cancer. At a premenopausal age, a history of breast pain that is cyclic and improves significantly after the onset of menses is reassuring. If there are no other findings on physical

Table 1: Categories of Mammography Results—BI-RADS American College of Radiology

0	Assessment incomplete; additional imaging or comparison with previous imaging needed
1	Negative
2	Benign finding
3	Probably benign: short-interval follow-up suggested
4	Suspicious abnormality; biopsy should be considered
5	Highly suggestive of malignancy

BI-RADS, Breast Imaging Reporting and Data System, 4th edition (http://acr.org).

examination or on routine screening studies, no further active evaluation is necessary. However, pain that is noncyclic, of new onset at a postmenopausal age, or associated with a mass or other physical or radiologic abnormality requires further diagnostic evaluation, similar to the evaluation of a mass noted earlier. Common benign causes of focal persistent breast pain include cyst, abscess, and mastitis.

Skin Changes

Skin changes that may be associated with cancer include dimpling, nipple retraction, nipple excoriation or scaling, and skin thickening with erythema. These findings should prompt evaluation to rule out a cancer and can include mammogram and ultrasound, with biopsy as indicated by these studies. If the radiologic evaluation is negative, a skin punch biopsy may be necessary to rule out malignancy. Benign skin changes may include erythema as a sign of infection or rash reflecting dermatitis. Most breast infections are exquisitely painful and present with significant erythema and warmth. If infection is clinically suspected, ultrasound can be a simple way to clarify whether an abscess is present.

Abnormal Screening Mammogram

With increased use of routine screening mammography, many abnormalities are reported, most of which prove to be benign. The most important issue to be addressed is whether the screening finding represents a cancer. The American College of Radiology describes six categories of mammography results to guide further action (Table 1). A screening mammogram with a new density or increasing or new cluster of microcalcifications requires evaluation by a radiologist specializing in breast imaging and usually requires focused diagnostic mammographic views, including spot compression or magnification views, as well as diagnostic ultrasound. If the lesion is concerning, a radiologic-guided core biopsy is usually the most appropriate method for biopsy. Correlation of the mammographic finding with the physical examination is important because it is sometimes possible to detect subtle physical changes if attention is directed to the vicinity of the mammographic finding.

MANAGEMENT OF BENIGN BREAST LESIONS

Fibroadenoma

Fibroadenomata are common throughout the reproductive years. The majority are small, benign, and asymptomatic or minimally symptomatic. Their identity can usually be confirmed by ultrasound-guided core biopsy, after which most can be left in place and observed over time with serial ultrasound. A fibroadenoma may require excision if it grows over time, is large (>2 or 3 cm) at diagnosis, or is painful. If there is some doubt about the diagnosis, either because of a question of atypia on the core biopsy or increased cellularity of the lesion, the lesion should be excised to rule out a small associated cancer and to rule out a phyllodes tumor.

Cysts

Cysts are a common cause of breast pain or focal mass; they are common in the reproductive years but can occasionally occur in postmenopausal women as well. A simple cyst, as determined by imaging evaluation, without associated solid component is unlikely to be associated with a cancer. Simple cyst aspiration may be appropriate for cysts that are large or symptomatic. Cyst fluid that is bloody should be sent for cytopathology; otherwise it may be discarded. A cyst that is complex or associated with a solid component must be biopsied, usually as a targeted core biopsy. If the aspirate is bloody or the cytology is atypical, an excision may be necessary to rule out a cancer.

Fibrocystic Changes

Most women have some element of fibrocystic changes, and most are entirely benign. Fibrocystic changes can present as breast pain with or without vague, masslike thickening. The pain is often cyclic in premenopausal women. If the diagnostic evaluation is complete with no suspicious lesion found, simple reassurance and clinical follow-up is often the most appropriate management strategy.

Diabetic Mastopathy

This uncommon, dense, fibrous lesion usually occurs in persons aged between 30 and 50 years with a long history of type I diabetes, particularly those with microvascular complications, although it has been described in type II diabetics as well. Presentation is with a dense, hard mass; both the physical examination and radiologic studies may appear suspicious for carcinoma. In the correct clinical setting, a core biopsy may be diagnostic, with excisional biopsy occasionally needed for confirmation. No active intervention is needed beyond confirmation of the diagnosis.

Infection

Breast infections are common and can be painful and difficult to clear. Acute mastitis is common in the postpartum period in lactating women. The most common causative agent is *Staphylococcus*. Antibiotics chosen empirically should have good staphylococcal coverage and can be changed to more specific agents if culture sensitivity later becomes available. Complete resolution of uncomplicated mastitis may take a few weeks. If a discrete abscess is present, drainage is indicated; the traditional method is an open incision and drainage. Deep sedation is usually necessary for deep-seated or loculated abscesses, given the severe pain that can be associated with this process. Select cases with limited nonloculated abscesses may be adequately managed by serial aspiration, antibiotics, and close follow-up. Mastitis and breast abscesses can usually be treated on an outpatient basis. One occasional exception is in diabetic patients in whom severe breast infection can be accompanied by systemic sepsis and may require intravenous antibiotics and hospitalization.

Lipoma

Lipomata can be found in the breast as elsewhere. If large or symptomatic, they can be managed with simple excision.

Fat Necrosis

Fat necrosis in the breast can be the result of injury to the soft tissues. Typical radiologic changes include rounded density with or without calcifications. Radiologic characteristics often cannot distinguish fat necrosis from cancer, and a targeted core biopsy may be necessary for definitive diagnosis. Fat necrosis can form a focal, hard mass, and some patients prefer to have it excised.

Lesions Benign by Core Biopsy That May Require Excision

Today most initial breast biopsies are radiologic-guided core biopsies. Most core biopsies of benign lesions are definitive, and no excision is required. However, some findings on core biopsy imply a risk of concurrent cancer in the surrounding tissue and warrant formal excisional biopsy to rule out a cancer. Atypical ductal hyperplasia, lobular carcinoma in situ, papilloma, radial scar, and mucin-producing lesions are each associated with a small chance of associated early breast cancer; if found on a core biopsy, excision of the lesion for complete diagnosis is warranted.

Benign Changes Associated with Elevated Breast Cancer Risk

Some benign breast changes can be associated with elevated cancer risk. Variants of fibrocystic change including proliferative changes without atypia, such as sclerosing adenosis, papillomatosis, and usual ductal hyperplasia are associated with only a small increase in breast cancer risk. Appropriate ongoing routine screening is the only necessary management. However, atypical hyperplasia (either ductal or lobular) is associated with a moderate increase in breast cancer risk, especially if there is a history of breast cancer in a first-degree relative. Some high-risk patients may consider risk reduction measures or ongoing screening through a high-risk clinic. Chemoprevention with tamoxifen has been shown to reduce risk of breast cancer in high-risk women; other risk-reducing agents are likely to be approved in the future.

■ SPECIAL CIRCUMSTANCES

Male Breast Complaint

Changes suggestive of cancer in the male breast include skin or nipple changes, particularly nipple retraction or nipple discharge, and a firm, painless mass. Male breast cancer is rare, but gynecomastia is common. Gynecomastia has frequently been associated with estrogen excess or testosterone deficiency. It may be associated with cirrhosis of the liver; primary hypogonadism; testicular tumors; obesity; and numerous drugs including steroids, estrogens, flutamide, ketoconazole, digoxin, spironolactone, phenothiazines, and marijuana. Gynecomastia usually presents with a firm, sometimes painful thickening of the subareolar tissues and may be bilateral or unilateral, even if caused by systemic factors. Radiologic evaluation includes diagnostic mammography and ultrasound. Mammography may be helpful to rule out findings such as abnormal microcalcifications that may suggest cancer. If a discrete mass can be seen by ultrasound, it can be targeted for a core biopsy. If evaluation is consistent with benign gynecomastia and implicates a specific drug, discontinuation of that drug with reevaluation in 3 to 6 months may be reasonable. Gynecomastia can also sometimes regress spontaneously. A persistent mass, particularly if painful, may be most appropriately managed by excisional biopsy for definitive diagnosis and symptom relief.

Pregnancy and Lactation

Changes associated with pregnancy and lactation may make cancer detection difficult. Most pregnancies occur in healthy young women, and any physical changes are likely to be benign. Common benign breast changes include fibroadenomata, which may enlarge in response to the stimulation of pregnancy-related hormones, and lactating adenoma, a benign, well-circumscribed mass. Either may be diagnosed with ultrasound and core biopsy during pregnancy. In the event that an excisional biopsy is necessary during pregnancy, local anesthesia can be used for most cases. If a biopsy must be performed during the months a woman is lactating, a milk fistula may occur regardless of whether the biopsy is an excisional biopsy or a core needle biopsy, particularly if the biopsied area is central within the breast. Some women choose to continue to lactate and manage the fistula locally during that time, knowing that it will close after lactation ceases. It should also be noted that with increased use of reproductive technologies, more women are pregnant in their late 30s and in their 40s, when the incidence of breast cancer begins to rise. Attention to abnormal physical breast changes is particularly important because such women will not be receiving screening mammography during that time, and the changes of pregnancy may mask the early physical signs of cancer.

SCREENING RECOMMENDATIONS

Evaluation of benign breast complaints can be an opportunity to remind patients of appropriate screening guidelines and provide a risk estimate. With the general population of women in the United States at a one-in-eight lifetime risk of breast cancer, all women are considered at risk, even in the absence of family history of breast cancer or specific predisposing factors. Assessment of individual risk can be calculated with a number of models. The most commonly used is the Gail model, which applies to women 35 years or older who have never been diagnosed with breast cancer (including in situ breast cancer) and results in an individual's risk of invasive breast cancer over the subsequent 5 years and up to age 90. This risk assessment model may be less accurate for non-white populations and for women with a known deleterious gene mutation; further research and development of other models are necessary. A simple risk assessment tool that is based on the Gail model is available online at http://www.nci.nih.gov/bcrisktool/.

The value of self-examination is unknown: randomized studies have failed to show improvement in breast cancer–related survival in populations who have been educated in self-examination techniques. Nonetheless, self-examination is to be encouraged because many women detect their own cancers between clinical screening intervals. Appropriate screening for women of average risk includes clinical breast examination every 1 to 3 years from age 20 to 40 and annual clinical breast exam beginning at age 40. Annual screening mammography should begin no later than age 40 and should continue as long as a woman is relatively healthy. Many societies have published screening guidelines: the National Comprehensive Cancer Network updates guidelines yearly at http://www.nccn.org/professionals.

SUGGESTED READINGS

Cady B, Steele GD, Morrow M, and others: Evaluation of common breast problems: guidance for primary care providers, *CA Cancer J Clin* 48:49, 1998.
Morrow M: The evaluation of common breast problems, *Am Fam Physician* 61:2371, 2000.
Santen RJ, Mansel R: Benign breast disorders, *N Engl J Med* 353:275, 2005.
Seltzer M: Breast complaints, biopsies, and cancer correlated with age in 10,000 consecutive new surgical referrals, *Breast J* 10:111, 2004.
Smith RL, Pruthi S, Fitzpatrick LA: Evaluation and management of breast pain, *Mayo Clin Proc* 79:353, 2004.

SCREENING FOR BREAST CANCER

Lisa K. Jacobs, MD

Breast cancer is the most common malignancy occurring in women in the United States, with an estimated 212,920 breast cancers diagnosed in 2006, accounting for 31% of all malignancies. It is the second most common cause of cancer death in women, with an estimated 40,970 cancer deaths—15% of all cancer deaths. Because of this high incidence of breast cancer in the United States, population screening and early detection are important public health measures. Although incidence rates of breast cancer continue to rise, the annual death rate from breast cancer has decreased by 2.3%. Early detection is likely to be the reason for this decrease. The 5-year survival rate for breast cancer has increased from 75% in 1974 to 1976 to 88% in 1995 to 2001; today 63% of all patients are diagnosed with localized breast cancer, 29% with regional spread, and 6% with distant disease. Trials looking at the effectiveness of mammography for screening have demonstrated a statistically significant reduction in mortality of 20% to 35% from breast cancer. Population-based studies conducted in countries such as Sweden, where mammography was not available and was subsequently made available, revealed a reduction in mortality after routine screening mammography was instituted. Since the institution of annual screening mammography in the United States, there has been a decrease in the T-stage of the primary tumor. We are now diagnosing progressively smaller tumors and diagnosing more women at an in situ (Tis) tumor stage. Now approximately 20% of all breast cancers are diagnosed as in situ with a good prognosis. Before screening mammography, in situ tumors were diagnosed only when they became palpable.

SCREENING RECOMMENDATIONS

The American Cancer Society (ACS) annually releases guidelines for early detection of cancer. Its recommendations for breast cancer screening were last updated in 2003 and include a three-part assessment of the patient: clinical breast examination, counseling to raise awareness of breast symptoms, and regular mammography beginning at age 40. These recommendations are summarized in Table 1. It is during the clinical examinations that a discussion of

Table 1: American Cancer Society Recommendations for Breast Cancer Screening

Age	Clinical Examination	Mammography
20–39	Every 3 years	None
≥40	Annual	Annual

family history of breast cancer, early detection, and the importance of regular mammography should be addressed. The ACS has deleted its recommendation for women to conduct a breast self-examination but continues to recommend informing patients about breast self-examination including benefits, limitations, and harms. There is no set age at which mammography should be discontinued; it should continue as long as the woman is a candidate for breast cancer treatment. It is important to recognize that screening recommendations are based on disease incidence and the reliability of the screening method in a sorted population; for this reason, routine screening mammography is not recommended for women younger than age 40, and the recommendations change for the high-risk population.

SCREENING MODALITIES

Clinical Breast Examination

The importance of clinical breast examination is based on the fact that 10% to 20% of all breast cancers are not visible on screening mammography. Therefore the only mechanism to identify breast cancer in those patients is by clinical breast examination. All suspicious palpable lesions should be evaluated with an ultrasound and biopsy performed, even if the mammogram is normal.

Mammography

The second component of screening is annual mammography. The ACS recommends annual mammography starting at age 40. Other organizations recommend the first baseline mammogram at 35 and then annual mammography at 40. There is some controversy in women between ages 40 and 50 as to the sensitivity of the test; this is due to increased breast density in women in this age range. Increased breast density not only decreases the sensitivity of mammography but is associated with an increased risk of breast cancer. Annual screening mammography is performed with two-view images: the craniocaudal view and the medial lateral oblique views. It is estimated that only 50% of women who are recommended for screening actually undergo annual screening mammography.

The use of computer-assisted diagnosis (CAD) with either digital or film screen mammography has been shown to improve the sensitivity and specificity. In this technique, the film is scanned and analyzed by a computer algorithm for changes from the prior examination, essentially completing a second read of the mammogram. The films are placed into the CAD machine, and the computer algorithm identifies new lesions, which are flagged by the program. The radiologist then reviews the films to determine whether the lesions identified by CAD are suspicious. A second read by either CAD or a second radiologist improves the diagnostic accuracy of mammography. Digital mammography has recently been compared with analogue mammography for routine screening. A study of more than 40,000 women found that film screen mammography was equivalent to digital mammography in all patients except the following subcategories: age older than 50, premenopausal or perimenopausal, and increased breast density.

Reporting of mammography results has been standardized by the American College of Radiology using Breast Imaging Reporting and Data System (BI-RADS) classifications, defined in Table 2. The BI-RADS classification has provided uniformity in reporting and interpretation of the reports and useful guidelines for management and follow-up. It is also important to correlate physical examination and biopsy results with the mammographic findings. Discordant findings are those in which the physical examination or biopsy results do not correlate with the mammographic result. For example, a needle biopsy result of fibrocystic change

Table 2: Breast Imaging Reporting and Data System (BI-RADS) Classification of Breast Imaging

BI-RADS Class	Findings	Action	Risk of Malignancy
0	Incomplete exam	Additional imaging	
1	Normal	Routine screening	
2	Benign finding	Routine screening	
3	Probably benign finding	Repeat imaging in 6 months	<2%
4	Suspicious abnormality	Biopsy recommended	Widely variable
5	Highly suggestive of malignancy	Biopsy recommended	>95%
6	Known biopsy proven malignancy		

on a BI-RADS 5 mammogram is considered discordant. In this case, repeat biopsy should be considered.

If a screening mammogram is abnormal, a number of additional diagnostic tools can be employed. Additional mammographic images include magnification views and compression views, which are used to differentiate whether the lesion is considered suspicious. Other imaging modalities such as ultrasonography or magnetic resonance imaging (MRI) may also be completed before biopsy. The method of biopsy should be by core needle biopsy if at all possible, as recommended by the National Comprehensive Cancer Network (NCCN) guidelines.

OTHER IMAGING MODALITIES

Ultrasonography

The standard use of ultrasonography in breast imaging is for palpable abnormalities or mammographic abnormalities that can be further characterized by ultrasound. Microcalcifcations identified on mammography are not generally well visualized; however, ultrasound is commonly employed in this situation to identify whether a mass is present in conjunction with those calcifications. In addition, any patient with a clinically suspicious palpable abnormality but normal mammography should have ultrasonography to further characterize the abnormality. Directed ultrasonography to an area of abnormality may give additional characteristics that are suggestive of malignancy, such as a lesion that is taller than it is wide, has indistinct borders, has solid rather than cystic characteristics, and has posterior acoustic shadowing.

Whole-breast screening sonography is another mechanism of breast cancer screening. Whole-breast screening ultrasound is indicated in women with an increased risk of development of breast cancer, women who have a difficult-to-image breast because of increased breast density, or women younger than age 40 who are at increased risk. In these situations, whole-breast ultrasound is performed.

Magnetic Resonance Imaging

At this time, MRI is not commonly used as a screening tool. Certain high-risk populations may be considered for MRI screening, but as a population-screening tool, it is not a useful technique because of the high false-positive rate and the cost per examination. MRI imaging of the breast is useful if an abnormality is identified on physical examination but cannot be imaged by either mammography or ultrasound. It is also a potentially useful tool in women with dense breast tissue.

High-Risk Screening

Routine screening recommendations in the United States follow ACS guidelines. However, a number of populations in the United States are at increased risk for development of breast cancer. These populations include individuals with a family history of breast cancer in a first-degree relative, patients with a prior breast cancer diagnosis, patients with germ-line mutations in the BRCA-1 or BRCA-2 genes, prior radiation therapy field that included the breast, or a prior diagnosis of cellular atypia or lobular carcinoma in situ. In this group of patients, modifications to the standard recommendations for screening apply. All patients with a strong family history of breast cancer in a first-degree relative at a premenopausal age should initiate screening 5 to 10 years before the youngest age of diagnosis of breast cancer in the family cohort. Patients with a BRCA mutation should begin screening at age 25.

Women in all categories of increased risk may potentially benefit from clinical breast exam performed every 6 months. Little evidence suggests that increasing the rate of mammography screening is beneficial. In women who are at particularly increased risk or BRCA-1 and BRCA-2 mutation carriers, the use of whole-breast

ultrasound and MRI for screening is currently being evaluated in research studies.

The NCCN guidelines estimate that approximately 5% to 10% of all breast cancers are a result of a specific hereditary mutation. NCCN guidelines for patients with a known gene mutation for hereditary breast or ovarian cancer recommend that screening include training in regular monthly self-examination starting at age 18, a clinical breast examination semiannually starting at age 25, and mammography and breast MRI screening starting at age 25. Consideration of chemoprevention for breast and ovarian cancer is recommended. Participation in investigational imaging and screening studies when available is encouraged.

Men with a personal history of breast cancer are recommended to have clinical breast examination every 6 months and consideration for genetic testing. The presence of a known mutation in the BRCA1 or BRCA2 genes in men is managed with monthly breast self-examination, a semiannual clinical breast examination, and annual mammography.

Suggested Readings

Daly MB, Axilbund JE, Bryant E, and others: Genetic/familial high-risk assessment: breast and ovarian, *J Natl Comp Cancer Netw* 4156, 2006.
NCCN Breast Cancer Screening and Diagnosis Guidelines. National Comprehensive Cancer Network Guidelines (website), www.nccn.org. Accessed April 20, 2007.
Smith RA, Cokkinides V, Eyre HJ: American Cancer Society guidelines for the early detection of cancer, *CA Cancer J Clin* 56:11, 2006.

Cellular, Biochemical, and Molecular Targets in Breast Cancer

Helen Krontiras, MD, and Kirby I. Bland, MD

Since the late 1980s a considerable amount of data have been published regarding the molecular and genetic pathways involved in breast carcinogenesis. This increased understanding has enabled physicians to alter or interfere with the multiple steps involved in the development of breast cancer. This chapter focuses on some of the scientifically proved and current clinically applicable factors.

CELLULAR MARKERS OF PROLIFERATION

Proliferation is the growth of a tumor by cell division that exceeds tumor cell death. There are a number of ways to determine the proliferative activity of a tumor. Histologic assessment of tumor grade is one method. Several grading systems have been evaluated in the breast oncology literature. The American Joint Committee on Cancer (AJCC) recommends the Nottingham combined histologic grade system, which is a modification of the Scarff-Bloom-Richardson (SBR) grading system. Cell mitosis, tubule formation (degree of architectural differentiation from normal breast tissue), and nuclear pleomorphism are essential components. Although intraobserver variability exists, histologic grade is well recognized for its prognostic

significance in cases of primary operable invasive breast carcinoma and is a predictor of overall survival for both lymph node-negative and lymph node-positive patients.

Several other measures of proliferation exist, but most are impractical for routine use. Some of the more common measures include mitotic index, S-phase fraction, and proliferation-associated antigens. Mitotic index is simply the number of mitotic bodies per high-powered field. S-phase fraction measures the number of cells in the DNA synthesis phase of the cell cycle. It is determined using DNA flow cytometry on fresh or fresh/frozen samples. Proliferation-associated nuclear antigens (Ki67, cyclin A, proliferating cell nuclear [PCNA], Ki-S1) are widely used as measures of proliferation and are found in cells in the proliferative phases of the cell cycle. Most common is the evaluation of Ki67, which is performed via the monoclonal antibodies Ki67 (used on fresh/frozen tissue) and MIB 1 (used on fixed, paraffin-embedded tissue) that stain this nuclear antigen in proliferating cells. Ki67 correlates significantly with modified SBR grading system, S-phase fraction, and mitotic index. Patients with high Ki67 percentages have a worse overall and disease-free rate of survival, but lack of independent significance limits its prognostic ability and thus its routine use.

ESTROGEN AND PROGESTERONE RECEPTORS

Beatson in the late 1800s treated breast cancer by removing ovaries in premenopausal breast cancer patients after observing that rabbits that had ovaries removed stopped producing milk, indicating a relationship between the breast and the ovary. However, not all breast cancer patients responded to oophorectomy. It was not until the 1970s, when the estrogen receptor (ER) was discovered, that the reason became known. Jensen developed the hypothesis that some breast cancers contain the estrogen receptor and others do not. Those that did not have the receptor would not respond to endocrine manipulation. Since that time, the ER has been extensively studied, and endocrine therapy remains an important modality in breast cancer treatment.

The ER is actually two receptors. The estrogen alpha receptor (ER-α) is a class I nuclear receptor located on chromosome 6q, and estrogen receptor beta (ER-β) is located on chromosome 14q. Both are members of the steroid receptor family of proteins and both share common structural and functional domains, except that ER-β lacks a portion of the C-terminal domain. They bind with high affinity to the ligand estrogen. Estrogen binds the receptor, causes dimerization, and facilitates interaction of the receptor with promoter regions in the DNA. These regions are termed *estrogen response elements;* the activation or repression of gene transcription ensues. Currently little is known about the role of ER-β in breast cancer, but lack of the C-terminal domain may be important in antiestrogen therapy.

Approximately 70% to 80% of all invasive breast cancers and nearly all intraductal breast cancers express the ER-α protein (ER positive). Traditionally ER positivity has been measured quantitatively with immunohistochemistry. Approximately 60% of ER-positive tumors are also progesterone receptor (PR) positive. Although patients with ER-positive tumors have a better prognosis than ER-negative patients, expression of the estrogen receptor is more useful as a predictor for response to endocrine therapy. In patients with ER-positive/PR-positive tumors, 70% respond to endocrine therapy. In addition, 50% of ER negative tumors express PR, perhaps indicating a functional ER, and of these 30% respond to tamoxifen therapy. Approximately 5% to 10% of patients with ER-negative/PR-negative tumors respond to endocrine therapy.

Selective estrogen receptor modulators (SERMs) are ER agonists and ER antagonists with differing activity in different tissues. Tamoxifen is the most widely used SERM for breast cancer treatment. Tamoxifen competitively inhibits the binding of estradiol to estrogen receptors, thus antagonizing the effect of estrogen on a variety of growth regulatory genes, including transforming growth factor B (TGFb) and insulin-like growth factor 1 (IGF-1).

Given in an adjuvant setting, tamoxifen reduces the risk of breast cancer recurrence and death in premenopausal and postmenopausal women with ER-positive disease by approximately 50%. It is given daily (20 mg) for 5 years. The side effect profile is notable in some women for symptomatic hot flashes and vaginal dryness or discharge related to the antiestrogenic effect of the medication on the central nervous system and vagina. More worrisome but rare side effects related to estrogenic properties of tamoxifen include an increased risk for the development of uterine cancer and thromboembolic events in postmenopausal women. Tamoxifen treatment may also offer beneficial estrogenic side effects in postmenopausal women, including an improvement in bone density and lipid profile. An increased risk for cataracts in women treated with tamoxifen is probably not related to its endocrine effects.

Tamoxifen is also recommended for breast cancer chemoprevention in women at increased risk for breast cancer. Tamoxifen can reduce the risk of invasive or preinvasive breast cancer by approximately 50% in women at increased risk of breast cancer. The short-term absolute risk of developing breast cancer must be weighed against the potential side effects. Tamoxifen is generally recommended for premenopausal women at increased risk, postmenopausal women without a uterus at moderate risk, and postmenopausal women with a uterus at high risk. A second-generation SERM, raloxifene, is currently used for osteoporosis treatment. It is similar to tamoxifen in its effects, with less of an estrogen agonist effect on the uterus. Studies have indicated a potential role for breast cancer risk reduction. A recently published initial report of the National Surgical Adjuvant Breast and Bowel Project (NSABP) STAR trial (tamoxifen vs. raloxifene) in postmenopausal women at increased risk for breast cancer shows that both drugs equally reduce the incidence of invasive breast cancer, but the

preliminary data suggest fewer adverse side effects with raloxifene compared with tamoxifen. Patient-reported symptoms and quality of life were similar for both drugs.

Newer endocrine agents, termed *aromatase inhibitors,* slow down conversion of adrenally produced androgens to estrogen by the aromatase enzyme, thus suppressing estrogen levels. This is the last step in steroid conversion to active hormones and does not interfere with production of corticosteroids or mineralocorticoids. Production of estrogen in the ovary is not suppressed, however, and aromatase inhibitors are currently indicated only for postmenopausal women with ER-positive breast cancer. Recent data demonstrate that aromatase inhibitors are superior to tamoxifen for adjuvant use in postmenopausal women with ER-positive breast cancer. Adjuvant studies include direct comparison of aromatase inhibitors with tamoxifen and switching after initial treatment with tamoxifen. Preliminary data also suggest that the side effect profile of aromatase inhibitors is also superior to tamoxifen, particularly with regard to thromboembolic events and endometrial cancer. Frequently observed side effects seen in women treated with aromatase inhibitors are decreased bone density and musculoskeletal complaints.

EPIDERMAL GROWTH FACTOR RECEPTOR

The epidermal growth factor receptor (EGFR) family is made up of four receptors: HER1 (erbB1/EGFR), HER2 (erbB-2), HER3 (erbB-3), and HER4 (erbB-4). These receptors are transmembrane proteins with three cellular domains and primarily function as tyrosine kinases. When activated by a ligand, homodimers or heterodimers are formed, resulting in cell cycle progression, cellular proliferation, angiogenesis, and tumor metastasis. Known ligands are transforming growth factor alpha (TGF-α), EGFR, and heregulins.

Perhaps the best characterized of the EGFR family receptors is HER2. HER2 overexpression is an early event in breast cancer development. HER2 is overexpressed or its gene amplified (or both) in approximately 20% to 30% of breast cancers. Patients with overexpression of HER2 often have high-grade tumors, axillary lymph node involvement, and decreased expression of estrogen and progesterone receptors. These characteristics are associated with an increased risk of recurrence and decreased survival; however, HER2 overexpression is also independently associated with poor prognosis. HER2 overexpression is determined using immunohistochemical or fluorescence in situ hybridization analysis of the breast cancer tumor.

Trastuzumab (Herceptin; Genentech, South San Francisco, CA) is a recombinant monoclonal antibody targeting the extracellular domain of the HER2 protein. Binding of the antibody with the receptor activates an immune response and decreases HER2 phosphorylation, phosphatidylinositol 3-kinase (PI3K)/Akt activity, and vascular endothelial growth factor levels. Randomized controlled trials of trastuzumab in the adjuvant setting have demonstrated that trastuzumab given in combination with chemotherapy to patients with tumors overexpressing HER2 significantly improves overall survival compared with chemotherapy alone. Cardiac toxicity occurs in approximately 3% to 4% of patients taking trastuzumab, compared with 1% with anthracycline-based standard chemotherapy. Those with tumors with low or negative levels of expression or amplification are not likely to benefit from treatment with trastuzumab. Studies evaluating optimal duration and sequencing are ongoing. Targeting of other EGFR/tyrosine kinase inhibitors also show promise in preclinical and clinical trials of metastatic breast cancer.

ANGIOGENESIS

Angiogenesis is essential for tumor growth and metastasis. Tumors with volumes less than a few cubic millimeters exist in a prevascular state with a continued cycle of proliferation and cell death,

Table 1: Classes of Antiangiogenic Drugs in Clinical Development

Class of Drugs	Mode(s) of Action
Matrix metalloprotease (MMP) inhibitors	Inhibits MMP2 and MMP9
Vascular endothelial growth factor (VEGF)	Inhibits binding of VEGF to receptor
Anti-VEGF antibody	Blocks the VEGF receptor
Anti-integrin antibodies	Causes endothelial apoptosis
Vascular targeting agents	Fixes complement and causes vasculitis

receiving oxygen and nutrients through diffusion. Tumor angiogenesis is the proliferation of a network of blood vessels that penetrate into cancerous growths, supplying nutrients and oxygen and removing waste products. Angiogenesis, or neovascularization, is a multistep process controlled by angiogenic and angiostatic factors. The exact mechanism that allows a tumor to convert from the pre-vascular state to an angiogenic state ("angiogenic switch") is still unknown.

After the angiogenic switch is thrown, angiogenic factors activate endothelial cells and prompt the activation and secretion of factors, including matrix metalloproteases, which precipitate the breakdown of the basement membrane. The endothelial cells can then invade the surrounding tissue. Eventually the endothelial cells begin to organize into hollow tubes that become a mature network of blood vessels. Vascular endothelial growth factor (VEGF) and its receptors are important for sustaining tumor growth. VEGF is synthesized inside tumor cells and then secreted into the surrounding tissue, binds to receptors, and activates a series of proteins that transmit a signal into the nucleus to initiate new endothelial cell growth, differentiation, and apoptosis. In addition, VEGF mediates vascular permeability and allows deposition of angiogenic proteins into the surrounding tissue, perpetuating angiogenesis.

Early studies by Dr. Judah Folkman demonstrated that inhibiting angiogenesis could inhibit cancer growth. This led to the development of agents to inhibit angiogenesis for therapeutic intention. Table 1 lists classes of anti-angiogenic drugs in clinical development.

Bevacizumab (Avastin; Genentech) is a humanized monoclonal antibody that inhibits VEGF. Several phase III studies in metastatic breast cancer patients demonstrate improved overall and progression-free survivals. Trials of bevacizumab in the adjuvant setting are ongoing in combination with other chemotherapy and endocrine regimens. Rare side effects include bowel perforations, thromboembolic events, and hemorrhage. VEGF inhibitors may increase toxicity of radiation therapy and can affect the function of organs with a fenestrated endothelium, such as the kidney and thyroid. To date, no surrogate markers have been identified that consistently predict which patients will respond to anti-VEGF therapy.

GENE EXPRESSION PROFILING

Although evaluation of individual gene expression may be useful for prognosis and predicting response to therapy, the interaction of multiple genes with each other may be more informative. Gene expression analysis of individual tumors is a promising approach to determine likelihood of recurrence and response to chemotherapy. The 21-gene reverse-transcriptase polymerase chain reaction assay (Oncotype DX; Genomic Health, Redwood City, CA) is performed on paraffin-embedded tissue and evaluates Ki67, STK15, survivin or BIRC5, CCNB1 or cyclin B1, MYBL2, GRB7, HER2, ER, PGR (http://www.jco.org/cgi/content/full/24/23/3726 - GLOSS#GLOSSBCL2), SCUBE2, MMP11

or stromelysin 3 (http://www.jco.org/cgi/content/full/24/23/3726), GLOSS#GLOSSCTSL2 or cathepsin L2, GSTM1, CD68, and BAG1 and five reference genes (ACTB or beta-actin, GAPDH, GUS, RPLPO, and TFRC). The 21-gene signature has been validated and is commercially available for newly diagnosed stage I or II breast cancer patients who have node-negative disease and whose tumors are estrogen-receptor positive, with the assumption that these patients will be treated with endocrine therapy. The results are provided as a recurrence score. If the recurrence score indicates a low-risk category, hormone therapy alone may be recommended; if the recurrence score indicates a high-risk category, chemotherapy followed by hormonal therapy may provide a better outcome. Initial studies indicate that this assay may also predict the magnitude of benefit from chemotherapy. Studies are ongoing with this and similar assays.

FACTORS RELATED TO BREAST CANCER PREDISPOSITION

The majority of breast cancers that occur are sporadic; however, approximately 5% to 10% of breast cancers are related to an inherited susceptibility. Hereditary breast and ovarian cancer syndrome (HBOC) comprises the majority of these inherited breast cancers and is due to deleterious mutations in BRCA1 or BRCA2. Other familial cancer syndromes comprise less than 5% of the inherited breast cancers (Table 2). BRCA1 and BRCA2 are inherited in an autosomal-dominant fashion. More than 70% of the identified mutations in BRCA1 or BRCA2 are frameshift mutations. In addition, a number of founder mutations have been documented, three of which are prevalent in those with Ashkenazi Jewish ancestry.

BRCA1, first described in 1994, is located at 17q21. BRCA1 functions in DNA damage repair, cell-cycle-checkpoint control, ubiquitylation, and chromatin remodeling. BRCA2 is located at 13q12 and is also involved in DNA repair via homologous recombination or "crossing over." Women with a deleterious mutation in BRCA1 or BRCA2 have a lifetime risk of developing breast cancer of 50% to 85%. There is a higher lifetime risk of developing ovarian cancer with BRCA1 (20%–40%) than BRCA2 (10%–27%). In male carriers of BRCA2, there is a 6% lifetime risk of breast cancer. BRCA2 is also associated with an increased risk of pancreatic and prostate cancers.

The breast cancer phenotype differs between BRCA1 and BRCA2. BRCA1-associated breast cancers offer have more adverse clinicopathologic features than BRCA2-associated breast cancers.

Table 2: Other Breast Cancer–Associated Familial Cancer Syndromes

Li-Fraumeni syndrome	Early-onset breast cancer, sarcoma, leukemia, brain tumors, and adrenocortical tumors	TP53; more recently CHEK2
Cowden syndrome	Multiple harmartomatous lesions: skin, mucous membranes, breast and thyroid tumors	PTEN
Peutz-Jeghers syndrome	Melanocytic macules of the lips, gastrointestinal hamartomatous polyps, increased risk for neoplasms of the breast and gastrointestinal tract	STK11 (LKB1)
Ataxia telangiectasia	Breast cancer, lymphoma, leukemia	ATM

Table 3: Family History Features Consistent with a BRCA Mutation

First-degree relatives with breast cancer, one of whom received the diagnosis at age 50 years or younger
A combination of three or more first- or second-degree relatives with breast cancer regardless of age at diagnosis
A combination of both breast and ovarian cancer among first- and second-degree relatives
A first-degree relative with bilateral breast cancer
A combination of two or more first- or second-degree relatives with ovarian cancer regardless of age at diagnosis
A first- or second-degree relative with both breast and ovarian cancer at any age
A history of breast cancer in a male relative
Ashkenazi Jewish ancestry

BRCA1-associated breast cancers tend to be higher grade and ER/PR-negative and HER2 negative ("triple negative"). Family history features suggestive of a deleterious mutation of BRCA1 and BRCA2 are listed in Table 3.

Genetic testing should be considered only in individuals who have a personal or family history consistent with a genetic susceptibility for breast cancer. Computational tools are available to assist with probability prediction of a deleterious mutation. Pretest and posttest counseling, including a discussion of risks and benefits, is important. In addition, it is important that the test is adequately interpreted and that the result will influence medical or surgical management of individuals at risk.

Women with increased risk for breast cancer secondary to an inherited predisposition can be managed with increased surveillance and chemoprevention or prophylactic surgery. Breast examination by a clinician is recommended semiannually beginning at age 25 and annual mammography beginning 5 to 10 years younger than the age of onset of the youngest affected relative. In addition, recent data suggest that magnetic resonance imaging may be useful as an adjunct to mammography for screening women at high risk for inherited breast cancer. Currently tamoxifen is the only Food and Drug Administration–approved medication for reducing breast cancer risk in high-risk populations. Prospective data regarding use of tamoxifen in asymptomatic BRCA1 or BRCA2 mutation carriers is lacking; however, prophylactic oophorectomy can reduce breast cancer risk by 50% in mutation carriers, indicating a potential benefit from tamoxifen therapy in these women. Prophylactic surgery to include bilateral prophylactic mastectomy and or bilateral prophylactic oophorectomy may be considered. Bilateral prophylactic mastectomy can reduce the risk of developing breast cancer by at least 90%. Prophylactic oophorectomy reduces the risk of ovarian cancer but can also reduce the risk of breast cancer in premenopausal women at increased risk of inherited breast cancer.

Suggested Readings

Esteva FJ, Gabriel N: Prognostic molecular markers in early breast cancer, *Hortobagyi Breast Cancer Res* 6:109, 2004.

Narod SA, Foulkes WD: BRCA1 and BRCA2: 1994 and beyond, *Nat Rev Cancer* 4:665, 2004.

Paik S, Shak S, Tang G, and others: A multigene assay to predict recurrence of tamoxifen-treated, node-negative breast cancer, *N Engl J Med* 351:2817, 2004.

Schneider BP, Miller KD: Angiogenesis of breast cancer, *J Clin Oncol* 23:1782, 2005.

BREAST CANCER: SURGICAL THERAPY

Marshall M. Urist, MD

INTRODUCTION

With an ever-increasing complexity of treatments for breast cancer, the surgeon's role remains central. This role requires an understanding of all treatment modalities currently applied to breast cancer care. Not only is surgical decision making important, the surgeon must also determine the optimal timing of surgery in relation to these other modalities. This chapter reviews the principle steps in evaluation and surgical care. Many other important details are described in the accompanying breast disease chapters of this text.

DIAGNOSIS, INITIAL EVALUATION, AND INFORMED CONSENT

The surgeon's first contact with the patient is because of breast symptoms, signs on physical examination, or findings on a screening radiological examination. In all cases, the evaluation begins with a complete history and physical examination. Breast imaging studies should include a bilateral mammogram with ultrasound to evaluate masses or densities. Magnetic resonance imaging (MRI) can provide additional information to define the extent of the tumor within the breast and multicentricity. MRI often identifies the site of origin when patients present with axillary adenopathy and no evidence of a primary tumor on mammogram and ultrasound.

The histologic diagnosis of breast cancer is, for the most part, a presurgical procedure. Core needle devices reliably yield representative samples of masses and areas of calcification using handheld or stereotactic techniques. This provides a definitive diagnosis (histologic type and grade in addition to hormone receptor status and gene expression) and is key in treatment planning. Surgical biopsy for diagnosis is now limited to situations in which tissue cannot be obtained by core needle biopsy or there is a discrepancy between the mammographic appearance and the core biopsy report. Fine needle aspiration (FNA) is limited to a cytologic diagnosis and is most effectively used in conjunction with ultrasound to diagnose axillary nodal metastases.

After the histologic diagnosis of breast cancer has been made, staging x-rays and scans seldom provide evidence of metastatic disease unless the patient has symptoms, a large primary tumor, or extensive axillary adenopathy. For this reason a complete metastatic workup is often unnecessary.

Surgical decision making is a complex issue for both the surgeon and the patient. The surgeon's challenge is to help the patient develop an understanding of the disease and the rationale for and benefits and risks of each surgical option. The surgeon has an obligation to give the patient a recommendation in addition to a list of options. Because this process can require time, patients should not be rushed into making a decision and beginning therapy. Multiple large randomized trials with long-term follow-up have confirmed that breast conservation surgery (BCS) and mastectomy are equivalent forms of treatment. By consensus, BCS is the preferred form of treatment. In early breast cancer, patients who remain undecided about surgical options are well served by undergoing tumor resection, sentinel lymph node biopsy, and reassessment in the context of the pathologic findings.

NONINVASIVE BREAST CANCER

Ductal carcinoma in situ (DCIS) and lobular carcinoma in situ (LCIS) are noninvasive pathologic conditions with contrasting appearances and natural histories. DCIS is commonly detected as mammographic calcifications, whereas LCIS is most often unexpectedly diagnosed after biopsy of a palpable mass or radiologic abnormality. DCIS is a precursor of invasive ductal carcinoma (IDC), and LCIS is considered to be a risk factor for the subsequent appearance of both ductal and lobular carcinomas. The mass or density containing LCIS should be completely excised to rule out the presence of an associated invasive malignancy. The treatment of DCIS is complete excision with histologically normal margins. If the diagnosis has been made by core needle biopsy, every effort should be made to have the first excision result in negative margins. This requires preoperative and intraoperative consultation with the radiologist and close communication with the pathologist postexcision. A complete discussion of in situ carcinoma is found in Chapter 12.10.

INVASIVE BREAST CANCER

Planning the surgical treatment of invasive breast cancer begins with a review of the history, physical examination, imaging studies, and pathology. Because of the effective use of screening mammography, the average primary tumor diameter has been steadily decreasing for decades. Consequently many patients are candidates for BCS. National consensus conferences have concluded that BCS is the preferred form of treatment. If there are no contraindications to BCS (previous radiation therapy to the breast or chest wall, some collagen vascular diseases, multicentricity, or the inability to achieve negative margins with a satisfactory cosmetic result), the discussion with the patient should include both BCS and mastectomy (Table 1). In patients with a normal axillary examination, sentinel lymph node biopsy has become the standard method for lymphatic staging for both BCS and mastectomy.

BREAST CANCER IN PREGNANCY

Pregnant patients who develop breast cancer can present with mastodynia, swelling, skin changes, a mass, or enlarged regional nodes. Initially, the breast and axilla are best evaluated by ultrasound. The diagnosis is made by core needle biopsy of a suspicious area or FNA

Table 1: Contraindications to Breast Conservation Therapy

1. Inability to obtain negative margins and preserve adequate cosmesis after lumpectomy
2. Suspicious or indeterminate calcifications remaining after lumpectomy
3. Previous radiation therapy to the breast, or chest wall, or both
4. Collagen vascular disease

of an enlarged axillary node. For many years, modified radical mastectomy was considered the procedure of choice for all pregnant patients. This remains true for those in the first trimester of gestation. In the second and third trimesters, patients who meet the criteria for BCS can undergo lumpectomy with axillary staging. In these trimesters, lymphoscintigraphy can be used; however, there is insufficient evidence to define the safety of using blue dye for mapping. Adjuvant chemotherapy can be administered after the first trimester and radiation therapy is given postpartum. The prognosis for pregnant patients is the same as nonpregnant patients who share equivalent stages of disease.

SURGICAL TECHNIQUES

Breast Conservation Surgery

The procedure by which a primary cancer is removed from the breast has been labeled with many terms depending on how much tissue is removed: lumpectomy, tumorectomy, tylectomy, partial mastectomy, segmentectomy, or quadrantectomy. The common goal in these procedures is to remove the tumor with margins containing histologically normal tissue. The minimal acceptable margin is one that is histologically free. Wider margins (≥ 1 cm) are desirable for lobular carcinomas and IDC associated with extensive DCIS to minimize the risk of local recurrence. Detailed preoperative planning is based on mammographic, ultrasound and possibly MRI findings. Ultrasound is useful even in cases in which the tumor is palpable because it can show the shape and relationship of the tumor to the skin and underlying muscle. The operative note should accurately describe the extent of the resection and relationship of the tumor to surrounding structures.

The incision is placed directly over the primary tumor site in most instances. Keeping the incision central in the breast aids in cosmesis, but this should not compromise the surgeon's ability to see the field and obtain negative margins of resection. The orientation of the incision can be concentric with the areola unless it is necessary to excise overlying skin. When skin is included on the specimen, a radial incision may create less distortion. An alternative to simple lumpectomy is a more comprehensive excision that incorporates a full-thickness resection of breast tissue to obtain wider margins. This approach is called *oncoplastic surgery* because it uses plastic surgical principles to achieve a cosmetically desirable appearance (see Anderson and colleagues). This procedure may result in a reduction in breast size that necessitates a contralateral mammoplasty to achieve symmetry.

In BCS, care should be taken to manipulate the specimen as little as possible because breast tissue is friable, especially in older women. Designation of margins on the specimen is extremely important, and the surgeon can do this most accurately. Several orientation techniques have been used with success: touch preparations directly from the specimen for cytology, sutures placed on at least two faces of the specimen, painting of the six surfaces with various colors, and surgical resection of separate pieces of tissue for each margin. This last technique can be performed by harvesting separate sections from the specimen itself or from the breast cavity walls after the specimen is removed. Applying ink to the surface of breast tissue may create the false impression of a positive margin because of color penetration of crushed or torn tissue.

In cases in which x-ray or ultrasound localization has been used, the specimen should be imaged to confirm successful resection of the abnormal area (Fig. 1). When the specimen radiograph shows extension of a mass or calcifications to a margin, additional tissue resection can be performed at the same procedure. Careful preoperative and intraoperative planning reduces the need for secondary procedures.

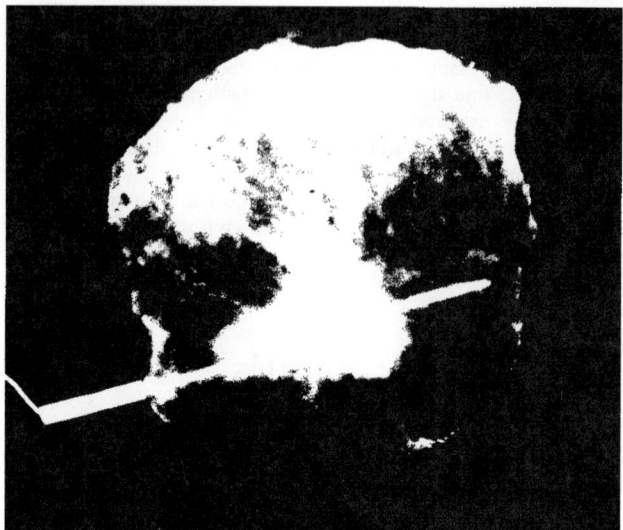

Figure 1 Lumpectomy specimen radiograph showing the mass (invasive component) and calcifications (ductal carcinoma in situ).

Techniques for closure of the wound depend on the size of the cavity, location within the breast, and quality of the glandular tissues of the breast. In early breast cancer, it is often not necessary to reapproximate the walls of the lumpectomy cavity; however, the long-term cosmetic result may be improved by reducing the size of the defect as long as the surrounding skin surface is not distorted in the process.

Finally, a detailed operative note is essential because it can aid in the interpretation of the pathology report, guide the radiation oncologist in treatment planning, and assist the radiologist in reading the follow-up mammograms.

Mastectomy

Total mastectomy is the procedure of choice when BCS is not an option or the patient prefers complete removal of the breast. Preoperative planning is important to determine the amount of skin to be removed. If reconstruction is not planned, skin flaps should be drawn to enable reapproximation of the skin with minimal tension. When an excisional biopsy has been performed, the scar of the biopsy is excised en bloc with the specimen. If the tumor extends to within 1 cm of the surface, it may also be necessary to include the overlying skin to ensure negative margins. Skin-sparing mastectomy is performed when reconstruction is planned. In most cases this procedure leaves all of the breast skin except the nipple and areola. In some centers, nipple- and areola-preserving mastectomies are being performed when there is no danger of leaving tumor in the subareolar tissue that is retained with this operation. A separate biopsy is taken from this area to ensure a negative margin and minimize the risk of local recurrence.

Lymphatic Mapping and Sentinel Lymph Node Biopsy

Lymphatic mapping and sentinel lymph node biopsy is a valuable technique that has improved the accuracy of lymphatic staging and reduced the morbidity associated with axillary dissection. Lymphoscintigraphy is performed preoperatively by the subareolar or peritumoral injection of ^{99m}technetium (^{99m}Tc) sulfur colloid agents to label the node(s) receiving primary drainage from the

breast. After the induction of anesthesia, isosulfan blue dye is also injected in the central area of the breast. At axillary exploration, all radioactive and blue-colored nodes are resected. Any visibly or palpably abnormal nodes are also submitted. A detailed discussion appears in Chapter 12.7.

The term *completion axillary dissection* refers to performing a regional dissection after a sentinel lymph node has been found to contain a metastasis. Reports from many centers have shown that the remaining axillary contents are free of additional metastases in approximately 50% of cases. A debate has ensued over the value of resecting more normal tissue when the risk of finding cancer is low. A definitive answer to this problem awaits further research. Unfortunately, no combination of variables has been found to predict zero risk of finding additional positive nodes. In the interval, it is possible to estimate the risk of finding additional positive nodes by using a nomogram reported by Van Zee and colleagues. The nomogram is useful in guiding discussions between patients and physicians as they weigh the value of complete lymph node resection.

Sentinel lymph node biopsy has also been performed for patients with DCIS. In a small percentage of cases, node metastases have been found despite the absence of an invasive focus in the breast. Fortunately, this finding has not been shown to be prognostic of a poor outcome. Therefore sentinel lymph node biopsy is not recommended for patients with DCIS who are undergoing BCS. When total mastectomy is being performed for extensive DCIS, sentinel node biopsy is recommended in the event that a focus of invasive carcinoma is discovered. Even under these circumstances, it is uncommon to find a nodal metastasis.

Axillary Lymph Node Dissection

Axillary lymph node dissection is the procedure of choice for patients with biopsy-proved positive nodes. With the widespread application of sentinel lymph node biopsy in patients with a normal axilla (physical examination and ultrasound), there has been a marked reduction in the need for complete axillary dissection. In this procedure, the patient is positioned supine with the ipsilateral upper extremity wrapped and prepped free into the field to allow the optimal exposure to the upper levels. The incision is placed transversely in the midaxilla and not carried anteriorly past the pectoralis major margin unless there is extensive adenopathy. After the margins of the dissection are defined, the interpectoral tissues are dissected to expose the lateral border of the pectoralis minor. Division of the clavipectoral fascia medially along this border and transversely in line with the coracobrachialis muscle releases the specimen and allows immediate exposure of the axillary vein. The median pectoral nerve is seen and readily preserved in most cases. As the inferior branches of the axillary vein are divided, the specimen is released to allow blunt dissection of the remaining attachments along the serratus and subscapularis muscles. Upper intercostal nerves can often be preserved, but normal sensation may not return after mobilization and retraction of these branches. The long thoracic and thoracodorsal nerves are identified and preserved. Local tissue reaction from a sentinel lymph node biopsy may result in a more difficult dissection along the thoracodorsal vessels and nerve.

Breast Reconstruction

Breast reconstruction should be discussed with patients undergoing total mastectomy. This procedure can be performed under the same anesthetic as the mastectomy or as a delayed operation. Immediate reconstruction is not recommended when there is a possibility of radiation therapy being used in the postoperative period. Compared with tissue implants, autogenous tissue reconstruction techniques have better durability but carry the higher risks associated with long periods of anesthesia.

ADJUVANT THERAPIES

Treatment advances in the long-term outcome of breast cancer therapy have come from early detection and systemic therapy. The high incidence of this disease has provided the opportunity for large randomized trials to detect significant increases in patient survival. It is important for the surgeon to keep up to date with the standards of adjuvant therapy because major trials are published several times per year. These results of adjuvant trials are rapidly incorporated into the National Comprehensive Cancer Network guidelines, which are available online at http://www.nccn.org. The decision to apply adjuvant therapy is based on an analysis of tumor size, lymph node status, and tumor markers such as estrogen and progesterone receptors and gene expression. Web sites are available on which patients and physicians can calculate the benefit of adjuvant therapy. Traditionally this decision has been made after surgical therapy is complete; however, there may be enough information available at presentation to warrant consideration of starting with chemotherapy. This is termed *neoadjuvant chemotherapy*. The advantage to the patient is a reduction in tumor size and the possibility of BCS. Neoadjuvant chemotherapy has not been shown to have a survival advantage over standard postsurgical adjuvant therapy. A complete discussion of this important subject is found in the chapter beginning on page 662.

CONCLUSIONS

Surgeons play a central role in the multidisciplinary care of breast cancer patients. Only through knowledge of all components of care can this role be effectively carried out. Using information obtained by minimal access techniques, options can be defined and a treatment plan designed in collaboration between the patient and her care team. Breast conservation and systemic adjuvant therapy are appropriate treatment for a rising proportion of patients and have resulted in an increase in the quality and quantity of life for women with this disease.

SUGGESTED READINGS

Anderson BO, Masetti R, Silverstein MJ: Oncoplastic approaches to partial mastectomy: an overview of volume-displacement techniques, *Lancet Oncol* 6:145, 2005.

Lyman GH, Giuliano AE, Somerfield MR, and others: American Society of Clinical Oncology guideline recommendations for sentinel lymph node biopsy in early-stage breast cancer, *J Clin Oncol* 23:7703, 2005.

National Comprehensive Cancer Network Guidelines for management of all phases of breast cancer care (online). (These are consensus-based guidelines from major institutions and are promptly updated as new evidence is published.)

Silverstein MJ, Lagios MD, Recht A, and others: Image-detected breast cancer: state of the art diagnosis and treatment, *J Am Col Surg* 201:586, 2005.

Van Zee KJ, Mannasseh DM, Bevilacqua JL, and others: A nomogram for predicting the likelihood of additional nodal metastases in breast cancer patients with a positive sentinel node biopsy, *Ann Surg Oncol* 10:1140, 2003.

ABLATIVE TECHNIQUES IN THE TREATMENT OF BENIGN AND MALIGNANT BREAST DISEASE

V. Suzanne Klimberg, MD

INTRODUCTION

Although the goal of breast conservation surgery (BCS) is to achieve better cosmesis without compromising local recurrence or survival, the treatment often results in deformity at the lumpectomy site, which causes significant psychological distress. The deformity occurs because margins are often positive and require reexcision. Current research seeks alternative breast cancer treatments that yield superior cosmesis and are more acceptable to patients.

Ablation is commonly used in the treatment of hepatic tumors and hepatic metastases. Surgeons have also explored the use of percutaneous ablation (most commonly with cryosurgery, laser ablation, and radiofrequency ablation (RFA); see Table 1) , rather than open surgical excision, to treat both benign and malignant breast abnormalities, including fibroadenomas and small breast cancers. Potential advantages of percutaneous ablation include outpatient treatment, short treatment times, low rates of treatment-related complications, and relatively lower costs than traditional therapy. Although promising, these techniques also carry several disadvantages. Treatment with percutaneous ablation may increase

Table 1: Comparison of Ablative Techniques Used in Breast Cancer

Cryoablation	Laser Ablation	Radiofrequency Ablation
Freezes lesion	Heals lesion	Heals lesion
Uses real-time US visualization	Requires precise targeting with MRI or stereotaxis	Uses real-time US visualization
Approved for fibroadenomas	Limited to tumors 1.5 cm	Ablation zone may be expanded to 3–7 cm
Size of cryoprobe may affect ability to freeze larger lesions		

MRI, Magnetic resonance imaging; *US,* ultrasound.

patient anxiety about the presence of tumor cells in the breast because there is no certainty that all of a tumor has been ablated, highlighting the inadequacies of present imaging capabilities. In addition, the ability to obtain full histologic status may be impaired, including margin status, pathologic tumor size, tumor grade, lymphovascular invasion, and biologic tumor markers including hormone and HER-2/neu protein status.

CRYOABLATION

Cryoablation creates an elliptical ice ball with argon gas that surrounds the lesion. The duration of freezing depends on the size of the lesion; the freezing, its proximity to the skin, and muscle tissue

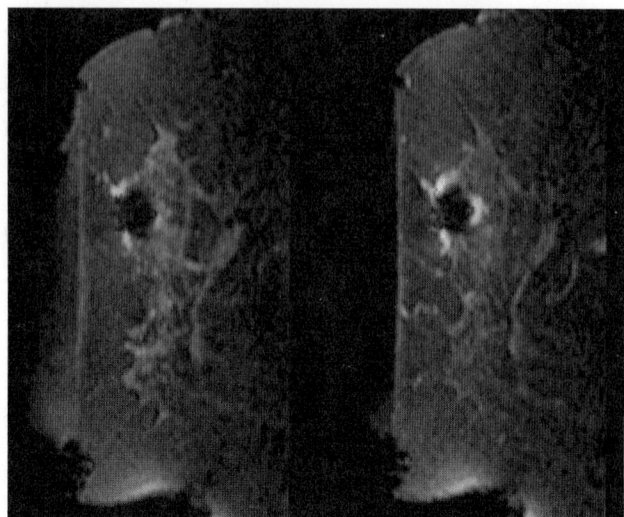

Figure I Ultrasound demonstrating a cryoprobe development of an ice ball. As the ice ball approaches skin, saline can be injected between the skin or chest wall to protect it.

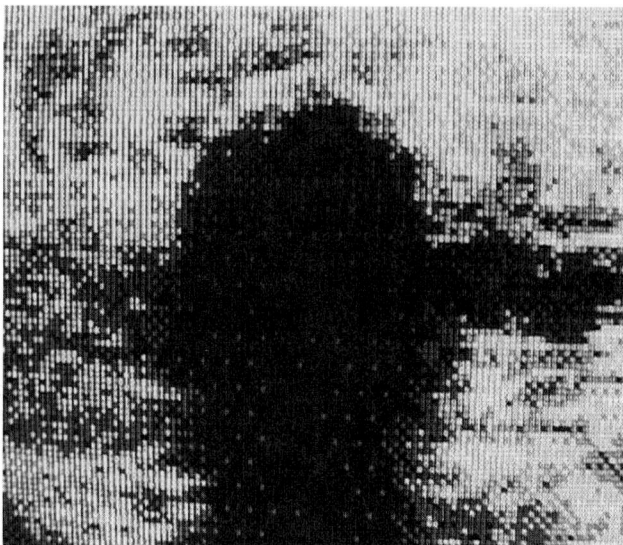

Figure 2 Magnetic resonance imaging section through the breast demonstrating laser ablation of a tumor *(black hole)* with slight hyperemic area around it.

are visualized with real-time ultrasound (US). The only Food and Drug Administration (FDA)-approved use of cryoablation is the treatment of core biopsy–proved fibroadenoma. Cryoablation effectively and safely treats fibroadenoma in an office setting with local anesthesia. Following treatment, lesions shrink over time and may take 12 months or longer to resolve completely. However, results from the FibroAdenoma Cryoablation Treatment registry show that of 444 patients entered into the registry, 35% still had palpable lesions at 12 months. Before any ablative process, a biopsy is obtained for pathologic concordance. Percutaneous excision via vacuum-assisted biopsy can be accomplished during the same biopsy and visit in approximately 15 minutes; this seems to have preempted any ablative technique for benign purposes.

Trials of cryoablation in small invasive breast cancers have yielded varying results but suggest that the size of the cryoprobe used may influence outcome. In a trial conducted by Pfleiderer and colleagues, 31% of tumors 16 mm in diameter were completely ablated, whereas no tumors 23 mm in diameter were completely ablated. Cryoprobes have also been used as an alternative to needle localization when nonpalpable lesions are excised. The cryoprobe freezes the lesion together with 5 to 10 mm of surrounding breast tissue, creating a palpable ice ball and obviating needle localization (Fig. 1). Furthermore, inclusion of a margin of normal breast tissue reduced to 6% the need for reexcision because of positive margins. However, cryoablation hinders further tumor assessment or special staining and as used here is merely a localization procedure.

LASER ABLATION

In laser ablation, a specific wavelength of light in a narrow beam of high-intensity light-containing energy generates heat at the tip of the laser, inducing apoptosis. Laser ablation requires precise targeting with either magnetic resonance imaging (MRI) or stereotaxis, and the treatment area is limited. In a trial by our group, MRI-guided laser was used to ablate tumors before surgery in 12 patients (Fig. 2). Simultaneous laser fibers were used to create composite zones of ablation to treat larger lesions, successfully ablating lesions in three cases and partially ablating lesions in nine cases. The primary objective of this trial was not to achieve complete ablation of tumors but to perform laser guidance and to evaluate the usefulness of MRI in assessing outcome.

Using stereotactic guidance to laser-ablate small breast cancers detected by mammography, Dowlatshahi and colleagues achieved a

success rate of 93%. The laser fiber was inserted into the center of the lesion, which was stereotactically identified, and a multisensor thermal needle at the periphery of the lesion monitored tissue temperature; temperatures of 50° to 55°C induced cell death (Fig. 3). Treatment is limited to tumors 1.5 cm in diameter. Laser ablation typically yields a coagulative zone of 2.5 to 3.0 cm in diameter, with a 0.5-cm negative margin surrounding the lesion (Figs. 4 and 5). Our group has found laser to be less predictable.

RADIOFREQUENCY ABLATION

The most intense ongoing research on ablation techniques focuses on RFA. In RFA, frictional heat generated by intracellular ions moving in response to an alternating high-frequency current results in tissue coagulation, causing cell death and the destruction of solid tumors. An RFA probe, consisting of a tube with retractable prongs, is positioned and monitored under US guidance. RFA may be performed in either of two modes, temperature or power. Increasing the area of current conduction can affect an ablation zone of 3 to 7 cm in diameter in a variety of tissues. RFA is currently approved by the FDA for ablation of subcutaneous tissue and unresectable tumors.

Current Experience with Radiofrequency Ablation in Breast Cancer

Percutaneous Radiofrequency Ablation

The rationale for using RFA in breast cancer is based on promising results seen in several other tumor types, including liver, bone, brain, kidney, pancreas, and prostate. Several trials of RFA in patients with breast cancer have also yielded promising results (Table 2). Complete coagulative necrosis was noted in select patients 86% to 100% of the time. Treatment was well tolerated, with few treatment-related complications noted and excellent cosmesis.

Jeffrey and colleagues first demonstrated the feasibility of using RFA in intact human breast tumors in five women with locally advanced breast cancer. Assessment of ablated tissue margins following mastectomy revealed zones of ablation measuring 0.8 to 1.8 cm in diameter. Initial results of a pilot trial of US-guided RFA in 26 patients with T1/2 breast carcinoma conducted by Izzo

Figure 3 Stereotactic localization of the tumor with clips placed around the tumor and a second thermal probe next to it. *Image courtesy Kambiz Kowlatshahi, MD. From Kepple J, VanZee KJ, Dowlatshahi K, Henry-Tillman RS, Israel PZ, and Klimberg VS: J Am Coll Surg 199(6):961, 2004.*

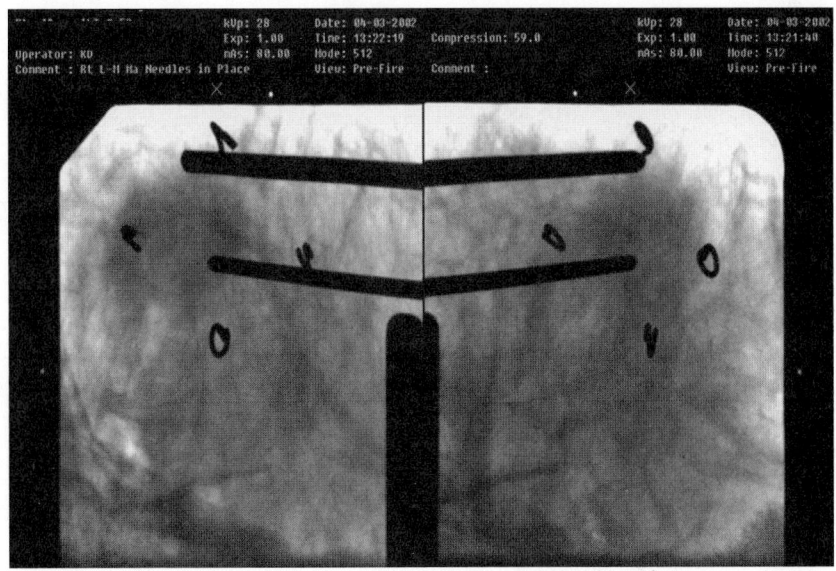

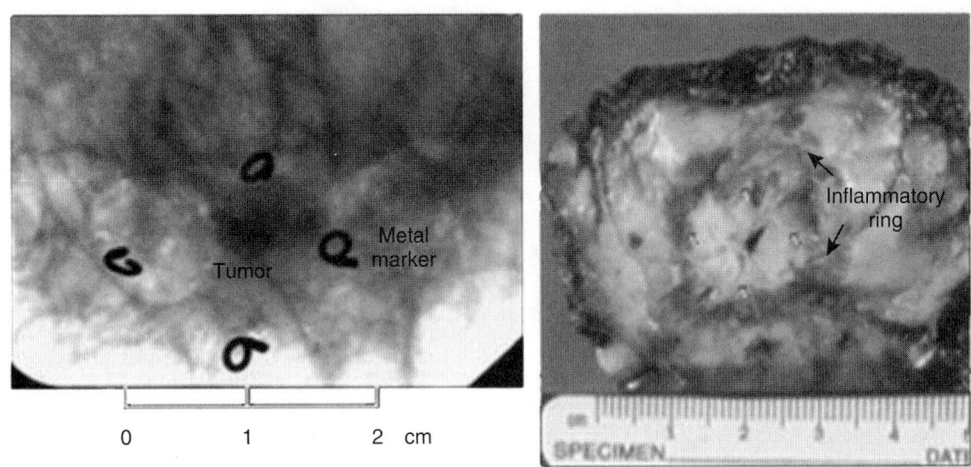

Figure 4 Subsequent stereotactic image to that in Figure 3A showing tumor ablation to markers and Figure 3B shows gross ablation of the tumor via laser.

Figure 5 Before and after mammograms of mass and ablation zone.

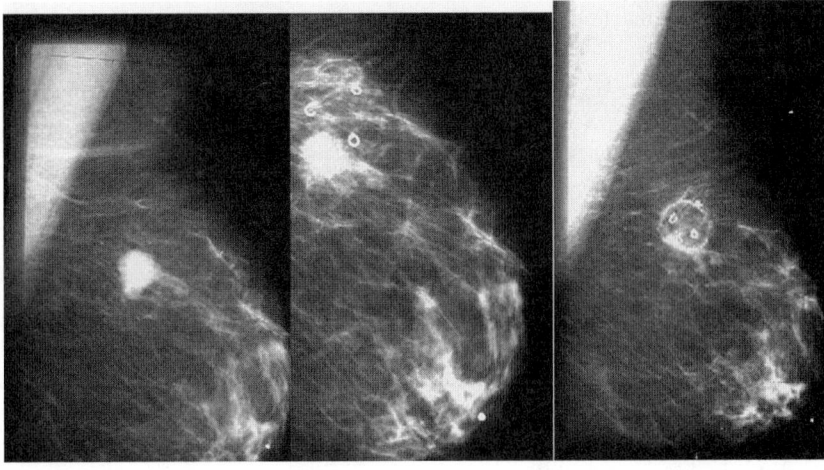

Table 2: Trials of RFA in Breast Cancer

Trial	Patients	N	Treatment	Outcome
Jeffrey and others, 1999 (feasibility)	Locally advanced disease	5	RFA → mastectomy	Ablation zones 0.8–1.8 cm in diameter
Izzo and others, 2001 (pilot)	T1/2	26	US-guided RFA (margin of ≥5 mm)	Complete coagulative necrosis in 25/26 patients*
Fornage, 2004	Tumor ±2 cm in diameter	21	RFA → surgery	Complete coagulative necrosis in all patients†
Burak and others, 2003	Tumor ≤2 cm in diameter	10	RFA → surgery (1–3 weeks later)	No residual lesions detected on MRI in 8/9 patients‡
Hayashi and others, 2003	Tumor ≤3 cm in diameter (T1)	22	RFA → surgery (1–2 weeks later)	Complete coagulative necrosis in 19/22 patients
Singletary, 2002	T1	30	Intraoperative RFA → excision	Complete ablation in 87% of patients

MDACC, MD Anderson Cancer Center; *RFA*, radiofrequency ablation.
*Full-thickness burn reported in one patient with tumor close to the skin.
†Included patients from Singletary multicenter trial.
‡Minimal breast ecchymosis was the only treatment-related complication reported.

and colleagues showed promising efficacy. Complete coagulative necrosis of the tumor was achieved in 25 of 26 patients, with only one treatment-related complication (a full-thickness burn in a patient whose tumor was immediately beneath the skin).

A multi-institutional trial conducted by Singletary and colleagues assessed the use of intraoperative RFA followed by surgical excision. The trial enrolled 30 patients with T1 breast carcinoma. Complete ablation, assessed with nicotinamide adenine dinucleotide staining, was achieved in 87% of patients. The investigators suggested that incomplete ablation in four patients was likely due to the inability to determine adequately the size of the tumor with standard preoperative imaging or due to inappropriate US targeting during RFA. When the MD Anderson Cancer Center reported their experience alone, which included patients from the multicenter trial, all of the 21 treated patients demonstrated complete coagulative necrosis of the tumor and margin, with no treatment complications. Burak and colleagues employed both pre-RFA and post-RFA breast MRI and more accurately assessed the extent of local disease preoperatively, while also enabling visualization of the zone of ablation, which differs in intensity from residual carcinoma.

To date, the RFA trials conducted in breast cancer provide promising results and suggest an important role for this new technique in managing early-stage disease. Together these results suggest that RFA may offer a more tolerable alternative to radiation therapy (XRT) following surgery, with excellent cosmesis and a high rate of negative margins. Nonetheless, several limitations of RFA must be addressed before the technique can be considered a definitive

treatment modality in breast cancer. Accurate three-dimensional pathologic reconstruction is necessary to ensure complete tumor ablation before treating breast carcinoma by in situ ablation only. In addition, follow-up imaging remains problematic. The ideal time to schedule imaging is unknown, and resolution of known scans (e.g., ±5–8 mm with MRI and positron emission tomography [PET]) and the costs associated with repeated scans may be prohibitive. Furthermore, posttreatment inflammatory changes cannot be differentiated from recurrence or untreated tumor.

Open Excision Followed by Radiofrequency Ablation

Open excision of tumor followed by RFA (eRFA) creates a tumor-free zone of breast subcutaneous tissue by ablation instead of surgical removal. eRFA overcomes imaging and targeting issues by removing the main tumor and using RF to ablate the margin only. RFA of margins also allows for this treatment to be performed in any size tumor that is eligible for lumpectomy to achieve better margins.

At our institution, we have combined two available and reliable techniques, lumpectomy and RFA, to provide full histology and clear margins with better cosmesis. Our strategy, eRFA, includes both excision of the cancer and ablation of the tumor bed at the excision site without removing large volumes of tissue, resulting in improved cosmesis. (Fig. 6) Furthermore, 1-cm circumferential ablation of the cavity may provide local control comparable to or better than that of brachytherapy (i.e., local XRT extending 1 cm in circumference around the tumor cavity).

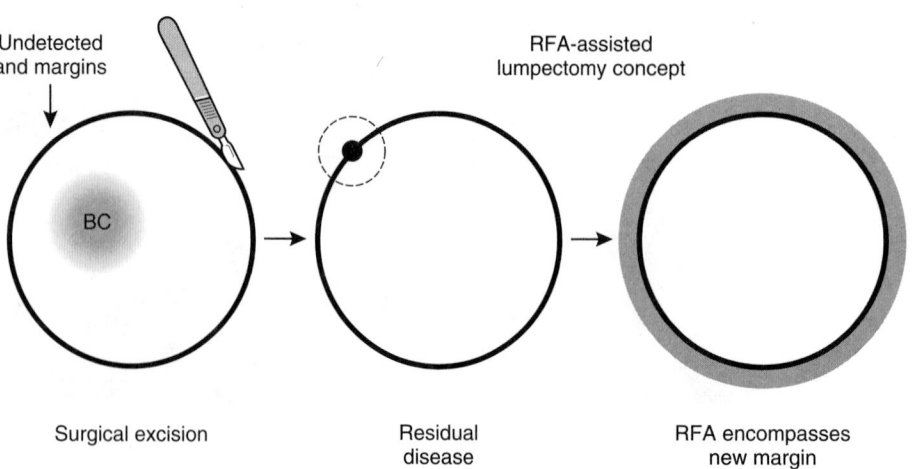

Undetected and margins

RFA-assisted lumpectomy concept

Surgical excision → Residual disease → RFA encompasses new margin

BC

Figure 6 Radiofrequency ablation–assisted lumpectomy concept.

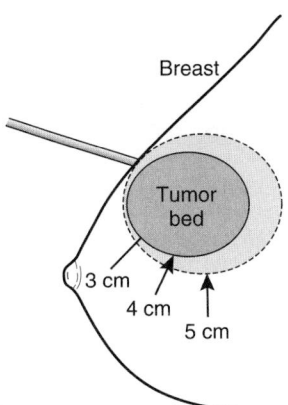

Figure 7 Diagram demonstrating deployment of the probe into the tumor cavity.

RFA-assisted lumpectomy avoids permanent external physical or cosmetic damage by completing RFA in the open wound following open lumpectomy at the time of the original operation. Immediately following standard surgical lumpectomy, a purse-string suture is used to reapproximate the cavity site (within 1 cm), and sutures are placed circumferentially around the wound to retract and protect the skin edges. The RFA probe is opened into the tumor cavity, and the prongs enter the bed of the tumor to a depth of 1 cm (Figs. 7 and 8). The temperature of the probe is gradually increased to the target temperature (100°C) over 1 minute, maintained for 15 minutes, and then cooled in the tumor bed for 1 minute. The suture around the cavity site is removed, and the probe is retracted from the cavity. The consistency and accuracy of this technique in ablating the lumpectomy cavity virtually extends margins beyond close or focally positive margins, thus avoiding repeat surgeries. This suggests that eRFA may yield outcomes comparable to brachytherapy. In the initial 68 patients undergoing eRFA at our institution, four required mastectomy for unresected calcification or grossly positive margins.

eRFA has the potential to expand the use of ablation therapy beyond the small population of patients currently treated with ablation (i.e., those with small, deep breast tumors). Standard treatment of patients with stage I/II breast cancer centers on successful surgical excision of the tumor and optimizing negative margins to reduce the risk of recurrence. A single excision yields the best outcome, both clinically and cosmetically. eRFA combines lumpectomy with intraoperative RFA, increasing the opportunity to gain clear

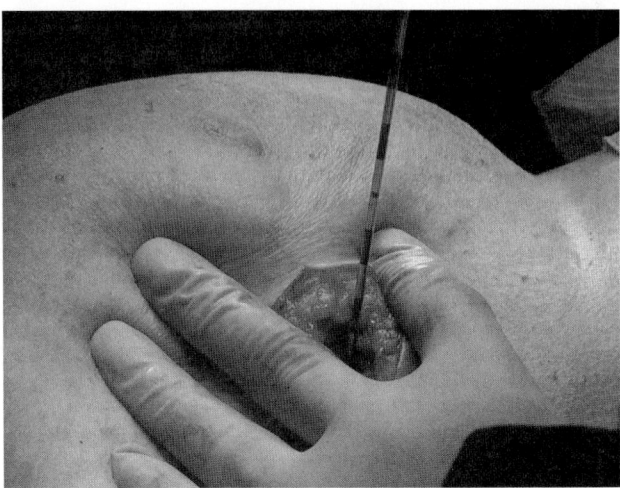

Figure 8 Actual deployment of the probe.

margins at the time of the original operation and perhaps overcoming the limitations in margin assessment of present-day pathology intraoperatively and postoperatively. In addition, the procedure may reduce the volume of excised tissue, improving cosmetic results. Further investigation is necessary to determine whether eRFA may be appropriate for patients eligible for BCS without XRT.

SUMMARY

Percutaneous excision of benign tumors seems unnecessary in light of newer methods of percutaneous excision. There is a clear need for improved, minimally invasive procedures to treat breast cancer. Advances in imaging will help this come to pass. eRFA or ablation after completing a standard lumpectomy for breast seems a more practical use at this time for the general surgeon or breast surgical oncologist to decrease reexcision rates.

SUGGESTED READINGS

Tafra L, Smith SJ, Woodward JE, and others: Pilot trial of cryoprobe-assisted breast-conserving surgery for small US-visible cancers, *Ann Surg Oncol* 10:1018, 2003.

LYMPHATIC MAPPING AND SENTINEL LYMPHADENECTOMY

Peter W. Henderson, MD, and Rache M. Simmons, MD

INTRODUCTION

Historically, every patient diagnosed with invasive breast cancer underwent an axillary dissection (ALND) to assess the metastatic status of the axilla. This procedure provided information regarding patient staging and prognosis and recommendations for subsequent adjuvant therapies. In the current age of mammographic screening and earlier detection, 70% of ALNDs do not yield axillary metastases, and thereby risk potential morbidity (including lymphedema, sensory disturbances, and future tendency toward infections) without any clinical benefit for the patient. Today sentinel lymph node biopsy (SLNB) offers a less invasive method of assessing the axilla for metastases compared with ALND and has been adopted as the standard of care in many surgical practices in this country and throughout the world.

SLNB is based on the concept that the lymphatic drainage from each breast first drains into one or several specific lymph node(s) before draining into more distal lymph nodes in the axilla. This first lymph node (or nodes) has been termed the "sentinel" lymph node (SLN) (Fig. 1). Multiple studies in the literature demonstrate that if an SLN is negative for metastatic disease, then the remainder of the axillary nodes are negative as well, and additional ALND is not warranted.

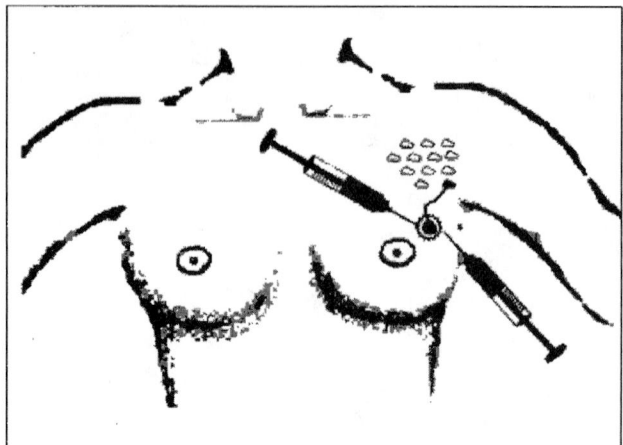

Figure 1 Uptake of isotope and blue dye from the breast to the sentinel lymph node.

SENTINAL LYMPH NODE BIOPSY TECHNIQUE

The first publication discussing the localization of the SLN is attributed to Cabanas, who in 1977 localized the SLN by palpation in a patient with penile cancer. Morton in 1992 described localizing SLN with blue dye in patients with melanoma, and Krag described localizing SLN with an injected radiolabeled material, also referred to as an isotope, in an animal model in 1993. Giuliano described the SLNB in breast cancer patients using blue dye in 1994.

To evaluate the SLN, it first must be identified and surgically removed. Most surgeons use a combination of isotope and blue dye to identify the SLN. The increased SLN identification rate using blue-dye in combination with isotope is well documented. This is particularly true for surgeons who are novices to the SLNB technique.

Although there is no consensus as to where the injections of the isotope should be given, considerable data suggest that intratumoral should be avoided and that the best uptake is achieved with intradermal or subdermal injections. The most commonly used isotope is [99m]technetium-labeled (^{99m}Tc) sulfur colloid particle. This product can be obtained both filtered and unfiltered, although filtered is more commonly used. The isotope is usually given in a single dose of 0.5 to1.0 mCi (18.5–37.5 MBq) in 1 to 8 ml of solution. There is also no consensus as to the optimal timing of isotope injection. If performed on the morning of surgery, it may cause delays in the operating room schedule. The alternative is to have patients receive the isotope injection on the day before SLNB. This way, the time allotted for the isotope uptake into the axilla does not conflict with the operating room schedule, and thus patients can have surgery at any time the following day, including as a first case.

Lymphoscintigraphy is a radiologic technique for visualizing isotope uptake after injection. Its utility is debatable, however. Some surgeons advocate its use because it provides a "road map" of the SLN and lymphatic system before the patient enters the operating room. Others, however, feel that its use is redundant because the sensitivity of the handheld intraoperative gamma probe allows SLN visualization even in patients in whom lymphoscintigraphy does not identify an SLN in the axilla.

The two most commonly used types of blue dye are isosulfan blue and methylene blue. It is documented that the two dyes have equivalent effectiveness in mapping the lymphatic drainage pattern. It has been suggested that methylene blue is a superior alternative to isosulfan blue on the basis of decreased risk of adverse reactions compared with isosulfan blue, as well as substantially decreased

cost. Common allergic reactions documented with isosulfan blue dye include urticaria, generalized rash, blue hives, or pruritus; isolated reports of anaphylaxis; and rare patient death. When using methylene blue, one must be aware that there is the potential for skin reaction (necrosis and epidermolysis) if the dye is injected superficially into the skin. These complications are eliminated when care is taken to avoid intradermal injection.

Most data suggest that localization of SLN is most successful when the injections are peritumoral, subareolar, or subdermal. To encourage drainage of the blue dye, many advocate brief breast massage to help direct the dye into the axilla. Typically 3 to 5 ml of blue dye is injected 5 to 10 minutes before the SLNB begins. SLNB is usually performed before simultaneous lumpectomy and can be performed at the beginning or end of a mastectomy depending on the surgeon's preference.

The handheld gamma probe can be used to direct placement of an axillary incision by finding the "hot" zone associated with the SLN. In the axilla, the surgeon identifies the SLN by visually tracing any blue dye tracts or using the handheld gamma probe (or both) to localize the area of highest radioactivity and precisely target the "hot" SLN. Electrocautery or blunt dissection is used to expose and then excise the SLNs. All SLNs that are blue or "hot" should be surgically excised for analysis. No data suggest that removal of more than five SLNs is unwarranted and unlikely to yield additional positive pathology.

After all obvious SLN(s) are excised, the 10-second count is performed of the radioactivity level by the gamma probe when the isotope technique is employed. As a general rule, if the remaining axilla shows more than 10% of the radioactivity count of the "hottest" SLN the surgeon should continue exploration to identify additional SLNs. It is also important that after the SLNs have been removed, the surgeon should palpate the axilla for any remaining palpable suspicious nodes and, if any are found, remove these as well for pathologic analysis. It is important to note that if no SLNB is identified by gamma probe or visualization of blue dye, ALND should be performed to allow pathologic assessment of the axilla for staging, prognosis, and treatment recommendations. For this reason, whenever a patient is consented for SLNB, she should be consented for possible ALND, as well.

After the SLNs have been removed, they are sent to surgical pathology for analysis. Whether the SLNs are subjected to immediate intraoperative frozen-section analysis or touch preparation cytology or await permanent sectioning is dependent on the preference of the surgeon and the institution. Many surgeons find benefit in performing an immediate completion axillary dissection for those patients with positive SLN.

The accuracy and clinical utility of SLNB is predicated by its ability to identify the SLNs (identification rate) and having the SLN accurately predicting the presence or absence of metastatic cells in the remaining axillary nodes (false-negative rate). In its consensus statement, the American Society of Breast Surgeons (ASBS) suggests that an acceptable identification rate is greater than 85% and an acceptable false-negative rate is less than 5%. As with all surgical procedures, SLNB has an appreciable learning curve. The ASBS also suggests that after a surgeon has performed 20 SLNBs followed by an axillary dissection (during residency, fellowship, or as a practicing surgeon), his or her identification and false-negative rates should meet the recommended acceptable rates, and SLNB may be performed alone.

CLINICAL IMPLICATIONS OF SENTINAL LYMPH NODE BIOPSY

Multiple studies in the literature have demonstrated that if an SLN is negative for metastatic disease, the remaining axillary nodes are negative as well, and additional axillary dissection is not warranted. The exceedingly low rate of reported axillary recurrences in SLN-negative patients also supports the clinical efficacy of SLNB.

In general, for patients with histologically hematoxylin and eosin (H&E)-positive SLN completion axillary dissection is recommended. However, it is debatable whether all patients with positive SLN require further axillary dissection. It has been documented that in 50% to 70% of patients, the SLN is the only positive node. The removal of additional negative axillary lymph nodes offers no clinical advantage and potential morbidity. Most surgeons today use completion axillary dissection selectively. Informational tools such as nomograms help surgeons determine each patient's risk of additional positive remaining axillary nodes, taking into account tumor type and nuclear grade, lymphovascular invasion, multifocality of primary tumor, estrogen-receptor status, number of positive SLNs, pathologic size, and method of detection of SLN metastases (Fig. 2). This information can be used in discussions between the patient and surgeon regarding further axillary dissection on an individual basis.

One topic on which there is considerable debate is the clinical significance of SLN micrometastases. In contrast to traditional ALND, SLNB affords the opportunity to extensively evaluate limited axillary nodes with more detailed analysis. Typically each SLN will be evaluated by serial sectioning with H&E and, at many institutions, additional immunohistochemistry (IHC) testing for the presence of metastatic disease on the basis of the presence of cytokeratin. In particular, IHC is able to identify micrometastases (0.2–2 mm) and isolated cancer cells (<0.2 mm), although the therapeutic implications of these results are currently unknown.

Current indications for SLNB (relative contraindications in italics):

Clinically node-negative T1-3 invasive breast cancer:
Prior breast surgery
Prior axillary surgery
Prior breast or axillary radiotherapy
Palpable axillary lymph nodes
Following neoadjuvant therapy
Pregancy

DCIS (when mastectomy required or microinvasive disease suspected)

Contraindications
Pathologically (FNA) proven positive axillary lymph nodes
Inflammatory breast cancer

Figure 2 Current American Society of Breast Surgeons indications for sentinel lymph node biopsy.

INDICATIONS FOR SENTINAL LYMPH NODE BIOPSY

According to the latest guidelines published by the ASBS, SLNB is currently indicated in virtually all patients with clinically node-negative T1–3 invasive breast cancer (Fig. 3). It was initially questioned whether SLNB would be accurate in multifocal and multicentric cancers because of concern that different areas of the breast may drain

---

Figure 3 Nomogram to predict likelihood of additional, non–sentinel lymph node *(non-SLN)* metastases in a patient with a positive SLN. *NUCGRADE,* tumor type and nuclear grade (ductal, nuclear grade I; ductal, nuclear grade II; ductal, nuclear grade III; lobular); *LVI,* lymphovascular invasion; *MULTIFOCAL,* multifocality of primary tumor; *ER,* estrogen-receptor status; *NUMNEGSLN,* number of negative SLNs; *NUMSLNPOS,* number of positive SLNs; *PATHSIZE,* pathological size, defined in centimeters; and *METHDETECT,* method of detection of SLN metastases *(frozen, routine hematoxylin and eosin stain [H&E], serial H&E, immunohistochemistry).* The first row *(Points)* is the point assignment for each variable. Rows 2 through 9 represent the variables included in the model. For an individual patient, each variable is assigned a point value (uppermost scale, *Points*) on the basis of the histopathologic characteristics. A vertical line is made between the appropriate variable value and the POINTS line. The assigned points for all eight variables are summed, and the total is found in row 10 *(Total Points).* After the total is located, a vertical line is made between Total Points and the final row, Row 11 *(Predicted Probability of +non-SLN).* See www.mskcc.org/nomograms.

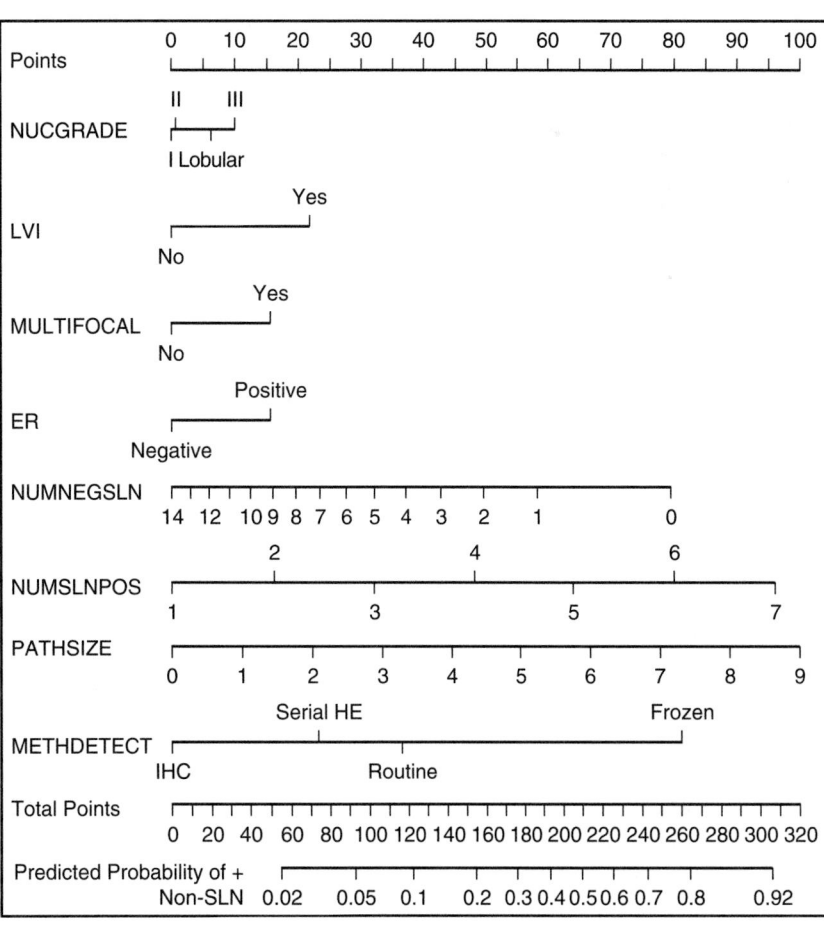

to different SLNs. SLNB, however, has been shown to be accurate in both unifocal, as well as multifocal and multicentric breast cancers.

By definition, ductal carcinoma in situ (DCIS) is not invasive disease and is not capable of metastasis. Nonetheless, studies have shown that 7% to 14% of patients with high-grade DCIS are SLN-positive. This probably represents patients who have underdiagnosed microinvasive disease. The recommendations on how to stage these patients and whether adjuvant therapy is indicated are debatable. Currently SLN is recommended in patients with DCIS who have high-grade disease as determined by core biopsy. It is also recommended when mastectomy is required because SLNB cannot be performed after mastectomy if occult invasive cancer is subsequently diagnosed.

Among those patients with T1–3 invasive breast cancer, relative contraindications may preclude some individuals as candidates for SLNB. The clinical situations that cause concern about the accuracy of SLNB because of the potential disruption of lymphatic drainage include extensive ipsilateral axillary surgery, previous SLNB/ALND, extensive upper outer quadrant resection, and ipsilateral radiation therapy. Series in the literature show that in all these situations and even in the setting of a previous SLNB or ALND, an SLNB can be attempted. The likelihood of identification of SLN can be less in these settings, but if a definite SLN is identified, it has been shown to be reliable.

Clinically palpable lymph nodes or those that are suspicious on ultrasound warrant further investigation via fine needle aspiration. If found to be positive, this indicates ALND without SLNB. If negative, these nodes should be considered indeterminate and evaluated by SLNB. It has been shown that clinically suspicious lymph nodes often do not represent metastatic disease and may instead represent benign reactive lymph nodes, especially in a setting of a diagnostic core biopsy.

The accuracy of SLN after neoadjuvant chemotherapy (NAC) is controversial. Recent data, however, suggest that SLN identification and false-negative rates may be equivalent in those patients who have received NAC, although more data are necessary before conclusions can be drawn. There has also been concern about the safety of SLNB in pregnant patients. There are limited data in this situation, but the information that is available does not demonstrate any increased risk to the fetus. If SLNB is considered in pregnancy, it should be discussed in detail with the patient with attention paid to fetal risk. Absolute contraindications include pathologically proved positive axillary lymph nodes and inflammatory breast cancer.

SUMMARY

SLNB offers most patients today an alternative to ALND as a less invasive technique with equally accurate staging information. The highest identification rate is found when using combined isotope and blue dye injection techniques. Whether to use immediate intraoperative assessment with frozen-section or touch preparation cytology is based on surgeon and institution preference and clinical experience. The clinical implication of IHC positivity in SLN is controversial. SLNB should be offered to most patients with T1–3 invasive breast cancer with few relative or absolute contraindications. Patients with negative SLN do not mandate further axillary dissection, and whether further axillary dissection is indicated in those patients with a positive SLN should be individualized and based on clinical judgment, additional information from tools such as nomograms, and patient-surgeon discussion.

Suggested Readings

American Society of Breast Surgeons consensus statement on guidelines for performing sentinel lymph node dissection in breast cancer (online), www.breastsurgeons.org. Accessed 2007.

Chu KU, Turner RR, Hansen NM, and others: Do all patients with sentinel node metastasis from breast carcinoma need complete axillary node dissection? *Ann Surg* 229:536, 1999.

Cody H, Borgen PI: State of the art approaches to sentinel node biopsy for breast cancer: study design, patient selection, technique, and quality control at Memorial Sloan-Kettering Cancer Center, *Surg Oncol* 8:85, 1999.

Kuerer HM, Newman LA: Lymphatic mapping and sentinel lymph node biopsy for breast cancer: developments and resolving controversies, *J Clin Oncol* 23:1698, 2005.

Newman LA: Lymphatic mapping and sentinel lymph node biopsy in breast cancer patients: a comprehensive review of variations in performance and technique, *J Am Coll Surg* 199:804, 2004.

Port ER, Fey J, Gemingnani ML, and others: Reoperative sentinel lymph node biopsy: a new option for patients with primary or locally recurrent breast carcinoma, *JACS* 195:167, 2002.

Simmons R, Thevarajah S, Brennan B, and others: Methylene blue dye as an alternative to isosulfan blue dye for sentinel lymph node localization, *Ann Surg Onc* 10:242, 2004.

Veronesi U, Paganelli H, Viale G, and others: A randomized comparison of sentinel-node biopsy with routine axillary dissection in breast cancer, *N Engl J Med* 349:546, 2003.

Advances in Adjuvant and Neoadjuvant Therapy for Breast Cancer

Lisa A. Newman, MD, MPH

INTRODUCTION

The benefits of adjuvant systemic therapy for breast cancer in reducing risk of distant relapse have been recognized for several decades. Early detection of breast cancer is essential for improving survival, yet 15% to 20% of patients with stage I disease ultimately experience treatment failure, despite having been diagnosed with small, node-negative lesions. The intent of adjuvant therapy is to eliminate the occult micrometastatic breast cancer burden before it progresses into clinically apparent disease. Successful delivery of effective adjuvant systemic therapy as a complement to surgical management of breast cancer has contributed to the steady declines in breast cancer mortality observed internationally over the past 2 decades. Multimodality treatment of invasive breast cancer is therefore essential to optimizing outcomes. Ongoing clinical and translational research in breast cancer seeks to improve the efficacy of systemic agents for use in the conventional postoperative (adjuvant) setting, as well as preoperatively (neoadjuvant).

ADJUVANT SYSTEMIC THERAPY FOR BREAST CANCER

The Early Breast Cancer Trialists Collaborative Group has published several pooled analyses of the worldwide experience with adjuvant systemic therapy, and its documentation of an associated 30% to

Table I: Summary of Worldwide Overview Analyses

Treatment Analyzed	No. Trials Analyzed	No. Women Analyzed	Proportional Reduction			Comments
			Relapse	Mortality	Contralateral Breast Cancer	
Tamoxifen for early-stage breast cancer	55	37,000	1 yr: 21% 2 yr: 29% 5 yr: 47%	1 yr: 12% 2 yr: 17% 5 yr: 26%	1 yr: 13% 2 yr: 26% 5 yr: 47%	• Risk of endometrial cancer doubled in trials of 1 or 2 yr and quadrupled in trials of 5 yr. • Approximately 8000 women had tumors with low/zero ER content; these patients had negligible benefit from tamoxifen for relapse and mortality. They are excluded from relapse and mortality data but are included in contralateral risk data.
Multiagent CTX for early breast cancer	47	18,000*	Aged <50 yr: 35% Aged 50–69 yr: 20%	Aged <50 yr: 27% Aged 50–69 yr: 11%	NR NR	• There was no significant survival advantage for more than approximately 3 mo of polychemotherapy. • Anthracycline-containing regimens better than CMF alone.
Ovarian ablation for early breast cancer	12	2102	18.5%	6.3%	NS	• Benefit of ovarian ablation was strongest in women not receiving CTX. • Menopausal status was not consistently defined in all studies; most were limited to women younger than 50 years.

CMF, Cyclophosphamide/methotrexate/fluorouracil; *CTX,* chemotherapy; *ER,* estrogen receptor; *NR,* not reported; *NS,* not significantly different.
*Including 6000 women in 11 trials of longer versus shorter CTX, and 6000 women in 11 trials of doxorubicin-containing CTX versus CMF.

50% reduction in odds of relapse has provided the foundation for consensus statements regarding selection of cases where adjuvant therapy is likely to be beneficial. Table 1 summarizes the results from these overview analyses of adjuvant systemic chemotherapy, as well as endocrine therapy, including ovarian ablation. The ovarian ablation trials have been more common in Europe than in the United States.

As additional prospective clinical trials mature and as the armamentarium of therapies and predictive and prognostic features expands, the algorithms for adjuvant therapy decisions have evolved accordingly. Hence in the 1980s it was commonplace to reserve any systemic therapy for patients who were node positive, but by the following decade, the National Cancer Institute recommended consideration of adjuvant systemic therapy for any woman whose invasive cancer is at least 1 cm in size. Indications for adjuvant therapy have broadened even further as a consequence of studies documenting the persistent risk of distant failure even in the selected population of T1b/node-negative cancer. The National Surgical Adjuvant Breast Project's (NSABP) pooled analysis of more than 1250 cases of node-negative cancers up to 1 cm in size (≈20% estrogen receptor [ER]-negative) revealed improved survival for cases treated with adjuvant tamoxifen, chemotherapy, or both. The most recent Overview Analysis documented improved outcomes at 15 years for breast cancer patients receiving polychemotherapy at all ages and regardless of ER status. The majority of invasive breast cancers therefore appear to harbor some risk of distant failure that can be modified by systemic therapy, but the absolute benefit will be a function of the patient's risk of relapse at the time of diagnosis (generally assessed by tumor size and nodal status). The toxicity of adjuvant therapy must be carefully balanced against this relapse risk. For example, adjuvant therapy that provides a 50% odds reduction in recurrence provides an absolute benefit of

15% to a stage IIB breast cancer patient with a 30% relapse risk; in contrast, the absolute benefit will be only 2.5% for patients diagnosed with a 0.5-cm node-negative, ER-positive breast cancer, for which the baseline relapse risk is only 5%. "Adjuvant! Online" (available free of charge at www.adjuvantonline.com) is a Web-based program that provides clinicians and patients with a detailed report of outcome risks of with-versus-without systemic therapy that is based on the clinicopathologic profile of the individual patient. This program's accuracy has been validated in external data sets.

As outlined by the St. Gallen International Consensus Conference, the primary cancer features that are necessary to assess adjuvant systemic therapy needs are as follows: size of primary tumor invasive component, nodal status, ER expression, progesterone receptor (PR) expression, and HER-2/neu expression. Additional characteristics that may influence systemic therapy decisions in borderline cases include histologic grade, presence versus absence of lymphovascular invasion, and primary histology (with metaplastic changes conferring an adverse risk). The data regarding isolated tumor cells in axillary lymph nodes (defined as metastatic foci no larger than 0.2 mm in diameter as per the American Joint Committee on Cancer Sixth Edition Staging System and staged as node negative) and the presence of circulating tumor cells in peripheral blood or bone marrow were not deemed to be mature enough to warrant taking these features into consideration for selection of adjuvant therapy.

The NSABP has developed a reverse-transcriptase polymerase chain reaction (RT-PCR)-based genetic profile that calculates a recurrence score for ER-positive, node-negative disease on the basis of a prospectively developed 21-gene assay. This assay (OncoType DX; Genomic Health, Redwood City, CA) is commercially available for application to paraffin-embedded tumor specimens; it has been shown to be prognostic for risk of relapse and predictive of benefit

Table 2: Systemic Adjuvant Therapy Options for Breast Cancer Patients Stratified by Risk of Relapse

Risk Category and Associated Features		Adjuvant Therapy Options
Low risk	Node-negative; *and* ER and/or PR positive; *and* T ≤1 cm; *and* grade I; *and* no LVI/PVI; *and* HER2/neu negative; *and* age ≥35 years	• None • Endocrine therapy only • Consider OncoType DX to confirm risk assessment via recurrence score
Intermediate risk	Node-negative *and* at least one of the following: • T >2 cm; *or* • Grade II/III; *or* • LVI/PVI present; *or* • Age <35 years; *or* • HER2/neu positive or amplified Node-positive (1–3 nodes); *and* HER2/neu negative	Endocrine-Responsive*†: • Endocrine therapy alone • CTX followed by ET • Consider OncoType DX to evaluate risk via recurrence score (OncoType DX appropriate for node-negative cases only) Not endocrine responsive*†: • CTX
High Risk	Node-positive (1–3 nodes); *and* HER2/neu positive Node positive (≥4 nodes)	Endocrine responsive*†: • CTX followed by endocrine therapy Not endocrine responsive*†: • CTX

CTX, Chemotherapy; *ER*, estrogen receptor; *LVI*, lymphovascular invasion; *PR*, progesterone receptor; *PVI*, perivascular invasion; *T*, tumor.

Note that these recommendations acknowledge the existence of varying degrees of risk within both endocrine-sensitive and endocrine-resistant breast cancer subtypes. Application of the algorithm suggested by this table therefore requires that the patient's disease be assessed first by nodal status and then by primary clinicopathologic features (age, histopathologic descriptors, molecular markers, etc.).

This table and the risk categories were adapted and modified from the risk categories described by Goldhirsch and colleagues; treatment options have been adjusted to reflect data regarding the OncoType DX genetic profiles and data regarding adjuvant trastuzumab therapy for HER2/neu overexpressing/amplified tumors.

*Include trastuzumab therapy if HER2/neu positive or amplified (however, note that trastuzumab is generally offered only to patients deemed to be at sufficiently high risk that CTX is indicated).

†Consider postmastectomy irradiation or extended-field-regional field irradiation if primary tumor is >5 cm or if 1 to 3 nodes are positive for metastatic disease.

from chemotherapy in addition to endocrine therapy, independent of primary tumor size and patient age. Preliminary studies reveal that ER-positive, node-negative breast cancer patients with a low recurrence score can be safely treated with endocrine therapy alone, even if they have a large primary tumor. In contrast, chemotherapy (in addition to endocrine therapy) should be considered for patients with T1a, node-negative disease if they have a high recurrence score. A prospective randomized clinical trial to evaluate management of patients with intermediate scores is currently under way. The St. Gallen experts acknowledge the potential value of this genetic profiling, but the test is costly and it was therefore not included as a routine component of their systemic therapy decision tree. Table 2 summarizes an algorithm that combines the risk stratification scheme of the St. Gallen experts with the associated options for adjuvant systemic therapy.

Selection of Patients Who Can Avoid Systemic Therapy Completely

In selected cases, patients with breast cancer have a sufficiently low risk for distant failure that local treatment alone will be adequate. Optimal characteristics of these low-risk cases include ER/PR positivity, node negativity, primary tumor size no more than 1 cm,

low grade, and with neither lymphovascular invasion nor HER2/neu overexpression. Tubular histology and older age are other favorable features that justify a modified approach to systemic adjuvant therapy recommendations. Hormone receptor-negative disease usually does not fall into this category unless it is associated with only a microinvasive, node-negative lesion.

Systemic Therapy for Endocrine-Responsive Breast Cancer

Breast cancer is expected to be sensitive to endocrine therapy if immunohistochemistry staining reveals at least 10% staining for the estrogen receptor within the invasive component. ER-negative tumors are also considered endocrine-responsive if they stain positive for the progesterone receptor (PR) because expression of the PR marker is dependent on the presence of intact ER machinery.

Endocrine Therapy for Postmenopausal Cases

Tamoxifen has been the mainstay of endocrine therapy for hormone receptor-positive breast cancer over the past 30 years. Tamoxifen was originally developed as an antifertility medication, and alternative uses in the oncology field were sought because of its dismal failure in antifertilization because of its ovulatory effects. As an effective antagonist of estrogen receptors on mammary tissue, however, it has remained extremely powerful as first-line adjuvant systemic therapy in breast cancer management. The selective ER activity of tamoxifen also yields estrogen agonist activity on the uterus, cardiovascular, cerebrovascular, and osseous tissues; this results in the mixed benefits and risks of uterine cancer, lowered cholesterol levels, vasomotor symptoms, and protection against osteoporosis. Tamoxifen decreases the odds of relapse in endocrine-responsive breast cancer by 3% to 50%. It also decreases the incidence of contralateral new primary tumors, and this benefit has resulted in its applications for chemoprevention in high-risk women. The NSABP B-14 trial randomized early-stage breast cancer patients to receive 5 versus 10 years of tamoxifen postoperatively and found that extended therapy resulted in higher rates of adverse events that were not outweighed by added protection.

Recent advances in the development of aromatase inhibitors (AIs) have expanded the options for postmenopausal women with endocrine-responsive disease. AIs result in near-complete shutdown of estrogen production by blocking peripheral conversion of adrenal gland–derived estrogen precursors by the enzyme aromatase. Following natural or induced menopause with loss of ovarian estrogen production, the majority of circulating estrogen is produced by adipocytes in body fat stores because this is the primary source of aromatase. The ATAC (Armidex, Tamoxifen, Alone or in Combination) trial was one of the first prospective randomized clinical trials to study an AI as adjuvant therapy for early-stage breast cancer. The ATAC trial randomized 9366 postmenopausal women to receive anastrazole versus tamoxifen versus the combination of anastrazole and tamoxifen. With a median follow-up of 3 years, anastrozole proved to be superior to both tamoxifen and the combination arm of the study.

Other large prospective randomized clinical trials have evaluated alternative AI's such as letrozole and exemestane and studied sequential therapy, with the AI given after 2 to 5 years of adjuvant tamoxifen therapy. These trials have consistently demonstrated added value for use of an AI in postmenopausal, ER-positive breast cancer; however, there is no consensus regarding which AI is superior; what the optimal sequence should be for tamoxifen and AI therapy; or whether an AI should completely replace tamoxifen.

The growing experience with AI therapy has been promising for improved outcomes in endocrine-responsive breast cancer, but the toxicity profile of AIs must still be considered. Unlike tamoxifen, AI therapy will not affect the uterus, but vasomotor symptoms occur in approximately 40% of cases; the most concerning risk associated with AI therapy is the potential for osteoporosis. Nonetheless, the American Society of Clinical Oncology has recommended that AI therapy be included as a component of managing postmenopausal endocrine-responsive breast cancer, either alone or in addition to tamoxifen.

Endocrine Therapy for Premenopausal Cases

Tamoxifen is the standard of care in managing endocrine-responsive breast cancer among women with functioning ovaries. Ongoing multicenter clinical trials are studying the potential benefits of ovarian suppression in combination with aromatase inhibition in premenopausal women; the optimal duration and long-term effects of ovarian suppression are currently undefined. Oophorectomy has been advocated as well, but concerns regarding the cardiovascular and osteoporotic risks of premature, permanent menopause have limited its popularity.

Adjuvant Chemotherapy in Addition to Endocrine Therapy for Endocrine-Sensitive Breast Cancer

Patients with node-positive breast cancer face a substantial increase in risk for disease relapse, and these women are therefore recommended to receive chemotherapy in addition to their endocrine treatment. Tamoxifen is known to be cytostatic (as opposed to cytotoxic), which potentially can interfere with chemotherapy effect on rapidly proliferating cancer cells; tamoxifen therapy is therefore usually sequenced to follow chemotherapy, and concurrent treatment is discouraged. AI therapy is generally recommended to follow chemotherapy as well. As noted previously, use of the OncoType DX recurrence score may also facilitate decision making regarding need for chemotherapy in endocrine-sensitive, node-negative breast cancer.

Systemic Therapy for Endocrine-Resistant Breast Cancer

Fewer options exist for this category of disease. Invasive breast cancers that are negative for both ER and PR can only be offered chemotherapy as adjuvant therapy, and trastuzumab (Herceptin; Genentech, South San Francisco, CA), discussed below, should be considered for those cases that overexpress HER2/neu. All node-positive cases are considered candidates for adjuvant chemotherapy and many node-negative cases (unless the disease is microinvasive). Tumors that overexpress the HER2/neu marker and that have been deemed appropriate candidates for chemotherapy are referred for trastuzumab therapy as well.

Selection and Dosing of Chemotherapy Regimen

Several chemotherapy regimens are accepted as comparable for management of breast cancer. The earliest studies of chemotherapy for breast cancer involved perioperative administration of medications that are considered inferior to the effective agents currently available, and the goal of these early investigations was to eliminate dissemination of cancer cells that might have occurred in conjunction with surgical manipulation of tumors. The NSABP B-01 trial (conducted nearly 40 years ago) therefore involved intravenous thiotepa versus placebo administered at the time of radical mastectomy and over the first couple of days postoperatively. Not surprisingly, this regimen failed to produce any improvements in outcome for the entire group of treated patients, but the subset of highest-risk women (those with four or more metastatic nodes) did experience some overall survival advantages. Subsequent trials conducted during the 1970s and 1980s revealed the power of cyclophosphamide and combination chemotherapy (CTX) regimens in reducing breast cancer relapse rates, as well as mortality risks.

Until recently, the two regimens of cyclophosphamide/methotrexate/fluorouracil (CMF), and cyclophosphamide/doxorubicin/fluorouracil (CAF), delivered in every-3-week cycles, were the most commonly employed regimens for adjuvant therapy of breast cancer. During the late 1990s, the taxanes emerged as an alternative and highly effective agent against breast cancer. Furthermore, the development of active and tolerable bone marrow–supportive therapy in the form of granulocyte colony stimulating factors has opened the door to dose-dense regimens, allowing safe delivery of higher cumulative CTX doses within shorter time frames. Collectively, the randomized controlled trial data show that adjuvant CTX regimens that include a taxane, as well as doxorubicin, are most reasonable for node-positive breast cancer patients. This conclusion is supported by findings from the CALGB 9344, NSABP B-28, and BCIRG 001 Phase III studies. These three trials all randomized node-positive patients to receive doxorubicin-based combinations versus doxorubicin CTX plus a taxane, and all three demonstrated an outcome advantage for the taxane arms. The CALGB 9741 and 9344 trials also revealed superiority of dose-dense therapy (9741), but no outcome advantage for increased doses of doxorubicin (9344). Questions regarding superiority of one taxane versus the other (paclitaxel versus docetaxel) remain unanswered.

Targeted Therapy for Breast Cancer with Trastuzumab (Herceptin)

Overexpression of the HER2/neu molecular marker is recognized as an adverse prognostic factor. The development of a trastuzumab, a monoclonal antibody that is administered intravenously and targets the HER2/neu marker, has proved to be effective in the management of metastatic breast cancer, and recently reported prospective randomized clinical trials have demonstrated its value as adjuvant therapy for early-stage disease as well. These trials have revealed an approximately 50% reduction in the odds of recurrence for these high-risk cancers. Breast cancer patients whose disease warrants chemotherapy will usually be offered one year of trastuzumab if the cancer overexpresses HER 2/neu. A phase III clinical trial comparing 1 versus 2 years of adjuvant trastuzumab is ongoing.

Adjuvant Systemic Therapy for Breast Cancer: Summary and Practical Considerations

Any invasive breast cancer is associated with some risk of distant organ micrometastatic disease, and the risk of breast cancer mortality is reduced by delivery of systemic therapy as adjuvant treatment after primary surgery. The absolute benefit from adjuvant therapy will depend on the patient's underlying risk of relapse. Patients with node-positive breast cancer therefore have the largest-magnitude benefit from adjuvant therapy. Conversely, patients with small, node-negative cancers must balance the toxicity of systemic therapy against the estimated risk of metastatic disease because some of these patients have an excellent outcome with primary surgery alone. Web-based computerized programs such as Adjuvant! Online provide patients and clinicians with a summary of calculated risks versus benefits from systemic therapy based on primary clinico-pathologic features. Genetic profiling and assignment of a recurrence score via the OncoType DX test can be helpful to determine benefit from adjuvant chemotherapy in addition to endocrine therapy for ER-positive, node-negative cases.

Endocrine-responsive breast cancer (ER- and/or PR-positive disease) usually requires tamoxifen or an aromatase inhibitor (or both) if the patient is postmenopausal. Chemotherapy is recommended for high-risk endocrine responsive disease (e.g., node-positive breast cancer) and for any endocrine-resistant breast cancer that is deemed appropriate for systemic treatment. Trastuzumab is indicated as targeted therapy to follow chemotherapy for HER-2/neu overexpressing cancers.

NEOADJUVANT CHEMOTHERAPY

Implementation of preoperative chemotherapy protocols (also commonly referred to as neoadjuvant or induction chemotherapy) revolutionized the management of locally advanced breast cancer (LABC) cases, and this approach is now considered the standard of care for patients with bulky breast or axillary disease (or both), usually staged clinically as stage III breast cancer. Patients with clinical stage II breast cancer (primary tumor 2–5 cm in size, and invasive primary breast tumors <2 cm but with metastatic axillary nodes) can also be considered candidates for neoadjuvant chemotherapy if tumor downstaging is expected to improve eligibility for breast-conserving surgery.

Early skepticism regarding the neoadjuvant therapy sequence was based on concerns that preoperative chemotherapy would adversely affect (1) surgical complication rates; (2) the prognostic value of the axillary nodal status; and (3) overall survival, as a consequence of delayed surgery. Nonetheless, the generally dismal results of treating LABC with primary surgery, radiation alone, or chemotherapy alone motivated investigations of multimodality therapy, and the benefits as well as the safety of preoperative downstaging of disease to improve resectability became apparent.

Broadwater and colleagues demonstrated comparable operative morbidity among nearly 200 LABC patients treated with mastectomy, approximately half of whom received preoperative doxorubicin-based chemotherapy. The induction chemotherapy patients in fact had a lower rate of postoperative seroma formation. Danforth and colleagues similarly reported that preoperative chemotherapy had no adverse effect on surgical complication rates and did not result in delayed delivery of any postoperative cancer care. Most patients are ready to undergo surgery approximately 3 weeks after the last chemotherapy treatment, when the absolute neutrophil and platelet counts have normalized (>1500 and 100,000, respectively).

McCready and colleagues confirmed that the axillary nodal status retains its prognostic value in the neoadjuvant chemotherapy setting. Their study of 136 LABCs undergoing modified radical mastectomy following induction chemotherapy revealed that patients with no axillary metastases in the postchemotherapy mastectomy specimen had an excellent outcome, with nearly 80% surviving 5 years. In contrast, less than 10% of patients with 10 or more positive nodes survived 5 years, and patients with an intermediate number of residual metastatic nodes had an intermediate survival rate.

The third issue, regarding induction chemotherapy and its relative impact on breast cancer survival compared with conventional postoperative adjuvant therapy, remains controversial. It is clear, however, that preoperative treatment and deferral of surgery do not increase rates of unresectability. On the contrary, approximately 80% of patients have at least 50% shrinkage of the primary tumor mass, and only 2% to 3% have signs of progressive disease. Fears that the surgeon will lose a "window of opportunity" to resect chest wall disease are therefore unfounded, and preoperatively treated patients are likely to be rendered improved operative candidates. A surgical resection is essential to accurately document chemotherapy response and achieve durable locoregional control of disease because the clinical assessment of response overestimates the actual pathologic extent by twofold to threefold.

The induction CTX benefits of tumor downstaging and the ability rapidly to identify chemoresistant disease by in vivo observation motivated expanded applications of this treatment to the setting of early-stage disease. Accordingly, the outcomes from prospective clinical trials have now been reported in which preoperative chemotherapy has been compared directly with postoperative chemotherapy in women with LABC, as well as early-stage disease. Some of these phase III clinical trial results are shown in Table 3. All have demonstrated overall survival equivalence for the two treatment sequences, confirming the oncologic safety of the neoadjuvant approach.

Subset analyses of the phase III studies, however, reveal that patients found to have a complete pathologic response (pCR) do have a statistically significant survival benefit, substantiating the concept that primary breast tumor response is a reliable surrogate for chemo-effect on micrometastases. In the NSABP B-18 trial, patients with stages I–III breast cancer who were randomized to receive four cycles of doxorubicin and cyclophosphamide for injection (Cytoxan; Baxter Healthcare, Deerfield, IL) preoperatively and who experienced a pCR had a 5-year overall survival of 86%, which was statistically superior to the outcome seen in all other study participants. Similarly, the University of Texas M.D. Anderson Cancer Center reported an overall survival rate of 89% for pCR patients treated on preoperative chemotherapy protocols designed specifically for LABC, and this outcome also represented a statistically significant benefit compared with patients who had a lesser response. Unfortunately, both studies found that only 12% to 13% of patients experience a pCR when treated with a doxorubicin-based regimen, and this proportion is simply insufficient in yielding a survival benefit for the entire pool of preoperatively treated patients.

Table 3: Randomized Trials of Neoadjuvant versus Adjuvant Chemotherapy for Breast Cancer

Study	Accrual Years	N	Stages	Median F/U (mos.)	BCT Rate PreOp CTX (%)	BCT Rate PostOp CTX (%)	Local Recurrence after BCT Preop CTX	Local Recurrence after BCT PostOp CTX (%)	Overall Survival at Median F/U PreOp CTX (%)	Overall Survival at Median F/U PostOp CTX (%)
Institut Bergonie	1985-1989	272	II–IIIA (T >3cm)	124	63.1	0	XRT: 34% L/ALND/XRT: 23	NA	55*	55*
Institut Curie	1983-1990	414	IIA–IIIA	66	82	77	24	18	86	78
Royal Marsden	1990-1995	309	I–IIIB	48	89	78	3[†]	4[†]	80*	80[a]
NSABP	1988-1993	1523	I–IIIA		60	68	10.7	7.6	69[‡]	70[‡]
EORTC	1991-1999	698	I–IIIA	56	37	21	NR	NR	NR	NR
ECTO	--2001	892	I–IIIA	23	71	35	NR	NR	NR	NR
ABCSG	1991-1996	423	I–IIIB	NR	67	60	NR[§]	NR[§]	NR[§]	NR[§]

ABCS, Austrian Breast and Colorectal Study Group; *ALND*, axillary lymph node dissection; *ECTO*, European Cooperative Trial in Breast Cancer; *EORTC*, European Organization for Research and Treatment of Cancer; *FU*, follow-up; *L*, lumpectomy; *NA*, not applicable; *NR*, not reported; *NSABP*, National Surgical Adjuvant Breast Project; *S*, surgery; *XRT*, radiation.

*Rate estimated from graph.

[†]Local recurrence rates reported for lumpectomy and mastectomy patients combined.

[‡]Overall survival rate at 9 years.

[§]Recurrence and survival rates not reported, but relapse-free survival noted to be lower in neoadjuvant CTX arm, and overall survival was similar for the two study arms.

Predictors of a pCR include relatively smaller size primary breast tumors, estrogen receptor negativity, and high-grade lesions. The latter two features probably characterize rapidly cycling tumors that may be particularly sensitive to chemotherapy effects.

The ability to downsize the primary breast tumor, thereby facilitating attainment of a margin-negative lumpectomy with a smaller-volume lumpectomy, is a major advantage of the neoadjuvant CTX sequence. A feasibility study reported by Singletary and colleagues addressed many of the concerns that induction CTX might leave a field of microscopic satellite lesions, with a resulting increased risk of margin failure or excessive local recurrence rates. The Singletary study involved a pathology review of the mastectomy specimens in 143 LABC cases that had been treated with preoperative CTX; approximately one quarter had adequate shrinkage of tumor and adequate eradication of disease in surrounding breast tissue and skin, such that they would have been candidates for successful lumpectomy. Table 3 demonstrates the overall comparability of local recurrence rates in subsequent clinical trials of women receiving breast-conserving therapy (BCT) with versus without neoadjuvant CTX.

The NSABP B-18 trial randomized more than 1500 women with stages I–IIIA breast cancer to receive preoperative versus postoperative chemotherapy. This study demonstrated a statistically significant increase in BCT use for the preoperative chemotherapy arm (68% vs. 60%). With a median follow-up of 72 months, the local recurrence rates were 7.9% and 5.8% (no statistically significant difference) following BCT in the preoperative and postoperative chemotherapy arms, respectively. The conversion rate to BCT eligibility was greatest in the patients with T3 tumors at diagnosis. The NSABP also reported that local recurrence was somewhat higher in the subset of lumpectomy patients who were downstaged to become BCT eligible compared with the BCT patients who were BCT candidates at presentation. However, this subset of downstaged BCT cases comprised predominantly T3 tumors, and because local recurrence is one manifestation of underlying tumor biology, it would be expected that the more advanced-stage lesions might have increased local recurrence rates regardless of surgery type and treatment sequence. Furthermore, radiation boost doses were not consistently used in the lumpectomy patients, and tamoxifen therapy was used only in patients aged older than 50 years. Both of these interventions, if implemented uniformly, might have influenced local recurrence rates in downstaged tumors. Lastly, the NSABP requires that margin-negative lumpectomies be free of any tumor cells at an inked margin; a more aggressive approach to margin control might be necessary for lumpectomies in tumors that have been downsized by preoperative CTX.

Newman and colleagues analyzed a series of 100 patients treated at the M.D. Anderson Cancer Center in a prospective protocol of preoperative sequential Taxotere (Sanofi-Aventis US, Bridgewater, NJ) and Adriamycin (Pharmacia, Milan, Italy)-based chemotherapy in patients with stages I–III breast cancer. These investigators reported that 34% of patients initially ineligible for BCT were converted to lumpectomy candidates with this preoperative chemotherapy regimen. Final surgical pathology review revealed that clinical assessment of BCT eligibility following induction chemotherapy was inaccurate for invasive lobular cancers, multicentric disease, and diffuse microcalcifications. Difficulties with assessment of chemoresponse in lobular cancers have also been noted by Mathieu and colleagues and Cristofanilli and colleagues.

Selection of the optimal induction CTX regimen is a topic of ongoing research. The earliest NSABP trials used doxorubicin and Cytoxan, but efforts to increase the response rates have motivated studies evaluating alternative regimens. Addition of a taxane to a doxorubicin-containing neoadjuvant regimen will increase the pathologic complete response rate from 13% to nearly 30%; unfortunately, however, these higher response rates have not yet translated into an improvement in survival. Preoperative trastuzumab for HER2/neu overexpressing cancers has been shown in pilot studies to increase pCR rates to more than 60% and will be studied in a larger cohort through an NSABP trial. Neoadjuvant endocrine therapy is also promising as a strategy for using targeted therapy in the preoperative setting. Neoadjuvant tamoxifen, as well as neoadjuvant

Table 4: Studies of Sentinel Lymph Node Biopsy Performed after Neoadjuvant Chemotherapy

Study	T Status	N		Sentinel Node ID Rate	False-Negative Rate	Metastases Limited to Sentinel Node(s)
Breslin 2000	2,3	51		85% (42/51)	12% (3/25)	40% (10/25)
Nason 2000	2,3	15		87% (13/15)	33% (3/9)	≥11%* (≥1/9)
Haid 2001	1–3	33		88% (29/33)	0% (0/22)	50% (11/22)
Fernandez 2001	1–4	40		90% (36/40)	20% (4/20)	20% (4/20)
Tafra 2001	1,2	29		93% (27/29)	0% (0/15)	NR
Stearns 2002	3,4	T4d	8	75% (6/8)	40% (2/5)	24% (5/21)
		NI	26	88% (23/26)	6% (1/16)	
Julian 2002	1–3	34		91% (31/34)	0% (0/12)	42% (5/12)
Miller 2002	1–3	35		86% (30/35)	0% (0/9)	44% (4/9)
Brady 2002	1–3	14		93% (13/14)	0% (0/10)	60% (6/10)
Piato 2003	1,2	42		98% (41/42)	17% (3/18)	0% (0/18)
Balch 2003	2–4	32		97% (31/32)	5% (1/19)	56% (10/18)
Schwartz 2003	1–3	21		100% (21/21)	9% (1/11)	64% (7/11)
Reitsamer 2003	2,3	30		87% (26/30)	7% (1/15)	53% (8/15)
Mamounas 2005	1–3	428		85% (363/428)	11% (15/140)	50% (70/140)
Tanaka 2006	2,3	70		63/70 (90%)	5% (1/24)	42% (8/19)
Jones 2005	2,3	36		29/36 (81%)	15% (2/13)	NR

NI, Noninflammatory; *T*, tumor.

aromatase inhibitors, have been studied in relatively small studies, and this strategy is feasible, but the clinical response tends to be slower compared with preoperative chemotherapy.

Neoadjuvant Chemotherapy and Sentinel Lymph Node Biopsy

There is ongoing debate regarding the optimal method for integrating sentinel node staging of the axilla into induction CTX protocols. The standard treatment sequence for neoadjuvant CTX patients involves a percutaneous needle biopsy for establishment of the cancer diagnosis, delivery of chemotherapy, breast/axillary surgery, followed by irradiation in selected cases, and endocrine therapy for hormone receptor-positive disease. It was therefore logical for initial investigations to evaluate the results of sentinel lymph node biopsy (SLNB) performed after the delivery of preoperative CTX and concomitantly with the breast surgery. Concerns arose early in these discussions that the lymphatic mapping concept might be compromised by

1. Lymphatic obstruction by tumor emboli from the relatively larger tumors that are more likely to be managed with neoadjuvant CTX,
2. CTX effect on axillary metastases might not be uniform, or
3. CTX might obliterate intramammary lymphatic channels.

Any combination of these factors could result in higher rates of sentinel node nonidentification or false negativity. Studies reported by Bedrosian and colleagues and Chung and colleagues documented the accuracy of lymphatic mapping for T2 and T3 breast cancers. Breslin and colleagues reported the first series of patients undergoing SLNB and completion ALND after neoadjuvant CTX in a 2000 study from the M.D. Anderson Cancer Center, and these investigators demonstrated that the lymphatic mapping technology is indeed feasible in these cases, but accuracy rates are optimized when the surgical team has progressed through the learning curve of mapping in the setting of CTX-treated axillary tissue.

As shown in Table 4, several other investigators have now reported varying success rates with lymphatic mapping performed after delivery of neoadjuvant CTX. Identification rates range from 85% to 97%, and false-negative sentinel nodes are identified in 0% to 33% of cases. One feature supporting the biologic rationale for this approach is the persistent observation that even after neoadjuvant CTX, the sentinel node is frequently the isolated site of axillary metastases. A meta-analysis of reported studies conducted by Xing and colleagues revealed an overall sensitivity of 88% for SLNB in this setting.

The inconsistent results associated with the post-neoadjuvant CTX SLNB have prompted many surgeons to perform SLNB for axillary staging before delivery of neoadjuvant CTX. The disadvantage to this approach is that some women will be subjected to unnecessary ALNDs because the node-positive patients identified at presentation will be committed to a completion ALND after induction CTX, despite the fact that the sentinel node(s) may have been the only sites of disease for some cases, and for others the CTX may have eliminated any residual axillary metastases. These advantages and disadvantages of the alternative sentinel lymph node/CTX approaches are summarized in Table 5.

Neoadjuvant Chemotherapy and Radiation Therapy

Decisions regarding locoregional irradiation also become more complicated among neoadjuvant chemotherapy patients. Consensus guidelines advocated by the American Society of Clinical Oncology and the American Society of Therapeutic Radiation Oncology state that postmastectomy radiation should be delivered to patients with T3 tumors (those >5 cm) and to patients with four or more metastatic axillary nodes. These guidelines are also followed in recommending extended-field (apical axillary, supraclavicular, and internal mammary) radiation in addition to breast radiation after lumpectomy. After neoadjuvant chemotherapy, however, the pathologic size of the primary tumor and the extent of nodal involvement are not definitively known. Findings from the NSABP suggest that

Table 5: Advantages and Disadvantages of Sentinel Lymph Node Biopsy Performed before versus after Delivery of Neoadjuvant Chemotherapy

	SNLB after	SLNB before
Advantages	• More studies reported on results of SLNB performed after neoadjuvant CTX has been delivered • Surgical sequence consistent with conventional neoadjuvant CTX regimens	• Significance of nodal status is better understood when axillary staging is performed at presentation • Preferred by many medical and radiation oncologists • More surgical experience with SLNB performed in the primary surgery, pre-CTX sequence

Disadvantages	• *False-negative rates not yet optimized (range, 0%–40%)*
	• *Significant learning curve*
		• *Potential for unnecessary ALNDs*
		   ○ *Patients with a metastatic SLN before neoCTX are committed to undergoing completion ALND, but*
		   ○ *Metastatic disease limited to the excised SLN in 30%–50%, and*
		   ○ *CTX sterilizes 25%–30% node-positive patients*
		• *Requires an additional surgical procedure*

ALND, Axillary lymph node biopsy; *CTX,* chemotherapy; *neoCTX,* neoadjuvant chemotherapy; *SLNB,* sentinel lymph node biopsy.

radiation therapy needs should be defined on the basis of the final, postchemotherapy pathology results. Patient care is clearly optimized when the multidisciplinary approach is proactively used; candidates for neoadjuvant therapy should be evaluated by the medical, surgical, and radiation oncologists before treatment is started so that a comprehensive plan can be outlined in advance.

A final controversy regarding use of the neoadjuvant chemotherapy sequence is related to patients undergoing mastectomy and whether they can be safely offered immediate breast reconstruction. Both autogenous-tissue (e.g., transverse rectus abdominis myocutaneous [TRAM] flap; latissimus dorsi flap) and tissue expander-implant reconstructions have been shown to be technically feasible for these patients. Delivery of postmastectomy radiation therapy can, however, substantially compromise the aesthetics achieved with immediate breast reduction. Up to half of radiated implants require explantation because of recurrent infections or severe contracture, and autogenous tissue reconstructions become subject to delayed adverse effects, with severe contracture and asymmetry becoming apparent more than 1 year after the surgery. Because of these issues, many plastic surgeons prefer to avoid any risk of reconstruction irradiation and defer breast reconstruction until after all of the breast cancer treatment has been delivered. An interesting alternative approach, delayed-immediate reconstruction, has been suggested by Kronowitz and colleagues. Delayed-immediate reconstruction involves the insertion of a saline-filled tissue expander as a "placeholder" after a skin-sparing mastectomy while pathology processing of the surgical specimen is completed. If the results indicate that postmastectomy radiation is not necessary, the patient is promptly returned to the operating room for definitive autogenous tissue reconstruction. If the patient does require radiation, the expander is deflated, radiation is delivered, and then the expander is reinflated after radiation treatment is completed in preparation for the subsequent autogenous tissue reconstruction. This strategy is offered with the hope of preserving as much skin as possible because chest wall radiation is well known to decrease skin elasticity.

Neoadjuvant Systemic Therapy: Summary and Practical Considerations

Induction chemotherapy is considered the standard of care for patients with locally advanced breast cancer. It is a reasonable and safe treatment approach for patients with early-stage invasive breast cancer, if the clinician is certain that chemotherapy would be recommended in the postoperative setting. The risk of overtreatment can be minimized by obtaining multiple diagnostic core biopsy specimens to confirm that a lesion is predominantly invasive because it would clearly be inappropriate to treat large-volume or palpable ductal carcinoma in situ tumors (with or without microinvasion) with CTX in any setting.

Primary tumor downstaging with neoadjuvant chemotherapy can improve lumpectomy eligibility. Patients presenting with multiple tumors or extensive calcifications on initial mammogram should be counseled that preoperative chemotherapy will not convert them to BCT eligibility, regardless of the extent of their primary tumor shrinkage. If the tumor is not associated with any microcalcifications, a radiopaque clip should be inserted (preferably under ultrasound guidance) either before delivery of the neoadjuvant CTX or within the first couple of cycles. For those patients who have a complete clinical response to the preoperative chemotherapy, this clip serves as the target for subsequent mammography-assisted wire localization lumpectomy when the patient is ready for surgery. Lesions associated with microcalcifications have an inherent target for subsequent localization.

Approximately 80% of cases experience a clinical response to neoadjuvant chemotherapy, and progressive disease occurs rarely. A complete pathologic response is a powerful positive prognostic feature. Induction chemotherapy with a doxorubicin-containing regimen yields a complete pathologic response in 12% of cases; adding a taxane can double this rate. Patients with estrogen receptor–negative, high-grade, and nonlobular carcinomas are more likely to respond to neoadjuvant chemotherapy. Studies of neoadjuvant endocrine therapy or neoadjuvant trastuzumab for estrogen receptor–positive or HER-2/neu overexpressing cancers, respectively, are ongoing.

Neoadjuvantly treated patients are monitored by clinical evaluation, and final surgical decisions are based on preoperative mammography and ultrasound imaging. The final preoperative imaging is essential for evaluation of the lumpectomy target and to rule out unmasking of microcalcifications or multicentric disease that might affect lumpectomy eligibility. The role of magnetic resonance imaging to evaluate response to neoadjuvant chemotherapy is not well defined because studies thus far have yielded inconsistent results.

Lymphatic mapping and SLNB in neoadjuvant chemotherapy cases is controversial. Prechemotherapy SLNB provides accurate staging information but may negate some of the downstaging benefits of preoperative systemic therapy because patients found to be node positive before treatment are committed to undergoing completion ALND when they have their definitive breast surgery.

SNLB performed after neoadjuvant chemotherapy is feasible and can minimize the number of women facing the morbidity of the completion ALND, but accuracy of lymphatic mapping in preoperatively treated patients is uncertain.

Decisions regarding locoregional radiation in patients who have been downstaged by neoadjuvant chemotherapy are also controversial. Patients with extensive residual disease (four or more metastatic lymph nodes and/or breast tumor at least 5 cm in size) are definite candidates for postmastectomy irradiation or for regional radiation in addition to standard postlumpectomy breast radiation. Patients with less residual disease should be evaluated by the radiation oncology team regarding the possible benefits of this treatment. Because radiation can adversely affect the cosmesis of breast reconstruction, and radiation needs may not become apparent until the final surgical pathology is available, most neoadjuvant chemotherapy patients undergoing mastectomy are discouraged from undergoing immediate breast reconstruction.

SUGGESTED READINGS

Early Breast Cancer Trialists' Collaborative Group (EBCTCG): Effects of chemotherapy and hormonal therapy for early breast cancer on recurrence and 15-year survival: an overview of the randomized trials, *Lancet* 365:1687, 2005.

Goldhirsch A, Glick JH, Gelber RD, and others: Meeting highlights: international expert consensus on the primary therapy of early breast cancer 2005, *Ann Oncol* 16:1569, 2005.

Kuerer HM, Newman LA, Smith TL, and others: Clinical course of breast cancer patients with complete pathologic primary tumor and axillary lymph node response to doxorubicin-based neoadjuvant chemotherapy, *J Clin Oncol* 17:460, 1999.

Newman LA, Buzdar AU, Singletary SE, and others: A prospective trial of preoperative chemotherapy in resectable breast cancer: predictors of breast-conservation therapy feasibility, *Ann Surg Oncol* 9:228, 2003.

Paik S, Shak S, Tang G, and others: A multigene assay to predict recurrence of tamoxifen-treated, node-negative breast cancer, *N Engl J Med* 351:2817, 2004.

INFLAMMATORY BREAST CANCER

S. Eva Singletary, MD

BACKGROUND AND CLINICAL DESCRIPTION

Inflammatory breast cancer (IBC) is a highly angiogenic and angioinvasive form of cancer that is characterized by rapid progression and aggressive behavior from the onset. Although it comprises less than 3% of all microscopically confirmed breast malignancies, IBC accounted for 7% of breast cancer mortality in the United States between 1988 and 2000, with a median survival time of 3 to 4 years, and a 15-year overall survival rate of 20% to 30%. It tends to occur in younger women compared with locally advanced breast cancer (58.8 years vs. 61.7 years, respectively) and is more common in African American women than in white women (3.1% vs. 2.2%, respectively). In more than half of patients with IBC, tumors are estrogen receptor negative, compared with approximately 20% in patients with noninflammatory breast cancer. From 20% to 35% of patients will have distant metastases at the time of presentation, and 60% to 85% will have metastases to the axillary or supraclavicular lymph nodes. In almost one third of patients, no discrete mass is detectable, although nonspecific changes such as increased skin thickness and diffusely increased tissue density resulting from edema may be apparent on mammography. According to the sixth edition of the AJCC Cancer Staging Manual, IBC is classified as stage IIIB/C (in the absence of distant metastases) or stage IV (in the presence of distant metastases).

IBC is a clinicopathologic entity, and diagnosis is based primarily on clinical characteristics, supported by biopsy confirmation of the presence of carcinoma (Table 1). The most distinctive aspects of the clinical presentation—diffuse erythema and peau d'orange, wheals or ridging of the skin—are the result of tumor emboli within dermal lymphatics. These changes in the breast skin typically show a rapid onset. Dermal lymphatic plugging can frequently be observed on skin biopsy, but this finding is not a necessary component of the diagnosis. IBC is often confused with bacterial mastitis, and a definitive diagnosis can be significantly

Table 1: Clinical Characteristics Commonly Used in the Diagnosis of Inflammatory Breast Cancer

Physical Appearance of Breast

Erythema, associated with increased heat

Edema or peau d'orange

Wheals or ridging of the skin

Involves the majority of the skin of the breast

Medical History

Rapid onset (<3 months)

Young age (mean 58.8 years vs. 61.7 years for LABC)

Negative for bacterial infection

Physical Examination

No discrete palpable mass in ≈30% of patients

Lymphadenopathy common

Nipple retraction possible

Biopsy

Diagnosis of carcinoma confirmed

Dermal lymphatic plugging by tumor emboli (common but not necessary for diagnosis)

Mammographic findings (in order of likelihood)

Skin thickening

Diffusely increased density

Discrete mass

Axillary lymphadenopathy

Trabecular thickening

Architectural distortion or focal asymmetric density

Malignant-appearing calcifications

LABC, Locally advanced breast cancer.

delayed while patients are treated with antibiotics in an attempt to clear the "infection." (One third of patients in a national IBC registry were initially diagnosed with an infection and received antibiotics for up to 10 months before a proper diagnosis was reached.) The differential diagnosis for IBC also includes leukemia; lymphoma; sarcoma; postradiation or nonspecific dermatitis; or a neglected, locally advanced breast cancer late in the course of the disease. At the time of diagnosis, photographs should be taken to document the secondary changes of the disease so that treatment results can be easily tracked.

MANAGEMENT OF INFLAMMATORY BREAST CANCER

Staging Workup

For the patient who has received a clinical diagnosis of IBC, additional procedures are used to assess prognostic factors and to screen for metastatic disease (Table 2). The staging workup begins with a thorough history and physical examination, routine serum chemistry, and bilateral mammography. The regional nodal basins are examined by ultrasonography, with fine needle aspiration used to assess suspicious areas. Material obtained from the diagnostic biopsy can be used to determine estrogen-receptor (ER) status and progesterone-receptor status, as well as human epidermal growth factor receptor-2 (HER-2) status. Baseline measurement of the tumor-specific markers carcinoembryonic antigen and cancer antigen (CA) 15–3 are useful for monitoring the subsequent course of the disease. Breast cancer commonly metastasizes to the bone, lung, liver, and brain (in that order), necessitating a full-body bone scan, chest x-ray, liver function tests, computerized tomography (CT) scan of the abdomen or ultrasound of the liver, and CT of the brain (when neurologic symptoms are present).

Neoadjuvant Chemotherapy

The multidisciplinary protocol currently in use at the University of Texas M.D. Anderson Cancer Center for the treatment of patients with IBC is shown in Figure 1. The most important component of this protocol is neoadjuvant chemotherapy. Clinical response to neoadjuvant therapy is highly predictive of both disease-specific and disease-free survival. With standard treatment protocols, approximately 12% of patients experience a clinical complete remission (CR), 62% experience a partial remission (PR), and 26% experience less than a partial remission. Patients who achieve a clinical CR have an expected 5-year disease-specific survival rate of 70%, compared with 44% in patients with a clinical PR, and 12% in patients with no significant response.

Table 2: Screening for Metastatic Disease in Inflammatory Breast Cancer

- History and physical examination
- Bilateral mammography
- Ultrasonography of regional nodal basins with FNA of suspicious areas
- Routine serum chemistry
- Tumor markers (carcinoembryonic antigen, CA 15–3)
- Chest x-ray and complete bone scan, with CT follow-up of abnormalities
- Liver function tests
- CT of abdomen or ultrasound of liver, especially in patients with elevated liver function tests
- CT of brain, if neurological symptoms are present

CA, Cancer antigen; *CT,* computed tomography; *FNA,* fine needle aspiration.

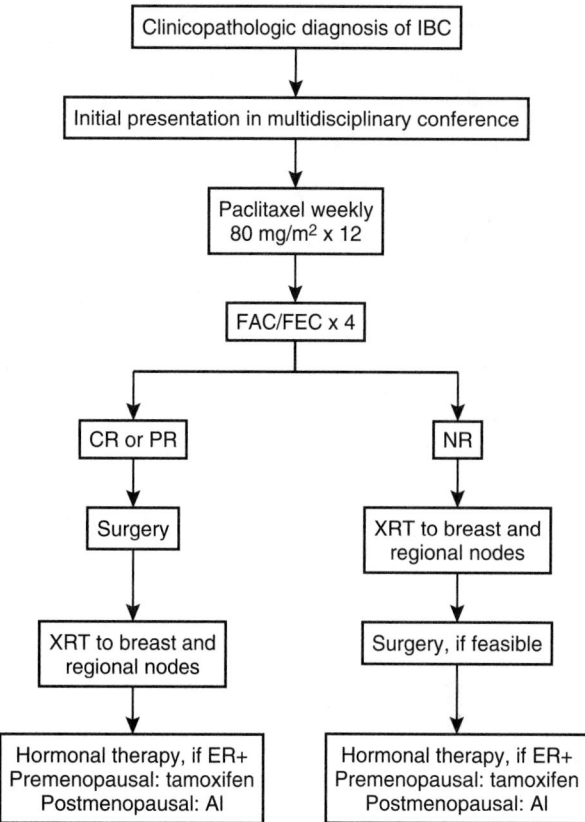

Figure 1 Treatment algorithm for inflammatory breast cancer at the University of Texas M.D. Anderson Cancer Center. *AI,* aromatase inhibitor; *CR,* clinical complete response; *ER,* estrogen receptor; *FAC/FEC,* 5-fluorouracil, Adriomycin (Pharmacia, Milan, Italy)/epirubicin, cyclophosphamide; *IBC,* inflammatory breast cancer; *NR,* no response or minimal response; *PR,* clinical partial response; *XRT,* radiation therapy.

After initial presentation and review in a multidisciplinary conference, patients receive a sequential regimen of weekly standard-dose paclitaxel (80 mg/m²) for 12 weeks followed by four cycles of 5-fluorouracil, doxorubicin/epirubicin, and cyclophosphamide (FAC/FEC). After the completion of the anthracycline-containing therapy, patients are evaluated for clinical response. If a discrete mass was detected by physical examination or mammography before chemotherapy, the mass should have resolved completely (for complete remission) or by more than 50% (for partial remission). In addition, the initial erythema and other skin changes should have resolved either completely or by more than 50%, as judged by visual comparison with photographs taken before treatment. In patients who had no detectable mass before chemotherapy, judgment of level of response is made on the basis of resolution of skin changes only. Those patients who have a complete or partial response to neoadjuvant chemotherapy are recommended for mastectomy, followed by radiation therapy to the breast and regional nodes. Patients who have less than 50% response to neoadjuvant chemotherapy are recommended for neoadjuvant radiotherapy, and then for mastectomy if the disease becomes resectable. Regardless of response to radiotherapy, ER-positive patients receive hormonal therapy.

The paclitaxel-anthracycline sequence was initially adopted on the basis of older studies indicating that this combination improved outcomes in noninflammatory, locally advanced disease compared with anthracyclines alone. The addition of paclitaxel to anthracyclines for treatment of IBC does not improve objective response rates of the primary disease, but it does lead to improved long-term outcomes, and the improvement is significant for patients with ER-negative disease. In addition, recent work at our institution indicates that the addition of paclitaxel significantly increases the likelihood of a pathologically complete remission in the axillary lymph nodes, a development that is associated with significantly better overall survival and relapse-free survival.

Surgical Approaches in Inflammatory Breast Cancer

The overwhelming trend in the management of noninflammatory breast cancer has been toward less invasive surgery. Axillary lymph node dissection with its often-significant morbidities has been largely replaced by sentinel lymph node biopsy, and breast-conservation therapy is now the standard of care for all but the most advanced cancers. Unfortunately, these less invasive approaches are usually not appropriate for the management of IBC.

Sentinel lymph nodes, which can be successfully identified in almost 90% of patients with locally advanced breast cancer, can be found in only 75% of patients with IBC; in those patients, the reported false-negative rate is as high as 25%, compared with less than 15% in other breast cancer patients. It is likely that because IBC infiltrates the dermis and lymphatics, the underlying architecture is disrupted, making correct identification and assessment of sentinel nodes difficult. In addition, the overall level of nodal involvement in IBC is high, and axillary lymph node dissection is the standard treatment in patients with involved nodes. If surgery is performed on a patient with IBC, it should include a full axillary dissection.

Surgery for the local treatment of IBC originally fell into disfavor because it appeared to have no effect on patient outcome. In early protocols that used mastectomy alone, survival rates were less than 5%, with a median survival of 12 to 32 months. However, subsequent studies have shown that surgery can improve disease-free and overall survival in patients who show a clinically complete or partial response, reduced pathologic tumor size as a result of neoadjuvant chemotherapy, or both. Even in patients who have less than a 50% response to chemotherapy, the use of surgery can reduce the incidence of local recurrence. For patients who do not respond at all to neoadjuvant chemotherapy, surgery may still be used as a palliative, tumor-debulking procedure.

The recommended surgical approach for local treatment in IBC is mastectomy. An advantage to mastectomy is that it allows a lower dose of radiation to be delivered to the chest wall, avoiding some of the late complications from radiotherapy. (Breast-conserving surgery has been attempted in a limited number of IBC patients, but the results have been unsatisfactory, with high rates of local recurrence and significant acute complications from the high-dose radiotherapy used after surgery.) Mastectomy is typically performed 2 to 3 weeks after the completion of induction chemotherapy, to allow blood counts and physiologic status to normalize. A primary concern in surgery planning is that the operative field must be wide enough to encompass all of the secondary skin changes. This is true even if surgery is undertaken only as a palliative measure. If this is not possible, additional chemotherapy may be considered. A related concern is the importance of obtaining negative excision margins. Although as much skin as necessary should be removed, tension must be avoided in closing the skin flaps because this would make the site unsuitable for radiotherapy. If necessary, repair with living autologous tissue should be used to ensure a healthy, flat chest wall. This is usually a latissimus dorsi myocutaneous flap, unless extremely broad coverage is necessary.

A major problem in surgical planning for IBD is the difficulty in determining the extent of surgical resection necessary in a patient with a significant clinical response to neoadjuvant chemotherapy. Clinical response as judged by physical examination or imaging may underestimate the extent of residual disease in more than 60% of patients. Clearly new technologies are necessary to close this

gap. Developments in imaging technology, including contrast-enhanced magnetic resonance imaging or functional positron emission tomography/CT scanning, may be useful. New approaches based on infrared imaging of nanoparticles or molecular fingerprinting of neoplastic tissue may also be adapted to visualize residual disease more accurately.

In patients with noninflammatory breast cancer who receive a mastectomy, immediate reconstruction provides a good cosmetic outcome with little or no effect on long-term treatment outcomes. However, these patients do not routinely receive the postsurgical radiation treatment that is recommended for patients with IBC. Although several small studies have shown that immediate reconstruction can be used in IBC patients postmastectomy, some technical issues may arise related to the extent of radiotherapy used after surgery for IBC. There are concerns about delaying adjuvant radiotherapy, and there may be difficulties in wound healing if radiotherapy is not delayed. We generally advise waiting until 6 to 12 months after the completion of radiotherapy before attempting a reconstruction.

Radiation Therapy

Radiation therapy is recommended following surgery in patients with a complete or partial response to neoadjuvant chemotherapy or before surgery for additional tumor debulking in patients with less than a partial response. Radiation therapy is primarily given for local control because the magnitude of its effect on survival for patients with inflammatory breast cancer is unknown. It is typically delivered to the chest wall, axillary lymph nodes, supraclavicular lymph nodes, and (if involved) internal mammary nodes.

Hormonal Therapy

Although hormonal therapy has not been shown to affect outcomes in patients with inflammatory breast cancer, it is usually recommended for patients with ER-positive disease. Tamoxifen has been shown to significantly reduce the rate of recurrence and of contralateral breast cancer in patients with noninflammatory disease and is usually recommended for premenopausal women with IBC. For postmenopausal women, an aromatase inhibitor such as anastrozole is recommended.

THE FUTURE OF INFLAMMATORY BREAST CANCER TREATMENT

Although multidisciplinary therapy has improved outcomes for patients with IBC since the early 1980s, the prognosis remains grim, with only approximately one third of patients surviving long term. The major problem to be resolved in improving outcomes for patients with IBC is the low rate of significant response to neoadjuvant chemotherapy, with approximately 25% of patients having less than a partial remission. For these patients, several alternatives to standard chemotherapy regimens are being tried, and new biologic therapies hold promise for successful treatments in the future.

Alternative Dosing Regimens

Theoretical models suggest that dose-dense chemotherapy may be more effective than standard dosing schedules because the time for tumor recovery between treatments is reduced. Although preliminary reports from studies involving patients with noninflammatory breast cancer showed great promise, follow-up reports indicate that the improvement in patient outcome may not be as dramatic as had been hoped. Nonetheless, several small studies have shown improved outcomes in IBC patients treated with dose-dense chemotherapy, and the current protocol used at M.D. Anderson recommends a dose-dense schedule for paclitaxel.

The use of high-dose chemotherapy with autologous bone marrow transplantation, although still considered experimental, may be useful in selected patients. Originally, the significant morbidity associated with this approach made clinicians extremely cautious about recommending it for their patients. Better strategies for the management of side effects are causing them to reconsider high-dose chemotherapy, especially in patients who have had limited response to standard dosing regimens.

Targeted Biologic Therapies

Targeted biologic therapies may hold the greatest promise for significant improvement in outcome for IBC patients. Therapies already in use involve specific inhibition of the transmembrane tyrosine kinase receptors ErbB1 (or EGFR) and ErbB2 (or HER2/neu) or of a vascular endothelial growth factor (VEGF) required for angiogenesis. Trastuzumab, a monoclonal antibody that blocks ErbB2, has shown remarkable results when combined with paclitaxel as neoadjuvant therapy for patients with HER2-positive noninflammatory locally advanced disease. Two recent reports (one case study and one uncontrolled descriptive study with 49 patients) suggest that this approach may also hold promise for IBC. Lapatinib is a potent reversible inhibitor of both ErbB1 and ErbB2. An ongoing clinical trial at M.D. Anderson is using daily lapatinib as monotherapy followed by 12 weeks of daily lapatinib in combination with weekly paclitaxel for patients with IBC whose tumors overexpress ErbB1 with or without overexpression of ErbB2. Bevacizumab, a monoclonal antibody against vascular endothelial growth factor 2, has shown a direct inhibitory effect on angiogenic markers in IBC cells.

The combination of two biologic agents with differing mechanisms may provide a treatment option with increased potency and a low side effects profile. For example, at the 2005 San Antonio Breast Cancer Symposium, Dr. Dennis Slamon presented promising results from a pilot study that was based on the observation that more than 75% of patients with HER2-positive disease are also VEGF-positive and that the combination is associated with a poor outcome. Patients with HER2-positive/VEGF-positive advanced breast cancer were treated with a combination of trastuzumab and bevacizumab. Five of nine patients showed a significant clinical response (two complete remissions), and two additional patients had stable disease for longer than 6 months with no additional chemotherapy and no serious side effects.

Continuing work in the molecular biology of breast cancer is revealing other potential targets for biologic therapies in IBC. These targets fall into the general classifications of oncogenes, tumor suppressor genes, and angiogenesis modulators. One of the most interesting targets currently under investigation is RhoC guanosine triphosphatase. This molecule is overexpressed in 90% of IBCs, and preclinical studies have shown that this overexpression is specifically implicated in the production of angiogenic factors by IBC cells. Therapeutic agents directed against this target have shown decreased angiogenesis in animal studies, and it seems likely that they could also be useful clinically.

Suggested Readings

Cariati M, Bennett-Britton TM, Pinder SE, and others: Inflammatory breast cancer, *Surg Oncol* 14:133, 2005.

Giordano SH, Hortobagyi GN: Inflammatory breast cancer: clinical progress and the main problems that must be addressed, *Breast Cancer Res* 5:284, 2003.

Greene FL, Page DL, Fleming ID, and others, editors: *AJCC cancer staging manual*, ed 6, New York, 2002, Springer.

Hance KW, Anderson WF, Devesa SS, and others: Trends in inflammatory breast carcinoma incidence and survival: the Surveillance, Epidemiology, and End Results Program at the National Cancer Institute, *J Natl Cancer Inst* 97:966, 2005.

Hennessy BT, Gonzalez-Angulo AM, Hortobagyi GN, and others: Disease-free and overall survival after pathologic complete disease remission of cytologically proven inflammatory breast carcinoma axillary lymph node metastases after primary systemic chemotherapy, *Cancer* 106:1000, 2006.

Wedam SB, Low JA, Yang SX, and others: Antiangiogenic and antitumor effects of bevacizumab in patients with inflammatory and locally advanced breast cancer, *J Clin Oncol* 24:769, 2005.

Ductal and Lobular Carcinoma In Situ of the Breast

Armando E. Giuliano, MD, and Helen Mabry, MD

INTRODUCTION

Both ductal carcinoma in situ (DCIS) and lobular carcinoma in situ (LCIS) are "in situ" lesions of the breast. Neither the proliferating malignant cells within the ducts in DCIS nor the cells filling and distending the lobules of the breast (LCIS) has invaded the basement membrane. The two lesions behave differently and have different demographics, but both are low threat to a patient's life. Because of the lack of potential for metastases, treatment goals for these preinvasive lesions have focused on preventing local recurrence and understanding the prognosis for future development of invasive lesions. DCIS is more common than LCIS, accounting for 85% of in situ breast lesions diagnosed from 1998 to 2002. DCIS incidence increases with age. LCIS is diagnosed most frequently in premenopausal patients between ages 40 and 50; 61,980 new cases of in situ breast lesions were expected to occur among women in 2006, of which 85% were expected to be DCIS.

DUCTAL CARCINOMA IN SITU

The term DCIS represents a heterogenous group of histologic changes with varying malignant potential. The entire group is characterized by proliferation of malignant epithelial cells within the breast ducts without invasion through the basement membrane.

The incidence of DCIS has been rising corresponding to the increasing use of screening mammography. According to Surveillance Epidemiology and End Results (SEER) data from 1983 to 1998, the incidence of DCIS increased 7.2-fold (4/100,000 to 37/100,000), but then it plateaued, increasing only 1.1-fold from 1997 to 2001. Over the same time period, rates of invasive ductal carcinoma have remained relatively constant. DCIS represents approximately 20% of all newly diagnosed breast cancers.

Pathophysiology

DCIS is classified by several histologic patterns (papillary, micropapillary, cribriform, solid, and comedo) and a low, intermediate, and high grading system based on nuclear features. Papillary and micropapillary types have multiple projections with fibrovascular stalks. Papillary projections fuse to form Roman bridges across the duct lumen. Most of these types have low nuclear grade. Cribriform has tumor cells arranged in a sievelike pattern with multiple small round glands growing within a gland or duct. These glands are confluent without fibrous walls. Sometimes they have one layer of fibroblasts between them. Most of these tumor cells have low nuclear grade. Solid-type DCIS is characterized by tumor cells filling the ducts as solid sheets. Nuclear grade is usually intermediate or high. Focal necrosis may be present in this type. Comedo type usually has a solid growth pattern with central necrosis as a prominent feature. Calcification occurs within the central necrotic cellular debris. Comedo tumors have high nuclear grade. DCIS may be broadly characterized as comedo and noncomedo. Noncomedo DCIS refers to all subtypes that lack central necrotic cellular debris. Comedo necrosis correlates with increased risk of local recurrence and invasion.

The nuclear features of DCIS cells are used to classify lesions as low, intermediate, or high grade. Nuclear size of 1.0 to 1.5 times the size of a red blood cell, uniform size and shape of nuclei, fine granular chromatin, small nucleoli, and low mitotic activity correspond to low nuclear grade. Intermediate grade consists of nuclear size up to two times the size of red blood cell, mild to moderate variation in nuclear size and shape, coarsely granular chromatin with even distribution, nucleoli small to medium sized, and mitotic activity between low and high grade. High-grade DCIS is characterized by nuclear size more than two times the diameter of a red blood cell, marked variation in nuclear size and shape, coarsely granular chromatin unevenly distributed, large and multiple nucleoli, and high mitotic activity.

DCIS exists within a spectrum of tissue alteration from atypical ductal hyperplasia (ADH) to invasive cancer. Features that distinguish ADH from well-differentiated, low-grade DCIS are cellular monotony with uniform nuclei approximately the size of a red blood cell, as well as a micropapillary, cribriform or solid growth pattern. When a few cells penetrate the basement membrane with no focus greater than 1 mm, the lesion is classified as "microinvasive" DCIS, which is no longer pure DCIS but an early invasive cancer.

Natural History

Current understanding of DCIS is that it is a precursor of invasive breast cancer. Not all DCIS will become invasive breast cancer, but the longer it is present and untreated, the more likely this becomes. Sanders and colleagues studied a group of 28 women with low-grade DCIS who were treated with biopsy only. These were excisional biopsies, but no attempt was made to obtain clear margins. These patients were recognized retrospectively when conducting a large review of surgical pathology at institutions associated with Vanderbilt University. Eleven of these 28 women developed invasive breast cancer, and all were in the same breast and quadrant as the DCIS biopsy. Seven were diagnosed within 10 years, one at 12 years, and three between 23 and 42 years. Most women with low-grade DCIS left untreated will eventually develop an invasive cancer at the same site, but it may take decades to happen.

Treatment

DCIS was treated by modified radical mastectomy in the past. With the advent of breast conservation for invasive breast cancer, randomized trials were initiated to determine the outcome of breast conservation for DCIS. When invasive breast cancer began to be treated with breast-conserving surgery, it seemed counterintuitive that noninvasive breast cancer should require a more aggressive operation. Subgroup analysis of National Surgical Adjuvant Breast Project (NSABP) B-06 suggested that breast-conserving surgery might be safe for DCIS.

Subsequently, NSABP B-17 randomized 818 women with DCIS between 1985 and 1990 to lumpectomy alone versus lumpectomy followed by radiation therapy. At 12 years, the incidence of invasive ipsilateral recurrence was reduced from 21.1% to 8.1% in the group treated with lumpectomy followed by radiation versus lumpectomy alone. Noninvasive recurrence was reduced from 18.3% to 8.9%. These data led to the recommendation for all patients with DCIS treated with breast-conserving surgery to receive radiation therapy postoperatively. The incidence of local, regional recurrence and distant metastases in both groups (2.2% lumpectomy alone vs. 2.8% lumpectomy plus radiation therapy [RT]) were similar. There was no difference in survival. After 8 years, the risk of invasive cancer in the ipsilateral breast, 3.9%, was equal to the risk in the contralateral breast, 3.5%. With the observation that tamoxifen decreased contralateral breast cancer and ipsilateral recurrence in patients with invasive cancer, NSABP B-24 was designed to compare treatment of DCIS by lumpectomy followed by radiation therapy with either tamoxifen or placebo.

NSABP B-24 randomized 1804 women with DCIS treated by lumpectomy and radiation to either tamoxifen or placebo for 5 years. For women aged 49 years and younger, the ipsilateral breast recurrence rate was 33.3/1000 per year with placebo and 20.8/1000 per year with tamoxifen. For women 50 and older, the ipsilateral breast recurrence rate was 13.0/1000 per year with placebo and 10.2/1000 with tamoxifen. Tamoxifen therapy decreased the rate of local recurrence but did not improve survival. At 5 years, the incidence of new invasive or noninvasive breast cancer in either breast was reduced 37%. The incidence of invasive breast cancer in either breast was reduced from 7.2% to 4.1% with tamoxifen.

The European Organization for Research and Treatment of Cancer (EORTC) studied 1111 women randomized between 1986 and 1996 with mammographically detected DCIS of less than 5 cm. They were randomized to lumpectomy or lumpectomy followed by RT. No tumor present at the margins was the only requirement for adequate lumpectomy. At 10-year follow-up, 26% of patients treated with lumpectomy alone had a recurrence; 15% of patients treated with lumpectomy followed by RT had a recurrence. Half of the recurrences in both groups were invasive. Similar to the B-17 trial, there was no difference in the distant disease-free or overall survival rates.

Diagnosis

DCIS is usually found by the presence of microcalcifications seen on screening mammography. Rarely it may present as a palpable mass, a mammographic mass, Paget's disease of the nipple, or a bloody nipple discharge. Calcifications that represent DCIS usually have a linear or branching pattern. Suspicious or indeterminate calcifications are further characterized by magnification views. Diagnosis may be confirmed by stereotactic core needle biopsy or wire-localized excisional biopsy. Needle biopsy is an improvement over wire-localized excisional biopsy because it avoids an operation and the potential deformity of surgical biopsy, as well as allowing for better surgical planning. Stereotactic core needle biopsy cannot be performed in some cases when the lesion is too superficial, deep, close to implants or there is too little breast tissue for compression.

Several issues are controversial in DCIS management: excision of the lesion, margin size, radiation, tamoxifen use, the questions of when sentinel node is appropriate—if ever—and whether mastectomy should be considered. Silverstein and colleagues devised

Table 1: University of Southern California–Van Nuys Prognostic Index (USC-VNPI)

	1	2	3
Size	<15 mm	16–40 mm	>40 mm
Margin	>10 mm	1–9 mm	<1 mm
Grade	Not high grade, without comedo	Not high grade with comedo	High-grade with comedo
Patient age	>60	40–60	<40

the Van Nuys Prognostic Index (VNPI; Table 1) to correlate the risk of local recurrence with pathologic features (size, margin, and grade). Later the index was modified to include patient age. The scores correlate with risk of recurrence. In a series of 583 patients treated with breast conservation and followed for an average of 83 months, the percent recurrence for USC-VNPI scores 4, 5, and 6 was 2%, 0% invasive. USC-VNPI scores of 7, 8, and 9 had a recurrence of 22%, of which 46% were invasive. USC-VNPI scores of 10, 11, and 12 had a recurrence of 52%, of which 43% were invasive. On the basis of these findings, treatment of lumpectomy alone was recommended by this group for 4, 5, and 6; lumpectomy followed by radiation for 7, 8, and 9; and mastectomy for 10, 11, and 12. Mastectomy was recommended for patients with a greater than 50% chance of recurrence. These criteria have not been validated prospectively by others.

Ideal margin width around DCIS is unknown. The wider the margins, the less likely local recurrence is. The USC-VNPI requires extensive pathologic analysis of the specimen. This may not be available in all settings.

Mastectomy may be indicated for DCIS when multicentric disease is present; when there are large lesions, i.e., greater than 4 cm; in the case of central disease, persistent positive margins when attempting breast-conserving surgery, or patient preference; or when radiation is contraindicated. Sentinel node biopsy is generally unnecessary for DCIS, but in some cases in which a core biopsy has secured the diagnosis of DCIS, there may be as much as a 20% chance of finding an invasive cancer on removal of the lumpectomy specimen. Sentinel node biopsy may be performed at the time of lumpectomy if the patient wishes to avoid a second operation. DCIS treated by mastectomy may be another indication for sentinel node biopsy because if an invasive tumor is found in the specimen, an axillary node dissection will be required and may be difficult if reconstruction has been completed.

LOBULAR CARCINOMA IN SITU

LCIS has traditionally been regarded as a diffuse change in both breasts that represents a "marker" for increased risk of developing breast cancer. Women with this diagnosis have been offered bilateral prophylactic mastectomies or close surveillance including clinical examination every 6 months with annual mammography. LCIS is usually found incidentally after excisional or core needle biopsy when the procedure is performed for another reason. Breast cancer has an equal risk of developing in either breast. The average time for invasive breast cancer to develop is 10 to 15 years. Invasive lobular carcinoma is more likely to develop in patients with a history of LCIS than in the general population, but invasive ductal carcinoma is still the most common histologic type of breast cancer in these women. LCIS rates have increased 2.6-fold from 1980 to 2001 and 1.1-fold from 1997 to 2001.

Pathophysiology

Histologic features of LCIS include a uniform population of cells that fill all the acini in at least one lobular unit, and half the acini must be expanded. Pagetoid spread into ducts is common. There are two distinct types: classic and pleomorphic. Classic LCIS is characterized by small round nuclei with fine chromatin, small nucleoli, and infrequent mitotic features. Pleomorphic LCIS has moderately large nuclei with coarse chromatin, prominent nucleoli, and mitotic figures, and central necrosis may be present. LCIS can be distinguished from atypical lobular hyperplasia (ALH), in which not all of the acini of a lobular unit are completely filled or less than half of the acini in the lobular unit are expanded. E-cadherin immuno stain can be used to differentiate cells of lobular origin from cells of ductal origin. Cells of lobular origin are E-cadherin negative, and cells of ductal origin are positive.

Natural History

The incidence of invasive breast cancer (IBC) after LCIS diagnosis and 10 years of follow-up was 7.1% for all patients based on SEER data of 4853 women with LCIS. In this study, the frequency of ipsilateral and contralateral IBC was equal: 23.1% had invasive lobular carcinoma (ILC), and 49.7% had invasive ductal carcinoma. The incidence of lobular histology (ILC) in the general population is 6.5%, and women with a previous diagnosis of LCIS are more likely to develop a lobular invasive cancer.

Treatment

The management of LCIS includes counseling the patient that she has an increased risk of developing an invasive cancer and such a cancer is more likely to be of lobular histology than for a woman without LCIS, although she is still more likely to develop an invasive ductal cancer. Options include bilateral prophylactic mastectomies with or without reconstruction or close observation with physical examination every 6 months, annual mammography, and possibly chemoprevention.

Some groups advocate surgical excision after a core needle biopsy of LCIS or ALH. Elsheikh and colleagues studied 33 cases of core biopsies (20 ALH and 13 LCIS) followed by surgical excision. Four of the 13 (31%) LCIS surgical excisions had invasive lobular carcinoma. Surgical excision of the tissue surrounding a core biopsy of ALH revealed 4 DCIS and one invasive lobular carcinoma. Underestimation of the disease present when a core biopsy showed ALH or LCIS occurred in 20% of the ALH patients and 31% of the LCIS patients. On the basis of this small study, surgical biopsy may be indicated for core needle biopsies showing ALH and LCIS. There is no need to obtain negative margins in patients with surgical excisions with LCIS present at the margin.

Chemoprevention of both invasive and noninvasive breast cancer has been studied in high-risk women, including women with LCIS in the NSABP P-1 trial and Study of Tamoxifen and Raloxifene (STAR) trial. In the P-1 trial, 13,388 high-risk women were randomized to receive either 20 mg tamoxifen or placebo daily for 5 years. High risk was defined by Gail model prediction or a diagnosis of LCIS (6% of the study group had a diagnosis of LCIS; 615 women were randomized to placebo and 581 to tamoxifen). After 7 years, the risk of invasive breast cancer was reduced from 42.5/1000 in the placebo group to 24.8/1000 in the tamoxifen group. The risk reduction for noninvasive breast cancer was decreased from 15.8/1000 in the placebo group to 10.2/1000 in the tamoxifen group. Among patients with a diagnosis of LCIS, the rate per 1000 women decreased from 11.7 with placebo to 6.27 with tamoxifen (relative risk [RR] 0.54). This effect was more pronounced than the benefit to high-risk women without a diagnosis of LCIS (RR 0.58).

The STAR trial enrolled 19,747 high-risk women; 9% (893) of these women had a diagnosis of LCIS. Women who participated in STAR were postmenopausal, at least 35 years old, and had an increased risk of breast cancer as determined by their Gail model risk estimation based on age, family history of breast cancer, personal medical history, age at first menstrual period, and age at first live birth or diagnosis of LCIS. They were randomized to tamoxifen or raloxifene daily. The numbers of invasive breast cancers in both groups were statistically similar. In the raloxifene group, 167/9745 women developed invasive breast cancer, compared with 163 of 9726 women in the tamoxifen group. Women in the tamoxifen group had a slightly higher incidence of endometrial cancer compared with the raloxifene group. Women in the raloxifene group had 29% fewer deep vein thromboses and pulmonary embolisms than women in the tamoxifen group. The number of strokes occurring in both groups of women was statistically equivalent: 53 of 9726 women in the tamoxifen group and 51 of 9745 women in the raloxifene group had a stroke during the trial. There was no difference in deaths from strokes: 6 of 9726 women in the tamoxifen group and 4 of 9745 women in the raloxifene group died from this event. Among the women with a history of LCIS, the rate per 1000 of the tamoxifen group was 9.83, and in the Raloxifene group, it was 9.61. The two drugs were equally effective for prevention of invasive breast cancer in women with a history of LCIS.

Although tamoxifen has been shown to reduce by half the incidence of LCIS and DCIS, raloxifene did not have an effect on these diagnoses. Of the 9726 women taking tamoxifen, 57 developed LCIS or DCIS, compared with 81 of 9745 taking raloxifene.

On the basis of these findings tamoxifen or raloxifene can be used in high-risk women with LCIS to reduce the risk of developing an invasive cancer. However, raloxifene may not decrease the development of DCIS or LCIS.

SUGGESTED READINGS

Fisher B, Costantino JP, Wickerham DL, and others: Tamoxifen for the prevention of breast cancer: current status of the National Surgical Adjuvant Breast and Bowel Project P-1 study, *J Natl Cancer Inst* 97:1652, 2005.

Fisher B, Dignam J, Wolmark N, and others: Tamoxifen in treatment of intraductal breast cancer: National Surgical Adjuvant Breast and Bowel Project B-24 randomized controlled trial, *Lancet* 353:1993, 1999.

Fisher ER, Land SR, Fischer B: Pathologic findings from the National Surgical Adjuvant Breast and Bowel Project: twelve-year observations concerning lobular carcinoma in situ, *Cancer* 100:238, 2004.

Silverstein MJ: The University of Southern California/Van Nuys prognostic index for ductal carcinoma in situ of the breast, *Am J Surg* 186:337, 2003.

Vogel VG, Costantino JP, Wickerham DL, and others: Effects of tamoxifen vs. raloxifene on the risk of developing invasive breast cancer and other disease outcomes: the NSABP Study of Tamoxifen and Raloxifene (STAR) P-2 Trial, *JAMA* 295:2727, 2006.

MANAGEMENT OF RECURRENT AND DISSEMINATED BREAST CANCER

Theodore N. Tsangaris, MD

INTRODUCTION

Breast cancer is the most common malignancy in women. It was estimated that for 2006 there would be more than 210,000 newly diagnosed breast cancers in the United States. Cancer of the breast is the second leading cause of cancer death in women after lung cancer. More than 40,000 women die annually of the disease. Although the incidence of breast cancer continues to increase, mortality has been decreasing. Advances in screening and adjuvant therapy together have led to this relatively recent and modest decrease in the rate of death from breast cancer. However encouraging our treatment advances against the disease might be, women will still present with locally recurrent and metastatic disease.

Because of the increased use of breast conservation as the primary local therapy for breast cancer, clinicians can expect to see a rise in locally recurrent disease. Surgery offers an opportunity to have an impact on these ipsilateral breast tumor recurrences. However, systemic therapy in addition to local therapy is warranted for many patients.

Metastatic disease, on the contrary, is almost always incurable. The main goals in the treatment of these patients are to control the disease, improve quality of life, and prolong life. Currently there are no absolute treatment approaches that work for all women.

Generalized recommendations should be tailored to the patient and her individual circumstances. Clinical studies are defining the roles of endocrine therapy, chemotherapy, biological therapy, and other novel approaches for treating metastatic disease.

SURVEILLANCE

Introduction

The availability of diagnostic testing for breast cancer patients has increased. Traditionally, breast cancer follow-up employed a conservative approach on the basis of clinical examination and mammography. There is, however, marked variation in practice patterns. This can significantly affect the cost of delivering breast care. Equally important is the fact that excess or abuse of available diagnostic tools has never been shown to improve disease-free or overall survivals.

Recommended Breast Cancer Surveillance

History and Physical

All women should have a careful history and physical examination every 3 to 6 months for the first 3 years after primary therapy, every 6 to 12 months for the next 2 years, and then annually.

Breast Self-Examination

All women should be instructed on how to perform monthly breast self-examinations.

Mammography

Mammography should be initiated approximately 6 months after definitive radiation therapy for women treated with breast conservation. Subsequent mammograms should be obtained every 6 to 12 months while establishing stability. Annual mammograms should follow when stability is achieved.

Coordination of Care

Continuity of care for the breast cancer patient is recommended and should be undertaken by a physician experienced in the surveillance of cancer patients and breast examination. Familiarity and a level of comfort in the examination of the irradiated breast are important. Primary care physicians (PCPs) may assume follow-up care provided that they meet the aforementioned requirements. The PCP should be expected to achieve similar results as the breast specialist. A "shared-care" model of patient follow-up has been suggested and may be more appropriate, depending on the stage of disease or requirements of long-term treatment such as adjuvant endocrine therapy.

Pelvic Exam

A regular annual gynecologic follow-up is recommended for all women. Patients on tamoxifen therapy should report any vaginal bleeding because of the increased risk for developing endometrial cancer.

Breast Cancer Surveillance Testing Not Recommended

The following tests are not recommended for routine breast cancer surveillance. Complete blood count, blood chemistries, chest x-rays, bone scans, ultrasounds of the liver, computed tomography (CT), positron emission tomography scans, breast magnetic resonance imaging, and breast cancer tumor markers (cancer antigen [CA] 15–3, CA27.29, and carcinogenic embryonic antigen).

Management of High-Risk Women

Women at high risk for familial breast cancer should be referred for genetic counseling. Women at high risk include those with the following history or characteristics:

1. Ashkenazi Jewish heritage
2. Ovarian cancer at any age in patient or any first- or second-degree relative
3. Any first-degree relative with a history of breast cancer diagnosed before age 50 years
4. Two or more first- or second-degree relatives diagnosed with breast cancer at any age
5. Patient or relative with bilateral breast cancer
6. History of breast cancer in a male relative

Table 1 summarizes current screening recommendations.

LOCOREGIONAL RECURRENCE

Ipsilateral Breast Tumor Recurrence

The use of breast conservation as the local treatment of choice for most early-stage breast cancers continues to increase. It would be expected and has been observed that there would be a 5% to 15% increase in ipsilateral breast recurrences. These recurrences are emotionally taxing to the patient and her health care providers but definitely treatable. Most women who have had lumpectomy and radiation are best treated with completion mastectomy. Simple reexcision of the recurrence may be appropriate in select patients and under special circumstances.

The significance of an ipsilateral breast tumor recurrence (IBTR) appears to go beyond the immediate problem and anxiety of treating the local recurrence. Meta-analysis suggests that an IBTR is not the instigator of a patient's demise but a prognosticator of future systemic disease. Therefore strong consideration should be given to providing these patients with systemic therapy in addition to treating to the visible local disease.

Table 1: Summary of Recommendations for Breast Cancer Surveillance

History and Physical

- By specialist or shared with primary care physician
- Every 3–4 months for 3 years
- Every 6–12 months for 2 years
- Every 1 year after 5 years

Mammography

- New baseline 6–12 months after definitive radiation therapy
- Ipsilateral breast every 6 months until stability is established, then every 1 year
- Contralateral breast every 1 year

Breast Self-Examination

- Every month

Pelvic Examination

- Routine yearly examination

Routine Blood Tests

- No

Routine Imaging

- No

Routine Tumor Markers

- No

Routine Positron Emission Tomography Scan

- No

Routine Breast Magnetic Resonance Imaging

- No

Chest Wall Recurrence

There is no question that local recurrence of the chest wall, after initial mastectomy, caries a far more ominous significance than an in-breast tumor recurrence after breast conservation. The active search for metastatic disease is appropriate and unfortunately often results in a positive finding. Systemic therapy is often used in this scenario. The presence of other metastatic sites, disease-free interval, prior treatment history, and performance score are all important when considering the multidisciplinary approach to these patients. Nothing is more devastating than uncontrolled local chest wall disease. Therefore when possible, a local resection with clear margins and radiation therapy should be used. If complete resection with clear margins is not possible, obtaining tissue through needle, or core biopsy, is important to facilitate systemic therapy. Incisional or partial resections should be avoided because retained tumor at the surgical site can make healing difficult if not impossible.

Regional Nodal Recurrence

In the past, a level I and II axillary dissection was employed with a lumpectomy, making resampling of the axilla for IBTR unnecessary and futile. However, the advent of the sentinel lymph node biopsy (SLNB) as the standard of care has challenged this dogma.

It may be appropriate to perform an axillary dissection in IBTR for patients with a prior SLNB. The more intriguing question may be the appropriateness and utility of a repeat SLNB as a substitute to a formal level I and II dissection in these patients. An increasing volume of experience is reported in the literature of successful and accurate SLNB for local recurrence of breast cancer after breast conservation therapy. The absolute number of lymph nodes removed during the initial axillary sampling, representing a surrogate marker for extent of surgical manipulation and alteration of the lymph node basin, seems to be important when considering a repeat SLNB. Studies suggest that reoperative SLNB was more successful when fewer than 10 lymph nodes were removed in previous surgeries. Variation in the dye migration times and drainage pathways were also seen with increasing lymph node numbers. In addition to the ipsilateral axilla, lymphoscintigraphy revealed drainage to the internal mammary chain, the interpectoral nodes, supraclavicular nodes, and the contralateral axillary basin. For this reason, preoperative lymphoscintigraphy should be used before any approach to the axilla. However, as with primary breast cancer, restraint should be implemented when sampling of the axilla will not affect systemic treatment or radiation therapy.

Internal mammary and supraclavicular lymph nodes are usually not addressed surgically. However, knowledge of their involvement could be important in prognosticating and planning systemic therapy and radiotherapy. Figure 1 summarizes the approach and treatment of locoregional recurrences.

DISTANT METASTASES

Introduction

The appearance of metastatic breast cancer is always devastating and almost never curable. Yet even in light of that disease dynamic, clear goals exist for managing patients with metastatic breast cancer.

The treatment goals of metastatic breast cancer are as follows:

1. Cure
2. Improve overall survival
3. Improve time to progression
4. Improve symptoms related to the disease
5. Improve quality of life

In reality, the main goals in the treatment of metastatic disease are to control the disease, improve quality of life, and prolong life.

As with adjuvant treatment, the clinician dealing with recurrent and metastatic disease must assess the patient for prognostic and predictive factors. Prognostic factors include an estimation of outcome independent of systemic treatment. This would be reflected in factors such as (1) tumor biology, (2) site of disease, (3) extent of disease, (4) time to recurrence, and (5) prior therapy. Predictive factors would reflect a relative resistance or sensitivity to a specific therapy such as estrogen receptor (ER) status or human epidermal growth factor receptor 2 (HER2) status. Patient characteristics should also be considered, including the following: (1) age, (2) menopausal status, and (3) performance status. Finally, balancing toxicity and efficacy is always a concern for the patient and her health care team.

Clinical studies are constantly looking at the roles of endocrine therapy, chemotherapy, and biological therapy in patients with metastatic breast cancer. Therapy options include the following:

1. Endocrine therapies
2. Chemotherapy
3. Novel therapies
4. Supportive therapy

These modalities are discussed separately in further detail.

Endocrine Therapy

Sixty-seven percent of recurrent breast cancers will express ER or progesterone receptors (PR). More than half of these women benefit from interventions that modulate ER or reduce estrogen content. Therefore endocrine intervention should be considered as first-line therapy in women with newly diagnosed hormone receptor-positive breast cancer. A number of endocrine agents are currently available for use against metastatic breast cancer. The following is a list of the classes of hormonal agents and other endocrine-based treatments.

1. Selective estrogen receptor modulators (SERMs)
2. Aromatase inhibitors
3. Estrogen receptor inhibitors
4. Progesterones
5. Ovarian ablation

Tamoxifen is a SERM and is effective in premenopausal and postmenopausal women. Although tamoxifen has traditionally been the first-line treatment of choice for metastatic breast cancer, the arrival of aromatase inhibitors (AIs) has challenged tamoxifen as the drug of choice in many situations. Several AIs have compared favorably with or even shown an advantage over tamoxifen. It should be noted that AIs are effective only in the absence of ovarian function. Therefore in premenopausal women for whom tamoxifen is not appropriate, the reduction of circulating estrogen should use ovarian suppression with or without an AI. Postmeno-

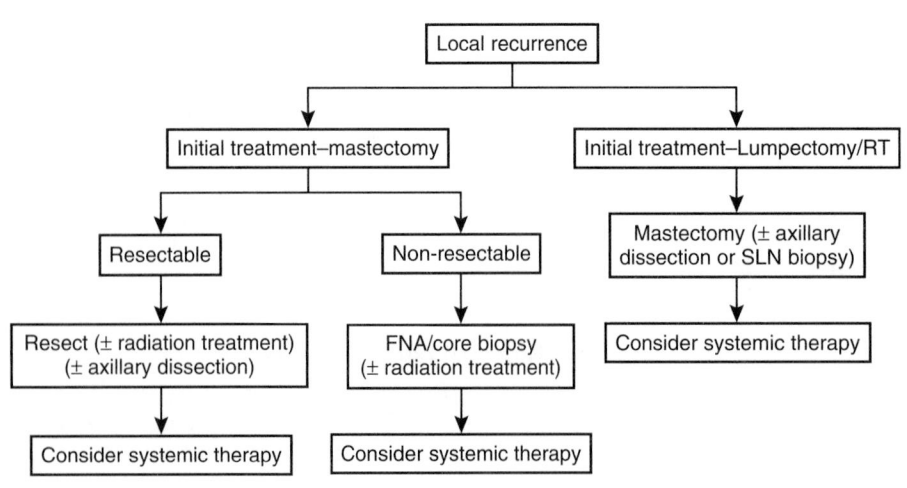

Figure 1 Algorithm for the approach and treatment of locoregional recurrences.

pausal women should be placed on an AI. Anastrozole, exemestane, and letrozole have all shown equivalence or superiority to tamoxifen in several studies for both clinical response and time to progression.

Fulvestrant is a selective ER down-regulator that acts as a pure antiestrogen. Administered intramuscularly on a monthly basis, it has been compared favorably to anastrozole in clinical trials. There are no significant differences in clinical response or time to progression. Fulvestrant has also been compared with tamoxifen as first-line treatment for metastatic breast cancer. Although the two drugs compared favorably with regard to time to progression and objective response, clinical benefit was greater for tamoxifen. The circle of contradictions among SERMs, AIs, and ER down-regulators only emphasizes the complexity of hormone therapy and the fact that there are several choices from which to choose. Thus in principle, the sequential use of hormone therapy is warranted. Studies are under way to examine combining agents such as anastrozole and fulvestrant compared with their sequential use.

Chemotherapy (Nonendocrine Therapy)

Indications for considering nonhormonal therapy include the following:

1. Hormone-negative breast cancer
2. Rapidly progressing visceral metastasis regardless of hormonal status
3. Hormone-positive disease that is refractory to sequential endocrine therapy
4. Short disease-free interval following adjuvant treatment

Several factors must be considered when choosing chemotherapy for patients with metastatic breast cancer. First, as discussed earlier, the relative benefits and toxicities of the various options for the individual patient must be considered. There are multiple options of treatment to consider, including combination versus single-agent chemotherapy, the role of dose-intense or dose-dense therapy, and biologically targeted therapy. In choosing an appropriate therapy, quality of life issues must be kept in perspective. Several single-agent chemotherapy options have been effective as first- or second-line therapies. Of the popular classes of agents, taxanes and anthracyclines have been the most effective. With the increased use of these drugs in the adjuvant setting, the newly diagnosed metastatic patient presents the clinician with a therapeutic dilemma. If the patient has received an anthracycline or taxane in the past 6 to 12 months, it might be preferable to begin treatment with a different class of drugs. However, if a longer time has passed, retreatment with an anthracycline or taxane might be considered. New forms of anthracyclines, such as epirubicin and the liposomal anthracyclines, have decreased concerns of cardiotoxicity and made retreatment with this class of drug for metastatic disease more feasible.

The question of sequential, single-agent therapy versus combination chemotherapy for the treatment of metastatic breast cancer remains an important issue. Combination therapy seems to improve response rates and time to progression. However, these benefits must be weighed against the greater toxicity. It has also been difficult to prove improved overall survival. Following are popular classes of drugs used as single and combination therapies:

Alkylating agents
Antimetabolites
Vinca alkaloids
Anthracyclines
Taxanes
Nucleoside analogues

Part of the difficulty in determining the benefits of single versus combination therapy is the comparison of apples to oranges. Many studies have compared one agent with a combination of different agents rather than comparing the same agents either in sequence or in combination. A recent Eastern Cooperative Oncology Group study, 1193, did contain a crossover design that has allowed for the direct comparison of sequential, single-agent treatment and combination therapy. The objective response and time to progression were higher for the combination therapy. Again no significant difference in overall survival was noted. Also encountered, however, were increases in grade 3 and 4 toxicities. The correct choice of single versus combination might rest with the clinical needs of the patient. If a significant response is clinically necessary, combination therapy is warranted. If the concern is toxicity without compromising survival or quality of life, sequential therapy may be more appropriate.

Novel Therapies

Novel therapies to metastatic disease include trastuzumab, lapatinib, and bevacizumab. Trastuzumab, a humanized antibody, targets and binds to HER2 in tumor cells. HER2 is a tyrosine kinase transmembrane growth factor receptor localized to chromosome 17q. Amplification or overexpression is seen in up to 30% of breast cancers. It is correlated with worse survival compared with HER2-negative tumors. HER2-positive tumors have increased cell proliferation, increased cell migration, and are resistant to apoptosis. By down-regulating the HER2 receptor and reducing tumor cell proliferation, trastuzumab is effective as a single agent when used as a first-line therapy against HER2-positive cancers. Data also exist to suggest that there are synergies between trastuzumab and certain chemotherapeutic agents such as cisplatin, docetaxel, thiotepa, and etoposide. Cardiotoxicity is again a concern with combination therapy of trastuzumab and anthracyclines and less so with trastuzumab and paclitaxel. Ongoing trials investigating the combination of trastuzumab and liposomal anthracyclines are showing encouraging reductions in toxicity while maintaining promising response rates. Additional trials exploring the flexibility of dosing trastuzumab and the continuation of trastuzumab after first-line therapy are also under way.

Lapatinib binds to intracellular adenosine triphosphate binding sites of HER2 and epidermal growth factor receptor (ErbB-1) blocking downstream signaling. This dual blockade of signaling may be more effective than the single-target inhibition provided by agents such as trastuzumab.

In a phase I trial of lapatinib and capecitabine the drug was well tolerated and showed clinical activity. Lapatinib is active in trastuzumab-resistant breast cancer in cell lines and in clinical trials.

Tumor growth is dependent on angiogenesis. Bevacizumab is a humanized monoclonal antibody directed against vascular endothelial growth factor. Bevacizumab appears to have activity in patients with refractory metastatic breast cancer.

The emergence of new and novel treatments is exciting and encouraging for both patients and clinicians. Patients who would benefit from systemic treatments for metastatic breast cancer should be encouraged to participate in clinical trials when appropriate. Fig. 2 summarizes the approach and treatment of systemic disease.

BISPHOSPHONATES

Pamidronate or zoledronic acid are drugs that bind to the bone matrix and reduce the number of adverse events associated with bony metastasis. They also prolong the time to the first event. Patients with bone disease and pain have a clinically relevant

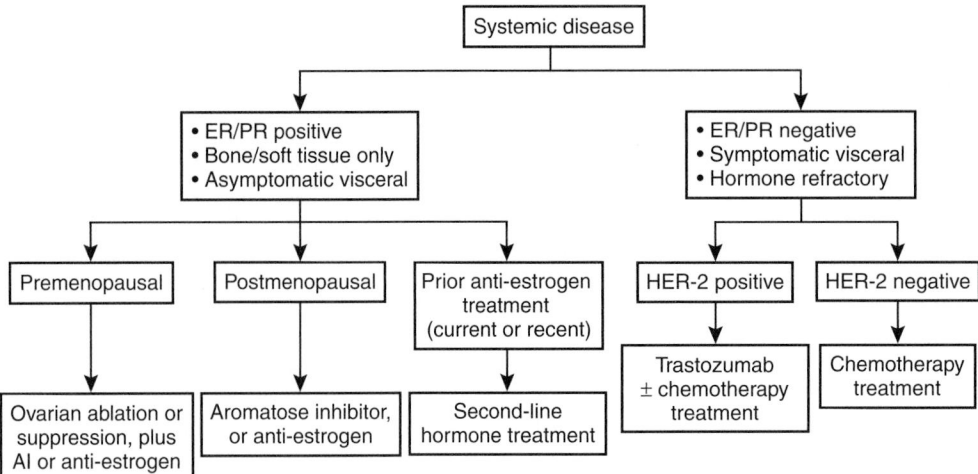

Figure 2 Algorithm for approach and treatment of systemic disease.

analgesic effect with these drugs. Therefore these drugs should be given in addition to hormone therapy or chemotherapy for patients with bone metastasis or patients with a reasonable expected survival. These drugs should be administered with calcium and vitamin D.

There are toxicities with these drugs. Renal toxicities have been observed and good renal function with close monitoring of creatinine clearance is important. Osteonecrosis of the jaw has been reported during long-term use of bisphosphonates.

SURGERY FOR DISTANT DISEASE

The role of the surgical oncologist or other surgical specialist in cases of distant metastatic disease is generally one of palliation. Although the decision to intervene surgically for palliation often has merit, the patient must understand that cure is rarely possible. Risks and benefits of any surgical intervention should be thoroughly explored by the patient and her health care team. Isolated liver metastasis has traditionally been considered a poor prognostic group, with median survival rates of less than 6 months. Several institutions have reported on the surgical approach to these situations. In studies with limited numbers of patients, morbidity and mortality are relatively low with modest gains in survival. Factors that are favorable in these patients are hormone status of tumor, histologic grade, number of other metastatic organ sites, performance scores, and time to developing initial liver metastasis. Again, although some have advocated metastasectomy in select cases of isolated lesions with reported improved survival rates, these scenarios are the exception and should be rigorously scrutinized on a case-by-case basis.

RADIATION THERAPY FOR DISTANT DISEASE

As with surgery, the role of radiation therapy for distant disease is largely one of palliation. It may be preferable to surgery, however, because of its ability to achieve the desired effect on the disease quickly and to avoid the morbidity of surgery. Brain metastases have increased in frequency, probably as a result of advances in palliative care. In patients with good performance scores and in the absence of multiple metastatic sites, intensified local treatment with systemic therapy appears to influence time to progression and

overall survival. The following are clinical situations in which surgery or radiation (or both) may provide significant palliation:

1. Brain metastases
2. Leptomeningeal disease
3. Choroid metastases
4. Pleural effusion
5. Pericardial effusion
6. Biliary obstruction
7. Ureteral obstruction
8. Impending pathologic fracture
9. Pathologic fracture
10. Cord compression
11. Localized painful bone or soft-tissue disease
12. Chest wall disease

It should be reemphasized that the decision to perform surgery or administer radiation therapy for palliation should be undertaken only after careful consideration of the risks and benefits to the patient.

PALLIATIVE CARE

Statistics suggest that more than 85% of patients with advanced cancer will ultimately die of their disease. Although palliative care is now considered integral to the care of these patients, most patients are referred too late to get the full benefit of available treatment. Unfortunately, many patients are never referred at all. The World Health Organization recommends that palliative care should be initiated at the same time as therapy for disease is implemented.

The National Comprehensive Cancer Network Palliative Care Guidelines were developed to facilitate the appropriate integration of palliative care into oncology practice. Included in the guidelines are procedures for screening, assessment, interventions, reassessment, and after-death care. The needs of the family during this time and after death should also be addressed using these guidelines.

SUGGESTED READINGS

Carlson RW, Anderson BO, Burstein HJ, and others: *NCCN clinical practice guidelines for breast cancer*, V.l. 2007. 2006, www.nccn.org/professionals/physician_gls/default.asp.

Fisher B, Anderson S, Fisher ER, and others: Significance of ipsilateral breast tumor recurrence after lumpectomy, *Lancet* 338:327, 1991.

Gralow JR: Optimizing the treatment of metastatic breast cancer, *Breast Cancer Res Treat* 89 (suppl): s9–s15, 2005.

Khatcheressian JL, Wolff AC, Smith TJ, and others: American Society of Clinical Oncology 2006 update of the breast cancer follow-up and management guidelines in the adjuvant setting, *J Clin Oncol* 31:5091, 2006.

Levy MH, Back A, Bazargan S, and others: *NCCN Clinical Practice Guidelines for palliative care* V. l. 2006, http://www.nccn.org/professionals/physician_gls/PDF/palliative.pdf.

Luini A, Galimberti V, and others: The sentinel node biopsy after previous breast surgery: preliminary results on 543 patients treated at the European Institute of Oncology, *Breast Cancer Res Treat* 89:159, 2005.

Taback B, Nguyen P, and others: Sentinel lymph node biopsy for local recurrence of breast cancer after breast-conserving therapy, *Ann Surg Oncol* 13:1099, 2006.

Male Breast Cancer

Kenneth A. Kern, MD, MPH

INTRODUCTION

Epidemiology

As a former surgical oncologist and breast surgeon, I can say from experience that the very existence of male breast cancer (MBC) surprises patients and surgeons alike. It is a rare disease, with only 1 case of breast cancer in male patients for every 150 cases in female patients. In essence, less than 1% of all breast cancers occur in men. Current U.S. estimates of yearly incidence rates of MBC are 1.2 cases per 100,000 men (compared with 150 per 100,000 women), leading to a projected annual case rate of 1450.

The peak age of incidence of MBC is 71 years, more than 15 years later than the initial rise in breast cancer rates in female patients. Women with breast cancer have a bimodal peak age distribution of cases (52 and 72), the earlier age peak possibly being related to estrogen "surges" just preceding menopause (age 50). In contrast, the single peak incidence at age 71 in males is consistent with the absence of estrogen in the male hormonal life cycle. It is important to remember that both in situ and invasive breast cancer have been reported in males as young as 16 to 22 years. The malignancies presented in these young men as isolated breast masses and were initially diagnosed and treated as "simple gynecomastia." These patients had no breast imaging or diagnostic testing beyond a physical examination of the breast.

Treatment Paradigm

The treatment paradigms for MBC are similar to those for female breast cancer. The infrequency of MBC means that there are no large, randomized, controlled clinical trials of male breast cancer from which to derive evidence-based treatment algorithms. Nonetheless, the treatment of MBC may be thought of as similar to treating a subset of female breast cancer that is (1) ductal-invasive in origin, (2) strongly estrogen-receptor positive, and (3) usually later in stage. Ultimately, this means that patients with MBC present with isolated breast masses, require more extensive surgery, and are treated adjuvantly with hormonal therapy.

RISK FACTORS IN MALE BREAST CANCER

Many surgeons harbor the impression that long-standing gynecomastia increases the risk of breast cancer. However, recent studies have shown that it is hyperestrogenemia, rather than gynecomastia itself, that is associated with increased rates of breast cancer in males. Hyperestrogenemic states that increase the risk of MBC include Klinefelter's syndrome (47 XXY instead of the normal 46 XY), testicular dysgenesis, low testosterone, obesity, and alcoholism resulting in cirrhotic liver impairment. The risk of breast cancer in these individuals is 20- to 50-fold higher than in other men. Obesity alone doubles the risk of male breast cancer because of increased conversion of adrenal androgens and testosterone to estrogen in peripheral adipose tissues. Each of these conditions should be kept in mind and ruled out in the initial office evaluation of a male with possible breast cancer.

Both extrinsic causes of genetic damage and inherited genetic alterations can increase the rate of MBC. The most common extrinsic cause of genetic damage to breast cells is radiation exposure to the chest wall resulting from mantle radiation in the treatment of Hodgkin's disease.

In terms of inherited predisposition to MBC, one in five patients (20%) with MBC has a first-degree relative with breast cancer. Whereas 7% to 8% of female breast cancer is associated with *BRCA1* or *BRCA2* mutations, the data for MBC are unclear (estimated to be between 4% and 40%). *BRCA2* mutations are thought to be the dominant genetic alteration in males, although whether the two forms of *BRCA* mutations are equally distributed among MBC patients remains controversial. Comparative genomic hybridization studies on both male and female breast cancer have shown them to harbor similar patterns of chromosomal imbalances. Typically these imbalances result from loss or chromosomal gains in the short and long arms of chromosomes 8, 13, 16, and 17. Given these common chromosomal alterations in male and female breast cancer, it appears that similar progression in genetic alterations leads to the malignant phenotype.

PRESENTATION

Nearly three quarters of patients with MBC present with an isolated breast mass, almost always self-detected. Rarely MBC will present with bilateral breast masses, and this presentation should immediately trigger a workup for hereditary breast cancer. That MBC presents as a mass, rather than diffuse breast enlargement, is consistent with its histopathologic features. MBC virtually always involves infiltrating, ductal (scirrhous) carcinoma (>95% of cases) and involves lobular invasive carcinoma only in less than 5% of cases. Ductal invasive carcinoma is described as "scirrhous" because it consists of a mass of hard, fibrotic, or indurated tissue. In comparison, lobular carcinoma usually consists of single files of cells diffusely present throughout one region of the breast. Because of this morphology, lobular invasive carcinoma may be ill defined, soft, and difficult to diagnose from physical examination. Whereas lobular invasive carcinoma may be present in up to 20% of women (and present as apparent breast enlargement or diffuse fibrocystic changes), it is a true rarity in men.

The remaining one quarter of patients with MBC present with nipple inversion or nipple discharge. Rarely nipple skin erosion may occur because of Paget's disease (invasive ductal carcinoma invading breast epithelium in the nipple-areolar complex). The rarity of fibrocystic changes in the male breast makes a benign diagnosis of a true breast mass or nipple-associated symptoms extremely unlikely. Any of these findings (true breast mass, discharge, nipple inversion) in a male breast must be treated with extreme suspicion of malignancy. A thorough workup to rule out breast malignancy of either the in situ or invasive type is mandatory.

OFFICE WORKUP OF MALE BREAST SYMPTOMS

The workup of a true breast mass or nipple-associated symptom in males follows a similar pattern to that in females, except that the index of suspicion for malignancy in males should be markedly increased. In essence, any of the following three physical findings in male patients should be thought of as signs of malignancy until proved otherwise: (1) a true, isolated mass (proven by image detection, to confirm that it is not simply unilateral breast enlargement); (2) nipple discharge; or (3) nipple inversion.

The busy clinical surgeon will be asked to evaluate many males with breast masses, both young and old. As in the evaluation of female breast masses, the workup begins with a careful family and treatment history to decide whether risk factors are present. Following this evaluation, physical examination is undertaken with a focus on whether a true breast mass is present in one or both breasts. Diffuse, symmetrical enlargement of both breasts in the absence of a palpable isolated mass in one breast can be clinically determined to be gynecomastia but is not definitive. From my own clinical experience, I urge the use of diagnostic breast ultrasound to rule out any masses in patients referred for breast evaluation or in those presenting with a self-discovered breast mass. Although unilateral gynecomastia is the rule in males, it is my opinion that relying on physical examination alone is inadequate to confirm the absence of a breast mass in a patient referred (or self-referred) for evaluation. Particularly in older males, it can be extremely difficult to differentiate a benign subareolar mound of firm, long-standing gynecomastia from potential breast malignancy presenting as a mass within this tissue.

I urge the use of high-resolution, whole-breast ultrasound in the evaluation of all cases of possible breast mass in males because the sonographic determination of breast lobules and ducts connected to the nipple, without a sonographic cystic or sold lesion, secures the diagnosis of gynecomastia.

Any sonographically determined solid or complex-cystic mass in the breast should be approached for immediate diagnosis by needle-core biopsy, rather than fine needle aspiration cytology (FNAC). The false-negative rate of FNAC is simply too high to use as a dependable diagnostic tool. In particular, in the setting of gynecomastia, normal breast cells may be extremely difficult to aspirate, whereas the core biopsy dependably returns glandular tissue. Intracystic papillary carcinoma of the male breast has been reported and presents as a complex cystic-solid mass on breast ultrasound. These types of complex lesions should be biopsied to prevent being mistaken for "simple cysts" or "cysts with protein debris." I have had personal experience with fluid aspiration of complex cysts initially being interpreted as "reactive atypia" but later returning as ductal

carcinoma in situ (DCIS) or low-grade invasive malignancy on core biopsy. I do not recommend the use of FNAC as a diagnostic tool in anything but a sonographically determined simple cyst (thin-walled, no internal debris, no wall irregularities).

Diagnostic mammography should play a secondary role in the diagnosis of MBC because it is far less frequently informative than in female breast cancer. For example, male breast cancers are spiculated less often than female cancers. In addition, microcalcifications are less frequently seen in male breast cancer compared with female cases. Rarely breast magnetic resonance imaging (MRI) may be used in suspected hereditary cancer to rule out bilateral breast cancer. The MRI features (using a dynamic contrast-enhanced technique) appear comparable in male and female breast cancer.

The differential diagnosis of isolated masses in the male breast include (1) invasive or noninvasive malignancy; (2) vascular tumors (cavernous hemangiomas, pseudo-angiomatous hyperplasia); or (3) metastatic disease (head and neck, e.g., parotid, hypopharyngeal, lung, lymphoma, leukemia). Only biopsies by FNAC (not recommended), core needle, or open technique are reliable methods to determine the true diagnosis of a breast mass. As a clinical example, I was asked to evaluate and remove a breast mass in a patient with acute lymphocytic leukemia. At biopsy the mass proved to be a metastatic deposit of high-grade leukemia, something that surprised all clinicians caring for the patient.

In a male patient, nipple retraction or bloody nipple discharge should be an immediate clue to a likely underlying breast malignancy. In males, retraction caused by chronic fibrocystic changes or bloody nipple discharge caused by benign intraductal papilloma are virtually unknown events. Later in this chapter, I describe a 56-year-old male patient who presented with spontaneous bloody-nipple discharge, which proved to be DCIS on subsequent biopsy.

The diagnosis of breast cancer initiates a discussion with the patient involving the clinical and radiologic findings and histopathology, followed by a workup for metastatic disease. From these findings, a clinical stage can be determined and prognosis estimated. Subsequent removal of the malignancy along with node sampling allows for a final determination of pathologic staging, and this information directs the need for adjuvant therapy.

PATHOLOGY

Unlike female breast cancer, male breast cancer is virtually always ductal-invasive in origin. Because lobular differentiation in the developing breast requires estrogen stimulation, male breast cancer involves lobular differentiation in less than 5% of cases. This means that clinical breast malignancies are likely to present in males as firm, isolated breast masses (typical of ductal invasive cancer) and not as the diffuse, poorly defined tumors typical of invasive lobular carcinoma.

Males may present with DCIS in less than 5% of cases. I treated a patient who was a 56-year-old male with spontaneous bloody nipple discharge from the left nipple and a subareolar thickening. He had no risk factors and no other symptoms, physical findings, or radiologic abnormalities. An excision of the subareolar mass revealed DCIS of 8 to 9 mm without invasion. Males have also been reported to have breast cancer histologies that span the same range of types as in females, such as papillary, medullary, mucinous, Paget's, lobular, and inflammatory carcinoma. All of these histopathologies occur with less than a 1% to 2% incidence rate.

The rate of hormone-receptor positive disease in male breast cancer is extremely high: 93% estrogen-receptor positive, 87% progesterone-receptor positive, and 87% androgen receptor position. Male breast cancers rarely overexpress the human epidermal growth factor receptor (HER-2), compared with nearly one third of women. These factors have important implications for the choice of postoperative adjuvant therapy or primary therapy of metastatic disease because they demonstrate that male breast cancer should be treated like a differentiated, hormonally sensitive form of female breast cancer.

STAGING AND PROGNOSIS

Similar to female breast cancer, axillary nodal status and tumor size are the most important independent prognostic factors in MBC. The age- and stage-matched rates of survival for MBC are also similar to that of female breast cancer. For MBC, the 5-year overall survival (OS) for all stages is approximately 73%, and the 5-year disease-free survival (DFS) is approximately 45%. For stages 0 to IIA, the 5-year OS and DFS are 100% and 71%, respectively. For stages IIB to IV, the 5-year OS and DFS are 71% and 20%, respectively.

The American Joint Committee on Cancer stage and its components (tumor size, nodal status, and presence of metastases) are the most important predictors of survival in MBC. Survival in MBC tends to be worse than that in female breast cancer because males have a 15% increase in late-stage at presentation (stage III or IV) compared with females (see Table 1). It has been assumed that this problem is related to delay in diagnosis by clinicians, with median delays in diagnoses reported between 4 and 12 months. However, it is unclear whether male breast cancer is truly delayed in diagnosis or is accompanied by more advanced features of disease because the tumors have more limited space in which to grow. Given the confined area of the male breast, extension into the nipple-areolar complex or chest wall is more likely in males. Because the nipple-areolar complex harbors a rich lymphatic plexus directly connected to axillary lymph nodes, the increased rate of node-positive disease in males is not surprising. These anatomic factors might explain the paradox that although two thirds of patients with MBC have tumors less than 2 cm, 55% have lymph nodes positive for metastases.

PREOPERATIVE WORKUP OF MALE BREAST CANCER

Following the diagnosis of breast cancer, a male is evaluated and staged using the TNM staging system (in which T = primary tumor, N = regional lymph nodes, and M = distant metastasis), in a similar fashion to that of females (Fig. 1). All available histopathologic data are accumulated. Clinical evidence for tumor size, nodal status, and the presence of metastatic disease is compiled. This involves a careful physical examination of the primary tumor, the draining nodal basins, distant nodal basins, lung, and liver. Radiologic evidence for local and metastatic disease is then obtained, involving bilateral mammograms (often uninformative) and only a chest radiograph in cases of small, low-risk lesions. Mammograms for screening the opposite breast are particularly useful in a case of suspected hereditary breast cancer or a patient confirmed to be a BRCA2 mutation carrier.

In larger tumors or more advanced cases with regional extension, a more wide-ranging search for local and metastatic disease may be indicated, involving regional computed tomography scans or positron emission tomography imaging. Serum chemistries and hematologic values should be obtained to determine whether any suggestion of liver or bone marrow involvement exists. Laboratory evidence for metastatic disease is followed by focused radiologic studies with possible image-directed biopsy. A bilateral breast MRI may be of value in suspected hereditary MBC.

TREATMENT

Surgical

Because male breast cancers grow within the rudimentary breast tissue located directly beneath the nipple-areolar complex, successful resection of these tumors with a negative margin virtually always requires a total mastectomy. A successful lumpectomy is almost never possible, except perhaps in an extremely enlarged male breast with a small tumor that might allow for a central lumpectomy. If successful breast preservation is achieved, radiation therapy is indicated, similar to the treatment of female breast cancer. This is the exception to the rule, however, and total mastectomy with some form of node sampling or dissection is the standard of care.

Sentinel lymph node biopsy (SLNB) or complete axillary lymph node dissection (ALND) are both acceptable options for early-stage disease male breast cancer. Mastectomy and concomitant SLNB is a safe option for well-selected breast cancer patients. Patients with a positive SLN undergo completion axillary lymph node dissection. The patient should be prepared for the definition of a "positive sentinel node," so as not to be surprised if a delayed, second procedure to complete the initial lymph node dissection is recommended.

ALND without initial SLNB would be required for more advanced cases, typically presenting as advanced tumors, significant nipple retraction, or palpable adenopathy. Recent clinical studies have shown that patients with MBC may be staged accurately with SLNB, with a success rate equivalent to that seen in female breast cancer. A negative axillary node status is the most important prognostic sign for prolonged DFS and OS in patients with MBC.

The enlarged breast and small tumor size in most cases of MBC usually allow for a successful primary skin closure of the mastectomy. However, some cases of MBC may not be amenable to primary skin closure and require skin grafting or complex rotational flaps. This issue should be considered preoperatively, and a

Table 1: Differences between Male and Female Breast Cancer

Factor	Male Breast Cancer	Female Breast Cancer
Peak age at presentation	71 years	51 and 72 years
Mean age at diagnosis	65 ($\pm$ 13) years	61 ($\pm$ 15) years
Age distribution	Unimodal	Bimodal
Hereditary gene	BRCA2	BRCA1, BRCA2
Histologic types	>95% ductal invasive	80% ductal, 20% lobular
Stage at presentation	>40% III/IV	25% III/IV, 75% <II
Incidence rate (per 100,000)	1.2	150
Case rate (2004)	1450	215,000
Proportion DCIS	9%	12%
Proportion ER (+)	95%	75%
Proportion HER2 (+)	<5%	33%
Type of resection required	Total mastectomy with SLNB or ALND	Breast preservation or total mastectomy with SLNB or ALND

ALND, Axillary lymph node dissection; DCIS, ductal carcinoma in situ; ER, estrogen receptor; HER2, human epidermal growth factor receptor; SNLB, sentinel lymph node biopsy.

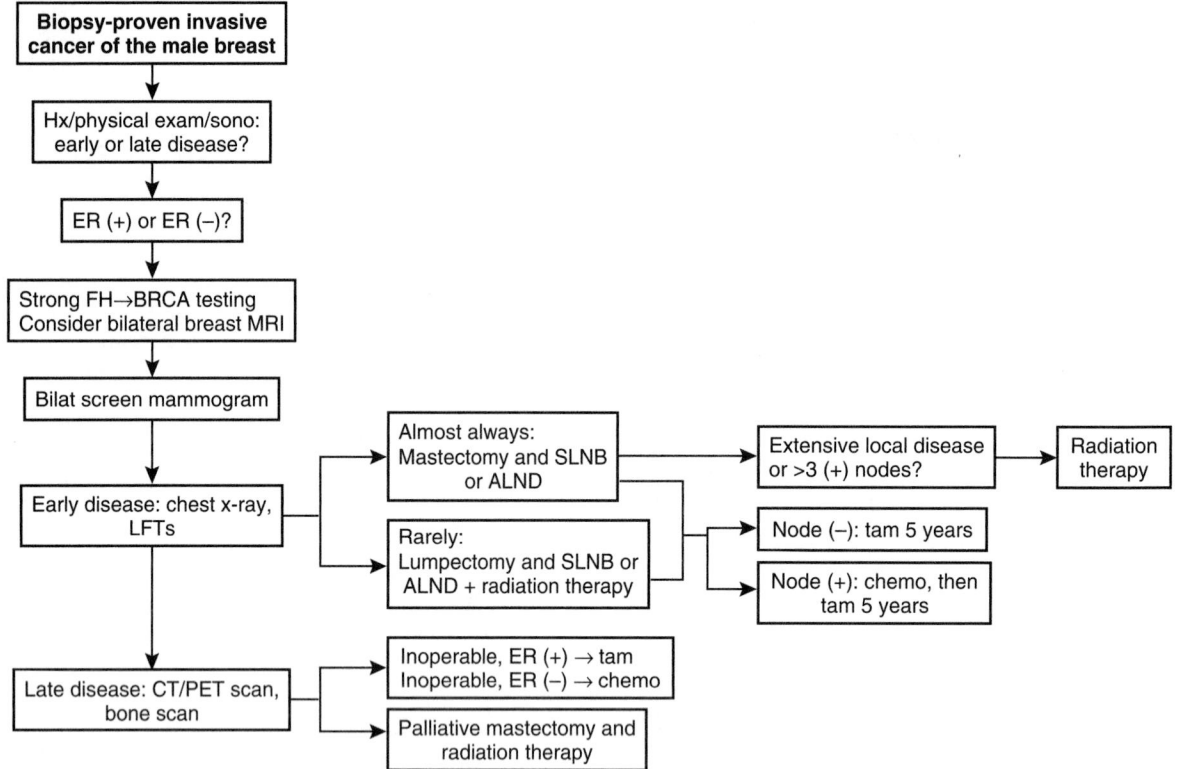

Figure 1 Treatment algorithm for male breast cancer.

reconstructive surgery consult should be obtained if problems with a primary closure might occur.

Radiation Therapy

Because lumpectomy is not the preferred surgical approach to MBC, radiation therapy is usually used in MBC in postmastectomy cases accompanied by poor prognostic signs (advanced tumor stage or nodal status). These signs are similar to those seen in female breast cancer and include close or regional involvement in high-grade disease or involvement of more than three axillary lymph nodes. The use of postmastectomy radiation is more common in men than women for the reasons discussed in the section on staging.

Adjuvant Therapy

The systemic treatment of male breast cancer is similar to that of female breast cancer, a strategy made easier by the fact that the overwhelming majority of cases are estrogen-receptor positive. It is recommended that MBC patients who have tumors greater than 1 cm and who are lymph node negative should receive anti-hormonal therapy for 5 years postoperatively. Although this treatment now involves tamoxifen, the role of newly developed aromatase inhibitors or estrogen-receptor down-regulators remains an unexplored option. Because testosterone and adrenal androgens undergo peripheral conversion to estrogen, orchiectomy is another

therapeutic option for patients with advanced or metastatic disease who are refractory to antihormonal therapy.

For cases of lymph-node positive disease, adjuvant therapy with anthracycline-based chemotherapy, in addition longer-term maintenance therapy with hormonal agents, has been suggested to improve survival.

Suggested Readings

Cimmino VS, Degnim AC, Sabel MS, and others: Efficacy of sentinel lymph node biopsy in male breast cancer, *J Surg Oncol* 86:74, 2004.

Fentiman PS, Fourquet A, Hortobagyi GN: Male breast cancer, *Lancet* 367:595, 2006.

Giordano SH, Perkins GH, Broglio K, and others: Adjuvant systemic therapy for male breast carcinoma, *Cancer* 104:2359, 2005.

Goodman MT, Tung K-H, Wilkins LR: Comparative epidemiology of breast cancer among men and women in the US, 1996 to 2000, *Cancer Causes Control* 17:127, 2006.

Goss PE, Reid C, Pintilie M, and others:: Male breast carcinoma: a review of 229 patients who presented to the Princess Margaret Hospital during 40 years: 1955–1996, *Cancer* 85:629, 2006.

Hill TD, Khamis HJ, Tyczynski JE, Berkel HJ: Comparison of male and female breast cancer incidence trends, tumor characteristics, and survival, *Ann Epidemiology* 15:773, 2005.

Kern KA: The delayed diagnosis of symptomatic breast cancer. In Bland K, Copeland E, editors: *The breast. Comprehensive management of benign and malignant diseases* ed 3, St Louis, MO, 2002, WB Saunders.

Vetto J, Jun SY, Paduch D, and others: Stages at presentation, prognostic factors, and outcome of breast cancer in males, *Am J Surg* 177:379, 1999.

Breast Reconstruction following Mastectomy: Indications, Techniques, and Results

Michele A. Manahan, MD, and Navin Singh, MD, MBA

INTRODUCTION

Breast cancer affects more than 1 of every 10 women in the United States, requiring large numbers of women to undergo breast surgery. Many women who are appropriate candidates will choose to undergo breast-conserving therapy (BCT), comprising lumpectomy with postoperative radiation, which has been shown to have equivalent survival rates to the more disfiguring mastectomy. However, certain absolute and relative contraindications to BCT exist, making approximately 25% of patients with stage I or II disease medically more appropriate for mastectomies. More severe cancers are also more appropriately managed with mastectomies. Additionally, approximately 20% of patients who are candidates for BCT opt for mastectomy on the basis of personal choice. Furthermore, some women with a strong family history of malignancies including maternal lineage breast cancer are considered at high risk for developing breast cancer. They may chose to undergo genetic testing for *BRCA1* or *BRCA2* mutation as well. Many of these patients select bilateral prophylactic mastectomy with reconstruction and oophorectomy. Some patients choose to have no breast reconstruction, whereas others choose either immediate or delayed reconstructions. Overall, close to 75,000 women undergo breast reconstruction each year.

Women undergoing immediate or early reconstructions comprise less than 20% of mastectomy patients. However, this number is on the rise, partially as a result of the Women's Health and Cancer Rights Act of 1998, which mandates that medical insurance companies cover the costs associated with reconstruction of the affected breast, as well as procedures to the contralateral breast to enhance symmetry. As more women undergo mastectomies and seek reconstructions, the reconstructive options available have expanded. Patients currently may choose between reconstruction with implants of several varieties and reconstruction with autologous tissue from the back, buttocks, or abdomen, either as pedicled flaps to preserve blood supply or as free tissue transfers.

ONCOLOGIC SURGERY

Optimal postoperative results occur when the oncologic, ablative surgeons work in concert with the aesthetic, reconstructive surgeons. Although the primary goal during a mastectomy should first and foremost always be eradication of tumor, several current trends facilitate breast reconstruction. Skin-sparing mastectomies, preservation of the inframammary fold, and conservation of blood vessels within the remaining subcutaneous and chest wall tissue play important roles in improving the appearance of the reconstructed breast.

In patients who have tumors of limited size without inflammatory characteristics or frank involvement of the overlying skin, the sacrifice of as little skin around the nipple areolar complex as possible allows greater leeway in reconstructive options. In certain circumstances, this can eliminate the need for tissue expansion before placement of a permanent implant or can allow for complete camouflage of breast scarring within the confines of a reconstructed nipple areolar complex. Preserving the integrity of the residual skin and subcutaneous tissue flaps by gentle handling, maximizing thickness, and minimizing electrocautery trauma will also promote postoperative aesthetics by decreasing skin loss, fat necrosis, scarring, and contracture of the native chest tissue.

The inframammary fold (IMF) is one of the most crucial landmarks of the breast, visibly defining its boundaries to a large extent, and slight discrepancies of placement of the IMF between sides of a patient can lead to poor approximation of aesthetic ideals. In some patients, these differences exist preoperatively and necessitate specific manipulation of the area during breast reconstruction because surgery on the breast may often unmask or emphasize abnormalities that were previously camouflaged by breast tissue, unnoticed by the patient or unimportant to the patient's self-esteem. The IMF must also be reconstructed when its boundaries are violated to ensure optimization of the oncologic portion of the breast procedures. However, manipulation of the IMF is difficult and prone to complications and poor results, and thus preservation of the IMF when possible greatly enhances the ease of breast reconstruction.

Conservation of blood vessels from the internal mammary artery and vein that perforate the chest wall and supply the subcutaneous tissue left behind after adequate mastectomy also facilitates reconstruction. Most notably, these vessels can be useful as recipient vessels in microvascular anastamoses that are necessary for free tissue transfer and may be used to augment blood supply in pedicled procedures as well. Other options exist should these vessels be sacrificed or be found to be of inadequate size; however, their preservation also ensures optimal vascularity and therefore health of the native breast flaps that will surround any reconstructive effort.

TIMING OF RECONSTRUCTION

As previously mentioned, breast reconstruction may be performed either immediately postmastectomy or as a delayed procedure. Often this decision is left to patient preference. It is no longer believed that patients must live with a mastectomy defect to be able to decide whether they would benefit from reconstruction. However, certain medical reasons occasionally lead health care providers to recommend delayed rather than immediate reconstructions. Patients who will require extensive postoperative radiation therapy are often counseled to delay breast reconstruction. Additionally, patients with advanced local disease or nodal metastases who will be enrolled in chemotherapy protocols must understand that any reconstructive complication that delays wound healing could delay institution of necessary, life-preserving chemotherapy. Additionally, certain patients are not optimal candidates for breast reconstruction because of concomitant medical illnesses. These patients may be counseled regarding the possibility of reassessment at a later date.

As a whole, patients undergoing immediate versus delayed reconstructions are all still candidates for the entire spectrum of reconstructive options. However, patients undergoing delayed procedures do present a unique set of challenges. The most striking of these is reduction in the breast skin envelope. Following mastectomy without reconstruction, the skin of the chest will contract, necessitating tissue expansion before implants or larger skin islands in autologous repairs. Additionally, scarring makes the tissue planes more difficult to appreciate and preserve during recreation of a breast pocket for placement of the volume of the breast substitute. These are well-known phenomena that may be controlled with adequate preoperative planning.

RECONSTRUCTIVE GOALS

The goal of any breast reconstruction is to imitate the contralateral natural breast as closely as possible. Breast reconstructions are judged on size, shape, symmetry, softness (or texture), and sensuality. Different patients have different expectations. Some will strive only to look balanced while fully clothed. Others will expect a breast that looks and feels natural when nude. It is essential that the reconstructive surgeon be involved as early as possible in the preoperative planning period to counsel the patient regarding reconstructive outcomes. Figures 1 through 5 detail various options for reconstructive surgery.

Although reconstructions can often achieve all goals, certain breasts are more difficult to reconstruct. Recreation of particularly large breasts may be beyond the plastic surgeon's reconstructive capabilities. Older patients often display significant ptosis and involutional changes on the unaffected side. Reconstructions are rarely able to mimic adequately the aged breast, so patients requesting symmetry must be prepared for operations on the contralateral breast, which can add to the scar burden but will likely result in overall rejuvenation of the breast appearance. Additionally, patients must understand the risk of complications from the additional procedures, which are largely specific to each reconstructive technique.

IMPLANT RECONSTRUCTION

Some patients will choose or be counseled to choose implant reconstruction. This involves placement of a liquid- or gel-containing prosthetic into the breast cavity. Implants are often recommended for patients who are thin and thus have insufficient autologous donor tissue on their abdomen, back, or buttocks; who are medically ill and unable to undergo lengthy autologous reconstruction; who are averse to additional scarring on other parts of their bodies; and who are not candidates for or prior recipients of radiotherapy.

The implants currently available include permanent saline prostheses, postoperatively adjustable saline prostheses, and both permanent and postoperatively adjustable silicone prostheses. Also available are implants with a silicone shell around a central saline core. Each variety has specific advantages and disadvantages. Silicone implants have a more natural texture when placed on the chest wall, but they have been shown to have higher rates of postoperative capsular contracture. Additionally, despite copious evidence to the contrary, certain elements of the public are still concerned about the risk for systemic illness as a result of silicone breast implants. Saline implants are less natural feeling to the touch and are more prone to wrinkling, which may be visible as rugae beneath the skin.

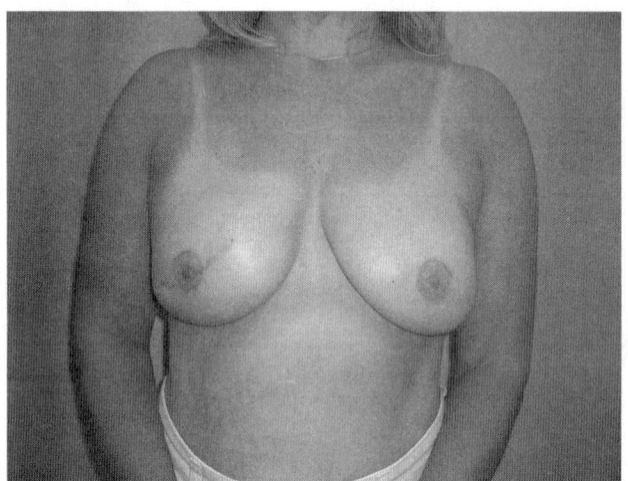

Figure 1   Right-sided implant based reconstruction after mastectomy. Left-sided deep inferior epigastric perforator flap–based reconstruction after mastectomy.

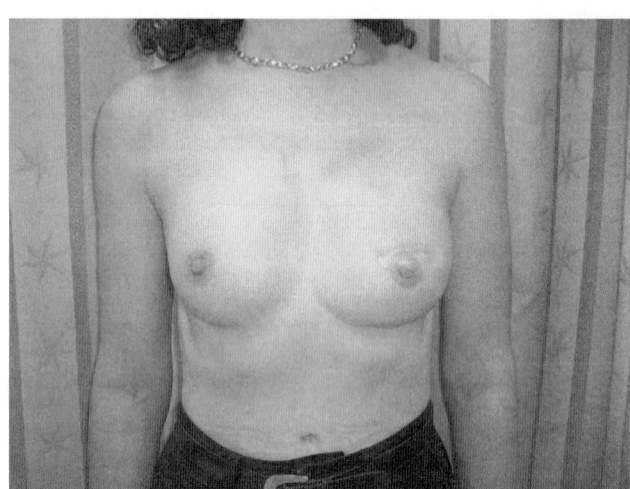

Figure 3   Left implant reconstruction.

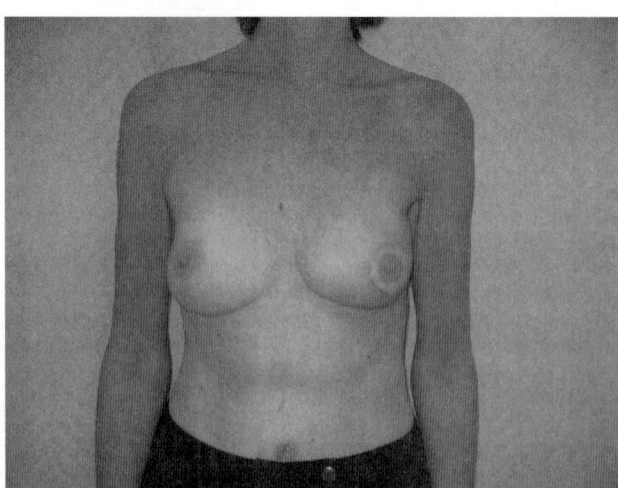

Figure 2   Left-sided deep inferior epigastric perforator flap.

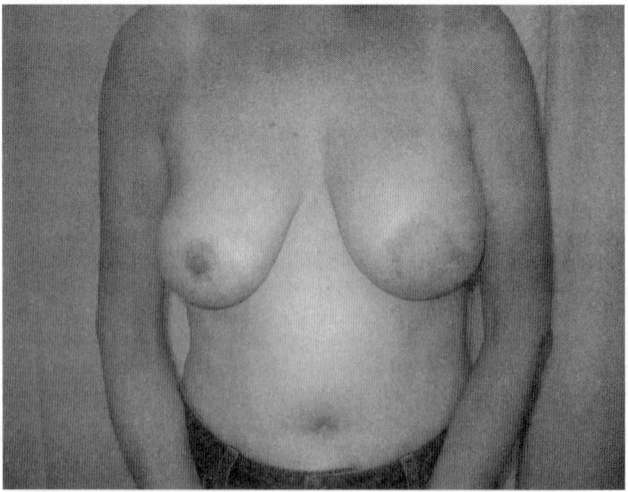

Figure 4   Left latissimus flap reconstruction with implant.

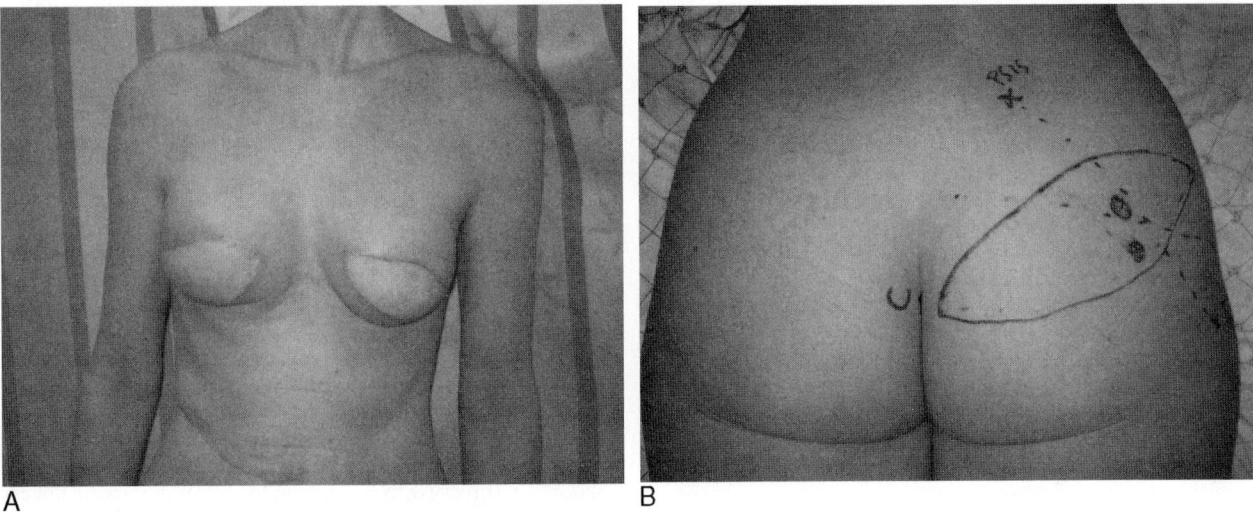

A   B

Figure 5 Bilateral superior gluteal artery flap reconstruction and buttock markings.

All implants have a significant risk of rupture—approximately 1% per year—and it is generally believed that 10% rupture by 10 years. Other risks include implant migration and "bottoming out," capsular contracture (as previously mentioned), infection, and (rarely) extrusion. Patients who have undergone or will undergo radiation therapy are much more likely to experience complications from breast implants compared with nonirradiated women. Patients must understand that as a result of these complications, most implants require reoperation for adjustment or replacement with time.

In general, implant reconstruction is the quickest type of reconstruction available in terms of length of operation. Most postmastectomy implants are placed subpectorally because the alternative subglandular method is not an option when the breast gland has been removed. Following mastectomy, the pectoralis major is dissected free from the chest wall along its inferior border. The subpectoral plane is then dissected, leaving intact the superior attachments and varying portions of the medial and lateral attachments on the basis of implant size. Because of the larger size implants that are often required to attempt to match the contralateral breast (rather than the relatively smaller implants that are used in purely cosmetic procedures to augment the preexisting breast tissue), a significant portion of the implant is often exposed without pectoralis major coverage. To increase the strength of tissue between the skin and the implant and to better support the implant along the IMF, acellular dermal matrices may be used to create a sling between the IMF and the detached inferior pectoralis muscle—the most common used being Alloderm (LifeCell, Branchburg, NJ).

Patients who have insufficient existing skin, either as a result of tumor biology requiring larger skin resection or because of skin contraction associated with delayed reconstructions, require tissue expansion. Adjustable implants incorporate a port for infusion of volume following surgery. Patients usually receive tissue expansion in the outpatient office weekly for 6 to 8 weeks. Some ports may remain permanently, whereas others should be removed as a separate procedure, often performed under local anesthesia. These devices provide an alternative to the more traditional method of temporary tissue expander placement followed by a second surgery through the mastectomy incision to replace the expander with a permanent implant.

AUTOLOGOUS RECONSTRUCTION

Breast reconstruction may also be accomplished with autologous tissue harvested from another region of the patient's body. The most widely used donor site is the abdomen. Current techniques include the pedicled transverse rectus abdominis myocutaneous (TRAM) flap, free TRAM flap, free deep inferior epigastric perforator (DIEP) fasiocutaneous flap, and free superficial inferior epigastric artery (SIEA) fasiocutaneous flap. When patients are not candidates for harvest from the abdomen because of insufficient tissue or prior abdominal procedures that may have eliminated necessary collateral blood supply, the latissimus dorsi muscle from the back can be used as pedicled or free tissue transfer. A further modification allows the thoracodorsal artery and vein perforators to be used to carry the soft tissues of the back while leaving the latissimus muscle intact and functional (TDAP flap). The skin and fat from the superior gluteal area can be harvested as a free tissue transfer from a perforating branch of the superior gluteal artery (SGAP flap).

The most basic distinction between types of autologous reconstruction is the use of pedicled versus free tissue transfer. Pedicled flaps require maintenance of the existing blood supply to the tissue that is transferred to the breast. This is accomplished by sacrificing the collateral, supplemental blood supply to the tissue while elevating a significant portion of the tissue mass. This is then shifted or rotated to the breast, but the tissue surrounding the remaining blood supply is left intact. Free tissue transfer is a more technically challenging procedure requiring (in addition to harvest of the donor tissue as in a pedicled procedure) isolation of the dominant blood supply to the donor tissue, dissection of these vessels for some distance along their course, division of the vessels, and reanastamosis under loupe or operating microscope magnification to recipient vessels in the breast pocket, which must also be located and dissected free from surrounding tissue.

Before the widespread use of microsurgery, the pedicled TRAM procedure was the autologous reconstruction of choice in breast surgery. This method requires a low transverse abdominal incision similar to that of an abdominoplasty, which is used to harvest abdominal skin and underlying subcutaneous tissue of sufficient volume to reconstruct the breast. The anterior rectus sheath is harvested, as is the majority of the rectus abdominis muscle. The deep inferior epigastric vessels are identified and sacrificed, and the rectus muscle is dissected free from its posterior sheath (or peritoneum below the arcuate line). The muscle serves as a conduit to protect the perforating vessels from the superior epigastric vessels that supply the skin and fat that are crucial to the breast reconstruction. This tissue must then be tunneled under the upper abdominal skin and subcutaneous fat and into the breast pocket, necessitating extensive undermining of the skin and fat of the entire anterior abdominal wall. This undermined tissue is then advanced inferiorly to allow closure of the abdominal defect, with relocation of the umbilicus as in a cosmetic abdominoplasty.

The pedicled TRAM procedure is acceptable for bilateral reconstructions but it may also be used for unilateral reconstructions. For unilateral procedures, tissue from either the contralateral or ipsilateral side may be used to recreate the breast. Use of contralateral tissue leaves a postoperative midline substernal bulge because of the bulk of the tissue protecting the blood supply, whereas ipsilateral tissue use effaces the inframammary fold in smaller-breasted women, again because of the bulk of the tissue around the pedicle. In addition to the suboptimal contour irregularities associated with the pedicled TRAM, it can be difficult to achieve final symmetry using this technique. Intraoperatively, the rectus abdominis muscles accounts for a significant portion of the bulk of the newly reconstructed breast. With time, however, this muscle will atrophy because of denervation, leaving a smaller breast. The amount of atrophy, and hence the final appearance of the reconstruction, can be difficult to estimate intraoperatively.

Certain patients are not ideal candidates for the pedicled TRAM procedure. Diabetic patients, smokers, and obese patients with extremely thick subcutaneous fat layers may experience more fat necrosis of both the breast flap and the extensively undermined areas of the abdomen. This results from insufficient blood supply to support the quantity of adipose tissue transferred and can lead to areas of wound breakdown and increased scarring, hardness that may mimic cancer recurrence and decrease the adequacy of the texture of the reconstruction, and contour irregularities that are aesthetically displeasing.

Patients who require a more robust blood supply to the reconstructed breast tissue are more appropriate candidates for free tissue transfer. The free TRAM procedure, similar to the pedicled TRAM, requires harvest of a significant portion of the rectus muscle and its fascia to protect the perforating branches of the blood vessels that supply the overlying skin and fat. However, in direct contrast to the pedicled TRAM reconstruction, free tissue transfer usually sacrifices the superior epigastric vessels, making the tissue dependent on the deep inferior epigastric vessels, which are isolated and dissected for a distance proximally along their course.

After these vessels have been adequately dissected, they must be divided and reconnected to recipient vessels in the chest. Axillary vessels such as the thoracodorsals or thoracoacromials, internal mammary perforators, and the internal mammary vessels themselves (ipsilateral or contralateral, following rib resection) are all possible candidates. These vessels, too, must be meticulously identified and dissected free from their surroundings to facilitate microscopic anastomosis.

In an effort to minimize morbidity associated with the procedure, most free TRAM procedures are now performed with minimal amounts of harvested muscle. Despite repair or reconstruction of the anterior rectus sheath following either pedicled or free TRAM harvest, studies have shown postoperative abdominal bulges in this area that are displeasing to the patients. Authors have also reported significantly decreased functionality of the abdominal wall following harvest of the majority of, or even a limited portion of, rectus abdominis muscle. Other authors feel that the functional limitations following rectus harvest are limited to specific activities such as performance of sit-ups, which may be considered superfluous in the majority of the target population.

Because the abdominal wall morbidity of the TRAM procedure can be considered significant, the use of the free DIEP flap has recently been on the rise. This procedure is more technically challenging than the free TRAM. It requires identification of a dominant deep inferior epigastric perforator artery and vein as they pierce the anterior rectus sheath and enter the subcutaneous fat of the abdominal wall. After an appropriate candidate perforator bundle has been identified, these vessels must be dissected free from the surrounding rectus muscle along their entire course until they meet the deep inferior epigastric vessels, increasing the risk of injury to the vessels during the procedure. This procedure allows for preservation of the entire rectus muscle and its sheath, thereby minimizing abdominal wall complications. To facilitate identification of these perforators, some centers use Doppler or three-dimensional computed tomography angiograms to preoperatively map perforators.

The free SIEA flap is another alternative reconstructive technique aimed at avoiding damage to the abdominal wall. This procedure depends on identification of the superficial inferior epigastric artery and vein within the subcutaneous tissue of the abdominal wall. As with the other free tissue transfers, these vessels are then freed along their course, harvested with the fat and skin they supply, and anastamosed to recipient vessels in the chest. However, these vessels are found to be missing or of inadequate size in more than half of patients, making this an unreliable initial reconstructive plan.

As previously mentioned, women who have no abdominal pannus or who have had prior abdominoplasty procedures or extensive abdominal surgery with multiple abdominal wall scars are not candidates for autologous reconstruction using the abdomen. In these circumstances, the latissimus dorsi muscle and overlying skin and fat may be transferred as a pedicled or free flap based on the thoracodorsal artery and vein. Loss of this muscle is well tolerated and leads to minimal functional impairment. However, seromas are frequent at the donor site, and the tissue is often of insufficient bulk to create a breast of sufficient size, necessitating use of an implant in addition to the autologous tissue. A modification of the latissimus flap using perforator techniques developed in the abdominal harvest of DIEP flaps allows a thoracodorsal artery perforator to be dissected in continuity with the overlying skin and fat while sparing the entire latissimus muscle. The TDAP flap requires meticulous dissection but is applicable in those patients with higher shoulder-girdle demand, such as avid swimmers, golfers, and tennis players.

The skin and subcutaneous tissue overlying the superior gluteal region can also be harvested as a free tissue transfer from perforating branches of the superior gluteal artery and vein. Unfortunately, the harvest of these vessels is technically challenging. Additionally, the vessels are often short, sometimes necessitating vein grafts as conduits to provide sufficient length between the recipient chest vessels and the donor vessels arranged to provide optimal breast shape.

Any free tissue transfer is an extremely complex procedure and carries significant risks, including total flap loss. Intraoperative anticoagulation and varying regimens of postoperative anticoagulation are aimed at preventing arterial and venous thrombosis. Either complication can lead to necrosis of the transferred tissue, thus intensive postoperative monitoring of the tissue and of the patient's fluid status and hemoglobin levels is necessary to minimize complications. If changes become evident in the flap, immediate return to the operating room may salvage the tissue in certain circumstances, but not all. Given the complexity of the technique, longer operating times are required, and frequent use of the internal mammary vessels prevents later cardiac revascularization with these vessels. Therefore free tissue transfer is not always considered a viable option in the older or sicker mastectomy patients.

SECONDARY PROCEDURES

Following reconstruction of the volume of the affected breast, women often undergo reconstruction of the nipple approximately 6 weeks postoperatively. This may be accomplished with myriad local flaps designed to create a small projection and is often performed under local anesthesia. Small adjustments to the reconstructed breast, including axillary liposuction, scar revision, and dog-ear resection, can also be performed at this time. Tattooing of the areolar complex is usually performed in the outpatient setting 6 weeks after creation of the nipple papillae.

Symmetry can be difficult to achieve with even the best breast reconstruction if the native breast is extremely large or aged and ptotic. Contralateral mastopexy, reduction mammaplasty, or mastopexy with augmentation are all treatments that may be applied to the native breast to achieve symmetry. However, these procedures do lead to additional scarring. Rearrangement of the breast tissue or augmentation may also be a concern to patients who are considering cancer surveillance. Reduction mammaplasty has not been shown to impair mammography, and special techniques are employed to perform mammograms on augmented breasts. However, areas of scarring or fat necrosis may be evident on mammograms and necessitate biopsies and further workup.

CONCLUSIONS

Given the large numbers of women affected by breast cancer, breast reconstruction is a frequently performed procedure for which there will likely be increased demand with time. Many studies have shown that women benefit physically and psychologically when given the option to undergo breast reconstruction following mastectomy. There is currently a wealth of techniques available to the reconstructive surgeon, but new frontiers remain to be explored to optimize the form and function of the reconstructed breast.

SUGGESTED READINGS

Disa JJ, McCarthy CM: Breast reconstruction: a comparison of autogenous and prosthetic techniques, *Adv Surg* 39:97, 2005.

Elliott LF, Hartrampf CR Jr: Breast reconstruction: progress in the past decade, *World J Surg* 14:763, 1990.

Granzow JW, Levine LJ, Chiu ES, and others: Breast reconstruction using perforator flaps, *J Surg Oncol* 94:441, 2006.

Kronowitz SJ, Juerer HM: Advances and surgical decision-making for breast reconstruction, *Cancer* 107L893, 2006.

Nahabedian MY, Dooley W, Singh N, and others: Contour abnormalities of the abdomen after breast reconstruction with abdominal flaps: the role of muscle preservation, *Plast Reconstr Surg* 109:91, 2006.

Spear SL, Ducic I, Low M, and others: The effect of radiation on pedicled TRAM flap breast reconstruction: outcomes and implications, *Plast Reconstr Surg* 115:84, 2005.

CHEST WALL, MEDIASTINUM, TRACHEA

CHEST WALL TRAUMA

Paul Freeswick, MD, and B. Robert Gibson, MD

GENERAL CONSIDERATIONS

The chest wall, comprising the ribs, spine, manubrium, and shoulder girdle, along with their associated soft tissues, performs two critical functions. The first is to provide protection for the underlying vital structures: the heart, great vessels, and lungs. The second is to provide an airtight structure capable of maintaining negative inspiratory pressure generated by the diaphragm in ventilating the lungs. Trauma to the chest wall should thus be assumed to involve at least one of these functions, and usually there is substantial involvement of both.

INCIDENCE AND ETIOLOGY

Chest wall trauma is second only to head injury as the leading cause of trauma-associated death. Worldwide there are more than 12 million reported cases per year, with approximately 10% of these occurring in the United States. Overall, chest wall trauma is responsible for 25% of trauma mortality and is a contributing factor in another 25%. Up to 30% of these injuries require hospitalization (≈400,000/year in the United States) and, given the often life-threatening nature of chest wall and associated injuries, they use a disproportionate amount of available health care resources.

Approximately 80% of chest wall trauma in the United States is secondary to a blunt mechanism of injury, with the preponderance involving motor vehicle collisions (70%–80%), followed by motorcycle crashes, falls, recreational injury, workplace injury, and assault. The overall U.S. experience has been that 20% of chest wall trauma is attributable to penetrating causes, most commonly gunshot and stab wounds. This ratio of 80% blunt to 20% penetrating trauma is only a generalization and will fluctuate with the referral area of a trauma center and the demographics within that area. Urban centers typically see a larger proportion of penetrating injuries and rural/suburban a larger proportion of blunt.

ASSOCIATED INJURIES

Up to 25% of patients presenting with a chest wall injury may have one or more associated injuries. It is important to process all the information available because missed concomitant injuries can lead to significant morbidity and mortality. Data obtained at the scene of a motor vehicle accident by the emergency response team can be helpful. Information such as the following are all correlates of a high-energy impact and help to notify the trauma team that there is an increased likelihood of associated injury mode of impact (head-on, side, or rollover), airbag deployment, significant intrusion (>24 inches) into the passenger compartment, prolonged extrication time, whether the patient was thrown from the vehicle, whether the patient was wearing a seatbelt, and on-scene fatality. Penetrating injuries, although dramatic, require operative intervention in less than 15% of cases. The mechanism of injury is paramount. Stab wounds in general carry a better prognosis than gunshot wounds, and among the latter, injury caused by low-velocity missiles (handguns) is usually less involved than injury arising from high-velocity (rifle) injuries. This relates to the disproportionate amount of kinetic energy imparted by projectile velocity as opposed to projectile mass (KE = mv2). In penetrating injuries, the size and location of the visible wound may not relate to the amount of internal damage, and the worst-case scenario should be considered.

Beyond the historical data, there are some specific fractures to the chest wall that may be associated with an increased likelihood of particular injuries, the most significant of these being first rib, second rib, and scapular fractures. In the trauma literature, it has been maintained that any of these fractures is associated with a great vessel injury. With time and further analysis, this association has not proved true, although these injuries do indicate a high level of energy involved in the trauma and rarely occur in isolation. Up to 75% of these patients have significant associated injuries including the chest, abdomen, or extremities. Given the associated morbidity and mortality of these injuries, a careful and thorough secondary survey is crucial.

Lateral midshaft rib fractures that occur in a direction away from the pleural cavity reflect anterior-posterior compression mediated injury, which frequently does not involve the pulmonary parenchyma. On the other hand, direct impact injuries with rib fracture are often associated with pulmonary contusion and may involve intercostal artery laceration. Sternal fractures may be associated with cardiac contusion and posterior dislocation of the sternoclavicular joint, which may impinge on the vessels and nerves of the thoracic inlet.

Special consideration must be given to patients from either extreme of age. In the elderly, there is a progressive change in the structure and strength of the thorax. Progressive kyphosis and osteoporosis occur, leading to mechanical and protective disadvantages. Concomitant underlying cardiorespiratory changes result in a reduced physiologic reserve, making this population ill equipped to handle the stress of even minor trauma. A low threshold for admitting and observing this patient populace is therefore highly recommended, with the goal of admission being aggressive management of pulmonary toilet and pain. Further consideration is also warranted with regard to the workup of these patients. As patients age, the likelihood of significant comorbidities increases; therefore clinically relevant comorbidities should be aggressively sought during the history and physical examination. Certain common conditions in the elderly, such as atrial fibrillation and hypertension, should lead one to ask about possible anticoagulant therapy or beta-blocker therapy, which could lead to increased bleeding or a blunted reflex tachycardia, respectively.

The pediatric population is unique in that its ribcage is extremely pliable; therefore the absence of rib fracture or superficial soft-tissue injury should not be interpreted as reflecting a lack of underlying pathology. Consideration to mechanism of injury and increased clinical suspicion are always prudent when evaluating this patient population. Furthermore, children have a greater cardiovascular reserve than adults and are capable of compensating for large physiologic insults while maintaining relatively normal vital signs in the face of catastrophic injury. Patients in this compensated state may be misinterpreted as being stable when in reality they are prone to a subsequent precipitous decline in status. Therefore an expeditious workup is warranted, even in the apparently "stable" pediatric patient.

INITIAL MANAGEMENT

Patients with chest wall injuries undergo the same triage and initial management as any other trauma patient. An adequate airway must be ensured, breathing established, and circulation supported (the ABCs). One caveat to the approach of the chest-injured patient, especially when significant pulmonary contusion is suspected, would be to consider restricting intravenous fluid administration. Only in the face of intact circulation and adequate organ perfusion should this algorithm be considered. This may be useful to reduce the physiologic impact of pulmonary contusion that frequently accompanies chest wall injuries. Supplemental oxygen should be placed on all patients until the workup is complete.

PHYSICAL EXAMINATION

Inspection of the entire skin surface to delineate abrasions, contusions, lacerations, and deformity is mandatory in all patients brought to the attention of the trauma service. Chest wall symmetry, even expansion and contraction, paradoxical movement, and splinting should be noted. Although the absence of paradoxical motion does not rule out flail segment (because patients may be able to splint during the initial exam), its presence signifies a potentially life-threatening injury. Palpation may reveal point tenderness associated with rib fractures and crepitus associated with pneumothorax or lung injury. The presence of lower lateral rib (9–12) tenderness on the right or left may signify liver or spleen injury, respectively. Auscultation may reveal decreased or absent breath sounds associated with pneumothorax or hemopneumothorax. Bruits or murmurs may accompany great vessel or cardiac injury.

Serial physical examinations must be performed to detect ongoing physiologic changes. Flail segment and pneumothorax may present in a delayed fashion. Pulmonary contusion may not "blossom" for 24 to 48 hours. Vigilance can be key to making the diagnosis for those who make a delayed presentation.

RADIOLOGY AND LABORATORY TESTS

A chest radiograph should be obtained in all trauma patients as soon after admission as possible. Good imagery of the skeletal structures of the chest wall is as important as imaging the heart, lungs, and great vessels. Again, scapular or first and second rib

fractures represent a high-energy mechanism of injury and are associated with other injuries approximately 75% of the time. Lower rib fractures may be associated with liver or spleen injuries, sternal fractures with cardiac contusion, and posterior sternoclavicular dislocation with injury or compression of the vessels and nerves of the thoracic outlet. Multiple rib fractures and flail segments (at least three consecutive ribs fractured in two separate places) may also be associated with underlying hemopneumothorax and pulmonary contusion.

Recently there has been growing support for whole body imaging in blunt multisystem trauma, even in patients without obvious signs of injury. There is no question that computed tomography (CT) scans are more sensitive and specific than traditional radiology. The advent of extremely sophisticated and fast multidetector array CT scanners with high resolution and immediately available multiplanar reconstructions may indeed be a valuable tool in the future. For instance, even in patients with no evidence of chest trauma, up to 20% may have abnormalities.

Laboratory analysis should include the usual trauma laboratory tests; in addition, an arterial blood gas test may be useful for determination of the A-a gradient in the elderly and patients exhibiting respiratory compromise, but it is not necessary for those without signs or symptoms of respiratory difficulty. Cardiac enzymes have fallen out of favor as a routine test for cardiac contusion. However, serial enzymes may be useful in patients who are symptomatic or who have documented electrocardiographic changes suggestive of a myocardial event. In this situation, inpatient observation and cardiac monitoring are warranted.

SPECIFIC INJURIES

Sucking Chest Wound

The most dramatic injury to the chest wall is the sucking chest wound. This occurs when a defect in the chest wall allows for preferential air entry through the chest wall as opposed to the tracheobronchial tree on initiation of a negative pressure breath. The defect can be as small as 2 cm, and immediate treatment is vital. Wound coverage using an occlusive dressing taped on three sides is required. This dressing forms a valve that allows air from the pleural cavity to escape while preventing ingress of air during inspiration. Care must be taken to avoid making a totally occlusive dressing because a tension pneumothorax may result if there is an underlying lung injury. Larger defects in the chest wall involving significant tissue loss may require rotational muscle flaps or prosthetic material for definitive treatment.

Flail Chest

Flail chest results when external force results in multiple rib fractures with two or more fractures within each rib. The classic definition is three or more consecutive ribs fractured in at least two places. Patients with this injury may not present with the classical paradoxical chest wall motion (collapse on inspiration and protrusion on expiration) of the affected segment. Of note, delayed presentation of this injury is common because patients are often able to splint the injury with intercostal muscle spasm, and this can lead to a delay in presentation as late as 9 days following the initial injury. Although it is true that the "bellows" action of the rib cage is compromised, ventilatory and oxygen deficits are most likely secondary to underlying lung injury and not due to an overall decrease in tidal volume.

More than 50% of these patients have a concomitant pulmonary contusion. Treatment of this injury is heavily centered on pain management and pulmonary toilet to prevent subsequent atelectasis and pneumonia. Positive pressure ventilation may be required in up to 50% of cases. Intercostal nerve blocks (both sides of fracture plus one rib above and one below) along with intrapleural catheters delivering long-acting local anaesthetics are frequently beneficial. For fractures in the lower rib cage (T5 or below), a continuous epidural catheter often is a helpful adjunct (provided the patient does not have a concurrent axial skeletal injury). Narcotic use is almost always necessary. Pulmonary toilet via incentive spirometry, nasotracheal suction, and chest physiotherapy are mandatory. Despite intensive therapy, up to 50% of these patients progress to pneumonia, and up to 25% develop pleural effusions. Bronchoscopy along with thoracentesis and appropriate antibiotic therapy covering gram-negative organisms should be employed. Long-term sequelae include chronic chest wall pain, chest deformity on chest film, and dyspnea on exertion in up to 70% of patients.

Simple Rib Fracture

This injury occurs as a result of chest wall compression on direct impact. The diagnosis is frequently clinical because routine radiography misses up to 50% of fractures. Point tenderness and pain on respiration are diagnostic. Computerized tomography or a designated "rib series" of plain films are more sensitive but rarely necessary because the management required for a rib fracture is the same. Underlying pulmonary contusion is infrequent. It is important to consider injury to the spleen or liver when the lower ribs in the lateral position are the site of fracture. Again, management is focused on pain control and pulmonary toilet to prevent subsequent atelectasis and pneumonia. Infrequently, rib blocks or narcotic analgesia may be necessary. After the initial evaluation, pain in many patients can be managed with nonsteroidal anti-inflammatory medications. Overall, prognosis is good; however, patients should be counseled that the pain associated with rib fracture can persist for months, not weeks, and that pain management and pulmonary toilet are directed toward preventing atelectasis and the increased pneumonia risk associated with decreased diaphragmatic excursion. Therefore the cornerstone of management is adequate analgesia and pulmonary toilet.

▮ STERNAL FRACTURE

Sternal fractures occur in approximately 5% of patients who experience blunt force chest trauma. Typically these injuries occur via sudden deceleration or by a direct blow to the anterior chest. Sternal fractures typically occur at the body or manubrium and are often missed on plain or chest radiography. Frequently they are picked up on subsequent chest CT when the patient undergoes completion of trauma workup. It was previously thought that cardiac contusion or other cardiac injury was commonly associated with sternal fractures. This is not necessarily the case, particularly in fractures that are minimally displaced. Currently the extent of cardiac workup indicated following sternal fracture alone would be limited to a 12-lead electrocardiograph. If there is no ectopy or change in rhythm from baseline, the workup is complete. If there is ectopy or a change in rhythm, 24 hours of observation on telemetry may be warranted. The use of cardiac enzymes in this context has been found to have minimal clinical utility. In an asymptomatic patient, there is little justification for a more extensive workup beyond a 12-lead electrocardiogram. Sternal fracture is associated with other injury, particularly rib fracture, which can be found in up to 40% of patients. Generally pain control is adequate management for minimally displaced fractures. Cases of severe displacement and instability may require operative fixation.

Clavicle Fracture

Clavicle fractures are common, and the majority (75%) occur at the middle third of the bone. The injury usually occurs after a fall or lateral force directed toward the shoulder. The majority of these injuries may be managed by a simple figure of eight splint and pain management. Infrequently, severe displacement or malunion may occur, which may require operative fixation.

Scapular Fracture

As previously stated, scapular fractures can be indicative of high-energy trauma and are associated with other significant injury in up to 75% of cases. Typically these fractures are managed nonoperatively. However, a fracture through the glenoid, acromion, or the coracoid process may require open reduction and internal fixation to preserve normal shoulder girdle function.

Sternoclavicular Dislocation

Sternoclavicular dislocation, although uncommon, represents a significant high-force injury to the chest wall. It is associated with other chest injuries in up to two thirds of patients. Anterior dislocations far outnumber posterior dislocations and are diagnosed most commonly on physical examination. There is pain with shoulder movement and a palpable bony protuberance. Anterior dislocations are generally managed with conscious sedation and closed reduction. Posterior dislocation, although far less common, may be associated with injury or compression of the vessels, nerves, or other structures of the thoracic inlet. These injuries are often occult, being identified on CT scan, and require operative reduction and internal fixation when discovered.

Chest Wall Contusion

Chest wall contusion represents injury to the deep soft tissues of the chest wall. Care must be taken to look for associated injuries. In female patients, involvement of the breast may lead to a significant tense, tender breast wall hematoma. Management generally consists of wound care and pain management. Judicious use of operative intervention is warranted if skin necrosis may be impending. More often than not, operative findings reveal diffuse tissue bruising with no identifiable drainable collection or bleeding site.

Traumatic Asphyxia

Traumatic asphyxia occurs with significant compression and crush injury to the chest wall. It is frequently associated with intra-abdominal injuries as well. The syndrome is characterized by a constellation of upper extremity, torso and facial cyanosis, edema, and petechial hemorrhages. This occurs secondary to superior vena cava compression and frequently also results in cerebral edema. Altered mental status and seizures commonly occur. Treatment is supportive and, barring associated injuries, outcome is generally good. Cerebral symptoms commonly resolve in 24 to 48 hours.

Blast Lung Injury

With the recent increase in global terrorism and military conflict, injury to the lung resulting from terrorist attacks is unfortunately rising. Blast lung injury is a major immediate cause of death at the scene of these attacks. It results from a pressure wave that causes acute compression of the chest wall, resulting in an acute transient rise in intrathoracic pressure. This compressive wave results in alveolar rupture and capillary disruption with resultant hemorrhage and edema. All patients will have concomitant injuries, including 100% with ruptured tympanic membranes and 50% with burn injury. Fractures, amputations, and intra-abdominal (particularly hollow viscus) injuries are also common and are due both to the initial concussive blast and to secondary projectiles. Diagnosis is based on clinical symptoms and presentation and the classic "butterfly" sign on chest film. This is seen as a progressive infiltrate from the pulmonary hilum spreading out distally in a butterfly pattern. Treatment is supportive with mechanical ventilation and pulmonary toilet. Mortality approaches 5%. Posttreatment, most patients revert to normal or nearly normal lung function.

SUGGESTED READINGS

Avidan V, Hersch M, Armon Y, and others: Blast lung injury: clinical manifestations, treatment, and outcome, *Am J Surg* 160:945, 2005.

Kent R, Lee SH, Darvish K, and others: Structural and material changes in the aging thorax and their role in crash protection for older occupants, *Stapp Car Crash J* 49:231, 2005.

Mayberry JC, Wanek S: Blunt thoracic trauma: flail chest, pulmonary contusion, and blast injury, *Crit Care Clin* 20:71, 2004.

Salim A, Sangthong B, Martin M, and others: Whole body imaging in blunt multisystem trauma patients without obvious signs of injury, *Arch Surg* 141:468, 2006.

Trinkle JK, Richardson JD, Frank JL, and others: Management of flail chest without mechanical ventilation, *Ann Thorac Surg* 19:355, 1975.

Yee WY, Cameron PA, Bailey MJ: Road traffic injuries in the elderly, *Em Med J* 23:42, 2006.

PRIMARY CHEST WALL TUMORS

Leora B. Balsam, MD, and Richard I. Whyte, MD, MBA

INTRODUCTION

Tumors of the chest wall include both primary and metastatic lesions. Metastatic lesions from primary carcinomas and sarcomas comprise nearly half of chest wall tumors; the remainder arise primarily from the chest wall structures. Primary chest wall tumors are rare and constitute only 1% to 2% of all primary tumors and 5% of all thoracic neoplasms. They can be categorized into two dominant types on the basis of the tissue of origin: (1) bony and cartilaginous tumors and (2) soft-tissue tumors. Nearly half of primary chest wall tumors are benign lesions; the other half are malignant. The most common benign lesions are chondromas and fibrous dysplasia (which presents as a mass but is not, technically, a neoplasm), and the most common malignant lesions are chondrosarcoma in the adult population and Ewing's sarcoma in the pediatric population. A survey of benign and malignant primary chest wall tumors is provided in Table 1. The mean age at presentation is 26 years for benign tumors and 40 years for malignant tumors. With the exception of desmoid tumors, primary chest wall tumors are twice as frequent in males than females.

These tumors present unique diagnostic and therapeutic challenges on the basis of their biological behavior and anatomic location. The general diagnostic approach and the surgical principles of chest wall resection and reconstruction are discussed in this chapter.

PRESENTATION AND DIAGNOSTIC EVALUATION

Primary chest wall tumors present in three ways. The majority present as painless enlarging chest wall masses. A smaller group presents with pain, often a late finding caused by pathologic bone fractures or compression of structures by the expanding tumor. Pain is more common with malignant tumors, although one third of benign tumors result in pain as well. A third group of patients presents asymptomatically with tumors that are discovered incidentally on imaging studies performed for other reasons.

Table 1: Primary Chest Wall Tumors

Benign
Chondroma
Fibrous dysplasia
Osteochondroma
Lipoma
Fibroma
Neurilemmoma
Eosinophilic granuloma
Aneurysmal bone cyst
Osteoid osteoma
Osteoblastoma
Giant cell tumor

Malignant
Chondrosarcoma
Osteosarcoma
Liposarcoma
Malignant fibrous histiocytoma
Rhabdomyosarcoma
Angiosarcoma
Fibrosarcoma
Neurofibrosarcoma
Ewing's sarcoma and primitive neuroectodermal tumor
Plasmacytoma

Imaging studies are a useful adjunct in the diagnostic process and are an absolute necessity for surgical planning. Typical studies include standard radiographs of the chest, as well as computed tomography (CT) and magnetic resonance imaging (MRI). Because many benign and malignant chest wall tumors have characteristic radiographic appearances, these studies may help in the diagnostic process. CT is used to evaluate tumor extent and identify pulmonary metastases, whereas MRI is particularly useful for identifying invasion into contiguous structures. Bone scans have a limited role but are helpful in the differentiation of solitary plasmacytoma from multiple myeloma and in the identification of polyostotic fibrous dysplasia.

After they are identified, primary chest wall tumors require a histologic diagnosis. Excisional biopsies are preferred for tumors less than 4 cm in diameter, whereas incisional biopsies may be performed for larger tumors. In the case of incisional biopsies, several principles must be followed. One should avoid raising skin flaps because seeding of malignant cells has been reported. Moreover, the biopsy incision should be positioned in a manner that allows for reexcision if pathologic analysis demonstrates malignancy. Core needle biopsies may be used as an alternative to incisional biopsies, although seeding of the biopsy tract may occur and tissue may be insufficient for diagnosis. For cartilaginous tumors, excisional biopsy is preferred for both small and large lesions because the histologic appearance of the tumor may not be uniform—that is, because some areas may be bland and others malignant, a limited incisional biopsy may result in a misdiagnosis.

TREATMENT APPROACH

Most primary chest wall tumors are treated with wide local excision. Acceptable margins of excision for benign lesions are 2 cm or less, whereas most malignant chest wall tumors should be resected with 4-cm margins. Many of these tumors are locally aggressive, and the incidence of tumor recurrence correlates with the presence of positive surgical margins. Negative margins 4 cm in size are associated with significantly lower local recurrence rates than margins 2 cm in size. One study reported a 56% 5-year freedom from recurrence in patients with malignant primary chest wall tumors resected with 4-cm margins, compared with 29% in a cohort resected with 2-cm margins. Given the location of chest wall tumors, it may be difficult to obtain wide surgical margins circumferentially; adjuvant external beam irradiation or intraoperative radiation therapy has been used in these cases to improve local control.

A small group of malignant chest wall tumors is treated nonoperatively (with chemotherapy and/or radiation) or with combined modality therapy (consisting of chemotherapy, surgery, and radiation therapy). These include plasmacytomas, which are treated with radiation, and the small round cell tumors (Ewing's sarcoma and primary neuroectodermal tumors), which are treated with a combination of chemotherapy and radiation.

BENIGN PRIMARY CHEST WALL TUMORS

In this section, features of the most common benign primary chest wall tumors are discussed. Treatment is primarily surgical.

Chondroma

Chondromas are benign cartilaginous tumors that typically arise anteriorly from cartilage at the costochondral junction and are the most common benign chest wall tumor. Radiographically, they appear as lobulated, well-demarcated osteolytic lesions with well-defined sclerotic margins. There is a 1% to 2% incidence of malignant transformation to chondrosarcoma. Radiographically, it may be difficult to differentiate between chondromas and chondrosarcomas; consequently, treatment is with local excision.

Fibrous Dysplasia

Fibrous dysplasia is a disorder in which osteoblasts fail to undergo normal differentiation and maturation. The result is a benign tumor that is monostotic in 70% to 80% of cases and polyostotic in 20% to 30% of cases. Fibrous dysplasia constitutes approximately 30% of benign chest wall tumors. It usually occurs in the posterior or lateral aspect of the rib and may be associated with a prior

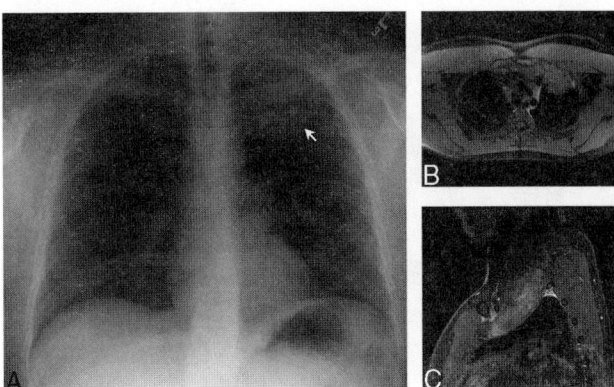

Figure 1 Fibrous dysplasia of the chest wall. Chest radiograph **(A)** and T1-weighted magnetic resonance axial **(B)** and sagittal images **(C)** demonstrating left chest wall fibrous dysplasia.

history of trauma. Most cases present in the second and third decade of life. Most patients are asymptomatic, although occasionally the tumor may lead to a pathologic fracture and resultant pain. Radiographic findings include a fusiform mass with amorphous or irregular calcification and cortical thickening (Fig. 1). Ground-glass appearance in the central aspect of the rib is characteristic. Local excision is performed for symptomatic painful enlarging masses and is curative. Excision of an asymptomatic rib lesion is generally not necessary; however, it may be appropriate in other locations to prevent deformity or pathologic fracture.

Osteochondroma

These tumors are cartilage-capped bony growths that usually occur anteriorly at the costochondral junction. The peak incidence is in the second decade of life. Radiographic features include a pedunculated osseous protuberance with cortical and medullary continuity with the bone of origin. Osteochondromas may lead to pathologic fractures or nerve compression. Malignant degeneration is rare but should be suspected in patients with new onset of pain at the lesion site and thickening of the characteristic cartilage cap documented on imaging studies. Treatment of osteochondromas is with local excision.

MALIGNANT PRIMARY CHEST WALL TUMORS

In this section, features of the most common malignant primary chest wall tumors are discussed. Surgery is the mainstay of treatment for the sarcomas, whereas multimodality therapy is the standard for small round cell tumors. Plasmacytomas are treated with high-dose radiation therapy.

Chondrosarcoma

Chondrosarcomas are the most common malignant primary chest wall tumor. These tumors constitute 50% of all malignant primary chest wall tumors and 25% of all primary chest wall tumors. They typically present between ages 30 and 60 years and may develop de novo or in previously benign cartilaginous tumors. They arise anteriorly from the ribs in 80% of cases and from the sternum in 20% of cases. Radiographically, the typical appearance of a chondrosarcoma is one of a lobulated mass arising from the medullary portion of a rib or the sternum, often with associated cortical bone destruction (see Fig. 2). Treatment consists of wide local

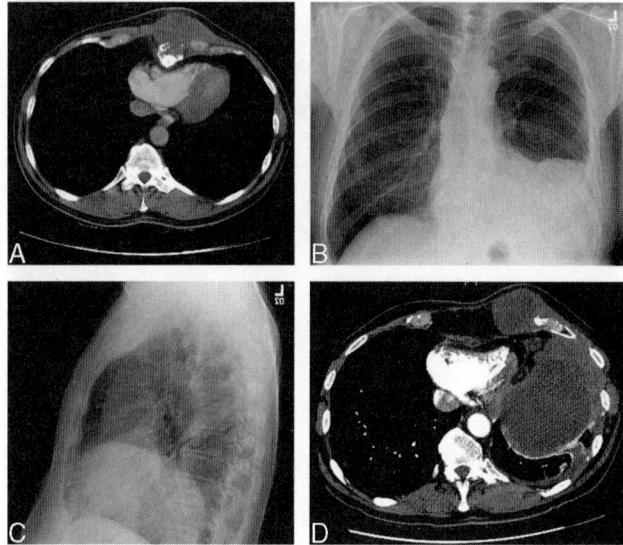

Figure 2   Chondrosarcoma of the sternum. Computed tomography (CT) scan **(A)** demonstrates a chondrosarcoma of the lower sternum and xiphoid. This tumor recurred 4 years after resection. Chest radiograph **(B and C)** and CT scan **(D)** of recurrent chest wall chondrosarcoma.

excision. For tumors that originate in the sternum, sternectomy with excision of bilateral costal arches is indicated. Chondrosarcomas are relatively chemoresistant and radioresistant, although postoperative radiation therapy has been used for local control for resections with positive margins. Five-year survival after surgical resection is 60% for all patients and 80% for patients without evidence of metastatic disease. Local recurrence rates for all patients are approximately 20%. Recurrence in patients with adequate surgical margins was reported as 10% in one series, compared with 75% in those with inadequate margins. Furthermore, mortality at 5 years was twofold higher in the patients with local recurrence in this series. Metastatic disease, when it occurs, most frequently involves the lung. Poor prognostic factors for chondrosarcomas include high tumor grade, large tumor size, incomplete resection, local recurrence, presence of metastatic disease, and age older than 50 years.

Osteosarcoma

Although osteosarcomas commonly originate from the metaphysis of long bones, occasionally they originate from a rib, scapula, or clavicle. Most chest wall osteosarcomas present in young adults as a painful mass. Less often, they may present in the elderly in association with prior irradiation, Paget's disease, or chemotherapy. Radiographic findings include a classic sunburst pattern of new periosteal bone formation. A multimodality treatment strategy is used, beginning with preoperative chemotherapy and followed by wide local excision. Long-term survival for patients with chest wall osteosarcomas is poor, with only a 15% reported 5-year survival. Of the 70% of patients who develop metastases, 5-year survival is 0%. Poor prognostic factors include poor response to preoperative chemotherapy and multifocal disease.

Soft-Tissue Sarcoma

Fifty percent of primary chest wall sarcomas are soft-tissue sarcomas. This diverse group of tumors includes liposarcomas, malignant fibrous histiocytomas, rhabdomyosarcomas, angiosarcomas, and fibrosarcomas. Each has characteristic radiographic features.

Wide local excision is the mainstay of treatment, although adjuvant radiation therapy may be useful for inadequate margins of resection and recurrences. Chemotherapy is also used in the treatment of rhabdomyosarcoma in which protocols of neoadjuvant chemotherapy followed by surgical excision confer a survival advantage at 5 years of 70% compared with 25% for surgical excision alone. Poor prognostic factors for chest wall soft-tissue sarcomas include high tumor grade, positive surgical margins, and presence of metastatic disease.

Desmoid Tumors

These locally aggressive tumors are actually considered to be low-grade fibrosarcomas, but they have unique characteristics that warrant further discussion. Whereas 50% of desmoids arise in the abdomen, the chest wall is the most common extra-abdominal site of origin (10% to 20%). Desmoids present most often in women of reproductive age. Predisposing factors include a history of trauma (present in 25% of cases), Gardner's syndrome, and estrogen exposure. These tumors are characterized by local invasion and frequent recurrences; they do not metastasize. Wide local excision is the primary treatment. Radiation may be used as an adjunct for incomplete resection. Anecdotal studies on the use of antiestrogen therapy have also been reported. A recent report from the Mayo Clinic demonstrates a 37.5% 5-year probability of local recurrence after resection. Recurrence occurred in 89% of cases with positive margins of excision and in 18% of cases with negative margins.

Ewing's Sarcoma and Primitive Neuroectodermal Tumor

Ewing's sarcoma and primitive neuroectodermal tumor (PNET or Askin's tumor) are small round-cell tumors with local and systemic manifestations. Both are associated with a translocation between chromosomes 11 and 22 and occur predominantly in children and young adults. Ewing's sarcoma arises from the chest wall in 15% of cases and is the most common primary chest wall malignancy in children. Presentation is with a painful mass and associated systemic signs, including fever and malaise. Characteristic radiographic findings are a chest wall mass with bony destruction and an onion-peel appearance caused by multiple layers of new periosteal bone formation. Treatment requires a multidisciplinary approach, including neoadjuvant multidrug chemotherapy followed by wide surgical excision. Radiation is often used for additional local control, and adjuvant chemotherapy may prevent or treat metastases. A recent study found a 5-year event-free survival (defined as freedom from disease progression, death, or diagnosis of second malignant neoplasm) of 56% using a multimodality treatment strategy. Overall 5-year survival has been reported as 50% to 65% in various single-institutional studies.

Plasmacytoma

Solitary plasmacytomas, tumors of plasma cell origin, constitute 10% to 30% of primary chest wall malignancies. They occur most frequently in the rib, followed by the clavicle and sternum. Evaluation includes excisional biopsy, imaging studies, and serum and urine electrophoresis to rule out multiple myeloma. The radiographic appearance is of a multicystic expansile mass or an osteolytic mass without expansion. After the diagnosis is established, treatment consists of high-dose irradiation to 5000 cGy. Late progression to multiple myeloma occurs in 35% to 55% of cases and correlates with a worse prognosis. Overall 5-year survival following treatment is 25% to 37%.

Chest Wall Resection and Reconstruction

With appropriate planning and preoperative evaluation, chest wall resection can be performed with limited morbidity and mortality to the patient. Preoperative evaluation should include pulmonary function assessment, cardiac evaluation, and appropriate imaging studies. In the current era, respiratory failure secondary to paradoxical ventilation can be avoided with appropriate skeletal reconstruction.

Surgery for malignant chest wall tumors proceeds in three phases: resection, skeletal reconstruction, and soft-tissue reconstruction. The patient is intubated with a double-lumen endotracheal tube and positioned in either a supine or lateral decubitus position, depending on tumor location. Resection proceeds with wide local excision, preferably with 4-cm margins circumferentially, to achieve local control of the tumor. For tumors that do not involve the skin, an incision is made overlying the tumor mass; skin flaps are raised, and skeletal and soft-tissue resection are performed. If a prior biopsy scar is present, the scar is excised. Because of the possibility of extension of the tumor within the bone marrow, resections for malignant rib tumors should include all involved ribs in their entirety, as well as one rib above and below the tumor. For anterior rib tumors, the anterior costal cartilage should also be excised. Malignant sternal tumors require either partial or total sternectomy along with excision of the contiguous bilateral costal cartilages. For tumors in the lower sternum, the manubrium can be preserved. A subtotal sternectomy with preservation of the upper 2 cm of the manubrium and clavicles is performed for tumors of the sternal body. For tumors in the manubrium, preservation of the lower sternum is feasible. Tissues adherent to the tumor, including lung, thymus, pericardium, and diaphragm, should be resected en bloc with the tumor.

Skeletal reconstruction is the next phase of the procedure. The goal of skeletal reconstruction is to reestablish stability of the rib cage and maintain adequate lung function. Skeletal reconstruction prevents paradoxical respiration and is necessary for most defects greater than 5 cm in diameter. Smaller lesions or those located under the scapula above the level of the fourth rib only require soft-tissue reconstruction. High posterior defects that extend to the tip of the scapula require skeletal reconstruction to prevent painful or bothersome herniation of the scapular tip into the chest cavity (alternatively, the lower portion of the scapula can be resected). In some cases of previous resection or prior irradiation, scarring of the lung to the parietal pleura will prevent the development of pneumothorax, and skeletal reconstruction after chest wall resection is not necessary.

In general, skeletal reconstruction is achieved by suturing prosthetic mesh to the chest wall under tension, creating a drum-tight chest wall prosthesis. A variety of materials have been used to achieve this effect (see Table 2); these include Marlex mesh (Chevron Phillips Chemical, The Woodlands, TX), Prolene mesh (Ethicon, Somerville, NJ), and polytetrafluoroethylene (PTFE; Gortex) patches. A sandwich of two sheets of Marlex mesh lined with methyl methacrylate has been used to create a more rigid prosthesis that preserves the chest wall contour and prevents paradoxical respiration. Anecdotally, the rigid Marlex–methyl methacrylate prosthesis, although associated with an excellent cosmetic appearance, is often associated with a mildly uncomfortable subjective sense of chest wall

Table 2: Prosthetic Options for Skeletal Reconstruction

Polytetrafluoroethylene (Gortex)
Marlex mesh
Prolene mesh
Marlex/methyl methacrylate composite
Steel mesh
Alloderm

rigidity and noncompliance. Prosthetic reconstruction is contraindicated in infected wounds; in these cases, skeletal reconstruction is either delayed or acellular dermal matrix (Alloderm; LifeCell, Branchburg, NJ) can be used in place of the prosthetic material.

Reconstruction of the anterior chest wall after complete sternal resection requires a rigid prosthesis for chest wall stabilization—that is, prevention of paradoxical respiration and protection of underlying mediastinal structures. Various materials have been used, including Marlex mesh supported by moldable titanium metal plates, sandwiched Marlex and stainless steel mesh, and Marlex mesh–methyl methacrylate composites. For partial sternal resections, Marlex mesh or PTFE prostheses alone may be sufficient to prevent paradoxical respiration. Resection of the manubrium and its associated costal cartilages does not typically result in paradoxical respiration, so soft-tissue reconstruction alone (without prosthetic reconstruction) is sufficient.

Factors that affect soft-tissue reconstruction include the location and size of the defect, local wound conditions (including prior irradiation, residual tumor), nutritional status, and overall prognosis. Soft-tissue defects can be reconstructed with rotational or free myocutaneous flaps, muscle alone, or omentum. In general, rotational flaps based on an axial blood supply are used most often. The choice of flap depends on the location and size of the defect. Commonly used soft-tissue flaps are illustrated in Figure 3. Latissimus dorsi is the largest flat muscle on the thorax and can cover defects anterolaterally, as well as posteriorly. A previous non-muscle-sparing posterolateral thoracotomy compromises the ability to use a latissimus dorsi flap. Pectoralis major is well suited for coverage of anterior chest wall defects. Rectus abdominus can be used for coverage of lower sternal wounds, and the harvest site can typically be closed primarily. Other muscle sources that are used include serratus anterior, external oblique, and trapezius. When

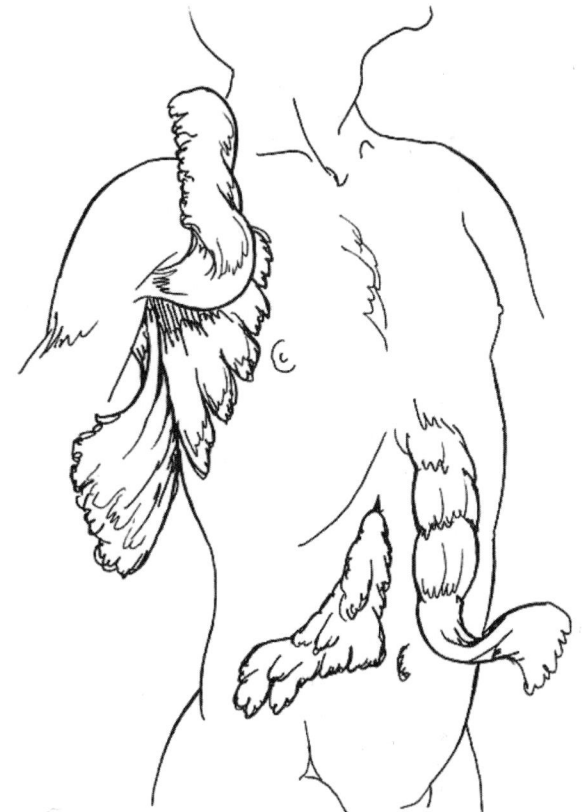

Figure 3 Pectoralis, serratus, latissimus dorsi, and rectus abdominus muscle flaps, as well as omental flaps, can be used to provide soft-tissue coverage for chest wall reconstruction.

rotational flaps are not adequate, soft-tissue reconstruction can be achieved with a free flap or omentum.

In summary, chest wall tumors comprise a heterogeneous group of lesions that require a fairly consistent diagnostic and therapeutic approach. A histologic diagnosis, obtained without compromising future treatment, must be obtained. The most common lesions are treated surgically with such operations comprising both ablative and reconstructive components. Appropriate excisional margins must be obtained to minimize the chance of local recurrence, and subsequent reconstructions may use simple prosthetic replacement or more complex tissue transposition techniques.

SUGGESTED READINGS

Abbas AE, Deschamps C, Cassivi SD, and others: Chest-wall desmoid tumors: results of surgical intervention, *Ann Thorac Surg* 78:1219, 2004.

Athanassiadi K, Kalavrouziotis G, Rondogianni D, and others: Primary chest wall tumors: early and long-term results of surgical treatment, *Eur J Cardiothorac Surg* 19:589, 2001.

Briccoli A, Manfrini M, Rocca M, and others: Sternal reconstruction with synthetic mesh and metallic plates for high grade tumours of the chest wall, *Eur J Surg* 168:494, 2002.

Deschamps C, Tirnaksiz BM, Darbandi R, and others: Early and long-term results of prosthetic chest wall reconstruction, *J Thorac Cardiovasc Surg* 117:588, 1999.

Fong YC, Pairolero PC, Sim FH, and others: Chondrosarcoma of the chest wall: a retrospective clinical analysis, *Clin Orthop Relat Res* (427):184, October 2004.

Haraguchi S., Hioki M, Hisayoshi T, and others: Resection of sternal tumors and reconstruction of the thorax: a review of 15 patients, *Surg Today* 36:225, 2006.

Incarbone M, Pastorino U: Surgical treatment of chest wall tumors, *World J Surg* 25:218, 2001.

King RM, Pairolero PC, Trastek VF, and others: Primary chest wall tumors: factors affecting survival, *Ann Thorac Surg* 41:597, 1986.

Sabanathan S, Shah R, Mearns AJ: Surgical treatment of primary malignant chest wall tumours, *Eur J Cardiothorac Surg* 11:1011, 1997.

Shamberger RC, LaQuaglia MP, Gebhardt MC, and others: Ewing sarcoma/primitive neuroectodermal tumor of the chest wall: impact of initial versus delayed resection on tumor margins, survival, and use of radiation therapy, *Ann Surg* 238:563, 2003.

TRACHEOSTOMY: TIMING, TECHNIQUES, AND OUTCOMES

Allan Philp, MD, and Thomas M. Scalea, MD

INTRODUCTION

Tracheostomies are among the oldest recorded surgical procedures, being referenced in Egyptian tablets as early as 3600 B.C. The first clearly documented case was performed by Asclepiades in 124 B.C., but successful tracheostomies were rarely performed until the nineteenth century, probably secondary to a combination of misunderstanding of the anatomy and lack of available treatments for the underlying disorders leading to airway compromise. In 1883, Trousseau reported a 25% success rate for surgical airway access in diphtheria, the later stage being otherwise fatal. By 1909, Chevalier Jackson had improved this to a 3% mortality rate, describing more modern indications and techniques using a standardized approach at the anterior second or third tracheal ring.

Tracheostomy remains among the most common procedures performed in intensive care unit (ICU) patients, and recent decades have shown an evolution of surgical approaches. Although conceptually simple, the surgical airway remains fraught with potentially devastating complications, and therefore a thoughtful approach and familiarization with multiple techniques is advisable.

INDICATIONS

The initial indications for the exchange of an orotracheal or nasotracheal tube for a surgical tracheostomy centered on issues of airway obstruction. These included facial trauma, bulky neoplasms, and edema secondary to burns or allergic reactions. Indications for tracheostomy were later broadened to include inherent or acquired pulmonary dysfunction and ventilator dependence.

Patients with no specific anatomic or pulmonary pathology but with an inability to protect the airway or perform pulmonary toilet, most notably severe traumatic brain injury, high spinal cord injury, or stroke victims, also are candidates for a tracheostomy. The placement of a tracheostomy facilitates weaning by lessening dead space ventilation and by allowing lower levels of sedation. It also lessens the risk of upper airway injury associated with prolonged intubation and allows improved patient comfort and oral and nasal hygiene. Tracheostomy provides a more secure airway in patients with difficult tracheal access. Overall the indications for tracheostomy are the same regardless of the technique used.

TIMING

Despite the frequency with which tracheostomy is performed, significant controversy remains regarding the most appropriate timing of the procedure. There is little argument that in cases in which mechanical ventilation is likely to extend beyond 14 to 21 days or the underlying inability to protect the airway is unlikely to rapidly improve (strokes, traumatic brain or spinal cord injury), tracheostomy is a reasonable option.

A number of emerging studies suggest that "early" tracheostomy (at 1 week or less) improves outcomes with regard to ventilator days, hospital stay, and nosocomial infections. Several smaller series suggest that very early tracheostomy (48−72 hours from admission) may also reduce mortality. Unfortunately, predicting prolonged ventilation remains an imperfect science, and practitioners are loath to commit to an unnecessary procedure in cases in which the duration of ventilation seems unclear. Larger studies must be carried out to clarify the issue of how early is "early," but the trend toward tracheostomy at less than 1 week from admission has gained support in the literature.

Another consideration is that of the level of ventilatory support that might preclude safe tracheostomy. During tracheostomy, the trachea is open to atmosphere for a period of time in which patients lose the effect of positive pressure. This allows alveolar derecruitment. Bronchoscopic guidance requires a time during which the airway lumen is compromised by the endoscope, and suctioning for clarity may also lead to derecruitment. The data are not clear, but our general practice has been to proceed with positive end expiratory pressure levels of less than 20 or mean airway pressures less than 30 in open lung ventilation methods.

METHODS

Open Tracheostomy

A standard open tracheostomy should be within the skill set of any practicing surgeon. It may be performed either in the operating room or a well-equipped ICU, if adequate instrumentation, lighting, and cautery are available at the bedside. The patient is placed supine with a shoulder roll in place, if possible, to allow neck extension and better exposure of the region of the second and third tracheal rings. After preoxygenation with 100% O_2 and adequate anesthesia, a 2- to 3-cm skin incision is made. This may be horizontal or vertical, according to the surgeon's preference. The platysma and strap muscles are divided on the midline, and dissection is carried down to the level of the trachea, where the pretracheal fascia is cleared sharply because the use of the cautery in the setting of an open trachea and 100% oxygen risks flame generation. The cricoid and tracheal rings should be clearly identified to allow appropriate placement of the tracheal incision. Stay sutures may be placed around the lateral aspects of the chosen ring to facilitate tube placement, and then either an H-shaped incision created or a ring excised. Alternatively, a Bjork flap may be created by using only the lower portion of the "H" tracheal incision and suturing the flap to the inferior skin edge. Superior placement of the tracheotomy may result in increased risk of stenosis, whereas more caudal positioning increases the risk of tracheoinnominate fistula.

The endotracheal tube cuff is then deflated and the tube withdrawn under direct visualization, after which the tracheal opening is dilatated if necessary and the tracheostomy tube positioned. Placement should be confirmed by end tidal CO_2, returned tidal volumes, and bilateral breath sounds. A #No. 8 cuffed tube is appropriate for most adults, although a particularly small trachea may require a correspondingly smaller tube. In instances of tracheostomy unrelated to positive pressure ventilation, an uncuffed tube might be considered. Large or obese individuals (discussed later) may also benefit from an extra long tracheostomy tube to minimize the risk of postoperative dislodgement. The tube is then secured with sutures and tracheostomy ties. Several series have shown that a postprocedural chest film is not necessary unless clinically indicated by conditions such as hypoxia, tachypnea, or asymmetric breath sounds.

Percutaneous

The initial impetus to perform bedside tracheostomies arose from the identification of the higher risk of airway and hemodynamic compromise during the transport of critically ill ICU patients. This led to efforts to simplify the procedure. In 1955, Sheldon and colleagues described a percutaneous technique using a slotted needle and trocar. In 1969, Toye and Weinstein employed a single tapered dilatator with recessed cutting blade in a similar approach. Unfortunately, a number of complications resulting from other practitioners' use of these techniques caused the percutaneous approaches to lose favor.

In 1985, Ciagli and colleagues demonstrated a Seldinger-based sequential blunt dilatation approach with outcomes and complications similar to open surgical tracheostomies but at lower cost and without the need to move the patients from the ICU setting (Fig. 1). At this point, enthusiasm was renewed for the percutaneous procedure and a variety of alternative techniques (described later) were developed. Although early series excluded patients from the percutaneous group on the basis of bleeding disorders, prior tracheostomy, higher ventilatory support levels, or obesity, more recent data suggest that the open and percutaneous approaches have similar outcomes and complications even in these more difficult populations when performed by experienced clinicians.

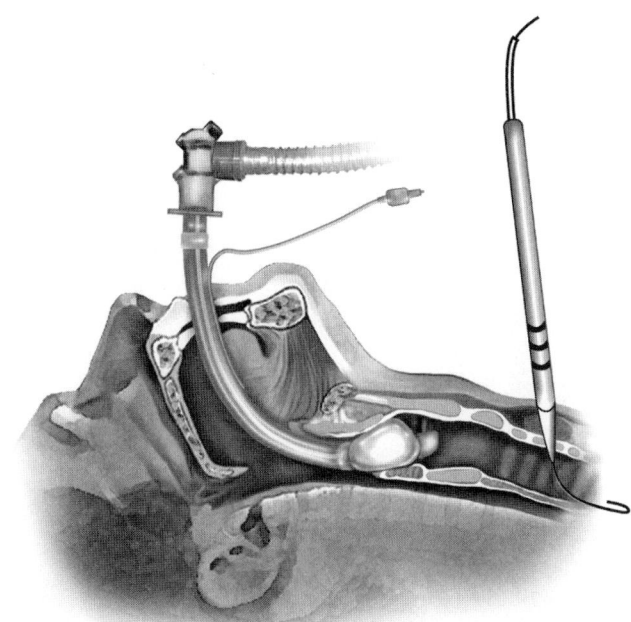

Figure 1 Seldinger-based dilational tracheostomy technique.

Dilatational (Multiple, Single, and Screw)

The dilatational approaches all essentially require cannulation of the trachea with a needle, threading of a guidewire through this access into the distal trachea, and then dilatation of the tract to the point that a tracheostomy tube with an obturator may be inserted into the airway. The initial technique described by Ciagli and colleagues used a variant of an Amplatz renal dilatator set, employing a graduated series of individual dilatators produced by Cook Critical Care (Bloomington, IN). Variants of multiple dilatator sets are also available as the Per-fit Percutaneous Trachesotomy Introducer Set (Smiths Medical, Kent, UK), which uses a Portex (Smiths Medical) instead of Shiley (Mallinckrodt, Hazelwood, MO) tracheostomy tube. A later modification in 1998 (Blue Rhino Percutaneous Tracheostomy Introducer Kit, Cook Critical Care) simplified the process using a single larger, sharply tapered dilatator with a lubricating hydrophilic coating (Fig. 2). This is the most widely used kit in the United States at present.

A more recently available modification of the dilatational technique uses a similar Seldinger process to access the trachea with a needle and guidewire but then employs an insertional dilatator resembling a large threaded screw. This engages the anterior tracheal wall as it dilatates, theoretically avoiding tracheal compression. A tracheostomy tube is then positioned over an insertion dilatator placed over the guidewire into the trachea. Early reports with this technique were promising, but case reports of complications suggest that further information is necessary. Most of the large series have used either the multiple dilatator or single tapered dilatator approaches.

Translaryngeal

The translaryngeal approach, also known as the Fantoni technique, was first published in 1993 and is based on a retrograde wire placement and subsequent antegrade pulling of a tube into position. Under bronchoscopic guidance, the endotracheal tube (ETT) is partially withdrawn and the trachea cannulated with a needle. A wire is passed either through or adjacent to the ETT, and the tube

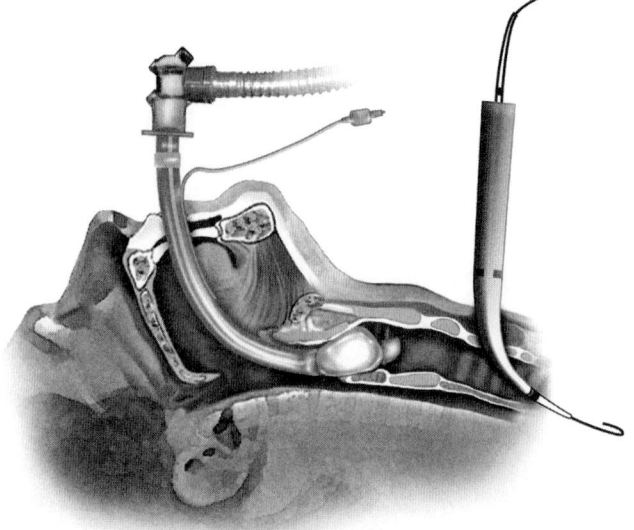

Figure 2   Single dilator tracheostomy technique.

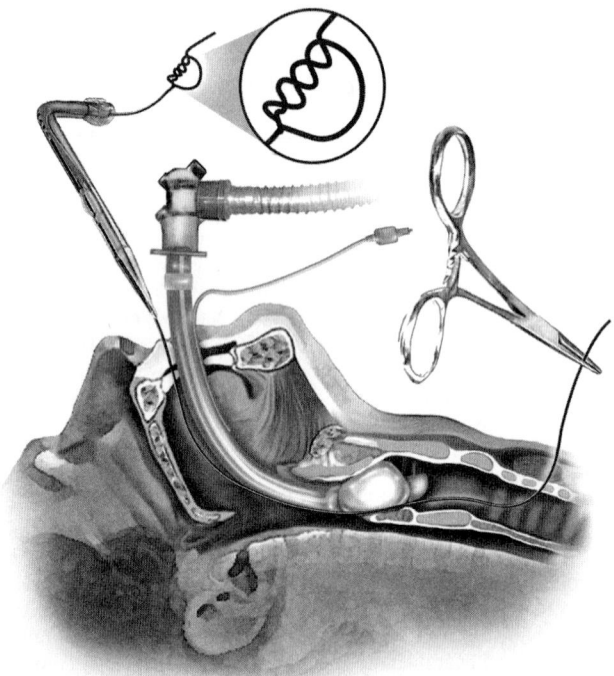

Figure 3   Translaryngeal tracheostomy technique.

COMPLICATIONS

Airway Compromise

The most common complication resulting in mortality during tracheostomy is loss of airway control while the endotracheal tube is being manipulated. Periods of hypoxia or hypercarbia may also result in cardiovascular instability, particularly given the critically ill population in which tracheostomies are often performed. This is especially a concern in percutaneous procedures in which lack of direct tracheal visualization makes urgent airway placement more challenging. Although the initial descriptions of percutaneous tracheostomy used only aspiration of air into the needle to confirm endotracheal placement, the use of endoscopic guidance during percutaneous tracheostomy has been shown to decrease the risk of airway loss to levels similar to that of open procedures. We advise the use of routine bronchoscopy to familiarize the surgeon with its utility (Figs. 4 and 5).

If an airway is lost during an open procedure and difficulty placing a tracheostomy tube is encountered, lateral stay sutures, further dilatation of the tracheal incision, or use of an airway exchange catheter as a guide may be useful. In percutaneous procedures, the bronchoscope usually can be readvanced into the airway even

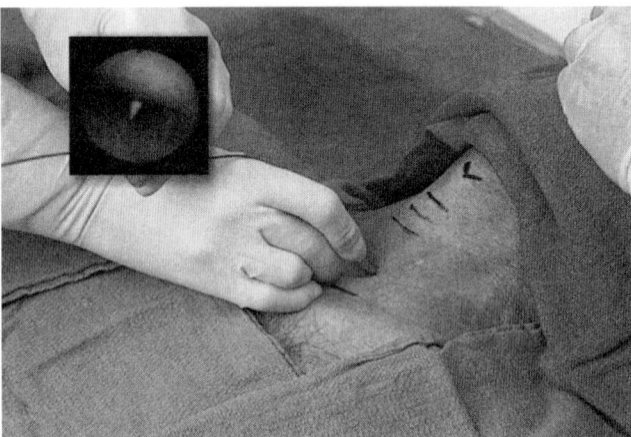

Figure 4   Bronchoscopic visualization of wire placement.

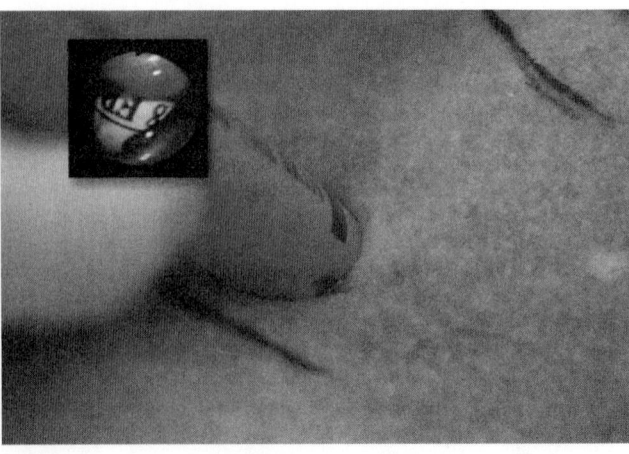

Figure 5   Bronchoscopic visualization of dilation.

is withdrawn (requiring a period of loss of airway control). A specially designed, smaller, cuffed endotracheal tube is positioned that allows work alongside it to proceed, and a tracheostomy tube with a conical distal portion is drawn through the mouth and into the airway using the wire (Fig. 3). After it is pulled through the skin, the tube is cut to size and rotated 180 degrees into position, then further advanced if necessary. An outer flange is placed to secure the tracheostomy tube, and the small orotracheal tube is removed after confirming placement.

if it is accidentally dislodged. Furthermore, if the wire has already been positioned, rapid dilatation and tracheostomy tube placement can be quickly accomplished. It should be noted that a default to conventional modes of orotracheal or nasotracheal intubation and airway control or a rapid surgical crichothyroidotomy may be appropriate if airway compromise is unlikely to be rapidly remedied with tracheostomy.

A risk of airway loss also exists early in the postoperative period, particularly in percutaneous cases in which the tract may not be well formed. Reinsertion of a tracheostomy tube may result in false passages, posterior tracheal laceration, bleeding, or other difficulties. In this case, an airway exchange catheter or cut nasogastric tube may serve as a guide for a Seldinger type insertion. Alternately, if a percutaneous tracheostomy kit is available and the wire may be passed, a replacement using the standard obturator is possible.

The safest method to resume the airway is endotracheal intubation. With the airway secure, the tracheostomy tube can be reinserted. Although an experienced surgeon may be able to reinsert a dislodged tracheostomy tube, this is ill advised if a junior surgeon is at the bedside. Depending solely on using the stay sutures to expose the tracheal opening to help reinsert the tube risks pulling them through the tracheal wall with loss of airway, hypoxia, and death.

Bleeding

As with any surgical procedure, minor bleeding is common with tracheostomies. Small subcutaneous vessels, anterior jugular or thyroidal veins, or enlarged thyroid tissue may all bleed. The vast majority can be controlled with patience and pressure or packing. Larger vessels may require ligation with an absorbable suture. Significant bleeding requires reintubation from above, removal of the tracheostomy, and exploration in the operating room. Recent literature shows that the rates of bleeding complications are at least equivalent between open and percutaneous techniques, and may even be less in the percutaneous group secondary to the smaller field of dissection and presence of some tamponade effect.

A delayed bleeding complication that may be rapid and devastating is that of tracheoinnominate fistula formation. Low placement of the tube, duration of cannulization, and overinflation of the cuff are believed to be risk factors for erosion into the innominate artery. A "herald bleed" often occurs first. Thus even small bleeding from the tracheostomy mandates investigation. Jones and colleagues suggested that in tracheostomies in place for 2 days or more that bled more than 10 ml, 50% had developed tracheoinnominate fistulae.

Because a small-volume herald bleed and fistula may be difficult to discern on angiography, operative investigation is wise. The tracheostomy should be slowly withdrawn over a bronchoscope until it is entirely removed and the trachea inspected for areas of irritation, erosion, or erythema. In cases of brisk bleeding, placing a cuffed tube distal to the bleeding helps to prevent the patient from drowning. A finger placed through the tracheostomy wound may serve to compress the vessel anteriorly against the sternum until surgical control may be obtained. In most cases, the local inflammation makes direct repair unsuccessful. Ligation with extra-anatomic reconstruction is usually necessary. A vascularized pedicle can also be placed over the tracheal repair to protect the inflamed area.

Tube Misplacement

The most common scenario resulting in tube misplacement is a technical error generating a false paratracheal passage into which the tube is placed. Less commonly, it can be placed into the esophagus or transtracheally into the mediastinum. Therefore confirmation of placement during the procedure with end tidal CO_2, returned tidal volumes, bilateral breath sounds, and bronchoscopy (if used for the procedure) should be considered mandatory.

Pneumothorax and Pneumediastinum

The low occurrence rate of these complications (<1%) makes routine postprocedure chest x-ray unnecessary unless the patient develops clinical signs of respiratory compromise.

Tracheolaryngeal Injury

The incidence of subglottic stenosis is similar in open and percutaneous tracheostomies, but at least one series indicates that percutaneous approaches are more likely to result in high tube placement, making the stenosis more proximal and potentially more difficult to correct. Bronchoscopic guidance during placement can facilitate an appropriate needle insertion at the second or third tracheal ring and centered in the midline. It can also decrease the incidence of posterior tracheal wall injury from needle placement or forceful blind dilatation.

Infection

This is a relatively uncommon complication given the nature of the tracheostomy tract as an open wound and can in most instances be managed with intravenous antibiotics if cellulitis develops. However, uncontrolled infection can contribute to tracheal erosion, which can progress to the point of requiring complex flap reconstruction. This is often heralded by increasing cuff pressures required for airway seal.

Tracheoesophageal Fistulae

Tracheoesophageal fistulae, although occurring in less than 1% of tracheostomies, are among the more complex problems to treat. Acutely, these are secondary to technical errors. Delayed fistulae are likely related to cuff erosion. High cuff pressures and an indwelling rigid nasoenteric tube are also contributing factors. The presenting symptoms may be subtle, including cough, recurrent aspiration, or persistent cuff air leaks. Endoscopy should be performed to confirm the diagnosis, and if present, distal feeding combined with a longer tracheostomy tube (to move the cuff below the site of injury) should be initiated. Ultimately, a surgical repair and local flap coverage may be required to repair the tissue defects.

CURRENT CONTROVERSIES

Open versus Percutaneous Placement

Several prospective trials have now demonstrated that the rates of complications of the two procedures are at least equivalent, varying from 4% to 10%. Several actually suggest a lower incidence of bleeding and infection in the percutaneous group (presumably because of a tamponade effect and smaller field of dissection). Bronchoscopic guidance seems to decrease the incidence of several types of potential complications in the percutaneous group, and so the routine practice at our facility is to use that technique. It also seems in several studies that complications follow a learning curve, with rates improving after 20 to 30 cases. Thus we also advocate the guidance of an experienced clinician during percutaneous tracheostomies.

Choice of Percutaneous Technique

Multiple techniques, described previously, exist for percutaneous tracheostomy placement. Rates of complications seem similar between the single dilatator methods and a translaryngeal approach.

The single dilator kit offers the potential benefit of a shorter learning curve compared with a translaryngeal approach and is slightly more rapid than serial dilator techniques. Thus practitioner experience and level of comfort should likely guide the choice within those three approaches.

High-Risk/Obese Patients

There is controversy as to the risk of percutaneous tracheostomy in higher-risk patients, including those with coagulopathies, thrombocytopenia, or obesity. The risk of complications related to bleeding appears similar when compared with the open approach. However, the data on obese patients are mixed. Earlier work indicated an increased risk of complications, including loss of airway, with percutaneous procedures. More recent series, largely using bronchoscopic guidance, showed equivalent safety between the open and percutaneous approaches. Because endoscopic guidance seems virtually to eliminate the most common operative complication of paratracheal or transtracheal placement of the tube, we have routinely performed percutaneous procedures in even the morbidly obese with good results. It should be noted, however, that the standard tracheostomy tube is sometimes replaced with an extra-long version if the amount of subcutaneous tissue would preclude proper positioning of the balloon without herniation into the tracheal opening.

Cost

It is clear that a bedside percutaneous tracheostomy using an available inclusive kit is both less expensive and less time consuming than an open procedure in the operating room. When both are perfomed in the ICU at the bedside, however, the added expense of bronchoscopy (and the staff to perform it) makes open bedside tracheostomy the more cost-effective procedure (at $307 vs. $965).

OUR PRACTICE

At our tertiary care trauma center, we perform tracheostomy across a broad spectrum of demographics and injury classes in several hundred patients per year. In general, bronchoscopically guided bedside tracheostomy in the ICU is our preference, using a single dilator technique. In patients on high levels of ventilatory support who have failed to improve in a reasonable amount of time, we favor open tracheostomy. It can be performed with a shorter period of airway compromise because the trachea is open for only a short time, and there is no need for a bronchoscope, which impairs gas flow mechanically.

Local wound complications such as tracheal erosion are addressed with intravenous antibiotics if cellulitis exists, coupled with a tube exchange to a longer and possible foam cuffed tube. We also refrain from routine tracheostomy tube exchange in the first week after a percutaneous placement, and, if necessary, perform this over an airway exchange catheter with skilled airway management personnel available.

SUGGESTED READINGS

Angel L, Simpson C: Comparison of surgical and percutaneous dilational tracheostomy, *Clin Chest Med* 24:423, 2003.

Antonelli M, Michetti V, Di Palma A, and others: Percutaneous translaryngeal versus surgical tracheostomy: a randomized trial with 1-yr double-blind follow-up, *Crit Care Med* 33:1015, 2005.

Bardell T, Drover J: Recent developments in percutaneous tracheostomy: improving techniques and expanding roles, *Curr Opin Crit Care* 11:326, 2005.

Barquist E, Amortegui J, Hallal A, and others: Tracheostomy in ventilator dependent trauma patients: a prospective, randomized intention-to-treat study, *J Trauma* 60:91, 2006.

Blankenship D, Kulbersh BD, Courin CG, and others: High-risk tracheostomy: exploring the limits of the percutaneous tracheostomy, *Laryngoscope* 11:987, 2005.

Freeman B, Isabella K, Lin N, and others: A meta-analysis of prospective trials comparing percutaneous and surgical tracheostomy in critically ill patients, *Chest* 118:1412, 2000.

Grover A, Robbins J, Bendick P, and others: Open versus percutaneous dilational tracheostomy: efficacy and cost analysis, *Am Surg* 67:297, 2001.

Johnson J, Cheatham ML, Sagraves SG, and others: Percutaneous dilational tracheostomy: a comparison of single- versus multiple-dilator techniques, *Crit Care Med* 29:1251, 2001.

Kost K: Endoscopic percutaneous dilational tracheotomy: a prospective evaluation of 500 consecutive cases, *Larnygoscope* 115:1, 2005.

McWhorter A: Tracheostomy: timing and techniques, *Curr Opin Otolaryngol Head Neck Surg* 11:473, 2003.

Rumbak J, and others: A prospective, randomized, study comparing early percutaneous dilational tracheotomy to prolonged translaryngeal intubation in critically ill medical patients, *Crit Care Med* 32:1689, 2004.

PNEUMOTHORAX

S. Rob Todd, MD, Gary A. Vercruysse, MD, and Frederick A. Moore, MD

ETIOLOGY AND PATHOPHYSIOLOGY

Pneumothorax, or the abnormal presence of air in the intrapleural space with secondary lung collapse, is commonly encountered in the practice of surgery. There are multiple etiologies, which may be categorized into four general classes.

Primary Spontaneous Pneumothorax

Primary spontaneous pneumothorax is defined as a spontaneously occurring pneumothorax in an individual without evidence of underlying lung disease. Patients are typically tall, slender male individuals younger than 40 years of age and have a history of cigarette smoking (91%). The relationship is dose dependent with regard to smoking. Primary spontaneous pneumothoraces are theorized to occur secondary to distal airway inflammation and obstruction. This obstructive pattern results in emphysematous-like changes (i.e., bullae), the rupture of which result in a pneumothorax. Less common associations include acupuncture, Marfan's syndrome, high-risk occupations, and menses-related thoracic endometriosis resulting in a catamenial pneumothorax.

Secondary Spontaneous Pneumothorax

Secondary spontaneous pneumothoraces occur in the presence of underlying lung disease (i.e., chronic obstructive pulmonary disease [COPD], malignancy, tuberculosis, idiopathic pulmonary fibrosis, cystic fibrosis, and sarcoidosis). Patients are generally older (60–65 years) than those experiencing primary spontaneous pneumothoraces. Secondary spontaneous pneumothorax is thought to be caused by a ruptured bulla greater than 2.5 cm in diameter.

Traumatic Pneumothorax

Traumatic pneumothorax results from both penetrating and blunt thoracic trauma. These injuries may be further classified into occult and nonoccult pneumothoraces. In contrast to nonoccult pneumothoraces, occult pneumothoraces are seen on computed tomography (CT) scans alone, and not on chest x-rays. With the increased use of CT in trauma, occult pneumothoraces are increasing in incidence (2%–12% of patients). In the setting of trauma, tension pneumothoraces develop when injured tissues form a one-way valve, allowing air to enter the pleural space while preventing the air from escaping naturally.

Iatrogenic Pneumothorax

Iatrogenic pneumothoraces are complications of medical management or invasive procedures. The incidence ranges from 3% to 20%. The most common cause documented in the literature is positive pressure mechanical ventilation. Other causes include central venous catheter insertion, thoracentesis, transthoracic pleural biopsy, bronchoscopy with transbronchial biopsy, and inadvertent right mainstem bronchus intubation.

CLINICAL PRESENTATION

The clinical manifestations of pneumothoraces range from mild to severe. Spontaneous pneumothoraces often occur at rest and are not associated with trauma or stress. Patients typically complain of acute chest pain or sudden dyspnea, both symptoms being present 64% of the time. Less common complaints include anxiety, cough, general malaise, and fatigue. Presenting dyspnea is more severe with secondary pneumothoraces secondary to decreased pulmonary reserve.

On physical examination, tachycardia is the most common finding. Patients are frequently tachypneic and may present diaphoretic, cyanotic, or a combination of these. Other findings include asymmetric lung expansion, distant or absent breath sounds, and hyperresonance on chest wall percussion. These subjective findings have varying diagnostic capabilities. In the presence of a tension pneumothorax, patients may experience tachycardia over 135 beats per minute, hypotension, and jugular venous distention. Patients requiring mechanical ventilation often manifest a pneumothorax with high peak airway pressures and difficulty with hand bagging.

DIAGNOSIS

The chest x-ray is the diagnostic tool most commonly used to confirm the presence of a pneumothorax. Erect posteroanterior (PA) and lateral radiographs are best. Radiographic findings include a lack of lung markings peripheral to the visceral pleural line, a mediastinal shift toward the contralateral lung, or a small pleural effusion. On supine chest x-ray, a pneumothorax is often depicted as a deep sulcus sign (a wide, deep radiolucency along the costophrenic angle). This is because when a patient is recumbent, a pneumothorax will be trapped anteriorly, resulting in diaphragmatic depression. Although expiratory films are requested for diagnostic purposes, Seow and colleagues demonstrated that inspiratory and expiratory upright x-rays are equally sensitive for pneumothorax detection. CT scans are not routinely recommended for pneumothorax detection or confirmation; however, occult pneumothoraces are often identified on neck, chest, or abdominal CT scans ordered for other reasons.

MANAGEMENT

Pneumothorax management depends on a number of factors including etiology, size, and number of occurrences. The treatment options are observation, simple aspiration, tube thoracostomy, immediate needle decompression, pleurodesis, video-assisted thoracoscopic surgery (VATS), thoracotomy, and other less commonly used modalities.

Observation

Observation is appropriate for patients who are asymptomatic and have a pneumothorax of less than 20% on chest x-ray or one visualized by CT alone. In this population, we order supplemental oxygen and a 6-hour delayed chest film. Pleural air resorbs at a rate of approximately 1.5% per day. This rate increases with supplemental oxygen. Nitrogen is the greatest component of the atmosphere and is not metabolized. Thus the partial pressure gradient between the air in the pleural space and capillary blood is small. If the nitrogen content is decreased by increasing the inspired oxygen concentration, the resorption rate will increase. We use this strategy most commonly in patients with primary spontaneous or blunt traumatic pneumothoraces.

Simple Aspiration

Simple aspiration of the air in the intrapleural space is another treatment option. In a pilot study, Noppen and colleagues documented that simple aspiration is as effective as tube thoracostomy in patients sustaining primary spontaneous pneumothoraces. It is safe, well tolerated, and feasible in an outpatient setting. Others have described simple aspiration following the development of iatrogenic pneumothoraces. We do not advocate this treatment modality.

Tube Thoracostomy

Tube thoracostomies are the most commonly performed procedures in the management of pneumothoraces. Despite this fact, the associated complication rate is as high as 21%. Potential complications include improper tube placement, pneumonia, empyema, and postremoval complications (i.e., recurrent pneumothorax). The following is our tube thoracostomy technique.

First, tube thoracostomies are extremely painful procedures. Therefore adequate pain control and sedation are critical for successful placement. We prefer conscious sedation via intravenous fentanyl and midazolam. This should be followed by appropriate local anesthesia (1% lidocaine infiltration of the skin, subcutaneous tissue, intercostal muscles, and rib periosteum). Furthermore, pain associated with the procedure often causes patients to contaminate the operative field with their hands. Secondary to this, we routinely restrain the patient's hands.

Next sterile technique is critical in preventing infectious complications. This includes the use of sterile gowns, gloves, and surgical masks and hats, regardless of where the procedure is performed. There has been debate as to the efficacy of antibiotics in preventing infectious morbidity; however, class I and II data in the trauma literature support the use of prophylactic antibiotics in patients receiving a tube thoracostomy following thoracic trauma. We routinely use one dose of cefazolin before thoracostomy tube placement, independent of the etiology. Following these steps, the tube thoracostomy field must be appropriately prepared and draped.

For isolated pneumothoraces, we use a 20- or 24-F thoracostomy tube; however, if there is an associated hemothorax or pleural effusion, we prefer a 32- or 36-F tube. We do not routinely use trocar thoracostomy tubes. For the insertion site, we prefer the nipple level (fifth intercostal space), just anterior to the midaxillary line. Routine "tunneling of the thoracostomy tube" is not necessary, except in occasional instances of extremely thin or emaciated patients. Following the skin incision, blunt dissection is performed through the subcutaneous tissues and intercostal muscles just over the rib via a Kelly clamp. The pleura is punctured with the clamp, followed by 360-degree digital inspection of the surrounding thoracic cavity to ensure that there are no pleural adhesions. Next the thoracostomy tube is inserted with or without the assistance of a Kelly clamp. The tube should be directed to the site of the pneumothorax (or posteriorly if an associated hemothorax or pleural effusion is present). On placement, look for "fogging" of the tube to confirm its intrathoracic location. The thoracostomy tube is then connected to a closed-chest drainage system (i.e., Pleur-evac; Genzyme Surgical Products, Fall River, MA) applied to wall suction, secured in place with a No. 2 nylon suture, and dressed appropriately. Alternatively, the closed chest drainage system may be applied without suction initially, but suction should be applied if the lung fails to reexpand. Placement should be confirmed immediately with a chest radiograph.

Thoracostomy tube removal is always variable. We maintain wall suction for 24 hours following reexpansion of the lung and the cessation of an air leak. Prospective randomized trials in the trauma population recommend a short trial of water seal (6–8 hours) before removal so that occult air leaks may become clinically or radiographically apparent. We adhere to this recommendation. Additionally, the thoracic surgery literature addresses the drainage volume per day at which thoracostomy tube removal is safe. In patients undergoing thoracic operations, Bell and colleagues concluded that increasing the threshold of daily drainage to 200 ml per 24 hours could be recommended for thoracostomy tube withdrawal decision in patients with uninfected pleural fluid or no evidence of an air leak. Despite this literature, we do not remove thoracostomy tubes until the drainage is less than 150 ml in 24 hours in cases in which there is a concurrent hemothorax or pleural effusion. Finally, on the basis of the trauma literature, we can conclude that complications (postremoval pneumothorax) following thoracostomy tube removal at either end-expiration or end-inspiration are statistically equivalent. We routinely remove tubes at end-inspiration.

Heimlich Valves

The Heimlich chest drain valve is a unidirectional, rubber flutter valve designed to replace the closed-chest drainage system. The proximal end attaches to most thoracostomy tubes, whereas the distal end connects to a drainage bag or suction device. It is 85% successful, particularly in cases of iatrogenic or primary spontaneous pneumothoraces, and allows for the outpatient treatment of pneumothoraces. Outpatient follow-up should be arranged within 48 hours.

Immediate Needle Decompression

Tension pneumothorax is a surgical emergency. If the diagnosis is suspected, needle decompression should be performed immediately to allow the air to escape and thus relieve the underlying pressure. Prior to performing the procedure, locate the anatomic landmarks and prepare the area. We prefer the second intercostal space at the midclavicular line. Insert a large-bore (i.e., 14- or 16-gauge) needle/catheter and listen for "a rush of air." Following decompression, a thoracostomy tube should be inserted in a timely fashion.

Pleurodesis

Pleurodesis entails the obliteration of the intrapleural space and thus the prevention of recurrent pneumothoraces. Both chemical and surgical techniques produce a moderate to severe pleural inflammation that promotes intrapleural adhesions. Many chemicals have been used (via a thoracostomy tube), the most common being talc,

bleomycin, and tetracycline and its derivatives (doxycycline). Chemical pleurodesis is a painful procedure; therefore patients should be premedicated with an intravenous sedative and intrapleural local anesthetic. Recurrence rates vary from 13% to 25% for tetracycline and 8% for talc in comparison with 41% for simple drainage alone. Surgical pleurodesis may be performed via VATS or thoracotomy and often includes mechanical pleural irritation. We generally limit pleurodesis to patients who wish to avoid surgery, are at an increased surgical risk (i.e., bleeding diathesis), or have a poor prognosis secondary to their underlying disease process.

Surgical Indications

The recurrence rate for primary spontaneous pneumothoraces is approximately 28% over 5 years and 43% for secondary spontaneous pneumothoraces over 5 years. This rate increases to 50% following the second episode. Most recurrences occur during the first 6 months to 3 years. The American College of Chest Physicians Delphi Consensus Statement, "Management of Spontaneous Pneumothorax," recommends surgical intervention following the second occurrence of a primary spontaneous pneumothorax and the first occurrence of a secondary spontaneous pneumothorax. It likewise advocates surgical intervention in instances of a persistent air leak for greater than 4 days.

Additional relative indications for surgical intervention include high-risk occupations (i.e., airline pilots, divers), a contralateral pneumothorax, bilateral pneumothoraces, and patients with acquired immune deficiency syndrome (AIDS) (secondary to extensive underlying necrosis).

Video-Assisted Thoracoscopic Surgery

Historically, open thoracotomy was the procedure of choice in the surgical management of a pneumothorax, with excellent results. More recently, VATS has surpassed the open thoracotomy. Numerous studies have attempted to document the superiority of VATS over thoracotomy; however, the results have been contradictory. We routinely perform VATS. The following is our technique.

Under general anesthesia, double-lumen intubation is performed. The patient is positioned, prepared, and draped for a posterolateral thoracotomy. Contralateral single-lung ventilation is performed throughout the procedure as tolerated. Proper port placement is critical to provide access to the entire thoracic cavity. The initial port site is positioned below the tip of the scapula at the sixth to seventh intercostal space. Next, the pleura is punctured with a Kelly clamp, followed by 360-degree digital inspection of the surrounding thoracic cavity to ensure that there are no pleural adhesions. A thoracoscope is inserted, and under direct visualization two additional working ports are positioned in a triangulated fashion. These port locations are determined on the basis of the patient's morphology.

If a single large bulla is identified, it is best resected with an endoscopic linear stapler. If multiple bullae are visualized, we attempt to identify the location of the air leak and resect that bulla. We do so by instilling saline into the thoracic cavity and looking for air bubbles during mechanical ventilation. Bulla resection should be followed by pleural abrasion or subtotal parietal pleurectomy.

CONCLUSION

Pneumothoraces are commonly encountered in surgical practice. The clinical presentation may vary from insignificant to hemodynamic instability, often correlating with the degree of lung collapse. The diagnosis is best confirmed by chest x-ray. There are a wide variety of management options that vary according to the underlying etiology.

SUGGESTED READINGS

Baumann MH, Strange C, Heffner JE, and others: Management of spontaneous pneumothorax. An American College of Chest Physicians Delphi Consensus Statement, *Chest* 119:590, 2001.

Beauchamp G, Ouellette D: Spontaneous pneumothorax and pneumomediastinum. In: Pearson FG, Cooper JD, Deslauriers RJ, and others, editors: *Thoracic surgery,* ed 2, Philadelphia, 2002, Churchill Livingstone, p. 1195.

de Lassence A, Timsit J-F, Tafflet M, and others: Pneumothorax in the intensive care unit, *Anesthesiology* 104:5, 2006.

Sawada S, Watanabe Y, Moriyama S: Video-assisted thoracoscopic surgery for primary spontaneous pneumothorax. Evaluation of indications and long-term outcome compared with conservative treatment and open thoracotomy, *Chest* 127:2226, 2005.

Younes RN, Gross JL, Aguiar S, and others: When to remove a chest tube? A randomized study with subsequent prospective consecutive validation, *J Am Coll Surg* 195:658, 2002.

HEMOTHORAX

Russell L. Gruen, MBBS, PhD, and
Gregory J. Jurkovich, MD

INTRODUCTION

Hemothorax is defined as blood in the pleural space, occurring most commonly as the result of blunt or penetrating injury. Intercostal or internal mammary vessels are the usual sources, followed by the lung parenchyma, heart and great vessels, or, rarely, intra-abdominal sources when a concomitant diaphragmatic injury is present. Following blunt thoracic trauma, the incidence of hemothorax ranges from 6.7% in patients with no rib fractures to 25% in patients with two rib fractures to 81% in patients with more than two rib fractures. The acute clinical manifestations are the consequences of intravascular hypovolemia, altered lung mechanics, or both, and the goals of initial management are arrest of bleeding, evacuation of the pleural space, volume resuscitation, and ventilatory support.

Nontraumatic hemothorax is much less common, resulting from a variety of thoracic cavity pathologies. Spontaneous pneumothoraces and rupture of pleural blebs can be accompanied by pleural vessel bleeding. Tumors of the thoracic cavity or severe lung infections with tissue necrosis may bleed spontaneously. Coagulopathies and bleeding diatheses predispose to nontraumatic hemothorax. In rare circumstances, subdiaphragmatic pathology such as pancreatic disease or ruptured aneurysm may also manifest as intrapleural bleeding.

This chapter discusses common and important clinical presentations of hemothorax (mild to moderate hemothorax, acute massive hemothorax, ongoing hemothorax), the delayed complications of hemothorax (retained hemothorax, with or without empyema or fibrothorax, and delayed hemothorax), and management techniques (tube thoracentesis, thoracotomy, and minimally invasive approaches).

CLINICAL SITUATIONS

Initial Management

Hemothorax presents in a spectrum of clinical scenarios ranging from a stable patient who sustained relatively minor thoracic trauma to a hemodynamically unstable patient with multiple injuries. The diagnosis of hemothorax can occasionally be made on clinical examination alone (e.g., a patient in shock with unilateral diminished breath sounds and dullness to percussion) or, more commonly, by the initial chest x-ray revealing unilateral opacity. In the supine patient's chest x-ray, minor or moderate hemothorax may be difficult to appreciate and requires a high index of suspicion. Chest computed tomography (CT) is sensitive for diagnosing hemopneumothorax, but real danger exists in isolating the unstable patient in the CT scanner, and imaging studies should complement and never interfere with resuscitation.

When hemothorax is diagnosed or suspected in the emergency department, the most prudent management plan is immediate tube thoracostomy. The unstable trauma patient with diminished breath sounds and evidence of a thoracic injury should undergo immediate tube thoracostomy (before imaging), along with securing of the airway, supporting ventilation, and replacing circulatory volume. In this setting, the chest tube is both diagnostic and therapeutic for tension pneumothorax, massive hemothorax, or monitoring ongoing pleural space bleeding. Small hemothoraces seen only on CT without pneumothorax in a stable and spontaneously breathing patient may simply be observed, but this is clearly an exception.

Sorting out the source of bleeding in a patient with multiple injuries from blunt trauma requires consideration of multiple body regions. Recognition of thoracic hemorrhage has high priority in the primary survey because it can involve all components of the ABCs of trauma resuscitation: airway, breathing, bleeding control, and circulatory restoration. Chest imaging and diagnostic tube thoracostomy are key maneuvers that help assess the severity of pleural space bleeding and ventilatory compromise. Diagnosing intra-abdominal and pelvic bleeding is more challenging and should follow assessment of the thorax. Computed tomography of the head and the diagnosis of intracranial injury is next, with particular attention given to identifying the patient with lateralizing signs of an epidural or subdural hematoma. Particularly vexing is the presence of critical injuries in more than one major anatomic locale. In general, exsanguinating hemorrhage control comes first, most commonly from intra-abdominal or intrathoracic vessels, but occasionally from retroperitoneal pelvic vessels. If both chest and abdomen are sources, it is usually prudent to prepare both cavities for exploration, beginning with the abdomen because intraperitoneal hemorrhage with associated diaphragmatic injury may be the source of thoracic blood.

Acute Massive Hemothorax

Indications or guidelines for thoracotomy for control of intrathoracic hemorrhage are an initial chest tube output exceeding 1500 ml (20 ml/kg) or a continued hourly output of more than 200 ml (3 ml/kg) for 4 consecutive hours. Delay or procrastination in operative control of bleeding are to be avoided because the volume of blood loss has been shown to correlate with mortality in patients undergoing early thoracotomy for either blunt or penetrating wounds.

The source of hemorrhage may be heart, lung, aorta or other great vessels, or chest wall, intercostal or internal mammary vessels; hence a formal posterior lateral incision in the fourth or fifth intercostal space usually affords the best exposure. Endotracheal intubation with a double-lumen tube is ideal. In the situation of diffuse chest wall bleeding from blunt trauma in the presence of coagulopathy, many experienced surgeons attempt a trial of positive end-expiratory pressure (PEEP) control ventilation, warming, and correction of coagulopathy even in the face of ongoing hemorrhage. The problem, however, is that it is impossible to tell without a thoracotomy whether chest wall bleeding is the true source. Early operation has the advantages of evacuation of clot and full lung expansion, aiding in cessation of bleeding, particularly when coagulopathy is reversed and body temperature is normalized. We advocate thoracotomy for hemorrhage whenever the total output exceeds 1500 ml in a 24-hour period, with signs of continued bleeding regardless of injury mechanism. This allows patients to reach the operating room in a more stable condition, with more options for thoracoscopy and improved outcome. We have not found angiography appropriate in this setting.

Ongoing Hemothorax

Ongoing hemothorax caused by unrecognized exsanguinations and inadequate chest drainage may be fatal, particularly in multiply injured patients. Initial chest tube drainage may cease because of a clotted or loculated chest tube, providing a false assessment that thoracic hemorrhage has ceased. For this reason, we advocate placing a second chest tube (see Fig. 1) if more than 10 ml/kg of blood is drained within a few minutes from the first chest tube and if the patient is not a candidate for immediate thoracotomy. This second tube promotes adequate pleural drainage and minimizes the risk of clotted blood occluding the single chest tube and obscuring any ongoing hemorrhage.

A second chest tube may be sufficient to allow lung expansion and tamponade of bleeding. If hemorrhage continues but the patient remains relatively stable, thoracoscopy may be useful to evacuate the pleural space, identify a bleeding source, and apply clips to an intercostal vessel, for example. Unstable patients with ongoing bleeding should undergo urgent thoracotomy.

Retained Hemothorax

In stable, nonventilated patients who have not had a chest tube inserted, small effusions that are diagnosed late will usually resolve without sequelae. However, in patients who have undergone tube thoracostomy, the tube fails to evacuate the hemothorax completely in approximately 5% of cases. These patients are at risk of empyema and fibrothorax, especially if prolonged mechanical ventilation, pneumonia, or other infectious sites are present. The typical scenario is a patient with a prolonged intensive care unit stay, with chest x-ray abnormalities, and retained hemothorax determined

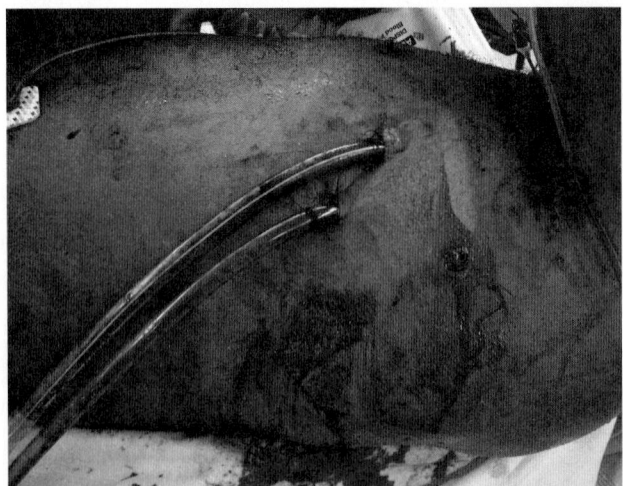

Figure 1 Use of second chest tube to optimize evacuation of hemothorax.

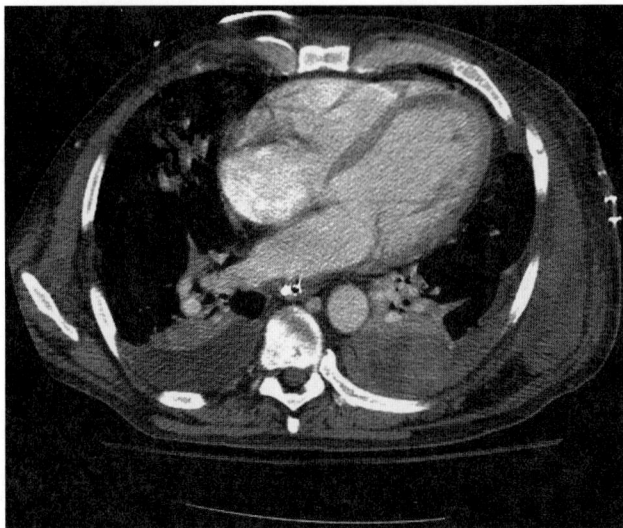

Figure 2 Computed tomography (*CT*) of retained right hemothorax despite tube thoracostomy for 10 days. Advantages of CT in evaluating residual chest fluid. This CT image displays bilateral atelectasis, right low-density pleural effusion (to contrast with hemothorax), and left mixed high- and intermediate-density hemothorax.

by subsequent chest CT (Fig. 2). Elevated fever and white blood count in the absence of other sources strongly suggests developing empyema. Aggressive drainage is indicated in these high-risk patients, although the timing of operative evacuation and the use of video assisted thoracostomy (VATS) with or without hemolytic agents injected into the pleural space remains controversial.

Although it is tempting to simply insert another chest tube into a retained hemothorax, a second chest tube inserted more than 24 hours after injury will fail to evacuate the hemothorax in more than 40% of cases. In comparison, early thoracoscopic drainage and decortication allows removal of all clot without the morbidity of a formal thoracotomy and reduces the duration of tube thoracostomy, hospital stay, and overall cost. Alternatively, a mini-thoracotomy approach may be sufficient to deal with localized collections and pleural rind. Intrapleural streptokinase, or urokinase lyses clot in 65% to 90% of cases without significant rebleeding risk, but kinases may cause pain and fever, take longer to act than operative approaches, and are ineffective for breaking down loculations.

Delayed Hemothorax

Rarely hemothorax may occur up to a week after injury, heralded by the onset of new chest pain and dyspnea. A previously normal chest x-ray or CT differentiates it from retained hemothorax. The differential diagnosis includes pulmonary embolism, and chest CT angiography may make the diagnosis.

TECHNICAL ISSUES

Tube Thoracostomy

A large (32 F or greater) chest tube is inserted at the fourth or fifth intercostal space, level with the inframammary crease, just anterior to the midaxillary line. The tube should not be inserted through traumatic wounds. Sterile technique is used. The skin, periosteum, subpleural space and parietal pleura are infiltrated with 10 ml of 1% lidocaine via a 23-gauge needle over the top of the fifth or sixth rib. The needle is used to identify the place for subsequent passage of the tube over the top of the rib to avoid the intercostal neurovascular bundle running along the inferior borders of the ribs. Subcutaneous tunneling over a rib from a skin incision one rib space below facilitates an airtight and watertight seal. A skin incision is made parallel to the ribs large enough to admit the operator's finger. A large, curved hemostat or a pair of curved Mayo scissors is inserted through the skin incision, directed cranially and over the selected rib into the intercostal space and the intercostal muscles, and parietal pleura are punctured. Because this may take some force with the hemostat (vs. snipping with the scissors), placement of the index finger on the hinge of the forceps may prevent sudden and hazardous plunging of the forceps into the chest. The intercostal muscles are spread with the hemostat or scissors, which are then removed, and a finger is inserted into the pleural space to confirm appropriate position by palpating smooth parietal pleura with the pulp of the examining finger. The chest tube is clamped at its external end, and a large curved forceps is used to guide the tube toward the apex of the pleural space. If a second tube is required, it may be placed posterobasally. In adults, approximately 10 cm of tube should lie inside the chest between the last side-hole and the chest wall. If correctly placed, the tube should "fog" with expiration. Spinning the tube between fingers ensures that it is not kinked within the chest. The tube is then secured in place with size 0 Prolene (Ethicon, Somerville, NJ), nylon, or silk suture that is wrapped tightly and tied to give the tube a "waist." An underwater seal drain is immediately attached, and the clamp is removed. All connections are taped, and the drain is placed on 20-cm water suction. The skin is closed with an additional vertical mattress suture if necessary. An airtight dressing is applied, and the tube secured to the chest wall to reduce the chance of accidental removal. A postoperative chest x-ray is obtained to confirm position and assess for residual hemopneumothorax.

The most common complication of tube placement is pain, which may lead to splinting, atelectasis, and pneumonia. Other complications include visceral or diaphragmatic injury, extrapleural or intraparenchymal placement, and inadvertent removal. These all constitute technical errors, and a hospital quality assurance program should track these errors and take steps to ensure that the incidence is less than 5%. Empyema occurs in 2% to 10% of patients who undergo emergency department tube thoracostomy, for which the primary risk factor is retained hemothorax. Other contributing factors include poor and unsterile placement technique, shock, pneumonia, and extrathoracic infections. There is little evidence that prophylactic antibiotic administration reduces rates of empyema, but this remains a controversial subject. We do not routinely use prophylactic antibiotics for chest tubes.

Tubes should be removed when they have ceased to function or the air leak has ceased and fluid drainage is no more than 150 ml per 24 hours. Recurrent or new pneumothorax can be a troublesome technical complication, occurring in 6% to 8% of patients. It is generally considered a complication of improper tube removal but occasionally is the result of the tube lacerating parietal pleura on removal. Evidence supports the benefit of an observation trial off suction and on water-seal before tube removal. Although the timing of tube removal (end-expiration vs. end-inspiration) remains controversial, we advocate rapid chest tube removal at the end of full inspiration and Valsalva maneuver, with simultaneous placement of prepared watertight and airtight dressing of Vaseline gauze, four by fours, and tape. The dressing is left in situ for at least 48 hours before changing, at which time Opsite (Smith & Nephew, Memphis, TN) can be applied. We have not been satisfied with U-stitches around the chest tube insertion site cinched tightly at time of removal.

Thoracotomy

Thoracotomy for massive hemothorax in the acute setting is best approached via a posterolateral incision with the patient in a full lateral decubitus position. This provides the best exposure for the most common causes of thoracic hemorrhage. In blunt trauma, and occasionally in the setting of transdiaphragmatic penetrating trajectories, access to the peritoneal cavity is also required. If laparotomy is performed first, access to the chest is usually obtained via an anterolateral thoracotomy without repositioning the patient. Exposure is improved by placing a roll behind the side of interest, by rotating the arm across the table, or by positioning the patient with both arms extended above the head to allow a formal clamshell approach.

Ideally a double-lumen endotracheal tube is used to allow single-lung ventilation of the contralateral lung. The incisions should be placed in the fifth intercostal space for both anterolateral and posterolateral approaches. As little muscle as possible should be incised. Exposure may be improved and postoperative pain reduced by removal of an entire rib or a posterior rib segment.

Intercostal vessel injury is the most common cause of hemothorax, but the surgeon must be prepared for the entire spectrum of thoracic cavity injuries. It is not uncommon in patients undergoing thoracotomy to find visceral or great vessel bleeding. Twenty to thirty percent of patients undergoing thoracotomy after trauma require some form of lung resection. Following penetrating trauma, simple suture and nonanatomic wedge resection using staplers may be sufficient for hemorrhage control. Tractotomy is used either to define deep injuries or to treat peripheral injuries that pass through the parenchyma. Blunt trauma, on the other hand, tends to be associated with significant diffuse parenchymal destruction and sheer injury, which may be salvageable only with more extensive resections. Emergency lobectomy and pneumonectomy after trauma are associated with mortality rates of 3% to 50% and 70% to 100%, respectively, but may occasionally be lifesaving when major pulmonary vessels are bleeding. Temporary control of the hilum can usually be obtained by first incising the inferior pulmonary ligament to free the lower lobe, then grasping the hilum between fingers or using a large vascular clamp or, in desperate situations, rotating the hilum 180 to 360 degrees to pinch off the vessels.

Irrigation systems can be considered when there is extensive contamination or when significant residual clot is anticipated. Obtaining pleura-to-pleura apposition, aided by tissue sealants if necessary and available, minimizes air leak. Simple oversewing of entrance or exit wounds in lung parenchyma is discouraged because the resulting closed-space fluid or air collections may cause unrecognized bleeding, air emboli, or eventual lung abscess.

Abbreviated Thoracotomy

In unstable patients, abbreviated closure of the thoracotomy incision can be employed, with plans to return to the operating room for completion of the damage control operation as the patient's physiology allows. Such an approach may be necessary if the facilities or time are not available to perform definitive surgery or in unstable patients in whom the "lethal triad" of coagulopathy, hypothermia, and acidosis are present. The goals are control of hemorrhage and massive air leak and not definitive repair or closure. Any source of bleeding should be addressed, if possible. The apices, posterior gutters, and lateral wall may be packed while avoiding the medial sites that might cause cardiac or vena caval compression. Closing the chest wall helps tamponade bleeding, but ischemia reperfusion may cause the heart and lung to swell, preventing closure or subsequently leading to a "thoracic compartment syndrome," with impaired venous return and cardiac arrest. Occasionally a sternal retractor must be temporarily left in place. The chest wall musculature can be sutured together or simply packed before the skin is closed or, if that is not possible, a steridrape is applied.

Emergency Room Resuscitative Thoracotomy

The term *emergency room resuscitative thoracotomy* (ERRT) should be restricted to a thoracotomy performed on a patient in extremis outside the operating room. Variable use of the term has made comparing survival rates difficult. It is generally agreed that ERRT may be beneficial and indicated only for blunt trauma patients who have detectable vital signs on arrival to the hospital or who have lost vital signs within 5 minutes of arrival. With penetrating mechanisms, the opportunity for rapid repair and resuscitation are more likely, hence the criteria are expanded for those who have sustained an isolated penetrating chest injury to include patients with signs of life at any time in the field. Survival rates have been reported to be as high as 38% in penetrating trauma (stab greater than gunshot), but only 1% to 2% in blunt trauma.

Minimally Invasive Approaches

Minimally invasive approaches are useful for controlling modest bleeding, evacuating retained hemothorax, and decorticating limited empyema and fibrothorax. They include mini-thoracotomy with visualization using a mediastinoscope, and VATS. The main advantages are smaller incisions and less pain, as long as sufficient local anesthetic is administered and port introducers are used as little as possible. The patient must have a double-lumen endotracheal tube and be able to tolerate single-lung ventilation. Thoracoscopy is contraindicated in hemodynamically unstable patients.

Usually the initial insertion site of the telescope is the tube thoracostomy site. After a pristine area of pleural cavity is entered, a second port is inserted under vision and the lung is taken down from the chest wall with sharp and blunt dissection. The pleural surfaces and the diaphragm are then carefully inspected with insertion of additional 5-mm ports in a 180-degree arc. Clot is evacuated using irrigation and suction, and rind is decorticated best using ring forceps introduced through a port site.

SUGGESTED READINGS

Bell RL, Ovadia P, Abdullah F, and others: Chest tube removal: end-inspiration or end-expiration? *J Trauma* 50:674, 2001.

Bilello JF, Davis JW, Lemaster D: Occult traumatic hemothorax: when can sleeping dogs lie? *Am J Surg* 190:841, 2005.

Cothran CC, Moore EE: Emergency department thoracotomy for critically injured patients: objectives, indications and outcomes, *World J Emerg Surg* 1:4, 2006.

Gruen RL, Jurkovich GJ, McIntyre LK, and others: Patterns of errors contributing to trauma mortality: lessons learned from 2594 deaths, *Ann Surg* 244:371, 2006.

Hunt PA, Greaves I, Owens WA: Emergency thoracotomy in thoracic trauma—a review, *Injury* 37:1, 2006.

Karmy-Jones R, Jurkovich GJ: Blunt chest trauma, *Curr Probl Surg* 41:205, 2004.

Karmy-Jones R, Jurkovich GJ, Nathens AB, and others: Timing of urgent thoracotomy for hemorrhage following trauma: a multi-center study, *Arch Surg* 136:513, 2001.

Karmy-Jones R, Jurkovich GJ, Shatz DV, and others: Management of traumatic lung injury: a WTA multicenter review, *J Trauma* 51:1049, 2001.

Martino K, Merrit S, Boyakye K, and others: Prospective randomized trial of thoracostomy removal algorithms, *J Trauma* 46:369, 1999.

Simon BJ, Chu Q, Emhoff TA, and others: Delayed hemothorax after blunt thoracic trauma: an uncommon entity with significant morbidity, *J Trauma* 45:673, 1998.

Wilson RF, Nichols RL: The EAST practice management guidelines for prophylactic antibiotic use in tube thoracostomy for traumatic hemopneumothorax: a commentary, *J Trauma* 48:758, 2000.

MEDIASTINAL MASSES

J. Timothy Sherwood, MD, and John D. Mitchell, MD

When one is confronted with a patient harboring a mediastinal mass, a logical and systematic approach is essential to providing tissue diagnosis, as well as therapeutic intervention. Typically patients with mediastinal masses are asymptomatic, and chest x-ray findings are subtle. Computed tomography (CT) of the chest is the most valuable imaging tool available to the clinician, and the location of the mass, the morphologic characteristics, and the relation to other mediastinal structures allow one to define more precisely the nature of the lesion. The decision regarding whether to primarily resect the mass for diagnostic and therapeutic purposes versus performing a biopsy of the mass can commonly be made on the basis of the CT characteristics. Magnetic resonance imaging (MRI) is sometimes necessary to assist with this decision-making process. Several approaches to the mediastinum can be used for access to these lesions. Finally, because the mediastinum contains cardiovascular structures, airway and alimentary tract tissue, lymphatic and neural tissue, and germ cell elements, a wide variety of tumors are possible.

ANATOMY

The mediastinum is defined by the parietal pleura laterally, the posterior aspect of the sternum anteriorly, and the vertebral bodies posteriorly. It is contained superiorly by the thoracic inlet and inferiorly by the diaphragm.

The anterior mediastinal compartment is defined anteriorly by the undersurface of the sternum and posteriorly by the anterior surface of the great vessels. Its lateral borders are the phrenic nerves. The anterior mediastinum contains the thymus gland, lymph nodal tissue, and pericardial fat. The visceral compartment or middle mediastinum has anatomic borders consisting of the pericardium and great vessels anteriorly and the vertebral bodies posteriorly. Contents of this compartment include the heart, pericardium, phrenic nerves, trachea and main bronchi, the hila of the lungs, the esophagus, and the vagus nerve. The paravertebral sulcus or posterior mediastinum is bounded anteriorly by the vertebral bodies, extends posteriorly to the ribs and is bound by the paravertebral gutters. This compartment contains the nerve roots of the thoracic spinal cord, the sympathetic chain, the thoracic duct, the azygous venous system, and the descending thoracic aorta. Although primary and metastatic disease involving mediastinal lymphatics can involve any or all of the three mediastinal compartments, primary mediastinal tumors tend to be located consistently within one of these anatomic zones.

DIAGNOSTIC TECHNIQUES

Should the Mass Be Biopsied?

Certain goals should be considered when contemplating a biopsy of an anterior mediastinal mass, and routine biopsy should be avoided. One should avoid biopsy of an early-stage thymoma because this could potentially result in capsule disruption with tumor dissemination. Conversely, one should avoid a potentially morbid major resection when a diagnosis of lymphoma or germ cell tumor is suspected because treatment is likely to be nonsurgical. Additionally, if a thymoma is suspected and is large or invasive, biopsy should be performed because neoadjuvant therapy may be given before surgical resection. Therefore the choice to proceed with biopsy should be based on what is believed to be the likely tumor pathology with consideration for the tumor stage. Well-circumscribed mass with no evidence of invasion and no associated lymphadenopathy can usually be resected primarily, serving both diagnostic and therapeutic purposes. This includes tumors such as early-stage thymomas, teratomas, mesenchymal tumors, or benign cysts. If lymphoma is suspected, biopsy is mandatory for adequate tissue typing and flow cytometry. Tumors that appear invasive should also be biopsied before initiation of any treatment. Biopsies of tumors in the anterior mediastinum should be performed with the least amount of morbidity and are often amenable to core needle biopsy via a parasternal approach, typically with CT or ultrasound guidance. Fine needle aspiration biopsy may be performed; however, the tissue volume obtained is usually not adequate to make a diagnosis of lymphoma, and its use in any situation can be called into question. If image-guided core needle biopsy expertise is not available, an anterior mediastinotomy (Chamberlain procedure) on the left or the right is appropriate. Mediastinoscopy provides access to the paratracheal. Thoracoscopy provides access to all compartments of the mediastinum; however, one must consider the risk of seeding the pleural space with tumor when this approach is used, as well as the postoperative pain and short hospital admission associated with its use. Cervical mediastinoscopy does not allow access to the anterior mediastinum but may provide diagnostic tissue should accessible paratracheal precarinal and subcarinal areas appear pathologic in the setting of a mediastinal mass.

Because the majority of middle mediastinal masses are malignant, representing lymphoma or metastatic disease, biopsies are usually the procedure the surgeon is called on to perform. One should be cautious if the mass represents a cyst because this should be excised rather than biopsied. Paravertebral sulcus or posterior mediastinal tumors can be biopsied, however, because the majority of these tumors are benign, and primary resection without preoperative diagnosis is acceptable provided the tumor appears resectable on preoperative imaging studies. If neoadjuvant therapy is contemplated, biopsy with transthoracic or transesophageal biopsy is warranted.

Tumor Markers

Serum tumor markers can be helpful in making a diagnosis of certain tumor types. Measurement of alpha feto-protein and human chorionic gonadotropin are especially helpful when one suspects a germ cell neoplasm. If a thymoma is present and one suspects a diagnosis of myasthenia gravis on the basis of clinical symptoms, measurement of anti-acetylcholine antibodies may help to establish the diagnosis. Other tumor markers or hormone levels are seldom useful in making a diagnosis of a mediastinal mass.

◼ ANTERIOR MEDIASTINAL MASSES

Anterior mediastinal masses comprise the most common tumors of the mediastinum. The anterior compartment contains the thymic gland and associated fatty and lymphatic tissue. This compartment is contiguous with the thoracic inlet, and therefore descending masses from the neck may also be seen in the anterior mediastinum. Classically referred to as the "Four Ts," 95% of all tumors of the anterior mediastinum include thymic neoplasms, teratoma or germ cell tumors, "terrible" lymphoma, and thyroid goiter. Less common tumors include thymic carcinoma, thymic carcinoid, and parathyroid adenoma.

Thymic Tumors

Tumors originating from thymic tissue include thymoma, thymic carcinoma, thymic carcinoid, and thymolipoma. The thymic gland is relatively large at birth and continues to grow until puberty, after which time the gland degenerates and becomes progressively replaced with fatty tissue. In elderly patients, the gland is barely identifiable. CT scan imaging reflects this change in size, and one should be familiar with normal thymic anatomy at various stages of life. Younger individuals up through at least the third decade of life have physiologic thymic uptake on fluorodeoxyglucose positron emission tomography (FDG-PET), and these findings should be correlated with radiologic anatomy and clinical course. Additionally, increased FDG-PET uptake resulting from chemotherapy-induced thymic hyperplasia has also been reported.

In adults, thymomas are the most common anterior mediastinal tumor, with an average age at presentation of 40 to 60 years. There is no sex predilection, and only approximately half of patients are symptomatic. Vague symptoms such as cough or dull chest pain are present in approximately one third of patients. Only 15% of patients with myasthenia gravis actually have a thymoma; however, 30% to 50% of patients with a thymoma have myasthenia gravis. Therefore a careful history should be taken in a patient with a newly discovered anterior mediastinal mass. More than 50% of patients with myasthenia present with symptoms of diplopia or ptosis, and roughly 15% present with bulbar symptoms such as dysarthria, dysphagia, and fatigable chewing. Any of these symptoms should raise suspicion of the diagnosis of myasthenia, and some clinicians advocate measuring serum antiacetylcholine receptor antibodies in all patients with thymoma, regardless of symptoms. In 5% to 10% of patients with a thymoma, paraneoplastic syndromes such as red cell aplasia, hypogammaglobulinemia, systemic lupus, Cushing's syndrome, or syndrome of inappropriate antidiuretic hormone are present. In patients with red cell aplasia, approximately 50% will have a thymoma. Patients with thymoma and myasthenia should be medically optimized before resection.

Thymomas are neoplasms that originate from epithelial cells, although the tumors may contain infiltrating nonneoplastic lymphocytes and reticular cells as well. The epithelial neoplastic cell is usually slowly growing and lacks cytologic characteristics of malignancy. On the basis of the proportion of each component, thymomas are subclassified as predominantly epithelial, predominantly lymphocytic, or mixed lymphoepithelial. Two types of neoplastic cells are encountered, the polygonal and the spindle-cell type.

CT with intravenous contrast remains the best imaging modality for the characterization of anterior mediastinal masses. Well-circumscribed, round masses are usually early-stage thymoma. Thymomas may sometimes be lobulated or occasionally have calcifications. Irregularly shaped, invasive masses are more likely to be advanced-stage thymoma or other neoplasms such as germ cell tumors or lymphoma. The presence of other associated lymphadenopathy should raise the suspicion of lymphoma, which is the usual competing diagnosis. Patients with invasive, seemingly nonresectable tumors should have a biopsy performed to obtain a tissue diagnosis. In the case of thymoma, the patient may benefit from neoadjuvant therapy before resection; in the case of lymphoma or germ cell tumor, medical therapy is the initial or sole therapy. Attention should be paid to the pericardium, lung parenchyma, and pleural space to assess for evidence of advanced or metastatic disease. There is no well-defined role for nuclear medicine imaging studies to evaluate thymic masses. Thallium-technetium scanning may identify an intrathymic parathyroid adenoma, and an octreotide scan can identify a neuroendocrine tumor such as a thymic carcinoid. FDG-PET has been reported to show high uptake of FDG in thymic cancer but not in thymoma. This is probably due to its slow growth and low glucose uptake. Carbon-11 acetate-PET has been reported to be of clinical value for the diagnosis and imaging of thymoma. MRI may sometimes be helpful to assess for evidence of vascular invasion.

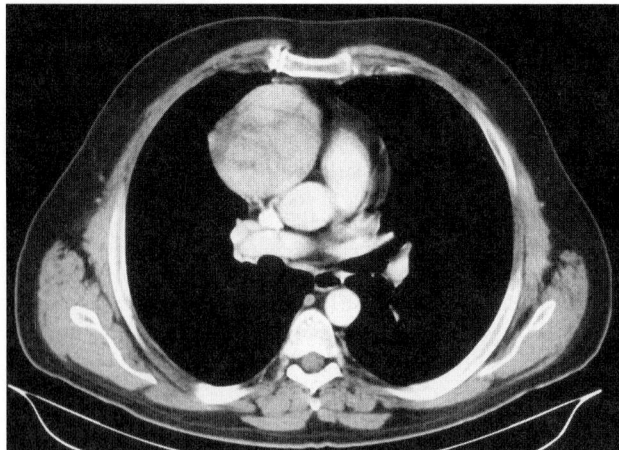

Figure 1   A large, 10-cm lobulated anterior mediastinal mass in a 50-year-old male patient that did not show any vessel invasion on magnetic resonance imaging. A median sternotomy was performed revealing a completely encapsulated Masaoka stage I thymoma.

Anterior mediastinal masses suspicious for thymoma without evidence of invasion can undergo primary surgical resection for diagnostic, as well as therapeutic, purposes. In general, small tumors less than 5 cm are usually encapsulated and are amenable to surgical resection with minimal morbidity. If the mass appears to be resectable, avoidance of tumor seeding via needle or open biopsy is thereby avoided. A full median sternotomy (Fig. 1) provides the best access to the anterior mediastinum for resection of a thymoma. A partial sternotomy does not allow for optimal exposure for resection of all thymic tissue and associated fat, and a transcervical approach is an inappropriate incision for resection of a tumor. Although some surgeons advocate video-assisted thoracoscopic surgery (VATS) or a thorascopic approach, this is a potentially hazardous approach because rupture of the thymoma capsule could lead to devastating consequences associated with tumor seeding. VATS may be an acceptable approach for small, stage I thymomas.

The operative goal for thymoma resection involves removal of the mass and all associated thymic tissue and pericardial fat, as well as en bloc resection of any adjacent areas of involvement such as pleura, pericardium, lung, and great veins. All thymic tissue from the cervical thymic extensions down to the diaphragm and laterally to the phrenic nerves should be resected. After the resection is completed, skeletonization of the pericardium and anterior mediastinum should be achieved. If the tumor involves the phrenic nerve on either side, this can be resected en bloc with the mass. However, if both phrenic nerves are involved, only one phrenic nerve should be sacrificed, and the other should be carefully preserved and marked with metallic clips for adjuvant radiation therapy. The patient may require diaphragm plication in the future, and some surgeons may elect to perform diaphragm plication at the time of initial phrenic nerve sacrifice. If the tumor invades resectable structures such as the pericardium, great veins, superior vena cava (SVC), pleura or lung, these should be resected en bloc along with the tumor. Reconstruction of the SVC should be performed if resection leads to significant decrease in diameter that in turn leads to stenosis. Resection of the innominate vein is usually well tolerated.

The staging system for thymoma is not standardized. The most widely used is the Masaoka staging system, which incorporates the presence of invasion and the anatomic extent of involvement, as defined both clinically and histopathologically. Because of the absence of histologic features of malignancy, thymomas should not be characterized as "malignant" but rather as "invasive." Stage I tumors have completely encapsulated macroscopically and no capsular invasion microscopically. Stage II tumors have macroscopic

invasion into surrounding fatty tissue or mediastinal pleura or microscopic invasion into the capsule. Stage III tumors have macroscopic invasion into neighboring organs, that is, pericardium, great vessels, or lung. Stage IVa tumors have pleural or pericardial dissemination, and stage IVb tumors have lymphogenous or hematogenous metastases. The Masaoka staging system correlates well with 5-year survival, with stage I having a 94% to 100% survival, stage II an 86% to 95% survival, stage III a 56% to 69% survival, and stage IV an 11% to 50% survival. Independent predictors of survival and freedom from recurrence also include tumor size (<11 cm), spindle cell, or lymphocyte predominance versus epithelial predominance or thymic carcinoma and completeness of resection.

Adjuvant and neoadjuvant therapy have a role in the treatment of thymoma. Chemotherapy and radiation therapy should be considered for locally advanced or metastatic unresectable disease, microscopic or macroscopic residual disease after incomplete surgical resection, and following complete resection of an invasive thymoma. In one study of patients with completely resected stage II or III thymomas, adjuvant radiotherapy reduced the rate of local recurrence from 28% to 5%. In another study, patients undergoing surgery for stage IVa thymoma followed by adjuvant radiotherapy had a higher 5-year disease-free survival (62 vs 18%). Some oncologists recommend postoperative adjuvant cisplatin-based chemotherapy for any stage thymoma with cortical differentiation. Neoadjuvant therapy should be considered in patients with pathologically confirmed thymoma that is considered unresectable because of invasion (Masaoka stage III or IV) because this therapy may make an unresectable tumor resectable. The M.D. Anderson Cancer Center group has recently reported its experience with induction chemotherapy using cyclophosphamide, doxorubicin, cisplatin, and prednisone followed by surgical resection. These patients then received postoperative radiation therapy and consolidative chemotherapy. Induction chemotherapy produced major responses in 17 (77%) of the 22 patients, including 3 (14%) complete responses and 14 (67%) partial responses. Of the 21 patients undergoing surgical resection, 16 (76%) had complete resections. The overall survival rate was 95% at 5 years and 79% at 7 years. The progression-free survival rates were 77% at 5 years and 77% at 7 years. Although the sample size was small in this study, these results mandate a thoughtful approach to patients who are considered unresectable or who have larger tumors and are likely to have invasion on the basis of preoperative CT scans.

Thymic carcinomas are tumors of thymic epithelial origin; however, they are distinguished from thymomas by malignant cytologic features and clinically more malignant behavior. Cells have marked atypia and increased proliferative activity. Radiographically they are indistinguishable from thymomas, but the presence of early regional lymph nodes and distant metastases is highly suggestive of thymic carcinoma. These tumors are usually invasive and have marked metastatic potential, making them refractory to medical and surgical therapy. PET scanning may be helpful to assess metastatic disease, with metastatic sites including lymph nodes, lung, liver, and bone. There is no standardized staging system, and because of the rarity of the tumor, no standardized treatment protocol exists. Surgical resection followed by radiation therapy can be performed for localized, noninvasive disease. However, tumors that are locally advanced should be treated with cisplatin-based chemotherapy and radiation alone. Survival rate in general is determined on the basis of histologic grade of the tumor, and prognosis is poor, with an overall median survival of less than 24 months.

Thymic carcinoid is a rare endocrine tumor of thymic origin. These tumors are rarely associated with the classic carcinoid syndrome but instead frequently produce adrenocorticotropin (ACTH) or a variety of other hormones. They are associated with the multiple endocrine neoplasia (MEN)-1 syndrome approximately 20% of the time. Most patients present with symptoms of cough, chest pain, or dyspnea, and 30% to 40% of patients have Cushing's syndrome. These tumors are aggressive locally and frequently associated with metastases. This is in stark contrast to carcinoid tumors found elsewhere in the body. The imaging of carcinoid tumors with FDG-PET is usually limited by slow tumor metabolism. [111]Inoctreotide scanning is therefore superior to PET for detection, staging, and characterization. Surgery is the primary treatment modality; however, most recur locally or with metastases despite "complete" resection. Because these tend to be slow-growing tumors, some centers advocate repeated resection of locally recurrent and metastatic disease. Radiation is indicated for primary and adjuvant therapy of carcinoid tumors and has been associated with improvement of paraneoplastic syndromes associated with these neoplasms.

Thymolipoma is a benign, slow-growing neoplasm that can grow to a large size. It is composed of both mature adipose tissue and thymic tissue. Most patients are asymptomatic, and there is a weak association with myasthenia gravis. Imaging may be diagnostic, with CT scan showing a well-defined fatty tumor with strands of soft-tissue attenuation representing normal thymic tissue. This tumor reliably conforms to adjacent structures. T2-weighted MRI images demonstrate low attenuation fatty tissue with bright thymic tissue. Surgical resection is usually curative.

Thymic cysts are rare tumors and may be associated with inflammation or with an inflammatory neoplasm such as Hodgkin's lymphoma. Congenital cysts are thought to be remnants of the thymopharyngeal duct. CT scanning usually demonstrates a well-circumscribed mass, but in general, internal architecture is difficult to assess. MRI with T2-weighted imaging shows homogenous high-signal intensity within the lesion and also may reveal internal septations. Complex cysts may be difficult to distinguish from malignant tumors, but if the clinical diagnosis is clear, these lesions may be observed. Otherwise surgical resection confirms the diagnosis.

Lymphoma

Lymphoma in general is not a surgical disease, and the major role of the surgeon in this clinical entity is to provide adequate tissue for diagnosis. The surgeon should be able to identify the characteristics of lymphoma in imaging studies that will allow one to avoid misguided attempts at resection of a malady that should be treated medically.

Primary mediastinal lymphomas are rare, with large-cell lymphomas representing 2% to 3% of all non-Hodgkin's lymphoma (NHL) and 6% to 12% of all diffuse, large-cell lymphomas. Lymphoblastic lymphomas represent less than 5% of all NHL. More than half of patients with lymphoblastic lymphoma present with mediastinal masses, and primary pulmonary lymphomas are rare, originating from mucosa-associated lymphoid tissue of the bronchus. Hodgkin's lymphoma is much less common than NHL and frequently involves mediastinal structures. Hodgkin's disease accounts for 50% to 70% of mediastinal lymphomas, with nodular sclerosing HD being the most common subtype, often manifesting with an anterior mediastinal mass. HD is rarely limited to the mediastinum, however, and therefore peripheral lymph node tissue is usually available for diagnostic purposes.

Clinical presentation is usually attributable to mass effect in the chest, with patients complaining of chest pain or pressure, cough, or dyspnea. Superior vena cava (SVC) syndrome may be seen, and occasionally pericardial effusions or cardiac tamponade is observed. Many patients may have completely asymptomatic bulky mediastinal adenopathy.

Because adequate tissue sample is essential for making a diagnosis, from time to time the surgeon is asked to provide surgical expertise. The surgeon should perform a complete physical examination, including assessment of cervical, axillary, and inguinal lymphadenopathy because this may uncover pathologic lymphadenopathy that is more safely and easily accessed than obtaining mediastinal tissue. Fine needle aspiration (FNA) (rarely) and preferably core needle biopsy under ultrasound or CT guidance are less invasive methods for obtaining tissue. In general, lymphoma represents the tumor diagnosis that requires the most tissue volume because special stains and flow cytometry are usually necessary to make a complete diagnosis.

FNA provides only cytologic material and does not allow for assessment of architectural detail, nor does it give adequate tissue for immunophenotyping. HD and NHL lymph nodes in particular typically have a significant fibrotic component, and therefore larger sample sizes are necessary for diagnosis. Lymphoblastic lymphoma is one subtype that may not require more tissue than that obtained with FNA. Core needle biopsy allows for larger tissue sampling and assessment of lymph node architecture. Typically this involves an 18-gauge needle through a parasternal route into the anterior mediastinum with CT or ultrasound guidance. In one study, the success rate did not depend on the size of the needle used, with 14-, 18-, and 20-gauge needles having similar diagnostic yield. Multiple passes of the needle should be performed to maximize tissue volume. If core needle biopsy is not successful, various surgical approaches may be entertained. Anterior mediastinal tumors are ideally accessed for biopsy via an anterior mediastinotomy (Chamberlain procedure). This can be performed on the left or right side, typically in the second or third intercostal space immediately adjacent to the sternum. Typically a short transverse incision is made over the interspace, and dissection is carried down to the costal cartilage, splitting the pectoralis muscle fibers. The costal cartilage may be removed, and the internal thoracic artery may be ligated if necessary. The pleura is then dissected laterally, and the mass is encountered. A mediastinoscope is helpful for retracting tissue and providing adequate lighting. This approach allows access to anterior mediastinal masses, as well as anterior-posterior window masses or lymphadenopathy. It does not provide access to the visceral compartment. Paratracheal, middle mediastinal, tracheobronchial angle, or subcarinal lymph nodes may be sampled with mediastinoscopy. Although a transthoracic thoracoscopic approach allows access to the anterior mediastinum, aortopulmonary window, and paratracheal and subcarinal areas, this should be reserved for situations in which lymphoma is high on the differential or no other route is available for biopsy to avoid inadvertent seeding of the pleural space. In summary, if needle biopsy is unsuccessful, the next least morbid approach is mediastinoscopy if the patient has involvement of paratracheal or subcarinal lymph nodes. Anterior mediastinotomy provides access to the anterior mediastinum but is more invasive than mediastinoscopy. If lymphoma is high on the differential, a VATS procedure is acceptable. Finally, frozen section should be obtained before completion of any of these procedures to ensure that diagnostic tissue has been sampled.

Patients with HD have neoplastic proliferation of Reed-Sternberg cells, and HD is subdivided into four distinct pathologic groups: (1) nodular sclerosing, (2) nodular lymphocyte predominant, (3) mixed cellularity, and (4) lymphocyte depleted HD. Nodular sclerosing is the most common subtype of mediastinal HD. Most patients with HD present with asymptomatic peripheral adenopathy. The adenopathy is usually contiguous, involving the cervical, supraclavicular, and mediastinal lymph nodes, with two thirds of patients having mediastinal adenopathy. Some patients may have large, bulky mediastinal masses. Isolated mediastinal involvement is usually seen in young female patients. Systemic symptoms such as fever, night sweats, or unexplained weight loss occur in 25% of patients but are uncommon in early-stage disease. Generalized pruritus is common. Patients with bulky mediastinal masses generally have a worse prognosis. Treatment involves mantle radiation and chemotherapy, with newer regimens providing better toxicity profiles. Primary mediastinal large B cell lymphoma is an aggressive lymphoma and is more common in younger patients, with a median age in the fourth decade. The tumor usually presents as an anterior mediastinal mass originating in the thymus and is locally invasive, with contiguous spread to the pleura, lung, pericardium, and chest wall. These patients may present as an oncologic emergency with a rapidly enlarging mass causing SVC syndrome or airway compression. Treatment is usually combined chemotherapy and radiation therapy, and overall survival of 70% to 90% at 2 to 5 years is seen with some regimens. Lymphoblastic lymphoma is cytologically similar to acute lymphoblastic leukemia (ALL). The majority of patients have a large mediastinal mass, and rapid tumor growth may result in airway compression or SVC syndrome. This is the most likely NHL to present as a medical emergency. Treatment is with multiagent chemotherapy and radiation therapy, and tumor responses are rapid, usually with complete resolution a few days after initiation of treatment.

Residual mediastinal masses may be present after therapy. Secondary malignancies related to radiation therapy, relapses of HD, or degeneration into another lymphoma may occur, and occasionally the surgeon may be asked to provide biopsy material of a new mediastinal mass or new or residual lymphadenopathy. One should keep in mind that surgical risk may be increased because of radiation-induced cardiac or pulmonary disease. Needle biopsy via a percutaneous or transbronchial route should be contemplated as an initial approach. Mediastinoscopy may be difficult because of mediastinal fibrosis and scarring, and other approaches such as with thoracoscopy or thoracotomy may be safer.

Germ Cell Tumors

Germ cell tumors are neoplasms that usually arise in the gonads; however, a small proportion do arise primarily in the anterior mediastinum, which is the most common extragonadal site. These comprise roughly 10% to 20% of all anterior mediastinal masses. Malignant transformation of germ cell elements within the thymus gland or the anterior mediastinum is the likely explanation for the occurrence of germ cell tumors in this area. Several studies have demonstrated only occasional synchronous testicular tumors in patients with mediastinal tumors; conversely, patients with primary testicular germ cell tumors only rarely have metastases to the mediastinum.

Germ cell tumors of the mediastinum are classified as being teratoma, seminomatous, or nonseminomatous. The nonseminomatous germ cell tumors include yolk sac tumors, choriocarcinomas, embryonal carcinomas, and mixed germ cell tumors. Most of these tumors occur in adolescents and young adults, and males almost exclusively develop the malignant variety. Benign teratoma is the most common tumor, accounting for approximately 70% of total cases, and seminoma tends to be the most common malignant variety. Benign tumors tend to be asymptomatic, whereas malignant tumors produce symptoms in more than 80% of patients. Symptoms usually consist of chest pressure, cough, or dyspnea and are usually a consequence of compression of adjacent structures.

CT with intravenous contrast is the best imaging modality for germ cell tumors. Benign tumors tend to be spherical and demonstrate slow growth on serial examination. The presence of calcification is a helpful sign; however, it is not specific and may be seen with other tumors such as thymoma or thyroid goiter. Benign teratomas may demonstrate bone or tooth elements, and the presence of a fat-fluid level or combination of fluid, soft tissue, and calcification is highly specific for a benign teratoma. Seminomas are usually large, homogenous masses with smooth margins, whereas nonseminomatous tumors tend to be large, inhomogeneous masses with necrosis, hemorrhage, or both. In general, malignant tumors are larger, more lobulated, and faster growing than benign tumors and tend to demonstrate mediastinal invasion with obliteration of fat planes, lymphadenopathy, and metastatic disease to the lung, pleura, or chest wall. The malignant tumors also tend to have areas of necrosis or hemorrhage, probably because of their rapid growth rates.

When one suspects that an anterior mediastinal mass represents a germ cell tumor, analysis of serum tumor markers is an essential component of the workup and provides diagnostic, as well as prognostic information. Alpha-fetoprotein (AFP) and human chorionic gonadotropin B (B-HCG) levels should be obtained before any attempt at biopsy or surgical intervention. Benign teratomas do not have any elevation of either of these proteins, whereas seminomas can be associated with low-level elevation of B-HCG (usually <100 mIU/ml), but any elevation of AFP indicates a nonseminomatous tumor. More than 80% of patients with a nonseminomatous germ cell tumor have elevated AFP, and 30% to 50% have elevation of B-HCG. Lactate dehydrogenase elevation is seen in 80% to 90% of nonseminomatous tumors, and this is directly related to tumor volume. When AFP levels are elevated, treatment may be initiated without confirmatory tissue biopsy. If tumor markers are not elevated, or if only the B-HCG is elevated, a biopsy of the mass is necessary. CT-guided core needle biopsy can be used to make the diagnosis; however, the sample size may be insufficient, and a Chamberlain procedure or thoracoscopic approach is necessary.

The diagnosis of teratoma is usually made clinically on the basis of presentation and radiographic appearance. FNA or core needle biopsy may be difficult to interpret because of the multiple tissue types and may not be required before planned resection. Treatment of teratoma is surgical excision, which is usually curative, and there is no role for adjuvant chemotherapy or radiotherapy. The surgical approach is most often from a median sternotomy, although a lateral thoracotomy or anterior thoracotomy combined with a sternotomy may be necessary for tumors that are lateral in the mediastinum. These tumors can be bulky and adherent to adjacent tissues, sometimes necessitating resection of pericardium, nonvital vascular structures, or lung tissue. A thoracoscopic approach may be used for small, well-circumscribed tumors. If any rib spreading is necessary, the perceived benefit of the VATS approach is usually lost, given the rapid recovery after a median sternotomy. Special consideration should be given to patients who wish to avoid the cosmetic defect associated with a median sternotomy.

Mediastinal seminomas are rare, slow-growing tumors that occur almost exclusively in males. Only pure seminomas reside in this category, and therefore mixed tumors are considered with the nonseminomatous classification. These usually become large before symptoms appear and the patient seeks medical advice. Sixty to seventy percent of patients have metastatic disease at the time of diagnosis, most commonly to the lungs, bone, or liver. Initial staging involves CT scanning of the chest, abdomen, and pelvis. Although these tumors are usually gallium avid, scanning is typically not indicated. Seminomas are exquisitely sensitive to radiation and cisplatin-based chemotherapy, although there is no standardized treatment algorithm. There is little if any role for surgery, even with early, well-circumscribed disease. Primary surgical debulking has never been shown to provide therapeutic benefit.

Primary chemotherapy with cisplatin, bleomycin, and etoposide is the most common treatment regimen for these mediastinal seminomas. Because of the potential for radiation pneumonitis, further pulmonary toxicity may be avoided by using ifosfamide instead of bleomycin. This regimen can result in remission rates of more than 90% and overall 5-year survival as high as 88%. Primary radiotherapy can be considered in patients who do not have bulky or metastatic disease. This can result in a high primary tumor cure rate; however, many patients relapse with distant metastatic disease, and the 5-year survival is only 60% to 70%. These patients can receive salvage chemotherapy; however, the data suggest that these patients have a worse 5-year survival than those who received primary chemotherapy.

The presence of a residual mass after primary chemotherapy or radiation therapy is concerning to the patient and the physician. Some studies have shown residual viable tumor to be present in up to 30% of tumors greater than 3 cm in diameter. As expected, surgical resection of these masses can be technically hazardous, and needle biopsy is subject to considerable sampling error, given the extensive necrosis and desmoplastic reaction in the tumor. Options therefore include resection of masses greater than 3 cm, or, depending on patient physiology, tumor location or, according to patient preference, surveillance CT scanning with intervention should the tumor mass grow. Confirmatory biopsy should be obtained before radiation therapy to these masses should they turn out to be teratomas. Salvage chemotherapy may be considered as well.

The nonseminomatous germ cell tumors (NSMGCT) are less common than seminomatous germ cell tumors and carry a far worse prognosis. These include yolk sac tumors, choriocarcinoma, embryonal carcinoma, endodermal sinus tumor, and teratocarcinoma (malignant teratoma). As stated earlier, any mixed seminomatous tumors are classified as NSGCT. These are rare tumors occurring in men in their 20s or 30s and are usually symptomatic on presentation. More than 80% of patients have metastatic disease at the time of presentation. Gynecomastia can develop as a result of B-hCG secretion, and 20% of the patients have Klinefelter syndrome. Overall these tumors carry a far worse prognosis than any other germ cell tumors, and patients are at risk for developing fatal hematologic disorders because of shared cytogenetic abnormalities. CT findings demonstrate large, lobulated tumors in the anterior mediastinum with evidence of mediastinal invasion or lymphadenopathy, as well as metastatic disease in the lungs, pleurae, or chest wall. The NSMGCTs tend to have areas of necrosis and hemorrhage and spiculated margins. Most patients present with an elevated AFP, and the majority have elevation of B-hCG. Because any elevation of AFP indicates an NSMGCT, many centers initiate therapy in the setting of an anterior mediastinal mass without a tissue diagnosis. Approximately 10% of patients have no serum marker elevation, and this group requires tissue for diagnosis.

Standard treatment of NSMGCT includes chemotherapy with bleomycin, etoposide, and cisplatin. Approximately 20% of patients have a complete radiographic and serologic response to chemotherapy. Pathologic complete response rates are as high as 50%, and up to 45% of patients are long-term disease-free survivors. Serial monitoring of AFP and B-hCG is useful to assess response to therapy. Salvage chemotherapy rarely results in any improvement in survival, and therefore surgical resection is recommended for residual masses after initial chemotherapy. This includes patients with normalization of tumors markers, as well as those who continue to have some elevation of serologic markers. Patients with progressive disease or those with extrathoracic disease should not undergo resectional therapy. Because these residual masses are usually associated with intense fibrosis, excellent surgical exposure is necessary, and this is usually accomplished via a median sternotomy or a clamshell incision. Patients may require a partial pericardiectomy in addition to a pulmonary resection to remove the tumor completely. Unilateral phrenic nerve resection may be necessary. Postresection histology can be variable and include persistent germ cell tumor, teratoma, or necrosis. All teratoma elements should be resected lest they grow back. This is observed in the face of normal serologic markers and is known as the growing teratoma syndrome. Patients with persistent germ cell tumors usually receive further cycles of chemotherapy; however, outcomes in this patient population are poor.

Thyroid

Almost as a rule, thyroid tissue in the mediastinum is a consequence of caudal migration from the normal anatomic location in the neck caused by tumor or benign enlargement. Only a few reports of isolated thyroid tissue in the mediastinum exist, unlike the ectopic parathyroid glandular tissue that may more commonly be seen because of the common embryologic origin with the thymus. Thyroid masses must descend through the thoracic inlet,

which consists entirely of the visceral mediastinum, and therefore most thyroid masses technically lie in this compartment anteriorly, rather than the anterior mediastinum. The perception that these lie in the anterior mediastinum is usually a consequence of displacement of the great vessels posteriorly. Because of constraints imposed by the pretracheal fascia, these never truly lie in the anterior compartment unless the patient has had prior surgery that would disrupt this plane.

Approximately half of patients with an intrathoracic thyroid mass have a multinodular goiter, and approximately 40% have a follicular adenoma. One review demonstrated the incidence of malignancy to be 8.3%. The majority of patients with substernal thyroid masses have symptoms, usually related to airway or recurrent nerve compression. Most patients are euthyroid, with hyperthyroidism found in 5% to 20% of patients. Chest radiograph demonstrates lateral deviation of the trachea in almost all cases, with the deviation beginning above the thoracic inlet. CT usually demonstrates a heterogeneous intrathoracic mass located superiorly on the left in continuity with the cervical pretracheal thyroid. Occasionally the mass descends posteriorly along the trachea. Clearly defined borders and punctuate calcifications are common, and the mass usually enhances with iodinated contrast. The great vessels are usually displaced laterally and anteriorly.

Treatment involves surgical resection, and there is no role for medical therapy in alleviating the compressive nature of the mass. Airway management is critical, and many patients have some degree of tracheomalacia or airway compression, making rapid sequence intubation essential. Awake fiberoptic intubation should be considered, and a rigid bronchoscope should be readily available should control of the airway be difficult. Note that if the patient's neck is flexed during a CT scan, this position may cause the mass to be pushed into the intrathoracic compartment. However, in the operating room, positioning the patient with a shoulder roll and neck extension may cause the mass to devolve out of the thorax, facilitating exposure and resection via a collar incision alone. Initially, a low collar incision should be used because these masses can be resected without a sternotomy more than 90% of the time. A partial sternal split to the third or fourth intercostal space may be used, with a "T" incision coming down from the initial collar incision. A full median sternotomy is unnecessary. Because of the high incidence of recurrent laryngeal nerve injury, a posterolateral thoracotomy should be avoided unless it is used in conjunction with a cervical incision when attempting to remove a posteriorly located mass.

VISCERAL MEDIASTINUM AND MIDDLE MEDIASTINUM

The visceral mediastinal compartment contains paratracheal and parabronchial lymph nodes, the trachea and main bronchi, major blood vessels, the heart and pericardium, and the esophagus. Tumors or masses involving the middle mediastinum or visceral compartment include lymph node enlargement; cysts arising from the esophagus, pericardium, or airway; and benign or malignant neoplasms arising from the esophagus or the airway.

Lymphadenopathy is the most commonly seen abnormality in the visceral mediastinum and may be secondary to a diverse group of malignant and nonmalignant entities. Lymph node enlargement secondary to metastases from lung or airway tumors, esophageal cancer, and head and neck cancer may be seen. Lymphoma, described earlier, may have significant middle compartment involvement and is most often seen with HD, usually in association with anterior mediastinal adenopathy. Bulky tumor is defined as either a single mass of tumor tissue exceeding 10 cm in largest diameter or a mediastinal mass exceeding one third of the maximal transverse transthoracic diameter measured to the inside of the ribs on a standard posteroanterior chest x-ray and is considered as a prognostic factor. Other entities that can sometimes be confused with lymphoma include atypical lymphoid proliferations. The most common are processes referred to as "reactive" or "atypical" lymphoid hyperplasia, and patients present with localized or disseminated lymphadenopathy associated with an underlying process related to drug therapy (anticonvulsants), autoimmune disease such as rheumatoid arthritis or systemic lupus erythematosus, viral infections, or bacterial infections. Castleman's disease, also known as giant lymph node hyperplasia, is a rare entity that may also be confused with lymphoma, although this disease may evolve into lymphoma over time. Most patients classically present with a focal area of lymph node enlargement, but a generalized form is also recognized. Treatment is reserved for symptomatic patients, and surgical resection in patients with localized disease is usually curative. Certain forms of the disease have extreme vascularity, and careful surgical resection should be performed to avoid massive hemorrhage. The generalized form is usually treated with steroids.

Sarcoidosis is a multisystem granulomatous disease that is characterized by the presence of noncaseating granulomas in involved tissues. Although sarcoidosis most commonly affects the lung, some patients may only have hilar or paratracheal lymphadenopathy. Granulomatous infections such as histoplasmosis or coccidiomycosis may also result in mediastinal lymph node enlargement and are most commonly associated with residents of the Ohio River Valley or San Joaquin Valley regions. Calcifications tend to be present in these lymph node tissues.

Mediastinal lymphadenopathy is usually diagnosed with needle biopsy through a transbronchial or transesophageal approach. Endoscopic ultrasound is helpful to improve the accuracy of both of these methods. A percutaneous approach is technically not possible, and therefore obtaining a core needle biopsy is not an option. Should the surgeon be called on to obtain diagnostic tissue, biopsy of paratracheal or subcarinal adenopathy is best performed with mediastinoscopy. Alternatively these areas can also be accessed via a thorascopic approach, usually from the right side, where access to the upper mediastinum is not hindered by the aortic arch (Fig. 2). The larger biopsy specimens obtained with these surgical techniques are also valuable when lymph node architecture is critical to establishing a specific diagnosis of lymphoma.

Cysts arising from the esophagus, pericardium, or airway are among the most common masses seen in the mediastinum. These cysts arise during embryonic development and grow in size during the course of development. Bronchogenic cysts are the most common mediastinal cysts and may be located anywhere along the course of lung development, from the mediastinum to the lung parenchyma. In the mediastinum, they most commonly occur in the subcarinal area but may be seen adjacent to the pericardium, esophagus, or sternum. Most recent reports have found that the majority of patients harboring these cysts eventually become symptomatic if they are not so at the time of diagnosis, presenting with airway complaints such as cough, wheezing, dysphagia, or airway obstruction. Sometimes symptoms are positional in nature. An infected cyst may cause symptoms such as fever, malaise, or chest pain. Bronchogenic cysts are best imaged using CT, which usually reveals a smooth rounded or oval structure of homogeneous soft-tissue density intimately associated with the tracheobronchial tree. Calcifications are rare, and water density is common. MRI may be helpful because all mediastinal cysts are hyperintense on T2-weighted imaging. If the diagnosis is in doubt, transtracheal or transesophageal aspiration may be diagnostic, demonstrating mucoid material. Bronchogenic cysts may be observed if asymptomatic, although many eventually become symptomatic or infected, and some may contain malignant tissue.

Esophageal cysts may be similar to bronchogenic cysts but are much less common. They are usually defined by being attached to the esophagus, with epithelial tissue representative of some layer of the gastrointestinal tract and sometimes containing two layers of muscularis propria. Most are asymptomatic but may present with dysphagia or pain. Infection and hemorrhage into the cyst has been reported, the latter being more common in children. Diagnosis is usually based on CT characteristics similar to bronchogenic cysts and characteristic hyperintensity with T2-weighted MRI. Because gastric mucosa lines the lumen approximately 50% of the time, a ^{99m}technetium (^{99m}Tc) pertechnetate scan may be positive. Differentiation from a leiomyoma can be accomplished by CT attenuation. Transesophageal biopsy should be avoided because infection may result.

Pericardial cysts are usually located at the right cardiophrenic angle or along the diaphragm but may be found in the mediastinum related to the right or left heart border or even the superior mediastinum. These cysts can be confused with a foramen of Morgagni hernia or the pericardial fat pad, and MRI may help to distinguish one from the other. Patients are rarely symptomatic, and resection is not usually necessary because they have no known malignant potential. Percutaneous aspiration may be therapeutic.

Removal of cysts may be accomplished via a VATS approach, although a thoracotomy may be necessary. Reports exist of removal with mediastinoscopy. The surgeon should attempt to remove all epithelialized tissue to avoid recurrence. If this is not technically possible or safe, fulguration of any residual secreting epithelial tissue should be performed. Care should be performed when excising foregut cysts because resection may leave a small defect in the esophageal mucosa.

POSTERIOR (PARAVERTEBRAL SULCUS) MEDIASTINAL TUMORS

Structures in the paravertebral sulcus include the autonomic ganglia, as well as the proximal intercostal nerves, arteries, and veins. Because there is minimal lymphatic tissue associated with this compartment, neurogenic tumors represent the vast majority of tumors arising from this area. Neurogenic tumors arise from the peripheral nerves, the sympathetic ganglia, or the paraganglionic cells, and the incidence of tumor type and degree of malignancy depends strongly on age. In children, tumors are more likely to be malignant, most arising from the autonomic ganglia. In adults, the overwhelming majority of paravertebral sulcus tumors are benign tumors arising from the nerve sheath.

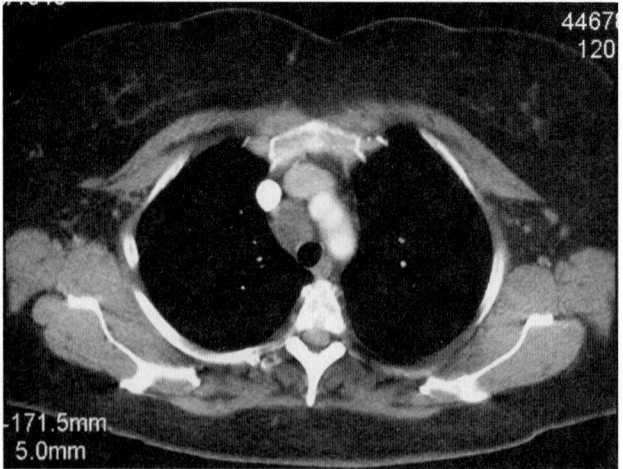

Figure 2 A visceral mediastinal paratracheal mass that was removed via a right thorascopic approach. Pathologic examination demonstrated this to be a mesothelial cyst.

Benign tumors include tumors originating in nerve sheath such as Schwannoma (neurilemoma or neurinoma), neurofibroma, melanotic schwannoma, or granular cell tumors. Ganglioneuroma, chemodectoma, and pheochromocytoma are benign tumors arising from the autonomic nervous system ganglia. Malignant tumors include malignant schwannoma or neurofibrosarcoma, malignant melanocytic schwannoma, neuroblastoma, ganglioneuroblastoma, and pigmented neuroectodermal tumors. The only known risk factor for benign or malignant neurogenic tumors is the presence of von Recklinghausen's neurofibromatosis; in these patients the benign neurofibroma is most common.

The posterior mediastinum along the paravertebral sulcus is the most common site for neurogenic tumors, and intraspinal extension can occur in up to 10% of tumors. CT scanning helps to define tumor characteristics and relation to adjacent tissues; however, MRI should be performed on all patients to identify any extension into the neural foramen. Presence of this finding changes the operative planning significantly.

Peripheral Nerve Origin

Benign nerve sheath tumors are the most common neurogenic tumors in the mediastinum, and more than 90% of these are schwannomas (neurilemmomas) or neurofibromas. Mediastinal benign schwannomas, which comprise 75% of nerve sheath tumors, originate from Schwann cells and affect patients predominantly in the third and fourth decade of life. Neurofibromas, which represent 25% of all nerve sheath tumors, can be multifocal in patients with neurofibromatosis (von Recklinghausen's syndrome). Benign nerve sheath tumors are slow growing and typically asymptomatic, but patients may present with symptoms such as back pain or signs of nerve compression or paralysis (with intraspinal extension), Pancoast's syndrome, or Horner's syndrome. Brachial plexus compression may be seen as well. Many times these tumors are incidental findings on chest x-rays or CT. Typical CT findings include a smooth, well-circumscribed, rounded mass lying in the paravertebral sulcus, with a propensity for the upper mediastinum (Fig. 3). Focal calcifications and cystic changes are frequent. Neurilemmomas and neurofibromas are radiographically indistinguishable. Notation should also be made as to the relationship with adjacent organs such as the aorta, esophagus, and spinal cord. MRI of the spine should be performed on all masses located in the paravertebral sulcus at the costovertebral angle because these may represent "dumbbell" tumors with extension into the neural foramen. Dumbbell tumors may occur with nerve sheath tumors or tumors arising from the sympathetic ganglia. Histologically, schwannomas may comprise spindle cells with twisted nuclei and nuclear palisading or have loose and myxoid connective tissue containing a random arrangement of cells. Neurilemmomas are S-100 positive. Neurofibromas are characterized by a disorganized proliferation of all nerve elements and may or may not be S-100 positive.

Neurofibrosarcoma (malignant schwannoma) is rare and most commonly associated with neurofibromatosis, affecting 2% to 5% of these patients. It is thought that these tumors may be the result of malignant degeneration of a neurofibroma. Malignant schwannomas are also associated with radiation exposure. CT findings of necrosis, hemorrhage, or cystic degeneration suggest malignancy. These tumors are often associated with local invasion and distant metastases. Surgical resection with negative margins is essential for long-term survival, otherwise local recurrence usually occurs despite adjuvant chemoradiation. Outcome is poor, with 5-year survival approximately 50% in nonneurofibromatosis patients, decreasing to 10% to 15% in patients with neurofibromatosis.

Sympathetic Ganglion Origin

Ganglioneuroma, ganglioneuroblastoma, and neuroblastoma arise from the sympathetic ganglia. The majority of these tumors occur in children and young adults. There is considerable overlap in their histopathology, as well as a broad range of clinical behavior from benign to highly malignant. The benign, well-differentiated ganglioneuroma occasionally secretes vasoactive intestinal peptide resulting in diarrhea symptoms; however, most are asymptomatic. Radiographically these tumors are well circumscribed and typically oblong. Intraspinal extension through the intervertebral foramen is common, and therefore, as with other paravertebral tumors, MRI is essential for preoperative planning. Complete resection is curative, with local recurrence uncommon. Ganglioneuroblastomas make up approximately one third of autonomic ganglion tumors and are more likely to have invasion of adjacent structures, but grossly the tumor usually remains encapsulated. Complete resection is usually possible, with an overall 5-year survival rate of 88%. Neuroblastoma is the most malignant-acting tumor of the sympathetic ganglion, with extension into the spinal canal or local invasion common at presentation. Staging of ganglioneuroblastoma and neuroblastoma is based on the extent of local invasion, lymph node involvement, and the presence of metastases. Well-circumscribed tumors can be cured with surgical resection alone; however, those with locally invasive tumors or tumors extending across the midline, as well as those with lymph node involvement, should receive adjuvant chemoradiation therapy.

Parasympathetic Ganglion Origin

Pheochromocytomas and chemodectomas, both of which are derived from paraganglionic tissues, are the least common tumors in the paravertebral sulcus. Both of these tumors tend to be highly vascular and are usually unencapsulated and infiltrative. Pheochromocytomas tend to be hormonally active, and only 10% of these behave in a malignant fashion, similar to those found in the retroperitoneum. Symptoms result from direct invasion of the tumor or as a consequence of catecholamine secretion, which may cause hypertension, diabetes, or hypermetabolism. Localization of the tumor can be achieved using I-131 metaiodobenzylguanidine scintigraphy in combination with CT. Complete excision is the mainstay of therapy, with preoperative use of alpha-adrenergic blockade essential for blood pressure control in metabolically active tumors. These tumors tend to be resistant to chemotherapy and radiation therapy. Chemodectomas tend to be hormonally inactive, and because of their highly vascular nature, preoperative angioembolization is advocated. If surgical resection is not feasible, radiation therapy can be used for tumor control.

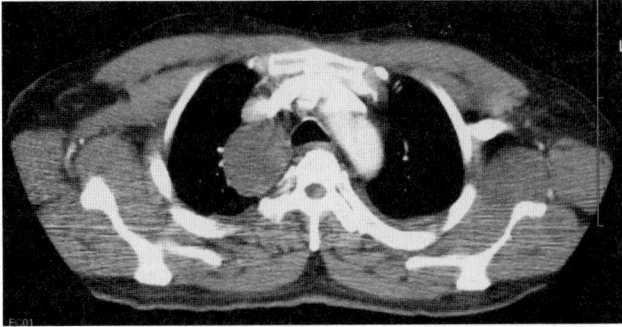

Figure 3 A round, homogeneous 7-cm mass in the paravertebral sulcus. This appeared bright on T2-weighted magnetic resonance imaging, suggesting a cyst, and was removed via a right thorascopic approach. Pathologic examination demonstrated a foregut cyst.

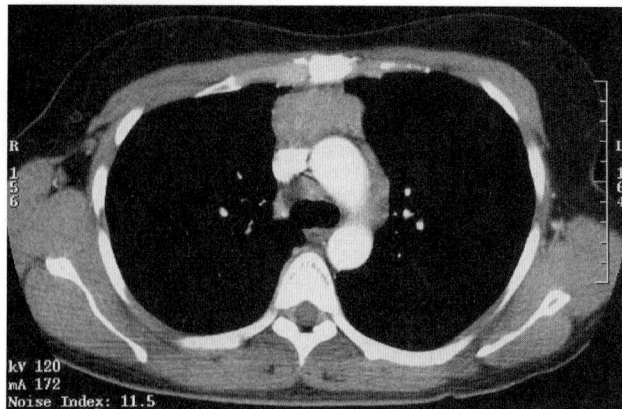

Figure 4   A heterogenous anterior mediastinal mass with irregular borders and associated paratracheal adenopathy in a 38-year-old female patient. Core needle biopsy demonstrated a B-cell lymphoma.

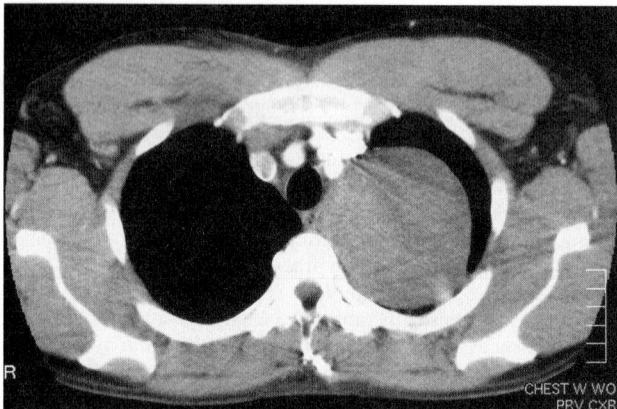

Figure 5   This 10-cm paravertebral sulcus tumor was an incidental finding on a chest x-ray in a 40-year-old male patient. When queried, the patient reported ipsilateral facial anhidrosis for greater than 6 years. A core needle biopsy was performed because of the unclear anatomic location of the mass. A high left thoracotomy was performed to remove this schwannoma, which was involved with heavy adhesions to the parasympathetic chain and chest wall.

Surgical resection is the mainstay of therapy for virtually all neurogenic tumors. Most well-circumscribed neurogenic tumors are cured with surgical resection, and smaller discrete tumors in the paravertebral sulcus may be removed with a thorascopic or VATS minimally invasive technique. Larger tumors or those with evidence of adherence or invasion may require a lateral or posterolateral thoracotomy for resection. Because the sympathetic chain lies in close proximity to the proximal nerve root, the tumor is usually adherent, and sacrifice of the ganglion is usually necessary. Chest wall resection or vertebral body resection is unusual. With large tumors in the upper mediastinum, great care should be made to avoid injury to the phrenic or vagus nerves during resection.

It is important to identify tumors with invasion into the neural foramen before surgical intervention is planned because the operative approach is more complex. A two-incision approach is performed, with an initial posterior approach to perform a laminectomy to separate the tumor from the dura of the spinal cord and proximal neural foramen. The second stage of the operation involves transthoracic resection of the tumor in the same setting.

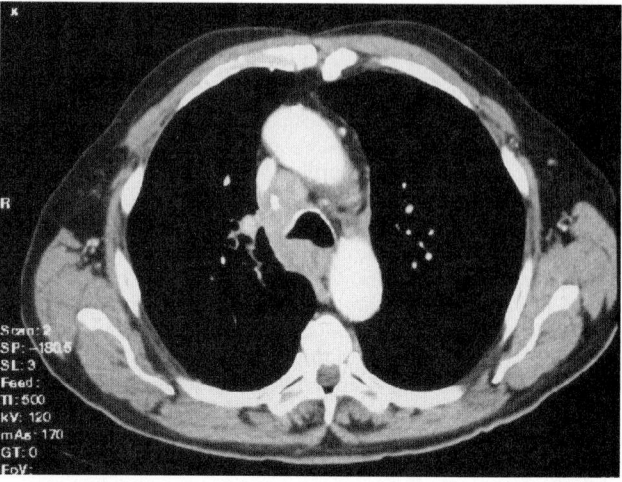

Figure 6   This paratracheal mass shows multiple enlarged lymph node areas in the visceral mediastinum. Note the area of calcification, which is likely related to old granulomatous disease. Biopsies using mediastinoscopy revealed a B-cell lymphoma.

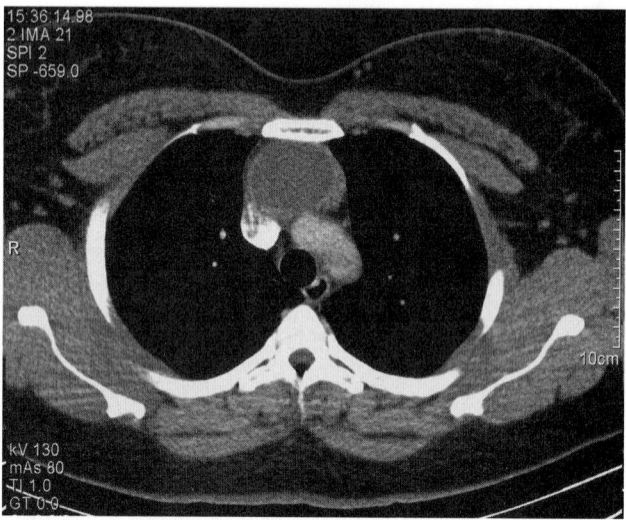

Figure 7   This round mass in the anterior mediastinum was seen in a 43-year-old woman who developed persistent chest pain after a minor automobile accident. A median sternotomy was performed that demonstrated a solid, densely adherent mass that was completely resected. Pathologic examination revealed a unilocular thymic cyst filled with organizing thrombus. It is likely the trauma resulted in hemorrhage, and her symptoms were a consequence of rapid expansion of the cyst.

SUGGESTED READINGS

Alavi A, Gupta N, Alberini JL, and others: Positron emission tomography imaging in nonmalignant thoracic disorders, *Sem Nucl Med* 22:293, 2002.

Kelemen JJ 3rd, Naunheim KS: Minimally invasive approaches to mediastinal neoplasms, *Sem Thorac Cardiovasc Surg* 12:301, 2000.

Kim ES, Putnam JB, Komaki R, and others: Phase II study of a multidisciplinary approach with induction chemotherapy, followed by surgical resection, radiation therapy, and consolidation chemotherapy for unresectable malignant thymomas, *Lung Cancer* 44:369, 2004.

Wright CD, Kessler KA: Surgical treatment of thymic tumors, *Sem Thorac Cardiovasc Surg* 17:20, 2005.

Primary Tumors of the Thymus

Kenneth A. Kesler, MD

The thymus gland is derived from the third brachial cleft and descends during embryogenesis into the anterior mediastinum while retaining bilateral cervical poles. The right and left thymic lobes, lying anterior to the great veins and pericardium, constitute the bulk of the gland. Both lobes extend to the phrenic nerves laterally and then usually contiguous with the pericardiophrenic fat inferiorly. The thymus gland occupies the vast majority of anterior mediastinal compartment, and therefore cells contained within the gland represent the origin of most anterior mediastinal neoplasms. The differential diagnosis for neoplasms originating in the anterior mediastinal compartment is simplified by the "4-T" mnemonic, which includes thymoma, "terrible" lymphoma, teratoma, and thyroid lesions. These four conditions represent more than 90% of all anterior mediastinal masses. A more specific list of tumors arising within the thymus is given in Table 1.

Table 1: Tumors Arising from Cells Contained within the Thymus Gland

Thymic Disease

Thymoma

Thymic carcinoma

Thymic neuroendocrine tumors

Thymolipoma

Thymic cysts

Thymic hyperplasia

Lymphoma

Hodgkin's

Non-Hodgkin's

Germ Cell Tumors

Teratoma

Seminoma

Nonseminomatous

Thyroid Lesions

Parathyroid adenoma

Aberrant thyroid

Mesenchymal Tumors

Lipoma

Fibroma

Lymphangioma

Hemangioma

THYMOMA

Clinical Presentation

Thymomas represent the most common mediastinal neoplasm, as well as the most common anterior mediastinal compartment neoplasm, occurring in the adult population. The overall incidence of thymoma is rare, however, estimated to be 0.15 cases per 100,000 population. Thymoma is an epithelial tumor generally considered to have an indolent growth pattern but malignant nonetheless because of potential for local invasion, pleural dissemination, and even systemic metastases. Most patients are between the ages of 30 and 60 years at the time of diagnosis, with an equal gender distribution. Approximately one third of patients with localized disease at presentation are symptomatic, most commonly reporting cough or vague chest discomfort. With increasing use of routine CT screening, higher percentages of patients are anticipated to present with asymptomatic disease. Patients demonstrating either locally advanced or disseminated thymoma at the time of presentation are usually symptomatic with significant chest pain, shortness of breath from lung or pleural involvement, phrenic nerve paralysis, pleural effusions, and/or superior vena cava (SVC) syndrome. Of unique interest, several immune disorders have been associated with thymoma. Myasthenia gravis is the most common, occurring in 30% to 40% of patients presenting with thymoma. Neurologic consultation should be considered if there is suspicion of myasthenia, particularly for any patient being evaluated for diagnostic or therapeutic surgical intervention because severe respiratory morbidity can be minimized with appropriate perioperative management. Up to 30% of thymoma patients present with an immune disorder other than myasthenia gravis; the most common include red cell aplasia and hypogammaglobulinemia.

Diagnosis

Chest computed tomography (CT) scanning with intravenous contrast is the radiographic examination of choice for evaluation of all masses in the anterior mediastinal compartment. CT imaging not only precisely defines size, density characteristics, and relationship to surrounding intrathoracic organs such as the great vessels, lungs, pericardium, and heart but also the presence of parietal pleural deposits or so-called droplet metastases most frequently found in the posterior basilar pleural space and diaphragm. Because this tendency to metastasize in the posterior basilar pleural space is rather unique to thymomas, the radiographic presence of both an anterior compartment mass and "droplet" metastases is highly suggestive of the diagnosis. In general, the differential diagnoses of patients presenting with a mass in the anterior mediastinal compartment are initially guided by patient's age, gender, associated symptoms, and CT findings. Malignant nonseminomatous germ cell tumors occur primarily in male young adults and can essentially be ruled in or out by simply obtaining serum tumor marker levels of alpha-fetoprotein (AFP) and the beta subunit of human chorionic gonadotropin (B-HCG). Thyroid lesions involving the anterior mediastinal compartment are readily identified on CT scan as contiguous with the thyroid gland. Iodine-131 nuclear medicine scans can be used to confirm a thyroid origin in cases in which CT scanning is equivocal or ectopic thyroid tissue suspected.

The two main differential diagnoses of most anterior mediastinal compartment masses are therefore lymphoma and thymoma. In general, thymoma patients are older compared with patients presenting with lymphoma originating in the anterior mediastinal compartment. Constitutional symptoms such as night sweats, fever, weight loss, and malaise are more consistent with lymphomas. Physical examination including careful palpation of lymph-bearing areas such as the neck, axillae, and groins for lymphadenopathy

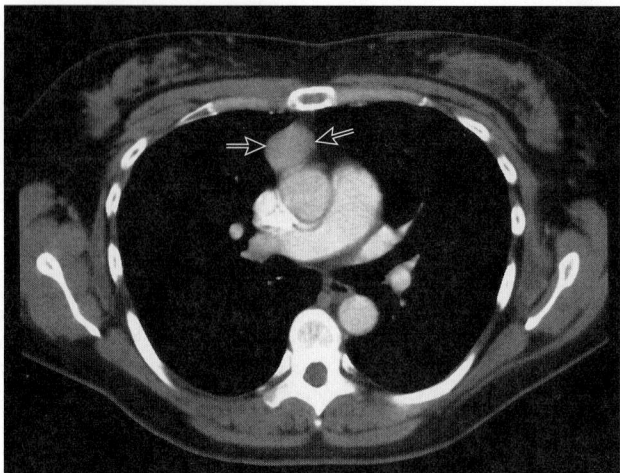

Figure 1 A small, lobulated mass in the anterior mediastinum identified in a patient with recently diagnosed myasthenia gravis on screening chest computed tomography. Because a Masaoka stage I or II thymoma was suspected, mediastinal dissection with complete en bloc thymectomy was performed through a median sternotomy approach. A stage I thymoma was pathologically confirmed. *From Kesler KA, Wright CD, Loehrer PJ: Sem Neurol 24:47, 2004. Used with permission.*

amenable to excisional biopsy, which might establish a diagnosis of lymphoma, is indicated. Along these same lines, any anterior mediastinal mass that is associated with surrounding lymphadenopathy is usually a lymphomatous process and should be biopsied rather than excised for diagnosis. In contrast, smaller lobulated anterior mediastinal masses in patients 30 to 60 years of age have a high likelihood of representing an early-stage thymoma; therefore surgical removal in any low-risk patient can be justified. Similarly, an anterior mediastinal compartment mass in a patient with a history of an associated immune disorder has a high probability of representing a thymoma (Fig. 1). In general we believe that wide surgical excision including en bloc thymectomy without biopsy is justified in most patients with an anterior mediastinal mass that is clinically determined most likely to represent an early-stage thymoma. The role of positron emission tomography (PET) scan for thymoma is currently being evaluated. Although not considered useful to differentiate thymoma from lymphoma, PET with 2-deoxy-2- [^{18}F] fluoro-D-glucose tracer can demonstrate hypermetabolic activity in pleural-based masses identified on CT scan, which would be highly suggestive of metastatic thymoma.

For larger or invasive anterior mediastinal masses suspected of representing locally advanced thymoma or a lymphomatous process, it must be emphasized that cytology obtained from CT-guided fine needle aspiration (FNA) may not only lack sensitivity to establish a diagnosis of thymoma but can occasionally be misleading with respect to differentiating thymomas and lymphomas. Moreover, a substantial tissue sample for genetic marker studies including flow cytometry is considered optimal before treatment for lymphoma. In our experience, CT-guided core needle biopsy can usually be safely performed for larger masses in the anterior mediastinal compartment, particularly if a large-bore needle can be passed into the mass without traversing lung parenchyma. If core needle biopsy is not possible, then two surgical options exist for further diagnostic evaluation. We consider anterior mediastinotomy (Chamberlain procedure) the next diagnostic procedure of choice. An anterior mediastinotomy may be performed on either side of the sternum and at any level that best provides access to the anterior mediastinal tumor. Standard cervical mediastinoscopy does not provide access to the anterior compartment and therefore should be avoided unless significant paratracheal lymphadenopathy suspicious of metastatic disease is present. Video-assisted thoracic surgery (VATS) provides

excellent exposure to the anterior compartment to accomplish a minimally invasive biopsy; however, the pleural space is traversed, and if thymoma is a diagnostic possibility, pleural space seeding could theoretically occur during VATS biopsy efforts.

Staging

Many histologic classifications have been described for thymoma. Most recently the World Health Organization (WHO) reached a consensus on histologic classification on the basis of both morphology and lymphocyte-to-epithelial-cell ratio (Table 2). Masaoka initially proposed an anatomic classification on the basis of the presence or absence of capsular invasion and the presence or absence of metastases, with subsequent revision in 1994 (Table 3). Several studies have attempted to correlate histologic staging systems with tumor invasion and prognosis. It appears that medullary (WHO A) and mixed histology (WHO AB) tumors are typically less invasive and therefore usually correspond to Masaoka stages I and II. Conversely, cortical (WHO B1, 2, or 3) thymomas tend to be invasive and present more commonly as stage III and IV lesions. The Masaoka anatomic staging system remains as the most widely accepted on which current management recommendations are based.

Surgical Therapy

Stages I and II

Although it is typically difficult, if not impossible, to differentiate Masaoka stages I and II by CT imaging, complete surgical resection

Table 2: World Health Organization (2002) Histologic Classification for Epithelial Thymic Tumors*

WHO Type	Pathologic Characteristics
A	Medullary
AB	Mixed medullary/cortical
B1	Predominately cortical
B2	Cortical
B3	Well-differentiated carcinoma
C	Carcinoma

*Currently the most commonly utilized classification system.

Table 3: Masaoka Anatomic Thymoma Staging as of 1994 Modifications

Masaoka Stage	Diagnostic Criteria
Stage I	Macroscopically and microscopically completely encapsulated
Stage II	A. Microscopic transcapsular invasion B. Macroscopic invasion into surrounding fatty tissue or grossly adherent to but not through mediastinal pleura or pericardium
Stage III	Macroscopic invasion into neighboring organs (i.e., pericardium, great vessels, lung) A. Without invasion of great vessels B. With invasion of great vessels
Stage IV	A. Pleural or pericardial dissemination B. Lymphogenous or hematogenous metastasis

is recommended for both stages, making preoperative differentiation irrelevant. The basic tenets of surgery include careful exploration of the entire mediastinum, complete en bloc thymectomy, and removal of all surrounding mediastinal fat with avoidance of phrenic nerve injury or intrapleural spread. Capsular invasion can be microscopic and therefore not grossly identified at the time of surgery, hence the tumor should not be shelled out but removed with surrounding tissue intact. A median sternotomy approach provides excellent access to the anterior mediastinum for total thymectomy and en bloc removal of adjacent structures, which are found to be involved during mediastinal exploration. Attention should also be paid to the preoperative CT scan with regard to abutment of the tumor to the underlying pericardium. If there is a fat plane between the two, simple removal of the tumor and surrounding fat is indicated. If there is no fat plane between the tumor and pericardium, the underlying pericardium probably should be resected en bloc. Small pericardial defects are usually of no consequence. If there is believed to be any potential for postoperative cardiac herniation, however, prosthetic patch reconstruction is indicated. With the advent of minimally invasive thoracic surgical techniques, several reports have recently appeared regarding the feasibility of excising early-stage thymomas using a VATS approach. With not only the completeness of resection but also the avoidance of pleural seeding being of prime importance, careful long-term follow-up is necessary to demonstrate whether these minimally invasive techniques will result in cure rates comparable to standard open surgical approaches.

Excellent long-term survival is anticipated following complete surgical excision for a pathologic stage I thymoma, and there appears to be no benefit of adjuvant radiation therapy following resection. For stage II thymomas, with capsular invasion pathologically demonstrated, adjuvant radiotherapy following complete surgical excision has previously been considered the standard of care despite the lack of prospective clinical trials. More recent retrospective studies have found no outcome difference in patients treated with or without postoperative radiotherapy following complete resection of stage II thymoma. To avoid the potential morbidity and costs associated with thoracic radiation, we currently reserve postoperative radiotherapy for stage II patients in whom adjacent organs are within a millimeter or so of the surgical margin as determined by the pathologic and intraoperative findings. The WHO histology classification should probably also be taken into account when considering postoperative radiotherapy. For example, we would typically not recommend radiation for a close margin in a WHO A tumor but would recommend postoperative radiotherapy for a similar WHO B3 tumor.

Operable or Potentially Operable Stages III and IVA

Similar to the difficulty encountered in clinically differentiating stage I from II thymomas by CT imaging, it can be difficult to identify invasion of adjacent organs, establishing a stage III status before treatment. Subtle invasion of the adjacent organs, such as underlying pericardium or adjacent lung, may be identified only at the time of mediastinal exploration. Proceeding with complete surgical resection is recommended in these cases, including en bloc pulmonary wedge, pericardial or left innominate vein resection, or a combination of these, with little additional surgical risks. Unilateral phrenic nerve resection can be performed if frank neural invasion is present and is usually well tolerated. Consideration should be given to ipsilateral diaphragmatic plication at the time of surgery in these cases. In contrast, bilateral phrenic nerve resection is not recommended because of the severe respiratory morbidity that would result.

Invasion of local organs can be apparent on CT imaging and can establish stage III status before treatment (Fig. 2). Larger masses (>10 cm) that do not obviously demonstrate frank invasion on CT are likely at least to be adherent to adjacent organs and

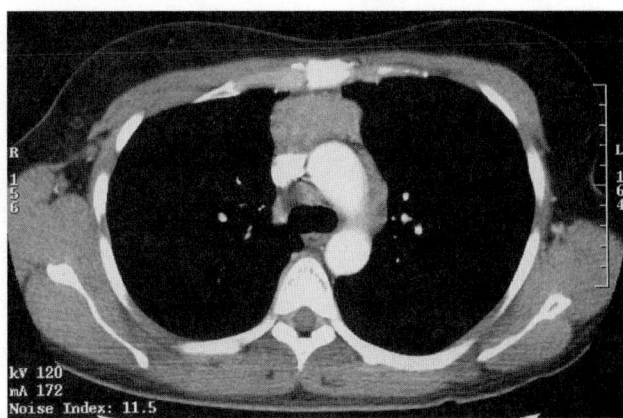

Figure 2 Thymoma with encasement of left innominate vein consistent with Masaoka stage III disease. The patient was treated with platin-based chemotherapy followed by en bloc surgical extirpation through a median sternotomy approach. Postoperative radiation therapy was also given. *From Kesler KA, Wright CD, Loehrer PJ: Sem Neurol 24:47, 2004. Used with permission.*

therefore should probably also be treated as stage III disease. We believe that patients presenting with or suspected of having potentially operable stage III disease are best treated with induction chemotherapy followed by repeat CT imaging for reassessment and consideration of surgical therapy. Most invasive thymomas have been found to be sensitive to cisplatin-based combination chemotherapy regimens with objective response rates from 80% to 100% and subsequent resectability rates ranging between 35% and 70%. Unlike early-stage disease in which establishing a preoperative histologic diagnosis of thymoma is not mandatory, either CT-guided core needle or surgical biopsy is necessary before considering induction chemotherapy. Postoperative radiation therapy should also be considered after resection of a stage III thymoma to control any local microscopic disease. For patients who otherwise have excellent performance status presenting with stage IVA disease, cisplatin-based combination chemotherapy followed by repeat CT scan to assess resectability of residual disease is not unreasonable and may occasionally result in durable disease-free survival (Fig. 3, *A* and *B*). Cisplatin-based combination chemotherapy is otherwise recommended for patients with unresectable stage IV disease. Octreotide and steroids have been successfully used in select patients as second-line chemotherapy.

PROGNOSIS

Anticipated 5- and 10-year survival rates for Masaoka stage I thymomas are approximately 95% and 85%; stage II, 80% and 75%; and stage III, between 40% and 60% and 20% and 30%, respectively. Reports of 10-year survival after treatment of stage IVA disease range from 0% to 40%.

Other Thymic Tumors

Tumors that less commonly originate in the thymus include carcinomas and neuroendocrine tumors. Thymic carcinomas (WHO C) are rare but unequivocally malignant by histology and, unlike thymomas, often present with pleural or pericardial effusions (or both). Most thymic carcinomas appear large and poorly defined and frequently encase other mediastinal organs or great vessels on CT scan. Aggressive multimodality therapy with neoadjuvant cisplatin-based combination chemotherapy with or without radiation therapy followed by surgical extirpation of residual disease can

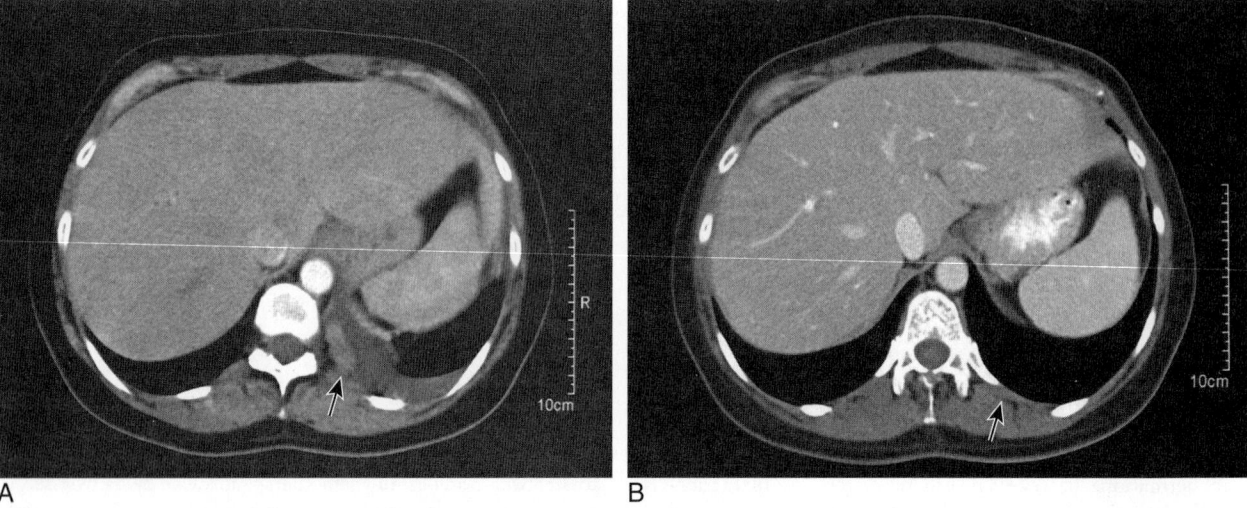

A   B

Figure 3   **(A)** Pleural "droplet" metastasis in patient with a large anterior mediastinal mass highly suspicious for Masaoka stage IVA thymoma. Computed tomography CT-guided biopsy of the pleural-based mass confirmed the diagnosis and stage. The patient was treated with cisplatin-based chemotherapy with CT resolution of the pleural-based mass. **(B)** Exploratory left thoracotomy was performed, and 10 to 12 small (2-mm) droplet metastases not visualized on postchemotherapy CT scan were identified in the posterior inferior recess of the pleural space. A pleurectomy was therefore performed in addition to resection of the residual anterior mediastinal mass, removing all visible evidence of disease.   *From Kesler KA, Wright CD, Loehrer PJ: Sem Neurol 24:47, 2004. Used with permission.*

occasionally result in cure; however, the prognosis is usually poor, and palliative chemoradiation therapy is frequently the only reasonable treatment option. Thymic neuroendocrine tumors are also rare and histologically identical to neuroendocrine tumors originating in the respiratory and gastrointestinal tracts. Current histologic classification is also similar to grade I—low grade ("typical" carcinoids). Grade II—intermediate ("atypical" carcinoids), and grade III—high grade (large or small cell neuroendocrine carcinoma). Neuroendocrine tumors tend to occur predominantly in males and may be associated with endocrinopathies such as Cushing's and multiple endocrine neoplasia syndromes. The classic "carcinoid syndrome" is rare, however. Surgical excision is the treatment of choice for neuroendocrine tumors confined to the anterior mediastinum, with good to excellent cure rates after complete resection of grade I and II histologic subtypes. Grade III neuroendocrine tumors usually present with local invasion or metastatic disease, which precludes surgical therapy. Thymic cysts, thymolipomas, and mesenchymal tumors are also uncommon. All are benign, and most have typical CT appearances; thus the diagnosis is established without biopsy. Surgical extirpation is typically offered to good-risk patients with an excellent prognosis anticipated. Thymic hyperplasia, although not a neoplasm per se, represents abnormal thymic growth that can be difficult to distinguish on CT imaging from stage II or early-stage III thymoma. Careful CT follow-up is usually not unreasonable in patients suspected of benign thymic hyperplasia because FNA is typically difficult and not helpful in distinguishing hyperplasia from thymoma. Patients at risk for thymic hyperplasia are characteristically younger, with autoimmune disorders or following chemotherapy.

LYMPHOMA

Lymphomas constitute the second most common anterior mediastinal compartment neoplasm in adults 20 to 40 years of age and are the most common neoplasm in the pediatric population. Lymphomas may present as isolated mediastinal disease but more frequently as generalized disease. Hodgkin's disease, in particular the nodular sclerosing subtype, is the most common type of mediastinal lymphoma with predilection for the anterior mediastinal compartment. Non-Hodgkin's lymphoma may present in the anterior or middle mediastinal compartment in all age groups with an overall prognosis that is statistically less favorable than Hodgkin's lymphomas. The most important non-Hodgkin's subtypes are poorly differentiated lymphoblastic, diffuse lymphocytic, and diffuse histiocytic. A primary mediastinal B-cell lymphoma has been defined as a separate entity primarily affecting young adults. These lymphomas typically present as a rapidly enlarging anterior mediastinal mass and carry a poor prognosis. Because the treatment for all Hodgkin's or non-Hodgkin's lymphomas is nonsurgical, the principal role of the surgeon is to direct diagnostic efforts in any patient suspected of having a lymphomatous process. As previously mentioned, careful physical examination often reveals palpable lymph nodes, which are easily removed for diagnostic purposes. CT-guided core needle biopsy is otherwise frequently possible because these tumors are typically large and in proximity to the anterior chest wall. If lymphoma is suspected and CT imaging demonstrates pathologic lymphadenopathy in the paratracheal space, transcervical mediastinoscopy is another diagnostic procedure to consider. If these less invasive diagnostic approaches fail or are deemed not possible, either an anterior mediastinotomy or VATS approach is recommended. In unusual cases in which a small anterior mediastinal tumor is completely resected and found pathologically to represent a lymphoma, adjuvant chemotherapy or radiation therapy is typically recommended. Hodgkin's disease limited to the mediastinum is associated with a 5-year survival of 75%.

GERM CELL TUMORS

Benign teratomas, seminomas (PMSGCT), and nonseminomatous (PMNSGCT) germ cell tumors arising in the anterior mediastinum are a heterogeneous group of benign and malignant neoplasms thought to originate from primordial germ cells that fail to complete migration from the urogenital ridge during embryogenesis.

Benign Teratoma

"Mature" or benign teratomas are the most common germ cell tumor arising in the anterior mediastinum, representing 60% to 70% of all mediastinal germ cell tumors. Mature teratomas are usually characterized by the presence of mature tissues derived from all three germinal layers: ectoderm, endoderm, and mesoderm. Unlike malignant germ cell tumors, which almost uniformly occur in the male population, mature teratomas occur with equal frequency in both genders. Although reported in all age groups, the vast majority present in infancy or childhood, with chest pain being the most common symptom, followed by dyspnea and cough. Occasionally, a cystic component can become infected, producing local or systemic symptoms. Rarely cyst contents may rupture into the pleural space or tracheobronchial tree, the latter resulting in the expectoration of hair or sebum. Asymptomatic or minimally symptomatic tumors, which are most common in the adult population, can be incidental findings on chest x-rays or CT scans. The diagnosis of benign teratoma can almost uniformly be made on the basis of CT scan findings alone. CT scan usually demonstrates a multilocular but well-circumscribed cystic anterior mediastinal mass containing fluid and fat density. Approximately half of these tumors radiographically demonstrate calcification, and on occasion recognizable bone or teeth are present. Serum tumor markers should be obtained but are usually normal with these radiographic findings.

Benign teratomas are not responsive to radiation or chemotherapy. Complete surgical excision is therefore recommended without biopsy. Because these tumors are usually large, exposure for surgical excision is usually optimally accomplished through a median sternotomy approach. A posterior lateral thoracotomy approach can be used for smaller tumors, tumors that are more lateralized, or for better cosmesis in younger patients. Excision using minimally invasive VAT has also been reported for smaller tumors. Even smaller benign teratomas usually require a large incision to remove the tumor from the chest cavity, negating any advantage a minimally invasive approach may offer. Moreover, although benign, surrounding soft tissues are not infrequently adherent to the tumor mass, making mediastinal dissection difficult through a minimally invasive approach.

During surgical extirpation, great care should be taken to avoid phrenic nerve injury. If either phrenic nerve is found to be adherent to the tumor, all efforts should be made to preserve the nerve carefully without resection. Most adherent lung can be freed from the tumor mass without resection as well, although in rare cases of bronchial fistulization, pulmonary lobectomy is usually necessary. An excellent long-term prognosis is anticipated following surgery, and no specific long-term follow-up is necessary. Occasionally, elements of undifferentiated fetal tissue, or a so-called "immature teratoma, are identified on final pathologic examination. The overall prognosis remains good, and adjuvant chemotherapy or radiation therapy is not advised in these cases, although clinical and radiographic follow-up should be considered because there is some potential for local recurrence or metastases.

Seminomatous Germ Cell Cancer

Primary mediastinal seminomas constitute slightly less than half of all malignant primary mediastinal germ cell tumors. Similar to PMNSGCT, PMSGCT occurs almost exclusively in young adult males, 20 to 40 years of age. Seminomas are typically slow growing and therefore usually become quite large before the symptoms, such as chest pain, dyspnea, and cough, develop. Chest CT characteristically reveals a bulky, lobulated but homogenous mass with only occasional invasion of adjacent structures. Sixty to seventy percent of patients have metastatic disease at the time of diagnosis, most commonly to bone, lungs, liver, spleen, or brain. Scrotal exam and ultrasound along with CT of the abdomen and pelvis are indicated to rule out a testicular primary neoplasm, as well as for staging purposes. Patients with pure PMSGCT usually have normal serum tumor markers; however, B-HCG levels are mildly elevated (<100 ng/ml) in approximately 10% of cases. Any elevations in AFP above normal levels or significant B-HCG elevations indicate

a nonseminomatous germ cell component, and the patient should therefore be treated with cisplatin-based chemotherapy followed by surgical extirpation of residual disease even in the absence of identifiable nonseminomatous elements demonstrated in pretreatment biopsies. Because these neoplasms are typically large, FNA or core needle sampling under CT guidance can usually be diagnostic without the need for surgery.

Although radiation therapy has historically been the treatment of choice for PMSGCT, radiation does not control systemic metastases, which are frequently present and additionally subject these relatively young patients to the long-term morbidity associated with mediastinal radiation. Cisplatin-based combination chemotherapy regimens such as BEP (bleomycin/etoposide/cisplatin), which have been extensively used in the treatment of nonseminomatous germ cell cancer, are now considered the first-line treatment of choice for PMSGCT. Cisplatin-based chemotherapy alone has been reported to result in up to a 100% response rate and 85% 5-year survival even in the presence of metastatic disease. In contrast to PMNSGCT, any residual anterior mediastinal mass following chemotherapy usually represents nonviable germ cell tumor, and surgery therefore is not indicated. Serial radiographic and clinical follow-up only is recommended. If local growth of a residual mass is demonstrated during long-term follow-up, second-line platin-based chemotherapy is usually offered, with surgery or radiation therapy considered only as "salvage" therapy on rare occasions after failure of second-line chemotherapy. The role of surgery in patients with pure PMSGCT is therefore usually negligible.

Nonseminomatous Germ Cell Cancer

Presentation and Diagnosis

Nonseminomatous germ cell cancers comprise somewhat more than half of the malignant germ cell tumors arising in the mediastinum. It has been well established that although histologically and serologically identical to their more commonly occurring nonseminomatous testicular cancer counterparts, PMNSGCTs have a distinctly worse prognosis. The relatively worse prognosis is perhaps best attributed to the fact that the histology of residual disease after cisplatin-based chemotherapy is benign in approximately 90% of testicular nonseminomatous germ cell tumors, compared with only 60% of PMNSGCTs. Additionally, up to 10% of patients with a PMNSGCT will unfortunately demonstrate radiographic and serologic progression of malignant disease during chemotherapy, rendering the patient inoperable and incurable; this rarely occurs in the treatment of testicular cancer. This distinct biology is finally reflected in the findings that up to 20% of PMNSGT patients have Klinefelter's syndrome and a unique risk for fatal hematologic dyscrasias after treatment, whereas these problems are not observed in patients with nonseminomatous testes cancer.

The vast majority of PMNSGCTs occur in men 20 to 40 years of age, with extremely rare cases of PMNSGCT occurring in females. Most patients present symptomatic with chest pain, cough, SVC syndrome, and shortness of breath secondary to a rapidly growing anterior mediastinal mass. CT scans usually demonstrate a large heterogeneous mass, with occasional evidence of necrosis and hemorrhage. Local invasion into lung, left innominate vein, SVC, or pericardium is common, and even direct cardiac chamber/great artery involvement can occasionally be present. Associated pericardial and pleural effusions are also common but typically not malignant in nature. As previously stated, for any male young adult presenting with a mass in the anterior compartment, obtaining serum tumor markers is an essential component of clinical evaluation because significant elevation of either marker is diagnostic of PMNSGCT. Cytologic confirmation with CT-guided FNA is optimal in these cases and necessary in patients with only marginally elevated or normal serum tumor markers before initiating chemotherapy. If

CT-guided FNA is not possible, proceeding directly with chemotherapy, on the basis of significant serum marker elevation alone, is recommended because open biopsy only delays chemotherapy and makes surgery following chemotherapy more difficult.

PMNSGCTs demonstrate at least one of three nonseminomatous histologic subtypes: yolk sac carcinoma, embryonal carcinoma, or choriocarcinoma in order of frequency. Other histologies occasionally found on pretreatment biopsy include mature teratoma; seminomatous germ cell cancer; and degenerative malignancies such as sarcoma, primitive neuroectodermal tumor, and adenocarcinoma. Metastatic disease is present in 20% to 25% of cases before chemotherapy, with lung being the most common site of metastases, followed by neck, retroperitoneum, liver, bone, and the central nervous system (CNS). Chest and abdominal CT scans are standard imaging tests for staging, with other radiologic studies including PET scan, nuclear bone scan, and CNS MRI obtained on an individual basis. Scrotal exam and ultrasound are also recommended during evaluation. In our experience, an isolated metastasis to the anterior mediastinum from a testes nonseminomatous cancer is distinctly rare, however.

Chemotherapy

After diagnosis and staging, primary surgical therapy for PMNSGCT is inappropriate. PMNSGCTs are usually large and infiltrative neoplasms. Surgical resection as initial therapy therefore rarely achieves local control and does not treat metastatic disease when present. Appropriate therapy begins with four cycles of cisplatin-based chemotherapy, usually BEP, followed by reevaluation with serum tumor markers and CT imaging for consideration of surgical extirpation of residual disease. BEP is administered with careful monitoring of pulmonary diffusing capacity. Bleomycin is decreased or discontinued when any reduction of pulmonary function is noted. If pulmonary resection is anticipated following chemotherapy, we have increasingly used non-bleomycin-containing regimens such as vinblastine, ifosfamide, and cisplatin, or alternatively withholding bleomycin for the final two cycles to minimize pulmonary toxicity before surgery. Following chemotherapy, there is typically a reduction in tumor dimensions with resolution of pleural and pericardial effusions. Optimally, serum tumor markers normalize and surgery is planned after adequate functional and hematologic recovery, which usually occurs between 4 and 6 weeks. Previously, patients with persistently elevated serum tumor markers were treated with second-line chemotherapy before surgery was considered. With relatively poor specificity of mild-to-moderate serum marker elevation after chemotherapy for viable residual malignancy and also the unsatisfactory results of second-line chemotherapy in the treatment of PMNSGCT, it is our current practice that surgery should be undertaken if the residual disease is deemed operable after first-line chemotherapy. Adjuvant cisplatin-based chemotherapy should, however, be considered if there is pathologic evidence of viable germ cell cancer in the resected specimen. Patients demonstrating rising serum tumor markers after first-line chemotherapy represent an unfortunate subset of patients with an exceptionally poor prognosis. High-dose platin-based chemotherapy or "desperation" surgery (or both) can be offered but have a low cure rate. Occasionally, patients demonstrate the so-called growing teratoma syndrome, with paradoxical growth of a cystic mass associated with normalization of serum tumor markers during chemotherapy. In these cases, chemotherapy should be discontinued and surgery undertaken because a mature teratoma is not sensitive to chemotherapy.

Surgery

In light of the high-risk nature of PMNSGCT, any residual mediastinal mass after chemotherapy should be surgically removed. The surgical approach is selected to optimize exposure of technically difficult areas of dissection anticipated during removal. Because the majority of residual masses are located directly behind the sternum without significant lateral extension, a median sternotomy is the most common approach. For residual masses that are more lateralized, a posterior lateral thoracotomy provides optimal exposure to phrenic nerves and pulmonary hilum. The "clamshell" incision (bilateral thoracosternotomy) offers excellent exposure to both the anterior mediastinum and pulmonary hilum for significantly larger residual masses. Surgical removal involves en bloc dissection of the residual mass, thymus, and surrounding involved structures. Because the majority of postchemotherapy masses pathologically demonstrate benign residual disease, a balanced surgical approach, sparing critical structures such as phrenic nerves, main pulmonary arteries, great veins, and cardiac chambers in which the residual mass abuts but does not invade, with liberal use of intraoperative frozen-section examination of the surgical margin, is appropriate. These surgical procedures are challenging from not only decision-making but also technical standpoints because chemotherapy typically results in marked fibrosis at the interface between the residual mass and surrounding mediastinal tissues. The overall surgical risk is reasonably low at experienced centers but significantly increases following high-dose bleomycin, particularly in patients requiring large pulmonary resections.

Prognosis

Overall survival following surgery has been reported to range between 30% and 60%. We have found that the "worst" pathology identified in the residual mass following chemotherapy is independently predictive of long-term survival. Patients who demonstrate complete tumor necrosis with no evidence of viable tumor cells have an excellent long-term prognosis. Patients with pathologic evidence of mature teratoma, with or without necrosis, demonstrate intermediate-to-good long-term survival. Long-term follow-up in patients pathologically demonstrating a component of teratoma should not only include serial serum tumor marker measurements but CT imaging because surgery for early recurrence of teratoma has a high success rate. On the other hand, teratoma has a propensity to degenerate into malignant histology over time, and this carries a significantly worse prognosis despite aggressive surgery. Aggressive "salvage" surgical therapy in cases with viable germ cell cancer or degenerative malignancy pathologically identified in the residual mass after chemotherapy results in relatively worse but still possible long-term survival.

CONCLUSION

Tumors arising in the thymus represent a wide spectrum of pathologic processes, with thymoma predominating. The surgeon's role in evaluating patients presenting with an anterior mediastinal mass begins with a thorough knowledge of the differential diagnoses, which can frequently be narrowed down by considering the patient's age, gender, associated symptoms, presence of palpable lymphadenopathy, CT findings, and serum tumor marker status. Ultimately, planning an approach for diagnostic biopsy or surgical extirpation (or both) is required in most cases.

SUGGESTED READINGS

Kesler KA: In Pearson FG, Cooper JD, Deslauriers J, and others, editors: *Thoracic surgery*, ed 2, Philadelphia, 2002, Churchill Livingstone, Chap 130.

Kesler KA, Wright CD, Loehrer PJ: Thymoma: current medical and surgical management, *Sem Neurol* 24:47, 2004.

Okumura M, Ohta M, Tateyama H, and others: The World Health Organization histologic classification system reflects the oncologic behavior of thymoma: a clinical study of 273 patients, *Cancer* 94:624, 2002.

Strollo DC, Rosado de Christenson ML, and others: Primary mediastinal tumors. Part I: tumors of the anterior mediastinum, *Chest* 112:511, 1997.

Management of Tracheal Stenosis

Robert E. Merritt, MD, and Douglas J. Mathisen, MD

INTRODUCTION

Diseases of the trachea that require surgical resection and reconstruction encompass idiopathic tracheal stenosis and postintubation injuries. Idiopathic tracheal stenosis describes an entity that involves the exclusion of all known and defined causes of nonneoplastic inflammatory stenosis, which occurs predominately in women. Patients with idiopathic tracheal stenosis must be screened for connective tissue disorders such as Wegener's granulomatosis. Tracheal stenosis secondary to Wegener's is usually treated with dilatation and steroid therapy. Tracheal stenosis is the most common postintubation injury to the trachea. These injuries occur at the level of the tracheal stoma or at the level of tracheal cuff. Both of these injuries result from proliferative and cicatric response to tracheal injury. Patients with tracheal stenosis have signs and symptoms of upper airway obstruction: dyspnea on exertion, wheezing, stridor, and obstructive pneumonia. The presentation of tracheal stenosis is often confused with adult-onset asthma; therefore steroid therapy is often initiated before the correct diagnosis is ascertained.

PREOPERATIVE ASSESSMENT

Before tracheal resection and reconstruction is undertaken, the definitive diagnosis of the underlying pathology of the airway must be established. A preoperative assessment should include a history and physical, radiologic imaging, and bronchoscopy. Relatively simple radiologic techniques without use of contrast delineate most pathologic conditions of the trachea. X-rays can demonstrate the location of a lesion, its linear extent, extratracheal involvement, and the amount of normal trachea. A lateral neck view, using soft-tissue technique with the patient swallowing and hyperextension of the neck brings the trachea above the clavicles and defines the anatomy of the upper trachea. Computed axial tomography offers little advantage over standard radiologic techniques for benign disease.

Bronchoscopy is invaluable in determining the extent of airway disease preoperatively. The initial evaluation should be performed with a rigid bronchoscope carefully inserted through the vocal cords just proximal to a point of stenosis. The rigid bronchoscope can be used to measure the length of a stenotic segment of trachea, as well as to access the mucosa for inflammatory changes and granulation tissue. Crucial to the management of tracheal stenosis is the ability to control the airway. Control of the airway is best accomplished in the operating room with an assortment of rigid bronchoscopes. Attempting to pass a large rigid bronchoscope beyond a tight inflammatory stricture is usually difficult and can result in tracheal rupture or total airway obstruction from bleeding and edema. Graduated rigid bronchoscopes can be used effectively to dilatate postintubation strictures serially. Racemic epinephrine and steroids are often administered for 24 to 48 hours to minimize postdilatation edema.

ANESTHESIA AND AIRWAY MANAGEMENT

Anesthesia for tracheal reconstruction is best administered by halothane or enflurane inhalation. A slow and gradual induction is usually necessary if there is a high degree of airway obstruction. This approach is preferable and safer than paralysis of respiration with consequent urgent need to establish an airway. The surgeon should be available with an array of rigid bronchoscopes during induction of anesthesia to control the airway. Total intravenous anesthesia is also well suited for tracheal resection. This process decouples ventilation and the delivery of anesthesia and prevents the contamination of the operating room with inhalation agents. Total intravenous anesthesia is advantageous because it blunts airway reflexes well and its effects wear off quickly at the completion of the operation. Remifentanil and propofol are delivered by infusion and are excellent agents commonly used with total intravenous anesthesia.

During resection of the trachea, the airway is divided, and the distal end of the trachea can be directly intubated with an armored, flexible endotracheal tube (Tovell tube) by the surgeon on the surgical field. Sterile connecting tubes are passed off the surgical field to the anesthesiologists. This technique allows ventilation during reconstruction of the trachea. Before completion of the tracheal anastomosis, the oral endotracheal tube is retrieved from the proximal trachea and passed distal to the suture line. Ideally it should be possible for the patient to be extubated and breathe spontaneously at the conclusion of the operative procedure. It is not desirable to have even a low-pressure cuff in close contact with the anastomosis for any period of time. If the patient does require intubation after surgery, a small, uncuffed endotracheal tube is preferred. The tube should be removed within 48 to 72 hours. If the airway is still a concern, a small tracheostomy should be placed two rings below the anastomosis. The innominate artery and the tracheal anastomosis should be protected by a strap muscle flap that is carefully sutured to the trachea.

INDICATIONS FOR TRACHEAL RESECTION

In general, any patient who has airway obstruction as a result of tracheal stenosis should have a tracheal resection and reconstruction. Absolute contraindications are few and include nonreconstructable airway, severe comorbidities, and prolonged need for mechanical ventilation. Relative contraindications include a history of radiation to the trachea, active trachea mucosal inflammation, and active steroid therapy.

SURGICAL TECHNIQUE FOR TRACHEAL RESECTION

The cervical or upper cervicomediastinal approach is used for benign strictures of the trachea at any level. The patient is usually anesthetized by inhalation agents, and a rigid bronchoscope is passed. A stricture less than 6 mm in diameter is dilatated under direct vision with rigid pediatric bronchoscopes. If the stricture is more than 6 mm, an endotracheal tube may be placed proximal to the lesion. If the tracheal stenosis is located in the subglottic area, the lesion usually requires dilatation to allow passage of a small endotracheal tube.

The trachea is explored through a collar incision, which may encompass an existing tracheal stoma (Fig. 1, *A*). Skin flaps

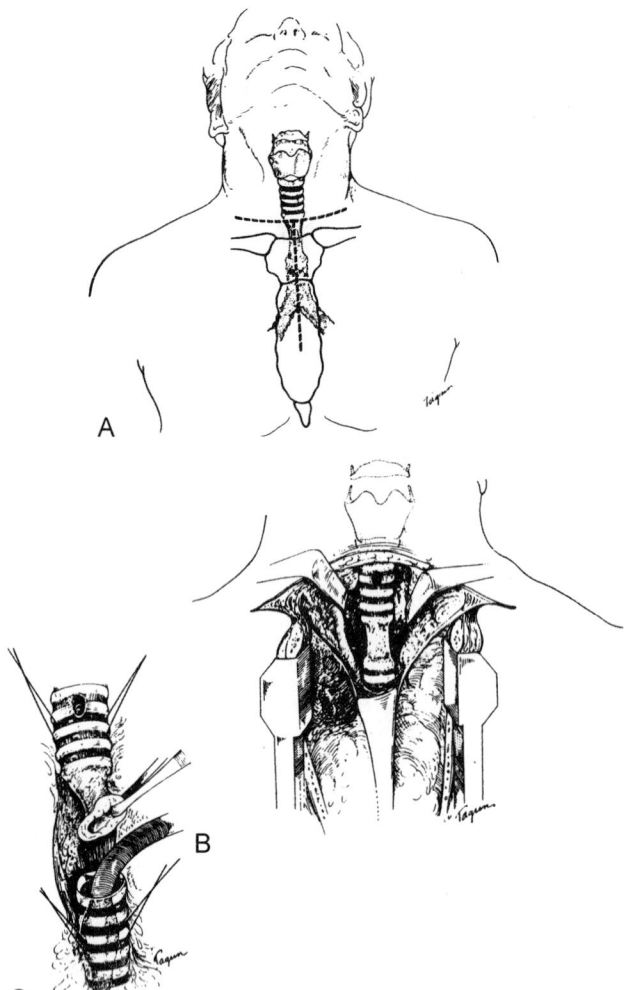

Figure 1 Tracheal resection and reconstruction for postintubation stenosis. **(A)** A collar incision provides access for many upper tracheal lesions. For a wider access to the upper thoracic inlet and the mediastinum, a partial sternotomy is performed. Usually the incision is not carried more than 1–2 cm below the angle of Louis. This provides exposure even for the supracarinal benign stenosis. **(B)** Partial sternotomy with retraction of innominate vein and artery without their exposure. The pretracheal plane is dissected only. Circumferential dissection is performed only just below the lesion. **(C)** After placement of lateral traction sutures above and below the points of the tracheal transection and after circumferential dissection around the distal trachea just below the lesion, the specimen is divided from the trachea. Upward traction on the specimen permits safe dissection of the esophagus and lateral tissues away from the specimen without injury to esophagus or recurrent laryngeal nerves. Eventually the specimen is transected above the level of stenosis. *From Mathisen DJ: Curr Probl Surg 35:453, 1998.*

are raised with platysma to the cricoid cartilage superiorly and the sternal notch inferiorly. The medial margins of the strap muscles are elevated, and the anterior surface of the trachea is exposed from the cricoid cartilage to the carina. The thyroid isthmus is divided, dissected from the trachea, and retracted laterally with sutures. It is essential to keep the dissection close to the trachea to avoid injury to the back wall of the innominate artery. If the innominate artery is adherent to the trachea and requires dissection, a strap muscle flap should be interposed between the artery and tracheal anastomosis. For lesions that are too far below the sternum to be accessible through a collar incision, the exposure can be increased by making a T incision in which the vertical arm extends downward to a point

1 cm below the sternal angle (Fig. 1, *A*). The sternum is divided to that point and separated with a pediatric chest spreader (Fig. 11, *B*). No additional useful exposure is obtained by full median sternotomy because the carina lies at the level of the angle of Louis and the great vessels obstruct access from an anterior approach. The upper sternal division provides access to the lower trachea. The innominate vein, which lies anterior and caudal to the dissection, is not divided. The tissues containing the innominate artery are dissected away from the trachea without exposing the wall of the artery. The anterior carina and the right and left tracheobronchial angles are can be exposed as needed.

In cases of tracheal stenosis, the dissection is made meticulously along the lateral borders of the involved trachea and posteriorly approximately 1 cm below the lesion (Fig. 11, *C*). If there is difficulty in identifying the level of the lesion, intraoperative bronchoscopy may be necessary to localize the lesion. The position of the bronchoscope light is identified at the upper and then the lower end of the lesion while an assistant pushes a 25-gauge needle through the tracheal wall for precise localization. These levels are marked with fine sutures. Dissection close to the tracheal wall avoids injury to the recurrent laryngeal nerves, which lie in the tracheoesophageal groove on either side. The recurrent laryngeal nerves are vulnerable to injury and are best not exposed by keeping the dissection close to the tracheal wall. This is particularly important if the stenosis lies just below the cricoid cartilage because the recurrent laryngeal nerves enter the larynx just medial to the inferior cornua of the thyroid cartilages. As the trachea is dissected circumferentially, great care must be taken to avoid perforation of the esophagus or the membranous wall of the trachea posteriorly. After the circumferential dissection of the trachea is completed, a tape is passed beneath the trachea for traction on the airway.

Before the division of the trachea, sterile anesthesia equipment is assembled on the field, and sterile corrugated tubing is passed off the table to the anesthetist. Lateral traction sutures of 2–0 Vicryl (Ethicon, Somerville, NJ) are placed on either side of the trachea in the midlateral position approximately 1 cm below the anticipated level of transection. These sutures pass vertically through the full thickness of the tracheal wall and around one or more rings (Fig. 11, *C*). The trachea is opened anteriorly just distal to the lesion, staying close to the lesion if it is a benign stricture. Healthy cartilage should be present at the cut edge of the trachea. Transection of the trachea is generally above the ring, but it is acceptable to make the incision in the cartilage. When the airway is open, continuous suctioning prevents seepage of blood into the distal airway. After transection, an assistant holds tension on the two lateral traction sutures and holds the flexible armored Tovell tube in the distal trachea. This maneuver draws the distal trachea and the ventilating tube away from the dissection. Circumferential dissection of the remaining proximal and distal trachea is limited to no more than 1 cm to protect the segmental blood supply, which enters laterally. Devascularization of the healthy trachea that will be anastomosed invites possible necrosis and anastomotic dehiscence.

To test the ease with which the tracheal ends can be brought together, the anesthetist flexes the patient's neck, and the surgeons draw on the crossed proximal and distal traction sutures, bringing the tracheal ends together. An experienced surgeon should be able to judge whether the tension is excessive. The length of trachea that may be safely removed obviously should be determined before division of the trachea. The feasibility of resection is based on radiologic and endoscopic examinations made before the operation. The length of trachea that can be safely removed is influenced by the patient's age and body habitus, by the anatomy of the trachea, and by previous treatments. After it has been demonstrated that the tracheal ends will come together without excessive tension, the neck is hyperextended again. The first anastomotic suture (4–0 coated Vicryl) is placed in the posterior midline with the knots on the outside. The sutures are carefully clipped to the drapes (Fig. 2, *A*). The next suture is placed lateral to this and clipped to the drapes just caudad to the previous one. The sutures are placed serially until a point is reached

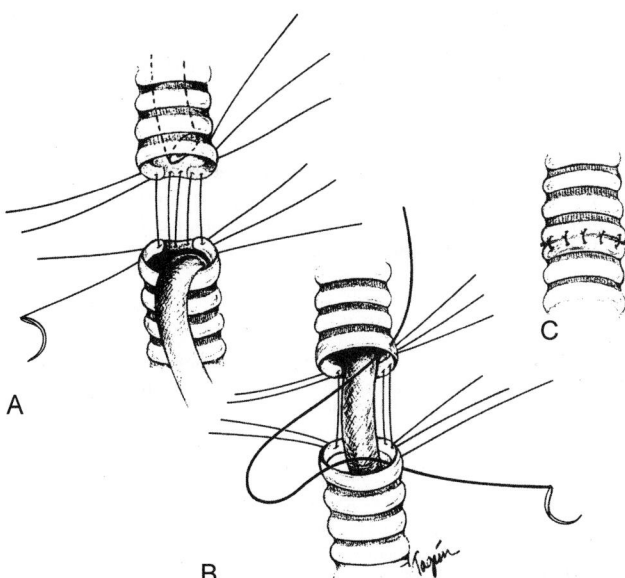

Figure 2 **(A)** Tracheal anastomosis. Sutures are placed individually beginning in the midline posteriorly and ranging anteriorly on either side. **(B)** After the sutures are placed on either side up to the level of the midlateral traction sutures, the anterior sutures are then placed. Frequently, the endotracheal tube is not advanced from above until after all sutures have been placed. **(C)** The neck is placed in the flexed position, and the lateral traction sutures are tied on either side (not shown) to remove tension from the anastomotic sutures. After this, anastomotic sutures are tied from anterior to posterior on either side. The completed anastomosis is airtight. *From Mathisen DJ: Curr Probl Surg 35:453, 1998.*

just posterior to the midline to the midlateral tracheal traction suture (Fig. 2, *B*). The same placement of sutures is now carried out on the opposite side, from the posterior midline to the midlateral suture. Serial sutures are similarly placed anteriorly, proceeding from the lateral traction sutures to the midline. The sutures are placed through the cartilage approximately 4 mm from the cut edge of the trachea and 4 mm apart. When all of the sutures are placed, the oral endotracheal tube is advanced from above until the tip is visible in the wound. The distal trachea is suctioned, and the endotracheal tube is advanced further, resuming ventilation through the original oral endotracheal tube. Care must be taken not to entangle the endotracheal tube in the anastomotic sutures. The patient's head is firmly supported on blankets in full flexion. The crossed lateral traction sutures are pulled together on either side and tied with surgeon's knots apposing the tracheal ends.

The anterior anastomotic sutures are tied first without tension, and the ends are cut after each suture is tied. The assistant then rotates the trachea by carefully drawing medially on the traction sutures on the surgeon's side of the table. The surgeon ties the suture just behind the lateral traction suture and ties sutures in the direction of the posterior midline. This same technique is repeated on the opposite side (Fig. 2, *C*). The cut traction sutures are left in place to guard against tension on the anastomotic sutures. The integrity of the anastomosis is checked by submersing the wound in saline solution, deflating the tube cuff, and insufflating to between 20 and 30 cm H_2O of pressure. The sternohyoid muscle or the thyroid isthmus is used to cover the suture line. If there is any concern of scar tissue involving the innominate artery, a pedicled strap muscle can be interposed between the innominate artery and the trachea. Flat suction drains are placed in the pretracheal and substernal spaces, and the strap muscles are approximated in the midline. After the incision is closed, a heavy suture is placed through the submental skin crease beneath the chin and

through the presternal skin. This suture is tied with the patient's neck in moderate flexion to prevent sudden hyperextension of the neck in the first week after the operation.

If it is determined after neck flexion that excessive anastomotic tension exists, maneuvers should be performed to reduce tension. The most helpful maneuver for the upper and mid-trachea is the Montgomery suprahyoid release. This can be performed by exposing the hyoid through a small horizontal incision just over the hyoid. The muscles inserting on the superior aspect of the hyoid between the lesser cornu are divided. The hyoid bone is divided just lateral to the lesser cornu on both sides. This release maneuver usually gives between 1 and 2 cm of additional mobility of the trachea.

After tracheal resection, patients are usually extubated as they awaken from anesthesia. If the airway is not satisfactory at this point, it is not likely to improve later unless the problem is caused by laryngeal edema. A small endotracheal tube with the cuff deflated can be left in place for 48 hours while the laryngeal edema resolves. The patient should be given 24 to 48 hours of steroids (Decadron [dexamethasone; Merck, Whitehouse Station, NY], 4 mg intravenously every 6 hours), fluid restricted, and have the head elevated in bed to reduce edema. We prefer to return the patient to the operating room at the end of the 48 hours and extubate under anesthesia. If there is still a problem, a small tracheostomy tube is placed two rings below the anastomosis. A pedicled strap muscle flap should be employed to cover the anastomosis if not already performed.

COMPLICATIONS OF TRACHEAL SURGERY

Complications after tracheal surgery are similar regardless of the problem for which resection and reconstruction is performed. The most in-depth analysis of complications after tracheal surgery was reported by Grillo and colleagues in patients with postintubation stenosis. The complications reported in this series of 503 patients are summarized in Table 1. Granulation tissue formed at the site of tracheal anastomosis in 49 patients in the series. After 1978, only

Table 1: Complications of Operations for Postintubation Tracheal Stenosis

	Major	Minor	Total
Granulations	11	38	44
Before 1978	10	34	44
After 1978	1	4	5
Dehiscence	28	1	29
Laryngeal dysfunction	11	14	25
Malacia	10	0	10
Hemorrhage	5	0	5
Edema (anastomosis)	3	1	4
Infection			
Wound		7	
Pulmonary	5	14	19
Myocardial infarction	1	0	1
Tracheoesophageal fistula	1	0	1
Pneumothorax	0	3	3
Line infection	0	1	1
Atrial fibrillation	0	1	1
Deep venous thrombosis	0	1	1
Totals	82	82	164

five such cases have occurred when the suture material was switched from nonabsorbable Tevdek (Deknatel, Mansfield, MA) to absorbable Vicryl. Thirty-eight of these patients were treated with bronchoscopic removal of granulation tissue, and five other patients required reoperation with a second tracheal resection. Four patients required tracheostomy, and two patients were treated with T-tubes.

A total of 29 patients had anastomotic dehiscence or restenosis. Seven patients with this complication died, and two patients also had erosions into the innominate artery, resulting in death. Eight patients with anastomotic dehiscence were treated with repeat tracheal resection with either good or satisfactory results. Four other patients were treated with permanent tracheostomy, and another five patients were treated with TT-tubes, three of which were temporary. Three patients developed a dehiscence of a small portion of the anastomosis. Two patients required reoperation and primary closure, and one patient was treated with cervical wound drainage and antibiotics. An additional two patients required repeated dilatations.

A total of 25 patients had varying degrees of laryngeal dysfunction (aspiration or vocal cord dysfunction) after tracheal resection and reconstruction. Fourteen of these patients had temporary laryngeal dysfunction that required no specific intervention. Eleven cases presented with more severe laryngeal dysfunction requiring either tracheostomy or T-tube. Two patients in this series required

gastrostomy tube feedings for persistent aspiration as a result of glottic dysfunction.

Other complications included tracheal malacia and hemorrhage. Ten patients were found to have residual tracheal malacia requiring either a second tracheal resection or tracheostomy. Five patients developed bleeding from the innominate artery that resulted in three mortalities. Infectious complications occurred in 34 patients, which included 15 wound infections and 19 cases of pneumonia or bronchitis. There were 12 perioperative deaths, 7 of which were related to the complication of anastomotic dehiscence.

SUGGESTED READINGS

Ashiku SK, Grillo HC, Mathisen DJ, and others: Idiopathic laryngotracheal stenosis: effective definitive treatment with laryngotracheal resection, *J Thorac Cardiovasc Surg* 127:99, 2004.

Gaissert HA, Grillo HC, Mathisen DJ: Long-term survival after resection of primary adenoid cystic and squamous cell carcinoma of the trachea and carina, *Ann of Thorac Surg* 78:1889, 2004.

Grillo HC, Donahue DM, Mathisen DJ, and others: Postintubation tracheal stenosis: treatment and results, *J Thorac Cardiovasc Surg* 109:486, 1995.

Montgomery WW: Suprahyoid release for tracheal anastomosis, *Arch Otolaryngol* 99:255, 1974.

THE MANAGEMENT OF ACQUIRED ESOPHAGEAL RESPIRATORY TRACT FISTULA

Cameron D. Wright, MD

Acquired esophageal respiratory tract fistulae are commonly separated into two types on the basis of etiology: malignant and benign. The presentation is similar: coughing with eating or drinking, aspiration pneumonia, and difficulty ventilating a patient on mechanical ventilation. Small fistulae may be hard to diagnose and are usually not life threatening. Large fistulae (>1 cm) are often life threatening and are readily diagnosed. Suspected small fistulae are best diagnosed with a barium swallow. Suspected large fistulae are usually best diagnosed with bronchoscopy and esophagoscopy.

MALIGNANT ESOPHAGEAL RESPIRATORY TRACT FISTULA

Esophageal and lung cancers are the most common tumors that cause airway fistulae because of their proximity to each other. These fistulae cause the rapid demise of the patient from aspiration pneumonia. Patients characteristically have a constant cough because of ongoing aspiration that drains the patient both physically and emotionally. The cough is not suppressed by usual measures and requires palliation. Burt and colleagues reported in 1991 a large series of 207 patients with malignant airway fistulae from 1926 to 1988. The median survival was only 5 weeks. Shin and

colleagues recently reported 60 patients with malignant airway fistulae treated by stents. The median survival was 13 weeks. These dismal survival results indicate that quick, effective palliation is required in these patients because their limited life expectancy precludes large operations that have substantial risk of major complications. Esophageal diversion and exclusion are largely historic operations that have little role today, given their high operative mortality and morbidity.

ESOPHAGEAL STENTS

Thin-walled, expandable, covered metallic stents that are easy to place endoscopically are now available. They effectively palliate dysphagia and fistulae caused by esophageal cancer. There must be a stricture present at the fistula site on which the stent must seat to prevent migration. For this reason esophageal stents are usually used only when esophageal cancer is causing both malignant obstruction and a fistula.

PLACEMENT OF EXPANDABLE ESOPHAGEAL STENTS

Although local anesthesia with sedation can be used, I prefer general anesthesia because it is most comfortable for the patient. Fluoroscopic guidance is used, and thus a proper bed must be used as well. Endoscopy is performed to obtain landmarks and delineate the fistula. If the stricture is especially tight, I dilatate it first so that the stent can readily pass the stricture. It should be underdilatated because the stricture helps to hold the stent in place. I place radiopaque markers (commonly large safety pins on the patient's gown) to mark the distal and proximal extent of the fistula under direct endoscopic and fluoroscopic guidance. A long guidewire is then placed in the stomach and the endoscope removed. The stent and applicator are threaded over the guidewire and inserted distally to span the fistula. The radiopaque markers here are key to ensure that the middle of the covered portion of the stent (i.e., at its center) exactly spans the fistula. The stent is then deployed and the applicator and guidewire removed. Repeat endoscopy confirms proper stent placement and fistula coverage. If necessary, balloon dilatation of the stent is performed to reduce luminal narrowing. Again, it is better to underdilatate because quick, large dilatations are more prone to perforate and more likely to cause pain. Stent expansion continues to occur as the stent warms to body temperature. I commonly perform a bronchoscopy at the conclusion of the procedure because patients invariably have a large amount of inspissated secretions. If possible, I prefer to obtain a barium swallow to confirm fistula occlusion before allowing the patient to eat.

TRACHEOBRONCHIAL STENTS

Thin-walled, expandable, covered metallic stents are now available that are easy to place endoscopically. They are commonly placed if the fistula is not associated with esophageal cancer that produces a malignant stricture. These stents often cause troublesome granulation tissue at the two ends; this is of concern in patients with benign disease but not usually those with advanced malignant disease. They also can be placed as a second stent in difficult-to-close fistulae in which the esophageal stent has not completely occluded the fistula. Like esophageal stents, they can also palliate airway narrowing caused by the associated cancer.

PLACEMENT OF AIRWAY STENTS

There are many possibilities in placing airway stents. Again, local anesthesia with sedation or general anesthesia may be used, but I prefer general anesthesia. Fluoroscopy can be used, but I rarely find it necessary because I deploy stents under direct endoscopic control. If desired, the airway can be controlled with a rigid bronchoscope and the stent deployed through the lumen (as well as the flexible bronchoscope to help guide the placement of the stent). Alternatively, intermittent apneic spells can be used to place a stent if it can be achieved expeditiously. A preliminary bronchoscopy is performed to map out the location of the fistula and clean up the airway. The airway is dilatated if there is a tight stenosis. A guidewire can be used if desired, but I rarely find it necessary because I place the stent under direct bronchoscopic control. When the stent is in proper position, it is deployed. It is best to adjust the position of the stent partway through deployment rather than waiting until full deployment because it is easier to move when it is only partially deployed. I usually try to seat the stent firmly by performing balloon dilatation of the stent after it is deployed. A chest x-ray is obtained at the conclusion of the procedure to search for pneumothorax and document the position of the stent. Again, I prefer to obtain a barium swallow to confirm occlusion of the stent.

RESULTS OF PALLIATIVE TREATMENT WITH COVERED, EXPANDABLE METALLIC STENTS

Success rates of 80% to 100% have been reported with sealing of malignant fistulae. Fistulae may reopen after initial successful closure because of stent migration or fistula enlargement. Successful fistula occlusion is associated with longer survival (15 vs. 6 weeks) in the recent series by Shin and colleagues. Complications include migration, perforation, erosion into a vascular structure, recurrent fistulization, and food impaction with esophageal stents.

BENIGN ESOPHAGEAL RESPIRATORY TRACT FISTULA

Most tracheoesophageal fistulae (TEFs) result from long-term ventilation with either an endotracheal tube or, more commonly, a tracheostomy tube. The mechanism of injury is usually ischemic necrosis from an overinflated cuff. TEFs may also result from injudicious oral intubation or placement of a tracheostomy tube (by either the traditional technique or percutaneous dilatation). Other causes include trauma, iatrogenic injury, caustic ingestion, infection, granulomatous inflammation, and impacted esophageal foreign bodies. Essentially all benign fistulae should be closed because spontaneous closure is rare.

POSTINTUBATION TRACHEOESOPHAGEAL FISTULA

Most postintubation TEFs are diagnosed while the patient is still receiving mechanical ventilation. The most common sign is a loss of returned tidal volume with a resultant difficulty in maintaining satisfactory ventilation. The cuff is commonly inflated more, which temporarily improves the situation but also enlarges the fistula. Other signs are an increase in secretions, distention of the stomach, and aspiration of tube feeds. Many patients have an indwelling hard nasogastric tube rather than a soft feeding tube or a gastrostomy. The diagnosis is easily made by bronchoscopy with the tracheostomy tube removed. The fistula size should be measured, the position of the fistula in relation to the rest of the airway should be measured, and the status of the surrounding trachea should be ascertained. In almost all cases the patient should be weaned from ventilation before definitive repair to maximize the possibility of success. It makes no sense to ventilate a fresh tracheal suture line if spontaneous ventilation is also possible. A long tracheostomy tube can usually be inserted so that the cuff is well below the fistula, effectively excluding the fistula. I prefer tracheostomy tubes that can be custom made in various lengths (Bivona; Smiths Medical, Kent, UK) with large foam cuffs that seal the airway well yet do not cause further tracheal damage. The nasogastric tube should be removed and a draining gastrostomy and feeding jejunostomy performed. When the patient is in reasonable condition, a definitive repair should be undertaken. Several techniques have been used to close a TEF: lateral division and closure, methods that involve esophageal division/exclusion, various muscle flaps, and an anterior approach with tracheal resection. The anterior approach is most common and usually leads to good results.

TRACHEAL RESECTION AND RECONSTRUCTION WITH ESOPHAGEAL FISTULA CLOSURE

Grillo popularized the anterior approach to repair of postintubation TEF in large part because of the frequent presence of concomitant tracheal stenosis and malacia at the fistula site. The anterior approach has been extended to include patients with a normal trachea because division of the trachea at the fistula site provides the best exposure to a satisfactory esophageal repair. The trachea is then reapproximated in the standard fashion. The patient is placed supine with the back elevated and the head extended as far as possible. A low collar incision, usually encompassing the stoma, is performed. Subplatysmal flaps are elevated. The strap muscles are separated in the midline. The thyroid isthmus is divided. The anterior aspect of the airway is exposed from the cricoid to the carina. The fistula site is identified, usually by bronchoscopy performed on the field to mark precisely the limits of the fistula. This is easily achieved with 25-gauge needles placed through the trachea under bronchoscopic control. A decision must be made about the stoma: will it be resected with the fistula, or, if too far away, will it be closed or left open to close at a later date? Circumferential dissection is then performed at the resection site, staying right on the tracheal wall to avoid injury to the recurrent nerve. The nerve should never be sought in the dense scar around the fistula site because the risk of injury is high. The trachea is then divided above and below the fistula. Intermittent ventilation is carried out with a sterile endotracheal tube inserted in the distal trachea while the native endotracheal tube is pulled back in the proximal trachea. The esophagus is dissected off the undersurface of the trachea above and below the tracheal transection site to allow ready closure of the esophagus. The esophagus is then closed in two layers with fine interrupted sutures with the first layer inverting with knots on the inside. A pedicled strap muscle is then sutured over the repair site along all edges to buttress the repair and separate it from the tracheal suture line. Stay sutures (2–0 Vicryl; Ethicon, Somerville, NJ) are placed at 3 and 9 o'clock positions one ring back and around one ring to reduce tension on the finer sutures. The tracheal sutures are then placed starting at the posterior membranous wall in a circumferential fashion with knots to be tied on the outside. Fine 4–0 Vicryl sutures are used. The sutures are placed approximately 4 mm from the cut edge and are approximately 5 mm apart. After all the sutures are placed, the native endotracheal tube is advanced across the anastomosis, and the stay sutures are tied after the neck is slightly flexed to reduce tension. If there is excessive tension, a suprahyoid laryngeal release is performed. Thereafter the fine sutures are tied, starting anteriorly and proceeding posteriorly. If the anterior tracheal suture line is adjacent to the innominate artery, it is covered with another pedicled strap muscle. The stoma is closed or covered with a strap muscle if it was not resected. The wound is closed in layers over a suction drain. The patient is always extubated at the end of the procedure so that positive pressure is not placed on the suture line.

RESULTS OF REPAIR OF POSTINTUBATION TRACHEOESOPHAGEAL FISTULA

Repair of postintubation TEFs (Figures 1–4) has been successful with the anterior approach along with tracheal

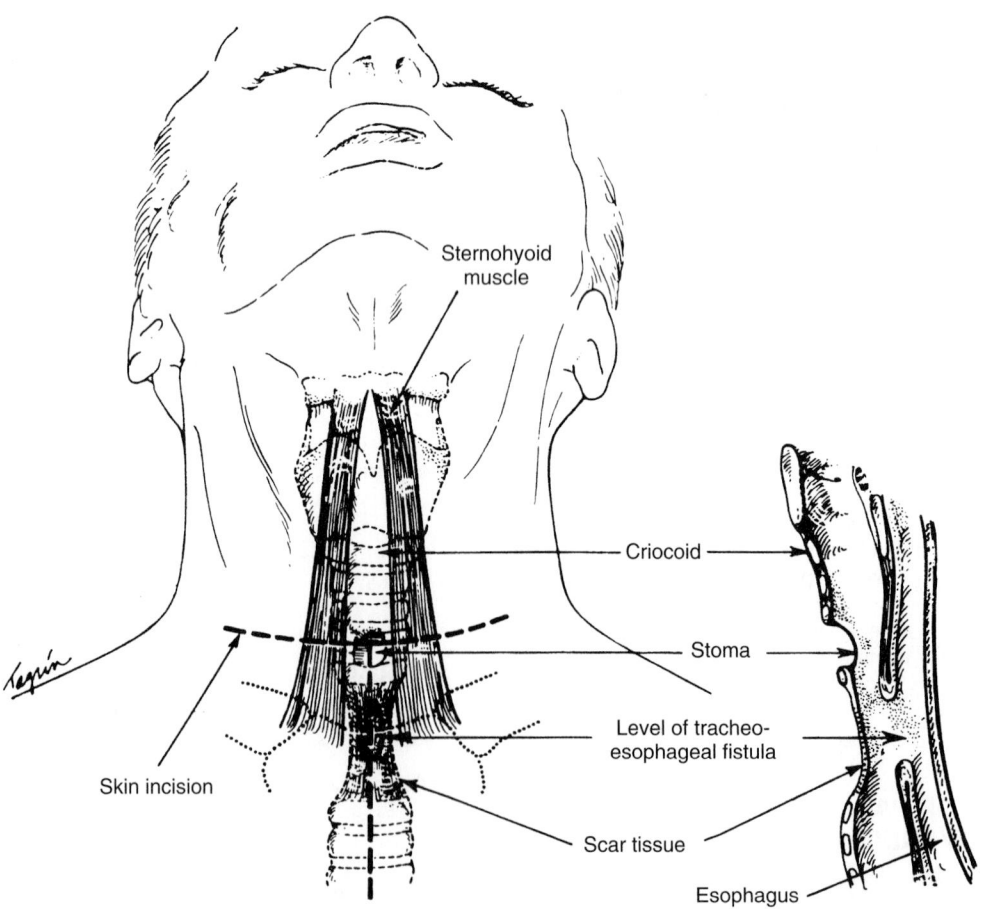

Figure 1 Anterior approach for postintubation tracheoesophageal fistula. Most high fistulae can be repaired through a simple collar incision. For lower fistulae, the manubrium can be divided in the midline to give excellent exposure. *From Mathisen DJ, Grillo HC, Wain JC, and others: Ann Thorac Surg 52:759, 1991.*

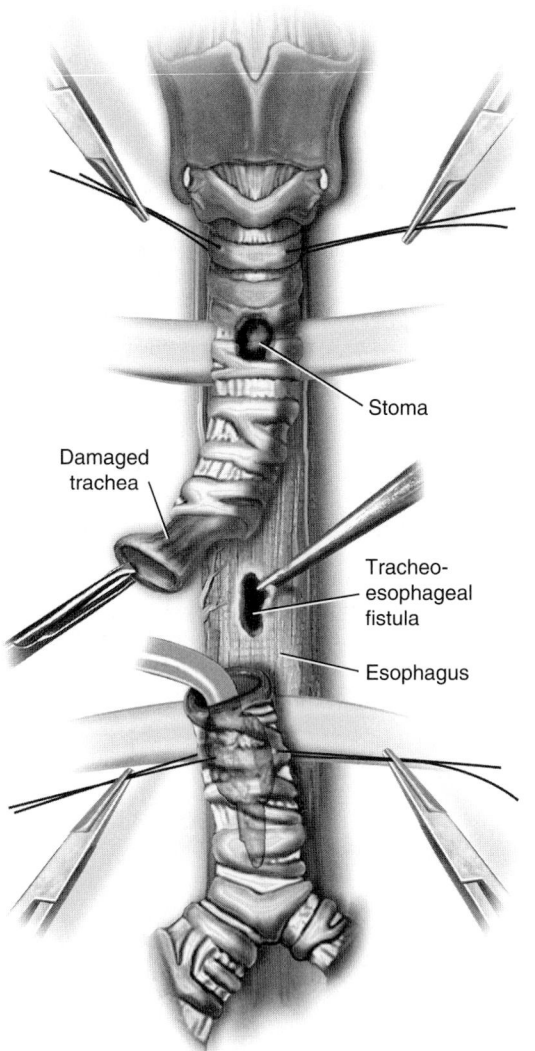

Figure 2 The trachea is divided below the fistula, providing excellent exposure to the esophageal fistula. The distal trachea is intubated with a sterile endotracheal tube for ventilation. *From Mathisen DJ, Grillo HC, Wain JC, and others: Ann Thorac Surg 52:759, 1991.*

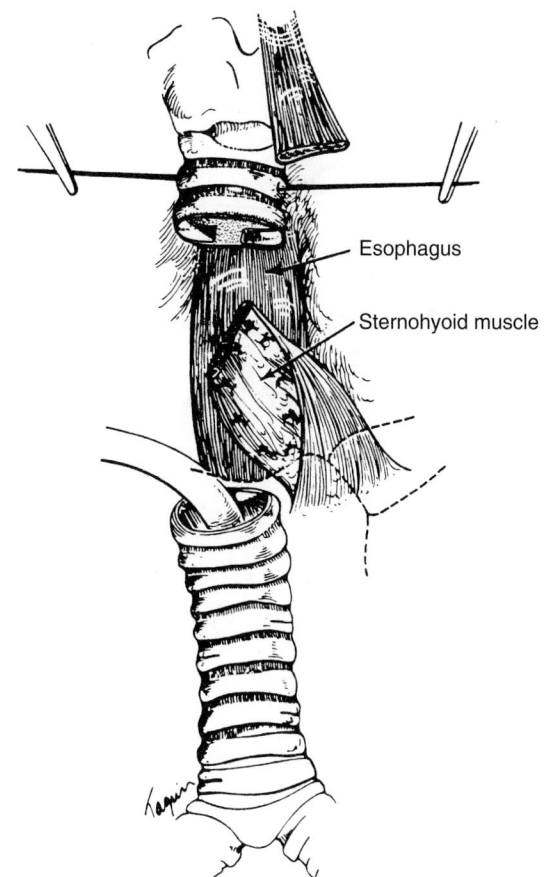

Figure 3 The esophagus is closed, and a pedicled strap muscle is carefully sutured around the edges to provide a reinforcing layer and to separate the two suture lines. *From Mathisen DJ, Grillo HC, Wain JC, and others: Ann Thorac Surg 52:759, 1991.*

resection. Couraud and colleagues reported on 17 patients with a 70% success rate. Macchiarini and colleagues reported on 14 patients treated by tracheal resection and esophageal closure with few complications (7%) and excellent long-term results (93% good or excellent). Mathisen and colleagues reported on 38 patients with simple division and closure in 9 patients and tracheal resection and esophageal closure in 29 patients. They achieved success in 89% of patients.

ACQUIRED BRONCHOESOPHAGEAL FISTULA

Most bronchoesophageal fistulae (BEFs) are due to lung or esophageal cancer and are treated with stents. Rarely, patients present with benign acquired BEF, usually with a chronic cough. The causes of a BEF include postsurgical complication, histoplasmosis, silicosis, foreign body, lye ingestion, and bronchogenic cyst. The diagnosis is made with a barium swallow and endoscopy. Almost all patients should undergo repair of the BEF. For most patients the surgeon operates through a right thoracotomy with exposure and division of the fistula. The bronchus and the esophagus are then closed and covered (and separated) with local tissue transposition. An intercostal muscle is the favored tissue flap because of the ease of harvest and ready location. Mangi and colleagues recently reported success in 12 of 13 patients with benign BEF.

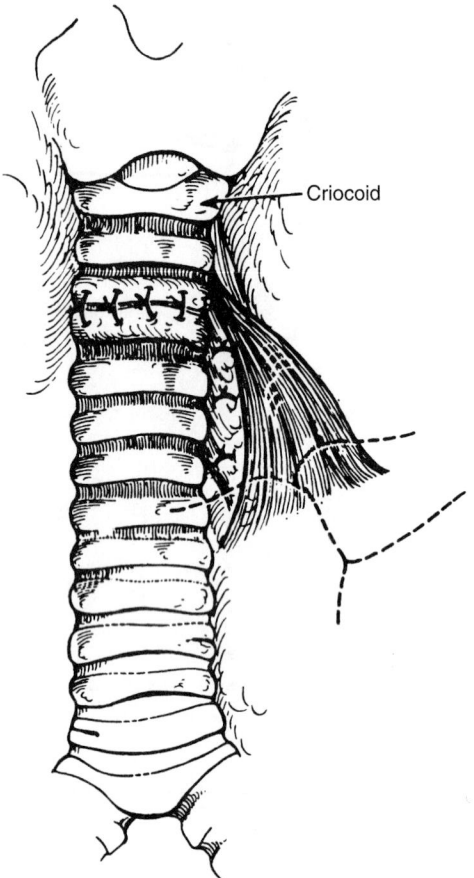

Criocoid

Figure 4   The tracheal repair is complete, and the pedicled strap muscle is seen separating the two suture lines.   *From Mathisen DJ, Grillo HC, Wain JC, and others: Ann Thorac Surg 52:759, 1991.*

SUGGESTED READINGS

Burt M, Diehl W, Martini N, and others: Malignant esophagorespiratory tract fistula: management options and survival, *Ann Thorac Surg* 52:1222, 1991.

Couraud L, Ballester MJ, Delaisement C: Acquired tracheoesophageal fistula and its management, *Sem Thorac Cardiovasc Surg* 8:392, 1996.

Macchiarini P, Verhoye JP, Chapelier A, and others: Evaluation and outcome of different surgical techniques for postintubation tracheoesophageal fistula, *J Thorac Cardiovasc Surg* 119:268, 2000.

Mangi AA, Gaissert HA, Grillo HC, and others: Benign broncho-esophageal fistula in the adult, *Ann Thorac Surg* 73:911, 2002.

Mathisen DJ, Grillo HC, Wain JC, and others: Management of acquired nonmalignant tracheoesophageal fistula, *Ann Thorac Surg* 52:759, 1991.

Shin JH, Song HY, Ko Gy, and others: Esophagorespiratory fistula: long-term results of palliative treatment with covered expandable metallic stents in 61 patients, *Radiology* 232:252, 2004.

VASCULAR SYSTEM

ABDOMINAL AORTIC ANEURYSM: OPEN REPAIR

Michael A. Curi, MD, MPA, and Brian G. Rubin, MD

Since Matas's first infrarenal aortic ligation for the treatment of an abdominal aortic aneurysm (AAA) in 1923, the surgical treatment of AAA has undergone several major advances. In 1951, Dubost first described aneurysm resection with homograft reconstruction of the abdominal aorta. The development of Vinyon "N" by Vorhees and the pioneering work of DeBakey, Cooley, and Blakemore ushered in the era of routine elective repair with interposition prosthetic graft placement. Although modern endovascular techniques afford less invasive options for treatment, open surgical repair remains the gold standard by which all other modalities are judged. Over the past half century, refinements in technique, investigations regarding natural history, improvements in perioperative care, development of new radiologic testing and endovascular aneurysm repair have all significantly affected surgical decision making regarding AAA management. The majority of AAAs are infrarenal in location; therefore repair of infrarenal aneurysms is the primary focus of this chapter.

INDICATIONS FOR REPAIR

The indication for repairing an AAA is based on the premise that surgical repair (open or endovascular) prevents aneurysm rupture, a condition that carries an 80% to 90% mortality rate. However, autopsy studies have shown that the majority of patients with aneurysms die from some other cause, most notably cardiovascular disease. Most aneurysms are asymptomatic, and the repair itself is associated with significant morbidity, mortality, and prolonged recovery. Thus there has been a significant effort to characterize both the natural history of AAAs and the morbidity and mortality associated with repair to delineate indications for treatment. Currently there are no distinctions in indications for open versus endovascular repair.

Symptomatic Aneurysms

Aneurysms are infrequently associated with symptoms, but when they occur, these symptoms can be classified into three categories: rupture or impending rupture, embolic/thrombotic complications, or mass effect. Clearly each category confers different risks and demands different levels of treatment and expediency.

Classically, the symptoms of back, flank, or abdominal pain in a patient with known aneurysm or palpable pulsatile mass represent AAA rupture or impending rupture unless proved otherwise. Because only a minority of patients with a known AAA and abdominal pain actually have a rupture or impending rupture, a careful history and physical examination can aid in making the diagnosis. With the widespread availability of spiral CT scanning, which can image the abdomen and pelvis in a matter of seconds, CT or other radiologic imaging is often performed to confirm the diagnosis and plan surgical intervention. In the presence of hypotension without another obvious explanation, prompt surgical intervention is indicated for AAA rupture. In the absence of hemodynamic changes, these symptoms in combination with the physical finding of a tender aneurysm on palpation may represent impending rupture, inflammation/infection in the aneurysm wall, or an inflammatory aneurysm. In this case, CT scanning and further workup are indicated in planning for repair.

Although distal embolization is an uncommon finding in AAA (2%–5%), it must always be considered, and spontaneous embolization represents an indication for repair. Other symptoms related to abdominal aortic aneurysms may be those related to mass effect. Symptoms such as back pain from vertebral erosion or urinary symptoms from ureteral obstruction are the result of mass effect and may require urgent but not emergent repair. Some unusual indications for emergent repair include aortic rupture into an adjacent lumen such as a "herald bleed" before massive hemorrhage in primary aortoenteric fistula or rupture into the vena cava (aortocaval fistula).

Asymptomatic Aneurysms

Despite AAAs being found in 3% of men older than 60 years and up to 12% in elderly hypertensive smokers, a large percentage of these patients remain asymptomatic and die from other causes. Through the early work by Estes, Wright, Szilagyi, and others, we know that risk of rupture is related to aneurysm size and rate of expansion (Table 1). The ADAM trial (Aneurysm Detection and Management Veterans Affairs trial) and the UK Small Aneurysm trial were large randomized trials conducted in the 1990s comparing early repair versus surveillance for small AAAs (<5.5 cm). Both trials found no difference in survival between patients undergoing immediate repair and patients followed biannually with surveillance and operative repair reserved for those AAAs becoming symptomatic, expanding rapidly, or enlarging to 5.5 cm in maximal diameter. In both trials, there was a dearth of female subjects, and some studies, including the UK Small Aneurysm trial, have suggested that female gender is an independent risk factor for rupture of aneurysms greater than 5.0 cm in diameter. Therefore the generally accepted threshold

Table 1: Rupture Risk of Stable Asymptomatic Abdominal Aortic Aneurysms by Diameter

Greatest Diameter (cm)	Annual Rupture Risk (%)
3.0–5.5	0.6
5.6–5.9	5–10
6.0–6.9	10–20
7.0–7.9	20–30
>8.0	30–50

for treating small AAAs is 5.5 cm in men. For women, the data are less clear, but typically a 5.0-cm diameter represents the surgical threshold in women. In addition, rapidly expanding AAAs, defined as growth by more than 1 cm in diameter over 12 months or 0.5 cm over 6 months, is an indication for repair. These guidelines require that patients with aneurysms that do not meet these criteria be able to undergo surveillance biannually. These are general guidelines, and surgeons must be prepared to tailor decision making on the basis of a risk versus benefit analysis individualized for each patient.

Open versus Endovascular Repair

The relative indications for open repair versus endovascular repair (EVAR) have been in a constant state of evolution since Juan Parodi performed the first EVAR. Currently the indications for aneurysm repair are those stated earlier, and the choice of open repair versus EVAR is left to the physician and patient. Two randomized prospective multicenter trials compared EVAR with open repair, the DREAM trial (Dutch Randomized Endovascular Aneurysm Management trial) and EVAR-1 trial from the United Kingdom, demonstrated lower perioperative mortality with EVAR that did not translate into differences in overall survival at 2 and 4 years, respectively. Although EVAR devices continue to evolve, the application of this technology to more patients with challenging anatomy continues to grow. Whereas proximal aneurysmal extension to the renal arteries and above has classically been an indication for open repair, fenestrated and branched devices have enhanced the pool of patients in whom EVAR technology can be applied. At this time, branched and fenestrated endografts are not commercially available in the United States.

PREOPERATIVE PREPARATION

Preoperative preparation of patients with symptomatic aneurysms is determined by the urgency for repair. In ruptured aneurysms, large-bore intravenous (IV) access and rapid transport and preparation are of utmost importance. Resuscitation should be conducted under direct supervision of the surgical staff because patients who are neurologically intact do not require normalization of blood pressure, which may hasten hemorrhage. Because most patients with a ruptured aneurysm have had a CT scan before arrival in the operating room, the patient's candidacy from endoluminal repair may have been determined. Endoluminal repair of a ruptured aneurysm can be performed on anatomically and physiologically selected patients, under local anesthesia if necessary. Induction of general anesthesia should be delayed until the patient is positioned and prepared to allow for rapid entry and aortic control in case induction precipitates cardiovascular collapse. Ruptured aneurysms are performed using the transperitoneal rather than retroperitoneal approach. With a near 50% mortality for patients surviving long enough to undergo surgery, the choice to operate is always weighed against the risk of significant life-altering morbidity, especially in elderly and significantly debilitated patients, and this decision is made in consultation with the patient or family. Overall only 10% to 20% of all patients will survive AAA rupture, and many of these will live with life-altering morbidity or significant reductions in functional capacity or quality of life.

In elective repair, the risk of surgery can be stratified on the basis of the presence of preoperative conditions and comorbidities characterized as low-, intermediate-, and high-risk factors. According to these risk factors, a patient's risk of perioperative mortality ranges from 1% to 2% in the low-risk category to at least 5% to 10% for patients with multiple high-risk factors (Tables 2 and 3). Patients with multiple high-risk factors must have a clear understanding of the potential for adverse outcomes before embarking on this procedure.

Although some risk factors such as age are not amenable to modification, preoperative preparation with medical optimization may reduce the risk of mortality in open aneurysm repair. Some evidence suggests that the use of beta-blockers for blood pressure and heart rate control, cessation of smoking, and possibly even statin use may reduce perioperative cardiovascular events, but the exact details of which drugs and which patients will benefit from these therapies remain to be delineated. Because nearly 15% of patients experience cardiovascular complications associated with open AAA repair, many patients previously would have been recommended to undergo preoperative coronary revascularization as a prophylactic measure. However, the recently completed randomized U.S. Veterans Affairs trial, the Coronary Artery Revascularization Prophylaxis (CARP) trial, challenges that concept.

Table 2: Risk Stratification for Open Abdominal Aortic Aneurysm Repair

Risk Factor	Low Risk	Intermediate Risk	High Risk
Age	Before eighth decade	Eighth decade	Ninth decade or later
Functional Status	Active regular physical exercise	Sedentary but otherwise independent	Minimally able to accomplish daily activities
Cardiac	No or minor ACC clinical predictors	Intermediate ACC clinical predictors	Severe ACC clinical predictors
Pulmonary	No clinical disease	Mild COPD, FEV1 > 1 L/sec	O₂ dependent, forced expiratory volume-1 <1 L/sec
Renal	Normal renal function	Creatinine 2.0–3.0	Creatinine >3.0
Other	Noninflammatory infrarenal AAA	Juxtarenal or suprarenal or inflammatory AAA	Pugh-Child's class B or C liver failure

AAA, Abdominal aortic aneurysm; *ACC*, American College of Cardiology; *COPD*, chronic obstructive pulmonary disease.

Table 3: Risk Factors for Operative Mortality Following Elective Abdominal Aortic Aneurysm Repair

Risk Factor	Multivariate Odds Ratio	Univariate Odds Ratio
Renal insufficiency (creatinine >1.8 mg/dl)	3.47	3.07
Congestive heart failure	5.94	2.83
Resting ECG ischemia	5.57	2.73
History of myocardial infarction	4.48	2.07
COPD, dyspnea, prior pulmonary surgery	2.32	1.83
Age (per decade)	2.67	1.79

Modified from Steyerberg EW, Kievet J, del Mol Van Otterloo JC, and others: Arch Intern Med 155:1998, 1995.
COPD, Chronic obstructive pulmonary disease; ECG, electrocardiography.

CARP investigators found no difference in perioperative mortality or long-term survival for coronary revascularization compared with maximal medical management in patients before vascular surgery. CARP trial patients had stable coronary artery disease involving at least one 70% stenosis (not including left main coronary). Additional guidelines regarding preoperative cardiac assessment have been published by the American College of Cardiology and the American Heart Association, which have developed consensus recommendations regarding the preoperative cardiac evaluation of patients with vascular disease.

Patients with aortic aneurysms are prone to aneurysms in other locations, and thus preoperative physical examination to evaluate the femoral and popliteal arteries should be routine. If necessary, a duplex scan of the femoral-popliteal system can differentiate diffuse arteriomegaly from focal aneurysmal degeneration. Finally, the chest x-ray should be reviewed to detect the presence of a thoracic aneurysm.

■ OPERATIVE THERAPY

A successful operation starts with an anesthesia team that is familiar with the volume shifts and hemodynamic changes inherent to the procedure and can communicate effectively with the surgeons involved. Epidural anesthesia has been shown to improve postoperative pain control, decrease the frequency of postoperative pulmonary complications, and possibly shorten the length of postoperative ileus following open AAA repair. The intraoperative cell salvage machine (cell saver) should be in the room and ready for use. Sufficient wide-bore IV access; arterial line placement; and, in patients with significant cardiac disease, central hemodynamic monitoring are standard. For EVAR patients, the intraoperative course is typically stable, with only minimal hemodynamic changes. EVAR can be conducted under general, regional, or local anesthesia.

Choosing an Approach for Open AAA Repair

Exposing the aorta and aneurysm repair can be accomplished though either a transperitoneal/transabdominal (TPA) or retroperitoneal approach (RPA). Clearly the anatomy of the aneurysm; renal, iliac, and femoral arteries; and left renal vein must be understood before deciding which approach is best for each patient. With up to 85% of AAAs now being repaired via EVAR, the AAAs undergoing open repair are more commonly juxtarenal or suprarenal or have other challenging aspects to their aortic neck anatomy. We routinely use the RPA for all aneurysms unless specific aspects of anatomy require TPA. The ability to gain control of bleeding safely and expeditiously is of utmost importance, and thus a fundamental tenet of aortic surgery is to obtain arterial exposure to ensure adequate proximal and distal arterial control.

Retroperitoneal Approach

The relative indications for RPA include the presence of severe chronic obstructive pulmonary disease (COPD), a history of previous abdominal surgery, the presence of a horseshoe kidney or an inflammatory aneurysm, and the presence of an abdominal wall stoma. Relative contraindications for RPA include a history of previous left retroperitoneal surgery and the need to perform mesenteric, nonostial right renal artery revascularization, or right iliac artery aneurysmal disease. Although some authors state that the TPA approach should be used when aortobiiliac or bifemoral bypass is necessary, we find that with proper positioning and dissection, RPA can afford adequate proximal to mid-right iliac exposure and access to the entire right femoral artery via a counterincision in the right groin.

After the patient is under anesthesia, he or she is positioned on a vacuum-operated beanbag positioner extending from the axilla to midthigh. Exposure of the aorta is facilitated if the patient is positioned so that the kidney rest is halfway between the costal margin and iliac crest, with left shoulder rotated roughly 60 degrees off the table. The hips are allowed to fall back as parallel to the table as possible. The left arm is rested on an "airplane hanger" or padded Mayo stand, the legs are padded with pillows, and all pressure points are well cushioned. The kidney rest is maximally elevated, the table is flexed into a jackknife position to allow maximal opening of the space between ribs and iliac crest, and the patient is strapped to the table (Fig. 1).

The location and extent of the incision depend on the body habitus and operation planned. For standard infrarenal aortic reconstruction, an incision starting at the lateral rectus border slightly below the level of the umbilicus and extending to the tip of the twelfth rib gives excellent exposure to the infrarenal aorta, proximal right common iliac, and entire left iliac arterial system. The incision can be extended posteriorly or the twelfth rib resected for more exposure. In more obese patients or those requiring suprarenal or supraceliac clamping, the incision should be carried into the tenth or eleventh intercostal space, which may result in entrance into the pleural cavity. The lateral edge of the rectus may be partially divided for more medial exposure if necessary.

After incising skin and subcutaneous tissue, the retroperitoneal space at the junction of the lateral border of the rectus is entered, and the peritoneum is mobilized off the undersurface of the flank muscles, with the plane of dissection initially developed with a

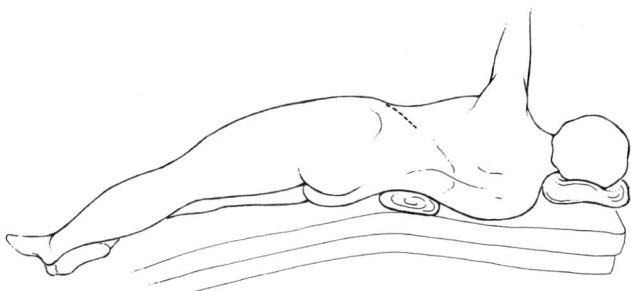

Figure 1   Proper positioning for left retroperitoneal approach to the aorta.

fingertip moving gently in the direction of the left iliac crest. The flank muscles are divided with cautery, and the peritoneum further mobilized posteriorly, medially, and superiorly until the left gonadal vein and ureter are visualized. The surgeon should take care when working to free the peritoneum because it becomes extremely thin and is easily torn as it courses along the undersurface of the abdominal wall musculature. With minimal dissection and manipulation, the ureter is encircled, including the periureteral fat that contains the blood supply, and mobilized and protected. The avascular space between Gerota fascia and the peritoneum is entered, allowing posterior displacement of the left kidney, exposure of the renal vein, and ligation of the left gonadal vein at the inferior border of the renal vein (Fig. 2). Care must be used during dissection along the iliac

arteries bilaterally to avoid injury to the overlying ureter. Also, limited or no dissection, if feasible, along the left posterolateral aortic wall and proximal left common iliac artery may minimize the risk of postoperative erectile or ejaculatory dysfunction. The left renal vein may be retroaortic in 2% to 3% of patients and circumaortic in 0.5% to 1.0%, and failure to recognize these anomalies can result in significant hemorrhage. Other vessels emptying into the renal vein are the left second lumbar vein medially and posteriorly and the left adrenal vein superiorly, which also may require ligation to prevent avulsion. Depending on the level required for aortic clamping, the kidney may be mobilized anteriorly for improved access to the suprarenal aorta (Fig. 3). Similarly, the fibers of the diaphragm envelop the suprarenal aorta and must be divided for suprarenal aortic exposure.

The left and right common iliac arteries are identified low in the wound and can be exposed for clamping. If clamping distally is not feasible because of concomitant iliac occlusive disease, inflammatory aneurysm, or a large obscuring aneurysm, balloon occlusion-irrigation catheters can be used to control backbleeding from one or both iliac arteries after the aneurysm is opened. This maneuver may also be employed to control and perfuse the renal arteries in an RPA approach if a suprarenal clamp is necessary.

Before clamping, systemic heparinization is initiated with 60 to 70 U/kg IV bolus. Clamps should be positioned distally on the iliac arteries before placing the proximal clamp (or even test clamping) to reduce the risk of distal embolization. The neck of the aneurysm is exposed with gentle finger dissection around the aorta. The proximal clamp should be positioned so that the handle is out of the operative field and secured with umbilical tape or silastic tubing to prevent dislodgement. Clamps with atraumatic inserts may slip more easily from the pulsating stump and should be used selectively in this location.

After the aorta is clamped and there is no pulsation within the aneurysm, it is opened longitudinally and the thrombus extirpated. The ligation of back-bleeding lumbar arteries and the inferior mesenteric artery (IMA) is performed with silk sutures from inside the aneurysm sac. Ligation of the IMA away from its origin risks compromising sigmoid and left colic collaterals; therefore oversewing of the IMA orifice from within the open AAA sac is recommended. The longitudinal opening is lengthened and T-incised proximally to leave a neck suitable for sewing. There must be 1 cm

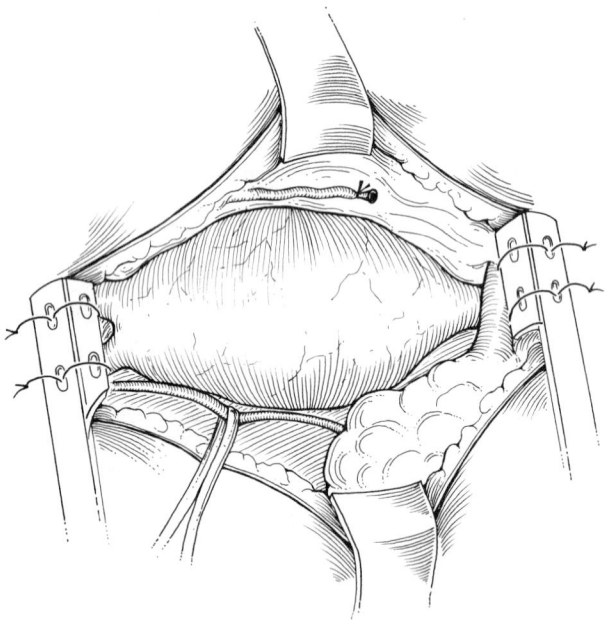

Figure 2 Appearance of the aortic aneurysm after retroperitoneal exposure. Note that the left gonadal vein has been ligated and divided and the left ureter marked with a vessel loop.

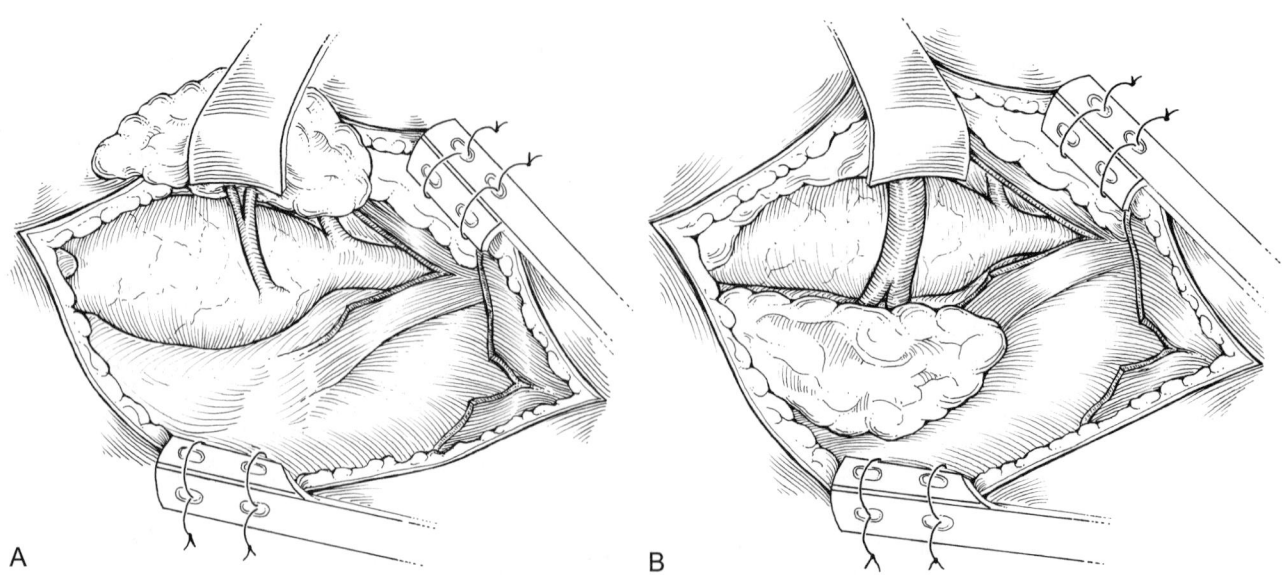

A   B

Figure 3 Appearance of the aortic aneurysm after retroperitoneal exposure for juxtarenal or suprarenal aortic clamping. Depending on the plan for surgical repair, the left kidney may be mobilized anteriorly **(A)** or left posteriorly **(B)**. Note that the aortic crus of the diaphragm is incised to gain exposure to the visceral aortic segment and the left thorax has been entered.

of normal aorta below the clamp (or the orifice of the renal arteries if the clamp is suprarenal) to permit adequate bites of tissue and sealing of the anastomosis. An appropriate-diameter prosthetic graft is chosen (using sizers if necessary). The choice of material varies with the surgeon's preference, with no clear advantage for Dacron or polytetrafluoroethylene (Teflon). Bifurcated grafts are used when there are concomitant iliac artery aneurysms (aortobiliac) or significant iliac occlusive disease (aortobifemoral). The proximal anastomosis is performed using a 2–0 or 3–0 polypropylene suture in a running fashion, starting along the posterior wall. When complete, the graft is clamped and the proximal clamp is gently released but not removed to test the anastomosis. The aorta can be reclamped should the anastomosis require revision. After hemostasis is achieved, the graft is flushed out from above and clamped just beyond the anastomosis. If IMA or renal artery reimplantation is required, backbleeding from these branch vessels can be controlled with a balloon-irrigation catheter while they are reimplanted into the aortic graft with a Carrel patch. The kidney can be cooled with ice slush before aortic clamping and infused with cold, heparinized plasma-lyte solution via the occlusion-irrigation catheter while the proximal aortic anastomosis is performed. The distal anastomosis either at the aortic bifurcation or to the common iliac arteries is performed in the same fashion as the proximal anastomosis. Before completing the distal anastomosis, the anesthesiologist is notified to prepare for the possibility of declamping hypotension and the anastomoses are flushed proximally and distally to remove any remaining plaque or thrombus. The clamps are removed and distal pulses verified. The aneurysm sac may be closed over the graft, but this is not essential in the RPA approach. The wound is irrigated, hemostasis confirmed, and the incision is closed in two facial layers and the skin closed with staples. Closure is facilitated by returning the bed to a flat configuration and lowering the kidney rest.

Transperitoneal Approach

Transperitoneal approach affords the most flexibility for exposure of the infrarenal aneurysm, renal arteries, and both iliac and femoral systems. Specifically, patients with right iliac artery aneurysms or ectasia requiring a graft limb anastomosed distal to the proximal right common iliac artery are best served by a transabdominal approach. However, the TPA makes it difficult to obtain suprarenal aortic exposure and necessitates dealing with problems such as adhesions resulting from previous abdominal surgery, horseshoe kidney, or other intra-abdominal pathology. This approach may be made through a midline or transverse incision, and the peritoneal cavity examined for any pathology. The transverse colon and omentum are retracted cephalad, and the small intestine eviscerated to the right. The posterior peritoneum is incised longitudinally over the aorta from the aortic bifurcation to the ligament of Treitz. Dissection should occur to the right of the inferior mesenteric vein but taking care to leave enough tissue adjacent to the duodenum to close the retroperitoneum at the conclusion of the procedure. As dissection is carried cephalad, the renal vein is encountered crossing the aorta at the neck of the aneurysm, which can be bluntly dissected on the lateral edges. Distally the iliac arteries are dissected only along their lateral walls for clamp placement because circumferential dissection carries risk of iliac vein injury. Care should be taken to identify the ureter and to minimize dissection of the aortic bifurcation and left common iliac artery to avoid damage to the parasympathetic nerve plexus responsible for erectile and ejaculatory function.

The aortic reconstruction is performed in a fashion similar to that described for the RPA. The aneurysm is then closed over the graft, the retroperitoneum is closed, and the abdominal contents replaced. The fascia is closed in the usual fashion and the skin closed with staples. Patients with aneurysms are at increased risk for developing incisional hernias, and thus care to obtain adequate tissue bites at the time of fascial closure is essential.

Postoperative Care

Patients can be extubated in the operating room unless there are extenuating circumstances such as massive blood loss, hypothermia, coagulopathy, or significant cardiopulmonary compromise. Most patients are followed in the surgical intensive care unit for proper response to hemodynamic changes and fluid shifts. Standard postoperative intensive care unit monitoring and routine blood work are performed. A chest x-ray should be performed to confirm endotracheal tube and central line placement. Because cardiac-related complications occur in approximately 15% of patients after elective aneurysm repair, electrocardiograms should be performed daily and compared with preoperative baseline. Routine serial troponin measurement is controversial, and the current clinical recommendations suggest routine "rule-out myocardial infarction" evaluation in patients characterized as being at high or intermediate risk during preoperative risk stratification.

Beta-blockade should be continued with IV formulations in patients taking them preoperatively or as part of a perioperative risk management strategy. Perioperative antibiotics are discontinued after 24 hours. Stress ulcer and deep vein thrombosis prophylaxis with sequential compression devices are indicated until the patients are eating and ambulatory, respectively. Importantly, adequate pain control via epidural or patient-controlled analgesia must be achieved to allow for adequate pulmonary toilet and incentive spirometry.

Early postoperative complications in addition to the cardiopulmonary complications include hemorrhage; renal and lower-extremity embolism; and, rarely, colonic ischemia. Although full-thickness colonic necrosis mandates immediate exploration for resection of the involved colon, ischemic colitis confined to the mucosa can be observed. This differentiation can occasionally be made with flexible sigmoidoscopy with biopsy, and any patient with bloody rectal discharge, fever, unexplained leukocytosis, or left lower-quadrant pain and diarrhea after AAA repair regardless of IMA ligation or reimplantation should be evaluated with sigmoidoscopy.

The most frequent late complications of open AAA repair are sexual dysfunction and incisional hernias. Retrograde ejaculation results from injury to the superior hypogastric plexus as it crosses the aortic bifurcation and proximal left common iliac vessels. Incisional hernias occur more frequently in AAA patients than age-matched aortic reconstructions for occlusive disease. Flank bulges from RPA incisions are less common than ventral hernias and are usually asymptomatic; they do not carry the same risk of intestinal strangulation. They are not true hernias and are thought to result from denervation and atrophy of the muscle layers in the flank. Anastomotic pseudoaneurysms may occur at the aortic (<0.5%), iliac (1%), or femoral (3%) level after 5 years but may be significantly more common 15 years after repair. Pseudo-aneurysms usually represent continued arterial degeneration with resultant anastomotic disruption. Late graft infections are rare and usually associated with instrumentation (i.e., cardiac catheterization). Secondary aortoenteric fistula formation after AAA repair is rare (<1%) and usually develops approximately 5 years after repair. These almost always involve the duodenum at the proximal anastomosis and may present with either massive gastrointestinal bleeding (aortoenteric fistula) or sepsis and more modest hemorrhage (aortoenteric erosion) associated with graft infection. Graft thrombosis or graft-limb thrombosis is also a rare late complication, usually occurring in the setting of severe iliac occlusive disease. With 5- and 10-year survival after AAA repair of 75% and 45%, we currently recommend follow-up visits and a routine CT scan at 5 years after repair.

Suggested Readings

Blankensteijn JD, de Jong SE, Prinssen M, and others: Dutch Randomized Endovascular Aneurysm Management Trial G. Two-year outcomes after conventional or endovascular repair of abdominal aortic aneurysms. [see comment], *N Engl J Med* 352:2398, 2005.

Eagle K, Berger PB, Calkins H, and others: Perioperative cardiovascular evaluation for noncardiac surgery update (online), Available at http://www.acc.org/qualityandscience/clinical/guidelines/perio/update/periupdate_index.htm. Accessed August 3, 2007.

EVAR trial participants.: Endovascular aneurysm repair versus open repair in patients with abdominal aortic aneurysm (EVAR trial 1): randomised controlled trial [see comment], Lancet 365:2179, 2005.

Lederle FA, Wilson SE, Johnson GR, and others: Immediate repair compared with surveillance of small abdominal aortic aneurysms, N Engl J Med 346:1437, 2002.

McFalls EO, Ward HB, Moritz TE, and others: Coronary-artery revascularization before major elective vascular surgery, N Engl J Med 351:2795, 2004.

Sicard GA, Reilly JM, Rubin BG, and others: Transabdominal versus retroperitoneal incision for abdominal aortic surgery: report of a prospective randomized trial, J Vasc Surg 21:174, 1995.

The UK Small Aneurysm Trial Participants: Mortality results for randomised controlled trial of early elective surgery or ultrasonographic surveillance for small abdominal aortic aneurysms, Lancet 352:1649, 1998.

The United Kingdom Small Aneurysm Trial Participants: Long term outcomes of immediate repair compared with surveillance of small abdominal aortic aneurysms, N Engl J Med 346:1445, 2002.

ENDOVASCULAR TREATMENT OF ABDOMINAL AORTIC ANEURYSMS

Mahmoud B. Malas, MD

Although open repair remains the gold standard treatment for abdominal aortic aneurysm (AAA), endovascular aneurysm repair (EVAR) has become an acceptable treatment option. Since its introduction by Juan Parodi in the early 1990s, this minimally invasive approach has undergone an intense refinement in technique and device design. This has resulted in impressively lower morbidity and mortality compared with the traditional open repair.

INDICATION

There are no data to support various indications for EVAR other than those already established for open repair. Two prospective randomized trials, the United Kingdom Small Aneurysm Trial and the U.S. Veterans Affairs Aneurysm Detection and Management trial (ADAM trial), showed no survival benefit of treating aneurysms between 4.0 and 5.5 cm in diameter over medical management. It is safe to follow these patients with ultrasound or computed tomography (CT) scans at 6-month intervals until the aneurysm reaches 5.0 to 5.5 cm in diameter. Exceptions to this rule are rapidly expanding aneurysms (>0.6 cm in 1 year) and symptomatic aneurysms (back or abdominal pain). Table 1 outlines analysis by experts for estimated rupture risk on the basis of aneurysm diameter. Independent risk factors not related to size that increase the rate of rupture include female patients who tend to rupture at smaller diameters (threefold increase in rupture rate), chronic obstructive pulmonary disease (COPD; 1.6 times per each liter reduction in forced expiratory volume [FEV]1), hypertension (1.02 times per each 1 mm Hg increase in mean arterial pressure), and smoking (1.5 times). Other, less significant, nonindependent risk factors that increase rupture rates include the number of first-degree relatives with AAA (10%–25% increase), the ratio of the AAA diameter to the native aorta diameter, and the shape of the aneurysm. Saccular (eccentric) aneurysms have an increased focal point of wall stress and tend to rupture at a higher rate than the more symmetrical fusiform aneurysms with concentric distribution of wall stress.

Table 1: Expert Consensus on Estimated Rupture Risk per Year According to Abdominal Aortic Aneurysms Diameter Only

Diameter (cm)	Experts Consensus (%)
<4.0	0
4–4.9	0.5–5
5–5.9	3–15
6–6.9	10–20
7–8.0	20–40
>8.0	30–50

PREOPERATIVE IMAGING

Spiral CT scans should be obtained with and without intravenous contrast and without oral contrast and collimated at 2-mm cuts. This has replaced angiography for most experienced surgeons. The noncontrast images help to evaluate vessel calcification. Avoiding oral contrast reduces artifacts. A three-dimensional (3D) reconstruction of the scan provides an excellent tool for graft sizing and detailed evaluation of the anatomy.

SIZING AND ANATOMIC CONSIDERATIONS

The proximal neck of the aneurysm is the relatively normal segment of the aorta that extends from the lowest renal artery to the beginning of the aneurysm (Fig. 1). The long-term durability of the endovascular repair is highly dependant on proper fitting of the proximal portion of the device in the neck. A favorable anatomic neck is 10 to 15 mm in length, less than 32 mm in diameter, and less than 60 degrees in angulation. We tend to oversize the device by 10% to 20% of the actual neck diameter to help fixation. The largest device diameter approved by the U.S. Food and Drug Administration (FDA) today is 36 mm. Thus the largest neck we can treat at present is 32 mm in diameter. Iliac arteries are the access vessels to deliver the device and provide the distal fixation site. Similar to proximal neck, the iliac arteries should provide at least 1 to 2 cm of proper fixation, preferably proximal to the internal iliac artery (IIA) to preserve the pelvic circulation. Because the largest iliac limb approved by the FDA is 24 mm, the iliac diameter should not exceed 20 mm. The smallest delivery system is 20 F (3-F is approximately equivalent to 1 mm). Thus the iliac diameter should be at least 6 to 7 mm. Distance from the lowest renal artery to the aortic bifurcation and each IIA is measured. Three-dimensional reconstruction of the CT scan provides accurate measurements of aneurysm, neck, and iliac diameter, as well as neck angulation and length measurement using centerline technology (Fig. 2). Using a chart specific to each device,

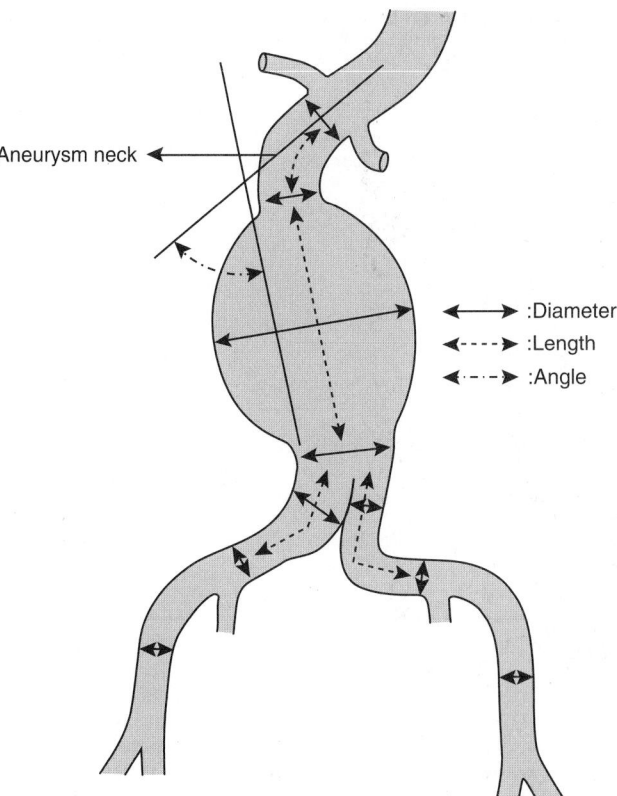

Figure 1 Diameter and length measurements required to size the appropriate endograft. Neck diameter and angulation. Common and external iliac arteries diameter. Length from the lowest renal to the aortic bifurcation and to each internal iliac artery. *From Ohki T, Mahmoud M: Endovascular treatment of abdominal and thoracic aneurysms. In Casserly I, Sachar R, Yadav JS, editor: Manual of peripheral vascular intervention, Philadelphia, 2005, Lippincott Williams & Wilkins. Reprinted with permission.*

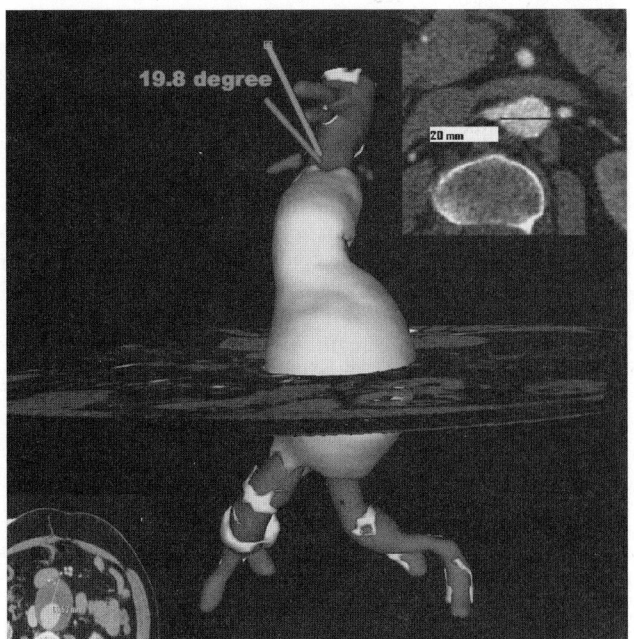

Figure 2 The benefits of three-dimensional (3D) computed tomography scan reconstruction in preoperative planning. Accurate measurement of aortic neck diameter and angulation with centerline technique by using 3D imaging along with axial slices. *From M2S The fusion of clinical data and 3D imaging, West Lebanon, NH.* **(See color insert Figure 32.)**

the length and diameter measurement determines the endograft size required for the repair.

CONTRAINDICATIONS

1. High-grade stenosis or occlusion of the superior mesenteric and celiac arteries with the inferior mesenteric artery (IMA) provides essential collateral circulation to the bowel. In this situation, covering the IMA would result in bowel ischemia with poor outcome. One approach for patients who cannot tolerate aortic cross clamping is to perform an external iliac to superior mesenteric artery (SMA) or celiac bypass (or both) 3 weeks before EVAR.

2. Neck angulation greater than 60 degrees (Fig. 1 and 2), diameter greater than 32 mm, or severe calcification with lining of the neck with circumferential mural thrombus all increase the chance of future graft migration and failure of the repair. A flared neck or reverse tapered neck (the diameter increases or decreases, respectively, more than 10%) is associated with higher incidence of endoleak.

3. Iliac arteries with severe calcification and tortuosity or with smaller than 7 mm diameter are associated with significant intraoperative complications. Attempting to force the delivery system through such arteries would result in iliac artery torsion or complete transection. At the end of the repair, while the surgeon is pulling the sheath, a segment of the artery would be pulled with the sheath, i.e., "iliac on a stick." To avoid this catastrophic complication, the surgeon could sew a conduit (10-mm Dacron graft) end to side to the common iliac artery through a small retroperitoneal incision. The endograft would be delivered through the conduit, bypassing the tortuous, calcified, small external iliacs.

4. Renal insufficiency is an obvious contraindication to intravenous contrast. Elevated creatinine is associated with significant increase in open repair morbidity and mortality. An experienced endovascular surgeon may perform EVAR with CO_2 angiography using selective catheterization of the renal and internal iliac arteries with gadolinium injections, avoiding a high load of contrast.

DEVICE PRESCRIPTION

Four devices are approved by the FDA for the U.S. market (Table 2). These are the Zenith (Cook, Bloomington, IN), Excluder (W.L. Gore, Flagstaff, AZ), AneuRx (Medtronic, Santa Rosa, CA), and Powerlink system graft (Endologix, Irvine, CA). All of these devices are self-expanding, modular (multicomponent) endografts consisting of a bifurcated main body and iliac limb extensions. The endografts are made of fabric that is either expanded polytetrafluoroethylene (ePTFE) (Excluder and Powerlink) or woven polyester (Zenith and AneuRx). To increase the structural support of the endografts and provide proximal and distal fixation, a stent is attached to the fabric. The stent is made of stainless steel (Zenith and Powerlink) or Nitinol (AneuRx and Excluder). The stent is an exoskeleton (AneuRx and Zenith), endoskeleton (Powerlink), or embedded in PTFE (Excluder). By oversizing the endograft (10%–20% of the diameter of the native vessel) at the proximal and distal fixation sides, the stent expands and firmly apposes to the wall of the aorta and iliac arteries. The Zenith graft has an additional bare metal suprarenal stent and 10 to 14 barbs, depending on the graft diameter, to provide additional fixation.

Table 2: FDA-Approved Endografts: Description, Length and Diameter Availability

Company	Device	Main Body		Iliac Leg		Delivery System Profile		Fixed Location	Stent Material	Graft Material
		Length (cm)	Diam. (mm)	Length (cm)	Diam. (mm)	OD	ID			
Cook	Zenith	7.4, 8.8, 10.3, 11.7, 13.2	22, 24, 26, 28, 30, 32, 36	3.7, 5.4, 7.1, 8.8, 10.5, 12.2	8, 10, 12, 14, 16, 18, 20, 22, 24	20, 22, 24 F	18, 20, 22 F	Suprarenal	Stainless steel	Woven polyester
Edologix	Powerlink	8,10	25, 28, 34	4,55	16	21 F		Infrarenal or suprarenal	Stainless steel alloy	ePTFE
Gore	Excluder	14, 16, 18	23, 26, 285, 31+	10, 12, 14	12, 145, 16, 18, 20	20 F	18 F	Infrarenal	Nitinol	ePTFE
Medtronic	AneuRx	13.5, 16.5	20, 22, 24, 26, 28	85, 115	12, 13, 14, 15, 16	21 F		Infrarenal	Nitinol	Woven polyester

Diam., Diameter; *ePTFE,* expanded polytetrafluoroethylene; *FDA,* U.S. Food and Drug Administration; *ID,* inner diameter; *OD,* outer diameter.

OPERATIVE TECHNIQUE

The procedure can be performed under general, epidural, or local anesthesia. Although a few centers perform this procedure in the interventional suites, the majority of cases take place in the operating room. A mobile C-arm with vascular imaging and digital subtraction with a fluoroscopy-compatible floating table are more than adequate for imaging. A wall-mounted unit with large image intensifier provides more detailed imaging. Intravenous antibiotic is given 30 to 60 minutes before incisions are made. The procedure can be performed percutaneously using a percutaneous closure device (Prostar XL; Abbott Vascular, Abbott Park, IL). This device delivers percutaneously two 3.0 braided polyester sutures placed through the arterial wall with four nitinol needles. The FDA has approved this device to close up to 10-F arterial holes. It has been used to close up to 22-F arteriotomy for percutaneous EVAR. The femoral arteries should be free of calcification and plaque. I prefer a cutdown because it is associated with less postoperative hematoma and pseudoaneurysm complications, especially because the majority of patients have significant atherosclerosis and calcification. Bilateral cutdowns on the femoral arteries are performed through transverse incisions along the inguinal ligament. This should be a few centimeters above the skin fold of the abdomen. An incision made farther down would be covered by the skin fold, especially with obese patients, who are more susceptible to sweating, are more difficult to clean, and have higher infection rates. The common femoral arteries are dissected free for approximately 2-cm-long segments, and vessel loops are placed proximally and distally. The arteries are inspected, and a soft area is chosen for puncture with an 18-gauge single wall needle. If the artery is particularly calcified, further proximal dissection is carried out under the inguinal ligament by freeing the ligament medially and laterally and retracting it superiorly. The lateral femoral vein, which crosses over the junction with the external iliac, is carefully dissected free, double ligated, and transected. The vein can easily be torn off the common femoral vein and cause excessive bleeding that is difficult to control. After puncturing the anterior wall of the common femoral or external iliac artery with the needle, a Benston wire (Boston Scientific, Natick, MA; 0.035-inch diameter hydrophobic 150 cm long) is inserted through the needle under fluoroscopy guidance.

A bilateral 7-F, 23-cm-long sheath is exchanged with the needle over the wire and placed through the iliac vessels into the aneurysm. A pigtail diagnostic catheter is placed over the wire under fluoroscopy guidance to the level of the renal arteries (L1–2). A diagnostic angiogram is performed using a power injector to establish the level of the renals and the length to the aortic bifurcation and to the level of IIAs. This helps to confirm the appropriate length of endograft to use. The angiogram is not helpful to determine the diameter of the vessels because it cannot evaluate the difference between the lining mural thrombus and the actual wall, and thus a preoperative CT scan is more accurate for diameter measurements. Intravenous heparin is given (80–100 units per Kg bolus) 5 minutes before advancing the large delivery sheath. The device should be delivered on the side with less tortuous, less calcified, and larger-diameter iliacs. Consideration for aorta and proximal neck angulation should be taken so that the device is placed from the side that results in minimal kinking and tension on the endograft. A Super Stiff wire (Boston Scientific/Medi-Tech, Watertown, MA) is positioned through the sheath into the aortic arch under fluoroscopy to avoid placement into the left ventricle or the arch breaches. A sudden-onset arrhythmia should alert the surgeon to migration of the wire into the ventricle. The 7-F sheath is removed after clamping the distal artery with a soft clamp and controlling the proximal artery by squeezing the artery gently with the surgeon's fingers. The main body delivery sheath is advanced over the Super Stiff wire while applying back tension on the wire (Fig. 3, *A*). There is no need to perform an arteriotomy because the newer sheath has a smooth, tapered end that gently dilatates the original opening with the 7-F sheath. Resistance encountered while advancing the device should not be overcome by forceful pushing, which will result in rupturing the iliac artery. Instead, a gentle push (on the delivery sheath) and pull (on the Super Stiff wire) technique should help with safely advancing the sheath. If a stenosis is found in the iliac arteries, an angioplasty without stenting would help. Changing the plan to use the contralateral side is another helpful maneuver. A small retroperitoneal incision and suturing an end-to-side 10-mm Dacron conduit to bypass a tortuous calcified external iliac is also helpful. After the device is delivered to the infrarenal aorta, a second angiogram with magnification is performed to mark the level of the renal arteries. The sheath is withdrawn while maintaining the upper end of the device just below the lowest renal artery (Fig. 3, *B*). Each

Figure 3 Steps in endovascular aneurysm repair. **(A)** Introduction of the delivery system over a stiff wire from the ipsilateral femoral artery. **(B)** Deploying the endograft after confirming the level of the renal arteries followed by cannulation of the short limb of the endograft from the contralateral iliac artery. **(C)** Advancing the iliac limb extension from the contralateral femoral artery over a stiff wire. **(D)** Final step of deploying the contralateral iliac limb extension. *From Ohki T, Mahmoud M: Endovascular treatment of abdominal and thoracic aneurysms. In Casserly I, Sachar R, Yadav JS, editor: Manual of peripheral vascular intervention, Philadelphia, 2005, Lippincott Williams & Wilkins. Reprinted with permission.*

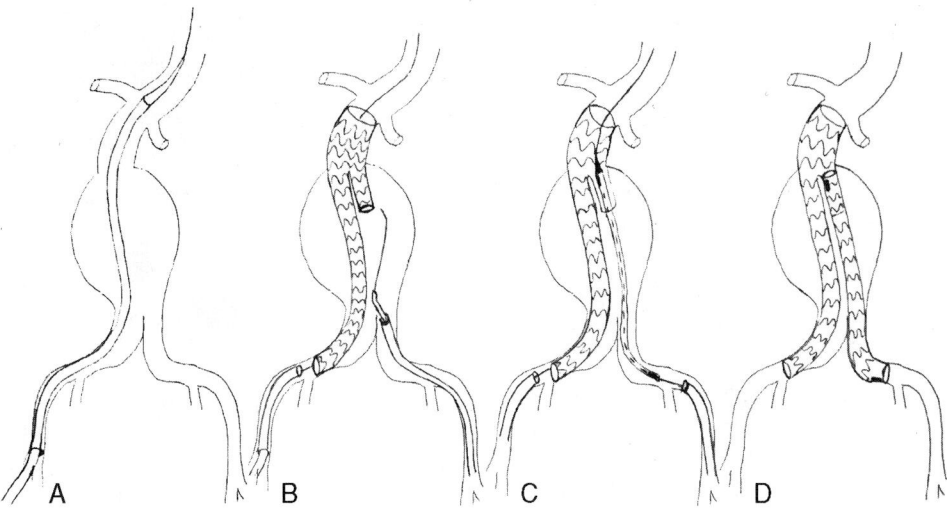

device has a different marker to orient the surgeon to keep the contralateral limb of the main body oriented to deploy in an anterior lateral position toward the contralateral iliacs. A directional catheter and guidewire are used to cannulate the contralateral limb through the 7-F sheath under fluoroscopy guidance (Fig. 3, *B*). This is one of the more technically demanding parts of the procedure. If not successful, advancing a wire from the ipsilateral sheath over the main body bifurcation (flow divider) and snaring it from the contralateral sheath is a helpful maneuver. Alternatively, the wire can be advanced from a separate puncture, and 4-F sheaths can be placed through the brachial artery. With a directional, long, guiding catheter (vertebral, or angled glide), the wire is advanced into the contralateral limb and snared from the contralateral sheath. After the cannulation has been established, a diagnostic angiogram is performed by advancing a pigtail catheter into the main body over the wire from the contralateral femoral sheath. This confirms filling of both renals and the main body with contrast. The pigtail catheter should also turn freely inside the main body. If the wire and catheter are between the endograft and the aortic wall, the pigtail will not turn freely and the contrast will fill the aneurysm first before the retrograde filling of the endograft. To extend the iliac limb on the contralateral side, an angiogram is performed with the appropriate oblique view (left anterior oblique for the right iliacs and right anterior oblique for the left iliacs). This helps to open the common iliac artery (CIA) bifurcation and obtain an accurate measurement on the length. The iliac limb is advanced over a stiff wire and overlapped at least 2 cm with the short contralateral limb of the main body (Fig. 3, *C*). The limb is deployed in a similar fashion (Fig. 3, *D*). The distal end of the iliac limb should be proximal to the IIA. An iliac extension might be required on the ipsilateral side, depending on the length and diameter of the common iliac. Ideally 1 to 2 cm of distal fixation is sufficient. My preference is to cover the entire CIA for added security. If a CIA aneurysm is extending to the IIA, the first step is percutaneous coiling of the latter. The EVAR should be delayed 3 to 4 weeks to allow collateralization from the contralateral IIA. During EVAR, the iliac limb is extended to cover the orifice of the coiled IIA, excluding the CIA aneurysm. The main side effect is buttock claudication, which is well tolerated and improved with walking exercises. We have covered both IIAs in cases of bilateral CIA aneurysms or insufficient landing zone in the CIAs. There are reports of less than a 1% incidence of sigmoid colon ischemia. Hence every effort should be made to preserve the pelvic circulation with at least one IIA. Gentle ballooning of the main body and iliac limb at the proximal and distal seal and overlap zones is performed to ensure good apposition of the endograft against the

vessel wall. A completion angiogram is performed to evaluate complete exclusion of the aneurysm and patency of renal and internal iliac arteries, and to rule out an endoleak. All wires and sheaths are withdrawn under fluoroscopy guidance, and both femoral arteriotomies are closed with running 5.0 Prolene (Ethicon, Somerville, NJ) sutures. In case of a calcified diseased femoral, a limited endarterectomy patch angioplasty with a Dacron patch might be required to maintain flow. Wounds are irrigated with antibiotics and closed with at least a four-layer closure to obliterate the dead space and reduce lymphocele, hematoma, and infection rate. The skin is closed with long-term absorbable sutures in a subcuticular fashion. The patient is extubated and transferred to a monitored subacute unit for 24 hours. Patients can eat the same day, be mobilized, and discharged within 24 hours.

FOLLOW-UP

Plane films (anteroposterior, lateral, and oblique views), as well as duplex scans, are obtained before discharge. Plane films are helpful to establish the level of the endograft in relation to the lumbar vertebrae. Color duplex, in the hands of an experienced operator, can document an endoleak. Pulsatile flow is seen within the sac outside the endograft, correlating well with the cardiac cycle. Two-millimeter cut CT scans with and without intravenous contrast are obtained at 1, 6, and 12 months, and every year thereafter.

ENDOLEAK

Type I (Fig. 4) endoleak is defined as leakage around the proximal neck (IA) or the distal iliac end (IB). This leak is usually identified at the completion angiogram during the procedure. The first step in management is to balloon the endograft again. If this is unsuccessful, an extension aortic cuff is placed proximally (IA) or an iliac limb extension is placed distally (IB). This usually helps when the endograft is deployed away from the renal artery. In situations in which the proximal end of the endograft is right at the renal arteries, a large, balloon-mounted Palmaz bare metal stent (Cordis, Miami Lakes, FL) is deployed over the proximal end of the endograft with some of the stent covering the renals. This stent will dilatate to any size of balloon on which it is mounted. If all of these options fail and the leak is large, converting to an open procedure may be the only solution. Late type IA leaks are seen more

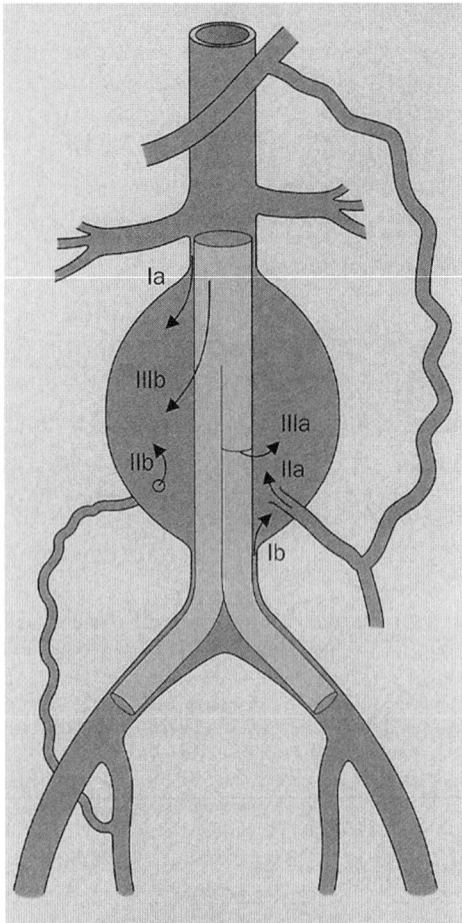

Figure 4 Endoleak types. Type Ia around the proximal end of the endograft and Ib around the distal iliac limb. Type IIa from a patent inferior mesenteric artery and IIb from a patent lumbar artery. Type IIIa at the overlap between the main body and iliac limb extension and IIIb through a defect in the graft material.

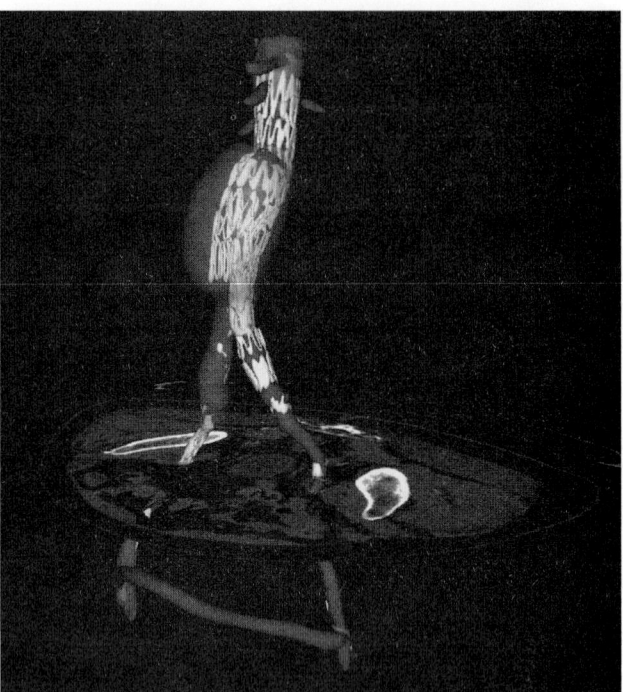

Figure 5 Repair of migrating endograft with resulting large type I endoleak. Three-dimensional model shows an aorto-uni-iliac endograft placed through the left iliacs. Left to right femorofemoral bypass is performed. *From M2S the fusion of clinical data and 3D imaging, West Lebanon, NH.* (*See color insert Figure 33.*)

with tube endografts from early experience with EVAR. A new device has been approved by the FDA (Zenith Renu) to treat these leaks resulting from migration of prior endografts. It consists of an aorto-uni-iliac endograft with suprarenal stent and is placed through the prior endograft or next to it if the tube graft has completely dislodged to the sac. The contralateral iliac is occluded with an occluder. A femorofemoral bypass is performed (Fig. 5).

Type II endoleak (Fig. 4) is the most common. It is associated with a patent inferior mesenteric artery (IIa) or lumbar (IIb). Usually there are at least two vessels: one acts as an entry channel and the second as an exit channel (Fig. 6). These leaks are seen commonly at the completion angiogram. Early on, we were aggressive about treating type II endoleaks, but we have learned that the majority resolve spontaneously and can be followed safely if the sac is not expanding. If the sac continues to expand on the first postoperative CT scan, the second scan is obtained earlier, at 2 to 3 months. If the sac further expands, treatment options include coiling of the leaking vessel through branches of the external iliac artery or SMA or translumbar approach (Fig. 7). Laparoscopic clipping of the lumbar artery has been described with less success.

Type III endoleak (Fig. 4) is leakage from overlap sites (IIIa) or through a defect in the endograft material (IIIb). This leak is becoming uncommon because of the continuous improvement in device design and because we now know that at least 2 to 3 cm of overlap are required.

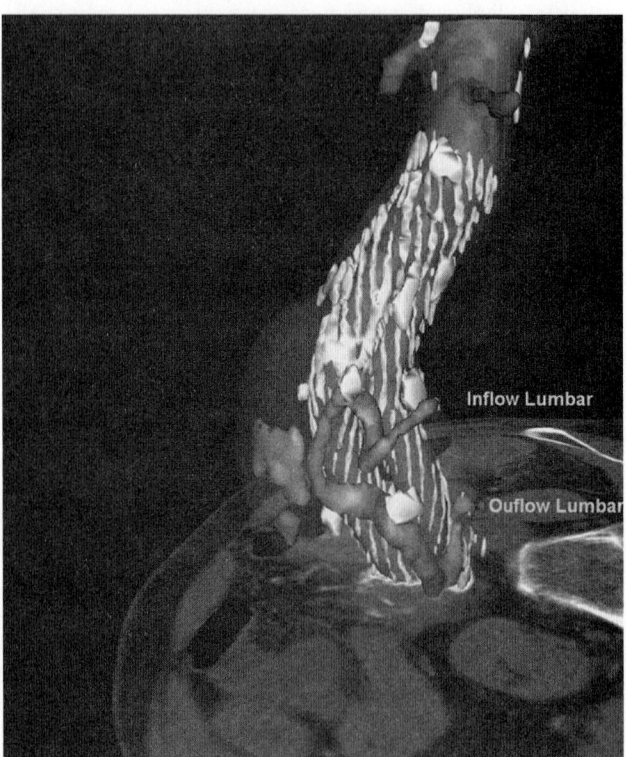

Figure 6 Three-dimensional model of type II endoleak with two lumbar arteries, one acting as inflow and the second as the outflow channel. *From M2S the fusion of clinical data and 3D imaging, West Lebanon, NH.* (*See color insert Figure 34.*)

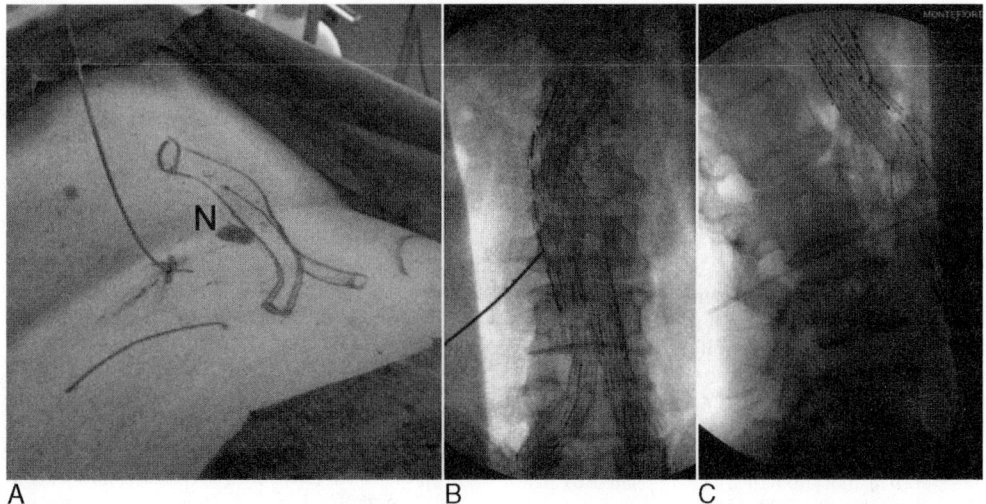

Figure 7   Translumbar coil embolization of endoleak. **(A)** The patient is placed in the prone position. The iliac crest and the device are marked on the patient's back with fluoroscopy guidance. From the axial cut of the computed tomography scan and the three-dimensional model the nidus *(N)* of the endoleak is located and marked on the patient skin in relation to the device. **(B, C)** Percutaneous access of the aneurysm sac with fluoroscopic guidance (using several views).   *From Ohki T, Mahmoud M: Endovascular treatment of abdominal and thoracic aneurysms. In Casserly I, Sachar R, Yadav JS, editor: Manual of peripheral vascular intervention, Philadelphia, 2005, Lippincott Williams & Wilkins. Reprinted with permission.*

Type IV endoleak (or *endotension*) occurs when the sac continues to expand without any of the previously described endoleaks on thin-cut CT scan and angiogram. This happens when the endograft acts as a filter, allowing serum to leak through and filtering most of the cells. This is similar to conventional open PTFE or Dacron grafts. It is uncommon for aneurysms to rupture with this type of endoleak. Usually open conversion is performed because of compression on the bowel or ureters, leading to early satiety/vomiting or urinary retention and abdominal pain. The sac is opened without clamping the aorta after checking sac pressure with a needle to confirm the absence of other types of endoleak. The lymphocele is evacuated. Dacron tube graft is cut longitudinally and wrapped tightly and resutured around the endograft. The sac is closed again over the Dacron as with conventional open AAA repair. The long-term durability of this repair is unknown because of the rarity of these cases. Type IV endoleaks were seen mostly with the Gore Excluder device. The newer-generation Excluder device with an added layer of PTFE has 1-year follow-up with no reportable type IV endoleaks.

Three-dimensional models can help to detect endoleaks and measure the aneurysm sac and endoleak volume. Follow-up studies will determine whether the volume is decreasing or increasing.

A new technology is under investigation that uses a wireless sensor called EndoSure (Cardiomems, Atlanta, GA) placed in the aneurysm sac outside the endograft while performing the EVAR. Pressure can be obtained wirelessly during the procedure. The sac pressure drops 70% from the systemic level after successful exclusion of the aneurysm. If the pressure continues to be similar to the systemic level, the surgeon should look for a significant endoleak. Postoperative pressure is measured wirelessly at the transabdominal wall. A trial is ongoing to evaluate the long-term comparison among CT scan, arterial duplex, and pressure measurements to identify a correlation between endoleak and established pressure level. The concept is to avoid repeating CT scans at 1, 6, and 12 months and then annually to preserve renal function, especially in patients with renal insufficiency.

RESULTS

Operative mortality has decreased to 1.7%. Respiratory and cardiac morbidity is less than 1%. Wound complications, including infection, seroma, and pseudo-aneurysm are 1% to 3%. Long-term follow-up (15 years) shows a remarkable decrease in endoleaks and reintervention rates to 10% (from 20%). The majority of reintervention procedures are performed percutaneously or through a small groin incision. Long-term aneurysm-related mortality is 0.3%. Device migration (any movement of the device on future follow-up imaging) is mainly related to oversizing (more than 20%) and fixation (below the renals). Migration incidence has decreased from 20% to 5%. Proximal neck dilatation is associated with further aortic degeneration and the constant radial force imposed by the self-expanding, oversized endograft on the aortic wall. If the radial force is greater than the aortic wall recoil force (elastic recoil of the vessel wall), the proximal neck will continue to dilatate. This might result in migration. Balloon expandable endografts (not yet approved by FDA) are not oversized and have an impressive 0% neck dilatation and migration. We now know that aneurysm-related mortality and rupture post-EVAR is associated with migration much more often than with endoleak. Each 1 mm the device is deployed away from the lowest renal artery is associated with a 5% increase in future migration.

ENDOVASCULAR ANEURYSM REPAIR VERSUS OPEN REPAIR

EVAR is associated with a 30% to 70% reduction in morbidity. The average length of hospital stay is reduced by 80%. This is not surprising given the following facts:

1. Avoiding aortic clamping results in significant reduction in cardiac strain and postoperative myocardial infarction (MI).
2. Reducing the blood loss by 70% (average estimated blood loss during EVAR is 200–300 ml) also reduces cardiac morbidity.
3. Avoiding the peritoneal cavity eliminates postoperative ileus and allows same-day feeding.
4. Small groin incisions have minimal postoperative pain (compared with the large midline, transverse, or retroperitoneal incisions for open repair). The patient is walking and discharged within 24 hours of the procedure.
5. Because patients have less incisional pain and can breathe and walk much earlier than with open repair and because intubation

time is limited to the procedure (2–4 hours) or completely avoided, the incidence of postoperative respiratory complication (atelectasis, pneumonia) is small.

Sexual dysfunction following EVAR is approximately 1% (even with coiling of the IIA), compared with 30% to 50% following open repair. This striking difference is mainly related to avoiding dissection along the pelvic nerves.

The operative mortality is reduced from 4.7% (open repair) to 1.7% (EVAR) in two European prospective randomized trials: Endo-Vascular Aneurysm Repair trial (EVAR I) and the Dutch Randomized Endovascular Aneurysm Management trial (DREAM). The U.S. Open versus Endovascular Repair trial (OVER) is ongoing. The operative mortality of open repair is significantly increased in patients with chronic renal insufficiency (creatinine >1.8), congestive heart failure (New York Heart Association Classification NYHA III, IV), recent MI (electrocardiogram-shown ischemic changes), COPD (FEV1 <1L), and in patients older than 75 years. A significant portion of the operative mortality in EVAR is related to iliac artery torsion while advancing the delivery system. This can be avoided with good preoperative planning and sizing. Using a conduit when necessary will bypass the tortuous calcified iliacs. The long-term aneurysm-related mortality is similar in both treatment modalities.

The decisions of whether to treat an AAA and between open versus EVAR must be made by a nonbiased surgeon who is well experienced with both approaches. The patient and family members should also be well educated about the risk of rupture and the morbidity and mortality of each approach to participate actively in the decision-making process. Patients should understand that long-term follow-up is necessary and be aware of the 10% incidence of endoleak and possible reintervention. Proper patient selection for EVAR, preoperative planning, and surgeon training minimize the perioperative and long-term morbidity and mortality.

SUGGESTED READINGS

Brewster DC, Cronenwett JL, Hallett JW, and others: Guidelines for the treatment of abdominal aortic aneurysms report of a subcommittee of the Joint Council of the American Association for Vascular Surgery and Society for Vascular Surgery, *J Vasc Surg* 37:1106, 2003.

Chaikof EL, Blankensteijn JD, Harris PL, and others: Reporting standards for endovascular aortic aneurysm repair, *J Vasc Surg* 35:1048, 2002.

Greenhalgh RM and the EVAR trial participants: Comparison of endovascular aneurysm repair with open repair inpatients with abdominal aortic aneurysm (EVAR trial 1), 30-day operative mortality results: randomized controlled trial, *Lancet* 364:843, 2004.

Malas MB, Ohki T, Veith FJ, and others: Absence of proximal neck dilatation and graft migration following endovascular aneurysm repair with balloon expandable stent-based endograft, *J Vasc Surg* 42:639, 2005.

Ohki T, Malas MB: Endovascular treatment of abdominal and thoracic aneurysms. In Casserly I, Sachar R, Yadav JS, editors: *Manual of peripheral vascular interventionm.* Philadelphia, 2005, Lippincott Williams & Wilkins.

RUPTURED ABDOMINAL AORTIC ANEURYSM

Brian G. DeRubertis, MD, and Peter L. Faries, MD

Rupture of an abdominal aortic aneurysm (AAA) occurs as a sudden, unheralded event that is lethal in up to 90% of patients.

Approximately 15,000 persons die each year from aneurysm rupture, making it the thirteenth leading cause of death in the United States. An additional 300,000 persons die each year from unexplained sudden death, and autopsy series suggest that approximately 5% of these, or an additional 15,000 cases, are due to aneurysm rupture. Recent studies have implicated increased matrix-metalloproteinase activity and focal shear stress as potentially important factors in rupture risk. However, it remains true that aneurysm rupture is generally related to size and rate of growth, with increased rates of rupture in patients with aneurysms greater than 5.0 cm in diameter or enlarging by greater than 0.5 cm per year. The fact that many patients with ruptured aneurysms had no prior knowledge of the aneurysm highlights the need for increased screening for high-risk populations, particularly men older than age 65 with a history of tobacco use or family history of AAA. The widespread use of screening in appropriate populations may lead to a decrease in mortality related to aneurysm rupture, which currently has not paralleled the decreasing rates seen in patients undergoing elective aneurysm repair.

PRESENTATION AND DIAGNOSTIC WORKUP

Patients presenting with ruptured AAA can generally be divided into two distinct groups on the basis of the presence or absence of hypotension. This distinction has important diagnostic and treatment implications (Fig. 1).

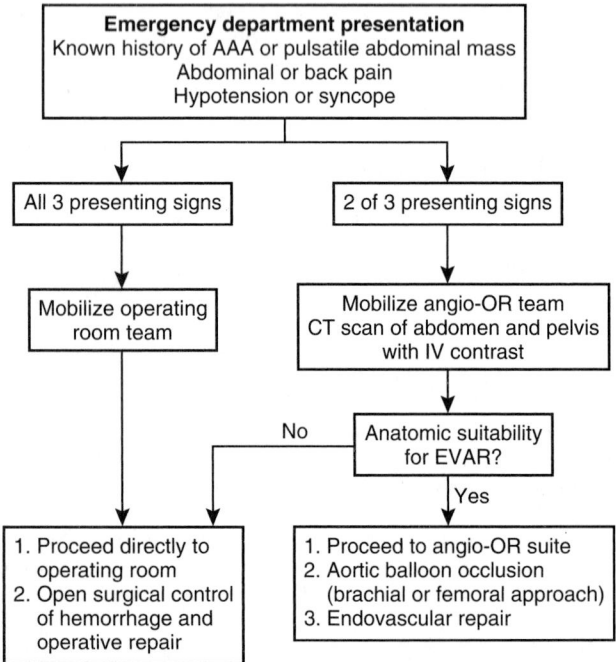

Figure I Algorithm for potential endovascular repair for a patient presenting with known aneurysm or pulsatile mass, abdominal pain, and hypotension. Patients with all three presenting symptoms require immediate operative repair. Hemodynamically stable patients with two of the three symptoms should undergo computed tomography scan to establish the diagnosis and evaluate for potential endovascular repair.

Patients with a known history of AAA or with a pulsatile mass on examination who present with abdominal or back pain associated with hypotension represent a true surgical emergency and should be transported to the operating room for immediate control of hemorrhage and operative repair. These patients most likely represent those with free intraperitoneal rupture and require rapid and efficient care if successful outcomes are to be achieved. In trauma centers, the activation of the hospital trauma system can expedite mobilization of resources, including anesthesiologists and support staff, blood product availability, and critical care services. Emergency department treatment should consist only of obtaining emergency consultation with the treating surgeon and establishing large-bore intravenous access.

A second subset of patients present with a clinical picture consistent with a rupture contained within the retroperitoneum. These patients may have a posterolateral rupture into the retroperitoneum that has led to tamponade of hemorrhage and stabilization of hemodynamics. This includes patients with a pulsatile mass and abdominal pain without hypotension or whose hypotension responded to initial small-volume resuscitation. It can also include patients who are found to have a contained rupture of an aneurysm on a computed tomography (CT) scan performed for evaluation of an alternative diagnosis, such as renal calculi or other intra-abdominal pathology. Although these patients require prompt treatment before intraperitoneal rupture and exsanguination occurs, their hemodynamic status usually allows for emergent CT scan of the abdomen and pelvis to establish definitively the diagnosis and plan for potential endovascular repair.

OPEN SURGICAL REPAIR OF RUPTURED ABDOMINAL AORTIC ANEURYSM

When open surgical repair is chosen for patients diagnosed in the emergency room with ruptured AAA, no diagnostic tests or invasive monitoring devices should delay immediate transfer to the operating room. Hemodynamic monitoring, nasogastric intubation, urinary catheterization, electrocardiogram, and blood draw for type and cross matching and routine laboratory tests can be performed in the operating room. Judicious fluid administration with type O negative blood and crystalloid should be instituted after large-bore peripheral intravenous access is obtained.

Hypotensive resuscitation may be considered in the treatment of patients with ruptured AAAs. In this technique, intravenous fluids are administered to maintain below-normotensive blood pressures that are still adequate to perfuse vital organs. Although there are no prospective studies of hypotensive resuscitation in humans, experimental animal model data and retrospective studies in trauma patients suggest that this approach may be preferable to aggressive immediate resuscitation until surgical control of bleeding can be achieved. This technique should be employed with considerable caution, however, to prevent underresuscitation and worsening of acidosis.

In the operating room, the patient should be positioned supine and prepared with antiseptic solution from the neck to the knees and table line to table line. The patient should be prepared and draped with the surgeon scrubbed and prepared for immediate entry into the abdomen or the left chest in the event of hemodynamic collapse at the induction of anesthesia. Intravenous fluids and blood should be warmed with a level I rapid transfusion system, and operating room ambient temperature should be increased to reduce the risk of hypothermia and resultant coagulopathy and arrhythmia. An autotransfusion device may be used when available.

The most important initial step in the repair of a ruptured AAA is control of hemorrhage by proximal aortic occlusion. This may be rapidly achieved by supraceliac compression or clamping of the aorta. In the patient who suffers cardiac arrest before incision, left

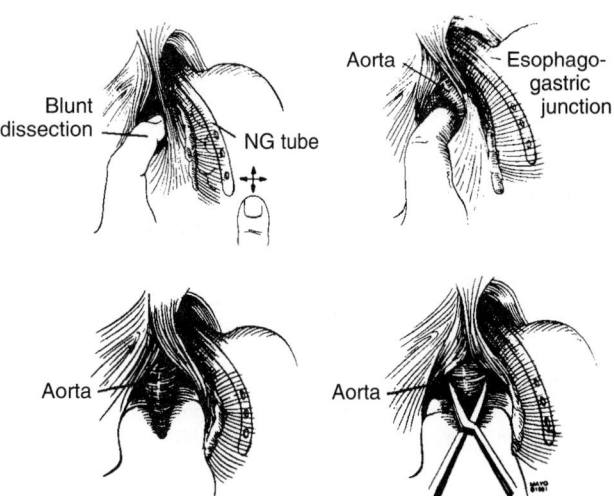

Figure 2 Technique of supraceliac aortic control includes mobilization of the left lobe of the liver, palpating the nasogastric tube lying within the esophagus, and then locating the aorta slightly medial between the crura of the diaphragm. The aorta is mobilized primarily by blunt dissection and then clamped with a large curved aortic clamp. *NG,* Nasogastric. *From Veith FJ, Gupta S, Daly V: Surg Gynecol Obstet 151:497,1980.*

lateral thoracotomy with aortic cross clamping in the chest followed by open cardiac massage can be instituted. In most cases, however, equally expedient aortic control can be obtained by midline incision from xiphoid to pubis and clamping of the aorta at the diaphragmatic hiatus (Fig. 2). The left lobe of the liver is mobilized by incising the left triangular ligament. The lesser sac is entered through the lesser omentum, and the esophagus is mobilized to the left to expose the aorta. Identification of the esophagus may be aided by palpation of the nasogastric tube, especially when the aorta no longer has a palpable pulse. The gastrohepatic ligament is then incised to reveal the crus of the diaphragm and the supraceliac aorta. Access to the aorta may be obtained by division of the crus of the diaphragm. Rapid partial control may be obtained by bluntly spreading the muscle fibers of the crus. Circumferential dissection of the aorta is unnecessary, and after the surgeon's index and middle finger can be inserted on either side of the aorta down to the vertebral column, a clamp can be placed. Exposure during this dissection is primarily achieved with the surgeon's free hand, although two large Richardson retractors placed on either side of the apex of incision can increase visualization.

After supraceliac control is achieved, self-retaining retractors are positioned and dissection of the infrarenal aorta to the level of the left renal vein is performed to move the aortic cross clamp to the infrarenal location. When the retroperitoneal hematoma makes identification of the infrarenal aortic neck difficult, its identification may be performed from within the aneurysm lumen after distal control of the iliac arteries is achieved. Intravenous mannitol (25 g) may be given to preserve renal function before aortic clamping. Although intravenous heparin may be administered before cross clamping, it may potentiate hemorrhage and should be used cautiously in patients with shock. After proximal and distal aortic control have been obtained and the lumbar arteries have been oversewn, a prosthetic graft is sewn into position. A tube graft configuration can be used in most cases; however, a bifurcated graft is employed when extension to the iliac or femoral arteries is necessary.

Intestinal edema from large-volume fluid resuscitation and hematoma from the initial rupture can make it difficult or impossible to close the abdomen in some patients. When the abdomen is closed, high intra-abdominal pressures can result in abdominal compartment syndrome, characterized by cardiovascular, renal, and respiratory compromise. These pathophysiologic effects have largely been attributed to impaired venous return and distorted respiratory mechanics, ultimately leading to oliguria, hypotension, and respiratory failure. Intra-abdominal pressure may be assessed by urinary bladder pressure measurement, and normal pressures range from subatmospheric to 0 cm H_2O. A bladder pressure above 25 cm H_2O combined with unexplained oliguria or elevated airway pressures is considered diagnostic for abdominal compartment syndrome and is an indication for surgical decompression. Decompression should be expedient because untreated abdominal compartment syndrome is almost universally fatal, whereas appropriate treatment often leads to rapid resolution of organ dysfunction. In unstable patients, the peritoneum can be opened in the intensive care unit. Consideration should be given to leaving the abdomen open prophylactically in patients who are deemed high risk for developing abdominal compartment syndrome at the time of operation. Patients who have been shown to be high risk for this syndrome include those with severe hemorrhage, prolonged shock, perioperative cardiac arrest, large-volume resuscitation, and long operative times. Options for managing the open abdomen include sewing a Vicryl (Ethicon, Somerville, NJ) mesh to the fascia and then sequentially tightening this mesh at the bedside over the ensuing days or by simply placing sterile towels, sump drains, and a large adhesive drape over the open abdomen and bringing the patient back to the operating room for abdominal wall closure after sufficient stabilization and diuresis.

OUTCOMES FOLLOWING OPEN REPAIR OF RUPTURED ABDOMINAL AORTIC ANEURYSM

Postoperative complications following repair of ruptured AAA are common and contribute to the overall 50% mortality associated with this procedure. Preexisting comorbidities, intraoperative factors, and postoperative development of abdominal compartment syndrome and other physiologic derangements typical of the postoperative period lead to a number of potential complications (Table 1). Most commonly, patients suffer respiratory failure, renal insufficiency (especially with suprarenal cross clamping), sepsis, and myocardial infarction.

Outcome analysis has identified specific risk factors for poor outcome following repair of ruptured AAA. Factors that have been shown to carry increased risk in multiple studies include presence of hypotension on presentation, underlying pulmonary disease, chronic renal insufficiency, incorrect initial diagnosis or extended delay before surgery, and inexperienced surgeon. Although overall perioperative mortality remains approximately 50%, it can range

Table 1: Postoperative Complications following Ruptured Aneurysm Repair

Complication	Incidence (%)	Mortality (%)
Respiratory failure	48	34
Renal failure	29	76
Sepsis	24	45
Myocardial infarction/CHF	24	66
Bleeding	17	90
Stroke	6	50
Ischemic colitis	5	67
Leg ischemia	3	17
Paraplegia/paresis	2	50

From Jones CE: In Cameron JL, editor: Current surgical therapy, *ed 6, Philadelphia, 1998, Mosby.*
CHF, Congestive heart failure.

from close to 30% in patients with only favorable risk factors to more than 90% in patients with multiple adverse risk factors. These high mortality rates, especially in patients with poor prognostic signs, further illustrates the importance of screening to establish the diagnosis and allow repair prior to rupture.

ENDOVASCULAR REPAIR OF RUPTURED ABDOMINAL AORTIC ANEURYSM

Because of the high morbidity and mortality associated with open repair of ruptured AAA, there has been considerable interest in an endovascular alternative for these patients. For elective surgery, endovascular AAA repair has been shown in randomized trials to have superior short-term results to open repair in selected patients. It has been hypothesized that the minimally invasive nature of this procedure may lead to a reduction in the cardiovascular, pulmonary, and renal complications that commonly accompany open repair of ruptured AAA. In addition, endovascular repair prevents the release of tamponade and resultant shock that can be seen on opening of the abdomen during open repair. Although this less invasive modality holds potential advantages for the treatment of ruptured AAA compared with conventional open repair, the application of endovascular techniques encounters logistic and practical barriers that must be overcome to provide such therapy. These include the need for an operating room equipped with adequate fluoroscopic imaging instrumentation and a radiolucent operating table, an easily mobilized endovascular team, a surgeon with appropriate endovascular experience, the availability of a range of endovascular device sizes, and the potential for treatment delays owing to the need for a preoperative CT scan for the assessment of aortic anatomy.

As with open repair, workup before intervention should be minimal. Preoperative CT scans, when unavailable from referring institutions, should be obtained only in hemodynamically stable patients. Initial proximal aortic control may be achieved by placement of an intra-aortic occlusion balloon. The balloon is advanced into position in the aorta proximal to the aneurysm over an angiographic wire introduced either through the femoral or the brachial artery. This may be performed percutaneously under local anesthesia if hypotension mandates more expeditious control of hemorrhage. Because balloon occlusion of the aorta interferes with further angiographic imaging, the balloon may be positioned but not inflated in the hemodynamically stable patient. These patients then undergo aortography to facilitate endovascular stent graft positioning and deployment. Suitability for endovascular repair is dependent on the length, diameter, and angulation of the infrarenal proximal implantation zone, as well as the tortuosity and size of the iliac arteries through which the device must traverse. Stable patients may be treated with bifurcated stent grafts, which are commercially available for aneurysms with neck diameters up to 32 mm. When a proximal occlusion balloon is used in patients treated with a bifurcated graft, the balloon can be replaced distally within the stent graft body after deployment of the main body to restore perfusion to the mesenteric and renal circulation. The contralateral limb is then deployed in the standard fashion, and after completion of graft deployment, the occlusion balloon is deflated and completion aortography is performed (Fig. 3).

Patients who become unstable can be treated by deployment of an aortouniiliac (AUI) device followed by femorofemoral bypass. After performing exclusion of the aneurysm with an AUI, the contralateral iliac artery is interrupted by endoluminal occlusion or open ligation. If deployment of a bifurcated device has already begun when the onset of hemodynamic instability occurs, the modular bifurcated stent graft can be converted to an AUI by deployment of a converter device across the flow divider of the main body of the stent graft.

Figure 3 Abdominal computed tomography scans **(A)** preexclusion and **(B)** postexclusion in a patient with a contained aneurysm rupture who was effectively treated with an endovascular repair using a modular bifurcated stent graft. Note resolution of adjacent hematoma **(C)** 6 months postoperatively.

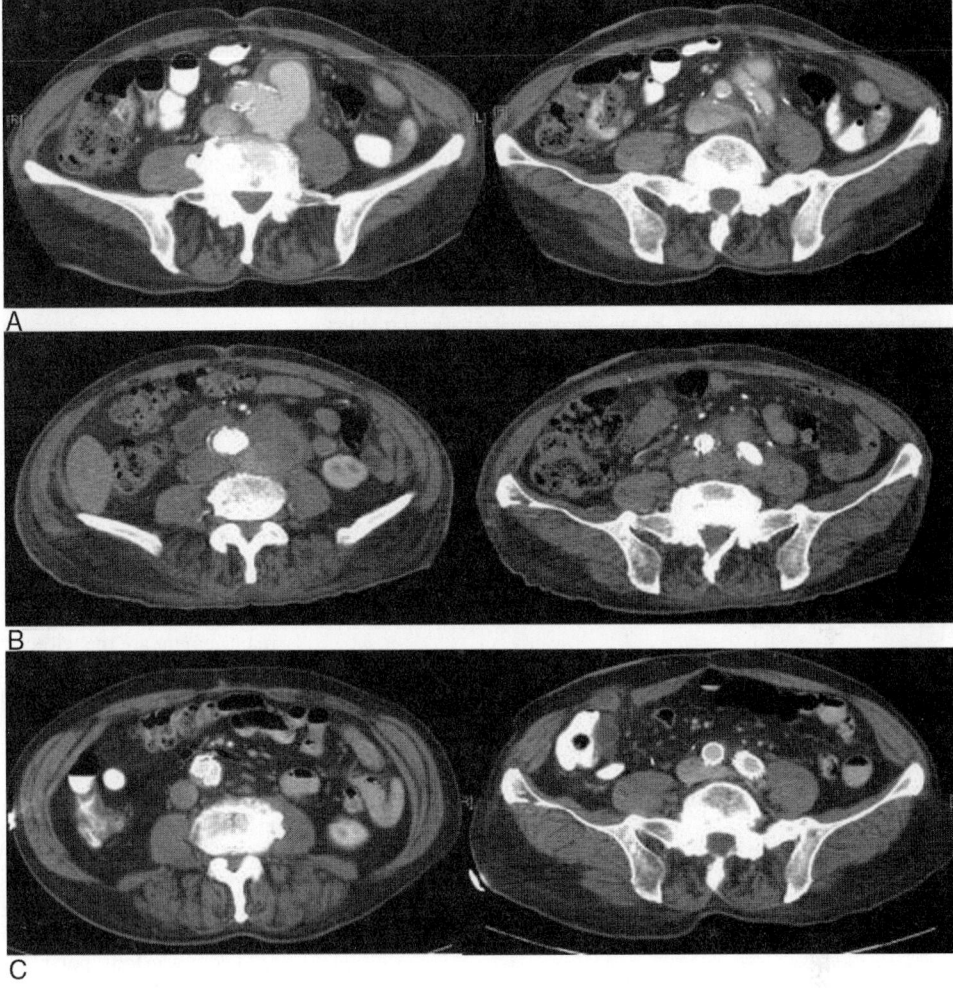

As with open repair, abdominal compartment syndrome can result from endovascular repair of ruptured AAA. In a retrospective review of 30 ruptured aneurysms treated by endovascular aneurysm repair, a 20% incidence of abdominal compartment syndrome was identified in these patients. This complication was associated with a mortality of 67%, whereas patients without abdominal compartment syndrome had a mortality of only 13%. Factors determined to lead to increased risk of abdominal compartment syndrome in patients undergoing endovascular repair included use of an aortic occlusion balloon, massive transfusion requirement, coagulopathy, and conversion from a bifurcated graft to an AUI device. It is likely that these factors also contributed to the high mortality rate observed in these patients.

OUTCOMES FOLLOWING ENDOVASCULAR REPAIR OF RUPTURED ABDOMINAL AORTIC ANEURYSM

An endovascular approach to ruptured AAA avoids many of the problems that are associated with open repair, including increased blood loss associated with release of tamponade, hazardous retroperitoneal dissection, coagulopathy, and hypothermia. Several institutions with expertise in endovascular techniques have reported promising results with endovascular repair of ruptured AAA. However, these outcomes have been derived from small, single institutional retrospective or prospective clinical series performed at specialized vascular centers. A clear understanding of the overall impact of this technique on mortality and adverse events in general practice is lacking.

In an attempt to represent an unbiased cross section of surgical practice in the United States, the in-hospital outcomes of endovascular and open surgical repair for ruptured AAA in a population-based sample of patients were compared using the hospital discharge databases from 2000 through 2003 for four states with a combined population that represents almost a third of the U.S. population. These data indicated that the overall mortality rate for the 4-year period was significantly lower for endovascular versus open repair (39.3% vs. 47.7%, $p = .005$). Moreover, compared with open repair, endovascular repair resulted in a significantly lower rate of pulmonary, renal, and bleeding complications. Survival after endovascular repair also correlated with hospital experience, ranging from 45.9% from small-volume hospitals to 26% for high-volume hospitals. Ultimately, well-designed, large-scale, multicenter randomized trials will be necessary to verify these promising results and to clarify to what extent the improved survival in ruptured AAA patients can be attributed to the endovascular approach rather than the selection of low-risk patients.

CONCLUSION

Although advances in the treatment of AAA have occurred in recent years, ruptured AAA continues to carry high morbidity and mortality rates. Successful outcomes rely on establishing the correct diagnosis expediently and rapidly instituting surgical treatment while optimizing management of associated comorbidities. The crucial step in patients who present with hypotension is interruption of ongoing hemorrhage by emergent operation and aortic cross clamping. Endovascular repair may be considered, particularly in hemodynamically stable patients, provided that appropriately skilled surgeons, support staff, and hospital systems are available. The most likely way to reduce aneurysm-related death remains increased screening, aneurysm detection, and elective repair of aneurysms before rupture.

Suggested Readings

Dardik A, Burleyson GP, Bowman H, and others: Surgical repair of ruptured abdominal aortic aneurysms in the state of Maryland: factors influencing outcome among 527 recent cases, *J Vasc Surg* 28:413, 1998.

Greco G, Egorova N, Anderson PL, and others: Outcomes of endovascular treatment of ruptured abdominal aortic aneurysms, *J Vasc Surg* 43:453, 2006.

Mehta M, Darling RC 3rd, Roddy RC, and others: Factors associated with abdominal compartment syndrome complicating endovascular repair of ruptured abdominal aortic aneurysms, *J Vasc Surg* 42:1047, 2005.

Ouriel K, Geary K, Green RM, and others: Factors determining survival after ruptured aortic aneurysm: the hospital, the surgeon, and the patient, *J Vasc Surg* 11:493, 1990.

Rasmussen TE, Hallett JW Jr, Noel AA, and others: Early abdominal closure with mesh reduces multiple organ failure after ruptured abdominal aortic aneurysm repair: guidelines from a 10-year case-control study, *J Vasc Surg* 35:246, 2002.

Abdominal Aortic Aneurysm and Unexpected Abdominal Pathology

David P. Kuwayama, MD, and Glen S. Roseborough, MD

The prevalence of abdominal aortic aneurysm (AAA) increases with age. They are extremely rare in men and women aged 25 to 44 but found in up to 14.4% of men and 4.3% of women aged 65 and older. Because many other intra-abdominal surgical conditions are also more prevalent among the elderly, the likelihood of finding unexpected concomitant disease (CD) at the time of aneurysmorrhaphy is elevated. In one recent study of almost 1000 patients undergoing elective AAA repair, 7.1% had additional intra-abdominal pathology meriting synchronous or staged surgical attention, illustrating the significant prevalence of CD. Encountering such pathology presents the surgeon with the need to make rapid but prudent patient management decisions.

The increasing availability and resolution of advanced imaging modalities such as magnetic resonance imaging (MRI) and computed tomography (CT) scanning has decreased the chances of encountering unexpected CD at exploration. When CD is identified preoperatively, a multidisciplinary team involving the relevant specialists should be assembled to develop a plan for management of the CD before aneurysm repair is undertaken. Nevertheless, a host of lesions, including small gastrointestinal (GI) masses, metastatic lesions, and biliary calculi, are nearly transparent to such imaging and therefore may only be first recognized intraoperatively. In addition, patients with an acute abdomen may undergo emergency laparotomy without any preoperative imaging.

The potential utility of simultaneous correction of AAA and CD was first suggested in 1960 by Oshner, Cooley, and DeBakey, who showed no increased mortality with simultaneous surgery in a series of 804 patients. However, in 82% of those patients, the nonvascular surgery performed was either a prophylactic appendectomy or a sympathectomy, minor operations that are no longer considered to be surgically indicated. The concerns with simultaneous treatment of AAA and CD include the increased perioperative morbidity and mortality that may result from a combined operation, as well as the long-term risk of graft infection if it is contaminated during treatment of the CD. The concerns with staged management are that either the patient will suffer serious complications from the untreated CD if its treatment is deferred or the patient will experience rupture of the AAA if its treatment is deferred. Fortunately, technological advances in laparoscopy, transluminal endoscopy, and percutaneous technology have expanded the therapeutic options for managing abdominal pathology. The past decade has also witnessed major steps forward in the minimally invasive management of aneurysms. The emergence of endovascular aneurysm repair (EVAR) as a safe and effective modality for the treatment of AAA has also created additional opportunities for near-synchronous management of both AAA and CD while minimizing the insult to patient homeostasis.

There are four potential clinical scenarios in which one may encounter an aortic aneurysm with CD:

1. An elective operation for aortic pathology, with incidental finding of asymptomatic nonvascular pathology
2. An emergent operation for (presumed) symptomatic aortic pathology, with incidental finding of nonvascular pathology
3. An emergent operation for nonvascular pathology, with incidental finding of an aortic aneurysm
4. An elective operation for nonvascular pathology, with incidental finding of an aortic aneurysm

ELECTIVE ABDOMINAL AORTIC ANEURYSM REPAIR AND ASYMPTOMATIC CONCOMITANT DISEASE

Most published studies deal with this scenario because it is the most common. Patients undergoing elective transperitoneal AAA repair frequently have other, ongoing intra-abdominal processes discovered during routine examination of the peritoneal cavity at laparotomy. The most commonly encountered concomitant nonvascular pathology is cholelithiasis, found in between 5% and 20% of laparotomies for AAA. On one hand, the possibility exists that gallstones left untreated could lead to a future episode of cholecystitis, biliary obstruction, or gallstone pancreatitis, thereby elevating the patient's risk of perioperative mortality. On the other hand, resection of the gallbladder at the time of AAA repair violates biliary continuity and risks seeding the peritoneal cavity with biliary microorganisms. Graft infection with such flora would represent a devastating complication entailing additional vascular procedures and a high risk of mortality.

Some small studies suggest a significant risk of biliary complications when cholelithiasis is left untreated at the time of open AAA repair. In 1984, String followed 17 patients with cholelithiasis identified at the time of open AAA repair in whom cholecystectomy was not performed; 53% of them developed symptomatic cholelithiasis over the next 2 weeks to 108 months. A similar study by Ouriel of 11 patients with cholelithiasis undergoing aneurysmorrhaphy without cholecystectomy found a postoperative incidence of acute cholecystitis of 82% over 2.9 years. Two of these events (18%) occurred in the immediate postoperative period, and one of these patients (9%) died from biliary sepsis. The conclusion of both of these publications was that simultaneous cholecystectomy should be performed when cholelithiasis is encountered incidentally.

In contrast, a study from the Mayo Clinic reported a complication rate of 38% after simultaneous cholecystectomy and aneurysmorrhaphy, and other studies have documented subsequent graft infection rates of up to 5.6%. In addition, both of the studies advocating simultaneous treatment were published before the advent of laparoscopic cholecystectomy and minimally invasive techniques for managing biliary sepsis, such as percutaneous cholecystostomy, transhepatic biliary stenting, and endoscopic retrograde cholangiopancreatography.

In light of the low but significant risk of graft infection in patients undergoing simultaneous cholecystectomy, as well as the relative ease with which symptomatic choledocholithiasis can be managed in the modern era, we generally avoid prophylactic cholecystectomy at the time of open repair and believe that the patient ought to be managed expectantly with a low-fat diet and possibly medication such as ursodiol in the postoperative period. However, any development of abdominal symptoms or laboratory abnormalities consistent with a biliary source should be viewed with an increased index of suspicion and the threshold for performing laparoscopic cholecystectomy in the postoperative period should be low.

GI malignancies are usually not detectable on CT; therefore these lesions are occasionally discovered incidentally at laparotomy. Most data on concomitant AAA and GI tract malignancy focus on colorectal cancer (CRC). Estimates of concomitant CRC range between 0.5% and 1.4% of all patients with known AAAs. Resecting the AAA first may significantly delay the treatment of CRC, and the effect of this delay on cancer progression is unknown. Operating on the CRC first potentiates the risk of a postoperative aneurysm rupture. Unfortunately there is a lack of prospective data comparing initial elective AAA repair with initial elective CRC repair; the preferable order of resection has been widely debated. Nevertheless, the classic recommendation has been for a staged approach of some type, rather than a synchronous approach, given the potential magnitude of a combined operation.

In 2002, Baxter published the largest retrospective review on the topic. Of 83 patients with synchronous AAA and CRC, 64 had their colorectal cancer treated first. Of those with AAAs smaller than 5 cm, there were no postoperative aneurysm ruptures. However, of those with AAAs 5 cm or larger, there was a 10% postoperative rupture rate. Seven patients underwent AAA repair first; however, this caused a significant delay to eventual CRC surgery (median of 122 days). Twelve patients had simultaneous operations for AAA and CRC, with no significant increase in morbidity or mortality and a 0% rate of graft infection. These data support the idea that in patients with AAAs larger than 5 cm and concomitant CRC, a synchronous operation may be the best approach, whereas those patients with AAAs smaller than 5 cm and concomitant CRC might best be treated with colonic resection first , followed by staged AAA repair. An applied decision analysis performed by Velanovich and Anderson supported this theory, concluding that patients with aneurysms larger than 5 cm, a colonic tumor with greater than 75% chance of obstruction or perforation, and a projected operative

mortality of less than 10% would benefit more from a combined operation than from staged management.

Combined with other small case series, the bulk of the data appears to support the safety of performing combined operations for AAA and CRC when necessary. We believe that those patients with AAAs larger than 5 cm would benefit from a combined operation. Good bowel preparation, preoperative antibiotics, and meticulous technique to minimize cross contamination of the surgical fields serve to further lower the risk of vascular graft infection. Benefits of a combined operation include the elimination of risks from delayed treatment of aneurysmal or colorectal disease and a significant reduction in the likelihood of a second, potentially hostile laparotomy. In patients with aneurysms smaller than 5 cm, however, the benefits are less pronounced, and we would advocate a staged approach entailing colonic resection first.

If the decision is made to proceed with immediate colon resection, one should enlist the assistance of a colorectal surgeon if necessary to ensure that a curative oncologic procedure is performed. One should also review the preoperative imaging of the patient's aneurysm and give further consideration to endovascular repair of the aneurysm, particularly if the patient has significant comorbidity. An Austrian group recently compared their experience with staged management of CD and AAA by endovascular aneurysm repair (EVAR) to their experience with simultaneous management of CD and AAA by open repair. They experienced no mortality in 49 patients who were managed with staged EVAR and CD surgery, compared with three mortalities in 33 patients who had simultaneous AAA and CD surgery. All three of these mortalities occurred in a subset of 22 patients who were ASA (American Society of Anesthesiologists) class III or IV, for a mortality of 13.6% in this high-risk group. This was statistically significant from the 0% mortality in the 48 EVAR patients who were ASA class III or IV. Another long-term benefit of EVAR is the ability to address both aortic and nonaortic lesions without violating the integrity of the natural barriers separating the two, thereby minimizing or eliminating the risk of direct aortic graft infection. Almost all graft infections occur by direct exposure of the graft to skin flora or infected surgical site effluent, and this likely accounts for the significantly increased risk of infection in open versus endovascular repairs.

Although the Velanovich study focused solely on colorectal cancer, the principles it enumerated, combined with favorable results from other small case series, are probably applicable to other GI malignancies. Although they are rare, reports exist of small bowel tumors, such as carcinoids, being resected along with AAAs. Multiple reports suggest that gastric tumors may be safely resected along with aneurysms. Reports of both subtotal and total gastrectomies have been published, with no reported cases of associated subsequent graft infections. Presumably, management considerations for these lesions are similar to those used for management of a colorectal malignancy. Under elective conditions, those patients with large aneurysms and a GI tumor might best be managed with synchronous resection. Those with smaller aneurysms should probably undergo gastrectomy or enterectomy immediately, followed by aneurysmectomy at a later date. The staged vascular procedure could later be performed via a retroperitoneal approach, maintaining surgical site exclusion and minimizing graft infection risk.

The strongest case for synchronous resection of AAA with a concomitant intra-abdominal malignancy can be made for renal carcinoma. Case series consistently support the safety of combined operations for AAA and renal malignancy. Given the low risk of infection in a nephrectomy basin, there should be little or no risk of bacterial cross contamination. Furthermore, because both lesions reside in the retroperitoneum, no surgical site exclusion is technically possible. The benefits of simultaneous nephrectomy include elimination of the need for future operation and for a second retroperitoneal dissection. In particularly difficult cases secondary to aneurysm morphology or decreased baseline renal function, however, a staged approach may be preferable. When planning, it helps to remember that simultaneous resection of large, left-sided renal tumors and AAAs may be best performed through a retroperitoneal approach.

The management of bladder cancer and prostate cancer is more debatable because resection of these lesions risks the potential of contaminating the peritoneal cavity with infected urine. Treatment for invasive bladder cancer often requires creation of urinary diversion with GI tract segments, thereby entailing the additional risk of intraperitoneal contamination with gastrointestinal flora. Despite these risks, some investigators have recommended simultaneous operation. A small prospective study by Greggo comparing simultaneous aneurysmectomy and radical cystoprostatectomy with a staged approach found no statistically significant difference in outcome, although there was an early trend toward increased mortality in the group undergoing simultaneous procedures. This trend was attributed to moderate preoperative renal insufficiency in the patients who died, reinforcing the importance of considering renal function before embarking on combined vascular and genitourinary procedures. The authors' interpretation was that combined operations were generally safe in suitable candidates. Other studies have noted that a major benefit of combined operation, from the urologic perspective, is the avoidance of retroperitoneal desmoplastic reaction from a preceding aneurysmectomy, thereby significantly facilitating ureteral dissection. Despite this advantage, most surgeons still advocate a staged approach because of the infectious risk. We believe that patients with aneurysms larger than 5 cm ought to have the aneurysm addressed first, whereas those with smaller aneurysms ought to undergo the urologic procedure first.

Case reports of simultaneous resection of AAAs and other solid organ tumors including liver masses, adrenalectomies, and splenectomies appear to document the safety of these procedures. Generally, additional procedures not involving opening a hollow viscus or risking bacterial contamination appear to be safe when performed in patients able to tolerate the additional physiologic insult and extended operative time. The benefit of elective resection of the appendix or a Meckel's diverticulum at the time of AAA repair appears to be small, and given the potential morbidity from such an intervention, in the absence of evidence of inflammatory disease elective resection of these structures is not advised.

EMERGENT ABDOMINAL AORTIC ANEURYSM REPAIR AND ASYMPTOMATIC/SYMPTOMATIC CONCOMITANT DISEASE

A symptomatic or rupturing aortic aneurysm represents a life-threatening situation. Depending on the urgency of the presentation, the surgeon may be with or without the benefit of an imaging study to guide preoperative planning: the classical teaching is that shock associated with a pulsatile abdominal mass should be treated immediately without further imaging. If the preoperative diagnosis of a ruptured AAA (rAAA) is confirmed, AAA repair should proceed expeditiously, regardless of other findings. Given the high mortality of open surgical repair of rAAA (50%), all but the most lethal coincidental abdominal pathology should be observed and all efforts should be devoted to getting the patient out of the operating room and to the intensive care unit for further resuscitation. A temporary laparostomy may be indicated, and if the patient improves, CD can be addressed when the patient is returned to the operating room for washout and closure of the abdomen. Experience with abdominal trauma has shown that even when a prosthetic vascular graft is grossly contaminated with enteric material, the long-term risk of graft infection is low.

There are now many centers employing EVAR to treat rAAA, and early published studies show that mortality is decreased compared with open surgical repair of rAAA. In this case the CD would be identified radiographically and clinically, rather than by observation at laparotomy. At this time, there are no published studies concerning CD and rAAA repaired by EVAR, but it would be reasonable to assume that laparotomy for CD could proceed soon or even immediately after EVAR for rAAA. This may even be beneficial to the management of the rAAA because complications such as ileus and postrenal failure have been caused by large, undrained retroperitoneal hematomas after EVAR for rAAA. Such a hematoma could be evacuated during the laparotomy for CD.

If the AAA is not ruptured but symptomatic, with the findings of periaortic edema, the decision to treat or observe CD is not as clear. Although the mortality of treating a symptomatic AAA is not as high as that for a ruptured AAA, it is still much higher than that of elective AAA repair. In this case, one may consider either treating the incidental pathology simultaneously if it is felt to be a threat postoperatively (i.e., acute cholecystitis, appendicitis) or treating it primarily, followed by immediate repair of the AAA by either a retroperitoneal approach or EVAR.

The hemodynamic instability thought to be due to a ruptured aneurysm could be due to sepsis caused by cholangitis, appendicitis, or diverticulitis or bleeding caused by a ruptured ovarian cyst or bleeding ulcer. Similarly, abdominal pain presumed to be due to a symptomatic AAA could be caused by pancreatitis, biliary colic, or renal colic. Therefore unexpected findings can occur in these and other scenarios, and it is possible that symptoms presumed to be due to a symptomatic or even ruptured aneurysm could be the result of other pathology. One should always review all preoperative studies critically and not necessarily accept a diagnosis provided by a referring physician or institution. The authors have had an experience with one patient who was transferred to our institution with abdominal pain and a CT scan that was interpreted to show a ruptured AAA, but on careful review, she actually had an intestinal tumor with a desmoplastic reaction in the small bowel mesentery, causing a partial small bowel obstruction. Laparotomy was deferred altogether by the vascular surgeon, and the patient was referred to a surgical oncologist.

However, if it turns out that the patient's symptoms are due to CD that is present in association with an asymptomatic AAA, that pathology should be addressed first and AAA treatment should be deferred because these patients are already at high risk for complications. The exception to this practice would be a massive AAA. Swanson and colleagues reported on 10 cases of asymptomatic AAAs that ruptured within 36 days of laparotomy. All but one of these aneurysms were greater than 6 cm, and the mean diameter of this group was 9.4 cm; two of these patients experienced rupture 1 day after laparotomy. In this case, combined open surgery, possibly with a retroperitoneal approach to the AAA to prevent contamination or immediate EVAR, would be appropriate. Obviously the decision to proceed with AAA repair supposes that the patient is stable enough to tolerate further surgery, and there is the expectation that the patient will survive his or her CD.

EMERGENT LAPAROTOMY FOR SYMPTOMATIC CONCOMITANT DISEASE WITH INCIDENTAL ASYMPTOMATIC ABDOMINAL AORTIC ANEURYSM

This situation is similar to those described earlier, but in this case the correct diagnosis of symptomatic nonvascular pathology is made preoperatively and the surgeon may or may not be aware of the associated aneurysm. The operating surgeon is most likely a GI surgeon, urologist, or gynecologist. In such an instance, a vascular surgeon should be consulted and the same algorithm followed. Few studies have addressed the management of concomitant asymptomatic AAA and acute nonvascular pathology. Small studies of combined AAA repair with acute inflammatory conditions such as appendicitis, diverticulitis, and cholecystitis have shown that it is a safe alternative without significant increase in vascular graft infection rates when the patient is hemodynamically stable and deemed able to tolerate the physiologic burden of a combined operation. In the majority of cases, we still advocate a staged approach whereby the acute nonvascular pathology is addressed first and the aneurysm addressed at a later date, preferably by EVAR to decrease morbidity to the patient.

Intestinal obstruction or perforation caused by hernia, malignancy, or adhesive disease requires immediate management. In simple cases of nonperforated obstruction caused by herniated but noninfarcted bowel or adhesive bands, it may seem feasible to proceed with AAA repair after the obstructing lesion has been addressed. However, given the general degree of dehydration in most patients with recent obstruction, it is probably advisable to defer aortic operation when possible in favor of resuscitation and recuperation. In cases of complicated obstruction requiring intestinal resection or gross perforation with intraperitoneal spillage of succus, staged or endovascular management of the aortic lesion would be most appropriate. When contamination is frank or visible, no open operation on the aorta can be considered safe.

Pancreatitis most often occurs in association with gallstones in the aneurysm patient population. This is probably best treated with endoscopic retrograde cholangiopancreatography and sphincterotomy before AAA repair. After amylase and bilirubin levels have returned to normal, aneurysm repair may proceed safely. Pancreatitis has been rarely described as a causative factor in the development of infrarenal aortic pseudo-aneurysms, likely because of the proximate location of the structures within the retroperitoneum. Management of such a situation represents a clinical challenge. Resection of necrotic pancreatic tissue is deferred when possible unless such tissue demonstrates evidence of infection, at which point open debridement becomes mandatory. Operating on both an aneurysm and infected pancreatic necrosis would predispose to an exceptionally high risk of graft infection, given the inability to separate the two compartments; such a situation would best be managed with EVAR combined with prompt open pancreatic debridement. Thankfully, the combination of infected pancreatic necrosis and aortic aneurysm is rare.

ELECTIVE LAPAROTOMY FOR CONCOMITANT DISEASE WITH INCIDENTAL ASYMPTOMATIC ABDOMINAL AORTIC ANEURYSM

When patients with AAA undergo elective laparotomy for CD, their AAA usually has been diagnosed preoperatively through previous history, physical examination, or–most frequently–radiology study performed to evaluate the CD. Consequently, an incidental finding of AAA at the time of elective laparotomy is rare. Nevertheless, it is still possible that the presence of an AAA could be missed by those interpreting the preoperative imaging or that the diagnosis is not communicated to the treating surgeon. This situation is the inverse of the first scenario described earlier and represents the most

favorable situation for the patient and surgeon. Therefore the same logic would apply, and one can extrapolate from the analysis of Velanovich and Anderson, which would suggest that AAAs larger than 5 cm undergo simultaneous repair with the CD surgery, either by open repair or EVAR. However, consideration should again be given to staged repair by EVAR after the CD is treated. This approach would allow the treating surgeon to obtain informed consent before the AAA surgery and clear up confusion regarding this new, unexpected diagnosis. Aneurysms smaller than 5 cm may be observed safely in favor of proceeding with an originally planned, nonvascular operation. In either event, intraoperative consultation with a vascular surgeon is critical to assess not only the size of the aneurysm but its suitability for EVAR.

CONCLUSIONS

The surgeon's approach to concomitant disease depends on the scenario in which it is encountered. Suspected aneurysmal rupture always mandates consideration superseding that of any other lesion. Indolent nonvascular pathology discovered during emergent aneurysmectomy is best left to delayed repair or conservative management to minimize the operative burden and decrease the chance of an aortic graft infection. In open, elective AAA repairs, unexpected nonvascular pathology generally should be left alone, except in certain cases of malignancy in which combined operations may be advisable. Incidental AAA discovered during operation for acute nonvascular pathology ought to take priority when it is found to be large. Any AAA repair combined with treatment of CD should be performed meticulously to minimize the chance of graft infection. The introduction of EVAR has simplified the management of AAA and CD and in many instances allows for closely staged but separate operations to treat AAA and CD safely with improved outcomes.

SUGGESTED READINGS

Baxter NN, Noel AA, Cherry K, and others: Management of patients with colorectal cancer and concomitant abdominal aortic aneurysm, *Dis Colon Rectum* 45:165, 2002.
Bickerstaff LK, Hollier LH, Van Peenen HJ, and others: Abdominal aortic aneurysm repair combined with a second surgical procedure—morbidity and mortality, *Surgery* 95:487, 1984.
Ouriel K, Ricotta JJ, Adams JT, and others: Management of cholelithiasis in patients with abdominal aortic aneurysm, *Ann Surg* 198:717, 1983.
Prusa AM, Wolff KS, Sahal M, and others: Abdominal aortic aneurysms and concomitant diseases requiring surgical intervention: simultaneous operation vs staged treatment using endoluminal stent grafting, *Arch Surg* 140:686, 2005.
String ST: Cholelithiasis and aortic reconstruction, *J Vasc Surg* 1:664, 1984.
Swanson RJ, Littooy FN, Hunt TK, and others: Laparotomy as a precipitating factor in the rupture of intra-abdominal aneurysms, *Arch Surg* 115:299, 1980.
Thomas JH, McCroskey BL, Iliopoulos JI, and others: Aortoiliac reconstruction combined with nonvascular operations, *Am J Surg* 146:784, 1983.
Velanovich V, Andersen CA: Concomitant abdominal aortic aneurysm and colorectal cancer: a decision analysis approach to a therapeutic dilemma, *Ann Vasc Surg* 5:449, 1991.

Transperitoneal Versus Retroperitoneal Approach to the Aorta

G. Melville Williams, MD

The approach to abdominal aneurysm repair is largely trumped by increasingly encouraging results of endovascular techniques. It is likely that 75% of aortic pathology can be treated with catheter-based techniques that clearly have a major role in the treatment of our elderly population with coexisting morbidities. Recent graduates from training programs are comfortable with endovascular aneurysm repair, and, largely because of inexperience with open cases, fearful of employing what used to be standard methods for treating aneurysms and occlusive disease. However, surgeons employing endovascular techniques should be familiar with the three main open surgical approaches—namely, the transabdominal, the anterior retroperitoneal, and the posterior retroperitoneal—to provide optimal treatment for patients and to extricate themselves from acute or chronic problems with stent grafts. Skilled surgeons recognize which approach best fits their patients and recommend appropriate therapy.

INDICATIONS FOR OPEN SURGERY

The clearest indication for open surgery is failure of endovascular therapy. This includes patients with occlusions of iliac stents or the limbs of endografts, continued expansion of the aneurysm sac despite attempts to stop endoleaks, and errors in the placement of aortic endografts. Anatomic issues are also important, and these include extension of the aneurysm above the renal arteries; a large tortuous, plaque-filled aorta at the proposed fixation site below the renal arteries; occluded iliac arteries; and a large inferior mesenteric artery demonstrating collateral to the midcolic or superior mesenteric artery. There are also gray areas in which the surgeon may push the limits of current endovascular technology because the patient is "too sick" to undergo open surgery. Because our long-term success rates for endografts remain unknown as new generations of graft are brought to market, I advocate open aortic surgery for any woman younger than 70 years for both aneurysmal and diffuse occlusive disease unless there are striking comorbidities. Women have smaller vessels less likely to remain patent after angioplasty and stent and do not have postoperative problems of impotence or retrograde ejaculation experienced by sexually active men following open operations on the aorta. Men younger than age 70 must be counseled about these potential problems. Some will opt for aortic stent grafts and some will want a procedure with a known, fairly benign long-term outcome free of anxiety produced by computed tomograph (CT) monitoring of the repair every 6 months.

TRANSABDOMINAL APPROACH

Anatomic Considerations

Most vascular surgeons favor using a long midline incision for aneurysm repair and aortofemoral bypass. This is the way they were taught; they are more familiar with the anatomy displayed this way and point out correctly that no study has shown differences in mortality between this and the retroperitoneal methods. After opening the peritoneum, the viscera are displaced superiorly, the duodenum mobilized from the aorta, and the aorta controlled just below the left renal vein. The aorta is surrounded by veins, and venous injury is one of the most feared complications of aortic surgery. To avoid this, sharp dissection and ligation of the areolar and lymphatic tissue surrounding the infrarenal aorta are advocated. The transabdominal approach is clearly indicated to treat recurrent occlusive disease of the right renal artery associated with aortic aneurysm. To expose the right renal artery, the right colon and duodenum are mobilized medially. The transabdominal approach is also the best method for exposure and repair of right common, internal, and external iliac aneurysms.

Ruptured Aneurysms

Although many vascular centers treat aortic aneurysm rupture by placing endografts, on occasion appropriate sizes are not immediately available. Furthermore, small hospitals may not believe they can justify maintaining the suitable, expensive inventory necessary for stent graft repair, mandating open repair in patients presenting in shock. Resuscitation and the placement of arterial and venous catheters must wait until the bleeding is controlled. Although the aorta may be controlled just as quickly through a flank incision, access to sites for monitoring lines and blood replacement is hampered. Therefore patients in shock require immediate laparotomy and manual control of the aorta at the diaphragm. The aneurysm sac is entered through the hematoma. Standing on the patient's right side, I favor inserting my left thumb into the aneurysm, pushing its tip proximally and thereby occluding the aorta at the base of the thumb while allowing some perfusion of the kidneys and viscera. The sac is opened widely, allowing catheter (a Foley catheter will do) placement into the iliac arteries to control backbleeding. This provides stability and is the time for blood replacement. The proximal aortic dissection should proceed carefully as the thumb controls the bleeding and defines the location of the more normal aorta. When the aorta is exposed well, a clamp takes over hemostatic duties.

Patients presenting with pain, a pulsating abdominal mass, and stable vital signs should have a rapid CT scan to confirm the diagnosis and define the location and extent of the aneurysm. If the aneurysm extends superior to the renal arteries, the flank approach is justified. Right iliac involvement tips the scale to the midline.

RETROPERITONEAL APPROACHES

Anterior Retroperitoneal Approach

The anterior retroperitoneal space is that plane anterior to the left kidney and ureter and posterior to the left colon, spleen, and pancreas (Fig. 1). This approach was pioneered by Rob and is certainly useful for repair of small distal aneurysms and for access to the visceral vessels. However, proximal exposure of the aorta is limited by the crossing renal vein, and this reduced exposure leads to less versatility in managing the aneurysmal disease. It is surprising to me that many surgeons continue to use this old approach as the "standard" with which to compare outcomes of the transabdominal method.

Nevertheless, one venous anomaly, a retroaortic left renal vein, is best managed with this approach. In this situation, the main left renal vein runs beneath the aorta, occupying the position usually taken by the lumbar branch of the left renal vein. Developing the plane anterior to the left kidney provides optimal exposure.

Figure 1 The anterior retroperitoneal plane is demonstrated. This display of anatomy is possible by making the incision in the tenth intercostals space. Note that the left renal vein still hampers exposure in the juxtarenal area. However, when there is a retroaortic left renal vein or when occlusive disease of the visceral arteries demands attention, the exposure is ideal. Minimizing the incision and placing it in the eleventh intercostals space allow adequate exposure of the infrarenal aorta, which is the approach used by many surgeons. A, Artery; *Inf*, inferior; *v*, vein; *vess*, vessicle(s).

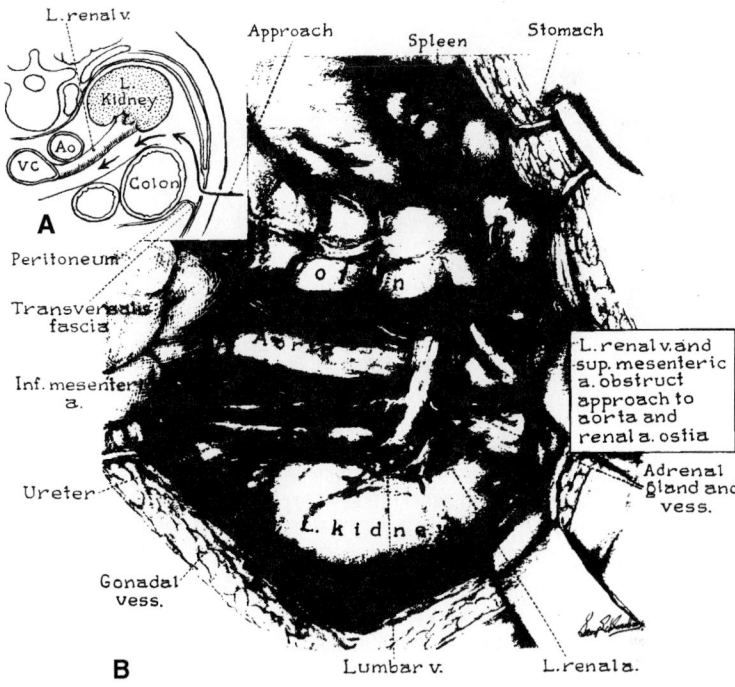

It places the renal vein in the position where sharp dissection displaces it easily from the lateral and posterior walls of the aorta.

Posterior Retroperitoneal Approach

The retroperitoneal planes are developed through a flank incision beginning at the tip of the twelfth rib and extending obliquely 15 to 20 cm in the direction of the ribs. It is vitally important to place the incision between the eleventh and twelfth intercostal nerves to prevent denervation of the flank muscles and a disfiguring bulge. To develop the posterior plane, the peritoneum is swept away, keeping the kidney with the peritoneum anteriorly. The ureter is also displaced anteriorly with the peritoneum. The left renal artery can be palpated superiorly in the majority of patients, defining the starting point for ligating and dividing the lymphatic and areolar tissue on the left side of the aorta. The lumbar branch of the renal vein is ligated and divided in the process. After the lateral surface of the aorta is exposed for 3 to 4 cm, gentle finger dissection anteriorly and posteriorly allows control of the aorta. Having anteriorly displaced the ureter, the kidney, and the renal artery, there are no structures of consequence guarding the aorta and left iliac artery. The only issue is the management of the right common iliac artery. When this artery is aneurysmal, the incision should be extended in the same direction medially. If exposure remains inadequate, further dissection should be deferred until the aortic aneurysm is decompressed. If exposure is still inadequate, the surgeon must oversew the iliac artery and extend the right limb of the graft to the femoral artery. When a tube replacement of an aneurysm is performed, it is easier to control the right iliac artery with a balloon catheter, thereby limiting the length of the incision.

▮ THE MANAGEMENT OF SPECIFIC CONDITIONS

Juxarenal Aneurysms

Venous injuries are the major complications of hurried attacks on aneurysms addressed from the midline or instances in which the aneurysm extends to the renal arteries. The left renal vein and its branches form a collar enclosing the anterior left lateral side of the aorta. The lumbar branch of the left renal vein is adjacent to the aorta on the left side and tethers the renal vein posteriorly. The left gonadal vein holds it inferiorly, and the left adrenal vein pulls it superiorly and laterally. This network is not a major problem when the aorta is normal in diameter at the level of the renal vein. However, when the aorta is large, the renal vein is stretched flat, raising the pressure in its distal branches. For this reason, great care must be taken to dissect the venous structures away from the aorta to allow clamping. Some surgeons advocate division of the renal vein, but it is not always benign and this must be achieved before the collateral veins are ligated. For this reason, aneurysms extending to or beyond the renal arteries are best managed by posterior retroperitoneal exposure. With this approach, the lumbar branch of the renal vein is divided, allowing the whole complex of veins to be moved out of the way anteriorly. As shown in Figure 2, control of the aorta just below the renal artery is far easier from the side when there is a huge aneurysm.

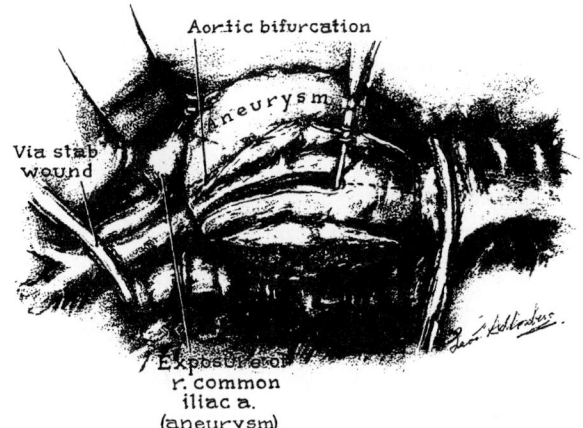

Figure 2 As shown, huge aneurysms are much easier to manage from the retroperitoneal approach. A, Artery.

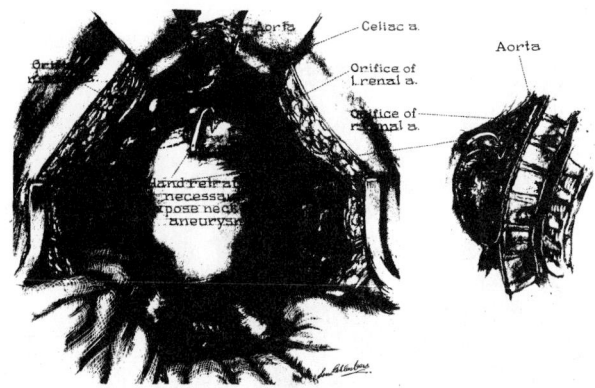

Figure 3 The posterior retroperitoneal plane is developed by dissection posterior to the left kidney, allowing exposure of the entire abdominal aorta. Note that the vascular clamp on the left common iliac artery is passed through a stab wound to keep the handle out of the surgeon's way. As illustrated, it is best not to attempt to control the right common iliac artery until the large aneurysm is decompressed.

The second major advantage of the posterior approach to repair extensive aneurysms is the ease of exposing and controlling the aorta superiorly (Fig. 3). The left crux of the diaphragm crosses the left side of the aorta at the level of the left renal artery. After this is cut, the rest of the crux can be divided in the direction of its fibers, allowing visualization of the entire abdominal aorta. To accomplish this division, the flank incision must extend into the eleventh interspace and carried to the erector spinae posteriorly.

The "Hostile Abdomen"

Most surgeons agree that endovascular repair or the retroperitoneal approaches are strongly indicated in patients who have had multiple intra-abdominal operations. However, the retroperitoneum may become scarred after a left colectomy and the pelvis may be difficult to dissect following irradiation. Thus endovascular aneurysm repair (EVAR) is clearly indicated unless there are strong anatomic barriers. In the latter case, the retroperitoneal route is the appropriate choice.

The Redo Aneurysm

Degenerative aneurysms and false aneurysms developing at suture lines or stent graft fixation points are best managed by additional stent grafts placed as extensions to seal the aneurysm from systemic pressure. When the aneurysm is at the proximal fixation site of a stent graft, there may not be room below the renal arteries to place an extension. Here the posterior retroperitoneal approach is best applied because of the ease of obtaining high proximal control.

Renal Anomalies

The presence of horseshoe or "pancake" kidney presenting with an aortic aneurysm is a prime indication for the posterior retroperitoneal approach. The isthmus of the kidney is commonly supplied by anomalous arteries that are not readily restored by endovascular means. Approaching the aneurysm from the posterior flank turns a difficult operation though the midline into a simple one. In the majority of cases, these kidneys have multiple arteries, generally arising from the anterior inferior part of the aneurysm. Proceeding retroperitoneally, the surgeon is posterior to the crossing kidney.

Control is achieved as for simple aneurysms, and a button or several buttons of aorta containing the openings of the branches to the kidney may be sewn into the graft with ease.

Inflammatory Aneurysms

The etiology of inflammatory aneurysms remains unknown. This chronic inflammatory and fibrotic process is generally most intense in the pelvis and generally ends at the renal arteries. Patients may have chronic flank and back pain, which in some cases is related to ureteral entrapment and hydronephrosis. The fibrous mass overlying the aorta may resemble a rupture on the CT scan. The duodenum is glued to the anterior surface of the aneurysm in most cases. It is not known whether EVAR manages to stifle the inflammatory process. It certainly does not accomplish ureterolysis. When left flank pain and left hydronephrosis are present, the retroperitoneal approach should be chosen. Because the process wanes superiorly, the proximal clamp can be placed on normal aorta comfortably without the need to dissect the duodenum from the anterior surface. After the aorta is clamped, the ureter can be freed with confidence that the aneurysm, if broached, will not result in profound bleeding. However, it is important to emphasize that the entire ureter must be freed, particularly as it crosses the common iliac artery. With this approach, the adherent duodenum is never even visualized.

Left-Sided Vena Cava

This anomaly is rare. The vena cava arises to the left of the aortic bifurcation and courses over the anterior side of the aorta at the location usually occupied by the left renal vein. Irrespective of which open approach is used, the vena cava must be mobilized where it crosses the aorta to enable placement of the proximal aortic clamp. For this reason, it is best to employ EVAR. If there is an anatomic contraindication to EVAR, the retroperitoneal approach is best because the vena cava is directly in front of the surgeon, aiding in the exposure and ligation of branches and mobilization of the cava. The proximal anastomosis is performed with the vena cava retracted anteriorly, the distal anastomoses with the cava freed posteriorly.

The Obese Patient

Endovascular repair is best suited for the obese patient. Here, however, it is important to place oblique incisions for femoral artery exposure in the fat superior to the groin crease. Incisions so placed heal much better than those buried by the overhanging pannus. When EVAR cannot be performed, the retroperitoneal approach offers a benefit to the surgeon that is perhaps greater than that gained by the patient. Using the flank approach, the surgeon does not have to deal with a huge omentum and abundant mesenteric and retroperitoneal fat. The basic landmarks are the same as those found in the thin patient. However, much larger incisions are required to achieve equivalent exposure. In a recent study, we found that obesity and incision length were independent risk factors for developing the postoperative bulge.

GENERAL CONSIDERATIONS

Virtually all of the specific indications and contraindications to the methods for the treatment of aortic disease are recognized by a preoperative thin-slice CT scan or magnetic resonance angiography, which should be performed in all cases. The reader will note that EVAR has more applications than the other alternatives. Indeed, this is why I apply it to routine cases in elderly patients. The flank approach provides the surgeon with the best alternative to EVAR.

The advantages of eating and leaving the hospital sooner are significant to the patient. Although the comfort level of my patients with small flank incisions is clearly better than those with midline incisions, neither can be compared with the patient who has small groin incisions. Their comfort level during the first week is so much superior that justification for randomized trials rests only with long-term performance and expense.

There is one significant drawback to the flank incision that deserves mention: a postoperative bulge. This occurs when the intercostal nerves are injured. When we first began using this approach, we made large incisions and faced patients who appeared to have footballs in their flanks. With greater experience, the huge bulges are rare, but 30% of patients have protrusions between 1 and 2 inches at 1 year even when we have used our best technique. In a recent study, we made a conscious effort to minimize incision length and keep within the line projected by the direction of the ribs to keep from dividing or cauterizing intercostals nerves. We found that obesity strongly influenced incision length but was also significant independently. Body mass index greater than 23 mg/kg^2 correlated strongly with bulge ($p = .018$ with an odds ratio of 16.9). However, incision length was equally if not more impressive. Patients developing bulges had mean incision lengths of 24 cm compared with 16.3 cm in those who did not ($p = 6 \times 10 - 5$). Extension of the incision into the eleventh interspace was not found to be significant independently, nor were any of the other 37 variables studied. It is important to counsel patients, particularly those carrying too much weight but also those with extensive disease that they have one chance in three of developing a moderate flank bulge.

CONCLUSIONS

The posterior retroperitoneal approach remains a valuable technique for the management of aneurysmal disease of the aorta (Table 1). In my mind there are only two strong remaining indications for the transabdominal approach, and both have a caveat: acute endograft failure with hemorrhage and repairs of ruptured aneurysms. The caveat is that both of these conditions may be treatable by additional means using endovascular techniques that have assumed first choice. When EVAR cannot be applied, the aneurysmal disease is best treated by the retroperitoneal approach. Conditions treated by EVAR as first line include simple abdominal aortic aneurysm (AAA) in the elderly, ruptured AAA, venous abnormality, hostile abdomen, coincidental renal or visceral artery stenosis, inflammatory aneurysm, AAA with bleeding diastasis,

Table 1: Indications for Various Approaches

EVAR—Strong Indications

Standard infrarenal AAA in women
Standard infrarenal AAA in men >70 years
AAA plus renal artery stenosis
AAA with venous anomalies
Obesity
Hostile abdomen
Bleeding diastasis

EVAR—Relative Indications

AAA in sexually active men
Inflammatory AAA without hydronephrosis
Ruptured AAA

Transabdominal—Strong Indications

Acute control of errors during EVAR

Transabdominal—Relative Indications

Ruptured AAA

Anterior retroperitoneal—Strong Indications

Juxtarenal AAA with retroaortic left renal vein
Failed angioplasty/stent of visceral vessels

Posterior retroperitoneal—Strong Indications

Juxtarenal and suprarenal AAA
Horseshoe kidney
Chronically failing EVAR
AAA with connective tissue disorder
Inflammatory aneurysms with hydronephrosis

and obesity. The conditions best treated by the retroperitoneal approach include horseshoe kidney, AAA with connective tissue disorder, chronically failing endovascular procedures, juxtarenal and suprarenal aneurysms, and inflammatory aneurysms with left ureteral entrapment and pain.

THORACIC AND THORACOABDOMINAL AORTIC ANEURYSMS

James H. Black, III, MD

INTRODUCTION

Descending thoracic aortic aneurysms are estimated to affect 10 of every 10,000 elderly adults with 30% to 40% of these aneurysms being limited to the thoracic aorta. Repair of thoracic aortic aneurysms (TAAs) and thoracoabdominal aortic aneurysms (TAAAs) remains a formidable surgical operation. Although traditionally viewed as less threatening and less demanding from a technical standpoint than the more extensive thoracoabdominal aneurysms, TAA repair also presents the surgeon with a multitude of technical and cognitive challenges extending through the perioperative period. Repair was first described in 1952 by Bahnson as a lateral resection of a saccular aneurysm of the thoracoabdominal aorta. Actual homograft replacement of the TAAA was reported by Etheridge soon thereafter in 1955. The modern era of complex aortic surgery was ushered in by Dr. Stanley Crawford, who greatly simplified the operation for extensive aneurysms of the thoracic and thoracoabdominal aorta. His experience both laid the foundation of TAAA repair and highlighted the challenges of visceral, renal, and spinal cord protection during the conduct of the operation. Since then, the work of many groups has further lowered the risk of renovisceral and spinal cord complications associated with repair of complex aortic aneurysms. As such, the attendant morbidity of TAA and TAAA repair had been admirably reduced in many series from "centers of excellence."

This chapter defines indications, preoperative stratification, and the surgical approaches to TAA/TAAA with adjunctive methods to decrease end-organ ischemia and spinal cord injury. New data from prospective registries elucidate the challenges yet to be overcome in the management of patients with aneurysms of the descending thoracic aorta. In addition, the proper selection of patients suitable for endovascular repair of TAA is reviewed. Lastly, the premise and development of "hybrid" open and endovascular techniques to address TAAA are elucidated.

INDICATIONS FOR SURGERY AND PREOPERATIVE RISK STRATIFICATION

The risk of operative repair of TAAAs is standardized by the Crawford Classification (Fig. 1). Extent type II TAAAs are traditionally considered most threatening because of the need for both extensive intercostal/spinal and visceral revascularizations; experimental evidence suggests that molecular ischemia/reperfusion events in the gut may compound spinal injury and drive spinal neuron apoptosis. There exists no standardized schema for aneurysm isolated to the thorax alone, yet it is generally assumed that the greater the extent of TAA, particularly encroaching on the T8–T12 segment, the greater the assumed risk of spinal cord injury.

Juvonen and coworkers reported on 114 patients with TAAAs managed without surgery and followed over a mean interval of 28 months. Most of the study population did not have large-extent TAAAs, but because the threshold for surgery was maintained at 7 cm, the data have important implications. Aneurysm rupture occurred in 23% of their patients, and another 20% met compelling indications for operation (e.g., pain, leak). Relatively modest mean diameters of 5.8 cm were appreciated in the ruptured TAA patients, and on analysis, pain and chronic obstructive pulmonary disease were associated with an elevated risk of rupture. Given the significant rupture rates with a treatment threshold of 7 cm, this diameter is likely too conservative. In a separate study, the natural history of TAA dictated a 30% 5-year risk of rupture when a TAA exceeds 6 cm, and thus the general recommendation of 6 cm as an appropriate size for repair seems warranted in acceptable-risk patients.

Given the variety of operative approaches employed in the treatment of TAA/TAAA, there are consistent themes with regard to the clinical variables that influence both the overall risk of the operation and the risk of cord injury. Balancing these risks represents a clinical dilemma for the aortic surgeon, and a thoughtful, logical risk analysis of the individual patient presentation is clearly warranted before repair of the TAA or TAAA. Preoperative testing should include cardiac, pulmonary, and renal evaluation. Because aortic aneurysms are considered as markers of coronary atherosclerotic disease, preoperative cardiac testing is mandatory in the elective setting. Indeed, most long-term reports of TAAA results indicate that the majority of mortality is related to cardiovascular events. Echocardiography, performed transthoracic or transesophageal, is important to screen for valvular and ventricular function that may be adversely affected by afterload increases during aortic cross clamping. Nuclear stress testing may also determine whether major areas of myocardium are at risk and require revascularization. Renal function is most often screened by serum creatinine. Should an elevated serum level be noted, angiography to delineate the offending lesion should be performed, and if necessary, revascularization should occur preoperatively (often by percutaneous stenting) or at the time of open repair by surgical bypass or endarterectomy. Because open repair of TAA or TAAA mandates single-lung ventilation, pulmonary function testing is recommended to identify patients who may not tolerate such technique. Generally, those patients with a forced expiratory volume 1 (FEV1) of 1.0 L or more or a PCO_2 of 45 mm Hg or less are considered suitable for open repair. Patients who do not meet such criteria may be offered a trial of medical therapy or be considered for the "hybrid" procedures, discussed later.

With regard to operative risk, mortality in circumstances other than elective operation is essentially doubled. Interestingly, the explanation for this is not as simple as hemodynamic instability because most patients are stable during their preoperative preparation. Regardless, the association of nonelective operation and perioperative mortality is verified in many series. Secondly, renal failure, whether dialysis dependent or not, has been consistently noted as a predictor of early death. Advanced age has also been associated with adverse outcomes in TAA or TAAA repair. In my view, the patient's overall functional status appears to be more important than the chronologic age. In support, Huynh and colleagues recently reported acceptable perioperative mortality in 63 octogenarians who underwent TAA repair. Balancing these risks is a common dilemma in clinical decision making in patients, and the perception of unacceptable risk leading to denial of open treatment has, in part, driven the demand for further refinement of surgical technique and alternative therapies for TAA and TAAA such as endovascular repair.

ANESTHESIA MANAGEMENT AND CONSIDERATIONS

The anesthetic management for the repair of TAA and TAAA varies across institutions, but standard approaches include invasive hemodynamic monitoring with arterial lines and pulmonary artery catheters, double-lumen endotracheal tubes for one-lung ventilation, and rapid infusers for volume resuscitation. Choice of anesthetic may be influenced by the need for neuromonitoring of motor-evoked potentials to maintain basal motor function for assessment.

Cerebral spinal fluid drainage (CSFD) is perhaps the best-studied and most widely accepted strategy employed in prevention of paraplegia in thoracic aortic surgery. Experimental data suggest that CSF pressure (CSFP) may rise with proximal aortic clamping and reducing this pressure may improve spinal perfusion pressure. As such, placement of a drainage catheter into the subarachnoid space to allow efflux of fluid during the operation and in the postoperative period may serve to benefit the fragile circulation of the spinal cord. Generally, the fluid is able to drain when CSFP exceeds 10 mm Hg as measured from the level of the spine. Coselli and colleagues demonstrated the beneficial effect of CSF drainage in a randomized trial that compared repair of types I and II TAAA performed with or without CSFD. A total of 145 patients underwent

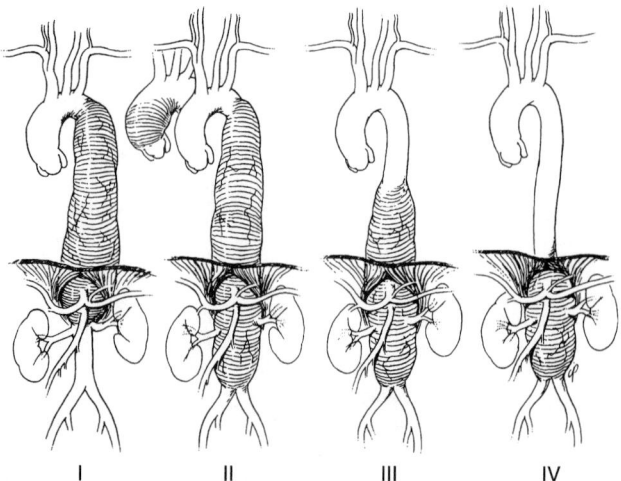

Figure 1 Crawford classification of thoracoabdominal aortic aneurysms.

I   II   III   IV

repair, with 76 receiving CSFD and the other 69 undergoing repair without CSFD. Aortic clamp times, left heart bypass (LHB) use, and number of intercostal artery reattachments were similar between groups. Nine patients (13.0%) in the control group suffered paraplegia or had paraparesis; in contrast, only two patients in the CSFD (2.6%) had deficits. Overall, CSFD delivered an 80% reduction in the risk of postoperative spinal ischemic complications after type I and II TAAA repair. The combined spinal and visceral ischemia encountered in type II TAAA repair likely confers a higher spinal cord complication threat because the spinal ischemic injury may be compounded by the concomitant visceral ischemia. Yet in this series, 3 of the 11 patients with deficits were only type I TAAA repairs, and all underwent CSFD. Because CSFD catheter placement is not risk free, it is generally accepted that CSFD is clearly of benefit in operations in which aortic topography may mandate combined spinal and visceral ischemia—most TAA and type I TAAA and all type I TAAA.

OPEN SURGICAL MANAGEMENT OF THORACIC AND THORACOABDOMINAL AORTIC ANEURYSMS

In general, the strategies to decrease the incidence and severity of end-organ injury and spinal cord injury after TAA repair have fallen into two categories. The first of these is aimed at maintaining visceral and spinal cord blood supply during the course of the operation and includes both shunts and bypasses for distal aortic perfusion, preoperative identification of critical intercostal vessels, cerebrospinal fluid drainage, and reconstruction of intercostal arteries. The basic premise for distal aortic perfusion is the ability to maintain blood flow to visceral and spinal aortic branch vessels, usually accomplished via partial LHB. Clearly the efficacy of distal aortic perfusion is a function of TAA extent. Those lesions truly isolated to the descending thoracic aorta are clearly amenable to continuous distal perfusion throughout the cross-clamp interval, whereas those lesions that involve the visceral segment—or portions thereof—disallow the same unless a scheme of "octopus" catheters is employed. The balance of femoral inflow and the visceral octopus perfusion catheter inflow may invite problematic pressure-to-volume relationships. Full cardiopulmonary bypass involves significant increases in need for heparinization and the threat of significant blood turnover. LHB via a centrifugal pump carries the advantage of less need for anticoagulation, as well as the ability to control distal perfusion pressure. Apart from distal perfusion techniques to prevent the most dreaded complication of paraplegia, strategies have been developed to protect the cord from spinal blood flow interruption. Epidural cooling using an iced saline infusion into the intrathecal space attempts to produce a temperature of 25° to 28° Celsius in the spinal canal, thereby decreasing neuronal energy requirement. The flow rate into the epidural space may be limited by the measured CSFP; as a target CSF perfusion pressure (mean arterial pressure − CSFP) should be kept above 40 mm Hg. Admirable paraplegia rates (6%) were reported from the Massachusetts General Hospital in their series of more than 300 thoracoabdominal repairs with adjunctive epidural cooling. This series included a substantial number of ruptures and acute presentations that are clearly associated with elevated risk. As stated by Cambria and colleagues, the application of local hypothermia avoids the need for systemic moderate hypothermia and the associated coagulopathy. Besides cooling, other mechanisms have been explored to lower spinal metabolism. Acher and colleagues reported the use of naloxone therapy and barbiturate-based anesthetic to decrease energy expenditure during the critical interval of spinal blood flow interruption. As reported in their series of 110 thoracic aortic repairs, an admirable 1.6% paraplegia rate was observed in

this strategy, which also included the deliberate oversewing of intercostal arteries in the critical thoracolumbar zone.

Intraoperative management of the fragile spinal cord circulation can be approached in several ways. For the critical zone of T8 to L2 in which most patients have a dominant intercostal/lumbar contribution to the thoracolumbar spinal cord, it is prudent to salvage intercostal circulation to the extent possible. Most experts aggressively pursue reimplantation of the T9 and T10 button because more than 75% of patients have an artery of Adamkiewicz originate at this level. In particular, those intercostals that appear patent but backbleed sluggishly may indicate poor collateralization to that level and mandate revascularization. Jacobs and coworkers have used motor-evoked potentials (MEPs) to provide online assessment of cord integrity and guarantee cord perfusion with excellent results in 70 type II TAAAs (early paraplegia rate 4.9%; Fig. 2). As a premise of this technique, the anterior spinal artery derives its circulation from the thoracoabdominal aorta. In turn, the anterior spinal artery perfuses the motor horns on the anterior spinal cord. Thus by eliciting MEPs (usually at the calf musculature after transcranial stimulation), such motor pathways could be demonstrated as functional intraoperatively. In Jacob's series, MEPs were successfully monitored in all patients, and in 17% (19 patients), MEPs decreased during cross clamping. Intercostal or lumbar revascularization by implant, bypass, or endarterectomy of occluded intercostals successfully restored MEPs in all but three patients, all of whom had deficit.

JOHNS HOPKINS APPROACH TO OPEN THORACIC AORTIC REPLACEMENT

Our approach to type I and II TAAA and TAA has been to employ LHB and active moderate hypothermia (30°-32° Celsius) via a heat exchanger on a Biomedicus (Boston Scientific, Natick, MA) centrifugal pump. CSFD is performed routinely and is placed 1 day preoperatively in case difficult passage mandates fluoroscopic assistance by neuroradiology. In emergent cases, CSFD tubes are placed if feasible. MEPs are monitored during sequential clamping, and intercostal reattachment is performed on the basis of MEPs, clinical inspection of patent intercostals, or as dictated by preoperative arteriographic localization of the artery of Adamkiewicz. For suprarenal, or type III and IV TAAA, LHB is rarely employed because no data exist to support its salutary effect in these groups. Infrequently, LHB is used in lesser extent TAAAs if significant aortic valvular disease is identified on screening.

RESULTS OF OPEN REPAIR OF THORACIC AND THORACOABDOMINAL AORTIC ANEURYSMS

The results of several series of TAA and TAAA repair are summarized in Tables 1 and 2. As expected, the overall complication rate is less with the TAA repair compared with TAAA. Among TAAAs, overall complication rates per series are heavily influenced by the number of patients presenting acutely or as a function of the more extensive repairs required that risk combined spinal and visceral ischemia (type I and type II TAAA). Advances in surgical technique have favorably affected the morbidities encountered after TAAA repair since Svensson's report of Crawford's experience in 1993.

The University of Michigan group identified greater hospital and surgeon volume-related outcomes as contributing to improved outcomes; 1542 patients were identified in the National Inpatient Sample (NIS) from 1988 to 1998, which represents approximately 20% of U.S. hospitals. Overall mortality for TAAA repair was 22.3% but did improve over time. High-volume surgeons (≥3 cases

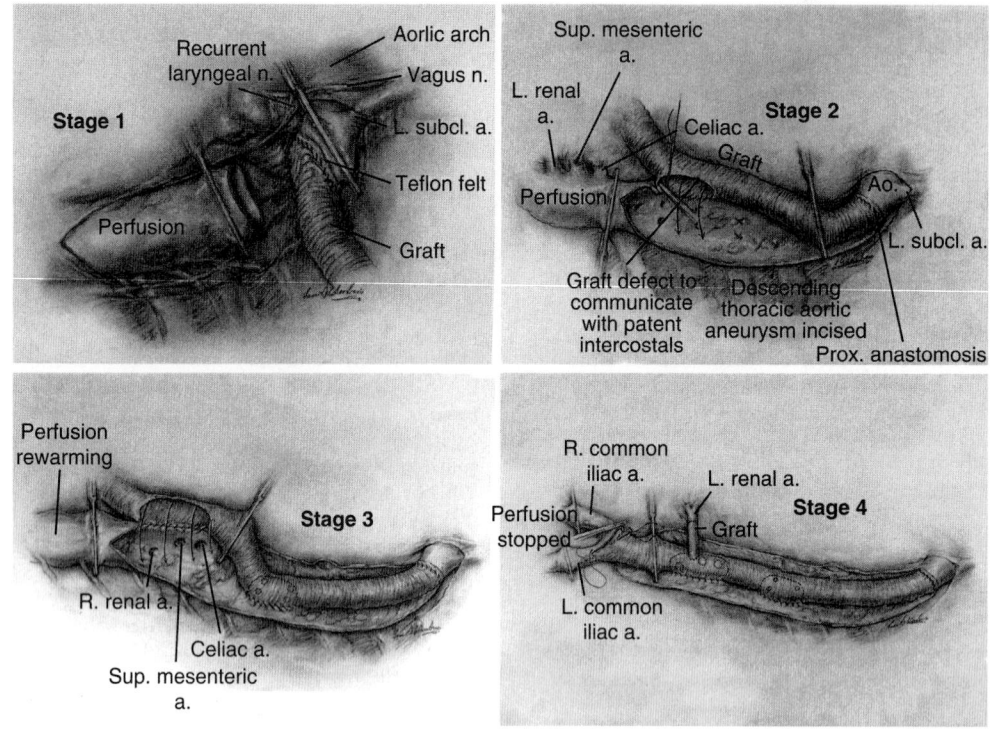

Figure 2 Repair of type II TAAA is performed with sequential clamping to maintain distal aortic perfusion with adjunctive cerebral spinal fluid drainage and moderate hypothermia. If aneurysm topography does not allow separate intercostal interrogation and continued visceral perfusion (i.e., stage 2 and 3 must be concurrent), a temporary 22-F venous cannula can be connected to the proximal graft (with a ⅜ – ⅜ connector and 8- to 10-mm Dacron graft) and secured into the superior mesenteric artery orifice with a Romel tourniquet while the intercostal button is created. During visceral reconstruction, additional iced saline perfusion is maintained into each renal orifice for renal protection. *A,* Artery; *n,* nerve; *Prox,* proximal; *subcl,* subclavian.

Table 1: Results of Open Thoracic Aneurysm Repair

Author, Year	Patients (N)	Elective/Urgent (%)	30-Day Mortality (%)	Renal Failure (%)	Paraplegia %	Technique*
Coselli, 2004	387	329/58 (17)	2.8	7.4	2.6	LHB, C&S
Estrera, 2001	182	182/34 (18)	8.8	NA	2.7	LHB, CSFD
Galloway, 1996	78	78/16 (20)	10.3	NA	3.8	LHB, C&S
Verdant, 1995	366	351/15 (4)	12	2.4	0	Gott

*Adjunctive techniques: *C&S,* "Clamp and sew" technique; *CSFD,* cerebrospinal fluid drainage; *Gott,* 9-mm Gott shunt for distal perfusion; *LHB,* left heart bypass with distal perfusion.

Table 2: Results of Open Thoracoabdominal Aortic Aneurysm (TAAA) Repair

Author, Year	Patients (N)	Elective/ Urgent (%)	Type I/II TAAA (%)	30-Day Mortality (%)	Renal Failure (%)	Paraplegia (%)
Svensson, 1993	1509	937/572 (37)	820 (54)	8	18	16
Safi, 1998	339	311/28 (18)	178 (52)	NA	NA	8.5
Coselli, 2000	1220	1108/112 (9)	794 (65)	4.8	11	4.6
Cambria, 2002	337	255/82 (25)	151 (44)	8.3	13.5	6.6
Jacobs, 2006	112	107/5 (4)	112 (100)	NA	1.8	4.2

NA, Not available.

per year) were compared with low-volume surgeons for mortality and complications after TAAA repair; operative mortality was 25.6% for low-volume surgeons versus 11.0% for high-volume surgeons ($p < .001$). Because greater hospital and surgeon volumes were associated with improved outcomes for length of stay, mortality, and cardiopulmonary complications, the authors champion regionalization as a method to improve delivery of care to patients with complex aneurysms.

Clearly open thoracic aortic replacement for TAA or TAAA remains a formidable operation that is associated with significant risk and use of resources. In part because of the gravity of risk, and perhaps the resources demanded of the institutions that perform complex aortic repairs, there has been increasing application of endovascular repair of thoracic aortic disease. Regardless, open surgical repair of TAA and TAAA remains the gold standard that refinements in technique will continue to affect favorably and to which endovascular technique will be compared.

OVERVIEW OF ENDOVASCULAR REPAIR OF THORACIC AORTIC ANEURYSMS

First-generation stent grafts for thoracic endovascular repair (TEVAR) were bulky, handmade devices that employed pressed Dacron material hand sewn onto Gianturco (Cook Medical, Bloomington, IN) stents. The packaging of these handmade devices required large-diameter sheaths (26-F) and stiff delivery systems, all of which made accurate delivery and deployment difficult. In addition, the large-caliber devices often required conduits to be sewn onto the iliac vessels or abdominal aorta to accommodate the diameter of the delivery. Newer-generation devices offer improved flexibility with small introducer systems. With these advances, the U.S. Food and Drug Administration (FDA) approved the first endovascular device for treatment of degenerative thoracic aneurysms in late 2004.

The current FDA-approved device (as of June 2006) is manufactured by W.L. Gore (Flagstaff, AZ) and labeled the Excluder Thoracic Endoprosthesis (Fig. 3). This device consists of a series

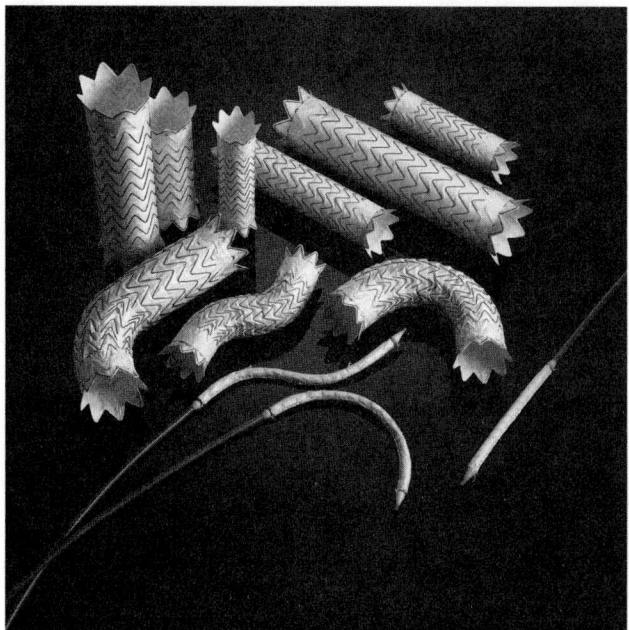

Figure 3 Thoracic aortic endoprostheses are sized for aortic diameters. *Courtesy WL Gore & Associates, Inc.*

of self-expanding nitinol stents affixed to a polytetrafluoroethylene (PTFE) membrane. The outer diameter of the sheath for delivery of the largest-diameter endoprosthesis (40 mm diameter) is 9.2 mm. The device is available in lengths of 10, 15, and 20 cm, and device diameters range from 26 to 40 mm. The device is constrained in a PTFE membrane that is removed by withdrawing a "rip cord" to deploy the device from the middle toward the ends. Currently undergoing investigation are thoracic devices manufactured by Cook (Bloomington, IN) labeled the Zenith TX2 thoracic endograft and by Medtronic Vascular (Santa Rosa, CA) called the Talent Endoluminal Stent-Graft. The Zenith TX2 device employs woven polyester affixed by suture to stainless steel Z stents. Barbs are oriented off the ends of the device to promote fixation to the aortic seal zone. Device diameters ranging from 28 from 42 mm are under trial. The Talent graft features an uncovered proximal stent to cross arch vessels and aid fixation. The device is deployed by withdrawing the introduction sheath to allow self-expansion of the endograft into the aorta.

PATIENT SELECTION FOR THORACIC ENDOVASCULAR REPAIR

Endovascular repair of thoracic aortic pathology requires facility with interpretation of axial imaging such as computed tomography angiography and magnetic resonance angiography to inspect aortic topography for device insertion and fixation. In addition, planning of thoracic aortic endografting may be aided by conventional diagnostic arteriography using both subtracted and unsubtracted techniques, especially when three-dimensional imaging cannot be obtained via available axial data (Fig. 4). A key tenet of thoracic aortic endovascular repair is the understanding that device selection and operative planning should be confirmed and verified to the greatest extent possible preoperatively. Furthermore, independent review of available data for device planning should occur by separate physicians because errors in device measurements often translate into immediate treatment failures.

Endovascular device insertion planning requires a thorough understanding of the aortic diameters at the proximal and distal sealing sites as measured from outer wall to outer wall. For the FDA-approved Gore device, an aortic diameter of no less than 23 mm to no greater than 37 mm allows for implantation using the range devices (26–40 mm) to yield an oversizing of graft to aorta of 10% to 20%. Oversizing the graft too aggressively may place undue force on the aortic endograft and result in migration or collapse of the entire graft. The length of proximal fixation should be longer than 20 mm, with an acceptable aortic diameter throughout this seal zone. If an adequate proximal fixation length is not immediately obtainable, the left subclavian artery can be crossed and excluded with little consequence to the patient (mean left arm pressure decreased with few symptoms); if the patient has a prior left internal mammary to coronary bypass, then left carotid to left subclavian bypass is required to maintain coronary circulation before coverage. Further encroachment into the arch generally requires salvage of the left common carotid circulation by prior carotid-carotid bypass. If excessive tortuosity is encountered in either fixation zone, a longer seal length of up to 30 mm may be necessary to prevent blood from escaping around the ends of the stent (type I endoleak). When multiple devices are required to cover long lengths of aortic pathology, each piece should be made to overlap 3 to 5 cm with the neighboring endograft. The distal aortic seal zone is usually cephalad to the celiac axis.

A common theme to complications of aortic endografting, whether abdominal aortic or thoracic aortic techniques, is the occurrence of damage to access vessels such as the common femoral or iliac arteries. Therefore if the measured diameter of an intended access vessel is demonstrated to be less than 8 mm, serious

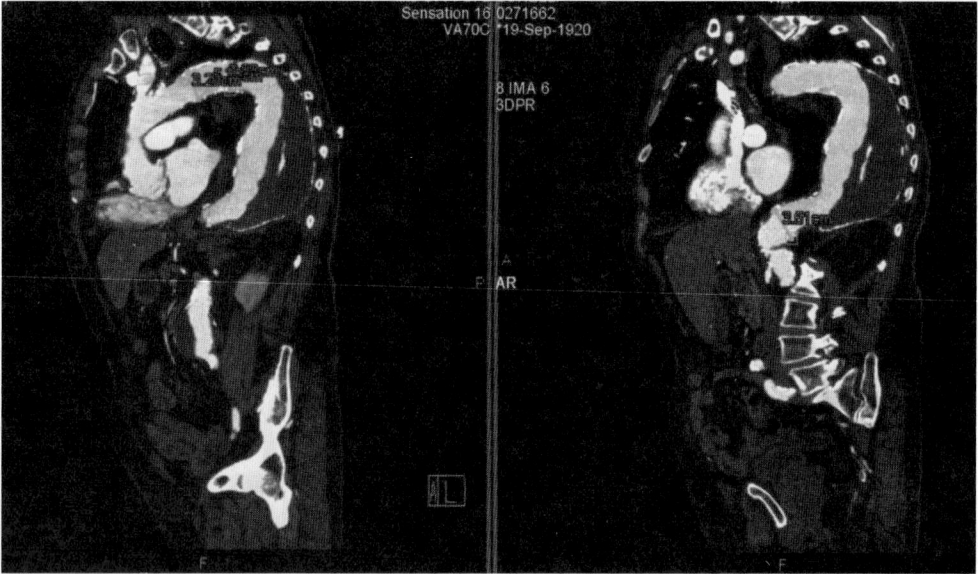

Figure 4   Three-dimensional reconstructions of computed tomography angiograms allow measurement of intended zones for "sealing" of the thoracic endografts. Tortuosity of the aortic segment may affect delivery of the device to the zone, as well as deployment.

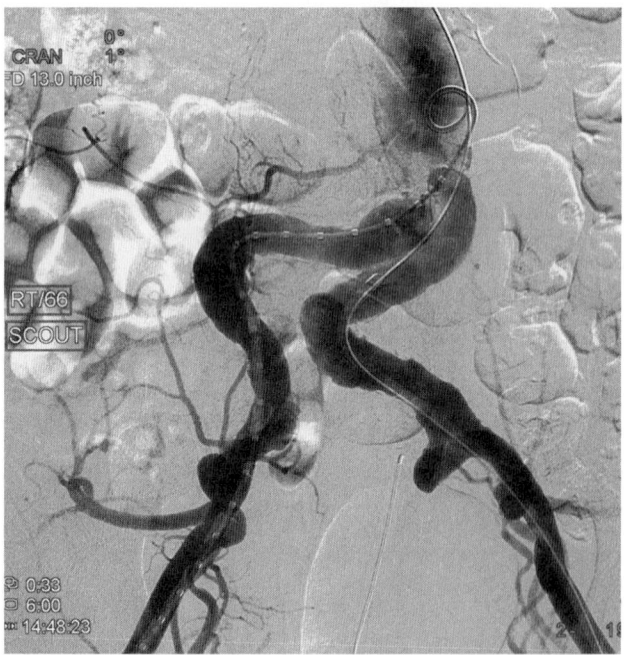

Figure 5   Tortuosity of iliac vessels may necessitate placement of Dacron conduits (to the common iliac or distal aorta) to introduce large-diameter sheaths necessary for device introduction. Calcification, particularly in a tortuous segment, may predispose to dissection and rupture.

consideration should be given to a surgical conduit. The 10-mm Dacron conduits are generally anastomosed to the common iliac or abdominal aorta through a miniflank incision with retroperitoneal exposure of the vessel (Fig. 5). In particular, severe calcification of an access vessel may elevate the risk of tear, perforation, dissection, or frank rupture. It is not uncommon for such iatrogenic injuries to become obvious when the device sheath is being withdrawn rather than with sheath insertion. As the device sheath is removed, the obturation of the injury is relieved and hemorrhage ensues.

PROCEDURAL TECHNIQUE OF THORACIC ENDOVASCULAR REPAIR

The procedure of aortic endografting for thoracic aortic pathologies should be performed in an operating room with a mandatory high-resolution digital imaging system and radiolucent table. Choice of anesthetic is generally based on preoperative cardiac risk stratification and may include local, epidural, or general anesthesia. The application of CSF drainage should be strongly considered when coverage of the entire thoracic aorta is planned or if a prior AAA repair has been performed. Grafts are inserted via cutdown on the intended access vessel—most commonly the right common femoral artery. Following this surgical exposure, systemic anticoagulation is achieved using heparin to maintain an activated clotting time greater than 250 seconds. An angiographic catheter is inserted percutaneously via the opposite common femoral artery or brachial artery to the level of the aortic arch. Using digital subtraction angiography, aortic arch or thoracic aortic angiography is performed to determine the approximate positioning of the endoprosthesis. To view the landing areas in the arch, it is often necessary to view the arch with a 45- to 90-degree left anterior oblique projection (Figs. 6 and 7).

To view the distal seal zone, a similar steep, near lateral projection will best depict the level of the celiac axis. To minimize manipulation, particularly in the arch, the final diagnostic studies before deployment should be performed with the device nearly in place; the stiffness of the wires and delivery systems may alter the aortic arch course and affect landmarks being used to mark the proximal limits of deployment. "Road-mapping" techniques or "fluoro-fade" may improve operator accuracy in proximal fixation. Maneuvers to minimize stroke during device delivery in proximity to the great vessels include flushing of all air from the device sheaths and lumens carefully. Manipulation of stiff wires into and from the arch should also be performed carefully under fluoroscopic guidance. After deployment, fixation should be improved using a large-diameter, compliant, occlusion balloon to maximize apposition of the stent graft to the aortic seal zones and regions of device overlap in a distal to proximal order. The access sheath is removed carefully with attention to mean arterial pressure as an early indicator of hemorrhage from iatrogenic

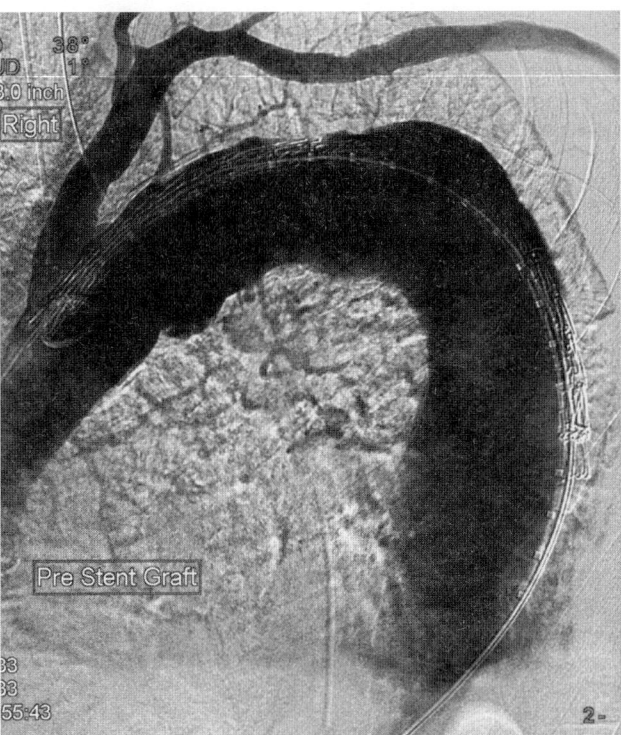

Figure 6 High-resolution angiography is key to proper placement of endografts to avoid inadvertent coverage of critical aortic branch vessels. Steep projection angles "lay out" the arch in most patients; the 38-degree left anterior oblique in this arch aortogram facilitates placement of first prosthesis.

insertion injury. If a tear in a vessel is suspected, the sheath can be reintroduced to obturate the injury. If the sheath will not pass, an occlusion balloon can be passed proximal to the injury and inflated to achieve vascular control. Frank transections usually require a flank incision and reconstruction, whereas small tears or dissections are often salvaged for endovascular stent placement without conversion.

JOHNS HOPKINS APPROACH TO THORACIC AORTIC STENT GRAFTING

Noting the preponderance of iatrogenic access injuries in industry trials, we liberally apply retroperitoneal conduits via a flank incision if iliac diameters are questionable (approximately 15%-20% patients). Most patients undergo general anesthesia both for flexibility of access approach and to avoid patient movement at critical imaging moments. The operations are performed in an endovascular operating room with a ceiling-mounted imaging device.

FUTURE DIRECTIONS OF THORACIC AND THORACOABDOMINAL AORTIC ANEURYSM REPAIR: "HYBRID PROCEDURES"

Impressive reductions in morbidity and mortality have been realized in the arena of complex aneurysm repair, especially in centers of excellence. However, diffusion and adoption of open surgical techniques of TAAA across centers has been difficult and may

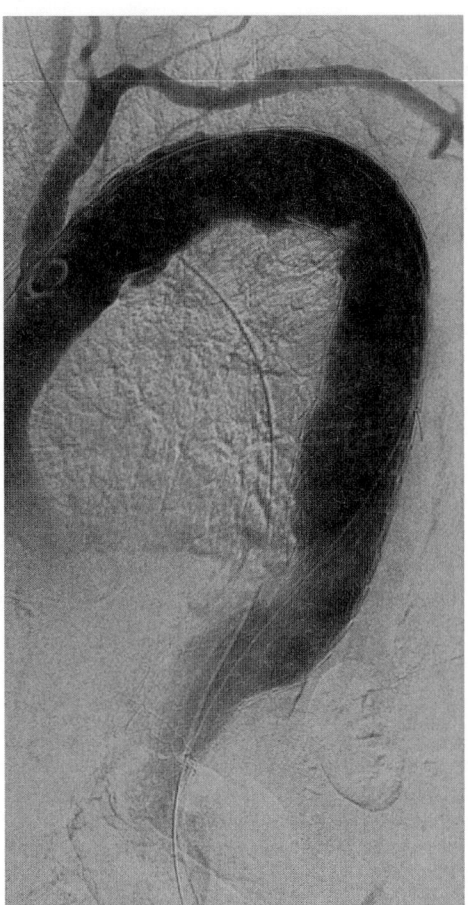

Figure 7 Completion angiogram of a thoracic aortic endovascular repair of a thoracic aortic aneurysm extending from left subclavian artery to the distal third of the thoracic aorta.

indicate that less stellar results are the norm. Indeed, audited data in the United Kingdom Cardiac Surgical Register, presented by Black and colleagues, revealed mortality for replacement of the descending thoracic aorta approaching 34%. The application of stent graft repair to the more complex TAAAs has been limited by the origin of the visceral vessels off the aneurysm itself. Single-center reports are now emerging that detail open techniques to ensure end-organ perfusion via surgical bypasses and subsequent stent-graft coverage of significant lengths of thoracoabdominal aorta. The results of these studies are summarized in Table 3. The key surgical aspects of the "hybrid" exclusions are the performance of individual bypasses to the visceral branches with ligation of the origins to prevent type II endoleak (branch vessel perfusion of aneurysm sac). In either the same procedure as the surgical revascularization or in a staged fashion days later, the endograft is inserted to cover the aneurysmal thoracoabdominal aorta. In reference to endovascular exclusion, proper fixation zones and substantial overlap of endoprostheses are mandatory to withstand the substantial hemodynamic forces present. In the series of Flye and Black, it was not uncommon for four to seven pieces to be placed in a single patient. As such, the occurrence of more type III endoleaks (perfusion into aneurysm sac between overlapping devices) can be expected, yet most of these would seem correctable with secondary "nonsurgical" endovascular procedures. Clearly, long-term data regarding device durability of this creative approach to extensive TAAAs are lacking, yet the complication rates (particularly spinal injury) compare favorably with series detailing open TAAA repair (Fig. 8).

Table 3: Results of "Hybrid" Thoracoabdominal Aortic Aneurysm (TAAA) Revascularization and Endovascular Repair

Author, Year	Patients (N)	Extent	F/U (mo)	30-Day Mort.	Type I or III Leak (%)	Complications (N)	Paraplegia (%)
Flye, 2004	3	III, IV, patch	11–21	0	33	TIA (1)	0
Fulton, 2005	10	IV (n = 2) jAAA (n = 8)	0–13	0	10% (I)	CV (7); pulm (9); GI (1)	0
Black, 2005	29	I (n = 3) II (n = 18) III (n = 7) IV (n = 1)	2–28	15%	23% (I) 4% (III)	CV (7); pulm (9); renal 4; GI (3)	0

CV, Cardiovascular; *GI*, gastrointestinal; *mo*, months; *mort.*, mortality; *pulm*, pulmonary; *TIA*, transient ischemic attack.

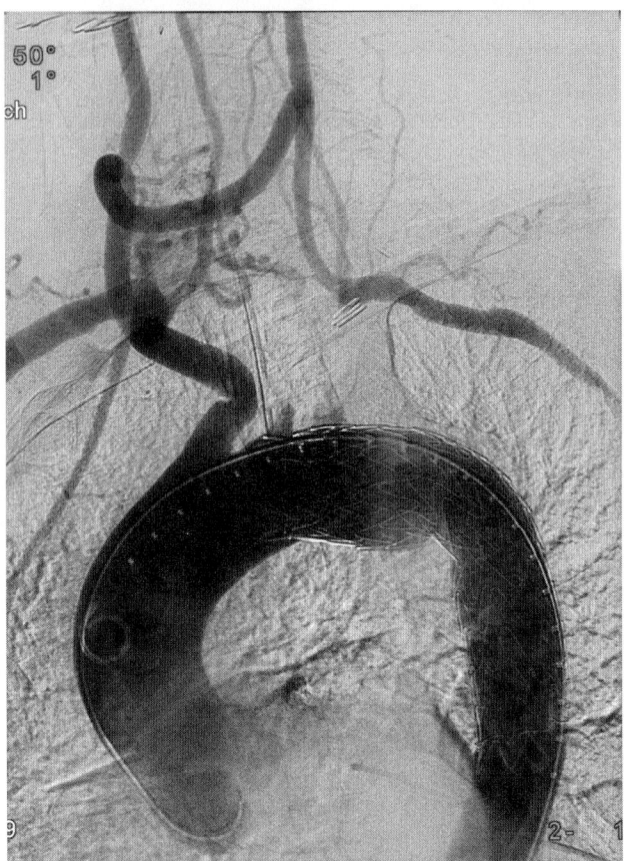

Figure 8 Completion angiography of a "hybrid" open/endovascular procedure to stent graft a thoracic aortic aneurysm involving the distal half of the aortic arch. Carotid-carotid and left-carotid-to-subclavian transposition isolates segment of arch for "seal" of proximal graft.

SUMMARY

Open surgical repair of TAA and TAAA is known to be durable with a low incidence of secondary aortic interventions. Graft-related complications per se, such as infection or anastomotic aneurysm, are rare; secondary aortic interventions occur in approximately 10% of patients after TAAA repair and are usually located in non-contiguous aortic segments. Although considerable progress has been made in diminishing the incidence and severity of renovisceral complications and spinal cord injury after TAA or TAAA repair, no strategy to date has eliminated these complications. Stent-graft therapy of the spectrum of thoracic aortic pathologies is a rapidly developing and emerging technology. Given satisfactory early and midterm results combined with the obvious avoidance of major cavitary incisions and the recovery thereafter, it is likely that thoracic aortic stent grafting will assume a role as primary therapy for aneurysms, dissections, and traumatic lesions or penetrating ulcers, particularly when isolated to the thoracic aorta. Not only have endovascular surgeons recognized the advantages of thoracic stent grafts, patients are now demanding consideration for such "minimally invasive" options. Open TAA repair may become reserved for cases in which anatomy and topography eliminate the viability of graft implantation. Requisite for any surgeon who desires to apply this technology to benefit patients are appropriate preoperative planning and imaging; a solid base of fundamental skill with catheter-based interventions; and the recognition of a need for regular, lifelong surveillance of all patients treated by thoracic aortic endografts. As comparative studies of open TAA repair and stent-graft repair emerge, endovascular repair will likely continue to demonstrate admirable reductions in overall perioperative morbidity and mortality with an assumed increased need for secondary aortic interventions. However, for some patients with TAAA at high risk for complications, variations in open surgical techniques to maintain end-organ perfusion and achieve "hybrid" endovascular reconstruction of TAAA may be a viable option in the future.

SUGGESTED READINGS

Black JH, Cambria RP: Current results of open surgical repair of descending thoracic aortic aneurysms, *J Vasc Surg* 43 (suppl A):6A, 2006.

Black JH, Davison JK, Cambria RP: Regional hypothermia with epidural cooling for prevention of spinal cord ischemic complications after thoracoabdominal aortic surgery, *Semin Thorac Cardiovasc Surg* 15:345, 2003.

Black SA, Wolfe JH, Clark M, and others: Complex thoracoabdominal aortic aneurysms: endovascular exclusion with visceral revascularization, *J Vasc Surg* 43:1081, 2006.

Cambria RP, Clouse WD, Davison JK, and others: Thoracoabdominal aneurysm repair: results with 337 operations performed over a 15-year interval, *Ann Surg* 236:471, 2002; discussion 479.

Clouse WD, Marone LK, Davison JK, and others: Late aortic and graft-related events after thoracoabdominal aneurysm repair, *J Vasc Surg* 37:254, 2003.

Coselli JS, Lemaire SA, Köksoy C, and others: Cerebrospinal fluid drainage reduces paraplegia after thoracoabdominal aortic aneurysm repair: results of a randomized clinical trial, *J Vasc Surg* 35:631, 2002.

Coselli JS, Lemaire SA, Miller CC 3rd, and others: Mortality and paraplegia after thoracoabdominal aortic aneurysm repair: a risk factor analysis, *Ann Thorac Surg* 69:409, 2002.

Cowan JA, Dimick JB, Jenke PK, and others: Surgical treatment of intact thoracoabdominal aortic aneurysms in the United States: Hospital and surgeon volume-related outcomes, *J Vasc Surg* 37:1169, 2003.

Elefteriades JA: Natural history of thoracic aortic aneurysms: indications for surgery, and surgical versus nonsurgical risks, *Ann Thorac Surg* 74:S1877, discussion S1892, 2002.

Safi HJ, Estrera AL, Miller CC, and others: Evolution of risk for neurologic deficit after descending and thoracoabdominal aortic repair, *Ann Thor Surg* 80:2173, 2005.

Svensson LG, Crawford ES, Hess KR, and others: Experience with 1509 patients undergoing thoracoabdominal aortic operations, *J Vasc Surg* 17:357, discussion 368, 1993.

ACUTE AORTIC DISSECTION AND ITS COMPLICATIONS

Thomas Reifsnyder, MD, and Robert Garvin, MD

INTRODUCTION

Acute aortic dissection ranges from a relatively benign, medically treated condition to one that can be rapidly fatal even when diagnosed and treated expeditiously. With aortic arch involvement, the mortality rate approaches 1% per hour, mandating rapid assessment and management. Although the treatment of acute ascending aortic dissection frequently requires the skill set of the cardiothoracic surgeon, the general or vascular surgeon may be called on to manage acute descending aortic dissections or to treat ischemic complications of the cerebral or visceral vessels or those of the extremities. Coincident with a better understanding of this disease, novel, minimally invasive therapies have evolved to treat both the dissection process itself and the resultant malperfusion syndromes. The appropriate selection and use of medical therapy, surgical intervention, and endovascular techniques are leading to improvements in the morbidity and mortality of this challenging disease process.

CLASSIFICATION

There are two frequently used classification systems for acute aortic dissections: DeBakey and Stanford. The DeBakey classification uses four categories determined by the origin and extent of the dissection (Fig. 1). DeBakey types I and IIIB most frequently lead to branch vessel complications. The Stanford system classifies dissections into those that do or do not involve the ascending aorta. Stanford type A (DeBakey I and II) dissections involve the ascending aorta and comprise approximately 60% of all dissections. The other 40% are type B (DeBakey IIIa and IIIb), which begin in the descending thoracic aorta distal to the left subclavian artery and extend distally.

PRESENTATION AND DIAGNOSIS

Acute aortic dissection is accompanied by the abrupt onset of the "worst pain ever" in nearly 90% of cases. Type A dissections more commonly present with anterior chest wall pain, whereas type B dissections typically present with midscapular or back pain. In either case, the pain is most often described as sharp, ripping, or tearing. On presentation, up to 30% of patients have symptoms of a malperfusion syndrome involving the cerebral, spinal or visceral vessels or those of the extremities (Fig. 2). Patients who present with acute stroke have a particularly devastating outcome, with 45% to 100% mortality in selected series even with expedient surgical intervention. Nearly three fourths of patients with type B dissections present with hypertension, compared with approximately 25% of patients with type A dissections. Occasionally patients may present with hypotension, an ominous sign that indicates one or more of the following: acute aortic rupture, aortic valve regurgitation, acute coronary occlusion, or pericardial tamponade.

In a patient suspected of harboring an acute aortic dissection, evaluation of the entire aorta using thin-slice computed tomography (CT) with intravenous contrast is the study of choice. The current generation of multidetector helical CT scanners makes possible rapid and accurate localization of the origin and extent of the dissection. The identification of a crescent-shaped

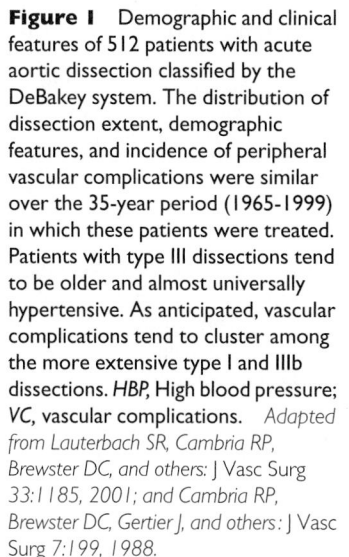

Figure 1 Demographic and clinical features of 512 patients with acute aortic dissection classified by the DeBakey system. The distribution of dissection extent, demographic features, and incidence of peripheral vascular complications were similar over the 35-year period (1965-1999) in which these patients were treated. Patients with type III dissections tend to be older and almost universally hypertensive. As anticipated, vascular complications tend to cluster among the more extensive type I and IIIb dissections. *HBP*, High blood pressure; *VC*, vascular complications. *Adapted from Lauterbach SR, Cambria RP, Brewster DC, and others: J Vasc Surg 33:1185, 2001; and Cambria RP, Brewster DC, Gertier J, and others: J Vasc Surg 7:199, 1988.*

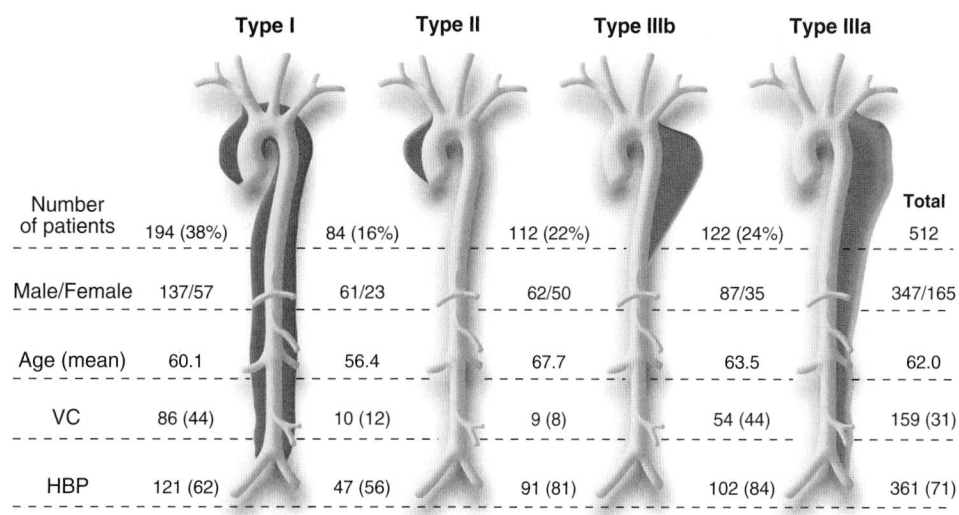

	Type I	Type II	Type IIIb	Type IIIa	Total
Number of patients	194 (38%)	84 (16%)	112 (22%)	122 (24%)	512
Male/Female	137/57	61/23	62/50	87/35	347/165
Age (mean)	60.1	56.4	67.7	63.5	62.0
VC	86 (44)	10 (12)	9 (8)	54 (44)	159 (31)
HBP	121 (62)	47 (56)	91 (81)	102 (84)	361 (71)

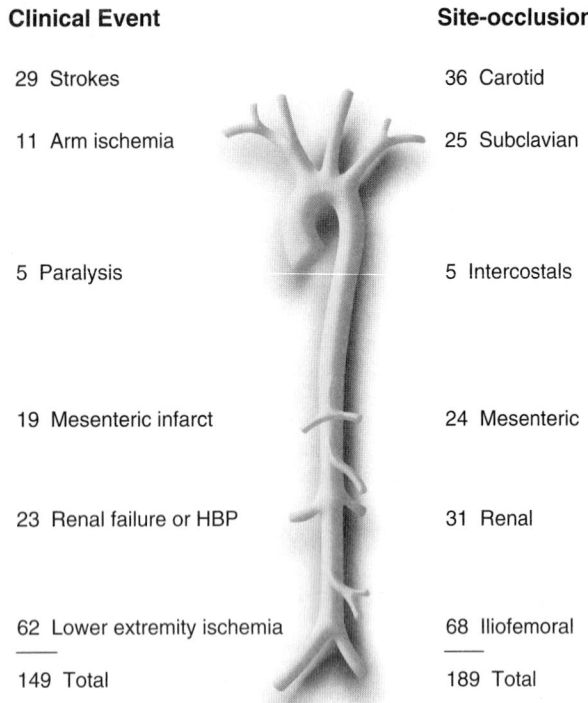

Clinical Event	Site-occlusion
29 Strokes	36 Carotid
11 Arm ischemia	25 Subclavian
5 Paralysis	5 Intercostals
19 Mesenteric infarct	24 Mesenteric
23 Renal failure or HBP	31 Renal
62 Lower extremity ischemia	68 Iliofemoral
149 Total	189 Total

Figure 2 Distribution of peripheral vascular complications in 512 patients over 35-year period (1965-1999). Peripheral vascular complications are classified by aortic branch site. Differences between site occlusions and clinical events represent asymptomatic occlusions. *HBP,* High blood pressure. *From Rutherford RB:* Vascular surgery, *ed 6, Philadelphia, 2005, Elsevier.*

septation with a narrow, slitlike true lumen (true-lumen-diameter-to-false-lumen-diameter ratio <0.4) increases the likelihood of a malperfusion syndrome. Identification of aortic root involvement, aortic valve regurgitation, pericardial tamponade, coronary artery involvement, and aortic arch involvement is crucial and sometimes requires the adjunctive use of transesophageal echocardiography (TEE). However, TEE should be reserved as an adjunct to CT and is best employed intraoperatively. Although aortography was at one time the gold standard for diagnosis, it is currently used only in conjunction with endovascular treatment and has been abandoned in the acute setting in lieu of rapid and accurate assessment by CT.

MEDICAL MANAGEMENT OF DISSECTIONS

Any patient with a tentative diagnosis of acute aortic dissection should be started immediately on aggressive antihypertensive therapy. Intravenous beta-blockers are administered first to lower the heart rate, decrease the force of ventricular contraction, and blunt the catecholamine response. After successful beta-blockade, a vasodilator such as sodium nitroprusside should be added. Data from the IRAD (International Registry of Acute Aortic Dissection) study reveals a mortality rate of 58% for medically treated type A dissections, and thus a surgical approach is mandated in the treatment of these patients. In the same study, type B dissections treated medically had an overall mortality of 10.7%, but this figure increased to 31.4% for the subgroup of patients with type B dissections that required operative intervention.

MANAGEMENT OF TYPE A DISSECTIONS

Details of the operative approach, which are outside the scope of this chapter, can be found in most cardiothoracic texts. Traditionally, patients have been placed on cardiopulmonary bypass with severe hypothermic (15°-20°C) circulatory arrest. The operative goal is to replace the ascending aorta and aortic arch with reimplantation of the arch vessels; resection of the area of intimal tear; elimination of false lumen flow distally; and, if necessary, replacement of the aortic root and aortic valve with reimplantation of the coronary vessels. Large series have shown that aortic valve replacement can be avoided in 80% of type A repairs. In cases of type A dissection that present with malperfusion syndromes, recent reports indicate that the best results are obtained by a staged approach with revascularization of the compromised viscera first, followed by reconstruction of the arch. Although earlier reports suggested that proceeding directly to arch repair could improve malperfusion of the viscera by eliminating the point of intimal tear and false lumen flow, current data suggest that this is a risky maneuver and should be avoided.

MANAGEMENT OF TYPE B DISSECTONS

Patients with type B dissections should be started on immediate medical therapy with beta-blockers and vasodilators. Patients should be admitted to an intensive care unit and should have continuous invasive blood pressure monitoring. Approximately 65% of patients will initially be refractory to medical management of hypertension, raising the suspicion for renal artery compromise; however, studies have shown true compromise of the renal arteries to be uncommon, and continued aggressive antihypertensive medication is warranted until adequate blood pressure control is achieved. Serial examinations and laboratory data are used to monitor the patient for complications of dissection, including acute aortic rupture and malperfusion syndromes. Patients often experience relief of their pain after appropriate pharmacologic management is instituted. Patients who have return of pain after initial response to medical therapy or who fail to achieve adequate pain relief should be reevaluated with helical CT to rule out progression of the dissection process. About 65% of patients with type B dissections will have return of pain, prompting further imaging. However, without evidence of extension of the dissection on CT, continuing nonoperative therapy is warranted.

Despite optimal medical management, approximately 30% of patients fail medical therapy. There are three firm indications for operative therapy in patients with type B dissections: malperfusion syndrome, aortic rupture or impending rupture, and dissection in the setting of a preexisting degenerative aneurysm. Overall the mortality rate for patients with type B dissections who are treated surgically remains high and can approach 20% in contemporary series. Recent published series of endovascular repair of type B dissections have demonstrated marked improvements in operative and 30-day mortalities.

The approach to open surgical therapy depends on the indication for surgery. For acute aortic rupture or impending rupture (acute aneurysm formation at the point of intimal tear), the operative approach is directed at tube graft replacement of the involved segment of descending thoracic aorta through a left posterolateral thoracotomy. The distal aorta can be perfused using left heart bypass or femorofemoral bypass to prevent ischemia to the spinal cord and viscera during aortic cross clamping. Tacking of the distal flap using felt pledgets on both the intimal and adventitial sides should suffice to limit flow in the false lumen (Fig. 3). It is unnecessary to attempt replacement of the entire involved aorta

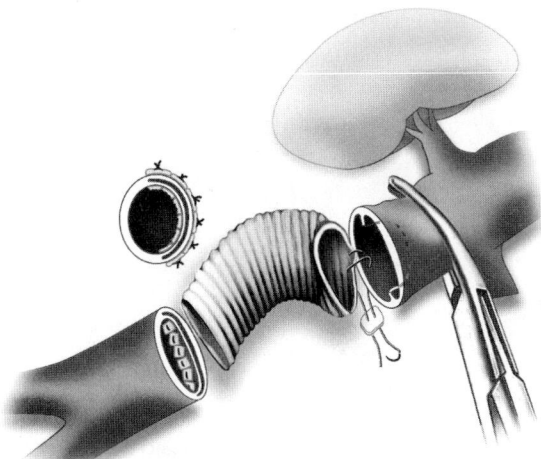

Figure 3 Technique of surgical abdominal aortic fenestration. When confined to the infrarenal aortic segment, the septum is excised up to the aortic cross clamp. The proximal anastomosis is performed with pledgetted 4-0 sutures as the anastomosis is extended to the remaining adventitia over the dissection aortic circumference. The distal anastomosis is created by reconstituting the distal aortic layers with a felt composite. *From Rutherford RB: Vascular surgery, ed 6, Philadelphia, 2005, Elsevier.*

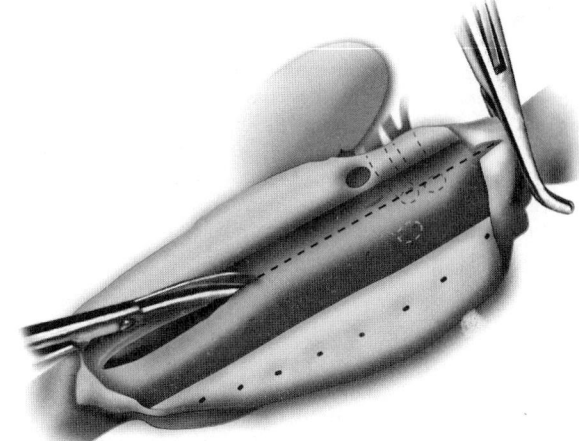

Figure 4 If static obstruction of the renal or visceral vessels is suspected on the basis of axial imaging studies, the fenestration can be carried onto the visceral aortic segment. The left kidney has been swept anteriorly, and the left renal artery is perfused from the false lumen. The septum is incised to expose the origins of the celiac/superior mesenteric/right renal artery perfused via the true lumen. *From Rutherford RB: Vascular surgery, ed 6, Philadelphia, 2005, Elsevier.*

because this is associated with increased mortality with no clear benefit to the patient. If the indication for surgery is a malperfusion syndrome, the operative approach consists of wide access to the thoracoabdominal aorta through a left thoracoabdominal incision. The patient is placed on partial bypass, and the involved aortic segment is opened with a long aortotomy (Figs. 4, 5, and 6). Using this approach, the dissected intimal flap is excised to allow unfettered perfusion to the visceral vessels.

MANAGEMENT OF MALPERFUSION SYNDROMES

When acute aortic dissections are complicated by branch vessel compromise, morbidity and mortality rates increase, particularly in the face of mesenteric ischemia. Management of these complications should take priority over other concerns. There are two mechanisms that contribute to the diminution of flow to branch vessels. The first is a process called *static obstruction,* in which the false lumen dissects into the branch vessel. This process may

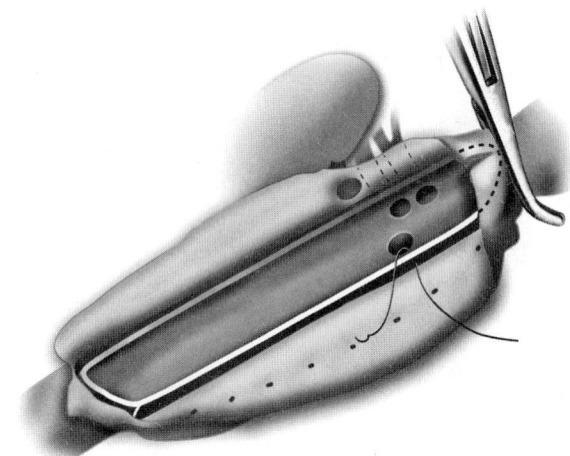

Figure 5 Direct suture repair of the vessel ostium may be required, here shown at the right renal origin, the orifice of which abuts the circumferential terminus of the dissection. *From Rutherford RB: Vascular surgery, ed 6, Philadelphia, 2005, Elsevier.*

Figure 6 After septectomy in the visceral segment, the outer aortic wall is closed over Teflon felt and the clamp is moved to the infrarenal aorta, which is most conveniently reconstructed with a tube graft. *From Rutherford RB: Vascular surgery, ed 6, Philadelphia, 2005, Elsevier.*

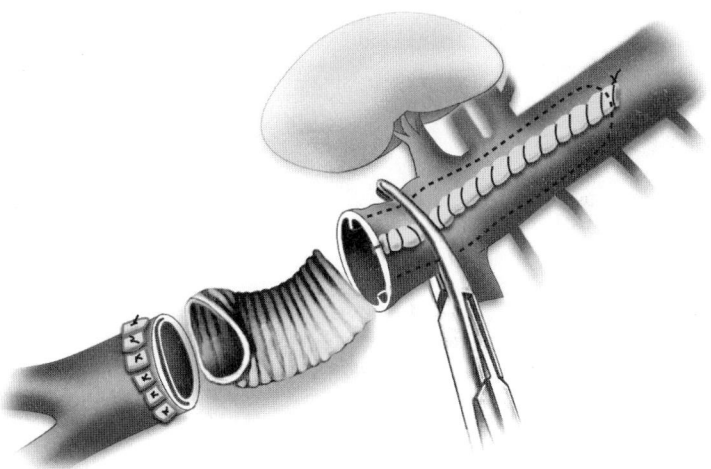

partially obstruct the lumen or completely occlude it, with resultant thrombosis (Fig. 7). The second mechanism, called *dynamic obstruction,* is a process that occurs when the inherent forces in the dissected vessel wall favor radial expansion of the false lumen, thereby reducing the diameter of the true lumen. This process essentially creates a flap valve that covers the branch vessel orifice (Figs. 8 and 9). Diagnosis of this process can be difficult because the malperfusion phenomenon becomes subject to change as the hemodynamic parameters of the patient change. The goal of treatment of malperfusion syndromes is to restore flow to the compromised vessels expeditiously. This can be accomplished surgically, as described earlier, or by using endovascular techniques.

ENDOVASCULAR THERAPIES

At the time of this writing, dramatic changes are being made in the management paradigm of acute type B dissections. The first two reports of endovascular treatment of aortic dissection were published in 1999. The current body of literature is small but points toward effectively treating type B dissections with covered

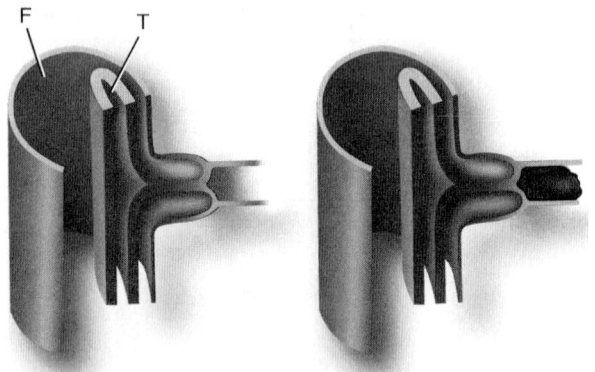

Figure 7 Near-complete circumferential dissection with static obstruction; the cleavage plan of the dissection extends into the ostium and compromises inflow. Thrombosis beyond the compromised ostia may worsen perfusion further. *From Rutherford RB: Vascular surgery, ed 6, Philadelphia, 2005, Elsevier.*

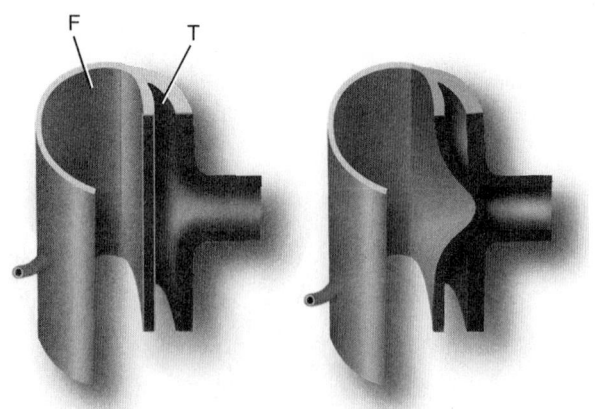

Figure 8 Mechanisms of aortic branch obstruction in acute dissection. In dynamic obstruction, the septum may prolapse onto the vessel ostium during the cardiac cycle, and the compressed true lumen flow is inadequate to perfuse branch vessel ostia, which remain anatomically intact. *From Rutherford RB: Vascular surgery, ed 6, Philadelphia, 2005, Elsevier.*

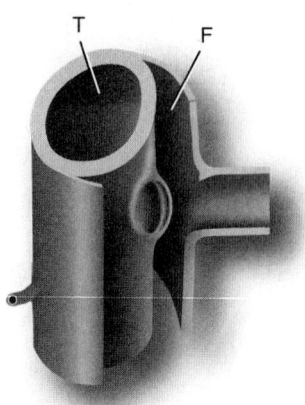

Figure 9 Spontaneous perfusion of aortic branches perfused from the false lumen occurs if the dissection process tears the ostia away from the true lumen. Such spontaneous "fenestrations" may account for persistent false lumen flow. *F,* False lumen; *T,* true lumen. *From Rutherford RB: Vascular surgery, ed 6, Philadelphia, 2005, Elsevier.*

stents or a combination of covered and bare metal stents. The first objective is to stop false lumen flow by sealing the proximal intimal tear with a covered stent or thoracic endograft. The remainder of the aorta may require formal thoracic endografting. However, when there has been no aneurysm formation, the effective use of bare metal stents distal to the sealed intimal tear is currently being investigated. Accurate localization of the intimal tear may require adjunctive use of intravascular ultrasound in addition to high-quality arteriography. In addition, both femoral and brachial artery access is frequently required to gain access to the true lumen. Occasionally the orifice of the left subclavian artery must be sacrificed to cover adequately the point of intimal tear. Sacrificing flow to the left subclavian artery can be safely achieved if the contralateral vertebral artery is patent. If not, a left carotid-subclavian bypass should precede placement of the endograft. Benefits of endovascular treatment of type B dissections include improved short-term morbidity and mortality compared with open techniques, as well as an anticipated lower risk of subsequent aneurysmal degeneration of the false lumen, which otherwise occurs in up to 40% of patients treated medically.

Endovascular therapies may also be used to treat malperfusion syndromes; however, treatment of the proximal intimal tear site and dissected thoracic aorta may obviate the need for direct treatment of the compromised visceral or lower extremity vessels. If treatment of compromised branch vessels is necessary, the two main techniques used are stenting and fenestration. Both of these are technically challenging, and liberal use of multiple arterial access sites is required. For stenting, the proximal nondissected aorta should be accessed through a brachial approach into the true lumen to identify compromised flow in the aortic side branches of interest. After it is identified, wire access should be obtained and secured into the compromised vessel, followed by stent deployment. Endovascular fenestration of the intimal flap will then equalize the pressure in both the true and false lumens. Fenestration can be accomplished using large angioplasty balloons expanded over a wire that has been used to perforate the intimal flap. Alternatively, the scissors technique can be used. This technique involves passing stiff wires into both lumens from a single femoral approach. A single stiff sheath is then advanced over both wires simultaneously to tear the intimal flap carefully in linear fashion. Although these techniques can be used to restore flow to compromised vessels, the long-term outcome is uncertain because of continued false lumen flow and the potential for subsequent aneurysmal degeneration.

With the current explosion of minimally invasive endovascular techniques, the treatment algorithm for uncomplicated acute descending thoracic aortic dissections is under assault. The standard of care has been aggressive antihypertensive medical therapy as initial intervention, reserving surgical intervention as salvage therapy for medical treatment failure. However, even when successful, medical treatment leads to a substantial incidence of late aneurysm formation. Endovascular repair in the acute phase of the initially uncomplicated dissection can re-create the normal integrity of the thoracic aorta and may prevent both early and late complications. A prospective randomized trial of early endovascular repair versus medical management is necessary to ultimately determine the optimal therapy.

CONCLUSIONS

Acute aortic dissection remains a highly challenging disease. Traditionally, surgical intervention has been reserved for involvement of the ascending aorta and for medical treatment failure or complications of descending aortic dissections. These operations are highly demanding and even in the best hands have considerable morbidity and mortality. With the advent of advanced endovascular techniques, the treatment of type B dissections is changing radically. We may be approaching the time when we preemptively treat type B dissections with endovascular techniques instead of reserving surgical and endovascular interventions for salvage therapy in patients who have failed medical management. Furthermore, early minimally invasive intervention may prevent delayed aneurysm formation.

SUGGESTED READINGS

Black JH, Cambria RP: Aortic dissection: perspectives for the vascular/endovascular surgeon. In Rutherford RB, editor: *Vascular surgery*, ed 6, Philadelphia, 2005, WB Saunders, p. 1512.

Greenberg RK: The management of acute aortic dissections. In Zelenock GB, Huber TS, and others, editors: *Mastery of vascular and endovascular surgery*, Philadelphia, 2006, Lippincott Williams & Wilkins, p. 95.

Iyer VS, Kent SM, Tse LW, and others: Early outcomes after elective and emergent endovascular repair of the thoracic aorta, *J Vasc Surg* 43:677, 2006.

Lauterbach SR, Cambria RP, Brewster DC, and others: Contemporary management of aortic branch compromise resulting from acute aortic dissection, *J Vasc Surg* 33:1185, 2001.

Roseborough G, Burke J, Sperry J, and others: Twenty-year experience with acute distal thoracic aortic dissections, *J Vasc Surg* 40:235, 2004.

POPLITEAL AND FEMORAL ARTERY ANEURYSMS

William C. Krupski

Popliteal and femoral artery aneurysms are the most common sites for peripheral arterial aneurysms. The incidence of all types of these aneurysms in hospitalized men is 7.4 per 100,000 persons and 1.0 per 100,000 persons in hospitalized women. Improved and increased use of imaging modalities along with aging of the population has led to increased recognition of these disorders. In recent series, that ratio of abdominal aortic aneurysms (AAAs) to peripheral aneurysms ranges between 15:1 and 8:1 Approximately 3% of individuals with aortoiliac aneurysms have peripheral aneurysms. Whereas the male to female ratio for AAAs is approximately 5:1, that ratio for peripheral aneurysms is greater than 30:1. Prevalence of peripheral arterial aneurysms peaks during the sixth and seventh decades of life. As with all aneurysms, complications include thrombosis, embolization, compression of adjacent structures, and rupture.

For practical purposes, both the popliteal and femoral arteries are considered to be aneurysmal if their external diameter exceeds 2 cm. True aneurysms involve all vessel wall layers, whereas false (pseudo-) aneurysms develop from a defect in the arterial wall or the site of an anastomosis; false aneurysms are encapsulated hematomas that communicate with the arterial lumen. Degenerative (previously termed *atherosclerotic*) popliteal artery aneurysms account for 70% of such peripheral lesions. Approximately one half of popliteal artery aneurysms are bilateral, and an AAA is present in one quarter to one third of patients with a unilateral popliteal aneurysm, and in up to one half of patients with bilateral popliteal aneurysms.

Although the femoral artery is the third most common location for degenerative peripheral aneurysms, this is nevertheless a rare condition. However, when all types of aneurysms are considered (true, false, infected, and nonspecific), the femoral artery is the most common site for this ailment. True femoral artery aneurysms are isolated to the common femoral artery approximately 40% of the time, involve the femoral bifurcation slightly more than half the time, and are isolated to the superficial or profunda femoris arteries less than 5% of the time. The incidence of bilateral femoral aneurysms ranges widely from 20% to 70%. Approximately 85% of patients with a true aneurysm of the femoral artery have a coexistent AAA, and one half of patients with a femoral artery aneurysm have a coexistent popliteal aneurysm. The high frequency of contemporaneous aneurysms justifies ultrasound screening of patients with a peripheral aneurysm for other central or peripheral aneurysms. Although degenerative femoral aneurysms are unusual, as diagnostic and therapeutic percutaneous interventions via the femoral artery have become increasingly common, iatrogenic pseudoaneurysms have become commonly encountered problems. Anastomotic aneurysms of the common femoral artery are also common. Finally, use of the femoral artery for injection of illicit drugs may lead to infected (mycotic) aneurysms; the femoral artery has replaced the central arteries as the most common site of an infected aneurysm.

POPLITEALANEURYSMS

Popliteal aneurysms have a long and colorful history. This condition often affected coachmen in eighteenth century England, and because they were easily accessible for palpation and surgical exposure, they were the first aneurysms to be diagnosed and treated in contemporary medical history. After observing regeneration of deer antlers and changes in blood flow associated with molting, John Hunter applied the principles of collateral blood vessel development to the treatment of popliteal aneurysms by ligation of the arteries above and below the aneurysm. During past centuries, management has evolved from ligation, intraluminal wiring, endoaneurysmorrhaphy, excision with sympathectomy, exclusion or bypass using autologous or prosthetic grafts, and endovascular repair with endoluminal stent grafts.

Pathogenesis

Patients with degenerative popliteal artery aneurysms commonly have generalized dilatation and elongation of their arteries, suggesting a systemic abnormality. Although atherosclerosis is usually present in these patients, this may be a coincidental factor in the age group affected rather than etiologic. If atherosclerosis is causative, it may be related to atrophy of atherosclerotic plaques, producing thin arterial walls that fail to resist increasing wall tension leading to aneurysm development; indeed, aneurysms occur in an experimental primate model of regression of atherosclerotic plaques when dietary cholesterol is reduced. Increased proteolytic activity of elastase and collagenase has also been implicated. Additional hypotheses relate to genetic factors (e.g., male predominance) or mechanical features of the artery (e.g., arterial wall vibration because of fixation at the adductor hiatus or extrinsic stress from knee flexion and extension). Nonspecific popliteal aneurysms may occur because of collagen vascular disorders, popliteal entrapment syndrome, and blunt or penetrating trauma.

Clinical Presentation

One third to one half of patients are asymptomatic at the time of diagnosis. When patients become symptomatic, they most commonly present with acute lower extremity ischemia caused by thrombosis or embolism. Occasionally, patients describe progressive claudication caused by recurrent thromboembolism. The so-called "blue toe syndrome" can occur because of recurrent embolization to the digital arteries (Fig. 1). Less commonly, patients present with local symptoms such as sensation of a mass, compression of adjacent veins with swelling or deep venous thrombosis, impingement of nearby nerves, or impaired mobility of the knee joint. Acute expansion and rupture occur in less than 5% of popliteal aneurysms, and hemorrhage is usually confined to the popliteal space and is typically limb threatening but not life threatening. Symptoms of acute rupture are usually nonspecific and consist of severe pain, local skin discoloration, peroneal nerve palsy, lower extremity ischemia, and swelling caused by accumulation of blood in conjunction with vein compression or deep venous thrombosis. A history of smoking, hypertension, and cardiac disease is often present in patients with popliteal artery aneurysms.

Diagnosis

Because the popliteal pulse is somewhat difficult to appreciate in most normal individuals, a popliteal aneurysm should be suspected when prominent pulsation can be felt in the popliteal or subsartorial space during physical examination. If the popliteal artery has occluded, a firm pulseless mass may be found behind the knee, often in the presence of a contralateral palpable popliteal aneurysm with good pedal pulses. Imaging studies are necessary to confirm existence of a popliteal aneurysm, to exclude other pathology such as a Baker's cyst, and to provide critical information about the size, extent, presence of mural thrombus, and condition of runoff vessels. Plain roentgenograms of the knee are not often useful, although they occasionally demonstrate calcium in the aneurysm wall. Color duplex scanning is a rapid, inexpensive, and accurate study that is ideal for serial measurements of size and thrombus when observational management is selected (Fig. 2). Computed tomography and magnetic resonance imaging provide similar information but are more expensive and unsuitable for screening tests. As for all aneurysms, arteriography may not confirm the presence of popliteal aneurysms because they reveal only the lumen of the artery that can appear relatively normal when mural thrombus is present (Fig. 3). However, contrast arteriography or magnetic

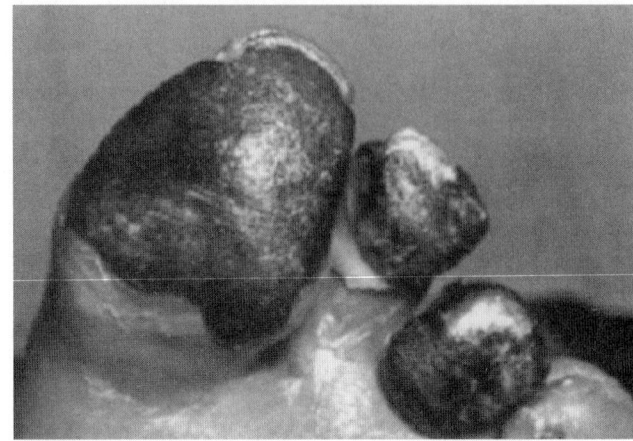

Figure 1 Gangrene of distal toes after embolization of debris from a popliteal aneurysm (the evolution of the "blue toe syndrome").

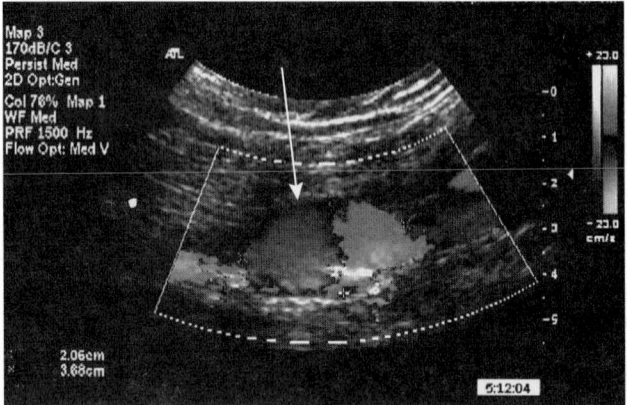

Figure 2 Color duplex scan of 3.5-cm fusiform popliteal aneurysm (*arrow*); color change indicates turbulent blood flow.

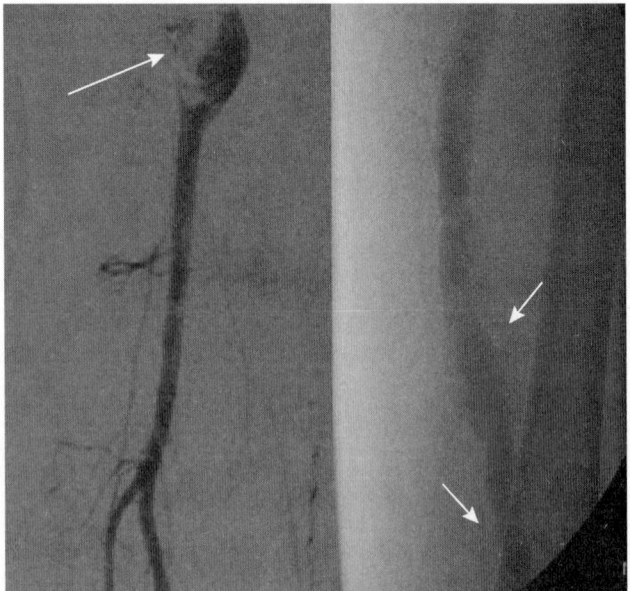

Figure 3 (**A**) Discrete fusiform aneurysm of proximal popliteal artery with interaluminal thrombus (*arrow*) but good runoff vessels. (**B**) Diffuse aneurysmal change of superficial femoral and popliteal arteries; *arrows* point to thin rim of calcium present in aneurysm wall, which is substantially larger than intraluminal contrast.

resonance arteriography (MRA) is essential for planning surgical repair or catheter-based interventions.

Natural History

In contrast to AAAs, there are few reliable natural history studies for popliteal aneurysms. Most published series consist primarily of popliteal aneurysms treated surgically. Rates of thromboembolic complications vary widely, ranging from 8% to 100%. A Markov decision tree constructed for popliteal aneurysms suggests that asymptomatic lesions become symptomatic at a rate of 14% per year, but this is based on extrapolated data. Another collective review of 29 reports in the English literature reviewing 2445 popliteal aneurysms in 1673 patients reported a mean of 35% of patients developed complications when followed by observation, and mean amputation rate was 25% despite attempted repair. In one retrospective study, 42 patients with asymptomatic popliteal artery aneurysms were followed by observation alone to identify variables predicting the risk of complications. The average size of the aneurysms was 3.1 cm; 18 of the 42 limbs in which an asymptomatic popliteal aneurysm was present had abnormal ankle-brachial indices (ABIs). Average follow-up was 6.2 years. Twenty-five patients (60%) developed complications at a mean observation time of 18 months. Three patients lost the limb, eight developed claudication, two required fasciotomy and one had a peroneal nerve palsy. The cumulative risk of developing some complication during follow-up was 24% at 1 year, rising to 68% at 5 years; however, the long-term major amputation rate was only 16%—or 2.4% per year. Another 20-year review of 147 popliteal aneurysms reported a 50% death rate at 5.7 years compared with 14 years for an age-matched population. Surgical intervention for popliteal aneurysms is often associated with general and local morbidity, including cardiac and pulmonary complications in these older individuals. Adverse outcomes after surgery include chronic edema, neuropathic pain, phlebitis, and graft thrombosis, sometimes producing limb-threatening ischemia in a previously asymptomatic individual.

Management

Asymptomatic Popliteal Aneurysms

Because the natural history of popliteal aneurysms is uncertain, management of asymptomatic lesions is controversial. Advocates of observational management emphasize the older age of most patients with this disorder; the many comorbidities encountered in such patients; their shortened life expectancies; reported patency rates for bypasses in these patients of 70% to 94% (average 80%), with subsequent profound ischemia in previously *asymptomatic* individuals (*primum non nocere*); relatively rare occurrence of *severe* sequelae (amputation rates of only 2.4% per year); and the high success rate of thrombolytic therapy combined with revascularization *if* thromboembolism occurs. Traditionally, a threshold size of 2 cm was considered by many to warrant operative intervention in good-risk asymptomatic patients, but even that benchmark has been questioned. Several recent reports have found that popliteal aneurysms less than 3 cm in diameter can safely be observed because very few (or in some accounts, no) popliteal aneurysms less than 3 cm thrombosed or became symptomatic. Anticoagulation of patients with popliteal aneurysms has not been effective in preventing complications.

Advocates of operative repair of asymptomatic popliteal aneurysms justify their aggressive approach by highlighting the eventual development of *some* symptoms in up to one third to one half of asymptomatic patients in several series, high complication and amputation rates once symptoms develop, and 5-year patency rates of only 65% (range 50% to 80%) for bypasses in symptomatic patients, which are inferior to patency rates in asymptomatic patients.

A compromise between serial observation and routine operative repair is a *selective* approach for patients with asymptomatic popliteal aneurysms. When life expectancy is low or operative risk is extremely high, a conservative approach is chosen. Availability of adequate and good-quality autogenous conduit for bypass or interposition grafting is also taken into account. Then, an attempt is made to identify aneurysms at high or low risk for development of complications. Features warranting consideration of operative repair include diameter greater than 3 cm, large amounts of mural thrombus or unstable thrombus on real-time duplex imaging, evidence of silent embolization with loss of runoff vessels, aneurysms with a great deal of distortion, distortion of popliteal arteries above or below the aneurysm, or evidence of unstable biologic behavior by complications that develop in one of two bilateral aneurysms. To date, however, these guidelines have not been substantiated in prospective studies.

Symptomatic Popliteal Aneurysms

When popliteal aneurysms become symptomatic, the likelihood of limb loss increases and operative repair should be undertaken. The most imperative surgical indication is acute ischemia from thrombosis or embolization. Any manifestation of peripheral thromboembolism (e.g., progressive claudication, blue toe syndrome) is an indication for exclusion and bypass of the aneurysm. Patients with compression of adjacent nerves and veins also should be treated surgically, as should patients with proven or suspected infected aneurysms. When patients present with stable compensated peripheral arterial insufficiency caused by an occluded popliteal aneurysm, operative aneurysm exclusion is not required because the risk of additional deterioration from thromboembolism is gone.

Operative Technique

As with all vascular reconstructions, the operative strategy must be individualized and tailored to the patient's anatomy. The extent, location, and patency of the aneurysm must be determined by appropriate preoperative imaging studies. When patients present with acute ischemia caused by thrombosis or thromboembolism, preoperative percutaneous intraarterial thrombolysis with tissue plasminogen activator or urokinase, sometimes in combination with catheter-based mechanical thrombectomy devices ("clot busters"), can improve limb salvage and graft patency. Most authorities believe catheter-based thrombolysis and percutaneous thrombectomy are better than operative thrombectomy using a Fogarty catheter. There is some evidence that thrombolysis produces more gradual reperfusion of the lower extremity and may result in fewer instances of compartment syndrome. Adverse outcomes associated with this approach relate to the large clot burden within the aneurysm leading to prolonged intraarterial infusion times, requirements for large amounts of lytic agents, bleeding complications, and secondary embolization, which may not respond to lysis and prevent reperfusion of the foot. Percutaneous thrombolysis is successful in one half to two thirds of such cases.

In patients with motor and sensory deficits caused by thrombosis or embolism of popliteal arteries, there is insufficient time to attempt catheter-based therapy and operative exploration with thrombectomy of the popliteal artery and the tibial and peroneal runoff vessels is indicated. In this setting, intraoperative instillation of thrombolytic agents into the runoff vessels has often been both safe and efficacious. Most reports have employed urokinase for intraoperative thrombolysis using bolus doses up to 500,000 units; a randomized, blinded, and placebo-controlled trial of intraoperative intraarterial urokinase during lower extremity revascularization has shown beneficial regional and systemic effects. Following these

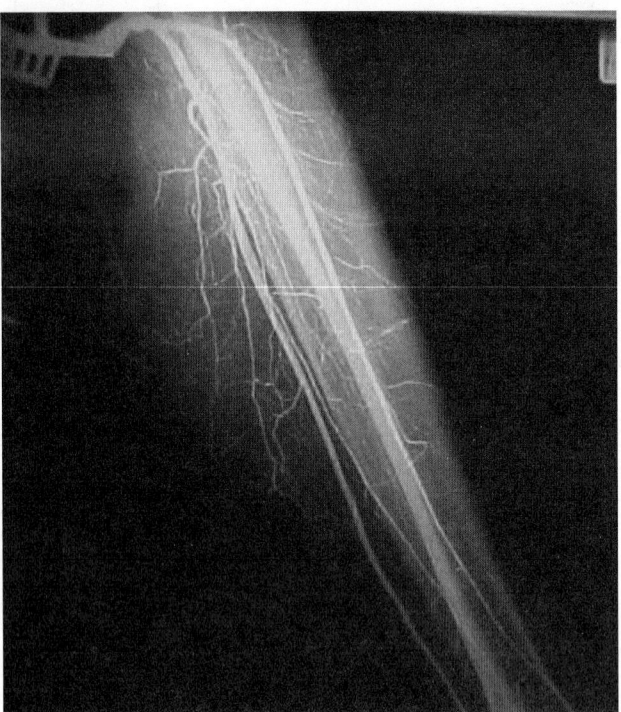

Figure 4 Intraoperative arteriogram after thromboembolectomy of outflow vessels using a Fogarty balloon catheter. Complete extraction of thrombi and emboli is demonstrated with three-vessel outflow.

maneuvers, intraoperative arteriography is essential to identify outflow vessels and plan optimal revascularization (Fig. 4). Operative thrombectomy should be performed by isolating the so-called popliteal "trifurcation" (which is actually a "bi-bifurcation") and directing thrombectomy catheters down all three main calf arteries; "blind" exploration of pedal arteries for attempted retrograde thrombectomy almost never produces successful limb salvage.

The operative plan for revascularization depends on several concerns, including the vessels available for inflow and outflow, extent of the aneurysm, elimination of the embolic source, relief of compression of adjacent structures, and prevention of continued enlargement after surgery (Fig. 5). A medial approach to the popliteal artery with the patient supine is generally recommended because this affords the most extensive exposure to the upper popliteal artery and the distal outflow vessels; the supine position also permits easy exposure of the femoral arteries, which may be required as an inflow source and allows harvest of the greater saphenous vein in the upper thigh, which is generally a better size-matched conduit than the saphenous vein near the popliteal incision(s) or the lesser saphenous vein. Either a continuous or two separate incisions on the thigh and calf may be used. For small aneurysms located directly behind the knee joint, a posterior approach with the patient prone is advantageous; some surgeons favor an S-shaped incision whereas others use a longitudinal incision directly in the posterior midline of the lower extremity bridging the joint. For a medial approach, the semimembranosus and semitendinosus tendons can be transected without producing knee instability or weakness in most patients.

If the popliteal aneurysm is not infected or producing compressive symptoms, resection is not necessary and the aneurysm should be left in situ to avoid injury to adjacent veins and nerves that are often tenaciously adherent. Very rarely, a small saccular aneurysm may be excised with mobilization of the popliteal artery above and below the aneurysm for end-to-end arterial anastomosis. In general, however, exclusion and bypass are the principles of treatment (see

Fig. 5, *B*). The location of the proximal anastomosis depends on the extent of aneurysmal degeneration of the superficial femoral and popliteal arteries; in general, the graft length is kept as short as possible, but all significant aneurysmal disease should be bypassed (see Fig. 5, *D*). The distal anastomosis should be performed to the most suitable target distal artery, balancing optimal runoff with a satisfactory anastomotic site. Autogenous saphenous vein is superior to prosthetic conduits, although ringed PTFE is a reasonable alternative for short bypasses when there is absent or inadequate autogenous vein. For testing the vein conduit for leaks and assessing its diameter, we gently distend it with a special "cocktail" that is less injurious to endothelium than heparinized saline, which has a slightly acidic pH; the solution, which is kept cold on ice, consists of 60 ml of the patient's whole blood, 5 ml unfractionated heparin (1:1000), 2 ml papaverine (30 mg/ml), 5 ml 1% lidocaine hydrochloride (without epinephrine), and 20 ml dextran-40. There is often significant size discrepancy between ectatic native arteries and the saphenous vein; thus whereas end-to-end anastomoses are hemodynamically preferable, end-to-side anastomoses may be required. Completion or early postoperative arteriography is useful to ensure technical excellence because the anastomoses are often difficult to perform deep within the leg (Fig. 6). Generally, the vein is positioned along the course of the inflow artery for a comfortable distance, but the conduit is best routed in a more superficial plane rather than directly in the popliteal space to avoid compression by the aneurysm. Care must be taken to avoid twisting the vein conduit, particularly when a skin bridge or deeper tunneling precludes inspection of the vein for much of its course (Figs. 7 and 8). Ligatures placed above and below the aneurysm generally ensure eventual thrombosis, but the aneurysm may be perfused by collaterals and remain patent under low pressure; on rare occasions this can lead to late expansion and rupture.

When the aneurysm is large and producing symptoms attributable to compression of adjacent structures or when a ruptured aneurysm is encountered, it should be decompressed and opened to evacuate thrombus, branches oversewn from within, and a portion of the redundant wall resected. An interposition graft is then placed within the aneurysm sac, much like the standard technique for AAA repair (see Fig. 5, *A*). Complete resection is required only for infected popliteal aneurysm (see Fig. 5, *C*).

As for AAAs, endoluminal graft repair for popliteal aneurysms is gaining increased popularity. Various types of covered stent grafts have been used successfully for exclusion of aneurysms and preservation of luminal flow. Advantages of this approach include minimal invasiveness, reduction of wound complications, conservation of the saphenous vein for other uses, and cost savings with respect to length of hospital stay (although procedural and device costs are expensive). Initial success rates of 100% have been described, and 1-year patency rates are approximately 70%. However, no long-term results have been reported and, traditionally, durability of prosthetic grafts placed across the knee joint is inferior to autogenous conduits.

Results

Outcomes after popliteal artery aneurysm repair depend on clinical presentations. Overall, operative mortality rates are approximately 1.5%, ranging from 0% for asymptomatic patients to 2.1% for symptomatic patients, presumably a consequence of emergency operations required for acutely ischemic extremities. Patency and limb salvage rates for repairs of popliteal artery aneurysms are superior to arterial reconstructions for standard atherosclerotic occlusive disease. Contributing factors for this finding may include shorter bypass grafts, larger arteries, and better runoff vessels, although this latter feature is not always applicable in the presence of recurrent embolization. Five-year patency rates for autogenous conduits in asymptomatic patients range from 50% to 100% (average approximately 85%); analogous statistics for prosthetic grafts are 29% to

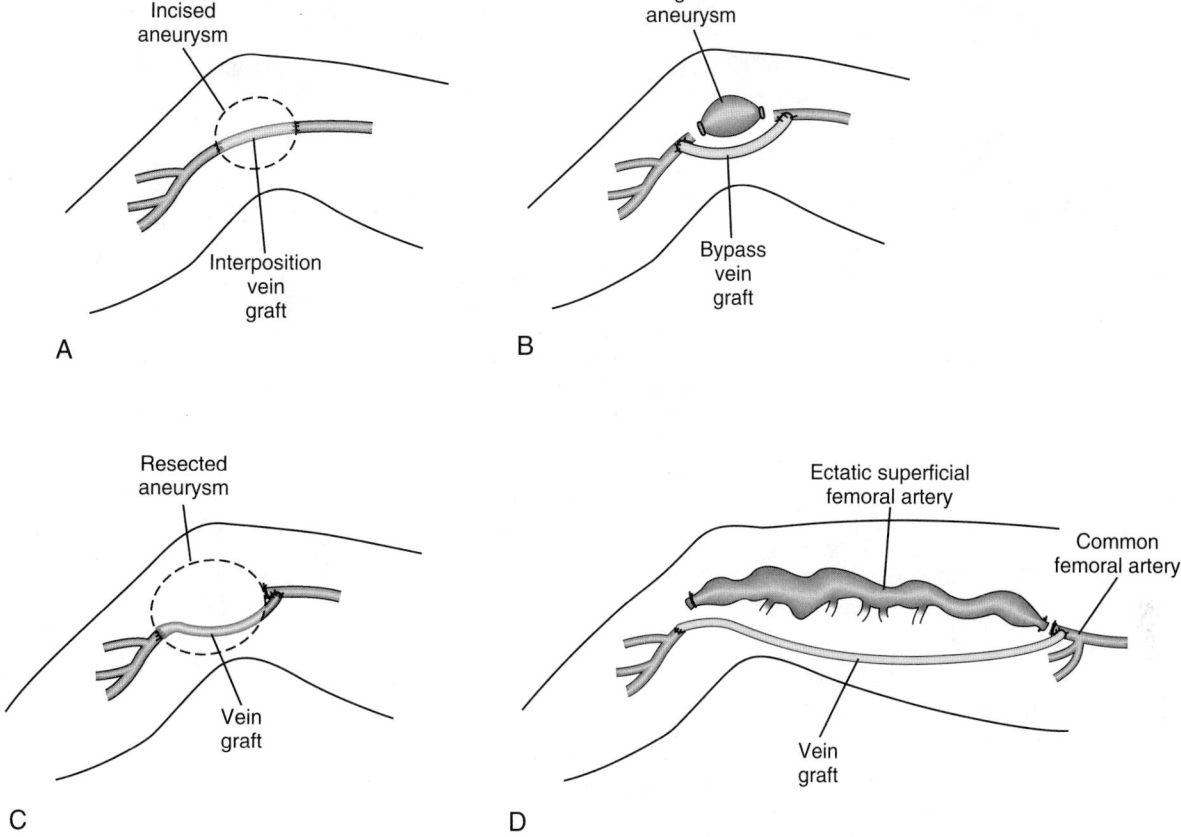

Figure 5 Diagram demonstrating operative strategies for popliteal artery aneurysms. (**A**) Interposition graft after decompression of the aneurysm by incising it and oversewing branches from within. (**B**) Exclusion of aneurysm by ligation above and below with bypass using vein conduit. (**C**) Excision of infected aneurysm with vein interposition graft (**D**) Common femoral to distal popliteal artery bypass for diffusely aneurysmal superficial femoral and popliteal artery (see Fig. 3, B).

80% (average 50%). In symptomatic patients, average 5-year patency rate falls to approximately 60%. Long-term limb salvage rates in asymptomatic patients average 98%, whereas only 60% to 80% of acutely symptomatic patients achieve long-term preservation of limbs. Not surprisingly, perioperative morbidity is substantially greater for acutely symptomatic aneurysms than for asymptomatic ones, including persistent ischemia, tissue loss, compartment syndrome, wound complications, seromas, hemorrhage from thrombolysis or anticoagulation, and neuropathies. Life expectancy is reduced compared with age- and sex-matched controls, averaging 60% and 40% at 5 and 10 years, respectively. Survival rates are further reduced in patients with multiple aneurysms, and in addition to a high prevalence of coexistent other aneurysms at the time of diagnosis, surviving patients are at increased risk for the development of new aneurysms. In a longitudinal study of patients with popliteal aneurysms, one third developed additional aneurysms (thoracoabdominal, femoral, and contralateral popliteal) during a mean follow-up of 5 years. These findings underscore the importance of lifelong surveillance of patients after popliteal aneurysm repair, although published protocols for the frequency of reevaluation are lacking.

FEMORAL ARTERY ANEURYSMS

Degenerative aneurysms of the femoral arteries are even more commonly associated with bilaterality and aneurysms in additional locations than the popliteal variety. Eighty-five percent of patients with true common femoral artery aneurysms have AAAs, as many as 70% have bilateral femoral aneurysms, approximately half have popliteal artery aneurysms, and more than 5% have thoracic aortic aneurysms. Femoral aneurysms involve the common femoral artery most commonly, and in approximately one half of cases, the profunda femoris artery (PFA) is involved. Fewer than 100 isolated aneurysms of the profunda femoris artery and the superficial femoral (SFA) artery have been reported in the medical literature. Although femoral aneurysms produce limb-threatening ischemia less commonly than popliteal aneurysms, their importance relates to their association with other life- and limb-threatening aneurysms. *Anastomotic* femoral pseudoaneurysms occur after arterial reconstructions or repairs; loss of structural integrity results from suture material fatigue, prosthetic graft degeneration, technical errors during graft placement, progressive disease in the host vessel, and infection. Risk factors for anastomotic aneurysms include local wound complications after the initial operation, female gender, and history of a previous anastomotic aneurysm. Accidental intraarterial injection of drugs leading to vascular complications was first reported because of unintentional infusions by nurses and physicians, but sequelae are now most often associated with illicit drug use. Pseudoaneurysms from drug injections are almost always infected. *Iatrogenic* pseudoaneurysm after percutaneous arterial access is a consequence of hemostatic failure after arterial decannulation.

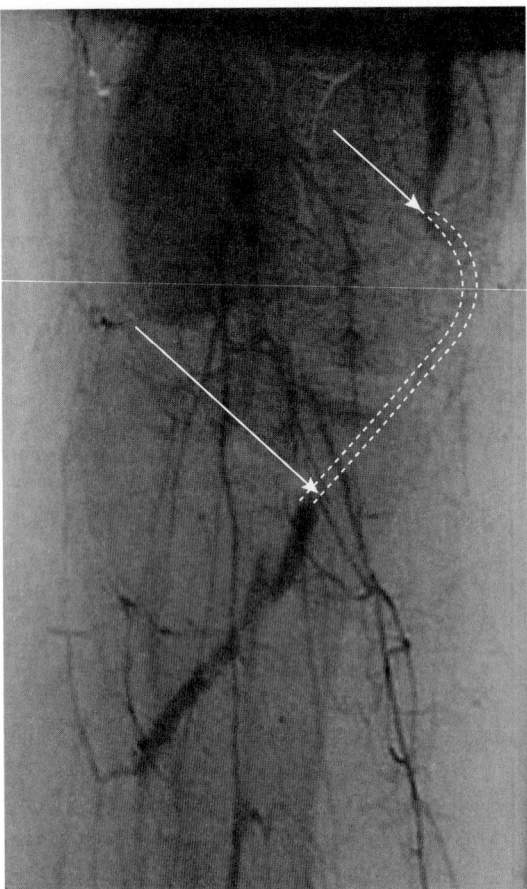

Figure 6 Postoperative arteriogram showing reduced flow through a vein interposition graft that has a 90-degree "twist" within the tunnel; the *dotted lines* outline the midbody of the vein graft, the *short arrow* points to proximal portion of the vein graft, and the *long arrow* points to the distal portion vein graft.

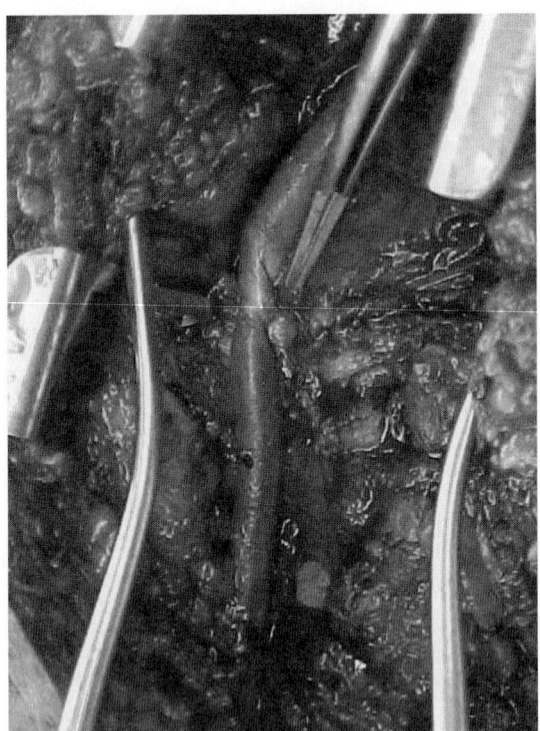

Figure 7 In this intraoperative photograph, forceps point to the "twist" in the interposition vein graft used for bypass of a popliteal aneurysm (see Fig. 6).

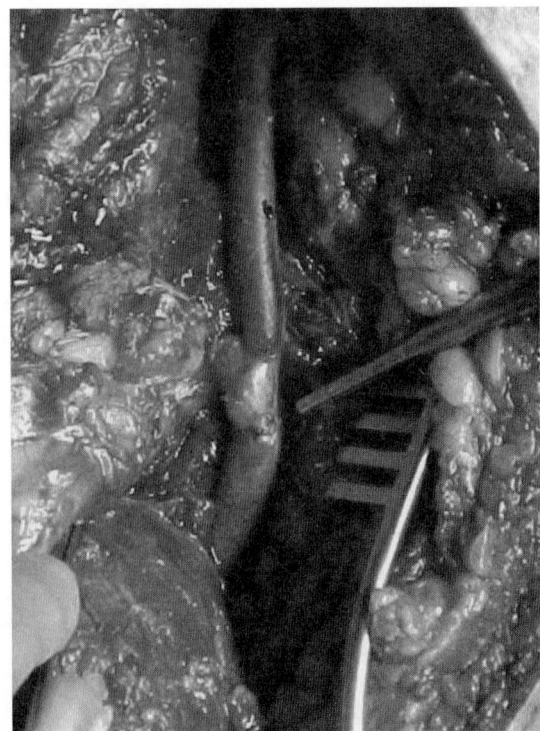

Figure 8 In this intraoperative photograph, the "twist" in the vein graft has been repaired by transection of the vein and end-end venovenostomy; note the methylene blue "stripe" on the graft to ensure proper orientation.

Clinical Presentation

Most patients with degenerative femoral aneurysms are asymptomatic or present with concern about the presence of a pulsatile mass, local discomfort, swelling from femoral vein compression, or neuropathy from femoral nerve impingement. Complications such as thrombosis, thromboembolism, or rupture are unusual manifestations, occurring in less than one fifth of patients; complications of superficial femoral artery aneurysms are exceptions to the typical presentations of femoral aneurysms, for one third of such lesions present with rupture and one fourth produce thromboembolic events. Iatrogenic false aneurysms after punctures occur more commonly than the degenerative variety, and they are more commonly associated with pain, progressive swelling, and ecchymosis. In addition, hemodynamically significant bleeding usually occurs only in traumatic pseudoaneurysms; hemorrhage can track into the retroperitoneum and produce shock and death without obvious local signs in the groin. In contrast, anastomotic false aneurysms generally are slow to enlarge and usually found on physical examination in asymptomatic patients. Infected (mycotic) femoral aneurysms are most often caused by needle puncture for illicit drug delivery. Patients have a suggestive history, other needle tracks, pain, signs of a local infectious process, and a systemic septic picture.

Diagnosis

Except in obese patients, the femoral artery is readily available for palpation on physical examination, which discloses the presence of most common femoral aneurysms of any etiology. Color-flow Doppler scanning is the best screening test; with a 95% sensitivity and specificity, it confirms the diagnosis, defines the size and presence of luminal thrombus, establishes the presence of associated aneurysms in other arteries, and can be effective for compression therapy of acute false aneurysms. Computed tomography and magnetic resonance imaging may also characterize morphology of the aneurysm, the presence of perigraft fluid, and integrity of surrounding structures (Fig. 9). As for other aneurysms, contrast arteriography and magnetic resonance arteriography may underestimate the size of femoral aneurysms but are useful to disclose coexistent occlusive disease and to delineate the anatomy of the inflow and outflow vessels adjacent to the lesion to plan surgical reconstruction.

Management

Degenerative Femoral Aneurysms

The natural history of asymptomatic femoral aneurysms less than approximately 3 cm in diameter is usually benign. In one study of 105 degenerative aneurysms followed during a mean of 28 months, only three produced limb ischemia. In another study of 19 patients monitored during an average of 52 months, no complications were encountered. Yearly serial ultrasound examination is appropriate for observational management of such lesions. The behavior of femoral aneurysms with substantial intraluminal thrombus is uncertain. Such aneurysms may pose increased thromboembolic risks; however, because the amount of thrombus correlates with increased size, the effect of these two variables is difficult to separate. The optimal threshold diameter for elective repair of asymptomatic femoral aneurysms has not been precisely determined. Repair is often recommended in good-risk patients with aneurysms greater than 3 cm containing substantial intraluminal thrombus to prevent local and thromboembolic complications.

Operative repair is indicated for all symptomatic, complicated, or rapidly enlarging aneurysms. Urgent repair is indicated for limb-threatening complications caused by embolism, thrombosis,

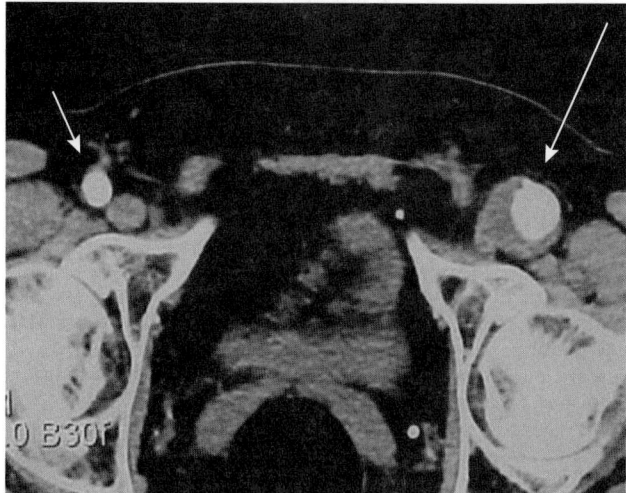

Figure 9 Computed tomography scan (with intravenous contrast) demonstrating a 3-cm degenerative left common femoral aneurysm containing a moderate amount of thrombus (*long arrow*) compared with normal right common femoral artery (*short arrow*).

or rupture. Although size and risk of rupture are thought to be related, because most femoral aneurysms thrombose rather than rupture, there is no convincing evidence that size correlates with limb-threatening ischemia.

Anastomotic Femoral Pseudoaneurysms

Anastomotic aneurysms occur most often after prosthetic bypasses. Before 1967, when silk sutures were widely used, up to one fourth of anastomoses between prosthetic grafts and femoral arteries resulted in pseudoaneurysm formation, but there has been a decline in the incidence of this disorder owing to improvements in technique, graft design, and suture durability; in addition, as interventional treatment employing percutaneous transluminal angioplasty (PTA) and stents for aortoiliac disease has exceeded operative intervention, anastomotic false aneurysms have become less common. Several reports have emphasized an infectious etiology for anastomotic aneurysm, often caused by low-virulence coagulase-negative staphylococcal organisms (e.g., *Staphylococcus epidermidis*); in surgically treated anastomotic aneurysm with no clinical evidence of infection, as many as 60% are culture-positive when meticulous bacteriologic recovery techniques are employed. Serial ultrasound surveillance is appropriate for most asymptomatic anastomotic aneurysms, but aneurysms larger than 2 to 3 cm warrant consideration for repair before they produce complications in good-risk patients; almost all symptomatic or complicated anastomotic aneurysms merit elective reconstruction.

Infected Femoral Pseudoaneurysms

The treatment of infected (mycotic) aneurysms is challenging. These lesions behave more unfavorably than anastomotic aneurysms contaminated with low-virulence organisms. Approximately 75% of all admissions for accidental intraarterial drug injections involve the lower extremities, most commonly resulting in pseudoaneurysm formation. Arteriovenous fistulae are second in frequency of complications. Associated findings often include overlying cellulitis, distal embolization, septic arthritis, endocarditis, vasospasm, arterial occlusion, compartment syndrome, lymphedema, and numerous neurologic sequelae. The predominant infecting organism is methicillin-sensitive *Staphylococcus aureus*, but other species of staphylococci, streptococci, gram-negative organisms, fungi, and a combination of organisms may be present. Infected femoral pseudoaneurysms have a virulent natural history and necessitate operative resection, wide débridement, and appropriate antibiotic therapy in all instances.

Femoral Pseudoaneurysms often Percutaneous Arterial Access

The natural history of false aneurysms after femoral artery punctures is generally benign. Multiple reports have documented an 85% to 90% incidence of spontaneous thrombosis/regression within 2 or 3 months of follow-up. Nonoperative management is recommended in most cases. In addition, both ultrasound-guided compression and local injection of thrombin are alternatives to surgical repair, but enthusiasm for the high success rate of these interventions must be tempered with the favorable results of observation alone. Although 90% to 95% success rates with both techniques have been reported in more than 700 cases, these procedures are often time consuming, difficult, and painful. Intravenous sedation and repeated trials are often required, and complications include arterial thrombosis, distal embolization, rupture, femoral nerve injuries, and recurrence. Absolute indications for surgical intervention are active hemorrhage and expansion, shock, compartment syndrome, femoral neuropathy, infection, embolization and distal ischemia, skin necrosis and breakdown, and severe pain. Relative indications for surgical therapy include size greater than 3 cm, short or wide "neck," coexistent arteriovenous fistula, requirement for chronic systemic anticoagulation, and poor compliance with follow-up.

Operative Technique

Surgical strategy for femoral artery aneurysms and pseudoaneurysms must be individualized based on the etiology of the disorder, symptoms, coexistent aneurysms elsewhere, and specific anatomic features. In asymptomatic patients with multiple aneurysms, a staged approach is best; the potentially life-threatening aortic aneurysm is usually treated first, followed by therapy for limb-threatening popliteal aneurysms and, finally, by femoral aneurysm repair as appropriate.

Degenerative Femoral Aneurysms

Concomitant involvement of the superficial (SFA) and profunda femoris (PFA) arteries determines the surgical plan for treatment of an isolated femoral artery aneurysm. Occasionally, for large and extensive aneurysms, proximal external iliac arterial control must be obtained through a retroperitoneal "transplant-type" incision. Alternatively, adequate exposure can be achieved using a long longitudinal groin incision; the inguinal ligament is incised to expose the distal external iliac artery for inflow control. Surgical exposure and control of the SFA and PFA are optimal but may not be feasible without risking injury to the vessels, adjacent nerves, veins, or lymphatic. Once the artery is opened, the back-bleeding from distal vessels can be controlled by insertion of intraluminal temporary balloon catheters.

Common femoral degenerative aneurysms isolated to the common femoral artery are best replaced with an interposition graft of polytetrafluoroethylene (PTFE) or Dacron (usually 8 to 10 mm in diameter) anastomosed end to end to the distal external iliac or proximal common femoral artery above the aneurysm and to the distal common femoral artery above the femoral bifurcation (Fig. 10, A). Saphenous vein can be used as a conduit if it is of adequate size, but there is no distinct advantage to prosthetic material in this location in the absence of documented infection. When degenerative aneurysms extend into the PFA or the SFA, repair is performed by anastomosis of the interposition graft to the uninvolved artery with reimplantation of the remaining artery (Fig. 10, B). Alternatively, the superficial femoral and profunda femoris arteries can be sewn together (creating a new distal common femoral bifurcation, a process called syndactylization). In addition, a prosthetic graft side limb can be placed between the new interposition graft and the PFA. If the SFA is diffusely aneurysmal in conjunction with a common femoral degenerative aneurysm, the SFA should be detached and excluded, placing a saphenous vein graft for improved lower extremity blood flow (Fig. 10, C). When the SFA is chronically occluded, the distal anastomosis is performed end to end of the PFA, and a vein bypass graft is interposed between the new PTFE and a distal target artery (Fig. 10, D).

Anastomotic Femoral Pseudoaneurysms

Anastomotic aneurysms involving the femoral arteries are challenging because of scar from previous surgery and difficulty in isolating the native iliac artery located deep to the graft. Often the suture line is completely disrupted and the entire graft is separated from native arteries with structures held together only by the fibrous capsule of the false aneurysm. The same principles described previously apply to surgical management of anastomotic aneurysms with direct control of as many branches as possible and intraluminal balloon catheter control from within the aneurysm when circumferential dissection is hazardous. Uncommonly, localized disruption of the suture line occurs, and after adequate

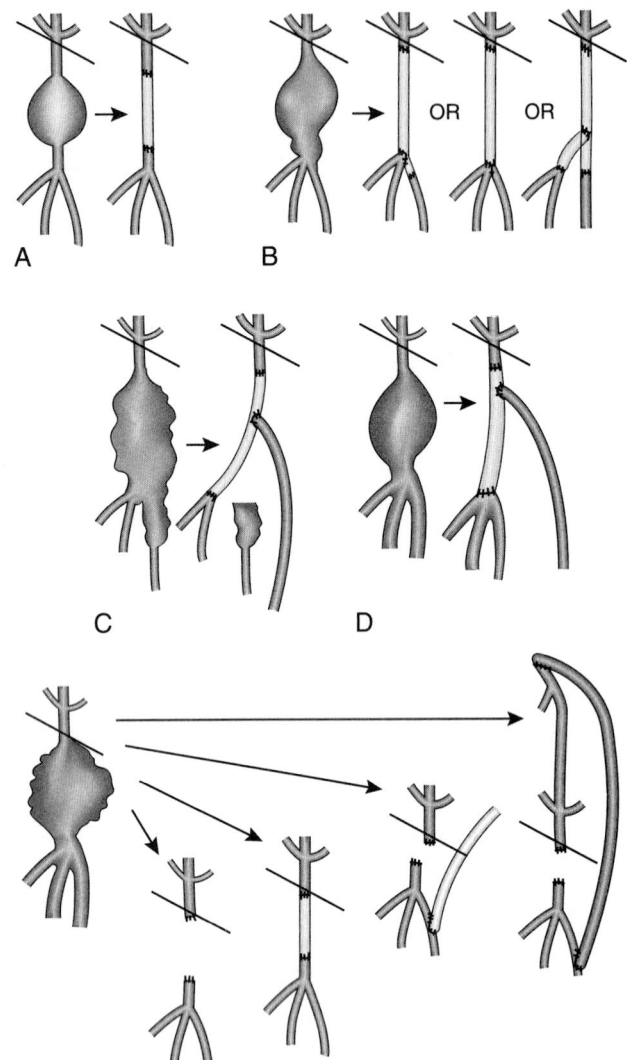

Figure 10 Diagram demonstrating operative management strategies for femoral artery aneurysms. **(A)** Interposition prosthetic graft for degenerative common femoral artery aneurysm. **(B)** Options for repair of a femoral artery aneurysm that involves the superficial and profunda femoris arteries; arterial continuity is restored using an interposition prosthetic graft to the superficial femoral artery with reimplantation of the profunda femoris artery, syndactylization of the superficial and profunda femoris arteries, or a side limb to the profunda femoris artery. **(C)** When both the common femoral artery and superficial femoral arteries are diffusely aneurysmal, an interposition prosthetic graft is anastomosed to the profunda femoris artery with a vein graft bypass to the popliteal artery. **(D)** In a patient with a femoral aneurysm and significant lower extremity ischemia caused by an occluded superficial femoral artery, an interposition prosthetic graft is anastomosed to the profunda femoris artery with a vein graft bypass to the popliteal artery. **(E)** Options for treatment of an infected femoral artery pseudoaneurysm include excision of the aneurysm with preservation of flow through collaterals and conservation of contiguity of the profunda and superficial femoris arteries; excision of the aneurysm and restoration of flow with an extraanatomic graft to the midthigh superficial femoral artery using inflow from the contralateral common femoral artery; excision of the aneurysm and restoration of flow with an extraanatomic graft to the midthigh superficial femoral artery using inflow from the ipsilateral common iliac artery with a vein graft conduit—alternatively a prosthetic graft can be routed through the obturator foramen.

débridement of the artery, simple reanastomosis of the old graft to the artery or patch angioplasty is satisfactory. Usually, however, the distal portion of the old graft should be resected and a new interposition graft sewn end to end to the old graft. Then, the new graft can be anastomosed to the previous arteriotomy if the artery is of good quality. Often a segment of artery must be excised to accomplish sufficient débridement; in this instance, the distal external iliac artery may be ligated and the new graft sewn end to end to the common femoral artery. Techniques shown in Fig. 10 are often required for repair of extensive and complex pseudoaneurysms. Because infection may play a role in development of anastomotic aneurysms, segments of tissue and portions of thrombus should be sent for cultures and sensitivities. Administration of longterm antibiotics is generally successful for low-virulence organisms, but all-autogenous reconstructions are sometimes required to eradicate persistent infections.

Infected Femoral Pseudoaneurysms

Excision of infected artery and graft with revascularization using autogenous conduits or prosthetic grafts placed in extraanatomic locations are the principles for surgical management of mycotic aneurysms (Fig. 10, *E*). Antibiotic therapy, usually administered intravenously for at least 6 weeks, is guided by blood and tissue cultures and sensitivities. All infected tissue must be resected and the surrounding area débrided. Monofilament suture is used to oversew inflow and outflow arteries. Blood flow is restored by routing autogenous vein grafts or prosthetic grafts originating from the contralateral femoral artery routed around the affected groin and anastomosed to the more distal superficial femoral artery, the distal profunda femoris artery, or even the popliteal artery on occasion. Occasionally, the ipsilateral iliac artery can be used as an inflow site using autogenous vein grafts or prosthetic grafts routed through the obturator foramen.

The optimal management of infected pseudoaneurysms caused by intravenous drug abuse (IVDA) is controversial. In up to three quarters of cases, it is possible to débride and oversew the affected arteries without revascularization; collateral blood flow is sufficient to maintain viability of the lower extremity, and this approach avoids recurrence of the same problem in individuals who practice IVDA. When this operative strategy is chosen, the proximal branches of the profunda femoris must be preserved to optimize collateral flow and the profunda and superficial femoral arteries should remain in contiguity to maximize distal flow. If there is no Doppler ultrasound signal at the foot and clinical signs of severe ischemia are present after resection of a mycotic femoral artery aneurysm, immediate revascularization is necessary. Despite IVDA, most of these patients have a greater saphenous vein in midthigh that is potentially suitable for a conduit for arterial reconstruction. When in situ autogenous reconstruction is not feasible or is inappropriate because of local conditions, an extraanatomic bypass may be required to route the graft through the obturator foramen or from the contralateral femoral artery to the midsuperficial femoral artery. In all instances, the wound must be débrided of all gross infection and the conduit should be covered with a well-vascularized sartorius muscle flap.

Femoral Pseudoaneurysms after Percutaneous Arterial Access

Observation alone is appropriate for most iatrogenic femoral artery aneurysms because of the favorable natural history. If ultrasound-guided compression treatment is selected, the ultrasound scanning head is used to localize the pseudoaneurysm or the arteriovenous communication. Using the B-mode image, the head is then compressed against the false aneurysm, limiting flow into it without occluding arterial flow. Typically, initial compression is performed for 20 to 30 minutes. If flow into the pseudoaneurysm is not eliminated, a subsequent compression for a similar period is often successful. Compression of acute pseudoaneurysms

is painful, especially when there is considerable surrounding hematoma, and patients require intravenous sedation to tolerate the procedure. Recurrence of false aneurysms occurs in approximately 10% of patients, so follow-up scanning the next day is indicated. Injection of thrombin to obliterate iatrogenic false aneurysms is performed by first localizing the aneurysm using duplex scanning. Approximately 0.5 to 1.5 ml of thrombin (1000 U/ml) is injected into the pseudoaneurysm with a micropuncture needle under indirect visualization using ultrasound. Color-flow duplex ultrasound documents cessation of flow in the aneurysm as thrombosis occurs. Care must be exercised to avoid injecting thrombin directly into the adjacent femoral artery or vein. Patients with arteriovenous fistulae, short aneurysm necks, or multiple puncture sites are poor candidates for this procedure.

When nonoperative management of pseudoaneurysms from percutaneous punctures of the femoral artery is unsuccessful or operative indications are present (see previous), operative repair consists of a vertical groin incision and proximal arterial control obtained at the inguinal ligament. Because distal control is usually difficult, it is usually best to clamp the proximal artery, open the hematoma/aneurysm, and use direct finger pressure to control back-bleeding. The distal vessel is then exposed and clamped, and the traumatic arterial opening is oversewn with a figure-of-eight suture. The artery must be inspected for additional punctures. The hematoma is evacuated, a closed suction drain is brought out through a separate stab wound incision, and meticulous wound closure is accomplished because of the potential for significant wound complications.

Results

Results of operative intervention for femoral artery aneurysms depend on the etiology of the aneurysm and the presence of coexistent vascular disease. Elective surgery for degenerative femoral artery aneurysms and anastomotic aneurysms produces excellent outcomes. Long-term patency and limb salvage rates approach 100%. Wound complications, lymphoceles, and recurrent aneurysms occur rarely. Not surprisingly, the results of emergency surgery for rupture or acute thrombosis of femoral aneurysms are less favorable, and both amputation and death ensue on occasion. Approximately one quarter of patients presenting with rupture or acute ischemia have adverse outcomes.

Complications of operative repair are more common when femoral artery aneurysms are caused by infection or iatrogenic punctures. IVDA patients who require revascularization rather than simple resection of mycotic femoral artery aneurysms commonly experience complications including hemorrhage, residual infection, graft thrombosis leading to limb loss, and residual or recurrent infections; major amputations are required in approximately 25% of these patients. Morbidity after operative repair of iatrogenic aneurysms is most often related to the underlying cardiac problems that required the percutaneous femoral artery puncture and wound complications associated with hematoma and tissue injury, which is most common in obese patients.

Suggested Readings

Dawson I, Sie RB, van Bockel JH: Atherosclerotic popliteal aneurysm, *Br J Surg* 84:293, 1997.

Diwan A et al: Incidence of femoral and popliteal artery aneurysms in patients with abdominal aortic aneurysms, *J Vasc Surg* 31:863, 2000.

Duffy ST et al: Popliteal aneurysms: a 10-year experience, *Eur J Endovasc Surg* 16:218, 1998.

Galland RB, Magee TR: Management of popliteal aneurysm, *Br J Surg* 89:1382, 2002.

Gourny P et al: Limb salvage and popliteal aneurysms: advantages of preventive surgery, *Eur J Vasc Endovasc Surg* 19:496, 2000.

Howell M et al: Wallgraft prosthesis for the percutaneous treatment of femoral and popliteal artery aneurysms, *J Endovasc Ther* 9:76, 2002.

Krupski WC, Nehler MR: Iatrogenic vascular injuries. In Pearce W, Yao J, editors: *Current trends in vascular surgery.* Chicago, 2003, Chicago Precept Press.

Nehler MR, Krupski WCA: Femoral artery aneurysm. In Cronenwett J, Rutherford RB, editors: *Decision making in vascular surgery.* Philadelphia, 2000, WB Saunders.

Paulson EK et al: Treatment of iatrogenic femoral arterial pseudoaneurysms: comparison of US-guided thrombin injection with compression repair, *Radiology* 215:403, 2000.

Sarcina A et al: Surgical treatment of popliteal artery aneurysm: a 20 year experience, *J Cardiovasc Surg* 38:347, 1997.

FALSE ANEURYSM AND ARTERIOVENOUS FISTULA

Kevin E. Taubman, MD, and David C. Han, MD

INTRODUCTION

False aneurysms (FAs), or pseudoaneurysms, are distinguished from true aneurysms by involvement of fewer than all three histologic layers of the arterial wall. FAs most frequently occur as a result of traumatic injury to the arterial wall and have become more common in current clinical practice with the increased use of percutaneous femoral and upper extremity access to perform diagnostic and interventional procedures.

Noniatrogenic trauma accounts for a significant portion of FAs as well. Both blunt and penetrating trauma can lead to disruptions of the arterial wall, creating an aneurysm constrained only by an outer wall of connective and fibrous tissue. Breakdown of anastomotic or patch suture lines can also lead to FA formation. These may or may not be associated with an underlying infection. More commonly, infected FA can be seen in patients with a history of intravenous drug abuse in whom inadvertent, or sometimes purposeful, arterial trauma occurs. Rarely, systemic vasculitides such as periarteritis nodosa or Bechet's disease present with an FA in any one of a number of vascular beds (Table 1).

Table 1: Etiology of False Aneurysm

Traumatic

Iatrogenic
    Vascular access for diagnostic or therapeutic intervention
Noniatrogenic
    Penetrating
        Gunshot wound
        Stab wound
    Nonpenetrating
        Stretch injury
        Injury from adjacent fracture

Anastomotic

Infectious

At site of previous anastomosis or patch
Traumatic from intravenous drug abuse

Vasculitis

Arteriovenous fistulae (AVFs) are abnormal direct connections between an adjacent artery and vein. AVFs are either congenital or acquired. This chapter focuses on acquired AVFs, which typically occur as a result of iatrogenic or noniatrogenic trauma. Another less common but clinically important cause of AVF is erosion from an artery into an adjacent vein, such as an aortic or iliac aneurysm rupturing into the vena cava or iliac vein.

DIAGNOSIS

Several diagnostic modalities exist with regard to FA and AVF. A thorough history is vital because these conditions do not necessarily present immediately after the inciting event. The insidious onset of heart failure, limb swelling, or claudication can be the initial presentation of an AVF from a percutaneous intervention days, months, or even years earlier. During physical examination, the presence of an FA may be suspected because of a palpable pulsatile lump at the site of previous access or injury and an audible bruit or palpable thrill may be present in either an AVF or FA. Bradycardia that occurs with compression of an AVF is known as the Nicoladoni-Branham sign. A complete pulse examination including ankle brachial indices should be performed and underscores the need to obtain this information before any percutaneous intervention. A loss of distal circulation or excoriation of the overlying skin from expansion of an FA represents a need for expeditious evaluation and treatment.

Noninvasive Methods

Duplex Ultrasound

Duplex ultrasound (DU) is typically the initial test used to diagnose FA or AVF. Gray-scale imaging can suggest the presence of an FA, but color-flow and spectral waveform analysis are diagnostic. Characteristic flow patterns of an FA include swirling within the FA as pulsatile blood flows in and then out, as well as a to-fro pattern in the pedicle as blood flows in one direction into the FA during systole, and then in the other direction as blood flows out of the FA during diastole (Fig. 1, *A* and *B*). In an AVF, spectral analysis shows high velocities in diastole consistent with the low-resistance venous bed. This low resistance is seen in the artery as it nears the fistula, then within the fistula itself (Fig. 1, *C*).

In addition to being noninvasive, the advantages of DU include its portability, rapidity, and accuracy. Limitations include the need for a well-trained technician, as well as difficulty with the morbidly obese or uncooperative patient. In the case of noniatrogenic FAs, awkward locations such as the subclavian artery or the visceral vessels may be difficult to image.

Magnetic Resonance Imaging

At this time, magnetic resonance imaging (MRI) and magnetic resonance angiography (MRA) play a limited role in the evaluation of FA and AVF. In those situations in which DU is inadequate, other imaging techniques, discussed later, currently provide the necessary cross-sectional and vascular imaging necessary to plan percutaneous

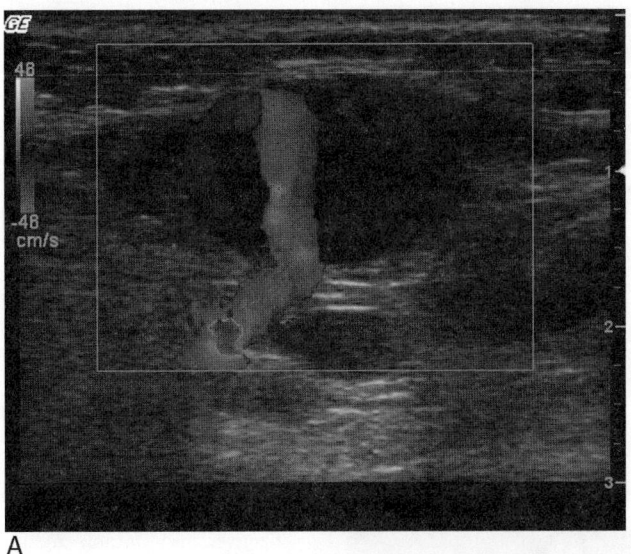

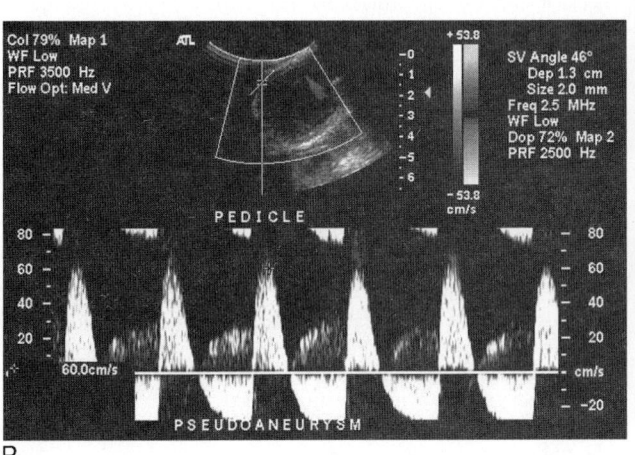

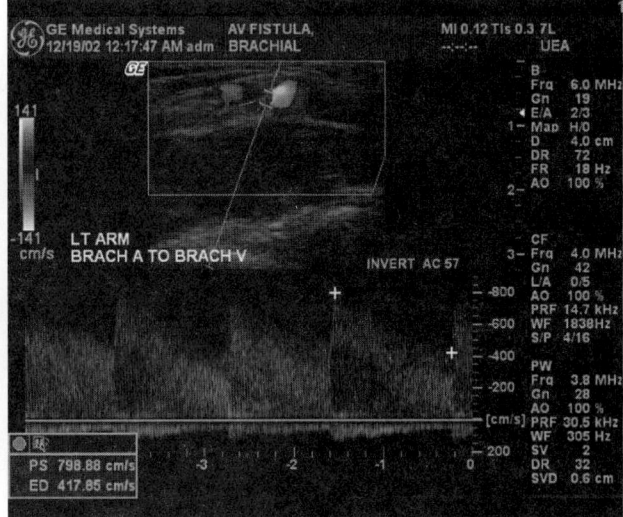

Figure 1 **(A)** Duplex ultrasound of femoral pseudoaneurysm. **(B)** Spectral analysis of pedicle showing to-fro signal. (*See color insert Figure 35.*)

or open interventions. In the future, however, as the capabilities of MRI and MRA advance, the ability to avoid administration of nephrotoxic intravenous contrast may make this modality more appealing.

Invasive Methods

Angiography

Digital subtraction angiography (DSA) has traditionally played a vital role in the diagnosis and treatment of FA and AVF, particularly in the planning of operative therapy. Identification of feeding vessels, as well as delineation of outflow vessels, can aid in determining the type and extent of repair. Invasiveness and the need for intravenous contrast are known drawbacks, especially in a patient with an iatrogenic FA who has recently received large volumes of dye.

Computed Tomography Scan

Thin-slice contrast-enhanced CT scanning in the arterial phase, or CT arteriography (CTA), represents an ideal method to detect FA and AVF and is often the first study used to diagnose and plan treatment (Fig. 2). Improvements in speed and postprocedure processing allow three-dimensional imaging that is equivalent, and in

some cases superior, to angiography. CT scanning performed for other reasons may lead to the incidental discovery of an AVF or FA. For treatment of FA involving the thoracic or abdominal aorta and the iliac vessels, CTA can provide valuable anatomic detail to aid in operative planning. As with angiography, the additional intravenous contrast required for CTA can be of significant concern in patients who have recently undergone a dye load.

TREATMENT

Indications and methods to treat FA and AVF must be individualized. Although in most situations treatment of symptomatic FA and AVF is indicated, different methods are appropriate depending on the clinical situation. Less invasive percutaneous methods are generally preferred when feasible.

False Aneurysms

Symptomatic FA may present as a painful pulsatile mass or with symptoms related to compression of adjacent structures such as neuropathic pain or venous thrombosis. For those FAs that are

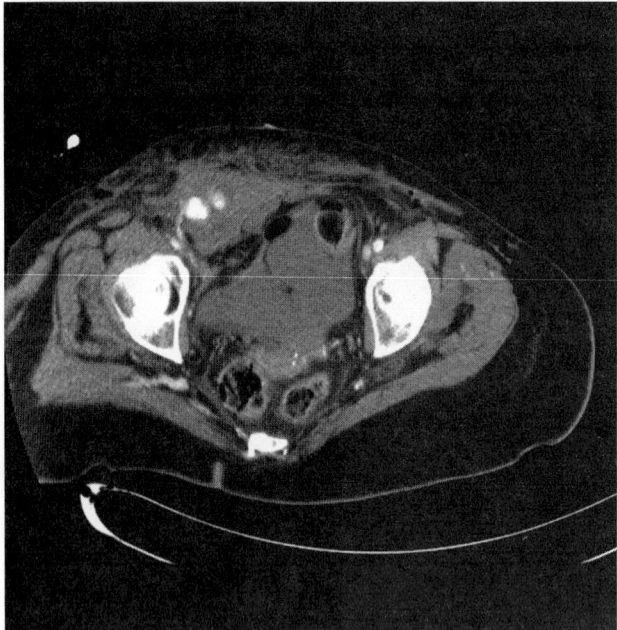

Figure 2 Computed tomography scan showing contrast actively filling a pseudoaneurysm *(arrow)* from a high puncture of the right common femoral artery.

the result of anastomotic degeneration or infection, open repair is typically required. In the case of penetrating or blunt trauma, standard indications and methods to intervene in the patient with symptomatic signs or symptoms of arterial compromise should be followed. Skin compromise from acute expansion of the FA is another indication for open surgical repair.

Asymptomatic FAs most often occur after iatrogenic trauma. An expanding hematoma or the presence of a thrill or bruit most often leads to ultrasound examination, at which time the diagnosis is made. Most are not truly asymptomatic in that there is typically pain from the associated hematoma. Although small (<1.0 cm) FAs may spontaneously thrombose, many of these patients are placed on anticoagulant therapy as part of their original percutaneous intervention. Less invasive methods of treatment should be considered depending on the location and ease of accessibility of the FA, as well as the experience of the surgeon.

Percutaneous Methods

Ultrasound-Guided Repair

The goal of ultrasound-guided treatment of FAs is to induce thrombosis of the FA without causing thrombosis of, or introducing thrombus into, the underlying feeding vessel. Ultrasound-guided compression has been used with moderate success but should be considered a second-line therapy to thrombin injection. Compression therapy uses ultrasound imaging to guide the operator such that the FA is compressed but the underlying vessel remains patent. Although there is no standard protocol, most reports and experienced operators suggest compression for up to an hour, with repeated episodes of compression sometimes required to achieve success. Because of the significant discomfort, conscious sedation of the patient may be necessary, and this procedure can be tiresome for the operator. Success rates are variable, and with the availability of thrombin injection, compression should not be considered as an initial therapy.

Ultrasound-guided thrombin injection (UGTI) is a safe, rapid, effective, and durable method to treat iatrogenic FAs (Fig. 3). After localization of the FA, with ultrasound, the skin is prepared and local anesthetic injected. The ultrasound transducer is oriented in a medial-lateral plane, visualizing the FA, as well as the pedicle or neck. Generally speaking, the FA is best approached laterally, approximately 2 to 3 cm from the lateral edge of the transducer. Either a 21- or an 18-gauge spinal needle is then introduced, with the stylet in place. Although a 21-gauge needle can be used without the need for local anesthetic, an 18-gauge needle is more easily seen. Some transducers may have an attachable guide that allows identification of the anticipated path of the needle. Turning off the color flow allows for optimal visualization of the needle. As the needle is seen to enter the FA, the stylet is withdrawn. If there is no return of pulsatile blood, the needle is not in the FA. Color flow is turned back on, and a prepared solution of bovine thrombin (1000 U/ ml) in a 1-ml tuberculin syringe is then injected slowly (over 2–3 seconds) into the FA. Cessation of flow is seen as the color flow disappears. Typically 600 to 800 U of thrombin are required; however, with larger or multilobulated FAs more may be required. Great care should be taken to avoid injecting directly in or around the neck of the FA because this will increase the chances of thrombus entering the underlying artery.

The results of UGTI are excellent, with success rates greater than 95% in most reported series. Major risks of UGTI include thromboembolization of the underlying artery; this can be

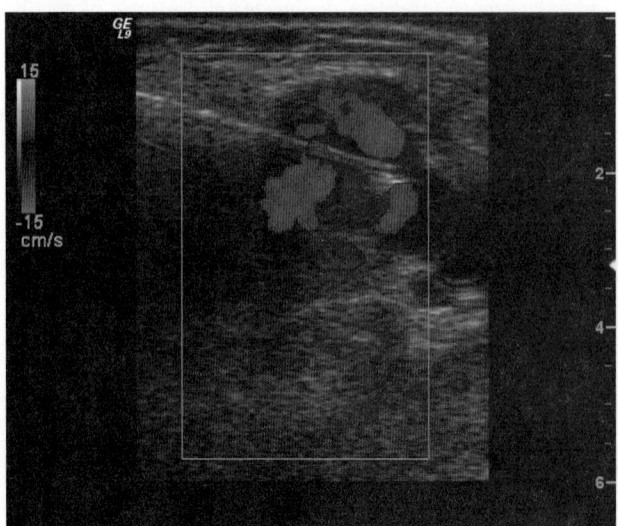

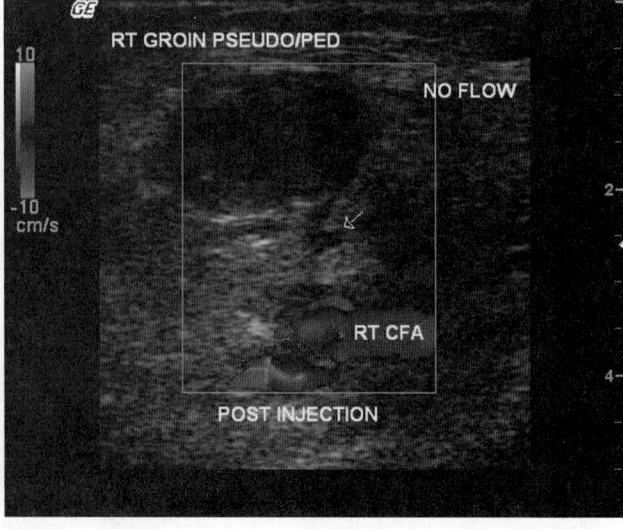

Figure 3 **(A)** Placement of needle within femoral false aneurysm. **(B)** Successful thrombin injection of femoral pseudoaneurysm.

avoided by injecting away from the pedicle and avoiding UGTI in FAs that have short, wide pedicles. Preprocedural and post-procedural ankle brachial indices should always be documented. Because anaphylactic reactions to thrombin have been reported, ready availability of standard resuscitation supplies is recommended. Multilobulated FAs may require multiple injections. In the case of a small, residual FA after injection, supplemental ultrasound-guided compression may be helpful. The need for and duration of immobilization of the limb and for follow-up imaging after UGTI is not well defined. Given that many of these patients are already observed overnight for the original intervention, bed rest and an ultrasound examination the following morning to confirm resolution of the FA are appropriate.

Endovascular Repair

Traumatic injury to the visceral and pelvic vessels can lead to FAs that are often best treated with percutaneous methods, including microvascular coils or thrombotic agents or particles. Injuries to larger vessels, where thrombosis of the vessel is not an option, are more suited to treatment with commercial, investigational, or homemade covered stents. In these cases, treatment must be individualized. Blast injuries to the aorta may be treatable with a device typically used for endovascular repair of true aneurysms but run the risk of infection in the setting of concomitant hollow viscus injury. Similarly, iatrogenic injury to the femoral vessels may be treated quickly using a covered stent with rapid cessation of hemorrhage (Fig. 4). This is highly advantageous in the

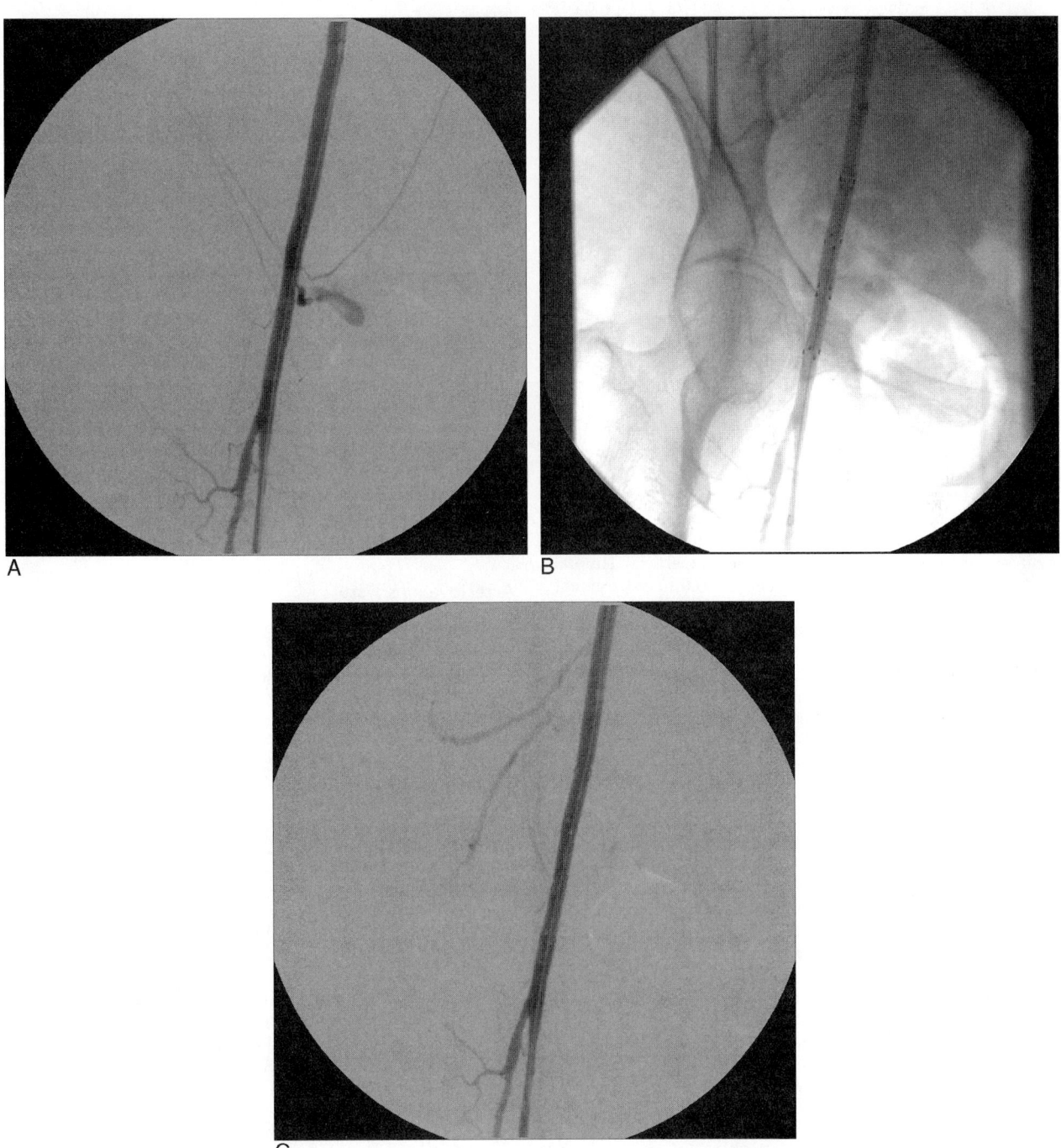

Figure 4 **(A)** Digital subtraction angiogram showing extravasation from the distal right external iliac/proximal common femoral artery. **(B)** Covered stents successfully deployed across the injury. **(C)** Final arteriogram showing resolution of a false aneurysm.

morbidly obese patient in whom rapid proximal and distal control would be difficult in an open setting. This also avoids the potential morbidity from large incisions. Placement of a stent across a joint, however, may lead to occlusion and subsequent open revision.

Certain anastomotic aneurysms can be treated through an endovascular approach. The primary requirement is suitable landing zones for anchoring of the device. In the case of aneurysms at the proximal anastamosis of an infrarenal abdominal aortic graft, there is often insufficient healthy aorta below the renal arteries. Distal anastomotic aneurysms at either the aortic bifurcation or the iliac arteries can often be treated using endovascular techniques, except in the case of infectious etiologies.

Open Repair

Traumatic False Aneurysms

Although UGTI has become widely used for iatrogenic femoral FA, open surgical repair remains the gold standard against which less invasive methods should be compared. In those patients with symptoms from the FA, such as skin necrosis or compression of the adjacent nerve or vein, thrombosis of the FA with thrombin injection is unlikely to relieve the symptoms and open repair is indicated. Also, in patients undergoing exploration for an open fracture or other associated injuries from blunt or penetrating trauma, open repair of the FA can often be accomplished at the same setting.

Wide skin preparation is essential to allow the surgeon access for proximal and distal control in areas remote from the injury. A retroperitoneal approach is often required to obtain control of the external iliac artery for injuries to the common femoral artery at the groin. Additionally, preparation of an uninjured limb for vein harvesting is preferable. After obtaining proximal and distal control, the FA is entered and the site of injury is identified. In many cases, simple suture repair is all that is necessary, but in those vessels with significant underlying atherosclerotic occlusive disease, endarterectomy and patch angioplasty may be required. In these patients, thromboembolic complications are more likely to be encountered. In those patients with an injury near the femoral bifurcation and a chronically occluded superficial femoral artery (SFA), profundaplasty using an endarterectomized segment of the SFA is a good option. Interposition grafting, if required, is ideally performed with autogenous vein; however, Dacron or polytetrafluoroethylene (PTFE) can also be used. In these more complex cases with underlying occlusive pathology, the primary goal is to restore the circulation to the preinjury state and attempts to make significant circulatory improvements (extensive endarterectomy, concomitant bypass) in this setting are generally ill advised.

Anastomotic False Aneurysms

For femoral anastomotic FAs, open surgical repair is the procedure of choice. In the typical setting of a graft inflow limb and up to three outflow vessels (common, superficial, and deep femoral arteries) in an area that crosses a joint, endovascular repair is not an attractive choice. Preoperative assessment of anastomotic FAs should include a plan to deal with an underlying infection even if one is not clinically apparent. Evaluation of these patients includes CT scan and angiography to delineate the extent of the FA, as well as all potential options for inflow and outflow.

Reoperation in the groin can be tedious and hazardous. Many of these patients have had multiple groin operations, and extensive scarring can displace structures from their usual anatomic locations. Proximal and distal control may be most easily obtained through incisions remote to the groin. Retroperitoneal control of the inflow graft is often helpful, especially if the FA extends up to or above the inguinal ligament. An incision in the proximal to

midthigh to identify the superficial or deep femoral artery, followed by subsequent dissection back into the groin, is a useful technique.

After obtaining proximal and distal control, systemic heparin is given and the FA entered. Any fluid encountered should be sent for Gram stain and culture, and it is often helpful to send a portion of the excised graft. Interposition grafting is most commonly required. Debridement of the atheromatous debris and intimal hyperplasia is necessary to identify proper sites for anastamoses. After fashioning the proximal anastamosis, several options exist for reconstructing the superficial and deep femoral arteries, including use of a bifurcated graft, placing an additional interposition graft from the graft to the second outflow vessel, or reimplanting the second outflow vessel onto the graft. In noninfectious settings, Dacron or PTFE are both reasonable choices.

Infectious False Aneurysms

FAs can become infected primarily or secondarily. The typical primary infection results from multiple injections by an intravenous drug abuser. Anastomotic aneurysms can become secondarily infected from a remote source. Both require an appreciation of the standard surgical principles of ligation of the involved vessels, wide debridement of the wound, and allowing healing through granulation. In the case of infected femoral FA, restoration of blood flow is most often accomplished through an extra-anatomic bypass (EAB) such as an axillary-to-superficial femoral artery bypass or an obturator bypass, both of which avoid tunneling through the infected groin. Staging of these procedures with EAB followed by FA excision runs the risk of secondarily infecting the EAB. Additionally, restoration of flow may not be necessary after ligation and excision of the infected FA.

Although some infectious FAs can be treated with *in situ* graft replacement, this carries the same hazards as in situ graft replacement of infected aortic grafts, including anastomotic blowout. Several algorithms exist to determine the likelihood of success of *in situ* replacement, including assessing the timing of infection relative to original graft implantation and identification of the causative organism. If in situ replacement is chosen, autogenous vein is the conduit of choice, although PTFE or rifampin-soaked Dacron have been used with limited success. Rotational muscle flaps are often helpful to provide vascularized tissue coverage of the repair.

Arteriovenous Fistula

Although symptomatic acquired AVF typically should be repaired regardless of size, asymptomatic, small AVF can initially be observed. The natural history of the small AVF is difficult to assess, given the number of undiagnosed small AVFs that likely exist. Nonetheless, it appears that most small AVFs spontaneously close. For those that require repair, both open and endovascular options exist.

Traumatic Arteriovenous Fistula

A traumatic AVF associated with an FA often resolves with treatment of the FA; however, care should be exercised in performing UGTI in the setting of communication with a large vein because of the risk of venous thromboembolism. Endovascular options are appealing in those locations that are difficult to access surgically. Covered stents can be placed in the artery feeding the AVF and have met with good results in the carotid, subclavian, iliac, and superficial femoral arteries.

Open surgical repair, especially in a chronic AVF, can be hazardous because of the friable nature of the involved vessels. Preoperative imaging, including angiography, is vital to document the relevant anatomy. At exploration, proximal and distal control of the arterial and venous segments is obtained, and optimal treatment includes obliteration of the fistula and restoration of arterial and venous flow (Fig. 5). This can be accomplished by division of the fistula primarily or through an arteriotomy or venotomy at the site of communication. Interposition grafting or patch angioplasty is not typically necessary but should be considered if primary

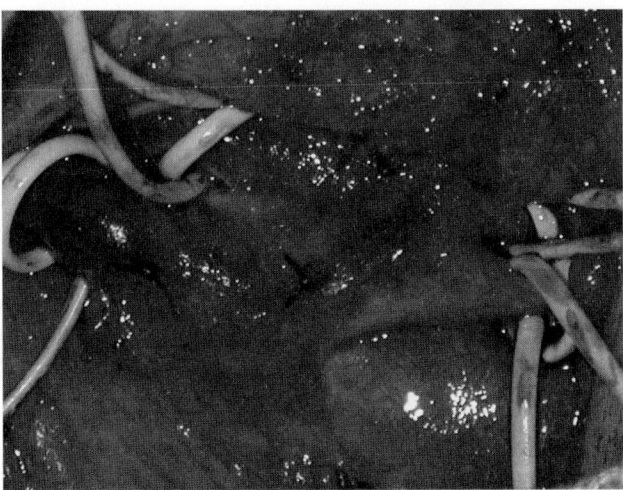

Figure 5 Brachial artery to brachial vein arteriovenous fistula with proximal and distal control of artery and vein.

repair leads to significant (>50%) narrowing of the vessel lumen. Autogenous vein is preferred and should be harvested from an unaffected extremity.

In some cases, restoration of arterial and venous flow may not be practical or possible. Repair of small-caliber veins such as tibial veins are unlikely to stay patent and are appropriately ligated. In dire circumstances, four-vessel ligation is necessary as a lifesaving maneuver. Subsequent bypass grafting from vessels remote to the AVF can be accomplished in a staged fashion.

Nontraumatic Atriovenous Fistula

An acquired, nontraumatic AVF can occur from erosion or rupture of an arterial aneurysm into an adjacent vein, typically the vena cava or the iliac or renal veins. Although the classic clinical triad is pain, a pulsatile abdominal mass, and a machinery-like abdominal bruit, all three findings may in fact be present in only 20% of patients. Other preoperative findings suggestive of AVF include

rapid onset of congestive heart failure, renal insufficiency, or hematuria, which can occur as a result of direct renal injury from elevated renal vein pressure. Preoperative CTA can also aid in the diagnosis by identifying a more round rather than oval shape of the vena cava or by revealing a dilatated vena cava with the same contrast intensity as the aorta. The fistula can also be discovered intraoperatively when a large volume of venous blood is encountered after the aneurysm sac is opened.

Surgical repair is challenging. Closure of the defect can be performed from within the aneurysm sac. Small fistulae may be addressed with simple suture repair, or an autogenous or prosthetic patch may be required for larger defects. Preoperative transfemoral placement of a venous occlusion balloon may be helpful. The balloon can be inflated as the aneurysm is entered. Close communication with the anesthesia team is vital, given the abrupt cessation of venous return that occurs from digital control of the fistula. Although thrombus will almost inevitably enter into the venous system, a preoperative vena cava filter does not appear necessary, given the low reported incidence of clinically significant pulmonary embolism after repair of aortocaval fistulae. Given the likelihood of large-volume blood loss, cell saver and rapid infusion devices are highly recommended. Several recent case reports have shown satisfactory results with endovascular grafting, with no increase in type II endoleak despite the presence of the aortocaval fistula.

SUGGESTED READINGS

Calton WC, Franklin DP, Elmore JR, and others: Ultrasound-guided thrombin injection is a safe and durable treatment for femoral pseuoaneurysms, *Vasc Surg* 35:379, 2001.

Gloviczki P, Baker WH, Kalman PG, and others: Expert exchange: the management of primary aortocaval and ilio-iliac arteriovenous fistulae, *Perspect Vasc Surg* 12:133, 1999.

Mansour MA, Baker WH: Arteriovenous fistulae of the aorta and its major branches. In Rutherford RB, editor: *Vascular surgery*, ed 6, Philadelphia, 2005, WB Saunders.

Morgan R, Belli AM: Current treatment methods for postcatheterization pseudoaneurysms, *J Vasc Inter Radiol* 14697, 2003.

van den Akker PJ, Brand R, van Schilfgaarde R, and others: False aneurysms after prosthetic reconstructions for aortoiliac obstructive disease, *Ann Surg* 210:658, 1989.

CAROTID ENDARTERECTOMY

Louis L. Nguyen, MD, MBA, MPH, and
Michael S. Conte, MD

Carotid endarterectomy (CEA) is one of the most frequently performed vascular surgery procedures, although its role in stroke prevention has been, and continues to be, the subject of much clinical investigation. Since the early 1990s, the results of several large prospective randomized trials have validated the role of CEA, as performed by surgeons, with low complications rates, in suitable patients with appropriate lesions. Improved efficacy of newer cardiovascular drugs may change the relative outcome advantage of CEA versus medical management. More recently, with the development of angioplasty and stenting techniques, a new debate is under way to determine the appropriate role

of CEA in the treatment of carotid artery stenosis. However, CEA still remains a well-established surgical treatment option with a proven track record of safety, efficacy, and anatomic durability in the treatment of carotid atherosclerosis.

INDICATIONS

The data that establish the efficacy of CEA for treatment of extracranial carotid artery stenosis emanate from a number of large, prospective, multicenter trials. The North American Symptomatic Carotid Endarterectomy Trial (NASCET) and the European Carotid Surgery Trial (ECST) demonstrated that CEA with medical management is superior to medical management alone for patients with symptomatic, high-grade, internal carotid artery (ICA) stenosis. For patients with severe lesions (70%–99% stenosis) in NASCET, the 2-year ipsilateral stroke risk was 9% for CEA versus 26% for medical therapy alone. The absolute risk reduction of 17% corresponds to a number-needed-to-treat (NNT) of six. For more moderate lesions (50%–69% stenosis) in symptomatic patients, the benefit of CEA over medical therapy remained statistically significant, but the risk reduction was notably smaller (22% vs. 16% at

5 years; NNT ≈15). Asymptomatic carotid disease has been the subject of several large, randomized studies. The Asymptomatic Carotid Atherosclerosis Study (ACAS) demonstrated benefit of CEA and medical management over medical management alone for asymptomatic patients with high-grade carotid stenosis. For patients with greater than 60% stenosis, the 5-year stroke and mortality risk was 5.1% for CEA and 11% for medical therapy. Although these results were statistically significant, the benefit was not manifest until 3 years after randomization and was notably less in women (17% relative risk reduction for women vs. 66% for men). More recently, the larger Asymptomatic Carotid Surgery Trial Group (ACST; $N = 3120$ patients) confirmed that CEA reduced the 5-year incidence of all strokes (6.4% CEA vs. 11.8% for medical therapy) and fatal or disabling strokes (3.5% vs. 6.1%) in patients with ICA lesions of 60% or greater. The larger size of ACST permitted a more robust subgroup analysis; accordingly, the advantage of CEA appeared to extend across age, sex, and degree of stenosis subgroups. It is critical to note that the superiority of CEA over medical therapy in these studies hinges strongly on the excellent perioperative outcomes achieved by these investigators (30-day combined stroke/death rate of 2.1% in ACAS, 5.8% in NASCET).

Based largely on the level I evidence provided by these trials, current guidelines from the American Heart Association (AHA) and American Stroke Association Council on Stroke recommend CEA for patients with transient ischemic attack or stroke within the last 6 months and ipsilateral 70% to 99% carotid artery stenosis, with CEA performed by a surgeon with perioperative morbidity and mortality rate of less than 6%. For patients with symptoms and 50% to 69% stenosis, CEA is recommended on the basis of patient-specific factors such as age, gender, comorbidities, and symptom severity. For patients with asymptomatic disease, AHA guidelines recommend risk factor reduction and suggest that CEA may be considered selectively in patients with 60% to 99% ICA stenosis if performed by a surgeon with stroke/mortality rate under 3%. Patient selection for treatment of asymptomatic disease should be guided by comorbidities, life expectancy, patient preference, and other individual factors.

Although the aforementioned randomized trials provided rigorous evidence supporting the role of CEA for selected patients, several criticisms have been raised and continue to be debated. The extrapolation of results from randomized clinical trials to everyday clinical practice must be approached with caution. Institutions and surgeons were selected to participate in the trials on the basis of expertise with CEA. Thus the extension of the perioperative outcomes from these trials to the general practicing community may not be valid, particularly because there seem to be volume-associated outcomes for CEA. Given that the risk-to-benefit ratio favoring CEA is substantially greater for symptomatic patients, the focus of this controversy primarily relates to the treatment of asymptomatic disease.

DIAGNOSIS

The diagnosis and treatment of carotid atherosclerosis is facilitated by the predilection for the disease to occur focally at the carotid bifurcation. Most often, carotid duplex examination, as performed in an accredited vascular laboratory, is the only imaging modality required to evaluate the carotid arteries before surgery. However, performing carotid duplex examination requires that the vascular laboratory programmatically validate its ultrasound results with angiographic results from the same institution. Duplex not only evaluates the degree of luminal narrowing but also gives information about surface characteristics (e.g., ulceration) and lesion composition (e.g., lipid vs. fibrous components) that may influence plaque stability. Limitations of duplex include suboptimal imaging in some patients because of neck obesity or immobility, calcium

shadowing, and high carotid bifurcations. In these cases, magnetic resonance angiography (MRA) or computed tomography angiography (CTA) may corroborate duplex findings. These modalities are also useful to assess the proximal aortic arch and supra-aortic trunks, the intracranial circulation, and the brain parenchyma. Cerebrovascular angiography provides outstanding anatomic definition, but it is costly, invasive, and associated with potential procedural complications, including stroke. Currently it is reserved for cases in which noninvasive imaging is inconclusive (e.g., uncertainty between subtotal versus total ICA occlusion) or when carotid artery stenting is planned.

It is commonly accepted that approximately 20% to 30% of ischemic strokes may be secondary to carotid atherosclerosis. In patients presenting with an acute deficit, the diagnosis of ischemic stroke is established by brain imaging (CT or MRI), and investigation of the carotid arteries by duplex ultrasound is indicated as part of the workup. The timing of CEA after ipsilateral stroke is controversial. Early studies suggested that waiting 6 weeks after completion of the stroke is favorable, whereas a number of others indicated that this wait is unnecessary and may be deleterious. A more recent large institutional review suggests that a delay of 4 weeks was associated with a decreased rate of perioperative stroke. Current AHA recommendations are that if CEA is indicated, it should be performed within 2 weeks of the initial symptoms. Factors that may affect the timing of CEA following cerebral infarction include the degree of disability, the size of the infarct, the amount of cerebral edema, and the presence of peri-infarct hemorrhage. Serial brain imaging (CT or MRI) is usually employed to document the presence or resolution of these findings before CEA.

OPERATIVE TECHNIQUE

Preparation and Positioning

Preoperative evaluation for CEA, as for other vascular surgery procedures, is focused on cardiovascular risk reduction. The cornerstones are a careful clinical assessment and optimization of medical therapies before surgery. In comparison with aneurysm repair and lower extremity bypass, the risk of myocardial infarction following CEA is relatively low but should not be ignored. However, preoperative stress testing or other provocative cardiac studies are performed only in patients whose clinical assessment suggests potential high risk. Appropriate use of cardioprotective medications, particularly beta-adrenergic antagonists, is critical for reducing the risk of perioperative complications. Treatment of hypertension is particularly important because poor blood pressure control preoperatively may translate into dangerous lability in the immediate postoperative period. Patients undergoing CEA should be on aspirin for at least 1 day before the procedure, including a dose on the morning of surgery. Patients on clopidogrel, ticlopidine, warfarin (Coumadin; Bristol-Myers Squibb, New York, NY), or fractionated heparin should be switched to aspirin, unless otherwise strongly contraindicated, for example by the presence of a recent coronary stent. A dose of intravenous antibiotic is given in the preoperative holding area.

CEA can be performed using various anesthesia modalities, depending on the experience and preferences of each surgeon, anesthesiologist, and institution. Regional anesthesia via a cervical block allows the patient to be awake during the procedure and permits ongoing neurological evaluation. However, patients have different preferences and tolerances for major surgery while awake and may not be cooperative. General anesthesia results in a still patient and more relaxed operating room environment. With general anesthesia, other modalities to assess and ensure adequate cerebral perfusion must be used (as discussed subsequently), such as electroencephalogram (EEG) monitoring, carotid back-pressure measurement, or routine carotid shunting. When EEG monitoring is used, multiple scalp electrodes are placed either before or immediately after induction of anesthesia, and multilead recordings are monitored continuously throughout the case by a trained neurophysiology technician.

After the induction of anesthesia, the patient is placed in the supine position, and the operating table is flexed to the modified semi-Fowler position (head up with hips and knees flexed), which also results in slight neck extension. The head is supported on a padded donut and gently turned to the contralateral side, and the arms are secured to the side of the patient. In some patients, a small posterior roll between the scapulae may be useful to achieve slight neck extension. The patient is prepared and draped to include the ipsilateral neck, lower jaw, ear lobe, and supraclavicular space.

Incision and Exposure

A longitudinal skin incision is made along the anterior border of the sternocleidomastoid (SCM). Electrocautery is used to divide the platysma and dissect through the deeper soft tissues while retracting the SCM posterolaterally to expose the carotid sheath. Often a common (transverse) facial vein is encountered and should be ligated to facilitate internal jugular vein dissection and lateral retraction. The common carotid artery (CCA) is first dissected and isolated at the level of the omohyoid muscle. Care must be taken to identify the vagus nerve, which usually courses posterior and deep to the carotid artery, although anatomic variation can occur. Dissection of the artery in the correct periadventitial plane ensures that the nerve is not ensnared in a catheter tourniquet or subsequently clamped. The dissection is then carried distally toward the bifurcation. Often the ansa cervicalis is seen crossing the field in a loop. Proper identification of the ansa cervicalis can be made by retracing its anterior descent from the hypoglossal nerve. Keeping the dissection posterior to the ansa facilitates sweeping the hypoglossal nerve anteriorly and away from the ICA. If necessary, the ansa can be divided, but only after the vagus nerve and hypoglossal nerve are clearly identified. If sinus bradycardia occurs during dissection around the bifurcation, 1 to 2 ml of 1% lidocaine can be injected into the tissues between the ICA and external carotid artery (ECA) to block the carotid sinus.

The carotid dissection is carried along the ICA to reach a point beyond the visible disease. Proceeding distally along the ICA, the surgeon will see the hypoglossal nerve traversing the field, limiting further dissection. If more distal ICA access is necessary, several maneuvers can be used. (1) The hypoglossal nerve is usually tethered by branches of the occipital artery and vein to the SCM. Division of these small branches with ties will allow the nerve to be swept anteriorly away from the ICA. (2) The posterior belly of the digastric muscle can be divided, visualizing and protecting the hypoglossal nerve during this maneuver. (3) The mandible can be subluxed; however, this maneuver is required only in extremely rare instances. Care should be taken to avoid vigorous upward retraction of the soft tissues against the mandible, which may injure the mandibular branch of the facial nerve coursing below the mandible. The ECA is dissected to its first branch, the superior thyroid artery. Modified Rumel tourniquets with umbilical tapes are positioned around the carotid arteries. After the dissection is complete, intravenous heparin (70 U/kg) is given to the patient.

Cerebral Perfusion

As mentioned earlier, several methods can be used to determine cerebral perfusion during carotid cross clamping. If the patient is awake and under regional anesthesia, he or she is asked to talk and move the contralateral arm and leg during a 3-minute test clamp period. For patients under general anesthesia, one of several

techniques can be employed: EEG monitoring, back-pressure measurement, or routine shunting. We favor continuous EEG monitoring using a multilead system with real-time waveform analysis. The EEG is monitored by a trained technician actively communicating with the anesthesia staff and surgical team. Changes in the depth of general anesthesia, as well as global hypoperfusion (e.g., secondary to hypotension), will affect the waveforms in a generally symmetric fashion. An ipsilateral change in cerebral activity beyond several standard deviations is considered significant. Back-pressure measurement uses a 22-gauge needle connected to pressure tubing and monitor. The needle is inserted into the CCA proximal to the ICA lesion and distal to a clamp on the CCA. A second clamp is placed on the ECA, resulting in a static column of blood through the length of the ICA. Even though the needle is proximal to the ICA stenosis, pressure equalizes on both sides of the stenosis because there is no flow. Patients with back-pressure measurements of less than 25 mm Hg receive shunts.

Carotid shunting maintains flow through the clamped carotid artery. However, carotid shunts can result in complications, such as embolism, damage to the distal arterial intima, and poor distal ICA endpoint treatment. Thus shunting is reserved for occasions in which cerebral perfusion during test clamping is inadequate or when perfusion monitoring is not available. We prefer to use straight Silastic shunts, although T-shaped and balloon occlusion shunts are also available options. Before the shunt is placed, the steps of shunt placement should be reviewed with the operative team, and a shunt is preselected to match the size of the distal ICA. The shunting process begins with clamping of the carotid arteries. A longitudinal arteriotomy is made in the CCA and extended through the lesion into the ICA. The distal end of the shunt is placed in the ICA and allowed to backbleed through the shunt. The proximal end of the shunt is placed in the CCA, and the CCA is allowed to forward flush. Flow through the shunt is confirmed with Doppler assessment, and the shunt secured by tightening the Rumel tourniquet.

Endarterectomy Techniques

The carotid endarterectomy is begun at the lesion where a natural cleavage plane exists between the diseased intima and fibers of the media. The endarterectomy is carried proximally and circumferentially into the CCA. A right-angle clamp is used to complete the circumferential dissection so that the same plane can be maintained throughout. The atheromatous plaque is then sharply divided at the proximal limit of the CCA. The plaque dissection is carried to the ECA where the plaque is excised by eversion of the artery until a natural breakpoint is reached. The last part of the dissection is performed by mobilizing the plaque distally up the ICA with the spatula. With gentle downward traction, the plaque will usually taper and detach from the less-diseased intima distally. Thorough inspection of the endpoint for a smooth transition must be performed, and the arteriotomy should be extended if necessary. Some surgeons routinely tack down the leading edge with suture, although we prefer to create a smooth and tapered endpoint and tack it selectively. The intimal edge at the CCA does not require tacking if it is a flush transition point because forward flow will not favor flap formation. The endarterectomized artery is generously flushed with heparinized saline solution, and all residual debris or loosely attached intima is removed using fine forceps and loupe magnification.

Eversion carotid endarterectomy is an alternative method to conventional CEA, with distinct advantage in cases in which the ICA is redundant. Instead of making a longitudinal arteriotomy, the ICA is obliquely transected from the CCA and an eversion endarterectomy of the ICA is performed. Open endarterectomy of the anteriorly spatulated CCA is performed in conjunction with limited eversion endarterectomy of the ECA. The posteriorly spatulated ICA is then reimplanted onto the CCA. A review of several controlled clinical trials comparing the two methods suggested improved restenosis (defined as >50%) rates for eversion endarterectomy compared with CEA (2.5% vs. 5.2%, respectively), although no statistical difference was seen in a subgroup analysis of conventional CEA with patch angioplasty versus eversion endarterectomy.

Arterial Closure and Intraoperative Assessment at Completion

Closure of the endarterectomy can be performed primarily or with patch angioplasty. We prefer patch angioplasty closure using bovine pericardium and a continuous 6-0 polypropylene suture starting at the distal apex. Evidence supports patch angioplasty in reducing recurrent restenosis, although not enough evidence exists to demonstrate benefit with one type of material (vein, polytetrafluoroethylene, Dacron, bovine pericardium) over another. Before the completion of the closure, the arterial clamps are briefly released to flush each vessel sequentially, and the vessel is forcefully rinsed with heparinized saline to remove air and debris. On completion of the closure, flow is restored first to the ECA to allow any possible debris to enter that vessel and avoid the ICA.

Flow in all vessels should be confirmed by Doppler examination. We routinely perform an intraoperative color duplex ultrasound study as our preferred method of ensuring technical success. A 10-MHz transducer with a sterile cover is used. The CCA, ICA, and ECA are scanned in both transverse and longitudinal planes, using gray-scale, color, and Doppler spectral analysis. Ultrasound allows for excellent visualization of the entire endarterectomy site and confirms vessel patency with low resistance flow in the ICA (Fig. 1). Flaps, residual debris, or abnormal flow velocities or waveforms may be detected. Reopening of the artery is considered for a visualized wall abnormality (flap or mobile plaque >2 mm) or a significant flow disturbance (peak systolic velocity >125 cm/sec). Completion angiography is another acceptable method to verify the technical results. Hemostasis is then meticulously achieved using ligatures and electrocautery. The heparin may be reversed with protamine. Depending on surgical preference, a drain may be placed in the field and is connected to bulb suction. Closure of the wound is performed with absorbable sutures to the platysma and continuous absorbable suture to the subcuticular layer.

POSTOPERATIVE CARE AND COMPLICATIONS

We prefer to wake and extubate the patient in the operating room while keeping the instrument table sterile. A general neurologic examination is performed on the patient to assess for deficits. New neurologic finds are generally an indication for immediate reexploration of the artery. In some cases, an immediately available imaging study such as duplex ultrasound or head CT may be appropriate, depending on the nature of the deficit, its timing, and the intraoperative completion study that was performed. Stable patients are transferred to the recovery room with the head of the bed at 30 degrees. Blood pressure should be closely monitored and kept at a systolic pressure of between 100 and 150 mm Hg. Many patients develop asymptomatic transient hypotension immediately postprocedure and may require minimal vasopressor support. Care must be taken to avoid hypertension and resulting cerebral edema.

Patients who develop a significant postoperative neck hematoma should be reexplored in the operating room to rule out ongoing hemorrhage and avoid airway compromise. The patients are observed overnight in a monitored setting with blood pressure and neurologic assessment. The drain is removed the following morning, and the patient is discharged from the hospital that day if neurologically intact, without significant headache, and capable of normal activity.

Other complications of CEA include nerve injury, infection, hyperperfusion syndrome, and development of late pseudo-aneurysm. The incidence of cranial nerve injury after CEA is estimated to be approximately 5.1%, with most being transient and only a few (0.5%) persisting at 4 months. Injury to the hypoglossal nerve results in deviation of the tongue to the ipsilateral side; injury to the marginal mandibular nerve results in asymmetry and drooping of the ipsilateral lower lip; vagus or recurrent laryngeal nerve injury results in ipsilateral vocal chord paralysis manifested as weakened voice. Clinical suspicion of nerve injury should be assessed with comprehensive speech evaluation, video fluoroscopy, and contrast testing for aspiration when appropriate. Patients with persistent vagus or recurrent laryngeal nerve injury may benefit from medialization of the paralyzed vocal cord and cricopharyngeal myotomy to restore swallowing and alleviate aspiration. Infection of the CEA closure (and often the resulting pseudo-aneurysm) is associated with use of prosthetic material, although the overall incidence is rare and estimated to be less than 1%. Hyperperfusion syndrome is a rare but potentially devastating complication that may occur days after the procedure, generally presaged by severe headache and seizure activity. Thought to result from failure of autoregulation in the intracranial vessels, it is more commonly seen in patients with high-grade, preocclusive lesions and may result in intracranial hemorrhage and cerebral edema. Prompt and aggressive treatment measures to control blood pressure and minimize brain swelling are required with intensive neurologic monitoring.

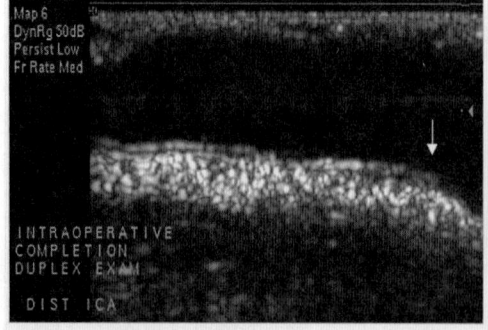 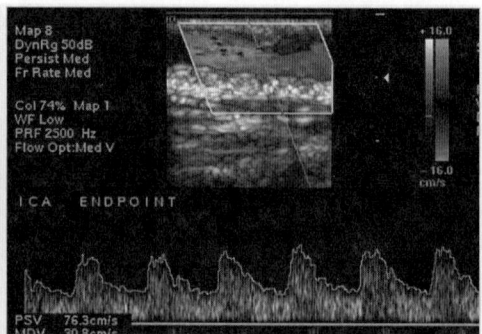

Figure I Intraoperative Duplex examination of carotid endarterectomy and patch angioplasty. The distal endarterectomy interface *(left panel)* and velocity measurements *(right panel)* are shown.

LONG-TERM SURVEILLANCE AND CAROTID RESTENOSIS

Analogous to graft surveillance for peripheral bypass patients, CEA patients require surveillance to detect midterm and long-term carotid restenosis (CR). Duplex examination is the most commonly used surveillance modality. Velocity criteria similar to those used to interpret de novo stenosis are used to interpret CR. Midterm CR, defined as diameter reduction of 60% or more and occurring from 3 to 18 months after surgery, is attributed to intimal hyperplasia and has been reported in 7.6% of patients in one study. Long-term CR, occurring beyond 18 months after CEA, is attributed to progression of atherosclerosis disease and has an estimated annual incidence of 1.9%. Regression of CR may occur in 10% of cases, emphasizing the importance of serial duplex examination for moderate lesions. Current practice is to survey by ultrasound at 6 and 12 months, followed by annual examinations thereafter. Better clinical data are necessary to estimate the frequency of CR and subsequently determine the most cost-effective surveillance plan. The use of patch angioplasty, especially in women, has reduced the apparent incidence of CR.

The clinical significance of CR is debated because the estimated incidence of symptoms related to these lesions is low, ranging from 0% to 8%. For symptomatic CR, most advocate intervention with lesions of 50% or greater stenosis; for asymptomatic lesions, the intervention threshold is 80% or greater. The operative management of CR is similar to primary CEA, with a greater use of patch angioplasty. The incidence of cranial nerve injury and wound hematomas is generally believed to be higher in redo CEA. The lack of uniform follow-up data on redo CEA makes the long-term outcomes difficult to estimate. Carotid artery stenting is currently considered a viable option for CR despite lack of long-term results, largely because of the presumed advantage of stenting for avoiding local complications such as cranial nerve injury and hematomas.

SUMMARY

CEA is a frequently performed procedure with a long history of reported outcomes. Clinical investigation has established the role of CEA for high-grade stenosis in symptomatic and asymptomatic patients. The benefits of CEA hinge on excellent surgical results, which are achievable in diverse practice settings by careful attention to preoperative, intraoperative, and postoperative management and technique. With the advent of new medical and technological strategies, CEA is again undergoing investigation to redefine its role in stroke prevention.

Suggested Readings

AbuRahma AF, Lim RY: Management of vagus nerve injury after carotid endarterectomy, *Surgery* 119:245, 1996.

Bond R, Rerkasem K, Naylor AR, and others: Systematic review of randomized controlled trials of patch angioplasty versus primary closure and different types of patch materials during carotid endarterectomy, *J Vasc Surg* 40:1126, 2004.

Cao P, De Rango P, Zannetti S: Eversion vs conventional carotid endarterectomy: a systematic review, *Eur J Vasc Endovasc Surg* 23:195, 2002.

Cowan JA Jr, Dimick JB, Thompson BG, and others: Surgeon volume as an indicator of outcomes after carotid endarterectomy: an effect independent of specialty practice and hospital volume, *J Am Coll Surg* 195:814, 2002.

Cunningham EJ, Bond R, Mayberg MR, and others: Risk of persistent cranial nerve injury after carotid endarterectomy, *J Neurosurg* 101:445, 2004.

European Carotid Surgery Trialists' Collaborative Group: MRC European Carotid Surgery Trial: interim results for symptomatic patients with severe (70–99%) or with mild (0–29%) carotid stenosis, *Lancet* 337:1235, 1991.

Executive Committee for the Asymptomatic Carotid Atherosclerosis Study: Endarterectomy for asymptomatic carotid artery stenosis, *JAMA* 273:1421, 1995.

Goldstein LB, Adams R, Alberts MJ, and others: Primary prevention of ischemic stroke: a guideline from the American Heart Association/ American Stroke Association Stroke Council: cosponsored by the Atherosclerotic Peripheral Vascular Disease Interdisciplinary Working Group; Cardiovascular Nursing Council; Clinical Cardiology Council; Nutrition, Physical Activity, and Metabolism Council; and the Quality of Care and Outcomes Research Interdisciplinary Working Group, *Circulation* 113:e873, 2006.

Halliday A, Mansfield A, Marro J, and others: Prevention of disabling and fatal strokes by successful carotid endarterectomy in patients without recent neurological symptoms: randomised controlled trial, *Lancet* 363:1491, 2004.

Healy DA, Zierler RE, Nicholls SC, and others: Long-term follow-up and clinical outcome of carotid restenosis, *J Vasc Surg* 10:662; discussion 668, 1989.

Hobson RW 2nd, Goldstein JE, Jamil Z, and others: Carotid restenosis: operative and endovascular management, *J Vasc Surg* 29:228; discussion 235, 1999.

Lattimer CR, Burnand KG: Recurrent carotid stenosis after carotid endarterectomy, *Br J Surg* 84:1206, 1997.

Mansour MA, Kang SS, Baker WH, and others: Carotid endarterectomy for recurrent stenosis, *J Vasc Surg* 25:877, 1997.

Mehta M, Roddy SP, Darling RC 3rd, and others: Safety and efficacy of eversion carotid endarterectomy for the treatment of recurrent stenosis: 20-year experience, *Ann Vasc Surg* 19:492, 2005.

Moore WS, Kempczinski RF, Nelson JJ, and others: Recurrent carotid stenosis: results of the asymptomatic carotid atherosclerosis study, *Stroke* 29:2018, 1998.

Naylor AR, Payne D, London NJ, and others: Prosthetic patch infection after carotid endarterectomy, *Eur J Vasc Endovasc Surg* 23:11, 2002.

North American Symptomatic Carotid Endarterectomy Trial Collaborators.: Beneficial effect of carotid endarterectomy in symptomatic patients with high-grade carotid stenosis, *N Engl J Med* 325:445, 1991.

O'Hara PJ, Hertzer NR, Karafa MT, and others: Reoperation for recurrent carotid stenosis: early results and late outcome in 199 patients, *J Vasc Surg* 34:5, 2001.

Rockman CB, Maldonado TS, Jacobowitz GR, and others: Early carotid endarterectomy in symptomatic patients is associated with poorer perioperative outcomes, *J Vasc Surg* 44:480, 2006.

Sacco RL, Adams R, Albers G, and others: Guidelines for prevention of stroke in patients with ischemic stroke or transient ischemic attack: a statement for healthcare professionals from the American Heart Association/American Stroke Association Council on Stroke: co-sponsored by the Council on Cardiovascular Radiology and Intervention: the American Academy of Neurology affirms the value of this guideline, *Circulation* 113:e409, 2006.

MANAGEMENT OF RECURRENT CAROTID STENOSIS

Adnan H. Siddiqui, MD, PhD, and
Robert H. Rosenwasser, MD

Carotid artery stenosis is responsible for up to 20% of cerebrovascular ischemic events. Screening for carotid stenosis is now an established integral component of the diagnostic workup for patients presenting with both transient ischemic events and stroke. Carotid stenosis is also routinely evaluated through auscultation for carotid bruits during physical examination for patients with risk factors for atherosclerotic disease. Evaluation includes noninvasive modalities such as Doppler ultrasonography and magnetic resonance angiography, as well as minimally invasive modalities such as computed tomographic angiography. Patients who are deemed to have carotid stenosis on the basis of findings on these modalities often undergo confirmatory digital subtraction angiography before intervention.

Prospective randomized studies have established the superiority of carotid endarterectomy (CEA) to best contemporary medical therapy for carotid stenosis detected on routine screening for asymptomatic patients (Asymptomatic Carotid Surgery Trial, Asymptomatic Carotid Atherosclerotic Study, Veteran Affairs Study), as well as for symptomatic patients (North American Symptomatic Carotid Endarterectomy Trial, European Carotid Surgery Trial) presenting with cerebrovascular events. The benefit of endarterectomy is greater for symptomatic patients with 70% to 99% stenosis, resulting in an absolute risk reduction (ARR) of 17%. This benefit is less pronounced for symptomatic patients with 50% to 69% stenosis (ARR 6.5%). The benefit for surgery is lost for stenosis less than 50%. In patients with asymptomatic disease and stenosis exceeding 60%, endarterectomy resulted in an ARR of 5.9% at 5 years. These studies catapulted CEA as one of the most common surgical procedures performed nationwide. These studies resulted in the establishment of guidelines that procedural morbidity (stroke) and mortality should be below 6% and 3% for symptomatic and asymptomatic carotid stenosis, respectively, to realize the benefit of surgery over medical management alone.

A by-product of the increased performance of CEA for carotid stenosis and increased survival in patients with atherosclerotic risk factors is recurrent carotid stenosis or restenosis after endarterectomy. These are well-recognized sequelae, affecting 3% to 7% of patients on protracted follow-up. The presentation of carotid restenosis is identical to primary disease or de novo carotid artery disease, with symptomatic disease presenting with cerebrovascular ischemic events, whereas asymptomatic disease is discovered on routine postendarterectomy clinical and radiologic follow-up.

Restenosis after CEA can be ascribed to three causes. First, there is the spectrum of inadequate decompression of the original stenosis with resultant residual disease, which leads to persistent stenosis and is identified on immediate postoperative imaging, as well as on follow-up imaging. Second is the spectrum of fibrointimal or myointimal hyperplasia, which is a proliferative inflammatory response encountered after CEA. This type of restenosis presents with early recurrent narrowing within the endarterectomized segment of the carotid artery, typically within the first year. Third is atherosclerotic plaque development within or at the ends of the endarterectomized carotid artery segment, representing new plaque secondary to underlying atherosclerotic risk factors.

Regardless of the cause for the restenosis, reoperation poses unique challenges for the surgeon. The loss of tissue planes secondary to the natural postoperative fibrotic response results in increased difficulty for identification of vascular structures and subsequent risk of vascular injury. In addition, the carotid bifurcation region is particularly well endowed with critical neural structures, which are routinely involved in postoperative fibrosis; therefore surgery poses an additional risk of cranial neuropathy affecting the vagus and hypoglossal nerves. This enhanced risk is well established in the literature, with an absolute risk of stroke and death of 4.4%. AbuRahma and colleagues published their results from a single center and a single vascular surgeon employing patch angioplasty for both recurrent (124) and primary (265) CEAs and reported a 4% versus 0.8% stroke rate, respectively, with no deaths in either category. In addition, the rate of cranial neuropathy was 17% for reoperation versus 5.3% for primary endarterectomy. However, the rate of long-term stroke-free survival was similar for both categories.

The higher operative risk for redo CEA has created the need for evaluation of alternative strategies for management of recurrent or residual disease. It has formed the basis for the evaluation of carotid angioplasty and stenting (CAS) as a viable alternative to redo CEA. The development of CAS has lagged significantly behind that of coronary and peripheral angioplasty and stenting. This is due in part to a fear of distal embolization but also to the technology's lagging behind that used in the coronary and peripheral vascular trees. Several recent European and U.S. studies have begun to show that CAS is both safe and effective. A recent analysis of prospective data by Coward and colleagues suggested no difference in the rates of 30-day or 1-year stroke, myocardial infarction (MI), or death for reoperation compared with angioplasty and stenting. However, the incidence of cranial neuropathy was obviously significantly lower with endovascular treatment. Although endovascular treatment was associated with an increased rate of restenosis (14% vs. 4%) at 1 year, there was no correlation with stroke rates as far out as 3 years postintervention. More recently, patients considered high surgical risk because of restenosis, anatomic considerations, and comorbidities were evaluated in Boston Scientific EPI: A Carotid Stenting Trial for High-Risk Surgical Patients (BEACH). For this cohort of 747 patients, the 30-day rates of 4.4% for stroke, 1.0% for MI, and 1.5% for death compared favorably with results reported previously for these cohorts.

At the Thomas Jefferson University Hospital for Neuroscience, we have therefore followed the development of CAS as a viable alternative and currently routinely employ CAS as the principal strategy for the management of recurrent carotid stenosis.

INDICATIONS

Indications for treatment of carotid restenosis are similar to those for the management of primary disease. They can, however, be divided into three categories, according to the underlying cause.

Early Restenosis Secondary to Residual Disease

Early restenosis such as that discovered following an early postoperative cerebrovascular event within days to a few weeks of the endarterectomy or during the initial postoperative radiologic screening indicates inadequate decompression during the primary surgical procedure. If the patient is symptomatic, this is certainly ground for an early return to the operating room for redo CEA. However, if the discovery is delayed until asymptomatic postoperative radiologic evaluation a few weeks after surgery, a more deliberate consideration can be made on the basis of the anatomic features of the residual lesion. If there remains a high-grade stenosis, certainly reexploration in the operating room is considered appropriate because of the inherent risks of both embolic and thrombotic disease. However, if the disease is mild, a cautious, frequent, radiographic follow-up is considered prudent.

Restenosis Secondary to Myointimal Hyperplasia

The second category of recurrent disease is discovered at 6 months to 1 year following initial radiologic studies that have suggested an excellent decompression. This is typically an asymptomatic presentation for an inflammatory response of the hyperplastic intima within the operated segment. The resulting hyperplastic response of the intimal layers presents a rubbery stenotic lesion that can either remain stable or be rapidly progressive and result in thromboembolic disease. Early detection (i.e., during the course of routine post-CEA follow-up imaging or ultrasonography) of recurrent stenosis after initial adequate decompression within the first year is a strong indication of intimal hyperplasia. If the patient is asymptomatic with mild to moderate stenosis, a more frequent radiographic follow-up is considered appropriate. However, if progression of disease is clearly demonstrated or if the patient is symptomatic, intervention should be considered. Certainly, reoperation is a viable option; however, as mentioned earlier, the intimal response complicates surgical decompression because of the difficulty associated with establishing planes between the rubbery lesion and the adventitia. Typically such an operation requires patch angioplasty with minimal removal of the occlusive lesion to restore flow without further irritation of the intima. However, depending on the location of the lesion, surgical resection of the affected segment with an interposition tubular graft reconstruction of the carotid artery and sacrifice of the external carotid may be necessary. In our experience, these patients are ideal candidates for CAS. Restenosis following CEA after radiation to the neck may result in similar surgical dilemmas that are again well addressed through CAS.

Restenosis Secondary to Recurrent Atherosclerotic Plaque

The final category of recurrent stenosis is detected on routine surveillance or following cerebrovascular events many years after the original surgery. This type of disease is reflective of recurrent atherosclerotic plaque development either within the bed or at the ends of the prior endarterectomy site. This is essentially continuation of the original disease because of underlying risk factors, either de novo within the operative bed or progression at the ends of the operated segment. Indications for treatment of this disease are identical to those for primary stenosis, with consideration based on the degree of arterial narrowing and the patient's symptoms. The principal surgical options for reoperation consist of redo endarterectomy with or without patch angioplasty or interposition tubular graft reconstruction (or both). In our experience, CAS is an excellent means to address this type of recurrent carotid stenosis.

■ TECHNIQUES

Surgical or interventional management of this condition is tailored to the underlying cause.

Early Reoperation for Residual Disease

Early restenosis from residual disease that is detected soon after the primary operation is best addressed through a reoperation. Patients are symptomatic either before discharge or soon thereafter. If asymptomatic, they are noted to have considerable, severe narrowing of the endarterectomized arterial segment on initial postoperative ultrasonography.

We perform CEA under general anesthesia with continuous intraoperative cerebral monitoring by electroencephalography (EEG) and somatosensory-evoked potentials (SSEPs). The patient is positioned supine with a small roll under the shoulders, and the head is turned away from the side being operated. The previous operative incision is marked with a sterile marker, and the patient is prepared and draped in the usual fashion. The prior skin incision is reopened, as is the underlying platysmal incision (Fig. 1). The medial border of the sternocleidomastoid is developed to expose the carotid sheath. Early reoperation is typically performed before the onset of significant postoperative fibrotic response; thus critical neural structures, principally the vagus and hypoglossal nerves, are easily identified and preserved.

Similar to primary surgery, the proximal common carotid and distal internal carotid arteries are dissected circumferentially for

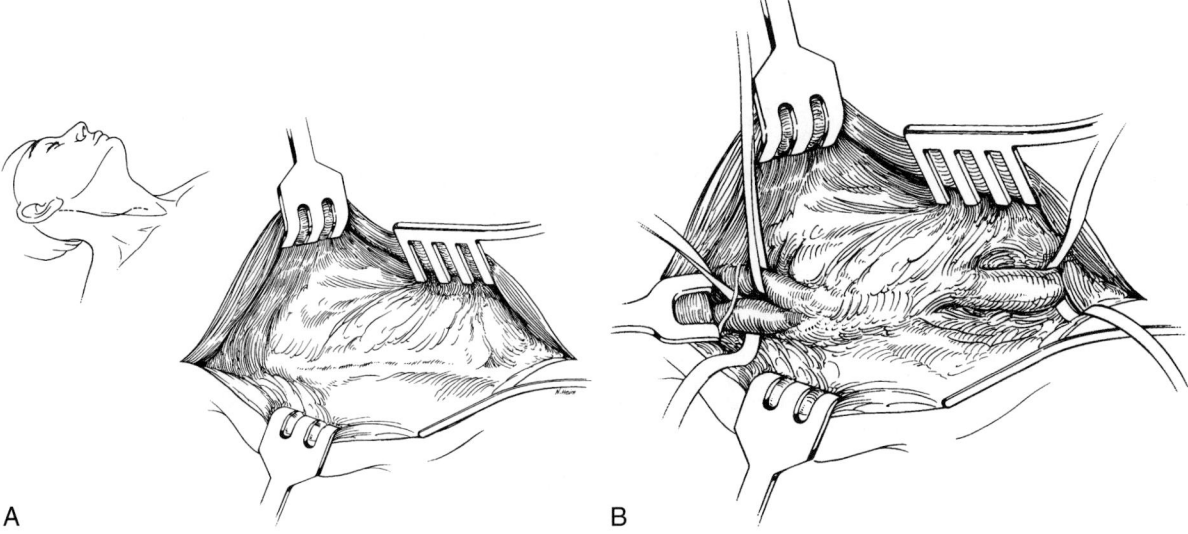

A   B

Figure 1 Surgical technique of carotid re-endarterectomy. **(A)** The initial incision is extended proximally and distally. **(B)** This allows the exposure of normal vessel proximal and distal to the old scar.

(continued)

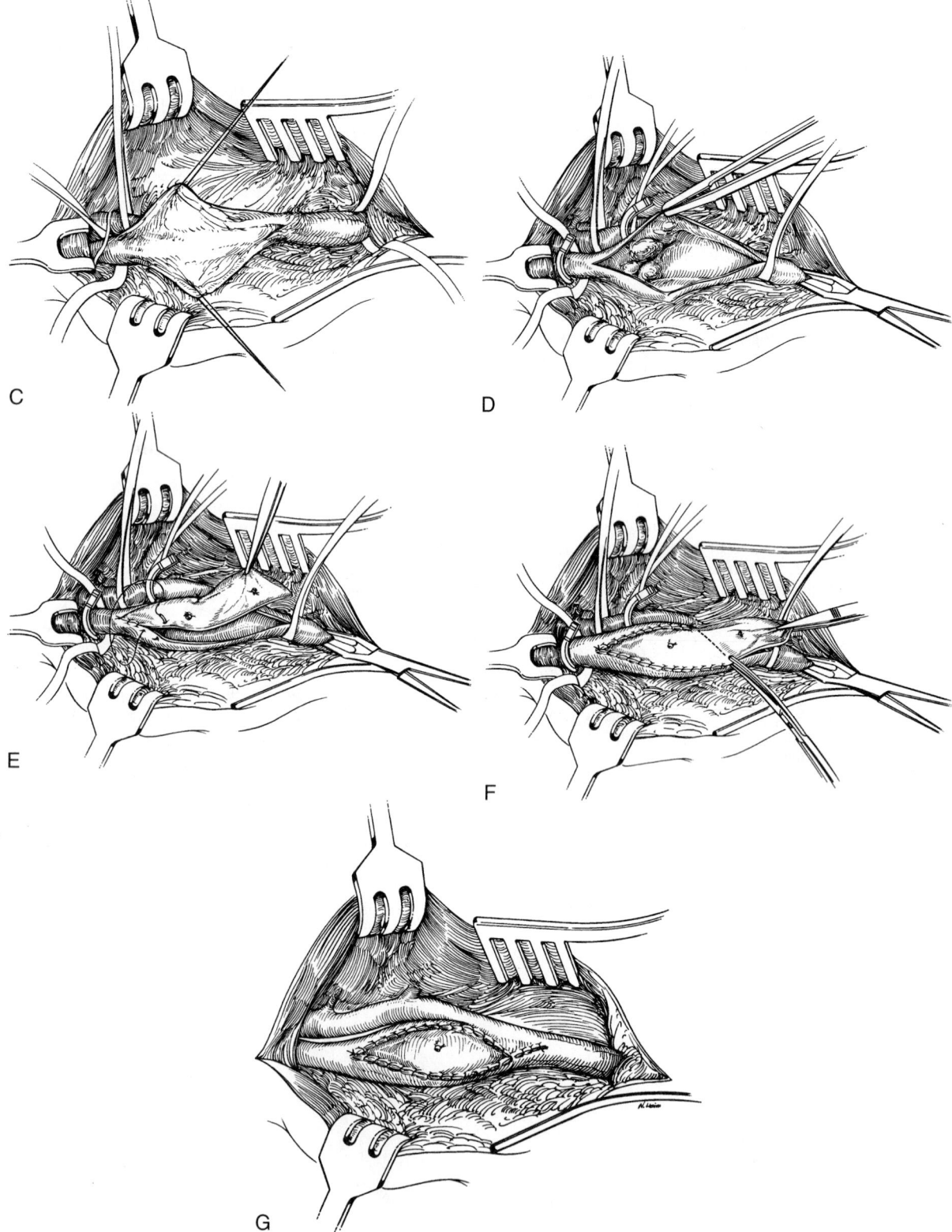

C

D

E

F

G

Figure 1   Cont'd—(C) Further dissection through the scar is performed after such proximal and distal control. **(D-G)** Re-endarterectomy and patch arterioplasty are subsequently performed according to the routine technique described in the text.   *From Awad A: Techniques in Neurosurgery 3(1): 61,1997* (Figure 2 , by permission).

proximal and distal control and secured with vascular loops. The external carotid artery is then dissected and secured with vascular loops. At this point, the patient is given an intravenous bolus dose of heparin. The superior thyroid artery is secured with temporary aneurysm clips or bulldog clamps. It is critical that the area of residual stenosis is determined preoperatively and clearly identified during surgery through palpation or with intraoperative Doppler imaging within the surgically exposed vessel. The vessels are clamped in order, with the internal carotid artery clamped first, and a period of 5 minutes is allowed to pass while the EEG and SSEP signals are carefully scrutinized to assess for collateral circulation. It is likely that if the patient required placement of a shunt during the primary operation, a similar placement would be required during reoperation. The second vessel clamped is the common carotid artery, followed by the external carotid artery.

After the vessels are clamped, the prior arteriotomy is reopened and the residual plaque identified, dissected, and peeled off. The carotid artery is then carefully inspected for intimal flaps. If they are found and cannot be peeled off, we suture them in an inside-out fashion with 6-0 prolene sutures. We routinely use Dacron grafts for patch angioplasty during reoperation. The patch is sewn in with a 6-0 Prolene (Ethicon, Somerville, NJ) suture in a running fashion. Before completion of the suture line, we allow the internal carotid artery to backbleed until patency is established and then it is reclamped. We then replace the internal carotid artery clamp and remove the external carotid artery clip, followed by removal of the common carotid artery clamp. A few seconds later, the internal carotid artery clamp is removed. Again, careful attention is placed on the EEG and SSEP signals during this period. Doppler ultrasonography is performed to assess arterial patency. If there is any concern in this regard, an intraoperative angiogram under fluoroscopy is performed via a direct common carotid artery puncture. The wound is closed in layers with a Jackson-Pratt drain placed above the carotid sheath. The drain is removed on postoperative day 1.

Carotid Angioplasty and Stenting for Intermediate or Delayed Restenosis

In patients who present with restenosis more than 3 months after the original operation and meet the indications outlined earlier, we routinely prefer to perform CAS. These patients are maintained on 81 mg of aspirin and 75 mg of clopidogrel for at least 1 week before the procedure.

The patient is positioned supine on the biplanar angiography table. Large-bore intravenous lines, a Foley catheter, and a radial arterial line are established. Transcutaneous pacer pads are placed across the chest. The patient is then placed under conscious sedation, with hemodynamic monitoring performed by anesthesiologists. Scalp EEG electrodes are placed. The transcutaneous pacer is tested. The groin region is prepared and draped bilaterally. The femoral head is fluoroscopically identified, and a 5-F femoral sheath is placed percutaneously between the inguinal ligament and the femoral artery bifurcation.

A femoral angiogram is performed to confirm the location of the sheath and its caliber for subsequent catheterization and eventual possible placement of an access site closure device. A pigtailed 5-F catheter is advanced into the aortic arch, and an angiographic run is performed to assess the angiographic anatomy and arch type (Fig. 2). The particular arch type and vessel selected for catheterization determine the choice of arterial sheath and guide catheters. Selective catheterization with a 5-F angled-tip Berenstein catheter is performed on the desired common carotid artery, and a biplanar angiogram is performed to obtain measurements of the internal and common carotid arteries, as well as the total length of the lesion to assess for

balloon and stent diameters and lengths. If catheterization of the affected common carotid artery is noted to be challenging, an exchange-length 0.38-inch glide wire is placed in the ipsilateral external carotid artery, typically the occipital artery.

The catheter and 5-F sheath are removed as a unit over the glide wire, and an 8-F femoral sheath is placed. The patient receives a bolus dose of intravenous heparin that is sufficient to produce an activated coagulation time (ACT) greater than twice the baseline value. An 8-F guide catheter is then advanced into the ipsilateral common carotid artery. Baseline cervical and cerebral biplanar angiography is performed.

Currently the majority of commercially available CAS systems are based on a 0.014-inch rapid-exchange monorail-over-the-wire delivery system. This system typically consists of a distal protection device, predilatation balloon, stent delivery device, postdilatation balloon, and distal protection retrieval device. All these are sequentially prepared and organized for a fluid procedure. After confirmation that the ACT exceeds twice the baseline value, the distal protection device is advanced over the rapid-exchange monorail system and, under road-map guidance, is used to cross the lesion at the bifurcation. The distal protection device is positioned in the upper segment of the cervical carotid artery, with the end of the wire typically in the petrocavernous internal carotid artery. It is critical that after the embolic protection device is deployed, further manipulations do not cause major transitions of the protection device within the internal carotid artery because of the risk for carotid intimal injury and dissection. The predilatation balloon (typically, a 4-mm balloon) is then advanced over the monorail wire and positioned within the stenotic segment. It is imperative that, in addition to road mapping, a careful inspection is made of adjacent vertebral radiographic anatomy to optimize placement of the balloon and stent. The balloon is inflated typically only to subnominal pressures to assist with stent passage. The balloon is then deflated and removed, followed by advancement of the selected stent.

Stents used for CAS are typically straight or tapered, varying in diameter from 6 to 10 mm and in lengths from 30 to 40 mm. The stent is positioned under road-map guidance within the chosen segment, which is confirmed through visualization of adjacent vertebral artery anatomy. The stent is then deployed according to the manufacturer's instructions, and the stent delivery device is removed. A biplanar cervical angiogram is performed to assess the extent of the stent deployment, as well as residual stenosis and the need for postdilatation.

If postdilatation of the lesion is required, an appropriately sized balloon is chosen on the basis of the nonstenosed distal cervical internal carotid artery diameter and advanced over the wire. Typically during this insufflation, patients develop bradycardia. To manage this potential adverse event, some interventionists use transcutaneous pacing; others simply pretreat patients with intravenously administered anticholinergic agents, such as atropine (0.5–1.0 mg) or glycopyrrolate (0.4 mg). It is imperative to inform the anesthesiologist and nursing staff about the impending insufflation. After the balloon is deflated, a follow-up cervical angiogram is performed to assess for residual stenosis and the need for additional angioplasty or stenting. After the balloon is removed, the embolic protection retrieval device is advanced, and the protection device retrieved.

A final cerebral angiogram is performed to ensure the presence of all preprocedural angioarchitecture and no "vessel dropout," as well as the absence of perfusion defects. The 8-F femoral sheath is left in place as the therapeutic effect of the heparin is allowed to wear off, and the patient is taken to the intensive care unit. The sheath is removed and a percutaneous closure device placed a few hours later, when the partial thromboplastin time has normalized. Patients are maintained on aspirin (81 mg daily) and clopidogrel (75 mg daily for 6 weeks, after which it is discontinued).

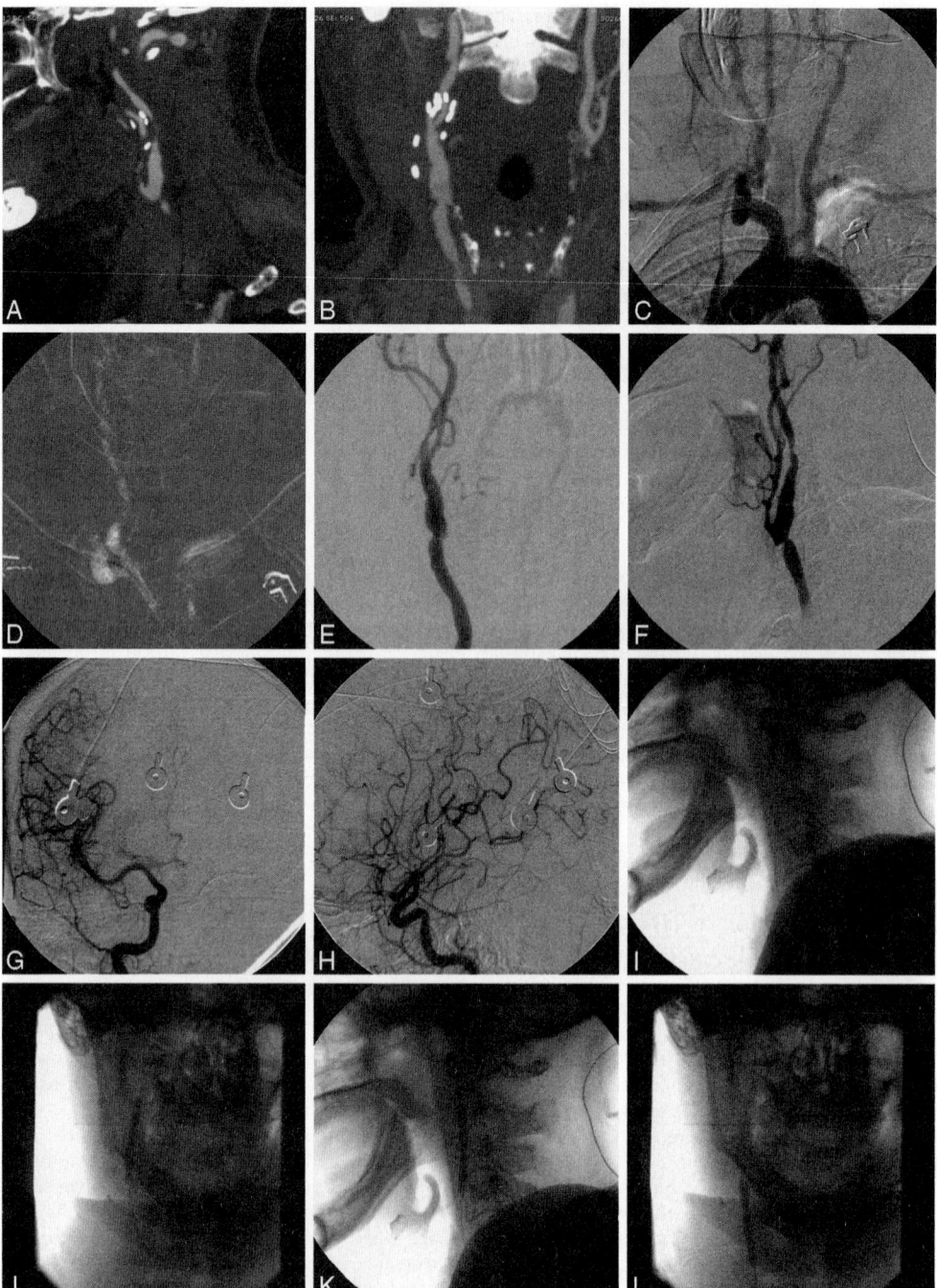

Figure 2   This 59-year-old woman presented with recent history of transient ischemic attacks affecting the left arm. She had previously undergone right CEA for asymptomatic stenosis and, subsequently, cervical radiation for laryngeal malignancy. Wherever possible, both anterior-posterior and lateral views are provided for this figure. Workup including computed tomographic angiogram of the neck confirmed restenosis **(A, B)**. A diagnostic aortic arch angiogram revealed a bovine arch **(C)**. Using roadmap assistance, an 8-French guide catheter was placed in the right common carotid artery **(D)**. Cervical carotid angiograms were performed to measure the dimensions of the diseased segments **(E, F)**. Cerebral angiography was also performed to assess baseline cerebral angioarchitecture **(G, H)**. A distal protection device mounted on a microwire was used to cross the distal stenosis and positioned in the high cervical internal carotid artery **(I)**. An angioplasty balloon was prepared and used to dilate the distal **(J, K)**, followed by the proximal, stenotic segments of the internal carotid artery **(L, M)**.

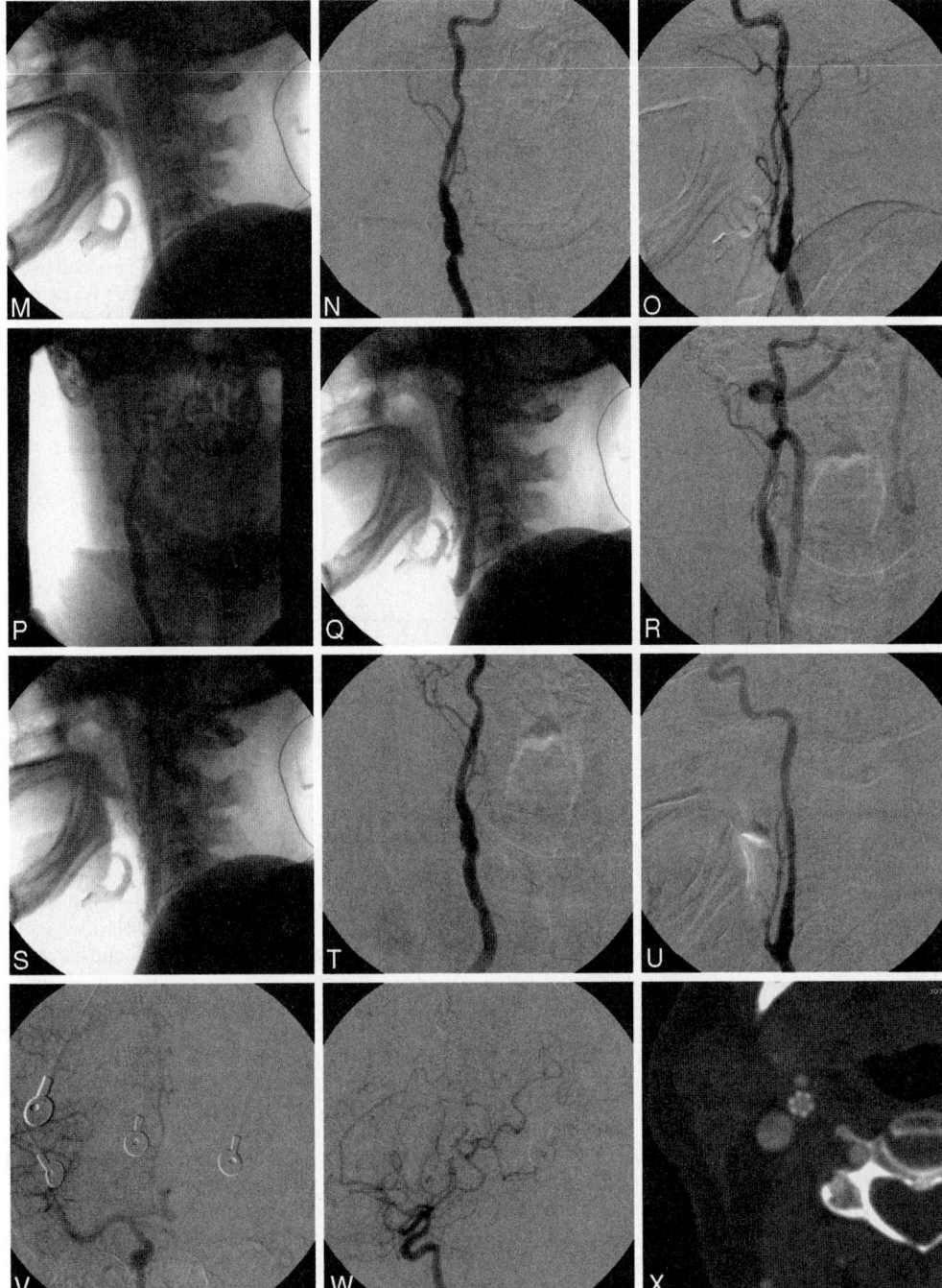

Figure 2 Cont'd—Postangioplasty cervical angiography was used to confirm widening of stenotic segments for ease of passage of stent delivery devices **(N, O)**. The carotid stent was first deployed across the distal segment **(P, Q)**, followed by a cervical angiogram to confirm adequate placement **(R)**. Subsequently, a second carotid stent was deployed across the proximal stenotic segment **(S)** and angiography used to confirm adequate placement and measure residual stenosis **(T, U)**. Cerebral angiography was then performed to confirm patency of all cerebral vessels without perfusion defects. At 6 weeks, an axial computed tomographic angiogram scan revealed excellent decompression of the stenotic segments **(X)**.

In patients for whom vascular access is an issue secondary to severe aortoiliofemoral disease, there are two options. One option is to perform a redo operation. The second involves exposure of the cervical common carotid artery proximal to the prior surgical site and placement of an arterial sheath in the operating room, which is secured through dual purse-string sutures within the common carotid artery; angioplasty and stenting are subsequently performed.

Reoperation for Carotid Restenosis

As outlined earlier, currently we routinely use endovascular techniques for the management of intermediate or delayed restenosis. Previously, however, for cases of reoperation after CEA, anesthesia, positioning, monitoring, and preparation and draping were performed in a fashion similar to the original operation. For

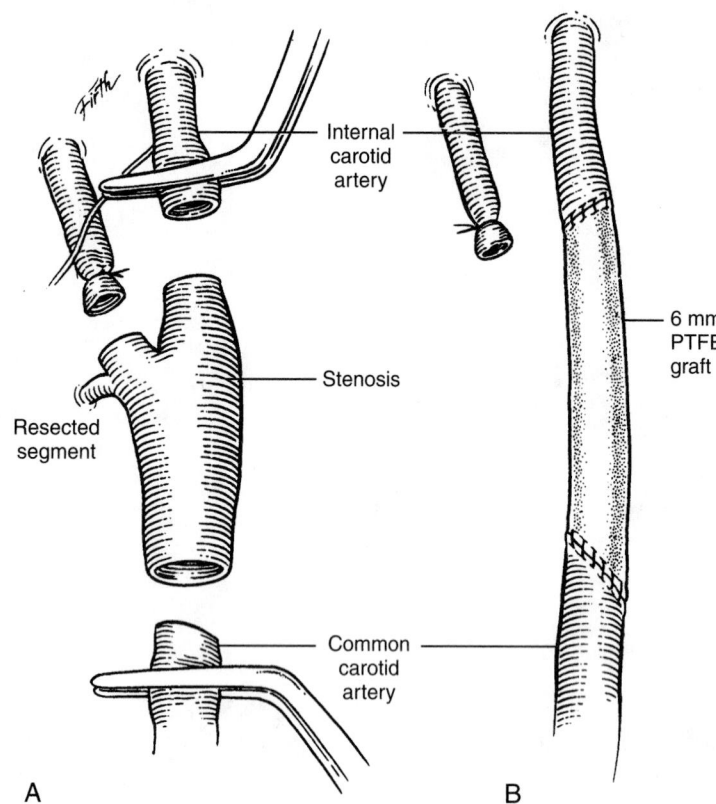

A   B

Figure 3 **(A)** Diseased segment of the carotid bifurcation, which will be resected. **(B)** The repair with an interposition polytetrafluoroethylene (PTFE) graft that has been appropriately beveled at both the proximal and distal anastomotic sites to conform to the size differences between the common and internal carotid artery using a graft of 6.0-mm diameter PTFE. *From Moore WS: Recurrent carotid stenosis. In Cameron JL, editor: Current surgical therapy ed 8, Philadelphia, 2004, Elsevier, p. 754 (figure 5).*

completeness, we are including a description of the reoperation in this chapter.

The previous incision is marked with a marking pen, deliberately extending the incision rostral and caudal along the medial sternocleidomastoid border. The incision is carried through the skin and platysma to identify the medial sternocleidomastoid border. The common carotid artery is identified proximal to its entry into the scar from prior surgery and secured with vascular loops. Second, the internal carotid artery is identified distal to its emergence from the prior surgical scar and secured following circumferential dissection within vascular loops. At this time, we attend to identification of the hypoglossal nerve before its entry into the prior endarterectomy scar, which invariably envelops the nerve in its trajectory across the internal carotid artery.

After these three structures are identified, sharp dissection is undertaken with a number 15 blade (rather than with a scissors), proceeding from caudal to rostral over the common carotid artery, to identify the carotid bulb and, in most cases, the prior endarterectomy suture line. The takeoff of the external carotid artery is then identified, and the plane of dissection is carried toward the internal carotid artery. At this point, we use sharp dissection to elevate the hypoglossal nerve, along with its adherent scar, off the internal carotid artery and connect the postendarterectomy segment with the bulb. A systemic heparin bolus is administered during this phase of dissection.

After the whole segment is exposed and confirmed to extend beyond the region of the plaque, every attempt is made to reopen the vessel along the previous endarterectomy scar. In cases in which myointimal hyperplasia is noted to be the major contributor to restenosis, we restrict dissection of the fibrous plaque off the carotid artery because of the absence of a well-defined border between the hyperplastic myointimal rubbery plaque and its adjacent adventitia. Instead, a generous patch angioplasty with Dacron, polytetrafluoroethylene (PTFE), or saphenous vein graft is performed. However, if there is recurrent atheromatous plaque, we proceed with

dissection of the plaque in a fashion similar to the original operation. However, this dissection can often be treacherous and result in arterial injury or incomplete removal of the plaque. In such cases, we ligate the external carotid artery at its takeoff. Next, the diseased segments of the common and internal carotid artery are resected in toto. An interposition graft using PTFE or saphenous vein is then beveled at both edges, and a primary end-to-end anastomosis is performed (Fig. 3). The challenge in these cases can arise if shunting is required because of EEG signal changes that do not respond to significant elevation of systolic arterial blood pressure. In these cases, the shunt is placed after the interposition segment is resected. The prepared graft is then secured at both ends, and after the graft is sown to the extent that the shunt becomes an encumbrance, the shunt is removed and the arteriotomies are rapidly closed. Drains are placed, and the wound is closed in layers after confirming patency with intraoperative Doppler ultrasonography and sometimes, if concerns remain, through intraoperative angiography.

RESULTS

We treated 23 vessels with CAS in 22 patients who developed intermediate and delayed restenosis after CEA. The mean age of these patients was 71 years. All patients had high-grade stenosis (>80%). All patients presented with symptomatic ipsilateral disease, except one with contralateral asymptomatic disease. There were no periprocedural neurologic or cardiac complications. There was one complication related to femoral artery access that resulted in a retroperitoneal hematoma requiring transfusion and delayed hospital discharge. No recurrent neurologic ischemic events occurred in the 22 patients during 3 years of clinical follow-up. One patient (4%) developed recurrent asymptomatic stenosis at 14 months that was discovered on 6-month Doppler ultrasonography surveillance. This patient was treated with balloon angioplasty without complications.

Similarly favorable results have been reported in BEACH. In this multicenter prospective enrollment registry for high-risk patients, 34.2% of 480 patients in the pivotal group were treated for recurrent stenosis following CEA. The 30-day composite major adverse event rate for the entire cohort of 747 patients was 5.8%, with death in 1.5%, stroke in 4.4%, and MI in 1%. Within this cohort, patients who were enrolled secondary to restenosis following CEA had a 30-day major adverse event rate of 3.8%. These results certainly compare favorably with those of AbuRahma and colleagues, who reported rates of 4.8% for perioperative stroke alone and 17% for cranial nerve injury following redo CEA for restenosis.

Surgery for carotid restenosis following previous CEA is a challenging operation in the best of circumstances and in the most experienced of hands. Carotid angioplasty and stenting is rapidly providing an effective and safe alternative with favorable results for treatment of this difficult disease.

SUGGESTED READINGS

AbuRahma AF, Bates MC, Wulu JT, and others: Redo carotid endarterectomy versus primary carotid endarterectomy, *Stroke* 32:2787, 2001.

Coyle KA, Smith RB 3rd, Gray BC, and others: Treatment of recurrent cerebrovascular disease. Review of a 10-year experience, *Ann Surg* 221:517, 1995.

Hertzer NR, O'Hara PJ, Mascha EJ, and others: Early outcome assessment for 2228 consecutive carotid endarterectomy procedures: the Cleveland Clinic experience from 1989 to 1995, *J Vasc Surg* 26:1, 1997.

Koebbe CJ, Liebman K, Veznedaroglu E, and others: Carotid artery angioplasty and stent placement for recurrent stenosis, *Neurosurg Focus* 18:e7, 2005.

Maxwell JG, Maxwell BG, Brinker CC, and others: Carotid endarterectomy reoperations in a regional medical center, *Am Surg* 66:773, 2000.

White CJ, Iyer SS, Hopkins LN, and others: Carotid stenting with distal protection in high surgical risk patients: the BEACH trial 30 day results, *Catheter Cardiovasc Interv* 67:503, 2006.

BALLOON ANGIOPLASTY AND STENTS IN CAROTID ARTERY OCCLUSIVE DISEASE

E. Lynne Kelley, MD, and Jean Pierre Becquemin, MD

Table 1: Potential Advantages of Carotid Stenting versus Carotid Endarterectomy

Less invasive technique	Ability to treat difficult lesions
Less discomfort	Postradiation treatment stenoses
Faster recovery time	Restenosis after endarterectomy
Avoidance of cranial nerve injury	Hostile neck (tracheostomy, prior surgery)
Avoidance of general anesthesia	High bifurcation stenoses

BACKGROUND

Stroke is the third leading cause of death in the United States and the number one cause of disability in adults, according to the American Heart Association. Approximately 25% of strokes are caused by carotid artery occlusive disease. Ischemic strokes occur either when small particles of atherosclerotic plaque become dislodged from the diseased artery wall or the stenosis progresses to occlusion, blocking all flow. More than 700,000 Americans have new (500,000) or recurrent (200,000) strokes each year, and approximately 280,000 die. The lifetime cost of stroke exceeds $90,000 per patient in the United States. The human and economic impact is enormous. In an effort to decrease the risk of stroke, both surgical and interventional treatments have been developed and refined.

The first surgical carotid endarterectomy (CEA) was reported by Pickering, Eastcott, and Robb in 1953. This procedure has been widely accepted, to the point that more than 120,000 CEAs are performed each year in the United States. Early concern over the efficacy of this procedure prompted critical evaluation through large, prospective, multicenter randomized trials. CEA has been validated with level I evidence as the gold standard for stroke prevention. During the early 1990s, the North American Symptomatic Carotid Endarterectomy Trial (NASCET) and the Asymptomatic Carotid Atherosclerosis Study (ACAS), as well as the European and Veterans Administration (VA) trials, established CEA as the standard of care in patients with high-grade obstruction. There was a clear reduction in the incidence of stroke over time compared with medical therapy standards in place when the trials occurred. The benefit of CEA was determined to be proportional to the degree of stenosis and the presence of symptoms. However, the NASCET and ACAS trials had extensive exclusion criteria, and many patients with comorbidities may have higher morbidity and mortality rates than these trials demonstrated. In addition, the highly selective inclusion process of trial centers may make the results less referable to patients whose operations are performed by lower-volume surgeons. Complications associated with CEA include stroke, death, transient ischemic attack (TIA), cranial nerve injury, hematoma, and infection, as well as the cardiac risks associated with general anesthesia. Although CEA continues to be an effective treatment for the majority of subjects with carotid occlusive disease, an endovascular treatment option is now available as well. This use of a minimally invasive carotid procedure as an alternative to open surgery had its roots in the established treatment of narrowing of the arteries that supply the heart, kidneys, and extremities. The number of carotid artery stenting (CAS) procedures has increased dramatically since 1998, actually doubling to more than 7500 in 2005. Theoretically endovascular treatment could eliminate the risks of cranial nerve injury, incisional complications, and the need for general anesthesia. However, to be preferred to CEA, the risk of stroke and TIA for CAS must be equivalent to the rates observed when CEA is performed. The overall objective of treating carotid stenosis is the same regardless of mode of treatment: to reduce the risk of stroke in patients with demonstrated anatomic occlusive disease. Table 1 compares advantages of CAS and CEA.

CAROTID ANGIOPLASTY

Carotid angioplasty (CAS) was first reported in 1980 by Kerber using direct carotid puncture and dilatation of a common carotid web in the setting of a standard CEA. In the following decade, other interventionalists started thinking about endovascular treatment of carotid disease. Initially this innovation was met with skepticism, which was reinforced by early termination of two clinical trials for safety reasons. Complications associated with CAS included stroke, death, TIA, access site issues, bleeding, and bradycardia. As technique and devices improved, single-center reports and registry case series began to sway thinking that CAS may be a viable alternative to open surgery, with acceptable safety and efficacy profiles, particularly in poor surgical candidates. The development of purpose-built stents for carotid lesions and the availability of embolic protection devices have contributed to the decrease of morbidity and mortality rates associated with CAS and have further increased enthusiasm for the procedure as a viable alternative to CEA. The use of stents minimizes plaque embolization, intimal dissection, and elastic recoil. Embolic protection devices are aimed at capturing particles and preventing TIAs and strokes.

CAS has been studied extensively in the patient population deemed at high risk for surgical intervention. These risk factors have included anatomic factors such as surgically inaccessible lesions at or above C2, previous neck or head radiation therapy, presence of laryngeal palsy or laryngectomy, presence of a tracheostoma, spinal immobility of the neck caused by cervical disorders, a contralateral total occlusion, or restenosis after a previous CEA (Fig. 1). Additional comorbid risk factors deemed high risk for CEA include congestive heart failure (New York Heart Association class III/IV), low left ventricular ejection fraction, unstable angina, chronic obstructive pulmonary disease, a requirement for staged coronary or peripheral vascular surgery, advanced age (≥75 years), recent myocardial infarction, or known coronary artery disease.

The majority of CAS trials conducted to date have been either single-center nonrandomized (Table 2) or industry-sponsored multicenter trials designed to gain U.S. Food and Drug Administration (FDA) approval for a specific stent system (Table 14.2-3). CAS procedures have been increasing in volume since 1998; Guidant's Acculink/Accunet in 2004 was the first system to gain FDA approval. To date, multiple CAS trials have been presented and published with acceptable (30-day, 1-year) morbidity and mortality rates (Tables 2 and 3; Fig. 2). A recent Cochran systematic review by

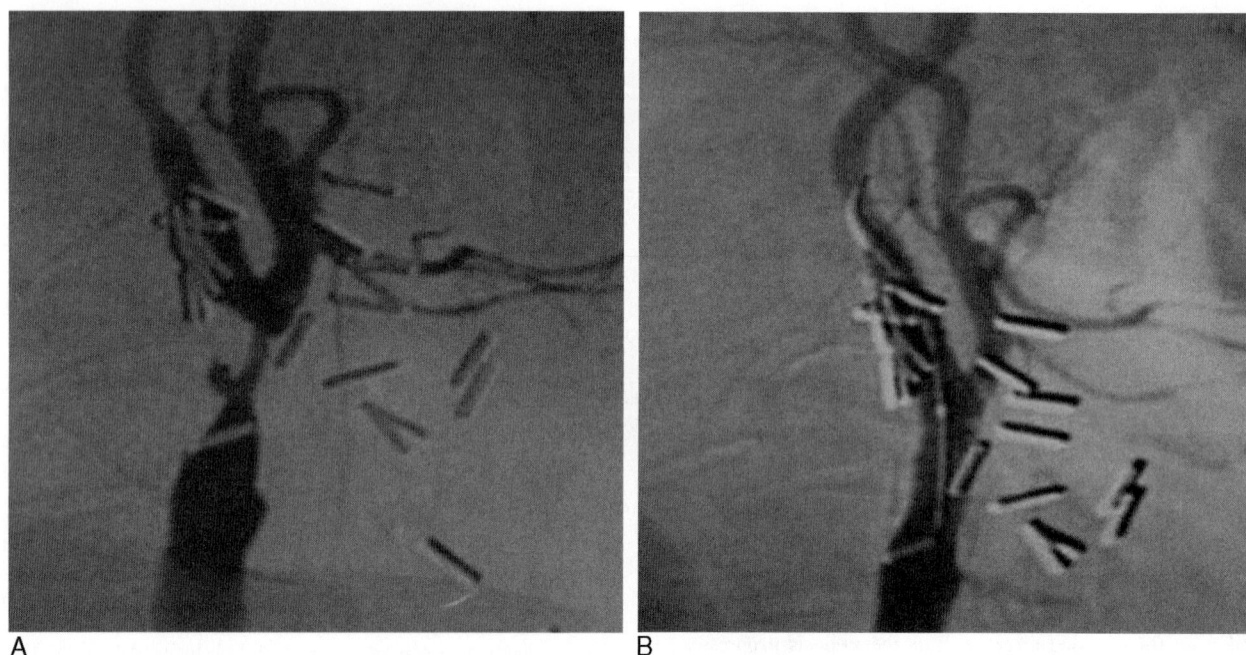

Figure 1 Patient with history of thyroid cancer and greater than 85% stenosis of distal common carotid artery. **(A)** Prestent. **(B)** Poststent.

Table 2: Single-Center Carotid Stenting Trials

Study	Pts./ Stent (N)	Asymp. (%)	Tech. Success (%)	30-Day—Morb. and Mort. (%)	Deaths (n)/ Mort (%)	Stroke—Major/ Minor (%)	Restenosis (Time; %)
Roubin 1996	146/210	37	99	NS	1/0.6	1.3/4.6	6 M; <5
Diethrich 1996	110/129	72	99.1	7.3	2/1.8	2.0/4.5	NS
Yadav 1997	107/189	36	100	NS	1/0.9	1.9/6.5	6 M; 4.9
Vozzi 1997	22/19	55	96	NS	1/4.5	4.5/4.5	NS
Criado 1997	33/NS	27	100	NS	0/0	0/0	8 M; 3.0
Wholey 1997	108/NS	44	95	NS	2/1.9	1.8/1.8	1.0
Henry 1998	163/178	35	99.4	NS	0/0	1.8/1.2	6 M; 2.3
Teitelbaum 1998	22/31	32	96.2	27.7	1/4.5	13.6/9.0	6 M; 14.3
Waigand 1998	50/56	72	100	2.0	1/2.0	2.0/2.0	8 M; 8.7
Bergeron 1999	99/99	42	97	2.0	0/0	0.0/1.0	13 M; 4.2

Asymp., Asymptomatic; *M*, month; *Morb.*, morbidity; *Mort.*, mortality; *NS*, not stated; *Tech.*, technical.

Table 3: Multicenter Carotid Stenting Trials

Trial	Design	Year	Patient Type	N	30-Day—Morb./ Mort.	1-Year—Morb./ Mort.	Primary Endpoint
ICCS (CAVITAS II)	Rand.	2001	High risk	723 (1500 planned)	NA	NA	Death/disabling stroke at 30 days
CARESS	Rand. 2:1	2003	Symp., Asympt.	397	2.1%	NA	Death/stroke at 30 days
SECURITY	Nonrand.	2003	High risk	305	7.2%	NA	Death/stroke/MI at 30 days; ipsilateral stroke at 1 year
ARCHER 1	Nonrand.	2004	High risk	158	7.6%	8.3%	Death/stroke/MI at 30 days; ipsilateral stroke at 1 year
ARCHER 2	Nonrand.	2004	High risk	278	8.6%	NA	Death/stroke/MI at 30 days; ipsilateral stroke at 1 year
ARCHER 3	Nonrand.	2004	High risk	145	8.3%	NA	Death/stroke/MI at 30 days; ipsilateral stroke at 1 year
MAVERIC I	Nonrand.	2004	High risk	99	5.1%	5.1%	Death/stroke/MI at 30 days; ipsilateral stroke at 1 year
MAVERIC II	Nonrand.	2004	High risk	399	5.3%	NA	Death/stroke/MI at 30 days; ipsilateral stroke at 1 year
SAPPHIRE	Rand.	2004	High risk	334	3.8%	12.2%	Death/stroke/MI at 30 days; ipsilateral stroke at 1 year
BEACH	Nonrand.	2005	High risk	747 (438 pivotal)	5.4%	9.1%	1-year composite
CABERNET	Nonrand.	2005	High, low risk	454	3.8%	4.5%	Death/stroke/MI at 30 days; ipsilateral stroke at 1 year
ACT I	Rand.	NA	Asymp.	1540	NA	NA	Major adverse events at 30 days; ipsilateral stroke at 1 year
CREST	Rand.	NA	Symp., Asymp.	789 (2500 planned)	4.6%	NA	Death/stroke/MI at 30 days; ipsilateral stroke at 30 days
EVA-3S	Rand.	NA	Symp.	300 (900 planned)	8.6%	NA	Death/stroke at 30 days; ipsilateral stroke 2-4 years

Asymp., Asymptomatic; *MI,* myocardial infarction; *NA,* not available; *nonrand.,* nonrandomized; *rand.,* randomized; *Symp.,* symptomatic.

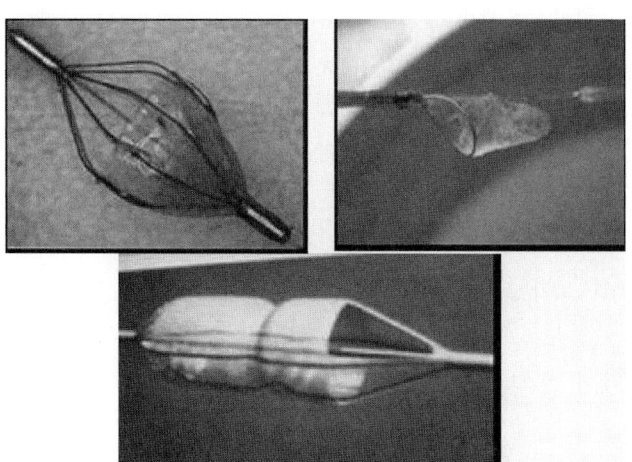

Figure 2   High-risk carotid artery stenting trials: 30-day composite endpoints.

Coward and colleagues analyzed five randomized trials involving 1269 patients. Although noting heterogeneity among trials, the authors concluded that there were no significant differences between CEA and CAS at either 30-day or 1-year endpoints. In addition, in an analysis of nonrandomized reports of aggregate 5000 or more CAS patients, the average 30-day stroke or death rate was 4.7%.

INDICATIONS FOR CAROTID STENTING

Proper patient selection is essential to the outcome of carotid stenting. Current indications are those patients who are considered high risk for surgical endarterectomy. In addition, patients must meet specific inclusion and exclusion criteria if the success reported in clinical trials is to be replicated. Finally, operator experience must be considered because there is a learning curve for CAS.

TRAINING

CAS is unique in that several subspecialty groups are laying claim to the procedure, including vascular surgeons, neurosurgeons, interventional cardiologists, and interventional radiologists. In an effort to improve training and performance of CAS, multiple professional societies have collaborated on the development of recommendations for stroke management, as well as training and credentialing for carotid angioplasty and stenting.

The performance of carotid stenting requires a thorough knowledge of cervical and cerebral anatomy, including anatomic variations; superior interventional catheter and balloon techniques; an understanding of the natural history of carotid stenosis including stroke risk; and a strategy for neurorescue should thrombosis, embolism, or spasm occur. The decision of whether to perform carotid stenting or carotid endarterectomy for stroke prevention should be made on a per-patient basis and depends on an analysis of the individual's risks and benefits.

TECHNIQUE OVERVIEW

Patients are admitted the day of procedure. If they have not been taking antiplatelet medication for at least 3 days before the procedure (aspirin 325 mg/day and clopidogrel 75 mg daily), they are given a loading dose (325 mg aspirin and 300 mg of clopidogrel). Alternatively, ticlopidine 250 mg/bid or 500 mg load can be administered with the aspirin. A neurologic examination is performed with documentation of preprocedure status, preferably by a trained neurologist. Preprocedure imaging such as computed tomographic angiography (CTA) or magnetic resonance angiography (MRA) can provide information on the type of the aortic arch, as well as other anatomic variations that can affect the procedure. Cardiac pacing patches are placed before positioning the patient, ensuring that they do not interfere with the fluoroscopic images, and pedal pulses are documented. The patient is administered light conscious sedation, and arterial access is gained, typically via the femoral artery with a sheath placed to protect the vessel. If no preprocedure CTA or MRA is available, four-vessel arch aortography is performed with a 5-F pigtail catheter. Full documentation of the status of the two carotids and the vertebral arteries and the hemispheric circulation should be available before initiating stenting. Images are obtained of the carotid bifurcation with the standard anteroposterior (AP), lateral, and antero-oblique projections. The intracranial circulation is evaluated with both AP and lateral views. Biplanar imaging can reduce both radiation exposure and contrast dose. The patient is anticoagulated throughout the procedure, and activated clotting times (ACT) are measured with a target of 250 seconds.

A variety of catheters can be employed to engage the carotid artery, depending on the tortuosity. For straightforward anatomy, a Berenstein catheter (USCI, Billerica, MA) may be all that is necessary with a soft, floppy-tip guidewire. For more tortuous anatomy, a reverse curve Simmons or a Vitek catheter (Cook, Bloomington, IN) can assist in selective cannulation. After the diagnostic angiogram has been obtained, the wire can be exchanged for a stiff 0.035-inch exchange wire that is positioned into the external carotid, avoiding the stenosis. A flexible sheath (6–7 F) or stiffer guide catheter (8–10 F) is advanced into the common carotid artery over the 0.035-inch wire, the choice being dependent on the difficulty of the anatomy. The lesion is crossed, and an occlusive balloon or a filter is positioned. Predilatation is performed only if it is believed that the filter or the stent cannot be advanced without it. A dedicated self-expanding stent is selected, taking into consideration the need for 1–2 mm oversize of the unstretched diameter. The stent is sized to the common carotid unless it is to remain exclusively in the internal carotid. The stent is normally positioned across the origin of the external carotid artery, leaving liberal margins to cover the lesion proximally and distally. Postdilatation is performed only if there is a significant residual stenosis. Balloon inflation at any time may precipitate bradycardia and hypotension, which are usually resolved with deflation of the balloon or with atropine (0.5 mg) if necessary. After a satisfactory result has been obtained, the filter or balloon embolic-protection device is removed. Final angiography is performed, including confirmation of an intact intracranial circulation. A postprocedure neurologic examination is documented. Antiplatelet medication is continued for a minimum of 1 month. Postprocedure cerebral MRA is recommended in all cases and obligatory if there have been any neurologic events.

Periprocedural Management

Cerebral Protection

Perhaps the single most important development in the evolution of CAS has been the innovation of methods with which to trap embolic debris during the procedure to prevent cerebral embolic events and potential strokes. Prior to embolic protection, complication rates were unacceptably high. Three distinct systems have been invented: permeable filters, which allow blood to flow through while trapping embolic particles; a balloon occlusion system that prevents emboli from traveling distally and allows aspiration out of the circulation before the balloon is deflated to restore flow (Fig. 3); and the Parodi reversal of flow system, which requires the creation of an arteriovenous circuit and uses a proximal occlusion balloon. Patients with contralateral occlusion may not tolerate balloon occlusion and are better served with a filter. Prospective randomized data are necessary to determine which system provides the best protection with the least complication risk.

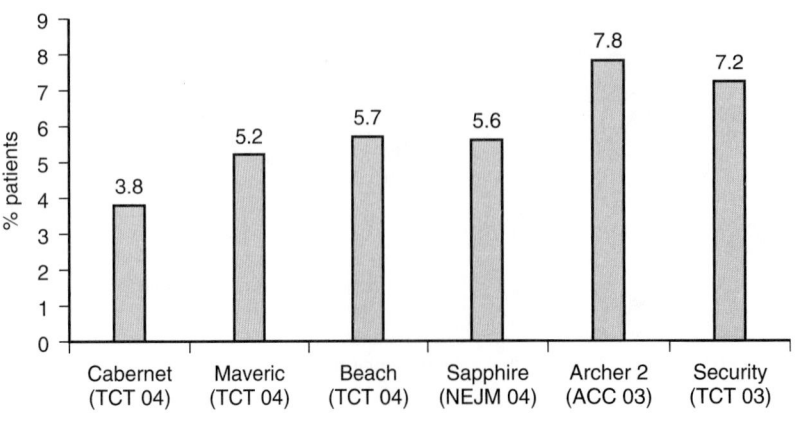

Figure 3 Embolic-protection devices.

Hemodynamic Instability

Procedural bradycardia is seen in up to 25% of cases, most commonly upon balloon inflation, and may be coincident with asystole and hypertension. There seems to be a decreased incidence in patients undergoing CAS for recurrent carotid stenosis caused by previous disruption of the neural pathways. Treatment consists of atropine 0.5 to 1.5 mg intravenously (IV), with cardiac pacing patches available. Postprocedural hypertension is seen in up to 35% of patients, with almost half requiring antihypertensive medications postprocedure. Significant predictive factors were female gender, history of hypertension, intraprocedural hypertension, previous ipsilateral carotid endarterectomy, and pre-CAS elevated diastolic blood pressure. Treatment consists of intravenous labetalol, hydralazine, or nitroglycerine drip. The major concern is the development of cerebral hyperperfusion syndrome in which the vessels in the brain, having been maximally dilatated because of the flow restriction from the stenosis, are not able to adjust rapidly to the increased perfusion pressure. Vessel rupture and intracranial hemorrhage can result with significant morbidity and mortality rates. The median time of onset is 10 hours postprocedure. Finally, poststenting hypotension can develop, which requires treatment with pressors. This may be secondary to the continued expansion that occurs with the nitinol stents.

Vasospasm

The internal carotid artery is prone to vasospasm, which can be precipitated by a guidewire or the embolic-protection device. It is often self-limited with removal of the filter or balloon. Resistant vasospasm can be broken with nitroglycerine (IV or paste) or calcium channel blockers.

Acute Changes in Neurologic Function

Stroke and death, although rare, are devastating complications of any carotid intervention. Intracranial hemorrhage is the most catastrophic result of hyperperfusion syndrome. Careful blood pressure control can partially limit this complication. Embolic events can occur during almost every step of the procedure because of disruption of atherosclerotic plaque or platelet aggregation. The consequences can range from asymptomatic intracranial lesions to TIAs and, finally, to stroke. Improved technique and cerebral-protection devices have decreased the number of embolic particles. This is evidenced by transcranial Doppler studies, as well as improved clinical results. A thorough knowledge of intracranial lytic therapy with an established protocol must be established before carotid stenting.

Follow-Up Care

Patients who undergo carotid stenting should be followed at 1 month, 6 months, and annually thereafter unless there is evidence of contralateral disease or recurrent stenosis that requires more frequent evaluation. The visit should include a neurologic examination and a duplex ultrasound. CAS has demonstrated a rate of approximately 4% of restenosis at 2 years when a threshold of more than 70% was used. In-stent restenosis is usually treated effectively with repeat balloon angioplasty. Carotid artery occlusive disease

does not usually occur in isolation. Physicians must always be concerned with coronary artery disease symptoms, hyperlipidemia, and hypertension and ensure that these comorbidities are under control. Smoking cessation must also be emphasized.

CONCLUSIONS

The treatment of carotid artery occlusive disease has evolved significantly over the past decade to include standard surgical endarterectomy, as well as lesser invasive carotid angioplasty and stenting. Current practice with clinical trial results supports CAS only for those patients considered to be at high risk for carotid surgery. Both CEA and CAS have their merits; some patients clearly benefit from one or the other method because of anatomic factors or comorbidities, whereas others may potentially be treated equally well with either. The results of ongoing trials such as CREST and others will help to define these groups. Every effort should be made to participate in these trials so that level 1 evidence is available for CAS. For those individuals who are candidates for either CEA or CAS, it is critical to discuss with the patient and the referring physician the risks and benefits of both methods so that an informed decision can be made. Although CAS is performed by interventional cardiologists and radiologists, it is only endovascular surgeons who can provide an unbiased view of which is the better treatment for an individual patient. Patient selection and planning is crucial to the success of this procedure. Finally, only physicians with extensive and proved endovascular skills should perform CAS.

SELECTED READINGS

Coward LJ, Featherstone RL, Brown MM: Safety and efficacy of endovascular treatment of carotid artery stenosis compared with carotid endarterectomy: a Cochrane systematic review of the randomized evidence, *Stroke* 36:905, 2005.

Cremonesi A, Manetti R, Stetacci F, and others: Protected carotid stenting: clinical advantages and complications of embolic protection devices in 442 consecutive patients, *Stroke* 34:1936, 2003.

Hobson RW 2nd, Brott TG, Roubin TG, and others: Carotid artery stenting: meeting the recruitment challenges of a clinical trial, *Stroke* 36:1314, 2005.

Kerber CW, Cromwell LD, Loehden OL: Catheter dilatation of proximal carotid stenosis during distal bifurcation endarterectomy, *Am J Neuroradiology* 1:348, 1980.

Naylor AR, Bolia A, Abbott RJ, and others: Randomized study of carotid angioplasty and stenting versus carotid endarterectomy: a stopped trial, *J Vasc Surg* 28:326, 1998.

Phatouros CC, Higashida RT, Malek MA, and others: Carotid artery stent placement for atherosclerotic disease: rationale, technique, and current status, *Radiology* 217:26, 2000.

Qureshi AI, Luft AR, Janardhan V, and others: Identification of patients at risk for periprocedural neurological deficits associated with carotid angioplasty and stenting, *Stroke* 30:2086, 1999.

SCAI/SVMB/SVS: Clinical competence statement on vascular medicine and catheter-based peripheral vascular interventions, *J Vasc Surg* 41:160, 2005.

Yadav JS, Wholey MH, Kuntz RE, and others: Protected carotid-artery stenting versus endarterectomy in high-risk patients, *N Engl J Med* 351:1493, 2004.

BRACHIOCEPHALIC RECONSTRUCTION

Ali F. AbuRahma, MD, and Patrick A. Stone, MD

The origin of the great vessels of the aortic arch rarely requires intervention compared with the number of extracranial carotid arterial procedures performed annually. Although the need for revascularization of the supraaortic vessels is infrequent, it has been a challenging area for most surgeons. The Joint Study of Extracranial Arterial Occlusion of more than 6000 patients demonstrated that only 17% had more than 30% luminal reduction of innominate or subclavian arteries. Additionally, the indications for interventions are less clear than the indications for extracranial carotid interventions. Furthermore, the management strategy is more convoluted because multiple routes of revascularization are possible: direct reconstruction/bypass (intrathoracic), cervical or extra-anatomic, and now endovascular solutions.

Atherosclerosis predominates as the most frequent indication for supra-aortic intervention (Fig. 1, *A* and *B*). Risk factors are similar for other atherosclerotic beds, with nearly 100% of patients having a smoking history. All of the nonatherosclerotic pathologies

of the supra-aortic trunk account for less than 20% of those requiring surgical therapy. They include Takaysu's arteritis, aortic dissection, aneurysmal degeneration, and complications of radiation to the head/neck and mediastinum for various cancers.

The treatment focus of supra-aortic vessel disease has historically been surgical. Yet since the mid 1990s, as seen in other vascular beds, there has been a growing trend toward endovascular intervention. Transpositions and bypass procedures for these vessels have declined in most institutions as a result of the increased use of endoluminal therapy. However, the prevalent use of thoracic endografts and the accompanying requirement of more proximal arch landing have increased the need for debranching of the supra-aortic vessels.

CLINICAL PRESENTATION

An evaluation of a patient with symptoms in the cerebrovascular system or upper extremities may identify pathology of the innominate, subclavian, vertebral, or proximal carotid arteries. Although cerebrovascular symptoms typically occur as a result of bifurcation disease, ostial lesions can produce identical symptoms because of both flow reduction and atheroemboli. Vertebrobasilar insufficiency may present with symptoms including: vertigo, ataxia, binocular visual symptoms, and drop attacks. Upper extremity ischemia may manifest as absent, diminished, or asymmetrical pulses in the arm, with limb fatigue with exercise or routine activities. Also, embolic

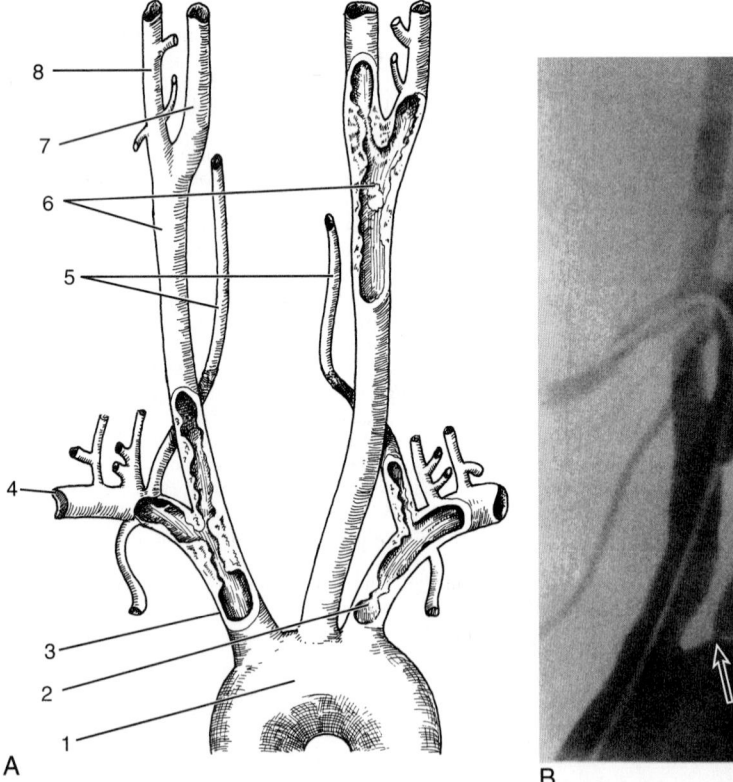
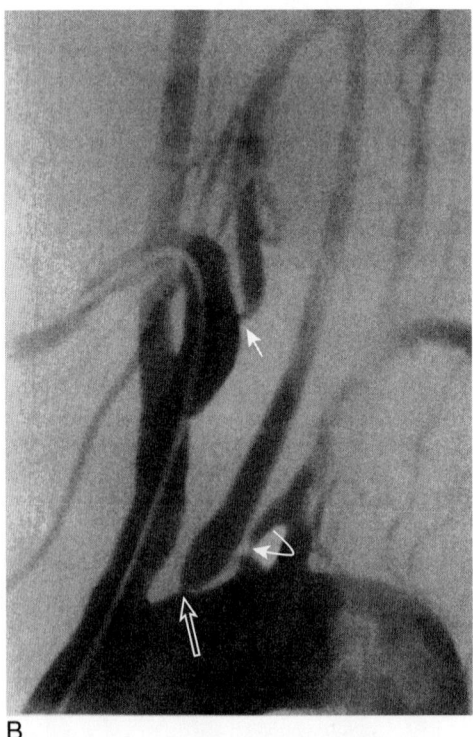

Figure I **(A)** Sites of atherosclerosis of brachycephalic vessels. *1*, Aortic arch; *2*, left subclavian artery; *3*, innominate artery; *4*, right subclavian artery; *5*, right and left vertebral arteries; *6*, right and left common carotid arteries; *7*, right internal carotid artery; *8*, right external carotid artery (note atherosclerosis at left subclavian, left vertebral, innominate with proximal right common carotid and subclavian arteries and left carotid bifurcation). **(B)** Arch aortogram showing the left vertebral artery originating from the arch of the aorta with tight stenosis at its origin *(curved arrow)* and the right vertebral artery (coming off the right subclavian artery) with a tight stenosis at its origin *(straight arrow)*. *From AbuRahma AF, Bergan JJ, editors: Noninvasive vascular diagnosis, Springer, 2000, London. (A) Fig. 5.22, chap. 5, p. 62. (B) Fig. 5.2, chap. 5, p. 52.*

complications may present as ulcerations or nonhealing wounds of the digits. Rarely, patients with aneurysmal disease of an aberrant right subclavian artery aneurysm may present with dysphagia.

With the widespread use of duplex examinations for bruits detected on physical examination, an increased number of asymptomatic patients will also be seen in referral for evaluation. Duplex evaluation will often show flow reversal in the vertebral artery or asymmetric upper extremity pulse evaluation at the time of examination. Duplex evaluation can also suggest proximal lesions secondary to dampened waveforms and low velocities in the common carotid artery.

DIAGNOSIS

History and physical examination are the backbone of diagnosing pathology of the brachiocephalic vessels. Palpation and auscultation of the carotids and evaluation of the upper extremity pulses should be performed at the initial evaluation. Inspection of the upper extremity for signs of embolic insult, including digital ulcerations, and ischemic changes of the hand and digits should be performed. Brachial artery blood pressures should be performed and compared, with a difference of more than 15 to 20 mm Hg between the two extremities considered a significant finding. A complete neurologic examination should also be performed to evaluate for previous stroke. Additionally, if patient history suggests vasculitis or collagen vascular disease, a comprehensive examination should include serologies.

Duplex examination should be the first line of investigation. With suspected carotid artery lesions, a standard evaluation of the extracranial carotid vessels should be performed. A dampened common carotid waveform with low velocities suggests proximal disease. The vertebral arteries also should be evaluated for antegrade and retrograde flow. Reversal of flow suggests high-grade subclavian or innominate disease. Transcranial Doppler ultrasound can also provide additional data, leading one toward a diagnosis of disease of the supra-aortic arteries.

Magnetic resonance arteriography and computed tomography continue to improve in their ability to diagnosis supra-aortic disease, but arteriography continues to be the gold standard. Imaging should include arch views in both left and right obliques and four-vessel selective injections. In patients with concomitant coronary artery disease, these evaluations should also be performed during the workup. Additionally, if arch reconstruction is planned, a combined approach prevents a redo sternotomy.

INDICATIONS FOR TREATMENT

Unfortunately, no prospective randomized trials have compared medical, endovascular, and surgical treatment modalities for supra-aortic disease. Therefore the indications for treatment are not as readily defined as those for carotid bifurcation disease. Patients with classical hemispheric symptoms with a corresponding lesion or lesions can be treated by the appropriate arterial reconstruction. Treatment for asymptomatic patients is controversial at the least. For patients with proximal carotid artery disease and no carotid bifurcation disease, treatment is recommended for lesions with luminal encroachment greater than 75%. When combined carotid bifurcation and proximal disease is present, endarterectomy and proximal repair is recommended, including carotid-subclavian transposition, bypass, or retrograde proximal stenting at the time of endarterectomy.

For lesions involving the proximal vertebral arteries, if atheroembolism is the suspected source, then stenosis greater than 75% should be treated. If, however, vertebrobasilar insufficiency is suspected as the source of symptoms, then the status of the contralateral vertebral is imperative. This includes a unilateral stenosis

greater than 75% and a contralateral vertebral artery that has similar luminal narrowing or is hypoplastic or absent.

It is not uncommon for patients with diffuse atherosclerotic disease to also have subclavian artery disease with associated vertebral flow reversal. However, in the absence of symptoms these lesions should not be treated. Rarely, a patient with bilateral proximal subclavian artery occlusion may require transposition or carotid-subclavian bypass. Mainly this would be performed to ensure accurate measurement of central arterial pressure for hypertension management or in patients with planned coronary artery revascularization in which the internal mammary artery is to be used as a conduit.

TECHNICAL PRINCIPLES

The goal of reconstruction of the brachiocephalic vessels is normalization of arterial perfusion. Several surgical and endovascular methods can achieve this, including endarterectomy, transposition, bypass, or endoluminal stent placement.

Reconstruction of the supra-aortic trunks can be accomplished through the chest (direct routes) or through cervical incisions. Direct repairs are usually preferred in younger patients who have complex lesions, for example, innominate artery lesions or multiple lesions, including innominate and the left common carotid artery. The direct approach is also indicated in patients who require combined coronary artery bypass and brachiocephalic reconstruction. The direct approach requires a median sternotomy for lesions of the innominate and left common carotid arteries, and a left thoracotomy for proximal left subclavian artery disease. Direct approach should also be indicated for patients with aneurysms or traumatic disruptions of these major vessels. These direct procedures include endarterectomy of the innominate artery, bypass grafting from the ascending aorta to the innominate artery, or carotid/subclavian grafting. Cervical repairs are usually selected in older patients, who are at high-risk of thoracotomy, and in those who have had previous transsternal procedures. They are also recommended for patients with single arterial lesions, other than the innominate artery. These indirect or cervical operations can be performed through transverse supraclavicular or cervical incisions, which are easily tolerated, even in high-risk patients. Although the cervical procedures have excellent results and low morbidity and mortality rates, advances in perioperative management, including contemporary surgical and anesthetic techniques, have made direct transthoracic repair nearly as safe as cervical repairs.

Shunting during proximal repair is infrequently necessary, unless the contralateral carotid artery has a hemodynamically significant stenosis. Transcranial Doppler ultrasound and cerebral oximetry can help to identify those patients who are at risk for cerebral malperfusion during surgical repair. Endovascular principles for treatment of proximal common carotid lesions should be similar to those widely used for bifurcation disease. This includes the use of a filter wire for embolic protection when approaching from the femoral artery. When a retrograde approach with concomitant endarterectomy is used, the common carotid can be controlled during proximal endovascular treatment. Most centers use balloon expandable stents for more accurate placement and place the proximal stent 1 to 2 mm in the aortic arch.

Innominate Artery Reconstruction

The direct transthoracic approach is generally recommended for certain innominate artery lesions, including aneurysms, traumatic disruptions, or dissections. These are generally performed through a full-length sternotomy. If the innominate lesion is suspected to be embolizing, as shown by grossly irregular ulcerative plaque, the

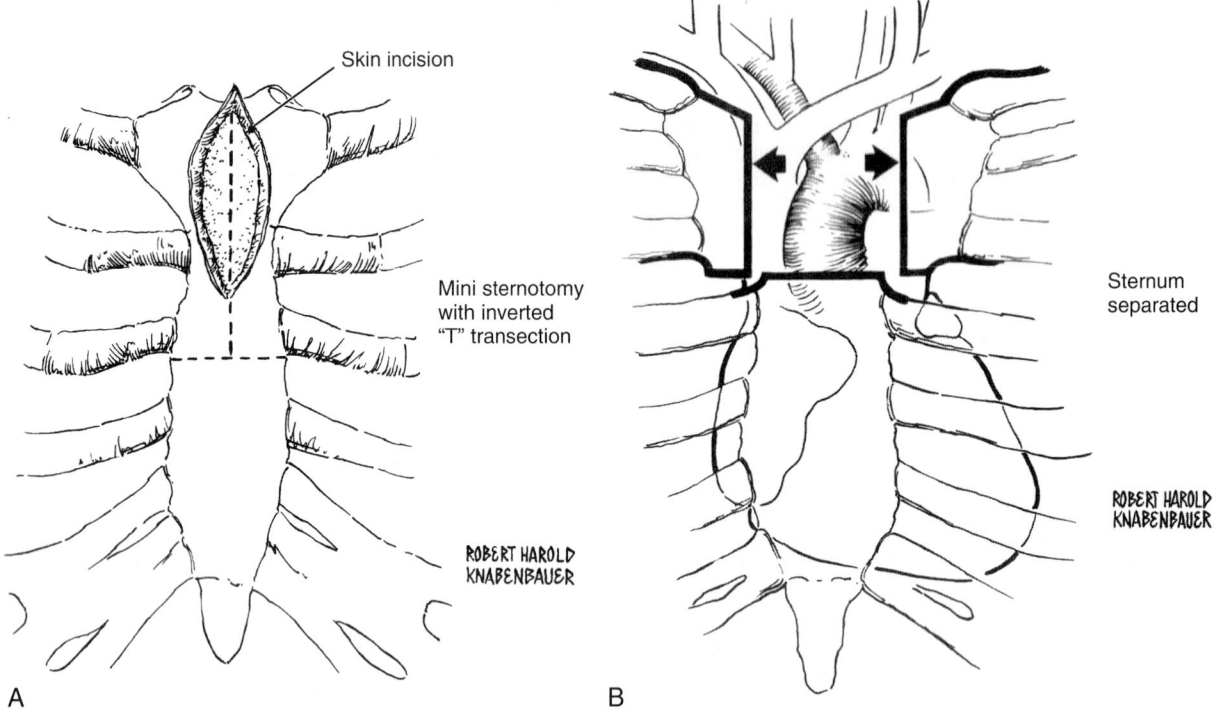

Figure 2   **(A)** Artist's rendering of skin incision and ministernotomy sternal division. **(B)** Upper sternum is divided and separated *(arrow)*, exposing the ascending aorta and arch vessels.   *From Sakopoulos AG, Ballard JL, Gundry SR: J Vasc Surg 31:200, 2000.*

distal innominate artery should be ligated or excluded at the completion of the remote bypass procedure. This may not be feasible using the cervical supraclavicular approach and may necessitate sternotomy.

Although the most widely accepted direct surgical route to either the innominate or proximal left common carotid artery is a full median sternotomy, a minimally invasive approach for aortic branch reconstruction can be achieved through a mini-sternotomy with inverted "T" transection. In this approach, a limited skin incision of approximately 7 to 8 cm is made in the midline, extending from the sternal notch to just past the angle of Louis. The manubrium and upper sternum are divided in the midline down to the third intercostal space with a narrow blade mounted on a redo sternotomy oscillating saw (Stryker, Kalamazoo, MI). The sternum is then transected transversely at the third intercostal space, creating an upside down "T" incision (Fig. 2, *A*). A small or pediatric sternal retractor is placed to open the upper sternum. This incision allows good exposure of a piece of the heart and arch vessels (Fig. 2, *B*). Innominate and left common carotid artery reconstruction can then be performed by either endarterectomy or bypass grafting in the usual fashion.

Extensive calcification of the ascending aorta or the aortic arch at the base of the innominate is a relative contraindication for an endarterectomy because of the risk of fracturing the plaque and producing distal embolization. It is also necessary to have space between the left common carotid artery and the innominate during clamping to prevent clamping of the left carotid artery, which may cause left cerebral ischemia. Overall, bypass grafting is performed more commonly than endarterectomy of the innominate, permitting revascularization of two or more distal arteries. These grafts generally originate from the lateral aspect of the ascending aorta. A bifurcation or single-limb graft can be used for the distal anastomosis made to the innominate artery, common carotid arteries, or subclavian arteries. Clamping of the innominate artery does not generally require shunting for cerebral perfusion.

Cervical repairs can also be considered for innominate reconstruction where grafting can be made from the left common carotid artery, axillary, or subclavian artery to the right subclavian or right common carotid artery, or both.

Common Carotid Artery Reconstruction

Stenoses of the proximal left common carotid artery are relatively common and the second most common lesions beyond the left subclavian artery. Most of these lesions are asymptomatic. These lesions can also be approached by direct transthoracic approach through a median sternotomy, similar to the innominate lesions or, preferably, by indirect cervical repairs. The common carotid artery can be revascularized by means of subclavian or carotid bypass grafts, preferably from the ipsilateral side; however, it can also be performed from the left subclavian to the right carotid artery or even by left carotid to right carotid cervical arterial bypass. If the stenotic lesion of the common carotid artery is at its origin, transposing the midportion of the common carotid artery, if healthy, to the subclavian artery may be a better alternative than a subclavian-to-carotid bypass grafting. This requires only one anastomosis, without the need of prosthesis.

Subclavian Artery Stenosis or Occlusion

Subclavian artery reconstruction is generally indicated to correct a symptomatic subclavian steal-arm ischemia secondary to a proximal subclavian lesion, to revascularize the subclavian artery before an internal mammary-to-coronary-artery bypass grafting, or to transpose the left subclavian to the left common carotid artery before extending a thoracic stent graft across its origin. Subclavian artery reconstruction can be accomplished by carotid-subclavian bypass or carotid-subclavian transposition. If the subclavian lesion is the source of thromboembolization, the prevertebral subclavian artery must be ligated at the time of the bypass. In certain high-risk patients, axillary-to-axillary artery bypass can be a simple alternative. Subclavian-to-subclavian artery bypass can also be used for patients with symptomatic subclavian artery disease.

Brief Technical Notes of Commonly Performed Cervical Procedures

Carotid-Subclavian Bypass Grafts

A transverse supraclavicular incision is made. The subcutaneous tissue, platysma, and clavicular head of the sternocleidomastoid muscle are incised. The sternal head of the sternocleidomastoid is retracted medially, and the common carotid artery exposed and isolated. The scalenus anticus muscle is transected after isolation of the phrenic nerve. The subclavian artery is exposed and isolated. The graft is sutured to the subclavian artery in end-to-side fashion. The distal end of the graft is then anastomosed end-to-side of the common carotid artery (Fig. 3).

Prosthetic polytetrafluoroethylene (PTFE) grafts are generally preferable to autogenous vein grafts in this location and usually have higher long-term patency rates. Kinking is less likely with prosthetic grafts than with autogenous vein grafts. This bypass can also be combined with carotid endarterectomy, if indicated. The carotid bifurcation endarterectomy is performed in the usual fashion, and the distal end of the subclavian-to-carotid bypass graft is fashioned to cover the arteriotomy in the form of a patch.

Carotid-Subclavian Transposition

An alternative approach to common carotid to subclavian bypass is transposition of the subclavian artery into the left common carotid artery. This technique requires more extensive mobilization of the common carotid artery and the subclavian artery (Fig. 4). One major advantage of this technique is the avoidance of prosthetic grafts and the small risk of potential infection.

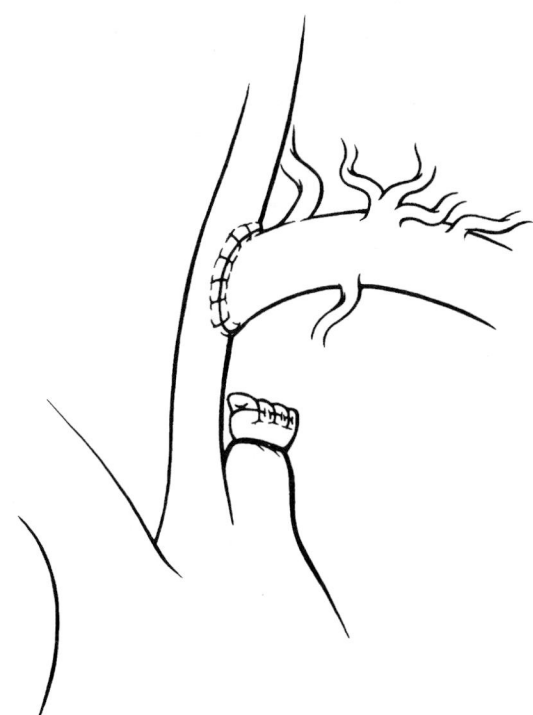

Figure 4 Transposition of the left subclavian artery to the left common carotid artery. *From Berguer R: Surgical reconstruction of the supra-aortic trunks and vertebral arteries. In Moore WS, editor: Vascular and endovascular surgery: a comprehensive review, ed 7, Philadelphia, 2006, Saunders, Elsevier, p. 659, Fig 36–5.*

Subclavian-Subclavian Artery Bypass

This technique is rarely performed; however, it can be considered for patients with an innominate lesion who may be at high risk for other repairs. The incision is supraclavicular on both sides, and the second, or rarely third, portion of the subclavian artery is exposed in a similar fashion to that which was described earlier. The graft is placed behind the sternocleidomastoid muscle and as low as possible.

Axillary-to-Axillary Artery Bypass Grafting

Two transverse incisions are made over the deltopectoral grooves. The incision is deepened to expose the axillary artery, axillary vein, and brachial plexus. The second portion of the axillary artery is isolated. An 8-mm Gortex graft is sutured in place in end-to-side fashion. The graft is placed underneath the pectoralis major and then through a tunnel, which is made in the presternal subcutaneous tissue to the contralateral axilla. The contralateral end of the graft is also placed under the pectoralis major. The distal end of the graft is then sutured to the other axillary artery in end-to-side fashion.

Carotid-to-Carotid Artery Bypass

In this technique, one carotid is used to revascularize the contralateral carotid, the origin of which is in the mediastinum or is severely diseased proximally. The common carotid artery is exposed in the usual fashion bilaterally. The bypass usually lies low in the midline, partially hidden by the upper edge of manubrium. The bypass can be tunneled across the neck through the retropharyngeal space, which is a shorter and straighter path.

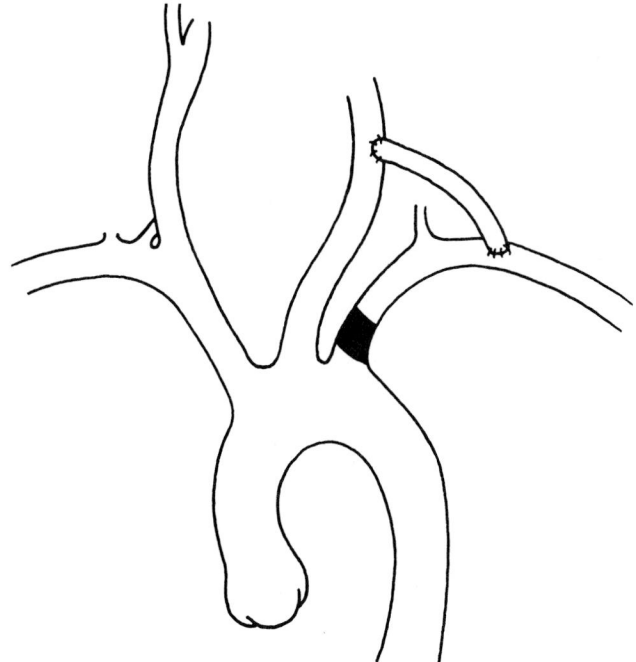

Figure 3 Carotid-to-subclavian bypass graft. *From AbuRahma AF, Lawton WE Jr: W VMed J 79:120, 1983; Fig. 4.*

CLINICAL EXPERIENCE AND RESULTS OF BRACHIOCEPHALIC RECONSTRUCTION (OPEN REPAIR)

Several studies reported satisfactory outcomes for various brachiocephalic reconstruction procedures. Berguer reported on his experience with supra-aortic trunk reconstruction from 1982 to 1998 on 282 patients (182 cervical repairs and 100 transthoracic repairs). The most frequent indication for cervical repair in his practice was single-trunk disease (carotid or subclavian artery) or history of myocardial revascularization). All innominate artery lesions were performed through a direct chest incision. He reported an incidence of 3.8% of transient ischemic attacks (TIAs) or stroke and 0.5% death rate for patients with cervical repairs, in contrast to 8% of TIAs or stroke and 8% death rate for the thoracic repairs. Uurto and colleagues reported on the long-term outcome of surgical revascularization of the supra-aortic vessels. Eighty surgical revascularizations were performed on 76 patients with subclavian or innominate artery disease. These included 38 bypasses (28 carotid-subclavian, four aorto-subclavian, three aorto-innominate, and three subclavian transpositions) and 42 endarterectomies. The perioperative mortality was 2.5% (0% for bypasses and 5% for endarterectomies). They reported an overall patency rate of 95% for both procedures at 1 and 5 years; 91% at 10 years (89% for bypasses and 93% for endarterectomies); and 89% (87% for bypasses and 90% for endarterectomies) at 15 years. Most of the patients (84%) were satisfied with the clinical results in the long term. They concluded that all of these surgical techniques had good and durable long-term outcome.

Cinà and colleagues reported their experience of subclavian carotid transposition and bypass grafting. They performed 27 subclavian carotid transpositions, 4 for aneurysmal disease and 23 for occlusive disease. A subclavian carotid transposition was performed in conjunction with an endarterectomy of the carotid artery in 12 patients (52%), an endarterectomy of the subclavian artery in 7 patients (30%), and an endarterectomy of the vertebral artery in 6 patients (26%). Two surgeries (9%) were complicated by a lymph leak. All patients improved clinically, and all reconstructions were patent by Doppler ultrasound scanning at a mean follow-up of 25 ± 21 months. In a systematic review of the literature from 1966 to 2000, 516 patients who underwent carotid subclavian bypass grafting and 511 patients who underwent subclavian carotid transpositions were reported. Patency rates were 84% and 98%, respectively (p <.0001), and the rates of freedom from symptoms were 88% and 99%, respectively, at a mean follow-up of 59 ± 17 months.

Takach and colleagues also reported on the results of brachiocephalic reconstruction, operative versus endovascular management of single-vessel disease. Their study included 391 consecutive patients with single-vessel brachiocephalic disease who were treated with either operative bypass (group A; $n = 229$) or percutaneous transluminal angioplasty/stenting (group B; $n = 162$). All patients were asymptomatic after surgery or endovascular intervention. Group A and group B patients had similar operative mortality (0.9% vs. 0%) and stroke (1.3% vs 0%) rates. However, five years after the procedure, group A had significantly better freedom from graft or intervention failure (92.7% ± 2.1%) than did group B (83.9% ± 3.7%; $p = .03$). They reported that endovascular intervention involved less initial cost (mean savings, $8787 per procedure), was less invasive, and did not necessitate general anesthesia. On satisfaction questionnaires, 96.5% of patients receiving an endovascular intervention and 95.1% of patients receiving operative bypass for single-vessel brachiocephalic disease subjectively rated their treatment as "good" or "very good." Takach and colleagues concluded that operative bypass and endovascular intervention for single-vessel brachiocephalic disease are both associated with acceptably low operative morbidity and mortality. Operative bypass produces significantly better midterm freedom from graft or intervention failure than endovascular intervention and produces excellent long-term freedom from

failure. Endovascular intervention offers tangible benefits regarding cost, level of invasiveness, and subjective patient satisfaction.

Takach and colleagues also reported on their experience of brachiocephalic reconstruction, the operative and long-term results for complex disease. One hundred fifty-seven consecutive patients with innominate artery or multivessel brachiocephalic disease underwent operative reconstruction using either a transthoracic approach (group A, $n = 113$) or a less invasive, extrathoracic approach (group B, $n = 44$). Reconstruction required multiple distal anastomoses in 70 patients (44.6%), concomitant coronary artery bypass grafting in 36 patients (23.6%), and concomitant carotid endarterectomy in 26 patients (16.6%). They reported that no significant differences were found between groups A and B when operative mortality (2.7% vs. 2.3%) and stroke rates (2.7% vs. 6.8%) were analyzed. However, 10 years after surgery, freedom from graft failure was significantly better in group A (94.4% ± 4.4%) than in group B (60.3% ± 13.4%, $p = .002$). They concluded that transthoracic arch reconstruction for complex brachiocephalic disease can be achieved with acceptably low morbidity and mortality similar to those of a less invasive, extrathoracic approach. Furthermore, the transthoracic approach is associated with significantly better long-term freedom from graft failure, possibly because it preserves aortic inflow to the great vessels.

We previously reported on brachiocephalic revascularization, comparing carotid subclavian artery bypass and axilloaxillary artery bypass. This study included 67 patients: 36 with carotid-subclavian bypass (CSBP) (28 CSBPs only and 8 with carotid endarterectomy) and 31 with axilloaxillary artery bypass using PTFE grafts and followed for a mean of 69.2 and 71.9 months, respectively. Indications for surgery in the CSBP group included hemispheric TIA/cerebrovascular accident in 5, nonhemispheric TIA in 7, upper extremity ischemia in 15, and combined TIA and arm ischemia in 9 patients. In the axilloaxillary artery group, 2 patients had hemispheric TIA, 5 had nonhemispheric TIA, 12 had upper extremity ischemia, and 12 had combined TIA and arm ischemia. Graft patency was determined clinically and confirmed by segmental Doppler pressures, duplex ultrasonography, or angiography. The 30-day mortality rate was approximately 3% in both groups. The 30-day complication rate was 3% for the axilloaxillary artery group and 8% for the CSBP group (not statistically significant). Relief of symptoms was achieved in 100% of patients in both groups; however, 20% of the patients in the axilloaxillary artery groups had a recurrence of symptoms, in contrast to 5.6% in the CSBP group. The cumulative 10-year primary and secondary patency rates, calculated by life-table analysis, were 66% and 84.6% for the axilloaxillary artery procedures and 93.8% and 93.8% for the CSBP procedures, respectively (statistically significant). Concomitant carotid endarterectomy with CSBP did not influence graft patency. We concluded that both bypasses had comparable morbidity and mortality rates; however, the CSBP has a statistically significantly better primary patency rate than the axilloaxillary bypass. Therefore CSBP should be the procedure of choice, and the axilloaxillary artery bypass should be restricted to high-risk patients.

We also recently reported on our 20-year experience of CSBP procedures, using PTFE grafts, for symptomatic subclavian artery stenosis or occlusion. Fifty-one patients with symptomatic subclavian artery disease (40 occlusions and 11 stenoses) who were treated with CSBPs using PTFE grafts were analyzed. The indications for surgery were arm ischemia in 34 (67%), vertebrobasilar insufficiency (VBI) in 27 (53%), and symptomatic subclavian steal in 7 (14%). A combination of arm ischemia and VBI occurred in 17 (33%). The mean follow-up was 7.7 years. The 30-day morbidity rate was 6%, with no perioperative stroke or mortality. Immediate relief of symptoms was achieved in 100% of patients; however, 4 patients (8%) had late recurrent symptoms (3 with VBI). The primary patency and secondary patency rates at 1, 3, 5, and 10 years were 100%, 98%, 96%, 92%, and 100%, 98%, 98%, and 95%, respectively.

The symptom-free survival rates at 1, 3, 5, and 10 years were 100%, 96%, 82%, and 47%, respectively. The overall survival rates at 1, 3, 5, and 10 years were 100%, 98%, 86%, and 57%, respectively. The mean hospital stay was 3.5 days in the late 1970s and 1980s and 2.1 days in the 1990s ($p < .001$). We concluded that CSBP using PTFE grafts for subclavian artery disease is safe, effective, and durable and should remain the procedure of choice, particularly in good-risk patients.

ENDOVASCULAR REPAIR

Although conventional open surgical reconstruction is the gold standard for the management of brachiocephalic intervention, most centers have evolved to first-line management of lesions by angioplasty and stent placement, particularly in the management of subclavian and proximal carotid artery pathology. Approach to either can be through a retrograde or antegrade fashion.

Indications for intervention should be similar to those for open repair. Liberal use of subclavian artery stenting of patients with asymptomatic subclavian steal diagnosed by noninvasive studies should be discouraged. In addition, endovascular repair of occlusions, heavily calcified lesions, and those suspected of embolizations, as well as lesions that extend into the origin of the vertebral artery, are not recommended. Stent placement distal to the vertebral artery should also be discouraged because the thoracic outlet can damage the integrity with repetitive movements. Lesions ideal for endovascular treatment are short-segment stenoses and in cases in which the patients are at high risk for surgical reconstruction. Patients considered ideal for endoluminal solutions include those with limited cardiopulmonary reserve for general anesthesia, previous median sternotomy, radiation injury, and body habitus that makes surgical exposure more difficult.

In the experience of our center, with more than 100 subclavian artery stents placed for symptomatic disease, we have reported a 5-year overall patency of 72% with no major perioperative complications and no deaths. In comparison, the primary 5-year patency of prosthetic carotid-subclavian bypass was 96%, with a 6% perioperative complication rate but no strokes or deaths.

With the increasing use of catheter-based therapy for extracranial carotid artery disease, acceptance of proximal lesion treatment has followed. Isolated proximal carotid stenosis can be treated via a femoral approach with adjunct embolic protection in cases of absent carotid bifurcation disease. In patients with combined proximal and bifurcation stenosis, we advocate the use of open repair and simultaneous retrograde proximal stenting. Others have shown impressive results with these proximal lesions, reporting expected patencies greater than 90% at 5 years. The benefits are obvious in that median sternotomy is prevented in those advocating direct reconstruction and there is no exposure to the risks of a subclavian carotid bypass.

Endovascular management of vertebral artery stenosis should be limited. The vertebral artery is prone to dissection, and complications are often severe when they occur. Direct reconstruction is associated with minimal operative morbidity and excellent patency. In high-risk patients, however, some centers have performed small series of interventions with acceptable results.

One area of continued interest is the management of trauma patients with endovascular therapies. Endoluminal repair can avoid the risks of urgent thoracotomy or median sternotomy, as well as eliminating the risk of dissection in patients with ongoing hemorrhage. Limited experience is available at present but is increasing in the literature. Durability reports are also limited, but endoluminal repair appears to be a reasonable option for the management of traumatic arterial injuries in brachiocephalic vessels.

SUGGESTED READINGS

AbuRahma AF, Robinson PA, Jennings TG: Carotid-subclavian bypass grafting with polytetrafluoroethylene grafts for symptomatic subclavian artery stenosis or occlusion: a 20-year experience, *J Vasc Surg* 32:411, 2000.

AbuRahma AF, Robinson PA, Khan MZ, and others: Brachiocephalic revascularization: a comparison between carotid-subclavian artery bypass and axilloaxillary artery bypass, *Surgery* 112:84, 1992.

Bates MC, Broce M, Lavigne PS, and others: Subclavian artery stenting: factors influencing long-term outcome, *Catheter Cardiovasc Interv* 61:5, 2004.

Cinà CS, Safar HA, Laganà A, and others: Subclavian carotid transposition and bypass grafting: consecutive cohort study and systematic review, *J Vasc Surg* 35:422, 2002.

Sakopoulos AG, Ballard JL, Gundry ST: Minimally invasive approach for aortic branch vessel reconstruction, *J Vasc Surg* 31:200, 2000.

Takach TJ, Duncan JM, Livesay JJ, and others: Brachiocephalic reconstruction II: operative and endovascular management of single-vessel disease, *J Vasc Surg* 42:55, 2005.

Takach TJ, Reul GJ, Cooley DA, and others: Brachiocephalic reconstruction I: operative and long-term results for complex disease, *J Vasc Surg* 42:47, 2005.

Uurto I, Lautamatti V, Zeitlin R, and others: Long-term outcome of surgical revascularization of supra-aortic vessels, *World J Surg* 26:1503, 2002.

MANAGEMENT OF ANEURYSMS OF THE EXTRACRANIAL CAROTID AND VERTEBRAL ARTERIES

Virginia L. Wong, MD, and Jerry Goldstone, MD

Aneurysms of the extracranial carotid and vertebral arteries are rare. Contemporary reports suggest that only 0.2% to 5% of all carotid procedures are performed for this diagnosis. Therefore large or randomized studies do not exist, and smaller, single-institution case series must be used to guide management and predict outcomes.

CAROTID ARTERY ANEURYSMS

Etiology

The majority of extracranial carotid artery aneurysms are atherosclerotic, or degenerative, in nature. This etiology accounted for one third to one half of all cases reported by the two largest published series of carotid artery aneurysms from Houston: Texas Heart Institute (THI, 67 cases) and Baylor College of Medicine (BCM, 42 cases). Pseudoaneurysm following prior carotid endarterectomy (CEA) was also responsible for a large number of the patients in both series, but only approximately 15% of all reported extracranial carotid aneurysms are pseudoaneurysms. Less frequently cited etiologies include local injury and dissection following trauma (blunt, penetrating, and iatrogenic), fibromuscular dysplasia (FMD), and infection. Rare causes include radiation injury and Behçet's or other collagen vascular disease.

Presentation and Diagnosis

Patients are frequently asymptomatic at presentation. A pulsatile neck mass is the most frequently encountered sign, described in more than 90% of the BCM patients (Fig. 1). Symptoms vary depending on the size, location, and etiology of the aneurysm. They usually consist of hemispheric neurologic events such as transient ischemic attacks, cerebral vascular accidents, and amaurosis fugax caused by embolic phenomena. However, compressive symptoms from the aneurysm itself, such as cranial nerve palsy, Horner's syndrome, headache or facial pain, hoarseness, and dysphagia have also been described. Patients presenting with infection may exhibit fever, leukocytosis, and peritonsillar abscess or cervical cellulitis. Rupture with frank hemorrhage is a rare event but may occur into the pharynx or to the outside via a draining sinus, as may be seen with infected pseudoaneurysm following CEA. The differential diagnosis includes carotid arterial redundancy (kink, coil, loop), carotid body tumor, cervical lymphadenopathy, neoplasm, peritonsillar abscess, and branchial cleft cyst. A condition frequently misdiagnosed as a carotid aneurysm is a tortuous common carotid and subclavian artery that presents as a pulsatile mass at the base of the neck, almost always on the right side in middle-aged, hypertensive women.

Carotid duplex ultrasound is the recommended initial diagnostic modality. It can determine size, extent, flow characteristics, and presence of thrombus or dissection. However, lesions that are located high in the neck or at the base of the skull cannot be interrogated by ultrasound and may be missed altogether with this modality. The same is true for aneurysms of the vertebral artery. Computed tomography (CT) or magnetic resonance imaging (MRI) is useful to visualize these lesions and surrounding structures, as well as to identify preoperative cerebral infarction. In some centers, CT or MR angiography (CTA, MRA) with three-dimensional reconstruction provides high-quality and detailed images for defining arterial anatomy and planning intervention without the risk of stroke that can be associated with conventional angiography. However, traditional catheter-based angiography remains the study of choice in most centers to obtain anatomic information about the aortic arch and its branch vessels and about cerebral arterial supply. Additionally, carotid artery back-pressure measurement, balloon occlusion testing, and endovascular repair of the aneurysm can all be accomplished during this procedure.

Indications for Intervention

Intervention for carotid artery aneurysm is certainly indicated for the relief of symptoms caused by local compression and for the treatment of rupture that, although rare, is associated with high morbidity and mortality. However, the primary indication for intervention is to prevent new or recurrent neurologic events associated with embolism of aneurysm contents into the cerebral circulation. In a classic publication by Winslow in 1926, nonoperative management resulted in a 70% mortality rate resulting from thrombosis, embolism, and rupture. Some recent reports suggest that anticoagulation and observation may be appropriate for certain asymptomatic patients with small and high aneurysms resulting from spontaneous or traumatic dissection. Follow-up imaging has demonstrated stabilization or resolution without clinical complications in at least some of these lesions. Close monitoring of this patient subset is essential, and lesions that enlarge or become symptomatic should be repaired to prevent devastating neurologic sequelae.

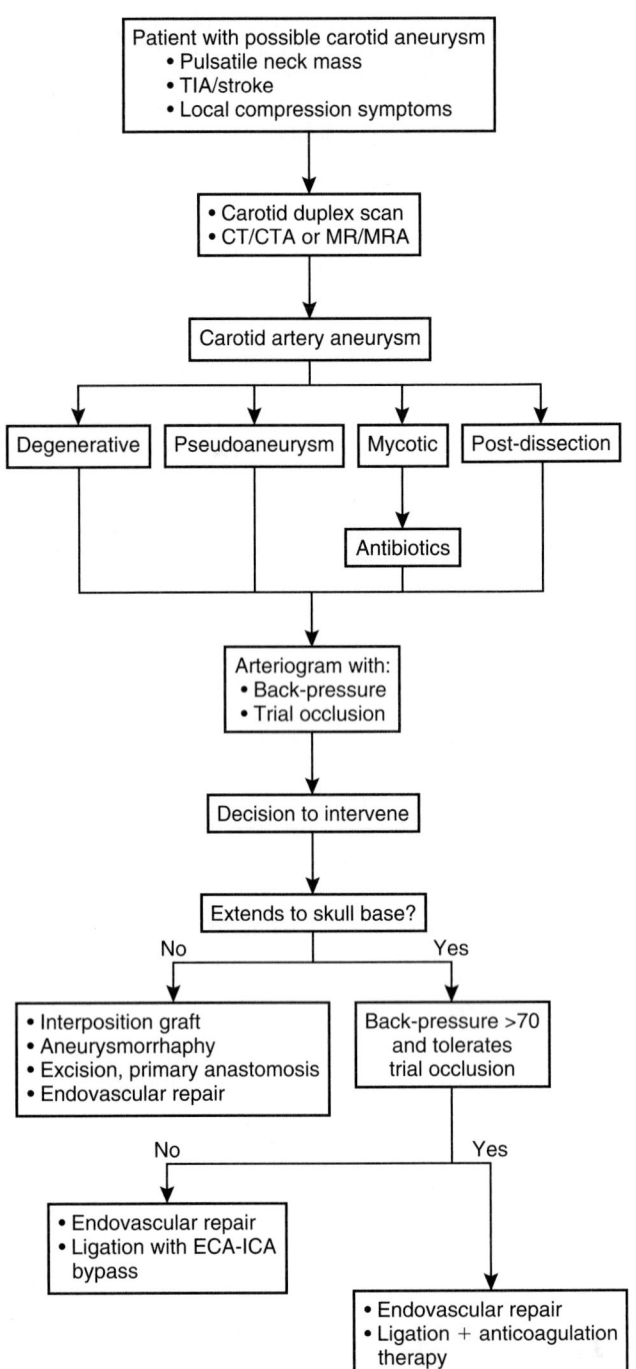

Figure I Algorithm for diagnosis and treatment of carotid aneurysms. *CT/CTA,* Computed tomography/CT angiography; *ECA,* external carotid artery; *ICA,* internal carotid artery; *MR/MRA,* magnetic resonance/ MR angiography; *TIA,* transient ischemic attack. *Modified from Rothstein J, Goldstone J. In Cronenwett JL, Rutherford RB, editors: Decision making in vascular surgery, Orlando, 2001, WB Saunders, p. 54.*

Treatment

Before undertaking repair by any method, a baseline neurologic evaluation should be performed, and cardiac performance should be optimized. Patients with atherosclerotic carotid artery aneurysms are also at risk for coronary disease and perioperative cardiac complications, and thus appropriate cardiac evaluation is prudent. The need for intraoperative cerebral perfusion monitoring and protection should be considered because cross-clamp times are generally long. Electroencephalogram, transcranial Doppler, carotid stump back-pressure measurement, and routine shunt use have all been described. Although carotid endarterectomy is successfully performed under local (regional) anesthesia, most authors prefer the use of general anesthesia for carotid aneurysms because of the difficult dissection through inflamed perianeurysmal tissue and the need for extensive distal cervical exposure and complex arterial reconstruction.

The location of carotid artery aneurysms varies with etiology. Atherosclerotic aneurysms most commonly occur at or near the common carotid bifurcation, as do pseudoaneurysms following CEA (Figs. 2, 3). Injuries from blunt trauma and dysplastic lesions typically occur much higher on the internal carotid artery (ICA), toward the base of the skull. Proximal exposure of the carotid artery and its bifurcation can be achieved through a standard longitudinal cervical incision along the anterior border of the sternocleidomastoid muscle (SCM), extending behind the ear, if necessary, to gain more distal exposure. Care must be taken to avoid manipulation of the aneurysm itself and dislodgement of material before application of a distal cross clamp. Cranial nerves VII, IX, X, XI, and XII may be encountered in the operative field and should be protected from injury. Their usual courses may be altered because of growth of the aneurysm, or they may be densely adherent to its surface. More distal exposure of the ICA may require division of the digastric muscle; anterior traction, subluxation, or division of the mandible; elevation of the parotid gland; division of the styloid process; or division of SCM from the mastoid. These maneuvers are facilitated by nasotracheal, rather than orotracheal, intubation. Control of distal backbleeding may also be achieved using an intraluminal balloon catheter instead of a cross clamp. However, if higher exposure to the base of the skull is required for reconstruction, removal of the petrous temporal bone with division of the mastoid and external auditory canal may be necessary and should be undertaken with assistance from an otolaryngologist or neurosurgeon experienced in skull-base surgery.

Open reconstructive options include ligation, resection with patch repair, or resection with reconstruction of arterial continuity using conduits. Ligation is technically less demanding and may be the only option for high lesions for which distal access to the ICA

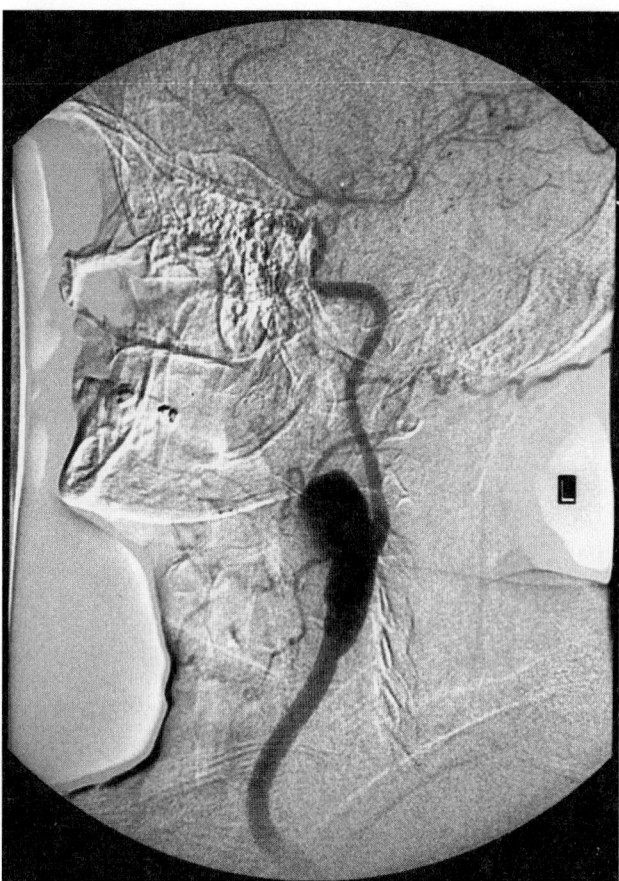

Figure 3 Digital subtraction angiogram showing pseudoaneurysm of left carotid bifurcation at site of previous carotid endarterectomy.

cannot be achieved or for rapid control of exsanguination from rupture or trauma. Unfortunately, ligation is associated with a high rate of stroke and mortality (30%–60%). Selection of patients who will tolerate ligation may be accomplished by performing a balloon occlusion test at the time of carotid angiography. After heparinization, a balloon is inflated in the ICA to occlude antegrade cerebral flow for approximately 30 minutes. The patient's neurologic response is monitored for changes. Carotid back pressures of 70 mm Hg or higher indicate adequate cerebral collateral perfusion pressure to allow carotid ligation if necessary. Patients who fail this occlusion test may be considered for extracranial to intracranial (EC-IC) carotid bypass before ligation. Consideration should also be given to postligation anticoagulation to prevent propagation of thrombus distal to the point of ligation. Aneurysm resection and patch repair of the ICA is appropriate for small-necked, saccular aneurysms, or pseudoaneurysms. The use of greater saphenous vein (GSV) and prosthetic material for patches and conduits has been well described, but if the possibility of infection as etiology for the aneurysm exists, autogenous materials must be used. Complete resection of the aneurysm with reconstruction of arterial continuity is the preferred method of open repair for fusiform or wide-based aneurysms. During this approach, ICA redundancy can be mobilized and primarily reimplanted or interposition grafting performed using GSV or prosthetic graft (Fig. 4). In some patients, the external carotid artery can be transected and used to bridge a short distance to the end of the resected internal carotid artery. Use of a shunt is facilitated by threading it through the interposition graft while the distal anastomosis is completed and then removing

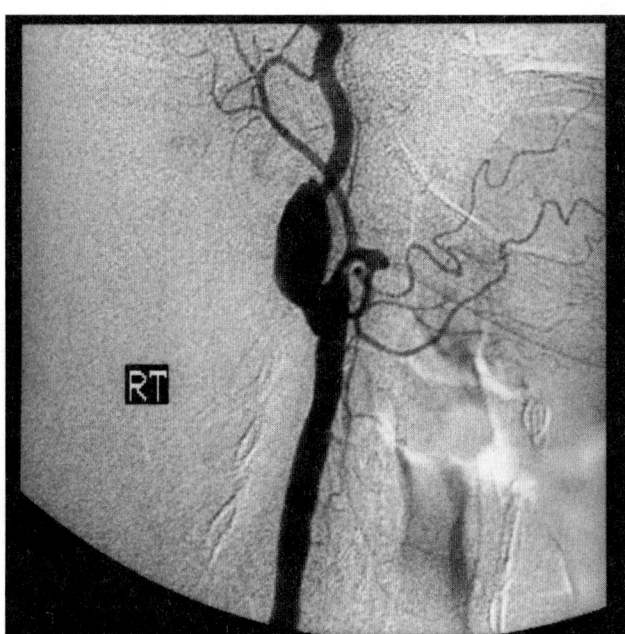

Figure 2 Digital subtraction angiogram showing aneurysm of right internal carotid artery.

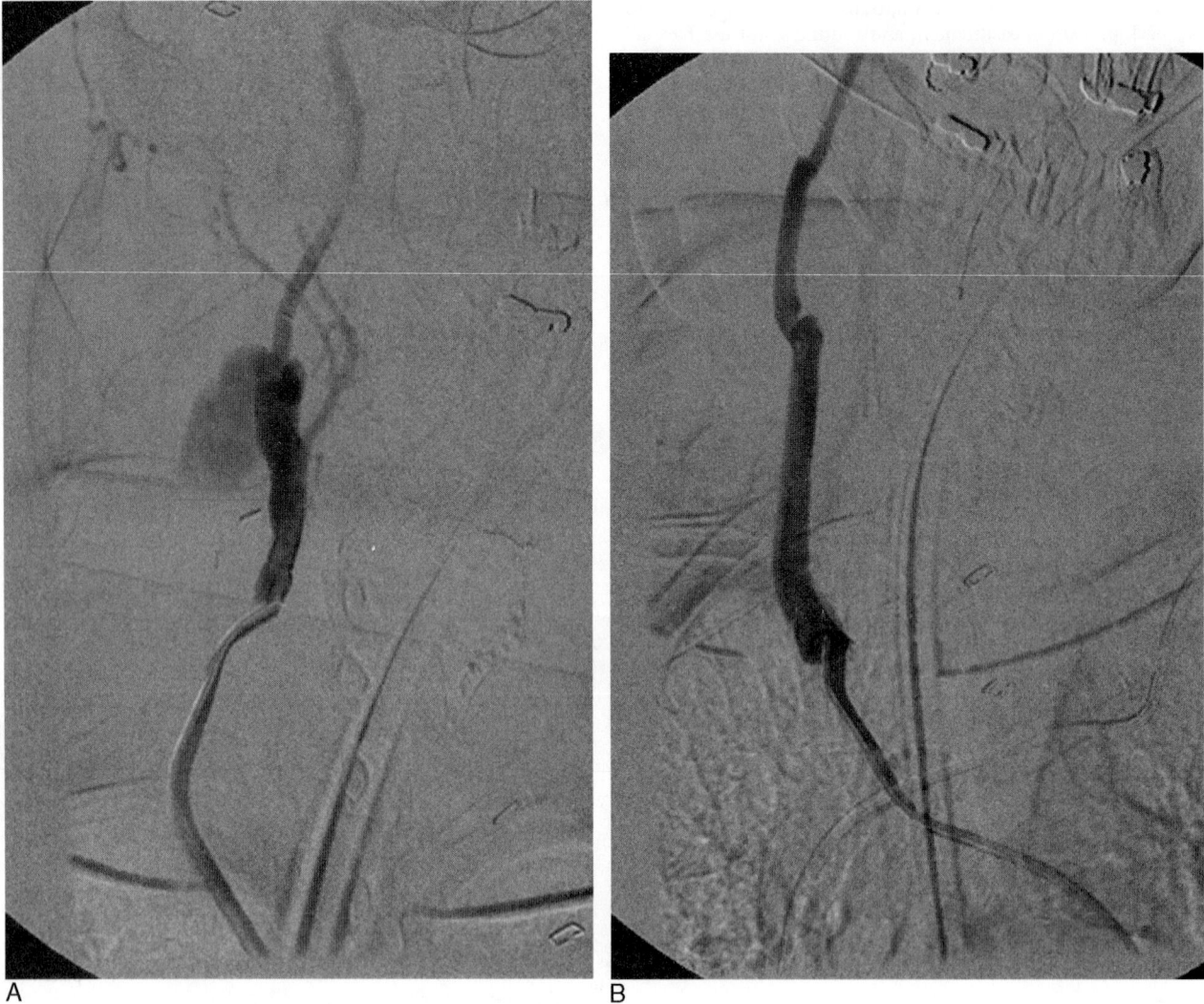

Figure 4 Digital subtraction angiogram of carotid aneurysm before **(A)** and after **(B)** repair with interposition vein graft. *Courtesy of Wei Zhou, MD, Baylor College of Medicine.*

it just before completion of the proximal anastomosis. For cases involving infectious processes, broad-spectrum intravenous antibiotics should be initiated before surgery. The procedure should include wide debridement of nonviable material, reconstruction of arterial flow through uninvolved tissue planes using autologous conduit, and coverage with viable tissue, such as the sternocleidomastoid muscle. Intraoperative cultures should be obtained, and long-term antibiotic therapy subsequently tailored according to organism sensitivity. These latter maneuvers are especially important if methicillin-resistant *Staphylococcus aureus* is known or suspected of being the causative organism.

Endovascular treatment of carotid artery aneurysms has become more common because of advances in endovascular equipment and growing endoluminal experience treating carotid occlusive disease. Multiple case reports populate the literature. In the BCM series, 70% of patients in the more recent treatment group (1995–2004) were treated with endovascular techniques. This method of treatment requires experienced staff and an available imaging suite with appropriate equipment, including embolic protection devices. Suitable patients for this approach have aortic arch anatomy that can accommodate stable, selective catheterization of the common carotid artery with a large-caliber long

sheath. Preferential consideration for endovascular treatment may be given to a surgically inaccessible lesion, a hostile operative field (prior radiation or cervical surgery), or a patient who is unfit for a lengthy general anesthetic. Treatment techniques generally use a transfemoral approach; however, transaxillary and transcarotid approaches have been described. Following heparinization and selective catheterization of the common carotid artery with a long sheath over a supportive wire, an embolic protection device is deployed in the ICA, distal to the aneurysm. A covered stent (stent graft) may be deployed across the aneurysm to exclude it from arterial flow, thereby preventing expansion and rupture or emboli from entering the flow channel. This technique requires accurate sizing of appropriate landing zones proximal and distal to the aneurysm for seal and may occlude side branch flow (e.g., external carotid artery [ECA]). A bare metal stent can be used to tack down a dissection entry point (flap) or cover a small aneurysm neck (pseudoaneurysm) enough to impede flow and cause sac thrombosis while preserving branch vessel flow. Both types of stent can treat concomitant carotid stenosis. Thrombogenic materials such as coils, detachable balloons, glue, and synthetic particles can be injected directly into the aneurysm sac to cause thrombosis; however, care must be taken not to allow the escape of such materials into the parent artery, leading to thrombosis or distal embolization. One technique that has been described is to first place a bare metal stent across the aneurysm neck and then direct coils through a microcatheter into the sac through the interstices of the stent to ensure sac thrombosis.

Results

As mentioned earlier, no randomized or controlled data for the treatment of carotid artery aneurysms are available. The results of observation with or without anticoagulation follow the natural history of the disease, with a 50% to 70% stroke and mortality rate. Ligation also results in a high rate of stroke and mortality (30% to 60%), but patient selection may reduce this risk substantially. Results of operative reconstruction in the THI series and an average from 13 single-center series reviewed in that same publication show that repair can be accomplished with approximately 10% combined stroke and mortality. Results vary with the size, location, and etiology of the lesion. The average rate of cranial nerve injury, which is more common in repairs involving the distal ICA, is much higher, approximately 30%. Fortunately, many of these deficits are temporary. Long-term results from these series are generally favorable, with most deaths occurring from cardiovascular disease or diagnoses not related to the carotid aneurysm repair. Surgical reconstructions remained patent in most patients subsequently imaged; occluded repairs were reportedly asymptomatic.

For endovascular treatment of carotid aneurysm, initial technical success rates are high. Periprocedural stroke and mortality are acceptably low in these small series. Cranial nerve injury, wound complication, and length of hospital stay appear markedly decreased with endovascular treatment compared with open reconstruction. Short-term and midterm results for up to 4.5 years after treatment are encouraging, with persistent exclusion of the aneurysm and patency of the reconstruction noted on follow-up examinations. With increasing use of endovascular techniques for treatment of carotid aneurysm, more data regarding long-term results should become available.

VERTEBRAL ARTERY ANEURYSMS

Aneurysms of the extracranial vertebral artery are extremely rare. Blunt and penetrating traumas are the most frequently cited causes, resulting in pseudoaneurysm or true aneurysmal dilatation after intimal dissection. Iatrogenic manipulation (chiropractic, vascular catheterization), fibromuscular dysplasia, prior radiation, and collagen vascular disease have been described as causes of vertebral artery aneurysm. Patients may present with pulsatile neck mass or with symptoms of vertebrobasilar insufficiency. Contrast angiography remains the gold standard diagnostic study; however,

CT and MR are helpful to visualize surrounding structures and provide important anatomic information that may influence the interventional approach. More than 80% of lesions resolve spontaneously, and therefore patients are often managed nonoperatively with anticoagulation. However, in cases of hemorrhage, continued neurologic symptoms, aneurysm enlargement, or contralateral vertebral artery absence or insufficiency, intervention may be best.

Surgical exposure of the vertebral artery can be challenging given its course deep in the posterior neck, through the transverse processes of the cervical vertebrae. Access to the proximal vertebral artery is achieved through a transcervical incision, exposing it from its subclavian artery origin to its entrance into the transverse process at C6 (V1 segment). Repair options include ligation, resection with repair, transposition onto the carotid artery, or bypass from the subclavian artery. The more distal portions of the vertebral artery including the intraosseous course from C6 to C2 (V2 segment), from the top of C2 to the atlantooccipital membrane (V3 segment), and the intracranial portion (V4) are more difficult to access. A posterior cervical approach may be necessary and repair accomplished by carotid or subclavian bypass or transposition to the carotid circulation. Endovascular access and repair by covered stent-graft placement or embolization have been reported for lesions at all levels of the vertebral artery and may be most useful for surgically inaccessible areas.

Ligation or endovascular sacrifice of the vertebral artery is well tolerated in the presence of a normal contralateral vertebral artery. Ultrasound or angiography may be used preprocedurally to look for atresia, hypoplasia, or occlusive disease in this vessel. A dominant vertebral artery aneurysm is best treated by a method designed to maintain its patency and prevent distal embolism.

Suggested Readings

Berguer R, Flynn L, Kline RA, and others: Surgical reconstruction of the extracranial vertebral artery: management and outcome, *J Vasc Surg* 31:9, 2000.

Bush RL, Lin PH, Dodson TF, and others: Endoluminal stent placement and coil embolization for the management of carotid artery pseudoaneurysms, *J Endovasc Ther* 8:53, 2001.

El-Sabrout R, Cooley DA: Extracranial carotid artery aneurysms: Texas Heart Institute experience, *J Vasc Surg* 31:702, 2000.

Longo GM, Kibbe M: Aneurysms of the carotid artery, *Sem Vasc Surg* 18:178, 2005.

Rosset E, Albertini JN, and others: Surgical treatment of extracranial internal carotid artery aneurysms, *J Vasc Surg* 31:713, 2000.

Rothstein J, Goldstone J: Carotid artery aneurysms. In Cronenwett JL, Rutherford RB, editors: *Decision making in vascular surgery*, Orlando, FL, 2001, WB Saunders, p. 54.

Zhou W, Lin PH, Bush RL, and others: Carotid artery aneurysm: evolution of management over two decades, *J Vasc Surg* 43:493, 2006.

NONOPERATIVE TREATMENT OF CLAUDICATION

H. Alden Kirk, MD, and Charles S. O'Mara, MD

Lower-extremity peripheral artery disease (PAD), which is caused by atherosclerotic occlusive disease in large arteries, is revealed objectively by a diminished Doppler-derived ankle-brachial pressure index (ABI). PAD occurs in approximately 20% of patients 55 years of age and older, thus affecting approximately 10 million people in the United States alone. An increasing public awareness of PAD is being fueled in part by a medically astute aging population, by market forces, and by expanding interest in peripheral vascular disease by multiple medical specialties.

CLINICAL CONSIDERATIONS

The most common symptom of PAD is intermittent claudication (IC), defined as cramping muscle pain or weakness produced by walking and relieved promptly by rest. IC is associated with lower-extremity hemodynamic alterations after ambulation that are demonstrable after treadmill walking by a temporary reduction in ABI. The cramping pain or weakness after walking involves muscles located distal to the arterial obstruction. Therefore superficial femoral artery occlusion produces claudication in the calf and occasionally the foot muscles. Likewise, aortoiliac occlusive lesions typically result in claudication of the buttock, hip, or thigh muscles, but they can also affect the more distally located calf muscles. Paresthesias in the lower extremities sometimes occur along with the muscular symptoms of IC.

Many patients with PAD are asymptomatic, primarily because the walking distance in their daily routine is not far enough to elicit symptoms. Sometimes a distinction must also be made clinically between vasculogenic claudication and neurogenic claudication caused by lumbar stenosis. The latter is characterized by inconsistent symptoms, a requirement for sitting or lying after walking to achieve complete relief of symptoms, and a normal treadmill-walking test. The occasional need to make this distinction emphasizes the importance of a careful and detailed history of IC to include location of the cramping pain, distance at which pain begins, distance at which the patient typically must stop to rest, and time required for resolution of symptoms.

Of equal importance is the performance of a thorough vascular examination, including auscultation of the abdomen and both groins for bruits, performance of Doppler-derived ABIs even when pulses are palpable, and realization that IC can occur in the setting of palpable pedal pulses and a normal ABI. When the diagnosis of vasculogenic claudication is questionable, we use a standard treadmill-walking test to verify hemodynamic changes. A variety of lower-extremity arterial imaging studies are now available, including magnetic resonance imaging, computed tomographic angiography, and conventional arteriography. However, imaging studies are rarely used in nonoperative management of IC and instead are used only when intervention is being considered.

ASSOCIATED RISK FACTORS

Because PAD and IC are manifestations of generalized atherosclerosis, they have a strong association with cardiovascular risk factors, such as cigarette smoking, diabetes mellitus, hypertension, and hyperlipidemia. Likewise, patients with IC often have other problems attributable to atherosclerosis, such as occlusive disease of the coronary, carotid, and renal arteries. In addition, approximately 9% of patients with significant limb ischemia have an abdominal aortic aneurysm. Sixty-three percent of deaths in patients with PAD result from coronary occlusive disease, 9% result from stroke, and 8% from other cardiovascular events, such as ruptured aneurysms. The simple and isolated finding of a diminished ABI has been shown to be an independent predictor of high mortality (5-year survival of only 55%-65% for ABI between 0.4 and 0.6).

These data emphasize the importance of a thorough evaluation regarding other systemic vascular diseases in patients with IC. They also underscore the need for IC management to be directed not only toward symptom relief but also toward prevention of secondary vascular complications that encompass major morbidity and mortality potential. Management of patients with IC can be usefully categorized into the following topics: (1) efforts that provide beneficial lifestyle and risk-factor alterations and (2) pharmacologic therapy. Both of these categories include overlapping elements that reduce atherosclerotic risk and improve claudication symptoms.

LIFESTYLE AND RISK-FACTOR MODIFICATION

Smoking Cessation

Cigarette smoking is the most important risk factor for the development and clinical progression of PAD. In young adults with premature lower-extremity atherosclerosis, smoking is the most prevalent risk factor. In older adults, the estimated risk of developing IC is up to 16-fold higher among smokers than among nonsmokers. In patients with PAD who continue to smoke, the 5-year mortality rate is greater than 60%, primarily because of myocardial infarction. Observational data strongly suggest that smoking cessation is associated with decreased rates of myocardial infarction and stroke compared with patients who continue to smoke. If PAD progresses to the point of requiring surgery, former smokers have improved patency of peripheral arterial reconstructions and decreased amputation rates compared with current smokers. Benefits of smoking cessation also include symptom relief with improvement in treadmill walking distance. For all of these reasons, complete cessation of smoking should be the primary goal of treatment for every patient with IC.

Strategies to accomplish smoking cessation should begin with informing the patient, through direct conversation, about the specific harmful effects of cigarette smoking, as well as the benefits of smoking cessation. We present to the patient a detailed list of the various components of cigarette smoke in a printed format that allows their deleterious effects to be clearly understood. We also emphasize the importance of complete cessation of smoking by others in the patient's household.

Nevertheless, the rate of spontaneous smoking cessation is disappointingly low even for smokers who have a true desire to quit, and additional help and support usually prove necessary. Nicotine replacement therapy, administered via either chewing gum or transdermal patch, has been shown to be a safe and effective aid for smoking cessation. In addition, the antidepressant bupropion is helpful in relieving nicotine withdrawal symptoms. Standard dosage of bupropion is 150 mg orally twice daily for 7 to 12 weeks. These agents are effective only when accompanied by the patient's firm resolve and strong will to stop smoking completely.

Exercise Therapy

The inverse relationship of previous level of physical activity to risk of PAD suggests a protective effect of exercise. In addition, trials have documented that walking capacity is increased by exercise training in patients with claudication and that regular exercise together with lifestyle modification, especially smoking cessation, is the cornerstone for nonoperative treatment of claudication symptoms. Increased exercise capacity of ischemic and nonischemic muscle after an exercise program is explained by improved oxygen uptake and extraction, as well as increased muscle enzyme activity. Moreover, exercise augments collateral flow around an occluded segment of artery in an ischemic limb and also provides systemic cardiovascular benefit. Exercise significantly improves maximal walking time and overall walking ability in patients with stable intermittent claudication. Walking distance can be increased in claudicant patients who engage in intermittent ambulation to near-maximal pain over a period of at least 6 months. Systematic reviews have shown that the effects of exercise are even superior to those of angioplasty or antiplatelet therapy and are equivalent to those of surgical intervention.

Walking exercise programs have been shown to be most effective when conducted in a supervised, structured environment. However, logistic considerations and lack of funding for such supervised programs usually make them impractical. We advise patients with IC to engage in a structured but self-monitored regimen in which they walk past the point of claudication, stop and rest to allow relief of discomfort, and then repeat the cycle multiple times in succession for a total of 30 to 60 minutes per day over at least 6 months. Patients should be reassured that walking through the pain of claudication is not deleterious and that this regimen is in fact helpful in achieving the goal of increasing their walking distance. Patients who are compliant with this regimen are often rewarded with a doubling of their walking distance within 6 weeks.

Control of Hypertension

Hypertension is an independent risk factor for PAD and can increase the risk of claudication twofold to threefold. Aggressive treatment of hypertension in patients with PAD is now advocated to achieve a target blood pressure at or below 130/80 mm Hg. In the past, physicians were reluctant to use beta-adrenergic blockade in patients with PAD because of the possibility of making claudication symptoms worse. However, a meta-analysis of 11 random controlled trials found no adverse effects of beta-blockers on IC.

Angiotensin-converting enzyme (ACE) inhibitors have shown benefit beyond lowering of blood pressure in high-risk patients. The Heart Outcome Prevention Evaluation (HOPE) study showed that ramipril significantly reduced the rate of cardiovascular death, myocardial infarction, and cerebral vascular accidents in patients at high risk of cardiovascular death. Subset analysis of this study showed that ramipril was effective in lowering the risk of fatal and nonfatal events in patients with PAD. This effect, however, could not be explained by a reduction in blood pressure, which in the study group averaged only approximately 2 mm Hg. It is important to remember that ACE inhibitors should be used with caution in patients with either renal failure or renal artery stenosis.

Diabetic Management and Glucose Control

In the Framingham study, patients with diabetes had a threefold to fivefold increase in the risk of developing IC compared with nondiabetic patients. These diabetic patients have worse lower-extremity function than those with PAD alone. PAD in diabetics is more aggressive in terms of both early large-vessel involvement and microangiopathy. Diabetic patients with IC have a 35% risk of sudden limb ischemia and a 21% risk of major amputation, compared with 19% and 3%, respectively, in nondiabetic patients. Furthermore, several large trials have clearly shown that maximizing control of blood glucose in patients with diabetes results in a significant reduction in both microvascular and macrovascular complications, as well as improvement of symptoms in those with IC.

Current consensus recommendation is that the glycated hemoglobin (HgA1c) level in diabetic patients should be maintained below 6.5%, even if institution of insulin therapy proves necessary to achieve that goal. In addition, evidence is now convincing that intensive multifactorial treatment of diabetics with stepwise implementation of behavior modification and pharmacologic therapy to treat hyperglycemia, hypertension, dyslipidemia, and microalbuminuria, along with aspirin therapy, is effective in reducing cardiovascular death, nonfatal myocardial infarction, nonfatal stroke, need for limb revascularization, and amputation.

Dietary Discretion

Many studies have confirmed the cardiovascular benefits of dietary discretion. Current logical dietary recommendations include limiting intake of calories, sugar, saturated fat, processed foods, and cholesterol, and understanding the benefits of consuming whole grains, lean meat, fish, omega-3 fats, and fresh fruits and vegetables. We encourage our patients to adopt the concept of lifelong healthy eating habits, rather than embracing trendy "low-this and high-that" diets. This concept affords the patient the best chance of achieving weight reduction along with other cardiovascular benefits that are sustainable over most of a lifetime.

The majority of our patients with IC are overweight. To convey clearly the impact of a patient's weight on symptoms of claudication, we often ask a patient to imagine the additional difficulty of walking with the burden of a 20- to 30-pound backpack. The patient can then better appreciate the anticipated improvement in walking that would occur after losing the same amount of weight through regular exercise and proper dietary habits, both of which are essential for weight control in most people.

Pharmacologic Therapy

Medications used in management of IC can be grouped into those that focus on cardiovascular risk-factor reduction and those that are used for symptomatic improvement. Specific agents, along with their standard doses and efficacy, are listed in Table 1.

Antiplatelet Agents

In patients at high risk for occlusive arterial disease, the Antithrombotic Trialist's Collaboration meta-analysis of 195 trials demonstrated that antiplatelet therapy reduces the risk of myocardial infarction, stroke, or cardiovascular death by approximately one fourth. In a subset analysis of patients with PAD, similar risk reduction was documented.

Aspirin has not been shown to improve claudication, but it appears to delay the rate of progression of symptoms. The effectiveness of different doses of aspirin has not been clearly established, but Antithrombotic Trialist's Collaboration meta-analysis suggests that 75 to 150 mg daily is at least as effective as higher doses and less likely to produce gastrointestinal and bleeding complications.

Clopidogrel selectively inhibits the binding of adenosine diphosphate to platelet receptors and the subsequent mediated

Table 1: Pharmacologic Management of Claudication

Indication	Drug	Dose	Efficacy
Risk factor reduction	Aspirin	81 mg/d	25% CV risk reduction over placebo in patients with history of MI or stroke
	Clopidogrel	75 mg/d	24% risk reduction over aspirin 325 mg/day
	Ticlopidine	250 mg BID	Efficacy similar to clopidogrel
	Ramipril	10 mg/d	20% CV risk reduction over placebo
	Simvastatin	40 mg/d	24% CV risk reduction over placebo; effective even in PAD with no prior history of MI or stroke; effective even if baseline LDL cholesterol <116 mg/dl
IC symptom relief	Pentoxifylline	400 mg TID	0%-25% improvement in absolute walking distance on treadmill
	Cilostazol	50–100 mg BID	50% improvement in absolute walking distance on treadmill

BID, Twice daily; *CV,* cardiovascular; *IC,* intermittent claudication; *LDL,* low-density lipoprotein; *MI,* myocardial infarction; *PAD,* peripheral artery disease.

action of the glycoprotein IIb/IIIa complex, thereby inhibiting platelet aggregation. In the Clopidogrel versus Aspirin in Patients at Risk for Ischemic Events (CAPRIE) trial, 5795 patients with PAD were randomized to clopidogrel 75 mg daily and 5797 patients to 325 mg aspirin daily. The annual incidence of vascular death, nonfatal myocardial infarction, and nonfatal stroke was 3.7% with clopidogrel versus 4.9% with aspirin, a 24% significant decrease. These data indicate that clopidogrel may be more effective than aspirin in lowering cardiovascular risk in patients with PAD; however, its higher cost is often prohibitive, and recent information suggests a higher complication rate with clopidogrel.

Lipid-Lowering Therapy

Dyslipidemias, manifested biochemically by elevated low-density lipid (LDL) cholesterol, decreased high-density lipid (HDL) cholesterol, and increased triglyceride levels, contribute to peripheral atherosclerosis. Over the past few years, HMG Co A (3-hydroxy-3 methglutaryl coenzyme A) reductase inhibitors, known as statins, have become the mainstay for pharmacologically reducing LDL cholesterol and increasing HDL cholesterol. Moreover, evidence suggests that statin therapy stabilizes plaque and reduces inflammation in the vessel wall. In the PAD group of the Heart Protection Study, 6748 patients with PAD treated with simvastatin had a 19% relative reduction and 6.3% absolute reduction in the risk of major vascular events. Similarly, in a subgroup analysis in the Scandinavian Simvastatin Survival Study, reduction in cholesterol level by simvastatin was associated with a 38% reduction in the risk of new or worsening symptoms of IC. Consensus holds that hyperlipidemia should be treated to achieve a target LDL level of less than 100 mg/dl.

Drugs for Symptomatic Benefit

Pentoxifylline, a methylxanthine derivative that increases cyclic adenosine monophosphate (cAMP), is approved by the U.S. Food and Drug Administration (FDA) for the treatment of IC. This agent favorably influences red blood cell morphology, lowers fibrinogen levels, and decreases platelet aggregation. All of these effects would theoretically relieve symptoms in patients with IC. Early trials evaluating pentoxifylline in claudicant patients showed improved maximal walking distance. However, more recent trials have not shown uniformly beneficial results. Usual treatment with pentoxifylline is 400 mg orally three times daily. Symptomatic improvement, when it occurs, develops gradually over 1 to 2 months.

Cilostazol, a phosphodiesterase inhibitor with antiplatelet and vasodilatatory capacity, was the second drug to gain FDA approval for treating IC. Cilostazol inhibits cyclic adenosine monophosphate phosphodiesterase, an effect that leads to vascular smooth muscle relaxation and inhibition of platelet aggregation. Several randomized, placebo-controlled trials have shown a 40% to 50% increase in walking distance in patients with IC on cilostazol after 12 to 24 weeks of therapy. The standard cilostazol dosage of 100 mg orally twice daily provides the most efficacy; however, this dosage should be reduced to 50 mg twice daily if side effects such as headache, dizziness, loose stools, or palpitations occur. In fact, we advise our patients to use this lower dose for the first week of treatment to minimize risk of experiencing side effects. Cilostazol is contraindicated in patients with congestive heart failure because of its chemical similarity to other oral phosphodiesterase inhibitors. Cilostazol should not be taken along with grapefruit juice, which causes drug inactivation, an effect not caused by other citrus products.

Pentoxifylline and cilostazol improve symptoms in some patients with IC, but these agents do not alter underlying vascular pathology. In those patients who receive benefit, symptom status usually returns to baseline after discontinuation of the medication. Long-term therapy is expensive and not without bothersome side effects. For these reasons, drug therapy for relief of IC symptoms is used selectively in our practice.

CONCLUSION

All patients with PAD should be evaluated for secondary preventive strategies because of the systemic nature of atherosclerosis. These specific strategies include treatment of blood pressure to 130/80 mm Hg, management of diabetics to a HgA1c below 6.5%, complete abstinence from cigarette smoking, and lowering of LDL cholesterol level to less than 100 mg/dl. All patients should be given an antiplatelet drug, usually aspirin 81 mg daily. In addition, dietary discretion and healthy eating habits are emphasized.

After systemic risk factors have been addressed, attention is focused on improvement of claudication symptoms. An exercise program, preferably supervised, with the patient walking up to and past his or her point of claudication several times daily, is initiated. Next a 6-week to 3-month trial of cilostazol should be considered, although its limitations should be kept in mind and disclosed fully to the patient. Following these steps, if symptomatic claudication continues to interfere significantly with activities of daily living, endovascular or surgical intervention should be entertained.

Suggested Readings

Hankey GJ, Norman PE, Eikelboom JW: Medical treatment of peripheral arterial disease, *JAMA* 295:547, 2006.

Hiatt WR: Pharmacologic therapy for peripheral arterial disease and claudication, *J Vasc Surg* 36:1283, 2002.

Khan S, Clanthis M, Smout J, and others: Life-style modification in peripheral arterial disease, *Eur J Vasc Endovasc Surg* 29:2, 2005.

Regensteiner JG, Hiatt WR: Current medical therapies for patients with peripheral arterial disease: a critical review, *Am J Med* 112:49, 2002.

AORTOILIAC OCCLUSIVE DISEASE

Rabih A. Chaer, MD, Brian G. DeRubertis, MD, and K. Craig Kent, MD

DIAGNOSIS

The primary clinical manifestation of aortoiliac occlusive disease (AIOD) is intermittent claudication. Although claudication symptoms in the buttock or thigh confirm that the level of occlusive disease is in the aorta or iliac arteries, calf claudication is the most frequent manifestation of AIOD. Chronic and isolated aortoiliac obstruction is rarely the cause of a limb-threatening condition. However, the combination of AIOD with obstruction of the infrainguinal vessels can be associated with rest pain, ulceration, or tissue loss. In its advanced stage, aortoiliac atherosclerosis may also result in total occlusion of the abdominal aorta or common iliac arteries and lead to a constellation of symptoms known as Leriche syndrome, which includes gluteal or thigh claudication, atrophy of the leg muscles, impotence, and diminished or absent femoral pulses.

Evaluation of patients with AOID includes a standard history and physical examination, including a thorough vascular evaluation. Physical examination usually demonstrates diminished or absent femoral pulse and, consequently, absent popliteal and pedal pulses. Dependent rubor and pallor with elevation are seen with severe disease, and ultimately ulceration or gangrene may become apparent in patients with advanced ischemia. The clinician should gain a thorough understanding of the patient's cardiovascular risk factors because they affect the success of intervention, as well as the patient's long-term survival. A more objective evaluation of the severity of disease can then be obtained in the vascular laboratory using noninvasive testing. This includes measurement of the ankle-brachial pressure index (ABI), segmental pressures, and pulse volume recordings. A subset of patients with symptoms suggestive of claudication has normal femoral pulses and normal resting ABIs. Exercise testing in these individuals can elicit a reduction in peripheral pulses and diminution in ABI.

Noninvasive imaging can be used for preoperative planning and includes such modalities as duplex ultrasonography, magnetic resonance angiography (MRA), and computed tomography angiography (CTA). Direct imaging with duplex ultrasound can be performed in the iliac circulation, although imaging of the proximal iliac segments is limited and dependent on patient body habitus and technician experience. MRA is particularly useful for patients with renal insufficiency or an allergy to contrast agents, although the quality of MRA does appear to be operator dependent. CTA is useful for defining aortoiliac disease but can be limited by calcification, which is commonly present in patients with atherosclerosis. The gold standard remains conventional angiography, which can be both diagnostic and therapeutic in the setting of a planned endovascular intervention.

INDICATIONS FOR TREATMENT AND LESION CLASSIFICATION

The indication for intervention in symptomatic patients with AIOD includes claudication that reduces quality of life sufficiently to justify revascularization. Revascularization is mandatory for all patients with critical limb ischemia manifested by rest pain, ischemic ulceration, or gangrenous skin changes. Less frequent indications for treatment include allowing access for coronary interventions or intra-aortic balloon pump placement or increasing inflow before a distal surgical bypass procedure. In the early 1990s, a system of classification, the TransAtlantic Inter-Society Consensus (TASC), was generated for lesions in the aortoiliac circulation. The development of this system was prompted by the observation that the response to treatment, particularly for angioplasty, varied with the extent of the lesion. For example, technical success and patency rates for long-segment occlusions of the iliac circulation treated with angioplasty are reduced compared with outcomes in short-segment stenoses. The TASC group devised a classification scheme recognizing four types of lesions (A–D) of increasing severity and stratified treatment recommendations on the basis of lesion type. Endovascular intervention was recommended for type-A lesions (stenoses <3 cm only) and surgical revascularization for type-D lesions (including bilateral external iliac artery occlusion, ipsilateral common and external iliac artery occlusion, or diffuse disease involving the aorta and both iliac arteries). TASC-B lesions include unilateral common iliac occlusion, whereas TASC-C lesions include unilateral external iliac or bilateral common iliac occlusion. Although an endovascular approach was suggested for TASC-B lesions and surgery for TASC-C lesions, the panel believed that more evidence was necessary to define further the best treatment modality for these two intermediate lesion grades. Table 1 provides average patency and complication rates for various aortoiliac revascularization techniques.

MEDICAL THERAPY

The aim of treatments for AIOD is to improve symptoms of claudication or prevent amputation. However, patients found to have AIOD are also at increased risk of cardiovascular morbidity and mortality. Risk-factor modification may not only improve leg symptoms but also increase longevity and reduce associated cardiovascular events such as myocardial infarction or stroke. Risk factor modification includes complete cessation of smoking together with tight control of hypertension, as well as serum glucose in diabetic patients. In addition, low-density lipid (LDL) cholesterol level should be reduced to less than 100 mg/dL with diet modification and lipid-lowering agents. In addition, patients with AIOD should receive lifelong antiplatelet therapy, which has been shown to reduce the risk of myocardial infarction, ischemic stroke, and vascular death.

Participation in a walking exercise program has been shown in several prospective randomized clinical trials to improve walking distance and symptoms of claudication. In addition, pharmacotherapy may afford symptom relief in some patients. Pentoxifylline is a

Table 1: Average Patency and Complication Rates for Various Techniques for Aortoiliac Revascularization

	5-Year Patency	Complication Rate	Reported Mortality
Aortobifemoral bypass	85%–90%	5%–8%	2%–5%
Axillobifemoral bypass	50%–80%	5%–15%	5%–10%
Femorofemoral bypass	70%–80%	5%	0%–5%
Iliofemoral bypass	80%–85%	—	0%–5%

	3-Year Patency Primary (Secondary)	Complication Rate	Reported Mortality
Iliac angioplasty and stenting	76%	1%–5%	0%–2%
TASC A	>80% (>90%)	—	—
TASC B	78% (95%)	—	—
TASC C	73% (93%)	—	—
TASC D	80% (83%)	—	—

TASC, TransAtlantic Inter-Society Consensus.

methylxanthine derivative that acts as a rheologic agent. It is effective in only a fraction of patients and only modestly improves walking distance compared with placebo. Cilostazol is a phosphodiesterase III inhibitor and has been shown to be more effective than either pentoxifylline or placebo in relief of claudication. Symptom relief may not persist after drug discontinuation, however.

ENDOVASCULAR INTERVENTION

As balloon angioplasty and endovascular stenting technologies have evolved, endovascular intervention for revascularization is proving to be the predominant method of treatment of aortoiliac disease. These procedures are lower risk when compared with open surgery and have allowed expansion of traditional indications for intervention. Combined or hybrid interventions involving endovascular and open procedures performed either successively or simultaneously are becoming increasingly popular with vascular surgeons facile with endovascular techniques. The results of aortoiliac percutaneous interventions are difficult to compare with surgical outcomes because randomized studies have been infrequent and the technology for percutaneous treatments continues to evolve and improve. Although the original TASC consensus document recommended percutaneous therapy primarily for types A and B iliac lesions, recent studies report encouraging results with angioplasty and stenting in patients suffering from TASC types C and D iliac disease.

Preprocedural planning includes determination of renal function and review of the clinical and noninvasive evaluation to better direct the approach and sequence of intervention. Patients with baseline renal insufficiency should be pretreated with oral acetylcysteine. Gadolinium, an alternative to iodinated contrast agents, is less nephrotoxic and can result in acceptable angiographic imaging. Arterial access can be achieved via puncture of the brachial or contralateral femoral artery, although the ipsilateral common femoral artery is most commonly used and is preferred in patients with

proximal iliac stenosis or occlusion. Ultrasound guidance is invaluable in situations in which there is an absent or diminished femoral pulse. After accessing the artery with an 18-gauge puncture needle, a 0.035-inch guidewire is passed into the vessel and used to direct a 5-F sheath and a multisidehole catheter (pigtail or OmniFlush [Angiodynamics, Queensbury, NY]) into the aorta for the initial diagnostic angiogram. With the catheter positioned in the upper abdominal aorta between the first and second lumbar vertebrae, digital subtraction angiography is performed to visualize the renal arteries and the aorta. The catheter is then retracted to the level of the aortic bifurcation, where imaging of the common, internal, and external iliac arteries is performed, potentially using left and right anterior oblique views to prevent overlap between the internal and external iliac vessels. If the degree of stenosis or the physiologic significance of a stenosis cannot be determined by standard imaging techniques, then additional adjuncts can be used, including intravascular ultrasound (IVUS) or pullback pressures across the stenotic lesions, with or without a vasodilator such as 30 mg of papaverine. A pressure gradient of 10 to 15 mm Hg indicates a stenosis diameter greater than 50%.

Iliac Angioplasty

After imaging, a hydrophilic angled guidewire is used to navigate across the lesion. An angled glide or equivalent catheter can supply support and directionality for the wire. After the lesion is crossed, options for treatment include primary stenting versus angioplasty and selective stenting. With a selective stenting approach, a stent is considered after angioplasty when there is a residual stenosis of more than 30%, a persistent pressure gradient across the lesion, or a flow-limiting dissection. Although the optimal approach has not been clarified, a randomized trial from the Netherlands suggested that the outcome of angioplasty with selective stenting was equivalent to that of perfunctory stenting. Commonly used stent diameters in the common and external iliac arteries range from 6 to 10 mm and can be estimated either using a calibrated catheter or inferred from the balloon used to predilatate the lesion. Self-expanding nitinol stents are generally used, especially across tortuous vessels. Conversely, balloon-expandable stents can be useful in heavily calcified lesions or when lesions are encountered at the origins of the common iliac arteries.

Bilateral common iliac artery lesions adjacent to the aortic bifurcation should be treated with a kissing-balloon technique in which balloon angioplasty of both common iliac arteries is performed simultaneously through bilateral femoral access. As the ipsilateral lesion is treated, the contralateral iliac artery is protected by a simultaneously inflated balloon. In a similar fashion, if stenting is required, a kissing-stent technique is used. Patency rates for lesions involving the common iliac arteries range from 76% to 92% at 3 years.

Iliac occlusions are more complex and challenging to treat via endovascular means (TASC-C and -D lesions). These lesions, however, are found in a significant proportion of symptomatic patients with aortoiliac occlusive disease. Recanalization of these lesions can be accomplished via either luminal or subintimal passage of a hydrophilic wire using an antegrade, retrograde, or brachial approach (Fig. 1). Stenting is relatively routine after recanalization of chronic total occlusions (Fig. 2). The use of catheter-directed thrombolytic therapy can also play an important role in treating iliac occlusions. Thrombolysis may dissolve thrombus superimposed on atherosclerotic stenoses and improve early success and 1-year patency rates when used before or in conjunction with percutaneous transluminal angioplasty (PTA). Thrombolysis should be considered in patients suspected of having subacute in situ thrombosis as the underlying cause of their symptoms. In some circumstances, disease involving the external iliac vessels extends across the inguinal ligament and into the common femoral arteries. Angioplasty and

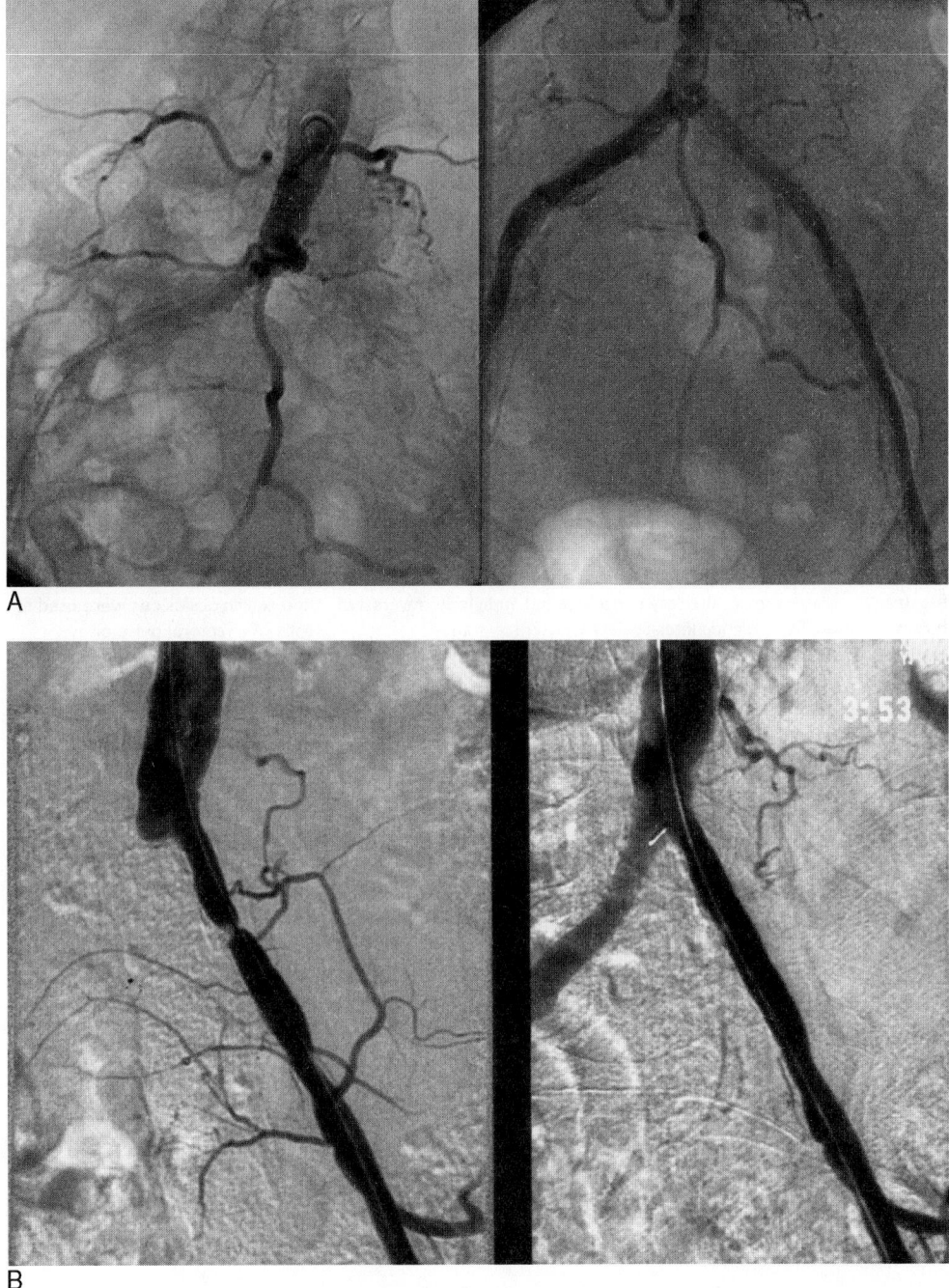

Figure I   Complete occlusions of the common and external iliac arteries (TransAtlantic Inter-Society Consensus grade-D lesions) are increasingly being treated by endovascular techniques. **(A)** Stenting is commonly employed after recanalization and balloon angioplasty of total occlusions. **(B)** Isolated stenoses (left common iliac artery) may be treated by angioplasty alone if minimal residual stenosis or dissection remains.

stenting across the inguinal ligament is not advised because movement with hip flexion can result in stent fracture and occlusion. In this circumstance, a combination of common femoral endarterectomy under local anesthesia followed by angioplasty and stenting of the more proximal iliac disease has been successfully employed.

Early technical success for endovascular interventions for AIOD, whether treatment is angioplasty or stent, is defined as a less than 30% residual stenosis and a systolic pressure gradient less than 10 mm Hg across the treated artery. Successful results have recently demonstrated in a number of series of patients with TASC-C and -D lesions, with reported 3-year primary and secondary patencies and limb salvage rates of 76%, 90%, and 97%, respectively. Although long-term outcomes associated with endovascular

repair may be somewhat diminished relative to standard bypass, the morbidity associated with the endovascular approach is markedly less. This has led some authors to conclude that the initial approach to all aortoiliac disease should be endovascular, with open surgical repair reserved for those patients in whom an endovascular approach has not been successful.

Infrarenal Aortic Stenosis

Good patency rates can be achieved with angioplasty and stenting of focal lesions involving the infrarenal aorta. Technical success has been reported to be as high as 94%, and 5-year patency rates

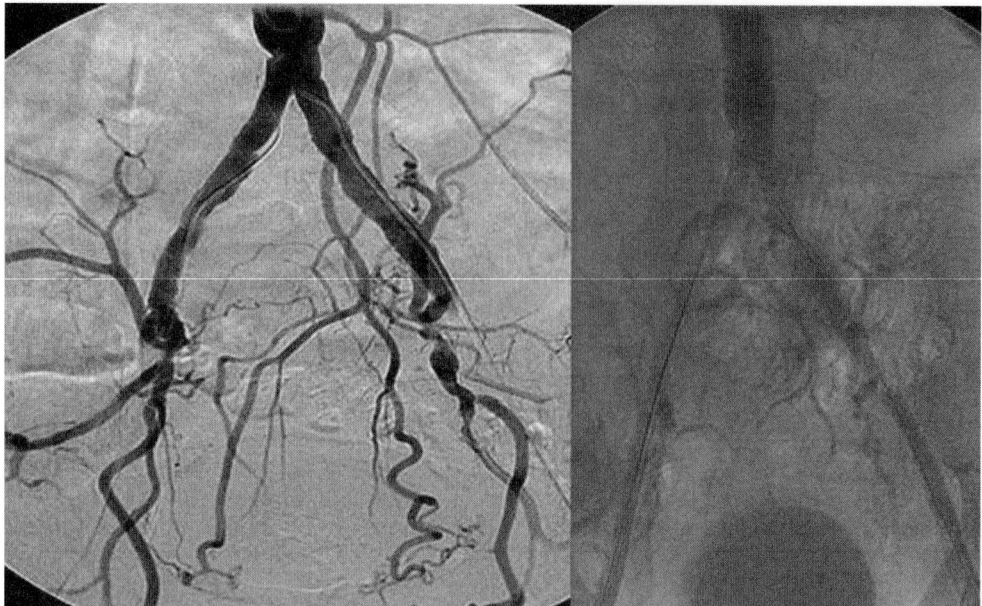

Figure 2 Bilateral femoral artery punctures and antegrade traversal of external iliac occlusions were used to recanalize these TransAtlantic Inter-Society Consensus grade-D lesions. Absence of a femoral pulse or Doppler signal sometimes mandates a brachial puncture and antegrade approach to recanalization of iliac lesions.

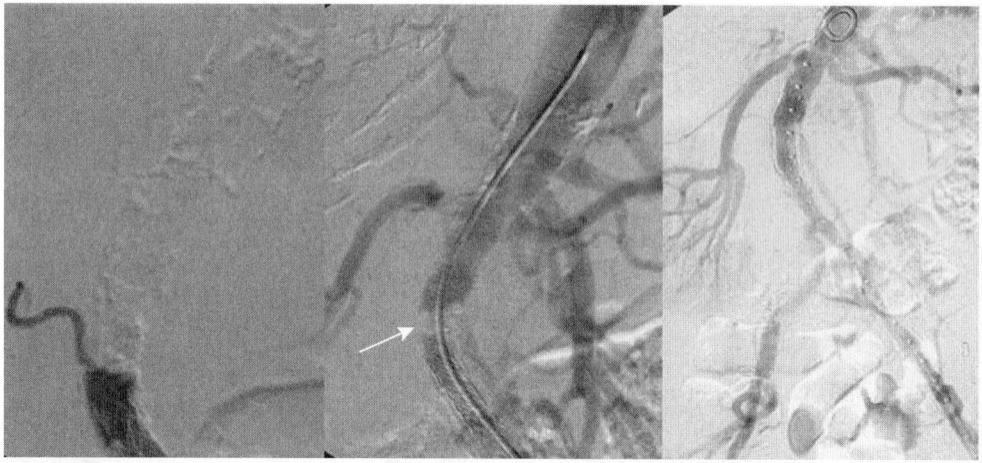

Figure 3 Self-expanding nitinol stents can be used for stenoses in the infrarenal aorta, although circumferentially calcified lesions *(arrow)* may necessitate balloon-expandable stainless steel stents.

approach 70%. Thrombolysis has also been used in patients with chronic aortic occlusion before PTA and stent placement. This approach may limit the risk of retrograde renal embolization with PTA. Techniques used for the treatment of aortic and iliac lesions are similar except that primary stenting is generally indicated and may decrease the rate of restenosis and the incidence of distal embolization. Large, self-expanding nitinol stents are available and can be successfully used in the infrarenal aorta (Fig. 3). Concentric calcified lesions, however, may require the use of balloon-expandable stainless steel stents, which produce greater radial force. A large Palmaz stent (Cordis, Miami Lakes, FL) can be mounted on an angioplasty balloon (diameter required usually ranges from 12 to 18 mm), which is inflated after positioning. If an aorta is thought to be at high risk for rupture during PTA, as might be the case with concentric calcified lesions in a small aorta, covered stents can be used. However, the effectiveness of covered stents in preventing hemorrhage in this situation has not been definitively proven.

Complications of Aortoiliac Angioplasty and Stenting

Access-site complications (at the site of the groin or arm puncture) occur in approximately 1% to 2% of patients and correlate with the size of the sheath used for intervention and the use of anticoagulation. Complications include bleeding, pseudoaneurysm formation, arteriovenous fistula, or thrombosis. The use of closure devices has not decreased the incidence of these complications; however, their use can decrease the time to ambulation following the procedure. Major systemic complications or death occur in approximately 1% of patients and are usually secondary to postprocedure coronary events or contrast-induced nephropathy. Complications at the site of angioplasty or in the distal vasculature include dissection, rupture, pseudoaneurysm formation, thrombosis, infection, or retrograde aortic dissection. Intimal hyperplasia following stent placement also occurs in more than 20% of patients within 2 years of intervention. Although the effects of intimal hyperplasia are less significant in the iliac circulation because of the large caliber of these vessels, routine surveillance duplex ultrasound provides early noninvasive recognition of this problem and allows prompt secondary intervention, which helps to maintain patency.

SURGICAL THERAPY

Surgical treatment of AIOD, although infrequently employed, is well established and provides excellent long-term outcomes. Aortobifemoral bypass is considered to be the definitive and most durable treatment option but is associated with a higher incidence of perioperative cardiovascular morbidity and mortality than the other available alternatives. Iliofemoral bypass is another alternative for disease isolated to the external iliac vessels. Extra-anatomic bypasses, including femorofemoral bypass or axillofemoral bypass, are less morbid procedures but not as durable as in-line reconstructions. Although percutaneous interventions are becoming the mainstay of therapy for most patients with AIOD, open reconstruction may be considered the favored primary approach in patients with flush aortic occlusion at the level of the renal arteries, individuals with diffusely small and diseased iliac arteries, or individuals with severe aortoiliac disease and heavy calcification involving the aortic bifurcation and iliac vessels.

Preoperative workup for surgical procedures includes a careful evaluation for coexisting cardiac, pulmonary, and renal disease. Under most circumstances, treatment of significant myocardial insufficiency takes precedence over limb revascularization. However, in the setting of acute limb-threatening ischemia, less morbid interventions such as the extra-anatomic bypasses may be undertaken without coronary revascularization. Clinical indications for surgical intervention are well established and are limited primarily to lifestyle-limiting claudication and limb-threatening ischemia.

Aortobifemoral Bypass

The reported 5-year patency rates for an aortobifemoral bypass are excellent at 85% to 90%, and the 10-year patency rates are 70% to 75%. Operative mortality for aortoiliac reconstruction ranges from 1.6% to 3.3%, with an aggregated systemic morbidity of 8.3%. Frequently, morbidity and mortality are related to coronary artery disease, which is clinically present in as many as 50% of these patients. The aortobifemoral bypass remains the gold standard with which all other interventions for AIOD, including angioplasty, are compared.

Femoral artery exposure through bilateral groin dissection is usually performed first to lessen the time that the peritoneal cavity is open. The transabdominal approach is used for the majority of patients, with the retroperitoneal approach reserved for patients who have had prior abdominal procedures or who have significant pulmonary disease. Aortic exposure is performed just below the origin of the renal arteries; it is limited to the segment of aorta below the renal arteries but above the inferior mesenteric artery. Tunneling to the groins is then bluntly performed along the anterior surface of the iliac arteries and posterior to the ureters. A knitted Dacron prosthetic graft, often collagen coated, is most frequently used for the bypass. Controversy remains regarding the optimal configuration of the proximal aortic anastomosis (end-to-end versus end-to-side). Proponents of the end-to-end anastomosis (Fig. 4) maintain that this approach results in superior hemodynamics and thus improved patency; excludes the distal aorta, thus preventing embolization or aneurysm formation; is less likely to become kinked or cause an aortoduodenal fistulae because of its lower profile; allows easier thrombectomy in the

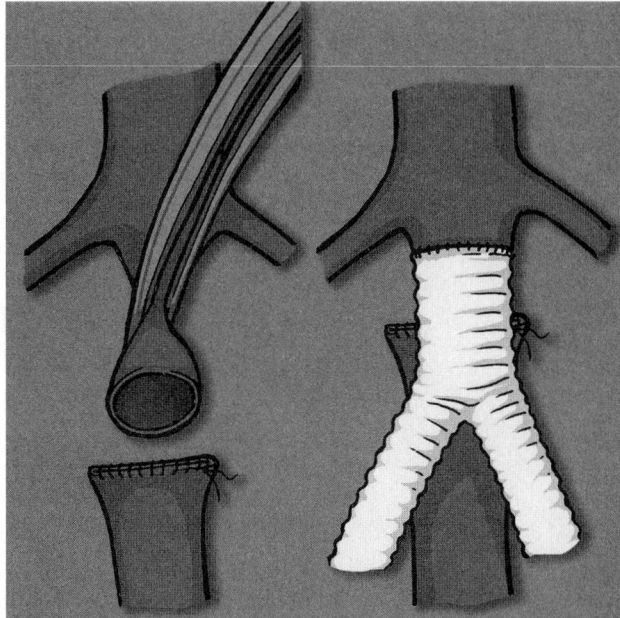

Figure 4   An end-to-end aortic anastomosis for aortobifemoral reconstruction is preferable in patients with coexisting aneurismal disease or complete occlusion extending to the renal arteries.

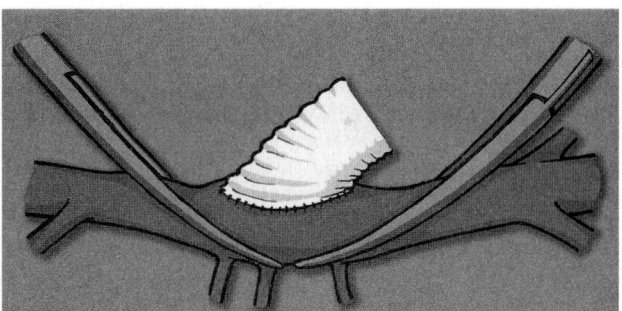

Figure 5   The end-to-side technique has the advantage of preserving inferior mesenteric and hypogastric flow while requiring less dissection.

case of graft occlusion; and avoids competition of flow between the graft and the native aorta. Those who favor an end-to-side anastomosis (Fig. 5) argue that it requires less dissection, can be more rapidly performed, provides a larger anastomosis, and preserves flow to the distal aortic branches (e.g., the hypogastric artery, inferior mesenteric, and accessory renal arteries), thereby reducing the potential of impotence, colon ischemia, and paraplegia. Moreover, aortic flow returns to baseline if the graft occludes or must be removed secondary to infection. Although there are few data to support one technique over the other and ultimately both approaches are effective, there are circumstances in which one technique is preferable. An end-to-end technique is preferred in patients with coexisting aneurysmal disease or a complete aortic occlusion extending to the renal arteries. Alternatively, patients in whom maintenance of flow to the hypogastric or mesenteric arteries (or both) is essential should be treated with an end-to-side technique. The distal anastomosis can be performed in an end-to-side fashion to the external iliac vessels or the femoral

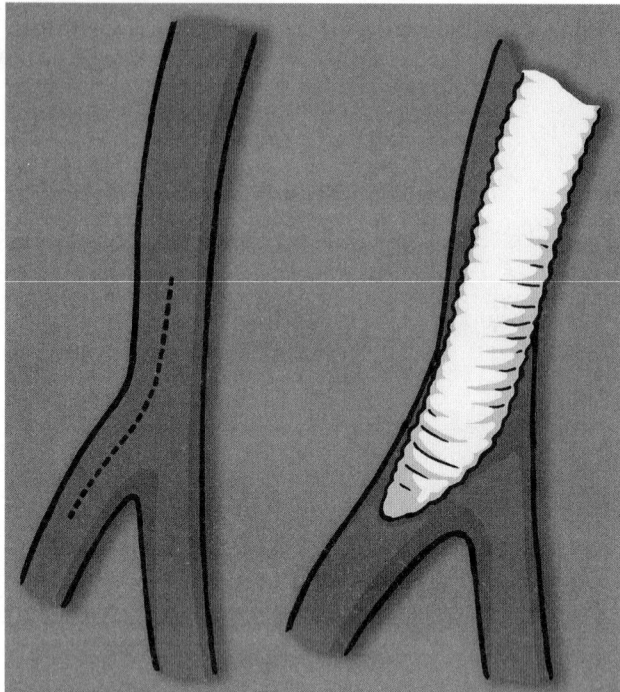

Figure 6 The femoral anastomosis should be carried onto the profunda femoris, thus preventing graft loss should progression of disease result in occlusion of the common femoral artery.

arteries (depending on the distal extent of disease). The femoral anastomoses should be made into the origin of the profunda femoris artery, which prevents graft occlusion from subsequent development of common femoral artery disease (Fig. 6). Aortobiliac bypass (with distal anastomoses to the iliac arteries) offers certain advantages in that it avoids all of the complications associated with grafting through a groin incision (lymph leak, a higher risk of infection, and anastomotic aneurysm). However, the later development of disease in the distal external iliac or common femoral vessels can lead to failure of this bypass.

Closure of the retroperitoneum and posterior parietal peritoneum to separate the graft and suture lines from abdominal contents is then performed and minimizes the occurrence of an aortoduodenal fistula or infectious complications.

Aortoiliac Endarterectomy

Aortoiliac endarterectomy has been used in patients with occlusive disease localized to the distal aorta and proximal common iliac arteries. A primary advantage of this procedure is that it avoids the use of a prosthetic graft, with its inherent risks, and therefore provides particular benefit for those at high risk for infection. The procedure is usually performed through a transperitoneal approach and involves an extensive endarterectomy through the distal aorta and iliac arteries, with or without the use of a patch for arteriotomy closure. This procedure is mentioned primarily for historical reasons because it carries a complication rate similar to that of an aortobifemoral bypass without equivalent patency rates. Furthermore, the sophistication of current techniques for angioplasty and stenting allows lesions comparable to those that were previously treated with aortic endarterectomy to now be treated by an endovascular approach.

Iliofemoral Bypass

Unilateral iliofemoral bypass is a therapeutic option for the patient with iliac occlusive disease isolated to the external iliac artery. A retroperitoneal approach through an obliquely oriented "transplant" incision in the lower quadrant allows exposure of the distal common iliac artery. A vertical groin incision is used to dissect out the common, superficial, and profunda femoral arteries. After systemic heparinization, a 6- to 8-mm Dacron graft is sewn to the distal common iliac artery in an end-to-side fashion. The graft is tunneled under the inguinal ligament to the groin, and the distal anastomosis is sewn to the proximal profunda femoris artery. Five-year patency of unilateral iliofemoral bypass is at least equivalent and perhaps superior to that of femorofemoral bypass, generally exceeding 80%. However, this procedure is uncommonly used because only a small proportion of patients have unilateral iliac disease that spares the common iliac artery.

Extra-Anatomic Bypass

Extra-anatomic bypass grafting for aortoiliac occlusive disease is a reasonable alternative for patients in whom endovascular techniques are not appropriate and a traditional in-line bypass is contraindicated. This includes patients with significant comorbidities that preclude a major arterial reconstruction or those with relative contraindications to laparotomy (e.g., multiple previous procedures or an ostomy). Removal of an infected intra-abdominal bypass is an additional indication for an extra-anatomic reconstruction. The most frequently used of these reconstructions are the axillofemoral and the femorofemoral bypasses. Less commonly used techniques include bypass from the axillary to popliteal arteries or an iliofemoral bypass through the obturator foramen.

Axillofemoral Bypass

The axillofemoral bypass passes in a subcutaneous plane between the axillary artery just below the clavicle and the femoral artery in the groin. Revascularization of the contralateral groin can be achieved with a concomitant femorofemoral bypass. This procedure results in minimal systemic stress and can even be performed under local anesthesia with sedation. The long-term patency of this bypass is related to several factors, but the status of the outflow vessels appears to be the most significant of these. If the superficial femoral artery is occluded, the patency of this bypass decreases significantly. In evaluating patients for axillofemoral bypass, the blood pressure in both arms should be determined to rule out disease in the ipsilateral "donor" subclavian artery (subclavian disease is more frequent on the left). Graft patencies up to 80% at 5 years are achievable if there is good inflow and outflow for the bypass; however, patencies can be as low as 50% to 60% at 5 years if the outflow is poor. The perioperative mortality is usually less than 5% in high-risk populations. The surgical technique includes exposure of the first portion of the axillary artery through an infraclavicular incision placed two fingerbreadths below the middle third of the clavicle. The pectoralis major muscle is retracted, and the pectoralis minor is reflected laterally. The axillary artery medial to the pectoralis minor is exposed and manipulated carefully because it is thin walled and can be easily injured. A 6- or 8-mm externally supported polytetrafluoroethylene (PTFE) graft is the conduit of choice, and it is routed through a subcutaneous tunnel developed along the midaxillary line. A counterincision in the lateral abdominal wall may occasionally be required.

The distal anastomosis is constructed in an end-to-side fashion to the common femoral artery, incorporating the origin of the profunda femoris artery. The proximal anastomosis of the femorofemoral crossover graft, if performed in conjunction with this procedure, is made to the hood of the axillofemoral bypass just proximal to the distal anastomosis.

Femorofemoral Bypass

The traditional indication for a femorofemoral bypass, which is performed through bilateral groin incisions, is unilateral iliac artery occlusive disease. Indications can range from claudication to limb-threatening ischemia. A second and now relatively common reason to perform a femorofemoral bypass is as an accompaniment of an aortouni-iliac endograft performed for repair of an abdominal aortic aneurysm. Similar to the axillofemoral bypass, femorofemoral bypasses have a higher patency rate (up to 80% at 5 years) when associated with robust distal runoff. It is imperative to ensure that there is normal inflow from the donor iliac artery, which should be evaluated preoperatively by duplex ultrasonography, MRA, or contrast angiography if necessary. Femoral exposure is preferentially performed via a longitudinal incision to better expose the profunda femoris artery, although transverse incisions can be used as well. We use externally supported PTFE grafts routed in a C configuration through a bluntly created suprapubic subcutaneous tunnel developed anterior to the rectus muscles. The proximal anastomosis is placed on the medial aspect of the common femoral artery, and the graft is allowed to take a gentle C-shaped course toward the recipient femoral artery.

Complications

Complications in patients undergoing reconstruction of the aorta or iliac vessels are similar to those for all major vascular reconstructions. Many of these patients have coexisting myocardial disease, and cardiac complications can be diminished by performing a thorough preoperative evaluation with the use of cardiac intervention preoperatively, when appropriate. The preoperative use of cardioprotective drugs such as beta-blockers has been shown to be beneficial. Renal dysfunction can complicate up to 10% of aortic reconstructions, particularly intra-abdominal procedures, and can be minimized by hydration, avoidance of hypotension, and minimization of aortic cross-clamp time. Colonic ischemia can occur with aortoiliac reconstructions, especially with disruption of pelvic collaterals from the hypogastric artery or interruption of or embolization through the inferior mesenteric artery. Prompt evaluation with flexible sigmoidoscopy in patients who develop early postoperative diarrhea or acidosis or sepsis can allow early therapy that ranges from treatment with antibiotics and optimization of cardiac output to colectomy. If colectomy becomes necessary, mortality is as high as 50%. Graft-related complications include infection, thrombosis, and anastomotic pseudoaneurysm formation. Wound complications include infection, hematoma, and lymphatic leak. These can be minimized with adequate hemostasis, gentle handling of tissue, and ligation of all lymphatics before a layered closure. There is currently no evidence that continuing antibiotic therapy beyond the preoperative prophylactic dose prevents infectious complications. Moreover, such complications are much more frequent in patients afflicted with a hematoma or lymphatic leak.

LAPAROSCOPIC AORTOILIAC SURGERY

Although laparoscopic aortoiliac surgery offers a minimally invasive alternative to open repair for patients with AIOD with advances in catheter-based techniques, this procedure is rarely performed. A number of centers have championed this technique. In the operating room, patients are placed in the supine position with the left side slightly elevated and a 10-mm trocar is introduced at the umbilicus, which serves as a port for a viewing laparoscope. Three additional trocars are inserted in the midline: one halfway between the symphysis pubis and the umbilicus and the other two evenly distributed between the umbilicus and the xiphoid process. When an aortobifemoral bypass is performed, a Dacron bifurcated graft is inserted through the left lower port, and each limb is tunneled using a laparoscopic clamp inserted from separate femoral incisions. Simple mobilization of the left and sigmoid colon is usually sufficient to provide adequate exposure of the aorta and both common iliac arteries. There are data to suggest that a laparoscopic approach is less invasive than conventional open aortic surgery and results in shorter hospital stays and recovery time and fewer perioperative complications. However, these procedures are time consuming and require significant expertise. Despite the minimally invasive nature of this procedure, its indications remain to be defined in an era when angioplasty and stenting for iliac occlusive disease are applicable in the vast majority of circumstances.

CONCLUSION

Treatment for AOID has undergone a paradigm shift over the past several years with the proliferation of endovascular technology. As reflected by the diminishing number of open aortoiliac reconstructions currently performed, it is clear that percutaneous interventions are replacing surgical alternatives because they offer near equivalent outcomes with less morbidity and mortality. Nevertheless, certain patients with complex disease still benefit from surgical reconstruction. An array of surgical alternatives, ranging from aortobifemoral bypass to a variety of extra-anatomic bypasses, provides a durable option for these patients.

SUGGESTED READINGS

Dion YM, Griselli F, Douville Y, and others: Early and mid-term results of totally laparoscopic surgery for aortoiliac disease: lessons learned, *Surg Laparosc Endosc Percutan Tech* 14:328, 2004.

Klein WM, van der Graaf Y, Seegers J, and others: Dutch iliac stent trial: long-term results in patients randomized for primary or selective stent placement, *Radiology* 238:734, 2006.

Leville CD, Kashyap VS, Clair DG, and others: Endovascular management of iliac artery occlusions: extending treatment to TransAtlantic Inter-Society Consensus class C and D patients, *J Vasc Surg* 43:32, 2006.

Management of peripheral arterial disease (PAD). TransAtlantic Inter Society Consensus (TASC), *J Vasc Surg* 31: (suppl): 1, 2000.

FEMOROPOPLITEAL OCCLUSIVE DISEASE

David Rosenthal, MD

Atherosclerosis is the most common cause of chronic arterial occlusive disease involving the femoral artery and its branches.

Symptoms of ischemia develop because of a reduction of blood flow in the lower limb during exercise or, in extreme cases, at rest. Depending on the severity of femoropopliteal occlusive disease, various clinical conditions may occur, including (1) asymptomatic occlusive disease; (2) intermittent claudication; and (3) critical limb ischemia, manifested as rest pain, ulceration, and gangrene.

Intermittent claudication is a common symptom of lower extremity arterial occlusive disease. The word *claudication* is derived from *claudicadio*, meaning "to limp." It is believed to have originated when physicians studying arterial pressure ligated the femoral arteries of horses and, after measuring pressures, observed them limping before stopping intermittently as they ran in the fields. The term *intermittent claudication* has thus come to mean leg pain sufficient to cause a patient to stop, which is induced by exercise, relieved by rest, and caused by arterial occlusive disease. Epidemiologic studies indicate that 5% of men and 2.5% of women 60 years and older have symptoms of intermittent claudication. In the natural history of intermittent claudication, it is generally benign and at 10-year follow-up, 70% of patients have symptoms that remain unchanged, 20% have progressive symptoms, and only 10% require amputation.

DIAGNOSIS

A careful history and pulse examination in the patient with suspected lower extremity ischemia are important. The strength of the pulse as assessed by an experienced practitioner is a valuable indicator of the arterial circulation. Pulses should be graded from 0 to 4+. A 0 pulse cannot be felt, a 1+ pulse is present but diminished, 2+ and 3+ pulses are normal intensity, and a 4+ pulse is abnormally strong and may indicate an aneurysm or aortic insufficiency. The value of a carefully performed physical examination cannot be overemphasized. It provides a basis for comparison if the disease progresses and is a simple means of assessing the arterial circulation in the lower extremities.

Physical examination is an indicator of what type of approach may be required to save a threatened foot. For example, if a patient has a gangrenous toe lesion and a palpable pedal pulse, local treatment without reconstructive arterial surgery should heal the foot. If, however, the patient has an ischemic foot lesion with no pedal or popliteal pulse, some form of infrapopliteal or small-vessel bypass is necessary to heal the foot.

NONINVASIVE VASCULAR LABORATORY TESTS

Pressure Measurements

Ankle-Brachial Index

Doppler ankle pressure measurement is a standard laboratory test that should be performed in patients suspected of having arterial occlusive disease. This test provides a baseline against which changes can be measured and allows a rough localization of the occlusive lesion and its severity. The ankle-brachial index (ABI) is determined by dividing the systolic blood pressure measured at the ankle with the brachial artery pressure and allows an objective method to grade ischemia. Asymptomatic arterial occlusive disease is defined by an ABI at rest ranging from 0.80 to 0.97. In patients with claudication the ABI at rest is often in the range of 0.50 to 0.60, whereas in patients with critical ischemia the ABI is less than 0.30. In calcified arteries, however, such as those seen in patients with diabetes mellitus, a falsely high reading may be observed because of the inability to compress the distal arteries. After an infrainguinal bypass, a change in the ABI of more than 0.15 is indicative of progressive occlusive disease or possible compromise of the bypass graft.

The ABI in concert with the flow-velocity waveforms at the femoral, popliteal, and pedal arteries defines the site and severity of the occlusive disease in virtually all patients. Flow-velocity waveforms are a valuable adjunct when evaluating diabetic patients with noncompressible arteries because a monophasic waveform at the pedal level, despite an elevated ABI, indicates more proximal occlusive disease.

Exercise Testing

To determine the severity of lower limb ischemia, Doppler treadmill exercise testing may be performed. Measurements of ankle blood pressure are made before and after standardized treadmill exercise. As the patient walks on the treadmill at a standardized incline, speed, and duration, ankle systolic pressure measurements are obtained. The patient walks until the onset of claudication, when ankle systolic pressure should fall precipitously, often to unrecordable levels. Ankle blood pressure may then take several minutes to return to baseline; an abnormal exercise response is defined by more than a 20% fall from the original baseline value, and more than 3 minutes are required for recovery to baseline.

Toe Systolic Pressure Index

Recording toe pressure is useful in patients with calcific diabetes mellitus occlusive disease. Toe pressures are obtained by strain gauge, photoplethysmograph, or Doppler. The toe pressure index is expressed as a ratio of pressure recorded from the arm to the toe systolic pressure. Normally the toe pressure index should be above 0.60. When the absolute pressure is lower than 30 mm Hg, it indicates severe ischemia, and a toe amputation or other foot operation will not heal without revascularization.

Ultrasonic Duplex Scan

Color-flow duplex ultrasonography is invaluable for examining peripheral arteries and autogenous infrainguinal bypass grafts. Estimations in the degree of stenosis depend on changes in peak systolic velocity that occur along the blood vessel or graft. Color-flow duplex ultrasonography is most useful in patients who have undergone saphenous vein lower extremity bypasses to detect areas of compromise caused by valvulotome injury, valve leaflet hypertrophy, or myointimal hyperplasia. Color-flow ultrasonography is also helpful in following the patient who has undergone balloon or stent angioplasty and endarterectomy.

Arteriography

Before surgery, high-quality arteriography is essential to delineate the inflow (aortoiliac), the deep femoral (profunda femoris) artery, and the runoff (popliteal, "trifurcation," and distal arteries). Oblique views may be required to completely visualize the origin and proximal portion of the deep and superficial femoral arteries. A detailed radiologic examination of the pedal arch is essential when the distal anastomosis will be placed at the infrapopliteal location. If a contraindication for contrast administration is present (e.g., renal impairment), carbon dioxide arteriography or gadolinium-enhanced magnetic resonance arteriography (MRA) is a useful alternative. Contrast arteriography using digital subtraction techniques, from the infrarenal aorta to the pedal arteries, however, remains the gold standard diagnostic study.

THERAPY

The presence of femoropopliteal occlusive disease is a "marker" for systemic atherosclerosis. Therefore therapy for femoropopliteal occlusive disease is directed toward relieving symptoms, which must be balanced against the potential risk of cardiovascular complications such as stroke, myocardial infarction, and death. Before an invasive treatment modality is initiated, a complete assessment of risk factors versus improvement in lifestyle or potential for limb salvage must be made. Many patients with intermittent claudication do not require intervention. Operations for disabling claudication must be individualized and should take into consideration bilaterality, the severity of the claudication, the patient's age and profession, and other risk factors. Conversely, when critical ischemia is present, the surgeon must reduce the systemic risk of mortality in this patient population (e.g., impaired cardiac function, renal or respiratory failure) before surgery.

Medical Treatment of Intermittent Claudication

Modifiable risk factors for peripheral arterial disease include smoking, diabetes mellitus, obesity, hyperlipidemia, hypertension, and homocysteine elevation. Risk factor modification, especially cessation of smoking, remains the mainstay of medical treatment of intermittent claudication. Smoking cessation is the most critical step in managing intermittent claudication. Patients who continue to smoke have a greater likelihood of myocardial infarction, stroke, limb loss, and death. Convincing data from controlled, randomized trials have demonstrated that a walking program in concert with risk factor modification is the most consistent and effective medical treatment for claudication. Unless patients have debilitating pulmonary or cardiac disease, within 3 months of instituting a walking program most patients report an increase in walking distance. Exercise programs include simple walking regimens, dynamic and static leg exercises, and a treadmill exercise program 3 to 4 times weekly.

Various vasoactive pharmacologic agents have been advocated for treating intermittent claudication. However, no pharmacologic agent alone has proved efficacious enough to gain widespread use. Several drugs have been promoted for the treatment of intermittent claudication, including rheologic agents (pentoxifylline, cilostazol) and vasodilators (nifedipine, nylidrin). Antiplatelet drugs (aspirin) are advocated to prevent death from stroke and myocardial infarction. The pharmacologic treatment of intermittent claudication has uncertain efficacy and best serves as adjunctive therapy.

Interventional Radiologic Procedures

In recent years the use of interventional radiologic procedures in treating arterial occlusive disease has increased significantly. The use of percutaneous transluminal angioplasty with or without stent placement, intraarterial thrombolytic therapy, and "endograft" placement has been reported with varying results.

Balloon angioplasty has been advocated for treating superficial femoral artery short-segment (< 3 cm) occlusive lesions. However, most symptomatic patients have long segmental occlusions and therefore are not candidates for angioplasty. Stenting improves the technical success in cases of residual pressure gradient, dissection, or elastic recoil after angioplasty; however, restenosis caused by intimal hyperplasia in the stented segment is common and the role of stents in the femoropopliteal vessels is uncertain. Thrombolytic therapy is best used for patients with sudden onset of symptoms from an acute thrombosis or embolic event. The advantage of thrombolytic therapy is its ability to uncover a short-segment critical stenosis, which would be amenable to balloon angioplasty. However, most patients have a protracted history of claudication and therefore are not candidates for thrombolytic and interventional radiologic procedures. Peripheral endovascular prosthetic stent-grafts have been developed, which offer the possibility of lining the superficial femoral artery after balloon angioplasty. Early primary patency reports are encouraging; however, long-term results are necessary to validate this new technology.

SURGICAL THERAPY

The indications for operation are disabling claudication, after a trial of medical therapy, and critical ischemia.

Choice of Surgical Procedure

Operations to improve distal circulation include profunda femoral artery reconstruction (i.e., profundaplasty) and infrainguinal bypass. In general, for patients with critical ischemia (i.e., tissue loss or gangrene), an infrainguinal bypass graft is necessary. For patients with mild rest pain or claudication, correction of a hemodynamically significant profunda stenosis alone, or in combination with an inflow procedure, is sufficient to relieve ischemic symptoms. Infrainguinal bypass should be considered when the superficial femoral or popliteal artery is occluded and the popliteal artery distal to the occlusion has luminal continuity with any of its three terminal branches. Infrainguinal bypass can be performed with either prosthetic material or autogenous vein. The bypass graft can be constructed in the following manner:

1. Reversed saphenous graft
2. In situ saphenous vein technique
3. Translocated in situ vein graft consisting of contralateral saphenous vein anastomosed to the inflow artery in a nonreversed manner
4. A composite sequential graft in which the proximal segment consists of a prosthetic graft (polytetrafluoroethylene [PTFE] or Dacron) anastomosed from the femoral artery to a patent popliteal segment (above or below knee) with a separate vein segment then anastomosed from this graft to a distal tibial or peroneal artery
5. A composite graft of prosthetic material anastomosed end to end to autogenous saphenous vein when vein length is inadequate

Bypasses for limb salvage to arteries beyond the popliteal artery are performed to the posterior tibial (74%), the anterior tibial (70%), or the peroneal (62%) arteries in order of preference to yield the best 5-year patency rates. A tibial artery generally is used only if its lumen is without obstruction onto the foot, although more recent reports indicate that these "do-or-die" grafts may remain patent for up to 3 years. The peroneal artery is used only if it is continuous with one or two terminal branches that anastomose with named arteries of the foot. Absence of a plantar arch and vascular calcification are *not* considered contraindications to distal vessel bypasses.

Choice of Graft Material

Autogenous vein grafts offer the best long-term patency rates for distal popliteal and tibial reconstructions. Therefore every effort must be made to use the saphenous vein in this setting. However, if the saphenous vein has been removed or is not suitable for use and a distal bypass is contemplated, other veins, such as the short saphenous, basilic, or cephalic vein, may be harvested as a substitute.

When performing an above-knee short-segment bypass, some surgeons prefer to use prosthetic material (e.g., Dacron, ePTFE, tanned human umbilical vein) to save the saphenous vein for potential distal reconstruction or coronary bypass in the future should the need arise. In general, above-the-knee prosthetic bypasses are performed for claudication, and a 5-year patency rate approaching 65% may be anticipated, regardless of the conduit used.

Surgical Technique

Surgical technique consists of exposing the inflow and outflow arteries, harvesting (reversed vein graft) or exposing (in situ vein graft) the long saphenous vein, and performing a tunneling maneuver for prosthetic vein grafts. In general, the proximal anastomosis is performed at the common femoral artery level; however, if the length of saphenous vein is limited, the proximal anastomosis may be performed to the profunda femoral or superficial femoral artery. If the superficial femoral artery is occluded, a short-segment endarterectomy offers an appropriate inflow vessel. The location of the distal anastomosis depends on preoperative arteriography; however, if preoperative arteriography fails to provide adequate visualization of the runoff vessels, an on-table arteriogram may select a suitable distal artery.

A vertical incision is used to expose the common femoral artery at the groin. Within the same incision, the saphenofemoral junction is dissected to divide the saphenous vein for proximal anastomosis. Care must be taken to preserve the lymphatic tissue between the saphenous vein and the common femoral artery. A medical approach is used to expose the popliteal (above or below the knee), peroneal, and posterior tibial arteries (Fig. 1). For exposure of the popliteal artery below the knee, division of the semitendinosus and gracilis tendons is necessary to expose the distal popliteal artery. The peroneal and posterior tibial arteries below the trifurcation are best

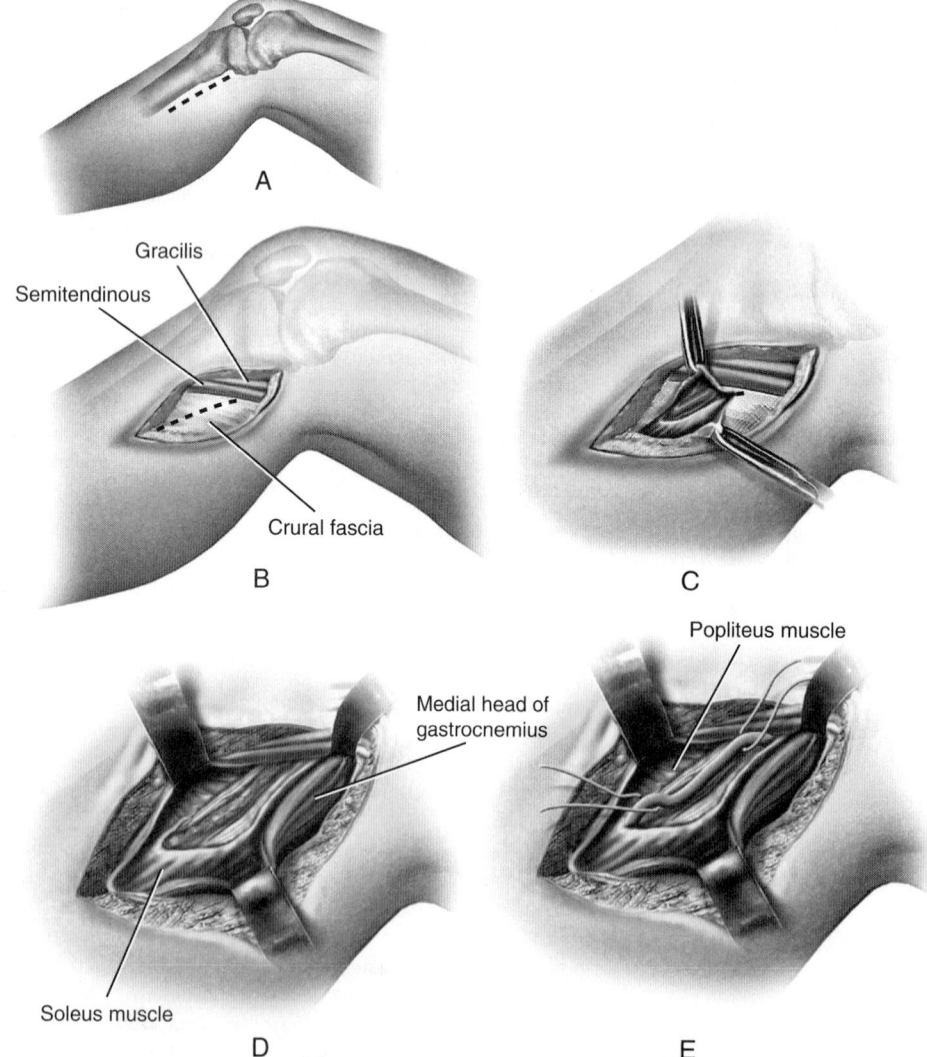

Figure 1 Medial exposure of distal popliteal. **A,** Position of limb, knee flexed, and line of skin incision. **B,** Exposure of crural fascia and line of skin incision. **C,** Fascia incised, exposing vascular bundle. **D,** Exposure of distal popliteal vessels and arcade of soleus muscle. **E,** Popliteal freed and mobilized. *From Haimovici H: Vascular surgery: principles and techniques,* ed 3, New York, 1992, McGraw-Hill.

Figure 2 Anterolateral exposure of the proximal anterior tibial artery. **A**, Line of skin incision. **B**, Exposure of neurovascular bundle.   *From Haimovici H: Vascular surgery: principles and techniques, ed 3, New York, 1992, McGraw-Hill.*

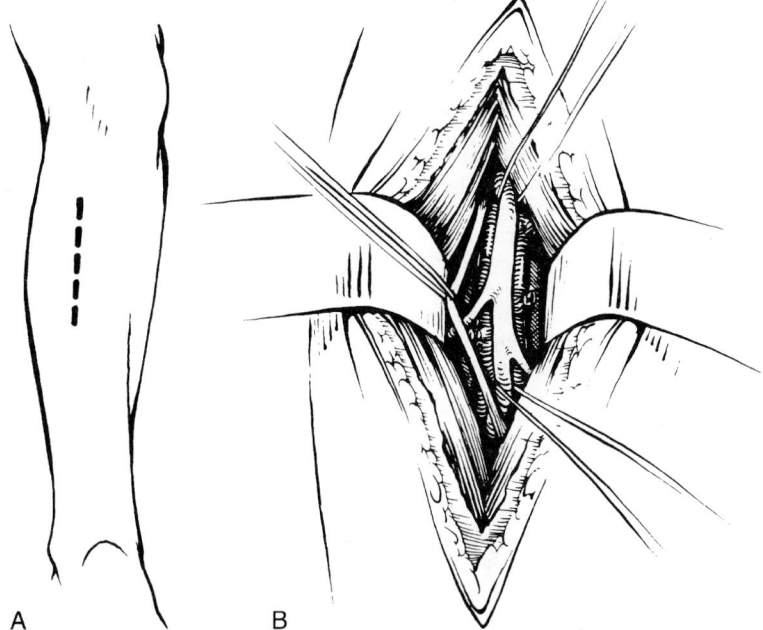

A   B

exposed by detaching the soleus muscle from the tibia. For the anterior tibial artery, a longitudinal skin incision two finger-breadths wide lateral to the tibial border between the anterior tibialis and extensor digitorum longus muscles allows exposure of the artery (Fig. 2). After the "target" vessel has been exposed, if a reverse vein graft is planned, the saphenous vein is harvested. The vein is reversed and distended with a saline, heparin (1000 IU/L), papaverine (50 mg/L) solution. The graft may lie in the subcutaneous tissue or be tunneled subsartorially in the thigh and through the normal popliteal space between the two heads of the gastrocnemius muscles to the distal target artery. For in situ vein grafts, a full-length exposure is preferred. After the proximal anastomosis the vein is arterialized and a valvulotomy is performed through the vein side branches with a Mills valvulotome or with a retrograde cutter-type valvulotome (i.e., LeMaitre, Hall). Recent reports detailing endoscopic saphenous vein harvest and endovascular side-branch occlusion techniques for in situ vein bypass are promising minimally invasive techniques. After completion of any infrainguinal bypass, a completion arteriogram or color-flow ultrasound interrogation should be performed to document patency of the bypass and distal arterial pathology or to identify residual fistulae after an in situ bypass.

Immediate Postoperative Care

Most early bypass graft occlusions occur within the first 24 hours after operation. Therefore careful pulse examination and Doppler ankle pressure measurements at regular intervals are mandatory to monitor patency of the bypass graft. If the bypass was performed in a patient with acute, severe ischemia, monitoring of the lower leg compartment pressures must be performed to prevent compartment syndromes. In patients for whom the bypass was performed with a marginal vein or to a compromised outflow vessel, postoperative heparin and dextran may improve patency, but bleeding complications can occur.

Operative Results

Many reports concerning the results of infrainguinal bypass grafts have accumulated. In general, prosthetic grafts fare less well than

Table 1: Classification of Types of Aortic Dissection

Location of the Tear		
Ascending	Arch	Descending
——Stanford A——		
		——Stanford B——Š——DeBakey I, extending——
——DeBakey II——		
		——DeBakey III——
		IIIa——
		IIIb extending to abdomen

saphenous vein grafts (Table 1). The site of distal anastomosis, the number and quality of runoff vessels, the size of the saphenous vein, and the presence/absence of risk factors (e.g., cigarette smoking, diabetes mellitus, chronic renal failure) all affect the outcome of the bypass graft. Table 1 is a meta-analysis summary of 5-year patency rates reported in the literature.

Antithrombotic Therapy

Perioperative heparin, low-molecular-weight dextran, warfarin sodium (Coumadin; Bristol-Myers Squibb, New York, NY), and antiplatelet drugs (ticlopidine, aspirin, dipyridamole) appear to be appropriate adjuncts in the high-risk patient with a small-caliber vein, poor runoff, or a prosthetic graft placed to the infrapopliteal arteries. Recent randomized trials conducted to ascertain the value of antithrombotic agents after infrainguinal bypass grafts have been reported, and the use of Coumadin in infrapopliteal vein grafts appears to enhance patency. In these patients perioperative intravenous heparin is recommended, followed by Coumadin; however, the surgeon must be prepared to follow these patients closely because wound complications (hematomas and seromas) are common.

Patient Follow-Up

Patients who have undergone infrainguinal bypass must undergo serial follow-up examination. After a prosthetic bypass grafting, physical examination and Doppler ankle pressure measurements to monitor graft patency are appropriate. However, if the ABI decreases by more than 0.2, arteriography is indicated to rule out the possibility of a failing graft. After a saphenous vein graft (in situ, transposed, or reversed), a surveillance program of duplex color-flow imaging is mandatory and should be performed 1 month after operation, every 6 months for the first year, and annually thereafter. Focal sites of increased flow velocity or a mean graft velocity decrease signify a vein graft stenosis that may be caused by neointimal hyperplasia, hyperplasia at a valve leaflet, or a residual arteriovenous fistula. Vein graft stenosis has an ominous prognosis, and arteriography is again warranted to correct the problem before graft failure occurs.

Suggested Readings

Bergqvist D, and others: Auditing surgical outcome: ten years with the Swedish Vascular Registry, *Eur J Vasc Surg* 164:suppl:23, 1998.

Dalman RL, Taylor LM: Basic data related to infrainguinal revascularization procedures, *Ann Vasc Surg* 4:309, 1990.

Hiatt WR: Current and future drug therapies for claudication, *Vasc Med* 2:257, 1997.

Hunink MGM et al: Patency results of percutaneous and surgical revascularization for femoropopliteal arterial disease, *Med Decis Making* 14:71, 1994.

Yao JST, Pearce WH, editors: *The ischemic extremity: advances in treatment* Norwalk, CT, 1994, Appleton and Lange.

Management of Tibioperoneal Arterial Occlusive Disease

Spence M. Taylor, MD, Dwight C. Kellicut, MD, Dane E. Smith, MD, and Jerry R. Youkey, MD

The management of tibioperoneal peripheral arterial disease (PAD) remains a significant problem in the modern landscape of vascular surgery. The ability to treat tibioperoneal PAD effectively requires an understanding of the disease process, appropriate patient selection, surgical technique, and outcome. The knowledge required to attain this understanding is not the result of an isolated event but rather a continuum of medical and surgical advances over time. Lower-extremity PAD has been present in humans since antiquity. The current understanding of tibioperoneal PAD has its lineage rooted in the early descriptions of lower-extremity gangrene nearly 180 years ago by Cooper and Curveilhier. In the early 1900s, Carrel pioneered the vascular anastomosis using his Nobel Prize–winning triangulation technique. Nearly 40 years later, Linton introduced the reverse saphenous vein graft for infrainguinal bypass, and in 1961, Palma described the use of vein grafts to the tibial vessels. This technique, however, was abandoned until the late 1970s and early 1980s, when in Albany Leather and Karmody reintroduced in situ saphenous vein bypass to the tibial vessels as an effective means of achieving limb salvage for patients with critical limb ischemia and occluded femoral and popliteal arteries. Simultaneously in Oregon, Porter and associates demonstrated similar technical success and effective limb salvage with tibial artery bypass using reverse saphenous vein. Advances in diagnostic imaging using duplex ultrasonography pioneered by Bandyk and others have produced postoperative surveillance and treatment protocols that have yielded successful long-term patency and successful limb salvage for patients with tibioperoneal PAD.

The management of tibioperoneal PAD is currently in a state of flux because vascular surgeons have developed an interest in catheter-based intervention. Although significant technologic advances have occurred that make tibial artery angioplasty feasible, tibial artery bypass with saphenous vein remains the gold standard for tibioperoneal PAD except in specifically selected cases. At our institution, we have managed and registered the results of nearly 2000 patients treated for PAD of the lower extremities since 1992. This chapter highlights some of the lessons learned over these years, examining five areas considered important to optimizing the successful treatment of patients with tibioperoneal PAD: (1) the general diagnostic approach to the patient with lower-extremity PAD, (2) the preoperative preparation, (3) important operative strategies, (4) the postoperative follow-up strategy, and (5) the management in desperate situations.

INITIAL APPROACH TO THE PATIENT WITH CHRONIC LOWER-EXTREMITY PERIPHERAL ARTERIAL DISEASE

General Considerations

The therapeutic options for treatment of lower-extremity PAD seem straightforward: medical treatment by risk-factor modification or restoration of circulation using either angioplasty or open bypass surgery. However, choosing the most appropriate therapy can be confusing and requires a thoughtful approach that begins by establishing the correct diagnosis and, when present, the anatomic distribution of the atherosclerotic disease. Multiple diagnostic modalities are available to help determine the cause of lower-extremity pain. These include duplex ultrasonography, computed tomography (CT) angiography, magnetic resonance imaging (MRI), and contrast angiography. However, before these expensive tests are performed, the experienced clinician usually can make the diagnosis of PAD, determine the general anatomic pattern of the disease, and devise a tentative treatment plan at the bedside.

Patients with lower-extremity PAD generally present with complaints of either intermittent ambulatory pain (claudication) or tissue ulceration/gangrene and rest pain (critical limb ischemia). It is important to realize that not all pain or ulceration of the lower extremities is vascular in origin. Leg pain can be divided into three general etiologic categories: vasculogenic claudication, arthritic pain, and neurogenic claudication. Patients who present with vasculogenic claudication experience discomfort in the muscles of the legs with walking or exercise that is relieved with rest. This discomfort is sometimes described as a burning fatigue and is consistent in onset every time the patient walks. Patients with vasculogenic claudication are typically older than age 50 and have a history of tobacco use, diabetes, or both. Sometimes the diagnosis can be complicated by concomitant symptoms of arthritis and neurogenic leg pain. Typically arthritic pain is associated with point tenderness on examination or pain with passive flexion of joints. Inflammation is often present. Most clinicians are able to distinguish vasculogenic claudication from arthritis at the bedside without difficulty. Patients with neurogenic leg pain can be more difficult to discern. Although nerve root compression from radiculopathy is usually distinctive, manifested by resting pain that radiates down the posterior leg, spinal cord compression from spinal stenosis is more difficult to differentiate from vascular disease. Such neurogenic symptoms often mimic aortoiliac occlusive disease, presenting with hip and thigh pain and muscle weakness. Symptoms occur after walking or standing and are not quickly relieved by rest. Relief is usually obtained only after changing position or by lumbar spine flexion. Lumbosacral MRI scan is often necessary to exclude neurospinal claudication. Lastly, diabetic peripheral polyneuropathy can often mimic ischemic rest pain. Neuropathic pain is frequently described as a burning pain involving the entire foot and ankle in a stocking distribution, whereas ischemic rest pain usually involves the forefoot and is positional in nature, improved in the dependent position. As well, it is important to remember that patients who present with leg discomfort may have multiple overlapping etiologies.

After the diagnosis of PAD is confirmed, a bedside assessment of the patient should be made (Table 1). From this assessment, it is usually possible to determine the anatomic extent of lower-extremity atherosclerotic disease (Fig. 1). The bedside evaluation of PAD requires knowledge of four clinical elements: two from the history and two from the physical examination. From the history, one must first define the presenting symptoms (claudication or critical limb ischemia). Second, one must ascertain the presence of comorbid risk factors (presence of diabetes,

history of tobacco use, or both). From the physical examination, one must determine the status of lower-extremity pulses. Subsequently, the ankle-brachial pressure index must be calculated. Patients with claudication and no evidence of critical limb ischemia typically have less severe anatomic atherosclerotic disease. Cigarette smokers typically have atherosclerotic disease that affects the lower-extremity vessels cephalad to the tibial arteries. Diabetics often have atherosclerotic involvement isolated to the tibial vessels. On physical examination, the femoral, popliteal, and pedal pulses should be palpated. It is important to remember that a Doppler-derived systolic blood pressure of 90 mm Hg at the ankle is usually necessary to palpate a pulse. Likewise, a systolic blood pressure of 50 mm Hg in nondiabetics and a systolic blood pressure of 90 mm Hg in diabetics are generally required to heal a foot ulcer. Therefore if a diabetic patient presents with a forefoot ulceration and a nonpalpable pedal pulse, it can be deduced (assuming the absence of calcified vessels) that the ankle pressure is less than 90 mm Hg and that an intervention to improve circulation will most likely be necessary to attain healing.

When considering PAD, involvement of the lower extremities can be divided into three anatomic levels: the aortoiliac (AIOD) level, the femoropopliteal level, and the tibioperoneal level. Determining the anatomic pattern of involvement is important. There are significant treatment and prognostic implications related to which level of disease is involved. Generally the severity of presenting symptoms increases, the technical outcomes worsen, and the

Table 1: The Bedside Assessment of Chronic Lower Extremity PAD

History		Physical Examination	
1. Presenting symptoms A. Claudication? B. CLI?	2. Medical comorbidity A. Cigarette smoking? B. Diabetes?	1. Pulse: qualitative assessment	2. ABI: quantitative interpretation
A. Claudication: pain that occurs with exercise and is relieved by rest in the muscle group one joint level below the arterial blockage	A. Cigarette smokers 1. AIOD and/or femoral popliteal distribution B. Diabetes	Qualitative assessment 1. Absent femoral pulses means significant AIOD 2. A palpable pedal pulse requires an ankle pressure ≈90 mm Hg	Quantitative interpretation 1. Normal = 1.07 ± 0.15 2. An ABI <0.92 suggests clinically significant PAD
1. AIOD, hip and thigh	1. Tibioperoneal distribution 2. Noncompressible vessels, when present, generally occurs in diabetic patients	3. An ankle pressure of 50 mm Hg is required to heal a foot ulcer in nondiabetics 4. An ankle pressure of 90 mm Hg is required to heal a foot ulcer in diabetics	3. An ABI > 1.22 suggests noncompressible vessels 4. Mild claudication may manifest with a drop in ABI with exercise only
2. SFA stenosis, calf	3. Diabetic patients with tibial vessel occlusion only, do not claudicate	**Caveat:** A foot ulcer in a diabetic with nonpalpable pedal pulses usually requires vascular intervention	
B. CLI, chronic ischemia (ankle pressure <50–70 mm Hg)	**Caveat:** A history of neither diabetes nor smoking suggests nonvascular etiology of pain		
1. Ischemic ulcers, moderate disease			
2. Rest pain (forefoot), severe multisegmental disease			
3. Gangrene, severe multilevel disease (not all gangrene is from CLI)			

ABI, Ankle-brachial pressure index; *AIOD*, aortoiliac occlusive disease; *CLI*, critical limb ischemia; *PAD*, peripheral arterial disease; *SFA*, superficial femoral artery.

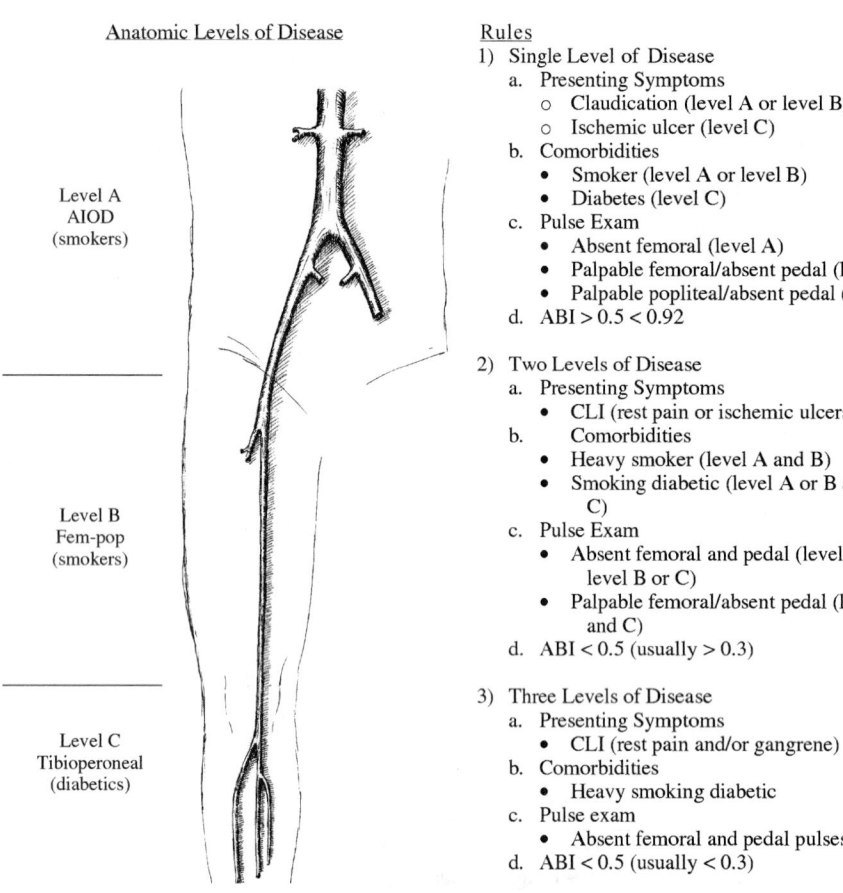

Anatomic Levels of Disease

Level A
AIOD
(smokers)

Level B
Fem-pop
(smokers)

Level C
Tibioperoneal
(diabetics)

Rules

Rules

1) Single Level of Disease
   a. Presenting Symptoms
      ○ Claudication (level A or level B)
      ○ Ischemic ulcer (level C)
   b. Comorbidities
      • Smoker (level A or level B)
      • Diabetes (level C)
   c. Pulse Exam
      • Absent femoral (level A)
      • Palpable femoral/absent pedal (level B)
      • Palpable popliteal/absent pedal (level C)
   d. ABI > 0.5 < 0.92

2) Two Levels of Disease
   a. Presenting Symptoms
      • CLI (rest pain or ischemic ulcers)
   b. Comorbidities
      • Heavy smoker (level A and B)
      • Smoking diabetic (level A or B and level C)
   c. Pulse Exam
      • Absent femoral and pedal (level A and level B or C)
      • Palpable femoral/absent pedal (level B and C)
   d. ABI < 0.5 (usually > 0.3)

3) Three Levels of Disease
   a. Presenting Symptoms
      • CLI (rest pain and/or gangrene)
   b. Comorbidities
      • Heavy smoking diabetic
   c. Pulse exam
      • Absent femoral and pedal pulses
   d. ABI < 0.5 (usually < 0.3)

Exceptions to the Rules

1) The Degree of Chronicity dictates symptom severity
   ○ Acute blockage = worse symptoms
   ○ Chronic = milder symptoms

2) In the presence of an SFA occlusion, a profunda stenosis may mimic two levels of infrainguinal disease (level B and C) despite normal tibials

Figure 1 The bedside diagnosis of lower extremity peripheral arterial disease on the basis of anatomic level. *ABI,* Ankle-brachial pressure index; *AIOD,* aortoiliac occlusive disease; *CLI,* critical limb ischemia; *Fem-pop,* femoral-popliteal artery; *SFA,* superficial femoral artery.

preferred method of intervention changes from endovascular to open surgery when the predominant anatomic level of disease changes from proximal (AIOD) to distal (tibial). Disease involving only one anatomic level typically presents with claudication of the muscle group one joint level below the arterial blockage. With one level of disease, ankle-brachial indices are typically less than 0.92 and greater than 0.5. On the other hand, critical limb ischemia usually involves two or three anatomic levels of disease and is associated with ankle-brachial indices less than 0.5. Figure 1 summarizes the history and physical findings associated with the specific anatomic levels and the number of levels involved by PAD. Using the history and physical examination, the surgeon should be able to make an immediate anatomic assessment of disease and then be able to determine the most likely treatment course required to address the specific symptoms.

Tibioperoneal Occlusive Disease

Patients with pure tibioperoneal PAD are usually diabetic and often do not claudicate. The circulation to the level of the geniculate vessels is usually normal. Therefore the calf muscles are often well perfused. Claudication, if it occurs, is usually confined to the muscles of the foot. Diabetics, because of the presence of diabetic polyneuropathy, often have no foot claudication symptoms. These patients most often present with nonhealing, ischemic, infected neuropathic ulcers. Is important to remember that although atherosclerosis is prevalent in the tibial vessels of diabetics, the foot

vessels and toe digital vessels are usually spared of disease. This anatomic pattern is amenable to successful pedal bypass, resulting in limb salvage in most cases. It is not uncommon to encounter diabetic smokers who present with lifestyle-limiting claudication and an anatomic pattern of disease involving the femoropopliteal and tibial vessels. With rare exception, tibial artery bypass should not be performed for claudication. These bypasses often fail to perfuse geniculate vessels that provide the circulation to the calf necessary to alleviate the symptoms of calf claudication, are technically demanding, and are generally associated with poorer long-term outcomes.

Preoperative Preparation

Strategy regarding the preoperative preparation of patients with critical limb ischemia should be directed by two concerns. First is to identify preoperative medical conditions that must be addressed before surgery. Second is to evaluate the symptomatic limb to plan optimal management. Medical assessment should address the treatment of acute illness and the management of chronic illness. Tibioperoneal PAD most commonly presents with limb-threatening foot infection and underlying chronic ischemia. Therefore the most important initial concern is to control any foot sepsis. Despite the presence of chronic ischemia, it is imperative to drain operatively all purulence and debride all nonviable tissue from the foot. Liberal use of toe amputation to enhance drainage of the foot is often necessary. These wounds obviously are left open. Broad-spectrum intravenous antibiotics capable of treating gram-positive cocci, gram-negative rods, and anaerobes should be administered. Revascularization to heal the open wounds should be performed only after all systemic sepsis and signs of local soft-tissue foot infection have been eradicated. Any other acute medical problems should be addressed before surgery.

A great deal of controversy exists regarding the cardiac evaluation of patients requiring tibial artery bypass for limb-threatening ischemia. Although there is little debate that acute cardiac symptoms at presentation should be addressed, it is unclear whether prophylactic evaluation for occult coronary artery disease decreases the perioperative morbidity. Clearly occult disease exists in the majority of these patients. In a recent review of 841 patients undergoing intervention at our institution, overall survival at 5 years was only 41.9%. The majority of deaths occurred because of complications of atherosclerotic cardiac disease. Although preoperative cardiac stress testing in these patients is often positive, the treatment options for the coronary artery disease detected are often limited. Unlike patients undergoing elective aortic surgery, these patients usually present with open foot wounds and limb-threatening ischemia, which increase the risk of infectious complications of coronary artery bypass surgery. Furthermore, any significant worsening of the critical foot ischemia during recovery from coronary artery bypass grafting will too often eliminate the possibility of limb salvage even with subsequently successful lower-extremity revascularization. Because of this, we have long adopted a policy of medical optimization of the asymptomatic or stable patient, assuming that significant coronary artery disease is probably present and then proceeding with lower-extremity revascularization without formal elective coronary risk assessment. Using this approach, we have achieved a perioperative mortality of less than 5% in more than 500 tibial artery bypass procedures performed.

Preoperative anatomic evaluation of the ischemic leg includes diagnostic arteriography and ultrasound-guided vein mapping of the saphenous vein. Judicious use of foot arteriography is mandatory and often necessary to determine the most appropriate target vessel for bypass. Other emergency diagnostic modalities include CT angiography. Patients with chronic renal insufficiency and thus a contraindication for nephrotoxic contrast agents can be studied using CO_2 angiography or MR angiography of the tibial vessels. Alternatively, duplex ultrasound mapping of tibial runoff and intraoperative on-table arteriography with small amounts of contrast injected directly into targeted runoff vessels has been successfully employed in some cases of critical ischemia from tibial occlusive disease associated with chronic renal insufficiency.

OPERATIVE STRATEGIES

Tibial artery bypass procedures are generally performed using epidural anesthesia. Arterial line placement is mandatory, and prophylactic antibiotics are routinely administered. Both lower extremities are prepped from the umbilicus to the toes. If vein mapping suggests that the saphenous veins are inadequate, then at least one arm with adequate cephalic vein identified by preoperative vein mapping is prepared as well. Tibial artery bypasses are performed using autogenous vein as the bypass conduit. Optimally a vein with a diameter of at least 3 mm after gentle dilatation with chilled, heparinized saline is preferred. The vein of choice is the ipsilateral greater saphenous vein. If this vein is inadequate, the contralateral greater saphenous vein is used. If this conduit is inadequate, arm vein or lesser saphenous vein is used. When using this approach, it is extremely unusual not to find enough autogenous conduit for bypass, even though it sometimes requires spliced segments. In the rare case in which no vein is available, a composite conduit using polytetrafluoroethylene (PTFE) and autogenous vein is constructed. The vein conduit can be left in the in situ configuration with valve lysis or can be used as a reversed vein graft. The vast majority of bypasses performed at our institution use a reversed vein conduit configuration. We have been impressed that the number of patients presenting with an intact greater saphenous vein amenable to an in situ technique is increasingly uncommon. It has long been our philosophy that tibial artery bypass using reverse vein can be used for all patients, a claim that cannot be made for the in situ technique. Although video-assisted endo-vein harvest techniques have been advocated as ways to reduce vein harvest incision morbidity, we have abandoned this technique because of an increased rate of intrinsic vein graft stenoses observed in intermediate follow-up. We currently use skip incisions to minimize the vein harvest wound length when possible.

The inflow and outflow vessels chosen for bypass are determined by the arteriogram. It has been repeatedly shown that the "weak link" of tibial artery bypass is the quality of the venous conduit. Philosophically, we therefore strive to perform the shortest bypass possible without compromising our goal of foot perfusion. Although the common femoral artery is considered to be the classic inflow source for most bypasses, we routinely bypass from the lowest open inflow vessel to the first open tibial vessel with collateralization to the foot. This includes the peroneal artery. In cases in which the conduit is limited and shorter bypasses are necessary, an alternative distal inflow vessel is used. Assuming that the severity of the proximal atherosclerosis is mild (<40% stenosis), long-term bypass patency is excellent when using alternative inflow sources. We have been impressed that bypasses rarely thrombose as a consequence of inflow disease progression. In our published series of 450 consecutive infrainguinal grafts performed, we observed no graft failures resulting from progression of inflow stenosis, including 11 cases of bypass patency despite complete proximal inflow occlusion. Alternative inflow vessels commonly used include the distal profunda femoris artery, the popliteal artery, the proximal tibial arteries, and the endarterectomized superficial femoral artery.

Although we enthusiastically endorse using alternative inflow sources as a means to compensate for a short vein conduit and avoid composite bypass, we strongly caution against compromising the integrity of the outflow vessel to achieve the same goal. Vein graft patency is dependent on a low-resistant, disease-free, outflow tibial vessel. As well, a disease-free outflow vessel is necessary to achieve pulsatile blood flow to the foot, a generally accepted requirement for healing. All attempts should be made to place the bypass to a disease-free distal target. A policy of "accepting" some outflow arterial disease to compensate for a short conduit usually results in a failed bypass.

The anterior tibial artery is generally exposed through an incision over the anterior compartment of the shin (Fig. 2). The dissection is carried down between the tibia and the anterior tibialis muscle. A medial exposure is used to expose the posterior tibial artery and the proximal peroneal artery. A lateral fibulectomy is used to expose the distal third of the peroneal artery. When using a reversed vein graft conduit, we have often used a technique described by Kunlin in which the proximal anastomosis incorporates a venous side branch into the anastomotic hood to avoid stenosis at the heel of the proximal vein graft anastomosis (Fig. 3). After the proximal anastomosis is performed, the vein conduit is tunneled anatomically or subfascially, with care taken not to twist the graft. Distal anastomoses are usually performed with loupe magnification using 7.0 polypropylene sutures. Completion arteriography (Fig. 4) is used liberally to visualize the conduit, the distal anastomosis, and the runoff bed to the foot. Technical abnormalities observed are corrected immediately before completion of the operation.

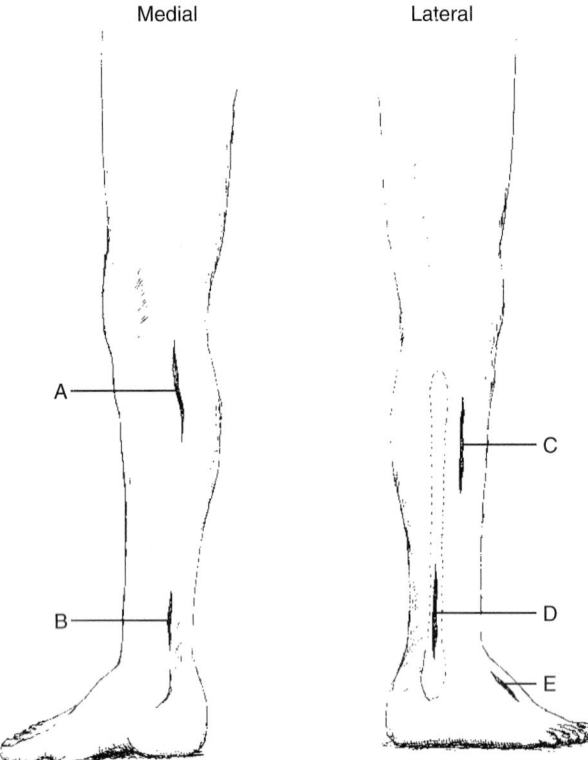

Figure 2 Common incision sites used to expose the tibioperoneal vessels. *(A)* Proximal posterior tibial and peroneal; *(B)* distal posterior tibial; *(C)* proximal anterior tibial; *(D)* distal peroneal; *(E)* Dorsalis pedis.

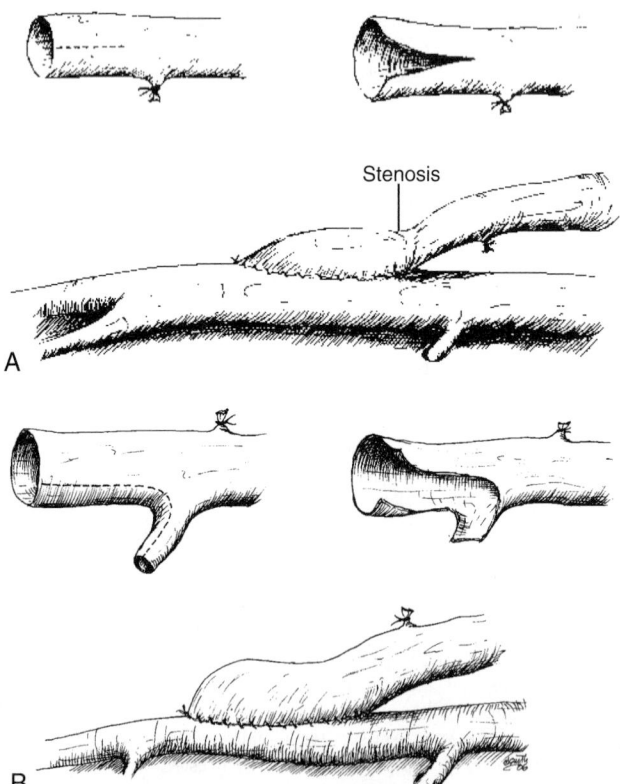

Figure 3 **(A)** An example of a proximal anastomotic heel stenosis caused by the use of a small reversed saphenous vein. **(B)** An example of incorporating a small venous side branch into the proximal anastomosis of a reversed saphenous vein graft to avoid a heel stenosis.

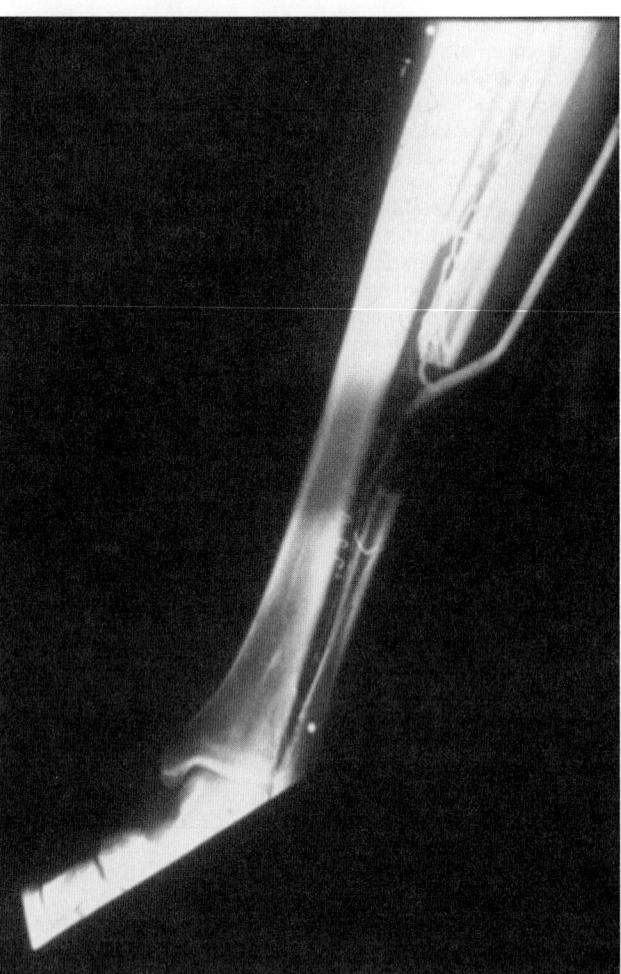

Figure 4 An on-table completion arteriogram of a femoroperoneal bypass after lateral fibulectomy.

POSTOPERATIVE FOLLOW-UP

On completion of the operation, patients are observed in a monitored setting for 6 to 23 hours. Perioperative ambulation using physical therapy is encouraged. Early complications commonly encountered include myocardial infarction and wound complications. Wound complications, usually from vein harvest incisions, are especially common, occurring in up to 25% of cases.

The most common late complication is graft thrombosis. Graft thrombosis, when it occurs, can be etiologically divided according to time of thrombosis. Early thrombosis can occur in up to 20% of cases and is usually the result of technical or judgmental error (poor conduit or compromised outflow vessel). Thromboses from 1 month to 2 years typically occur because of neointimal hyperplastic intrinsic vein graft stenoses. Late thromboses usually occur because of recurrent atherosclerosis distal to the graft. By far the most common cause of graft thrombosis is the progression of a neointimal hyperplastic intrinsic vein graft stenosis. Graft-threatening intrinsic vein graft stenoses can occur in up to 35% of all bypasses. Meaningful long-term patency can therefore be achieved only by detection and correction of these lesions. Stenoses that are found before thrombosis (i.e., the failing graft) can be treated to prevent graft failure. Long-term patency is excellent after correction of these graft lesions, assuming that thrombosis has not occurred. However, if graft thrombosis occurs, long-term graft patency is substantially reduced, by as much as 30% to 40% at 3 years. This compromise in patency is independent of the method used to clear the thrombus from the clotted graft, i.e., balloon embolectomy or thrombolytic therapy. It is postulated that thrombosis of the graft causes permanent endothelial cell damage that irreversibly compromises the integrity of the conduit. The detection and correction of these intrinsic vein graft stenoses before thrombosis is therefore imperative.

On the basis of this discussion, our bypass grafts are surveilled using duplex ultrasonography before discharge. Patients are followed weekly until wounds are healed. Routine graft surveillance using history and physical examination, ankle-brachial indices, and duplex-derived graft low velocities are obtained at 1 month and every 3 months for the first 18 months. Grafts are followed every 6 months thereafter. Any subjective evidence of recurrent symptoms, a drop in ankle-brachial index greater than 0.15, or any abnormal graft flow velocity is investigated with contrast angiography. Ideally, graft flow velocities should possess a triphasic Doppler-derived waveform, a velocity greater than 45 cm per second and less than 180 cm per second. Focal graft flow velocities of 180 cm per second or greater are usually associated with discrete stenoses of at least a 50% diameter reduction. Critical vein graft stenoses have velocities greater than 300 cm per second or velocity ratios (peak systolic velocity per normal systolic velocity) greater than 4 and are particularly ominous when accompanied by a drop in ankle-brachial index or a distal graft flow velocity of less than 45 cm per second. All critical vein graft stenoses should be repaired. At our institution, focal stenoses are usually treated initially with percutaneous transluminal angioplasty. Diffuse, long-segment stenoses are treated with surgical vein bypass.

Using this protocol, primary graft patency of 66% at 5 years can be expected. With an aggressive surveillance protocol, graft-threatening lesions can be detected and repaired. Assisted primary patency rates from 75% to 80% at 5 years can be expected. When considering all infrainguinal bypasses, graft patency is strongly influenced by the indication for bypass. Patency rates in grafts for claudication exceed patency rates in grafts for critical limb ischemia. Femoropopliteal grafts achieve higher patency rates than tibial bypass. Limb-salvage rates typically exceed patency rates in most series.

MANAGEMENT IN DESPERATE SITUATIONS

As the population ages, the physiologic reserve of patients presenting with critical limb ischemia will no doubt become progressively poor. Patients with multiple medical problems and functional comorbidities who are unsuitable for open surgery will become more prevalent. In these cases, goals of therapy should be modified. The notion of graft patency and limb salvage as measures of success should be replaced with outcomes such as meaningful survival, maintenance of ambulation, and maintenance of independent living status. In our series of 1000 limbs in 841 patients treated for critical limb ischemia, we found that functional outcome postoperatively was most often determined by intrinsic patient comorbidities at the time of presentation. The most important independent predictors of poor functional outcome were impaired ambulatory ability at the time of presentation and the presence of dementia. These factors were more important than eventual limb loss itself. The ideal treatment for patients with these comorbidities is unclear. We have increasingly employed less morbid percutaneous transluminal angioplasty in many of these cases. Although long-term patency of these interventions is often inferior to open bypass, this type of intervention is frequently sufficient to meet the goals of

therapy—namely, to increase circulation enough to promote healing and maintain functionality. Angioplasty for critical limb ischemia in our series resulted in a limb salvage of greater than 60% of cases at 1 year.

Advocates for angioplasty to treat critical limb ischemia rationalize that although the outcomes are inferior to open bypass, limb salvage, and thus improved functionality, are generally superior to no treatment at all. However, in a recent review of 533 patients undergoing major limb amputation at our institution, maintenance of ambulation with a prosthesis at 3 years was 44% and maintenance of independent living status at 5 years was 72%; this is surprisingly similar to results after angioplasty, which yielded a maintenance of ambulation of 59% and a maintenance of independent living status of 66%. The role of angioplasty for critical limb ischemia is therefore not precisely defined. What can be concluded, however, is that as the population ages, we will encounter more patients who possess medical comorbidities that may potentially blunt any benefit associated with limb salvage. Identification of these patients will be essential. Specific treatment plans should be geared toward palliation and optimal functional status. To that end, more studies looking at functional outcome in high-risk patients are necessary.

Finally, there are situations in which saphenous vein bypass to the tibial vessels is not possible because of the lack of adequate autogenous vein. Although many have advocated long grafts with PTFE and a distal anastomotic vein patch, we are impressed that these operations provide intermediate-term patency, at best, and afford little benefit compared with aggressive angioplasty alone. As well, we have observed an increased rate of prosthetic graft infection rate when these grafts are used in the setting of open, infected, ischemic ulcers of the foot. Technical advances for the percutaneous intervention of critical limb ischemia using procedures such as subintimal angioplasty have broadened the treatment horizons of this technique. Therefore in most cases of critical limb ischemia in which saphenous vein is unavailable, percutaneous angioplasty is our initial alternative therapy.

In summary, tibioperoneal arterial disease should be treated in the presence of critical limb ischemia only. Tibial artery bypass using autogenous saphenous vein is the treatment of choice. Although future studies are necessary to determine the best role of percutaneous transluminal angioplasty for the treatment of critical limb ischemia, patients best suited for this less morbid technique appear to be those who possess medical comorbidities or technical limitations that preclude open bypass.

SUGGESTED READINGS

Hunink MG, Wong JD, Donaldson MC, and others: Patency results of percutaneous and surgical revascularization for femoropopliteal arterial disease, *Med Decis Making* 14:71, 1994.

Mills JL: Infrainguinal bypass. In Rutherford RB, editor: *Vascular surgery*, ed 6, Philadelphia, 2005, Elsevier Saunders.

Mills JL, Fugitani RM, Taylor SM: The characteristics and anatomic distribution of lesions that cause reverse vein graft failure: a five-year prospective study, *J Vasc Surg* 17:195, 1993.

Mills JL, Taylor SM, Fujitani RM: The role of the deep femoral artery as an inflow site for infrainguinal revascularization, *J Vasc Surg* 18:416, 1993.

Taylor SM, Kalbaugh CA, Blackhurst DW, and others: Determinants of functional outcome after revascularization for critical limb ischemia: an analysis of 1000 consecutive vascular interventions, *J Vasc Surg* 44:747, 2006.

Taylor SM, Mills JL, Fujitani RM, and others: Does arterial inflow failure cause distal vein thrombosis? A prospective analysis of 450 infrainguinal vascular reconstructions, *Ann Vasc Surg* 8:92, 1994.

Transatlantic Inter-Society Consensus (TASC) Working Group. Management of peripheral arterial disease, *J Vasc Surg* 31: (suppl): 5168, 2003.

PROFUNDA FEMORIS RECONSTRUCTION

Jimmy Pak, MD, and Christopher Zarins, MD

INTRODUCTION

The profunda femoris artery is the major source of blood flow to the thigh muscles, and the superficial femoral artery is the primary source of circulation to the calf muscles and distal extremity. When the superficial femoral artery is diseased or occluded, the profunda femoris becomes the major blood supply to the lower extremity through multiple collateral vessels. Although superficial femoral artery disease can cause symptoms of severe and limiting claudication, limb loss is rare unless there is significant concomitant profunda disease. Maintenance of normal blood flow into the profunda and its collaterals is a critical factor in avoiding amputation in patients with peripheral vascular disease. The purpose of this chapter is to review the anatomy of the profunda femoris artery, as well as the techniques and strategies of maintaining blood flow in the profunda.

ANATOMY

The profunda is one of the two main branches of the common femoral artery. It exits the common femoral artery posterolaterally approximately 3 to 5 cm below the inguinal ligament and is crossed anteriorly by the circumflex femoral vein (Fig. 1). It then tracks deep to the sartorius and vastus medialis muscles. An extensive network of collaterals via the medial and lateral circumflex femoral arteries anastomoses with branches of the internal iliac artery and posteriorly with the sciatic artery. The profunda provides retrograde flow to the pelvis in circumstances of internal iliac artery or external iliac artery occlusion. Additionally, the profunda supplies the lower extremity in cases of superficial femoral artery and popliteal artery occlusion. Branches of the profunda communicate with the popliteal artery through the geniculate arteries around the knee.

DIAGNOSIS AND IMAGING

The profunda should be imaged on all evaluations for peripheral vascular disease. Imaging modalities include duplex ultrasound, computed tomography (CT) angiography, magnetic resonance (MR) angiography, and angiography. Duplex ultrasound can provide not only an anatomic description of the artery in terms of the location of the stenotic areas but can also help to determine the severity of the stenosis. Duplex examination can become less reliable in cases of severe calcification. CT angiography can provide detailed information but requires an intravenous contrast load and close image sequencing. Angiography is considered the gold standard for imaging. Typically, angiography is performed with a lateral oblique projection of 30 to 45 degrees to best visualize the profunda. Figure 2 demonstrates the increased separation of superficial femoral and profunda femoral arteries with lateral oblique imaging.

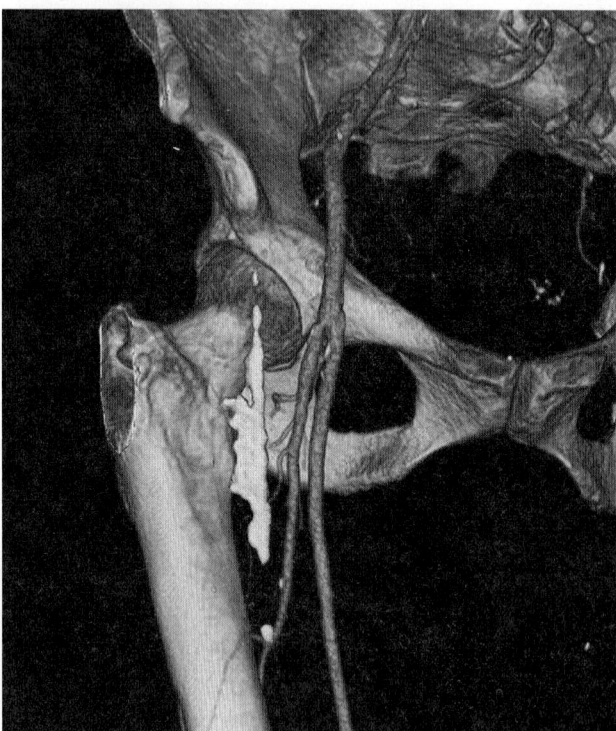

Figure I   The profunda femoris artery originates from the common femoral artery in the groin and courses posterolaterally to supply the muscles of the thigh. *Image courtesy Dr. Dominik Fleischmann.*

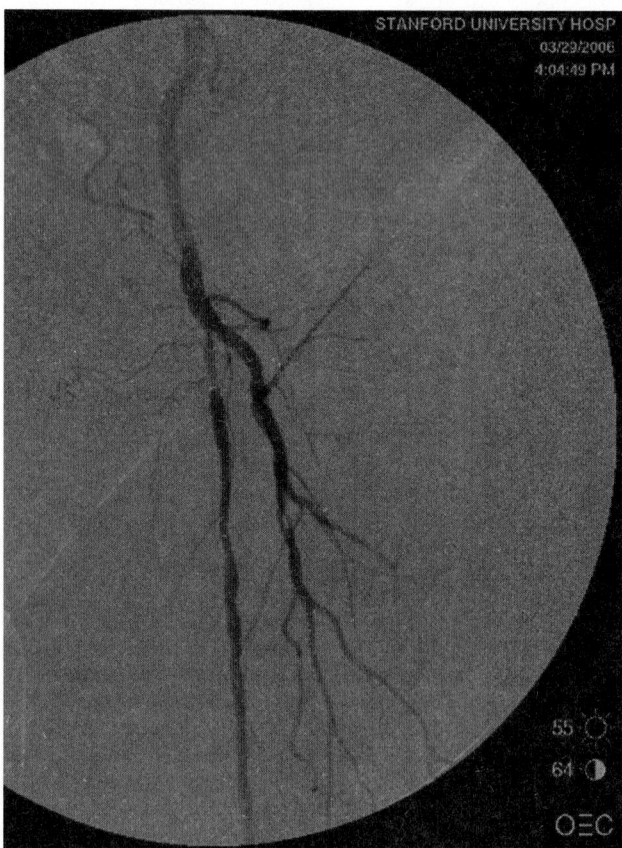

Figure 2   Angiogram of the femoral artery demonstrating the increased separation of the superficial and profunda femoral arteries with a lateral oblique projection of the image intensifier.

INDICATIONS AND SELECTION OF PATIENTS

Patients with profunda stenosis or occlusion and lower-extremity ischemia may benefit from profunda reconstruction. However, resolution of ischemic symptoms is rarely accomplished by profundaplasty alone but usually requires aortoiliac inflow or femoropopliteal outflow reconstruction. In certain circumstances of severe profunda stenosis in which there is no inflow disease and no treatable superficial femoral or popliteal disease, isolated profundaplasty may provide significant improvement of lower-extremity perfusion. Symptoms of rest pain are usually relieved, and claudication is improved. However, isolated profundaplasty is unlikely to heal ischemic ulcerations in the foot and gangrenous lesions on the toes.

Patients with severe profunda stenosis and superficial femoral artery occlusion may benefit from profunda reconstruction by revascularization of the extensive network of collaterals. The lower extremity is fed through collaterals from the deep femoral branches to the geniculates. Figures 3 and 4 demonstrate the extensive collateral that develops with superficial femoral artery (SFA) occlusion from the deep femoral branches. This is important in patients who do not have distal bypass targets and also in patients who may not tolerate a longer bypass procedure because of medical comorbidities. Also patients without suitable vein conduit may be helped by profundaplasty because of the unfavorable long-term outcome of long prosthetic bypasses to tibial vessels. In patients with gangrene who are not candidates for distal bypass, profunda reconstruction may significantly improve lower-extremity blood flow so that below-knee rather than above-knee amputation can be performed.

PROFUNDAPLASTY

Profundaplasty is most commonly performed in combination with either an inflow or outflow revascularization procedure. The profunda femoral artery is versatile and can be used as an inflow or outflow vessel.

Inflow

The profunda femoris can be used as the inflow source for a femoropopliteal or femorotibial artery bypass. Endarterectomy of the common femoral artery and profunda orifice may be necessary with patch angioplasty of the proximal profunda. If the bypass fails at a later date, the profundaplasty may provide adequate perfusion of the lower extremity. Although the patient may experience claudication, the ischemic foot lesions may have healed and reoperation or amputation may be avoided. In the case of severe common femoral artery disease with proximal stenosis of the profunda and superficial femoral artery occlusion, femoral endarterectomy and profundaplasty alone may relieve symptoms of rest pain. More proximal iliac stenoses can often be treated with balloon angioplasty and stenting, thus avoiding aortofemoral bypass surgery.

Outflow

The profunda femoris artery is an essential outflow vessel for aortoiliac reconstruction procedures such as aortofemoral, axillofemoral, iliofemoral, and femorofemoral bypass. The profunda ensures long-term patency of such bypass grafts by providing outflow when there is superficial femoral artery disease and ensuring long-term patency in the event of progression of disease in the superficial femoral artery. If there is stenosis of the orifice of the profunda artery, the stenosis should always be corrected at the time of aortofemoral bypass by endarterectomy or extension of the bypass graft onto the proximal profunda as a patch angioplasty. Failure to correct a profunda stenosis may reduce the long-term patency of aortofemoral, axillofemoral and femorofemoral bypass

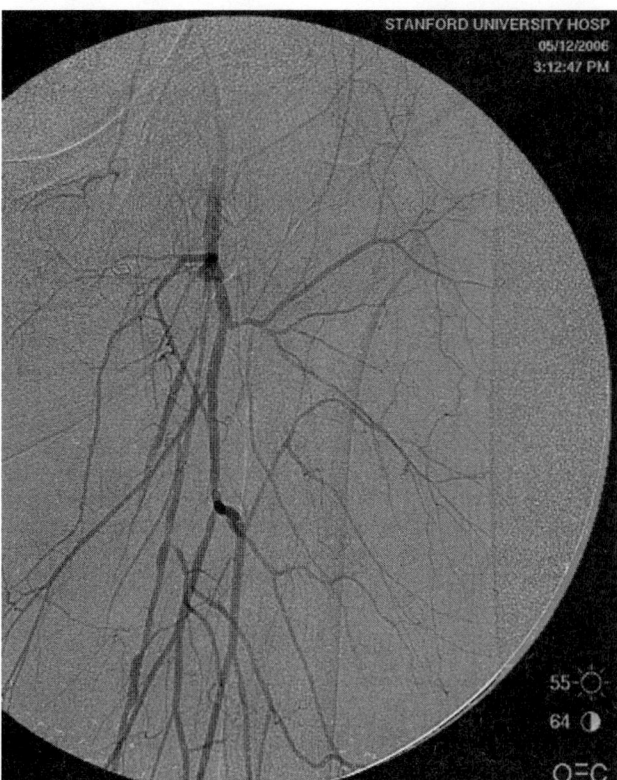

Figure 3 Angiogram demonstrating an extensive network of collateral branches from the profunda femoral artery with diffuse stenosis of the superficial femoral artery.

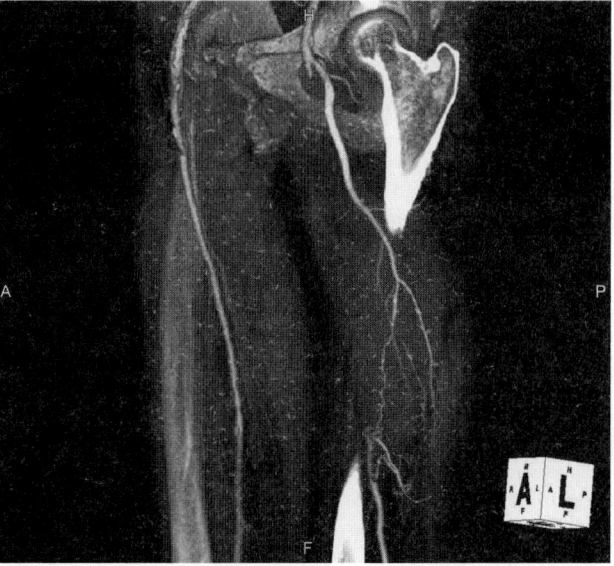

Figure 4 Computed tomography angiogram with three-dimensional reconstruction demonstrates collaterals from the profunda femoral artery reconstituting the popliteal artery with total occlusion of the left superficial femoral artery. *Image courtesy Dr. Dominik Fleischmann.*

procedures. Profundaplasty will also provide outflow for endovascular procedures such as iliac angioplasty and stenting.

Exposure of the profunda femoris artery is obtained by dissection of the common femoral artery and its bifurcation into the superficial femoral and profunda branches. In cases in which there have been multiple previous groin operations, scarring may make dissection of the femoral artery difficult. In these circumstances, if the proximal profunda is patent without stenosis, the distal profunda may be

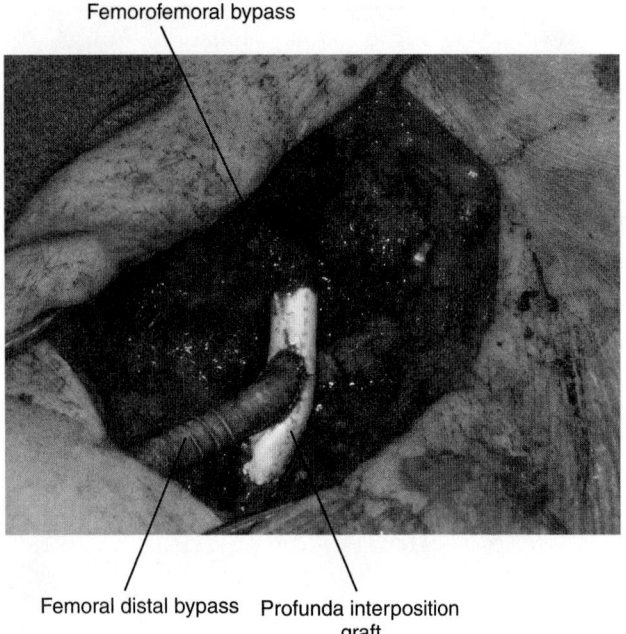

Figure 5 An interposition graft to the left profunda femoris artery provides outflow for a femorofemoral bypass and serves as the inflow source for a left femorotibial bypass graft. (*See color insert Figure 36.*)

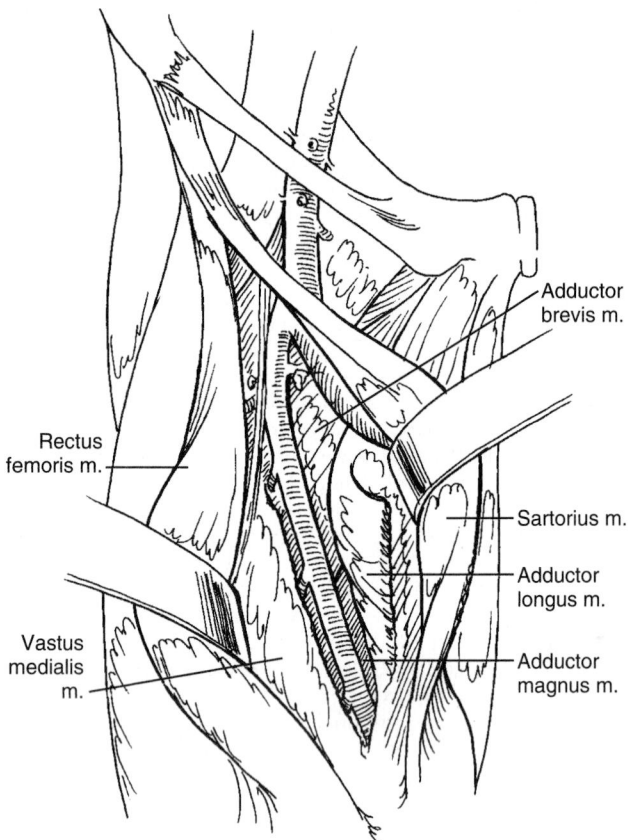

Figure 6 Operative exposure of the distal profunda femoral artery. *m*, Muscle. *From Valentine RJ, Wind GG: Anatomic exposures in vascular surgery, ed 2, Baltimore, 2003, Lippincott Williams & Wilkins, p. 429.*

exposed through new, more lateral dissection planes and used as the inflow source for more distal bypass procedures. This avoids reoperating in the area of the groin crease, avoids the scarred areas, and may reduce the risk of infection. The profunda femoral artery can be used as an inflow vessel, thus shortening the length of vein necessary for lower bypass procedures. An additional 10 to 15 cm can be gained by placing the proximal anastomosis of a distal bypass graft on the profunda femoris artery instead of the common femoral artery. This may facilitate the use of autogenous vein for the distal bypass rather than a prosthetic graft, which has a significantly lower patency rate.

In some cases, the profunda can perform both inflow and outflow functions. In the case shown in Figure 5, a new interposition prosthetic graft to the profunda provides outflow from a femorofemoral bypass while also serving as the inflow source for a femorotibial bypass graft.

Techniques

The profunda femoris artery is exposed by dissection distal of the bifurcation of the common femoral artery. The transition in the diameter of the common femoral artery to the superficial femoral artery is a reliable marker of the location of the origin of the profunda femoral artery. This transition point is typically several centimeters inferior to the inguinal ligament. The profunda femoris artery usually emerges posterolateral to the common femoral artery. However, one should be aware that the lateral and medial circumflex branches of the deep femoral artery may originate from the common femoral artery or close to it. Incomplete dissection and control of the profunda femoris artery and its branches will interfere with vascular reconstruction because of retrograde bleeding from uncontrolled circumflex branches. Haphazard dissection can result in injured profunda branches with significant bleeding and the need to obliterate important profunda outflow branches. The lateral circumflex femoral vein crosses over the anterior surface of the proximal profunda and should by ligated and divided to ensure good exposure. Exposure of the distal profunda is facilitated by dissection of the superficial femoral artery with gentle retraction medially to reveal the underlying profunda. Operative exposure of the distal profunda through a lateral approach is shown in Figure 6.

Profunda femoris reconstruction may be performed using autogenous or prosthetic graft material. The most favorable autogenous material is saphenous vein, but this is rarely used for profunda reconstruction because autogenous saphenous vein is usually preserved for use in lower-extremity bypass or coronary bypass procedures. In cases in which the superficial femoral artery is occluded, a segment of endarterectomized superficial femoral artery may be used as a profundaplasty patch material. However, the endarterectomized superficial femoral artery is prone to restenosis, and thus there is no advantage over prosthetic patch materials. Long segments of endarterectomized profunda can be successfully patched using Dacron or polytetrafluoroethylene (PTFE) patch materials. This requires careful and extensive dissection of the profunda with preservation of all the profunda branches to provide good outflow. Segmental interposition grafts in the profunda with ligation of branch vessels is suboptimal because important collateral branches are sacrificed. Polypropylene sutures, usually 6-0 for anastomoses and patching and 7-0 for tacking uplifted intima, are most commonly used.

Reconstruction of the profunda as an outflow vessel for aortofemoral or iliofemoral bypass can be accomplished by extending the hood of the bypass graft onto the profunda, past the level of the profunda orifice plaque. Such an anastomosis is preferable to extension of the hood of the graft onto the orifice of the superficial femoral artery because there often is progression of disease in the superficial femoral. Extension of the bypass onto the profunda is facilitated by extending the common femoral arteriotomy laterally onto the profunda and avoiding the bifurcation of the femoral artery. Because most profunda femoral disease occurs at the most proximal portion of the artery, it is not necessary to dissect the profunda femoral artery far but it must be far enough to be well past the plaque (Fig. 7). Care must be taken to avoid a dissection plane in the artery with potential intimal flaps. In rare cases, the limb of an aortofemoral bypass can be anastomosed end-to-end to the

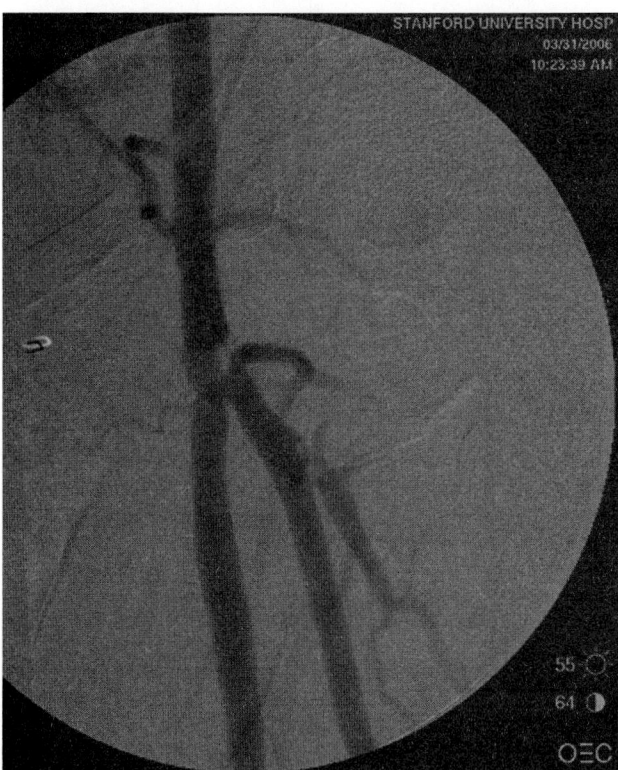

Figure 7 This angiogram demonstrates a focal stenosis of the profunda femoral artery at its origin. Note the lack of disease distally.

profunda, provided that important collateral branches such as the lateral circumflex femoral branch are preserved.

Endovascular treatment of profunda femoris stenosis can be achieved by balloon angioplasty through a contralateral femoral artery approach. Although balloon angioplasty, particularly of anastomotic stenoses, has been successful, the use of stents in this area is hazardous because of possible compression of the stent as a result of flexion in the groin. Percutaneous puncture of the contralateral femoral artery allows retrograde access to the aorta and antegrade introduction of a guidewire and crossover sheath into the external iliac artery. The image intensifier is angulated 20 to 25 degrees laterally to separate the profunda femoral artery from the superficial femoral artery, and the guidewire is advanced into the profunda femoris artery under fluoroscopic control. Balloon angioplasty can successfully dilatate local focal profunda orifice stenoses; however, there is danger of dissection. In addition, balloon angioplasty of a profunda lesion may result in occlusion of the superficial femoral artery orifice. Kissing-balloon techniques to dilatate simultaneously the origins of the profunda and superficial femoral arteries have been used successfully. Long-segment profunda lesions are not likely to benefit from an endoluminal procedure.

Results

The utility of isolated profundaplasty has been debated extensively over the past several decades. In 1988, McCarthy reported his experience with 17 patients over a 10-year period. Only four patients had objective evidence of improvement with an increase in ankle-brachial pressure index (ABI > 0.15). Four patients required subsequent amputation, and two patients required femoral-to-peroneal bypasses. Perioperative mortality rate was 5.9%.

Fugger reported 181 patients treated with isolated profundoplasty with subjective improvement in 111 (61%) and improved ABI (> 0.12) in more than half of the patients. However, operative mortality was 8%, and 25% of patients required major amputation, which reflects the critical nature of their ischemia.

Both the older and newer series suggest only moderate improvement from isolated profundaplasty, with documented improvement

in ABI in only 25% to 50% of patients. These figures confirm that isolated profundaplasty should be considered as a primary procedure on only rare occasions and only in patients who have no other revascularization treatment options. Patients considered for isolated profundaplasty as the only treatment option are almost uniformly in a limb-salvage situation and have multiple comorbidities, thus making them poor operative candidates, even for a relatively small groin procedure. Nonetheless, regional or general anesthesia is usually necessary and contributes to operative mortality rates of 5% or higher.

The possibility of endovascular treatment is an attractive alternative for such high-risk patients with critical limb ischemia. Silva reported on 31 consecutive patients with critical limb ischemia treated with endovascular profundaplasty: the procedure was successful in 91% of patients, with a mean increase in ABI from 0.5 to 0.7 $\pm$ 0.2 ($p < .01$). During a mean follow-up of 34 months, no additional amputations were necessary, three patients required repeat revascularization, and five patients died. The profunda lesion treated was located in the proximal profunda before the lateral circumflex branch in 88% of patients; 62% of patients had concomitant occlusion of the SFA. These results of endovascular treatment are promising, but direct comparison with other published series of profundaplasty is not possible because of differences in patient-selection criteria. Nonetheless, these results suggest that endovascular strategies to treat the profunda femoris deserve consideration.

Diehm reported a less favorable experience in 20 patients with critical limb ischemia and long-segment femoropopliteal occlusions unsuitable for a bypass procedure. Despite a 100% technical success rate with profunda angioplasty in 14 patients and surgical profundaplasty in 6 patients, healing of ischemic lesions occurred in only 1 patient. At 12 months, 55% of patients had died, 36% had major amputations, and 49% had repeat revascularization efforts. These results reaffirm the poor response of isolated profunda revascularization, regardless of technique, in patients with ulcerated and gangrenous ischemic lesions.

Moore found in his 18-year experience with 281 aortofemoral bypass grafts that the primary cause of late graft failure was profunda disease. Occlusive disease of the profunda femoral artery was believed to be the primary cause of graft failure among 54 patients who experienced aortofemoral graft limb occlusion. Repair of graft limb occlusion consisted of profunda angioplasty and proximal thrombectomy. No deaths were reported, and patency after the reconstruction was 100% at 30 days. In Moore's experience, long-term patency following thrombectomy and profunda reconstruction was best in nondiabetic patients who underwent patch profundaplasty using autogenous vein as the patch material. Others have experienced similar good long-term results using prosthetic profundaplasty patches. Kalman reported favorable long-term results when profundaplasty is combined with aortofemoral bypass, with a 5-year patency of the aortofemoral bypass of 97 $\pm$ 1.3%.

CONCLUSIONS

The profunda femoris artery is a major source of blood supply to the lower extremity and is critical to maintaining limb viability in patients with peripheral occlusive disease. Severe profunda stenosis should be corrected with profundaplasty in all patients with symptomatic peripheral occlusive disease who are undergoing either inflow or outflow procedures in the groin. Isolated profundaplasty has limited usefulness as a primary procedure for the treatment of claudication or critical limb ischemia. The role of endovascular treatment of profunda stenosis is unsettled.

SUGGESTED READINGS

Diehm N, Savolainen H, Mahler F, et al: Does deep femoral artery revascularization as an isolated procedure play a role in chronic critical limb ischemia? *J Endovasc Ther* 11:119, 2004.

Fugger R, Kretschmer G, Schemper M, et al: The place of profundaplasty in the surgical treatment of superficial femoral artery occlusion, *Eur J Vasc Surg* 1:187, 1987.

Harward TR, Bergan JJ, Yao JS, et al: *Am J Surg* 156:126, 1988.

Kalman PG, Jolustor KW, Walker PW: The current role of isolated profundaplasty, *J Cardiovasc Surg* 31:107, 1990.

Malone MM, Goldstone J, Moore WS: Autogenous profundaplasty: the key to long-term patency in secondary repair of aortofemoral graft occlusion, *Ann Surg* 188:817, 1978.

Silva JA, White CJ, Ramee SR, and others: Percutaneous profundaplasty in the treatment of lower extremity ischemia: results of long-term surveillance, *J Endovasc Ther* 8:75, 2001.

Valentine RJ, Wind GG: Anatomic exposures in vascular surgery, ed 2, Baltimore, 2003, Lippincott Williams & Wilkins, p. 429.

AXILLOFEMORAL BYPASS

Evan C. Lipsitz, MD

INTRODUCTION

Although atherosclerosis is a diffuse process, distinct disease patterns of arterial occlusive disease can be identified. One such pattern is disease within the aortoiliac segment. Classic symptoms are those of thigh or buttock claudication and impotence in male patients, known as Leriche syndrome. This pattern can be found in isolation or in combination with infrainguinal occlusive disease, in which the presentation is frequently more severe. The diagnosis of aortoiliac occlusive disease is made on the basis of history and physical examination, with findings of diminished or absent pulses throughout the lower extremities. These findings can be confirmed with a number of diagnostic tests. Pulse-volume recordings, a plethysmographic evaluation of lower extremity arterial circulation, show decreased waveforms in all segments, including thigh tracings, distinguishing aortoiliac occlusive disease from infrainguinal disease, in which thigh tracings are largely preserved. Arterial duplex mapping can be used to assess noninvasively the degree of stenosis or occlusion (or both) within the aortoiliac segment and can also be used to plan intervention. Traditional angiography, especially in the setting of concomitant infrainguinal disease, provides detailed anatomic information and permits assessment of the abdominal, pelvic, and lower-extremity arterial tree. If warranted, intervention may be performed at the same time as the diagnostic procedure. In the setting of aortoiliac occlusive disease, femoral artery access may be difficult or impossible, and the use of alternative access sites, such as the brachial artery, may be required. Computed tomography (CT) angiography is also a useful modality for defining aortoiliac anatomy and has the added advantage of providing evaluation of the degree and extent of calcification within the aortoiliac segment. This modality may be especially useful in patients who have undergone previous arterial surgery in that nonfunctioning grafts are well visualized by this method, and knowledge of their locations is helpful in planning subsequent interventions. A potential limitation of CT angiography is its difficulty in evaluating tibial vessels when infrainguinal disease is present. Magnetic resonance angiography can also be used to evaluate aortoiliac and lower-extremity arterial anatomy but may also have limitations in the evaluation of the distal circulation.

Axillofemoral bypass was first introduced in the early 1960s as an alternative to direct aortoiliac reconstruction in patients with aortoiliac occlusive disease (Fig. 1). This extra-anatomic bypass, so called because the reconstruction does not course along the normal anatomic path of the vessels, permits placement of the graft in a superficial and largely subcutaneous position, reducing physiologic stress on the patient during the perioperative period, compared with direct reconstruction, which requires abdominal dissection and clamping of the aorta. Because of the long length of conduit required, these procedures are usually performed with prosthetic grafts.

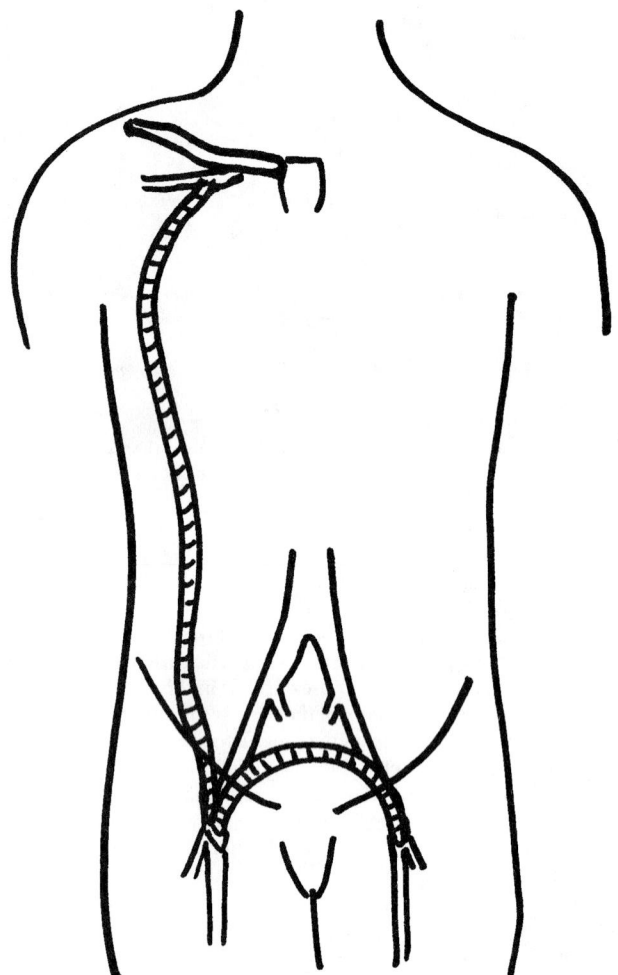

Figure 1 Typical configuration of a right axillobifemoral bypass.

INDICATIONS

Patients requiring axillofemoral bypass generally have chronic arterial insufficiency, manifest as disabling claudication, rest pain, ischemic ulceration, or gangrene. Axillofemoral bypass is infrequently required in the setting of acute occlusion. The timing of intervention depends on the indication for operation, as well as the overall health status of the patient. The primary indication for axillofemoral bypass is a patient with severe aortoiliac disease who is unable to undergo aortofemoral bypass for any number of reasons. These include anatomic considerations such as heavy aortic calcification; hostile abdomen or the need for peritoneal dialysis; medical comorbidities such as severe cardiopulmonary, renal, or hepatic disease; or the presence of intra-abdominal infection as a result of infected grafts, mycotic aneurysms, or aortoenteric fistula (Table 1). Another indication is the placement of a temporary

Table 1: Indications for Axillofemoral Bypass

Anatomic

Heavy aortic calcification

Hostile abdomen

    Previous surgery

    Extensive scarring

    Pelvic irradiation

Peritoneal dialysis

Comorbid conditions

Severe cardiopulmonary disease

Severe renal or hepatic disease

Otherwise unfit for major surgery

Infectious

Infected intra-abdominal graft

Other intra-abdominal infection

Mycotic aneurysm

Aortoenteric fistula

Temporary

Need for temporary visceral and renal perfusion during major aortic reconstruction

---

axillofemoral bypass for visceral and renal artery perfusion during complex thoracoabdominal aortic reconstruction.

The development and advancement of endovascular therapies has and will continue to affect the treatment of aortoiliac occlusive disease. In the early 1990s, reports showing the efficacy and relative durability of iliac angioplasty and stenting for focal stenoses (TransAtlantic Inter-Society Consensus [TASC] A and B lesions) led many patients to undergo this treatment as their primary mode of therapy, reducing the overall need for aortofemoral reconstruction or other surgical intervention. Since the mid 1990s, advancements for crossing total occlusions (TASC-C and -D lesions), including the development of subintimal angioplasty, have made the treatment of an even greater number of patients with endovascular methods possible. As such, many patients who finally do come to surgical therapy are older with more significant comorbid disease and thus are not candidates for direct aortic reconstruction; therefore they require axillofemoral bypass.

A small subset of patients presenting with aortoiliac occlusive disease will also have associated abdominal aortic aneurysms. Axillofemoral bypass is not the preferred treatment for this group of patients unless the aneurysms are particularly small or the patient is believed to be a prohibitive surgical risk. These patients require aortofemoral bypass to address the aneurysmal component of the disease process.

In patients in whom the abdominal aorta is unsuitable for inflow, another alternative for direct reconstruction is to use the supraceliac or distal thoracic aorta for inflow, gaining exposure through a transperitoneal incision with medial visceral rotation, a retroperitoneal incision, or a thoracotomy. In patients with combined aortoiliac and infrainguinal occlusive disease, the aortoiliac segment should be restored first, and the infrainguinal component treated subsequently as needed. Such an approach depends on disease severity and may not be possible in the setting of severe limb-threatening ischemia. In these cases, concomitant axillofemoral and infrainguinal reconstructions may be required. When the common femoral artery is occluded, patients undergoing axillofemoral bypass require alternative outflow to the profunda femoral artery, superficial femoral artery, or the popliteal artery.

In patients with combined aortoiliac and infrainguinal occlusive disease (multilevel disease) requiring intervention, decisions regarding the extent of reconstruction are based on the patient's clinical status. For patients with claudication, rest pain, or minor tissue lesions,

restoration of inflow to the femoral level alone should be sufficient to achieve relief of symptoms while minimizing surgical risk. For patients with extensive gangrene, a multilevel reconstruction may be required, with the attendant increase in potential complications.

PREOPERATIVE EVALUATION

Patients should undergo a thorough preoperative evaluation. Many patients are selected for axillofemoral bypass on the basis of their comorbid conditions and as such should be medically optimized to the greatest degree possible before surgery.

The choice of donor axillary artery depends on a number of factors. The axillary arteries can be evaluated by a number of invasive and noninvasive methods. Most simply, blood pressure measurements are taken in both arms and compared. If there is a significant gradient between the two sides (e.g., >20–30 mm Hg), the arm with the higher pressure is chosen for inflow. The presence of any gradient in the upper extremities may itself prompt further evaluation. Upper-extremity pulse-volume recordings or Doppler waveforms of the brachial arteries (or both) are similarly useful for guiding therapy. Direct duplex of the subclavian arteries can be used to identify proximal stenoses. Digital subtraction angiography provides detailed anatomic information of the upper-extremity circulation. In patients undergoing arteriography, views of the aortic arch and great vessels should be obtained. Although this is an invasive procedure, there is the opportunity to address any lesions with angioplasty and stenting before the bypass procedure. Finally, the inflow can be evaluated with CT angiography or magnetic resonance angiography, as noted earlier.

All else being equal, the right axillary is usually chosen for inflow because of the somewhat higher propensity of the left subclavian artery to develop stenosis. This choice is frequently made despite the fact that most patients are right handed. Some authors advocate choosing the ipsilateral axillary artery to the side with the more severe lower-extremity symptoms. Grafts should not be based off an upper extremity with significant distal arm ischemia or where a dialysis access is present. Additional anatomic considerations include the presence of thoracic outlet syndrome, breast cancer, the presence of an ostomy, abdominal hernias, or other previous surgeries that may complicate graft positioning. Finally, in patients undergoing axillofemoral bypass for intra-abdominal sepsis with previous transperitoneal surgery and who may in the future be candidates for aortic reconstruction via a left retroperitoneal approach, the right axillary artery should be used for inflow to avoid interference of a left-sided graft with a retroperitoneal procedure.

TECHNIQUES

The room is kept warm to prevent hypothermia, given the large body surface area that is exposed, although the importance of this measure is not as great as in open abdominal procedures. General anesthesia is preferred. Although the procedure can be performed with local anesthesia and sedation, large volumes of anesthetic are required and even then the desired analgesia may not be achieved. Preoperative antibiotics are given in the operating room. Patients are positioned supine on a fluoroscopy table with an attached, flexible arm board and the shoulder of the inflow arm abducted to 90 degrees. A rolled towel is placed between the scapulae to facilitate exposure to the medial-most portion of the axillary artery, as well as for the creation of a lateral body wall tunnel. The chest, abdomen, pelvis, and thighs are prepared and covered with an impervious, sterile, plastic dressing. This permits wide exposure should thoracotomy or celiotomy be required. The right or left arm is prepared circumferentially, and an impervious stocking may be placed to the level of the mid upper arm. This facilitates passive movement of the arm during the procedure, permitting the surgeon to confirm by direct inspection that undue tension has not been placed on the axillary anastomosis.

A transverse, infraclavicular incision is made approximately one fingerbreadth below the lateral third of the clavicle, and the dissection

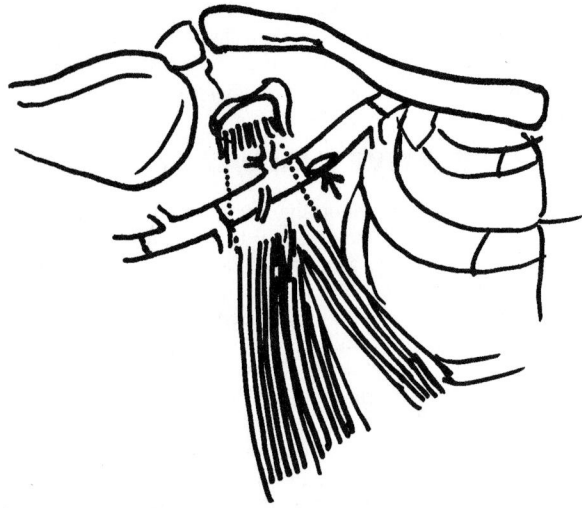

Figure 2 Following division of the pectoralis major. Shows the approximate position of the axillary anastomosis at the distal most first portion of the axillary artery (arrow). The divided pectoralis minor is indicated by the dashed lines and overlies the second portion of the axillary artery.

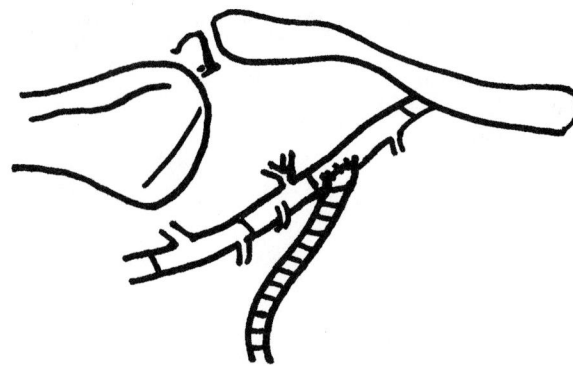

Figure 3 Showing acute angle of the graft at the axillary anastomosis with the axillary artery.

is carried down through the clavipectoral fascia. The pectoralis major muscle fibers are split in the horizontal plane, exposing the deep fascia with the investing fat of the axillary artery, vein, and brachial plexus below. Our approach is to divide the pectoralis minor to improve exposure and reduce the risk of kinking postoperatively, although not all authors perform this maneuver. The first portion of the axillary artery is then exposed and encircled with Silastic loops. The axillary vein overlies the artery, and care must be taken to avoid injuring this structure. Frequently, venous tributaries are ligated to provide adequate exposure. Branches of the axillary artery are controlled with Silastic loops under gentle tension or with removable microclips. Division of these arterial branches is rarely required. Because of the proximity of brachial plexus structures, it is best to avoid excessive electrocautery in the vicinity of the vessels (Fig. 2).

The femoral arteries are exposed through bilateral longitudinal groin incisions. This approach allows flexibility in the placement of the femoral anastomoses and facilitates the performance of any adjunctive procedures that may be required, such as femoral endarterectomy. Oblique groin incisions may be beneficial for wound healing, especially in obese patients, but limit flexibility for the performance of adjunctive procedures, as noted earlier. The anastomoses are generally placed at the distal-most common femoral artery, over the takeoff of the profunda femoris artery. When the superficial femoral artery is occluded, the anastomosis can be made onto the common femoral artery, provided that there is no stenosis of the profunda femoris artery. If there is an orificial stenosis, the anastomoses can be made with the heel on the common femoral artery and the toe on the profunda femoral artery, that is, the distal anastomosis is used to create a profundoplasty. In the case of common and superficial femoral artery occlusions, the anastomosis can be fashioned directly to the deep femoral artery as proximally as possible. If the common, deep, and superficial femoral arteries are all occluded, direct reconstruction to the popliteal artery may be performed.

With the vessels exposed, a long, standard tunneling device is used to create a tunnel between the axilla and the groin. The graft begins by taking a lateral course away from the anastomosis before heading caudally along the midaxillary line. The tunnel extends under the pectoralis major and along the outer chest wall, then subcutaneously along the lateral abdominal wall before coursing in an anterior direction above the iliac crest and over the inguinal ligament to the groin. The use of a counterincision below the inferior aspect of the pectoralis major on the chest wall facilitates tunneling along the abdominal wall, thereby avoiding inadvertent injury to the abdominal contents. Some

authors do not use a counterincision because of the small risk of local wound infection at this site. A suprapubic tunnel for the crossover graft is then made in the subcutaneous space over the inguinal ligaments with either the tunneling device or a large aortic clamp.

An externally supported polytetrafluoroethylene (PTFE) or Dacron prothesis is selected. An 8-mm graft is preferred, but a 6-mm graft may be used in patients with small arteries without a negative effect on patency. The graft is passed through the tunnels, and the patient is systemically heparinized. The graft is then cut to the appropriate length, with care taken not to make the graft too short to prevent the tension on the anastomosis and not to make it too long to prevent redundancy and possibly kinking of the graft. We prefer to leave external ring supports to within 1 cm of anastomosis as a further protection against kinking.

The axillary anastomosis is fashioned such that it is less than perpendicular to the axillary artery, with the acute angle on the lateral side of the anastomosis (Fig. 3). It is sewn using a 5-0 or 6-0 polypropylene suture beginning in the midpoint of the posterior aspect of the anastomosis. The knot may be tied inside the anastomosis, facilitating sewing of the posterior suture line. Both ends of the suture are then run away from the knot toward the heel and toe of the anastomosis. A single suture can be used to complete the anastamosis or additional sutures can be started at the heel or toe (or both) and run over the anterior aspect of the anastamosis. If a single suture is used, care must be taken to avoid pulling up too hard on the suture and "purse-stringing" the anastomosis. The axillary artery is generally soft and delicate and should be handled with care during both dissection and suturing to avoid tearing of the vessel. Finally, care should be taken to ensure that the posterior suture line is secure and without gaps because this area is difficult, if not impossible, to repair after the suture line is completed. The femoral anastomosis is sewn in standard fashion, beginning with the heel and proximal half of the anastomosis and then placing the toe and completing the distal half of the anastomosis. In either case, the sutures may be tied at the ends or approximated using a "parachute" technique, depending on the surgeon's preference.

The incisions are closed using absorbable polypropylene sutures. We prefer to use a subcuticular closure for the axillary incision, as well as for the groin and counterincisions. Staples or staples and exposed suture tend to catch on clothing, and this technique eliminates the need for dressings until the sutures or staples are removed. Confirmation of the patient's pulse status, both lower and upper extremities, is performed before leaving the operating room. In patients with superficial femoral artery occlusions, it may difficult to palpate even the femoral pulse because pulses may be obscured by the external rings of the graft.

GRAFT CONFIGURATIONS

Multiple possible graft configurations can be used when constructing axillofemoral bypass, depending on the surgeon's preference and the patient's anatomy (Fig. 4). The order in which the

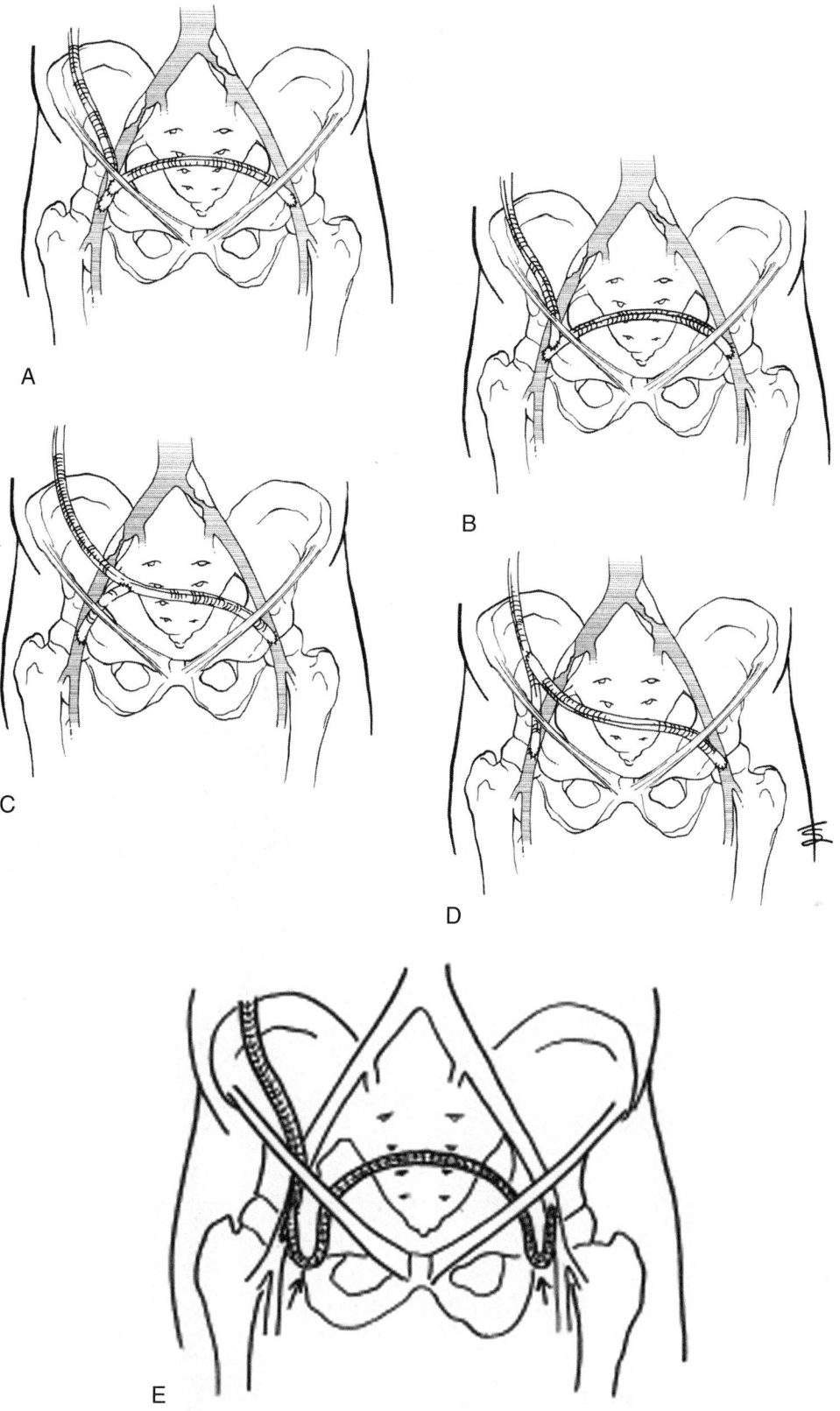

Figure 4 Standard outflow configurations for axillobifemoral grafts. **(A)** "C" Configuration: axillofemoral graft precedes femorofemoral graft (author's preference). **(B)** Alternate "C" configuration: femorofemoral graft precedes axillofemoral graft. **(C)** "Rutherford" configuration. **(D)** "Lazy S" configuration. **(E)** "Ram's Horn" configuration: stress is displaced from the anastomosis to the inferior curve of the graft *(arrows)*, reducing the risk of disruption (preferred in obese patients). Can be used with either the "C" or alternate "C" configuration.

anastomoses are created depends on the graft configuration chosen and the number of operators. It is advantageous to have two teams such that the anastomoses can be performed simultaneously, reducing operative and total anesthesia time.

RESULTS

The overall 5-year patency rates for axillobifemoral grafts, once as low as 30% to 40%, are now in the 60% to 80% range since the introduction of externally supported grafts. These external rings prevent compression on the grafts when patients lie on their sides. Although this effect has not been proven by direct comparison, externally supported grafts have been widely adopted on the basis of the theoretical advantages, outlined earlier. There does not appear to be any difference in externally supported Dacron versus PTFE. The actual patency rates achieved vary according to the indication for operation, patient selection, and extent of disease. Patients undergoing operation for infected abdominal grafts originally placed for aneurysmal disease and without occlusive disease can be expected to have better patency than patients for whom the grafts were placed for severe occlusive disease. Similarly, patients in whom grafts are placed for claudication can expect better patency than patients with rest pain or gangrene on the basis of less overall severe disease. Axillobifemoral grafts have better 5-year patency than axillounifemoral grafts, presumably because of the approximately double flow rate in the axillary limb of the bifemoral graft.

In the event of graft thrombosis, patency can frequently be reestablished with thrombectomy performed under local anesthesia. We prefer to perform these procedures under fluoroscopic guidance for several reasons. First, the chance of injury to the native vessels is reduced by preventing overdistention of the balloon thrombectomy catheters. Second, it allows the surgeon to identify and sometimes treat any underlying inflow or outflow lesions with an endovascular approach. Third, should a revision be required, angiogram defining the patient's anatomy can be obtained.

When comparing reports in the literature regarding axillofemoral bypass grafts, it is important to note that there is considerable variability in the technique used and the outcome measures defined, that is, primary versus secondary patency and whether various graft components are considered separately in patency calculations, for example, the axillofemoral and femorofemoral components counted as distinct grafts.

COMPLICATIONS

Potential complications of the procedure include the standard risks of bleeding and wound infection seen in all surgical procedures. The risk of graft infection is especially problematic because the majority of patients undergoing these procedures already have both limited reconstructive options and significant medical comorbidities. Another potential complication is injury to intrathoracic or intraabdominal organs during tunneling of the graft. Injury to the lung, colon, liver, or spleen can occur and may go initially undetected. As noted earlier, care must be taken to avoid injury to other neurovascular structures such as the axillary vein and brachial plexus.

CONCLUSIONS

Axillofemoral bypass is an important and valuable option in the treatment of patients with aortoiliac occlusive disease. For many reasons, it may be the preferred, and sometimes the only viable, option in patients with anatomic or medical comorbidities that preclude more standard treatments. Axillofemoral bypass can be performed with acceptable morbidity, mortality, and long-term results even in high-risk patients. For these reasons, surgeons should be familiar with the indications and application of this technique.

SUGGESTED READINGS

Johnson WC, Lee KK: Comparative evaluation of externally supported Dacron and polytetrafluoroethylene prosthetic bypasses for femoro-femoral and axillofemoral arterial reconstructions, *J Vasc Surg* 30:1077, 1999.

Landry GL, Moneta GL, Taylor LM Jr, and others: Axillofemoral bypass, *Ann Vasc Surg* 14:296, 2000.

Musicant SE, Giswold ME, Olson CJ, and others: Postoperative duplex scan surveillance of axillofemoral bypass grafts, *J Vasc Surg* 37:54, 2003.

Schneider JR, Golan JF: The role of extraanatomic bypass in the management of bilateral aortoiliac occlusive disease, *Sem Vasc Surg* 7:35–44, 1994.

Seeger JM, Preetus HA, Wellborn MB, and others: Long-term outcome after treatment of aortic graft infection with staged extra-anatomic bypass grafting and aortic graft removal, *J Vasc Surg* 32:451, 2000.

PERIPHERAL ARTERIAL OCCLUSIVE DISEASE: ANGIOPLASTY, STENTING, AND ENDOVASCULAR GRAFT TREATMENT

Juan Carlos Jimenez, MD, and Samuel S. Ahn, MD

Since the mid 1990s, the development of newer endovascular techniques has revolutionized the approach to treatment of peripheral arterial occlusive disease (PAOD) by vascular surgeons. Refinements in the development of percutaneous balloons, stents, and guidewires, coupled with increased training in endovascular techniques, have expanded the vascular surgeon's armamentarium for treating critical limb ischemia. Thus the demand for endovascular procedures to treat arterial disease continues to increase. Using data from a large national database over a 10-year period (1990–2000), Anderson and colleagues found that although there was a moderate decrease in the number of open surgical revascularizations for PAOD, this decline corresponded with a nearly 1000% increase in the number of catheter-based interventions over the same time period. At our institution, endovascular procedures have become the initial treatment of choice for most symptomatic peripheral arterial occlusive lesions, and we have noted a dramatic increase in the number of infrainguinal, percutaneous interventions coupled with high technical success and limb-salvage rates (Fig. 1). During this same time period, the number of open procedures has remained relatively constant and this traditional technique is being used to treat increasingly complex lesions and failures of endovascular therapy.

Despite improvements in risk-factor modification, PAOD currently affects approximately 5 million adults. According to census

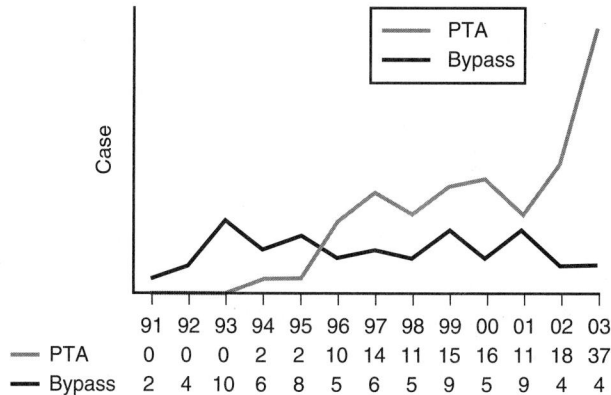

	91	92	93	94	95	96	97	98	99	00	01	02	03
— PTA	0	0	0	2	2	10	14	11	15	16	11	18	37
— Bypass	2	4	10	6	8	5	6	5	9	5	9	4	4

Figure I Number of endovascular versus open procedures over a 12-year period at the University of California at Los Angeles. A single surgeon's experience.

population projections, close to 7 million people aged 40 and older will have PAOD by 2020. This disease is common among elderly patients, affecting almost 10% of men by age 65 and 20% of men and women who are 75 years of age or older. At least one traditional cardiovascular disease risk factor—such as current smoking, diabetes, hypertension, and hypercholesterolemia—is present in 95% of persons with PAOD, and a particularly high prevalence is present among current smokers, diabetic patients, persons with renal insufficiency, and non-Hispanic African-Americans. Patients with low ankle-brachial pressure indices (ABI) demonstrate a significant, progressive decline in overall functional outcomes such as walking performance and velocity compared with patients who have normal ABI. Symptoms range from mild, lifestyle-limiting claudication to severe, limb-threatening ischemia. Proper diagnosis and treatment require an understanding of the arterial pathology, including anatomic disease patterns and physiologic considerations, knowledge regarding noninvasive and angiographic testing, and skill sets for both surgical revascularization and catheter-mediated therapies.

As patients have become more familiar with minimally invasive approaches for managing medical conditions, they often request that the less-invasive option be performed initially. The treating physician is therefore obligated to understand the issues pertinent to both open surgical and catheter-mediated therapies, including outcomes and specific, device-related techniques.

DIAGNOSTIC EVALUATION

Asymptomatic patients with nonpalpable pulses should be evaluated using noninvasive arterial testing to document the extent of disease and provide guidance and counseling. ABI; segmental arterial pressures of the thigh, calf, and ankle; toe plethysmography; and duplex arterial scans are usually obtained before treatment. Doppler ultrasound waveforms should also be evaluated in limbs with falsely increased ankle pressures caused by severe arterial calcification. All symptomatic patients presenting with claudication, rest pain, tissue loss, or gangrene should undergo noninvasive testing initially. Patients with renal insufficiency (creatinine > 1.5 mg/dl) may undergo magnetic resonance angiography with gadolinium enhancement to define the arterial anatomy before invasive testing. Computed tomographic angiography, another modality for three-dimensional reconstruction of the arterial anatomy, is usually not necessary before treatment of critical limb ischemia but may serve as an alternative diagnostic modality, especially with aortoiliac occlusive disease.

At our institution, we perform all invasive angiograms at the time of intended treatment through either an ipsilateral or contralateral femoral approach by using various sizes of introducer sheaths, ranging from

5- to 9-F. In cases in which contralateral femoral access is used, a Balkin sheath (Cook, Bloomington, IN) is introduced and positioned in the contralateral iliac artery for added stability. Heparin sodium is administered (100 U/kg) before crossing arterial lesions with a guidewire. Occlusions and stenoses are passed with a 0.014- to 0.035-inch hydrophilic guidewire. (Terumo Glidewire, Boston Scientific, Natick, MA). Percutaneous transluminal angioplasty (PTA) is performed with standard noncompliant angioplasty balloons (2–10 cm in length and 2–10 mm in diameter), selected to match the length of the lesion and the diameter of the artery. The balloon is generally inflated between 8 and 16 atm and is routinely and repeatedly inflated at the same segment two to four times. If the primary angioplasty resulted in residual stenosis, inflation is repeated with a balloon 1 mm larger than the previous one. Stents are placed if there is residual stenosis or flow-limiting dissection. Patients are usually placed on clopidrogel (Plavix; Bristol-Myers Squibb, New York, NY) following the procedure if there are no contraindications.

The technique of subintimal angioplasty is useful in clinical scenarios in which a complete intraluminal arterial occlusion is present. Using an angled hydrophilic wire and a 5-F KMP catheter (Cook), a dissection plane proximal to the occlusion between the intimal core and the adventitial layer of the arterial wall is purposely created and the lesion is traversed in the subintimal plane. After the wire tip is distal to the lesion, it is redirected back into the true lumen distally. The recanalized segment is then balloon dilatated to profile using an appropriately sized, noncompliant balloon catheter. Stenting is reserved for persistent flow-limiting stenosis and arterial dissection. Covered stent grafts are used, in rare cases, for perforation.

Aortoiliac Disease

Patients with aortoiliac occlusive disease present with buttock, thigh, and calf claudication that can be lifestyle limiting. Associated sexual dysfunction may also be seen in patients with atherosclerotic disease of one or both hypogastric arteries. Dilatational angioplasty in the iliac arteries was first introduced by Charles Dotter in the 1960s and has progressively supplanted aortobifemoral bypass as the initial treatment option for patients with iliac occlusive disease. At our institution, we perform angioplasty with selective stenting of iliac lesions that demonstrate residual stenosis (> 30%), a brachio-femoral pressure (> 5 mm Hg), or acute dissection. Although placement of intraluminal stents reduces the risk of immediate restenosis or obstructive plaque dissection, a tendency for in-stent hyperplasia may predispose to late reocclusion. In a review of our experience over 11 years, 151 iliac lesions in 104 patients were treated by PTA. According to TransAtlantic Inter-Society Consensus (TASC) classification, 26% were type A, 47% were type B, 24% were type C, and 3% were type D. Indications for treatment were disabling claudication (Society for Vascular Surgery clinical category 2 or 3) 50%, rest pain (category 4) 25%, and ulcer/gangrene (category 5), 25%. Twenty-three percent of patients required stent placement for primary PTA failure. The initial technical success rate was 99%. The cumulative primary patency rates at 1, 3, and 5 years were 76%, 59%, and 49%, respectively. The cumulative primary assisted and secondary patency rates at 7 years were 98% and 99%, respectively. Limb-salvage rates at 7 years were 93%. Thus although primary patency rates with iliac angioplasty were not high, assisted primary and secondary patency rates were excellent using selective stenting. TASC type C/D iliac lesions, a stenotic ipsilateral superficial femoral artery, ulcer/gangrene, smoking history, and chronic renal failure with hemodialysis were found to be significant independent predictors for adverse outcomes and thus should be considered indicators for primary stenting.

With the publication of the TASC consensus statement in 1999, classification of aortoiliac and femoral-popliteal lesions was stratified by lesion length and morphology (Tables 1 and 2). In general, for TASC-A lesions, initial endovascular treatment was

Table 1: TASC: Morphologic Stratification of Iliac Lesions

Classification	Lesion Morphology	Recommended Treatment
A	Single <3 cm stenosis of common iliac artery and/or external iliac artery	Endovascular
B	Single 3–10 cm stenosis, not extending into common femoral artery Two <5-cm stenoses in common iliac artery and/or external iliac artery Unilateral common iliac artery occlusion	Insufficient evidence
C	Unilateral external iliac artery stenosis or occlusion not extending into common femoral artery Bilateral common iliac artery occlusion	Insufficient evidence
D	Diffuse, multiple stenoses any iliac artery segment (>10 cm) Unilateral occlusion of both segments Bilateral external iliac artery occlusions Diffuse disease involving aorta and iliac arteries Associated aneurysmal or other disease requiring aortoiliac surgery	Open surgery

TASC, TransAtlantic Inter-Society Consensus.

Table 2: TASC: Morphologic Stratification of Femoropopliteal Lesions

Classification	Lesion Morphology	Recommended Treatment
A	Single <3 cm stenosis (unilateral or bilateral)	Endovascular
B	Single 3–5 cm stenosis not involving the popliteal artery Heavily calcified stenosis up to 3 cm in length Multiple lesions each <3 cm (stenoses or occlusions) Single or multiple lesions, in the absence of tibial runoff to improve inflow for infrageniculate bypass	Insufficient evidence
C	Single stenosis or occlusion >5 cm, not involving popliteal artery Multiple stenoses or occlusion, each 3–5 cm	Insufficient evidence
D	Complete occlusion of the common femoral artery or superficial femoral artery or popliteal + proximal crural arteries	Open surgery

TASC, TransAtlantic Inter-Society Consensus.

strongly recommended and, likewise, for TASC-D lesions, open reconstruction was recommended. In recent years, however, several authors have published increasingly high patency and limb-salvage rates using endovascular techniques, even for complex TASC-D lesions. These results have been mirrored at our institution as well. Leville and colleagues reviewed results of 89 consecutive patients with symptomatic iliac occlusions at the Cleveland Clinic and noted an 86% initial technical success rate for TASC-D lesions. Technical failure was defined as the inability to completely cross the occluded segment or reenter the native artery distally following intraplaque or subintimal passage of a hydrophilic wire. Primary patency for the entire cohort was 76% and did not vary with TASC stratification. Secondary patency for TASC-D lesions was 83% and, likewise, not statistically different from TASC-A, -B, and -C lesions. The limb-salvage rate was 95% for all patients with TASC-D lesions. With improving technology, the results for PTA and stenting of iliac lesions continue to improve. Despite TASC classification and its recommendations, even the most complex iliac lesions may be amenable to endovascular treatment.

Femoropopliteal Disease

Occlusive disease of the femoropopliteal segment occurs most commonly at the adductor canal where the superficial femoral artery passes into the popliteal fossa. Common symptoms include calf claudication, which limits walking distance and is relieved at rest. Patients with mild claudication are at low risk for limb loss and have been traditionally treated with a conservative program of walking, smoking cessation, and antiplatelet medications such as cilastozol. Mild claudication usually requires no interventional treatment. Patients with severe, lifestyle limiting claudication, rest pain, or tissue loss are candidates for interventional treatment, as are patients who have persistent claudication despite medical management. Advantages of endovascular therapy for femoropopliteal arterial occlusive disease include patient preference for a minimally invasive procedure, a lack of autogenous conduit, multiple comorbidities that place the patient at high risk for open surgery, or infection at the proposed site of bypass. In addition, failure of endovascular treatment does not necessarily negate the ability to proceed with open bypass.

The TASC classifications for lesions in the femoropopliteal segment are shown (Table 1). Traditionally, the use of routine stenting in the superficial femoral has not been supported by randomized trials. However, emerging stent design and technology have continued to evolve rapidly, and the benefits of stents in the superficial femoral artery (SFA) remain controversial. Surowiec and colleagues reviewed the results of 380 total limbs in 329 patients treated with PTA with and without stenting of the superficial femoral artery over an 18-year period. TASC lesion grades were A (48%), B (18%), C (22%), and D (12%). Sixty-three percent of lesions were treated with angioplasty alone. Primary technical success rate was 93%, and there was one periprocedural death. Primary patency rates were 86% at 3 months and 52% at 60 months. Statistically, higher preoperative ABI and angioplasty alone without stenting were associated with higher patency. Primary patency rates in this series were highly dependent on TASC classification, whereby TASC-A and -B lesions compared favorably with prosthetic and venous femoropopliteal bypass. Surgical bypass was superior to PTA and stenting for TASC-C and -D lesions.

This finding has been disputed by other series. In their review of 95 patients who underwent angioplasty-based infrainguinal percutaneous interventions at the Massachusetts General Hospital, Black and associates found that increasing complexity of femoropopliteal lesions was not a reliable predictor of PTA failure. Mean follow-up was 14 months. Although there was no statistical difference in patency results between TASC-A and -B lesions compared with TASC-C and -D lesions, the presence of two or more runoff vessels below the knee was a strong predictor of vessel patency. In our own experience, we have noted high limb-salvage rates (93%) at 3 years following femoropopliteal angioplasty with selective stenting for critical limb ischemia, despite a relatively low primary patency of approximately 50%. Stenting was limited to lesions that did not respond to balloon dilatation secondary to elastic recoil, arterial dissection, or both. Thus we advocate that in patients with claudication refractory to conservative management, nonhealing wounds or rest pain, if intraluminal guidewire access across the lesion is safely possible, balloon angioplasty should be the initial treatment of choice. Surgical bypass should be reserved for treatment failures.

Tibioperoneal Disease

Historically, primary amputation was the sole alternative in high-risk patients with nonhealing wounds who were not candidates for surgical bypass because of severe tibioperoneal occlusive disease. The advent of aggressive endovascular management for arterial occlusive disease below the knee has shifted this paradigm, and we are observing improved limb-salvage rates for even the most complex below-knee lesions. Since the mid 1990s at our institution, more aggressive treatment of tibial lesions has been instituted, including extension of treatment toward more distal, diffuse lesions and complete occlusions. Routine duplex ultrasonography is obtained in our vascular ultrasound lab, and changes in flow velocities are carefully measured. Distal below-knee lesions are identified following runoff angiography. Heparin sodium is routinely administered (100 U/kg) before crossing arterial lesions with a guidewire. A 0.14- or 0.18-cm guidewire is typically used to traverse the arterial lesion, and exchange length (260–300 cm) wires are usually required, especially if arterial access is obtained through the contralateral femoral or brachial arteries. The most distal lesions are treated initially with progression to proximal lesions if indicated. Successful angioplasty is usually accomplished using a 2- to 4-mm noncompliant balloon of 2 to 10 cm in length selected to match the length of the lesion and the diameter of the artery. The use of subintimal angioplasty is often required at this level for complete intraluminal occlusions.

Although no randomized trials comparing tibial angioplasty to surgical bypass for critical limb ischemia are present in the literature, retrospective series have noted excellent primary technical success and limb-salvage rates. Dorros and colleagues observed a clinical success rate (defined as relief of rest pain or improvement of lower extremity blood flow) of 95% in 270 limbs that underwent tibioperoneal vessel angioplasty for limb-threatening ischemia. Clinical 5-year follow-up demonstrated that only 8% of patients required surgical bypass and only 9% of patients required significant amputation. The limb-salvage rate in this cohort was 91%. Three years later, Tefera and colleagues reviewed the results of tibial angioplasty performed in patients deemed poor surgical candidates secondary to absence of distal target vessels, the presence of severe comorbid conditions (i.e., recent myocardial infarction, symptomatic coronary artery disease, renal insufficiency, or chronic obstructive pulmonary disease), or lack of autogenous vein for distal bypass. The technical success rate was 82.5%, and the major amputation rate was 19.3% at 33-month follow-up. In a 10-year review of our experience at University of California at Los Angeles with tibioperoneal angioplasty, our limb-salvage rate at 3 years was 77.3% despite poor primary

patency rates (23.5%). Fifty-one percent of patients demonstrated continued clinical improvement at 3 years, and low complication rates (2%) were observed. Significant risk factors for adverse outcomes included hypertension, multiple segment lesions, more distal lesions, and TASC-D lesions. A possible explanation for low amputation rates in the face of poor primary patency may be that the improved perfusion is necessary early postprocedure, resulting in enhanced wound healing. However, skin integrity can remain despite vessel reocclusion. Another possibility is that slow restenosis of treated arteries allows collateral circulation to form. The importance of strict, long-term follow-up in these patients cannot be understated. Routine follow-up at our institution includes a postoperative visit at 1 to 2 weeks; every-3-month visits for the first postoperative year, and every-6-month visits thereafter. ABI or duplex ultrasound examinations (or both) are performed at each follow-up visit. Recurrent stenosis greater than 60% by duplex ultrasound or persistent symptoms are indications for repeat intervention.

NEW DEVELOPMENTS

Several new devices for endovascular management of peripheral arterial occlusive disease have shown early promise despite a lack of evidence validating their efficacy. Cutting balloon angioplasty involves inflation of a noncompliant balloon equipped with three to four atherotomes or microsurgical blades positioned longitudinally on its surface. The radial direction of the blades creates incisions within the atheromatous plaque, which is subsequently dilatated with inflation of the balloon. This mechanism has been associated with enhanced cross-sectional plaque reduction, decreased elastic vessel recoil, and barotraumas compared with conventional angioplasty. Technical success and limb-salvage rates have compared favorably with traditional balloon angioplasty and bypass rates despite the lack of level I evidence justifying its use over conventional techniques. Disadvantages include vessel rupture and need for larger introducer sheaths to accommodate the atherotomes located on the balloon surface.

Cryoplasty (PolarCath Peripheral Dilatation System, Boston Scientific) is a method that allows for simultaneous angioplasty and cooling of the atheromatous plaque and is believed to decrease the rate of neointimal proliferation largely through the induction of cellular apoptosis. The saline and radiopaque contrast medium used to inflate conventional angioplasty balloons is replaced with nitrous oxide, which dilatates and cools the balloon. Advocates of this technique have demonstrated less arterial dissection, reduced vessel wall recoil because of freeze-induced alteration of elastin fibers, and reduced neointima formation. In a review of 70 patients treated with femoropopliteal cryoplasty for symptoms of intermittent claudication, the clinical patency rate was 83.2% and 75% at 300 days and 3 years, respectively. Further long-term studies are necessary to justify efficacy and cost-effectiveness.

Excimer laser-assisted angioplasty (Spectranetics, Colorado Springs, CO) involves the application of light energy directly to the arterial plaque in short pulse durations, allowing penetration depth of 50 umol/ml and improving the ability to maneuver guidewires across complex lesions and complete occlusions. Thus balloon angioplasty for generally inaccessible lesions can be achieved. Although technical success and long-term patency rates compare favorably with historical angioplasty data, further studies are necessary to analyze long-term patency rates.

Newer-generation percutaneous directional atherectomy catheters such as the Silverhawk Plaque Excision System (Foxhollow, Redwood City, CA) facilitate removal of intraluminal atheromatous plaque from the arterial wall using small rotating blades housed within a catheter, which is passed repeatedly through the lesion. Atherosclerotic remnants are collected within a nosecone reservoir, which can be removed and cleaned before subsequent plaque removal. Although short-term patency rates and safety have been favorable in limited retrospective studies, long-term patency and limb salvage rates are unknown.

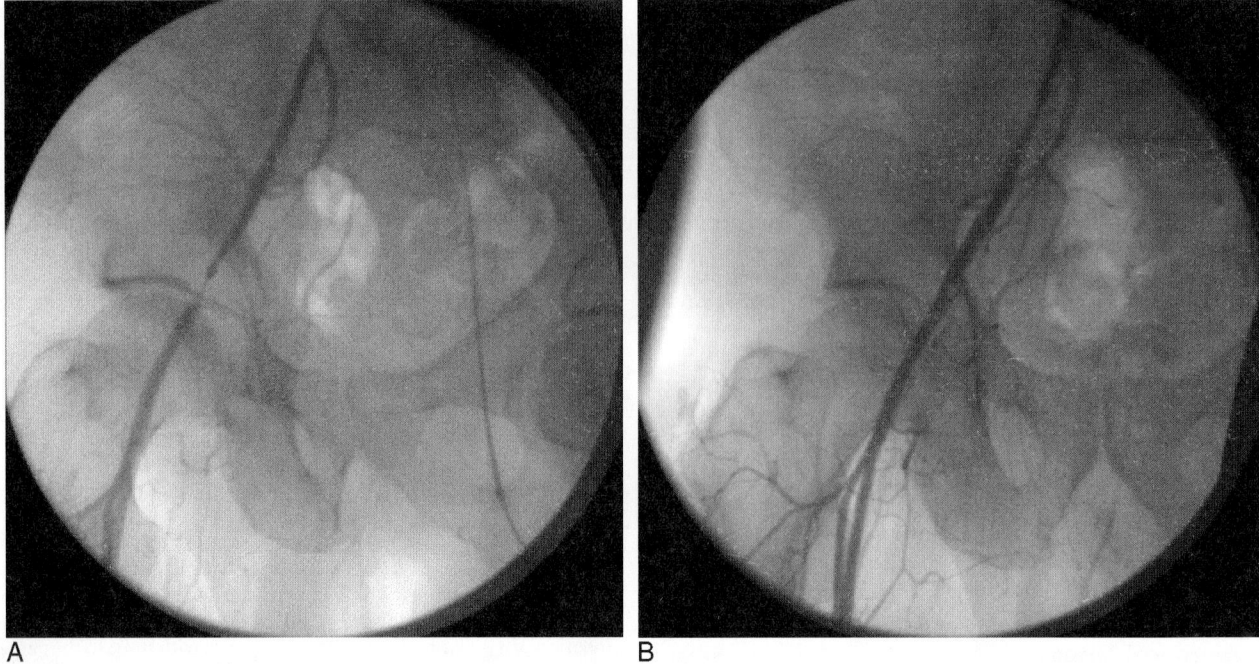

Figure 2   Angioplasty of severe stenosis of left external iliac artery.

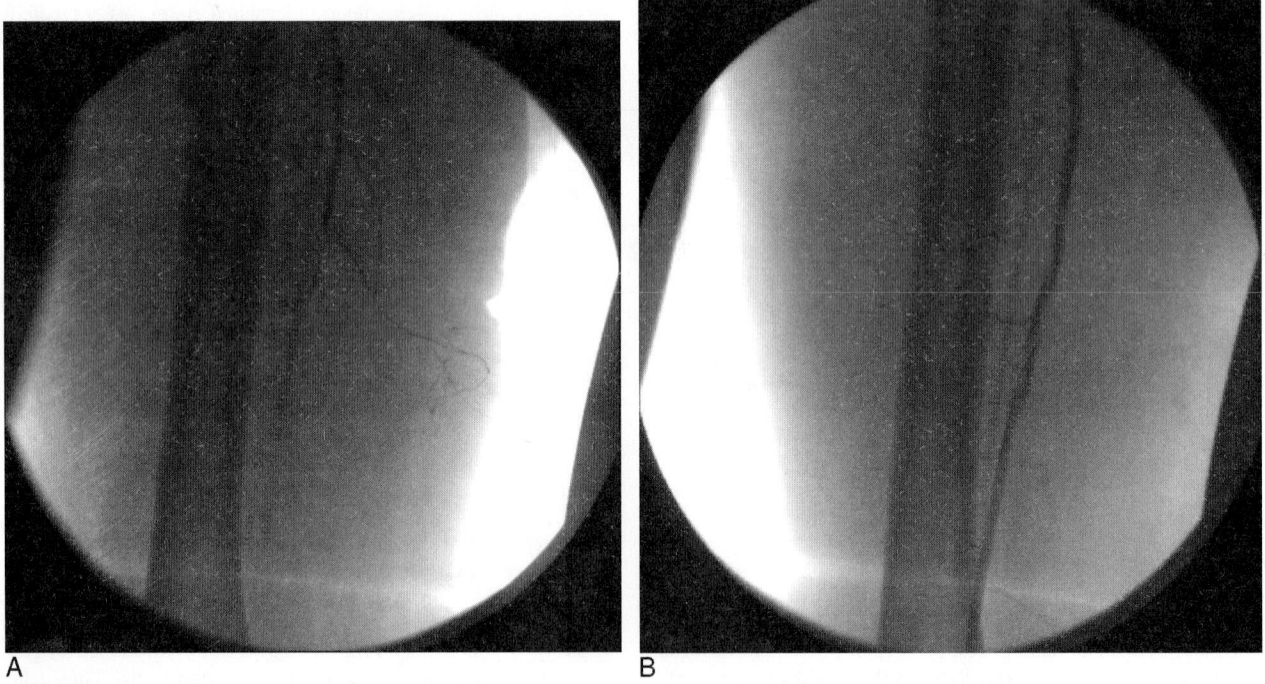

Figure 3   Subintimal angioplasty of complete occlusion of superficial femoral artery yields an excellent technical result.

Suggested Readings

Anderson PL, Gelijns A, Moskowitz A, and others: Understanding trends in inpatient surgical volume: vascular interventions, 1980–2000, *J Vasc Surg* 39:1200, 2004.

Black JH 3rd, LaMuraglia GM, Kwolek CJ, and others: Contemporary results of angioplasty-based infrainguinal percutaneous interventions, *J Vasc Surg* 42:932, 2005.

Dorros G, Jaff MR, Dorros AM, and others: Tibioperoneal (outflow lesion) angioplasty can be used as primary treatment in 235 patients with critical limb ischemia: five-year follow-up, *Circulation* 104:2057, 2001.

Kudo T, Ahn SS: Long-term outcomes and predictors of iliac angioplasty with selective stenting, *J Vasc Surg* 42:466.e1, 2005.

Kudo T, Chandra FA, Ahn SS: The effectiveness of percutaneous transluminal angioplasty for the treatment of critical limb ischemia: a 10-year experience, *J Vasc Surg* 41:423, 2005.

Leville CD, Kashyap VS, Clair DG, and others: Endovascular management of iliac artery occlusions: extending treatment to TransAtlantic Inter-Society Consensus class C and D patients, *J Vasc Surg* 43:32, 2006.

Ruef J, Hofmann M, Haase J, and others: Endovascular interventions in iliac and infrainguinal occlusive artery disease, *J Interven Cardiol* 17:427, 2004.

Selvin E, Erlinger TP: Prevalence of and risk factors for peripheral arterial disease in the United States: results from the national health and nutrition examination survey, 1999–2000, *Circulation* 110:738, 2004.

Surowiec SM, Davies MG, Eberly SW, and others: Percutaneous angioplasty and stenting of the superficial femoral artery, *J Vasc Surg* 41:269, 2005.

Treiman GS, Treiman R, Whiting J: Results of percutaneous subintimal angioplasty using routine stenting, 43:513, 2006.

Treiman GS, Whiting JH, Treiman RL, and others: Treatment of limb-threatening ischemia with percutaneous intentional extraluminal recanalization: a preliminary evaluation, *J Vasc Surg* 38:29, 2003.

Upper Extremity Arterial Occlusive Disease

Alexander D. Shepard, MD, and Robert R. Slater, MD

Upper-extremity arterial occlusive disease is much less common than its lower-extremity counterpart. The causes of upper-extremity ischemia are diverse, ranging from vasospasm to autoimmune disease. Because of extensive collateral channels around the shoulder and elbow, many patients remain asymptomatic despite significant lesions. However, when ischemic symptoms of the hands and digits do manifest, the loss of function can lead to significant disability and limitation. Given these factors, the diagnosis and treatment of upper-extremity ischemia can be significantly more complex than the management of lower-extremity ischemia.

ETIOLOGY

The causes of upper-extremity ischemia are diverse. Table 1 offers a broad, conceptual categorization that is far from exhaustive. The most common cause is vasospasm, but this is rarely severe and is almost always managed medically (see chapter on Raynaud's syndrome). Large-artery vasospasm is rare but can be caused by ergot poisoning, most often from migraine medications containing ergotamine (Fig. 1).

Intrinsic Arterial Disease

Atherosclerosis can affect the upper-extremity vasculature but is usually limited to the more proximal brachiocephalic arteries. The origin of the left subclavian artery is the most frequently involved segment. Prior radiation, most commonly for lymphoma or lung/breast cancer, can accelerate this process. Involvement of the distal extremity vasculature occurs in patients with end-stage renal disease, of which a particularly virulent form, azotemic arteriopathy, can lead to critical limb ischemia.

A number of inflammatory diseases can affect the upper extremity arteries. Connective-tissue disorders such as scleroderma, CREST (calcinosis, Raynaud phenomenon, esophageal dysmotility, sclerodactyly, and telangiectasia) syndrome, lupus, and rheumatoid arthritis are frequently associated with small-artery occlusive disease, affecting the palmar and digital arteries (Fig. 2). A similar small-vessel disease pattern can be seen with a variety of relatively rare medical disorders (e.g., cryoglobulinemia or hepatitis-associated vasculitis), which should be looked for only after connective-tissue diseases have been excluded. In the absence of an

Table 1: Causes of Upper-Extremity Ischemia

Vasospasm

Raynaud's disease

Ergot poisoning

Medication induced—beta-blockers, vasopressors

Intrinsic Arterial Disease

Atherosclerosis (innominate-subclavian)

Radiation arteritis (innominate-axillosubclavian)

Azotemic arteriopathy (radial/ulnar, palmar, digital)

Inflammatory Diseases

Connective tissue disorders (palmar/digital)

Hypersensitivity angiitis (palmar/digital)

Thromboangiitis obliterans (Buerger's disease) (radial/ulnar, palmar, digital)

Takayasu's arteritis (innominate, subclavian)

Temporal arteritis (axillobrachial)

Medical Diseases (Palmar and Digital Arteries)

Thrombophilic states

Myeloproliferative disorders

Cold injury

Hepatitis-associated vasculitis

Cryoglobulinemia

Vinyl chloride exposure

Embolism

Cardiac (brachial)

Arterial source

    Thoracic outlet syndrome (subclavian is source)

    Peripheral aneurysm

    Atheroembolism

Trauma

Blunt/penetrating trauma

Iatrogenic—catheter-associated

    Cardiac catheterization (distal brachial)

    Diagnostic arteriography (proximal brachial)

    Arterial monitoring lines (radial, brachial)

Hypothenar hammer syndrome (ulnar)

Vibration (palmar/digital)

Sports/athletic injury (axillosubclavian)

Arteries most commonly involved in the disease process are listed in parentheses.

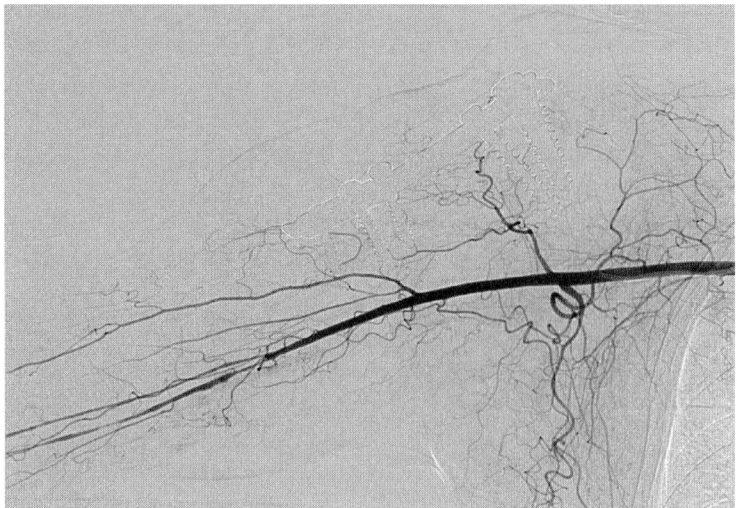

Figure 1 Right upper-extremity angiogram of a 65-year-old woman who developed acute ischemic symptoms in her right hand. Careful questioning revealed a long-standing history of migraine headaches, which the patient treated with daily doses of an ergotamine formulation. Note the profound vasoconstriction of the proximal brachial and deep brachial arteries.

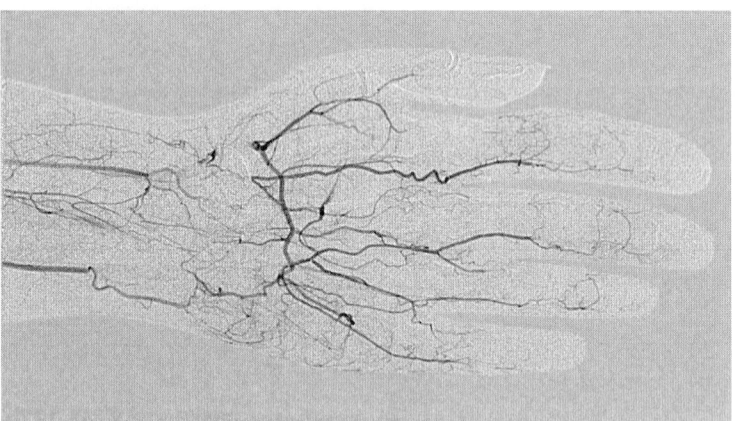

Figure 2 Left-hand angiogram of a patient with scleroderma and small-artery occlusive disease, producing multiple occlusions of the distal forearm, palmar, and digital arteries. The patient presented with severe Raynaud's syndrome and nonhealing fingertip ulcerations.

identifiable cause, which occurs in approximately one third of cases, such small-artery occlusive disease is termed *hypersensitivity angiitis.*

Thromboangiitis obliterans, or Buerger's disease, is a segmental, inflammatory, obliterative disease of the medium and small arteries of the extremities seen in heavy smokers (see chapter on Buerger's disease). It frequently affects the forearm and palmar/digital arteries, with sparing of the more proximal arteries. Takayasu's disease and temporal arteritis are large-vessel vasculitides that can affect the proximal upper-extremity vasculature. Both are frequently associated with an initial inflammatory stage (myalgias, arthralgias, elevated erythrocyte sedimentation rate) and produce characteristic smooth, tapering stenoses (Fig. 3). Takayasu's disease affects young women and usually involves the innominate, subclavian, and proximal axillary arteries. Temporal arteritis, on the other hand, is a disease of women older than age 60 that usually affects the branches of the external carotid artery. Although the subclavian and axillary arteries can be affected by temporal arteritis, the most common site of upper-extremity involvement is the proximal brachial artery. We have seen two patients since the mid 1990s with temporal arteritis, the primary presentation of which was upper-extremity ischemia.

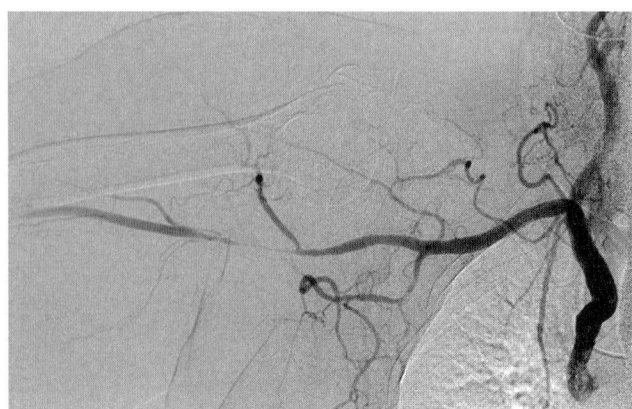

Figure 3 Right upper-extremity angiogram of a 57-year-old woman with temporal arteritis showing a classic, smooth, tapering stenosis in the proximal brachial artery. The patient's primary presenting complaint was forearm effort fatigue.

Embolism

Twenty percent of all emboli involve the upper extremities. Most cardiac emboli lodge in the brachial artery, either at its bifurcation into the ulnar/radial or just proximal to the takeoff of the deep brachial artery. Emboli usually present as acute episodes of forearm/hand ischemia in patients with an underlying cardiac condition but may present more chronically in elderly or debilitated patients who do not use their upper extremities enough to induce symptoms. Most distal arterial emboli (palmar/digital) are usually due to an arterial source. The most common lesion is an aneurysm or ulcerative lesion within the subclavian artery associated with thoracic outlet syndrome (see chapter on thoracic outlet syndrome). In this situation, repetitive compression of the subclavian artery by anomalous myofascial bands attached to a cervical rib (or other osseous anomaly) leads to a focal stenosis. Poststenotic dilatation/aneurysm and/or intimal ulceration result in mural thrombus formation. Subsequent embolization of luminal debris can produce both large and small artery occlusions distally. Unilateral Raynaud's syndrome is a common presentation. Degenerative aneurysms of the subclavian artery or posttraumatic aneurysms of other upper-extremity arteries (e.g., crutch-induced axillary artery aneurysms) are other rare causes of ischemia and produce symptoms either through distal emboli or, less commonly, by in situ thrombosis. Ulcerative atherosclerotic plaques within the aorta or proximal brachiocephalic arteries can also, rarely, lead to emboli.

Trauma

Undiagnosed or neglected arterial injuries are a well-recognized cause of upper-extremity occlusive disease. Although bleeding and significant ischemia are obvious manifestations of arterial injury requiring treatment in the acute setting, intimal injuries from both penetrating and blunt trauma may lead to arterial thrombosis with less dramatic symptomatology. Iatrogenic injuries are particularly common. Brachial artery injuries are a well-recognized complication of cardiac catheterization procedures performed via this approach. Such occlusions may go undetected in the acute setting because of the abundant collaterals around the elbow. The only manifestation may be the development of effort fatigue in the forearm on resumption of normal activities.

Cumulative occupational trauma can also lead to significant vascular injury. Hypothenar hammer syndrome results from repetitive blunt trauma to the terminal portion of the ulnar artery in Guyon's tunnel (formed by the pisiform, the hook of the hamate, and the transverse carpal ligament in the proximal palm). This injury is caused by repetitively striking objects with the base of the palm. Segmental occlusion or aneurysm formation of the ulnar artery, with or without distal digital artery embolism, can result. Vibration-induced injury to the digital arteries occurs after prolonged exposure of the hands to vibratory tools or machinery. The tools most commonly implicated are pneumatic tools and chainsaws. Patients initially present with neurologic complaints (i.e., numbness or paresthesias) in the affected hand and digits. As the syndrome progresses, Raynaud's phenomenon develops. Tissue loss is rare. Sports-related trauma is a rare cause of ischemia but can occur in individuals who use an upper extremity with a fixed repetitive motion in competitive athletic endeavors. Axillary and subclavian artery injuries in baseball pitchers are the most frequently encountered.

▋ EVALUATION

Given the diverse etiologies of upper-extremity vascular disease, a thorough history and careful physical examination are critical to accurate diagnosis. Presenting symptoms can range from color changes, coolness, numbness, weakness, or effort-induced fatigue (claudication) to rest pain and tissue loss. Raynaud's syndrome can result from pure vasospasm but is also a frequent manifestation of fixed occlusive lesions. The classic tricolor digital changes (white to blue to red—pallor to cyanosis to hyperemic rubor) in response to cold or emotional stress are uncommon. Most patients note only one or two of the three phases. Exercise-induced fatigue in the arm musculature is usually due to large-vessel disease, whereas symptoms in the hand or digits may be due to large-vessel disease, small-vessel disease, or a combination. Digital tissue loss is nearly always associated with small-artery occlusive disease with or without more proximal involvement. Concomitant posterior cerebral circulation symptoms (e.g., dizziness, ataxia, diplopia) should be sought and, if present, suggest involvement of the subclavian or innominate artery, proximal to the takeoff of the vertebral artery. Bilateral upper-extremity symptoms suggest the presence of a systemic cause, such as a connective tissue disease, whereas unilateral complaints often indicate localized arterial pathology (e.g., arterial thoracic outlet syndrome).

Atherosclerotic risk factors, including dyslipidemia, diabetes, smoking, family history, and renal failure, must be catalogued. Symptoms suggestive of atherosclerotic disease involving other tissue beds (e.g., coronary artery disease or lower-extremity occlusive disease) should be elicited. Patients should also be questioned about possible underlying connective-tissue disorders or associated symptoms—tight skin or dysphagia in scleroderma, facial rash in lupus, or joint complaints in rheumatoid arthritis. Past medical history should also address the presence of possible hypercoagulable states, renal insufficiency, cardiac arrhythmias/disorders, or drug abuse. A history of surgical or catheter-based procedures in the upper extremity should be sought. A prior vascular access graft may hint at steal syndrome, graft thrombosis, or azotemic arteriopathy. Any antecedent trauma to the neck or upper extremity should be identified and specific injuries noted. Details concerning medication history, occupational or environmental exposures, and athletic activities may also be important. The family history should focus on connective-tissue disorders, hypercoagulable states, and premature atherosclerotic disease.

A complete pulse examination of the neck and upper extremities is essential and remains the primary modality for diagnosing upper-extremity occlusive disease. The superficial temporal, carotid, subclavian, axillary, brachial, radial, and ulnar pulses should be carefully examined. A decreased or absent pulse indicates a proximal high-grade stenosis or occlusion. A normal pulse does not completely exclude proximal disease, particularly in the setting of a chronic occlusion, because of the rich collateral pathways present in the upper extremity. An irregular pulse should prompt a more detailed cardiac examination to identify atrial fibrillation or other arrhythmias that may predispose to cardioembolism. Supraclavicular tenderness may be present in patients with thoracic outlet syndrome. Auscultation for bruits over all major arteries should be performed. The skin envelope of the digits is examined for signs of color or temperature difference, tissue loss, or trophic changes. In patients with unilateral complaints, the asymptomatic extremity should be carefully examined for occult disease. Allen's test to identify patency of the palmar arch is helpful in patients with digital ischemia. A number of provocative tests (e.g., Adson's maneuver) have been suggested for diagnosing arterial thoracic outlet syndrome but are of limited usefulness secondary to their high false-positive rates.

Noninvasive Vascular Assessment

All patients with ischemic symptoms should undergo bilateral upper-extremity segmental pressure testing. Such testing provides objective, reproducible data to identify fixed obstructions or inducible vasospasm and to determine the degree of associated ischemia. Serial examinations can assess disease progression and evaluate the effectiveness of therapeutic interventions. Bilateral brachial, upper forearm, and wrist systolic pressures are obtained along with associated waveforms. The normal pressure differential between arms should not exceed 15 mm Hg, and a pressure drop of 20 mm Hg or more between levels indicates an intervening hemodynamically significant lesion. Reduced brachial pressures bilaterally, particularly when associated with blunted or monophasic waveforms, should prompt thigh pressure measurements to exclude the possibility of bilateral proximal disease. Although digital pressures and waveforms are notoriously temperature dependent, they can be extremely helpful in documenting the presence of small-artery occlusive disease or vasospasm. An absolute digital pressure less than 70 mm Hg, a wrist/digital gradient over 30 mm Hg, or an interdigital gradient over 15 mm Hg are all considered abnormal. The finding of normal or near-normal digital pressures with vasospastic waveforms is helpful in establishing a diagnosis of Raynaud's syndrome. Duplex scanning can provide even more information than segmental pressures but has limited utility proximally because of the bony structures of the thoracic outlet. We have found it most useful when dealing with suspected lesions in the axillary, brachial, and forearm arteries.

Angiography

Angiography remains the mainstay for diagnosis of upper-extremity arterial diseases but is usually reserved for patients with critical limb ischemia or debilitating symptoms with evidence of proximal disease amenable to intervention. Biplanar arch aortography is necessary to rule out brachiocephalic disease. Selective studies of both upper extremities should be obtained because many disease processes affect both arms. Digital subtraction technology helps to minimize the radiocontrast load. Concomitant administration of vasodilators, such as tolazoline or nitroglycerin, is frequently necessary to adequately visualize the arteries of the hand and fingers. Magnetic resonance angiography (MRA), although helpful in patients with renal insufficiency, frequently lacks sufficient detail to be diagnostic. Computed tomography angiography (CTA) is useful for imaging the aorta and large proximal arteries but does not currently provide enough detail of the distal vasculature to be of use when disease of these segments is suspected. Despite advances in the resolution of MRA and CTA, contrast angiography remains the gold standard and, with the proliferation of endoluminal techniques, can offer the opportunity for simultaneous intervention.

Laboratory Testing

Specific laboratory studies are obtained on the basis of the index of suspicion and are most useful when dealing with distal small-artery occlusive disease. Routine chemistries, blood counts, and coagulation profiles should be drawn when the diagnosis is unclear. If a hypercoagulable state is considered, patients should be checked for factor V Leiden, antithrombin III deficiency, protein C and S deficiencies, antiphospholipid antibodies, the prothrombin gene mutation, and hyperhomocystinemia. Testing for connective-tissue disorders should include rheumatoid factor, antinuclear antibodies, complement levels, and a sedimentation rate (arteritis). Additional tests looking for cryoglobulinemia, hepatitis, or myeloproliferative disorders may be helpful if the other, more common causes of small-artery occlusive disease have been excluded. When a cardioembolic source is suspected, electrocardiography is obtained to document the presence of an arrhythmia. Similarly, plain films of the neck looking for a cervical rib are useful to exclude most thoracic outlet problems.

MANAGEMENT

Appropriate treatment of upper-extremity occlusive disease depends on the etiology. Operative intervention is neither indicated nor helpful for many of the causes of upper-extremity ischemia. With occasional exceptions, revascularization is reserved for patients with critical ischemia (tissue loss or rest pain) or debilitating symptoms (effort fatigue) secondary to large- or medium-vessel occlusions. Single-level, large-artery atherosclerotic disease, most commonly a short-segment proximal subclavian stenosis or occlusion, is frequently associated with minimal symptomatology and is best managed with risk factor modification. On the other hand, embolic and traumatic occlusions should usually be treated when diagnosed, regardless of symptom and perfusion status, because of their frequent and unpredictable progression to significant symptomatology. Regardless of the indication, increased care is necessary when operating on the upper-extremity vasculature. Because of a size similarity, there is a tendency to treat the axillary and subclavian arteries like the common femoral artery. Proximal upper-extremity arteries, however, lack the thick muscular layer of the femoral artery and are easily torn if handled roughly. The forearm arteries are also problematic because of their extreme vasoreactivity. Avoidance of excessive manipulation is critical.

Operative reconstruction is most useful for treating atherosclerotic occlusive disease of the proximal arteries. Bypass is the most common technique because the overwhelming majority of lesions are not amenable to endarterectomy. Intrathoracic procedures to treat innominate and subclavian artery occlusive disease are covered in the chapter on brachiocephalic reconstruction.

Subclavian Artery

The most frequently performed procedures for proximal subclavian disease are carotid subclavian bypass and subclavian transposition. Although bypass is technically simpler, we prefer transposition whenever feasible because of its superior long-term patency. Both procedures require preoperative confirmation that the common carotid artery is disease free. The patient is placed on the operating table in a semi-Fowler's position, with the head of the table elevated 20 to 30 degrees. A roll is placed under the shoulders to allow for extension of the neck, and the head is rotated slightly away from the operative side. A transverse incision is made approximately one fingerbreadth (2 cm) above the clavicle, extending from the sternoclavicular joint to the midportion of the clavicle. Subcutaneous tissues and platysma are divided, and the clavicular head of the sternocleidomastoid is transected. The underlying uscalene fat pad is mobilized superiorly, exposing the anterior scalene muscle. We do not routinely ligate the thoracic duct or right lymphatic duct if encountered unless they are injured. The phrenic nerve is identified (coursing lateral-to-medial along the surface of the anterior scalene) and carefully mobilized and retracted to allow division of the anterior scalene from its tubercle on the first rib. Care is taken not to injure the underlying subclavian artery and adjacent brachial plexus. The subclavian artery can then be dissected free. If a bypass is planned, only a short segment (4–5 cm) of the artery just distal to the thyrocervical trunk must be mobilized. Small branches can and should be ligated to improve exposure. As previously outlined, care should be taken when retracting the subclavian artery to avoid inadvertent injury.

Exposure of the carotid artery is accomplished through the medial portion of the incision. Injury to the vagus nerve and internal jugular vein is avoided by retracting them laterally. If exposure of the carotid bifurcation is necessary (e.g., for concomitant endarterectomy), a separate incision can be made along the medial border of the sternocleidomastoid. For both bypass and transposition, we create a tunnel posterior to the internal jugular vein. Systemic heparin is administered, and a 4- to 5-cm segment of the common carotid artery is clamped proximally and distally. Electroencephalographic monitoring is not routinely used. A short, vertical arteriotomy is made along the lateral wall of the carotid. A 7- to 8-mm prosthetic graft or a large-caliber saphenous vein graft is anastomosed to the carotid in an end-to-side fashion with running 5-0 cardiovascular sutures. Although there is limited evidence in the literature that prosthetic grafts have superior patency in this position compared with saphenous vein, our experience suggests that vein may actually be slightly better, as long as it is of adequate caliber. The proximal end of the graft should be transected with a 20- to 30-degree bevel to promote a slightly downward course to the graft. Following appropriate venting and restoration of carotid flow, the graft is tunneled laterally. The subclavian artery is next clamped proximally and distally, and a short longitudinal arteriotomy is made along the superior surface of the artery at the highest point of its arc above the clavicle. An end-to-side anastomosis is then constructed with a 5-0 suture.

Transposition is a more complicated procedure than bypass and is not suitable for a subclavian artery with plaque extending more than a few centimeters beyond its origin. Transposition requires mobilization of the subclavian artery as far proximally as possible. Small branches are divided, but an effort should be made to preserve the vertebral and internal mammary arteries. To minimize the risk of embolization, the distal subclavian, vertebral, and internal mammary arteries are clamped before ligating the proximal subclavian artery. The subclavian is transected proximally, tunneled posterior to the jugular, and anastomosed in end-to-side fashion to the carotid artery as described previously for bypass. If additional mobilization of the subclavian artery is required to avoid kinking, it may be necessary to divide the internal mammary branch. Flow is restored after appropriate venting.

Both carotid subclavian bypass and subclavian transposition have low morbidity and excellent long-term patency (75%–80% at 5 years for bypass and almost 100% for transposition). Complications include injury to adjacent nerves (brachial plexus, phrenic nerve, and sympathetic chain) and lymphatic structures (thoracic and accessory thoracic ducts). Nerve injuries are usually self-limited. Lymphatic injuries can be problematic and, if drainage is significant or persistent, are best treated by reexploration and thoracic duct ligation.

Endoluminal therapy is being used with increasing frequency for proximal subclavian disease in patients with significant symptoms. Stenting of short-segment proximal stenoses or occlusions can be performed relatively easily through a femoral approach. If femoral access is a problem, the lesion can also be approached in retrograde fashion from the brachial artery. A potential complication of this procedure, vertebral artery embolization is, fortunately, rare, probably because of reversed flow in the vertebral artery distal to a significant subclavian stenosis. Although the technical success rate of this procedure in properly selected patients is high, long-term patency is currently inferior to open revascularization.

Axillary Artery

Occlusive lesions of the axillary artery are extremely unusual. Trauma or neglected emboli are probably the most common causes. Bypass procedures originating from or terminating on the axillary artery are also relatively rare. In the past, axilloaxillary bypass was advocated as an alternative procedure for dealing with subclavian disease when the ipsilateral carotid was an unsuitable inflow site. This bypass has been largely abandoned, however, because of its superficial location and reduced patency. Carotid-axillary bypass has been used to manage extensive subclavian disease, whereas axillobrachial bypass has been implemented for distal axillary or proximal brachial occlusions.

To expose the first and second portions of the axillary artery, the arm should be positioned at the patient's side (a narrow armboard is helpful). Significant abduction must be avoided because this position stretches the axillary artery. A transverse incision is made one fingerbreadth below the clavicle, extending from 2 cm lateral to the sternum to the deltopectoral groove. The fibers of the pectoralis major muscle are split, and the underlying clavipectoral fascia incised. Large crossing branches of the axillary vein are divided and traced back to the axillary vein, which lies inferior and slightly anterior to the artery. If encountered, the crossing medial and lateral pectoral nerves should be preserved to avoid postoperative atrophy of the pectoralis muscles. It is usually necessary to divide a branch or two of the thoracoacromial artery to gain exposure. The artery is located just above the vein, with the cords of the brachial plexus lying superiorly and posteriorly. As with the subclavian artery, care should be taken when mobilizing this thin-walled artery, which frequently has small posterior branches. The head of the pectoralis minor can be divided to facilitate exposure laterally (second portion of the axillary artery). Saphenous vein is the conduit of choice for bypasses originating from or terminating on the axillary artery. Bypasses from the carotid to the axillary (or brachial artery) are tunneled under the clavicle.

Brachial Artery

Brachial artery lesions are rare and most commonly due to emboli and trauma. Temporal arteritis is a rare cause of proximal brachial occlusive disease. For brachial artery exposure, the arm is abducted and the hand supinated on an arm board. The proximal brachial artery is exposed through a longitudinal incision along the medial aspect of the upper arm in the bicipital groove. Dissection along the posterior aspect of the muscle belly reveals the artery, accompanied by the median and ulnar nerves. The proximal brachial/distal axillary artery can be exposed through a hockey–stick-shaped extension of this incision along the lateral border of the pectoralis major. Brachial exposure immediately proximal to the elbow is achieved through an incision along the bicipital groove extended laterally across to the antecubital fossa. The median nerve lies immediately medial to the artery at this level. Alternatively, the distal brachial artery and its bifurcation into the radial and ulnar arteries can be exposed by making a longitudinal incision in the antecubital fossa just distal to the elbow crease and dividing the bicipital aponeurosis. If more distal exposure is required, the incision can be carried inferiorly along the volar aspect of the forearm. If the entire brachial artery at the elbow requires exposure, a standard "lazy-S" incision is used to avoid scar contracture across the elbow crease. Autogenous vein is the only conduit suitable for bypasses involving the brachial and more distal arteries.

Radial and Ulnar Arteries

Bypass to the forearm arteries is rarely necessary and is most often used for trauma and neglected embolic occlusions. In dialysis patients, these arteries can be affected by a particularly aggressive form of atherosclerosis that is rarely amenable to revascularization. Buerger's disease is another cause of forearm occlusive disease that is usually not reconstructable. Exposure of theses arteries at the wrist is relatively straightforward, but more proximal exposure requires a thorough understanding of forearm anatomy. Topical papaverine or nitroglycerin is helpful to combat vasospasm. Hypothenar-hammer syndrome can be treated by an interposition vein graft of the involved segment of ulnar artery in the proximal hand. A dorsal foot vein provides the best size match.

Embolism

The management of large artery embolism is covered in more detail in the chapter on peripheral artery embolism. Because of increased vasoreactivity and the inevitable resulting vasospasm, multiple passages with balloon embolectomy catheters must be avoided with upper extremity emboli. For this reason, we have a lower threshold for obtaining preoperative angiography when dealing with acute arterial occlusions of the upper extremity, even with a good clinical story for embolism. Angiography confirms the diagnosis and allows a more directed approach, a particularly important concept when dealing with emboli in the axillary and subclavian arteries. Although retrograde removal of such proximal clots can usually be performed through a brachial approach, we sometimes prefer to expose the occluded segment directly if there is significant clot burden. This approach minimizes the number of catheter passages necessary to extract the embolus and avoids stripping off clot into patent branches of the segment between the arteriotomy and the occlusion. Although most macroemboli originate from the heart, an arterial source can sometimes be responsible and, if identified, must be addressed. Treatment of arterial thoracic outlet syndrome requires not only excision of the compressive thoracic outlet elements but also some type of arterial reconstruction (discussed in more detail in the chapter on thoracic outlet syndrome).

Trauma

As outlined previously, most traumatic occlusions should be fixed at the time of diagnosis. Isolated radial or ulnar artery occlusions are an exception because they are usually well tolerated. Iatrogenic occlusions can usually be relieved with a thrombectomy alone. For more significant injuries, reconstruction is required. Resection with end-to-end anastomosis can sometimes be performed, but in the majority of cases, interposition grafting with saphenous vein of appropriate caliber is most appropriate. A more detailed description of how to manage traumatic occlusions is available in the chapter on vascular trauma.

Small-Artery Occlusive Disease

Treatment of occlusive disease affecting the small arteries of the digits and hands can be challenging. After a proximal embolic source has been ruled out, attention is focused on identification and treatment of any underlying causative disease states. Patients with Buerger's disease frequently experience significant improvement with successful smoking cessation. Vibration-induced injury will respond to avoidance of the causative vibratory machinery. The rare patient with cryoglobulinemia or hepatitis-associated vasculitis will respond to appropriate therapy. Unfortunately, in the majority of cases, no specific therapy is available. In our practice, these are patients with an associated connective-tissue disorder, hypersensitivity angiitis, or renal failure. For these individuals, care is focused on supportive measures. Abstinence from tobacco and avoidance of cold are routinely advised. Antiplatelet therapy (aspirin or clopidogrel) and hemorrheologic agents (cilostazol or pentoxiphylline) are usually prescribed. Vasodilators, primarily calcium channel blockers, can be used to treat associated vasospasm with variable success. Areas of tissue loss are treated with local wound care and debridement as indicated. Sympathectomy, both cervicothoracic and digital, can lead to a temporary improvement in skin blood flow but has such limited durability (approximately 6 months) that most authorities have abandoned it except in highly selected patients with residual ischemia following revascularization.

CONCLUSION

Upper-extremity arterial occlusive disease is an uncommon problem with diverse etiologies. Accurate diagnosis depends on a thorough history and physical examination supported by noninvasive vascular testing. Angiography remains the primary modality of diagnosis. Treatment depends on the nature of the disease process and the severity of the ischemia. Patients with embolic/traumatic occlusions and significantly symptomatic proximal large-artery disease can usually undergo vascular reconstruction with good results. Revascularization options for patients with distal small-artery occlusive disease, on the other hand, are extremely limited. In this setting, after a careful search for treatable causes, management is primarily supportive. Progression to limb loss is, fortunately, rare. The role of endoluminal therapies is unclear at this time but has shown some promise in the treatment of large-artery disease.

SUGGESTED READINGS

Edwards WH Jr, Tapper SH, Edwards WH Sr, and others: Subclavian revascularization—a quarter century experience, *Ann Surg* 219:673, 1994.

Fujitani RM, Mills JL: Acute and chronic upper extremity ischemia. I. Large vessel arterial occlusive disease, *Ann Vasc Surg* 7:106, 1993.

Fujitani RM, Mills JL: Acute and chronic upper extremity ischemia. II. Small vessel arterial occlusive disease, *Ann Vasc Surg* 7:195, 1993.

McLafferty RB, Edwards JM, Taylor LM, and others: Diagnosis and long-term clinical outcome in patients diagnosed with hand ischemia, *J Vasc Surg* 22:361, 1995.

Mesh CL, McCarthy WJ, Pearce WH, and others: Upper extremity bypass grafting—a 15-year experience, *Arch Surg* 128:795, 1993.

MANAGEMENT OF INFECTED VASCULAR GRAFT

Bruce A. Perler, MD, MBA

It has been estimated that approximately 450,000 vascular grafts are implanted annually in the United States. At a time of rapid progress and innovation in the diagnosis and treatment of peripheral vascular disease, vascular graft infection remains a serious and potentially limb- and life-threatening problem for the patient, as well as a challenging management problem for the surgeon. The true incidence of this complication depends on how one defines the problem (graft infection or graft exposure in a nonhealing wound), the anatomic location of the bypass (aortoiliofemoral or infrainguinal), the graft material (autogenous vein, Dacron, or polytetrafluoroethylene [PTFE]), the duration of the follow-up, and other factors (Table 1). However, most recent series document an incidence ranging from just under 1% to as high as 6%, with an overall incidence of approximately 4%. In addition to its considerable morbidity, it is estimated that the cost of caring for a patient with an infected vascular graft currently averages $40,000. Furthermore, in view of the rapid growth of the elderly segment of our population in whom peripheral vascular disease predominates and the associated

Table 1: Risk Factors of Vascular Graft Infection

Prosthetic > autogenous conduit
Femoral-popliteal-tibial > aortoiliofemoral bypass
Groin incision
Reoperative incision
Wound infection
Lymphorrhea
Emergency operation
Prolonged operative time
Depressed host immunity

increased number of major vascular reconstructions, as well as the introduction of endovascular stent-graft technology, it is likely that the number of patients presenting with graft infection will increase in the future.

PREVENTION

Although graft infection may become clinically manifest from a few days to as late as several years after implantation of the bypass, the preponderance of evidence suggests that in the majority of cases bacterial seeding of the conduit at the original operation was the cause. This observation affords the surgeon the potential to minimize the incidence of this complication by careful attention to a few fundamental principles of patient management during that critical perioperative period. Prophylactic broad-spectrum antibiotics, usually a cephalosporin, should be administered intravenously before the skin is incised. Although there is no compelling evidence that antibiotic use prevents frank graft infection, there is good evidence that the incidence of surgical site infection is decreased, and wound infections are an important contributor to the development of graft infection in some cases. The duration of antibiotic therapy postoperatively is somewhat controversial. Although the evidence to support the practice is not conclusive, it is reasonable to continue antibiotic administration for 24 hours postoperatively. On the other hand, there is no convincing evidence to support continuing antibiotic therapy until the urinary drainage catheter and all intravascular lines are discontinued, as was the practice for many years. Because skin flora is an important source of graft contamination, the operative field should be widely cleansed with a bactericidal solution such as povidone-iodine, and ischemic or infected ulcerations in the limb should be carefully isolated. Excessive use of the cautery should be avoided. Lymphatics are another potential route of graft inoculation, and thus lymphatic tissues should be ligated and sharply divided.

The potential benefit of antibiotic-bonded Dacron and PTFE grafts to resist infection has been investigated for many years. Although encouraging results have been reported in animal models, it is unclear whether this will translate into a clinically valuable modality. Most work has focused on the use of rifampin-bonded prosthetic grafts. These grafts have been shown to elute the antibiotic at the implantation site for only a few days, possibly limiting overall clinical utility. Although there is some evidence that they are effective against *Staphylococcus epidermidis* and *Staphylococcus aureus,* they may have more limited benefit in resisting infection caused by methicillin-resistant *Staphylococcus* and gram-negative organisms.

Before closure, the incision(s) should be copiously irrigated with topical antibiotic solution, both for its bactericidal and mechanical benefits in removing devitalized tissue from the wound. It is important to achieve absolute hemostasis before closing because a wound hematoma provides an excellent environment for bacterial growth. I prefer to avoid leaving a drain, except in the exceptional case or when postoperative formal anticoagulation is mandatory. The wound should be closed in layers, taking care to obliterate dead space while avoiding tissue devitalization.

Because the reoperative groin incision is a documented risk factor for graft infection (Table 1), avoidance of the previously operated groin is an important strategy to expedite healing and minimize the risk of this complication. One may construct the proximal anastomosis of an infrainguinal bypass graft to the superficial femoral artery (SFA) or distal profunda femoris artery because if flow is not compromised at this level, long-term graft patency is comparable to what has been reported for grafts originating from the common femoral artery. Similarly, in the patient undergoing thrombectomy of an infrainguinal bypass graft, I prefer to approach the conduit at least initially through a new incision just distal to the groin. In placing an aortic graft for aneurysmal disease, the incidence of graft infection is probably lower when the distal anastomoses are constructed to the common or external iliac, as opposed to the femoral, arteries. Furthermore, although endovascular stent grafts for aortic aneurysms are increasingly being placed in the nonoperating room catheterization laboratory venue, it is critically important that the strict principles of sterile technique are compulsively followed in this setting as they would be if the grafts were placed in the operating room.

THERAPEUTIC OPTIONS

Historically, the high rates of mortality (25%-75%) and limb amputation (8%-75%) associated with vascular graft infection have been attributed, at least in part, to delayed diagnosis. The difficulty in establishing a correct diagnosis has reflected the diverse spectrum and nonspecific nature of clinical signs and symptoms associated with graft infection (Table 2). The clinical presentation in the individual patient depends on the anatomic location of the graft, its age, and the causative organism. A number of diagnostic modalities are helpful (Table 3). Computed tomography (CT) scanning is the most useful diagnostic modality for establishing the presence and extent of graft infection, particularly in the aortoiliac position. Key radiographic findings indicative of infection include perigraft fluid, soft-tissue inflammation, perigraft gas, pseudoaneurysm formation, focal bowel wall thickening, and hydronephrosis. Perigraft fluid is not unusual for the first month after graft placement but is worrisome for infection beyond 3 months postoperatively. CT can also facilitate fluid aspiration for culturing. Magnetic resonance imaging (MRI) provides comparable

Table 2: Signs and Symptoms of Vascular Graft Infection

Fever
Leukocytosis
Malaise
Weight loss
Incisional erythema
Incisional drainage
Incisional hemorrhage
Gastrointestinal hemorrhage
Septic emboli
Pulsatile mass
Hydronephrosis

Table 3: Diagnosis Modalities

Blood cultures
Sinogram
Ultrasound
Computer tomography
Magnetic resonance imaging
Radionuclide scans
Endoscopy
Arteriography

information to CT scanning and may allow differentiation of a hematoma from a perigraft fluid collection more indicative of infection.[111] Indium-labeled and[67] gallium-labeled scans provide evidence strongly suspicious of graft infection, albeit with relatively high false-positive rates, especially within the first several weeks postoperatively. Ultrasound is most useful for evaluating the distal and proximal anastomoses in patients with aortofemoral and femorodistal bypass grafts, respectively.

GRAFT EXCISION AND EXTRA-ANATOMIC BYPASS

The conventional management of the infected vascular graft is predicated on the notion that infection involving a foreign body can be eradicated only by complete removal of the foreign body. The fundamental tenets of management therefore include complete removal of the graft, wide soft-tissue debridement, restoration of adequate distal arterial perfusion, and long-term antibiotic therapy. Although infected infrainguinal vein grafts may be an exception, especially when low-virulence organisms are involved, when infection involves the entire extent of a prosthetic infrainguinal bypass graft (especially in the setting of systemic sepsis, septic emboli, or anastomotic disruption) or the body of an aortoiliofemoral, bypass graft, typically the graft has been completely removed. Revascularization is performed, if necessary, through clean, extra-anatomic tissue planes. A number of extra-anatomic methods of arterial reconstruction are available, depending on the location of the infection (Table 4).

INFRAINGUINAL GRAFT INFECTION

The patient with an infected prosthetic infrainguinal bypass should be prepared and draped to isolate the infected wound. Proximal arterial control should be initially obtained, usually in the

Table 4: Extra-Anatomic Revascularization Options

Aortoiliofemoral Graft Infection

Axillobifemoral bypass
Bilateral axillosuperficial femoral bypass
Bilateral axilloprofunda femoris bypass
Bilateral axillopopliteal bypass

Femoral-Popliteal-Tibial Graft Infection

Ilioprofunda femoris obturator bypass
Ilial-popliteal-tibial obturator bypass
Lateral bypass

retroperitoneum, and a new graft proximal anastomosis performed, typically to the external iliac artery. The graft may then be tunneled through the obturator foramen or through a lateral, more superficial plane to the intended site of the distal anastomosis. After construction of the distal anastomosis, the incisions are closed, and then the infected graft is directly explored and excised. The original arterial anastomotic site should be debrided and carefully repaired, typically as a patch angioplasty, using either autogenous vein or endarterectomized occluded SFA to preserve collateral flow. An ankle systolic pressure greater than 40 mm Hg determined by Doppler ultrasound is a reasonable criterion of the adequacy of perfusion after graft excision.

In general, infection of an infrainguinal prosthetic bypass graft has been associated with a lower mortality rate but a higher amputation rate compared with an infected aortic graft. Although several reports have documented mortality rates ranging from 10% to 30% and limb amputation rates from 10% to 70% among patients undergoing graft excision, one recent series of 33 consecutive cases documented no operative deaths and an amputation rate of only 12%. Limb loss among survivors typically results from the inability to perform an adequate revascularization procedure or early/recurrent thrombosis of the extra-anatomic arterial bypass.

AORTOILIOFEMORAL BYPASS

Management of aortic graft infection has historically been associated with the highest mortality rates and considerable risk of limb amputation. However, several recent large series have demonstrated a significant improvement in outcomes, with mortality rates ranging from 10% to 17% and limb amputation rates ranging from 4% to 12%. A common denominator underlying this improved outcome has been the staging of operative management. Whereas formerly the infected graft was explored and resected as the initial step and then extra-anatomic bypass performed, current evidence supports preceding graft excision with extra-anatomic revascularization. This reduces the duration of peripheral ischemia, operative blood loss, and association complications. One can stage the procedure by one or several days. Although there is little evidence that the new extra-anatomic graft will experience thrombosis because of competitive flow or become secondarily infected during the interval, I favor proceeding with graft excision under the same anesthetic in the stable and good-risk patient. Conversely, in the patient who is bleeding or unstable because of active sepsis, the initial step should be exploration and removal of the infected graft.

If the aortic graft had been placed via a transperitoneal midline incision, I prefer to use the right axillary artery for inflow to allow aortic exposure via the extended left retroperitoneal approach. Incision into the tenth intercostal space will allow rapid supraceliac aortic exposure and clamping, which expedites securing an adequate aortic stump closure. The aortic suture line must be excised back to viable aortic tissue and oversewn in two layers with polypropylene suture, using omentum or prevertebral fascia to support the suture line. If necessary, one or both renal arteries may have to be sacrificed to obtain a satisfactory aortic stump closure, and splenorenal or hepatorenal bypass (or both) is carried out as needed. Aortic stump blowout may occur from days to months postoperatively, has occurred in nearly 10% of cases, and is almost universally fatal. In two recent series, 43% and 71% of late deaths, respectively, resulted from aortic stump rupture. The periaortic tissue should be cultured and aggressively debrided.

ENDOVASCULAR STENT GRAFTS

There has been no reason to believe that endovascular stent grafts would be immune from septic complications, particularly because these procedures are increasingly being performed outside of the formal operating room setting and by nonsurgical vascular specialists. To date, reports of stent graft infection have been anecdotal. However, in a recent review of 40 centers, 65 cases of infected aortic stent grafts were identified, yielding an incidence of 0.43%. These patients were treated with removal of the conduit and either extra-anatomic or in situ bypass. The operative mortality was 16% after extra-anatomic bypass and 5.8% after in situ reconstruction.

GRAFT EXCISION AND IN-SITU BYPASS

Although improvements in medical and surgical management have reduced operative morbidity among patients undergoing excision of infected grafts and extra-anatomic bypass, especially in the aortic position, this conventional management still conveys significant risk. Operative morbidity remains considerable, and as noted earlier, the risk of potentially fatal aortic stump disruption is ongoing. In addition, there is evidence that until a protective pseudo-intima develops, the new graft is susceptible to secondary bloodborne infection. Infection of the extra-anatomic graft has occurred in 5% to 20% of cases long term. Finally, limb viability is dependent on an extra-anatomic conduit that is subject to early and recurrent thrombosis. In view of these limitations, in recent years considerable enthusiasm has developed for, and experience accumulated with, the somewhat more conservative approach of infected aortic or infrainguinal graft excision and in situ anatomic bypass with a variety of conduits (Table 5).

Endarterectomized, occluded, autogenous arteries such as the SFA, often in combination with autogenous peripheral veins, may be used for restoring flow after excision of the infected infrainguinal graft. For managing aortic graft infection, the deep and superficial veins of the lower extremities have been used to perform in situ revascularization. In the largest series reported to date, only 12% of patients required fasciotomy procedures acutely. The 5-year primary patency rate was 83%. Graft stenoses occur much more frequently in superficial veins, thus deep veins should be preferentially used in this setting. Significant limb edema has occurred in approximately 10% of cases and can be avoided by preserving the profunda femoris and greater saphenous veins. These are long and arduous cases and ideally should be performed with a two-team surgical approach.

Fresh or cryopreserved allografts represent another option for in situ replacement of the infected graft in the aortoiliac or infrainguinal position. Freshly harvested aortic allografts may offer better resistance to recurrent infection and provide an excellent size match when replacing an infected aortic graft. The availability of tissue banks has rekindled interest in the use of cryopreserved saphenous vein conduits. Cryopreserved grafts are tissue typed and screened for potential viral contaminants. The experience with cryopreserved allografts to manage infected vascular grafts has yielded imperfect results. In a registry of aortic cryopreserved allografts, including 31 centers, there was a major complication rate of 20% with a mean follow-up of just 5.3 months. Significant problems included pseudoaneurysm formation, graft thrombosis, persistent infection, and anastomotic bleeding. Similar problems have been recognized when cryopreserved allografts are used in the infrainguinal position as well. I argue that cryopreserved conduits should be used cautiously in the presence of virulent gram-negative bacteria such as *Pseudomonas aeruginosa* because exogenous proteases are capable of digesting the structural integrity of tissue grafts. In addition, these grafts appear prone to develop aneurysmal degeneration and recurrent thrombosis. However, they may serve an important temporizing function, allowing complete eradication of infection until a more suitable prosthesis can be placed in the field.

Finally, infection with *S. epidermidis* appears to be a special case in which in situ replacement with a prosthetic conduit is a reasonable option. These patients typically present months to years after graft placement and lack signs of systemic infection. Moreover, perigraft fluid specimens may show only white blood cells on Gram stain and are often culture-negative. When routine cultures are negative, sonication of the aspirate, the use of liquid as opposed to agar media, and maintaining the culture for 14 days may identify this organism. In the absence of available autogenous tissue, replacement of the infected graft with a PTFE conduit, given its documented lower rate of bacterial adherence compared with Dacron, is advised. Nevertheless, a recurrent infection rate of 22% has been reported in one series.

GRAFT SALVAGE

The most controversial strategy for managing vascular graft infection is aggressive local wound care with prevention of most, or all, of the involved graft. Although contrary to conventional surgical dogma, numerous reports since the 1970s have indicated that when the graft infection is localized at presentation, drainage of all gross infection, extensive soft-tissue debridement, repetitive wound dressing changes, and the administration of antibiotics both topically and parenterally may effect sterilization of the wound and allow healing to occur by secondary intention. Although traditionally used in the management of peripheral graft infection, local care may also be carried out in patients with infected aortic prostheses. Although it avoids the morbidity inherent in excising the original graft and performing arterial ligation and repair in an infected field and obviates the necessity to perform an extra-anatomic bypass that is susceptible to recurrent thrombotic episodes, there are several disadvantages to this approach. A protracted period of hospitalization is generally required at considerable financial cost, and during this interval, the graft and patient are vulnerable to a number of potential secondary complications such as anastomotic hemorrhage, thrombosis, and superinfection by more virulent organisms.

A recent addition to our therapeutic armamentarium in managing graft infection locally has been the use of a vacuum-assisted closure (VAC) system. To date, VAC therapy has been used to treat patients with groin wounds after infected pseudoaneurysm repair, in patients with groin infections after femoral endarterectomy and synthetic patch closure, and to treat groin wounds with exposed vein grafts. In a recent series, four patients with exposed synthetic bypass grafts in the groin who were considered too infirm to undergo more definitive therapy underwent VAC therapy. Healing was achieved in all cases; and, with a mean follow-up of 18 months, there have been no recurrent infections. It has been reported that VAC therapy reduces the bacteria count in open wounds; removing excess fluid in the wound may stimulate lymphatic and blood flow and increase oxygen concentration, thereby killing bacteria. Further experience is necessary to evaluate fully the potential for VAC therapy to manage graft infections in the groin.

Table 5: In Situ Graft Replacement: Potential Conduits

Autogenous arteries
Autogenous veins
Cryopreserved veins
Venous homografts
Arterial homografts
Polytetrafluoroethylene
Antibiotic-bonded grafts

ROTATIONAL MUSCLE FLAPS

The use of muscle tissue to cover vascular structures is not a new concept. Local sartorius transfer has been performed for years in the management of difficult groin wounds and in fact has been the most frequently used muscle to treat graft infection in the groin. In addition to its mechanical benefits of covering the graft and filling the wound, there is considerable experimental evidence suggesting that well-vascularized muscle tissue may actually help to eradicate the infection process through its potential to raise the oxygen tension in, and deliver a high level of immunocompetent cells and antibiotics to, the local wound. Although local sartorius transfer is easy to perform and leaves the patient without function deficit, I believe that creating a formal rotational muscle flap, whereby a muscle is rotated from a separate, clean bed and based on a pedicled blood supply that is independent of the site of infection, ensures maximal vascularity and is preferable. A number of muscles are available for graft coverage in the groin or at any anatomic site in the body (Table 6). The muscle selected depends on the location and size of the infected wound and the underlying arterial anatomy in the individual patient.

Although this approach is most appropriate for the patient with infection involving a single limb of an aortofemoral or infrainguinal bypass graft, I have also successfully used it to manage graft infection in the chest and neck. The involved graft limb must be patent, and systemic sepsis must be controlled. Historically, anastomotic disruption was an absolute contraindication to attempted graft preservation. However, my experience has demonstrated that even if there is anastomotic breakdown, if the anastomosis can be repaired primarily or by placement of a new short interposition conduit, ultimate graft salvage is possible with muscle flap coverage. Over a 7-year period at the Johns Hopkins Hospital, 22 rotational muscle flap procedures have been performed to close 19 wounds in 18 patients with infections involving 21 prosthetic grafts, including 3 patients who presented after previous failed coverage with local sartorius transfer. There was one (5.8%) operative death, and wound healing was achieved in the 17 survivors. Recurrent infection developed in three (16%) patients from 12 to 22 (mean: 18) months after wound closure, and one of these patients underwent a successful secondary muscle flap procedure with graft sal-

vage. In total, 15 (88%) of the original operative survivors had healed wounds with functional grafts, with a mean follow-up of 30 months.

ANTIBIOTIC THERAPY

Culture-specific antibiotic therapy is a fundamental component of the management of vascular graft infection. The absolute duration of antibiotic therapy is not well defined by evidence-based study. Clearly the virulence of the responsible organism, the extent of infection, and the surgical strategy used will factor into this judgment. On balance, it appears that 6 weeks of intravenous antibiotic therapy is reasonable, and some would then continue with oral antibiotics for another 3 to 6 months following definitive surgical intervention. Lifelong antibiotics have been advocated in selected cases, such as with residual synthetic or in situ synthetic graft replacement. Some have advocated measurement of the erythrocyte sedimentation rate or C-reactive protein levels (or both) to guide antibiotic therapy.

SUMMARY

Management of the patient with an infected vascular graft must be individualized because no two patients are exactly alike. The graft material and location, the bacterial species involved and quantitative bacteria counts, the patient's nutritional and immunologic status, and other factors influence the potential for successful eradication of infection. The surgeon's challenge is to eradicate all signs of infection and preserve limb viability through a strategy that minimizes the risk to the patient's life. None of the approaches discussed here represents a perfect solution to the problem. What has become clear in recent years, however, is that although many patients with extensive graft sepsis will continue to require complete graft removal, an increasing number of autogenous and allograft options are available that offer the opportunity to maintain in-line anatomic arterial perfusion and preserve long-term limb viability. In addition, the use of muscle flap coverage allows some grafts that were previously believed to require excision to be salvaged. Finally, because graft infection may fester indolently for years, the patient undergoing operation for graft infection by any of these strategies must be closely followed for life.

Table 6: Potential Rotational Muscle Flaps

Rectus abdominis
Rectus femoris
Tensor fascia lata
Gracilis
Gastrocnemius
Soleus
Pectoralis major
Latissimus dorsi
Sternocleidomastoid
Flexor digitorum sublimis

SUGGESTED READINGS

Castier Y, Francis F, Cerceau P, and others: Cryopreserved arterial allograft reconstruction for peripheral graft infection, *J Vasc Surg* 41:30, 2005.

Clagett GP, Bowers BL, Lopes-Viego MA, and others: Creation of a neo-aortoiliac system for lower extremity deep and superficial veins, *Ann Surg* 218:239, 1993.

Perera G, Fujitani RM, Kubaska SM: Aortic graft infection: update on management and treatment options, *Vasc Endovasc Surg* 40:1, 2006.

Perler BA: The case for conservative management of infected prosthetic grafts. In Cameron JC, editor: *Advances in surgery*–vol 29, Mosby-Year Book, 1996, Chicago, p. 17.

Perler BA, Vander Kolk CA, Manson OM, and others: Rotational muscle flaps to treat prosthetic graft infection: long-tern follow-up, *J Vasc Surg* 18:358, 1993.

GANGRENE OF THE FOOT

Juan Carlos Jimenez, MD, and Peter F. Lawrence, MD, FACS

INTRODUCTION

Gangrene refers to the end product of cellular destruction following a complex, morphologic chain of events. Gangrene of the foot is the result of both denaturation of proteins within the cell, referred to as *coagulative necrosis*, and lysosomal enzymatic digestion, referred to as *liquefaction necrosis*. The most common cause of coagulative necrosis is hypoxia following ischemic injury. Cell architecture can be preserved for a period of time but eventually deteriorates from hypoxia. In the presence of inflammatory cells following bacterial or fungal infection, liquefaction necrosis occurs. Tissue death leads to two forms of gangrene: dry gangrene results when slow tissue death occurs, exclusive of proteolytic enzymatic breakdown. It presents with tissue desiccation and mummification. The alternative form, wet gangrene, occurs when the devitalized tissue becomes infected and extensive liquefaction necrosis and purulence are present.

Immediate evaluation and treatment of patients presenting with gangrene of the foot is necessary to halt further tissue destruction, preserve existing tissue and function, and remove irreversibly injured or dead tissue. Advances in imaging and endovascular procedures have added new options to treatments traditionally used to treat patients with gangrene of the foot.

EVALUATION

History and Physical Examination

The determination of the cause of a gangrenous foot requires an in-depth assessment of the patient's medical history and a complete physical examination. Common risk factors for atherosclerotic lower-extremity vascular disease include smoking, diabetes, hypertension, and hyperlipidemia, which must be addressed and modified with optimal medical treatment. The most common cause of acute, dry gangrene is lower-extremity occlusive vascular disease. Progression to wet gangrene of the foot frequently occurs with chronic infection secondary to neuropathic trauma in diabetics. One must also consider remote sources of atheroemboli, including the heart, thoracic aorta, and upper and lower abdominal aorta. In addition, various medical conditions including vasculitis and other autoimmune conditions may also be underlying causes of acute gangrene of the foot. Massive venous occlusive disease is an infrequent etiologic factor. During the initial assessment, care must be taken to determine whether underlying infection is present. Care must be taken to assess for signs of possible deep-space abscesses or compartment abscesses. Signs of accompanying generalized sepsis must also be ruled out.

A complete vascular examination, including palpation of peripheral pulses, is critical in all patients, as is evaluation of the extent and nature of gangrene. Flexion of joints in the leg and foot; evaluation of the patient's ability to ambulate; determination of the presence of rubor, pallor, and sensatory loss; and motor function are all important signs and findings that must be assessed. Assessment for cellulitis, lymphangitis, osteomyelitis, and deep-space tissue infections must be performed. Deep wounds can be probed and explored with cotton applicators. A complete examination identifies the presence of gangrene, but the extent of gangrene frequently requires further testing.

Noninvasive Testing

Ankle-brachial pressure index (ABI), segmental pressures, pulse volume recordings, toe plethysmography, and arterial duplex scanning are all used for assessment of peripheral arterial disease. The ABI is obtained by dividing the systolic blood pressure measured at the ankle by the brachial systolic blood pressure. An ABI of less than 0.9 is indicative of a hemodynamically significant arterial stenosis; an ABI of less than 0.4 is consistent with ischemia. Advantages of ABIs include reproducibility, simplicity, and the ability to perform them quickly at the bedside; however, falsely elevated values occur in diabetic patients with calcified, noncompressible peripheral arteries. When "stiff arteries" are present, Doppler waveform analysis and toe pressures are often the most reliable measures of limb perfusion.

Segmental pressures at the upper and lower thigh, calf, and ankle can provide more specific information regarding the level of arterial disease. Pulse-volume recordings with waveform analysis can also help to localize the specific level of arterial disease, as well as provide an overall assessment of collateral circulation in the diseased limb. Analysis of arterial waveforms in the toes using digital plethysmography also provides a physiologic overview of the degree of proximal arterial obstruction and is used in conjunction with other noninvasive diagnostic studies.

Arterial duplex scanning has become a powerful tool in the noninvasive evaluation of patients with lower-extremity ischemia and gangrene. This modality provides gray-scale B-mode imaging, color flow, and pulsed-Doppler spectral waveform analysis. Measures of flow velocity through diseased and nondiseased segments can be used to estimate the degree of diameter reduction within the vessel wall and identify sites of arterial stenosis and occlusion. Accuracy of this technique is operator dependent, especially in the distal arteries of the lower extremity, and must be performed by experienced ultrasound technologists and clinicians with knowledge of the relevant anatomy and physiology of the underlying disease process.

Transcutaneous measurement of the partial pressure of oxygen (TcPO2) can be used in patients with critical limb ischemia and lower-extremity gangrene to measure the metabolic state of the surrounding tissue. TcPO2 measurements may help to determine the likelihood of success with conservative management versus revascularization and may also be useful in establishing the proper level of amputation required for wound healing. Patients with a resting TcPO2 of 30 mm Hg or greater should be treated with conservative measures, including local wound care, wound debridement, and minor amputation. All patients with a resting TcPO2 less than 30 mm Hg should undergo arteriography and revascularization. In one study using this approach, 86% of patients treated conservatively healed without the need for intervention, whereas 83% of patients with TcPO2 levels less than 30 mm Hg healed following angioplasty or vascular reconstruction. Thus TcPO2 determination serves as an effective, noninvasive, and inexpensive method of determining the severity of tissue ischemia in patients with limb-threatening arterial disease.

Imaging

Computed tomography with intravenous contrast (CT angiography, or CTA) and magnetic resonance angiography (MRA) are frequently used as the initial imaging modalities in patients with abnormal, noninvasive arterial studies and lower-extremity gangrene. Both modalities have improved significantly over the past several years with enhanced speed and image quality. Principles of CTA involve arterial scanning during the peak administration of an intravenous contrast bolus. The development of newer multislice CT scanners has added to the speed and accuracy with which these studies can be performed. Advantages of CTA include the ability to obtain delayed three-dimensional reconstructions and relatively fast scan

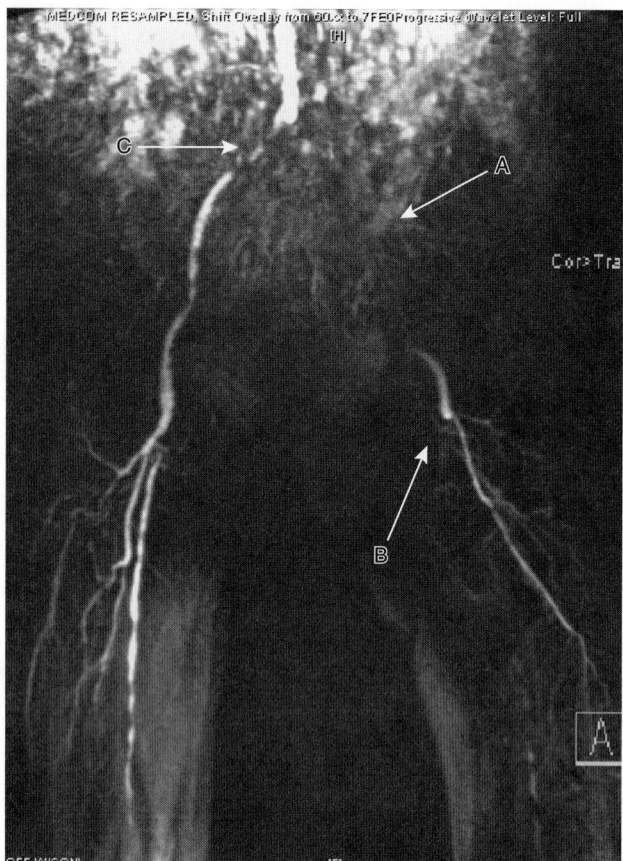

Figure 1 Magnetic resonance angiography demonstrating a complete occlusion in the left common and external iliac arteries *(A)* and ipsilateral superficial femoral artery *(B)*. Note artifact from prior stent placement *(C)* in right common iliac artery.

times compared with MRA. Contrast administration is achieved via a peripheral intravenous line without the need for arterial cannulation. Disadvantages include the need for modest doses of ionizing radiation and nephrotoxic iodinated contrast agents. The presence of arterial calcification and metallic implants may create artifacts in the final image, diminishing study accuracy. CTA is most useful in evaluating larger vessels above the popliteal artery but is less useful for infrapopliteal arterial evaluation.

MRA uses applied magnetic fields in conjunction with small volumes of gadolinium-based contrast agents to obtain three-dimensional images of the peripheral arterial system and associated atherosclerotic lesions. Advantages of MRA over CTA include the absence of nephrotoxicity and lower incidence of contrast allergy using gadolinium compared with iodinated contrast. Disadvantages include longer scan times compared with CTA. The presence of arterial stents creates artifacts in the final image, making MRA an unsuitable modality for evaluation in these selected patients. MRA is also contraindicated in patients with implanted metallic devices, including certain pacemakers, defibrillators, and prosthetic heart valves. MRA is extremely valuable in assessing arterial flow and vessels below the inguinal ligament (Fig. 1).

TREATMENT

Dry Gangrene

Following evaluation of the vascular system using noninvasive testing, MRA or CTA, the extent of the arterial occlusive disease and

the potential for revascularization will be evident. However, contrast angiography remains the gold standard for delineation of arterial anatomy and determining the presence and extent of occlusive lesions and is currently used in conjunction with interventions. Most vascular surgeons perform all invasive angiograms at the time of intended treatment through an ipsilateral or contralateral femoral approach.

With the publication of the TransAtlantic Inter-Society Consensus (TASC) statement in 1999, classification of aortoiliac and femoropopliteal lesions was stratified by lesion length and morphology, and guidelines for either endovascular or surgical management were recommended. In general, patients with short focal lesions in the aortoiliac and femoropopliteal segments or patients with multiple medical comorbidities who are poor candidates for surgery should be treated with angioplasty. Selective stenting of aortoiliac lesions should be reserved for patients who demonstrate residual stenosis (>30%), a brachiofemoral pressure (>5 mm Hg), or acute dissection following balloon angioplasty. Patients with long (>5 cm) lesions, multiple stenoses, or complete occlusions are treated with surgical revascularization; however, in many institutions, more aggressive treatment of superficial femoral, popliteal, and tibial lesions with angioplasty, atherectomy, and stenting is being used, including extension of treatment into more distal, diffuse lesions and occlusions. Decisions regarding endovascular versus open management should be determined on an individual patient basis, according to lesion morphology, surgical risk, and patient preference.

Debridement and amputation of dry gangrene secondary to lower-extremity arterial occlusive disease should be avoided before maximization of perfusion to avoid poor subsequent wound healing in the ischemic limb. Following revascularization, clinical evidence of skin perfusion by physical examination, along with TcPO2, should be used to assess the appropriate level of amputation for optimal healing.

In the face of a stable, nonprogressively dry lesion without associated ischemic problems, local treatment may be adequate. The foot or digit should be kept dry, and the spaces between the toes should be protected from maceration with lamb's wool or cotton swabs. Treated in this fashion, these lesions may remain dormant for long periods. If perfusion is adequate, a local digit or ray amputation should be performed.

Acute Wet Gangrene

When devitalized tissue progresses to infection, this is referred to as *wet gangrene* and represents a life- and limb-threatening emergency. Extensive liquefaction, purulence, and suppuration are frequently encountered. Rapid extension of the infectious process may occur if prompt debridement and amputation of devitalized tissues is not quickly performed. This may result in loss of further salvageable tissue, deep-space abscesses or compartment abscesses, and generalized sepsis. Because these infections are frequently polymicrobial, broad-spectrum antibiotics covering gram-positive, gram-negative, and anaerobic organisms should be instituted promptly. Effective coverage for *Pseudomonas* and *Clostridium* species is especially important.

For wet gangrene of the foot, aggressive debridement to the level of normal tissue with appropriate drainage of all deep spaces is imperative. Intraoperative wound cultures should be obtained. In cases of extensive, necrotizing, soft-tissue gangrene, open amputation with delayed wound closure is the only acceptable approach; primary skin closure is inappropriate. Delayed amputation at the appropriate level is then performed after revascularization and when signs of wound sepsis subside. The viability of the skin adjacent to the gangrene is often the determining factor in wound closure, so all viable skin should be preserved, with delayed debridement staged until all nonviable tissue is removed.

Patients with acute limb ischemia frequently have myonecrosis with hyperkalemia and myoglobinuria, requiring acute potassium reduction measures, volume loading, and alkalinization of the urine. In these patients with partial or entire limb gangrene who are too unstable for transport to the operating room for guillotine amputation, cryoamputation at the bedside should be performed. Techniques for guillotine amputation and cryoamputation are described later in this chapter.

Following debridement of all infected, gangrenous tissues, evaluation of the lower-extremity arterial system should be repeated using noninvasive and imaging studies as previously described. Angiogram followed by endovascular or surgical revascularization should be performed before definitive reamputation and wound closure. Determination of the appropriate level of amputation should be determined only after revascularization.

AMPUTATIONS

Forefoot Amputations

Digit and Ray Amputation

Digital amputation is indicated when one or more toes are gangrenous and still have viable skin at the base of the phalanx. Ray amputation of the digit includes removal of the proximal metatarsal head. In these instances, excision of the toe can be carried out without loss of function. If the necrosis is confined to the distal toe, the proximal phalanx can be preserved by interphalangeal disarticulation. If the skin at the base of the phalanx is not viable, the incision is carried more proximally to include the head of the metatarsal. Patient adaptation to ambulation is usually excellent following toe amputation as long as the proximal metatarsal head remains.

The operative technique includes an elliptical incision at the base of the digit (Fig. 2). If the metatarsal head is to be removed, the elliptical incision is carried onto the dorsum of the foot, proximal to the metatarsal head. This allows for tension-free closure. When the great toe is amputated, the proximal incision is carried to the midpoint of the first metatarsal (tennis racquet incision). This provides good exposure for the more extensive bone resection that is often necessary with the first metatarsophalangeal joint.

Transmetatarsal Amputation

Gangrene that extends to multiple digits, as well as to the distal dorsum of the foot, is the most common indication for a transmetatarsal amputation. Although removing the entire forefoot disrupts proprioceptive sensation, the remaining broad-based platform provided by the proximal metatarsal bones, as well as the tarsometatarsal joints, allows for an excellent functional stump, as long as the "parabolic" shape of the foot is preserved. When walking ability is augmented by an orthotic shoe with a molded distal filler, patients often ambulate without a limp. If extensors of the foot are divided, Achilles tendon lengthening may be required to maintain a normal gait.

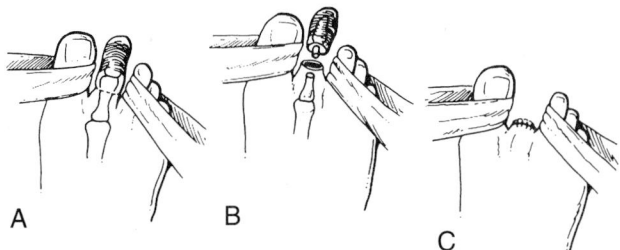

Figure 2 Toe amputation. *Adapted from Moore WS, editor: Vascular and endovascular surgery. Philadelphia, 2005, WB Saunders.*

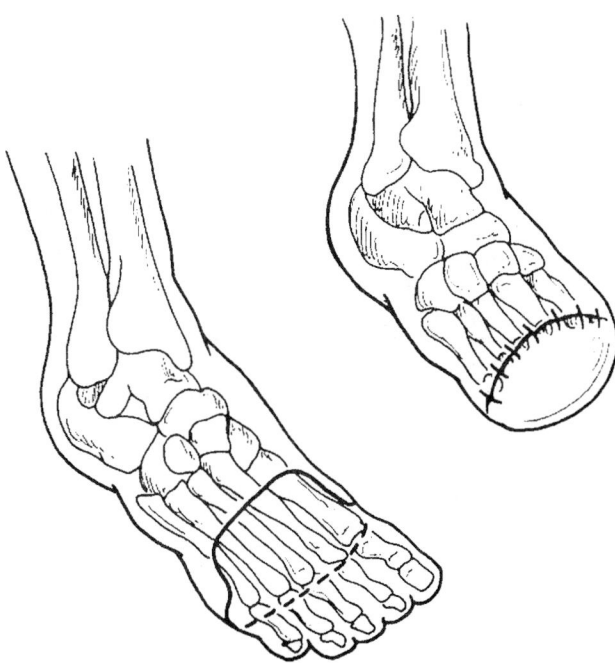

Figure 3 Transmetatarsal amputation. *Adapted from Moore WS, editor: Vascular and endovascular surgery. Philadelphia, 2005, WB Saunders.*

The principle factor in selecting a transmetatarsal amputation is the viability of the plantar skin and fat pad. This surface must be free of ischemic changes proximal to the line of the metatarsal heads to allow for flap coverage of the divided metatarsal components.

The technique for a transmetatarsal amputation involves placing the dorsal incision as a curved, parabolic line proximal to the area of ischemia, with the plantar incision at the metaphalangeal skin crease (Fig. 3). This allows preservation of as much length as possible. This is important because the flap closure line is ideally placed on the upper surface of the stump end. The toes are extended to stretch the flexor tendons, which allows for proximal retraction after division. The metatarsal bones are divided in a parabola without undermining of the skin flaps. Good hemostasis of soft tissues must be obtained to avoid postoperative hematoma. Closure is limited to the skin edges, which are approximated using interrupted nylon sutures in simple or vertical mattress fashion. Care must be taken to approximate, but not strangulate, the tissue.

When there is a large necrotic area on the lateral side of the foot, a partial lateral transmetatarsal amputation can often be performed. This often includes removal of most of the third, fourth, and fifth metatarsal and digits. Although this results in a foot with deformed appearance, the remaining presence of the first two digits and metatarsophalangeal joints offers an adequate push-off platform and balance surface. The operation is performed by excising the devitalized tissue on the lateral foot and preserving as much dorsal and plantar skin as possible. The lateral one, two, or three metatarsals are excised proximal to the area of ischemia. The plantar fat pad is carefully debrided of any necrotic fat. Wound closure is carried out in the long axis of the foot over a drain.

Amputations of the Midfoot

Chopart's and Lisfranc Amputation

The critical element in performing midtarsal procedures is the availability of a well-perfused long plantar flap to allow for a full, tension-free closure. The Lisfranc amputation involves disarticulation of the tarsometatarsal joints and disruption of the tendinous attachments of the midfoot. The disadvantage of this technique is the frequent development of a severe equinus deformity, which often leads to poor functional outcomes and ambulation.

Chopart's amputation is performed by division of the talonavicular and calcaneocuboidal joints, debridement of all remaining cartilaginous tissue, and complete removal of the midfoot and forefoot. Care must be taken to avoid shifting of weight from the residual calcaneus to the amputation stump. Aggressive rehabilitation and physical therapy, as well as appropriate patient selection, shorten time to ambulation.

Achilles tendon lengthening should be performed in patients with Chopart and Lisfranc amputations to reduce the severity of equinovarus deformity following midfoot amputations. This technique is performed with multiple posterior stab incisions to the Achilles tendon, increasing its overall length and improving the degree of ankle dorsiflexion in these patients.

Amputations at the Ankle Level

Symes Amputation

The Symes amputation is the most commonly performed amputation at the ankle level and provides a weight-bearing end stump covered with an anteriorly rotated heel flap. The Symes amputation involves complete removal of the talus and calcaneus in conjunction with resection of the malleolar heads. This procedure requires heel sensation, so it is a poor choice for diabetics. Advantages of this procedure include a durable, although cosmetically bulky, stump end pad. Disadvantages include the need for a patent posterior tibial artery to perfuse the heel pad, possible posterior migration of the heel pad secondary to lack of bony fixation, and a high failure rate.

Amputations Proximal to the Ankle Level

Below-Knee Amputation

The below-knee amputation (BKA) is indicated when the extent of distal gangrene is proximal to the level appropriate for midfoot or ankle amputations. Preservation of the knee joint in the BKA is associated with decreased energy expenditure for ambulation compared with above-knee amputation (AKA). However, BKA has a higher incidence of failure, occasionally prompting operative revision or conversion to an AKA. In a recent series, 25% of patients who underwent BKA for critical ischemia required operative revision, mostly conversion to AKA. Healing for BKA at 100 days was 83%.

Major amputation is associated with significant morbidity and mortality at both the above-knee and below-knee levels. Aulivola and colleagues, who reviewed 959 consecutive major, lower-extremity amputations (704 BKA and 255 AKA), reported an overall 30-day mortality for BKA and AKA, respectively, of 5.7% and 16.5%. Despite increased ease of ambulation with prosthetics following BKA compared with AKA, a significant percentage of patients remain nonambulatory. In Nehler's series, 35% of patients remained nonambulatory following their BKAs, compared with 71% in the nonambulatory AKA group.

Major amputation is not a benign procedure. The operative risk associated with lower-extremity revascularization may increase with cardiac and pulmonary comorbidities. Multiple medical and social factors must be analyzed before proceeding with major lower-extremity amputation, including extent of disease, rehabilitation potential, and patient preference.

Technique: Below-Knee Amputation

In patients with distal ischemia, BKA is ideally performed by creating a long, posterior, myocutaneous flap. The optimal tibial bone length is 8 to 10 cm below the tibial tuberosity. The anterior skin flap should extend at least 2 cm lower than the bone. Meticulous operative technique is imperative to maintain optimal flap viability. When adequate posterior skin or muscle is present, another alternative is the creation of anterior and posterior flaps that are equal in length ("fishmouth incision"). One disadvantage of this technique is the placement of the incision at the distal weight-bearing portion of the stump as opposed to a more anterior position provided by a long posterior flap. However, current prosthetics are not end-weight bearing, so this is primarily a theoretical concern.

The incision for the anterior skin flap should measure two-thirds the circumference of the leg, and the posterior flap must measure one-third the diameter of the leg (Fig. 4). These incisions are connected by a longitudinal incision on the medial and lateral leg. Sharp dissection is used to divide the skin and muscular fascia. The incision is extended through the muscles of the anterior and lateral compartments with electrocautery. The anterior tibial artery and vein are ligated and divided. The peroneal nerve is retracted and divided sharply. The tibia is then divided using an electric saw. An anterior bevel of 45 to 60 degrees should be used to prevent superficial stump erosion, and the edges should be rounded. The fibula should be divided 1 cm proximal the level of the tibial stump and rounded. Ligation and division of the peroneal and posterior tibial vessels and nerves are then performed. The posterior flap is then fashioned using either a sharp amputation knife or electrocautery and trimmed to match the anterior flap. All nerves should be retracted before cutting to avoid painful neuromas. The myoplasty is performed as the two fascial edges are then approximated and closed in layers with polydioxane (PDS) interrupted sutures to minimize dead space. Suction drains may be placed. We close the skin using interrupted nylon sutures in a vertical mattress fashion. Care is taken to approximate, but not strangulate, the skin edges to minimize necrosis.

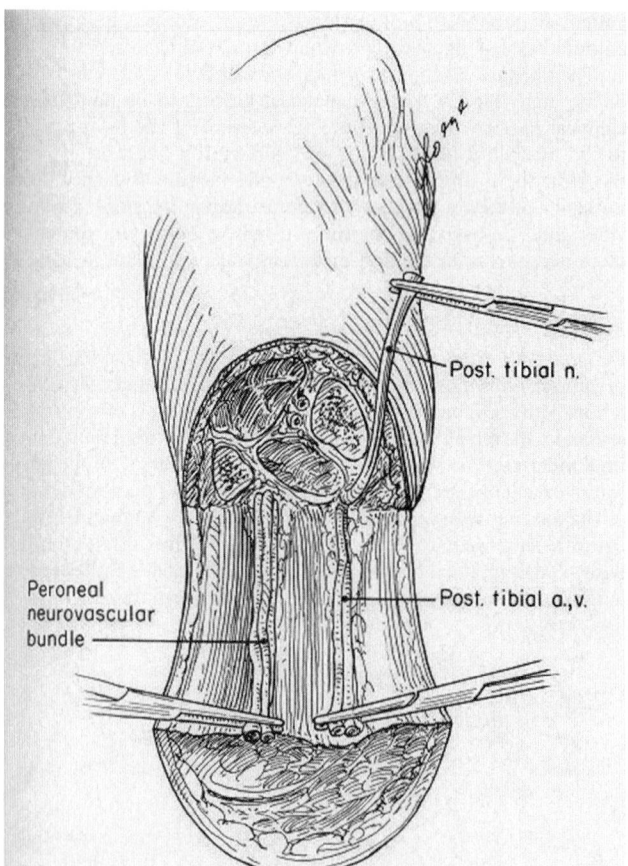

Figure 4 Below-knee amputation. *a*, Artery; *n*, nerve; *v*, vein. *Adapted from Moore WS, editor:* Vascular and endovascular surgery. *Philadelphia, 2005, WB Saunders.*

Above-Knee Amputation

In cases in which the level of ischemia would leave a below-knee stump without viable skin or muscle coverage, the transfemoral above-knee amputation is indicated. AKA is associated with significant morbidity and mortality, with 5-year survival in some recent series as low as 22%. The ultimate goal of the AKA is to preserve as much length of the femur as possible. Preservation of femur length facilitates ambulation in patients postoperatively; however, it is more difficult to heal long than short above-knee stumps in patients with severe ischemia.

In AKA, equal anterior and posterior skin flaps are used (fishmouth technique) (Fig. 5). The anterior and posterior muscle bundles are divided in beveled fashion with electrocautery to match both flaps. The femur is transected and rounded with an anterior bevel, using an electric saw, at a level proximal enough to provide padded closure. Care must be taken to avoid shortening of the femur to a point that a floppy stump is created. The myoplasty is performed by approximating anterior and posterior muscles in multiple layers using absorbable suture to reduce dead space and prevent bone herniation. Myodesis may be used to reduce the probability of bone herniation. Subcutaneous tissue and skin are approximated carefully, with care taken to avoid undue tension and resulting stump necrosis. The stump is dressed with a bulky protective dressing, and a light compression bandage is placed.

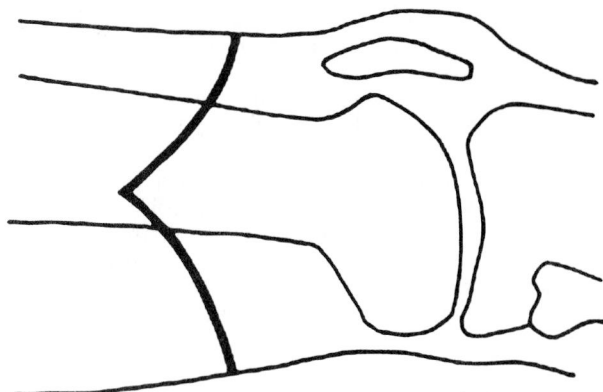

Figure 5 "Fishmouth" incision for above-knee amputation. *Adapted from Moore WS, editor: Vascular and endovascular surgery. Philadelphia, 2005, WB Saunders.*

Two-Stage Amputation

Guillotine Amputation and Cryoamputation

In situations when the patient presents with signs of advanced local wound or systemic sepsis, a two-stage amputation is often necessary to halt the extent of life-threatening infection (Fig. 6, *A*). Immediate, definitive amputation has a high failure

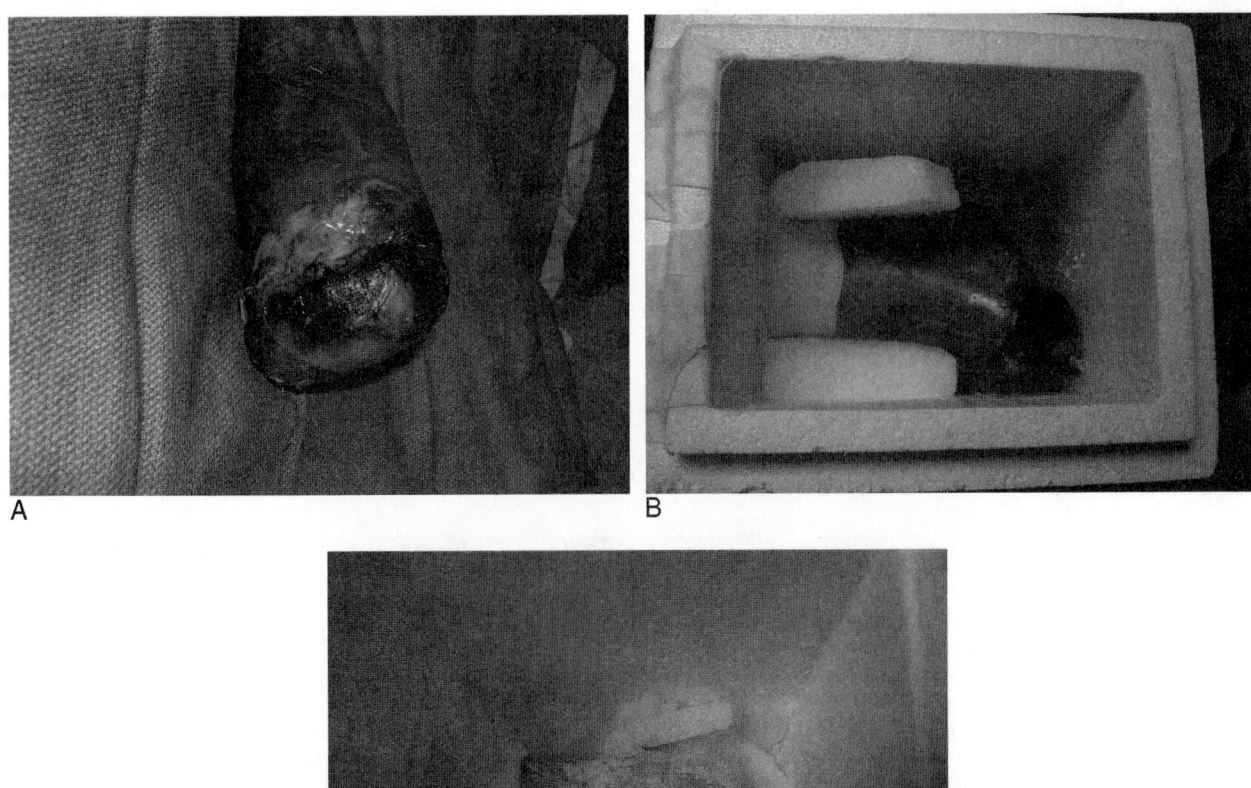

A

B

C

Figure 6 **(A)** Acute, wet gangrene following infection at site of transmetatarsal amputation. **(B and C)** Cryoamputation with dry ice for treatment of acute, wet gangrene in a patient with systemic sepsis.

rate, so a staged procedure is often preferable. Although necrotizing soft-tissue infections of the lower extremity are frequently polymicrobial, *Streptococcus* and *Clostridium* species are frequently implicated. Thorough debridement of all affected tissue and drainage of all affected muscle compartments are imperative. The guillotine amputation is traditionally performed at the transmalleolar level for patients with advanced wet gangrene of the proximal forefoot when foot salvage is not possible. The proximal extent of the amputation, however, should be determined individually to remove all affected tissue. The wound is typically left open for adequate drainage and packed with antibiotic-soaked gauze. Reevaluation of the wound must be performed frequently because further debridement may be necessary before subsequent definitive amputation.

In a series of 75 patients undergoing BKA for advanced wet gangrene of the foot, McIntyre and colleagues noted that 97% of patients who had a guillotine amputation followed by staged BKA healed without the need for further revision. In contrast, 78% of patients who underwent a one-stage BKA healed without subsequent revision. Similar findings were noted in a randomized prospective trial by Fisher and colleagues. In their series, 21% of patients in the one-stage group had wound complications, compared with no wound complications in the two-stage group.

In septic patients who are hemodynamically unstable, physiologic cryoamputation may be performed at the bedside to limit the proximal progression of systemic gangrene and allow hemodynamic improvement. Physiologic amputation involves temporary freezing of the affected extremity with dry ice to avoid emergency operation. Elective BKA or AKA is then performed after systemic signs of sepsis are ameliorated. Winburn and colleagues reported an overall mortality rate of 11% in a series of 320 cryoamputations. Further revision following subsequent amputation was required in 9% of limbs.

Cryoamputation: Technique

See Figure 6, *B* and *C*, for illustration. The leg proximal to the affected area is wrapped in gauze, and a tourniquet and heating pad may or may not be placed at this level. The leg may then be placed in a simple Styrofoam cooler filled with large blocks of dry ice. Periodic replenishment of dry ice is required, as is frequent evaluation of the foot and proximal amputation margin. The timing of elective definitive amputation is determined following hemodynamic stabilization and improvement in systemic signs of sepsis. Legs have been kept "frozen" for up to 10 days before definitive amputation.

SUGGESTED READINGS

Aulivola B, Hile CN, Hamdan AD, and others: Major lower extremity amputation: outcome of a modern series, *Arch Surg* 139:395, 2004.

Ballard JL, Eke CC, Bunt TJ, and others: A prospective evaluation of transcutaneous oxygen measurements in the management of diabetic foot problems, *J Vasc Surg* 22:485, 1995.

Fisher DF Jr, Clagett GP, Frye RE, and others: One-stage versus two-stage amputation for wet gangrene of the lower extremity: a randomized study, *J Vasc Surg* 8:428, 1988.

Kreitner KF, Kalden P, Neufang A, and others: Diabetes and peripheral arterial occlusive disease: prospective comparison of contrast-enhanced three-dimensional MR angiography with conventional digital subtraction angiography, *AJR Am J Roentgenol* 175:1188, 2000.

McIntyre KE Jr, Bailey SA, Malone SA, and others: Guillotine amputation in the treatment of nonsalvageable lower-extremity infections, *Arch Surg* 119:350, 1984.

Mueller MJ, Sinacore DR, Hastings MK, and others: Effect of Achilles tendon lengthening on neuropathic plantar ulcers. A randomized clinical trial, *J Bone Joint Surg Am* 85-A:1436, 2003.

Winburn GB, Wood MC, Hawkins ML, and others: Current role of cryoamputation, *Am J Surg* 162:647, 1991.

MANAGEMENT OF PERIPHERAL ARTERIAL EMBOLISM

Deepak Nair, MD, and Elliot L. Chaikof, MD PhD

Peripheral arterial embolization is associated with varying degrees of end organ hypoperfusion, and treatment directed at restoration of arterial blood flow may be accomplished by thrombolysis, surgical or percutaneous embolectomy, or bypass with an autologous or prosthetic graft. An understanding of the pathophysiology of this entity and an appreciation of the significant medical comorbidities that are often associated with this patient population are essential before embarking on treatment. Thorough diagnostic evaluation, selection of an appropriate intervention, and careful attention to the details of perioperative management are the determinants of optimizing outcome.

CLINICAL PRESENTATION

In the patient who presents with the acute onset of extremity pain, the history and physical examination should confirm the presence of acute arterial occlusion, differentiate among other presentations that may masquerade as an acute embolus (Table 1), identify the site of occlusion and potential source of the embolus, and determine the extent of ischemia and potential for revascularization. Current symptoms should be explored relative to the onset and severity of the ischemia, information gathered to determine potential etiology, and the presence of significant concurrent disease determined. Patients presenting with an embolus are often able to

Table 1: Differential Diagnosis of an Acutely Ischemic Extremity

Embolus
Thrombosis caused by
• Atherosclerosis
• Thrombosed aneurysm
• Vasculitis (e.g., giant cell arteritis)
• Vasospasm (e.g., ergotism)
• Low flow state
• Vascular graft occlusion
• Thrombophilia
Arterial dissection
Intra-arterial drug administration
Compartment syndrome
Extrinsic compression

pinpoint the exact time at which the abrupt onset of severe ische-mic symptoms began, whereas patients with acute thrombosis typically describe preexisting symptoms of chronic ischemia, such as intermittent claudication, which suddenly worsen. Moreover, patients who present with a profoundly ischemic lower extremity and a normally perfused contralateral extremity are likely to have experienced an embolus, whereas acute thrombosis is often associated with stigmata of chronic arterial insufficiency in both lower extremities, and a history of vascular intervention is common. In the presence of abdominal or flank pain, emboli in visceral or renal arteries should be considered, and acute paralysis and anesthesia of the lower extremities can be caused by an aortic saddle embolus and initially confused with a primary neurologic process. In considering the differential diagnosis for acute ischemia, arterial dissection should be suspected in the patient who complains of coexistent chest pain and is hypertensive on examination, whereas phlegmasia cerulea dolens can be diagnosed by the presence of edema and the absence of a femoral Doppler venous signal.

Although the heart is the most common source of arterial emboli (85%), other sources include peripheral aneurysms and atherosclerotic lesions (Table 2). Until the latter half of the twentieth century, rheumatic valvular heart disease was the cause of the majority of cardiogenic emboli. Currently, atrial fibrillation, recent myocardial infarction, or ventricular aneurysm are common underlying etiologies of emboli arising from the heart. Aortic and other peripheral arterial aneurysms, as well as focal mural ulcers or atherosclerotic thrombi, are additional sources for peripheral emboli. Finally, although venous thrombosis is a more common presentation of familial or acquired thrombophilia, a hypercoagulable state may lead to an acute arterial embolism. Of note, up to 5% of emboli have no identifiable source.

During the course of physical examination, all peripheral pulses should be evaluated, including the external iliac, axillary, and subclavian arteries. Arterial emboli typically lodge at bifurcation points, with the common femoral artery the most frequent site, followed by the common iliac artery, the terminal aorta ("saddle embolus"), and the popliteal artery (Table 3). A femoral artery occlusion can be established by recognizing the presence of a pulse, which may have a "water hammer"–type character, in the external iliac artery just proximal to the inguinal ligament. Likewise, upper-extremity emboli often lodge at the bifurcation of the

Table 3: Distribution of Acute Arterial Emboli

Femoral	47%
Iliac	20%
Aortic	16%
Popliteal	12%
Brachial	3%
Visceral	2%

brachial artery and cause ischemic symptoms of the hand. However, upper-extremity limb loss is less common because of abundant collateral circulation. As such, the status of collateral circulation, the extent of thrombus propagation from the site of the embolus, and the magnitude of preexisting atherosclerotic disease dictate the degree of ischemic symptoms. Multiple emboli are common, and in 10% of patients more than one limb may be involved. "Silent emboli" may occur in tissue beds with well-developed collateral blood supply, such as the spleen.

The degree and extent of ischemia at the time of presentation, the duration of symptoms, and time to revascularization are the most important determinants of clinical outcome. The cardinal features of acute arterial occlusion in an extremity include pain, pallor, paresthesia, paralysis, pulselessness, and poikilothermia, but it is the presence of diminished or absent sensation, proprioception, and motor function that characterize a true vascular emergency. A reporting scheme has been described for clinical stratification of the severity of acute ischemia and risk of limb loss (Table 4). Significantly, patients categorized as class IIb or early class III (Rutherford and colleagues, 1997) require expeditious revascularization because they are considered at high risk for tissue injury or limb loss should reperfusion be delayed beyond 6 hours. Late class III patients have major, irreversible, neuromuscular damage at the time of presentation that precludes limb salvage despite revascularization. Embolectomy should not be performed unless removal of an embolus might improve proximal limb perfusion and ensure subsequent healing of an amputation site. After the decision for amputation has been made, the procedure should be performed as soon as possible to avoid the metabolic consequences of prolonged tissue ischemia.

Table 2: Etiology of Arterial Emboli

Cardiogenic (85%)

- Atrial fibrillation
- Mural thrombus after myocardial infarction
- Diseased or prosthetic heart valve
- Left ventricular aneurysm
- Atrial myxoma

Noncardiac (10%)

- Aortic or peripheral aneurysm
- Aortic mural thrombus
- Ulcerative plaque
- Paradoxical embolus
- "Shaggy" aorta

Iatrogenic (2%–5%)

- Intravascular catheter or wire manipulation

Foreign body (0.5%–1%)

Indeterminate (2%–5%)

◼ MANAGEMENT AND TECHNIQUE

All patients with an acute arterial occlusion should be given anticoagulant medication promptly to prevent further embolization or propagation of the thrombus and to minimize clotting in the stagnant arterial circulation distal to the embolus. Heparin should be administered intravenously at a dose of 100 U/kg. Although intervention should generally follow shortly thereafter, continuous heparin infusion at 10 to 15 U/kg/hour can be instituted to maintain the partial thromboplastin time 2.5 times control or a systemic heparin concentration of either 0.2 to 0.4 U/mL by protamine titration or 0.3 to 0.7 U/mL by antifactor Xa analysis.

Vascular imaging, performed by either conventional or CT angiography, may be helpful if diagnostic uncertainty exists and to assist in treatment planning. However, imaging should be conducted in a manner that minimizes any delay in intervention. Significantly, the increasing availability of high-quality fluoroscopy units in the operating room provides an opportunity to acquire important diagnostic information without an inherent delay in revascularization. Typical angiographic findings of an arterial embolus include a sharp cutoff of contrast without significant collateral circulation, which, if present, suggests an acute thrombosis of a chronic atherosclerotic lesion.

Table 4: Clinical Stratification of an Ischemic Extremity

Grade	Description	Motor	Sensory Loss	Arterial Doppler Signals	Venous Doppler Signals	Capillary Return	Prognostic Implications	Therapeutic Implications
Class I	Intermittent pain	None	None	Present	Present	< 4 sec.	Viable limb	Elective angiography
Class IIa	Numbness and paresthesias	None	Mild	Absent	Present	Delayed	Limb is threatened	Urgent angiography
Class IIb	Persistent ischemic pain with any motor loss	Mild	Present	Absent	Weakly Present	Delayed	Limb is threatened	Emergent revascularization
Class III early	Profound anesthesia and paralysis	Paralysis	Anesthetic	Absent	Absent	Delayed	Increased risk of irreversible tissue loss	Emergent revascularization
Class III late	Muscle rigor and skin marbling	Paralysis with rigor	Anesthetic	Absent	Absent	None	Limb not salvageable	Amputation

From Rutherford RB, Baker JD, Ernst C, and others: J Vasc Surg 26:517, 1997.

Surgical Embolectomy

Balloon-catheter thromboembolectomy performed remotely via an open surgical incision and arteriotomy was first reported by Thomas J. Fogarty in 1963. In the case of an aortic or saddle embolus, bilateral transfemoral embolectomy is required, whereas an iliofemoral or popliteal embolism can often be treated via ipsilateral transfemoral embolectomy. As a routine, the common femoral, superficial femoral, and deep femoral arteries are isolated and an incision situated to allow embolectomy of both superficial and profunda femoral arteries. A transverse arteriotomy minimizes the risk of narrowing of the artery on closure, but a longitudinal arteriotomy facilitates bypass should embolectomy prove unsuccessful. Typically, the balloon catheter is advanced beyond the embolus, inflated, and retracted to remove the clot. A 3-F catheter is used for embolectomy of the profunda femoral artery, a 4-F catheter for a femoral-popliteal-tibial embolectomy, and a 5-F catheter for aortoiliac embolectomy. As a routine, the entire leg should be prepared and draped in the field should embolectomy not restore blood flow and a bypass becomes necessary or a fasciotomy is required. In addition, an additional site of arterial inflow, such as the contralateral common femoral artery or ipsilateral axillary artery, should be included in the field to provide an alternative source of inflow, if required.

For an embolus located at or distal to the popliteal trifurcation, initial passage of a balloon catheter through a femoral arteriotomy may successfully extract the clot. Because the catheter usually enters the peroneal artery, bending the tip of the catheter before its introduction and then rotating the catheter or bending the knee as it passes distally may facilitate its passage down the anterior or posterior tibial arteries. If removal of popliteal or tibial thrombus has been unsuccessful, options include the passage of a coaxial over-the-wire Fogarty catheter under fluoroscopic guidance into the infrageniculate vessels or direct popliteal artery exposure with arteriotomy and tibioperoneal embolectomy. On occasion, thromboembolectomy via direct exposure of the dorsalis pedis and posterior tibial arteries at the ankle may be required using a 2-F catheter. Passage of the embolectomy catheter is repeated until further embolic material is no longer removed. Pathologic examination of the embolus should be considered if atrial myxoma or a tumor embolus is suspected. If embolectomy is uneventful, extensive thrombus removed, excellent backbleeding and prograde flow established, and palpable pulses restored, no further measures are necessary. However, if these conditions are not strictly met, operative angiography should be performed to assess possible residual arterial occlusion. If thrombus remains in the distal circulation, additional passages of the balloon catheter can be performed. In addition,

adjunctive intraoperative lytic therapy with 2 to 5 mg of tissue plasminogen activator (tPA) or 250,000 units of urokinase over 15 to 20 minutes followed by repeat embolectomy may be helpful.

Thrombolytic Therapy

Catheter-directed thrombolysis (CDT) was initially introduced in the 1980s as a possible alternative to surgical embolectomy, particularly in the high-risk patient who presented with mild or moderate limb ischemia. Urokinase and tPA are examples of some of the currently available lytic agents. Important advantages of CDT include the potential to remove thrombus from small vessels that may be inaccessible to balloon-catheter thrombectomy and, in the case of an acute thrombosis, identify coexistent lesions. However, limitations of this approach include delayed reperfusion, which may result in irreversible tissue injury, and the ineffectiveness of lytic agents to dissolve emboli that are well-organized, either having developed at their site of origin months previously or being composed of atherosclerotic material or a myxomatous fragment. Other potential problems with lytic therapy include bleeding and embolization of clot fragments into the distal circulation. In addition, absolute contraindications that preclude thrombolytic therapy are recent stroke, craniotomy, surgery or percutaneous procedure, as well as active bleeding, pregnancy, or recent delivery. Advanced age, known coagulation disorder, or uncontrolled hypertension are relative contraindications. The recent development of recombinant thrombolytic agents such as alfimeprase and plasmin, which are active within the thrombus but rapidly inactivated by physiologic inhibitors in the plasma, provides an opportunity to deliver high local doses for rapid clot dissolution while avoiding bleeding complications. Clinical trials to establish efficacy in acute limb ischemia are ongoing.

Percutaneous Mechanical Thrombectomy Devices

Percutaneous mechanical thrombectomy using aspiration devices, such as the Angiojet (Possis Medical, Minneapolis, MN), Hydrolyzer (Cordis, Miami Lakes, FL), or Oasis (Boston Scientific, Natick, MA) thrombectomy catheters or cerebrovascular clot extraction devices, such as the Merci Retrieval System (Concentric Medical, Mountain View, CA), is an evolving strategy for thrombus removal, often used in conjunction with local thrombolytic therapy. In principle, these devices offer the potential to minimize the duration and total dose of thrombolytic therapy, thereby decreasing complication rates, reducing time to revascularization, and improving outcomes. However, the current experience with these devices among patients who present with an acute peripheral embolus is limited, and documented experience remains, at this time, largely confined to case reports.

POSTOPERATIVE CARE AND MANAGEMENT

Adjunctive fasciotomies should be considered in any instance of profound ischemia, particularly if revascularization has been delayed beyond 6 hours after the onset of symptoms. However, if fasciotomy has not been carried out at the initial operation, the patient must be monitored for signs of compartment syndrome. In the sedated patient, compartment pressures should be measured at regular intervals and prompt fasciotomy performed if the pressure exceeds 50% of diastolic blood pressure or if signs of neurologic compromise occur. The metabolic consequences of sudden reperfusion of a limb that has suffered prolonged severe ischemia include hyperkalemia, myoglobinuria causing renal failure, and acidosis. Hyperkalemia can be controlled acutely by diuresis or infusion of insulin and glucose. Myoglobinuria with an attendant risk of acute renal failure can be reduced by alkalization of the urine and intravenous hydration and mannitol to maintain a brisk diuresis. Metabolic acidosis is treated with bicarbonate. Postoperative anticoagulation with heparin should be instituted to prevent a recurrent embolic episode and may be initiated within 4 to 8 hours after surgical thromboembolectomy.

During the postoperative period, detection and treatment of the underlying source of the embolus should be pursued to avoid recurrent episodes. A thorough evaluation typically includes electrocardiography and Holter monitoring to assess for arrhythmia, as well as echocardiography to exclude a mural thrombus, valvular vegetations, and septal defects, such as a patent foramen ovale. Transesophageal echocardiography is more sensitive than transthoracic echocardiography and should be performed if conventional echocardiography fails to identify a cardiac source. If a cardiogenic source is not apparent, evaluation of the aorta and peripheral arteries is indicated. CT angiography is an effective technique for detecting aortic mural thrombus, irregular atherosclerotic plaque, penetrating ulceration, and aneurysmal disease. Conventional contrast aortography remains helpful in evaluating iliac and femoropopliteal vessels for focal irregular atherosclerotic plaque that can be a source of distal embolization. Depending on location and extent, these lesions can be addressed by either open surgical or endovascular approaches. Unless a source of embolization is identified and repaired, the risk of recurrent embolization remains and anticoagulation with oral warfarin is required to prevent another event.

Unfortunately, operative mortality after embolectomy has not changed significantly in the past several decades and remains 10% to 15%, with concomitant amputation in 10% of patients. These disappointing results are related to the presence of significant comorbid medical conditions, the underlying disease state that produced the embolic event, and delays in treatment. Further reductions in limb loss and perioperative mortality will be dependent on earlier diagnosis and treatment, as well as improved strategies for management of related medical problems in these high-risk patients. It is hoped that evolving percutaneous technologies and a new generation of thrombolytic agents will have a positive impact on these results.

ATYPICAL CLINICAL CIRCUMSTANCES

Atheromatous microembolization, which has been referred to as blue toe syndrome, cholesterol embolization, atheroembolism, and pseudo-vasculitis, is invariably due to thrombus fragments, cholesterol crystals, or platelet aggregates from established atherosclerotic or aneurysmal arterial disease. Trauma, vascular surgery, angiographic procedures, anticoagulation, and thrombolysis are common precipitating factors, but atheroembolization may occur spontaneously in 20% of cases. There is often a strong association with thrombocytosis, myeloproliferative disorder, collagen vascular disease, neoplasm, and polycythemia.

As opposed to an embolus arising from a cardiogenic source, embolic events arising from either aneurysm or irregular atherosclerotic plaque are characterized by diffuse microembolization, often with skin manifestations such as livedo reticularis, which presents as a blue-red mottling over the buttocks, thighs, or legs, as well as blue toes or digits. The *blue toe syndrome* manifests as the sudden appearance of a cool, cyanotic, and painful toe in the presence of palpable distal pulses, whereas patchy areas of foot discoloration have been referred to as *trash foot*. Therapy should include administration of an antiplatelet agent, pain control, and conservative local wound care before consideration of digital or forefoot amputation. Heparinization is often initiated, but reperfusion is difficult to achieve through use of anticoagulant, antiplatelet, or thrombolytic therapy. The embolic source should be eliminated to prevent recurrent events that will lead to even greater tissue loss.

Although upper-extremity emboli are usually cardiogenic, 10% to 15% may arise from lesions in the subclavian artery that may arise because of generalized atherosclerosis or thoracic outlet syndrome. Most upper-extremity emboli lodge at the brachial artery bifurcation, with the axillary artery the next most common location. Embolectomy in the upper extremity can be readily accomplished via a distal brachial arteriotomy under local anesthesia. Principles for treating upper-extremity emboli and the underlying lesion are generally the same as those for the lower extremity.

Paradoxical embolization should be suspected in any patient with an arterial embolus who presents with deep vein thrombosis or pulmonary embolism. Characteristically, a venous embolism passes through a patent foramen ovale or ventricular or atrial septal defect to the arterial circulation. The presence of the cardiac defect can be documented by transesophageal echocardiography with bubble test. Warfarin therapy and placement of an inferior vena cava (IVC) filter have been established methods of management, with surgical closure reserved for the patient with a recurrent event despite adequate anticoagulation and an IVC filter. However, the recent development of percutaneous closure devices now offers a minimally invasive approach for definitive management of intracardiac defects. As the long-term durability, safety, and efficacy of these devices is established, it is anticipated that they will be applied with increasing frequency.

An infected heart valve and on occasion an infected aortic graft or aneurysm may produce septic emboli that can manifest as both a macroscopic embolus and subtle microembolic splinter hemorrhages. Patients typically present with fever and findings related to the primary source of infection. In addition to treatment of the embolus, appropriate antibiotic therapy and removal of the underlying source of infection are critical components of therapy.

Suggested Readings

Becquemin JP, Kovarsky S: Arterial emboli of the lower limbs: analysis of risk factors for mortality and amputation, *Ann Vasc Surg* 9:suppl:S32, 1995.

Chaikof EL, Campbell BE, Smith II IRB: Paradoxical embolism and acute arterial occlusion: rare or unsuspected, *J Vasc Surg* 20:377, 1994.

Costantini V, Lenti M: Treatment of acute occlusion of peripheral arteries, *Thrombosis Res* 106:285, 2002.

Cwikiel W, Midia M, Williams D: Nontraumatic vascular emergencies: imaging and intervention in acute arterial conditions, *Eur Radiol* 12:2619, 2002.

Eliason JL, Wainess RM, Proctor MC, and others: A national and single institutional experience in the contemporary treatment of acute lower extremity ischemia, *Ann Surg* 238:382, 2003.

Rutherford RB, Baker JD, Ernst C, and others: Recommended standards for reports dealing with lower extremity ischemia: Revised version, *J Vasc Surg* 26:517, 1997.

BUERGER'S DISEASE (THROMBOANGIITIS OBLITERANS)

Carl-Magnus Wahlgren, MD, and Bruce L. Gewertz, MD

INTRODUCTION

Thromboangiitis obliterans (TAO) or Buerger's disease is a non-atherosclerotic, segmental, inflammatory disease that affects the small and medium-sized arteries and veins of the extremities. Patients are mostly young male tobacco smokers who present with distal-extremity ischemia, ischemic ulcers, or gangrene. Buerger's disease has a worldwide distribution, but it is more prevalent in the Mediterranean, the Middle East, and Asia. Recently the prevalence of disease seems to have declined in the United States and Europe. In the United States, the prevalence of disease was 104 cases per 100,000 patient registrations in 1947 and dropped to 12.6 cases per 100,000 patient registrations in 1986. Whether this is a true decline attributed to the decline in smoking or an adoption of more uniform, stricter diagnostic criteria is unclear. There has been an increase in the incidence in women, who constitute up to 20% of patients in certain series. This relative rise in incidence in women is undoubtedly due to the increase in cigarette smoking among women.

Although the etiology of Buerger's disease is unknown, the condition is strongly associated with heavy tobacco use. Smoking is considered by most to be an absolute requirement for diagnosis, and progression is closely linked to continued use. However, a causal relationship has not been conclusively demonstrated. There have been reports of the presence of TAO in cigar smokers and in users of smokeless tobacco products such as chewing tobacco and snuff. The disease is classified pathologically as a vasculitis. Features that distinguish TAO from other types of vasculitis include highly inflammatory thrombus with relative sparing of the blood vessel wall, normal acute phase reactants, and no serum markers of immunoactivation.

CLINICAL PRESENTATION

Buerger's disease typically begins with ischemia of the distal small arteries and veins. More proximal arteries may be involved when the disease progresses, but involvement of large arteries is unusual. The onset of symptoms usually occurs before the age of 40 to 45 years. Patients may present with claudication of the feet, legs, hands, or arms. Two or more limbs are always involved; all four limbs are affected in approximately 40% of patients. Intermittent symptoms are initially localized to the forefoot or the arch of the foot because of the distal nature of the disease, as opposed to patients with peripheral atherosclerotic disease, who first experience symptoms in the calves. Progression of the inflammatory disease leads to development of ischemic rest pain and ulcerations in the distal portion of toes or fingers. In most series, approximately three quarters of patients present with ischemic ulcers. Raynaud's phenomenon and superficial migratory thrombophlebitis are manifestations that are commonly encountered.

Although Buerger's disease predominantly affects the vessels of the extremities, a few instances of aortic, cerebral, coronary, mesenteric, pulmonary, and renal involvement have been reported in the literature. Mesenteric Buerger's disease is extremely rare and is associated with a poor prognosis. Patients with known Buerger's disease presenting with gastrointestinal manifestations should be urgently evaluated for bowel ischemia; early surgical intervention is recommended.

DIAGNOSIS

Physical examination often reveals cyanotic and erythematous extremities. Sensory abnormalities (burning, hypoesthesia, numbness, and tingling) caused by ischemic neuropathy are common, as is cold sensitivity that may be related to ischemia or to increased sympathetic nerve activity. Absent distal pulses in the presence of normal proximal pulses are typical in patients with the disease. Involvement of both the upper and lower extremities is common. Dry punctuate ischemic lesions are often seen on both the hands and feet.

Although a definitive diagnosis of TAO can be made only with a vessel biopsy showing cellular thrombus and the classic acute-phase lesion involving all layers of the vessel wall, the physical examination and history are often classic. As a consequence, biopsies are rarely necessary unless a patient presents with unusual characteristics, such as large-artery involvement or an age older than 45 years.

There are no specific laboratory tests to confirm the diagnosis, but several serologic tests should be included in the workup to rule out other diseases that mimic TAO, including scleroderma, CREST (calcinosis, Raynaud's phenomenon, esophageal dysmotility, sclerodactyly, and telangiectasia) syndrome, mixed connective-tissue disease, systemic lupus erythematosus, and hypercoagulability disorders. We routinely obtain a complete blood count with differential, electrolytes, renal and liver function tests, fasting blood glucose, urinalysis, sedimentation rate and C-reactive protein, and a complete hypercoaguability screen including antiphospholipid antibodies. Serologic markers that should be obtained include antinuclear antibody, rheumatoid factor, complement measurements, and serologic markers for CREST syndrome and scleroderma (SCL-70 and anticentromere antibody). Patients with giant cell arteritis or Takayasu's arteritis usually present with more proximal vascular involvement and more frequently have elevations of acute-phase reactants.

Standard arteriography is not essential for the diagnosis. Noninvasive imaging such as gadolinium-enhanced magnetic resonance angiography (MRA) and computed tomographic angiography (CTA) are good alternatives. Four-limb segmental arterial pressures and digital plethysmography (waveform, digital pressure measurement, or both) are useful to document distal occlusive disease. When suggested by unilateral involvement, a proximal source of emboli should be excluded with echocardiography.

Arteriography should be performed in patients with threatened limb loss. A number of angiographic findings are suggestive of TAO, but there are no pathognomonic findings (Table 1). The angiographic appearance of TAO may be identical to other types of small-vessel vasculitis or toxic arterial responses related to amphetamine, cannabis, or cocaine abuse. If a nonsmoking patient presents with signs consistent with Buerger's disease, it is advisable to obtain a toxicology screen for these drugs.

Given the relatively young age of most patients, the possibility of popliteal artery entrapment syndrome, cystic adventitial disease, or politeal artery aneurysm should be considered. The presence of diabetes mellitus, end-stage renal disease, or significant risk factors for atherosclerosis argues against a diagnosis of Buerger's disease.

Table 1: Angiographic Findings in Thromboangiitis Obliterans (Buerger's Disease) (See Figs. 1 and 2)

- Involvement of small and medium-sized vessels: palmar, plantar, tibial, peroneal, radial, and ulnar arteries, as well as digital arteries of fingers and toes
- Normal extremity arteries proximal to the popliteal and distal brachial levels
- Proximal atherosclerosis and vascular calcification are absent
- No source of thrombus
- Abrupt transition from a normal and smooth proximal artery to an area of occlusion
- Symmetrical and segmental arterial involvement
- Tortuous "corkscrew" collaterals are suggestive, but not pathognomonic, of Buerger's disease

TREATMENT

The main and most effective treatment for Buerger's disease is total abstinence from tobacco products. Smoking is closely related to exacerbation and remission of the disease. Even smoking a few cigarettes a day or using smokeless tobacco or nicotine replacement may keep the disease active. It was initially thought that smoking cessation was not possible in patients with Buerger's disease. Our experience and that of others would suggest that this is unduly pessimistic; up to a third of our patients have successfully discontinued tobacco use with proper counseling and support.

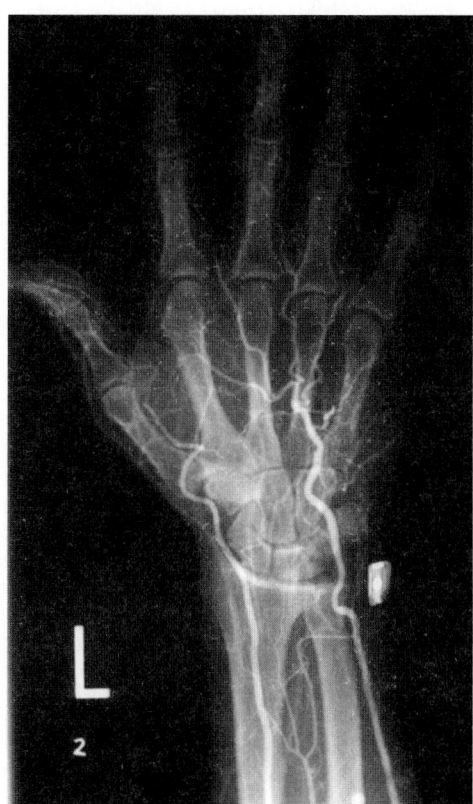

Figure 1 Hand angiogram of patient with Buerger's disease illustrates involvement of the digital arteries with several occlusions and collaterals.

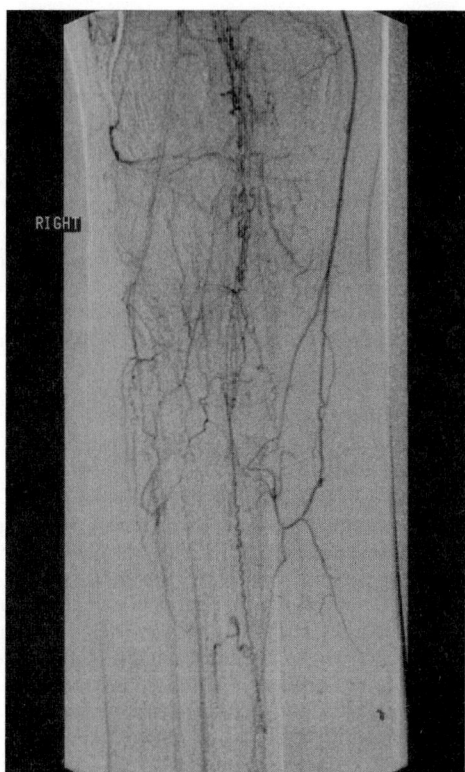

Figure 2 Lower-extremity angiography of patient with Buerger's disease demonstrates multiple occlusions and "corkscrew" collaterals.

There is a correlation between continued smoking and limb amputation. If patients discontinue tobacco use, they can be reassured that the disease will often remit and amputation can be avoided as long as ischemic ulcers have not already occurred. That said, patients with already significant occluded arterial segments might continue to experience intermittent claudication or Raynaud's phenomenon.

In patients whose disease progresses despite smoking cessation, effective therapeutic options are limited (Table 2). Initial enthusiasm for infusion of the prostaglandin analogue iloprost has not been borne out by further trials or experience. Anticoagulants, antiplatelet drugs, and rheologic agents seem to be ineffective. Calcium channel blockers are only helpful if significant vasospasm is present.

Table 2: Treatment Options in Thromboangiitis Obliterans (Buerger's Disease)

Cessation of tobacco products
Local wound care
Arterial reconstruction with vein graft
Therapeutic options:
   Prostaglandin analogue iloprost or treprostinil sodium
   Cilostazol
   Hyperbaric oxygen therapy
   Calcium channel blockers (i.e., amlodipine or nifedipine, if vasospasm)
   Intermittent pneumatic compression pump
   Implantable spinal cord stimulator
   Therapeutic angiogenesis
Amputation

Intra-arterial thrombolytic therapy is not effective and has not been used in our practice.

Unfortunately, arterial reconstruction is usually not an attractive option because of the diffuse segmental involvement and distal nature of the disease. As well, the concomitant inflammatory venous disease often renders the saphenous veins unsatisfactory for use as conduits. However, if conservative treatment fails in patients with severe ischemia and nonhealing ischemic ulcers of the lower extremities, revascularization should be considered. The distal arteries must be thoroughly evaluated by arteriography for optimal preoperative planning. If surgical exploration reveals a diminutive receiving vessel, bypass should be abandoned.

Although less invasive endovascular approaches might be attractive in this population, the diffuse, distal, and segmental involvement of the lesions confounds the currently available techniques.

As with many interventions for occlusive vascular disease, limb-salvage rates usually exceed graft patencies. Although patency for distal bypass is no more than 50% even in the small number of patients with Buerger's disease who can undergo bypasses, limb-salvage rates frequently exceed 75%. In these well-selected patients, even limited periods of revascularization provide a sufficient interval to heal ischemic ulcers in the feet.

Sympathectomy as a primary or adjunctive treatment option has been tried in a large number of patients with Buerger's disease without encouraging results. This lack of success reinforces the obstructive rather then vasospastic nature of the disease. Nonetheless, in some patients, spinal cord stimulation can have a salutary effect through pain reduction.

Amputations are inevitable in patients with extensive gangrene or sepsis. The goal is to remove all nonviable tissue, preserve optimal residual function, and minimize surgical morbidity. Application of these principles may result in unconventional amputation levels with a preponderance of multiple digital or distal amputations.

PROGNOSIS

In general, the prognosis for many patients with Buerger's disease is surprisingly good. Despite the considerable morbidity, life expectancy for patients approaches that of an age-matched population. This could possibly be explained by the young age of presentation and the lack of coronary involvement in the disease process.

Even though ischemic ulcers are already present in the majority of patients presenting for medical care, the overall limb amputation rate is less than 50%. It seems that occurrence of necrotic lesions subsides in patients older than 60 years. Nonetheless, follow-up of patients with TAO shows frequent hospitalization and surgical procedures. Major amputation and prolonged hospitalization markedly influence quality of life, with many patients losing any opportunity for productive jobs.

SUMMARY

Thromboangiitis obliterans (TAO) or Buerger's disease is a non-atherosclerotic, segmental, and inflammatory disease. It is characterized by the development of segmental thrombotic occlusions of the medium and small arteries and veins of the extremities.

It occurs in young smokers who present with distal extremity ischemia, ulcers, or gangrene. The most important diseases to exclude are atherosclerosis, emboli, and autoimmune diseases. The only effective treatment is complete and permanent abstinence from tobacco products. Several medical and surgical therapies are palliative.

SUGGESTED READINGS

Mills JL Sr: Buerger's disease in the 21st century: diagnosis, clinical features, and therapy, *Semin Vasc Surg* 16:179, 2003.

Ohta T, Ishioashi H, Hosaka M, and others: Clinical and social consequences of Buerger disease, *J Vasc Surg* 39:176, 2004.

Olin JW: Thromboangiitis obliterans (Buerger's disease), *N Engl J Med* 343:864, 2000.

Olin JW, Shih A: Thromboangiitis obliterans (Buerger's disease), *Curr Opin Rheumatol* 18:18, 2006.

PERIPHERAL ARTERIAL AND BYPASS GRAFT OCCLUSION: THROMBOLYTIC THERAPY

Anthony J. Comerota, MD, and Santiago Chahwan, MD

BACKGROUND

Few patient care problems challenge the clinical acumen of the vascular surgeon more than the patient who presents with acute limb ischemia. This clinical scenario threatens the limb in all patients and the life of many, especially the elderly.

This chapter focuses on patients with acute lower-extremity arterial occlusion and bypass graft occlusion, with an emphasis on the appropriate application of catheter-directed thrombolysis.

Proper application of any therapy is guided by an understanding of the underlying pathology and its natural history. In patients with acute arterial occlusion, successful treatment is determined in large part by properly identifying the underlying etiology. Is the patient presenting with acute arterial thrombosis or acute embolic occlusion? Was there a recent intravascular intervention or trauma? Is acute dissection a possibility? Patients should be queried for prior symptoms of intermittent claudication and undergo an evaluation of the contralateral limb for occlusive disease, as well as a thorough investigation for a possible source of emboli.

Classically, acute limb ischemia presents with the six P's: pain, pulselessness, pallor, poikilothermy, paresthesias, and paralysis. The presence of these findings and the levels of severity are variable and are influenced by the severity and duration of ischemia. For example, ischemic pain may resolve either as collateral circulation is recruited and the ischemia lessens or as a result of nerve dysfunction as ischemia worsens. Obvious neurologic deficits suggest an advanced state of ischemia, with sensory deficits preceding motor deficits. Fixed mottling of the skin with muscle necrosis and induration implies an unsalvageable limb (Table 1).

Table 1: Classification of Acute Limb Ischemia

Category	Description/Prognosis	Findings		Doppler Exam	
		Sensory Loss	Muscle Weakness	Arterial	Venous
I. Viable	Not immediately threatened	None	None	Audible	Audible
II. Threatened					
a. Marginally	Salvageable if promptly treated	None or minimal (toes)	None	Inaudible	Audible
b. Immediately	Salvageable with immediate revascularization	More than toes, associated with rest pain	Mild, moderate	Inaudible	Audible
III. Irreversible	Major tissue loss, permanent nerve damage inevitable	Profound, anesthetic	Profound, paralysis (rigor)	Inaudible	Inaudible

From Rutherford RB, Baker JD, Ernst C, and others: J Vasc Surg 26:517, 1997. Reprinted with permission.

Despite the obvious clinical findings, a formal system of stratifying acute limb ischemia is required to guide evaluation and management and to define prognosis. An acutely ischemic limb should be described as viable, threatened, or irreversibly ischemic according to currently accepted reporting standards (Table 1). Experienced clinicians can fine-tune these guidelines. Threatened limbs are reversibly ischemic and are salvageable with timely intervention, whereas irreversibly ischemic limbs generally require amputation because major neuromuscular damage has occurred and is not reversible with revascularization. That is not to say that concomitant revascularization is unnecessary because it may be valuable in reducing the level of amputation.

The degree of ischemia is determined by a number of factors, including the level of obstruction, the adequacy of collateral circulation, the degree of thrombus propagation, the etiology of obstruction, and the patient's underlying cardiac output. The peripheral nerves and muscles are most sensitive to hypoxic injury, whereas the skin and subcutaneous tissues tolerate a longer duration of ischemia. Complete cessation of blood flow produced by tourniquet-induced ischemia, which interrupts both axial and collateral perfusion, is associated with histologic evidence of striated muscle injury at 2 hours and extensive necrosis by 6 hours. Although a period of 6 hours has been historically accepted as the maximal interval before revascularization for acute limb ischemia, the tolerance of skeletal muscle to clinical ischemia is variable because most patients do not have complete cessation of blood flow in both their axial and collateral vessels and acceptable results have been achieved with revascularization after substantially longer periods. In practice, the degree of ischemia is more important than the absolute duration of ischemia, and patients must be assessed on an individual basis and in an expedient fashion.

In patients with acute lower-extremity graft thrombosis, the initial indication for the bypass must be established. The preoperative and completion arteriograms should be examined to evaluate for clues leading to graft failure. The quality of the underlying conduit, especially in the case of a saphenous vein graft, should be assessed. Catheter-directed thrombolysis is designed to eliminate the thrombus and reveal the underlying cause of the graft occlusion. Therefore it is assumed that the underlying etiology of graft occlusion is reversible. An important consideration is whether the graft is worth salvaging. It should be determined whether additional segments of the arterial tree are thrombosed and contributing to the patient's ischemia and whether disease of the inflow or outflow vessels contributed to the graft thrombosis. Ultimately a decision must be made as to whether the patient requires revascularization at all following graft thrombosis.

The severity of limb ischemia is used to guide decision making and the timing of intervention (Table 2). Patients who are asymptomatic at rest (grade I) require no intervention for limb salvage, and one must consider seriously whether any form of revascularization should be attempted. Patients with mild symptoms at rest (grade IIa) can be managed with the full spectrum of treatment options, including catheter-directed thrombolysis or operative

Table 2: Differential Diagnosis and Etiology of Acute Limb Ischemia

Conditions Mimicking Acute Limb Ischemia

- Heart failure (especially if associated with chronic occlusive disease)
- Acute deep vein thrombosis
- Acute compressive neuropathy

Nonatherosclerotic Causes of Acute Limb Ischemia

- Arterial trauma
- Aortic/arterial dissection
- Arteritis with thrombosis (e.g., giant cell arteritis, thromboangiitis obliterans)
- Spontaneous thrombosis associated with a hypercoagulable state
- Popliteal cyst with thrombosis
- Popliteal entrapment with thrombosis
- Vasospasm with thrombosis (e.g., ergotism)

Causes of Acute Limb Ischemia in Patients with Atherosclerosis

- Thrombosis of an atherosclerotic stenosed artery
- Thrombosis of an arterial bypass graft
- Embolism from heart, aneurysm, plaque, or critical stenosis upstream (including cholesterol or atherothrombotic emboli secondary to endovascular procedures)
- Thrombosed aneurysm (especially popliteal aneurysm)

revascularization. Patients with more severe ischemia (grade IIb) traditionally have been managed with operative approaches. However, with the development of pharmacomechanical thrombolysis and rapid, direct-acting clot-dissolving drugs (alfimeprase and plasmin [now in clinical trials], which do not act via plasminogen activation), patients with grade IIb ischemia will increasingly be considered for percutaneous, catheter-directed revascularization procedures. Patients who present with grade III ischemia having rigor, neurologic dysfunction, and paralysis may be best served with primary amputation.

GOOD CANDIDATES FOR CATHETER-DIRECTED THROMBOLYSIS

Patients who have acute arterial or graft occlusion are the patients most likely to have successful reperfusion following thrombolytic therapy. Choosing patients who will have a lower complication rate with catheter-directed thrombolysis compared with operative revascularization is the ultimate goal of good clinical judgment. Patients considered good candidates for catheter-directed thrombolysis include those with (1) acute embolic or thrombotic occlusion of arteries relatively inaccessible or requiring involved surgical exposure for operative thromboembolectomy; (2) leg wounds, which would compromise operative revascularization; (3) a thrombosed bypass graft with thrombus extending into additional segments of the arterial tree, causing more severe ischemia than the original indication for the bypass; (4) acute thrombosis of a popliteal aneurysm, causing limb-threatening ischemia, usually associated with thrombosis of the infrapopliteal arteries; (5) acute arterial thrombosis, especially in proximal arteries; and (6) thrombosed saphenous vein grafts that have been functioning for 1 year or more (suggesting a good vein graft that has occluded because of a segmental lesion).

POOR CANDIDATES FOR CATHETER-DIRECTED THROMBOLYSIS

Patients whose underlying condition is associated with a low likelihood of success or a high complication rate from catheter-directed thrombolysis or whose surgical options are associated with better success rates and fewer complications are considered poor candidates for catheter-directed thrombolysis. Among them are patients with the following conditions: (1) acute embolic occlusion of a large artery easily accessible via a limited operative procedure, (2) acute postoperative bypass graft thrombosis, (3) modest ischemia following bypass graft occlusion (intermittent claudication), and (4) severe limb ischemia in which viability is imminently threatened, although these patients are also at high risk for operative management. (This may be modified with the newer pharmacomechanical devices that more rapidly restore perfusion and with the development of more rapidly acting clot-dissolving agents, i.e., alfimeprase and plasmin.)

Early postoperative graft thrombosis is most often associated with technical error, poor conduit, or poor patient selection for the bypass. Technical errors require operative correction. A poor conduit will rethrombose unless the conduit itself is replaced. Poor patient selection generally results in rethrombosis regardless of the mechanical or pharmacologic therapy offered; therefore additional intervention with lytic agents poses needless risk without potential gain. The combined complication and failure rate of thrombolysis in these patients is unreasonably high. Patients with severe limb ischemia in which viability is imminently threatened are the most challenging patients requiring the most experienced clinical judgment.

OUTCOMES OF PATIENT CARE

The ultimate goal of patient care is to provide safe and effective revascularization that is durable and free of complications. Recurrent ischemia and treatment-related morbidity and mortality are common in these patients.

Patients with acute embolic occlusion are the most likely to have a successful outcome from catheter-directed thrombolysis. This would include patients with distal emboli, multivessel occlusion as a result of fragmentation of emboli, or multiple embolic episodes. However, patients with a large-artery embolus who have an easily accessible vessel through a limited operative approach are best managed with surgical embolectomy.

Although randomized trials have failed to demonstrate benefit of catheter-directed lytic therapy in patients with acute arterial thrombosis, a robust clinical experience with proper patient selection has demonstrated the multiple benefits of this approach, especially in patients presenting with classic acute occlusion who have a history of intermittent claudication, suggesting that segmental arterial occlusive disease was present before arterial thrombosis.

Dissolving the thrombus and identifying and correcting the underlying stenosis can be associated with long-term success (Fig. 1).

In patients who present with lower-extremity bypass graft occlusion, the initial indication of the bypass is reviewed, as are the duration of patency and the type of graft used. An autogenous vein graft that has functioned for 1 year or more is worthy of aggressive attempts at revascularization using catheter-directed thrombolysis because a focal lesion is frequently responsible for graft failure. After the thrombus is lysed and the lesion has been unveiled and corrected, secondary patency of these grafts is quite good. Prosthetic grafts, on the other hand, have poor secondary patency rates, with several studies demonstrating that the majority of the patients rethrombosed within 1 year. A new bypass is often better than attempting to salvage the thrombosed prosthetic. If the initial indication for the graft was limb salvage, and after graft thrombosis the patient's limb is not threatened, most patients should be treated with nonoperative, noninterventional management.

Frequently, when a prosthetic graft thromboses, the thrombus extends into additional segments of the arterial tree, causing more severe ischemia than the original indication for the bypass. In these cases, catheter-directed thrombolysis offers significant advantage compared with operative revascularization alone. In the Surgery and Thrombolysis in Ischemia of the Lower Extremity (STILE) Trial, the subset of patients with acute graft thrombosis randomized to catheter-directed thrombolysis had significantly better amputation-free survival at 1 year than those randomized to operative revascularization.

DIFFERENTIAL DIAGNOSIS OF NATIVE ARTERIAL OCCLUSION

Acute arterial occlusion may result from an embolus, arterial thrombosis, trauma (iatrogenic or accidental), or spontaneous arterial dissection (Table 2). Excluding trauma, acute upper extremity ischemia is almost always of embolic origin, whereas thrombosis of underlying atherosclerotic lesions in addition to emboli is common in the lower extremities. The relative frequencies of embolic occlusion versus arterial thrombosis vary according to patient populations and referral patterns, the inclusion of vascular graft occlusions, and errors in diagnosis. Depending on these considerations, embolism may vary from single-digit percentages to the majority of patients with acutely ischemic limbs. The lower frequency of embolic occlusion in recent reports is most likely due to the declining incidence of rheumatic heart disease, more widespread use of anticoagulation, the treatment of patients with myocardial infarction and atrial fibrillation with anticoagulation, and an increasing number of patients with arterial grafts for limb salvage being treated with anticoagulation.

Although many reports of patients with acute limb ischemia include both embolic and thrombotic occlusions, distinction is important because the management and natural history are substantially different. Acute embolic occlusions are associated with higher rates of limb salvage but also higher mortality than arterial thrombosis. Furthermore, embolic occlusions often can be managed with mechanical or pharmacologic removal of the embolus alone, whereas acute thrombosis resulting from underlying arterial occlusive disease requires arterial reconstruction for ultimate success. Misdiagnosis and inadequate treatment of arterial thrombosis with only thrombus extraction has been associated with high rates of limb loss, reoperation, and death.

A patient presenting with acute limb ischemia who has a history of intermittent claudication, with physical findings of occlusive disease, and a reduced ankle-brachial pressure index (ABI) in the contralateral limb without atrial fibrillation or a recent myocardial infarction most likely has acute arterial thrombosis. Arteriographic findings include evidence of underlying atherosclerosis with established collateral circulation and frequently contralateral disease.

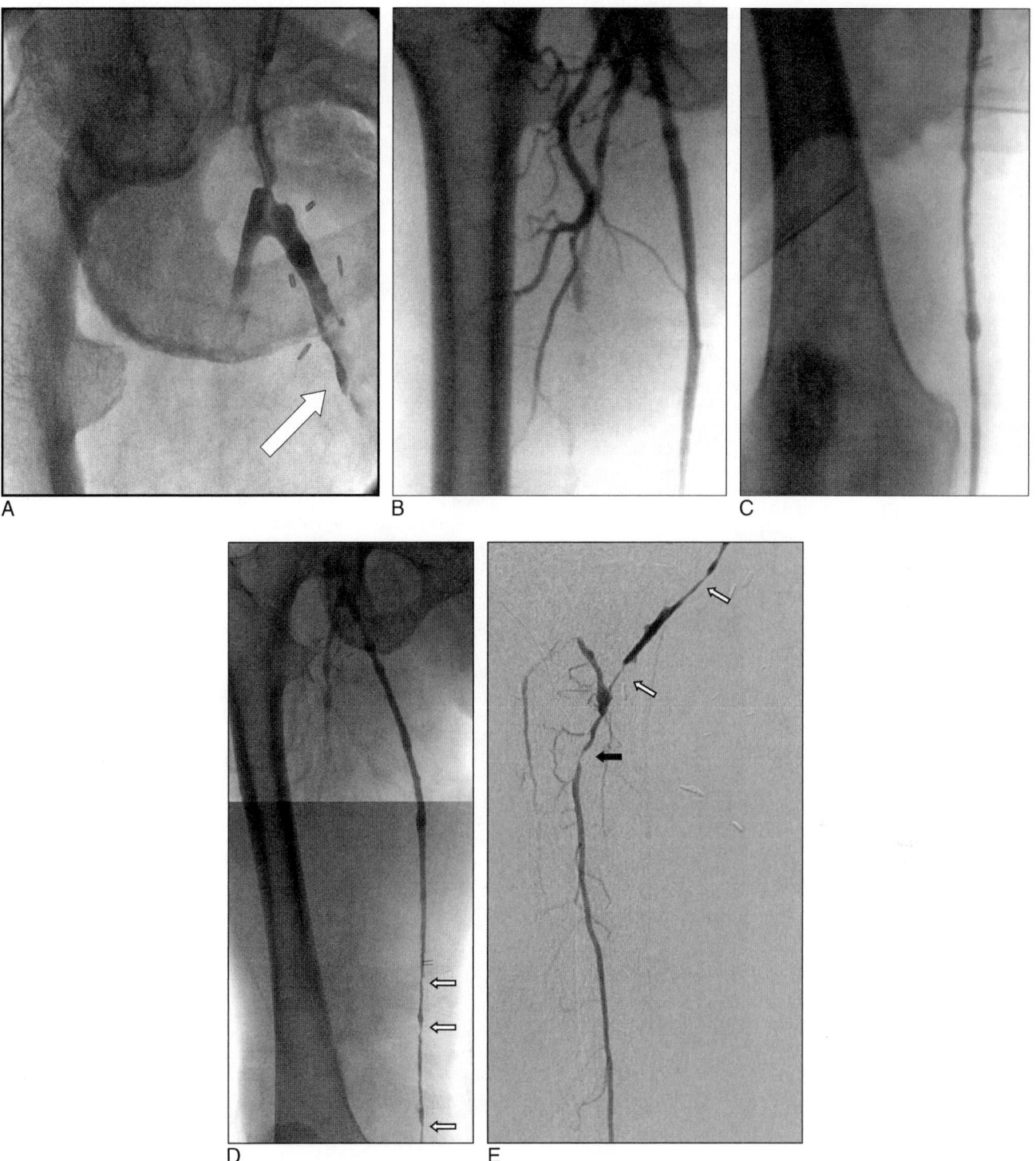

Figure I **(A)** Arteriogram of a patient presenting with a pulseless, painful, cool right leg 2 years after a femoral-tibioperoneal in situ bypass. Arrow shows point of occlusion. A guidewire was passed through the graft, and a 4-F catheter was advanced into the thrombus. rt-PA was infused at the rate of 1.2 mg/hr. After 18 hours, flow was restored through the graft **(B, C)**, although several moderate-to-severe stenoses remained in the mid- and distal sections of the graft **(D, E, white arrows)**. A high-grade stenosis of the peroneal artery is noted *(black arrow)*. Angioplasty was performed with good results, restoring perfusion to the patient's limb.

On the other hand, patients without any history suggestive of occlusive disease complaining of sudden onset of symptoms with normal physical findings on the contralateral extremity often have a history of arrhythmia or myocardial infarction and characteristically have embolic occlusion. Arteriographic signs of embolic occlusion include abrupt arterial occlusion, usually at bifurcations associated with a meniscus sign. Multiple sites of occlusion suggest fragmentation of peripheral emboli. Often the distinction between embolic and thrombotic occlusion may be difficult to establish. Some have suggested that the mere presence of atrial fibrillation in a patient with sudden arterial occlusion is evidence enough to suggest an embolic etiology. The usual risk factors for atherosclerosis have not proved useful in distinguishing thrombosis from embolism because only 40% of patients with acute arterial thrombosis have a history of intermittent claudication.

TECHNIQUE OF CATHETER-DIRECTED THROMBOLYSIS

All of the available thrombolytic agents function by activating plasminogen to form plasmin. Plasminogen bound to fibrin within the clot is particularly susceptible to activation, and the plasmin that is then produced is protected from rapid neutralization by circulating antiplasmins. The plasmin can then act within the thrombus to break down fibrin and lyse clot. It follows that the most effective means of achieving thrombus resolution is by delivering the plasminogen activator directly into the occluding thrombus. In addition to being an intuitively proper approach, intrathrombus delivery has been shown to be significantly more effective than systemic infusion. Recommended dosage and infusion rates for thrombolytic agents are shown in Table 3.

Success rates of 80% to 90% can be anticipated in properly selected patients. A contralateral approach to the arterial graft occlusion is most common, although an antegrade ipsilateral approach in some patients might be preferable. It is often difficult to pass the guidewire into an occluded bypass graft or native artery using the antegrade approach if the level of occlusion is at the common femoral artery or high on the superficial femoral artery because the wire or catheter preferentially enters the profunda femoris artery. If one is dealing with a distal superficial femoral artery (SFA) or popliteal thrombosis, or if the graft originates from a more distal location, an ipsilateral approach might be appropriate.

Aspirin is initiated (or continued) in all patients on presentation. The urgency of intervention depends on the severity of the patient's ischemia. Anticoagulation is immediately initiated to prevent thrombus propagation. Following a complete arteriogram, which usually includes the infrarenal aorta and both the iliofemoral systems and complete runoff of the leg in question, the diagnostic catheter is replaced with an appropriate infusion catheter and threaded around the aortic bifurcation. Generally, a 5-F multi-side-hole catheter is used, with an infusion distance appropriate to the length of the occlusion. The first and the last holes of the catheter should be positioned within the proximal and distal portions of the thrombus. A tip-occluding wire is useful to prevent the majority of the thrombolytic agent from flowing out of the end hole rather than the smaller side holes. Multihole and diagnostic flush catheters are inappropriate for lytic therapy because the endhole cannot be occluded and thrombolysis is often less effective.

Coaxial systems with infusion through an outer catheter and an inner infusion wire are often useful when two separate sites require simultaneous infusion. Small, segmental, distal-vessel (tibial/peroneal) occlusions can often be treated with a single-endhole catheter. The smallest possible introducer sheath that will accept the infusion catheters is chosen. Occasionally, with a prolonged infusion, the additional introducer sheath requires upsizing because catheter manipulation enlarges the arterial puncture site and produces bleeding around the sheath.

A variety of methods of catheter-directed thrombolysis have been used in attempts to increase the speed of lysis. *Thrombus lacing* refers to the infusion of greater amounts of plasminogen activator along the length of the thrombus as the catheter is withdrawing from distal to proximal thrombus. This technique uses a concentrated form of lytic agent and is intended to saturate the thrombus with the plasminogen activator.

Intrathrombus, intermittent, high-pressure infusion refers to the pulse-spray technique of delivering the thrombolytic agent. This technique forcefully injects the plasminogen activator into the thrombus; this might fragment the thrombus and increase the surface area available for enzymatic action by the plasminogen activator. The purpose of this technique is to accelerate lysis and shorten treatment time. It is accepted that when antegrade flow is established, there is no benefit from additional pulse-spray infusion compared with the continuous infusion technique.

Rheolytic thrombectomy is gaining popularity in efforts to further speed therapy. Experimental studies have objectively demonstrated that which clinicians have observed in practice. The use of high-pressure rheolytic catheters without the addition of a plasminogen activator can achieve reperfusion, but with a significant added risk of distal emboli. Adding a plasminogen activator to the rheolytic solution reduces time to reperfusion, improves the completeness of thrombus dissolution, and reduces the amount and size of emboli debris. Catheter-directed lysis without using power injection requires a significantly longer duration of infusion; however, the size and number of distal emboli are significantly reduced.

Segmental pharmacomechanical thrombolysis is an increasingly popular method in patients with acute arterial and graft occlusion (Fig. 2). A catheter with distal and proximal balloons (Trellis; Bacchus Vascular, Santa Clara, CA) is inserted into the occluded vessel with a plasminogen activator infused between the two occluding balloons. The intervening catheter then assumes a spiral configuration with the insertion of a distribution wire and rotates at 15,000 rpm, distributing the plasminogen activator and fragmenting the thrombus. After 15 to 20 minutes, the particulate debris and dissolved thrombus are then aspirated and a repeat arteriogram is performed. The process is repeated if necessary. A longer-duration infusion of a high-volume dilute plasminogen activator (1–2 mg rt-PA in 50–100 ml saline) can follow to lyse residual thrombus. Preliminary observations suggest more rapid reperfusion with much less risk of distal embolization.

Another pharmacomechanical technique takes advantage of ultrasound waves generated from transducers built into the infusion catheter to accelerate thrombus dissolution. The Lysus catheter system (EKOS, Bothell, WA) has been used for these patients with favorable results.

Table 3: Recommended Dosage and Infusion Rate of Thrombolytics*

	Alteplase	Reteplase	Tenecteplase
Dosage/ solution	10 mg in 500 ml NSS	10 U in 250 ml NSS	5 mg in 400 ml NSS
Bolus	0–5 mg	0.5–2.0 U	1–5 mg
Infusion rate	1–2 mg/hr, not to exceed 100 mg/24 hr	0.5 U/hr; may be adjusted up to 1 U/hr	.25–.5 mg/hr

NSS, Normal saline solution.

*Intrathrombus bolus or lacing is variable; however, it is generally approximately 4 to 6 times the hourly infusion dose in a concentrated solution.

NEW DIRECT-ACTING FIBRINOLYTIC AGENTS

Two new direct-acting fibrinolytic agents that show great promise for the management of patients with acute arterial and bypass graft occlusion are under investigation. Alfimeprase and plasmin are in a new class of pharmacologic lytic agents that act directly on the thrombus (not via the plasminogen enzyme system), appear to act much more rapidly than traditional plasminogen activators, and are immediately neutralized on entering the systemic circulation. Alfimeprase is immediately neutralized by alpha-2 macroglobulin upon entry into the systemic circulation, whereas plasmin is neutralized by circulating antiplasmins. Preliminary observations suggest that both agents act more rapidly and are associated with fewer bleeding complications than traditional plasminogen activators, although the results of controlled trials are not yet available.

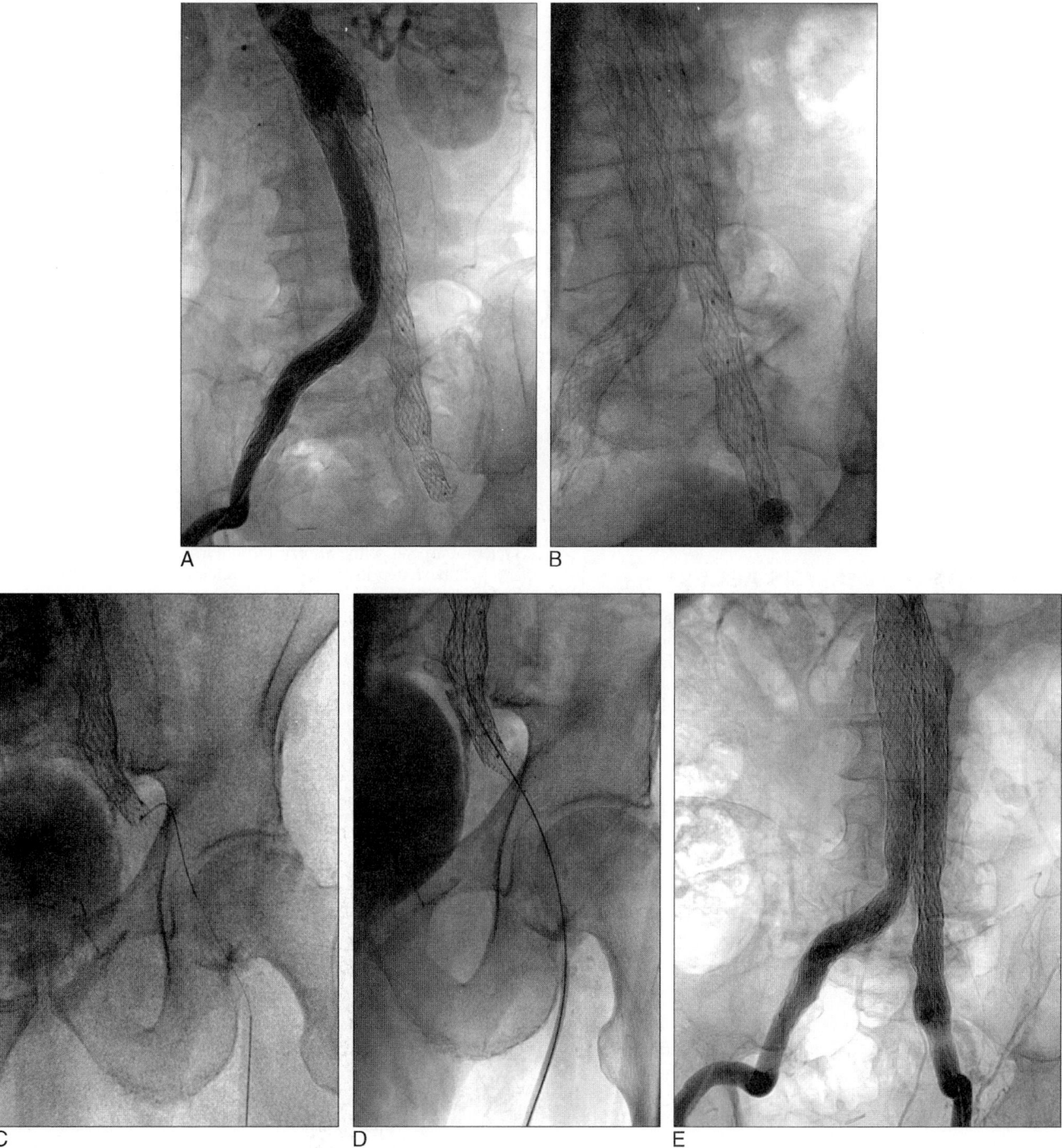

Figure 2   A patient presented with acute ischemia of the left lower extremity one month after endovascular aneurysm repair (EVAR) with no pulse in the left leg. **(A)** An arteriogram showed occlusion of the left limb of the stent-graft. **(B)** A Trellis catheter was placed with the occluding balloons inflated, and segmental pharmacomechanical thrombolysis was performed using 4 mg of rt-PA. An acute angle (kink) at the end of the left iliac limb **(C)** was treated with a self-expanding nitinol stent **(D).** A completion arteriogram shows successful reperfusion through the graft **(E),** and the patient had normal distal pulses.

SUGGESTED READINGS

Ariani M, Fishbein MC, Chae JS, and others: Dissolution of peripheral arterial thrombi by ultrasound, *Circulation* 84:4:1680–1688, 1991.

Comerota AJ: Intra-arterial catheter-directed thrombolysis. In Rutherford RB, editor: *Vascular surgery,* ed 6, Philadelphia, 2005, Elsevier Saunders.

Comerota AJ, Weaver FA, Hosking JD, and others: Results of a prospective, randomized trial of surgery versus thrombolysis for occluded lower extremity bypass grafts, *Am J Surg* 172:105, 1996.

Ouriel K, Cynamon J, Weaver FA, and others: A phase I trial of alfimeprase for peripheral arterial thrombolysis, *J Vasc Interv Radiol* 16:8:1075, 2005.

Shortell CK, Ouriel K: Thrombolysis in acute peripheral arterial occlusion: predictors of immediate success, *Ann Vasc Surg* 8:1:59, 1994.

VASCULAR ACCESS

Michael J. Costanza, MD, and Vivian Gahtan, MD

Vascular access surgery has a simple goal that is challenging to achieve. The goal is to create a reliable conduit to deliver a high rate of blood flow to and from the dialysis machine. The challenge lies in creating and maintaining an access that is durable, dependable, and resistant to complications. The number of patients receiving hemodialysis increases each year, and the 2004 data from the U.S. Renal Data Systems recorded more than 335,000 patients on hemodialysis. The cost of placing and maintaining vascular access in these patients exceeds $3 billion, and vascular access dysfunction continues to be one of the leading causes of hospitalization for patients with kidney failure. The Dialysis Outcome Quality Initiative (DOQI) guidelines provide a valuable resource for optimizing vascular access care. These evidence-based recommendations address all aspects of vascular access and form the basis of this chapter.

TEMPORARY DIALYSIS ACCESS

Patients who require immediate dialysis require the insertion of a double-lumen catheter into the internal jugular, femoral, or subclavian vein. Noncuffed catheters can be used if dialysis is expected to be of short duration (<3 weeks); however, these should be removed within 3 weeks. Noncuffed femoral catheters should be removed within 5 days to avoid infection and other complications (e.g., thrombosis and venous stenosis).

Temporary access longer than 3 weeks in duration warrants placement of a tunneled, cuffed catheter. The preferred site for cuffed catheters is the right internal jugular vein. If possible, the catheter should be placed contralateral to an extremity with a maturing fistula. Subclavian vein catheters should be avoided because they increase the incidence of subclavian vein stenosis and thrombosis, either of which can make the extremity useless for future permanent access. Ultrasound guidance facilitates percutaneous catheter placement and minimizes insertion complications. Fluoroscopy directs placement of the catheter tip at the caval atrial junction to maximize flow rates.

PREOPERATIVE ASSESSMENT

Successful hemodialysis access depends on selecting the most suitable type of access for each patient. This selection process begins with the history and physical examination. The history should search for any conditions that could lead to access failure or complications. Often a patient questionnaire or preprinted history form ensures that all relevant aspects of the patient's history are covered. The physical examination should focus on the patient's venous, arterial, and cardiopulmonary systems. Table 1 includes some of the most relevant aspects of the history and physical examination.

The next step in the patient's evaluation involves duplex ultrasound vein mapping of the upper extremities. Duplex imaging provides a noninvasive method for evaluating the patency of the deep and superficial venous system of the upper extremities. It can also assess the superficial veins for evidence of previous phlebitis (e.g., wall thickening, filling defects, multiple tributaries, tortuosity). Continuous vein segments greater than 3 mm in diameter are usually considered suitable targets for autogenous access. Because the duplex examination does not require contrast, it is the ideal

Table 1: Important Elements of History and Physical Examination for Vascular Access Surgery

Consideration	Relevance
Patient History	
History of previous central venous catheter	Associated with central venous stenosis
Dominant arm	Use of the nondominant arm is preferred
History of implanted pacemaker or defibrillator	Associated with central venous stenosis
History of severe congestive heart failure	Access may alter hemodynamics
History of arterial or venous peripheral catheter	May have damaged target vasculature
History of PICC line, upper extremity DVT, superficial thrombophlebitis, IV drug abuse, frequent venous punctures	May severely damage superficial veins of the upper extremity, making them unsuitable for use in access
History of vascular access	Previously failed vascular accesses will limit available sites; if still present, the cause of a previous failure may influence planned access
History of previous arm, neck, or chest surgery/trauma	May limit viable access sites
Physical Examination	
Character of peripheral pulses, supplemented by Doppler evaluation	The quality of the arterial system will influence the choice of access site
Results of Allen test	Abnormal arterial flow pattern to the hand may contraindicate the creation of a radial-cephalic fistula.
Bilateral upper extremity blood pressures	Pressures determine suitability of arterial access in upper extremities.
Evaluation for edema	Edema can indicate venous outflow problems
Assessment of arm size comparability	Differential arm size may indicate venous obstruction
Tissue loss on fingers or hands	Indicative or arterial insufficiency
Examination for collateral veins	Indicative of venous obstruction

IV, Intravenous; *DVT,* deep vein thrombosis; *PICC,* peripherally inserted central catheter.

Table 2: Indications for Preoperative Venography

Edema in the extremity in which an access site is planned

Collateral vein development in any planned access site

Differential extremity size, if that extremity is contemplated as an access site

Current or previous subclavian catheter placement of any type in venous drainage of planned access

Current or previous transvenous pacemaker or defibrillator in venous drainage of planned access

Previous arm, neck, or chest trauma or surgery in venous drainage of planned access

History of intravenous drug abuse

Multiple previous accesses in an extremity planned as an access site

Table 3: Order of Preference for Vascular Access

1. Radio-cephalic primary AV fistula
2. Brachial-cephalic primary AV fistula
3. Either of the following is acceptable:
   a. Forearm loop prosthetic AV graft (for dialysis-dependent patients)
   b. Brachial-basilic primary AV fistula (for patients who have not started dialysis)
4. Upper arm AV graft
5. Chest wall (axilloaxillary) or groin AV access

AV, Arteriovenous.

preoperative study for patients who have residual renal function and have not yet started hemodialysis.

The use of duplex ultrasound vein mapping has virtually eliminated the need for routine preoperative venography. Venography is now reserved for specific conditions associated with venous impairment (Table 2). The evaluation of central venous structures often requires venography because these veins are poorly imaged by duplex examinations. Formal arterial evaluation in the form of Doppler ultrasound or arteriography is required only when extremity pulses are markedly diminished.

■ TIMING OF PERMANENT HEMODIALYSIS ACCESS

Appropriately timed access surgery can maximize the use of autogenous fistulae and reduce the need for temporary catheters. Autogenous arteriovenous fistulae require 2 to 3 months to mature and should be placed well in advance of a patient's projected need for hemodialysis. The DOQI guidelines state that patients with chronic kidney disease should be evaluated for vascular access when their creatinine clearance falls below 25 ml/minute and their serum creatinine rises above 4 mg/dl, or 1 year in advance of anticipated initiation of dialysis. In diabetic patients, a lower threshold (serum creatinine >2.5 mg/dl) for access referral may be appropriate. Prosthetic arteriovenous (AV) grafts should be reserved for patients in whom dialysis is imminent or has already begun through a temporary catheter. Although prosthetic AV grafts can be used within 1 month after placement, their limited durability and ongoing infection risk makes them undesirable for patients who are not dialysis dependent.

■ ORDER OF PREFERENCE FOR HEMODIALYSIS ACCESS

A primary AV fistula in the nondominant arm represents the first choice for permanent AV access (Table 3). This fistula can be constructed at the wrist (radial-cephalic) or the elbow (brachial-cephalic), depending on the patient's venous and arterial anatomy. The second tier of preference remains somewhat controversial. The next autogenous option is a brachial-basilic vein fistula, which requires transposition of the basilic vein. Reports demonstrate mixed findings with respect to maturation and longevity of brachial-basilic fistulae compared with other autogenous access configurations. Dialysis-dependent patients who cannot have a standard wrist or elbow fistula may be better served with a prosthetic arteriovenous

graft. The prosthetic AV grafts offer the advantage of relatively quick and reliable maturation and generally less extensive operative incisions than a brachial-basilic vein fistula.

Radial-Cephalic Arteriovenous Fistula

A radial-cephalic fistula at the wrist is simple to create and preserves more proximal vessels for future access placement. A longitudinal incision at the wrist halfway between the palpable radial pulse and the visible cephalic vein provides access to both vessels. Careful dissection will avoid injury to the median nerve and flexor carpi radialis tendon. Mobilizing the cephalic vein as far distally as possible facilitates a tension-free, end-to-side anastomosis with the radial artery. This configuration is superior to a side-to-side anastomosis, which can result in symptomatic venous hypertension in the hand. Compared with other configurations, the radial-cephalic fistula has a lower blood flow rate and this represents its primary drawback. Approximately 30% of radial-cephalic fistulae fail to mature, and elderly patients may have a disproportionately high rate of maturation failure. Wrist fistulae that do not support adequate hemodialysis within 4 months should be abandoned for an alternative permanent access.

Brachial-Cephalic Arteriovenous Fistula

A brachial-cephalic fistula at the elbow provides higher blood flow and more reliable maturation than a wrist fistula. The cephalic vein is exposed through a longitudinal incision starting at the antecubital fossa that is placed directly over the vein. After the cephalic vein has been mobilized, a shorter, medial incision is made over the palpable brachial pulse and a subcutaneous tunnel is made to connect the two incisions. The cephalic vein is then divided near the antecubital fossa, delivered through subcutaneous tunnel, and anastomosed end-to-side to the brachial artery (Fig. 1). The parallel incisions offer the advantage of more proximal exposure if the antecubital segment of the vein is fibrotic because of repeated blood draws or previous intravenous (IV) sites. Alternatively, the cephalic vein and brachial artery can be exposed through a single, oblique, transverse incision just proximal or distal to the antecubital fossa. This incision also can be used if it becomes necessary to convert to an AV graft. Because of its more proximal location and greater blood flow, a brachial-cephalic fistula has a slightly higher incidence of arm edema and hemodynamic steal syndrome.

Basilic Vein Transposition

The deep location of the upper arm basilic vein protects it from phlebotomy and IV catheter injuries. The basilic vein is often the only

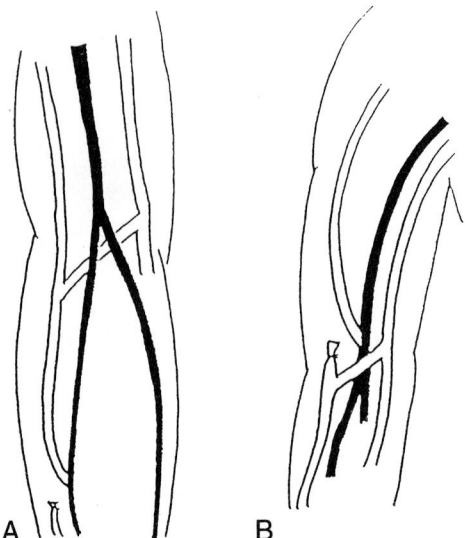

Figure 1 Arteriovenous fistulae. **(A)** Brescia-Cimino (radial-cephalic) fistula performed at the level of the wrist. **(B)** Brachial-cephalic fistula performed proximal to the antecubital fossa. *From Rutherford RB: Vascular surgery, ed 5, Philadelphia, 2001, WB Saunders.*

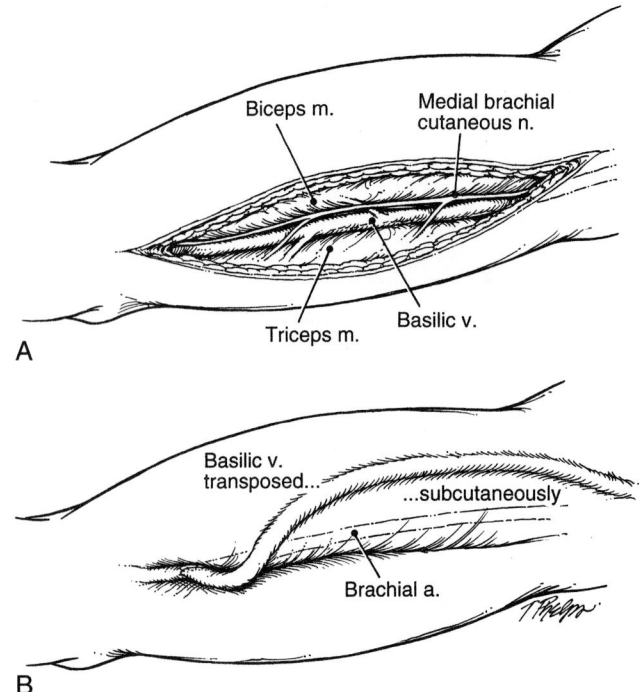

Figure 2 Anatomy of basilica vein transposition. **(A)** Basilic vein in situ. **(B)** Basilic vein transposition after mobilizing and tunneling laterally.

upper-extremity superficial vein that remains patent in patients with multiple previous access procedures or indwelling intravenous catheters. Preparing for a basilic vein transposition should include the axilla and shoulder. A short, longitudinal incision is made on the patient's medial upper arm. After the basilic vein has been identified, the incision is extended proximally and distally, and the natural orientation of the vein is noted and marked before extensive mobilization. Achieving maximal length for the fistula requires dissecting the vein from the antecubital fossa to the axilla. Transposition of the mobilized basilic vein can be performed in one of two ways. A subcutaneous tunnel from the axilla to the distal brachial artery can be created. The basilic vein is then passed through the tunnel and anastomosed end-to-side to the brachial artery (Fig. 2). Alternatively, the mobilized vein can be connected to the brachial artery with an end-to-side anastomosis and then allowed to assume its natural configuration on the upper arm. After superficial skin flaps are developed on each side of the incision, the deep soft tissue is closed under the basilic vein and the skin is closed over the transposed vein. Usually a closed suction drain is placed in the dissected bed of the basilic vein and brought out through a separate stab incision. The skin-flap method maximizes the usable length of the fistula and avoids unnatural configurations or kinking. The primary drawback of this technique is its susceptibility to wound complications.

For patients with duplex evidence of an adequate-caliber basilic vein down to the wrist, transposition of the basilic vein in the forearm has been described. After the vein is mobilized through a medial incision, it is passed through a subcutaneous tunnel on the anterior forearm and either connected end-to-side to the radial artery or put in a loop configuration to the brachial artery.

Prosthetic Arteriovenous Graft

Prosthetic AV grafts provide hemodialysis access for patients who cannot have a primary AV fistula. Although prosthetic AV grafts offer technically easy cannulation and a short lag time from insertion to maturation, these advantages are offset by a higher rate of thrombosis and infection compared with autogenous fistulae. A variety of materials have been used in the construction of AV grafts. Polytetrafluoroethylene (PTFE) is the most commonly used material and has proved superior to biologic grafts; however, direct comparisons between PTFE and human umbilical cord vein grafts and other

synthetic polymers have not been made. Consensus has not been reached on the ideal location or configuration for prosthetic AV grafts. Distally placed grafts preserve the proximal extremity at the cost of lower blood flow rates. In general, patient anatomy often determines graft location, and the configuration of the graft is designed to maximize surface area for cannulation. The most commonly employed prosthetic AV grafts are the forearm loop graft and the upper-arm curved or looped graft. Maturation of AV grafts occurs when arm swelling subsides and the course of the graft can be easily palpated. This process generally takes at least 2 weeks, and grafts should ideally be allowed to mature for 3 to 6 weeks before cannulation.

Forearm Loop Arteriovenous Graft

The forearm loop AV graft is based in the antecubital fossa, with the brachial artery providing arterial inflow. Venous outflow can employ the cephalic, basilic, median antecubital, or brachial veins. An incision is made 1 to 2 cm distal to the antecubital fold, taking care to preserve superficial veins and tributaries for potential use as venous outflow. After the brachial artery and a suitable vein have been isolated, a 2-cm counterincision is made on the distal anterior forearm to create the loop. Using a semicircular sheath tunneler to pass the graft minimizes the risk for graft kinking and creates a uniform and smooth subcutaneous tunnel. After placement in the tunnel, PTFE grafts do not require expansion with saline under pressure because this practice may predispose the grafts to excessive serous leaking ("sweating"). After controlling the outflow vein, the venotomy should be directed toward the side to prevent a twist or rotation of the vein at the anastomosis. An arteriotomy that is less than approximately 1 cm in length is used to construct the end-to-side arterial anastomosis.

Upper Arm Arteriovenous Graft

A variety of configurations are possible in the upper arm, depending on the patient's arterial and venous anatomy. The antecubital brachial artery, proximal brachial artery, and axillary artery can provide arterial inflow, and venous outflow sites include the proximal cephalic vein, upper arm basilic vein, brachial vein, and axillary vein. Both loop grafts and curved grafts should be placed anterolaterally on the patient's arm to make them easily accessible for cannulation. Although upper-arm grafts have high blood flow rates, they also have a higher rate of hemodynamic steal syndrome compared with AV fistulae and forearm grafts.

Alternative Sites for AV Access

A "necklace" AV graft uses the axillary artery for inflow and the contralateral axillary vein or jugular vein for venous outflow. Because these grafts cross over the anterior chest wall, they are not ideal for patients who may require a sternotomy for cardiac revascularization in the future. Groin AV access sites have a higher incidence of infection and ischemia and should be used only if all other sites have been exhausted. A prosthetic loop graft between the common femoral artery and the saphenous or common femoral vein represents the most common configuration. The graft should be tunneled onto the anterior thigh to enhance its accessibility. Vein transpositions using the femoral vein in the thigh require an extensive incision and dissection to mobilize the vein, and wound complications are common. Although saphenous vein transpositions have been described, they are rarely used because the saphenous vein does not tend to dilatate beyond its original diameter.

MONITORING AND SURVEILLANCE OF ARTERIOVENOUS ACCESS

Most AV fistulae and grafts are lost because of thrombotic events that cannot be resolved. Monitoring and surveillance protocols can extend the patency of AV grafts and fistulae by detecting and treating problems before access thrombosis occurs. In prosthetic AV grafts, surveillance techniques in the dialysis unit detect decreased graft blood flow or increased intra-access pressure, which are indicative of venous outflow stenosis. Physical findings predictive of venous outflow stenosis include edema of the extremity, prolonged bleeding after venipuncture, and changes in the pulse or thrill in the graft. Trends of decreasing flow and increasing pressure mandate further evaluation with graft contrast studies and possible endovascular or surgical intervention.

Primary AV fistulae typically fail as a result of inadequate flow. Surveillance techniques that measure fistula flow are useful, and recirculation studies can help to detect failing AV fistulae that are patent but do not provide adequate flow for dialysis.

COMPLICATIONS

Vascular access is unique among vascular surgical procedures. AV grafts and fistulae are intentionally placed in superficial locations and subjected to percutaneous punctures three times a week. It is therefore not surprising that AV access has a wide range of complications, and dysfunctional vascular access remains one of the leading causes of hospitalization among dialysis patients.

Stenosis

Significant vascular access stenosis (>50%) requires treatment when it is associated with previous access thrombosis, decreased access flow, or inadequate dialysis. Endovascular therapy and surgical revision both offer reasonable choices in the treatment of AV access stenosis, and neither has proved to be superior to the other in terms of patency rates or complications. Percutaneous balloon angioplasty has a high initial technical success rate but may have be repeated

within 6 to 12 months because of restenosis. Patients who require more than two angioplasty interventions in less than 3 months should be referred for surgical revision. Surgery to treat access stenosis can involve patch angioplasty or jump grafts farther up the arm. Surgical revisions offer longer durability at the expense of a more invasive procedure that can use up more veins in the extremity.

Thrombosis

Ideally, a thrombosed prosthetic graft should be treated promptly to preserve the access and minimize the need for temporary catheters. Satisfactory treatment of AV graft thrombosis involves three components: (1) complete thrombus removal, (2) total graft imaging, and (3) identification and correction of all significant stenoses.

For clot removal, equivalent results have been attained with surgical thrombectomy, percutaneous mechanical thrombectomy, and thrombolysis. The overall success of the procedure depends on what happens after the thrombus is removed. More than 85% of graft thrombotic events are associated with underlying venous stenosis, and failure to identify and treat these lesions will result in repeat thrombosis.

Thrombosis of a primary AV fistula presents a more difficult problem. Although thrombectomy techniques for fistulae have been described, the success rate is generally lower than the success rate for treatment of thrombosed AV grafts. Although thrombolysis is an option, it has not become a uniformly accepted practice. Because of a lack of sufficient clinical data, treatment guidelines for thrombosed AV fistulae remain undeveloped.

Infection

The treatment of AV graft infection depends on the extent of the infection and the age of the graft. A superficial infection that does not involve the graft can often be initially treated with broad-spectrum antibiotics; the spectrum can then be narrowed according to culture results. A focal graft infection that does not involve the anastomoses can be managed with segmental resection of the infected graft and rerouting a new piece of PTFE through uninvolved tissue planes. Success of this treatment strategy depends on the absence of purulence and adequate incorporation of the noninvolved graft. Newly established grafts (<30 days old) are by definition not incorporated into the surrounding tissue and cannot be treated with segmental resection. Therefore signs of infection in a newly constructed AV graft usually mandate removal of the entire graft. Graft infection involving the anastomoses also requires complete graft removal, even if the graft appears to be incorporated, because of the hemorrhagic risk.

Infection of a primary AV fistula occurs infrequently, and treatment usually consists of 6 weeks of antibiotics. Ligation of an infected AV fistula is necessary only when it is the source of septic emboli.

Steal

The presence of an AV fistula or graft provides a high-flow, low-resistance circuit that always reduces perfusion to the distal extremity. Usually arterial collaterals and peripheral vasodilation maintain adequate distal perfusion, and patients remain asymptomatic or report only subjective extremity coolness. Ischemic steal syndrome occurs when these compensatory mechanisms are insufficient and blood flow distal to the fistula does not satisfy the metabolic requirements of the extremity. Symptoms range in severity from hand coolness and vague neurosensory changes to ischemic rest pain, tissue loss, and motor impairment. Mild symptoms that occur in the early postoperative period often resolve, whereas more severe symptoms warrant prompt investigation and intervention. The incidence of ischemic steal is 1.6 to 8.0%, and risk factors include female gender, age older than 60 years, diabetes, multiple previous operations on the same limb, and use of the brachial artery as the donor vessel.

In symptomatic patients, noninvasive tests such as digital photoplethysmography, duplex ultrasound, and Doppler waveforms document low digital blood flow, which increases with compression of the fistula.

Although ligation of the AV access always cures ischemic steal syndrome, the goal of treatment is to resolve distal ischemia while preserving uninterrupted vascular access. Banding or plication of the fistula attempts to improve peripheral perfusion by increasing the resistance in the fistula. Unfortunately, the increased resistance in the fistula creates a low-flow state, which ultimately results in thrombosis of the access. Distal revascularization and interval ligation (DRIL) provides a more physiologically sound solution to ischemic steal. The DRIL procedure involves creation of a bypass graft (typically reversed saphenous vein) between the artery proximal to the fistula and the artery distal to the fistula. A ligature is then placed on the arterial segment between the fistula inflow anastomosis and the distal anastomosis of the bypass graft (Fig. 3). The bypass graft acts as a low-resistance collateral that increases distal perfusion, and the interval ligation prevents retrograde flow from the distal extremity into the low-resistance fistula. Pressure measurements during preoperative arteriography are necessary to determine the location of the proximal arterial pressure sink. The pressure sink is the area of low pressure immediately proximal to the fistula inflow anastomosis. To be effective, the bypass graft must originate proximal to the pressure sink. Usually the location of the proximal anastomosis is 3 to 5 cm proximal to the fistula, but occasionally the pressure measurements demonstrate a much more extensive pressure sink and mandate a more proximal anastomosis.

Aneurysms

Aneurysms are common in long-standing primary AV fistulae and warrant treatment only if they involve or compromise the arterial anastomosis. Pseudoaneurysms of prosthetic AV grafts can be repaired by resection of the aneurysm and placement of an interposition graft or patch angioplasty. Treatment indications for pseudoaneurysms include infection, rapid size expansion, size greater than twice the graft diameter, threatened viability of the overlying skin, and bleeding. Needle insertion into aneurysms and pseudoaneurysms should be avoided to prevent hemorrhagic complications.

Other Complications

Symptoms from venous hypertension can range from mild edema to ulceration and, rarely, hand loss. When reflux through incompetent valves causes venous hypertension (uncommon), the treatment involves limiting retrograde flow by ligating tributary veins to the access. Venous hypertension caused by venous outflow obstruction (common) can be treated with endovascular or surgical interventions. Balloon angioplasty for central venous lesions has limited durability and may require repeated treatments. Surgical techniques to correct subclavian stenosis include the internal jugular vein turndown and subclavian-vein-to-internal-jugular-vein bypass.

The most common causes of neuropathy in vascular access patients are uremia, diabetes, and anatomic compression (carpal tunnel). A rare neuropathy termed *ischemic monomelic neuropathy* (IMN) represents steal syndrome involving only the nerves of the distal extremity. IMN affects older diabetic patients with access arising from the brachial artery and presents with acute pain, weakness, or paralysis of the muscles of the hand and forearm within hours of access placement. IMN requires immediate treatment with access ligation, and failure to recognize and treat IMN can result in irreversible, profound neurologic deficits in the affected extremity.

CONCLUSION

For the patient with kidney failure, every vascular access surgery is a life-prolonging procedure. Keeping this in mind often tempers some of the frustration and discouragement engendered by complicated vascular access cases. The DOQI recommendations offer sound principles for the creation and preservation of vascular access. The guidelines can help surgeons choose the appropriate access, avoid predictable pitfalls, and manage access complications.

ACKNOWLEDGEMENT

The authors acknowledge Dr. Nowokere Esemuede for creating Figure 14.28-28.

SUGGESTED READINGS

Ascher E, Hingorani A, Gunduz Y, and others: The value and limitations of the arm cephalic and basilic vein for arteriovenous access, *Ann Vasc Surg* 15:89, 2001.

Davidson IJA: *Access for dialysis: surgical and radiologic procedures* ed 2, Austin TX, 2002, Landes Biosciences.

National Kidney Foundation.: K/DOQI clinical practice guidelines for vascular access, 2000, *Am J Kidney Dis* 37:suppl 1:S137, 2001 www.kidney.org/professionals/kdoqi/guidelines_updates/doqi_uptoc.html#va.

Wixon CL, Hughes JD, Mills JL: Understanding strategies for the treatment of ischemic steal syndrome after hemodialysis access, *J Am Coll Surg* 191:301, 2000.

Wolford HY, Hsu J, Rhodes JM, and others: Outcome after autogenous brachial-basilic upper arm transpositions in the post-National Kidney Foundation Dialysis Outcomes Quality Initiative era, *J Vasc Surg* 42:951, 2005.

DISTAL REVASCULARIZATION INTERVAL LIGATION

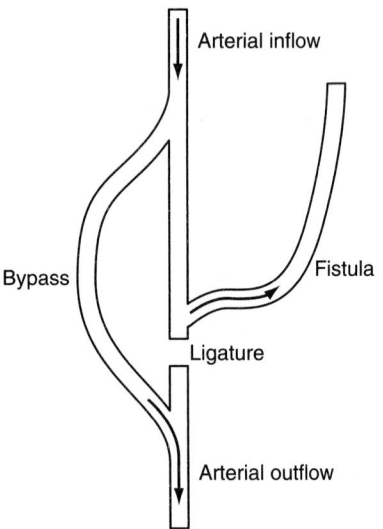

Arterial inflow

Bypass

Fistula

Ligature

Arterial outflow

Figure 3 This drawing demonstrates a representative layout for the distal revascularization and interval ligation procedure, with an arterial bypass with the proximal anastomosis proximal to the arteriovenous fistula anastomosis. To prevent retrograde flow from the bypass back to the fistula, an interval ligation is performed, encouraging preferential flow to the hand.

ATHEROSCLEROTIC RENOVASCULAR DISEASE

R. Eugene Zierler, MD

Atherosclerosis is by far the most common cause of renovascular disease, accounting for approximately 90% of cases. These lesions are typically located at the origins or in the proximal segments of the renal arteries and are found in patients older than 50 years of age with significant coronary, carotid, and peripheral artery atherosclerotic disease. Hypertension affects approximately 50 million individuals in the United States, and the proportion with a renovascular etiology is in the range of 1% to 6%. However, the prevalence of renovascular hypertension in patients with severe hypertension (diastolic blood pressure > 105 mm Hg) may be as high as 30% to 40%. Ischemic nephropathy is characterized by a progressive decline in renal function secondary to global renal ischemia. On this basis, it has been estimated that 60,000 to 120,000 patients in the United States have azotemia, and ischemic nephropathy may account for 5% to 15% of the patients who develop end-stage renal disease each year and require renal replacement therapy.

Despite the clinical significance of atherosclerotic renovascular disease, the optimal approach to management has not been established. There are still no definitive results from prospective, randomized trials comparing medical, endovascular, and open operative treatment. This chapter reviews the current status of diagnosis, indications for intervention, therapeutic options, and outcomes for patients with atherosclerotic renovascular disease.

CLINICAL PRESENTATION AND DIAGNOSIS

Prevalence and Natural History

Renal artery stenosis is relatively common, particularly in patients with atherosclerosis in other arterial segments. In a study of 395 patients undergoing routine arteriography for peripheral arterial disease, a renal artery stenosis of more than 50% diameter reduction was found in 38% with abdominal aortic aneurysms, 33% with aortoiliac occlusive disease, and 39% with lower extremity arterial occlusive disease. Renal artery disease has also been documented in 30% of patients undergoing cardiac catheterization. In a population-based study of 834 subjects 65 years of age or older, the overall prevalence of significant renovascular disease by duplex ultrasound was only 6.8%. However, in another study involving 629 hypertensive individuals screened for renovascular disease, the prevalence of significant renal artery stenosis or occlusion among patients 60 years of age and older with diastolic blood pressure greater than or equal to 110 mm Hg was 52%. When severe hypertension was associated with elevated serum creatinine, the prevalence of significant renovascular disease increased to 71%.

Atherosclerotic renal artery stenosis is a progressive disease. In retrospective studies, progression of disease severity has been observed in 36% to 71% of patients, with renal artery occlusion in 16%. Prospective natural history studies indicate that risk factors for renal artery disease progression include severity of renal artery disease, hypertension, and diabetes. Renal atrophy, as indicated by a decrease in pole-to-pole kidney length, has also been associated with renal artery stenosis.

Diagnostic Evaluation

The rationale for diagnostic testing in patients with suspected renal artery stenosis is to identify those individuals who are most likely to benefit from renal artery interventions for management of hypertension or renal insufficiency. However, because many patients are found to have unilateral or bilateral renal artery stenosis without major clinical abnormalities, it is clear that not all renal artery lesions are physiologically significant. To be most useful, diagnostic tests therefore must address both the anatomy and physiology of renovascular disease. Some general features that suggest the presence of clinically significant renovascular disease are sudden or recent onset of severe hypertension, resistance to standard antihypertensive therapy with multiple medications, and acute azotemia during treatment with angiotensin-converting enzyme inhibitors. Historically, a variety of tests have been used to detect significant renal artery disease. Peripheral plasma renin assays, rapid-sequence intravenous pyelography, and isotope renography all lack sufficient sensitivity to be clinically useful. Captopril renal scintigraphy is based on the pathophysiology of renovascular hypertension and has been advocated as a valid screening test.

Contrast arteriography remains the gold standard for the anatomic diagnosis of renal artery disease, but it is unsuitable for use as a screening test because of its high cost and the nephrotoxicity of iodinated radiographic contrast. Spiral computed tomography (CT) and magnetic resonance angiography (MRA) are also being used as screening tests for renal artery disease. Although sensitivities and specificities of greater than 90% have been reported for detection of main renal artery stenoses by spiral CT, this approach is not suitable for some patients because it requires relatively large volumes (up to 150 ml) of iodinated contrast. MRA does not require injection of iodinated contrast and can produce images that appear similar to standard arteriograms. Gadolinium is a nonnephrotoxic contrast agent that may enhance the ability of MRA to identify accessory renal arteries. Excellent sensitivities and specificities have been reported for imaging main renal artery stenoses by MRA. The main disadvantage of MRA is that it may overestimate the severity of stenosis and produce false-positive results. As with all magnetic resonance studies, the test cannot be performed on patients who have pacemakers, stents, or other metal devices.

In many centers, duplex ultrasound has become the screening imaging method of choice for both renovascular hypertension and ischemic nephropathy. The principal advantage of ultrasound is that it provides anatomic information and an assessment of the hemodynamic significance of renal artery lesions, as well as information on kidney size and the status of the renal parenchyma, without requiring iodinated contrast or radiation exposure. The challenge in renal duplex scanning is to locate the vessels and obtain satisfactory B-mode and pulsed Doppler information. Through continued experience and improvements in technology, renal ultrasound has identified hemodynamically significant main renal artery lesions with a 93% sensitivity, 98% specificity, and 96% overall accuracy. However, renal duplex does not reliably identify lesions in accessory renal arteries or the segmental branches. The relevance of this limitation depends on the indication for study. Ischemic nephropathy results from global renal ischemia; thus there must be hemodynamically significant lesions in both main renal arteries (or in a single main renal artery in patients with a solitary kidney) for this condition to be present. Consequently, if one or both main renal arteries is shown to be widely patent, ischemic nephropathy can be ruled out. When renovascular hypertension is suspected, the status of the main renal arteries and any accessory or polar arteries must be evaluated because hypertension can result from isolated accessory renal artery stenosis. In this situation, failure to detect a stenosis in an accessory renal artery could result in a false-negative screening test. Therefore additional imaging studies should be considered when a duplex scan shows nonstenotic main renal arteries and there is a strong clinical suspicion for renovascular hypertension.

When a hemodynamically significant renal artery stenosis is confirmed, functional studies may be indicated to determine whether the lesion is truly responsible for the clinical problem. This can be accomplished by either renal vein renin determinations or split renal function studies. However, both of these methods are complex and invasive. The most commonly used approach is to measure the renin concentration in blood sampled from each renal vein to detect unilateral renin hypersecretion. The test is considered positive if there is a ratio of at least 1.5 to 1.0 when the stenotic and nonstenotic sides are compared. Split renal function studies are infrequently used and require cystoscopy with ureteral catheterization to measure urine flow and urinary concentration from each kidney. Unfortunately, these functional studies have numerous sources for error and the results are not uniformly reliable, particularly in the presence of bilateral renal artery disease or renal artery stenosis involving a solitary kidney. Therefore the decision to intervene is often based on the severity of the renal artery lesions, the severity of hypertension, and the degree of associated renal insufficiency.

INDICATIONS FOR INTERVENTION

The goal of treatment for atherosclerotic renal artery disease is the prevention of major cardiovascular events and end-stage renal disease. Because hypertension is a major risk factor for all cardiovascular events, this is usually the initial focus of therapy. Most hypertensive patients with normal (or nearly normal) renal function can be managed by medication alone. However, those hypertensive patients who do not respond to multiple drug therapy or whose renal function deteriorates should be considered for renal revascularization. Patients with renovascular disease and renal insufficiency are at increased risk for end-stage renal disease and cardiovascular death. Therefore renal revascularization should also be considered for patients with deteriorating renal function, particularly when the renal artery lesions are bilateral or involve the artery to a solitary kidney. Selected patients with hemodynamically significant renal artery disease and recurrent, unexplained congestive heart failure or sudden onset of pulmonary edema may benefit from renal revascularization. Natural history studies suggest that earlier intervention, before renal function is severely impaired, may lead to better outcomes. Renal artery intervention in the setting of severe renal insufficiency and atrophy is clearly not beneficial. Similarly, revascularization is not indicated for unilateral renal artery stenosis and renal failure because these patients have advanced renal parenchymal disease.

APPROACHES TO RENAL REVASCULARIZATION

After the threshold for intervention is reached, the options for renal revascularization include percutaneous transluminal angioplasty (PTA), with or without stenting, and a variety of open surgical procedures. Before the availability of stents for use in the renal arteries, the relatively poor results of PTA alone for orificial and proximal atherosclerotic renal artery lesions made open surgery the preferred approach. However, most patients with atherosclerotic renal artery disease have multiple comorbidities that increase their risk for major, open, vascular surgery, and a less invasive option would clearly be valuable. Experience with PTA and stenting suggests that this is the initial procedure of choice for most patients with atherosclerotic renal artery stenosis. Surgical approaches to renal revascularization should be considered in those patients undergoing open repair of aortic or other abdominal vascular pathology. However, prophylactic repair of renal artery lesions in the absence of hypertension or renal insufficiency is not recommended. Open repair of a renal artery lesion is occasionally required after a failed PTA procedure, which cannot be salvaged using catheter-based techniques.

Percutaneous Transluminal Angioplasty and Stenting

In 1978, Grüntzig described the use of PTA for treatment of renal artery stenosis, but the results of PTA alone for atherosclerotic renal artery disease were generally poor because of elastic recoil, residual stenosis, and dissection. The use of self-expanding and balloon-expandable metallic stents was reported in 1991 as a technique for overcoming the limitations of renal artery PTA alone. Subsequent experience has shown that the use of stents provides better anatomic results, particularly for ostial renal artery lesions. Primary PTA was compared with primary stenting in a prospective study of 163 patients with 200 treated renal artery atherosclerotic lesions, including ostial, proximal, and isolated truncal stenoses. The primary patency rates at 12 months for PTA alone were 34% for ostial stenoses, 65% for proximal stenoses, and 83% for truncal stenoses. The corresponding primary patency rates for the stented renal arteries were 80%, 72%, and 66%. A significant reduction in the rate of restenosis for the stented renal arteries was observed for the ostial stenoses.

In a meta-analysis of published studies on primary renal artery PTA and renal artery stenting, the initial technical success rate for the predominantly ostial stenoses was 77% for PTA alone and 98% for stenting. Restenosis was found in 17% of the stented renal arteries and 26% of the arteries treated by PTA alone after follow-up ranging from 6 to 29 months. Renal artery stenting is indicated when a residual stenosis is noted immediately after PTA alone or when there is a complication of a primary PTA such as an intimal flap or dissection. Alternatively, a renal artery lesion may be stented primarily when the risk of technical complications is considered to be high, particularly with ostial lesions. Late restenosis following primary renal artery PTA can also be treated by repeat PTA with stenting.

Open Surgical Techniques

Whenever technically possible, all hemodynamically significant renal artery disease should be corrected. Direct aortorenal reconstructions are preferred over extra-anatomic methods because concomitant atherosclerotic stenosis of the celiac axis is present in up 50% of patients. Intraoperative assessment of the repair by duplex scanning is strongly recommended to identify any immediate technical problems that could lead to failure of the reconstruction. After they are identified, defects can be viewed in multiple image planes during conditions of pulsatile blood flow. In addition, important hemodynamic information is obtained from spectral analysis of the pulsed Doppler signals proximal and distal to the anatomic defect. Hemodynamically significant defects are revised before completion of the operation.

Antihypertensive medications should be reduced during the preoperative period to the minimal number and doses necessary for blood pressure control because patients often have reduced requirements while hospitalized. Vasodilators and selective beta-adrenergic blockers are the agents of choice. If a patient's diastolic blood pressure exceeds 120 mm Hg, operative treatment is postponed until the pressure is brought under control. During the procedure, mannitol is administered intravenously in 12.5-g doses repeated before and after periods of renal ischemia, up to a total dose of 1 g/kg patient body weight. Just before renal artery cross clamping, 100 units/kg of heparin is given intravenously, and appropriate follow-up doses are given to maintain anticoagulation until all arterial clamps are removed. Unless required for hemostasis, protamine is not routinely administered for reversal of heparin at the completion of the operation.

The basic operative approaches to renal revascularization include aortorenal bypass, reimplantation, thromboendarterectomy, and extra-anatomic bypass. Each method has advantages and limitations, and no single approach provides optimal repair for all patterns of renal artery disease. Aortorenal bypass, preferably with autogenous saphenous vein, is the most versatile and commonly applied technique. When the renal artery is sufficiently redundant, reimplantation is simple and expeditious. Thromboendarterectomy can be useful for ostial atherosclerotic lesions involving multiple renal arteries or in cases in which the perirenal aorta is opened for other reasons. Extra-anatomic bypass using the hepatic or splenic arteries for inflow may be necessary when the infrarenal aorta is unavailable because of infection, occlusion, or multiple prior procedures.

Aortorenal Bypass

Autogenous saphenous vein is used preferentially for aortorenal bypass (Fig. 1). When the vein is small or sclerotic, the hypogastric artery or a synthetic graft, such as 6-mm thin-walled polytetrafluoroethylene (PTFE), are acceptable alternative conduits. In most instances, an end-to-end anastomosis between the graft and the renal artery is performed. A 6-0 or 7-0 monofilament polypropylene suture is employed. In creating both the proximal and distal anastomoses, the length of the arteriotomy should be at least three times the diameter of the smaller conduit to avoid late suture-line stenosis. The native infrarenal aorta serves as the inflow source in most cases. When the aorta is replaced by a Dacron graft for treatment of aneurysmal or occlusive disease, this prosthetic graft can be used as the inflow source. Rarely, a common iliac artery is the most appropriate inflow source for the renal artery bypass graft.

Reimplantation

When the renal artery is sufficiently redundant following complete mobilization, the artery can be transected and reimplanted into the aorta at a slightly lower level. This requires spatulation of the renal artery and removal of a portion of the aortic wall. Although this is not routinely possible, it requires no graft material and only a single anastomosis.

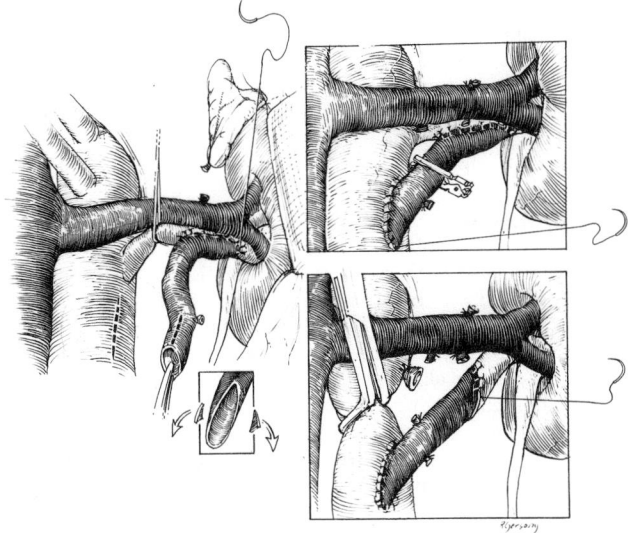

Figure 1 Aortorenal bypass grafting with end-to-side and end-to-end anastomoses. An end-to-end anastomosis between the graft and the native renal artery is generally preferred. *From Benjamin ME, Dean RH: Ann Vasc Surg 10:306, 1996. Used with permission.*

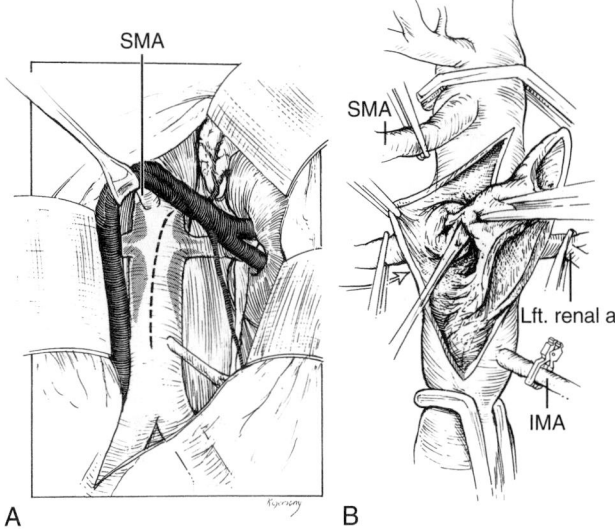

Figure 2 Transperitoneal approach for a longitudinal transaortic endarterectomy. **(A)** Dotted line shows the location of the aortotomy. **(B)** The plaque is transected proximally and distally, and the renal arteries are everted to remove the atherosclerotic plaque from each renal ostium. The aortotomy is closed with a running 4-0 or 5-0 monofilament polypropylene suture. *IMA,* Inferior mesenteric artery; *SMA,* superior mesenteric artery. *From Benjamin ME, Dean RH: Ann Vasc Surg 10:306, 1996. Used with permission.*

Thromboendarterectomy

Thromboendarterectomy can be performed by either a transaortic or transrenal technique. In cases of bilateral atherosclerotic involvement of multiple renal arteries, the transaortic technique is preferred (Fig. 2). The endarterectomy is performed through a longitudinal aortotomy, with sleeve endarterectomy of the aorta and eversion endarterectomy of each renal artery orifice. When combined with aortic replacement, the endarterectomy is performed through the transected aorta. In either instance, it is important to mobilize the renal arteries to enable an eversion of the vessel into the aorta. These techniques are most effective when the visible and palpable renal artery atheroma ends within 1 cm of the renal artery origin. Aortic control is required proximal to the origin of the superior mesenteric artery. Less commonly, a transrenal approach may be possible for endarterectomy of a focal atherosclerotic renal artery lesion. This involves a longitudinal incision in the renal artery, sometimes with an extension onto the adjacent aorta, and closure with a prosthetic or autogenous vein patch. As with endarterectomy in general, renal thromboendarterectomy is contraindicated in the presence of aneurysmal degeneration of the aorta and transmural calcification.

Extra-Anatomic Bypass

When the aorta or an aortic graft is not available as inflow sources for renal revascularization, alternative extra-anatomic sources may be considered. This most often involves the splanchnic arteries in the form of hepatorenal and splenorenal bypass grafts. However, because these procedures are not as durable as direct aortorenal reconstructions, they should be used only when other approaches are not possible. Both hepatorenal and splenorenal bypasses can be performed through either midline or subcostal incisions. In the case of hepatorenal bypass, a saphenous vein graft is preferred (Fig. 3). The proximal anastomosis is usually in the common hepatic artery, with a distal end-to-end renal artery anastomosis. A splenorenal bypass can often be created with the transected splenic artery, obviating the need for saphenous vein graft.

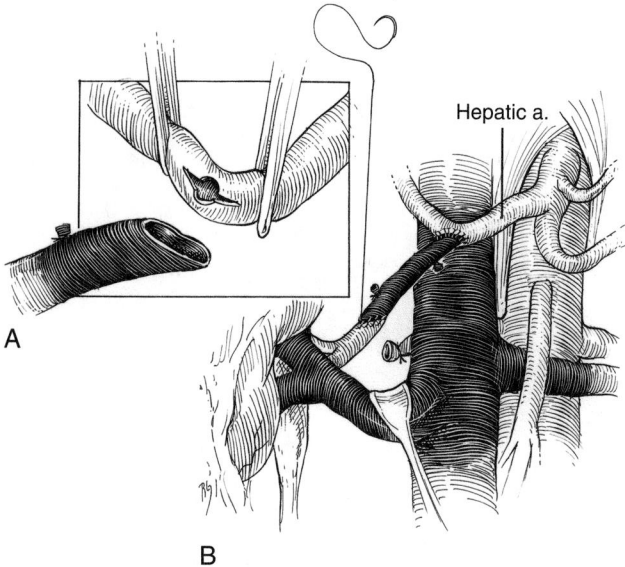

Hepatic a.

A

B

Figure 3 Extra-anatomic approaches to renal revascularization include hepatorenal and splenorenal bypass grafts. In this figure, a vein graft is anastomosed end-to-side to the hepatic artery **(A)** and end-to-end to the right renal artery **(B)**. *From Benjamin ME, Dean RH: Ann Vasc Surg 10:409, 1996. Used with permission.*

Nephrectomy

Nephrectomy is reserved for those rare patients with unreconstructable disease in a renal artery to a nonfunctioning kidney ($\leq$10% function by radionuclide renography). In the case of an occluded renal artery, reconstruction can still be performed when a patent distal renal artery is found at the time of surgery. Although outcomes are difficult to predict, the clinical response to revascularization of small ($\leq$8 cm in length) kidneys with high parenchymal resistance to flow is likely to be poor with regard to blood pressure and renal function. In these cases, a more favorable blood pressure response may be obtained by nephrectomy.

RESULTS OF TREATMENT

In a randomized study comparing PTA with surgical reconstruction for treatment of patients with hypertension and atherosclerotic renal artery stenosis, 58 patients were randomized (28 in each group). There was no significant difference in the initial technical success rate for the PTA group (83%) and the surgical group (97%). For technically successful cases, the primary patency rate at 24 months was 75% for the PTA group and 96% for the surgical group. However, secondary patency was 90% in the PTA group and 97% in the surgical group, with 4 PTA patients requiring surgery and 1 surgical group patient having a PTA. After the secondary interventions, there was no significant difference in blood pressure or renal function between the two treatment groups. Hypertension was cured or improved in 90% of the PTA patients and 86% of the surgical patients; the corresponding proportions for improved or unchanged renal function were 83% and 72%, respectively. On the basis of these observations, the authors recommended PTA as the intervention of first choice, as long as it was combined with close follow-up and aggressive reintervention.

In a series of 500 patients who had open surgical repair for atherosclerotic renovascular disease, there were 254 women and 246 men, with a mean age of 65 years. Mean blood pressure for the entire group was $200 \pm 35/104 \pm 21$ mm Hg, with a mean duration of hypertension of 15 years. On the basis of a serum creatinine of 1.3 mg/dl or greater, 78% were considered to have at least mild

renal insufficiency, and 49% had a serum creatinine of 1.8 mg/dl or greater and were considered to have ischemic nephropathy. Forty of the patients were dialysis dependent. Angiography showed bilateral renal artery disease in two thirds of the patients, and 16% demonstrated renal artery occlusions. The stenotic lesions were considered to be ostial in 97% of kidneys.

Among a total of 720 renal artery reconstructions, aortorenal bypass was performed in 384 patients, including 204 vein grafts, 159 PTFE grafts, and 21 Dacron grafts. Renal artery reimplantation was performed in 56 patients, renal artery thromboendarterectomy in 267, and nephrectomy in 56, for a total of 776 kidneys that underwent operation. During these 776 repairs, 8% required an intraoperative revision on the basis of the completion duplex scan. In addition, 177 patients required simultaneous repair of clinically significant aortic disease. Perioperative mortality (death in-hospital or within 30 days of surgery) occurred in 23 patients or 4.6%. Mortality after isolated renal artery repair (0.8%) was significantly less than mortality after combined aortic and renal repair (6.9%). Perioperative mortality also showed a significant association with advanced age and congestive heart failure.

When the blood pressure response for all surgical survivors was assessed at least 1 month after surgery, 85% were considered cured or improved and 15% were considered treatment failures. Hypertension cure was significantly associated with increased dialysis-free survival. A significant change in renal function was defined as a change in estimated glomerular filtration rate of at least 20% obtained 3 or more weeks after surgery. Fifty-eight percent of the patients in the ischemic nephropathy group (serum creatinine of 1.8 mg/dl or greater) were considered improved, including 30 patients who were removed from dialysis. Of the remaining ischemic nephropathy patients, 35% remained unchanged and 7% had worsened renal function. Analysis of patients with serial preoperative measurements of renal function suggested that the more rapid the rate of decline in renal function before surgery, the better the chance for recovery of function after operation. Improvement in renal function was significantly associated with the extent of both the renal artery disease and the repair: complete repair of bilateral renovascular disease was associated with the greatest incremental increase in renal function.

There were 171 patient deaths at a mean follow-up of 56 months. Only a cured blood pressure response was associated with improved survival, compared with patients considered as improved or failed. The renal function response to repair influenced both survival and progression to dialysis dependence. Patients with improved renal function had significantly increased survival compared with patients with unchanged or worsened renal function. Improved renal function was also associated with a significantly decreased risk for dialysis dependence. Patients with unchanged renal function demonstrated a relative risk of dialysis dependence and death that was similar to those who had worsened renal function after surgery.

SUMMARY

Atherosclerosis is the most common cause of renovascular disease and is associated with both renovascular hypertension and ischemic nephropathy. Diagnosis of clinically important renal artery disease requires documenting the presence of renal artery lesions that are both hemodynamically and physiologically significant. Although this remains challenging, duplex ultrasound provides a method for assessing the anatomy and physiology of the renal arteries and kidneys. Spiral CT and MRA are alternative methods for anatomic screening. Invasive contrast arteriography is generally reserved for those patients who require intervention, and the initial procedure of choice for most patients with atherosclerotic renal artery stenosis is PTA and stenting. Surgical approaches, such as aortorenal bypass, direct reimplantation, thromboendarterectomy, and extra-anatomic bypass, should be considered in those patients undergoing open repair of aortic disease or after a failed catheter-based intervention.

Percutaneous and open surgical repair of atherosclerotic reno-vascular disease can improve blood pressure control and renal function in selected patients. Patients with hypertension cure show increased dialysis-free survival compared with patients who are improved or unchanged. For patients with ischemic nephropathy and poor preoperative renal function, improved postoperative renal function is associated with increased dialysis-free survival compared with those who have unchanged or worsened renal function.

SUGGESTED READINGS

Caps MT, Perissinotto C, Zierler RE, and others: Prospective study of atherosclerotic disease progression in the renal artery, *Circulation* 98:2866, 1998.

Cherr GS, Hansen KJ, Craven TE, and others: Surgical management of atherosclerotic renovascular disease, *J Vasc Surg* 35:236, 2002.

Hansen KJ, Cherr GS, Craven TE, and others: Management of ischemic nephropathy: dialysis-free survival after surgical repair, *J Vasc Surg* 32:472, 2000.

Hirsch AT, Haskal ZJ, Hertzer NR, and others: *ACC/AHA 2005 Practice Guidelines for the management of patients with peripheral arterial disease (lower extremity, renal, mesenteric, and abdominal aortic): a collaborative report from the American Association for Vascular Surgery/Society for Vascular Surgery, Society for Cardiovascular Angiography and Interventions, Society for Vascular Medicine and Biology, Society of Interventional Radiology, and the ACC/AHA Task Force on Practice Guidelines (Writing Committee to Develop Guidelines for the Management of Patients With Peripheral Arterial Disease)*, *Circulation* 113:463, 2006.

Zierler RE: Update on renal stent trials. In Pearce WH, Matsumura JS, Yao JST, editors: *Trends in Vascular Surgery 2003*. Chicago, 2003, Precept Press.

Zierler RE: Vascular diagnosis of renovascular disease. In Mansour RE, Labropoulos N, editors: *Vascular Diagnosis*. Philadelphia, 2005, Elsevier Saunders.

RAYNAUD'S SYNDROME

Ravi Veeraswamy, MD, and Gregorio A. Sicard, MD

INTRODUCTION

The hallmarks of Raynaud's syndrome are its inciting factors and reliable symptomatology. Exposure to cold temperature or emotional stress is the most common preceding events. Patients typically describe discoloration beginning in one or several fingers and spreading to involve both hands. The duration of the attack varies and a tricolor pattern with white and blue digits eventually developing hyperemia with red digits before resolution of the attack is classic. The majority of patients present in the second or third decade of life, but the pediatric population is also susceptible. Women are more commonly affected than men in all age groups. Geographic areas with colder temperatures have a higher incidence, and patients have more frequent attacks in the winter months.

PRIMARY AND SECONDARY RAYNAUD'S

Raynaud's syndrome is subdivided into primary Raynaud's phenomenon (PRP) and secondary Raynaud's. It is often difficult to classify patients, and a number of patients with PRP will ultimately manifest their underlying disorder and fall into the secondary category with long-term follow-up. Nail-fold capillary microscopy, carotid artery elasticity, erythrocyte sedimentation rate and antinuclear antibody assays can be used to differentiate primary from secondary disease. In primary Raynaud's, all of these factors are normal, whereas secondary Raynaud's is associated with abnormalities with each assay. PRP is a purely vasospastic disorder, whereas the secondary form has an underlying arterial occlusive component of varying etiology ranging from systemic sclerosis to atherosclerotic disease. PRP is first seen in adolescence, and patients present with a long history of mild to moderate attacks. It is unusual to have tissue damage caused by digit ischemia in PRP, and pain is an infrequent symptom. Secondary Raynaud's is most commonly associated with mixed connective-tissue disorder or systemic sclerosis but can be seen with a variety of other causes (see Table 1). Patients are generally older than

Table 1: Common Underlying Etiologies of Secondary Raynaud's

Autoimmune disease
   Scleroderma
   CREST syndrome
   Systemic lupus erythematosus
   Undifferentiated/mixed connective
     tissue disease
Polyarteritis nodosa
Sjögrens syndrome
Hepatitis induced vasculitis
Reiter's syndrome
Arteriosclerosis
Occupational disease
   Arm-hand vibration syndrome
   Hypothenar hammer syndrome
Medications
   Beta-blockers
   Bleomycin
   Cisplatin
   Vinblastine
Myeloproliferative/hematologic disorders
   Leukemia
   Polycythemia vera
   Cold agglutinins
   Cryoglobulinemia
   Multiple myeloma
   Disseminated intravascular coagulation
Reflex sympathetic dystrophy
Chronic renal failure
Neurofibromatosis

CREST, Calcinosis, Raynaud phenomenon, esophageal dysmotility, sclerodactyly, and telangiectasia.

age 30 and describe intense, painful, and asymmetric attacks. Importantly, digital ulcers and severe gangrene can be seen with the secondary form of Raynaud's and present a significant morbidity for the patient.

PATHOPHYSIOLOGY

The precise etiology of Raynaud's remains elusive. Multiple theories have been invoked, including altered sympathetic neurotransmitters, increased platelet serotonin release, and increased sensitivity of alpha-2 receptors to norepinephrine, but none have proved conclusive. Current investigation is focused on the biology of endothelial cells and how they regulate vascular tone using an array of mediators. For example, nitric oxide, prostacyclin, and leukotrienes relax the vascular smooth muscle, and endothelin, angiotensin II, and thromboxane II lead to vasoconstriction. It has been hypothesized that vascular smooth muscle cells have a varied response to the endothelial cell stimuli, depending on the vascular bed. Thus the interplay between these two cell types may result in pathologic vasoconstriction that manifests as the physical findings of Raynaud's.

DIAGNOSIS

Establishing the diagnosis of Raynaud's begins by obtaining an appropriate history of symptoms. It is generally difficult to replicate these symptoms in an office setting even with the use of known triggers. A thorough pulse examination of the upper extremity, including an Allen's test, should be performed. For the surgeon, it is important to perform a thorough vascular evaluation to exclude proximal sources of emboli such as atherosclerotic disease or aneurysms. Other etiologies that can mimic Raynaud's include thoracic outlet syndrome and carpal tunnel syndrome, and these must be excluded by appropriate measures. Buerger's disease in its early presentation can be confused with Raynaud's, but the progression to ischemic digits and strong association with tobacco in Buerger's help to distinguish the two. Historically, clinical assessment by the physician or patient has served as the sole method of recording the symptoms of the disease and response to treatment. Newer techniques aim to quantitate blood flow to the digits during episodes of vasospasm. Nailfold capillaroscopy has high specificity for Raynaud's. Laser Doppler imaging is being developed to measure blood flow through Doppler scanning across the palmar surface of the hand. This technology shows promise as a tool for quantitating microcirculatory blood flow.

LIFESTYLE MODIFICATION

Nonpharmacologic management involves avoiding stimuli that trigger an attack. Thus cold exposure should be avoided, and stressful or anxiety-provoking situations should be minimized. Cigarette smoking has not been directly linked to attacks, but it should be strongly discouraged because of the deleterious effects of smoking on digital circulation.

PHARMACOLOGIC THERAPY

A variety of medications have been used to treat Raynaud's, most with modest success. These are outlined in Table 2.

Calcium channel blockers (CCBs), especially nifedipine, are established as the most commonly used and effective therapy for Raynaud's. A meta-analysis of 18 studies using CCBs showed that the number and severity of attacks in both primary and secondary Raynaud's were reduced. Although individual responses may vary, CCBs have the most consistent record as an effective treatment for Raynaud's phenomenon. Dosages can vary greatly and must be individualized; side effects of flushing and headache can be prohibitive in some patients.

Prostaglandin infusion is being increasingly studied as a possible therapy for the vasospasm of Raynaud's. Its therapeutic benefit lies in its vasodilatory effects, as well as its ability to inhibit platelet aggregation. Several small trials have confirmed the benefits of repeated intravenous infusion of several drugs in this class, including iloprost, alprostadil, and prostin. Oral administration has not been shown to be beneficial. Side effects of systemic prostaglandin administration such as headache, flushing, and nausea can be significantly reduced by using catheter-directed arterial infusion. Current trials are focusing on measuring the duration of physiologic effects and whether this translates into clinical efficacy and identifying which specific agent within this class is most useful.

Sildenafil, a phosphodiesterase inhibitor, has recently been used to treat vasospastic disorders such as pulmonary hypertension and Raynaud's. A trial of 18 patients found that sildenafil promotes healing of digital ulcers and reduces the number, duration, and severity of attacks. These newer agents are awaiting validation in larger studies.

Several investigators have used low-level irradiation via laser therapy. Randomized trials with more than 40 patients who received treatments over a several-week period found some benefit from this therapy. The mechanisms underlying this modality are poorly understood, however, and it is unclear how clinically effective laser therapy will be in limiting the symptoms of Raynaud's. Finally, as our understanding of vascular biology increases, targeted therapies are being developed, including Rho-kinase inhibitors, alpha-adrenergic blockers, and endothelin blockers.

SURGICAL TREATMENT

Surgical treatment of Raynaud's has consisted of cervicothoracic sympathectomy by supraclavicular, transaxillary, posterior, or thorascopic means. The sympathetic chains of the T2 and T3 ganglia must be resected. The initial increase in cutaneous blood flow is transient. Poor long-term results are the norm, with relapses occurring by 12 months. Complications can include injury to the thoracic duct, azygous vein, peripheral nerve roots, and transient or permanent Horner's syndrome. Given the potential complications and the limited efficacy of sympathectomy, its popularity as a therapy for Raynaud's has waned. Most surgeons consider it as a measure of last resort, useful for healing ulcers refractory to all medications but not as a durable therapy.

Palmar or digital sympathectomy, arteriolysis of the radial and ulnar vessels, and ulnar artery reconstruction have all been mentioned in recent years as useful modalities for managing the symptoms of Raynaud's, but they have been used infrequently. Reports in the literature involve fewer than 10 patients, and follow-up is limited.

CONCLUSION

Raynaud's phenomenon is an episodic vascular disease resulting in digital ischemia. Although the current role for surgical intervention is limited, it is possible that catheter-directed vasodilatory therapies will become more important in managing these patients and will require surgeons with endovascular expertise. Furthermore, it is important for the surgeon to be familiar with this entity to exclude other surgically correctable conditions that can mimic it.

Table 2: Pharmacologic Treatment of Raynaud's Phenomenon

Agent	Dose	Side Effects	Comments
Calcium-channel blockers			
Nifedipine	10–30 mg 3 times daily orally	Tachycardia, edema, flushing, headache, dizziness, constipation, orthostatic hypotension	Placebo-controlled trials indicate benefit
Sustained-release nifedipine	30–120 mg/day orally		
Amlodipine	5–20 mg/day orally		
Felodipine	2.5–10 mg twice daily orally		
Isradipine	2.5–5.0 mg twice daily orally		
Diltiazem*	30–120 mg 3 times daily orally		
Sustained-release diltiazem*	120–300 mg/day orally		
Sympatholytic agent			
Prazosin	1–5 mg twice daily	Syncope, postural hypotension, dizziness, and palpitations possible after first dose	Efficacy often transient, may wane after several weeks
Angiotension II–receptor type I antagonist			
Losartan	25–100 mg/day orally	Dizziness, headache, fatigue, diarrhea	One placebo-controlled trial indicated benefit
Selective serotonin-reuptake inhibitor			
Fluoxetine	20–40 mg/day orally	Insomnia, nausea, diarrhea, tremors	One placebo-controlled trial indicated benefit
Vasodilator			
Nitroglycerin	¼–½ in. of 2% ointment applied topically per day	Headache, tachycardia, syncope, angina, rash, impotence, nausea, rebound hypertension	Popular therapy but little controlled data to support its use
Other vasoactive drug			
Pentoxifylline	400 mg 3 times daily orally	Dyspepsia, nausea, vomiting	Popular therapy but little controlled data to support its use
Prostaglandins			
Epoprostenol†	0.5–6 ng/kg of body weight/min intravenously for 6–24 hr for 2–5 days	Flushing, diarrhea, headache, hypotension, rash	Used for critical ischemia; in-hospital infusion recommended
Alprostadil	0.1–0.4 μg/kg/min intravenously for 6–24 hr for 2–5 days		
Iloprost‡	0.5–2 ng/kg/min intravenously for 6–24 hr for 2–5 days		

*Dilriazem is not as effective as the dihydropyridine class of calcium-channel blockers.
†The Food and Drug Administration has approved the use of epoprostenol for the treatment of pulmonary hypertension.
‡Iloprost is not available in the United States.

SUGGESTED READINGS

Boin F, Wigley FM: Understanding, assessing and treating Raynaud's phenomenon, *Curr Opin Rheumatol* 17:752, 2005.
Cooke JP, Marshall JM: Mechanisms of Raynaud's disease, *Vasc Med* 10:293, 2005.
Fries R, Shariat K, von Wilmowsky, and others: Sildenafil in the treatment of Raynaud's phenomenon resistant to vasodilatory therapy, *Circulation* 112:2980, 2005.
Kahaleh MB: Raynaud phenomenon and the vascular disease in scleroderma, *Curr Opin Rheumatol* 16:718, 2004.
Wigley FM: Clinical practice. Raynaud's phenomenon, *N Engl J Med* 347:1001, 2002.

THORACIC OUTLET SYNDROMES

David J. Caparrelli, MD, and Julie A. Freischlag, MD

INTRODUCTION

Thoracic outlet syndrome (TOS) manifests in three forms according to the structures involved: arterial, venous, and neurogenic. Although controversy remains regarding the existence, diagnosis, and treatment of neurogenic TOS, compression within the thoracic outlet is the main etiologic factor in the arterial and venous forms of this disease. Early recognition, a comprehensive workup, and appropriately timed surgical interventions result in excellent clinical results and an improved quality of life for most. A thorough understanding of the workup and, often, multidisciplinary therapeutic approach to all three forms of thoracic outlet syndrome are vital to the successful treatment of this disease.

ANATOMY

Although a number of anatomic anomalies can predispose patients to TOS, the normal anatomy can itself be responsible for the syndrome. The thoracic outlet has been described as a triangle, with the apex pointing toward the manubrium and the first rib and clavicle as its lower and upper limbs. The point at which these two structures overlap serves as a fulcrum where dynamic changes occur during arm movement that can lead to injury of the nerves, artery, and vein that run through the thoracic outlet (Fig. 1). Moving medial to lateral, the subclavian vein is positioned adjacent the apex of the anatomic triangle where the first rib and clavicle come together. Lateral to the vein is the anterior scalene muscle, which inserts on the first rib. The subclavian artery is then found lateral, deep, and cephalad to the anterior scalene. The C4–C6 (oriented superiorly) and C7–T1 (oriented inferiorly) nerve roots of the brachial plexus are the next structures encountered. The middle scalene inserts on the first rib posterior and lateral to the plexus. It is through this muscle that the long thoracic nerve travels on its way to the serratus anterior muscle (Fig. 2). Other structures in the thoracic outlet, including the dorsal scapular and phrenic nerves, the stellate ganglion, the thoracic duct, and the cupola of the lung, are important when planning surgical intervention but are less frequently involved with the presentation of the thoracic outlet syndromes.

PATHOPHYSIOLOGY

Although particular anatomic configurations predispose patients to develop each form of TOS, there can be variability in the presentation and considerable overlap with regard to symptomatology in these disorders. Found in approximately 0.5% of the general population, a cervical rib is the most obvious bony abnormality contributing to the neurovascular compressive syndromes of the thoracic outlet. Whether completely formed or rudimentary, cervical ribs tend to displace structures forward. Although there are several other bony abnormalities that can result in TOS, the majority of cases are associated with a number of soft-tissue anomalies, first described by Roos in 1976. Moreover, hypertrophy of otherwise normal structures such as the pectoralis minor muscle, subclavius

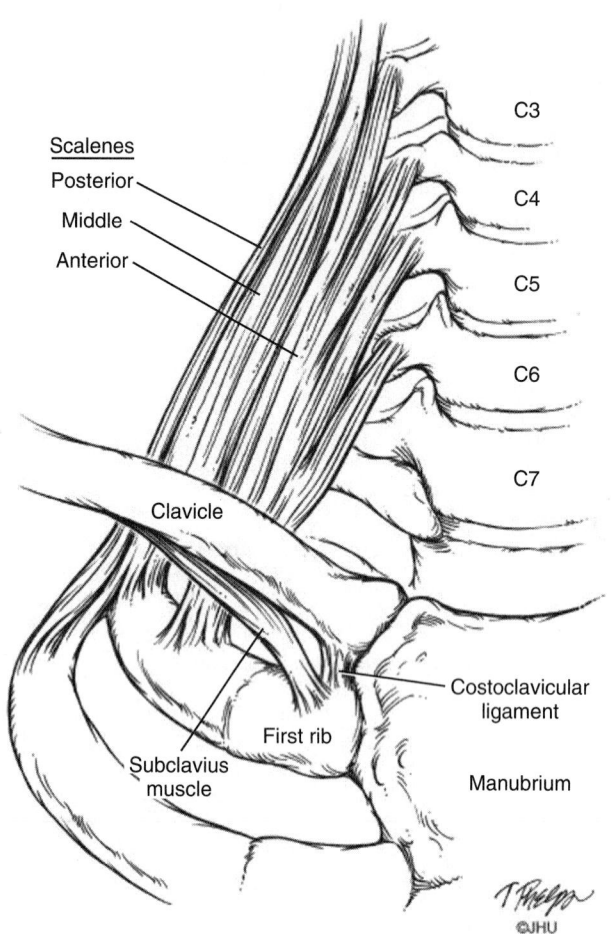

Figure 1 The thoracic outlet has been described as a triangle, with the apex pointing toward the manubrium and with the first rib and clavicle as its lower and upper limbs. The point at which these two structures overlap serves as a fulcrum where dynamic changes occur during arm movement that can lead to injury of the nerves, arteries, and vein that run through the thoracic outlet. *Copyright The Johns Hopkins University.*

tendon, and scalene musculature have been implicated as etiologic factors in TOS. In a series published by Machleder and colleagues, 34% of patients had no identifiable anatomic abnormality, 8.5% had a cervical rib, 10% had a scalenus minumus muscle, 19.5% had an abnormality of the subclavius tendon, and 43% of patients had a developmental or insertional defect in the scalene musculature. Trauma to the neck and shoulder has also been reported to cause TOS. In one review of operative TOS patients with neurogenic symptoms, 86% reported a history of trauma. This is, however, considerably higher than other reports in the literature.

DIAGNOSIS

There is no generally accepted set of tests to confirm the diagnosis of TOS. To begin, an extensive history and physical examination are required to delineate the duration and severity of the symptoms. Next cervical spine films to rule out disk disease and a chest x-ray to evaluate for bony abnormalities are required before any further testing should be considered. With respect to the initial findings,

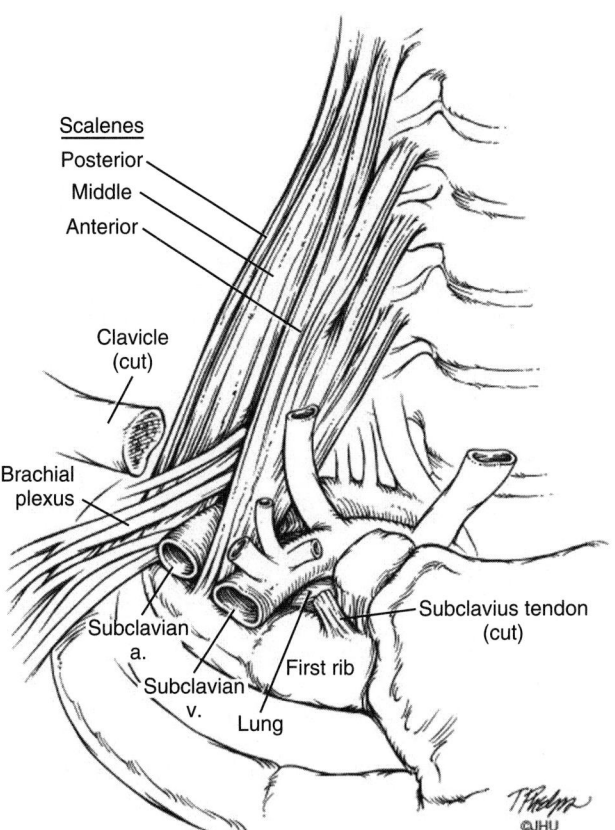

Figure 2 Moving medial to lateral, the subclavian vein *(v)* is the first structure encountered. It is usually positioned adjacent the apex of the anatomic triangle where the first rib and clavicle come together to form a fibrocartilaginous joint with the manubrium. Lateral to the vein is the anterior scalene muscle. The subclavian artery *(a)* is then found deep, lateral, and cephalad to the anterior scalene and subclavian vein. The C4–C6 (oriented superiorly) and C7–T1 (oriented inferiorly) nerve roots of the brachial plexus are the next structures encountered. Posterior and lateral to the plexus, the middle scalene inserts on the first rib. *Copyright The Johns Hopkins University.*

a number of other diagnostic tests can be performed on the basis of the clinical scenario or in cases for which there is diagnostic uncertainty. However, the utility of these tests is highly dependent on the level of expertise at each institution, and therefore their use varies greatly among specialists.

Patients with arterial TOS have the most widely varied presentations of the three syndromes because compression of the subclavian artery can result in a number of distinct injuries. These patients often present with cold intolerance or hypersensitivity, Raynaud's phenomenon, hand edema, or a combination of these. Easy fatigability or crampy arm pain with exercise can also be seen with complete occlusion of the axillosubclavian artery. Often misdiagnosed with collagen-vascular disease, patients with arterial TOS are often young, healthy, active individuals (manual laborers, athletes, etc). On physical examination, patients may demonstrate diminished radial or ulnar pulses. Punctate lesions at the paronychial area may be seen from embolic debris showered from an intraluminal ulcer at the site of compression. When aneurysmal, the subclavian artery can often be appreciated as a pulsatile mass in the neck or supraclavicular region.

Venous thoracic outlet syndrome or Paget-Schroetter syndrome is most often a disease of young, active, otherwise healthy men and women. The most common presenting complaint is sudden, severe swelling of one extremity, accompanied by cyanosis or rubor. Patients may also report the development of collateral veins around the shoulder or lateral pectoral region. On physical examination, patients presenting acutely are straightforward, and there is rarely a need for provocative testing to elicit symptoms. Patients presenting after the symptoms of the initial venous thrombosis have resolved often demonstrate symptoms only with physical activity such as push-ups. Swelling, easy fatigability, and vasomotor changes such as pallor and sweating are common in this situation and are exacerbated by any situation that causes vasodilation, such as warm weather.

Neurogenic TOS also usually presents in young to middle-aged adults with no major comorbidities. Patients can present with a wide variety of motor and sensory symptoms ranging in severity from mild to severely disabling. Weakness is the most common motor defect, and gross upper-extremity dysfunction is rare. The most common sensory finding in patients with neurogenic TOS is paresthesia, reported in up to 90% of patients. Pain is also a common symptom of neurogenic TOS and can originate anywhere in the upper extremity. Back and shoulder pain are most common, but pain can radiate to the arm, neck, and face. Headaches associated with neurogenic TOS are often first misdiagnosed as migranes. When the arm is involved, symptoms can be attributed to the C5-C7 plexus, the C8-T1 plexus, or both. Lower (C8-T1) plexus symptoms in the ulnar distribution are thought to be more common. Patients often report that their symptoms began after a traumatic event or give a history of a chronic repetitive motion injury, as with manual labor or athletics (e.g., baseball pitchers). Ipsilateral hyperhidrosis from irritation of the sympathetic chain is a rare symptom of neurogenic TOS and is always accompanied by other upper-extremity complaints.

A thorough physical examination is vital to the diagnosis of neurogenic TOS. Besides a standard neurologic examination evaluating both motor and sensory nerve distributions, symmetry of muscle groups and strength should be noted. Deep-tendon reflexes and pulses should be assessed as well. Tenderness over the anterior scalene muscle is frequently associated with brachial plexus entrapment, and percussion over the clavicle can reproduce the pain and paresthesias seen in patients with neurogenic TOS. The elevated arm stress test and the abduction and external rotation are the two most frequently used provocative tests used to diagnosis TOS.

The first diagnostic tests that should be undertaken in the workup of TOS are cervical spine and chest x-rays, as previously mentioned. It is important to rule out cervical disease as a cause of neurologic symptoms before entertaining the diagnosis of TOS. Chest x-ray can often identify the bony abnormalities (cervical ribs, elongated C7 transverse processes, old fractures) that can contribute to compression in the thoracic outlet.

Because arterial thoracic outlet syndrome can present with a wide variety of signs and symptoms, the diagnostic algorithm is not straightforward. If TOS is suspected, digital plethysmography or, more commonly, arterial duplex of the upper extremity is usually undertaken. Because these tests may or may not indicate abnormality on the basis of the severity of the arterial lesion, arterial compression at the thoracic outlet in almost all cases requires arteriography. Particular attention should be paid to the axillosubclavian artery at the thoracic outlet with the arm at the patient's side, as well as at a 90-degree angle to the chest wall. Both the degree of stenosis and aneurysmal dilatation can be evaluated; however, this diagnostic modality can underestimate the luminal irregularities subsequently found at the time of operation.

Acute axillosubclavian venous occlusion (Paget-Schroetter syndrome) can often be identified by history and physical examination alone. However, a number of tests can be used to confirm the diagnosis. Workup usually begins with noninvasive duplex ultrasonography and dynamic phlebography (or both) with the arm at the patient's side and at a 90-degree angle to the chest wall. Most patients with Paget-Schroetter syndrome then go on to have a diagnostic venogram, which is the gold standard for the diagnosis of venous thrombosis of the axillosubclavian vein and is often followed by thrombolytic therapy.

Unfortunately, because most currently available electrophysiological tests evaluate larger myelinated nerve fibers and not the injured smaller fibers that mediate the pain associated with neurogenic TOS, these tests have met with only modest success. Furthermore, these tests lack both sensitivity and specificity in the diagnosis of TOS. Despite these shortcomings, nerve conduction studies, electromyography, F-wave analysis, and somatosensory evoke potentials can play an important adjunctive role in the workup of patients suspected of suffering from neurogenic TOS.

TREATMENT

Decompression of the thoracic outlet is the mainstay of surgical treatment for TOS. Before proceeding with operative intervention, however, a number of factors should be considered. First, the timing of surgery is dependent on the variant of TOS. Although arterial and venous TOS tend to require a prompt surgical response, most experts recommend at least 6 weeks of conservative management with physical therapy for neurogenic TOS before considering surgical decompression because the majority of patients have substantial improvement without surgery. Second, the need for adjuvant therapy must be considered. Endovascular therapeutics such as thrombolysis and venoplasty play an important role in the treatment of venous TOS (Paget-Schroetter syndrome) and are used both before and after surgery, depending on the clinical situation. Third, consideration must be given to the surgical approach and its effect on the vascular reconstructive options. Although we recommend the transaxillary approach to first rib resection and scalenectomy in uncomplicated TOS, the need for arterial reconstruction may necessitate another approach for proximal vascular control.

As mentioned earlier, the arterial variant of TOS can present with a wide variety of signs and symptoms. Although cold intolerance, pain, and easy fatigability can be debilitating, these symptoms do not pose an immediate threat to the affected limb. Complete thrombosis of the subclavian artery, aneurysm formation, and distal embolization from intraluminal lesions, on the other hand, require a more expeditious approach to therapeutic intervention. Distal embolization poses the greatest threat to limb viability because ongoing embolization can obliterate the outflow vessels in the arm, severely limiting the options for revascularization. Acute limb-threatening ischemia must be addressed immediately and can be treated with a combination of standard open and endovascular therapies. Symptoms secondary to chronic ischemia can be addressed on a more elective basis. The mainstay of treatment for arterial TOS is decompression of the thoracic outlet with the addition of arterial reconstruction when necessary. Decompression and arterial reconstruction can be undertaken as separate operations or as one combined procedure. When staging the procedures or when revascularization is not necessary, we recommend a transaxillary approach to first rib resection and scalenectomy. This approach, however, does not provide adequate exposure for arterial reconstruction. For distal lesions, a variety of supraclavicular and infraclavicular approaches can be used, whereas proximal lesions may require a high thoracotomy (left) or median sternotomy (left or right) to obtain vascular control. Prosthetic material (polytetrafluoroethylene or Dacron), vein, and arterial grafts have all been used with success and rarely require anticoagulation therapy.

As with arterial TOS, presentation of acute axillosubclavian venous thrombosis should be treated aggressively. Current therapeutic protocols stress catheter-directed thrombolysis, maintenance of vein patency with systemic anticoagulation, and correction of the anatomic abnormality contributing to the thrombosis. At the time of diagnostic venogram, tissue plasminogen activator, urokinase, and streptokinase have all been used successfully to lyse the obstructing clot, reestablishing venous outflow to the affected limb. Systemic anticoagulation is then instituted to maintain patency until surgical intervention can be undertaken. Although traditional protocols mandated a 3-month period of oral anticoagulation with warfarin sodium (Coumadin; Bristol-Myers Squibb, New York, NY) before first rib resection, some groups now advocate early surgical decompression of the thoracic outlet following thrombolysis during a single hospital admission.

For those patients presenting with chronic axillosubclavian venous thrombosis, it is often difficult if not impossible to reestablish flow through the vein because of organized thrombus and severe scarring. In this subset of patients, decompression of the thoracic outlet should precede any attempt at recanalization or balloon angioplasty of the vein. Two weeks after surgical decompression, venography with thrombolysis and venoplasty is undertaken, if necessary. Three months of oral anticoagulation is recommended in this setting, after which patients can discontinue the warfarin sodium with only rare instances of recurrent or chronic symptoms.

SURGICAL APPROACH

In most instances of uncomplicated TOS, the transaxillary resection of the first rib and scalenectomy is our procedure of choice because of anatomic visualization of the area, effectiveness of decompression, and the excellent published long-term results. Induction of general anesthesia is undertaken with short-acting paralytics or none. The patient is positioned in a lateral decubitus position, and the entire arm and chest wall are prepared and draped in a standard fashion. A number of devices are available that can be used to elevate the arm to expose the contents of the thoracic outlet; however, we prefer the Machleder retractor. The retractor is attached to the operating room table, and the arm is positioned in the retractor such that it is abducted at a right angle to the chest wall (Fig. 3). Care is taken to generously pad the forearm and antecubital fossa before securing the arm to the retractor with an elastic wrap. After it is secured to the retractor, the arm can be raised for visualization of the thoracic outlet and lowered to allow periods of increased blood flow and decreased tension of stretched nerves. Incision is made approximately 1.0 cm below the hairline in the axilla between the border of the pectoralis and latissimus muscles, and dissection of the subcutaneous tissues down to the chest wall is accomplished with electrocautery. In patients with longstanding venous occlusion, care must be taken to preserve the often-large collateral veins during this dissection. After the chest wall is reached, the retractor is raised on the vertical support, providing an excellent view of the thoracic outlet. With minimal blunt

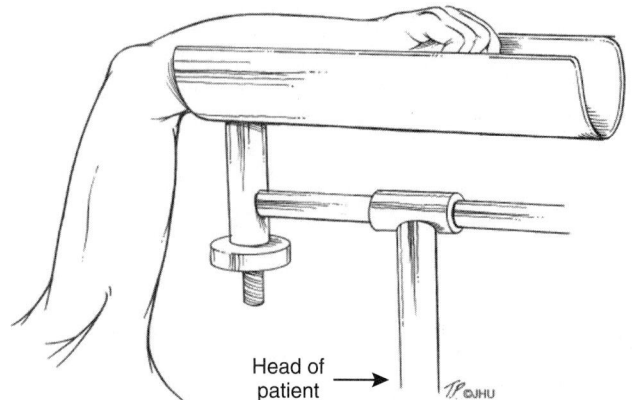

Head of patient →

Figure 3 The patient is placed in a decubitus position with the nonoperative side down. Ample sterile towels are used for padding (not shown), and the arm is secured in the retractor with a combination of gauze and elastic wraps (not shown). *Copyright The Johns Hopkins University.*

dissection, the vein is identified medially, and the subclavian artery and nerve roots are located right behind the first rib. After these structures are identified, the inferior aspect of the first rib is gently dissected from the surrounding connective tissue using a periosteal elevator. Care must be taken while freeing the underside of the rib because this can result in a pneumothorax. Next a right-angle clamp is used to isolate the anterior scalene muscle and subclavius tendon from the artery and nerve (Fig. 3, *A*). The muscle

and tendon are then divided with scissors or a scalpel. Then the middle scalene is bluntly dissected off the rib with a periosteal elevator, and the first rib is divided with a bone cutter. No more than 2 to 4 mm of the rib should remain at the costovertebral articulation, whereas the entire rib and costochondral cartilage is removed at the costosternal junction (Fig. 4, *B*). If there are any compressive bands of tissue present after removal of the rib, they are divided before closure. The wound is irrigated as the

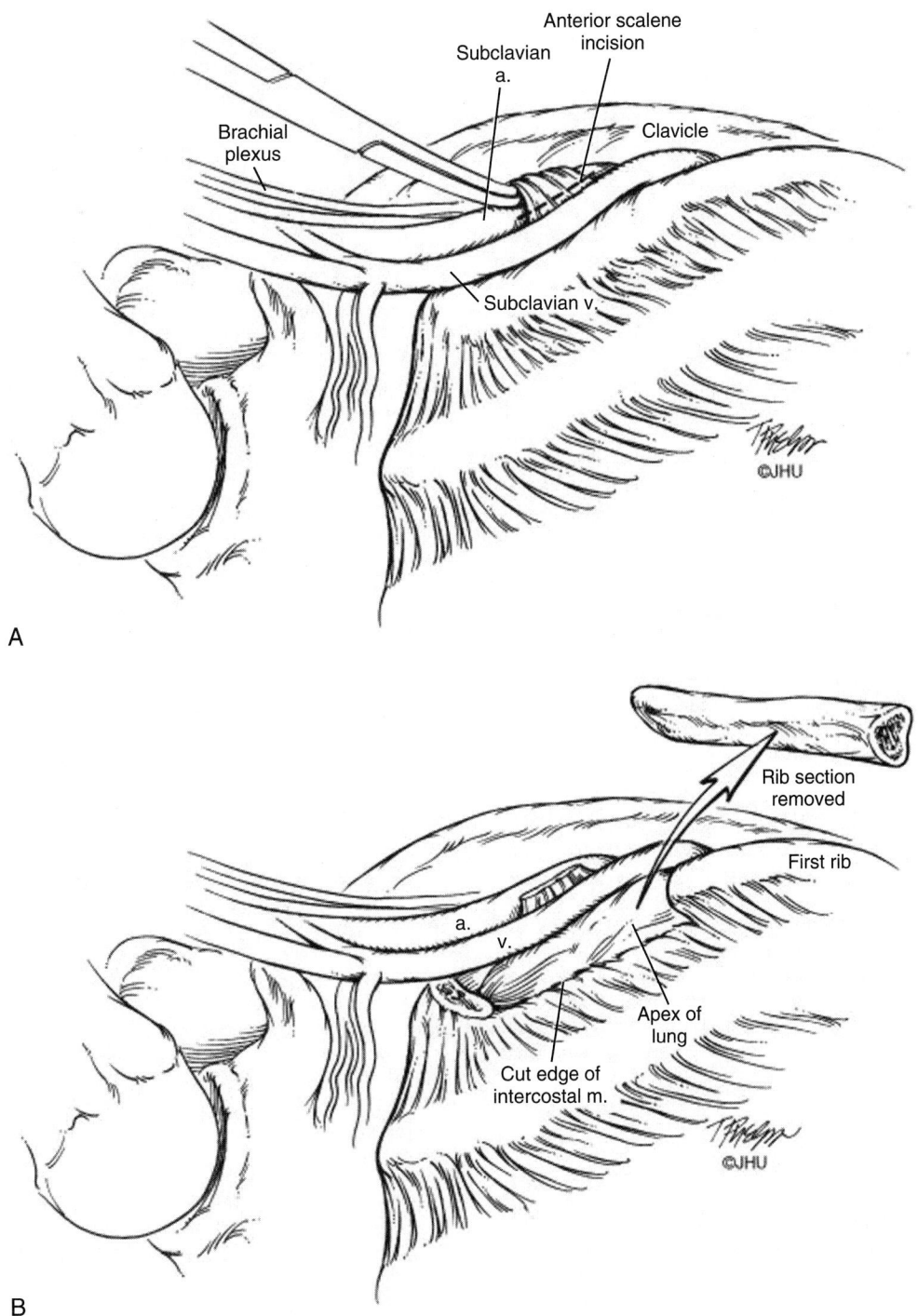

Figure 4 **(A)** Depicted is the right-angle clamp that is passed behind the anterior scalene muscle to protect the subclavian artery *(a)* and brachial plexus during division of the muscle in the transaxillary approach. The subclavian vein *(v)* is also depicted medial to the anterior scalene muscle. **(B)** Subclavian artery *(a)*, subclavian vein *(v)*, muscle *(m)* with rib removed. *Copyright The Johns Hopkins University.*

anesthesiologist gives several large breaths to check for pneumothorax. A chest x-ray should always be obtained in the recovery room. Closure is in two layers with absorbable sutures. Postoperatively, the arm is placed in a sling and pain managed overnight with intravenous narcotics administered by a patient-controlled analgesia pump. Patients are routinely discharged 1 day postoperatively with oral analgesics. When systemic anticoagulation is necessary, as is usually the case for axillosubclavian venous thrombosis, low-molecular-weight heparin and warfarin sodium are instituted at home on the third postoperative day because immediate anticoagulation therapy, in our experience, significantly increases the risk of postoperative bleeding.

Supraclavicular scalenectomy with or without first-rib resection is also an effective approach for decompression of the thoracic outlet. In fact, some believe that it is safer than the transaxillary procedure and that anomalous anatomy such as a cervical rib can be dealt with more effectively with a supraclavicular incision. Moreover, when the patient's symptoms are particularly suggestive of upper-brachial plexus involvement (as opposed to the more common lower plexus), it is reasonable to use a supraclavicular incision so that these nerves can be more directly decompressed. For patients who have undergone inadequate transaxillary scalenectomy, the supraclavicular approach avoids the scar tissue usually present in the previous operative field. Finally, when patients require arterial reconstruction, this approach provides better access to the proximal vasculature for arterial control.

Although advocates of the supraclavicular approach believe that scalenectomy alone provides adequate decompression of the thoracic outlet, resection of the first rib can be accomplished through this incision. Again, a short-acting paralytic agent or none is used on induction of anesthesia so that nerve function can be assessed during the procedure. The patient is placed in the semi-Fowler position, with the head turned away from the operative side. An incision is placed 2 fingerbreadths above the clavicle, extending from the external jugular vein to the sternocleidomastoid (SCM) muscle (Fig. 5, *A*). The SCM is mobilized medially, and the omohyoid muscle is usually transected. The scalene fat pad is carefully divided, taking care to avoid the underlying phrenic nerve. Underlying the nerve is the anterior scalene muscle (Fig. 5, *B*). This is divided inferiorly at its insertion on the first rib. Any adhesions between the muscle and the subclavian artery and brachial plexus must be lysed, and the proximal end of the muscle is divided medially to expose the C5–C7 roots. The subclavius muscle is then divided. At this point, the five roots should be completely cleared and tested using a nerve stimulator (Fig. 5, *C*). If the operation is to include first-rib resection, the middle scalene muscle must also be divided. The rib is divided posteriorly, and a finger used to dissect it from the pleura. The subclavian artery must be freed from the anterior portion of the rib before it is divided. As with the transaxillary procedure, the wound is filled with irrigation to assess for pleural leak. If present, a soft, closed suction drain can be positioned so that the tip drains the pleural space. The postoperative algorithm is the same as with the transaxillary approach.

COMPLICATIONS

Surgical decompression of the thoracic outlet is safe; however, as with any surgical intervention, complications can occur. The most common complication during thoracic outlet decompression is violation of the pleural space, which occurs in up to 30% of patients. This is, however, easily recognized and evacuated at the time of operation without the need for a chest tube, resulting in a 5% incidence of postoperative pneumothorax. Major injuries to the subclavian artery and subclavian vein are extremely rare and can often be detected and dealt with at the time of surgery. Injuries to the brachial plexus, although sometimes identified at the time of surgery,

are more often a result of excessive traction on the nerves from the retractor. These injuries are thought to be secondary to stretching of the perineurium, leading to ischemia, and can be prevented by intermittently relieving traction on the arm. Besides the brachial plexus, other nerves can be injured during thoracic outlet decompression. Both the long thoracic nerve and the phrenic nerve can be injured, more frequently through the transaxillary and supraclavicular approaches, respectively. A number of other complications are extremely rare but warrant mention. Postoperative causalgia, Horner's syndrome, thoracic duct injuries, and injury to the laryngeal nerve have all been reported and are far more common in the reoperative setting. With a thorough understanding of the anatomy and structures surrounding the thoracic outlet, most of these complications can be avoided.

RECURRENT THORACIC OUTLET SYNDROME

Published rates of recurrence for TOS range from 2% to 20%, with recurrent symptoms most often seen in patients who presented initially with the neurogenic variant of the disease. A variety of studies have implicated long, posterior, first-rib stumps; missed cervical ribs; and incomplete scalene resection, but none has shown good correlation with symptoms. Scar formation has also been implicated in persistent or recurrent neurogenic symptoms, but no quantifiable measure allows for correlations to be drawn. With adequate decompression of the thoracic outlet and adequate adjuvant therapies (arterial reconstruction, thrombolysis, venoplasty), recurrence of the arterial and venous forms of TOS is rare.

The workup and initial treatment for recurrent TOS is essentially the same as the initial workup of previously undiagnosed disease, with an emphasis on ruling out other disease processes. When reoperation is deemed appropriate, there are a variety of ways to approach the postsurgical thoracic outlet. Although using the same incision is possible, we typically elect to approach the thoracic outlet through a new incision and previously undissected tissues (e.g., supraclavicular incision if the initial operation was completed transaxillary). If the first operation did not include a first-rib resection, this procedure should be performed as part of the second surgical intervention. Finally, whether through a supraclavicular or transaxillary incision, most surgeons also add some form of neurolysis to the reoperation.

REHABILITATION AND FOLLOW-UP

In most cases, patients are discharged home on postoperative day 1 or 2 with oral narcotics. Regardless of the variant of TOS or the approach to thoracic outlet decompression, physical activity is limited for the first 2 weeks postoperatively, and the arm is maintained in a sling. A program of physical therapy is then instituted. Even with adequate decompression, the ultimate success or failure of treatment is heavily dependent on patient compliance with this physical therapy regimen (especially in patients with neurogenic TOS). In Paget-Schroetter syndrome (axillosubclavian vein thrombosis), patients are instructed not to resume anticoagulation therapy until postoperative day 3, and low-molecular-weight heparin is generally used. All Paget-Schroetter patients then undergo a follow-up venogram 2 to 3 weeks postoperatively with further endovascular therapy (lysis or angioplasty as necessary), followed by 3 months of anticoagulation with warfarin. After 3 months, follow-up duplex ultrasound scanning is performed and anticoagulation discontinued if the patient is asymptomatic and no abnormality is identified. Patients who have undergone a vascular reconstruction of the subclavian artery along with decompression usually require antiplatelet therapy with aspirin alone for 3 months regardless of the conduit used (vein or prosthetic). More aggressive oral anticoagulation

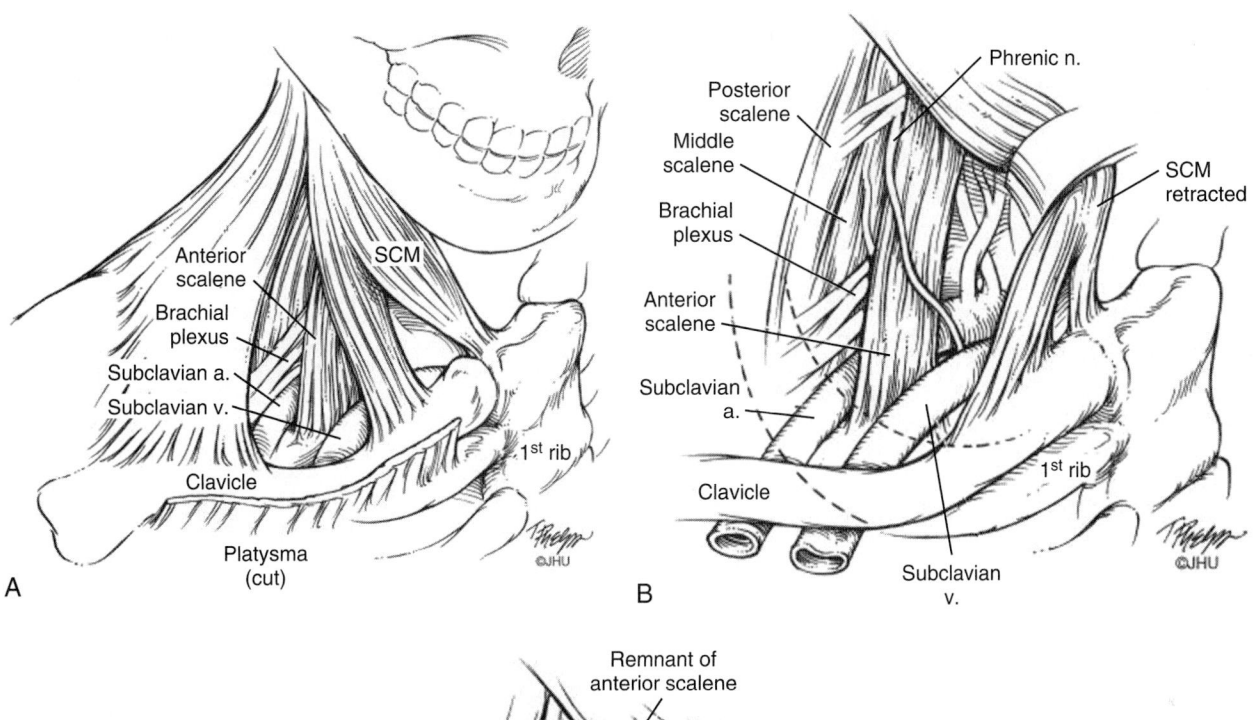

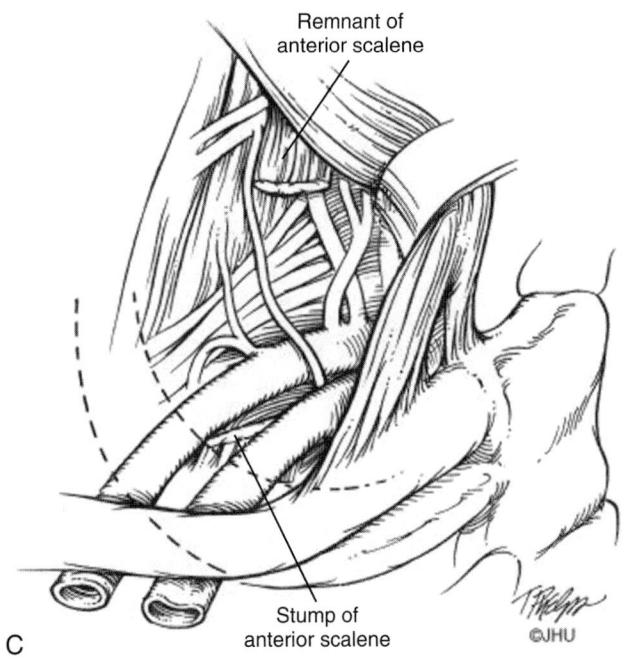

Figure 5 **(A)** The patient is placed in the semi-Fowler position, with the head turned away from the operative side. An incision is placed 2 fingerbreadths above the clavicle, extending from the external jugular vein to the sternocleidomastoid *(SCM)* muscle. Depicted is the musculoskeletal anatomy with the scalene fat pad removed. Artery *(a)*; vein *(v)*. **(B)** The scalene fat pad (not shown) is divided, taking care to avoid the underlying phrenic nerve *(n)*. Underlying the nerve is the anterior scalene muscle and the structures of the thoracic outlet. Artery *(a)*; vein *(v)*. **(C)** The anterior scalene muscle is resected, leaving the subclavian vein, artery, and nerve roots well visualized. The subclavian vein, artery and nerve roots of the brachial plexus are all well visualized. The first rib is often left intact in this approach; however, it can be resected if necessary. *Copyright The Johns Hopkins University.*

therapy with warfarin sodium is used only in rare situations to help maintain patency of collaterals when repeated embolic events have severely compromised arterial outflow.

SUMMARY

The three variants of TOS can present in dramatically different ways, depending on the structures involved. Early recognition, a comprehensive workup, and appropriately timed surgical interventions result in excellent clinical results and a substantially improved quality of life for most patients. Therefore it is important to be able to recognize these disorders and be comfortable with the workup of and often-multidisciplinary approach to the treatment of TOS.

SUGGESTED READINGS

Angle N, Gelabert HA, Farooq MM, and others: Safety and efficacy of early surgical decompression of the thoracic outlet for Paget-Schoretter syndrome, *Ann Vasc Surg* 15:37–42, 2001.

Caparrelli DJ, Freischlag J: A unified approach to axillosubclavian venous thrombosis in a single hospital admission, *Semin Vasc Surg* 18:153, 2005.

Green RM, McNamara J, Oriel K: Long-term follow-up after thoracic outlet decompression: an analysis of factors determining outcome, *J Vasc Surg* 14:739, 1991.

Machleder HI: Thoracic outlet syndromes: new concepts from a century of discovery, *Cardiovasc Surg* 2:137, 1994.

Perler BA, Mitchell SE: Percutaneous transluminal angioplasty and transaxillary first rib resection. A multidisciplinary approach to the thoracic outlet syndrome, *Am Surg* 52:485, 1986.

Roos DB: Transaxillary approach for first rib resection to relieve thoracic outlet compression syndrome, *Ann Surg* 163:354, 1966.

Roos DB: Congenital anomalies associated the thoracic outlet syndrome: anatomy, symptoms, diagnosis and treatment, *Am J Surg* 8:183, 1976.

ACUTE MESENTERIC ISCHEMIA

Heitham T. Hassoun, MD

Acute mesenteric ischemia (AMI) is an uncommon but life-threatening clinical condition. Despite improvements in our basic understanding of the pathophysiology of AMI and in our ability to treat critically ill patients adequately, there has been little change in the significant morbidity and mortality associated with this clinical problem over the past several decades. Although the reasons for this are multifactorial, failure to recognize symptoms on presentation remains the most likely cause for the persistently high mortality associated with this syndrome. After the diagnosis is considered, prompt diagnostic study followed by therapeutic intervention is paramount to prevent the deadly cascade of local and remote organ injury and inflammation.

Although AMI can result from a number of pathophysiologic conditions, the clinical syndrome can be divided into four distinct presentations: (1) embolic occlusion of the superior mesenteric or celiac arteries (or both), (2) acute thrombosis of one of these mesenteric arterial vessels, (3) nonocclusive mesenteric ischemia (NOMI) and (4) mesenteric vein thrombosis (MVT). This chapter focuses on the clinical presentation, diagnostic evaluation, surgical and non-surgical management, and contemporary outcomes for these clinical conditions. A detailed overview of the pathophysiology of mesenteric ischemia/reperfusion (I/R) injury is beyond the scope of this chapter, but selected references can be found in the Suggested Reading section.

CLINICAL PRESENTATION

The sine qua non of patients presenting with AMI is the sudden onset of severe midabdominal pain that is disproportional to the physical findings. This presentation is particularly classic for patients who present with superior mesenteric artery (SMA) embolus and is frequently associated with immediate bowel evacuation, either forceful emesis or diarrhea. When peritoneal signs are present, they are usually indicative of advanced ischemia and likely intestinal infarction.

Patients with embolic occlusion of the mesenteric circulation typically have a history of recent cardiac events such as arrhythmia (i.e., atrial fibrillation) or recent myocardial infarction. In addition, paradoxical SMA embolism can occur in patients who have cardiac defects with a right-to-left shunt such as an atrial septal defect or patent foramen ovale. Approximately one third of patients who present with an acute SMA embolism have a prior history of arterial embolus. In contrast, patients with AMI secondary to SMA thrombosis typically have other manifestations of diffuse atherosclerotic occlusive disease or a previous history of chronic mesenteric ischemic symptoms.

Patients with NOMI typically present in a somewhat different fashion. These patients usually report pain that is not sudden in nature but rather that occurs in a waxing and waning fashion and is diffuse in nature. AMI in these patients typically results from vasospasm or vasoconstriction in the mesenteric circulation. Although this condition can occur in ambulatory patients taking vasoconstrictive drugs such as ergot alkaloids or digitalis, most patients with NOMI are critically ill in an intensive-care setting undergoing treatment for systemic illnesses such as sepsis or cardiogenic shock.

Patients presenting with MVT usually have nonspecific complaints of abdominal pain that is frequently associated with nausea, vomiting, or diarrhea. In general, symptoms are not sudden in onset, and the diagnosis is frequently made after obtaining a noninvasive diagnostic study such as a computed tomography (CT) scan. Risk factors for MVT include a known hypercoagulable state, use of oral contraceptives, smoking, and a previous history of deep vein thrombosis or pulmonary embolism.

DIAGNOSIS

The diagnosis of AMI relies heavily on a thorough history and physical examination. No basic laboratory studies are diagnostic for AMI, but various studies can alert the physician to the diagnosis. Laboratory tests generally indicate systemic inflammation; the white blood cell count is frequently elevated and often greater than 20,000/mm^3. Although not validated by level-one clinical evidence, other markers of systemic inflammation such as C-reactive protein and serum cytokines (i.e., interleukin-6, tumor necrosis factor-alpha) are likely elevated. In addition, patients frequently have signs of metabolic acidosis such as an increased base deficit or elevated serum lactate levels.

After a diagnosis of AMI is suspected, several noninvasive imaging modalities are available for diagnosis. Although abdominal plain films cannot confirm or exclude the diagnosis of AMI, x-rays may reveal signs that are consistent with the diagnosis. For instance, bowel thumbprinting along with a generalized pattern of ileus can be suggestive of AMI. In more advanced cases, plain films may reveal air in the bowel wall, portal vein, or both. Abdominal plain films are mostly helpful for excluding other potential causes for abdominal pain, such as bowel obstruction, perforation of a hollow viscus, or kidney stones.

CT angiography (CTA) and magnetic resonance angiography (MRA) are frequently used to confirm a diagnosis of AMI. CTA, particularly with the newer multislice, multiarray helical CT scan technologies with three-dimensional (3D) reconstruction, has become the diagnostic test of choice in patients with normal renal function (Fig. 1). In addition, CT scans are helpful to evaluate the presence of bowel necrosis or other potential causes of abdominal pain such as pancreatitis or diverticulitis. Furthermore, CTA with delayed films plays a valuable role in the diagnosis of MVT and has become the diagnostic test of choice for this condition.

Advances in MR technology such as contrast-enhanced 3D MRA have made this test an excellent imaging modality for the diagnosis of AMI. Fast imaging techniques using intravenous (IV) administration of gadolinium over a single breath hold can provide quality

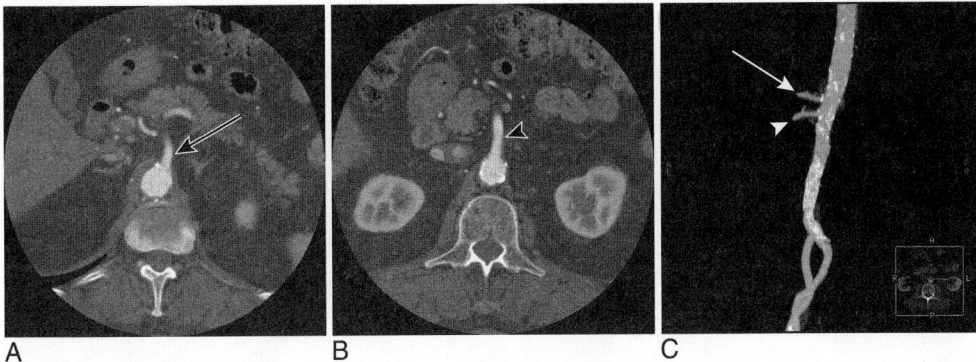

Figure 1 Evaluation of mesenteric arterial occlusive disease with CT imaging. Shown are axial images of patent celiac **(A)** and superior mesenteric **(B)** arteries. Lateral projection of three-dimensional reconstructed images from same patient **(C)** demonstrates more acute takeoff of celiac artery *(arrow)* from the aorta when compared with the superior mesenteric artery *(arrowhead).*

3D images with the advantage of being significantly less nephro-toxic than other contrast agents used for CT scans or traditional contrast angiography.

Contrast angiography remains the gold standard for imaging the visceral vessels. The procedure can be performed from a transfemoral or transbrachial approach using a modified Seldinger technique and should be performed in both anterior-posterior and lateral views to identify the proximal segments of the celiac, superior mesenteric, and inferior mesenteric arteries. Classic angiographic patterns can distinguish AMI caused by SMA embolism versus thrombosis. The SMA is by far the most likely visceral vessel for an embolism because its takeoff from the aorta is at a much less acute angle than the celiac or inferior mesenteric arteries. SMA emboli usually lodge distal to the middle colic and proximal jejunal branch, whereas SMA thrombosis usually occurs at the origin of the vessel where there is forma-tion of atherosclerotic plaque (Fig. 2). Angiographic findings in patients with AMI secondary to NOMI include narrowing of the origins of SMA branches, alternate narrowing and dilatation of branch vessels, generalized spasm of distal arteries, and absent filling of distal intramural branches (Fig. 3).

MANAGEMENT

Specific treatment for acute mesenteric ischemic depends on the etiology and patient presentation. The goals of treatment are (1) to restore normal pulsatile flow to the abdominal viscera, (2) to resect any nonviable intestine, and (3) to perform second-look laparotomy when viability of the intestine is questionable. The ther-apeutic approach to patients with AMI depends on the underlying etiology and is outlined in this section.

Superior Mesenteric Artery Embolus

SMA embolus is the cause of AMI in approximately 50% of patients with this condition. The treatment is embolectomy, and this proce-dure should be performed before resection of any compromised intestine. After initial resuscitation with intravenous fluids, systemic heparinization, and antibiotics, the patient is taken to the operating room, where a midline incision is performed for abdominal explo-ration. The transverse colon is then reflected superiorly and the small bowel is reflected laterally to the patient's right. The ligament of Treitz is fully incised, and the root of the mesentery is then mobilized. The SMA is easily palpated by placing four fingers of the surgeon's hand behind the root of the mesentery with the thumb opposite and anterior to the root. The SMA is easily identi-fied as a firm, tubular structure that may or may not have a palpa-ble pulse. Alternatively, the SMA can also be identified by following the middle colic artery through the transverse colon until it enters the SMA at the root of the mesentery. Proximal and distal control of the SMA is then obtained by sharp dissection, exposing the artery from its surrounding mesenteric tissue. Patients with the diagnosis of SMA embolus will usually have an identifiable pulse proximally in the root of the mesentery with absent pulse distally. After proximal vascular control is obtained, an arteriotomy, either transverse or longitudinal, is performed. A Fogarty balloon embo-lectomy is performed both proximally and distally. The embolus is usually removed with restoration of both backbleeding and inflow. After adequate backbleeding is obtained, the arteriotomy is closed primarily or with a patch angioplasty.

At this point, a handheld, continuous-wave Doppler ultra-sound can be used to detect the adequacy of intestinal blood flow. After restoration of mesenteric perfusion is attained, an assessment

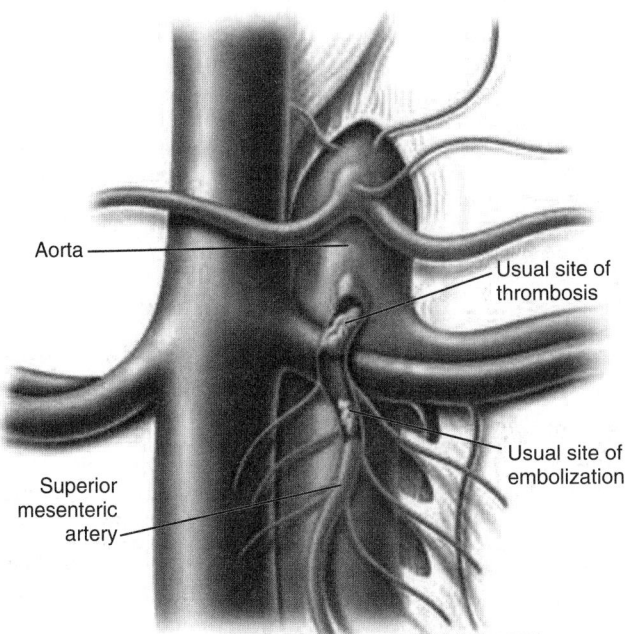

Figure 2 Depiction of usual sites of superior mesenteric artery embolus versus thrombosis. Note sparing of proximal jejunal branches with more distal lodgment of an embolus. *From WebMD, 2006.*

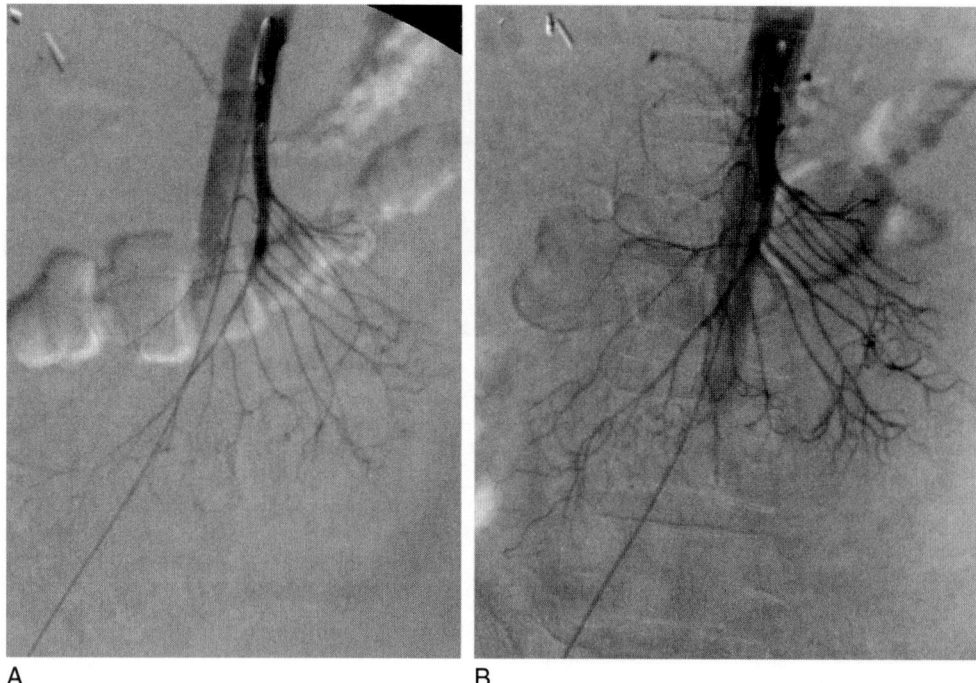

Figure 3 Selective superior mesenteric artery *(SMA)* angiogram in a patient with nonocclusive mesenteric ischemia before **(A)** and after **(B)** treatment with catheter-directed papaverine infusion. Note improved filling of more distal SMA branches after treatment. *From WebMD, 2006.*

of bowel viability is performed. Clearly necrotic or nonviable intestine should be resected at the time of initial exploration. For cases of SMA embolism, the distal small bowel and the proximal colon are typically affected, and the proximal jejunum and transverse colon are usually spared. Nonetheless, determination of bowel viability of marginally perfused intestine can be difficult even in the most experienced hands. Continuous-wave Doppler ultrasound of the antimesenteric border, intraoperative IV administration of fluorescein, and transcutaneous oxygen measurements have been used, but none of these modalities is sensitive or specific for predicting ultimate bowel viability. Therefore if any areas of intestine are questionably viable at the end of revascularization, the patient should be scheduled for a second-look laparotomy within 24 to 48 hours for further resection of nonviable intestine. The decision to perform second-look laparotomy should be made at the initial operation and adhered to strictly. Often patients respond to fluid resuscitations and correction of acid-base imbalance but still harbor necrotic bowel that must be removed to prevent systemic sepsis.

Superior Mesenteric Artery Thrombosis

AMI secondary to acute SMA thrombosis occurs in approximately 25% of patients with this condition. It most commonly occurs in patients with a history of atherosclerotic occlusive arterial disease, and in this situation the entire midgut is usually involved. After diagnosis is reached and the patient is adequately resuscitated with intravenous fluids, systemic heparinization, and antibiotics, the patient is taken to the operating room for midline abdominal exploration and surgical revascularization. Rapid revascularization of the mesenteric circulation by the most expeditious means is the goal of the operation, via either an antegrade or retrograde approach (Fig. 4). The decision regarding the optimal method is often made intraoperatively on the basis of the quality of the required inflow vessels and patient condition. In the setting of intestinal necrosis, the conduit of choice is generally autogenous

greater saphenous vein. There are several inflow options for revascularization of the SMA, including the supraceliac aorta, the infrarenal aorta, and the iliac arteries. Although an antegrade bypass graft from the supraceliac aorta to the SMA tunneled behind the pancreas is the optimal anatomic configuration because of its lesser susceptibility to kinking, retrograde bypass from either the infrarenal aorta or iliac artery may be easier to perform in the acute setting, when rapid revascularization is the ultimate goal. However, many of these patients have severe aortoiliac disease, making a retrograde bypass essentially impossible; therefore the surgeon should be ready to perform revascularization from either approach.

Patients with severe comorbidities and without signs of peritonitis who present with an acute SMA thrombosis superimposed on chronic mesenteric ischemia can occasionally be treated with catheter-directed thrombolysis followed by percutaneous angioplasty and stenting (Fig. 5). However, this treatment modality should be performed selectively and patients monitored closely for the need to undergo surgical exploration.

Nonocclusive Mesenteric Ischemia

NOMI accounts for 15% to 20% of patients with AMI. Management is generally nonoperative, and optimal results require early diagnosis and treatment, of the underlying pathophysiology. This generally requires optimization of patient hemodynamics, elimination of vasopressor treatment, and correction of any systemic factors contributing to shock. After the diagnosis is reached, either by history and physical examination or through noninvasive imaging, the patient should undergo angiography, including selective catheterization of the SMA. This allows for potential direct treatment with papaverine either as a single bolus or continuous infusion (30–60 mg/hr), which can be employed for 24 to 48 hours. Repeat angiography should be performed at established intervals to determine the effectiveness of therapy, and this treatment algorithm is reserved for patients who are hemodynamically

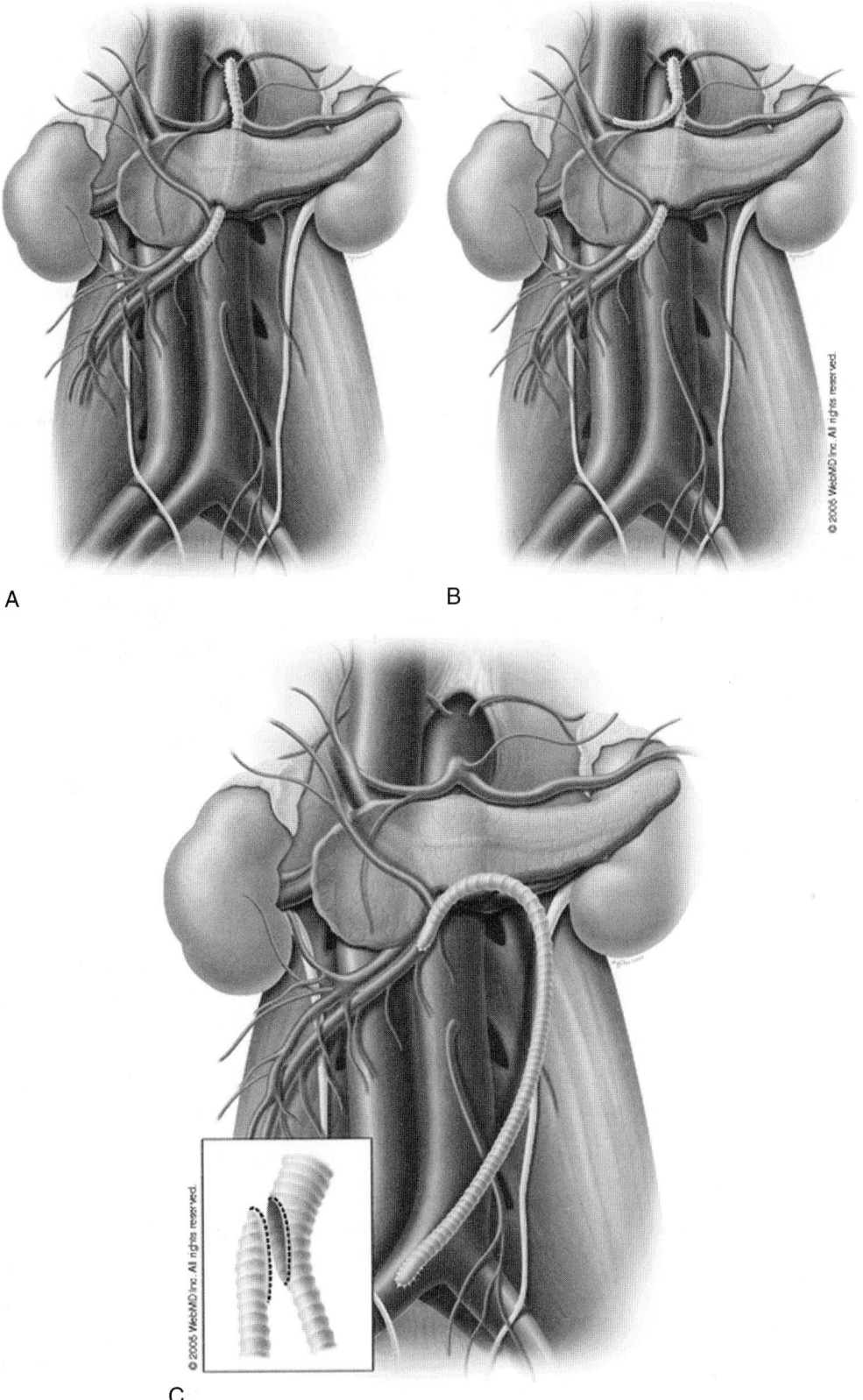

A

B

C

Figure 4   Depiction of arterial reconstruction options for mesenteric occlusion with synthetic bypass graft.
(A) Single antegrade retropancreatic bypass from supraceliac aorta to superior mesenteric artery *(SMA)*.
(B) Antegrade bypass to both celiac artery and SMA. **(C)** Retrograde bypass from right iliac artery to SMA
with a C-loop configuration.   *From WebMD, 2006.*

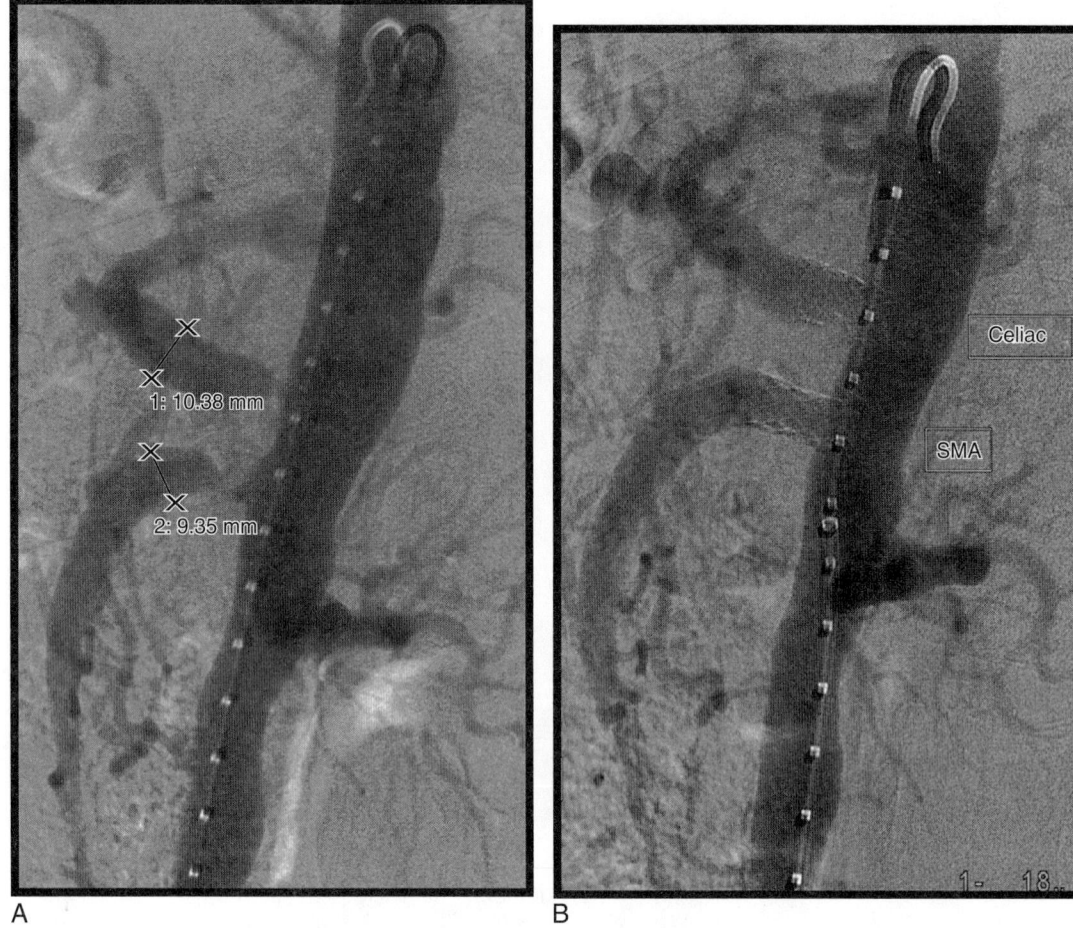

Figure 5   Before **(A)** and after **(B)** aortogram demonstrating potential treatment of a nearly occluded celiac artery and superior mesenteric artery *(SMA)* with balloon-expandable stents via retrograde femoral access.

stable and continue to have evidence of mesenteric ischemia. Occasionally patients present with peritoneal signs on examination or evidence of bowel necrosis on CT scan. Surgical exploration is mandatory in these patients to remove any source of sepsis, and second-look laparotomy should be performed routinely as outlined earlier.

Mesenteric Vein Thrombosis

MVT accounts for 5% to 10% of patients with AMI. The treatment of MVT is generally systemic anticoagulation therapy. Similar to patients with mesenteric ischemia secondary to NOMI, these patients should be monitored closely for signs of worsening bowel ischemia, peritonitis, and systemic inflammation. Up to one third of patients with MVT require exploration for resection of necrotic bowel. These patients should undergo second-look laparotomy as outlined earlier to assess viability of marginally perfused bowel. In addition, patients with MVT should undergo a hypercoagulable workup in an effort to identify any underlying etiology that would necessitate lifelong anticoagulation therapy.

SURGICAL OUTCOMES

Despite effective surgical management of acute mesenteric ischemia, significant morbidity and mortality remain. This is largely due to the effects of mesenteric I/R injury on local and systemic inflammation and subsequent progression to multiple organ failure (MOF). At the cellular level, oxidative stress leads to proinflammatory gene expression and activation of circulating neutrophils that cause remote organ injury and early MOF. This activation of proinflammatory genes may also cause local gut dysfunction characterized by ileus and increased intestine epithelial and microvascular permeability, leaving the patient susceptible to endotoxemia, sepsis, and MOF.

Most large studies have demonstrated significant 30-day mortality of 32% to 60% and a dismal 5-year survival rate ranging from 18% to 50% after an episode of AMI. The mortality and morbidity associated with this condition largely depend on the underlying etiology. For instance, a systematic review of 45 observational studies that included more than 3600 patients was recently conducted by Schoots and colleagues. This study identified that mortality varied substantially according to the cause of AMI. Overall, mortality was lowest with AMI secondary to MVT (44% mortality) and greatest with the underlying etiologies of NOMI (73%) and SMA thrombosis (77%). It is apparent that AMI is associated with significant morbidity and mortality, and it is likely that the only way to achieve any meaningful improvement in outcomes will be to rapidly diagnose and treat the underlying etiology. In addition, we must expand our knowledge of the early molecular pathways involved in the activation and proliferation of both local and systemic inflammation in this disease process.

ACKNOWLEDGMENT

The author acknowledges the editorial assistance of Tracey Stinney in completing this chapter.

SUGGESTED READINGS

Hassoun HT, Moore FA: The role of gut hypoperfusion in multiple organ failure. In Yao JST, Pearce WH, editors: *Current techniques in modern vascular surgery*, New York, 2000, McGraw-Hill, p. 419.

Kibbe MR, Hassoun HT, and others: 16 Acute mesenteric ischemia. 5 Vascular system. In Souba WW, Fink MP, Jurkovich GJ, editors: *ACS surgery: principles & practice*, 2005, WebMD, p. 1.

Park WM, Gloviczki P, Cherry KJ Jr, and others: Contemporary management of acute mesenteric ischemia: factors associated with survival, *J Vasc Surg* 35:445, 2002.

Schoots IG, Koffeman GI, Legemate DA, and others: Systematic review of survival after acute mesenteric ischaemia according to disease aetiology, *Br J Surg* 91:17, 2004.

MANAGEMENT OF CHRONIC MESENTERIC ISCHEMIA

Kaj H. Johansen, MD, PhD, and Sanjiv Parikh, MD

INTRODUCTION

Chronic mesenteric ischemia (CMI) is a syndrome characterized by abdominal pain and weight loss resulting from markedly diminished arterial perfusion to the intestine. CMI results when blood flow to the gut via the main visceral arteries—the celiac artery (CA), the superior mesenteric artery (SMA), and the inferior mesenteric artery (IMA)—is critically reduced and cannot be maintained by collateral splanchnic arterial sources.

The lesions that obstruct intestinal blood flow and result in the symptoms and signs of CMI are almost always atherosclerotic and are thus commonly focal and proximal in the main arteries supplying the small and large intestine. Only in extremely unusual circumstances—various forms of inflammatory arteritis, for example, or the consequences of abdominal irradiation or aortic dissection—does CMI result from a nonatherosclerotic cause.

Because atherosclerosis is centrally relevant to the etiology of CMI, these patients warrant constant vigilance regarding concurrent cardiac and cerebrovascular comorbidity. Previously described as a disease of the elderly, it is no longer uncommon for CMI to be seen in younger individuals with vascular pathology, primarily related to smoking. Indeed, the major risks associated with the management of CMI result from coexistent cardiopulmonary and cerebrovascular comorbidities in these patients. For example, patients with CMI may show evidence of myocardial ischemia, renovascular hypertension, extracranial carotid disease, or other manifestations of systemic atherosclerosis.

Another critical feature in the management of patients with CMI involves their sometimes-profound nutritional depletion. Because eating predictably results in abdominal pain ("intestinal angina"), patients quickly develop behavioral patterns that limit nutritional intake ("food fear"). Weight loss, sometimes to a degree reminiscent of that seen in patients with terminal visceral cancer, is commonplace and has an obviously deleterious impact on the ability of surgical wounds to heal in such patients.

INDICATIONS FOR INTERVENTION

Mesenteric arterial insufficiency should be managed when weight loss, postprandial pain, and food fear are clearly evident. When such a circumstance is present, critically reduced splanchnic blood flow can be intimated; because collateral perfusion is maximal in such a circumstance, no increase in postprandial splanchnic arterial perfusion is possible, and the likelihood of worsened symptoms (and occasionally acute thrombosis resulting in catastrophic bowel infarction) is predictable. In this regard, mesenteric arterial insufficiency differs from lower-extremity arterial insufficiency, for example caused by superficial femoral artery occlusion, in which distal ischemic symptoms may initially be severe but tend to stabilize or even diminish over time as deep femoral artery collaterals are enhanced.

As noted earlier, the diagnosis of chronic mesenteric arterial insufficiency may initially be obscure. An extensive but unrevealing workup for upper gastrointestinal tract problems, inflammatory bowel disease, or occult abdominal malignancy will frequently have been completed before the explanation for the patient's symptoms is clarified.

Significant symptoms arising from malperfusion in certain vascular beds may respond well to various forms of pharmacologic management. For example, the use of certain rheologically active agents can significantly improve lower-extremity claudication caused by superficial femoral artery occlusion; various antihypertensive medications often satisfactorily control hypertension arising from renal artery stenosis. However, no equivalent pharmacologic or other noninterventional therapy is demonstrably useful in mitigating either the symptoms or the nutritional and metabolic effects of chronic mesenteric arterial insufficiency.

SURGICAL REVASCULARIZATION

The first arterial reconstructive procedure to treat chronic mesenteric arterial insufficiency was carried out in 1957 by Shaw and Maynard. Over the next 3 decades, various surgical means of reperfusing the gut were explored, initially involving the creation of bypass grafts from the aorta to the CA and SMA using autogenous or prosthetic conduits. Wylie and colleagues popularized the concept of direct transaortic endarterectomy, with eversion disobliteration of the various visceral arteries, as an alternative approach to reconstructing the gut and the abdominal/renal viscera.

It has been axiomatic that, to develop symptoms of sufficient significance to warrant surgical intervention, at least two of the three main visceral arterial vessels must be occluded or highly stenotic. However, almost one fifth of contemporary patients present with single-vessel disease in the SMA, their symptoms presumably arising because of inadequate development of collaterals from the gastroduodenal artery and the inferior mesenteric artery (IMA) (marginal artery of Drummond and arc of Riolan). Reconstruction of as many of these vessels as possible, either by bypass grafts off the infrarenal aorta, the iliac arteries, or the supraceliac aorta, seemed optimal. Success rates with such procedures are high, although coexistent coronary and cerebrovascular problems in these patients result in a nontrivial 5% to 20% perioperative mortality rate.

The Oregon Health Sciences University group published data in 2000 refuting the concept that revascularization of both of the two main visceral arterial vessels—the CA and the SMA—is necessary, in view of the robust gastroduodenal and pancreaticoduodenal arterial collaterals that often connect these two arterial trunks.

Although the IMA is likely dispensable in most clinical scenarios, Schneider and others have demonstrated the utility of revascularization of this important collateral contributor.

As for other settings in the body, the success rate of intervention has appeared to be higher with autogenous graft material than with prosthetic conduits, although for mesenteric revascularization, no compelling patency difference can be assumed.

ENDOVASCULAR RECONSTRUCTION FOR CHRONIC MESENTERIC ISCHEMIA

Because of the accessibility of the ostia of the visceral arteries to diagnostic catheters placed in the aorta, cannulation of the proximal CA, SMA or IMA has long been available. Following the introduction of therapeutic endovascular reconstruction by Dotter and Gruntzig, interventionalists were quick to exploit their increased catheter skills in treating proximal visceral arterial stenoses—balloon angioplasty first being used by Furrer and Gruntzig and colleagues in 1980 and stenting of the SMA by Finch in 1993. Impetus for such an approach has arisen from the substantial perioperative risk incurred by CMI patients undergoing open surgical repair and by the demonstrable efficacy, safety, and relative durability of endovascular treatment for arterial occlusive disease, particularly for focal atherosclerotic stenoses in first-order arterial branches of the aorta.

Several large series—including our own—of endovascular treatment for CMI have been presented. These experiences appear to suggest that endovascular reconstruction for CMI is predictably technically successful; has an early efficacy of CMI symptoms of 80% to 90%; results in periprocedural mortality and morbidity of 1% to 5% and 5–15%, respectively; and has reasonable durability, with 70% to 95% primary patency at 2-year follow-up. The morbidity in most cases is related to puncture-site issues, especially when the approach is brachial.

Technical aspects of catheter-directed visceral arterial reconstruction have been well summarized. In our view, the most effective access to all three of the main visceral arteries is via an ultrasound-guided, left transbrachial arterial approach. This is because of the downward angle of the CA, and particularly the SMA, relative to the horizontal plane, that becomes more conspicuous as age advances. A left brachial approach, unlike the right brachial, avoids crossing three brachiocephalic arteries and provides direct access to the descending thoracic and abdominal aorta. The rate of puncture-site complications with the brachial approach is undeniably higher than with a femoral approach; on the other hand, the transfemoral approach may preclude adequate stent coverage of the ostium, and the aortic component of the disease is more likely to cause dissection at the vessel origin during manipulation.

Our standard protocol is to perform an abdominal aortogram to characterize flow in the trunk and branches of visceral arteries and also to establish the status of splanchnic collaterals. The dominant collateral cascade is via the gastroduodenal artery and pancreaticoduodenal arteries between the CA and SMA and the arc of Riolan (meandering artery) and via the marginal artery of Drummond between the IMA and SMA. Delayed imaging is imperative to establish collateral circulation. A lateral abdominal aortogram is performed to characterize the ostia of the CA and SMA. After a wire has crossed the lesion, a tapered 6-F sheath is "traversed" through the lesion, and in most cases primary stenting is performed unless the stenosis/occlusion precludes passage of a sheath through the lesion. The procedure is performed with therapeutic anticoagulation

and small aliquots of nitroglycerine administered intra-arterially to prevent vasospasm. The typical balloon-expandable stent sizes used are 6 to 8 mm in diameter and approximately 20 to 30 mm in length.

THERAPEUTIC DECISION MAKING

As previously indicated, intervention for CMI is governed by the presence and severity of symptoms. Attention to general cardiovascular risk-factor modification in patients with CMI should be carried out in parallel with specific efforts directed toward restoration of splanchnic perfusion. In particular, smoking cessation and the institution of various validated adjunctive pharmacologic treatments—aspirin, statins, angiotensin-converting enzyme inhibitors, and beta-blockade—should be ensured. Attention must be paid to concurrent coronary, cerebrovascular, or lower-extremity arterial occlusive disease.

Because the necessity to manage CMI is not common—in our regional, tertiary-level cardiovascular institute, we see only approximately 6 to 10 such patients annually—it seems likely that such patients should be managed in major centers offering appropriate patient care and technologic resources plus substantial experience with both open surgical and transcatheter techniques directed toward the visceral arteries.

Open surgical reconstruction capabilities remain crucial as a fallback mechanism for management of CMI, although they are used uncommonly. This is because approximately 10% of individuals requiring intervention for CMI are not reconstructible by catheter-directed means and necessarily require visceral artery bypass grafting or endarterectomy. Having surgical expertise available as a backup for the occasional acutely thrombosed or a dissected SMA is obligatory.

That stated, the vast majority of individuals with CMI can be treated effectively, safely, and durably through endovascular means. Symptom relief is immediate, and regaining of lost weight is predictable over the following weeks to months.

Over the 5-year period 2001 to 2006, we carried out interventional or surgical treatment for 49 patients with CMI. Of this group, four underwent a surgical intervention and 45 underwent catheter-based therapy. The technical success rate of surgical revascularization was 4 of 4 (100%); the mortality rate was 25%. Reintervention, in all cases by catheter-directed means for diagnostic or therapeutic purposes, was required in 20% of patients during follow-up averaging 2.3 years.

Among 63 catheter-directed interventions, technical success was achieved in 97%, and primary patency at 2 years was 70%. Twenty percent of patients have required a repeat intervention, all of them endovascular and involving angioplasty, cutting-balloon angioplasty, or restenting. Mortality among this group of patients was 8% (1 patient died following surgery after repeat intervention was not successful in chronic total occlusion recanalization).

SUMMARY

Although uncommon, chronic mesenteric arterial insufficiency can result in substantial morbidity and occasional mortality. Recognition and timely management can be lifesaving. Principles of management involve restoration of physiologic arterial perfusion by relief of proximal stenoses or occlusions—almost always atherosclerotic—of the major visceral arteries. Such management historically involved open surgical reconstruction such as aortomesenteric bypass or, on occasion, transaortic endarterectomy. In almost all such contemporary patients, CMI can be managed effectively, safely, or durably by catheter-directed endovascular means—angioplasty or stenting, with primary stenting being a preferred approach. With further refinement and development of new, low-profile, flexible delivery systems and stents, the clinical outcome and safety of percutaneous interventions is likely to improve further in the future. Surgical reconstructive capabilities remain important in backup for endovascular therapy for CMI, as well as for the small number of CMI patients whose proximal visceral arterial occlusive disease proves unreconstructible by endovascular means.

SUGGESTED READINGS

Brown DJ, Schermerhorn ML, Powell RJ, and others: Mesenteric stenting for chronic mesenteric ischemia, *J Vasc Surg* 42:268, 2005.

Cho J-S, Carr JA, Jacobson G, and others: Long-term outcome after mesenteric artery reconstruction: a 37-year experience, *J Vasc Surg* 35:453, 2002.

English WP, Pearce JD, Craven TE, and others: Chronic visceral ischemia: symptom-free survival after open surgical repair, *Vasc Endovasc Surg* 38:493, 2004.

Evans DC, Murphy MP, Lawson JH: Giant cell arteritis manifesting as mesenteric ischemia, *J Vasc Surg* 42:1019, 2005.

Finch IJ: Use of the Palmaz stent in ostial celiac artery stenosis, *J Vasc Interv Radiol* 3:633–635, 1992.

Foley M, Moneta GL, Abou-Zamzam AM, and others: Revascularization of the superior mesenteric artery alone for treatment of intestinal ischemia, *J Vasc Surg* 32:37–47, 2000.

Furrer J, Gruntzig A, Kugelmeier J: Treatment of abdominal angina with percutaneous dilatation of the arteria mesenterica superior stenosis, *Cardiovasc Intervent Radiol* 3:43, 1980.

Harward TR, Brooks DL, Flynn TC, and others: Multiple organ dysfunction after mesenteric artery revascularization, *J Vasc Surg* 18:459, 1993.

Israeli D, Dardik H, Wolodiger F, and others: Pelvic radiation therapy as a risk factor for ischemic colitis complicating abdominal aortic reconstruction, *J Vasc Surg* 23:706, 1996.

Jiminez JG, Huber TS, Ozaki CK, and others: Durability of antegrade synthetic aortomesenteric bypass for chronic mesenteric ischemia, *J Vasc Surg* 35:1078, 2002.

Neri E, Sassi C, Massetti M, and others: Nonocclusive intestinal ischemia in patients with acute aortic dissection, *J Vasc Surg* 36:738, 2002.

Parikh SR, Johansen K: Angioplasty/stenting for chronic visceral arterial occlusive disease. Presented at the seventeenth annual meeting of the Western Vascular Society, Newport Beach, CA, September 22, 2002.

Park WM, Cherry KJ, Chua HK, and others: Current results of open revascularization for chronic mesenteric ischemia; a standard for comparison, *J Vasc Surg* 35:853, 2003.

Schneider DB, Nelken NA, Messina LM, and others: Isolated inferior mesenteric artery revascularization for chronic visceral ischemia, *J Vasc Surg* 30:51, 1999.

Sharafuddin MJ, Olson CH, Sun S, and others: Endovascular treatment of celiac and mesenteric arterial stenoses: applications and results, *J Vasc Surg* 38:692–698, 2003.

Shaw RS, Maynard EP: Acute and chronic thrombosis of the mesenteric arteries associated with malabsorption: a report of two cases successfully treated with thromboembolectomy, *N Engl J Med* 258:874, 1958.

Siegelman SS, Warren A, Veith FJ, and others: The physiologic response to superior mesenteric angiography, *Radiology* 96:101, 1970.

Silva JA, White CJ, Collins TJ, and others: Endovascular therapy for chronic mesenteric ischemia, *J Am Coll Cardiol* 47:944, 2006.

Steinmetz E, Tatou E, Favier-Blavoux C, and others: Endovascular treatment as first choice in chronic intestinal ischemia, *Ann Vasc Surg* 16:693, 2002.

Stoney RJ, Wylie EJ: Surgical management of lesions of the thoracoabdominal aorta, *Am J Surg* 126:157, 1973.

DIABETIC FOOT

Dennis F. Bandyk, MD, and Patrick A. Stone, MD

Foot-related disorders, including infection, ulceration, and gangrene, are the most frequent indication for hospitalization of diabetic patients. The diabetic population in the United States continues to increase, and in 2006 it was estimated to be more than 20 million. It is projected that up to 20% of these patients will require hospitalization with a diabetic foot condition. The development of skin ulceration in the foot of a diabetic is a serious condition that, if not healed promptly, can lead to amputation. Annually, nonhealing diabetic foot wounds account for 80,000 amputations, and in 60% of patients the inciting event was a foot ulcer. The societal impact of the diabetic foot is significant in terms of individual disability, ensuing hospitalizations, and health care costs—estimated to be in excess of $1 billion annually. The development of multidisciplinary care programs that include surgeons can reduce both the number and extent of lower-extremity amputations. The prevalence of diabetic foot problems is expected to increase because of the aging U.S. population and the problem of obesity in the population with its concomitant development of type II diabetes. Thus surgeons must remain informed with updated data on the pathophysiology, diagnostics, management, and prevention of the diabetic foot problems.

PATHOPHYSIOLOGY

A triad of neuropathy, trauma with secondary infection, and arterial occlusive disease account for the pathophysiology of the diabetic foot. Peripheral neuropathy produces intrinsic muscle atrophy, leading to functional anatomic changes of hammertoe formation and the development of "high-pressure" zones on the plantar surface of the foot at the metatarsal heads (Fig. 1). Repetitive trauma with walking, in concert with decreased sensation and proprioception, predisposes to skin injury by producing atrophy and dislocation of protective plantar fat pads, leading to ulceration and infection with inadequate skin protection or improper footwear. Inattention to skin care, such as failing to use moisturizing creams or to promptly recognize dermal trauma (redness, blister formation), can lead to ulceration and the development of an invasive soft-tissue infection. If not promptly treated, tissue breakdown will continue, especially if the individual continues to walk. Risk for ulceration increases dramatically (by 32 times) in the presence of neuropathy, foot deformity, or prior digit amputation. Eventually the destructive processes of trauma and infection penetrate the deep fascia, enabling infection to extend into the midfoot muscles and joints, and along tendon sheaths. Infection accounts for half of major (above- or below-knee) lower-extremity amputations in diabetic patients.

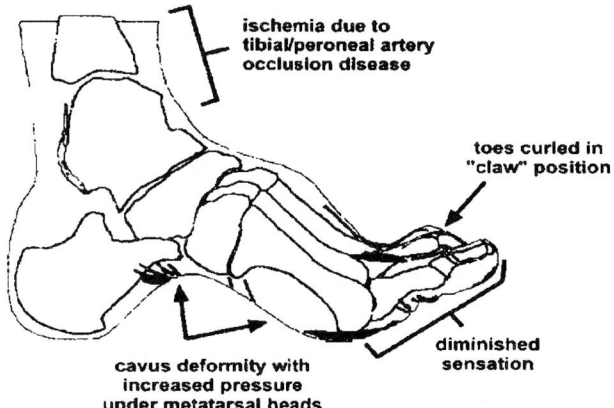

Figure 1   Mechanisms involved in diabetic foot disorders.

ischemia due to tibial/peroneal artery occlusion disease

toes curled in "claw" position

diminished sensation

cavus deformity with increased pressure under metatarsal heads

Neuropathy

The neuropathy produced by diabetes mellitus is a symmetric poly-neuropathy in which motor, sensory, and autonomic functions are affected to varying degrees. In some patients, the peripheral myelin motor fibers are affected in a length-dependent pattern, with the longest nerves affected first, resulting in a "stocking" distribution of sensory-motor loss. Loss of the Achilles reflex is the earliest sign of these changes. With atrophy of the lumbricales and interosseous muscles, the anatomy of foot arch changes, with a relative increase in extensor tendon forces producing a "claw" deformity of the toes. A shift to extrinsic muscle-tendon function contributes to depression of the metatarsal heads, hammertoe contracture of the digits, and equine ankle deformity.

In addition to the motor fiber dysfunction, sensory loss involving type A myelin fibers causes impaired gait and a loss of proprioception, pressure sensation, and vibratory perception. Destruction of the type-C sensory fibers leads to an inability to appreciate painful stimuli. As a result of these impaired sensations, the diabetic patient can experience repetitive foot trauma, including blister formation or even metatarsal bone fracture, without an appreciation of foot discomfort. Neuroarthropathy or Charcot's foot involves extensive destruction of the midfoot, with collapse of the arch and loss of foot stability. The warmth and swelling of the inflammatory stage of neuroarthropathy can mimic infection. Subluxation or dislocation of tarsal bones produces a bowed, "rockerbottom" appearance of the foot, which is susceptible to "high-pressure" ulceration. Autonomic system dysfunction, with impaired microvascular thermoregulation and anhidrosis, further adds to the motor and sensory disturbances. The skin becomes dry and prone to fissuring, diminishing its effectiveness as a barrier to microorganism invasion, and therefore becomes susceptible to dermal infection (i.e., cellulitis).

Arterial Insufficiency

Hyperglycemia and associated changes in glucose metabolism produce endothelial injury; hyperlipidemia; increased platelet viscosity and activity; and, with time, atherosclerosis. The distribution of lower-extremity atherosclerotic disease in diabetic patients differs from that in nondiabetic patients and preferentially involves the infrageniculate leg arteries (posterior and anterior tibial arteries), with less common involvement of the femoropopliteal arterial segment (superficial femoral, popliteal) and often sparing of the aortoiliac artery segment. With the development of diffuse tibial artery occlusive disease or more proximal arterial occlusion, perfusion of the foot below a level adequate to maintain skin integrity can result and an ischemic ulcer or gangrene can develop. Typically the peroneal and dorsalis pedis artery are less involved with atherosclerosis, allowing limb revascularization via vein bypass grafting from the popliteal or a more proximal artery to restore foot perfusion and achieve ulcer or foot (digit, transmetatarsal) amputation healing.

Infection

The nature of diabetic foot infection can range from uncomplicated cellulitis to limb- and life-threatening necrotizing fasciitis. Intervals of poor glycemic control produce immunologic dysfunction with impaired leukocyte activity and complement functions that facilitate development of invasive tissue infection. In the presence of damaged or poorly perfused skin and soft tissues, rapid bacteria penetration deep to fascia can occur, producing a foot-threatening infection and sepsis. Polymicrobial (*Staphylococci, Streptococci, Enterococci, Escherichia coli,* and other gram-negative bacteria) infections are common, as is the presence of antibiotic-resistant bacterial strains, especially methicillin-resistant *Staphylococcus aureus* (MRSA), which is present in 30% to 40% of patients. Amputation risk increases when the diabetic foot infection involves resistant bacterial strains, which are often the result of repeated or prolonged antibiotic usage. Gas-forming infections, present in approximately one third of patients, are caused by *Clostridium* species or a mixed infection of anaerobic *Streptococcus* and *E. coli.*

EVALUATION OF THE DIABETIC FOOT

A thorough patient history and physical examination, with special consideration for coexisting renal and cardiac conditions, initiate a comprehensive assessment of foot anatomy, neurosensory dysfunction, and vascular perfusion. The patient should be queried regarding recent foot trauma—including the possibility of a foreign body being present—and the duration and prior treatment of an ulcer or foot wound. Both lower extremities should be inspected for skin trauma (redness, induration, edema), ulceration, and foot or toe deformity, and popliteal and ankle (posterior tibial, dorsalis pedis) pulses should be palpated. When pulses are not palpable, arterial flow assessment using a handheld, continuous-wave (5–7 MHz) Doppler ultrasound should be performed to verify pulsatile flow in the pedal and digital arteries. The site(s) of inflammation should be evaluated for crepitus or tenderness along tendon sheaths, which indicate involvement of deep structures. Probing a plantar wound to verify penetration of deep fascia to bone is highly predictive (>90%) of osteomyelitis.

Neurologic examination includes: testing of vibratory (128-Hz tuning fork) sense; sensation to light touch (Semmes-Weinstein 5.07 microfilament); pinprick; temperature (tuning fork placed in warm or iced water and then applied to dorsum of foot); positional sense in the toes; and assessment of deep tendon (Achilles) and patellar reflexes. Loss of these neurologic functions is predictive of foot ulceration, with the annual risk increasing to more than 6% if all are abnormal. Laboratory examinations should include: complete blood count with differential; hemoglobin A_{1C}; urinalysis; and metabolic panel of serum electrolytes, creatinine, blood urea nitrogen, and glucose level.

Noninvasive arterial testing of limb and foot perfusion should be performed in all patients without palpable pulses and should include measurements of ankle and toe pressure in combination Doppler or plethysmographic waveforms. The normal ankle-brachial systolic pressure index (ABI) is 0.9 to 1.3, and toe systolic pressure should be 80% of the ankle pressure. Artery wall calcification producing incompressibility to external cuff pressure can falsely elevate ankle pressure measurements and should be suspected when the ABI is greater than 1.3 but abnormal arterial waveforms or toe pressure (<80% of brachial pressure) measurements are recorded. An ankle systolic pressure greater than 65 mm Hg or toe pressure of 40 mm Hg or greater is required for healing a superficial ulcer or digit amputation. Transcutaneous oximetry testing also is predictive of healing when transcutaneous partial pressure of oxygen (TcPO2) level is greater than 30 mm Hg.

Anatomic Imaging Studies

Plain x-rays of the foot (anterior-posterior and lateral views) are the initial imaging studies to evaluate for fracture, osteomyelitis, artery wall and soft-tissue calcifications, foreign bodies, edema, or tissue air produced by a gas-forming infection. Presence of cortical-bone erosion or periosteal elevation is indicative chronic infection of more than 14 days. Three-phase bone scans are highly sensitive for osteomyelitis but are prone to error in the presence of severe arterial occlusive disease and following amputation. Magnetic resonance (MR) imaging is highly diagnostic (sensitivity and specificity >80%) in determining the presence and extent of soft-tissue infection, plantar abscess, and osteomyelitis (characterized by altered bone-marrow signal). Simultaneous MR angiography of the lower limb can also be performed to image the femoropopliteal and tibial arteries for patency, presence of occlusive disease, and communication with the pedal arch. Duplex ultrasonography can also be used to assess artery patency, determine extent and severity of occlusive disease, and identify lesions amenable to endovascular intervention. Digital subtraction angiography has a risk of producing contrast–media-induced nephropathy, and thus its use in diabetics with renal insufficiency (serum creatinine >2 mg/L) should be limited or avoided if possible. When it is necessary to evaluate patients with multilevel occlusive disease or to monitor an endovascular intervention, using carbon dioxide gas as a contrast agent supplemented by small volumes (10–15 ml) of contrast media (when necessary) minimizes renal toxicity, especially if the patient has received oral Mucomyst (acetylcysteine; Roberts, Eatontown, NJ) 600 mg and intravenous fluids before the angiogram procedure. The risk of radiocontrast nephropathy may also be reduced by an intravenous infusion of fenoldopam (Corlopam; Abbott, Abbott Park, IL), a potent vasodilator of the renal circulation that produces an increase in renal blood flow and prevents a rise in serum creatinine in patients with preexisting renal dysfunction.

MANAGEMENT

The goals of diabetic foot treatment are to achieve tissue healing while maintaining adequate function and weight bearing for ambulation. The essential management principles are antibiotic treatment of invasive infection in conjunction with tissue debridement or amputation and off-loading foot pressure until healing is achieved. In patients presenting with advanced ischemia, control of infection takes precedence over limb revascularization. A multidisciplinary team that includes the primary physician, diabetologist, nurse educator, prosthetist, and home care nurse is indispensable to assist the surgeon in treating patients presenting with invasive foot infections, neuropathic ulcers, or tissue ischemia with and without gangrene.

Specific adjunctive therapies such as topical antimicrobial ointments (silver sulfadiazine, Murpicin), wound growth factors, biologic dressings, negative pressure wound therapy, and hyperbaric oxygen treatments have been shown to aid in ulcer and wound healing. Wound-healing rates must be optimized in clinics that provide specialized treatments in conjunction with pressure off-loading techniques.

Invasive Foot Infection

Acute foot sepsis can develop from a site-chronic infection or following acute trauma. Antibiotic therapy is based on the extent of foot infection, expected pathogens, and presence of arterial occlusive disease (Table 1). Hospitalization with parenteral antibiotic therapy is recommended when the infection penetrates to the deep fascia with or without the presence of pedal pulses. Patients with chronic ulcers, prior antibiotic treatment, and recurring infection should be assumed to have MRSA infection, and empiric treatment should be instituted.

Soft-tissue erythema—swelling with overlying skin gangrene—indicates a deep-space infection and the need for surgical exploration in the operating room for abscess drainage; debridement of necrotic tissue; and, if necessary, resection of bone or digit amputation to establish open drainage of infected tissue planes. Wounds should be left open and may require serial debridements to ensure adequate control of infection. Culture of deep tissue should be performed to guide antibiotic therapy.

In patients presenting with erythema and swelling but in whom clinical response to antibiotic therapy is not evident within 24 to 36 hours, additional diagnostic imaging such as MR should be performed to exclude presence of deep-space infection or osteomyelitis. For advanced foot infections with exposed joint spaces or gangrenous digits, prompt surgical debridement is necessary, including toe and corresponding metatarsal amputation to drain the infection adequately and facilitate tissue debridement. On occasion, an ankle disarticulation may be necessary to remove the septic foot when surgical exploration confirms invasive infection involving the mid and hindfoot. These patients commonly present with septic shock, requiring monitoring in the intensive care unit, fluid resuscitation, insulin infusion to control hyperglycemia, and broad-spectrum antibiotic therapy to include anaerobe coverage.

Table 1: Empiric Antibiotic Therapy for Diabetic Foot Infection

Extent of Infection	Pathogens	Antibiotic Regimen
Ulcer without infection	Colonizing skin flora	No antibiotic therapy
Superficial ulcer with ≤2 cm of inflammation; pedal pulses present	*Staphylococcus aureus* (assume MRSA) *Streptococcus* sp. (*S. pyogenes* predominate)	Oral therapy: Trimethoprim/sulfamethizole-DS or minocycline, or amoxicillin/clavulanic acid; plus linezolid
Ulcer with >2 cm of inflammation with extension to fascia; pedal pulses present	As above plus coliforms	Oral therapy: Trimethoprim/sulfamethizole-DS plus amoxicillin/ clavulanic acid; plus linezolid or clindamycin *or* ciprofloxacin or levofloxacin; plus linezolid
Extensive local inflammation plus systemic toxicity *or* ulcer/gangrene with penetration of fascia and absent pedal pulses	As above plus anaerobic bacteria	Parenteral therapy: Daptomycin plus piperacillin/tazobactam or imipenem cilastatin or meropenem *or* linezolid or vancomycin plus ciprofloxacin or levofloxacin or aztreonam If *Clostridia* sp. or gas gangrene is suspected, add penicillin G and/or clindamycin

Adapted from Gilbert DN, Moellering RC, Eliopoulos GM and others: The Sanford guide to antimicrobial therapy, Hyde Park, VA, 2006, Antimicrobial Therapy, Inc.

Neuropathic Ulceration

Diabetic foot ulceration may be caused by neuropathy, ischemia, or both etiologies. When arterial circulation is confirmed to be normal by pedal pulse palpation and pressure measurement, management of the neuropathic ulcer includes debridement of nonviable tissue and callus, antibiotics if inflammation is present, and off-loading of skin pressure. Treatment is site specific, with off-loading techniques tailored to prevent focal high-pressure zones, and includes walking with the assistance of specially formed orthotic insoles, an Aircast walker (Aircast, Vista, CA), Bledsoe boot, or total contact casting. With a diagnosis of neuropathic ulcers on the plantar foot surface, the metatarsal head is typically the culprit, and healing at this site may require metatarsophalangeal joint resection via a ventral incision to remove protruding bone and achieve skin healing. Treatment may require 3 months of off-loading therapy to achieve healing and longer in the noncompliant patient. When healing is not progressing as determined by serial assessment of ulcer size and depth, patients should be reevaluated for surgical intervention to achieve a more functional weight-bearing plantar surface.

Amputation

Dorsal skin ulceration on a hammertoe or osteomyelitis involving a digit may require digit amputation if healing does not occur promptly. Digit-metatarsal amputation for neuropathic ulcer is performed to redistribute plantar surface pressure to a larger area and is used in conjunction with prescription orthotic shoes to prevent recurrence. More proximal foot amputations (transmetatarsal, transtarsal) may be required to treat advanced plantar space infection or following revascularization in patients presenting with ischemia forefoot gangrene. Ankle systole pressure greater than 100 mm Hg or toe pressure greater 50 mm Hg has a positive predictive value of 80% for healing of midfoot amputations, but decreased healing rates occur in the diabetic patients with end-stage renal disease. Aggressive measures for foot salvage are justified in diabetic patients because ambulation rate of 90% and limb salvage rate of 60% to 70% at 5 years is possible after a transmetatarsal or midfoot (Lisfranc, Chopart) amputation. It is essential to perform an adjunctive Achilles tendolysis to prevent development of an equine deformity, and patients ambulate using an orthotic, padded shoe and ankle brace or clamshell prosthesis.

In diabetic patients with total bony collapse of the ankle and arch, or advanced Charcot foot deformity involving the tarsal bones with nonhealing ulceration, a below-knee amputation should be recommended. In selected diabetic patients, arch reconstruction may be possible. When providing counsel to the diabetic patient before amputation, it should be emphasized that patients who are ambulatory at the time of amputation are likely to retain ambulatory status following major limb amputation because of advances in prosthetic limb technology.

Ischemic Ulceration or Gangrene

Tissue ischemia manifested as dependent rubor with rest pain, ulceration, or gangrene requires prompt evaluation for correctable arterial occlusive disease to improve perfusion and achieve limb salvage. Invasive infection should be controlled before open arterial bypass. In general, all patients with foot lesions and vascular testing demonstrating an ankle pressure less than 100 mm Hg or toe pressure less than 55 mm Hg should undergo arterial imaging studies to identify occlusive lesion amenable to endovascular or surgical intervention. Nearly all patients are candidates for arterial intervention using advanced endovascular techniques, including recanalization of chronic arterial occlusion or bypass grafting to tibial or pedal arteries. Often these services are available only at tertiary referral vascular centers. When bypass grafting is required, an autogenous venous conduit should be used. Foot salvage can be expected in more than 90% of diabetic patients requiring concomitant arterial intervention and minor foot amputation, with failure related to graft- or angioplasty-site thrombosis, recurrent foot infection, or persistent forefoot ischemia. In the absence of end-stage renal disease, outcomes after arterial intervention are similar in diabetic and nondiabetic patients.

PREVENTION AND PATIENT EDUCATION

The importance of patient education in techniques of meticulous foot care and appropriate footwear cannot be overstated. A multidisciplinary approach that includes annual (3-month intervals in high-risk patients) assessments by primary care physicians, a podiatrist, or vascular specialist to evaluate arterial perfusion is imperative. The diabetic patient with peripheral neuropathy should be instructed to perform routine self-examination of the skin and foot and be educated in skin hygiene and footwear use. Self-examination and education are the cornerstones of a prevention and surveillance program. Education of diabetic patients and their families or caregivers should include the following: instructions for foot hygiene, proper footwear use, and the importance of prompt evaluation of any new skin lesion or foot pain. Diabetic patients with peripheral neuropathy, foot deformity, absent pedal pulses or toe pressure less than 40 mm Hg, and prior ulceration are at high risk for development of a diabetic foot condition and would benefit from a multidisciplinary diabetic foot-care program. Prospective studies have demonstrated the risk for diabetic ulcer formation to be 5 in 100 person-years.

Suggested Readings

Akbari CM, LoGerfo FW: Diabetes and peripheral vascular disease, *J Vasc Surg* 30:373, 1999.

American Diabetes Association: Consensus development conference on diabetic foot wound care, *Diabetes Care* 22:1354, 1999.

Boulton AJM, Kirsner RS, Vileikyte L: Neuropathic diabetic foot ulcers, *N Engl J Med* 351:48, 2004.

Boyko EJ, Ahron JH, Cohen V, and others: Prediction of diabetic foot ulcer occurrence using commonly available clinical information, *Diabetes Care* 29:1202, 2006.

Frykberg RG: Diabetic foot ulcers: pathogenesis and management, *Am Fam Physician* 66:1655, 2002.

Sumpio BE: Foot ulcers, *N Engl J Med* 343:787, 2000.

DIAGNOSIS OF VENOUS DISEASE

George Manis, MD, Nicos Labropoulos, PhD, and Peter J. Pappas, MD

Chronic venous disease (CVD) is the most common vascular disorder. Approximately 10% to 35% of all adults show some form of the disease, ranging from venous telangiectasias and small varicosities to venous ulcerations. Age, gender, height, obesity, race, pregnancy, occupation, posture, and heredity are some of many proposed predisposing factors. Moreover, the number of operations performed for this disorder rank CVD as one of the costliest disease processes in the Western world. It is estimated that in the United States alone yearly treatment costs exceed $3 billion, which comprises up to 3% of the total health care budget. The average hospital stay may average 5 to 7 days and may total $15,000.

There are profound ramifications to society, with an estimated 2 million working days lost per year. The disease produces a wide range of physical sequelae, including prominent varicosities, edema, skin pigment changes, and chronic ulcerations. These sequelae affect between 3% and 11% of the population, and the prevalence of ulcer disease is approximately 1% in the Western world. A British population study showed that the median duration of an ulcer was 9 months. In 20% of these, the ulcer was not healed in 2 years and 66% of patients had ulcerations lasting 5 years or longer. The negative impact on quality of life, body image, and physical functioning is substantial.

Veins are thin-walled conduits that return blood flow to the heart. They operate as a low-pressure system and thus rely on muscular contractions to propel blood antegrade against gravity to the heart. A series of intraluminal valves prevents retrograde flow with gravity to the distal lower extremity. The venous system in the lower extremity is composed of the superficial, deep, and perforating veins.

The importance of the interrelationship among these three groups of veins cannot be underestimated in the understanding of CVD. The methods of diagnosis, classification, and treatment of chronic venous disease that are discussed in this chapter stem from the similarities, differences, and interrelationships among these veins.

ETIOLOGY

The most common etiology of venous hypertension in the lower extremity is venous reflux. Other important causes include venous obstruction and calf-muscle pump dysfunction. Reflux alone is found in 80% of limbs, whereas venous obstruction results in 2% of all cases. A combination of reflux and obstruction involves the remaining 17% of cases of CVD. These latter cases are associated with a higher classification, as evidenced by concomitant skin damage and ulceration of the affected limb, and have a worse prognosis. There is a higher prevalence of deep vein thrombosis (DVT) in these limbs that is consistent with deep vein involvement.

Reflux

Reflux is retrograde flow through the veins of the lower extremity that occurs when the valves are malfunctioning. Vein wall dilation, inflammation, and thrombosis are the causes associated with valve damage. Primary reflux is associated with the first two causes, and secondary reflux is due to thrombosis.

The morphologic changes to the valve include tearing, thinning, and adhesion. These lead to inflammation of the valve leaflet with a concomitant influx of mononuclear cells and other inflammatory infiltrates. There is an overproduction of type I collagen and a degradation of extracellular matrix, leading to a decrease in the elasticity of the vein wall. A significant increase in the collagen-to-elastin ratio of the venous wall occurs. The elastic network decreases and becomes dystrophic. This results in a disorganization of the wall by fibrosis and a breakdown of the structure of the muscular layers. The result is an incompetent valve and a stiffer venous wall, leading to a rise in ambulatory venous pressure as blood pools in the dependent lower extremity. Furthermore, the absence of competent venous valves attenuates the efficiency of the calf-muscle pump.

Reflux progresses in most patients with CVD; however, its natural history is not well established because most reports are cross-sectional. In a recent longitudinal and prospective study of 113 limbs with CVD, 12% of patients experienced reflux extension and 15% developed reflux in previously normal venous segments. The progression of reflux was found to occur in an antegrade and a retrograde direction, as well as in both directions. The majority of changes occurred in the great saphenous and perforating veins.

Venous Obstruction

The sequelae of deep venous thrombosis account for 18% to 28% of limbs with CVD. The resultant edema and skin changes are called *postthrombotic syndrome*. Thrombus formation at venous confluences and valve pockets leads to activation of neutrophils and platelets. The subsequent production of inflammatory cytokines leads to infiltration of the vein wall by leukocytes, with subsequent inflammation leading to vein wall fibrosis and valvular destruction. After an episode of thrombosis, the vein may be fully or partially recanalized or remain occluded. Functional obstruction may result from inadequate recanalization and collateralization. Postthrombotic syndrome, characterized by edema, skin changes, and ulceration, has an incidence of 20% to 30% over 8 years. Ipsilateral, recurrent DVT increases the risk for postthrombotic signs and symptoms by a factor of six. A combination of venous reflux and obstruction also increases the chance by a factor of three. It has been shown that after a first episode of DVT, reflux developed in the affected limbs in 17% at 1 week, 37% at 1 month, and 69% at 1 year. The rate of recurrent DVT was 25% at 5 years and 30% at 8 years, and the incidence of postthrombotic syndrome was 30% at the same time.

Superficial vein thrombosis that affects the saphenous veins has been shown not to be a benign process. A French study that followed 427 patients with superficial vein thrombosis found that over a period of 3 months, 18% of the patients developed venous thrombotic complications, including DVT, pulmonary embolism, or recurrence or extension of the thrombus to the deep system. Most of these patients were male and had severe chronic venous disease. The incidence of pulmonary embolism (PE) was 4%, with severe chronic venous disease being the only predictive factor in regression analysis.

Muscle Pump Dysfunction

The venous valves of the lower extremity constitute a series-parallel arrangement of reciprocating pumps. The blood is in the reservoir of the capillaries of the muscles themselves. The tight, investing fascia creates a counteracting squeezing force when the muscle contracts, forcing blood upward.

Patients with severe CVD are often debilitated. As the patient becomes less ambulatory, the calf-muscle pump loses its effectiveness, and a vicious cycle of edema and ulceration can occur. The importance of maintaining the calf-muscle pump system can be shown in a study of 31 patients with severe CVD (skin changes or ulceration) randomized to calf-muscle–strengthening exercises or no exercise. At the end of 6 months, the exercise group showed an improvement in muscle pump function and calf-muscle strength, with a concomitant decrease in symptoms. Other conditions that limit the muscle pump function such as arthritis, spinal cord injury, and trauma worsen the severity of CVD.

CLINICAL EVALUATION

CVD is a multifactorial disease with patient-specific historical and anatomic clues to its etiology. The clinical presentation may differ over time and after therapy. The clinician must be skilled at obtaining the subtle, yet readily identifiable clues that point to a disease process that is in constant evolution. A combination of history, physical examination, and specific tests available in the vascular laboratory allow for the accurate classification of the disease and stratification of available treatment and provide valuable follow-up information of disease progression.

History and Physical Examination

A documented episode of thrombosis and conditions during which a thrombosis could occur, such as surgery, major illnesses requiring prolonged bed rest, and trauma to the extremity should be noted. The presence of an inferior vena cava (IVC) filter and anticoagulant use should alert the examiner to look for a previous thrombosis. A family history of hypercoagulable syndromes and CVD should be obtained. Increasing age, Caucasian race, prolonged standing, and pregnancy are recognized risk factors.

The majority of patients with CVD relate an aching tiredness and discomfort in the legs that is relieved by sitting and leg elevation. These symptoms are exacerbated by long periods of standing and are often worse at the end of the day. Women will display symptoms during their menstrual cycles, and many relate the onset of their symptoms during pregnancy.

The pain is usually identified at the site of the varicosities. Iliofemoral obstruction may produce pain on exercise that is not relieved by rest. This "venous claudication" is due to the sudden development of venous hypertension from the hyperemia in the setting of high outflow resistance. In a study of 39 patients with iliofemoral DVT, 44% developed venous claudication that impaired their quality of life.

An intense itch or burning sensation may be present before any skin changes are evident. In a study of 100 patients evaluated with a prospective questionnaire, the prevalence of itch was found to be 66%. Concomitant itch and burning or itch and pain were noted in almost half of the patients. The intensity of the itch was noted to have a negative impact on quality of life.

The findings on the physical examination of a patient with CVD vary from nothing to ulceration. The ubiquitous venous varicosity appears in only 20% of patents. The extremities are evaluated in the standing position because the signs and symptoms are more apparent. A complete arterial pulse examination, as well as an ankle-brachial index, should be performed to elucidate the presence of arterial disease.

An accurate height and body mass index (BMI) should also be obtained. Morbidly obese patients may have a higher incidence of CVD symptoms. In a retrospective review of 20 patients with morbid obesity and CVD, a correlation was found between rising BMI and clinical, etiologic, anatomic, and pathophysiologic (CEAP) clinical class. The pathologic mechanism is believed to be secondary to increased intra-abdominal pressure being transmitted through incompetent femoral veins to the extremity.

Table 1: Typical Signs of Chronic Venous Disease

Edema	Malleolar regions Worse at the end of the day Spares the foot Asymmetric
Ulceration	Full thickness defect of the skin Medial malleolus Associated with skin changes of chronic venous disease
Skin changes	
Atrophie blanch (white atrophy)	Localized atrophic areas white in color Surrounded by dilatated capillaries and hyperpigmentation
Corona phlebectatica (malleolar flare)	Fan-shaped pattern of small veins on the medial or lateral aspects of the ankle or foot
Eczema	Erythematous dermatitis that may present as blistering, weeping, or scaling of the dermis, usually located near varicose veins
Lipodermatosclerosis	Localized scarring and contracture of the skin secondary to fibrosis from chronic inflammation
Pigmentation	Brownish skin discoloration secondary to extravasated blood and deposition of hemosiderin, typically in the ankle region
Veins	
Varicose veins	Large, dilatated, tortuous veins in the subcutaneous tissues, ≥ 3 mm
Reticular veins	Tortuous veins <3 mm
Telangiectasias	Small, ectatic vein clusters that represent a confluence of dilatated intradermal venules <1 mm in caliber

The typical signs of CVD include edema, ulceration, skin changes, and visible veins. A recent publication on the classification of CVD defined these signs in a consensus statement (Table 1).

Laboratory Evaluation

In conjunction with a careful physical examination, the vascular laboratory offers many methods of diagnosing CVD. These methods are used for assessing both reflux and obstruction and are most useful in stratifying patients for treatment and evaluating the progression of disease following therapy. Both invasive and noninvasive techniques are available. Invasive tests for venous reflux are rarely used today but include phlebography and pressure measurements. Noninvasive tests are the procedures of choice, offering diagnostic sensitivity and maximal patient safety and comfort. Noninvasive testing can be separated into physiologic tests and ultrasound testing.

Physiologic Testing

Physiologic testing provides quantitative measurements of venous dynamics. They include ambulatory venous pressure measurements, strain-gauge plethysmography, light-reflection rheography, photo plethysmography, air plethysmography, and foot volumetry. They do not provide an anatomic evaluation; therefore the extent and distribution of the disease are not known. For this reason, treatment cannot be provided on the basis of the information from these tests alone.

The measurements obtained can help to evaluate the severity of reflux through the refilling time from the supine to standing position or after exercise: The shorter the refilling time, the worse the severity of reflux. Obstruction can be estimated from the venous outflow curves or from the pressure measurements at rest during hyperemia. The calf-muscle pump function is evaluated by measuring the ejecting ability of the calf and the volume of blood remaining at the end of the exercise. These tests are useful to evaluate the overall effect of treatment in the limbs.

Duplex Ultrasound

Duplex ultrasound (DU) is inexpensive, quick, and noninvasive. Several studies have shown DU to be superior to venography. Valuable information regarding etiology can also be obtained using the B-mode imaging coupled with Doppler velocity measurements. The superficial, deep, and perforating systems may all be evaluated at one sitting. All this information may be obtained with minimal discomfort to the patient. Thus DU is now regarded the test of choice to diagnose venous reflux and its response to treatment.

Both reflux and obstruction can be determined. Reflux is identified by compressing the veins distal to the area of imaging followed by sudden release of the compression. A short duration of retrograde flow after the release is normal because the valves close rapidly. The best cutoff value of reflux in the femoropopliteal veins was greater than 1000 milliseconds. In the superficial, deep femoral, and deep calf axial and muscular veins, it was greater than 500 milliseconds. In the perforating veins, it was greater than 350 milliseconds.

The velocity of reflux and its duration have been used to characterize severity of the disease. The severity of the CVD increases with a rise in velocity, duration, and anatomic vein segments involved. However, in the literature this has been applied in a simplistic fashion, and thus it is difficult to make any meaningful conclusions because there are many other factors that contribute to the severity of the disease.

Obstruction is identified by the noncompressibility of the vein and the filling defects when the color mode is used. The characteristics of a chronic thrombus include a bright echogenicity within the lumen of the vessel. Partial recanalization of the lumen with filling defects and reflux may be present. In fully recanalized veins, wall thickening with luminal reduction may be seen. The affected vein will be smaller, and dilatated collateral vessels can be seen.

Invasive Tests

Noninvasive testing has supplanted invasive venous tests. However, these are still deemed necessary to identify specific anatomic sites of disease as a preoperative workup and help to guide treatment. They are especially useful in demonstrating venous obstruction.

Phlebography

These methods involve the direct injection of contrast dye into the veins of the affected limb with examination under fluoroscopy. In ascending phlebography, the contrast is injected in the foot and followed proximally. It is routinely used in the iliofemoral veins and IVC for thrombolysis, angioplasty, and stenting. During this procedure, pressure measurements can be obtained across a stenosis to evaluate its significance and the outcome of interventions. The site of injection in descending phlebography is the common femoral vein. The contrast is followed distally, and the competency, location, and morphology of the valves are assessed.

Intravascular Ultrasound

This is the best method currently available to evaluate venous stenosis. It allows a 360-degree view of the vein lumen from the shortest possible distance. The high-resolution ultrasound can detect pathology in the lumen, venous wall, and the immediate perivenous area. Unlike phlebography, intravascular ultrasound (IVUS) can clearly visualize intraluminal webs, wall thickening, and extrinsic compression. IVUS is the best method to size the balloon and stent and allow the optimal stent apposition to the wall.

Clinical, Etiologic, Anatomic, and Pathophysiologic Classification System

Great variation in the reporting standards existed in the world literature on the reporting of venous disease. At the Fifth Annual Meeting of the American Venous Forum, a suggestion was made that a classification system analogous to the TNM (T, primary tumor; N, regional lymph nodes; M, distant metastasis) classification for cancer be adopted for venous disease. In 1994, the CEAP classification system was proposed and adopted by the forum in the form of a consensus document.

The consensus detailed two segments consisting of a classification of CVD and a severity scoring system. The classification system, or CEAP, consists of six symptoms and 17 anatomic sites, involving three etiologic and pathophysiologic categories. It includes a numbered scale for C (clinical), E (etiology), A (anatomic distribution), and P (pathophysiologic) findings. The C classification can be readily discerned in many nonspecialty clinics on physical examination. The addition of the E, A, and P classifications defines the presence of venous disease as the cause for the observed clinical findings out of a fairly large differential diagnosis.

The clinical section of CEAP grades the severity of CVD in seven classes, numbered 0 to 6. The severity of the clinical signs equates with a higher number. Class 0 = no signs of disease, class 1 = telangiectasias, class 2 = varicose veins, class 3 = edema without skin changes, class 4 = hyperpigmentation/lipodermatosclerosis, class 5 = healed ulceration, and class 6 = active ulceration. There is no association between CEAP class and the presence of symptoms, but the severity of symptoms is related to the stage of the disease. There is a significant association between ascending severity and risk factors.

The anatomic distribution of the clinical classes was studied in 1000 consecutive limbs evaluated at a single center (Fig. 1). Approximately 90% of limbs had an involvement of the superficial veins and approximately 30% the deep veins. Reflux was most frequently present in the veins and tributaries of the saphenous system. Deep vein reflux alone was uncommon even in patients with ulceration. Patients with reflux in the lower classifications have their reflux limited to the superficial system, whereas those in the higher classes involve both the deep and superficial systems. The number and size of incompetent perforator veins increased with class severity.

Venous Clinical Severity Score

In this system, known as the VCSS, the clinical features of CVD are graded from 0 to 3 as absent, mild, moderate, and severe. A maximum of 30 points describes the most severely affected limb.

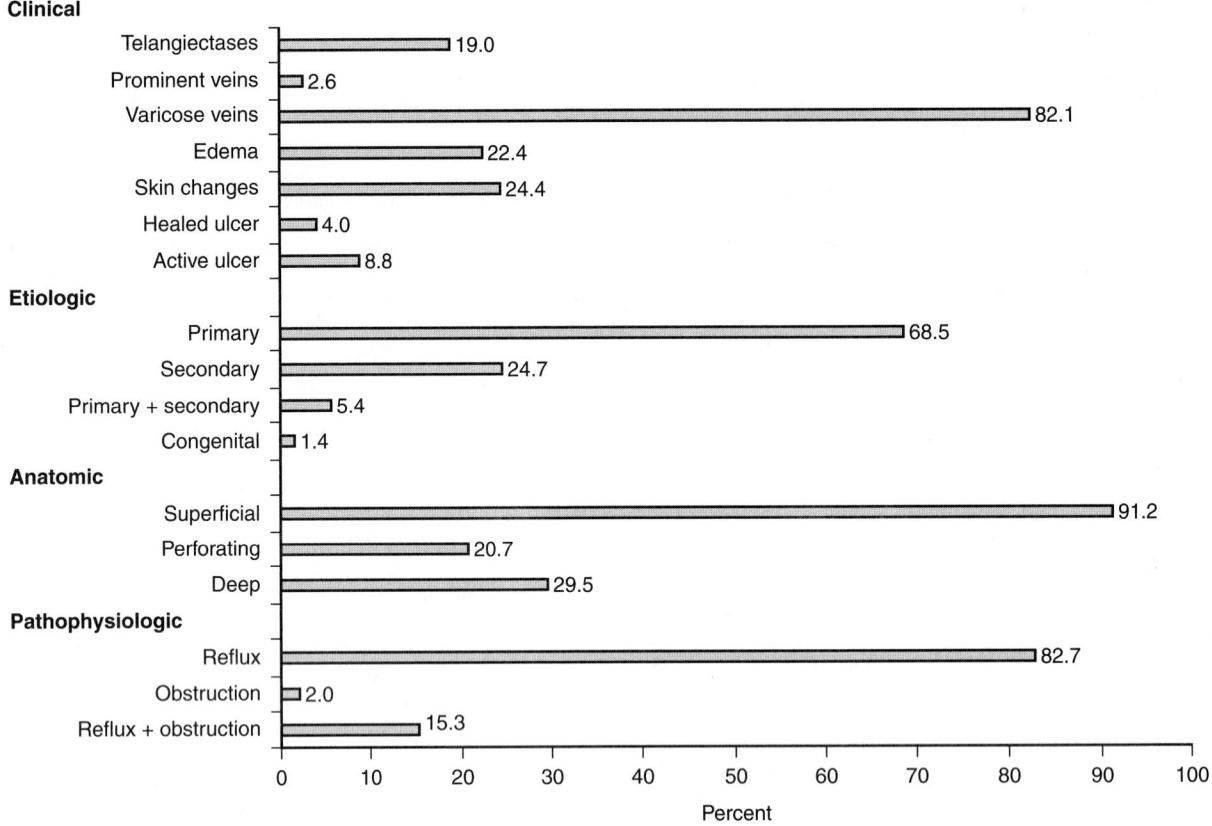

Figure 1 Anatomic distribution of clinical cases in 1000 consecutive limbs.

The VCSS was validated in observational studies to demonstrate good correlation with anatomic extent. A venous disability score (VDS) was also added that takes into account symptoms during an 8-hour workday and the ability to perform the activities of daily living.

THERAPY AND FOLLOW-UP

A good initial clinical examination combined with noninvasive study information leaves the practitioner with good knowledge for the initiation of therapy. This information, coupled with the CEAP/VCSS evaluation, allows the clinician to treat symptomatic individuals in a way that provides the most benefit and the least harm.

Localized venous disease as manifested by isolated varicose veins or telangiectasias may be treated with local noninvasive therapy, such as compression stockings. However, if the VCSS is high, indicating discomfort for the patient, sclerotherapy may be offered. A duplex study that reveals reflux in the superficial system may be treated with complete or partial vein stripping. Newer endovascular techniques of saphenous vein ablation that use radiofrequency or laser energy to "close" the saphenous vein have been developed and have replaced open surgery in many centers. These procedures are being performed with ultrasound guidance.

After the procedure is complete, the patient may be assessed in appropriate follow-up intervals with clinical examination and DU. Residual or recurrent disease can be identified and treated. The recurrence rate after surgery has been demonstrated to be 20% to 80% depending on the definitions and the time of the follow-up.

Combined angioplasty and stenting is a proven method to treat iliocaval obstruction. The patency is 75% over 3 years. However, not all patients have anatomy that is amenable to endovascular technique and reocclusions can be difficult to manage endovascularly. Open surgery is usually reserved for these patients. These large operations involve a laparotomy and construction of complex native conduits, such as spiral vein grafts and arteriovenous fistulae, to ensure good, long-term patency. Although these procedures are labor intensive, patency rates of 67% over a 3- to 5-year period can be achieved.

CONCLUSION

The care of the patient with lower-extremity venous disease is a satisfying practice. Competency in the diagnosis and treatment of the disease is multifaceted. The practitioner must be skilled in both traditional history taking and physical examination. These observations are supported and assisted by the technology of the vascular laboratory. Finally, the VCSS/CEAP integrates the information obtained into a manageable algorithmic approach that allows tailoring of therapy to each individual patient. Patients may be followed throughout life and can take comfort in knowing that a diagnosis and treatment option will be available to relieve them of this morbid disease.

SUGGESTED READINGS

Almeida JI, Raines JK: Radiofrequency ablation and laser ablation in the treatment of varicose veins, *Ann Vasc Surg* 20:547, 2006.

Arfvidsson B, Eklof B, Balfour J: Iliofemoral venous pressure correlates with intraabdominal pressure in morbidly obese patients, *Vasc Endovasc Surg* 39:505, 2005.

Bergan JJ, Schmid-Schonbein GW, Smith PD, and others: Chronic venous disease, *N Engl J Med* 355:488, 2006.

Callam MJ, Harper DR, Dale JJ, and others: Chronic ulcer of the leg: clinical history, *Br Med J (Clin Res Ed)* 294:1389, 1987.

Delis KT, Bountouroglou D, Mansfield AO: Venous claudication in iliofemoral thrombosis; long-term effects on venous hemodynamics, clinical status, and quality of life, *Ann Surg* 239:118–126, 2004.

Duque MI, Yosipovitch G, Chan YH, and others: Itch, pain, and burning sensation are common symptoms in mild to moderate chronic venous insufficiency with an impact on quality of life, *J Am Acad Dermatol* 53:504, 2005.

Eklof B, Rutherford RB, Bergan JJ, and others: American Venous Forum International Ad Hoc Committee for Revision of the CEAP Classification. Revision of the CEAP classification for chronic venous disorders: consensus statement, *J Vasc Surg* 40:1248, 2004.

Guex JJ: Foam sclerotherapy; an overview of use for primary venous insufficiency, *Semin Vasc Surg* 18:25, 2005.

Johnson BF, Manzo RA, Bergelin RO, and others: Relationship between changes in the deep venous system and the development of the postthrombotic syndrome after an acute episode of lower limb deep vein thrombosis: a one- to six-year follow-up, *J Vasc Surg* 21:307, 1995.

Jost CJ, Gloviczki P, Cherry KJ Jr, and others: Surgical reconstruction of iliofemoral veins and the inferior vena cava for nonmalignant occlusive disease, *J Vasc Surg* 33:320, 2001.

Kistner RL, Ferris EB, Randhawa G, and others: A method of performing descending venography, *J Vasc Surg* 4:464, 1986.

Labropoulos N: CEAP in clinical practice, *Vasc Surg* 31:224, 1997.

Labropoulos N: Hemodynamic changes according to the CEAP classification, *Phlebolymphology* 40:130, 2003.

Labropoulos N, Delis K, Nicolaides AN, and others: The role of the distribution and anatomic extent of reflux in the development of signs and symptoms in chronic venous insufficiency, *J Vasc Surg* 23:504, 1996.

Labropoulos N, Leon L, Kwon S, and others: Study of the venous reflux progression, *J Vasc Surg* 41:291, 2005.

Labropoulos N, Patel PJ, Tiongson JE, and others: Patterns of venous reflux and obstruction in patients with skin damage due to chronic venous disease, *Vasc Endovasc Surg* 41:33, 2007.

Labropoulos N, Tiongson J, Pryor, and others: Definition of venous reflux in lower extremity veins, *J Vasc Surg* 38:793, 2003.

Leon L, Giannoukas AD, Dodd D, and others: Clinical significance of superficial vein thrombosis, *Eur J Vasc Endovasc Surg* 29:10–17, 2005.

Lurie F, Creton D, Eklof B, and others: Prospective randomized study of endovenous radiofrequency obliteration (closure) versus ligation and vein stripping (EVOLVeS): two-year follow-up, *Eur J Vasc Endovasc Surg* 29:67, 2005.

Markel A, Manzo RA, Bergelin RO, and others: Valvular reflux after deep vein thrombosis: incidence and time of occurrence, *J Vasc Surg* 15:377, 1992.

Meissner MH, Natiello C, Nicholls SC: Performance characteristics of the venous clinical severity score, *J Vasc Surg* 36:889, 2002.

Neglen P, Raju S: In-stent recurrent stenosis in stents placed in the lower extremity venous outflow tract, *J Vasc Surg* 39:181, 2004.

Neglen P, Raju S: Intravascular ultrasound scan evaluation of the obstructed vein, *J Vasc Surg* 35:694, 2002.

Neglen P, Raju S: Proximal lower extremity chronic venous outflow obstruction: recognition and treatment, *Semin Vasc Surg* 15:57, 2002.

Nicolaides AN: Investigation of chronic venous insufficiency: a consensus statement (France, March 5–9, 1997), *Circulation* 102:E126, 2000.

Padberg F Jr, Cerveira JJ, Lal BK, and others: Does severe venous insufficiency have a different etiology in the morbidly obese? Is it venous? *J Vasc Surg* 37:79, 2003.

Padberg FT Jr, Johnson MV, Sisto SA: Structured exercise improves calf muscle pump function in chronic venous insufficiency; a randomized trial, *J Vasc Surg* 39:79, 2004.

Perrin MR, Labropoulos N, Leon LRJr: Presentation of the patient with recurrent varices after surgery (REVAS), *J Vasc Surg* 43:327–334, 2006.

Prandoni P, Lensing A, Cogo A, and others: The long-term clinical course of acute deep venous thrombosis, *Ann Intern Med* 125:1, 1996.

Quenet S, Laporte S, Decousus H, and others: STENOX Group. Factors predictive of venous thrombotic complications in patients with isolated superficial vein thrombosis, *J Vasc Surg* 38:944, 2003.

Raju S, Hollis K, Neglen P: Obstructive lesions of the inferior vena cava: clinical features and endovenous treatment, *J Vasc Surg* 44:820–827, 2006.

Rutherford RB, Padberg FT Jr, Comerota AJ, and others: Venous severity scoring: an adjunct to venous outcome assessment, *J Vasc Surg* 31:1307, 2000.

Sansilvestri-Morel P, Rupin A, Jaisson S, and others: Synthesis of collagen is dysregulated in cultured fibroblasts derived from skin of subjects with varicose veins as it is in venous smooth muscle cells, *Circulation* 106:479, 2002.

Tassiopoulos AK, Golts E, Oh DS, and others: Current concepts in chronic venous ulceration, *Eur J Vasc Endovasc Surg* 20:227, 2000.

Woodside KJ, Hu M, Burke A, and others: Morphologic characteristics of varicose veins: possible role of metalloproteinases, *J Vasc Surg* 38:162, 2003.

Deep Venous Thrombosis

John Byrne, MCh, Sean P. Roddy, MD, and R. Clement Darling, III, MD

INTRODUCTION

Most physicians are familiar with the management of acute deep venous thrombosis (DVT); they know that clinical assessment is unreliable and that venous duplex is the gold standard for diagnosis. With the advent low-molecular-weight heparins, treatment for many patients can be accomplished in an outpatient setting with transition to oral warfarin.

Surgeons are consulted when simple algorithms no longer suffice: is there a role for thrombolysis? Or thrombectomy? Is a vena caval filter insertion beneficial? What is the management of phlegmasia cerulea or alba dolens? Or superficial vein thrombosis or thrombus in the internal jugular or subclavian veins? In this chapter, we review these conditions and try to supply the answers.

"SIMPLE" DEEP VENOUS THROMBOSES

Natural History

DVTs may be asymptomatic. They may also result in fatal pulmonary emboli regardless of presentation. A cause of major morbidity is postthrombotic syndrome (PTS) (see Fig. 1). PTS covers a

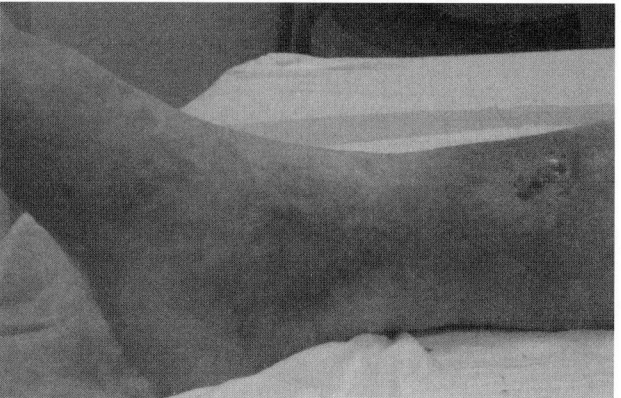

Figure I Consequences of previous deep venous thrombosis: the postphlebitis limb.

spectrum from leg heaviness and swelling to frank ulceration, caused by DVTs that fail to dissolve, convert to a chronic scar, and thereby cause venous outflow obstruction. Alternatively, they may resolve but render valves incompetent. Reflux within the deep veins leads to venous hypertension and its associated inflammatory changes. Untreated DVTs of the iliac and femoral veins result in fatal pulmonary emboli in 11% to 23% cases. Even in treated patients, 20% to 30% will progress to skin pigmentation changes, and 3% to 5% to ulceration. "Clot burden" is clearly important because extensive iliofemoral thromboses are more pernicious than isolated calf vein clots. Heparinoids and warfarin do not cause clot lysis. They act to prevent further clot propagation. Clot dissolution occurs through endogenous fibrinolysis.

Prevention

It is useful to consider patients in terms of low, moderate, and high risk for DVT (see Table 1). Low-risk patients require early ambulation after surgery. High-risk patients require thromboprophylaxis, usually low-molecular-weight heparin such as fondaparinux, enoxaparin, or tinzaparin, as well as TED (thromboembolism-deterrent) stockings and sequential compression devices that provide rhythmic external compression at 35–40 mm Hg for 10 seconds every minute. Many surgeons worry that DVT prophylaxis with anticoagulants will cause bleeding; however, bleeding complications resulting from prophylaxis occur less than 3% of the time.

Diagnosis and Treatment

Diagnosis is rapid and straightforward with duplex interrogation of the suspected limb. D-dimer elevation is an indicator of endogenous fibrinolysis. If it is negative, it is unlikely that the patient has a venous thrombosis. However, it will be elevated in any situation in which fibrinolysis is taking place, such as following surgery. Thus false positives are common. Its main use is as a screening tool when a panel of blood investigations is ordered. It cannot be used reliably to diagnose a DVT. Venograms are now rarely used and have a small, but real, chance of causing a clot.

Distal (Isolated Calf Vein) Thrombosis

Clots confined to the *gastrocnemius* and *soleus* veins are usually benign. Untreated, 3% will propagate to the popliteal and femoral veins, usually in oncology patients who are often inherently hypercoagulable. They rarely cause pulmonary emboli. By 3 months, many will have disappeared. Thromboses isolated to the peroneal or posterior tibial veins are almost as benign, with propagation in 8% of untreated patients (the anterior tibial vein is almost never affected by isolated thrombosis). All clots will have dissolved by 3 months. Again, pulmonary embolism is rare. Up to 11% will develop overt PTS with leg swelling and, rarely, ulceration, but approximately one third will develop deep venous reflux by 3 years. Therefore most specialists would advise anticoagulation therapy for isolated calf thromboses for at least 6 weeks, especially because outpatient treatment is now relatively straightforward. The alternative, for patients in whom anticoagulation is not feasible, is to repeat their duplex scans within 14 days to ensure that a clot has not propagated proximally.

Proximal (Iliac and Femoropopliteal) Thromboses

Compared with patients who have isolated calf DVTs, patients with proximal thromboses fare much worse. Clot dissolution is slower. Deep venous reflux is seen in almost all these patients at 5 years. Approximately 42% will develop symptoms of PTS as described earlier. Overall, 4% of patients will develop frank ulceration on long-term follow-up. For patients with proximal thromboses and a precipitating factor such as recent surgery or leg immobilization, the duration of therapy should be 3 to 6 months. In patients with

Table 1: Risk Stratification and Prophylaxis for Patients Undergoing Surgery

Risk Stratification

Low risk	Uncomplicated surgery in patients aged ≤40 years with minimal immobility postoperatively and no risk factors
Moderate risk	Any surgery in patients aged 40–60 years, major surgery in patients <40 years and no other risk factors, minor surgery in patients with one or more risk factors
High risk	Major surgery in patients aged >60 years, major surgery in patients aged 40–60 years with one or more risk factors
Very high risk	Major surgery in patients aged >40 years with previous venous thromboembolism, cancer or known hypercoagulable state, major orthopaedic surgery, elective neurosurgery, multiple trauma, or acute spinal cord injury

Prophylaxis

Low risk	**Early mobilization**
Moderate risk	5000 IU every 12 hours starting 2 hours before surgery or low-molecular-weight heparin <3400 anti-Xa IU daily,* or compression elastic stockings, or intermittent pneumatic compression
High risk	Low-molecular-weight heparin >3400 anti-Xa IU daily[†] plus compression elastic stockings, or unfractionated heparin 5000 IU every 8 hours starting 2 hours before surgery plus compression elastic stockings, or intermittent pneumatic compression if anticoagulation is contraindicated
Very high risk	Perioperative warfarin (INR 2–3), low-molecular-weight heparin >3400 anti-Xa IU daily[†] plus compression elastic stockings, or prolonged low-molecular-weight heparin therapy plus compression elastic stockings

From Turpie AG, Chin BS, Lip GY: BMJ 325(7369):887, 2002.
INR, International normalize ratio; Xa, activated factor X.
*Dalteparin 2500 IU once daily starting 2 hours before surgery.
[†]Dalteparin 5000 IU once daily starting 10–12 hours before surgery.
Enoxaparin 20 mg once daily starting 2 hours before surgery.
Nadroparin 3100 IU once daily starting 2 hours before surgery.
Tinzaparin 3500 IU once daily starting 2 hours before surgery.
Danaparoid 750 IU twice daily starting 1 to 2 hours before surgery.
Enoxaparin 40 mg once daily starting 10–12 hours before surgery.
Tinzaparin 50 IU/kg once daily starting 2 hours before surgery.

Table 2: Duration of Therapy for DVT

Recommended Duration of Therapy	Type of DVT and Risk Factors
DVT *with* Identifiable Risk Factor (Hospitalization, General Anesthesia, 3 Days of Bed Rest, Leg Fracture with or without Plaster Immobilization, All within 3 Months)	
6 weeks	Isolated distal DVT (posterior tibial/peroneal/calf veins)
3 months	Proximal DVT
6 months	Proximal DVT and identified thrombophilia; concomitant cancer with a normal functional status; inferior vena cava filter; patient preference
DVT *without* Risk Factor ("Spontaneous")	
3 months	High risk for bleeding; isolated distal DVT; patient preference
6 months	Minor reversible risk factor (estrogen therapy, prolonged travel [4 hours or more], treated hyperhomocysteinemia); moderate risk of bleeding; patient preference
Long-term therapy*	More than one episode of idiopathic DVT; active cancer, identifiable thrombophilia, severe immobilization; PE; pulmonary hypertension; severe postthrombotic syndrome; inferior vena cava filter; low risk of bleeding; patient preference

From Kearon C: Circulation 107:(Suppl 1):122, 2003.
DVT, Deep vein thrombosis; PE, pulmonary embolism.
*No upper limit to duration of anticoagulation. Decision to continue anticoagulant therapy may be changed if risk of bleeding increases or at patient's request.

no precipitating factor, treatment should be for 6 months or even for life (see Table 2). For patients on anticoagulation therapy, bed rest does not reduce risk of pulmonary embolism.

Therapy

For decades, treatment of deep venous thrombosis was unchanged. Patients were hospitalized and placed on a heparin drip with bridging to oral warfarin. Heparin and warfarin are both idiosyncratic drugs, with dose adjustments differing significantly between patients. Low-molecular-weight heparins, on the other hand, are much more predictable. They act by inhibiting factor Xa. They have a long half-life, and many of them can be administered as a once-daily subcutaneous injection. Therefore they are ideal for outpatient treatment. A word of caution: Precisely because they have a long half-life (and have no antidote), they should be used with care in patients at risk of bleeding.

Newer anticoagulants are also on the horizon but not yet commercially available. Idraparinux is an inhibitor of activated factor X (Xa). It is currently undergoing phase III clinical trials. Its half-life is 80 hours (the half-life of warfarin is 42 hours), meaning that once-weekly subcutaneous injections are sufficient with no need for monitoring. Ximelagatran is even more promising because it is the first oral direct-thrombin inhibitor. It has a rapid onset of

action and thus could be used acutely in place of the current subcutaneous agents. Up to 13% of patients develop elevated serum transaminase levels, which usually revert to normal. However, more concerning, given the recent cyclooxygenase 2 inhibitor scare, is that coronary events are more frequent in patients treated with ximelagatran.

"COMPLICATED" DEEP VENOUS THROMBOSES

Surgeons are consulted for difficult DVTs. As surgeons become more adept with catheters, they may be called on to assess patients for possible catheter-directed interventions or, rarely, to provide surgery.

Is There a Role for Surgical or Percutaneous Mechanical Thrombectomy?

Surgical thrombectomy has never really received widespread acceptance. It is invasive, involves a degree of blood loss, and does not obviate the need for anticoagulation. The few studies demonstrating benefit emphasize that surgery must be performed within the first 3 to 7 days. After that, conservative therapy is just as effective. Many patients undergoing surgical thrombectomy still develop PTS. The role of surgical thrombectomy today may be in young patients with isolated iliac thromboses and phlegmasia cerulea dolens.

Percutaneous mechanical thrombectomy catheters have been available for some time. There are two main types: (1) rotational, a high-speed, rotating basket breaks up the clot, and the resulting debris travels to the pulmonary circulation; and (2) rheolytic (based on the Venturi effect), high-speed, saline jets fragment the thrombus, and the material is then aspirated into the device. However, when these devices are used alone, only 24% of patients have total or near-total clot extraction, although most will notice an improvement in symptoms. Therefore the role of percutaneous devices *alone* is limited to those with contraindications to anticoagulation or thrombolysis. Where there really is a role for these devices, however, is when they are combined with catheter-directed thrombolysis (discussed subsequently).

Is There a Role for Systemic or Catheter-Directed Thrombolysis?

Systemic thrombolysis is used successfully in acute myocardial ischemia and in acute stroke. It has also been used for DVTs. Compared with standard anticoagulation, it reduces PTS. However, it has a four-fold bleeding risk and may predispose to early pulmonary embolism. As with acute arterial thrombosis, systemic thrombolysis has been abandoned in favor of a catheter-directed approach. This allows the thrombolytic drug to be directed at the clot, thereby increasing its efficacy. It results in significantly better patency rates in patients with iliofemoral thrombosis than anticoagulation alone (72% vs. 12%). Nevertheless, bleeding complications requiring blood transfusion occur in 11% of patients. Fatal hemorrhagic strokes have also been reported. The technique is labor intensive for both physicians and nurses. To reduce time, many now recommend percutaneous thrombectomy to reduce clot burden followed by catheter-directed thrombolysis to the residual clot. In theory, "pharmacomechanical" therapy reduces the dose of agent required and lysis time.

Inferior Vena Cava and Superior Vena Cava Filters

The Greenfield filter, introduced in 1973, was the first percutaneous device. The function of an inferior vena cava (IVC) filter is to prevent fatal pulmonary embolism. It does not prevent or treat a DVT and does not prevent small emboli from reaching the lung. The most common indication (75%) for IVC filter placement is a contraindication to systemic anticoagulation such as pregnancy, major trauma, active internal bleeding, or recent major surgery. The rest (25%) are placed in patients who have bleeding complications or those who have pulmonary emboli while undergoing adequate anticoagulation therapy. Filters are used in patients with free-floating iliofemoral thrombi because they have high rates of embolization. Those with established DVTs who undergo surgery in which anticoagulation will be stopped for a period of time also require an IVC filter. Filter technology has come a long way since 1973. However, there can be problems. Earlier filters resulted in insertion-site thrombosis and filter embolization. This is now rare. Caval penetration occurs but is seldom symptomatic. PST resulting from IVC thrombosis is now the main worry. This has led to the development of "temporary" or "retrievable" IVC filters. These stay in place for up to 4 weeks and are then removed. Many patients do not require filters beyond this time. If they do, the filters can be left in place throughout life. Hence, they are also referred to as "optional" filters.

Superior vena cava (SVC) filters are different. Arm and internal jugular DVTs have a lower risk of embolization, in the range of 5% to 10%. Therefore fewer patients require SVC filters. Consideration of the anatomy of the SVC will confirm the shortness of the "landing zone" for a filter in this territory. Insertion is via the femoral vein. In our center, SVC filters comprise less than 1% of all filters deployed.

Phlegmasia Alba/Cerulea Dolens

The two clinical syndromes associated with extensive iliofemoral thrombosis are *phlegmasia alba dolens* ("milk leg syndrome," so-called because of the leg's pallor) and the more malignant *phlegmasia cerulea dolens*. In *phlegmasia alba*, the iliac vein is occluded but the hypogastric and collateral veins remain patent. The patient has moderate to severe swelling and leg tenderness but no ischemia. Management is either anticoagulation or catheter-directed lysis in good-risk patients. *Phlegmasia cerulea dolens* occurs in patients with extensive clots of the iliac and femoral veins. Collateral circulation is lost, and clot propagation is fast. Half of patients will progress to venous gangrene (see Fig. 2). More than 90% of patients have an underlying malignancy. It is occult at time of presentation in 50% of patients. Patients typically have pain, coolness, and cyanosis of the affected foot but often have palpable pulses. Management is systemic anticoagulation, intravenous fluid, and leg elevation. Catheter-directed thrombolysis is emerging as an effective option.

Surgical thrombectomy and systemic thrombolysis have been abandoned because of poor results. Palliative care is appropriate for those with disseminated malignancy.

Internal Jugular Vein Thrombosis and Subclavian Vein Thrombosis

Catheters are the most common cause of thromboses of the head and neck veins. In young patients with spontaneous subclavian and axillary vein thromboses, Paget-Schroetter's syndrome must be considered. Treated with anticoagulation alone, these patients are often left with pain and swelling of the arm that will affect them for the rest of their lives. On the other hand, aggressive management with catheter-directed thrombolysis followed by thoracic-outlet decompression and first-rib resection either immediately (during same admission) or later (6 weeks) provides excellent functional results. As always, awareness of the diagnosis is key. Patients without evidence of Paget-Schroetter's syndrome can be treated with heparinoids and warfarin, although consideration should be given to thrombolysis in good-risk patients.

Thrombus in the internal jugular veins is usually due to catheter insertion. Intravenous drug abuse is also now a risk factor. Less usual causes are head and neck cancers and thrombophilias. A feared complication is secondary infection of the thrombus by a local oropharyngeal infection (*Lemierre syndrome*), usually by anaerobes or methicillin-resistant *Staphylococcus aureus*. Management of internal jugular vein thrombosis caused by catheters is catheter removal followed by anticoagulation. Septic complications are managed by intravenous antibiotics. Rarely, surgical excision of all the infected tissue may be necessary.

Superficial Vein Thrombosis

The majority of episodes of superficial vein thrombosis in the leg occurs in patients with varicose veins and usually affects branches of the greater saphenous vein (GSV). This is treated with rest and nonsteroidal anti-inflammatory drugs. When the main trunk of the GSV is affected, propagation to the femoral vein occurs in 5% to 10% of patients. Such patients should have a follow-up duplex scan. If clot propagates to within 5 cm of the femoral vein, saphenofemoral junction ligation should be performed. If the junction itself is involved, the patient should receive anticoagulation therapy for at least 3 months.

■ CONCLUSION

The management of DVT is generally straightforward. Newer anticoagulants may simplify matters further. However, not all DVTs are equal, and some require more consideration than others. As many of the more complex scenarios occur in perioperative and trauma patients, all surgeons ought to be intimately acquainted with DVT management. In the future, regulating authorities will probably use thromboprophylaxis as an indicator of quality of care.

Suggested Readings

Creech O Jr: The surgical treatment of acute iliofemoral thrombophlebitis, *Circulation* 33:833, 1966.

Ganger KH, Nachbur BH, Ris HB, and others: Surgical thrombectomy versus conservative treatment for deep venous thrombosis; functional comparison of long-term results, *J Vasc Surg Eur J Vasc Surg* 3:529, 1989.

Greenfield LJ, McCurdy JR, Brown PP, and others: A new intracaval filter permitting continued flow and resolution of emboli, *Surgery* 73:599, 1973.

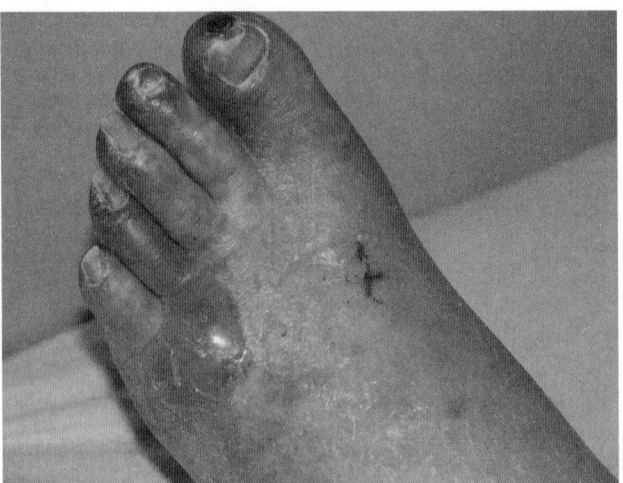

Figure 2 Phlegmasia cerulea dolens leading to venous gangrene.

Hingorani A, Ascher E, Lorenson E, and others: Upper extremity deep venous thrombosis and its impact on morbidity and mortality rates in a hospital-based population, *J Vasc Surg* 26:853, 1997.

Johnson BF, Manzo RA, Bergelin RO, and others: Relationship between changes in the deep venous system and the development of the post-thrombotic syndrome after an acute episode of lower limb deep vein thrombosis: a one- to six-year follow-up, *J Vasc Surg* 21:307, 1995.

Junger M, Diehm C, Storiko H, and others: Mobilization versus immobilization in the treatment of acute proximal deep venous thrombosis: a prospective, randomized, open, multicentre trial, *Curr Med Res Opin* 22:593, 2006.

Kasirajan K, Gray B, Ouriel K: Percutaneous AngioJet thrombectomy in the management of extensive deep venous thrombosis, *J Vasc Interv Radiol* 12:179, 2001.

Kearon C: Duration of therapy for acute venous thromboembolism, *Clin Chest Med* 24:63, 2003.

Kearon C: Natural history of venous thromboembolism, *Circulation* 107: (suppl 1):I22, 2003.

Leon L, Giannoukas AD, Dodd D, and others: Clinical significance of superficial vein thrombosis, *Eur J Vasc Endovasc Surg* 29:10, 2005.

Leonardi MJ, McGory ML, Ko CY: The rate of bleeding complications after pharmacologic deep venous thrombosis prophylaxis: a systematic review of 33 randomized controlled trials, *Arch Surg* 141:790; discussion 797, 2006.

Macdonald PS, Kahn SR, Miller N, and others: Short-term natural history of isolated gastrocnemius and soleal vein thrombosis, *J Vasc Surg* 37:523, 2003.

Markel A: Origin and natural history of deep vein thrombosis of the legs, *Semin Vasc Med* 5:65, 2005.

Masuda EM, Kessler DM, Kistner RL, and others: The natural history of calf vein thrombosis: lysis of thrombi and development of reflux, *J Vasc Surg* 28:67; discussion 73, 1998.

Milne AA, Stonebridge PA, Bradbury AW, and others: Venous function and clinical outcome following deep vein thrombosis, *Br J Surg* 81:847, 1994.

Mohr DN, Silverstein MD, Heit JA, and others: The venous stasis syndrome after deep venous thrombosis or pulmonary embolism: a population-based study, *Mayo Clin Proc* 75:1249, 2000.

Semba CP, Razavi MK, Kee ST, and others: Thrombolysis for lower extremity deep venous thrombosis, *Tech Vasc Interv Radiol* 7:68, 2004.

Strandness DJ, Langlois Y, Cramer M, and others: Long-term sequelae of acute venous thrombosis, *JAMA* 250:1289, 1983.

Turpie GG, Chin BS, Lip GY: ABC of antithrombotic therapy: venous thromboembolism: pathophysiology, clinical features, and prevention, *BMJ* 325:887, 2002.

Weitz JI: New anticoagulants for treatment of venous thromboembolism, *Circulation* 110:(suppl 1):I19, 2004.

PULMONARY THROMBOEMBOLISM

Stephen T. Smith, MD, and G. Patrick Clagett, MD

Deep venous thrombosis (DVT) and pulmonary thromboembolism (PE) are a continuum of the disease known as venous thromboembolism. This is an entity of great importance that crosses multiple specialties and occurs worldwide. The incidence at autopsy has varied from 1% in the general population to 30% in patients dying from major trauma, burns, or fractures. PE causes 100,000 deaths annually in the United States and contributes to another 100,000 deaths. DVT and PE often go unsuspected clinically because of the nonspecific signs and symptoms. The incidence of DVT and PE are highest in hospitalized medical and surgical patients. However, appropriate prophylaxis of venous thromboembolism remains underutilized. Given these considerations, fatal PE may be the most common preventable cause of hospital death. A high index of suspicion must be maintained to make the correct diagnosis and initiate appropriate therapy.

PATHOGENESIS AND EPIDEMIOLOGY

More than 95% of all PEs arise from thrombi within the deep veins of the lower extremities—popliteal, femoral, and iliac veins. Acute thrombus may be soft and fragile and break off from weak attachments to the vein wall, resulting in PE. Large macroemboli may lodge in the main pulmonary artery or its major branches, precipitating right heart strain and sudden death. Smaller microemboli can travel out to the peripheral vessels and may cause infarction. Pulmonary infarctions, which occur in the minority of PEs, are wedge-shaped consolidations visible on chest radiographs. Rarely, an embolus may pass through an atrial or ventricular septal defect and present as an arterial embolus (paradoxical embolism). Hypercoagulability has been increasingly diagnosed as a cause of venous thromboembolism (Table 1). The most common hypercoagulable states are factor V Leiden, the G20210A mutation in the prothrombin gene, and homozygous C677T mutation in the methylenetetrahydrofolate reductase gene, causing mild to moderate elevations in homocysteine levels.

Patients can be organized as having low, moderate, and strong risk factors for venous thromboembolism (Table 2). Patients at highest risk of venous thromboembolism include those with major fractures, hip or knee replacements, major general surgical operations, and major trauma or spinal cord injuries. Moderate risk factors include malignancy, previous venous thromboembolism, central venous catheters, and estrogen therapy. Other risk factors include bed rest or prolonged immobility, obesity, and increasing age. These risk factors are used to guide the level of prophylaxis for venous thromboembolism.

DEEP VENOUS THROMBOSIS PROPHYLAXIS

The rationale for prophylaxis of DVT is based on the clinically silent nature of the disease. The diagnosis of DVT and PE is often difficult, with few specific signs and symptoms. More than half of patients with DVT are asymptomatic. Even worse, the first manifestation of the disease may be a fatal PE. Intensive screening of asymptomatic, high-risk patients with duplex ultrasound or impedance plethysmography has shown only moderate sensitivity and positive predictive value for diagnosing DVT. Therefore prophylaxis is the best method to prevent DVT. Prevention of DVT has been shown to prevent PE.

Application of effective prophylaxis should be adapted to specific clinical risk factors for individual patients. These risk factors are based on large epidemiologic studies of general groups of patients. An effective strategy is to classify a patient's risk for venous thromboembolism as low, moderate, high, or highest risk.

Recommendations for prophylaxis based on the level of risk can be found in Table 3. In low-risk general surgery patients who are undergoing minor operations and are younger than age 40 years with no clinical risk factors, no prophylaxis other than early ambulation is necessary. In moderate-risk general surgery patients who are older than age 40 years and undergoing major operations but have no clinical risk factors, low-dose unfractionated heparin (5000 units subcutaneously [SC] every 12 hours) or mechanical calf-compression devices should be used. In high-risk general surgery patients with additional risk factors, unfractionated heparin

Table 1: Hypercoagulable States

Inherited

Common

G1691A factor V Leiden mutation

G20210A mutation in the prothrombin (factor II gene)

Homozygous C677T mutation in the methylenetetrahydrofolate reductase gene (moderate hyperhomocysteinemia)

Rare

Antithrombin III deficiency

Protein C deficiency

Protein S deficiency

Very Rare

Dysfibrinogenemia

Homozygous homocystinuria

Probably inherited

Increased levels of factor VIII, factor IX, or fibrinogen*

Acquired

Heparin-induced thrombocytopenia

Cancer

Myeloproliferative disorders

Pregnancy and the puerperium

Use of oral contraceptives or hormone-replacement therapy

Resistance to activated protein C that is not due to alterations in the factor V gene

Antiphospholipid antibodies

Mild-to-moderate hyperhomocysteinemia from folic acid, vitamin B6 and B12 deficiencies

Modified from Seligsohn U, Lubetsky A: N Engl J Med 344:1222, 2001.
*Levels of factor VIII and fibrinogen may also increase as part of the acute phase response.

Table 2: Strong, Moderate and Weak Risk Factors for Venous Thromboembolism

Strong Risk Factors

Fracture (hip or leg)

Hip or knee replacement

Major general surgery

Major trauma

Spinal cord injury

Moderate Risk Factors

Arthroscopic knee surgery

Central venous lines

Chemotherapy

Congestive heart or respiratory failure

Hormone replacement therapy

Malignancy

Oral contraceptive therapy

Paralytic stroke

Pregnancy/postpartum

Previous deep venous thrombosis/pulmonary embolism

Thrombophilia

Weak Risk Factors

Bed rest >3 days

Immobility from sitting (prolonged car or air travel)

Increasing age

Laparoscopic surgery (e.g., cholecystectomy)

Obesity

Pregnancy/antepartum

Varicose veins

From Anderson FA Jr, Spencer FA: Circulation 107:I, 2003.

(5000 units SC every 8 hours) or low-molecular-weight heparin (LMWH) should be used for prophylaxis of DVT. For the highest-risk general surgery group, including major trauma and spinal cord injury patients, the most effective pharmacologic prophylaxis (SC heparin every 8 hours, fondaparinux, or LMWH) should be combined with mechanical compression devices and begun preoperatively. In selected very-high-risk patients, perioperative warfarin (international normalized ratio [INR] 2.0–3.0) should be considered. In patients undergoing total hip or knee replacement or hip fracture surgery, LMWH given subcutaneously twice daily, fondaparinux, or postoperative warfarin (INR 2.0–3.0) combined with mechanical compression devices should be used.

CLINICAL PRESENTATION

DVTs may be clinically silent, have minimal symptoms, or present with incapacitating and obvious symptoms and signs. Symptomatic patients usually exhibit leg swelling distal to the site of the venous obstruction. Venous hypertension in the calf may cause pain with passive dorsiflexion at the ankle (Homans's sign). However, this sign is neither sensitive nor specific for DVT. Symptoms may also include warmth, erythema, and tenderness. Patients may complain of leg heaviness that worsens with exercise (venous claudication). Up to 50% of patients with symptomatic proximal (iliofemoral) DVT also have silent PE at the time of diagnosis.

The symptoms of PE are nonspecific, but patterns may be recognized that suggest the diagnosis. Common signs and symptoms are presented in Table 4. PE may be silent or present with respiratory compromise resulting from nonperfused, ventilated pulmonary segments, or hemodynamic compromise resulting from the obstruction of pulmonary blood flow. Sudden onset of symptoms may be suggestive of PE, but symptoms may also develop over hours to days. Dyspnea and chest pain are the two most common presenting symptoms. Chest pain is often pleuritic but may also mimic angina pectoris. Cough is a common symptom but is nonspecific. Signs and symptoms of DVT in a patient with new onset of respiratory symptoms are highly suggestive of PE.

Two of the most common signs in patients presenting with PE are tachypnea and tachycardia (Table 5). An electrocardiogram (ECG) typically shows sinus tachycardia, and the presence of right heart strain strongly suggests PE. Tachypnea and tachycardia are common in both medical and surgical illnesses, and an index of suspicion must be maintained. After PE is suspected, it should be investigated with an imaging study. If there is a high clinical suspicion, anticoagulation should begin while the diagnosis is being confirmed.

DIAGNOSIS

After DVT or PE is suspected, effort should be made to secure the diagnosis. When a patient has signs or symptoms of DVT, a duplex examination and laboratory evaluation are performed. For patients

Table 3: Classification of Level of Risk

Level of Risk	Calf	DVT(%), Proximal	PE(%), Clinical	Fatal	Successful Prevention Strategies
Low Risk Minor surgery in patients aged <40 with no additional risk factors	2	0.4	0.2	<0.001	No specific prophylaxis; early mobilization
Moderate Risk Minor surgery in patients with additional risk factors Surgery in patients aged 40–60 with no additional risk factors	10–20	2–4	1–2	0.1–0.4	LDUH (every 12 hours), LMWH (≤ 3400 U daily), GCS or IPC
High risk Surgery in patients aged >60, or aged 40–60 with additional risk factors (prior DVT/PE, cancer, molecular hypercoagulability)	20–40	4–8	2–4	0.4–0.1	LDUH (every 8 hours), LMWH (≤3400 U daily), or IPC
Highest Risk Surgery in patients with multiple risk factors (aged >40, cancer, prior VTE) Hip or knee arthroplasty, hip fracture Major trauma, spinal cord injury	40–80	10–20	4–10	0.2–0.5	LMWH (≤3400 U daily), fondaparinux, oral VKAs (INR 2–3), or IPC/GCS + LDUH/LMWH

DVT, Deep venous thrombosis; *GCS*, graded compression stocking; *LDUH*, low-dose unfractionated heparin; *LMWH*, low-molecular-weight heparin; *INR*, international normalized ratio; *IPC*, intermittent pneumatic compression (calf); *PE*, pulmonary thromboembolism; *VKAs*, vitamin K antagonists; *VTE*, venous thromboembolism.
From Clagett G, Anderson F, Heit J, and others: Chest 108:312, 1995.

Table 4: Symptoms and Signs in Patients with Acute PE without Preexisting Cardiac or Pulmonary Disease

Symptoms	Patients (%)	Signs	Patients (%)
Dyspnea	73	Tachypnea (≥20/min)	70
Pleuritic pain	66	Rales (crackles)	51
Cough	37	Tachycardia (>100 bpm)	30
Leg swelling	28	Fourth heart sound	24
Leg pain	26	Increased pulmonary component of second sound	23
Hemoptysis	13	Deep vein thrombosis	11
Palpitations	10	Diaphoresis	11
Wheezing	9	Temperature ≥38.5 °C	7
Angina-like pain	4	Wheezes	5
		Homans's sign	4
		Right ventricular lift	4
		Pleural friction rub	3
		Third heart sound	3
		Cyanosis	1

From Stein PD, Fowler SE, Goodman LR, and others: Chest 100:598, 1991.
PE, Pulmonary thromboembolism.

exhibiting symptoms of PE, a chest radiograph, ECG, laboratory tests, and an imaging study are usually performed. For patients with high clinical suspicion and no contraindication, anticoagulation should begin while the tests are in progress.

Table 5: Indications for Vena Cava Filter Placement

Absolute Indications

Recurrent DVT or PE despite adequate anticoagulation

DVT or PE in a patient with contraindication to anticoagulation

Complications of anticoagulation

Chronic PE in patients with pulmonary hypertension

After pulmonary embolectomy

Relative Indications

Large free-floating iliofemoral thrombus

DVT in patients with poor cardiopulmonary reserve

Propagating iliofemoral thrombus despite adequate anticoagulation

Protection during iliofemoral mechanical thrombectomy

DVT, Deep venous thrombosis; *PE*, pulmonary thromboembolism.

Initial Testing

The D-dimer assay is a laboratory test that measures a specific product from the breakdown of cross-linked fibrin. A variety of D-dimer assays are available, but the quantitative enzyme-linked immunosorbent assay (ELISA) test may be the most sensitive for the presence of thrombosis. A negative ELISA D-dimer in the presence of a low clinical suspicion effectively rules out the diagnosis of venous thromboembolism. However, in surgical or trauma patients the D-dimer is often positive and thus lacks specificity. A positive D-dimer should then be followed with a confirmatory test.

Because of hypoxemia, arterial blood gases (ABGs) are often obtained when PE is suspected but are of little value in the diagnosis of PE. The test lacks specificity because hypoxemia can be secondary to a variety of cardiopulmonary disorders. In addition, the ABGs may be normal in up to 20% of patients with PE.

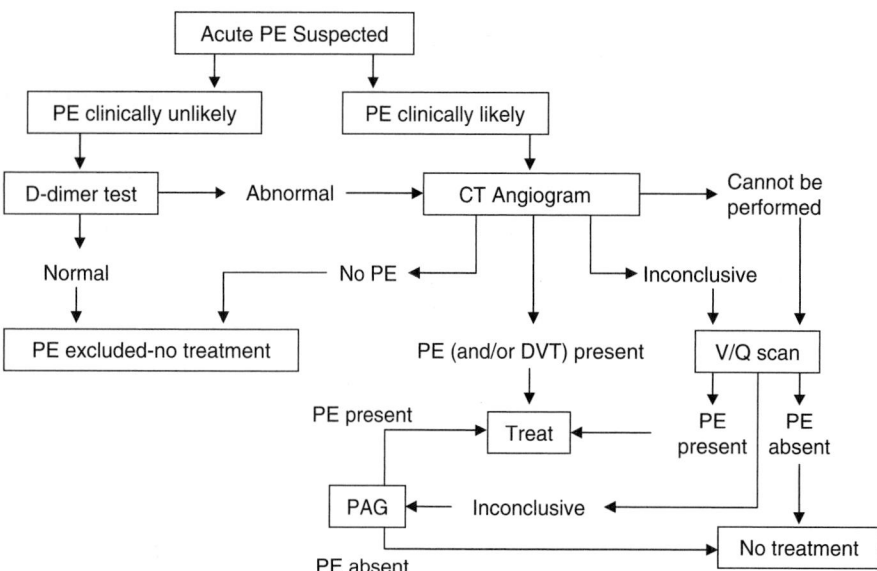

Figure I Algorithm for the diagnosis of pulmonary embolus. *PAG,* Pulmonary arteriogram; *PE,* pulmonary thromboembolism; *V/Q,* ventilation and perfusion. *From Tapson VF: Dis Mon 51:86, 2005.*

An ECG is also regularly ordered when evaluating a patient with signs and symptoms of PE. The most common finding is sinus tachycardia, but this is obviously not specific for the diagnosis of PE. A more specific sign may be right heart strain, but this is present only when there is significant obstruction to the pulmonary outflow. More important, an ECG may help to diagnose other conditions that present in a similar manner, such as myocardial infarction.

A chest x-ray is standard in the workup of patients with pulmonary complaints. This test is rarely diagnostic for PE but may have findings suggestive of it. Hampton's hump is a peripheral, wedge-shaped consolidation that suggests pulmonary infarction. Westermark's sign is a zone of peripheral oligemia caused by obstruction of a pulmonary artery branch. A chest x-ray is more commonly helpful in diagnosing other cardiopulmonary conditions that may be causing the patient's symptoms.

Diagnostic Imaging for Suspected Pulmonary Thromboembolism

Pulmonary arteriogram is the traditional gold standard for the diagnosis of PE. However, this test is invasive and has been largely replaced by CT angiography (CTA). Ventilation and perfusion (V/Q) scanning is noninvasive and detects a mismatch between ventilation and perfusion in a pulmonary segment. This has been the mainstay of diagnostic imaging for many years. However, there are several sources of error with V/Q scans. False-positive tests can result from underlying lung diseases or previous PE. The results are usually reported as normal, low, intermediate, or high probability for PE. A normal result, although unusual, excludes the diagnosis of PE. A high-probability scan is specific for the presence of a PE. However, the most limiting feature of V/Q scanning is the frequency of intermediate probability, nondiagnostic results. The associated clinical suspicion for PE is an important component for interpreting the results of the V/Q scan. A high clinical suspicion for PE with a nondiagnostic result should prompt further testing.

Contrast-enhanced spiral CT pulmonary arteriography (CTA) is the imaging test most commonly used for diagnosis of acute pulmonary embolus. The limitation of CT angiography is the lower sensitivity for detection of smaller peripheral emboli. A recent prospective multicenter trial for the diagnosis of PE (PIOPED II) provides information about the accuracy of this test. The sensitivity of CTA for pulmonary embolism is 90%, with a specificity of 95%. CTA has a high negative predictive

value, and a normal CTA virtually excludes the diagnosis of PE. For the detection of emboli in segmental vessels, the clinical suspicion for PE is important. In patients with high clinical suspicion, CTA has a positive predictive value of 95% for the diagnosis of PE. With an intermediate suspicion, there is a high (79%) probability of detecting segmental PE. For patients with a low suspicion, the probability of detecting segmental PE is low (33%), and the false-positive rate is high (42%). When findings contradict clinical suspicion, CTA has a low diagnostic value. As the newer, advanced-generation devices with increasing multidetector rows and improved spatial resolution become available, CTA for the diagnosis of PE should become even more accurate. An algorithm for the diagnosis of PE using CTA as the primary imaging modality is presented in Figure 1.

▮ MANAGEMENT

After the diagnosis of venous thromboembolism is made, the mainstay of treatment is anticoagulation. This accomplishes the goals of preventing recurrent DVT or PE, limiting extension of thrombosis, and possibly reducing the complications from the postthrombotic syndrome. A variety of approaches can be used to provide anticoagulation therapy to patients with venous thromboembolism.

Anticoagulation

The initial treatment of venous thromboembolism involves heparin therapy and transitioning to warfarin. Hospitalized patients can be treated immediately with intravenous (IV) heparin (80 U/kg bolus followed by 18 U/kg/hr). Monitoring of the activated partial thromboplastin time (aPTT) and platelet counts is traditional, with the aim of maintaining the aPTT 1.5 to 2.5 times control values. However, evidence suggests that aPTT values do not correlate with adequacy of anticoagulation or bleeding risk because aPTT results are dependent on the types of reagents used, as well as the type of coagulometer. A randomized study (*JAMA* 296:935, 2006) comparing weight-based subcutaneous heparin and LMWH showed no difference in recurrent venous thromboembolism or bleeding risk. The dose of unfractionated heparin administered subcutaneously was 333 U/kg initially, then 250 U/kg every 12 hours. Thus unmonitored, weight-based, subcutaneous, unfractionated heparin can be safely administered in an outpatient setting.

LMWH has a more predictable pharmacokinetic profile and greater bioavailability than unfractionated heparin. These features allow LMWH to be administered in once or twice daily subcutaneous doses without laboratory monitoring. The therapeutic dose for treatment of DVT and PE with enoxaparin is 1.0 mg/kg SC twice daily or 1.5 mg/kg SC daily. Several randomized trials and meta-analyses have showed equivalence of LMWH and IV unfractionated heparin in terms of bleeding risk and prevention of recurrent venous thromboembolism. The advantage of LMWH is that it can be delivered in an outpatient setting without monitoring, but it is significantly more expensive than unfractionated heparin. LMWH may be more effective than warfarin for treatment of venous thromboembolism in patients with cancer. Patients with DVT/PE and cancer should be treated indefinitely or until the cancer is resolved, and the first 3 to 6 months of treatment should be with LMWH.

Patients with acute venous thromboembolism require long-term anticoagulation because of the high frequency (15%-50%) of recurrent thrombosis and thromboembolism. An oral vitamin K antagonist such as warfarin is the preferred approach to long-term treatment in patients with venous thromboembolism. Warfarin therapy is initiated at the time heparin is started in dosages of 5 to 7.5 mg daily. Large loading doses of warfarin are no longer used because they can precipitate a sudden drop in protein C levels and cause a paradoxical hypercoagulable state. Laboratory monitoring of the anticoagulant effect (INR to 2.0–3.0) and dose adjustment is required because of the wide variation of anticoagulation response and the many drug and diet interactions with warfarin therapy. The recommendation for patients with DVT or PE secondary to a reversible risk factor, such as the postoperative state, is 3 months of warfarin. Patients with a documented hypercoagulable state or idiopathic venous thromboembolism should be treated for 6 to 12 months and considered for lifelong anticoagulation. Patients with two or more documented episodes of venous thromboembolism should receive anticoagulation therapy indefinitely.

Thrombolysis

Anticoagulation with heparin for acute PE should be considered the mainstay of therapy. For selected patients who are hemodynamically unstable and at low risk of bleeding, thrombolysis can be considered. In a review of nine trials of thrombolysis versus anticoagulation, thrombolysis showed improved resolution of angiographic and hemodynamic abnormalities but no difference in death rate or clinical symptoms. Thrombolysis is associated with a 1% to 2% risk of intracranial bleeding. When promptly diagnosed and treated with anticoagulation, the mortality from PE is approximately 2%. Because of the favorable results with anticoagulation alone, thrombolysis should be reserved for patients with hemodynamic instability who are at low risk for bleeding. Streptokinase and tissue plasminogen activator (tPA) have shown similar efficacy, but tPA has shorter duration of administration. These drugs have the potential to lyse fibrin anywhere in the body and cause bleeding at that site. Catheter-directed delivery of thrombolytics may therefore increase bleeding risk at the puncture site without an increase in efficacy.

Thrombectomy

A variety of mechanical thrombectomy devices have been developed for the treatment of severe symptomatic DVT and PE. These percutaneous techniques fragment and aspirate the clot and improve blood flow. The distal pulmonary vasculature can accommodate multiple smaller emboli as the larger embolus is removed from the main pulmonary arteries, improving cardiac output. The technique may be improved with the addition of a small amount of thrombolytic agent that can help to soften and break up the clot. Mechanical thrombectomy shows promise in treating massive PE, but there is insufficient experience to make recommendations regarding its use. Patients in whom mechanical thrombectomy should be considered are highly selected, compromised patients who are unable to receive thrombolytic therapy or whose critical status does not allow sufficient time for infusion of thrombolysis.

Open pulmonary thrombectomy has been used when more conservative measures have failed. These situations usually include massive PE with hemodynamic instability despite heparin and resuscitation and failure of or a contraindication for thrombolytic therapy. This procedure requires cardiopulmonary bypass and is associated with a high mortality rate. The most appropriate patients for open pulmonary thrombectomy may be patients with chronic PE and associated pulmonary hypertension, those who require closed cardiac massage to maintain blood pressure, or those in whom thrombolytic or catheter thrombectomy procedures fail to improve cardiac output.

Inferior Vena Cava Filters

Anticoagulation is effective in the majority of patients with venous thromboembolism. The major rationale for treatment with an inferior vena cava (IVC) filter is in patients who have a contraindication for or complication of anticoagulation and who are at risk for recurrent PE. These filters are placed percutaneously from jugular or femoral vein access. Removable devices are available and have been retrieved successfully many months after implantation. Patients with contraindications to IVC filters include venous anatomic abnormalities, pregnancy, or thrombosis proximal to the intended point of placement. In a randomized trial of 400 patients, IVC filters decreased the incidence of PE at 12 days over anticoagulation alone, but the incidence of recurrent DVT was higher. There was no prolonged early or late survival. IVC filters are recommended for patients with proximal DVT or PE with contraindications for anticoagulation, complications of anticoagulation, or recurrent venous thromboembolism despite adequate anticoagulation. Table 5 lists the indications for IVC filter placement.

Suggested Readings

Christopher Study Investigators: Effectiveness of managing suspected pulmonary embolism using an algorithm combining clinical probability, d-dimer testing, and computed tomography, *JAMA* 295:172, 2006.

Geerts WH, Pineo GF, Heit JA, and others: Prevention of venous thromboembolism, *Chest* 126:(suppl):338S, 2004.

Kearon C, Ginsberg J, Julian J, for the Fixed-Dose Heparin (FIDO) Investigators: Comparison of fixed-dose weight-adjusted unfractionated heparin and low-molecular-weight heparin for acute treatment of venous thromboembolism, *JAMA* 296:935, 2006.

Stein PD, Fowler SE, Goodman LR, and others, for the PIOPED II Investigators: Multidetector computed tomography for acute pulmonary embolism, *N Engl J Med* 354:2317, 2006.

INFERIOR VENA CAVA FILTERS

Christos S. Georgiades, MD, PhD, and Kelvin Hong, MD

INTRODUCTION: EPIDEMIOLOGY OF DEEP VENOUS THROMBOSIS AND PULMONARY EMBOLISM

The rationale for inferior vena cava (IVC) interruption by means of filter placement is to decrease the risk of pulmonary embolism (PE) from thrombus originating in the deep veins of the pelvis or lower extremities. Deep venous thrombosis (DVT) is a major cause of morbidity and mortality in the United States with an annual incidence of approximately 2 million. The incidence of clinically significant PE in the United States is reportedly between 150,000 and 600,000, with 25% to 40% of patients presenting with sudden death. The remaining patients, if properly diagnosed, will be treated with either systemic anticoagulation or placement of IVC filter and rarely with surgical or catheter-directed thrombectomy. Even without anticoagulation, patients who receive an IVC filter alone show a significantly reduced PE-related mortality. As a result, the use of IVC filters has dramatically increased over time. From 1980 to 2000, the number of filters placed increased from 2000 to approximately 50,000 per year. The first IVC filter was marketed in the late 1960s. Before that,

surgical ligation of the IVC, first described by Armand Trousseau in 1865, was the only option for prevention of PE in high-risk patients. Since their introduction, a number of IVC filters have been marketed with improved designs and capabilities, including retrievability. Figure 1 shows the six filter types available in the United States today, and Table 1 describes their features. The majority of IVC filters are placed in patients who have a contraindication to anticoagulation (56%), for prophylaxis in high-risk patients (27%), and in patients with recurrent PE despite anticoagulation (15%). Despite improvements in design that make filters safer and retrievable, there are still filter-associated risks. Therefore the indications for filter placement and choice of appropriate filter must be carefully followed.

INDICATIONS AND CONTRAINDICATIONS FOR INFERIOR VENA CAVA FILTER PLACEMENT AND RETRIEVAL

The standard of treatment for DVT and PE is systemic anticoagulation. A major misconception is that systemic anticoagulation with warfarin, heparin, low-molecular-weight heparins (LMWH), or argatroban treats existing thrombus. The goal of systemic anticoagulation is to prevent extension of existing clot or recurrence of DVT or PE (or both). Six-month systemic anticoagulation reduces the 2-year risk of recurrent DVT or PE by 50%, from 18% to 9%. However, not all patients have the same risk for developing thromboembolic disease, nor do all patients have the same pulmonary reserve. Therefore treatment should be tailored according to individual risk and ability to sustain a thromboembolic event. First-time DVT or PE patients with idiopathic disease and normal pulmonary reserve should be treated with systemic

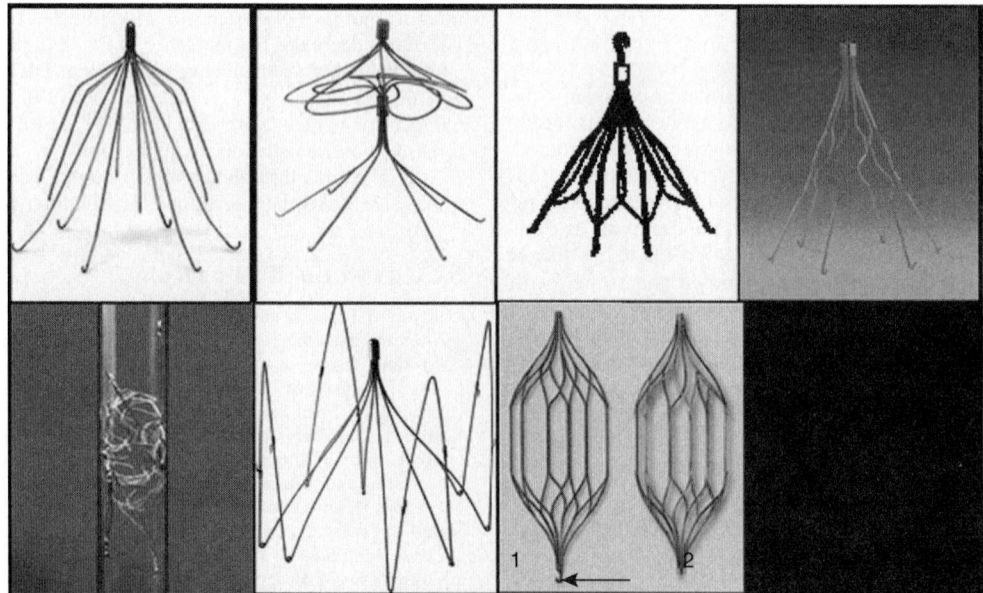

Figure 1   The six types of inferior vena cava *(IVC)* filters available in the United States are: *(A)* G2 (C.R. Bard, Murray Hill, NJ); *(B)* Simon Nitinol (C.R. Bard); *(C)* Günther-Tulip (Cook Medical, Bloomington, IN); *(D)* Greenfield (Boston Scientific, Natick MA); *(E)* Bird's Nest (Cook Medical); *(F)* VenaTech (B. Braun Medical, Bethlehem, PA); *(G)* OptEase (Cordis J&J, Roden, The Netherlands), *(1)* (retrieval hook, *arrow*); and TrapEase (Cordis, Miami Lakes, FL) *(2)*. There is no prospective, randomized study that compares the safety and efficacy of these filters. Therefore the choice is made simply on the basis of operator preference, technical feasibility (diameter of IVC), and the need for retrievability. The Günther-Tulip *(C)* and OptEase *(G1)* have Food and Drug Administration indication for retrievability. Studies have shown this to be feasible up to 3 to 4 weeks postplacement. Beyond that, epithelial overgrowth may increase the risk of IVC injury if removal is attempted. The G2 filter *(A)*, although not approved for retrievability, technically can be removed because it is the same design as its G1 predecessor, which had approval for indefinite retrieval.

Table 1: Features of the Six IVC Filter Types Available in the United States

Company	Filter	Max. IVC Diameter (mm)	Sheath Size (F)	Jugular Placement	MR Compatible	Retrievable/Time
C.R. Bard (Murray Hill, NJ)	G2	28	10	Yes	Yes	No FDA indication, but technically retrievable
C.R. Bard	Simon Nitinol	28	7	Yes	Yes	No
B. Braun Medical (Bethlehem, PA)	VenaTech LGM	28	10	Yes	Yes	No
B. Braun Medical	VenaTech LP	35	7	Yes	Yes	No
Boston Scientific (Natick, MA)	Greenfield	28	12	Yes	Yes	No
Cook Medical (Bloomington, IN)	Günther-Tulip	30	7	Yes		Yes
Cook Medical	Gianturco-Roehm Bird's Nest	40	12	Yes	Yes, 6 weeks post-placement	No
Cordis (Miami Lakes, FL)	TrapEase	30	6	Yes	Yes	No
Cordis J&J (Roden, The Netherlands)	OptEase	30	6	Yes	Yes	Yes, 4 weeks

FDA, U.S. Food and Drug Administration; *IVC*, inferior vena cava; *max.*, maximal; *MR*, magnetic resonance (imaging).
The choice of filter depends primarily on need for retrievability. If a retrievable filter is desired, the choices are OptEase, Günther-Tulip, and G2. If the filter is expected to remain in place for longer than 1 month, a G2 should be placed. For vena cavas with a diameter >30 mm, the only choice is a Bird's Nest filter, which is permanent. One can, of course, deploy two retrievable filters, one each in right and left common iliac vein, to allow for possible retrieval. However, this may be associated with an increased risk of in situ thrombosis, and retrieval is technically challenging. All available filters are MRI compatible. Although they are unlikely to move during MR imaging, all filters will cause local artifact.

anticoagulation alone. This group represents the majority of patients. However, a large number of patients cannot receive anticoagulation for a variety of reasons, and still others have comorbid conditions that increase their risk of recurrence, limit their tolerance to another event, or altogether prevent them from receiving anticoagulation therapy. These are the patients who should be considered for an IVC filter. Table 2 summarizes the indications for IVC filter placement.

■ INDICATIONS FOR PLACEMENT

Deep Venous Thrombosis and Pulmonary Embolism with Contraindication to Anticoagulation

This category includes patients who have a high risk of complications from anticoagulation. Some patients may declare themselves as high risk with a recent history of gastrointestinal hemorrhage (GIH), intracranial hemorrhage (ICH), or other hemorrhage. Others have comorbid conditions that make them high risk for anticoagulation, such as intracranial neoplasm, vascular neoplasm in critical locations, or recent surgery or trauma. This group represents the majority of patients (56%) who receive an IVC filter.

Patients at High Risk

A smaller percentage of patients (19%-27%) receive a filter because they are considered high risk for DVT or PE (or both). This category includes the following patients.

Trauma: Severe, multiorgan injury is a major risk factor for DVT and PE. In addition, when these patients suffer a PE, their mortality risk is much higher compared with non–trauma-related PE patients. PE is thought to contribute or be the direct cause of death in at least 85% of trauma patients with PE. Therefore prevention is crucial for a positive outcome. Because of their trauma, most of these patients cannot be placed on systemic anticoagulation, leaving IVC filters as the only option to prevent PE from DVT.

Paralysis: Asymptomatic DVTs have been reported in 60% to 80% of patients with permanent spinal cord injury, whereas symptomatic DVT is reported in less than 20%. Therefore IVC filter placement in patients with paraplegia or tetraplegia should not be routine but reserved for patients with documented, symptomatic DVT or for those who cannot or will not receive lifelong systemic anticoagulation.

Surgery: Major surgery raises the risk for DVT and PE for many reasons. Prolonged immobilization of the patient is common, especially after major abdominal, neurologic, and orthopedic surgeries. The risk of DVT/PE is increased, albeit less so, even in minor surgeries. Transient dehydration is another factor predisposing patients to the formation of clot, as is surgery-associated vascular injury or extrinsic compression. All patients undergoing surgery should receive some form of prophylaxis for DVT/PE. In most cases, pneumatic compression stockings are adequate because recovery from surgery is relatively short. When recovery is prolonged and the risk of DVT/PE is high, chemical anticoagulation has been shown to reduce the risk of DVT/PE. However, many postsurgical patients are not candidates for anticoagulation. Until recently, placing an IVC filter in these patients was avoided because of the transient nature of the risk for DVT/PE. Since the advent of retrievable filters, however, their use in the perioperative period has increased because they can be removed after the risk normalizes.

Free-floating IVC clot: Although commonly discussed, a free-floating clot in the IVC or pelvic veins is extremely rare. If identified incidentally, a prophylactic filter is indicated, as is anticoagulation. Free-floating clots are usually fresh clots and thus are vulnerable to anticoagulation. If the patient does not require long-term prophylaxis with a filter, a retrievable filter is indicated and removed when the clot resolves.

Hypercoagulable states: Congenital (i.e., sickle cell disease, protein C or S deficiency, anti-thrombin III deficiency, factor VI Leiden mutation, prothrombin 20210A, hyperhomocysteinemia)

Table 2: Indications and Contraindication for IVC Filter Placement and Retrieval

Indications for Placement	Clinical Frequency (%)	Contraindications to Placement (Relative)	Indications for Retrieval	Contraindications for Retrieval (Relative)
PE or DVT with contraindication to anticoagulation	56	Hypercoagulable state	Filter no longer necessary Risk for DVT baseline Patient can receive anticoagulation therapy	Nonretrievable filter
PE or DVT despite therapeutic anticoagulation	15	Bacteremia	Active bacteremia (Replacement)	Clot within filter (>1 cm^3)
High risk for PE and limited pulmonary reserve (i.e., pulmonary hypertension, chronic thromboembolic disease)	<1		Hypercoagulable state diagnosed after filter placement (if risk of IVC thrombosis is deemed greater than PE)	Persistent clot in pelvis/lower extremities
High-risk patients Severe multitrauma Paralysis High-risk surgery Hypercoagulable state Free-floating IVC thrombus	19–27		Migrated/fractured/ineffective filter	
Paradoxical embolism	<1			

DVT, Deep venous thrombosis; *IVC,* inferior vena cava; *PE,* pulmonary embolism.
Despite their proven benefit in preventing PE and saving lives, IVC filters are associated with periprocedural and long-term complications. Therefore these indications and contraindications should be followed carefully. In rare cases, the risk cannot be properly ascertained; therefore multidisciplinary input may be required, especially in cases of a hypercoagulable state, which can be both an indication and contraindication.

or acquired hypercoagulable disorders (i.e., antiphospholipid syndrome, cancer, pregnancy, nephritic syndrome, diabetes, smoking, oral contraceptive pill, heparin-induced thrombocytopenia) are common in clinical practice and present a difficult therapeutic challenge. On one hand, the underlying disease predisposes the patient to DVT and thus to an increased risk for PE; on the other hand, the filter itself may be the cause of focal clot formation and subsequent IVC thrombosis. Even in patients with contraindication to anticoagulation, filter placement should be considered carefully and only with input from the hematology service. Patients who, despite their hypercoagulable state, do not have a DVT or PE should generally not receive a filter. On the other end of the spectrum are patients with DVT and recurrent PE who cannot receive anticoagulation and should receive a filter. The gray zone between these poles is more common, and the decision to place a filter should be based on a careful, multidisciplinary risk-benefit analysis.

Recurrent Deep Venous Thrombosis and Pulmonary Embolism on Anticoagulation

A smaller percentage of patients receive an IVC filter because of recurrent PE while they are on anticoagulation therapy (15%). Simply being on anticoagulation therapy and having a PE does not represent failure of anticoagulation. One must ensure that the measure of the efficacy of anticoagulation (international normalized ratio [INR] for warfarin, activated partial thromboplastin time ratio [APTTr] for heparin) was within the therapeutic range when the PE occurred. If not, the dose should be adjusted so that the outcome measure is within therapeutic range. Only then should a filter be considered. The risk of PE recurrence for patients while on therapeutic anticoagulation is 5% to 10%.

Limited Pulmonary Reserve or Chronic Pulmonary Hypertension

This is a rare condition of unknown cause, although chronic thromboembolic events have been postulated to be the main

culprit. Along with etiology, treatment is controversial. It does not present a serious medical problem from an epidemiologic standpoint because only 500 to 2500 new cases are reported each year. However, given the limited pulmonary reserve in these patients, prevention of further embolic events is crucial for survival. Although no prospective, randomized study exists to show any benefit from routine IVC filter placement in such patients, the majority of centers treating such patients recommend routine IVC filter placement for the prevention of new embolic events.

CONTRAINDICATIONS FOR PLACEMENT OF INFERIOR VENA CAVA FILTER

Technical contraindications include a thrombosed or occluded IVC, clot in the intrahepatic IVC, no available venous access, and megacava (IVC >32 mm diameter). The last contraindication is relative because for megacavas, a Bird's nest–type filter can be used if available. Clinical contraindications include active bacteremia and severe prothrombotic state.

If a filter is considered clinically necessary, a retrievable one may be placed in cases of active bacteremia, assuming it will be removed as soon as it is not required or replaced as soon as bacteremia resolves. A prothrombotic state increases the risk for in situ filter clot formation; however, it should not prevent filter placement if protection against potentially lethal PE is necessary. Input from a hematology specialist is important to screen these patients and to develop a plan of action related to type of filter used, duration of protection, retrieval, and possibly concurrent systemic anticoagulation.

INDICATIONS FOR FILTER RETRIEVAL

Any filter that can be retrieved and is no longer required or effective should be removed as soon as possible. If the patient's underlying risk for PE has returned to baseline or if the patient has become a candidate for anticoagulation, the filter should be removed. If the filter itself is ineffective (migrated, kinked, fractured), it should be removed and, if necessary, replaced. Active bacteremia is a strong relative contraindication to filter placement. Nevertheless, in some cases of active bacteremia, a filter may become necessary. The filter should be considered a source of infection (even if blood cultures are negative) and removed or replaced as soon as it is no longer required or bacteremia resolves.

CONTRAINDICATIONS FOR FILTER RETRIEVAL

A clotted filter cannot be removed because it creates the risk of sending the clot to the lungs. Thus many filters that are labeled as retrievable will become permanent. Another contraindication to filter removal is persistence of clot in the pelvic or lower-extremity veins unless the patient can now receive anticoagulation therapy. Unless the risk for PE normalizes and the patient is still not a candidate for anticoagulation, the filter cannot be removed. A nonretrievable filter is designed to stay in place, and thus removal, although technically possible in experienced hands, creates a risk for IVC rupture.

COMPLICATIONS

Complications related to IVC filters are periprocedural or delayed (Table 3). Periprocedural complications include filter malpositioning, migration, iatrogenic pulmonary embolism, groin hematoma, or infection. All of these complications can be avoided with experience and proper patient preparation. Meticulous technique and experience can prevent malpositioning; choice of appropriate filter can prevent migration; and proper technique and patient care can prevent hematoma and infection. The rates of these complications are listed in Table 3 and range from 0% to 6%. The most feared complication of IVC filters is filter thrombosis, with subsequent IVC occlusion and possible PE. IVC thrombosis after filter placement is reportedly between 2% and 19%; however, the risk increases with time, and long-term risk is unknown.

TECHNIQUE

The role of an IVC filter is to minimize the risk for PE. Optimal performance requires catheter expertise, proper venous access selection, appropriate filter type selection, and proper location and orientation of filter. First, the clinical indication for IVC filter

Table 3: Complications from IVC Filter Placement

Complication Type	Rate (%)
Filter thrombosis	2–19
Filter migration/ malposition	2–6
Groin hematoma	3–4
Groin infection	<1
Iatrogenic pulmonary embolism	1

IVC, Inferior vena cava.
With the exception of in situ filter thrombosis, the associated risks are minimal (1%-6%). However, inferior vena cava thrombosis can lead to considerable morbidity, including pulmonary embolism and symptoms of lower-extremity venous stasis. Long-term follow-up of patients with filters is limited, and the true risk of IVC thrombosis is unknown. Removal of a filter that is no longer needed or is ineffective (kinked, fractured, source of pulmonary embolism in upper extremities) is indicated to minimize this risk.

placement should be confirmed. Then review of imaging studies and physical examination of the patient dictate appropriate venous access selection. For example, common femoral vein thrombosis precludes use of this vein for access lest an iatrogenic PE is caused. Next, the choice of filter becomes crucial. If permanent anticoagulation is required, one may place a permanent or retrievable filter. If there is any question as to whether it will be necessary to retrieve the filter, a retrievable one should be placed. The Günther-Tulip (Cook Medical, Bloomington, IN) and OptEase (Cordis J&J, Roden, The Netherlands) filters are the only filters that carry an indication for retrievability. Technically they can be removed up to 3 or 4 weeks after placement because epithelial overgrowth sets at that time. Interestingly, even though the G2 filter (C.R. Bard, Murray Hill, NJ) is not approved for retrievability, it is technically retrievable indefinitely. Its predecessor, the G1, did have U.S. Food and Drug Administration approval for indefinite retrievability, and it has the same design. An IVC venogram before filter placement is necessary to ensure the following:

1. the IVC is not thrombosed,
2. the IVC is 30 mm or less (otherwise use Bird's Nest filter [Cook Medical, Bloomington, IN]),
3. there is no duplicated IVC, and
4. the filter is deployed below renal veins.

Figure 2 shows the critical aspects of IVC filter deployment. Filter retrieval is more challenging and requires more extensive

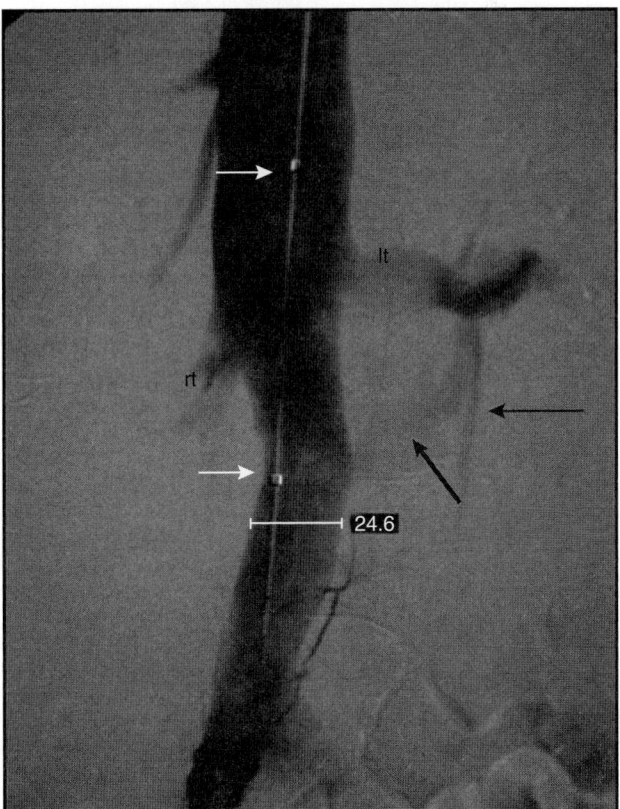

Figure 2 Prefilter deployment inferior vena cava *(IVC)* venogram from a jugular approach. The sheath markers *(white arrows)* are used as calibration and are 5 cm apart. The right *(rt)* and left *(lt)* renal veins are noted, as is a normal variant left circumaortic renal vein *(block arrows)*. The filter must be placed below that, otherwise a clot may bypass the filter via the left circumaortic drainage. The IVC diameter was measured to be 24.6 mm, allowing for secure filter deployment. The black arrow points to the left gonadal vein draining into the left renal vein.

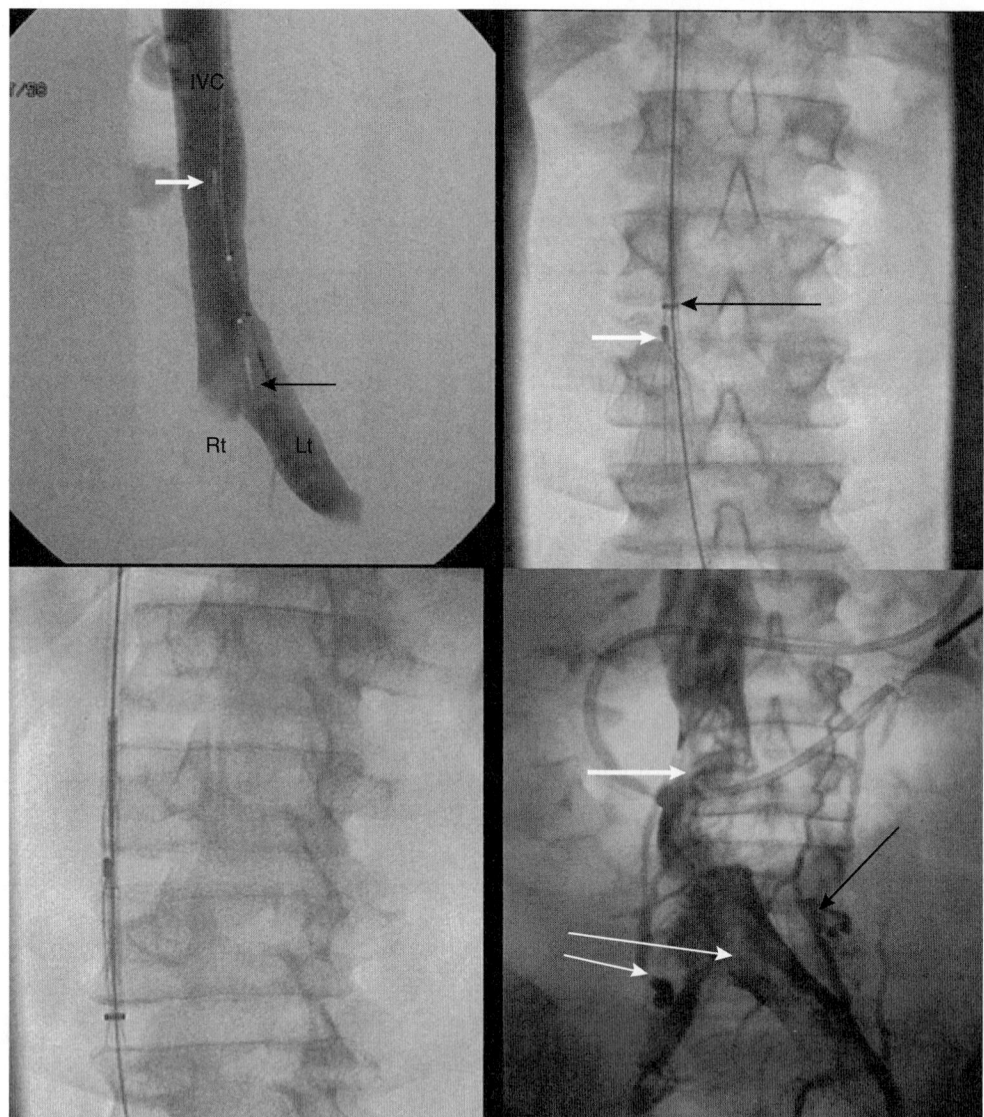

Figure 3 Retrieval of G2 filter. A preretrieval venogram **(A)**, performed via the catheter placed in the *(arrow)*, excludes clot in the right *(rt)* and left *(lt)* common iliac veins and in the IVC. The filter tip is indicated by block arrow. **(B)** The sheath is advanced over the conical retrieval system *(arrow)*, which grabs the cephalad tip of the filter *(block arrow)*. The filter is pulled into the sheath, and both are then removed en block **(C)**. Preretrieval IVC venogram in another patient **(D)** shows a large burden of clot in the filter *(block arrow)* and iliac vein *(white arrows)*, as well as collateral drainage *(white arrow)* precluding filter removal.

skills. First, one must ensure that filter removal will not leave a patient with increased risk for PE for lack of protection. Proper access depends on the type of filter used. The G2 and Günther-Tulip filters are removed via a jugular approach, the OptEase via a femoral approach. IVC and iliac venograms are required to exclude residual clot. Figure 3 shows the steps for removal for a G2 filter.

Special Considerations: Suprarenal Inferior Vena Cava Filter

The ideal location of any IVC filter is such that the filter is properly centered (not skewed), with its cephalad tip at or a few millimeters below the lowest renal vein. Placing the filter too low may result in a higher rate of IVC thrombosis because of the turbulent flow caused by the filter. Placing the filter above or across the renal veins

may result in renal failure if the filter thromboses and the resulting clot obstructs the renal vein drainage. Rarely, however, placing a filter in a suprarenal location is necessary despite this higher risk. Indications for suprarenal IVC filter placement are tabulated in Table 4. Whatever the indication, if feasible any suprarenal IVC filter should be removed as soon as the risk of PE returns to baseline. Therefore retrievable filters are preferred in this location.

DISCUSSION

IVC filters have demonstrated efficacy in preventing PE and saving lives. However, as with any other medical device, there are associated risks in both the immediate and long term. In addition, there has been an explosive increase in IVC filter use since the mid-1990s that is likely to continue with the advent of more versatile filters and increased incidence of DVT. It is therefore prudent to select patients properly and

Table 4: Indications for Suprarenal IVC Filters

Indications for Suprarenal IVC Filter Placement	Notes
Renal vein thrombosis	Consider catheter directed thrombolysis and filter removal
Pregnancy	Uterine compression may dislodge infrarenal filter
IVC clot above renal veins or above IVC filter	Consider catheter-directed thrombolysis and filter removal
PE from gonadal vein thrombus	May coil embolize gonadal vein and avoid filter
Duplicated IVC	May instead place two infrarenal filters
Short infrarenal IVC	May instead place two common iliac filters

IVC, Inferior vena cava; *PE,* pulmonary embolism.
Suprarenal IVC filters have a higher risk for IVC thrombosis and possible subsequent renal-vein obstruction and renal failure. On occasion, however, such a filter may be indicated. Clinical scenarios that call for suprarenal IVC filters are uncommon and are shown in the table. The most common indication is IVC clot extending above the renal veins. Whatever the indication, every effort should be made to retrieve the filter if it is no longer clinically indicated.

ensure that placing an IVC filter is truly indicated. The clinical scenario for each patient is different, affecting the choice of filter, retrievability, location, duration, and associated risks. When the interventional radiologist is unsure about the duration of required protection, a retrievable filter should be selected. Any filter that is no longer providing its intended benefit—whether because the underlying risk for PE has returned to baseline or the filter is ineffective—should be removed as soon as possible. The longer a filter remains, the more likely it will become permanent because of clot formation or endothelialization.

Suggested Readings

Audibert G, Faillot T, Vergnes MC, and others: Thromboprophylaxis in elective spinal surgery and spinal cord injury, *Ann Fr Anesth Reanim* 24:928, 2005.

Bick RL: Heredity and acquired thrombophilia: preface, *Semin Thromb Hemost* 25:251, 1999.

Capstick T, Henry MT: Efficacy of thrombolytic agents in the treatment of pulmonary embolism, *Eur Respir J* 26:864, 2005.

Crane C: The Mobin-Uddin inferior vena cava filter, *Arch Surgery* 103:661, 1971.

Dovrish Z, Hadary R, Blickstein D, and others: Retrospective analysis of the use of inferior vena cava filters in routine hospital practice, *Postgrad Med J* 82:150, 2006.

Garcia D, Ageno W, Libby E: Update on the diagnosis and management of pulmonary embolism, *Br J Haematol* 131:301, 2005.

Goldhaber SZ: Prevention of recurrent idiopathic venous thromboembolism, *Circulation* 110:(suppl 1):IV20, 2004.

Hann CL, Streiff MB: The role of vena cava filters in the management of venous thromboembolism, *Blood Rev* 19:179, 2005.

Heit JA: The epidemiology of venous thromboembolism in the community: implications for prevention and management, *J Thromb Thrombolysis* 21:23, 2006.

Jamieson SW, Nomura K: Indications for and the results of pulmonary thromboendarterectomy for thromboembolic pulmonary hypertension, *Semin Vasc Surg* 13:236, 2000.

Johns JS, Nguyen C, Sing RF: Vena cava filters in spinal cord injuries: evolving technology, *J Spinal Cord Med* 29:183, 2006.

Kucher N, Rossi E, Rosa M, and others: Massive pulmonary embolism, *Circulation* 113:577, 2006.

Linsenmaier U, Rieger J, Schenk F, and others: Indications, management, and complications of temporary inferior vena cava filters, *CardioVasc Inter Rad* 21:464, 1998.

Lopez JA, Kearon C, Lee AY: Deep venous thrombosis, *Hematology Am Soc Hematol Educ Program* 439, 2004.

Piazza G, Goldhaber S: Acute pulmonary embolism. Part I: epidemiology and diagnosis, *Circulation* 114:28, 2006.

Sing RF, Camp SM, Heniford BT, and others: A timing of pulmonary emboli after trauma: implications for retrievable vena cava filters, *J Trauma* 60:732, 2006.

Stein PD, Kavali F, Olson RE: Twenty-one year trends in the use of inferior vena cava filters, *Arch Intern Med* 164:1541, 2004.

Tapson VF, Humbert M: Incidence and prevalence of chronic thromboembolic pulmonary hypertension: from acute to chronic pulmonary embolism, *Proc Am Thorac Soc* 3:564, 2006.

Thabut G, Thabut D, Myers RP, and others: Thrombolytic therapy of pulmonary embolism: a meta-analysis, *J Am Coll Cardiol* 40:1660, 2002.

PREVENTION OF VENOUS THROMBOEMBOLISM

Eric Peden, MD, and Alan B. Lumsden, MD, ChB

INTRODUCTION

Prevention of perioperative complications is one of the most important aspects of patient surgical care. Venous thromboembolism (VTE) continues to be a major risk in the perioperative period of surgical patients. Observational studies have documented that nearly half of patients diagnosed with deep venous thrombosis (DVT) in the hospital were not treated with prophylaxis. Autopsy studies have shown, as well, that for the majority of cases of confirmed pulmonary embolism (PE), the diagnosis was not considered before death. PE accounts for up to 10% of hospital deaths and has been targeted as the most preventable cause of hospital deaths by the Agency for Healthcare Research and Quality, highlighting the importance of this topic. VTE prophylaxis has been shown to be efficacious, with reduction of deep venous thrombosis by 70% or more. It is widely accepted that reducing DVTs reduces the incidence of PE. Furthermore, prophylaxis is cost effective. Studies continue to show, however, underutilization of prophylaxis. This underutilization appears to be related to perception of VTE as a low-incidence event, a lack of acceptance of the importance of VTE prophylaxis, and concerns in surgical patients about hemorrhagic complications. Orthopedic patients, in particular those requiring hip or knee replacement, have the highest incidence of VTE (40%-60%) if no prophylaxis is used, and consequently educational efforts have resulted in this being the patient population most consistently treated with prophylaxis.

One of the best sources of information on VTE continues to be the reports from the American College of Chest Physicians (ACCP) Conference on Antithrombotic and Thrombolytic Therapy, most recently published in 2004. This group reviews published literature and performs detailed analysis, allowing evidence-based guidelines and recommendations.

INCIDENCE

In studies in which venography or duplex ultrasound was used for screening, DVT has been estimated to occur in up to 40% of general surgical patients if no prophylaxis is used. Twenty-five percent of those DVTs are proximal deep veins that are much more likely to cause symptoms and result in PE. Most cases discovered by screening are asymptomatic calf DVTs. Ten to twenty percent of calf DVTs, however, are thought to progress to more proximal DVTs. It has been estimated that half or more of DVTs begin intraoperatively, but certainly not all. Several of these clots resolve spontaneously, and addition of postoperative prophylactic agents facilitates this resolution. For patients at greatest risk, longer duration of prophylaxis correlates with further reductions in DVT incidence, adding evidence to the concept that many DVTs develop later in the course. The majority of symptomatic DVTs related to hospitalizations become evident after discharge. The diagnostic test of choice continues to be duplex ultrasound, with the hallmarks of acute DVT being noncompressibility with venous distention and a hypoechoic lumen, as seen in Figure 1. The 1-year mortality rate of DVT has been found to be 16% to 30%, with most deaths occurring within the first month, and this is at least three times as high as age-matched control patients without DVT, although this likely reflects increased comorbidity in this cohort.

CONSEQUENCE

The consequence of DVT continues to be a major clinical problem despite advances in medicine. The potential complications of DVT include: worsening acute venous symptoms, with development of phlegmasia and potential limb loss; pulmonary embolism and subsequent death; recurrent thromboembolic events; and the development of chronic venous insufficiency caused by postthrombotic syndrome. The development of postthrombotic syndrome is a function of the extent of thrombosis, its subsequent effect on venous valvular competence, and long-term residual obstruction. The consequences of postthrombotic syndrome and chronic venous insufficiency are severe, with persistent edema, pain, and recurring skin problems including ulcerations. These problems lead to decreased quality of life and considerable economic burden. The annual costs of postthrombotic syndrome are estimated at more than $1 billion in the United States, underlining the importance of this disease process.

RISK FACTORS

Several risk factors have been identified for DVT and are listed in Table 1. More than a century since the original description by Virchow of the triad of risk factors—stasis, hypercoagulability, and endothelial injury—most risk factors can still be attributed to these categories. Previous prophylaxis recommendations were based on risk assessment models assigning varying degrees of weight to the different risk factors; however, this is cumbersome. Current prophylactic recommendations from the ACCP are generalized to type of surgery, with considerations of additional risk factors.

PROPHYLACTIC MODALITIES

Because the incidence of asymptomatic DVT is higher than symptomatic DVT or PE, the studies on which recommendations can be based relied principally on DVTs found on screening studies for the primary endpoint. Clearly the least costly and for many patients a highly effective prophylactic method is early mobilization. For patients who are medically and physically able to get out of bed and at low risk for VTE, this is sufficient. Patients at higher risk, however, require more active means of VTE prophylaxis.

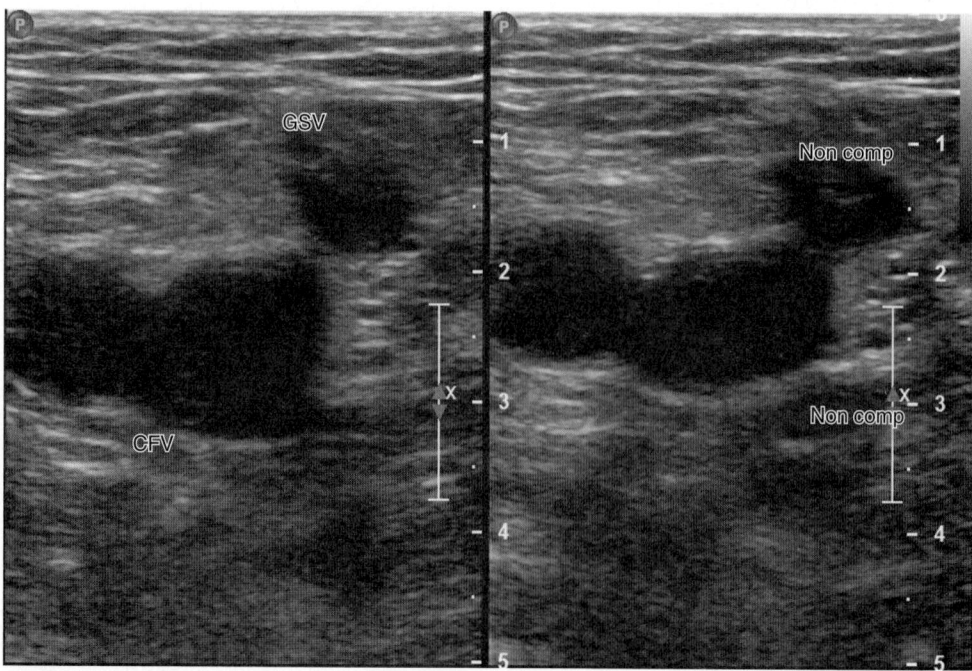

Figure 1 Duplex ultrasound.

Table 1: Risk Factors for VTE

Previous VTE
Hypercoagulability states
Malignancy
Increasing age
Immobility
Paralysis/paraplegia
Trauma
Surgery
Estrogen-based contraception and replacement therapy
Obesity
Smoking
Indwelling venous catheters
Acute medical illness
Cardiopulmonary system failure
Inflammatory bowel disease
Nephrotic syndrome
Paroxysmal nocturnal hemoglobinuria

VTE, Venous thromboembolism.

Mechanical

Mechanical means of DVT prophylaxis include graduated compression stockings, sequential compression devices (SCDs), and venous foot pumps. The mechanism of action is reduction in stasis and perhaps a local increase in fibrinolytic activity. The attraction of using mechanical prophylaxis is the lack of any anticoagulant activity and thus no increased bleeding concerns. It is therefore most useful in patients who are deemed to be at high risk of bleeding complications from pharmacologic prophylaxis. In direct comparison studies, mechanical prophylaxis has been found to be better than no prophylaxis but less effective than pharmacologic means. Compression stockings should be used with caution in patients with significant arterial insufficiency because there are reports of worsening limb ischemia and tissue loss. Perhaps the biggest problem with mechanical prophylaxis, however, is compliance. First, stockings must be adequately sized and properly fitted. Compression devices work only when used properly, but in clinical practice they commonly are found at the foot of the bed or on the floor in the patient's room. This compliance issue has been discussed and studied in the literature. It appears that outside of clinical trials in which compliance is carefully maintained, day-to-day use proves less reliable and is less efficacious. Most encouraging for mechanical prophylaxis is the finding that when combined with pharmacologic prophylaxis, there is enhanced protection over pharmacologic treatment alone. This additive effect is predictable given the approach of both relieving venous stasis and correcting or preventing hypercoagulability.

Pharmacologic

The most effective single modality of prophylaxis for VTE in surgical patients is pharmacologic. Although an in-depth discussion of the pharmacologic mechanism of the various agents is beyond the scope of this chapter, a brief review of the mechanisms of action is in order to understand the various drugs and their unique properties.

Low-dose, unfractionated heparin (UFH) has been in clinical use for many years. In general surgery patients, UFH has been shown to reduce VTE by 70%. UFH works by binding to antithrombin (formerly referred to as antithrombin III) and greatly enhancing its activities. The effects are predominately against activated factor X (Xa) and thrombin. Additional antithrombotic effects include

release of a tissue factor pathway inhibitor and some binding of platelets. UFH is cleared by both the liver and the kidneys, although the majority seems to be hepatic clearance, and it is the first-pass hepatic clearance that leads to a shorter half-life, compared with the low-molecular-weight heparins (LMWHs). A downside to UFH is the somewhat unpredictable treatment response in terms of dosing for full anticoagulation. This variability appears to be due largely to UFH binding to plasma proteins, endothelial cells, and macrophages. It is principally the binding to plasma proteins that leads to problems with predictability. This problem is most evident when therapeutic anticoagulation is desired and there is considerable variability, which necessitates frequent laboratory monitoring. It is also this binding to plasma proteins, specifically platelet factor 4, that can lead to heparin-induced thrombocytopenia (HIT). The standard prophylactic dosing regimens for UFH are 5000 U subcutaneously 1 to 2 hours preoperatively and then continued two or three times daily until the patient is ambulatory or is discharged home. The more frequent dosing seems to be somewhat more effective without increased complications noted. Bleeding risk from UFH in prophylactic doses has been shown to be 2% higher than placebo, but most of these instances are wound hematoma because major bleeding has not been found to be higher than placebo.

LMWH compounds have been thoroughly tested in surgical patients. LMWHs work by binding to and markedly enhancing the activity of antithrombin. In contrast to UFH, there is much more specificity against activated factor X with little effect against thrombin. Decreased binding to plasma proteins translates into increased bioavailability and longer half-life, enabling daily dosing. It is this more predictable availability and activity that allow weight-based dosing without monitoring. In contrast to UFH, LMWH is cleared almost entirely by the kidneys. It is therefore less predictable in patients with severe renal insufficiency, defined in most studies as a creatinine clearance of less than 30 ml/min. This is particularly important in therapeutic dosing of LMWH for VTE. In those cases, monitoring with anti-Xa levels is prudent. Also in morbidly obese patients, defined as body mass index (BMI) greater than 50, dosing of LMWH is less predictable and requires monitoring during full anticoagulation. Decreased binding to plasma proteins, specifically platelet factor 4, results in a decreased incidence of HIT. Even so, patients with HIT should not receive LMWH because cross reactivity with UFH does occur. Another benefit of LMWH is that long-term dosing is associated with decreased rates of osteoporosis compared with UFH. Common prophylactic dosing regimens for LMWH include enoxaparin 40 mg subcutaneously daily, enoxaparin 30 mg subcutaneously twice a day, and dalteparin 2500 to 5000 U daily, depending on the level of risk of VTE. LMWH has been shown to be equally efficacious to UFH in general surgical patients, with no consistent benefit and similar rates of bleeding. In higher-risk patients, such as cancer patients, trauma patients, and joint replacement patients, LMWH has been shown to be more efficacious than UFH. LMWH is more expensive than UFH, and this must be considered in the choice of agents.

Warfarin (Coumadin; Bristol-Myers Squibb, New York, NY) is an oral anticoagulant commonly used for treatment of VTE. It is a competitive inhibitor of production of vitamin K–dependent clotting factors in the liver. In general surgery, it is not used for perioperative VTE prophylaxis. In some orthopedic procedures, however, it is commonly used as a prophylactic anticoagulant. Its delayed onset of action allows for resolution of any perioperative bleeding tendencies prior to full effect.

Aspirin therapy is considered ineffective for VTE prophylaxis. Original support came from collections of small studies with small numbers of patients, conducted some time ago. More modern studies involving aspirin have shown considerable inferiority to LMWHs and UFH. Additionally, aspirin has been linked to increased bleeding, leading to further discouragement of its use.

Fondaparinux is a relatively new synthetic agent that contains the pentasaccharide sequence common to both UFH and LMWH. It has been approved for thromboprophylaxis in hip and knee joint replacement surgery. It has better bioavailability and a greater half-life than LMWH. Results in joint surgery patients suggest that it is somewhat more effective than LMWH but associated with a higher incidence of bleeding complications.

Ximelagatran is a direct thrombin inhibitor that is taken orally and has predictable bioavailability because no food or drugs have been shown to affect its absorption. It has been studied for VTE prophylaxis in orthopedic patients and appears to be equally efficacious as LMWH. At present, however, it has not yet received U.S. Food and Drug Administration approval but is potentially an exciting drug in the future because of its oral administration and the fact that it does not require routine laboratory monitoring.

RECOMMENDATIONS FOR VENOUS THROMBOEMBOLISM PROPHYLAXIS

The ACCP recommendations for general surgery patients can be broken down to four levels of risk as seen in Table 2, which is adapted from the latest report from that conference. Clearly, the type and length of surgery are directly related to the incidence of VTE. In general, UFH and both LMWHs work better than mechanical prophylaxis, and LMWH-treated patients have fewer asymptomatic DVTs; overall, however, symptomatic DVT, PE, risk of death, and complications are similar between the two agents.

In the low-risk group of patients, no specific prophylaxis is required, given the extremely low incidence of VTE in this patient population. This recommendation includes patients undergoing relatively minor procedures such as laparoscopic cholecystectomy. In this instance, however, the ACCP recommendations differ from the European Association for Endoscopic Surgery (EAES) and the Society of American Gastrointestinal Endoscopic Surgeons (SAGES), which recommend prophylaxis for laparoscopy, at least in the form of SCDs.

It is recommended that moderate-risk patients be treated with prophylaxis that can consist of UFH at twice-daily dosing or LMWH. It is recommended that high-risk patients be treated with prophylaxis that consists of UFH at three times daily dosing or LMWH. It is recommended that highest-risk patients be treated with prophylaxis that consists of UFH at three times daily or LMWH, combined with compression stockings, SCDs, or both. In select general surgery patients at highest risk, such as those undergoing cancer surgery, consideration should be given to prolonged prophylaxis after hospital discharge, up to 1 month.

Interestingly, vascular surgery patients appear to be at low risk for VTE. Randomized trials have demonstrated no benefit over placebo, although the numbers are small. The ACCP recommends no specific VTE prophylaxis unless additional risk factors are present, in which case it recommends UFH or LMWH. Preoperative dosing is rarely necessary because most of these patients receive UFH

intraoperatively, but postoperative treatment should be considered for those who remain at bed rest for a prolonged period.

Trauma patients—in particular, those with spinal cord injury, severe brain injury, pelvic fracture, and others with lengthy periods of immobilization—are at especially high risk for VTE, demonstrated to be 60% or greater. In studies of this group, LMWH has been found to be superior to UFH, with 60% less proximal DVTs. Therefore it is recommended that these patients be treated with LMWH. If the patients cannot be treated with LMWH because of bleeding concerns, mechanical prophylaxis should be initiated and then LMWH started after the risk of bleeding is reduced. For patients with prolonged immobility, the ACCP recommends prophylaxis until discharge, including any period of inpatient rehabilitation. Burn patients are also at risk for VTE and are recommended to have prophylaxis with UFH or LMWH.

Prophylactic Inferior Vena Cava Filters

Placement of prophylactic inferior vena cava (IVC) filters is effective for prevention of PE. Naturally, there is no impact on incidence of DVT because filters are not a DVT-prophylactic measure. Accepted indications for IVC filters are patients with PE despite anticoagulation, patients with DVT or PE and a contraindication to anticoagulation or a complication of anticoagulation, and patients requiring pulmonary embolectomy for PE. Relative indications have included patients with large DVTs (free-floating, iliofemoral DVTs), problems with compliance with anticoagulant therapy, and those with VTE and limited cardiopulmonary reserve. Although incidence of complications is small, IVC filters do pose some risk of caval thrombosis and by some reports increase the chance of future DVT. These factors and the fact that many patients are at greatest risk for PE for a relatively short period of time have led to the development of retrievable IVC filters. The relatively recent development of these retrievable IVC filters and their demonstrated safety of removal as long as 1 year after implantation has encouraged the placement of these filters in a large number of patients. Prophylactic, retrievable filters have been most commonly placed in patients considered to be at high risk for VTE in whom anticoagulation is not advisable or is contraindicated, such as trauma patients with spine or brain injuries and patients undergoing morbid obesity procedures. Review of the literature, however, shows no strong evidence to support those practices, likely because even in those patient groups, PE is still an uncommon occurrence. The indications for placement of retrievable filters therefore remains in evolution and is currently based on individual or regional practice patterns until large trials are available to provide evidence to support specific recommendations.

Table 2: American College of Chest Physicians Recommendations for General Surgery Patients

Low risk	Minor procedure with age <40 and no additional risk factors
Moderate risk	Minor procedure in patients with additional risk factors Major procedure with age 40–60 and no additional risk factors
High risk	Age >60 or age 40–60 with additional risk factors Prior VTE, malignancy, hypercoagulability
Highest risk	Surgical patients with multiple risk factors Major trauma, hip or knee replacement, spinal cord injury

VTE, Venous thromboembolism.

CONCLUSIONS

Probably the most important factor in VTE prophylaxis is simply the recognition of its necessity. Multiple studies now have demonstrated that a computer prompt increases use of VTE prophylaxis and in some studies has significantly reduced rates of VTE. Clearly there is an ongoing need for continuing education about the importance of VTE prophylaxis. Choice of prophylactic modality is best made on the basis of risk-group assessment, with individual adjustment based on certain high-risk groups, such as in patients with previous VTE. Mechanical and pharmacologic prophylactic measures will continue to predominate modern practice. Pharmacologic prophylaxis remains the most effective method, and UFH offers protection equivalent to LMWH in relatively low-risk surgical patients at a reduced cost. In high-risk patients, LMWH is more efficacious, and the highest-risk patients should be treated with both LMWH and mechanical devices. Future developments will likely include the approval of oral agents with greatly improved ease of administration. It is hoped that the role for removable filters will become better defined with further study.

Suggested Readings

Alastair J, and others: Low-molecular-weight heparins, *N Engl J Med* 337:688, 2006.

Geerts WH, Pineo GF, Heit JA, and others: Prevention of venous thromboembolism, *Chest* 126:338S, 2004.

Kaufman J, Kinney TB, Streiff MB, and others: Guidelines for the use and retrievable and convertible vena cava filters: Report from the society of interventional radiology multidisciplinary consensus conference, *J Vasc Int Rad* 17:449, 2006.

Kucher N, Koo S, Quiroz R, and others: Electronic alerts to prevent venous thromboembolism among hospitalized patients, *N Engl J Med* 352:969, 2005.

LYMPHEDEMA

Julie E. Park, MD, Paul N. Manson, MD, and E. Gene Deune, MD

PATHOPHYSIOLOGY

Lymphedema occurs when there is impaired uptake of lymphatics, resulting in an accumulation of protein-rich fluid in the interstitium of affected limbs or body parts. The increased protein concentration in the subcutaneous tissues raises the interstitial oncotic pressures. This increases the egress of fluids out of the vasculature, worsening the edema in the interstitium.

The remaining lymphatics develop massive dilatation and valvular incompetence. Subsequently, fibrosis of lymphatic walls and fibrinoid thrombi accumulation in the lumen obliterates the lymphatic channels. Lymph nodes harden, shrink, and lose normal architecture. The protein and fluid accumulation leads to increased inflammation. The increased macrophage activity leads to the destruction of elastic fibers and production of fibrosclerotic tissues. Fibroblasts migrate into the interstitium and deposit collagen.

Pitting edema progresses to brawny, nonpitting edema. The thickened skin can manifest peau d'orange from congested dermal lymphatics. The epidermis develops thick, scaly deposits of keratinized debris and verrucosis, creating cracks and furrows as entry ports for bacteria, leading to cellulitis or lymphangitis. The local immunologic surveillance is suppressed. The tissues are susceptible to chronic infections.

Lymphedema may progress to malignant degeneration to lymphangiosarcoma. This rare (0.07%-0.45%) condition, also known as Stewart-Treves syndrome, was reported first in postmastectomy patients with chronic upper-extremity lymphedema (Fig. 1). Presenting with reddish purple discoloration or nodule that tends to form satellite lesions, it may be confused with Kaposi sarcoma or traumatic ecchymosis. Treatment involves radical amputation and has extremely poor prognosis.

ETIOLOGY

Lymphedema is categorized as either primary or secondary. Primary lymphedema is congenital, with a genetic inheritance pattern, whereas secondary lymphedema is acquired. There are three types of congenital lymphedema, grouped according to the age of the patient when then lymphedema presents, although secondary lymphedema may have multiple etiologies (Table 1).

Lymphedema I, or Milroy's disease, is present at birth and typically affects the dorsum of the foot. Although chronic, the lymphedema typically is not progressive. Histologically, superficial or subcutaneous lymphatic vessels are aplastic or hypoplastic. There tends to be a 2:1 preference for females. Representing approximately 10% of primary lymphedemas, this is a genetic disorder that is autosomal dominant with variable penetration. The mutations

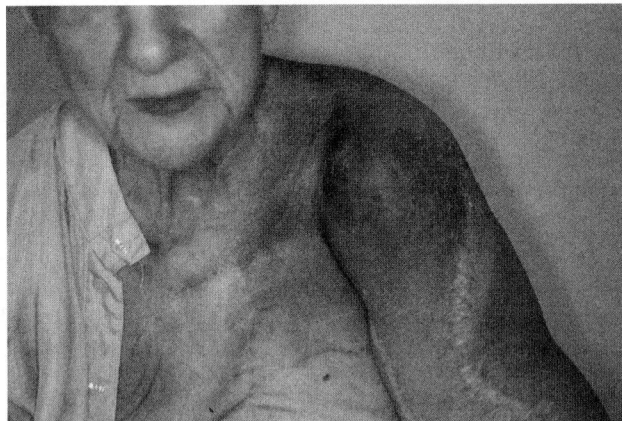

Figure I Stewart-Treves syndrome: malignant degeneration of long-standing lymphedema. This lymphangiosarcoma has a rare incidence but a poor prognosis.

Table I: Classifications of Lymphedema

Primary
● Birth
● Puberty
● Midlife

Secondary
● Parasitic
● Cancer
● Surgical—lymphadenectomy
● Metastasis
● Radiation
● Recurrent infections
● Obesity

for the gene for *VEGF-3*, a tyrosine receptor kinase, mapped to chromosome 3, have been implicated.

Lymphedema II, also called *lymphedema praecox* or *Meige's disease*, frequently presents approximately at puberty, but between the ages of 15 and 35. This is the predominant form of primary lymphedema (65%-80%). Typically affecting the lower extremities, the majority of these lymphedemas are unilateral, although bilateral involvement has been reported. The peripheral lymphatics are hypoplastic with dilatation of lymphatic trunks. Again, there is a predilection for females, and the inheritance is autosomal dominant. The *VEGFR-3* and *FOXC-2* genes are involved.

Lymphedema III is also called *lymphedema tarda* and presents itself in midlife, or after the age of 35. Again the lower extremities are targeted, and women are more often affected. The lymphatics

Table 2: Classifications of Degrees and Progression of Lymphedema

Stages	Grades
Latency—lymphatic capacity reduced • No visible/palpable edema • Subjective complaints	Grade 1—mild edema • Distal—forearm and hand or lower leg and foot • Difference in circumference <4 cm • Other tissue changes not yet present
Stage I—reversible lymphedema • Accumulation of protein rich fluid • Pitting edema • Reduces with elevation (no fibrosis)	Grade 2—moderate edema • Entire limb or quadrant of trunk • Difference in circumference >4 cm, <6 cm • Tissue changes apparent (pitting) • Infections
Stage II—spontaneously irreversible lymphedema • Accumulation of protein-rich fluid • Pitting becomes progressively more difficult • Connective tissue proliferation (fibrosis)	Grade 3a—severe edema • One limb + associated trunk quadrant • Difference in circumference >6 cm • Significant skin changes (cornification, keratosis, cysts, fistulae) • Repeated infections Grade 3b—massive edema • Two or more extremities affected
Stage III—lymphostatic elephantiasis • Accumulation of protein-rich fluid • Nonpitting • Fibrosis and sclerosis (severe induration) • Skin changes (papillomas, hyperkeratosis, etc.)	Grade 4—gigantic edema • Elephantiasis • Affected extremities large because almost complete blockage of lymph channels • May also affect head and face

Table 3: Risk Factors

• Lymph node surgeries
• Infections
• Deep, invasive wounds
• Radiation
• Morbid obesity
• Burns
• Parasitic infections
• Family history of primary lymphedema

are hyperplastic, tortuous, and increased in caliber and number. The valves are incompetent or absent. The *FOXC-2* gene is involved.

Secondary lymphedema is acquired, resulting as a sequela of infection, cancer, or morbid obesity. Worldwide the most common cause of lymphedema is infection with the parasite *Wuchereria bancrofti,* a nematode that is spread by a mosquito vector and resides in the lymphatic systems of infected patients, causing blockage and scarring.

In developed nations, lymphedema is usually secondary to cancer, resulting from surgical extirpation of cancer, lymphadenectomy, radiation, or lymphatic obstruction from metastatic disease. For the purposes of this chapter, the nonparasitic forms of lymphedema are discussed in terms of management and prognosis. Another rising cause of lymphedema is morbid obesity, which seems to cause obstruction by crushing lymphatics with the excessive weight.

The degree of lymphedema can be classified by either stages or by grades that compare the involved limb with a normal limb (see Table 2). The risk factors for lymphedema are outlined in Table 3.

DIAGNOSIS

The workup for lymphedema starts with a basic history and physical examination. Other causes for edema must be ruled out. These include, but are not limited to, cardiac, venous, renal, and hepatic causes and iliac compression syndrome. Imaging studies may be of some value. Historically lymphangiography was used to visualize the lymphatic channels. However, it became apparent that the procedure itself sclerosed lymphatic channels and often exacerbated the lymphedema. This

procedure has mostly been abandoned in favor of lymphangioscintigraphy, a nuclear medicine study that shows uptake and clearance of tracer. It does not, however, delineate specific lymphatic channels.

TREATMENT

Conservative Management

Treatment options are divided into conservative and surgical management. Conservative management involves various therapeutic modalities and pharmacology. The goal of conservative therapies is to avoid the stagnation of protein-rich edema in the interstitium and to stop the positive feedback cycles of inflammation, infection, and fibrosis. Most cases of lymphedema can be managed with conservative therapy, but this is completely dependent on strict patient compliance. Furthermore, the therapies are chronic and lifelong. Many of them are time-consuming, cumbersome, and uncomfortable. Psychosocial support in the form of counseling and support groups is also valuable to help increase patient compliance.

The therapies range from lifestyle modifications to compression pumps. Therapy starts simply with basic skin care and hygiene. Meticulous management of even minor traumas and rigorous use of moisturizers helps to maintain a supple skin barrier to minimize ports of entry for bacteria and fungus.

The patients must also work closely with a physical therapist for various forms of exercise, massage, and compression garments and wraps. Exercise is important for two reasons: facilitating weight loss and also increasing the return of lymphatics by the contraction of skeletal muscles. Various protocols exist for massage therapies or manual decompressive therapies with the goal of increasing lymphatic drainage by recruitment of existing, nondamaged lymphatics.

Compression is available in various forms of garments and wraps that are important adjuncts to these therapies. Low-stretch wraps or compression garments may be used. The pressure gradient should go from distal to proximal. Compression garments may require refitting as therapy continues and limb sizes change. Pneumatic compression devices may also be used. Elevation of the affected limb, especially at night, is also effective. Lifestyle modifications include avoidance of constrictive clothing and meticulous surveillance for skin trauma or breakdown.

Pharmacologic Therapy

The pharmacologic treatments for lymphedema play a secondary role in overall therapy. Antibiotics are valuable to control recurrent bouts of infection—both prompt treatment with oral and topical antibiotics to superficial skin infection and intravenous antibiotics for more serious cases of cellulitis and lymphangitis. Benzopyrenes are a family of drugs used to increase proteolysis of proteins in the edema in the interstitium to facilitate their absorption into the bloodstream and decrease the oncotic pressure in the interstitium. There are conflicting data in the literature regarding the efficacy of benzopyrene usage. Finally, diuretics have been used, the idea being that hemoconcentration might help to draw more fluid out of the interstitium. The benefits of long-term usage for lymphedema management are questionable.

Surgical Management—Excisional Procedures

Surgical therapies can be divided into debulking procedures and physiologic procedures. Debulking procedures are aimed at reducing the size and weight of the affected limb. The Charles procedure involves a radical excision of all subcutaneous tissues down to and including the fascia. A full-thickness skin graft is harvested from the excised tissue and is used to cover the muscle (Fig. 2). Historically, split-thickness skin grafts have been used for coverage, but over time this may lead to problems such as wound breakdown, ulcerations, and hyperkeratosis. Some consider the Charles procedure to be radical, with a high aesthetic morbidity. However, it still has a role in treating some cases of lymphedema in which limbs recalcitrant to conservative therapy have gained such a girth and weight as to make the patient bedridden.

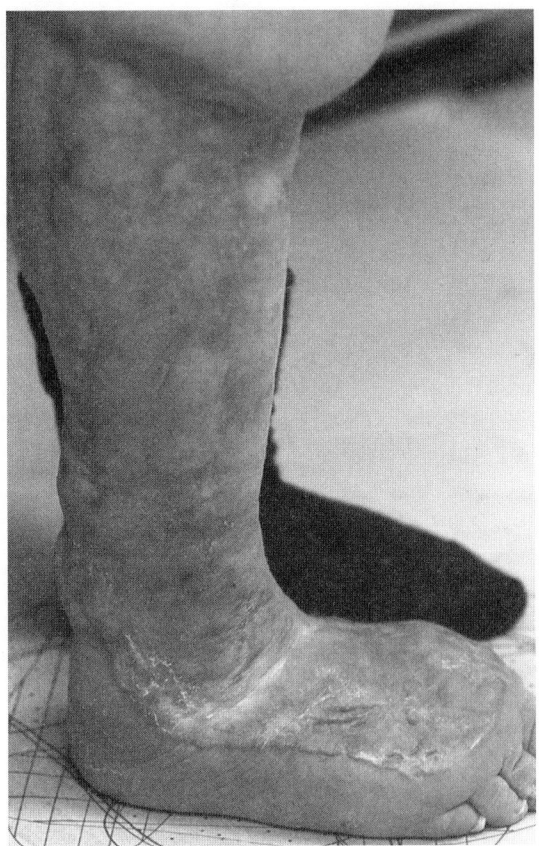

Figure 2 Lower extremity after Charles procedure.

The Thompson procedure can be described as both a debulking and a physiologic procedure. It involves excision of subcutaneous tissues, with the creation of de-epithelialized dermal flaps that are buried in the deep muscle. The theory behind this maneuver is to create a bridge between the superficial and deep lymphatic tissue in an attempt to improve lymphatic drainage. Although Thompson had fair long-term successes with his patients who had this procedure, it was most likely attributable to the excisional component of the procedure rather than the physiologic component because no evidence of bridging was ever found.

Sistrunk (1918) advocated using staged excision. This was then popularized in the United States by Homan (1936) and revisited again by Miller (1998). This technique involves staged, subcutaneous excisions of lymphedematous tissues beneath dermal flaps. Seventy percent of patients have 50% reduction in size at 8-year follow-up. Some of the complications include a 6% incidence of postoperative ischemic necrosis and a loss of sensation of 2 to 3 cm on either side of the incision. It is also not as effective in upper extremities.

Liposuction has been used as both a therapy and an adjunct to aid in debulking lymphedema. Described first in lymphedema of the upper extremity after mastectomy, it has also been cited in the literature as case reports for the lower extremity.

Surgical Management—Physiologic Procedures

The physiologic procedures are based on trying to reestablish lymphatic flow. Many various techniques have been tried, including insertion of threads and other foreign bodies to act as capillaries for lymphatic flow (which obviously failed). Flaps of omentum were also used without real success and led to potential complications such as hernia or obstruction.

Creation of lymphovenoshunts has also achieved varying rates of success. Rivero (1966) created lymph–node-venous shunt that had 100% obstruction at 3 months. In the late 1980s, O'Brien employed microsurgical techniques to create lymphovenous and lympholymphatic anastomosis. The long-term clinical effectiveness of microsurgical correction of lymphedema is mixed. More recently, applying the developments of supermicrosurgery (anastomosis of vessels 0.8 mm in diameter), some success has been reported in Asia.

Koshima (1996) studied the histology of the lymphatics of lymphedematous limbs. He found that the endothelial cells and smooth muscle cells in the proximal levels of the lymphatic trunks were damaged. The destruction of the smooth muscles cells leads to the loss of the tunica media and dilatation of thinned lymphatic wall. However, the small lymphatics of the distal limb tend to remain patent. These are also a better match for smaller, subdermal venules, the intravenous pressures of which are less than cutaneous veins, which are also more sensitive to external pressures. Therefore instead of anastomosing proximal, larger lymphatics and veins, Koshima favors creating lymphovenoanastomosis distally with smaller, patent lymphatics and venules.

An algorithm for conservative management of lymphedema is described in Table 4. Decompression of lymphedematous limbs first

Table 4: Treatment Algorithm

- Skin care
- Manual lymphatic drainage
- Compression bandaging
- Exercise
- ± Benzopyrene treatment
- Occupational therapy
- Psychological consultation/support group
- Nutrition counseling, weight loss
- Compression garment
- Home maintenance program

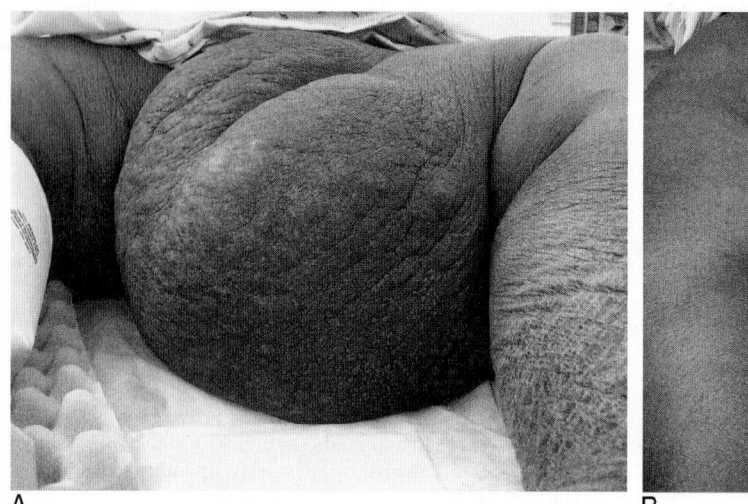
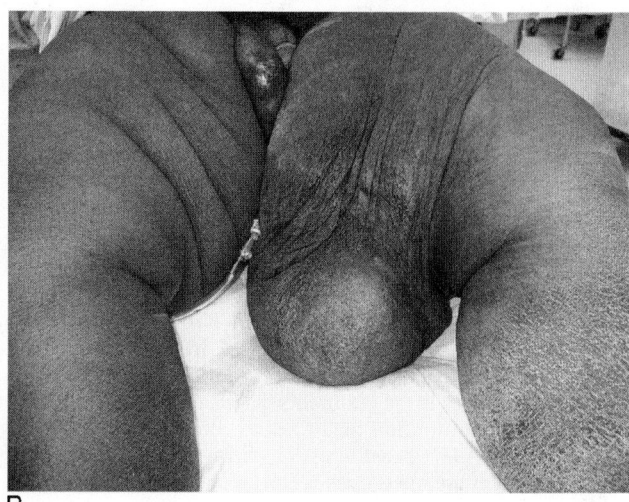

Figure 3 **(A)** Right lower-extremity lymphedema caused by obesity. **(B)** Debulking and skin softening after physical therapy, decompressive message, and compression garments. Subsequent surgical excision was carried out. Wound-healing complications are frequent.

Table 5: Surgical Indications

- Size and weight
- Lymphorrhagia
- Recurrent lymphangitis
- Abscess
- Fistula
- Malignant degeneration
- Failure of conservative measures
- ± Early microsurgical intervention

with compressive therapies can be effective to prepare for excision of excess tissues (Fig. 3). Frequently, wound-healing complications occur along the incision. Vacuum-assisted closure is useful in management of wound breakdown. Surgical indications are reviewed in Table 5.

CONCLUSIONS

Lymphedema is a chronic condition. Conservative measures aim at breaking the positive-feedback cycle of protein-rich fluid stagnation and inflammation. Surgical procedures attempt to either debulk tissues or reestablish physiologic conditions to drain lymph fluid. Patient motivation and psychosocial support are key elements in prognosis. Recent developments in identifying genes related to lymphedema lead to potential gene therapies in future.

SUGGESTED READINGS

Brennan MJ, Miller LT: Overview of treatment options and review of the current role and use of compression garments, intermittent pumps, and exercise in the management of lymphedema, *Cancer* 83:2821, 1998.

Koshima I, Kawada S, Moriguchi T, and others: Ultrastructural observations of lymphatic vessels in lymphedema in human extremities, *Plast Reconstr Surg* 97:397, 1996.

O'Brien BM, Mellow CG, Khazanchi RK, and others: Long-term results after microlymphaticovenous anastomoses for the treatment of obstructive lymphedema, *Plast Reconstr Surg* 85:562, 1990.

Miller TA, Wyatte LE, Rudkin GH: Staged skin and subcutaneous excision for lymphedema: a favorable report of long-term results, *Plast Reconstr Surg* 102:1486, 1998.

Nagase T, Gonda K, Inoue K et al: Treatment of lymphedema with lymphaticovenular anastomoses, *Int J Clin Oncol* 10:304, 2005.

TRAUMA AND EMERGENCY CARE

AIRWAY MANAGEMENT IN THE TRAUMA PATIENT

Robert C. Mackersie, MD, and Julin F. Tang, MD, MS

INTRODUCTION

Airway management is one of the most critical elements in the overall management of the severely injured patient. It is included as the first step in protocols for the management of the trauma patient, including those in advanced trauma life support (ATLS), and is incorporated into the ABCs of initial patient management (i.e., secure the airway, stabilize breathing, and obtain control of hemorrhage [circulation]). These ABCs are not a simple or convenient mnemonic but represent the fundamental philosophy of prioritizing the most critical aspects of care in a manner that reflects the potential consequences of delay or error.

Airway management is often thought of as primarily the technical act of placing a plastic tube in a patient's trachea. Airway management, however, encompasses a great deal more and involves a comprehensive array of elements designed to facilitate and improve oxygenation, ventilation, and the establishment and maintenance of a secure airway. These elements may include maneuvers as basic as a chin lift or the administration of oxygen or as technically complex as fiber-optic intubation or double-lung ventilation. Airway management also may involve the initiation and early management of mechanical ventilation during the resuscitation phase of trauma care. Regarding airway management as mostly a technical exercise involving endotracheal intubation will lead to errors and adverse outcomes in the management of a number of conditions and specific injury types encountered at the major trauma centers.

The decision to actively intervene or to not intervene in establishing a definitive airway is perhaps the most critical decision made early in the management of the trauma patient. As injury severity increases, so does the chance for precipitous and often unexpected clinical deterioration. In many circumstances, there is considerable unpredictability of the clinical course of certain types of injuries (clinical "trajectory") and critical risks associated with the loss of airway, oxygenation, or ventilation. In these cases, prophylactic intubation as a means of risk reduction may be a prudent decision. The use of prophylactic intubation as a risk reduction strategy weighs the potential complications of endotracheal intubation against the risks of clinical deterioration in the absence of a controlled airway and regulated oxygenation and ventilation.

CLINICAL GOALS

The therapeutic goals of airway management must consider the context of the type and severity of injury. Therapeutic goals generally pertain to acute deficits in oxygenation, ventilation, or the durable ability to maintain a patent airway (Table 1). In addition, the prophylactic use of airway management, including tracheal intubation, is often required to reduce the risk of potential deterioration in oxygenation, ventilation, or airway patency.

Often, the most common cause of airway obstruction encountered in a trauma population involves the loss of the normal airway reflexes associated with severe traumatic brain injury (TBI). The risk for airway compromise and that of secondary brain injury from hypoxia or hypercapnia increases as the Glasgow Coma Score (GCS) decreases. A GCS below 9 (attributable to TBI) is associated with a higher incidence of more severe cerebral injury and usually mandates the establishment of a secure airway and controlled oxygenation and ventilation. Deficiencies in oxygenation, often caused by direct lung injury or aspiration, may be mitigated by the delivery of high concentrations of O_2, as well as by the application of end-expiratory pressure. Deficiencies in ventilation and ventilatory capacity may occur in a variety of shock states as physiologic dead space increases and diaphragmatic blood flow decreases, as well as with direct injury to the chest wall, with or without associated diaphragmatic or abdominal injuries. Ventilatory insufficiency and airway compromise may be compounded by exogenous drugs, including alcohol and narcotics.

Perhaps the most common error made with regard to airway intervention during initial resuscitation is the failure to recognize patients at high risk for subsequent respiratory failure or progressive airway compromise. The issue is essentially one of patient safety and involves weighing the risks of planned rapid sequence induction/intubation (RSI) against the risks of subsequent (and usually untimely) patient deterioration and need for delayed "crash" intubation in radiology, transit, or elsewhere. Airway management, including tracheal intubation, should be viewed as a risk-reduction strategy in many circumstances, and there should be little hesitation in initiating these interventions in the setting of appropriate risk factors, including injury type, age, diagnostic uncertainty, and clinical trajectory.

CLINICAL AND PHYSIOLOGIC CONSIDERATIONS

Initial Clinical Assessment

The fundamentals of airway assessment are well described in a number of protocols, including ATLS. The presence of impeded or altered phonation, subjective dyspnea, tachypnea, hoarseness, respiratory stridor, hemoptysis, paradoxic breathing, chest wall

Table 1: Therapeutic Goals of Airway Management in the Trauma Patient

Therapeutic Goals	Clinical Situations
Augment airway protection ("secure" airway)	Relief from airway obstruction: edema, stenosis, external compression, direct injury, or airway hemorrhage. Loss of normal airway reflexes caused by depression in level of consciousness.
Augment oxygenation	Blunt chest trauma, pulmonary confusion, endobronchial hemorrhage, aspiration.
Augment ventilation	High cervical spine injuries, disrupted chest wall mechanics, specific abdominal trauma plus ruptured diaphragm, elderly patients with little reserve. Ability to regulate P_{CO_2} (severe traumatic brain injury).
Control Pa_{O_2} and Pa_{CO_2} within prescribed guidelines (certain injury types)	In traumatic brain-injured patients, must maintain cerebral oxygenation and prevent cerebral vasospasms or vasodilatation.
Risk reduction: prophylactic airway management	Anticipated or observed progressive deficiencies in oxygenation, ventilation, or progressive airway or anticipated airway obstruction (e.g., burns). Clinical need for risk reduction (to patient and/or providers) in cases of refractory agitation or belligerence when more severe injuries exist.

retractions, nasal flaring, cyanosis, and altered or absent breath sounds are commonly used to assess possible impairments in airway or breathing. Objective measures such as pulse oximetry, infrared capnography, or arterial blood gases may provide additional objective assessment. Although the presence of these clinical signs and symptoms may be important in determining the need for active airway intervention, the absence of these findings does not provide a high degree of negative prediction because many patients will develop progressive deficits in airway, oxygenation, or ventilation resulting from their underlying injuries.

Specific Injuries and Situations

Discussions of airway management often focus on the technical details of tracheal intubation, which can be an understandable source of performance anxiety (Will I be able to get the tube in?) for the clinician. This is in spite of the fact that the overwhelming majority (98%-99%) of acute tracheal intubations in the trauma patient are uncomplicated and straightforward. In most cases,

errors and complications result not from an inability to place a tube in the trachea but from a failure to consider the physiologic effects of airway management, including RSI and positive pressure ventilation, and to tailor airway management and timing to the physiologic needs and risks of a given clinical situation.

Intubation with positive pressure ventilation is rarely the definitive treatment for a given injury but rather a critical adjunctive measure that can have profound positive and negative physiologic effects. The positive effects have been discussed earlier in the context of achieving specific clinical goals. The negative effects are related to the pharmacologic agents used in RSI (discussed later) and the ability of positive pressure ventilation to cause physiologically profound decreases in venous return, cardiac preload, end-diastolic volume, and ultimately blood pressure in certain circumstances. A detailed discussion of injury pathophysiology related to intubation and positive pressure ventilation is beyond the scope of this chapter, but it is important that clinicians involved with airway management recognize the negative and positive effects of RSI and positive pressure ventilation and use this information in developing a plan for airway management (Table 2).

Table 2: Risks and Airway-Related Management Options in Specific Injuries

Risk	Suggested Management
Traumatic Brain Injury	
Loss of normal airway reflexes, ability to maintain patent airway, cerebral sensitivity to hypoxia (worse outcomes), or inappropriate cerebral vasoconstriction (low PA_{CO_2}) or cerebral vasodilatation (high PA_{CO_2})	Patients with a Glasgow Coma Score of 8 or less are at increased risk for having increased intracranial pressure and being more susceptible to changes in oxygenation or ventilation. Tracheal intubation and definitive airway control are indicated for most of these patients. RSI should avoid hypotension and involve agents designed with a neuroprotective effect in mind (see next section).
Spinal Cord Injury	
Majority of patients with C6 and above spinal cord injuries will require eventual intubation and even tracheostomy for definitive airway management, pulmonary toilet, and long-term care. Ventilatory insufficiency is produced by abdominal and thoracic wall muscular weakness and by diaphragmatic weakness with higher (C3-C5) cervical spine injuries. Normal swallowing reflexes may be impaired as well, leading to increased risk of aspiration.	Carefully controlled tracheal intubation (oral route preferred initially) followed by formal revision to a tracheostomy as dictated by the clinical situation (usually complete C6 levels and above). High thoracic and lower cervical (C7) injuries may not require tracheal intubation in the absence of other indications. Patients needing nonemergent intubation and having a high degree of mechanical instability of the cervical spine may require fiber–optic-assisted intubation.

Massive Facial Injury

Progressive edema leading to airway obstruction, oropharyngeal bleeding leading to massive bronchial aspiration of blood and secretions, a need for an operative intervention.	Tracheal intubation, oral route preferred if possible; emergent cricothyroidotomy necessary in many patients with more severe injuries all by elective conversion to formal tracheostomy.

Blunt Chest Trauma

Pulmonary contusion leading to severe oxygenation deficits, endobronchial bleeding. Disruption of chest wall leading to progressive ventilatory incapacity secondary to pain, with geriatric patients at much higher risk.	Management should be selective on the basis of the degree of oxygenation deficits or demonstrable acute ventilatory insufficiency. Directed analgesia (epidural) may provide pain relief sufficient to reduce the risk of subsequent ventilatory deterioration from more straightforward blunt chest wall trauma; obviate "prophylactic" intubation in these patients.

Shock, Hypotension

Dead space ratio increases with progressive hypovolemia, thereby increasing minute volume requirements. Lactic acidosis from shock may compound need for compensatory hyperventilation. Although blood flow to the diaphragm is conserved, more severe shock results in decreased diaphragmatic perfusion and secondary decreases in ventilatory capacity may lead to a need for intubation. There is a risk of exacerbating hypotension associated with positive pressure ventilation.	Hypovolemia/shock per se not an automatic indication for tracheal intubation. Decision whether to intubate should be made on the basis of the specific or presumed injury type producing the hypovolemia, observed patient response to fluid resuscitation, and expectations for immediate correction and need for definitive care (i.e., angiography, operating room). Full intubation should proceed in accordance with volume resuscitation.

Penetrating Lung Injuries

Respiratory distress may be caused by pneumothorax/tension pneumothorax, massive endobronchial bleeding, or hypovolemia (as described above). A small risk of air embolism may be associated with positive pressure ventilation in patients with more central penetrating lung injuries.	Pneumothorax/tension pneumothorax is managed by tube thoracostomy (not tracheal intubation, which may exacerbate both of these conditions). Massive endobronchial hemorrhage from penetrating lung injuries may be an indication for intubation both for oxygenation and to enable control of endobronchial hemorrhage (see section below). Decision whether to intubate is most often made on the basis of need for emergent operative intervention (thoracotomies) in these patients.

Tracheobronchial Injuries

Massive subcutaneous emphysema and secondary loss of airway (ballooning of soft tissues). Refractory lung collapse.	Acute respiratory distress from airway obstruction (vs. pneumothorax) may require emergent intubation. Fiber-optic assisted intubation may be necessary in some patients. Definitive treatment directed at "venting" the bronchial leak using pleural or, rarely, mediastinal tubes and effecting full lung reexpansion. Proximal tracheobronchial injuries may require operative repair.

Penetrating Cardiac Injury

Increased pericardial pressure leading to decreased end-diastolic volume leading to hypotension abnormal perfusion leading to respiratory embarrassment through the mechanisms described above. A very high risk from institution of positive pressure ventilation and subsequent diminution in pre-load precipitating further hypotension or even cardiac arrest.	Volume augmentation; rapid transport to OR; intubation performed in conjunction with the surgical team (after patient is prepared and draped), who are prepared to undertake immediate pericardial decompression repair. Severely hypotensive patients who require intubation in the emergency department often will require immediate resuscitative thoracotomy at that time. If possible, RSI/intubation should be deferred to the OR after the patient is prepped, draped, and the surgical team ready to perform immediate pericardial decompression.

Neck Injury (Blunt and Penetrating)

Neck bleeding causing secondary airway obstruction, endotracheal and secondary endobronchial bleeding, direct laryngeal trauma, causing stridor respiratory embarrassment.	Oral tracheal intubation preferred, and may require fiber-optic assist. This is best performed in the OR if patient's condition will tolerate this, and should be carried out in conjunction with the surgical team, who are prepared to perform an emergent cricothyroidotomy. Less severe cases can be transported to the OR and undergo conscious fiber-optic intubation with the surgical team on standby.

(continued)

Table 2: Risks and Airway-Related Management Options in Specific Injuries—Cont'd

Risk	Suggested Management
Geriatric Patients	
Elderly patients have decreased ventilatory capacity and less cardiac vascular reserve and may present with precipitous hypotension and more fragile chest walls. The effect of shock on ventilatory function may be pronounced in the geriatric population. Increased abdominal pressure resulting from abdominal hemorrhage or pelvic fractures may produce secondary respiratory embarrassment more frequently in this group.	Prophylactic intubation should be strongly considered in patients who will require any operative intervention or those requiring angioembolization for pelvic fractures. Patients with pulmonary contusions demonstrable on initial chest x-ray with any degree of respiratory embarrassment or deficiencies in gas exchange should usually undergo tracheal intubation.
Burns	
Airway edema caused by direct burn injury to the face and neck, massive volume resuscitation, or inhalational injury.	Suspected major inhalational injury, burns over more than 20% body surface area, those requiring early operative debridement, and patients with more focused but severe neck and facial burns should undergo early tracheal intubation.
Situational Control	
Altered behavior resulting from TBI, drugs, or psychiatric illness that creates a risk either to the patient or to the medical staff, interfering with patient care in life- or limb-threatening situations, or creating unnecessary risks to the medical staff.	RSI with tracheal intubation (oral route preferred) to facilitate resuscitation, control dangerous behavior, and institute life- or limb-saving therapy. Agitation may be an early sign of hypoxia or traumatic brain injury (e.g., frontal lobe contusion).

OR, Operating room; *RSI,* rapid sequence induction; *TBI,* traumatic brain injury.

Rapid Sequence Induction/Intubation in the Prehospital Setting

The relative risks and benefits of prehospital intubation remain somewhat controversial. Benefits of establishing and maintaining a secure airway with augmentation of oxygenation and ventilation must be weighed against the risks of the transient hypoxia, aspiration, and unrecognized esophageal intubation, particularly in settings in which individual prehospital providers may not have ongoing experience with difficult airway management. Perhaps the most common clinical scenario is one involving the patient with TBI. In this selected population, the risks and benefits of intubation, often requiring RSI, are amplified. Secondary brain injury may result from hypotension, prolonged hypoxia, or a significantly low or high $PaCO_2$. The safety of prehospital intubation or RSI for victims of TBI has been questioned recently in studies demonstrating adverse outcomes in this patient cohort when compared with historical or concurrent controls. This effect may be related to the tendency, in a poorly monitored situation, toward hyperventilation and induced hypocapnia, causing cerebral vasoconstriction and ischemia. An association between prehospital RSI, hyperventilation, and mortality has been reported. Additional work in this area suggests that when rigorous protocols for prehospital RSI are implemented and coupled with focused training programs and monitoring, the benefits of RSI for TBI patients may outweigh the risks.

Despite the relatively low incidence of unrecognized esophageal intubation and tube displacement during transport, every patient undergoing prehospital tracheal intubation must have the tube position confirmed immediately on hospital arrival. This is best accomplished by direct laryngoscopy, but alternatives such as chest x-rays, infrared capnography, and tube position may be used also.

Airway management in the trauma patient begins in the prehospital setting, and it is important that trauma programs maintain some degree of oversight over this activity, including provisions for ongoing training in airway management techniques for prehospital staff and the use of "rescue" intubation techniques, such as the use of the Combitube (Tyco-Kendall, Mansfield, MA), discussed later. Results of prehospital airway interventions, including the incidence of unrecognized esophageal intubations, should be monitored and compared with established benchmarks for purposes of performance improvement.

RAPID SEQUENCE INDUCTION

RSI is an organized, stepwise approach to endotracheal intubation designed to facilitate tube placement and minimize the risk of aspiration. It is often the definitive maneuver in emergency situations, including trauma. In addition to the placement of an endotracheal tube, RSI requires the administration of drugs to provide amnesia or unconsciousness, muscle relaxation, analgesia, and the reduction of undesirable autonomic reflex reactions to endotracheal tube placement. Although used in the majority of trauma patients requiring emergent intubation, RSI is not indicated or needed for patients arriving in profound shock without airway reflexes or those in cardiac arrest. In addition, high-risk patients with partial airway compromise, potentially depending on maintenance of upper airway muscle tone to maintain even partial airway patency, may be better served by conscious nasal intubation or fiber-optic intubation rather than risk loss of airway with RSI and the need to convert to a surgical or needle cricothyroidotomy.

The steps to performing RSI are outlined in Table 3. Most well-equipped emergency departments will stock the equipment and instruments required to perform and monitor RSI. Teamwork and preparation are critical, as are the decision and timing regarding the overall strategy of the trauma resuscitation. Close collaboration and clear communication among the physicians responsible for airway management and the resuscitation team leader will minimize complications related to the physiologic effects of RSI and positive pressure ventilation, as described earlier.

In the "heat of battle" during critical resuscitations, preoxygenation is sometimes neglected or minimized in the interest of immediate tube placement. Preoxygenation creates an oxygen "reservoir" in the airspaces that potentially allows a 3- to 6-minute period of apnea during RSI before significant desaturation occurs. It also may reduce CO_2 in the hypercapnic patient, an important consideration when dealing with patients with TBI.

Table 3: Steps for Performing Rapid Sequence Induction

Preparation and equipment	• Universal precautions • Airway equipment; laryngoscopes, endotracheal tubes, LMAs, needle cricothyrotomy kit, surgical airway kit • Oxygen source, suction device • Medications (hypnotics, muscle relaxants, pressors) • Tracheotomy tray, electrical defibrillator • Additional experienced assistants • Discussion with trauma team leader regarding timing
Monitoring	ECG monitoring, recurrent BP monitoring (often automated BP cuffs, pulse oximeter, in-line capnography).
Positioning (in-line stabilization of the cervical spine)	Requires an assistant to maintain gentle in-line stabilization and prevent neck extension in *all* patients at risk, based on mechanism or clinical findings, for cervical spine injury.
Preoxygenation	Administration of 100% O_2 by sealed face mask, with or without assisted ventilation. Prevents hypoxia during period of RSI-associated apnea.
IV access	Essential for the administration of RSI agents.
Cricothyroid pressure (Sellick maneuver)	All trauma patients should be considered to have full stomachs. Essential for compression of the esophagus posteriorly and reducing risk of aspiration.
Administration of hypnotic agents	Etomidate now the standard and most commonly used agent (see Table 4).
Administration of neuromuscular blocking agents	Succinylcholine remains the standard and most commonly used agent for RSI (see Table 5).
Placement of the endotracheal tube	Miller (straight) or MacIntosh (curved) blade. Visualization of the tip of the ETT passing through the vocal cords. Typical tube position: 21 cm at the incisors (women) or 23 cm (men). Placement at incisors for children approximately age (yrs)/2 + 12.
Manual ventilation and confirmation of physiologic response	Observed symmetric chest rise, auscultation with breath sounds over both lungs, fogging of the ETT with expiration, ballotable ETT balloon at suprasternal notch, normal ETco_2 tracing on capnography.

BP, blood pressure; *ECG,* electrocardiogram; *ETT,* endotracheal tube; *IV,* intravenous; *LMA,* laryngeal mask airway; *RSI,* rapid sequence induction/intubation.

The application of pressure on the anterior portion of the cricoid cartilage has become part of the standard of care during RSI. This maneuver, also called the *Sellick maneuver,* uses the 360-degree ring of the cricoid cartilage to compress the esophagus, located directly posterior, thereby preventing reflux pulmonary aspiration of gastric contents during RSI and tracheal intubation. The recommended amount of compressive force (30 N) is considerable, approximating the equivalent weight of 3 kg; it must be applied before the administration of the induction agent and remain in place until successful placement of the endotracheal tube is confirmed.

In the induction phase of RSI, anesthesia and unconsciousness are produced by the rapid (vs. titrated) administration of hypnotic agents. (Table 4) The risks of causing or exacerbating hypotension in brain-injured or hypovolemic patients make

thiopental and propofol less attractive in the trauma setting. Etomidate has become the agent of choice because of its relatively rapid onset of action, lack of cardiovascular depressant effects, and salutary effects on intracranial pressure and cerebral oxygen consumption.

To facilitate visualization of the vocal cords and endotracheal tube placement, chemical paralytics are given immediately following administration of the induction agent. (Table 5) Succinylcholine remains the agent of choice for most acute trauma situations. In the rare situations in which succinylcholine, a depolarizing neuromuscular blocking agent, is undesirable, rocuronium may be substituted. Confirmation of endotracheal tube placement may use a variety of elements, the most reliable being visualization of the tube passing between the cords and a capnographic tracing consistent with tracheal tube placement.

Table 4: Hypnotic Agents Used for Rapid Sequence Induction

Name	Dose	Onset	Duration	Advantages	Disadvantages
Thiopental	3–5 mg/kg	30 sec	7–10 min	Decreased ICP	Hypotension
Propofol	2 mg/kg	20 sec	15 min	Decreased ICP	Hypotension
Etomidate	0.3 mg/kg	30 sec	10 mg	No CV effect, (Decreased ICP)	Adrenal insufficiency
Ketamine	2 mg/kg	<1 min	20 min	Asthma patient	Increased ICP

CV, Cardiovascular; *ICP,* intracranial pressure.

Table 5: Neuromuscular Blocking Agents Used for Rapid Sequence Induction

Name	Dose	Onset	Duration	Advantages	Disadvantages
Succinylcholine	1.5 mg/kg	40 sec	10 min	Immediate onset	Hyperkalemia
Rocuronium	0.6 mg/kg	60 sec	40 min	Short onset	Long duration
Vecuronium	0.1 mg/kg	3 min	30 min	Short onset	Longer onset, longer duration
Cis-atracurium	0.15 mg/kg	2–3 min	75 min	Safer in pregnancy	Longer duration

AIRWAY MANAGEMENT: TECHNICAL CONSIDERATIONS

Anatomic Maneuvers and Airway Stents

Simple anatomic maneuvers (chin lift and jaw thrust) are often the first step in airway management. These maneuvers are designed to open an otherwise occluded airway by lifting the tongue up off of the posterior pharynx and may be accompanied by the removal of foreign bodies or material and the use of Yankauer suction for blood, vomitus, or excessive secretions. In-line cervical immobilization is maintained at all times for patients at risk for cervical spine injuries (virtually all major-mechanism blunt-trauma patients).

Oropharyngeal and nasopharyngeal plastic or rubber stents are used as adjuncts in assisting bag valve mask (BVM) ventilation or in facilitating spontaneous ventilation. Both of these airway "stents" are designed to overcome airway obstruction caused by displacing the tongue anteriorly, producing relief of airway obstruction. Although relatively easy to insert, these devices have their disadvantages, which include causing gagging, vomiting, and aspiration in a marginally conscious patient and causing nasopharyngeal bleeding, particularly in a patient with maxillofacial injuries.

Bag-Valve-Mask and Assisted Ventilation

BVM ventilation is one of the most important, straightforward, and sometimes difficult means of assisting or providing ventilation to a nonintubated patient. The most difficult aspect of BVM ventilation is obtaining a good mask seal with one hand while providing positive pressure ventilation with the other hand. Facial hair, maxillofacial anatomy, mandibular fractures, and combativeness are all factors that make BVM ventilation either difficult or impossible. In many cases it is preferable for BVM ventilation to be performed by two people; however, this is not often practical in the field setting outside of the emergency department. In the acute trauma setting, BVM ventilation is most commonly used to provide preoxygenation before RSI.

Tracheal Intubation

Orotracheal intubation using rapid sequence induction is the most common method of establishing a secure airway in the trauma patient. The criticality of most trauma patients requiring airway management mandates that orotracheal intubation be performed by individuals with sufficient training and experience, often acquired in more elective settings, so that intubation is accomplished without delay and without causing secondary injury. Using either a Macintosh- (curved) bladed or Miller- (straight) bladed laryngoscope, the treating physician gently sweeps the tongue to the left, retracts the epiglottis anteriorly, and visualizes the cords (Fig. 1). In most cases, the vocal cords are easily visualized and tracheal intubation confirmed by visualization of the passage of the endotracheal tube between the vocal cords.

The principal advantages of nasotracheal intubation are that it can be performed without direct visualization of the cords (blind intubation), making it feasible in a conscious, cooperative patient and possible when anatomic- or injury-related conditions make orotracheal intubation difficult or impossible. The disadvantages of nasotracheal intubation are considerable and include potential for tube misplacement; the disruption or worsening of patients with occult nasal or maxillary injuries; increased risk of significant

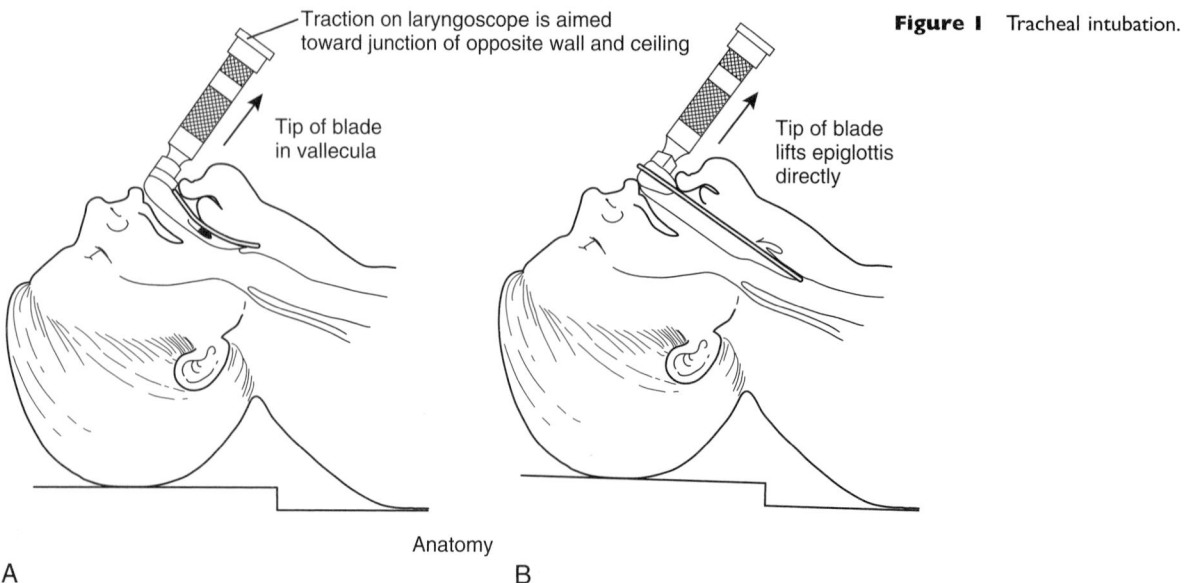

Traction on laryngoscope is aimed toward junction of opposite wall and ceiling

Tip of blade in vallecula

Tip of blade lifts epiglottis directly

Figure 1 Tracheal intubation.

Anatomy

A   B

Figure 2 Laryngeal mask airway and insertion.

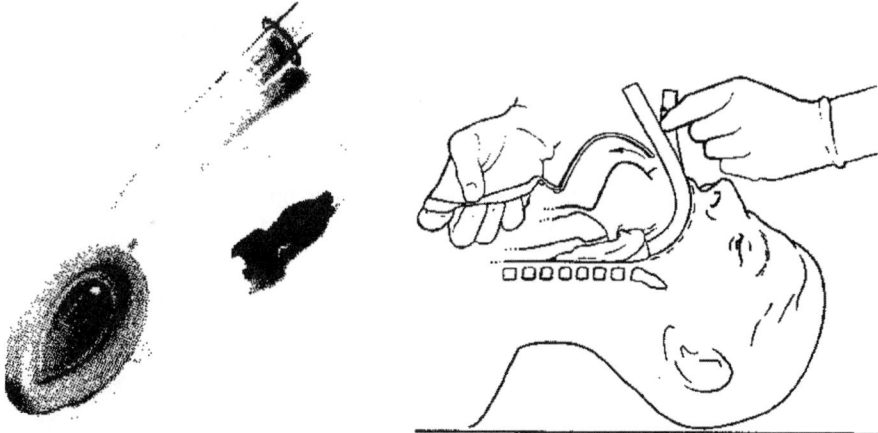

epistaxis; and the longer-term risk of obstruction of sinus drainage with the tube and subsequent hospital-acquired sinusitis in the intensive care unit (ICU) setting, which predisposes to ventilator-associated pneumonia. Because of these risks, nasotracheal intubation is not the preferred route and should be used only when conditions mandate tracheal intubation but make orotracheal impractical or impossible.

Alternatives: Laryngeal Mask Airways and Combitubes

The two most important alternative airway devices that can be used in combination with positive pressure ventilation are the laryngeal mask airway (LMA) and the Combitube. These devices are not generally regarded as adequate substitutes for conventional endotracheal intubation in the trauma patient but can be used as an adjunct to tracheal intubation in the prehospital setting or occasionally for rescue of ventilation when endotracheal intubation fails. These devices allow positive pressure ventilation and have the advantage of ease of insertion. The LMA is used principally in the

operating room in situations in which endotracheal intubation is not required. It consists of a soft rubber flange or "mask" on the end of the tube, designed to form a seal around the glottic opening (Fig. 2). LMA placement is blind, with insertion being relatively easy. It has the disadvantage of requiring fairly precise fit (requiring the selection of the proper sizes), and there is an associated risk of aspiration.

The Combitube is a large, double-lumen tube designed to be placed blindly into either the esophagus or the trachea. The Combitube consists of two separate ports, one distal and the other more proximal, either of which can be used to provide positive pressure ventilation. In most cases (>95%), the distal portal will be placed into the esophagus, thereby mandating tracheal ventilation using the more proximal port (Fig. 3). Advantages of the Combitube include ease of placement and less risk of aspiration. In addition, comparative studies have suggested that the tube has an 85% to 90% success rate for rescue intubation and an overall success rate of 98%. Patients arriving in the emergency department with Combitubes in place need them replaced eventually with conventional endotracheal tubes. The need, however, is rarely emergent for properly placed tubes, particularly if oxygenation and ventilation are adequate.

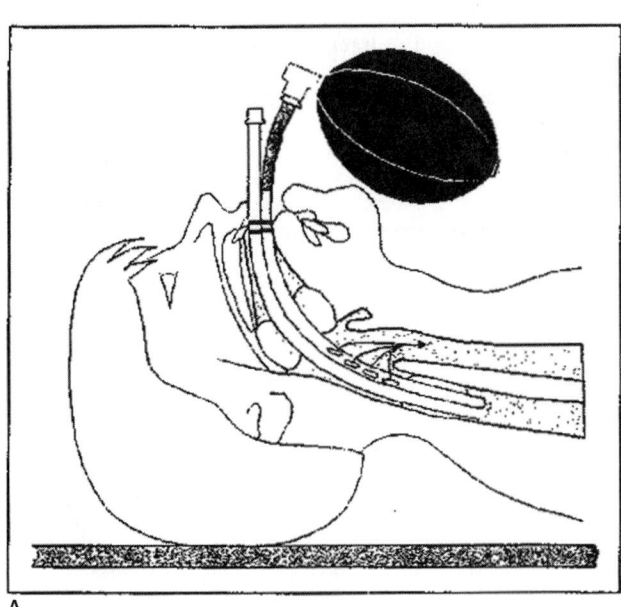

A

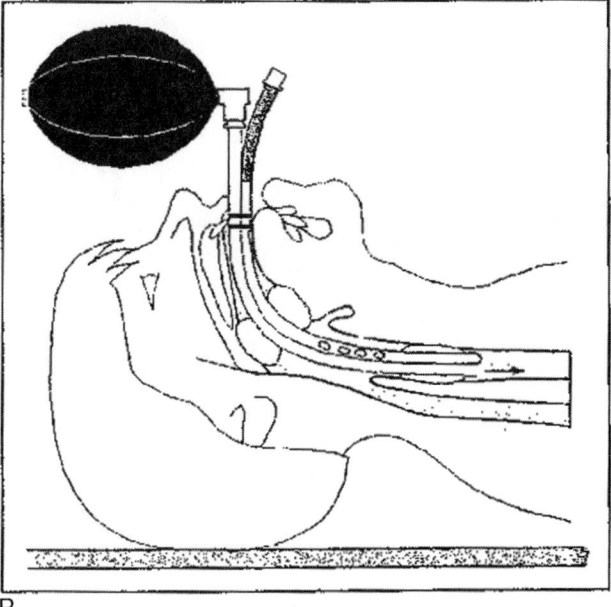

B

Figure 3 **(A)** Combitube with esophageal intubation and ventilation through laryngeal (proximal) port. **(B)** Combitube with tracheal intubation and ventilation through tracheal (distal) port.

Transtracheal Intubation (Surgical and Percutaneous Airways)

Formal tracheostomy, typically performed via the second tracheal ring, is rarely indicated in an emergent situation for the trauma patient because of the difficult nature of the procedure. Occasionally, direct laryngeal or tracheal trauma will require a more formal approach to surgical airway, but cricothyroidotomy has the advantage of greater ease and speed of airway placement. A surgical airway should be contemplated in situations in which the need for definitive tracheal intubation has been established and nasal or oral routes have proved to be impossible. Typical situations for tracheostomy involved massive craniofacial injuries or direct laryngeal, airway, or tracheal injuries. Occasionally, hemorrhagic lesions such as penetrating carotid injuries will produce airway distortion such that orotracheal intubation is impossible.

The conduct of surgical cricothyroidotomy involves preparing and draping the patient and the administration of local anesthesia as the situation allows. A midline vertical incision (in emergent settings) is made directly over the cricothyroid membrane, palpated just between the thyroid cartilage and the cricoid cartilage. The incision is carried down, remaining always in the midline, through underlying fat, fascia, and the cricothyroid membrane (Fig. 4). In many cases, the easiest airway to place through a cricothyroidotomy is not a rigid tracheostomy tube but a 6-mm, cuffed endotracheal tube.

Cricothyroidotomies of short-term duration, less than 10 to 14 days, need not be converted to formal tracheostomy and may simply be removed. Patients who are anticipated to require endotracheal intubation for longer than 10 to 14 days should undergo formal conversion of the cricothyroidotomy to either formal tracheostomy or orotracheal intubation (often via fiber-optic adjuncts).

Percutaneous transtracheal intubation has been applied increasingly in the ICU setting for the past several years and is applicable to the emergency setting, as well. The technique uses a Seldinger-type approach, in which a needle is inserted through the cricothyroid membrane until free air is obtained. A small, flexible guidewire is passed through the needle; a skin incision is made at the entry site of the wire; and a small tracheotomy tube is passed, via an introducer, over the wire and into the airway. The advantages of this method are that it may be easy and fast for nonsurgeons who been specifically trained in its use. Insofar as there are no definitive data suggesting the superiority of open (surgical) versus percutaneous cricothyroidotomy, the choice of methods should be determined on the basis of the user's experience.

Fiber-Optic Adjuncts to Tracheal Intubation

The time and equipment required for fiber-optic intubation limit its use in the acute trauma setting. The use of this technique in patients with temporarily or partially patent airways needing urgent tracheal intubation, however, may prevent the need for a surgical airway. Patients with adequate oxygenation and ventilation and mechanically unstable cervical spine injuries, neck hematomas, or suspected tracheobronchial injuries with subcutaneous air and those with suspected laryngotracheal injuries may benefit from this approach. Ideally, most fiber-optic intubation procedures should be performed in the operating room, with surgical and anesthesia teams in attendance, allowing more complete access to instrumentation and monitoring. Then, in the event of fiber-optic failure or sudden loss of airway, surgical or percutaneous airway instruments are readily available. Facial or airway trauma with hemorrhage precludes the use of a fiber-optic scope because of the difficulties in suction and visualization of the vocal cords.

▓ TROUBLESHOOTING IN AIRWAY MANAGEMENT

For the majority of trauma patients, RSI with orotracheal intubation is a fairly straightforward procedure that is associated with a high degree of reliability and relatively few complications. However, a number of problems can arise, particularly in patients with severe injuries (see Table 2). Troubleshooting during airway management will usually follow the basic and well-described ABC mnemonic used in trauma resuscitation. Reconfirmation of the position and patency of the endotracheal tube and replacement, if necessary, are often the first maneuvers, which include an assessment of the movement of air into and out of the chest. Assessment of hypoxia and an estimate of $Paco_2$ are provided via pulse oximetry and capnography. Hemodynamic compromise, as well as deficits in gas exchange, may be caused by tension pneumothorax, cardiac tamponade, or malpositioned endotracheal tubes, and the window of opportunity to diagnose and correct these problems is often measured in seconds or minutes. Although major adverse pharmacologic effects are uncommon, RSI drugs such as succinylcholine can cause bradycardia, leading to asystole. To avoid bradyarrhythmia altogether during RSI and intubation, atropine can be preadministered. A high dose of rocuronium, 0.9 mg/kg, can also be substituted for succinylcholine to facilitate the intubation procedure. Troubleshooting the malfunctioning devices necessitates vigilant, real-time physical examination and accurate differential diagnosis of the patient. Close monitoring of the patient's physiologic status becomes crucial to the success of resuscitation. Errors in identifying malfunctioning devices and delay in correcting the patient's underlying pathophysiology are two examples of problems encountered in the daily practice of trauma airway management in the emergency department. Other scenarios are outlined in Table 6.

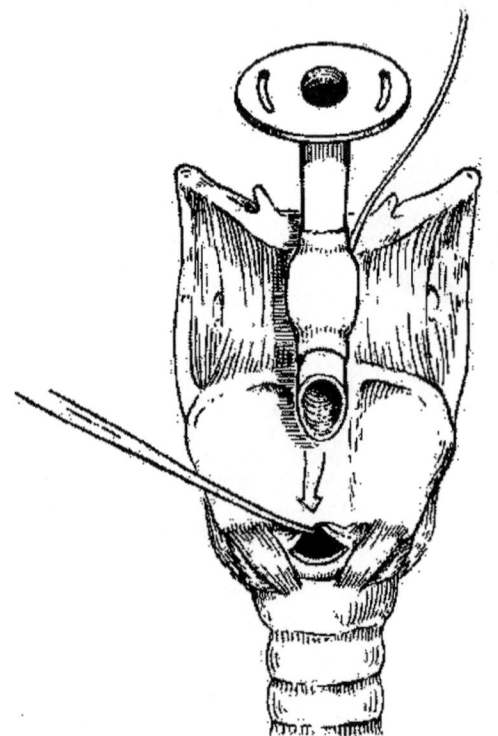

Figure 4   Cricothyroidotomy. *From Moore EE, Eiseman B, Van Way CE: Critical decisions in trauma, St Louis, 1984, CV Mosby, p. 502.*

Table 6: Problems Encountered in the Course of Airway Management in the Trauma Patient

Problem/Complication	Possible Causes	Management
Inability to place oro- or nasotracheal tube	Anatomic injury, inadequate paralysis to allow for proper visualization	Reestablish mask ventilation, LMA, "intubating" LMA, cricothyroidectomy, fiber-optic intubation
Inability to ventilate	Tension pneumothorax, inadequate paralysis, abdominal compartment syndrome, severe bronchospasm, ETT obstruction, malposition, and cuff damage	Recheck ETT placement, ETT suction or replacement, CXR, treat underlying problems, bronchodilators
Hypoxia (inability to provide adequate oxygenation)	Aspiration, esophageal intubation, pulmonary edema, pneumothorax, abdominal compartment syndrome	Recheck ETT placement, CXR, treat underlying problems, apply PEEP if BP is stable
Cardiac arrest—PEA	Air embolism, cardiac tamponade, profound hypovolemia, hypoxia from malpositioned ETT	Recheck ETT placement, initiate ACLS, treat underlying problems
Hypotension	Shock, inadequate preload, tension pneumothorax, cardiac tamponade	Recheck ETT placement, treat underlying problems, avoid PEEP
Hyperventilation, hypoventilation	Delivered wrong minute ventilation, inadequate ET_{CO_2} monitoring, malpositioned ETT	Recheck ETT placement, apply 6–10 ml/kg Vt, vent rate adjustment per ET_{CO_2}
No ET_{CO_2} tracing	Esophageal intubation, ETT obstruction, no cardiac output, severe hypothermia, severe bronchospasm, device malfunction	Recheck ETT placement, ACLS, recheck device, treat underlying problems
Bradycardia	Hypoxia, hypercapnia, succinylcholine	Recheck ETT placement, ACLS, CXR, ABGs, treat underlying problems

ABG, Arterial blood gases; *ACLS,* advanced cardiac life support; *CXR,* chest x-ray; *ET_{CO_2},* end-tidal carbon dioxide; *ETT,* endotracheal tube; *LMA,* laryngeal mask airway; *PEA,* pulseless electrical activity; *PEEP,* positive end-respiratory pressure.

SUGGESTED READINGS

American College of Surgeons: *Advanced trauma life support (ATLS),* ed 7, Chicago, 2004, American College of Surgeons.

Bulger EM, Copass MK, Sabath DR: The use of neuromuscular blocking agents to facilitate prehospital intubation does not impair outcome after traumatic brain injury, *J Trauma* 58(4): 718, 2005.

Davis DP, Stern J, Sise MJ, and others: A follow-up analysis of factors associated with head-injury mortality after paramedic rapid sequence intubation, *J Trauma* 59(2): 486, 2005.

Davis DP, Valentine C, Ochs M, and others: The Combitube as a salvage airway device for paramedic rapid sequence intubation, *Ann Emerg Med* 42(5): 697, 2003.

Krafft P, Schebesta K: Alternative management techniques for the difficult airway: esophageal-tracheal Combitube, *Curr Opin Anaesthesiol* 17(6): 499, 2004.

Sakai T, Planinsic RM, Quinlan JJ, and others: The incidence and outcome of perioperative pulmonary aspiration in a university hospital: a 4-year retrospective analysis, *Anesth Analg* 103:941, 2006.

Zed PJ, Abu-Laban RB, Harrison DW: Intubating conditions and hemodynamic effects of etomidate for rapid sequence intubation in the emergency department: an observational cohort study, *Acad Emerg Med* 13(4): 378, 2006.

INITIAL ASSESSMENT AND RESUSCITATION OF TRAUMA PATIENTS: A PRACTICAL, EFFICIENT, AND EVIDENCE-BASED MEDICINE APPROACH

Norman E. McSwain, Jr., MD

INTRODUCTION

The care of the trauma patient does not begin as the patient arrives in the emergency department (ED) or in the operating room (OR). Therefore the surgeon's involvement with the care of the trauma patient should begin not at either one of these points, but with the education of the prehospital provider who will be managing the trauma patient. The physician should be sure that the ambulances are correctly designed, staffed, and equipped to manage the severe injuries that occur on the streets, on highways, in buildings, and in homes.

The education of the emergency medical technician (EMT) should include those important aspects of airway management, hemorrhage control, and rapid transportation of the patient to the appropriate hospital (trauma center, if available) to adequately manage the patient.

Although emergency physicians and others have taken an active part in the education of the EMT, trauma is a surgical disease from beginning to end. The critical first 30 to 45 minutes of patient care in the field should not be abdicated by the surgeon.

Prehospital Care

Care of the patient in the field is similar to care of the patient in the ED in that the principles are the same; only the situation differs, along with preferences or choices of management techniques.

In the management of any patient care situation, the provider must distinguish between principles and preferences. *Principles* are a defined characteristic of patient care that must be carried out. *Preferences* are means by which the principles are achieved. As an example, one principle is that a patient's airway must be secured. The preference is how it is secured: via an oral airway, a nasal airway, or an endotracheal tube.

Factors in the field such as rain, snow, darkness, potential fire, unruly bystanders, and toxic chemicals or gases influence the technique that is used for management of the principles of patient care. Prehospital providers must be taught all methods of patient care management and to let their knowledge of and experience with the technique, situation, and environment dictate which of these techniques is used.

Another principle is hemorrhage control. Generally, only external hemorrhage control can be obtained outside the hospital. Internal hemorrhage control must be obtained in the hospital and in the OR. Therefore it is important that the severely injured patient be transported to a trauma center, if one is available in the immediate area, as quickly as possible. There should be no delay in the field (e.g., no performing of unnecessary tasks); neither should there be a delay in transporting the patient to the correct hospital.

The principles of prehospital care therefore include proper assessment (primary and secondary) and proper management of life-threatening or potentially life-threatening injuries through proper packaging of the patient for rapid transportation to the appropriate medical center (trauma center).

Prehospital Education

Prehospital management of the patient is divided into three phases: acquisition of the patient, field care, and transportation. Ambulances should be distributed so that they can access any point within the community (unless rural) within 6 to 8 minutes. Field time to assess a patient's injuries, establish life-threatening injury management, and package and load the patient should require no more than 10 minutes. Transportation to the closest appropriate trauma center also should require less than 10 minutes. This is a total of almost 30 minutes, which constitutes half of the "Golden Hour," as described by R Adams Cowley. Therefore this time should be spent as efficiently as possible. Physician involvement and training are necessary to ensure that these principles are carried out.

Similar to the American College of Surgeons' (ACS) Advanced Trauma Life Support (ATLS) course, which is directed at the in-hospital care within the first hour, the Prehospital Trauma Life Support (PHTLS) course, developed by the National Association of EMTs in cooperation with the Committee on Trauma (COT) of the ACS, is devoted to the care of the patient in the field and en route to the hospital. The patient care principles established by the ATLS program are used in the PHTLS program but with an emphasis on the kind of care required in the field.

The principles of airway (with cervical spine immobilization), breathing and ventilation, circulation and hemorrhage control, neurologic assessment, and total patient assessment are the principles used both in the hospital and in the field.

These principles do not change. The only change is the preferences or the situations that require different methods of management in-hospital versus prehospital.

KINEMATICS OF INJURY

The correct interpretation of the history of the incident (kinematics, or mechanism of the trauma) allows the physician to identify 95% of the likely injuries before he or she ever touches the patient. (Details are available in the PHTLS course 2006.)

IN-HOSPITAL CARE

Introduction

Proper patient care cannot be carried out without an adequately designed resuscitation room, appropriately trained resuscitation personnel, and adequate equipment. The ACS Optimal Care document has identified those personnel who should be immediately (or quickly) available to the resuscitation room and to the in-house care of the patient. These include the surgeon, the emergency physician, anesthesiologist (or Certified Registered Nurse Anesthetist), trauma-trained nurses, radiographic technicians, blood bank personnel, and respiratory therapists. Supervision in individual duties of the personnel present varies according to the resources of the hospital (teaching hospital or nonteaching hospital) and with prior agreement of the department of emergency medicine and the department of surgery. Resuscitation should not be run without both surgery and emergency medicine personnel present and without adequate planning and discussion regarding the jobs that each person should carry out. Figure 1 demonstrates the design of a proven resuscitation room and personnel positioning in a trauma center in a teaching hospital.

Rapid access to a properly equipped OR is critical to the survival of a critically injured patient. The patient should not be carried to a major hospital without immediate access to the OR (within 10 minutes). Just as we have taught the EMS personnel that prolonged field times are detrimental (as indicated by Frank

Lewis, MD), the same applies to the ED. A hypotensive, severely injured patient should not remain the in ED for longer than 10 minutes. For the same reason that prolonged prehospital time is harmful (ongoing blood loss), so, too, is prolonged time in the ED (ongoing hemorrhage). An efficient, well-trained emergency care team can complete the necessary intravenous lines, intubation, chest tubes, and radiographs of the chest and abdomen within 10 minutes and move the patient into the OR, where the abdomen or chest can be quickly opened and hemorrhage controlled. This implies that the surgeons and anesthesiologists and OR staff are either in-house or can rapidly respond when the ED is notified that such a patient is en route. Each major community

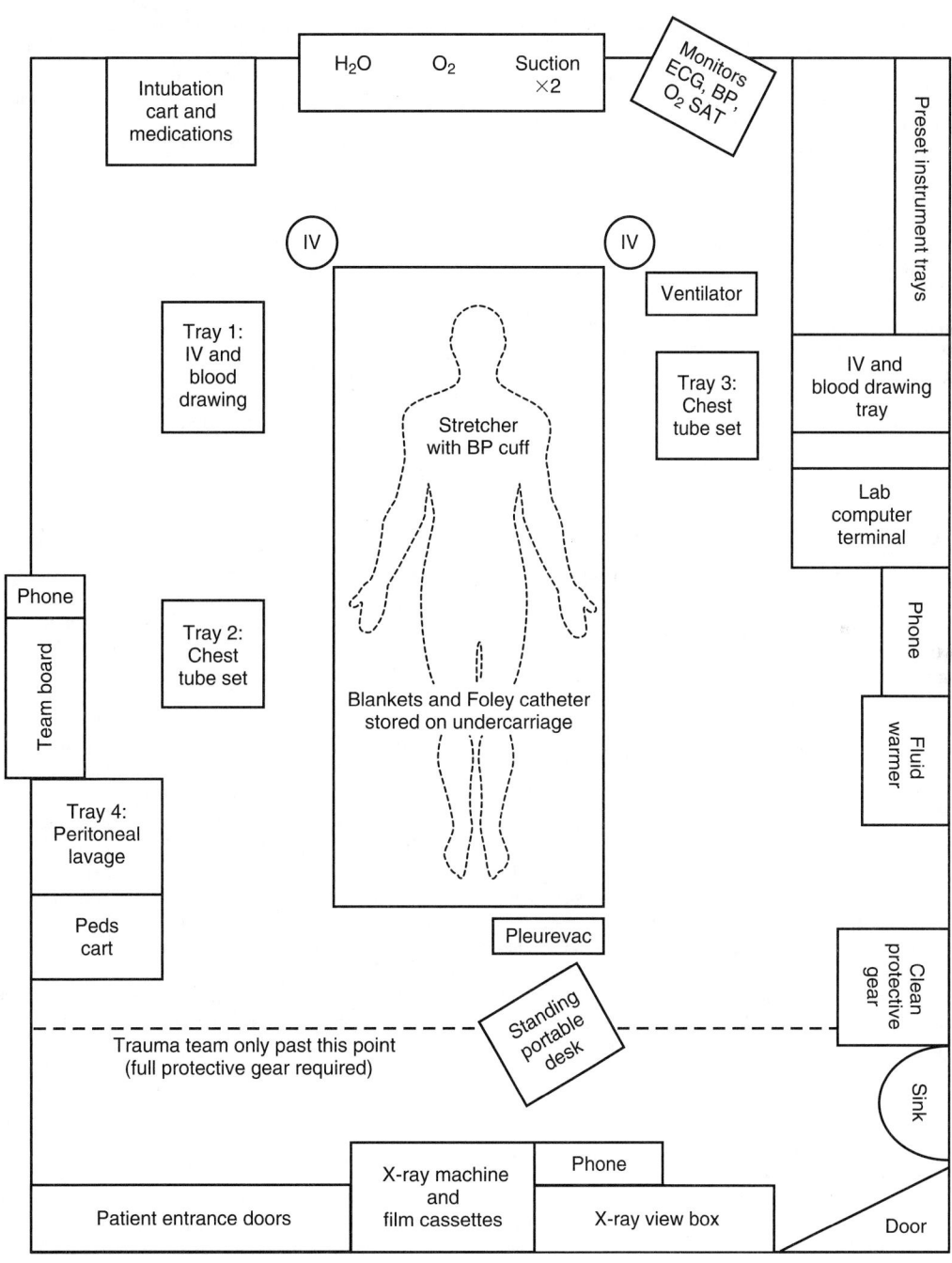

Figure 1 Trauma Bay setup.

should have an available trauma facility. Facilities that are not so equipped should be bypassed by the EMS system, and the patient should be taken to a facility that is properly prepared to manage major trauma.

In smaller communities where the trauma volume is too low to require in-house personnel or personnel available within 10 to 15 minutes, meeting the Level I or Level II criteria of the ACS, there should be an established Level III hospital with appropriate response times or a mechanism of directing the EMS system, either by ground or by air, to bypass the hospitals in the smaller community and go directly to a city in which such capabilities are available.

The readers are directed to the "Green Book" (2006 edition of *Resources for Optimal Care in the Injured Patient*, published by the ASC/COT).

To correctly understand the principles of management of an acutely injured patient, each principle must be considered individually. Our brains do not work this way, however. The brain can multitask, assessing many different signs and symptoms at the same time, and the process should not confuse the examiner. Information is simultaneously processed by using the eyes, ears, hands, mouth, and nose to assess a patient, although learning must be linear to understand the information received.

The other critically important factor in resuscitation is that someone MUST be in charge. Not everyone can be a worker bee, and not everyone can direct the resuscitation. The supervisor must have an overview of the patient and also must see everything else that is going on and take care of everything. If there is a task that must be handled by the senior surgeon in the room, then his or her supervisory control must be given to someone else.

Initial Assessment

Scene Assessment

The first step is to survey the scene. The EMT will note hazards in the field: fire, toxic fumes, criminal perpetrators still on the scene, precarious position of a vehicle, environmental conditions, and so forth. For the physicians in the ED, a similar scene assessment is important: is the patient still armed? Did the perpetrators come to the ED posing as "family?" Is the resuscitation room cold? Are all the caregivers organized? Are there enough people in the room to provide care? Are the blood bank personnel present? Where are the security personnel, if needed? Is the necessary equipment available, if needed?

Patient Assessment

Patient assessment is divided into three stages. The first stage is observation as the patient is rolled down the hall into the trauma resuscitation room and offloaded onto the resuscitation stretcher. The second assessment (primary survey) is a brief head-to-toe examination of the patient, concentrating on conditions that are life threatening, and then an assessment of the general condition of the patient. The third assessment (secondary survey) is a head-to-toe detailed examination. There are occasions when the level of shock is so severe and there is significant ongoing hemorrhage that this secondary survey is not completed until the patient has been taken to the OR for hemorrhage control.

The first assessment (*quick view assessment*) is cursory: cardiopulmonary resuscitation in progress; obvious blood on the sheets; high epinephrine level; endotracheal tube in place; activity of the patient; eyes of the patient. Are the EMTs bringing the patient in quickly or slowly? Are the patient's clothes burned? Is blood running out onto the floor? What happened *to* that patient before you ever *saw* the patient? Once an EMT has decided what the scene is all about and has an overview of the patient, then the assessment is directed to the specific problems of the patient.

The first full patient care assessment is the *primary survey*, which is the identification of life-threatening injuries and simultaneous resuscitation of the patient, if necessary. Some patient conditions require care within the OR before the secondary assessment can be performed. This is especially true when extensive radiographic assessment is required or when hemorrhage is ongoing. The primary survey is divided into steps that are familiar to most physicians because a primary assessment is performed every day on ward rounds. "Hello Ms. Jones. How are you doing this morning?" "I'm doing fine. My belly hurts." The patient's airway is open. The level of the patient's mental process is evident. The patient is ventilating. A quick feel of the pulse identifies the cardiac status, the perfusion of the skin (warm or dry, the pulse character, and the capillary refill time). The primary survey is completed within 15 seconds of entering the patient's room.

In a primary assessment of a trauma patient, the steps are the same as those for an in-hospital patient. The difference is that the trauma patient is new, so more information is required.

A - Airway (with cervical spine control)
B - Breathing
C - Circulation with hemorrhage control
D - Disability (mental function)
E - Expose (examine every part of the patient)

A: Airway

In the trauma patient, one must be concerned not only with the airway but also with the technique used to open the airway. Because of the possibility of a cervical spine (C-spine) injury, hyperextension of the neck is not a possibility. The airway must be opened by bringing the mandible forward while maintaining the positioning of the C-spine. The sniffing position of the C-spine used in the OR to place the endotracheal tube will hyperextend C1 and C2 and hyperflex C5 and C6. Those are the two most common places where C-spine fractures occur. This does not mean that the airway is not opened or that an endotracheal tube is not placed. It simply means that the airway is secured without manipulating the C-spine.

The jaw thrust maneuver moves the mandible forward. The tongue is attached to the mandible, so the tongue follows forward and opens the posterior pharynx. The most common cause of airway obstruction is the tongue becoming lax and falling back to occlude this area. The jaw lift is another easy mechanism to achieve this process. A mechanical airway, such as an oral airway or a nasal airway, can then be inserted to keep it open. Mechanical airways simply hold the tongue out of the way while you do other things, and then you can put in the endotracheal tube (ET) if you want.

Maintaining the position of the C-spine is important. The principle is in-line immobilization of the C-spine. The two preferences for achieving this are (1) from the front of the patient placing the palms of the hands on the patient's ears and the forearm on the clavicles and (2) squatting below the patient's head and holding it steady while the operator inserts the ET tube, moving only the mandible toward the feet and the ceiling at the same time.

In a small percentage of patients (probably <½ of 1%) the ET cannot be inserted and a surgical airway will be necessary. Contrary to popular opinion, most patients with facial injuries do not fall into this category. It is frequently easier to place an ET in a patient with massive facial injuries because a stable mandible is not in the way.

The principle is this: below the larynx, opening and tube insertion. The preferences are a percutaneous insertion, a cricothyroidotomy, and a tracheostomy (the surgical airways). I prefer the percutaneous insertion simply because it is quicker and safer and does not require any equipment other than a large-bore needle (≥14-G) and a female/female oxygenation administration tube with a hole cut in the side to control oxygenation inflation of the lungs.

B: Breathing (Ventilation)

Adequacy of ventilations can be assessed by counting the number of chest movements per minute and noting their depth. This will provide a gross assessment of ventilation. Assessment of ventilation is not assessment of respiration. It is common to use the term *respiration*, but this is not correct. Respiration is a process of use of oxygen in metabolism and not just the external movement of air in and out of the lung.

In the primary survey, everything is gross. Everything gives a general impression but no specifics. Lord Kelvin once said that if you can speak of something in numbers, your knowledge is very great. If you cannot speak of it in numbers, your knowledge is very meager indeed. This is partially true of the primary survey. Even though the numbers are not specific, it does give a picture of the immediate condition of the patient and allows planning for the next few minutes of patient care. Numbers can be added in the secondary survey.

In the management of the airway and using this to assess respiration and metabolism, it is not just getting air into the patient's lungs that is important; also important is the amount of oxygen, as measured by the fraction of inspired oxygen (Fio_2). The Fio_2 is determined partially by the flow rate but more importantly by the device that is being used to deliver the oxygen. Table 1 provides assistance in determining the amount of oxygen to deliver to the patient.

Nasal prongs, in general, provide minimal oxygen enhancement for the trauma patient. During the initial resuscitation period, a non-rebreathing mask with two valves should be used. Even if the initial indication is that a patient has no airway or ventilation issues, that is no reason not to provide full oxygenation until definitive data indicate that oxygen is not beneficial for the patient in question. Table 2 provides some guidance.

Table 1: Fio₂ from o₂ Administration Devices

Device	Fio₂
Nasal prongs	≈0.24
Nasal canula	≈0.30
Ventimask	0.35–0.45
Non-rebreathing mask (1 valve)	0.75
Non-rebreathing mask (2 valves)	0.85
ET tube with accumulator	0.40
ET tube with ventilator	1.00

ET, Endotracheal tube; *Fio₂*, fraction of inspired oxygen.

Table 2: Management for Abnormal Spontaneous Ventilation

Spontaneous Ventilations per Minute	Management
0–8	Bag valve mask with accumulator device; possible intubation
8–20	Observation
20–30	Supplementation oxygenation; possible assisted ventilation
>30	Assisted ventilation; possible intubation
GCS <8	*Immediate intubation with assisted ventilation*

GCS, Glasgow Coma Score.

The presence of a pneumothorax, or the major suspicion of one, requires immediate insertion of a chest tube on the affected side. Delay to obtain a chest radiograph in a shock patient with decreased breath sounds is not appropriate.

C: Cardiac

1. Control hemorrhage to reduce red cell mass loss.
2. Ensure that an adequate amount of blood is circulating in the cardiovascular system.

To oxygenate the tissue cells of the body, the red cells must deliver oxygen to those cells. This is the basis of the Fick principle. This, of course, means an adequate red cell mass (control of hemorrhage and replacement of red cells). Resuscitation with crystalloid solution without control of hemorrhage leads to a rapid dilution of the remaining red cell mass as hemorrhage continues and the volume is replenished by non–oxygen-carrying fluid. On the basis of the Bernoulli principle, continued raising of the blood pressure without hemorrhage control increases the rate of hemorrhage (intraluminal pressure vs. extraluminal pressure). The solution to this dilemma is

1. intraoperative hemorrhage control,
2. reduction of mean arterial pressure to minimal level of 80–90 mm Hg systolic, or
3. increase of extraluminal pressure (pneumatic anti-shock garment).

The above, along with the Bernoulli principle, is the basis for the controversy of full fluid resuscitation, limited fluid resuscitation, or colloid resuscitation. This is discussed in detail in the resuscitation section of this chapter.

The time-honored method of initial hemorrhage control both inside and outside of the hospital is compression, followed as soon as possible with factor XIV (suture ligature). Compression dressings for extremity injuries in the prehospital period and in the ED have been used for quite some time and are still used successfully. However, the experiences of the military in Iraq and the assessment of extremity injuries, as studied by Champion and Holcomb, have shown the benefit of tourniquets. A review of the autopsies performed on bodies that have come back from Iraq identified that one of the major causes of death in the field is compressible hemorrhage that was not compressed or a hemorrhage suitable for application of tourniquet that was not stopped. The Tactical Combat Casualty Care Committee (TCCC) has recommended that all combatants carry one hand tourniquet and that these be used when direct pressure fails or the tactical situation makes it impossible or difficult to apply (see *PHTLS Prehospital Trauma Life Support: Military Version*, ed 6). Although the need and usefulness of this device in civilian medical care is less than in a military situation, nonetheless it is not the disparaged device of the past.

Noncompressible hemorrhage (torso) is an indication to take the patient immediately to the OR.

The modern definition of the shock patient is decreased energy (adenosine triphosphate [ATP]) production on the cellular level. The etiology is most likely anaerobic metabolism secondary to hypoperfusion with oxygenated red blood cells. The symptoms of shock or decreased perfusion and anaerobic metabolism in the ED are hypothermia (shivering), tachycardia, hypotension, decreased capillary refilling time, and perhaps decreased level of consciousness.

Too often the physician managing the patient ignores hypothermia because the room is cold (or totally discounts the shivering as coming in from the outside environment). A recent study from Tulane/Charity Hospital indicates that hypothermia less than 35 °C in the ED is a predictor of nonsurvival in patients with traumatic shock. The cold resuscitation room will contribute to the hypothermia, but it is not the cause. Decreased ATP production secondary to anaerobic metabolism is the cause.

D: Disability

Cerebral function must be assessed, including blood flow to the brain and cerebral oxygenation. Causes of disability are hypoxia, cerebral injury, overdose on alcohol or drugs, or metabolic conditions.

E: Expose

The patient must be examined completely from head to toe.

RESUSCITATION

The first step toward resuscitation of a patient is identifying life-threatening abnormalities during the primary survey. In addition, as indicated in the ATLS guidelines from the ACS/COT, appropriate lines and tubes should be placed. The decision made at this point is the subsequent care and assessment in the OR, the intensive care unit, or the radiology suite. There are three approaches to fluid replacement: (1) a large volume of saline (white blood) at three times the blood loss, developed by Shires during the Viet Nam conflict; (2) colloid resuscitation, propagated by Holcroft and others; and (3) restricted fluid resuscitated prior to hemorrhage, researched and taught by Mattox. All three have their advocates. The difficulty of deciding which method to follow is that there has never been a randomized, prospective large multi-institutional study comparing all three methods. Such a study will never happen because of the arcane rules of research on the acutely injured and shock patient. The unfortunate outcome is that the patient is not able to benefit from the latest research.

This study must be carried out, separating the patient with uncontrolled hemorrhage from the patient with controlled hemorrhage. The key pathophysiology in the process is the patient with uncontrolled hemorrhage. If increasing the blood pressure to the "normal" levels of systolic pressure, 120 mm Hg, increases blood loss, according to the Bernoulli principle, then the use of both large-volume resuscitation and colloid resuscitation will increase the loss of the remaining red cell mass into the tissue or the abdominal or thoracic cavities. This would mean that the restricted fluid method, as described by Mattox, is the only correct method of management. Many surgeons believe this to be true, but there is no study to support a definitive answer.

The Tactical Combat Casualty Care Committee (TCCC) has recommended for tactical combat care that the pulse be used as the gauge for fluid replacement. If the character of the pulse is normal and the patient is alert, resuscitation consists of two canteens of water orally. If the injured combatant is without a head injury but not alert or the pulse is weak and thready, then 500 ml of Hextend (HES [hydroxyethyl starch]; Hospira, Lake Forest, IL) is given intravenously. If there is no response in the pulse within 30 minutes, another 500 ml of Hextend is given. This meets the need of a volume expander that can be carried out within a small volume yet stays in the vascular system much longer than a larger and heavier volume of crystalloid.

Secondary Assessment

Ongoing assessment for life-threatening injuries following primary evaluation is critical for injury identification and proper triage of resources. Adjuncts to evaluation, such as urinary and gastric catheters, should be considered as the secondary survey ensues, especially if the patient is considered unstable or has been intubated. The secondary survey is best performed as a second, rapid, but more detailed, head-to-toe inspection of the patient, including rectal examination. Findings during this survey should be communicated to the team leader so that diagnostic studies can be initiated when needed. Chest and pelvis

radiographs, as well as a torso ultrasound examination (focused assessment with sonogram in trauma [FAST] examination) can be used if the patient's clinical state warrants expeditious delineation of sites of hemorrhage.

History/Date Accrual

Again, ATLS provides a simple mnemonic for the purpose of history assessment, the AMPLE method:

Allergies
Medications
Past illnesses/**P**regnancy
Last meal
Events/**E**nvironment related to the injury

Prehospital personnel can provide invaluable help with reconstructing mechanisms of injury. Certain mechanisms may impart a greater risk to anatomic structures (e.g., motor vehicle collision with rollover increases the risk of axial spine injury).

Physical Examination

The physical examination portion of the secondary survey is a second, concise yet global look at the trauma patient. Radiographs and ultrasound examination may be performed after this head-to-toe evaluation, or simultaneously, if necessary, based on patient physiology.

Head

A thorough examination of the head involves quick incorporation of many senses. Palpation and inspection for cephalohematoma or laceration that may be hidden by hair need to be completed early so that ongoing or delayed hemorrhage from a scalp wound can be prevented. Pupillary examination and tympanic membrane examination may reveal hidden clinical signs of intracranial hypertension or basilar skull fracture. Midface instability and mandibular fractures need to be elucidated quickly because they constitute a separate category of airway compromise and control that may not readily present itself during the primary examination.

Neck

Neck examination must be performed with a team approach so as to maintain cervical spine immobilization if needed. The cervical collar should not be allowed to hinder a thorough examination; experienced personnel can easily maintain in-line stabilization and perform examination of the trachea and neck without endangering the patient. Neck vein distention may mark impending hemodynamic instability from cardiac tamponade. Tracheal deviation may suggest the need to decompress a tension pneumothorax. Laceration or other penetrating injuries can be investigated and recorded according to external neck zones of penetration. Any hematoma requires repeated examination for expansion or ongoing blood loss. The posterior neck may be more easily examined during the log roll.

Chest/Cardiac

The examination of the chest requires careful inspection and constant attention to early diagnostic modalities, primarily chest x-ray (CXR), and possible therapies. Breath sounds, although insensitive as single data points, can aid enormously if decreased on one side in a patient with hypotension. Anterior torso injury can present as crepitus over rib fractures, subcutaneous emphysema from decompressing pneumothorax, or paradoxical motion overlying flail chest. Signs of blunt high-energy transfer in conjunction with a mechanism of injury related to rapid deceleration denotes an injury complex in which aortic disruption must be considered and ruled out, especially if findings on CXR are suspicious. Penetrating injuries with cardiac or great-vessel proximity should be noted and addressed according to a patient's hemodynamic stability. With the advent of ultrasound, rapid interrogation of cardiac injury and possible tamponade has become feasible and routine.

Abdomen

Examination of the abdomen commences with a general palpation and assessment for peritonitis. If the patient has extreme tenderness with peritoneal signs, the examination generally warrants exploratory laparotomy. In the absence of peritonitis, a formal but rapid abdominal evaluation is necessary. The margins of the abdomen stretch from the fourth intercostal space to the pelvis and include the diaphragm and the retroperitoneum. Confounding variables such as rib and pelvis fractures make the diagnosis and triage of abdominal injuries difficult. Physiology must play a significant role in the diagnostic strategy of potential abdominal injury. Unstable patients must have intra-abdominal hemorrhage rapidly ruled out with bedside ultrasound or diagnostic peritoneal lavage (DPL). More stable patients can be evaluated with serial abdominal examinations or computed tomography (CT) scan.

Back

Patients should be rolled over to permit assessment for injury related to back, spine, and flank. All of these increase the risk for retroperitoneal injury. The rectal examination can be performed during the log roll. Rectal examination offers the opportunity to assess for pelvic fracture after blunt trauma (by palpating the location of the prostate gland) and rectal injury after penetrating trauma.

Pelvis

The pelvis should be examined for bony instability and tenderness. Both hip joints should also be ranged to rule out dislocation and to aid in diagnosing occult pelvic fractures. Pelvic x-ray is always indicated in any patient who presents as hemodynamically unstable or with tenderness to palpation during examination. The vagina and perineum should also be examined at this time.

Musculoskeletal

Inspection of the upper and lower extremities for evidence of penetrating or blunt trauma is also performed. Anatomic positioning such as internally rotated and foreshortened lower limbs should be noted—these may point toward hidden injury such as posterior hip dislocation or proximal fracture. Deformities should be assessed for distal neurovascular integrity. Formal splinting should be performed at this time. Peripheral pulses are assessed, and a more focused neurologic assessment of each limb is performed to further elucidate extremity injury.

Secondary Studies

As stated earlier, patient physiology should dictate the timing and sequence of secondary testing to augment injury identification. Presentation of an injured patient with hemodynamic instability necessitates the immediate application of secondary studies aimed at identifying sources of hypotension (usually from hemorrhagic shock) after trauma. Only after secondary testing is applied and hemorrhage determined to be absent are other etiologies, such as neurogenic shock from cervical spinal injury, entertained.

The secondary testing arsenal related to hemodynamic instability offers a few constant choices. In evaluation of a chest injury, early CXR can accomplish visualization of the internal chest architecture and localize injury to one hemithorax. Hemodynamic instability should prompt earlier intervention. In agonal patients, tube thoracostomy may become both a diagnostic test (searching for tension pneumothorax or hemothorax) and a therapeutic modality.

Another important secondary study is ultrasound. With growing education and availability, ultrasound has now become an accepted adjunct to assess the hypotensive trauma patient. A FAST examination may be considered the modern method for examining the peritoneal cavity and pericardium for fluid (i.e., blood). FAST examination offers a four-quadrant view of the abdomen. Views of three quadrants—right upper, left upper, and bladder—are obtained to interrogate dependent portions of the peritoneum for free fluid. FAST offers the added advantage of visualizing the pericardial space (fourth view) to help diagnose tamponade. A FAST examination can be performed quickly and can be repeated as indicated. One must be reminded that FAST examines for fluid only and does not offer reliable examination of the retroperitoneum or pelvis or rule out hollow viscus injury.

DPL has been used reliably for years and is a good technique when indicated. The procedure involves the percutaneous or open insertion of a catheter into the peritoneal cavity. DPL is considered positive if gross aspiration from the catheter reveals 10 ml of gross blood. For blunt trauma, if after the instillation of 1L of crystalloid within the peritoneal cavity the effluent reveals a red blood cell count greater than 100,000/ml, a white blood cell count greater than 500/ml, amylase higher than 20 U, or the presence of bacteria or vegetable matter, the test is considered positive for intraperitoneal injury. Penetrating trauma has similar indications, although cell-count triggers are lowered (e.g., red blood cells > 10,000/ml). Supraumbilical DPL should be used for patients with pelvic fractures or suspected pregnancy. DPL is useful in the triage of hypotensive patients with pelvic fractures. In addition, it may play a role in diagnosing hollow viscus injury.

A pelvic x-ray should always be considered when the patient is unstable. Injury complexes such as an open-book pelvis fracture are clearly amenable to pelvic ring closure devices (e.g., external fixation or temporary pelvic orthotic device) and may indicate a retroperitoneal source of hemorrhage. C-spine radiograph assessment should be obtained to rule out spinal cord injury as a source of hypotension if prior workup fails to identify the source of hemorrhage.

When patients present in stable condition, the secondary testing algorithm shifts from urgent cavitary triage looking for hemorrhage to injury identification and maintenance therapy with resuscitation. CT scan for blunt trauma has proven to be invaluable and cost effective. CT scanning has a negative predictive value that has been repeatedly found to equal 100%. Thus it can easily be used to discharge patients home who have normal findings on CT scan. Abdominal CT scan is quite useful for detecting solid-organ injury and triaging patients to the OR; the intensive care unit, for higher levels of care; or the medical floor, for observation. In this era of ever-growing nonoperative management of solid-organ injury, the CT scan has quickly replaced most other modalities of imaging the stable injured patient. CT scan has recently enjoyed an explosion in technologic advancement, such that modern multidetector imaging capability and new software allow increasingly rapid scan times and higher resolution. The sequence of CT scan is in part dictated by the team leader's concerns, but generally follows a logical course. CT scan of the brain should be obtained first, followed by CT scans of the chest, and abdomen, and pelvis, as needed. Because of the prolonged processing time, spine evaluation continues to require more time than standard imaging of the head and torso. Formal CT scanning of the spine (when indicated) is usually performed after internal organ injury and brain injury have been ruled out. As familiarity with CT scan interpretation grows, this modality is minimally accurate for injury identification of penetrating injury.

CONCLUSION

The management of acute trauma can be reduced to ATP production at the cellular level. The solution is early hemorrhage control and replacement of the lost red cell mass and vascular volume.

SUGGESTED READINGS

Advanced trauma life support for doctors, ed 7, Chicago, American College of Surgeons, 2005.

McSwain NE Jr: Prehospital care from Napoleon to Mars: the surgeon's role, *J Am Coll Surg* 200(4): 487, 2005.

National Association of Emergency Medical Technicians: *PHTLS prehospital trauma life support: military edition,* ed 6 St Louis, 2007, Mosby.

EMERGENCY DEPARTMENT THORACOTOMY

Jay Menaker, MD, and Thomas M. Scalea, MD

INTRODUCTION

Little is as controversial as the use of emergency department thoracotomy (EDT) following injury. EDT has the ability to immediately salvage patients who would otherwise certainly die. Advances in prehospital care and care in the intensive care unit make some patients, who in the past would have died, now potentially salvageable. EDT can be an important part of this early resuscitative scheme; however, EDT is a surgical procedure and must be performed properly if it is to be valuable. Few centers see a sufficient number of patients who are true candidates for EDT. Thus there are important issues related to EDT, such as adequate training for both surgical and emergency medicine residents.

The concept of thoracotomy as a resuscitative measure was first described with Schiff's promotion of open cardiac massage. The potential application of a thoracotomy for cardiac injury was first suggested by Block in 1882, when it was used to repair a canine heart laceration. At about the turn of the 20th century, Rehn performed the first successful suture repair of a cardiac wound using a thoracotomy. EDT was first described in 1966, when Beall and colleagues described the procedure as a component of the resuscitation of moribund patients with penetrating chest trauma.

INDICATIONS AND CULTURE

All would agree on certain indications for EDT, such as the patient with penetrating chest trauma who suffers cardiac arrest in the resuscitation bay. Other indications will vary by institution. In our institution, the operating room (OR) is located immediately adjacent to the resuscitation area. Patients who are marginal can be transported to the OR rather than undergo EDT. In other institutions, where the OR is located a distance from the resuscitation area, however, it may be wise to perform EDT rather than risk having the patient go into cardiac arrest in transport.

The outcome of EDT will also vary with the indications. If one performs EDT on every patient who presents with cardiac arrest, regardless of mechanism, the outcome will be dismal, particularly if that institution sees a preponderance of blunt trauma. In addition, survival should not be the only meaningful end point. Resuscitating a patient who ends up neurologically crippled from anoxic encephalopathy can be considered only a marginal success.

Discussion of the rational use of EDT suffers from lack of clear definition of terms. We define the presence of vital signs as patients who have recordable blood pressure, a palpable pulse, and spontaneous respirations. Patients without recordable vital signs may still have signs of life if they have electrical cardiac activity, respiratory effort, or at least pupillary reactivity. Patients without have signs of life no detectable blood pressure, pupillary activity, respiratory effort, or electrical activity. It is tempting to use the term *pulseless electric activity* to describe the patient without a palpable pulse who has electrical cardiac activity. In fact, this is probably not accurate. Most of these patients have mechanical cardiac activity but are simply so vasoconstricted that they do not have a palpable pulse or recordable blood pressure. The use of bedside ultrasound can be extremely helpful to diagnose cardiac tamponade, as well as to define the presence or absence of mechanical cardiac activity.

Overall, the reported survival rate of EDT is 5% to 10%. Factors that generally contribute to the outcome are mechanism of injury, location of major injury, and presence of signs of life. For instance, survival rates after penetrating injury are close to 10% but they are approximately 1% for blunt trauma. Survival for patients with thoracic injuries is significantly better than for those with abdominal injuries or those with injuries to multiple body cavities. Success rates are highest for cardiac injury, particularly if located in a single chamber. Outcome is better if there is a clear presence of signs of life on patient presentation. Prognosis is much worse if signs of life are not present, especially if none was present in the field. Other factors that clearly affect outcome include patient age and presence or absence of preexisting conditions.

Thus the perfect patient for EDT is the patient who presents with recordable vital signs and a single anterior thoracic stab wound with a single-chamber cardiac injury with pure cardiac tamponade. This patient has not lost a significant amount of blood and has very little physiologic deficit. Survival in that patient should be approximately 30% to 40%.

A number of authorities have commented on decisions to perform EDT. The Advanced Trauma Life Support Course says that EDT may be indicated for patients with penetrating thoracic injuries who arrive pulseless but with myocardial activity. Patients who sustain blunt trauma and arrive without a pulse but with myocardial electrical activity are not candidates for resuscitative thoracotomy.

Biffl and colleagues categorize the indication for EDT into "clear" and "relative."

Clear indications include:

1. salvageable postinjury cardiac arrest, for example, patients sustaining witnessed cardiac arrest with a high likelihood of isolated intrathoracic trauma, particularly penetrating cardiac wounds;
2. persistent severe postinjury hypotension (systolic blood pressure <60 mm Hg) resulting from:
   a. cardiac tamponade,
   b. intrathoracic hemorrhage,

c. air embolism, or

d. active intra-abdominal hemorrhage.

Relative indications include

3. refractory moderate postinjury hypotension (systolic blood pressure <60 mm Hg) resulting from:

a. cardiac tamponade,

b. intrathoracic hemorrhage,

c. air embolism, or

d. active intra-abdominal hemorrhage.

Biffl and colleagues clearly state that these recommendations must take into account a patient's age, preexisting disease, signs of life, mechanism of injury, and the logistics of proximity to the operating room, as well as personnel availability.

In 2000, Rhee and colleagues classified the indication for EDT into three categories:

1. Indicated: patients with penetrating thoracic injuries and signs of life (SOL), defined as those with cardiac electrical activity, respiratory effort, or pupillary response in the field who do not respond to fluids and are losing their vital signs in the resuscitation area.

2. Relative indication: patients with penetrating abdominal injury with at least one clear SOL in the field, and blunt trauma patients who lose SOL in the hospital or immediately before arrival.

3. Contraindication: patients with no SOL in the field from either penetrating or blunt trauma.

PROCEDURAL TECHNIQUE

EDT is performed as part of the resuscitation and should occur simultaneously with the initial assessment and evaluation, including endotracheal intubation, intravenous access, and rapid volume infusion. A left anterolateral thoracotomy is the incision of choice. Advantages of the incision include its rapid access, the ability to perform it in the supine patient, and the ready extension into the right hemithorax (clamshell) for additional exposure. An orogastric tube helps to differentiate the aorta and esophagus. Extending the patient's left arm parallel to the head and neck will facilitate proper exposure.

The entire area is rapidly prepped with antiseptic solution prior to the incision. The incision should begin at the lateral border of the left sternocostal junction inferior to the nipple and is continued to the latissimus dorsi. Some physicians prefer to start the incision above the sternum; however, this increases the risk of transecting the internal mammary artery. The incision should be placed at the fourth or fifth intercostal margin, just below the nipple in a male or the inframammary fold in a female (Fig. 1). In women, the breast should be retracted superiorly to make this space more accessible. The proper level of the incision should correspond with the inferior border of the pectoralis major muscle. It is important to curve the incision to follow the fourth or fifth rib. A common mistake is to bring the incision straight down to the xiphoid. This becomes problematic if one must convert to a clamshell thoracotomy.

The incision is rapidly carried through skin, subcutaneous tissue, and the serratus anterior muscle until the intercostal muscles have been reached. To expose the thoracic cavity, the intercostal muscles are then cut using a scalpel, Mayo scissors, or Metzenbaum scissors. The incision should course the superior margin of the rib to avoid injuring the intercostal neurovascular bundle. Care should be taken to prevent lacerating the lung or heart while entering the thoracic cavity. A Finochietto retractor is then placed to spread the ribs (Fig. 2). Extension of the incision to the right hemithorax, if necessary, can be quickly accomplished using a Lebsche knife (Fig. 3). The internal mammary arteries must then be ligated.

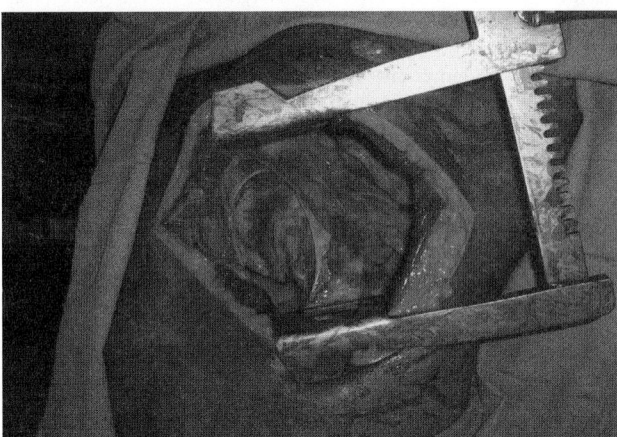

Figure 2 Finochietto retractor placement. The Finochietto rib retractor is placed to gain access to the thoracic cavity. The handle should be placed laterally as to allow extension of the incision to the right chest, if necessary.

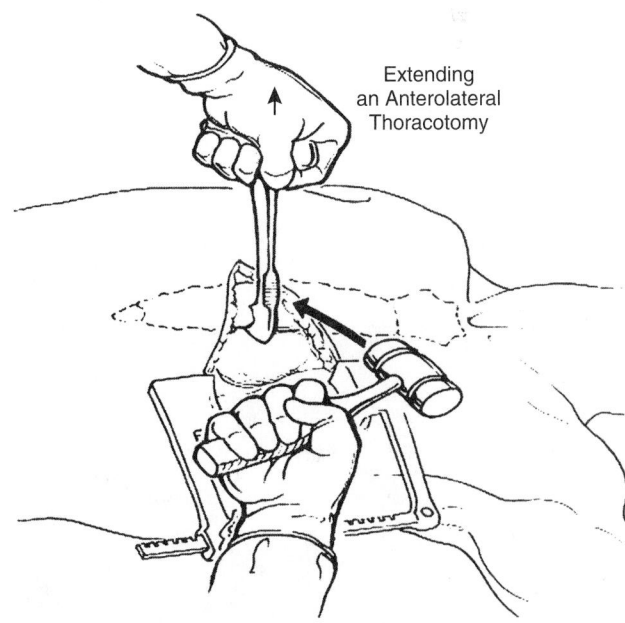

Extending an Anterolateral Thoracotomy

Figure 3 Extending anterolateral thoracotomy. A Lebsche knife and mallet are used to extend a left lateral thoracotomy across the sternum for additional exposure. When the sternum is transected, the internal mammary vessels must be ligated. Extension into the right thoracic cavity, "clamshell," gives wide exposure to both pleural cavities.

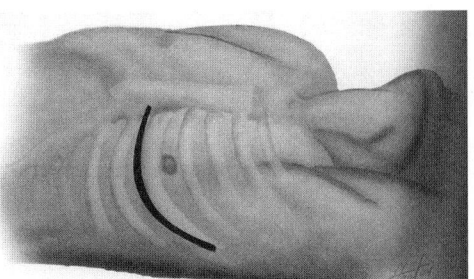

Figure 1 Incision at the fourth or fifth intercostal margin. A left anterolateral thoracotomy is initiated at the level of the fourth or fifth intercostal space. Generally, the incision is just inferior to the nipple in the male and the inframammary fold in the female. It is the preferred incision for resuscitation of the acutely injured patient in extremis. It provides the best access to the heart and great vessels.

PERICARDIOTOMY

In a traumatic cardiac arrest, the pericardium should be opened routinely because one cannot visually rule out cardiac tamponade. The pericardium is incised anteriorly and opened parallel to the left phrenic nerve (Fig. 4). The excision should extend superiorly to the aortic root and then inferiorly to the apex of the heart. Making a T incision at the pericardium inferiorly increases exposure to the heart. Blood clots should be removed, and the myocardium should be thoroughly examined for injury. Cardiac bleeding should be controlled immediately with digital pressure while preparing for better temporizing measures. Inserting a Foley catheter, blowing up the balloon, and using gentle traction can also achieve temporary control of hemorrhage (Fig. 5). Excessive pressure on the Foley, however, may cause the balloon to tear through the myocardium, creating a much larger injury. We prefer to use intestinal Allis clamps for temporary control in all chambers of the heart except the left ventricle. The clamps may be sequentially stacked to appose the cut edges of the injured heart. These sutures can be run under the clamps as a temporary repair. Staples, temporary sutures, and vascular clamps are all potential techniques used to stop acute hemorrhage while preparing definitive repair in the operating room.

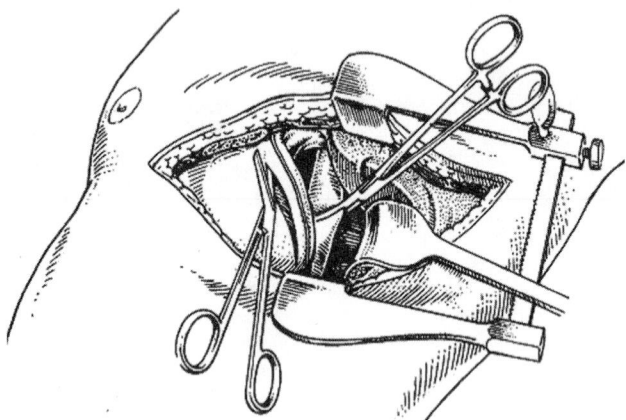

Figure 4 Opening the pericardium. Pericardial tamponade cannot be excluded using visual inspection alone. The pericardium is opened anterior to the phrenic nerve using a longitudinal incision.

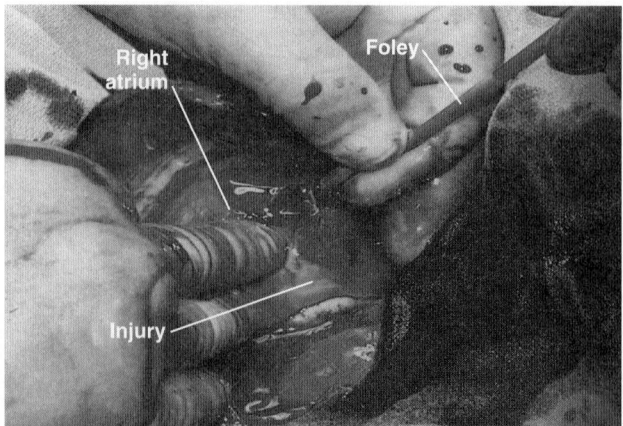

Figure 5 Foley catheter placement into the heart. Gentle traction on an inflated Foley catheter assists with control of hemorrhage. Saline, rather than air, is used to inflate the balloon to avoid a possible air embolism if the balloon ruptures.

AORTIC CROSS-CLAMPING

The aorta lies immediately anterior to the vertebrae, actually lying on the bodies themselves. To expose the descending aorta, the lung is elevated anteriorly and superiorly. At this point the inferior pulmonary ligament should be taken down for improved exposure and access to the aorta. The aorta and esophagus are both covered by the mediastinal pleura on the anterolateral surface. The pleura must be bluntly dissected away, separating the esophagus and aorta. Palpating the nasogastric tube may help to differentiate the aorta from the esophagus because this may be difficult in a hypotensive patient. After the esophagus is separated anteriorly and the prevertebral fascia posteriorly, the left hand is used to encircle the aorta while a clamp is applied with the right hand (Fig. 6). Blind placement of a cross-clamp without aorta isolation usually results in the clamp slipping off.

Aortic cross-clamping makes intuitive physiologic sense by preferentially shunting blood to the most important areas, that is, the brain and myocardium. However, it simultaneously occludes blood flow, distally causing ischemia in those regions. Although blood pressure may transiently rise after cross-clamping of the aorta, clamping may in fact be quite toxic to cardiac performance. Placement of an aortic cross-clamp radically increases afterload and can place an enormous strain on the left ventricle. In a situation of near arrest or full cardiac arrest, cardiac output is undoubtedly quite low already; thus the additional strain of aortic cross-clamping may be more detrimental than helpful.

Aortic cross-clamping can provide transient help. Unfortunately, areas distal to the clamp are now rendered completely ischemic. A "declamp shock" occurs if the aortic cross-clamp is left in place too long. When the clamp is removed, the reperfusion injury may result in profound hypotension, cardiac arrest, or both. There is little that can be done to prevent this devastating consequence of the aortic cross-clamp. Although it is unclear exactly how long a clamp may be left in place, most experienced clinicians believe that 20 to 30 minutes is the maximum. Unfortunately, in most institutions, resuscitation, transport to the operating room, and definitive repair of complex injury cannot be accomplished in that amount of time. Although some surgeons at our institution continue to use aortic cross-clamping, our preference, in fact, is to not use this technique.

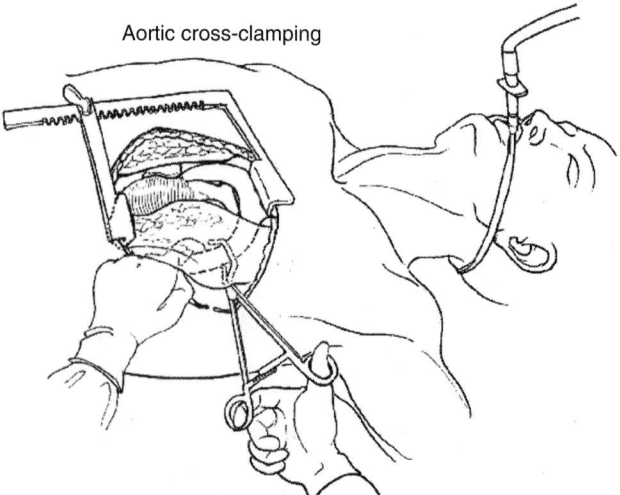

Aortic cross-clamping

Figure 6 Aortic cross-clamping. The aorta lies immediately anterior to the vertebrae. The lung is elevated anteriorly and superiorly for improved exposure and access to the aorta. Palpating the nasogastric tube may help differentiate the aorta from the esophagus, as this may difficult in a hypotensive patient. The left hand is used to encircle the aorta while a clamp is applied with the right hand.

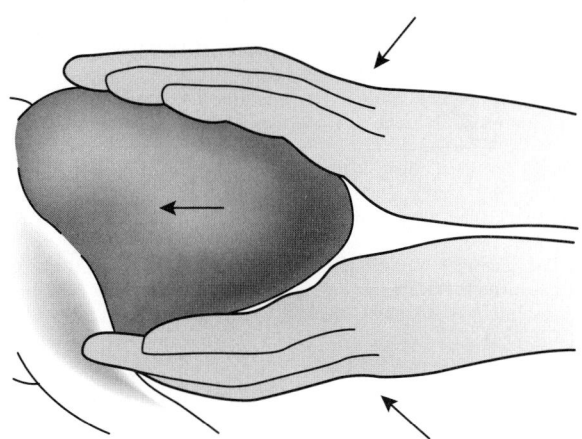

Figure 7 Bimanual cardiac massage. Open cardiac massage using the preferred bimanual technique. The palmar surfaces of the fingers act in a clapping motion compressing the heart. Fingertip pressure should be avoided at all times.

CARDIAC MASSAGE

Bimanual internal cardiac massage should begin immediately if there is true cardiac arrest. The preferred method is a hinged clapping motion with the wrists apposed and ventricular compression proceeding from the apex to the base of the heart. This is best accomplished by cupping the left hand and placing it over the right ventricle. The fingers of the right hand are held tightly together to form a flat surface supporting the left ventricle (Fig. 7). The right hand compresses the flat surface against the cupped surface supported by the left hand.

CONTROLLING NONCARDIAC HEMORRHAGE

Occasionally, one encounters a massive hemothorax of noncardiac etiology at the time of resuscitative thoracotomy. The chest should be evacuated and an immediate search for the source of the hemorrhage undertaken. Temporary hemorrhage control is essential. If this is from a mediastinal great vessel such as subclavian or nominate, repair in the emergency department is almost impossible. Direct pressure, resuscitation, and transport to the OR are the only rational course. Occasionally, a proximal aortic injury can be digitally controlled and at least temporarily repaired in the emergency department.

Figure 8 Twisting at the hilum. Isolated pulmonary hemorrhage can be controlled with either a Duvall clamp or a vascular clamp. If simple clamping does not achieve hemostasis, blood flow may be occluded by twisting the lung on its hilum. This eliminates aeration of the lung as well.

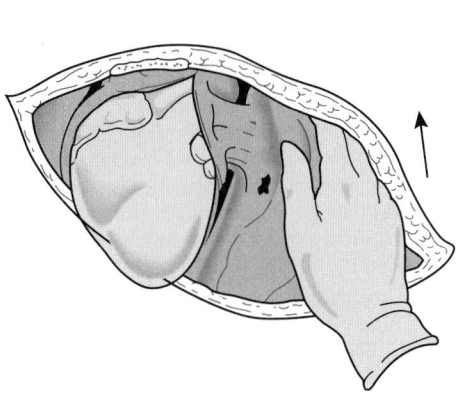

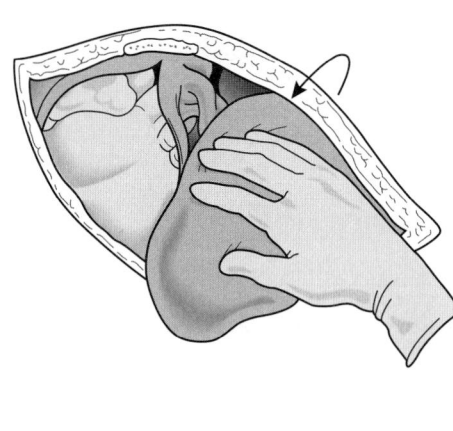

Pulmonary hemorrhage represents another potential source of bleeding. Occasionally, bleeding from the lung can be controlled with either a Duvall clamp or a vascular clamp. More attempts should not be made to dissect the lung out and perform definitive hemostasis in the emergency department.

If simple clamping does not achieve hemostasis, there are several other methods available. Occluding flow of the pulmonary hilum has the advantage of achieving complete inflow control. This can be accomplished by mobilizing the inferior pulmonary ligament and simply twisting the lung on the hilum (Fig. 8). This occludes blood flow and also eliminates aeration of the lung. Another method is to simply place a vascular clamp across the hilum. One should avoid dissecting the hilum structures because this risks inadvertent injury to the bronchus or other adjacent structures. The final possibility is to pass an umbilical tape around the hilum and occlude the hilum with it.

Hilar control can provide immediate hemostasis for major hemorrhage from the lung. Unfortunately, this maneuver radically increases pulmonary vascular resistance and may produce profound right ventricular failure and, subsequently, significant hypotension, often leading to cardiac arrest. Nevertheless, this is an important maneuver to remember if other methods fail.

COMPLICATIONS

Potential complications of EDT include those of a technical manner, as well as those of postoperative sequelae. Common technical complications include damage to intercostal vessels and the internal mammary. Those less commonly reported include laceration to the heart (including damage to coronary arteries), damage to phrenic nerve, and damage to lung tissue. Postoperative morbidities include infection, bleeding, pericarditis, acute respiratory distress syndrome, and post-pericardotomy syndrome.

CONCLUSION

EDT remains a highly debated topic; however, it may be invaluable in the resuscitation of a patient in profound shock. It is probably the most dramatic procedure performed in the emergency department, if not hospital wide. With the growing incidence of penetrating trauma coupled with the advances in prehospital care, the number of patients who may benefit from an EDT has increased. The procedure has the best results when used on patients with penetrating cardiac injuries and witnessed SOL. The survival rates decrease for those with abdominal hemorrhage, those with blunt trauma, or those who never had SOL. A traditional left anterior thoracotomy is performed by quickly making an incision from the lateral border of the sternum to the axilla. The ribs are spread, and the thoracic cavity is entered. The pericardium is then opened by making a longitudinal incision, avoiding the phrenic nerve and releasing any clotted blood. Cardiac injuries may be repairable in the ED. Other injuries should be temporary controlled, and the patient taken to the OR for definitive repair.

SUGGESTED READINGS

American College of Surgeons Committee on Trauma: *Advanced trauma life support for doctors,* ed 7, Chicago, 2004, American College of Surgeons.

Bartlett RL: Resuscitative thoracotomy. In Roberts JR, Hedges JR, editors: *Clinical procedures in emergency medicine,* ed 3, Philadelphia, 1998, Saunders.

Beall AC Jr, Diethrich EB, Crawford HW, and others: Surgical management of penetrating cardiac injuries, *Am J Surg* 112:686, 1966.

Beck CS: Wounds of the heart, *Arch Surg* 13:205, 1926.

Biffl WL, Moore EE, Johnson JL: Emergency department thoracotomy. In Moore EE, Feliciano DV, Mattox KL, editors: *Trauma,* ed 5, New York, 2004, McGraw-Hill.

Blatchford JW III: Ludwig Rehn: The first successful cardiorrhaphy, *Ann Thorac Surg,* 39:492, 1985.

Hemreck AS: The history of cardiopulmonary resuscitation, *Am J Surg* 156:430, 1988.

Rhee PM, Acosta J, Bridgeman A, and others: Survival after emergency department thoracotomy: Review of published data from the past 25 years, *J Am Coll Surg* 190:288, 2000.

COAGULOPATHY IN THE TRAUMA PATIENT

Peter Rhee, MD, MPH, and Kenji Inaba, MD

INTRODUCTION

In the bleeding trauma patient, hemostasis remains the primary goal. Following surgical or endovascular control of bleeding, the detection and aggressive correction of systemic coagulation defects remain critical. The bleeding trauma patient is at high risk of developing an acquired coagulopathy. Platelets and coagulation factors are lost during hemorrhage and are consumed for hemostasis locally and systemically. Other contributing factors during the resuscitation process that can lead to coagulopathy include the dilution of factors from volume replacement, hypothermia, and acidosis. In elderly patients, the use of preinjury anticoagulants may also contribute to this problem. The major goal of correcting an acquired coagulopathy in the trauma patient is to reduce nonsurgical blood loss in traumatized tissue and to limit further functional damage in specific clinical scenarios such as intracranial hemorrhage. A secondary goal is to reduce the use of allogeneic blood products and thereby reduce the risk of potentially fatal, transfusion-associated adverse events such as ABO hemolytic reaction, transfusion-related acute lung injury, anaphylaxis, or infection. As understanding of the association of blood transfusion with conditions such as sepsis, systemic inflammatory response syndrome, and multisystem organ dysfunction syndrome increases, the importance of limiting transfusion in the overall management of critically ill trauma patients is becoming more evident. Rapidly correcting this acquired coagulopathy remains an integral part of resuscitation and the ongoing management of acutely injured patients.

ETIOLOGY

The coagulopathy seen in trauma is multifactorial in origin and not uncommon. In fact, several retrospective reviews have shown that up to one fourth of severely injured patients arrive at the hospital with an initial laboratory panel showing coagulation system defects, including a prolonged prothrombin time (PT) and activated partial thromboplastin time (aPTT). It has also been shown that the incidence of this abnormality is higher with increased severity of injury and is an independent predictor of mortality. Although this coagulopathy may be partially explained by preinjury anticoagulant medications, the exact underlying mechanism by which this coagulopathy occurs is not yet completely understood.

After care is initiated, the hemorrhagic loss of both coagulation factors and platelets is accentuated by dilution with resuscitation fluids, which have no clotting factor activity, and component therapy with packed red blood cells (PRBCs), which have only minimal residual plasma content. In addition to this loss and dilution, the tissue injury results in local consumption of coagulation factors and platelets as the body attempts to naturally stop bleeding. Systemically, thromboplastin exposure from traumatic brain injury can result in a consumptive disseminated intravascular coagulopathy.

Severely injured trauma patients are also at high risk of hypothermia and acidosis. Hypothermia is a known independent risk factor for death in trauma patients and has a detrimental effect on coagulation. The coagulation process relies on a variety of temperature-dependent enzymatic reactions that are slowed by hypothermia. Experimental studies have demonstrated that at a temperature of 33 °C, the functional factor deficiency is approximately 50%. Clinically, the magnitude of this effect is underrepresented because blood samples in the laboratory are routinely warmed to 37 °C for testing and will not accurately reflect the actual in vivo status. Platelet adhesion is also impaired by hypothermia. In fact, at milder levels of hypothermia, the depression in core body temperature will have a greater effect on platelets than on the enzymatic clotting cascade. Although not as well defined as hypothermia, acidosis may also have a detrimental effect on the coagulation cascade. The exact mechanism by which this occurs has not been well elucidated; however, it is postulated that primarily the pH-sensitive enzymatic reactions central to the coagulation cascade are affected. Both hypothermia and acidosis remain important contributors to the coagulopathy seen in trauma patients. It should be remembered that the underlying triad of coagulopathy, hypothermia, and acidosis is caused by bleeding, and after surgical bleeding has been addressed, the other factors will usually reverse in due time.

Finally, as the population ages and continues to live increasingly active lives, the at-risk population for injury will include a significant cohort of older patients. This segment of the population will have concomitant medical problems that may require antiplatelet or anticoagulant agents. These pharmacologic agents potentiate any coagulopathy that develops as a result of the injury. Because many of the most critically ill patients with active bleeding may not be able to communicate a coherent medical history, the early detection and aggressive reversal of preinjury pharmacologic anticoagulation is important. One recent study in the elderly has shown that rapid empiric infusion of fresh frozen plasma improves functional outcome and survival in elderly trauma patients with intracranial hemorrhage.

TREATMENT—GENERAL

In the acutely bleeding trauma patient, surgical or endovascular control of hemorrhage remains the primary goal; however, aggressive steps should be taken early to detect and treat coagulopathy.

HYPOTHERMIA

Hypothermia is common in patients with major blood loss because of the decreased cellular metabolism during hemorrhagic shock. This topic warrants a brief discussion. When metabolic rate is below normal, as during hemorrhagic shock, the body will not generate enough adenosine triphosphate (heat) to maintain normal temperature and will thus fall to ambient temperature. The primary measure to treat blood–loss-associated hypothermia is to stop blood loss. In most circumstances, if the source of blood loss has been controlled then the associated hypothermia is not necessarily detrimental and will self-correct. However, in many circumstances, such as in blunt trauma, the source of hemorrhage is multiple and not easily controllable because fractures and tissue injury will continue to bleed. In these cases, in addition to resuscitating with warmed fluids, other causes of heat loss should be addressed. This includes removal of wet clothing and sheets. The patient should be immediately dried and covered to keep the ambient temperature around the patient warm. Adjuncts include heating pads, Bair Huggers (Arizant Healthcare, Eden Prairie, MN), and warming of humidified air from ventilators. The transfer of heat through air (convection) is extremely inefficient, and thus the main goal here is to prevent heat loss. Although warming of the operating room technically reduces the gradient between the patient and the ambient temperature, the few additional degrees to which the room can be elevated are not that helpful, especially if the patient is mostly covered, and can make the operating room staff inefficient. The transfer of heat through fluids is via conduction and is the most efficient means to transfer heat because the circulation reaches all aspects of the body. However, because the fluids can be only a few degrees higher than 37 °C at best when infused, the amount of heat transferred is minimal, so the goal here again is prevention of heat loss by warming the fluids and blood from room temperature or from refrigerator temperature (4 °C). Patients warmed with these means take an average of up to 4 hours to warm from 34 °C to 37 °C. Active warming using arteriovenous or venous-venous shunts can warm patients more rapidly, but its practice is not always used nor is it standard. Cardiopulmonary bypass is the most effective method of heating but is not relevant to this scenario.

TREATMENT—WHOLE BLOOD

For the routine care of trauma patients, blood component therapy with PRBCs rather than whole blood transfusion is the current standard of care. Whole blood is rarely available in most hospitals in the United States and is vastly different from fresh whole blood, which is readily available in the military setting, with the use of the walking blood bank. Extensive experience has been gained from military surgeons who have used the walking blood bank to infuse warm, fresh, cross-matched whole blood minutes after donation. There are specific clinical situations, however, when whole blood use may be considered. In the civilian setting, the autotransfusion of scavenged, shed, intracavitary blood that is not contaminated should always be used. This is performed by adding approximately 100 ml of citrate phosphate dextrose per 500 ml of whole blood. The binding of calcium by the citrate keeps the blood from coagulating in the collection device, and because there is an ample supply of calcium in the body, the infused citrate is of minimal concern. If the blood collected for autotransfusion has not been anticoagulated, the blood can still be used because the blood transfusion filter will remove clots and particulates.

The coagulation defects expected with whole blood replacement differ from PRBC transfusion. Provided that whole blood has not been refrigerated after collection, it is rich in all coagulation factors and platelets. With refrigerated storage, however, concentrations of the two labile factors (V and VIII) are depressed (FVIII much more than FV), and platelets become dysfunctional. From a practical standpoint, even if factor VIII levels were to drop to zero in banked whole blood, this should not be problematic because there is an endogenous burst of circulatory factor VIII in stress situations. The ex vivo preservation of platelets requires stringent storage conditions. Although ongoing research into cold storage, surface glycoprotein modulation to decrease circulatory clearance, and external pathogen detection and removal appears promising, practically, under optimal conditions, the current room temperature storage life span for platelets is only 7 days, and most U.S. blood banks still employ platelet-storage techniques that limit the platelets to a 5-day life span. In whole blood the functional life span of platelets is even shorter, with the functional platelet population rapidly degrading to effectively be zero within 1 to 2 days. In summary, although whole blood is not indicated solely for factor or platelet replacement, whole blood that is not refrigerated and immediately transfused is replete with coagulation factors and platelets. In clinical situations in which replacement occurs with older or refrigerated whole blood, there will be a coagulation defect with a profile that differs from PRBC replacement. Fresh, whole blood is usable for up to 24 hours if kept at room temperature or 7 to 10 days if refrigerated. The earliest defect requiring treatment will be the platelet deficit and not a prolonged PT, international normalized ratio (INR), or aPTT.

COMPONENT THERAPY—PLASMA

As with red blood cell replacement, coagulation products have been broken down into component parts for replacement. Plasma is produced from whole blood separation or apheresis and is frozen within 8 hours (called *fresh frozen plasma* [FFP]) or 24 hours (called *FP24*) to preserve the labile factors and can be stored frozen for up to 1 year. This frozen plasma is packaged in 200- to 600-ml aliquots, and by convention each ml contains 1 International Unit of all coagulation factors. The FFP and FP24 can then be thawed for use in approximately 30 minutes and used as A, B, O, or AB type-specific plasma without the need for Rh matching or cross matching prior to infusion. If not used immediately, the plasma can be stored refrigerated for up to 5 days. After the first 24 hours, the "fresh frozen" label is removed, and the resulting plasma is now known to be deficient in the labile factors V and VIII. At our center, the LAC+USC (Los Angeles County and University of Southern California) Medical Center blood bank maintains a ready thawed-plasma supply. This allows us immediate access to 8 units of type O or type A plasma at all times. At our institution, we have found that 85% of the patients are either group O or group A. Because 10% of the remaining patients are group B and 5% group AB, only 2 units of thawed B plasma are routinely kept as liquid stock. Additional units of group B and group AB plasma are thawed on demand. Although this plasma is theoretically stored for more than 5 days, in practice the units are continuously being exchanged so that the plasma issued is less than 24 hours old and complete with all labile and nonlabile factors. This practice drastically reduces the need to wait for the initial set of plasma that requires infusion. As the thawed plasma is issued, the thawing process for replacement frozen units is immediately initiated.

COMPONENT THERAPY—PLATELETS

Platelets are available through centrifugation separation or, increasingly, as apheresis single-donor units. They are stored at room temperature for up to 5 days. Platelets require an ABO/Rh match. One traditional unit will provide approximately 5.5×10^{10} platelets suspended in 40 to 70 ml of plasma. Transfusion of 1 unit should result in an increase of 5 to 10,000 platelets per microliter, and these platelets should last in the systemic circulation for 3 or 4 days. With apheresis platelets, 1 unit contains greater than 3×10^{11} platelets suspended in 200 to 300 ml of plasma. Therefore, 6 to 10 units of traditional platelets are equivalent to 1 unit of apheresis platelets and constitute a standardized dose. Apheresis platelets are used at LAC+USC Medical Center for all trauma patients and aid in the logistics of rapidly infusing the platelets.

COMPONENT THERAPY—CRYOPRECIPITATE

Cryoprecipitate is the cold, soluble precipitate that is recovered at 1 °C to 6 °C during the FFP thaw process. This will contain, on average, 80 International Units of factor VIII and 250 mg of fibrinogen, as well as factor XIII, von Willebrand factor, and fibronectin. In the trauma patient, it is rare to acutely deplete fibrinogen in the absence of a global factor depletion or massive diffuse intravascular coagulation because there is 200 to 300 mg of fibrinogen in every 100 ml of FFP. Should fibrinogen depletion occur, however, cryoprecipitate is available as a supplement. Cryoprecipitate offers the advantage of delivering a large dose of fibrinogen (1.5 and 2.5 g per 10 bags pooled) in a volume that is less than that of a single unit of FFP. However, it is rarely necessary to minimize volume in trauma.

TREATMENT—INDICATIONS

The indications and optimal replacement strategy for plasma components and platelets in the acutely bleeding trauma patient are unknown. Ideally, factor and platelet loss would be quantitated and the deficit replaced. However, quantifying the deficit is challenging because even the best estimates of the magnitude of the blood loss are inaccurate. Standard washout equations factoring in the additional effect of dilution are mostly inaccurate and clinically irrelevant. The main reason is that the underlying estimate of blood loss is inaccurate, and the theory of a fixed, single blood compartment does not apply to the actively bleeding trauma patient. This leaves two clinical approaches to correcting the coagulopathy in the acutely bleeding patient: (1) empiric replacement and (2) laboratory–result-guided replacement.

Unlike laboratory–result-driven replacement, empiric replacement therapy applies to situations in which there is massive and rapid ongoing hemorrhage. Obtaining laboratory-based therapy in this scenario is often not feasible. Component therapy is largely arbitrary because the dynamic status of the bleeding patient is not accurately reflected by the traditional laboratory results. Because of the difficulties in quantifying the magnitude of component loss, its replacement is tied to the volume of PRBC that is infused. At some institutions, this has been standardized so that for every X units of PRBC, X units of plasma and platelets are infused concurrently, without waiting for laboratory results. Although protocols have been written and are followed, there are no ASA class 1 data to support this practice. Not surprisingly, institutional protocols and individual practices vary widely in their fixed ratio replacements, ranging from 1 to 10 units of FFP for every 10 units of PRBC. The usage of platelets ranges from 1 to 2 units for every 6 to 10 units of PRBC. This lack of a standardized approach is due to the difficulty of systematically studying this group of severely injured patients, where most of the efforts are devoted to lifesaving efforts. When massive, ongoing bleeding is being replaced with crystalloids and PRBCs, empiric factor and platelet replacement are justifiable and required. Although it was previously felt that platelet replacement was the earliest and most common deficit, this was based on evidence from earlier studies using coagulation–factor-rich, platelet-poor whole blood replacement. It has become clear, however, that with PRBC resuscitation, both factor and platelet replacement is required. In fact, computer modeling has demonstrated that the earliest defect is in the PT and that a platelet deficit comes later, likely because of the physiologic recruitment of platelets from a sequestered supply. Figure 1 shows the massive transfusion protocol that is currently used in our institution.

Laboratory–result-guided treatment requires the measurement of PT (INR), aPTT, platelet count, and fibrinogen and uses these results to detect component deficits and trigger replacement. The best test for the efficacy of replacement therapy is bleeding time, and although this is not practical in the bleeding patient, the surgeon's estimate of the wound and its ability to coagulate should not be underestimated and is often used as a "poor man's bleeding time." In general, a PR ratio greater than 1.5, aPTT greater than 1.5 times normal, platelet count less than 50–70,000/ml (assuming normal function), and a fibrinogen level less than 100 mg/dl are all clear indications for

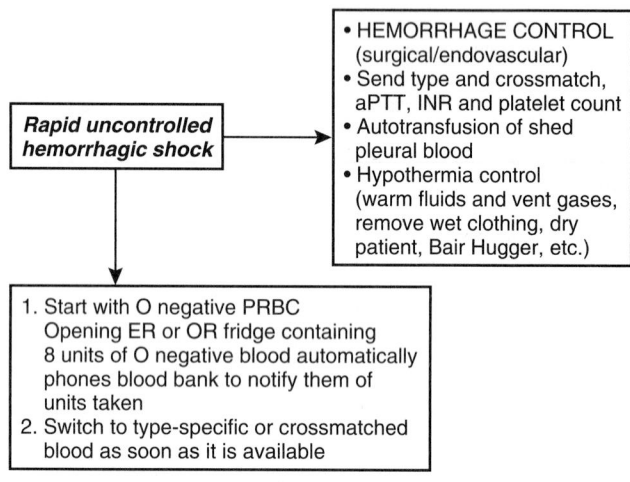

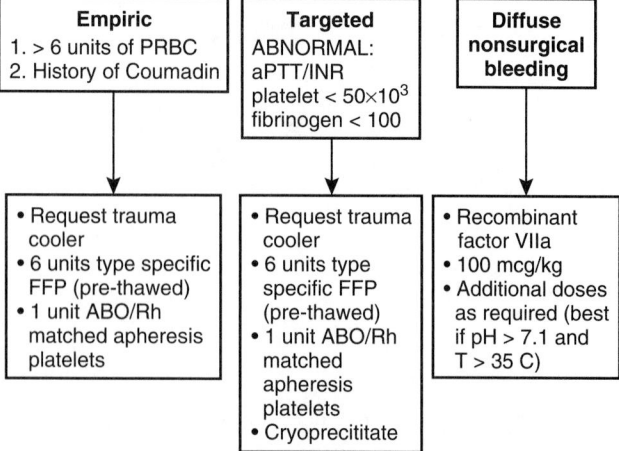

Figure 1 Transfusion protocol at Los Angeles County, University of Southern California.

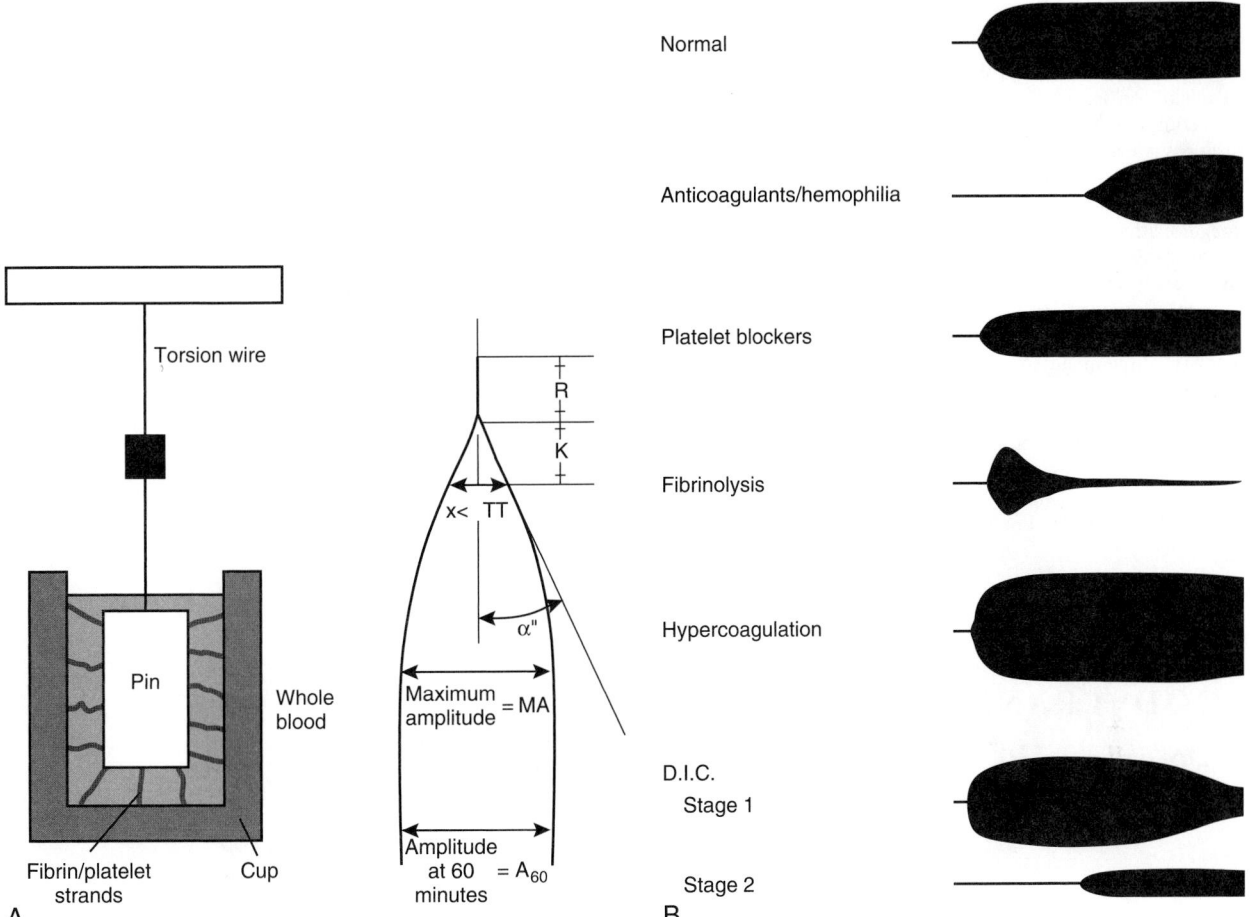

Figure 2 Measurements taken by the thromboelastogram (TEG) determine the component that is required to treat coagulopathy.

plasma or platelet replacement in the bleeding patient. This result-guided approach is ideal in slow, smaller-volume bleeds in which there is time available to obtain and react to laboratory results.

There is currently a push in trauma care to use the thromboelastogram (TEG). In some sophisticated trauma centers, this technology is available and gaining popularity because it can determine the component that is required to treat coagulopathy. Briefly, the TEG machine inserts a metal probe into a vial of whole blood and moves back and forth. As the clot is formed, the resistance to the movement of the probe is graphed and the data can be easily shown on a portable computer. From the shape of the graph, the deficient component—whether it is plasma, platelets, or fibrinogen—can be determined more accurately. TEG measurements include R value (time to initial fibrin formation), K value (time at which amplitude of tracing reaches 20 mm), MA value (maximal amplitude reflecting absolute strength of clot), and alpha angle (the rate of clot formation) (Fig. 2). It can also calculate a clotting index, which evaluates overall coagulation function. The TEG machine is relatively inexpensive and portable, adding to its desirability. This technology is currently being used by the military at some larger field hospitals where blood banking is available.

ACTIVATED RECOMBINANT FACTOR VII

To date, several case series and a large, multinational, randomized, placebo-controlled, double-blinded trial have been published that document the results of recombinant activated Factor VII (rFVIIa NovoSeven; Novo Nordisk Health Care AG, Princeton, NJ) in trauma. The multinational trial was performed with two arms: one in blunt-trauma patients and one in penetrating trauma patients. In the blunt-trauma trial there was a significant reduction in both red cell transfusion and the need for massive transfusion (defined as >20 units of PRBC per 48 hours). A smaller, nonsignificant trend in both of these outcome measures was seen in the penetrating-trauma trial. Although an improvement in mortality was demonstrated, this was not statistically significant because the study was not designed or powered to demonstrate survival as an endpoint. A major finding in both of these trials was that adverse events such as thromboembolic complications were similar between the placebo group and the rFVIIa treatment group. Although rFVIIa was originally designed to treat various forms of hemophilia, the numerous case series being reported demonstrate that the use in trauma is gaining popularity in the United States. The major downside of this systemic drug therapy to treat coagulopathy is that the drug is extremely expensive. The cost is approximately $1 per microgram, which equates to approximately $7,000 per dose if 100μgm/kg dose is used. In addition, because the drug does not have approval from the U.S. Food and Drug Administration for use in trauma, the uses in trauma are "off label." A major, multicenter, randomized, placebo-controlled, double-blinded trial with survival as a primary endpoint has been initiated and is currently under way at this time. In this trial, rFVIIa is to be infused between the fourth and eighth unit of PRBC.

SUMMARY

Coagulopathy is a common problem in the acutely bleeding trauma patient. The cause of this coagulopathy is multifactorial and involves component loss, consumption, and dilution from resuscitation fluids. Coagulation is also affected by temperature, acidosis, and preinjury medications. The complexity of the etiologic factors during massive blood loss and the difficulty in quickly quantifying the coagulopathy make calculating component therapy difficult. If time is available, laboratory–value-guided treatment is optimal. In massive transfusion for which laboratory data cannot accurately and dynamically reflect ongoing coagulopathy, empiric replacement is warranted. Although many massive transfusion protocols are in place today, surgeon judgment remains integral to initiating and monitoring the adequacy of replacement protocols. As understanding of the complex pathophysiology of coagulopathy evolves and treatment options expand, a multidisciplinary approach to diagnosis and treatment involving blood banking and laboratory specialists, anesthesiologists, and surgeons is imperative. Advances in point of care testing in the operating room, such as TEG and platelet function assays, may allow more accurate replacement and monitoring in the future, even in patients with rapid ongoing bleeding.

Suggested Readings

American Association of Blood Banks, America's Blood Centers, American Red Cross, Accessed August 11, 2007: *Circular of information for the use of human blood and blood components.* http://www.fda.gov/cber/gdlns/crclr.pdf.

Boffard KD, Riou B, Warren B, and others: Recombinant factor VIIa as adjunctive therapy for bleeding control in severely injured trauma patients: two parallel randomized, placebo-controlled, double-blind clinical trials, *J Trauma* 59(1):8, 2005.

Ivascu FA, Howells GA, Junn FS, and others: Rapid warfarin reversal in anticoagulated patients with traumatic intracranial hemorrhage reduces hemorrhage progression and mortality, *J Trauma* 59(5):1131,2005.

Schreiber MA: Coagulopathy in the trauma patient, *Curr Opin Crit Care* 11(6):590,2005.

Spahn DR, Rossaint R: Coagulopathy and blood component transfusion in trauma, *Br J Anaesth* 95(2):130,2005.

Blood Transfusion Therapy

Melissa M. Cushing, MD, and Paul M. Ness, MD

Blood transfusion is an integral component of the practice of medicine with significant applications in trauma, general surgery, and emergency care treatment plans. Advances in transfusion medicine have addressed many issues concerning the safety of the blood supply and the frequency and severity of transfusion reactions. Although the emergence of new blood-borne infectious diseases will always threaten the integrity of the blood supply, a combination of improved management practices and technological advances has significantly decreased the transmission of known infectious diseases. This chapter provides an overview of today's transfusion practice, with specific attention to surgeons, emerging transfusion technologies, and the current risks of transfusion.

BLOOD DONATION

Allogeneic Blood Components

All blood donors in the United States are volunteers; conversion to an all-volunteer donor system in the 1960s accounted for the single greatest advancement in blood safety. Molecular testing methods, such as polymerase chain reaction, markedly decrease the risk of transmission of some viral diseases by shortening the "window period," the period of time when a donor is infectious but does not have any detectable markers of viral infection. All blood components are subjected to a battery of infectious disease tests (Table 1), and all blood donors undergo a private interview and complete a questionnaire that focus on social, travel, and medical risk factors associated with exposure to blood-borne pathogens. All blood components are tested and labeled with ABO group and Rh(D) type. A screen for red cell antibodies is performed on all donors.

In addition to the required infectious disease testing, blood components must adhere to rigorous quality control standards. Storage requirements vary by product and are intended to preserve the principal elements of the component for as long as acceptable function can be maintained (Table 2).

Red Blood Cells: The hemoglobin of an allogeneic donor must be at or above 12.5 g/dL. Red blood cells are stored between 1°C and 6°C at a hematocrit of approximately 55% in an additive preservative solution. In a nonbleeding patient, 1 unit of red cells can be expected to raise the hemoglobin by 1 g/dl or the hematocrit by 3%.

Platelets: Platelets (collected from whole blood) must have a minimum of 5.5×10^{10} platelets per unit in approximately 50 ml plasma. Platelets pheresis (prepared by apheresis) must have a minimum of 3.0×10^{11} platelets in approximately 200 ml plasma. In storage, platelets last for 5 days and must be maintained at a pH higher than 6.2. Recently, blood centers have been given clearance by the U.S. Food and Drug Administration (FDA) to collect platelets that may be stored for 7 days. This practice is not yet widespread, but it may help to alleviate platelet shortages. One unit of platelets should raise the total platelet count by 5,000 to 10,000/μL (whole-blood derived), or 30,000 to 60,000/μL (platelets pheresis).

Plasma: Fresh frozen plasma (FFP) must be frozen within 8 hours of collection. Plasma can also be frozen within 24 hours of collection, with marginally lower levels of factor V and factor VIII. Plasma should be used to treat patients with documented or anticipated coagulopathy and not for volume expansion.

Cryoprecipitate: Cryoprecipitate ("cryo") is the cold-insoluble portion of FFP. Each unit is required to contain at least 150 mg of fibrinogen and 80 International Units of factor VIII in a 10- to 15-ml volume. Because there is little factor V or IX in cryo, it should not be used alone to treat disseminated intravascular coagulation (DIC) or hemophilia B. Plasma should be used to treat DIC with the addition of cryo if the patient has documented hypofibrinogenemia.

Autologous Blood

Despite significant progress in reducing the risk associated with allogeneic transfusions, autologous blood donation continues to play an important role in transfusion medicine. Patients often ask about autologous blood donation and should be made aware of

Table 1: Transfusion-transmitted Pathogens and Risk in United States

Infectious Disease	Test Method	Risk of Transfusion Transmission (per unit transfused)
HIV	HIV I/II Ab (EIA) HIV RNA (PCR)	1:1,525,000
HCV	HCV Ab (EIA) HCV RNA (PCR)	1:1,390,000
HBV	Hepatitis B core Ab (EIA) Hepatitis B surface antigen (EIA)	1:144,000
HTLV	HTLV I/II Ab (EIA)	1:1,208,000
Syphilis	RPR	Not a significant risk
Bacterial contamination of platelets	Various methods used (pH, aerobic blood culture, etc.)	1:100,000–250,000 (fatality)
West Nile Virus	WNV RNA (PCR) implemented July 2003	Regional and seasonal variation
Babesiosis	Not currently screened	1:1800 (endemic areas)
Malaria	Not currently screened	1–2 cases transmitted annually
Creutzfeldt-Jakob disease	Not currently screened	No known transmission in the United States

EIA, Enzyme immunoassay; *HBV*, hepatitis B virus; *HCV*, hepatitis C virus; *HIV*, human immunodeficiency virus; *HTLV*, human T-cell leukemia/lymphoma virus; *PCR*, polymerase chain reaction; *RPR*, rapid plasma reagin.

Table 2: Blood Product Storage Times and Temperatures

Blood Product	Storage Time	Storage Temperature
Red cells	42 days	1°–6 °C (additive solutions)
	35 days	1°–6 °C (CPDA-1)
Platelets	5–7 days	20°–24 ° C
Frozen plasma	1 year	≤−18 °C
Thawed plasma	5 days	1°–6 °C
Cryoprecipitate	1 year	≤−18 °C
Thawed and pooled cryoprecipitate	4 hours	20°–24 °C

CPDA-1, Citrate phosphate dextrose with adenine.

Table 3: Contraindications to Autologous Blood Donation

Evidence of infection or risk of bacteremia

Surgery to correct aortic stenosis

Unstable angina

Active seizure disorder

Myocardial infarction or cerebrovascular accident within 6 months of donation

Patients with significant cardiac or pulmonary disease that have not yet been cleared for surgery

High-grade left main coronary heart disease

Uncontrolled hypertension

its advantages and disadvantages. Autologous blood donation can address the supply shortage in patients with rare blood phenotypes or alloantibodies. It reduces the risk of transfusion-transmitted diseases, avoids sensitization to allogeneic blood-related antigens, and limits transfusion-related immune modulation.

As a group, patients are less suited for blood donation than volunteer donors. The frequency of a severe donor reaction requiring hospitalization, although quite low, is significantly higher in autologous donors than in allogeneic donors. Blood collection centers will defer autologous donors with high risk for an adverse event (Table 3). If an autologous unit is not used by the intended patient, it is discarded because blood bank standards do not permit allogeneic transfusion of unused autologous units (i.e., crossover).

The criteria for autologous donors are not as stringent as those for allogeneic donors. Standards require that an autologous donor's hemoglobin level be no less than 11.0 g/dL or the hematocrit 33% before each donation. Patients may donate 10.5 ml/kg per donation in addition to testing samples. Patients should be stable and scheduled for surgical procedures in which blood transfusion is likely. In some cases, the donor is given supplemental iron or erythropoietin to prevent anemia. There are no age or weight limits.

Pediatric patients are able to provide autologous donations with suitable volume adjustments, parental participation, and adequate reassurance.

Autologous donations may be scheduled once per week (or as frequently as every 72 hours in an urgent situation), but the last donation should occur no less than 72 hours before surgery to allow time for the restoration of intravascular blood volume and testing of the donated blood. This is usually accomplished by beginning the donation series 4 to 6 weeks before the scheduled surgery.

Some patients and their families ask for directed blood donations, hoping to select blood donors that are known to them and presumably have less risk. This practice has not been shown to have any medical benefit, may cause reduced or delayed blood availability, and should not be considered a worthwhile transfusion alternative.

SURGICAL PRACTICE ISSUES

Transfusion Trigger

Transfusion is rarely indicated when the hemoglobin concentration is greater than 10 g/dL and is almost always indicated when it is less than 6 g/dL, especially when the anemia is acute. For all intermediate values, an absolute hemoglobin "trigger" for transfusion is not recommended. Instead, the patient's ability to tolerate inadequate oxygenation should be assessed. Factors such as tachycardia, age, underlying disease, type of surgery, and cardiac status should be taken into consideration. The indications for transfusion of autologous red blood cells may be more liberal than for allogeneic red cells.

Emergency Release Blood

Red blood cells may be necessary emergently during surgery without time for complete blood typing and antibody identification. In such a situation, different degrees of compatible blood are available depending on the level of urgency. If there is no time for ABO/Rh typing or no specimen is available, group O red blood cells can be issued. If there is a patient specimen and sufficient time, ABO and Rh type-specific blood can be issued. If the patient specimen demonstrates a positive antibody screen but the antibody has yet to be identified, transfusion medicine specialists will assess the situation and issue the most compatible red cells available (e.g., antigen-matched or crossmatch-compatible). Transfusion medicine specialists, surgeons, and anesthesiologists should discuss the risk of emergency transfusions versus delayed transfusions.

Transfusion-Related Immunomodulation

There is some clinical evidence that transfusions may have immunosuppressive effects. Early reports of immunosuppression were based on unfiltered red blood cells, and these reports described decreased renal transplant rejection in patients transfused preoperatively. This effect is thought to be related to the presence of white blood cells in blood products, and some studies have reported reduced cancer recurrence or postoperative bacterial infection in surgical patients receiving leuko-reduced red cells rather than unfiltered products. In addition, some multicenter observational studies suggest that patients receiving fewer transfusions have improved patient survival compared with patients receiving more transfusions. Despite a number of randomized controlled trials, no overwhelming clinical evidence is available to establish the existence of a transfusion-related immunomodulation (TRIM) effect that relates allogeneic blood transfusion to postoperative infection or cancer recurrence. Further studies must be performed to elucidate the biology of TRIM.

Perioperative Bleeding

Excessive perioperative bleeding remains a major complication of surgery. The main risks include an undetected bleeding disorder, coagulopathy arising from massive blood loss, or causes related to the surgery procedure itself (e.g., failure to control bleeding vessels, cardiopulmonary bypass, orthotopic liver transplant, and so forth). Identifying patients at risk by means of a good history and clinical examination remains one of the most important strategies in managing perioperative bleeding (Table 4).

Pharmacologic interventions should be considered to reduce the quantity of allogeneic blood products transfused. Anti-fibrinolytic agents such as aprotinin, epsilon amino caproic acid, and tranexamic acid have been found in several trials to decrease bleeding and transfusion requirements. The use of these agents, particularly aprotinin, should be restricted to excessive bleeding in view of recent safety concerns regarding increased risk of renal, cardiac, or cerebral events. Desmopressin increases activity of von Willebrand factor and improves platelet function. It is useful in reducing perioperative blood loss in patients with von Willebrand's disease and functional platelet disorders, including aspirin-induced platelet dysfunction.

Table 4: Patients at Risk for Perioperative Bleeding

Drugs
Antiplatelet drugs
Warfarin
Heparin
Acquired
Vitamin K deficiency
Liver dysfunction
Renal disease
Sepsis
Shock
Thrombocytopenia
Disseminated intravascular coagulation
Inherited
Quantitative and qualitative platelet disorders
von Willebrand's disease
Coagulation factor defects

NSAIDs, Nonsteroidal anti-inflammatory drugs.

Massive Blood Transfusion for Trauma

In situations in which a patient receives a massive transfusion with banked blood products, there will be several predictable pathophysiologic effects. The degree to which these effects will have an impact on the patient's condition depends on the severity and type of injuries sustained from trauma. Prior attempts to standardize protocols, through algorithms based on ratios of blood components or screening coagulation tests, have not adequately defined the optimal clinical response, requiring case-by-case judgment.

Hypothermia, metabolic acidosis, thrombocytopenia, thrombocytopathy, and hypofibrinogenemia appear to be the parameters that predispose patients to continued bleeding and microvascular hemorrhage. A large part of the impaired hemostasis is due to a consumptive coagulopathy in addition to the dilution of the hemostatic elements.

Recombinant Factor VIIa

Recombinant factor VIIa is approved by the FDA for the treatment and prevention of bleeding in hemophiliacs with inhibitors, as well as patients with congenital factor VII deficiencies. Many anecdotal reports have been published on the use of recombinant factor VIIa for off-label clinical indications. NovoSeven (Novo Nordisk HealthCare AG, Princeton, NJ), activated recombinant factor VIIa, has seen increasing use for uncontrolled bleeding in the trauma and surgery settings when conventional methods to control bleeding have failed. However, this drug is not without risks, and large, well-designed clinical trials are required to demonstrate both efficacy and safety in the treatment of patients with perioperative or trauma-related bleeding. Many institutions require that clinicians consult with the transfusion service before proceeding with NovoSeven therapy.

TRANSFUSION REACTIONS

There are several instances in which a transfusion results in an adverse event in a patient. Transfusion reactions can occur acutely (within 24 hours) or after a significant delay (from days to years after transfusion). These reactions can be subcategorized into immunologic and nonimmunologic types (Table 5). For purposes of this chapter, we have focused on those transfusion reactions notable for severity or frequency in trauma and surgical settings. Clinicians must be aware of the risk of transfusion reactions; fortunately, the most frequent transfusion reactions are the least severe.

Acute Hemolytic Transfusion Reactions

Most fatal hemolytic reactions are the result of ABO incompatibility. ABO incompatibility can result from three types of errors: (1) misidentification of the intended patient during blood draws at the bed side, (2) misidentification of patient samples or blood components within the blood bank, or (3) misidentification of the patient at the time of blood administration. The results of such errors can be life threatening.

ABO hemolysis begins by intravascular, complement-mediated red cell lysis. As hemolysis accelerates, the reaction manifests clinically as fever, hypotension, severe shock, and DIC. Renal failure often occurs in acute hemolytic reactions as a result of acute tubular necrosis secondary to hypotension, arteriole thrombi deposition, and direct inflammatory effects on the kidneys. Hemoglobin and its derivatives may precipitate in the renal tubules, especially under acidic conditions. Binding of bacterial endotoxin and nitric oxide by free hemoglobin exacerbates renal failure. Acute hemolytic reactions can also cause pulmonary dysfunction and acute respiratory distress.

Table 5: Transfusion Reactions

Acute Reactions		Incidence per Unit Transfused
Immunologic	Acute hemolytic	1:50,000
	Anaphylactic	1:40,000
	TRALI	1:2500–5000
	Febrile nonhemolytic	1:200
	Urticarial	1:100
Nonimmunologic	Bacterial contamination of platelets	1:2000
	Bacterial contamination of red plates	1:1,000,000
	Circulatory overload	1:2000
	Thermal/mechanical hemolysis	—

Delayed Reactions

Immunologic	Delayed hemolytic	1:5000
	Alloimmunization	—
	TA-GVHD	Only 200 cases reported
	Posttransfusion purpura	—
Nonimmunologic	Hemochromatosis	>50–100 units transfused
	Transfusion-transmitted pathogens	See Table 4

TA-GVHD, Transfusion-associated graft-versus-host disease; *TRALI*, transfusion-related acute lung injury.

Although less common, acute hemolytic reactions can occur with other red cell antigen-antibody incompatibilities besides ABO, such as the Rh, Kell, Kidd (Jk^a greater than Jk^b) and Duffy (Fy^a greater than Fy^b) antigen systems.

CLINICAL AND LABORATORY FEATURES: Signs and symptoms include fever, chills, hemoglobinemia, hemoglobinuria, anxiety, shock, DIC, dyspnea, chest pain, flank pain, and oliguria. During surgery, only oliguria, hemoglobinuria, and diffuse bleeding from DIC may be recognized.

TREATMENT: The implicated transfusion should be stopped as soon as symptoms are identified. Treatment for a hemolytic reaction is supportive and includes blood pressure support, maintenance of urine output (=100 ml/hour) with adequate hydration, and monitoring of oxygen delivery, including additional red-cell transfusions if necessary. Patients experiencing intravascular hemolysis may be unstable, and intensive care monitoring should be considered. Both the renal and the coagulation status should be monitored closely. Early initiation of dialysis may be critical.

Delayed Hemolytic Transfusion Reactions

In contrast to acute hemolysis, delayed hemolytic reactions are much more common and are caused by extravascular hemolysis occurring usually in the spleen. Delayed hemolysis typically presents 3 days to 2 weeks after a transfusion. Most delayed hemolytic reactions are discovered in the blood bank when an antibody screen reveals a previously undetected antibody. Complicated clinical situations are often resolved in consultation with the blood bank or hematology service.

CLINICAL AND LABORATORY FEATURES: Decreasing hemoglobin, hyperbilirubinemia, elevated lactate dehydrogenase, a positive direct antiglobulin (Coombs) test, and fever are the most commonly reported features in delayed hemolytic transfusion reactions.

TREATMENT: Supportive care with maintenance of renal function and adequate oxygenation is sufficient until hemolysis subsides. The patient should be notified to avoid subsequent reactions; this could be problematic for future surgical procedures.

Febrile Nonhemolytic Transfusion Reactions

Febrile nonhemolytic transfusion reactions (FNHTRs) are mediated by leukocytes or the cytokine by-products of leukocytes in donor blood. Most transfusion services have moved toward universal leuko-reduction of blood products to reduce the incidence of FNHTRs. Although prestorage leuko-reduction has greatly decreased the incidence of these reactions, they remain common (1 in 200 units transfused).

FNHTRs are a diagnosis of exclusion—all other causes of fever (transfusion or nontransfusion related) must first be ruled out, especially those with more severe complications, such as hemolytic or septic transfusion reactions.

CLINICAL AND LABORATORY FEATURES AND TREATMENT: Febrile reactions usually occur during or shortly after a transfusion but may occur up to 6 hours after the end of the transfusion. Pretreatment with antipyretics can prevent recurrent FNHTRs in susceptible patients. In a patient with a history of previous FNHTRs, subsequent transfusions should be leuko-reduced.

Transfusion-Related Acute Lung Injury

Transfusion-related acute lung injury (TRALI) describes a range of clinical and laboratory features seen within 6 hours of the transfusion of plasma-containing blood products. TRALI results from two situations: (1) transfused blood products containing antibodies directed against patient white blood cell antigens (human leukocyte antigens or human neutrophil antigens) or (2) activation of the patient's granulocytes by metabolites released during blood storage.

The clinical presentation of TRALI is identical to adult respiratory distress syndrome. The initial symptoms are caused by the onset of pulmonary edema, which may be seen first in the dependent area of the lungs but is often more generalized within a few hours. It is important to rule out congestive cardiac failure or transfusion-associated circulatory overload before initiating treatment for TRALI. TRALI has a mortality rate of between 5% and 8%. If the patient survives, the episode of TRALI is generally limited to 24–48 hours. TRALI does not generally recur.

CLINICAL AND LABORATORY FEATURES: Patients with TRALI have respiratory distress symptoms requiring oxygen support or mechanical ventilation. The onset of symptoms is within the first 2 to 6 hours after initiation of blood transfusion. Hypotension, tachycardia, cyanosis, and fever are also seen in the majority of cases. Chest roentgograms initially show a patchy, dependent, interstitial, and alveolar process that progresses to a radiologic picture often described as "white out." Auscultatory findings are rarely observed. Anesthesiologists may note a copious, frothy fluid oozing from the endotracheal tube or may notice that the lungs "feel heavy" and are difficult to ventilate. TRALI does not cause an increase in the pulmonary capillary wedge pressure.

TREATMENT: Management of TRALI is supportive and includes intubation and mechanical ventilation in approximately 70% of patients. Small tidal volume settings should be used for optimal ventilatory care. All patients will require oxygen support. Hypotension is often managed with intravenous fluids alone, but vasopressor agents may also be necessary in severe cases. The use of corticosteroids has been described in case reports, but there are no convincing data to support the efficacy of this treatment. The donors of the implicated units can be evaluated for antibodies to white blood cell antigens, but this information is not usually available for several weeks. If such antibodies are found, the donor will be permanently deferred.

Allergic or Anaphylactic Reactions

Allergic transfusion reactions are generally related to the volume of plasma transfused and the rapidity with which it is administered. Blood products with higher plasma content, such as FFP and platelets, are more likely to trigger these reactions than products with lower plasma content, such as red blood cells. Although mild allergic reactions are common (1:100 transfusions), severe anaphylaxis is uncommon.

Immunoglobulin A (IgA) deficiency is one recognized cause of allergic transfusion reactions. Patients with IgA deficiency can naturally produce immunoglobulin E (IgE) anti-IgA without previous exposure. If a patient has received previous transfusions that were not associated with anaphylaxis, IgA deficiency can usually be ruled out. Patients with IgA deficiency and a history of anaphylaxis can receive plasma only from IgA-deficient donors, but platelets and red cells can be extensively washed to remove IgA. IgA-deficient donors are rare (1:1000). Fortunately, most severe allergic reactions are not related to IgA deficiency and will not recur with repeated transfusions.

CLINICAL AND LABORATORY FEATURES: Patients with moderate-to-severe allergic reactions may present with hypotension, bronchospasm, decreased oxygen saturation, and chest tightness with or without tachycardia.

TREATMENT: Treatment for mild urticarial reactions consists of histamine (H_1) blockers such as diphenhydramine, either as a single agent or in combination with steroids, or H_2 blockers. Administration of vasopressors for blood pressure support may be required in severe reactions. Although (non-IgA mediated) anaphylactic reactions do not usually recur, additional transfusions should be undertaken with caution, and resuscitative support should be readily available. If moderately severe non-IgA reactions do recur, consideration should be given to administering washed red blood cells (RBCs) and platelets in the future. IgA deficiency with the presence of antibody should be ruled out in any patient experiencing anaphylaxis with a first transfusion.

Infectious Complications

Transfusion-Transmitted Viral Infection

With recent advances in molecular diagnostics, the science of viral infectious disease testing in transfusion medicine has improved dramatically. Blood collection centers now routinely employ polymerase chain reaction and enzyme immunoassay techniques to screen donated blood for dangerous, known viruses (see Table 1). Other potential pathogens transmitted by transfusion include cytomegalovirus (CMV), Epstein-Barr virus, and parvovirus B19.

CMV is especially dangerous in immunosuppressed patients. Because leuko-reduction is effective in reducing CMV harbored in donor white blood cells, leuko-reduced or CMV-seronegative products should be issued to patients at risk for CMV infection. Leuko-reduced products are more available than CMV-seronegative screened units and are a good choice for patients in need of protection against CMV in the acute care setting. FFP and cryoprecipitate carry a minimal risk of CMV transmission because of the small number of leukocytes present.

Bacterial Contamination

Progress in laboratory testing over the past several decades has greatly reduced the risk of viral infection via allogeneic blood. As a result of these efforts, attention has shifted to bacterial contamination of blood products as the greatest residual source of transfusion-transmitted disease.

PLATELETS: Because they are stored at 20 °C to 24 °C to preserve function and survival, platelets are an excellent growth medium for bacteria: 1 in 1000–2000 platelet units are bacterially contaminated. Two thirds of the organisms grown from platelets are gram positive, such as *Staphylococcus epidermidis* and *Bacillus cereus*, and one third are gram negative. The gram-negative organisms are more likely to cause fatal septic reactions. Blood banks have focused on reducing this risk, recently requiring implementation of methods to limit and detect bacterial contamination in all platelet components.

RED BLOOD CELLS: Bacterial contamination in RBCs is much less common because they are stored at 1 °C to 6 °C. *Yersinia enterocolitica* and *Serratia* species are typically isolated from contaminated RBCs because of their ability to grow in colder temperatures.

CLINICAL AND LABORATORY FEATURES: Patients with septic transfusion reactions present with high fevers, rigors, hypotension, shock, nausea, vomiting, and possibly DIC. A culture or Gram stain of the remainder of the residual product should demonstrate the same organism that is growing in the patient's blood.

TREATMENT: When transfusion-related sepsis is suspected from the patient's clinical presentation, immediate administration of broad-spectrum antibiotics may be lifesaving. Blood cultures may take days to become positive, and false-negative Gram stains are common. Patients experiencing septic reactions should be monitored for at least 24 hours in an intensive care setting because they may rapidly destabilize despite supportive care and appropriate antibiotics.

Metabolic Complications

Rapid infusion of blood products stored in citrated plasma (FFP and platelets) can produce citrate toxicity manifested by acute hypocalcemia. This condition commonly presents symptoms of acral or perioral paresthesias, lightheadedness, a metallic taste, abdominal cramping, and nausea and may progress to involuntary muscle tremors, chest pain, seizures, and electrocardiogram changes. In severe cases, convulsions and shock may occur. Treatment includes supplemental calcium therapy that should not exceed a total dose of 1 g unless signs of hypocalcemia persist.

Transfusion-induced hyperkalemia can occur in massively transfused patients but is quite rare. The potassium concentration in 1 unit of red blood cells can increase up to 40–70 mEq/L after 35 to 40 days of storage. This additional potassium can be tolerated in most patients, but patients in shock or with preexisting renal failure who receive more than 6 to 10 units of older RBCs may show symptoms of hyperkalemia. Pediatric patients may also be affected because of their smaller blood volume. Severe cases may require dialysis or a transvenous pacemaker.

PATHOGEN REDUCTION AND BLOOD SUBSTITUTES

To address the remaining risks in the integrity of the blood supply, extensive research has focused on pathogen reduction technologies and blood substitutes. Pathogen inactivation technologies have all but eliminated the infectious risks of plasma-derived protein fractions, but no technique is currently licensed for traditional blood components. Traditional methods of mechanical removal, such as washing and filtration, are ineffective in reducing the risk of cell-associated agents, and sterilization methods have caused unwanted toxicities in either the product itself or in the recipient. Several countries have licensed solvent-detergent treatment and methylene blue addition to reduce infectious transmission by plasma and cryoprecipitate, but both methods have major limitations and are not available at this time in the United States. There are a number of promising methods that have recently entered clinical testing.

Three different RBC substitutes are in advanced clinical testing at this time. These products suffer from critical shortcomings, such as short in vivo half-life, that make them more suitable for short-term gaps (e.g., acute blood loss or ischemia) than long-term solutions. Bovine-derived products introduce additional safety hurdles, such as immunogenicity and fear of prion contamination. We are still several years away from an FDA-approved product available for clinical use.

CONCLUSION

Transfusion medicine has made significant progress to improve the safety of the blood supply and reduce the risks associated with transfusion reactions. Ongoing research in transfusion medicine, such as pathogen inactivation, may soon eradicate many of the remaining risks from clinical practice. Longer-term blood substitutes may address both product shortages and the immunosuppressive effects of transfusions. Although the decision to transfuse a patient involves less risk than ever before, clinicians must assess the benefits and risks of transfusions for their patients on a case-by-case basis. Transfusion specialists are trained to support the use of blood products in clinical settings and are available for consultation.

Suggested Readings

Dodd RY: Current safety of the blood supply in the United States, *Int J Hematol* 80:301, 2004.
Goodnough LT, Brecher ME, Kanter MH, and others: Transfusion medicine. First of two parts—blood transfusion, *N Engl J Med* 340:438, 1999.
Goodnough LT, Brecher ME, Kanter MH, and others: Transfusion medicine. Second of two parts—blood conservation, *N Engl J Med* 340:525, 1999.
Hillyer CD, Silberstein LE, Ness PM, and others: *Blood banking and transfusion medicine.* Philadelphia, 2003, Churchill Livingstone.

HEAD INJURIES

Jon David Weingart, MD

The management of head injuries involves rapid evaluation of the extent of injury followed by rapid intervention to halt ongoing injury and to prevent additional secondary injury. The overall goal of treatment is to maintain intracranial pressure (ICP) at a normal level. Elevated ICP results in decreased blood flow to the brain and subsequently to irreversible brain injury. Treatment includes surgical interventions to remove space-occupying mass lesions, primarily hematomas, and nonsurgical treatments to reduce brain tissue volume.

EVALUATION

The evaluation of a patient with a head injury is multidisciplinary. All patients must undergo a complete trauma evaluation because patients with severe head injuries secondary to nonpenetrating trauma are likely to have injuries to other systems. Assurance of cervical spine stability is an important aspect of the initial evaluation. The neck should be immobilized with a cervical collar until

the stability of the cervical spine has been cleared. A lateral cervical plain film and an odontoid view plain film are used to evaluate the cervical spine. The C7-T1 disk space must be visualized on the lateral film to clear the cervical spine. If the C7-T1 disk space is not visualized, a computed tomography (CT) scan through the C7-T1 disk space is obtained.

Ideally, the extent of the head injury is assessed before the patient is given any medications that will alter the central nervous system (CNS). When this is not possible because of cardiovascular instability or other unstable injuries, short-acting muscle relaxants should be used. The initial evaluation of the patient's CNS function is aimed at assessing for global brain dysfunction (i.e., level of consciousness) and for focal brain dysfunction (i.e., unilateral signs such as hemiparesis). The Glasgow Coma Scale (GCS) is an excellent, rapid way to evaluate for global or focal brain dysfunction. The GCS involves three parameters: eye opening, verbalization, and motor responses (Table 1). The GCS score is also reproducible and can be used to follow a patient's neurologic status over time. Other aspects of the neurologic examination are papillary responses, corneal responses, and gag responses. These reflexes are used to evaluate brainstem function in an unresponsive patient with severe head injuries.

After the initial stabilization and evaluation are complete, the patient is taken as quickly as possible for a noncontrast brain CT scan. In the patient with a severe head injury, the brain CT should be obtained as quickly as possible because the CT determines whether a mass lesion, which requires surgical evacuation, is present.

Table 1: Glasgow Coma Scale

Parameters for Evaluation of Global or Focal Brain Dysfunction	Points
Best Eye Opening	
Spontaneous	4
To speech	3
To pain	2
None	1
Best Verbal Response	
Oriented	5
Confused	4
Inappropriate	3
Incomprehensible	2
None	1
Best Motor Response	
Obeys	6
Localizes to pain	5
Withdraws to pain	4
Flexor response	3
Extensor response	2
None	1

The CT scan should be evaluated for (1) presence of blood extra-axial or intra-axial, (2) mass effect or effacement of the lateral ventricle, (3) midline shift, and (4) presence or absence of cerebrospinal fluid in the basal cisterns. A patient with a mass lesion and a GCS score of 8 or less should undergo rapid surgical decompression.

SURGICAL TREATMENT

Acute Subdural Hematoma

All patients with severe head injury (GCS score of 3–8) should be initially approached as if they have an acute subdural hematoma that is causing increased ICP. The patient should be intubated and hyperventilated to a Pco_2 of 28 to 30 mm Hg before the head CT is obtained. Mannitol 1 g/kg should be given intravenously over 15 minutes. Throughout this phase of the evaluation, intravascular volume should be maintained. Hypotension leads to decreased cerebral perfusion and therefore should be treated if it occurs.

Early evacuation of acute subdural hematomas (within 4 hours of injury) has been shown to reduce mortality. Patients with subdural blood greater than 1 cm associated with shift of the midline structures should be taken to the operating room immediately for evacuation. Patients with thin subdural hematomas (≤ 5 mm) and mild neurologic symptoms can be observed and treated medically because small subdural hematomas can resolve on their own. These patients should be followed with serial CT scans until the blood has resolved.

Patients with large subdural hematomas are taken directly from the CT scanner to the operating room. While the anesthesiologist is preparing the patient, the surgeon is positioning the head. The head can be positioned on a donut or horseshoe cushion, but we prefer to stabilize the head with head pins and the Mayfield head clamp (SchaererMayfield USA, Cincinnati, OH). The entire half of the head is shaved. The location of the incision depends on the size

of the subdural hematoma. The incision must be large enough to allow for the entire subdural to be included in the craniotomy. For a subdural hematoma that is primarily frontal and temporal, a standard frontotemporal incision may be adequate. For a more posteriorly located subdural hematoma, a linear incision may be adequate. For a large subdural hematoma involving the frontal, temporal, and parietal areas, the incision is a large trauma or hemicraniotomy incision. The incision begins anteriorly in the midline and extends posteriorly to the lambdoidal suture, where it is curved forward to above the ear and around to the root of the zygoma.

After the area is prepared and draped, the incision is quickly opened through the galea, with Raney clips placed on the skin edge to control bleeding. The temporalis muscle is incised with the cautery in line with the scalp incision. Cautery and periosteal elevators are used to dissect the pericranium off the skull with the skin flap. The skin and temporalis muscle are held back with towel clips or suture and a rubber band. The power perforator is used to quickly place burr holes in the temporal fossa at the root of the zygoma. If the dura seen through the burr hold appears blue, the dura should be opened at this point to allow for partial decompression. Several additional burr holes are placed frontally, along the midline, and posteriorly. The dura is stripped off the inner table, and a power craniotome is used to evaluate the craniotomy flap. At this point, several holes are placed in the flap and on the intact skull, through which size 0 Tevdek (Deknatel, Mansfield, MA) sutures are passed. The Tevdek sutures are readied in case the bone flap must be replaced quickly, as in the case of malignant brain swelling. At this point, the dura is opened in a cruciated fashion, allowing the ICP to extrude the hematoma. Normal saline irrigation is used to wash the clot off the brain. At the edge of the dural opening, cotton strips are placed and handheld brain spatulas are used to gently depress the brain. With use of irrigation again, the residual clot is washed off the cortex and evacuated. This is particularly important in the anterior frontal and temporal areas. Along the midline, the surgeon should be cautious when removing small clots, which may be tamponading a torn bridging vein. While the hematoma is being washed out, any source of bleeding—veins or arteries—is controlled with bipolar coagulation.

After evacuation of the convexity hematoma, the medical temporal lobe and uncal herniation over the tentorium should be relieved. This is accomplished by retracting and lifting the anterior temporal lobe off the floor of the middle fossa. If the anterior temporal lobe is contused and hemorrhagic, the anterior temporal lobe can be resected, which will allow for improved vision. The brain spatula elevating the temporal lobe is advanced until the edge of the tentorium is identified. An attempt is made to lift the herniated medical temporal lobe back into the supratentorial space if the tissue looks viable. If the surgeon is unable to reduce the herniation or if the medial temporal lobe appears contused and nonviable, a subpial resection of the tissue should be carried out using suction and bipolar coagulation. Arachnoid attachments from the ambien cistern to the temporal lobe should be cut. A gush of cerebrospinal fluid is often seen when the temporal lobe has been reduced and the brainstem decompressed.

After the medial temporal lobe has been decompressed, the operative field is irrigated to check for any additional bleeding. The dura is closed primarily if possible. If the closure appears to strangulate the brain because of brain swelling, a pericranial graft is used to cover the brain. Gelfoam (Pfizer, New York, NY) is placed in the epidural space, and the bone flap is attached with sutures or titanium plates.

At the end of the procedure, an ICP monitor should be placed on the opposite side. The ICP measurement is critical to managing a patient with poor findings on neurologic examination. Medical management is directed toward maintaining the ICP in a normal range. This ensures adequate blood flow to the brain and minimizes secondary injury. If, while ICP is being monitored, a patient develops a rapid increase in the ICP measurement, a repeat head CT should be obtained to look for development of a new hemorrhagic mass lesion.

All patients with acute subdural hematomas should have a follow-up head CT within 24 hours of surgery to have a baseline picture of the brain and to see what was accomplished at surgery. It is not unusual for small remnants of the hematoma to remain or for there to be a new accumulation of a small amount of blood. This baseline head CT scan is invaluable when trying to interpret follow-up head CT scans 2 to 5 days after surgery.

Two scenarios that can occur in the setting of a subdural hematoma are (1) the presence of a large intraparenchymal hematoma and (2) malignant brain edema. If a large intraparenchymal hematoma is present and is contributing to the mass effect in the brain, it should be decompressed. The hematomas usually come to the surface, and it is not difficult to enter them and to evacuate the blood clot. The goal is to decompress the brain and not to remove every small piece of hematoma. Intraparenchymal hematomas should be removed using irrigation and gentle suction. Aggressive removal of the clot in the wall of the hematoma cavity can produce bleeding that is difficult to stop. If this occurs, different hemostatic agents can be used to achieve hemostasis because bipolar cauterization is often ineffective. Hemostatic agents include thrombin-soaked cotton balls, thrombin-soaked Gelfoam, Avitene (fibrillar collagen; Davol, Cranston, RI), and as a last resort, cotton balls soaked in half-strength hydrogen peroxide.

The second scenario to be aware of is the development of malignant brain edema and swelling, which occurs after the dura is open. When this occurs, the brain begins to swell out of the dural opening. This is a poor prognostic sign and probably reflects a severe diffuse brain injury. When met with this situation, the surgeon should quickly approximate the dura and attach the bone flap.

Epidural Hematoma

Epidural hematomas occur in the potential space between the dura and the inner table of the skull. Because the dura is strongly adherent to the cranial sutures, epidural hematomas typically respect the sutures and do not cross them. On a head CT, an epidural hematoma has a convex shape. Epidural hematomas usually occur in the setting of blunt trauma to the head and, in most cases, are associated with a skull fracture. Classically, the history of a patient with an epidural hematoma is a transient loss of consciousness after a head injury, followed by a lucid phase and then neurologic deterioration. Five different clinical courses have been described in patients with epidural hematomas: (1) unconscious-conscious-unconscious, (2) unconscious throughout, (3) conscious-unconscious, (4) unconscious-conscious, and (5) conscious throughout. Occasionally, a patient with an initial normal head CT will, after some delay, develop an epidural hematoma. Regardless of how the patient presents, the key issue for patients with epidural hematomas is that prompt treatment before loss of consciousness results in excellent outcomes. Because of the excellent prognosis with rapid treatment, all patients with impairment in consciousness following head trauma should have a head CT to rule out the presence of an epidural hematoma.

The treatment for an epidural hematoma that is causing alteration in consciousness or alteration in the patient's neurologic function is evacuation of the hematoma. Patients can deteriorate quickly, so they should have surgery immediately. The general surgical approach involves adequate exposure of the hematoma and obliteration of the epidural space with dural tack-up sutures.

Patients can be positioned with the head on a horseshoe pad or in a three-point fixation head-holding device. The craniotomy should be large enough to completely expose the hematoma. Because epidural hematomas are commonly in the temporal area, a standard frontotemporal incision with or without posterior extension of the incision behind the ear is often used. As the burr

holes are placed, the epidural hematoma will be encountered immediately beneath the burr hole and a partial evacuation can be carried out quickly. After the bone flap is elevated, the hematoma is evacuated and the source of the bleeding, if found, is controlled. Middle meningeal and other dural branches are the most common cause of epidural hematomas. The dura around the craniotomy edge is tacked up to the skull. Similarly, multiple tack-up sutures serve to obliterate the epidural space and reduce or eliminate the risk of recurrence. If, on the basis of the head CT, a question of a concomitant subdural hematoma exists, the subdural space is explored before replacing the bone flap. A linear dural incision allows for exploration of the subdural space to rule out a subdural component. If a subdural hematoma is encountered, the dura can be opened widely to drain the hematoma. In patients with GCS scores of 8 or less, an ICP monitor is placed at the end of the hematoma evacuation. Postoperative management of increased ICP is the same as for patients with an acute subdural hematoma.

Epidural hematomas near the midline or in the posterior fossa should be approached with a plan to control a hole or tear in a venous sinus. A skull fracture typically is seen crossing the sinus. As long as there is no concern for the patency of the venous sinus, the bone flap should extend up to the sinus but not across it. Any sinus bleeding can be controlled with tack-up sutures located along the sinus. Gelfoam and Avitene can be useful to control sinus bleeding.

Penetrating Injuries and Gunshot Wounds

Gunshot wounds to the head are evaluated and treated in the emergency department the same way as blunt head trauma. The entrance site and an exit site, if present, should be identified on the scalp. Once stabilized, patients are taken immediately for a head CT to evaluate the trajectory and the areas of brain affected by the missile. The two major issues in management of these types of injuries are (1) the presence of a hematoma, extra-axial or intra-axial, causing mass effect and increased ICP; and (2) the risk of infection because of the bone fragments and other debris carried into the brain by the force of the bullet. Although unusual, a hematoma causing mass effect and neurologic compromise should be surgically removed.

The standard treatment for patients with gunshot wounds to the head remains controversial. Some surgeons believe that debridement of the bullet track in the brain leads to better outcomes. Bone chips, hair, and bullet fragments, along with necrotic brain tissue, are removed. The craniotomy is carried out using standard techniques to adequately expose the bullet entry point. The dura is opened in a crucial fashion and the bullet track debrided. All hemorrhagic and devitalized brain tissue should be removed until normal-appearing white matter is present. Handheld brain spatulas or a speculum can be used to provide exposure to permit debridement of the bullet track. Irrigation flushed down the bullet track will help to debride in the deeper portions of the bullet track. An attempt to remove all bone fragments should be made. Once the track has been debrided and hemostasis achieved, the dura is closed in a watertight fashion to prevent postoperative cerebrospinal fluid leaks and infections. Usually, a pericranial tissue graft is necessary to achieve dural closure. Both the bone and skin also should be debrided. In addition, it is important to get good closure of the scalp with healthy viable tissue. Postoperatively, patients are placed on broad-spectrum antibiotics, although the most common pathogens are gram-positive *cocci*.

Most studies evaluating the treatment of gunshot wounds have arisen out of wartime experiences. Because of the high incidence of infection in these series, debridement became the standard approach. However, recent experiences have demonstrated that local debridement and closure of the entry site followed by intravenous antibiotics is also effective at preventing infectious complications of the gunshot wound. Although this more conservative treatment course may not be appropriate for all patients, it is appropriate for patients with poor neurologic function and poor prognosis. Poor prognosis is associated with bullet wounds that cross the midline or pass through the ventricle.

In addition to antibiotics, these patients are started on an anticonvulsant and given a tetanus toxoid shot. Steroids are not indicated.

DECOMPRESSIVE CRANIECTOMY

The role of decompressive craniectomy in the management of medically intractable intracranial hypertension remains controversial. Clinical studies to date are poorly controlled, results are inconsistent, and thus firm conclusions are difficult to derive. Patients with prolonged elevation of ICP despite maximal medical therapy would be potential candidates for these procedures. The most common decompressive procedures are: (1) a hemicraniectomy with duraplasty and (2) a bifrontal craniectomy. The bone can be removed in one or more pieces and is placed in the bone bank for later replacement. For the hemicraniectomy, the bone flap should extend back to the occipital region. The dura should be opened in a cruciate fashion to allow the swollen brain to expand outward. Large pieces of bovine pericardium are used to cover the brain so that a plane of dissection will exist between the galea and the brain when the bone is replaced at a later date.

The goal of these procedures is to limit the secondary damage caused by extended intracranial hypertension. There is some suggestion in the clinical studies available that these procedures have more impact on outcome when performed earlier in the course of the injury.

NONSURGICAL MANAGEMENT

The nonsurgical management of patients with head injuries includes that of the postoperative patient and the management of patients for whom surgery was not indicated. The primary management issue is control of the ICP. The result of controlling ICP in a normal range is to maintain adequate cerebral perfusion and oxygenation and thus limit ongoing secondary injury.

In l993 a task force established by the Brain Trauma Foundation looked at 12 issues related to the medical management of patients with severe head injures. Within each category, treatments were designated as *standards* when the treatment represented principles of patient management that reflect a high degree of clinical certainty, guidelines when the treatment represented a particular strategy or range of management strategies that reflect a moderate clinical certainty, and options for remaining management strategies for which there is unclear clinical certainty.

Of the 12 categories evaluated, only 3 met the standards criteria:

1. Chronic prolonged hyperventilation therapy ($Paco_2 \leq 25$ mm Hg) should be avoided after severe traumatic brain injury.
2. The use of glucocorticoids is not recommended to improve outcome or reduce ICP in patients with severe head injury.
3. Prophylactic use of phenytoin carbamazepine or phenobarbital is not recommended for preventing late posttraumatic seizures.

Medical Management of Increased ICP

Who Should Be Monitored?

Most of the 12 guidelines addressed by the task force involve decisions to monitor ICP and the interventions to take to reduce ICP when it is elevated. Although the indications to monitor ICP did not reach standard criteria, the data in the literature strongly support ICP monitoring in the patient with a GCS score of 3 to 8 and an abnormal CT scan. This includes the postoperative patient and the nonoperative patient. These patients have a high likelihood of increased ICP, and intervention to lower ICP can prevent secondary brain injury.

In patients with GCS scores of 3 to 8 and normal head CT scans, the risk of increased ICP is less. However, it has been shown that in this patient group, if patients demonstrated two of three adverse features (age >40 years, unilateral or bilateral motor posturing, or systolic blood pressure < 90 mm Hg), then the risk of increased ICP was similar to that of patients with abnormal head CT scans. Therefore patients meeting these criteria should also be monitored.

How Should Patients Be Monitored?

The two ways to monitor ICP are with a ventriculostomy, which is placed into the cerebrospinal fluid ventricular space, or with a device that measures pressure only. The advantage of the ventriculostomy is that drainage of the cerebrospinal fluid can be used to decrease ICP. Therefore in patients in whom monitoring is recommended, a ventriculostomy should be placed when possible.

What Intracranial Pressure Is Considered High?

Although an absolute threshold of ICP at which point treatment should be initiated does not exist, current data support 20 to 25 mm Hg as an upper threshold for the point at which steps to lower ICP should be initiated.

How Should Elevated Intracranial Pressure Be Treated?

Osmotic diuretics such as mannitol have been used over the years to reduce ICP. Mannitol has become the most commonly used osmotic diuretic. Although its exact mechanism is still debated, it is effective at decreasing ICP. Mannitol can be used as a large bolus (1 g/kg) when ICP increases above a threshold such as 25 mm Hg, or it can be used as small boluses (0.25 g/kg) every few hours regardless of the ICP. Serum osmolarity should be followed closely and kept below 320 mOsm. If mannitol is used for several days continuously, the patient must be weaned off slowly because abrupt cessation can lead to increased ICP.

An alternative to mannitol is hypertonic saline; a solution of 7.5% given in a 30-ml bolus is effective at acutely decreasing ICP. Treating patients with continuous infusions of 3% saline also can control ICP. The goal of hypertonic saline is to raise the sodium levels to 155 to 160. One advantage of the hypertonic saline treatment is that the patient's intravascular volume is maintained at a normal level, which is advantageous for maintaining cerebral perfusion. As with mannitol, patients must be weaned off the hypertonic saline infusions slowly.

In patients with a ventriculostomy in place, ICP can be controlled with constant cerebrospinal fluid drainage. However, often it is not possible to place a ventriculostomy in a trauma patient because of the compression of the ventricular space secondary to the brain injury.

For patients in whom osmotic or hypertonic saline therapy is ineffective, barbiturates are the next option. Barbiturate therapy is an option in patients who are hemodynamically stable. A loading dose of pentobarbital is given as a bolus, 10 mg/kg over 30 minutes, followed by 5 mg/kg every hour for three doses. This is then followed by a l mg/kg/hr maintenance infusion. The correlation between serum levels and therapeutic effect is poor. For this reason, all patients should have electroencephalographic monitoring with the goal of inducing burst suppression. Near-maximal reduction in cerebral metabolism and cerebral blood flow occurs when burst compression is present. After several days of pentobarbital coma, the drug is discontinued and the effect allowed to wear off this can take days. When the pentobarbital has disappeared from the patient's system, the patient is reevaluated by a neurologic examination, ICP measurement, and head CT.

MANAGEMENT OF MILD TO MODERATE HEAD INJURIES

Many patients sustain head injuries that do not necessitate surgery and ICP monitoring. The extent of the injury can vary from a patient who has alteration in neurologic function with a normal head CT scan to a patient with an abnormal head CT scan with the usual finding of subarachnoid blood or a brain contusion. Brain contusions caused by trauma are often located at the frontal and temporal poles. On the initial head CT, contusions appear low density, often with punctuated hemorrhages within the low density. These contusions can change over several days into large, consolidated hemorrhages, which can produce a mass effect. Patients can have neurologic deterioration when these contusions change into hematomas.

The management of these patients centers on close observation and frequent neurologic checks. Because these patients have neurologic examinations that can be followed, any changes occurring within the brain will be reflected in the neurologic function of the patient. If a change in the patient's examination is noted, a head CT is obtained. If a new mass lesion has appeared, surgical evacuation may be indicated, depending on the size of the mass and its effect on the surrounding brain.

When admitted, patients with mild to moderate head injuries should be placed on two-thirds maintenance fluid restriction. If intravenous fluids are given, normal saline should be used. The goal of this therapy is to increase the serum osmolality, which results in decreasing brain volume and ICP. Some patients may require an intensive care setting for observation and for receiving hypertonic saline or mannitol regularly over the first few days after the head injury. Steroids and anticonvulsants are not given routinely to these patients. If a patient has a seizure, anticonvulsants are started. All patients admitted with abnormal head CT scan following trauma should have a repeat head CT scan 24 hours after the trauma. Patients with large contusions, especially temporal lobe contusions, should have several head CT scans over the first week while in the hospital to check for delayed development of an intraparenchymal hematoma.

COMMENTS

The prognosis for patients with severe head injuries is generally poor. The damage sustained at the moment of the trauma is irreversible. However, with rapid evaluation and treatment aimed at maintaining ICP in a normal range, ongoing and secondary injury can be halted and reversed.

SUGGESTED READINGS

Guidelines for the management of severe head injury, New York, 1995, Brain Trauma Foundation.

Guidelines for the surgical management of traumatic brain injury, *Neurosurgery* 58(suppl): S2–S1, 2006.

Kaufman HH: Civilian gunshot wounds to the head, *Neurosurgery* 32:962, 1993.

Marshall LF, Gautille T, Klauber MR, and others: The outcome of severe closed head injury, *J Neurosurg* 75:SS28, 1991.

Seelig JM, Becker DP, Miller JD, and others: Traumatic acute subdural hematoma: major mortality reduction in comatose patients treated within four hours, *N Engl J Med* 304:1511, 1981.

Wilberger JE, Harris M, Diamond DL: Acute subdural hematoma: morbidity, mortality, and operative timing, *J Neurosurg* 74:212, 1991.

THE SURGEON'S USE OF ULTRASOUND IN THORACOABDOMINAL TRAUMA

Christopher J. Dente, MD, and Grace S. Rozycki, MD, RDMS

For nearly 15 years, surgeons in American trauma centers have successfully performed, interpreted, and taught ultrasound examinations of patients who are injured or critically ill. Real-time imaging allows the surgeon to receive instantaneous information about the clinical condition of the patient and therefore helps to expedite the patient's management. In many trauma centers, ultrasound machines are owned by surgeons and are part of the standard equipment in the trauma resuscitation room. Although diagnostic peritoneal lavage and computed tomography (CT) scanning are valuable diagnostic tests for the detection of intra-abdominal injury in patients, ultrasound is faster, as well as noninvasive and painless. As such, it is an examination that is well tolerated not only by adults but also by children. Moreover, the portability of the ultrasound machine makes it useful not only in the hospital setting but also in more austere settings.

As an extension of the physical examination, ultrasound is routinely used by surgeons in the acute setting to determine the presence or absence of fluid in the peritoneal cavity, the pericardium, and the pleural cavities. Additional uses of this modality include the detection of pneumothoraces and sternal fractures. What follows is a discussion of the use of ultrasound in blunt and penetrating thoracoabdominal trauma with an additional discussion of the use of ultrasound in forward settings and in space exploration.

FOCUSED ASSESSMENT FOR SONOGRAPHIC EVALUATION OF THE TRAUMA PATIENT

Developed for the evaluation of injured patients, the *F*ocused *A*ssessment for the *S*onographic Evaluation of the *T*rauma Patient (FAST) is a rapid diagnostic examination to assess patients with potential injuries to the thorax or abdomen. The test sequentially surveys for the presence or absence of fluid in the pericardial sac and in the dependent abdominal regions, including the Morison's pouch region of the right upper quadrant (RUQ); the left upper quadrant (LUQ) behind the spleen; between the spleen and kidney; and the pelvis posterior to the bladder.

The FAST is performed in a specific sequence. The pericardial area is visualized first so that blood within the heart can be used as a standard to set the gain. Most modern ultrasound machines have presets so that the gain does not need to be reset each time the machine is turned on. Occasionally, if multiple types of examinations are performed with different transducers, the gain should be checked to ensure that intracardiac blood appears anechoic. This maneuver ensures that the hemoperitoneum will also appear anechoic and will be readily detected on the ultrasound image. The *abdominal* part of the FAST should begin with a survey of the RUQ, which is the location within the peritoneal cavity where blood most often accumulates and is most readily detected with the FAST. In fact, in a multicenter trial of 275 trauma patients from the 1990s who had blunt or penetrating injuries, investigators found that regardless of the injured organ (with the exception of those patients who had an isolated perforated viscus), blood was most often identified on the RUQ image of the FAST. This can be a time-saving measure: when hemoperitoneum in the RUQ view is identified on the FAST examination of a hemodynamically unstable patient, that image alone, in combination with the patient's clinical picture, is sufficient to justify an immediate abdominal operation. In a stable patient, following the examination of the RUQ, the LUQ and pelvis are visualized.

Technique

Ultrasound transmission gel is applied on four areas of the thoracoabdomen, and the examination is conducted in the following sequence: the pericardial area, RUQ, LUQ, and the pelvis (Fig. 1). Abdominal structures are best imaged with a lower-frequency probe, which allows for deeper penetration into tissues (sacrificing some resolution). Most ultrasound probes are now capable of imaging in multiple frequencies, allowing the sonographer to achieve the best balance of resolution (higher frequency) and tissue penetration (lower frequency) on the basis of an individual patient's body habitus.

To begin the examination, a 3.5-MHz convex transducer is oriented for sagittal or longitudinal views and positioned in the subxiphoid region to identify the heart and to examine for blood in the pericardial sac. The normal and abnormal views of the pericardial area are shown in Fig. 2. The subxiphoid image is usually not difficult to obtain, but a severe injury to the chest wall, a narrow subcostal area, subcutaneous emphysema, or morbid obesity can prevent a satisfactory examination. Both of the latter conditions

are associated with poor imaging because air and fat reflect the wave too strongly and prevent penetration into the target organ. If the subcostal pericardial image cannot be obtained or is suboptimal, a parasternal ultrasound view of the heart should be performed.

Next, the transducer is placed in the right anterior or midaxillary line between the eleventh and twelfth ribs to identify a sagittal section of the liver, kidney, and diaphragm (Fig. 3). The presence or absence of blood is sought in Morison's pouch and in the right subphrenic space. Next, attention is turned to the LUQ, and with the transducer positioned in the left posterior axillary line between the tenth and eleventh ribs, the spleen and kidney are visualized and blood is sought between the two organs and in the left subphrenic space (Fig. 4). The splenic window is often the most difficult, and the probe should be placed significantly more posterior (posterior axillary line) and superior (one to two rib spaces higher) than with the RUQ window.

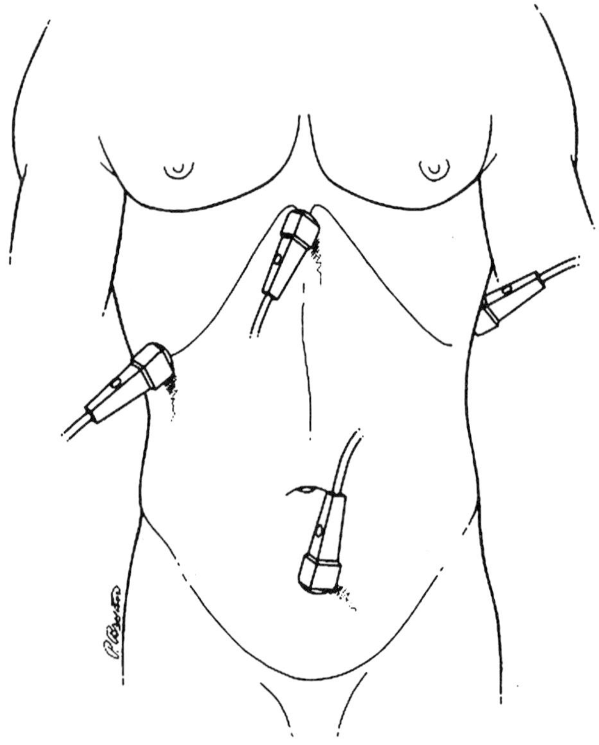

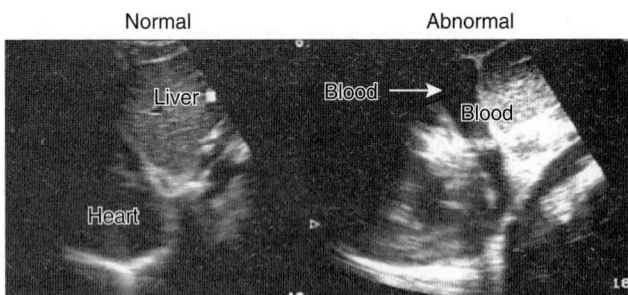

Figure 2 *Left,* Sagittal view of pericardial area showing pericardium as single echogenic line (normal). *Right,* Sagittal view of pericardial area showing separation of visceral and parietal areas of pericardium with blood *(arrow)* that appears anechoic.

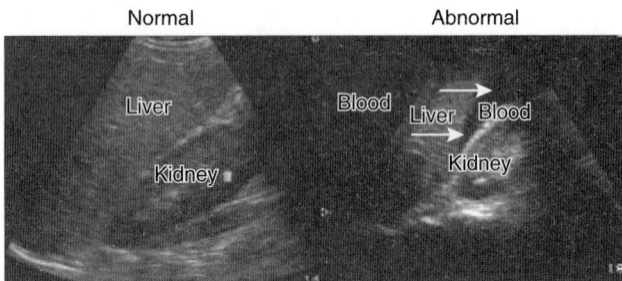

Figure 3 *Left,* Normal sagittal view of liver, kidney, and diaphragm. Note Gerota's fascia is hyperechoic. *Right,* Abnormal sagittal view of liver, kidney, and diaphragm. Note fluid (blood) between liver and kidney *(arrows)*.

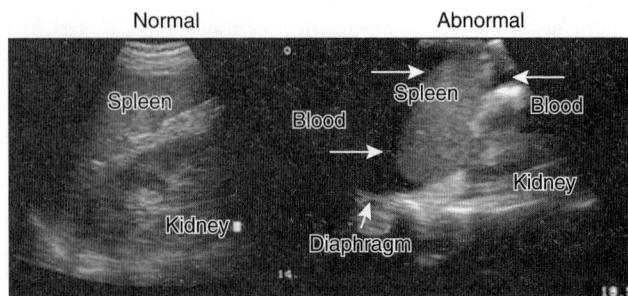

Figure 4 *Left,* Normal sagittal view of spleen, kidney and diaphragm. *Right,* Abnormal sagittal view of spleen, kidney, and diaphragm with fluid (blood) in between spleen and kidney and above the spleen in the subphrenic space.

Figure 1 Schematic diagram of transducer positions for FAST: pericardial, right upper quadrant, left upper quadrant, and pelvis.

Normal | Abnormal

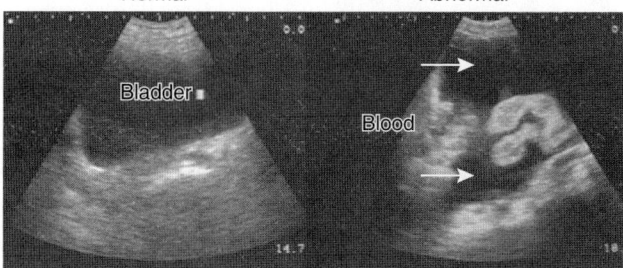

Figure 5 *Left,* Normal coronal view of full urinary bladder. *Right,* Abnormal coronal view of full bladder with fluid in pelvis. (Note the bowel floating in fluid.)

Finally, the transducer is directed for a transverse view and placed approximately 4 cm superior to the symphysis pubis. It is swept inferiorly to obtain a coronal view of the full bladder and the pelvis, which are examined for the presence or absence of blood (Fig. 5).

Accuracy of the Focused Assessment for the Sonographic Evaluation of the Trauma Patient

Improper technique, inexperience of the examiner, and inappropriate use of ultrasound have long been known to adversely affect ultrasound imaging. More recently, the cause of injury, presence of hypotension on admission, and select associated injuries have also been shown to influence the accuracy of this modality. Failure to consider these factors has led to inaccurate assessments of the accuracy of the FAST by inappropriately comparing it with a CT scan and not recognizing its role in the evaluation of patients with penetrating torso trauma. Both false-positive and false-negative pericardial ultrasound examinations have been reported to occur in the presence of a massive hemothorax or mediastinal blood. Repeating the FAST after the insertion of a tube thoracostomy improves the visualization of the pericardial area and decreases the number of false-positive and false-negative studies. Notwithstanding these circumstances in which false studies may occur, a rapid, focused, ultrasound survey of the subcostal pericardial area is an accurate method to detect hemopericardium in most patients with penetrating wounds in the "cardiac box." In a recent large study of patients who sustained either blunt *or* penetrating injuries, the FAST was 100% sensitive and 99.3% specific for detecting hemopericardium in patients with precordial or transthoracic wounds. Furthermore, the use of pericardial ultrasound has been shown to be especially helpful in the evaluation of patients who have no overt signs of pericardial tamponade. This was highlighted in a study in which 10 of 22 patients with precordial wounds and hemopericardium on the ultrasound examinations had admission systolic blood pressures higher than 110 mm Hg and were relatively asymptomatic. On the basis of these signs and the lack of symptoms, it is unlikely that the presence of cardiac wounds would have been strongly suspected in these patients, and therefore this rapid ultrasound examination provided an early diagnosis of hemopericardium before the patients underwent physiologic deterioration.

The FAST is a focused examination for the detection of fluid in dependent areas of the abdomen and is designed to answer the simple question of "fluid or no fluid." Therefore its results should not be compared with those of a CT scan because the FAST does not readily identify intraparenchymal or retroperitoneal injuries. Therefore select patients considered at high risk for occult intra-abdominal injury should undergo a CT scan of the abdomen regardless of the results of the FAST examination. These patients include those with fractures of the pelvis or thoracolumbar spine, major thoracic trauma (pulmonary contusion, lower-rib fractures), and hematuria.

Recent Advances and Organ Specificity

As surgeons have become more facile with ultrasound examinations and as technology has improved, extensions of the FAST examination have been described. Again, it is noted that the standard FAST examination is designed to accurately answer two simple questions: whether there is fluid in the peritoneal cavity and whether there is fluid in the pericardial sac. The use of ultrasound for more complex diagnostic interventions is described later, but these areas are less well studied and beyond the purview of the traditional FAST examination.

A recent prospective, multicenter trial conducted by the Western Trauma Association reported on the use of ultrasound to serially evaluate patients with documented solid organ injuries (SOI) after trauma. The so-called BOAST examination, or the *B*edside *O*rgan *A*ssessment with *S*onography after *T*rauma, was performed by a limited number of experienced surgeon-sonographers in 126 patients with 135 SOI in four American trauma centers. This study, performed over nearly 2 years, was designed to be a more thorough abdominal ultrasound examination, with multiple views obtained of each solid organ (kidneys, liver, and spleen). Criteria for enrollment included normal hemodynamics, absence of peritonitis or other need for urgent laparotomy, and lack of excessive blood transfusion, in the attending physician's judgment. All patients were victims of blunt trauma, with a mean injury severity score of nearly 15.

Overall, only 34% of injuries to solid organs were seen, with BOAST yielding an error rate of 66%. None of the 34 grade I injuries was identified, and only 13 (31%) of the grade II injuries were identified. Sensitivities for grade III and grade IV injuries ranged from 25% to 75%, and only one grade V injury (to the liver) was examined and positively identified. It is noted, however, that 11 patients developed 16 intra-abdominal complications (8 pseudoaneurysms, 4 bilomas, 3 abscesses, and 1 necrotic organ), of which 13 (81%) were identified by the sonographers. This study emphasizes that ultrasound, in most surgeons' hands, should not be considered a reliable modality for diagnosis and grading of SOI, although it may be acceptably accurate in the diagnosis of posttraumatic abdominal complications in patients with SOI managed nonoperatively.

In Europe, preliminary work using power Doppler ultrasonography to identify specific organ injuries has been published in recent years. Many of these examinations include the use of a sonographic contrast agent injected peripherally during the scan. In one study, the authors were able to document contrast extravasation in 20 of 153 patients (13%). Extravasation was seen not only from the spleen, liver, and kidney after trauma, but also in postoperative patients (aortic aneurysm repair, postsplenectomy) and in a patient with a ruptured aortic aneurysm. In 9 of 20 cases, CT scan was performed, and all 9 confirmed contrast extravasation. In the 133 patients without extravasation, the absence of active bleeding was inferred by a subsequent CT scan in 82 patients, surgical data in 13 patients, and clinical follow-up in 38 cases, with no cases of active bleeding missed by ultrasound. Thus the addition of ultrasonic contrast agent and power Doppler may be of some benefit in the diagnosis of specific injuries. It should be emphasized again, however, that the FAST examination in most American trauma centers is used simply as a screening tool to identify the presence or absence of hemoperitoneum or hemopericardium in a trauma patient.

TRAUMATIC HEMOTHORAX

A focused thoracic ultrasound examination was developed by surgeons to rapidly detect the presence or absence of a traumatic hemothorax in patients during the Advanced Trauma Life Support secondary survey. A test that promptly detects a traumatic effusion or hemothorax is worthwhile because it dramatically shortens the interval from the diagnosis of a hemothorax to the insertion of a thoracostomy tube.

Technique

The technique for this examination is similar to that used to interrogate the upper quadrants of the abdomen in the FAST and also uses the same type and frequency transducer. In fact, it is performed one to two rib spaces higher than the RUQ and LUQ FAST views using the same probe. Ultrasound transmission gel is applied to the right and left lower thoracic areas in the mid to posterior axillary lines between the ninth and tenth intercostal spaces (Fig. 6). The transducer is slowly advanced cephalad to identify the hyperechoic diaphragm and to interrogate the supradiaphragmatic space for the presence or absence of fluid (Fig. 7), which appears anechoic. In the positive thoracic ultrasound examination, the hypoechoic lung can be seen "floating" amid the fluid. The same technique can be used to evaluate a critically ill patient for a pleural effusion.

Accuracy

Surgeons at Grady Memorial Hospital have examined the accuracy of the focused thoracic ultrasound examination in 360 patients with blunt and penetrating torso injuries. They compared the time and accuracy of ultrasound with that of the supine portable chest x-ray and found them to be very similar: 97.4% sensitivity and 99.7% specificity observed for thoracic ultrasound versus 92.5% sensitivity and 99.7% specificity for the portable chest x-ray. Performance times, however, for the thoracic ultrasound examinations were statistically much faster ($p < 0.0001$) than those for the portable chest x-ray. Although it is not recommended that the thoracic ultrasound examination replace the chest x-ray, its use can expedite treatment in many patients and decrease the number of chest radiographs obtained.

▍ PNEUMOTHORAX

Ultrasound examination is useful to the surgeon who is evaluating a patient for a potential pneumothorax if (1) bulky radiology equipment is not readily available, (2) inordinate delays for obtaining a chest x-ray are anticipated, or (3) numerous injured patients (mass casualty situation) must be rapidly assessed and triaged. In addition to using ultrasound for pneumothorax detection in the trauma resuscitation area, surgeons may also find it helpful in detecting a pneumothorax in a critically ill patient who is on a ventilator, after a thoracentesis procedure, or after discontinuing the suction on an underwater seal device.

Technique

A 5.0- to 7.5-MHz linear array transducer (the higher frequency allows for better resolution of superficial structures) is used to evaluate a patient for the presence of a pneumothorax. The examination may be performed while the patient is in the erect or the supine position. Ultrasound transmission gel is applied to the right and left upper thoracic areas at approximately the third to fourth intercostal space in the mid-clavicular line, and the presumed unaffected thoracic cavity is examined first. The transducer is oriented for longitudinal imaging, is placed perpendicular to the ribs, and is slowly advanced medially toward the sternum and then laterally toward the anterior axillary line. The normal examination of the thoracic cavity identifies the rib (seen as black on the ultrasound

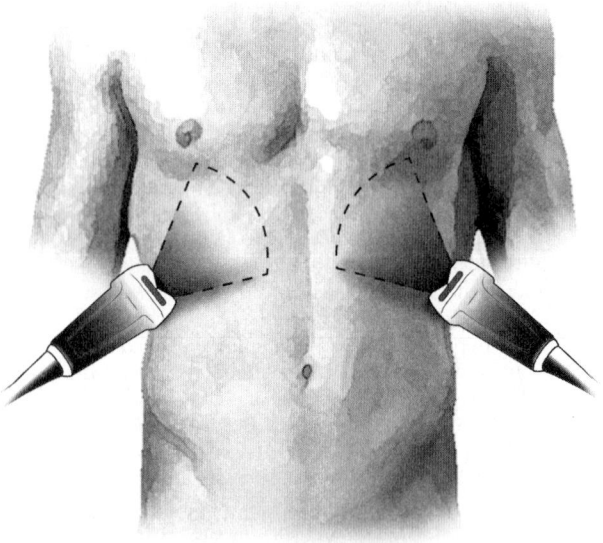

Figure 6 Transducer positions for thoracic ultrasound examination (detection of hemothorax).

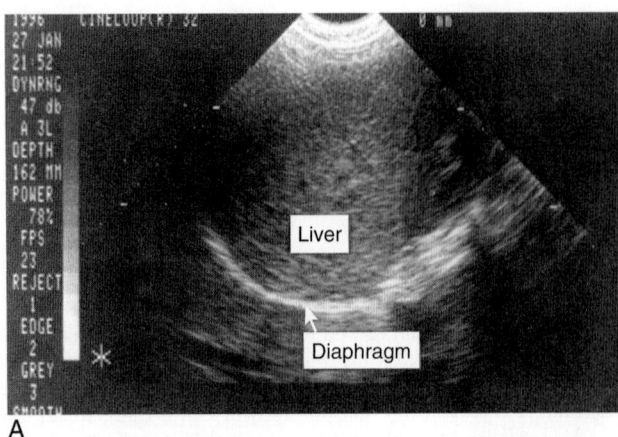

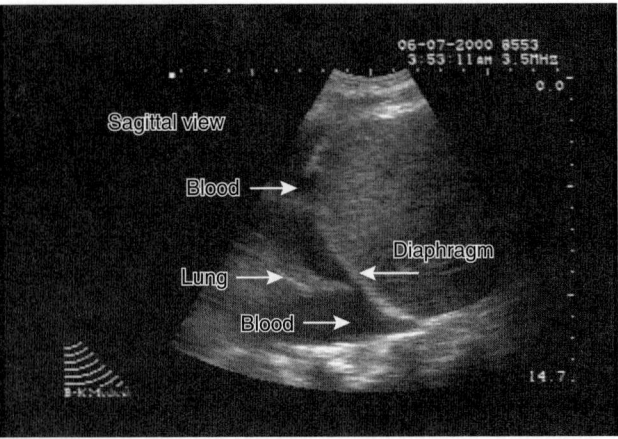

Figure 7 **(A)** Sagittal view of liver, kidney, and diaphragm. Note supradiaphragmatic (lung) area but absence of pleural effusion. **(B)** Sagittal view of right supradiaphragmatic space. The right hemithorax contains fluid (blood) that appears anechoic.

image because it is a refraction artifact), pleural sliding, and a comet-tail artifact. *Sliding* is the identification of the visceral and parietal layers of the pleura, which are seen as hyperechoic superimposed pleural lines moving upon each other with respiration. When a pneumothorax is present, air becomes trapped between the visceral and parietal pleura and does not allow for the transmission of the ultrasound waves. Therefore, the visceral pleura are not imaged and pleural sliding is not observed. The comet tail artifact is generated because of the interaction of two highly reflective opposing interfaces, that is, air and pleura (Fig. 8). When air separates the visceral and parietal pleura, the comet tail artifact is not visualized. The examination may be repeated with the transducer oriented for transverse views, with images obtained with the probe parallel to the ribs.

Accuracy

Several studies have documented the sensitivity and specificity of ultrasound for the detection of a pneumothorax. Dulchavsky and colleagues from Detroit Receiving Hospital showed that ultrasound can be successfully used by surgeons to detect a pneumothorax in injured patients. Of 382 patients (362 trauma; 18 spontaneous) evaluated with ultrasound, 39 had pneumothoraces, and ultrasound successfully detected 37 of them, yielding 95% sensitivity. Pneumothoraces in two patients could not be detected because of the presence of significant subcutaneous emphysema. The authors recommended that when a portable chest x-ray cannot be readily obtained, the use of this bedside ultrasound examination for the identification of a pneumothorax can expedite the patient's management. In our experience, ultrasound is extremely sensitive for the detection of pneumothorax, and we have detected many that were seen only on subsequent thoracic CT scan (i.e., not identified by chest x-ray). Thus, this test may be useful not only to rapidly diagnose and treat a pneumothorax in an unstable patient but also to avoid unnecessary chest tubes in a patient who becomes hypotensive for unclear reasons.

STERNAL FRACTURE

Fractures of the sternum are visualized on a lateral x-ray view of the chest, but this film may be difficult to obtain in a multisystem injured patient. An ultrasound examination of the sternum can rapidly detect a fracture while the patient is still in the supine position, thereby obviating an x-ray.

Technique

The ultrasound examination of the sternum is performed using a high-frequency linear array transducer that is oriented for sagittal or longitudinal views. Ultrasound transmission gel is applied over the sternal area while the patient is in the supine position. Beginning at the suprasternal notch, the transducer is slowly advanced in a caudad direction to interrogate the bone for a fracture, and then the examination is repeated with the transducer oriented for transverse views. The examination of the intact sternum is shown in Figure 9. A sternal fracture is identified on the ultrasound examination as a disruption of the cortical reflex (Fig. 10). Investigators have found that the use of ultrasound for this diagnosis is as accurate as, and much more rapid than, a lateral x-ray view of the chest.

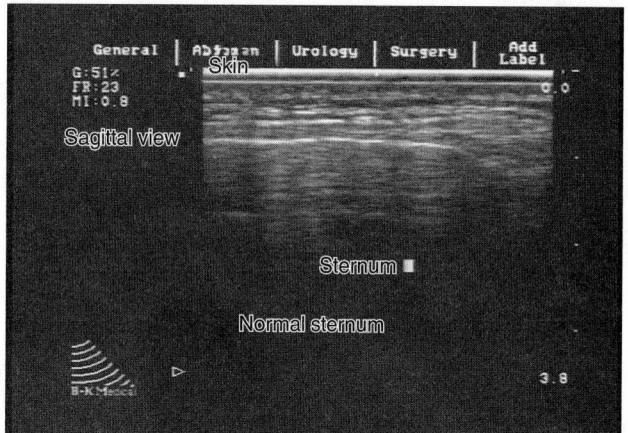

Figure 9 Sagittal view of sternum. Normal findings.

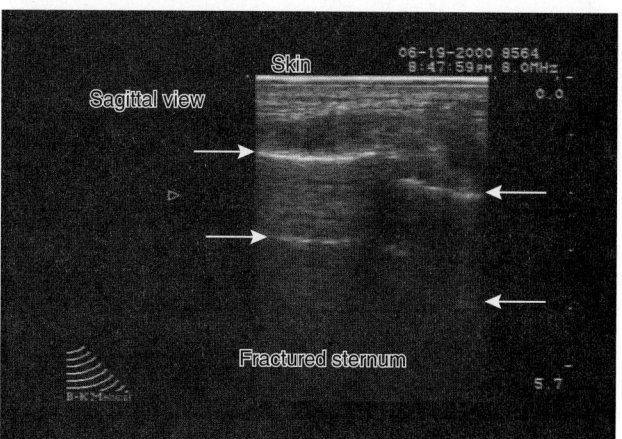

Figure 10 Sagittal view of sternum illustrating fracture (interruption of hyperechoic line).

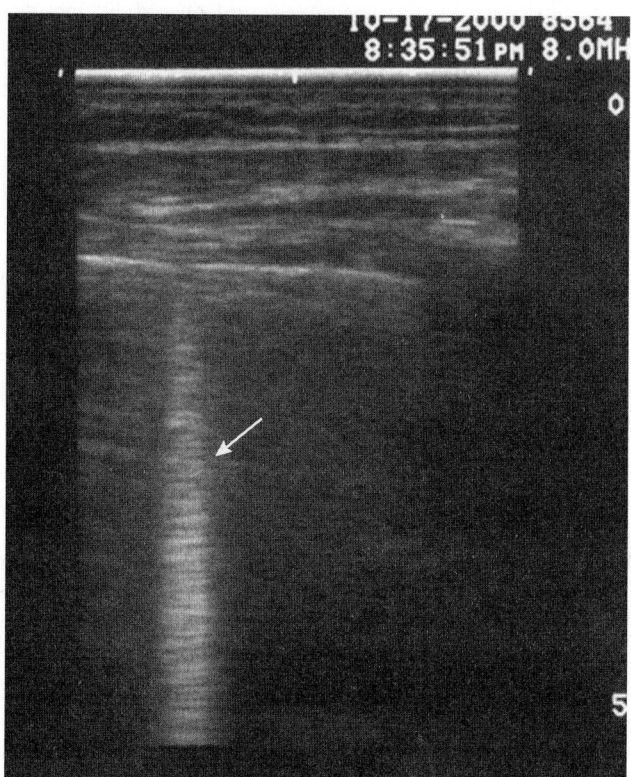

Figure 8 Comet tail artifact (*arrow*).

SPECIAL SITUATIONS

Ultrasound in the Pregnant Trauma Patient

Ultrasound would seem to be an ideal method of evaluating a pregnant patient with suspected blunt abdominal trauma because it is portable, noninvasive, and free of ionizing radiation. Indeed, the Advanced Trauma Life Support (ATLS) course teaches that unrecognized abdominal trauma is one of the leading causes of morbidity in the pregnant trauma patient. Concerns over changes in abdominal anatomy leading to difficulty in obtaining images have not been supported by objective evaluation. Goodwin and colleagues reported on their 8-year experience with the FAST examination in 127 pregnant patients, of which 5 of 6 patients with hemoperitoneum were found to have fluid on FAST examination (sensitivity 83%). Of the 120 without abdominal injury, 117 had a true negative FAST (specificity 98%), with three false-positive examinations resulting from serous intraperitoneal fluid. Furthermore, Brown and colleagues reported on their experience with a more extensive ultrasound examination in 101 stable, pregnant patients with suspected blunt abdominal trauma. Median gestational age was just over 24 weeks, and these patients underwent an official abdominal ultrasound by a certified technician that included images of the fetus and placenta. The sensitivity was 80%, and injuries identified included 1 placental abruption, 2 splenic lacerations, 1 liver laceration, and 1 kidney injury. None of the 96 patients with a negative ultrasound had injuries discovered later in their hospital course (specificity 100%). Thus it would seem that ultrasound remains a good screening tool for the pregnant patient with blunt abdominal trauma and has the advantages of repeatability and a lack of radiation exposure.

Ultrasound in Penetrating Trauma

Ultrasound for diagnosis of injuries after penetrating trauma has been studied much less extensively than ultrasound use after blunt trauma. Several of the larger, well-known series have included patients with penetrating trauma and, as stated earlier, ultrasound of the pericardium has been shown to be accurate for diagnosis of injury in patients with penetrating injury to the "cardiac box." In a recent study of 32 patients with penetrating anterior chest trauma, ultrasound was used to diagnose 8 pericardial effusions with a reported 100% accuracy (8 true-positive and 24 true-negative examinations). Eight other patients were noted to have intraperitoneal fluid and underwent therapeutic exploration, including repair of five diaphragm injuries, three liver lacerations, three splenic lacerations, three gastric injuries, two small bowel injuries and one adrenal injury. No false-positive or false-negative examinations of the peritoneum were reported. Other studies have shown that the accuracy of FAST after penetrating trauma is somewhat less, with one study reporting sensitivity for abdominal injury after penetrating trauma as low as 67%.

A recent report by Murphy and colleagues looked at the utility of ultrasound to diagnose fascial penetration after anterior abdominal stab wounds. In this study, 35 patients underwent ultrasonic evaluation of their anterior abdominal fascia with an 8.0-MHz linear array probe followed by a local wound exploration. Although ultrasound had only 59% sensitivity (13/22 patients), it did have 100% specificity with no false-positive studies. Thus, if fascial penetration is noted on ultrasound, a more invasive wound exploration is probably not necessary; however, a negative ultrasound evaluation is clearly less helpful and does not preclude peritoneal penetration.

USE OF ULTRASOUND IN AUSTERE SETTINGS

Ultrasound on Deployment

The portability of ultrasound makes it ideal for use in forward settings. In fact, training courses are in place to teach military surgeons the use of the FAST examination, and handheld ultrasound is now routinely deployed within the British Defence Medical Services. Indeed, in a survey of surgeons reviewing potential preventable casualties in Vietnam, ultrasound was the fourth most commonly mentioned advancement in technology (after modern ventilators, CT scanners, and modern antibiotics) that may have assisted in better patient salvage.

Although up to 90% of war wounds are penetrating, ultrasound may allow quicker, more accurate triage decisions because patients with penetrating abdominal trauma with no or minimal hemoperitoneum may be transferred to the next echelon, where the ultrasound may be repeated or additional diagnostic maneuvers taken. In a study from the Croatian conflict in 1999, FAST was shown to have a sensitivity of 86%, a specificity of 100%, and an accuracy of 97% when applied to 94 casualties evaluated over a 72-hour period. This was comparable to the accuracy achieved by the same authors in their civilian experience with FAST in more than 1000 patients over the 3 years preceding the conflict. In a recent small series, FAST was used with excellent results in a British military hospital in Iraq. Fifteen casualties were evaluated with serial FAST examinations, and fourteen had negative examinations at admission and again after 6 hours. One patient underwent laparotomy on the basis of trajectory and had no intraperitoneal fluid, but two small holes were discovered in the cecum that required repair. The other 13 patients recovered without sequelae. One examination was positive and led to immediate laparotomy in a patient with a grade V liver injury after a motor vehicle collision.

Because ultrasound is sufficiently portable for use in active combat situations, research is ongoing to evaluate the best method to teletransmit images obtained in the field. Several different satellite transmission systems have been evaluated, and high-quality images were obtained in the majority of cases, although the balance between the weight of the system and the minimal image quality has still not been completely achieved. It is noted, however, that images can be transmitted from up to 1500 feet from the antennae without significant degradation. As technology advances, one would expect imaging systems to continue to become smaller and lighter with improved image quality, making ultrasound even more appealing as a modality for use in the forward setting.

Ultrasound in Outer Space

Many of the same qualities that make ultrasound appealing for use in combat make it equally appealing as a diagnostic modality in space, where an injury might require abortion of a multimillion dollar mission. Indeed, ultrasound is one of the only feasible diagnostic modalities on space missions, given size and weight restrictions. Also, ultrasound examinations are easily taught, and images can be relayed with minimal delay to physicians on the ground. ATLS procedures are also feasible in space, and lifesaving procedures could be performed on the basis of ultrasound findings.

Ultrasound has been used in space for several decades. Indeed, it was ultrasound technology that taught us much about the physiologic effects of microgravity, especially the fluid shifts associated with space travel. As early as 1982, cardiac ultrasound was used to evaluate left ventricular systolic function and cardiac chamber size in cosmonauts. The first American ultrasound

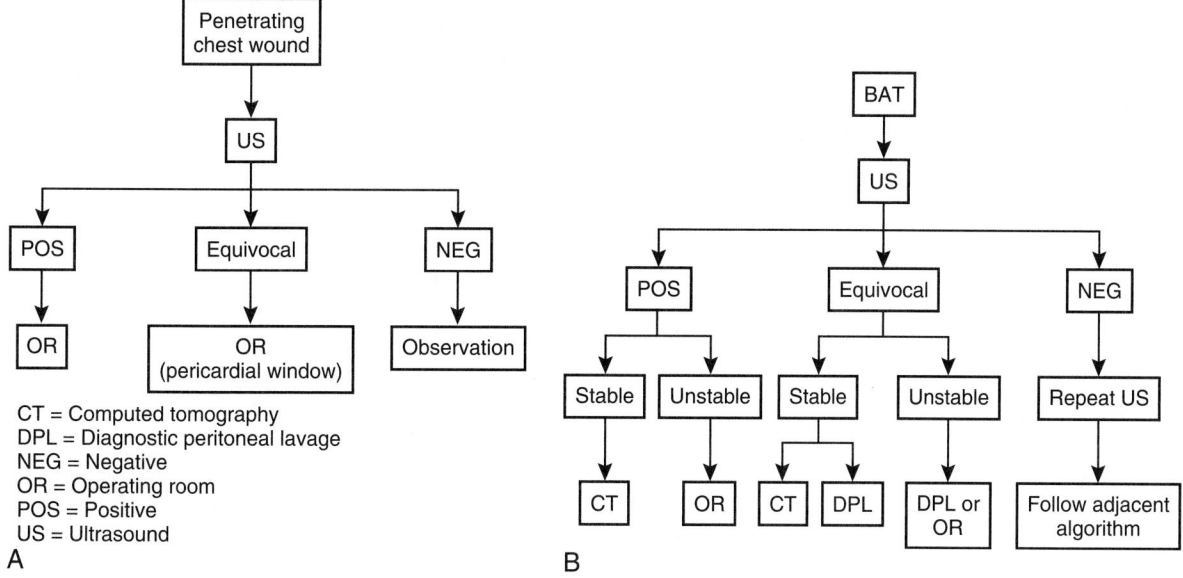

Figure 11 **(A)** Algorithm for the use of ultrasound in patients with penetrating chest wounds. **(B)** Algorithm for the use of ultrasound in patients with blunt abdominal trauma.

system in space was the American flight echograph from Advanced Technology Laboratories (Bothell, WA), which first flew in 1984 and eventually was capable of three-dimensional images using a tilt frame device. Currently, the Human Research Facility aboard the International Space Station (ISS) is equipped with a state-of-the-art Philips HDI 5000 (Philips Medical, Bothell, WA).

Because surface tension and capillary action are the principal physical forces in space, scientists questioned whether images obtained on the standard FAST examination would be useful in microgravity. There are now several published studies of ultrasounds performed on parabolic flights onboard the NASA Microgravity Research Facility, a KC-135 aircraft. This aircraft can generate 25- to 30-second intervals of weightlessness using serial parabolic trajectories. A porcine model of intra-abdominal hemorrhage was created on the ground and studied during parabolic flights. More than 2000 ultrasound segments were recorded, with 80% of these considered feasible for diagnosis of the presence or absence of abdominal fluid. The sonographers felt the examination was no more difficult than one performed on the ground as long as the sonographer and patient were adequately restrained. For the intraperitoneal portion of the examination, a fourth view (the midline "abdominal sweep") was added, and with this addition, the FAST examination was able to reliably detect even relatively small amounts of intraperitoneal fluid. The Morison's pouch view remained the most sensitive window for fluid detection. Further study using a similar model revealed that ultrasound can also reliably detect both hemothorax and pneumothorax in microgravity.

Recently, astronauts aboard the ISS performed FAST ultrasounds that were transmitted with a 2-second satellite delay to directors on the ground, who were able to provide them with real-time instructions for probe position and system adjustments. Examinations were completed in approximately 5 minutes, with adequate images obtained in all views. Astronauts have also been able to perform comprehensive ocular ultrasounds aboard the ISS with the same real-time feedback.

In summary, ultrasound fulfills all the necessary criteria for a diagnostic modality in space. It is sufficiently portable, teletransmittable, teachable, and accurate. It will likely continue to be the only feasible technology to assist with medical diagnoses on space missions in the near future.

SUMMARY

As the role of the general surgeon continues to evolve, the surgeon's use of ultrasound will surely influence practice patterns, particularly for the evaluation of patients in the acute setting. With the use of real-time imaging, the surgeon receives instantaneous information to augment the physical examination, narrow the differential diagnosis, or initiate an intervention. Algorithms for the suggested use of ultrasound in penetrating trauma and blunt abdominal trauma are shown in Figure 11.

The advantages of ultrasound are easily seen in each of the following clinical scenarios. As a *noninvasive, nonionizing radiation* modality, ultrasound can be used to evaluate the injured pregnant patient and simultaneously identify the fetal heart so that its rate can be recorded. For the patient with multiple fractures who is in traction, the *portable* machine is wheeled to the patient's bedside, and FAST is performed without having to move the patient. If hypotension or an unexpected decrease in hematocrit occurs, an ultrasound examination can be easily *repeated* to exclude hemoperitoneum as the source of hypotension. When several patients with penetrating thoracoabdominal injuries present simultaneously to the emergency department, a *rapid* FAST examination with thoracic views can help the surgeon to assess for pericardial effusion, massive hemothorax, or hemoperitoneum within seconds. This information helps the surgeon to prioritize resources and triage patients. Finally, this *painless*, noninvasive modality is well accepted, even by children, because it is performed at the bedside and is not intimidating.

As surgeons become more facile with ultrasound, it is anticipated that other uses will develop to further enhance its value for the assessment of patients in the acute setting.

SUGGESTED READINGS

Ballard RB, Rozycki GS, Newman PG, and others: An algorithm to reduce the incidence of false-negative FAST examination in patients at high-risk for occult injury, *J Am Coll Surg* 189:145, 1999.*

*One of two large series that focus on indications for CT scan after a normal FAST examination.

Kirkpatrick AW, Hamilton DR, Nicolaou S, and others: Focused assessment with sonography for trauma in weightlessness: a feasibility study, *J Am Coll Surg* 196:833, 2003.
One of a series of articles by these authors establishing the role of ultrasound as one of the primary diagnostic modalities for space travel.
Rozycki GS, Ballard RB, Feliciano DV, and others: Surgeon-performed ultrasound for the assessment of truncal injuries: Lessons learned from 1,540 patients, *Ann Surg* 228:557, 1998.[†]

Rozycki GS, Feliciano DV, Schmidt JA, and others: The role of surgeon-performed ultrasound in patients with possible cardiac wounds, *Ann Surg* 223:737, 1996.[‡]
Zagzebski JA , editor: *Essentials of ultrasound physics*, St Louis, 1996, Mosby.[§]

[†]One of the largest early series establishing the FAST examination as a reasonable and accurate diagnostic modality.

[‡]One of the original series on diagnosis of hemopericardium with ultrasound.
[§]A clinically oriented and readable textbook for those interested in understanding more about ultrasound physics.

BLUNT ABDOMINAL TRAUMA

Anna M. Ledgerwood, MD, and Charles E. Lucas, MD

HISTORICAL PERSPECTIVE

The approach to blunt abdominal injury (BAI) has changed in the past 50 years. This reflects the more frequent use of invasive diagnostic tests, improved imaging studies, and a more conservative decision tree. The history and physical examination (PE) remain the gold standard of diagnosis, focusing on signs of hemoperitoneum, determined by vital signs, and hollow viscus injury, determined by tenderness and guarding. In the past, suspected hemoperitoneum or peritonitis led to exploratory laparotomy, in which exploration was completed and treatment provided. Standard chest and abdominal films were seldom helpful except for diagnosis of a specific injury such as a ruptured diaphragm or hollow viscus perforation with pneumoperitoneum.

Diagnostic Paracentesis

Diagnostic paracentesis (DPC) performed just lateral to the recti muscles was introduced in the 1950s. This procedure, performed with a 10-ml syringe and a 20-gauge needle, requires less than 1 minute. When any blood is aspirated, significant hemoperitoneum is present because of a probable liver, splenic, or mesenteric injury. DPC was seldom helpful in diagnosing a hollow viscus injury; observation for the signs and symptoms of peritonitis would continue if the DPC were negative. The DPC, however, is not sufficiently sensitive to identify significant hemoperitoneum in some patients for whom laparotomy is indicated.

Diagnostic Peritoneal Lavage

Diagnostic peritoneal lavage (DPL) was introduced in the 1960s. This test can be performed in 5 minutes by inserting a multihole catheter through an infraumbilical stab wound toward the pelvis and infusing 1 liter (10 ml/kg for children) crystalloid solution; the fluid is siphoned out by gravity. With experience, a positive test for significant hemoperitoneum was defined by an effluent with greater than 100,000 red blood cells (RBCs) per milliliter, a hematocrit over 1%, or inability to read newsprint through clear intravenous infusion tubing. A positive test for hollow viscus perforation was defined as an effluent with a white blood cell (WBC) count greater than 500/ml, the presence of stool or particulate matter, or an elevation in amylase and alkaline phosphatase. Positive DPL, however, led to many nontherapeutic laparotomies in patients with major pelvic fractures, and this in turn led to a redefinition of a positive DPL in these patients to a hematocrit of 3%. When the DPL was performed too soon after injury, the inflammatory response from a hollow viscus perforation would not have fully evolved so that the WBC count would be less than 500; animal studies demonstrated that a 2-hour interval from the time of perforation until the performance of the DPL eliminates this false-negative result.

Abdominal Computed Tomography

Computed tomography (CT) for abdominal trauma was introduced in the 1970s and was routinely used in the 1980s; this permitted earlier anatomic diagnoses of solid viscus injuries to the liver and spleen. With twenty–first-century scanners, CT can be performed within 5 minutes. The addition of oral contrast helps with diagnoses of hollow viscus injury to the small bowel and duodenum. The addition of intravenous contrast eliminated the need for intravenous pyelography for evaluation of hematuria. Although we do not use it, rectal contrast is sometimes recommended to assess for colon injury. By the mid-1980s, routine abdominal CT after BAI had identified many liver and spleen injuries, thereby promoting earlier laparotomy. Many of these laparotomies were nontherapeutic; better discrimination regarding which injuries should be explored came later. Routine CT after BAI led to many patients being transported to the CT suite while still being resuscitated. This often resulted in cardiovascular collapse and death because ongoing monitoring and resuscitation were compromised during scanning. Criteria for abdominal CT had to be modified to avoid this catastrophic event.

Abdominal Ultrasonography

Although ultrasonography for BAI has been used in Europe for many years, the real advent of the *F*ocused *A*ssessment for the *S*onographic Evaluation of the *T*rauma Patient (FAST) in North America occurred in the 1990s. This examination, which assesses for pericardial fluid, subhepatic fluid, perisplenic fluid, and pelvic fluid, can be performed within 5 minutes during resuscitation. Intraperitoneal fluid can be seen early after injury in unstable patients who therefore are not candidates for CT. A positive FAST in stable patients can be followed by CT to identify the specific causes for the intraperitoneal fluid. Currently, the FAST examination is not being used to assess retroperitoneal injuries.

Laparoscopy

The advent of widespread laparoscopic procedures in the early 1990s rekindled its use in the trauma patient; its greatest benefit is in patients with altered mentation in whom serial PE is not reliable. Retroperitoneal organ injuries are not well seen with this technique.

Nonoperative Therapy of Abdominal Organ Injury

In the past, many patients with hemoperitoneum, as defined by a positive DPL, FAST or CT, underwent nontherapeutic laparotomies for minor liver or splenic injuries. Splenectomy was often performed when blunt splenic ruptures were not bleeding. The most important historical event in patients with BAI is the recognition that laparotomy is not indicated for all solid organ injuries. This important milestone began sporadically in the 1970s but did not really gain widespread acceptance until the 1980s. We have practiced the nonoperative therapeutic approach to patients with blunt liver or splenic injury for more than 25 years; major injuries to the liver or the spleen are treated nonoperatively if vital signs are stable and no RBC replacement is necessary.

THE TWENTY-FIRST CENTURY APPROACH TO BLUNT ABDOMINAL INJURY

Knowledge of history facilitates the application of appropriate diagnostic and therapeutic aids, thereby maximizing the likelihood for a good outcome after BAI. The benefits and risks of each procedure must be integrated with the patient's clinical course. Most BAIs result from motor vehicle crashes, falls from heights, or physical assault; consequently, multiple injuries should be suspected.

Refractory Hemorrhagic Shock from Hemoperitoneum

When the patient presents with hemorrhagic shock, resuscitative and diagnostic efforts are initiated. Refractory hemorrhagic shock from hemoperitoneum requires prompt laparotomy with direct hemostasis or temporary damage control. In contrast, a nontherapeutic laparotomy for severe refractory hemorrhage from elsewhere aggravates the underlying insult and very likely will contribute to the patient's death. Bilateral DPC just lateral to the recti muscles can be performed in 30 seconds; when the DPC is positive, prompt laparotomy is indicated. When a DPC is negative, bleeding is likely from an extra-abdominal source; a more sensitive FAST or DPL is indicated. When FAST or DPL is negative, the life-threatening hemorrhage is not intra-abdominal and the surgeon should look elsewhere.

Responsive Hemorrhagic Shock

When the patient responds promptly to the resuscitation, identification of the site of bleeding can be achieved in a more deliberate manner. The FAST or DPL should be performed. When one or both is negative, the prior shock is not from an intraperitoneal source. A positive FAST or DPL points to bleeding from the liver, spleen, or bowel mesentery, or from two or even all of these organs. The stable patient with a positive FAST or DPL should have a contrast CT to identify the severity of the liver or spleen injury and to determine whether there is any evidence of hollow viscus perforation. The CT will also document the extent of hemoperitoneum and retroperitoneal injuries. Although major hepatic and splenic injuries with an Abbreviated Injury Score (AIS) of 4 or 5 in association with diffuse pelvic blood will likely require exploratory laparotomy for hemostasis, many such patients stop bleeding spontaneously and can be treated successfully without undergoing surgery. The gold standard continues to be serial PE, with the decision to operate determined by vital signs and response to therapy. The current policy of letting the hemoglobin drift below 10 g in a patient who

has stopped bleeding allows for a significant bleed to occur without need for operation or blood transfusion. When a patient with injury to the liver or spleen requires RBC replacement, however, laparotomy with definitive organ repair remains the safer course. A course of continued observation of a patient requiring RBC replacement should be followed only under those special circumstances in which the risk of operation would outweigh the risk of additional blood replacement.

The stable patient admitted for nonoperative therapy can be observed on the open surgical floor as long as there are no significant comorbidities demanding specialized care. When the patient has continued abdominal discomfort, bed rest is recommended; once the discomfort has gone, frequent ambulation is encouraged. When bowel function has returned, the patient should be started on a liquid diet and, if the diet is tolerated, he or she should be discharged home; diet is advanced at home. Rebleeding during observation is a failure of therapy, and the patient should undergo exploratory laparotomy. This will occur in less than 10% of patients with liver or spleen injury (or both) if the guidelines discussed earlier are followed (Fig. 1). When rebleeding occurs after discharge, prompt exploratory laparotomy is indicated; this rarely occurs. Patients who are successfully treated nonoperatively do not require repeat imaging studies; multiple studies over past years have demonstrated that the major organ injuries defined by CT require many days and often weeks to disappear and have no bearing on the clinical decision-making process.

The subgroup of patients who respond to treatment, remain stable, and have hemoperitoneum on FAST or DPL, but no liver or spleen injury, likely have a mesenteric tear. These patients, if explored, are likely to have a therapeutic laparotomy with surgical control of mesenteric bleeding, closure of a small bowel perforation, or resection of ischemic bowel. Successful nonoperative therapy may occur in these patients, but there should be a low threshold for exploratory laparotomy. Hemoperitoneum by itself seldom causes tenderness beyond 6 hours; small bowel injury or compromise should be suspected if tenderness persists.

The decision to institute nonoperative therapy in patients with minor injuries to the liver or spleen (AIS 1–3) but major associated injuries, especially to long bones, requiring RBC replacement is more problematic. Is the need for RBC replacement due to the associated injuries or to the known intra-abdominal injuries? A major pelvic fracture predictably causes 3 or more units of blood loss, whereas a major femur fracture often causes a 2-unit loss; the

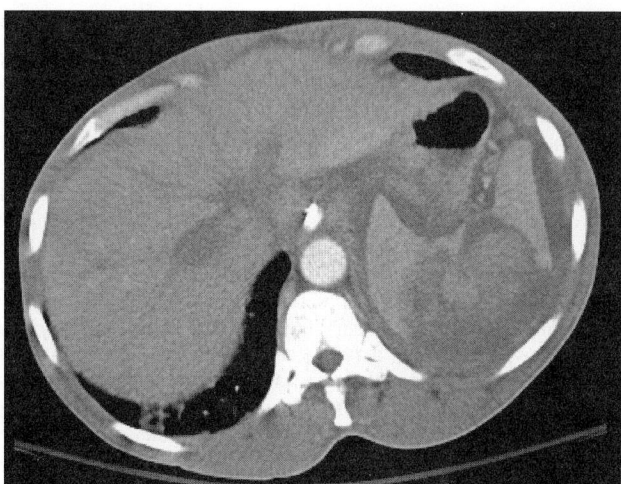

Figure 1 This 36-year-old woman presented 4 days after assault with multiple rib fractures, abdominal distention, left upper-quadrant pain, and symptomatic anemia (Hg = 4.1 g/dl); successful treatment included rib blocks and two blood transfusions.

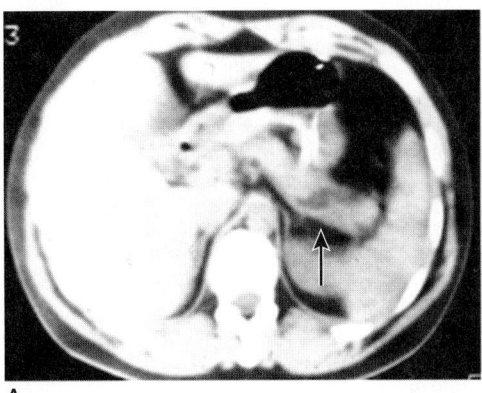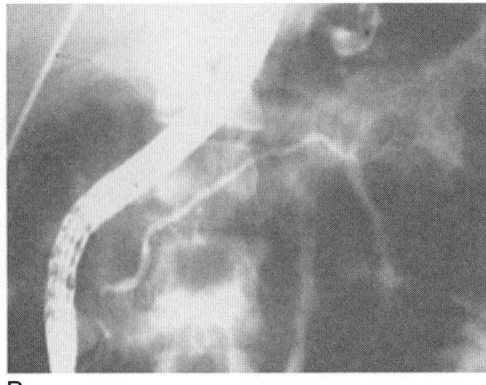

A   B

Figure 2 **(A)** CT scan suggesting transsection of pancreas after blunt abdominal injury in patient with multiple injuries but minimal abdominal symptoms; **(B)** endoscopic retrograde cholangiopancreatogram showing normal primary, secondary, and tertiary ductal radicals. Patient was successfully treated nonoperatively.

ranges may be quite extensive. A nontherapeutic laparotomy in a patient with associated multisystem injuries aggravates the potential for recovery, whereas prolonged observation before a therapeutic laparotomy aggravates the hemorrhagic shock insult and potentiates the development of multiorgan failure. An old surgical maxim applies, namely, "Sins of commission are less hazardous than sins of omission." Another maxim also applies: "When in doubt, operate." When the stable patient with severe pelvic fracture also has a large perineal laceration, laparotomy is indicated to perform a proximal colostomy to prevent retroperitoneal sepsis.

The decision regarding laparotomy for patients requiring blood replacement must be modified when coagulopathy from antiplatelet medications, warfarin therapy, or prior treatment with fractionated heparin exists. These medications are more frequently used in the elderly population, including patients involved in motor vehicle collisions, the most common cause for severe BAI. Any patient with injuries that require admission should be treated with fresh frozen plasma as the bleeding times and clotting times are corrected; the amount of blood required before the coagulopathy is corrected should not be the determinant regarding observation or laparotomy. Any blood replacement required after the coagulopathy has been corrected, however, is an indication for exploration.

Retroperitoneal Hemorrhage

The kidneys and pancreas are the most common retroperitoneal solid organs that are injured after BAI. DPC, DPL, and the FAST provide no benefit for diagnosing these injuries. Renal injury typically causes hematuria, which may be microscopic. The extent of renal injury in the stable patient is best determined by contrast CT, which also assesses ureteral integrity. Most minor renal injuries (AIS 1–3) are treated expectantly; some major renal injuries (AIS 4–5) can also be observed. The decision to explore for renal injury should be made on the basis of lack of renal perfusion, perinephric extravasation, or worsening vital signs thought to be from renal hemorrhage. When the CT shows lacking or impaired perfusion of one kidney in a stable patient, angiography will define the vascular anatomy; when renal artery occlusion is identified soon after injury, operative repair of the renal artery may preserve renal function. We have observed a number of patients in whom this diagnosis was made several hours after injury, and the patients were treated nonoperatively; late hypertension did not develop and late imaging studies showed extensive collateralization with preserved renal perfusion. Exploration for major renal injuries (AIS 4–5) that are not causing hypotension often leads to nephrectomy, even when proximal vascular control is initially obtained.

The decision to explore pancreatic injuries is difficult because the best imaging study, namely, the abdominal CT, is often imprecise, and clinical symptoms may be slow to evolve. We recommend that serum amylase be part of the trauma panel after BAI; although the initial serum amylase may be normal, a progressive rise at 6 and 12 hours is strong evidence for a pancreatic injury. Once the pancreatic injury is identified by CT, the patient with abdominal pain or tenderness should be explored. When the CT strongly suggests a pancreatic injury in an asymptomatic patient, an emergency endoscopic retrograde cholangiopancreatogram (ERCP) will define the ductal anatomy. Patients with a normal ERCP and no abdominal symptoms despite an abnormal CT can be successfully observed (Fig. 2). Patients with any extravasation on ERCP, even from peripheral pancreatic ductules, require exploration for definitive treatment and drainage.

INTRAPERITONEAL HOLLOW VISCUS INJURIES

In order of frequency, the most common intraperitoneal hollow viscus injuries are to the small bowel, stomach, and colon. Peritoneal soilage with sulcus entericus causes early pain and tenderness in patients not mentally impaired. A positive FAST in a patient with pain and tenderness is an indication for exploration. When the FAST is equivocal, a positive DPL with leukocytosis mandates exploration. When both the FAST and DPL are negative, the surgeon should question whether the pain and tenderness are truly related to peritonitis. Associated injuries to the lower ribcage with fractures often cause somatic pain referred along the corresponding intercostal nerves to an upper quadrant of the abdomen. An intercostal nerve block proximal to the fractures will alleviate the pain and confirm that the pain is of somatic origin. These patients should be admitted for serial observation. The stable patient with an equivocal DPL and FAST is a candidate for a CT, which is usually helpful in showing extraluminal extravasation. Unfortunately, a small number of patients will have a false-negative FAST, DPL, and CT despite intraperitoneal hollow viscus rupture. Over-reliance on these studies often leads to an inordinate delay in exploration and definitive treatment. Consequently, the serial PE remains the gold standard. When the patient does not improve over the first 12 hours, a repeat DPL or CT may define the intraperitoneal extravasation. The objective of this chapter is to define the diagnostic approach to intra-abdominal injuries rather than the technical aspects of treatment. However, we strongly recommend that patients with delay in exploration and with need for small bowel resection undergo a two-layer hand-sewn anastomosis with generous seromuscular bites to accommodate for the thickened and edematous bowel wall. The stapling devices were not constructed to deal with the excessive thickness seen in the inflamed bowel wall.

Full-thickness gastric perforations are almost always identified early after BAI because of the large discharge of both blood and gastric content into the peritoneal cavity. These patients are explored early for peritonitis. Intraperitoneal colon injuries are much less common and may be partial thickness. Pneumoperitoneum is uncommon. The full-thickness injuries cause early peritonitis, which leads to exploration.

Retroperitoneal Hollow Viscus Injury

The most frequent retroperitoneal hollow viscus injuries are to the duodenum, ascending and descending colon, and rectum. The FAST and DPL are not helpful. Plain flat and upright films of the abdomen are no longer routinely taken, with the result that the classic findings of obfuscation of the right psoas muscle, scoliosis concave to the right, and small air bubbles superimposed on the kidney are no longer valuable signs for making an early diagnosis of blunt duodenal injury. These findings, of course, are present on the CT, but they are subtler and often overlooked. The diagnosis is usually made on contrast CT showing extraluminal extravasation. Serial PE remains the gold standard in a patient with persistent abdominal symptoms more than 6 hours after BAI. When the diagnosis of duodenal rupture has been delayed until extensive retroperitoneal inflammation has ensued, we recommend that the patient undergo duodenal diverticulization consisting of antrectomy, gastrojejunostomy, layered repair of the duodenal perforation, and wide drainage.

Blunt rupture to the retroperitoneal ascending or descending colon is rare and usually is seen in association with major pelvic fractures involving the iliac wing. The diagnosis may be suspected on the basis of CT. More often, however, the diagnosis is suspected because of tenderness over the lateral abdomen; the greatest point of tenderness is over the abdominal musculature near the perforation rather than at the associated fracture of the iliac wing. Blunt rectal rupture, in the absence of sexual toys, is also rare. This injury is seen in patients with disruption of the sacroiliac joint or extensive injury to the sacrum itself. The diagnosis is suspected on the basis of retroperitoneal air in the deep pelvis and confirmed by digital examination.

CRYPTIC INJURIES DIAGNOSED LATE

Certain injuries after BAI are often missed. These include liver injury with late hemobilia, contusion of the fundus of the gallbladder with mural ischemia and delayed rupture, contained extrahepatic biliary duct rupture with delayed jaundice and sepsis, major liver injury with hemoperitoneum and delayed biliary leakage, and focal devascularized mural injuries to the small bowel or colon. Hemobilia typically occurs when a major liver injury (AIS 4–5) develops a contained hematoma that decompresses approximately 4 to 14 days after BAI into the biliary system, leading to pain and hematemesis. The diagnosis is made by hepatic arteriography (Fig. 3).

Although most gallbladder injuries have rupture of the dome with early peritonitis or avulsion from the hepatic fossa and hemoperitoneum, some patients develop an ischemic contusion of the fundus, which ruptures at 2 to 4 days when the intraluminal pressure rises after diet is reinstituted. This rupture may occur after discharge. The patient will then return with bilious ascites, tenderness, and jaundice. Patients with contained extrahepatic biliary duct ruptures often have associated injuries that require laparotomy. Some patients, however, will have isolated injuries, especially to the left hepatic duct, with no associated injuries. Minimal findings are present initially; later jaundice and bilious ascites may occur.

Endoscopic retrograde ductography will define the injury and guide treatment. Major liver injuries are often observed; when the patient develops sepsis after 24 hours, intrahepatic bile duct rupture with leakage should be expected. Biliary scintigraphy will confirm the diagnosis and prompt laparotomy. The focal avascular injury to the antimesenteric portion of the small bowel or colon presumably represents a partial blowout injury in which the intraluminal stretch disrupts the capillaries, thus creating ischemia without perforation (Fig. 4). When identified early during exploration for other intraperitoneal injuries, the ischemic area can be inverted. When the patient has no other indications for early laparotomy, this area will rupture, often after diet has been started. Awareness of these cryptic injuries permits the surgeon to explore early when new symptoms appear. This is one reason why the patient with multiple injuries from blunt trauma should remain on the trauma service while the associated injuries are being treated by the surgical specialists.

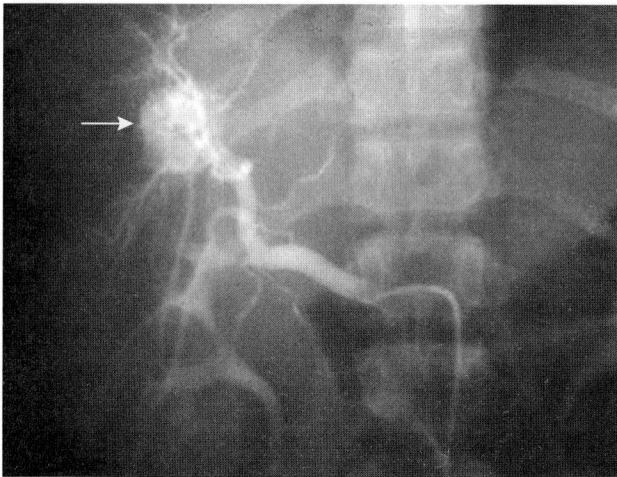

Figure 3 This patient presented with abdominal pain and hematemesis 9 days after a motor vehicle crash and discharge from another trauma center. Hemobilia from this arterial bilious fistula was treated with hepatotomy and ligation of the partially severed artery.

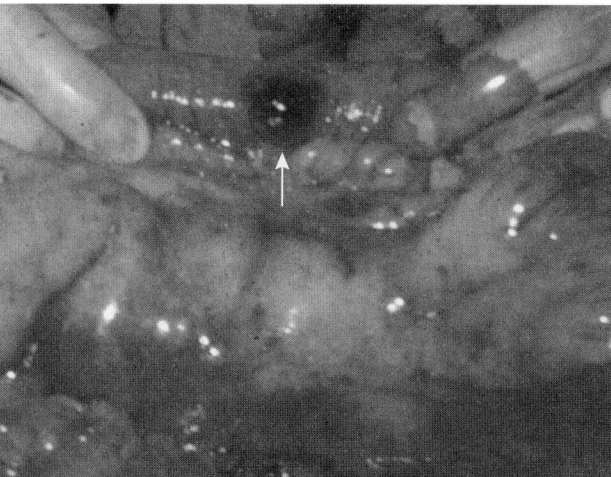

Figure 4 This area of focal necrosis of the small bowel was identified at the time of laparotomy, performed for other reasons; successful treatment consisted of inversion of this ischemic area with seromuscular sutures. These lesions may rupture late after discharge.

Suggested Readings

Kirkpatrick AW, Baxter K, Germann E, and others: Intra-abdominal complications after surgical repair of small bowel injuries: an international review, *J Trauma* 55(3): 399, 2003.

Lucas CE: Splenic trauma: choice of management, *Ann Surg* 213:98, 1991.

Lucas CE, Ledgerwood AM: Injuries to the stomach, duodenum, pancreas, small bowel, colon, and rectum. In Wilmore DW, Cheung LY, Harken AH, and others, editors: *ACS surgery principles and practice*, New York, 2003, WebMD.

Ross SE, Cobean RA, Hoyt DB, and others: Blunt colonic injury: a multicenter review, *J Trauma* 33:379, 1992.

Shorr RM, Greaney GC, Donovan AJ: Injuries of the duodenum, *Am J Surg* 154:93, 1987.

Stone A, Sugawa C, Lucas CE, and others: The role of endoscopic retrograde pancreatography (ERP) in blunt abdominal trauma, *Am Surg* 56:715, 1990.

Penetrating Abdominal Trauma

L.D. Britt, MD, MPH, and G.D. Rushing, MD

HISTORICAL PERSPECTIVE

Although aggressive surgical intervention has been challenged recently, the cornerstone of penetrating abdominal trauma management has been early operative intervention. This approach was firmly established during the World War II and Korean military campaigns after it had been determined during World War I that there was a high mortality rate associated with nonoperative management (the treatment plan often chosen). The emphasis on nonoperative management of penetrating trauma preceded World War I. In the nineteenth century, gunshot wounds to the abdomen were managed nonoperatively. As depicted in Table 1, the international community advocated supportive care for this type of injury. With implementation of mandatory exploration, there was a precipitous decline in both morbidity and mortality rates. This management paradigm was adopted in the civilian setting, with routine laparotomies being performed for both stabbings and gunshot wounds to the abdomen. This was the standard of care until 1960, when the concept of "selective conservatism" was initially introduced by G. W. Shaftan and subsequently endorsed by Carter Nance. Because of the inordinately high negative exploration rate (especially with stab wounds

to the abdomen), Shaftan and Nance advocated expectant management (selective observation) for those patients with penetrating injuries to the abdomen who were essentially asymptomatic. This radical departure from what was considered the gold standard of management of penetrating abdominal injuries received limited approval in the surgical community. Although the selective approach was eventually embraced for stab wounds to the abdomen, the debate over the role of more selective management of patients with gunshot wounds to the abdomen in cases in which the missile has clearly traversed the abdominal cavity continues today. E. E. Moore and others have advocated mandatory exploration for gunshot wounds penetrating the abdomen because of their findings of a 98% to 99% risk of significant intra-abdominal injury with such injuries.

Even with the advent of diagnostic modalities such as high-speed, helical computed tomography (CT) scanners and abdominal ultrasound (*F*ocused *A*ssessment for the *S*onographic Evaluation of the *T*rauma Patient [FAST] examination), the controversy continues regarding the efficacy of selective nonoperative management for gunshot wounds that have penetrated the abdominal cavity.

GENERAL PRINCIPLES

The essential principles of the initial assessment in the Advanced Trauma Life Support (ATLS, American College of Surgeons) directives are just as applicable to penetrating abdominal injuries as for any other injury. The ATLS-directed primary survey, with its mandatory emphasis on the ABCs (airway, breathing, and circulation), resuscitative efforts, and secondary survey are all imperative in the optimal management of penetrating abdominal injuries. A definitive airway, preferably a translaryngeal endotracheal intubation, should be performed for establishment of a secure airway if there are doubts about airway stability. On the rare occasion that a translaryngeal airway cannot be established in an emergency setting, a surgical airway (cricothyroidotomy) should be the next option for a more definitive airway. Associated life-threatening complications, such as pneumothorax, hemothorax, or tension pneumothorax, can occur with penetrating abdominal injuries when there is a missile (or weapon) trajectory into the thorax or thoracoabdominal regions. Such associated injuries necessitate prompt recognition and pleural space decompression. Circulatory assessment and stabilization are required after appropriate airway and ventilatory management. In the case of a hemodynamically unstable patient with abdominal injury, such assessment and stabilization should be performed in the operative theater, for it is likely that injury involves a vascular structure that will require optimal exposure with, if possible, proximal and distal control. With a team approach, these life-saving measures can often be performed simultaneously. For the hemodynamically stable patients who have undergone the primary survey and the necessary resuscitative interventions, a history (if feasible) along with a thorough but expeditious physical examination should be conducted during the secondary evaluation to detect any occult injuries or other penetrating wounds. At no time should

Table 1: Management of Gunshot Wounds to the Abdomen

Historical Perspective

1800s	Surgical dogma: nonoperative management of gunshot wounds to the abdomen
1880	J. Marion Sims, a Southern surgeon, advocated operative management
1880s	Paul Reclus, a French surgeon, enthusiastically endorsed supportive care only
1881	President James A. Garfield shot through the abdomen. No surgical exploration performed. Supportive care only ("Garfield's death watch"). J. Marion Sims openly criticized this nonoperative approach.
1890s	Sir William McCormick, chief army surgeon for the British troops, highlighted the following aphorism: "If a man undergoes surgery after being shot, he dies and lives if left in peace."

wounds be probed, except in the operating room under direct visualization.

All knife and bullet wounds should be identified and marked with a paper clip or some other radiopaque marker before abdominal plain radiography to assist in determining localization and possible trajectory of a bullet. For example, two bullet wounds detected on abdominal inspection could represent a through-and-through injury by a single bullet or two entry wounds resulting from two missile injuries. With a penetrating abdominal gunshot wound, no visualization of a foreign body when there is no evidence of an exit wound is suggestive of a possible bullet embolism via the vascular system. Also, being shot or stabbed does not preclude a patient from sustaining blunt injuries. Pertinent history should always include the mechanism and time of injury, whether loss of consciousness occurred, and whether significant blood loss was noted at the scene. This vital information usually can be obtained from the prehospital personnel or, at times, friends or family.

Irrespective of the specific mechanism of injury, indications for emergency laparotomy for penetrating abdominal injuries are highlighted in Table 2. High-velocity bullets travel 2500 to 3250 feet per second, whereas low-velocity missiles travel less than 1000 feet per second. The civilian armamentarium (handguns, rifles, and shotguns) causes mostly low-velocity injuries. However, a close-range shotgun blast can result in high–velocity-type tissue destruction. Because of the extensive intra-abdominal injuries resulting from expanding tissue cavitation, high-velocity injuries mandate surgical exploration.

Although often not a top priority, all missiles should be removed, if readily accessible, to prevent the potential for infection, bullet embolism, or lead poisoning if the missile is located in some body fluids (e.g., synovial fluid).

If a surgical approach is taken, the basic "operative plan" (Table 3) remains the same no matter what the mechanism of injury happens to be.

Table 2: Penetrating Abdominal Injuries

Indications for Emergency Laparotomy

Peritoneal signs

Hemodynamic liability

Evisceration

Blood from any natural orifice

Extensive bleeding from the wound

Positive radiologic sign (e.g., pneumoperitoneum)

Impaled object

High-velocity missile injury

Table 3: Surgical Approach

The "Operative Plan"

- Control hemorrhage
- Control gross spillage and cross-cavity contamination
- Meticulous exploration*
  Mobilization techniques
  Adequate assessment of all holes/hematomas
- "Damage control"
- Definitive repair of intra-abdominal injuries and closure of diaphragmatic rents*

*"Damage control" management will likely preclude all aspects of this specific operative plan being performed at the original operation.

THORACOABDOMINAL INJURIES

The thoracoabdominal region is defined as the area between the nipples and the costal margins (Fig. 1). Penetrating injuries in the central area of this region always necessitate ruling out a possible cardiac injury. Clinical presentation and findings on physical examination such as hypotension, distended neck veins, and muffled heart sounds can heighten the suspicion for a cardiac injury with associated tamponade. Among the diagnostic studies helpful in determining a possible cardiac injury as a result of a penetrating thoracoabdominal wound include the FAST examination (specifically of the xiphoid window) or pericardiocentesis performed in the operating room. Often labeled the "ultimate blind spot," the thoracoabdominal region can easily hide diaphragmatic injuries resulting from penetrating trauma. Even with the liberal use of diagnostic modalities such as CT, diagnostic peritoneal lavage, FAST examination, or plain radiography, definitive documentation of a full-thickness diaphragmatic tear cannot always be achieved. Given the fact that diaphragmatic herniations can have a delayed presentation (in one series up to 20 years), determining the integrity of the diaphragm (especially the left diaphragm) is imperative. Until 1992, when Ivatury and colleagues proposed using diagnostic laparoscopy for evaluation of thoracoabdominal injuries, exploratory laparotomy was the only definitive method to rule out a diaphragmatic injury, and thus for potential intra-abdominal injuries. Although Feliciano recommended CT scan evaluation and observation for patients with right upper-quadrant gunshot wounds associated with right-sided pneumothoraces, McQuay and Britt highlighted the importance of also diagnosing right diaphragmatic injuries. In their study, the majority of penetrating thoracoabdominal injuries necessitated therapeutic intervention. McQuay and Britt proposed the algorithm depicted in Figure 2. Currently, there are those who advocate both diagnostic and therapeutic laparoscopy for penetrating thoracoabdominal injuries in which a diaphragmatic laceration has been confirmed. With the necessity to perform a thorough exploration after diagnosing a full-thickness diaphragmatic injury and the fact that the missed injury rate has been reported to be as high as 77%, an open laparotomy should still be considered the standard of care for this type of injury. However, with more trauma surgeons developing complex

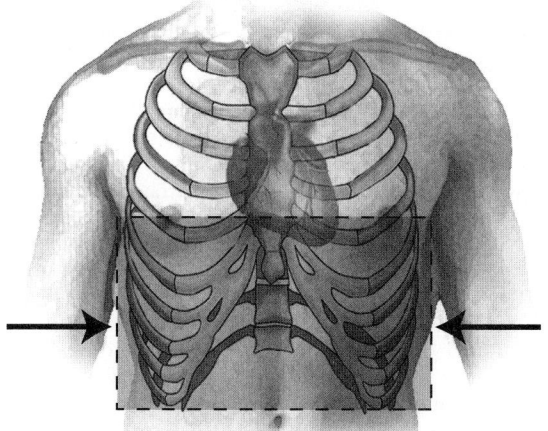

Figure 1

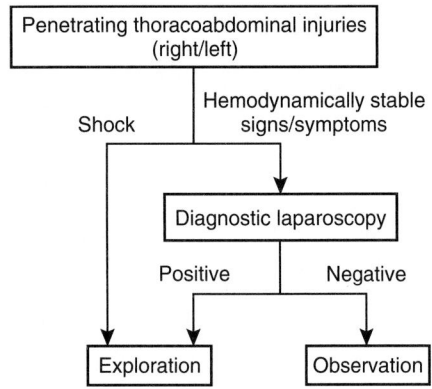

Figure 2

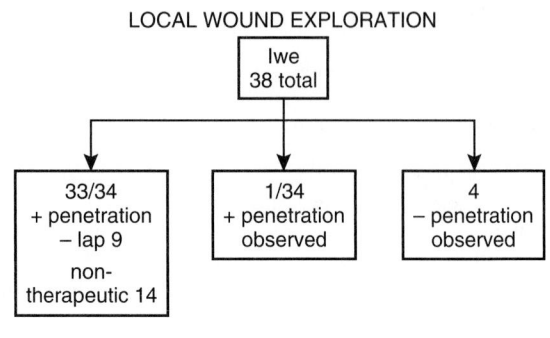

Figure 3

laparoscopic skills and with the advancement of technology in this area (microinstruments, microcameras, advanced staplers, and suction-irrigation dissection systems), the next-generation trauma surgeon will likely be highly competent in therapeutic laparoscopy.

In the acute setting of penetrating thoracoabdominal injuries, there are few (if any) indications for performing diagnostic thoracoscopy to determine the integrity of the diaphragm. Such an intervention will likely require a double-lumen endotracheal tube insertion and a lateral decubitus positioning of the patient. If a diaphragmatic through-and-through injury is actually confirmed (especially on the left side), the patient would need to be repositioned in the supine position and prepared and draped for a celiotomy. Therefore, performing a diagnostic laparoscopy is more appropriate and efficient management.

ANTERIOR ABDOMEN

The boundaries of the anterior abdomen include the costal margin (superiorly), the symphysis pubis and bilateral inguinal ligaments (inferiorly), and the anterior axillary line (laterally). As discussed earlier, controversies still exist regarding the management of penetrating abdominal injuries. Perhaps the most heated debate is that which revolves around whether there should be a nonoperative, selective management approach to gunshot wounds that clearly traverse the abdominal cavity without any indication for mandatory exploration. Although most trauma surgeons would adopt a nonoperative, selective management approach to a penetrating injury that appears to be superficial and tangential, the majority of trauma surgeons would still advocate mandatory celiotomy for gunshot injury that has penetrated the abdominal cavity, even when the patient is essentially asymptomatic and hemodynamically stable. With the expectation of avoiding an unnecessary laparotomy, surgeons have used CT to assist in determining the trajectory of the missile. The sensitivity and specificity of such a diagnostic modality are considered less than optimal. Also, with the risk of intra-abdominal injuries requiring therapeutic intervention, many continue to adopt the policy of mandatory exploration. Velmahos and Demetriades have been the most fervent proponents of nonoperative management for gunshot wounds to the abdomen. Their rationale for opposing surgical exploration in patients with gunshot wounds traversing the abdominal cavity is that 90% of the data supporting mandatory exploration are derived from the military setting, with the civilian data demonstrating only a 30% to 74% injury rate for gunshot wounds to the abdomen. A recent review of our institutional experience shows some similarity to the military data in that

90% of patients shot in the abdomen had significant injuries that required operative management. Velmahos and Demetriades also reported a complication rate, as a result of unnecessary (nontherapeutic) laparotomies, of 22% to 41%. At our institution, the complication rate is less than 10%. This debate will likely continue. Nevertheless, the standard of care for gunshot wounds of the abdomen in which the missile has penetrated the abdominal cavity is operative intervention. However, selective nonoperative management is currently being practiced.

At some institutions, patients with stab wounds to the anterior abdomen who have no indication for abdominal exploration are currently managed selectively. For this cohort of patients, there are many who advocate local wound exploration; if the posterior fascia and the peritoneum are found to be penetrated, celiotomy is performed. There are some who adhere to the original diagnostic evaluation by Thal and Carrico, who recommended local wound exploration. They recommended performing a diagnostic peritoneal lavage if it was found that the posterior fascia/peritoneum had been penetrated. Positive results (100,000 mm³ RBC count) dictated that patients be subsequently explored. Our data for local wound exploration are shown in Figure 3. Sixty-seven percent of the patients had unnecessary operations as a result of local wound explorations; this prompted our institution to question the efficacy of this diagnostic maneuver. Because of the high false-positive rate, there is a growing interest in expectant management (i.e., observation only) for those patients who have an anterior abdomen stab wound and no obvious indication for surgery. The disappointing results with local wound exploration are not surprising, given the fact that, of the variables used to predict a need for laparotomy (shock, peritonitis, intra-abdominal bleeding, and peritoneal penetration), peritoneal penetration has the lowest specificity (21.2%). A simple algorithm for penetrating abdominal trauma is shown in Table 4.

FLANK AND BACK

The flank region is defined as the area within the inferior tip of the scapula and the iliac crest (inferiorly) and between the anterior and posterior axillary lines. The back is the area between the posterior axillary lines. Because of the substantial musculature in these regions, local wound exploration is not an option and could be hazardous because of the risk of bleeding and inadvertent entry into the retroperitoneum. The indications for mandatory exploration remain the same. However, if these indications are not present, the patient who sustains a flank or back penetrating injury should undergo selective management, which requires a triple-contrast (intravenous, via nasogastric tube, and via rectal) abdominal CT to determine whether there are any occult injuries.

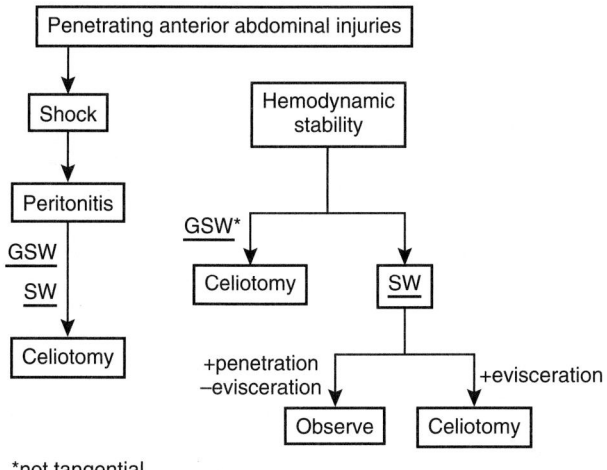

*not tangential

Figure 4 *GSW,* Gunshot wound; *SW,* stab wound.

SPECIFIC INJURIES

When abdominal exploration is required, it is imperative to be knowledgeable about the full spectrum of operative options and the potential outcomes (Table 4).

RETROPERITONEAL HEMATOMAS

Retroperitoneal zones are classified as Zones I (central), II (perinephric or lateral), or III (pelvic). Retroperitoneal hematomas resulting from penetrating injuries are major, vascular, or renal injuries (Zone II) unless proven otherwise. Even if the retroperitoneal hematoma is not pulsatile or expanding, the zones in the retroperitoneum should be explored (obtaining proximal and distal control when possible). This management is in contrast to stable retroperitoneal hematomas resulting from a blunt trauma mechanism (Table 5). Only the central retroperitoneal hematoma should be routinely explored.

Table 4: Penetrating Abdominal Trauma

Organ	Incidence	Diagnosis	Specific Management	Results
Small bowel	Highest incidence of injury of the intra-abdominal organ	• Physical examination • Cannot rely on tenderness/peritoneal signs in the early stage of injury • Plain radiography • FAST exam: free fluid with CT scan demonstrating no solid organ injury • CT scan High false-negative rate Pneumoperitoneum Free fluid	• Preoperative antibiotics • Primary closure of simple lacerations • Segmented resection of complex injuries with functional end-to-end tensionless anastomosis • One (or double) layer closure/anastomosis or stapled anastomosis • Exploration of large expanding mesenteric hematomas	• Outcome is good Negligible leak rate even in contaminated field
Colon	Stab wounds 5% Gunshot 25%	• Physical examination Tenderness/peritoneal signs Gross blood on rectal examination	• Preoperative antibiotics • Primary closure of simple injuries (avoid narrowing the lumen) • Segmental resection and fecal diversion of complex colonic wounds	• Overall, favorable outcome • Complications Low leak rate Wound infection Intraperitoneal abscess
Liver	Most commonly injured solid organ	• Physical examination right upper-quadrant tenderness • Plain radiography Nonspecific Pneumothorax if there is associated pleural space entry as a result of the penetrating injury • FAST examination Can be unreliable • CT scan If necessary for diagnostic study should only be performed in the hemodynamically stable patient	• Preoperative antibiotics • Depending on the severity of the injury (grade) and the hemodynamic status of the patient, the management armamentarium is as follows: Expectant (observation) Drainage Hepatorrhaphy (including Argon beam coagulation) Debridement/resection Packing Angiography/embolization	• Outcome—variable (depending on the degree of hepatic injury, grade I-VI) Grade I and II mortality unlikely Grade III ≈ 25% Grade IV ≈ 50% Grade V 80% Grade VI lethal

(continued)

Table 4: Penetrating Abdominal Trauma—Cont'd

Organ	Incidence	Diagnosis	Specific Management	Results
Spleen	Less common injury rate than with a blunt trauma mechanism	• Physical examination LUQ tenderness/ peritoneal signs Referred pain to left shoulder (Kehr's sign) • Plain radiography Nonspecific Associated pneumothorax • FAST examination Unreliable • CT scan If necessary, should only be performed in the hemodynamically stable patient	• Preoperative antibiotics • Operative management armamentarium Expectant Splenorrhaphy (including Argon beam coagulation) Partial splenectomy Splenectomy • Postsplenectomy immunization vaccines Streptococcus pneumoniae Haemophilus influenza Meningococcus	• Overall, good outcome with all the management choices • Infrequent complications Pleural effusion Pneumonia Subphrenic abscess Thrombocytosis Overwhelming postsplenectomy infection (rare)
Diaphragm	6% of all intra-abdominal injuries resulting from penetrating trauma	• Physical examination Chest pain and shortness of breath Scaphoid abdomen Bowel sounds on auscultation of the hemithorax • Plain radiography Hollow viscus noted in the left hemithorax Nasogastric tube in the left hemithorax • FAST examination Unreliable • DPL Inconclusive; high false-negative • CT scan Inconclusive • Laparoscopy, the diagnostic modality of choice	• Preoperative antibiotics • Primary closure is the preferred definitive management • With documentation of a diaphragmatic rent (laceration), exploratory laparotomy is necessary	• Associated injuries dictate morbidity and mortality
Stomach	More common injury in penetrating trauma than blunt 10% of penetrating injuries of the abdomen	• Physical examination - epigastric tenderness - peritoneal signs - bloody gastric aspirate • Plain radiography - free air under the diaphragm • FAST examination - unreliable • DPL - + lavage RBCs WBCs Gross contamination • CT scan - pneumoperitoneum • Laparoscopy - operator dependent	• Preop antibiotics • Debridement when necessary • Primary closure (two layers)	• Associated injuries dictate morbidity and mortality

Duodenum/ Pancreas	• Isolated injuries are uncommon • High percentage of associated injuries	• Physical examination - abdominal tenderness - peritoneal signs • Plain radiography - free air - retroperitoneal air • FAST • DPL • CT scan	• Preop antibiotics • Duodenal operative armamentarium - primary repair - primary repair with gastrostomy retrograde jejunostomy; feeding jejunostomy - pyloric exclusive • Pancreas operative armamentarium - drainage - debridement - partial resection - pancreaticoduodenectomy	• Highly lethal due to associated injuries • Increased mortality with delayed diagnosis of duodenal injury
Biliary	• Extrahepatic biliary injury Infrequent	• Physical examination - abdominal tenderness - peritoneal signs • Plain radiography - nonspecific findings • FAST • DPL • CT scans	• Preoperative antibiotics • Operative armamentarium - cholecystectomy (for gallbladder injuries) - biliary duct reconstruction (e.g., choledochojejunostomy)	• Cholecystectomy - negligible morbidity • Biliary duct reconstruction - bile leak - possible stricture
Kidney	• 20% of renal injuries result from penetrating trauma	• Physical examination - penetrating wound or trajectory in close proximity to the kidney - hematuria • Plain radiography - nonspecific • FAST • DPL • CT scan (if peritoneal penetration not suspected in a gunshot wound) - perinephric hematoma - extravasation	• Preoperative antibiotics • Operative armamentarium - primary repair with viable tissue buttress - partial nephrectomy - nephrectomy	• Mortality related to the associated injuries
Bladder	• Usually an occult injury found during intraoperative abdominal exploration	• Physical examination - penetrating wound or trajectory in close proximity to the bladder - hematuria • Plain radiography - nonspecific • FAST • DPL • CT scan (if peritoneal penetration not suspected) - extravasation of contrast agent	• Preoperative antibiotics • Multilayer closure with absorbable sutures with indwelling bladder catheter	• Excellent outcomes • Morbidity and mortality relate to associated injuries
Ureter	• Infrequent injury in penetrating trauma	• Usually an intraoperative diagnosis	• Preoperative antibiotics • Management armamentarium Primary repair/stenting Delayed repair and suprapubic cystostomy Diverting nephrostomies	• Good outcome if no major associated injuries

CT, Computed tomography; *DPL,* diagnostic peritoneal lavage; *FAST,* focused assessment for the sonographic evaluation of the trauma patient; *LUQ,* left-upper quadrant; *RBCs,* red blood cells; *WBCs,* white blood cells.

Table 5: Retroperitoneal Hematomas

Zone	Blunt	Penetrating
1 (Central)	Explore	Explore
2 (Perinephric)	Observe	Explore
3 (Pelvic)	Observe	Explore

SUMMARY

With advancing technology and surgical expertise in both the open and minimally invasive arena, the management of penetrating abdominal trauma will continue to evolve. Evidence-based practice, not emotion or surgical dogma, should be the paramount driving force guiding decision making in the management of penetrating abdominal trauma.

SUGGESTED READINGS

Asensio J, Feliciano DV, Britt LD, and others: Management of duodenal injuries, *Curr Probl Surg* 30(11): 1023, 1993.

Britt LD, McQuay N, Jr: Laparoscopy in the evaluation of penetrating thoracoabdominal trauma, *Am Surg* 69(9):788, 2003.

Brown C, Velmahos GC, Neville AL, and others: Hemodynamically "stable" patients with peritonitis after penetrating abdominal trauma, *Arch Surg* 140:767, 2005.

Nance FC, Wennar MH, Johnson LW, and others: Surgical judgment in the management of penetrating wounds in the abdomen: experience with 2,212 patients, *Ann Surg* 179:639, 1974.

Shaftan GW: Indication for operation in abdominal trauma, *Am J Surg* 99:657, 1960.

Velmahos GC, Demetriades D, Toutouza KG: Selective nonoperative management in 1,856 patients with abdominal gunshot wounds, *Ann Surg* 234:395, 2001.

Welch CE: War wounds of the abdomen, *N Engl J Med* 237:156, 1947.

Renz BM, Feliciano DV: Gunshot wounds to the right thoracoabdomen: a prospective study of nonoperative management, *J Trauma* 37(5): 737, 1994.

ABDOMINAL COMPARTMENT SYNDROME

Horacio Hojman, MD, and Reuven Rabinovici, MD

INTRODUCTION

Abdominal compartment syndrome (ACS) is a clinical condition in which increased pressure concealed within the abdominal cavity leads to multisystem dysfunction by reducing abdominal organ perfusion and by compressing the respiratory and cardiovascular systems.

ACS is caused by the accumulation of fluid and gas (or both) in the intraperitoneal and retroperitoneal cavity (or both). Because these cavities are surrounded by the less compliant facial planes and skin, intra-abdominal pressure (IAP) inevitably increases with the rising volume of intra-abdominal contents. Acute compartmental hypertension subsequently is generated, compromising tissue perfusion and organ function when it rises above a critical level.

Many different etiologies can lead to fluid or gas accumulation in the abdominal cavity. These include direct mechanisms associated with injury, disease, or abdominopelvic surgery, including: traumatic abdominal bleeding, peritonitis, pancreatitis, ascites, hollow viscus perforation, colonic pseudo-obstruction, liver transplantation, and abdominal packing for uncontrolled bleeding. Abdominal fluid accumulation can also result from indirect or remote mechanisms. Prime examples of such etiologies are shock fluid resuscitation with resultant retroperitoneal and bowel edema, as well as systemic interstitial edema caused by sepsis, multiple organ failure, or burns.

Unless promptly diagnosed and treated, ACS severely attenuates resuscitation efforts in critically ill patients and is highly lethal. Thus every surgeon should be aware of this grave condition and its timely diagnosis and management. This chapter provides a brief overview of ACS, with special emphasis on its pathophysiology, clinical presentation, diagnosis, and treatment. Furthermore, the review outlines controversial issues critical to the understanding and treatment of this syndrome.

HISTORICAL PERSPECTIVE

For more than a century, the medical literature has documented that elevation of IAP can produce serious pathologic derangements. Although the respiratory, hemodynamic, and renal consequences of increased IAP were already delineated in the 1950s and 1970s, they were generally ignored by both medical and surgical communities. Since the mid 1980s, a large number of experimental and clinical studies rediscovered the concept that increased IAP may cause a series of pathophysiologic changes, termed *ACS*. This syndrome was extensively characterized and recognized as a common significant entity in critically ill patients.

INCIDENCE

The exact incidence of ACS is difficult to estimate and varies from 5.5% to 35%. Many factors account for this variability, including diverse patient populations, different levels of acuity, and inconsistent diagnostic criteria.

ETIOLOGY

Primary Abdominal Compartment Syndrome

Primary ACS results from intra-abdominal and retroperitoneal (or both) disease processes or extensive surgical procedures, which lead to accumulation of intracavitary or interstitial fluid or gas. A typical example for this condition is massive traumatic or nontraumatic bleeding that occurs after a major retroperitoneal vascular injury or after liver transplantation, respectively. In these patients, the ACS further exacerbates preexisting hypovolemic shock state. The evolution of damage control approach to severely injured trauma patients, which includes temporary abdominal packing to achieve hemostasis, also contributes to the rapid buildup of abdominal hypertension and to the increased incidence of ACS.

Primary ACS has been also reported in patients undergoing major abdominal, retroperitoneal, or pelvic operations, such as aortic, gynecologic, and urinary tract procedures. In addition, primary ACS was described in association with abdominal distention caused by megacolon or fecal impaction, as well as in critically ill cirrhotic patients with ascites.

Secondary Abdominal Compartment Syndrome can follow systemic medical emergencies that are remote from the abdominal cavity (secondary ACS). For example, ACS has been demonstrated in polytrauma patients who develop massive bowel edema and ascites in the absence of any intra-abdominal injury. Although the pathogenic mechanisms that cause fluid accumulation in this condition are still obscure, several factors have been implicated. These include shock-induced bowel hypoperfusion, resuscitation-driven ischemia-reperfusion injury, and systemic inflammatory response.

Secondary ACS is a well-established complication of massive fluid resuscitation. Other medical conditions in which capillary permeability defects lead to extravasation of intravascular fluid and "third spacing" have been shown to produce ACS. For example, the incidence of ACS in patients with greater than 20% body surface area burns was reported at 20% and 90% when IAPs of 25 mm Hg and 15 mm Hg, respectively, were used as diagnostic endpoints. Significant risk for developing ACS was also documented in patients with sepsis and multiple organ failure.

PATHOPHYSIOLOGY

Central Nervous System Dysfunction

A particular concern in patients with traumatic brain injury and elevated IAP is worsening intracranial pressure (ICP) associated with decreased cerebral perfusion pressure. The proposed pathogenic mechanism for this relationship is decreased venous return (discussed later).

There have been several reports of trauma patients with concomitant refractory intracranial hypertension and increased IAP in whom abdominal decompression resulted in a markedly improved ICP. Similar results were reported recently in 17 patients who underwent abdominal fascial release solely for the treatment of traumatic brain injury with uncontrolled ICP. Nevertheless, it should be emphasized that none of these patients had clear signs of ACS at the time of decompression and that the mean IAP was 27.5 ± 5.2 mm Hg only.

Pneumoperitoneum has been reported to elevate ICP in humans. Although it is unclear whether elevated ICP is associated with decreased cerebral perfusion pressure (CPP) in normal patients, this potential adverse effect of pneumoperitoneum remains a concern in head injury patients undergoing diagnostic laparoscopy.

Respiratory Dysfunction

ACS affects the lungs by exerting external pressure through the diaphragm. This transmitted pressure has several intrathoracic effects. First, the elevated diaphragm increases intrathoracic pressure, which restricts lung expansion. Second, in mechanically ventilated patients, there is an increase in peak airway pressure and peak inspiratory pressure. Third, the external pressure decreases the dynamic compliance of the lung. Subsequently, alveoli and lung vessels are compressed, lung segments collapse, and ventilation-perfusion mismatch develops, with increased intrapulmonary shunting and dead space.

Cardiovascular Dysfunction

The adverse cardiovascular consequences of ACS are also produced by pressure transmitted from the abdomen. Clinical and experimental data suggest several pathogenic mechanisms, which together lead to hemodynamic collapse. Most importantly, the increased abdominal and thoracic pressures compress the low-pressure, thin-walled vena cava, with a dramatic reduction in venous return and cardiac output combined with increased extremity venous pressure and edema. These observations are supported by reports of patients and animals undergoing laparoscopic surgery that demonstrated a dose-response relationship between inferior vena cava (IVC) pressure and diameter and IAP during the pneumoperitoneum. It should be noted that despite the decreased venous return, the elevated intra-abdominal pressure transmitted to the chest causes a spurious increase in central venous pressure (CVP) and pulmonary capillary wedge pressure (PCWP). These false-positive values complicate hemodynamic monitoring and require adjustments to better evaluate the patient's volume status (discussed later). Another pathogenic mechanism that compromises cardiovascular status is pressure-induced rise in both systemic and pulmonary resistance, possibly through mechanical compression of the capillary beds. Last, the elevated diaphragm displaces the heart from its native position, compromising diastolic filling. All of these mechanisms are accentuated in the presence of hypovolemia.

Renal Dysfunction

Oliguria is often the result of increased IAP, even in the presence of adequate hemodynamics, and abdominal decompression usually results in immediate diuresis. Several factors contribute to the development of abdominal hypertension-induced oliguria. Renal blood flow and glomerular filtration rate are reduced because of the cardiovascular effects of increased IAP, direct compression of renal parenchyma, and decreased renal outflow secondary to increased renal vein pressure. In addition, animal data suggest that ACS elevates plasma renin and aldosterone levels. Interestingly, compression of the ureters does not seem to play a pathogenic role because ureteral stenting does not prevent oliguria in ACS patients. It should be noted that increased IAP seems to be an independent marker of renal dysfunction.

Bowel Dysfunction

Bowel dysfunction is a central component of ACS. Several experimental models demonstrated a significant decrease in splanchnic blood flow at an IAP greater than 20 mm Hg and mucosal ischemia at an IAP of 15 mm Hg. These unfavorable consequences of increased IAP occurred despite maintaining normal mean arterial pressure with intravenous fluid administration. Clinical studies reported the presence of mucosal ischemia in patients undergoing laparoscopic cholecystectomy and laparotomy closure. It was speculated that this pressure-induced bowel ischemia may be partially responsible for the increased rate of anastomotic breakdown observed in trauma patients with ACS. It was also hypothesized that bowel hypoperfusion and mucosal ischemia in patients with ACS led to bacterial translocation, which may have a role in the development of multiple organ failure.

Musculoskeletal Dysfunction

Decreased blood flow to the abdominal wall was reported in a porcine model of progressively increased IAP. This could explain the high incidence of wound complications seen in trauma patients with ACS.

In a recent publication, one out of six patients with secondary ACS was reported to develop compartment syndrome of the lower extremities requiring fasciotomy in the absence of orthopedic or vascular injuries. It was suggested that global ischemia and reperfusion combined with IVC compression played a role in the evolution of this condition.

DIAGNOSIS

The clue to the diagnosis of ACS is a high index of suspicion and awareness. After this syndrome is considered, its actual diagnosis is not complicated and usually involves the identification of patients at risk and clinical manifestations combined with measurement of IAP. Less commonly, radiologic imaging is used to establish the diagnosis of ACS.

Predisposing Factors

The presence of predisposing conditions such as critical traumatic or general surgery disease processes, which require massive fluid resuscitation and staged damage control laparotomy (or both), is useful for the diagnosis of increased IAP and ACS. These conditions were described earlier in this chapter.

Physical Examination

The hallmark of physical examination in patients with ACS is a tensely distended abdomen. However, this finding is not always reliable because ACS can occur with normal abdominal examination or with a tensed but nondistended abdomen. Furthermore, the administration of paralytic and sedative agents (or both) can modify the physical examination. Thus, more objective methods are required to diagnose increased IAP and ACS.

Measurement of Intra-abdominal Pressure

The measurement of IAP is the most significant diagnostic tool for ACS. It can be measured directly or indirectly. Direct methods use a catheter connected to a pressure transducer and placed in the peritoneal cavity. Whereas this method is used during laparoscopic surgery, it is less practical in the intensive care setting and is more invasive compared with the various indirect methods.

The most popular and easiest indirect method of IAP monitoring, which has been shown to correlate with the clinical presentation and treatment of ACS, is the determination of bladder pressure. This technique involves the infusion of 50 to 100 ml of sterile saline into an empty bladder via a Foley catheter, which is then clamped and connected to a transducer or a manometer. At this volume, the urinary bladder wall acts as a passive diaphragm that transmits the IAP without imparting any additional pressure from its own. The zero reference point is the top of the symphysis pubis with the patient supine. Measurements should be established after a 30- to 60-second stabilization period to allow detrusor muscle relaxation. Because the bladder serves as a passive transducer, factors that might limit its wall motility, such as neurogenic or contracted bladder, can compromise the accuracy of this method. However, because these factors are uncommon, bladder pressure determination can be obtained in the vast majority of patients. Interestingly, pelvic fractures associated with hematoma do not affect the accuracy of pressure readings. Nevertheless, any concern regarding the accuracy of bladder pressure measurements should prompt the consideration of alternative indirect methods. These include the insertion of a catheter into the stomach or IVC (through the femoral vein), which have been shown to correlate well with bladder pressure determinations.

A grading system for IAP was introduced in the mid 1990s. This system, which is based on indirect IAP measurements, established treatment recommendations for various IAP levels, as described in Table 1. Notably, this grading methodology confirmed an IAP of 25 mm Hg as an indicator to surgically decompress the ACS and defined abdominal hypertension as a sustained IAP of 12 mm Hg. Furthermore, this grading system correlated organ dysfunction with the magnitude of IAP (Table 2). However, it should be emphasized that patients do not respond

Table 1: Grading System for Intra-Abdominal Pressure

Grade	Bladder Pressure (mm Hg)	Recommendation
I	10–15	Maintain normovolemia
II	16–25	Hypervolemic resuscitation
III	26–35	Decompression
IV	>35	Decompression and reexploration

From Meldrum DR, Moore FA, Moore EE, and others: Am J Surg 174:667, 1997, used with permission from Excerpta Medica, Inc.

Table 2: Percentage of Patients with Respective Organ Dysfunction per Intra-Abdominal Pressure Grade

Grade	UO <0.5	PAP >45	SVR >1,000	DO$_2$I <600
I	0	0	0	0
II	0	40	20	20
III	65	78	65	57
IV	100	100	100	100

From Meldrum DR, Moore FA, Moore EE, and others: Am J Surg 174: 667, 1997, used with permission from Excerpta Medica, Inc.
PAP, Peak airway pressure (cm H$_2$O); DO$_2$I, oxygen delivery index (ml O$_2$/min/m^2); SVR, systemic vascular resistance (dyne/sec/cm^{-5}); UO, urine output (ml/kg/hr).

uniformly to similar IAP levels, and therefore the diagnosis (and treatment) of ACS must be based on the physiologic response to increased IAP.

More recently, the use of abdominal perfusion pressure (mean arterial pressure minus the IAP) was proposed as a criterion for the diagnosis and treatment of ACS. For example, abdominal perfusion pressure of greater than or equal to 60 mm Hg was defined as intra-abdominal hypertension, and a value greater than 60 mm Hg was proposed as a target endpoint for resuscitation. Although conceptually attractive, the use of abdominal perfusion pressure rather than IAP in the management of ACS did not gain popularity in the surgical and critical care communities and requires further validation.

Finally, it should be emphasized that in different studies, IAP was measured using either mm of Hg or cm of H$_2$O. Thus, caution is necessary when evaluating different reports and when applying their proposed practice guidelines.

Diagnostic Imaging

Chest radiographs in patients with ACS show clear but small lung fields and elevated hemidiaphragms. Plain kidney, ureter, and bladder radiographs can demonstrate either significant small or large (or both) bowel dilatation or paucity of gas patterns caused by fluid-filled bowel loops and ascites.

Although the diagnosis of ACS is usually made on the basis of the clinical picture and confirmed by bladder pressure measurements, some patients with this syndrome undergo abdominal computed tomography (CT) scan examination as part of their evaluation. A recent report of CT scan findings in patients with ACS identified several characteristics. Most importantly, the ratio of anteroposterior-to-transverse abdominal diameter at the level of the left renal vein (0.85) was significantly higher in patients with

ACS compared with controls (0.7). The study proposed a 0.8 value for 100% sensitivity and 94% specificity in diagnosing ACS. Other CT scan findings included extrinsic compression of the IVC with distal distention, compression of the kidneys, and abnormal bowel wall thickening with enhancement.

Summary

Standard diagnostic criteria, as well as a grading system for ACS, have not yet been established. Nevertheless, most physicians contemplate this diagnosis in patients with intra-abdominal hypertension associated with abdominal distention and clinical evidence of organ dysfunction unresponsive to aggressive resuscitation.

▌ TREATMENT

The first established treatment aim for ACS is prevention. This is achieved by avoiding abdominal wall closure and by using temporary closure techniques when elevated abdominal pressure is present or expected. A detailed discussion of these methods, which include a variety of vacuum-assisted closures (VACs) and mesh closures,

is beyond the scope of this chapter. Our practice has been to temporarily close the abdomen using a VAC dressing technique. The abdominal contents are protected with a bowel bag (Steri-Drape Isolation Bag; 3M Pharmaceuticals, St. Paul, MN) placed over the peritoneal surface (Fig. 1, *A*). Two large Jackson-Pratt drains (Baxter Healthcare, Deerfield, IL) are placed over the bowel bag along both wound edges and exteriorized in a cephalad direction (Fig. 1, *B*). Antimicrobial incise drape (Ioban 2; 3M Pharmaceuticals) is then used to tightly cover the entire area (Fig. 1, *C*). To maintain a watertight seal, it is useful to embed the drains within an elevated Ioban fold, which creates a "mesentery" (Fig. 1, *D*). This method allows for abdominal decompression, suctioning of blood or peritoneal fluid while containing all abdominal contents, and maintaining the sterility of the peritoneal cavity. Within 24 to 48 hours, the temporary closure is removed at the bedside or in the operating room, packs are removed (if present), and the abdomen is copiously irrigated. If the factors responsible for the elevated IAP (such as bowel and retroperitoneal edema) persist, a new VAC dressing or a Vicryl mesh (Ethicon Endosurgery, Somerville, NJ) is applied. Primary abdominal closure could be attempted if these factors have regressed. In this case, all potential physiologic consequences of ACS, as well as bladder pressure, must be closely monitored, and evidence of recurrent ACS should immediately prompt reopening of the abdomen.

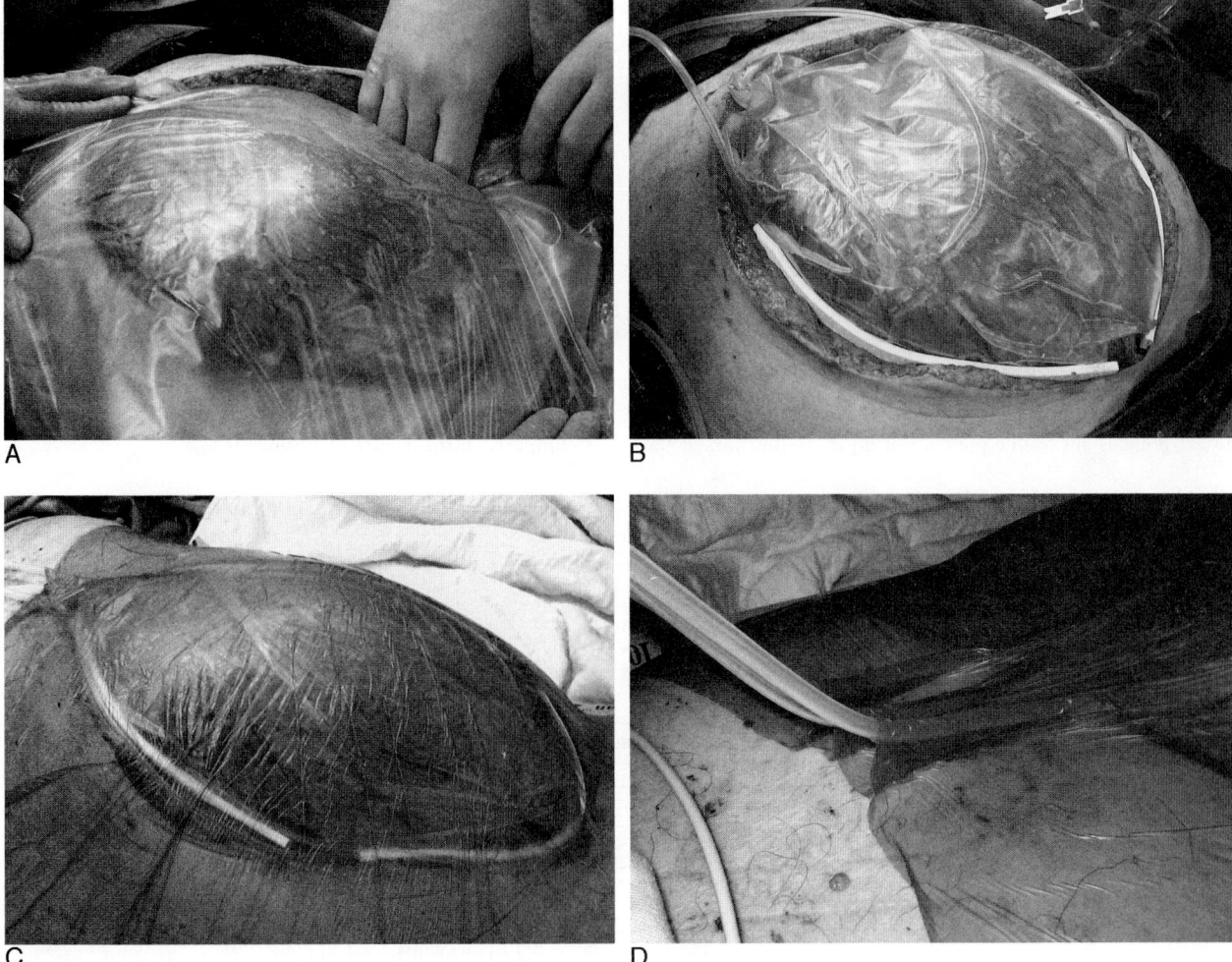

Figure I A method for temporary vacuum abdominal wound closure. Abdominal organs are protected with a bowel bag (Steri-Drape Isolation Bag; 3M Pharmaceuticals, St. Paul, MN) placed over the peritoneal surface and pushed under the wound edges **(A).** Two large Jackson-Pratt drains are placed over the bowel bag along both wound edges and exteriorized in a cephalad direction **(B).** Antimicrobial incise drape (Ioban 2; 3M Pharmaceuticals, St. Paul, MN) dressing is then used to tightly cover the entire area **(C).** Please note that embedding of the drains within an Ioban "mesentery" drape is helpful to maintain a watertight seal **(D).**

After the syndrome develops, the treatment for intra-abdominal hypertension is decompressive laparotomy. However, as outlined earlier, there is no consensus on the IAP level at which ACS occurs or when to intervene. Some investigators suggest that IAP of 20 to 25 mm Hg warrants intervention (see Table 15.10-1), whereas others recommend abdominal decompression for IAP between 25 to 35 mm Hg. More commonly, surgeons interpret IAP measurement in light of organ dysfunction and do not perform decompressive laparotomy solely for intra-abdominal hypertension. Thus a high index of suspicion should be maintained in those patients who are at risk, and laparotomy should be performed with any combination of elevated IAP and system failure.

It should be noted that experimentally significant organ hypoperfusion with mucosal ischemia and bacterial translocation can occur with IAP as low as 10 mm Hg. However, there are no clinical data that support surgical intervention for such a low value.

Several other measurements are available for treating ACS. Aggressive fluid resuscitation is recommended because hypervolemia can partially compensate for the deleterious cardiovascular effects of increased IAP. Fluid resuscitation should be monitored, preferably with a Swan-Ganz catheter or using right-ventricular end-diastolic volume determinations. The surgeon must be mindful that elevated IAP transmitted to the chest may falsely increase both central venous pressure (CVP) and pulmonary capillary wedge pressure (PCWP). This phenomenon, which is similar to the impact of high positive end-expiratory pressure (PEEP) levels, is particularly problematic because most patients with ACS have a diminished venous return caused by mechanical compression or hypovolemia (or both). Some investigators suggested subtracting the intrathoracic pressure, measured with an esophageal balloon, to determine the real CVP and PCWP. An alternative endpoint of resuscitation in patients with ACS is the determination of right-ventricular end-diastolic volume with a volumetric pulmonary artery catheter. This method has been shown to better correlate with cardiac output in the presence of increased PEEP.

Muscle relaxants may also be used in an attempt to reduce the IAP, especially when a prompt resolution of the initiating factor is expected (e.g., overly resuscitated cirrhotic patients or patients with secondary ACS). The IAP of patients treated with complete paralysis usually decreases by an average of 10 mm Hg.

Although there are no clear guidelines for the treatment of ACS, we use a general algorithm to manage this condition (Fig. 2). The start point is always the presence of organ dysfunction. If the patient's condition does not improve in spite of aggressive resuscitative efforts, a diagnosis of ACS must be considered and IAP measured. Patients with a bladder pressure lower than 25 mm Hg can be observed with repeated IAP measurements. In contrast, a bladder pressure greater than 25 mm Hg suggests the need for an emergent operative decompression. If, however, it is estimated that the underlying condition can be quickly reversed, temporizing with fluid resuscitation and paralytic agents can be an option. The management of patients with organ dysfunction who respond positively to resuscitation is dependent on the presence or absence of predisposing factors. If such factors are present, IAP should be measured, and the same algorithm described for unresponsive patients must be followed. On the other hand, if no risk factors for ACS exist, the likelihood that this syndrome is responsible for organ dysfunction is low and no specific actions are necessary.

One clinical scenario associated with decompression of ACS is a reperfusion syndrome, consisting of severe hypotension, coagulopathy, and even asystole. The syndrome is attributed to the sudden washout into the circulation of multiple inflammatory mediators and anaerobic metabolism by-products. Its incidence was estimated at 12% to 25%, although more recent series indicate a much lower rate, which probably reflects an increased awareness of this problem with early intervention. Treatment includes volume expansion to maintain preload, pressor support, and sodium bicarbonate.

Finally, there is some debate whether prophylactic abdominal decompression should be performed in a carefully selected group of critically ill patients undergoing massive fluid and blood product resuscitation. Although there are no data to support this approach, it may potentially improve resuscitation and prevent the dramatic opening of the abdomen in the intensive care setting.

OUTCOME

Because most patients with ACS are critically ill with severe underlying pathologies or injuries, it is difficult to determine the net effect of the syndrome on outcome. Nevertheless, the mortality in this group of patients is high, with reported rates of 42% to 71%. Even with early recognition and treatment, most patients with ACS have a high incidence of multiple organ dysfunction triggered by the initial physiologic insult. Because ACS presents a second severe pathology for these patients, without urgent abdominal decompression the chance of survival is low.

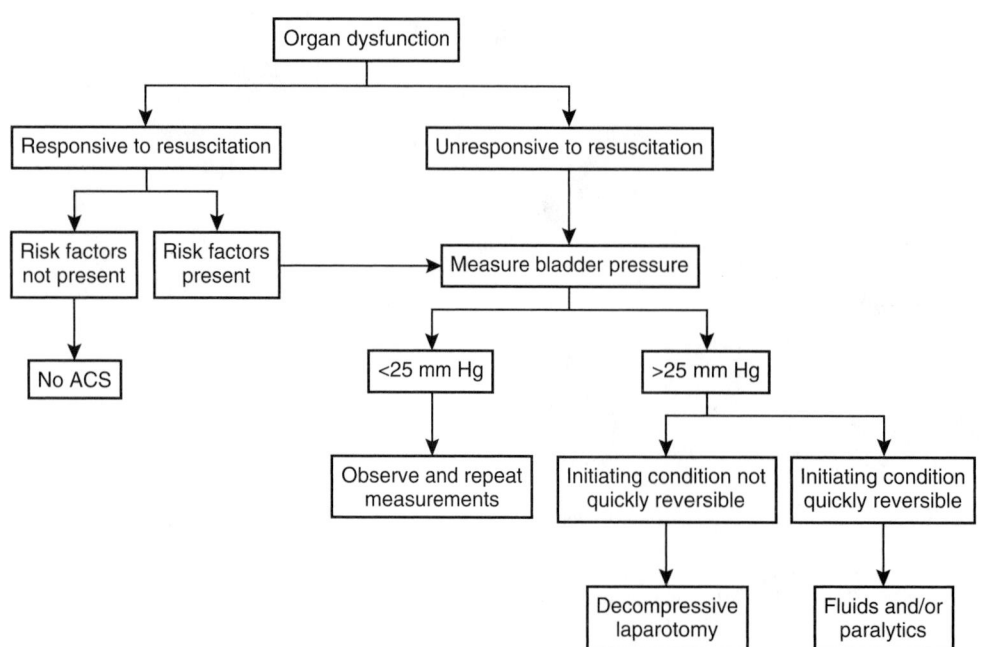

Figure 2 Algorithm for the treatment of abdominal compartment syndrome (see text for details).

SUGGESTED READINGS

Biffl WL, Moore EE, Burch JM, and others: Secondary abdominal compartment syndrome is a highly lethal event, *Am J Surg* 182(6): 645, 2001.

Britt RC, Gannon T, Collins JN, and others: Secondary abdominal compartment syndrome: risk factors and outcomes, *Am Surg* 71(11): 982, 2005.

Burch JM, Moore EE, Moore FA, and others: The abdominal compartment syndrome, *Surg Clin North Am* 76(4): 833, 1996.

Cheatham ML, Nelson LD, Chang MC, and others: Right ventricular end-diastolic volume index as a predictor of preload status in patients on positive end-expiratory pressure [see comments], *Crit Care Med* 26 (11): 1801, 1998.

Ivatury RR, Sugerman HJ: Abdominal compartment syndrome: a century later, isn't it time to pay attention? [editorial], *Crit Care Med* 28(6): 2137, 2000.

Ivy ME, Atweh NA, Palmer J, and others: Intra-abdominal hypertension and abdominal compartment syndrome in burn patients [see comments], *J Trauma* 49(3): 387, 2000.

Maxwell RA, Fabian TC, Croce MA, and others: Secondary abdominal compartment syndrome: an underappreciated manifestation of severe hemorrhagic shock, *J Trauma* 47(6): 995, 1999.

Nathens AB, Brenneman FD, Boulanger BR: The abdominal compartment syndrome, *Can J Surg* 40(4): 254, 1997.

Sugrue M: Abdominal compartment syndrome, *Curr Opin Crit Care* 11(4): 333, 2005.

DIAPHRAGMATIC INJURIES

Udo Rudloff, MD, and H. Leon Pachter, MD

INTRODUCTION

Recognition and management of diaphragmatic injuries remain a challenge to the trauma surgeon. Traumatic diaphragmatic ruptures occur in 3% to 4% of patients with abdominal trauma who present to trauma centers in the United States. Timely diagnosis is imperative to prevent the potentially fatal sequence of enlargement of the diaphragmatic defect, herniation, strangulation, and perforation of displaced visceral organs. Thus appropriate and timely surgical intervention constitutes the focus of modern trauma management of these injuries.

For the hemodynamically unstable patient, immediate operative exploration should be undertaken without delay. In stable patients, a delay of several hours or days has not been associated with a worse prognosis under selected circumstances. The judicious use of noninvasive and invasive investigative techniques is the most common approach to determine the need and optimal timing for operative intervention. Diaphragmatic rupture is considered an indication for repair because acute and chronic complications are not insignificant, including the potential for strangulation of herniated abdominal viscera and the high incidence of missed associated injuries.

Although chest radiographs, helical computed tomography (CT) scanning with three-dimensional reconstruction, and magnetic resonance imaging (MRI) have all found their place in the diagnostic workup of patients with suspected diaphragmatic injuries, videothoracoscopy and thoracoscopy have become the imaging modalities of choice in stable patients for these injuries in recent years. Laparoscopy and thoracoscopy have now progressed in patients with diaphragmatic injuries from the diagnostic to the therapeutic arena, including repair of acute diaphragmatic lacerations with sutures, staples, or the application of prosthetic mesh. However, diagnosis and treatment management depend on a high index of suspicion, as well as persistence on the part of the trauma surgeon in pursuing the correct diagnosis of these challenging injuries.

EPIDEMIOLOGY

Traumatic diaphragmatic injuries occur in approximately 3% of all abdominal injuries, with a rate that varies from 0.8% to 8%.

The exact incidence of penetrating versus blunt traumatic diaphragmatic injuries is presently unknown. Considering left-sided penetrating thoracoabdominal and flank trauma only, incidence rates of diaphragmatic injuries have been reported as high as 24% to 53%. A review of diaphragmatic injuries secondary to blunt abdominal trauma revealed an incidence rate that varied between 0.8% and 5%. Interestingly, up to 90% of diaphragmatic ruptures resulting from blunt traumatic injuries occur in young men involved in motor vehicle accidents. Overall, diaphragmatic injuries resulting from penetrating trauma are considerably more common than those resulting from blunt trauma; however, statistics may be biased and relative to whether the receiving institution is located in an urban or rural location.

PATHOPHYSIOLOGY

Mechanism of Injury

Mechanisms of injury include lateral impacts, which distort the chest wall and shear the diaphragm, and direct frontal impacts, which lead to an abrupt increase in intra-abdominal pressure (Fig. 1). A sudden and abrupt increase in the transdiaphragmatic pleuroperitoneal pressure gradient has been implicated as one of the main pathogenetic factors of diaphragmatic disruption.

During quiet respiration, the intraperitoneal pressure fluctuates between -5 and -10 cm H_2O, and the intraperitoneal pressure between $+2$ and $+10$ cm H_2O. This results in a pleuroperitoneal pressure gradient of $+7$ to $+20$ cm H_2O under resting conditions. With maximal inspiratory efforts, pleuroperitoneal pressure gradients can reach $+100$ cm H_2O; and with sudden increases in intra-abdominal pressures, gradients exceeding $+150$ cm H_2O have been observed. The kinetic energy of blunt abdominal trauma, which is transmitted in a perpendicular fashion, causes a sudden rise in the pleuroperitoneal pressure gradient. This gradient might be several times higher than that under physiologic conditions, causing diaphragmatic disruption. Following tearing of the diaphragm, the height and persistence of the pleuroperitoneal pressure gradient will determine speed and timing of transdiaphragmatic migration and herniation of abdominal viscera, including the possible enlargement of the diaphragmatic defect. Thus any untreated form of intra-abdominal hypertension will likely propagate and facilitate the development of complications of unrecognized diaphragmatic injuries.

Transdiaphragmatic migration of herniating abdominal viscera can restrict ventricular filling secondary to kinking of mediastinal venous structures. Diminished end-diastolic volumes secondary to impaired ventricular filling lead to decreased stroke volumes; diminished cardiac outputs; and, without intervention, cardiogenic shock. Displaced abdominal viscera may also compromise ventilation, initially of the ipsilateral and in its late stage on the contralateral lung. Analogous to the pathophysiology of tension pneumothorax, herniation of abdominal organs into the thorax leads to cardiorespiratory distress. Studies in animal models have confirmed that an increased pleuroperitoneal pressure gradient secondary to abdominal hypertension has a detrimental influence

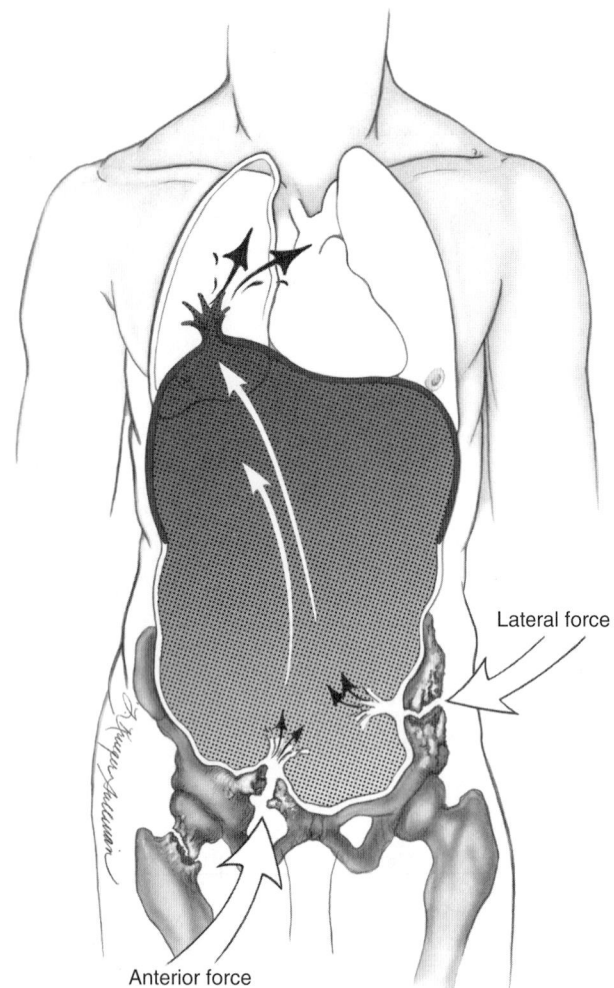

Figure 1 Diaphragmatic injuries secondary to blunt trauma are usually caused by a sudden rise in the transdiaphragmatic pleuroperitoneal pressure gradient. The high-energy transfer from the initial impact explains the common association with other abdominal and thoracic injuries and pelvic fractures.

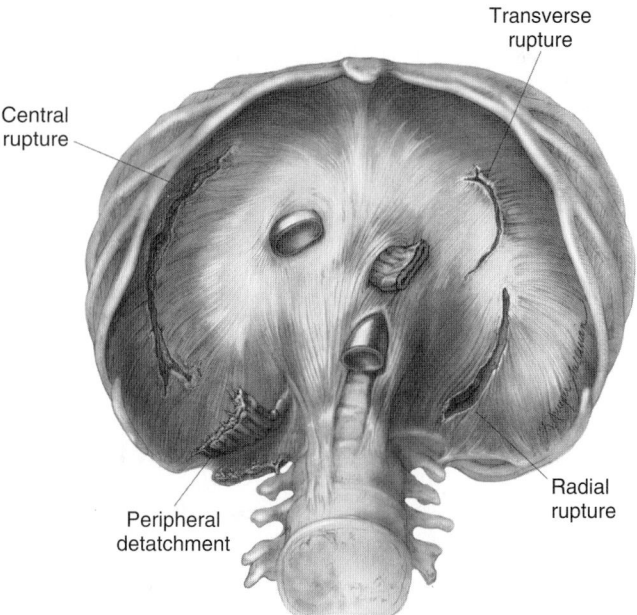

Figure 2 Anatomic location of diaphragmatic injuries. **(A)** Ruptures following a radial course occur most commonly. **(B)** Transverse rupture. **(C)** Central injury. **(D)** Peripheral detachments are least frequent.

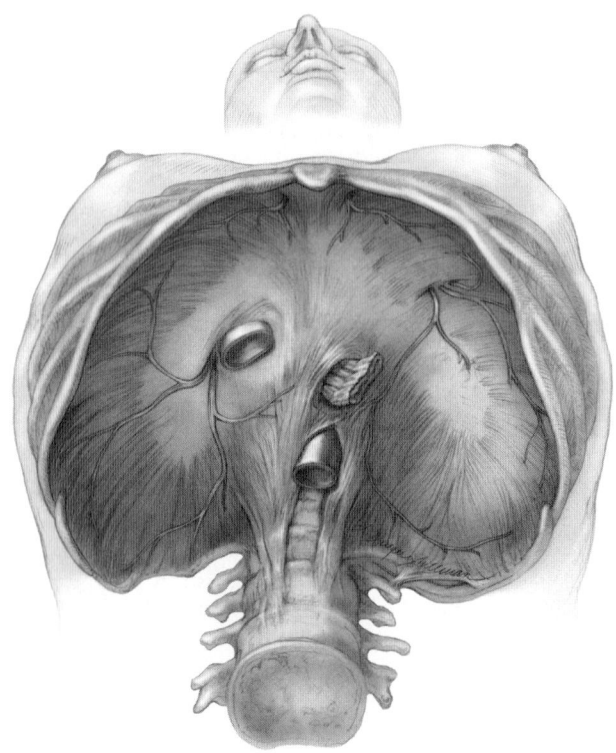

Figure 3 The course of phrenic nerve divisions on the diaphragm follows a "double-handcuff" pattern.

on cardiopulmonary function in the presence of diaphragmatic injuries. Keeping the intra-abdominal pressure at a minimum before operative reduction and repair is essential in patients with suspected or proven diaphragmatic injuries.

Anatomic Location of Injuries

Most ruptures are longer than 5 cm and occur at the posterolateral aspect of the diaphragm between the lumbar and intercostal attachments and spread centrally in a radial direction (Fig. 2). In decreasing frequency, ruptures following a transverse and central course occur; least frequently noted are peripheral detachments.

Knowledge of the relation of these injuries to the natural course of the phrenic nerve and its branches is essential for repair. The phrenic nerve, running along the posterolateral mediastinum, divides into four branches either at the level of the diaphragm or 1 to 2 cm above it. It gives off an anterior branch toward the sternum, a posterior (crural) branch, and two lateral divisions (anterior and posterolateral) (Fig. 3). These branches are the main components of the nerve and result in a pattern that is best described as a "double handcuff." The radial course of most of the phrenic nerve divisions might increase the risk of inadvertent

injuries to the nerve supply of the diaphragm when radial ruptures are being repaired.

In blunt abdominal trauma, injuries to the left hemidiaphragm occur three times more frequently than injuries to the right side, likely because of a buffering effect of the liver on the right hemidiaphragm. Given the assumption that any kinetic energy from severe blunt abdominal trauma is distributed equally throughout the peritoneal cavity, a decreased incidence of right hemidiaphragmatic disruption seems plausible when taking the superior energy-absorbing capacity of the liver compared with the less bulky stomach and spleen into account. Postmortem investigations compared the tensile strength of both hemidiaphragms and found increased resistance of the right hemidiaphragm against axial tension. Whether this finding plays a significant role in keeping the right hemidiaphragm intact is, at present, conjectural at best.

Penetrating injuries such as gunshot wounds or stab wounds are more randomly distributed and produce smaller diaphragmatic defects that are often overlooked. A recent analysis of penetrating injuries to the left lower chest found the incidence of diaphragmatic injuries to be similar for anterior, lateral, and posterior injuries. When gunshot injuries are present, the extent of tissue necrosis can initially be difficult to ascertain. Inadequate debridement plays a significant role in the breakdown of diaphragmatic repair. Penetrating injuries involving the diaphragm had a slightly greater incidence of concomitant hemothorax and pneumothorax compared with those without diaphragmatic injuries.

The natural course of diaphragmatic injuries caused by penetrating trauma is poorly defined. Retrospective case series indicate that diaphragmatic injuries are diagnosed in approximately 18% of blunt and 32% of penetrating trauma cases in a delayed fashion representing occult or missed injuries. Although these findings suggest a significant proportion of patients who either never develop symptoms or heal without intervention, the validity of data on the natural course of diaphragmatic ruptures is hampered by the retrospective nature and high dropout rates of these studies. The majority of symptoms in these patients developed more than 3 years after the initial trauma, and the period of time between the initial injury and presentation for repair has been reported to be as long as 41 years. These observations are contrary to findings in animal models. Experimentally, spontaneous healing of the vast majority of stab wounds to either the muscular or tendinous portion of the diaphragm has been described. Extrapolation of this observation to human diaphragmatic injuries, however, may not be valid.

Associated Injuries

The anatomic location, its close proximity to adjacent intrathoracic and intra-abdominal organs, and the severity of the traumatic impact necessary to cause disruption of the integrity of the diaphragm account for the frequency of associated injuries in 52% to 100% of patients with diaphragmatic tears. Ruptures of the right hemidiaphragm are more commonly associated with blunt abdominal trauma than disruption of the left hemidiaphragm. Studies of blunt abdominal trauma and diaphragmatic injuries describe a 100% rate of other visceral organ injuries in cases of right hemidiaphragmatic disruption, compared with a 77% incidence of associated intra-abdominal injuries on the left side. This observation

adds further evidence to the protective effect of the liver on the right hemidiaphragm. For rupture of the right diaphragm to occur, an enormous amount of kinetic energy must be transferred. As a result there is an increased likelihood of associated visceral injuries when compared with injuries of the left side. The overall median Injury Severity Score (ISS) of right diaphragmatic injuries was 21 (range, 9–50). The median time (range) spent in the intensive care unit was 2 days. The trauma surgeon should be alert to the possibility of encountering multivisceral organ involvement in cases of right hemidiaphragmatic disruptions. Because injuries to the diaphragm are seldom isolated injuries, and in view of the frequent association with severe intracavitary injuries often involving multiple organs, diaphragmatic injuries should also be considered as an occult marker of serious associated injuries. The presence of diaphragmatic rupture therefore demands an aggressive search for concomitant injuries.

Table 1 gives an overview of the incidence of associated injuries with blunt diaphragmatic rupture. Despite demonstrating a relationship between the presence of these associated injuries and diaphragmatic rupture, individually none of them proved to be more than a moderately sensitive measure for identifying a diaphragmatic rupture. Some of these associated injuries did, however, provide exceptional specificity, most notably thoracic aortic injury (96.6%), spleen and liver injury (88.0%), and pelvic fractures (86.4%). Of note is the triad of severe pelvic fractures, thoracic aortic rupture, and diaphragmatic injury. This injury pattern reflects the massive thoracoabdominal force required to simultaneously disrupt the pelvic ring and cause a massive increase in the intra-abdominal pressure, leading to disruption of the diaphragm and blunt injury of the aortic wall. Overall, the frequency of associated injury patterns requiring transmission of significant amounts of kinetic energy, as well as the frequent occurrence of diaphragmatic disruption in polytraumatized patients, underscores the severity of the initial impact to cause disruption of the diaphragm.

The occurrence of associated injuries in patients with diaphragmatic injuries secondary to penetrating trauma is more variable and dependent on the nature, velocity, and pattern of the weapon or projectile. Table 2 gives on overview of associated thoracic and abdominal injuries in patients with diaphragmatic rupture secondary to penetrating wounds.

Course of Injury

Diaphragmatic injuries follow a course divided into three phases: (1) acute, (2) latent, and (3) obstructive. The acute phase starts at the time of injury and ends with control of bleeding and gastrointestinal spillage, as well as stabilization of the patient. All diaphragmatic injuries identified during initial operative exploration should be classified according to the American Association for the Surgery of Trauma Organ Injury Scale (AAST-OIS) for diaphragmatic injuries (Table 3) and repaired. In cases in which a nonoperative approach for other injuries is initially pursued, detection rates of diaphragmatic injuries during the initial phase might be as low as 25%.

Table 1: Associations between Diaphragmatic Injury and Specific Associated Organ Injuries in Blunt Thoracoabdominal Trauma

Injury	Diaphragm Rupture (%)	No Diaphragm Rupture (%)	OR (95% CI)	Sensitivity	Specificity
Pulmonary contusion	3,7770 (44.9)	87,183 (22.4)	2.8 (1.9–4.2)	44.9	77.6
Rib fracture	5,368 (63.9)	209,940 (54.0)	1.5 (0.9–2.5)	63.9	46.0
Thoratic aorta	1,294 (15.4)	13,083 (3.4)	5.2 (2.2–12.5)	15.4	96.6
Spleen	4,483 (53.4)	46,844 (12.1)	8.4 (3.9–17.8)	53.4	88.0
Liver	3,048 (36.3	46,740 (12.0)	4.2 (1.7–10.6)	36.3	88.0
Pelvic fracture	3,565 (42.5)	52,960 (13.6)	4.7 (2.7–8.0)	42.5	86.4

From Reiff DA, McGwin G Jr, Metzger J, and others: J Trauma 53:1139, 2002.

Table 2: Associated Injuries of Diaphragmatic Rupture in Penetrating Abdominal Trauma

Organ	Gunshot Wound	Stab	Blunt	Total
Liver	57	21	7	85
Stomach	18	22	5	45
Spleen	18	6	5	29
Lung	19	9	1	29
Colon	19	5	4	28
Kidney	12	6	2	20
Small bowel	10	4	2	16
Heart	2	6	3	11
Other	103	38	6	147
Total	258.0	117.0	35.0	410.0
Average	2.9	1.8	3.2	2.5

From Wiencek RG, Wilson RF, Steiger Z: J Thorac Cardiovasc Surg 92:989, 1986.

Table 3: American Association for the Surgery of Trauma Organ Injury Scale for Diaphragmatic Injuries

Grade	Description
I	Contusion
II	Laceration $\leq$ 2 cm
III	Laceration 2–10 cm
IV	Laceration > 10 cm with tissue loss 25 cm^2
V	Laceration with tissue loss >25 cm^2

Unrecognized or untreated diaphragmatic ruptures at the initial exploration enter the latent phase of diaphragmatic injuries. The injured diaphragm, as a muscle, starts to retract and begins to atrophy rapidly, setting the stage for herniation. The latent phase is variable, with the majority of complications developing more than 3 years after the initial trauma. Vague, intermittent abdominal pain and upper gastrointestinal distress are the predominant symptoms. Intermittent incarceration of herniated abdominal viscera through the enlarging diaphragmatic defect may cause strangulation of abdominal organs, partial small bowel obstruction, and formation of chronic adhesions. The development of symptoms caused by chronic incarceration marks the transition from the latent phase to the obstructive phase. The obstructive phase, or phase 3, is caused by vascular compromise of the incarcerated and strangulated abdominal organs or by intestinal obstruction of herniated gut. Symptoms may be vague and range from nonspecific pleuritis and chest pain to frank sepsis resulting from free intestinal perforation into the abdominal or thoracic cavity. On the left side, the colon, small bowel, stomach, and spleen are the predominant organs prone to herniation. Spillage of intestinal contents into the peritoneal cavity will result in peritonitis, and empyema, respiratory compromise, sepsis, and death may follow contamination of the pleural cavity.

DIAGNOSIS

Clinical Features

The diagnosis of diaphragmatic rupture is challenging. The difficulty in confirming or refuting the possibility of diaphragmatic disruption preoperatively is largely due to the lack of a sensitive and specific imaging test. Therefore the trauma surgeon often has to judge the likelihood of diaphragmatic injuries from the mechanism of injury, clinical presentation, and radiographic imaging.

In cases of blunt abdominal trauma secondary to motor vehicle accidents, a retrospective review of the National Automotive Sampling System has identified independent factors in the history predictive of diaphragmatic injury. Findings of vehicular intrusion or significant deceleration (measured as change in velocity, ΔV)—or both—in the history of the accident in combination with specific injuries identified during primary and secondary surveys can be highly suggestive of diaphragmatic rupture. For example, the combination of vehicular intrusion greater than 30 cm or ΔV greater than 40 kph with the presence of a splenic injury or pelvic fracture (or both) had sensitivity greater than 85% to detect diaphragmatic rupture (Table 4). Knowledge of collision characteristics, such as velocity at impact and vehicular intrusion, combined with the finding of visceral or orthopedic injuries (or both), should raise the suspicion of an occult diaphragmatic injury.

Further pertinent information suggesting the possibility of diaphragmatic injury includes any history of crush injury, direct impacts on the thoracoabdominal area, or falls from great heights. The presence of accompanying severe intestinal, orthopedic, or neurologic injuries should alert the trauma surgeon of a significant transfer of energy and should, even in the absence of external signs, mandate an aggressive search for diaphragmatic disruption.

In the case of diaphragmatic injuries secondary to penetrating trauma, injury to the diaphragm should be readily suspected in any injury to the lower chest, upper abdomen, or any midtorso- traversing injury. Significant tissue destruction might be encountered in close-range shotgun injuries. These injuries might be associated with

Table 4: Associations between Diaphragmatic Injury and Collision Characteristics Combined with Splenic Injury and/or Pelvic Fracture*

Combined Characteristics	Diaphragm Rupture (%)	No Diaphragm Rupture (%)	OR (95% CI)	Sensitivity	Specificity
Intrusion $\geq$ 30 cm or $\Delta V \geq$ 40 kph	6,980 (83.1)	163,316 (42.0)	6.8 (4.3–10.7)	83.1	58.0
Spleen injury or pelvic fracture or intrusion $\geq$ 30 cm	7,148 (85.1)	138.168 (35.5)	10.4 (7.1–15.2)	85.4	64.5
Spleen injury or pelvic fracture or $\Delta V \geq$ 40 kph	7,395 (88.1)	160,717 (41.3)	10.5 (5.3–20.6)	88.1	58.7
Spleen injury or pelvic fracture or intrusion $\geq$ 30 cm or $\Delta V \geq$ 40 kph	7,653 (91.1)	200,051 (51.5)	9.7 (4.0–23.5)	91.1	48.5

*Data from the National Automotive Sampling System.
From Reiff DA, McGwin G Jr, Metzger J, and others: J Trauma 53:1139, 2002.

large diaphragmatic or chest wall defects and may present with organ herniation, tension viscerothorax, or respiratory or cardiovascular failure.

Physical examination of trauma victims harboring diaphragmatic injuries can be completely unrevealing. Overall, the diagnostic accuracy of physical findings in detecting diaphragmatic injuries is disappointing. Often diaphragmatic injuries produce no abnormal physical signs, and large series reported normal physical findings in 53% of diaphragmatic ruptures caused by blunt injuries and 44% caused by penetrating injuries. In patients with significant diaphragmatic injuries following penetrating trauma, 30% of patients who sustained stab wounds and 20% of patients with gunshot wounds had no abnormal physical findings at presentation. In patients with abnormal findings, clinical signs of diaphragmatic injury can be divided into thoracic and abdominal symptoms. Common symptoms include decreased breath sounds, associated rib fractures, and hemopneumothoraces but can range to overt chest wall disruptions in the form of central or peripheral flail chests. Visceral herniation might be occasionally detected by the presence of bowel sounds on auscultation or, on occasion, by tympany on percussion. Abdominal symptoms usually reflect associated visceral injuries and can range from overt peritonitis secondary to hollow viscus perforation to progressive distention in the case of massive hemoperitoneum. Overall, the presence of clinical symptoms is generally closely linked to an increased ISS and the presence of associated injuries.

Imaging

Table 5 lists noninvasive and invasive imaging modalities employed in patients suspected to have traumatic diaphragmatic injuries.

Chest Radiographs

Despite the technical limitations of chest x-rays, such as supine positioning and limited patient cooperation, plain chest films remain essential in the acute phase for the detection of diaphragmatic injuries and are the most commonly performed radiologic study for such injuries.

Specific diagnostic findings of diaphragmatic tears on chest radiographs include: (1) intrathoracic herniation of a hollow viscus (stomach, colon, small bowel), with or without focal constriction of the viscus at the site of the tear (collar sign); or (2) visualization of a nasogastric tube above the hemidiaphragm on the left side. Chest radiographic findings depicting elevation of the hemidiaphragm, distortion or obliteration of its outline, and contralateral shifting of the mediastinum are the most commonly observed findings of diaphragmatic disruptions but are not specific for diaphragmatic tears. Many other conditions can display similar findings, and the aforementioned observations on chest radiographs as such cannot be relied on as being specific to diaphragmatic injuries. Differentials related to trauma include hemopneumothorax, with or without

Table 5: Current Imaging Modalities to Diagnose Diaphragmatic Injuries

Noninvasive	Invasive
Chest roentgenography	Diagnostic peritoneal lavage
Contrast studies	Laparoscopy
Upper gastrointestinal series	Thoracoscopy
Barium enema	
Computed tomography	
Magnetic resonance imaging	

traumatic pleural effusion; pulmonary contusion or laceration; atelectasis; or phrenic nerve palsy. Nontrauma-related pulmonary abnormalities might be due to nontraumatic pleural effusion, disease process of the lung parenchyma, or congenital eventration of the diaphragm. Overall, initial radiographs allow the diagnosis of diaphragmatic rupture in 27% to 60% of left-sided injuries and in 17% of right-sided injuries. Between 40% and 50% of initial chest radiographs obtained in patients with confirmed diaphragmatic rupture are reported as normal, and the majority of positive abnormal radiographic findings consist of nonspecific, minor findings, such as fractured ribs, small pneumohemothoraces, or elevation of the hemidiaphragm. The overall diagnostic accuracy of chest x-rays for diaphragmatic injuries ranges from 13% to 93%, and the rate of missed diaphragmatic injuries has been reported as high as 66%. The diagnostic accuracy of chest radiographs for traumatic diaphragmatic injuries is further diminished in patients on positive pressure ventilation. A recent report confirms that diaphragmatic injuries cannot be confidently excluded if the patient is ventilated with positive end-expiratory pressure. Late diagnosis can be facilitated if chest radiographs are reviewed in sequence as ventilator support is decreased. The diagnostic value of chest x-rays for traumatic diaphragmatic rupture is also diminished in elderly patients. Compared with younger patients, elderly trauma victims with blunt diaphragmatic injuries had significantly higher rates of initial normal chest radiographic findings. This higher rate of missed diaphragmatic injuries in elderly trauma patients has been attributed to earlier intubation and ventilation of elderly trauma victims, which makes detection of occult diaphragmatic tears more difficult and also is associated with higher rates of delays before surgical intervention.

Contrast Studies

Contrast studies are rarely obtained in the acute phase of diaphragmatic injuries because they require cooperative and hemodynamically stable patients. Upper gastrointestinal (GI) series and barium enema have good sensitivities to detect herniated stomach or colon in the thoracic cavity. Their role is more focused to investigate, in the latent phase, stable patients suspected of harboring an occult and missed diaphragmatic tear. Because contrast studies have high sensitivity, some surgeons suggest performing them routinely in all patients with serious body injuries and suspected diaphragmatic involvement before hospital discharge.

Ultrasonography

Despite occasional, favorable, single-institutional reports, sonography has failed to play a significant role in the detection of diaphragmatic injuries. And, despite the increase in frequency and familiarity with the FAST (Focused Assessment for the Sonographic Evaluation of the Trauma Patient), no large series to date has substantiated its usefulness in the diagnosis of diaphragmatic rupture.

Computed Tomography

Initial reports of the ability of CT to accurately and consistently demonstrate diaphragmatic injuries were disappointing. Sensitivity of conventional CT has been reported to vary between 14% and 61% and specificity between 76% and 99% for the diagnosis of diaphragmatic rupture. The introduction of helical CT, new array detector technology, and three-dimensional reconstruction in the late 1990s has improved the diagnostic accuracy of diaphragmatic tears substantially.

CT findings suggestive of hemidiaphragmatic tears include the following:

1. Direct discontinuity of the hemidiaphragm. Although an apparent diaphragmatic defect appears to be the most sensitive sign,

the diagnosis of diaphragmatic rupture should not be made on the basis of this CT finding alone.

2. Intrathoracic herniation of abdominal contents has a sensitivity of 100%. The stomach and the colon are the most frequently detected viscera to herniate on the left side, and the liver the most common viscus on the right side.

3. The collar sign is a constriction of the herniating organ at the entrance through the diaphragmatic tear. It can appear at the right side as subtle as a small, focal indentation of the liver (Fig. 4, *A*) and is best appreciated after analysis of axial cuts and sagittal or coronal multiplanar reformatted images (Figs. 4, *B-D*).

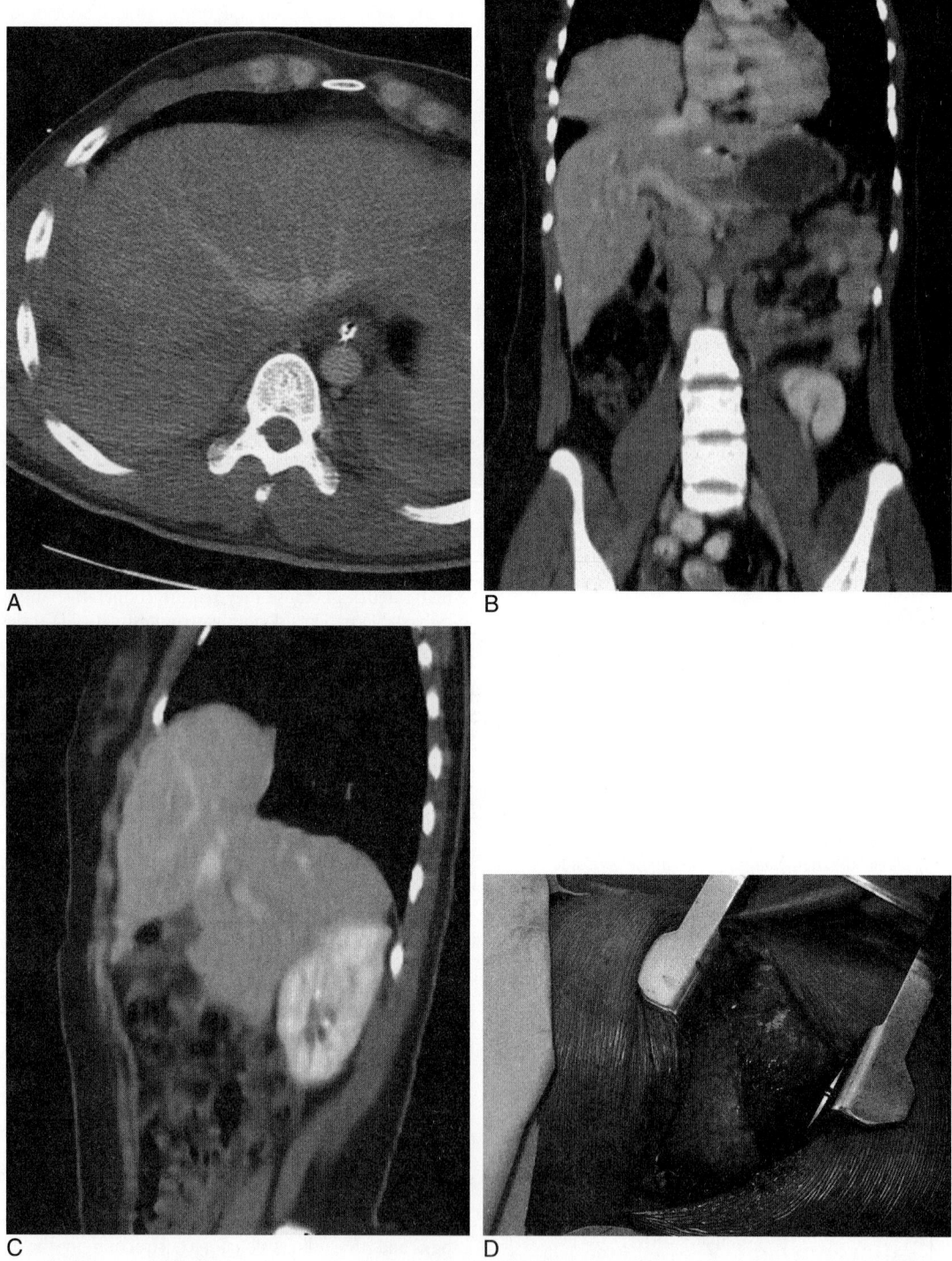

Figure 4   Computed tomography (CT) appearance of right diaphragmatic disruption in a 46-year-old man after motor vehicle accident. **(A)** Helical CT scan (direct axial section) shows a focal indentation at the lateral aspect of the liver (*arrow*) with a contusion, a subtle finding suggestive of a right diaphragmatic tear. **(B)** Coronal reformatted images show intrathoracic herniation with a waistlike constriction of the liver (collar sign). **(C)** Sagittal reformatted images confirm anterolateral herniation of the liver. **(D)** Image from right anterolateral thoracotomy shows the intrathoracic herniation of the liver and the diaphragmatic tear.   *Courtesy Dr. M. Marcari, Department of Radiology, New York University Medical Center.*

4. The dependent viscera sign is present when the herniated viscera are no longer supported posteriorly by the injured diaphragm and fall into a dependent position against the posterior ribs or retroperitoneum. This obliteration of a normally unoccupied space is best seen in reformatted axial images that show abutment of the posterior ribs by stomach, bowel, or spleen on the left side and by the liver on the right side. The dependent viscera sign has been said to be an early indicator of a diaphragmatic tear or injury.

Despite these recent advances and improvements in CT imaging technology, the detection of diaphragmatic injuries on the basis of this imaging modality alone is associated with pitfalls. False-positive findings of diaphragmatic defects not related to traumatic diaphragmatic ruptures are seen in 6% of asymptomatic adults. These defects represent congenital, asymptomatic hernias and do not require further interventions. In addition, congenital eventration can mimic diaphragmatic rupture, as can motion artifacts secondary to respiration. Small tears, on the other hand, can be missed in the absence of herniation of intra-abdominal organs in the setting of thoracic trauma because pleural effusions may prevent exact delineation of the diaphragmatic contours.

Magnetic Resonance Imaging

The use of MRI shows promise in the evaluation of diaphragmatic injuries but in practice is applicable only to hemodynamically stable trauma patients. New gradient-echo sequences and faster imaging sequences reduce study time but maintain the superior soft-tissue resolution of MRI compared with CT. Because of its muscular and fibrous nature, the normal diaphragm appears as a hypotense band on both T1- and T2-weighted sequences. MRI signs of diaphragmatic tears include herniation of abdominal fat or viscera and disruption of its dome-shaped contour (Fig. 5). Currently, MRI is underused

in the acute trauma setting and reserved for patients with an uncertain CT diagnosis or delayed signs of diaphragmatic rupture.

Diagnostic Peritoneal Lavage

The use of diagnostic peritoneal lavage (DPL) as the initial invasive technique directed at detecting a suspected diaphragmatic rupture is mainly of historical interest. DPL is notoriously inaccurate in detecting isolated diaphragmatic tears. Although DPL may still play a role in the treatment of a patient with multiple injuries, its use to detect diaphragmatic injuries should be discouraged.

Videolaparoscopy and Video-Assisted Thoracoscopic Surgery

Videolaparoscopy and video-assisted thoracoscopic surgery (VATS) are the most recent imaging modalities used in the evaluation and treatment of abdominal trauma and lower thoracic trauma. During the past decade, both laparoscopy and VATS have been recognized as critical tools in the evaluation of patients with suspected diaphragmatic injuries. The role of these two modalities is likely to expand with continuous refinement in technology. Several studies endorse laparoscopy and thoracoscopy as optimal methods in resolving the diagnostic dilemma of diaphragmatic injuries in patients who are hemodynamically stable and who have no immediate need or indication to undergo laparotomy or thoracotomy. It is predominantly among this group of patients that the diagnosis of traumatic diaphragmatic hernia remains a challenge because of the lack of sufficiently sensitive and accurate diagnostic tools. Occult injuries missed by conventional workup and chest radiograph may occur in as many as 30% of patients who sustain stab wounds to the left lower chest. This delay in diagnosis and treatment contributes to

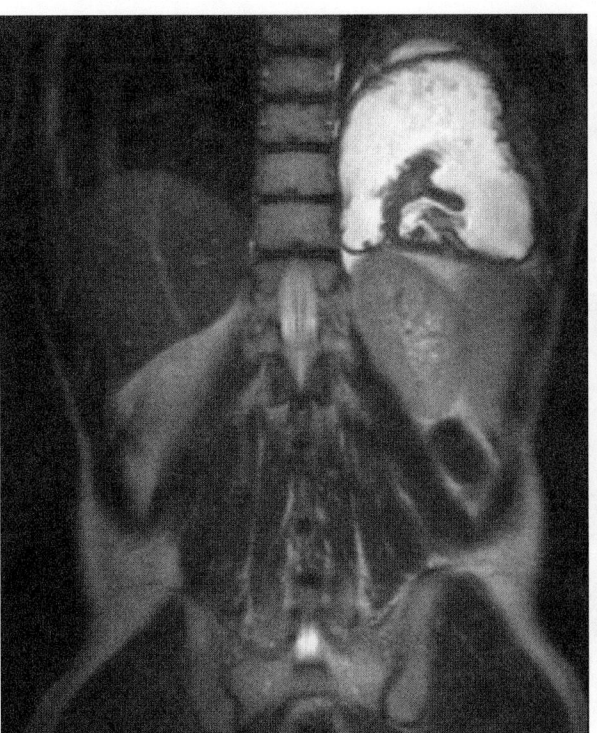
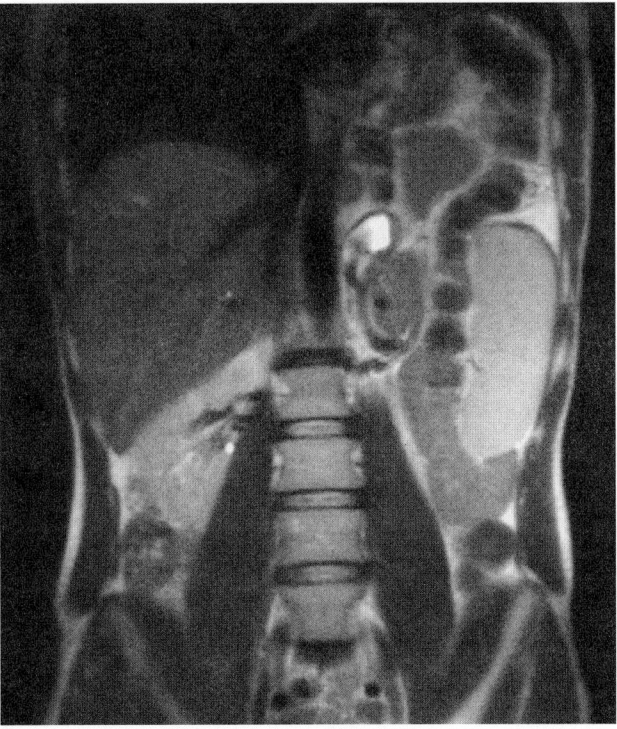

A   B

Figure 5 Magnetic resonance image (MRI) of a left diaphragmatic tear in a 65-year-old patient after blunt trauma. Coronal T2-weighted, fast-gradient MRI shows intrathoracic herniation of stomach and colon. *Courtesy Dr. M. Marcari, Department of Radiology, New York University Medical Center.*

significant late morbidity and mortality. Because of the unreliability of noninvasive diagnostic studies, an aggressive approach for early identification of these injuries has been advocated.

Laparoscopy has been evaluated in the detection of diaphragmatic rupture resulting from both blunt and penetrating injuries. In a landmark study on 119 consecutive patients with left-sided thoracoabdominal trauma, the overall incidence of diaphragmatic injuries was 42%. Compared with conventional studies, laparoscopy detected an additional 26% of occult diaphragmatic injuries later confirmed at laparotomy. This study's findings show the value of laparoscopy because 31% of patients with diaphragmatic injuries had no abdominal symptoms, 40% had a normal chest x-ray, and only 49% had associated hemopneumothorax. This pivotal role in the detection of occult diaphragmatic injuries in patients who otherwise have no indication for undergoing laparotomy has been reproduced in other study populations who had stab or gunshot wounds to the left lower chest. Adequate visualization of the entire diaphragm requires a 35- or 45-degree laparoscope, visceral mobilization, retraction, and patient positioning in steep Trendelenburg. As tension pneumothorax may occur, a CO_2 insufflation pressures should not exceed 12 mm Hg during laparoscopy in the presence of diaphragmatic injury. The surgeon must be prepared to immediately decompress the left pleural space, initially by needle decompression of the second intercostal space followed by insertion of a chest tube in the already prepared lower chest.

VATS has been shown to be an accurate method for identifying diaphragmatic injuries. Indications for VATS in hemodynamically stable patients include those patients in whom (1) the mechanism of injury suggests predominant involvement of the thoracic cavity, (2) abdominal injuries have been ruled out, and (3) laparoscopy cannot be safely performed because a hostile abdomen is present. VATS has recently been shown to significantly improve the sensitivity, specificity, and accuracy of identifying diaphragmatic injuries after penetrating chest trauma. Five independent risk factors for finding diaphragmatic injuries in penetrating chest trauma have been identified: (1) abnormal chest x-ray, (2) entrance wound inferior to the nipple or scapula, (3) associated intra-abdominal injuries, (4) high-velocity mechanism of injury, and (5) right-sided entrance wound (Table 6). A diagnostic algorithm for stable patients following penetrating chest trauma was recently established. Patients whose physical examination reveals two or more predictors of diaphragmatic injuries should undergo VATS to exclude occult diaphragmatic tears (Fig. 6). Patients with fewer than two independent

Table 6: Independent Predictors of Diaphragmatic Injury after Penetrating Chest Trauma

Variable	Odds Ratio	95% Confidence Interval	p Value
Abnormal chest radiograph	21.3	5–91	< 0.01
Entrance wound inferior to nipple line	7.0	2–24	< 0.01
Intra-abdominal injuries	6.1	3–13	< 0.01
High-velocity mechanism	2.9	2–6	< 0.01
Right-side entrance wound	2.5	1–5	< 0.01

From Freeman RK, Al-Dossari G, Hutcheson KA, and others: Ann Thorac Surg *72:342, 2001.*

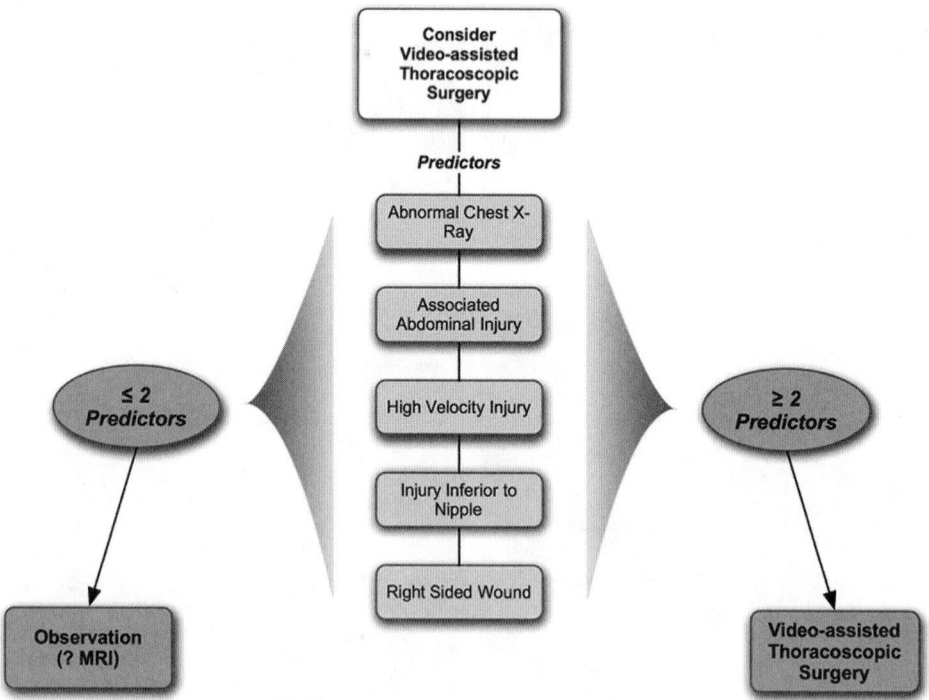

Figure 6 Diagnostic algorithm for diaphragmatic injuries following penetrating chest trauma. Patients whose history and physical examinations reveal two or more predictors of diaphragmatic injury should undergo VATS to exclude an occult diaphragmatic injury. *From Freeman RK, Al-Dossari G, Hutcheson KA, and others:* Ann Thorac Surg *72:342–347, 2001. **Abd,** Abdomen; **CXR,** chest x-ray; **MRI,** magnetic resonance imaging; **VATS,** video-assisted thoracoscopic surgery.

predictors have a risk too low to justify the routine use of VATS. Because the finding of diaphragmatic laceration on thoracoscopy or thoracotomy usually necessitates abdominal exploration to rule out intestinal injury, laparoscopy remains the minimally invasive procedure of choice to diagnose occult diaphragmatic injuries.

TREATMENT OF DIAPHRAGMATIC INJURIES

Principles of the Abdominal Approach

Patients with suspected diaphragmatic injuries should undergo primary and secondary surveys as outlined in the Advanced Trauma and Life Support (ATLS) manual of the American College of Surgeons. Principles of injury prioritization are followed, and patients with life-threatening thoracic or abdominal injuries are expeditiously explored via thoracotomy, laparotomy, or both.

As part of the initial assessment, a nasogastric tube is inserted. Resistance may be encountered in cases of distortion of the esophagogastric junction caused by gastric herniation. The tube should not be forced because there is a risk of iatrogenic perforation. The tube should be left in the distal esophagus and suction applied because the esophagus may evacuate swallowed air. If there has been visceral herniation with resultant respiratory compromise, it might be necessary to intubate the patient. If there is an associated pneumothorax, digital exploration of the pleural cavity should be performed before chest tube placement to avoid iatrogenic injury to the herniated abdominal viscera.

Acute injuries are best approached through an abdominal incision. This approach affords the surgeon the advantage of being able to assess and treat any associated abdominal injuries. Because chest injuries, which occur more frequently in blunt thoracoabdominal trauma than abdominal injuries, can often be managed nonoperatively, the need for thoracotomy and a second operation is frequently avoided.

The abdomen is entered through an upper midline incision from the xiphoid process to the umbilicus following a wide prep from the proximal thighs to the neck. Intraperitoneal blood and clots are rapidly evacuated, and the abdominal cavity is packed to control ongoing hemorrhage. Thorough exploration of the peritoneal cavity and retroperitoneum will prevent missed injuries. Blood loss is controlled, and gross spillage is limited by closing any hollow viscus perforation. The diaphragm is then evaluated by visual inspection and palpation.

Herniated viscera are reduced from the thoracic cavity by gentle traction. Releasing negative intrapleural pressure via a nasogastric tube passed alongside the herniated organs might facilitate reduction by releasing a vacuum (Fig. 7). Another maneuver to reduce herniated viscera is to carefully guide a nasogastric tube with digital manipulation through the diaphragmatic constriction of the stomach, decompressing the upper intestines. The decompressed stomach can then be reduced with the nasogastric tube acting as a stent. Ultimately, the surgeon might need to extend the diaphragmatic defect to allow reduction. To avoid postoperative diaphragmatic dysfunction, knowledge of the natural course of the phrenic nerve and its branches is essential. In general, lateral extensions in a radial fashion are safe for central ruptures, whereas medial and parahiatal defects are best extended anteriorly to avoid phrenic nerve injuries (see Figs. 2 and 3).

The rate of missed diaphragmatic injuries, even after explorative laparotomy, has been reported as high as 11%. This high rate has been attributed to inadequate exposure of both hemidiaphragms during initial exploration. Exposure of the right diaphragm should start with transaction of the falciform ligament followed by division of the anterior coronary and left triangular ligaments (Fig. 8, A). After division of the right triangular ligament and the posterior hepatic attachments, the liver is gently pulled downward and rotated medially. This exposes the entire right hemidiaphragm, suprahepatic IVC, right adrenal gland, and anterior surface of the right kidney (Fig. 8, B).

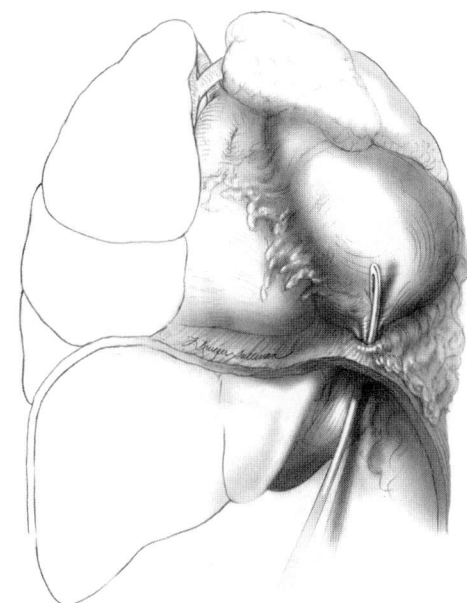

Figure 7 Reduction of transdiaphragmatic herniated viscera can be facilitated by releasing negative intrapleural pressure via transdiaphragmatic passage of a nasogastric tube.

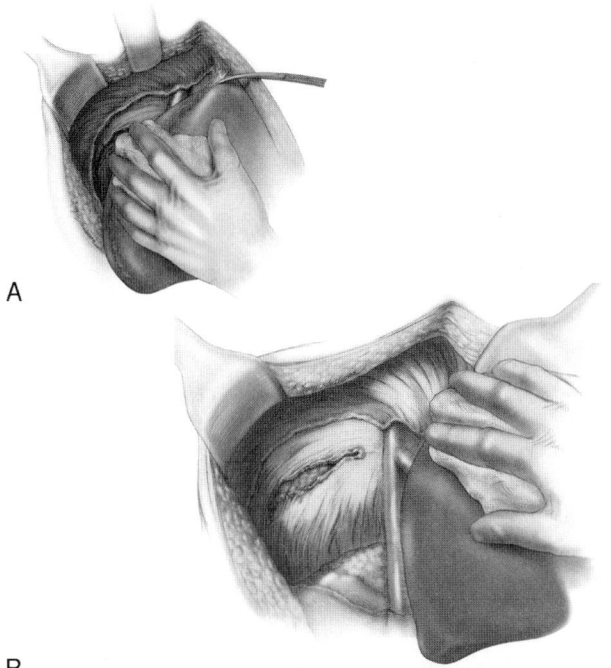

Figure 8 Exploration of the right hemidiaphragm. **(A)** Division of the triangular and coronary ligaments. **(B)** Medial rotation of the liver exposes the right hemidiaphragm.

On the left side, exploration of the left hemidiaphragm begins by dividing the lienophrenic ligament and mobilization of splenic flexure interiorly. Occasionally, small feeding arteries run in these splenic attachments, thus adequate hemostasis must be assured. The spleen, splenic flexure of the colon, and body of the stomach are then carefully moved medially. By applying gentle, downward traction on the spleen and the greater curvature of the stomach, the entire left hemidiaphragm can be assessed (Fig. 9).

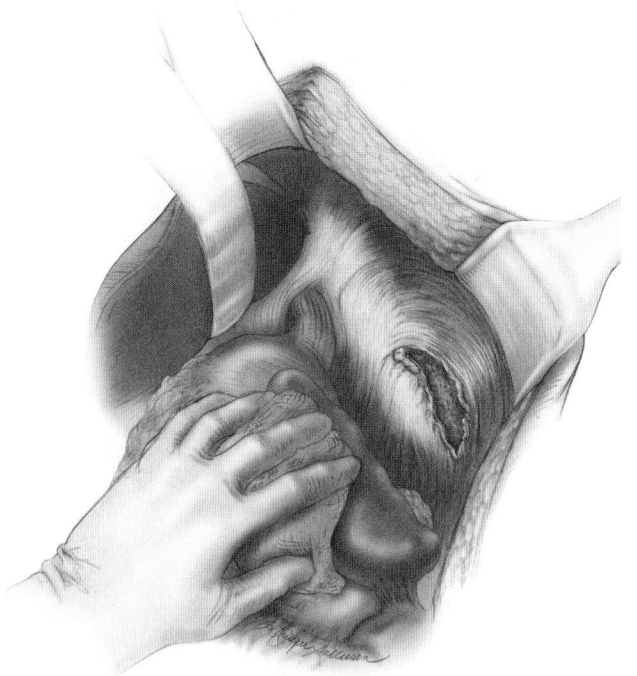

Figure 9 The left hemidiaphragm is exposed by retracting the spleen and body of the stomach medially.

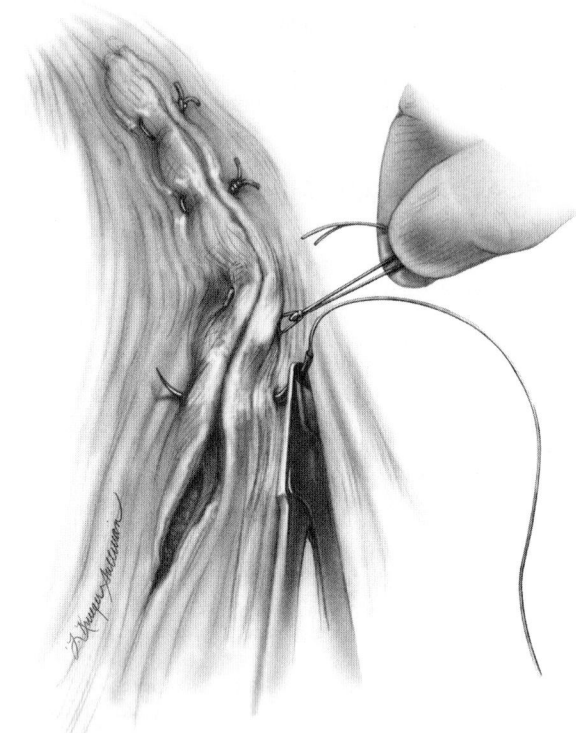

Figure 10 Diaphragmatic single-layer repair using interrupted horizontal mattress sutures. The tail of the previous suture can be used as a handle to facilitate repair of the posterior portion of the defect.

All identified injuries of the diaphragm should be repaired. Repair starts with careful debridement of nonviable tissue. In particular, devitalized edges of lacerations caused by missile injuries should be trimmed into healthy tissue. The laceration is gently spread with the use of Babcock forceps or Allis clamps to inspect the ipsilateral pleural cavity. After evaluating for any ongoing hemorrhage from associated thoracic injuries and cross-contamination between the abdominal and thoracic cavities, the pleural space is thoroughly irrigated with warm saline to remove retained blood and clot. Diaphragmatic closure is accomplished with interrupted figure-of-eight or horizontal mattress sutures of size 0 or 2-0 monofilament sutures. Closure should be performed in an everting fashion. The tail of the previously placed suture is used as a handle to provide exposure, facilitating correct suture placement during repair of the posterior portion of the defect (Fig. 10). For lacerations longer than 5 cm, recommendations are either closure with a running suture or a two-layer repair. With this approach, the inner layer of interlocking horizontal mattress sutures serves to evert the edges of the laceration and is then reinforced with a running 2-0 or 3-0 polypropylene suture. For repairs in which closure appears to be tenuous, Teflon pledgets may be used to buffer the repair.

When tube thoracostomy has not been performed preoperatively and no underlying lung injury is present, residual air and fluid can be aspirated from the pleural space, thereby eliminating the need for postoperative chest tube. A 24F red rubber catheter is placed through the final mattress suture into the chest (Fig. 11). Air and fluid are evacuated with suction from the pleural cavity. With the lungs held in full inspiration, the catheter is removed while the final mattress suture is tied. At the completion of diaphragmatic closure, the repair should be tested with full expansion of the lung using large tidal volumes. The upper quadrant is filled with warm saline and the maneuver is repeated. Emerging bubbles or air from the suture line should trigger reinforcement of the repair. Usually, additional figure-of-eight sutures are sufficient, and it is not necessary to take down the repair.

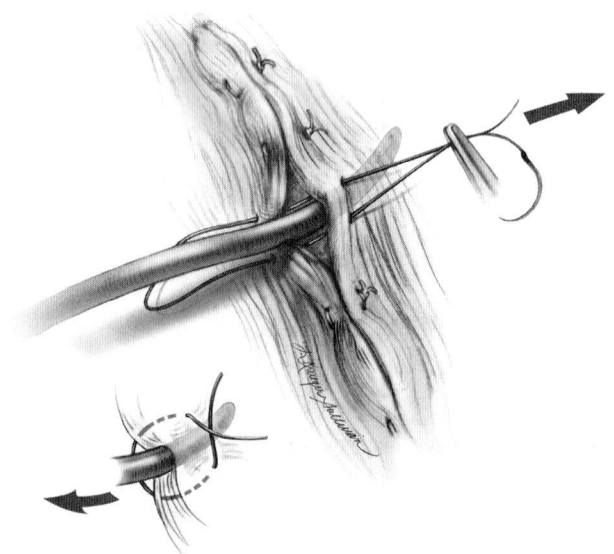

Figure 11 Evacuation of residual pneumothorax with a 24F red rubber catheter. The catheter, which is connected to continuous suction, is removed as the final mattress suture is tied.

Laparoscopic Repair

A more thorough preoperative workup and the shift toward nonoperative management of many injuries in stable trauma patients has led to a significant reduction in the need for immediate operative exploration when diaphragmatic injuries are suspected. This development, together with the firm establishment of laparoscopy as the procedure of choice to diagnose diaphragmatic injuries, has frequently led to the detection of diaphragmatic injuries in stable patients without other injuries necessitating laparotomy. Several studies have now confirmed that acute diaphragmatic injury detected by laparoscopy can safely be repaired in selected patients using intracorporeal suturing and, less often, staples. Laparoscopy has evolved from the diagnostic to the therapeutic arena. In recent years, numerous examples of therapeutic maneuvers in selected patients in the trauma setting have been documented. These include suturing of GI perforations; hemostasis of low-grade splenic and liver lacerations; autotransfusion of collected blood from the hemoperitoneum; and repair of diaphragmatic lacerations with staples, sutures, or the insertion of prosthetic mesh. However, laparoscopy has pitfalls in the management of trauma patients; these became evident with the transition from the diagnostic phase to the therapeutic phase. A small group of patients developed tension pneumothorax because of occult diaphragmatic lacerations. Small bowel injuries were missed on laparoscopic examinations in several series. Cost effectiveness was also a matter of concern. However, despite these pitfalls, the benefits offered by minimally invasive surgery, particularly in terms of avoiding negative or nontherapeutic laparotomies and decreasing hospitalization, are believed to be sufficient enough to accept the aforementioned shortcomings.

Our laparoscopic approach to traumatic diaphragmatic hernias is depicted in Figure 12. The patient is placed in Lloyd-Davis position with reversed Trendelenburg tilt. A 30-degree, 10-mm telescope is used through a port placed between the xiphisternum and the umbilicus slightly to the left of the midline. Diagnostic explorative laparoscopy is performed and includes, depending on the patient's presentation and preoperative findings, running of the entire small intestines, mobilization of the right and left colon, a laparoscopic Kocher maneuver, and exploration of the lesser sac. Exposure of the right diaphragm is obtained with the same ligamentous divisions as described for the open approach. A 5-mm triangular liver retractor is used for medial rotation of the liver. Similarly, exposure of the left hemidiaphragm follows the same divisions as in open surgery. The initial steps are performed in a steep right tilt to facilitate mobilizing the spleen and exposing the lienophrenic attachments. Atraumatic forceps are used to exert gentle, downward traction of the spleen and stomach. The edges of the defect are grasped with endoscopic Allis forceps and debrided as needed. The tear is closed in an everting manner using nonabsorbable, polypropylene sutures, and the knots are tied intracorporeally (Fig. 13). Aspiration of residual pneumothorax can be performed with a smaller, red rubber catheter or a 12F nasogastric tube placed laparoscopically, similar to the open technique. The catheter is withdrawn as the final suture is tied. If the defect is too large for primary closure, a suitably sized polypropylene mesh (margins of the mesh at least 3 to 4 cm beyond the edges of the defect) can be used and fixed with spiral tacks (ProTack; Tyco Healthcare, Princeton, NJ) or nonabsorbable autosutures (Fig. 14).

Massive Cross-Contamination between the Pleural and Peritoneal Cavities

In the past, the routine performance of an anterolateral thoracotomy in cases of massive cross-contamination between the two

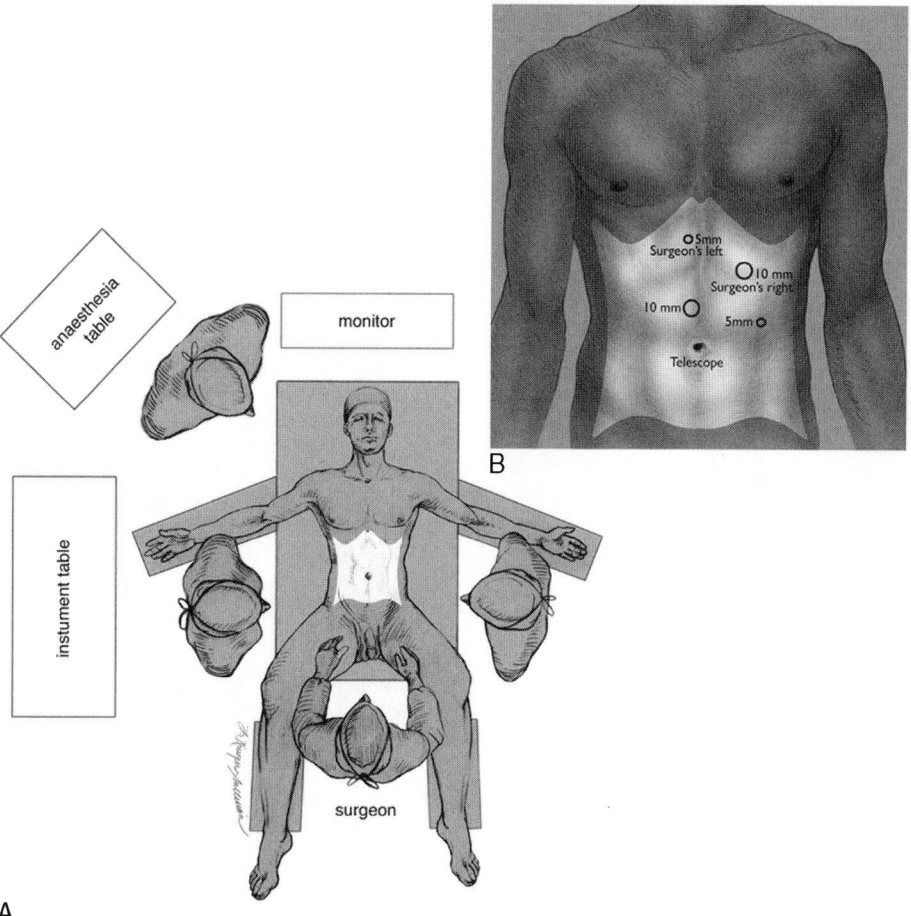

Figure 12 Explorative laparoscopy for suspected diaphragmatic injury. **(A)** Operating room layout. **(B)** Port placements.

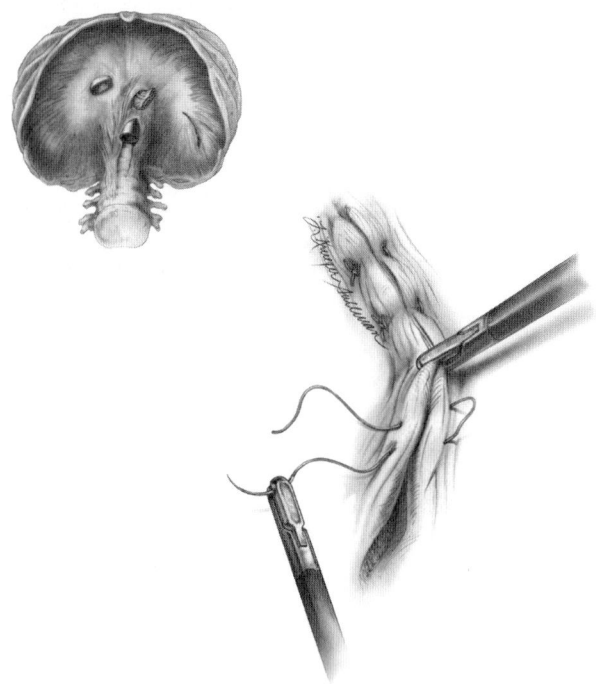

Figure 13 Laparoscopic diaphragmatic repair with interrupted horizontal mattress sutures.

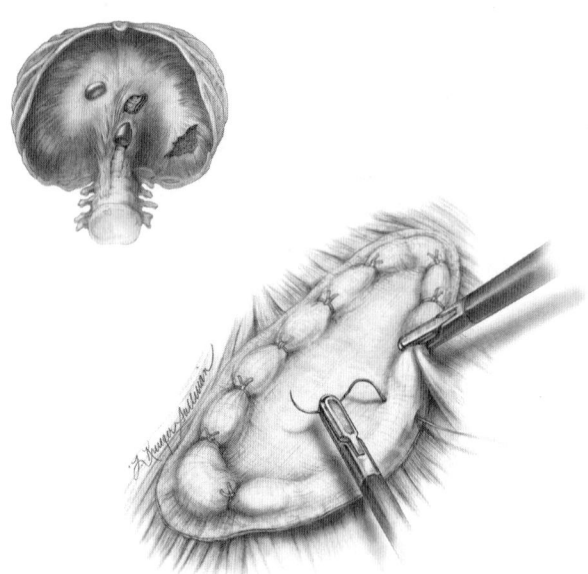

Figure 14 Laparoscopic placement of a polypropylene mesh for repair of large diaphragmatic defect.

cavities has been advocated. Medical professionals in favor of such an aggressive approach argued that thorough inspection and evacuation of all contaminating material can be effectively accomplished only via thoracotomy. This procedure also allows precise placement of a second chest tube, which helps drainage and reduces subsequent risk of empyema formation. Using 10-mm ports in the midclavicular and posterior axillary line of the fifth intercostal space, we have successfully used VATS in this circumstance. The pleural cavity is copiously irrigated, and any remaining clots are removed under direct vision. Both thoracotomy and VATS are safer and more efficient in the management of a heavily soiled pleural

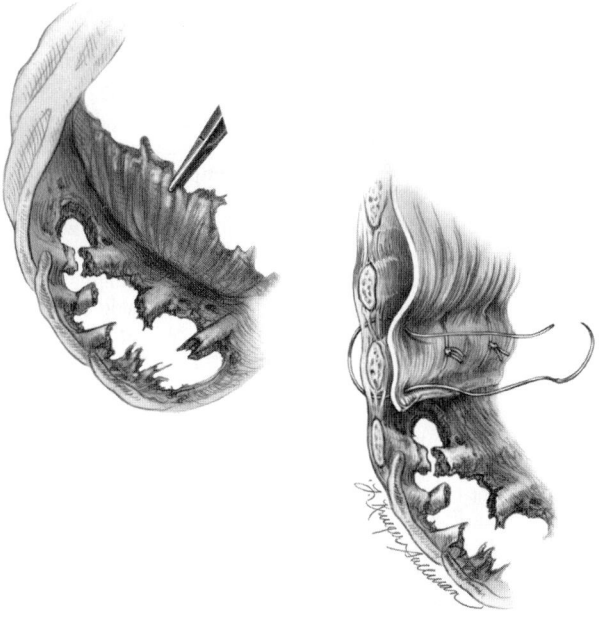

Figure 15 Reattachment of diaphragm. The diaphragm is resutured with interrupted mattress sutures encircling the entire rib.

cavity than any extensive manipulations through the diaphragmatic defect. The intentional or inadvertent enlargement of the diaphragmatic laceration may cause iatrogenic injury to the phrenic nerve or its branches and may permanently impair diaphragmatic function.

Massive Diaphragmatic Destruction

Severe, blunt, thoracoabdominal trauma or, more commonly, a thoracoabdominal shotgun injury may cause significant tissue loss of the chest wall, diaphragm, or both, as well as avulsion of the diaphragm from the rib cage. Definite reconstruction of the diaphragm or closing the chest wall defect might not be immediately possible. Converting an initially nonreconstructible complex chest wall defect functionally into an abdominal defect amenable to delayed reconstruction may be the only option, requiring detaching the diaphragm and relocating it to a higher level. The affected hemidiaphragm is detached anteriorly, laterally, and posteriorly and reattached one or two ribs higher to permit closure without tension. The diaphragm is resutured to the intercostal muscles with interrupted mattress sutures placed around the entire rib (Fig. 15). The abdominal wall defect is managed with local wound care in anticipation of further reconstruction at a later date.

MORTALITY

Mortality in patients with traumatic diaphragmatic rupture is ultimately determined by the associated injuries. Mortality rates reported in the literature range from zero to 41%. The largest series on traumatic diaphragmatic rupture quotes an overall mortality rate of 23%. The mortality rate of 10% was lower in traumatic diaphragmatic ruptures with associated abdominal injuries compared with those associated with concomitant thoracic injuries. It should be noted, however, that patients in the former group were not as severely injured. The highest mortality rate (36%) was reported in the combined thoracic and abdominal injury group. The most significant independent predictors of mortality in patients with traumatic diaphragmatic ruptures were the Revised Trauma Score,

Table 7: Multivariate Analysis of Factors Affecting Mortality in Diaphragmatic Injuries

Variable	X^2	p Value
Revised Trauma Score < 5	24.57	0.0000
Thoracotomy	18.19	0.0000
pRBC transfusion ≥ 10	17.02	0.0000
Operating Room Systolic Blood Pressure < 100	5.38	0.0203
Number of organs injured	4.00	0.0454
Abdominal venous injury	3.68	0.0551
Injury Severity Score > 25	1.94	0.1634
Abdominal artery injury	0.88	0.3487

From Williams M, Carlin AM, Tyburski JG, and others: Am Surg 70:157, 2004.

the need for thoracotomy, transfusion requirements greater than 10 units of packed red blood cells, and hemodynamic instability within the operating room (defined as systolic blood pressure <100 mm Hg) (Table 7). The mortality rates of predominantly blunt diaphragmatic injuries tend to be higher, with some series reporting mortality rates for diaphragmatic ruptures caused by penetrating trauma as low as 4.9%. Overall, the initial physiologic presentation of the patient and the severity of hemorrhagic shock are the primary determinants for survival.

SUGGESTED READINGS

Asensio JA, Petrone P, Demetriades D: Injuries to the diaphragm. In Moore EE, Feliciano DV, Mattox KL, editors: *Trauma,* ed 5, New York, 2004, McGraw-Hill.

Freeman RK, Al-Dossari G, Hutcheson KA, and others: Indications for using video-assisted thoracoscopic surgery to diagnose diaphragmatic injuries after penetrating chest trauma, *Ann Thorac Surg* 72:342, 2001.

Iochum S, Ludig T, Walter F, and others: Imaging of diaphragmatic injury: a diagnostic challenge? *RadioGraphics* 22:S103, 2002.

Reiff DA, McGwin G Jr, Metzger J, and others: Identifying injuries and motor vehicle collision characteristics that together are suggestive of diaphragmatic rupture, *J Trauma* 53:1139, 2002.

Thal ER, Provost DA: Traumatic rupture of the diaphragm. In Baker RJ, Fischer JE, editors: *Mastery of surgery,* ed 4, Philadelphia, 2001, Lippincott Williams & Wilkins.

Wiencek RG, Wilson RF, Steiger Z: Acute injuries of the diaphragm: an analysis of 165 cases, *J Thorac Cardiovasc Surg* 92:989, 1986.

Williams M, Carlin AM, Tyburski JG, and others: Predictors of mortality in patients with traumatic diaphragmatic rupture and associated thoracic and/or abdominal injuries, *Am Surg* 70:157, 2003.

LIVER INJURY

Christopher J. Sonnenday, MD, MHS

The appropriate management of hemorrhage from the liver and its associated vasculature remains a daunting challenge in general surgery. Missteps in judgment or technical blunders can quickly turn a serious but manageable problem into a life-threatening one. Careful consideration must be given to when to operate, when to consider nonoperative therapies, how much to do in the operating room, and when to convert to damage-control strategies to avoid the ominous downward spiral of ongoing hemorrhage, coagulopathy, and hypothermia.

Blunt, penetrating, and iatrogenic mechanisms can lead to a diverse set of injuries that may require markedly different strategies for management. Moreover, the typical general surgery practice may not involve the routine dissection of the liver and its vasculature that is necessary to manage complex hepatic injuries. All surgeons managing a hepatic injury, whether in the trauma bay or the operating room, should give immediate consideration to consulting the most experienced hepatobiliary surgeon at their center. The wisdom and additional pair of hands that such a specialist brings to the table can prove invaluable in these situations.

As trauma systems have evolved, it has been clearly demonstrated that the majority of blunt injuries to the liver can be managed nonoperatively. Large retrospective and single-center prospective studies have documented that as many as 85% of liver injuries may be managed successfully without an operation. Injuries that may appear remarkable by cross-sectional imaging can often be managed without operation in stable patients (Fig. 1). The addition of

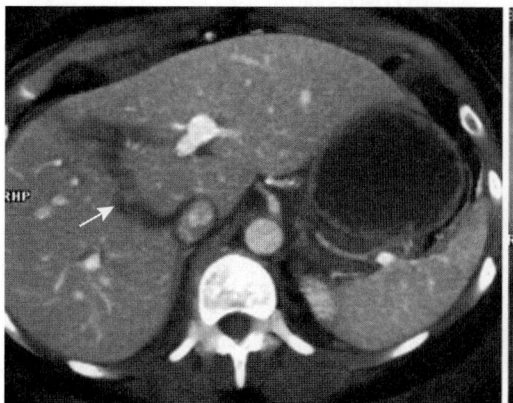 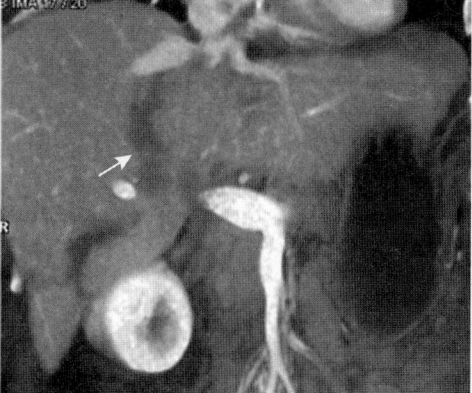

Figure 1 Axial (*left*) and coronal (*right*) views of high-resolution abdominal computed tomography with intravenous contrast of a 50-year-old female driver who was wearing a seat belt in a high-speed motor vehicle accident. A grade IV laceration may be seen extending into Couinaud segments 5, 6, and 8. The patient was successfully managed nonoperatively and required no transfusions or other interventions.

interventional radiologists and skilled endoscopists to the trauma center has allowed many injuries that previously posed significantly morbid intraoperative challenges to be managed in a rather routine manner by nonoperative means. Selection of such patients requires a comprehensive understanding of the spectrum of injuries encountered following blunt trauma.

Penetrating injuries to the liver are more likely to require an operative approach. Whereas injuries confined to the peripheral hepatic parenchyma may require little more than electrocautery or direct pressure, more central injuries or perihepatic vascular trauma require a specialized and well-executed strategy. In highly selected cases, penetrating injuries isolated to the liver occurring in hemodynamically stable patients with a reliable abdominal examination and no evidence of peritonitis may be managed nonoperatively. In such cases, computed tomography (CT) often clearly documents the missile's trajectory.

INITIAL EVALUATION AND MANAGEMENT

The patient with a hepatic injury often presents in the context of a significant mechanism of blunt trauma that may involve multiple organ systems. A thorough and systematic trauma evaluation is necessary to rule out associated injuries to other solid organs in the abdomen; gastrointestinal injuries; and other life-threatening injuries to the head, thoracic organs, and extremities. Advanced Trauma Life Support protocols should dictate initial care and resuscitation efforts. Hemodynamically stable patients should undergo a thorough radiographic evaluation to rule out associated injuries before efforts are focused on the hepatic injury.

High-resolution CT with intravenous contrast enhancement is essential for the evaluation of the hemodynamically stable patient at risk for a solid organ injury of the abdomen. Furthermore, a high-quality CT scan serves as the gold standard test for the initial evaluation of a patient with trauma to the liver. Caution should be taken in the evaluation of patients found by CT to have a liver laceration and free fluid in the abdomen, particularly following trauma with a significant deceleration mechanism. Gastrointestinal injuries must always be considered, and the importance of being able to follow a reliable abdominal examination is central to being able to effectively manage such patients nonoperatively.

Hepatic trauma can be graded on the basis of CT findings, allowing communication between trauma teams and centers and establishing some prognostic information (Table 1). The demonstration of a blush of contrast from the liver parenchyma or adjacent vessels is a fairly reliable marker of an injury that may produce significant, ongoing hemorrhage and require angiographic or operative evaluation. Hemodynamically stable patients with evidence of contrast extravasation in the liver or adjacent to it and without associated injuries that require immediate operative management should be evaluated emergently by angiography. Injuries to the hepatic arterial tree within the liver parenchyma are best treated with embolization with metallic coils or thrombogenic materials (e.g., Gelfoam; Pfizer, New York, NY) (or both) by an experienced interventional radiologist (Fig. 2). If such a specialist is not available to assist in the management of an otherwise stable patient, this constitutes an indication for an emergent transfer to a regional trauma center with such capabilities.

The management of the hemodynamically unstable patient with CT evidence of a significant parenchymal injury to the liver or contrast extravasation (or both) is best accomplished in the operating room. The prompt realization and execution of this decision can be life saving in such a patient. In highly specialized trauma centers at which angiography and a skilled interventionalist are immediately available, this may constitute an initial strategy for evaluation of such a patient. Ideally, the procedure should be performed in a multimodality operating room, where a laparotomy can be

Table 1: Liver Injury Scale

Grade		Description of Injury
I	Hematoma	Subcapsular, <10% surface area
	Laceration	Capsular tear, <1 cm parenchymal depth
II	Hematoma	Subcapsular: 10% to 50% surface area Intraparenchymal: <10 cm in diameter
	Laceration	1–3 cm parenchymal depth, <10 cm in length
III	Hematoma	Subcapsular: >50% surface area or expanding, ruptured subcapsular or parenchymal hematoma Intraparenchymal: hematoma >10 cm or expanding
	Laceration	>3 cm parenchymal depth
IV	Laceration	Parenchymal disruption involving 25% to 75% of hepatic lobe or 1–3 Couinaud segments within a single lobe
V	Laceration	Parenchymal disruption involving >75% of hepatic lobe or >3 Couinaud segments within a single lobe
	Vascular	Juxtahepatic venous injuries (retrohepatic vena cava, central major hepatic veins)
VI	Vascular	Hepatic avulsion

From The American Association for the Surgery of Trauma, www.aast.org. Derived originally from Moore EE, Cogbill TH, Jurkovich GJ, and others: J Trauma 38:323, 1995.

performed immediately if endovascular means of arresting ongoing bleeding are unsuccessful. The trauma team, including the trauma surgeon, absolutely must accompany the patient to angiography so that a decision to abandon the angiography and convert to operative management can be made and executed immediately, if necessary. In addition, having the trauma surgeons and nurses at the bedside allows the interventional radiology procedure to occur without interruption of the patient's resuscitation, which may require ongoing administration of significant volumes of blood products with careful monitoring and correction of any associated coagulopathy.

PRINCIPLES OF NONOPERATIVE MANAGEMENT

Hemodynamically stable patients who have parenchymal liver injuries and no other injuries that require operative intervention may be managed nonoperatively. Safe nonoperative management of a patient with a hepatic injury can be performed only in a dedicated trauma unit, with appropriate monitoring and a dedicated team of trauma nurses and physicians trained to serially evaluate these patients. The lack of such a dedicated unit is an appropriate indication for urgent transfer of the patient with a hepatic injury. The trauma unit should have immediate access to the trauma surgeons, operating room, blood bank, and interventional radiology. The level and intensity of care of these patients can change rapidly, and such a unit must be able to accommodate patients who require critical care. Most trauma centers maintain such units either within or parallel to their surgical intensive care units.

The importance of serial monitoring of vital signs, physical examination, and hemoglobin levels cannot be overemphasized. A dedicated trauma team should evaluate this patient as frequently as hourly or more often until stability is established. In addition to

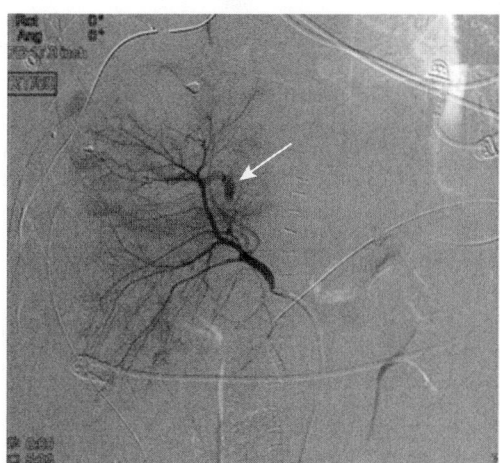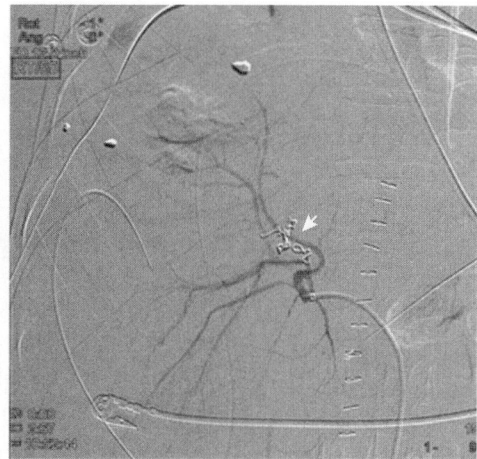

Figure 2 Angiographic images of a 26-year-old male who sustained multiple gunshot wounds to the abdomen, thorax, and extremities. The patient was initially managed operatively, and a large liver laceration was controlled with packing in a damage-control fashion. After definitive closure, the patient underwent a computed tomography scan of the abdomen in evaluation of a fever. There was minimal free fluid in the abdomen, but a clear blush of contrast visualized in the right hepatic lobe. The left panel shows a traumatic arterial-venous fistula that was closed successfully by embolization with multiple metallic coils (*right*). The patient recovered uneventfully without further intervention.

evidence of ongoing, delayed, or recurrent hemorrhage, other associated injuries may be detected. Any changes in the patient's hemodynamics, physical examination, or fall in hemoglobin should lead to an immediate reassessment of the strategy of observation. Liberal use of reimaging or additional evaluation with angiography should be encouraged. In addition, the trauma surgeon should be available immediately and able to make the decision to convert to an operative strategy.

The length of intensive monitoring and length of hospitalization necessary for patients with hepatic injuries may be approximated by the grade of injury (Table 2), although individual trauma centers often have varied protocols for nonoperative management of solid-organ injuries. Obviously, consideration must be given to each patient, his or her likelihood of compliance with activity restrictions, and associated injuries. For trauma patients on extended bedrest protocols in which anticoagulation for deep vein thrombosis prophylaxis is not possible, graded elastic stockings and sequential compression devices should be strictly maintained. Patients should be observed in the hospital for 24 hours or more

Table 2: Suggestions for Nonoperative Management of Blunt Hepatic Trauma

Grade of Injury	Length of ICU or Monitored Trauma Unit Stay (Hours)	Length of Hospitalization or Bed Rest (or Both) (Days)	Period Free from Strenuous Activity or Contact Sports (or Both) (Months)
I	<24	2	1
II	24	4	2
III	48	4–5	3
IV or V*	48–72 or longer	5 or longer	3 or longer

ICU, Intensive care unit.

*Successful nonoperative management in patients with grade IV or V injuries is less common, and decisions regarding management should be made on an individual basis considering associated injuries, bleeding risk, and other factors.

after their bedrest restrictions are lifted so that they can be observed for delayed bleeding. On hospital discharge, patients should be counseled extensively about the importance of paying attention to changes in their condition, the avoidance of significant physical activity, and compliance with follow-up care. The routine use of follow-up imaging studies after hepatic injury has not been shown to be effective in detecting ongoing problems in the absence of clinical signs and is not recommended.

OPERATIVE MANAGEMENT

As with any significant intra-abdominal traumatic injury, liver trauma requires a disciplined intraoperative approach, with continuous reassessment of the operative strategy and the patient's stability. When a major hepatic or perihepatic vascular injury is encountered, the initial goals should be to obtain control of major bleeding and to assess the resources available to address the injuries involved. Early consideration should be given to involving the most experienced hepatobiliary surgeon available. Ancillary treatment modalities that may not be immediately available in every operating room should be obtained and available. Examples include: an argon beam coagulator (ABC); versatile retractor systems such as an Omni or Thompson; synthetic procoagulants such as FloSeal hemostatic matrix (Baxter Healthcare, Deerfield, IL) or Tisseel VH fibrin glue (Baxter Healthcare); vascular sutures; appropriate stapling devices with vascular (2.5 mm) loads; and large vascular clamps. The critical nature of the patient's injuries should be communicated to the anesthesia team, and ample help at the head of the bed should be ensured as well. The room should be warmed, adequate venous access placed, rapid infusers and blood warmers obtained, and a second suction setup or cellsaver (if no enteric contamination exists) established.

A midline celiotomy is the most appropriate initial incision for the trauma laparotomy. Extension to a median sternotomy or right thoracotomy may be considered in those rare cases in which exposure and vascular control is not adequate or those in which injuries involve multiple cavities. Sequential four-quadrant packing with laparotomy pads should be performed, with brief inspection of each quadrant for a source of ongoing, life-threatening hemorrhage. Packing the liver is most effectively accomplished by packing pads above the liver under the costal margin and under both the right and left hepatic lobes. The surgeon can control nearly all significant liver bleeding with packs and manual compression. Associated injuries to the aorta, infrahepatic vena cava, iliac vessels, spleen, and mesentery should be excluded or addressed. Ongoing sources of enteric contamination should be quickly controlled.

When the liver is identified as the source of intra-abdominal hemorrhage, a quick determination should be made (after stepwise removal of packs) about the degree of ongoing bleeding. Sometimes horrific-appearing lacerations of the liver parenchyma can be associated with little ongoing bleeding. Venous bleeding often can be stopped with a prolonged period of packing and compression (10–15 minutes), with the ABC or direct vascular sutures used to control any remaining bleeding. Adjuvant agents such as fibrin glue or other hemostatic matrix may be helpful in controlling diffuse bleeding from raw surfaces of the liver parenchyma. Small lacerations or punctures may be packed with hemostatic agents such as Gelfoam (Pfizer, New York, NY) or Surgicel (Johnson & Johnson, New Brunswick, NJ). Transcapsular liver sutures should probably be avoided in all but the most peripheral lacerations because they may lead to further ischemia of already devascularized segments.

When brisk, ongoing bleeding from a hepatic or perihepatic injury is encountered, packs should be replaced and rapid efforts made to mobilize the liver and control inflow. The Pringle maneuver can be accomplished immediately, initially by placing the surgeon's left second and third fingers through the Foramen of Winslow and using the thumb to compress the portal vein and hepatic artery. The lesser omentum can be opened bluntly or with electrocautery; this should be a reminder to look for a replaced or accessory left hepatic artery running through the gastrohepatic ligament that will not be included in the Pringle maneuver (it can be easily controlled with a small vascular clamp or vessel loop). The surgeon's hand can then be replaced with an umbilical tape and Rummel tourniquet, which has the advantage of being able to be released slowly, as opposed to the alternatives of a Satinsky clamp or Penrose drain. An effective Pringle will often convert unmanageable bleeding to tolerable levels, allowing inspection of the field and consideration of treatment strategies. Ongoing bleeding that is not significantly affected by a Pringle maneuver is diagnostic of a major injury to the central hepatic veins or to the retrohepatic vena cava. In this case, the Pringle should be left in place while packs and the surgeon's hand are used to directly compress the area of injury, or in the case of a retrohepatic injury, compression of the liver dorsally onto the vena cava. This maneuver will slow the hemorrhage notably, allowing the anesthesiologist to proceed with resuscitation and providing time to obtain additional surgical hands if necessary. Subsequent moves in this dangerous scenario often must be performed in brief episodes, with dissection performed quickly and intermittently with breaks for compression, blood evacuation from the field, and resuscitation.

The ability to address complex injuries to the hepatic veins or retrohepatic cava is dependent on rapid and complete mobilization of the liver's ligamentous attachments using electrocautery. The ligamentum teres and falciform ligament should be divided and then followed back toward the suprahepatic vena cava. A rolled lap pad can then be packed between the suprahepatic vena cava and the diaphragm. The left lateral segment should be released from the attachments of the left triangular ligament to the diaphragm. This allows the left lateral segment to be rotated toward the right hepatic lobe. This maneuver, in combination with opening the gastrohepatic ligament, allows exposure of the left side of the vena cava and caudate lobe. Laparotomy pads may be packed along the cava and the left lateral segment and then compressed dorsally while the right lobe is mobilized. The right lobe is mobilized by first releasing the inferior attachments of the right coronary ligament from the hepatic flexure and right kidney. This move, combined with an extensive Kocher maneuver, allows exposure of the intrahepatic vena cava and right aspect of the caudate lobe. Packs may be placed in this region while the right lobe is then rotated toward the

patient's left by the surgeon. An assistant should then release the posterior attachments of the right lobe to the diaphragm, exposing the right side of the vena cava and continuing until the lateral aspect of the right hepatic vein is identified. Again, packs can be placed along the vena cava and between the liver and the diaphragm. After this mobilization has been completed, the liver should be surrounded with laparotomy pads and returned to an anatomic position. Again, manual compression of the liver toward the retroperitoneum will allow control of most of venous bleeding.

An important decision should then be made about the necessity of surgically repairing large vascular injuries versus leaving the liver packed in a damage-control strategy. Diffuse bleeding from raw, injured surfaces of the hepatic parenchyma, particularly in the setting of a cold, coagulopathic patient who has received multiple blood products, will not be stopped easily. Such a patient is best served by packing as described and closing the abdomen in a temporary fashion. Aggressive resuscitation, warming, and correction of coagulopathy are then best accomplished in an intensive care unit setting.

Ongoing bleeding from an obvious laceration to the hepatic veins, a portal venous or hepatic arterial branch, or the vena cava should be addressed as efficiently as possible. Significant bleeding within a laceration of the parenchyma can be oversewn with nonabsorbable 3-0 or 4-0 suture placed carefully with Pringle occlusion. The surrounding parenchyma should then be thoroughly treated with the ABC and then observed as the Pringle is released. Again, in an unstable patient, time should not be wasted controlling anything but large-caliber vessels. Packing will likely stop less significant bleeding from small parenchymal vessels. Extrahepatic injuries to the portal vein or hepatic artery should be repaired primarily, when possible. A lobar or sublobar branch of either the portal vein or hepatic artery can be ligated, although a second-look operation should be considered to assess for nonviable segments of the liver parenchyma. More complex vascular reconstructions in the portal triad (i.e., the main portal vein or proper hepatic artery) should not be attempted without the assistance of an experienced hepatobiliary or transplant surgeon, if possible. Individual hepatic veins or their larger branches that are not controlled by compression may be ligated as long as other hepatic veins are intact.

A major injury to the retrohepatic vena cava can be an intimidating surgical challenge. Historical options for control and repair have included a cavoatrial shunt or emergent veno-veno bypass. A more quickly executed strategy is that of total hepatic vascular exclusion, achieved by Pringle maneuver and clamping of the intrahepatic and suprahepatic cavae with large vascular clamps. This decompresses the retrohepatic cava of all but occasional posterior thoracolumbar veins. This allows visualization and repair of lacerations to the cava and provides control in the rare case that a cava replacement or hepatic vein reimplantation (or both) is necessary (best accomplished with an 18- to 20-mm ringed polytetrafluoroethylene graft). Total vascular exclusion may also be the only way to diagnose and control significant bleeding from the posterior right hepatic or caudate lobes. These areas can be controlled with direct suture ligation of larger vessels, ABC, use of adjuvant hemostatic agents, with or without packing. More cranial injuries that cannot be controlled with a suprahepatic clamp should prompt a median sternotomy and opening of the pericardium.

In rare circumstances, a significant peripheral segment of hepatic parenchyma may be lacerated in such a manner that it is devascularized. In such a case, a nonanatomic resection of the compromised segment may be performed. The residual attachments of such a segment may be divided with electrocautery, clamps and ligatures, or an endovascular stapler with 2.5-mm staple-size load. It is not wise to attack more extensive anatomic resections in the acute setting, and these are rarely if ever indicated. They are best accomplished at a second-look operation when that becomes necessary because of significant parenchymal destruction with large devitalized segments. It should be emphasized that large lacerations that may effectively appear to divide the hepatic parenchyma into two or more discrete segments may not require further intervention as long as major vascular pedicles are intact.

Repair of biliary injuries may be necessary when more central injuries are encountered. Injuries to the hepatic ducts or common bile duct may be primarily repaired over a T-tube or internal Silastic stent (pediatric feeding tube) when tissue is not significantly devitalized. Roux-en-Y hepaticojejunostomy may be used in the rare cases in which primary repair is not possible. Such a procedure can be performed at a second-look procedure when the patient is hemodynamically stable and resuscitated and other injuries have been addressed. When definitive abdominal closure is performed in the setting of large parenchymal lacerations without active bleeding, placement of intra-abdominal drains adjacent to the laceration may be considered to detect and drain biliary leaks that may not be evident at the original procedure.

DIAGNOSIS AND MANAGEMENT OF COMPLICATIONS FOLLOWING HEPATIC TRAUMA

A high index of suspicion for the delayed presentation of associated injuries or complications is essential. The occurrence of fever, sepsis, leukocytosis, increased pain or tenderness, or elevation of liver biochemistries should prompt evaluation for complications. High-resolution CT with oral and intravenous contrast is the best initial test for evaluation of patients with these symptoms.

Significant intra-abdominal collections or intraparenchymal demarcated fluid in patients with evidence of infection, pain, or elevated serum total bilirubin or alkaline phosphatase should prompt further evaluation with aspiration and percutaneous drainage.

Demonstration of a significant biloma or bilious ascites should prompt evaluation of the biliary tree with cholangiography. Endoscopic retrograde cholangiopancreatography (ERCP) is the preferred modality in these patients when anatomically possible. Magnetic resonance cholangiopancreatography (MRCP) may be considered as an alternative diagnostic tool, but it is not a functional study that allows real-time demonstration of what may be subtle biliary leaks from peripheral biliary radicles. Furthermore, endoscopic sphincterotomy and stenting may be therapeutic in even the most peripheral and high-volume biliary leaks. Decompression of the sphincter of Oddi, in association with fastidious drainage of bile collections, is usually sufficient to allow healing of even high-output biliary fistulae (Fig. 3). Percutaneous transhepatic cholangiography (PTC) and percutaneous biliary drainage (PBD) should be reserved for biliary fistulae that cannot be controlled or navigated by ERCP. In some cases, biliary injuries may be complicated by the later development of biliary strictures, hepatic abscess, and atrophy of chronically obstructed or poorly drained segments. These conditions may require PTC and cholangioplasty, with partial hepatectomy or hepaticojejunostomy (or both) reserved for recalcitrant cases.

Hepatic abscess may also present as a delayed complication of hepatic trauma when a devascularized segment of hepatic parenchyma necroses and is secondarily infected as it liquefies.

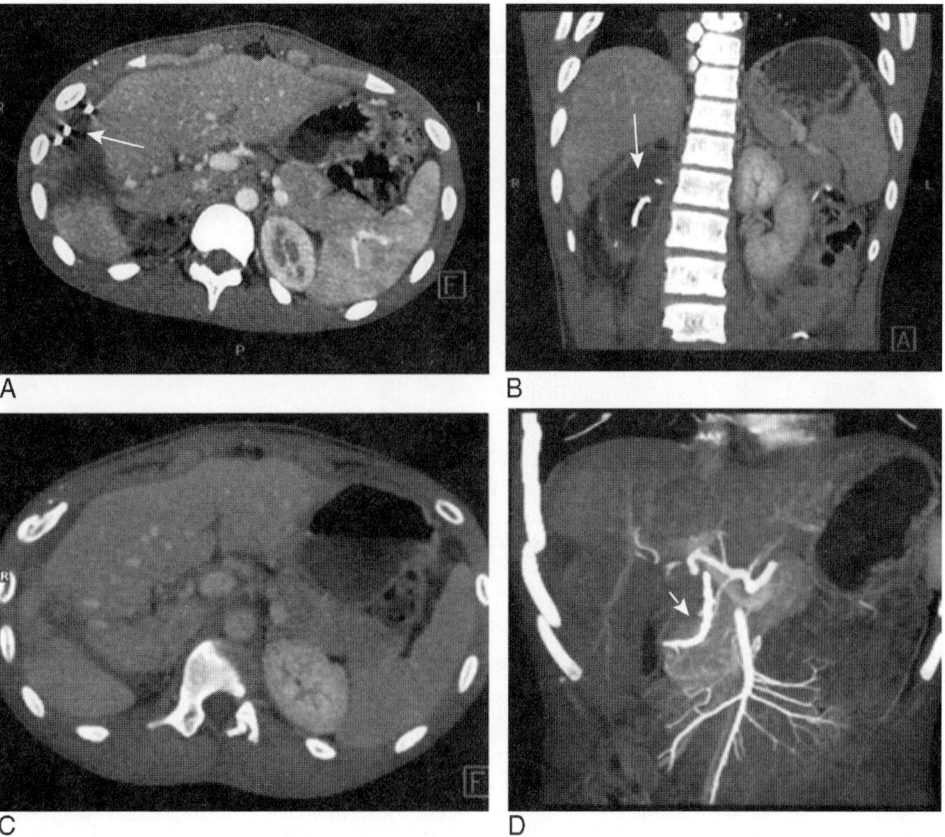

Figure 3 Sequential computed tomography images of a 16-year-old male treated for multiple gunshot wounds. He initially underwent a laparotomy, damage-control packing of the liver, and a bowel resection. He subsequently underwent removal of packs and abdominal closure but developed two large bilomas that required placement of two percutaneous drains (*long arrows,* **A, B**). Despite drainage of initially more than 1 liter of bile per day from his drains, his biliary leak sealed and his bilomas resolved **(C)** after endoscopic sphincterotomy and endostent placement (*arrow,* **D**).

Percutaneous drainage and an extended course of antibiotics are usually sufficient to address this complication, with debridement of an ischemic liver reserved for rare cases. Injury to a segment of the hepatic arterial tree also may be associated with pseudoaneurysm formation, which can present with delayed bleeding either within the abdomen or after formation of an arteriobiliary fistula, presenting with hemobilia. Gastrointestinal bleeding following hepatic trauma, without another obvious source (e.g., an associated enteric injury or repair) should prompt an urgent move toward angiography.

Among patients with high-grade (grades III–V) injuries managed nonoperatively, approximately 10% to 25% of patients will develop complications requiring additional interventions. Among patients with grade V injuries, more than 50% will require additional therapy, although many can be managed without a laparotomy. The most common complications are related to biliary leaks, with necrosis of ischemic liver segments occurring more commonly in grade IV and V injuries. Despite the relatively high incidence of associated complications, experienced trauma centers have documented less than 5% mortality among patients with high-grade injuries treated initially nonoperatively.

CONCLUSIONS

Despite improved clinical outcomes in recent series, liver trauma remains a clinical problem that requires the full expertise and resources of an experienced trauma center. The majority of patients with liver injuries may be managed nonoperatively, although they require meticulous observation and a continuous reevaluation of the necessity for operative therapy or other interventions. Complications are common but may be managed efficiently. Among the most challenging of intra-abdominal emergencies are those patients requiring operative therapy. A disciplined approach, with careful selection of patients most appropriate for damage-control strategies, can allow patients with devastating injuries to be salvaged.

SUGGESTED READINGS

Cornwell EE III, Chang DC, Phillips J, and others: Enhanced trauma program commitment at a level I trauma center: effect on the process and outcome of care, *Arch Surg* 138:838–843, 2003.

Kozar RA, Moore JB, Niles SE, and others: Complications of nonoperative management of high-grade blunt hepatic injuries, *J Trauma* 59:1066–1071, 2005.

Stein DM, Scalea TM: Nonoperative management of spleen and liver injuries, *J Intensive Care Med* 21:296–304, 2006.

Trunkey DD: Hepatic trauma: contemporary management, *Surg Clin N Am* 84:437–450, 2004.

Velmahos GC, Toutouzas KG, Radin R, and others: Nonoperative management of blunt injury to solid abdominal organs, *Arch Surg* 138:844–851, 2003.

PANCREATIC AND DUODENAL INJURIES

Michael F. Rotondo, MD, and Mark A. Newell, MD

The diagnosis and management of injuries to the pancreas and duodenum are complex for many reasons. Damage to these organs is uncommon, occurring in less than 5% of patients sustaining abdominal injuries. The infrequency of these injuries limits opportunities to acquire individual or institutional expertise. Associated injuries frequently occur and contribute markedly to the morbidity and mortality resulting from pancreatic and duodenal injury. The juxtaposition of major solid (liver, spleen, kidneys), hollow (stomach, colon), and vascular (inferior vena cava, portal vein, superior mesenteric vessels) structures puts these adjacent organs at risk when injury to the pancreas and duodenum has occurred (Fig. 1). Injury to the pancreas and duodenum can be life threatening, especially if diagnosed in a delayed fashion. The retroperitoneal location of the pancreas and duodenum protects the organs but also masks symptoms when they are injured. The fragile nature and tenuous blood supply of these organs create management dilemmas. Therefore because of all the complexities outlined, a systematic approach to these challenging and vexing injuries is the key to effective management.

DIAGNOSIS

A high index of suspicion is necessary to make the diagnosis of injury to the pancreas and duodenum. Certain injury patterns

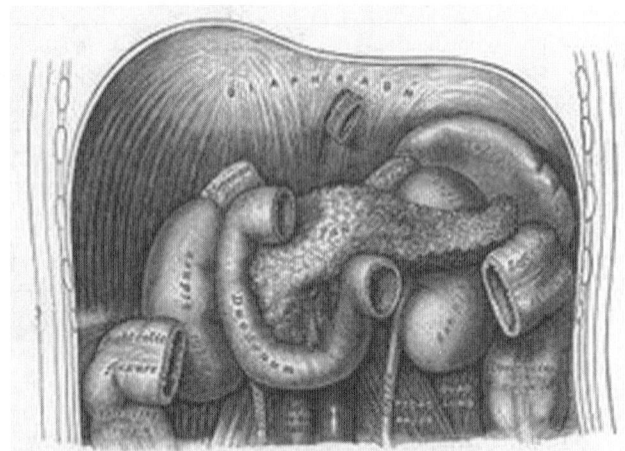

Figure 1 Adjacent organs to pancreas and duodenum.

should raise the awareness regarding the potential of a pancreaticoduodenal injury. Deceleration injuries with blunt force to the epigastrium and crush injuries that appose the anterior abdominal wall with the spinal column commonly involve the pancreas or the duodenum (or both). Although the retroperitoneal location of these organs may limit physical examination findings, persistent abdominal pain and tenderness should prompt efforts to rule out intra-abdominal injury. Eliciting peritoneal signs, although not specific for injury to the pancreas or duodenum, mandates exploratory laparotomy, thereby optimizing injury identification.

Diagnostic studies aid in detecting the presence of pancreatic or duodenal injury. Although not specific, diagnostic peritoneal lavage fluid analyzed for amylase may suggest injury to the pancreas or duodenum. Focused assessment for the sonographic evaluation of the trauma patient (FAST) contributes little to the definite diagnosis of pancreaticoduodenal trauma because of the retroperitoneal location of these structures. Computed tomography (CT) scan, more effective at imaging the retroperitoneum, provides clues to injury of these structures. Injury to the pancreas is suggested by parenchymal laceration, intrapancreatic or retroperitoneal hematomas, peripancreatic fluid, phlegmon or fluid between the pancreas and splenic vein (Fig. 2). Bowel wall thickening, extraluminal gas and fluid, and contrast extravasation on CT indicate duodenal injury (Fig. 3). Endoscopic retrograde cholangiopancreatography is sensitive and specific for delineating pancreatic duct injury. Its preoperative and intraoperative use in the trauma setting is limited, but postoperatively it may reveal missed pancreatic duct injury, albeit in a delayed fashion. Magnetic resonance pancreatography, a noninvasive means of determining duct integrity, is rarely used in the acute setting.

Other adjuncts used to diagnosis pancreatic and duodenal injuries include an analysis of serum amylase and lipase. Management decisions based on a single normal or high value are fraught with problems. An elevated amylase value may occur in trauma scenarios without injury to the pancreas or duodenum. Conversely, injury to the pancreas or duodenum (or both) may be present in the setting of a normal amylase, especially if analyzed less than 3 hours from injury. As hyperamylasemia ultimately develops in nearly all patients with pancreaticoduodenal trauma, repeat measurements increase the sensitivity and specificity of the test.

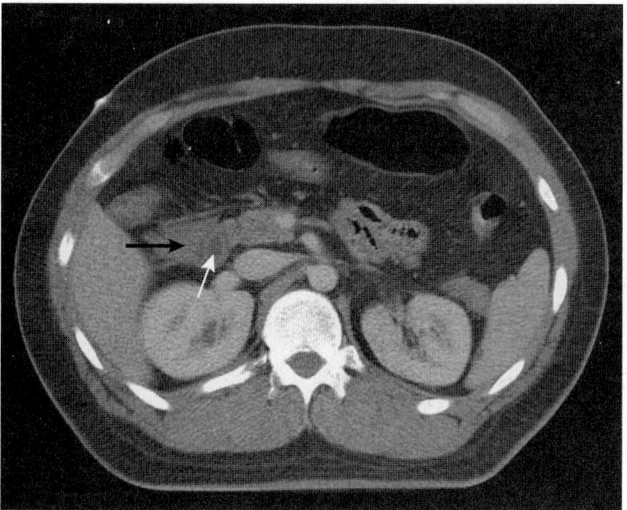

Figure 2 Duodenal injury. Duodenum *(white arrow)*; periduodenal fluid *(black arrow)*.

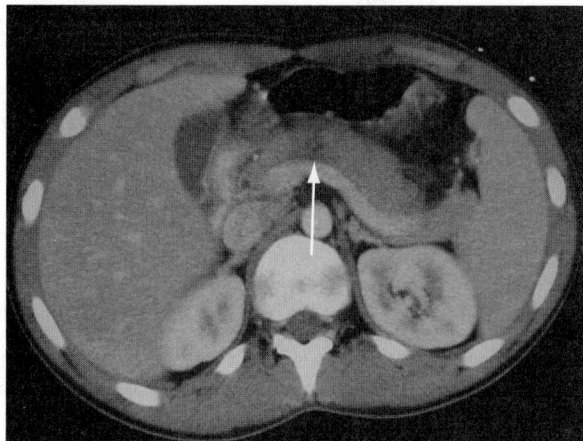

Figure 3 Pancreatic injury. Pancreatic transaction *(arrow)*.

MANAGEMENT

Duodenal Injury

Ultimately, diagnosis of a duodenal injury may take place in the operating room. This is facilitated by adequate mobilization and exposure of the duodenum, assessing for suggested injury to the duodenum that includes central retroperitoneal hematomas, bile, or air. These findings mandate full exposure of the duodenum to exclude injury. Exposure of the duodenum is accomplished using several maneuvers (Table 1). Dissecting the hepatic flexure medially away from its retroperitoneal attachments allows for the anterolateral aspect of the duodenum to be visualized. The lateral attachments of the duodenum are dissected sharply and bluntly in the Kocher maneuver, allowing for upward and medial mobilization of the first and second portions of the duodenum. This allows inspection of the anterior and posterior aspects of these segments of the duodenum to be assessed for injury. A Cattell-Braasch maneuver facilitates the exposure of the second, third, and fourth portions of the duodenum by mobilizing the posterior parietal attachments of the ascending colon and small bowel and medially rotating the viscera en bloc to the midline. Transecting the ligament of Treitz and rotating the duodenum allows the anterior and posterior surfaces of the fourth portion of the duodenum to be viewed. Full visualization of the first portion of the duodenum is aided by transection of the gastroduodenal artery.

After full exposure of the duodenum has been achieved, the organ can be adequately assessed for injury. The American Association for the Surgery of Trauma Organ Injury Scale (AAST/OIS) classifies injury to the duodenum on the basis of a grading scale from I to V (Table 2). Duodenal hematomas may be diagnosed preoperatively and treated expectantly with nasogastric decompression and parenteral nutrition for up to 2 to 3 weeks if signs of improvement are seen. Oral intake is resumed with decreased nasogastric output or duodenography demonstrating the unobstructed passage of contrast through the duodenum. If the resulting obstruction is unresolved after 3 weeks of expectant management, surgical intervention may be necessary. When duodenal hematomas are diagnosed during the course of exploratory laparotomy for trauma, the serosa should be incised and the hematoma evacuated if 50% of the lumen is involved. Hemostasis should be ensured. The resulting partial-thickness defect can be repaired primarily. Closed-suction drainage adjacent to but not abutting any duodenal repair, as well as a nasojejunal feeding tube, is recommended.

Approximately 75% to 85% of all full-thickness duodenal injuries can be repaired primarily (duodenorrhaphy) (Table 3). Repair consists of debridement of devitalized tissues and two-layer closure of the defect using absorbable, inner-suture and nonabsorbable, outer-suture materials. The closure should be oriented in a

Table I: Five Ways to Visualize the Duodenum during Exploratory Laparotomy

1. Hepatic flexure mobilization—anterolateral visualization of the first and second portions of the duodenum

2. Kocher maneuver—full anterolateral and posterior visualization of the first and second portions of the duodenum

3. Cattell-Braasch maneuver—visualization of the second, third, and fourth portions of the duodenum

4. Transection of the ligament of Treitz—visualization of the fourth portion of the duodenum

5. Transection of the gastroduodenal artery—full visualization of the first portion of the duodenum

Table 2: American Association for the Surgery of Trauma Organ Injury Scale (AAST/OIS) Duodenum Injury Scale

Grade*	Type of Injury	Description of Injury	ICD-9	AIS-90
I	Hematoma	Involving single portion of duodenum	863.21	2
	Laceration	Partial thickness, no perforation	863.21	3
II	Hematoma	Involving more than one portion	863.21	2
	Laceration	Disruption <50% of circumference	863.31	4
	Laceration	Disruption 50%-75% of circumference of D2	863.31	4
III		Disruption 50%-100% of circumference of D1, D3, D4		
IV	Laceration	Disruption >75% of circumference of D2	863.31	5
		Involving ampulla or distal common bile duct	863.31	5
V	Laceration	Massive disruption of duodenopancreatic complex	863.31	5
	Vascular	Devascularization of duodenum	863.31	5

AIS, Abbreviated Injury Scale; *D1,* first position of duodenum; *D2,* second portion of duodenum; *D3,* third portion of duodenum; *D4,* fourth portion of duodenum; *ICD,* International Classification of Diseases.
*Advance one grade for multiple injuries up to grade III.

Table 3: Pancreas and Duodenal Injury Management Scheme

	Duodenum	Pancreas	Distal Common Bile Duct	Combined
Drainage	CS—All but most simple repair DC—Tube duodenostomy†	ALL*	ALL Red rubber choledochostomy or T-tube	ALL
Diversion	←————————— Pyloric exclusion Diverticulization —————————→			
Definitive repair/ reconstruction	Primary repair* Resection and repair Thal patch Jejunal graft Roux-en-Y	Distal pancreatectomy† Pancreaticoenteric anastomosis Duct ligation	Primary repair (T-tube) Choledochoduodenostomy Choledochojejunostomy*	Whipple*
Adjuncts	←————————— Omental flap Peritoneal flap Feeding tube Endoscopic retrograde cholangiopancreatography Nasoduodenal tube Nasojejunal tube —————————→			

CS, Closed suction; *DC,* damage control.
*Most common.
†Less common.

transverse direction unless the defect is greater than 50% the circumference of the lumen. The omentum is used to buttress the repair. Nasoduodenal stenting allows for luminal decompression.

Many adjuncts to duodenorrhaphy have been described to reduce the incidence of suture line dehiscence and duodenal fistula formation (see Table 3). Tube duodenostomy, whether antegrade or retrograde, has been used. Although initially touted to reduce duodenal fistula rates, subsequent studies showed no difference in suture line dehiscence after duodenorrhaphy with or without tube duodenostomy. Duodenal diverticulization consists of duodenorrhaphy, antrectomy, truncal vagotomy, gastrojejunostomy, and duodenostomy, choledochostomy, and feeding jejunostomy tubes. The concept of the procedure involves complete diversion of gastric and biliary contents away from the duodenal repair. This is a cumbersome procedure that necessitates the removal of uninjured stomach and is

not recommended. Pyloric exclusion, another means of diversion, is performed either by oversewing the pylorus through a gastrostomy or stapling the pylorus. A gastrojejunostomy is created and diverts gastric contents until the pylorus reopens within 3 months. However, neither this procedure nor any of the other adjuncts has been proven to enhance the integrity of the initial repair. For tenuous duodenal repairs, omental buttressing or peritoneal flap reinforcement is recommended with the addition of closed-suction drainage.

A minority of duodenal injuries may not be amenable to duodenorrhaphy because of the inability to create a tension-free repair. Defects larger than 50% of the luminal circumference may fit this category (see Table 3). Large proximal and distal duodenal injuries may be repaired by resection and duodenoduodenostomy. Thal patches and jejunal interposition grafts, although described, are rarely used. The second and third portions of the duodenum, because of their intimate relationship with the ampulla and pancreas, may not allow for the mobilization necessary for duodenorrhaphy or duodenoduodenostomy. These injuries, if they are without ampulla or common bile duct (CBD) involvement, are repaired via Roux-en-Y duodenojejunostomy.

Complex Duodenal and Combined Pancreaticoduodenal Injuries

Other injuries to the duodenum, because of their complexity, require great foresight to manage. These injuries include duodenal injury with ampulla, CBD, or pancreas involvement (or a combination of these injuries) (see Table 15.13-3). Because lacerations to the second portion of the duodenum may in turn injure the ampulla, this area must be assessed for ampullary injury. A knowledge of the anatomy of the ampulla helps with this assessment. The ampulla is a dilatation of the common pancreatobiliary channel adjacent to the duodenal papilla, located on the posteromedial wall of the second portion of the duodenum. Visualization can be improved by attempting to express bile through the ampulla by palpation of the CBD. If, in fact, the ampulla is injured, the ampulla may be primarily repaired or reimplanted into the duodenum or a Roux loop of the jejunum. An injury that cannot be reconstructed may necessitate pancreaticoduodenectomy.

Similarly, distal CBD injury complicates injury to the duodenum. Exploration of the posterior pancreatic head enhances visualization of the injury. Injuries to the CBD less than 50% of the circumference can be repaired over a stent. Larger defects or involvement of the intrapancreatic or intraduodenal CBD require reimplantation of the CBD or pancreaticoduodenectomy.

Combined injuries to the duodenum and pancreas should be managed separately unless there is injury to the head of the pancreas. Duodenal injuries without extensive tissue loss associated with nonductal pancreatic injuries are treated with duodenorrhaphy and closed-suction drainage. More extensive duodenal injuries with major pancreatic duct injury may require duodenal repair, as described earlier, along with distal pancreatectomy. As mentioned, pyloric exclusion may be considered, but omental buttressing of the repairs is recommended. Closed-suction drainage is provided.

Because of the shared blood supply to the pancreas and duodenum from the superior and inferior pancreaticoduodenal arteries, massive destruction or devascularization of the organs necessitates pancreaticoduodenectomy. This procedure is discussed in more detail later.

Pancreatic Injury

Pancreatic injuries can be missed intraoperatively; therefore a thorough and meticulous exploration is necessary to establish

Table 4: Five Ways to Visualize the Pancreas during Exploratory Laparotomy

1. Through the root of the transverse mesocolon
2. Through the hepatogastric omentum
3. Through the gastrocolic omentum
4. Cattell-Braasch maneuver—for pancreatic head visualization
5. Mattox maneuver—for pancreatic tail visualization

the presence or absence of a pancreatic injury. The pancreas may be visualized five ways (Table 4). In patients without significant intra-abdominal fat, the pancreas may be visualized through the transverse mesocolon. Dissection of the lesser sac through the greater and lesser omentum provides an inspection of the pancreas. The Cattell-Braasch maneuver is used for visualizing the pancreatic head, and the Mattox maneuver is used to visualize the tail of the pancreas. Exposure of the pancreas is incomplete without mobilizing the superior and inferior borders, making sure that the posterior aspect of the pancreas is felt for defects.

After the pancreas has been fully exposed, it can be assessed for injury (Table 5). Three types of treatment strategies can be used for pancreatic injury: drainage, resection, and reconstruction (see Table 3). Approximately 60% to 70% of injuries to the pancreas can be managed by closed-suction drainage. Pancreatic injuries without major duct involvement can be treated with simple, closed, external drainage. Drainage effluent can be tested for amylase in the postoperative period. When the drain amylase level is less than that of the serum, the drain can be discontinued.

Major and minor injuries to the pancreas are differentiated by the integrity of the main pancreatic duct. Ductal injury can be anticipated on the basis of knowledge of pancreatic ductal anatomy. The main pancreatic duct runs just superior to a line bisecting the pancreas into upper and lower halves. Injuries above or below this level are less likely to have injured the pancreatic duct. Other predictors of main pancreatic duct injury include near-total or complete gland transection, central gland perforation, and ductal injury visualization (Table 6).

Intraoperative pancreatography (IOP) can be used to make the diagnosis of pancreatic duct injury. The simplest method of performing IOP is via needle cholecystocholangiography. The injection of water-soluble contrast through the gallbladder under fluoroscopic visualization allows a complete pancreatogram to be obtained. Intravenous opiates may improve pancreatic duct visualization by causing sphincter of Oddi contraction. Iatrogenic injury to the pancreas and duodenum to facilitate cannulation of the pancreatic duct via distal pancreatectomy or the ampulla by way of a duodenotomy has fallen out of favor.

Table 5: American Association for the Surgery of Trauma Organ Injury Scale Pancreas Injury Scale

Grade*	Type of Injury	Description of Injury	ICD-9[†]	AIS-90
I	Hematoma	Minor contusion without duct injury	863.81–863.84	2
	Laceration	Superficial laceration without duct injury		2
II	Hematoma	Major contusion without duct injury or tissue loss	863.81–863.84	2
	Laceration	Major laceration without duct injury or tissue loss		3
III	Laceration	Distal transection or parenchymal injury with duct injury	863.92–863.94	3
IV	Laceration	Proximal[‡] transection or parenchymal injury involving ampulla	863.91	4
V	Laceration	Massive disruption of pancreatic head	863.91	5

*Advance one grade for multiple injuries up to grade III.
[†]863.51, 863.91, head; 863.99, 862.92, body; 863.83, 863.93, tail.
[‡]Proximal pancreas is to the patient's right of the superior mesenteric vein.

Table 6: Predictors of Main Pancreatic Duct Injury

1. Complete transection of the pancreas
2. Visualization of ductal injury
3. Central pancreatic gland perforation
4. Laceration of pancreas $\geq$50% of gland
5. Severe pancreatic gland maceration

Adapted from Heitsch RC, Knutson CO, Fulton RL, and others: Surgery 80:523–529, 1976.

Confirmed or highly suspicious pancreatic duct injuries to the left of the superior mesenteric vessels are treated with distal pancreatectomy. The spleen may or may not be preserved, depending on the hemodynamic stability of the patient. The pancreas is transected just proximal to the level of injury, the pancreatic duct is ligated if visualized, and the remaining pancreatic tissue closed with nonabsorbable suture. Alternatively, a TA-55 stapler (US Surgical, Norwalk, CT) with a 4.8-mm staple can be used for transection and closure of the pancreatic remnant. Closed external drainage is performed. Placement of a nasojejunal feeding tube is recommended as an adjunct for all pancreatic injuries.

Pancreatic duct injury to the right of the superior mesenteric vessels may similarly be treated with distal pancreatectomy. However, given the amount of pancreatic tissue loss, the likelihood of pancreatic insufficiency with the resection of $\geq$80% of the pancreas is significant. In this situation, wide external drainage is recommended when there has not been complete destruction or massive devascularization of the pancreatic head. A resultant fistula will either close spontaneously or require subsequent pancreatic resection or pancreaticoenteric anastomosis, which may be facilitated by the chronicity of the fistula.

With massive destruction of the pancreatic head and unreconstructable main pancreatic duct injury or uncontrollable retropancreatic bleeding from adjacent associated vascular injuries, pancreaticoduodenectomy may be performed. Because this procedure carries with it extensive morbidity and mortality, the necessity to perform it is, fortunately, rare. In the scenario of massive hemorrhage, a staged pancreaticoduodenectomy may be necessary after an initial damage-control laparotomy. Although the pylorus-sparing pancreaticoduodenectomy has been described, few centers have adapted this procedure for use in trauma patients. Simple pancreatic duct ligation and interval cystenterostomy have also been suggested, but the combined procedure has shown an excessive rate of fistula formation that renders it prohibitive except in the most extreme circumstances.

COMPLICATIONS

The interval from injury to operation has a significant impact in determining morbidity and mortality from duodenal injury. There is a threefold increase in mortality in patients undergoing surgery 24 hours after injury compared with those treated within 24 hours. Associated injuries also contribute to mortality. Fistula formation is the most common complication after duodenal injury, followed by duodenal obstruction. Fistulae are managed with external drainage and strict attention to correction of fluid and electrolyte abnormalities. Pyloric exclusion with gastrojejunostomy may be necessary for persistent fistulae. Duodenal obstruction is managed expectantly for 3 to 4 weeks if there is partial obstruction. Complete obstruction may necessitate earlier operative intervention.

Associated injuries also affect mortality in pancreatic trauma. Whereas early death from pancreatic injury occurs secondary to exsanguination, late deaths result from sepsis, usually because of pancreatic fistulae. Pancreatic fistulae may close spontaneously over time. Somatostatin, although not shown to influence fistula closure rates, does diminish fistula output. Postoperative pancreatic abscesses are treated with CT-guided drainage.

Suggested Readings

Asensio JA, Demetriades D, Berne JD, and others: A unified approach to the surgical exposure of pancreatic and duodenal injuries, *Am J Surg* 174:54, 1997.

Carrillo E, Richardson JD, Miller FB: Evolution in the management of duodenal injuries, *J Trauma* 40:1037, 1996.

Ivatury RR, Nassoura ZE, Simon RJ, and others: Complex duodenal injuries, *Surg Clin North Am* 76:797, 1996.

Patton JH, Fabian TC: Complex pancreatic injuries, *Surg Clin North Am* 76:783, 1996.

Patton JH, Lyden SP, Croce MA, and others: Pancreatic trauma: A simplified management guideline, *J Trauma* 43:234, 1997.

Injuries to the Small and Large Bowel

J. David Richardson, MD

Most recent series of blunt trauma patients have an incidence of bowel injuries of 1% to 5%. Although seat belts and air bags have been dramatically effective in preventing many types of serious injuries caused by motor vehicle crashes, the incidence of bowel injuries has not diminished (and may have actually increased) with their use. The incidence of bowel injuries in penetrating trauma of the anterior abdomen varies greatly depending on the location of the injury, type of wounding agent, trajectory of the injury, and body habitus of the victim. Penetrating wounds to the flank and back may result in bowel injuries, and historically it has been taught that any gunshot wound below the nipples should have consideration for abdominal penetration that could result in an injury to the bowel.

The conundrum for the clinician managing potential or suspected bowel injury involves several generally accepted premises: (1) the treatment of small and large bowel injuries is generally straightforward if diagnosed promptly; (2) however, there is no single diagnostic test, maneuver, or algorithm that is totally accurate in confirming or excluding these injuries, except laparotomy; but (3) routine laparotomy, even in patients with a high index of suspicion for bowel injury, is often nontherapeutic and carries considerable ongoing morbidity when negative.

Thus surgeons caring for trauma patients should not be deluded into believing there is only one "standard of care" in the diagnostic evaluation of such patients. Time-honored methods such as clinical judgment and maintaining a high index of suspicion augmented by other diagnostic tests will usually be required.

DIAGNOSIS ON BLUNT INJURIES

The diagnosis of intra-abdominal injury on the basis of traditional clinical evaluation is fraught with problems, and the specificity of physical examinations alone is rarely greater than that obtained by a coin toss. Alcohol intoxication, illicit drug use, and head injuries may obscure physical findings. Many seriously injured patients are chemically paralyzed and intubated in the field and are not able to actively participate in an abdominal examination. Patients may have abdominal tenderness, mimicking peritoneal signs, which is elicited on physical examination because of associated rib or pelvic fractures or because of abdominal wall contusion or hematomas despite an absence of intraperitoneal injuries. There are several associated signs that should alert the clinician to assess the patient for blunt intestinal injury. These include abdominal wall ecchymoses (lap belt sign), Chance's fracture with lumbar spine hyperflexion, unexplained hyperamylasemia, leukocytosis, and an unexplained base deficit. Given the prevalence of nonoperative management of many solid-organ injuries and the difficulty of diagnosing blunt intestinal injuries, various diagnostic adjuncts are required to aid in the assessment of these patients.

The most commonly used diagnostic modality for patients with blunt abdominal trauma is computed tomography (CT) scanning. Late-generation scanners allow for high-resolution imaging of the bowel and mesentery. Although studies have compared the attenuation coefficients (Hounsfield units) of fluid within abdomen and noted that blood and small-bowel contents have different attenuation levels (average of 45 HU and 10 HU-20 HU, respectively), we have not found such information helpful in our trauma unit. If the patient has lower attenuation fluid, one must be concerned about the possibility of extravasation of enteric contents. However, if the patient has blood in the abdomen without solid organ injury, that blood could come from a devascularizing mesenteric injury that renders the bowel ischemic with delayed perforation. Additionally, bowel perforations may lead to a mixture of blood and enteric contents, confounding the use of attenuation coefficients. We have an extremely high index of suspicion for any diagnostic abnormality (even subtle ones) of the bowel manifested on CT scans (Table 1). If the patient has pneumoperitoneum or contrast extravasation, the decision for operative treatment is straightforward, but, in fact, these clear-cut findings are rather unusual. More commonly, subtle signs are present. In our unit, subtle signs of bowel or mesenteric injury generally are evaluated further by an operation. The risk life-threatening peritonitis resulting from delayed diagnosis is so great that we feel operation is justified. Depending on the clinical setting, diagnostic laparoscopy or exploratory celiotomy is performed. If laparoscopy is chosen, one must be careful to inspect the viscera carefully, and evaluation of the small bowel is mandatory. If the abdomen is pristine and no fluid or edema of the bowel is noted, then the procedure is terminated. Even a subtle finding on laparoscopy mandates a celiotomy.

The management of free fluid in patients without evidence of solid-organ injury on CT scan is even more controversial. The question the clinician must answer is whether this free fluid represents succus or intestinal contents or blood from a mesenteric injury that

Table 1: Small or Large Bowel Injury: Diagnostic Abnormality of CT Scans

- Fluid in abdomen
- Bowel wall thickening or edema
- Edema or thickening of mesentery
- Pneumoperitoneum
- Contrast extravasation

CT, Computed tomography.

could devitalize the intestine. There are several options in this clinical scenario because free intraperitoneal fluid is not always associated with a bowel injury requiring treatment. These options include continued observation, especially if the patient is able to cooperate with a physical examination, repeat CT scanning, diagnostic peritoneal lavage (DPL), diagnostic laparoscopy, or exploratory celiotomy. Brownstein and colleagues reported in 2000 on practice patterns of trauma surgeons gleaned from a survey of members of the American Association of the Surgery of Trauma. A minority indicated that they would perform DPL in patients with free fluid and alterations in levels of consciousness even though DPL is frequently recommended on algorithms for management of suspected small bowel injury.

If patients are unable to be evaluated by physical examination and have free fluid as the only CT finding, our practice has been to perform some type of invasive diagnostic "test." That test may be DPL, diagnostic laparoscopy, or celiotomy, depending on the clinical scenario.

Even though DPL is used only occasionally in our trauma unit, it is still a valuable tool in some clinical circumstances if applied and interpreted correctly. If a surgeon is to rely on DPL for the evaluation of bowel injuries, certain caveats should be considered. The erythrocyte (red blood cell) count (RBC) is probably less important than the leukocyte count. In the past, when the RBC count was used to diagnose solid-organ injury, it was the value that seemed most important. However, extravasation of enteric contacts should produce an intraperitoneal inflammatory response manifested by an elevated leukocyte count in the recovered lavage fluid. It is mandatory that the effluent be examined for an increased leukocyte count. The value of 500 leukocytes per mm^3 of fluid is the traditional number used to define an elevated count. Second, the experimental studies of Root and associates on DPL demonstrated that several hours of exposure to enteric contents were necessary to elicit an inflammatory peritoneal response. Therefore DPL studies performed immediately following injury could produce a false-negative leukocyte count. The third area in which a potentially false-negative DPL could occur is with a mesenteric vascular injury that renders the bowel wall ischemic. A DPL performed several hours following injury could demonstrate a mildly increased RBC count resulting from minor bleeding from the vascular injury and fail to demonstrate an increased leukocyte count because the bowel wall had not yet become sufficiently ischemic to incite a peritoneal reaction. Our unit recently treated an intubated, head-injured patient with a "negative" DPL performed for free fluid on CT in the absence of a solid-organ injury. Twenty hours later the patient exhibited leukocytosis to 24,000 and a mild base deficit with a soft abdomen on physical examination. Celiotomy disclosed an 18-cm segment of necrotic jejunum secondary to a mesenteric injury that devitalized the intestine. The patient had a complicated postoperative course secondary to the delay in diagnosis. Such cases illustrate the fact that there is no single diagnostic test or approach, short of celiotomy, that is uniformly used to exclude bowel injuries.

The use of diagnostic ultrasound has gained widespread acceptance for the evaluation of blunt abdominal trauma. Our unit employs the focused abdominal ultrasound examination routinely in blunt trauma patients. However, we have found its role in the evaluation of bowel injuries to be limited. Surgeons not experienced in the technique would certainly not be able to use it on a sporadic basis, even with radiologic consultation, to make decisions about bowel injuries.

Although the earlier discussion has focused on the presence of free fluid on CT in the absence of solid organ injury, bowel injuries occur with regularity in patients with solid organ injuries. The incidence of small bowel injury in patients with blunt hepatic trauma is approximately 2% to 8%. Isolated splenic injury has a lower, albeit real, association of intestinal injuries. Virtually every large series of solid-organ injuries treated nonoperatively will have a few patients with intestinal injuries in whom the diagnosis was made in a delayed manner. These delays almost always result in increased morbidity and may result in mortality. For this reason, blind reliance on a "negative" CT scan is not appropriate, and a high index of suspicion must be maintained in patients who exhibit any features other than the expected course with nonoperative treatment. Finally, a surgeon should not apologize for using an operation as the ultimate diagnostic test in patients with such worrisome features after blunt trauma.

PENETRATING INJURIES

All discussions on the diagnostic or therapeutic approach to penetrating abdominal trauma must be initiated by an acknowledgment of the pivotal role of hemodynamic instability in the decision analysis for patients with those injuries. Patients with truncal penetrating trauma who are hemodynamically unstable should be transported to the operating suite on an emergent basis. In such patients, ancillary diagnostic studies are usually not feasible. Stable patients may be able to undergo appropriate diagnostic tests depending on the mechanisms of injury and the likelihood of sustaining serious injury. In our unit, patients with gunshot wounds thought to have entered the peritoneal cavity are rapidly evaluated with a goal of urgent operation even if they are hemodynamically stable.

Many clinicians tend to lump all penetrating wounds into a broad category for diagnostic purposes, but we distinguish wounds according to the mechanism of injury (e.g., stab wounds vs. gunshot wounds). Our unit practices selective management of patients with stab wounds liberally, but we are much more likely to practice routine exploration for most patients with gunshot wounds thought to have entered the peritoneal cavity. As with blunt trauma, there is no single gold standard for the evaluation of patients with penetrating wounds.

In patients with stab wounds, there are several elements of the history that aid in the diagnostic evaluation, including type of weapon, blade length, number of injuries, and location of entrance wounds. Patients who have peritoneal signs or evisceration of bowel on omentum should undergo celiotomy. Patients who are alert and able to be clinically evaluated by physical examination may be followed by serial examinations. In trauma centers or teaching hospitals at which there are several experienced surgeons to evaluate the abdomen, it is often difficult to perform timely serial examinations if the unit is busy and surgeons have multiple patients requiring urgent attention. In a nontrauma center or hospital at which surgical coverage may be more limited, serial physical examinations may not be practical. In such scenarios a more active diagnostic approach may be prudent.

Local wound exploration may be used to determine whether there is fascial penetration, which would heighten the concern for possible visceral injury. DPL has been advocated as a means of detecting abdominal penetration. If DPL is used, there is no standard of what constitutes a "positive" cell count, particularly for erythrocytes. Generally, low counts, in the range of 5000 to 10,000, are "positive" because an intestinal injury could occur and result in very little blood loss within the abdomen. Our unit formerly used DPL regularly for penetrating wounds but now does so infrequently. Likewise, we have not found a role for ultrasound examinations in the routine evaluations of penetrating abdominal trauma.

Diagnostic laparoscopy is used frequently for several types of penetrating trauma, whether from stab or gunshot wounds. Laparoscopy can usually determine whether the peritoneal cavity has been entered. It is particularly useful for thoracoabdominal wounds and some flank wounds to assess the presence of injuries and avoid unnecessary celiotomy. However, because retroperitoneal injuries may occur with some flank and many back wounds, detection of these injuries by laparoscopy may be difficult. The evaluation of back wounds and most flank wounds is initiated by CT scanning. With left-sided wounds, triple-contrast CT is accurate for the assessment of colon injuries.

TREATMENT OF SMALL BOWEL INJURIES

If a small bowel injury is detected at laparoscopy, I recommend a celiotomy to thoroughly assess the entire small bowel. Full-thickness wounds to the intestinal wall should be closed, preferably with sutures. A single layer of nonabsorbable sutures placed in a horizontal manner by the Lembert technique is acceptable. I prefer a two-layer closure with an inner layer of absorbable sutures and an outer layer of 3-0 nonabsorbable seromuscular sutures to invert the closed mucosa. Although this is a time-honored method, there are no data in humans in clinical situations that demonstrate the superiority of one technique over another. I do not recommend stapled closure on anastomosis of the small bowel in trauma patients. Whereas such techniques are clearly safe in elective cases, they may be less reliable in situations with severe bowel edema.

Some clinical papers have indicated a high failure rate with stapled repairs in patients with bowel edema. Because resuscitation may be necessary in trauma patients, I recommend suture repair.

One question that frequently arises in celiotomy for blunt trauma is whether to oversew areas of bruising of the small bowel (grade I small bowel injury in the American Association for the Surgery of Trauma grading system). I recommend oversewing such injuries. Undoubtedly, the conversion of "bruises" to full-thickness perforations is an uncommon event. However, experienced trauma surgeons can frequently recount an instance in which a patient with a "negative" celiotomy developed peritonitis secondary to an intestinal injury several days after operation. Rather than postulate a "missed" injury, I suspect that some contusions undergo full-thickness bowel wall ischemia and perforate. It would be impossible to prove the negative, that is, that suture imbrication prevented such occurrences, but imbrication is rapid and relative risk free.

If multiple perforations are present, the surgeon's judgment must dictate whether to close individual holes by enterorrhaphy or to resect the area of perforations and perform a primary anastomosis. Factors influencing this judgment might include number of perforations, circumference of bowel wall involved, amount of intestine removed by resection, and degree of mesenteric injury. Multiple wounds that are in close proximity are usually treated by resection and reanastomosis with the two-layer suture technique. Large circumferential defects can usually be closed primarily in the small bowel by horizontal enterorrhaphy. Small-bowel narrowing of 50% is certainly well tolerated, and some surgeons suggest that even 30% of remaining lumen is satisfactory.

Mesenteric injuries are occasionally problematic and may present the surgeon with no option that is satisfactory. Some mesenteric defects can be closed to prevent internal bowel herniation with little fear of compromising intestinal viability. If there is any evidence of ischemia, the bowel should be resected and anastomosed primarily. Major bleeding from the mesentery can usually be temporarily controlled with digital compression and then by clamping or oversewing bleeding vessels. Large, mesenteric hematomas may be particularly problematic. Should these be left intact or opened? Does the presence of a large hematoma mandate bowel resection? If the hematoma is small and nonexpanding, it should probably be left intact. Expanding hematomas should be opened, and bleeding vessels controlled. Occasionally, a large hematoma is present that is not closely associated with the bowel. If it is at the base of the mesentery and is not expanding, I generally do not open it. When the hematoma extends to the medial intestinal wall, it is imperative that a perforation be excluded.

The prognosis of small bowel wounds is generally excellent if these injuries are detected and repaired promptly. Statistically, it is difficult to detect a difference in outcome among patients with a single, small perforation closed primarily and those with multiple holes requiring a bowel resection. This reemphasizes the crucial nature of early diagnosis and repair.

MANAGEMENT OF COLONIC INJURIES

The options for treatment of colonic wounds are outlined in Table 2. The evolutionary nature of primary repair is worth noting. Military experience in World War II mandated colostomy for virtually all colon wounds, and this was transferred to civilian experience. A few surgeons advocated primary repair for most civilian colon injuries. Studies then demonstrated the safety of primary repair in the absence of shock, operative delay, major blood loss, and heavy fecal contamination. Subsequently, even the majority of these circumstances were not felt to be a contraindication to primary repair. Further advances have been made in the area of resection and primary anastomosis. Reconstruction was initially practiced safely with right-colon injuries, and a randomized study and nonrandomized experiences have shown that left-colon wounds can be repaired safely as well.

The necrotic edges of wounds to be primarily closed should be excised beforehand. Wounds near the mesentery must be adequately visualized to ensure that all of their margins can be examined and securely closed. I close larger defects in two layers when feasible and generally perform a single-layer closure for smaller defects.

In our unit, most right-sided injuries are reconstructed by an ileocolostomy if primary repair is not feasible. It is always beneficial to avoid an ileostomy, with its large fluid loss, in addition to other benefits associated with primary repair. We perform left-colon reconstruction when technically feasible in stable patients. Several trauma units have consistently extended the indications for resection and reconstruction and avoidance of an ostomy. However, several recent experiences have suggested it may be advantageous to consider colostomy in the patient who is badly injured and not fully resuscitated. This has been my personal experience and recommendation. A recent report also showed a high failure rate of suture-line closure from transverse colon wounds treated by immediate reconstruction, attributable to a less consistent blood supply in this area.

Several studies in the literature are important to note in considering a strategy for management of destructive colon wounds that require either colostomy or reanastomosis following resection. Miller proposed that patients with risk factors consisting of blood transfusion greater than 5 units and major comorbidity receive an ostomy, whereas all others should undergo primary repair or reconstruction. Under these criteria, only 7% of patients required ostomy. A nonrandomized trial by American Association for the Surgery of Trauma members included 297 patients with 197 colon wounds treated by resection and reanastomosis. Eighty-four of

these (42%) involved the left colon. The authors noted that patients with severe fecal contamination, greater than 4 units of blood transfused, and single-agent antibiotic therapy had higher complications. However, the method of management of the colon injury itself was not related to outcome.

Because the study was nonrandomized, it is difficult to discern patient factors that prompted one operation to be chosen over another. Much has been made of the morbidity of colostomy takedown and reconstruction, but relatively little has been written about the morbidity and potential mortality from the creation of the stoma itself. Although stoma creation has been advocated as the "safest" approach in some patients, the formation of an ostomy may be difficult in obese patients. A short, thick mesentery and thick abdominal wall may pose extreme difficulties in ostomy creation. Necrotic ostomy from vascular compromise may predispose to necrotizing fasciitis or intra-abdominal abscess. The risks of ostomy creation and takedown must be balanced against that of primary reconstruction, particularly in the obese. In patients with central obesity who require a colostomy, which might be difficult to create, the use of a left-transverse colostomy may be helpful.

There are some associated injuries in which it may be preferable to avoid a primary repair or reconstruction. If the risk of failure of repair of an injury compromises the repair of another, a colostomy remote from the area of the second repair might be useful. A pancreatic wound in proximity to a primary colon repair might lead to suture-line failure if an amylase-rich fistula develops. A left-side colon reconstruction adjacent to a reconstructed left iliac artery and vein might place the vascular repair at considerable risk if the colon anastomosis leaks. It is difficult to prove the relative dangers inherent in these judgments, but an occasional anecdotal case has suggested that these situations should be avoided.

INTESTINAL INJURIES IN DAMAGE-CONTROL CELIOTOMY

The concept of the damage-control celiotomy, which was initially applied primarily to liver injuries, has been extended to a variety of traumatic wounds, many of which may involve intestinal disruption. If hemodynamic instability or coagulopathy renders the patient a poor candidate for definitive operation, there are several methods of temporization of intestinal injuries. Injuries may be rapidly closed via suture or staples with definitive, more secure repair at a later time. Devastating injuries may be resected with the bowel ends left stapled. The timing of definitive closure, intestinal reconstruction,

Table 2: Options for Treatment of Colonic Wounds

Treatment Method	Indication	Comment
Primary repair, colorrhaphy	Used to treat most wounds less than 50% of bowel circumference, even when multiple.	Shown to be safe in most conditions associated with trauma.
Exteriorization of repair	The repair itself is brought externally to the abdominal cavity to observe its healing before return to abdomen in 3–5 days.	Primarily of historical interest. It is difficult to envision clinical circumstances that would dictate its use.
Colostomy	This was mandated treatment for military wounds from World War II to recently; used for civilian wounds as "standard of care" until 1980s; still useful in irreparable or devastating wounds and in patients with shock, large blood loss, or heavy contamination (or both).	Whereas primary repair has emerged as the dominant treatment, colostomy is still a frequently performed operation at busy trauma units; usually chosen for patients with shock, increased blood transfusion, major associated injuries, or major contamination (or a combination of these factors).
Colostomy proximal to resection/anastomosis	Not standard practice but might be useful for distal colorectal reconstruction.	Judgment decision for surgeon; no data to support widespread use in trauma.
Primary resection/ reanastomosis	Now used in appropriate clinical circumstances in right- and left-sided injuries.	Nonrandomized data suggest it can be safely applied in many patients.

or ostomy formation depends on clinical circumstances such as proper resuscitation and reversal of coagulopathy. It is our goal to deal with the intestinal problems within 24 to 48 hours. Several recent reports have indicated that a patient can have intestinal reconstruction performed immediately at the initial reoperation if he or she is well resuscitated and the bowel is not overly edematous.

Although some reports suggest all colon wounds can be primarily repaired by colorrhaphy or anastomosis following resection, caution should be taken when attempting aggressive reconstruction in patients with major injuries and shock.

RECTAL INJURIES

Rectal wounds occur less frequently than intra-abdominal intestinal injuries. Mechanism of injuries may include penetrating trauma, impalement injuries, and blunt trauma. The diagnosis is made by proctosigmoidoscopic examination in patients with a suspicious mechanism of injury or by the presence of blood on rectal examination.

Patients with intraperitoneal rectal injuries can generally have primary repair along guidelines similar to that for left-colon wounds. Generally, extraperitoneal wounds diagnosed by sigmoidoscopy are difficult to repair primarily, and opening of retrosacral hematomas is not recommended. If the defect can be identified and closed primarily with minimal dissection, this may be advantageous to subsequent reconstruction. Low-lying rectal injuries can often be repaired transrectally and should be attempted in stable patients.

Complete diversion is indicated in most extraperitoneal rectal wounds. Diversion may be accomplished by end colostomy with Hartmann's pouch creation or by a loop colostomy with a stapled distal segment. Historically, the literature advised that presacral, retrorectal drainage be used in all rectal injuries to prevent the development of an abscess in the area (or at least to provide egress for purulence, should it occur). This was accomplished by performing a curvilinear incision between the tip of the coccyx and anus and attempting to enter the presacral space from which drains were brought out. After many years in trauma practice, I came to doubt the necessity and wisdom of this approach and abandoned it as a routine. Subsequent studies have come to similar conclusions. Another tenet of management of rectal injuries was that stool in the rectum should be removed and a rectal "washout" performed. There were no data to suggest the value of this approach at its inception, and none has been produced in subsequent decades. On the other hand, it is difficult to conceive how this question could be the subject of a randomized trial. If the patient is stable and in the operating room, surgeons in our unit may perform a rectal washout, but it is not considered mandatory.

SUGGESTED READINGS

Brownstein MR, Bunting T, Meyer AA, and others: Diagnosis and management of blunt small bowel injury: a survey of the membership of the American Association for the Surgery of Trauma, *J Trauma* 48:402, 2000.

Brundage SI, Jurkovich GJ, Hoyt DB, and others: Stapled versus suture gastrointestinal anastomosis in the trauma patient: a multicenter trial, *J Trauma* 51:1054, 2001.

Chappuis CW, Frey DJ, Dietzen CD, and others: Management of penetrating colon injuries. A prospective randomized trial, *Ann Surg* 213:492, 1991.

Demetriades D, Murray JA, Chan L, and others: Penetrating colon injuries requiring resection: diversion or primary anastomosis? An AAST prospective multicenter study, *J Trauma* 50:765, 2001.

Dente CJ, Patel A, Feliciano DV, and others: Suture line failure in intra-abdominal colonic trauma: is there an effect of segmental variations in blood supply on outcome? *J Trauma* 59:358, 2005.

Gonzalez RP, Falimirski ME, Holevar MR: The role of presacral drainage in the management of penetrating rectal injuries, *J Trauma* 45:656, 1998.

Miller PR, Fabian TC, Croce MA, and others: Improving outcomes following penetrating colon wounds: application of a clinical pathway, *Ann Surg* 235:775, 2002.

Sasaki LS, Allaben RD, Golwala R, and others: Primary repair of colon injuries: a prospective randomized study, *J Trauma* 39:895, 1995.

RECTAL INJURIES

Jordan A. Weinberg, MD, and Timothy C. Fabian, MD

The management of traumatic rectal wounds evolved from wartime surgical experience, particularly during World War II and the Vietnam War. The principles of rectal wound management advocated by military surgeons included mandatory colostomy; repair of the wound, when possible; distal rectal washout (lavage of the rectum); and drainage of the retrorectal space. As experience with the management of these injuries has increased in civilian practice, the relative value of each of these principles has been challenged, resulting in variations in management from surgeon to surgeon and institution to institution. In this chapter, we present our approach to the diagnosis and management of rectal injuries.

ETIOLOGY

Owing to its relatively well-protected position in the bony pelvis, the rectum is an uncommonly injured viscus. The majority of traumatic rectal injuries are the result of a penetrating mechanism: primarily gunshot wounds and, less often, stab wounds. In our most recently reported experience with penetrating rectal injuries, 96% were a result of gunshot wounds. Injury may also occur as a result of blunt mechanism in the setting of pelvic fracture, usually as a result of bone shards lacerating the rectum, or transrectal impalement with a blunt instrument, often in the setting of assault.

DIAGNOSIS

The recognition of a rectal injury requires a high degree of diagnostic vigilance on the part of the surgeon. Any patient with a penetrating wound to the groin, perineum, buttock, or upper thigh should be evaluated for rectal injury. Digital examination for the presence of rectal blood is mandatory, but the absence of blood does not rule out injury. Rigid proctoscopy should be performed whenever there is suspicion of rectal injury, even when the digital rectal examination is negative. The rectal injury may be well visualized with the proctoscope, but visualization is often obscured by stool or blood (or both) in the rectal vault. Identification of blood, however, confirms the diagnosis of rectal laceration in the setting of penetrating injury. Thus visualization of the injury itself is not essential. Computed tomography and contrast enema have been recommended by others as additional diagnostic tests for equivocal cases. It has been our experience that such investigations are cumbersome and unrewarding. In the case of an equivocal rectal injury, it is best to assume the presence of injury and manage the patient accordingly.

TREATMENT

It has become our practice to classify rectal injuries according to anatomic criteria, which then direct management decisions. The anatomy of the rectum is notable for variation in the pattern of serosalization (Fig. 1). The anterior and lateral sidewalls of the upper two thirds of the rectum are serosalized, and injury in this region is classified as intraperitoneal. The upper two thirds of the rectum posteriorly and the lower one third circumferentially are not serosalized, and injury in this region is classified as extraperitoneal. Furthermore, distinction may be made between proximal extraperitoneal injuries, which involve the nonserosalized posterior aspect of the rectum proximal to the peritoneal fold, and distal extraperitoneal injuries, which are relatively more difficult to expose from an abdominal approach. Our clinical pathway for the management of rectal injury according to anatomic criteria is presented in Figure 2.

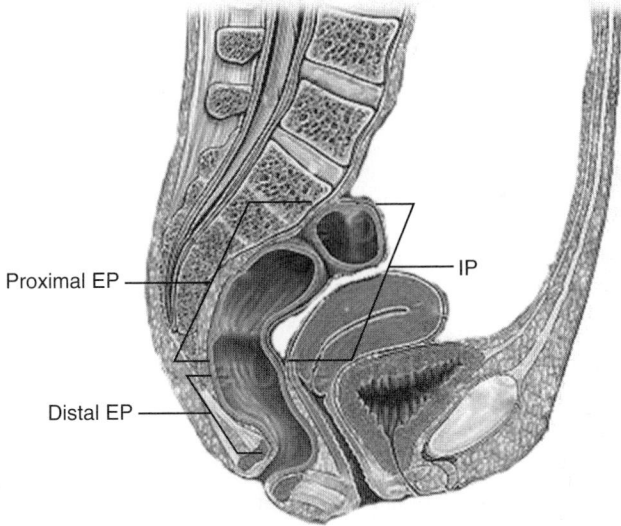

Figure 1 Intraperitoneal (IP) and extraperitoneal (EP) divisions of the rectum.

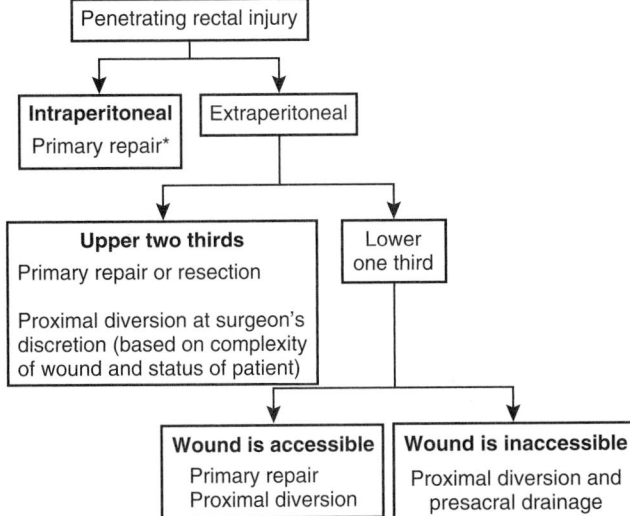

Figure 2 Clinical pathway for the management of penetrating rectal injury at the University of Tennessee Health Science Center, Memphis, Tennessee. *Primary repair is performed for nondestructive wounds or destructive wounds in the absence of blood transfusion >6 units or medical comorbidities. Otherwise, resection and colostomy are performed.

Intraperitoneal Wounds

Wounds to the intraperitoneal rectum are essentially no different than colon wounds and are managed similarly. In the absence of significant tissue loss or devascularization of the bowel segment, primary repair may be safely performed. It is our practice to close these wounds in two layers, using a full-thickness running absorbable suture followed by interrupted silk seromuscular sutures. Colostomy is not performed. In the presence of significant tissue loss or devascularization of the bowel segment, resection of the injured segment is generally required. The decision to then proceed with anastomosis versus colostomy is determined by the condition of the patient. Should the patient be in shock, require a transfusion greater than 6 units, or have an underlying medical comorbidity such as diabetes or liver disease, colostomy is recommended. This is easily accomplished with end colostomy and rectal stump closure (Hartmann's procedure), but anastomosis with proximal loop colostomy is an acceptable alternative. In the absence of such comorbidity, anastomosis without diversion may be performed, although this scenario is encountered infrequently because destructive rectal wounds are often associated with significant blood loss, given the proximity of large vessels.

If a solitary rectal gunshot wound is encountered, it is important to consider the presence of an associated wound (to complete the "through-and-through" type of injury). Although a solitary proximal rectal gunshot wound may truly be tangential (or the projectile may be intraluminal), a distal extraperitoneal wound is often present. Following repair of the intraperitoneal wound, if a distal wound cannot be ruled out with certainty, its presence should be assumed, and management should then be directed toward the extraperitoneal wound as described later.

Proximal Extraperitoneal Wounds

Wounds involving the proximal extraperitoneal rectum are generally amenable to exposure and repair with a limited amount of rectal dissection. Such wounds are often intraperitoneal with extension into the proximal extraperitoneal rectum or, less often, exclusively extraperitoneal but evident from a mesorectal hematoma. Primary repair of these injuries is recommended, with a two-layer technique as described earlier. Proximal diversion may be performed at the surgeon's discretion, taking into account the relative complexity of the repair and the patient's general condition. Destructive extraperitoneal wounds require diversion and are usually managed with Hartmann's procedure.

Distal Extraperitoneal Wounds

Wounds to the lower third of the rectum may present a difficult challenge, given the relative difficulty of exposure in the pelvis, which is often fat laden and, in males, narrow. For cases with favorable anatomy, dissection may be performed relatively easily and safely to allow identification and repair of the rectal wound. Often, however, unfavorable anatomy and anatomic distortion from the injury preclude safe exposure, risking injury to the associated neurovascular and genitourinary structures.

It has been well demonstrated that low-velocity, extraperitoneal rectal wounds may be managed without repair; good results have been achieved with proximal diversion and drainage of the retrorectal space alone. Diversion is often most easily achieved with the construction of a loop sigmoid colostomy. Care should be taken to ensure that the loop of colon is tension free to avoid postoperative stoma complications. To achieve complete fecal diversion with the loop construction, it is important that the posterior wall of the loop be maintained above the level of the skin. This is accomplished primarily by avoiding tension on the loop but also by the placement of a Silastic rod or red rubber catheter to support the loop. Drainage of the retrorectal space (presacral drain placement) is performed with the patient in the lithotomy position (Fig. 3). A curvilinear incision is made in the

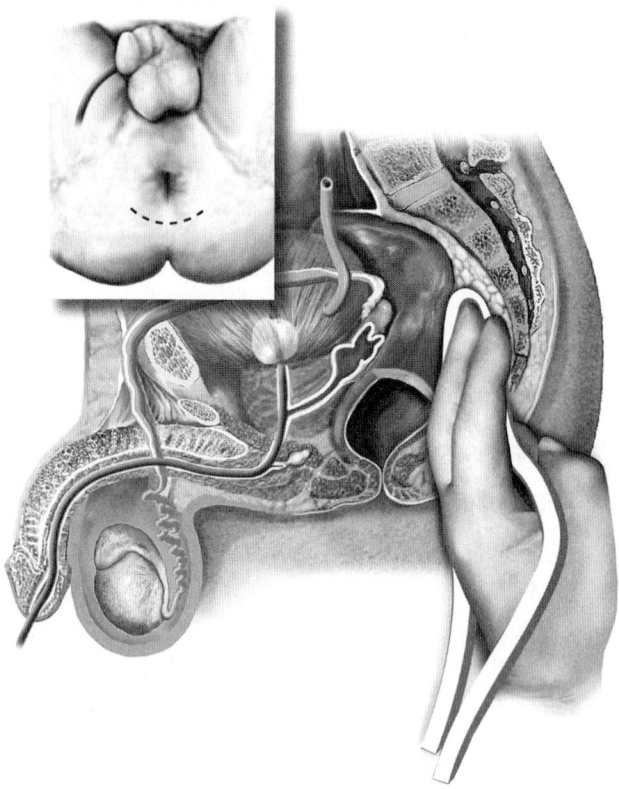

Figure 3 Access to the presacral space is provided through a curved incision midway between the anus and the tip of the coccyx. With blunt dissection, two fingers are inserted between the rectum and the hollow of the sacrum. A Penrose drain is inserted and sutured to the skin. *Reproduced from Weinberg JA, Fabian TC: Injuries to the stomach, small bowel, colon, and rectum. In Souba WW, Fink MP, Jurkovich GJ, and others, editors: ACS surgery: principles and practice, New York, NY, 2005, WebMD.*

skin between the coccyx and anus, and blunt dissection is employed to penetrate Waldeyer's fascia and gain entry into the presacral space. A 1–inch-diameter Penrose drain is then placed in this space and gradually withdrawn between postoperative days 5 and 7.

The efficacy of presacral drain placement has been challenged. There are published prospective data from Gonzalez and colleagues to suggest that drainage does not lessen morbidity; however, their study did not make a distinction between wounds that were exposed and repaired versus those that were not, and it was also statistically underpowered. It is our contention that presacral drainage should be performed selectively. For inaccessible extraperitoneal wounds, presacral drainage is recommended to prevent retroperitoneal abscess formation, which results from fecal contamination of a relatively closed space and can produce significant morbidity in the form of retroperitoneal infection (discussed later). Accessible extraperitoneal wounds that are explored and repaired become effectively intraperitonealized, and presacral drainage is not required for these injuries.

Wounds that are confined to the anterior portion of the distal rectum will not benefit from the creation of a posterior outflow tract via presacral drain placement. Precise localization of the wounds, however, is often difficult, as described earlier, and it is prudent to assume the presence of a posterior wound unless visualization with proctoscopy is excellent.

Distal Rectal Washout

Distal rectal washout involves lavage of the distal rectum in an attempt to decontaminate the injured portion (Fig. 4). Typically, 3 to 6 liters of irrigant is flushed through the distal limb of a loop

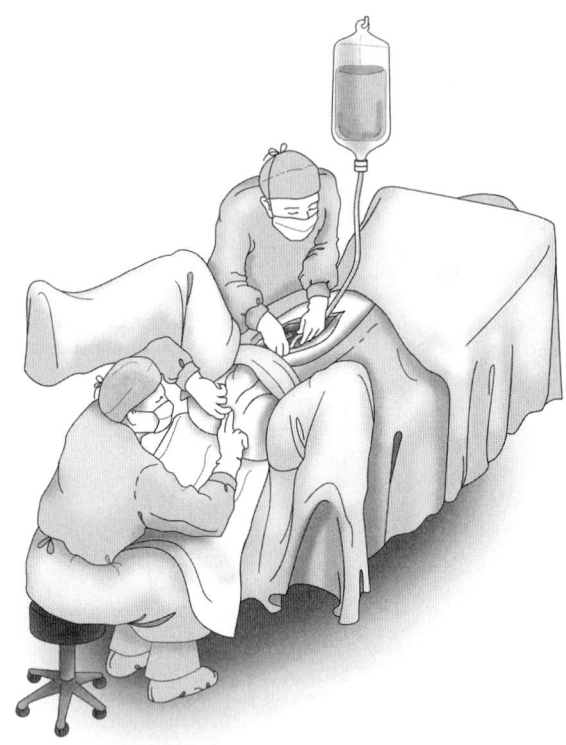

Figure 4 Distal rectal washout. *Reproduced from Burch JM, Feliciano DV, Mattox KL: Ann Surg 209:600, 1989.*

colostomy. The irrigant may be saline or an antiseptic solution. Digital rectal dilatation is simultaneously performed by an assistant to facilitate drainage of the irrigant. Although advocated on the basis of salutary experience from the Vietnam War, the reports of civilian experience have not demonstrated any effect on outcome, and distal rectal washout is no longer practiced routinely by most surgeons, including our group. It may still have utility, however, for severe wounds from high-velocity, military-type firearms or explosives.

Anorectal Trauma

Wounds of the anal sphincter complex or distal rectum (or both) may result from transpelvic gunshot wounds but are often associated with sexual assault or erotic misadventure. Uncomplicated lacerations of the anus are often amenable to suture repair alone, but more extensive wounds likely benefit from proximal diversion as well. Assault by transanal penetration with a blunt object may result in full-thickness proximal rectal injury; these injuries are identified by physical examination and proctoscopy and are managed according to the guidelines described earlier.

Colostomy Closure

If colostomy is performed, it will eventually become the preference of most patients to have reversal performed. We typically perform colostomy reversal 2 to 3 months after hospital discharge to allow time for the resolution of the dense inflammatory adhesions that form following laparotomy. Before the procedure, a contrast enema is obtained to confirm that the rectum has healed without complication. Some have recommended early closure (within 2 weeks) over the traditional interval, reporting a shorter operating time and less intraoperative blood loss. To date, however, this practice has not garnered enthusiasm among most practicing surgeons.

COMPLICATIONS

Although reported complications following rectal wound management include intra-abdominal abscess, wound infection, and necrotizing abdominal wall infection, the only major complication that is directly attributable to a rectal injury (as opposed to other associated injuries) is retrorectal infection. Often identified by computed tomography during the course of an evaluation of postoperative fever, the infection may present as a relatively simple presacral abscess, amenable to percutaneous drainage, or a more complex retroperitoneal abscess that may even track downward into the thighs. With such complex infections, the patient often is septic, requiring resuscitation, monitoring in the intensive care unit, and operative drainage. It has been our experience that such morbid retroperitoneal sepsis has occurred exclusively in cases of distal extraperitoneal injury managed by diversion alone. It is our bias that the presence of a presacral drain allows for an outflow tract, precluding the occurrence of a potentially disastrous closed-space infection and resulting in, at worst, a drain tract infection requiring drain manipulation and irrigation.

Suggested Readings

Burch JM, Feliciano DV, Mattox KL: Colostomy and drainage for civilian rectal injuries: is that all? *Ann Surg* 209:600, 1989.

Gonzalez RP, Falimirski ME, Holevar MR: The role of presacral drainage in the management of penetrating rectal injuries, *J Trauma* 45:656, 1998.

Lavenson GS, Cohen A: Management of rectal injuries, *Am J Surg* 122:226, 1971.

Weinberg JA, Fabian TC, Magnotti LJ, and others: Penetrating rectal trauma: management by anatomic distinction improves outcome, *J Trauma* 60:508, 2006.

Injury to the Spleen

Rebecca D. Edmonds, MD, and
Andrew B. Peitzman, MD

INTRODUCTION

The spleen is the most commonly injured intra-abdominal organ in patients with blunt-trauma injuries. More than 90% of cases result from a blunt mechanism, with motor vehicle collisions accounting for 58% of splenic injuries. Penetrating injuries are much less common, accounting for 7% of splenic injuries. Patients with injury to the spleen from blunt mechanism should be managed on the basis of their hemodynamic status, classified as follows: (1) Patients are hemodynamically normal (never hypotensive or tachycardic), (2) responsive (one or two episodes of tachycardia or hypotension but vital signs are normalized with fluid resuscitation), or (3) unstable (hypotensive or tachycardic patients who do not respond or transiently respond to fluid resuscitation).

DIAGNOSIS

The diagnosis of splenic injuries relies on a high index of suspicion on the basis of the mechanism of injury. Although history and physical examination are neither sensitive nor specific, there are a number of findings that should raise suspicion for splenic injury. Patients may complain of either generalized abdominal pain or pain that localizes to the left upper quadrant. The presence of subdiaphragmatic blood may cause pain referred to the left shoulder (Kehr's sign). Lower-left rib fractures (ribs 9 through 12) are associated with splenic injuries in 20% to 25% of adult patients.

Because of the lack of sensitivity and specificity of physical examination, additional diagnostic studies are usually necessary to diagnose splenic injury. The choice of study is guided by the patient's hemodynamic status. Patients with tachycardia or hypotension refractory to fluid challenge (unstable patients) are treated using a different algorithm from that used for patients with normal heart rate and blood pressure. The presence of peritonitis, significant abdominal tenderness, or a distended abdomen in a patient with unstable vital signs warrants immediate laparotomy. If the etiology of hypovolemia is uncertain, rapid evaluation of the abdomen in the trauma bay to assess for hemoperitoneum is mandatory. Focused assessment for the sonographic evaluation of the trauma patient (FAST) or diagnostic peritoneal lavage (DPL) can be rapidly performed at the bedside to detect the presence of hemoperitoneum. FAST is an excellent screening tool in patients with blunt-trauma injuries. In the unstable patient, a positive FAST will validate the necessity for prompt laparotomy. In an unstable patient, an indeterminate or negative FAST should be followed by DPL. In patients with normal hemodynamics, computed tomography (CT) is the study of choice for diagnosis of solid visceral injury.

FAST is an ultrasound examination of the abdomen performed at the bedside to assess for the presence of free intraperitoneal fluid. Sagittal views of Morison's pouch and the splenorenal recess and a transverse view of the pelvis are obtained. Free fluid, which presumably represents hemoperitoneum, appears anechoic compared with adjacent structures. FAST is widely used because it can be performed rapidly and has a sensitivity of 70% for diagnosing the presence of hemoperitoneum. However, FAST does not diagnose injury to a specific organ. Its usefulness is limited by significant variability among users, with a false-negative rate of 15% to 40%.

DPL is a rapid and accurate means of diagnosing the presence of hemoperitoneum; accuracy is 98.5%. After access to the peritoneal cavity is accomplished by placement of a catheter through a small supraumbilical or intraumbilical incision, peritoneal contents are aspirated. The presence of 10 ml of gross blood or enteric contents such as bile or succus constitutes a positive DPL. If the DPL is not grossly positive, 1 L of isotonic fluid is infused into the peritoneal cavity and allowed to drain by gravity. The effluent is then sent to the laboratory for cell count and Gram stain. The presence of more than 100,000 red blood cells or 500 white blood cells per mm^3 or bacteria shown by Gram stain meets the criteria for positive DPL. A positive DPL is an indication for laparotomy. DPL has a sensitivity of 97%, but, similar to FAST, it confirms only the presence of hemoperitoneum and not specific organ injury. The incidence of nontherapeutic laparotomy performed on the basis of positive DPL is as high as 27%. It is not useful in the identification of retroperitoneal injuries. Because of its relative invasiveness, the role of DPL is limited to hemodynamically unstable patients.

CT has revolutionized the diagnosis and treatment of blunt-trauma injuries to the spleen. Contrast-enhanced CT has become the standard of care for diagnosis of blunt splenic injury in hemodynamically stable patients. It is widely available and is both sensitive and specific. CT allows for identification of specific organ injuries. The American Association for the Surgery of Trauma organ injury scale provides a standardized grading system for splenic injuries that is based on size of hematoma or laceration and degree of vascular injury (Table 1).

Table 1: Spleen Organ Injury Scale—1994 Revision by the American Association for the Surgery of Trauma

Grade		Injury Description	AIS-90
I	Hematoma	Subcapsular, <10% surface area	2
	Laceration	Capsular tear, <1 cm parenchymal depth	2
II	Hematoma	Subcapsular, 10%-50% surface area; intraparenchymal, <5 cm in diameter	2
	Laceration	1–3 cm parenchymal depth that does not involve a trabecular vessel	
III	Hematoma	Subcapsular, >50% surface area or expanding; ruptured subcapsular or parenchymal hematoma Intraparenchymal hematoma >5 cm or expanding	3
	Laceration	>3 cm parenchymal depth or involving trabecular vessels	3
IV	Laceration	Laceration involving segmental or hilar vessels producing major devascularization (>25% of spleen)	4
V	Laceration	Completely shattered spleen	5
	Vascular	Hilar vascular injury that devascularizes spleen	5

AIS, Abbreviated Injury Scale.

MANAGEMENT

Management of splenic injuries can be broadly categorized as non-operative or operative. Historically, splenectomy was the standard of care for all injuries to the spleen, with the first successful splenectomy for blunt trauma reported in 1892. In the mid-1900s, recognition of overwhelming postsplenectomy infection prompted the development of spleen-preserving treatment strategies, including splenorrhaphy and partial splenectomy. Nonoperative therapy was first described in 1971 in a study of children with suspected splenic injuries who were patients at the Hospital for Sick Children in Toronto. A healed transection of the spleen was found at autopsy in a child with a suspected splenic injury. On the basis of this observation, the authors of that study subsequently described their experience with 16 children with high likelihood of splenic injuries who were treated with close monitoring. Presently, approximately 60% of adults and 90% of children with blunt-trauma splenic injuries are successfully managed nonoperatively.

Successful nonoperative management relies on appropriate patient selection. Candidates for nonoperative therapy must have normal hemodynamics, and there must be no other indication for laparotomy. Other factors such as age, injury severity score, and degree of hemoperitoneum have been debated in the literature. In addition to appropriate candidate selection, nonoperative therapy mandates immediate availability of a surgeon and operating room, as well as the ability to admit the patient to a monitored or intensive care unit. Patients should be placed on bed rest, undergo serial abdominal examination, and have serial hematocrit follow-ups.

Nearly all children with blunt splenic injury are hemodynamically normal and can be observed; the necessity for splenectomy is uncommon. Management of blunt splenic injury in adults has been more controversial. In a multicenter study published in 2000, Eastern Association for the Surgery of Trauma (EAST) investigators sought to identify factors associated with failure of nonoperative management of blunt splenic injury in adults. They retrospectively reviewed 1488 adult patients with splenic injuries admitted to 27 trauma centers in 1997. Failure of nonoperative management was defined as any patient who was admitted with diagnosis of splenic injury with planned nonoperative management who later required laparotomy. The most common indications for failure of nonoperative management included falling hematocrit (36%), change in CT findings (21.6%), abdominal pain (16.5%), and hypotension (15.5%). Failure of nonoperative management increased significantly by grade of splenic injury. Nonoperative failure was reported in 5% of grade I injuries, 10% of grade II, 20% of grade III, 33% of grade IV, and 75% of grade V injuries. The necessity for laparotomy (either on admission or as failure of nonoperative management) also increased with increasing grade of splenic injury. Seventy-five percent of grade I splenic injuries were amenable to nonoperative management. In comparison, 77 of 78 (98.7%) of grade V injuries required laparotomy; 74 of these patients went directly from the emergency department to the operating room; and 3 of the remaining 4 patients as failure of observation.

Before the EAST study was conducted, there were conflicting data regarding the usefulness of quantity of hemoperitoneum as a prognostic marker for success of nonoperative management. Because the great majority of patients with spleen injury undergo CT scan, prognostication based on CT findings should be useful. Quantity of hemoperitoneum was described based on CT or intraoperative findings. Small hemoperitoneum was described as perisplenic blood or blood in Morrison's pouch. Blood in either of the paracolic gutters defined moderate hemoperitoneum, whereas blood in the pelvis defined large hemoperitoneum. Initially, 85.5% of patients with small hemoperitoneum were treated nonoperatively, with a 6.3% failure rate. A total of 62.4% of patients with moderate hemoperitoneum initially underwent nonoperative management, with a 19% failure rate. Of the 35.3% of patients with large hemoperitoneum who were treated nonoperatively, 22.3% failed. Overall, nonoperative management was successfully employed in 80.1% of patients with small hemoperitoneum, 50.6% of patients with moderate hemoperitoneum, and 27.4% of patients with large hemoperitoneum. This study demonstrates that increasing quantity of hemoperitoneum is associated with higher rate of failure of nonoperative management and that the ultimate management strategy correlates with the degree of hemoperitoneum. When degree of hemoperitoneum is considered as a function of grade of injury, the EAST study showed that successful nonoperative management declined as the quantity of hemoperitoneum increased within each injury grade.

The overall failure rate reported in the EAST study for nonoperative management was 10.8%; 61% of these patients failed within the first 24 hours. Another multicenter study by EAST, published in 2005, sought to identify common variables in patients who failed nonoperative management. Of the 97 patients in the EAST study who failed nonoperative management, charts of 78 patients were reviewed to determine common variables. Patients were categorized on the basis of heart rate and blood pressure data obtained from prehospital and emergency department records. Group 1 consisted of hemodynamically stable patients (normal) who never had a systolic blood pressure less than 90 mm Hg or a heart rate greater than 112 beats per minute (44% of total). Group 2 included patients with one or two periods with systolic blood pressure less than 90 mm Hg or heart rate greater than 112 beats per minute (31% of total), but who then stabilized with fluid resuscitation (responsive). Group 3 was composed of patients with three or more

Table 2: Criteria for Nonoperative Management of Blunt Splenic Injury

No indication for laparotomy on the basis of physical examination or diagnostic tests

Hemodynamically normal or normal vital signs with minimal fluid resuscitation

No transfusion requirement that is attributed to the splenic injury

Constant availability of surgical and critical care resources

Table 3: Criteria for Failure of Nonoperative Management of Blunt Splenic Injury

Increasing or persistent fluid requirements to maintain normal hemodynamic status

Failed angioembolization of arteriovenous fistula/pseudoaneurysm

Transfusion requirement to maintain hematocrit and hemodynamic stability

Increasing hemoperitoneum associated with hemodynamic instability

Peritoneal signs/rebound tenderness

episodes of hemodynamic instability (25% of total) (unstable). Thus hemodynamically unstable patients were admitted with the intent to manage them nonoperatively. Two thirds of the patients in group 3 (unstable) underwent laparotomy within 12 hours of admission, and 100% required laparotomy within 72 hours. In comparison, 82% of patients in group 1 and 78% of patients in group 2 underwent laparotomy within 72 hours. Mortality was significantly different among the three groups: group 1 (3%), group 2 (8%), group 3 (37%). In this study of patients who failed nonoperative management, overall mortality was 12%. The majority (60%) of deaths were from delayed treatment of intra-abdominal injuries. This study provides convincing evidence that the risk of failure of nonoperative management of blunt splenic injury in adults includes mortality. This study furthermore emphasizes the absolute necessity to appropriately select patients for nonoperative management because most of the preventable deaths occurred in unstable patients (Table 2).

The role of arteriography/embolization of blunt splenic injury is an evolving process and is quite variable among institutions. When used in the patient in a stable or responsive group with a demonstrable arterial blush on CT, the failure of nonoperative management is less (Table 3). Recent data have reemphasized that pseudoaneurysms that are not seen on initial CT often are seen on follow-up CT of the abdomen at 48 hours. It is important to keep in mind that 10% to 15% of patients who undergo angioembolization will rebleed, with splenectomy generally indicated at that point.

OPERATIVE MANAGEMENT

As mentioned earlier, laparotomy is indicated in patients with persistent hypotension, evidence of ongoing hemorrhage, peritonitis, or evidence of hollow viscus injury. The patient is placed on the operating table in supine position, and general anesthesia is administered. The areas from the neck to the knees and from table to table are prepared and draped in the usual sterile fashion. A generous midline incision is used to enter the peritoneum. Free blood is quickly evacuated, and all four quadrants are packed. If packing does not adequately control hemorrhage, the source of bleeding should be identified and controlled. Next, obvious contamination by enteric contents is controlled. The abdomen is then inspected in a systematic fashion.

The spleen is best visualized with the aid of a subcostal retractor. The nondominant hand of the operating surgeon mobilizes the spleen inferiorly and medially into the field of view. Following the ligation and division of splenocolic ligament, the avascular splenorenal and splenophrenic attachments are divided sharply. The spleen is further mobilized by blunt dissection from the retroperitoneum in the plane posterior to the tail of the pancreas. The hilar vascular structures can then be controlled with digital compression. The gastrosplenic ligament is ligated and divided. Particular attention should be paid to dividing the short gastric arteries as close to the spleen as possible to avoid ischemia to the stomach. At this point, the surgeon should be able to adequately mobilize the spleen into the operative field to permit close inspection. In the stable patient without other, competing needs for intervention, splenorrhaphy may be employed. With the promulgation of nonoperative management, splenorrhaphy is infrequently an option. If splenectomy is indicated, the splenic artery and vein are divided close to the spleen and the spleen is removed from the field. The tail of the pancreas must be avoided and protected. After adequate hemostasis is obtained, the left upper quadrant is thoroughly inspected, with particular attention to the tail of the pancreas. Closed-suction drains are indicated only if there is concern for injury to the pancreas because the use of drains has been associated with an increased incidence of subphrenic abscess formation.

As mentioned, splenic salvage in the form of splenorrhaphy or partial splenectomy may be considered in a select group of patients. Absolute contraindications to spleen salvage include intraoperative hemodynamic lability, significant associated injuries, and grade V spleen injuries. Hemostasis can be obtained using topical agents, mesh wraps, electrocautery, argon beam coagulation, or suture repair.

POSTINJURY CARE

Follow-up care for patients managed nonoperatively remains controversial. Some surgeons advocate follow-up CT scan within 48 hours of injury. The current practice at our institution is to repeat CT in 48 hours in all patients with grade III and IV injuries. Lower-grade injuries are managed without follow-up imaging, and essentially all grade V injuries are managed operatively. The role of follow-up CT after discharge from the hospital is less clear. Although there are no available data in the literature on adult injuries, data from the pediatric literature suggest that CT scan after discharge is not necessary. Splenic cysts and splenic abscesses may result from nonoperative management. These patients are generally symptomatic from these complications.

All patients who undergo splenectomy should be vaccinated against the encapsulated organisms (*Streptococcus pneumoniae*, *Neisseria meningitidis*, and *Haemophilus influenzae*). The vaccines should be administered before the patient is discharged from the hospital, primarily to ensure the patient receives his or her vaccines. The *S. pneumoniae* vaccine should be readminstered in 3- to 5-year intervals. The necessity of revaccination against *H. influenzae* and *N. meningitidis* is not clear.

SUGGESTED READINGS

Davis KA, Fabian TC, Croce MA, and others: Improved success in nonoperative management of blunt splenic injuries: embolization of splenic artery pseudoaneurysms, *J Trauma* 44:1008, 1998.

Peitzman AB, Harbrecht BG, Rivera L, and others: Failure of nonoperative management of blunt splenic injury in adults: variability in practice and adverse outcomes, *J Amer Coll Surg* 201:179, 2005.

Peitzman AB, Heil B, Rivera L, and others: Blunt splenic injury in adults: multi-institutional study of the Eastern Association for the Surgery of Trauma, *J Trauma* 49:177, 2000.

Richardson JD: Changes in management of injuries to the liver and spleen, *J Amer Coll Surg* 200:670, 2005.

RETROPERITONEAL INJURIES: KIDNEY AND URETER

Steven B. Brandes, MD, and
Robert F. Buckman Jr, MD

TRAUMATIC RENAL INJURIES

External trauma to the kidneys occurs in 1% to 5% of all trauma cases. Both kidneys are at equal disposition for injury. Depending on the trauma center, the mechanism of kidney injury is 80% to 90% blunt trauma and 10% to 20% penetrating trauma. At some inner-city trauma centers, penetrating renal injuries are more common (up to 30%). Blunt trauma includes falls from height; motor vehicle and motorcycle accidents; and direct blows to the abdomen, flank, and back. Children (<16 years old) are more prone to renal injury because of the relatively large size of the kidney, scant perirenal fat, underdeveloped Gerota's fascia, and incomplete ossification of the lower ribs.

Penetrating renal injuries are the results of gunshots and stab wounds. Of penetrating abdominal wounds, approximately 10% involve the kidney. Conversely, of penetrating renal trauma, 77% to 100% have associated injuries. The majority of renal injuries are American Association for the Surgery of Trauma (AAST) grade I. Such injuries heal spontaneously and without adverse events and require no imaging or active treatment. Only 4% of blunt traumas and 67% of penetrating traumas are significant renal injuries (AAST grades II–V). Proper radiographic staging of renal injuries (grades II–V) is essential to determine whether an injury is a candidate for nonoperative management. Table 1 shows the AAST injury scale for the kidney.

Initial Evaluation

Hematuria is the hallmark of renal injury. The degree of hematuria, however, does not correlate well with the extent of injury. The first voided or catheterized urine should be analyzed for blood. Dipstick urinalysis is adequate for the detection of microscopic hematuria. Significant microhematuria is typically defined as greater than 5 red blood cells per high-power field (RBC/HPF). An important caveat is that a small percentage of renal injuries, and up to 40% of renal pedicle injuries, will not present with hematuria.

Blunt Trauma

A history is gathered to quantify the forces involved in the renal injury, such as the speed of the vehicle or the height of the fall. Falls from a height or high-speed motor vehicle accidents imply deceleration injury and warrant evaluation for renal pedicle and ureteropelvic junction (UPJ) injury.

All patients with severe multiple trauma to the flank, abdomen, or lower chest should be suspected of having a renal injury, regardless of the presence or absence of hematuria. Indicators of blunt renal injury on physical examination are flank ecchymoses, lower (eleventh and twelfth) rib fractures, and transverse process fractures. Furthermore, seemingly minor trauma that results in a significant renal injury usually occurs in a congenitally abnormal kidney (typically to the chronically hydronephrotic UPJ kidney).

Table 1: American Association for the Surgery of Trauma Injury Scale for the Kidney

Grade*	Type	Description
I	Contusion	Microscopic or gross hematuria, urologic studies normal
	Hematoma	Subcapsular, nonexpanding without parenchymal laceration
II	Hematoma	Nonexpanding perirenal hematoma confirmed to renal retroperitoneum
	Laceration	<1 cm parenchymal depth of renal cortex without urinary extravasation
III	Laceration	<1 cm parenchymal depth of renal cortex without collecting system rupture or urinary extravasation
IV	Laceration	Parenchymal laceration extending through renal cortex, medulla, and collecting system
	Vascular	Main renal artery or vein injury with contained hemorrhage
V	Laceration	Completely shattered kidney
	Vascular	Avulsion of renal hilum, which devascularizes kidney

Data from Moore EE, et al: J Trauma 29:1664, 1989 (appears online at www.aast.org/injury/injury.html).
*Advance one grade for bilateral injuries up to grade III.

Penetrating Trauma

Information on the type of firearm used and the caliber of the bullet is helpful to differentiate between high-velocity and low-velocity missiles. The entrance and exit wound sites should be noted with radiopaque markers. High-velocity missiles (>2200 ft/sec) cause both entrance and exit wounds, extensive soft-tissue injury, and often delayed tissue necrosis (caused by a "blast" effect). Low-velocity missiles generally do not cause severe renal injuries unless the missile passes through the renal hilum or collecting system.

Site of the stab wound in relation to the anterior axillary line (AAL) is important. Entrance wounds anterior to the AAL and below the nipple line are often associated with intra-abdominal injuries. Wounds posterior to the AAL are less likely to have associated intraperitoneal organ injury, and thus these renal injuries can often be managed conservatively. It is also important to note knife blade length, so as to help predict the degree or depth of injury.

Hemodynamically Stable Patient

Indications for Renal Imaging

1. **Blunt trauma and gross hematuria.** Hematuria is the hallmark of renal injury. However, hematuria does not correlate and cannot predict the degree or extent of renal injury. Hematuria is absent in up to 40% of renal vascular injuries.
2. **Blunt trauma, microscopic hematuria, and shock.** Significant microscopic hematuria is greater than 5 RBC/HPF in the first voided or catheterized specimen. Shock is considered as a systolic blood pressure less than 90 mm Hg during transport or on arrival in the emergency department.

3. **Major acceleration or deceleration injury**, such as a fall from height, high-speed motor vehicle accident, or pedestrian-versus-motor-vehicle accident.
4. **Microscopic or gross hematuria after penetrating** flank, back, or abdominal trauma; or when the missile path or the entrance and exit sites are in line with the kidney.
5. **Pediatric (<16 years) trauma patient with any degree of significant hematuria.**
6. **Associated injuries/physical signs** suggesting underlying renal injury (e.g., flank ecchymosis/tenderness, lumbar spine fractures, eleventh or twelfth posterior rib fractures).

B. Imaging Studies

Intravenous Urogram

In stable patients, abdominal computed tomography (CT) has replaced the intravenous urogram (IVU) in the trauma setting. However, in undeveloped countries where CT may not be available, IVU with nephrotomography can be a useful tool to outline cortical borders and thus demonstrate more clearly any cortical lacerations, intrarenal hematomas, or areas of poor vascular perfusion. An obscured renal outline, loss of the ipsilateral psoas margin, or displacement of the bowel or ureter (or a combination of these factors) suggests significant perirenal hematoma. Furthermore, failure to visualize an enhancing kidney, persistence of the renal nephrogram, or segmental parenchymal enhancement suggests significant renal parenchymal or pedicle injury. An abnormal or equivocal IVU generally warrants further imaging or surgical exploration.

Computed Tomography

CT is the imaging study of choice for evaluating the stable abdominal trauma patient. CT is the gold standard for demonstrating kidney contusions, segmental parenchymal infarcts, parenchymal lacerations, urinary extravasation, the size and location of the retroperitoneal hematoma, or associated intra-abdominal organ injuries (or a combination of these injuries). CT can also accurately evaluate injuries to the hilum and great vessels. As with splenic injuries, "blush" noted in the arteriographic phase suggests a major arterial kidney bleed and will typically require aggressive therapy, namely, selective embolization in the angiography suite or celiotomy. Renal vein injuries, however, are often difficult to detect, but they can be inferred by the presence of hematoma medial to the kidney that displaces the renal vasculature. Renal artery occlusion and renal infarct are noted by lack of parenchymal enhancement or by a persistent "cortical rim sign." The classic rim sign, however, is usually not seen until more than 8 hours after injury.

Contemporary helical CT imaging scanning times are quick. In order not to understage renal injuries, images into the arterial and nephrographic phases are needed to detect renal parenchymal and vascular injuries, whereas delayed images (2–10 minutes later) are needed to distinguish urine (collecting system injury) from blood extravasation.

Ultrasound

Ultrasound (US) is a relatively inexpensive, safe, rapid, portable, and noninvasive method for imaging the abdomen. FAST (focused assessment for the sonographic evaluation of the trauma patients) is an accepted method for evaluating the blunt-trauma patient for possible intra-abdominal injuries. In properly trained hands, US is sensitive and specific for detecting hemoperitoneum (suggesting intra-abdominal injury). The true value to FAST is evaluating for blood in the pericardial sac, hepatorenal fossa, splenorenal fossa, and the pelvis. Because the kidney is a retroperitoneal organ, renal trauma blood and urine (free fluid) are confined to Gerota's fascia and the retroperitoneum. With kidney trauma, associated free fluid

is absent up to half the time. Free fluid noted with renal injuries is more likely due to associated intra-abdominal injuries than from the kidney injury. Furthermore, US imaging can be severely limited by obesity, subcutaneous air, and previous abdominal operations, and it is operator dependent. Further limitations of US are its inability to distinguish between a urine leak and blood or to reliably assess kidney vascularity. Thus US can be a valuable tool for triaging the unstable trauma patient, but when it comes to evaluating the injured kidney, US is not the optimal mode of imaging.

Arteriography

Arteriography and superselective embolization have important roles in the evaluation and treatment of posttraumatic, delayed renal bleeding or arteriovenous fistulae. In recent anecdotal reports, arteriography and endoluminal stent placement have also been successful in managing renal artery intimal tears and subsequent arterial thrombosis from blunt trauma.

Hemodynamically Unstable Patient

Imaging

Classically, the one-shot IVU has been advocated for the unstable trauma patient before the exploration of a retroperitoneal hematoma discovered on laparotomy. The IVU was supposed to demonstrate the function of the noninjured (contralateral) kidney; the presence and extent of any urinary extravasation; and, in penetrating injuries, the likely course of the missile. In the rare instance that an IVU is necessary, 2 ml/kg of body weight of standard 60% intravenous contrast is typically injected, followed by a single abdominal radiograph 10 minutes later. Scout or other films are unnecessary. In children, 2–3 ml/kg of nonionic contrast is preferred.

Although performing a one-shot IVU seems to makes sense, we do not advocate its use for the hemodynamically unstable or penetrating-trauma patient with hematuria. There is mounting evidence in the literature that one-shot IVU provides little additional information, the images are typically of poor quality (faint and delayed), and it expends precious time. A useful method that we employ to assess whether there is a functional contralateral kidney is to place an occlusive vessel loop on the ureter of the injured (ipsilateral) kidney, administer indigo carmine intravenously, and await blue urine from the contralateral side. Blue urine indicates the presence of a functional contralateral kidney. The other often-cited method is to palpate the contralateral retroperitoneal space for a kidney of normal size and consistency. Although this is often reliable for the experienced surgeon, in inexperienced hands a hypertrophied Psoas muscle can be mistaken for a palpable kidney.

Injury Scaling

The Organ Injury Scaling Committee of the AAST has classified five grades of traumatic renal injuries (see Table 1), ranging from least to most severe (I to V). Grades I and II renal injuries are considered minor and are commonly managed expectantly. Grade III injuries are those with deep parenchymal lacerations that do not involve the collecting system. Grade IV injuries have deep parenchymal lacerations, urinary extravasation, or confined renal arterial and venous injuries. Grade V injuries are life threatening— namely, pedicle avulsion or totally shattered kidney.

Indications for Renal Exploration

It is obvious that the vast majority of renal injuries, no matter how severe anatomically, can be safely managed nonoperatively. This is because the mechanism of injury is typically blunt and Gerota's fascia remains substantially intact. Even if there are breaches in Gerota's fascia, the retroperitoneal fibroareolar tissue and overlying peritoneum confine or contain blood and urine leaking from the injury. Confined or contained injuries can be managed nonoperatively, but injuries that have breached the spontaneous containment and decompressed into the peritoneal cavity are the ones that typically require operation (such as injuries caused by high-energy gunshot wounds and, rarely, by violent crushing, deceleration, or impalement). In general, kidney injuries do not result in such massive hemorrhage; thus approximately 3 of 4 renal gunshot wounds, 1 of 2 renal stab wounds, and only 2% of blunt renal injuries demand exploration.

Absolute Indications

Persistent and potentially life-threatening renal bleeding is an indication for renal exploration. Signs of continued renal bleeding are the presence of a pulsatile, expanding, or unconfined/uncontained retroperitoneal hematoma. Such retroperitoneal hematomas should be explored. Stable and contained retroperitoneal hematomas can be safely observed, as long as proper preoperative or intraoperative radiographic studies document a renal injury that can be observed safely. Grade V injuries involve avulsion of the main renal artery or vein or a shattered kidney with massive tissue destruction. By definition these injuries are life threatening and demand surgical exploration.

Relative Indications

Devitalized Parenchyma

A major devitalized renal segment (>25%) is a relative indication. When associated with colon or pancreatic injuries, urinary extravasation, extensive renal injury, or a large retroperitoneal hematoma, the subsequent abscess rate is higher and thus the threshold for renal exploration should be lower.

Urinary Extravasation

AAST grade 4 renal injury does not necessarily demand surgical exploration. More than 75% of the time, extravasations will resolve spontaneously (usually within 72 hours). Extravasations that worsen or develop a urinoma can be successfully managed percutaneously (drain the urinoma) or endoscopically (place a ureteral stent). UPJ avulsion injuries, however, typically do not heal spontaneously and are best managed by prompt surgical repair. In all blunt renal injuries it is vital that delayed CT images are obtained for visualization of contrast distal to the UPJ. Medial extravasation of contrast suggests UPJ injury, whereas lack of contrast distal to the UPJ suggests avulsion injury.

Incomplete Staging

Complete staging of the renal injury by appropriate imaging studies permits the selection of nonoperative management. Incomplete staging demands either further imaging or renal exploration.

Arterial Thrombosis

Renal artery occlusion usually occurs from a major deceleration injury in which the main renal artery is stretched, the less elastic intima torn, the vessels thrombose, and the kidney infarcts. Renal salvage is remote after 12 hours of ischemia. If the contralateral kidney is normal and diagnosis prompt, it is controversial to attempt revascularization because chances are poor that any significant renal function can be preserved. In only 20% to 56% of such cases is there more than 17% of differential function preserved. In such circumstances, it has not been our practice to attempt revascularization or exploration. We typically leave the devascularized kidney in situ because it rarely leads to late complications and usually just involutes. Blood pressure should be periodically monitored for the exceedingly rare incidence of persistent, renally induced hypertension. Revascularization should be

reserved only for bilateral renal artery occlusion or unilateral occlusion in a solitary kidney, regardless of the ischemic time.

Penetrating Renal Injuries

Theoretically, grade for grade, renal injuries should be managed the same, regardless of mechanism. This is particularly true for penetrating AAST grade 1 and II renal injuries, which can be managed conservatively. Penetrating AAST grade III and IV renal injuries, however, particularly stab wounds, are generally managed surgically because of a high rate of delayed bleeds (24%) and the necessity to explore for associated intra-abdominal injuries. There is mounting support in the literature, however, that when the penetrating kidney injury is isolated and no major intra-abdominal structure has been injured, it is safe to manage these injuries conservatively. Stab wounds to the kidney posterior to the anterior axillary line are less likely to have associated visceral injuries and thus are more likely to undergo successful conservative management of the renal injury. The conservatively managed penetrating trauma patient must undergo frequent serial abdominal examinations, particularly in the first 12 hours. Any changes in the physical examination warrant abdominal exploration.

Management

Surgical: Methods of Retroperitoneal Exploration and Renal Reconstruction

Retroperitoneal Exploration

The injured kidney is best exposed through a standard trauma laparotomy midline transperitoneal incision from the xiphoid process to the symphysis pubis. In the stable trauma patient, associated intra-abdominal injuries should be systematically examined and repaired before the kidney injury is explored. However, when renal bleeding is massive or persistent (as in a renal hilar injury), the kidney should be explored first.

The location of the retroperitoneal hematoma often dictates the operative approach. Zone 1 hematomas—namely, midline supramesocolic or midline inframesocolic from a blunt or penetrating mechanism—demand exploration. Zone 2, lateral perinephric hematomas, should be selectively explored for penetrating trauma and typically observed for blunt trauma.

In the stable patient with a zone 1 injury supramesocolic hematoma, the right colon is medially rotated to gain proximal control of the lower thoracic aorta by cutting the crus of the diaphragm. To prevent potential backbleeding, we also obtain aortic control above the bifurcation. Injuries to the aorta between the celiac and renal arteries are particularly lethal. Penetrating injury to the proximal renal artery is essentially a sidehole in the aorta, and its management is detailed later. Injury to the proximal supramesocolic aorta is another unforgiving situation that presents with a zone 1 supramesocolic hematoma.

Exsanguinating retroperitoneal injuries Two conditions are generally required for exsanguination from a retroperitoneal wound: (1) a full-thickness injury of a significant blood vessel, usually an artery; and (2) failed effective or spontaneous containment or tamponade of the bleeding. These circumstances occur much more commonly in penetrating trauma, particularly with high-energy gunshot wounds or the most extreme variants of blunt trauma. Unfortunately, injudicious actions taken by a surgeon to open a tense, contained hematoma and thereby defeat the natural containment, without proper precautions being taken, can result in the same form of exsanguinating hemorrhage. The clinical scenarios in which exsanguination from a renal or renal-artery injury is present will also have patterns and mechanisms likely to be associated with hemorrhage from other vessels and viscera.

Table 2: Methods for Managing Massive Retroperitoneal Bleeding

1. Manually compress the aorta at the hiatus.
2. Scoop and sponge blood from the peritoneal cavity.
3. Locate and manually compress any sources of uncontained hemorrhage.
4. Resuscitate the circulation with manual control in place.
5. Obtain proximal vascular control while manual compression is held.
6. Prove the function of the opposite kidney.
7. Open Gerota's fascia and deliver the kidney.
8. Repair or resect the damaged structures.

Because of these general facts, uncontained renal artery or hilar injuries are the most dangerous (potentially lethal) wounds that can involve the kidney and its proximal collecting system. Immediate manual control of hemorrhage and vigorous resuscitation are the keys to saving the life of the exsanguinating patient (Table 2). All maneuvers to get clamps on vessels and to expose renal or other injuries for resection or repair should be deferred until the patient has been properly resuscitated. After the patient has been resuscitated, time can be taken to place a vascular clamp on the aorta, if necessary, and to obtain renal artery control at a point proximal to the suspected injury. Manual control of bleeding is maintained during these maneuvers. If there is a wound in the hilum of the kidney, control of the renal artery is obtained near the aorta so that the manual compression does not have to be interrupted to permit encirclement and clamping. The kidney should not be allowed to bleed while proximal control is being obtained. After the renal artery is clamped and the aortic clamp has been removed, there is no hurry to deliver the kidney because it is no longer capable of further hemorrhage. A technique we commonly perform here to prove the function of the contralateral kidney is to administer indigo carmine intravenously while the blood supply to the damaged kidney is occluded. Blue appearance to the urine proves the function of the opposite kidney. Then the kidney can be delivered, the extent of damage assessed, and repair or resection decided. Most kidney injuries capable of causing massive, uncontained hemorrhage, especially those involving the hilum, will require nephrectomy. Complex and exotic repairs are not justified if a functioning opposite kidney has been demonstrated.

Rapidly mobilizing the right or left colon medially gives rapid access to the retroperitoneal kidney. It is important to incise Gerota's fascia laterally and then lift the kidney out of its bed, leaving the perinephric fat behind. It is essential to approach the kidney laterally and to avoid accidentally bluntly dissecting the kidney subcapsular, stripping the capsule off the kidney. The capsule of the kidney is fairly fibrous, and its preservation is important for placing sutures that will hold for renorrhaphy. Without the renal capsule, the kidney is more like a friable spleen, in which sutures can easily pull through. The perinephric hematoma typically accomplishes the dissection, around the kidney. Thus the traumatized kidney is often easily and rapidly mobilized anteriorly and medially, after Gerota's fascia is opened. After the kidney is mobilized, the hilum can be compressed manually, followed by careful placement of a vascular clamp. Unfortunately, in inexperienced hands, rapidly delivered kidneys tend to be judged irreparable and removed. Moreover, this approach often results in the removal of the damaged kidney before the function of the opposite kidney has been proved.

Renovascular injuries Injuries to the renal hilar vessels are less common and more challenging than most textbooks indicate. A penetrating injury to the right renal hilum will often also injure the pancreatoduodenal complex, the right renal artery, and the right renal vein. The right renal vein is wide and short, and thus such injuries are often just a sidehole in the vena cava. Such

right-sided hilar injuries can result in life-threatening hemorrhage. On the left, if the injury to the left renal vein is proximal to the gonadal and adrenal branches, the renal vein can be ligated. This maneuver cannot be performed contralaterally because the right renal vein has no branches. When repairing an injured renal artery, we usually intermittently perfuse the kidney with iced, heparinized saline and perform the simplest repair possible (i.e., end-to-end anastomosis). If a graft is necessary, our first choice is a reversed saphenous vein. However, the most expeditious method is to use a polytetrafluoroethylene conduit and anastomose the artery to a convenient lateral aspect of the infrarenal aorta (end-to-side).

Stable retroperitoneal injuries For the stable trauma patient without an exsanguinating bleed, ongoing controversy exists regarding the best method to obtain vascular control of the injured kidney. Classic teaching dictates that vascular control take place before a retroperitoneal hematoma is explored. The efficacy of consistent proximal vascular control of the renal pedicle before opening Gerota's fascia is demonstrated (by retrospective data) by the reduction in the nephrectomy rate, from the usual 31% to 56% to a low of 11% to 15%. Obtaining proximal renal arterial control is typically time consuming, often taking 10 or more minutes, particularly for the right kidney. Therefore the advantages of proximal primary renal arterial control may be of value in the stable trauma patient but much less so for the unstable patient. Furthermore, when the injured kidney is repaired, temporary occlusion of the renal artery is usually not required (<17%). Instead, bleeding from the cut edge of the injured kidney usually can be controlled simply by digital compression, with no need for arterial occlusion. Hilar vascular control is necessary in patients with renal vascular injuries, those in shock, and those with large or expanding retroperitoneal hematomas.

In the stable patient with a zone 1 midline inframesocolic retroperitoneal hematoma, the classic description of proximal vascular control requires displacing the small bowel along the root of the mesentery to the right and lateral. The important anatomic landmarks here are the inferior mesenteric vein and the ligament of Treitz (Fig. 1). First take down the ligament of Treitz and reflect the fourth portion of the duodenum laterally, then dissect between these two structures onto the infrarenal aorta. Regardless of the size of the hematoma, the inferior mesenteric vein (IMV) is a constant landmark and the aorta can at least be palpated. Move up along the aorta until the left renal vein is identified crossing the aorta. Note that in less than 5% of patients, the renal vein will run retroaortic, so this important landmark will be missing. Gentle traction on the left renal vein with a vein retractor will permit access to the left renal artery, which is usually slightly cephalad to the vein and coming off the lateral aspect of the aorta. The right renal artery is more difficult to identify. After the left renal vein is looped, it is dissected out medially toward its origin off the lateral vena cava. With cephalad retraction of the left renal vein and interaortocaval dissection, the right renal artery can be identified and controlled. The origin of the right renal artery is slightly cephalad to the left renal artery. This is particularly time consuming.

However, if the inframesocolic hematoma extends cephalad and totally obscures the ligament of Treitz instead of obtaining vascular control at the level of IMV, it is safer to obtain supraceliac control through the lesser omentum above the stomach, either by manually compressing the aorta against the spine or by clamping through the crus of the diaphragm.

Reconstruction

In the absence of persistent hemodynamic instability or coagulopathy, kidney reconstruction can be safe and effective. The method of kidney reconstruction is dictated by the degree and location of the injury and not by the associated intra-abdominal injuries. Even a concomitant pancreatic or colonic injury with frank fecal contamination is not a contraindication to renal reconstruction. However,

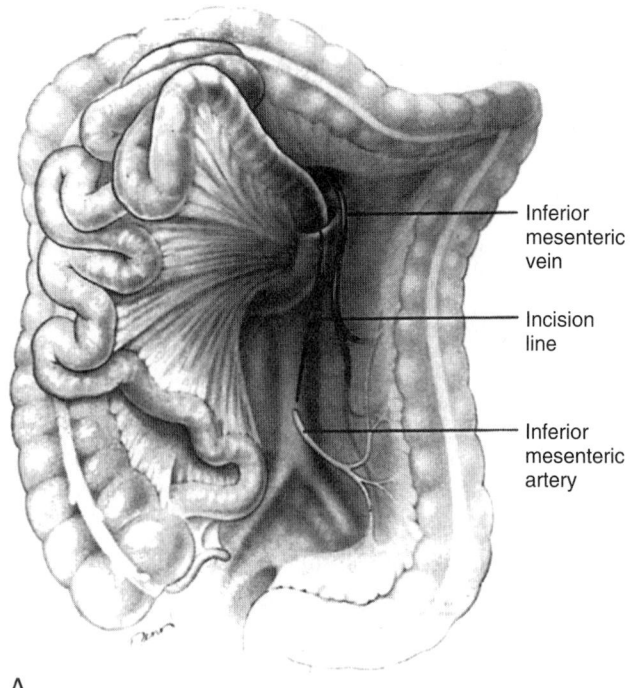

A

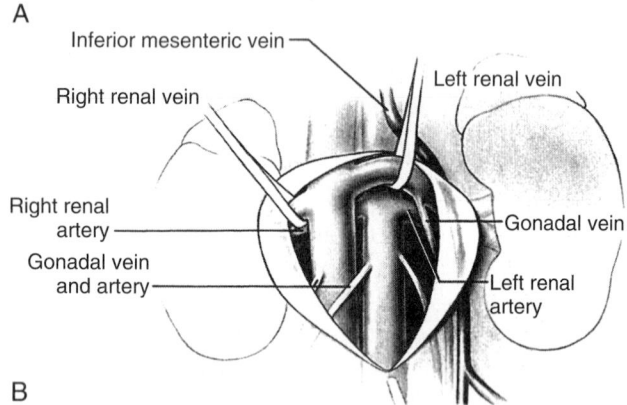

B

Figure 1 Technique of exposure of renal vessels. **(A)** Exposure of the root of the mesentery to visualize the aorta. **(B)** Relationship of the renal veins and arteries after incision of the posterior peritoneum over the aorta. *From Cameron, JL, editor: Current surgical therapy, ed 7, 1998, Mosby, p. 1124.*

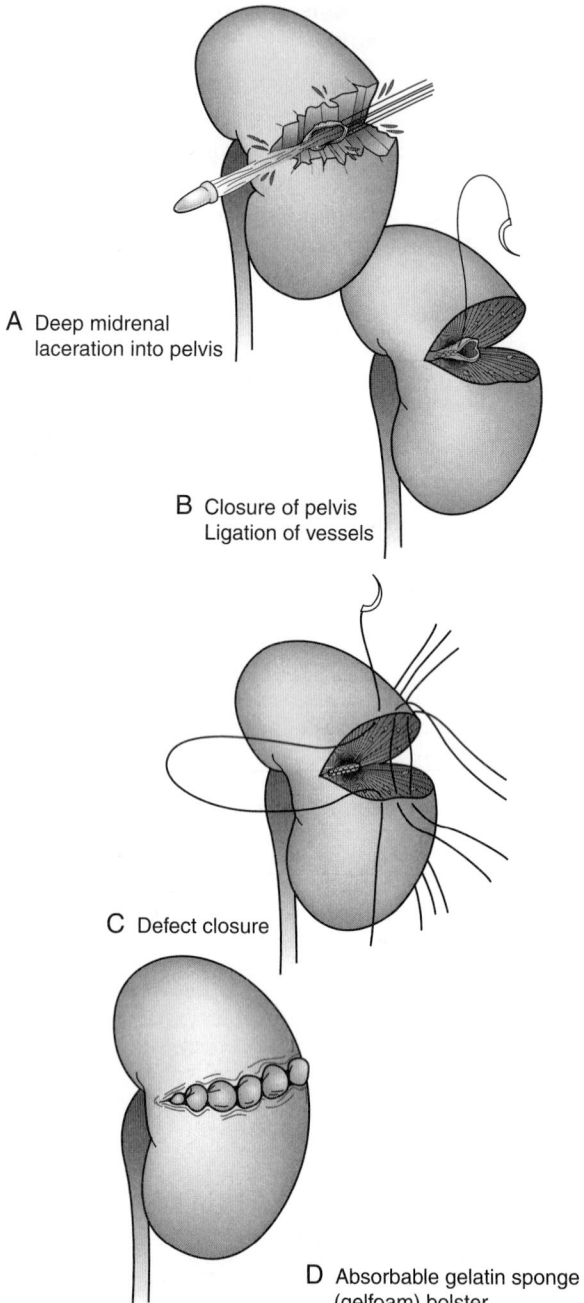

Figure 2 Suture repair of the renal pelvis and parenchyma over bolsters. *From Cameron, JL, editor: Current surgical therapy, ed 8, Philadelphia, 2004, Elsevier Mosby, p. 977.*

the resulting complication rates are slightly increased. The reconstructive principles for renal injures are the following:

1. Broad exposure of the kidney and injured area
2. Temporary vascular occlusion for brisk renal bleeding, when not well controlled by manual compression of the parenchyma
3. Sharp excision of all nonviable parenchyma.
4. Meticulous hemostasis
5. Watertight closure of the collecting system
6. Parenchymal defect closure by approximation of the capsular edges over a Surgicel (Johnson & Johnson, New Brunswick, NJ) or Gelfoam (Pfizer, New York, NY) bolster or coverage with omentum, perinephric fat, peritoneum, or polyglycolic acid mesh (Fig. 2)
7. Interposition of an omental pedicle flap among associated vascular, colonic, or pancreatic injuries and the injured kidney (Fig. 3)
8. Ureteral stent placement for a renal pelvis or ureteral injury
9. Retroperitoneal drain

Nonoperative/Conservative Management

Properly staged and selected renal injuries can be successfully managed conservatively as follows:

1. Strict bed rest until the urine visibly clears
2. Close monitoring of vital signs
3. Hematocrit blood drawn every 6 hours until patient is stable
4. Prophylactic antibiotics
5. Transfusions to keep the hematocrit stable

The confined spaces of the retroperitoneum and Gerota's envelope can tamponade and limit bleeding. Transfusion requirements of more than4 to 6 units in 24 hours demand repeat imaging and possible arteriography/embolization or surgical exploration. For grade IV renal

Figure 3 Partial nephrectomy with omental patch. *From Cameron, JL, editor: Current surgical therapy, ed 8, Philadelphia, 2004, Elsevier Mosby, p. 978.*

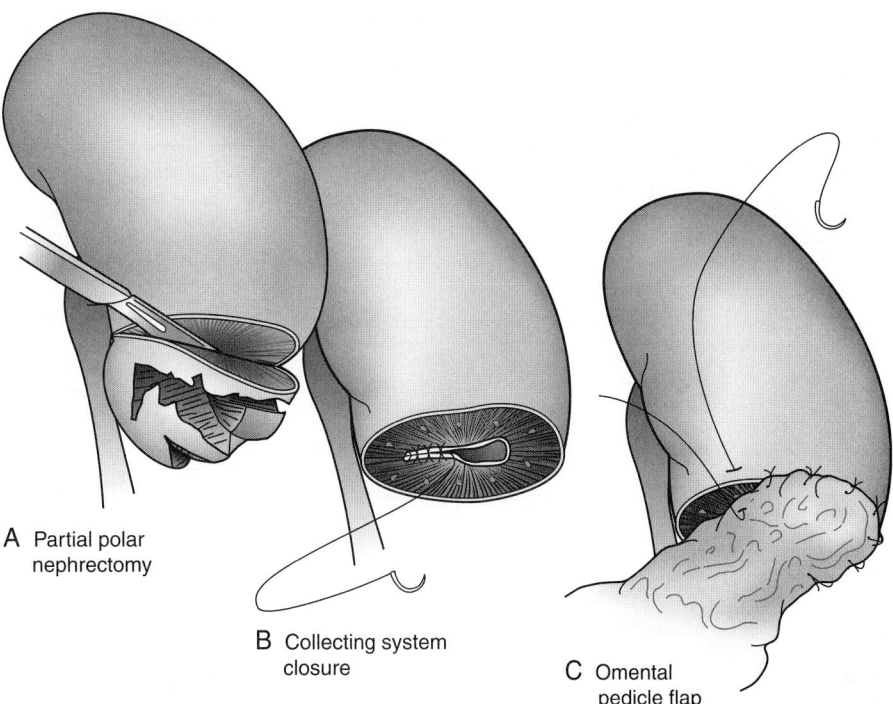

A Partial polar nephrectomy

B Collecting system closure

C Omental pedicle flap

injuries, the kidney should be reimaged by CT with intravenous contrast and delayed images (3 to 5 days after initial injury) to assess for persistent urinary leakage. Worsened or unimproved leak warrants ureteral stent placement of urinoma drain placement.

Damage Control

One obvious method to control damage is to avoid exploring zone 2 retroperitoneal hematomas. It is reasonable to leave the nonexpanding, contained, and nonpulsatile hematoma alone. If the hematoma is zone 2 and the Gerota's fascia is oozing but not massively bleeding, we pack the kidney. If the hematoma is expanding or pulsatile or there is significant bleeding from the hole in Gerota's, then the hematoma and kidney should be explored. If the kidney has sustained irreparable vascular or parenchymal injuries or if the patient has persistent hemodynamic instability or other associated life-threatening injuries, then a rapid damage-control nephrectomy can be a lifesaving maneuver.

Complications after Renal Trauma

Complications are dependent on the grade of the initial renal injury and the method of management and usually occur within 1 month of injury.

Early Complications

Prolonged urinary extravasation is the most common complication after renal trauma. Urinomas occur in less than 1% of renal trauma cases. Small, uninfected, and stable collections do not require intervention. Large collections (typically >4 cm) are prone to abscess formation and sepsis and are usually managed by percutaneous catheter drainage.

Other potential complications include shock from massive blood loss, renal infarction, and abscess formation.

Late Complications

Other complications include delayed bleeding, arteriovenous fistula, abscess, urinary fistula, and hydronephrosis. In general, complications are usually of minimal long-term morbidity, can be successfully managed by minimally invasive means, and do not significantly prolong the length of stay. At 3 to 6 months after a renal injury, follow-up renal imaging should be obtained to evaluate for delayed hydronephrosis, vascular compromise, or renal atrophy.

Hypertension

Renal vascular hypertension after renal trauma is usually transient. Sustained or delayed hypertension, such as by a Page or Goldblatt kidney, are renin mediated and rare events (<1%). Nevertheless, blood pressure should be monitored carefully for several months after injury.

Hydronephrosis

Perinephric fibrosis that involves the UPJ is usually seen after a lower-pole kidney injury and can result in hydronephrosis. To prevent such occurrences, interposition of perirenal fat or omentum between the injured kidney and the ureter is effective.

URETERAL AND RENAL PELVIS INJURIES

Mechanisms of Injury

External trauma

Penetrating ureteral injuries are rare, with only 2.5% of all abdominal gunshot wounds (GSWs) involving the ureter. Overall, the mechanism of ureteral injuries is 95% penetrating and 5% blunt (e.g., rapid acceleration or deceleration, as in falls from a height or motor vehicle accidents). GSWs in proximity to the ureter can result in severe ureteral contusion and delayed necrosis caused by a blast effect. This more commonly occurs with high-velocity missiles because of more surrounding tissue and delayed tissue injury. After a deceleration injury, the kidney is often dislocated and tears can occur at its fixation points, namely, the UPJ and hilar vasculature. Another mechanism for injury is hyperextension of the back, where stretching by the lumbar and lower thoracic vertebral bodies avulses the ureter. This classically occurs in child-pedestrian-versus-motor-vehicle accidents because children are limber.

Iatrogenic trauma

Ureteral injuries usually occur during difficult or bloody pelvic operations. Overall, the ureter is injured in only 0.5% to 1% of pelvic operations. Iatrogenic injuries commonly occur during the course of the following surgeries:

> Urological procedures: ureteroscopy, vesicourethral suspension, and radical prostatectomy
> Gynecological procedures: hysterectomy, salpingo-oophorectomy, and cystocele repair
> Colorectal surgery: abdominoperineal resection
> Vascular surgery: aortic and iliac graft surgery.

Of all surgeries, iatrogenic ureteral injury most commonly occurs during transabdominal hysterectomy. Sites of common ureter injury are at the uterine vessels and the cardinal and uterosacral ligaments.

Diagnosis of Ureteral Injury

Successful surgical management of collecting-system injuries requires a high index of suspicion, early diagnosis, a low threshold for urinary-tract imaging, and an intimate knowledge of ureteral anatomy and blood supply.

Preoperative Diagnosis

Hematuria (gross or microscopic) is not a reliable sign and is absent in 23% to 45% of penetrating ureteral injuries and in 31% to 67% of blunt UPJ injuries. In the absence of hematuria, a high index of suspicion is required to diagnose ureteral injuries reliably.

Intraoperative Diagnosis

The majority of penetrating ureteral injuries are diagnosed intraoperatively. Direct exploration is the most accurate method for diagnosis. Ureteral peristalsis is not a reliable indication of viability or of adequate vascularity. The most reliable way to determine ureteral viability is by incision and monitoring for a bleeding edge. Intravenous indigo carmine is also helpful in identifying ureteral injury by extravasation of blue dye from the injury site. Cystotomy and retrograde injection of indigo carmine by pediatric feeding tube is another method of testing ureteral integrity.

Missed Ureteral Injury Diagnosis

Ureteral injuries are morbid and potentially lethal when they are unrecognized and present in a delayed fashion. Clinical signs of a missed injury usually do not become obvious for days. Early physical signs are usually nonspecific and include prolonged ileus, elevated blood urea nitrogen, persistent flank or abdominal pain, palpable abdominal mass, prolonged drainage from drain sites, urinary obstruction, sepsis, and abscess or peritonitis.

Imaging

Intravenous Urography

IVU is the primary imaging study used to evaluate ureteral integrity. Accuracy in diagnosing a ureteral injury is variable and thus considered unreliable. IVU findings suggestive of ureteral injury are incomplete visualization of the entire ureter, ureteral deviation or dilatation, urinary extravasation, hydronephrosis, and delayed visualization or nonvisualization of the injured renal unit. One-shot IVU has little value for assessing ureteral integrity.

Retrograde Pyelography

Although accurate in demonstrating the site, presence, and location of extravasation, retrograde pyelography is both time consuming and cumbersome. It thus has little role in the acute trauma setting.

Computed Tomography

CT has been used with increasing frequency to evaluate ureteral trauma. Medial perirenal extravasation of contrast is the most common finding of renal ureteropelvic injury. The use of quick-imaging, spiral CT scanners demands delayed images with intravenous contrast, and the presence of hypotension or significant renal injury can make opacification of the collecting system poor and thus decrease overall imaging sensitivity. On CT, avulsion of the UPJ can be inferred by the presence of medial perirenal contrast extravasation and no filling of the ipsilateral ureter. Lacerations of the UPJ also have medial contrast extravasation; however, contrast is seen in the ipsilateral ureter distal to the UPJ.

Classification

Ureteral injuries are typically classified by location of the ureteral injury; mechanism and manner of injury (e.g., avulsion [UPJ], contusion, transection, devascularization, crush, ligation, resection, or fulguration). Table 3 shows the AAST Injury Scale for the Ureter.

Associated Injuries

Patients with penetrating ureteral injuries also have associated multi-organ system injuries. More than 90% have concomitant injuries of the bowel, iliac vessel, liver, and vena cava... Patients with blunt ureteral trauma also commonly suffer from associated injuries (up to 77%), for example, to the liver, long bones, head, and diaphragm.

Management

General considerations are the patient's overall physical condition, presence of associated injuries, any delay in diagnosis, and the level and full extent of ureteral injury. Promptly diagnosed ureteral injuries should be explored and reconstructed through a midline transperitoneal incision. Lack of bleeding from the cut edge suggests ischemia and warrants ureteral debridement until viable tissue is reached.

At a minimum, ureteral contusions or bruising caused by proximity to blast injury should be stented and a retroperitoneal drain placed. With severe contusions, the ureter should be segmentally resected, debrided, and reanastomosed over a stent. If the blast-injured ureter is not resected, then a double-J stent and

Table 3: American Association for the Surgery of Trauma Injury Scale for the Ureter

Grade*	Type	Description
I	Hematoma	Contusion or hematoma without devascularization
II	Laceration	<50% transection
III	Laceration	≥50% transection
IV	Laceration	Complete transection with <2 cm of devascularization
V	Laceration	Avulsion with >2 cm of devascularization

Data from Moore EE, et al: J Trauma 33:337, 1992.
*Advance one grade for bilateral up to grade III.

retroperitoneal drain adjacent to the area of concern should be placed. The segment in major, iatrogenic, ureteral crush injuries should be excised and formal reconstruction performed, depending on the location of the injury. Minor crush injuries require a stent placed either endoscopically or through a cystotomy.

The surgical principles for successful ureteral repair are careful ureteral mobilization preserving the adventitia; debridement of nonviable tissue to a bleeding edge; mucosa-to-mucosa, spatulated, tension-free, and watertight anastomosis; ureteral stenting/urinary diversion; isolation of repair from associated injuries (e.g., omental interposition for associated bowel, vascular, or pancreatic injuries); and lastly, a retroperitoneal drain.

Distal Ureteral Injuries (below the Iliac Vessels)

Ureteroneocystostomy

For low transections without significant ureteral loss (after the proximal end of the ureter is debrided to viable tissue and spatulated), a simple refluxing ureteral reimplantation into a fixed (floor/trigone) rather than mobile area of the bladder (dome) is preferred. A tunneled nonrefluxing reimplant is generally unnecessary and slightly increases the chances for ureteral stenosis. Ureteral stenting is for 4 to 6 weeks.

Psoas Hitch

With greater distal ureteral loss, the gap is bridged by hitching (sewing) the apex of bladder to the ipsilateral psoas minor tendon (Fig. 4). The contralateral superior vesical pedicle is often divided to improve bladder mobilization. Care is taken not to entrap the genitofemoral nerve. The ureter is then reimplanted over a ureteral stent, and a suprapubic tube is placed. Rarely is the Psoas hitch used during acute trauma, but more typically is reserved until a planned, staged repair is performed by a urologist.

Transureteroureterostomy

Except in a few select circumstances, transureteroureterostomy (TUU) is a procedure that should not be performed in the acute

trauma situation. As an alternative, the ureter can be treated in a damage-control approach by temporarily diverting the urine over a ureteral stent, with planned definitive reconstruction in a staged fashion (typically by a urologist). TUU seems particularly useful when there are associated rectal, major pelvic vascular, or extensive bladder injuries. Relative contraindications to a TUU are a prior history of urothelial cancer, genitourinary tuberculosis, nephrolithiasis, pelvic irradiation or infection, retroperitoneal fibrosis, or chronic pyelonephritis.

Midureteral Injuries

Ureteroureterostomy

The majority of complete transections, regardless of mechanism, can be repaired by primary ureteroureterostomy. Both ureteral segments are spatulated, and a watertight, tension-free anastomosis is performed over a double-J ureteral stent (Fig. 5).

Upper Ureteral Injuries

Ureteroureterostomy

Injuries to the upper third of the ureter are best repaired by primary ureteroureterostomy.

Ureteropelvic Junction Injuries

UPJ injuries are usually avulsions after blunt trauma. Avulsion of the UPJ is the most common blunt ureteral injury and occurs primarily in children (<16 years). Complete UPJ tears (avulsion) will not resolve spontaneously and demand primary surgical repair, ureteral stenting, and a retroperitoneal drain. Incomplete UPJ lacerations can often be successfully managed expectantly.

Large Ureteral Loss

Large segment of ureter loss requires aggressive and time-consuming surgical reconstruction that is best performed in a staged fashion and not during an acute trauma. Ileal interposition, Boari flap,

Figure 4 Psoas hitch provides additional length for low uretal injuries for creation of a tension-free reimplantation of the ureter. *From Cameron, JL, editor: Current surgical therapy, ed 8, Philadelphia, 2004, p. 979.*

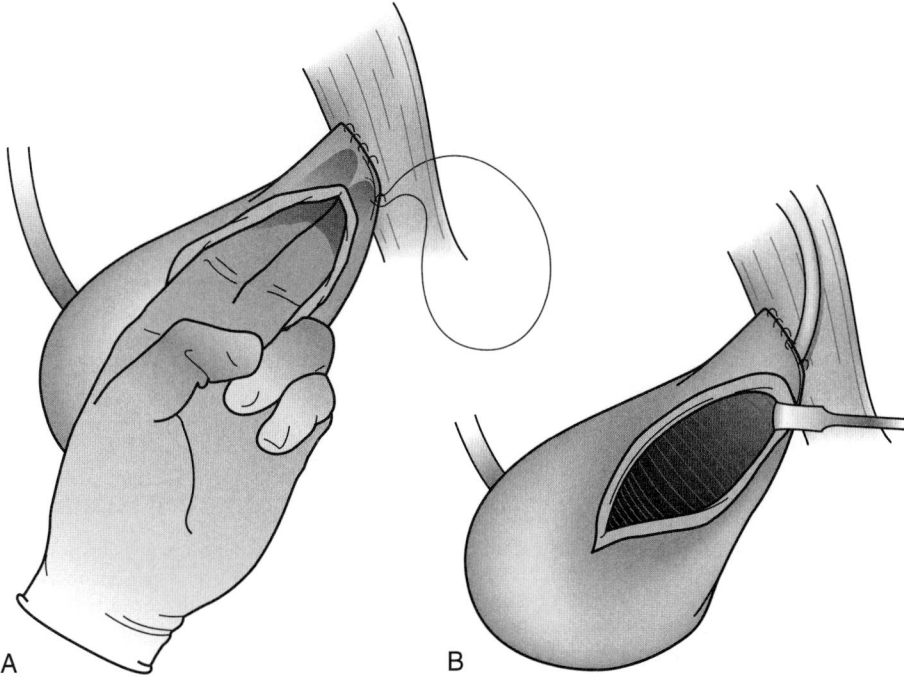

A   B

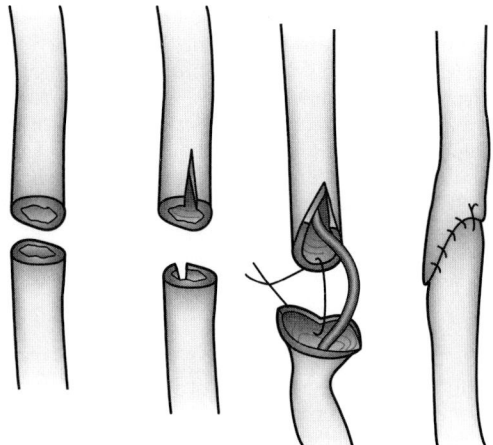

Figure 5 Ureteroureterostomy requires debridement, spatulation, stenting, and anastomosis with absorbable interrupted sutures. *From Cameron, JL, editor: Current surgical therapy, ed 8, Philadelphia, Elsevier Mosby, p. 978.*

renal displacement, urinary ileal conduit, and autotransplantation are complex procedures that are best performed by urologists and in a staged and delayed setting.

The Unstable Patient and Damage Control

When the patient is too unstable to undergo lengthy ureteral reconstruction, a damage-control approach of temporary cutaneous ureterostomy over a single-J ureteral stent or pediatric feeding tube should be performed. Time should not be wasted mobilizing the ureter fully to bring it to the skin, but rather a tie should be placed around the distal ureter and stent and then the stent is brought to the skin. An alternative method of last resort is ureteral ligation, proximal to the injury, followed by a percutaneous nephrostomy tube when the patient becomes stable. Intraoperative placement of a nephrostomy tube is time consuming and difficult and should not

be performed. Definitive reconstruction is delayed until the patient has stabilized from his or her other injuries. Such delayed reconstructions are typically time consuming and best left to urologists.

Management of Complications and Delayed Diagnosis

Delayed recognition of ureteral injuries is common, occurring in up 60% of cases. Significant morbidity, including sepsis, abscess formation, hydronephrosis, and loss of renal function occurs in up to 50% of such patients. Other complications include ureteral stricture and fistula, urinary extravasation/urinoma formation, infection, and loss of renal function.

Ureteral injuries that are diagnosed within 2 weeks of initial trauma and have no significant infection should be surgically explored and repaired. If iatrogenic ligation of the ureter is found, the suture should be removed and the ureter stented. Injuries that are diagnosed after 10 to 14 days should undergo proximal urinary diversion by percutaneous nephrostomy tube; percutaneous drainage of any urinoma or abscess; and, when possible, antegrade stent placement across the injured ureter. Definitive ureteral reconstruction is usually delayed for at least 3 months.

SUGGESTED READINGS

Boone TB, Gilling PJ, Husman DA: Ureteropelvic junction disruption following blunt abdominal trauma, *J Urol* 150:33, 1993.

Brandes SB, Chelsky MJ, Buckman RF, and others: Ureteral injuries from penetrating trauma, *J Trauma* 36:766, 1994.

Brandes SB, McAninch JW: Reconstructive surgery of the injured upper urinary tract, *Uro Clin North Am* 26:183, 1999.

Carroll PR, McAninch JW, Klosterman P, and others: Renovascular trauma: risk assessment, surgical management, and outcome, *J Trauma* 30:547, 1990.

Eastman JA, Wilson TG, Ahlering TE: Urological evaluation and management of renal-proximity stab wounds, *J Urol* 150:1771, 1993.

Haas CA, Dinchman KH, Nasrallah PF, and others: Traumatic renal artery occlusion: A 15-year review, *J Trauma* 45:557, 1998.

Holcroft JW, Trunkey DD, Minagi H, and others: Renal trauma and retroperitoneal hematomas—indications for exploration, *J Trauma* 15:1045, 1975.

DAMAGE CONTROL IN THE TRAUMA PATIENT

Aurelio Rodriguez, MD, and Adrian W. Ong, MD

INTRODUCTION

Damage control in trauma surgery refers to a situation in which the surgeon controls life-threatening bleeding and contamination but deems the patient so critically ill that the less urgent phases of the operation are not finished. Definitive surgical treatment is postponed in favor of optimizing resuscitation, addressing other life-threatening injuries, and performing urgent diagnostic or therapeutic tests (or both). The concept of damage control started to gain popularity in the late 1970s when there was a resurgence of the practice of packing for bleeding liver injuries. In 1979 Calne and colleagues described three patients who underwent surgery for exsanguinating liver trauma who were temporarily packed

during initial laparotomy and then transferred to a tertiary care center with good outcomes. Stone and colleagues in 1983 showed improved outcomes when the technique of abbreviated laparotomy was adopted. The term *damage control* was used by Rotondo and colleagues in 1993 to describe the continuum of treatment through the three phases of (1) surgical control of hemorrhage and contamination, (2) correction of hypothermia and coagulopathy in the intensive care unit (ICU), and (3) reoperation with definitive surgical management of intra-abdominal injuries. This concept has been further extended to thoracic, vascular, and orthopedic trauma and is now an established approach in the care of any patient with complex injuries.

PATHOPHYSIOLOGY AND RATIONALE

The onset of hypothermia and acidosis in a hypotensive severely injured patient marks the development of life-threatening coagulopathy. Studies have shown altered platelet function and coagulation enzyme activity below 34°C. Transfusions of red blood cells and acellular resuscitation fluids also exacerbate coagulopathy by a dilutional effect. There are several criteria well described in the literature that have been associated with the development of coagulopathy and increased mortality: a temperature of less than 34°C, pH of less than 7.20, base deficit of −12 or greater, need for more than 10 units of blood, initial systolic blood pressure of 70 mm Hg or less, need for resuscitative thoracotomy, and number and type of intra-abdominal injuries. Although all of these variables are markers of poor outcome and may not all be controllable by the surgeon, they offer the surgeon certain criteria for terminating the operation quickly in favor of further resuscitation. The ideal scenario occurs when the surgeon recognizes the previously mentioned physiologic derangements and terminates the operation *before* the onset of coagulopathy.

Other indications to abbreviate operative procedures include (1) the need for further urgent diagnostic or other therapeutic procedures (e.g., pelvic angiography to control surgically inaccessible bleeding, urgent head computed tomography [CT] in a comatose patient, need to control bleeding from multiple other body sites); (2) the need for reassessment of intra-abdominal contents; and (3) the inability to reapproximate fascia primarily because of tissue edema.

PHASE I: INITIAL OPERATION

General Considerations

The operating room should be heated to minimize heat loss, and an autologous blood recovery system should be prepared. Chest tube drainage systems should be positioned at the head of the bed before draping so that the anesthesiologist can assess the blood loss easily. When large amounts of blood products are required, our institution has a "massive transfusion protocol" that *initially* provides for 10 units of uncross-matched packed red cells, 4 to 6 units of fresh frozen plasma, and one platelet transfusion. Activating a hospital-wide transfusion protocol simplifies communication with the blood bank and enables rapid acquisition of blood products in the operating room.

Thorax

Resuscitative thoracotomy via a left anterolateral approach provides quick access for resuscitation and for assessing thoracic injuries in the patient who is in extremis. A right-chest tube should be placed simultaneously to evaluate for right-chest bleeding when thoracotomy is performed. If there is significant right-chest bleeding, the incision should be extended to the right chest across the sternum. Left-lung expansion with ventilation is confirmed, correct endotracheal tube placement is verified, and open cardiac massage is performed. The pericardium is then opened anterior and parallel to the phrenic nerve to evaluate for cardiac injuries and hemopericardium. Lung parenchymal injuries are controlled temporarily with clamps to the parenchyma or hilum. The descending thoracic aorta may be cross-clamped to aid in resuscitative efforts. With evidence of improvement in organ perfusion, the immediate disposition of the patient depends on the mechanism of injury, injury complex, and hemodynamic stability.

In instances in which resuscitative thoracotomy is not necessary, assessment in the emergency department continues in accordance with Advanced Trauma Life Support principles, using focused assessment for the sonographic evaluation of the trauma patient (FAST) to assess for pericardial effusion. In the hypotensive patient sustaining penetrating trauma to the chest, the patient should proceed directly to the operating room after these initial interventions. The choice of incision(s) will depend on the location of wounds, chest tube outputs, and the presence or absence of pericardial effusion as revealed by the FAST.

Lung Injuries

Nonanatomic lung resection with staplers offers a rapid way to control bleeding and air leaks. For a through-and-through penetrating injury with bleeding from the lung wounds, tractotomy or opening the tract with staplers and controlling individual bleeding vessels and air leaks allow for rapid hemostasis. Formal lobectomy using a stapler to fire across the hilum of the lobe may be necessary if the previously mentioned methods do not provide satisfactory control of bleeding.

Cardiac Injuries

Resuscitative thoracotomy provides for repair of cardiac injuries in the patient presenting in extremis. This may be extended to include a right anterolateral thoracotomy to obtain exposure to injuries of the superior vena cava, right heart, and right hilum. Typically, a laceration is repaired with 3-0 Prolene (Ethicon, Somerville, NJ) suture with pledgets, or staples, using the surgeon's finger to occlude bleeding as sutures or staples are placed. Large destructive wounds may require repair with a heavier suture on a large needle. They may also be temporarily occluded with a urinary catheter with its balloon inflated as the patient is being transported to the operating room.

Tracheobronchial Injuries

Tracheal injuries, which are uncommon, are best served with primary repair in the unstable patient. Bronchial injuries are treated with debridement and primary repair, if the injuries are not extensive. In cases in which extensive injury has occurred, lobectomy rather than repair with anastomosis may be preferable in the unstable patient.

Vascular Injuries in the Chest and Neck

In patients sustaining penetrating injuries with profuse external bleeding, tamponade of bleeding by inserting a urinary catheter into the wound and then inflating the balloon may be performed in the emergency department before the patient is transported to the operating room (Figs. 1 and 2). Whereas the majority of vascular injuries in the chest and neck are treated with primary repair, interposition graft, or bypass, ligation of the subclavian, external carotid, and internal carotid arteries has been

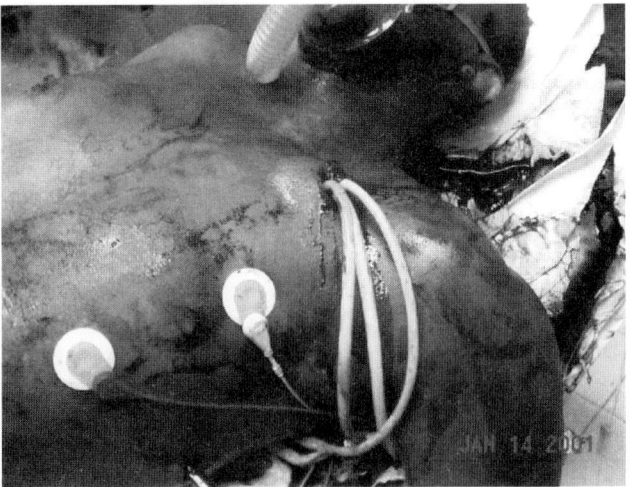

Figure I   Balloon tamponade of a bleeding chest wound. *Picture courtesy of Ricardo Ferrada, MD.*

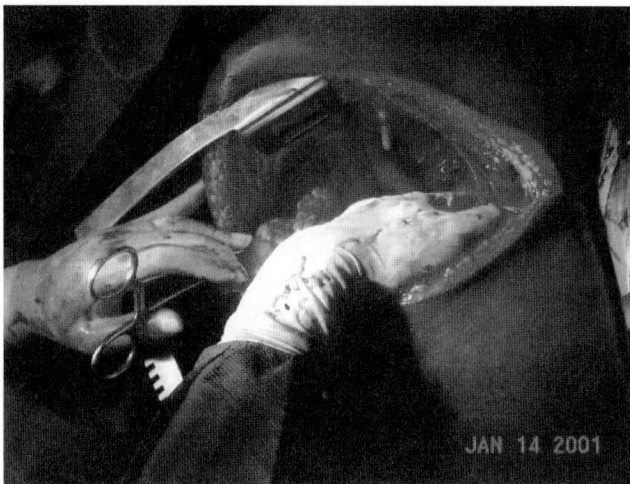

Figure 2 Same patient with tamponade by Foley catheter seen at thoracotomy (*arrow*). *Picture courtesy of Ricardo Ferrada, MD.*

reported. The rare injury to the vertebral artery, being difficult to expose and repair, is treated by proximal and distal ligation.

In the patient with blunt mechanism of injury, we make every effort to perform CT of the chest, supplemented if necessary with arteriography to evaluate for injuries to the thoracic great vessels. Occasionally, when the patient requires emergent laparotomy and CT is not possible, depending on the surgeon's index of suspicion, intraoperative transesophageal echocardiography may be used to evaluate for blunt aortic injury. If an injury is found that requires operative management, the laparotomy is abbreviated.

Neck injuries are initially evaluated using Roon and Christensen's classification of the level of the entrance wound into three neck zones. Angiography is a modality that is used in selected patients with penetrating zone I and zone III injuries to rule out the presence of vascular injuries and to plan operative management. This approach allows for endovascular treatment of injuries that could be difficult to expose operatively (e.g., vertebral artery injuries).

Abdomen

After the abdomen has been accessed through a midline laparotomy, the four quadrants are packed with laparotomy sponges and excess blood is evacuated. Liver and splenic injuries are packed, and fecal contamination is addressed quickly. Intestinal perforations are temporarily controlled with clamps or umbilical tapes without resection, and attention is turned toward dealing with the source of major blood loss.

Splenic Injuries

Splenic conservation techniques are not used in damage control. Splenectomy is preferred.

Liver Injuries

The liver is initially packed and manually compressed to allow volume resuscitation by the anesthesiologist if the patient is in extremis. Attempts to control bleeding from the depths of the liver wound without allowing time for the anesthesiologist to "catch up" will result in a vicious cycle of exsanguination. There are a variety of techniques described in the literature to approach liver parenchymal bleeding and juxtahepatic venous injuries that are beyond the scope of this chapter. After controlling liver bleeding,

the injury is packed. Packing may also be used to control hemorrhage when all else fails, but "desperate packing" is associated with a high mortality rate. Packing may be successful occasionally in retrohepatic venous injuries that are difficult to control and repair. After rapid termination of the laparotomy, hepatic angiography may be considered as a valuable adjunct to optimally control bleeding from the liver. Some have also advocated angioembolization as the primary means for treatment of liver bleeding instead of laparotomy. We believe that such an approach should be undertaken only in select patients who are hemodynamically stable and in situations in which the concept of damage control does not necessarily apply.

Biliary Tract Injuries

Primary closure is indicated in simple lacerations of the bile duct in which the injury occupies less than 50% of the circumference. A T-tube is placed through a separate incision for biliary drainage. A more extensive injury will require choledochojejunostomy or hepaticojejunostomy, neither of which is performed during the initial operation in the damage-control setting. In this instance, the bile duct is ligated and a T-tube or cholecystostomy placed for biliary drainage.

Pancreaticoduodenal Injuries

Minor pancreatic lacerations or contusions to the left of the superior mesenteric vessels are drained during the initial laparotomy. Major lacerations or injuries involving the main pancreatic duct to the left of the superior mesenteric vessels are best treated by distal pancreatectomy with splenectomy. Lacerations to the right of the superior mesenteric vessels are usually drained, with endoscopic retrograde pancreatography or intraoperative pancreatography performed at a later date for evaluation of the main pancreatic duct. Control of bleeding at the head of the pancreas may be extremely challenging and may require supraceliac aortic control before exposure. Transection of the neck of the pancreas may be necessary to facilitate access to the portal vein and superior mesenteric vessels.

Duodenal injuries are usually treated with primary closure. If there is doubt about the integrity of the repair, the pylorus may be closed by a heavy running suture through a gastrotomy, and the stomach decompressed with tube suction. For destructive injuries to the pancreaticoduodenal complex with extensive devitalization or injury to the ampulla of Vater, poorly controlled bleeding from the pancreatic head, or poorly visualized retropancreatic bleeding, pancreaticoduodenectomy may be indicated if less radical measures fail to stop the bleeding. Reconstruction is deferred to the subsequent reexploration after stabilization of the patient. During the initial operation, the common bile duct is ligated and the biliary system decompressed via a T-tube. The duodenal bulb and the pancreatic neck remain stapled.

Intestinal Injuries

Intestinal spillage is controlled initially with clamps or umbilical tapes. After life-threatening bleeding has been addressed, small perforations may be debrided and closed primarily, and larger perforations or devitalized segments are resected with staplers. Anastomoses are deferred to reexploration.

Renal and Ureteral Injuries

Ureteral injuries are rare and are almost always due to penetrating trauma. Primary repair of these injuries is best left to the reoperative phase. Some advocate stent placement through the injury proximally to the kidney to exteriorize urinary drainage.

A zone II retroperitoneal hematoma is not explored in the blunt-trauma patient if the hematoma is not expanding or pulsatile and if there is no visualized urinary extravasation. In penetrating trauma, zone II hematomas should be explored. If the perirenal hematoma is explored and there is an injury to the renal artery, assessment of the patient's physiologic status and the time between injury and laparotomy will determine whether revascularization is feasible, but when abbreviated laparotomy is contemplated, nephrectomy is usually performed. When the decision to perform nephrectomy is made, evaluating the function of the contralateral kidney via intravenous pyelogram does not alter management because the patient would not be expected to tolerate a complex renovascular reconstruction.

If exploration of a zone II retroperitoneal hematoma is not required during initial laparotomy, CT is performed for evaluation when the patient is in the intensive care unit (ICU). If there is evidence of a major renovascular injury with clinical signs of ongoing bleeding, it may be necessary to return the patient to the operating room. Because the patient is usually critically ill in this scenario, nephrectomy is performed. A viable alternative is angiography with endovascular techniques to achieve the dual goals of cessation of bleeding and renal salvage: proximal artery injuries may be excluded by stenting, and injuries to the distal branches may be embolized.

Abdominal Vascular Injuries

Ligation of the celiac artery and inferior mesenteric artery may be performed to control bleeding from injuries to these vessels. Ligation of the superior mesenteric artery is not well tolerated, and therefore the artery should be repaired. There are few reports of shunting of this artery. Injuries to the iliac arteries should be repaired, if possible, with temporary shunting or ligation as options. If the iliac artery is ligated, fasciotomy is recommended and planned in-situ reconstruction or extra-anatomic bypass is almost always required later because of limb ischemia.

Injuries to the major veins are usually best treated with primary repair. Occasionally, the infrarenal vena cava and portal vein may be ligated to control bleeding. To prevent renal insufficiency, avoid ligating the suprarenal vena cava, if possible.

Pelvic and Extremity Injuries

If surgical stabilization of long-bone fractures is required beyond splinting with plaster, external fixation is expeditiously applied. In unstable patients with pelvic fractures showing pubic symphysis widening ("open-book" fractures), a commercially available pelvic binder is applied to reduce the fracture in the resuscitation bay. With this intervention, emergent external fixation is almost never required. Urgent angiography with embolization is frequently required for ongoing bleeding after adequate volume resuscitation and is effective in more than 90% of cases.

If there is a large pelvic hematoma and continued hemodynamic instability possibly originating from the pelvis when laparotomy is performed for blunt abdominal trauma, the abdomen is packed and pelvic external fixation performed concomitantly, if indicated. We prefer to proceed then to angiography. In penetrating trauma, pelvic hematomas should be explored to prevent missing a major vascular injury. A particularly challenging injury is the open pelvic fracture with exsanguinating bleeding. Rapid packing into the depths of the wound is necessary to staunch the bleeding, thus allowing for volume resuscitation and urgent angiography.

The approach to extremity vascular trauma uses the same techniques as vascular torso injuries. If the patient is unstable and the common femoral or popliteal arteries are ligated, planned reconstruction should follow to prevent the necessity for subsequent amputation. The superficial femoral artery may be ligated without reconstruction in selected cases, given the presence of collateral flow through the deep femoral artery. Injuries to the vessels below the knee level are treated with ligation as long as a single vessel runoff is preserved.

For extremity fractures with vascular compromise, the options are to perform rapid stabilization with external fixation of the fracture, followed by revascularization, or to perform revascularization first. The decision depends on the duration and degree of limb ischemia. If revascularization is necessary to restore flow before orthopedic stabilization is achieved, a temporary shunt may be placed to prevent the possibility of disruption of a vascular repair with subsequent manipulation of the fracture. Definitive repair can be accomplished after fracture stabilization or after ICU resuscitation during reoperation, depending on the physiologic status of the patient. Amputation as a damage-control procedure is justified if the limb is clearly nonviable as a result of a prolonged period of ischemia; if there is loss of motor nerve function with signs of vascular injury; or if the patient would not be expected to tolerate further blood loss, prolonged general anesthesia, or reperfusion (e.g., an elderly patient with ischemic changes on electrocardiogram following major trauma). The potential for inducing life-threatening arrhythmias during reperfusion of a limb with advanced ischemia must be considered in the already acidotic, multiply injured patient.

Closure of Chest and Abdominal Incisions after Initial Operation

We use a "vacuum-assisted closure" technique in which a nonadherent, plastic, fenestrated dressing (bowel isolation bag) is placed over the abdominal contents. One or two laparotomy towels are then folded and placed over the isolation bag. One or two tubes (Kendall Argyle Salem sump tubes; Tyco Healthcare, Princeton, NJ) are placed within the folded laparotomy towels to drain off excess fluid. A sterile, adhesive, transparent drape (Ioban; 3M Pharmaceuticals, St. Paul, MN) is then placed over all of the dressings and the abdominal wound. The Salem sump tubes are connected to wall suction in the ICU. Other authors have advocated closing the skin with sutures, towel clips, suturing mesh, or nonexpandable material (i.e., plastic, intravenous fluid bags) directly to the skin edges or fascia to create a "silo." We do not favor these techniques because of the risk of precipitating abdominal compartment syndrome.

At the end of the initial operation, we usually close the chest with rib sutures, followed by a mass closure of skin, muscle, and fascia because there is typically significant bleeding from cut muscle and skin during initial thoracotomy. The thoracic cavity is usually not packed because this may interfere with lung ventilation and cardiac function. Some surgeons have used the technique of suturing a "silo" or bag to the thoracotomy incision (Fig. 3). Others have reported taking the patient back to the ICU with the aorta cross-clamped, with subsequently successful weaning from the clamp, but we have not had similar success.

PHASE II: RESUSCITATION IN THE INTENSIVE CARE UNIT

The patient is then taken back to the ICU, where rewarming is performed, coagulopathy corrected, and acidosis monitored. Both active and passive rewarming techniques are necessary, using

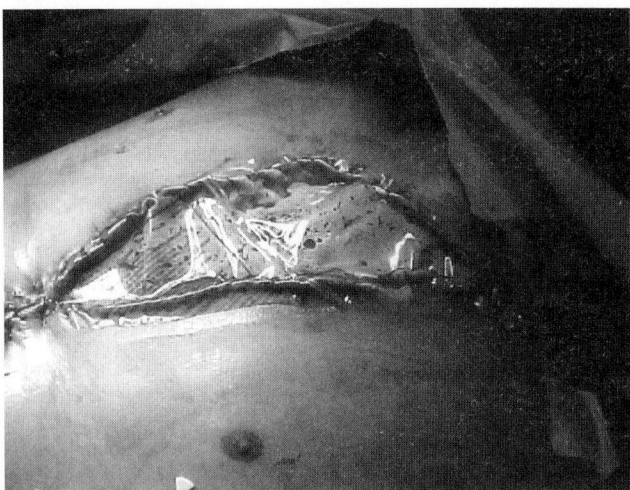

Figure 3 Temporary closure of a thoracotomy wound with a plastic sheet. *Picture courtesy of Ricardo Ferrada, MD.*

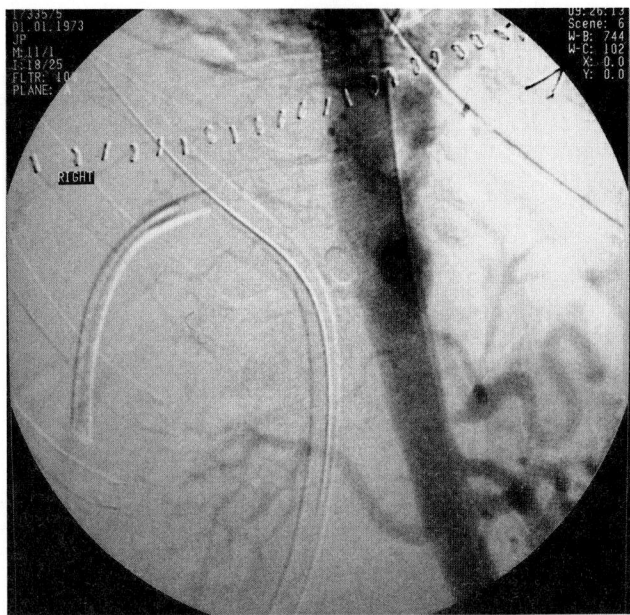

Figure 4 After sustaining a thoracoabdominal gunshot wound, this patient underwent laparotomy and right thoracotomy for a large right hemothorax and liver injuries. An injury to the aorta at the level of the hiatus was not appreciated during initial operation. Postoperative angiography showed the injury, which was treated with stenting, which resolved the hemodynamic instability.

intravenous fluid-warming devices and warming blankets. To reverse coagulopathy, in addition to using fresh frozen plasma (FFP) and platelets, we have used recombinant activated factor VII in patients with recalcitrant coagulopathic bleeding; results have been mixed. The international normalized ratio (INR) and platelet count are laboratory tests commonly used to guide transfusion therapy. However, it should be remembered that in the hypothermic patient, these values might not correlate with coagulopathic bleeding clinically. Also, in the patient requiring ongoing packed red blood cell (PRBC) transfusions, recent literature suggests that the dilutional effect of red cell component therapy requires an FFP-to-RBC transfusion ratio of as much as 1:1. To prevent the vicious cycle of coagulopathy, it is therefore prudent to initiate early plasma transfusions in the operating room or ICU rather than be guided by delayed laboratory tests. An ongoing dialogue between the surgeon and the anesthesiologist in the operating room is essential to minimize the occurrence of transfusion-related coagulopathy.

An unplanned return to the operating room may be necessary before optimizing the patient's physiologic status if the surgeon sees clinical evidence of ongoing bleeding (e.g., bloody output from drains, hemodynamic instability, persistent lactic acidosis). This may happen if there is inadequate control of surgical bleeding caused by inadequate exposure of significant injuries, failure to recognize bleeding from other cavitary sources, or iatrogenic injury during initial laparotomy. Resuscitation in the ICU will not produce clinical improvement because the patient will require ongoing transfusions of blood products and remain coagulopathic. It is sometimes unclear whether the surgeon has missed a source of surgical bleeding or whether coagulopathy has produced a vicious cycle of bleeding and transfusions. During relaparotomy, if an obvious source is not found after unpacking, signifying coagulopathic bleeding, the abdomen is repacked and the patient is returned to the ICU for further resuscitation.

Angiography with endovascular treatment of injuries is required in selected instances as a lifesaving therapeutic modality, complementing the initial damage-control efforts. These scenarios usually involve surgically inaccessible bleeding (e.g., liver, pelvic injuries) or evaluation for suspected vascular injuries not appreciated during initial operation (Fig. 4). The patient is sometimes taken from the operating room directly to the radiology department for angiography, depending on the circumstances. The risks of taking a patient to the angiography suite, which is usually geographically remote from the ICU, and the difficulty of performing further

resuscitation in the angiography suite (should that become necessary) must be weighed against the potential therapeutic benefits. It is often difficult to muster adequate resources and personnel for resuscitation in the radiology department.

Another scenario in which unplanned reexploration is necessary is the development of abdominal compartment syndrome in the ICU, signified by intra-abdominal hypertension with clinical signs of compromise in organ perfusion; increased difficulty with ventilation and oxygenation; and occasionally, increased intracranial pressure. Elevated bladder pressures usually signify intra-abdominal hypertension. If the patient is not expected to tolerate transport back to the operating room, bedside laparotomy with decompression is necessary. To prevent the occurrence of compartment syndrome, the skin and fascia should be left unapproximated after initial laparotomy. Because we leave the abdomen open using the previously described techniques, we have not had to perform decompressive laparotomy for abdominal compartment syndrome.

PHASE III: DEFINITIVE SURGERY

The definitive phase of the damage-control sequence involves removal of packing; more precise evaluation of injuries; the establishment of bowel, biliary tract, and genitourinary tract continuity; the development of an ileostomy or colostomy, if indicated; reassessment of hemostasis; definitive vascular repair; and debridement of devitalized tissues. The decision to perform these procedures should be made as soon as there is evidence of improvement in end organ perfusion and resolution of hypothermia, coagulopathy, and lactic acidosis. In general, this happens within 24 to 48 hours after initial operation. Relaparotomy should not be delayed because there is a risk of subsequent intra-abdominal infection if packs are left in the abdomen for more than 72 hours. During reoperation, packing should be removed carefully to prevent rebleeding. Because the packs are fairly adherent to viscera and omentum, the abdominal cavity is soaked for a few minutes, and the packs are then removed slowly "under water." If hemorrhage recurs after pack removal, the abdomen must be repacked and the patient must undergo another operation. Insertion of a nonadherent plastic drape between packs and viscera at the time of initial laparotomy helps to prevent this problem.

OUTCOME

Given the obvious difficulty of performing randomized trials, there are retrospective data showing improved outcome with the adoption of damage-control techniques. In one study of patients requiring transfusions of 50 or more units of packed RBCs in a 48-hour period, there was improved survival compared with historical controls. Significant factors identified were more frequent use of damage-control procedures, faster rewarming, and more aggressive correction of coagulopathy. In another study, comparing patients who underwent damage-control surgery with historical controls undergoing similar procedures, improved survival was seen. This was attributed to increased awareness of adverse physiologic conditions during initial laparotomy, prevention of abdominal compartment syndrome, and use of adjunctive interventional radiologic techniques.

Despite few studies showing improved outcome, surgeons worldwide have developed a greater appreciation for the indications and techniques used in damage control. Although there is a broad general consensus among surgeons caring for trauma patients regarding physiologic and anatomic considerations in the decision to abbreviate operative procedures, it is possible that there are certain instances when spending more time achieving hemostasis and fascial closure rather than terminating the operation too early may result in a better outcome for the patient, thereby possibly reducing transfusion requirements, as well as circumventing the open abdomen and its associated complications and morbidities (i.e., enterocutaneous fistula, abscess, prolonged bedrest, and mechanical ventilation). We believe that more prospective studies on selecting patients to undergo damage control are necessary.

Suggested Readings

Hirshberg A, Mattox KL, editors: Damage control surgery, *Surg Clin North Am* 77, 1997.

Johnson JW, Gracias VH, Schwab CW, and others: Evolution in damage control for exsanguinating penetrating abdominal injury, *J Trauma* 51:261, 2001.

Malone DL, Hess JR, Fingerhut A: Massive transfusion practices around the globe and a suggestion for a common massive transfusion protocol, *J Trauma* 60:S91, 2006.

Roon AJ, Christensen N: Evaluation and treatment of penetrating cervical injuries, *J Trauma* 19(6):391, 1979.

Rotondo MF, Schwab CW, McGonigal MD, and others: "Damage control": an approach for improved survival in exsanguinating penetrating injury, *J Trauma* 35:375, 1993.

Moore EE, Burch JM, Francoise RJ, and others: Staged physiologic restoration and damage control surgery, *World J Surg* 22:1184, 1998.

Stone HH, Strom PR, Mullins RJ: Management of the major coagulopathy with onset during laparotomy, *Ann Surg* 197:532, 1983.

THE ABDOMEN THAT WON'T CLOSE

Rao R. Ivatury, MD, Ajai K. Malhotra, MD, Michel B. Aboutanos, MD, and Thérèse M. Duane, MD

Closing the abdomen under tension is a practice that is still widely prevalent in various forms (the classic culprit is retention sutures), despite the warnings of many thoughtful clinician-scientists of the nineteenth century. Marey in 1863 and Henricus in 1890 commented on the adverse effects of increased intra-abdominal pressure. In 1951 Baggot, an anesthetist from Dublin, suggested that forcing distended bowel back into the abdominal cavity of limited size might kill the patient from abdominal wound dehiscence ("abdominal blow-out") and coined the term *acute tension pneumoperitoneum*. Since that time, the concept of intra-abdominal hypertension (IAH) and the ensuing abdominal compartment syndrome (ACS) has been emphasized, neglected, resurrected, and forgotten again. Only in the twentieth century did the "open abdomen" approach become a widely recognized clinical technique. Multisystem injuries, exsanguination, massive fluid resuscitation volumes, and damage-control celiotomy have thrust IAH, ACS, and the open abdomen approach to the forefront. It is not enough to use this approach in cases in which the abdomen won't close. There are strong clinical data to suggest that the open abdomen approach, when used for patients at risk for IAH and ACS, has tremendous implications for reduced morbidity and mortality. In our opinion, fascial closure under tension, that is, resorting to retention sutures, is a technique that should be condemned.

The broad indications and rationale for the open abdomen approach are the following:

1. For the prophylaxis and treatment of ACS in high-risk patients. *Rationale:* Prevention of the syndrome and treatment by early recognition has been shown in multiple studies to reduce the incidence of multiorgan failure and mortality.
   The groups at risk are those who have the following types of conditions:
   a. Extrinsic: reduction of large hernias (loss of domain); retention sutures
   b. Intraperitoneal: gastric dilatation, intestinal obstruction, ileus, neglected peritonitis, damage-control celiotomy with coagulopathy and intra-abdominal packing, ascites
   c. Retroperitoneal: bleeding, tumors, pancreatitis, abscess
   d. Miscellaneous: morbid obesity, multisystem trauma with large-volume resuscitation
2. Diffuse peritonitis in a compromised host: delayed treatment, the old, debilitated, and immunocompromised. *Rationale:* The infectious process may be so extensive (fecal peritonitis,

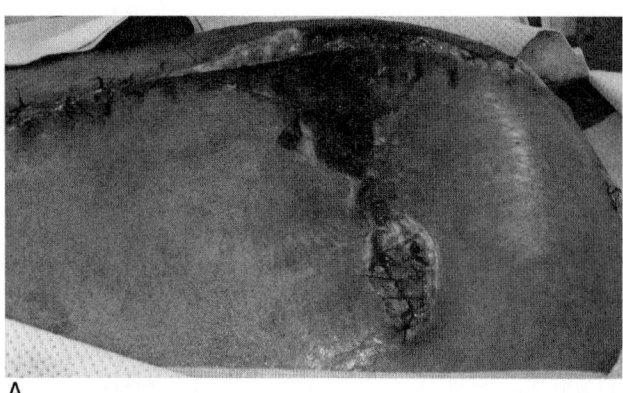

A

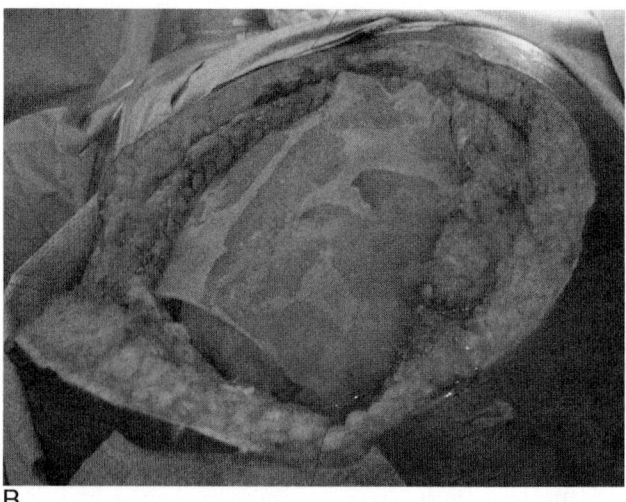

B

Figure 1 **(A)** Necrotizing fasciitis of the abdominal wall, requiring radical debridement and an open abdomen. **(B)** Radical debridement and application of temporary abdominal closure.

extensive purulence, infected exudate that cannot be easily debrided, etc.) and the host so compromised that one laparotomy may not be able to control the infection.

3. Intra-abdominal vascular catastrophes leading to resection of necrotic bowel and the decision for a second look has been made. *Rationale:* Second-look laparotomy is facilitated by the open abdomen, and the fascia is preserved for subsequent closure without violation at the first operation.

4. Abdominal wall necrotizing infections (postoperative or de novo) leading to extensive debridement and loss of abdominal wall. *Rationale:* Familiarity and comfort with the open abdomen technique will facilitate adequate, uncompromised debridement of all dead tissue (Fig. 1, *A,B.*).

5. Extensive abdominal trauma in an unstable patient: Damage-control approach. *Rationale:* The open abdomen technique will facilitate a rapid abbreviation of the celiotomy to resuscitate the patient.

The potential advantages of open abdomen in this setting are the following:

1. Allows rapid truncation of laparotomy in extremely sick patients and allows transport of patient to the intensive care unit (ICU) for correction of hypothermia, acidosis, and coagulopathy

2. Facilitates radical debridement of all dead tissue without worries about closure

3. Protects the abdominal fascia from repeated suturing and opening when subsequent laparotomy is performed

4. Enlarges the abdominal cavity in situations of massive bowel and tissue edema and may prevent IAH and ACS

5. In high-risk patients, will facilitate rapid decompression of the abdomen and expansion of the abdominal cavity in the ICU as an urgent treatment for IAH

6. Reduction in the frequency of multiple-organ failure in extensively injured patients, probably by several mechanisms:
   a. Prevention of IAH and ACS and also allows rapid decompression, should these complications occur
   b. Maintenance of adequate splanchnic perfusion and integrity of the gut mucosa and prevention of cytokine activation from sequential insults of hemorrhagic shock and IAH

7. Occasionally may facilitate rapid control of sudden intra-abdominal hemorrhage in patients with severe abdominal injuries

8. Subsequent operations on the open abdomen are surprisingly easy, with very flimsy adhesions between the bowel loops and between the bowel and the skin

The disadvantages of the open abdomen approach are as follows:

1. Aesthetically unappealing
2. Fluid losses from the exposed bowel and the peritoneum
3. Nursing difficulties
4. Increased need for ventilation in some patients
5. Enteroatmospheric fistulae (in the open abdomen)
6. Secondary peritonitis
7. Difficulty in closing the abdominal fascia
8. Need for abdominal wall skin grafting
9. Development of a hernia and the need for subsequent operations

The majority of these pitfalls are currently minimized because of better techniques of temporary closure of the open abdomen.

TEMPORARY CLOSURE OF OPEN ABDOMEN

The goals of temporary abdominal closure (TAC) are as follows:

1. To have a tension-free closure without elevating intra-abdominal pressure
2. To prevent evisceration, control third-space losses, lower bacterial counts, and minimize desiccation and damage to the viscera
3. To minimize the risks of increasing intra-abdominal pressure and developing an ACS
4. To minimize trauma to the abdominal wall and fascia, facilitate closure of the abdomen, and quantify third-space losses
5. To allow for rapid reexploration at the bedside

The various methods of TAC are summarized in Table 1.

Many surgical centers now prefer to use some variant of the vacuum-pack technique. The steps in applying this technique are described here:

Step 1: The bowel is covered by a plastic sheet (e.g., fluid-warmer bag) and tucked between the bowel and inner lining of the peritoneum. The goal is to prevent adhesion between the bowel and the abdominal wall. Multiple holes are then cut in the exposed portion of the plastic sheet (Fig. 12, *A,B*).

Table 1: Various Methods of Temporary Abdominal Closure

Closure Technique	Description	Advantages	Disadvantages
Skin only (towel clip closure, running suture of skin) (Fig. 2)	Serial application of towel clips or suture	Rapid	Does not prevent IAH; damage to clips may interfere with subsequent radiography (e.g., angiography)
Bogota bag (Fig. 3)	3-L IV bag, Steri-drape (3M, St. Paul, MN), Silastic bag, plastic bag rapidly sutured to skin	Inexpensive, inert, nonadherent	Risk of evisceration, loss of abdominal domain, risk for IAH
Dexon mesh (Davis & Geck, Danbury, CT) (Fig. 4); Vicryl mesh (Ethicon, Somerville, NJ) (Fig. 5)	Suturing of absorbable mesh to skin or fascial edges	Can be applied directly over bowel; allows for drainage of peritoneal fluid	Rapid loss of tensile strength (in the setting of infection), potentially large-volume losses Later ventral hernia development risk for bowel fistula when mesh is absorbed
Polypropylene mesh (Fig. 6)	Suturing of the mesh to the fascial edges	Good tensile strength, allows for drainage of peritoneal fluid	Risk of intestinal erosion when applied directly over bowel, potentially large-volume losses, high risk of mesh infection and hernias, difficult to remove
Polytetrafluoroethylene (PTFE) mesh (Fig. 7)	Suturing of the mesh to the fascial edges	Good tensile strength	Potential fluid accumulation underneath the mesh, limited tissue integration and granulation tissue formation over the mesh, risk of mesh infection, expensive
Wittmann patch, (Star Surgical, Burlington, WI) (Fig. 8)	Suturing of artificial burr (i.e., Velcro) to fascia, staged abdominal closure by application of controlled tension	Good tensile strength, allows for easy reexploration and eventual primary fascial closure	Poor control of third-space fluid, adherence of bowel to abdominal wall, potential for fistulae
Human acellular dermal graft (Alloderm; LifeCell, Branchburg, NJ) (Fig. 9)		Effective and safe in contaminated wounds. Can be used as a permanent prosthesis.	Limited experience, long-term results not yet known; may require multiple pieces sown together
Vacuum-pack closure (Fig. 10)	Bowel covered with plastic sheet and towel or Kerlix (KCI, San Antonio, TX) rolls; flat drains attached to wall suction	Inexpensive, uses material found in operating rooms, moderate control of fluid, high success in fascial closure	Inability to quantify suction
Negative pressure therapy; V.A. C. Abdominal Dressing System (KCI, San Antonio, TX) (vacuum-assisted closure device) (Fig. 11)	Reticulated polyurethane foam dressing over the plastic covering of the bowel. The negative pressure is controlled with a computer-controlled vacuum pump that applies a constant, regulated pressure to the wound surface and a sensing device to prevent uncontrolled fluid (e.g., blood) drainage.	Increase in blood flow, a reduction on abdominal wall tension, reduction in size of the abdominal wall defect, decreased bowel edema, and potential removal of inflammatory substances that accumulate in the abdomen during inflammatory states. Edema and third-space losses can be controlled and abdomen closed in a timelier manner.	Expensive

IAH, Intra-abdominal hypertension; *IV,* intravenous.
Adapted from Kaplan M, Banwell P, Orgill DP, and others: Guidelines for the management of open abdomen. Recommendations from a multidisciplinary expert advisory panel, Wounds: a compendium of clinical research and practice *17(suppl):1, 2005.*

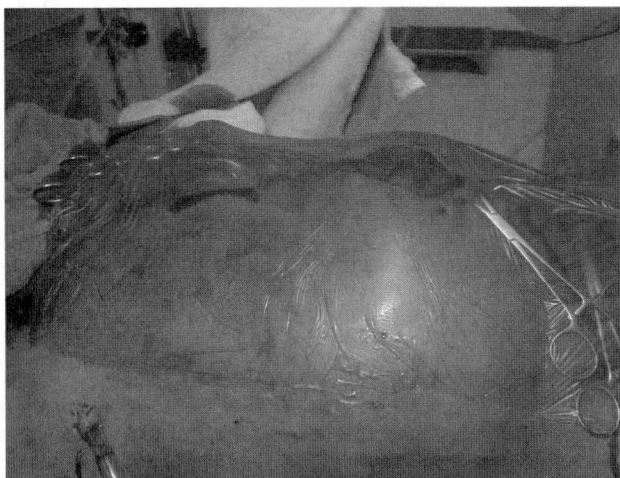

Figure 2 Temporary abdominal closure with serial applications of towel clips to the skin edges.

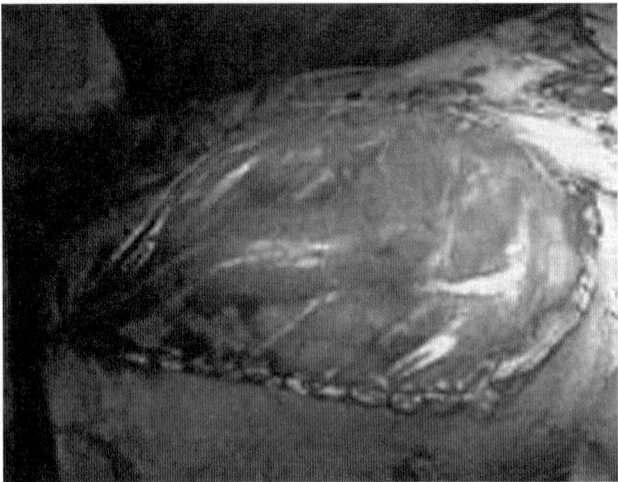

Figure 3 Temporary abdominal closure with a plastic bag (sometimes called "Bogota bag") sutured or stapled rapidly to skin.

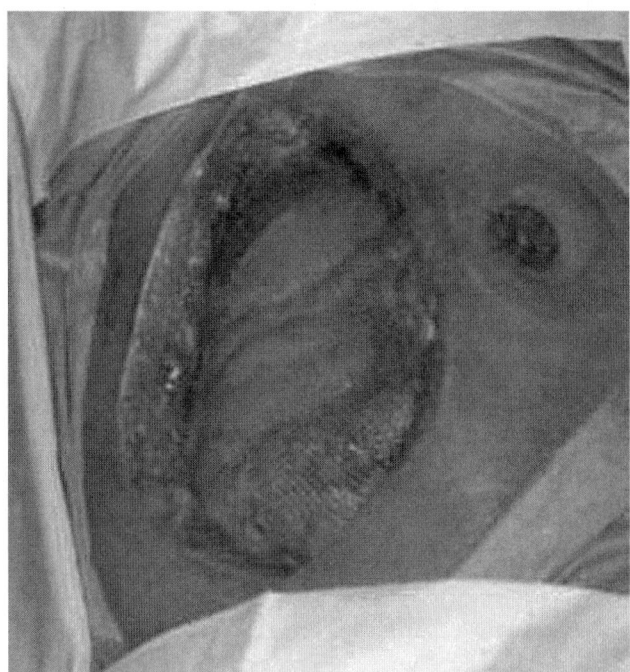

Figure 4 Dexon (US Surgical, Norwalk, CT) mesh for temporary abdominal closure.

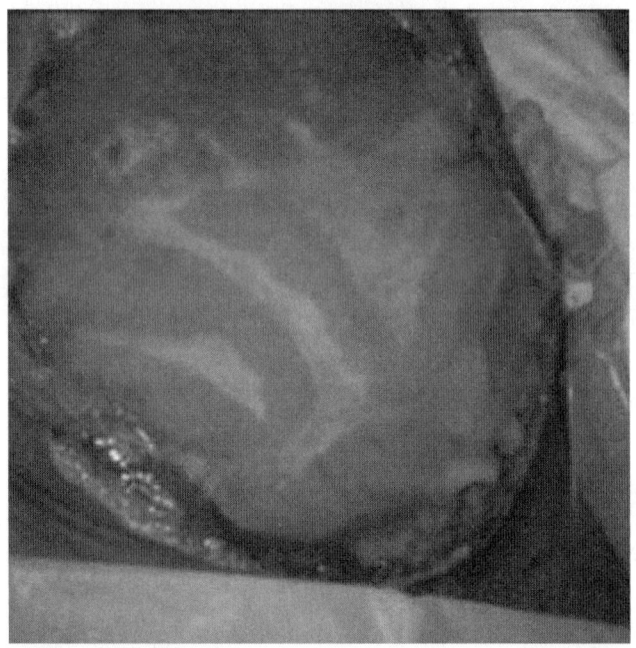

Figure 5 Vicryl (Ethicon, Somerville, NJ) mesh for temporary abdominal closure.

Step 2: Wet Kerlix (Kendall-LTP, Chicopee, MA) rolls are used to cover the plastic sheet, two flat Jackson-Pratt drains are placed on the Kerlix, and another roll of Kerlix is draped on top of the drains (Fig. 13).

Step 3: The skin on the abdominal wall is then dried thoroughly. Tincture of Benzoin is helpful.

Step 4: A wide piece of Ioban (3M Pharmaceuticals, St. Paul, MN) is then firmly placed on the abdominal wall to close the open abdomen in an airtight fashion. A tight seal is extremely important, and particular attention should be paid to the suprapubic region (see Fig. 13).

Step 5: The Jackson-Pratt drains are connected to moderate wall suction. Immediate collapse of the entire dressing indicates a watertight seal.

The advantages of this method are constant suction of the intra-abdominal fluid, prevention of leak of fluid onto the patient's bed, ability to quantitate the amount of fluid (and blood) losses from the abdomen, and maintenance of a lower intra-abdominal pressure.

SUBSEQUENT MANAGEMENT OF THE OPEN ABDOMEN

In the ICU, the patient is resuscitated to optimize tissue perfusion and to control coagulopathy, acidosis, and hypothermia. Intra-abdominal pressure is monitored by measurement of bladder pressure every 4 to 6 hours. Persistent elevation above 20 mm Hg should prompt reexploration to evacuate blood and clots. Fluid balance is monitored carefully, and over-resuscitation is avoided.

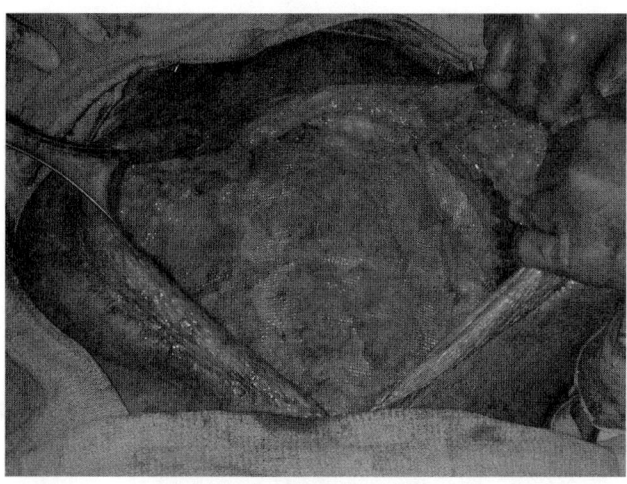

Figure 6 Polypropylene mesh as fascial substitute.

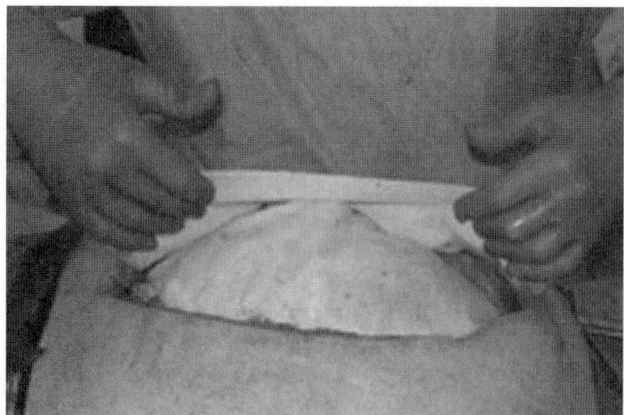

Figure 8 Wittmann (Star Surgical, Burlington, WI) patch for temporary abdominal closure. *From www.surgicalproductsmag.com*

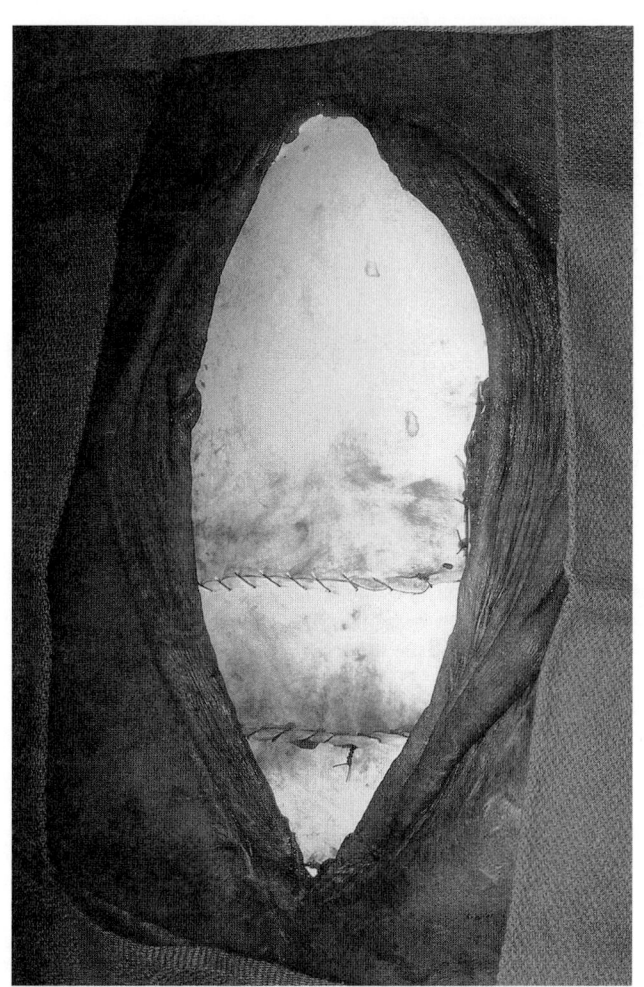

Figure 7 Polytetrafluoroethylene (PTFE) mesh for temporary abdominal closure.

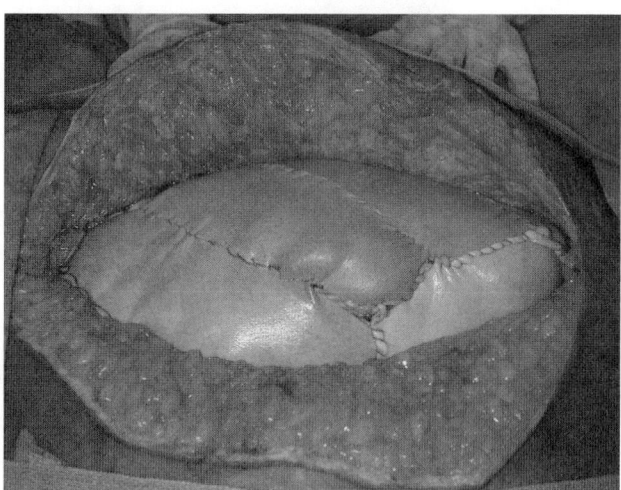

Figure 9 Human acellular dermal matrix (Alloderm; LifeCell, Branchburg, NJ) graft for fascial defects.

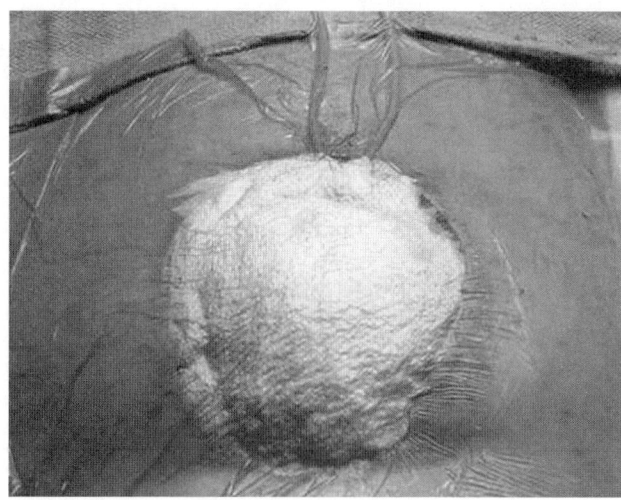

Figure 10 Vacuum-pack technique.

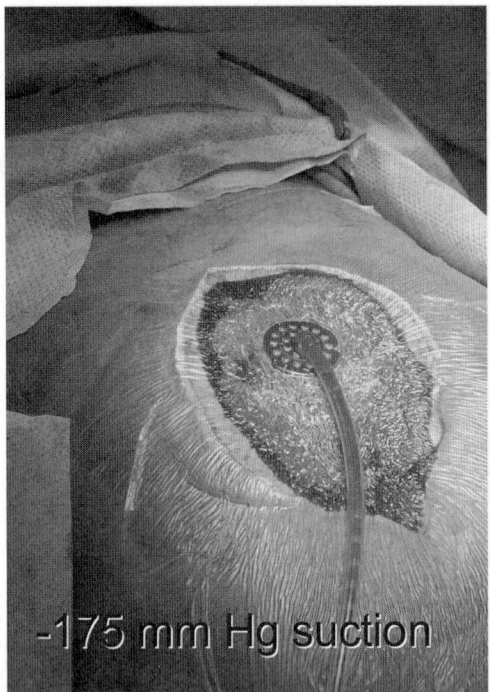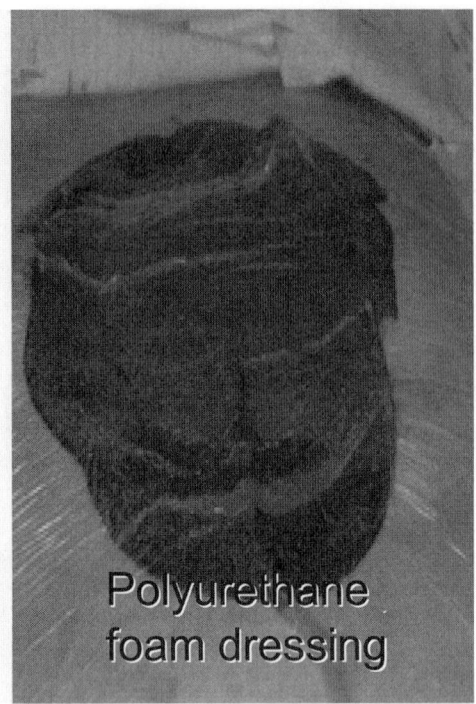

Figure 11 V.A.C. (KCI, San Antonio, TX) Abdominal Dressing System. Polyurethane sponge applied to the open wound and V.A.C. suction device applied.

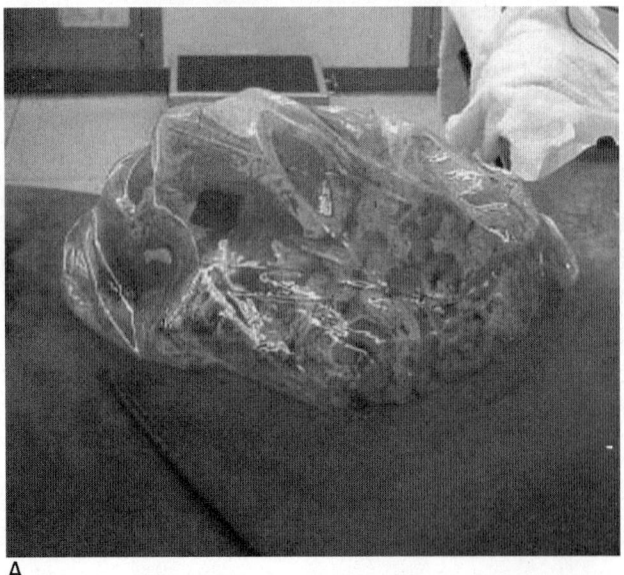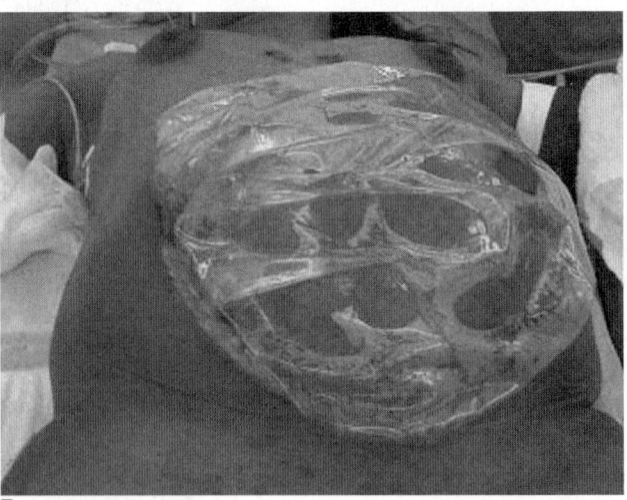

A B

Figure 12 **(A, B)** Application of a vacuum-pack dressing. The bowel is separated by the plastic sheet (e.g., fluid-warmer bag) from the peritoneum; multiple holes are cut in the sheet.

Careful use of diuretics may be considered to reduce third-space fluid accumulation.

At 2- to 3-day intervals, the patient is returned to the operating room, where the abdomen is irrigated and necessary therapeutic maneuvers (bowel anastomosis, drainage of purulent collections, etc.) are accomplished. At each operation, fascia is brought together by tension-free sutures (Fig. 14). If tension-free fascial closure cannot be completely reapproximated, the "poor-man's vac" (vacuum-assisted closure [VAC]) is repeated. Another option is to apply the VAC abdominal dressing at this second operation; we prefer the V.A. C. Abdominal Dressing System (KCI, San Antonio, TX). By the third or the fourth visit, fascial approximation is usually possible in a high

percentage of patients (Fig. 15). Several series are now available to document a high rate of success (>75%) with negative pressure therapy, with a mean time to closure of 7 to 9 days.

If, after these maneuvers, the fascia still cannot be approximated without tension after 1 to 2 weeks, it is unlikely that fascial approximation is a real possibility. In the absence of continuing systemic inflammatory syndrome, the abdominal wound begins to fill with granulation tissue (Fig. 16). At this point, skin flaps on either side of the midline should be raised and sutured together (accepting a large fascial defect that can be repaired at a later date) (Fig. 17, A-C). Next, a composite fascial prosthesis is used with an outer, nonabsorbable mesh and an inner,

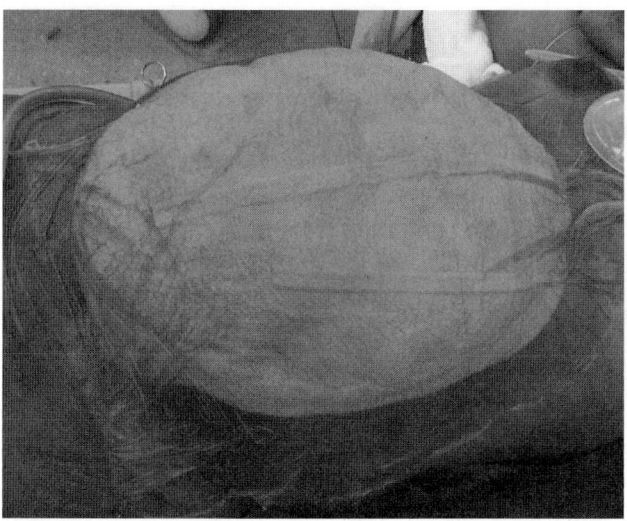

Figure 13 Wet rolls of gauze (e.g., Kerlix;Kendall-LTP, Chicopee, MA) are placed on the sheet and covered over two flat Jackson-Pratt drains, which are connected to wall suction. An airtight seal is applied with Ioban (3M Pharmaceuticals, St. Paul, MN).

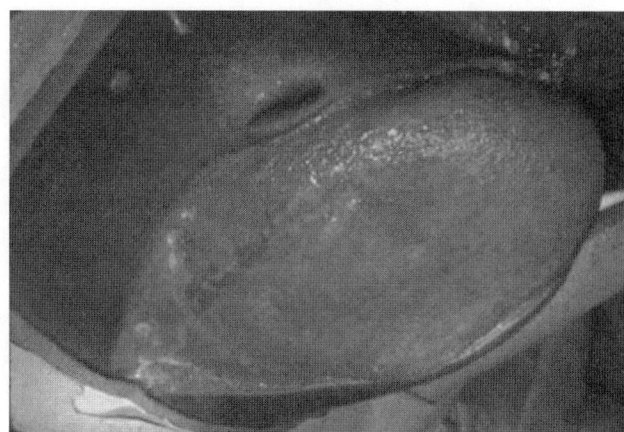

Figure 15 Fascial reapproximation is possible in approximately 75% of patients.

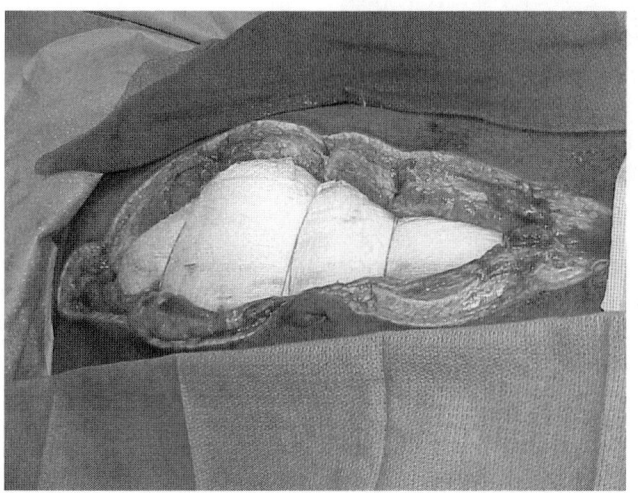

Figure 14 Sequential approximation of fascia in stages.

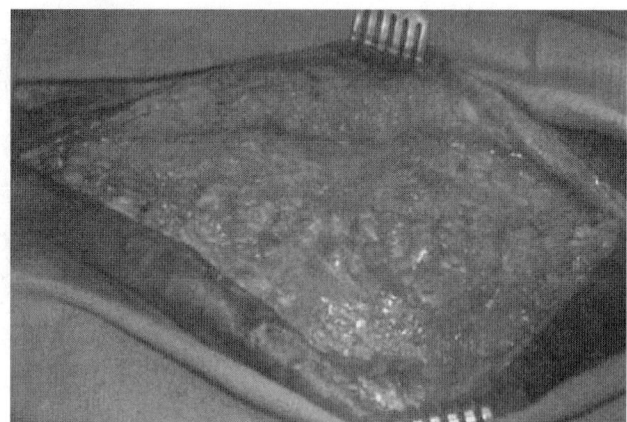

Figure 16 Open abdomen covered with healthy granulation tissue.

absorbable mesh to prevent dense adhesions, which usually occur with nonabsorbable mesh. Alternatively, a mesh prosthesis such as Alloderm (LifeCell, Branchburg, NJ) can be used. A split-thickness skin graft should be applied to the granulating surface of the bowel (Figs. 18 and 19), the components of the abdominal wall separated, and the defect by fascial transposition closed (Fig. 20).

A useful algorithm for the open abdomen is presented in Figure 21.

The following is a list of important technical aspects to keep in mind:

1. Try to avoid drains and stomas in the open abdomen. If unavoidable, bring them out as laterally in the flanks as possible. This will preserve enough normal abdominal wall for subsequent mobilization and closure.
2. Always use the omentum to cover the bowel loops when leaving the abdomen open.
3. Airtight seal in the vacuum-pack dressing is essential to maintain suction. Special attention must be given to the suprapubic

area. This can be confirmed when the entire abdominal dressing is "sucked in" as soon as suction is applied to the Jackson-Pratt drains. If this does not happen, the Ioban drape is removed, the skin is dried, and the Ioban is reapplied.

4. If using a V.A.C. dressing over exposed bowel, use the V.A.C. abdominal dressing. If not, a nonadherent interface must be placed between the bowel and the polyurethane sponge to prevent fistula formation.
5. In resuscitation phase, avoid over-resuscitation. Consider diuresis to minimize bowel edema after the patient has been resuscitated.
6. Continuing edema of the bowel and abdominal wall signifies systemic complications (systemic inflammatory response, intra-abdominal sepsis, multiorgan dysfunction syndrome, etc.). This problem is more common when the original indication for the open abdomen is abdominal sepsis. Under these circumstances, it is unlikely that the abdomen will be amenable to closure. Continued exposure of the edematous bowel is an invitation to fistulization. It is best to cover the bowel with skin-only closure, ignoring the fascia, or to suture an

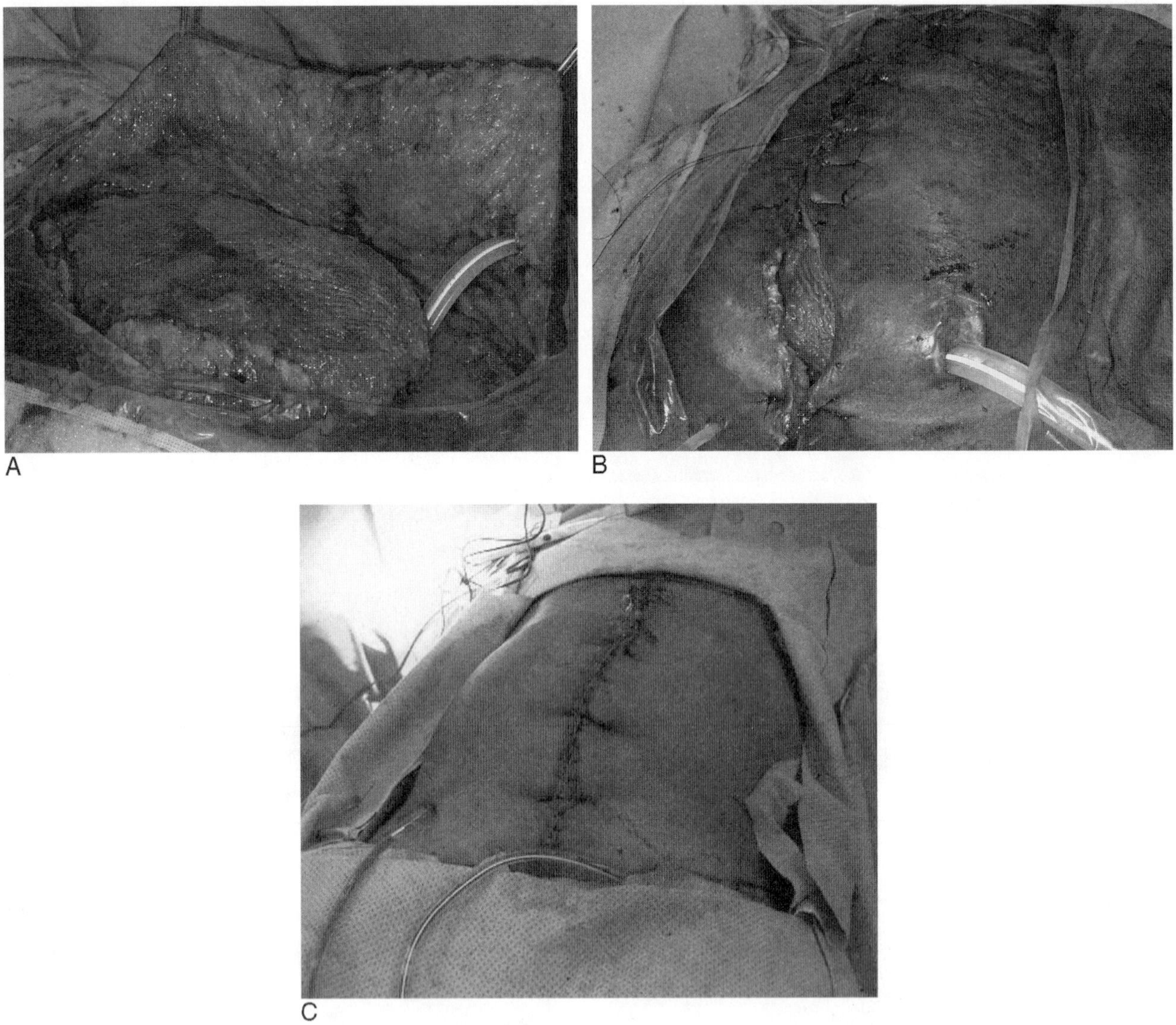

A

B

C

Figure 17 **(A, B, C)** Skin flaps may be mobilized on either side of the defect and sutured in the midline.

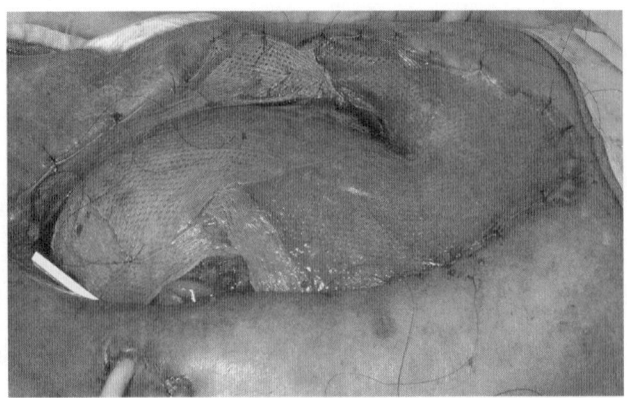

Figure 18   Split-thickness skin grafting may be applied to the granulating surface as seen in the operating room.

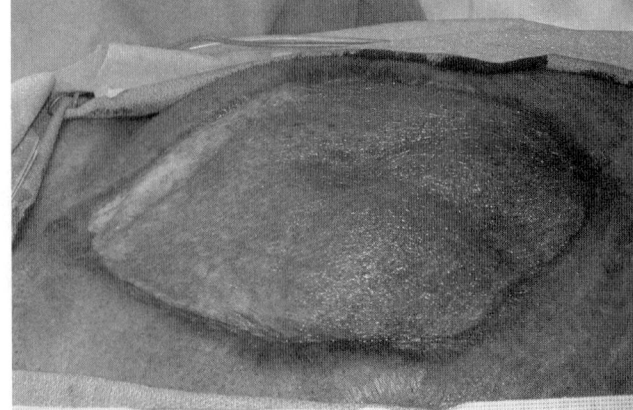

Figure 19   The skin graft after a few weeks. The large ventral hernia may be repaired at a later stage.

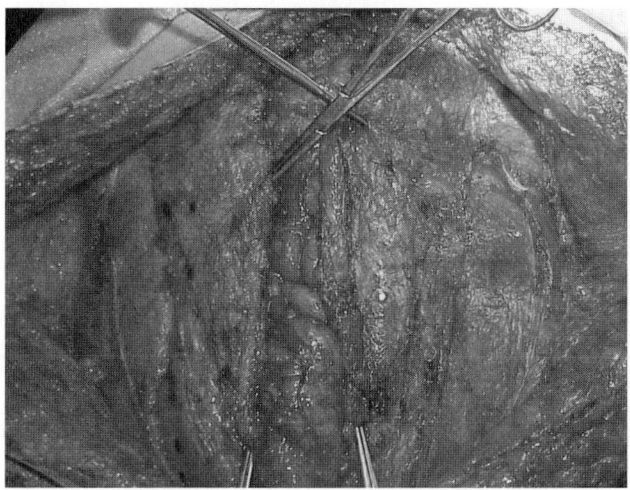

Figure 20 Component separation of the abdominal wall on either side may facilitate mobilization of the fascia and reapproximation in the midline.

absorbable mesh (e.g., Vicryl; Ethicon, Somerville, NJ), allowing the open abdomen to granulate. When granulation tissue begins to spread over the bowel, it may be skin that grafted or the skin that closed after flaps were mobilized.

7. Care must be taken to keep the dressings moist to wet. During dressing changes of the open abdomen, especially with edema of the bowel, it is easy to cause serosal tears by rough handling and these tears usually progress to a fistula.

8. Exquisite critical care of these severely ill patients is an integral part of managing the open abdomen.

SUMMARY

Many options are available for management of the abdomen that cannot close or that should not be closed. Open abdomen management has proven benefits. Its disadvantages and pitfalls are being resolved through the development of modern principles and techniques. Application of these principles is highly recommended for clinicians taking care of these desperately ill patients.

Figure 21 Algorithm for management of open abdomen. *ARDS,* Adult respiratory distress syndrome; *IAP,* intra-abdominal pressure; *MOF,* multi-organ failure; *V.A.C.,* vacuum-assisted closure.

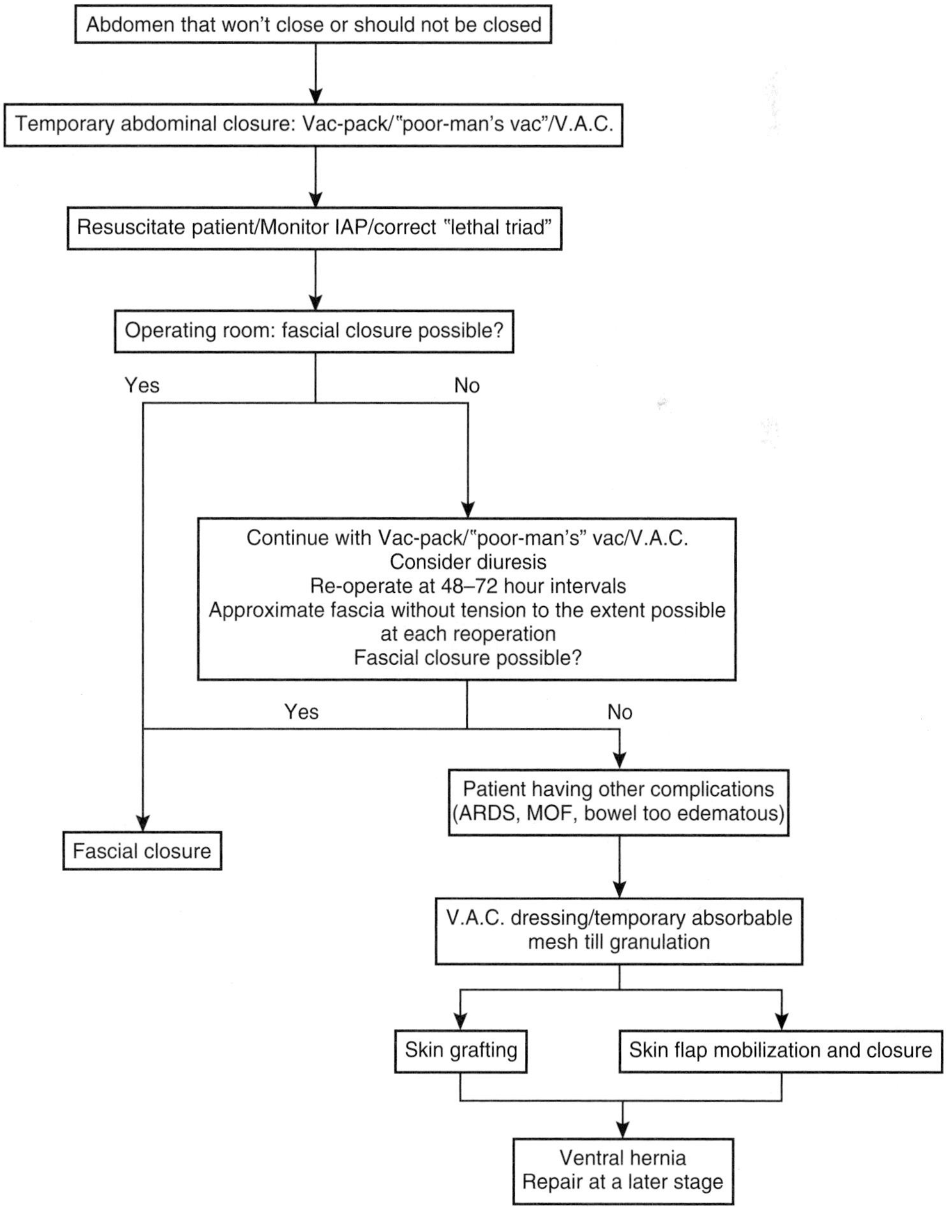

```
┌─────────────────────────────────────────────────┐
│ Abdomen that won't close or should not be closed │
└─────────────────────────────────────────────────┘
                        │
                        ▼
┌───────────────────────────────────────────────────────────┐
│ Temporary abdominal closure: Vac-pack/"poor-man's vac"/V.A.C. │
└───────────────────────────────────────────────────────────┘
                        │
                        ▼
┌─────────────────────────────────────────────────┐
│ Resuscitate patient/Monitor IAP/correct "lethal triad" │
└─────────────────────────────────────────────────┘
                        │
                        ▼
┌─────────────────────────────────────────────────┐
│ Operating room: fascial closure possible?       │
└─────────────────────────────────────────────────┘
        Yes                          No
         │                            │
         │                            ▼
         │         ┌──────────────────────────────────────────┐
         │         │ Continue with Vac-pack/"poor-man's" vac/V.A.C. │
         │         │ Consider diuresis                          │
         │         │ Re-operate at 48–72 hour intervals         │
         │         │ Approximate fascia without tension to the  │
         │         │ extent possible at each reoperation        │
         │         │ Fascial closure possible?                  │
         │         └──────────────────────────────────────────┘
         │            Yes                          No
         │             │                            │
         ▼             ▼                            ▼
┌─────────────────┐              ┌──────────────────────────────────┐
│ Fascial closure │              │ Patient having other complications │
└─────────────────┘              │ (ARDS, MOF, bowel too edematous)  │
                                 └──────────────────────────────────┘
                                                 │
                                                 ▼
                                 ┌──────────────────────────────────┐
                                 │ V.A.C. dressing/temporary absorbable │
                                 │ mesh till granulation              │
                                 └──────────────────────────────────┘
                                      │                    │
                                      ▼                    ▼
                              ┌───────────────┐  ┌──────────────────────────────┐
                              │ Skin grafting │  │ Skin flap mobilization and closure │
                              └───────────────┘  └──────────────────────────────┘
                                            │
                                            ▼
                                 ┌──────────────────────┐
                                 │ Ventral hernia        │
                                 │ Repair at a later stage │
                                 └──────────────────────┘
```

SUGGESTED READINGS

Ivatury RR, Cheatham M, Malbrain M, and others, editors: Abdominal compartment syndrome. Georgetown, TX, 2006, Landes Bioscience.

Kaplan M, Banwell P, Orgill DP, and others: Guidelines for the management of the open abdomen. Recommendations from a multidisciplinary expert advisory panel, *Wounds: a compendium of clinical research and practice* 17(suppl): 1, 2005.

Miller PR, Meredith JW, Johnson JC, and others: Prospective evaluation of vacuum-assisted fascial closure after open abdomen: planned ventral hernia rate is substantially reduced, *Ann Surg* 239:608, 2004.

Schechter W, Ivatury R, Rotondo M, and others: Open abdomen after trauma and abdominal sepsis: a strategy for management, *J Am Coll Surg* 203:390, 2006.

Scott BG, Feanny MA, Hirshberg A: Early definitive closure of the open abdomen: a quiet revolution, *Scand J Surg* 94(1): 9, 2005.

THE MANAGEMENT OF VASCULAR TRAUMA

Ben L. Zarzaur, MD, MPH, and Martin A. Croce, MD

Before the development of trauma systems and the implementation of advanced prehospital care, victims of vascular trauma rarely survived transport to the hospital. Now, survival is more frequent and surgeons have the opportunity to care for patients with these challenging injuries. Advances in surgical techniques and perioperative critical care, the introduction of advanced hemostatic agents, and the use of emerging endovascular techniques have improved the overall survival of patients with severe vascular injuries. This chapter covers the indications for operation of the most common vascular injuries and offers suggestions for treatment of these injuries.

GENERAL CONSIDERATIONS

Cervical Vascular Injuries

Physical examination provides the most sensitive test for the detection of most vascular injuries that require immediate operation following penetrating injury. This is particularly true for penetrating injuries to the neck. Injuries that violate the platysma are serious in nature, given the density of vital structures in the neck. For patients with penetrating injuries and hard signs (Table 1) on physical examination, immediate operative intervention is indicated. However, for patients who are without hard signs, the management of penetrating neck injuries depends on the anatomic location of the injury. Zone I of the neck is often referred to as the "thoracic outlet" and is between the clavicles and the cricoid cartilage. Zone II is between the cricoid cartilage and the angle of the mandible. Zone III is the area superior to the angle of the mandible. For zone I injuries, hemodynamically stable patients should undergo arteriography to delineate the exact vessel injured because different incisions are necessary to gain access to vessels in the

thoracic outlet. Similarly, because of the difficulty of gaining distal control of vascular structures above the angle of the mandible, injuries to zone III should be investigated via angiography in stable patients. In some cases, endovascular techniques may be the only option available for the management of distal carotid injuries.

Penetrating injuries to zone II of the neck have historically been managed by mandatory exploration. In institutions without sufficient radiologic support, this is the preferred method of management. If the surgeon is well supported, a selective management approach may be used. Zone II injuries in patients without hard indications for the operating room can undergo cerebrovascular angiography, tracheobronchoscopy, and either esophagoscopy or barium swallow. If any of these tests reveal an injury, immediate operative exploration is indicated.

Blunt cerebrovascular injury has been an underdiagnosed and undertreated injury in the past. However, with adequate screening protocols, injuries can be promptly recognized and treated, and the significant morbidity and mortality that can result from blunt cerebrovascular injury can be prevented. The typical spectrum of injuries includes intimal dissection, pseudoaneurysm, and occlusion. Urgent cerebrovascular angiography is recommended for patients who present with a neurologic deficit that is not explained by findings on computed tomography (CT) of the brain. Patients who are candidates for treatment with anticoagulation or antiplatelet therapy should undergo semiurgent angiography if they have risk factors for cerebrovascular injury (Table 2). With advances in the hardware and software for CT and widespread use of multislice scanners, it is likely that CT angiography will replace conventional angiography as a screening test.

Thoracic Vascular Injury

Victims of penetrating thoracic vascular injuries often exsanguinate at the scene or en route to the hospital. For those who survive to arrival at the hospital, there are often obvious indications for immediate operative intervention, including cardiac tamponade, significant hemothorax with more than 2000 ml of blood on placement of

Table 1: Hard Signs for Penetrating Vascular Injuries to the Neck

Ongoing hemorrhage
Large-sized or expanding hematoma
Bruit
Massive blood loss at scene
Hemiparesis or hemiplegia
Stridor

Table 2: Criteria for Screening for Blunt Cerebrovascular Injury

High-energy transfer mechanism with:
Le Fort II or III fracture
Subluxation of cervical spine
Fractures through the transverse foramen of the cervical spine
C1–C3 fractures
Basilar skull fracture with carotid canal involvement
Diffuse axonal injury with a Glasgow Coma Score <6
Neurologic examination incongruous with head CT findings
Near hanging with anoxic brain injury

CT, Computed tomography.

a chest tube, or loss of pulse in an extremity. Emergency department thoracotomy may be indicated in patients with penetrating injury or injuries to the chest who have no vital signs but show signs of life (defined as spontaneous movement, pupillary response, eye movement, or spontaneous respirations) in the field or in the emergency department. Patients with prolonged transport times (>10 minutes) who had signs of life in the field but who no longer have a palpable pulse are unlikely to have a functional outcome following emergency department thoracotomy. Moreover, victims of blunt trauma rarely benefit from emergency department thoracotomy, and this procedure should not be performed unless pericardial tamponade (indicating blunt cardiac chamber rupture) is suspected and the patient loses vital signs in the emergency department.

The most feared thoracic vascular injury resulting from blunt trauma is blunt aortic injury. If this injury is missed and goes untreated, it results in nearly 100% mortality within 1 year. With an aggressive screening protocol, this poor outcome can be avoided. Patients who present after a decelerating type of injury are at highest risk of blunt aortic injury. However, up to 25% of patients with blunt aortic injuries have other mechanisms of injury. Findings on anteroposterior (AP) chest x-ray that are suggestive of—but not diagnostic of—blunt aortic injury include a widened mediastinum, blunting of the aortic knob, presence of a left pleural effusion, an apical cap, a first or second rib fracture, tracheal deviation, nasogastric tube deviation, and depressed left bronchia. A widened mediastinum is the finding most suggestive of a blunt injury to the aorta. CT is the screening test of choice for blunt aortic injury. Findings that are consistent with the presence of an injury include a periaortic hematoma or evidence of intimal or vessel wall disruption. Controversy exists regarding the optimal test for the definitive diagnosis of a blunt aortic injury. Earlier reports showed that CT is sensitive but lacks specificity for diagnosis of blunt aortic injuries. Lack of specificity may lead to cases in which severely injured patients are subjected to an unnecessary operation. More recent reports using helical CT scanning demonstrate improved accuracy and justify its use as a viable screening test. Aortography should be performed if the CT is equivocal.

Abdominal Vascular Injuries

Penetrating injuries to abdominal vasculature are rarely subtle in their presentation. Common presenting symptoms are hemodynamic instability and abdominal distention in the presence of a penetrating abdominal injury. Patients with these symptoms require immediate operative exploration. Blunt injuries to major intra-abdominal vessels are uncommon, but they do occur. Because the major abdominal vascular structures are located in the retroperitoneum, most injuries are coupled with a retroperitoneal hematoma. Midline retroperitoneal hematomas (zone I) are associated with injuries to the aorta and the vena cava, as well as their major branches. Lateral retroperitoneal hematomas (zone II) are associated with renal artery and vein injuries and kidney injuries. Pelvic retroperitoneal hematomas (zone III) are associated with pelvic fractures and injuries to the iliac vessels. In patients with penetrating injuries to the retroperitoneum, mandatory exploration is the safest option for zones I, II, and III. Exceptions may be made for hemodynamically stable patients with a nonexpanding, lateral, zone II hematoma from either stab wounds or low-velocity gunshot wounds. For patients with blunt abdominal injuries, a selective approach to retroperitoneal exploration may be followed. Patients with nonexpanding zone II hematomas and nearly all zone III hematomas do not require exploration. On the other hand, all zone I injuries resulting from blunt trauma require exploration.

Peripheral Vascular Injuries

Attention to physical examination findings is essential to the diagnosis of peripheral vascular injury. As in injuries to the neck, patients with

Table 3: Hard and Soft Signs for Penetrating Vascular Injuries to the Extremity

Hard Signs	Soft Signs
Absent as diminished distal pulses	Proximity of wound or blunt injury to artery
Pulsatile bleeding	Small nonpulsatile hematoma
Expanding or pulsatile hematoma	Extremity neurologic deficit
Palpable thrill or bruit	Prehospital arterial bleeding
Signs of distal ischemia; pain, pallor, paresthesia, paralysis, coolness	

hard signs of peripheral vascular injury (Table 3) require immediate operative intervention. Patients with soft signs of injury may need further evaluation with arteriography. To increase the diagnostic yield of arteriography in patients with soft signs of peripheral vascular injury, arterial pressure distal to the site of injury should be compared with the arterial pressure in the contralateral extremity. If the difference in pressure between the two extremities is more than 10%, arteriography should be performed for definitive diagnosis. For patients without hard or soft signs, there is no need for further evaluation.

TREATMENT

General Techniques

Vascular injuries resulting in significant bleeding should be temporarily controlled with direct digital pressure, if possible. An alternative is the placement of a Foley catheter into the bleeding wound and inflation of the balloon to tamponade the bleeding. This technique should be used only for wounds of the extremities. In the operating room an assistant should maintain temporary control of the bleeding with direct pressure while the patient is prepared and draped. The surgeon should prepare the field widely and should include an uninjured lower extremity in the operative field. This will allow ready access to the saphenous vein if it is needed as a conduit for an arterial repair or bypass.

While the operation is under way, extensile exposure of the injury is critical. This means that the surgeon should be able to extend the incision along the same axis as the original incision to gain better proximal or distal control. Although it should be obvious, many surgeons forget the importance of gaining proximal and distal control of the injured vessel. Digital pressure applied to the bleeding vessel proximally and distally is often all that is needed for temporary control. The surgeon can then sequentially move his or her fingers closer together to identify the site of injury. In some situations, a sponge stick works well for this maneuver. However, one should exercise caution when using sponge sticks to apply pressure to large veins because the sponge sticks have a tendency to tear the vein if used improperly.

After the injury is identified and the bleeding controlled, the surgeon should determine the extent of the injury. While dissecting along the vessel, the surgeon is likely to encounter a large hematoma within the tissue planes. Anatomy is frequently distorted within a large hematoma. By approaching most vessels anteriorly and by identifying the anterior perivascular plane, the surgeon can safely identify the vessel and dissect along its length. After the injury has been identified, the injured vessel should be debrided back to healthy uninjured tissue. Particular attention should be paid to the intima. Damaged intima is extremely thrombogenic and should be debrided; it may extend 1 to

2 cm from the obvious injury. When trimming the vessel, the surgeon must bevel the vessel to help prevent anastomotic stenosis. If the patient has no contraindications to systemic anticoagulation, heparin should be administered. If the patient will not tolerate systemic heparinization, use of heparinized saline (50 U/ml) injected into the proximal and distal ends of the injured vessel provides a safe alternative.

After identifying the extent of the injury, the surgeon must decide between definitive repair and damage control. The surgeon must consider the patient's entire burden of injury and the realistic time required for definitive repair. Extensive blood loss associated with soft-tissue injury, coagulopathy, hypothermia, and acidosis are indications that the patient may not tolerate an immediate attempt at repair. If this is the case, damage control should be considered. Temporary shunting of arteries is possible and can be accomplished quickly. Clot should be removed from the proximal and distal ends of the vessel using a Fogarty catheter, followed by flushing of both ends to remove any remaining clot. Carotid shunts, pediatric chest tubes, and pieces of nasogastric tubes have been successfully used for temporary shunts. The surgeon should choose a shunt with the largest diameter that will fit into the vessel. The distal end should be inserted first; then the shunt material is trimmed to the desired length and the proximal end inserted. Vessel loops can be used to secure the shunt in place.

If the patient is exsanguinating from an arterial or venous injury, ligation is an option. The only veins for which repair should be attempted, even in dire situations, are the superior vena cava, the perirenal inferior vena cava, and the portal vein. However, if any of these veins cannot be controlled and the alternative for the patient is exsanguination, ligation is the preferred choice. Surprisingly, the list of arteries for which repair or temporary shunting should be attempted is short: the carotid, innominate, brachial, superior mesenteric, proper hepatic, renal, iliac, femoral, popliteal, and the aorta.

If the patient's physiologic condition allows, an attempt at definitive repair should be made. Simple lateral repairs can usually be accomplished quickly and should be performed whenever possible. If lateral repair is not possible, primary end-to-end anastomosis is the next best option. The proximal and distal ends of the vessels should be mobilized to the fullest extent possible. Side branches may be taken to increase the length available so that an anastomosis can be performed without tension. If, after mobilization, the repair will still be under tension, an interposition graft should be used. The reversed saphenous vein is an ideal conduit for most situations. However, when dealing with injuries to the lower extremity, it is essential that the saphenous vein be taken from the contralateral lower extremity because the deep venous system in the injured leg may be damaged. When this is the case, the saphenous vein becomes an important means for venous outflow in the injured extremity.

Alternatives to using vein for repairs include transposition procedures at arterial branches (such as substituting the external carotid artery for an injured proximal internal carotid artery) or using polytetrafluoroethylene (PTFE) grafts. For larger vessels such as the aorta, a PTFE graft is one of the only options available to the surgeon for definitive repair. If PTFE must be used in a contaminated field, such as the abdomen with an associated gastrointestinal injury, the surgeon should make every effort to decontaminate the operative field as much as possible before manipulating the graft. The operative field should be liberally irrigated, and new instruments, gowns, gloves, and drapes should be used. After the anastomosis is completed, viable tissue should be used to cover the graft. In the abdomen, the omentum is a useful covering for the graft. Definitive repair of gastrointestinal injuries can be accomplished after the graft has been covered.

The surgeon should use standard vascular anastomotic techniques for definitive repair. When the vessel is not tethered, repair may be accomplished by continuous suture (for large vessels) or partial running suture (for most other vessels). This technique will minimize the chance of creating a "purse sting" anastomosis. Stay sutures are placed directly opposite one another. One is tied, and then a tail is used to sew half the anastomosis toward the other stay suture. This suture is then tied to itself and the continuous suture. The vessel can be rotated so that the other half of the anastomosis may be sewn. For smaller vessels, three stay sutures forming a triangle may be used. Alternatively, for vessels that are tethered, a parachute technique can be used as long as the surgeon keeps in mind that it is essential to maintain tension on both ends of the posterior suture line to prevent leakage after the anastomosis is completed. The size of suture used for repair should be the smallest size appropriate for the vessel; this will ensure close suture placement and prevent anastomotic leaks.

CONSIDERATIONS FOR SPECIFIC INJURIES

Cervical Vascular Injuries

For operative repair of the carotid arteries, exposure is easiest to obtain via an incision anterior to the sternocleidomastoid muscle. For extensive injuries to the internal carotid artery, transposition procedures can be useful because the external carotid artery can be readily ligated. When there is concern for injury on both sides of the neck, a collar-type incision can be used to gain access to both sides. However, more extensive exposure is obtained with bilateral anterior sternocleidomastoid incisions.

Increased screening for blunt cerebrovascular injuries will ultimately lead to an increased likelihood of finding injuries to these important vessels. Advanced-generation CT scanners will likely accomplish this screening role.

Data from Memphis and Denver indicate that an aggressive screening and treatment protocol will lead to a significant decrease in the stroke rate following blunt cerebrovascular injury. Treatment of blunt cerebrovascular injuries continues to evolve. After an injury has been identified, transections and occlusions that are operatively accessible should be repaired. For injuries that are not readily accessible, or for vessels with luminal irregularities, intimal injuries, or pseudoaneurysms (the vast majority of blunt injuries), systemic anticoagulation with heparin is the treatment of choice. The partial thromboplastin time should be kept between 40 and 50. Even patients with significant solid-organ injury who are 24 to 48 hours from the time of injury will typically tolerate systemic heparinization. Consultation with neurosurgery colleagues is essential before performing anticoagulation in patients with closed head injuries. For patients who have a contraindication to systemic heparinization, antiplatelet agents (either aspirin 325 mg/day or clopidogrel 75 mg/day) can be used. Endovascular stenting is gaining popularity for patients with blunt carotid injuries, especially for patients with pseudoaneurysms because these are unlikely to resolve.

Thoracic Vascular Injuries

The type of incision necessary to gain access to injuries of the thoracic vasculature is dependent on which vessel is injured. Median sternotomy provides the best exposure for the heart, ascending aorta, aortic arch, and the innominate artery and vein. The advantage of this incision is that it can be easily extended into the cervical region (for injuries to the proximal carotid arteries), the supraclavicular fossa (for injury to the proximal right subclavian artery), or a combined supraclavicular fossa and left anterolateral thoracotomy (for injury to the left subclavian artery). A left posterolateral incision is used to gain access to the descending thoracic aorta, the proximal left subclavian artery, and the left pulmonary hilum. A right posterolateral incision is made to gain access to the right pulmonary hilum and the azygous vein. Emergent control of exsanguinating hemorrhage from either subclavian vessel may be accomplished with an anterolateral thoracotomy through the third intercostal space.

Aggressive beta-blockade should be used for patients with blunt injuries to the descending thoracic aorta. This will decrease myocardial contractility and subsequent shear forces on the injured aorta. The target heart rate should be between 60 and 80 beats per minute, with a systolic blood pressure less than 110 mm Hg. Vasodilators are to be avoided before adequate institution of beta-blockade because unopposed vasodilatation will lead to increased contractile activity of the heart and a deleterious increase in wall tension in the injured aorta. Operative repair should be attempted as soon as practical for most patients. Significant controversy exists concerning the proper way to address this injury. Advocates for the "clamp-and-sew" technique argue that the increased time and potential morbidity resulting from the use of full or partial bypass for distal aortic perfusion is greater than the potential for paralysis resulting from a lack of blood flow to thoracic spinal vessels. Bypass advocates argue that the time needed to perform an adequate anastomosis is often greater than anticipated, and the risk for postoperative paralysis is too great to perform a clamp-and-sew technique. Large series confirm the safety and reduced paraplegia rates in patients who have been treated with distal aortic perfusion techniques.

Abdominal Vascular Injuries

The transverse mesocolon is an important landmark that helps the surgeon to decide how to approach a midline retroperitoneal hematoma. If the hematoma is supramesocolic, an injury to the suprarenal aorta, celiac axis, proximal superior mesenteric artery, or proximal renal artery should be suspected. The best exposure for this type of injury is a left-sided medial visceral rotation. Incising the left-lateral peritoneal attachments of the descending colon and carrying the incision past the splenic flexure allows the surgeon to complete this maneuver relatively quickly. The spleen is then mobilized from the lateral attachments to the abdominal wall. After this is completed, the colon, spleen, and pancreas are rotated medially to expose the aorta from the hiatus to the aortic bifurcation. The kidney can be mobilized with the rest of the left-sided organs but usually is left in situ. To obtain better control of the proximal aorta, the left crus of the diaphragm can be incised.

For inframesocolic midline retroperitoneal hematomas, injury to the infrarenal aorta or inferior vena cava should be suspected. This type of hematoma may be approached as one would in an elective abdominal aortic aneurysm repair. The transverse mesocolon is reflected cephalad, and the small bowel is eviscerated to the patient's right. The midline peritoneum is incised to expose the inframesocolic aorta inferior to the left renal vein. If the aorta appears intact or the hematoma appears to be emanating predominately from the right side, an injury to the inferior vena cava may be the source of bleeding. Although a portion of the inferior vena cava can be exposed by incising the midline peritoneum as just described, much better exposure can be gained by performing a right-sided medial visceral rotation (Cattell-Braasch maneuver). The peritoneum lateral to the ascending colon is incised and carried to the hepatic flexure. The ascending colon and the duodenum are widely mobilized medially. This allows for exposure of virtually the entire inframesocolic retroperitoneum.

For lateral retroperitoneal hematomas, it is likely that the kidney has been injured. Occasionally, a lateral retroperitoneal hematoma will indicate that an injury to the distal renal artery or vein has occurred. There is a fair amount of controversy regarding the optimal way to manage acute renal arterial injuries. In most cases of penetrating trauma, the patient is usually so physiologically compromised that attempted repair is not warranted. For patients with blunt renal artery injuries more than 3 hours from the time of injury, the outcome from attempted repair would likely be poor. However, it may be advantageous to proceed with renal arterial repair if the patient is within 3 hours of injury, can tolerate a potentially lengthy procedure, or has a nonfunctional or absent

contralateral kidney (or a combination of these factors). Unfortunately, a blunt renal artery injury is rarely diagnosed within this time frame. It is best to observe these patients because many will regain renal function via collateral vessels and most do not become hypertensive. Endovascular stenting in also an option for management of blunt renovascular injuries.

Large, right-sided retroperitoneal hematomas that appear to be above the area of the kidney usually are a sign of juxtahepatic venous injuries. If the hematoma is not actively expanding or if the patient is hemodynamically stable, the hematoma should not be opened. However, if it becomes necessary to approach this hematoma, the likelihood of a successful outcome is low. Total vascular isolation of the liver can be used to manage these severe injuries. Total hepatic vascular isolation is obtained by performing a Pringle maneuver, clamping the aorta at the hiatus, and clamping of the infrahepatic and suprahepatic inferior vena cava. After this has been accomplished, the liver can be mobilized and the venous injury exposed. Even with total hepatic vascular isolation, a significant amount of bleeding still occurs, making the repair difficult to perform. Additionally, many patients do not tolerate the sudden decrease in cardiac preload caused by clamping of the inferior vena cava. The atriocaval shunt has been devised as a way to supply the heart with preload while still providing the surgeon with a more controlled operative field through which to perform a vascular repair on an injured juxtahepatic vein. The atriocaval shunt is fashioned from a chest tube or a no. 9 endotracheal tube. It is placed into the infrarenal inferior vena cava, and the distal end is placed into the right atrium. This maneuver is difficult to perform correctly and is often an effort of final recourse for what is likely a poor outcome. The most prudent approach is early gauze packing of the injury, with temporary abdominal closure. Effective packing will tamponade these injuries and improve chances of survival.

The presence of a pelvic hematoma in patients with blunt trauma usually indicates that the patient has a significant pelvic fracture. Pelvic hematomas should not be explored routinely in patients with blunt trauma because releasing the tamponade will lead to diffuse and often uncontrollable bleeding. However, in patients with penetrating injuries, a pelvic hematoma may indicate an injury to the iliac artery or vein. To expose these vessels, the small intestine is eviscerated to the patient's right and the midline peritoneum is incised. Proximal control can usually be obtained just at the aortic bifurcation. If primary repair or interposition grafting are not possible, extra-anatomic bypass may be necessary. The adage "life over limb" must be kept in mind.

Peripheral Vascular Injuries

In patients with a single penetrating injury to an extremity, a preoperative arteriogram is rarely indicated if the patient has a hard sign for operative intervention. The location of the injury is most often at the level of the wound, and performing preoperative arteriography is unlikely to provide any additional information. However, in patients with soft signs of arterial injury or in patients with multiple wounds in the extremity, an intraoperative arteriogram might be helpful. Furthermore, in patients with lower-extremity injuries, serious consideration should be given to performing fasciotomies, particularly in patients who are already several hours from the time of injury. The edema caused by reperfusion can be significant and result in muscle necrosis if no fasciotomy is performed.

For injuries to the axillary artery, exposure is best obtained by an incision starting at the level of the clavicle and extending along the deltopectoral groove. An incision in the groove between the triceps and biceps muscles can expose the brachial artery. If the incision must cross the antecubital fossa, it should be S shaped. Injuries to the vessels in the forearm can be exposed via a longitudinal incision extending from the antecubital fossa and down the palmar surface of the forearm. If the injury involves only the radial artery or the ulnar artery and perfusion to the palmar arch is undisturbed, the injured vessel can usually be safely ligated.

Injuries to the common femoral, superficial femoral, and profunda arteries can be exposed by a longitudinal incision along the course of the vessels in the groin. The inguinal ligament can be incised to gain access to the unmolested retroperitoneum if there is a significant hematoma in the groin or if it is difficult to obtain proximal control of the vessels in the groin.

Injuries to the popliteal artery are often a challenge to manage. A multidisciplinary approach is necessary, with close communication between the orthopedic team and the trauma surgery team, particularly when patients have blunt popliteal injuries secondary to a fracture or dislocation involving the bones of the knee. Popliteal injuries can be managed in two ways. The artery can be approached directly by making an incision on the medial aspect of the thigh, just above the knee, in the groove between the vastus medialis and the sartorius muscles. After the incision has been made, the lower border of the femur can be palpated and the deep fascia incised, revealing the fatty tissue in the popliteal fossa. From this point, the artery should be identified. Next, an incision is made along the medial aspect of the leg below the knee approximately 1 cm posterior to the inferior border of the tibia. After the incision has been made, the deep fascia just below the tibial border should be incised to gain access to the below-knee popliteal segment. At this point, the surgeon can either expose the entire popliteal artery by incising the tendinous attachments of the posteromedial muscles of the thigh where they attach at the knee or he or she can perform a bypass and exclusion procedure. If the surgeon chooses to expose the entire popliteal artery, the injury can be approached directly. Occasionally, the artery can be primarily repaired. More commonly, a reverse saphenous vein graft is required to complete the repair. If the bypass and exclusion procedure is chosen, the injured segment is bypassed through use of a reverse saphenous vein graft by anastomosing the proximal end to the uninjured above-knee popliteal segment and the distal end to the below-knee popliteal segment. A tunnel for the graft can be created in the intercondylar space using blunt dissection. Four compartment fasciotomies should be performed.

ADJUNCTS TO OPERATIVE REPAIR

As endovascular techniques and equipment improve, they will find wider application in the field of trauma. Endovascular repair of blunt thoracic aortic injuries, distal internal carotid injuries, and retrohepatic caval injuries are but a few of the potential applications of emerging endovascular techniques used to treat the injured patient. Over the next few years it will be critical for surgeons, particularly those interested in the care of patients with significant injuries, to become familiar and proficient with endovascular techniques to provide optimal care for patients with these challenging injuries.

SUGGESTED READINGS

Biffl WL, Moore EE, Rehse DH, and others: Selective management of penetrating neck trauma based on cervical level of injury, *Am J Surg* 174:678, 1997.

Fabian TC, Davis KA, Gavant ML, and others: Prospective study of blunt aortic injury: helical CT is diagnostic and antihypertensive therapy reduces rupture, *Ann Surg* 227:666, 1998.

Frykberg ER, Crump JM, Dennis JW, and others: Nonoperative observation of clinically occult arterial injuries: a prospective evaluation, *Surgery* 109:85, 1991.

Johansen K, Lynch K, Paun M, and others: Noninvasive vascular tests reliably exclude occult arterial trauma in injured extremities, *J Trauma* 31:515, 1991.

Mattox KL, Holzman M, Pickard LR, and others: Clamp/repair: a safe technique for treatment of blunt injury to the descending thoracic aorta, *Ann Thoracic Surg* 40:456, 1985.

Miller PR, Fabian TC, Croce MA, and others: Prospective screening for blunt cerebrovascular injuries: analysis of diagnostic modalities and outcomes, *Ann Surg* 236:386, 2002.

THE MANAGEMENT OF EXTREMITY COMPARTMENT SYNDROME

David V. Feliciano, MD

First described by Richard von Volkmann (1830–1889) in 1881, extremity compartment syndromes result from a wide range of injuries and operative procedures. A *compartment syndrome* is defined as increased pressure within a closed fascial space that reduces capillary perfusion to a level less than that required for tissue viability. In truth, extremity compartment syndromes are similar to the other closed-space pressure problems seen in all areas of the body; for example, increased intracranial pressure resulting in cerebral herniation, increased pericardial pressure resulting in cardiac tamponade, and increased intra-abdominal pressure resulting in primary or secondary abdominal compartment syndrome. Of interest, the "dangerous" pressure levels reached when adverse sequelae begin to occur in all of these locations are essentially the same as one would expect.

ETIOLOGY AND PATHOPHYSIOLOGY

An extremity compartment syndrome results most commonly from increased content of a musculofascial compartment caused primarily by edema of the contained structures, hemorrhage into or around these structures, or chronic exercise that results in an increased muscle mass within the self-limiting musculofascial compartment (Table 1). Decreased volume of a musculofascial compartment is a less common cause of an extremity compartment syndrome (Table 2). The most common etiology is external compression of a compartment that already contains some edema or hemorrhage.

One unusual clinical entity recognized in the past 5 years has been the "secondary extremity compartment syndrome." This is a rare complication that is part of postresuscitation systemic inflammatory response (SIRS) and often occurs in uninjured extremities. Patients described in the original series from Grady Memorial Hospital in Atlanta, Georgia, had a mean Injury Severity Score of 29, a mean base deficit of −13 on presentation, and a mean of 3.1 extremities that developed compartment syndromes. Seven of the ten patients in this report died, and the secondary extremity compartment syndrome may simply be a marker of a systemic capillary leak syndrome preceding death. Secondary extremity compartment syndrome should be ruled out by measurement of compartment pressures (see Measuring Compartment Pressures, discussed later) in uninjured and injured extremities in patients with severe diffuse edema after resuscitation for multiple injuries or near-exsanguination (or both).

Table 1: Etiologies of Extremity Compartment Syndromes: Edema of Contents/Increased Content/ Hemorrhage into Compartment

Capillary leak syndrome
Near exsanguination
Systemic inflammatory response
Septic shock
Extravasation of intravenous fluids
Fracture of adjacent long bone
Increased muscle mass from exercise
Ischemia–reperfusion syndrome
Arterial occlusion
Low flow state
Obstruction of venous outflow
Edema of proximal extremity
Improper positioning in operating room
Venous ligation
Snakebite

Table 2: Etiologies of Extremity Compartment Syndromes: Decreased Volume of Compartment

Air splint
Elastic wraps
Pneumatic antishock garment
Premature closure of fasciotomy site
Tight cast

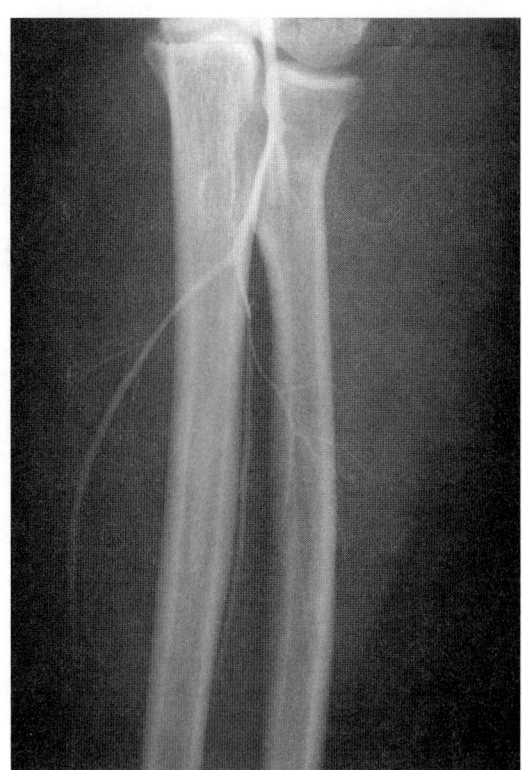

Figure 1 Crush injury to right forearm resulting in compartment syndrome with loss of collateral arterial flow on intraoperative arteriogram.

HIGH-RISK PATIENTS

Recognizing the variety of etiologies described earlier, there are certain generic elements of the patient's history, physical examination, and operation performed that should make the surgeon suspicious that an extremity compartment syndrome is likely to be present or will occur soon. A delay in treatment of an injured or ischemic extremity in the patient's history is an important risk factor because compression of venous outflow from the compartment may already be present or because an ischemia-reperfusion injury is likely to occur after a revascularization procedure.

On physical examination, the presence of shock on first evaluation is ominous because the low flow state causes ischemic edema of muscle tissue in the compartment and resolution of shock will, once again, lead to an ischemia-reperfusion injury. The presence of a crush injury is a high-risk factor because compression or loss of venous outflow and edema or hemorrhage of contained muscle are already present (Figs. 1 and 2). Swelling of a distal extremity after injury or ischemia is important to note on physical examination but remains a most imprecise marker for the presence of an extremity compartment syndrome. This is particularly true in the leg, where the small size of the anterior compartment between the tibia and fibula makes it difficult to assess and the deep posterior compartment behind the tibia cannot be palpated at all.

One operative procedure that significantly increases the likelihood that an extremity compartment syndrome will occur is simultaneous temporary occlusion of the common or superficial femoral *or* popliteal artery and vein. This occurs most commonly in patients

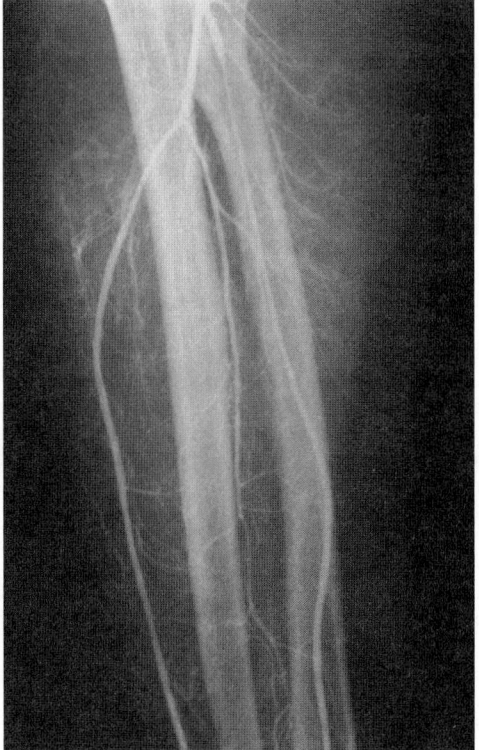

Figure 2 Same patient after superficial and deep flexor compartments of right forearm opened with a fasciotomy. Note restoration of collateral arterial flow on repeat intraoperative arteriogram.

with gunshot or shotgun wounds to the lower extremity. No matter which vessel is repaired first, the combination of ischemic edema, venous obstruction, and ischemia-reperfusion injury suggests to many trauma surgeons that a "prophylactic" below-knee fasciotomy is mandatory after vascular repairs have been completed. The other operative procedure that significantly increases the chance that an extremity compartment syndrome will occur is ligation of the infrarenal inferior vena cava or ipsilateral common iliac, external iliac, common femoral, superficial femoral, or popliteal vein. These veins are usually ligated only in exsanguinating patients with shock, and a postoperative extremity compartment syndrome will almost surely occur. For this reason, experienced trauma surgeons place thoracostomy tubes as temporary intraluminal vascular shunts in severely injured femoral or popliteal veins in patients with shock rather than perform ligation. In patients with ligation of the infrarenal inferior vena cava or ipsilateral common or external iliac vein, measurement of the below-knee compartment pressures is mandatory before the patient leaves the operating room.

SYMPTOMS AND SIGNS

Patients who are awake and have a periresuscitation or perioperative extremity compartment syndrome complain of severe pain in the distal extremity. The pain is out of proportion to that described by other patients with an injured or previously ischemic extremity but no extremity compartment syndrome. This severe pain in the extremity is often the first complaint of a patient on awakening from resuscitation or operation in the recovery room or in the intensive care unit. The patient may complain of numbness and tingling in the extremity, as well. Rather than increase the patient's dose of analgesics, the surgeon should immediately examine the painful extremity. A tight cast should be bivalved and constricting dressings removed to eliminate possible contributing causes and allow for a complete physical examination. Findings on physical examination when an extremity compartment syndrome is present include the following: tenderness or palpation of the involved compartment, pain on passive stretching of the muscle groups in the compartment, a sensory deficit (hypesthesia) in the area of a nerve passing through the compartment, and weakness of the muscles in the compartment. The latter two findings in a patient with the syndrome involving the anterior compartment of the leg, the most commonly affected compartment in all reviews, would be hypesthesia in the webspace adjacent to the first toe and weakness of dorsiflexion of the ankle. These findings suggest that permanent damage to the deep peroneal (anterior tibial) nerve or the tibialis anterior, exterior hallucis longus, exterior digitorum longus, or peroneus tertius muscles may already be present.

Because arterial pressure is significantly higher than the elevated compartment pressure associated with the syndrome, distal pulses in the involved extremity are always present. Therefore symptoms of a compartment syndrome associated with absent distal pulses are evidence of proximal arterial occlusion as the cause of the syndrome. Because venous pressure in the involved extremity is more affected by the elevated compartment syndrome, capillary refill may be delayed in some patients.

Because a patient with a traumatic injury to the brain or one who is undergoing general anesthesia during operation or is under sedation in the intensive care unit cannot speak, the symptoms and signs described here cannot be elicited. Reliance on the patient's history, superficial examination of the extremity (e.g., is a crush injury present or is the compartment tense to palpation?), and known operative procedures may be enough to diagnose a presumed extremity compartment syndrome in this group of patients. Confirmation of the presence of the syndrome in these patients and in conscious patients with classical symptoms and signs is by measurement of the compartment pressure.

MEASURING COMPARTMENT PRESSURE

Although "prophylactic" fasciotomies are often performed in high-risk patients with classical symptoms and signs, the disfigurement that accompanies a fasciotomy to decompress the involved compartment should always be considered. Confirmation of an elevated compartment pressure with a quick measurement preceding the performance of a fasciotomy is both medically and medicolegally appropriate and will prevent an unnecessary fasciotomy.

Pressures are generally measured in the anterior compartment or deep posterior compartment of the leg *or* in the superficial anterior (flexor) or posterior compartments of the forearm. The described techniques include measurement using an arterial transducer, a needle manometer, a wick catheter, a slit catheter, or a commercially available device.

Use of an *arterial transducer* is the easiest technique and can be performed in any operating room or hospital unit in which hemodynamic monitors are available. A 16-gauge needle connected to arterial pressure tubing and a monitor are held just above the compartment, and after flushing with saline to remove air, a "0" reading is obtained on the monitor. The needle is inserted through the skin and fascia over the compartment, and a direct reading of the intracompartmental pressure is available on the monitor. If the pressure is inconsistent with the clinical situation, it is worthwhile to flush the system and insert the needle to a deeper level and repeat the measurement at one or two other sites in the compartment.

Use of a *needle manometer* is an older technique in which a 16-gauge needle placed in the compartment is connected to a 20-ml syringe containing saline and air via a three-way stopcock. This pressure tubing beyond the three-way stopcock is attached to a standard mercury manometer. When the air-saline meniscus in the syringe is seen to move, the compartment pressure is read from the mercury manometer.

The *wick catheter* includes a piece of polyethylene 60 (PE 60) tubing into which a piece of absorbable suture material (polyglycolic acid) is inserted. After flushing with saline and calibration, the wick catheter is inserted at an acute angle into the compartment through a large needle or trocar, which is then withdrawn. The intracompartmental pressure is then read from the monitor. This technique allows for continuous measurement of the compartment pressure without a continuous saline infusion. The *slit catheter* is a related technique in which five 3-mm longitudinal slits are placed at the distal end of the PE 60 tubing. After the saline flush and calibration, the slit catheter is inserted into the compartment as described for the wick catheter.

The Solid-State Transducer IntraCompartmental Monitor System (Stryker Surgical, Kalamazoo, MI) is a handheld instrument system that contains a monitor, a disposable syringe containing fluid, and a disposable needle/catheter. After the system is assembled, flushed, and calibrated, the needle is inserted into the compartment and the pressure is read directly from the handheld monitor.

COMPARTMENT PRESSURE THAT SHOULD PROMPT FASCIOTOMY

The normal pressure in a musculofascial compartment of an extremity is up to 8 mm Hg, with the variation related to recent level of activity and to position. There has always been moderate debate regarding which compartment pressure should indicate fasciotomy. This is not surprising because an elevated compartment pressure alone is not the only factor that leads to adverse sequelae if fasciotomy is delayed. Numerous studies using microelectrodes in muscle, radiotracers, mass spectrometers, or tissue biopsy and histology have been performed in animals to define the factors that contribute to permanent tissue damage. These studies have documented that compartment pressure in combination with the patient's blood pressure, metabolic demands in the muscles of the compartment, length of time that the compartment pressure has been elevated, and individual susceptibility to an elevated pressure contribute to the final outcome.

With a capillary blood pressure of 25–30 mm Hg in humans, a compartment tissue pressure greater than this will compromise capillary flow and collapse venous outflow. For this reason, many authors have used a compartment pressure greater than 30 mm Hg as an indication for fasciotomy. There are, however, numerous clinical reports documenting that compartment pressures less than 45 mm Hg in patients not in shock are well tolerated by the muscles and nerves in a musculofascial compartment. I continue to use a compartment pressure in the range of 30–35 mm Hg as an indication for fasciotomy and recognize that some patients will undergo an unnecessary procedure.

Certain orthopaedic groups use the "differential pressure" as an indication for fasciotomy. This is defined as the patient's diastolic blood pressure minus the compartment pressure. The suggested differential pressures that should prompt fasciotomy range from 20 mm Hg to 30 mm Hg.

ALTERNATIVES TO FASCIOTOMY

A number of alternatives to fasciotomy for treatment of compartment syndrome have been studied. Elevation of the affected extremity lowers arterial pressure, reduces the local arteriovenous gradient, and reduces microcirculatory flow further; hence elevation is contraindicated. Neither the administration of free radical scavengers such as mannitol nor the use of hyperbaric oxygen treatment has been demonstrated to significantly affect outcome in studies to date.

TECHNIQUE FOR BELOW-KNEE FOUR-COMPARTMENT FASCIOTOMY

The three techniques described for decompression of the anterior, lateral, posterior, and deep posterior compartments of the leg are fibulectomy-fasciotomy, single-incision perifibular fasciotomy, and the double skin incision. Because the first two techniques are rarely used in general, trauma, or vascular surgery services, I describe only the third technique: the two-skin incision four-compartment fasciotomy (Fig. 3).

The *anterior compartment* of the leg contains the tibialis anterior, extensor hallucis longus, extensor digitorum longus, and

peroneus tertius muscles, the deep peroneal (anterior tibial) nerve, and the anterior tibial artery with its venae comitantes. This is a relatively tight compartment to begin with and has a blood supply that is angulated and passes through the interosseous septum in the proximal part of the leg. The *lateral compartment* of the leg contains the peroneus longus and peroneus brevis muscles and the superficial peroneal (musculocutaneous) nerve. These two compartments are approached through the same lateral, longitudinal, 30-cm skin incision 2 cm anterior to the upper border of the fibula. This long skin incision is necessary because the skin is part of the constricting envelope in a patient with an extremity compartment syndrome. Rake retractors are used to lift the anterior and posterior skin-subcutaneous tissue flaps off the underlying fascia for a width of 6–8 cm, and perforating vessels are ligated rather than coagulated with the electrocautery. A 25-cm longitudinal anterior compartment fasciotomy is made approximately 2 cm posterior to the anterior edge of the tibia. The intermuscular septum is palpated or visualized with a small, transverse cut in the fascia, and a 25-cm longitudinal lateral compartment fasciotomy is made approximately 1 cm posterior to the intermuscular septum. In the lower leg, the superficial peroneal nerve, which descends in front of the fibula, divides into cutaneous branches and should be avoided.

The *posterior compartment* of the leg contains the soleus and gastrocnemius muscles and the plantaris tendon. The *deep posterior compartment* of the leg contains the flexor hallucis longus, tibialis posterior, and flexor digitorum longus muscles; the tibial nerve; the posterior tibial artery and its venae comitantes; and the peroneal artery and its venae comitantes. These two compartments are approached through a 30-cm medial, longitudinal skin incision 2 cm posterior to the posterior border of the tibia. Rake retractors are once again used to lift the anterior and posterior skin-subcutaneous tissue flaps off the underlying fascia for a width of 6–8 cm. A 25-cm, longitudinal, superficial, posterior compartment fasciotomy is made 2 cm posterior to the posterior border of the tibia. To decompress the deep posterior compartment, the proximal soleus muscle is detached from the posterior edge of the tibia to allow for a 25-cm longitudinal fasciotomy 1 cm posterior to the tibia. This fasciotomy should be performed carefully in the lower leg to avoid the more superficially located posterior tibial artery and its venae comitantes.

TECHNIQUE FOR ABOVE-KNEE (THIGH) THREE-COMPARTMENT FASCIOTOMY

Compartment syndromes in the thigh are uncommon, but they can occur after a severe fracture of the femur, severe pelvic fracture, ligation of the ipsilateral common or external iliac vein, or ligation of the infrarenal inferior vena cava. The three compartments of the thigh (anterior or extensor, posterior or flexor, medial or adductor) are decompressed through two skin incisions. A 30-cm, anterolateral, longitudinal incision is made along the iliotibial tract (intertrochanteric space to lateral condyle of the femur). After mobilization of the anterior and posterior skin-subcutaneous tissue flaps, the fascia over the vastus lateralis muscle is opened with a 25-cm incision. By manually elevating the anterior leaf of the fascia, the remaining muscles of the quadriceps femoris group are decompressed. The vastus lateralis muscle is then freed from its posterior attachments and retracted superomedially. The thick intermuscular septum lying lateral to the posterior compartment is then incised for 20–25 cm to decompress the "hamstring" muscles of the posterior compartment. Decompression of these two compartments will often decompress the medial compartment, so the pressure in this compartment should be remeasured at this time. Should the medial compartment pressure still be significantly elevated, a 30-cm anteromedial longitudinal incision is made over the adductor-pectineus-gracilis muscle group, followed by the 25-cm fasciotomy.

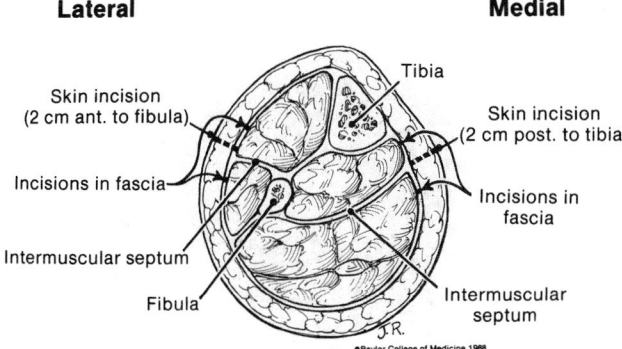

Lateral   **Medial**

Skin incision (2 cm ant. to fibula)
Incisions in fascia
Intermuscular septum
Fibula
Tibia
Skin incision (2 cm post. to tibia)
Incisions in fascia
Intermuscular septum

Figure 3 Two-skin incision four-compartment fasciotomy for decompression of musculofascial compartments of the leg. *Copyright Baylor College of Medicine, 1986. Used with permission.*

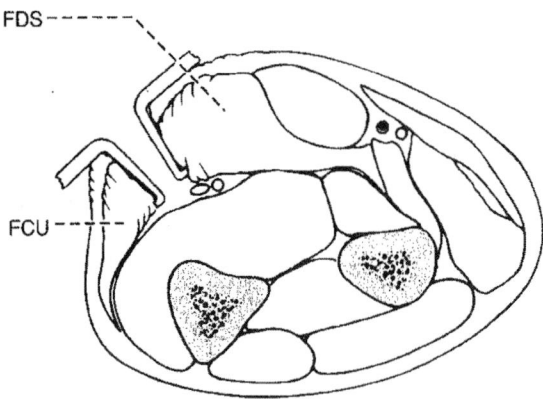

Figure 4 Access to the deep flexor compartment of the forearm by retraction of the flexor carpi ulnaris *(FCU)* and flexor digitorum sublimis *(FDS)* muscles. *From Amendola A, Twaddle, BC. In Browner BD, Jupiter JB, Levine AM, and others: Skeletal trauma, ed 3, Philadelphia, 2003, Saunders, p 282.*

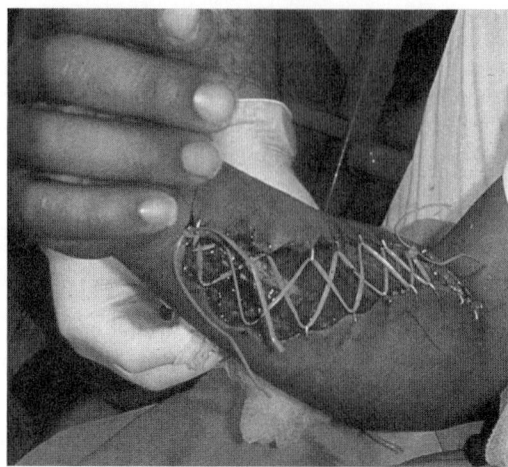

Figure 5 "Shoelace" technique for gradual closure of volar forearm fasciotomy site.

TECHNIQUE FOR BELOW-ELBOW THREE-COMPARTMENT FASCIOTOMY

Compartment syndromes in the forearm are uncommon (5 times less frequent than in the leg) and usually follow significant injury to the ipsilateral brachial, axillary, or subclavian vessels. There are different descriptions of the compartments of the forearm in the literature. Some authors describe superficial flexor, deep flexor, and extensor compartments. Others describe a flexor compartment with superficial and deep components, the mobile wad compartment containing the brachioradialis, extensor carpi radialis longus, and extensor carpi radialis brevis muscles, and an extensor compartment.

There are two different volar skin incisions described to decompress the flexor compartments of the forearm. I favor the volar-ulnar approach, in which the skin incision starts on the radial side of the proximal volar forearm, passes transversely and laterally distal to the antecubital fold, and then extends down the ulnar side of the volar forearm. At the wrist, the incision is carried medially and then curves across to the thenar crease of the hand. A longitudinal fasciotomy incision closer to the ulnar side of the volar forearm decompresses the superficial flexor compartment in the forearm and the carpal tunnel at the wrist. The space between the flexor carpi ulnaris and flexor digitorum sublimis muscles is separated with retractors, and the ulnar nerve and artery are visualized lying on the deep flexor compartment (Fig. 4). A longitudinal fasciotomy of this compartment is performed by retracting the vessel and nerve laterally. If there is continued tightness at the level of the wrist, both the median and the ulnar nerve tunnels should be divided. The mobile wad compartment can be decompressed by manually elevating the medial fascial flap resulting from the fasciotomy of the superficial flexor compartment.

Fasciotomy of the flexor compartments and the mobile wad compartment will often decompress the extensor compartment, so the pressure in this compartment should be remeasured at this time. Should it still be significantly elevated, the forearm is pronated. A longitudinal skin incision from the lateral epicondyle of the humerus to the midaspect of the posterior wrist is then made. The extensor compartment longitudinal fasciotomy is performed between the extensor carpi radialis brevis and extensor digitorum communis muscles.

WOUND MANAGEMENT AFTER FASCIOTOMY

Bleeders in the wound are ligated with ties to ensure hemostasis, especially in the presence of a coagulopathy. In a hemodynamically stable patient in whom there is only moderate bulging of the exposed muscles, vertical mattress skin sutures of 3-0 nylon are placed 1 cm apart but not tied. This is in anticipation of a delayed primary skin closure after 5 days of elevation of the extremity. Another approach, when there is only moderate bulging of the exposed muscles, is to use the "shoelace" technique, in which an elastic vessel loop is crossed repeatedly from one skin edge to the other edge under skin staples (Fig. 5). As edema resolves, tightening of the vessel loop will bring the skin edges together gradually until closure with skin sutures or staples is possible. The vacuum-assisted closure device V.A.C. (KCI, San Antonio, TX) can be used and, as with the open abdomen, suctions edema fluid out of the exposed muscle and skin-subcutaneous flaps of the incision. When marked edema of exposed muscle persists despite continuous elevation of the extremity, selective use of intravenous diuretics, and use of the techniques described earlier, the application of a split-thickness skin graft harvested from the thigh is appropriate. The need for skin-graft coverage has decreased to less than 25% of all fasciotomy sites in recent years.

WHEN FASCIOTOMY HAS BEEN PERFORMED TOO LATE

Pale muscle in a fasciotomy site that does not react to the stimulation of the electrocautery device should be debrided. Muscle that bleeds actively but does not react can be observed until a reoperation is performed. Debridement is performed cautiously so as not to denervate or devascularize any remaining viable muscles in the compartment. When viable muscle is reached, daily wet-to-dry dressing changes are performed until a split-thickness skin graft can be applied to the granulating bed. As muscles are debrided, appropriate splinting of the ankle and foot or hand and wrist is performed. For example, debridement of necrotic muscles in the anterior compartment of the leg should be followed by the application of a right-angle ankle splint to prevent an equinus deformity (footdrop).

A delay in the diagnosis of a compartment syndrome can also be a cause of rhabdomyolysis, in which myoglobin from disintegrating muscle passes through renal tubules that may then become occluded. The reabsorption of the myoglobin is thought to generate toxic oxygen radicals as well. Rhabdomyolysis should be suspected when the urine turns dark and the patient's serum creatine phosphokinase (CPK) is elevated. The diagnosis can be confirmed by documenting the presence of myoglobin in the urine. Attempts at prevention of a secondary renal injury include vigorous hydration and alkalinization of the urine via the administration of intravenous sodium bicarbonate. Hydration prompts a diuresis and clears tubules, whereas alkalinization is thought to decrease the formation of myoglobin casts. Patients with a significant risk of developing secondary renal failure usually have a CPK level greater than 5000 U/L, a creatinine level greater than 1.5, and a base deficit less than −4 when the rhabdomyolysis is first recognized.

Suggested Readings

Amendola A, Twaddle BC: Compartment syndromes. In Browner BD, Jupiter JB, Levine AM, and others, editors: *Skeletal trauma,* ed 3, Philadelphia, 2003, WB Sanders.

Blaisdell FW: The pathophysiology of skeletal muscle ischemia and the reperfusion syndrome: a review, *Cardiovacs Surg* 10:620, 2002.

Dente CD, Feliciano DV, Rozycki GS, and others: A review of upper extremity fasciotomies in a level I trauma center, *Am Surg* 70:1088, 2004.

Feliciano DV, Cruse PA, Spjut-Patrinely V, and others: Fasciotomy after trauma to the extremities, *Am J Surg* 156:533, 1988.

Matsen FA III: *Compartmental syndromes.* New York, 1980, Grune & Stratton.

McQueen MM, Court-Brown CM: Compartment monitoring in tibial fractures. The pressure threshold for decompression, *J Bone Joint Surg (Br)* 78-B:99, 1996.

Mubarak SJ, Hargens AR: *Compartment syndromes and Volkmann's contracture.* Philadelphia, 1981, WB Saunders.

Sharp LS, Rozycki GS, Feliciano DV: Rhabdomyolysis and secondary renal failure in critically ill surgical patients, *Am J Surg* 188:801, 2004.

Tremblay LN, Feliciano DV, Rozycki GS: Secondary extremity compartment syndrome, *J Trauma* 53:833, 2002.

Pelvic Fractures

H. Gill Cryer, MD, PhD

The management of severe pelvic fractures remains one of the most troublesome clinical problems in the treatment of injured patients. Pelvic-fracture patients have a wide spectrum of injuries, from solitary, nondisplaced, single, pubic rami fractures that require little treatment to pelvic crush injuries and multiple associated life-threatening injuries in other organ systems in hemodynamically unstable patients that tax the resources of even the best-equipped trauma center. More patients die from pelvic fractures than from any other skeletal injury, and survivors often suffer from prolonged disability. Improved resuscitation techniques and multidisciplinary management protocols addressing both the pelvic fracture and other life-threatening, associated injuries have substantially reduced morbidity and mortality rates in experienced trauma centers. Although the mortality rate in patients with pelvic fractures is high, the cause of that mortality frequently resides in an organ system other than that associated with the pelvis itself. Therefore the pelvic fracture serves as a marker of high-energy transfer to the patient as a whole, causing potentially severe injuries to all organ systems, and the management of these injuries must be appropriately prioritized to ensure an optimal outcome.

HISTORICAL LESSONS

The most common cause of death in patients with pelvic fracture is hemorrhage. Blood banking and modern resuscitation techniques have improved mortality rates because tamponade of bleeding from fracture fragments and laceration of the pelvic venous plexus usually occur after the retroperitoneal hematoma expands to fill the pelvis. However, if severe soft-tissue disruption occurs, the retroperitoneal hematoma escapes the pelvis without tamponading the bleeding. In the 1960s it was learned that direct operative attempts to control bleeding by exploration failed: surgeons failed to identify discrete bleeding sources and patients died by exsanguination. Direct attempts at bilateral hypogastric artery ligation had similar results. From these observations the principle developed that pelvic retroperitoneal hematomas associated with pelvic fracture should not be explored.

During the 1970s, three therapeutic modalities were developed to treat pelvic fracture hemorrhage without opening the pelvic hematoma: the pneumatic antishock garment (PASG), external pelvic fixation, and angiographic embolization. Despite considerable controversy over the order and timing of the use of these techniques and the variability in protocols among institutions, a general decline in mortality from pelvic fracture hemorrhage was achieved. During the 1980s and 1990s, it became clear that open reduction and internal fixation of pelvic fractures had markedly superior functional results compared with results of external pelvic fixation. Furthermore, external fixation and PASG were found to create skin blistering and pin-track problems that compromised the results. Several cadaver studies showed that the effect of external fixation on reducing pelvic volume was much less than previously thought, with the result that today the PASG is obsolete and external fixation has largely been replaced by a variety of temporary pelvic binders used only for the initial resuscitation phase of care. Interestingly, it has been found that with the use of multidisciplinary protocols, modern advances in resuscitation, invasive monitoring, and early angiography, most patients can be managed without pelvic binders or external fixation at all. The latest developments include the use of percutaneous pin techniques, which limit the morbidity of posterior approaches to the pelvis. As a result, the principal issues currently facing pelvic fracture care are prompt management of other, associated life-threatening injuries and limitation of morbidity from the pelvic fracture itself. The advances in computed tomography (CT) scan and ultrasound technology have vastly improved the ability to rapidly identify the site of bleeding in hemodynamically unstable patents with pelvic fracture. The most formidable challenge remaining is the frequent need to simultaneously treat bleeding in more that one site. A variety of recent protocols have used intraoperative angiography, operative pelvic packing of the extraperitoneal pelvic area through the space of Retzius, and angiographic embolization of multiple sites. The degree to which these techniques are employed varies among institutions, depending on available resources, and it remains to be seen which will work the best.

EPIDEMIOLOGY

Pelvic fractures are the third leading cause of death in motor vehicle accidents (MVAs), representing 3% of all fractures encountered and occurring in 5% of trauma victims requiring hospital admission. Reported mortality in recent series ranges from 2% to 16%, with an average of 8%. The most common mechanisms of injury for pelvic fractures are (in order of frequency of occurrence) MVAs, pedestrian injuries, falls, motorcycle accidents, crush injuries, and bicycle accidents.

PELVIC FRACTURE CLASSIFICATION

Numerous pelvic fracture classification schemes have been developed to provide guidance to the trauma team regarding the nature of primary bone fractures and associated injuries and to indicate the type and likelihood of the various management techniques that might be required. For the trauma surgeon interested in the initial management of the multiply injured patient, classification schemes structured on the basis of clinical characteristics such as hemodynamic stability are important, whereas the orthopaedist is more interested in whether the pelvic fracture is skeletally stable or unstable and whether it is amenable to external or internal stabilization. Perhaps the most useful fracture classification scheme today is the Burgess and Young modification of the Pennell and Sutherland classification (Table 1 and Figs. 1-7). This scheme takes into account both the force vector and an indication of increasing severity of fracture displacement. It is useful to the

Table 1: Burgess and Young Modification of the Pennell and Sutherland Classification of Pelvic Fractures

Anteroposterior Compression

Type I Disruption of pubic symphysis <2.5 cm of diastasis, no significant posterior pelvic injury

Type II Pubic symphysis disruption >2.5 cm with tearing of anterior sacroiliac, sacrospinous, and sacrotuberous ligaments

Type III Complete disruption of pubic symphysis and posterior ligament complexes with hemipelvic displacement

Lateral Compression

Type I Posterior compression of sacroiliac joint without ligament disruption, oblique pubic ramus fracture

Type II Rupture of posterior sacroiliac ligament, pivotal internal rotation of hemipelvis on anterior SI joint with crush of sacrum with an oblique pubic ramus fracture

Type III Findings in type II with evidence of anteroposterior compression injury to contralateral hemipelvis

Vertical Shear

Complete ligament or bony disruption of hemipelvic associated with hemipelvic displacement

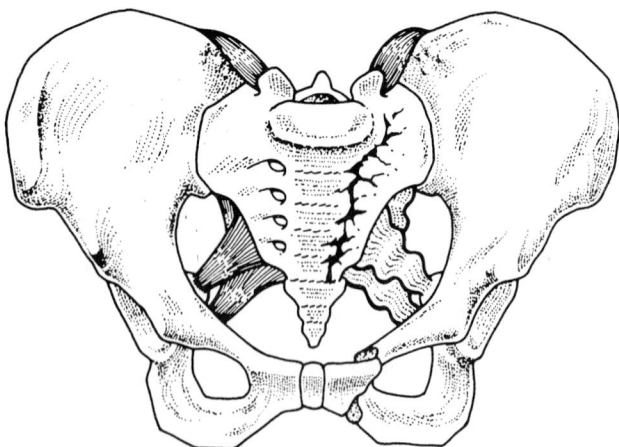

Figure 1 Pelvic fracture classification: lateral compression type I (LC-I).

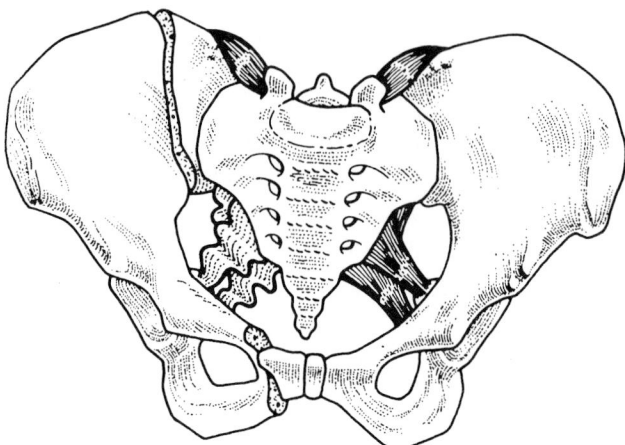

Figure 2 Pelvic fracture classification: lateral compression type II (LC-II).

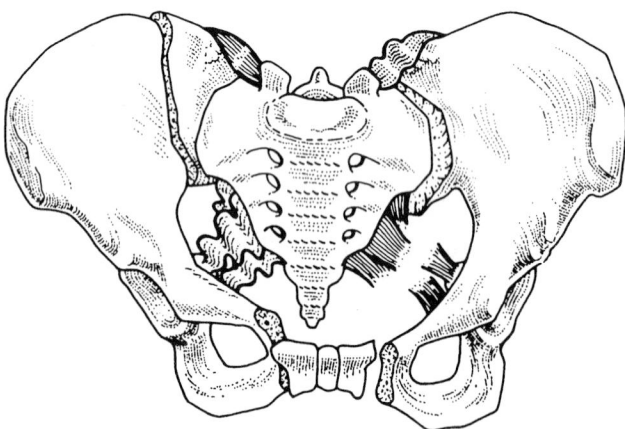

Figure 3 Pelvic fracture classification: lateral compression type III (LC-III).

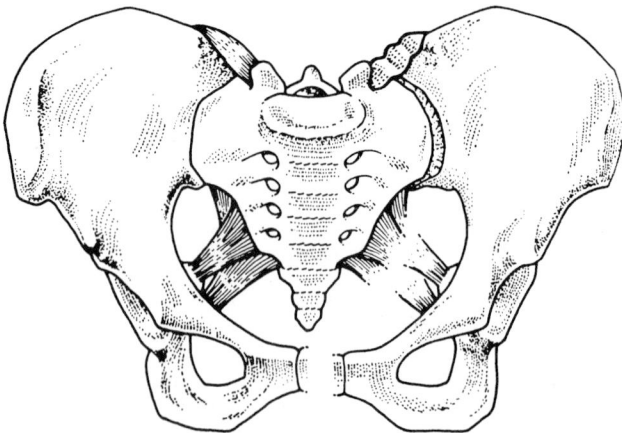

Figure 4 Pelvic fracture classification: anteroposterior compression type I (APC-I).

trauma surgeon because the fracture patterns correlate with certain patterns of injuries and complications that may be expected during patient management. In addition, the increasing severity of displacement correlates with the likelihood of associated intra-abdominal injuries and pelvic arterial bleeding. On the other hand,

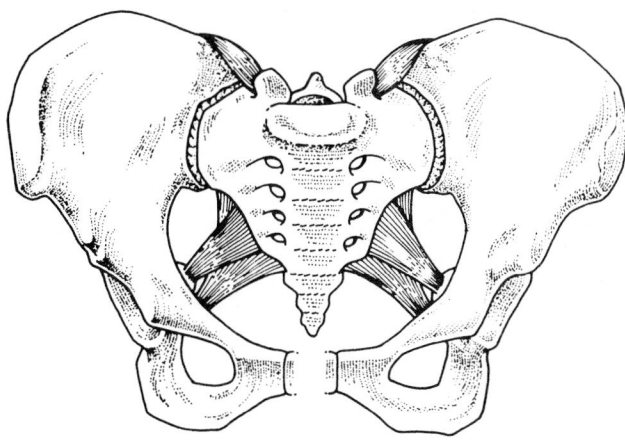

Figure 5 Pelvic fracture classification: anteroposterior compression type III (APC-II).

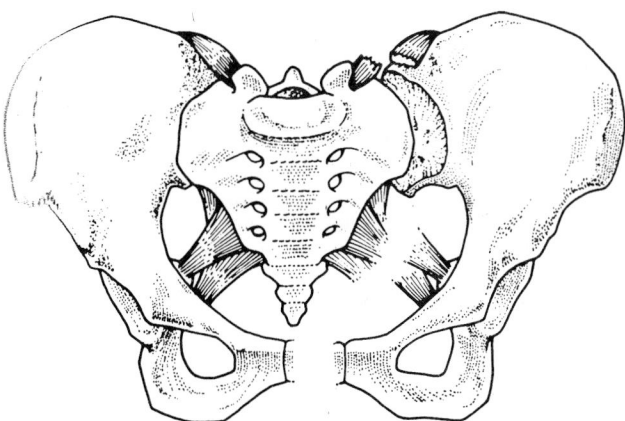

Figure 6 Pelvic fracture classification: anteroposterior compression type III (APC-III).

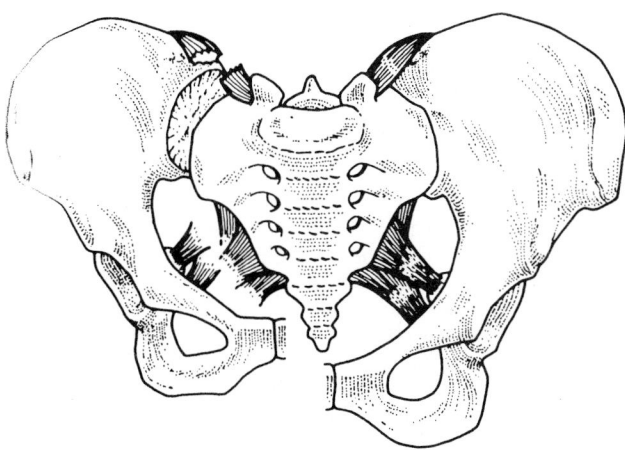

Figure 7 Pelvic fracture classification: VS (vertical shear).

intra-abdominal organ injury and pelvic arterial bleeding can also occur with the more common, minimally displaced fracture patterns. From the perspective of the orthopaedic surgeon, this classification is also helpful in evaluating pelvic instability and choosing among the various alternatives for pelvic fracture stabilization.

MANAGEMENT PRIORITIES

The most important principle in the management of pelvic fractures is the realization that the patient is the victim of high-energy transfer and that potentially life-threatening injuries in the pelvis and numerous other organ systems may be present. The initial priority in the multiply injured patient is the assessment of the ABCs of trauma resuscitation (i.e., airway, breathing, and circulation) and disability from neurologic injury. The second priority is to diagnose the pelvic fracture because it potentially adds an important source of hemorrhage and morbidity to the patient. The management priorities then become the control of free bleeding into the intraperitoneal or intrapleural space, identification and evacuation of subdural and epidural hematomas, identification and control of contained hemorrhage in the retroperitoneal or retropleural space, identification and repair of nonbleeding visceral injuries, and definitive fracture stabilization, in that order.

A presumptive diagnosis of pelvic fracture may be made by history and systematic physical examination. Gentle palpation of the iliac crest and anterior pubis and gentle inward manual compression of the iliac wings can elicit tenderness or pain suggestive of underlying bony injury in conscious patients. Vigorous attempts to elicit crepitus by movement of fracture fragments should be avoided because these are extremely painful to the patient and may aggravate bleeding or soft-tissue injury. Rectal and vaginal examinations are routinely performed, and if blood is noted, a proctoscopic and or vaginal speculum examination should be made with the patient under anesthesia, with care taken to minimize fracture fragment movement. It is also important to examine the perineum for evidence of laceration indicating an open pelvic fracture that may require fecal diversion and operative washout. In male patients, the location and consistency of the prostate gland should be assessed; if this is abnormal, it may indicate disruption of the urethra. If a urethral injury is suspected because of blood at the penile meatus, a scrotal hematoma, or inability to insert a Foley catheter, the patient should undergo a urethrogram. If the results are positive, the patient will require a suprapubic cystostomy.

The mainstay of pelvic fracture diagnosis is the anteroposterior supine pelvic radiograph, which has become routine, along with the portable cervical spine (C-spine) and chest x-ray film. These comprise the minimal radiographic examination during the secondary survey of major blunt trauma resuscitation. After a pelvic fracture has been identified on the anteroposterior x-ray film, additional radiographs are necessary to completely characterize the fracture. The timing of these depends on the hemodynamic stability of the patient and the presence of other, associated life-threatening injuries. However, after the patient has become hemodynamically stable and associated injuries have been repaired, a complete characterization of pelvic fracture stability, both clinically and roentgenographically, is necessary for the orthopaedic surgeon to treat the pelvic fracture definitively. The orthopaedic evaluation of pelvic injury involves assessment of pelvic stability by correlating the clinical examination with standard radiographs (anterior/posterior, inlet, outlet, Judet oblique views of the pelvis) and with two-dimensional and three-dimensional CT scans.

Even though early diagnosis is important, the initial management priority in patients with pelvic fractures is not the pelvic fracture itself. After an airway has been established and breathing ensured, the most immediate threat to life is hemorrhage. The diagnosis of a pelvic fracture during the secondary survey adds an important potential source of hemorrhage to the list. However, pelvic fracture hemorrhage is not the first priority. Free hemorrhage, either external or into the pleural or peritoneal cavity, takes precedence over contained hemorrhage in the retroperitoneum, extremity fascial compartments, and retropleural space. This does not minimize the risk of hemorrhage from the pelvic fracture. Even the hemodynamically stable patient with a pelvic fracture has the potential for ongoing hemorrhage that may become clinically significant over time. Free intrapleural bleeding is usually easily identified on the initial chest radiograph. In the hemodynamically unstable patient, prompt ultrasound examination in the resuscitation suite can rapidly identify free intraperitoneal hemorrhage. An ultrasound examination that demonstrates significant fluid in the peritoneal cavity should prompt immediate laparotomy in the operating room if the patient is too unstable to go to the radiology department for CT scan. If there is a large pelvic hematoma noted at the time of laparotomy, the patient will also require emergent angiographic embolization of pelvic arterial bleeding. If the ultrasound examination is negative for intraperitoneal fluid, it is presumed that the source of hemorrhage is the pelvis, and the patient should undergo immediate angiography and embolization of pelvic arterial bleeding. A recent consensus practice guideline has been suggested for hemodynamically unstable patients with pelvic fractures, defined as patients with class II or IV hemorrhage leading to a systolic blood pressure that had a transient or no response to initial fluid bolus or requiring more than 2000 ml of fluid in the prehospital or resuscitation suite. The authors of the guideline recommended that the site of hemorrhage be determined within 30 minutes and the patient taken to the radiology department for angiography or to the operating room within 45 minutes. Pelvic hemorrhage without evidence of intra-abdominal hemorrhage (negative focused assessment for the sonographic evaluation for the trauma patient [FAST] or diagnostic peritoneal lavage [DPL]) should be controlled by noninvasive pelvic stabilization and angiographic embolization. This guideline is evidence based and stresses the need to control bleeding quickly by getting the patient to the radiology department or operating room within a 45-minute time frame. On the other hand, the definition of hemodynamic instability in the guideline would result in too many patients being taken to the wrong department. Whereas a positive ultrasound examination is a good predictor of intraperitoneal bleeding, a negative ultrasound alone is a poor predictor of pelvic arterial bleeding. Furthermore, 8% to 10% of patients will need both laparotomy and angiographic embolization. Moreover, some patients will also require craniotomy for space-occupying brain injuries and some will require thoracotomy for a transected thoracic aorta. In a recent study, my colleagues and I found that 30% of hemodynamically unstable patients with pelvic fracture had active hemorrhage at two or more sites (Table 2). Therefore every effort should be made to stabilize the patient sufficiently to undergo CT scan if the ultrasound is negative. The CT scan findings of hemodynamically unstable patients with pelvic fracture in our recent study are shown in Table 3. With modern angiographic techniques, the CT scan can usually identify

Table 2: Sites of Active Bleeding

Active Bleeding Sites	Protocol n (%)	CT Scan n (%)	p Value
Pelvis ($n = 249$)	52 (57)	197 (64)	0.253
Abdomen ($n = 129$)	32 (35)	97 (31)	0.499
Extremity ($n = 50$)	13 (14)	37 (12)	0.558
Chest ($n = 29$)	10 (11)	19 (6)	0.118
Face ($n = 4$)	0 (0)	4 (1)	0.355
One site	31 (34)	176 (57)	0.001
Two sites	29 (32)	80 (26)	0.260
Three sites	6 (7)	7 (2)	0.022

Table 3: CT Results ($n = 309$)

	n	%
Pelvic hematoma	236	76
Free fluid	116	38
Extremity injury	105	34
Other intra-abdominal injury	94	30
Bladder injury	68	22
Splenic injury	47	15
Liver injury	36	12
Aortic injury	11	4

CT, Computed tomography.

active arterial bleeding or the lack of bleeding by the presence or absence of a contrast blush in the pelvic hematoma; it can also accurately identify intraperitoneal organ injury requiring laparotomy. If a decision is made to take the unstable patient to the radiology department for CT scan, it is imperative that the angiography team be called in so that no time is lost if they are needed. Another option, if ultrasound is not available or is equivocal, is the use of diagnostic peritoneal tap or DPL performed with the patient in the supraumbilical position to prevent the surgeon from entering the pelvic hematoma. If the DPL is grossly positive (aspiration of 10 ml or more of free blood), the patient should proceed directly to the operating room for laparotomy, and the angiography staff should be notified that they may be needed within the next hour. After intraperitoneal hemorrhage has been controlled by laparotomy, attention is turned to the pelvic hematoma. If this is large or expanding, the laparotomy should be completed as quickly as possible and the patient taken immediately to the angiography team for potential embolization of arterial bleeding.

Patients with both intraperitoneal and pelvic arterial hemorrhage are the most challenging and frustrating to deal with. They literally must be in two different places at the same time. Three recent approaches to dealing with this problem have been described over the past several years. The first is to take all patients to the radiology department for angiography first, if it is immediately available. The angiographer quickly studies the celiac axis looking for hepatic or splenic bleeding and the hypogastric arteries looking for pelvic arterial bleeding. Embolization of as many as three different sites has been described. Another approach is to have the angiography team come into the operating room and perform angiographic embolization of the pelvic arterial bleeding at the same time the surgeons are controlling intraabdominal bleeding with portable equipment. The third approach is to open the pelvic hematoma in the operating room through the space of Retzius and pack the retroperitoneum from there; angiographic embolization in the operating room (OR) or in the angiographic suite should follow. This prevents the decompressing of the pelvic hematoma into the peritoneal cavity. It should be mentioned that these techniques are relatively recent, with few patients reported, and they all require considerable forethought and organization before a patient needs them. Rarely, lacerations of the external or internal iliac artery or iliac veins cause such rapid bleeding that the patient cannot be resuscitated sufficiently to go to the angiography suite from the OR. If this happens, various angiographic techniques must be used in the OR to identify the bleeding site, and occasionally direct operative ligation of these major vessels is necessary even though it requires opening the retroperitoneal hematoma.

Hemodynamically stable patients with a pelvic fracture should undergo CT scan of the abdomen and pelvis to identify intraperitoneal hemorrhage, look for evidence of solid viscous injury, look for a pelvic hematoma, and characterize the fracture. Additionally, evaluation for any contrast extravasations in the pelvic hematoma should be performed to identify arterial bleeding. CT scan has replaced conventional angiography as a diagnostic tool. Patients with evidence of arterial blush or large pelvic hematomas (or both) on CT scan should undergo angiographic embolization. The threshold for performing angiography in patients who have responded to resuscitation and have moderate blood requirements is somewhat controversial. Most of these patients are bleeding from cancellous bone fragments or venous sources. Immediate external fixation or the use of pelvic binders has been recommended as a primary method to control pelvic fracture hemorrhage under these circumstances. The theory behind both the pelvic binder and external pelvic fixation is that pelvic fracture hemorrhage from cancellous bone fragments and lacerations of the pelvic venous plexus can be arrested by compression and immobilization of fracture fragments.

There are two philosophies regarding the use of pelvic fracture stabilization in the management of pelvic fracture bleeding. Some institutions use pelvic fracture stabilization as the initial treatment of ongoing hemorrhage, reserving angiography for patients who continue to bleed after pelvic fracture stabilization. Other institutions rely on angiography as the initial therapeutic maneuver and reserve pelvic fracture stabilization for patients who continue to bleed after angiography. The protocol chosen depends on the resources and track record of the individual institution. In those institutions at which early open reduction and internal fixation (ORIF) are performed, there is usually reluctance to place an external fixator because of the problems with pin-track infections and reluctance to use a pelvic binder for prolonged periods because of skin blistering, which compromises incision placement of ORIF. Interestingly, several recent series of pelvic fracture patients have shown a dramatic decrease in the number requiring pelvic fracture stabilization as a means of controlling hemorrhage.

PELVIC FRACTURE STABILIZATION

Long-term results of conservative treatment of displaced and unstable pelvic fractures are poor and include significant lifelong disability for the patient. Recent advances in operative stabilization of pelvic fractures have decreased this disability. Early aggressive fracture management using a combination of internal and external fixation techniques within the first 24 to 72 hours of patient injury is now becoming standard. Multidisciplinary protocols that control hemorrhage and manage other, associated injuries as rapidly as possible have made it possible to prepare most patients for orthopaedic stabilization of their pelvic fracture within 24 hours.

A stable pelvic fracture is treated with bed rest until the patient is tolerant of mobilization. Weight bearing may be started early on the affected side if the pelvic injury is stable. After pelvic instability has been diagnosed, the approach to definitive stabilization depends on the fracture pattern. Direct stabilization of the posterior pelvis restores pelvic stability and usually eliminates the need to provide further anterior ring fixation. Anterior pelvic fractures resulting from anterior/posterior compressive forces involving the pubic symphysis may be reduced and stabilized by either closing the "book" with an anterior external frame or plating the symphysis. Most iliac wing fractures associated with hemipelvic instability require plate osteosynthesis, through either a retroperitoneal approach or a lateral or posterior exposure to the iliac wing. Sacroiliac dislocation or sacroiliac joint fracture requires reduction of the hemipelvic displacement and correction of the rotational misalignment. These dislocations are stabilized in most cases with plate and lag screw techniques. Bilateral sacroiliac dislocations and sacral fractures may require significant exposure

and reduction techniques, followed by tension band plate stabilization using a posterior reconstruction plate placed on the external posterior aspect of the pelvis, with screw stabilization in both the iliac wings, in addition to iliosacral lag screw fixation. Other types of posterior fixation involve sacral bars, larger plate configurations, and combinations of posterior and anterior internal fixation.

OPEN PELVIC FRACTURES

Open pelvic fracture is an injury in which a break of skin or mucous membrane communicates into the area of the fracture. The mortality rate from open pelvic fractures is high, with free external hematoma and fecal or vaginal contamination of the retroperitoneal hematoma leading to death from hemorrhage and sepsis. Patients with open pelvic fractures who are hemodynamically unstable should be taken to the OR for hemorrhage control. Diffuse bleeding from decompression of the retroperitoneal hematoma often responds to packing followed by angiography if bleeding persists. This is one situation in which it is necessary to use an external fixator on the pelvis. Otherwise, the fracture fragments will move with the packing and there will be nothing to pack against. More problematic is rapid bleeding from a major arterial injury, which usually requires direct operative exposure and ligation. Open wounds in the buttock, perineum, or perirectal area act as a portal of entry for fecal bacteria to infect the pelvic hematoma, with resultant sepsis. If the patient has wounds in these areas, a diverting colostomy should be performed. The timing of this operation depends on the hemodynamic stability of the patient and other, associated injuries. It can safely be delayed for up to 48 hours. Open wounds of the rectum or vagina, on the other hand, represent ongoing contamination of the pelvic hematoma. These lacerations should be repaired, if possible, and widely drained. In the case of a rectal laceration, a diverting colostomy should also be performed and the distal rectum irrigated free of fecal material. After hemorrhage has been controlled and further contamination prevented, these patients require daily trips to the OR for continued irrigation and debridement of their frequently extensive wounds. Another important point is that the anal sphincters should be approximated at the first operation as much as possible to give the best chance for later fecal continence. Otherwise the wound is left open and irrigated daily until it will support a vacuum-assisted dressing. Many of these wounds require split-thickness skin grafting.

Pelvic hemorrhage with associated intra-abdominal hemorrhage is controlled by immediate laparotomy and pelvic stabilization in the operating room, followed by angiographic embolization. Indications for embolization at angiography include extravasations of contrast, false aneurysms, and arterial vasospasm. Rotationally unstable pelvic ring fractures should be initially stabilized with a noninvasive device.

Suggested Readings

Ballard RB, Rozycki GS, Newman PG, and others: An algorithm to reduce the incidence of false-negative FAST examinations in patients at high risk for occult injury. Focused assessment for the sonographic examination of the trauma patient, *J Am Coll Surg* 189:145, 1999.

Clayton JL, Robinson E, Tillou A, and others: CT scan improves diagnostic accuracy and mortality in hemodynamically unstable patients with pelvic fracture, *J Trauma* (submitted).

DiGiacomo JC, Bonadies JA, Cole FJ, and others: *Practice management guidelines for hemorrhage in pelvic fracture.* East Northport, NY, 2001, Eastern Association for the Surgery of Trauma.

Evers BM, Cryer HM, Miller FB: Pelvic fracture hemorrhage. Priorities in management, *Arch Surg* 124:422, 1989.

Heetveld MJ, Harris I, Schlaphoff G, and others: Guidelines for the management of hemodynamically unstable pelvic fracture patients, *ANZ J Surg* 74:520, 2004.

Smith WR, Moore EE, Osborn P, and others: Retroperitoneal packing as a resuscitation technique for hemodynamically unstable patients with pelvic fractures: report of two representative cases and a description of technique, *J Trauma* 59:1510, 2005.

Totterman A, Dormagen JB, Madsen JE, and others: A protocol for angiographic embolization in exsanguinating pelvic trauma, *Acta Orthopaedica* 77:462, 2006.

Velmahos GC, Chahwan S, Falabella A, and others: Angiographic embolization for intraperitoneal and retroperitoneal injuries, *World J Surg* 24:539, 2000.

Spine and Spinal Cord Injuries

Michael Pasquale, MD, and Mark Li, MD, PhD

The most common sites of spine injury are the cervical spine and the thoracolumbar junction. The incidence of spinal cord injury (SCI) is estimated to be approximately 40 new cases per million population per year, or roughly 11,000 new cases per year in the United States. SCI primarily affects young male adults, with the average age at the time of injury being 37.6 years. SCI is seen most commonly with injuries to the cervical spine and injuries at the thoracolumbar junction. The most frequent neurologic sequela is incomplete tetraplegia (34.5%), followed by complete paraplegia (23.1%), complete tetraplegia (18.4%), and incomplete paraplegia (17.5%).

INITIAL EVALUATION

A detailed neurologic examination must be performed and documented. This is crucial because subsequent changes in the examination will be determined on the basis of the initial assessment. Determining the neurologic level and the completeness of injury is the most accurate way to prognosticate recovery and functional outcome. Using the International Standards of Neurological and Functional Classification of Spinal Cord Injury, the examiner determines the motor and sensory level on the right and left and ascertains whether the injury is complete or incomplete. Five muscle groups each are tested in the upper and lower extremities. Each muscle group is supplied by two root levels, and each group is graded from 0 to 5 (Fig. 1). Using standard dermatomes and myotomes defined by the American Spinal Injury Association (ASIA), the motor level is defined as the most caudal segment to have a muscle grade of 3 (see Fig. 1). The sensory level is defined as the most caudal dermatome to have normal sensation to pinprick and light touch (see Fig. 1). In addition to the neurologic level, the completeness of injury must be determined (Fig. 2). A complete injury results in no motor or sensory function preserved in the sacral segments, ASIA A. There are four incomplete levels: ASIA B, C, D, and E. Incomplete injuries are defined as those that spare sensory or motor function (or both) below the neurologic level that includes the sacral (S4-S5) segments.

There are a number of incomplete SCI syndromes that manifest symptoms, depending on which part of the cord is affected. Central cord syndrome occurs in the cervical cord and produces greater weakness in the upper extremities. Brown-Séquard syndrome refers to a lesion that produces ipsilateral motor and proprioceptive loss and contralateral loss of pain and temperature perception. Anterior cord syndrome causes variable loss of motor function, pain, and temperature perception, while sparing proprioception, and is usually seen with injury to the anterior spinal artery at the thoracic level. Cauda equina syndrome occurs when lumbosacral nerve roots

---

ASIA IMPAIRMENT SCALE

☐ **A = Complete:** No motor or sensory function is preserved in the sacral segments S4-S5.

☐ **B = Incomplete:** Sensory but not motor function is preserved below the neurological level and includes the sacral segments S4-S5.

☐ **C = Incomplete:** Motor function is preserved below the neurological level, and more than half of key muscles below the neurological level have a muscle grade less than 3.

☐ **D = Incomplete:** Motor function is preserved below the neurological level, and at least half of key muscles below the neurological level have a muscle grade of 3 or more.

☐ **E = Normal:** Motor and sensory function are normal.

CLINICAL SYNDROMES

☐ Central cord
☐ Brown-sequard
☐ Anterior cord
☐ Conus medullaris
☐ Cauda equina

Figure 1 ASIA Impairment Scale. *From American Spinal Injury Association: International Standards for Neurological Classification of Spinal Cord Injury, rev ed, Chicago, American Spinal Injury Association, 2002.*

---

are injured and results in areflexic bladder, bowel, and lower limbs. In addition to the examination, application of effective spinal radiographic imaging remains the key to successfully completing the task of determining the presence of spinal injury.

SCREENING FOR CERVICAL SPINE INJURY

Cervical spine injury (CSI) is the most commonly missed severe injury with potentially catastrophic consequences for the patient and major medicolegal implications for the physician. In the blunt-trauma population, the published incidence for all types of cervical spine injury ranges from 2% to 4%. Importantly, 15% to 20% of the patients with CSI will have an associated spinal cord injury. Early recognition and management of cervical spine injuries is necessary to prevent detrimental neurologic outcomes. It is

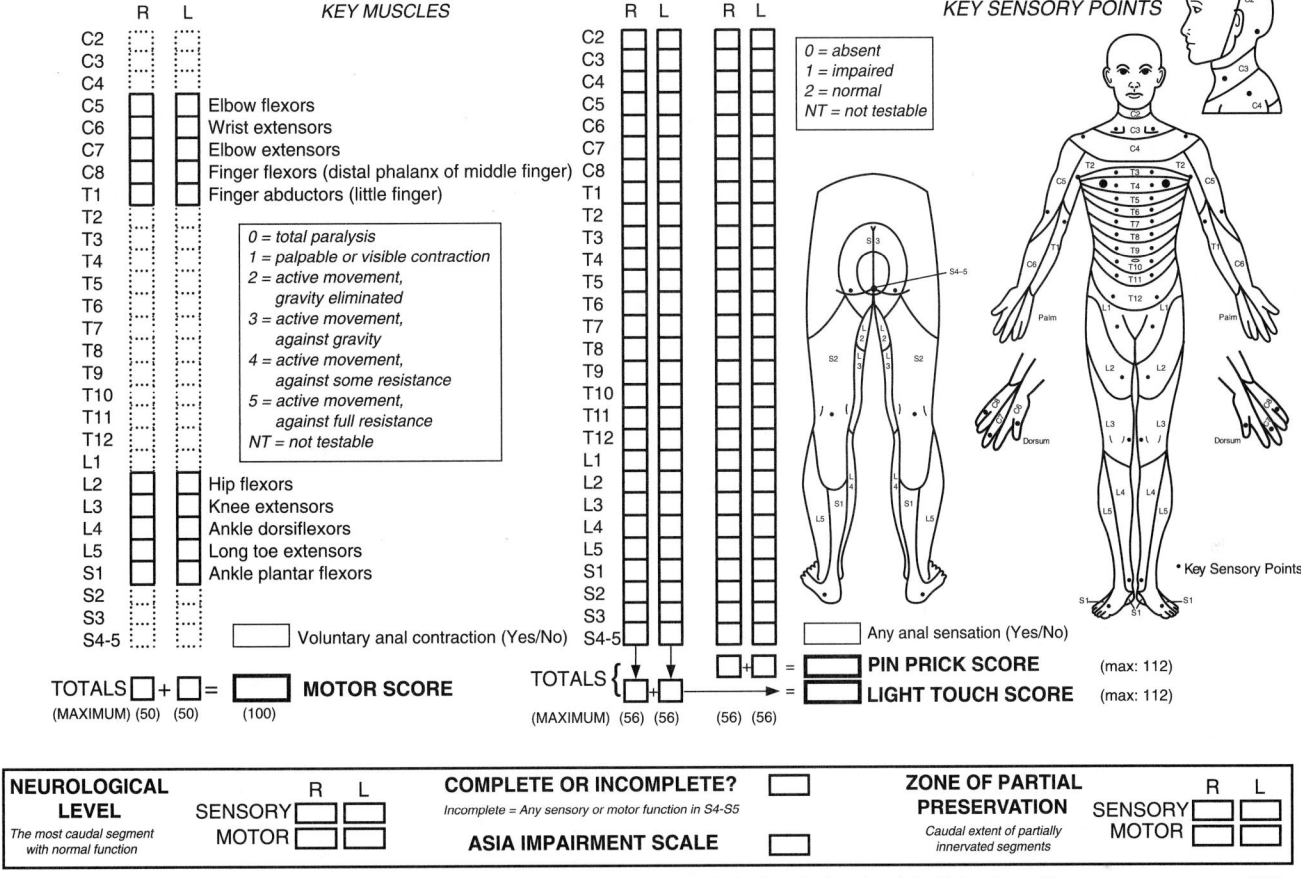

Figure 2 Standard Neurological Classification of Spinal Cord Injury. *From American Spinal Injury Association:* International Standards for Neurological Classification of Spinal Cord Injury, *rev ed, Chicago, 2002, American Spinal Injury Association.*

estimated that between 5% and 30% of CSIs are delayed or missed, most of which are related to technically inadequate plain films or misinterpretation of radiographs. Furthermore, up to 10% of patients who arrive at the emergency department with cervical spine injury will have worsening of their neurologic function because of delays in diagnosis or improper cervical spine precautions. Formulating an imaging approach to a patient with a potential cervical spine injury allows the care provider to achieve an accurate diagnosis in a timely manner with minimal risk to the patient.

Asymptomatic patients are those with no cervical spine tenderness at the posterior midline, no focal neurologic deficit, no evidence of intoxication, a normal level of alertness, and no clinically apparent distracting injuries. Asymptomatic patients do not require radiographic imaging of the cervical spine and can be clinically cleared, and their collars can be safely removed.

Symptomatic patients complain of neck pain, have cervical spine tenderness, or have symptoms or signs of a neurologic deficit associated with the cervical spine, or cannot be assessed for symptoms or signs (or both). These patients require radiographic study of the cervical spine to determine whether injury is present. The American Association of Neurologic Surgeons (AANS) found a 2.6% incidence of significant CSI in the symptomatic patient population following trauma. The AANS and the Eastern Association for the Surgery of Trauma (EAST) have published evidence-based guidelines regarding the radiographic clearance of cervical spine injuries, and on the basis of the available data it was concluded that a combination of imaging modalities (plain films, computed tomography [CT], magnetic resonance imaging [MRI]) will be required to rule out CSI in symptomatic patients. Plain films (three-view) and CT have been shown to be useful to determine the presence of bony injury; flexion-extension views and MRI have been shown to better diagnose the presence of soft-tissue injury; and MRI is superior for the assessment of spinal cord injury. It is recommended that an evidence-based cervical spine clearance protocol be developed at individual institutions to address the symptomatic population.

SCREENING FOR THORACOLUMBAR SPINE INJURY

Up to 4.4% of patients arriving at level I trauma centers have been reported to have fractures of the thoracolumbar spine, with 19% to 50% of these fractures being associated with spinal cord injury. Trauma patients who are awake, show no evidence of intoxication, and have normal mental status and normal examinations may be cleared clinically and do not need radiographic imaging of the thoracolumbar spine. In symptomatic patients, multidetector CT scan with reformatted axial collimation is superior to plain films for screening the thoracolumbar spine for bony injury and is recommended for patients requiring CT scans of the chest and abdomen as part of their evaluation. In patients not requiring CT scans as part of their evaluation, plain films of the thoracolumbar spine are adequate for evaluation. MRI is indicated for patients with neurologic deficits, abnormal CT scans, or clinical suspicion despite normal radiographic evaluation suggesting an unstable injury, although ligamentous injury without bony injury of the thoracolumbar spine is extremely rare.

INITIAL MANAGEMENT CONSIDERATIONS

Results from the National Acute Spinal Cord Injury Studies (NAS-CIS) suggest that all patients with acute spinal cord injury secondary to blunt trauma receive treatment with methylprednisolone. These trials have demonstrated that patients with acute SCI have improved recovery of neurologic function at 6 months after injury if treated with methylprednisolone within 8 hours of injury. The recommended dosage is a 30 mg/kg bolus followed by an infusion of 5.4 mg/kg/hr for 23 hours. Results from the third NASCIS concluded that patients treated within 3 hours of injury should receive 24 hours of steroid treatment, and those treated within 3 to 8 hours of injury should receive 48 hours of treatment. There appears to be no benefit to giving steroids to those patients who are examined or diagnosed more than 8 hours after injury.

Patients with complete injury, particularly those with high neurologic levels, may experience "spinal shock" after injury. During spinal shock there is temporary loss of all or most spinal reflexic activity below the level of injury, along with decreased sympathetic activity. It is imperative that adequate resuscitation be ensured with a combination of adequate volume loading and pressor support. Patients with spinal shock should have their filling pressures monitored to guide the resuscitation. Subsequent to the resuscitation, patients should be fitted for elastic stockings and abdominal binders to compensate for decreased vascular tone.

The degree of respiratory dysfunction is directly related to the level of spinal cord injury and the degree of completeness of injury. The higher the level of injury, the greater the degree of pulmonary compromise, and patients with C1 through C3 neurologic levels will require continuous ventilator support. The phrenic nerve, supplied by C3-C5 nerve roots, will be intact in patients with a C5 neurologic level and below, and these patients have a better chance of being liberated from the ventilator. As the level descends from midcervical to lower cervical and then to thoracic, there will be greater innervation to abdominal and intercostal muscles, thereby making the work of breathing easier. The primary objectives in early pulmonary management include prevention of hypoxemia, atelectasis, and aspiration, with a focus on ensuring adequate clearance of secretions.

Bladder management is initially accomplished with a Foley catheter because the bladder is often areflexic. The goals of bladder management are to prevent urinary retention, minimize the occurrence of urinary tract infections, and determine the best methods of facilitating independent bladder management. These methods may include use of an indwelling Foley catheter or placement of a suprapubic tube. Intermittent catheterization is appropriate for patients with use of their upper extremities. Male patients who have reflex voiding and detrusor hyperreflexia may require a sphincterotomy procedure or pharmacologic agents to reduce outflow resistance and allow the use of an external catheter. Bowel management

should include stool softeners with or without digital stimulation to prevent constipation and minimize incontinence.

Prevention of deep venous thrombosis (DVT) and pulmonary embolism (PE) is extremely important in the SCI population. Sequential compression devices should be used with or without elastic stockings to improve lower-extremity venous return. Pharmacologic prophylaxis should be initiated as soon as the bleeding risk is acceptable, ideally no longer than 72 hours after injury. Low-molecular-weight heparin is the current agent of choice for initiation of prophylaxis. Subsequent conversion to warfarin (Coumadin; Bristol-Myers Squibb, New York, NY) is recommended, and patients should be maintained with an international normalized ratio (INR) of 1.8–2.0 for approximately 8 to 12 weeks, depending on the degree of motor impairment and other DVT/PE risk factors (lower limb fractures, history of thrombosis, cancer, heart failure, obesity, and age older than 70 years). The current recommendation is to screen for DVT 1 to 2 weeks after injury and thereafter if symptoms of DVT/PE develop. Vena caval filter placement should be considered for prophylaxis in those SCI patients who cannot undergo pharmacologic prophylaxis.

NONSURGICAL AND SURGICAL MANAGEMENT CONSIDERATIONS FOR SPINE FRACTURES

Cervical spinal fractures comprise the majority of vertebral column fractures found in trauma (up to 75%). When forces are exerted on the head, injury to the cervical spinal column can result, including ligamentous injury or fracture. Stable fractures can generally be managed with external orthoses such as hard cervical collars, whereas unstable fractures require rigid immobilization via halo fixation or operative arthrodesis. Operative management of cervical fractures is based on achieving appropriate anatomic alignment and stabilizing the destabilized segment with hardware and bony fusion.

Upper Cervical Spine

The upper cervical spine is defined as the atlanto-occipital junction, C1, and C2. The atlanto-occipital junction is the articulation of the cranium onto C1, which is the most rostral part of the cervical spine. The most serious of injuries to this area is the atlanto-occipital dislocation, which derives from distraction of the head relative to the cervical spine; this type of injury is almost always fatal. Complex fractures of the articulating surfaces of the atlanto-occipital junction can cause mass effect from bony fragments that impinge from laterally onto the structures of the craniocervical junction. Injuries to the lower cranial nerves are common, as are injuries to the lateral aspect of the medulla. Operative management of this type of injury includes a far lateral approach, with identification and preservation of the vertebral artery, followed by decompression of the affected neural structures and then by atlanto-occipital fixation with posterior hardware. More common is the nondisplaced, unilateral, occipital condyle fracture, which can be treated with a hard cervical collar for 6 weeks (Fig. 3).

Traumatic axial loads to the upper cervical spine can lead to fractures of C1. The most common of these is a burst or Jefferson fracture. Most exhibit lateral migration of the lateral masses with relative preservation of the ligamentous structures. These fractures can be managed by halo immobilization until bony union is achieved. After 2 to 3 months, dynamic x-rays should be taken to look for ligamentous instability. Patients with greater than 7 mm of instability should be treated with a C1–2 arthrodesis.

Ligamentous injuries to the C1/C2 complex derive from the large amount of rotational motion between the odontoid process of C2 and the C1 ring. The ligamentous components of upper

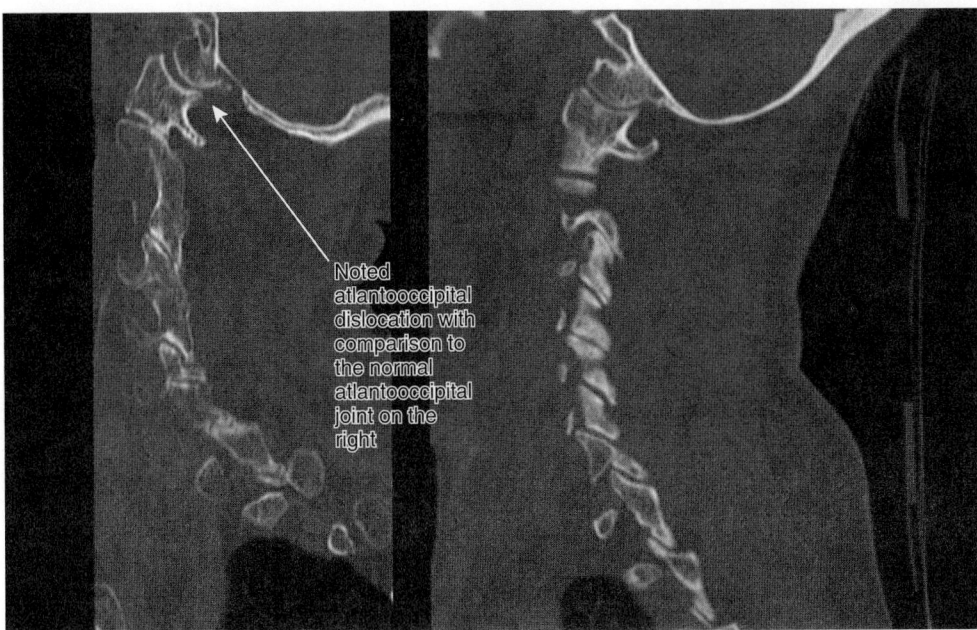

Figure 3 Atlanto-occipital dislocation.

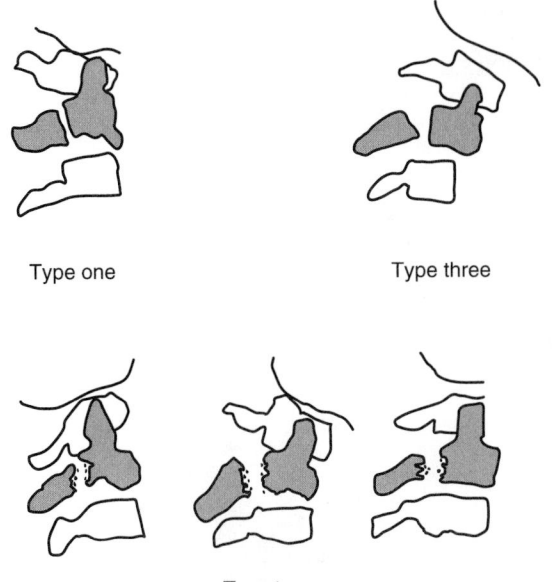

Type one   Type three

Type two

Figure 4 Types of odontoid fractures.

cervical spine are important to maintaining alignment and stability. Of particular importance is the atlantal or transverse ligament, which provides the primary force that restrains the atlanto-dens articular relationship. The alar and apical ligaments provide additional holding forces. Consequently, an abnormal relationship between the ring of C1 and the odontoid process, the atlanto-dens interval (ADI), suggests rupture of these ligaments and potential ligamentous instability. A 3- to 5-mm ADI implies interruption of the transverse ligament, whereas an ADI greater than 5 mm implies rupture of all three ligamentous structures. Persistent ligamentous instability after 12 weeks requires C1-C2 arthrodesis.

Two main types of fracture (odontoid and "hangman's") can occur at C2. Three types of odontoid fracture are shown in Figure 4. Type I is a fracture at the tip of the odontoid, which is a stable fracture and can be treated using a cervical collar (Fig. 5). A type II fracture occurs at the base of the odontoid

process and, because of the characteristics of the blood supply to C2, fractures of this area can lead to relative avascularity of the odontoid process and poor bony union. Up to 75% of these fractures will exhibit nonunion with simple cervical immobilization. Patients at increased risk of nonunion include age older than 55, nicotine use, and displacement greater than 5 mm. The treatment option for acute type II odontoid fractures is realignment followed by either arthrodesis or halo fixation. Care must be taken to assess the transverse and alar ligaments for injury. Type II fractures that are accompanied by ligamentous injury are prone to subluxation, even with bony union of the fracture, and consideration should be given to early C1-C2 arthrodesis. Type II fractures with intact ligamentous structures may be fixated using an odontoid screw, which is passed through the body of C2 into the odontoid process, capturing the fractured segment and pulling it tight to the body. Failure of fusion must be assessed after 3 to 6 months, and a C1-C2 arthrodesis may be necessary if nonunion persists (Figs. 6 and 7).

The hangman's fracture is a traumatic spondylolisthesis of C2 caused by a forceful flexion-distraction mechanism. The fracture is classically described as a bilateral fracture through the pars interarticularis of C2, potentially causing instability. Type I hangman's fractures display greater than 3 mm of displacement and can be treated with a hard cervical collar for 8 to 12 weeks. A type II hangman's fracture has greater than 3 mm translation, usually with the body of C2 subluxing anteriorly. These fractures are inherently unstable and must be realigned using cervical traction. Traction should be placed to enhance neck extension for anterior subluxation, and halo fixation can be used to immobilize the fracture site for 12 weeks. Type III hangman's fractures exhibit marked C2/C3 disk disruption, have perched or locked facets, and require operative reduction and arthrodesis via an approach from the anterior, posterior, or both.

Lower Cervical Spine

Fractures of the lower cervical spine are generally classified by the loading forces that cause them. Acute compression forces in the flexed position generally result in compression of the anterior column and distraction of the posterior elements. Milder forms of this type of injury result in anterior wedge fractures and evidence of edema in the interspinous ligaments on MRI scan (Fig. 8).

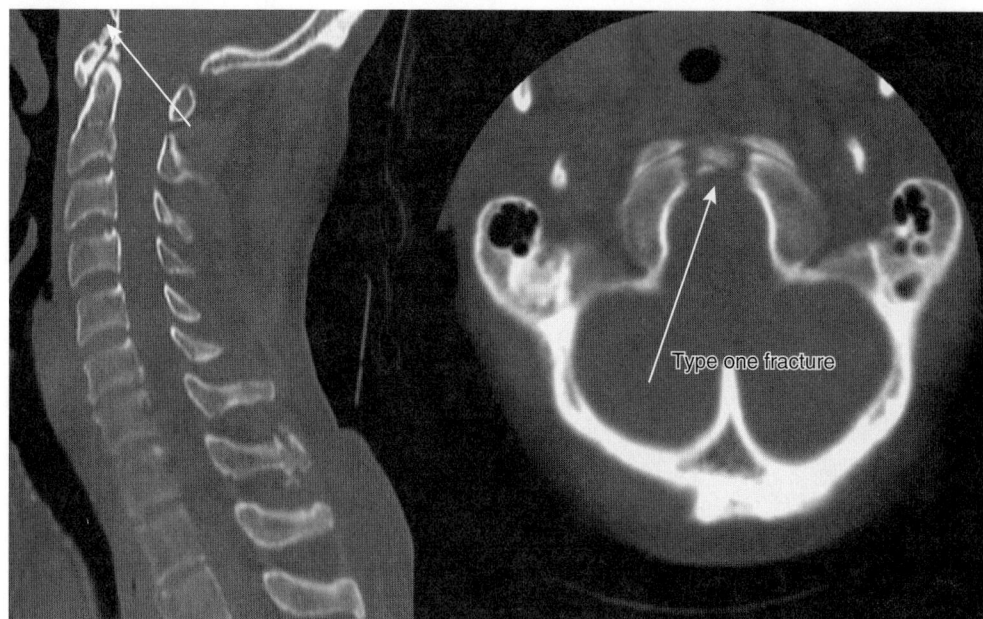

Figure 5 Type I odontoid fracture.

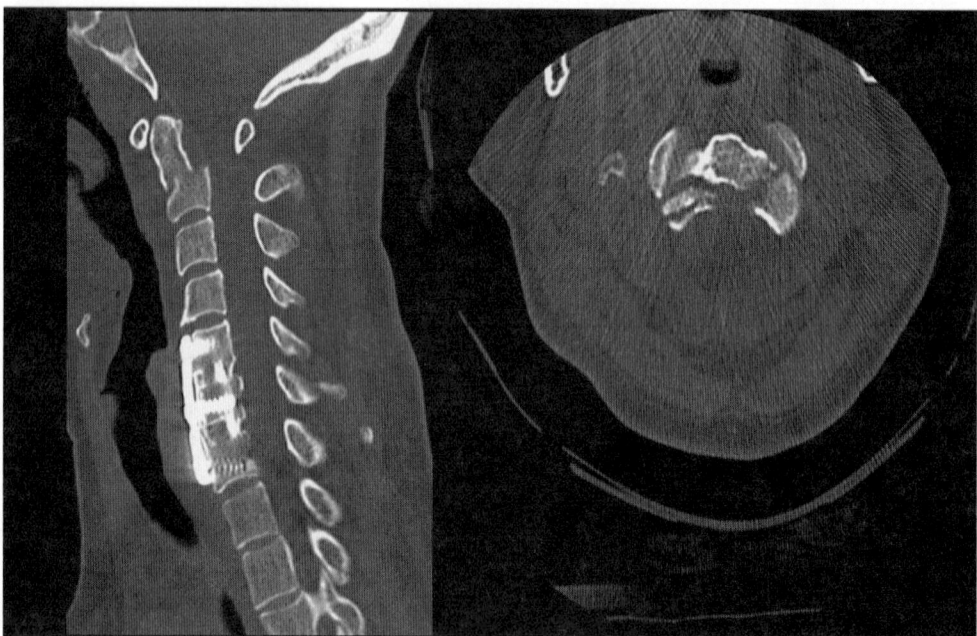

Figure 6 Type III odontoid fracture in patient with previous fixation of C5-7.

More severe forms of injury can result in an unstable fracture involving all three columns when the anterior column fails in flexion and the posterior column fails in tension. These fractures usually cause a split in the vertebral body anteriorly and retropulsion of the posterior aspect of the vertebral body into the spinal canal, sometimes resulting in devastating neurologic injury. These fractures must be reduced with Gardner-Wells tongs and require surgical intervention. At times, the fixation must span the injured segment.

Injuries resulting from hyperflexion usually cause disk and ligamentous injury. These injuries can cause enough ligamentous injury to disrupt the disk and cause facet perching or frank dislocation and "locking." In the case of locked facets, the facets from the rostral level can translate anterior to the facets of the caudal level, causing foraminal compromise and potential compromise to the spinal cord of the injured segment if severely angulated. Bilateral facet dislocations are associated with a high rate of neurologic injury. These types of injury must be treated immediately with reduction while assessing the conscious patient's neurologic condition. Gardner-Wells tongs may be used, assessing alignment using plain x-rays after each 10-lb increase in traction weight until alignment is achieved (up to 75 lb) (Fig. 9). If the locked facets cannot be reduced with tongs, operative reduction must be undertaken, followed by an arthrodesis (usually posterior) at the injured level (Fig. 10).

Hyperextension or lateral twisting forces may result in posterior element or lateral mass fractures. Most unilateral lateral mass fractures are relatively stable and can be managed using a hard cervical collar. With more forceful injury, the lateral mass can be avulsed and pushed into the neural foramen or spinal canal. These fractures

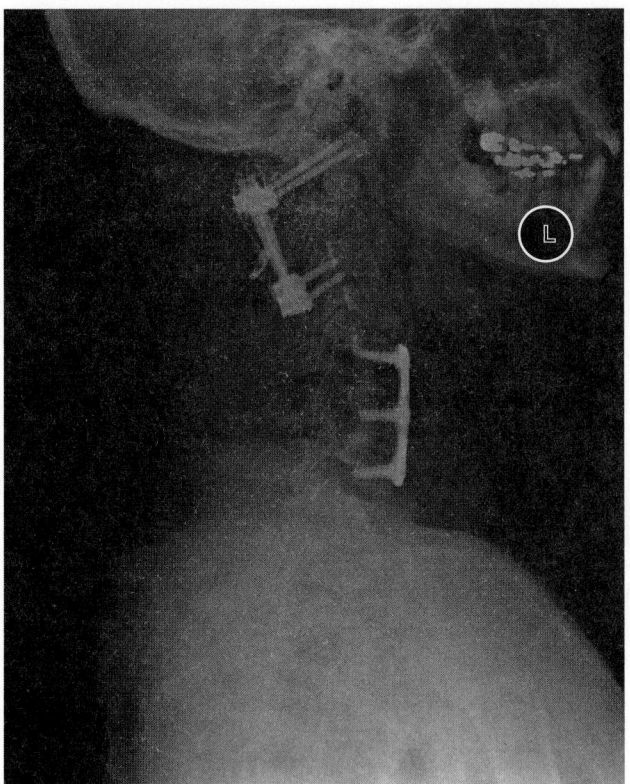

Figure 7 Fixation of C2 fracture.

must be operatively explored, removing all fragments from the neural foramen and spinal canal, followed by appropriate fixation and arthrodesis.

In general, surgery for lower cervical traumatic injuries uses anterior realignment and fixation for vertebral fractures and posterior fixation for facetal or ligamentous instability. The advent of lateral mass fixation has made posterior fixation safe and effective for posterior immobilization. In the case of fractures that involve significant posterior ligamentous instability combined with injury to the intervertebral disk, anterior and posterior fixation may be necessary. Current literature supports the careful examination of normal cervical

lordosis, and an attempt should be made to reestablish normal alignment. Failure to do so may result in later juxtafusional disk degeneration, progressive alignment abnormalities, or both.

Of note, the foramen transversarium houses the vertebral artery, which ascends through the bony cervical spine from C6 to C1/C2, where it then pierces the dura to become intracranial. In any fractures that involve the foramen transversarium, vertebral artery injury should be considered. Gadolinium-enhanced MR angiography (MRA) or multislice CT angiography can be used as a screening tool for vertebral dissection. Conventional angiography may be used if there is a high degree of suspicion for vertebral injury, or for frank symptoms related to vascular insufficiency or embolic phenomena in the vertebral artery distribution. Vertebral dissections should be treated with anticoagulation if not contraindicated.

Thoracic Spine Injury

Thoracic spinal injuries account for a minority of spine fractures (20%), but more than 50% of these fractures are accompanied by neurologic deficit. Because the thoracic spine has increased stability from its relationship to the costovertebral joints and ribs, relatively large forces are required to result in a fracture. More often, forces applied to a rigid thoracic spine are transferred to the next most mobile segment, resulting in fractures at the thoracolumbar junction.

Thin-section CT scan of the thoracic spine with reconstructions is the study of choice to evaluate thoracic fractures. Analysis of spinal stability is determined using the Denis three-column theory. The anterior column includes the anterior longitudinal ligament and the anterior half of the vertebral body and intervertebral disk. The middle column is composed of the posterior half of the vertebral body, the intervertebral disk, and the posterior longitudinal ligament. The posterior column includes the pedicles, lamina, ligamentum flavum, spinous processes, interspinous ligaments, transverse processes, and intertransverse ligaments. Frank instability is defined as any injury that involves two of the three columns, bony vertebral compression with more than 50% loss of height, greater than 2.5 mm of sagittal displacement, or greater than 20 degrees of angulation in the sagittal plane.

Treatment for thoracic fractures is determined by the type and stability of the injury. Stable fractures can often be treated with an external thoracic-lumbar-sacral orthotic until bony union is noted. Care must be taken with any such fracture to watch the patient for

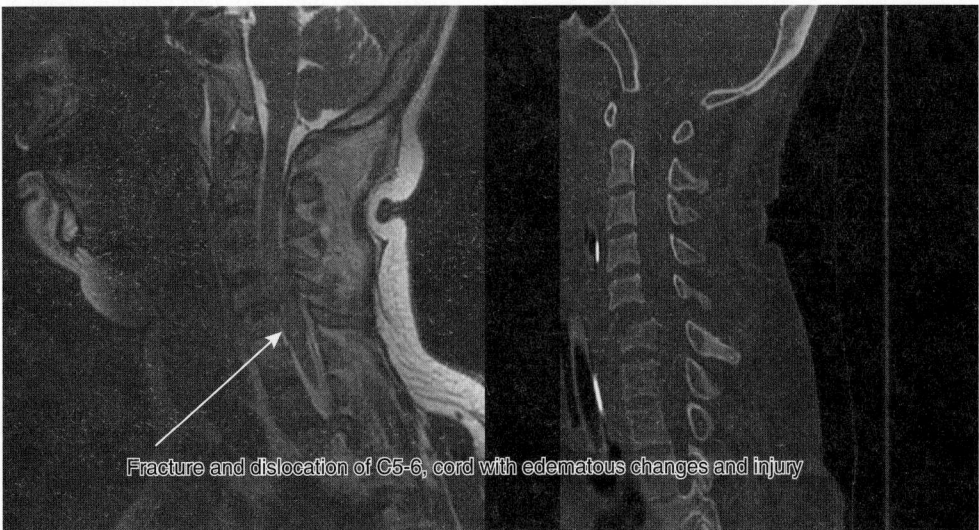

Fracture and dislocation of C5-6, cord with edematous changes and injury

Figure 8 Instability secondary to ligamentous instability.

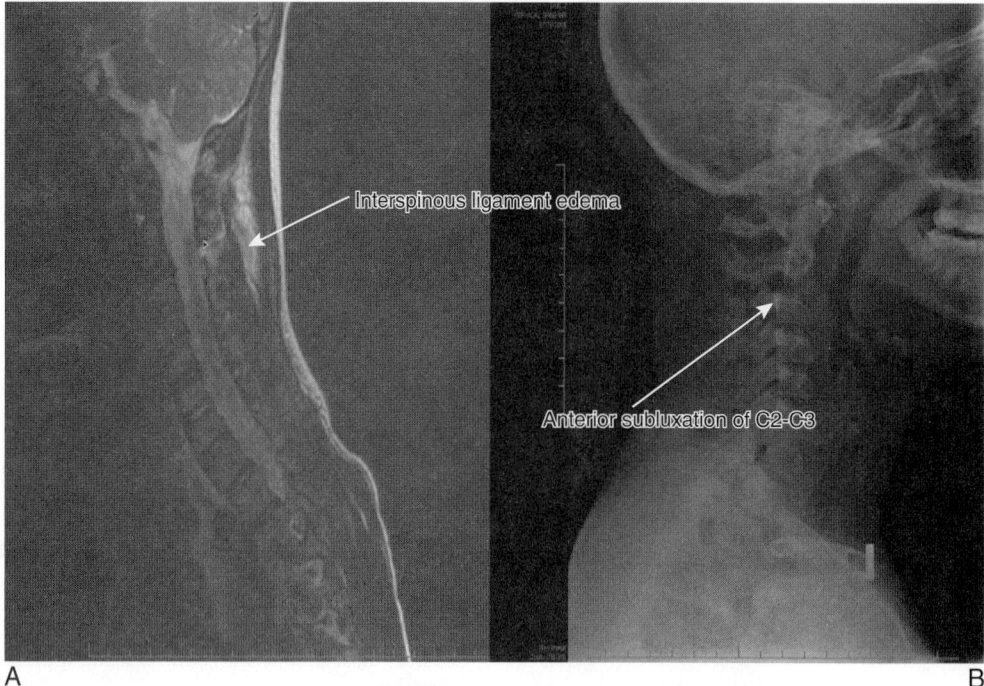

Figure 9 Complex fracture of C5 and C6 **(B)** with resultant cord edema **(A)**.

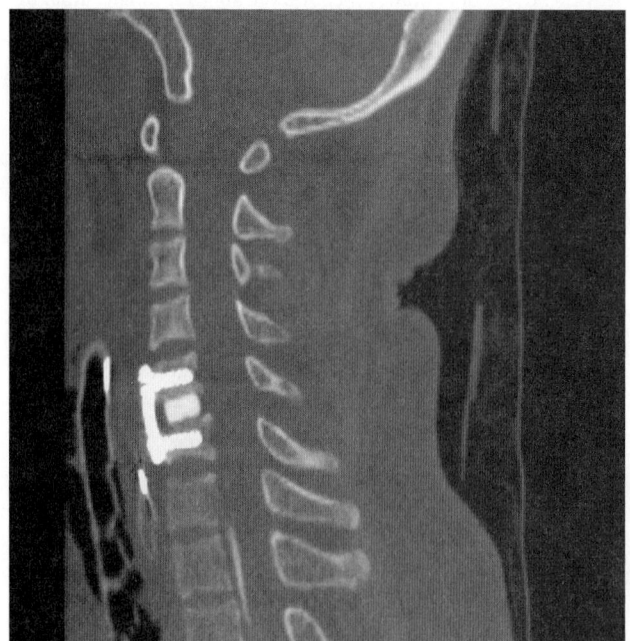

Figure 10 Fixation of C5-C6 with anterior diskectomy and allograft fusion.

progressive kyphosis. Frequently kyphotic changes can take place over the first several months, causing progressive back pain and neurologic symptoms. For unstable fractures, stabilization may be performed with posterior pedicle screw fixation if the overall sagittal alignment is satisfactory. If there is excessive angulation, an anterior approach may be required to achieve realignment. In patients with complete paraplegia, controversy exists regarding the utility of spinal fixation. Our practice has been to use spinal fixation early to allow for more rapid mobilization and rehabilitation (Fig. 11).

Thoracolumbar Fractures

Up to 60% of spinal fractures occur at the thoracolumbar junction (T12-L1). Because the spinal cord ends at this level, these fractures rarely result in neurologic injury unless the conus medullaris is directly injured. As with thoracic fractures, the Denis three-column injury is used to determine stability. The most common fracture at the thoracolumbar junction is the compression fracture, which involves the anterior column alone. As with thoracic fractures, 50% compression or 20 degrees of angulation (or both) is the threshold for surgical intervention. Otherwise thoracolumbosacral orthotic (TLSO) bracing can be used to maintain alignment until these fractures heal.

Axial loads can cause "burst" fractures of the thoracolumbar junction. These fractures involve both anterior and middle columns and have a high risk of neurologic injury from retropulsed bone from the superior half of the vertebral body. These fractures are characterized by loss of height involving both anterior and posterior columns, specifically the posterior vertebral cortex. In addition, the "burst" fracture widens the interpedicular distance, and bony retropulsion of the posterior vertebral wall between the pedicles can cause significant compromise of the spinal canal. Burst fractures can be treated with TLSO bracing unless there is greater than 50% compression, greater than 30% spinal canal compromise, and less than 20 degrees kyphotic angulation. Surgical correction and realignment in burst fractures yield a lower incidence of progressive angulation and progressive neurologic compromise. If the angulation is less than 30%, a posterior approach may be used to decompress the spinal canal and fixate the fracture in adequate alignment. The posterior approach results in shorter operative time and less blood loss and can be highly effective for the appropriate patient. If the degree of angulation is more significant, an anterior approach may be necessary, the advantages being complete decompression of the spinal canal under direct vision. Postoperative recovery time is slightly longer than that resulting from the use of a posterior approach because of the transthoracic and retroperitoneal dissection. However, in the appropriate setting, the anterior transthoracic approach allows for excellent realignment and good mechanical fixation with modern hardware (Fig. 12).

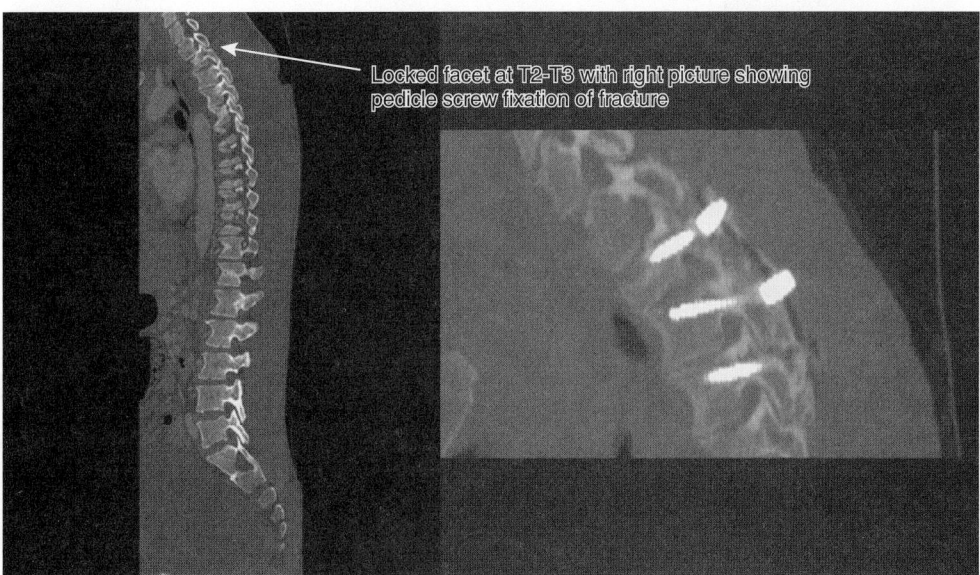

Locked facet at T2-T3 with right picture showing pedicle screw fixation of fracture

Figure 11 Locked facet in thoracic spine.

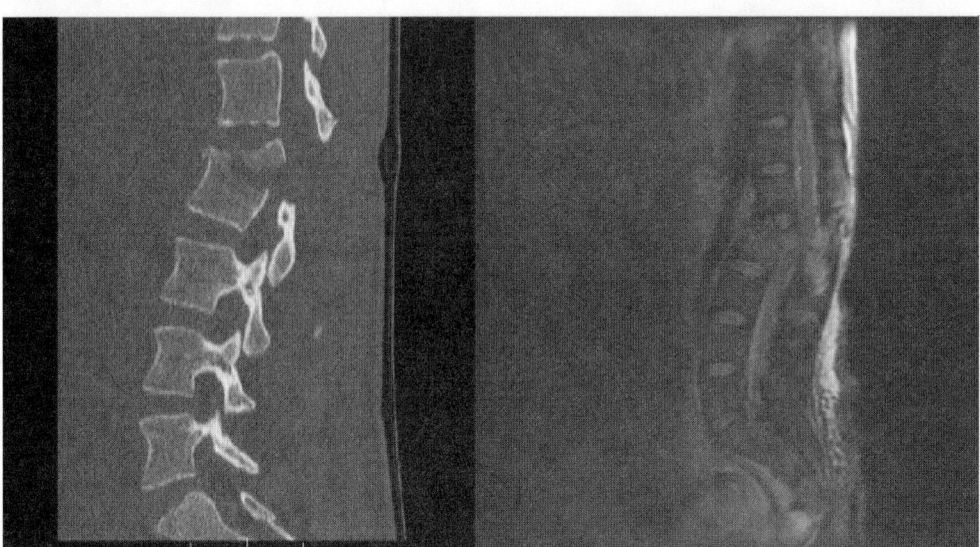

Figure 12 L2 burst fracture with associated distraction of L1 and L2 posterior elements and acute kyphosis.

Flexion distraction injuries result in the "Chance" fracture. These fractures involve the vertebral body, pedicles, and lamina (bony Chance fracture) or the intervertebral disk, ligamentum flavum, and interspinous ligaments (ligamentous Chance fracture). These fractures are highly unstable because of the involvement of two, or most commonly, all three columns. These fractures can be stabilized posteriorly if there is no anterior translation of the fracture fragments. If there is significant translation of the upper and lower vertebral segments in the sagittal plane, the fracture becomes a fracture dislocation, as opposed to a simple flexion distraction injury. These fractures have a 50% chance of complete paraplegia and are associated with much higher forces applied in flexion. Again, operative reduction and fixation must be used to achieve both stability and appropriate alignment.

Lumbar Fractures

Lower lumbar fractures are relatively rare compared with those fractures described earlier. Because of the load-bearing characteristics of the lower lumbar spine, combined with the presence of significant lumbar lordosis, the treatment of these fractures is highly controversial. Specifically, fractures of L4 and L5 often occur with no neurologic compromise but can be unstable using the Denis classification. Experience with these fractures is limited, but many recent reports show poor functional outcome with surgical fixation, especially if the surgical fixation includes the sacrum. For fractures of the lower lumbar spine, conservative therapy can be used to preserve relative motion at the lumbosacral junction as fusion to the sacrum can result in ongoing low back pain and difficulty with prolonged sitting (Fig. 13).

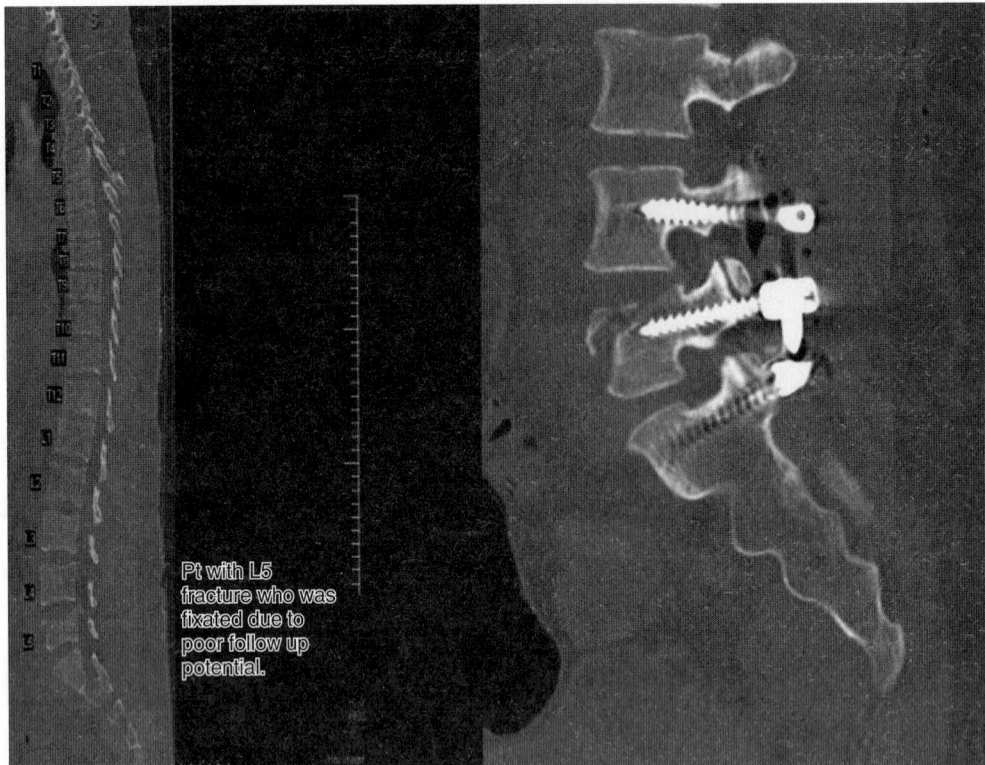

Pt with L5 fracture who was fixated due to poor follow up potential.

Figure 13 Lower lumbar fracture.

SUGGESTED READINGS

Amar AP, Levy ML: Surgical controversies in the management of spinal cord injury, *J Am Coll Surg* 188:550, 1999.

American Association of Neurological Surgeons and the Congress of Neurological Surgeons: *Radiographic assessment of the cervical spine in symptomatic trauma patients*, The Section on Disorders of the Spine and Peripheral Nerves of the American Association of Neurological Surgeons and the Congress of Neurological Surgeons, December 27, 2001.

American Spinal Injury Association: International standards for neurological classification of spinal cord injury (rev. 2002), Chicago, 2002, American Spinal Injury Association.

Barba CA, Taggert J, Morgan AS, and others: A new cervical spine clearance protocol using computed tomography, *J Trauma* 51:652, 2001.

Bracken MB, Shepard MJ, Collins WF, and others: A randomized, controlled trial of methylprednisolone in the treatment of acute spinal cord injury: results of the Second National Acute Spinal Cord Injury Study, *NEJM* 322:1405, 1990.

Bracken MB, Shephard MJ, Holford TR, and others: Administration of methylprednisolone for 24 or 48 hours or tirilazad mesylate for 48 hours in the treatment of acute spinal cord injury: results of the Third National Acute Spinal Cord Injury Randomized Controlled Trial, *JAMA* 277:1597, 1997.

Clagett GP, Anderson FA Jr, Geerts WH, and others: Prevention of venous thromboembolism, *Chest* 114(suppl): 531, 1998.

Consortium for Spinal Cord Medicine: *Clinical practice guidelines: prevention of thromboembolism in spinal cord injury*, ed 2, Washington, DC, 1999, Paralyzed Veterans of America.

Eastern Association for the Surgery of Trauma, Practice Management Guideline Committee: *Practice management guideline for the screening of thoracolumbar spine fracture*. East Northport, NY, 2006, Eastern Association for the Surgery of Trauma.

Eastern Association for the Surgery of Trauma, Practice Parameter Workgroup for Cervical Spine Clearance: *Practice management guidelines for identifying cervical spine injuries following trauma*, East Northport, NY, 1998, Eastern Association for the Surgery of Trauma. (Also published in Pasquale M, Fabian TC: Practice management guidelines for trauma from the Eastern Association for the Surgery of Trauma, *J Trauma* 44:941, 1998.)

Grossman MD, Reilly PM, Gillett T, and others: National survey of the incidence of cervical spine injury and approach to cervical spine clearance in U.S. trauma centers, *J Trauma* 47:684, 1999.

Hoffman JR, Mower WE, Wolfson AB, and others: National Emergency X-radiography Utilization Study Group. Validity of a set of clinical criteria to rule out injury to the cervical spine in patients with blunt trauma. National Emergency X-radiography Utilization Study Group, *N Engl J Med* 343:94, 2000.

Hoffman JR, Wolfson AB, Todd K, and others: Selective cervical spine radiography in blunt trauma: methodology of the National Emergency X-radiography Utilization Study (NEXUS), *Ann Emerg Med* 32:461, 1998.

National Spinal Cord Injury Statistical Center: *Facts and figures at a glance, September 25, 2007*: www.spinalcord.uab.edu Accessed MONTH DAY, YEAR.

FACIAL INJURIES

Paul N. Manson, MD

Facial injuries consist of damage to bone and soft tissue. The facial injury may be isolated or a part of a multiple-system injuries pattern. Multiple-system injuries that include a facial injury often require a coordinated effort by general surgeons and specialty teams.

EMERGENCY TREATMENT OF MAXILLOFACIAL TRAUMA

The presence of a facial injury implies a geographic (simultaneous) injury to the head, face, and neck region. Evaluation for brain injury, skull fracture, and cervical spine injury is required in any patient with a maxillofacial injury to exclude serious injuries in adjacent anatomic regions.

Maxillofacial trauma presents three life-threatening emergencies:

1. Airway obstruction
2. Hemorrhage
3. Aspiration

Airway Obstruction

Airway obstruction is expected in those patients with fractures of the upper and lower jaws and injuries that result in swelling or bleeding into the airway spaces (neck, pharynx, mouth, floor of the mouth, and nose). The onset of stridor, hoarseness, drooling, inability to swallow, and noisy respirations should prompt an alert clinician to urgently intubate the patient or perhaps perform a tracheostomy. Cricothyroidotomy is an emergency maneuver to access the airway through the cricothyroid membrane. It should always be converted to tracheostomy as soon as feasible.

Life-Threatening Hemorrhage

Life-threatening hemorrhage results from two categories of injury: (1) facial lacerations and (2) closed fractures of the sinus and midface.

Facial Lacerations

Bleeding from facial lacerations is usually the result of partially or fully transected major arteries. These are controlled by direct ligation, carefully avoiding branches of the facial nerve. The partially transected artery cannot retract and will continue to bleed.

Closed Fractures, Sinus Injuries, and Midface Injuries

Midface and orbital fractures produce hemorrhage from lacerations of arteries and veins in the walls the sinus cavities or adjacent to them. Generally, manual repositioning of the maxilla and anteroposterior nasal packing control the bleeding. The maxilla is best put at rest in intermaxillary fixation. Angiographic embolization is the usual method of control in those few patients (5%) who continue to bleed. Selective ligation of the internal maxillary artery (accessed through the posterior wall of maxillary sinus) or bilateral external carotid and superficial temporal artery ligation can be performed, but it is seldom necessary.

Aspiration

Aspiration of oral secretions, gastric contents, or blood frequently accompanies fractures of the middle and lower face, especially if there is cerebral injury. Rapid, noisy respirations, low arterial oxygen content, and a decrease in pulmonary compliance are seen. Intubation prevents aspiration and should be performed immediately when there is evidence that the airway is not being protected.

Occult Injuries

The possibility of occult injuries demands a thorough multisystem examination in every patient. Observation of other organ systems must be continued throughout the entire period of facial injury treatment.

EARLY MANAGEMENT OF MAXILLOFACIAL TRAUMA

The early management of maxillofacial trauma consists of the following:

1. Clinical examination
2. Appropriate diagnostic imaging
3. Definitive wound or fracture management

Clinical Examination

The diagnosis of most facial injuries is accomplished by a thorough clinical examination noting contusions, bruises, discoloration, crepitus, pain, localized tenderness, numbness, paralysis, malocclusion, diplopia, visual acuity loss, facial asymmetry, deformity, and changes in eye position and facial contour. One should assume that there is a fracture under any soft-tissue laceration, contusion, or bruise until proved otherwise. The physical examination should be both sequential and direct; an orderly examination of the facial structures in sequence from top to bottom is followed by a careful, redirected examination to those areas obviously injured; a double examination is thus performed. Palpation of all bony surfaces begins at the supraorbital rims around the orbit and extends to the infraorbital rims, includes the zygomatic arches and malar prominences, and concludes with an intraoral examination of the mandible, intraorally and externally in movement. Any malocclusion, crepitus, bone irregularity, or tenderness is noted. An evaluation of facial nerve and trigeminal motor nerve function compares the two sides of the face. Facial sensation is documented in the supraorbital, corneal, infraorbital, and mental distributions (anesthesia or hypesthesia). A search for occult lacerations in the ear canal, nose, mouth, and pharynx should be completed. The excursion of the jaws, the relation of the teeth in occlusion, and the ability of the teeth to occlude are noted, looking for irregular arch form and abnormalities of intercuspation of the teeth. Fractured or missing teeth, intraoral and gingival lacerations, gaps, or level discrepancies in the maxillary and mandibular dentition indicate the possibility of fractures. Lacerations of the lips, chin, and floor of the mouth often accompany anterior jaw fractures.

The function of the eyes should be evaluated. The range of extraocular motion, the presence of a field defect, diplopia, decrease in visual acuity, hyphema, pupil symmetry, speed of pupillary reaction, periorbital ecchymosis, or subconjunctival hematoma imply the possibility of an orbital fracture or globe injury.

Alginate impressions of the dentition are taken, and stone models are prepared to provide a dental record. At the close of the physical examination, any grossly displaced fractures can be manually repositioned, and if desired, intermaxillary fixation can be applied to the jaws to stabilize a fracture. The airway must be protected.

Radiographs

Plain roentgenograms are of little value in radiographic evaluation of facial injuries; the ideal examination is computed tomography (CT). Multiply injured patients should not be sent unmonitored for extensive radiographic evaluation. Radiographic studies supplement, but do not replace, the findings of a physical examination. For most fractures, the best radiographic evaluation consists of axial and coronal plane CT scans of the frontal sinus, nasoethmoidal, orbital, maxillary, and mandibular regions. If the patient cannot be positioned for direct coronal images, coronal images may less ideally be reconstructed from the axial CT format.

Wound and Fracture Management

Soft-Tissue Injuries

Soft-tissue injuries include lacerations, bruises, contusions, and hematomas. Cutaneous wounds are inspected for foreign material and assessed for depth and direction to predict deep structure involvement (probing with a cotton-tipped applicator) and to detect contamination or foreign material. Lacerations require inspection for damaged structures, then cleansing by scrubbing, pressure irrigation, and minimal but judicious sharp debridement of the contused tissue edge. One to two millimeters is usually a sufficient edge resection. A layered repair then achieves a flat wound, resulting in minimal scar formation. Antibiotics are indicated when a clean wound (defined by surgical debridement) cannot be created, especially in the presence of contamination, such as an animal bite. Direct primary closure of facial wounds is always preferred, with a "second look" procedure at 48-hour intervals if there is concern about infection or further devitalized tissue. Open wound management is not employed, with the possible exception of human bites. Debridement should be quite conservative in the region of the vermillion, oral commissures, eyelids, eyebrows, and distal nose. All foreign material (traumatic tattoo) *must* be meticulously removed at the time of the initial examination because it cannot be satisfactorily removed after healing. Postoperative wound hygiene is accomplished four times daily with a 50/50 peroxide-saline solution on cotton-tip applicators and the application of either bacitracin (facial sutures) or an ophthalmic ointment (periorbital sutures). Intraoral repairs are cleansed with mouthwash and tooth brushing three times daily.

Any localized facial hematoma should be drained by incision, and a soft compressive dressing should be applied. Localized hematomas most commonly occur in the ear region but may involve the forehead or buccal areas. Laceration of the lacrimal system should be suspected in any wound near the inner third of the eyelids. Eyelid or periorbital lacerations raise the possibility of globe rupture or penetrating injury.

Lacerations of the facial nerve and parotid duct are managed by direct repair using loupe magnification. Parotid duct lacerations are diagnosed by inserting a no. 22 Angiocath sleeve (Becton Dickinson, Franklin Lakes, NJ) into the duct orifice intraorally and irrigating with saline. The presence of saline in the wound implies duct laceration. Stensen's duct is a short structure that extends from the anterior margin of the parotid gland (1 in anterior to the tragus on a line between the tragus and floor of the nostril) to the second maxillary bicuspid. Ductal lacerations are almost always accompanied by buccal branch facial paralysis because the two structures are adjacent.

Cerebrospinal Fluid Rhinorrhea

Fractures involving the frontal or basilar skull may lacerate the dura, allowing cerebrospinal fluid (CSF) to exit from the nose (rhinorrhea) or may allow air to enter the intracranial area (pneumocephalus). Either condition permits entry of organisms through the meninges with the possibility of meningitis. Generally, prophylactic antibiotics are used on a pulse rather than a prolonged basis in these conditions; perioperative antibiotics accompany operative treatment. CSF rhinorrhea is detected by the presence of clear fluid exiting from the nose or pharynx. Often CSF is mixed with blood, making its detection difficult. The double ring sign (absorption of blood and CSF onto a paper towel) produces a small, central blood ring with a large, peripheral, clearer fluid ring surrounding it. A detailed CT scan is mandatory if CSF leak or pneumocephalus is suspected.

DEFINITIVE FRACTURE MANAGEMENT BY REGION

Nasal Fractures

Nasal fractures produce dislocation laterally or posteriorly. The diagnosis is suggested by epistaxis, bruising, swelling, lateral deviation, retrusion, and flattening of the nose in frontal impact injuries of the nasal pyramid (Fig. 1). Intranasal inspection shows dislocation, deviation, or laceration of the septum with difficulty breathing. Nasal and periorbital hematomas generally accompany nasal fractures, and at least one third have a small laceration over the nasal bridge.

Classically, the radiographic evaluation consists of plain films: a nasal series, a Water's view, and sinus films; they are not particularly definitive, and a CT scan is the best examination. The value of nasal radiographs is both medicolegal and clinical. Adjacent bony injuries are excluded, and the exact displacement of structures, including the septum, is identified.

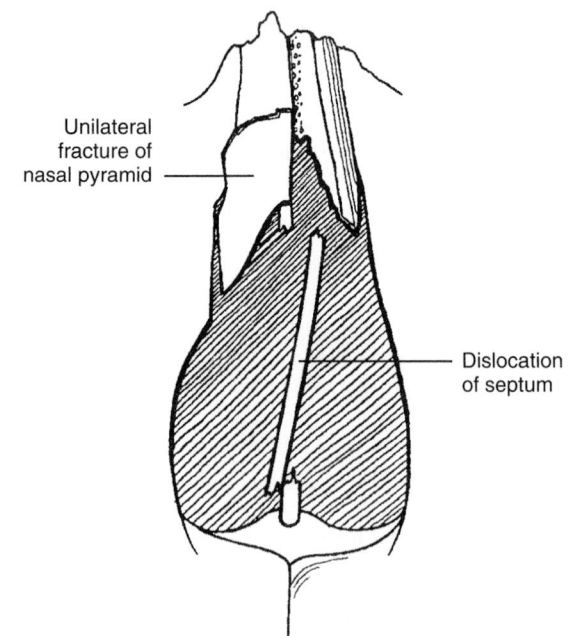

Unilateral fracture of nasal pyramid

Dislocation of septum

Figure 1 Nasal fractures are characterized by lateral or posterior displacement, or both. Both deformities require specific reduction maneuvers.

Treatment

Closed reduction of the septum and nasal pyramid are performed under anesthesia: less ideally, an external field block and intranasal topical Afrin (Schering-Plough, Kenilworth, NJ) are used. Laterally deviated nasal fractures are first completed by intranasal mobilization of the nasal pyramid and septum, restabilizing them in the midline and supporting them with external and internal nasal splints. The septum is straightened and centralized with an Asch forceps and supported with antibiotic-impregnated gauze packing. Frontal-impact nasal injuries produce varying degrees of nasal retrusion and may require open reduction and bone or cartilage grafting to restore projection and achieve the nasal support necessary to produce an adequate aesthetic result.

Zygomatic Fractures

The zygoma constitutes the malar prominence and forms the lateral and inferior walls of the orbit. The zygoma has five attachments to adjacent structures: laterally to the temporal bone, superiorly to the frontal bone, medially to the maxilla, inferiorly to the maxillary alveolus, and in the lateral orbit to the greater wing of the sphenoid (Fig. 2).

The diagnosis of a zygomatic fracture is suggested by the combination of a periorbital and subconjunctival hematoma. These are sensitive but nonspecific signs that may accompany any orbital fracture. If the frontal process of the zygoma is dislocated inferiorly, the lateral canthus is inferiorly displaced by its attachment at Whitnall's tubercle. Depression of the malar eminence accompanies posterior displacement of the zygoma. "Steps" or "level discrepancies" may be palpated in the bone forming the inferior orbital rim or at the zygomaticofrontal suture. Intraorally, a hematoma is present in the upper buccal sulcus, and irregularity intraorally of the maxillary buttress may be palpated. Unilateral epistaxis is secondary to hemorrhage exiting through the ipsilateral maxillary antrum. If the zygoma is posteriorly or medially dislocated, difficult or painful chewing or difficulty bringing the teeth into occlusion results from impingement of the zygomatic body or zygomatic arch on the coronoid process of the mandible or from bruising in the temporalis muscle. Orbital entrapment symptoms (diplopia) result from the orbital floor fracture component and depend on the degree of involvement of extraocular muscles, with limitation of their motion by entrapment in the fracture. Infraorbital nerve numbness accompanies most zygomatic fractures and is related to bruising or injury of the infraorbital nerve at the infraorbital foramen. In the case of a significant orbital fracture, globe dystopia, enophthalmos, and double vision may be present.

The definitive radiographic examination of the zygomatic fractures is an axial and coronal CT scan with bone and soft-tissue windows.

Indications for surgery include the functional symptoms produced by bone displacement, which include deformity, enophthalmos, double vision resulting from incarceration of an extraocular muscle or its surrounding fat; vertical malposition of the globe; loss of malar prominence; anesthesia of the infraorbital nerve (in medially dislocated zygomatic fractures that compress the nerve at the infraorbital foramen); radiographically extensive orbital floor fracture; and interference with the excursion of the coronoid process.

Treatment

Displaced fractures isolated to the zygomatic arch are treated by elevation through a "Gilles" approach. An incision in the temporal hair permits insertion of an elevator under the deep temporal fascia on the temporalis muscle to elevate the zygomatic arch. Because of periosteal continuity, medially displaced arch fractures are generally stable following closed reduction. Displaced zygomatic fractures not isolated to the arch are managed by open reduction and internal fixation with plate and screw fixation (Fig. 3). Incisions for zygomatic fracture reduction consist of lower eyelid incisions (subciliary, midtarsal, or infraorbital rim); gingivobuccal intraoral sulcus incisors; and, in extensive fractures, a coronal incision. Simple fractures may often be reduced with a single approach. Comminuted zygomatic fractures, especially those with lateral displacement of the zygomatic arch, require a coronal incision. Temporary alignment is initially achieved by placing interfragment wires at the zygomaticofrontal suture and infraorbital rim. The zygomaticomaxillary buttress, exposed through an intraoral gingivobuccal sulcus incision, is then stabilized by plate and screw fixation. The orbital floor is explored, and following retrieval of soft-tissue contents of the orbit from the antrum, the orbital floor is reconstituted either by alloplastic material or a thin, curved bone graft.

Nasoethmoidal-Orbital Fractures

Nasoethmoidal-orbital fractures are comminuted fractures of the central upper midface. They result either directly from a blow to the glabella and upper nasal area that shatters the medial orbital rims, nose, and frontal sinus or indirectly by the extension of other

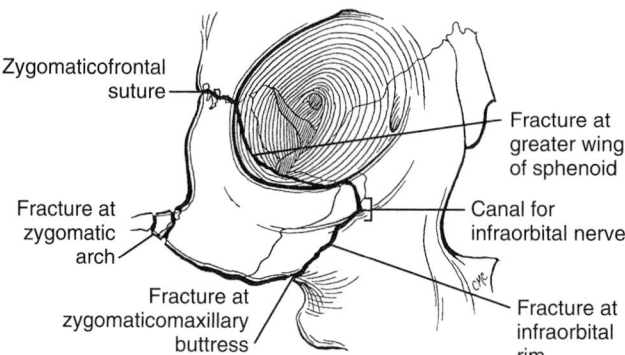

Figure 2 The zygomatic bone constitutes the lateral and inferior portion of the orbit and malar eminence. It attaches to the frontal bone superiorly, the temporal bone posteriorly, and the maxilla medially and inferiorly. In the orbit, the alignment of the orbital process of the zygomatic bone with the greater wing of the sphenoid provides an accurate clue to reduction.

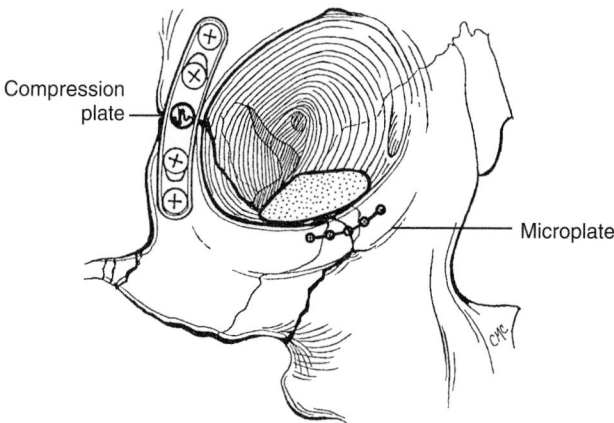

Figure 3 Rigid internal fixation of a zygomatic fracture has been performed by applying plates and screws to the junction of the zygoma with the frontal bone and maxilla. The bone is maneuvered into position and temporarily secured with interfragment wires before rigid internal fixation is applied.

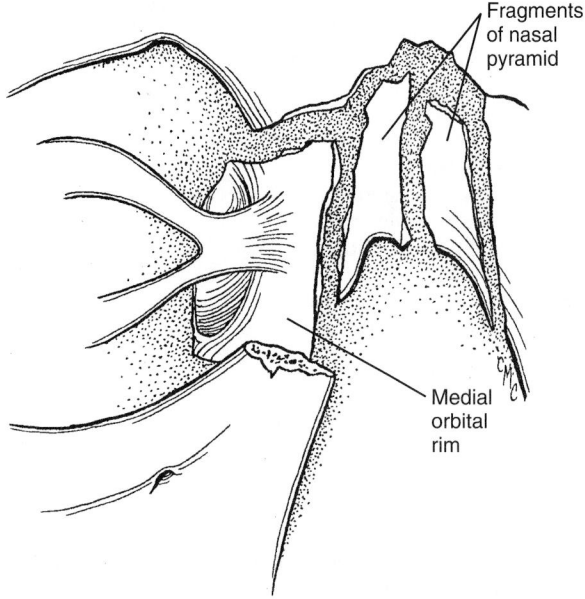

Figure 4 labels: Fragments of nasal pyramid; Medial orbital rim

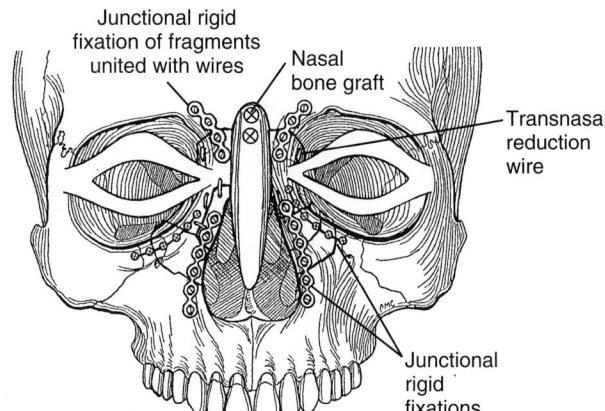

Figure 5 labels: Junctional rigid fixation of fragments united with wires; Nasal bone graft; Transnasal reduction wire; Junctional rigid fixations

Figure 5 Scheme for open reduction and internal fixation of a nasoethmoid orbital fracture. Initially, the fracture fragments are maneuvered into position and temporarily held with interosseous wires. Plate and screw fixation is then applied. The two frontal processes of the maxilla are linked by a transnasal reduction wire, passed from one frontal process of the maxilla to the other at the posterior and superior edge of the lacrimal fossa.

Figure 4 The central segment of a nasoethmoidal orbital fracture is the lower two thirds of the medial-orbital rim. Here the medial canthal ligament attaches to the frontal process of the maxilla. Dislocation of the frontal process of the maxilla dislocates the canthal ligament, producing canthal instability.

midface or frontal fractures. One third of these fractures are unilateral. Commonly, a nasoethmoid fracture exists with a midface Le Fort fracture. The sine qua non of this fracture is the presence of fractures that isolate the lower two thirds of medial orbital rim with the attached canthal ligament from adjacent bones, allowing canthal migration (Fig. 4).

The diagnosis is suggested by the presence of a depressed, comminuted, frontal-impact nasal fracture. Pain and tenderness are present with direct finger pressure over the medial canthal ligament. Unilateral or bilateral eyelid (spectacle) hematomas are present. Nasal lacerations are present in 50% of patients. Epistaxis invariably accompanies this injury. A foreshortened, depressed nose is usually accompanied by telecanthus. Crepitation is present on palpating the nose, and a CSF leak, pneumocephalus, or orbital emphysema may be present. Traumatic telecanthus is measured by an increase in the distance between the medial commissures of the eyelids. This distance normally equals the length of a palpebral fissure. A high index of suspicion is necessary to confirm the diagnosis in patients with minimal displacement or impacted fractures. Mobility of the medial orbital rim may also be detected on "bimanual examination" with simultaneous intranasal-extranasal examination. A palpating finger placed externally against the bone bearing the medial canthal ligament attachment detects movement of the bone produced by the tip of a clamp placed in the nose under the canthal ligament. Movement of the medial orbital rim confirms the presence of a fracture requiring open reduction.

The definitive radiographic examination consists of axial and coronal CT scans.

Treatment

Treatment should generally be accomplished within 96 hours because of the high frequency of associated CSF leaks, frontal sinus fractures, and pneumocephalus. The fracture is exposed with a coronal lower eyelid and gingivobuccal sulcus incisions so that the entire frontal-nasomaxillary buttress is visualized. Initially, fracture fragments are linked together with interosseous wires and then stabilized by plate and screw fixation (Fig. 5). Reconstruction of the integrity of the internal orbit and nose is accomplished by inserting bone grafts in the orbit and nose to replace orbital wall defects, reconstituting orbital volume, nasal height, contour, and projection. Bone grafts replace critical areas of structural bone loss. If the medial canthus is detached from the frontal process of the maxilla, it is reattached by a transnasal canthopexy posterior and superior to the lacrimal fossa.

Frontobasilar Fractures

Frontobasilar fractures include fractures of the frontal bone, frontal sinus, supraorbital rims, and anterior cranial base. Anterior cranial base fractures often accompany frontal vault skull fractures and supraorbital, nasoethmoid, and frontal sinus fractures. High Le Fort (II or III) fractures are often accompanied by a fracture of the frontobasilar region.

The diagnosis is suggested by frontal contusions and lacerations, periorbital hematomas or swelling (the spectacle hematoma is a classic symptom of an anterior cranial base fracture), the presence of CSF leak, pneumocephalus, hemotympanum, frontal lobe injury symptoms (confusion, coma, and somnolence), epistaxis, anosmia, and visual impairment.

The radiographic examination is an axial and coronal CT scan of the frontal bone, frontal sinus, and anterior cranial fossa.

Frontal Sinus Fractures

The frontal sinus consists of two asymmetric cavities separated by one or more bony partitions. The size of the frontal sinus is quite variable, from almost nothing to pneumatization of the entire frontal bone and orbital roof. The most common symptoms of a frontal sinus fracture are lacerations, contusion, or bruises in the forehead area. Often these are the only physical signs of a fracture, and their presence should prompt a CT scan. Epistaxis is usually present. In severe cases, a deformity or depression of the glabellar area may be seen, especially after resolution of the swelling. A CSF leak, pneumocephalus, or orbital emphysema may be noted.

Radiographic examination consists of axial and coronal CT scans.

Treatment

Nondisplaced fractures without duct obstruction require only observation if they are confined to the anterior wall. Depressed fractures of the anterior wall that do not obstruct patency of the nasofrontal duct (Fig. 6) can be treated by elevation and conservative mucosal debridement. Fractures blocking the duct are treated either by obliteration with bone or cranialization of the sinus cavity after removing the mucosa. Posterior wall fractures imply the possibility of a dural laceration. Nondisplaced posterior wall fractures can be observed if duct obstruction is not present. Posterior wall fractures displaced more than the thickness of the inner table require surgical exploration. If the posterior wall of the frontal sinus is fractured, the integrity of the dura must be confirmed.

In cases in which enough of the sinus is destroyed so that there is a chance the sinus will not function, sinus mucosa is removed both by stripping and light abrasion of the bony walls of the sinus cavity to eliminate microscopic invaginations of mucous membrane into the bone. Both nasofrontal ducts are then plugged with "formed-to-fit" calvarial bone grafts. The remainder of the sinus may then be obliterated with bone shavings or allowed to sclerose by the process of osteogenesis (the slow formation of scar tissue in the frontal sinus cavity containing small amounts of bone). The procedure of cranialization implies removal of the posterior wall, sealing the ducts with calvarial bone grafts following thorough removal of the mucosal membrane, and reconstruction of the anterior wall. In effect, the procedure of cranialization converts the sinus to a portion of the intracranial cavity (Fig. 7).

The anterior bony wall of the sinus may be reconstructed by bone grafts where appropriate.

Supraorbital Fractures

Supraorbital fractures are suggested by the presence of bruises or lacerations in the area, a depression of the supraorbital region, a

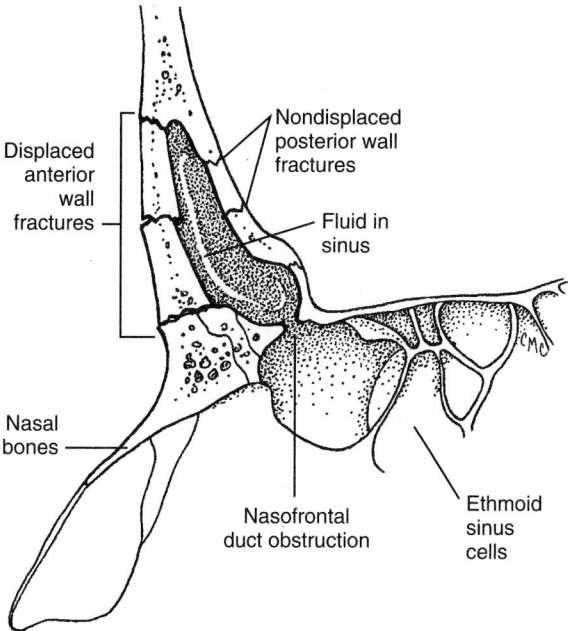

Figure 6 Depressed fractures of the anterior wall of the frontal sinus are treated by evaluation following mucosal debridement. Fractures blocking the duct are treated by obliteration of the sinus cavity. Absence of duct function would create an abscess. Fractures of the posterior wall of the frontal sinus imply the possibility of a dural laceration. Generally, displaced fractures of the posterior wall of the frontal sinus require surgical exploration.

downward and outward protrusion of the globe, ptosis, components of the superior orbital fissure or orbital apex syndromes, and superior gaze paresis (which may mimic inferior rectus entrapment) (Fig. 8). A "step" or bone discontinuity may be palpated in the supraorbital rim. Numbness may occur in the distribution of the supraorbital or supratrochlear nerves.

The radiographic examination consists of axial and coronal CT scans.

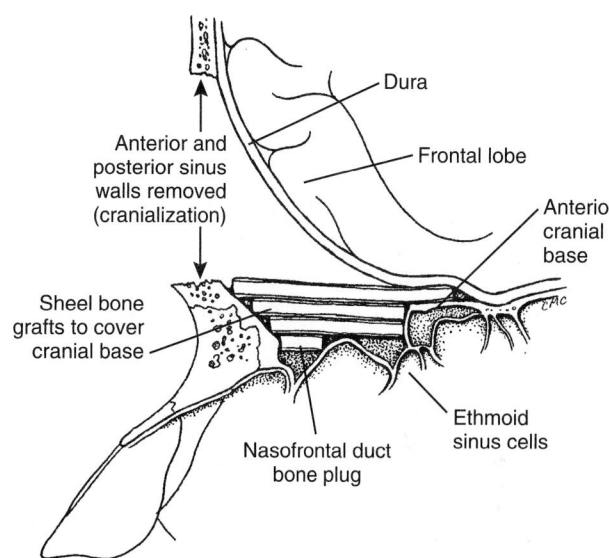

Figure 7 The procedure of cranialization of the frontal sinus involves removal of the posterior wall of the frontal sinus, removal of all of the mucosa, sealing the nasal frontal ducts with bone grafts, and bone grafting defects in the anterior cranial fossa (floor of the frontal sinus). The anterior wall of the sinus is then reconstructed either with the preserved fracture fragments of the anterior wall or with the bone grafts. Here, the sinus is being cranialized with the reconstruction of the anterior wall to follow.

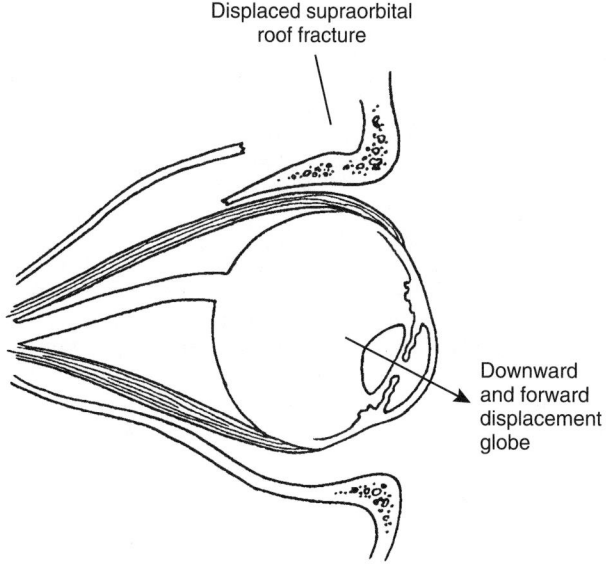

Figure 8 Displaced supraorbital fractures produce a downward deformity of the orbital roof. The globe is dislocated downward and forward producing exophthalmos; reduction of the fracture corrects the eye position.

Treatment

The treatment of displaced supraorbital fractures involves confirmation of the integrity of the dura and replacement of bone pieces into the proper position and direct stabilization by interosseous wiring or plate or screw fixation. Damaged segments of the orbital roof are replaced by repositioning or bone grafting. Frontal sinus involvement is frequent in supraorbital fractures and is managed as described. Exposure for operative reduction may occasionally be through a laceration but generally requires a coronal incision.

Fractures of the Orbit

Isolated fractures of the internal portion of the orbit are accompanied by globe injury in 10% of cases. The minimal visual screening examination consists of an assessment of visual acuity, confrontation fields, confirmation of the extent of extraocular motion, examination of the anterior and posterior chambers, and a determination of intraocular pressure. The pupillary size and reaction must be assessed and compared bilaterally. Subtle physical signs of an optic nerve injury are a sluggish pupil in reaction to bright light and reduced visual acuity.

Orbital Floor Fractures

The diagnosis of an orbital floor fracture is suggested by periorbital and subconjunctival hematomas. Anesthesia is invariably present in the infraorbital sensory nerve distribution, which produces cutaneous anesthesia of the ipsilateral nose, cheek, and upper lip and anesthesia of the anterior maxillary teeth. Diplopia is present on looking up or down by virtue of contusion or entrapment of the fascial system of the inferior rectus and inferior oblique muscles. Exophthalmos is often present initially, because of swelling, and is followed by enophthalmos when enlargement of the orbital cavity allows retrusion of the globe into the orbit as the swelling resolves. Inferior and medial displacement of the globe accompanies posterior displacement. Orbital emphysema and ipsilateral epistaxis are usually present. Topical anesthesia, instilled into the conjunctival sac, allows the performance of a forced-duction examination: the globe is manually rotated after grasping the insertion of the inferior rectus muscle through the conjunctiva with a forceps. More difficult rotation implies incarceration of the muscle or its ligament system, which would benefit from operative reduction.

The radiographic examination consists of axial and coronal CT scans with soft-tissue and bone windows.

The indications for surgery are enophthalmos, entrapment of a muscle (diagnosed by double vision in a field of gauze controlled by the muscle), forced-duction examination and CT confirmation, and vertical or anterior-posterior malposition of the globe. Anesthesia of the infraorbital nerve usually resolves without treatment. If massive destruction of an orbital floor is seen on CT scan, reconstruction of the orbit is indicated in the absence of globe malposition to prevent late globe malposition.

Treatment

Surgical treatment consists of an exploration through a lower eyelid incision (subciliary, midtarsal, or infraorbital rim) with a dissection of the orbital floor and removal of any incarcerated tissue from the maxillary sinus. The orbital floor is then reconstituted by alloplastic material (Silastic; Dow Corning, Midland, MI; Supramid; S. Jackson, Alexandria, VA; Medpor; Porex Surgical Products, Newnan, GA) or curved bone grafts harvested from the calvarium, rib, or iliac region. The calvarium is preferred because the head is a "self-contained reconstructive unit" (after Tessier).

Medial Orbital Wall Fractures

Medial orbital wall fractures are suggested by the presence of periorbital and subconjunctival hematoma, diplopia when looking laterally, orbital emphysema, epistaxis, enophthalmos, and medial displacement of the pupil. The radiographic examination consists of axial and coronal CT scans with both bone and soft-tissue windows.

The indications for surgery are radiographic entrapment of the medial rectus muscle with positive forced duction (medial-to-lateral rotation of the globe) and the presence of enophthalmos, either on physical examination or the prediction of such an occurrence on the basis of radiographic evidence of an extensive medial orbital wall fracture (Fig. 9).

Treatment

Surgical treatment is accomplished by a medial conjunctival or a coronal incision with removal of incarcerated tissue from the crushed ethmoid sinuses and reconstruction of the medial orbital wall with alloplastic material or bone grafts. Patients with orbital fractures should refrain from blowing their noses.

Le Fort (Maxillary) Fractures

Maxillary fractures are classified according to a pattern described by Rene Le Fort in 1901 (Fig. 10).

A Le Fort I fracture is a horizontal or transverse maxillary fracture separating the maxillary alveolus from the upper midfacial skeleton. A Le Fort II (pyramidal fracture) separates a central (pyramid-shaped) nasomaxillary segment from the zygomatic and orbital portions of the facial skeleton.

A Le Fort III fracture is a craniofacial dysjunction separating the facial bones from the cranial skeleton through the upper portion of the nose and the lateral and medial orbits. Most Le Fort II and III fractures are comminuted and consist of combinations of lesser Le Fort fragments such as simultaneous fractures at the Le Fort I, II and III levels. The injury is usually worse on one side than the other;

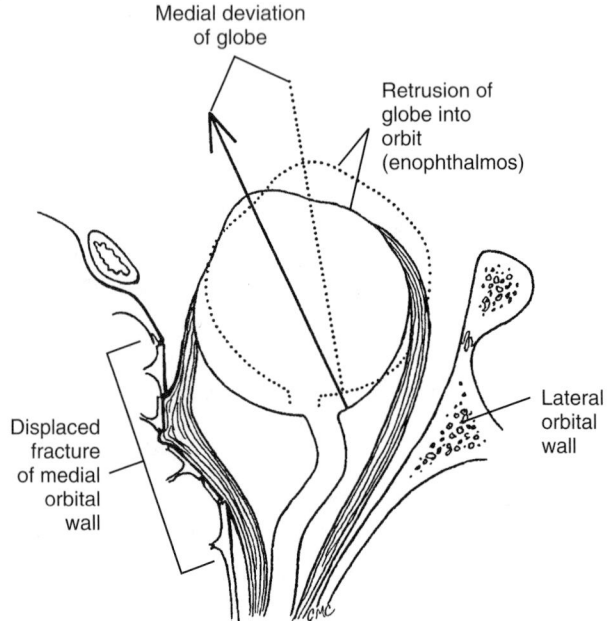

Figure 9 Displaced fractures of the medial orbital wall crush the ethmoid sinus and expand the orbital volume. The surgical treatment consists of inserting bone grafts to narrow the volume of the orbit. The soft tissue is removed from its prolapsed position into the fracture site.

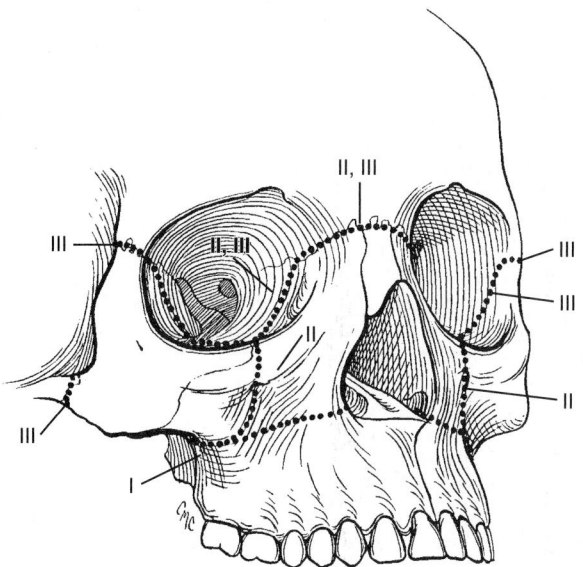

Figure 10 The Le Fort maxillary fracture classification. A Le Fort I fracture is a horizontal fracture separating the maxillary alveolus from the upper midfacial skeleton. The Le Fort II or pyramidal fracture separates a central, pyramid-shaped nasomaxillary segment from the upper midfacial skeleton. The Le Fort III fracture is a craniofacial disjunction where the midface is fractured through the upper portion of the orbits. Generally, Le Fort II and III fractures do not exist as single segments but display comminution.

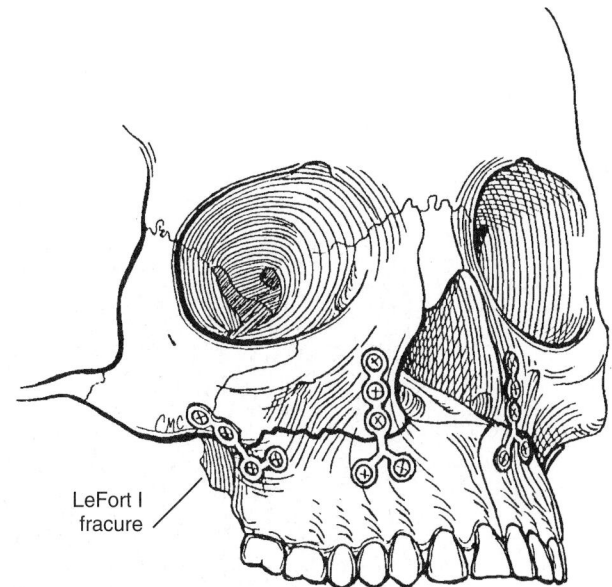

Figure 11 A Le Fort I fracture has been treated by plate and screw fixation at the four anterior buttresses of the maxilla at the Le Fort I level. The patient is initially placed in intermaxillary fixation. The fracture fragments are aligned and plate and screw fixation applied to stabilize the reduction. Postoperatively, the intermaxillary fixation can be released because of the stability of plate and screw fixation.

commonly, a Le Fort III superior-level fracture is seen on one side with a Le Fort II superior level fracture on the other. Single-fragment Le Fort III fractures are unusual and frequently are accompanied by bilateral eyelids hematomas, no maxillary mobility, and a slight malocclusion (1/2 cusp), reflecting the minimal displacement of the fracture. They are thus easily missed on physical examination. The presence of bilateral eyelid hematomas should always suggest the possibility of a Le Fort fracture. Also, if fluid is seen in both maxillary sinuses on CT scan, a Le Fort fracture should be suspected. The physical diagnosis of a Le Fort fracture rests on malocclusion and mobility of the maxillary alveolus in reference to the lower midfacial craniofacial skeleton. This mobility is confirmed by grasping the maxillary alveolus and testing for movement, holding the cranium stable with the contralateral hand. Upper Le Fort fractures possess signs of zygomatic, orbital, nasal, and nasoethmoidal fractures, depending on the level and extent of the injury. When Le Fort fractures are not treated, midfacial proportions change, and midfacial elongation and midfacial retrusion follow. Profuse nasopharyngeal bleeding initially accompanies Le Fort fractures; marked facial and eyelid swelling occur. CSF leak, pneumocephalus, and orbital emphysema occur less frequently in Le Fort II and III fractures, and 10% to 15% of Le Fort fractures are accompanied by palatal alveolar fractures that divide the maxillary alveolus in an anteroposterior plane ("sagittal fracture" of the maxilla), making treatment more complicated.

The radiographic examination consists of axial and coronal CT scans with bone and soft tissue windows.

Treatment

Treatment is accomplished by placing the patient in intermaxillary fixation in occlusion. Sagittal fractures of the maxilla are united by plate and screw fixation in the roof of the mouth and at the piriform aperture. The Le Fort I fracture is treated by plate and screw fixation at the four anterior buttresses of the maxilla (Fig. 11). Intermaxillary fixation may then be released postoperatively if rigid fixation has been employed. Otherwise, the patient is kept in intermaxillary fixation for a 6- to 8-week period to ensure bone healing.

The treatment of a Le Fort II fracture involves exposure through a lower eyelid incision (subciliary, midtarsal, or lower orbital rim), with a reduction of the orbital floor or medial orbital wall components of these fractures and open reduction of the central midface and nasoethmoidal area. A coronal incision may be required in upper Le Fort II fractures for an open reduction and internal fixation of the nasofrontal area. Upper Le Fort fractures are often accompanied by simultaneous fractures in the frontobasilar region.

Complex or Pan Facial Fractures

Pan facial fractures consist of combinations of frontal, midface, and mandibular fractures. The treatment consists of reconstructing the lower face as one unit and reconstructing the upper face as a separate unit, relating both units to the cranial base in their proper relationship. The "upper face" is then reconstructed to the "lower face" at the Le Fort I level. Both the horizontal and vertical portions of the mandible are stabilized with open reduction. The upper midface (consisting of the orbits and nasoethmoidal area) is stabilized to the frontal bone and cranial base and then linked to the stabilized lower face (mandible and Le Fort I segment) at the Le Fort I level. Previously, as an initial step, the maxilla is aligned with the mandible and the dental arches through intermaxillary fixation.

Mandibular Fractures

Mandibular fractures are one of the most common facial injuries. They are (in the horizontal mandible and the tooth-bearing area) usually compounded into the mouth. Less commonly, they are compounded through the skin. Fractured, loose, or broken teeth; bleeding from a tooth socket; and intraoral lacerations imply the presence of a mandible fracture. One third of mandibular fractures occur in the condylar-subcondylar area, one third occur in the region of the angle, and the other third occur in the body,

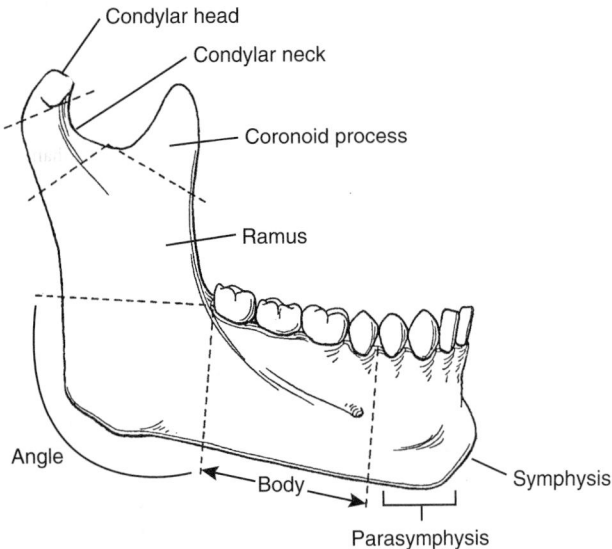

Condylar head
Condylar neck
Coronoid process
Ramus
Angle
Body
Parasymphysis
Symphysis

Figure 12 Anatomic region of the mandible includes the condylar and subcondylar areas, the angle, the body, and anteriorly the symphysis and parasymphysis areas. Weak areas are the subcondylar region, the angle (weakened by the third molar tooth), and the parasymphysis area (weakened by the long root of the cuspid tooth).

symphysis, and parasymphysis area (Fig. 12). These areas represent "weak" areas of the mandible. The angle is weakened by the presence of the third molar tooth and, anteriorly, the parasymphysis by the long root of the cuspid tooth and the mental foramen. The subcondylar area represents a thin region in the ramus. More than 50% of mandibular fractures are multiple. The presence of a single mandibular fracture therefore prompts a thorough search for a second or third fracture, often present contralaterally. Combinations such as parasymphysis and contralateral subcondylar, parasymphysis and contralateral angle, or symphysis with unilateral or bilateral subcondylar fractures are frequent. The diagnosis of a mandibular fracture is suggested by pain; swelling; abnormal occlusion; numbness in the distribution of the mental nerve (lower lip); swelling; bruises; extraoral or intraoral lacerations; bleeding from a tooth socket; fractured or missing teeth; trismus (pain on moving the jaw); inability to bring the teeth into occlusion (this may occur anteriorly, laterally, or bilaterally); abnormality or irregularity in dental arch form; or malocclusion of the teeth, steps, level discrepancies, or gaps detected either in the dentition or by palpating the mandible. Bleeding from the ear canal implies the possibility of a condylar fracture. In some cases, a segment of the dental alveolus is separated from the lower portion of the mandible and constitutes an alveolar fracture. Alveolar fractures may occur by themselves or in the presence of more extensive mandibular fractures. An unpleasant odor in the mouth is present soon after mandibular fractures occur.

The plain radiographic examination includes posteroanterior (PA), lateral oblique, and Towne plain films of the mandible. Seldom are plain x-rays taken, but a CT scan for the condylar, coronoid, and ramus areas and horizontal portion of the mandible is routine. The Panorex examination is the one helpful "plain film" and requires a cooperative patient able to stand. Often it cannot be obtained urgently. Occlusal and apical dental films are sometimes required to visualize specific areas of the teeth to examine for root fracture and apical or tooth root pathology.

Treatment

The treatment of mandibular fracture includes the application of arch bars to the teeth, placing the teeth of the mandible in intermaxillary fixation (IMF) in occlusion with the maxilla. IMF is continued for 4 to 8 weeks unless rigid internal fixation or the ability to spontaneously bring the jaws into proper occlusion permits immediate mobilization. Closed reduction is appropriate for many condylar, coronoid, and ramus fractures and those stable fractures in the angle that are not displaced. Displaced fractures in the horizontal mandible require open reduction with plate and screw fixation. Exposure is obtained intraorally. Intraoral exposure is preferred for the anterior portion of the horizontal segment of the mandible. Angle fractures may be treated intraorally if simple and extraorally if comminuted. Condylar and subcondylar fractures that require open reduction (those that would result in mechanical interference with mandibular motion or a loss of ramus height) are exposed with a preauricular, upper mesh, or intraoral ramus incision for fixation.

Patients requiring intermaxillary fixation are given a blenderized diet. The average patient with IMF loses 15 to 20 lb in 4 to 6 weeks.

The use of rigid internal fixation (plate and screw fixation) allows many patients to immediately move the mandible, to have better oral hygiene, and to take a soft diet. Occlusion must be observed at least weekly in these patients to detect any displacement.

GUNSHOT AND SHOTGUN WOUNDS

Gunshot wounds of low velocity may be managed as facial fractures with overlying lacerations. The soft-tissue injury is excised and closed. High-velocity gunshot or close-range shotgun wounds produce extensive soft-tissue and bone loss and damage. A zone of soft-tissue and bone loss and a separate zone of soft-tissue and bone injury are characterized. The bones present are immediately stabilized in anatomic position in all regions by rigid internal fixation. Areas of bone loss are stabilized, preserving the length-of-bone defects to achieve anatomic reconstruction of the bone fracture to normal dimensions. Soft-tissue closure is obtained either by advancement or skin-to-mucosa closure after conservative debridement. Serial, "second-look" procedures are required at 48-hour intervals until no further devitalized tissue is seen. Soft-tissue reconstruction may then be completed; usually, distant flap transfer is required for intraoral lining and sinus obliteration. At the time of flap transfer, composite replacement of bone and soft tissue may be considered, or soft-tissue reconstruction accomplished first and then bone reconstruction secondarily. The bone defects resulting from missing bone are maintained by rigid internal fixation until bone grafting can be performed.

LATE SCARRING FROM WOUNDS

Generally, it takes 1 to 2 years for a cutaneous scar to fully mature. A red, raised scar that is initially quite prominent and shows some soft-tissue contracture may resolve satisfactorily with time. Patients who understand the course of scar maturation can be patient through the healing process. Early scar revisions are not indicated unless there is malalignment of tissues or contracture of the type that causes functional problems such as ectropion and corneal exposure.

CONCLUSION

The face is of supreme importance in communication, nutrition, perception, and interpersonal relationships. The aesthetic attractiveness of an individual's facial features influences his or her personality and success. Although there are few facial emergencies, the literature has underemphasized the advantage of prompt, definitive reconstruction of facial injuries and the contribution of early anatomic skeletal reconstruction to superior aesthetic results. It is not unusual for a victim of a multiple injury to be principally concerned about residual facial deformity after life-threatening injuries have been resolved. The early definitive care of maxillofacial injuries is safe and possible and will repay the surgeon with superior results and grateful patients. A coordinated reconstruction is accomplished by interspecialty communication. All patients require counseling and rehabilitation, and psychologic dividends result from these efforts.

Suggested Readings

Clark N, Manson P: Complication in maxillofacial trauma. In Maull KI, Rodriguez A, Wiles CIII, editors: *Complications in trauma and critical care*, Philadelphia, 1996, WB Saunders.

David DJ, Simpson DA: *Craniomaxillofacial trauma*, New York, 1995, Churchill Livingstone.

Dufresne C, Manson P: Facial injuries in children (Chap 67, p. 381). In Mathes S, editor: *Plastic surgery*, vol 3, Part 2, New York, 2005, Elsevier,

Fonseca R, Walker R: *Oral and maxillofacial trauma*, Philadelphia, 1991, WB Saunders.

Manson P: Facial injuries (Chap 66, p. 77). In Mathes S, editor: *Plastic surgery*, vol. 3, Part 2, New York, 2005, Elsevier.

Manson P, Vander Kolk C, Dufresne C: Facial trauma. In Oldham K, Columbani P, Foglia R, editors: *Surgery of infants and children*, Philadelphia, 2005, Lippincott-Raven.

Manson PN: Reoperative facial fracture surgery. In Grotting J, editor: *Reoperative plastic surgery*. St Louis, 2006, Quality Medical Publishing.

Mueller RV: Soft tissue injuries (Chap 64, p. 1). In Mathes S, editor: *Plastic surgery*, Vol 3, Part 2, New York, 2005, Elsevier.

Williams JL, editor: *Rowe and Williams maxillofacial injuries*, Edinburgh, 1994, Churchill Livingstone.

Wolf A, Baker SA: *Facial fractures*, New York, 1993, Thieme.

Penetrating Neck Trauma

Carrie A. Sims, MD, and Patrick M. Reilly, MD

Penetrating neck trauma occurs in approximately 5% to 10% of all traumatic injuries. The lethality of the neck injury is directly related to the trajectory and energy transferred, with fatality rates ranging from 1% to 2% for stab wounds and up to 50% for rifle or shotgun blasts. Most injuries seen in the civilian sector are the result of stab wounds. Whereas at first glance these wounds may appear to be innocuous lacerations, they have potential to cause major damage if the platysma has been violated. Gunshot wounds are associated with more significant damage because of their higher kinetic energy. Weapons typically seen in civilian trauma use low-velocity missiles and tend to cause less severe damage than those seen in combat or hunting accidents.

Surprisingly, approximately 40% of all penetrating neck wounds do not result in injury to any major structure. When injury does occur, major venous injuries are more common than major arterial injuries. The pharynx or esophagus is injured in 5% to 15% of cases. Laryngotracheal injury occurs in 4% to 12% of cases. Although spinal cord injury is a relatively infrequent occurrence, gunshot wounds are associated with a 10% to 15% incidence of cord injury, making patients with this injury complex more vulnerable to cervical spine instability and neurogenic shock.

The treatment of penetrating neck injury was described as early as 1522, when Ambrose Pare ligated both carotids and an internal jugular vein in a wounded soldier. In 1956, Fogelman and Stewart demonstrated a significant improvement in mortality when penetrating neck injuries underwent prompt surgical exploration (6% vs. 35%). Their report of significant improvement in mortality ushered in the era of mandatory surgical exploration of all penetrating neck wounds. Mandatory exploration, however, is associated with a negative exploration rate that has been reported as high as 67% in some series. With improved radiographic imaging and endoscopy, a more selective approach to the management of penetrating neck injuries emerged in the 1980s. Proponents of selective management recommended evaluating stable penetrating neck injuries with angiography, radiologic studies, and endoscopy. If these techniques revealed an injury amenable to surgical repair, the patient

was explored. Using this selective approach, the incidence of negative neck explorations was reduced to 20%, with a negligible incidence of missed injury. More recently there has been a trend toward increased reliance on physical examination alone to make clinical management decisions regarding vascular injuries. Several studies have suggested that the absence of vascular hard signs can reliably exclude the presence of a major vascular injury. This approach, however, is not universally accepted and should be used with some degree of caution.

ANATOMY

The relatively unprotected neck accommodates vital vascular, aerodigestive, and nerve structures in a compact area. The neck is divided into separate compartments by major fascial planes. The superficial fascial plane lies just beneath the skin and encompasses the platysma. Underlying the platysma is the deep cervical fascia that is further subdivided into the investing, pretracheal, and prevertebral layers. The deep cervical fascial plane extends from the skull base deep into the mediastinum and provides a potential tract for infection. Hematomas developing within these tight fascial compartments can rapidly compress the airway and other vital structures with minimal external signs of hemorrhage.

Roan and Christensen described the neck as being divided into three anatomic zones (Fig. 1). Although the traditional landmarks used to demarcate these zones are anterior structures, the neck is a cylindric structure and the zones circumferentially include the anterior, lateral, and posterior neck. Moreover, depending on trajectory, an injury in one zone may easily traverse into another zone. Zone I is often referred to as the *thoracic outlet* and extends from the clavicles to the cricoid cartilage. Zone II extends from the cricoid cartilage to the angle of the mandible. This large, relatively exposed area includes the carotid arteries, jugular veins, vertebral vessels, larynx, trachea, esophagus, vagus nerves, recurrent laryngeal nerves, and spinal cord. Zone III includes a small area from the angle of the mandible to the base of the skull and is exceptionally difficult to access surgically.

DIAGNOSTIC EVALUATION

Physical Examination

A rapid and thorough physical examination should be performed, with particular attention paid to the airway (Table 1). Determining

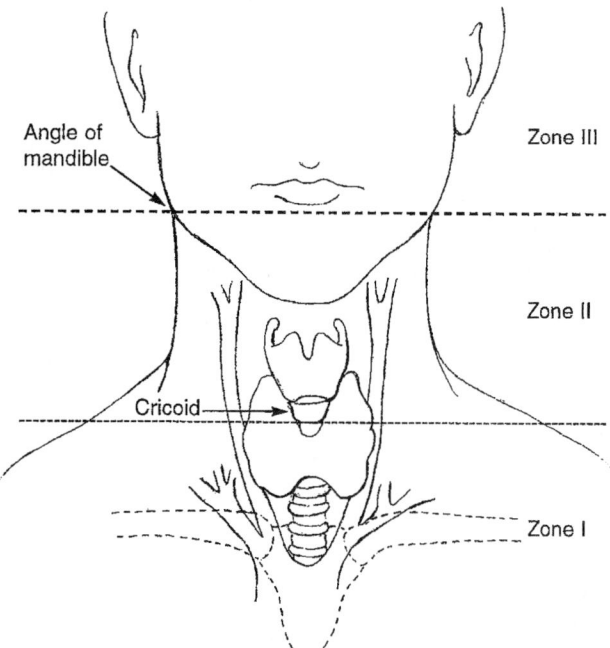

Figure 1 Zones of the neck. *From Maxwell RA. In Peitzman AB, Rhodes M, Schwab CW, and others, editors: The trauma manual, ed 2, Philadelphia, 2002, Lippincott Williams and Wilkins, with permission.*

Table 1: Clinical Signs and Symptoms of Surgically Significant Injury to the Neck

Respiratory	Vascular	Digestive
Tenderness in trachea, cricothyroid cartilage	Pulsatile or expanding hematoma	Hematemesis
Hoarseness	Absence or loss of pulses	Odynophagia
Hemoptysis	Active hemorrhage	Dysphagia
Dysphonia	Hemodynamic instability	Subcutaneous emphysema
Significant subcutaneous emphysema	Bruit Global neurologic deficit	Tracheal deviation
Acute airway obstruction		

whether or not the patient requires intubation to secure the airway is critical and should be established expeditiously during the initial assessment.

Physical examination of the injured neck is often deceptively benign despite underlying injuries to major vessels or the aerodigestive track. Physical findings that suggest a major vascular injury include active bleeding; a large, pulsatile or expanding hematoma; a bruit or thrill; or the presence of a central neurologic deficit. Any of these "hard" signs mandates vascular exploration. Patients with laryngeal trauma may complain of shortness of breath, tenderness, or changes in the quality of the voice. Injury to the aerodigestive tract can manifest itself as odynophagia, subcutaneous emphysema, air bubbling from the wound, hemoptysis, dyspnea,

stridor, or hoarseness. Esophageal perforations, however, may be difficult to appreciate initially. Most patients have no signs or symptoms suggestive of esophageal trauma on arrival at the hospital. If signs or symptoms are present, subcutaneous emphysema (19%) and dysphagia (7%) are most common.

A detailed neurologic examination should include an evaluation of the patient's mental status, cranial nerves, spinal cord, brachial plexus, and sympathetic nerves. If the patient requires emergent intubation, an abbreviated neurologic examination should be performed and gross motor function should be documented before medications are given.

Radiographic Imaging and Endoscopy

Chest and cervical radiographs and a single anteroposterior (AP) skull/head radiograph aid in the initial evaluation. Radiopaque markers (e.g., paperclips) placed over the wounds can assist in determining trajectory. Radiographic evidence of underlying injury may include the presence of a pneumothorax, pneumomediastinum, subcutaneous emphysema, retropharyngeal air, cervical spine fracture, tracheal deviation, or an apical cap. In stable patients, a CT scan of the neck may provide a three-dimensional determination of missile trajectory and its proximity to vital structures. The addition of intravenous contrast (CT angiogram) may further increase the positive predictive value (75%-93%) and negative predictive value (near 100%). Still, the routine use of CT is controversial, with concern that small esophageal injuries from stab wounds may not be appreciated.

Arteriography remains the gold standard for evaluating potential vascular injuries in the neck. This modality also allows for potential therapies such as embolization, balloon occlusion, and stent placement, especially in areas that are difficult to surgically access, expose, or repair. Duplex ultrasonography may provide a noninvasive diagnostic alternative to arteriography, with a reported 90% to 100% sensitivity and 85% to 100% specificity. The bony structures in zone I and zone III obscure sonographic visualization, however, limiting this modality to injuries in zone II.

Radiographic evaluation of the cervical esophagus is best performed using barium contrast esophagography. The reported sensitivity of esophagography ranges from 47% to 93%. The combination of esophagography and rigid esophagoscopy may increase the sensitivity to near 100%. With improved fiber-optic technology, flexible esophagoscopy has essentially usurped the role of rigid esophagoscopy. Flexible endoscopy can be used to evaluate the cervical aerodigestive track. Laryngoscopy, esophagoscopy, and bronchoscopy may be used either individually or in conjunction with radiographic contrast studies. In general, the possibility of a vascular injury should be explored before any endoscopic procedure is conducted. If endoscopy is performed using topical anesthesia, gagging and retching may restart bleeding from an unappreciated vascular injury.

INITIAL MANAGEMENT

General Considerations

The most pressing concern in the management of penetrating neck trauma is to ensure a secure airway. Injury to the larynx or trachea can result in blood pooling and airway obstruction. Maintaining the patient in an upright, slightly forward position, with suction readily available, may avoid a precipitous airway obstruction. Bleeding should be initially controlled with direct pressure. Intraoral bleeding can be more difficult to manage. Intraoral gauze packing can be attempted if the patient is intubated and sedated. Maneuvers that may induce retching or gagging (e.g., nasogastric

[NG] tube placement, intraoral packing) should be strictly avoided in the conscious, nonintubated patient to avoid disrupting any tamponade. Similarly, local exploration or probing of the wound should be avoided. Large hematomas may distort and compress the airway, making intubation potentially difficult. If endotracheal intubation is necessary, the surgeon must be prepared to provide an immediate surgical airway and control any ensuing hemorrhage. Routine cervical immobilization is unnecessary and potentially harmful following penetrating neck trauma. There is an extremely low likelihood of an unstable spine fracture in a fully awake patient with no spinal tenderness and a normal neurologic examination. The cervical collar prevents serial wound evaluation. In patients who are unexaminable following gunshot injuries to the neck, there is a small (<1%) risk of missing a cervical spine injury.

Unstable Patients

Massive hemorrhage from a major vascular injury can lead to profound hypotension. Hemodynamic instability can also result from the inability to ventilate the patient because of airway disruption or tension pneumothorax. Unstable patients require immediate intubation and operative exploration. Because the exact location and extent of underlying injuries may not be clear, the patient's neck and chest should be prepared and draped widely. Although the wound location may provide an educated guess regarding the initial operative exposure, the surgeon should be prepared to make another incision after the actual injuries are found (Fig. 2).

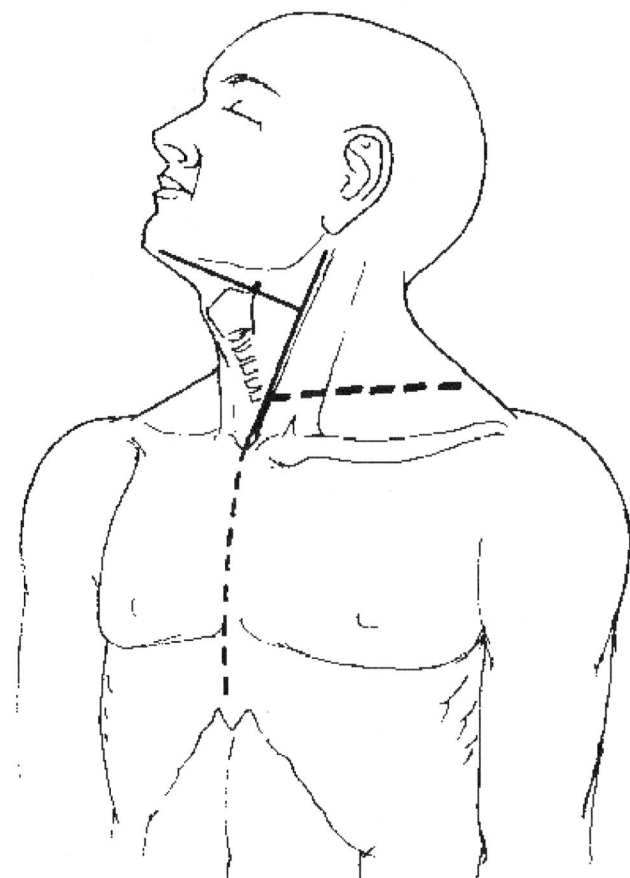

Figure 2 Neck incisions. *From Robbs JV, Keenan J: Exploration of the neck. In Rob and Smith's operative surgery: trauma surgery, pt 1, Boston, 1989, Butterworth, with permission.*

Stable Patient: Zone II

Stable patients with penetrating zone II injuries and hard signs of vascular injury should undergo immediate operative exploration. Similarly, evidence of obvious laryngotracheal injury warrants immediate surgical exploration. An incision along the anterior border of the sternocleidomastoid provides excellent exposure of the major vessels, trachea, and esophagus.

Stable patients with platysma penetration who do not have hard signs of vascular or aerodigestive injury may be safely managed in a number of ways, depending on the institutional resources available. Surgical exploration remains the safest approach if access to diagnostic imaging or endoscopy is limited. Selective nonoperative management algorithms rely on diagnostic studies to reliably rule out vascular, laryngotracheal, and esophageal injuries. The use of CT imaging, especially with gunshot wounds, may accurately determine trajectory and further direct or eliminate additional management. Although a growing body of literature suggests that the absence of hard signs effectively rules out the presence of a major vascular injury, many centers still obtain routine arteriography, especially in the setting of gunshot wounds. Simple, nonoperative observation without imaging may be acceptable, provided that the patient can be closely followed and emergently treated.

Nonoperative evaluation of the pharynx, larynx, and trachea can be performed using direct laryngoscopy and flexible bronchoscopy. It is unusual for airway injuries to occur in the absence of clinical or radiographic evidence of air leak. Esophageal injury should be investigated routinely following zone II injuries because patients with these injuries may not show early signs or symptoms. Because esophageal injuries carry such a high morbidity and mortality, any diagnostic workup should be pursued expeditiously.

Stable Patient: Zones I and III

Although there are a few studies that have examined the reliability of physical examination to rule out vascular injury in zones I and III, most agree that stable patients with injuries that penetrate the platysma in these areas should routinely undergo arteriography. These zones are fairly inaccessible, and injuries can be hidden within the thorax or near the base of the skull. Manifestations of vascular injury in these areas may be difficult to identify clinically. Even if the physical examination suggests vascular injury, arteriography can be used to localize the injury and potentially treat it endoluminally. Knowing the location of the injury can also assist in planning the most appropriate incision for exposure and control. With zone I injuries, esophagography or esophagoscopy should be routinely considered to evaluate the thoracic esophagus. CT imaging can aid in determining trajectory and further direct management.

OPERATIVE MANAGEMENT

Exposure: Zone I

Preoperative arteriography and diagnostic studies can help the surgeon to plan the most appropriate incision. A median sternotomy affords the most versatile exposure in the unstable patient with a zone I injury. A neck extension along the sternocleidomastoid or laterally under the clavicle on either side can provide exposure to most major vessels of the neck and upper chest. Exposure of the proximal left subclavian and descending aorta, however, may require a left clavicular incision and a counterincision along the third intercostal space to create a "trapdoor" exposure (see Fig. 2). The thoracic esophagus and distal trachea can be exposed and examined via these incisions.

In stable patients with preoperative diagnostic studies, the incision can be tailored to the identified injuries. The right subclavian artery, the subclavian veins, and distal left subclavian artery can be approached through a clavicular incision with or without resecting the medial clavicular head. The origins of the right subclavian, innominate, and proximal left carotid arteries are best exposed through a median sternotomy. A clavicular incision can be added for further exposure. Exposure of the proximal left subclavian artery can be challenging and is best accomplished through a left anterolateral thoracotomy.

Exposure: Zone II

Injuries in zone II can be easily exposed by extending the neck and rotating it away from the injury. Care should be taken during preparation to avoid rubbing the neck vigorously because this action may dislodge a clot. An incision is made anterior to the sternocleidomastoid. Visualization of the hypopharynx can be facilitated by retracting the omohyoid muscle anteriorly and the vessels posteriorly. The placement of an NG tube may facilitate esophageal exposure. During surgical exploration, an esophageal injury may be appreciated by insufflating air during esophagoscopy or by direct instillation of air via an NG tube. A collar incision 1 to 2 cm above the clavicular heads can be used to expose combined tracheal-esophageal injuries or in the setting of bilateral injuries. If necessary, an incision along the contralateral sternocleidomastoid can be created if further exposure is deemed necessary.

Exposure: Zone III

Zone III injuries are notoriously difficult to expose. The initial exposure is identical to that of zone II injuries. Improved exposure can be accomplished by dividing the omohyoid and digastric muscles, detaching the sternocleidomastoid from its skull base attachments, subluxing the mandible anteriorly, or by creating a vertical osteotomy of the mandibular ramus. The hypoglossal nerve crosses the internal and external carotid arteries approximately 1.5 to 3 cm cephalad to the bifurcation and should be preserved. Similarly, the spinal accessory nerve can be easily damaged during this exposure. This nerve can be identified as it enters the sternocleidomastoid 3 to 4 cm below the mastoid process.

▌ SPECIFIC INJURIES

Vascular Injury

The carotid artery should be repaired unless the vessel is completely occluded. Because of the theoretic concern for reperfusion injury, it was recommended in the past that patients in coma should undergo ligation rather than repair. The current consensus, however, is to repair the injury regardless of neurologic status if there is flow because it will result in overall improved morbidity and mortality. Proximal and distal control of the common, internal, and external carotid arteries should be accomplished before a repair is attempted. Distal control can be accomplished with a Fogarty catheter. Unless otherwise contraindicated, systemic heparinization should be considered. If backbleeding is poor, shunting may be advisable. A primary repair should be attempted when possible. For circumferential injuries, a primary end-to-end repair can be performed. The external carotid artery may be ligated and used as an in-continuity bypass graft for proximal internal carotid injuries. If an interposition graft is necessary, the saphenous vein is the preferred conduit. Although prosthetic grafts are a suitable alternative, especially in unstable patients, their use is associated with an increased risk of postoperative stroke. Although an extracranial-intracranial bypass from the carotid to the middle cerebral artery has been described for severe, distal, internal carotid injuries, this is rarely performed. Ligation of the external carotid artery may be performed with minimal concern.

Whenever possible, internal jugular vein injuries should be repaired. If a lateral venorrhaphy or end-to-end anastomosis cannot be performed easily or the patient is unstable, the internal jugular vein may be ligated unilaterally with little risk of morbidity. Bilateral internal jugular ligation, however, should be avoided.

Injury to the subclavian, common carotid, or innominate arteries should be repaired primarily. If necessary, these arteries may be bypassed with prosthetic grafts. In desperate situations, the injured subclavian artery may be ligated distal to the takeoff of the vertebral artery. The subclavian artery has a rich collateral circulation, and arm ischemia is a rare occurrence. If arm ischemia does develop, the stabilized patient can undergo an elective direct repair or a carotid-to-subclavian bypass. The subclavian vein can be ligated with little risk of morbidity.

The vertebral arteries are rarely injured as the result of penetrating neck trauma because they are enclosed within the cervical spine. The vertebral arteries can be ligated at the subclavian artery origin and via the C1-C2 vertebral interspace. Surgical access within the cervical spinal column is extremely difficult and should not be attempted. If active bleeding is encountered during the neck exploration, the vessel should be clipped or packed, and immediate arteriographic embolization performed.

Aerodigestive Tract Injury

Small, hypopharyngeal injuries can be managed nonoperatively with close observation, parenteral antibiotics, and cessation of oral intake. Shotgun and high-velocity gunshot wounds may result in larger defects that require extensive reconstruction.

Full-thickness esophageal injuries should be debrided and closed using a two-layer technique. If it is difficult to visualize the edges of the mucosal defect, a Foley catheter can be inserted through the injury into the pharynx. The balloon is then inflated and pulled back gently to bring the mucosal edges into view. The esophageal repair should be buttressed with a local muscle flap, such as the omohyoid, and the area should be drained. If there is a concurrent vascular repair, drainage of the neck should be established via the contralateral neck. With destructive esophageal injuries, primary repair may not be possible and a diverting cervical esophagostomy and esophageal exclusion procedure should be performed. In this situation, a draining gastrostomy and feeding jejunostomy should also be placed. Delayed diagnosis and treatment of esophageal injuries significantly increase the patient's morbidity and mortality. Contaminated tissues should be debrided and widely drained. It is imperative to ensure that any contamination has not entered the mediastinum. Mediastinitis carries an extremely high mortality and requires wide debridement and drainage via a thoracotomy. Following an esophageal repair, a barium swallow should be performed 5 to 7 days postoperatively before oral feedings are resumed.

Laryngotracheal Injury

Simple injuries to the trachea can be repaired with a single layer of interrupted absorbable suture. If resection is necessary, the anterior trachea can be mobilized for additional length, provided that the lateral blood supply is not disrupted. Following tracheal repair, the best results are obtained if a tracheostomy is avoided and the patient is immediately extubated. If a tracheostomy is necessary, it should be performed at least one tracheal ring distal to the injury. With combined tracheal-esophageal injuries, a well-vascularized muscle pedicle (e.g., intercostal or sternocleidomastoid) should be mobilized and placed between the two suture lines to decrease the risk of fistula formation. A tracheostomy is generally performed in the setting of laryngeal injury repairs.

Thoracic Duct Injury

Injuries in zones I and II can occasionally result in thoracic duct injury. A missed thoracic duct injury can cause persistent drainage and chylothorax, but if the injury is noticed at the time of exploration, simple ligation of the injured duct is sufficient. If diagnosed after the formation of a chylothorax, a tube thoracotomy should be placed and the patient should be started on a low-fat diet or total parenteral nutrition. If conservative management fails, the duct may require surgical ligation or embolization.

SUGGESTED READINGS

Asensio JA, Chahwan S, Forno W, and others: Penetrating esophageal injuries: multicenter study of the American Association for the Surgery of Trauma, *J Trauma* 50:289, 2001.

Barkana Y, Stein M, Scope AM, and others: Prehospital stabilization of the cervical spine for penetrating injuries of the neck—is it necessary? *Injury* 31:305, 2000.

Gracias VH, Reilly PM, Philpott J, and others: Computed tomography in the evaluation of penetrating neck trauma, *Arch Surg* 136:1231, 2001.

Nason RW, Assuras GN, Gray PR, and others: Penetrating neck injuries: analysis of experience from a Canadian trauma centre, *Can J Surg* 44:122, 2001.

Woo K, Magner DP, Wilson MT, and others: CT angiography in penetrating neck trauma reduces the need for operative neck exploration, *Am Surg* 71:754, 2005.

BLUNT CARDIAC INJURY

Elliott R. Haut, MD

Blunt cardiac injury (BCI) encompasses a wide range of pathology. The continuum spreads from patients with blunt cardiac rupture and immediate death to patients who are asymptomatic with only myocardial bruising. This disease entity has been simplified considerably by emphasizing only clinically significant cardiac injury. BCI is diagnosed in trauma patients with (1) hypotension in the absence of bleeding and neurogenic cause, (2) cardiac arrhythmias, (3) depressed cardiac index (< 2.5 L/min/m^2), or (4) anatomic abnormalities diagnosed on echocardiography.

The definitions of blunt cardiac injury have changed dramatically. Older terminologies such as *blunt cardiac trauma* and *myocardial* (or *cardiac*) *contusion* or *concussion* should no longer be used. The commonly accepted current classification scheme defines the injury on the basis of anatomic defects or physiologic derangements. The suggested categories include BCI with (1) septal rupture, (2) free wall rupture, (3) coronary artery thrombosis, (4) cardiac failure, (5) minor electrocardiogram (ECG) cardiac enzyme abnormality, or (6) complex arrhythmia.

INCIDENCE

The true incidence of blunt cardiac injury is difficult to discern. Rates ranging from as low as 10% to as high as 76% have been reported. This wide variety depends largely on the population studied. If only patients who survive to reach the hospital are examined, the incidence will be relatively low. To get the correct rate, all trauma patients must be considered because many patients with BCI die at the scene from either their cardiac injury or other injuries associated with massive blunt force trauma.

MECHANISM AND PATTERNS OF INJURY

Mechanism of injury from blunt cardiac injury usually involves high-energy blunt trauma. The most common mechanism is motor vehicle collision. Other blunt mechanisms include falls,

pedestrians struck by vehicles, assaults, blast injuries, and sports-related trauma. Anatomic injuries to the heart are caused by direct precordial impact, thoracic crush injury, deceleration or torsion causing the heart to tear, or hydraulic effects when abdominal compression leads to a large amount of fluid being returned to the right heart quickly and causing cardiac rupture resulting from rapidly elevated intracardiac pressure. Blunt trauma mechanisms can also cause penetrating cardiac trauma from fractured ribs or the sternum. As expected, patients with high-energy mechanisms have other significant associated injuries. At least three quarters of patients with BCI have other associated thoracic injuries (Table 1). Commonly associated extrathoracic injuries are seen involving the head, extremities, abdomen, and spine (see Table 1).

The right heart is the anatomic region most commonly injured in BCI because of its location directly behind the sternum. Rates of specific anatomic abnormalities reported also depend on the patient population studied (Table 2).

Table 1: Incidence of Associated Injuries in Patients with Blunt Cardiac Injury

Associated Injuries	Incidence of Findings in Patients with BCI (%)
Thoracic injury	
Chest pain	18–92
Rib fracture	18–69
Aortic or great vessel injury	20–40
Hemothorax	7–64
Pulmonary contusion	6–58
Pneumothorax	7–40
Flail chest	4–38
Sternal fracture	0–60
Head injury	20–73
Extremity injury	20–66
Abdominal solid organ injury	5–43
Spinal injury	10–20

BCI, Blunt cardiac injury.
Reprinted with permission from Schultz JM, Trunkey DD: Crit Care Clin *20(1):57, 2004.*

Table 2: Pattern of Blunt Cardiac Injuries in Reported Autopsy Series and Clinical Series

Cardiac Injury	Incidence of Injury in Autopsy Series of Patients with BCIs (%)	Incidence of Injury in Clinical Series of Patients with BCIs (%)
Myocardial contusion	60–100	60–100
Chamber rupture	—	—
Right ventricle	19–32	17–32
Right atrium	10–15	8–65
Left ventricle	5–44	8–15
Left atrium	1–7	0–31
Atrial septa defect	7	Case reports
Valve injury	5	Case reports
Ventricular septal defect	4	Case reports
Coronary artery injury	3	Case reports

BCI, Blunt cardiac injury.
Reprinted with permission from Schultz JM, Trunkey DD: Crit Care Clin 20(1):57, 2004.

In clinical studies of trauma patients brought to the hospital alive, patients with myocardial contusion alone predominate. In autopsy studies, more significant anatomic findings (i.e., chamber rupture, septal perforation, valve injury) are reported. At least 20% of patients with BCI have multiple anatomic injuries in the heart.

CLINICAL PRESENTATION

Accurate, early diagnosis of BCI is essential to treat patients effectively. Making the diagnosis always begins with having a high index of suspicion for BCI. Mechanism of injury should alert the physician. Specific patient complaints, findings on physical examination, and other associated injuries also prompt the consideration of BCI. Many tests are available to the clinician to help with this diagnosis; the most important decision is determining which tests to perform and in which order to perform them. There is no one definitive "gold standard" test to confirm or rule out BCI. Patients often are evaluated with a number of tests, and test outcomes are considered together.

Chest pain is a common finding in patients with BCI. However, it is often difficult to differentiate the chest pain from BCI from musculoskeletal thoracic trauma (i.e., sternum or rib fractures). Directed physical examination should be performed in which the physician looks for the commonly described physical findings of cardiac tamponade such as Beck's Triad (hypotension, muffled heart sounds, and elevated venous pressure/distended neck veins). However, distant heart sounds, extra heart sounds (e.g., S3), cardiac rubs, or murmurs are often quite difficult to discern in the loud and busy trauma resuscitation bay. Jugular venous distention may not be seen because of associated blood loss from other injuries.

The majority of patients with BCI are asymptomatic and fall into the category with only ECG or cardiac enzyme abnormalities. Alive patients with the other types of BCI are relatively rare and usually have signs and symptoms of shock. BCI must be included in the list of differential diagnoses of posttraumatic shock only after hemorrhagic shock from acute bleeding has been ruled out. Even

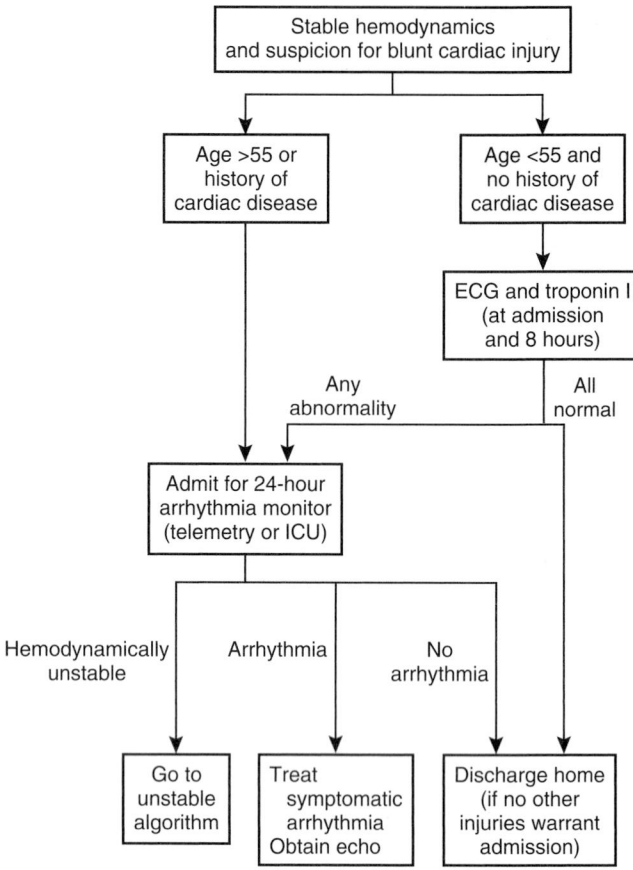

Figure 1 Algorithm for evaluation and management of hemodynamically stable patient with suspected blunt cardiac injury. ECG, *Electrocardiogram;* ICU, *intensive care unit.*

the rare case of neurogenic shock after spinal cord injury is more prevalent than shock from BCI.

All patients in whom BCI is considered should have an initial 12-lead ECG (Fig. 1) ECG is helpful in diagnosis of BCI but is neither sensitive nor specific. The major difficulty with using ECG for evaluation of BCI is that there are no classic or prototypical ECG findings. The most common ECG finding in patients with BCI is sinus tachycardia (which also has many other causes in trauma patients, such as bleeding and pain). Premature atrial or ventricular contractions are next on the list of most common arrhythmias found. Other abnormalities include nonspecific T wave changes, atrial fibrillation, atrial flutter, ST elevation or depression, conduction delays, ventricular dysrhythmias, and presence of Q waves. A normal ECG alone rules out clinically significant BCI and completes the workup in most patient populations. However, there are reported cases of delayed presentation of BCI up to 24 hours after injury. Patients at risk for BCI who are older than 55 years of age or have a history of cardiac disease should be admitted for continuous cardiac monitoring, even if they have a normal initial ECG (Fig. 1).

The role of cardiac enzymes in the diagnosis of blunt cardiac injury has changed significantly over the years. Historically, creatinine kinase (CK) with Mb fraction was the only serum biomarker available for evaluation of patients thought to be at risk for BCI. Most early studies performed using these serum markers to diagnose BCI suggested that there is no role or benefit of CK-Mb testing because of the lack of sensitivity and specificity. CK is found in other muscle sources injured in trauma. Guidelines from the Eastern Association of the Surgery for Trauma (EAST) for screening of BCI propose that CK and CK-Mb isoenzyme testing is not "useful in predicting which patients have or will have complications related to BCI."

Figure 2 Algorithm for evaluation and management of hemodynamically unstable patient with suspected blunt cardiac injury. *ASAP,* As soon as possible; *IABP,* intra-aortic balloon pump; *ICU,* intensive care unit; *PA,* pulmonary artery; *TTE/TEE,* transthoracic echocardiogram/transesophageal echocardiogram.

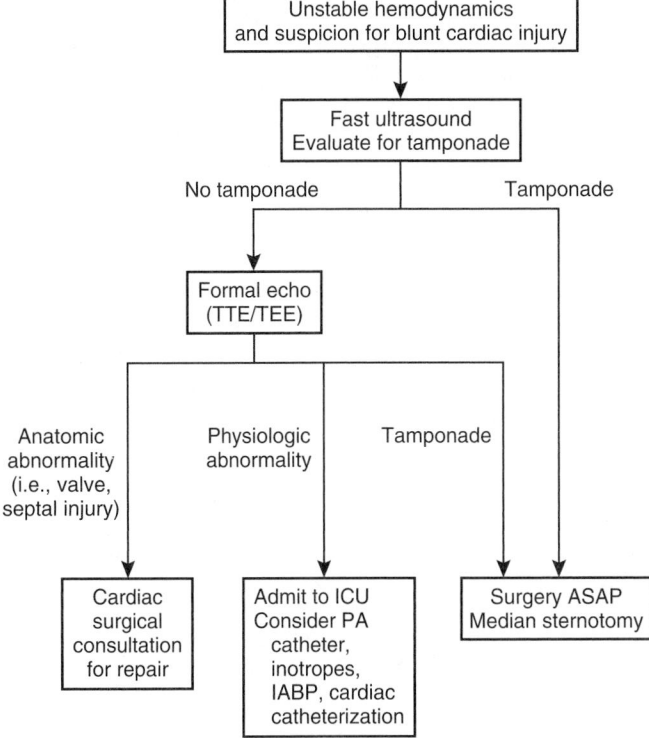

The introduction of newer cardiac specific enzymes such as cardiac troponin I has changed the role of serum markers in diagnosing BCI. The EAST guidelines (published in 1998) summarized the early studies of cardiac troponin I and concluded that it was no better than CK-Mb testing. More recently, however, multiple studies have shown that cardiac troponin I testing may have some benefit in diagnosing (and, more importantly, ruling out) BCI, especially when combined with ECG testing. Velmahos and colleagues have shown that the combination of a normal ECG and cardiac troponin I (at admission and repeated after 8 hours) has a 100% negative predictive value and rules out the diagnosis of significant BCI. Unless there are other reasons for admission, these patients can be safely discharged to home (see Fig. 1).

In hemodynamically unstable patients at risk for BCI, early echocardiography should be performed to rapidly evaluate cardiac function (Fig. 2). Clearly defining pericardial tamponade, valvular lesions, and wall-motion abnormalities will guide the clinician down an appropriate path of therapy. This is most expeditiously accomplished with bedside focused assessment for the sonographic evaluation of the trauma patient (FAST). This provider-performed ultrasound is commonly used by surgeons and emergency physicians in the early evaluation of trauma patients. FAST does not evaluate cardiac function, but it is highly sensitive and specific for diagnosing pericardial tamponade. Formal echocardiography, either transthoracic (TTE) or transesophageal (TEE), gives significantly more information than the FAST examination. Specific anatomic injuries or functional abnormalities can be more clearly identified. Noninvasive TTE is the initial test of choice. However, other chest injuries, pneumothorax with subcutaneous emphysema, pleural tubes, body habitus, and pain are significant barriers to its successful completion in the trauma patient. Studies have shown that nearly 20% of TTEs after trauma are nondiagnostic or suboptimal. In these cases, TEE may be necessary, even with its obvious drawbacks, including necessary sedation and possible intubation. TEE has higher sensitivity and specificity for BCI and is superior at identifying wall-motion abnormalities, septal and valvular lesions, and cardiac performance. TEE also gives the added benefit of examining the thoracic aorta to help diagnose (or rule out) cases of blunt aortic injury.

The advent of better echocardiographic imaging has made other diagnostic tools that were used in the past nearly obsolete. Nuclear medicine studies such as radionucleotide ventriculography, single photon emission computed tomography, and multigated acquisition are now rarely indicated. Pericardiocentesis had been the mainstay for diagnosis of pericardial tamponade; however, this has also fallen out of favor with the ready availability of echocardiography.

TREATMENT

Management of patients with BCI is dictated by specific patient symptoms. For patients with BCI and only minor ECG or cardiac enzyme abnormalities, "watchful waiting" in a monitored setting is the best approach. As long as these patients are closely observed in a monitored setting, these abnormalities usually resolve on their own within a 24-hour period. In patients with BCI and a complex arrhythmia, antiarrhythmic medications may become necessary for heart rate control or rhythm management. There are not enough of these patients to permit specific, evidence-based suggestions for treatment algorithms. Treatments have been described only in anecdotal reports.

Of particular note is the rare but devastating injury known as *commotio cordis.* Patients with this injury suffer lethal ventricular arrhythmias after what initially appears to be minimal chest trauma. Classically, these cases occur during ball sports (e.g., baseball) in which cardiovascular collapse is seen immediately after a minor blow to the chest. Prompt defibrillation is the only lifesaving therapy. Immediate resuscitation measures begun within 3 minutes of injury may have as high as a 25% survival rate. However, after the 3-minute period, survival is exceedingly rare.

Patients with pericardial tamponade and BCI require immediate surgical intervention. In hemodynamically stable patients, urgent median sternotomy is the treatment of choice. After the median sternotomy has been performed and the pericardium has been entered, the cardiac wound is usually easily identified. In patients surviving to urgent sternotomy, likely places to identify the injury are the right atrium, right ventricle, or the atriocaval junction. Temporary occlusion with a finger is the easiest first maneuver. Then more definitive (but still temporary) control can be obtained. For the right atrium, Allis clamps may be used to pull the wound edges together or a curved Satinsky clamp placed to occlude the opening. In the right ventricle, skin staples may have a role for cardiac wound closure (although these are more often used in penetrating trauma). The wound can be closed definitively in any number of fashions, depending on surgeon preference. Options include a running or interrupted suture that can be performed with or without felt pledgets. A qualified trauma or general surgeon can often repair these injuries without the use of cardiopulmonary bypass. Cardiothoracic surgical consultation is necessary in patients with internal cardiac injuries diagnosed by echocardiography (e.g., valve lesions, septal rupture, papillary muscle injury) because these lesions usually require cardiopulmonary bypass for their urgent (as opposed to emergent) repair.

Emergency department thoracotomy has only a limited role for treatment of patients with BCI. Emergency department thoracotomy is indicated for known or suspected BCI in patients in extremis or who lose vital signs; survival is rare, however. Blunt trauma patients with prehospital cardiac arrest have nearly 100% mortality, even with emergency department thoracotomy. In the event that a patient arrives alive with vital signs and then progresses to cardiac tamponade (diagnosed by FAST) with cardiac arrest, thoracotomy may be indicated. In this case, a left anterolateral thoracotomy is performed. The technical procedures will be similar to emergency department thoracotomy performed for penetrating thoracic trauma. Pericardotomy is performed to expose the heart and identify any area of bleeding. Cross-clamping the descending thoracic aorta may help to preferentially perfuse the heart and brain with any small amount of forward flow. If the patient truly suffered tamponade, release may allow the heart to fill and continue to beat. The hole in the heart must be temporarily occluded with a finger until the wound can be surgically repaired.

In patients with BCI and cardiac failure, intensive care unit admission is mandatory. Aggressive management based on symptoms, and physiology is crucial to get these patients over the initial insult. Patients with concomitant respiratory failure or hypoxia require mechanical ventilation. Volume resuscitation is necessary for preload to the injured heart and treatment of associated hemorrhagic shock from other injuries and ongoing bleeding. Pulmonary artery catheterization continues to have a role in diagnosing and guiding management of patients with BCI. It may help to guide inotropic support (e.g., dobutamine) in patients with low cardiac index and vasopressors (e.g., epinephrine) in cases of refractory hypotension. In patients with persistent cardiogenic shock, intra-aortic balloon pump (or even, rarely, ventricular-assisted device) placement may be necessary to improve cardiac output.

Coronary artery lesions are rare in patients with BCI. Coronary artery contusions, spasm, plaque rupture, dissection or laceration appear with signs and symptoms of myocardial infarction. In patients with these symptoms, cardiac catheterization with percutaneous angioplasty, stenting, or both, may be an option for restoration of blood flow to the distal target vessels. These lesions require prompt consultation with a cardiologist and a cardiothoracic surgeon.

FOLLOW-UP

Long-term follow-up of patients after BCI is not well described. Only a few small studies have tried to evaluate cardiac function after the acute injury period. These studies have shown that BCI resolves nearly uniformly. In general, after patients have recovered from their initial immediate hospitalization, their hearts heal and cardiac function returns to normal.

SUGGESTED READINGS

Elie MC: Blunt cardiac injury, *Mt Sinai J Med* 73(2): 542, 2006.
Mattox KL, Flint LM, Carrico CJ, and others: Blunt cardiac injury, *J Trauma* 33(5): 649, 1992.
Pasquale MD, Nagy K, Clarke J: *Eastern Association for the Surgery of Trauma (EAST) Practice Management Guidelines for Screening of Blunt Cardiac Injury.* http://east.org/tpg.html. Accessed June 28, 2006.
Schultz JM, Trunkey DD: Blunt cardiac injury, *Crit Care Clin* 20(1): 57, 2004.
Velmahos GC, Karaiskakis M, Salim A, and others: Normal electrocardiography and serum troponin I levels preclude the presence of clinically significant blunt cardiac injury, *J Trauma* 54(1): 45, 2003.

BURN WOUND MANAGEMENT

Richard L. Gamelli, MD, and Geoffrey M. Silver, MD

A burn injury occurs when some or all of the cells of the skin and other tissues are destroyed by scalding injuries, contact with hot objects or flames. Injuries to the skin can also result from radiation, radioactive exposure, electricity, friction, or chemicals. All of these wounds to the skin are considered to be burn wounds. The consequences of a burn injury may be local, that is, only within the injured tissues, or they may be associated with profound systemic responses. In addition to needing care of their burn wounds, patients with major burn injuries also require resuscitation for wound-related changes in fluid dynamics and the systemic response to the burn injury. Furthermore, the mechanism of the injury must be well understood so that associated injuries such as fractures, the most common nonburn-related injuries, are not missed. Patients may also need attention to the airway and require intubation, as well as ventilatory support to facilitate gas exchange and respiratory function related to an inhalation injury. Burn injury induces a profound change in the metabolic and nutritional needs of patients in association with a hypermetabolic state. Proper care of a burn wound requires not only attention to the wounds but also support of the patient's overall response to burn injury. The patient's preinjury health status can adversely affect patient outcome following a burn injury. In infants and elderly adults, the patient's limited physiology reserves require precise management of all aspects of care.

Substantial improvements in the outcome of critically injured burn victims are the consequences of advances in technology and the highly coordinated care process given in a burn center led by an experienced burn surgeon. This care is important for the acute management of the burn patient and his or her full rehabilitation and re-entry into society.

BURN WOUND PATHOPHYSIOLOGY AND THE SYSTEMIC RESPONSE

At the level of the burn wound, thermal injury causes coagulation necrosis resulting in a loss of capillary integrity in the affected tissues. This results in a loss of plasma volume from the intravascular compartment into the injured tissue interstitium. In patients with larger areas of cutaneous injury, similar intervascular volume shifts occur in nonburn tissues. The net effect is the necessity for fluid resuscitation in patients with larger burns. If the resuscitation is not effectively managed, hypovolemia and hypoperfusion can result in progressive local and systemic complication related to tissue ischemia. Fluid sequestered in the tissue space results in burn wound edema. The edema has minimal effects except in those circumstances in which the edema accumulation produces life-threatening and limb-threatening complications. The exuberant administration of resuscitation fluids can lead to over-resuscitation and subsequent edema. Circulation in the extremities can be compromised by significant edema formation, resulting in the development of a compartment syndrome. Patients with torso burns and burn wound edema may develop impaired respiration, and in the most severe circumstances, this can result in an abdominal compartment syndrome. Compartment syndromes involving the extremities or torso require surgical decompression to prevent further complications related to changes in circulation or ability to ventilate the patient. As a result of the burn injury, skin loses its barrier capacity and has a marked impairment in its ability to control loss of fluid and body heat into the environment. These events can add further to the complexity of managing the fluid needs of a burn patient.

INITIAL WOUND MANAGEMENT

After necessary lifesaving maneuvers have been completed, all reasonable attempts to preserve the remaining functional integrity of the burn-injured tissue are initiated. A well-managed resuscitation preserves the viability and functional integrity of injured areas. Shock, hypoxemia, hypothermia, and wound contamination may cause progression of the injury and further loss of function. At the time of initial resuscitation, and even at the scene of an injury, attention to such issues as smoldering articles of clothing, chemical decontamination, and removal of fuel-soaked clothing can have a positive effect on outcome. Failure to remove contaminated clothing before transport to the point of definitive care can extend both the depth and extent of the injury when transport times are prolonged.

Chemical decontamination procedures and removal of clothing may cause early wound contamination with potentially pathogenic organisms, but this a necessary risk dictated by patient and provider safety concerns. Hypothermia should be prevented from the outset. Placing a patient in cold, saline-soaked towels contributes to hypothermia and may cause local vasoconstriction and shunting of blood flow away from the injured area, thereby increasing the extent and depth of injury. Patients should be kept warm and in clean or sterile sheets until arrival at the point of definitive care.

In patients meeting transfer criteria to a burn unit, topical antimicrobial agents should not be applied until communication

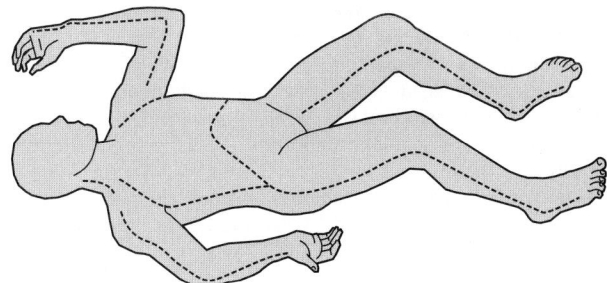

Figure 1

with the receiving unit is established. Application of some commonly used agents may preclude the use of biologic membrane dressings that are designed to adhere to a partial-thickness wound until closure. Premature application of a topical agent and occlusive dressing may impede the ability of the burn team to assess the depth and extent of an injury on arrival of the patient. Size and depth of the wound must be determined early in the course of the therapy. Accurate assessment of surface areas and depth aids in resuscitation and operative planning. Accordingly, dressings and agents applied before admission to the burn unit must be removed and the wound reassessed accurately. In children, occlusive dressings and opaque layers of topical agent may obscure subtle signs of abuse.

Early recognition of the necessity for escharotomy or fasciotomy (or both) on an injured extremity prevents necrosis of digits and loss of limb function in many patients. In most cases an escharotomy can and should be deferred until the patient arrives at the receiving institution. Many patients with circumferential extremity burns do not require an escharotomy; and, conversely, some patients with extremity injuries that are not circumferential do require this treatment. Patients at risk should be observed closely for signs of flow-limiting swelling by experienced personnel in an intensive care unit setting. Digital and distal extremity Doppler examinations and digital pulse oximetry are helpful tools in assessing limb blood-flow compromise.

A basic anatomic diagram of preferred escharotomy sites is shown in Figure 1, which illustrates the site and orientation of escharotomy incisions for each body part. The length of the incision should be adjusted to the patient's injury. Incisions must be sufficiently long and deep to completely release the burn wound constriction and should extend into uninjured tissue proximally and distally to avoid residual bands of eschar capable of impeding blood flow as the tissue swelling continues. When considering the patient's need for escharotomy before he or she is transferred to a burn unit, the medical team in the field should take into account both the transport time and the risk of the patient's developing limb-threatening ischemia during transport. The possibility of bleeding during transport from inadequate hemostasis or coagulopathy should also be considered. Torso burn wounds of sufficient surface area and depth may become difficult to ventilate, requiring higher-than-desirable airway pressures to deliver the necessary minute volume. This process tends to be progressive as the patient undergoes fluid resuscitation. Chest escharotomies should be performed if airway pressures cannot be effectively reduced by sedation, neuromuscular blockade, and manipulation of the ventilator mode.

NUTRITION

Early enteral delivery of sufficient calories and nitrogen to meet the patient's metabolic needs improves wound healing and decreases the incidence of infectious complications and associated graft loss. Patients with large burns need long-term enteral nutritional support and frequent reassessment of nitrogen balance and caloric intake to ensure that their metabolic requirements are being met. Patients who achieve positive nitrogen balance heal faster and have fewer septic complications, thereby improving their chances for a good outcome and a shorter hospital stay. The use of beta-blockade and oxandrolone in burned children and oxandrolone in adults has recently been shown to improve patient outcome.

TOPICAL ANTIMICROBIAL THERAPY AND INFECTION CONTROL

Burn injury–induced immunosuppression and loss of skin barrier function are associated causes of bacterial colonization and invasion of the burn wound. Wound sepsis used to be a common cause of mortality in patients with large burn wounds. Since the development of effective topical antimicrobial agents, the incidence of hemodynamically significant sepsis and death caused by infected burn wounds has been low. Nevertheless, in patients with large, open wounds, colonization of the wound with bacteria aggravates and perpetuates the burn-induced systemic inflammatory response. In patients with smaller wounds, high bacterial numbers in a grafted area may result in graft loss and significantly delay wound closure. In patients with extensive burns, infection in an area of meshed autograft or a donor site contributes to wound morbidity and, potentially, patient mortality. If donor sites must be reexcised to provide burn wound coverage, significant donor site loss or delayed reepithelialization may become a life-threatening event.

Prevention of wound sepsis by overgrowth of pathogenic bacteria with a topical antimicrobial agent is the standard of care. The advantages and disadvantages of several agents commonly in use are shown in Table 1. In patients with large burns, silver sulfadiazine and silver nitrate are preferred agents. Other agents include mafenide acetate cream, mafenide acetate solution, bacitracin, triple antibiotic ointment, and iodine-based ointments. Silver sulfadiazine cream and bacitracin ointment are the agents used most often in the outpatient setting. Alternative dressing techniques include silver-impregnated materials, which may offer some advantages as compared with silver nitrate solution and silver sulfadiazine cream. Silver-impregnated dressings are relatively easy to apply, and the antimicrobial properties are effective for several days, thereby decreasing the frequency of painful dressing changes necessary with other agents.

Patients with large wounds are prone to infection at sites distant from the wound. The presence of infections remote from the wound site adds to the metabolic burden and, if not the source of a fatal event, contributes to delayed burn wound healing and graft loss. Prevention of infectious complications leads to earlier wound closure and a better outcome.

EARLY ESCHAR EXCISION AND EARLY WOUND CLOSURE LEAD TO IMPROVED OUTCOME

Early eschar excision and wound closure, as demonstrated by Tompkins and Burke, is associated with improved survival. Removal of full-thickness eschar prevents the systemic manifestations of bacterial colonization of dead tissue. Direct invasion of adjacent tissue and bacteremic septic shock are also potential complications of wound colonization. Removing the burn eschar prevents many of the complications associated with wound infection. The limitation of this approach is that removal of eschar leaves an open wound that must be covered. A functional barrier must be restored if the desired goal of reducing the duration of exposure to bacterial by-products is to be achieved.

Autograft skin is the best solution if donor sites are available. In patients with large burns, cadaver allograft provides excellent temporary closure. The use of a dermal substitute can be applied to large surface areas. The advantage of this approach is that a barrier is restored while vascular ingrowth into the neodermis proceeds. After the neodermis matures, autografts or cultured endothelial cells can be applied. When combined with topical antimicrobial agents, early eschar excision followed by restoration of barrier integrity significantly reduces the incidence of fatal sepsis caused by bacterial colonization of the wound.

INDICATIONS FOR SURGICAL INTERVENTION

The depth of the wound is the essential factor involved in the decision to operate on a patient with a thermal injury. The delineation of burn wound thickness on the basis of histologic criteria is clear (Fig. 2); however, bedside determination of wound depth and early recognition of the need for surgical intervention are often difficult. Superficial partial-thickness burns are easily recognized and heal well without grafting. On the other hand, full-thickness

Table 1: Advantages and Disadvantages of Topical Antimicrobial Agents Currently in Use

Topical Agent	Advantages	Disadvantages
Silver sulfadiazine cream	Good gram-negative spectrum Active against yeast Easy application	Hypersensitivity Thrombocytopenia (rare) Neutropenia (rare)
Silver nitrate solution	Good gram-negative spectrum, gram-positive coverage, and yeast coverage No hypersensitivity Painless	Labor-intensive application Stains most surfaces Requires occlusive dressings Electrolyte abnormalities
Sulfamylon (Bayer HealthCare Pharmaceuticals, Montville, NJ)	Good gram-negative and gram-positive coverage	Painful on partial-thickness burns Can cause metabolic acidosis Hypersensitivity
Silver-coated dressing (Acticoat, Smith & Nephew, Memphis, TN)	Good gram-negative, gram-positive, and yeast coverage Needs less frequent application and is less labor intensive No hypersensitivity	Expensive

Figure 2

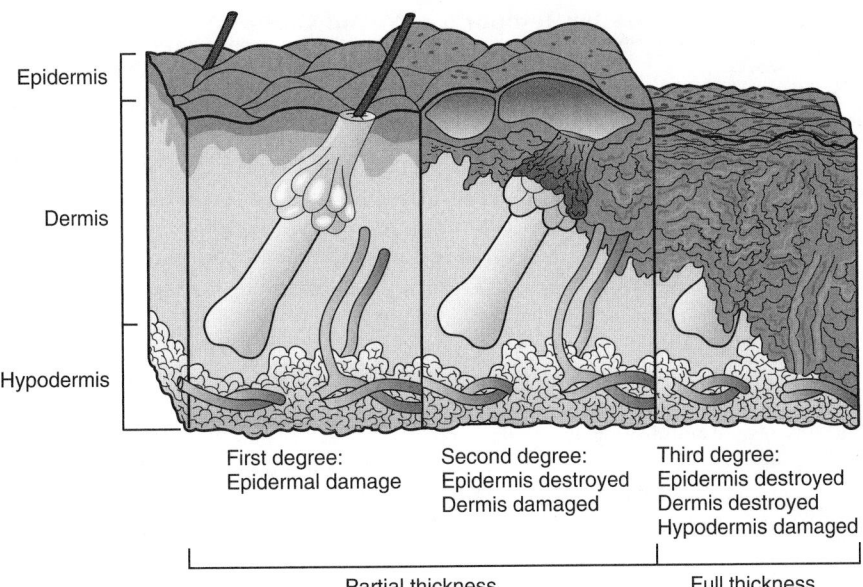

Epidermis

Dermis

Hypodermis

First degree:
Epidermal damage

Second degree:
Epidermis destroyed
Dermis damaged

Third degree:
Epidermis destroyed
Dermis destroyed
Hypodermis damaged

Partial thickness

Full thickness

injuries are also readily recognized and require surgical intervention unless they are quite small. The recognition and management of intermediate-to-deep, partial-thickness injuries are often difficult and depend on several factors, including the bedside assessment of depth and an educated prediction of the time to closure. In general, wounds that will likely require several weeks to close should be excised and grafted. Deeper wounds of significant size, although not of full thickness, often require several weeks of painful dressing changes in a hospital setting to heal and therefore should be excised and grafted. Intermediate-thickness injuries over joint surfaces may cause dysfunctional scarring and contracture. In these patients, grafting is often the best choice, with the goal of optimal return of function with less overall morbidity; however, in patients with coexisting diseases that pose an increased operative risk or prolonged wound healing, conservative management without grafting, despite potential dysfunctional scarring, may in the end be the appropriate plan.

CHOICE OF TECHNIQUE

Partial-thickness injuries that are deep enough to require grafting should be tangentially excised. A mounted single-edge razor (Weck) with removable metal templates (Goulian guard) of various sizes to control the depth of excision is commonly used for this purpose. With the appropriate-sized template, delicate areas of the hands and face can be excised with precision. An adjustable-depth dermatome can be used to tangentially excise large wounds to a uniform depth in a rapid fashion. Tangential excision of partial-thickness wounds can be associated with rapid and significant loss of blood. Blood conservation techniques, such as tourniquets or subeschar injection of dilute epinephrine solution, should be used when appropriate. The use of topical thrombin and epinephrine-containing solutions aids in hemostasis. Fibrin glue in spray form may also be of incremental value in achieving hemostasis.

After an injury has been identified as full thickness, the patient should be prepared for operative eschar excision and surgical closure. The technique used to excise the eschar depends on several factors, including depth beyond the dermis, location, and size. Very large and very deep injuries should be excised at the level of the deep fascia, thereby limiting blood loss and reducing operative time and time to wound closure. Wounds not deeply full thickness can be sequentially excised to viable subdermal fat. Although meshed

autografts placed directly on fatty tissue might take longer to close, graft take is usually excellent. Sparing a layer of viable fatty tissue helps to preserve the natural tissue contour and may prevent functional limitations imposed by fixing an autograft directly to a mobile muscle.

Autografts are harvested from donor sites using an adjustable-depth dermatome. The location of the donor site depends on many factors, including donor availability, recipient bed, required donor-skin thickness, color, and cosmetic acceptability. After harvesting, donor sites should be carefully managed to prevent trauma, infection, and painful exposure. A wide variety of dressings and techniques are used by various centers. The dressing used should protect the site from trauma and bacterial invasion while not contributing to discomfort. Other considerations include ease of application, adherence, support for epithelialization, minimal scarring, and cost.

LOCATION AND SURFACE AREA CONSIDERATIONS

In patients with smaller wounds and adequate available donor sites, preservation of function of the face and hands should be the highest priority. These areas should be grafted as soon as the need is identified. In patients with massive wounds, preservation of life at times supersedes the goal of optimal limb function. After survival has been achieved, other options for reconstruction and prostheses become available. Experience and judgment are required to balance the necessity for wound closure with functional outcome. Using a thick, unmeshed sheet graft to cover the dorsum of the hand is appropriate for smaller surface area or isolated hand injuries, whereas it is inappropriate if the patient's survival depends on closure of large surface areas, where donor sites are at a premium. Temporary closure with cadaver homograft or another biologic membrane dressing (Table 2) helps to preserve viable tissue and function until donor sites become available for definitive grafting. In all cases, preservation of function must be optimized by aggressive mobilization and splinting.

LARGE, SURFACE-AREA WOUNDS

In the past 30 years, the survival of patients with large burn wounds (more than 30% body surface area burn) has improved dramatically. Topical antimicrobial agents, aggressive nutritional support,

Table 2: Biologic Materials Currently in Use for Temporary Wound Closure

Description	Use	Advantages	Disadvantages
Cadaver homograft: cryo-preserved viable human cadaver skin	Temporary coverage of wound after eschar excision	Functional barrier coverage Good take rate	Limited duration of take because of rejection Potential transmission of cytomegalovirus
Xenograft: porcine	Temporary coverage of partial-thickness wounds	Good temporary coverage of partial-thickness burns of various depths	Suboptimal adherence; requires frequent observation for infection, limiting its application to inpatients except in small wounds after adherence is ensured
Integra (Integra, Plainsboro, NJ): bioengineered dermal substitute with collagen glycosaminoglycan matrix and disposable silicone membrane barrier	Coverage of excised wounds until autograft is available Neodermal layer is permanent	Excellent adherence, effective antimicrobial barrier, low infection rate, readily accepts autografts, improved functional and cosmetic results because of permanent dermal replacement Excellent long-term clinical results	Although vascularized "neodermis" is permanent, it still requires eventual autograft
Biobrane (Smith & Nephew, Memphis, TN): silicone membrane bound to nylon mesh coated with porcine collagen	Coverage of partial-thickness injuries and donor sites	Reduces painful dressing changes Can be used in outpatient setting	Suboptimal adherence
Transcyte (Smith & Nephew, Memphis, TN): cultured human neonatal fibroblasts on a collagen matrix with a silicone barrier Matrix contains fibronectin, tenascin, glycosaminoglycans, and multiple growth factors	Temporary coverage of partial-thickness wounds	Reduces painful dressing changes Can be used in outpatient setting	Cost effectiveness unknown

and early eschar excision have had the greatest survival impact in this group of patients. Although survival of patients with large wounds is no longer unusual, successful management of these patients is a tremendous clinical challenge. The improved survival rates reported by high-volume, experienced burn units are by no means universal. Functional survival and return to a productive existence with an acceptable quality of life after a massive injury are often limited to young, healthy patients. Survival is poor in older patients, in those with significant preexisting health conditions, and in the presence of inhalation injury.

In patients with large wounds, survival must often take precedence over function. Wound closure with the patient's own skin remains as the mainstay of burn surgery. Although cultured epithelial cell sheets are available (at high cost), attempts to cover large surface areas with the present technology have been of limited success to date. Because excision and reexcision can temporarily exhaust available donor sites, the surgeon must make choices regarding technique and timing that are required for survival but often at the expense of functional outcome. To cover large wounds, thinner wide-meshed autografts are employed. At operation, the graft is harvested at a thickness of 6/1000 to 10/1000 of an inch. The skin is meshed at 3:1, 4:1, and even 6:1 expansion ratios. With the higher expansion ratios, a large area can be covered by a given piece of skin. By using this technique, the surgeon can use relatively small areas of donor site to cover large wound areas. The downside of this approach is that large mesh interstices result in an open wound bed that requires a longer time to healing, and the amount of scarring and contracture is proportional to the expansion ratio used.

In patients with large burns, donor sites can become precious and must be nurtured and protected. If properly managed, donor

sites can be reexcised many times. This process is often required in patients with burns exceeding 60%. Unusual donor sites occasionally must be used to obtain enough skin to achieve closure. Donor sites become open wounds at the time of excision and have similar problems with healing and infection, as do partial-thickness burns. Therefore donor sites should be covered with a suitable dressing. Donor-site infection, albeit unusual, can be physiologically significant in a patient with large surface area burn. More often, donor-site infections can lead to temporary or permanent loss of a donor site. The incidence of donor-site loss to infection can be decreased by the use of dressings that prevent contamination and promote healing.

The development of cryopreservation techniques used by skin banks facilitates the availability of viable cadaver homograft. The ability to cover excised areas with homograft skin is a major advance that allows for continued eschar removal in the absence of available donor sites. Homograft can remain in place or be replaced if necessary until the donor sites are again available for harvesting.

Often in patients who have extensive injuries, areas that are partial thickness are managed without grafting. Temporary closure of such areas can be accomplished by using porcine xenograft or other biologic membrane dressings. Many wounds heal and reepithelialize underneath a xenograft or biologic membrane dressing. This approach often prevents or reduces the need for grafting large areas of partial-thickness injury.

The use of an artificial dermal substitute allows the creation of a functional barrier after eschar excision. Vascular ingrowth occurs within a reasonable time frame, and as soon as the blood supply is sufficient, the "neodermis" accepts an autograft with a high level of success. Long-term wound outcomes have been good, and this approach allows the use of thin autografts. It can be of particular benefit in patients with deep burns over critical structures and in the elderly and young children.

PROBLEM AREAS

The face has multiple and diverse functions of critical importance to an individual's ability to interact with the environment and communicate with other individuals. Therefore even small injuries can have a large impact on a patient's quality of life and ability to function. Therefore management of facial burns is a high-priority issue because early closure most effectively preserves function. Because facial skin is thick and the dermis is highly trabeculated, partial-thickness wounds often heal with excellent cosmetic and functional results. Full-thickness injuries should be tangentially excised and grafted as early as possible. Earlier grafting prevents much of the morbidity associated with delayed management. Optimally, facial burns should be grafted with unmeshed sheets taken from donor sites that most closely approximate the patient's normal skin tone, such as the scalp or inner thighs. Care should be taken to preserve complex contours by excising as little viable tissue as possible. Temporary placement of cadaver homograft before definitive autografting allows marginal tissue to demarcate without risking the loss of the patient's own skin from under-excised burns.

The neck is a difficult area to manage because it is often the site of major dysfunctional scarring and skin contracture, which can limit neck mobility, mandibular closure, and facial expression. The cause of scarring includes decreased graft take because of inadequate excision, contamination, and shearing. The neck is in constant motion related to swallowing, coughing, talking, and facial expression. All movements of the head involve the neck at some level of extremes of rotation and extension that can easily shear or lift a graft. In addition, postoperative compliance with physical therapy, splinting, and compression therapy is often poor because of patient discomfort. Early and late release of contractures is often necessary to maintain functional mobility and prevent progressive deformity.

Isolated partial-thickness injuries of the wrist and hands also pose a difficult problem. In many patients, early grafting of the hands leads to earlier hospital discharge; however, this does not necessarily lead to an earlier return to full function and to work. The preservation of function should guide the decision-making process. The goal is to identify those wounds that must undergo grafting and surgery early. Allowing a full-thickness injury to demarcate or separate only delays definitive closure and risks exposing viable tissues to local inflammation and infection. Mobilization and splinting to prevent contracture should begin at the time of admission and continue as long as needed to ensure an optimal functional result in both nonoperative and operative cases. Early management of dysfunctional scarring and prevention of contracture decrease long-term morbidity. This approach should be emphasized in children in whom normal bone growth and shape may be damaged by the limitations caused by dysfunctional scarring and contracture. Failure to manage these problems early may result in irreversible loss of function.

PSYCHOSOCIAL CONSIDERATIONS

Understanding the psychosocial consequences of a burn injury improves the effectiveness of burn care and overall outcome. In many patients, a preexisting psychiatric or social condition contributes directly or indirectly to injury. Recognizing this fact and acting appropriately to treat the underlying psychiatric disease enables the provider to treat an injury more effectively through improved patient compliance and motivation. Recovery from the burn injury requires more than simple wound closure for these patients.

Patients must adjust to new physical limitations and comply with long-term therapy to optimize their recovery. Depression, anxiety, stress, and substance abuse are detractors to recovery and should be prevented, if possible, and managed aggressively when they occur or if already present.

Abuse and neglect are common causes of thermal injuries in children and the elderly. Recognition of abuse requires a high index of suspicion. The reported history should be consistent with the injury pattern. Children who are victims of abuse or neglect are often underweight and not up to date with pediatrician visits and immunizations. Functional recovery from a thermal injury in abused children is problematic because these children cannot take care of themselves and must be protected from recurrent abuse. Recovery requires committed parents, relatives, or guardians who are able to take care of the many needs of an injured child and provide a safe environment.

OUTPATIENT MANAGEMENT

Many patients with thermal injuries can be managed as outpatients. In recent years the trend has been toward early hospital discharge or no hospital admission for burns of increasing size and depth. When deciding to discharge a patient with thermal injuries or to manage him or her as an outpatient, the clinician must consider several issues. The patient should be able to perform the required dressing changes or have assistance. Pain control should be adequate but not sedating. The wound should be at low risk for infection, and the patient should not to be at risk for reinjury, abuse, or neglect. Outpatient management requires a clinic that is capable of following the patient's progress and providing the necessary medical care, physical therapy, occupational therapy, and social services to achieve an optimal outcome.

CONCLUSION

Burns patients often require long-term follow-up. Burn wound care and treatment may be required for months to years following wound closure. The outpatient burn clinic provides patient access to the multidisciplinary team. The continuous availability of treatment and services provided by the burn surgeon, the reconstructive surgeon, physical and occupational therapists, social workers, and others is essential to the patient's ultimate recovery. Burn center hospitals have made long-term commitments to provide standards-based, quality patient care that goes beyond that of initial burn care.

Suggested Readings

Burke JF, Bondoc CC, Quinby WC: Primary burn excision and immediate grafting; a method of shortening illness, *J Trauma* 14:389, 1974.

Hartford CE: The bequests of Moncrief and Moyer: an appraisal of topical therapy of burns B 1981: American Burn Association presidential address, *J Trauma* 21:827, 1981.

Janzekovic Z: A new concept in the early excision and immediate grafting of burns, *J Trauma* 10:1103, 1970.

McManus WF, Mason AD, Jr, Pruitt BA, Jr: Excision of the burn wound in patients with large burns, *Arch Surg* 124:718, 1989.

Nissen NN, Gamelli RL, Polverini PJ, and others: Differential angiogenic and proliferative activity of surgical and burn wound fluids, *J Trauma* 54(6):1205, 2003.

Sheridan RL, Choucair RJ: Acellular allordermis in burn surgery: 1 year results of a pilot trial, *J Burn Care Rehabil* 19:528, 1998.

Thompkins RG, Remensnyder JP, Burke JF, and others: Significant reductions in mortality for children with burn injuries through the use of prompt eschar excision, *Ann Surg* 208(5):577, 1988.

Fluid Management and Nutritional Support of the Burn Patient

Stephen M. Milner, MBBS, BDS, Vijay A. Singh, MD, and Jennifer Eldred, MBBS, RD, LD, CNSD

FLUID MANAGEMENT

As early as 1931, experimental studies by Blalock demonstrated that burn shock was caused by loss of plasma from the circulation. A massive release of chemical mediators takes place in the burning process. These include histamine, complement, arachidonic acid, products of the coagulation cascade, cytokines, and oxygen free radicals, which produce an increase in vascular permeability and microvascular hydrostatic pressure. The net result is an imbalance of physical forces controlling fluid flux across the capillary as fluid passes from the vascular to the interstitial compartments. In burns greater than 25% total body surface area (TBSA) these changes are also seen in non-burned tissue. If fluid resuscitation is inadequate, the net result is hypovolemic shock with decreased cardiac output and hypotension.

In large burns, injury also occurs at the cellular level, and a progressively diminishing cell membrane potential and cellular shock may be the final common pathway to multiorgan failure and death.

Pharmacologic agents that can diminish capillary leakage by antagonizing or blocking the vasoactive mediators have been extensively studied. Documented benefit has been reported in the laboratory, and the use of high-dose vitamin C has been found to decrease total fluid requirements in one clinical trial. Currently, however, this approach remains a key research issue for the future.

As in the treatment of other forms of shock, the primary goal thus is to restore and preserve tissue perfusion. Resuscitation following thermal injury, however, is complicated because huge transvascular fluid shifts occur, and the resulting obligatory burn edema has attendant risks of increased vascular compromise, airway obstruction, and conversion of a viable, ischemic, deep, second-degree burn to a nonviable, full-thickness injury, increasing morbidity and mortality. Thus the basic principle of fluid resuscitation is to carefully titrate the fluids administered to provide the least amount necessary to maintain adequate organ perfusion.

Fluid Management (0–24 Hours)

Replacement of fluid sequestered should begin as soon as possible. Fluid requirements are directly related to the size of the burn, which can be estimated by the "rule of nines" or more accurately from a body–surface-area diagram, such as the Lund-Browder chart (Fig. 1). Intravenous fluid resuscitation is required for all

Figure 1 Lund-Browder Chart relative percentage of body surface area affected by growth.

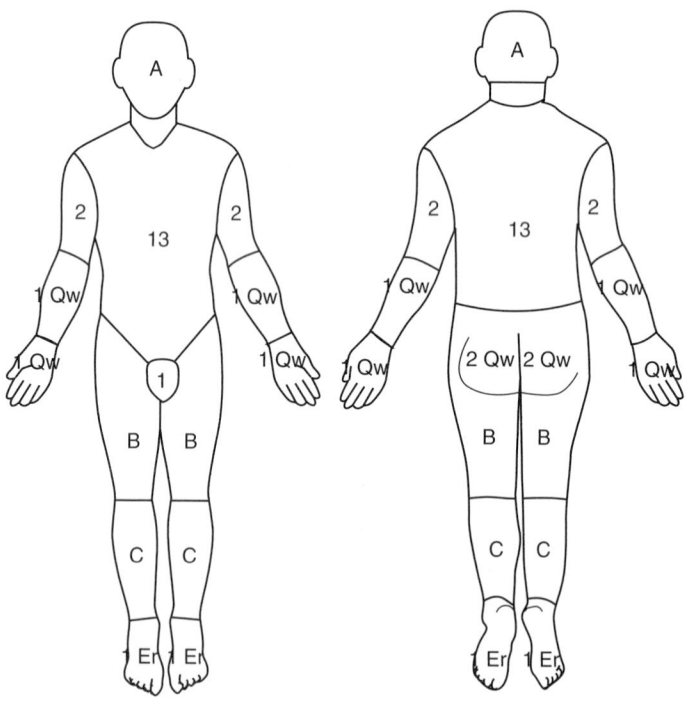

LUND-BROWDER CHART
Relative percentage of body surface area affected by growth

Age in years	0	1	5	10	15	Adult
A—head (back or front)	9 Qw	8 Qw	6 Qw	5 Qw	4 Qw	3 Qw
B—1 thigh (back or front)	2 Er	3 Qr	4	4 Qr	4 Qw	4 Er
C—1 leg (back or front)	2 Qw	2 Qw	2 Er	3	3 Qr	3 Qw

Table 1: The Parkland Formula

4 ml × weight (kg) × % TBSA burn = ml for the first 24 hrs.

One half of this total is administered over the first 8 hours, and the second half over the next 16 hours.

Calculation begins from the time of the burn and not the time of treatment.

TBSA, Total body surface area.

patients with second- and third-degree burns greater than 10% TBSA in patients younger than 10 or older than 50 years of age and for those with greater than 20% TBSA in all other age groups. Venous access is best obtained by large-bore (16-gauge) catheters, preferably placed percutaneously through nonburned skin, although central access may be necessary. These patients also require a Foley catheter and a nasogastric tube.

There are numerous formulae that can be used for successful fluid resuscitation; however, no prospective, randomized studies have been undertaken to enable comparison, and all formulae are only a starting point. The volume administered should be continuously titrated to the urine output to avoid over-resuscitation or under-resuscitation. Increased fluid requirements are seen following inhalation injury, after high-voltage electrical injuries, and in children. The most popular fluid used for resuscitation in the United States is lactated Ringer's solution, with a sodium concentration of 130 mEq/L. This solution is most commonly prescribed for adults, using the Parkland formula (Table 1), and was designed to produce a urine output of 0.5 to 1 ml/kg/h.

Pigmented urine resulting from the presence of hemochromogens is often associated with high-voltage electrical injuries (>1000 volts). To avoid injury to the renal tubules, the pigment should be cleared as quickly as possible. The rate of crystalloid infusion can be increased to produce a urine output of 2 ml/kg/h. Mannitol can be administered to facilitate the diuresis, and sodium bicarbonate can be used to alkalinize the urine to decrease the precipitation of myoglobin in the renal tubules. Rhabdomyolysis may be complicated by hyperkalemia, and serum potassium should be monitored frequently until the urine clears.

Monitoring

Early release of catecholamines can maintain arterial pressure despite hypovolemia. Thus measurement of arterial pressure is a poor guide to resuscitation. The pulse rate is more helpful, and a tachycardia in excess of 120 per minute is usually indicative of hypovolemia. If central monitoring is believed to be necessary, in most cases a central vein pressure line is adequate; Swan-Ganz catheters are not routinely used because they can cause complications, including venous thrombosis, emboli, sepsis, and endocarditis. Nevertheless, a right heart catheter may be a useful adjunct in patients not responding to resuscitation or in those who have cardiac or pulmonary disease.

Other Types of Resuscitation Fluid

Protein

The oncotic pressure generated by plasma proteins serves to maintain the intravascular volume. Following all resuscitative regimens, severe hypoproteinemia is seen following major burns, and this in turn potentiates further edema. The administration of colloid is therefore logical but controversial, and much debate exists as to when capillary integrity is established and whether infused protein stays within the vascular compartment.

Experimentally this has been shown to be at about 8 hours after the burn injury. Therefore colloids generally are prescribed in burns greater than 40% TBSA, after the first 8 hours, in patients with oliguria who are not responding to crystalloid resuscitation. The choice of protein solution is either fresh frozen plasma (0.5–1 ml/kg/%burn) or albumin, which can be conveniently given by adding 50 g of albumin to each liter of crystalloid. Fresh frozen plasma has the theoretical advantage of replacing clotting factors and fibronectin, an adhesion molecule and key fibroblast-derived signal protein, which initiates healing of the burn wound.

Hypertonic Saline

Hypertonic salt solutions may also be used to decrease fluid requirements. Rapid infusion produces serum hyperosmolarity, which extracts water from the cellular compartment. The administration of crystalloid with a sodium concentration of 250 mEq/L was used by Monafo, and a slightly hypertonic solution (180 mEq/L), made by adding sodium bicarbonate to lactated Ringer's solution, was advocated by Warden for large burns. Close monitoring of serum sodium levels is mandatory; they should not be allowed to increase to levels greater than 160 mEq/dL. However, there is no consensus on the use of hypertonic saline, which has not proved popular because of concerns over outcome.

Fluid Management (Greater Than 24 Hours)

After 24 hours, extravasation of fluid from the microcirculation is minimal, serum sodium levels are high, and protein is low. However, maintenance requirements may be high because there is continued evaporative loss from the raw surface of the burn wound. Thus urine output can be maintained by hypotonic solutions such as D5 1/2N Saline. The addition of dextrose is necessary because glucose stores are depleted by catecholamine release. Maintenance requirements can be calculated by the following formula: basal (1500 ml/m^2) + evaporative water loss of [(25 + %burn) × m^2 × 24]. Protein losses should be replaced to minimize further edema and restore blood volumes when albumin levels fall below 1.5 mg/L. The volumes of enteral nutrition, usually begun at approximately 6 hours, are factored into any calculations.

Pediatric Resuscitation

Fluid resuscitation requirements differ in children. When venous access cannot be accomplished, fluid can be delivered by cannulation of the bone marrow. A 16-gauge spinal needle can be inserted directly into the tibial plateau, medial malleolus, anterior iliac crest, or distal femur and used to deliver fluid rates of up to 100 ml/h. Because of their increased surface area-to-weight ratio, fluid losses are proportionally greater and the "rule of nines" is not accurate; thus burn charts are mandatory for TBSA calculation. Children are best resuscitated with formulae based on surface area rather than weight, such as the modified Carvajal formula used in Galveston (Table 2), and urine output should be titrated to 1 ml/kg/hr. Lactated Ringer's solution is prescribed for children older than 1 hr; however, infants younger than 2 years of age are prone to

Table 2: Total 24-Hour Fluid Requirements in Children

5000 ml × BSA* burned (m^2) [burn-related losses]
+ 2000 ml × TBSA(m^2) [maintenance fluids]

*Body surface area, obtained from a standard height-weight nomogram.
TBSA, Total body surface area.

hypoglycemia because of small glycogen stores and therefore should receive D5/LR.

In the following 24 hours, fluid requirements are 3750 ml/m^2 TBSA (to replace losses caused by evaporation from the wound) plus 1500 ml/m^2 TBSA (for maintenance).

Uncertainty and inaccuracy of mathematical calculations related to resuscitation formulae have been eliminated by use of the Burn Wheel. Developed for preparation for mass casualties in the First Gulf War (1990–1991), the Burn Wheel facilitates accurate prescription of fluids for children and adults by simply dialing the weight and TBSA into a circular revolving disc. This has proved invaluable for use by inexperienced personnel and in mass casualty situations.

BURN NUTRITION

It is important to initiate enteral feedings within the first 24 to 48 hours of admission and advance to goal as quickly as possible to preserve gut mucosal integrity, prevent bacterial translocation, and achieve nutritional goals. Thermal injuries pose important ramifications for nutritional support because of a persistent state of hypermetabolism. The sustained increase in energy consumption causes a parallel increase in energy demand and a shift in substrate use from glucose to amino acids as the preferred source of fuel. This promotes mobilization of amino acids and protein catabolism, which may translate into loss of muscle and other proteins required for organ structure and cell function. The hypermetabolic response is perpetuated by factors such as fever, pain, presence of burn eschar, multiple surgical procedures, and recurrent infection and may last for weeks or months until wound closure is achieved. The basic objective in meeting nutritional requirements following a burn is to provide adequate energy to attenuate the stress response, maximize immune competence, minimize the loss of lean body mass, and facilitate wound healing.

There are several methods or predictive equations that can be used to estimate a burn patient's total caloric requirements. We have found the use of the Ireton-Jones equation to be the most consistently applicable to our adult population in determining resting metabolic rate (see Table 2). The Curreri and Harris-Benedict equations have been found to overestimate and underestimate caloric requirements, respectively. Actual energy requirements are best determined by use of indirect calorimetry within the first 72 hours after the burn injury and weekly thereafter.

In larger burns (>20% TBSA), protein should be provided as 20% to 25% of the total calories, or 1.5 to 2.5 g protein per kg of body weight.

Numerous feeding formulations are commercially available, each with a variable content of carbohydrate, fat, and protein. In most cases, a calorically dense, high-protein formula containing less than 30% of total calories as fat is ideal. Final adjustments in the nutritional formula can be made by adding modular supplements and micronutrients. Parenteral nutrition, which is associated with higher mortality, should be avoided but may be indicated in isolated cases of enteral feeding intolerance.

Continuous monitoring and reassessment are essential for evaluating response to nutrition therapy, and adjustments are made thereafter on the basis of these laboratory tests and progression of wound healing. Approaches include biochemical assays, monitoring weights, intake and output records, indirect calorimetry, and overall progression of wound closure. Nitrogen balance studies should be conducted weekly to biweekly to assess the adequacy of protein provision. Elevated C-reactive protein (CRP) levels are indicative of the stress response and should be monitored in conjunction with prealbumin and transferrin because a decrease in CRP is associated with recovering levels of these transport proteins. Albumin does

Table 3: Recommended Daily Allowance (RDA)

Males		Females	
0–3 yr: kcal/day	= (60.9 × kg) −54	0–3 yr: kcal/day	= (61.0 × kg) −51
3–10 yr: kcal/day	= (22.7 × kg) + 495	3–10 yr: kcal/day	= (22.5 × kg) + 499
10–18 yr: kcal/day	= (17.5 × kg) + 651	10–18 yr: kcal/day	= (12.2 × kg) + 746

kcal, Kilocalories.

not reflect acute changes in nutritional status because of its sensitivity to fluid shifts, plasma leakage, and a longer half-life and therefore should not be used as a nutritional marker. Glucose control (80–110 mg/dL) has been associated with improved clinical outcomes, and insulin, being an anabolic hormone, may assist in nitrogen utilization and retention.

Despite appropriate enteral feeding prescriptions, tube feedings are frequently held for bedside procedures, nursing care, physical therapy, and surgical operations. Preoperative and interoperative feedings are becoming more acceptable practices to prevent cumulative caloric deficits.

Children necessitate greater caloric requirements per kilogram than adults. Additionally, they have baseline requirements to meet essential growth needs. The functional immaturity of a child's gastrointestinal tract and renal system poses a challenge to delivering nutrient dense products. Caloric needs for burned children may be calculated using the recommended daily allowance for age (Table 3). Protein requirements for children are generally 2.5 to 4.0 g protein per kg body weight or 20% of total caloric requirements. Monitoring renal function (blood area nitrogen/creatinine) is then critical in assessing protein tolerance.

Patients who sustain large burns are in a continuous catabolic state. The persistence of this prolonged catabolism causes severe muscle wasting and immune suppression. The result is poor wound healing and the recurrence of infections, which eventually can lead to sepsis, multiple organ failure, or death. Appropriate nutrition is essential and must be supplied to these patients to offset the complications associated with malnutrition. Early initiation and maintenance of an appropriate nutrient mix feeding (oral or enteral) will decrease protein losses, aid in wound healing, and enhance immune response. Frequent reassessments of nutrient requirements are crucial in providing adequate nutrition and achieving favorable outcomes.

Age in Years	0	1	5	10	15	Adult
A-head (back or front)	9½	8½	6½	5½	4½	3½
B-1 thigh (back or front)	2½	3¼	4	4¼	4½	4¾
C-1 leg (back or front)	2½	2½	2¾	3	3¼	3½

SUGGESTED READINGS

Curreri PW, Richmond D, Marvin J, and others: Dietary requirements of patients with major burns, *J Am Diet Assoc* 65:415, 1974.

Demling RH: The role of anabolic hormones for wound healing in catabolic states, *J Burns Wounds* 4e2 2005.

Milner SM, Hodgetts TJ, Rylah LT: The Burns Calculator: a simple proposed guide for fluid resuscitation, *Lancet* 342(8879): 1089, 1993.

COLD INJURY

Robert J. Spence, MD

Formerly considered almost exclusively a military problem, cold injury is a continuum of clinical syndromes that has become much more prevalent in the civilian population because of the increasing number of homeless people and increasing enthusiasm among the general population for outdoor activities such as climbing and skiing. Consequently, cold injury should be considered within the scope of a civilian physician's practice.

Cold injury can be divided into three major classifications: (1) slow, nonfreezing local tissue injury, such as trench foot and cold immersion foot; (2) freezing injuries, also known as *frostbite*; and (3) its generalized form, accidental hypothermia (Table 1).

PHYSICAL PRINCIPLES

The physical mechanisms of heat loss are important to understand in the prevention and treatment of cold injuries. The four primary means of heat loss are (1) conduction, (2) radiation, (3) evaporation, and (4) convection.

Conduction

Conduction is the transfer of heat between two masses in contact with one another. The rate of transfer is proportional to the temperature differential, the size of the contact area, and the thermal conductivity of the materials. Thermal conductivity is roughly equivalent to the insulating ability of the material. Gases are poor conductors, whereas metals and liquids are most conductive. Water has approximately 25 to 30 times more conductivity than air. For this reason, immersion in cold water and lying on a wet surface are among the fastest ways to lose body heat.

Radiation

Radiation is the transfer of heat by electromagnetic transmission. The rate of heat loss is dependent on the temperature gradient between the body temperature and the surroundings. Radiation is the primary mode of heat transfer when the body is fully exposed to the air. Radiation accounts for 55% to 65% of heat loss.

Evaporation

The conversion of liquid into vapor requires energy, most commonly in the form of heat. Evaporation from the body surface and the subsequent heat loss are functions of the change in vapor pressure from the body surface to the ambient air and the velocity of air movement. Typically, the greatest of evaporative heat loss from the body is through the saturation of inspired air in the lung. Evaporation from the body surface via perspiration is also a large component. Generally, evaporation accounts for 10% to 15% of total body heat loss.

Convection

Convection is the transfer of heat caused by the flow of liquids or gases over a surface. Clinically, it is proportional to the velocity of the flow and the differential in temperature between the body and the surrounding environment. Convection generally transfers energy poorly, but it becomes important when a patient is transported and can become a significant factor if the patient is not adequately covered. Convection is the primary component of wind chill. Exposed skin may suffer a similar injury in calm air at 0 °F or in a 15-mph breeze at 25 °F. Convection is used to the patient's advantage with the Bair Hugger system (Augustine Medical, Eden Prairie, MN), with which heat loss is minimized by surrounding the patient with flowing warm air. Note, however, that there is initial heat loss through evaporation if the patient is wet.

PHYSIOLOGIC THERMAL REGULATION

Normal body temperature is 32 °C at the skin, 37 °C under the tongue, 38 °C in the rectum, and 38.5 °C deep within the liver. Hypothermia is defined as a decrease in the body's core temperature to 35 °C (95 °F) or below. Maintenance of homeothermy is central for normal body functioning.

The central nervous system regulates thermal homeostasis. Core cooling causes hypothalamic-pituitary axis stimulation of catecholamine release, peripheral vasoconstriction, and inhibition of perspiration to conserve heat. Thyroid stimulation results in upregulation of oxidative metabolism and shivering with resultant heat production. The basal metabolic rate is further accelerated via *catecholamines*. *Shivering* can lead to a fivefold increase in heat production but fails after glycogen stores have been depleted. To conserve heat, skin blood flow can drop as low as 0.5 mm per minute per 100 ml of tissues with *vasoconstriction*.

PATHOPHYSIOLOGIC EFFECTS OF HYPOTHERMIA

Hypothermia has profound effects on the body's vital organ systems:

Central nervous system: There is a progressive decrease of cerebral blood flow at the rate of 6% to 7% for every 1 °C drop in core temperature. There are electroencephalogram abnormalities below 34 °C and loss of electrical activity between 19 °C and 29 °C. There is a variable but progressively diminished ability of the patient to speak, move, and mentate as body temperature diminishes.

Cardiovascular system: Hypothermia initially causes a sympathetic response resulting in tachycardia, vasoconstriction, and increased myocardial oxygen consumption. This is followed by bradycardia, which becomes severe at approximately 32 °C. Mean

Table 1: Cold Injury

Accidental Hypothermia	Local Cold Injury
1. Mild	1. Pernio or chilblain
2. Moderate	2. Trench foot (nontropical immersion foot)
3. Severe	3. Freezing injury/frostbite
	A. Frostnip
	B. Superficial frostbite
	C. Deep frostbite

arterial pressure and myocardial contractility and cardiac output fall dramatically. Both atrial and ventricular fibrillation can occur.

Full-body (including the head) immersion in cold water initiates the "diving reflex." The diving reflex involves apnea, bradycardia, increased total peripheral vascular resistance with decreased stroke volume, and cardiac output with an increased mean arterial pressure. The diving reflex and hypothermia cause decreased metabolic activity, which may explain prolonged submersion survival from the minimized cardiac work, vasoconstriction of all noncritical vascular beds, and resulting conservation of oxygen consumption.

Respiratory system: Hypothermia causes a fall in the respiratory rate, progressively resulting in hypoxia, carbon dioxide retention, and severe respiratory acidosis. Mucociliary function is also depressed, predisposing to pneumonia.

Renal: Hypothermia is associated with "cold diuresis," thought to be due to decreased sensitivity to antidiuretic hormone.

Hematologic system: There is a 2% increase in blood viscosity for every 1 °C drop in temperature. Hemoconcentration can also be related to secondary cold diuresis. As a result, the rheologic blood flow is suboptimal, which could potentiate sludging and thrombosis.

On the other hand, hypothermia results in decreasing platelet function and platelet count. Sequestration of platelets occurs primarily in the portal venous system. Enzymes involved in regulation are also affected, even with mild hypothermia. As much as 40% of coagulation enzymatic activity of coagulation factors can be lost with a temperature of 34 °C. A syndrome similar to disseminated intravascular coagulation with an increased propensity for thromboembolism can occur.

PREDISPOSING FACTORS

As with all thermal injury, the ambient temperature and the length of exposure are the primary determining factors for the degree of injury. Several predisposing factors potentiate the effect of low temperature in causing the various forms of cold injury. Wind chill and moisture such as in wet clothing are major contributing factors, as are other circumstances that may cause the rapid conduction of heat away from the exposed tissue (e.g., direct contact with cold objects such as metal). A multitude of host factors has been shown to contribute to the incidence and severity of cold injury. These include age and infirmity; substance abuse, especially alcohol; neurologic and mental factors, including psychiatric illness, fatigue, and apathy; and social factors, such as homelessness, lack of protective clothing, winter activities, and climbing. Both cold and high altitudes raise the viscosity of blood, slowing peripheral blood flow. These factors plus hypoxia make climbing at altitudes greater than 17,000 feet particularly dangerous. Concurrent factors such as cigarette smoking and peripheral vascular disease also contribute to the severity of the injury.

ACCIDENTAL HYPOTHERMIA

Accidental hypothermia can be subdivided into primary and secondary. Primary accidental hypothermia occurs in patients with normal thermoregulatory mechanisms that become hypothermic from extreme cold stress. Secondary accidental hypothermia occurs when the patient's thermoregulatory mechanisms are abnormal, and hypothermia results from being subjected to only relatively mild cold stress. The mortality rate associated with secondary hypothermia is much greater because of the comorbidities that affect the thermoregulatory mechanisms. These comorbidities include hemorrhage associated with trauma, stroke, hypoglycemia, intoxication, and hypothyroidism.

Hypothermia can also be classified according to its severity, as follows: *Mild hypothermia,* with core temperatures between 32°C and 35 °C; *moderate hypothermia,* with temperatures between 30 °C and 32 °C; and *severe hypothermia,* with temperatures below

30 °C. As already noted in the section on the systemic effects of hypothermia, various systemic events can be expected at different degrees of hypothermia. Humans become poikilothermic (i.e., behave as if cold blooded) at approximately 30 °C. At 23 °C, apnea commonly occurs. Asystole commonly occurs at 21 °C.

MANAGEMENT OF HYPOTHERMIA

The management of hypothermia consists of rapid rewarming with close monitoring and management of the effects of the hypothermia. Rewarming methods are classified as *passive* and *active* and are tabulated in Table 2.

It is exceedingly important to understand that a cold, cyanotic patient with no respiratory or cardiac activity may not be dead, and recovery might be possible. Rescue efforts should continue until rewarming is achieved so that the patient can be declared "warm and dead."

Prehospital Care

Prehospital care consists of removing the patient from the cold environment and eliminating all sources of heat loss such as cold, wet clothing. Ideally the patient should be dried off and clothed or covered with warm, dry coverings or at least with coverings that will prevent further heat loss. Any areas suspected of being frozen should not be thawed in the prehospital environment if there is a possibility that they may be exposed to cold again because secondary freezing adds further damage to the initial insult. Massage, friction rubbing, and manipulation should be minimized to avoid trauma to cold, stressed body parts. These parts should be immobilized, padded, and splinted.

Definitive Care

When the patient arrives at the treating facility, diagnosis should be confirmed with a thermometer that has an adequate scale to measure the extremes of cold. If shivering is present, mild hypothermia

Table 2: Rewarming Techniques for Hypothermia

Passive
Warm environment
Shivering
Blanket or clothing insulation

Active
External
Heating pad
Immersion in warm bath
External convection heaters
Internal
Heated intravenous solutions
Hemodialysis
Gastric/colonic lavage
Peritoneal lavage
Mediastinal lavage
Warmed inhalational agents
Extracorporeal circulation

From Bickel KD: In Cameron JL, editor: Current surgical therapy, *ed 6, St Louis, 1998, Mosby.*

is the probable diagnosis. The absence of shivering suggests more severe hypothermia.

The patient is approached, as with any trauma patient, by first ensuring the adequacy of airway, breathing, and circulation. Cardiopulmonary resuscitation is instituted in the absence of an effective cardiac rhythm. In general, cardiac drugs and fibrillation are withheld until rewarming to at least 28 °C is achieved because these measures probably would be ineffective at a lesser temperature. Large-bore intravenous access is established and a Foley catheter placed. Then blood is drawn and sent to the laboratory for routine tests, including drug toxicology and blood alcohol levels. Arterial blood gases, electrocardiogram, and a chest x-ray are obtained.

Severely hypothermic patients will require continuous monitoring in an intensive care setting along with serial blood tests to follow electrolytes for monitoring hyperkalemia and rhabdomyolysis. Cold diuresis or alcoholic diuresis can mislead the physician into thinking that the patient is adequately hydrated; thus urine output should not be the only measure of hydration that is closely followed. Pulmonary artery catheters are contraindicated because they might induce myocardial irritability. Cardiac disturbances occur during external warming as a result of a temperature difference that develops between the warmer epicardium and the cooler endocardium. Electric conduction is more efficient in warmer myocardial cells. The conduction fibers internally remain relatively cooler and conduct more slowly, leading to fibrillation.

Treatment of mildly-to-moderately hypothermic patients consists primarily of active external measures. Immersion in a warm bath is probably the most efficient. Use of external convection heaters, including devices such as the Bair Hugger and radiant heaters, is also helpful.

Severely hypothermic patients may require more aggressive, internal rewarming techniques. *Warmed intravenous solutions* are important but cannot be relied on to restore body temperature efficiently. The relatively small difference in temperature between the fluid and the body provides only modest additional heat to the relatively large body mass. It is most useful in those hypothermic patients who require a large volume of fluid resuscitation or if there is ongoing blood loss. *Body cavity lavage* is the circulation of warm fluid through the thoracic or abdominal cavities. When this is performed with warmed fluids in the thoracic cavity, direct cardiac rewarming occurs and may be the method of choice when arrhythmia is present. Similarly, lavage of the peritoneal cavity restores liver functions more quickly. The heat-exchange surface of the stomach, colon, and bladder is poor, and therefore lavage of these organs is inefficient in rewarming the body.

Cardiopulmonary bypass is the most efficient way of rewarming severely hypothermic patients. In medical centers that do not have open-heart surgery programs, continuous arteriovenous rewarming (CAVR), first described by Gentilello, should be considered. CAVR uses femoral arterial and venous lines to create an arteriovenous fistula that runs continuously through an external warming system using the patient's own blood pressure. Although CAVR is not as efficient as cardiopulmonary bypass for rewarming, it has the advantage of not requiring heparinization, as does bypass.

Clinical Spectrum

The various forms of localized cold injury are classified by their clinical presentation, the conditions in which they occur, and the degree of ultimate tissue injury. *Frostnip* is the earliest manifestation, least severe, and the only fully reversible one. It is characterized by pallor and numbness of the involved tissue. Warming of the tissues reverses the condition entirely and prevents tissue loss. *Pernio or chilblains* is another mild form of cold injury caused by repeated exposure to cold but not freezing temperatures in the presence of high humidity. There is no actual freezing of tissue. The lesions are red and pruritic and located on the feet and other similarly exposed areas. The condition is thought to be a chronic vasculitis rather than actual tissue destruction. Pernio is self-limited, and treatment consists of removal of the inciting cause, elevation, and application of moisturizers. *Frostbite* is the most severe of the localized forms of cold injury and is characterized by actual destruction of tissue.

Pathophysiology

Frostbite itself is a spectrum of injury severity that appears to have two distinct mechanisms of tissue destruction: (1) direct cellular destruction occurring at the time of exposure, and (2) progressive dermal ischemia resulting in further necrosis.

Direct cellular damage results from the freezing of the exposed tissue. Initially, extracellular ice crystals are formed, damaging the cell membrane and changing the osmotic gradient across it. Intracellular dehydration results, causing cell death. Continued decrease in temperature causes intracellular ice-crystal formation, leading to actual mechanical destruction of the cells. Immediate dermal ischemia develops, but initially it is moderated by alternating cycles of vasoconstriction and vasodilatation known as the *hunting reaction*. With the vasodilatation, a degree of thawing results. This process of partial thawing and refreezing with continued cold exposure appears to cause further cellular damage and, particularly, endothelial cell damage. This, in association with increasing viscosity of the blood with decreased temperature, causes a progressive thrombosis of the microcirculation.

In animal studies examining both types of injury, continued progressive necrosis seen in frostbite is similar to that seen in thermal burn injury. Inflammatory mediators such as prostaglandins and thromboxanes, bradykinin and histamine in edema formation, endothelial injury, and subsequent reduction and cessation of dermal blood flow apparently play a part. Furthermore, manipulation of these mediators has similar effects in both conditions in these models. These and other components of the inflammatory response to injury result in edema formation and endothelial cell damage, leading to the slowing and ultimate cessation of blood flow in the injured part. Rewarming of the area of frostbite necessary for treatment leads to ischemia/reperfusion injury, resulting in the obstruction of the microcirculation with leukocyte or platelet thrombi.

Clinical Manifestations

Frostbite classically has been classified into four degrees. *First-degree* frostbite is characterized by anesthetic, central, white plaque with peripheral erythema. *Second-degree* injury is diagnosed when blisters filled with clear or milky fluid surrounded by erythema and edema appear in the first 24 hours. Hemorrhagic blisters leading to black eschars over the course of 2 weeks represent *third-degree* damage. Complete necrosis and tissue loss is characteristic of *fourth-degree* frostbite. These levels of injury are diagnosed tentatively by the appearance after rewarming, but conclusively only by the clinical course of the injury after complete demarcation of the tissue loss. Therefore it is usually more helpful to consider frostbite injury in one of two general categories at the time of initial presentation: superficial or deep. These tend to predict outcome more accurately.

The patient's symptoms help to predict the severity of the injury. The patient usually describes numbness of the injured part. In the case of the hands, there will be a feeling of clumsiness and lack of fine motor control. With rewarming, the patient develops a throbbing sensation that may last several days or weeks. Later, these sensations may be replaced by tingling sensations with occasional electric–shock-type shooting pains.

On physical examination, the sensibility of the part should be tested. The ability to sense light touch and successively noxious stimuli will help to determine the prognosis of the injury. Favorable prognostic indicators suggesting superficial injury would be normal skin color on rewarming, or, if blisters form, the development of clear fluid in the blisters. Milky fluid suggests a superficial but deeper injury. The ability of the skin to deform under pressure is considered a sign of viability and therefore is favorable. Deep injury is suggested by dark color; hemorrhagic blisters; nonblanching cyanosis: and hard, nondeforming skin.

Ancillary laboratory tests have little to offer in the definitive diagnosis of the extent of injury early in its course. Clinical examination alone will frequently not establish the extent of tissue injury deep to the skin. Radionuclide scanning techniques have been described to attempt to delineate the blood flow of the injured part, but they are generally too vague to determine tissue viability accurately enough to guide early debridement. Arteriography can delineate flow in larger blood vessels but cannot accurately delimit ischemic or nonviable tissue. Magnetic resonance imaging may be a superior technique for this purpose because it can directly visualize blood vessels and give a more definite delineation of ischemic soft tissue. Laser Doppler flowmetry has been shown to quantify tissue blood flow in burn injuries, but there is minimal information about its use in frostbite. Presently, no technique is sufficiently accurate to guide excision of tissue in the early stages of frostbite to make it clinically useful.

Cauchy demonstrated that bone scans have excellent correlation with the extent of acral necrosis and ultimate level of amputation in frostbite injuries. The correlation was good when the bone scan was taken as early as 3 days. The correlation was even better when the scan was taken at day 7 or later.

Management of Frostbite

There are three phases of frostbite treatment: (1) prethaw, prehospital phase, (2) immediate hospital (rewarming) phase, and 3) postthaw care phase.

Prethaw, Prehospital Care

The prethaw, prehospital care takes place before reaching a health care center and consists primarily of protecting the injured part from mechanical trauma and avoiding thawing until definitive rewarming can be performed and the part can be kept warm. Rubbing the affected part with the warm hand or snow or placing it near a heat source should *not* be performed because the part may be further traumatized mechanically or by refreezing when the heat is withdrawn. Furthermore, slow rewarming in suboptimal conditions is not as beneficial as proper rewarming that can be performed in an adequate health care center.

Immediate Hospital Care (Rewarming)

Immediate hospital rewarming is performed rapidly at temperatures of 40 °C to 42 °C (104 °F-108 °F) in a waterbath containing a mild antibacterial agent such as 4% chlorhexidine gluconate (Hibiclens; Mölnlycke Health Care US, Norcross, GA) or povidone-iodine. This temperature range is important because lower temperatures have been shown to reduce tissue survival and higher temperatures might increase the injury through thermal damage. This rewarming should be continued for at least 15 to 20 minutes or until thawing is complete. A red or purple appearance and pliable texture of the involved part indicate the end of vasoconstriction and that rewarming can be discontinued. Active motion during rewarming is helpful, but massage may increase tissue damage. Rhabdomyolysis and subsequent renal failure have been reported in some cases of frostbite involving muscle and constitute another indication for intravenous fluids.

Postthaw Hospital Care

Postthaw care is directed to reducing the progressive dermal ischemia seen in frostbite injury. Work by McCauley and colleagues established a therapeutic approach that is based on current knowledge of pathophysiology (Table 3).

Table 3: Treatment Protocol for Frostbite

1. Admit frostbite patient to a specialist unit, if possible.

2. On admission, rapidly rewarm the affected areas in warm water at 40 °C to 42 °C (104 °F–108 °F) for 15 to 30 minutes or until thawing is complete.

3. On completion of rewarming, treat the affected parts as follows:

   a. Debride white blisters and begin topical treatment with aloe vera (Dermaide aloe cream; Dermaide, Chicago, IL) every 6 hours.

   b. Leave hemorrhagic blisters intact and begin treatment with topical aloe vera (Dermaide aloe cream) every 6 hours.

   c. Elevate the affected part(s) with splinting as indicated.

   d. Administer antitetanus prophylaxis (toxoid or immunoglobulin).

   e. Analgesia: opiate, intramuscularly or intravenously as indicated.

   f. Administer ibuprofen (400 mg orally every 12 hours).

   g. Administer benzyl penicillin (600 mg every 6 hours for 48 to 72 hours).

   h. Perform daily hydrotherapy for 30 to 45 minutes at 45 °C.

4. For documentation, obtain photographic records on admission, at 24 hours, and serially every 2 to 3 days until discharge.

5. Prohibit smoking.

From Murphy JV, and others: J Trauma 48:171, 2000; adapted from McCauley RL, Hing DN, Robson MC, and others: J Trauma 23:143, 1983.

White blisters are debrided to reduce the contact of the wound with the high levels of prostaglandin F2-alpha and thromboxane A2 in the blister fluid. The resulting wounds are treated topically with aloe vera every 6 hours. Hemorrhagic blisters suggest damage to the superficial dermal plexus and are best left intact to prevent desiccation by exposure if debrided. These are treated with aloe vera on the intact blisters. Aloe vera is used as a topical inhibitor of thromboxane. When used in conjunction with ibuprofen and penicillin or with the vasodilator oxpentifylline, aloe vera has been shown to reduce tissue necrosis. The affected part(s) is elevated and splinted as indicated. In this way, edema is reduced. Not only is edema associated with poor wound healing but it also has been implicated in the pathogenesis of progressive ischemic necrosis seen in frostbite and thermal injuries. Edema has also been found to inhibit the skin's streptococcicidal properties. Tetanus prophylaxis is administered. Analgesics are given along with ibuprofen 400 mg every 12 hours as an antithromboxane agent. Some use antibiotics prophylactically, whereas others prefer to use them for specific infectious complications. Daily hydrotherapy and wound care allow debridement of the wounds and encourage active and passive range of motion in an effort to preserve function.

A number of other therapeutic modalities have been investigated to determine whether they might reduce the progressive tissue damage seen in frostbite. These include infusion of low-molecular-weight dextran to reduce blood viscosity; anticoagulation (particularly with heparin to reduce thrombosis of the superficial dermal plexus); hyperbaric oxygen; and the use of vasodilators such as the intra-arterial use of reserpine. None of these has been conclusively shown to

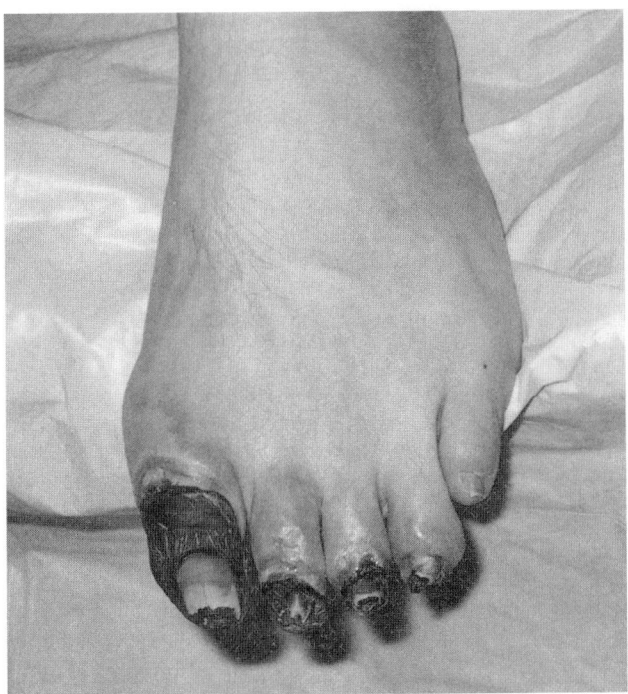

Figure 1   Demarcating deep frostbite, 2 months after injury.

improve tissue viability over that seen with rapid rewarming. Thrombolysis has shown definite promise in animal models and preliminary success clinically in reducing the extent of tissue loss in frostbite. Further clinical study is necessary.

Early surgical care consists of limited debridement of blisters and obviously necrotic tissue, and, rarely, escharotomy and fasciotomy if circulation is impaired or compartment syndrome develops. Amputation and more aggressive debridement are generally delayed until the progressive ischemia is complete and final demarcation is achieved (Fig. 1); these often take 1 to 3 months. However,

confirmation of the observations of Cauchy (discussed earlier) may lead to more rapid definitive therapy.

Late sequelae of frostbite injury include cold sensitivity, sensory loss, and hyperhidrosis affecting the injured part and may last for years. Growth-plate changes, osteoarthritis, chronic pain, and heterotopic calcification have all been reported as long-term effects of frostbite.

SUGGESTED READINGS

Bickel KD: Cold injury. In Cameron JL, editor: *Current surgical therapy,* ed 6, St Louis, 1998, Mosby.

Cauchy E, Chetaille E, Lefevre M, and others: The role of bone scanning in severe frostbite of the extremities: a retrospective study of 88 cases, *Eur J Nucl Med* 27:497, 2000.

Cauchy E, Marsigny B, Allamel G, and others: The value of technetium 99 scintigraphy in the prognosis of amputation in severe frostbite injuries of the extremities: a retrospective study of 92 severe frostbite injuries, *J Hand Surg [Am]* 25:969, 2000.

Gentilello LM, Cortes V, Moujaes S, and others: Continuous arteriovenous rewarming: experimental results and thermodynamic model simulation of treatment for hypothermia, *J Trauma* 30:1436, 1990.

Harari A, Regnier B, Rapin M, and others: Haemodynamic study of prolonged deep accidental hypothermia, *Eur J Intensive Care Med* 1:65, 1975.

Heimbach D, Jurkovich GJ, Gentilello LM: Accidental hypothermia. In Shoemaker WC, Ayres SM, Grenvik A, and others, editors: *Textbook of critical care,* ed 4, Philadelphia, 2000, WB Saunders.

McCauley RL, Hing DN, Robson MC, and others: Frostbite injuries: a rational approach based on the pathophysiology, *J Trauma* 23:143, 1983.

Morris SE: Cold-induced injury: frostbite. In Herndon DN, editor: *Total burn care,* ed 2, Philadelphia, 2002, WB Saunders.

Murphy JV, Banwell PE, Roberts AH, and others: Frostbite: pathogenesis and treatment, *J Trauma* 48:171, 2000.

Petrone P, Kuncir EJ, Asensio JA: Surgical management and strategies in the treatment of hypothermia and cold injury, *Emerg Med Clin North Am* 21:1165, 2003.

Singh NK: Cold injury. In Cameron JL, editor: *Current surgical therapy,* ed 8, Philadelphia, 2004, Mosby.

Tveita T, Mortensen E, Hevroy O, and others: Hemodynamic and metabolic effects of hypothermia and rewarming, *Arctic Med Res* 50(suppl 6): 48, 1991.

ELECTRICAL AND LIGHTNING INJURIES

Robert J. Spence, MD

Humans have always been injured by electricity due to exposure to lightning. The awesome power and destructive capability of electricity in this form led to deification of it from human's earliest history. The discovery and widespread use of electricity are much more recent. The first fatality from electricity was recorded in France in 1879.

Now, at the beginning of the 21st century, electrical injury causes in excess of 500 deaths per year in the United States. Most deaths occur in the workplace and represent 5% to 6% of all workers' deaths overall. There are more than 200 electrocutions (i.e., deaths by electricity) per year in the home. Lightning causes an average of 93 deaths per year in the United States.

Electrical injuries represent 3% to 4% of admissions to U.S. burn centers. "Electrocution" does not apply to living patients, as the term connotes death by electricity. Although many admissions represent short-term observation for possible cardiac effects, those that are a result of serious electrical injury average longer stays and greater expense than admissions for thermal injury.

Overall, electrical injuries account for 2% to 3% of all burns in children requiring emergency department care. Pediatric electrical injuries generally occur in the home, are associated with low-voltage electrical cords and wall outlets, and rarely require admission to intensive care units. An oral commissure burn from biting on an electrical cord causing a spark is a common presentation in young children. Older children are exposed in life-threatening high-voltage injury through climbing activities.

PHYSICS AND PATHOPHYSIOLOGY

Electricity is defined as the flow of electrons through a conductor from an area of electron excess (negative charge) toward an area of relative deficiency (positive charge). The flow of electrons (electrical current) is measured in amperes. The force that causes the flow is the potential energy caused by the relative difference in charge between the negative and positive poles. This force (voltage) is measured in volts. Anything that impedes the flow of electrons in the conductor is termed *resistance* and is measured in units called *ohms*. Materials that are the best conductors have the least resistance. With increasing resistance, more energy is expended in the form of heat.

Electrical power in common usage is generated at very high voltages, often exceeding one million volts. The voltage is gradually reduced through a series of transformers as power lines distribute the power for industrial and home use. The voltage in common use in the United States and Canada is 120/240 V, providing 240 V, for appliances requiring high power and 120 V for general use. The household current in most other countries is 220 V. The U.S. National Electrical Code defines less than 600 V as low voltage. Medically, the traditional distinction between high- and low-voltage electrical injury is defined as those caused by voltages more or less than 1000 V.

Electrical current exists in two forms. By far the most common is alternating current (AC) in which the electrons flow back and forth cyclically with a standardized frequency of 60 cycles per second (60 Hz). Direct current (DC) is the second form where the electrons flow in only one direction. This current is produced by batteries and from AC current using transformers. AC current is more efficient, but also more dangerous because it causes tetanic contractions that prevent a victim from releasing the electrical source and can alter the cardiac cycle, causing arrhythmias and cardiac arrest.

Electrical injury occurs when a person comes in contact with an electrical source with enough current to cause either tissue damage or electrical abnormalities within the body. The injury can be a direct or indirect effect of the electrical current. The direct damage is due to the actual effect of the current on the body tissues such as destruction by the conversion of the electrical energy into heat, causing thermal damage, or by direct electrical effects on the myocardium. Indirect injuries result from secondary effects such as muscle contraction, the electricity rendering the victim unconscious, or the ignition of clothing or nearby flammables by the arcing of the current.

Tissue damage is most obviously caused when electrical energy is converted to heat, causing a thermal burn. The heat and the subsequent damage are proportional to the square of the current multiplied by the resistance of the tissue (Joule's law: Power = I^2R). Tissues have different resistances innately and under different conditions. Dry skin has a much greater resistance than moist skin. The tissues with least resistance are nerves and blood vessels. Although damage to individual tissues resulting from bodily transmission of current is often considered as being relative to their individual resistance, more likely the body acts as a "single-block" resistance, particularly in the case of high-voltage injury. Greater destruction to deeper tissues is likely due to retained heat in the deep tissues such as in the interosseous spaces. Voltage across smaller areas of tissue causes greater damage because electric field strength is concentrated there. Field strength is the voltage difference per unit length. This explains why areas of smaller cross-sectional area such as the wrist and ankles tend to be most damaged in high-voltage transmission injuries. Even in low-voltage injuries, the highly concentrated field strength in the short distance between a child's two lips can create a devastating injury.

The thermal injury can be divided into three components, as follows: (1) that caused by direct conduction of current against tissue resistance resulting in heating of the tissues; (2) direct thermal burn from the intense heat of arcing (up to 5000 °C), which is caused when high-voltage current passes through the air from negative to positive points; and (3) direct thermal burn from ignited clothing and nearby combustibles.

Direct electrical damage to tissue exclusive of thermal injury occurs when current disrupts the cell membrane and the microelectrical gradient across it. This process is called *electroporation*. Other, less obvious effects may help explain why this type of electrical injury often seems to evolve with time. Cytokine release with thrombosis of the local microvasculature, late thrombosis of injured vessels, and circulatory obstruction from edema and infection most likely contribute.

Not all components are necessarily present in every electrical injury. The skin is usually the first point of contact. The skin is charred to a greater or lesser extent depending on its resistance and the current. In low-voltage injuries, the char causes the resistance to rise dramatically, limiting the further conduction of current. In high-voltage injuries, the increase in resistance is not significant, and the current passes to the deeper tissues where conduction takes place, heating the tissues to a greater or lesser extend depending on the magnitude of the current and the duration of time of conduction. The current escapes the body at some other contact point seen as a wound in the skin, frequently referred to as an "exit injury." Occasionally, even in a high-voltage situation, a simple flash or arcing of electricity without actual damaging internal current conduction can cause external thermal damage without the internal heating and deep tissue damage. It is therefore important to distinguish between "flash" injuries and the true "transmission" electrical injuries.

In a transmission injury, even after the current ceases, the energy, now in the form of heat, dissipates through the tissues, causing often extensive secondary injury. Extravasation of fluid causes fluid depletion, an enormous amount of edema, and increases in compartment pressures. Muscle necrosis can be extensive, releasing intracellular enzymes and myoglobin. Intravascular fluid depletion and myoglobin endanger renal function. Further secondary effects referred to above come into play over time, resulting in an apparently progressive injury and necrosis of tissue. Although the true progressive necrosis of tissue in electrical injury is controversial, clinically there clearly tends to be necrotic tissue that develops in debrided wounds for several days after the initial insult.

Because AC current causes 99% of these injuries with reversal of the direction of the current 120 times per second, that is, 60 cycles, the designation of entrance and exit points is academic at best. However, the positioning of these skin wounds suggests the pathway of the current. This pathway determines the number of organs that are affected by the current. A "vertical path" parallel to the axis of the body is most dangerous because it may affect all of the vital organs. A "horizontal path" from hand to hand may spare the brain but may still be fatal from its effect on the heart, respiratory muscles, and spinal cord. A path with contact points confined to a single extremity may cause extensive local damage, but not be lethal.

Immediate cardiac arrest and life-threatening arrhythmias may occur with the conduction of current across the heart. AC current tends to cause ventricular fibrillation, whereas DC current tends to cause asystole. Actual injury to the heart or the metabolic effects from injury elsewhere in the body (e.g., hyperkalemia) may result in delayed cardiac arrhythmias. Paralysis of the muscles of respiration can result in apnea. Effects on the spinal cord and brain can lead to immediate death or long-term neurologic abnormalities.

Lightning is a form of DC current and causes a unique type of electrical injury. It occurs when the massive electron buildup in a thundercloud causes such a huge voltage difference (more than one million volts) between it and the ground that it overcomes the resistance in the intervening air. The current of a lightning strike can be more than 200,000 amps, and the transformation of this electrical energy to heat can generate temperatures as high as 50,000 °F. However, the duration of this transmission is only 1 to 2 ms. As a result, the insulating function of the skin does not have time to break down. Actual charring of the skin with "entrance" and "exit" wounds is rare, as is the actual deep tissue conduction of electrical current seen in conventional electrical

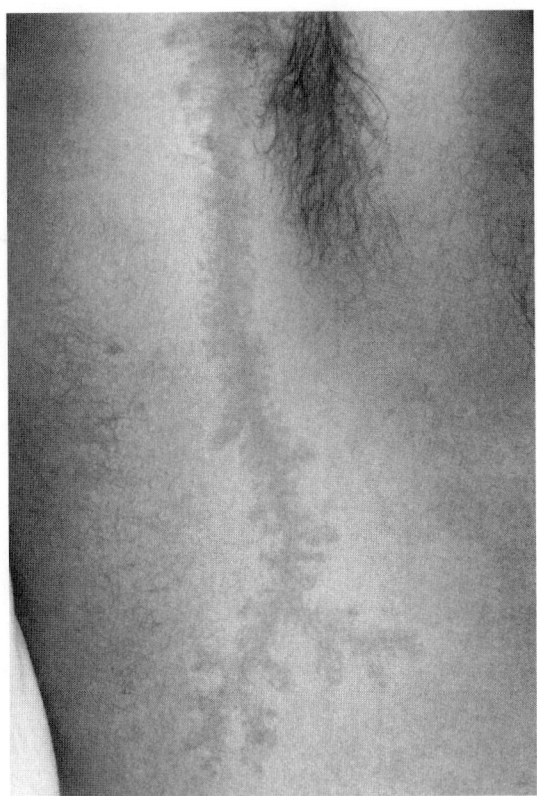

Figure 1 Keraunographic marking associated with lightning injury. *From Cohen MA: Acad Emerg Med 8:893, 2001.*

injury. The current tends to flow along the surface of the body, causing more or less serious burns depending on the heat, duration, and dissipation of the heat. There may be an explosive vaporization of the humidity on the skin surface that may blast away the victim's clothes.

Most commonly, the thermal burns are superficial from a direct strike in which nothing in contact with the patient ignites. A pathognomonic fernlike pattern on the skin called *Lichtenberg figures* or *keraunographic markings* may appear (Fig. 1). These markings are thought not to be actual burns, but the result of the electron flow over the body surface, and often disappear within 24 hours. Interestingly, similar markings can be seen on the ground around lightning strikes.

Actual lightning injuries may be caused by various mechanisms:

1. Direct strike
2. Side flash or "splash" that occurs when lightning hits a nearby object and jumps to the victim
3. Direct contact with an object that has been struck
4. Current flow through the ground with buildup of a potential difference between the extremities of the victim (step voltage)
5. Thermal burns through clothing or other heated material
6. Trauma caused by shockwave (e.g., ruptured tympanic membrane)
7. Injury caused by a fall

The most common causes of death from lightning injury are cardiopulmonary arrest and apnea. The interruption of the cardiac cycle caused by the DC results in asystole, but like a defibrillator, spontaneous cardiac activity resumes shortly thereafter. The apnea that results from the DC on the brain's respiratory center, however, is longer lasting and if left untreated will result in hypoxia, arrhythmias, and secondary cardiac arrest.

Another common injury associated with lightning injury is that on the central nervous system. Unconsciousness, paresis, paresthesia, and hypoesthesia all occur and are generally temporary, although long-term effects have been observed. Autonomic dysfunction with Horner's syndrome, papillary dilatation, areflexia, and anisocoria can occur. Cataracts, tympanic membrane rupture, and sensorineural hearing loss can all occur as long-term effects of lightning strike, some of which is attributed to the shockwave.

EVALUATION AND MANAGEMENT

In the Field

At the time of an electrical injury, any attempt to contact the victim while still in contact with the intact electrical circuit will likely result in injury to the rescuer. The first rule of electrical injury is to turn the power off. Once disconnected from the electrical source, life support measures are instituted if necessary. Apnea and cardiac asystole or arrhythmias are treated with cardiopulmonary resuscitation. Associated injuries from involuntary muscle contractures or falls must be considered immediately and treated accordingly when suspected or obviously present. Once stabilized, the patient is taken to a hospital for further diagnosis and treatment.

In the Hospital

Further evaluation in the hospital requires the removal of all clothing, and the entire skin surface must be examined. The scalp must be closely examined to find any occult points of contact that might suggest intracranial injury. Direct contact burns of the trunk must also raise the suspicion of intrathoracic or intraabdominal injuries. Significant burns of the scalp or trunk may warrant a computed tomography or magnetic resonance imaging scan to rule out underlying deep tissue damage. The extent of burns is documented using the Lund and Browder diagram giving the percentage of total body surface area (TBSA) injured. The history of the electrical injury is reviewed, and the injury is classified in terms of low or high voltage, whether actual transmission of high-voltage current was likely, and the likely path of that transmission.

A full physical examination is performed to discover other direct and indirect injuries. Careful baseline neurologic and ophthalmologic examinations are performed. Radiologic examination for fractures and to rule out spinal injury may be required. Based on the history and physical examination, a clear determination of whether the electrical source was low or high voltage is made. If the voltage was greater than 1000 V, determination of transmission through deep tissues upgrades the seriousness of the diagnosis with increased concerns of deep tissue necrosis, compartment syndrome, renal failure, and cardiac and neurologic sequelae.

Low-voltage electrical injuries are treated with topical antibiotic treatment of the usually small charred burn wounds at the points of contact, as well as cardiac monitoring. History of unconsciousness or dysrhythmia, abnormality of mental status on examination, or electrocardiographic abnormalities require admission for cardiac monitoring.

High-voltage flash injuries with no apparent transmission of high voltage can largely be treated as equivalent-sized thermal burns with regard to fluid resuscitation and wound management. Intravenous fluids are begun immediately or as soon as possible, and a urinary catheter is placed for the larger burns. All patients are placed on cardiac monitoring, and blood tests for cardiac enzymes and myoglobin are sent as a final check for transmission injury.

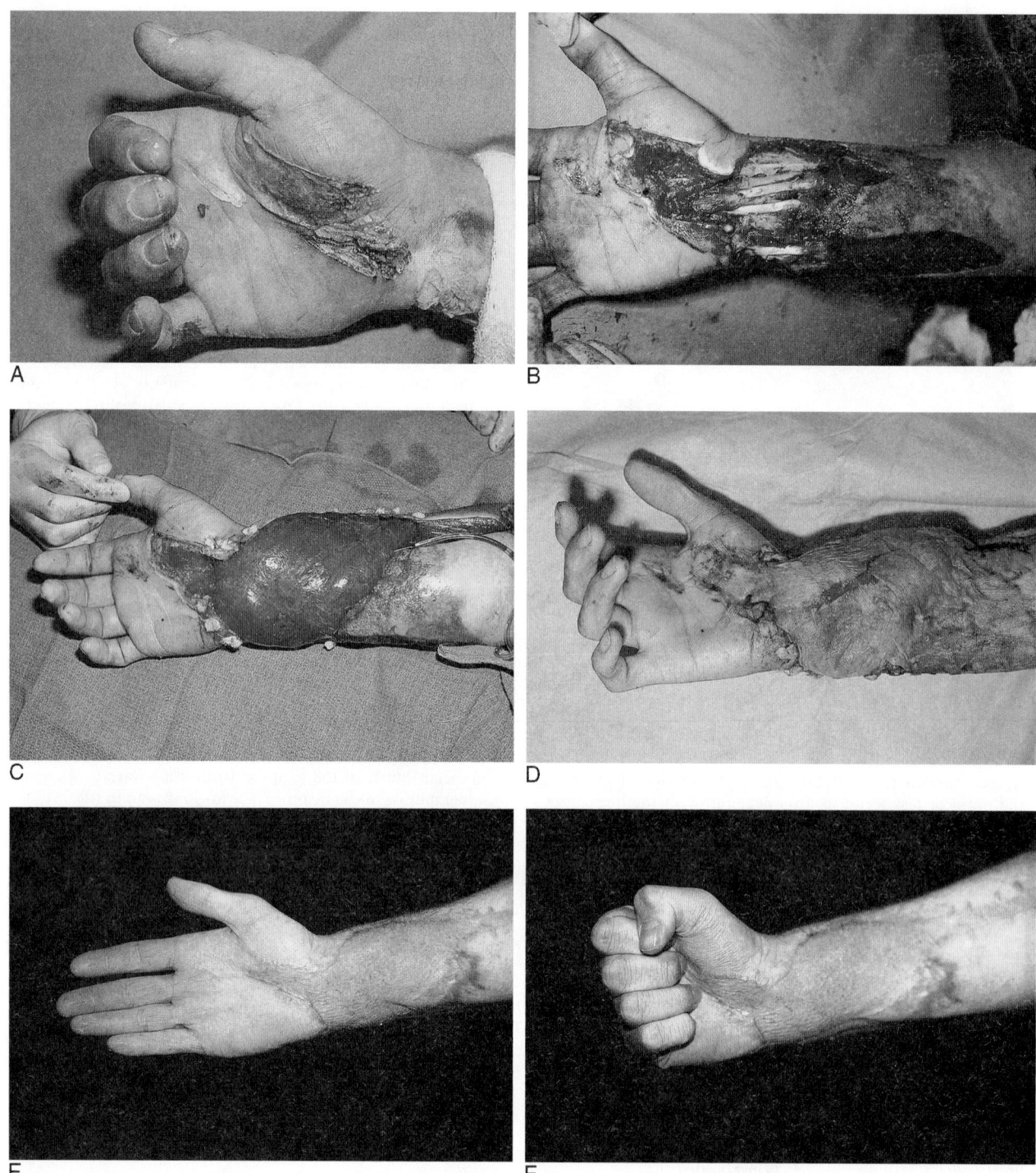

Figure 2 **(A)** Right hand and wrist component of 13,000-V transmission electrical injury on day of injury. **(B)** Serial debridement and sheet allograft closure. Note that tendons and nerves are left intact. **(C)** Wound closure with free gracilis muscle flap attached to vein grafts to proximal vessels outside of zone of injury 18 days after injury. **(D)** Autograft skin used to cover gracilis muscle flap. **(E)** Appearance 8 months after reconstruction with gracilis free flap. Note atrophy of gracilis muscle. **(F)** Appearance 8 months after reconstruction with gracilis free flap. Note tendon function. Nerve function also returned to near normal.

High-voltage transmission injuries, because of the often large extent of deep tissue injury, require special consideration. The following discussion focuses on the particular management of these injuries in our burn center. We concur with Luce who found that these injuries require an average of 9 ml of fluid per kilogram per percentage of TBSA injured, which is more than twice the amount of fluid resuscitation of equivalent-sized thermal burns. Urine output of 1.0 to 1.5 ml/kg per hour is used as a guide. Renal failure from dehydration and myoglobinuria is a danger in these injuries with major myonecrosis. Conventionally bicarbonate and diuretics such as mannitol have been used, along with fluid resuscitation in these cases. However, Luce found that hydration alone was sufficient to treat the myoglobinuria that accompanies the deep muscle necrosis and acidosis in these injuries.

Further immediate concerns include the circulatory status of the extremities and the high risk of compartment syndrome related to the deep tissue injury and swelling within the various extremity fascial muscle compartments. As with any thermal injury, circumferential eschar may also cause vascular compromise and require treatment. For these reasons particularly, patients with high-voltage transmission injuries routinely have their wounds explored in the operating room as soon as they are stabilized and within no more than the first few hours after injury.

In the operating room, obviously necrotic tissue is débrided. Large peripheral nerves are released, particularly in the carpal and tarsal tunnels when indicated. Fasciotomies are performed whenever any concern exists regarding deep muscle injury in the path of the high-voltage electrical current. Superficial muscle may be found viable and even appear uninjured by color and electrical stimulation with cautery. However, the muscle located deeply along the bone may be severely injured. Any questionably viable tissue is not débrided at the first exploration. Open wounds remaining at the end of the initial débridement are closed with sheet (unmeshed) skin allograft to provide the most optimal environment for the marginally viable tissues and to prevent bacterial contamination in the sterile wounds. If the patient's condition allows, any obviously deep thermal burns may also be tangentially excised and autografted.

The patient is returned to the operating room every 48 hours to reexplore the wounds, débride any necrotic tissue, and reclose with sheet skin allograft. This is continued until no more necrotic tissue is present and the wound has stabilized. This usually requires 6 to 8 days (i.e., three to four operative explorations). When the wound has stabilized, reconstruction is performed with appropriate techniques. With the wound closed with sheet allograft skin, edema resolves much more rapidly and the wounds remain sterile and without granulation tissue, unlike wounds dressed with gauze dressings. The loss of edema and absence of bacteria and granulation tissue often allows primary closure of fasciotomy wounds rather than having to autograft them. Exposed avascular structures such as nerves and tendons, when uninfected, can be covered with flaps with the expectation of return of some level of function for both (Fig. 2). For smaller areas of avascularity, synthetic dermal substitutes have been used as an initial cover before autografting.

Regrettably, high-voltage transmission extremity injuries often are so severe that amputation is necessary. Rarely performed at the first exploration to allow proper preparation of patient and family, moving to primary amputation early and often at the second exploration 48 hours after injury is common. This combined with sheet allograft coverage of other wounds provides rapid primary closure of all wounds to minimize pain, prevent fluid loss and bacterial contamination, reduce the length of the catabolic state, and speed rehabilitation.

Physical and occupational therapy, nutrition, and psychologic and social services are important in treatment of these severe wounds early in their course. Long-term sequelae of dysfunction and deformity are common, and minimizing these problems should be an important early goal.

Suggested Readings

Cohen MA: Clinical pearls: struck by lightning: cutaneous manifestation of lightning strike ("splash"), *Acad Emerg Med* 8:893, 2001.

Graber J, Ummenhofer W, Herion H: Lightning accident with eight victims: case report and brief review of the literature, *J Trauma* 40:288, 1996.

Jain S, Bandi V: Electrical and lightning injuries, *Crit Care Clin* 15:319, 1999.

Koumbourlis AC: Electrical injuries, *Crit Care Med* 30:S424, 2002.

Luce EA: Electrical burns, *Clin Plast Surg* 27:133, 2000.

Muehlberger T, Vogt PM, Munster AM: The long-term consequences of lightning injuries, *Burns* 27:829, 2001.

Purdue GF, Hunt JL: Electrical injuries. In Herndon D, editor: *Total burn care*, ed 2, London, 2002, WB Saunders.

SKIN AND SOFT TISSUE

SKIN LESIONS: EVALUATION, DIAGNOSIS, AND MANAGEMENT

Rebecca Kazin, MD, and Michele A. Shermak, MD

Surgeons are often asked to evaluate and treat growths arising in the skin. This chapter highlights the distinguishing features of benign and malignant cutaneous neoplasms and reviews techniques for surgical treatment.

BENIGN CUTANEOUS NEOPLASMS

Keratoses

Seborrheic keratoses (SKs) are benign skin tumors that are exceedingly common and typically found in the over-30 age group (Fig. 1). They can appear on any part of the body, particularly the face, chest, and arms, as flat, sharply demarcated brown macules that progress into polypoid papules with a warty "stuck-on" appearance. Color can vary from pale brown with pink hues to dark brown or black. *Actinic keratoses* (AKs), also known as *solar keratoses,* are the most common epithelial precancerous lesion among light-complected patients (Fig. 2). Risk factors include age, blue eyes, and childhood freckling. Immunocompromised patients and patients with genetic melanin disorders such as albinism and xeroderma pigmentosum have increased risk for AKs as well. The risk for an individual AK to progress to an invasive squamous cell carcinoma (SCC) is low, probably less than 1 in 1000 per year, with lifetime risk of SCC estimated to be 6% to 10%. AKs are typically flesh-colored to erythematous, ill-defined macules or papules with dry adherent scale, measuring a few millimeters to several centimeters in diameter. Some lesions may have exuberant hyperkeratosis and are called *hypertrophic AK* or *cutaneous horn.* Treatment options include cryotherapy, topical 5-fluorouracil (5-FU), and topical imiquimod. Photodynamic therapy (PDT) may treat large photo-damaged areas with numerous AKs.

Cutaneous horn is a clinical term for a firm, white to yellow, conical, hyperkeratotic protuberance ranging in size from a few millimeters to several centimeters. This can arise anywhere on the body, but the face and other sun-exposed sites are most common. Many lesions may give rise to a cutaneous horn, the most common being an AK. Up to 20% of cutaneous horns arise over SCCs. Other lesions at the base of horns include SKs and verrucae.

Keratoacanthomas (KAs) clinically and microscopically resemble SCCs (Fig. 3). Clinically, KAs present as nodules (typically greater than 1 cm in diameter) with a crater-like center that contains a keratin plug, often in hair-bearing sites of sun-exposed skin in older patients. Even though it is generally accepted that KAs are benign neoplasms, on the basis of their potential for spontaneous regression over a 4- to 8-week period after a 4- to 6-week period of rapid growth, excision of these lesions is critical for proper diagnosis and management.

Dermatofibroma is a common fibrohistiocytic tumor of the skin seen primarily in adults and frequently on the lower extremities (Fig. 4). They are firm, dome-shaped papules classically less than 1 cm in size and pink or brown in color. On palpation they feel attached to subcutaneous tissue, and pinching the lesion demonstrates the "dimple sign" with apparent downward movement of the tumor. Dermatofibromas may be biopsied or excised to exclude other diagnoses.

Neurofibromas are usually slow-growing, asymptomatic, solitary, flesh-colored, rubbery papulonodules. They often demonstrate the "buttonhole sign"—the tumor is easily invaginated with finger pressure. Neurofibromas can develop as solitary, sporadic lesions or as multiple lesions, as part of peripheral neurofibromatosis (NF-I) or von Recklinghausen's disease. Neurofibromas are benign tumors composed of a proliferation of neuromesenchymal tissue including Schwann, perineural, fibroblastic, and mast cells, as well as axons. Treatment involves simple excision and is required in lesions that have demonstrated growth to rule out neurofibrosarcoma.

Nevus sebaceous (Fig. 5) is a hamartoma of varying degrees of follicular, sebaceous, and apocrine differentiation. The clinical lesion commonly involves the scalp or face and is only slightly palpable at birth. Typically scalp lesions remain hairless, and during childhood they may thicken slightly and assume slightly yellow or orange hue. In adolescence, a progressive thickening and verrucoid change may occur. Classic teaching reports that basal cell carcinomas (BCCs) may develop in up to 10% of tumors over the course of 15 to 20 years. Excision has been justified by a risk for malignant transformation.

Benign Melanocytic Neoplasms

Common acquired nevi are well-circumscribed, round to ovoid lesions, typically 2 to 6 mm in diameter, that appear symmetric with regular, defined borders. There are three subtypes defined by histologic location of collections of nevus cells: *junctional, compound,* and *intradermal.* Whereas junctional nevi are macular and dark, compound nevi are variable in elevation and lighter, and intradermal nevi are usually more elevated and skin-colored or light brown.

Becker's nevus (Fig. 6) arises predominantly in males as an irregularly shaped tan-to-brown patch, typically located over the

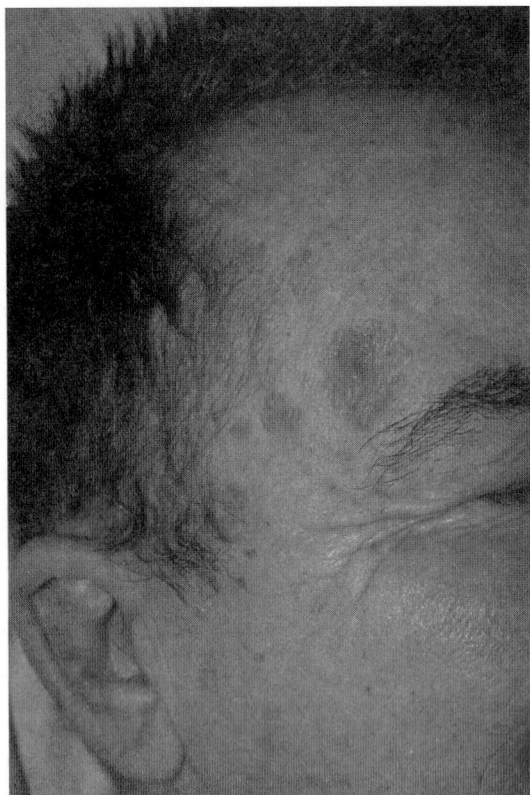

Figure 1   Seborrheic keratosis (SK) is often seen in large numbers, especially on the trunk, face, and arms of individuals older than 30 years of age. The SK typically presents as a sharply circumscribed, waxy, papillomatous plaque with a friable, hyperkeratotic surface, most often described as having a "stuck-on" appearance. (*See color insert Figure 37.*)

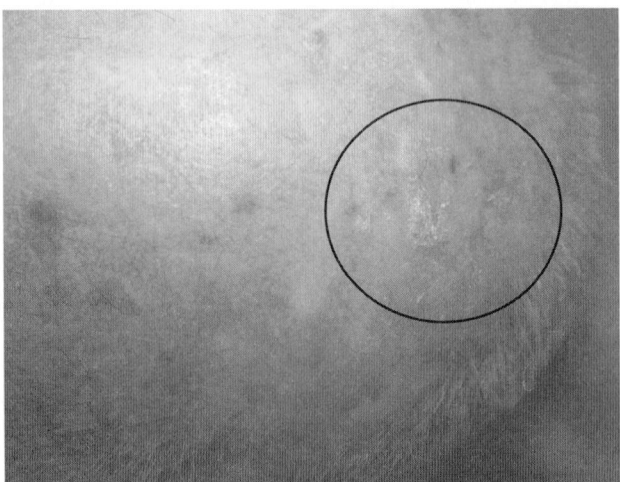

Figure 2   Actinic keratoses (AKs) are found primarily on exposed surfaces as rough, adherent hyperkeratosis that are skin-colored, yellow-brown or brown, possibly with a reddish tinge. They are often numerous in older adults. (*See color insert Figure 38.*)

shoulder, upper chest, or back. The nevus enlarges during the first several years as new, irregularly pigmented macules and patches develop at the periphery and coalesce with the larger patch. Hair may develop both within and in close proximity to the patch; however, hair density can be variable. Although it is considered benign, Becker's nevus has been associated with melanoma as discussed in a series of nine patients in whom both Becker's nevus and melanoma developed (Fehr and colleagues).

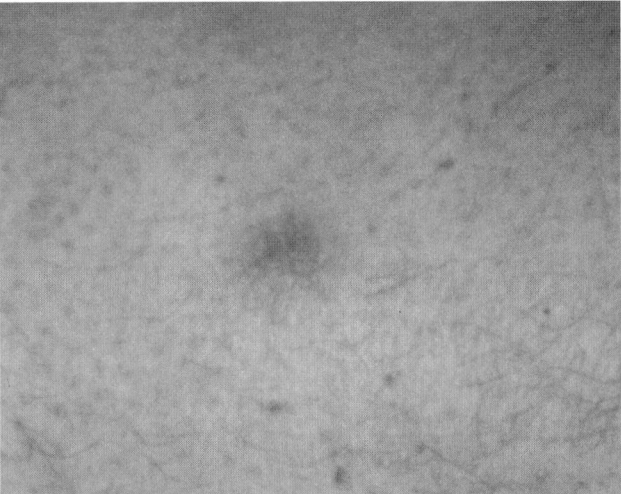

Figure 3   Dermatofibromas are firm, dome-shaped papules often found on the lower extremities. (*See color insert Figure 39.*)

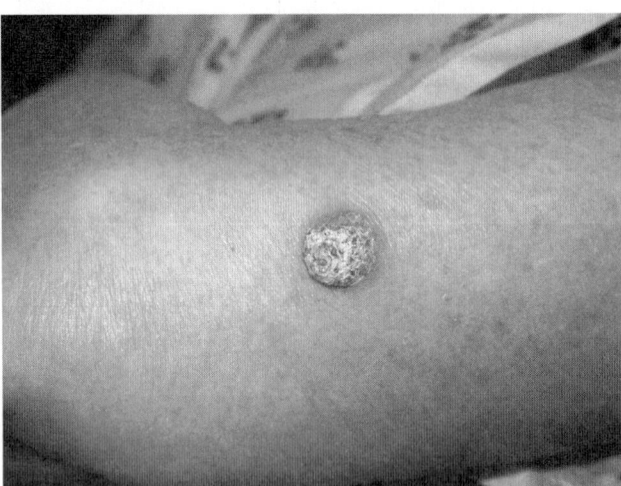

Figure 4   Keratoacanthomas are typically solitary neoplasms on sun-exposed skin that rapidly enlarge and spontaneously involute. Because of an appearance resembling squamous cell cancer, biopsy is recommended. (*See color insert Figure 40.*)

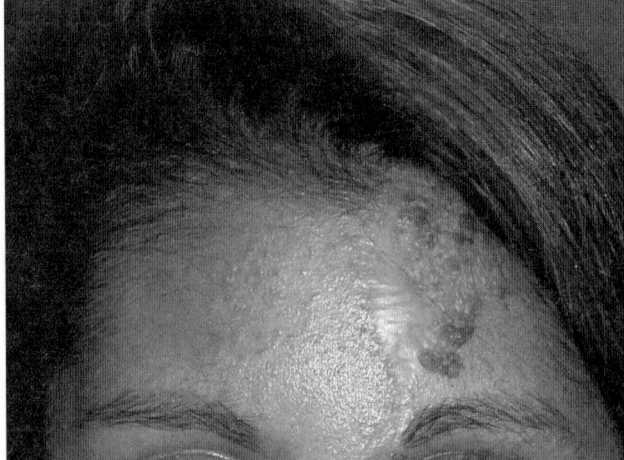

Figure 5   Nevus sebaceous is often diagnosed in children; it is found on the head and neck region and is reported to convert to basal cell cancer. In this case, serial excision was necessary because of the extensive surface area involved. (*See color insert Figure 41.*)

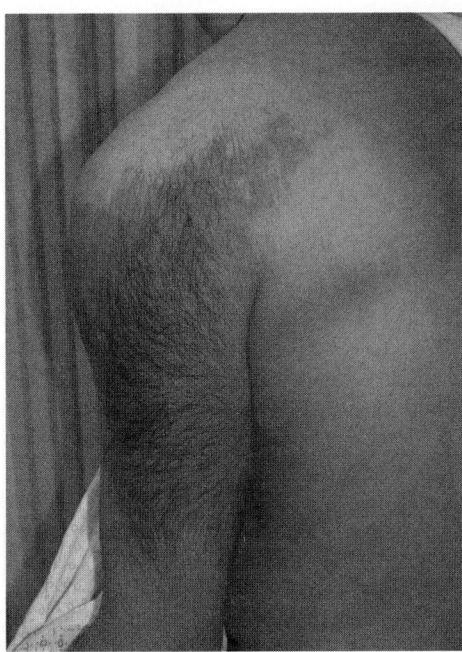

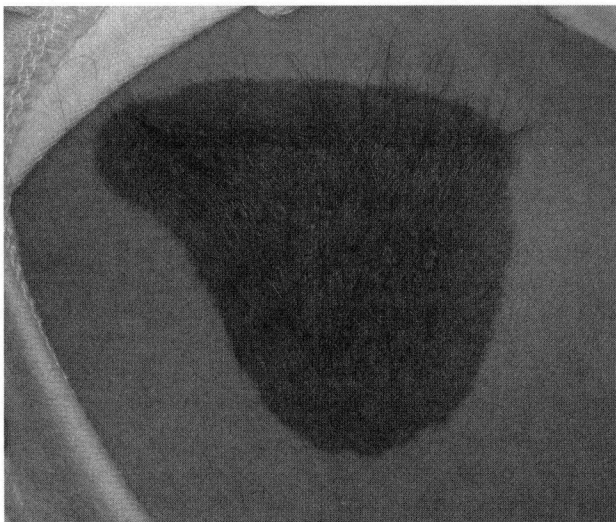

Figure 7 Giant congenital nevi present during childhood. Excision is recommended because of the risk of malignant transformation. (*See color insert Figure 43.*)

Figure 6 Becker's nevus occurs predominantly in males and presents as an irregularly shaped tan-to-brown patch, typically located over the shoulder, upper chest, or back. (*See color insert Figure 42.*)

Atypical melanocytic nevi (AMN) are thought to occupy an intermediate position on a continuum with common acquired nevi on one pole and malignant melanoma on the other. Features commonly observed in AMN include asymmetry, irregular or ill-defined borders, color variation, and diameter of 5 to 15 mm. AMN may be single or multiple and may arise "sporadically" without a history of familial melanoma or atypical nevi, or in patients with a family history of atypical moles and melanoma. In either setting, it appears that they mark an increase in melanoma risk.

Nevi that meet certain pathologic criteria are classified as having *architectural disorder* and may or may not have cytologic atypia. Management of atypical nevi involves complete excision with 2-mm margins to ensure complete histologic evaluation. If the lesion is "mildly atypical," no reexcision is required as long as the entire nevus is removed. If the lesion is "moderately atypical," reexcision with clear margins is recommended. "Severe atypia" should be reexcised with up to 5-mm margins. Patients with numerous atypical moles and a positive family history of many atypical nevi or melanoma (or both) have the *familial atypical mole melanoma* (FAMM) syndrome and should have close follow-up every 3 to 6 months with total-body mole photography, as well as photography of the most atypical nevi.

Spitz nevi are typically dome-shaped papules or nodules of homogenous pink-to-tan-to dark brown color with defined borders and average diameter of 8 mm: 50% are diagnosed in patients younger than 10 years, and 70% are diagnosed within the first 2 decades of life. Most lesions occur on head and neck regions. Histologically, Spitz nevi display nests of large epithelioid or spindle cells (or both), usually extending from the epidermis into the reticular dermis in an inverted-wedge or "raining down" configuration. Management of Spitz tumors involves complete excision to ensure proper histologic diagnosis and to protect against recurrence. Atypical Spitz tumors should be excised with 1-cm margins with follow-up every 6 to 12 months. Sentinel lymph node biopsy may be considered.

Common *blue nevi* are well-circumscribed, dome-shaped papules or nodules 5 to 10 mm in diameter that can occur anywhere, but approximately 50% are on the dorsa of hands and feet. Histology reveals dermal melanocytes believed to be of neural crest origin. Cellular blue nevi are blue-gray or black nodules or plaques, generally 1 to 3 cm in diameter, and in half of reported cases are located on the buttocks or sacrococcygeal area, followed in frequency by the scalp, face, and feet. The ratio of frequency of common blue-to-cellular nevus is 5:1. Malignant blue nevi are rare forms of malignant melanoma most commonly arising in cellular blue nevi. They grow as multinodular or plaquelike lesions typically on the scalp and often measure several centimeters in diameter. They can arise de novo or in preexisting, benign, cellular blue nevus or other dermal melanocytosis (nevus of Ito or Ota). Blue nevi that are less than 1 cm in diameter, clinically stable, and in a typical anatomic location do not require removal; however, excision is recommended for changing, de novo, multinodular, or plaquelike lesions. Cellular blue nevi should be excised completely to prevent recurrence and misdiagnosis as malignant blue nevus, and because of rare but documented risk for malignant transformation.

Congenital melanocytic nevi (CMN) are classified as small (<1.5 cm), intermediate (1.5 to 20 cm), or giant (>20 cm) (Fig. 7). Small and intermediate nevi generally can be primarily excised, whereas giant nevi often require staged excisions or complex reconstruction, possibly with tissue expansion and/or skin grafting. Although all CMN are susceptible to malignant transformation, the potential risk is related to the size of the nevus and is reportedly low, in the range of 3% to 10%.

MALIGNANT CUTANEOUS NEOPLASMS

Basal Cell Carcinoma

Basal Cell Carcinoma (BCC) (Fig. 8) is the most common type of skin cancer in whites, particularly in those with light skin color, inability to tan, blond or red hair, and childhood freckling. Even though ultraviolet light exposure has long been accepted as the principal risk factor for BCC, the causal relationship is less clear than for SCC. Although most BCCs develop on the head and neck, approximately 20% occur on non–sun-exposed areas.

Nodular BCCs are most common (60% of BCCs) and present as dome-shaped "pearly" papules with a telangiectatic surface with a rolled, raised border. Superficial BCCs are the second most common (15% of tumors) and typically appear on the trunk or extremities as pink to erythematous, minimally elevated papules or plaques with a thin telangiectatic border. Infiltrating BCCs account for 5% of tumors and are typically found on the head and

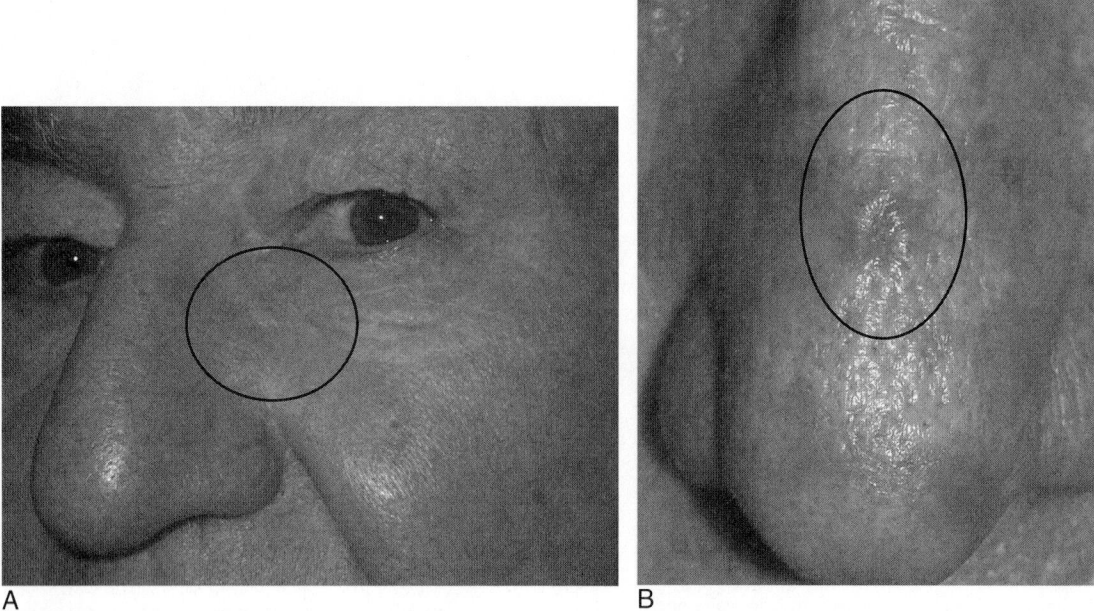

Figure 8   Nodular basal cell cancer, the most common form, presents as dome-shaped, "pearly" papules with a telangiectatic surface and a rolled, raised border on sun-exposed parts of the body, often on the head and neck. The basal cancers here are on the **(A)** face and **(B)** nasal dorsum. (*See color insert Figure 44.*)

neck of older patients. These lesions most typically resemble nodular BCCs, but they can also mimic morpheaform tumors. Morpheaform or sclerosing BCCs account for 3% of all tumors and present as indurated, whitish plaques with ill-defined borders, often mimicking a scar.

Histologically, BCCs may contain focal areas of individual dyskeratotic cells to keratin pearls. If a predominance of this mature, atypical keratinizing squamous component is seen, the tumor is termed *basosquamous carcinoma*. This tumor may have a capacity to metastasize more similarly to SCC.

If left untreated, BCC is rarely life threatening, but it does cause local tissue destruction; therefore the treatment goal is complete elimination of the primary lesion. In well-circumscribed tumors less than 2.0 cm in diameter, surgical excision with 4-mm margins can achieve complete removal in 95% of cases. BCCs that are recurrent, large, poorly defined, or display an aggressive histologic pattern may be treated with Mohs micrographic surgery. Additionally, radiation therapy may be used for very large lesions, for patients who cannot tolerate surgery, for challenging anatomic sites, and for cancers invading neurovascular structures.

Squamous Cell Carcinoma

Cumulative dosage of ultraviolet exposure is a major risk factor in the development of SCC (Fig. 9). SCCs can arise in a body

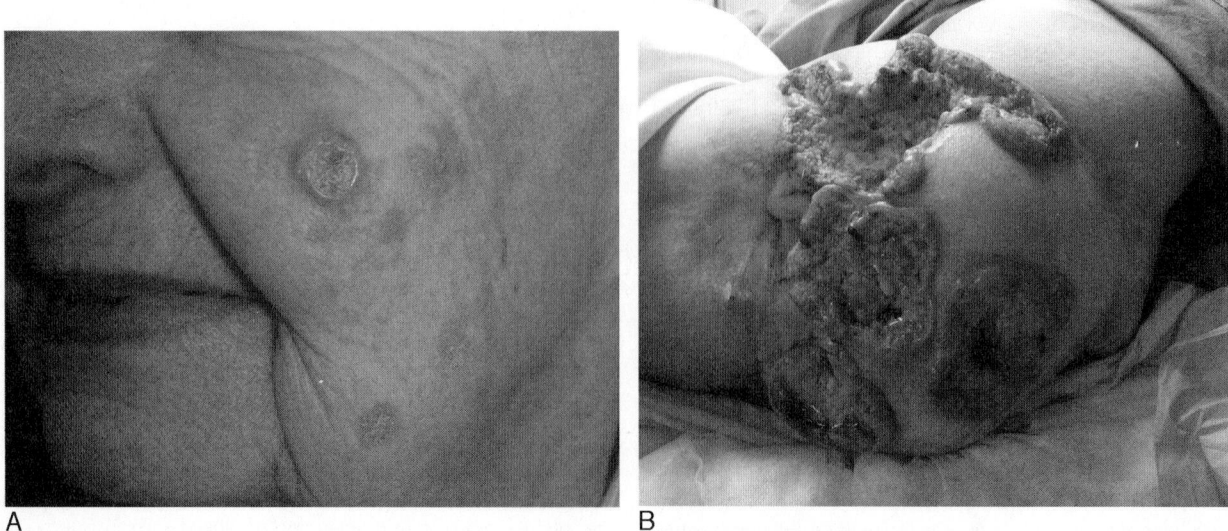

Figure 9   **(A)** Squamous cell carcinoma (SCCA) is associated with sun exposure, and is shown on the face with characteristics including hyperkeratosis and ulceration. **(B)** Marjolin's ulcers are chronic wounds that develop SCCA over the long term. (*See color insert Figure 45.*)

site lined by squamous epithelia (mouth, esophagus, vagina), but the biology of cutaneous SCC differs than that seen on noncutaneous sites. SCCs arising in chronically sun-exposed skin behave in a relatively indolent manner, with a less than 5% risk of metastasis; however, SCCs arising in mucocutaneous interfaces like lips, genitalia, and perianal areas appear to be more aggressive, with a higher risk of metastasis. SCC also arises in tissues where squamous cell metaplasia occurs (e.g., lung, cervix, and salivary glands). Two thirds of SCCs develop in non–sun-exposed sites, such as the legs, anus, and areas of chronic ulceration and scarring (Marjolin's ulcer). Lesions developing at these sites have a worse prognosis, with more aggressive behavior and more frequent metastases than those in sun-exposed skin. Squamous cell cancers appear hyperkeratotic, flesh-colored, and raised, with possible associated ulceration or erythema. Treatment consists of surgical excision with 4-mm margins. If there are concerns of high-risk SCCs secondary to location, size (>1 cm), or indistinct borders, Mohs micrographic surgery may be performed. Like BCC, SCC may be treated by radiation as a primary modality for the appropriate patient or adjuvantly for tumors with perineural invasion, for stage III (positive lymph node) SCCs, or for palliation for certain unresectable tumors.

Squamous cell carcinoma in situ (SCCis) (Fig. 10) comprises full-thickness epidermal involvement and includes entities such as

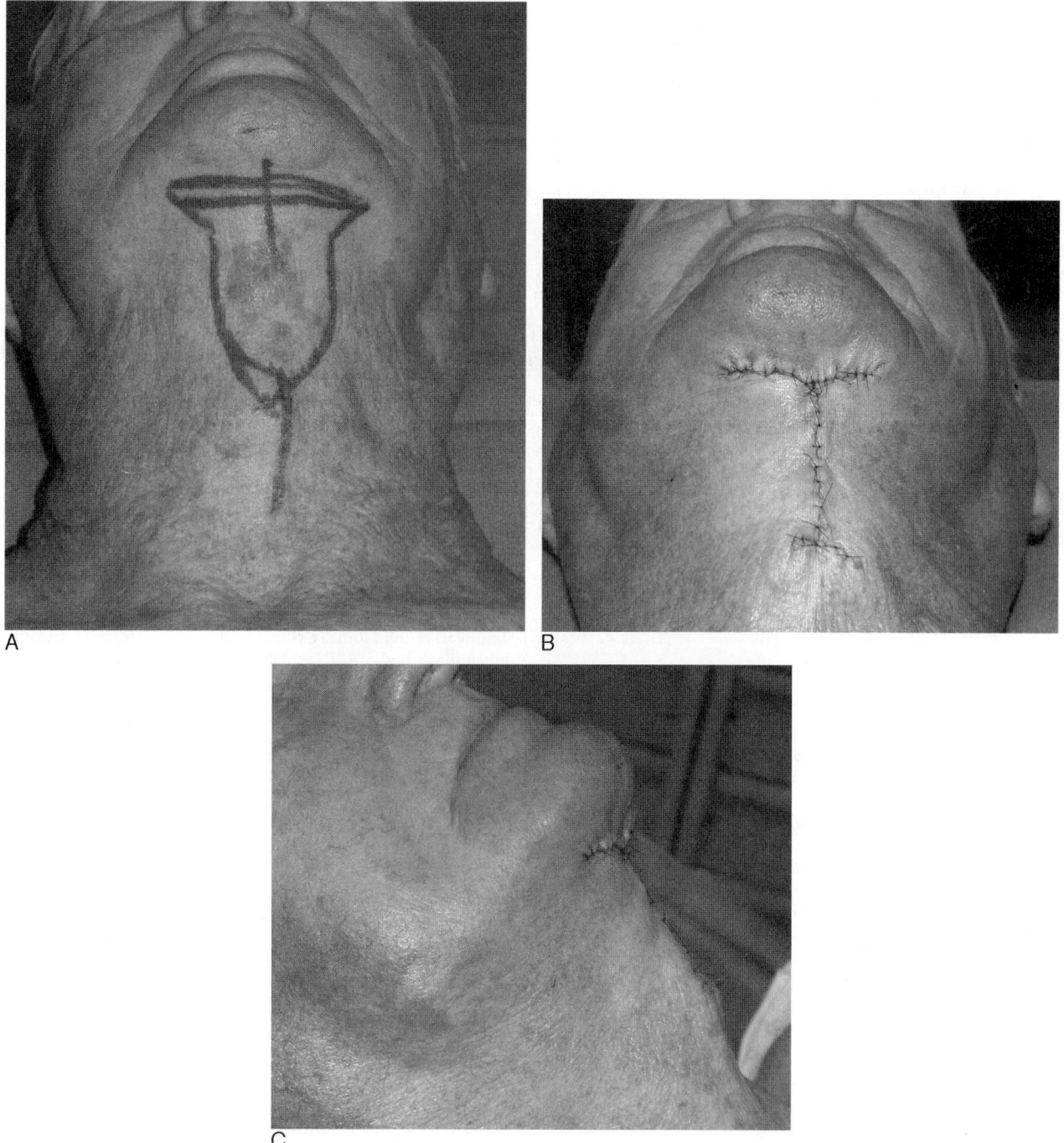

A

B

C

Figure 10 Squamous cell carcinoma in situ (SCCis), Bowen's disease, presents as poorly defined, scaly, erythematous plaques and is most common on the head and neck. Preoperative photograph of SCCis on the neck **(A)**, and frontal **(B)** and lateral **(C)** views after excision with advancement of lateral skin and working out of "dog ears" superiorly and inferiorly. (*See color insert Figure 46.*)

Bowen's disease and erythroplasia of Queyrat. Clinically, SCCis often presents as solitary, sharply demarcated, pink to red, scaly plaques that may resemble superficial BCCs or small patches of psoriasis or eczema. Most arise in sun-exposed skin. Typically the lesions grow slowly over years, seldom progressing to invasive carcinoma. Invasion of the dermis occurs in up to 26% of cases, according to some reports, and subsequent metastases occur in up to 16% of cases.

Bowen's disease describes SCCis involving hair follicles and may be precursor lesions to invasive adnexal carcinoma, whereas SCCis that does not involve follicular units is the precursor lesion to invasive SCC. Erythroplasia of Queyrat develops on the male genitalia, characteristically on the glans penis of uncircumcised men, and often relates to human papilloma virus infection. Mucosal SCCis is thought to have a greater likelihood of progression to invasive carcinoma than its counterpart in glabrous skin. SCCis can be treated much like superficial BCC, with electrodesiccation and curettage, topical chemotherapy (5-FU), or immune modulators (imiquimod); PDT is still under investigation.

Adnexal Tumors

Adnexal tumors arise from appendageal skin cells of hair follicles and from sebaceous, apocrine, and eccrine glands. Typically the lesions are flesh colored or yellowish papules that may have hair within them. Diagnosis typically requires histologic evaluation. Clustering of one type of adnexal tumor can be syndromic; thus a complete history and physical is recommended. If the histology reveals a benign hamartoma, no further treatment is necessary.

Adnexal adenocarcinomas are relatively uncommon. They can arise de novo or in preexisting lesions. Patients who report that a lesion recently grew rapidly or began to ulcerate or bleed require evaluation.

Microcystic adnexal carcinoma (MAC) is a slow-growing, low-grade adnexal carcinoma that presents in young to middle-aged adults, typically women, on sun-exposed areas of the face. Although MACs are classified as low-grade, there is a small risk of metastasis. Complete surgical excision is recommended.

Sebaceous carcinoma can be separated into ocular and extraocular types. They present as red nodules or plaques with crusting or ulceration and a yellowish coloration, commonly in the periorbital region. Surgical extirpation is the primary treatment.

Fibrous and Fibrohistiocytic Tumors

Atypical fibroxanthoma (AFX) is a low-grade sarcoma of older patients in sun-damaged skin of the head and neck. AFX usually presents as a rapidly growing, 1- to 2-cm pink nodule. Surgical excision is typically curative.

Dermatofibrosarcoma protuberans (DFSP) is a locally aggressive sarcoma of intermediate malignant potential in young to middle-aged adults. It is located on the trunk in 50% to 60% of cases. DFSP starts as a slow-growing, asymptomatic, skin-colored, indurated plaque that eventually develops into violaceous to red-brown nodules 1 cm to several centimeters in diameter. Complete surgical excision is the treatment of choice. DFSP is characterized by its local invasion and tendency to recur.

Neuroendocrine Carcinoma

Merkel cell carcinoma is a malignant proliferation of highly anaplastic cells that share structural and immunohistochemical features with various neuroectodermally derived cells, including the cutaneous Merkel cells. The tumor is a red-pink to violaceous, firm, solitary, rapidly growing nodule typically on the head and neck. Other sites include extremities and buttocks. Merkel cell carcinoma is characterized by its aggressive behavior, with 40% of patients developing distant metastases and 30% of patients dying of the disease in 5 years. Management is primarily surgical; however, adjuvant chemotherapy, immunotherapy, and radiation are often administered.

Malignant Vascular Neoplasms

Angiosarcomas are rare endothelial neoplasms that usually occur in adults, with approximately 70% of tumors occurring in patients older than 40 years of age and with the highest incidence in patients older than 70 years of age. In affected older patients, approximately 50% involve the face and scalp. Male-to-female ratio is approximately 2:1, and white patients are at highest risk. Lesions typically start as an ecchymotic-appearing patch with or without facial edema. The area expands, eventually covering large portions of the head and neck. Five-year survival rate is less than 15%. In 1948, Stewart and Treves described angiosarcoma in postmastectomy lymphedema patients. Greater than 90% of angiosarcoma associated with lymphedema is in postmastectomy and lymph node dissection patients. In these cases, the upper arm is the most common site of the classic coalescing violaceous nodules on a background of woody edema. Other risk factors are chronic or congenital lymphedema, chronic radiodermatitis, and immunosuppression. Surgical excision with wide excision of 5 cm is indicated; however, on the head and neck this is often difficult. Even with negative margins by histologic examination, the recurrence rate and chance of metastasis is high because the tumor demonstrates multifocality. Chemotherapy and radiation may be palliative but do not improve survival.

Cutaneous Metastases

The skin is an uncommon site for metastatic spread of an internal malignancy. Prompt recognition of cutaneous metastases is important but usually portends a poor prognosis. In men, cutaneous metastases are most commonly due to melanoma and carcinomas of lung, colon/rectum, oral cavity and larynx, and kidney. In women, breast carcinoma is most common, followed by melanoma and ovarian carcinoma. Cutaneous metastases are more uncommon in children and usually result from leukemia or neuroblastoma. Cutaneous metastases often present as painless, flesh-colored to pink, firm papules or nodules commonly in the general vicinity of the primary tumor. Scalp involvement is usually secondary to tumors of the breast, lung, stomach, pancreas, and kidney. Additional clinical presentations include inflammatory cutaneous metastases or "carcinoma erysipeloids" secondary to occlusion and dilatation of superficial lymphatics by tumor cells and "en cuirasse," which is a peau d'orange skin change of the chest wall caused by metastatic breast cancer encasing superficial lymphatics by dermal fibrosis.

Evaluation requires histologic examination, which generally resembles the primary malignancy. Treatment options include surgical excision, radiation, and chemotherapy.

SURGICAL EXCISION

In planning surgical removal of skin lesions, one must consider the possibility of malignancy. Even for those lesions that may appear to be benign, excisional biopsy is recommended to ensure complete diagnostic and therapeutic treatment. Excision within relaxed skin tension lines, particularly in the face, is recommended to ensure the most acceptable cosmetic scar.

Directionality of the incision must also be planned with the possibility of malignancy in mind in case reexcision becomes necessary. This is particularly important if the skin lesion is found to be a sarcoma, for which relatively large margins for reexcision are necessary. Rather than creating a transverse scar on an extremity, a longitudinal approach along the length of the limb is recommended to allow for elongating a scar if margins must be extended.

Adequate margins are important in effectively treating skin cancer, and the margins increase in size with the likelihood of later recurrence. The acceptable margin for basal cell cancer is 3 mm; for squamous cell cancer, 4 mm to 1 cm; and for sarcoma, 5 cm. Melanoma margins depend on the severity and stage of melanoma, generally ranging from 2 to 3 cm. If diagnosis is more severe than had been anticipated, then reexcision of the scar with appropriate margins is recommended. In cosmetically important areas, such as the face, margins may be modified. Referral to a dermatologic specialist who performs Mohs micrographic surgery may be considered for such areas. Immediate histologic evaluation at the time of excision makes Mohs surgery a valuable option to consider.

Reconstruction and Closure

Defects created by surgical excision are addressed in as cosmetic a manner as possible. One must be sure that "no bridges are burned" and that effective excision has been performed with negative permanent margins before embarking on a complex reconstruction involving movement of local or distant tissue. Local wound care or temporary coverage with allograft and delayed reconstruction are recommended if margins may be inadequate when primary closure or full-thickness skin grafting with good donor resources are not possible (Fig. 11).

The reconstructive ladder is important to follow in closing wounds after excision (Fig. 12). The lowest rung of the ladder is the simplest closure, whereas the top rung is the most complex. The ladder progresses from secondary healing to primary closure to closure with grafts, flaps, and free flaps. Tissue expansion of donor skin in adjacent or distant sites is another option for providing skin, fascia, or muscle to a tissue-deficient region.

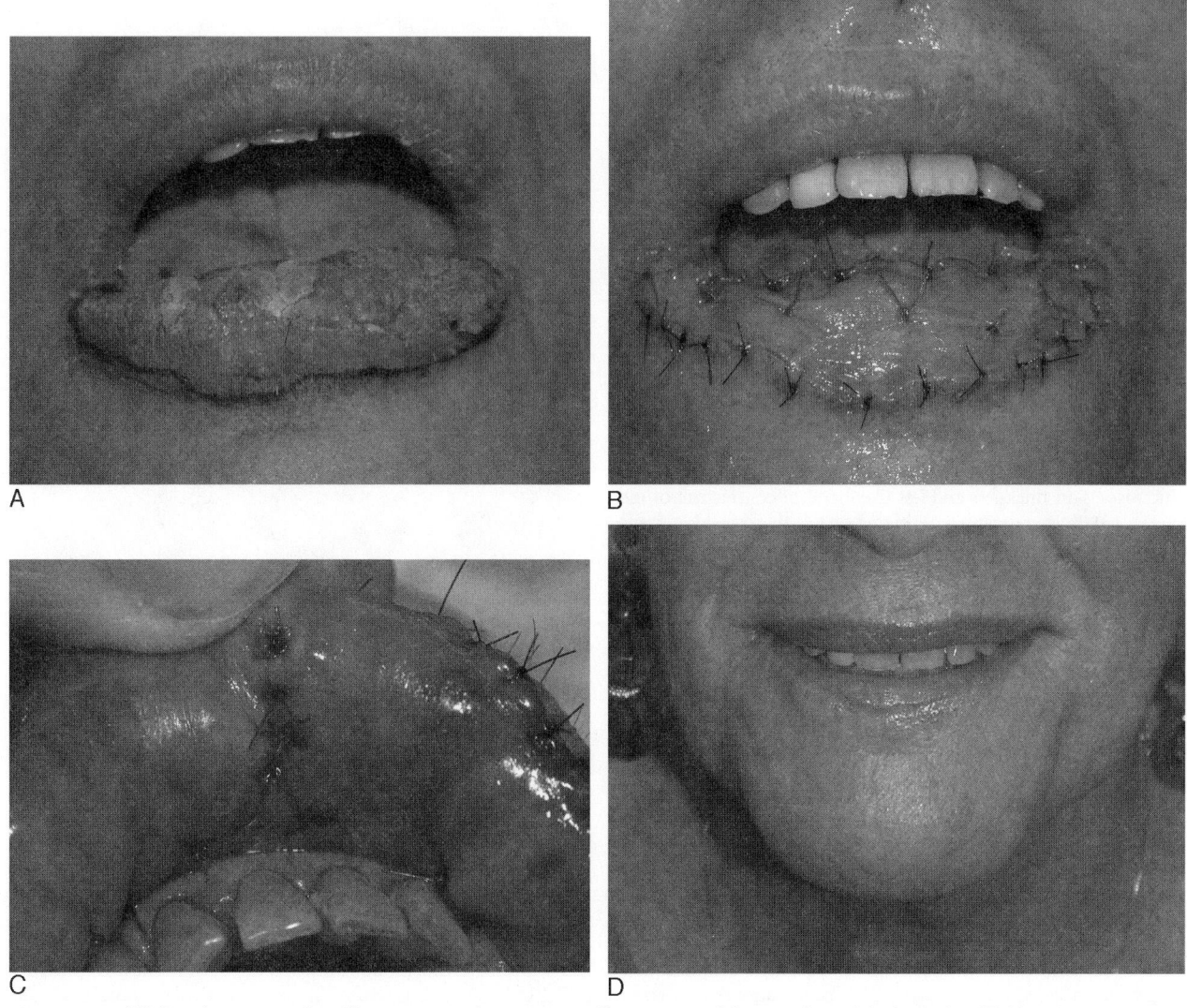

Figure 11   **(A)** Female patient in her 60s presents with squamous cell carcinoma of the vermilion of the lower lip. **(B)** Vermilionectomy was performed, and allografting was performed to allow wound closure while awaiting permanent analysis by pathology. **(C)** V-Y advancement was performed from buccal mucosa to reconstruct vermilion. **(D)** Postoperative result 1 year later. (*See color insert Figure 47.*)

Reconstructive ladder

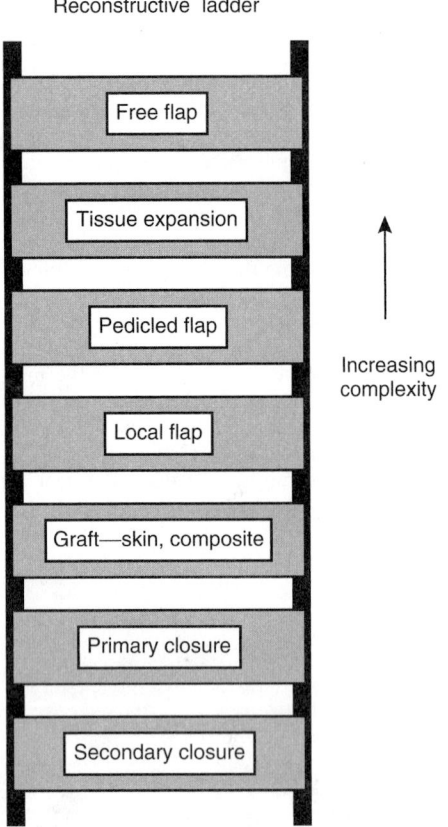

Figure 12 The reconstructive ladder guides the surgeon in closure of wound defects created with skin cancer excision. The surgeon should start with the least complex possibility and work up the ladder if lesser complex techniques do not apply.

Grafts may comprise only skin, split thickness or full thickness, or may be composite, including skin and other elements such as cartilage. Split-thickness skin grafts are used for large areas in cosmetically less important areas. Full-thickness skin grafts may be taken from around the ear, clavicle, or inguinal crease for reconstruction of defects requiring increased skin thickness and less likelihood of contracture of the graft (Fig. 13). Bolster dressings are placed on full-thickness skin grafts to prevent seroma and shear on the graft, which would impair healing. Composite grafts are limited by their size to bridging defects no greater than 1.5 cm. The classic example is use of ear helix skin and cartilage to reconstruct an alar rim defect of the nose.

Local tissue rearrangement is an excellent way to replace "like with like," which is the goal in more superior reconstructions. Random local flaps without a defined blood supply include Z-plasties and advancement flaps such as the V-Y advancement (see Fig. 11). Rotation flaps, including rhomboid, banner, and bilobed flaps, are particularly useful on the face, and specifically on the nose (Figs. 14 and 15). It is recommended in random flaps that length-to-width ratio not exceed 3:1.

Tissue expansion may be performed on adjacent skin for wounds too large to close primarily but inappropriate for skin grafting because of cosmesis. Generally this procedure is performed in stages, placing the tissue expander at an initial stage (Figure 16). This is followed by expansion, on an outpatient basis, in which saline is transcutaneously injected into a defined port connected to the expander. After adequate time has been allowed for expansion, the second surgical stage comprises skin cancer excision with immediate reconstruction with

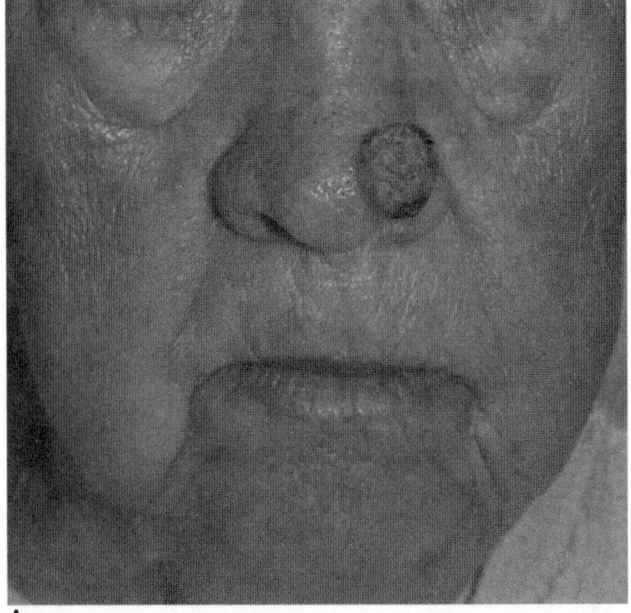

A

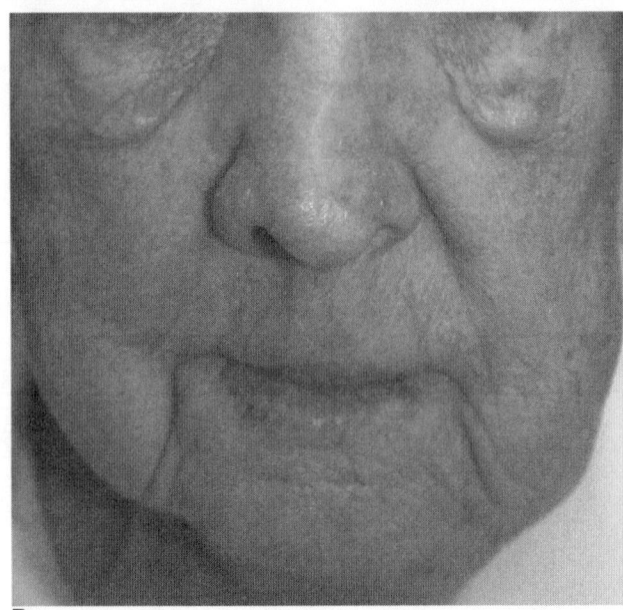

B

Figure 13 Full-thickness skin grafts (FTSGs) are useful in older patients and may be taken from around the ear or clavicle. **(A)** Squamous cell carcinoma of the left nasal ala. **(B)** Cosmetic result of FTSG reconstruction is satisfactory 6 months later. (*See color insert Figure 48.*)

adjacent expanded skin. Tissue expansion may also be performed in nonadjacent tissue that can be rotated on a known vascular supply, which is a pedicled flap, or to create more skin for grafting.

Pedicled flaps have a known blood supply and are an excellent way of importing well-vascularized tissue including skin, dermis, fascia, and muscle. Examples of such flaps include the forehead flap based on supratrochlear vessels for nasal reconstruction and the latissimus flap with the thoracodorsal blood supply for chest reconstruction (Fig. 17). Defects are often larger and missing more components when using pedicled flaps.

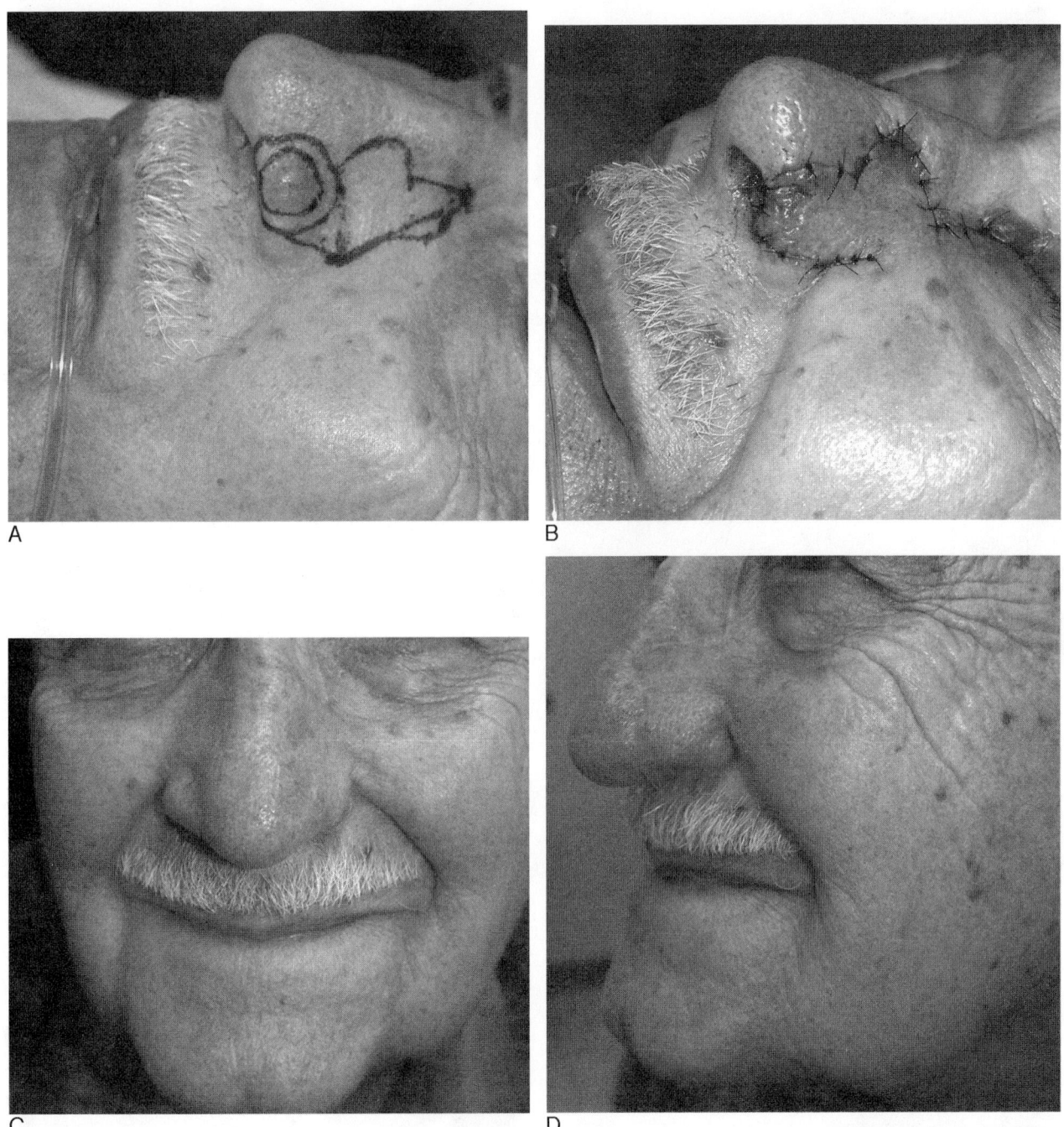

Figure 14 **(A)** Basal cell carcinoma of the left nasal ala, with markings designated for the Zitelli modification of the bilobed flap. This is a random rotation flap **(B)** The two lower lobes are rotated down to fill the wound defects, and the third flap defect is closed primarily. Frontal **(C)** and lateral **(D)** views demonstrating satisfactory aesthetic result. (*See color insert Figure 49.*)

Free flaps are the most complex form of reconstruction, whereby tissue is detached and moved from a distant location and then anastomosed to a vascular supply at the defect site. An example of this is reconstruction of a large scalp defect after sarcoma resection with a latissimus free flap covered by a split-thickness skin graft or with a fasciocutaneous flap such as the anterolateral thigh flap.

The various forms of reconstruction are not mutually exclusive and complement each other, particularly when replacing all tissue elements that have been removed. An example includes complex nasal reconstruction, in which the lining, support, and skin cover all must be reconstructed: local flaps can reconstruct lining, and a cartilage graft support may be placed, which is then covered with a free fascio-cutaneous flap.

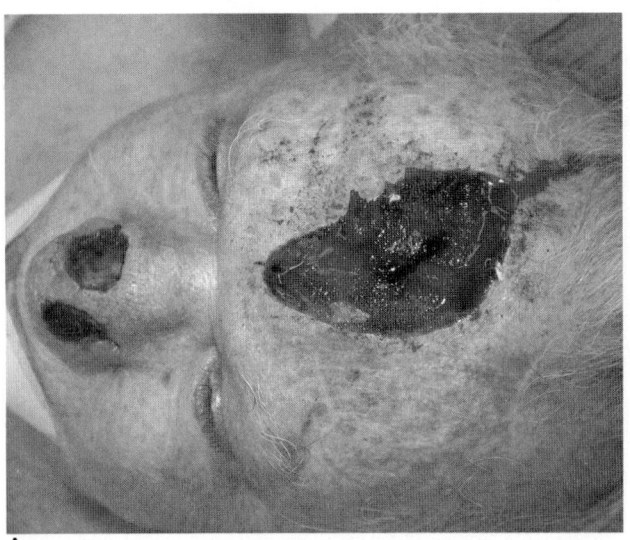

A

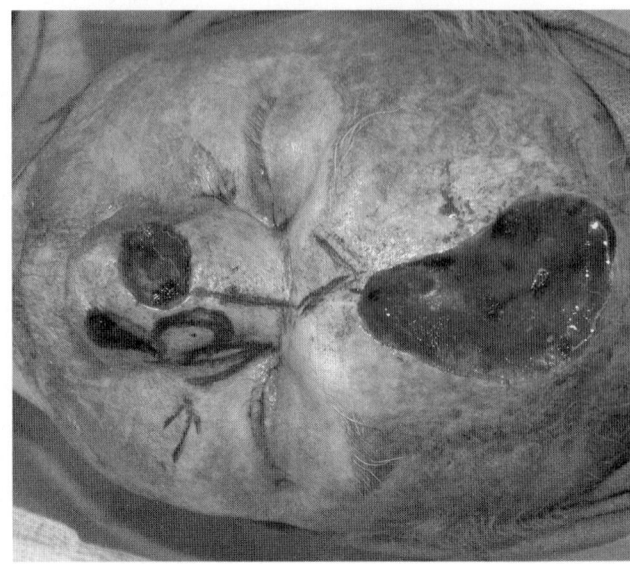

B

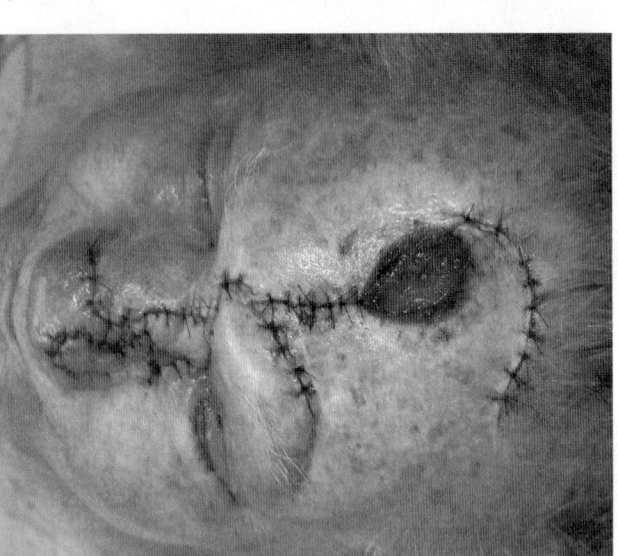

C

Figure 15 **(A)** Patient referred for reconstruction on the same day as her Mohs surgery, with defects of forehead, dorsal nose, and left ala. **(B)** Markings demonstrate Bishop-Mitre flap to reconstruct nasal dorsum and bilobed rotation advancement flap to reconstruct left ala. **(C)** Flaps are advanced and closed. An advancement of forehead skin was also performed along the brow and hairline, leaving the rest of the frontal defect to heal in secondarily. (*See color insert Figure 50.*)

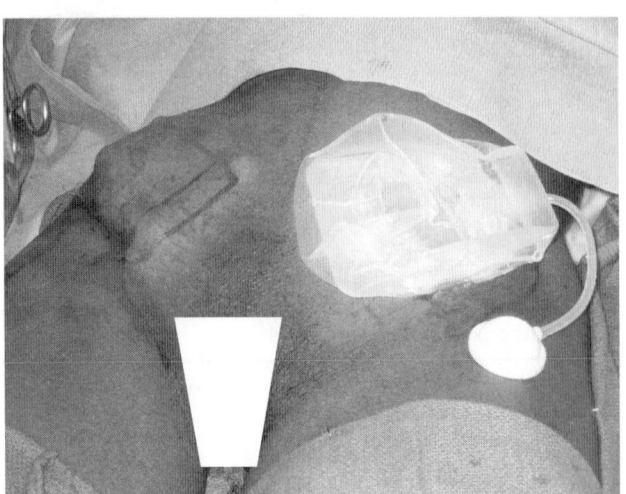

Figure 16 Tissue expander placement in the inguinal region to prepare full-thickness skin grafts. The right expander is already placed within its subcutaneous pocket. (*See color insert Figure 51.*)

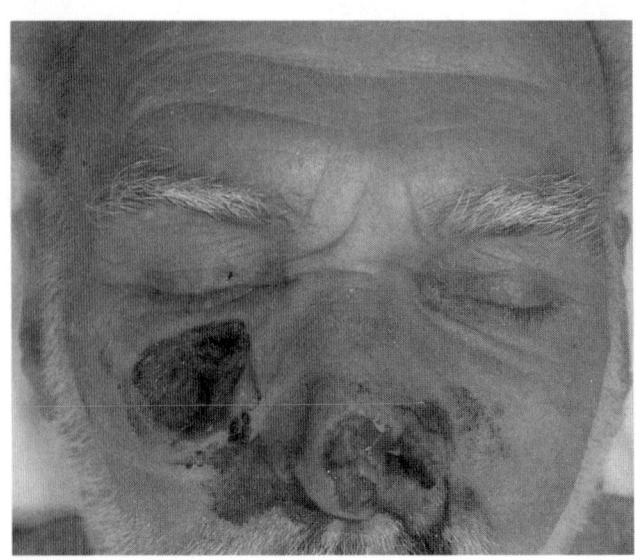

A

Figure 17 **(A)** Patient referred after Mohs surgery with dorsal nasal defect and right cheek defect. (*See color insert Figure 52.*)

(continued)

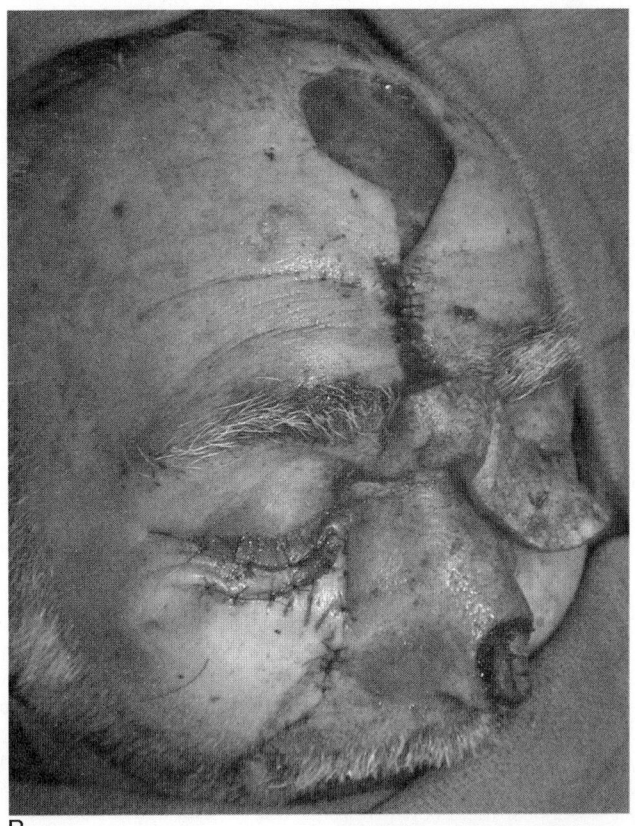

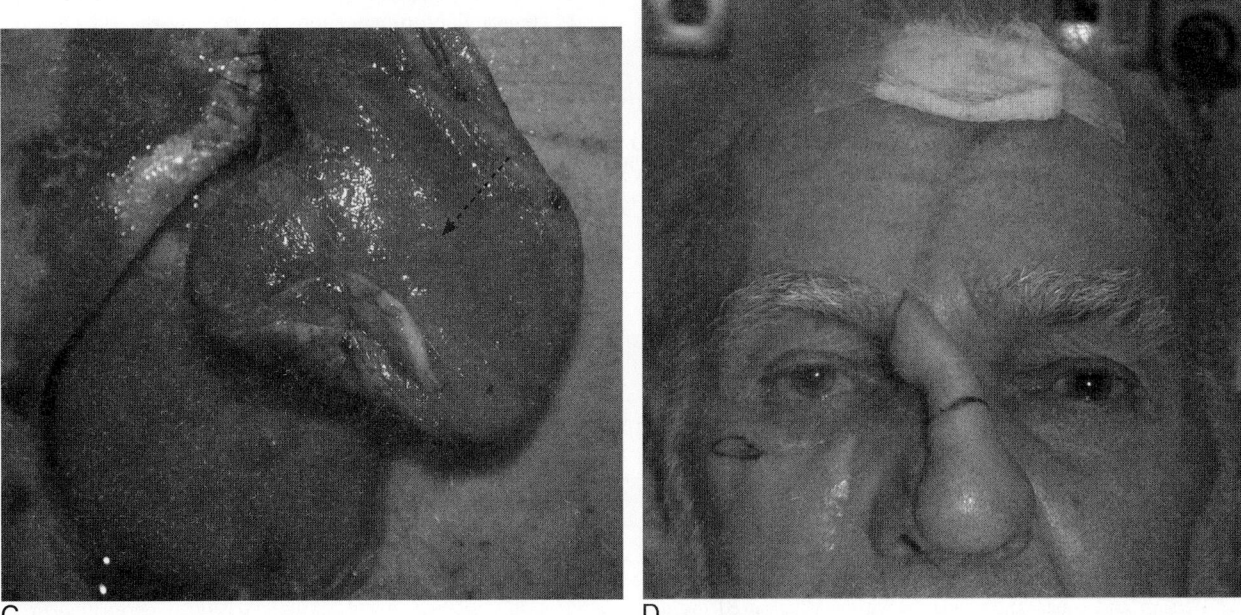

Figure 17 Cont'd—(B) Forehead flap based on supratrochlear vessels rotated down to cover nose. Right cheek advancement performed as well. **(C)** Forehead flap had cartilage graft *(arrow)* from ear concha to reconstruct resected alar cartilages. **(D)** Nasal flap just before division of pedicle 1 month later with forehead defect healing secondarily. "Dog ear" excision planned for cheek below the right eye. *(See color insert Figure 52.)*

SUGGESTED READINGS

Bolognia J, Jorrizo J, Rapini R, editors: *Dermatology,* 2003, Mosby Publishing.

Cohen B, Lehmann C: *Dermatology image atlas,* Baltimore, 2000, Johns Hopkins University. Available at www.dermatlas.org.

Fehr B, Panizzou RG, Schnyder UW: Becker's nevus and malignant melanoma, *Dermatologica* 182(2):77, 1991.

Freedberg I, Eisen A, Wolff K, and others: *Fitzpatrick's dermatology in general medicine,* ed 6, New York, 2003, McGraw-Hill Medical Publishing.

Schusterman MA, editors: Nonmelanoma skin cancer, *Clin Plastic Surg* 24(4):673, 1997.

Zarem HA, Lowe NJ: Benign growths and generalized skin disorders. In Aston SJ, Beasley RW, Thorne CH, editors: *Grabb and Smith's plastic surgery,* ed 5, Philadelphia, 1997, Lippincott-Raven, p. 141.

CUTANEOUS MELANOMA

Mark B. Faries, MD, and Donald L. Morton, MD

Table 1: Recommended Margins for Wide Local Excision of Primary Site

Thickness	Margin	Note
Melanoma in situ	5 mm	Head and neck: consider preoperative margin assessment
Melanoma < 1 mm	1 cm	
Melanoma 1 to 4 mm	2 cm	1 cm acceptable in limited anatomic locations
Melanoma > 4 mm	2 cm	Consider 3 cm if easily obtained

The incidence of melanoma is increasing at an alarming rate. The American Cancer Society estimated there would be more than 62,000 new cases of melanoma in 2006, with 7910 deaths. Because melanoma often strikes young people, it is one of the leading causes of lost years of life owing to malignancy. Fortunately, surgery can be curative in many patients with melanoma and is the only clearly effective treatment modality at any stage of disease.

Risk factors for melanoma include a family history, fair skin, a history of at least one previous blistering sunburn, and a large number of nevi. Suspicious pigmented lesions include those that are Asymmetric, have an irregular Border, have a variegated Color, or are large in Diameter (ABCD). Other suspicious findings include "ugly duckling" lesions (those that differ significantly from a patient's other nevi) and any changing lesion.

BIOPSY TECHNIQUES

The goal of any biopsy is to provide the pathologist with enough material to ensure complete evaluation of the lesion. For melanoma, this must include the deepest portion of the lesion so that the prognosis, dictated in part by the Breslow depth, can be determined. Excisional biopsies are the surest means of obtaining a complete and accurate specimen. The possible need for wide local excision must be considered when orienting the biopsy incision, which should be longitudinal on the extremities.

When complete excisional biopsies are not possible, as is the case for large (>2 cm) lesions in anatomic locations such as the face, scalp, or distal extremities, incisional (or punch) biopsies may be performed. These biopsies should include any areas of particularly dark pigment or palpable thickness. Patients should be counseled that the final pathologic diagnosis may differ from the biopsy results. Shave biopsies are acceptable in some circumstances but often fail to sample the deepest portion of the lesion. They are most appropriate when an atypical nevus or melanoma in situ is more likely than invasive melanoma. A shave biopsy must include the majority of the underlying dermis.

Finally, many melanocytic lesions are difficult for pathologists to interpret. Equivocal findings must be reviewed by a pathologist experienced in melanoma.

TREATMENT OF PRIMARY LESION

Complete treatment of a melanoma primary tumor consists of excision of all skin and subcutaneous tissue within a measured radius from the edge of the previous biopsy site or the widest area of associated pigment. In the past, 5-cm margins were used for all melanomas. However, randomized trials of narrower margins have reported no adverse effect on local recurrence or overall survival and substantial reduction in morbidity, including the need for skin grafting. Currently, the width of margins is determined by the maximal thickness of the primary lesion (Table 1).

Local recurrences result from one of two phenomena: radial extension of abnormal melanocytes or local dissemination (metastasis) of tumor cells through lymphatic channels. The latter of these two is classified as stage III disease (satellite or in-transit metastasis). The risk for this type of recurrence depends on the pathologic

characteristics of primary lesion, not the resection margin. A true local recurrence caused by radial extension probably carries only the prognostic significance of a primary lesion with similar pathologic characteristics. Another type of local recurrence occurs in the setting of desmoplastic melanoma with neurotropism. Spread along nearby nerves may extend beyond resection margins. Adjuvant radiation therapy may be considered in neurotropic, desmoplastic lesions in areas where wide margins cannot be reasonably obtained, such as the head and neck.

Subungual melanoma requires the same margin (based on depth) as lesions in other anatomic locations. Its removal generally requires amputation at the midproximal phalanx. Functional preservation of the remaining digit requires reimplantation of the flexor and extensor digitorum tendons by securing the cut ends of the tendon to the distal remaining phalanx using nonabsorbable suture. Failure to reimplant the tendons may lead to paradoxical movement of the digit and compromised function.

Care should be taken in planning excision margins in certain patients. Often older patients with lesions in chronically sun-exposed areas such as the head and neck will exhibit abnormal melanocytic proliferation well beyond the visible edge of the lesion. Preoperative margin assessment can involve a series of punch biopsies at the proposed margin. If there is no evidence of abnormality, the reconstruction can proceed with confidence that the primary lesion has been completely excised.

Reconstruction

Most wide excisions are closed with simple local advancement flaps. If the orientation of these flaps is clear before wide excision is performed, an elliptical excision can be planned. To close the wound without untoward tissue bunching at each end ("dog ears"), the resected specimen should have a length-to-width ratio of 3:1. If the optimal orientation of the flaps cannot be determined until after wide local excision, a circular excision is performed first and the final flaps oriented subsequently (Fig. 1).

If closure by rotational or advancement flaps is not possible, skin grafting generally provides good to excellent closure, although the healing process is extended. For the scalp and face, full-thickness grafting provides optimal cosmetic results. The graft is taken from an area of skin with similar color, such as the upper chest or postauricular neck. The donor skin must be trimmed of all subcutaneous tissue to the level of the dermis. Thicker grafts do not allow sufficient oxygenation to sustain the graft; loss of the epidermis or even of the entire graft may occur. Split-thickness grafts can cover larger areas, and the thin nature of these grafts makes survival more predictable in areas with suboptimal blood flow. The donor

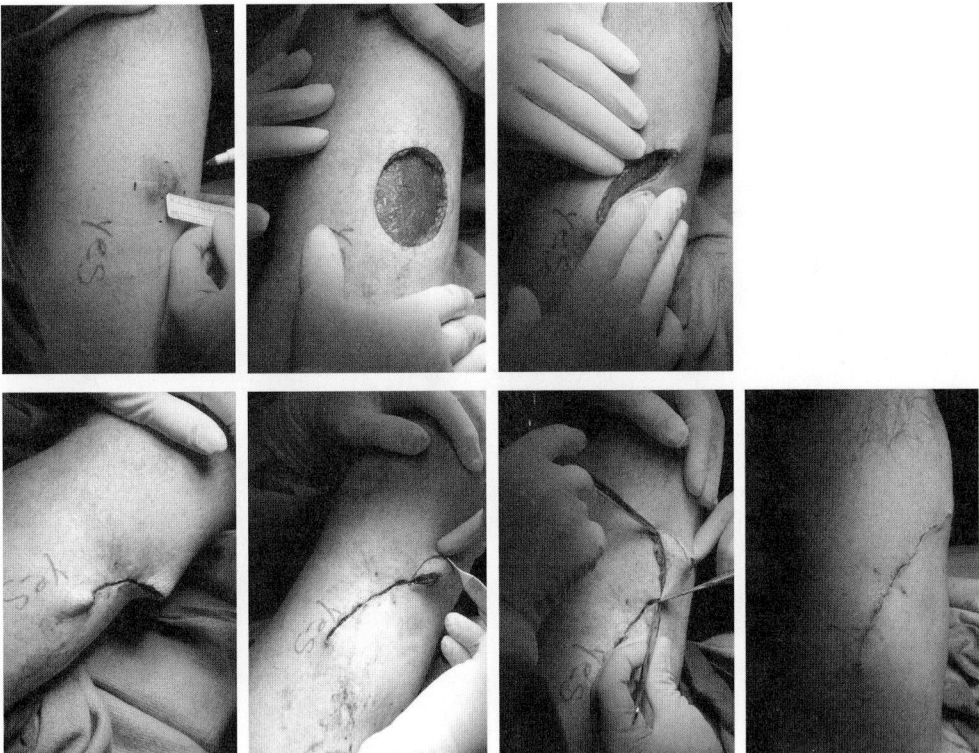

Figure 1 Wide local excision of an extremity melanoma. *Top row (left to right):* Measurement of circumferential margin; after excision; assessment of lines of tension. *Bottom row (left to right):* Wound closure after flap mobilization; marking of redundant skin; extension of redundant skin across wound; final closure.

area is usually the lateral thigh. For lower-extremity lesions, the contralateral thigh should be used because of the possible need for lymphatic procedures on the same side. More complex flap closures, such as Z-plasty or V-Y flaps, and pedicled or free flaps can be used in difficult situations. However, the requirement for such procedures is uncommon.

Wide local excisions of melanoma of the face present special reconstructive challenges. Reconstruction of wide excisions of the ear is dictated by the location of the lesion on the ear. For lesions on the top of the ear, a simple wedge excision is generally adequate and cosmetically successful. The cartilage is closed with interrupted, nonabsorbable sutures, and minimal subsequent mobilization of the skin allows for straightforward reapproximation of the skin edges using the surgeon's preferred technique. Defects of lower portions of the ear may be reconstructed using skin grafting or flaps constructed using adjacent skin of the postauricular neck. Lesions of the cheek can generally be reconstructed using a rotational flap (Fig. 2). Every reconstruction should be individualized to the location of the lesion and the preferences of the patient. Liberal consultation with plastic and reconstructive surgeons should be employed, but the margins of the excision should never be compromised for cosmetic reasons.

TREATMENT OF REGIONAL NODES

The most likely first site of melanoma metastasis is in regional lymph nodes. In the past, consideration was given for elective removal of all lymph nodes in the draining basin. However, because the regional nodes are not involved in the majority of cases, elective lymphadenectomy subjects many patients to a potentially morbid major operation without the possibility of benefit. The advent of lymphatic mapping and sentinel node biopsy has eliminated this issue by allowing identification of occult lymphatic metastases with a low-

morbidity procedure. It is indicated in all patients whose melanomas are at least 1 mm in thickness. For patients with occult nodal metastases, there is strong evidence that survival is substantially improved with early removal of the disease; nodal status is the most important prognostic factor for patients with clinically localized disease. If primary melanomas are thinner than 1 mm, selection is based on other clinicopathologic features (Table 2) associated with a higher risk of lymph node metastasis.

Sentinel node biopsy is conceptually simple but requires experience for optimal accuracy. The sentinel node is the first lymph node to receive lymphatic drainage from the primary tumor site. In melanoma, two tracers are used: radiocolloid and blue dye. We use technetium-sulfur colloid and isosulfan blue dye. In Australia, radiolabeled antimony is believed to be an excellent agent, but this agent is not generally available in the United States.

Patients undergo lymphoscintigraphy preoperatively, generally on the day of surgery, but injections may also be administered on the day before surgery. Imaging must include all potential drainage basins, including ectopic locations such as popliteal and epitrochlear basins and the intramuscular triangle of the upper back. These sites harbor a sentinel node approximately 10% of the time. The skin is marked over the identified sentinel nodes, and a lymphoscintigraph is sent with the patient to the operating room. The film should include an outline of the patient for orientation, and the lymphatic channels leading from the primary to the sentinel nodes should be visualized. There is generally a separate visible channel that is going to each sentinel node.

In the operating room, before the operative site is prepared, blue dye is injected at the biopsy site. The injection must be intradermal because there are relatively few lymphatic channels within the subcutaneous tissue. The rich investment of channels in the dermis allows for rapid transit of the tracer to lymph nodes using small amounts of dye (1 to 2 ml). Although gentle massage of the injection site increases lymphatic flow, we have not found this to be necessary.

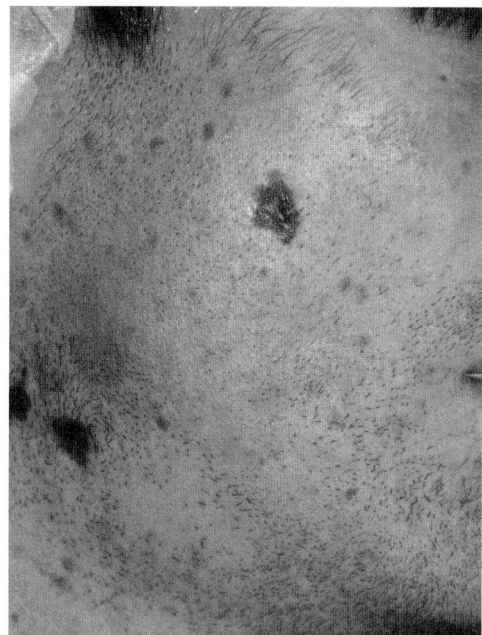
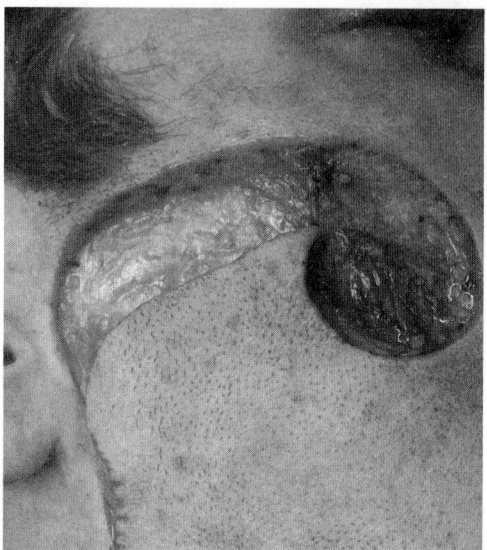
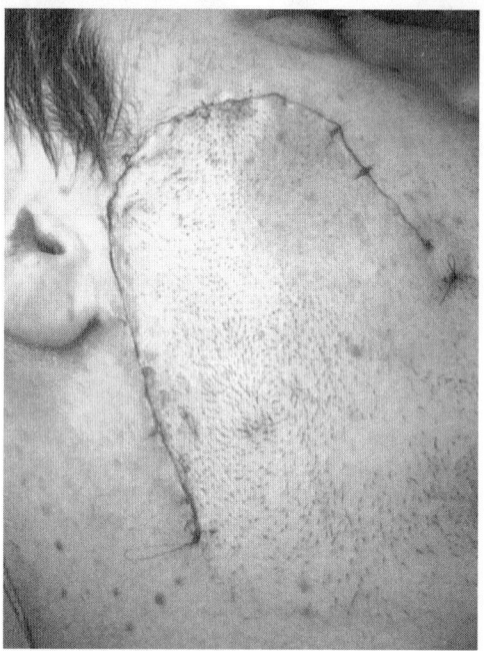

Figure 2 Rotational flap closure of cheek defect. *Top right:* The upper edge of the wide local excision line is extended laterally toward the ear and then inferiorly. The flap is created with dissection along the so-called facelift plane. Care must be taken to avoid penetrating too deeply and risking injury to the facial nerve. *Bottom:* The flap is then rotated into position, and any redundant skin at the inferomedial edge of the suture line removed. One potential difficulty with this reconstruction is downward tension on the lower eyelid. To avoid this, deep sutures can be used to secure the flap to underlying periosteum. (*See color insert Figure 53.*)

At the time of surgery, a gamma probe is used to confirm the location of the sentinel node and a small incision is made. Dissection can then be carried out using the probe intermittently for guidance. Sentinel nodes are identified by color or radioactivity and are removed. The point of greatest radioactivity of the node (where micrometastases are most likely to occur) should be identified and marked with a suture to assist the pathologist. The basin is then reexamined for significant residual radioactivity, blue-stained nodes, or palpably abnormal nodes. A commonly used rule is to remove any node with at least 10% of the counts of the "hottest" node in that basin. This rule can be difficult to apply because the actual counts within a node are not known until the node has been thoroughly dissected. We have found it to be extremely uncommon that a node that is neither the hottest node nor blue is the only node involved with tumor. Gloves and instruments are changed before undertaking wide local excision of the primary melanoma.

The pathologist also serves a critical role in the sentinel node procedure. Nodes are evaluated at multiple levels, using conventional

Table 2: Indications for Lymphatic Mapping and Sentinel Node Biopsy

Thickness	Note
Thin (<1 mm)	Consider if: young age, >0.75 mm, ≥Clark's IV, ulceration, regression, incomplete biopsy, high mitotic rate
Intermediate	Prognosis (most important), disease-free survival benefit, possible overall survival benefit
Thick (>4 mm)	Prognosis

Table 3: Recommended Number of Evaluated Nodes by Basin

Basin	No. of Nodes
Axillary	15
Inguinal, superficial	8
Inguinal, deep	6
Cervical, anterior	15
Cervical, posterior	15
Supraclavicular	6
Suprahyoid	4
Parotid	3
Popliteal	2–3

hematoxylin and eosin staining and immunohistochemistry with antibodies to several melanoma marker epitopes (S100, HMB45, MART-1). We do not recommend frozen section analysis of sentinel lymph nodes because of the limited accuracy of this technique and the loss of diagnostic material during processing of sections in the cryostat.

All of the components of this procedure must be performed well to ensure a low false-negative rate. The learning curve is long; during the first 50 cases, the false-negative rate is relatively high (10%), even at centers with an interest in lymphatic mapping. If all three components of the procedure cannot be confidently performed, referral to a specialized center is recommended.

Technical difficulties arise in certain situations, including mapping of melanomas of the head and neck, where lymphatic drainage is particularly unpredictable, and in any area where the primary lesion is close to the draining basin. In these situations it is important to communicate with the nuclear medicine physician to ensure evaluation of all potential nodal locations and to use the gamma probe intraoperatively to confirm identification of all pertinent sites. In addition, potential sentinel node locations should be reexamined with the probe after wide local excision. This reduces interference caused by high background radioactivity emanating from the primary injection site.

Complications of sentinel node biopsy are generally mild and temporary. They include wound seroma, hematoma, and infection. Depending on the location of the node, nerve injury is also possible and care must be taken to avoid inadvertent injury during the dissection. In the neck, particular attention must be paid to the marginal mandibular and spinal accessory nerves, which are frequently close to nodes. Finally, although significant lymphedema is uncommon with sentinel node biopsy for melanoma, it can occur, particularly in the setting of a wound infection. The surgeon should avoid unnecessary disruption of lymphatic channels and removal of nonsentinel lymph nodes. Limiting the morbidity of the procedure in this way may decrease the risk of limb swelling.

Complete Lymphadenectomy

Complete lymphadenectomy is the standard of care for all patients with nodal metastases. This operation is clearly more invasive than the sentinel node procedure and entails an increased risk of morbidity. Complete removal and pathology evaluation of an adequate number of lymph nodes is important (Table 3).

The first step in all anatomic sites is creation of skin flaps. Sharp dissection of flaps decreases thermal injury and should be considered when survival of the flap may be tenuous. Experience is important in determining the thickness of the skin flaps, which should be as thin as possible without compromising perfusion. In all anatomic areas, sacrifice of some sensory nerves is frequently necessary, but these structures should be preserved when the completeness of the dissection is not compromised. Electrocautery is useful for much of the dissection, but any visible lymphatic channels should be secured with ties or clips.

Closed-suction drains are placed through separate stab incisions and left in place until drainage is less than 25 ml/day for 2 consecutive days. Gentle range-of-motion exercises are advisable after complete dissection, but exercise should be avoided until drains have been removed and healing is complete. Then exercise can be gradually increased, taking care to avoid lymphedema caused by strenuous exercise before collateral lymphatic channels are fully developed.

Neck Dissection

The specific nature of a complete lymph node dissection in the neck is dependent on the clinical scenario indicating the need for the procedure. Dissections for clinically evident disease will differ from those for micrometastases, and there may be variation based on the site of the primary melanoma, as well. The presence of gross disease requires a more radical approach, rarely with removal of the internal jugular vein, spinal accessory nerve, and sternocleidomastoid if they are invaded by extracapsular invasion. In the setting of microscopic disease, such as a positive sentinel lymph node, all functionally important structures can generally be preserved. Dissections in patients with primary lesions of the trunk can spare the submandibular level I nodes. The parotid lymph nodes should be removed via superficial parotidectomy for patients with primary lesions of the face or scalp anterior to the coronal suture or for patients with evidence of preauricular drainage seen on lymphoscintigraphy.

Axillary Dissection

All three levels of the axilla should be included in the dissection. The superior border of the dissection is the axillary vein from the thoracic inlet (Halsted's ligament) to the latissimus dorsi tendon. Medially the dissection extends to the serratus anterior and intercostal muscles and should include any interpectoral (Rotter's) nodes if the primary lesion is on the anterior chest. The lateral border is the edge of the latissimus dorsi muscle, and the inferior border is the fourth intercostal space. The subscapularis forms the posterior border of the dissection. The pectoralis minor muscle may be transected or removed if necessary to ensure complete dissection of level III nodes. The lateral thoracic and thoracodorsal nerves should be preserved unless directly involved with tumor. Some branches of the intercostobrachial sensory nerves may need to be sacrificed, and patients should be counseled preoperatively regarding possible sensory changes in the posterior upper arm.

Inguinal Dissection

A superficial inguinal dissection extends 5 to 6 cm superior to the inguinal ligament, clearing tissue superficial to the abdominal fascia. The medial border is the adductor magnus, and the lateral border is the sartorius. The dissection extends inferior to the bottom of the muscular triangle formed by these muscles. All lymphatic tissue overlying or surrounding the femoral vessels should be removed.

The motor branches of the femoral nerve should be spared, but some sensory branches may need to be included. The patient should be advised of a possible area of numbness in the anterior thigh. The highest superficial lymph node (Cloquet's node) is taken from the femoral canal and sent for immediate frozen section analysis. The presence of tumor within this node mandates dissection of the deep inguinal basin, as does a palpable inguinal nodal metastasis.

Because a superficial dissection leaves the femoral vessels unprotected except for thin skin flaps, it is advisable to transpose the sartorius muscle over these vessels. The muscle is mobilized and transected at its origin. Horizontal mattress sutures secure the muscle to the inguinal ligament at the level of the vessels. At the time of wound closure, the skin edges should be trimmed if there is any question of viability so that well-perfused tissue is used for closure. Drains should exit proximal to the wound.

A deep inguinal dissection of the iliac, hypogastric, and obturator nodes should be performed if Cloquet's node contains tumor, if there is clinically evident disease in the superficial basin, or if more than three superficial lymph nodes are involved. One of two approaches is used. The superficial dissection incision can be extended superolaterally onto the lower abdomen and the inguinal ligament transected. Alternatively, a separate, muscle-splitting incision can be made obliquely along the lower abdomen, 5 cm above the inguinal ligament. The musculature of the abdominal wall is then split, and the retroperitoneal space entered anteriorly. The peritoneum is preserved and swept superiorly. The ureter is protected and kept with the peritoneum. This mobilization is generally easily accomplished with gentle, blunt dissection. The pelvic vessels are left exposed to allow dissection of all lymphatic tissue along the iliac, hypogastric, and obturator vessels.

Popliteal Dissection

The popliteal basin is bordered laterally and superiorly by the biceps femoris and medially and superiorly by the semimembranosus and semitendinosus muscles. The medial and lateral heads of the gastrocnemius form the inferior borders; the popliteus muscle is the deep limit. Ligation of the lesser saphenous vein is often necessary. This basin should be considered part of the inguinal basin, and positive lymph nodes in this location mandate dissection of the superficial inguinal nodes.

Ectopic Sentinel Nodes

The advent of lymphatic mapping has increased recognition of ectopic nodal sites, including epitrochlear nodes and nodes within the intermuscular triangle of the back. Popliteal nodes and nodes along the flank, inferior to the traditionally defined axilla, should also be included in this category. These locations should be treated as extensions of the adjacent lymphatic basin. Positive nodes within these sites should be treated with excision of those sites and dissection of the adjacent basin.

Adjuvant Radiotherapy

Although melanoma is classically considered to be radioresistant, evidence suggests that radiotherapy may decrease the risk of recurrence in dissected nodal basins with high-risk features such as multiple grossly enlarged metastases and significant extracapsular extension, or more than three tumor-involved nodes. The improvement in regional control must be balanced with increased morbidity related to radiation, such as a markedly increased risk of lymphedema. The risk-benefit ratio is most favorable in the cervical region, which also has a relatively high risk for regional nodal relapse. The surgeon's assessment of the extent of local disease and the risk for recurrence should be the basis for advising the patient regarding the potential role of radiation.

IN-TRANSIT METASTASES

Certain patients exhibit a pattern of metastatic disease that is peculiar to melanoma, in-transit metastases. These lesions result from foci of tumor cells that have spread via lymphatics without reaching lymph nodes and present as lesions of the dermis or subcutaneous tissue. The risk of in-transit metastasis is determined by characteristics of the primary melanoma and does not appear to be related to either the wide local excision margin or management of regional lymph nodes. Metastases may be extensive and management is often challenging. Limited numbers of lesions may be simply excised with a negative pathologic margin. However, this is often impossible because of the extent of disease, and recurrences are common. Among the several treatment strategies are isolated limb perfusion with a pump-oxygenator circuit and isolated limb infusion by a percutaneous approach. These techniques frequently lead to clinical responses but entail morbidity and are only possible when disease is limited to the extremity. Radiation has been employed, but it is often difficult to define an acceptable treatment field. Furthermore, radiation is not particularly effective for gross disease, but it can be effective in combination with other therapy to prevent or delay recurrence. Because laser ablation can effectively treat significant numbers of lesions with minimal morbidity, it is appropriate for dermal disease. Even fairly large defects heal well by secondary intention because of the limited damage of surrounding tissue.

We have used local immunotherapy effectively in most patients with in-transit disease. Techniques include injection of bacille Calmette-Guerin (BCG) or interferon-α and topical application of imiquimod cream (Aldara; 3M Pharmaceuticals, St. Paul, MN). These agents induce significant local inflammation and toxicities, including erythema, edema, and ulceration. BCG reportedly has also caused systemic toxicities and even deaths. We have not recently experienced this level of toxicity when using BCG dosing regimens based on purified protein derivative (PPD) skin test responsiveness. Approximately 80% of injected lesions regress after injection. Larger lesions and subcutaneous lesions have a lower response rate and should be excised after BCG injection.

TREATMENT OF DISTANT METASTASES

The presence of distant metastatic disease has traditionally been regarded as a contraindication for surgery. However, surgical resection of distant metastases is appropriate in carefully selected patients. Although systemic therapy in melanoma has never been associated with improved survival (response rates are low and 5-year survival is measured in single digits), a recent trial of postoperative adjuvant vaccine therapy after complete resection of distant melanoma metastases demonstrated nearly 40% 5-year survival, comparable to that after resection of hepatic metastases from colorectal cancer. Long-term survival has been seen after resection of melanoma metastatic to distant soft tissue, lung, and other visceral sites. Isolated small bowel metastases appear to have a particularly favorable prognosis.

Selection of appropriate patients for resection is important. Preoperative staging of disease should be based on computed tomography of the chest, abdomen, and pelvis, whole-body positron emission tomography and magnetic resonance imaging of the brain. Tumors with slow doubling times (>40 days) have the most favorable prognosis. Although a solitary metastasis carries the best prognosis, the number of lesions in patients with more than a single metastasis does not seem to have a major impact on outcome, as long as all disease can be removed.

SUGGESTED READINGS

Balch C, Buzaid AC, Soong SJ, and others: Final version of the American Joint Committee on Cancer staging system for cutaneous melanoma, *J Clin Oncol* 9:3635, 2001.

Cochran A, Roberts A, Wen DR, and others: optimized assessment of sentinel lymph nodes for metastatic melanoma: implications for regional surgery and overall treatment planning, *Ann Surg Oncol* 11:(3S):156S, 2004.

Morton DL, Thompson JF, Cochran AJ, and others: Multicenter Selective Lymphadenectomy Trial Group: Sentinel node biopsy versus nodal observation for primary melanoma, *N Engl J Med* 355:1307, 2006.

Morton D, Ollila DW, Hsueh EC, and others: Cytoreductive surgery and adjuvant immunotherapy: A new management paradigm for metastatic melanoma, *CA Cancer J Clin* 49:101, 1999.

Morton D, Wen DR, Wong JH, and others: Technical details of intraoperative lymphatic mapping for early stage melanoma, *Arch Surg* 127:392, 1992.

SOFT-TISSUE SARCOMA

Samuel Singer, MD, and Robert J. Canter, MD

S oft tissue sarcomas are tumors that show evidence of mesenchymal differentiation. There are more than 50 individual histologic types of sarcoma, and accumulating evidence suggests that sarcomas exhibit unique patterns of spread, recurrence, and prognosis, depending on histologic type. For clinical purposes, sarcomas are primarily divided among extremity, superficial truncal, retroperitoneal/intra-abdominal, visceral, and head and neck locations. Extremity sarcomas account for nearly 50% of adult sarcomas, while retroperitoneal/intra-abdominal sarcomas represent approximately 15% (Fig. 1).

Soft tissue sarcomas have an age-adjusted incidence of 2 per 100,000 and represent approximately 1% of adult malignancies and approximately 15% of pediatric malignancies. In the United States, there are approximately 10,000 cases per year, divided equally between males and females.

ETIOLOGY

Several genetic syndromes are associated with the development of sarcomas. Gardner's syndrome is associated with the formation of multiple desmoid tumors. Li-Fraumeni syndrome is a familial cancer syndrome associated with an increased risk of soft-tissue sarcoma, as well as osteosarcoma, breast cancer, acute leukemia, brain tumors, adrenocortical carcinomas, and gonadal germ cell tumors. This syndrome arises from a germline mutation in the p53 tumor suppressor gene. Neurofibromatosis I, or von Recklinghausen's disease, is an autosomal dominant disorder characterized by multiple

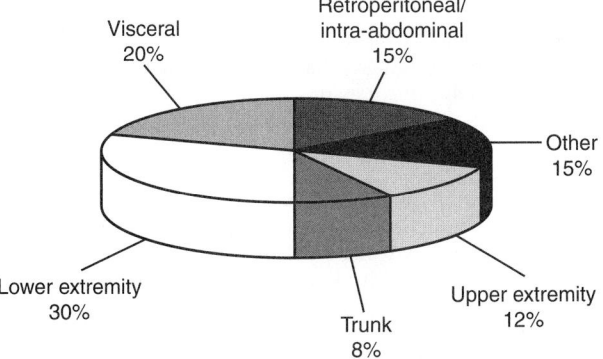

Figure 1 Anatomic distribution of all cases of soft-tissue sarcoma evaluated, treated, and followed prospectively at Memorial Sloan-Kettering Cancer Center over a 23-year period. ("Other" includes head and neck, thoracic, breast, and skin.)

neurofibromas and café au lait spots. These patients are predisposed to malignant peripheral nerve sheath tumors. Sarcomas have also been associated with other chromosomal alterations including amplification of chromosome 12 (well-differentiated and dedifferentiated liposarcoma) and the translocations TLS-CHOP (myxoid/round cell liposarcoma) and SSX-SYT (synovial sarcoma).

Environmental factors have also been linked to the occurrence of sarcomas. For example, exposure to herbicides has been postulated to predispose patients to an increased incidence of sarcoma, although a true causal relationship has not been firmly established. Previous exposure to radiation has clearly been shown to predispose patients to the development of subsequent soft-tissue sarcoma. There is generally a delay of 3 years or more between radiation exposure and onset of disease. However, once present, radiation-induced sarcomas tend to run a virulent course. Stewart-Treves syndrome is defined as the development of an angiosarcoma associated with lymphedema, classically in the arms of breast cancer patients following mastectomy and axillary lymph node dissection.

TREATMENT

The primary treatment modality for soft-tissue sarcomas in all locations and for the majority of histologic types remains wide, en bloc surgical resection. Accomplishing this goal frequently requires contiguous organ resection to achieve a complete resection. This is particularly true for retroperitoneal sarcoma, for which 30% of patients undergo additional organ resection. Astute surgical judgment is necessary to determine the appropriate extent of resection. Location, depth, proximity to critical anatomic structures, and histologic type are all important factors for the surgeon to evaluate.

The treatment of sarcoma has evolved considerably over the past 30 years. Although wide resection with adequate margins remains of critical importance, limb preservation and avoidance of major morbidity have received increasing attention. When complete resection would involve sacrifice of a major nerve or bony structure with risk of serious functional loss, the trend has been toward preservation of major neurovascular structures with the addition of appropriate radiation therapy. These considerations highlight the importance of coordinated, multimodality treatment of sarcoma patients at specialized, multidisciplinary centers. The involvement of surgeons, radiotherapists, medical oncologists, and reconstructive surgeons in the total care of these patients is essential.

EXTREMITY SARCOMAS

The clinical evaluation and treatment of sarcomas is dictated in large part by their location. Extremity soft-tissue sarcomas are considered first, followed by retroperitoneal and visceral sarcomas.

Diagnosis

Diagnosis begins with a comprehensive history and physical examination. During the early course of disease, clinical manifestations are infrequent, and a mass is the most common presenting complaint. Frequently, a trivial traumatic event may initially draw attention to the area, although there is probably no causal relation between a history of trauma and the development of a sarcoma.

When a suspicious mass is discovered, a biopsy is indicated. In centers having significant experience with sarcomas, a core needle biopsy is typically performed as the first step. This can diagnose the presence of sarcoma and the grade in greater than 80% of cases. For histologic type, the accuracy of core biopsy decreases to approximately 75%. In some institutions, an open biopsy remains the most reliable means of obtaining a diagnosis. Lesions smaller than 3 cm can be completely excised in one procedure, as long as such an approach would not compromise a subsequent reexcision. An incisional biopsy in a longitudinal orientation is the preferred approach for lesions larger than 3 cm. It is critical that the dissection, including the skin incision, is planned so that the biopsy tract can be excised completely in the final resection. The consequences of an inappropriately placed incision can be severe, requiring greater tissue dissection at reoperation and the need for a more complex wound closure with a resultant higher risk of postoperative wound complications.

Staging

After a tissue specimen has been obtained, the pathologist can determine the histologic type and grade of sarcoma. There are more than 50 different histologic types of sarcoma, and classification is based principally on the light microscopic appearance of the tumor, its presumed site of origin, and immunohistochemical and molecular markers. The most common soft-tissue sarcomas of the extremity in adults are liposarcoma and malignant fibrous histiocytoma (MFH) (Fig. 2), although several studies suggest that MFH may be further classified into myxofibrosarcoma and other undifferentiated, pleomorphic subtypes. In children, rhabdomyosarcoma and fibrosarcoma are the most prevalent types. Liposarcoma is subdivided into three main biologic groups including (1) well-differentiated/dedifferentiated, (2) myxoid/round cell, and (3) pleomorphic. The myxoid/round cell and pleomorphic subtypes are typically found on the extremity, whereas the well-differentiated/dedifferentiated subtype is more common in the retroperitoneum. Histologic type, grade, and size are the most important predictors of outcome and are used to select patients most likely to benefit from neoadjuvant or adjuvant therapies.

Cross-sectional imaging is invaluable before definitive resection of a sarcoma. The goal of these studies is to define the size and extent of the tumor so that an optimal resection can be designed and patients informed of the functional consequences of the planned procedure. The most commonly used imaging modalities for evaluation of soft-tissue sarcomas are computed tomography (CT) and magnetic resonance imaging (MRI). Although CT scanning is less expensive and easier to obtain, MRI typically provides better resolution of soft tissues. Bone scans and conventional angiography were previously used to delineate bony involvement and vascular anatomy but are now rarely necessary with the quality of current cross-sectional imaging modalities. Because the lungs are the most common site of distant disease, a CT scan of the chest is indicated, particularly in patients with high-grade lesions, to rule out metastasis.

The combination of histologic and radiographic information can then be used to stage the patient. Multiple staging systems have been developed. They are based on the histologic grade of the tumor, its size, and the presence of metastases in regional lymph nodes or distant sites. The American Joint Committee on Cancer (AJCC) produced a revised staging system in 2002. Histopathologic grade is divided into four categories: well differentiated (G1), moderately differentiated (G2), poorly differentiated (G3), and undifferentiated (G4). Tumors less than or equal to 5 cm in greatest dimension (T1) are separated from tumors greater than 5 cm (T2). The size classification is further subdivided into superficial and deep tumors as noted by the suffixes *a* and *b*, respectively. Stage IV disease is defined as the presence of regional lymph node metastases (N1) or distant metastases (M1).

Some experts disagree regarding the most accurate staging system. Although the AJCC staging system has overall been found to correlate with rates of local recurrence, disease-free survival, and overall survival, significant variability exists within respective stages in relation to prognosis, and many authors consider it to have little applicability to the care of patients with sarcoma. Long-term follow-up data from more than 2000 patients at the Memorial Sloan-Kettering Cancer Center have been used to develop a postoperative nomogram that predicts disease-specific death for individual patients with soft-tissue sarcoma (Fig. 3). This model has been validated in other large, single-institution sarcoma databases. It should complement, if not replace, other staging systems in patient counseling and stratification for clinical trials.

Surgical Treatment

Resection is the mainstay of treatment, although other modalities are important as adjuvants. Sarcomas are typically surrounded by a pseudocapsule. This cannot be used as a plane of dissection, in that microscopic disease extends beyond the pseudocapsule and will uniformly lead to local recurrence. Local recurrence rates decreased dramatically when this was recognized, and radical resection was often performed, with excision of entire muscle groups. Significant morbidity may be associated with this approach because it can lead to substantial impairment in limb function and even amputation. In patients who eventually will succumb to distant disease, the increased morbidity of compartmental resection seems unnecessary. Recent focus has therefore been placed on preservation of limbs and limb function by using wide local resection with selected application of adjuvant radiation.

A wide excision with 1- to 2-cm margins is the ideal surgical approach for all sarcomas. However, margins are sometimes limited by functional and anatomic constraints. For patients with low-grade sarcomas, wide excision alone with 1-cm or greater margins is sufficient treatment. External beam radiotherapy is selectively employed for certain histologic types of low-grade sarcoma excised with microscopically positive margins or margins less than 1 cm (without an intact fascial boundary). This can reduce the risk of local recurrence for low-grade tumors by approximately 20% and is appropriate if a subsequent local recurrence would result in sacrifice of a major neurovascular bundle or

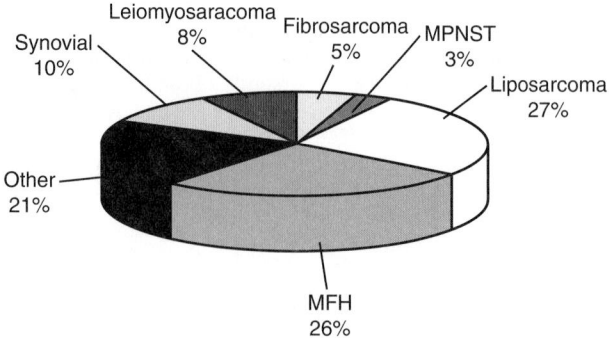

Figure 2 Histopathologic distribution of all cases of extremity soft-tissue sarcoma evaluated, treated, and followed prospectively at Memorial Sloan-Kettering Cancer Center over a 23-year period. ("Other" includes Ewing's sarcoma/primitive neuroectodermal tumor osteosarcoma, rhabdomyosarcoma, epithelioid sarcoma, chondrosarcoma, and clear cell sarcoma, among others.) *MFH,* Malignant fibrous histiocytoma; *MPNST,* malignant peripheral nerve sheath tumor.

Figure 3 Postoperative nomogram for 12-year sarcoma-specific death based on 2163 patients treated at Memorial Sloan-Kettering Cancer Center. Points are assigned for each variable to calculate a total number of points, which is then used to determine probability of disease-specific death. *Fibro,* Fibrosarcoma; *Gr,* grade; *Lipo,* liposarcoma; *Leiomyo,* leiomyosarcoma; *MFH,* malignant fibrous histiocytoma; *MPNST,* malignant peripheral nerve sheath tumor; *SSD,* sarcoma-specific death. *From Kattan MW, Leung DH, Brennan MF: Post-operative nomogram for 12-year sarcoma-specific death, J Clin Oncol 20(3):791, 2002, with permission.*

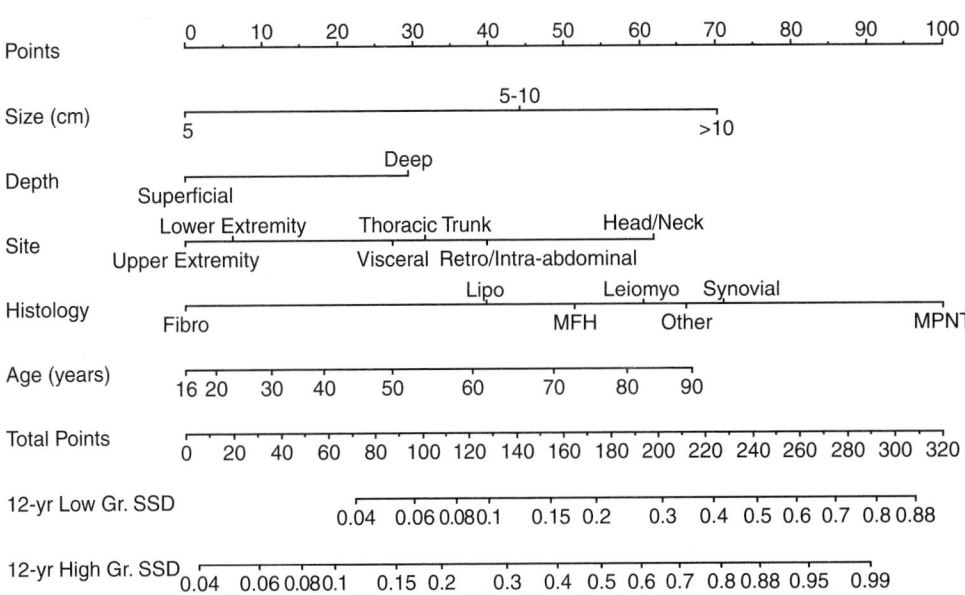

risk amputation. For atypical lipomatous tumors/well-differentiated liposarcoma of the extremity, the local recurrence rate following surgical resection is sufficiently low that postoperative external beam radiotherapy is rarely necessary even in cases with microscopically positive margins.

Dermatofibrosarcoma protuberans (DFSP) typically has finger-like extensions that extend radially from the main tumor mass. Initial excision with 2- to 3-cm lateral margins and excision of deep fascia with the specimen should be performed. DFSP with microscopically positive margins should be aggressively reexcised until clean margins are achieved. Radiotherapy is rarely indicated unless frank fibrosarcomatous degeneration is found.

In cases of high-grade sarcoma, equivalent disease-free and overall survival rates have been reported with limb-sparing procedures in conjunction with radiotherapy, as compared with amputation. In most specialized centers, amputation rates for primary tumors are currently 3% to 5% and are typically limited either to cases of distal tumors or advanced tumors in which it does not appear possible to perform a complete resection without compromising limb function. An algorithm for patient management on the basis of sarcoma grade, size, and surgical margin is depicted in Figure 4. Because histologic type in many cases defines grade and underlying biologic behavior, we foresee a time when this variable will ultimately dictate the overall treatment approach.

When tumors are close to neural or bony structures, close margins are accepted to avoid significant functional impairment. Tumors abutting major vascular structures may be carefully dissected free of the vessel while preserving a sufficient sheath around the tumor. Conversely, vascular resections can be performed if a clear dissection plane cannot be achieved because arterial reconstruction is possible with good results (Fig. 5). Venous reconstruction is rarely successful and typically unnecessary because of the development of collateral circulation. However, an effort should be made to preserve the greater saphenous vein when resection of the superficial femoral vein is performed. For distal tumors, every effort is made to minimize functional deficits and optimize wound healing while avoiding amputation by the liberal use of pedicled and/or free flap tissue reconstruction.

Adjuvant Therapy

Radiotherapy can be administered before, during, or after surgery. For patients with lesions smaller than 5 cm, adjuvant radiation

therapy adds little to complete surgical excision, except in cases of recurrent sarcoma. Conversely, all patients with lesions greater than 5 cm, particularly if these were excised with margins less than 1 cm, should be considered for adjuvant radiotherapy as a proven method for limiting local recurrence. It may be given as external beam radiation or in the form of brachytherapy. There have been no studies directly comparing these methods of administration, and no marked difference in local control has been noted when each method has been used separately for high-grade tumors. Each technique offers some advantages and disadvantages that may guide the physician's choice of administration, as well as timing with other treatment modalities. Preoperative radiotherapy has the advantages of requiring a smaller field of radiation exposure and a lower dose than postoperative radiation because of relative hypoxia at the resection site. However, it has been demonstrated to have a higher wound complication rate than postoperative radiation without a significant benefit in terms of local recurrence or survival. Therefore, preoperative radiotherapy is generally reserved for patients whose tumors are initially considered too large to resect with acceptable morbidity.

Brachytherapy involves intraoperative placement of catheters within the resection bed, followed by loading of the catheters with radioactive isotope 5 to 7 days postoperatively and treatment for a period of 5 to 6 days. Although this technique is associated with rates of wound complications similar to those of postoperative external beam radiotherapy (provided that therapy is delayed at least 5 days after surgery), it has the advantages of less radiation scatter and a much shorter duration of therapy. Brachytherapy is indicated only in the setting of high-grade lesions, whereas external beam radiation has been used for both high-grade and low-grade lesions.

Adjuvant systemic chemotherapy has also been used in patients with extremity sarcoma. Individual trials of postoperative chemotherapy have generally failed to demonstrate a survival benefit. A meta-analysis of data from previous randomized trials revealed statistically significant improvements in local recurrence, distant recurrence, and disease-free survival rates, ranging from a 6% to 10% absolute benefit at 10 years in patients who received doxorubicin-containing postoperative chemotherapy. However, the same analysis showed only a 4% improvement in overall survival, a rate that was not statistically significant. Therefore, postoperative chemotherapy cannot be considered standard therapy. The combination of doxorubicin and ifosfamide appears to have improved antitumor activity, with improvements in local control, disease-free survival, and overall

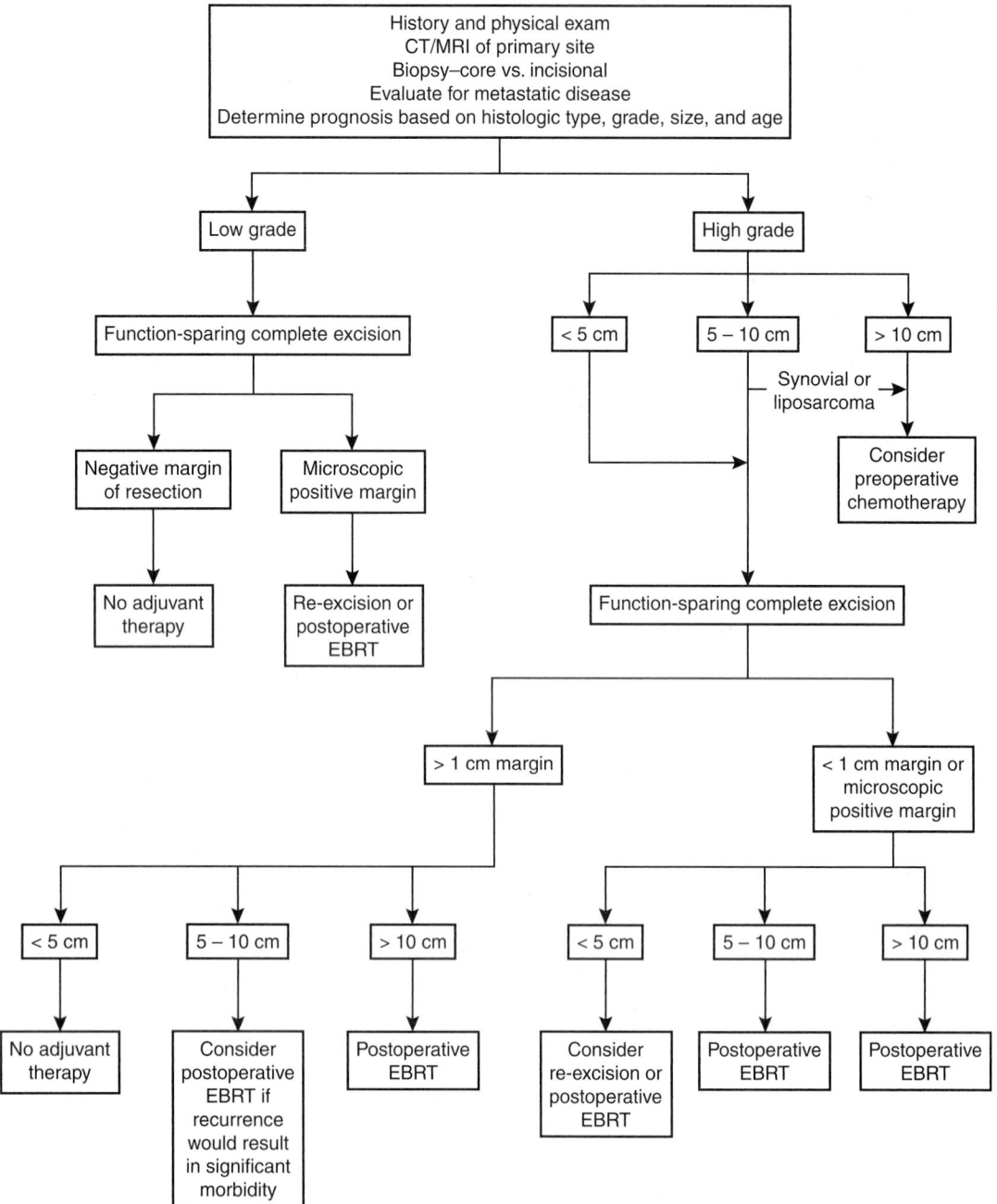

Figure 4 Algorithm for multimodality patient management based on sarcoma grade, size, and surgical margin. Perioperative brachytherapy can substitute for EBRT depending on physician and patient preference. *CT*, Computed tomographic scan; *EBRT*, external beam radiation therapy; *MRI*, magnetic resonance imaging. *Adapted from Brennan MF, Singer S, Maki RG, O'Sullivan B: Sarcomas of the soft tissues and bone. In De Vita V, Hellman S, Rosenberg S, editors: Cancer: Principles and practice of oncology, ed 7, Philadelphia, 2005, Lippincott Williams, and Wilkins, p 1602, with permission.*

survival, particularly for large, high-grade sarcomas. However, potential toxicity from these agents is substantial, and there remains little consensus regarding the indications for their use.

Given the high risk of recurrence in patients with tumors greater than 10 cm, these patients should be considered candidates for investigational approaches, especially neoadjuvant chemotherapy (see Figure 4). Preoperative chemotherapy has been shown to improve outcomes for patients with Ewing's sarcoma, rhabdomyosarcoma, and osteosarcoma. These results have prompted investigators to extend the use of preoperative chemotherapy to other histologic types of adult soft-tissue sarcoma. Advocates have emphasized several theoretical benefits, including an ability to assess tumor responsiveness to the given chemotherapeutic agents, early treatment of metastatic disease, and downstaging of the primary tumor. Since 1990, interest has focused on regimens combining systemic doxorubicin and ifosfamide. A recent retrospective stratified analysis of prospectively collected, multi-institutional data demonstrated an association between improved disease-specific survival (21% survival benefit at 3 years) and the use of neoadjuvant chemotherapy using combination doxorubicin and ifosfamide

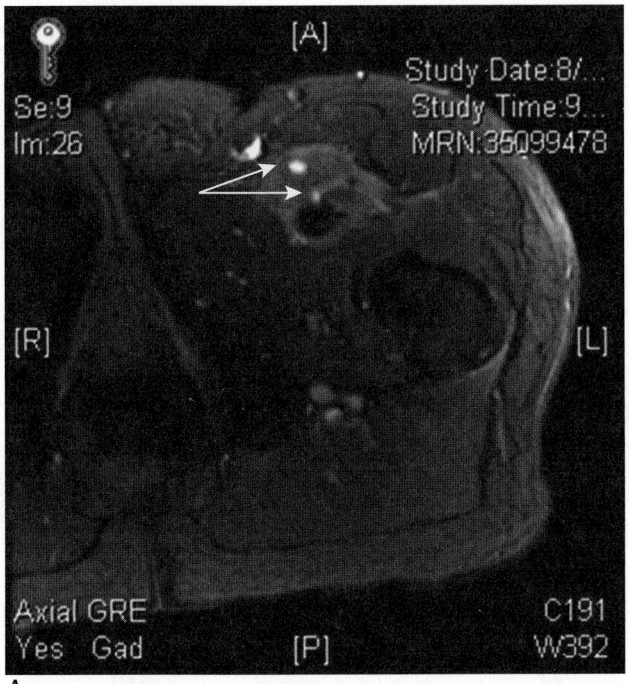

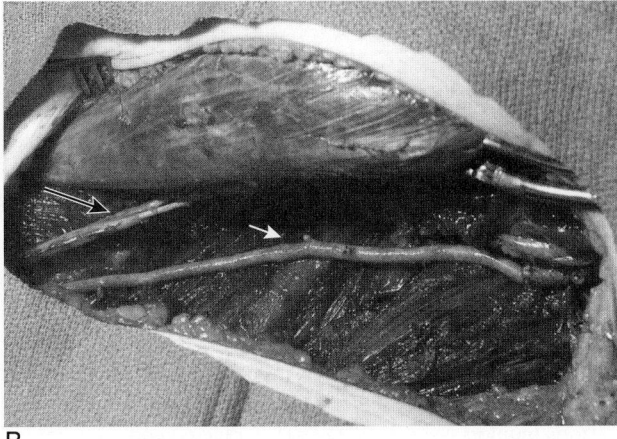

A   B

Figure 5 **(A)** Magnetic resonance imaging depicts a 5- × 4-cm extraskeletal osteosarcoma arising between the abductor longus and vastus medialis muscles, encasing the superficial and deep femoral vessels at their origin *(white arrows)*. **(B)** Intraoperative photograph following en bloc resection of proximal thigh sarcoma with the superficial femoral artery and vein. The artery was reconstructed with a reversed saphenous bypass graft *(thick arrow)*. The femoral nerve was skeletonized, and branches to the vastus lateralis muscle were preserved *(thin arrow)*. Tumor extended to this margin, but postoperative external beam radiotherapy was administered, and excellent limb function was maintained. *(See color insert Figure 54.)*

in patients with high-grade extremity sarcomas greater than 10 cm, extremity synovial sarcoma greater than 5 cm, and high-grade extremity liposarcoma greater than 5 cm.

Finally, regional therapy in the form of isolated limb perfusion (ILP) or isolated limb infusion (ILI) with chemotherapeutic agents such as melphalan in combination with tumor necrosis factor-α or interferon-γ can be used in cases in which local control or limb salvage is particularly challenging. Toxicity in the perfused limb is generally not severe and is often related to necrosis of the tumor. Systemic toxicity can be severe if there is a leak of perfusate into the systemic circulation. This technique provides only regional therapy; thus its application is limited to locally advanced disease that would otherwise require amputation for local control. ILP has demonstrated limb salvage rates of greater than 80%. In addition, ILP may be used to palliate patients with stage IV disease that is unresectable. This may preserve the function of the affected limb and quality of life over the anticipated short period of survival of these patients.

Sarcomas spread by a hematogenous route. Therefore regional lymph node involvement is unusual, and elective lymph node dissection is usually not indicated. Approximately 10% of patients with epithelioid sarcoma, synovial sarcoma, and rhabdomyosarcoma subtypes have metastases to regional lymph nodes. Nodal metastases are also seen in 5% of patients with malignant fibrous histiocytomas.

Local recurrence of sarcoma is associated with a poor prognosis. However, it has not been determined whether there is causal relationship between local recurrence and decreased survival. The site of recurrence may be a source for further metastasis, but randomized trials comparing wide local excision to amputation have shown no measurable difference in overall survival, despite a 25% to 30% difference in local recurrence rate. The size of the local

recurrence and the time interval to local recurrence are the critical determinants of subsequent sarcoma-specific survival. Local recurrences should be treated by aggressive reexcision encompassing previous drain sites and scars. Considerations for preservation of limb function are analogous to those in primary resections, and radiotherapy should also be considered. Even if the site has been previously irradiated, brachytherapy or intraoperative radiotherapy may be options for additional treatment. Neoadjuvant chemotherapy should be considered for patients with local recurrences of high-grade tumors, especially for those that are large in size and occur with a short, disease-free interval. Approximately two thirds of patients who undergo resections for local recurrences will experience long-term survival.

Patients who die of their disease generally succumb to distant metastases. Tumors with high histologic grade and size exceeding 5 cm have a greater probability of metastasizing. Longer intervals from the treatment of the primary tumor to the occurrence of metastatic disease are associated with a better prognosis. Pulmonary lesions should be resected, as long as a complete resection is possible and the patient can tolerate the operation. Survival at 5 years in patients with completely resected pulmonary metastases ranges from 15% to 30% in multiple series.

RETROPERITONEAL AND VISCERAL SARCOMA

Retroperitoneal and visceral sarcoma are less common than extremity sarcoma, comprising 34% of all cases. The most common histopathologic types in the retroperitoneum are liposarcoma (48%) and leiomyosarcoma (23%) (Figure 6). Approximately 55% of retroperitoneal liposarcomas are well differentiated and therefore low grade,

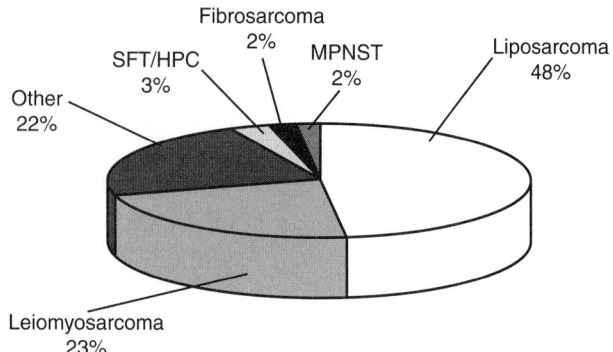

Figure 6 Histopathologic distribution of all cases of retroperitoneal soft-tissue sarcoma evaluated, treated, and followed up prospectively at Memorial Sloan-Kettering Cancer Center over a 23-year period. ("Other" includes rhabdomyosarcoma, synovial sarcoma, and Ewing's sarcoma/primitive neuroectodermal tumor, among others.) *MPNST,* Malignant peripheral nerve sheath tumor; *SFT/HPC,* solitary fibrous tumor/hemangiopericytoma.

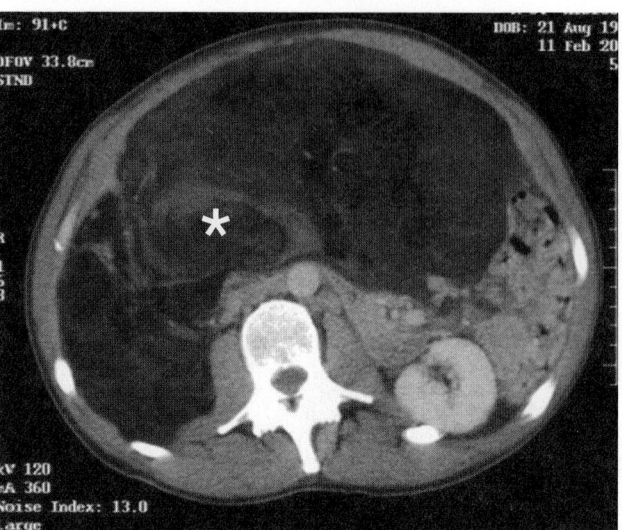

Figure 7 Computed tomographic scanning demonstrates a 34-cm tumor of the right retroperitoneum with involvement of perirenal tissue *(asterisk).* The tumor was resected en bloc with the right kidney. Pathologic analysis revealed well-differentiated liposarcoma with a close margin near the vena cava (0.03 cm). No postoperative therapy was administered.

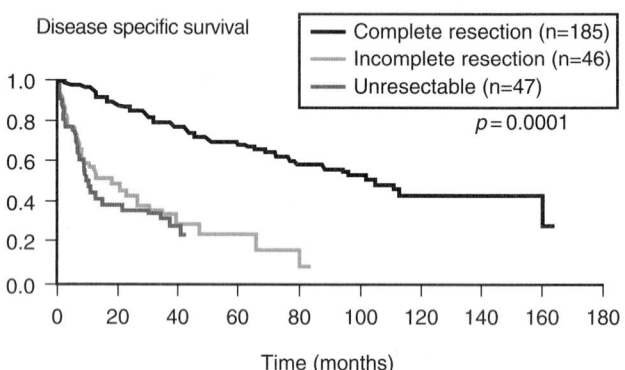

Figure 8 Incomplete resection provides no survival benefit for patients with retroperitoneal sarcoma. *From Lewis JJ, Leung D, Woodruff JM, and others: Retroperitoneal soft tissue sarcoma: analysis of 500 patients treated and followed at a single institution,* Ann Surg *228(3):355, 1998, with permission.*

while approximately 40% are dedifferentiated and therefore high grade at primary presentation. In the visceral location, gastrointestinal stromal tumors (GIST), leiomyosarcoma, and desmoid tumors are the most common histologic types. Overall, retroperitoneal and visceral sarcomas carry a worse prognosis because their central location often precludes wide resection, the delivery of effective doses of radiotherapy without bowel toxicity is difficult, and they are frequently not diagnosed until they have reached a relatively advanced stage.

Diagnosis

Most patients present with an abdominal mass (80%) and occasionally with lower-extremity neurologic symptoms (42%) or pain (37%). The majority of tumors are greater than 10 cm in diameter at the time of presentation. Occasionally, patients with leiomyosarcoma of the retroperitoneum can present with profound hypoglycemia and concomitant neuroglycopenic symptoms secondary to secretion of insulin-like growth factor by the tumor.

Evaluation of a suspected retroperitoneal sarcoma should include a CT scan of the chest, abdomen, and pelvis to evaluate the local extent of disease and the presence of hepatic or lung metastasis (see Figure 7). Percutaneous core biopsy is generally not performed before operation because of concerns of seeding the needle tract with malignant tumor cells or rupture of a suspected GIST. However, if lymphoma or a germ cell tumor is considered in the differential diagnosis, for example with a tumor in a para-aortic or paracaval location, then image-guided biopsy is indicated because these entities are treated primarily with chemotherapy. Similarly, preoperative biopsy is necessary before enrollment in trials of investigational neoadjuvant therapy.

Treatment

As with extremity sarcoma, surgery remains the critical component of therapy in retroperitoneal and visceral lesions. Multiple studies with large numbers of patients have consistently shown that complete surgical resection is the primary factor in outcome (Fig. 8). In contrast, chemotherapy has not been shown to be effective for retroperitoneal sarcoma, and radiation is limited by toxicity to adjacent structures, particularly the bowel. Preoperative radiation therapy with newer, more focused, image-guided technology has received attention as a strategy to potentially improve outcomes. However, a recent, randomized, phase III trial of preoperative external beam radiation versus surgery alone sponsored by the American College of Surgeons Oncology Group was closed early because of poor accrual. As a result, surgery offers the only proven effective treatment.

Complete gross resection is possible in approximately 80% of patients who present with primary disease and frequently requires resection of neighboring organs. Consequently, preoperative bowel preparation is important because resection of intestine is often necessary for technical reasons to achieve the goal of complete resection with negative margins. With retroperitoneal sarcoma, evaluation of renal function, particularly the kidney contralateral to the tumor, is important because ipsilateral nephrectomy is often necessary. Because actual renal parenchymal invasion by retroperitoneal sarcoma is rare, it is possible to preserve nephron mass by dissecting the renal capsule with the tumor and leaving the underlying kidney parenchyma in place. This technique may be more challenging than simple nephrectomy and requires careful attention to hemostasis because bleeding from the renal parenchyma can be troublesome. In patients with borderline renal function, this is an effective strategy that permits organ preservation without compromising oncologic outcome. In the left retroperitoneum, it may also be necessary to remove the spleen and the distal pancreas in order to achieve a complete resection. In addition, when operating on well-differentiated/dedifferentiated liposarcoma, we advocate removal of all the retroperitoneal fat from the ipsilateral pelvis to the diaphragm because involvement by liposarcoma may be multifocal and discontinuous.

Patients who have unresectable tumors on the basis of radiologic studies may be candidates for neoadjuvant chemotherapy and/or radiotherapy trials in an attempt to decrease tumor size to the point at which resection is possible. However, resection should be attempted only if a complete resection is anticipated because incomplete resection has not been shown to offer any survival benefit (see Figure 8). Approximately 25% of patients with complete gross resections will nevertheless have positive microscopic margins.

Patients with high-grade retroperitoneal sarcoma have a disease-specific rate of survival significantly worse than those with low-grade tumors (median survival 33 months versus 149 months). Approximately half of the patients with a local recurrence have disease that is grossly resectable. Resection is the only effective treatment for a local recurrence. Distant disease most frequently occurs in the liver (44%), lung (38%), or both (18%). If the distant disease is isolated, it should be considered for resection because long-term survival is possible following metastasectomy. Overall, however, patients with metastatic disease have only a 10-month median survival.

As with sarcomas of the extremity, locally recurrent retroperitoneal sarcoma can be a formidable clinical problem. Patients with retroperitoneal recurrence usually present with nonspecific symptoms, sometimes only after the lesion has reached a substantial size. Following an assessment of the extent of disease, patients with isolated local recurrence should undergo re-resection if possible. The most difficult decision in retroperitoneal liposarcoma is the timing of reoperation, and a period of close observation is often appropriate. When re-resection can be performed, two thirds of patients experience a durable survival benefit. Conversely, it is a reasonable strategy with locally recurrent retroperitoneal sarcoma that appears unresectable to wait for patients to develop symptoms referable to the sarcoma and then to perform a palliative resection. Patients can often be durably palliated, sometimes for years with well-differentiated liposarcoma, with debulking. After surgical options have been exhausted, systemic chemotherapy may be used. Tumor regression and improved, progression-free survival are possible in 30% to 50% of patients, but treatment is largely palliative and patients are rarely cured with this approach.

CONCLUSION

Primary therapy for soft tissue sarcoma is predicated on surgical resection with an adequate margin of normal tissue. For high-risk patients, neoadjuvant chemotherapy with doxorubicin and ifosfamide may improve 3-year survival, but the long-term benefit on outcome remains unclear. Local control is improved with adjuvant radiation therapy, particularly for patients with margins less than 1 cm. Local recurrence rates vary, depending on anatomic site. In extremity lesions, 10% to 30% of patients develop locally recurrent disease, with a median disease-free interval of 18 months. Outcomes for patients with isolated extremity local recurrence approach those for primary disease. Long-term survival is also possible following complete resection of pulmonary metastases. In patients with retroperitoneal and visceral sarcoma, en bloc resection remains the cornerstone of therapy. As opposed to extremity sites, local recurrence in this location is a common cause of death. Patients with unresectable disease typically have a poor prognosis. However, in selected cases, surgical resection can provide meaningful palliation.

It is hoped that the advent of improved molecular techniques will lead to a better understanding of the pathogenesis and biology of soft-tissue sarcoma. Future improvements in the care of these patients will come from the development of targeted therapies specific to histologic type. In the meantime, surgical resection will remain the principal treatment for patients with soft-tissue sarcoma.

Suggested Readings

Brennan MF, Singer S, Maki RG, and others: Sarcomas of the soft tissues and bone. In DeVita V, Hellman S, Rosenberg S, editors: *Cancer: Principles and practice of oncology,* ed 7, Philadelphia, 2005, Lippincott Williams & Wilkins.

Grobmyer SR, Maki RG, Demetri GD: Neo-adjuvant chemotherapy for primary high-grade extremity soft tissue sarcoma, *Ann Oncol* 15(11):1667:2004.

Kattan MW, Leung DH, Brennan MF: Postoperative nomogram for 12-year sarcoma-specific death, *J Clin Oncol* 20:3:791:2002.

Lewis JJ, Leung D, Woodruff JM, and others: Retroperitoneal soft tissue sarcoma: Analysis of 500 patients treated and followed at a single institution, *Ann Surg* 228(3):355:1998.

Singer S, Antonescu CR, Riedel E, and others: Histologic subtype and margin of resection predict pattern of recurrence and survival for retroperitoneal sarcoma, *Ann Surg* 238(3):358:2003.

Singer S, Demetri GD, Baldini EH, and others: Management of soft-tissue sarcomas: An overview and update, *Lancet Oncol* 1:75:2000.

Management of the Isolated Neck Mass

Wayne M. Koch, MD, and David E. Tunkel, MD

The management of an isolated neck mass requires a working familiarity with neck anatomy, an organized and thorough approach to differential diagnosis, and a decision tree driven by consideration of factors including the location of the mass, its physical features, timing of appearance and growth, and patient characteristics.

DIFFERENTIAL DIAGNOSIS

The differential diagnosis of a solitary neck mass can be organized in broad categories: congenital, inflammatory, benign and malignant neoplasms, and traumatic (Table 1). The construction of an exhaustive differential diagnosis may be an interesting intellectual exercise and is occasionally useful for the true diagnostic dilemma. Generally, however, a good surgeon will quickly prioritize the possibilities, arrive at a short list of most likely candidates, and institute a plan to confirm the true diagnosis. In accord with this strategy, this review does not attempt to be exhaustive, but rather descriptive of thought process, emphasizing the most important factors for consideration.

Locations within the neck may be described using anatomic place-names, such as *jugulodigastric* or *paratracheal,* or by Roman numeral of neck levels (I through VI) (Fig. 1). Certain entities are

Table 1: Differential Diagnosis of Isolated Neck Mass

Category	Entity	Location	Age Range (Years)	Physical Features
Congenital	Vascular malformation	Any	0–2	Compressible, blue/red
	Branchial apparatus	Lateral	2–40	Cystic, rounded, discrete
	Thyroglossal	Central	2–30	Cystic
	Epidermoid	Any	0–30	Cystic
Inflammatory	Viral, bacterial, fungal	Lateral	Any	Soft solid*
	Granulomatous (atypical mycobacterium)		1–20	Solid
Benign	Salivary		>15	Firm, solid
	Thyroid		>15	Firm solid
	Schwannoma	Lateral	>15	Hard solid
	Chemodectoma	Lateral	>30	Pulsatile, CN palsy
	Lipoma	Any	>20	Soft
Malignant	Salivary		>25	Firm solid
	Thyroid		>15	Firm solid
	Sarcoma		>25	
	Lymphoma	Lateral	>10	Firm solid*
Metastatic	Squamous	Lateral	>35	Firm solid/cystic
	Adenocarcinoma	Supraclavicular	>35	Firm solid
	Salivary gland	Lateral	>25	Firm solid
	Thyroid	Any	>15	Firm solid
Traumatic	Hematoma	Any	Any	Compressible-firm
	Pseudoaneurysm	Lateral	Any	Pulsatile
	Neuroma			Trigger point pain

*Usually multiple.
CN, Cranial nerve.

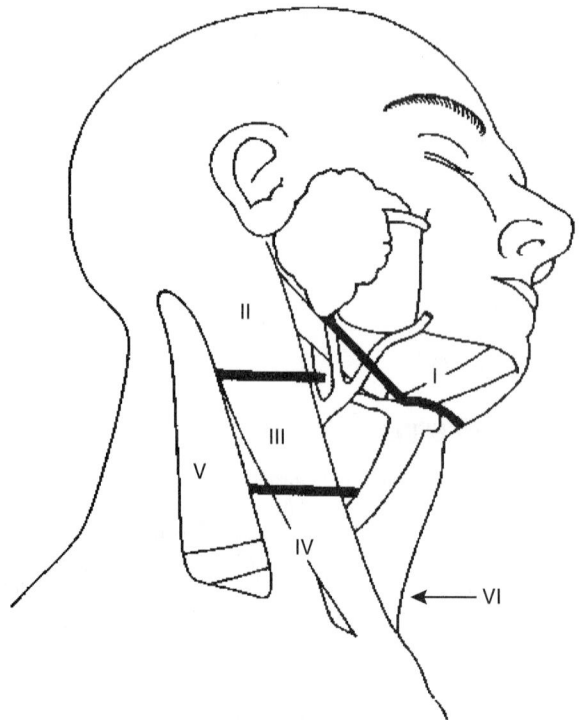

Figure 1   Regions of the neck are designated by Roman numerals as shown. Location of neck mass should be described accordingly.

found only in defined locations. For example, a thyroglossal duct cyst arises along the epithelial remnant left when the thyroid descends from tongue base to level VI during development, so these masses are found near the midline between hyoid bone and cricoid cartilage. Carotid body tumors splay the internal and external branches of the carotid just above the carotid bulb. Many normal structures that may be mistaken for isolated masses are suspected because of asymmetry of the hyoid, thyroid cartilage, or lateral processes of the cervical vertebrae. The distinctive location of these structures is one clue as to their identity. Similarly, the location of masses within the thyroid, submandibular, and parotid glands are consistent and will not be mistaken by experienced clinicians.

Some disease entities may occasionally present as isolated neck masses, such as lymphoma or reactive adenopathy from viral infection, but more typically present with more than one mass. Careful examination of the neck in an individual with lymphoma frequently leads to palpation of a second mass within the same nodal basin. Inflammatory nodes are rarely solitary because the other nodes within the drainage basin will be similarly affected. Therefore these entities are not considered further.

HISTORY

The timing of presentation and duration of a neck mass provides some clues as to its nature. Inflammatory processes cause nodes to hypertrophy contemporaneously. After the resolution of the underlying disorder, enlarged nodes may take weeks to regress and then may never return to original size. Most healthy individuals have several normal nodes less than two centimeters in diameter yet large enough to palpate. Congenital cysts may appear suddenly in young adults as a result of internal bleeding, lymphatic obstruction, or associated inflammation. Some benign neoplasms are very slow growing, presenting as a mass that may be reported as unchanged for many years. Malignant neoplasms have variable rates of growth and may fluctuate with inflammation, reducing in size after a course of antibiotics, but generally will have grown perceptibly over months.

Other matters of importance to note in the patient history include known risk factors for malignancy (alcohol and tobacco use, sexual history, family history); travel and exposure history (tuberculosis, cat scratch, histoplasmosis); and personal medical history (dental infection, constitutional symptoms).

PHYSICAL EXAMINATION

The size of the neck mass should be estimated during the physical examination. A caliper or flexible ruler can be used, if necessary. The width of the examining finger (usually approximately 2 cm) serves as a useful aid. A mass that rolls under the fingertip is likely to be less than 1 cm in diameter. Size can be confirmed by imaging. Other physical features are also useful. Are the edges of the mass easily discernible (discrete)? Does the mass move with respect to skin and surrounding structures such as sternocleidomastoid (SCM)? Assessment of the firmness (turgor) of a neck mass is subjective but useful. Is the mass compressible, ballotable, or firm?

RADIOLOGIC EVALUATION

Ultrasound, computed tomography (CT), and magnetic resonance imaging (MRI) are useful to delineate the size, extent, and physical characteristics of the mass. Some lesions have distinctive appearances, such as the high signal intensity on T2-weighted MRI imaging of neural sheath tumors, a cystic or necrotic center, contrast enhancement, calcification, or sharp or indistinct boundaries. Normal lymph nodes are characterized by ovoid shape and a fatty hilum. Each imaging modality has its own strengths. MRI provides more variable shading of soft tissues of different quality; CT demonstrates bone and calcification. Ultrasound evaluation of thyroid nodules provides information that can provide an index of suspicion for malignancy (internal complexity of echo, microcalcifications). Each of these modalities may also help to guide needle placement for fine needle aspiration (FNA). Positron emission tomography scanning is useful in the search for primary cancer site in the setting of metastatic disease of unknown primary and suspicious metabolic activity in small lymph node metastases.

HUMAN PAPILLOMAVIRUS–RELATED CANCER: A MODERN EPIDEMIC

An important factor to be considered when evaluating an adult with a solitary neck mass in the beginning of the twenty-first century is the marked increase in individuals presenting with head and neck squamous cell carcinoma (HNSCC) resulting from an epidemic of human papillomavirus (HPV)-related disease. This phenomenon violates longstanding demographic patterns of past decades in which more than 80% of people with HNSCC were smoker-drinkers older than 45 years of age. A typical scenario for HPV-related metastatic SCC is the abrupt discovery of a single firm neck mass in level II-III in individuals older than age 30 years with no known risk factors for head and neck cancer and no other signs or symptoms of disease. Often these neck masses are cystic, as demonstrated by radiographic imaging or on FNA biopsy (Fig. 2). A typical case is of an individual discovering his or her own neck mass, already more than 2 cm in size, while shaving or performing some other activity. Frequently, health care providers unfamiliar with the prevalence of HPV assume that these cases represent branchial cleft cysts and proceed to excision, only

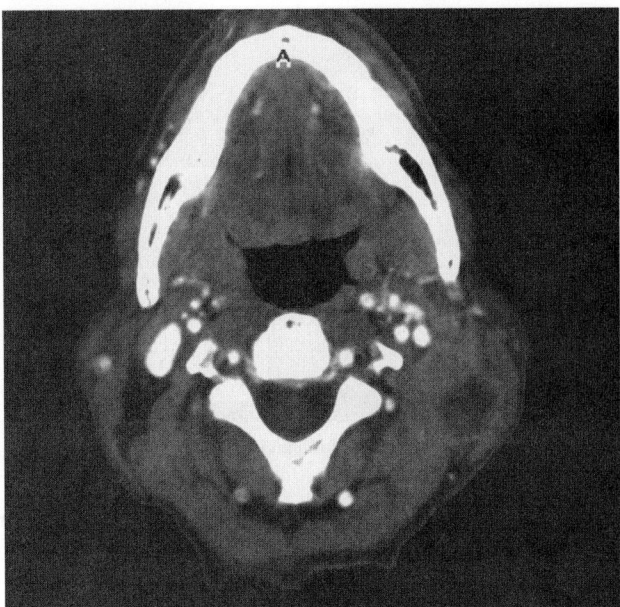

Figure 2 Axial computed tomography scan showing cystic degeneration in squamous cell carcinoma from tonsillar primary.

to be alarmed to find the diagnosis of cancer. It is critical to recognize that a unilateral cystic mass in a person older than age 30 years that was not apparent over a long period is metastatic cancer from a lymphoepithelial (lingual or palatine tonsil) primary site until proved otherwise. The diagnosis, once suspected, can be confirmed in many cases by FNA but a cytopathologic reading of benign squamous cells may be misleading, and surgeons must be ready to deal with cancer diagnosis at the time of excisional biopsy. Regardless of the cytology, the patient should be counseled regarding the possibility of cancer, and plans should be made to proceed from excisional biopsy to at least selective neck dissection, thoroughly removing the index mass together with nodal-bearing tissue within the dissected region. If frozen section indicates malignancy, a comprehensive neck dissection should be considered and a search made for the primary site. The palatine tonsils and tongue base should be palpated. A firm mass indicates the likely primary site. If none is apparent and palatine tonsils remain in place, these should be removed in tonsillectomy. If they are absent or if frozen section of tonsils is negative, directed biopsies of the tongue base lingual tonsillar tissue should be performed. If the frozen section is certain, these might all be accomplished at the same time using the same anesthetic. These measures are best managed by surgeons familiar with head and neck cancer diagnosis and management, suggesting the wisdom of referring such individuals early, as soon as the typical scenario is recognized.

BIOPSY

If the workup has focused concern on neoplastic disease, a biopsy is generally required before treatment selection. The benefits of FNA over open biopsy cannot be overemphasized. Cytologic evaluation of FNA specimens provides a correct diagnosis with sensitivity and specificity approaching 90%. Even when a precise diagnosis is not possible, the results often lead in a useful direction (low or high index of suspicion). Awareness of the benefits of FNA remains disappointingly limited within community settings where, all too often, incisional biopsy is performed instead. Incisional biopsy conveys a risk of spread of malignant cells within the wound bed and interference with the performance of eventual definitive surgery. It obscures assessment of the region when appropriate specialists are eventually enlisted, limits the selection of surgical approach, and endangers important structures in

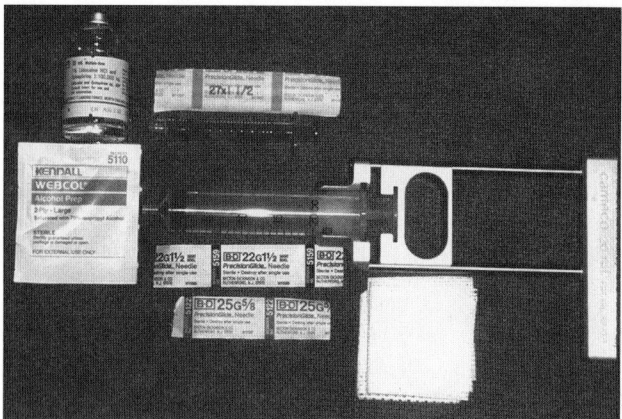

Figure 3 Equipment necessary for fine needle aspiration biopsy.

the region that must be reexposed and dissected. These factors are so compelling that the recommended step when an initial FNA is non-diagnostic (especially for insufficient, acellular specimen) often may be repeat FNA, perhaps engaging the help of image guidance; immediate cytopathologic evaluation to ensure adequacy of the specimen; and involvement of more experienced surgeons and pathologists.

When the neck mass is easily palpated, FNA can be performed in the clinician's office or by a cytopathologist, depending on institutional practice and policy. A 23- to 25-gauge needle attached to a 20-ml syringe with special control handle is used. Local anesthesia should be used to dull the discomfort of multiple needle insertions (Fig. 3). On-site evaluation by a cytopathologist provides immediate information as to the sufficiency of the sample procured. Aspiration attempts may be repeated as needed to obtain a useful specimen. When the presence of a cytopathologist is not available, we repeat the sampling aspiration three times in order to increase the likelihood of sufficient sample for successful diagnosis. The needle is inserted into the mass without pulling on the syringe and with careful direction by the palpating fingers of the nondominant hand. Subtle cues indicate the entry of the needle into the mass of interest (gritty texture, movement of the mass with small movements of the needle). After the mass is engaged, the plunger of the syringe is rapidly and repeatedly pulled back to engage a plug of tissue into the needle. Then, with constant suction applied, the needle may be moved back and forth within the mass, varying the angle slightly to obtain more solid tissue. Aspiration is discontinued with any return of cystic fluid or blood into the needle hub because these fluids will obscure the diagnostic tissue on the microscope slide. Suction is released before removing the needle from the neck to avoid pulling the tissue into the syringe. The needle is removed from the syringe, which is then filled with air. The needle is replaced on the syringe, and the air used to rapidly expel tissue from the needle onto a microscope slide. A smear is made immediately with a second slide, and both are placed quickly into ethanol to preserve the cells and avoid air drying. The needle and syringe are then rinsed with balanced salt solution or ethanol solution to collect remaining cells for cytospin.

When a deep or indistinct mass is present, ultrasound, CT, or MRI should be employed to ensure accurate placement of the FNA needle.

SURGICAL MANAGEMENT OF THE ISOLATED NECK MASS

Anesthesia

When FNA is not successful or tissue is required for tumor architecture (lymphoma), an open biopsy may be required. Even though

this may be accomplished with local anesthesia, lidocaine can abrogate nerve impulses, making precise localization of regional motor nerves (marginal mandibular branch of the facial nerve, spinal accessory nerve) difficult. Most neck masses reside deep to the platysma and may be deeper within the neck than would be judged by palpation. For these reasons, we prefer general anesthesia for most open neck biopsies.

Airway Considerations

Most neck masses will not adversely affect the airway, and standard endotracheal intubation should be sufficient for the maintenance of general anesthesia. If the mass shifts the airway, fiberoptic guidance for intubation may be required. Tracheotomy is best performed in situations in which the airway is markedly compromised or the management team is uncomfortable with intubation and postoperative extubation and monitoring.

Planning the Incision

Incisions should be placed within skin creases for best cosmetic result. Generally, this means that incisions in the neck are horizontal when favorably designed. The placement of incisions should be planned to permit their incorporation into longer incisions in case full neck dissection or other surgical procedure becomes necessary. Incisions should be long enough to permit accurate identification of landmarks (e.g., digastric muscle, submandibular gland fascia, posterior boundary of SCM) that are useful for precise identification of nerves that reside in deeper planes.

Prevention of Nerve Injury

Injuries to cranial nerves VII and XI are among the most common complications of neck surgery. The lower branches of the facial nerve course downward over the body of the mandible and then back up toward the lower lip at the commissure. The marginal mandibular branch generally remains just along the lower edge of the mandible, and platysma branches reside in the fascia of the submandibular gland (Fig. 4). The surgeon should avoid the region of the body of the mandible, descending two fingerbreadths below for incisions to reduce risk to the marginal mandibular branch. Flaps are then elevated just below platysma in the submandibular region or just above when approaching the parotid. Here, the platysma feathers out and attaches to the superficial musculoaponeurotic system. Fibers of cranial nerve VII lie deep to this layer. When dissecting in the submandibular region, the fascia of the gland should be elevated with the skin flap and the facial vein should be isolated and divided low, with constant attention given to scanning for nerve branches. All dissection should proceed with blunt technique spreading in the expected direction of the nerve.

Platysma is generally absent behind the posterior border of the SCM muscle, and the spinal accessory nerve (CN XI) may be superficial in this area. The spinal accessory nerve traverses level V (the posterior triangle) from a point behind the SCM muscle, 2 cm (one fingerbreadth) above Erb's point (the position of the great auricular and transverse cervical plexus nerve's emergence from deep tissues up and over the posterior SCM muscle) to enter the trapezius muscle 4 cm (two fingerbreadths) above the clavicle (Fig. 5). It tends to dive deeper into tissue as it descends. Supraclavicular branches of the cervical plexus have an appearance (caliber, trajectory) similar to that of cranial nerve XI, but they enter the deeper aspect of the neck inferior to the course of cranial nerve XI. Just behind the SCM muscle, cranial nerve XI may be crossed by a cervical plexus branch, making its precise identification difficult even with the assistance of a nerve stimulator because impulses may be transmitted through contiguous

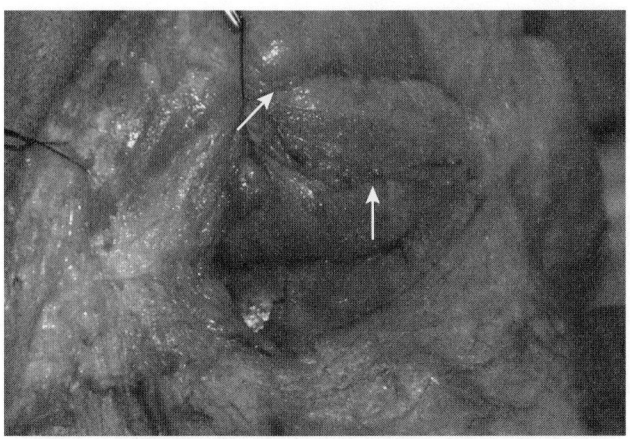

Figure 4 Preservation of marginal mandibular branch of facial nerve. Fascia overlying submandibular gland has been cut and elevated *(straight arrow)*; facial vein has been ligated *(suture retracted by instrument)*. Location of marginal mandibular nerve is indicated by curved arrow.

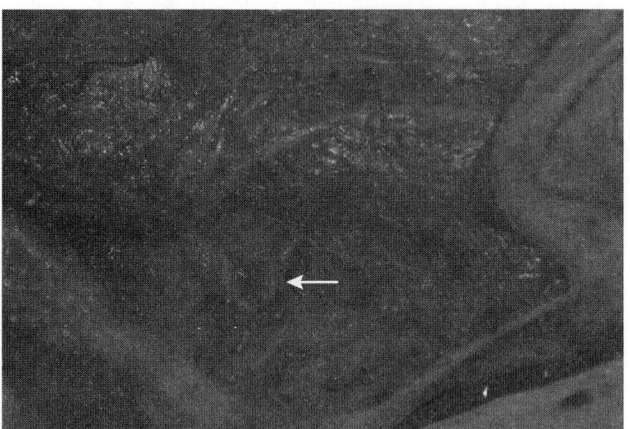

Figure 5 Location of spinal accessory nerve in posterior triangle of neck: Erb's point *(clamp)*, where sensory branches of the cervical plexus (transverse cervical and great auricular nerves) cross the posterior border of the sternocleidomastoid muscle, is one fingerbreadth (2 cm) below the point at which cranial nerve XI nerve *(arrow)* passes deep to the muscle border.

sensory branches to cranial nerve XI. It is best to avoid cutting any nerve of more than 2 mm diameter found in the posterior triangle during open biopsy procedures.

The superior (proximal) segment of cranial nerve XI must be considered when approaching a mass in level II under the SCM muscle. Here, cranial nerve XI descends from a point near the lateral process of C1 vertebra, deep to the posterior belly of the digastric muscle, and runs obliquely over the internal jugular vein to the undersurface of the SCM muscle, into which it generally penetrates.

The hypoglossal nerve (CN XII) traverses levels I and II deep in the neck tissues. It descends on the superficial surface of the carotid (between internal and external) before turning to run horizontally just behind and then under the posterior belly of the digastric. Here it is surrounded by a plexus of veins, the venae comitantes. Resection of most neck masses need not reach this depth, although carotid body tumors, metastatic squamous carcinoma, and branchial cleft anomalies may reside nearby.

The vagus nerve (CN X) runs vertically through the neck between the jugular vein and carotid artery, typically along their posterior surface. This deep location should not be encountered

in the resection of most isolated neck masses. Careful identification of cranial nerve X and separation from venous structures must be completed before ligation of the internal jugular vein.

The supraclavicular fossa contains many important structures, making dissection here hazardous. The thoracic duct lies deep in the inferomedial aspect of the left supraclavicular region, emerging from behind the common carotid artery several centimeters above the clavicle and turning downward to enter the internal jugular vein near its junction with the subclavian. It is best to avoid this region. If the thoracic duct must be approached, it is imperative to identify and preserve the phrenic and vagus nerves before beginning careful blunt dissection of soft tissue that may contain the duct. All tissue between phrenic and vagus nerves should be clamped, divided, and ligated.

The phrenic nerve and brachial plexus reside deep to the deep layer of the deep cervical fascia, with the phrenic nerve crossing from lateral to medial over the middle scalene muscle. The only common isolated neck mass that may require dissection this deep into the neck would be a neurogenic tumor such as schwannoma or neurofibroma.

Surgery for Suspected Malignancy

If epithelial malignancy is possible, dissection should aim for complete excision without violation of pseudocapsule and spillage of contents of the mass. Care should be taken to avoid penetration of cystic masses because complete removal is easier when the mass boundary is distinct. Lymphoma architectural studies require removal of a block of tissue but may not necessitate complete excision of a node. In this case, incision into the mass with removal of a wedge or cube of tissue is appropriate, avoiding unnecessary risk to surrounding structures.

When malignancy is suspected, the surgeon should be prepared to perform a dissection of surrounding lymph node–bearing tissues in case the malignant nature of the index mass is confirmed by frozen section histopathologic evaluation. The extent of dissection required (selecting specific "levels" or "comprehensive" dissection of all nodal bearing regions) depends on the type of malignancy, the feasibility of postoperative radiation, the size and location of the index mass, and the judgment and experience of the surgeon. After a region of the neck has been manipulated, particularly with the exposure of vital nerves, it is much more difficult and hazardous to reenter and resume dissection at a later date. For this reason, the surgeon should endeavor to complete whatever work is required in the vicinity at the time of resection of the isolated neck mass.

Details regarding surgical excision of specific neck masses are beyond the scope of this text; however, some guidelines can be provided for specific situations. Incisional/excisional biopsy of parotid masses is unwise because of the possibility of injury to the facial nerve. All but the most superficial, posterior, and inferior parotid masses should be removed with full superficial parotidectomy beginning with identification of the facial nerve trunk. Familiarity with the distribution of distal branches (e.g., the marginal mandibular nerve near the facial notch of the mandible, buccal branches near the parotid duct, and temporal branches 2 cm anterior to the tragus over the zygoma) may be useful in identifying key structures before excision of distal parotid masses, for which superficial parotidectomy is not desirable.

Carotid body tumors are among the most challenging of neck masses. These highly vascular tumors envelop and densely adhere to the wall of the carotid at the bifurcation. Nearby, the tenth and eleventh cranial nerves are at risk. Carotid body tumors should not be biopsied (either by needle or wedge). Fortunately, their appearance is characteristic and generally poses no diagnostic dilemma. Within 24 hours of the planned surgery, the vascular supply to the tumor may be diminished by selective angiography and embolization of feeding vessels. This useful procedure is potentially hazardous, requiring talented and experienced interventional neuroradiologists. The extirpative surgeon must make plans that include methods to maintain cerebral blood flow in case the internal carotid artery is injured. The availability of an experienced vascular surgeon prepared to graft the involved segment is highly encouraged.

Another special case is that of the mass caused by nontuberculous mycobacteria. These lesions tend to occur in young children and should be considered when an inflammatory etiology is suspected and a neck mass persists despite adequate antibiotic therapy. Because of the extensive inflammatory component of this entity, complete excision may not be safe. Subtotal resection by curettage of necrotic material may suffice to encourage the eventual resolution of these neck masses (Fig. 6).

Vascular lesions, including hemangiomas, vascular malformations, and lymphatic malformations, present difficult challenges to the pediatric neck surgeon. The lymphatic malformations (lymphangioma, cystic hygroma) are thin-walled masses that present near the time of birth as swelling anywhere in the neck. They can be well-defined large cysts or more diffuse microcysts and fluid-filled lymphatic channels that interdigitate with the normal muscles and nerves of the neck. Incomplete excision is often followed by recurrence. Occasional neck surgeons should not attempt to excise these challenging lesions.

SUGGESTED READINGS

Goldenberg D, Sciubba J, Koch WM: Cystic metastasis from head and neck squamous cell cancer: A distinct disease variant? *Head Neck* 28(7):633, 2006.

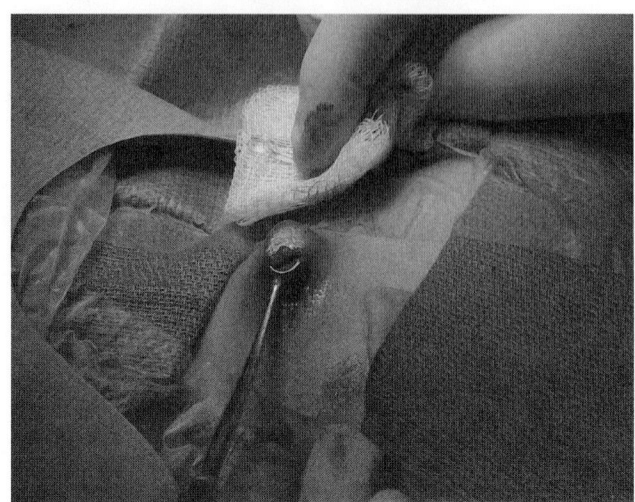

Figure 6 Curettage to remove necrotic tissue from a neck lesion of a child with granulomatous adenitis from *Mycobacterium avium* infection.

Koch WM: Complications of surgery of the neck. In Eisele DW, editors: *Complications in head and neck surgery*, ed 2, St. Louis, 1993, CV Mosby, p. 393.
Robbins KT, Samant S: Neck dissection. In Cummings CW, Frederikson JM, Harker LE, and others, editors: *Cummings otolaryngology head and neck surgery*, ed 4, vol 3, St Louis, 2005, Elsevier Mosby, p. 2614.
Tunkel DE, Kelly SM: Diagnosis and treatment of cervicofacial masses in children, *Adv Otolaryngol Head Neck Surg* 13:249, 1999.

NERVE INJURY AND REPAIR

Gedge D. Rosson, MD, and A. Lee Dellon, MD

Although the peripheral nervous system was described by Hippocrates in the fourth century BC, it was exceedingly rare for anyone to attempt nerve repairs before the nineteenth century. Unfortunately these nerve repairs were not commonly successful. It has only been in the past 40 years that surgeons have been routinely repairing nerves. This has been due mainly to the availability of surgical operating microscopes and has paralleled the advance of microvascular free flap reconstruction and digital replantations. Meticulous detail must be paid to the microsurgical operative techniques, and the physician must use both the science of peripheral nerve surgery and the art of peripheral nerve surgery to exercise judgment in correction of these difficult problems.

In addition, the patients must be well educated regarding realistic expectations. Microsurgical techniques can yield good functional outcomes; unfortunately, patients rarely obtain excellent results in terms of motor and sensory regeneration. The surgeon must exercise patience and care to appropriately direct sensory fibers into sensory end organs and motor fibers into appropriate muscles. Nerve repair is an exercise in delayed gratification in that it can take many months or years to achieve the final results.

GENERAL PRINCIPLES

Basic Anatomy

Before embarking on peripheral nerve surgery, it is critical to understand the basics of peripheral nerve anatomy and physiology. The most basic subunit of the peripheral nerve is the axon. Each axon is surrounded by endoneurium. Axons are grouped into fascicles, and these fascicles are surrounded by a thin perineurium. The grouped fascicles are also surrounded by interfascicular epineurium. The main nerve itself is surrounded by an external epineurial sheath. The external segmental blood supply to the nerve travels through a final layer of connective tissue referred to as the *mesoneurium*, which also allows nerve gliding during normal range of motion (Fig. 1).

Fascicular Topography

When performing nerve repairs, it is important to understand the difference between the fascicular topography in the proximal nerve trunk versus the fascicular topography in the distal nerve. Most nerves have a significant intermingling of sensory and motor fibers, with plexus formation in the nerve trunks proximally. At the more distal nerve, it usually will be observed that the fascicles have become groups of sensory fibers and groups of motor fibers. This partially accounts for the fact that more distal nerve repairs have better long-term functional outcomes than more proximal nerve repairs. For example, repair

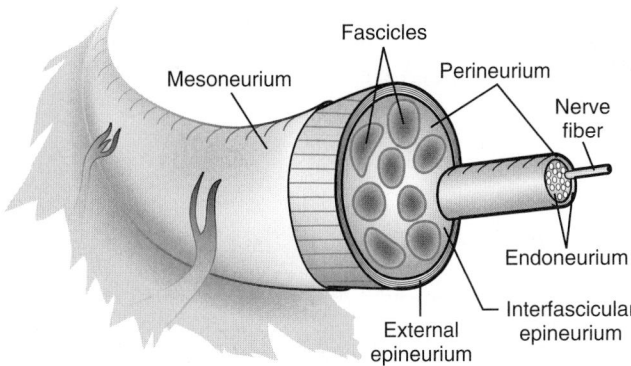

Figure 1 Schematic of the normal anatomy of the peripheral nerve.

of facial nerve injuries within the temporal bone often leads to significant, disabling synkinesis and dyskinesis owing to the lack of distinctive fascicular architecture in the proximal facial nerve trunk. This is in contradistinction to repair of the facial nerve in the parotid gland branches or distally because these fascicles are in their final configuration.

Physiology of Nerve Injury

Distinct physiologic changes occur within the nerve proximal to the site of injury versus the nerve distal to the site of injury. On the basis of the degree of injury to the nerve and the proximity of the injury to the nerve cell body, the amount of degeneration of the axons in the proximal nerve can be variable. With damage to the axon alone, the axon itself will just die back to the nearest node of Ranvier. After the injury has stabilized over the next several hours, the injured axon begins to grow. These axons form multiple "growth cones" and attempt to grow into the distal endoneurial tubes, if available. The segment of the nerve distal to the injury undergoes Wallerian degeneration. In this case, the myelin sheath and cellular debris are phagocytosed and the axon is completely replaced over 3 to 6 weeks. If the nerve damage is not too severe, endoneurial tubes can accept new axon sprouts from the proximal nerve. Most importantly, the distal nerve segment will still have viable axons that can transmit electrical stimulation for up to 72 to 96 hours. This is most important when repairing small motor nerves such as distal branches of the facial nerve. Thus when confronted with a sharp facial laceration with nerve injury, it is critical to bring the patient to the operating room within 72 hours, if possible, because the distal nerve endings can be located with electrical stimulation.

It has also been found that the changes in the innervated muscles are different from the changes in the sensory end organs. When muscles are denervated, they suffer from both disuse atrophy and denervation atrophy. Also, most of the motor endplates themselves will die within 12 months, and by 18 to 24 months they will all be gone. After that, the muscle cannot be reinnervated. The sensory end organs, on the other hand, are not known to die, and reports have been made of reinnervating sensory targets and improving sensibility even many years after the original injury.

Degree of Injury and Zone of Injury

As alluded to earlier, it is critical to understand the possible degree of injury and the potential extent of the zone of injury when managing nerve damage. It is nearly impossible to accurately detect the zone of injury during the initial exploration if there is any crush or avulsion component. A very clean injury to the nerve, such as that achieved with a scalpel, will have a small zone of injury, whereas

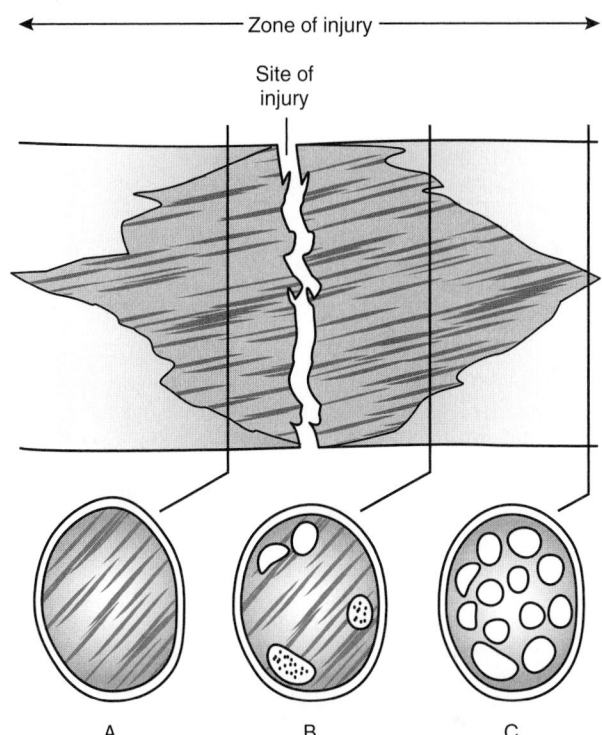

Figure 2 Following nerve injury, the zone of injury may extend well beyond the site of injury. **(A)** The nerve consists entirely of scar tissue. **(B)** Scar tissue and a fascicular pattern are seen in the more remote zones of injury. A fascicular pattern may be seen but may be scarred *(stippled)*. **(C)** Normal fascicle *(clear)* will protrude from the plane of the cut nerve because of increased endoneurial pressure.

avulsion nerve injury with a table saw will have a wide zone of injury (Fig. 2). Degree of nerve injury has been classified by Sedon as neurapraxia, axonotmesis, and neurotmesis. Neurapraxia ultimately leads to a complete recovery within days to months without intervention. Axonotmesis can result in a range from complete recovery to no recovery, depending on the degree of axonotmesis. In these cases, Wallerian degeneration takes place and the ultimate recovery is based on the degree of scar tissue that forms within the endoneurial or perineurial sheaths. Axons grow at a rate of approximately 1 inch per month, or 1 millimeter per day. Sedon's third classification is neurotmesis, in which there is no recovery and nerve repair or grafting will be required. Sunderland further delineated nerve injuries into first- through fifth-degree injuries, and Mackinnon and Dellon added a sixth degree, or combined, nerve injury; these are summarized in Table 1.

Timing

The appropriate timing of nerve repair and operative intervention is critical. Closed injuries must be treated differently from open injuries. In an open injury such as a stab wound, we prefer to explore the nerve immediately if the patient is stable. Certainly for lacerations of the face, as mentioned earlier, facial nerve branches are preferably repaired within 3 days because the distal branches can be more easily identified with intraoperative nerve stimulation. If the nerve injury is a clean laceration, the nerves can be primarily repaired at that time. The surgeon should always consider tagging the nerve ends and performing a definitive repair 3 weeks later if a significant crush or avulsion component is present. The scarred, damaged nerve ends are not readily apparent until 2 or 3 weeks after the injury. By waiting 3 weeks, the surgeon avoids suturing scarred nerve endings

Table 1: Degree of Injury Classification

Degree of Injury	Recovery	Rate of Recovery	Surgical Procedure
1st Neurapraxia	Complete	Fast	None
2nd Axonotmesis	Complete	Slow	None
3rd	Variable	Slow	None or neurolysis
4th	None	No recovery	Nerve repair or graft
5th Neurotmesis	None	No recovery	Nerve repair or graft
6th Combined	Variable	Dependent on combination of injury pattern	Variable

together; axons cannot regenerate through scar. A closed injury, on the other hand, may be a simple stretch-traction injury with neurapraxia and may regenerate well on its own. Therefore these patients must be followed closely. Patients must be followed up clinically every month, and sensation should be monitored by noninvasive neurosensory testing of the skin distal to the nerve injury. A formal nerve conduction study and electromyography should be performed at 6 weeks and 12 weeks following significant closed injury of a motor nerve. Motor nerves should be repaired within 4 to 6 months to give the regenerating axons time to grow into the target muscles. Gunshot wounds, although technically open, behave more like closed injuries because the nerve damage is more likely due to the blast effect than transection. This often results in neurapraxia or axonotmesis and may not need surgical repair.

OPERATIVE TECHNIQUE

Equipment

Before any nerve exploration or repair is attempted, proper equipment must be readily available. Nerve repairs should be performed only on medically stable patients. The surgical team should be well rested and well trained in microsurgical techniques. The equipment and room setup is similar to that for microvascular surgery, as needed for free flap reconstruction. A well-maintained and working operative microscope or a minimum of 4× loupe magnification should be available. Microsurgical instruments such as microforceps, microscissors, microbipolar, and microsurgical needle drivers are required, as are 9-0 or 10-0 nylon sutures. Heparinized saline solution is required if a nerve conduit will be used.

Positioning and Planning

Patients must be positioned on the operating room table in a manner that permits ease of access to both the site of injury and any potential donor sites if nerve grafting will be required. These areas should be simultaneously exposed and draped for availability. For nerve repairs in the upper extremities, the patient's arm is placed on an arm board and comfortable seating should be available. Nerve repairs of the lower extremities can also be performed with the surgeons seated, as long as the operating table is turned appropriately before the patient is placed on it, such that there is room beneath the legs for the surgeon and assistant to sit comfortably across from each other. Otherwise, the base of the table will be in exactly the position where the surgeon would like to place his or her knees. Common potential donor sites for nerve grafting include the sural nerve in the leg, the medial antebrachial cutaneous nerve and the lateral antebrachial cutaneous nerve in the upper extremity, or the greater auricular nerve in the head and neck.

The initial exploration should be under loupe magnification and tourniquet control, if possible. If the plan is to repair a motor

nerve within 72 hours of the original injury, it is critical to remember that tourniquet time greater than 30 minutes will cause ischemia of the distal nerve and then intraoperative nerve stimulation will no longer be possible. Thus the initial dissection must be well planned, focused, and directed to ensure that the putative distal nerve has been dissected out within 30 minutes or the tourniquet must be deflated.

After the proximal and distal nerve endings have been identified, dissection should be directed a few centimeters proximal and distal to these nerve endings. When working near an area with a known site of compression, such as the ulnar nerve near Osborne's band, it is indicated to also release the site of compression at this time. The regenerating nerve will become swollen during the regenerative phase, and potential future compression should be prophylactically removed.

Preparation of Nerve Endings

The most critical step is the preparation of the nerve endings. Adequate nerve resection is the most neglected technique in nerve repair. Care must be taken to sufficiently resect damaged nerve endings on the basis of the mechanism of injury and the zone of injury. If there is any crush or avulsion, then it may be wise to tag the nerve endings with a small Prolene suture (Ethicon, Somerville, NJ) and come back in 3 weeks to adequately assess the scar formation. If the nerve repair is undertaken 3 weeks or more after the original injury, then adequate assessment of the scarred nerve endings can be performed. Any neuroma and scar is excised sharply using a scalpel blade with the nerve placed on a flat, sterile, wooden tongue depressor. The nerve stumps should be sliced proximally and distally as if one is slicing a loaf of bread until a healthy fascicular pattern is visualized. This can be referred to as *les yeux d'escargot* (snail's eyes [Fig. 3]). This pattern of healthy

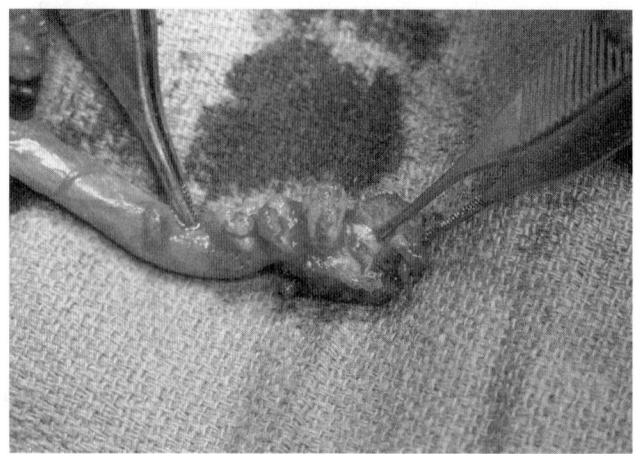

Figure 3   The damaged nerve ending, which in this case is a neuroma, is cut back until healthy fascicles are visualized: *les yeux d'escargot*.

fascicles protruding from the cut nerve endings is due to the pressure within the endoneurium. The fascicles that protrude past the cut nerve ending should be further divided until all the fascicles lie flush with the epineurial sheath. This is critical so that the fascicles do not overlap after the epineurium is sutured. Any overlap of fascicles will lead to failure of the axonal sprouts to find the distal endoneurial tubes.

Tension-Free Nerve Coaptation

Following meticulous preparation of the nerve endings, the tourniquet is usually deflated. Nerve coaptation is then performed using several interrupted 9-0 or 10-0 nylon sutures. Good results with fibrin glue have been reported, but interrupted nylon suture remains the standard. Nerves are generally repaired with an end-to-end coaptation; the pros, cons, and possible indications for end-to-side neurorrhaphy are beyond the scope of this chapter. It is *essential* that there be no tension whatsoever on the repair. The knowledge that nerve repair results drop off significantly if there is any tension on this repair has greatly advanced nerve repair techniques. It is more important to have a tension-free repair than to perform a primary nerve coaptation. If necessary, a nerve graft or interpositional bioabsorbable nerve conduit can be used. Some additional length on the nerve can be achieved for certain nerves such as the ulnar nerve at the elbow, which can be transposed anterior to the medial humeral epicondyle to provide several centimeters of extra length. Most nerves cannot be transposed to add length. It is essential to never use positioning of joints, such as flexion of the elbow, to give added length to the nerve. This will only result in stretching the nerve and poor outcome after the limb is straightened later.

Epineurial versus Grouped Fascicular Repair

For primary nerve repair, an epineurial repair is usually the most predictable (Fig. 4). It is often possible to line up the external epineurial vessels to ensure that the fascicles are appropriately aligned. Usually only two or three interrupted sutures are necessary to align and coapt the nerve ends. It is crucial at this stage to ensure that there is no overlapping of the fascicles (Fig. 5). The fascicles should just be gently coapted within the epineurium. It is also important to note that the needle passes through the epineurium only and does not catch a portion of one of the fascicles because this can lead to a small intraneural neuroma, and consequently this fascicle will not heal appropriately.

Occasionally it is appropriate to perform fascicular or grouped fascicular repairs. In a large nerve in which the fascicles are easily identifiable, it may be possible to suture the internal

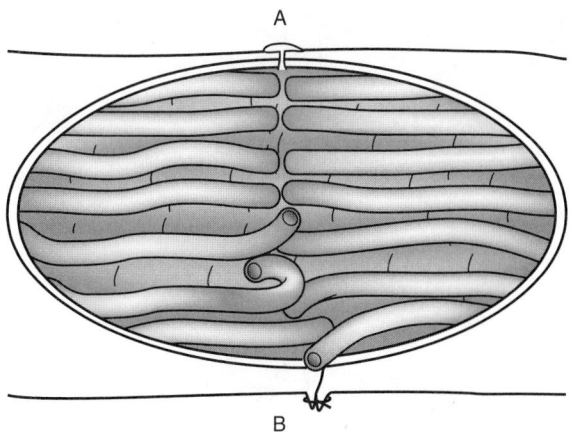

Figure 5 *(A)* Appropriately trimmed fascicles will lightly oppose when the epineurium is gently approximated. *(B)* Fascicular overlap and disorder may arise when fascicles have not been trimmed and protrude from the epineurium or when the epineurial repair is too tight.

epineurium between the fascicles with a few small, interrupted, nylon sutures and then perform the epineural repair. Knowledge of the internal topography of the fascicles of various nerves is beyond the scope of this chapter, but it is important if group fascicular repair were attempted. Some researchers have reported that grouped fascicular repair results in more intraneural scarring; thus most peripheral nerve surgeons continue to employ epineural repair.

Management of the Nerve Gap

Most often the resection of the scarred nerve endings will result in some amount of nerve gap. Nerve gaps require alternative methods of nerve repair such as interpositional nerve grafting or use of commercially available bioabsorbable nerve conduits. These bioabsorbable nerve conduits are excellent for gaps less than 3 cm (Fig. 6). Prospective double-blind trials have shown that use of the bioabsorbable nerve conduits actually results in better two-point discrimination than primary repair in digital injuries and nerve grafts less than 3 cm in digital injuries.

Use of the nerve conduit requires an entubulation technique. First, the nerve conduit chosen must have a diameter that is adequate to accept the nerve to be placed inside it. The length of the nerve conduit selected should be 10 mm longer than the nerve gap. Thus a nerve gap of 3 cm would require a 4-cm nerve tube. The entubulation technique entails placing the proximal end of the nerve 5 mm within one end of the nerve tube; the distal nerve ending should be placed 5 mm within the distal end of the nerve tube. This is accomplished using a horizontal mattress suture, entering the nerve conduit 5 mm from the ending, then performing a horizontal mattress suture in the epineurium of the nerve ending itself, pulling it within the nerve tube 5 mm, and finally tying the horizontal mattress suture on the outside of the nerve conduit. A few extra epineural interrupted sutures can then be placed from the epineurium to the end of the nerve tube. This should be performed without the tourniquet to ensure that perfect hemostasis has been achieved. Bleeding from the nerve ending must not be allowed to enter the nerve tube and cause coagulation within the nerve tube. The final step is to flush any blood or debris out of the nerve conduit with heparinized saline. If a synthetic, biodegradable nerve conduit is not available, an acceptable alternative is autogenous vein grafting. These do tend to collapse, however, and do not have as predictable a final result.

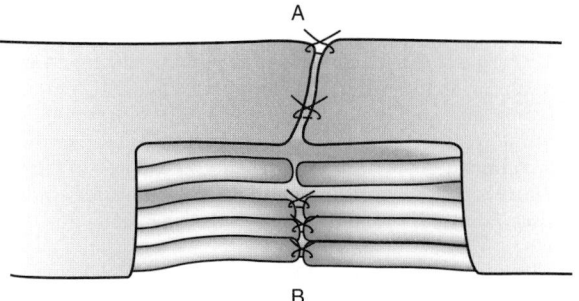

Figure 4 Schematic representation of nerve repairs. *(A)* Epineurial repair. Note that the visible fascicles under the epineurium are opposed without overlap. *(B)* Grouped fascicular repair.

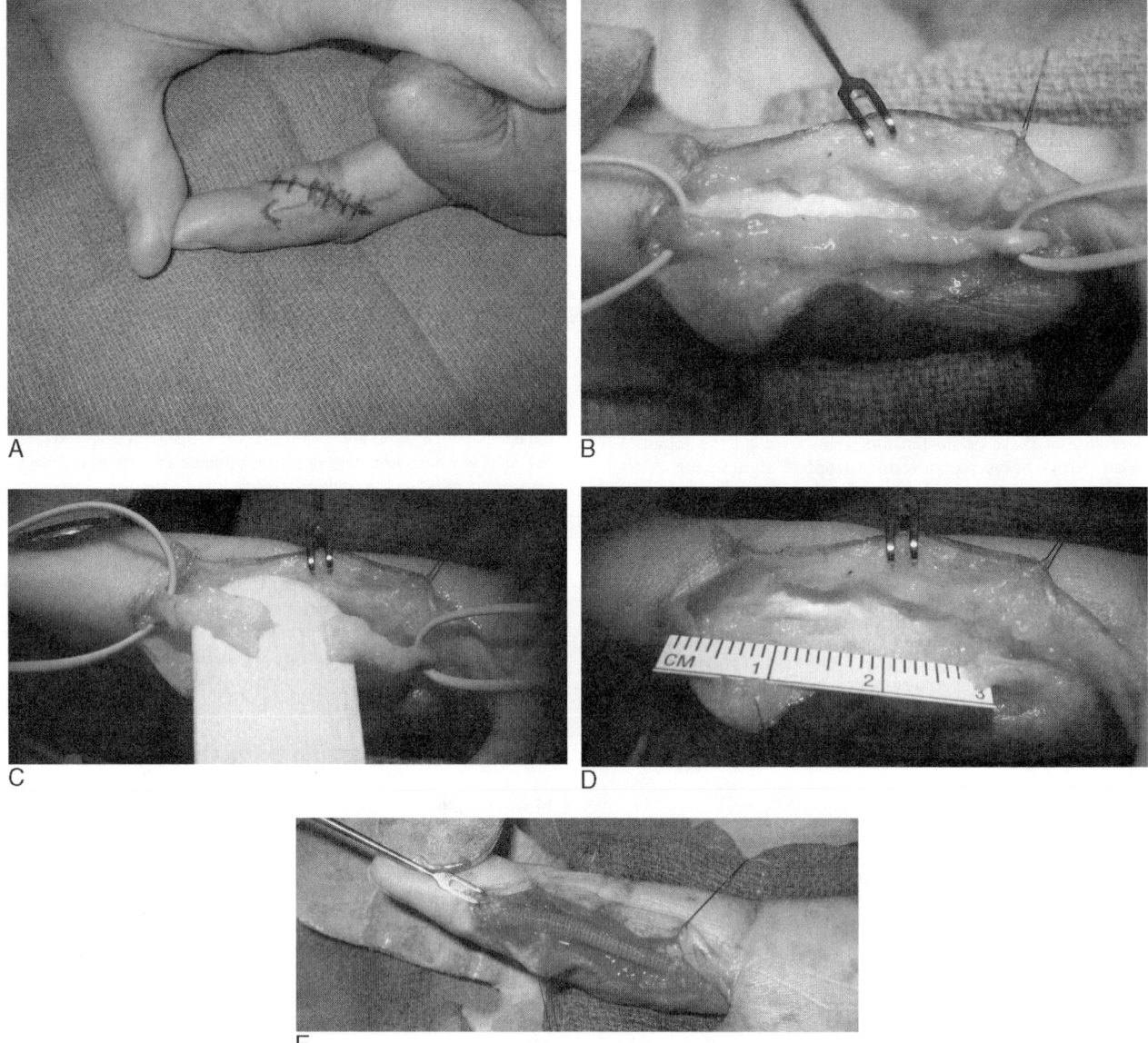

Figure 6 **(A)** Finger injury with painful neuroma in the old scar. **(B)** Neuroma. **(C)** Beginning to cut the nerve endings using a sterile wooden tongue depressor. **(D)** The resultant nerve gap is 3 cm. **(E)** Bioabsorbable nerve conduit made of a rigid, corrugated polyglycolic acid tube.

For nerve gaps greater than 3 cm, an interpositional nerve graft should be used. There are many potential donor sites for nerve grafts, and appropriate patient consent should be obtained preoperatively if the nerve graft is a possibility. The nerve graft should be sutured into place in a reversed fashion from its usual anatomic course. Thus the more distal end of the nerve graft should be sutured to the proximal end of the nerve gap that is being repaired, and the proximal end of the nerve graft should be sutured to the distal end of the nerve gap. This ensures that axons will not be lost through small side branches in the nerve graft as the axons grow through the graft. It is common that the diameter of the nerve at the site of repair is much larger than the diameter of the nerve graft, and thus grouped fascicular repair is used. As mentioned earlier, it is essential to know the appropriate anatomic topography of the fascicles in the nerve to guarantee that motor fascicles are grafted to motor fascicles and sensory fascicles are grafted to sensory fascicles.

Nerve Compression

Some nerve injuries do not result in interruption of the nerve or a neuroma-in-continuity, and thus there is no nerve scar to resect and reconstruct. Sports injuries and crush injuries to extremities can result in milder stretch-traction injuries and compression of nerves at the usual sites of compression. These nerve injuries do not require resection of the nerve with grafting but rather they can improve dramatically with appropriate decompression of the nerves with neurolysis. Detailed discussion of nerve compression syndromes following trauma is beyond the scope of this chapter.

Nerve Transfers

Certain proximal nerve injuries such as injuries to the proximal brachial plexus traditionally have poor outcomes. In many of these cases, improved outcome is seen with nerve transfers rather than actual repair of the damaged nerves; these nerve transfers are performed more distally and closer to the muscles in question. For example, an upper trunk brachial plexus injury would result in loss of flexion of the elbow. If the lower trunk is intact, redundant fascicles of the ulnar nerve to the flexor carpi ulnaris muscle can be transferred to either the brachialis or biceps motor nerve and, at the same time, some redundant fascicles from the median nerve going to superficial flexor muscles can be transferred to the brachialis or biceps motor nerve. This will result in faster reinnervation of the muscles than if a repair of the upper trunk of the brachial plexus were performed because it would take many months for the axons to grow all the way down into the arm.

POSTOPERATIVE MANAGEMENT

Postoperative management begins in the operating room, even before closing the skin. After the nerve has been repaired, the joints should go through full range of motion and must be observed for any nerve tension. It is critical at this stage to make sure that there is never any tension on the nerve repair; any tension will greatly diminish the functional outcome. After the skin closure is complete, the extremity should be placed in a well-padded, protective splint for 7 to 10 days. At this point, gradual protective range of motion can begin under the careful direction of a physical therapist or occupational therapist knowledgeable about nerve injuries. Range of motion should be gradually increased over the next 6 to 8 weeks. Physical therapists are integral to keeping the limb supple and free of contractures. Occasionally patients have a burning sensation or pain in the area of the neurosensory territories; this can be due to collateral sprouting from normal surrounding nerves or the actual nerve regeneration sending impulses to the cortical pain centers. During this phase of healing, Neurontin (Pfizer, New York, NY) or Lyrica (Pfizer) can be added to the medical management and the occupational therapist or physical therapist can begin desensitization programs.

Sensory and Motor Reeducation

Any sensory nerve repair can have an improved outcome if sensory reeducation regimens are implemented. The sensory reeducation encourages cortical plasticity for any sensory end-organ mismatch. Even if a digit is reinnervated by an inappropriate sensory fascicle, the patient can relearn over time to correctly localize stimulation of that digit. When motor nerves are repaired, it is essential for a physical therapist and occupational therapist to assist the patient with motor retraining as the muscles become reinnervated. On the other hand, if motor reinnervation does

Table 2: Principles of Nerve Repair

1. Medical stability of patient.
2. Preoperative and postoperative quantitative assessment of sensory and motor function.
3. Early surgical exploration if open injury for microsurgical repair with appropriate magnification, sutures, and instrumentation.
4. Bloodless field under tourniquet control, when possible.
5. Extent of zone of injury assessed appropriately. All scarred nerve must be resected.
6. Primary nerve repair when clinical and surgical judgment permits.
7. Secondary repair if zone of injury is indeterminate at initial exploration.
8. Tension-free nerve repair.
9. Interpositional nerve graft or bioabsorbable nerve conduit, if direct repair would result in tension.
10. Avoidance of positional or postural maneuvers to facilitate tension-free repair.
11. Epineurial repair unless intraneural topography dictates group fascicular repair.
12. Postoperative immobilization for 7 to 10 days, followed by early protected motion.
13. Postoperative sensory and motor reeducation.
14. Routine postoperative monitoring with noninvasive neurosensory testing.

not occur, various tendon transfers must be considered and can also improve functional outcome. The basic tenets of nerve repair are summarized in Table 2.

SUGGESTED READINGS

Dellon AL: Resection: Nerve repair's most neglected technique, *Plast Surg Techn* 1(3):191, 1995.
Dellon AL: *Somatosensory testing and rehabilitation*, Baltimore, 2000, Kirby Lithographic.
Mackinnon SE, Dellon AL: *Surgery of the peripheral nerve*, New York, 1988, Thieme.
Millesi H: The nerve gap. Theory and clinical practice, *Hand Clin* 2:651, 1987.
Seddon MS: Three types of nerve injury, *Brain* 66:237, 1943.
Sunderland S: A classification of peripheral nerve injuries producing a loss of function, *Brain* 74:491, 1951.
Weber RA, Breidenbach WC, Brown RE, and others: A randomized prospective study of polyglycolic acid conduits for digital nerve reconstruction in humans, *Plast Reconstr Surg* 106:1036, 2000.

HAND INFECTIONS

**Hugo St-Hilaire, MD, DDS, and
Richard J. Redett, MD**

Hand infections are common and can result in significant morbidity if not treated properly. A thorough understanding of hand and finger (Fig. 1) anatomy and knowledge of the bacteria commonly involved in infections of the upper extremity are required of the surgeon who will be caring for these patients. An understanding of the fascial boundaries of the hand will help to identify the extent of the infection and plan surgical incisions.

EVALUATION OF THE PATIENT WITH INFECTIONS AFFECTING THE HAND

A thorough history and physical examination should be performed. Emphasis should be placed on the patient's hand dominance, occupation, and the timing and type of injury or infection. Herpes simplex infections can be seen in dental and health care workers, *Vibrio vulnificus* and *Mycobacterium* in fisherman or marine workers, *Sporothrix schenckii* in gardeners, *Eikenella corrodens* in human bites, and *Pasteurella multocida* in cat and dog bites. Comorbidities including diabetes and immunosuppression should also be ascertained. Physical examination includes general observation of the skin color and the size and shape of the hand, as well as the presence or absence of wounds, ecchymosis, crepitus and erythema. A complete neurovascular and functional examination should be performed. Tenderness to palpation over a bone or joint may help to identify fractures. Tenderness over a flexor tendon may indicate underlying suppurative tenosynovitis. Plain radiographs of the affected area are obtained to rule out the presence of a foreign body or bony pathology. On the rare occasion when the history and clinical examination are unreliable, additional radiological tests such as computed tomography scan, ultrasound, or magnetic resonance imaging may be helpful.

Laboratory tests should include a complete blood count, CRP, and erythrocyte sedimentation rate. Blood cultures may be obtained, depending on the clinical scenario. If an open wound or purulent drainage is noted, cultures and Gram stain for aerobic and anaerobic bacteria, fungus, and mycobacteria should be obtained before administering antibiotics. Tetanus prophylaxis should be given if tetanus status is unknown or not current.

The initial history and physical examination will help to determine the presence of cellulites versus a deep or superficial abscess. The former can usually be treated with elevation, splinting, and antibiotics; the latter requires surgical drainage.

SURGICAL PRINCIPLES IN THE TREATMENT OF HAND INFECTION

Infection of the fingertip and other localized superficial infections can be treated effectively under local anesthesia. Anesthesia of the finger is obtained using a digital nerve block. A mixture of lidocaine and bupivacaine without vasoconstrictor is infiltrated on the radial and ulnar aspect of the affected finger through a dorsal puncture just distal to the metacarpophalangeal joint. Complicated or deep-space infections are more effectively treated under general anesthesia.

As with other surgical procedures involving the hand, incision and drainage can be performed under tourniquet control with either a Penrose-type drain wrapped carefully around the base of the finger or a pneumatic tourniquet placed proximally on the upper arm. Exsanguination of the affected limb is performed by elevation of the arm for approximately 5 minutes before inflation of the tourniquet. The use of an elastic bandage to exsanguinate the extremity is controversial in that it may lead to proximal spread of the infection.

Damage to motor and sensory nerves and to flexor or extensor tendons is avoided by using a careful combination of sharp and blunt dissection. Incisions are planned to allow for easy proximal or distal extension, if it becomes necessary. After the infected space has been entered, adequate debridement should be performed, including tenosynovectomy when indicated. Copious normal saline irrigation should then be used. Pulse lavage should be avoided in the hand to prevent damage to neurovascular structures. Continuous irrigation may be used for specific infections such as suppurative flexor tenosynovitis.

When an infection involves a joint space, evaluation of the articular surfaces is necessary. The quality of the articular cartilage and bone must be assessed. When bone is found to be soft and spongy, it should be debrided and sent for pathologic examination to confirm the diagnosis of osteomyelitis. The presence of osteomyelitis usually requires 6 weeks of antibiotic therapy.

COMMON INFECTIONS OF THE HAND

Paronychia

Acute *paronychia* is the most common infection of the hand and occurs when the soft tissue folds surrounding the lateral aspects of the fingernail become infected (Fig. 2). The usual pathogen is *Staphylococcus aureus*. An infection of the proximal nail fold is referred to as an *eponychia*. Common causes of paronychia include minor trauma from nail biting or manicure.

Symptoms

An acute paronychia presents with edema, erythema, and tenderness of the soft tissue surrounding the nail. Left untreated, a small abscess may form under the nail fold. Severe infections can spread proximally along the involved finger.

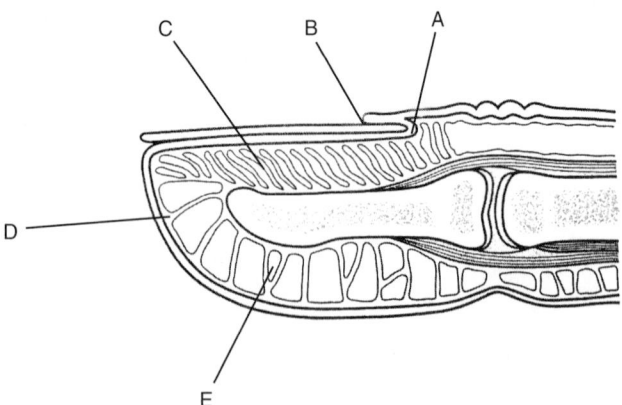

Figure 1 Anatomy of the fingertip. *(A)* Nail fold; *(B)* Eponychium; *(C)* Nailbed; *(D)* Hyponychium; *(E)* Vertical septa.

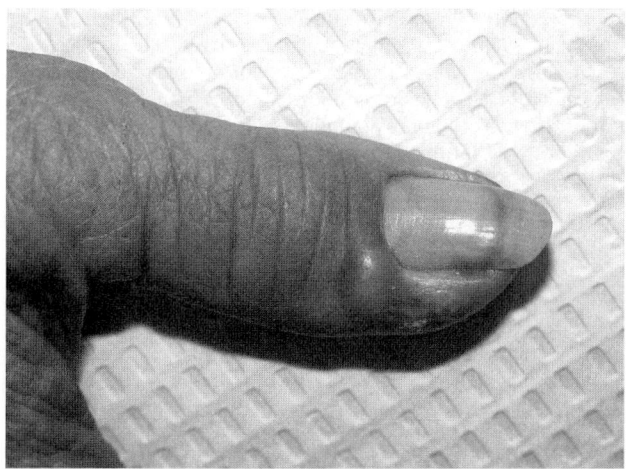

Figure 2 Acute paronychia of the thumb showing erythema and fluctuance.

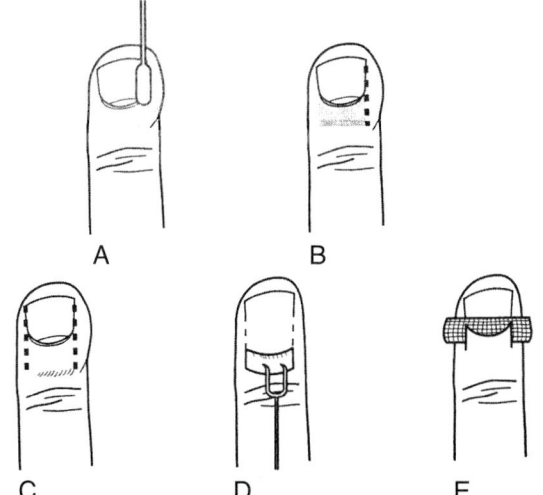

A   B

C   D   E

Figure 3 Surgical approaches for incision and drainage of acute paronychia. **(A)** Elevation of paronychial fold with scalpel or elevator. **(B)** Unilateral skin incision. **(C)** Bilateral skin incision. **(D)** Elevation of the entire eponychial fold and excision of the proximal on third of the nail. **(E)** Gauze packed underneath the eponychial fold prevents premature closure.

Treatment

Early paronychia can be treated with splint immobilization and oral antibiotics if no purulence is present. For more advanced infections, drainage can be performed under digital block anesthesia. A 15-blade scalpel is inserted under the infected paronychial fold and is gently swept back and forth to incise the abscess (Fig. 3, A). This lifts the fold off of the nail, thereby allowing drainage. More severe infections may require alternative incisions (see Figure 3, B to E). For an abscess found under the nail plate, a longitudinal section of nail may require removal for adequate drainage. A Penrose drain can be lightly wrapped around the finger as a tourniquet if necessary. Care must be taken to not wrap the Penrose too tightly and to remove it promptly after the procedure is over. After incision and drainage, the finger is bandaged for 1 to 2 days before starting daily warm soaks. Antibiotics are continued for 10 to 14 days. The patient can be seen for follow-up in 3 to 5 days or sooner, if necessary.

A chronic paronychia is usually the result of a candidal infection. The proximal nail plate and nail fold may separate. The eponychium may become indurated and rounded. The treatment of choice is marsupialization. A crescent-shaped excision of the thickened eponychium is performed. The excision should be performed to the level of the germinal matrix to prevent recurrence.

Felon

A *felon* is a painful infection involving the volar fingertip. Fibrous septa originating from the periosteum of the distal phalanx and inserting into the dermis help to contain the infection in the fingertip. However, left untreated, infection can track along these same septa down to the phalanx, leading to osteomyelitis, fat necrosis of the tip, and suppurative tenosynovitis. Penetrating trauma to the fingertip from a thorn, splinter, or needle is a common cause of felons. Radiographs of the fingertip are necessary to look for foreign body and evidence of osteomyelitis of the distal phalanx.

Symptoms

The patient usually presents with pain and tense swelling 1 to 2 days after a penetrating injury to the fingertip (Fig. 4). Felons are exquisitely tender to palpation because of the increased pressure within the septal compartments.

Treatment

Early felons can be treated with splinting, elevation, and antibiotics. One must have a low threshold to perform surgical drainage if symptoms worsen or fluctuance is identified. A digital block can be used for regional anesthesia. Multiple types of incisions have been described to drain a felon. The volar longitudinal incision allows for direct drainage of superficial felons without injury to the digital neurovascular bundle (Fig. 5, D). The incision is made 3 mm distal to the flexion crease and is extended toward the tip of the finger.

A J-incision can also be used to drain a deep felon, but it carries the risk of injuring the neurovascular structures (see Figure 5, B). The incision should be placed on the noncontact side of the fingertip (radial side of thumb and ulnar side of the fingers) and should be carried down to periosteum to release the septal compartments.

After incision and drainage, the cavity is irrigated and gently packed for 1 day before initiating warm soaks. Antibiotics are continued for 10 to 14 days. The patient should be seen in 2 to 3 days or sooner, if necessary, to make sure that the abscess is adequately drained. The incision can be closed after the infection clears.

Herpetic Whitlow

Herpetic whitlow is a painful infection of the hand usually involving one or more fingers. Herpes simplex virus 1 (HSV-1) and 2 (HSV-2)

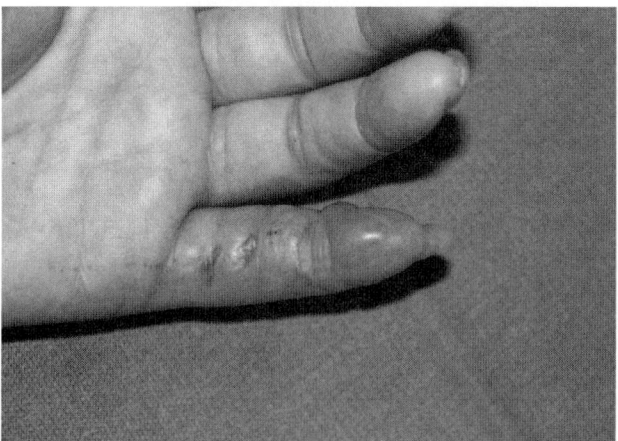

Figure 4 Acute felon of finger.

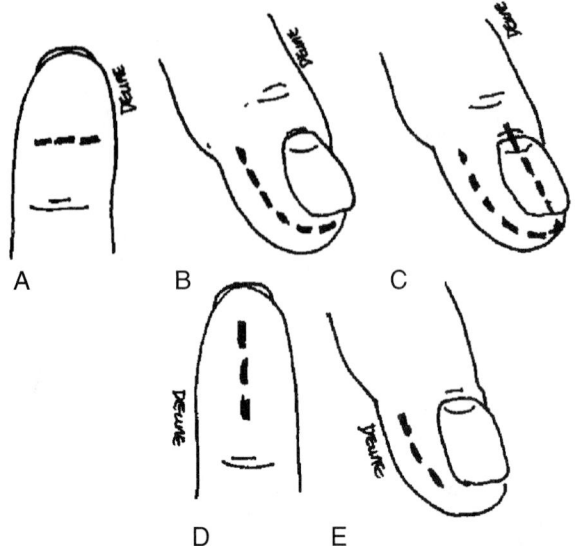

Figure 5 Surgical approaches to incision and drainage of a felon.

are the causative agents. The infection is initiated through viral inoculation from infected body fluids. The infection can be seen in dental or health care workers. Children usually obtain the infection from thumb sucking in the presence of primary oropharyngeal lesions. Adults can obtain the lesions from contact with genital herpes lesions.

Symptoms

The incubation period for herpetic whitlow is 2 to 14 days. Fever and malaise may precede pain, burning, or tingling of the affected digit. Within 7 to 10 days, small clear vesicles form and coalesce. These vesicles may rupture and ulcerate. This is a self-limiting infection; however, recurrence rates are as high as 50%.

Treatment

It is important to distinguish between a paronychia and herpetic whitlow in that the latter is not treated with incision and drainage. A Tzanck test, viral cultures, or rapid immunofluorescent antibody test can confirm the diagnosis. Because the disease is self-limiting, treatment is aimed at providing symptomatic relief. Blisters can be unroofed for pain relief, although this is usually not necessary. Topical or oral acyclovir can shorten the duration of symptoms and prevent recurrence. Antibiotics are used only to treat superimposed bacterial infection.

Suppurative Flexor Tenosynovitis

Most patients with suppurative flexor tenosynovitis present after having sustained a penetrating injury to the volar surface of the finger. Bacterial inoculation of the flexor tendon sheath between the first annular pulley (A1 pulley) at the metacarpal head and the insertion of the flexor digitorum profundus tendon (FDP) at the distal phalanx can infect this closed potential space. The proximal aspect of the tendon sheath of the thumb and small finger communicate with the radial and ulnar bursae, respectively, allowing for the proximal spread of infection. *Staphylococcus aureus* and *Streptococcus* are the most common causative organisms.

Symptoms

In 1925, Kanavel described the following four cardinal signs of flexor tenosynovitis, which are still used to make the diagnosis:

1. Symmetric enlargement of the affected finger (fusiform swelling) (Figure 6)
2. Semiflexed position of the finger
3. Pain along the flexor tendon sheath
4. Severe pain on passive extension of the finger along the tendon sheath

Treatment

Early diagnosis and treatment of suppurative flexor tenosynovitis is essential to prevent destruction and scarring of the gliding surfaces of the sheath and tendon. Early suppurative flexor tenosynovitis may be treated with intravenous antibiotics targeted at *S. aureus* and group A *Streptococcus,* splinting, and elevation. Delayed presentation or failure to improve after 24 to 48 hours of intravenous antibiotics necessitates surgical intervention. Limited incision of the A1 and A5 pulley with placement of an irrigation catheter is often effective when no gross purulence or tendon sheath necrosis is present. A fenestrated pediatric feeding tube or angiocatheter can be sutured

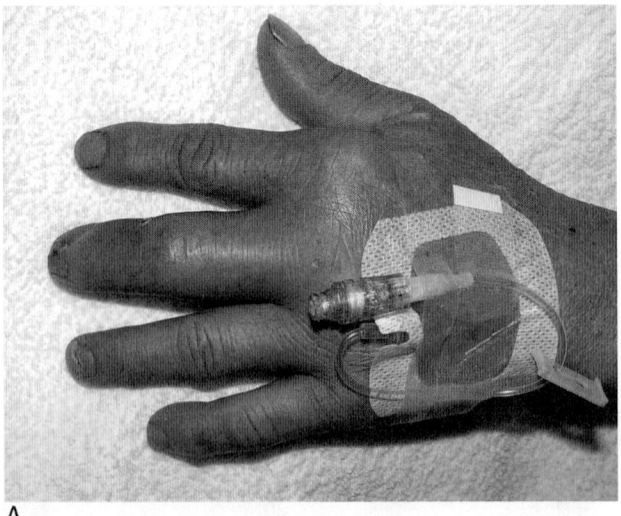

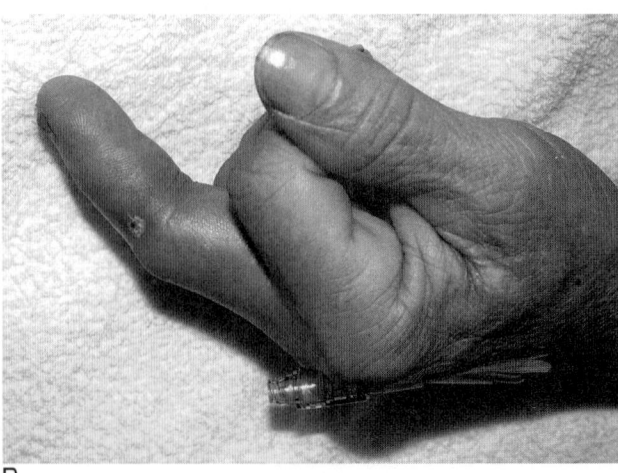

Figure 6 Dorsal **(A)** and lateral **(B)** views of pyogenic flexor tenosynovitis of the long finger showing edema and flexed position of the involved finger.

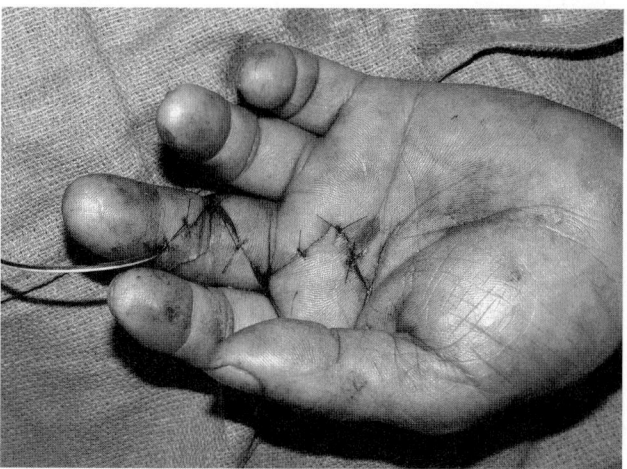

Figure 7 Brunner-type incision for the treatment of pyogenic flexor tenosynovitis. A pediatric feeding tube has been placed within the tendon sheath for continuous irrigation.

into position and continuously irrigated with 25 to 30 ml of saline every hour. The hand is loosely wrapped and splinted. After 48 hours, the splint can be removed and physical therapy initiated.

In the setting of gross purulence, necrosis of the tendon sheath, or failure to improve with catheter irrigation, a more extensive approach with exposure of the entire tendon sheath should be undertaken. Access to the tendon sheath is obtained using a Brunner incision (Fig. 7) placed along the volar surface of the digit or a straight midaxial incision placed alongside the finger. The cruciate pulleys can be incised to irrigate the sheath. Inflamed synovium can be carefully debrided without damaging the annular pulleys.

DEEP INFECTIONS OF THE HAND

Deep infections involve the subfascial spaces of the hand and forearm. There are six such areas: the thenar, hypothenar, midpalmar, interdigital space, dorsal subaponeurotic space of the hand, and Parona's space of the volar forearm (Fig. 8). Most deep-space infections occur as a result of penetrating injury. The most common organisms are *S. aureus* and *Streptococcus* species.

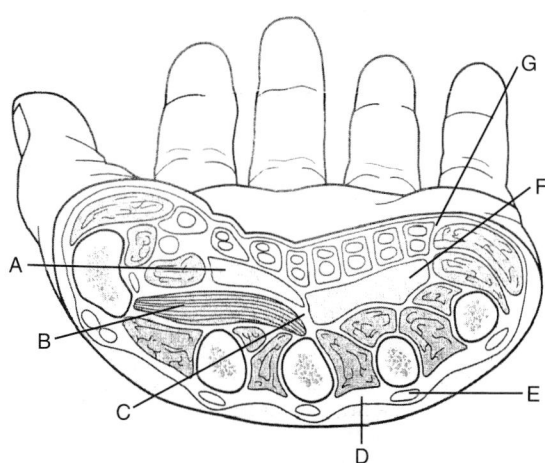

Figure 8 Cross-section anatomy of the hand. *(A)* Thenar space; *(B)* Adductor pollicis; *(C)* Midpalmar septum; *(D)* Dorsal subaponeurotic space; *(E)* Extensor tendon; *(F)* Midpalmar space; *(G)* Hypothenar space.

Interdigital (Web)-Space Infection

Web-space infections can occur through a break in the skin between the fingers, from a palmar callus that becomes secondarily infected, or from proximal spread of an infection in the subcutaneous area of the fingers.

Symptoms

Often the patient presents with painful swelling of the distal palmar region. Tenderness and fluctuance are usually present. The adjacent finger can be abducted when there is a large volar web-space collection. A "collar button" abscess forms when there is a volar and dorsal component to the web-space infection.

Treatment

Surgical incision and drainage can be performed through a volar, dorsal or combined approach to the web space. Access to the palmar space should be performed using a "zigzag" incision that starts at the edge of the web space and ends just distal to the distal palmar crease (Fig. 9, *A*). The subcutaneous tissue is bluntly dissected and retracted, and the palmar fascia and the transverse metacarpal ligament are incised to drain the collection. The digital neurovascular bundle should be identified and protected. When additional dorsal drainage is necessary, a longitudinal incision

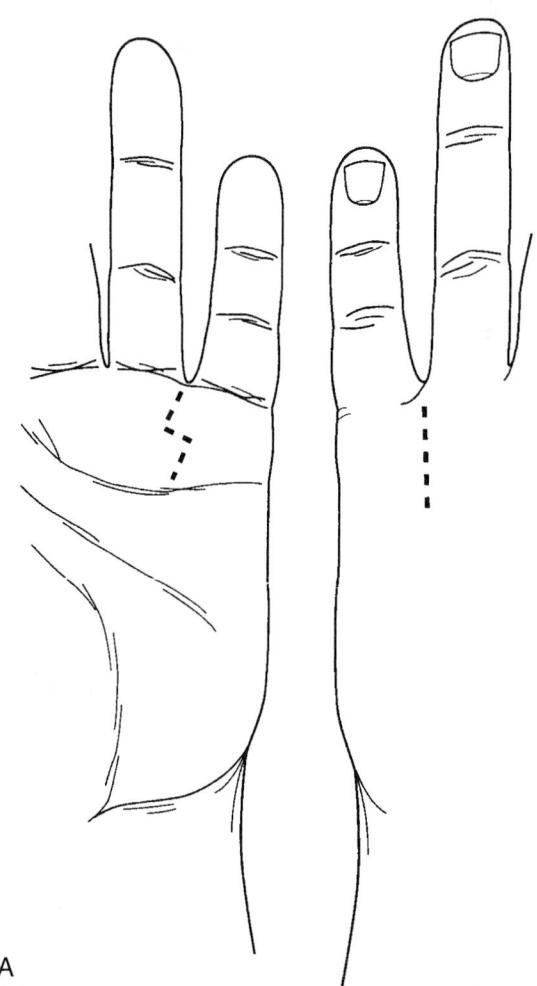

Figure 9 Palmar zigzag **(A)** and dorsal longitudinal incision **(B)** for drainage of a web space infection.

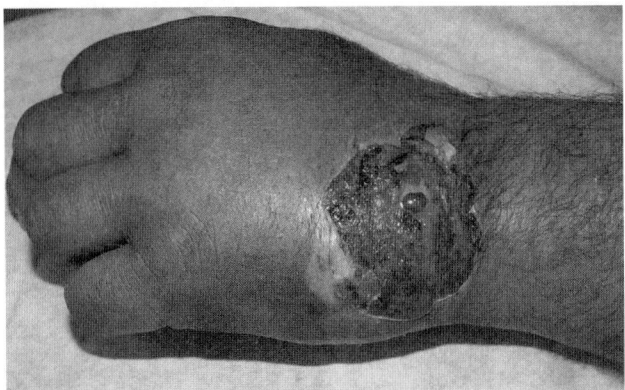

Figure 10 Infection of the dorsal subcutaneous and subaponeurotic space resulting from a puncture wound.

should be made from the metacarpal phalangeal joint level to the edge of the web space (see Figure 9, *B*). The incisions should be loosely closed over a Penrose drain and the hand splinted.

Dorsal Subcutaneous and Subaponeurotic Space

The dorsal subaponeurotic space lies deep to the extensor mechanism and superficial to the periosteum of the metacarpal bones and fascia of the dorsal interosseous muscles. Infections of the subaponeurotic and subcutaneous spaces usually result from a local, penetrating injury and are often seen in intravenous drug users.

Symptoms

Patients present with pain, erythema, and marked edema of the dorsum of the hand (Fig. 10). Because of the proximity of the extensor mechanism, tenderness is elicited on finger extension.

Treatment

Cellulitis of the dorsum of the hand can be treated with antibiotics, elevation, and splint immobilization. When fluctuance is noted, surgical drainage is performed through a dorsal longitudinal incision. The fascia between the extensor tendons is incised to enter the subaponeurotic space. On occasion, two parallel incisions are necessary to provide adequate drainage. Care should be taken when planning these incisions to ensure that the skin bridge has adequate blood supply. The wound can be left open or loosely closed over a Penrose drain. It is important to protect the extensor tendon paratenon from desiccation to prevent subsequent tendon adhesions. The hand is splinted. Physical therapy is initiated when the edema begins to resolve.

INFECTIONS INVOLVING THE PALMAR SPACES

Thenar Space

The thenar space is a triangular space defined by the interosseous muscles and abductor pollicis longus, the midpalmar septum, and the thumb metacarpal bone.

Symptoms

Thenar space infections are characterized by edema, pain with passive or active movement of the thumb, and exquisite tenderness to palpation of the thenar eminence and radial side of the palm. The thumb may be held in abduction when large abscess is present

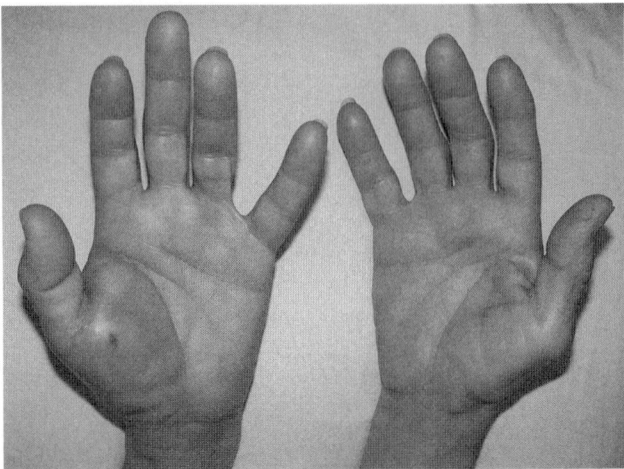

Figure 11 Thenar space infection resulting from a cat bite showing thenar edema and abduction of the thumb.

(Figure 11). The infection can spread dorsally through the adductor pollicis and first dorsal interosseous muscle to create a "dumbbell" or "pantaloon" abscess.

Treatment

Surgical drainage can be performed through a palmar incision along the thenar crease or a transverse incision proximal to the metacarpophalangeal crease in the distal area of the thenar musculature. When necessary, dorsal drainage is obtained through longitudinal incision of the first web space (Fig. 12).

Midpalmar space

The midpalmar space is located deep to the palmar fascia. It is bordered radially by the oblique septum and ulnarly by the hypothenar septum. Infection of the midpalmar space is uncommon and may result from a penetrating injury, following rupture of a pyogenic flexor tenosynovitis, or in association with a distal abscess that extends through the lumbrical canal.

Symptoms

Patients present with edema of the volar and dorsal surfaces of the hand. The normal palmar concavity may be effaced. The palm is tender to palpation, and passive flexion and extension of the fingers is painful.

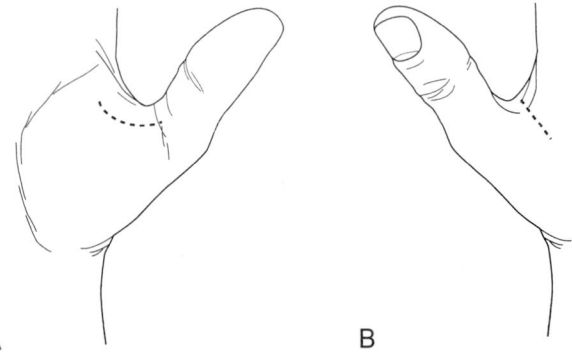

A   B

Figure 12 Surgical approach for incision and drainage of a thenar space infection. **(A)** Transverse incision. **(B)** Dorsal longitudinal incision.

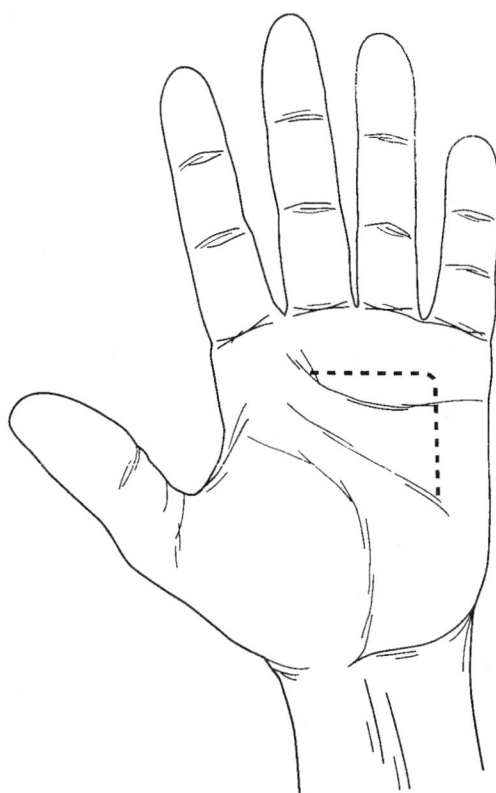

Figure 13 Combined longitudinal and transverse incision for drainage of midpalmar space abscess.

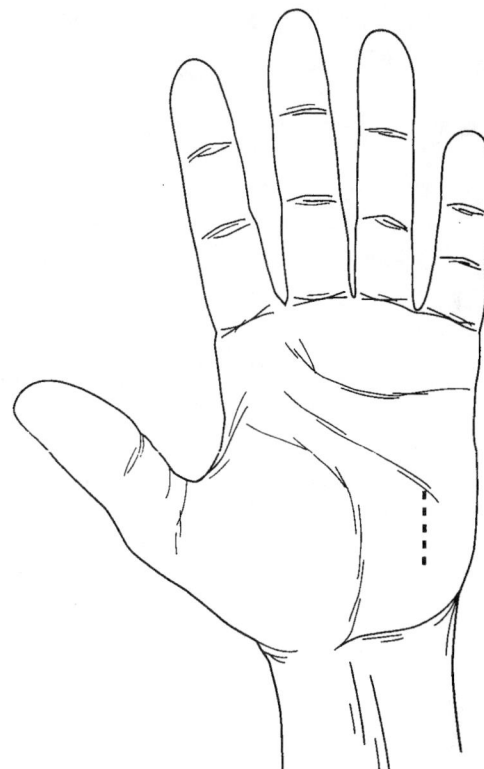

Figure 14 Longitudinal incision for drainage of a hypothenar space abscess.

Treatment

Drainage of this space is performed through a longitudinal or transverse palmar incision over the most prominent portion of the abscess (Fig. 13). The deep space is entered through blunt dissection while protecting the neurovascular bundles. As with other hand infections, the wound can be left open or loosely closed over Penrose drains. The hand should be splinted and elevated postoperatively. Therapy can be initiated when pain and swelling improve.

Hypothenar Space Infections

The hypothenar space is located between the hypothenar fascia and the hypothenar musculature. These infections are rare.

Symptoms

Hypothenar-space infections present with edema and tenderness of the hypothenar eminence. There is often pain with flexion of the small finger.

Treatment

The hypothenar space is accessed through an incision along the ulnar aspect of the palm beginning proximal and ulnar to the midpalmar crease (Fig. 14). The incision should not cross the wrist flexion crease. Blunt dissection is used to enter the deep space while protecting the ulnar nerve and artery.

Parona's Space

Parona's space is found deep to the flexor tendons of the forearm. The space communicates with the radial and ulnar bursa and midpalmar space and thus may become infected following deep hand infections or pyogenic flexor tenosynovitis.

Symptoms

Edema, tenderness, and fluctuance will be noted on the volar distal forearm (Fig. 15). Passive flexion of the wrist and fingers elicits pain.

Treatment

Access for drainage is provided by a longitudinal incision between the flexor tendons, ending proximal to the wrist crease.

SEPTIC ARTHRITIS

Septic arthritis is usually caused by penetrating trauma, bites, joint infection, or contiguous spread from adjacent infection. Early diagnosis and treatment is important because inflammatory reaction resulting from the infection can destroy the articular cartilage. Joint aspiration can confirm the diagnosis.

Symptoms

The affected joint is swollen and tender. Motion is restricted and painful. Fever and chills can be present.

Treatment

An arthrotomy through a dorsal longitudinal incision along the affected joint is the preferred method of drainage for the metacarpophalangeal or distal interphalangeal joint. The extensor tendon should be avoided. A midaxial incision is used for the proximal interphalangeal joint to prevent subsequent formation of a boutonniere deformity from damage to the central slip. Copious saline

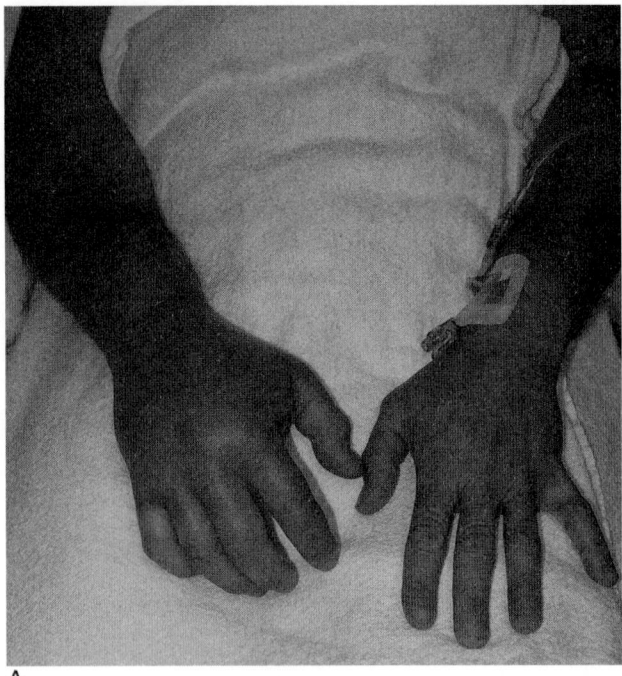

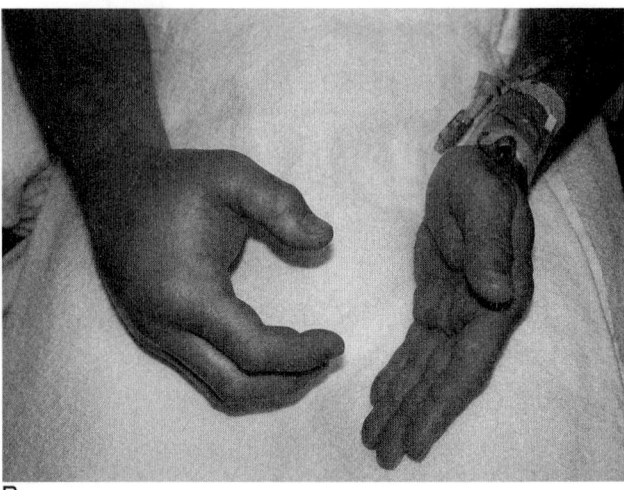

A   B

Figure 15   Dorsal **(A)** and lateral **(B)** view of an infection involving Parona's space in an intravenous drug user. This patient required volar and dorsal incisions to adequately drain and decompress his hand.

irrigation is used to clean the joint. The wound is closed over a Penrose drain, and the hand is splinted. Physical therapy is initiated after the pain has resolved.

Septic arthritis of the wrist can be drained and irrigated arthroscopically using small dorsal incisions.

OSTEOMYELITIS

Osteomyelitis usually results from a penetrating injury or, rarely, from hematogenous spread. The most common pathogen is *S. aureus*. It is

usually treated with debridement and long-term antibiotic therapy. Certain cases may require amputation of the affected finger.

BITES

Human bites are most commonly seen over the metacarpophalangeal joints, usually as a result of a clenched-fist blow to the mouth (Fig. 16, *A*). Communication with the joint space occurs in up to 60% of cases, resulting in septic arthritis. The most common organism cultured from this type of infection is *Eikenella corrodens*.

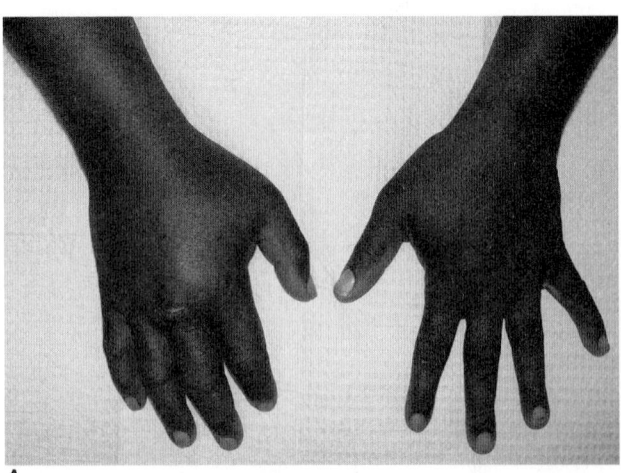

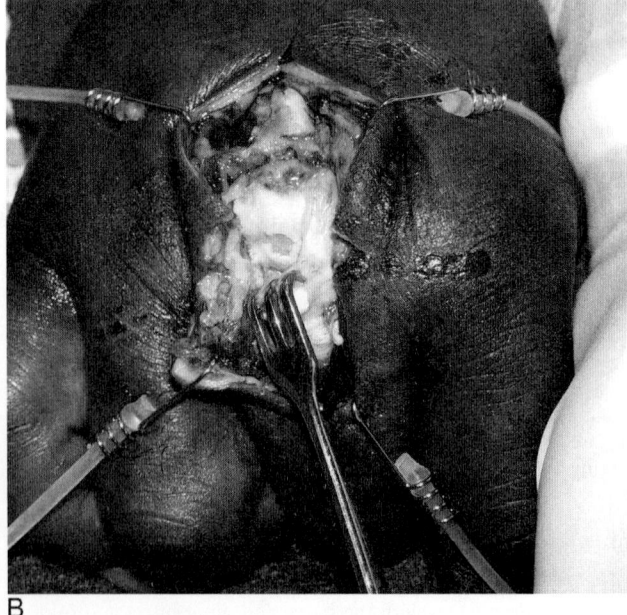

A   B

Figure 16   **(A)** Human bite to the metacarpophalangeal joint of the right long finger following a fight. **(B)** Surgery revealed a complete laceration of the extensor digitorum communis violation of the joint space and damage to the articular cartilage.

Streptococcus viridans and *S. aureus* are the two most common organisms found in infected dog-bite wounds. *P. multocida* is common bacteria found in infected cat bites. Dog bites can be accompanied by significant tissue destruction from tearing or crushing. The wound from a cat bite is usually a small puncture.

Treatment

A detailed hand examination should be performed. Larger wounds can be directly inspected for injury to deep structures. Tendon, nerve, or artery injury or the presence of significant injury or devitalized tissue necessitates treatment in the operating room.

Human bites can be irrigated clean and treated with oral antibiotics and close follow-up if treated soon after the injury. Human-bite joint infections are aggressive and should be treated accordingly with high-dose intravenous antibiotics and urgent incision and drainage. Irrigation with several liters of saline is required to adequately clean the wound. Advanced infections may require debridement of necrotic soft bone (see Fig. 16, *B*). The hand should be splinted and elevated. Physical therapy is initiated when pain begins to resolve. Tetanus prophylaxis should be considered if immunization status is unknown or not current.

Many animal bites can be treated in the emergency department. Lacerations from a dog bite can usually be closed after thorough irrigation and debridement of devitalized tissue. Lower-extremity dog bites have a higher rate of wound complication and infection. Forty percent of puncture wounds from a cat become infected. Oral antibiotics are given if indicated. All human and animal bites should be followed up closely to inspect the wounds for infection. Consider tetanus and rabies prophylaxis.

Suggested Readings

Benson LS, Edwards SL, Schiff AP, and others: Dog and cat bites to the hand: treatment and cost assessment, *J Hand Surg* 31A:468, 2006.

Clark DC: Common acute hand infections, *Am Fam Physician* 68:2167, 2003.

Haussman MR, Lisser SP: Hand infections, *Orthop Clinic North Am* 23:171, 1992.

Spann M, Talmor M, Nolan WB: Hand infections: Basic principles and management, *Surg Infect* 5:210, 2004.

Weinzweig N, Gonzalez M: Surgical infections of the hand and upper extremity, *Ann Plast Surg* 49:621, 2002.

Gas Gangrene of the Extremity

William C. Watson, and Peter Muscarella, II, MD

Gas gangrene is a rapidly progressive infection of soft tissues that results in high mortality if left untreated. Louis Pasteur initially identified a bacterial component to the infection when he described *Clostridium butyricum* in 1861. Later research identified other pathogenic microbes including, most notably, *Clostridium perfringens*. Epidemiologic and outcome studies of gas gangrene gained most notoriety during World War I, when this was a common wound infection, with systemic complications occurring in 6% of open fractures. Modern day incidence has been drastically reduced with the development of antibiotic therapies, evolving wound management strategies, and improved understanding of the disease process.

Gas gangrene has been divided into a number of classifications, including cellulitis, fasciitis, and myonecrosis, and these entities are often used interchangeably. These terms are useful to discriminate the depth of infectious invasion and to determine the extent of surgical debridement required. Although the term *gas gangrene* leads one to think of infection caused by clostridial species, more than half of the cases of necrotizing infections with gas occur as a result of multiple, nonclostridial organisms, including *Streptococcus* and *Staphylococcus* (Table 1). Fortunately, infections from gas-forming pathogens are relatively unusual and we encounter this problem infrequently during our surgical careers. The most common cause of gas accumulation within a wound is direct injection at the time of injury. Whenever gas is encountered within a wound, gas gangrene must be considered. Mortality in this patient population may range from 15% to 70%. The key to treating these

Table 1: Summary of the Differences and Similarities between Clostridial and Nonclostridial Extremity Infections

	Clostridial Infections	Nonclostridial Infections
Bacterial etiology	*C. perfringens, C. histolytica, C. septicum, C. bifermentan*	*β-hemolytic Streptococcus, S. aureus, Bacteroides sp., Peptostreptococcus sp.*
Toxins	Phospholipase C, collagenase, deoxyribonuclease	α-hemolysins, β-toxins, hyaluronidase, leukocidans, enterotoxins
Onset	Rapid, 8 to 12 hours	Slower
Symptoms	None, extremity heaviness, pain out of proportion to examination	Insensate, local pain
Signs	Crepitus, skin bronzing, hemorrhagic bullae	Subtle edema, tenderness
Antibiotic treatment	Penicillin G	Penicillin + lindamycin + aminoglycoside

infections is rapid diagnosis, early initiation of broad-spectrum antibiotic therapy, supportive care, and most importantly, timely and adequate surgical debridement.

CLOSTRIDIAL GAS GANGRENE

"Classic" clostridial gas gangrene is typically caused by *C. perfringens*. However, there are multiple clostridial species, including *C. histolytica, C. septicum,* and *C. bifermentans,* which are equally pathogenic. These saprophytic organisms are ubiquitous in soil but have been isolated from the gastrointestinal tract and the perineum of healthy persons. The clinical manifestations of clostridial soft-tissue infections result from the release of several exotoxins during periods of low oxygen tension that occur within the tissue after injury or in chronic low blood flow states (e.g., diabetes mellitus, surgical devascularization). More than 20 exotoxins have been isolated from *C. perfringens,* including α-toxin (phospholipase C), κ-toxin (collagenase), and ν-toxin (deoxyribonuclease). α-Toxin appears to be the most lethal and induces profound shock via direct cardiotoxicity, hemolysis, increased capillary permeability, and leukocyte dysfunction. Direct contamination of relatively hypoxic wounds with clostridial spores establishes the infection.

Clostridial gas gangrene has been associated with crush injuries, motor vehicle accidents, open fractures, wounds involving large muscle masses, high-velocity missiles, iatrogenic injuries during hip replacement surgery, abortions, and amputations for acute vascular ischemia. Interestingly, rare, nontraumatic clostridial gas gangrene has been described in patients with metastatic colorectal carcinoma, or as a primary infection of the scrotum or perineum. It is estimated that 30% to 60% of cases of gas gangrene occur as a result of poor wound hygiene. *C. perfringens* is a facultative anaerobe that can survive in 30% oxygen. At 100% oxygen, bacterial growth is arrested and exotoxins are inactivated.

Clinically, clostridial infections progress rapidly, occurring sometimes as soon as 8 to 12 hours after the initial injury. Shock can ensue rapidly, depending on the extent of the inoculum and local tissue oxygen tensions. Diagnosis is best made by clinical examination. Some patients may complain only of extremity heaviness. Others complain of pain out of proportion to examination findings. On physical examination, crepitus, edema, skin bronzing or necrosis, and hemorrhagic bullae formation (Fig. 1) may be identified. Crepitus may not be appreciated in all cases because of dense inflammation and edema. The wound often has an extremely foul or even sweet odor, suggesting progressive infection. As the infection progresses, systemic symptoms, including tachycardia, oliguria, and mental status changes, develop rapidly, indicating impending cardiovascular collapse. Radiographic evaluation of the affected area may reveal subcutaneous emphysema, but subcutaneous air in itself is not diagnostic of gas gangrene, particularly in a fresh wound. Few tests are necessary for diagnosis. Rapid detection tests of α-toxin or neuraminidases in infected tissue by enzyme-linked immunosorbent assay (ELISA) are not widely available and are unnecessary, but they do represent potential diagnostic tools in difficult situations. Definitive treatment should not be delayed pending ELISA results if clinical evidence of active infection exists. Gram stains of infected tissue may offer some additional evidence of gas gangrene, particularly if large gram-positive bacilli are identified. Again, treatment should not be delayed pending Gram-stain results.

Aggressive medical therapy should be instituted as soon as the diagnosis is entertained. This includes resuscitation with intravenous fluids, administration of broad-spectrum antibiotics, and possibly transfusion with blood products if there is evidence of hemolysis or coagulopathy from exotoxemia (or both). In cases of clostridial gangrene, high-dose intravenous penicillin G is the antibiotic treatment of choice. In cases in which nonclostridial gangrene is suspected, triple-antibiotic therapy is recommended until culture results have returned from the laboratory.

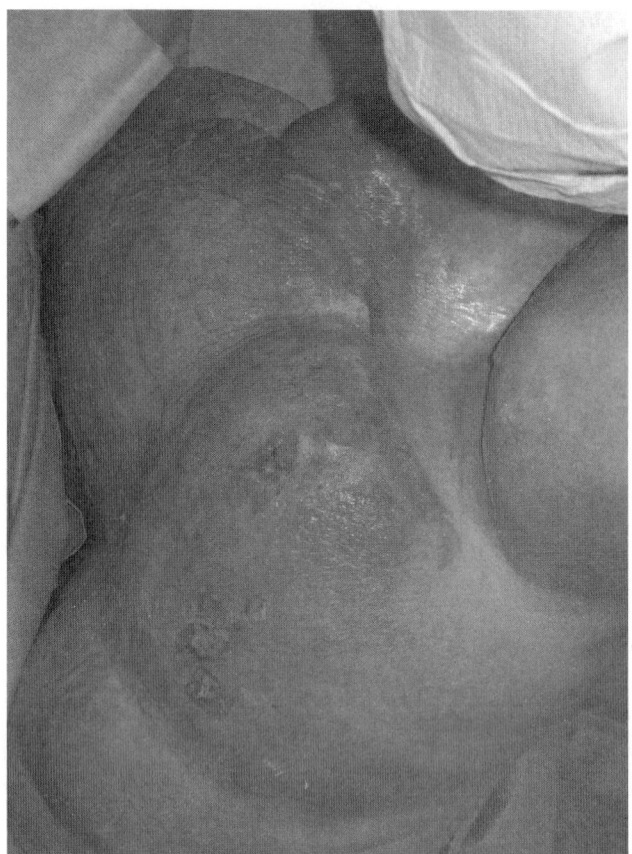

Figure I   Photograph of an obese, diabetic patient with lower-extremity gas gangrene that started from an animal scratch, characterized by edema, erythema, and bullae formation. The patient complained of extreme leg heaviness and numbness.

After the diagnosis is confirmed (or suspected) and the patient is properly resuscitated, the patient should be taken emergently to the operating room for extensive surgical debridement of all affected tissue (Fig. 2). Large amounts of subcutaneous tissue may require debridement. Limb sparing is acceptable if the disease is limited to the superficial layers of skin and soft tissue. Amputation may be required if the infection involves large muscle groups, is circumferential, or has progressed to advanced stages with systemic effects and hemodynamic collapse. Guillotine amputation across a joint space with open wound management is preferred when limb salvage is not deemed possible. If the diagnosis is uncertain, local wound exploration is warranted with evaluation of the involved soft tissue and muscle groups. Wide excision of all of the affected tissue is required. One should strive to avoid incision and drainage procedures without soft-tissue debridement in these patients. After debridement has been completed, patients require intensive care with close monitoring of urine output, hemodynamic parameters, and wound hygiene. Hemodynamic support with pressors is sometimes required, but should be avoided unless the patient has been adequately resuscitated with intravenous fluids. Antibiotic coverage can be tailored after Gram-stain and culture results are available. Wounds can be cared for using a number of techniques, including wet-to-dry saline dressing changes and the application of wound vacuum systems. Wound management at our institution typically consists of frequent saline-gauze dressings with close clinical monitoring. These patients are frequently maintained in the surgical intensive care unit because of the relatively labor-intensive dressing changes and the need for intravenous sedation and narcotics during dressing changes. We encourage the presence of a member of the

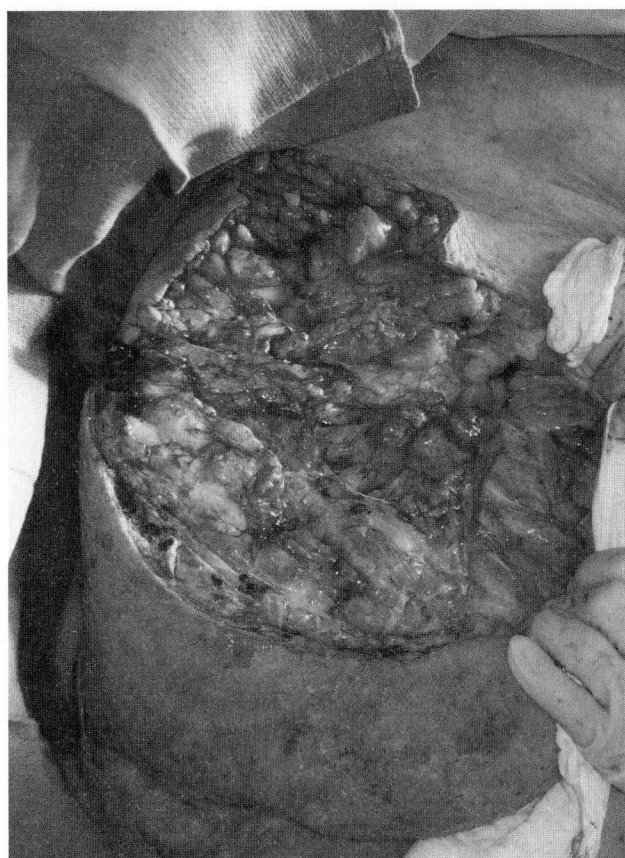

Figure 2 Photograph of the affected leg following surgical debridement. Note that the amount of soft tissue requiring debridement was much more than apparent on primary physical examination.

surgical team at the time of all dressing changes until the need for potential further debridement has essentially been eliminated. After granulation tissue is apparent and systemic signs of sepsis have resolved, the dressings may be converted to a vacuum-type dressing. Early consultation with plastic and reconstructive surgeons is also encouraged.

The development of wound vacuum systems marks a great advance in the care of acute and chronic wounds. The application of negative pressure via suction tubing embedded in polyurethane foam placed into the wound, covered by an occlusive dressing, results in removal of excess fluids, increased local blood flow, and decreased bacterial counts. Ultimately, this results in more rapid formation of granulation tissue and wound closure. An added benefit is decreased frequency of dressing changes. The dressing is changed every 72 hours instead of every 8 to 12 hours as with conventional wet-to-dry dressings. This benefit is somewhat offset by the added cost of the device and supplies. It is important to remember that the wound vacuum system should not be instituted too early after debridement, nor should it be used in place of prompt surgical debridement. The vacuum should not be used in grossly infected wounds.

There continues to be controversy regarding the role of hyperbaric oxygen in the treatment of gas gangrene. Recommendations for the use of hyperbaric oxygen in gas gangrene are limited and suggest that it be used only as an adjunct after surgical debridement. The results of small case series suggest that hyperbaric oxygen therapy may result in decreased mortality rates and decreased duration of antibiotic therapy. The therapeutic effects of hyperbaric oxygen therapy are thought to be mediated through a variety of mechanisms, including inhibition of α-toxin release, direct inhibition of bacterial replication, and improved tissue oxygenation. In animal studies of clostridial soft-tissue infection, overall survival was significantly improved in dogs treated with hyperbaric oxygen (95% versus 70%). If treatment is initiated, it should be started immediately following surgery and should be continued at least twice daily until evidence of toxin hemolysis subsides. If adequate surgical debridement is performed, the amount of toxin should be minimal and the need for hyperbaric oxygen limited. Hyperbaric oxygen should never be used as the primary or initial treatment for "classic" gas gangrene.

NONCLOSTRIDIAL GANGRENE

Nonclostridial necrotizing soft-tissue infections are more common than "classic" gas gangrene. These mixed infections may be increasing in frequency as the number of immunocompromised patients at risk increases. This infection is usually associated with diabetes mellitus, chronic lower-extremity vascular compromise, radiation exposure, cholecystitis, and following appendectomy. The most common isolates from these polymicrobial wounds include β-hemolytic *Streptococcus*, *Staphylococcus aureus*, *Streptococcus* species, *Bacteroides*, *Peptostreptococcus*, and aerobic coliform bacteria. *Candida* and *Mucormycosis* have also been cultured from the wounds of poorly controlled diabetics. Nonclostridial gangrene typically progresses slower than clostridial gangrene, but it requires the same prompt surgical attention. Preoperative resuscitation and preparation is the same as with clostridial gangrene. Antibiotic coverage must be more generalized because of the polymicrobial nature of the disease. We typically treat these patients with penicillin, clindamycin, and tobramycin. Clindamycin appears to work synergistically with penicillin, particularly against *Streptococcus*. In hemodialysis or previously hospitalized patients, vancomycin may be added to cover against methicillin-resistant *S. aureus*. Initial evaluation of the patient with nonclostridial gangrene may be more difficult than it is with patients who have clostridial gas gangrene. Skin changes are often subtle, with edema and mild color changes commonly being the only findings. The area may be insensate or nontender, confusing the diagnosis even further. Diagnosis is best made by local exploration and examination of the tissue. If necrosis or purulence is encountered, wide local debridement is indicated. Similar to clostridial gangrene, all nonviable tissue must be removed. If muscle groups are involved or extensive necrosis is present, amputation is an option. Postoperative care of the patient is identical to that provided for patients with clostridial gas gangrene. Although limited data exist to support its use, hyperbaric oxygen is rarely used in this patient population.

UNUSUAL INFECTIONS

Immunocompromised patients are more likely to contract unusual infections, and certain pathogens are more commonly seen in these patient populations. *Aeromonas hydrophilia*, an aerobic, gram-negative rod indigenous to fresh water, can cause cellulitis and an infection very similar to clostridial gangrene. The most common presentation in humans occurs as acute gastroenteritis. It has been reported to result from both wild and medicinal leech bites. Treatment consists of aggressive surgical debridement and gentamicin. *Vibrio vulnificus* is a gram-negative, motile, spiral bacterium found in marine environments. Similar to *Aeromonas*, it can induce a severe gastroenteritis when ingested from undercooked seafood, or a severe cellulitis and gangrene if the entry point is an open wound. Cirrhotic patients are particularly susceptible to infection with these bacteria and treatment is difficult. Antibiotics of choice are ceftazidime and doxycycline. Atypical mycobacteria cause a slow-growing, indolent soft-tissue infection in the immunocompromised patient. These are rare and difficult to treat, often requiring multiple drugs.

Other organisms that cause atypical infections that have been reported in children include *Apophysomyces elegans* and *Proteus* species. Standard treatment is surgical debridement and antibiotic therapy.

CONCLUSION

Necrotizing soft-tissue infections of the extremity are rarely seen but may potentially result in rapidly lethal outcomes. These infections are characterized by massive tissue destruction and systemic collapse from exotoxin release and bacterial overload. Treatment relies on rapid diagnosis and consists of fluid resuscitation, cardiovascular support, intravenous antibiotic therapy, and prompt surgical debridement of all devitalized tissues. Little workup other than clinical suspicion and examination is necessary for evaluating these patients. Mortality from gas gangrene may be improved with prompt recognition and therapy, but delays in treatment or inadequate surgical debridement may result in devastating consequences for affected individuals.

SUGGESTED READINGS

Brook I: Microbiology and management of infectious gangrene in children, *J Pediatr Orthop* 24(5):587, 2004.
Demello FJ, Haglin JJ, Hitchcock CR: Comparative study of experimental *Clostridium perfringens* infections in dogs treated with antibiotics, surgery, and hyperbaric oxygen, *Surgery* 73(6):936, 1973.
Hart GB, Lamb RC, Strauss MB: Gas gangrene, *J Trauma* 23(11):991, 1983.
Present DA, Meislin R, Shaffer B: Gas gangrene: A review, *Orthop Rev* 19(4): 333, 1990.
Sugihara A, Watanabe H, Oohashi M, and others: The effect of hyperbaric oxygen therapy on the bout of treatment for soft tissue infections, *J Infect* 48(4):330, 2004.
Titball RW: Gas gangrene. An open and closed case, *Microbiology* 151 (Pt 9):2821, 2005.
Weinstein L, Barza X: Gas gangrene, *N Engl J Med* 289(21):1129, 1973.

NECROTIZING SKIN AND SOFT TISSUE INFECTIONS

Michele A. Manahan, MD, Stephen M. Milner, MD, DDS, Paul Freeswick, MD, and John W. Harmon, MD

Skin and soft-tissue infections range in severity from mild cellulitis to rapidly progressive necrosis (up to 1 inch per hour) with early mortality. Necrotizing soft-tissue infections (NSTIs) afflict between 500 and 1500 patients yearly in the United States with necrosis of skin, subcutaneous fat, superficial fascia, deep muscular fascia, muscle, or any combination of these structures. Given the diversity of pathology, nomenclature can be confusing. *Necrotizing fasciitis, Fournier's gangrene, clostridial myonecrosis, gas gangrene, Meleney's ulcers,* and *flesh-eating infections* are all part of the same spectrum of disease, defined by rapidly progressive necrosis of soft tissue requiring early, radical excision to prevent the early onset of sepsis, multisystem organ failure, and death.

On the microscopic level, a variety of microorganisms infect susceptible soft tissues, promoting polymorphonuclear cell infiltration of the dermis and fascia. The microorganisms and inflammatory cells also invade blood vessels of the soft tissue, leading to obliterative endarteritis and necrosis of blood vessel walls and thrombosis of the small vessels passing through the soft tissues. Liquefactive necrosis of the fascia ensues, with concomitant necrosis and breakdown of skin, muscle, and surrounding tissues. Macroscopically, cellulitic skin often represents the "tip of the iceberg" in terms of extent of underlying soft-tissue necrosis.

A Confederate army surgeon, Joseph Jones, first described NSTIs in 1871 on the basis of his observations of 2642 infections during the Civil War, and he noted a 50% mortality rate at that time for "hospital gangrene." Fournier described necrotizing infections of the perineum in 1883. It was not until 1918 that the microbiologic etiology of these presentations became clear. F. L. Meleney is credited with the landmark papers from the 1920s and 1930s that provided what are still considered classic descriptions of skin gangrene caused by infections in the subcutaneous tissues, and he noted a 20% mortality rate. Wilson, in 1952, first used the term *necrotizing fasciitis* to describe the disease, on the basis of its most frequent early finding during gross examination of tissue specimens. Despite the length of time that the medical community has been struggling with this disease, morbidity and mortality remain largely unchanged.

MICROBIOLOGY

The majority of NSTIs (70%-80%) result from polymicrobial infections. Cultures obtained from patients demonstrate an average of three to four organisms per patient, but some reports have demonstrated up to 14 isolates in a single tissue sample. Gram-positive aerobes, gram-negative aerobes, anaerobes, and fungi are all found with significant frequencies, and these pathogens likely act synergistically to produce more severe destruction than would normally be expected on the basis of their individual virulences. Table 1 delineates some of the more common culprits, but it is by no means an exhaustive list of all causative factors. *Bacteroides* and *Streptococcus* are the most frequently cultured organisms. In cases attributable to single microorganisms, anaerobes such as *Clostridium* species (most commonly *C. perfringens*) are twice as likely as aerobes such as group A β-hemolytic *Streptococcus*. The severity of presentation in monomicrobial infections often results from the toxins produced by the pathogen (i.e., hemolysin, streptolysins O and S, and leukocidin by group A streptococci and α-toxin by *Clostridium perfringens*). Infections of the skin without deeper involvement are most likely monomicrobial.

DIAGNOSIS

Early diagnosis and treatment is the essential key to preventing extreme morbidity and high rates of mortality with NSTIs. Therefore a high index of suspicion must be maintained by health care providers encountering soft-tissue infections. Patients often cite fevers and pain, swelling, and erythema at the site that have progressed over the course of several days following trauma of some sort. Frequently reported inciting events include intravenous drug use, blunt or penetrating trauma, insect bites, surgical incisions or indwelling catheters, chickenpox vesicles, cutaneous infections or ulcers, and abscesses. In approximately 10% of cases, however, no identifiable portal of entry for microorganisms exists. Immunocompromised states predispose to NSTIs. Increased risk is associated with diabetes mellitus, human immunodeficiency virus/acquired immunodeficiency

Table 1: Causative Organisms in Necrotizing Soft-Tissue Infections

Gram-positive Aerobes	Gram-negative Aerobes	Anaerobes	Other
Staphylococcus species (*S. aureus,* coagulase-negative staph)	*Klebsiella, Escherichia coli, Enterobacter, Pseudomonas, Serratia, Citrobacter, Acinetobacter*	*Bacteroides fragilis*	Fungi (*Candida,* mucormycoses)
Streptococcus species (beta—all groups, alpha, and nonhemolytic)		*Clostridium perfringens*	
Enterococcus species (*E. faecium*)		*Peptostreptococcus*	
Gram-positive rods (*Corynebacterium, Bacillus, Lactobacillus*)			

syndrome (HIV/AIDS), alcohol abuse, peripheral vascular disease, medical immunosuppressants such as steroids or cancer chemotherapy, renal failure, cirrhosis, heart disease, old age, obesity, and malnutrition. The nonspecific nature of these aspects of the patient's history makes diagnosis of an NSTI from history alone difficult.

Physical examination remains the keystone in diagnostic efforts. Frank purulence is rare. Worrisome findings on physical examination include tense edema; ecchymosis; skin necrosis; bullae that may become hemorrhagic; crepitus (resulting from hydrogen, methane, and nitrogen gas produced mainly by anaerobes but also by coliforms); cutaneous numbness; and turbid, foul-smelling, brownish discharge known as "dishwater pus" (resulting from liquefactive necrosis of the fascia and subcutaneous tissue). However, these signs are not always present, and patients frequently present simply with erythema, edema, warmth, and tenderness, making it difficult to differentiate the symptoms from nonnecrotizing infections that do not require urgent operative intervention (Figures 1 through 3). NSTI patients are more likely to exhibit systemic toxicity and vital sign abnormalities and complain of symptoms out of proportion to initial appearance.

Because early diagnosis is a crucial first step toward early treatment to prevent extreme morbidity and death, and initial presentation can be nonspecific, adjunctive studies may be useful supplements. However, as with any test, abnormal findings are not always present. Absence of abnormal values should not prevent aggressive treatment if clinical suspicion is high, and therapy should not be delayed to obtain additional laboratory or radiologic evidence.

The literature remains controversial regarding specific laboratory abnormalities. Leukocytosis, hyponatremia, hypochloremia, elevated blood urea nitrogen and creatinine, hypocalcemia, hypoalbuminemia, anemia, thrombocytopenia, hyperglycemia, and coagulopathy have all been associated with NSTIs. These values are also deranged in severe systemic illnesses of other etiologies. Occasionally, fine needle aspiration may secure tissue for Gram stain (or silver stain for fungus), and frozen section analysis of tissue biopsies may be performed preoperatively. These can provide a definitive positive

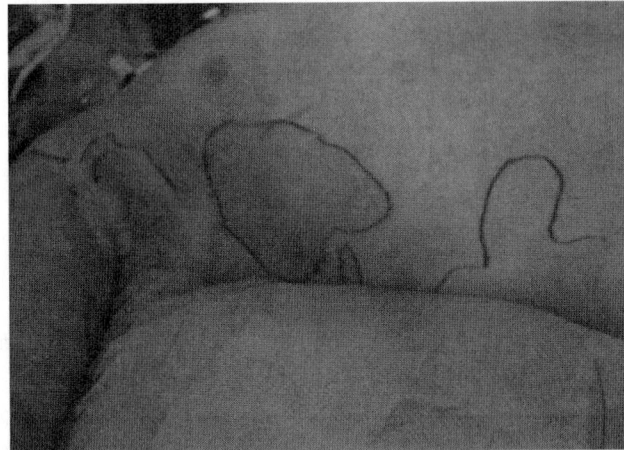

Figure 2   Initial presentation of necrotizing fasciitis of the arm and trunk.

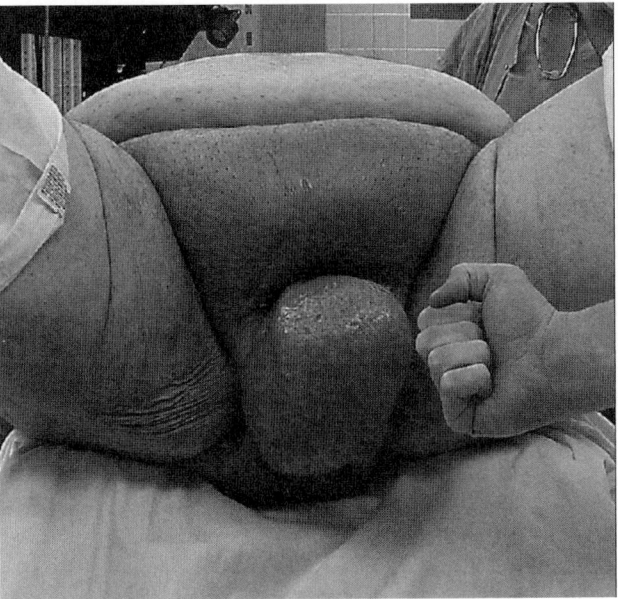

Figure 3   Initial presentation of necrotizing fasciitis of the perineum.

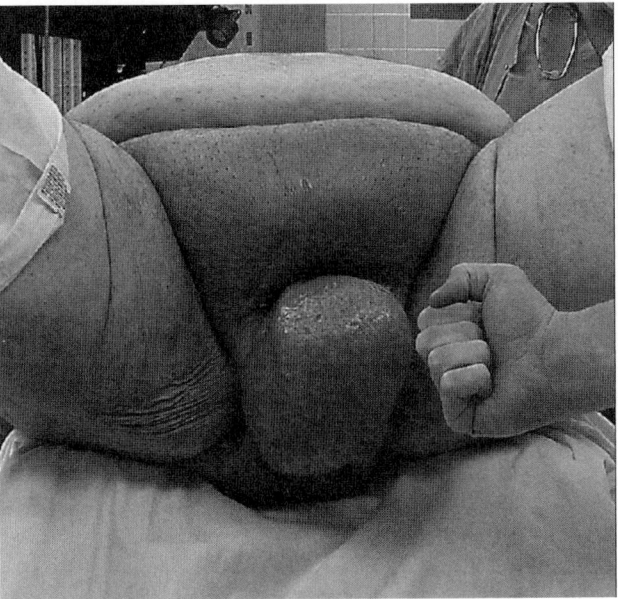

Figure 1   Initial presentation of necrotizing fasciitis of the leg.

diagnosis and may also allow identification of fungal species not identifiable quickly by fungal culture. However, analyses of the sections are observer dependent, making them unreliable. They also tend to underestimate disease and may delay diagnosis. There is an association in the literature between performance of frozen sections and improved survival, but this is likely confounded by a higher index of suspicion in patients undergoing pathologic examination of biopsy specimens.

Radiologic evidence may also confirm a diagnosis, but like other adjunctive studies, absence of positive findings should not be interpreted as absence of an NSTI. Plain radiographs may demonstrate gas within the soft tissue. In a majority of patients, computed tomography (CT) demonstrates abnormalities such as fascial thickening, fat infiltration, focal fluid collections, soft-tissue gas, and muscle involvement. Magnetic resonance imaging (MRI) has been demonstrated to have a high sensitivity for abnormal findings in cases of NSTIs. However, MRI tends to overestimate the extent of disease because of edema of surrounding tissues. This imaging modality also has a low specificity in that many nonnecrotizing infections also demonstrate similar findings, but experienced observers may be able to distinguish non-NSTIs from NSTIs. CT better demonstrates subcutaneous gas, but MRI more accurately reveals deep fascial fluid. The authors find a preoperative CT scan useful to help plan the extent of surgery. Once again, however, definitive treatment of suspected NSTIs should not be delayed while waiting for radiologic studies. Definitive diagnosis can be achieved only by findings of necrotic fat, fascia, or muscle on gross examination of the tissue in the operating room and subsequent histopathology. Microbiologic analysis from intraoperative cultures allows tailoring of antibiotic therapy.

TREATMENT

Definitive treatment of NSTIs requires operative intervention in an urgent fashion within 12 to 24 hours of presentation to limit mortality. Delay of more than 24 hours doubles the mortality rate. Wide excision of all infected tissue with margins of normal tissue both laterally and deep within the wound is necessary to ensure adequacy of the procedure. Evidence of swollen gray fascia and easy dissection between tissue planes signifies continued infection. Frozen sections may be used to determine presence of normal tissue in areas where unaffected tissue is at a premium. Repeated trips to the operating room every 24 to 48 hours are often necessary to confirm that all necrotic material is removed. Patients usually rapidly improve with regard to systemic toxicity after debridement is complete. Diversion of the fecal stream may be helpful in cases involving the perineum. Fig. 4 demonstrates the intraoperative appearance of necrotizing fasciitis. Fig. 5 and 6 demonstrate the appearance of the wounds following surgical debridement.

In concert with surgical excision, broad-spectrum antibiotics are essential and may be tailored as culture data become available. The standard regimen includes penicillin G (18–24 million units/day divided into 4 or 6 doses) or ampicillin (500 mg to 2 g every 4–6 hr) to treat gram-positive organisms such as clostridia, enterococci (not covered by penicillin G), and peptostreptococci; vancomycin for other gram-positive organisms such as resistant *Staphylococcus aureus* (1 g every 12 hr); clindamycin (900 mg every 8 hr) or metronidazole (1 g intravenous load then 0.5 g every 6 hr or 1 g every 12 hr) for anaerobic coverage; and gentamicin (2 mg/kg intravenous load then 5 mg/kg/day or 1.7 mg/kg every 8 hr) or another aminoglycoside to cover gram-negative organisms. Use of extended-spectrum pharmaceuticals (imipenem/cilastatin, piperacillin/tazobactam, and ampicillin/sulbactam) may be used as monotherapy if resistance is not likely, reducing the number of individual drugs received by the patient. Given the high concurrent rate of systemic toxicity in NSTI patients, intensive monitoring, hemodynamic resuscitation, and

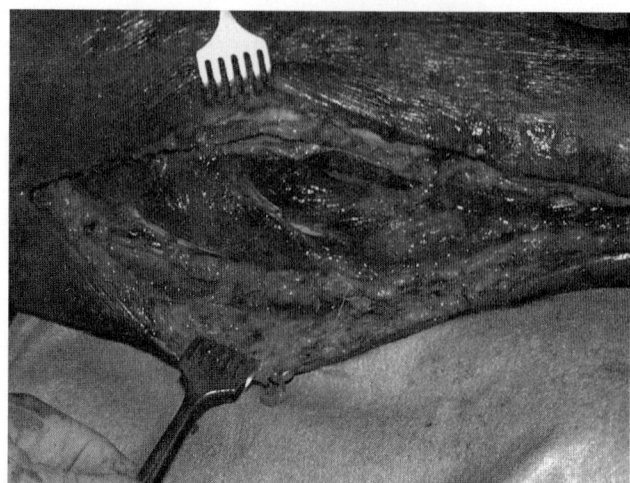

Figure 4   Intraoperative appearance of necrotizing fasciitis prior to complete surgical debridement.

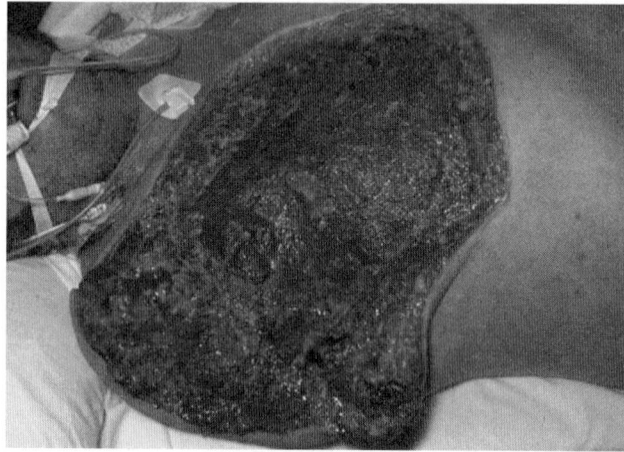

Figure 5   Appearance of necrotizing fasciitis wound following surgical debridement and extremity amputation.

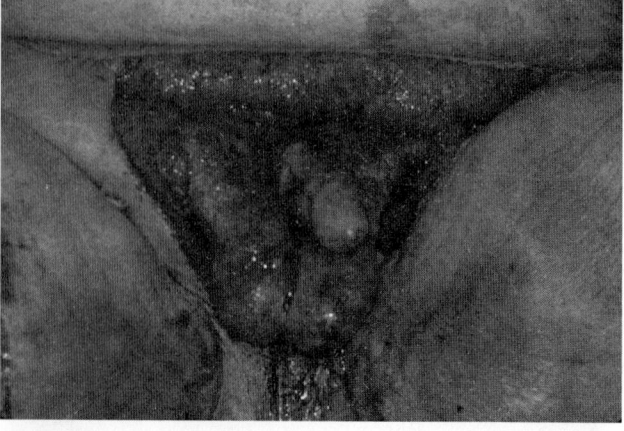

Figure 6   Appearance of necrotizing fasciitis wound of the perineum following surgical debridement.

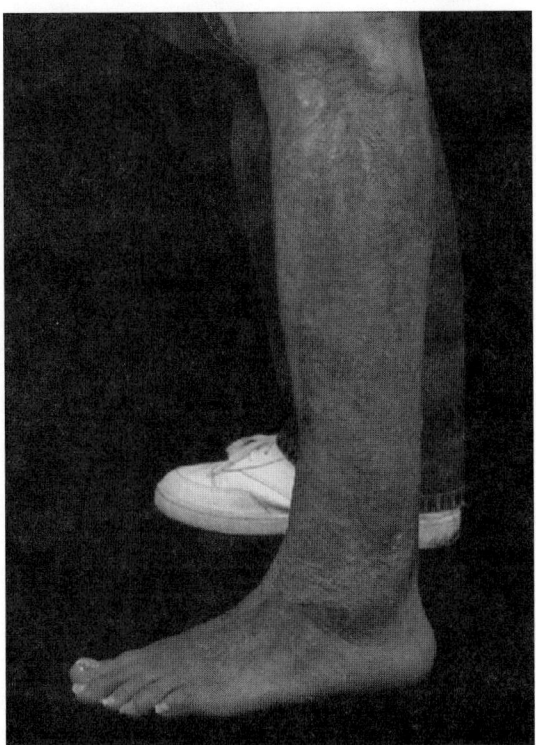

Figure 7 Appearance of necrotizing fasciitis wound of the lower extremity following skin graft reconstruction.

nutritional support are also critical and have been shown to decrease mortality.

Hyperbaric oxygen has no proven benefit in the treatment of NSTIs. Theoretical evidence for the usefulness of hyperbaric oxygen includes studies showing that increased oxygen tension in the tissues has direct antibacterial effect on anaerobic organisms, decreases endotoxin activity, increases leukocyte phagocytosis, increases antibiotic delivery, and increases fibroblast proliferation. No survival benefit has been found. Prospective, randomized, controlled clinical trials are necessary.

Often, successful treatment of NSTIs leaves patients with disfiguring and disabling defects. Following stabilization of the patient's status and confirmation of appropriate wound healing, reconstruction of several varieties may be considered. The reconstructive plan depends on the characteristics of the defect but may include skin grafting, as well as pedicled and free tissue transfer (Fig. 7). The timing of these reconstructions remains debatable and may be performed during the initial hospitalization, after wounds have stabilized, or in a delayed fashion.

PROGNOSIS

Mortality rates between 10% and 80% have been reported, but most authors quote a 30% to 40% rate for all cases. Delay in diagnosis is the most consistent prognosticator of poor outcomes (more operations and higher mortality) and has been shown to occur when patients are transferred between facilities for definitive management, admitted to a nonsurgical service, or demonstrate negative findings on adjunctive studies. Increased mortality has also been associated with greater extent of disease on presentation, older age (>50 years), comorbid illnesses (diabetes, atherosclerosis, renal failure, obesity), multiorgan system failure, malnutrition, bacteremia, and anatomic site of infection involving the trunk.

CONCLUSION

The term *necrotizing soft-tissue infection* encompasses a spectrum of infectious disease defined by its severity, rapidity of progression, significant morbidity, and high mortality rate. Early diagnosis and treatment is critical. Despite many pathognomonic findings, detection can be difficult because of infrequent presence of the pathognomonic evidence and somewhat benign, nonspecific initial appearance. Therapy includes aggressive, wide, surgical debridement to well within the limits of normal tissue in conjunction with broad-spectrum antibiotic therapy. Despite advances in medical science and a better understanding of the nature of NSTIs, prognosis is still poor, with a high incidence of disfigurement or death. Future study must aim to alter the outcomes of these diseases in a positive manner.

SUGGESTED READINGS

Bosshardt TL, Henderson VJ, Organ CH: Necrotizing soft tissue infections, *Arch Surg* 131:846, 1996.

Elliott DC, Kufera JA, Myers RAM: Necrotizing soft tissue infections: Risk factor for mortality and strategies for management, *Ann Surg* 224:672, 1996.

Elliott D, Kufera JA, Myers RAM: The microbiology of necrotizing soft tissue infections, *Am J Surg* 179:361, 2000.

Lille ST, Sato TT, Engrav LH, and others: Necrotizing soft tissue infections: Obstacles in diagnosis, *J Am Coll Surg* 182:7, 1996.

Malangoni MA: Necrotizing soft tissue infections: Are we making any progress? *Surg Infections* 2:145, 2001.

Taviloglu K, Cabioglu N, Cagatay A, and others: Idiopathic necrotizing fasciitis: Risk factors and strategies for management, *Am Surg* 7:315, 2005.

Tillou A, St. Hill C, Brown C, and others: Necrotizing soft tissue infections: Improved outcomes with modern care, *Am Surg* 70:841, 2004.

Wall DB, de Virgilio C, Black S, and others: Objective criteria may assist in distinguishing necrotizing fasciitis from nonnecrotizing soft tissue infection, *Am J Surg* 179:17, 2000.

Young M, Engleberg N, Mulla Z, and others: Therapies for necrotizing fasciitis, *Expert Opin Biol Ther* 6:155, 2006.

PREOPERATIVE AND POSTOPERATIVE CARE

FLUID AND ELECTROLYTE THERAPY

Jared M. Huston, MD, Soumitra R. Eachempati, MD, and Philip S. Barie, MD, MBA

Precise regulation of fluid and electrolyte balance is essential to maintain homeostasis. Surgery and surgical diseases can alter this dynamic equilibrium substantially. Therefore prompt identification and management of fluid and electrolyte disorders are integral parts of surgical practice. In this chapter we discuss the normal anatomic distribution and physiologic characteristics of fluids and electrolytes, strategies for managing fluid administration, and diagnosis and treatment for electrolyte disorders.

ANATOMY AND PHYSIOLOGY OF BODY FLUIDS

Total body water (TBW) comprises 50% to 70% of total body mass in kilograms. Individual variations in body water exist because muscle mass contains more water than adipose tissue. Lean, young males have higher percentages of TBW, whereas females and obese individuals have lower percentages of TBW. Total body water is distributed between intracellular (two thirds by volume) and extracellular (one third) compartments (Figure 1). The extracellular compartment can be divided further into intravascular (one fourth) and interstitial (three fourths) components. In theory, the different fluid compartments can be thought of as being separated by a semipermeable membrane, which restricts movement of electrolytes but allows water to diffuse freely to maintain osmotic forces. Sodium is the primary extracellular cation. Potassium and magnesium are the primary intracellular cations. Chloride is the primary extracellular anion, whereas bicarbonate, phosphate, and proteins are the predominant intracellular anions.

Movement of fluid between compartments is determined by hydrostatic and oncotic pressures, otherwise known as *Starling forces*. Net fluid movement is directed away from higher hydrostatic pressure and toward higher oncotic pressure. For example, systemic hypertension increases intravascular hydrostatic pressure and causes movement of water into the interstitial space, as can a low serum albumin concentration. In contrast, increased serum sodium or glucose concentrations will result in movement of water into the intravascular space. Normal net transvascular fluid movement is outward to the interstitial space, thus keeping tissues hydrated.

The various fluid and electrolyte compartments are not directly accessible, except for the intravascular space. However, many acute fluid disorders in surgical patients originate in the intravascular space and are treatable with direct fluid or blood product replacement. Examples include intraoperative bleeding and traumatic hemorrhage. In contrast, gastrointestinal losses caused by diarrhea, vomiting, nasogastric suctioning, enterocutaneous fistula, or ostomy drainage are also common sources of surgical fluid imbalance but do not originate directly from the vascular space. These fluid disorders can be corrected with intravenous (IV) therapy, albeit indirectly and more slowly.

The microcirculation is subject to damage via circulating inflammatory mediators and activated immune cells (e.g., neutrophils and monocytes/macrophages) released in response to infection, ischemia, or tissue injury. This systemic inflammatory response syndrome (SIRS) results in endothelial cell dysfunction, "leaky" microvessels, and loss of fluid into the "third space," an extravascular tissue compartment that does not participate in normal fluid equilibrium. Replacement of ongoing third space fluid deficits with aggressive IV therapy is necessary to preserve vital visceral organ perfusion or reverse tissue ischemia but can also result in a "reperfusion syndrome" caused by oxidant injury that is occasioned by reoxygenation of hypoxic/ischemic tissue. The result may be worsened tissue insult and microcirculatory derangements from additive injury. When the microcirculation is disrupted, massive tissue edema, pulmonary edema, and the abdominal compartment syndrome are potential sequelae of large-volume fluid administration. The key is to give enough fluid, but not too much, although so-called endpoints of resuscitation are difficult to define.

MAINTENANCE FLUIDS

All surgical patients have normal daily losses of water and electrolytes that require replacement. Daily water losses are divided into sensible (urine and stool) and insensible (lungs and skin) losses. Urine water loss ranges from 800 to 1500 mL/day and is the body's primary mechanism for maintaining water balance. Up to 250 mL of water is lost in the stool each day. Insensible losses vary between 0.5 and 1.0 L/day. Cutaneous insensible losses increase by 10% per day for every 1°C increase in body temperature above 37.2°C. Insensible losses are also increased with hyperventilation and hypermetabolism. Evaporative water loss may approach 1 L/hr from the open laparotomy or thoracotomy incision. Maintenance fluid volumes are calculated per 24-hour time period (100-50-20 rule) or hourly (4-2-1 rule), on the basis of patient body mass in kilograms (Table 1).

The electrolyte composition of maintenance fluids is based on daily losses. Daily sodium requirements average 1 to 2 mEq/kg, and potassium requirements are 0.5 to 1 mEq/kg/day. Electrolyte losses vary widely depending on a patient's condition, and daily

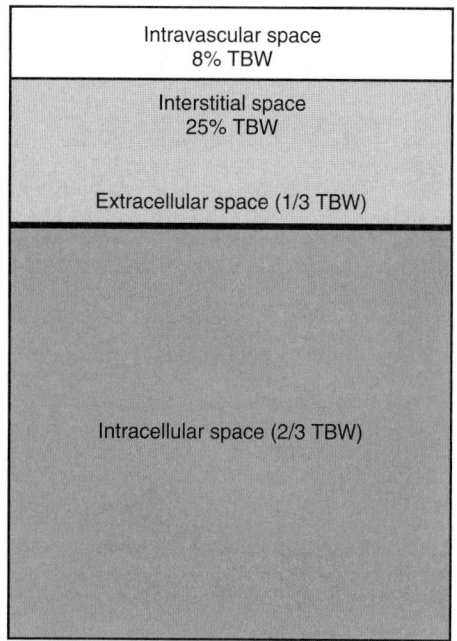

Figure 1 Body fluid distribution.

Table 1: Maintenance Fluid Requirements

Body Mass (kg)	Fluid Volume (mL/kg/hr)	Fluid Volume (mL/kg/day)
First 10 kg	4	100
Second 10 kg	2	50
Each kg > 20 kg	1	20
60 kg	100	2300

monitoring of electrolyte concentrations is recommended for critically ill patients. In addition to salt replacement, dextrose is added commonly to maintenance fluids for isotonicity and prevention of short-term proteolysis. For most adults, an IV solution composed of dextrose 5% (D_5) in half-normal saline (0.45% NaCl) with 20 mEq of KCl/L is an appropriate maintenance fluid. In children, D_5 0.2% NaCl with 20 mEq KCl/L is substituted because the kidneys may have difficulty excreting high sodium loads.

RESUSCITATION FLUIDS

In addition to maintenance requirements, surgical patients often have existing deficits or ongoing abnormal losses, including blood, gastrointestinal, or third space losses. The composition of gastrointestinal fluid losses depends on the source (Table 2). These

physiologic disorders present acutely as depletion of the extracellular fluid (ECF) space. Common signs and symptoms include mental status changes, excessive thirst, dry mucous membranes, poor skin turgor, tachycardia, hypotension, orthostatic changes in heart rate and blood pressure, oliguria, and recent weight loss. Infants may have a depressed fontanelle.

Diagnosis of ECF depletion is aided by laboratory monitoring of serum and urine osmolarity and electrolytes. Normal serum osmolarity ranges from 274 to 296 mOsm/L, and urine osmolarity can range from 50 to 1200 mOsm/L. Large increases in either serum or urine osmolarity are consistent with ECF depletion. Elevations in the hematocrit and plasma albumin concentration, a blood urea nitrogen (BUN)-to-plasma creatinine (Cr) concentration ratio greater than 20:1 (prerenal azotemia), and a low serum bicarbonate concentration are also consistent with ECF losses. The urine sodium concentration can reflect and provide clues to the underlying etiology of volume loss. A urine sodium concentration less than 20 mEq/L is consistent with gastrointestinal, third space, or evaporative losses, whereas a concentration greater than 40 mEq/L is observed with intrinsic renal disease, diuretic therapy, osmotic diuresis, or hypoaldosteronism. An alternative to measuring the urine sodium concentration is to calculate the fractional excretion of sodium (FE_{Na}) using the formula in Equation 1:

$$FE_{Na} = ([\text{Urine Na}] \times [\text{Plasma Cr}] / [\text{Plasma Na}] \times [\text{Urine Cr}]) \times 100 \qquad \text{(Eq. 1)}$$

The FE_{Na} is most useful in the differential diagnosis of acute renal failure with a low glomerular filtration rate resulting from substantial ECF losses. In these cases, a value under 1% is specific for hypovolemia.

A thorough knowledge of the composition of IV fluids is necessary to resuscitate surgical patients (Table 3). Lactated Ringer's solution (LR) and 0.9% NaCl are isotonic crystalloid resuscitation fluids with desirable attributes because of electrolyte concentrations that approximate those of the extracellular fluid (ECF). Whereas LR most closely approximates the ECF, the use of 0.9% NaCl may be preferable when there is an associated metabolic alkalosis. Conversely, large-volume resuscitation with 0.9% NaCl may precipitate or perpetuate metabolic acidosis because of the high chloride load. Colloid solutions such as albumin or synthetic colloids such as hydroxyethyl starch can also replace ECF losses and are theoretically advantageous because less fluid is required to correct the volume deficit. Colloids are also substantially more expensive than crystalloid solutions and have not been shown to improve patient outcome.

The rate of fluid administration is dictated by several factors, including the severity of the existing deficit, rate of ongoing losses, and physiologic reserve of the patient. Severe ECF losses associated with hemodynamic instability should be treated initially with IV boluses (10 to 20 mL/kg) of LR or 0.9% NaCl and repeated as needed until an adequate clinical response is observed. Assessment of urine output is an excellent measure of adequate volume resuscitation. A urine output of 0.5 mL/kg/hr for adults and 1 to 2 mL/kg/hr for infants and children is usually indicative of adequate volume replacement and tissue perfusion but can be unreliable with diuretic therapy, glycosuria, proteinuria, or after administration of

Table 2: Electrolyte Composition (mEq) of Gastrointestinal Fluids

Source	Daily Loss (mL)	Na$^+$	K$^+$	Cl$^-$	HCO$_3^-$
Saliva	1000	30-80	20	70	30
Gastric	1000–2000	60-80	15	100	0
Pancreas	1000	140	5-10	60-90	40-100
Bile	1000	140	5-10	100	40
Small bowel	2000–5000	140	20	100	25-50
Large bowel	200–1500	75	30	30	0

Table 3: Electrolyte Composition (mEq) of Parenteral Fluids

Fluid	Na$^+$	K$^+$	Cl$^-$	Ca^{2+}	HCO$_3^-$	Dextrose	pH
Extracellular fluid	142	4	103	5	27	0	7.4
Lactated Ringer's (LR)	130	4	109	2.7	28	0	6.5
Normal saline (0.9% NaCl)	154	0	154	0	0	0	4.5
½ Normal saline (0.45% NaCl)	77	0	77	0	0	0	4.5
¼ Normal saline (0.2% NaCl)	34	0	34	0	0	0	4.5
3% Saline	513	0	513	0	0	0	4.5
5% Dextrose in water	0	0	0	0	0	50 g	4.5
5% Albumin	145	0	0	0	0	0	7.4

radiocontrast media. Improved mental status, resolution of tachycardia, and normotension are also associated with a favorable response to fluid replacement.

Unfortunately, the standard clinical indices of adequate volume restoration and tissue perfusion are not useful for all patient populations. Individuals with preexisting cardiac, renal, or neurologic disease, or those receiving antihypertensive therapy, such as beta-blockers, may not manifest hypovolemia with classic signs of tachycardia, oliguria, or mental status changes. These patients require alternative means of determining their response to fluid replacement, such as invasive monitoring of central venous pressure (CVP), pulmonary artery occlusion pressure (PAOP), and mixed venous oxygen saturation (S$\sqrt{mv}$ $\sqrt{O_2}$). Although still somewhat controversial, consensus is emerging that restoration of acid-base status is the most reliable indicator of the adequacy of resuscitation.

DIAGNOSIS AND TREATMENT OF ELECTROLYTE DISORDERS

Sodium

Hyponatremia is defined as a serum sodium concentration less than 136 mEq/L. Severe hyponatremia, which can lead to seizures and permanent neurologic dysfunction, may occur at concentrations less than 120 mEq/L, especially if the change is acute. Hyponatremia is classified as *hypertonic, isotonic,* or *hypotonic.* Hypertonic hyponatremia is a result of increased circulating solutes, such as glucose or BUN, which exert oncotic pressure and cause water to shift from the intracellular to the extracellular space. Each 100-mg/dL increase in serum glucose concentration or 30-mg/dL increase in BUN produces a 1.5- to 2.0-mEq/L decrease in serum sodium concentration. Isotonic hyponatremia, also known as *pseudohyponatremia,* occurred in patients with hypertriglyceridemia or hyperproteinemia when sodium was measured with a flame photometry technique. Modern laboratory determinations of serum sodium have essentially eliminated this artifact.

Hypotonic hyponatremia is most common and is observed in patients who are hypovolemic, hypervolemic, or euvolemic. Hypovolemic hyponatremia often results from isotonic gastrointestinal (e.g., vomiting, diarrhea, fistulae), renal, or blood losses that are partially replaced with hypotonic IV fluids, leading to hypovolemia and hyponatremia. The urine sodium concentration can be used to distinguish between renal and extrarenal sources of sodium loss. A urine sodium concentration less than 20 mEq/L is consistent with extrarenal losses, whereas a concentration greater than 20 mEq/L may indicate inappropriate renal excretion. Euvolemic hyponatremia occurs in patients with the syndrome of inappropriate antidiuretic hormone (vasopressin) secretion (SIADH), hypothyroidism, or excessive water intake (psychogenic polydipsia). Increased vasopressin secretion occurs transiently in the early postoperative, trauma, and burn period, following injury of the central

nervous system, and as a paraneoplastic syndrome (especially with carcinoma of the lung). Excess vasopressin impairs renal function by inappropriately elevating urine osmolality and sodium concentration. Hypervolemic hyponatremia occurs in patients with congestive heart failure, chronic renal insufficiency, nephrotic syndrome, cirrhosis, or hypoalbuminemia. These disorders are characterized by a reduced effective circulating blood volume, which leads to retention of water via increased vasopressin secretion. Administration of hypotonic replacement fluids to patients with increased vasopressin secretion can exacerbate hyponatremia further.

Treatment of hyponatremia begins with an estimate of the body sodium deficit, which may be calculated using the formula in Equation 2:

$$\text{Sodium deficit (mEq)} = (140 - \text{serum Na}) \times 0.6 \\ \times \text{weight (kg)} \qquad \text{(Eq. 2)}$$

The aggressiveness of sodium correction depends on the patient's signs and symptoms (Table 4), and specifically the volume status. Hypovolemic patients require rapid volume replacement with isotonic 0.9% NaCl. Hypervolemic or euvolemic patients are usually treated with fluid restriction. Symptomatic patients, however, may require hypertonic saline (3% NaCl) administration, with or without loop diuretics, to increase serum sodium concentration by up to 2.0 mEq/L/hr in the short term to above the neurotoxic threshold (approximately 120 mEq/L). In general, the rate of sodium correction should not exceed 8 to 10 mEq/L in a 24-hour period to prevent development of permanent neurologic dysfunction (central pontine myelinolysis). It is reasonable to correct half the estimated sodium deficit within the first 24 hours and the remaining deficit over the next 24 to 48 hours. Frequent laboratory monitoring is necessary during rapid corrections of sodium deficits.

Hypernatremia is defined as a serum sodium concentration greater than 145 mEq/L. Hypernatremia occurs primarily in patients who lack free access to water combined with uncontrolled fluid losses, as with protracted vomiting, diarrhea, or forced diuresis. Infants, elderly patients, mentally impaired patients, and intubated patients are most likely to be affected. Clinical symptoms (see Table 4) are usually the result of neurologic dysfunction, but rarely occur at a sodium concentration less than 160 mEq/L.

Treatment of hypernatremia begins with an estimate of the free water deficit, which may be calculated using the formula in Equation 3:

$$\text{Free H}_2\text{O deficit (L)} = [(\text{serum Na} - 140) \div 140] \\ \times 0.6 \times \text{weight (kg)} \qquad \text{(Eq. 3)}$$

One half of the free water deficit should be given in the first 24 hours, and the remaining deficit over the next 24 to 48 hours. Serum sodium concentration should not be reduced by more than approximately 0.5 mEq/L/hr to prevent cerebral edema. Laboratory monitoring of sodium concentration is required during periods of rapid correction. Hypotonic fluids (0.45% NaCl) or free water can be used to correct the deficit and may be administered IV or enterally.

Table 4: Signs and Symptoms of Electrolyte Disorders

Disorder	Neurologic	Cardiovascular	Gastrointestinal	Renal	Other
Hyponatremia	Confusion, seizures, coma	Hypotension Hypertension	Salivation	Oliguria	
Hypernatremia	Confusion, seizures, coma	Fluid overload Edema	Thirst		Tachypnea
Hypokalemia	Fatigue, weakness	Atrial arrhythmias, flat T wave, U waves	Ileus	Nephrotoxicity	
Hyperkalemia	Confusion, paralysis, areflexia	Ventricular arrhythmias, peaked T wave, prolonged PR interval, wide QRS complex	Nausea, vomiting, abdominal pain		
Hypocalcemia	Paresthesia, perioral tingling, carpopedal spasm, Chvostek's sign	Ventricular arrhythmias, prolonged QT interval			Laryngospasm
Hypercalcemia	Confusion, fatigue, coma	Shortened QT interval	Abdominal pain	Renal stones Nephrogenic diabetes insipidus (long-term)	
Hypomagnesemia	Weakness, cramping, hyperreflexia	Atrial, ventricular arrhythmias (torsades de pointes)	Dysphagia		Refractory hypokalemia, hypocalcemia
Hypermagnesemia	Sedation, paralysis, areflexia	Atrial, ventricular arrhythmias	Diarrhea		
Hypophosphatemia	Confusion, seizures, weakness	Heart failure Respiratory failure			Bone pain
Hyperphosphatemia	Symptoms of hypocalcemia				

Potassium

Hypokalemia is defined as a serum potassium concentration less than 3.5 mEq/L. It most often occurs as a result of increased gastrointestinal or renal losses, rather than reduced intake. Serum potassium concentration also falls secondary to alkalosis, elevated catecholamine concentrations, and insulin administration. Because potassium is primarily intracellular (98%), small changes in serum concentration reflect large differences in total body stores. There is no reliable formula to estimate body potassium stores from the measured serum concentration.

Hypokalemia is treated with potassium administration. As with other electrolyte disorders, the route of replacement is guided by the patient's clinical condition (see Table 4). Oral replacement is safer and better tolerated than IV administration, and it is absorbed readily regardless of the specific preparation. Typical doses for treatment of mild hypokalemia (3.0 to 3.5 mEq/L) are 40 to 100 mEq daily in divided doses. For more severe forms (2.5 to 3.0 mEq/L), or if more modest hypokalemia is expected to persist or worsen if not treated aggressively (e.g., large-volume forced diuresis), 20 to 40 mEq/L can be given IV every 3 to 4 hours. IV administration of potassium is useful when oral therapy is not tolerated or in cases of severe hypokalemia (< 2.5 mEq/L). Cardiac monitoring and central venous access are essential during IV administration of greater than 10 to 20 mEq/hr. Serum potassium concentration should be monitored every 2 to 4 hours during aggressive IV potassium therapy.

Hyperkalemia is defined as a serum potassium concentration greater than 5.5 mEq/L. Chronic elevations in potassium, as observed in renal dialysis patients, are well tolerated, but rapid fluctuations can lead to fatal cardiac arrhythmias. Common causes of hyperkalemia include renal failure, acidosis, rhabdomyolysis, ischemia-reperfusion injury, cell lysis, and insulin deficiency. *Pseudohyperkalemia* occurs with hemolysis of red blood cells in the collection tube, resulting in a falsely elevated serum concentration that should not be treated. Pseudohyperkalemia can be detected easily by determination of the plasma potassium concentration. Thrombocytosis and leukocytosis can also yield falsely elevated potassium concentrations.

Hyperkalemia is the most dangerous electrolyte disorder because of the immediate danger to the cardiac conduction system. An electrocardiogram should be obtained immediately to search for changes consistent with hyperkalemia (e.g., peaked T waves, prolonged PR interval, widened QRS complex, and ventricular ectopy). Potassium-containing fluids and supplements should be removed simultaneously. Signs of cardiac instability (see Table 4) require emergent treatment with a 10% calcium gluconate bolus IV injection, which stabilizes the cardiac membrane by raising the activation threshold. The next step is to induce a transcellular shift of potassium into cells by administering 10 units of regular insulin IV along with 50 mL of 50% dextrose (D_{50}) to prevent hypoglycemia. This therapy will decrease serum potassium concentration by 1 mEq/L for approximately 60 minutes. Administration of 1 ampule (50 mEq) of 8.4% $NaHCO_3$ will also enhance the intracellular movement of potassium.

Whereas the above measures lower the serum potassium concentration temporarily, definitive therapy to remove excess potassium from the body should be instituted. Gastrointestinal excretion is augmented by administration of the sodium-potassium exchange resin sodium polystyrene sulfonate, either orally or via retention enema with sorbitol. One gram of this ion exchange resin will bind and permanently remove 1 mEq of potassium when excreted. Renal excretion of potassium is enhanced with loop diuretics, such as furosemide or bumetanide. Hemodialysis is effective in cases of renal failure.

Calcium

Hypocalcemia is defined as a total serum calcium concentration less than 8.4 mg/dL or an ionized calcium concentration less than 4.5 mg/dL. Circulating calcium exists either as the biologically active free ionized form (≈50%) or the biologically inactive protein bound form (≈50%). The serum albumin concentration can affect measurable total calcium because one half of circulating calcium is bound to protein (mostly albumin). The ionized calcium concentration is unaffected by the serum albumin concentration. The corrected total calcium level is calculated with the formula in Equation 4:

$$\text{Calcium (corrected)} = \text{Calcium (measured)} + (4.0 - \text{serum albumin}) \times 0.8 \quad \text{(Eq. 4)}$$

Serum calcium concentrations are regulated by parathyroid hormone (PTH) and vitamin D, and diseases that disrupt their normal function can lead to hypocalcemia. Examples include end-stage renal disease and hypoparathyroidism, particularly of iatrogenic cause after parathyroid or thyroid surgery. A serum calcium concentration should be checked after thyroid surgery to ensure intact parathyroid function. After parathyroidectomy, most surgeons place patients on prophylactic oral calcium carbonate supplementation the night of surgery. Other common causes of hypocalcemia include hyperphosphatemia, hypomagnesemia, acute pancreatitis, malnutrition, rhabdomyolysis, infusion of large volumes of fluid, and acute alkalosis secondary to hyperventilation. Patients with large transfusion requirements previously developed hypocalcemia from chelation of calcium by the citrate anticoagulant used in the storage of blood products, but this is no longer an issue with modern blood banking techniques.

Treatment of hypocalcemia involves calcium replacement and therapy of the underlying etiology. Calcium replacement is recommended for symptomatic patients (see Table 4) and patients with a corrected total serum calcium concentration less than 7.0 mg/dL, or an ionized calcium concentration less than 3.0 mg/dL. Symptomatic patients should receive IV calcium gluconate (9 mg elemental calcium/mL). Treatment with IV calcium boluses requires cardiac monitoring because of associated bradycardia and hypotension. Following IV calcium administration or in asymptomatic patients, oral calcium therapy (~4 g/day) is sufficient. Refractory symptoms may be treated with 1,25-dihydroxy vitamin D₃. Patients with concurrent hypomagnesemia or hyperphosphatemia should also receive appropriate therapy. When coexistent, hypocalcemia may be difficult to correct if hypomagnesemia persists.

Hypercalcemia is defined as a serum calcium concentration greater than 10.4 mg/dL or an ionized calcium concentration greater than 5.6 mg/dL. Malignant diseases cause the majority of cases of hypercalcemia in hospitalized patients, mostly from metastasis to bone. Hyperparathyroidism is the major cause of hypercalcemia in the general population. Other common causes include vitamin A and D overdose, thyrotoxicosis, immobilization, excess exogenous calcium intake, granulomatous diseases, familial hypocalciuric hypercalcemia, and medications such as thiazide diuretics and lithium chloride. The clinical presentation is usually related to the patient's underlying disorder, although symptoms related directly to hypercalcemia can occur with serum concentrations greater than 14.0 mg/dL or after a rapid increase.

Patients with symptoms of hypercalcemia (see Table 4) require rapid treatment with IV 0.9% NaCl to expand the intravascular volume, dilute the circulating calcium concentration, and increase filtration of calcium in the kidneys. Furosemide is then administered IV to increase renal calcium excretion. Patients with hypercalcemic crisis require inhibition of osteoclast-induced bone resorption with bisphosphonates, such as pamidronate (60-90 mg IV), for which the onset of action is between 24 and 48 hours. Calcitonin (4 IU/kg every 12 hours, subcutaneously) also inhibits bone resorption and decreases renal tubular reabsorption of calcium but works much more quickly than the bisphosphonates. Corticosteroids inhibit the action of vitamin D and are useful in treating patients with granulomatous diseases, vitamin D toxicity, multiple myeloma, lymphoma, solid tumor metastases, and other hematologic malignancies.

Magnesium

Hypomagnesemia is defined as a serum concentration less than 1.6 mg/dL. It occurs as a result of poor nutritional intake, particularly among alcohol abusers, or increased gastrointestinal or renal losses. The most common cause of hypomagnesemia is dilutional. Serum magnesium concentrations may not reflect total body stores because magnesium is found predominantly in the intracellular space. Hypocalcemia and hypokalemia often coexist with hypomagnesemia. Symptoms (see Table 4) rarely occur unless the serum concentration decreases below 1.0 mg/dL.

Treatment of hypomagnesemia involves replacement of losses, correcting the underlying cause, and treating associated electrolyte abnormalities. IV magnesium therapy is reserved for patients with serum concentrations less than 1.2 mg/dL. Magnesium sulfate (1 g = 8 mEq) may be given intermittently or as a continuous infusion. Hypotension can occur with infusions higher than 2 g/hr. Life-threatening arrhythmias associated with severe hypomagnesemia (e.g., torsades de pointes) are treated with bolus doses of magnesium sulfate (1 to 2 g over 3 to 5 minutes).

Hypermagnesemia is a rare disorder. It is defined as a serum concentration greater than 2.8 mg/dL. Patients with renal insufficiency or those receiving magnesium-containing antacids or laxatives are most commonly affected. Symptoms (see Table 4) are uncommon with a serum concentration less than 4.0 mg/dL. Initial treatment of hypermagnesemia is similar to that of hyperkalemia. IV calcium gluconate is used to stabilize the cardiac membrane. Renal excretion is enhanced with hydration with IV saline followed by administration of loop diuretics. Hemodialysis is reserved for severe, refractory hypermagnesemia.

Phosphorus

Hypophosphatemia is defined as a serum concentration less than 2.5 mg/dL. It results from decreased intestinal uptake resulting from vitamin D deficiency, malabsorption or use of phosphorus binders (e.g., aluminum, magnesium, iron salts), or increased renal excretion associated with diuretic therapy, alkalosis, or hyperparathyroidism. Hypophosphatemia is also caused by major hepatic resection or rhabdomyolysis. Signs and symptoms of hypophosphatemia (see Table 4) include respiratory and cardiac failure. Replacement is necessary when the serum concentration decreases below 2.0 mg/dL and can be administered as sodium or potassium phosphate (0.08 to 0.24 mmol/kg every 4 to 6 hours).

Hyperphosphatemia is defined as a serum concentration greater than 5.0 mg/dL. It occurs primarily in patients with renal insufficiency. Hyperphosphatemia is associated with hypocalcemia because of increased calcium precipitation (which may cause heterotopic ossification), decreased vitamin D production, and interference with parathyroid hormone-mediated bone resorption.

Symptoms of acute hyperphosphatemia (see Table 4) are due to the effects of hypocalcemia. Treatment involves enhancing renal excretion with IV 0.9% NaCl hydration followed by diuresis with acetazolamide (500 mg IV every 12 hours). Phosphate absorption is reduced with phosphate binders such as aluminum hydroxide. Iron and bile acid sequestrants are also available and are not associated with aluminum toxicity. Hemodialysis is reserved for severe refractory hyperphosphatemia.

SUGGESTED READINGS

Adrogue HJ, Madias NE: Hypernatremia, *N Engl J Med* 342:1493, 2000.
Adrogue HJ, Madias NE: Hyponatremia, *N Engl J Med* 342:1581, 2000.

Eachempati SR, Reed RL II, Barie PS: Serum bicarbonate concentration correlates with arterial base deficit in critically ill patients, *Surg Infect* 4:193, 2003.
Finfer S, Bellomo R, Boyce N, and others: A comparison of albumin and saline for fluid resuscitation in the intensive care unit, *N Engl J Med* 350:2247, 2004.
Holte K, Kehlet H: Fluid therapy and surgical outcomes in elective surgery: a need for reassessment in fast-track surgery, *J Am Coll Surg* 202:971, 2006.
Pestana C: *Fluids and electrolytes in the surgical patient*, ed 5, Baltimore, 2000, Lippincott Williams & Wilkins.
Rose BD: *Clinical physiology of acid-base and electrolyte disorders*, ed 5, New York, 2000, McGraw-Hill.
Tisherman SA, Barie PS, Bokhari F, and others: Clinical practice guideline: Endpoints of resuscitation, *J Trauma* 57:898, 2004.

NUTRITIONAL SUPPORT IN THE CRITICALLY ILL

Kevin P. Keating, MD, and William Marshall, DO

METABOLIC RESPONSE

Preexisting malnutrition has been estimated to be present in 30% to 50% of inpatient surgical admissions. Up to 80% of patients admitted to an intensive care unit will experience a deterioration of nutritional status during their hospital stay.

Hypometabolism characterizes nonstressed starvation. Lipolysis generates free fatty acids, which are converted by the liver to ketones, the primary substrate for metabolism in this state. A small amount of proteolysis to provide amino acids for gluconeogenesis provides the approximately 300 kcal/day required by the obligatory glucose-using tissue (central nervous system [CNS] before it adapts to ketones, kidney, formed blood elements). With adequate provision of water, the nonstressed starved state is sustainable for up to 90 days.

The stressed starved state seen in surgical patients differs significantly from the nonstressed state. After a brief, hypometabolic ebb phase, a prolonged hypermetabolic flow phase is entered. Initiated by the activated neurohumoral axis and amplified by cytokine release, the metabolic hallmarks of this phase are catabolism, proteolysis, and gluconeogenesis. The amplitude and duration of this hypermetabolic response is proportional to the degree of surgical stress or trauma. In the uncomplicated surgical patient, this flow phase lasts for approximately 7 days.

Because this hypermetabolic/hypercatabolic response is hormone and cytokine mediated, efforts at providing substrate to ameliorate the proteolysis are minimally effective unless provided in a way that can modulate the response.

ENERGY REQUIREMENTS

Energy requirements are expressed as nonprotein calories. Indirect calorimetry is the gold standard for determining energy requirements. This measure of oxygen consumption and carbon dioxide production provides values for measured energy expenditure (MEE), as well as a respiratory quotient (RQ). RQ (CO_2 production/O_2 consumption) provides valuable information on substrate use. The combustion of glucose as a fuel has an RQ of 0.9 to 1.0. Mixed substrate combustion has an RQ of 0.8 to 0.9. The use of fat as a primary fuel source has an RQ of 0.7 to 0.8. Overfeeding results in lipogenesis, which has an RQ of 8.0 and should be suspected whenever the measured RQ is greater than 1.1. The increased CO_2 production associated with overfeeding requires an increase in minute ventilation or the development of respiratory acidosis ensues, either of which has significant negative implications for critically ill patients. Patients may not be overfed on the basis of MEE but still have an elevated RQ with attendant respiratory acidosis or increased minute ventilatory requirements. This set of circumstances should make the clinician consider the possibility that the patient's maximal glucose use rate ($\approx$5 mg/kg/min) has been exceeded and an alteration in substrate composition to include or to increase lipid may be in order. Other patients, whose needs are being met as determined by MEE and with a normal RQ, may still have a respiratory acidosis or increased minute ventilation when their pulmonary pathophysiology inhibits their ability to handle a normal CO_2 load. This is another situation in which increasing the ration of fat to glucose calories may prove beneficial.

In the absence of indirect calorimetry, estimating energy expenditure (EEE) from the basal energy expenditure (BEE) using the Harris-Benedict equation is often accomplished as follows:

$$\text{(Male) BEE} = 66.5 + (13.8 \times \text{weight in kg}) + (5 \times \text{height in cm}) - (6.8 \times \text{age})$$

$$\text{(Female) BEE} = 655 + (9.6 \times \text{weight in kg}) + (1.7 \times \text{height in cm}) - (4.7 \times \text{age})$$

The BEE is then multiplied by activity factors (e.g., 1–1.1 for bed rest) and stress factors (e.g., 1.25 uncomplicated surgery, 1.5 major trauma, 2.0 major burn). A simple formula (25–35 kcal/kg) can be used if MEE or BEE is unavailable.

It should be remembered that the dextrose monohydrate in total parenteral nutrition provides 3.4 kcal/g. Ten percent intralipid emulsion provides 1.2 kcal/ml. Twenty percent intralipid emulsion provides 2.1 kcal/ml. Lipid calories should not exceed 60% of daily calories or 2.5 g/kg/day.

PROTEIN REQUIREMENTS

Nitrogen balance determinations are used frequently to determine protein requirements. Nitrogen balance = 24-hr nitrogen intake − 24-hr nitrogen output where:

$$24 - \text{hr nitrogen input(g)} = 24 - \text{hr protein intake(g)}/6.25.$$

$$24 - \text{hr nitrogen output(g)} = 24 - \text{hr urine urea nitrogen(g)} + 4 \text{ (nonurea nitrogen + nonurine nitrogen losses)}.$$

Protein administration is considered adequate when the nitrogen balance is greater than plus 3 g. In the absence of nitrogen balance studies, the provision of 1 to 2 g of protein per kilogram per day should prove adequate. Nonprotein-calorie-to-nitrogen ratios of 125–150:1 are recommended to achieve optimal nitrogen utilization. Recent studies advocate nonprotein-calories-to-nitrogen ratios as low as 80:1 for highly stressed patients.

MONITORING NUTRITIONAL SUPPORT

Potassium, sodium, and chloride should be determined daily until serum levels have stabilized. Calcium, magnesium, and phosphate (along with potassium) are primarily intracellular electrolytes. During anabolism, as the intracellular compartment expands, serum levels of the intracellular electrolytes may fall (refeeding syndrome) and clinically manifest as respiratory muscle weakness secondary to hypophosphatemia. Persistent hypercalcemia may be secondary to hypomagnesemia. Calcium, magnesium, and phosphate should be checked two to three times weekly in the critically ill.

A growing body of evidence suggests that strict glycemic control in the intensive care unit is associated with a decrease in adverse outcomes (e.g., nosocomial infections and mortality). Frequent monitoring of blood glucose with a low threshold for instituting insulin infusions to maintain blood glucose in near normal ranges (80-100 mg%) is gaining increasing acceptance. Serum triglyceride levels should be obtained for a baseline and monitored weekly in patients receiving daily lipid emulsion infusions. High triglyceride levels can have an immunosuppressive effect.

Visceral protein markers are used to assess the adequacy of nutritional support. Albumin, although common as a preoperative indicator of nutritional status, has little utility as a marker for nutritional repletion because of its long serum half-life (18-21 days) and variance with fluid shifts. Prealbumin, with a half-life of 3 to 5 days, is an earlier indicator of nutritional repletion, albeit limited in patients with renal failure in whom its serum value is elevated. Transferrin has a half-life of 7 to 10 days, with its utility limited by iron deficiency that elevates its serum levels.

ESSENTIAL NUTRIENTS

Vitamins and minerals are necessary for proper substrate metabolism and as cofactors for a variety of enzymatic reactions. There is no consensus on the requirements for these nutrients during acute stress. In general, water-soluble vitamins (B vitamins, vitamin C) are more apt to be depleted than fat-soluble vitamins (vitamins A, D, E, K). Because of accelerated use, malabsorption, and varying degrees of renal wasting, trace minerals (zinc, copper, chromium, manganese, and selenium) are routinely supplemented during acute stress. Zinc deficiency manifests as dermatitis, diarrhea, and alopecia. Copper deficiency manifests as anemia, leukopenia, and neutropenia. Insulin-resistant hyperglycemia is a hallmark of chromium deficiency. A reversible cardiomyopathy is associated with selenium deficiency.

Linoleic acid, an omega-6 polyunsaturated fatty acid (PUFA) that is a major constituent of cell membranes and serves as a substrate for prostanoid and leukotriene synthesis, cannot be synthesized by humans and is an essential fatty acid. Its deficiency, an early sign of which is dermatitis, can be prevented by its provision as either enteral fat or parenteral lipid emulsion in the amount of approximately 5% of total calories (in parenteral nutrition [PN]: 250 ml of 20% lipid emulsion, 2-3 times per week). The omega-3 PUFA, alpha linoleic acid, also cannot be synthesized in vivo. Its role in immune enhancement as a substrate for the synthesis of immunostimulatory prostanoids and leukotrienes is gaining increasing acceptance. There are currently no available parenteral forms of alpha linoleic acid. Enteral immune-enhancing formulas containing omega-3 PUFA are available.

Glutamine, although the most abundant amino acid in the body, is considered to be a conditionally essential amino acid.

Because of its instability in solution, it is not a component of standard PN solutions. It is a component of the protein in enteral formulas and is added in "free form" to specialized formulas. It is used by enterocytes as a primary fuel source and has a trophic effect on the gut mucosal barrier. Its proven utility is in bone marrow transplant and short-gut syndrome patients. Arginine is another amino acid considered by some to be conditionally essential. It functions as a secretagogue for growth hormone and enhances wound healing. It exhibits immune-enhancing effects by increasing T-cell responsiveness. Its clinical utility has been established in burn patients.

At this time, abundant evidence for the routine use of specialized, immune-enhancing formulas is lacking.

ROUTE OF SUPPORT—ENTERAL

Provision of substrate by the enteral route appears capable of modulating the stress response and therefore is the preferred route of early nutritional support. The mechanism by which this effect occurs is still unclear. It is thought to involve maintenance of gut mucosal barrier function with decreased activation of gut-associated lymphoid tissue, a rich source of proteolytic cytokines. When compared with PN, enteral nutrition is associated with lower costs of administration and a decreased incidence of postoperative septic complications. Absolute contraindications to enteral nutrition include complete intestinal obstruction. Relative contraindications include high-output intestinal fistulae, severe acute pancreatitis, severe acute inflammatory bowel disease, severe diarrhea, ileus, and massive gastrointestinal hemorrhage. Enteral feeding in patients with hemodynamic instability should be delayed until stable mesenteric perfusion has been restored.

Enteral nutrition by tube can be accomplished via several routes: nasogastric, nasoenteric, gastrostomy, jejunostomy, or gastrojejunal. Transnasal passage of a small-bore silicone feeding tube into the stomach or duodenum is the most common method of gaining enteral access. Contraindications to the nasogastric route include gastric aspirate greater than 600 ml/24 hr, known history of aspiration, lack of protective reflexes, and inability to be maintained in at least 30-degree reverse Trendelenburg. Prolonged gastric atony, present in at least 30% of critically ill patients, further limits nasogastric feedings. If these contraindications exist or the inability to achieve nutritional goals within 72 hours occurs, transpyloric placement of a nasogastric tube into the nasoenteric position should be attempted. Several techniques have been described to achieve this goal. We have achieved a spontaneous transpyloric tube placement rate of greater than 85% using an insufflation technique. This technique requires placement of a feeding tube into the stomach in a standard fashion. The patient is then rolled to the right lateral decubitus position and, with the stylet still in place, 500 cc of air is insufflated into the stomach. The feeding tube is then advanced until no more than 5 to 10 cm is external to the nares. The patient is then returned to the supine position, the stylet is removed, the tube is secured, and abdominal x-rays are obtained. If these techniques are unsuccessful, fluoroscopic placement of the tube into the postpyloric position should be undertaken. In patients in whom long-term enteral access is required, consideration should be given to open surgical, percutaneous endoscopic, or percutaneous radiologic gastrostomy or jejunostomy.

ROUTE OF SUPPORT—PARENTERAL

PN is indicated when nutritional needs cannot be met by the enteral route. It can be used as the sole source of calories and nitrogen or to supplement inadequate enteral intake. There is little evidence that PN is efficacious in the immediate perioperative period. PN solutions contain dextrose, amino acids, electrolytes, and trace minerals. "Three-in-one" formulas also contain lipid emulsion. Two routes can achieve parenteral nutrition: central parenteral nutrition (CPN) or peripheral parenteral nutrition (PPN).

CPN using a central venous catheter is the most frequently used form of PN. CPN formulations are usually hypertonic, with glucose concentrations greater than 10% and an osmolarity greater than 2000 mOsm/L, requiring infusion into a large-diameter central vein in which high flows cause rapid dilution.

PPN is administered via peripheral veins using fine-bore silicone or polyurethane peripheral venous catheters. PPN can be used with glucose concentrations of less than 10%, and total solution osmolarities less than 1000 mOsm. Concurrent use of intravenous lipid emulsion is necessary as a carbohydrate source and minimizes the incidence of thrombophlebitis. PPN is indicated in patients who require short-term (< 7-10 days) PN and is rarely used in critically ill patients.

CONDITIONALLY SPECIFIC SUPPORT

Renal Failure

Both parenteral and enteral renal failure formulas are designed as calorie-dense, low-protein, electrolyte-restricted solutions. The aim of these solutions is to meet nonprotein calorie needs with minimal volume, reduce ureagenesis, and prevent potential electrolyte imbalances. Formulas for both acute oliguric renal failure and chronic renal insufficiency are available. Patients receiving renal replacement therapy have higher protein requirements than nondialyzed chronic renal failure patients, with hemodialysis requiring 1 to 1.4 grams of protein per kilogram of body weight per day and continuous venovenous hemofiltration requiring 1.5 to 2.5 grams of protein per kilogram of body weight per day.

Hepatic Failure

The altered protein metabolism seen in hepatic failure results in decreased serum levels of branched chain amino acids and elevations in aromatic amino acids. This alteration in amino acid profile can lead to the synthesis of false neurotransmitters and be a mechanism of encephalopathy. Both parenteral and enteral hepatic failure formulas are designed with high branch-chain-to-aromatic-amino-acid ratios and have been shown to improve encephalopathy in up to 80% of hepatic failure patients.

Pulmonary Failure

The issue of lipid versus carbohydrate calories to decrease carbon dioxide production was addressed earlier. An enteral, low-carbohydrate, high-fat formula containing the omega-3 PUFA eicosapentaenoic acid and the omega-6 PUFA gamma linoleic acid plus antioxidants is available for patients with adult respiratory distress syndrome (ARDS). The substrates are intended to decrease the synthesis of proinflammatory prostanoids and decrease oxidant-induced microvascular permeability. Preliminary studies indicate some improvement in respiratory gas exchange and markers of inflammation. Further studies on clinical outcomes must be completed.

Cardiac Failure

The primary concerns in nutritional support of critically ill patients with congestive heart failure involve fluid restriction and sodium restriction. Calorie- and protein-dense enteral formulas are available for this purpose. In patients unable to be fed enterally, fluid-

restricted CPN solutions with high dextrose and amino acid concentrations can be used. The use of 20% parenteral lipid emulsions can also be used to limit volume in these patients.

Neurologic Injury

Head injury can result in a significant hypermetabolic/hypercatabolic response. Management of intracranial pressure frequently requires the use of sedatives, muscle relaxants, and paralytics, which can modulate this response to varying degrees. Associated injuries can further complicate this picture. Energy requirements are particularly difficult to estimate in these patients, and MEEs, if available, are quite useful. Early nutritional support can be achieved safely in these patients, but special attention must be directed to preventing hyperglycemia, which has been shown to exacerbate ischemic brain injury.

Burn Injury

Major burns are the most hypermetabolic/hypercatabolic of injuries and can double basal metabolic rate. The profound immunosuppression seen in these patients has prompted a great deal of the work on nutritional approaches to enhancing the immune response. Patients receiving enteral formulas containing arginine, omega-3 PUFA, and high doses of vitamins E and C demonstrated fewer infectious complications and increased graft survival compared with patients receiving standard formulas. Application of these formulas to the broader population of surgically critically ill patients has failed to show significant improvements in outcome, with the exception of some specific patient populations (e.g., upper gastrointestinal [UGI] malignancy). Oxandrolone is an oral anabolic steroid with minimal androgenic activity. Its Food and Drug Administration indications for use have been expanded to include its use as an adjunct to promote weight gain, lean body mass, and wound healing after extensive surgery, chronic infections, severe trauma, and burns. It should not be used in patients with malignancy.

Pancreatitis

Severe acute pancreatitis is not an absolute contraindication to enteral feeding. The goal of nutritional support is to provide adequate nutrition with limited pancreatic exocrine stimulation. This can be achieved with elemental (dextrose, crystalline amino acids, low fat) enteral formulas infused into the distal duodenum or proximal jejunum. If enteral formulas are not tolerated, parenteral formulas should be used. The use of intravenous lipid emulsions in the absence of hypertriglyceridemia is safe in these patients and may be a useful adjunct in the face of recalcitrant hyperglycemia. The use of dipeptide- and tripeptide-based enteral formulas has been associated with decreased pancreatic inflammation, especially in patients with chronic pancreatitis.

Obesity

Mean body weight has increased 10% since the mid 1980s in the United States, and clinical obesity (body mass index >30) has doubled to nearly one third of the adult population. Obesity has been determined to be an independent risk factor for increased mortality in the intensive care unit, largely because of an increased risk of infectious complications. Consensus on determining nutritional needs and optimal provision of substrate is difficult to come by, with some authors advocating hypocaloric nutritional support. Indirect calorimetry is especially useful in this patient population. The Harris-Benedict equation can be used by substituting an adjusted body weight (ABW) for the actual body weight according to the following formulas:

Ideal body weight (IBW) female = 45.5kg + 2.3 (inches > 60)

Ideal body weight (IBW) male = 50.0kg + 2.3 (inches > 60)

Adjusted body weight (ABW) = [(actual body weight −IBW)0.4] + IBW

For ventilated obese patients, a simple 21 cal/kg seems to be as accurate as some of the more complex equations. Glycemic control is both challenging and essential in these patients. Provision of substrate in a staged fashion, with early administration of protein followed by carbohydrate and then lipid, provides for anabolism and improves glycemic control.

Suggested Readings

Doig GS: Evidence-based guidelines for nutritional support of the critically ill: Results of a bi-national guideline development conference. Carlton, Australia: Australian and New Zealand Intensive Care Society (ANZICS), 2005. Available at www.guideline.gov.

Merritt R, editor-in-chief: The A.S.P.E.N. Nutrition Support Practice Manual, ed 2, Silver Spring, MD, 2005, American Society for Parenteral and Enteral Nutrition.

Quercia RA, Keating KP, Evasovich M: Nutrition in the hospitalized patient. In Shargel L, Mutnick AH, Sourney PF, and others, editors: *Comprehensive pharmacy review*, ed 6, Baltimore, 2007, Lippincott Williams & Wilkins.

Schulz MA, Santanello SA, Monk J, and others: An improved method of transpyloric placement of nasoenteric feeding tubes, *Int Surg* 78:79, 1993.

CATHETER SEPSIS IN THE INTENSIVE CARE UNIT

Carol R. Schermer, MD, MPH and Ben L. Zarzaur, MD, MPH

Intravascular catheter use places patients at risk for local infectious complications that include exit site infections and septic thrombophlebitis, and for systemic infectious complications that include catheter-related bloodstream infections (CRBSIs), endocarditis, and remote infections such as brain abscesses. Together, these local and systemic infectious complications are called *catheter-related infections* (CRI). Most hospital-acquired blood stream infections (BSIs) are associated with central venous catheter (CVC) use, and most serious catheter-related infections are associated with CVCs placed in patients in intensive care units (ICUs).

CRBSIs are responsible for much of the morbidity and mortality resulting from CRI. The mortality rates attributable to CRBSI range widely from 0% to 35%, but most studies report attributable mortality rates between 5% and 10%. The cost per CRBSI in an ICU is thought to exceed $25,000.

EPIDEMIOLOGY

The incidence of CRBSI varies by type of catheter, frequency of catheter manipulation, and underlying patient factors. Rates also vary by hospital size and by type of unit (Table 1) and are influenced by type and severity of illness, urgency of placement, and catheter type and position. National Nosocomial Infection Surveillance System (NNIS) BSI rates can be used as benchmarks by hospitals in quality assurance and performance improvement efforts. To improve comparability across studies and study sites and to use benchmark data, ICU BSI data should be expressed as number of CRBSIs per 1000 catheter days. Excluding high-risk nurseries, just over 4.1 million CVC ICU days were reported to the NNIS between 2002 and 2004. The average rate of CRBSI in the 2004 NNIS data was 4.9 per 1000 catheter days, which represents a slight decrease from 2002 (5.3 per 1000 catheter days). Nontunneled CVCs are the most commonly used central line in ICUs and account for more than 90% of CRBSIs.

Table 1: Central Venous Catheter–Associated Bloodstream Infections in Surgical Intensive Care Units

ICU Type	Mean Rate*	50th Percentile
Cardiothoracic	2.7	1.8
Medical-surgical		
Major teaching	4.0	3.4
All others	3.2	3.1
Neurosurgical	4.6	3.1
Surgical	4.6	3.4
Trauma	7.4	5.2
Burn	7.0	Not available

*(Number of CRBSI/number of CVC days) × 1000
CRBSI, Catheter-related bloodstream infection; *CVC*, central venous catheter; *ICU*, intensive care unit.
Adapted from National Nosocomial Infection Surveillance (NNIS) System Report, 2004.

Types of organisms involved in CRBSIs have changed over time and differ among units, but gram-positive organisms are the most prevalent. Formerly, coagulase-negative *Staphylococcus* (CNS) and *Staphylococcus aureus* were most frequently reported. Current NNIS data report *Enterococcus* spp. (many of which are vancomycin resistant) second to CNS infections. The NNIS also reports that more than 50% of all *S. aureus* isolates from ICUs are oxacillin resistant. Increases are also being seen in *Candida* species, many of which are resistant to fluconazole and of which nearly 50% are non-albicans species. Gram-negative bacilli accounted for approximately 15% of CRBSIs in the 1990s. There has been an increase in the frequency of *Enterobacteriaceae* that produce extended-spectrum beta-lactamases, and increases of *Klebsiella pneumoniae* resistance to third-generation cephalosporins are up nearly 50%. Although not all CRBSI organisms are associated with increased mortality rates, *S. aureus* BSI appears to be associated with increased mortality.

PATHOGENESIS

A CVC may become infected from extraluminal colonization, intraluminal colonization, hematogenous spread, and infusate contamination. The skin and catheter hub are the most common sources of colonization of intravascular catheters. *Extraluminal colonization* of CVCs occurs when skin flora invade and migrate along the cutaneous catheter tract. This is the most common route of infection for short-term, nontunneled, noncuffed catheters. *Intraluminal colonization* results from frequent manipulation and subsequent contamination of the catheter hub. The catheter hub is a more common source for cuffed, tunneled, silicone catheters and ports. Occasionally the catheter becomes infected via *hematogenous* spread from another focus or from *infusate contamination*. Infusate contamination should be strongly considered during epidemics of catheter infections.

When catheters become colonized, microorganisms can produce substances that facilitate adhesion to CVCs. These biofilms, which decrease antimicrobial susceptibility, are produced by coagulase-negative staphylococci, *S aureus, Enterococcus faecalis, K. pneumonia, Pseudomonas aeruginosa,* and *Candida albicans.* Microorganism adherence properties also are important. *S. aureus,* coagulase-negative staphylococci, and *Candida* can adhere to host proteins (fibronectin and fibrin) found in the fibrin–thrombin sheath surrounding the catheter. CNS readily adheres to polymer surfaces, and some strains produce "slime" (extracellular polysaccharide) that potentiates its pathogenicity by functioning as a barrier. Some *Candida* species in the presence of glucose-containing fluids produce a similar slime. Biofilms and fibrin sheaths make it difficult to eradicate CRIs without catheter removal.

PREVENTION

CVC infections can be prevented by a number of mechanisms, ranging from education of personnel to catheter and dressing type. Each prevention mode is described below. Table 2 lists five guidelines for preventing CVC infections.

Quality Assurance Programs

Insertion and maintenance of catheters by inexperienced staff increases risk for colonization and CRBSI, whereas infectious risk decreases following standardization of aseptic care. Specialized intravenous (IV) teams reduce the incidence of CRI-associated complications and cost.

Catheter Insertion Site

The density of skin flora at the insertion site is a major risk. In adults, lower-extremity sites are associated with higher risk for infection than are upper-body sites. Femoral catheters clearly have a high colonization rate in adults. The subclavian site appears to have a lower infectious risk than either the jugular or femoral site.

Table 2: Five General Guidelines for Preventing Catheter-Related Infections*

1. Education and training of health care providers who insert and maintain catheters: indications, proper procedures for insertion and maintenance, appropriate infection control measures

2. Use of maximal sterile barrier precautions during central venous catheter (CVC) insertion: mask, hat, gown, sterile gloves, large sterile drape

3. Use of 2% chlorhexidine preparation for skin antisepsis

4. Avoidance of routine replacement of CVC as a strategy to prevent infection

5. Use of antiseptic/antibiotic-impregnated short-term CVCs if infection rates are high despite adherence to items 1 through 3 above

*Adapted from Centers for Disease Control and Prevention: MMWR 51(RR10): 1, 2002.

Catheter Material

Catheters made of polyvinyl chloride or polyethylene are more susceptible to adherence of microorganisms than are catheters made of Teflon, silicone elastomer, or polyurethane. Recent studies show that Teflon and polyurethane catheters are associated with fewer infectious complications compared with polyvinyl chloride or polyethylene catheters. As a result, most catheters in the United States are now made of Teflon or polyurethane.

Aseptic Technique

Aseptic technique consists of good hand hygiene, skin antisepsis, and maximal sterile barrier precautions. Hand hygiene with a waterless, alcohol-based product or antibacterial soap and water contributes to decreased infection rates. Hand washing is necessary in addition to sterile gloves. Skin antisepsis studies demonstrate that 2% chlorhexidine gluconate dramatically reduces CRIs in comparison with 10% povidone-iodine and 70% alcohol. Lower concentrations (0.5%) of chlorhexidine may not be as effective. ChloraPrep (Enturia, Leawood, KS) is a readily available 2% chlorhexidine solution. For CVCs, maximal sterile barrier precautions, which include a cap, mask, sterile gown, sterile gloves, and a large sterile drape, reduce the incidence of CRBSI compared with sterile gloves and small sterile drapes.

Catheter Site, Dressing, and Dressing Change Frequency

In the ICU, CVCs in the subclavian position have the lowest incidence of CRBSI, followed by jugular and femoral lines. Transparent semipermeable polyurethane dressings are popular because they secure the device, permit easy visual inspection, permit bathing, and require less frequent dressing changes. Large studies show that transparent dressings have a 5.7% colonization rate, which is comparable with the 4.6% colonization rate of gauze and tape. A recent meta-analysis showed that neither is superior. If the patient is diaphoretic or if the site is bleeding or oozing, gauze dressing is preferable. For short-term catheters, the Centers for Disease Control and Prevention (CDC) recommends that gauze dressing be replaced every 2 days and transparent dressings every 7 days. The dressing should also be replaced when the dressing is damp, loosened, or soiled.

Antimicrobial/Antiseptic Impregnated Catheters and Cuffs

To date, all studied impregnated catheters have been triple-lumen, uncuffed catheters in adults and used less than 30 days. Catheters impregnated with chlorhexidine/silver sulfadiazine reduce CRBSI compared with standard noncoated catheters. However, their antimicrobial activity decreases over time. Resistance has not yet been determined. They are more expensive than standard catheters but still lead to cost savings in units where CRBSI risk is high (ICU, burns, neutropenia) and infection exceeds 3.3/1000 catheter days. Catheters impregnated with minocycline/rifampin have been compared with first-generation chlorhexidine-coated catheters. One study shows superiority of minocycline/rifampin. There has been no reported resistance. The advantage of minocycline/rifampin-impregnated catheters over chlorhexidine/silver sulfadiazine is a longer half-life of antimicrobial activity against *Staphylococcus epidermidis,* but further study is necessary. Other catheter trials include using platinum/silver, which does not appear to be superior to using chlorhexidine/silver catheters.

Topical antibiotic ointments should not be used except with dialysis catheters because they promote fungal infections and antimicrobial resistance. Although silver cuffs show no demonstrated efficacy, chlorhexidine-impregnated disk sponges appear to reduce the risk of catheter colonization and CRBSI. Their use is recommended if CRBSI rates exceed 5 per 1000 catheter days in the ICU.

Systemic Prophylactic Antibiotics

No studies demonstrate that prophylactic oral or parenteral antibacterial or antifungal agents reduce incidence of CRBSI among adults. In low–birth-weight infants, a reduction has been shown in CRBSI but not mortality. However, the risk of infection with vancomycin-resistant enterococci (VRE) appears to outweigh the benefit.

Anticoagulants

Flush solutions are widely used to prevent thrombosis. Thrombi and fibrin deposits may serve as a nidus for colonization; thus anticoagulants may help prevent CRBSI. Heparin decreases thrombus formation but does not clearly decrease CRBSI. The majority of pulmonary artery, umbilical, and CVCs are available with a coating of heparin bonded with benzalkonium chloride. They provide an antimicrobial and antithrombotic effect. Heparin-bonded pulmonary artery catheters have reduced microbial adherence and reduced CRBSIs compared with nonbonded catheters (5.5 vs. 2.6/ 1000 catheter days).

In-Line Filters and Administration Set Replacement

No good evidence exists that in-line filters decrease rates of CRI or CRBSI, likely because of the small proportion of infusate-related infections. Administration sets do not need to be replaced more frequently than every 72 hours after initiation. The indication for more frequent administration set changes occurs when the infusate enhances microbial growth (lipids, blood products) because these are independent risk factors for CRBSI.

Catheter Replacement

Catheters should be replaced for local or systemic complications and removed when no longer essential. The longer catheters are left in place, the greater the risk of infection. Although replacement of peripheral IV lines every 72 hours decreases colonization and thrombophlebitis, scheduled replacement of CVCs, percutaneously inserted central catheters (PICCs), and hemodialysis catheters does not lower CRBSI rates when compared with changing as needed. Guidewire change is associated with less discomfort and lower mechanical complication rates than new insertions. Scheduled guidewire changes do not decrease CRBSI rates. Guidewire change is unacceptable during suspected bacteremia episodes because the source of infection is usually the skin tract.

■ DIAGNOSIS

Diagnosis of CRI and CRBSI can be made by a number of methods. Common diagnostic methods include local site assessment, semiquantitative, and quantitative cultures of the catheter tip and the intracutaneous segment. Clinical findings are not particularly reliable for diagnosing CRBSI. Specificity is poor for fever, and the appearance of the exit site has reasonable specificity but poor sensitivity. Clinical data suggesting the catheter as the source of infection include absence of another source for the BSI, with isolation of a typical CRBSI organism (S. aureus, Candida spp.), and local catheter infection such as exit site inflammation, tunnel tract inflammation, or port pocket abscess with BSI.

Quantitative electron microscopy shows that most indwelling catheters become colonized after insertion. The roll-plate semiquantitative culture method established by Maki is the standard for diagnosis of CRBSI in many laboratories. This semiquantitative technique, however, cultures only the external catheter surface and does not retrieve internal organisms or those embedded within the biofilm. For long-term catheters in which the internal surface is the predominant source of colonization and BSI, more quantitative culture methods published by Sherertz, Brun-Buisson, and Cleri, such as vortex sonication or flushing the catheter lumen with broth, should be considered.

Many CVCs have been unnecessarily removed for suspected CRI or to obtain a diagnosis of CRI. The percentage of catheters removed for suspected CRBSI that ultimately yield no growth exceeds 50% in most series. Most of these catheters are removed for unexplained fever rather than for bacteremia from an unknown source. The Infectious Disease Society of America (ISDA) guideline for the diagnosis and treatment of CRI is that nontunneled CVCs should not be routinely removed from patients with unexplained fever and mild to moderate disease. The decision whether to remove a catheter should be made on the basis of the patient's clinical condition and the appearance of the catheter insertion site. Any short-term CVC with purulence at the insertion site should be removed. For patients with mild to moderate severity, without signs of exit-site infection, the ISDA recommends obtaining peripheral and line cultures, exit-site cultures, exchange of the catheter over a guidewire, or a combination of these procedures.

Newer diagnostic techniques do not require catheter removal. Simultaneous collections of quantitative blood cultures can be performed in which the number of microbes obtained through the CVC is at least fivefold greater than the number of microbes on peripheral culture.

Simultaneous cultures can also be collected and are considered positive if growth from the CVC shows up at least 2 hours earlier than simultaneously collected peripheral blood culture. This latter diagnostic technique is called *differential time to positivity*. An endoluminal brush method has also been described in which the lumen of the catheter is brushed and an acridine orange leukocyte cytospin test is performed on the blood drawn through the catheter.

For BSI to be determined as *catheter related*, the same organism must be isolated from peripheral blood and from the catheter by one of the following:

- ≥ 15 colony-forming units by semiquantitative (roll plate) technique.
- ≥100 colony-forming units by quantitative (vortex or sonication) techniques.
- Comparison of line and peripheral blood cultures by quantitative culture or by differential time to positivity. These are particularly helpful in situations in which catheter removal is problematic.
- Quantitative culture. Line blood cultures have a fivefold greater yield than peripheral blood cultures.
- Time to differential positivity. Growth from culture drawn through the line occurs 2 hours sooner than growth drawn from the peripheral culture specimen; the sensitivity of the catheter as the source is greater than 98%.

Other modalities that have been used to confirm catheter infections include swabbing the exit site of the catheter. A negative exit-site culture has excellent negative predictive value (80%-90%) and hence tells the clinician when a short-term CVC can be left in place because it is unlikely to be the source of infection. However, the positive predictive value is poor and cannot be used to definitively diagnose the infection.

■ TREATMENT

After peripheral blood cultures and catheter samples are obtained, appropriate empirical intravenous antibiotics should be given, depending on clinical signs, severity of the patient's illness, underlying disease, and potential pathogens. In ICUs with high rates of oxacillin-resistant *S. aureus*, empirical treatment should include vancomycin, linezolid, or quinupristin/dalfopristin. In units without high levels of resistance, nafcillin or oxacillin can be used. Severely immunocompromised patients should have additional empirical coverage for gram-negative rods, including *Pseudomonas*. When fungemia is suspected, patients should also be empirically covered with either amphotericin B or fluconazole. After the pathogen is identified, the antibiotic spectrum should be narrowed. Recommendations from the ISDA, the Society of Critical Care Medicine, and the American College of Critical Care Medicine are to *remove the CVC* for most cases of nontunneled CVC-related bacteremia and fungemia. The CVC should also be removed and cultured in a patient with unexplained sepsis and severe disease or with an erythematous or purulent exit site. If the removed catheter was changed over a guidewire for unexplained sepsis and a normal-appearing exit site but by culture it significantly colonized, the second catheter must be removed and another site used if a catheter is still necessary.

At this time, there are no good data to support duration of antimicrobial therapy for CRBSI. Complicated infections such as osteomyelitis, endocarditis, and suppurative thrombophlebitis certainly require longer courses of therapy than uncomplicated infections. Generally uncomplicated bloodstream infections without permanent indwelling intravascular prosthetic devices can be treated for 10 to 14 days. Infections with CNS do not require such long therapy, and 5 days after device removal may be sufficient. If bacteremia persists after device removal, 4 to 8 weeks of therapy may be necessary, depending on the diagnosis. Patients with positive line cultures but no growth on peripheral blood cultures can be observed for signs of infection. However, patients with valvular heart disease or neutropenia and a positive line but negative blood cultures should probably receive a short course (5–7 days) of antibiotics, particularly for *S. aureus* and *Candida*.

Guidewire changes should not be used in high-risk patients suspected of CRI. A low-risk CRBSI consists of a low-virulence organism (CNS) in a nontoxic patient. In a low-risk CRBSI, attempts can be made to treat the patient with systemic antimicrobials. Long-term catheters in patients without strict indications for

catheter removal may be considered for flushing with antimicrobial solutions or antibiotic lock techniques. Persistence of fever for more than 48 hours after appropriate treatment or hypotension are considered complicated CRBSIs and mandate catheter removal. Additional indications for catheter removal are septic thrombosis, septic emboli, or deep-seated infections such as endocarditis, and tunnel or pocket infections. Most recommendations include removing CVCs for bloodstream infections without a known source, erythema, induration or purulence at the insertion site, and hemodynamic instability caused by an unknown source. However, one recent study randomly assigned hemodynamically stable patients with suspected CRI to automatic catheter replacement versus watchful waiting. It showed that in hemodynamically stable patients with suspected CRI, catheters could safely be left in situ while the suspected infection was being treated. Persistent sepsis, bacteremia, or the development of hemodynamic instability were indications for eventual catheter removal. The patients in whom the catheters were left in place had three times fewer catheter changes, and this strategy resulted in outcomes similar to those for patients in whom catheters were automatically replaced on suspicion of CRI.

However, it cannot be overemphasized that clinically ill patients with CRBSI should in general not be considered for in situ treatment of infections. Catheter removal is also obligatory in *Candida* and *S. aureus* infections. Transesophageal echocardiography should be performed in patients with *S. aureus* or *Candida* BSI. Patients with persistent positive blood cultures more than 3 days after catheter removal should be evaluated for metastatic infections, endocarditis, and septic thrombosis.

Suggested Readings

Centers for Disease Control and Prevention: Guidelines for the prevention of intravascular catheter-related infections, *MMWR* 51(RR10): 1, 2002.

Mermel LS, Farr BM, Sherertz RJ, and others: Guidelines for the management of intravascular catheter-related infections, *Clin Infect Dis* 32:1249, 2001.

National Nosocomial Infection Surveillance (NNIS) System Report: Data summary from January 1992 through June 2004, issued October 2004, *Am J Infect Control* 32:470, 2004.

Preoperative Assessment of the Elderly Patient

Martin A. Makary, MD, MPH, Colleen Christmas, MD, and John R. Burton, MD

The population older than age 65 years in the United States is predicted to double within the next 40 years. This forecast has created increased attention on how health care and other needs will be provided for older adults. This demographic imperative has already elevated the Medicare and Social Security programs to the center of public debate. At the day-to-day level, most physicians in recent years have experienced an increasing proportion of older patients in their practices. In the surgical setting, the population growth phenomenon is further augmented by expanding indications to operate, given the increased safety of general anesthesia, improved perioperative medical care, and advanced surgical techniques. The result is a striking increase in the surgical volume of older patients, most notably among the very elderly. In a study translating the meaning of the increasing elderly population in the United States to surgeons, Etzioni and colleagues calculated that the average surgeon will experience a 31% growth rate in overall surgical volume in general surgery alone within 20 years (2001–2020). This forecasted increase is expected to strain the current surgical workforce.

An example of this change in surgical patterns is occurring at our own institution. At The Johns Hopkins Hospital, we have observed a marked increase in the proportion of Whipple operations being performed in the very elderly. As of March 2005, we have performed more than 200 Whipple operations on patients older than 80 years of age, with the vast majority of these being done in the past few years. Our recent experience and that of others performing an increasing number of thoracic and vascular operations in older adults confirm estimates of an exponentially expanding elderly population, with different and more complex perioperative considerations compared with their younger counterparts. Systems of care must adapt to meet these needs, if ideal outcomes are to be achieved.

Older patients are remarkably heterogeneous because of marked variations with aging of different organ systems, accumulated chronic diseases, life experiences, beliefs, and expectations. Understanding these variations is the challenge to the surgeon in formulating a management plan. Each patient's surgical care must be tailored to consider operative risk, physiologic reserves, quality of life, and personal values. Indeed, physicians are increasingly avoiding standardized diagnostic and treatment algorithms because of this heterogeneity. For example, a screening colonoscopy at age 85 years may carry a higher risk than potential benefit of discovery that will lead to a successful intervention and beneficial long-term outcome. Furthermore, most treatment guidelines address single diseases, whereas most geriatric patients who present for surgery have several concomitant comorbid conditions that may be affected by treatment guidelines. Uniform surgical management pathways, such as the National Institute of Health (NIIH) consensus statements on the criteria to remove an adrenal incidentaloma or an area of high-grade esophageal dysplasia, are not applicable to older patients because the natural history of these findings is not accurately predicted and the burden of surgery may well outweigh the benefit. Finally, older patients are at increased risk for hospital-acquired complications, and these risks must be considered with the patient and her or his family or caregiver. Complications, which confound surgical indications in older patients, include an increased risk of delirium, falls, infections, pressure sores, malnutrition, and functional impairment that may be long lasting. Strategies to identify and mitigate these risks are the basis of preoperative assessment and perioperative care.

SURGICAL DECISION MAKING

The decision to proceed with surgery should balance the patient's individualized surgical risk with the probability for survival and a meaningful quality of life as determined by the patient and, when appropriate, her or his family or caregiver. Thus there are no hard rules for management, only principles that are the core of the preoperative assessment. Age alone carries few additional risks to the patient. Rather, the complex constellation of the estimate of physiologic reserve, functional assessment, comorbid conditions, and severity of disease are the main determinants of risk and the likelihood of achieving desired outcomes. Despite patients' earnest requests, we have not offered surgery to patients in their 60s for small elective procedures such as hernia repairs because of several debilitating comorbidities, such as liver failure or impaired pulmonary function. Conversely, we have performed Whipple procedures in patients in their late 90s and have achieved good results for a significant period of time because their preoperative assessment did not reveal marked functional impairment, frailty, or severe comorbidities, and this approach was consistent with the patient's values and preferences.

Seeking an older patient's preferences is paramount because surgery can potentially result in a permanent disability and even accelerated death. The risk of a procedure in an older patient can be hard to estimate, given the paucity of data regarding elderly surgical patients with comorbidities. In presenting the probability of success of an operation while obtaining informed consent, it is important to recognize that there is a significant publication bias in the literature and that quoting a mortality rate from a best series may understate the true risk a patient may actually experience. In the meta-analysis of pancreatic surgery, we have found that published mortality rates in the literature underrepresented true mortality rate in the national inpatient sample and the Medicare databases by threefold to fourfold. Moreover, published complication rates in the literature are often based on younger cohorts and are not generalizable to a very elderly, frail patient—an important consideration when discussing surgical risk with a patient and family. There are few data on outcomes other than survival, and survival often is not the most important outcome to patients and their

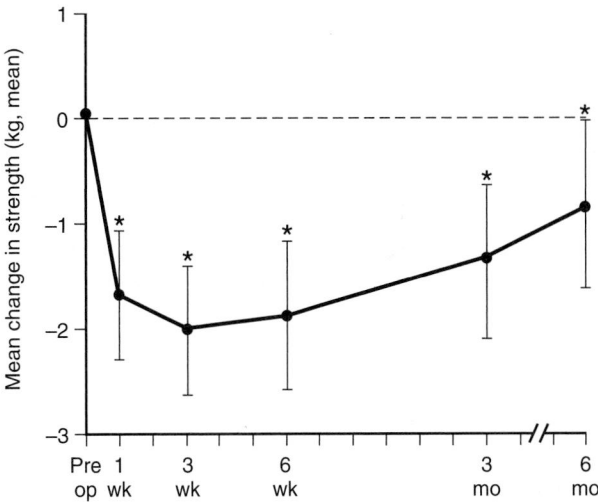

Figure 1 Postoperative strength following abdominal surgery among 372 older patients (strength measured as grip strength in kilograms). *From Lawrence VA, Hazuda HP, Cornell JE, and others: J Am Coll Surg 199:762, 2004.*

families. For example, a 92-year-old woman with severe valvular heart disease who is increasingly losing her independence from knee arthritis may be willing to accept a relatively high surgical risk for total knee replacement to avoid becoming dependent on others and to continue to live at home alone.

To better understand the increased risk of surgery in the very elderly, we reviewed our experience in performing the Whipple procedure in this population. We found that patients older than 80 years of age had an operative mortality rate of 4% compared with a historical operative mortality of 1.7% for all patients since 1970. There were no perioperative deaths among the 10 patients who were 90 years of age or older, and the 1-year survival for patients older than 80 years of age was 60% compared with an overall 1-year survival rate of 80% for patients of all ages. Overall, this study demonstrated that age as an independent variable was a minor contributor to perioperative mortality and morbidity and that postoperative outcomes were more closely associated with confounding comorbidities. Accordingly, age *alone* is not a contraindication for surgery, but only a context in which a risk-to-benefit ratio should be discussed.

Finally, postoperative function and quality of life are important aspects of survival. Recent data from a research team in San Antonio have demonstrated that surgery has a small but definite effect on long-term activities of daily living and strength, with a majority of patients still testing as "weak" at 6 months compared with their baseline preoperative strength (Fig. 1). Other studies have similarly shown that after an admission to the intensive care unit, patients have significant long-term disability that is usually underestimated by physicians.

RISK ASSESSMENT

Frailty

Although frailty increases with age, it is not a universal phenomenon in all older people. The determinants of this syndrome are now starting to be understood, but certainly its presence highly modifies an elderly patient's ability to handle stress such as a surgical procedure. Frailty represents a complex syndrome of sarcopenia, easy exhaustion, slow walking speed, and reduced functional activity. A frailty assessment has practical utility in that it allows

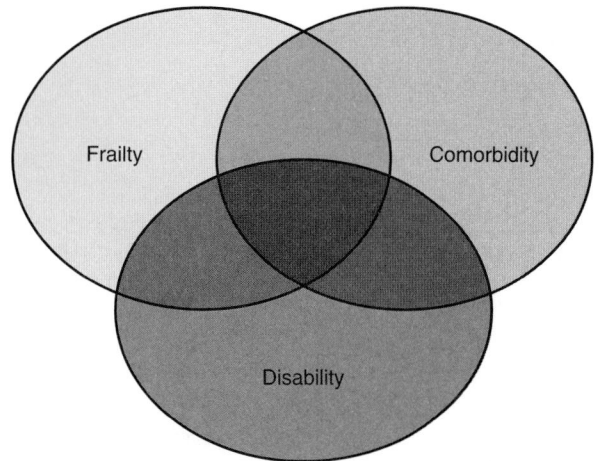

Figure 2 Factors in surgical decision-making in older patients.

clinicians to estimate a patient's physiologic reserve and thus the patient's ability to handle surgical stress.

Even though frailty may and often does coexist with comorbidity and disability (Fig. 2), it appears to be a distinctly independent surgical risk factor. For example, a patient may have minimal comorbidity and not be disabled yet meet the diagnostic criteria for being frail. The assessment of a patient to determine whether frailty is present is useful in considering the special needs of patients postoperatively to minimize complications. Examples of such postoperative risk modification strategies include delirium precautions, early ambulation, minimization of medications, and deep breathing—simple interventions that may make the difference between a long-term surgical failure and success. Thus a frailty assessment is a useful tool in estimating complication risk and planning postoperative care strategies.

Risk Factors for Surgery

Beyond an assessment for the presence of frailty, a focused history and physical examination, with specific attention to a few key items, can reveal valuable additional information about an older patient's operative risk (Table 1). Specifically, a history of low

Table 1: American Society of Anesthesiologists Classification System

ASA Class	Disease State
1	No organic, physiologic, biochemical, or psychiatric disturbance
2	Mild or moderate systemic disturbance that may or may not be related to the reason for surgery
3	Severe systemic disturbance that may or may not be related to the reason for surgery
4	Severe systemic disturbance that is life threatening with or without surgery
5	Little chance of survival; surgery is a last resort (resuscitative effort)
E	Emergency operation required

From American Society of Anesthesiologists: New classification of physical status, Anesthesiology 24:111, 1963.

serum albumin or a myocardial infarction within the past 3 months elevates a patient's operative risk for developing a complication. On physical examination, the finding of hemodynamically significant aortic stenosis or jugular venous distention similarly portends a high-risk postoperative course. Different preexisting comorbidities are associated with varying degrees of operative risk. The American College of Cardiology has categorized predictors of increased perioperative cardiovascular risk into major, intermediate, and minor risk factors. Using this stratum, major risk factors are unstable coronary syndromes, decompensated heart failure, significant arrhythmias, or severe valvular disease. Intermediate risk factors include mild angina pectoris, a past coronary event, compensated congestive heart failure, or diabetes mellitus. Minor risk factors include advanced age, abnormal electrocardiogram, a rhythm other than sinus, low functional respiratory capacity, stroke, or uncontrolled hypertension. Similarly, the American College of Physicians has identified the following risk factors associated with an elevated risk of postoperative pulmonary complications: advanced age, ASA class 2 status or higher, functional dependence in activities of daily living, chronic obstructive pulmonary disease, heart failure, general anesthesia, low serum albumin, type of surgery, and prolonged operative time. This authoritative group has identified deep breathing and other lung expansion techniques as having the most evidence in preventing postoperative pulmonary complications. They also conclude that although malnutrition is a risk factor for pulmonary complications, enteral or parenteral nutrition has not been shown to reduce this risk (Table 2).

Cognitive Status

The presence of dementia preoperatively is associated with an increased operative mortality (as much as 50% higher) and can complicate postoperative recovery and participation in rehabilitation. Falls, especially among anticoagulated patients, are a common cause of death and disability in elderly patients. Falls are closely associated with decreased cognitive status. For this reason, the decision to anticoagulate a patient should consider both the risk of fall and the estimated relative risk reduction of a major thrombotic event.

Table 2: Predictors of Poor Surgical Outcome

Parameter	Predictor
Age	Increased (>70 years)
Type of surgery	Emergent, contaminated, open abdominal, thoracic or aortic surgery, prolonged surgery
ASA	Greater than class 3
Cardiac	Presence of an S3 gallop, jugular venous distention, MI within 6 months, >5 PVC, aortic stenosis, unstable angina, absence of beta-blockade
Pulmonary	COPD, $FEV_1 < 1.0$ L, $Pao_2 < 60$, $Pco_2 > 50$, fatigue with walking (steps)
Neurologic	Impairment, decreased function, nonambulatory status
Renal	Decreased creatinine clearance, BUN > 50 mg/dL
Nutrition	Hypoalbuminemia, hypokalemia
Frailty	Weakness, early exhaustion, dependency

ADL, Activities of daily living; BUN, blood urea nitrogen; COPD, chronic obstructive pulmonary disease; FEV_1, forced expiratory volume in 1 second on pulmonary function testing; MI, myocardial infarction; PVC, premature ventricular contractions.
Creatinine clearance = (140 − age) × weight (kg) ÷ 72 × serum creatinine.

Postoperative delirium occurs in up to 40% of all elderly patients following surgery. It is associated with advanced age, underlying dementia, and the extent of surgery. The most common preventable causes of postoperative delirium are medication-induced, especially long-acting narcotics and benzodiazepines, undertreated pain, and environmental stressors such as noise or other interruptions to sleep and the application of mechanical restraints. The preoperative assessment alerts the clinician to the increased risk of delirium and should lead to the implementation of preventive strategies. Delirium usually occurs in the first 5 days postoperatively and lasts a few days to a few weeks, but it may be of long duration. In many older patients, this complication of surgery is associated with a lasting impact on quality of life and a significant long-term cognitive loss. The delirious state also places the patient at increased risk of falls and other life-threatening complications. Prevention, by minimizing medications—limiting in particular benzodiazepines and anticholinergic drugs—providing frequent orientation, allowing sleep at night, and judiciously treating pain (using nonnarcotic adjunctive therapies whenever possible), is far more effective than treatment after delirium has occurred. We have found that a quiet environment and the continuous presence of a reassuring, caring family member or hospital staff person are helpful.

Anticoagulation in Older Patients

"Polypharmacy" is a major problem in older patients. Medications such as clopidogrel and warfarin are associated with bleeding complications following surgery, so a careful review of the indication, in consultation with the prescribing physician, is important during the preoperative assessment. Although clopidogrel is widely used, evidence supports its use only for management of cardiovascular stents for 2 to 6 months following the placement of the stent, until an endothelial coat can form. Liberal use of anticoagulants for stroke prevention and intermittent leg claudication should be reconsidered because the indications here are less definitive and the bleeding consequences when these medications are administered at the time of surgery can be significant.

Perioperative Beta-Blockade

Beta-blocker agents have been shown to reduce the rate of in-hospital death following surgery in high cardiac-risk patients. Care should be taken to avoid bradycardia when starting beta-blockers for the first time in a patient. A patient who is taking a beta-blocker preoperatively should continue this medication. However, the general use of such agents in older patients is dangerous. Indeed, a 2006 report in the *New England Journal of Medicine* found that there was no benefit in initiating prophylactic perioperative beta-blocker drugs in low cardiac-risk patients (Revised Cardiac Risk Index score of 0 or 1); furthermore, there was a potential harm. Indeed, we and other centers have had a few asymptomatic, low-risk patients experience life-threatening bradycardia, at times requiring cardiac pacing during and after surgery, as a result of initiating a beta-blocker drug. The optimal dose, timing, and duration of preoperative beta-blockers is poorly understood and the subject of much debate. Elderly patients may be at particularly high-risk for arrhythmias caused by beta-blockers. For these reasons, we reserve beta-blockers for patients who have a cardiac history or have been on them previously. Until more definitive data

are available, we suggest avoiding initiation of a perioperative beta-blocker drug in low cardiac-risk patients.

Preoperative Interventions

Despite advances in medical and surgical care, interventions to improve operative risk are still limited. In an older patient with increased cardiac risk, the only correction that can truly optimize a patient is management of uncompensated heart failure, correction of abnormal electrolyte concentrations (e.g., hypokalemia or hyponatremia), or the addition of beta-blockade. Data are accumulating to support the finding that "statin" medications, clonidine, and aspirin reduce cardiovascular events after surgery. However, the evidence is limited currently, and until more definitive data are published, the prophylactic initiation in the perioperative period cannot be endorsed.

Preoperative exercise programs are likely to be of benefit in older patients preparing for elective surgery. However, several weeks or months of increasing exercise are necessary, so this practice is only occasionally applicable.

Almost all diagnostic cardiac procedures, such as a stress echocardiograph test, provide risk assessment information; however, rarely do the results lead to strategies that improve operative mortality. For this reason, we often limit preoperative stress cardiac testing to patients in whom the decision to proceed with surgery will be affected by the degree of operative cardiac risk. Many patients with malignancy, for example, are prepared to undergo surgery with an understanding of a general range of estimated risk, and they do not need a more precise measurement of risk. Conversely, a patient in whom a decision to proceed with surgery will be altered by a high cardiac-risk designation may be a good candidate for such preoperative testing. Age alone is not an indication for a preoperative cardiac evaluation in a patient without risk factors for heart disease. Finally, there is little role for preoperative cardiac catheterization because the risk of the catheterization procedure often approximates the risk of an operation. Evidence does not support the use of preoperative pulmonary function testing except in predicting recovery from lung resection surgery. Indeed, studies now indicate that even a routine preoperative chest x-ray study has little evidence of benefit, although such a procedure is still widely used. Because of new knowledge accumulating in the literature, most clinicians now have transitioned from focusing on preoperative risk assessment to concentrating on improving as much as possible a patient's multiple chronic medical problems before surgery.

Suggested Readings

Etzioni DA, Liu JH, Maggard MA, and others: The aging population and its impact on the surgery workforce, *Ann Surg* 238:170, 2003.

Eagle KA, Brundage BH, Chaitman BR, and others: *J Am Coll Cardiol* 27:918, 1996.

Eagle KA, Berger PB, Calkins H, and others: ACC/AHA guideline update for perioperative cardiovascular evaluation for noncardiac surgery, American College of Cardiology/American Heart Association, *J Am Coll Surg* 39:542, 2002.

Lawrence VA, Hazuda HP, Cornell JE, and others: Functional independence after major abdominal surgery in the elderly, *J Am Coll Surg* 199:762, 2004.

Lindenauer PK, Pekow P, Wang K, and others: Perioperative beta-blocker therapy and mortality after major noncardiac surgery, *N Engl J Med* 353:349, 2005.

Makary MA, Winter JM, Cameron JL, and others: Pancreaticoduodenectomy in the very elderly, *J Gastrointest Surg* 10:347, 2006.

PERIOPERATIVE CARE AND MONITORING OF THE SURGICAL PATIENT: EVIDENCE-BASED PERFORMANCE PRACTICES

Robert W. Thomsen, MD, Elizabeth A. Martinez, MD, and Brett A. Simon, MD, PhD

Whereas the care of the surgical patient encompasses a wide range of patient conditions and procedure complexities, there are a number of perioperative and intraoperative practices that apply to all patients and procedures. Increasingly, evidence-based measures are invoked to identify patients at risk for certain complications and to introduce processes designed to broadly reduce certain risks for large groups of patients. Some of these initiatives have been embraced by regulatory agencies to the point of inclusion in current or proposed performance standards. Together, these practices comprise an important component of the perioperative care and monitoring of the surgical patient with which every surgeon should be familiar.

EVIDENCE-BASED PERFORMANCE PRACTICES

Evidence-based measures to improve the quality of perioperative care have emerged as a driving force in American medicine. The 1999 Institute of Medicine report "To Err is Human: Building a Safer Health System" highlighted that the problem with medical errors is significant. Many caregivers associate medical errors as those instances of commission, for example, administration of the wrong medication or dose. However, errors of omission, such as failing to administer aspirin to a patient with an acute myocardial infarction, are also extremely important and contribute equally to morbidity and mortality. Two influential organizations, the Joint Commission on Accreditation of Healthcare Organizations (TJC) and the Centers for Medicare and Medicaid Services (CMS), have established regulatory policies supporting a culture of patient safety that include making certain that patients receive interventions that are evidence-based and are broadly accepted as the standard of care. TJC has incorporated quality care standards in its accreditation process. The Pay-for-Performance (P4P) initiatives proposed by CMS reflect many of these practices and are designed to promote streamlined delivery of rational therapeutic measures. A comprehensive understanding of these rules is essential to maintain facility accreditation, optimal reimbursement, and exceptional patient care.

During the past decade we have amassed a large body of clinical knowledge supported by rigorous experimental investigations. The state of the art of perioperative care continues to evolve, but our present understanding of those measures proven to affect morbidity and mortality should be understood by providers and incorporated into general practice as appropriate. The imminent implementation of P4P will also establish financial incentives to apply many of these quality care measures.

THE SURGICAL CARE IMPROVEMENT PROJECT

In 2003, the Surgical Care Improvement Project (SCIP) was initiated as a partnership of public and private organizations dedicated to the goal of reducing the incidence of surgical complications nationally by 25% by the year 2010. This multidisciplinary coalition provides a mechanism for generating a consensus evaluation of the evidence and, importantly, also educating providers and encouraging institutional leaders in the application of these processes. Although ultimately the outcomes of these various targeted interventions will be evaluated, initial efforts are directed at the implementation and compliance with the evidence-based *processes* that are anticipated to result in the improved outcomes (Table 1). Thus in the immediate future institutions will be focusing on collecting data on specific process measures, and performance indicated by quantitative compliance with these process measures is therefore a likely source of future P4P benchmarks. We outline the key perioperative measures that encompass the areas

Table 1: SCIP Process and Outcome Measures*

Process Measures

Surgical site infections
  On-time prophylactic antibiotic administration
  Appropriate selection of prophylactic antibiotics
  Discontinuation of prophylactic antibiotics within 24 hours
  Perioperative serum glucose $\leq$ 200 mg/dL in major cardiac surgical patients
  Appropriate hair removal
  Perioperative normothermia

Cardiovascular events
  Perioperative beta-blocker administration in noncardiac vascular surgery patients
  Perioperative beta-blocker administration in high-risk patients
  Continuation of beta-blockers in patients on preoperative therapy

Venous thromboembolism (VTE)
  Perioperative VTE prophylaxis (any) in all major surgery patients
  Appropriate perioperative prophylaxis based on surgical level of risk for VTE

Respiratory complications
  Ventilated patients with orders for head of bed elevated $\geq$ 30 degrees
  Ventilated patients with stress ulcer prophylaxis
  Surgical patients with order for ventilator weaning protocol

Proposed outcomes

Mortality within 30 days of surgery

Readmission within 30 days of surgery

30-day complication rates for:
  Postoperative wound infections
  Intraoperative or postoperative myocardial infarctions
  Intraoperative or postoperative cardiac arrest
  Intraoperative or postoperative pulmonary embolism
  Intraoperative or postoperative deep vein thrombosis
  Postoperative pneumonia

*See http://www.medqic.org/scip for most updated measures.

of infectious, cardiac, venous thromboembolism, and respiratory complications that are included in the SCIP measures, in addition to other key areas of impact.

PREVENTION OF SURGICAL SITE INFECTIONS

Appropriate Antibiotic Selection, Timing, and Discontinuation

Three SCIP measures are related to the appropriate use of prophylactic antibiotics in the perioperative period. For those procedures for which prophylactic antibiotics are recommended, these measures are (1) prophylactic antibiotic administration within 1 hour before incision, (2) appropriate antibiotic selection, and (3) discontinuation of prophylactic antibiotic within 24 hours after surgery end time. Those patients who have had a surgical intervention during the same hospitalization or are on preoperative antibiotics for treatment of a known or suspected infection are excluded from this measure.

Recommendations for the appropriate antibiotic selection for common procedures have been published, and these can be used to guide standardized management protocols. The antibiotic selected must be active against the major contaminating organisms, most commonly gram-positive skin organisms. In order to be effectively prophylactic against contamination of the wound with skin flora, the tissue concentration of the agent must be adequate at the time of incision. The best current evidence supports that this is achieved and maintained when the antibiotic is administered within 60 minutes before the time of incision. Studies have shown that, when the antibiotic is administered too early or too late, there is more than a twofold increase in the association with surgical site infections. The final measure is discontinuation of prophylactic antibiotics at 24 hours. There are no data to support the notion that antibiotics beyond the operating room are effective in decreasing the risk of perioperative infections, and continuation of these antibiotics increases the likelihood of drug-resistant organisms in case the patient develops an infection. However, given that the current practice of most surgical services is to continue antibiotics into the perioperative phase, the current quality measure is discontinuation of antibiotics at 24 hours. The one exception is for cardiac surgery, for which the recommendation is 48 hours postsurgery, and this recommendation is expected to change over time. A recent report on the national performance with these measures revealed compliances of less than 58% and 41% with antibiotic timing and discontinuation, respectively.

Appropriate Hair Removal

Shaving of hair before surgery has been shown to be associated with increased risk of surgical site infections. The biologic plausibility for this practice contributing to infections is that small microabrasions serve as a portal for skin flora to enter the bloodstream. In a recent Cochrane review, the authors reported that they found no difference in SSIs among patients who had hair removed before surgery and those who did not have hair removed. They also reported that if it is necessary to remove hair, the use of a clipper or depilatory results in fewer SSIs than the use of a razor. The relative risk of shaving versus using a clipper for hair removal is 2.02 (95% CI 1.21–3.36). Furthermore they found no difference in outcomes on the basis of the timing of hair removal (either day of or 1 day before surgery). For the SCIP measure, appropriate hair removal is defined as the percentage of patients with no hair removal or, if removed, removed with a clipper or depilatory and not with a razor. It is recommended that hair not be removed, but if it is to be removed, to limit the area of hair removal.

Maintenance of Normothermia

Anesthesia induces a state of poikilothermia. The mechanisms to protect core temperature are lost and there is a rapid redistribution of body heat, resulting in a fall in body temperature by 1 to 2 degrees centigrade. Impairment of thermoregulation is compounded by low ambient temperature in many operating rooms and exposed skin surfaces, especially during the surgical preparation. Hypothermia induces peripheral vasoconstriction, which decreases subcutaneous oxygen tension. This effect is magnified because hemoglobin binds oxygen more avidly at lower temperature and prevents its release to the tissues. Cutaneous tissues with reduced blood flow are also likely to have decreased antibiotic delivery. Hypothermia decreases the activity of nicotinamide adenine dinucleotide phosphate (NADPH) oxidase, an enzyme essential for the bactericidal action of neutrophils, and impairs leukocyte chemotaxis. Significant hypothermia will globally reduce enzyme function, which can precipitate coagulopathy. Hypothermia may also impair wound healing by impairment of collagen cross-linking. As thermoregulatory mechanisms return, the body is exposed to a period of intense physiologic stress. Colorectal surgery patients randomized to receive mild intraoperative hypothermia were significantly more likely to have wound infections, delayed wound healing, and prolonged hospitalization than their normothermic counterparts. The results of this study were sufficiently influential to prompt inclusion of perioperative normothermia in the Centers for Disease Control and Prevention (CDC)-CMS Surgical Care Improvement Project.

Furthermore, a 55% risk reduction in morbid cardiac events was found when patients with known coronary artery disease or risk factors for coronary artery disease were normothermic during major abdominal, thoracic, or vascular procedures.

Older adults are particularly at increased risk for developing perioperative hypothermia and the attendant complications, including wound infections and myocardial ischemia. Maintenance of normothermia is an essential component of a comprehensive surgical site infection strategy and will likely be viewed by Medicare as an important measure of quality care.

Although the current quality measure includes only patients undergoing colorectal surgery, it is anticipated, and expected, that this core measure will be expanded to a broader patient group. This intervention is low cost and carries low risk of harm to patients and should be considered to be widely adopted in operating suites (Table 2).

Glucose Management

Multiple clinical trials have identified hyperglycemia in the perioperative period and in critically ill patients as an independent risk factor for increased morbidity and mortality. Diabetic

Table 2: Interventions to Maintain Normothermia

Passive Interventions

Maintain ambient temperature greater than 21°C (69.8°F)
Cover exposed skin with thermal barriers
Heat–moisture exchangers (conserve respiratory heat and humidity)

Active Interventions

Infusate warming
Convective warming via forced air
Conductive warming via heating mat

patients who present for surgery have a higher incidence of wound infections, intensive care unit (ICU) admissions, and prolonged hospitalization than nondiabetics. However, the stress response associated with surgery and critical illness may induce hyperglycemia in nondiabetic patients. Catecholamines, insulin-like growth factor, glucocorticoids, and proinflammatory cytokines released in the perioperative period alter normal glucose homeostasis by promoting catabolic processes and creating peripheral insulin resistance. There are increasing data to support the concept that early perioperative glycemic control decreases the risk of perioperative infections. Critically ill patients who have experienced acute myocardial infarction or stroke have dramatically decreased morbidity and mortality when intensive insulin therapy is initiated. Cardiac surgery patients who were randomized to an intensive insulin regimen were significantly less likely to develop infection; were less likely to require postoperative pacing, inotropic support, or ventilatory support; and had shorter ICU and total duration of hospital stays compared with those patients managed with a standard sliding scale insulin therapy. Most importantly, the 2-year survival rate was significantly higher in the intensive therapy group.

Excellent evidence exists to support tight glucose control programs in critically ill patients during the postoperative period. Adequate resources must be available to administer a continuous insulin infusion, check frequent blood glucose measurements, and titrate the infusion on the basis of those measurements. The deleterious effects of hyperglycemia are likely relevant in the operating room, but intraoperative glycemic control needs further study before widespread adoption. The most concerning adverse event in these trials was hypoglycemia. The dynamic nature of the operating theater may increase the risk of hypoglycemic events. Furthermore, many clinical signs of neuroglycopenia will be masked by general anesthesia, and severe adverse events may occur.

Available evidence clearly supports the use of tight glucose control protocols in the postsurgical ICU environment, especially in cardiac surgical patients. The profound reduction in morbidity and mortality may drive its eventual inclusion into the P4P plan. However, attempts to extend this benchmark into the operating theater should be resisted until more evidence is available, along with rapid and reliable methods for determination of blood glucose in the operating room.

PREVENTION OF VENOUS THROMBOEMBOLISM

Venous thromboembolism prophylaxis is an important perioperative consideration because nearly all surgical patients have risk factors for deep venous thrombosis (DVT), and the presence of multiple risk factors confers additive risk. There is a high prevalence of DVT in the surgical population, and most of these are clinically asymptomatic. Whereas many DVTs remain silent, significant morbidity and mortality from pulmonary embolism can occur unexpectedly.

Mechanical methods for DVT prophylaxis are simple and inexpensive and do not increase the risk of bleeding. Compression stockings limit venous pooling in the lower extremities. Intermittent pneumatic compression devices may decrease venous stasis and promote elaboration of tissue thromboplastin. However, their efficacy is questionable and no study has demonstrated a reduction in pulmonary embolism or death.

Pharmacologic prophylaxis through the use of anticoagulant drugs remains the most efficacious therapy. Level 1a recommendations support the routine use of low-dose, unfractionated heparin in trauma patients; most patients in ICUs; and patients undergoing major abdominal operations, particularly those involving pelvic manipulation. Orthopaedic surgery patients are among patients with the highest risk for DVT, and level 1a recommendations include use of low-molecular-weight heparin or warfarin (Coumadin; Bristol-Myers Squibb, New York, NY) for prophylaxis. Furthermore, prophylaxis should be continued for 10 days postoperatively in patients undergoing hip or knee arthroplasty. Aspirin should not be used for DVT prophylaxis.

The greatest concern with the use of anticoagulant prophylaxis is bleeding. Wound hematoma formation is more likely if pharmacologic DVT prophylaxis is used, but serious perioperative bleeding is no different than with placebo.

The Medicare population is at high risk for venous thromboembolism (VTE) in that many older patients are debilitated and may present for hip fracture repair. However, anticoagulation may also increase the risk of bleeding complications for patients who are most at risk for falls or who have other conditions that predispose them to life-threatening hemorrhage. If DVT prophylaxis is incorporated into Medicare's initiative, special consideration should be given to exclusion of select patient groups or allow a reduced standard such as mechanical prophylaxis only.

PREVENTION OF VENTILATOR-ASSOCIATED PNEUMONIA

Ventilator-associated pneumonia (VAP) is a leading cause of morbidity and mortality in the critically ill. The cost associated with VAP is substantial, considering that patients who develop VAP require approximately 13 additional ICU days. Attributable mortality is estimated to be as high as 30%. Multiple strategies have been proposed to decrease the risk of VAP, and many of these measures should be considered perioperatively if prolonged mechanical ventilation is expected.

Aspiration of oral or gastric fluids is believed to be a major factor in the development of VAP. The semirecumbent position has been proven to reduce the incidence of clinically and microbiologically diagnosed VAP, likely by reducing gastroesophageal reflux. Level IIa recommendations support this safe, cost-free intervention. Similarly, subglottic suctioning decreases obstructive secretions and microbial inoculum. There is level IIa evidence to support this practice, but special endotracheal tubes used in these studies may limit widespread adoption.

To prevent stress ulcer formation, gastric prophylaxis is widely undertaken. Gastric microbial colonization, however, increases with increasing gastric pH. VAP rates are lowest in patients who do not receive stress ulcer prophylaxis. The substantial costs associated with a gastrointestinal bleed are significant, and some form of prophylaxis should be used in patients requiring prolonged ventilation. Level 1 evidence supports the use of sucralfate over H_2 receptor antagonists for stress ulcer prophylaxis because this therapy does not affect gastric pH. Patients who have multiple risk factors for gastric ulceration should continue to receive H_2 receptor antagonists or possibly proton pump inhibitors.

Selective decontamination of the upper digestive tract with topical antibiotics clearly reduces the rate of VAP. This practice is strongly discouraged, however, given the likelihood of altering bacterial antibiotic resistance patterns.

The body of evidence-based interventions that decrease the risk of this expensive and life-threatening complication continues to expand. Many of these interventions are inexpensive and require minimal resources. Given the potential for cost savings and decreased morbidity and mortality, there is a high likelihood that prevention of VAP will be incorporated into P4P.

The current campaigns for the prevention of VAP include the following interventions: elevation of head of bed 30 degrees; appropriate peptic ulcer disease (PUD) prophylaxis; appropriate VTE prophylaxis; appropriate sedation; and daily assessment of ability to be extubated. The first three measures are also Joint Commission on Accreditation of Healthcare Organizations (TJC) core measures.

BETA-BLOCKADE

Perioperative cardiovascular complications remain a leading cause of morbidity and mortality. It is estimated that approximately 1 million individuals experience a perioperative cardiac complication, ranging from 1% to as high as 30% of high-risk vascular surgical patients. There are data to support that perioperative beta-blockade reduces the incidence of perioperative myocardial ischemia and infarction and may also confer protection out to 2 years postoperatively.

Current recommendations from the American College of Cardiology and the American Heart Association Task Force include (1) perioperative beta-blockers for those patients who are in the highest risk categories; and, (2) importantly, continuation of beta-blockers for those who were on them preoperatively. Discontinuation of beta-blockers can result in rebound tachycardia and has been shown to actually increase the risk for perioperative ischemia. A recent retrospective study by Lindenauer and colleagues showed that there was no benefit to administering perioperative beta-blockers to patients with a revised cardiac risk index of 0–2 and that there was the potential of increased risk when they were administered to patients with a score of 0. This study was limited by its retrospective nature; however, it is generally widely accepted that beta-blockers are not indicated for low-risk individuals. For example, beta-blocker prophylaxis is not indicated for a young healthy trauma patient.

MEASURES OTHER THAN SURGICAL CARE IMPROVEMENT PROJECT

Prevention of Catheter-Related Bloodstream Infections

Central venous catheters are often a necessary adjunct in the management of surgical patients. Patients may require central access for administration of vasoactive agents, for administration of nutritional support, secondary to limited peripheral access in the setting of significant perioperative edema, or for monitoring of cardiovascular status. Central venous catheters are associated with bloodstream infections, which have been shown to be associated with a 10% increase in mortality in ICU patients. Although not an SCIP measure, prevention of catheter-related bloodstream infections (CRBSI) is important in the overall management of surgical patients.

Recent studies have reported the successful implementation of evidence-based practices in essentially eliminating CRBSIs. Key principles that should be adopted in the placement and management of central lines include the use of chlorhexidine skin preparation; full-barrier protection (use of sterile, full-body drape; all team members involved should be fully gowned, masked, and gloved with sterile gloves following appropriate hand washing); and use of sterile dressings over a dry and cleaned insertion site. Many ICUs have implemented a checklist to make certain that (1) all key steps are implemented and (2) if there is a breakdown in the sterile technique, any person observing can and should halt the placement of the line until the error is corrected. This approach has been successful in reinforcing the local efforts, which include a "zero tolerance" for a break in sterility, except in a true emergency.

When determining vascular access that is required to appropriately manage a patient, consideration should be given to (1) the number of lumens required (there is some evidence suggesting that multilumen catheters are associated with an increased risk of infection); (2) the site of the catheter placement (femoral lines are associated with an increased risk of infection); and (3) discontinuation of the catheter as soon as it is no longer needed. Additional adjuncts to maintenance of central lines are the use of antiseptic-impregnated dressings of coated catheters, which may be considered locally.

POSTOPERATIVE NAUSEA AND VOMITING

Postoperative nausea and vomiting (PONV) continues to be one of the most common adverse events associated with anesthesia. Up to 80% of outpatients report nausea in the postanesthesia care unit, and 35% of these patients complain of PONV after discharge from the hospital. PONV may cause patient discomfort and distress, increased pain, wound dehiscence, increased risk of bleeding, increased risk of aspiration and airway compromise, and electrolyte disturbances. These complications considerably increase the cost of health care and often require unplanned hospital admission and prolonged duration of hospitalization.

The risk of PONV is directly related to patient factors, type of surgery, and type of anesthesia. Patient factors associated with increased risk include nonsmokers, females, and those with a history of motion sickness or PONV. Surgical procedures associated with increased risk include those involving the head and neck or breast, gynecologic, intra-abdominal, and laparoscopic. Procedures lasting longer than 3 hours confer additional risk. Anesthetic factors include general anesthesia, the use of volatile anesthetics and possibly nitrous oxide, and postoperative opioid analgesia. The incidence of PONV in patients with no risk factors is approximately 10%. Each risk factor increases the chance of PONV by 20%. Maximal antiemetic therapy may be targeted for those patients with significantly increased risk, whereas patients at lower risk may not warrant such aggressive prophylaxis. PONV protocols based on risk stratification allow rational delivery of costly antiemetic therapies to those patients who are expected to receive the greatest benefit from them while minimizing total health care costs.

Reduction of PONV is a desirable goal, but even with maximal therapy, elimination of PONV is impossible. Some hospitals may use this as a performance measure, but PONV reduction is unlikely to be incorporated into the Medicare plan at this time.

PERIOPERATIVE PAIN MANAGEMENT

The American Pain Society has promoted pain as "the fifth vital sign" in an effort to increase provider awareness of patient discomfort and promote early intervention. Physicians involved in perioperative patient care should have a basic understanding of the tools used to assess pain and the treatment modalities available to them. Every patient should have a thorough pain history included in the initial evaluation and a comprehensive analgesia strategy formulated on the basis of previous experience with analgesic medications, comorbid medical conditions, and baseline pain levels. Patient concerns and questions regarding the risk of addiction after using opioid analgesics should be addressed early, and additional education regarding administration of postoperative analgesia should be provided. Validated pain quantification systems such as the visual analog scale (VAS) should be administered perioperatively so that treatment efficacy may be ensured.

The analgesic plan for each patient should be influenced by patient factors, provider experience, and institutional resources. Multimodal strategies may provide the highest quality analgesia with fewest side effects. Nonnarcotic pharmacologic therapies include acetaminophen, nonsteroidal anti-inflammatory agents, and membrane-stabilizing agents such as gabapentin. Opioid agonists provide potent analgesia, but side effects are common, including pruritus, nausea, constipation, hypoventilation, and sedation. The use of local anesthetics via field block, nerve block, or neuraxial techniques may greatly reduce or eliminate the need for agents with troublesome side effects.

Patient-controlled analgesia (PCA) should be provided to patients expected to experience moderate to severe postoperative pain. Multiple studies have demonstrated improved patient satisfaction, reduced pain scores and nursing calls, and lower total analgesic usage in patients with PCA compared with intravenous or intramuscular as-needed dosing.

The TJC mandates that all patients have the right to appropriate assessment and management of pain. We must integrate effective pain management systems in our hospitals or risk loss of hospital accreditation. Collaborative efforts among providers can increase the safety and efficacy of these plans and allow maximal patient satisfaction.

CONCLUSION

The implementation of evidence-based best practices should be a priority in all institutions providing perioperative care for surgical patients, whether or not there are externally imposed regulations or incentives for their implementation. These goals require real team efforts, with shared responsibility for making sure they are achieved. System improvements, including introduction of automated reminders, implementation of interdisciplinary protocols, readily available reference material (e.g., appropriate antibiotic choices), and monitoring of results with timely feedback of performance and successes to the care team, can assist in making these practices part of routine, excellent patient care.

SUGGESTED READINGS

American Society of Anesthesiologists Task Force on Pain Management: Practice guidelines for acute pain management in the perioperative setting, *Anesthesiology* 100:1573, 2004.

Apfel CC, Roewer N: Risk assessment of postoperative nausea and vomiting, *Int Anesth Clin* 41(4):13, 2003.

Collard HR, Saint S, Matthay M: Prevention of ventilator-associated pneumonia: An evidence-based systematic review, *Ann Intern Med* 138:494, 2003.

Fleisher LA, Beckman JA, Brown KA, and others: ACC/AHA 2006 guideline update on perioperative cardiovascular evaluation for noncardiac surgery: Focused update on perioperative beta-blocker therapy: A report of the American College of Cardiology/American Heart Association Task Force on Practice Guidelines, *Circulation* 113(22):2662, 2006.

Geerts WH, Pineo GF, Heit JA, and others: Prevention of venous thromboembolism: The seventh ACCP Conference on Antithrombotic and Thrombolytic Therapy, *Chest* 126:338, 2004.

Lindenauer PK, Pekow P, Wong K, and others: Perioperative beta-blocker therapy and mortality after major noncardiac surgery, *N Engl J Med* 353:349, 2005.

Mermel LA: Prevention of intravascular catheter-related infections, *Ann Intern Med* 132:391, 2000.

The Surgical Care Improvement Project (SCIP): Available at http://www.medqic.org/scip.

SURGICAL SITE INFECTIONS

Meghan A. Arnold, MD, and Adrian Barbul, MD

Surgical site infections cause significant morbidity and mortality in the postoperative period and are the second most common nosocomial infection in the United States. Overall, approximately 25% of all nosocomial infections in hospitalized patients are surgical site infections. Among surgical patients, however, surgical site infections are the most common nosocomial infection and occur in 2.6% of all surgical procedures performed. Patients with surgical site infections are more likely to need admission to an intensive care unit (ICU), have a longer length of stay, and are more likely to die than their counterparts without surgical site infections. Rather than treating all operative patients with broad-spectrum antibiotics in an effort to decrease the prevalence of surgical site infections, however, the emergence of widespread antibiotic resistance has required a more judicious use of antimicrobial prophylaxis.

This chapter reviews the definition of a surgical site infection and summarizes the patient, environmental, and operative risk factors for infection. The microbiology of surgical site infections is briefly reviewed as it relates to key strategies and recommendations for the prevention and treatment of this complication. Finally, the morbidity and mortality that result from surgical site infections are summarized.

DEFINITIONS

The Center for Disease Control and Prevention (CDC) National Nosocomial Infections Surveillance System (NNIS) was established in 1970 and monitors the incidence of surgical site infections among acute care hospitals in the United States. In an effort to standardize reporting, the NNIS clearly defined characteristics that must be present for a diagnosis of surgical site infection (Table 1). This nomenclature allows for consistent reporting among physicians and hospitals, enabling a more

accurate portrayal of the prevalence, prevention, and treatment of surgical site infections.

According to the NNIS, surgical site infections must occur within 30 days after the primary procedure unless an implant was placed, in which case the time limit for a procedure-related infection is extended to 1 year. Once diagnosed, surgical site infections are divided into those involving the incision itself ("incisional") and those involving the deeper tissues ("organ/space") involved in the procedure. In the former category, incisional surgical site infections are further characterized as "superficial" (involving only the skin or subcutaneous tissue of the incision) or "deep" (involving the fascial and/or muscle layers of the incision). Most surgical site infections are of the superficial incisional type. Organ/space surgical site infections are infections that involve any part of the spaces entered during the procedure or any organ involved in the procedure. Surgical site infections that involve more than one level are differentially categorized—incisional surgical site infections that involve any part of the fascia or muscle are considered deep incisional, and an organ/space surgical site infection that drains through the incision is also considered a deep incisional infection.

RISK FACTORS

Risk factors for surgical site infections are those factors that have been shown to have a significant, independent association with the development of infection following a specific procedure. Factors that have been shown to influence the development of surgical site infections have typically been divided into those specific to the patient, the environment, and the operative procedure or technique (Table 2). Surgical site infections occur within this complex milieu in which host defense mechanisms—both systemic and local—must function adequately to prevent the progression of incisional bacterial colonization to frank infection. Bacterial colonization of surgical wounds is a prerequisite for surgical site infection, with an inoculum of 10^5 colony-forming units per square centimeter of wound surface required for impaired healing.

To stratify the specific risk of infection in the setting of a variety of the patient and operative characteristics mentioned earlier, numerous risk classification schemes have been proposed and used

Table 1: Criteria for Defining a Surgical Site Infection

Superficial Incisional SSI

Infection occurs within 30 days after the operation; *AND*

infection involves only skin or subcutaneous tissue of the incision; *AND at least ONE of the following*:

1. Purulent drainage, with or without laboratory confirmation, from the superficial incision

2. Organisms isolated from an aseptically obtained culture of fluid or tissue from the superficial incision

3. At least one of the following signs or symptoms of infection *AND* superficial incision is deliberately opened by surgeon, *UNLESS* incision is culture negative:
   a. Pain or tenderness
   b. Localized swelling
   c. Redness
   d. Heat

4. Diagnosis of superficial SSI by the surgeon or attending physician

DO NOT report any of the following as SSI:

1. Stitch abscess (minimal inflammation and discharge confined to the points of suture penetration)

2. Infection of an episiotomy or newborn circumcision site (different criteria are used for these infections)

3. Infected burn wound

4. Incision SSI that extends into the fascial and muscle layers (see deep incision SSI)

Deep Incisional SSI

1. Infection occurs within 30 days after the operation of no implant is left in place; *OR*

2. Infection occurs within 1 year if implant is in place and the infection appears to be related to the operation; *AND*

3. Infection involves deep tissues (e.g., fascial and muscle layers) of the incision; *AND at least ONE of the following:*

4. Purulent drainage from the deep incision but not from the organ/space component of the surgical site

5. A deep incision spontaneously dehisces or is deliberately opened by a surgeon when the patient has at least one of the following signs or symptoms, *UNLESS* site is culture-negative:
   a. Fever (>38 °C)
   b. Localized pain or tenderness

6. An abscess of other evidence of infection involving the deep incision is found on direct examination, during reoperation, or by histopathologic or radiographic examination

7. Diagnosis of a deep incisional SSI by a surgeon or attending physician

Notes:

Infection that involves both superficial and deep incision sites should be reported as deep incisional SSI

Report an organ/space SSI that drains through the incision as a deep incisional SSI

Organ/Space SSI

1. Infection occurs within 30 days after the operation if no implant is left in place; *OR*

2. Infection occurs within 1 year if implant is in place and the infection appears to be related to the operation; *AND*

3. Infection involves any part of the anatomy (e.g., organs or spaces), other than the incision, which was opened or manipulated during an operation; *AND at least ONE of the following:*
   a. Purulent drainage from a drain that is placed through a stab wound into the organ/space
   b. Organisms isolated from an aseptically obtained culture of fluid or tissue in the organ/space

4. An abscess or other evidence of infection involving the organ/space that is found on direct examination, during reoperation, or by histopathologic or radiographic examination

5. Diagnosis of an organ/space SSI by a surgeon or attending physician

SSI, Surgical site infection.

in clinical surgical practice. The simplest classification was developed by the National Research Council (NRC) and divides procedures into clean, clean/contaminated, contaminated, and dirty, on the basis of the amount of bacterial contamination expected to occur during normal practice (Table 3). Use of this classification system has revealed a direct relationship between the amount of bacterial contamination and the subsequent rate of surgical site infection. Because of its ease of use and clinical utility regarding the choice of antimicrobial prophylaxis, the NRC classification is the clinical tool most widely used by surgeons today. A more complex classification scheme was developed by the NNIS and incorporates the NRC incision categories with the type of operation being performed, the patient's American Society of Anesthesiology class, and other factors that have been shown to influence the development of postoperative surgical infections (Table 4). This system, initially developed in the 1970s using a prospective analysis of voluntarily collected data from 60 hospitals across the United States, sought to identify the incidence, risk factors, and pathogens responsible for

Table 2: Risk Factors for Surgical Site Infection

Patient Characteristics	Operative Characteristics	Environmental Characteristics
Extremes of age	Preoperative antiseptic showering	Ventilation
Obesity	Preoperative hair removal	Routine cleaning of environmental surfaces
Nicotine use	Preoperative skin preparation	Sterilization of surgical instruments
Diabetes mellitus	Duration of preoperative scrub	Surgical attire and drapes
Malnutrition	Preoperative arm/forearm antisepsis	
Length of preoperative hospitalization	Management of infected or colonized surgical personnel	
Altered immune response	Antimicrobial prophylaxis	
Preoperative nares colonization with Staphylococcus aureus	Duration of procedure	
Concurrent infection in a remote body site	Foreign material in the surgical site	
	Surgical drains	
	Inadequate hemostasis	
	Failure to obliterate dead space	
	Tissue trauma	

Table 3: National Research Council Surgical Wound Classification

Class I/Clean

An uninfected operative wound with no inflammation

The respiratory, alimentary, genital, or uninfected urinary tract is not entered

Wound is primarily closed and, if necessary, drained with closed drainage

Includes operative incisional wounds that follow nonpenetrating (blunt) trauma

Class II/Clean-Contaminated

The respiratory, alimentary, genital, or urinary tracts are entered without unusual contamination

Operations involving the biliary tract, appendix, vagina, and oropharynx are included in this category

No evidence of infection or major break in technique is encountered

Class III/Contaminated

Open, fresh, accidental wounds

Operations with major breaks in sterile technique

Gross spillage from the gastrointestinal tract

Incisions with acute, nonpurulent inflammation

Class IV/Dirty-Infected

Old traumatic wounds with devitalized tissue or retained foreign material

Wounds with existing clinical infection/purulence

Perforated viscera

Table 4: National Nosocomial Infections Surveillance Risk Index for Surgical Site Infections

Operation Class	NNIS Risk Index (%)				Overall
	0	1	2	3	
Clean	1.0	2.3	5.4	–	2.1
Clean/contaminated	2.1	4.9	9.5	–	3.3
Contaminated	–	3.4	6.6	13.2	6.4
Dirty	–	3.1	8.1	12.8	7.1
Overall	1.5	2.9	6.8	13.0	2.8

The surveillance system has since expanded to include more than 300 hospitals, and the initial factors identified continue to accurately predict risk for nosocomial infection. The NNIS data have also clearly shown that the risk of developing a surgical site infection is directly proportional to the bacterial contamination of the wound and the number of risk factors present.

Patient-related factors that have been definitively shown to increase the risk of postoperative infection include diabetes mellitus, nicotine use, prolonged hospitalization before surgery, and being a preoperative carrier of *Staphylococcus aureus*. Diabetes has both short- and long-term effects on the risks of surgical site infections. Individuals with higher HbA1c levels have been shown to have increased surgical site infections following coronary artery bypass grafting. Glucose levels greater than 200 mg/dL in the first 48 hours following surgery may also be associated with an increased risk of postoperative infection. Nicotine retards wound healing and may consequently increase the likelihood of developing a surgical site infection. Likewise, current smoking is an independent risk factor for the development of a mediastinal or sternal infection following cardiac surgery. Carriers of *S. aureus* are at least twice as likely to develop a postoperative staphylococcal infection as are noncarriers. Given that approximately 30% of the population normally harbors this organism, the scope of the potential problem cannot be underestimated. Although mupirocin ointment eradicates *S. aureus* from the nares of colonized individuals, a randomized controlled trial recently demonstrated that although the administration of prophylactic mupirocin to *S. aureus* carriers decreased the rate of all nosocomial infections due to *S. aureus* in that population, prophylaxis did not reduce the rate of *S. aureus* surgical site infections, regardless of carrier status.

hospital-acquired infections. Points are assigned to patients according to presence of any of the following (one point each):

- A contaminated or dirty infection, NRC class
- A procedure that lasts 75% longer than all other operations of the same type
- An ASA class of 3 or greater

MICROBIOLOGY

The microbiology characteristic of surgical site infections has not changed dramatically since the mid 1980s (Table 5). Whereas gram-positive organisms tend to be the most common pathogens isolated from surgical site infections, procedures with any level of contamination are more likely to be complicated by infections with gram-negative organisms (Table 6). Regardless of the pathogen,

Table 5: Distribution of Pathogens Isolated from Surgical Site Infections*

Pathogen	Percentage of Isolates	
	1986–1989 (n = 16,727)	1990–1996 (n = 17,671)
Staphylococcus aureus	17	20
Coagulase-negative staphylococci	12	14
Enterococcus species	13	12
Escherichia coli	10	8
Pseudomonas aeruginosa	8	8
Enterobacter species	8	7
Proteus mirabilis	4	3
Klebsiella pneumoniae	3	3
Other Streptococcus species	3	3
Candida albicans	2	3
Group D streptococci (non-enterococci)	–	2
Other gram-positive aerobes	–	2
Bacteroides fragilis	–	2

*National Nosocomial Infections Surveillance, 1986–1996.

Table 6: Common Pathogens Isolated from Surgical Site Infections, by Operative Site

Operative Site	Common Pathogens
Gastrointestinal	
Oropharynx	Staphylococcus aureus, Bacteroides (except B. fragilis), peptostreptococci, Fusobacterium
Esophagus, gastroduodenal	Gram-negative bacilli, streptococci, Bacteroides (except B. fragilis), peptostreptococci
Hepatobiliary	Gram-negative bacilli, enterococci, Clostridia
Colorectal, small intestine, appendix	Gram-negative bacilli, B. fragilis, anaerobes
Gynecologic	Gram-negative bacilli, enterococci, anaerobes
Orthopedic	S. aureus, coagulase-negative staphylococci, gram-negative bacilli
Thoracic	S. aureus, Streptococcus pneumoniae, coagulase-negative staphylococci, gram-negative bacilli
Cardiovascular	S. aureus, coagulase-negative staphylococci
Urologic	Gram-negative bacilli

however, most surgical site infections are caused by the individual's endogenous bacteria. These endogenous organisms are influenced by the patient's concurrent medical condition (severe illness, immunocompromised state) and the necessity for prolonged hospitalization before a surgical procedure. Patients who have been hospitalized for as little as 48 to 72 hours begin to exhibit changes in their endogenous flora that are more representative of nosocomial and resistant pathogens.

An increasing number of surgical site infections are caused by antimicrobial-resistant pathogens. Methicillin-resistant *S. aureus* (MRSA) and resistant strains of *Candida albicans* have become prevalent, particularly among chronically ill and debilitated patients. MRSA, which was first identified in 1961, is ubiquitous in hospitals, with a prevalence of more than 50% among patients in intensive care units. Hospital-acquired MRSA infection is most likely in patients who require prolonged hospitalization, ICU patients, patients on prolonged antimicrobial therapy, and patients who undergo surgical procedures. Even though it is generally assumed that MRSA has had a negative impact on clinical outcomes, not all studies have been confirmatory. Regardless, knowledge of a specific institution's MRSA prevalence will aid in the prompt and appropriate treatment of surgical site infections.

PREVENTION AND ANTIMICROBIAL PROPHYLAXIS

The prevention of surgical site infections requires a multipronged approach. The Centers for Disease Control and Prevention published guidelines for the prevention of surgical site infection in 1999 (Table 7). These guidelines, which consist of category I and II evidence from experimental and nonexperimental studies, cover the important aspects of surgical site infection prevention—preoperative, intraoperative, and postoperative care of the patient, the use of appropriate antimicrobial prophylaxis, management of surgical and operating room staff, and guidelines for surgical site infection surveillance.

Current recommendations for antimicrobial prophylaxis emphasize a minimalist approach because widespread resistance, adverse events following administration, increased costs of hospitalization, and an increased chance for medical errors are the often underemphasized consequences of irrational antibiotic use. Single-dose prophylaxis with a first- or second-generation cephalosporin is typically adequate for most procedures (Table 8). Effective prophylaxis requires that adequate tissue levels of the drug be achieved before the procedure has begun—60 minutes for cephalosporins and 120 minutes for vancomycin or fluoroquinolones—and that they be maintained throughout the duration of the case. Antibiotics should be redosed if the operation continues beyond two half-lives after the first dose of the drug. An easier rule of thumb to follow is that redosing should be considered if the operation takes longer than 3 hours or if the blood loss exceeds 1.5 L. A preponderance of scientific evidence supports the conclusion that, for most procedures, continuing antibiotic prophylaxis after wound closure is unnecessary and may, in fact, be detrimental through increased nosocomial bloodstream infections, increased emergence of MRSA, and an increased risk of developing *Clostridium difficile* colitis. Exceptions to single-dose prophylaxis include vascular and cardiac cases, in which prophylaxis is recommended for 24 hours.

Recommendations for bacterial endocarditis prophylaxis have been simplified with the recognition that most cases of endocarditis are not caused by invasive interventions. Patients with mitral valve prolapse and a midsystolic click without thickened valve leaflets or regurgitation no longer require prophylaxis. In addition, it is no longer recommended that patients with pacemakers and defibrillators and those with an isolated atrial septal defect receive prophylaxis. The use of prophylaxis should be determined on a case-by-case basis according to the patient's cardiac risk and the risk of the procedure (Table 9).

Table 7: Guidelines for the Prevention of Surgical Site Infection*

Preparation of the Patient

1. Whenever possible, identify and treat all infections remote to the surgical site before elective operation and postpone elective operations on patients with remote site infections until the infection has resolved. *Category IA*

2. Do not remove hair preoperatively unless the hair at or around the incision site will interfere with the operation. *Category IA*

3. If hair is removed, remove immediately before the operation, preferably with electric clippers. *Category IA*

4. Adequately control serum blood glucose levels in all diabetic patients and particularly avoid hyperglycemia postoperatively. *Category IB*

5. Encourage tobacco cessation. At minimum, instruct patients to abstain for at least 30 days before elective operation from smoking cigarettes, cigars, pipes, or any other form of tobacco consumption (e.g., chewing/dipping). *Category IB*

6. Do not withhold necessary blood products from surgical patients as a means to prevent SSI. *Category IB*

7. Require patients to shower or bathe with an antiseptic agent on at least the night before the operative day. *Category IB*

8. Thoroughly wash and clean at and around the incision site to remove gross contamination before performing antiseptic skin preparation. *Category IB*

9. Use an appropriate antiseptic agent for skin preparation. *Category IB*

10. Apply preoperative antiseptic skin preparation in concentric circles moving toward the periphery. The prepared area must be large enough to extend the incision or create new incisions or drain sites, if necessary. *Category IB*

11. Keep preoperative hospital stay as short as possible while allowing for adequate preoperative preparation of the patient. *Category II*

Hand/Forearm Antisepsis for Surgical Team Members

1. Keep nails short and do not wear artificial nails. *Category IB*

2. Perform a preoperative surgical scrub for at least 2 to 5 minutes using an appropriate antiseptic. Scrub the hands and forearms to the elbow. *Category IB*

3. After performing the surgical scrub, keep hands up and away from the body (elbows in flexed position) so that water runs from the tips of the fingers toward the elbow. Dry hands with a sterile towel and don a sterile gown and gloves. *Category IB*

4. Clean underneath each fingernail prior to performing the first surgical scrub of the day. *Category II*

5. Do not wear hand or arm jewelry. *Category II*

6. No recommendation on wearing nail polish. *Category II*

Management of Infected or Colonized Surgical Personnel

1. Educate and encourage surgical personnel who have signs and symptoms of a transmissible infectious illness to report conditions promptly to their supervisory and occupational health service personnel. *Category IB*

2. Develop well-defined policies concerning patient-care responsibilities when personnel have potentially transmissible infectious condition. These policies should govern (a) personnel responsibility in using the health service and reporting illness, (b) work restrictions, and (c) clearance to resume work after an illness that required work restriction. The policies should identify persons who have the authority to remove personnel from duty. *Category IB*

3. Obtain appropriate cultures from, and exclude from duty, surgical personnel who have draining skin lesions until infection has been ruled out or personnel have received adequate therapy and infection has resolved. *Category IB*

4. Do not routinely exclude surgical personnel who are colonized with organisms such as *S. aureus* (nose, hands, or other body site) or group A *Streptococcus*, unless such personnel have been linked epidemiologically to dissemination of the organism in the health care setting. *Category IB*

Antimicrobial Prophylaxis

1. Administer a prophylactic antimicrobial agent only when indicated, and select it based on its efficacy against the most common pathogens causing surgical site infection (SSI) for a specific operation and published recommendations. *Category IA*

2. Administer by the intravenous route the initial dose of prophylactic antimicrobial agent, timed such that a bactericidal concentration of the drug is established in serum and tissues when the incision is made. Maintain therapeutic levels of the agent in serum and tissues throughout the operation and until, at most, a few hours after the incision is closed in the operating room. *Category IA*

3. Before elective colorectal operations, mechanically prepare the colon by use of enemas and cathartic agents. Administer nonabsorbable oral antimicrobial agents in divided doses on the day before the operation. *Category IA*

4. For high-risk cesarean section, administer the prophylactic antimicrobial agent immediately after the umbilical cord is clamped. *Category IA*

5. Do not routinely use vancomycin for antimicrobial prophylaxis. *Category IB*

Surgical Attire and Drapes

1. Wear a surgical mask that fully covers the mouth and nose when entering the operating room if an operation is about to begin or is already under way, or if sterile instruments are exposed. Wear the mask throughout the operation. *Category IB*

2. Wear a cap or hood to fully cover hair on the head and face when entering the operating room. *Category IB*

3. Do not wear shoe covers for prevention of SSI. *Category IB*

4. Wear sterile gloves if a scrubbed surgical team member. Put on gloves after donning a sterile gown. *Category IB*

5. Use surgical gowns and drapes that are effective barriers when wet (i.e., materials that resist liquid penetration). *Category IB*

6. Change scrub suits that are visibly soiled, contaminated, and/or penetrated by blood or other potentially infectious materials. *Category IB*

Asepsis and Surgical Technique

1. Adhere to principles of asepsis when placing intravascular devices (e.g., central venous catheters), spinal or epidural anesthesia catheters, or when dispensing and administering intravenous drugs. *Category IA*

2. Handle tissues gently, maintain effective hemostasis, minimize devitalized tissue and foreign bodies (i.e., sutures, charred tissues, necrotic debris), and eradicate dead space at the surgical site. *Category IB*

3. Use delayed primary closure or leave an incision open to heal by secondary intention if the surgeon considers the surgical site to be heavily contaminated (e.g., class III and class IV). *Category IB*

4. If drainage is necessary, use a closed-suction drain. Place a drain through a separate incision distant from the operative incision. Remove the drain as soon as possible. *Category IB*

Postoperative Incision Care

1. Incisions that have been closed primarily should be protected with a sterile dressing for 24 to 48 hours postoperatively. *Category IB*

2. Wash hands before and after dressing changes and any contact with the surgical site. *Category IB*

3. When an incision dressing must be changed, use sterile technique. *Category II*

4. Educate the patient and family regarding proper incision care, symptoms of SSI, and the need to report such symptoms. *Category II*

Surveillance

1. Use Centers for Disease Control and Prevention definitions of SSI without modification for identifying SSI among surgical patients and outpatients. *Category IB*

2. For inpatient case finding (including readmissions), use direct prospective observation, indirect prospective detection, or a combination of both direct and indirect methods for the duration of the patient's hospitalization. *Category IB*

3. When postdischarge surveillance is performed for detecting SSI following certain operations (e.g., coronary artery bypass graft), use a method that accommodates available resources and data needs. *Category II*

4. For outpatient case finding, use a method that accommodates available resources and data needs. *Category IB*

5. Assign the surgical wound classification upon completion of an operation. A surgical team member should make the assignment. *Category II*

6. For each patient undergoing an operation chosen for surveillance, record those variables shown to be associated with increased SSI risk (e.g., surgical wound class, ASA class, and duration of operation). *Category IB*

7. Periodically calculate operation-specific SSI rates stratified by variables shown to be associated with increased SSI risk (e.g., National Nosocomial Infections Surveillance risk index). *Category IB*

8. Report appropriately stratified, operation-specific SSI rates to surgical team members. The optimum frequency and format for such rate computations will be determined by stratified case load sizes (denominators) and the objectives of local, continuous quality improvement initiatives. *Category IB*

*Centers for Disease Control and Prevention, 1999.

DIAGNOSIS AND TREATMENT

Surgical site infections tend to present in the week following a procedure but can be diagnosed up to 30 days after the operation. In patients in whom an implant is placed, the diagnosis can be made up to 1 year following the initial procedure. The signs and symptoms of incisional surgical site infections include fever, incisional tenderness, erythema, and swelling. Drainage, fluctuance, or an elevated white blood cell count may not be present. Deep-tissue infections are characterized by fever, pain, erythema, swelling, and purulence with or without tissue necrosis.

Opening and cleaning the wound is the basic tenet in the treatment of surgical site infections. Specifically, staples and sutures are removed, the wound is opened to its fullest extent, and any purulent drainage or devitalized tissue is removed. If this is done properly, often only simple wound care two to four times daily is required for treatment and resolution of the infection. Severe cellulitis of the overlying skin or necrosis of the wound bed is an indicator of more severe infection requiring antimicrobial therapy. The choice of empirical therapy should be guided by the severity of the infection and the procedure it follows (Table 10). Routine swabs of affected skin or wound drainage are not recommended to guide antimicrobial therapy because contamination with skin flora is exceedingly high. If cultures are necessary for therapy, tissue specimens or an aseptic sample of pus is required for appropriate analysis.

Surgical site infections caused by *Clostridium perfringens* or *Streptococcus pneumoniae* (group A β-hemolytic *Streptococcus*) require special mention because they may occur within 2 days of surgery and are particularly aggressive. Wounds infected with these organisms are characterized by serous drainage with few overlying skin changes, and may progress quickly to a life-threatening, soft-tissue infection. In addition to antibiotic treatment, surgical debridement is the mainstay of therapy.

Table 8: Recommended Surgical Antimicrobial Prophylaxis, by Procedure

General Surgery

Colon Surgery or Whipple Procedure

Neomycin and erythromycin (or metronidazole), 1 g each PO at 1, 2, 11 PM day prior to surgery

Ampicillin/sulbactam 3 g IV preoperatively

Penicillin allergy: clindamycin 600 mg IV *AND* gentamicin 1.5–3.0 mg/kg IV preoperatively

Cholecystectomy (Open or Laparoscopic)

Prophylaxis only recommended for the following patients: age >60, previous biliary surgery, acute symptoms, jaundice

Ampicillin/sulbactam 3 g IV Preoperatively

Penicillin allergy: clindamycin 600 mg IV ± gentamicin 1.5–3.0 mg/kg IV preoperatively

Appendectomy (Uncomplicated)

Ampicillin/sulbactam 3 g IV preoperatively

Penicillin allergy: clindamycin 600 mg IV preoperatively

Appendectomy (Complicated)

Treat as peritonitis

Penetrating Abdominal Trauma

Ampicillin/sulbactam 3 g IV preoperatively; continue 3 g IV q6 hours for 24 hours

Penicillin allergy: clindamycin 600 mg IV *AND* gentamicin 1.5–3.0 mg/kg IV preoperatively

Inguinal Hernia Repair (Uncomplicated)

Prophylaxis not recommended

Inguinal Hernia Repair (Uncomplicated, Recurrent or Emergent)

Ampicillin/sulbactam 3 g IV preoperatively

Penicillin allergy: clindamycin 600 mg IV ± gentamicin 1.5–3.0 mg/kg IV preoperatively

Mastectomy

No prophylaxis recommended

Thoracic Surgery

Esophageal Procedures

Ampicillin/sulbactam 3 g IV preoperatively

Penicillin allergy: clindamycin 600 mg IV preoperatively

All Cases Except Esophageal

Cefazolin 2 g IV preoperatively

Penicillin allergy: clindamycin 600 mg IV preoperatively

Gynecologic Surgery

Cesarean Section (Uncomplicated)

No prophylaxis necessary

Cesarean Section (Complicated)

After cord clamping: cefazolin 2 g IV *OR* metronidazole 500 mg IV

Penicillin allergy: clindamycin 600 mg IV after cord clamping

Hysterectomy (Abdominal or Vaginal)

Ampicillin/sulbactam 3 g IV preoperatively

Penicillin allergy: clindamycin 600 mg IV preoperatively

Repair of Cystocele or Rectocele

Ampicillin/sulbactam 3 g IV preoperatively

Penicillin allergy: clindamycin 600 mg IV preoperatively

Dilatation and Curettage (Uncomplicated)

no prophylaxis necessary

Dilatation and Curettage (Complicated)

Cefazolin 2 g IV preoperatively

Penicillin allergy: clindamycin 600 mg IV preoperatively

Orthopedic Surgery

Open Reduction of Fracture

Cefazolin 2 g IV preoperatively, continue for 24 hours for closed hip fractures

Penicillin allergy: vancomycin 1 g IV preoperatively, continue for 24 hours

Open Fracture

Cefazolin 2 g IV q8 hours for 18 days

Joint Replacement

Cefazolin 2 g IV preoperatively

Penicillin allergy: vancomycin 1 g IV preoperatively *OR* clindamycin 600 mg IV

Lower Limb Amputation

Ampicillin/sulbactam 3 g IV preoperatively

Penicillin allergy: gentamicin 1.5–3.0 mg/kg IV *AND* clindamycin 600 mg IV preoperatively

Spinal Fusion

Cefazolin 2 g IV preoperatively

Penicillin allergy: vancomycin 1 g IV preoperatively

Arthroscopic Surgery

No data support prophylaxis

Laminectomy

Cefazolin 2 g IV preoperatively

Penicillin allergy: clindamycin 600 mg IV preoperatively

Urologic Surgery

Transperitoneal Prostate Biopsy, Urethral Dilatation

No prophylaxis needed if urine sterile

Prostatectomy (TURP or Peritoneal)

Sterile urine

Gatifloxacin 400 mg IV preoperatively only if patient is considered high-risk

Radical, Retropubic Prostatectomy

Cefazolin 2 g IV preoperatively

Penicillin allergy: clindamycin 600 mg IV preoperatively

Nephrectomy

Cefazolin 2g IV preoperatively

Penicillin allergy: clindamycin 600 mg IV preoperatively

Radical Cystoprostatectomy OR Anterior Exenteration

Ampicillin/sulbactam 3 g IV preoperatively

Penicillin allergy: gatifloxacin 400 mg IV preoperatively

Head and Neck Surgery

Major Procedure with Incision of Oral or Pharyngeal Mucosa

Clindamycin 600 mg IV ± gentamicin 1.5–3.0 mg/kg IV preoperatively

Alternative: cefuroxime 1.5 g IV preoperatively

Tonsillectomy, Rhinoplasty

No data support prophylaxis

Cardiac Surgery and Cardiac Procedures

Median Sternotomy

Cefazolin 2 g IV preoperatively and q2 hours intraoperatively; continue for 24 hours after procedure

Penicillin allergy: vancomycin 1 g IV preoperatively, continue for 24 hours

LVAD/BIVAD Placement

Vancomycin 1 g IV *AND* gatifloxacin 400 mg IV/PO *AND* fluconazole 400 mg IV/PO preoperatively; continue for 48 hours postoperatively

Pacemaker Placement

Cefazolin 2 g IV preoperatively

Penicillin allergy: clindamycin 600 mg IV preoperatively

Vascular Surgery

Any Procedure Except Carotid Procedure

Cefazolin 2 g IV preoperatively

Penicillin allergy: vancomycin 1 g IV preoperatively

Carotid Procedure

Prophylaxis not necessary unless risk of infection thought to be high

Neurosurgery

Craniotomy (Including Shunt Placement)

Cefazolin 2 g IV preoperatively

Penicillin allergy: clindamycin 600 mg IV preoperatively and one dose 4 hours later

Endoscopic Procedure

PEG Tube Placement

Ampicillin/sulbactam 3 g IV preoperatively

Penicillin allergy: clindamycin 600 mg IV *AND* gentamicin 1.5–3.0 mg/kg IV preoperatively

Interventional Radiology Procedures

Biliary procedures

Ampicillin/sulbactam 3 g IV preoperatively

Penicillin allergy: gatifloxacin 400 mg IV *AND* metronidazole 500 mg IV preoperatively

Urologic Procedures

Gatifloxacin 400 mg IV preoperatively

Placement of Implantable Access Port

Cefazolin 2 g IV preoperatively

Penicillin allergy: clindamycin 600 mg IV preoperatively

Placement of Tunneled Catheter

Prophylaxis not indicated

IV, Intravenously; *LVAD/BIVAD,* left ventricle assist device/biventricular assist device; *PO,* by mouth; *q,* every x hours.

▌ MORBIDITY AND MORTALITY

Surgical site infections have a dramatic impact on the morbidity and mortality of affected individuals. Whereas the mortality rate attributable to surgical site infections is less than 5%, when surgical patients with nosocomial surgical site infection die, a majority of deaths are attributable to the infection. Most deaths occur following organ/space infection.

The morbidity associated with surgical site infection is more difficult to quantify. Whereas superficial incisional infections may increase the length of hospitalization by only a few days, organ/space infections may result in a prolonged hospitalization and the need for additional procedures. In 2004, surgical site infections increased hospital length of stay an average of 6.5 days. Finally, individuals with substantial wounds following debridement may require discharge to a nursing facility or daily home visits by a skilled wound care nurse.

Table 9: Guidelines for Prophylaxis Against Bacterial Endocarditis

		Cardiac Risk	
Procedure Risk	High		Intermediate
High	Recommended		Recommended
Low	Unclear—use clinical judgment		Not recommended

Dental, Upper Respiratory Tract, Esophageal Procedures

Amoxicillin 2 g PO 1 hour before procedure

Penicillin allergy: clindamycin 600 mg PO *OR* clarithromycin 500 mg PO 1 hour before procedure

Gastrointestinal (Except Esophageal) or Genitourinary Procedures

High risk condition *AND* high risk procedure

Ampicillin 2 g IV *AND* gentamicin 1.5 mg/kg (not to exceed 120 mg) IV 1 hour before procedure

Penicillin allergy: vancomycin 1 g IV *AND* gentamicin 1.5 mg/kg (not to exceed 120 mg) IV 1 hour before procedure

Intermediate risk condition AND high risk procedure

Amoxicillin 2 g PO 1 hour before procedure

Penicillin allergy: vancomycin 1 g IV

IV, Intravenously; *PO,* by mouth.

Table 10: Empirical Therapy for Surgical Site Infection

Infection after Clean Procedures

Oxacillin 1–2 g IV q4 hours *OR* cefazolin 1 g IV q8 hours

Penicillin allergy: clindamycin 600 mg IV q8 hours

Infection after Contaminated Procedures

Patient not on broad-spectrum antibiotics at time of surgery and not severely ill

Cefoxitin 1 g IV q6 hours

Penicillin allergy: gatifloxacin 400 mg IV/PO q24 hours *AND* clindamycin 600 mg IV q8 hours

Patient on broad-spectrum antibiotics at time of surgery or severely ill

Piperacillin/tazobactam 3.375 g IV q6 hours

Penicillin allergy: gatifloxacin 400 mg IV/PO q24 hours *AND* clindamycin 600 mg IV q8 hours

Patient severely ill *AND/OR* deep fascia involvement—treat as necrotizing fasciitis

Operative Intervention

Piperacillin/tazobactam 3.375 g IV q6 hours *OR* cefepime 1 g IV q12 hours *WITH* clindamycin 600 mg IV q8 hours

Penicillin allergy: gatifloxacin 400 mg IV q24 hours *AND* clindamycin 600 mg IV q8 hours *OR* metronidazole 500 mg IV q8 hours

IV, Intravenously; *PO,* by mouth; *q,* every x hours.

CONCLUSION

Despite advances in operative technique and postoperative care, surgical site infections remain a common problem. Adherence to accepted guidelines for appropriate antimicrobial prophylaxis is essential to decrease the incidence of surgical site infection. Prompt recognition and proper treatment of surgical site infections requires an understanding of the risk factors involved and the microbiology characteristic of the disease.

SUGGESTED READINGS

Barie PS: Modern surgical antibiotic prophylaxis and therapy—Less is more, *Surg Infect* 1(1):23, 2000.
Barie PS, Eachempati SR: Surgical site infections, *Surg Clin N Am* 85:1115, 2005.
Bratzler DW, Houck PM, for the Surgical Infection Prevention Guidelines Writers Workgroup: Antimicrobial prophylaxis for surgery: An Advisory statement from the National Surgical Infection Prevention Project, *Clin Infect Dis* 38:1706, 2004.
Mangram AJ, Horan TC, Pearson ML, and others: Guideline for prevention of surgical site infection, 1999, Hospital Infection Control Practices Advisory Committee, *Infect Control Hosp Epidemiol* 20:250, 1999.

INTRA-ABDOMINAL INFECTIONS

Rahima Nenshi, MD, and John C. Marshall, MD

The spectrum of intra-abdominal infection encompasses a diverse and complicated group of disorders, from relatively benign processes such as acute appendicitis and cholecystitis to life-threatening conditions such as diffuse peritonitis and intestinal infarction. Their clinical presentation is equally diverse. Intra-abdominal infection in the ambulatory patient characteristically presents with the clinical manifestations of an acute abdomen; in contrast, in the hospitalized patient, the clinical picture evolves insidiously and atypically, often with unexplained organ dysfunction as the first sign. The degree of associated physiologic derangement is also variable: for patients whose clinical deterioration is severe enough to merit intensive care unit (ICU) admission, the mortality rate of intra-abdominal infection may be as high as 50%.

With the widespread availability of computed tomography (CT) scanning and increasing radiologic expertise in interventional procedures, the surgical management of intra-abdominal infections has changed significantly. However, the underlying management principles remain the same: timely recognition of the clinical syndrome, rapid initiation of appropriate antibiotics, and prompt anatomic diagnosis and effective source control, which may or may not include operative intervention. Prompt and adequate resuscitation, accompanied by successful source control and appropriate systemic antibiotic therapy, can attenuate the symptoms of acute inflammation, minimize the development of new organ dysfunction, and significantly reduce the risk of major morbidity and mortality.

PATHOGENESIS

Although the clinical presentation of intra-abdominal infection is variable, its pathogenesis reflects a characteristic series of events: passage of microorganisms from the lumen of the gastrointestinal (GI) tract into the peritoneal cavity, activation of local peritoneal defense mechanisms, and secondary induction of a systemic inflammatory response to the local infection and its physiologic sequelae.

The peritoneal cavity is a closed potential space created by a single layer of mesothelial cells that covers the abdominal viscera and reflects onto the anterior abdominal wall. Under normal conditions, the peritoneal cavity contains 50 to 100 ml of peritoneal fluid, including cells of the innate immune system—specifically macrophages, mast cells, and lymphocytes. Inflammatory stimuli within the peritoneal cavity trigger the exudation of a protein-rich

fluid, and the expression of tissue factor on the surface of peritoneal macrophages results in the deposition of fibrin around the inflammatory focus. Local activation of coagulation produces both the wall of an abscess and the fibrinous adhesions evident at laparotomy conducted for an acute abdomen. The inflammatory process also results in activation of the sympathetic nervous system, and in suppression of intestinal peristalsis, resulting in the clinical condition known as *ileus*. It is for this reason that one of the earliest clinical signs of intra-abdominal infection in ICU patients may be an increase in postfeed residuals. Because absorption through the wall of the bowel is impaired, fluid may be sequestered in the lumen of the gut, further aggravating a state of systemic hypovolemia triggered by systemic vasodilatation and increased capillary permeability. Impaired splanchnic perfusion further compromises function of the intestinal barrier and promotes bacterial translocation from the gut lumen into the peritoneal space.

Intra-abdominal infection commonly arises as a consequence of a mechanical disruption of the GI tract, with spillage of indigenous gut flora into the peritoneal space. Therefore, the presence of specific microbes often suggests the anatomic source of infection. For example, the stomach and proximal small bowel are sparsely colonized with gram-positive bacteria. The numbers and diversity of microorganisms increase with progression along the GI tract. The distal small bowel is populated predominately by gram-negative organisms, whereas in the colon, anaerobes vastly outnumber aerobes, and in excess of 500 distinct microbial species constitute the normal flora. However, because obtaining the results of cultures of an infectious focus can often take several days, specific microbial identification of bacteria is rarely used to guide initial antibiotic therapy. Nevertheless, it is important, particularly in the case of recurrent or nosocomial infection, to obtain reliable culture data to guide the rational selection of antimicrobial agents.

CLASSIFICATION

Intra-abdominal infections can be classified both anatomically and by mode of bacterial infection. An anatomic classification differentiates infections within the peritoneal cavity from those arising in the retroperitoneum and further classifies them with respect to viscus whose disruption is responsible for the bacterial spillage (Table 1). Such infections may result in a localized abscess or in diffuse peritonitis.

Peritonitis can also be classified as *primary*, *secondary*, or *tertiary* (see below). Independent of the classification used, the mortality risk is directly related to the extent of organ dysfunction at the time of diagnosis and treatment.

Primary peritonitis develops spontaneously in the absence of an anatomic breach of the GI tract. It is characteristically diagnosed in previously stable cirrhotic patients who develop otherwise unexplained acute deterioration. Peritoneal infection arises as a result of translocation of organisms from the gut lumen into the

Table 1: Intra-abdominal Infection: An Anatomic Classification

Anatomic Site	Example
Retroperitoneal	Infected peripancreatic necrosis/pseudocyst
	Pyelonephritis/abscess
	Psoas abscess
	Retroperitoneal perforation of GI tract
Intraperitoneal	Perforated gastric/duodenal ulcer
	Acute cholecystitis
	Cholangitis
	Small bowel perforation/infarction
	Appendicitis/appendiceal abscess
	Typhlitis
	Colonic perforation/infarction
	Diverticulitis/abscess
	Anastomotic leak
	Postoperative abscess
Pelvic	Tubo-ovarian abscess/PID
	Endometritis
	Prostatic abscess

GI, Gastrointestinal; *PID*, pelvic inflammatory disease.

peritoneal cavity, a consequence, in turn, of proximal gut microbial overgrowth and decreased antimicrobial activity of the ascitic fluid. The diagnosis is established by abdominal paracentesis and assessment of the ascitic fluid, which yields greater than 500 white cells/mm^3, increased lactate, and/or reduced glucose. Primary peritonitis is typically monomicrobial. Its management is supportive, based on antibiotic therapy directed against the bacteria most commonly encountered in a given geographic area, typically gram-negative aerobes and enterococci. Therapy is titrated to reduce the ascitic fluid polymorphonuclear leukocyte count to less than 250 cells per milliliter by 48 hours.

Secondary peritonitis arises as a consequence of a mechanical breach of the GI tract. The flora involved is typically polymicrobial and reflects the patterns of colonization of the involved level of the GI tract. The characteristic clinical presentation of secondary peritonitis is as abdominal pain with classic signs of peritoneal irritation on physical examination (either localized or diffuse). Diffuse pain suggests generalized peritonitis, whereas localized peritonitis usually suggests a walled-off process arising from an organ in the immediate anatomic vicinity (as is seen, for example, when rebound tenderness is elicited over McBurney's point in patients with acute appendicitis). The clinical presentation may be subtle in the older or hospitalized patient with concomitant illness, in whom the only sign of infection may be new onset, and otherwise unexplained organ dysfunction. Shortness of breath on the third day following a complex, elective, intra-abdominal procedure, for example, should suggest the possibility of a surgical complication producing intra-abdominal infection, before the diagnosis of pulmonary embolism is entertained.

The most common causes of secondary bacterial peritonitis in the ambulatory patient presenting de novo to the emergency department include perforation of a peptic ulcer (either gastric or duodenal), strangulating obstruction of the small bowel or acute enteric ischemia, acute appendicitis, acute diverticulitis, and infections of the biliary tree—either cholecystitis or cholangitis. A careful history and physical examination, combined with carefully selected radiographic imaging studies, usually establishes the diagnosis.

In the hospitalized patient, the most common causes of secondary peritonitis are postoperative complications and anastomotic leaks. Risk factors for an anastomotic leak include tension on the suture line, hematoma at the suture line, ischemia related to widespread vascular disease, devascularization of the bowel at the site of

the anastomosis, and technical errors in the creation of the anastomosis. Collections of bile or blood within the peritoneal cavity favor bacterial proliferation and contribute to postoperative intra-abdominal infection. Unrecognized intra-operative complications must also be considered, particularly inadvertent bowel injury occurring during dissection, manipulation, or abdominal closure. Postoperative peritonitis typically first becomes apparent on the third postoperative day as fluid retention, supraventricular tachydysrhythmias, or increasing dyspnea. Particularly in the older patient, an alteration in level of consciousness may also be a presenting symptom.

Tertiary peritonitis is that developing at least 48 hours after apparently successful treatment of primary or secondary bacterial peritonitis. The mortality rate of tertiary peritonitis typically exceeds 50%, and the syndrome is largely a disorder of the critically ill patient in the ICU. Response to antibiotics is poor, and source control may be challenging in that imaging studies often reveal multiple, poorly localized collections, the response of which, even to the most aggressive surgical approaches, is unsatisfying.

DIAGNOSIS

Although the clinical presentation of intra-abdominal infection in the ambulatory patient is usually characteristic, the signs and symptoms of intra-abdominal infection in hospitalized patients are subtle. Therefore the clinician must retain a high suspicion for intra-abdominal infection to make a timely diagnosis.

The history can usually focus subsequent investigations. In a known cirrhotic patient whose condition deteriorates, primary peritonitis should be high on the list of differential diagnoses. Prior abdominal surgery raises the possibility of an anastomotic leak, intra-abdominal infection, or an unrecognized complication such as an inadvertent small bowel injury. In the patient with known vascular disease or hypotension, or one who has recently undergone angiography, intestinal ischemia or infarction should be considered. Perforated duodenal ulcer should be considered in the patient who has had a major surgical intervention or who has been in the ICU. An intra-abdominal foreign body, such as a peritoneal dialysis cannula or biliary stent, is prone to infection, and so may serve as a nidus of intra-abdominal infection. Pancreatitis, initially a sterile process, can become secondarily infected. In older patients, perforated diverticulitis is a frequent cause of intra-abdominal infection.

In the ambulatory patient who can provide a reliable history and participate in physical examination, the presentation of intra-abdominal infection is characteristically dominated by abdominal pain, either diffuse or well localized, and may include a history of fever, chills, nausea or vomiting, and ileus or diarrhea. A thorough history including previous operative interventions; risk factors for or symptoms of malignancy, peptic ulcer disease, or diverticulosis; and a history of cardiac or vascular disease can lead to identifying the cause of intra-abdominal infection in most cases. In the ambulatory patient, an abdominal CT scan will often have been completed before referral to the surgeon and, in combination with the history and physical examination, will dictate the course of subsequent therapy.

The diagnosis of intra-abdominal infection in the older patient is often challenging. Physical findings may be minimal, and concomitant medical problems (including possible dementia) or an incomplete or inaccurate history may confound the initial clinical evaluation. The clinical history of the evolution of symptoms over time is of great importance, and every attempt should be made to obtain this information from caregivers and/or family members. Judicious resuscitation and timely imaging are essential to effective treatment. It is also important to involve a multidisciplinary care team—an internist, anesthetist and, if applicable, an intensivist—early in the course of illness to optimize the patient's condition preoperatively and to ensure appropriate postoperative management.

The diagnosis of intra-abdominal infection in the hospitalized patient requires a high level of clinical suspicion. This is particularly the case in sedated or intubated ICU patients who are unable to provide a history. Once again, new or unanticipated organ dysfunction is often the first sign of intra-abdominal infection in the hospitalized patient. Persistent fluid retention is also a common sign. Under normal circumstances, the trauma of surgery induces increased levels of antidiuretic hormone, leading to fluid retention. In the absence of factors promoting an ongoing stress response, this state should resolve by postoperative day 3, when vigorous diuresis, resulting in a net negative fluid balance, is expected. A persistently positive fluid balance and the associated clinical signs of fluid overload—tachypnea, hypoxemia, confusion, or new onset supraventricular dysrhythmia—should alert the clinician to the possibility of a complication such as intra-abdominal infection.

Although the clinical examination and history in an ambulatory patient typically suffice to establish a diagnosis of intra-abdominal infection and to define the site of origin, the advent of CT has made radiographic studies routine in the initial evaluation of abdominal pain. The widespread use of diagnostic imaging before surgical consultation does not eliminate the need for a thorough history and physical examination, but it can confirm clinical suspicion and aid in planning surgical treatment.

Radiographic studies are the mainstay of definitive diagnosis of intra-abdominal infection. Plain radiographs may disclose free intraperitoneal air, suggesting GI perforation in the patient presenting de novo. However, in the postoperative patient, radiologic evidence of intraperitoneal air can be present for up to 7 days. Abnormalities of the mucosal pattern, such as thumbprinting—a reflection of mucosal edema—can suggest ischemia. Both mechanical bowel obstruction and ileus can be diagnosed by plain films. Contrast studies are useful for identifying leaks or transition points in bowel obstruction. Ultrasonography is useful in evaluating the biliary tree and liver. CT is the most reliable imaging modality for evaluating the abdomen. A CT scan with oral and IV contrast can identify intraperitoneal or retroperitoneal collections and abscesses; typical findings include rim enhancement, air fluid levels, and inhomogeneity of the contents of the collection (Figure 1). Intestinal ischemia can be demonstrated by the absence of flow within a feeding vessel or visualization of clot within a vessel, as well as by gas in the wall of the intestine or within the portal vein (Figure 2). Radiographic imaging studies—particularly CT scanning—can also provide an anatomic map to facilitate image-guided drainage of a localized collection (Figure 3).

MANAGEMENT PRINCIPLES

Successful management of intra-abdominal infection is dependent on the prudent application of three principles:

1. Hemodynamic resuscitation and support of vital organ function
2. Early administration of antimicrobial agents
3. Anatomic diagnosis and implementation of source control measures

Most patients presenting with intra-abdominal infection will benefit from fluid resuscitation to restore intravascular volume and normal delivery of oxygen to the tissues. Resuscitation should be guided by serial clinical examination and monitoring of heart rate and blood pressure. Urinary output is an adequate and sensitive measure of intravascular volume and is readily monitored in an ICU patient or the elderly. An hourly output of 30 to 50 ml/kg should be the objective of therapy. Patients presenting with significant hemodynamic instability should be managed in an ICU setting.

Broad-spectrum systemic antibiotics should be initiated as soon as the suspicion of intra-abdominal infection is entertained. Animal studies indicate that anaerobic bacteria from the gut lumen

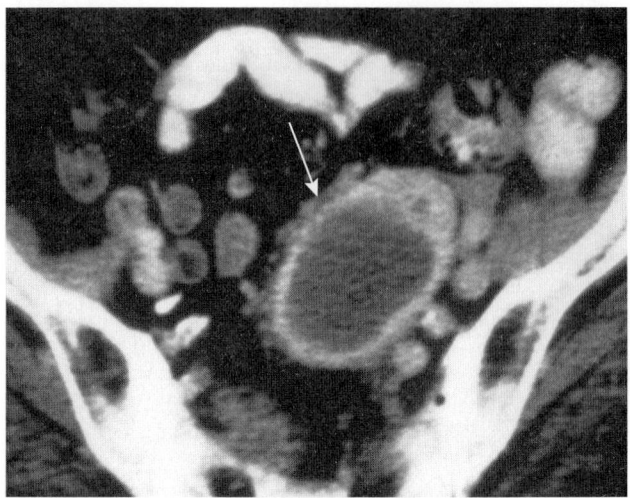

Figure 1 Diverticular abscess *(arrow)* as seen on computed tomography scan. Note characteristic features of rim enhancement and inhomogeneity of abscess contents.

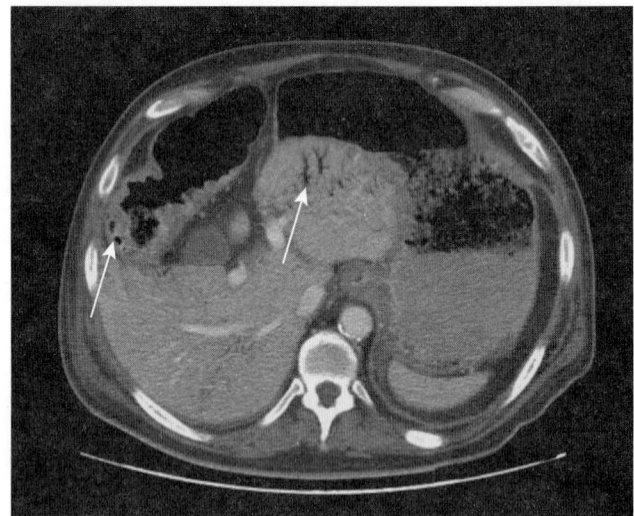

Figure 2 Intestinal ischemia and infarction as seen on computed tomography scan. Characteristic features include pneumatosis and disruption of the mucosa of the intestinal wall *(white arrow)* and portal venous gas *(black arrow)*.

promote abscess formation, whereas gram-negative aerobes are responsible for the lethality of peritonitis. Therefore empirical antibiotic therapy for intra-abdominal infection should provide adequate coverage for both gram-negative aerobes and anaerobes. There is no compelling evidence for the superiority of one agent or regimen over another; acceptable options are summarized in Table 2. Furthermore, there is no evidence of additional benefit for expanded coverage directed against gram-positive aerobes or fungi. Antimicrobial therapy should begin as soon as clinical diagnosis is made, without waiting for radiographic confirmation. There is controversy regarding the utility of obtaining cultures in patients with community-acquired intra-abdominal infection: results are typically polymicrobial, the number of species isolated reflecting more the patience of the microbiology laboratory than the composition of the infected fluid. On the other hand, cultures should always be obtained for nosocomial intra-abdominal infection because the GI flora in the hospitalized patient is significantly altered, and colonization with resistant organisms is the rule. When antibiotics are used in association with adequate source control, the duration of therapy can be short, and a maximal course of 5 to 7 days is considered appropriate.

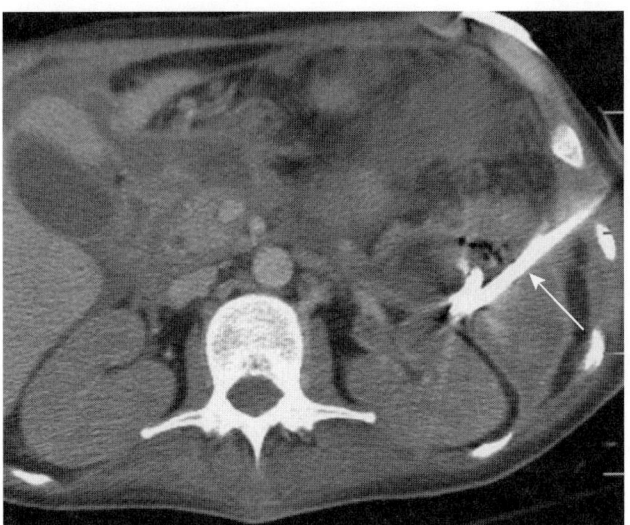

Figure 3 Percutaneous drainage of a pancreatic abscess. The percutaneously placed drain *(arrow)* permitted decompression of a complex retroperitoneal collection, and enabled subsequent minimally invasive debridement of the residual infected peripancreatic necrosis.

Table 2: Antimicrobial Options for Intra-abdominal Infection

Mild-Moderate Infection	Severe Infection
Single Agents	
Ampicillin/sulbactam Ticarcillin/clavulanic acid	Piperacillin/tazobactam
Ertapenem	Imipenem, meropenem
Combination Regimens	
Cefazolin or cefuroxime + metronidazole	3rd/4th-generation cephalosporin (Ceftriaxone, ceftazidime, cefotaxime, Ceftizoxime, cefepime) + metronidazole
Quinolone (ciprofloxacin, gatifloxacin, levofloxacin, moxifloxacin) + metronidazole	Ciprofloxacin + metronidazole Aztreonam + metronidazole

Source control encompasses all physical measures used to eliminate a focus of infection, to prevent ongoing contamination, and to restore functional anatomy. Source control measures include the drainage of abscesses or fluid collections, the debridement of necrotic infected tissue, and the excision, repair, or exteriorization of anatomic defects that led to peritoneal contamination. Subsequent needs for definitive or reconstructive treatment should be incorporated into the initial treatment planning, and as a general principle, the approach that accomplishes the source control objective with the least distress to the patient is the preferred one. For example, in a patient with CT-proven locally perforated diverticulitis, percutaneous drainage treatment can accomplish source control, obviating the need for a stoma and its subsequent closure, and leaving open the option of an elective sigmoid resection with primary anastomosis at a future date. If surgical management is indicated (e.g., because of diffuse peritonitis), a two-step approach—sigmoid resection and end-colostomy, followed by colostomy closure—is superior to a three-step approach (colostomy and drainage only, followed by resection and reconstruction). Indeed several recent studies suggest that primary resection and anastomosis may be the preferred approach, even in the presence of diffuse peritonitis. When a stoma is created, consideration should be given to its ultimate closure. Placing the two ends in close proximity, or performing a proximal diverting loop stoma, greatly simplifies the subsequent reconstructive procedure.

Drainage converts an abscess to a controlled sinus or fistula. This is most frequently achieved with percutaneous techniques guided by radiographic imaging. Factors that preclude percutaneous drainage are diffuse peritonitis, lack of localization of the infectious process, multiple collections, anatomic inaccessibility, or the concomitant presence of a diagnosis requiring surgery, such as intestinal infarction.

Debridement is the removal of necrotic or infected tissue, either operatively or, if the necrosis is superficial, by frequent dressing changes at the bedside. Debridement in the management of intra-abdominal infection includes the resection of necrotic intestine, the removal of feces or fibrin from the peritoneal cavity, or the excision of infected necrotic retroperitoneal fat in the patient with infected pancreatic necrosis. Successful debridement is dependent on clear demarcation between viable and nonviable tissue. For patients with intestinal ischemia, uncertainty as to the extent of necrosis should prompt a decision to undertake a second look laparotomy. In the case of infected peripancreatic necrosis, the plane between viable and nonviable retroperitoneal fat is not clearly defined until 3 to 4 weeks after the onset of the disease. Attempted debridement before adequate demarcation has occurred can lead to uncontrolled retroperitoneal hemorrhage.

CONCLUSION

Intra-abdominal infection is common; however, its etiology, clinical presentation, and prognosis vary widely. Effective treatment requires rapid diagnosis, resuscitation, antibiotic therapy, and source control. In hospitalized patients, attention should be focused on prior operative or invasive angiographic procedures that may suggest an etiology. An anatomic diagnosis can usually be established with radiographic studies, particularly CT; these studies are also invaluable in planning and even in effecting appropriate measures of source control. Broad-spectrum antibiotics are crucial adjuvant therapy, but source control remains the mainstay of definitive treatment. Diagnostic vigilance and a high index of suspicion leading to timely treatment can significantly alter morbidity and mortality.

SUGGESTED READINGS

Anaya DA, Nathens AB: Risk factors for severe sepsis in secondary peritonitis, *Surg Infect* 4:355, 2003.

Cinat ME, Wison SE, Din AM: Determinants for successful percutaneous image-guided drainage of intra-abdominal abscess, *Arch Surg* 137:845, 2002.

Hall JC, Heel KA, Papdimitriou JM, and others: The pathobiology of peritonitis, *Gastroenterology* 114:185, 1998.

Marshall JC, Innes M: ICU management of intra-abdominal infection, *Crit Care Med* 31:2228, 2003.

Marshall JC, Maier RV, Jimenez M, and others: Source control in the management of severe sepsis and septic shock, *Crit Care Med* 32(11):S513, 2004.

Mazuski JE, Sawyer RG, Nathens AB, and others: The Surgical Infection Society guidelines on antimicrobial therapy for intra-abdominal infections: An executive summary, *Surg Infect* 3:161, 2002.

Nathens AB, Rotstein OD, Marshall JC, Tertiary peritonitis: Clinical features of a complex nosocomial infection, *World J Surg* 22:158–163, 1998.

Roehrborn A, Thomas L, Potreck O, and others: The microbiology of postoperative peritonitis, *Clin Infect Dis* 33:1513, 2001.

Salem L, Flum DR: Primary anastomosis or Hartmann's procedure for patients with diverticular peritonitis? A systematic review, *Dis Colon Rectum* 47:1953, 2004.

ABNORMAL OPERATIVE AND POSTOPERATIVE BLEEDING

John J. Como, MD, and Charles J. Yowler, MD

The control of perioperative bleeding has taken on additional significance as surgeons have learned more about the detrimental effects of blood transfusions. Although the risks of viral transmission and transfusion reactions have long been known, the profound effects of blood transfusion on the immune system have only recently been recognized. Further studies are required to determine the exact impact of blood transfusions on postoperative morbidity, but it seems clear that the incidence of postoperative infections, organ failure, and intensive care unit (ICU) length of stay increases directly with the amount of blood transfused. Thus the deleterious effects of hemorrhage resulting from organ hypoperfusion are compounded by the organ dysfunction attributable to the blood transfusion. The purpose of this chapter is to outline an approach to the problem of perioperative bleeding that emphasizes preoperative recognition and correction of coagulopathy, intraoperative avoidance of conditions that promote bleeding (acidosis, hypothermia, dilution of platelets, and clotting factors), and use of appropriate transfusion triggers.

PREOPERATIVE ASSESSMENT

The goal of the preoperative assessment is to identify the patient with a preexisting bleeding disorder because treatments are available for most platelet function disorders and coagulation factor deficiencies. It is clear that routine preoperative screening tests of platelet and coagulation function are not cost effective if used in all patients. The key to the identification of the patient who will benefit from such an evaluation is a thorough history and physical examination (Table 1). The history may reveal a tendency to bleeding with minor trauma (epistaxis, gingival bleeding, and menorrhagia) or excessive bleeding with past surgical or dental procedures. The presence of significant renal impairment requires baseline chemistries to rule out uremia, whereas a history of hepatic disease requires a baseline hepatic and coagulation panel (Table 2).

A detailed drug history should be obtained, including the use of over-the-counter medications. Aspirin and other nonsteroidal anti-inflammatory drugs should be stopped 10 to 14 days before surgery and clopidogrel should be held for 5 to 7 days. Warfarin should be held for 4 days, assuming the international normalization ratio (INR) is within therapeutic range. The INR can be checked the morning of surgery; an INR of 1.5 or less is acceptable for surgery not involving the brain or spine. An INR of 1.3 or less is acceptable for all procedures.

The management of perioperative anticoagulation is more complicated if the patient is on warfarin for recent thrombolic disease. Elective surgery should be postponed for 1 month following an acute episode of venous thromboembolism. For urgent operative procedures that must be completed during this time period, heparin infusions should be given while the INR is less than 2.0 preoperatively and stopped 6 hours before surgery.

Table 1: Preoperative Evaluation of Hemostasis

History

Excessive bleeding after surgical or dental procedures (i.e., multiple transfusions, reexploration required)

Heavy menstrual bleeding

Recurrent epistaxis (particularly if requiring medical attention)

Excessive bruising/hematoma formation (particularly spontaneous)

Chronic iron deficiency or chronic iron supplementation

Renal or hepatic disease

Poor nutritional status

Medications (including nonprescription medications, dietary supplements, herbal remedies)

Family history of excessive bleeding

Physical Examination

Examine for petechiae, ecchymoses, mucous membrane bleeding, signs of liver disease (spider angiomas, jaundice, ascites, splenomegaly), isolated splenomegaly, joint laxity, evidence of impaired wound healing.

From: Streiff MB. In Cameron JL, editor: Current surgical therapy, *ed 8, St. Louis, 2004, Elsevier Mosby, p. 1122.*

Table 2: Preoperative Testing

Perioperative Screen	Planned Surgery	Recommended Tests
Negative	Minor	None
Negative	Major	Platelet count, aPTT, INR
Positive	Minor or major	Platelet count, aPTT, INR; consider hematology consult

aPTT, Activated partial thromboplastin time; *INR,* international normalization ratio.

Heparin infusion may be started 12 hours postoperatively at the preoperative maintenance rate without a bolus in patients with low risk of postoperative hemorrhage. An inferior vena cava filter may be considered in patients requiring surgery within 2 weeks of a thrombolic event.

In patients receiving warfarin for prevention of arterial thromboembolism (atrial fibrillation, mechanical heart valves), the risk of embolism is not sufficiently high to justify perioperative heparin infusion. Subcutaneous low-dose heparin or low-molecular-weight heparin is indicated in the perioperative period. Warfarin should be started following surgery with the expectation that the patient will be satisfactorily anticoagulated in 72 to 96 hours.

A family history of bleeding disorders may signify an inherited coagulation defect. The most common genetic defect in platelet function, von Willebrand disease (vWD), is inherited in an autosomal dominant pattern, whereas hemophilia A (factor VIII) and B (factor IX) are inherited in an X-linked recessive pattern.

The physical examination may reveal petechiae, scattered ecchymoses, purpura, hepatosplenomegaly, or evidence of malnutrition.

Preoperative laboratory studies may disclose unexpected iron-deficiency anemia and Hemoccult-positive (Beckman Coulter, Miami, FL) stools or microscopic hematuria. All of these findings require further testing of the coagulation system to rule out preexisting coagulation defects.

Selective screening of platelet and coagulation function is indicated if the history or physical examination is suggestive of a bleeding disorder. The prothrombin time (PT) assesses the function of factors V, VII and X, prothrombin, and fibrinogen. The activated partial thromboplastin time (aPTT) reflects the function of the intrinsic pathway (factors VIII, IX, XI, and XII). Platelet function may be evaluated by a platelet count and the bleeding time. Factor levels may be obtained in the rare case of a child who appears to have a bleeding disorder. Hematology consultation is useful if an inherited bleeding disorder is suspected.

PREOPERATIVE MANAGEMENT: COAGULATION DISORDER

Coagulation disorders may be classified as either congenital or acquired. The most common congenital disorder is hemophilia A (factor VIII deficiency). Its X-linked recessive transmission makes it almost universally a disease of males. It may be categorized as mild (factor level > 5%), moderate (1%-5%), or severe (<1%). Spontaneous bleeding occurs with levels less than 5%, whereas patients with mild disease might bleed only after minor trauma or surgery. A factor level of 30% should be maintained for 3 to 4 days in patients undergoing minor surgery and a level of greater than 80% in patients undergoing major procedures. Neurosurgical or cardiac procedures may require a level of 100% for 3 to 4 days, followed by levels of 80% for an additional week. Approximately 10% to 20% of hemophiliacs may have circulating inhibitors (IgG antibodies) to factor VIII that further complicate replacement therapy.

Preoperative preparation of a patient with severe hemophilia A includes checking for the presence of a circulating inhibitor and, in its absence, replacing with enough factor VIII concentrate to achieve the factor level desired for the proposed operation. A normal factor VIII level is 1 unit per milliliter of plasma. For example, a 70-kg patient with a blood volume of 5000 ml has a circulating plasma volume of 3000 ml. If the preoperative factor VIII level were less than 1%, the patient would need 3000 units of factor VIII concentrate to obtain 100% levels for major surgery. Appropriate transfusions of factor VIII must be repeated every 8 hours, although some experts prefer continuous infusions to maintain targeted plasma concentrations.

Hemophilia B, or Christmas disease, has an X-linked deficiency of factor IX, which results in a clinical condition similar to hemophilia A. Factor replacement guidelines are identical to those outlined earlier, although there have been reports of venous and arterial thrombosis with replacement to levels greater than 50%. Circulating inhibitors may also complicate management.

vWD is caused by a deficiency of von Willebrand factor (vWf), which normally is involved in the adhesion of platelets to damaged endothelium and which also stabilizes factor VIII in the blood. There are three types of vWD. Type I is due to a partial deficiency of vWf while type III refers to complete absence of the factor. Type II represents a defective factor that is present in normal quantity but is not functional.

Diagnosis may be difficult because of the lack of a specific screening test. Patients with type I or II vWD present with a history of recurrent mucosal (epistaxis, menorrhagia) bleeding, whereas patients with type III disease have a history of severe hemorrhage. The PT/PTT and bleeding time may be prolonged, and patients with types I and III disease will have decreased levels of vWf antigen and factor VIII coagulant (VIII:c). An in vitro platelet function analyzer is useful for rapid screening and may be used after treatment to confirm return of normal platelet function.

Administration of DDAVP causes release of vWf and factor VIII into the blood and is effective for type I disease. It can become ineffective after repeated dosing because of depletion of the endothelial stores of vWf and factor VIII. Its use is not indicated in either type III disease (because of the absence of vWf) or type II disease (because of the absence of effective vWf). Cryoprecipitate can be used in types II and III disease for minor procedures, and factor VIII-vWf concentrates are available for use during major procedures. Levels should be maintained at greater than 50% for 3 days for minor surgery and between 50% and 100% for 1 week for major procedures.

Several other rare congenital factor defects exist and may be identified with factor assays. They may be treated with fresh frozen plasma (FFP), which contains all the coagulation factors; cryoprecipitate, which contains factor VIII, vWf, fibrinogen, fibronectin, and factor XIII; or prothrombin complex concentrates, which contain the vitamin K–dependent factors: prothrombin and factors VII, IX, and X. Recombinant human activated VII (rhFVIIa) is now commercially available for patients with factor VII deficiency. Whichever product is used, daily trough levels must be obtained to confirm the adequacy of plasma concentrations.

Vitamin K deficiency results in deficiencies of prothrombin, factors VII, IX, and X, and protein C and S. This deficiency may be due to malnutrition, hepatic dysfunction, drugs, or malabsorption. Because vitamin K is a fat-soluble vitamin, factors that decrease bile salt secretion into the gut (biliary obstruction, cholestasis) can result in malabsorption. Prolonged antibiotic use can kill enteric bacteria that produce vitamin K. Warfarin interferes with hepatic production of the vitamin K–dependent factors. Oral or intravenous vitamin K may be administered to replete levels, whereas FFP is used for emergent surgery or active bleeding.

PREOPERATIVE MANAGEMENT: PLATELET DYSFUNCTION

Platelet disorders may be due to either low numbers of normally functioning platelets (quantitative) or normal numbers of dysfunctional platelets (qualitative). Quantitative disorders may be due to either decreased production or increased destruction of platelets.

Qualitative disorders may be classified as either congenital or acquired (Table 1).

Thrombocytopenia is defined as a platelet count of less than 100.000/mm^3. In general, a platelet count of 100,000/mm^3 is adequate for major procedures and 50,000/mm^3 is sufficient for minor procedures, including central line placement. Spontaneous bleeding seldom occurs with platelet counts greater than 20,000/mm^3 but becomes common with counts below 10,000/mm^3.

Decreased production of platelets may be secondary to drugs (ethanol, chemotherapy), tumor infiltrating the bone marrow (leukemia, multiple myeloma), aplastic anemia, or bone marrow suppression resulting from chronic illness or infection. Production defects secondary to marrow dysfunction are typically associated with anemia and leukopenia. Increased consumption may occur because of specific diseases (immune thrombocytopenic purpura [ITP], thrombotic thrombocytopenic purpura [TTP]), disseminated intravascular coagulation (DIC) secondary to infection or cancer, or hypersplenism. Heparin-induced thrombocytopenia (HIT) is a commonly recognized drug-induced immune thrombocytopenia, but many additional drugs may also be associated with thrombocytopenia.

Congenital platelet disorders are rare, and a hematologist should be consulted. In general, platelet transfusions should be reserved for major surgery or active bleeding because repeated platelet transfusions over time will result in the production of platelet alloantibodies that complicate future treatment.

Acquired platelet dysfunction generally is due to drugs or renal failure. Antiplatelet medication should be stopped preoperatively, as discussed earlier. If bleeding occurs during emergency surgery on a patient taking antiplatelet medication, DDAVP and platelet transfusions may be useful. Preoperative platelet transfusions should be considered for patients taking clopidogrel or ticlopidine who require emergency surgery or are actively bleeding. Renal failure decreases platelet adhesiveness and aggregation. These effects may be reversed with hemodialysis, DDAVP, cryoprecipitate, and conjugated estrogens. Hemodialysis is the most effective treatment in nonemergent situations.

INTRAOPERATIVE BLEEDING

Intraoperative bleeding may be classified as *surgical* or *coagulopathic*. Prevention of excessive surgical bleeding is essential because most intraoperative coagulopathies develop secondary to excess blood loss. Surgical bleeding occurs at the site of tissue dissection and must be appropriately addressed with cautery or ligature. The onset of bleeding at nonsurgical sites (e.g., intravenous access, endotracheal tube) or previously dry surgical sites heralds the onset of coagulopathy.

Coagulopathic intraoperative bleeding is due to dilution and dysfunction of platelets and coagulation factors. Massive transfusion results in dilution of both platelets and coagulation factors, but the dilutional thrombocytopenia appears to be the major factor in the clotting disorder. Hypothermia and acidosis that accompany the operative shock and organ hypoperfusion cause further dysfunction of platelets and coagulation factors.

The result is a cycle of bleeding, hypothermia, acidosis, and further bleeding. This cycle must be interrupted before the coagulopathy can be addressed.

Damage control procedures, first described in trauma patients with hemorrhagic shock and coagulopathy, have become increasingly used in patients with nontraumatic hemorrhage. Surgical bleeding from vessels is controlled with ligature or shunts, enteric wounds are temporarily handled with resection without anastomosis, and packing is applied to the areas of generalized microvascular hemorrhage. The patient is taken to the intensive care unit, where resuscitation continues with emphasis on rewarming and correction of acidosis. Platelets and FFP are transfused if necessary, but it is recognized that replacement of clotting factors is futile unless the acidosis and hypothermia are corrected.

Intraoperative cell salvage and autotransfusion involve the retrieval and reinfusion of blood lost at the time of operation. The blood is obtained in a suction canister, anticoagulated with heparin, and then washed. This yields a solution containing red blood cells but essentially no clotting factors. Care should be taken in the presence of a grossly contaminated field because the washing process does not remove bacteria completely. Broad-spectrum intravenous antibiotics should be given in this circumstance. Intraoperative cell salvage and autotransfusion should be considered in all cases in which there is a potential for massive blood loss. The goal is to increase the hemoglobin level above the trigger level for transfusion with the patient's own blood, thereby decreasing the need for blood transfusion.

The role of rhFVIIa in intraoperative hemorrhage remains controversial. Pharmacologic doses of factor VII form a complex with tissue factor (TF) to form active TF–factor VII complexes at the site of vessel injury. This results in increased thrombin formation and platelet plug formation at the site of injury. Originally used in hemophiliacs, rhFVIIa has been increasingly used for coagulopathic bleeding following massive transfusion in trauma patients. No randomized studies have shown statistically improved survival with its use, although one prospective randomized study revealed a trend toward reduction in mortality and complications. However, small case series have shown impressive results in massive hemorrhage

following trauma. It appears to be more effective if used before acidosis becomes severe. Surgeons contemplating its use should review the literature and establish guidelines for its use in their practice.

Diffuse intravascular coagulation (DIC) is another source of diffuse intraoperative bleeding. This disorder is due to diffuse activation of the coagulation system with fibrin deposition, platelet aggregation, and microvascular thrombosis. The resulting consumption of platelets and coagulation factors, coupled with systemic activation of fibrinolysis, results in bleeding and end-organ failure. Intraoperatively, it may occur because of bacteremia. Therefore it should be considered when diffuse microvascular bleeding develops during an infected procedure. Treatment includes rapid termination of the procedure and antibiotics. The diagnosis may be suggested by thrombocytopenia, decreased fibrinogen levels, and an increase in fibrin-split products. Platelets and coagulation factors should be transfused as needed. Antithrombin III levels are decreased in DIC, and administration of this factor has shown some efficacy in patients with DIC secondary to sepsis.

In summary, control of intraoperative bleeding starts with avoidance of factors that result in coagulopathy: uncontrolled surgical bleeding, hypothermia, acidosis, and dilution of platelets and coagulation factors. Damage control techniques have proven to be just as useful in general surgical procedures as they are in trauma cases. rhFVIIa has appeared useful in small series of patients, but its true value and indications for use await further randomized controlled studies.

ABNORMAL POSTOPERATIVE BLEEDING

It is important to emphasize that the most common causes of postoperative bleeding are technical in nature. Postoperative bleeding is a risk of all operations, and the first priority is to exclude a surgically correctable cause. A bleeding vessel or organ is much more likely to be the cause of a falling hematocrit than an endogenous hemostatic defect. This type of bleeding is not likely to respond to nonoperative management.

The first step in the diagnosis is the recognition that the patient might be bleeding. This, however, may not be obvious. Heart rate may remain normal until class II shock ensues (15%-30% blood loss), and blood pressure may remain normal until the patient is in class III shock (30%-40% blood loss). A fall in hematocrit may be wrongly attributed to hemodilution. Tubes and drains may become clogged or stop functioning for other reasons, giving the clinician a false sense of security. A high index of suspicion for bleeding requiring reoperation is necessary in any postoperative patient for these reasons. Delay in making the diagnosis will lead to increased blood loss and an increase in the need for and amount of transfusion, with its known complications. A bleeding vessel treated nonsurgically with blood products only (as if it were an endogenous hemostatic defect) is likely to have disastrous consequences for the patient.

The assessment of the patient who may be bleeding in the postoperative period begins with the history and physical examination. The anemic patient or the patient in frank shock may have an altered mental status or be obtunded, whereas other patients may have no complaints. It is important to review the operative report, with attention paid to the estimated blood loss and fluid and blood requirement. Vital signs should be evaluated. If the patient is hypothermic, aggressive rewarming is warranted. On examination, the patient may be pale or diaphoretic. Attention should be paid to operative sites and wounds for bleeding. Auscultation of the chest may reveal diminished breath sounds in the presence of massive hemothorax, but this examination may also be normal. The abdomen should be assessed for distention and flank ecchymosis. Extremities should be assessed for swelling. Note should be made of drain and thoracostomy tube outputs. Urine output, if low, may indicate postoperative bleeding. Complete blood count and coagulation studies are ordered. Chest radiograph may be helpful in ruling out hemothorax. Again, serial evaluations may be necessary.

Postoperative bleeding may be classified as *coagulopathic* or *surgical*, and a distinction must be made between these two types of bleeding. If the patient has bright red bleeding from any site and if the coagulation profile, platelet count, and temperature are normal, the site of bleeding must be found and surgically controlled. In the presence of active arterial bleeding, surgical control is performed emergently and the hematologic workup is performed simultaneously. In all patients, the physical examination is performed and decisions are made in conjunction with all other data points, including vital signs, urine output, central venous pressure, pulmonary artery catheter measurements, and laboratory values. These may need to be performed serially. In the postoperative period, technical reasons for bleeding often coexist with coagulopathic bleeding, and the pursuit of these is performed simultaneously.

Even after a technical cause of bleeding has seemingly been excluded, the possibility of surgical bleeding should be periodically reconsidered. In a patient who is underresuscitated, vasospasm may occur, causing tamponade of the bleeding point. After the patient has been resuscitated, this vasospasm may subside and bleeding may subsequently resume. Constant reassessment of the possibility of a technical source of bleeding is important for this reason. Only after excluding a technical source of bleeding be investigated.

The principles involved in the patient who is bleeding postoperatively are as follows. First the shock state must be identified and treated appropriately. Usually this involves the administration of fluid and consideration of blood transfusion. Vasopressors are contraindicated in the setting of hemorrhagic shock. Other life-threatening conditions should also be treated at the same time (i.e., cardiogenic or septic shock). If the problem is thought to be technical, the patient should undergo reexploration. Principles for management of intraoperative bleeding were addressed earlier. Clotting parameters should be simultaneously restored to normal with blood products or clotting factors. Platelet transfusions should be considered for thrombocytopenia. The hypothermic patient should be aggressively rewarmed. Serial assessment of hemoglobin, platelets, and clotting factors should be performed to assess for stability and should be corrected as needed. New or ongoing sources of blood loss should be monitored and corrected as quickly as possible. Treatable complications associated with the coagulopathic state should be identified and addressed (i.e., other bleeding sites, including intracranial hemorrhage).

Postoperative management of blood loss includes (1) monitoring the amount of blood loss, if possible; (2) monitoring hemoglobin or hematocrit; (3) monitoring for the presence of inadequate perfusion and oxygenation of vital organs (i.e., blood pressure, heart rate, urine output, base deficit, serum lactate); and (4) transfusion as needed (Table 3). In patients who are not bleeding but are anemic, a conservative transfusion trigger (hemoglobin = 6–7 g/dL) is recommended, but caution should be used in patients with significant cardiovascular disease. This may not be applicable to the actively bleeding patient. In the patient who is actively bleeding or who is in hemorrhagic shock, transfusion should be given more liberally. A target hemoglobin of 10 g/dL has been advocated in cases of major injury. The amount of blood to be given will depend on serial hemoglobin determinations. Red blood cell transfusions are usually unnecessary when the hemoglobin concentration is more than 10 g/dL.

The determination of whether intermediate hemoglobin levels will require red blood cell transfusion should take into account any indication of organ ischemia, the rate and magnitude of ongoing bleeding, the patient's intravascular volume status, and the patient's risk factors for complications of inadequate oxygenation. If oxygen-carrying capacity is thought to be insufficient to support necessary activities, transfusion should be considered. Signs and symptoms of this might include fatigue, light-headedness, angina, pallor, impaired mentation, postural hypotension, tachycardia, tachypnea, and decreased exercise capacity.

Table 3: Indications for Postoperative Transfusions

Otherwise stable patients with Hgb < 7 g/dL
Patients with cardiac disease with Hgb < 9 to 10 g/dL
Actively bleeding patients with projected Hgb levels below the above thresholds
Symptomatic anemia

Hgb, Hemoglobin.

If a patient is in hemorrhagic shock, blood pressure should be supported with crystalloids and colloids until criteria for blood transfusion are met. Because the patient is in the postoperative period, type-specific blood should be available. If not, type O blood should be given.

The literature does not supply the information needed to determine precisely the time when transfusion of a blood component should occur in the coagulopathic patient. Laboratory monitoring for coagulopathy should include the determination of platelet count, PT or INR, and aPTT (Table 4). Patients should rarely require a platelet transfusion when the platelet count is greater than 100×10^9/L and should usually receive a transfusion when the platelet count is less than 50×10^9/L in the presence of excessive bleeding. Platelet transfusion may be considered in the face of a normal platelet count if there is microvascular bleeding and known or suspected platelet dysfunction (i.e., the use of antiplatelet agents or cardiopulmonary bypass). When thrombocytopenia is due to excessive platelet destruction (i.e., HIT, TTP, ITP), platelet transfusion is ineffective and rarely indicated.

Transfusion of FFP is not indicated if PT, INR, and aPTT are normal. FFP transfusion is indicated for (1) correction of excessive microvascular bleeding in the presence of PT greater than 1.5 times normal or INR greater than 2.0, or an aPTT greater than 2 times normal; (2) correction of coagulopathy in patients transfused greater than one blood volume when a coagulation profile cannot be obtained in a timely fashion; (3) urgent reversal of warfarin therapy; (4) correction of known factor deficiencies when specific factor concentrates are unavailable; and (5) heparin resistance (antithrombin III deficiency) in a patient requiring heparin.

Administration of FFP will not correct the anticoagulant effect of either unfractionated or low-molecular-weight heparins. Reversal of the heparin effect, if desired, should be accomplished with protamine sulfate. Protamine should be used with caution because it has been reported to produce a hypercoagulable state. It should also be used with caution in diabetics. Remember that the aPTT does not reflect appropriately the anticoagulant effect of any of the low-molecular-weight heparins, such as enoxaparin. Direct thrombin inhibitors, such as lepirudin, can cause prolongation of the aPTT. If thrombin inhibition is no longer wanted, FFP must be given to reverse the aPTT. Because the inhibitor will bind to the prothrombin in the FFP, a larger amount of FFP than normally expected for a simple factor deficiency may need to be given in this situation.

Table 4: Postoperative Coagulopathy in Actively Bleeding Patients

Coagulation Tests	Treatment
Elevated INR, normal fibrinogen	Fresh frozen plasma
Fibrinogen < 125 mg/dL	Cryoprecipitate
Platelet count < 100,000	Platelets
Preexisting hepatic dysfunction	Vitamin K
Pathologic fibrinolysis	Aminocaproic acid
is suspected	

INR, International normalization ratio.

Coagulopathy resulting from warfarin administration may be corrected by giving vitamin K. If the patient is actively bleeding, vitamin K should still be given, but the primary corrective measure should be to give FFP. Caution should be exercised when giving vitamin K intravenously because anaphylactic reactions have been reported. Also, if the patient is to be anticoagulated with warfarin again in the near future, dosing may be difficult because the patient may exhibit resistance to warfarin for a variable period after receiving vitamin K.

Before the transfusion of cryoprecipitate is given, a fibrinogen concentration should be obtained, if possible. Transfusion of cryoprecipitate is rarely indicated if the fibrinogen concentration is greater than 150 mg/dL. Transfusion of cryoprecipitate is usually indicated (1) when the fibrinogen level is less than 80 to 100 mg/dL in the presence of excessive microvascular bleeding, (2) for correction of excessive microvascular bleeding in patients transfused greater than one blood volume when a fibrinogen level cannot be obtained in a timely fashion, and (3) for patients with congenital fibrinogen deficiencies. The determination of the need for cryoprecipitate in the patient with a fibrinogen level between 100 mg/dL and 150 mg/dL should be made on the basis of the potential for active and ongoing bleeding and the risk of bleeding into a confined space, such as the brain or eye.

When traditional measures for correcting diffuse microvascular bleeding in the postoperative period have been exhausted, rhFVIIa should be considered. The use of this product was discussed earlier.

SUGGESTED READINGS

American Society of Anesthesiologists Task Force on Perioperative Blood Transfusion and Adjuvant Therapies: Practice guidelines for perioperative blood transfusion and adjuvant therapies: an updated report, *Anesthesiology.* 105:198, 2006.

Boffard KD, Riou B, Warren B, and others: Recombinant factor VIIa as adjunctive therapy for bleeding control in severely injured patients: Two parallel randomized, placebo-controlled, double-blind clinical trials, *J Trauma* 59:8, 2005.

Dari TF: The management of postoperative bleeding, *Surg Clin N Am* 85:1191, 2005.

Kearon C, Hirsh J: Management of anticoagulation before and after elective surgery, *N Engl J Med* 336:1506, 1997.

McKenna R: Abnormal coagulation in the postoperative period contributing to excessive bleeding, *Med Clin N Am* 85:1277, 2001.

Owings JT, Gosselin RG: Approach to the patient with ongoing bleeding. In Souba WW, editor: *ACS surgery: Principles and practice.* New York, 2005, WebMD.

Streiff MB: Abnormal operative and postoperative bleeding. In Cameron JL, editor: *Current surgical therapy,* ed 8, St. Louis, 2004, Elsevier Mosby.

OCCUPATIONAL EXPOSURE TO HIV AND OTHER BLOOD-BORNE PATHOGENS

John G. Bartlett, MD

Human immunodeficiency virus (HIV) has been the subject of substantial progress after the introduction of highly active antiretroviral therapy (HAART) in 1996. This has substantially changed the prognosis for this disease. At present, HAART has added an average of 13 years to the life of the HIV-infected patients; for those who have achieved a virologic control, the benefit could be a normal life span. Thus these patients are likely to have the common medical problems that are found in the general population, including conditions requiring surgical intervention. Current projections are that, on the basis of the treatments that are currently available and those expected, patients with HIV infection will soon be in two categories: those who have good virologic control and live a relatively normal life and those who will not adhere to the medical regimen. This chapter reviews some of the progress that has had such a dramatic effect, but the main emphasis is on the management of blood-borne exposures, which is the component that is perhaps most important to surgeons.

PROGRESS IN THE FIELD

Acquired immunodeficiency syndrome (AIDS) was first described in 1981, the putative agent was described in 1983, serologic testing became available in 1985, and the effective therapy was established as zidovudine (AZT) in a trial that was completed in 1986. This was effective, but the results were temporary as a result of the rapid development of resistance. The beginning of effective therapy was the introduction of HAART with protease inhibitors, introduced in 1996-1997. Since then, we have seen a continuous evolution of new drugs, concepts of treatment, simplification of regimens, and at least 20 large databases to track population-based progress in the field. An assessment in 2006 indicated that the sum total of therapeutic benefit was an average addition of 13 to 24 years of life and 3 million life-years saved. The current recommendation for therapy is for three drugs, usually two nucleosides and a "third drug" that is either a nonnucleoside of reverse transcriptase inhibitor or a protease inhibitor. With this therapy, the expected response is for the HIV viral load, which averages 50,000 to 100,000 copies/ml (a copy equals 1 virion) at baseline to a level below the limits of detection with the standard assay (<50 copies/ml). There is good evidence that this level of viral control actually indicates a total shutdown of the virus, meaning no replication and consequently no sequence evolution with development of resistance. The result is total virologic control with no disease progression. Problems associated with this ideal response have been the toxicities associated with the drugs and lapses in adherence that often result in viral escape with mutations that confer resistance to the drugs. Medication changes are common, usually because of toxicity or resistance. There are at least 21 drugs that are currently available and 64 in development.

This information provides an optimistic view of HIV and the progress in management. Nevertheless, this is an infection that has not been cured, and we seem unlikely to achieve that goal with the drugs currently available and those in development. Another failure has been the ability to prevent transmission of HIV. Thus in the United States, there have been an estimated 40,000 new cases every year since 1990. It is now estimated that there are approximately 1 million people living with HIV infection in the United States, and that number is anticipated to increase by approximately 25,000/year with the dramatic decrease in HIV-related mortality and the continued rates of HIV transmission. Thus the epidemic seems destined to grow, but those who are treated have a good chance for normal life expectancy.

Table 1: Risk of Viral Transmission with Sharps Injury from Infected Source

Source	Prevalence: U.S.—General Population (%)	Risk/Exposure with Sharps Injury (%)
HIV	0.3	0.3
HBV		
HBsAg	0.1-0.3	1-6*
HBeAg	0.05-0.1	22-31*
HCV	1.8	1.9

*Unvaccinated health care worker.

HIV, Human immunodeficiency virus; *HBV,* hepatitis B virus; *HbeAg,* hepatitis B virus e antigen; *HbsAg,* hepatitis B virus surface antigen; HCV, hepatitis C virus.

OCCUPATIONAL EXPOSURE TO BLOOD-BORNE PATHOGENS

Three pathogens of major concern include HIV, hepatitis B virus (HBV), and hepatitis C virus (HCV). There is now a substantial database to document the risk of transmission from an infected host with exposure, usually by needlestick injury, but also with mucous membrane and skin exposure. The relative risk per exposure with "sharps" injury and the prevalence of each of these three viruses in the general population are noted in Table 1.

It should be noted that the prevalence of these infections in the general population does not represent their prevalence in hospitals in that all three should be substantially higher. Furthermore, with respect to hepatitis B, the data refer to the risk of an unvaccinated health care worker—a population that we hope is small.

HUMAN IMMUNODEFICIENCY VIRUS

Risk

Analysis of 23 studies of needlestick injuries to health care workers from an HIV-infected source showed HIV transmission in 20 of 6135 (0.33%). With mucosal membrane exposure, the rate was 1 in 143 exposures (0.09%), and there were no transmissions with 2712 exposures.

Through June 2004 there were 57 documented cases of occupationally acquired HIV infection in health care workers in the United States. This refers to patients who had a defined exposure and in whom subsequent seroconversion took place. There were also 138 cases of "possible occupational transmission" in which the health care worker had otherwise unexplained HIV infection. For obvious reasons, the best data are for those with documented exposure and seroconversion. In terms of the injuries that accounted for the 56 cases, 48 resulted from parenteral exposure, 5 had mucosal injuries, 2 individuals had both, and 1 had an unknown source of exposure. With regard to needlestick injuries, all transmissions have been with a hollow-bore needle; there is no record of HIV transmission with a suture needle, although the Centers for Disease Control and Prevention (CDC) recommends similar management of exposure with either needle type. The occupations of the 56 health care workers with documented exposure are summarized in Table 2.

It is noted that there are no documented HIV transmissions to surgeons and that the great majority of exposures have occurred in nurses or laboratory technicians.

Analysis of cases with transmission shows the following exposure-related factors that were correlated with the probability of HIV transmission:

- The depth or severity of the exposure
- The presence of visible blood on the device
- The history that the device had previously been used in the patient's vein or artery
- The fact that the source patient died within 60 days of exposure

A fifth factor that increased risk was the absence of prophylaxis with zidovudine. It should be noted that these data were collected in the early phase of the HIV epidemic; thus some of the results may have a somewhat different contemporary interpretation. For example, the poor prognosis of the source patient probably reflected a high viral load, and it is well known that the inoculum size of HIV, as with virtually all infectious diseases, correlates directly with the probability of transmission. Also, although this type of retrospective analysis is not necessarily good science, all of these observations make sense on the basis of what we know about the virus in terms of viral load in the source and the severity of the injury as important risks.

Efficacy of Zidovudine

Several lines of investigation support the role of antiviral agents with exposure to HIV infection.

1. Retrospective analyses of cases show a risk reduction of approximately 80% when standardized for the four variables noted earlier.
2. There is precedent for effectiveness of AZT in preventing HIV transmission according to the early studies of perinatal transmission; this trial showed that zidovudine reduced HIV vertical transmission by 67%. These data have now been substantiated by multiple studies that show consistent results with reductions in perinatal transmission rates from 27% in the absence of antiviral agents to less than 2% when there is virologic control in the maternal source at the time of exposure at birth.
3. There are supporting data from animal models using both zidovudine and tenofovir for 1 month starting either before exposure or after exposure up to 24 to 48 hours.
4. One notable case was in a child who inadvertently received transfusion with HIV-infected blood. This is associated with a risk approaching 100%, but the child was treated prophylactically and was not infected.

Despite these promising data on the effectiveness of postexposure prophylaxis (PEP), there are at least six cases in which PEP was not successful despite initiation of the treatment within 2 hours using regimens that are generally advocated. It should also be acknowledged that the number of occupationally acquired infections in the United States since 1996 has been reduced to 0-2/year.

Management of an Exposure

The first response must be decontamination as quickly as possible. Cutaneous injuries should be washed with soap and water. A visible

Table 2: Occupations of Health Care Workers with Occupationally Acquired HIV

Occupation	Documented Occupational Exposure	Possible Occupational Exposure
Laboratory technician	19	17
Nurse	23	35
Physician-surgeon	0	6
Nonsurgeon	6	12
Other	7	61
Total	56	138

HIV, Human immunodeficiency virus.

defect such as an incision wound should be irrigated with saline or a disinfectant. Mucosal surfaces such as the mouth or nose should be flushed with copious amounts of water. Ocular exposures should be irrigated with saline or water. For decontamination, the use of bleach, peroxide, iodophors, or other disinfectants with immediate wound care is satisfactory, but not viewed as necessarily an important priority.

Testing the Source

In the absence of recent positive tests, the source should be tested for all three blood-borne pathogens: HIV, hepatitis B virus (HBV), hepatitis B virus surface antigen (HBsAg), and hepatitis C virus (HCV) (anti-HCV). For HIV, a notable advance in the past several years has been the availability of rapid testing, which can provide results within 20 minutes. This has been an important development in our ability to efficiently manage HIV exposures. These tests have a sensitivity and specificity of approximately 99%. Positive results should be verified with a Western blot test for purposes of HIV management of the source, but this can be a presumed positive result so that management decisions can be made regarding an occupational exposure. If there is any suspicion that the patient has the acute retroviral syndrome (early HIV infection before seroconversion), the appropriate test is HIV viral load. Such cases are uncommon, but the issue occasionally comes up in a patient at risk who has typical symptoms of acute HIV infection. In the great majority of cases, negative serology virtually excludes this diagnosis. None of this screening is necessary in a patient known to have HIV infection. In that case, the review should note the recent viral load tests, resistance tests, and the medication record because these may alter drug decisions for antiviral prophylaxis.

The guidelines for HIV testing have undergone some substantial changes since the HIV test was introduced in 1985. Initially, there was substantial concern for stigma, there was no available treatment, and there was great concern for the confidentiality of medical records. As a consequence, the standard practice was to acquire signed informed consent, which was often problematic in patients who could not give informed consent because of medical conditions. In the United States, some states made allowances to permit obtaining blood from the source for HIV testing in the context of occupational exposure, but other states had no such legislation. More recently, the CDC has advocated "opt-out testing," which would treat HIV much like other tests. This means that the patient has the opportunity to decline the test, as with any test or procedure, but there is no requirement for the signed informed consent with counseling. This became an official CDC recommendation in 2006, although some states still had legislation that required signed informed consent with pretest and posttest counseling. Thus the method of obtaining blood from the source for HIV serology testing may show some substantial variation between states. The occupational health departments of hospitals clearly know the local rules.

Counseling

Health care workers must be informed about the risks involved in exposure to HIV. This includes the knowledge that the odds of HIV transmission from an HIV-infected source are approximately 3 in 1000, assuming that the source is not receiving therapy and that the health care worker does not accept antiretroviral therapy. As noted, the probability of transmission depends to a large extend on the inoculum size and the extent of injury. With the average type of needlestick exposure to a patient source who is receiving therapy and has a viral load below the limits of detection (i.e., <50 counts/ml) the risk is probably small—but it is not zero. This was demonstrated in the studies of perinatal transmission, which also

showed a direct correlation between the probability of transmission and the viral load. However, some transmission occurs even in women who had very low viral loads. Furthermore, PEP has documented benefit. Zidovudine seems to reduce the probability of seroconversion by 80%, but the current recommendation is for two or three drugs, and we expect that this would make the prophylaxis even more effective. However, the additional benefit cannot be quantitated.

Timing of Initiation of Antiretroviral Drugs

Studies in macaques show that the earlier treatment is initiated the more likely it is to be effective. The goal of PEP is to initiate treatment as quickly as possible, preferably within 1 to 2 hours of exposure. According to the CDC guidelines, the allowable window is 36 hours postexposure, but consensus is that earlier is better. In a review of 435 health care workers with HIV exposure, the median time from exposure to treatment was 1.8 hours. It should be emphasized that, even when the source HIV status is unknown, rapid HIV tests permit treatment to begin within the time frame of test results that verify potential exposure. Standard serologic tests usually take 3 to 7 days, although a negative enzyme immunoassay screening is usually available within 24 to 48 hours and is adequate for the decision to discontinue PEP when a rapid test is not available.

Health Care Worker Counseling

Health care workers should be informed about the following:

1. The risk of transmission according to the data provided earlier. This should include information regarding seroconversion rates based on available data, including risk assessment based on viral load in the source, severity of the injury, and the potential impact of PEP, which reduces risk by at least 80%, according to the best available data.
2. The impact of time delays in terms of PEP efficacy.
3. Methods to minimize the risk of secondary transmission. This usually means "safe sex" or abstention from sex until serology is negative at 6 months postexposure. The greatest risk is in the first 6 to 12 weeks, and many authorities recommend these precautions only through the 3-month test.
4. Description of the PEP regimens and the side effects of the drugs likely to be used.
5. Regardless of the PEP drug decision, there must be follow-up serology at 6 weeks, 3 months, and 6 months. The current recommendation is to repeat serology at 12 months in the health care worker who has acquired HCV with the injury as well, because this may delay the time of HIV seroconversion. Some occupational health departments perform a test at 1 year on all exposed health care workers because there are at least three who seroconverted between 6 and 12 months.
6. Female health care workers who are not pregnant and have childbearing capacity must be advised of the limited data regarding safety of many of the antiretroviral drugs, especially during the first trimester. Nevertheless, the only drug that is clearly contraindicated is efavirenz, a drug that is not usually advocated for PEP anyway. In terms of safety of other drugs, the pregnancy registry (www.apregistry.com) indicates birth defects in 110 of 4391 live births among HIV-infected women receiving antiretroviral drugs during pregnancy. This rate of 2.5/100 is not significantly different from the CDC population-based birth defects surveillance system, which indicates 3.1/100 live births.

7. Acute retrovirus syndrome. Health care workers should be advised of the possibility of this syndrome, which represents the initial clinical expression or first state of HIV infection. Many patients are asymptomatic, but others have an acute febrile syndrome that may resemble infectious mononucleosis. In that event, the health care worker should have medical evaluation, with an HIV viral load test as the best method to establish this diagnosis.

Postexposure Prophylaxis

Recommendations from the CDC include two types of PEP on the basis of risk assessment: a two-drug regimen considered the "basic" regimen and a three-drug regimen for patients at higher risk. The risk assessment includes evaluation of the source, as well as the nature of the injury. In general, risk in the source is determined by HIV viral load. The average for an untreated patient is 50,000 to 80,000 counts/ml, but this is often reduced to less than 50 counts/ml in patients receiving successful therapy. In the latter instance, the risk would be viewed as extremely low, but not zero. In terms of injury, the risks related to the extent of injury and inoculum size, discussed earlier, are the major indicators of high risk. Details are provided in Table 3, which separates the evaluations of "sharps" injuries and skin or mucous membrane exposures. The drugs used for the basic two-drug regimen include two nucleosides, usually zidovudine + lamivudine or tenofovir + emtricitabine. The former has the advantage of data showing the 80% reduction, but the disadvantages of zidovudine often being poorly tolerated and the combination requiring twice-daily administration. The combination of tenofovir + emtricitabine has excellent data in the primate model, is generally very well tolerated, and is given just once daily. When a "third drug" is necessary, the usual recommendation is for a protease inhibitor, often lopinavir, which is combined with ritonavir (Kaletra; Abbott Laboratories, Abbott Park, IL). All

Table 3A: HIV Postexposure Prophylaxis for Percutaneous Injuries

Exposure	Status of Source			
	Source HIV+ and low risk*	Source HIV+ and high risk*	HIV status of source is unknown
Not severe: solid needle, superficial	2-drug PEP[†]	3-drug PEP[†]	Usually none; consider 2-drug PEP[‡]
Severe: large-bore, deep injury, visible blood in device and/or needle in patient artery/vein	3-drug PEP[†]	3-PEP[†]	Usually none; Consider 2-drug PEP[‡]

*Low risk: asymptomatic HIV or viral load <1500 counts/ml. High risk: symptomatic HIV.
[†]Concern for drug resistance: Initiate prophylaxis without delay and consult an expert.
[‡]Consider 2-drug PEP if source is high risk for HIV or exposure is from an unknown source with where HIV-infected source is likely.
HIV, Human immunodeficiency virus; PEP, postexposure prophylaxis.

Table 3B: HIV Postexposure Prophylaxis for Prophylaxis for Mucous Membranes and Nonintact Skin Exposures*

Exposure	Status of Source		
	HIV+ and low risk[†]	HIV+ and high risk[†]	Unknown
Small volume (drops)	Consider 2-drug PEP	2-drug PEP	Usually no PEP; consider 2-drug PEP[‡]
Large volume (major blood splash)	2-drug PEP	3-drug PEP	Usually no PEP; consider 2-drug PEP[‡]

*Nonintact skin: dermatitis, abrasion, wound.
[†]Low risk: asymptomatic or viral load <1500 counts/ml; high risk: acute seroconversion or high viral load.
[‡]Consider if source has HIV risk factors or exposure from unknown source where HIV-infected source is likely.
HIV, Human immunodeficiency virus; PEP, postexposure prophylaxis

protease inhibitors are associated with some gastrointestinal intolerance, and all have extensive drug interactions with any concurrent medication that is a substrate or inducer of the P450 metabolic pathway. Some drugs that are commonly used in management of HIV-infected patients are ill advised for PEP. Nevirapine and abacavir are associated with relatively high rates of serious toxicity during the first weeks of treatment. Although these rates are acceptable for patients with HIV infection, who will be treated for a lifetime, they are unacceptably high for PEP, the transmission risk of which is usually substantially less than 3/1000, and taking into account the availability of many alternative drugs that are comparably effective. Serious hepatotoxicity, including the requirement for a liver transplant, has been reported with PEP using nevirapine. Even though efavirenz is perhaps the most frequently used agent in newly treated patients with HIV infection, many physicians are reluctant to prescribe it because some frequent central nervous system toxicities may interfere with function during the first 2 to 3 weeks of treatment.

The specific agents and comments about use are summarized in Table 4.

Follow-Up

Routine management of PEP includes baseline serologies for HIV, HBV, and HCV. With HIV exposure, serologic testing is repeated at 6 weeks, 3 months, 6 months, and occasionally, as discussed earlier, 1 year. The follow-up at 1 year is arbitrary and is best supported in health care workers who have transmission of hepatitis C, but there are also three to four cases of persons who had not seroconverted after 6 months. It is recommended practice to obtain a complete blood count and liver function test at each of the 2 weeks during the 4 weeks of antiviral treatment. Health care workers must be warned of side effects commonly associated with these drugs and the importance of adherence. The initial experience was that more than 75% of health care workers who took PEP experienced side effects. The most common were nausea, vomiting, abdominal pain, headaches, diarrhea, myalgias, malaise, and insomnia. The early results with the recommended PEP regimens resulted in less than 50% completing the full course. More recently there have been many additional options for medications, including regimens that are much better tolerated.

Table 4: Drugs for Postexposure Prophylaxis

Agent	Comment
Nucleoside Analogs	
Zidovudine	Only drug with established efficacy; note high rates of gastrointestinal intolerance, fatigue, and headache; monitor complete blood count
Lamivudine	In most regimens due to good tolerability, potency, and qd dosing; may need to check for 184V/I resistance in source
Stavudine	Potent; good short-term tolerability; avoid combining with AZT
Abacavir	Concern for potentially lethal hypersensitivity reaction (reported in 5% to 9%)
Didanosine	Concerns fasting requirement and gastrointestinal intolerance
Tenofovir	Well tolerated, effective in primate model, benefit of qd dosing
Emitricitabine	Similar to lamivudine
Nonnucleoside RTIs	
Efavirenz	Potent, but concern for short-term central nervous system toxicity in health care workers
Nevirapine	Avoid: Food and Drug Administration has reports of 22 postexposure prophylaxis recipients with serious reactions, including 12 hepatotoxicity cases (one requiring a liver transplant) and 14 skin reactions, including 3 with Stevens-Johnson syndrome
Protease Inhibitors	
Lopinavir	Potent and favored among protease inhibitors; warn of probable diarrhea
Atazanavir	Potent, well tolerated, qd dosing, boosted well with RTV; note food requirement, risk of jaundice, boosting requirement for TDF, multiple drug interactions including PIIs
Nelfinavir	Well tolerated except for diarrhea that usually responds to Imodium; note fatty food requirements and diarrhea
Fosamprenavir	Potent, relatively low pill burden, option of once-daily therapy; no food effect
Indinavir	Note need for q8h dosing unless boosted with RTV; note need for food and 1.5 L fluid/day or more and risk of nephrolithiasis
Sequinavir	Potent, option for once daily
Entry inhibitors	
Enfuvirtide	Some theoretical advantage with blocking entry, but no experience in postexposure prophylaxis and requirement for injections

PIIs, Protease inhibitors; *qd*, once daily; *RTI*, reverse transcriptase inhibitor; *RTV*, ritonavir; *TDF*, tenofovir; *VI*, resistance mutation.

Expert Opinion

The field of HIV infection has become extremely complicated with the rapid advances that have rapidly evolved since 1995. Many hospitals do not have the available expertise within the occupational medicine department to deal with the complexities of issues. Therefore a CDC recommendation is to frequently seek expert consultation. This includes the following situations:

- A delay in exposure report or decision for PEP beyond the 24- to 36-hour "window of opportunity"
- Unknown source of a "sharps" injury, which must be reviewed on a case-by-case basis
- Use of PEP regimens in pregnancy, potential pregnancy, or breast feeding
- Resistance of the source virus to antiretroviral drugs
- Toxicity of the PEP regimen in terms of symptom management or decision for different drug regimens

OCCUPATIONAL EXPOSURE TO HEPATITIS B

The risk of transmission is dependent on the vaccine status of the health care worker and the presence or absence of e antigen (HBeAg) in a patient with HBsAg. Recommendations for PEP are summarized in Table 5. Vulnerability in the unvaccinated health care worker is high, as indicated in Table 1, and is exceptionally high in those for whom the source is HBeAg positive. It is hoped that nearly all health care workers, including all surgeons, will have been vaccinated, but rates of protection are somewhat variable. Response to the vaccine is age related; it is 95% for persons vaccinated at 20 to 30 years of age, 86% at 40 to 50 years of

Table 5: HBV Postexposure Prophylaxis

Vaccination Status of Health Care Workers	Features of source	
	HBsAg Positive	**Source Unknown**
Unvaccinated	HBIG* + vaccine series (3 doses)	HBV vaccine (3 doses)
Vaccinated Responder†	No Rx	No Rx
Nonresponder	HBIG × 1 + vaccine series or HBIG × 2‡	Rx as source positive if high risk
Antibody status unknown	Test for anti-HBs • Anti-HBs >10 mlU/ml— no Rx • Anti-HBs <10 mlU/ml— HBIG × 1 + vaccine booster	Test for anti-HBs • Anti-HBs > 10 mlU/ml—no Rx • Anti-HBs >10 mlU/ml— HBV vaccine series with titer at 1 to 2 months

*Anti-HBs, Antibody levels; HBIG, hepatitis B immune globulin; dose is 0.06 ml/kg IM. Should be given as soon as possible and within 7 days.
†Responder defined by antibody to HBsAg of >10 mlU/ml.
‡HBIG + the vaccine series is preferred for nonresponders who did not complete the 3-dose series; HBIG × 2 doses is preferred if there were 2 vaccine series and no response.

age, and 45% for those older than 60 years of age. Titers of antibody decrease an average of 10% per year, but prior responders who had a demonstrated response with an antibody titer exceeding 10 U/ml are probably protected as a result of cell-mediated immunity. It is now common practice to measure antibody response at 1 to 6 months after completion of the three-dose series, but many programs did not do this when the health care vaccination programs were initially launched. Currently, for non-responders, the recommendation is to repeat the vaccination series, and nonresponders have a 55% probability of response with revaccination. The vaccine efficacy is approximately 80% to 95% for all vaccine recipients and 99% for those who have had a documented response.

On the basis of these data, health care workers are considered protected if they have been vaccinated and have documented antibody response at any time. If response was never measured, it should be done in the context of exposure in terms of subsequent decisions. If the antibody levels are greater than 10 U/ml, the health care worker is considered protected. If antibody levels were never measured and are now less than the stated threshold, the health care worker must be managed as a "nonresponder."

OCCUPATIONAL EXPOSURE TO HEPATITIS C

A review of 25 published studies from 1991 to 2002 indicated that the rate of HCV transmission after a "sharps" injury from an HCV-infected source was 44/2357 (1.9%). Cutaneous exposure with blood from a contaminated source with intact skin does not appear to confer risk. According to CDC guidelines, the management guideline for HCV PEP is as follows:

- Source testing: the source should be tested for anti-CV and positive results are confirmed with a virologic assay for HCV.
- The health care worker should have baseline testing for anti-HCV and alanine (ALT); these tests are repeated at 3 to 6 months. Any positive serology is confirmed with the test for HCV virus.
- The health care worker may be tested for HCV RNA to detect viremia before seroconversion. This could establish the diagnosis of acute HCV, which is usually asymptomatic but usually accompanied by an elevation of the ALT.
- No prophylaxis with immune globulin or antiviral agents is recommended
- It should be noted that the decision to withhold therapy following documented HCV transmission is somewhat arbitrary. There is a report from Germany of a high cure rate of HCV with treatment during acute HCV infection, and others have had similar success. Nevertheless, there are substantial concerns regarding drug toxicity for an infection that has a 20% to 40% probability of spontaneous clearance. Also, the long-term prognosis for persons with HCV and no additional risks appears to be favorable, and current guidelines for management of chronic HCV infection have shown substantial success for cure.

All of these are important issues for discussion and should be reviewed, preferably with an expert in HCV.

SUGGESTED READINGS

Beekmann SE, Fahrner R, Henderson DK, and others: Zidovudine safety and tolerance among uninfected healthcare workers: A brief update, *Am J Med* 102:63, 1997.

Branson BM, Handsfield HH, Lampe MA, and others: Revised recommendations for HIV testing of adults, adolescents, and pregnant women in health-care settings, *MMWR* 55:1, 2006.

Cardo DM, Culver DH, Ciesielski CA, and others: A case-control study of HIV seroconversion in healthcare workers after percutaneous exposure, *N Engl J Med* 337:1485, 1997.

Centers for Disease Control: Updated US Public Health Service guidelines for the management of occupational exposures to HIV and recommendations for postexposure prophylaxis, *MMWR* 54:RR-9, 2005.

Centers for Disease Control and Prevention: Updated US Public Health Service guidelines for the management of occupational exposures to HBV, HCV, and HIV and recommendations for postexposure prophylaxis, *MMWR Morb Mortal Wkly Rep* 50(RR-11):1, 2001.

Craven DE, Awdeh ZL, Kunches LM, and others: Nonresponsiveness to hepatitis B vaccine in healthcare workers. Results of revaccination and genetic typings, *Ann Intern Med* 105:356, 1986.

Connor EM, Sperling RS, Gelber R, and others: Reduction of maternal-infant transmission of human immunodeficiency virus type 1 with zidovudine treatment. Pediatric AIDS Clinical Trials Group Protocol 076 Study Group, *N Engl J Med* 331:1173, 1994.

Durlach R, Laugas S, Freuler CB, and others: Ten-year persistence of antibody to hepatitis B surface antigen in healthcare workers vaccinated against hepatitis B virus, and response to booster vaccination, *Infect Control Hosp Epidemiol* 24:773, 2003.

Gerberding JL: Clinical practice. Occupational exposure to HIV in health care settings, *N Engl J Med* 348:826, 2003.

Gerberding JL, Henderson DK: Management of occupational exposures to blood-borne pathogens: Hepatitis B virus, hepatitis C virus, and human immunodeficiency virus, *Clin Infect Dis* 14:1179, 1992.

Henderson DK: Managing occupational risks for hepatitis C transmission in the healthcare setting, *Clin Microbiol Rev* 16:546, 2003.

Henderson DK: Postexposure treatment of HIV—Taking some risks for safety's sake, *N Engl J Med* 337:1542, 1997.

Henderson DK, Fahey BJ, Willy M, and others: Risk for occupational transmission of human immunodeficiency virus type 1 (HIV-1) associated with clinical exposures. A prospective evaluation, *Ann Intern Med* 13:740, 1990.

Ioannidis JP, Abrams EJ, Ammann A, and others: Perinatal transmission of human immunodeficiency virus type 1 by pregnant women with RNA virus loads <1000 copies/ml, *J Infect Dis* 183:539, 2001.

Jaeckel E, Cornberg M, Wedemeyer H, and others: Treatment of acute hepatitis C with interferon alfa-2b, *N Engl J Med* 345:1452, 2001.

Johnson S, Chan J, Bennett CL: Hepatotoxicity after prophylaxis with a nevirapine-containing antiretroviral regimen, *Ann Intern Med* 137:146, 2002.

Katzenstein TL, Dickmeiss E, Aladdin H, and others: Failure to develop HIV infection after receipt of HIV-contaminated blood and postexposure prophylaxis, *Ann Intern Med* 133:31, 2000.

Martin LN, Murphey CM, Soike KF, and others: Effects of initiation of 3′-azido, 3′-deoxythymidine (zidovudine) treatment at different times after infection of rhesus monkeys with simian immunodeficiency virus, *J Infect Dis* 168:825, 1993.

Nettles RE, Kieffer TL, Kwon P, and others: Intermittent HIV-1 viremia (Blips) and drug resistance in patients receiving HAART, *JAMA* 293:817, 2005.

Oldach D: Multidose jeopardy: HCV transmission risk and management of acute HCV in hospital settings, *Hepatology* 36:1020, 2002.

Quinn TC, Wawer MJ, Sewankambo N, and others: Viral load and heterosexual transmission of human immunodeficiency virus type 1. Rakai Project Study Group, *N Engl J Med* 342:921, 2000.

Saltzman DJ, Williams RA, Gelfand DV, and others: The surgeon and AIDS: Twenty years later, *Arch Surg* 140:961, 2005.

Scotto G, Palumbo E, Fazio V, and others: Peginterferon alfa-2b treatment for patients affected by acute hepatitis C: Presentation of six reports, *Infection* 33:30, 2005.

Shackman BR, Gebo KA, Walensky RP, and others: The lifetime cost of current human immunodeficiency virus care in the United States, *Med Care* 44:990, 2006.

Shih CC, Kaneshima H, Rabin L, and others: Postexposure prophylaxis with zidovudine suppresses human immunodeficiency virus type 1 infection in SCID-hu mice in a time-dependent manner, *J Infect Dis* 163:625, 1991.

Sulkowski MS, Ray SC, Thomas DL: Needlestick transmission of hepatitis C, *JAMA* 287:2406, 2002.

Walensky RP, Paltiel AD, Losina E, and others: The survival benefits of AIDS treatment in the United States, *J Infect Dis* 194:11, 2006. Epub 2006 Jun 1.

Watts DH: Management of human immunodeficiency virus infection in pregnancy, *N Engl J Med* 346:1879, 2002.

Wang SA, Panlilio AL, Doi PA, and others: Experience of healthcare workers taking postexposure prophylaxis after occupational HIV exposures: Findings of the HIV Postexposure Prophylaxis Registry, *Infect Control Hosp Epidemiol* 21:780, 2000.

ANTIFUNGAL THERAPY IN THE SURGICAL PATIENT

Joseph S. Solomkin, MD

*C*andida infections have become common in surgical patients, affecting both general surgical and solid-organ transplant patients. The incidence of fungal infections, particularly with *Candida* species, increased substantially through the 1980s and 1990s, but has since leveled off. At many medical centers, *Candida* species remain the fourth leading cause of nosocomial bloodstream infection, preceded only by coagulase-negative staphylococci, *Staphylococcus aureus*, and enterococci. Furthermore, in infections that occur following previous intra-abdominal operation, *Candida* is seen in approximately 20% of the patients.

There have been substantial changes in notions of prevention and management of *Candida* infection syndromes in surgical patients, in large part driven by the availability of effective and non-toxic antimicrobial agents. This chapter reviews these changes and discusses indications for prophylaxis in surgical patients.

THE MICROBIOLOGY, INCIDENCE, MORBIDITY, AND MORTALITY OF *CANDIDA* INFECTION

Although there are more than 100 described species of *Candida*, only four are commonly associated with infection: *C. albicans, C. tropicalis, C. parapsilosis,* and *C. glabrata*. Of these, *C. albicans* has long been the most common (>60% of infections). The other three major species are seen at rates varying from 5% to 20%. *C. tropicalis* is a virulent organism, and mucosal colonization by this organism frequently leads to invasive infection.

An evolution of the epidemiology of candidiasis has been recently described, with a reduction in the incidence of *C. albicans* in favor of the non-*albicans* species, in particular *C. glabrata* and *C. krusei*. This appears to have occurred because of wide usage of fluconazole and is important because several strains of *C. glabrata* have reduced susceptibility to fluconazole. *C. krusei* is highly resistant to all triazoles.

CLINICAL ASPECTS OF *CANDIDA* INFECTION

Sources of *Candida* in the Surgical Patient

In humans, as well as in animals, the gastrointestinal (GI) tract is an important portal of entry for microorganisms, including yeasts, into the bloodstream. The passage of endogenous fungi across the mucosal barrier is referred to as *fungal translocation* (by analogy with bacterial translocation).

Although yeast cells have no intrinsic motility, they are able to translocate across the intestinal mucosa within a few hours of ingestion if present in sufficiently high concentration. That this mechanism is important in clinical disease is attested to by the finding of GI tract involvement and submucosal invasion in an autopsy study of patients with hematogenous candidiasis.

Colonization as a Major Risk Factor for Subsequent *Candida* Infection

In critically ill patients, colonization with *Candida* species precedes and leads to infection. If multiple body sites are colonized, the risk of severe infection in high-risk patients increases, and the chance of invasion can be predicted by the extent of preexisting colonization. The evidence for this is compelling and worth reviewing briefly.

Pittet and colleagues performed a 6-month prospective cohort study among patients admitted to surgical and neonatal intensive care units in a 1600-bed university medical center. Routine microbiologic surveillance cultures at different body sites were performed. A *Candida* colonization index was determined daily as the ratio of the number of distinct body sites (DBS) colonized with identical strains over the total number of DBS tested; a mean of 5.3 DBS per patient was obtained. Twenty-nine patients were found to be colonized; all were at high risk for *Candida* infection. Eleven patients (38%) developed severe infections (8 candidemia); the remaining 18 patients were heavily colonized, but never required intravenous antifungal therapy. *Candida* colonization always preceded infection with genotypically identical *Candida* species strain.

Even though it is commonly stated that antibiotic administration itself is an independent risk factor, this is not the case. In a case-controlled study, antibiotic administration was shown to be only marginally associated with candidemia and to be substantially less important than prior *Candida* colonization. There are many other factors that result in changes in the GI flora. These include ileus, antacid therapy, and contamination with a hospital flora. The particular concern is that appropriate anti-infective therapy for a bacterial infection should not be stopped because *Candida* is identified at one or more sites. In intra-abdominal infections, mixed flora infections involving *Candida* and bacteria are the norm rather than the exception.

Who Should Receive Antifungal Prophylaxis in the Intensive Care Unit?

The primary debate surrounding administration of *prophylaxis* concerns the risk of subsequent *Candida* infection in the particular patient. Unit-wide treatment policies, except in extremely unusual circumstances, are not appropriate. Although the incidence of candidemia among unselected intensive care unit (ICU) patients is only 0.5% to 2%, those with certain risk factors, such as recent abdominal surgery, GI tract perforation, dialysis, central venous catheterization, total parenteral nutrition, broad-spectrum antibiotic therapy, and colonization with *Candida* species, are at increased risk. That said, there is no doubt that the key risk factor is colonization. The other factors serve to increase the risk of colonization, the sine qua non of subsequent infection. Recently, two prospective studies have been reported. Taken together, the results of these two studies would argue that patients known to be at high risk of colonization should be placed on lower-dose fluconazole prophylaxis (100 mg/day).

SPECIAL POPULATIONS AT RISK OF CANDIDA INFECTIONS AND POSSIBLY MERITING PROPHYLAXIS

Transplantation

The incidence and mechanism of microbial entry vary in different groups of transplant recipients, depending on the organ transplanted, the donor source, the type of surgical procedure performed, and the recipient's age and general condition at the time of the procedure. Other influential factors are the conditioning regimen, the type and duration of immunosuppressive therapy, and the presence or absence of organ rejection and graft versus host disease. In heart transplant recipients, for example, *Aspergillus* infection is a major problem, whereas in other organ transplant recipients, most fungal infections are attributable to *Candida*. The infection is usually located at the site of the operation; an intra-abdominal abscess in liver or pancreas transplantation, the mediastinum or the lungs in heart or heart-lung transplantation, and the urinary tract in kidney transplantation; however, dissemination from the primary site is common.

Several studies have documented the efficacy of amphotericin B, liposomal amphotericin B, and fluconazole in preventing *Candida* infections. The incidence of *Candida* infection in patients not receiving prophylaxis varies between 10% and 20%, and prophylaxis is cost effective.

Acute Necrotizing Pancreatitis

Appreciation is increasing for the role of *Candida* in infections following acute pancreatitis. A large series of patients undergoing operation for infected pancreatic necrosis found *Candida* present in approximately 10% of the patients at their initial operation for infection. These patients had received prophylaxis with amoxicillin/clavulanate, a factor that might explain intestinal overgrowth and translocation of *Candida*. This is a particular issue because of the interest in the use of broad-spectrum antibiotics, especially imipenem/cilastatin, as prophylaxis for patients with necrotizing pancreatitis. The results of contemporary randomized clinical trials restricted to patients with prognostically severe acute pancreatitis have demonstrated improvement in outcome associated with antibiotic treatment.

We believe the appropriate strategy for such patients, a group similar to the population included in the Garbino study of patients receiving selective digestive decontamination, is to provide low-dose fluconazole enterally.

MANAGEMENT OF SPECIFIC INFECTIONS

Candidemia

Many if not most candidemias seen in the ICU are catheter associated. This is defined as *candidemia*, occurring in a patient with an intravascular catheter and no other obvious site of origin of infection after careful clinical and laboratory evaluation. Several

procedures have been developed to aid in the diagnosis of catheter-associated candidemia. If the catheter is removed, a quantitative culture of the tip should recover at least 15 colony-forming units of the same *Candida* species as that found in blood culture by the roll-plate technique, or at least 100 colony-forming units of the same *Candida* species as that found in blood culture by the sonication technique.

Antifungal Therapy

Fluconazole is now considered the primary treatment of choice for *Candida* infections in patients not previously exposed to antifungals, and particularly if their illness is caused by *C. albicans*. This recommendation is made on the basis of several recent comparative studies of amphotericin B and fluconazole. In each of these trials, efficacy was similar, and the incidence of dose-limiting toxicities was significantly lower in persons treated with fluconazole. Therefore fluconazole has supplanted amphotericin B as the primary treatment for uncomplicated candidemia.

The primary concern with the use of fluconazole for empirical therapy is regarding the possibility that a resistant strain may be present and the belief that amphotericin B, as a cidal agent, may be more efficacious in patients with shock or other evidence of a severe physiologic response to infection.

The use of amphotericin B is associated with frequent and potentially severe side effects, including infusion-related events such as fever, rigors, and hypotension, as well as metabolic derangements such as hypokalemia and nephrotoxicity. The frequency of occurrence of such events may be as high as 80%. Nephrotoxicity, the primary non–infusion-related toxicity, likely results from the nonselective cytotoxic interaction between amphotericin B and cholesterol-containing mammalian cells. An acute infusion-related reaction, consisting of fever, hypotension, and tachycardia, occurs in approximately 20% of patients.

Because of the high incidence of nephrotoxicity and other side effects with amphotericin B and the demonstrated efficacy of echinocandins, there is little role left for amphotericin and its various forms in surgical patients with suspected or documented *Candida* infections. Patients who have previously received fluconazole either for prophylaxis or therapy should be treated with an echinocandin. Otherwise, the decision should be based on the incidence of *C. glabrata*, typically not highly susceptible to fluconazole. An incidence greater than 20% would mandate therapy with an echinocandin.

Lipid Formulations of Amphotericin B

Lipid formulations of amphotericin B are less nephrotoxic. These preparations differ in the amount of amphotericin B and the type of lipid used as well as in the physical form, pharmacokinetics, and toxicities. Studies comparing lipid formulations of amphotericin to the parent compound have shown a reduction in nephrotoxicity. In addition, AmBisome (Astellas Pharma US, Deerfield, IL) appears to reduce the incidence of acute infusion-related adverse events and hypokalemia, and to be better tolerated than amphotericin B lipid complex. However, given the high cost of these formulations, their use should be restricted to patients with significant renal impairment or patients failing on amphotericin B therapy.

Newer therapeutic options have become available with the advent of the lipid-associated formulations of amphotericin B, which are less nephrotoxic than the parent compound. So far, three lipid products of amphotericin B have been marketed in Europe or the United States: Abelcet (amphotericin B lipid complex [Enzon, Fairfield, NJ]), Amphocil (amphotericin B colloidal dispersion [Intermune, Burlingame, CA]), and AmBisome (liposomal amphotericin B). A prospective randomized trial has shown that Abelcet was as efficacious as conventional amphotericin B in hematogenous candidiasis.

The Echinocandins

The echinocandins are large lipopeptide molecules that are inhibitors of beta-(1,3)-glucan synthesis, an action that results in disruption of the fungal cell wall and consequently in osmotic stress, lysis, and death of the microorganism. Two other echinocandins—anidulafungin and micafungin—have recently been approved for use by the U. S. Food and Drug Administration (FDA). In vitro and in vivo, the echinocandins are rapidly fungicidal against most *Candida* species. No drug target is present in mammalian cells. Adverse events are generally mild, including (for caspofungin) local phlebitis, fever, abnormal liver function tests, and mild hemolysis. Poor absorption after oral administration limits use to the intravenous route. Dosing is once daily, and drug interactions are few. The echinocandins are widely distributed in the body and are metabolized by the liver.

Results of studies of caspofungin in candidemia and invasive candidiasis suggest efficacy equivalent to amphotericin B, with substantially fewer toxic effects.

Choice of Agent and Dose Schedule

All patients with candidemia should receive antifungal therapy. We recommend the administration of fluconazole, 600 to 800 mg/day intravenously (IV) for 3 days, particularly if the infecting organism is known to be or is likely to be *C. albicans*. If the patient responds rapidly to this regimen, the dosage may be decreased to 400 mg/day and administered orally.

Duration of Therapy

Duration of therapy depends on the extent and seriousness of the infection. Therapy can be limited to 7 to 10 days for patients with catheter-related and low-grade fungemia without evidence of organ involvement or hemodynamic instability. On the other hand, patients with high-grade fungemia, evidence of organ involvement, or hemodynamic instability must receive antifungal therapy for 10 to 14 days after resolution of all signs and symptoms of infection (Figure 1).

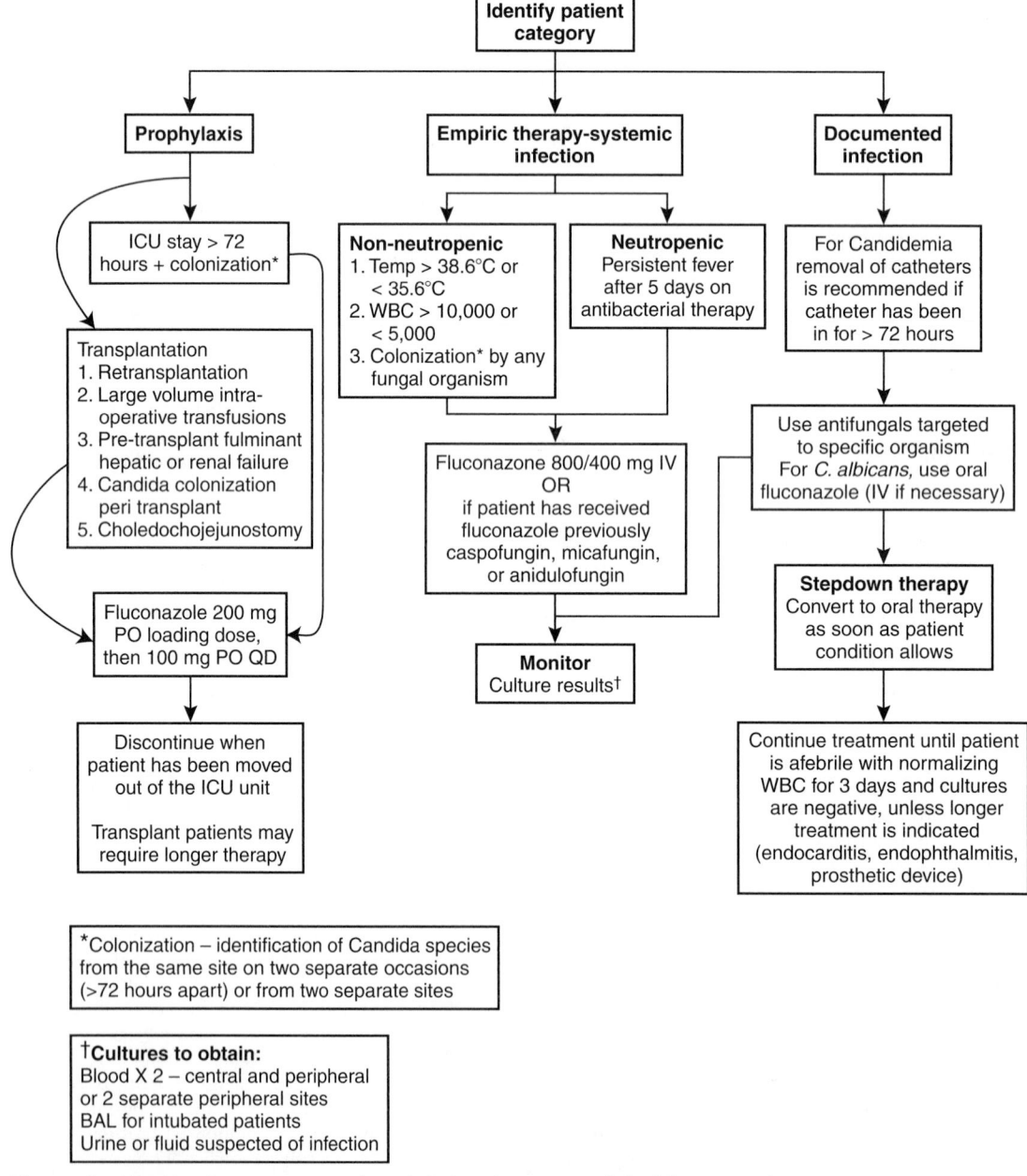

Figure 1   Algorithm for management of prophylaxis and treatment of *Candida* in surgical patients.

Suppurative Thrombophlebitis

A rare but serious consequence of candidemia is suppurative thrombophlebitis, which results from infection of a vessel traumatized by prolonged catheterization. Endothelial disruption exposes the basement membrane and leads to thrombus formation and propagation. Suppurative thrombophlebitis is particularly serious because intravascular infection results in a persistent, high-density fungemia. Management of this disease consists of high-dose antifungal therapy, removal of the central venous catheter, and excision of the infected vein, when possible. Typically, blood cultures remain positive for several days; sometimes they remain positive for as long as 3 to 4 weeks despite appropriate antifungal therapy, if the infected vein is not excised.

Superficial Mucosal Infection

Oral candidiasis (thrush) appears as a whitish, patchy pseudomembrane covering an inflamed oropharynx and commonly involves the tongue, the hard and soft palates, and the tonsillar pillars. Controlled trials have documented the efficacy of nystatin suspension, clotrimazole troches, oral ketoconazole, fluconazole, or itraconazole in eradicating the clinical symptoms of oral candidiasis.

Peritonitis and Intra-abdominal Abscess

A controversial aspect of *Candida* infectious syndromes in surgical patients is whether systemic therapy is required to eradicate *Candida* found within intra-abdominal abscesses, peritoneal fluid, or fistula drainage. *Candida* is frequently cultured from intra-abdominal infectious foci but should be considered a serious threat only in specific patient groups. Four risk factors for intra-abdominal *Candida* infection have been identified, including (1) failed treatment for intra-abdominal infection, (2) anastomotic leakage following elective or urgent operation, (3) surgery for acute pancreatitis, and (4) splenectomy.

The following four factors were independently associated with mortality resulting from *Candida* peritonitis: (1-2) APACHE II score and respiratory failure, which indicate severity on admission to the ICU; (3) upper GI tract origin of peritonitis; and (4) results of direct examination of peritoneal fluid that are positive for *Candida*. Although the pathogenicity of *Candida* was not investigated, our data suggest that the magnitude of the *Candida* inoculum is associated with mortality. This study raises the question of early antifungal treatment when direct examination of peritoneal fluid is positive versus delayed treatment when cultures are positive.

Systemic antifungal therapy should be provided for these patients found to have *Candida* at the site of recurrent of intra-abdominal infection or previous operation, and we would include patients with extensive areas of communication between the abdominal cavity and the external environment via either fistulae or drain tracts. Antibacterial therapy should be provided if bacteria are identified either by Gram stain or culture. Most of these patients have polymicrobial infection.

Occasionally, *Candida* species may cause acalculous cholecystitis or cholangitis. This problem is increasingly found in patients with percutaneously placed drainage catheters for malignancy. Such patients must be given systemic therapy for clinical evidence of infection, including candidemia, and the drainage catheter must be changed.

Because fluconazole is safe and capable of reaching high concentrations in peritoneal fluid, it is likely to be useful in the management of candidal peritonitis. Fluconazole should be given at a dosage of 100 to 200 mg/day orally for 2 to 6 weeks. Immediate removal of the peritoneal catheter has been recommended. In one study, however, seven of nine patients treated with oral flucytosine responded to therapy without catheter removal.

Urinary Tract Infection

The recovery of *Candida* species from the urinary tract most commonly results from contamination from the perirectal or the genital area. Colonization of the bladder is usually seen in patients who have undergone prolonged catheterization or who have diabetes mellitus or another disease that leads to incomplete bladder emptying. In addition, *Candida* species usually colonize ileal conduits. Persistent candiduria in the surgical ICU may, however, be an early marker of disseminated infection in critically ill high-risk patients. Alkalization of the urine with oral potassium-sodium hydrogen citrate is a simple and effective method of treating candiduria in patients with an indwelling catheter. Replacing or removing the bladder catheter is preferable. If *Candida* colonization persists, particularly if the patient has a risk factor for cystitis (e.g., diabetes mellitus or a disease that leads to incomplete bladder emptying) or for hematogenous dissemination (e.g., immunosuppression or manipulation of the genitourinary system), antifungal therapy should be considered. Amphotericin B bladder irrigation provides only temporary clearance of funguria, and systemic agents (single-dose IV amphotericin B or a 5-day course of oral fluconazole) are usually needed. Recently, a large, multicenter, prospective study has evaluated fluconazole versus amphotericin B bladder irrigations for this condition. This study included few ICU patients and thus was unable to specifically address the issue of progression to candidemia. Candiduria cleared by day 14 in 79 of 159 (50%) patients receiving fluconazole and 46 of 157 (29%) patients receiving placebo ($p < .001$). Fluconazole initially produced high eradication rates, but cultures at 2 weeks revealed similar candiduria rates among treated and untreated patients. Oral fluconazole was safe and effective for short-term eradication of candiduria, especially following catheter removal. Long-term eradication rates were disappointing and not associated with clinical benefit.

Fluconazole, 200 mg once daily, is a more attractive approach because of the convenience, low cost, and high drug concentrations achieved in the urine. Flucytosine is excreted in the urine in high concentrations and may be particularly useful against *C. glabrata* infection.

CONCLUSION

Continued progress in supportive care, including the development of antibiotics with increasingly broad spectra of activity, has resulted in an increasing frequency of fungal infections, particularly candidiasis. Because of the inadequacy of the available knowledge base, we do not fully understand the pathophysiology of these infections in surgical patients, nor can we always be certain precisely when prophylaxis and therapy should be administered.

Despite these limitations, sufficient information is available to justify an aggressive therapeutic approach to suspected *Candida* infections. Now that less toxic agents are available (the newer triazoles, particularly fluconazole, and the echinocandins), the clinical approach to presumed fungal infections in surgical patients has been made far simpler.

SUGGESTED READINGS

Eggimann P, Garbino J, Pittet D: Epidemiology of *Candida* species infections in critically ill non-immunosuppressed patients, *Lancet Infect Dis* 3:685, 2003.

Pappas PG, Rex JH, Sobel JD, and others: Infectious Diseases Society of America. Guidelines for treatment of candidiasis, *Clin Infect Dis* 38(2):161, 2004.

Pelz RK, Hendrix CW, Swoboda SM, and others: Double-blind placebo-controlled trial of fluconazole to prevent candidal infections in critically ill surgical patients, *Ann Surg* 233(4):542, 2001.

SURGICAL CRITICAL CARE

SURGICAL PALLIATIVE CARE

Geoffrey P. Dunn, MD

Surgical palliative care is the treatment of suffering and the promotion of quality of life for seriously or terminally ill patients under surgical care. The conceptual framework for surgical palliative care evolved from the hospice concept of care introduced by the late Dr. Cicely Saunders in the 1960s. The hospice concept was subsequently modified to apply to individuals with more favorable prognoses.

The twin core values of surgical culture, nonabandonment and preservation of hope, are consistent with the essence of palliative care as it has developed around the globe as a standard of care for advanced and terminal illness. The indication for palliative care in surgical practice is based on the patient's and the patient's family's desire for relief of distress in any of its forms, as well as the wish to improve the quality and promise of life regardless of diagnosis or prognosis. The choice of therapy is based on the ability of the treatment to meet the agreed-upon goals of care, not its impact on the underlying disease process.

In 2005, the American College of Surgeons' Board of Regents endorsed the *Statement of Principles of Palliative Care,* drafted by its Task Force on Surgical Palliative Care and Committee on Ethics (see Table 1).

The primary target for palliative intervention is distress, not disease. To dissect out this target consistently, a conceptual model for pain and suffering is necessary. Useful models of pain and suffering widely recognized in clinical palliative care are Cicely Saunders's model of "Total Pain" and Eric Cassell's concept of suffering. Saunders's model outlines four cardinal dimensions of pain (physical, social/economic, psychological, and spiritual) that in aggregate are referred to as "total pain" that contributes to suffering. Cassell described suffering as the feeling that arises from a threat to integrity (wholeness) of the person. The elements of personhood include the individual's past, present, and future—his or her social role, private life, and a transcendent dimension. Suffering is not relieved until the threat to personhood has passed or is diminished.

Principles of communication with individuals receiving palliative care are analogous to the right conduct of an operation: creation of the right physical and social context, assessment of the individual's preparedness, permission to proceed, definitive action, acknowledgment of the impact of the action on the recipient, closure, and follow-up.

Surgical palliative care assessment includes identification of: previous illness and treatments, sources of pain in all dimensions, sources of personal strength, liabilities, and individual values and wishes (see Table 2). Decision-making capacity, surrogacy, and advance medical directives are addressed at this time. *Relief of pressing symptoms should be given before or concurrently with assessment.* The patient's goals of care that emerge from this discussion set the parameters for the surgeon's involvement. In cases in which operative intervention is anticipated, preoperative anesthesiology consultation is helpful in planning intraoperative and perioperative analgesia (especially if use of an epidural catheter is desired), reviewing the patient's goals of care in light of what anesthesia expertise can offer, and reconsideration of existing "do not resuscitate" (DNR) orders.

As a general rule, physical symptom relief takes immediate priority of action over intervention for nonphysical distress even if nonphysical issues are ultimately more important to the patient. Symptom management is the work of palliative care and requires an interdisciplinary approach. A strong liaison with clinical pharmacists is particularly helpful because of the effectiveness of pharmacotherapy for the most common symptoms and the frequency of adverse drug reactions and costs that add to total symptom burden. Tables 3, 4, and 5 show medications and their conversions commonly used for control of major symptoms encountered during palliative care in the hospital setting. For nonphysical symptoms, the surgeon's role is to identify, triage, and refer appropriately and promptly.

The importance of collegiality with individuals entrusted with spiritual care of the individual cannot be overemphasized, particularly if spiritual anguish is the predominating form of the patient's distress. Despite differences in faith and values, "moral friendship," a concept proposed by cleric and surgeon, Daniel Hall, between surgeon and patient is usually possible and remains one of the worthiest goals of care. One can conceive of situations in which the moral perspectives of physician and patient are sufficiently opposed that a mutual accommodation might not be possible in the setting of the clinical relationship. For specific ethical concerns frequently encountered in surgical palliative care, see Table 6.

Palliative care service consultation should be actively sought to complement surgical expertise, especially when nonphysical symptom burden is high and clarification of goals is difficult in the face of rapidly progressing or critical illness. Palliative care consultation services, which are increasingly available in the United States, have been shown to improve symptom control, enhance patient and family satisfaction, lower costs, and even increase organ donations. Surgeons should be mindful of the option of hospice referral for patients with an estimated survival of 6 months or less if the illness(es) pursues its usual course without further attempts to reverse it. Referral can follow operative palliation of symptoms but should not be made until the patient or surrogate has had a chance to

Table 1: Statement of Principles of Palliative Care

- Respect the dignity and autonomy of patients, patients' surrogates, and caregivers.

- Honor the right of the competent patient or surrogate to choose among treatments, including those that may or may not prolong life.

- Communicate effectively and empathically with patients, their families, and caregivers.

- Identify the primary goals of care from the patient's perspective, and address how the surgeon's care can achieve the patient's objectives.

- Strive to alleviate pain and other burdensome physical and nonphysical symptoms.

- Recognize, assess, discuss, and offer access to services for psychological, social, and spiritual issues.

- Provide access to therapeutic support, encompassing the spectrum from life-prolonging treatments through hospice care, when they can realistically be expected to improve the quality of life as perceived by the patient (Table 8).

- Recognize the physician's responsibility to discourage treatments that are unlikely to achieve the patient's goals, and encourage patients and families to consider hospice care when the prognosis for survival is likely to be less than a half-year.

- Arrange for continuity of care by the patient's primary and/or specialist physician, alleviating the sense of abandonment patients may feel when "curative" therapies are no longer useful.

- Maintain a collegial and supportive attitude toward others entrusted with care of the patient.

From Dunn GP: Bull Am Coll Surg 2005;90:34.

Table 2: Palliative Care Staging

Domain	Assessment Questions to Ask the Patient
Illness/treatment summary	Tell me what you know about your illness. Could you give me an account about your illness and treatment you have had until now? Tell me what stands out in your memory … (about your illness, about treatment to date). I will review (have reviewed) your medical history in your chart, but I am really interested in hearing about it from your point of view.
Physical symptoms	How long have you had (symptom)? Are you having this (symptom) all the time or on and off? How would you describe what you are feeling? Is the (symptom) staying the same, getting better, or getting worse? Using a scale (provide a scale), what is the lowest you have been in the past day? The highest? Where are you now? In which number range would you be satisfied? Do you notice any change depending on what you are doing? Does anything make the (symptom) better? Worse? Is it (symptom) keeping you from sleeping (etc.)? To what extent does the (symptom) interfere with what you want to do? Is the (symptom) causing problems in your relations to others? Have any treatments helped your (symptom)? How much? What do you think is causing it (symptom)? What does it (symptom) make you think about? Does it (symptom) frighten you? Why?
Psychological symptoms	Does everything happening make any sense to you? What do you think will happen next? How has your illness affected your life? How would you describe your mood? What do you see as the biggest problem facing you now? What frightens you most about your illness? How well do you think you are coping now? Do you feel depressed? Have you ever thought of taking your life? Do you have a plan? Have you been sad? Frightened? Anxious? Are you afraid of being a burden to others? How have you handled tough times in your life previously? Whom do you turn to for support in tough times? Have you ever had problems with depression, alcohol, or other psychological difficulties before your illness? Did you ever have treatment for these? Are you afraid we won't be there when you need us?

Spiritual issues	Do you consider yourself a religious or spiritual person?
	How important is your faith or belief in your life?
	Do you belong to a community of faith?
	Is there a group of people particularly important to you?
	What sustains your hope?
	Do you have religious or spiritual beliefs that help you through difficulty?
	What gives your life meaning?
	Does your faith influence your feelings about your illness? Your surgery?
	Do you see any possible conflicts between your healthcare and your beliefs?
	Do you have any specific observances or rituals we should be mindful of during your care [here]?
Social context	Can you tell me about other people in your everyday life, at work, at home, etc.?
Communication preferences	Is it your preference to be alone or have someone close to you present when we discuss important matters?
	Is there anyone with whom you would like me to discuss your care?
	If I am approached by family members with questions about your situation, do I have your permission to discuss it? To what extent?
	Would an interpreter be helpful [professional interpreters, not family or friends, and definitely not children, are recommended]?
Decision making	Who will make decisions about your medical care if (when) you are not able to?
Practical concerns	When you are ready for home, will your home be ready for you?
Anticipatory planning	Have you given any thought to what comes after your hospitalization?
	What plans have you made for your future?
	Are there things you need to know right now for planning for the future?
	Would it be helpful for us to schedule a meeting with us and your family to plan your future treatment and care?

Nine dimensions of palliative care assessment identified. *From Whole Patient Assessment. In:* EPEC, the American Medical Association's Education for Physicians on End-of-Life Care Project, Trainer's Guide, *American Medical Association, Chicago, 1999.*

Table 3: Pharmacopoeia for Management of Persistent Pain

Symptom	Medication and *Usual* Starting Doses (Adults)
Mild persistent pain, VAS 1–3	Acetaminophen, 325–650 mg PO qid • Maximal dose = 3200 mg/24 hr; use less (<2400 mg) if concomitant use of alcohol or other hepatotoxic drugs (cytochrome P450 inducers). Care must be taken to identify total daily intake of acetaminophen in other prescription and nonprescription preparations. Aspirin, 600–1500 mg PO qid • Gastropathy, decreased platelet aggregation Choline magnesium trisalicylate (Trilisate; Purdue Pharma, Stamford, CT), 750–1500 mg PO bid • Little effect on platelet aggregation Ibuprofen (Advil [Wyeth Consumer Healthcare, Richmond, VA]; Motrin [McNeil Consumer Healthcare, Philadelphia, PA]), 200–400 mg PO qid • Maximal dose = 3200 mg/24 hr. Gastropathy, nephropathy, decreased platelet aggregation Naproxen (Naprosyn; Roche Pharmaceuticals, Nutley, NJ), 250 mg PO bid • Usual adult dose 500–1000 mg/24 hr (maximum: 1300 mg/24 hr) • Nonsteroidal anti-inflammatory drugs (NSAIDs) are most useful when there is an inflammatory component of pain and can be used concomitantly with opioids exploiting this property. All of these agents have a maximal therapeutic dose unlike opioids. They are not benign drugs, particularly for the elderly, and may be less safe than the use of opioids. Patients at increased risk of NSAID-induced renal dysfunction include the elderly, those with preexisting renal dysfunction, congestive heart failure, hepatic dysfunction, hypovolemia, and concomitant nephrotoxic drug use. Good hydration and dose reduction minimizes risk. • Major complications are not necessarily preceded by minor ones.

(continued)

Table 3: Pharmacopoeia for Management of Persistent Pain—Cont'd

Symptom	Medication and *Usual* Starting Doses (Adults)
Moderate to severe persistent pain, VAS 4–10	Hydrocodone (Vicodin [Abbott Laboratories, Abbott Park, IL]; Lortab [UCB, Brussels, Belgium]), 5–10 mg PO q3–4 hr

- Hydrocodone in tablet form is only available compounded with acetaminophen. Caution when escalating because of ceiling dose of acetaminophen.

7–10 = Pain Emergency!

Oxycodone, 5–10 mg PO q 3–4 hr (moderate pain), 10–30 mg PO q 4 hr (severe pain)
- Compounded form (Percocet [Endo Pharmaceuticals, Chadds Ford, PA]; Tylox [Ortho-McNeil, Raritan, NJ]) used only for *moderate* cancer pain because of dose-limiting toxicities of acetaminophen and aspirin (Percodan; Endo Pharmaceuticals). Single-entity oxycodone can be used for moderate and severe cancer pain because it has no ceiling dose.
- Available in immediate release (Roxicodone [Roxane Laboratories, Columbus, OH]) and controlled-release (OxyContin [Purdue Pharma]) forms.
- Immediate-release forms include a solution, concentrate (20 mg/ml), and tablet. IV form is not available.
- Slow-release form can be given rectally. Slow-release preparations should never be crushed or cut.

Morphine, 15 mg PO q 3–4 hr, 5–10 mg IV q 3–4 hr
- The gold standard. Most flexible opioid for dosing forms.
- Caution when using in elderly patients, patients with renal or hepatic insufficiency.
- Controlled-release forms (MS Contin [Purdue Pharma]; Oramorph [Thomson Healthcare, Montvale, NJ]; Kadian [Alpharma Pharmaceuticals, Piscataway, NJ]) available and can be given rectally. Kadian and Avinza (King Pharmaceuticals, Bristol, TN) can be opened and given via a PEG tube.

Hydromorphone (Dilaudid; Abbott Laboratories, Abbott Park, IL), 4 mg PO q 3–4 hr, 1.5 mg IV q 3–4 hr
- Useful in renal failure patients and for subcutaneous infusions.

Fentanyl (Duragesic; Janssen LP, Titusville, NJ), transdermal, 12 µg/hr patch q 72 hr
- Not for acute pain management. Should not use more than 12-µg patch on opioid-naive patients. Prolonged half-life may require close monitoring in case of accumulation.

Methadone, 5–10 mg PO q 6–8 hr, 2.5–5 mg IV q 6–8 hr
- Not a first-line agent, although effective, especially for pain with a neuropathic component. Inexpensive. Flexible: can be given PO, IV, SC, PR, SL, and vaginally.
- Its long half-life makes dosing more difficult than alternative opioids, and close monitoring is required when initiating.
- Numerous medications, alcohol, and cigarette smoking can alter its serum levels.
- Physicians who write methadone prescriptions *for pain* should specify this indication. Methadone use for drug-withdrawal treatment requires special licensure.
- Consultation with pain management, clinical pharmacists, or palliative care/hospice services skilled in methadone use is recommended for surgeons inexperienced with use of methadone.

General comments:
- Opioid analgesics are the agents of choice for severe cancer-related pain. Oral administration is the preferred route. There is *no reason* to use the painful and occasionally morbid intramuscular route.
- Respiratory depression is most likely to occur in the opioid-naïve and patients with significant pulmonary disease. It is always preceded by sedation. Reversal with naloxone should be reserved for life-threatening respiratory depression or hypotension, not sedation or confusion. Sedation is a common side effect when initiating opioid therapy. Tolerance to this usually develops within a few days.
- Initiate bowel stimulant prophylaxis for constipation when prescribing opioids unless contraindicated.
- Management of moderate to severe persistent pain requires familiarity with approximate equivalent doses of differing opioids. See Table 4 (e.g., morphine 30 mg orally is equinanalgesic to hydromorphone 7.5 mg orally), and the conversion between parenteral and oral dosing (e.g., morphine 30 mg PO is equianalgesic to 10 mg IV, IM, or SC)
- Adjuvant or coanalgesic agents are drugs that enhance analgesic efficacy of opioids, treat concurrent symptoms that exacerbate pain, or provide independent analgesia for specific types of pain (e.g., a tricyclic antidepressant for treatment of neuropathic pain). Coanalgesics can be initiated for persistent pain at any VAS level. Gabapentin is commonly used as an initial agent for neuropathic pain.

- *No place* for meperidine (Demerol [Bayer, Myerstown, PA]); propoxyphene (Darvon [Eli Lilly, Indianapolis, IN]; Darvocet [Xanodyne Pharmaceuticals, Newport, KY]; or mixed agonist-antagonist agents (Stadol [Magnum, Alexandria, VA]; Talwin [Sanofi-Aventis US, Bridgewater, NJ]) in management of persistent pain.
- Codeine is of limited use for persistent pain because of increasing untoward side effects for doses above 65 mg with plateau of analgesic effect. Seven percent of whites genetically lack capacity to convert codeine to morphine, which accounts for part of its analgesic effect. Compounding with acetaminophen imposes ceiling for use unlike uncompounded opioids.
- Invasive techniques (axial analgesia, neurolytic blocks) should be considered at the outset of pain management in pain emergencies (VAS 9–10).

Constipation prophylaxis	Docusate sodium (Colace;Purdue Pharma), 100 mg PO qd • Stool softener. Give with stimulant laxative and titrate up as needed. Increasing opioid dosage requires up-titration. Sennosides (Senokot [Purdue Pharma, Stamford, CT]), 15 mg PO qd • Combination products with docusate and sennosides are available (Senokot-S; Peri-Colace [Purdue Pharma]). Bisacodyl, 2 tablets PO qd or 1–2 suppositories qd Sorbitol, 70% solution 15 ml PO or PR qd • Use for exacerbations of constipation in patients already on bowel regimen. General: • Avoid bulk-forming laxatives because of their propensity to form bowel concretions in underhydrated, debilitated patients. • Nausea and anorexia are frequent presentations of opioid-induced constipation.

Bid, Twice daily; *IM,* intramuscular; *IV,* intravenous; *PEG,* percutaneous endoscopic gastronomy; *PO,* by mouth; *PR,* per rectum; *q,* every; *qid,* four times daily; *SC,* subcutaneously; *SL,* sublingually; *VAS,* visual analogue scale.

Selected dosing recommendations from: Miaskowski C, Cleary J, Burney R, and others: Guideline for the management of cancer pain in adults and children, *APS Clinical Practice Guidelines Series, No. 3, Glenview, IL, 2005, American Pain Society, pp. 51–68.*

The medications listed in the table are meant to give the surgeon a rough idea of the commonly used medications and their usual starting doses. These are not recommendations for specific patients.

Considerable variability of response requires individualizing dosing and titration to effect.

Table 4: Approximate Opioid Equivalences for Management of Moderate to Severe Pain

Analgesic	IM, SC, IV route (mg)	Oral route (mg)
Morphine	10	30
Hydromorphone	1.5	7.5
Oxycodone	Not available	20
Fentanyl	10 µg IV ≈ 1 mg IV morphine 25 µg/hr patch q 72 hr ≈50 mg oral morphine/24 hr	–
Methadone*	Ratios relative to methadone depend on the dose of the previous opioid	If daily morphine dose before switch is 30–90 mg, EDR = 4:1 (i.e., 4 mg morphine = 1 mg methadone); 90–300 mg morphine, EDR = 8:1; above 300 mg morphine, EDR = 12:1. Methadone has a variable and long half-life. Dosing interval every 8–12 hr.

EDR, Estimated dose ratio; *IM,* intramuscular; *IV,* intravenous; *PO,* by mouth; *q,* every; *SC,* subcutaneously.

From Ripamonti C, Bianchi M: Hematol Oncol Clin N Am *2002:16:543.*

These are not recommendations for specific patients. The interindividual and intraindividual variability to opioids requires individualizing dosing and titration to effect.

become aware of a prognosis of 6 months or less. (See Tables 6 and 7 for estimating prognosis and referral criteria for palliative care and hospice services.)

Palliative surgery is currently moving away from its earlier definition of noncurative intervention to the more affirmative concept of deliberate symptom control and restoration of quality of life. This transition has been guided by increased emphasis on determining personal relevance for symptom relief ("patient-centered"), minimizing morbidity, improving nonphysical domains, and maintaining symptom relief.

Considerations for palliative surgery include the expected course of the disease, the psychology of the patient, the effectiveness of the given operation, and the capacities of the surgeon. Therapeutic benefit from palliative surgery must achieve symptom control, durability of symptom control, and symptom control with minimal morbidity (including social morbidity of hospitalization of an individual during the last weeks of life) (Table 8). Major operative complications dramatically (Table 8). worsen the prospects of achieving durable symptom relief up to the time of death.

Table 5: Pharmacopoeia for Management of Selected Nonpain Symptoms

Dyspnea	Hydrocodone (Vicodin [Abbott Laboratories, Abbott Park, IL]; Lortab [UCB, Brussels, Belgium]), 5 mg PO q 4 hr
	• Use in opioid-naïve patient for mild dyspnea.
	• May use an equivalent dose every 1–2 hr for breakthrough dyspnea.
	• Syrup preparations of hydrocodone without acetaminophen (Hycodan; Bristol-Myers Squibb, New York, NY) are available. Hydrocodone compounded with acetaminophen limits its dosing because of the ceiling of acetaminophen.
	• Useful agent if cough accompanies dyspnea.
	Morphine, 5 mg PO q 4 hr, 1.5 mg IV q 4 hr
	• Use in opioid-naïve patient with severe dyspnea.
	• May use an equivalent dose every 1–2 hr for breakthrough dyspnea.
	• When 24-hr requirements are determined and stable can convert to a controlled-release formulation.
	Oxycodone, 5 mg PO q 4 hr
	• Use in opioid-naïve patient with severe dyspnea.
	• May use an equivalent dose every 1–2 hr for breakthrough dyspnea.
	• When 24-hr requirements are determined and stable can convert to a controlled release formulation.
	Hydromorphone, 2 mg PO q 4 hr, 0.3 mg IV q 4 hr
	• Use in opioid-naïve patient with severe dyspnea.
	• May use an equivalent dose every 1–2 hr for breakthrough dyspnea.
	General comments:
	• Doses can be titrated up 50%-100% every 24 hr as needed.
	• For patients already receiving opioids, increase baseline opioid dose by 25%-50% and titrate as with opioid-naïve patients.
	• In severe pulmonary disease, start with half of the above doses and up-titrate no more than 25% every 24 hr.
	• Extreme caution when using anxiolytics for dyspnea because of their sedating effect. Anxiety accompanying dyspnea often resolves with effective relief of dyspnea using opioids.
	• *Hypoxemia is not the same as dyspnea.* In situations when life prolongation is not desired, oxygen supplementation is not necessary in nondyspneic hypoxemic patients. Oxygen saturations and arterial blood gases are not necessary under these circumstances and confuse the goals of care. Oxygen supplementation should be given only if it relieves symptoms.
Nausea/vomiting	Prochlorperazine (Compazine; GlaxoSmithKline, Research Triangle Park, NC), 5–10 mg PO/IV/PR qid
	Promethazine (Phenergan; Wyeth Consumer Healthcare, Richmond, VA), 6.25–12.5 mg PO/IV/PR q 4 hr
	• Avoid; very sedating, increased risk of respiratory depression with other central nervous system depressants. Can cause dystonia.
	Metoclopropamide (Reglan; Wyeth Consumer Healthcare), 5–20 mg PO/IV/PR q 6 hr
	• Contraindicated in bowel obstruction. May be useful in reversing early, partial malignant bowel obstruction when used with other agents.
	• Avoid use with other agents with potential extrapyramidal side effects.
	Haloperidol (Haldol; Ortho-McNeil Consumer Healthcare, Raritan, NJ), 0.5 mg PO q 4–8 hr, 0.25 mg IV/SC q 4–8 hr
	• Can cause dystonia. For dystonia, use diphenhydramine (Benadryl; McNeil Consumer Healthcare) 1 mg/kg PO/IV or benztropine (Cogentin; Merck, Whitehouse Station, NY), 0.02–0.05 mg/kg PO up to 4 mg.
	• IV dosing can cause hypotension, although haloperidol is generally well tolerated by infirm patients.
	Odansetron (Zofran; GlaxoSmithKline), 0.15 mg/kg/dose PO/IV q 6 hr (max = 8 mg)
	• Expensive. Specific for chemotherapy-induced nausea. No evidence that its efficacy exceeds other antiemetics for other etiologies of nausea.
	Dexamethasone, 4–10 mg PO/SC/IV, loading; then 2–4 mg bid
	• Useful for nausea resulting from elevated intracranial pressure and has appetite-stimulating properties. Also helpful for reducing pain secondary to hepatic capsular distention.
	• Can be used as adjunct to pharmacologic management of malignant bowel obstruction.
	• Side effects (mood swings, gastrointestinal hemorrhage, myopathy) should not be overlooked, even in patients with limited prognosis.
	Scopolamine, 0.5 mg per transdermal patch, changed q 72 hr, 0.006 mg/kg/dose q 6 hr IV/SC
	• Useful for nausea and vomiting triggered by vestibular stimulation (motion sickness) or hypovolemia.
	• Helpful for reducing terminal secretions, i.e., "death rattle."
	• Anticipate dry mouth and, occasionally, confusion.

Malignant bowel obstruction "Pharmacologic nasogastric tube"	Antisecretory agent (glycopyrrolate, scopolamine, octreotide); centrally acting antiemetic (haloperidol, chlorpromazine); opioid (morphine, hydromorphone) • This combination of agents can be given to control the symptoms associated with inoperable malignant bowel obstruction (MBO) without nasogastric suctioning. For intractable symptoms on combination therapy, consider placement of PEG. Octreotide, which is expensive, is reserved for high-volume emeses and should be initiated only when opioid and a centrally acting antiemetic fail to control obstructive symptoms. Dexamethasone • May reverse early, incomplete MBO in conjunction with a peristaltic agent (metoclopromamide)
Anxiety/restlessness	Lorazepam (Ativan; Biovail Pharmaceuticals, Mississauga, Ontario), 0.5 mg PO q 4 hr PO/SL/PR
Delirium, moderate	Haloperidol (Haldol), start at 1–2 mg PO/SC q hr until calmer, then 1–2 mg PO/SC qid or bid Chlorpromazine (Thorazine; GlaxoSmithKline), 25–50 mg PO/IV/PR q hr until calmer, then 25–50 mg PO/IV/PR qid or bid • Benzodiazepines (diazepam, lorazepam) can worsen delirium. • Address and treat reversible causes of delirium (i.e., hypercalcemia, dehydration with opioid metabolite accumulation).
Delirium, severe, agitated	Haloperidol combined with midazolam as an hourly infusion • Requires monitoring. Chlorpromazine, 100 mg q hr PO/IV/PR Propofol (Diprivan; AstraZeneca, Wilmington, DE) is highly effective sedation, although its use is limited to closely monitored settings. General: • Sedation may worsen mental clouding seen in delirium but should be mentioned as the necessary cost of preventing bodily injury from thrashing or psychological distress of the patient and caretakers. • In rare cases of refractory, severe symptoms in the last hours/days of life, deliberate sedation to the point of unconsciousness (palliative sedation) can be considered in consultation with medical ethics and palliative care specialist.

IV, Intravenous; *PEG,* percutaneous endoscopic gastronomy; *PO,* by mouth; *PR,* per rectum; *q,* every; *qid,* four times daily; *SL,* sublingually.

Dosing recommendations from Storey P, Knight CF: UNIPAC Four: management of selected non-pain symptoms in the terminally ill, ed 2, Mary Ann Liebert, Publishers, 2003, New York, pp. 40–51.

The medications listed below are meant to give the surgeon a rough idea of the commonly used medications and their usual starting doses. These are not recommendations for specific patients. Considerable variability of response requires individualizing dosing and titration to effect.

Table 6: Common Ethical Issues in Surgical Palliative Care

Issue	Commentary
Disclosure of bad news	Broad legal and ethical consensus supporting disclosure of bad news *when permitted* by patient or surrogate. No evidence that disclosure of bad news "takes away hope" if conveyed gently and in the spirit of nonabandonment. Empathic truth telling fosters trust, which is the basis of hope.
Perioperative do-not-resuscitate (DNR) orders	The American College of Surgeons, the Association of Operating Room Nurses, and the American Society of Anesthesiologists position papers condemn policies requiring automatic cancellation of existing DNR orders for patient undergoing anesthesia based on the principle of patient autonomy. All recommend preoperative discussion ("required reconsideration") during which patient or surrogate confirms patient's treatment goals and limits of care including revision or implementation of a DNR order; risks of patient's care plan; and recommendations by anesthesiologist and surgeon. During this discussion the anesthesiologist and patient can set the parameters for resuscitation for the procedure itself and in the recovery room.
Withhold/withdraw of life support	The withholding and withdrawal of medical treatments are considered legally and ethically equivalent and are based on the right to bodily integrity. It is more difficult to withdraw a life-supporting treatment after it has been started than to not initiate it at all. A surrogate's persistent reluctance to consider termination of life support is usually related to their fear that they will be "killing the patient" or their fear that withdrawing life support will cause suffering. Legally and ethically, termination of undesired medical treatment of the properly informed patient/surrogate is not considered homicide or suicide.

(continued)

Table 6: Common Ethical Issues in Surgical Palliative Care—Cont'd

Issue	Commentary

Aggressive symptom management	• Aggressive symptom management of unbearable symptoms is a moral imperative if effective treatment is available, even at the risk of hastening or causing death, as long as causing death is not the intention of treatment. The risk of hastening death is present with any surgical treatment for serious illness, including attempts to cure.
	
	• In situations in which rapid escalation of dosing is necessary to relieve intractable severe symptoms (pain, dyspnea, agitated delirium) in the imminently dying patient, the Rule of Double Effect, broadly accepted by ethicists, is invoked. RDE is composed of these elements:
	  - The act must be good or morally neutral.
	  - Bad effects are foreseen but not intended.
	  - A good end cannot justify a bad means.
	  - The risk-to-benefit ratio must be reasonable.

Terminal sedation	Rarely indicated in palliative care. Reserved for severe, intractable symptoms when death is imminent. The goal of palliative sedation is to use the minimal amount of sedation necessary to relieve severe physical symptoms to the point of unconsciousness, if necessary, not deliberate induction of coma or hastening of death. Consultation with ethics committee, neuropsychiatric consultant (to determine competency), and palliative care specialist are recommended.

Table 7: Prognostic Indicators

General Indicators of Poor Prognosis

• Functional ability: single most important predictive factor

• Median survival of 3 months: Karnofsky ≤50 or Eastern Cooperative Oncology Group ≥3

• Additional evidence: unintentional progressive weight loss >10% over prior 6 months; serum albumin <2.5 gm/dl (not to be used in isolation from other factors)

Cancer-Related Indicators of Poor Prognosis

• Patients with solid tumors typically lose 70% of functional ability in last 3 months of life

• If >50% of time is spent sleeping or lying down and is increasing, median survival is 3 months, less with increasing symptoms, especially dyspnea

• Most solid tumors that progress through 2 rounds of chemotherapy: <6 months

• Hypercalcemia: 8 weeks (except newly diagnosed myeloma or breast cancer)

• Pericardial effusion: 8 weeks

• Carcinomatous meningitis: 8–12 weeks

• Multiple brain metastases: 1–2 months without radiation, 3–6 months with radiation

• Malignant ascites or pleural effusion: <6 months

• Most metastatic solid cancers, acute leukemias, high-grade lymphomas not on chemotherapy: <6 months

Table 8: Palliative Care Consultation Indications and Medicare Hospice Benefit Eligibility

Palliative Care Consultation

• Patient has an illness typified by progressive deterioration and worsening symptoms, often ending fatally.

• Patient has limiting/threatening conditions with declining functional status, mental or cognitive function.

• Suboptimal control of pain or other distressing symptoms.

• Patient/family would benefit from clarification of goals and plan of care, or resolution of ethical dilemmas.

• Patient/surrogate declines further invasive or curative procedures, preferring comfort-oriented symptom management only.

• Patients on medical/surgical or critical care units who are expected to die imminently or shortly following hospital discharge.

• Bereavement support of hospital workers, particularly after the death of a colleague under care.

Eligibility for Medicare Hospice Benefit

Courtesy Robert A. Milch, MD, FACS, Buffalo, NY.

Although life expectancy of less than 2 months has been suggested as a contraindication for palliative surgery, prognostication by physicians is notoriously inaccurate, especially if the symptom is the reason for loss of function rather than progression of disease.

For major palliative intra-abdominal procedures such as malignant bowel obstruction, generally agreed-upon relative contraindications include: diffuse intraperitoneal carcinomatosis, palpable multiple intra-abdominal masses, multiple liver metastases, extra-abdominal metastases, pleural effusions, multiple sites of partial obstruction or prolonged transit time of contrast on intestinal radiographs, ascites, cachexia or hypoalbuminemia, advanced age, poor performance status, recurrence following recent laparotomy for malignant obstruction, previous abdominal radiation therapy, and disease refractory to chemotherapy.

The availability of stenting, minimally invasive procedures, laparoscopic approaches, and improved adjuvant chemotherapy and radiation therapy have increased flexibility in relieving symptoms related to obstruction, pain, bleeding, fistula, and contaminated wounds. Many of the principles and interventions useful for the palliation of malignant disease can be applied to nonneoplastic disorders encountered in surgical practice, such as chronic pancreatitis, inflammatory bowel disease, and chronic liver failure.

Patient self-report is the gold standard for outcomes measurement following palliative treatment. Numerous validated measuring instruments exist, some of which offer multiple languages and disease-specific modules with ongoing updates. Some of the more commonly used questionnaires include the Functional Assessment of Cancer—General Version (FACT-G), the European Organization for Research and Treatment of Cancer Quality of Life Questionnaire-Core 30 (EORTC QLQ-C30), and the McGill Quality of Life Questionnaire (MQOL).

Access to bereavement services is a critical component of surgical palliative care, not only for patients and families but also for hospital caregivers. Hospital-based bereavement services, including pastoral care departments and family support services, have been shown to affect long-term psychosocial functioning of surviving family members and decisions about organ donation. Surgeons may also benefit from these services as they seek the balance between aloofness and overwhelming emotion in response to serial losses. Recognition that one's status as a surgeon does not inure one from loss is an essential step for adapting to the calling of surgical palliative care.

SUGGESTED READINGS

Dunn GP, Johnson AG, editors: *Surgical palliative care*, Oxford, UK, 2004, Oxford University Press

Baron TH, Dunn GP, editors: Palliative gastroenterology *Gastro Clin N Am*, 35:1, 2006.

Wagman LD, editor: Palliative surgery, *Surg Clin N Am*, 13:401, 2004.

Doyle D, Hanks G, Cherny N, and others: *Oxford textbook of palliative medicine*, ed 3, Oxford, UK, 2003, Oxford University Press.

Dunn GP, editor: The surgeon and palliative care, a monthly series in *J Am Coll Surg*, September 2001–September 2004.

Dunn GP, editor: Surgical palliative care, *Surg Clin N Am*, 2005.

ANALGESIA AND SEDATION IN CRITICAL CARE MEDICINE

Brad Winters, MD

The management of pain and agitation in patients requiring intensive care unit (ICU)–level treatment presents unique challenges to health care practitioners. These patients often have physiologic instability that, combined with their disease processes and frequently impaired communication abilities, puts them at risk for inadequate treatment of their pain or agitation as the clinician tries to balance these competing interests. Often clinicians may find themselves believing they must choose between one of two goals: stabilizing the patient versus providing adequate analgesia and sedation. However, the clinician may also find that pain and agitation are actually compromising his or her ability to stabilize the patient physiologically, making the two goals complementary.

Pain has extremely complex underlying mechanisms, and a thorough discussion of these mechanisms is beyond the scope of this chapter. Suffice it to say that most pain encountered in the ICU setting results from a noxious stimulus (i.e., surgical trauma) that activates peripheral nociceptors, leading to a central nervous system response that results in autonomic output, the sensation of discomfort, possibly agitation, and what is commonly referred to as suffering. Although abnormal and maladaptive pain syndromes such as reflex sympathetic dystrophy (RSD) may present in the ICU, they are uncommon, and their management is discussed elsewhere. In addition to causing agitation, pain may result in shallow breathing ("splinting"), which in turn is thought to promote atelectasis, secretion retention (poor cough), hypoxemia, and pulmonary infection. Pain also contributes to the perioperative stress response. This stress response is characterized by heightened sympathetic tone, increased secretions of catecholamines and catabolic hormones such as glucagon and cortisol, and at the same time depressing secretion of anabolic hormones such as insulin. The overall imbalance leads to a catabolic state that results in protein catabolism and loss of lean body mass and simultaneously contributing to hyperglycemia. Levels of antidiuretic hormone and aldosterone also increase, leading to retention of fluid and salt.

It is imperative that the physician assess for and differentiate between pain, agitation, and delirium. This differentiation is particularly difficult because in many patients in the ICU the ability to communicate is compromised by the process or severity of their disease or the necessity for both invasive and noninvasive mechanical ventilation, or both factors. These three differentials may also be interlinked. A patient may be agitated secondary to pain. Alternatively, agitation may simply result from dyssynchrony with a particular ventilator mode. Agitation may also be secondary to delirium, which is a condition characterized by altered sensorium, whereas pain is not. The ability to recognize the underlying problem allows for effective implementation of a treatment plan.

Assessment of pain and agitation in critically ill patients should include an evaluation of the patient's sensorium that is as thorough as possible. Because verbalization may be impaired, clinicians must be creative in their assessment to determine whether the patient's level of interaction with and awareness of their surrounding is appropriate. Delirium has many life-threatening causes and as such should not be mistaken for other conditions. Some of these causes are hypoxia, hypercarbia (usually secondary to hypoventilation), hypoglycemia, acidosis, electrolytes abnormalities, intoxications and toxicities, and drug and alcohol withdrawal. Although pain may also be associated with life-threatening conditions such as an acute abdomen, the evaluation and treatment of delirium requires a prioritization. After the clinician is certain that the patient's sensorium is not altered and that delirium is unlikely, assessment of pain and agitation is undertaken.

ASSESSMENT OF PAIN AND AGITATION

Pain management in hospitalized patients and ICU patients has been an area identified by several authors and organizations as a focus for improvement in patient quality of care. Several studies have highlighted the prevalence and the impact of pain on critically ill patients. The Support (Study to Understand Prognoses and Preferences for Outcomes and Risks of Treatments) Investigation, in studying more than 4000 conscious ICU patients, found that approximately 50% of these patients who died in the hospital had their pain rated as moderate to severe at least half of the time, as reported by family members. In separate studies, a majority of surviving patients in both surgical and medical critical care units surveyed after their stay reported experiencing pain. Nearly 50% of surgical patients in one study rated that pain as severe, whereas 95% of the house staff and 81% of nurses rated the same patients' pain as adequately controlled. Fifty-three percent of the house staff reported having never assessed the patients' pain relief directly by asking them. Sixty-eight percent of the patients reported that inadequate pain management impaired their ability to cough and clear secretions, and 55% reported that it impaired their ability to perform full inspiration exercises. Communication and disparities in perception were thought to explain the difficulties encountered. Clearly, patients and caregivers had completely different perceptions of how much pain the patients were experiencing. Interestingly, patients frequently reported that they had not requested more analgesia despite their pain being moderate to severe, and nearly one fifth of the patients reported a fear of becoming addicted to a narcotic. Physicians and nurses voiced concerns about adverse physiologic consequences of additional dosages of pain medication as one of their reasons for not providing more analgesia.

Improvements in these results can and should be made. One study demonstrated the effectiveness of a comprehensive program using a multiple-point action plan to provide education on the importance of pain and the use of visual pain scales as an assessment tool, having residents report pain scores on rounds and creating an expectation that a pain score above a certain value demonstrated inadequate quality of care. Use of the pain scoring system by nurses improved from 42% of the time to 70% over a 5-week period, and the incidence of patients having a pain score less that the threshold value rose from 59% preimplementation to 90% in the same time frame.

In light of this and other data, the Joint Commission for the Accreditation of Health Care Organizations (now known as The Joint Commission, or "TJC") has made pain management a priority and established standards that health care institutions must meet. This important organization, accreditation from which is necessary for hospitals to be eligible for Medicaid and Medicare reimbursement, has defined pain rated as equal to or greater then seven on a verbal or visual pain scale as a pain emergency requiring immediate intervention.

Several tools have been developed and validated for the assessment of pain and agitation, and some of these are amenable to use in critically ill patients. These include the Behavioral Pain Scale (BPS), the Numerical Rating Scale (NRS), the Ramsay Sedation Scale, the Wong-Baker Faces Pain Scale, and the Richmond Agitation Sedation Scale (RASS). The features and scoring for three of these (the RASS, BPS, and Ramsay Scale) are described in Figure 1. This is not an exhaustive list, and there is no gold standard for pain and agitation scales. Scales should, however, have good validation data supporting them before their implementation in everyday practice. Although thresholds for providing analgesia or sedation (or both) may vary, scores above 3 for the NRS, above 5 for the BPS, and above 1 for the RAS are usually used to trigger an intervention.

ANALGESIA

There are several modalities for providing analgesia in the ICU. One of the most commonly used is narcotics, usually in intravenous form. Opioids mediate analgesia by interacting with a variety of peripheral and central receptors, with agonism of the mu and kappa receptors being the primary ones for effecting analgesia. Each individual opioid has its own desirable and undesirable attributes. Morphine is known for causing histamine release, which may exacerbate hypotension in patients whose vascular tone or volume status is tenuous. Morphine is also metabolized to two active metabolites, morphine-6-glucuronides and 3-glucuronides, which may accumulate in critically ill patients with renal insufficiency. On the other hand, its pulmonary vascular dilatating properties may be of benefit in patients experiencing pulmonary vascular congestion. Meperidine is a narcotic notorious for the accumulation of a dangerous metabolite, normeperidine, in patients with renal disease. Accumulation of normeperidine may precipitate delirium and seizures. Other commonly used narcotics include fentanyl, hydromorphone, and methadone. All opioids can lead to hypotension in patients with intravascular volume compromise or reliance on the stress response of pain for sympathetic tone. Allergic reactions may also occur, but allergy to one narcotic does not correlate

with allergy to others. Nausea and vomiting are also common side effects, and slowing of peristalsis may occur.

The route of administration is important. Because of changes in volume of distribution, abnormalities of perfusion, and the tendency for critically ill patients to develop interstitial edema secondary to capillary leak, subcutaneous and intramuscular administrations should be avoided. Absorption of the drugs is unreliable under these conditions. Oral administration may also be unreliable in patients with abdominal pathology or ileus. The preferred route is intravenous for most critically ill patients. This may be performed as an intermittent dose, either on a schedule or as needed (prn), a continuous infusion, or if the patient is sufficiently conscious and able to manipulate a button, through patient-controlled analgesia (PCA). PCA allows patients to dose themselves when they perceive their pain to have reached a level at which they are uncomfortable. The dose, interval, and maximal dose per hour are set by the physician with the goal of preventing an overdose while providing adequate pain relief. The dosing schedule on such a device may or may not include a continuous background infusion. The dose and intervals may require adjustment periodically on the basis of the patient's condition and pain and agitation assessments.

Although narcotics often provide excellent pain relief, they are also commonly used for the purpose of sedation in the ICU even when the patient may not be experiencing pain. Sedation is a side effect of narcotics and not their primary benefit. Certainly when the patient is having pain or discomfort (e.g., the irritation of an endotracheal tube) and sedation is desirable, narcotics are an appropriate choice. However, if sedation is the primary goal and pain and discomfort are not thought to be a significant issue, other medications such as the benzodiazepines should be considered. The use of these drugs in treating agitation is discussed later. Of course, if the agitation is thought to be secondary to pain, narcotics are an appropriate first-line therapy.

Other medications may also be used for the treatment of pain in critically ill patients, including the nonsteroidal anti-inflammatory drugs (NSAIDs) such as ketorolac. Although this medication may provide significant pain relief and as such provide an opioid-sparing effect, its nonselective inhibition of cyclo-oxygenase (COX) may affect gastric mucosal perfusion, platelet aggregation, and renal perfusion in critically ill patients whose intravascular volume may be suboptimal. Bleeding risk becomes a significant concern in certain patient groups, particularly in patients with intracranial pathology. On the other hand, this drug has been shown to be well tolerated in thoracic patients and is commonly used in this population because it has essentially no respiratory depression, unlike the narcotics. Ketorolac must be used judiciously in patients with renal insufficiency, including the elderly, and its use should be limited to no more than 5 days' duration. Selective COX-2 inhibitors offered promising alternatives for pain relief in the ICU, especially as intravenous forms started to become available. Unfortunately recent evidence suggesting increased risk of myocardial events with this class of drugs and the subsequent litigation associated with this problem have left the future of these medications uncertain.

Analgesia may also be provided in the ICU through regional anesthetic techniques including nerve blocks (single injection or with continuous catheter placement), continuous or single-injection epidurals or spinals, and local infiltration or infusions such as intrapleural catheters. Patients may come to the ICU postoperatively with these in place or they may be placed in the ICU for any patient. Single-injection nerve blocks such as intercostal blocks for chest tube site pain are effective, but the effect lasts only for a few hours at best. If pain persists, the procedure may have to be repeated, exposing the patient to the procedure risks a second or third time. For this reason, placement of a continuous catheter is often desirable so that the patient may have uninterrupted pain relief over an extended period of time. One of the most popular techniques in the ICU is the epidural catheter. It may be used for a variety of pain problems, including postoperative management of thoracic, abdominal, and pelvic pain, as well as lower limb pain. It may also be placed to control the pain associated with multiple rib fractures in trauma patients to prevent splinting and improve ventilation. Placement of the epidural is dictated by the clinical situation. For

Behavioral Pain Scale (BPS)	Description	Score
Facial Expression	Relaxed	1
	Partially tightened (e.g., brow lowering)	2
	Fully tightened (e.g., eyelid closing)	3
	Grimacing	4
Upper Limbs	No movement	1
	Partially bent	2
	Fully bent with finger flexion	3
	Permanently retracted	4
Compliance with Ventilation	Tolerating movement	1
	Coughing but tolerating ventilation for most of the time	2
	Fighting ventilator	3
	Unable to control ventilation	4

Richmond Agitation Sedation Scale (RASS)		
Score	Term	Description
4	Combative	Combative or violent, immediate danger to staff
3	Very agitated	Pulls on or removes tubes(s) or catheter(s) or has aggressive behavior toward staff
2	Agitated	Frequent nonpurposeful movement or patient-ventilator dysynchrony
1	Restless	Anxious or apprehensive but movements not aggressive or vigorous
0	Alert and calm	
−1	Drowsy	Not fully alert, but has sustained (>10 seconds) awakens with eye contact to voice
−2	Light sedation	Briefly (<10 seconds) awakens with eye contact to voice
−3	Moderate sedation	Any movement (but no eye contact) to voice
−4	Deep sedation	No response to voice, but any movement to physical stimulation
−5	Unarousable	No response to voice or physical stimulation

Ramsay Level of Sedation Scale	
1	Anxious, agitated, or restless
2	Cooperative, oriented, tranquil
3	Awake, obey commands
4-6	Are based on response to loud auditory stimulus or light glabellar tap
4	Asleep but arousable and brisk response
5	Asleep but arousable, sluggish response
6	No response

Figure 1 Selected pain and agitation scoring scales.

postthoracotomy patients, midthoracic (T5–T8) placement is desired. These patients are usually given spare amounts of crystalloid in the operating room, and the sympathectomy that this may cause must be watched closely because profound hypotension may occur. Low-thoracic (T10–T12) or high-lumber (L1) catheters are used for upper abdominal pain. Lower-placed catheters (L2–L5) are used for lower abdominal or pelvic pain and for extremity pain. Typically this technique uses mixtures of a local anesthetic such as bupivacaine or ropivacaine combined with a narcotic such as fentanyl, although it may occasionally use only the local anesthetic agent. This combination of local anesthetic and narcotic provides for a synergistic effect through two mechanisms of action while also allowing for lower doses of either drug to minimize deleterious side effects. Local anesthetics work by blocking neural sodium channels, interrupting neural transmission, and have cardiac and neurotoxicity properties, whereas narcotics bind to the aforementioned mu and kappa receptors and cause respiratory depression. Fentanyl is the most common choice of narcotic for these mixtures secondary to its lipophilicity. This allows for its rapid absorption into the surrounding neural tissue at the site of infusion, localizing its effect. Narcotics such as morphine are relatively hydrophilic and as such tend to diffuse, which is thought to lead to cephalad migration in the neuroaxis, potentially contributing to delayed respiratory depression. This delayed respiratory depression is a particular concern when long-acting morphines such as Duramorph (Baxter Healthcare, Deerfield, IL) are injected intrathecally. Because most epidural catheters have the potential to blunt some or most of the thoracolumbar sympathetic output, close attention to intravascular volume and blood pressure must be maintained. Occasionally, low-dose pressors may be warranted to tolerate the vasodilating effects of this technique. Bradycardia may be a worrisome sign because it suggests that the cardioaccelerator centers of the upper thoracic region (T1–T4) are being affected. Without close attention to management, this, along with hypotension from the sympathectomy, may lead to end-organ hypoperfusion.

An additional use of these local anesthetic techniques is for treatment of poor distal perfusion in the extremities. The sympathectomy associated with techniques such as an epidural may be harnessed for its vasodilation to improve arterial inflow. This is part of the benefit that stellate ganglion blocks have for RSD of the upper extremity. In the ICU, they may be useful in a situation such as inadvertent intra-arterial injection of a compound, for example sodium thiopental, where severe vasoconstriction puts survival of the limb at risk. Stellate ganglion blocks or intra-axillary catheters may be used for the upper extremity, whereas placement of a lumbar epidural may be used for similar issues in the lower extremities.

The choice of modality for management of pain is greatly patient and situation dependent. Some data exist in the literature to assist in the decision process. One study performed a meta-analysis of randomized controlled trials of various therapies on pulmonary outcomes. Outcomes included atelectasis, pulmonary infection, and overall pulmonary complications, as well as spirometry measurements. Epidural opioids showed a statistically significant reduction in the incidence of atelectasis compared with systemic opioids but no benefit in terms of pulmonary infection or overall pulmonary complications. Epidural local anesthetic agents, however, showed a statistically significant reduction in pulmonary infections and overall pulmonary complications compared with systemic opioids. No significant differences were seen in forced vital capacity, forced expiratory volume in one second, or peak expiratory flow rate. Whether spirometry has validity in predicting the incidence of pulmonary infection, atelectasis, or overall pulmonary complications in this study or other situations is questionable.

Intrathecal narcotics have become a popular modality for postoperative pain management. This technique is hampered by the incidence of delayed respiratory depression, a complication that has led many institutions to require postoperative monitoring of these patients, using valuable ICU resources that may better be served for other patients. A study of lumbar spine fusion patients who received intrathecal morphine under direct visualization during the surgery in varying doses (0.2, 0.3, and 0.4 mg) found similar pain relief at the 0.3- and 0.4-mg doses but higher pain scores in the 0.2-mg group. Respiratory rate was found to be significantly lower in the 0.4-mg group compared with the other doses, and there was a trend toward higher $PaCO_2$ in the highest dose. Although this has led to some debate that as long as the dose is kept to no more than 0.3 mg, no monitored bed is necessary, this is not universally accepted. If the patient is already assigned to the ICU postoperatively, this modality has advantages. However, to take up an ICU or other monitored bed through the use of this technique without clear data on its superiority is probably not the best use of resources.

SEDATION

Anxiety and agitation can be disconcerting to both staff and family members. As mentioned previously, the life-threatening causes of agitation and delirium must be addressed immediately. These include hypoxia, hypercarbia, hypoglycemia, hypotension, metabolic abnormalities, toxicities, and withdrawal syndromes. Anxiety and agitation may be secondary to pain but also secondary to mechanical ventilation, restraints, and simply being critically ill. Agitation complicates dyssynchrony with mechanical ventilation, increases oxygen consumption, and increases sympathetic tone and the stress response, and it may place the patient at risk for inadvertent extubation or removal of other devices and catheters, with dire consequences.

Sedatives should be used to reduce anxiety and agitation to reduce the risk of these complications. Narcotics, although possessing sedative properties, should be used for pain management primarily, and if the anxiety or agitation is resulting from pain, both treatment goals may be realized with one agent. However, controlling anxiety and agitation often requires other medications. Benzodiazepines are the most commonly used medications for this purpose. Midazolam, lorazepam, and diazepam are often the drugs of choice, although this class includes a large number of options. The choice is usually driven by duration of action, concern about active metabolites, clearance in face of renal or hepatic insufficiency, and cost. They are usually administered intravenously, either intermittently or by continuous infusion. Accumulation can become a significant problem with large doses or long infusions. Patients have been known to require several days for emergence from sedation even when some of the shorter-acting choices are used. This is also true with the narcotics, particularly when narcotics and benzodiazepines are used together. Notably, benzodiazepines alone have been associated with patients developing delirium. This is especially true in the elderly, and these medications should be carefully titrated, particularly in vulnerable patients. This has been cited as a major reason to favor narcotics over benzodiazepines for sedation.

When agitation is associated with elements of delirium or hallucinations and the life-threatening causes of delirium have been ruled out, a commonly employed medication is haloperidol. The drug provides sedation with minimal respiratory depression and, because of its antipsychotic properties, it is effective at treating the hallucinations and delirium often encountered in the ICU. In fact, it has been long recognized that because of its alien nature and lack of normal environmental cues, coupled with the severity of the patient's conditions, the ICU may create delirium in patients in and of itself. Use of benzodiazepines and other medications may exacerbate this "ICU psychosis" or "ICU delirium." The elderly are also prone to this condition, even without administration of benzodiazepines, and "sundowning" is a well-recognized phenomenon that occurs when night falls and the risk of disorientation increases. In the ICU, sundowning may occur anytime, progressing to hallucinations and severe agitation. When using haloperidol in this clinical situation, the clinician should be watchful for side effects, especially prolonged QT interval, which may precipitate the ventricular tachycardia known as torsades de pointes. Close attention to repletion of magnesium and potassium may offset this risk.

Propofol is also a popular agent for sedation in the ICU. This drug is a general anesthetic induction agent, commonly used in the operating room for both induction and maintenance of general anesthesia. At lower doses, the drug functions as a sedative, allowing for exquisite titration of the depth of sedation and anesthesia. Other advantages of propofol include rapid clearance and awakening (especially high doses may take longer, however). The deleterious effects include pain at the injection site, thrombophlebitis, respiratory depression, so-called propofol syndrome (resulting from prolonged infusions and its requiring emulsification in a lipid mixture), and especially the ability of this emulsion to support rapid bacterial growth. Cases of lethal sepsis secondary to propofol have been reported, and careful aseptic technique must be rigorously observed with this agent, as must time limits for the emulsion after it has been started.

Dexmedetomidine is a centrally acting alpha-2 agonist that has generated much interest as a sedating agent, and its use in ICUs is becoming more widespread. It exerts its effects through the alpha-2 presynaptic receptors to decrease sympathetic output and provide sedation. Its advantages are that it is titratable and that respiratory depression is minimal. Cost remains a major barrier to its more widespread use. In the case of patients requiring mechanical ventilation, studies have shown that halting sedative medication on a daily basis to effect a "wake-up test" is associated with earlier weaning from mechanical ventilation. Thus one should consider using sedative medications in these patients that will facilitate this exercise. This generally will dictate use of shorter-acting agents and close titration. Other patients who may benefit from shorter-acting drugs are patients in whom frequent neurologic checks are necessary. Dexmedetomidine may turn out to be an appropriate choice. Overall it is important to titrate sedative medications to achieve a defined endpoint based on use of one of the available sedation scales.

CONCLUSION

Pain management and sedation are essential components of ICU care. Even though many patients have limited memory of their time in the ICU, good management of these issues has multiple benefits, including increased patient safety, reduction of the stress response and its deleterious effects, reduced suffering, increased patient and family satisfaction, and improved overall quality of care.

SUGGESTED READINGS

Ang P, Knight H, Matadial C, and others: Managing acute postoperative pain: is 3 hours too long? *J Perianesth Nurs* 19:312, 2004.
Ballantyne J, Carr D, de Ferranti, and others: The comparative effects of postoperative analgesic therapies on pulmonary outcome: a meta-analysis for randomized, controlled trials, *Anesth Analg* 8:598, 1988.
Booezaart A, Eksteen J, Spuy G: Intrathecal morphines: double blind evaluation of optimal dosage for analgesia after major lumbar spinal surgery, *Spine* 24:1131, 1999.
Chanques G, Jaber S, Barbotte E, and others: Impact of systematic evaluation of pain and agitation in an intensive care unit, *Crit Care Med* 34:1, 2006.
Erdek M, Pronovost P: Improving assessment and treatment of pain in the critically ill, *Int J Qual Health Care* 16:59, 2004.
Jacobi J, Farser G, Coursin D: Clincial practice guidelines for the sustained use of sedatives and analgesics in the critically ill adult, *Crit Care Med* 30:115, 2002.
Pandharipande P, Shintani A, Peterson J, and others: Lorazepam is an independent risk factor for transitioning to delirium in intensive care patients, *Anesthesiology* 104:21, 2006.

CARDIOVASCULAR PHARMACOLOGY

Paul R. Crisostomo, MD, Daniel R. Meldrum, MD, and Alden H. Harken, MD

INTRODUCTION

Although it sounds astonishingly simple, cardiovascular pharmacology is all about optimizing the function of a pump: if it is too fast, slow it down; if it is too slow, speed it up; if it is empty, fill it; if it is too full, help it empty. The tools that we use to "grease" the pump are best understood when learned in the context of the cardiac action potential.

CARDIOVASCULAR PHARMACOLOGY IN THE CONTEXT OF THE CARDIAC ACTION POTENTIAL

Five phases of the ventricular myocyte action potential may be targeted in the treatment of cardiac arrhythmias. Figure 1 shows the action potential of cardiac myocytes and the ionic shifts responsible for each phase and correlates these with the surface electrocardiogram. Antiarrhythmic agents influence cardiac electrical activity by their effects on ion channels. The predominant mechanism of action on the cardiac action potential serves as the basis of the modified Vaughan-Williams classification scheme (Table 1) for antiarrhythmic agents, as follows:

Phase 0: Rapid depolarization resulting from influx of sodium through the voltage-gated sodium channels. Class I antiarrhythmic agents (e.g., lidocaine, procainamide) block the sodium channel and depress phase 0 depolarization. Slowing phase 0 depolarization is useful for slowing rapid heart rates, such as ventricular tachycardia and atrial fibrillation.

Phase 1: Brief repolarization resulting from chloride influx and potassium efflux.

Phase 2: Plateau phase sustained by balance of calcium influx through L-type calcium channels and efflux of potassium. Calcium channel blockers (e.g., verapamil), class IV antiarrhythmic agents, inhibit slow L-type calcium channels and prolong the phase 2 plateau. Beta-blockers (e.g., metoprolol), class II antiarrhythmic agents, also indirectly blockade calcium channels. Prolonging phase 2 may be useful for supraventricular tachycardias.

Phase 3: Rapid membrane repolarization produced by potassium leaving the cell. Class III antiarrhythmic agents (e.g., amiodarone) block the potassium channel and delay phase 2 and 3 repolarization. By slowing repolarization, class III agents prolong refractoriness and therefore make the myocardium less irritable. This may be useful both in supraventricular arrhythmias and ventricular arrhythmias.

Phase 4: Resting membrane potential. Slow depolarization of pacemaker cells governed by slow influx of sodium. Slowing phase 4 depolarization may be useful in ventricular arrhythmias.

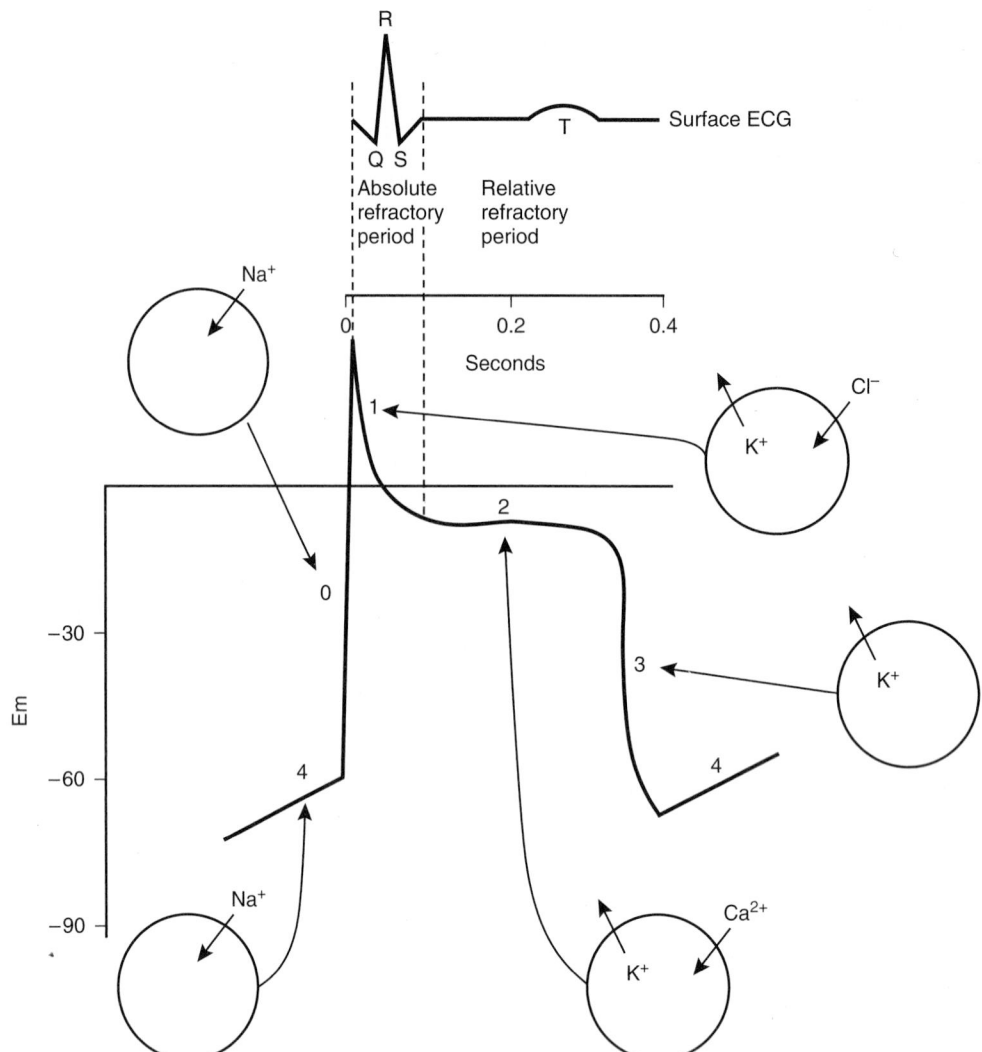

Figure 1 Cardiac action potential. *Phase 0:* Rapid depolarization resulting from influx of sodium through the voltage-gated sodium channels. Class I antiarrhythmic agents (e.g., lidocaine, procainamide) block the sodium channel and depress phase 0 depolarization. Slowing phase 0 depolarization is useful for slowing rapid heart rates such as ventricular tachycardia and atrial fibrillation. *Phase 1:* Brief repolarization caused by chloride influx and potassium efflux. *Phase 2:* Plateau phase sustained by balance of calcium influx through L-type calcium channels and efflux of potassium. Calcium channel blockers (e.g., verapamil), class IV antiarrhythmic agents, inhibit slow L-type calcium channels and prolong the phase 2 plateau. Beta-blockers (e.g., metoprolol), class II antiarrhythmic agents, also indirectly blockade calcium channels. Prolonging phase 2 may be useful for supraventricular tachycardias. *Phase 3:* Rapid membrane repolarization produced by potassium leaving the cell. Class III antiarrhythmic agents (e.g., amiodarone) block the potassium channel and delay phase 2 and 3 repolarization. By slowing repolarization, class III agents prolong refractoriness and therefore make the myocardium less irritable. This may be useful both in supraventricular arrhythmias and ventricular arrhythmias. *Phase 4:* Resting membrane potential. Slow depolarization of pacemaker cells governed by slow influx of sodium. Slowing phase 4 depolarization may be useful in ventricular arrhythmias. *From Meldrum DR, Cleveland JC Jr, Sheridan BC, and others: Ann Thorac Surg 61:1273, 1996.*

Table 1: Vaughan Williams Classification of Antiarrhythmic Agents

Class I agents interfere with the sodium (Na⁺) channel (phase 0).

Class II agents, beta-blockers, indirectly blockade calcium channels (phase 2).

Class III agents affect potassium (K⁺) efflux (phase 2 and 3).

Class IV agents, calcium channel blockers, block the atrioventricular node and inhibit slow L-type calcium channels (phase 2).

Class V agents work by other or unknown mechanisms.

TACHYCARDIC ARRHYTHMIAS

Atrial fibrillation and atrial flutter have been reported in up to 60% of patients in the early postoperative period following cardiac surgery. Amiodarone may be the most effective antiarrhythmic drug available and is the drug of choice for pharmacologic reversion of atrial fibrillation. Amiodarone (class III) primarily blocks the potassium ion channel, slows phase 2 and phase 3 repolarization, and prolongs refractoriness. However, its antiarrhythmic efficacy can also be derived from its multiple other effects on the action potential. It inhibits inactivated phase 0 sodium channels (class I), noncompetitively blocks the beta receptor (class II), and blocks L-type calcium channels (class IV). Consequently, amiodarone decreases myocardial irritability, inhibits sympathetic activity, slows atriovenous (AV) conduction, and has a low rate of proarrhythmia. Intravenous amiodarone begins with a 150-mg bolus over 10 minutes, followed by a continuous infusion of 1 mg/minute for 6 hours and 0.5 mg/minute thereafter. Repeated boluses can be given over 10 minutes every 10 to 15 minutes to a maximal total dose of 2.2 g in 24 hours. The best chance of reestablishing normal sinus rhythm is through an amiodarone load followed by electric cardioversion.

Rate control for atrial fibrillation is best achieved with beta-blockers (class II). Beta-blockers indirectly blockade calcium channel opening, prolong the phase 2 plateau, and block the proarrhythmic effects of postoperative catecholamines by attenuating adrenergic activation. Intravenous esmolol is particularly useful in the acute setting of atrial fibrillation because of its fast onset, short half-life, and beta-1 specificity. Verapamil, a calcium channel blocker (class IV), and digoxin (class V) are other AV nodal blockers that prevent unwanted supraventricular impulses in atrial fibrillation, but they are not more effective than beta-blockers. Verapamil prolongs the phase 2 plateau and slows the sinoatrial node pacemaker cell and AV conduction by direct blockade of L-type voltage-gated calcium channels.

The other predominant narrow complex tachycardia is paroxysmal supraventricular tachycardias. Adenosine (class V) is effective in terminating up to 99% of these cases and interacts with A1 receptors on the surface of cardiac cells, activating potassium channels, and shortening the phase 2 action potential plateau. Adenosine also indirectly reduces calcium influx into cells by antagonizing catecholamine-stimulated adenylate cyclase. The resulting effects include a slowing of the sinus rate and an increase in the AV nodal conduction delay. Adenosine is administered by rapid intravenous injection over 1 to 2 seconds followed by a normal saline flush at a peripheral site (initial dose 6 mg, up to 12 mg), or a central venous site (initial dose 1 mg, up to 3 mg). When paroxysmal supraventricular tachycardia is refractory to adenosine, calcium channel blockers, beta-blockers, or digoxin may work.

The more ominous sustained monomorphic or polymorphic ventricular tachycardia or ventricular fibrillation occur in less than 3% of postoperative patients but are associated with a significant increase in postoperative mortality. This increased mortality is due to cardiac arrest, enhanced myocardial oxygen demand, and exacerbation of ischemia. For patients who are hemodynamically stable during ventricular tachycardia, intravenous pharmacologic therapy should be tried before electrical cardioversion. In these cases, amiodarone and lidocaine work well. The key is to slow phase 0 depolarization, block the fast inward sodium current, and depress the rate of spontaneous phase 4 depolarization (automaticity). Lidocaine is given by intravenous push in a dose of 0.5 to 0.75 mg/kg; this dose is repeated every 5 to 10 minutes as needed. At the same time, a continuous intravenous infusion of 1 to 4 mg/minute is begun. The maximal total dose is 3 mg/kg over 1 hour. This can be followed by synchronized cardioversion if necessary. However, all antiarrhythmic drugs have the potential to induce or aggravate ventricular tachycardia, torsades de pointes, ventricular fibrillation, conduction disturbances, or bradycardia.

BRADYCARDIC ARRHYTHMIAS

Sinus bradycardia is prevalent after acute myocardial infarction (MI) and, when accompanied by symptoms or hemodynamic compromise, should be treated. Atropine is the preferred initial treatment for symptomatic bradycardia. Atropine increases the heart rate by inhibiting vagal and acetylcholine stimulation of sinus pacemaker cells and is given by intravenous push in a dose of 0.5 to 1.0 mg every 3 to 5 minutes to a maximal dose of 3 mg. However, atropine treatment is also accompanied by extracardiac acetylcholine inhibition of intestinal smooth muscles and glands. In acute instances, an external pacemaker is easy to use, is well tolerated, and can be lifesaving.

CARDIOVASCULAR PHARMACOLOGY IN THE CONTEXT OF THE FRANK STARLING MECHANISM

The Frank Starling Mechanism states that up to a point, the more blood that returns to the heart (preload), the greater the stroke volume and systolic pressure. In Figure 2, with increased filling (preload A to B), there is increased stroke volume (C to D) and increased stroke work (area inside A-B-C-D). Inotropes and vasopressors influence the location of the heart on the Frank Starling curve and further improve stroke work (increase the area inside A-B-C-D). Figure 2 also relates the Frank Starling curve to the pathophysiology of shock. Shock is a physiologic state in which a reduction in tissue perfusion and oxygen delivery leads to end-organ dysfunction. Three broad types of shock states are recognized: hypovolemic, cardiogenic, and distributive (or systemic vascular collapse). Hypovolemic shock is a reduction in preload (B to B′), either through blood loss or fluid loss such as diarrhea and vomiting. Hypovolemic shock (empty pump) is the most prevalent shock state, making volume replacement (filling it) a prerequisite before instituting cardiovascular pharmacologic therapy. Cardiogenic shock is a failure of the heart to pump effectively (lower Starling curve) through arrhythmias, mechanical abnormalities, obstructive disorders, or myopathies. If the pump is full (cardiogenic shock), empty it by using therapies that improve overall cardiac function (higher Starling curve). Distributive or vasodilatory shock is a reduction in systemic vascular resistance (SVR) resulting from a variety of causes such as sepsis, systemic inflammatory response, anaphylaxis, and neurogenic shock. Distributive shock is a "relative" hypovolemia; if the pump is empty because of relative hypovolemia (preload), fill it by tightening dilatated vessels.

DISTRIBUTIVE (SEPTIC/NEUROGENIC/ANAPHYLACTIC) SHOCK

Septic shock is characterized by a massive inflammatory response to infection mediated by cytokines and other factors, including prostaglandins, thromboxane A2, and nitric oxide (NO), resulting in

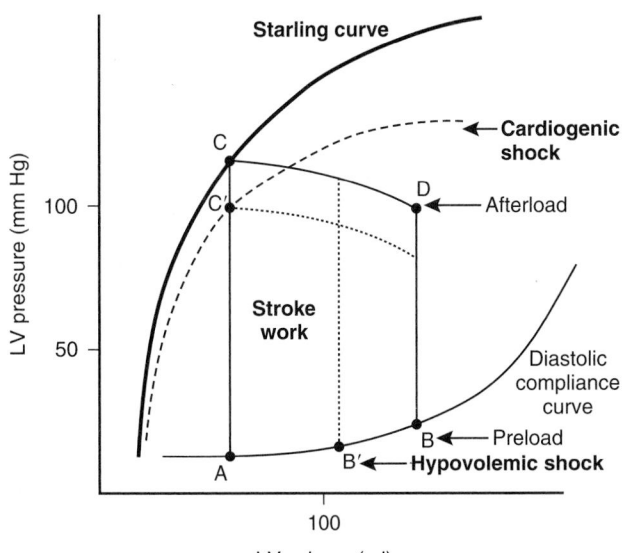

Figure 2 Frank-Starling Mechanism. *(A)* Atrioventricular valve opens and the ventricle fills to point B (preload). *(B)* Atrioventricular valve closes and the ventricle contracts, increasing pressure to point C. *(C)* Aortic valve opens after ventricular pressure is greater than aortic diastolic pressure (afterload). *(D)* Aortic valve closes and ventricular relaxation occurs and drops pressure to point A.

vasodilation, endothelial damage, and capillary leak. These endogenous responses to pathogen in addition to endotoxin itself cause a physiologic drop in systemic vascular resistance. Neurogenic shock and anaphylactic shock are also characterized by a profound decrease in systemic vascular tone. These forms of distributive shock eventually lead to tissue hypoperfusion despite fluid resuscitation and an otherwise normal heart. If the pump is empty because of a relative hypovolemia, fill it by tightening dilatated vessels with vasopressors.

Vasopressors, particularly those agents with vasoconstrictive properties, play an important role in addressing pathologic vasodilation (see Table 2). Norepinephrine (5 mcg/min up to 20 mcg/min) is the most potent vasoconstrictor and consequently is often the initial vasopressor of choice for septic shock. Norepinephrine is a potent alpha-adrenergic agonist with minimal beta-adrenergic agonist effects. (Table 3 highlights the adrenergic receptor agents.) This stimulation of alpha-1 adrenergic receptors (vascular smooth muscle contraction) and alpha-2 receptors (peripheral vasoconstriction) increases systemic vascular resistance without significantly increasing cardiac index. Dopamine (2–20 mcg/kg/min) is a precursor of norepinephrine and epinephrine and has varying effects according to the doses infused. At high doses (>10 mcg/kg/min), its alpha-adrenergic effects predominate, leading to arterial vasoconstriction and an elevation in blood pressure. However, this vasoconstriction at high doses is accompanied by a significant stimulation of beta-receptors, inducing an increase in heart rate, cardiac contractility, and myocardial oxygen consumption. These inotropic effects of dopamine may be undesirable in the early stages of sepsis, in which a normal heart is already maximally physiologically stimulated. Compared with norepinephrine, dopamine has greater inotropic effects but fewer vasoconstrictive properties.

Epinephrine (1–20 mcg/min), an alpha- and beta-adrenergic agonist, is recommended in patients unresponsive to other vasopressors. In distributive shock, epinephrine may be useful for treatment of pathologic vasodilation and results in a greater increase in SVR and vasoconstriction than dopamine and nearly the same level as norepinephrine. Epinephrine also has high affinity for the beta-1 receptor, resulting in increased cardiac index and stroke volume greater than either aforementioned vasopressor. These potent inotropic effects may preclude its use in early high-output sepsis. Further, administration of this agent is associated with an increase in systemic and regional lactate concentrations, a potential to produce

Table 2: Vasopressors and Inotropes

Agent	Alpha1	Alpha2	Beta1	Beta2	Dopa
Dopamine (dose)					
Low	0	0	+	0	+++
Middle	0	0	++	+	++
High	++	+	++	+	+
Dobutamine	+	+	+++	++	0
Norepinephrine	+++	+++	+	+	0
Epinephrine	+++	+++	+++	++	0
Isoproterenol	0	0	+++	+	0
Phenylephrine	+++	+	+	+	0

Table 3: Adrenergic Receptors

Alpha-1 adrenergic: vascular smooth muscle contraction
Alpha-2 adrenergic: vasodilation (central), vasoconstriction (peripheral)
Beta-1: inotropy, chronotropy
Beta-2: vasodilation, bronchodilation
Dopa: renal, coronary, and mesenteric vasodilation

myocardial ischemia, the development of arrhythmias, and a reduction in splanchnic flow.

Drotrecogin alfa is recombinant human activated protein C, an endogenous protein that modulates inflammation, decreases coagulation, and increases fibrinolysis. Specifically, it inhibits coagulation factors Va and VIIIa, which subsequently inhibit thrombin, and thus prevents microvascular thrombi. In addition, it indirectly inhibits tumor necrosis factor-alpha, interleukin (IL)-1, and IL-6, the mediators thought to play a major role in initiating the inflammatory response seen in sepsis. Activated protein C levels have been shown to be low in sepsis, and randomized phase 3 controlled trials suggest that drotrecogin alfa significantly lowers vasopressor requirements and decreases mortality.

CARDIOGENIC SHOCK

Cardiogenic shock is characterized by pump failure and myocardial damage, with subsequent tissue hypoperfusion and sustained hypotension despite adequate left ventricular filling pressure. Cardiogenic shock (a full pump) is treated by decreasing cardiac afterload and improving cardiac contractility (emptying it). Sympathomimetic inotropes and vasopressors are the cornerstone of acute pharmacologic therapy during cardiogenic shock.

Despite the complexity of its dose-dependent inotropic effects, dopamine is often a first-line agent in the treatment of cardiogenic shock. At low doses (2–5 mcg/kg/min), selective stimulation of dopamine receptors improves renal, mesenteric, and coronary blood flow; at medium doses (5–10 mcg/kg/min) preferential stimulation of beta-1 receptors results in inotropic (increased contractility) and chronotropic (increased heart rate) effects. However, in critically ill patients, marked interpatient variability in plasma clearance of dopamine may alter the latter dose specific effects. Further narrowing its therapeutic window in cardiogenic shock, high-dose dopamine increases vasoconstriction and afterload and should be avoided.

Dobutamine is a synthetic catecholamine that may also be used to support cardiac output. Dobutamine is a selective beta-receptor agonist and induces significant positive inotropy (beta-1), mild chronotropy (beta-1), and peripheral vasodilation (beta-2). This increase in myocardial contractility and decrease in afterload make dobutamine a drug of choice for cardiogenic shock. However, in the setting of acute MI, dobutamine may exacerbate infarct size because of increased myocardial oxygen consumption. Dobutamine may also produce unwanted effects in patients with moderate hypotension because of its vasodilatatory actions.

Isoproterenol is another synthetic catecholamine with selective beta-agonist properties. Its specific positive chronotropic effects (beta-1) have proved useful in maintaining heart rate status following heart transplantation or in selected patients with complete heart block. In parallel with dobutamine, isoproterenol is contraindicated in acute MI because of its marked increase in oxygen demand.

Although epinephrine is considered an inotrope and vasopressor, low-dose epinephrine results in vasodilation and inotropy, which may prove useful in cardiogenic shock. Vascular smooth muscle contains a large number of alpha-1 receptors (vasoconstriction) relative to beta-2 receptors (vasodilation), which oppose each other. However, epinephrine has a higher affinity for the beta-2 receptor relative to the alpha-1 receptor. Thus low-dose epinephrine produces a beta-2 mediated muscle relaxation and a decrease in peripheral resistance, whereas high-dose epinephrine produces an alpha-1-mediated vasoconstriction. As mentioned previously, caution remains regarding use of epinephrine because of elevated lactate concentrations and increased incidence of arrhythmias, and potential myocardial, splanchnic, and distal extremity ischemia.

Phosphodiesterase inhibitors (PDIs) such as milrinone and inamrinone are novel noncatecholamine inotropes with vasodilating properties. PDIs mediate their vascular effects via prolongation of the vasodilatory molecules cyclic guanosine monophosphate (cGMP) and nitric oxide (NO). The net benefit of this mechanism includes peripheral vasodilation (decreased afterload), pulmonary vasodilation (decreased LV preload), and increased myocardial contractility. The pulmonary vasodilation is a unique property of PDIs and has physiologic benefit in right ventricular afterload reduction. PDIs also differ from catecholamine inotropes by demonstrating longer half-lives, less tolerance, less tachycardia, and less myocardial oxygen demand. Although PDIs are beneficial in persons with cardiac pump failure, they may require concomitant vasopressor administration.

Morphine 3 to 5 mg given intravenously (IV) over 2 minutes may relieve severe chest pain, help to reduce elevated catecholamine levels, and reduce preload and afterload on the failing heart; the response must be closely monitored because morphine causes respiratory depression, is a venodilator, and may cause blood pressure to fall.

PERIOPERATIVE RISK REDUCTION

Beta-blockers appear to be the most useful medical therapy to reduce morbidity and mortality after major cardiac and noncardiac surgery. Several randomized and nonrandomized studies have demonstrated that beta-blockers reduce the risk of postoperative ischemia, myocardial infarct, atrial fibrillation, and death in selected patients. The Revised Goldman Cardiac Risk Index may be a useful stratification that separates patients who benefit (index >2) and those who do not (index 0–2), from beta-blocker therapy and identifies six independent predictors of postoperative cardiac complications: high-risk type of surgery, history of ischemic heart disease, history of heart failure, history of cerebrovascular disease, diabetes mellitus requiring treatment with insulin, and preoperative serum creatinine greater than2 mg/dL.

All studies that have reported a cardiovascular benefit of perioperative beta-blockers have used beta-1 cardioselective agents (e.g., metoprolol, atenolol, esmolol). Beta-1 blockers are competitive inhibitors of the sympathetic catecholamines norepinephrine and epinephrine at beta-1 adrenoreceptors in cardiac nodal tissue, the conducting system, and contracting myocytes, and thereby decrease contractility, heart rate, and conduction velocity. Ultimately, selective beta-blockers may mediate their protective effect by decreasing myocardial oxygen demand caused by increased stress and catecholamine release in the perioperative period. Despite their similarities in pharmotherapeutic effects, selective beta-blockers exhibit differing pharmacokinetic properties. Metoprolol, available in generic formulations, is metabolized by the liver but tends to have variable bioavailability and short plasma half-life. Atenolol is eliminated unchanged by the kidney, has less variance in bioavailability, and has a longer plasma half-life. Intravenous esmolol has a plasma half-life of 5 to 10 minutes because of its rapid metabolism by blood and hepatic esterases. This ultra-short-acting agent may prove useful in scenarios in which hypotension or heart failure (or both) are suspected. There are no data to recommend one beta-1 selective agent versus another in perioperative risk reduction.

Nonselective beta-blocking agents (propranolol) suffer the major disadvantage of blocking beta-2 receptors associated with airway or vascular smooth muscle and consequent exacerbation of airway or peripheral vascular disease. However, these agents demonstrate greater efficacy in the management of anxiety, migraines, esophageal varices, and thyrotoxicosis. It is not necessary for patients taking a nonselective beta-blocker chronically to change to a beta-1 selective agent perioperatively. Other side effects seen in beta-blockers include sedation, fatigue, sexual dysfunction, and impairment of mental function. Hypotension, bradycardia, and blunted glycopenic symptoms can occur. These agents may also increase triglycerides and decrease high-density lipid cholesterol. As stated earlier, nonselective agents (and selective agents at high doses) can increase airway reactivity and peripheral vascular vasoconstriction. Nevertheless, these symptoms should not preclude the use of beta-blockers in the perioperative period in selected patients with indications discussed herein.

SYSTEMIC HYPERTENSION

Postoperative hypertension is a ubiquitous phenomenon following cardiac and noncardiac surgery and may lead to serious neurologic, cardiovascular, or surgical-site complications. Any marked rise in blood pressure despite resuming chronic antihypertensive therapy and excluding causes such as pain, agitation, and bladder distention should be treated immediately.

Vasodilatators have proved to be effective mainstays in the management of acute postoperative hypertension and produce decreases in preload, afterload, or both. Sodium nitroprusside reduces both preload and afterload through its relaxation of arteriolar and venous smooth muscle. Nitroprusside is an unstable molecule that spontaneously decomposes into an active metabolite, NO, and a toxic metabolite, cyanide. Despite endogenous cyanide detoxification into thiocyanate, fatal poisoning may still occur, requiring careful limitations in dose (0.25 mcg/kg/min up to a maximal dose of 10 mcg/kg per minute) and length of treatment (usually <48 hours). In contrast, nitroglycerin predominantly reduces preload (venodilation) at therapeutic doses (start at 5 mcg/min) and reduces afterload (arteriodilation) only at high doses (maximum 100 mcg/min). Nitroglycerin is an organic nitrate that requires an enzymatic process to release NO from its structure. However, the organic nitrate predilection for collateral coronary vessel dilatation, coronary spasm relief, antiplatelet activity, and lack of cyanide accumulation make organic nitrates such as nitroglycerin an ideal antihypertensive first-line agent in patients with myocardial ischemia. Hydralazine (5–20 mg) directly reduces afterload with high specificity for arterial vessels and little or no effect on the venous circulation. Hydralazine may mediate arterial vasodilation through both NO-dependent and NO-independent mechanisms. However, hydralazine also results in indirect cardiac stimulation (tachycardia) because of activation of the baroreceptor reflex, necessitating caution in patients with underlying coronary disease or an aortic dissection. A beta-blocker may be given concurrently to minimize this reflex sympathetic stimulation.

The rapid onset of action for labetalol (5 minutes or less) makes this agent useful in the treatment of hypertensive emergencies. Labetalol, a combined alpha- and beta-adrenergic blocking agent, uniquely blocks alpha-1 receptors, as well as beta-1 and beta-2 receptors, with a potency ratio of 1:4. This dual alpha- and beta-blockade prevents the unopposed alpha-adrenergic activity seen in other nonselective beta-blockers and may allow greater safety in peripheral vasculopathology; however, caution still remains in patients with asthma, chronic obstructive pulmonary disease, congestive heart failure, bradycardia, and heart block. Labetalol may be given as an intravenous bolus (10–20 mg initially, followed by 10–80 mg every 10 minutes to a total dose of 300 mg) or infusion (0.5–2 mg/min).

It is widely accepted that diuretics, through their effects on sodium and water balance, increase urine output by the kidney, decrease blood volume, decrease venous pressure, and ultimately decrease cardiac filling (preload). However, there is some evidence that loop diuretics (Lasix, Sanofi-Aventis, Bridgewater, NJ) also cause transient venodilation via local vascular prostaglandin synthesis. This venodilator response may be blocked in the presence of nonsteroidal anti-inflammatory drugs.

PULMONARY HYPERTENSION

Pulmonary arterial hypertension (PAH) can develop postoperatively as a result of hypoxic vasoconstriction, decreased surface area of the pulmonary vascular bed, or right ventricular volume or pressure overload. The treatment of secondary PAH initially consists of specific interventions or specific medical therapies to correct the primary disease such as atrial septal defect or mitral stenosis. However, if reversal of the primary disease in secondary PAH is not possible or if the diagnosis is primary and idiopathic PAH, a variety of pharmacologic interventions aimed at pulmonary hypertension are required.

Although understudied, inhaled NO has the distinct advantage of delivery only to areas that are ventilated, thereby preserving ventilation-perfusion matching and limiting extrapulmonary activity. NO activates guanylyl cyclase, catalyzing the conversion of guanosine triphosphate to cGMP. cGMP activation of several cGMP-dependent kinases results in phosphorylation of several proteins, a decrease in intracellular potassium and calcium, and ultimately relaxation of vascular smooth muscle. In addition to its actions as an acute vasodilator, NO may also suppress smooth muscle proliferation and inhibit platelet aggregation. Inhaled NO has an effective half-life of 15 to 30 seconds, with a dose range of 5–80 ppm. Pulmonary vasodilation appears to be a threshold effect (with vasodilation occurring at concentrations of approximately 10 ppm), rather than a dose-response effect. However, an improvement in survival has not been demonstrated with this approach in patients with spontaneous pulmonary artery hypertension (SPAH).

Type 5 phosphodiesterase (PDE5) inhibitors have also found clinical benefit in pulmonary hypertension. Recent investigations reveal that PDE5, a vascular smooth muscle enzyme that hydrolyzes cGMP to its inactive form, is upregulated in PAH, contributing to increased pulmonary vascular resistance. Thus inhibition of PDE5 prolongs the vasodilatory effect of cGMP and NO. Three PDE5 inhibitors (sildenafil, vardenafil, tadalafil) are in clinical use and differ in their rate of onset (most rapid effect by vardenafil), duration of effect (most sustained by tadalafil), pulmonary vascular selectivity (sildenafil and tadalafil, but not vardenafil), and effect on oxygenation (improvement with sildenafil only). At this time, only sildenafil (20 mg orally three times daily) is approved for use in patients with PAH.

Bosentan (125 mg orally twice daily) is a novel, nonselective endothelin receptor antagonist that may have efficacy in PAH. Endothelin-1 is a potent vasoconstrictor that binds receptors expressed on both endothelial cells and vascular smooth muscle within the pulmonary circulation. Thus bosentan inhibits endothelin binding to its receptors and mediates pulmonary vasodilation. Randomized studies indicate that bosentan decreases mean pulmonary artery pressure and pulmonary vascular resistance. However, careful monitoring of liver function tests is necessary because elevation of serum aminotransferase enzyme levels has been noted.

CONCLUSION

Armed with a basic understanding of cardiovascular pharmacology, the critical care surgeon may better target the pathogenic physiology behind various perioperative disease processes. Further knowledge of the pharmacologic nuances of cardiovascular agents may enable the physician surgeon to optimize cardiovascular hemodynamics and ultimately patient care.

SUGGESTED READINGS

Harken AH: Evaluation and treatment of cardiac dysrhythmias. In: Harken AH, Moore EE, editors: *Abernathy's surgical secrets*, ed 5, Philadelphia, 2004, Mosby Elsevier.

Morrell ED, Tsai BM, Crisostomo PR, and others: Experimental therapies for hypoxia-induced pulmonary hypertension during acute lung injury, *Shock* 25:214, 2006.

POSTOPERATIVE RESPIRATORY FAILURE

Pedro Alejandro Mendez-Tellez, MD, and Todd Dorman, MD

Postoperative pulmonary complications (PPCs) are as common as cardiac complications and a major cause of overall perioperative morbidity and mortality in selected groups of patients and in those with high-risk surgical procedures. The reported frequency of PPCs ranges from 2% to 70%. Postoperative pulmonary complications include atelectasis, pulmonary infections such as bronchitis and pneumonia, prolonged mechanical ventilatory support and respiratory failure, and exacerbation of underlying chronic lung disease and bronchospasm.

Acute postoperative respiratory failure is not an uncommon complication. Excluding patients with chronic respiratory disease, circulatory disease, and obstetric or neonatal conditions, the incidence of postoperative respiratory failure is estimated to be 3.66 per 1000 elective surgery discharges. The lowest incidence rate (1.41 per 1000 elective surgery discharges) occurs in people aged 18 to 44, whereas the highest incidence rate (3.85 per 1000 elective surgery discharges) happens in people older than age 65.

Acute postoperative respiratory failure is defined as the acute onset of severe impairment of pulmonary gas exchange during the postsurgical period in quantities sufficient to cause severe organ dysfunction or to threaten life. Respiratory failure can affect either pulmonary ventilatory pump or the gas exchange function of the lung. Thus respiratory failure is often categorized as hypercapnic or ventilatory respiratory failure, manifested primarily by hypercapnia (PCO_2 >45 mm Hg) and respiratory acidosis or hypoxemic respiratory failure, which presents mainly as hypoxemia. *Hypoxemic respiratory failure* has classically been defined as an arterial PO_2 of less than 60 mm Hg. Often both hypoxemic and hypercapnic respiratory failure coexist.

Arterial hypoxemia is usually classified by five pathophysiologic mechanisms: (1) decreased inspired PO_2, (2) hypoventilation, (3) impaired diffusion, (4) ventilation-perfusion (V/Q) mismatch, and (5) right-to-left shunt. Hypoventilation presents clinically as hypercapnia and respiratory acidosis. Most critically ill patients with acute hypoxemic respiratory failure have some combination of V/Q mismatch and right-to-left shunt. Whereas hypoxemia from V/Q mismatch is responsive to supplemental oxygen, hypoxemia from a shunt is not responsive. Arterial hypoxemia can also be classified on the basis of whether the primary pathology is located in the air spaces, interstitium, heart and pulmonary vasculature, airways, or pleural space. Common causes of postoperative hypoxemic respiratory failure are listed in Table 1. Common causes of postoperative hypercapnic respiratory failure are listed in Table 2.

EFFECTS OF ANESTHESIA ON THE RESPIRATORY SYSTEM

General anesthesia is associated with marked alterations in respiratory drive, lung volumes, diaphragmatic movement, and inhibition of the hypoxic pulmonary vasoconstriction mechanism. General anesthetics are significant respiratory depressants. Inhalational anesthetic agents affect the ventilatory response to hypercapnia and hypoxia and the pattern of breathing. Inhalational agents shift the CO_2-ventilation response curve to the right and depress the slope in a dose-dependent manner; arterial PCO_2 increases with increasing concentration of these agents. Surgical stimulation

Table 1: Acute Hypoxemic Respiratory Failure

Alveolar Filling Disorders

- Pneumonia
- Posttraumatic (i.e., contusion)
- Atelectasis

Increased Pulmonary Capillary Pressure

- Cardiogenic pulmonary edema
- Intravascular volume expansion
- Pulmonary venous disease

Increased Pulmonary Capillary Permeability

- Acute respiratory distress syndrome
- Fat embolization
- Smoke inhalation
- Chemical inhalation

Unclear Mechanisms

- Neurogenic pulmonary edema
- High-altitude pulmonary edema
- Pulmonary embolus

Table 2: Hypercapnic Respiratory Failure

Central Nervous System Failure

- Drug overdose (opioids, sedatives, hypnotics)
- Cerebrovascular accident, neoplasms, infections
- Primary alveolar hypoventilation, obesity hypoventilation syndrome

Neural and Neuromuscular Junction Failure

- Neural transmission disorders (spinal chord trauma, Guillain-Barre syndrome, amyotrophic lateral sclerosis, phrenic nerve injury)
- Neuromuscular junction disorders (myasthenia gravis, botulism, tetanus, neuromuscular blocking agents)

Ventilatory Muscles Failure

- Primary myopathies: muscular dystrophy, polymyositis
- Critical illness polyneuropathy and myopathy
- Electrolyte disorders (hypophosphatemia, hypokalemia, hypermagnesemia)

Chest Wall and Pleural Disorders

- Chest wall disorders (kyphoscoliosis, trauma and flail chest, massive obesity)
- Pleural disorders (pneumothorax, pleural effusion, pleural thickening, malignancy)

Airway Disorders

- Upper airway obstruction (laryngospasm, tracheomalacia, tracheal obstruction)
- Acute bronchospasm (asthma, chronic obstructive pulmonary disease, allergic or transfusion reaction)
- Artificial airway problems (i.e., endotracheal tube obstruction, leak or displacement)

Increased CO_2 Production

- Hypermetabolism: hyperthyroidism, fever, sepsis
- Increased muscle activity: tetany, seizures, malignant hyperthermia, shivering
- Excessive calorie intake

increases minute ventilation and reduces arterial PCO_2. Additionally, the duration of anesthesia affects arterial PCO_2. The magnitude of respiratory depression induced by inhalational anesthetics is reduced after 5 to 6 hours. Similarly, inhalational anesthetic agents cause a profound reduction in the ventilatory response to hypoxemia, even when the inhalational concentration of these agents is low (0.1 minimal alveolar concentration [MAC]). A completely blunted hypoxic drive is observed at anesthetic concentrations of these agents. Lastly, inhalational anesthetics cause a dose-dependent increase in respiratory rate and a decrease in tidal volume, producing rhythmic, shallow respirations without intermittent sighs.

The resting lung volume (functional residual capacity [FRC]) is reduced from approximately 3.5 to 2.1 by changing body position from upright to supine and with induction of general anesthesia. The decrease in FRC seems to be related to loss of respiratory muscle tone, shifting the balance between the elastic recoil force of the lung and the outward forces of the chest wall to a lower chest and lung volume. Compliance of the respiratory system (lung and chest wall) is also reduced during anesthesia, from a mean of 95 to 60 ml/cm H_2O, mainly because of a decrease in lung compliance.

POSTOPERATIVE PULMONARY CHANGES

Intraoperative respiratory changes result from both anesthesia and the surgical procedure. In the postoperative period, changes in the respiratory system result from residual anesthetic effect, the surgical procedure itself and the effects of pain, and the premorbid conditions. Residual anesthetic effect and the use of opioids depress the respiratory drive during the postoperative period. Inhibition of cough and impairment of mucociliary clearance are also factors that contribute to the risk of postoperative infection. Other postoperative changes include mucus hypersecretion with airway closure; lung or chest wall restriction; respiratory muscle dysfunction, particularly diaphragmatic dysfunction; abnormal respiratory drive; and cardiac pump dysfunction. Diaphragmatic dysfunction appears to play an important role in these postoperative pulmonary changes. After thoracic and upper abdominal surgery, for example, a decreased tidal volume, loss of sighing breaths, and increase in respiratory rate are

common. Lung volumes are also decreased. Vital capacity (VC) is reduced by 50% to 60%, and FRC is reduced by approximately 30%. These changes in lung volumes recover gradually over 1 week. Reduction of the FRC below closing volumes contributes to the risk of atelectasis, pneumonia, and ventilation and perfusion (V/Q) mismatching. Microatelectasis results in areas of the lung that are perfused but not ventilated, leading to impaired gas exchange with consequent postoperative hypoxemia. Lower abdominal surgery is associated with similar changes but to a lesser degree. Reductions in lung volumes are not usually seen with surgery on the extremities.

RISK FACTORS FOR POSTOPERATIVE PULMONARY COMPLICATIONS

PPCs play a significant role in the risk for surgery and anesthesia (Table 3). The most important and morbid PPCs are atelectasis, pneumonia, respiratory failure, and exacerbation of underlying

Table 3: Risk Factors for Postoperative Pulmonary Complications

	Odds Ratio
Patient-Related Factors	
Advanced age	2.09–3.04
ASA class >II	2.55–4.87
Congestive heart failure	2.93
Functional dependency	1.65–2.51
COPD	1.79
Weight loss	1.62
Impaired sensorium	1.39
Cigarette use	1.26
Alcohol use	1.21
Procedure-Related Factors	
Aortic aneurysm repair	6.90
Thoracic surgery	4.24
Abdominal surgery	3.01
Upper abdominal surgery	2.91
Neurosurgery	2.53
Prolonged surgery	2.26
Head and neck surgery	2.21
Emergency surgery	2.10
Vascular surgery	1.83
General anesthesia	1.47
Laboratory and Ancillary Testing	
Albumin level <35 g/L	2.53
Chest x-ray	*4.81*

ASA, American Society of Anesthesiologists; *COPD*, chronic obstructive pulmonary disease.

chronic lung disease. PPCs are as prevalent as cardiac complications and contribute similarly to morbidity, mortality, and length of hospital stay. Pulmonary complications may also be more likely than cardiac complications to predict long-term mortality after surgery.

Patient-Related Risk Factors

Evidence shows that patient-related risk factors such as chronic obstructive pulmonary disease (COPD), age older than 60 years, American Society of Anesthesiologists (ASA) class of II or greater, functional dependence, and congestive heart failure increase the risk for postoperative pulmonary complications. Obesity and mild or moderate asthma are not significant risk factors for postoperative pulmonary complications.

Procedure-Related Risk Factors

Procedure-related risk factors are as important as patient-related factors in estimating risk for postoperative pulmonary complications. The following procedures have been associated with a higher risk for postoperative pulmonary complications: prolonged surgery (>3 hours), abdominal surgery, thoracic surgery, neurosurgery, head and neck surgery, vascular surgery, aortic aneurysm repair, and emergency surgery. General anesthesia and serum albumin

levels below 35 g/L are also a strong marker of increased pulmonary risk. Measurement of serum albumin should be considered in patients with at least one risk factor for perioperative pulmonary complications. Routine preoperative spirometry and chest radiography are not indicated for predicting pulmonary risk. Preoperative pulmonary function testing or chest radiography may be appropriate in patients with a previous diagnosis of chronic lung disease or asthma or reserved for patients who are thought to have an undiagnosed chronic lung disease.

STRATEGIES TO REDUCE POSTOPERATIVE PULMONARY COMPLICATIONS

Strategies to reduce postoperative pulmonary complications should generally be reserved for those at higher than average risk, such as patients with at least one risk factor undergoing upper abdominal or thoracic surgery (Table 4). Interventions to reduce the risk of postoperative pulmonary complications should begin in the preoperative period and continue through the postoperative period.

Preoperative Interventions

Potential preoperative strategies include cigarette cessation, optimization of underlying chronic lung disease, and appropriate antibiotic use.

Smoking Cessation

Current smokers have a modest increase of pulmonary risk even in the absence of chronic lung disease. Current smokers should be advised to stop smoking and receive nicotine replacement 6 to 8 weeks before surgery to lower pulmonary risk. Of interest, current smokers who attempt to reduce cigarette use shortly before surgery may be more likely to develop PPCs than those who continue usual smoking habits.

Table 4: Strategies to Reduce Postoperative Pulmonary Complications

Strategies of Proven Benefit

Lung expansion maneuvers (i.e., incentive spirometry, deep breathing exercises, and continuous positive airway pressure) after abdominal surgery

Strategies of Probable Benefit

Selective nasogastric tube decompression after abdominal surgery

Short-acting neuromuscular blocking agents

Strategies of Possible Benefit

Laparoscopic abdominal operations

Strategies of Unclear Benefit

Preoperative smoking cessation

Intraoperative epidural anesthesia and postoperative epidural analgesia

Strategies of No Benefit

Routine total parenteral or enteral hyperalimentation

Invasive perioperative monitoring with pulmonary artery catheterization

Chronic Obstructive Lung Disease

In patients with COPD, preoperative pulmonary optimization with a combination of bronchodilators, antibiotics, and systemic steroids lowers the rate of PPCs. In symptomatic COPD, inhaled ipratropium and beta-agonists should be initiated preoperatively. Perioperative steroids benefit patients with persistent symptoms and wheezing despite optimal bronchodilator therapy. On the other hand, theophylline should not be added in a stable patient in preparation for surgery.

Asthma

Poorly controlled asthma may be a risk factor for PPCs, but well-controlled asthma confers little additional risk. Symptomatic patients should receive inhaled beta-agonists. Systemic corticosteroids are indicated for asthmatics with wheezing, productive cough, chest tightness, or shortness of breath despite receiving their usual therapy. Systemic corticosteroids are also recommended for asthmatics who have a peak flow rate or forced expiratory volume in 1 second (FEV1) less than 80% of predicted or 80% of their personal best despite optimal therapy.

Preoperative Antibiotics

Only patients with a clinically apparent respiratory infection, including those with purulent sputum or a change in the character of sputum, should receive antibiotics. Antibiotics are not useful in those with stable COPD or asthma unless other disorders are present. Whenever preoperative antibiotics are used, consideration for delaying surgery should be entertained.

INTRAOPERATIVE INTERVENTIONS

Anesthesia Type

The selection of the type of anesthesia and neuromuscular blockade both may affect the incidence of PPCs. To date, however, the evidence supporting neuroaxial anesthesia, either spinal or epidural, to hasten recovery and reduce pulmonary risk is conflicting. In the past, several meta-analyses suggested that neuroaxial blockade would improve recovery and reduce pulmonary risk, but more recent, large, randomized trials have not confirmed these findings. On the other hand, long-acting neuromuscular blocking agents such as pancuronium are more likely to lead to postoperative residual neuromuscular blockade than intermediate-acting agents such as vecuronium and atracurium. Prolonged or residual postoperative neuromuscular muscular blockade may increase the risk of PPCs. Several prospective, nonrandomized and randomized studies have shown that PPC was up to four times more likely to develop in patients with pancuronium-induced, postoperative, residual neuromuscular blockade.

Duration and Type of Surgery

Surgical procedures lasting more than 3 to 4 hours are associated with a higher risk of pulmonary complications. Similarly, upper abdominal, aortic aneurysm repair, and thoracic operations carry the greatest risk of PPCs. Thus whenever feasible a different surgical procedure should be considered in very high-risk patients, for example, a percutaneous cholecystostomy instead of an open cholecystectomy in a critically ill, high-risk patient. To date, the evidence is not clear whether laparoscopic versus open procedures reduce the risk for clinically important pulmonary complications.

Postoperative Interventions

Risk reduction strategies continue into the postoperative period and include lung expansion maneuvers, adequate pain control, and appropriate use of nasogastric tube decompression after abdominal surgery.

Lung Expansion Maneuvers

Decreased lung volumes and atelectasis resulting from surgery-related shallow breathing, bed rest, diaphragmatic dysfunction, pain, and impaired mucociliary clearance may be the first events leading to PPC. Lung expansion maneuvers lower the incidence of PCPs in patients who are at higher than average risk for pulmonary complications. Techniques include incentive spirometry; deep-breathing exercises; chest physical therapy including deep breathing exercises, cough, postural drainage, percussion and vibration, suctioning, and ambulation; intermittent positive-pressure breathing; and continuous positive airway pressure (CPAP).

The goal of these maneuvers is to increase lung volumes through inspiratory efforts. Deep-breathing exercises and incentive spirometry appear to be equally effective and capable of reducing the risk of postoperative pulmonary complications by approximately one half of cases. Incentive spirometry may be the least labor intensive. Intermittent positive pressure breathing has been associated with more complications than other methods of lung expansion and should not be used for routine prophylaxis. CPAP offers the potential advantage of being effort independent but may be associated with gastric distention, hypoventilation, and barotrauma. It also requires special equipment and is costly. The use of CPAP has been recommended as a primary postoperative prevention strategy for patients who are unable to perform regular deep-breathing exercises or incentive spirometry and as a secondary intervention for refractory atelectasis. The available evidence suggests that for patients undergoing abdominal surgery, any type of lung expansion intervention is better than no prophylaxis at all. Overall, no modality seems to be superior, and combining modalities does not provide any additional risk reduction.

Pain Control

Adequate postoperative analgesia seems important in preventing postoperative pulmonary complications by encouraging earlier ambulation and improving the patient's ability to take deep breaths. Postoperative pain control has been consistently improved with epidural analgesia, although results have been mixed with regard to reduction in postoperative pulmonary complications. Randomized trials of combined intraoperative and postoperative anesthetic or analgesic regimens do not clearly indicate that a combined epidural approach prevents postoperative pulmonary complications. On the other hand, both postoperative epidural and patient-controlled intravenous analgesia are superior to on-demand delivery of opioids in preventing postoperative pulmonary complications. Furthermore, epidural analgesia may further reduce postoperative pulmonary complications.

Nasogastric Decompression after Abdominal Surgery

Routine use of nasogastric decompression (i.e., standard use until bowel function returns) has been thought to speed bowel recovery and decrease risk for aspiration. On the other hand, routine use of nasogastric tube (NGT) decompression postoperatively increases the risk of pulmonary complications. A systematic review comparing routine versus selective nasogastric decompression found that the routine use of an NGT significantly increased PPCs including pneumonia and atelectasis. A subsequent systematic review similarly found a trend toward increased pulmonary complications with routine postoperative use of an NGT.

Mechanical Ventilation

In patients with acute postoperative respiratory failure, mechanical ventilation can be lifesaving by reversing hypoxemia or respiratory acidosis (or both) refractory to more conservative measures. In addition, in patients with respiratory distress the action of the respiratory muscles may account for as much as 50% of total oxygen consumption. In such circumstances, mechanical ventilation decreases the excessive work of breathing, allowing for adequate resting of the respiratory muscle, decrease in oxygen consumption, and reversal of respiratory muscle fatigue.

Ventilator Modes and Settings

The most common ventilator modes are assist-control ventilation, intermittent mandatory ventilation, and pressure-support ventilation. With assist-control ventilation, the ventilator delivers a breath when triggered by a patient's inspiratory effort or independently if such an effort does not occur within a preselected period. With intermittent mandatory ventilation, the patient receives periodic breaths from the ventilator at a preset volume and rate, and between these mandatory breaths, the patient is allowed to breathe spontaneously. In pressure-support ventilation, the physician sets a level of pressure to augment every spontaneous inspiratory effort. Tidal volume is determined by the level of pressure set, the patient's effort, and pulmonary mechanics.

Newer methods of ventilatory support include high-frequency ventilation, inverse-ratio ventilation, airway-pressure-release ventilation, and proportional-assist ventilation. The purpose of these new modes of ventilation may be to enhance respiratory-muscle rest, prevent respiratory muscle deconditioning, improve gas exchange, prevent ventilator-associated lung damage, enhance synchrony between the ventilator assistance and the patient's respiratory efforts, and foster lung healing. Although these techniques are exciting from theoretical and physiologic viewpoints, there is no firm evidence that they improve outcomes in patients.

The most common way to improve oxygenation is through the use of positive end expiratory pressure (PEEP) with the intention of recruiting previously nonfunctioning lung tissue. In patients with adult respiratory distress syndrome, PEEP usually produces a substantial increase in PaO$_2$. This is primarily due to a reduction in intrapulmonary shunting as a result of a redistribution of lung water from the alveoli to the perivascular interstitial space. In patients with acute respiratory distress syndrome, selecting the right level of PEEP is sometimes difficult because the severity of injury varies throughout the lungs. PEEP can recruit atelectatic areas but may overdistend normally aerated areas, worsening the dead space ventilation. The addition of PEEP also influences lung mechanics. Patients with acute lung injury commonly have a decreased end-expiratory lung volume, and thus tidal breathing occurs on the low, flat portion of the pressure-volume curve. By shifting tidal breathing to a more compliant portion of the curve, PEEP can reduce the work of breathing.

AVOIDING VENTILATOR-ASSOCIATED COMPLICATIONS

Mechanical ventilation places patients at increased risk for additional complications, such as ventilator-induced lung injury (VILI), upper gastrointestinal bleeding, deep venous thrombosis, ventilator-associated pneumonia (VAP), and death.

Ventilator-Induced Lung Injury

Mechanical ventilation is associated with two primary types of lung injury: volutrauma and atelectrauma. Volutrauma occurs when the lung is overinflated and alveoli are overstretched. In a normal lung, inflation volumes necessary to cause overdistention injury are much larger than those commonly used clinically. However, in patients with acute lung injury and acute respiratory distress syndrome, the delivery of a "normal" tidal volume results in regional overinflation. Atelectrauma is caused by the repetitive opening and closing of recruitable alveoli. In the injured lung, positive-pressure ventilation can force open some airless alveoli, but on expiration, these same alveoli again collapse. This cycling between open and collapsed is often referred to as *recruitment-derecruitment* of alveoli. The shear stresses occurring during recruitment-derecruitment of alveoli are high and can cause trauma, resulting in disruption of the surfactant monolayer, which in turn affects the permeability of the alveolar-capillary barrier to proteins and other solutes.

Lastly, VILI is also associated with the production and release of inflammatory mediators and cytokines such as tumor necrosis factor-alpha, interleukin-6, macrophage inflammatory protein-2, platelet-activating factor, and thromboxane B2. These mediators exacerbate the local lung injury and the systemic inflammatory response, resulting ultimately in the multiple organ dysfunction syndrome. Strategies to alleviate VILI, termed *lung-protective strategies*, are aimed at reducing overstretching and shear stresses associated with repetitive alveolar collapse and reopening. Lower tidal volume mechanical ventilation, maintenance of PEEP, and high-frequency ventilation are the best-studied lung-protective strategies that appear to reduce VILI.

Ventilator Bundle

The ventilator bundle encompasses the implementation of a series of interventions on every mechanically ventilated patient aimed at reducing the rate of ventilator-associated complications, duration of mechanical ventilation, length of intensive care unit stay, and risk of death. The key components of the ventilator bundle are elevation of the head of the bed more than 45 degrees, stress ulcer prophylaxis, deep venous thrombosis prophylaxis, daily interruption of sedatives, and daily assessment of the "readiness to wean" from mechanical ventilation.

Discontinuation of Ventilatory Support

The timing and method of discontinuing mechanical ventilation, also termed *weaning*, continue to be a challenging clinical problem. Weaning ventilatory support is relatively easy in patients requiring short-term ventilatory support, but it can be difficult in patients recovering from severe respiratory failure and those patients requiring prolonged ventilatory support.

Weaning from mechanical ventilation requires careful timing. As previously noted, mechanical ventilation can result in life-threatening complications and therefore discontinuation should be attempted at the earliest possible time. However, premature attempts at discontinuation from ventilatory support may lead to failure and reinstitution of mechanical ventilation, which carries an increased risk of morbidity and mortality.

In general, discontinuation of mechanical ventilation is not contemplated until the patient is hemodynamically stable and gas exchange is satisfactory. All patients should be evaluated daily to determine whether they are candidates for discontinuation of mechanical ventilation. To be considered a candidate, at least four criteria should be met: (1) evidence of reversal or stability of the cause of acute respiratory failure, (2) hemodynamic stability, (3) ability to make an inspiratory effort, and (4) adequate oxygenation as indicated by PaO_2/FIO_2 greater than 150 to 200, PEEP in the range of less than 5 to 8 cm H_2O, FIO_2 0.4 or less to 0.5, and pH greater than 7.25.

The outcome of a weaning trial is best predicted by the ability of the respiratory muscles to adapt to an increased workload. Traditional predictors of successful weaning, such as maximal inspiratory pressure, vital capacity, and minute ventilation, frequently have limited predictive accuracy. A more reliable predictor is the ratio of respiratory frequency to tidal volume during 1 minute of spontaneous breathing (f/VT). An f/VT ratio of 100 best discriminates between successful and unsuccessful attempts at weaning, and an f/VT of 80 is associated with almost a 95% probability of successful weaning.

Several weaning methods have been used, including trials of spontaneous breathing several times a day using a T-tube circuit; gradual reductions in the level of intermittent mandatory ventilation or pressure-support ventilation; and single daily T-tube trials, lasting for up to 2 hours. Until recently, it was believed that all weaning methods were equally effective. The results of randomized, controlled trials indicate that trials of spontaneous breathing are superior when compared with either pressure support or intermittent mandatory ventilation weaning. If a weaning trial is successful, the patient is extubated after the ability to protect his or her upper airway and clear secretions have been evaluated. If the trial is unsuccessful, the patient is given at least a 24-hour period of respiratory muscle resting with full ventilatory support before the next weaning trial is attempted.

Suggested Readings

Acute Respiratory Distress Syndrome Network: Ventilation with lower tidal volumes for acute lung injury and the acute respiratory distress syndrome, *N Engl J Med* 342:1301, 2000.

Fan E, Needham DM, Stewart TE: Ventilatory management of acute lung injury and acute respiratory distress syndrome, *JAMA* 294:2889, 2005.

Qaseem A, Snow V, Fitterman N, and others: Clinical Efficacy Assessment Subcommittee of the American College of Physicians. Risk assessment for and strategies to reduce perioperative pulmonary complications for patients undergoing noncardiothoracic surgery: a guideline from the American College of Physicians, *Ann Intern Med* 144:575, 2006.

Tobin MJ: Advances in mechanical ventilation, *N Engl J Med* 344:1986, 2001.

Ware LB, Matthay MA: The acute respiratory distress syndrome, *N Engl J Med* 342:1334, 2000.

West JB: *Pulmonary pathophysiology: the essentials*, ed 5, Baltimore, 1998, Williams & Wilkins.

West JB: *Respiratory physiology: the essentials*, ed 5, Baltimore, 1995, Williams & Wilkins.

Acute Renal Failure

Richard J. Mullins, MD

INTRODUCTION

Normal glomerular filtration rates in healthy adults exceed 100 ml/min. Patients with acute renal dysfunction (ARD) have glomerular filtration rates between 30 and 100 ml/min. Patients with acute renal failure (ARF) have glomerular filtration rates less than 30 ml/min. Abrupt onset of ARF is a serious complication requiring that the patient be treated with renal replacement therapy. Timely and focused, effective interventions when renal function of seriously ill patients is declining can, in many circumstances, prevent ARF. Surgeons evaluating patients with renal dysfunction seek to identify the specific cause that will guide them in selecting the most effective intervention. Serum creatinine is not a reliable laboratory test for identifying a patient with declining renal function. In a patient with abrupt decline in glomerular filtration from normal to less than 30 ml/min, the serum creatinine doubles approximately every 24 hours. A fall in urine flow rates is typically the surgeon's first indication of a declining glomerular filtration rate. In an adult, urine flow rates less than 30 ml per hour warrant evaluation. Surgeons use urine flow rates to categorize patients who develop ARF. Adults have nonoliguric ARF if urine flow rates exceed 15 ml per hour. These patients have a prognosis that is superior to adults with oliguric ARF, defined as urine flow less than 15 ml per hour. Patients with profound ARF may produce less than 4 ml of urine per hour and are at highest risk for death. Sudden total arrest of urine flow should always prompt the surgeon to investigate for obstruction in ureters or urethra or drainage device, or acute renal artery thrombosis.

The prevalence of ARF is 4% to 8% among patients treated in surgical intensive care units. Surgical conditions commonly associated with ARF are septic shock, acute pancreatitis, cardiovascular surgery, hemorrhage, and intra-abdominal sepsis. More than half of patients who develop ARF die, a mortality rate unchanged for the past 4 decades. Among survivors, a substantial proportion of ARF patients recover sufficient renal function by the time they are discharged from the hospital that they no longer require renal replacement therapy.

RENAL REPLACEMENT THERAPY

Patients with ARF require renal replacement therapy, and they require it immediately if there is hyperkalemia. On electrocardiogram, peaked T waves indicate that the patient has significant hyperkalemia and that lethal cardiac arrhythmias are imminent. Temporary measures to reverse severe hyperkalemia are intravenous infusion of sodium bicarbonate and infusion of glucose and insulin, two interventions that shift the extracellular potassium into the intracellular fluid. Administration of potassium-binding resins such as sodium polystyrene sulfonate (Kayexalate [Sanofi-Aventis US, Bridgewater, NJ] 15 g 1 to 4 times daily) by oral or rectal routes can shift potassium in the extracellular fluid to the lumen of the gastrointestinal tract. Azotemia, acidemia, electrolyte abnormalities (hyperphosphatemia, hypercalcemia), and toxic elevations in the serum concentrations of drugs normally cleared by the renal function are additional complications that can quickly develop in patients with ARF. Definitive management of the toxicity of ARF is renal replacement therapy.

Three types of renal replacement therapies are available, and each has advantages and disadvantages. Intermittent hemodialysis (IHD) and continuous hemofiltration/dialysis (CHH) are two methods of renal replacement therapy that require extracorporeal circulation of blood. IHD can achieve rapid clearance of fluid and solutes from extracellular fluid, and for most patients a dialysis run can be completed in less than 4 hours. There are several techniques for performing CHH. However, all CHH methods are a slower means than IHD for clearance of extracellular fluid, and patients usually require continuous therapy over days. Because the blood of patients on IHD and CHH is in contact with dialytic membranes, anticoagulation is required. Outcomes are equivalent for patients with acute ARF treated with either IHD or CHH. The advantages and disadvantages of each method influence which is used in individual patients. IHD is the most rapidly effective method for removing water, potassium, and other uremia-related solutes; however, IHD is associated with hypotension. CHH is better tolerated in hemodynamically unstable patients but has the disadvantages of requiring continuous immobilization of the patient, sustained intensive nursing care, greater expense, and continuous anticoagulation. Debate continues whether renal replacement therapy should be implemented early in patients with ARD before they meet the laboratory criteria for ARF. Peritoneal dialysis (PD) is the third method of renal replacement therapy and is accomplished by alternating steps of dialysis fluid being infused and drained through a catheter inserted in the peritoneal cavity. PD is a slow method of renal replacement therapy but does not require anticoagulation. PD has value in infants and children with ARF in whom vascular access is difficult.

HYPOVOLEMIC PATIENTS

Patients in shock are at risk for ARF. The physiologic mechanism for shock can be intravascular hypovolemia following hemorrhage or shifts of fluid within the body, as in patients with burns or severe diarrhea. ARF occurs in patients with cardiogenic shock. The renal arteries of patients in shock constrict in response to elevated levels in blood of epinephrine, angiotensin II, and vasopressin. Tubule cells in nephrons during shock are stressed in proportion to the duration of inadequate oxygen delivery. If shock can be promptly reversed and renal blood flow restored, the tubular cells recover normal function. Delay in restoration of oxygen delivery severely damages the tubule cells, and days of renal replacement therapy are necessary. Associated conditions predispose patients in shock to progress to ARF. These conditions include older age (>60 years) preexisting renal dysfunction, diabetes mellitus, invasive infection, and heart failure. Infusion of a vasoconstrictor agent to raise the blood pressure by increasing vasoconstriction in a patient in shock is an intervention that increases the patient's systolic blood pressure but exacerbates the ischemic insult and risk of ARF.

Surgical patients who suddenly develop oliguria are managed in a two-step process. First, patients in hypovolemic shock are given intravenous infusion of fluid or, in patients who have hemorrhaged, blood products that restore intravascular volume and hemoglobin concentration. Expanding the blood volume preserves renal function because it enables cardiac function to increase systolic blood pressure and reduces endogenous vasoconstriction stimulated by baroreceptors. Patients in shock because of cardiac dysfunction require vasoactive drugs. Inotropic drugs improve perfusion pressure in a patient with impaired cardiac contractility. In patients with complex hemodynamic physiology, resuscitation is best guided by continuous invasive hemodynamic monitoring with arterial catheters and pulmonary artery catheters. In complex patients, the surgeon infuses intravenous fluids to achieve optimal ventricular end-diastolic filling pressures, adjusting the rate of inotropic drugs infusion to achieve both normal systolic blood pressure and cardiac output. The goal in adults is to produce a renal perfusion that sustains tubular cell function and urine flow rates. In many patients, surgeons can best prevent hypovolemia-related renal dysfunction by timely surgery that stops hemorrhage.

For decades, anecdotal reports in the clinical literature have reported that patients with oliguric ARF benefit from infusion of diuretics and dopamine that force an increase in urine flow. However, randomized control trials have demonstrated that neither medication is effective at preserving renal function in patients at risk for ARF from shock. Surgeons should infuse dopamine only as an inotropic agent.

SEPTIC SHOCK

A patient with a serious infection faces two threats: the microorganisms may progressively invade the infected organ, and the patient's exaggerated endogenous inflammatory response to the infection may damage healthy organs. Although toxins from microorganisms damage the infected organ, the pathophysiology of multiple organ dysfunctions, including renal failure, which occurs at sites remote from the infection, is attributed to the individual's inflammatory response. Patients with severe sepsis have hypotension; lactic acidemia; respiratory failure; altered mental status; and, commonly, oliguria. More than half of patients with severe sepsis deteriorate into *septic shock,* defined as hypotension unresponsive to resuscitation by intravenous infusion of isotonic saline infusions. Resuscitation of an oliguric septic patient begins with intravenous infusion of balanced electrolyte solution sufficient to expand blood volume. Surgeons can be guided during resuscitation of patients with severe sepsis or septic shock by concurrent measurement of pulmonary artery pressures, cardiac output, and calculated systemic vascular resistance. The most common hemodynamic abnormality in septic shock is vasodilation caused by excessive synthesis of the potent vasodilator nitric oxide. Patients in septic shock with a low systemic vascular resistance are treated with vasoconstrictor agents that restore mean arterial pressure to 60 mm Hg. Two vasoconstrictor agents reported in septic shock studies to be effective are norepinephrine or, when this alpha-adrenergic agonist fails, arginine vasopressin. Norepinephrine and arginine vasopressin induce vasoconstriction of perivascular smooth muscle cells through different mechanisms, and thus in some patients with septic shock, both drugs are used. In the patient with shock caused by vasodilation, drug-induced vasoconstriction in the circulation to skin and skeletal muscle shifts blood flow to vital organs of the heart, brain, and kidney. Septic shock patients with impaired cardiac contractility are treated by infusion of inotropic agents. Epinephrine, dobutamine, and dopamine are three drugs reported to increase myocardial contractility effectively.

Brisk urine flow and correction of acidemia are indications that septic patients have been adequately resuscitated. Supplemental therapies have been reported as effective at improving preservation of organ function in patients with septic shock. Intravenous infusion of recombinant human activated protein C (drotrecogin alfa), an antithrombotic (inactivates coagulation factors Va and VIIa), anti-inflammatory, and profibrinolytic agent, improves survival of hypotensive septic shock patients who had dysfunction of at least one organ system. Glucocorticoids and mineralocorticoids (hydrocortisone, 50-mg intravenous bolus every 6 hours; and fludrocortisone, 50-μg tablet once daily) improved the survival of patients in septic shock who had laboratory evidence of adrenal dysfunction. The most effective interventions for preserving organ function in patients with septic shock are definitive surgical interventions that control sites of infection.

ACUTE RENAL FAILURE SECONDARY TO ABDOMINAL COMPARTMENT SYNDROME

Abdominal compartment syndrome is an increase in the volume of the organs confined within the peritoneal cavity that, when compressed within a confined space, produce an increase in hydrostatic pressure, which causes venous hypertension.

Common specific causes for acute abdominal compartment syndrome are intra-abdominal hemorrhage, the rapid onset of ascites, visceral edema as a consequence of peritonitis, venous hypertension, and intravenous infusion of large volumes of balanced electrolyte solutions to resuscitate the patient from shock. Tight intraluminal distention of the stomach, small bowel and colon with fluid, infused enteric-tube feeding, or air can produce abdominal compartment syndrome. As the intra-abdominal pressure increases, venous compression produces venous hypertension that leads to a reactive vasoconstriction and impaired blood flow. ARD and ARF develop because abdominal compartment syndrome compresses retroperitoneal veins including the vena cava, raises renal vein pressure, and reduces glomerular filtration.

Typical clinical findings in patients with abdominal compartment syndrome are oliguria, respiratory distress leading to hypoventilation, and a tensely distended abdomen that is hard on palpation. In intubated and mechanically ventilated patients who develop abdominal compartment syndrome, an increase in peak inspiratory pressure is an early sign that abdominal pressures are progressing to a critical level. Bladder pressures should be measured in patients to determine whether the patient has abdominal compartment syndrome. An easy method for measuring bladder pressure is to measure the height above the pubic symphysis of a urine column in the tubing of the Foley catheter. A urine column exceeding 20 to 30 cm indicates that abdominal pressure is high and may contribute to renal dysfunction. Patients with bladder pressures that push the urine column to more than 30 to 40 cm have abdominal compartment hypertension (Fig. 1). A caution regarding interpreting abdominal compartment pressures is that in patients who are morbidly obese, there may be a substantial chronic elevation in abdominal compartment pressure.

Surgeons have several options for relieving abdominal compartment syndrome. Patients who are mechanically ventilated can be paralyzed with pharmacologic agents. Large volumes of ascites or blood in the abdominal cavity can be drained by inserting a peritoneal catheter to reduce pressure. Often for patients with abdominal compartment syndrome, the most immediately effective technique is to open the abdominal cavity and allow the swollen viscera to decompress through the wound. To achieve a tension-free closure of the open abdomen, surgeons use prosthetic materials that temporarily prevent evisceration while the primary problem resolves (Fig. 2).

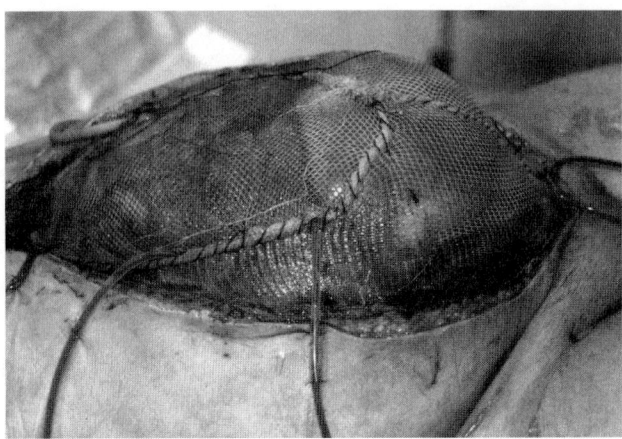

Figure 2 Open abdomen: this patient had substantial visceral edema following laparotomy for a gunshot wound to the vena cave, kidney, and duodenum. The abdomen was closed with an absorbable polyglycolic acid mesh because it enables controlled evisceration and avoids abdominal compartment syndrome. As the visceral edema resolved over days, the mesh was "pleated" by resuturing it until the fascia edges were reapproximated.

RHABDOMYOLYSIS AND MYOGLOBINURIA

Rhabdomyolysis is a pathologic process in which skeletal muscle cells are disrupted, releasing cell contents that include potassium, phosphate, and myoglobin. Myoglobin is toxic to renal tubule cells. Myoglobin circulating in plasma is filtered across the glomerular capillary membrane, and as the myoglobin concentration increases in renal tubular fluid, the ferrous species in heme generates toxic oxygen radicals that damage tubule cells. Skeletal muscle ischemia lasting for more than 4 hours followed by reperfusion is the most common cause of rhabdomyolysis in surgery patients. Rhabdomyolysis occurs when a major arterial occlusion to an extremity is repaired and blood flow returns to ischemic muscle. For example, rhabdomyolysis has developed when an extremity is compressed for hours beneath the debris of a collapsed building and then the victim is released, or postoperatively in obese patients whose back and buttock muscles were compressed against the hard surface of the operating table. In addition to ischemia and reperfusion injury, other causes of rhabdomyolysis encountered by surgeons are direct muscle injury and crush, invasive infection, intense exercise, and drugs (statins, corticosteroids, and nondepolarizing muscle-relaxing agents).

The risk of renal failure in patients with rhabdomyolysis increases in proportion to the amount of myoglobin released. The surgeon should suspect that renal toxic rhabdomyolysis has occurred in a patient who experiences skeletal muscle ischemia and reperfusion, and in the hours following the event, urine flow declines below 30 ml per hour and the urine acquires a dark "tea color." Three findings indicate that a patient has significant myoglobinuria and that treatment should be implemented immediately: 4+ positive reaction on the orthotolidine site of the urine "dipstick" test, a urine pH less than 6, and oliguria. Laboratory tests that measure the quantity of myoglobin take hours, and creatine kinase (CK), an enzyme located in skeletal muscle that is quickly assayed in blood samples, provides a reliable surrogate measure of the amount of myoglobin in plasma. Patients whose serum CK remains under 10,000 U/L will not develop renal failure. Patients whose serum CK exceeds 30,000 U/L are at a substantial risk for ARF. Patients whose peak serum CK is between 10,000 U/L and 30,000 U/L are principally at risk for ARD.

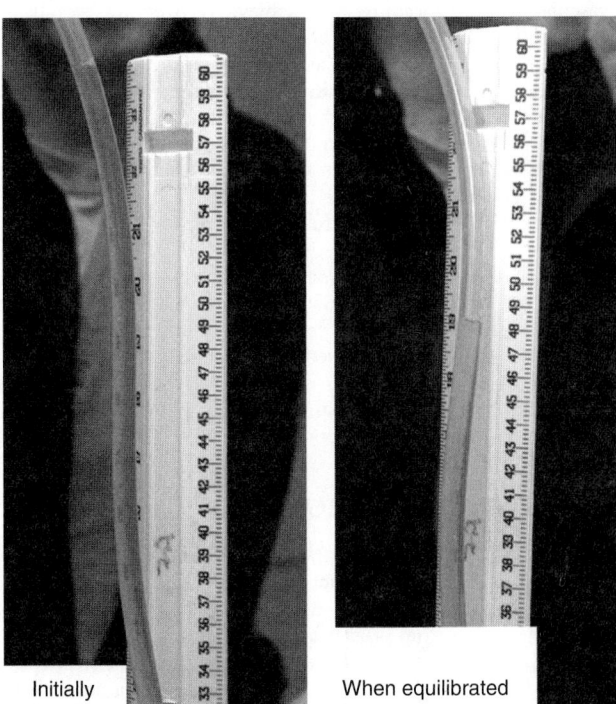

Initially   When equilibrated

Figure 1 Measuring bladder pressure: the column of urine in the Foley catheter tube provides a reliable indication of whether the patient has abdominal compartment syndrome. The tubing filled with fluid (in oliguric patients, 100 ml of saline may have to be instilled into the bladder) is elevated next to a ruler resting on the pubic symphysis. The remainder of the tube must be evacuated to avoid an airlock effect. The meniscus of fluid should descend from the initial location and then equilibrate at a level where it is observed to fluctuate with respirations. This patient's bladder pressure is 48 cm and indicates that the patient has abdominal compartment syndrome.

Table 1: Treatment of Rhabdomyolysis and Myoglobinuria in Adult*

Patients with CK elevation >20,000 U/L should receive the following:

1. Intravenous infusion of Ringer's lactate (10–20 ml/kg) over 1 to 4 hours to restore systolic blood pressure to normal

2. Intravenous infusion of sodium bicarbonate (1 mEq/kg) every 4 to 6 hours to achieve a urine pH >6.0

3. Intravenous infusion of mannitol (1–2 g/kg) as a bolus and 2–6 g/hr as a constant infusion, to achieve a urine flow rate over 200 ml/hr

Modulate infusions to maintain an alkaline diuresis, and discontinue when CK levels decline to <10,000 U/L

*In patients with cardiac dysfunction, infusions of fluids to induce alkaline diuresis are best monitored with central venous or pulmonary artery catheters.
From Malinoski DJ, Slater MS, Mullins RJ: Crit Care Clin 20:171, 2004.
CK, Creatine kinase.

The treatment for rhabdomyolysis and myoglobinuria is to induce an alkaline diuresis (Table 1). Urine flow rates should exceed 200 ml per hour within 1 hour of beginning treatment. Diuresis is best accomplished by intravenous infusion of mannitol. Loop diuretics are avoided because the mechanism by which these drugs effect diuresis results in a decline in urine pH. Patients with myoglobinuria receive intravenous infusion with enough sodium bicarbonate to produce a modest bicarbonate excess in arterial blood, which in turn induces the nephron to generate urine with a pH higher than 6.0. Prompt, brisk, alkaline diuresis is hypothesized to purge toxic myoglobin from tubules, preventing precipitation of casts and obstruction of the nephron. Patients are given carbonic anhydrase inhibitor (acetazolamide) if urine pH remains under 6.0 and the patient develops alkalemia on an arterial blood gas. Most patients with rhabdomyolysis have a 24- to 48-hour period of increasing serum CK, which then declines. When treating patients who have rhabdomyolysis with aggressive intravenous fluid infusions, the surgeon should remain aware that if myoglobin has precipitated in renal tubules, ARF is established, and severe fluid overload can occur because the patient can respond with a diuresis. The majority of patients who develop acute renal failure from rhabdomyolysis require days of renal replacement therapy before recovery of renal function.

IODINATED CONTRAST AGENTS INDUCED RENAL TOXICITY

Iodinated contrast agents (ICAs) are toxic to tubule cells. Patients who are given infusion of iodinated contrast agents risk developing renal failure that is proportional to the dose of contrast. Contrast for computed tomography (CT) scans is rarely the sole cause of ARF. Patients with highest prevalence of contrast-related nephropathy are those who have therapeutic intra-arterial angiograms. Renal dysfunction following exposure to contrast is more likely in patients with additional risk factors, including preexisting renal dysfunction; diabetes mellitus; hypertension; congestive heart failure; and shock from hypovolemia, sepsis, and abdominal compartment syndrome. Surgeons commonly face a dilemma. The contrast can be vitally important in radiographic studies essential in the diagnosis and treatment of critically ill patient. The majority of patients who have contrast nephropathy show a transient increase in serum creatinine that peaks between the second and sixth day following exposure before returning to normal. Less than 10% of patients with normal renal function show evidence of renal toxicity following exposure to iodinated contrast agents, and less than 5% of these patients progress and require renal replacement therapy.

Agents chemically engineered to have low osmolarity have less renal toxicity. Iso-osmolar, dimeric, nonionic contrast iodixanol (300 mOsm/L) has the lowest risk of renal toxicity in high-risk patients (diabetes and serum creatinine 1.5–3.5 mg/dL). Surgeons should ensure that adult patients are well hydrated with intravenous infusion of isotonic saline solution sufficient to produce a brisk urine flow before proceeding with radiographic studies that involve exposure to iodinated contrast. Substantial experimental evidence indicates that the renal toxicity of iodinated contrast agents can be attributed to oxygen radicals. The antioxidant N-acetyl cysteinate is a potent and clinically practicable drug that clinical investigators have reported to reduce risk of contrast nephropathy. Meta-analysis of all published studies testing in randomized control trials the effectiveness of N-acetyl cysteinate have led to the recommendation that evidence is equivocal on the effectiveness of N-acetyl cysteinate at preventing renal failure in high-risk patients. Further evidence from additional clinical studies is necessary before antioxidant therapy can be recommended.

ACUTE VASCULAR ISCHEMIA

Renal artery thrombosis occurs in patients who sustain blunt and penetrating trauma. Blunt-trauma patients develop renal artery thrombosis typically because the energy of a sudden blow to the torso is translated into a violent shift in the kidney that stretches the renal artery, disrupts the intima, and causes thrombosis. The warm time ischemia tolerance is less than 1 hour for the kidney before permanent damage occurs, and thus it is virtually never realistic that, following injury in which blood flow to the kidney stops abruptly, a surgeon can intervene and restore renal function with a revascularization procedure and achieve recovery of significant renal function. In contrast to acute occlusion of a normal renal artery caused by injury, when atherosclerosis slowly occludes the renal artery, collateral arterial flow can provide blood flow to the kidney sufficient to sustain its viability, even if glomerular filtration stops because of hypotension. In these circumstances, revascularization of the obstructed segment may recoup renal function when normal renal perfusion pressure is restored.

Patients with extensive atherosclerosis can have a specific form of renal ischemia that leads to ARF. Diffuse embolization of atheromatous material from the intimal surface of the aorta into afferent arterioles can occlude blood flow sufficiently that segments of the kidney infarct. Atheromatous embolization to the renal arteries occurs when catheters are passed through the aorta or when the aorta is cross-clamped in the suprarenal location for vascular surgery. The prognosis for renal recovery in patients who sustain atheromatous embolization is poor.

OBSTRUCTED UROPATHY

Surgeons work up patients with the abrupt termination of urine flow to identify a site of acute obstruction. Stones, tumor, or inadvertent ligation during a surgical procedure can obstruct ureters. Bladder outlet obstructions from prostatic hypertrophy or intravesicle blood clots are common causes of bladder outlet obstruction. Surgeons use ultrasound to evaluate the location of obstruction in a patient with the abrupt onset of anuria. A dilatated bladder is obviously an indication for insertion, or replacement, of a bladder catheter. Catheters can be blocked by a blood clot or kink or because the deflated balloon of a Foley catheter leads to the catheter tip's slipping out of the bladder into the urethra. Ultrasonography of the kidneys can identify dilatated intrarenal collecting systems or ureters and suggest the site of the obstruction. CT scans of the abdomen have superior precision at identifying the location of the obstruction in the urinary tract, but a decision must be made whether to give iodinated contrast to a patient with renal dysfunction. Urologists can evaluate and treat patients using cystography and a variety of techniques to reverse the obstruction, including transcutaneous nephrostomy tube insertion into the renal pelvis. However, surgeons manipulating the urinary tract of patients with chronic obstruction to urine flow should be wary that urine may be infected, often by resistant organisms, thereby putting the patient at risk for bacteremia during the manipulation of the urinary tract.

OTHER CAUSES

Nephrology textbooks contain long lists of specific potential causes for ARF that surgeons rarely encounter. Nephrotoxic drugs used by surgeons include the antibiotics aminoglycosides and vancomycin, nonsteroidal anti-inflammatory agents, angiotensin-converting enzyme inhibitors, and, in transplant patients, the calcineurin inhibitors cyclosporine and tacrolimus. Surgeons must remain acutely aware of the need to adjust drugs that depend on renal function for clearance. A specific syndrome of renal dysfunction and renal failure is hepatorenal syndrome. This highly lethal syndrome develops in patients with end-stage liver disease, cirrhosis, and ascites. Renal dysfunction occurs because of intense vasoconstriction of the afferent renal arteries as a physiologic consequence of a chronically and substantially contracted blood volume. Patients with cirrhosis and adequate renal function develop hepatorenal syndrome acutely following an initiating insult, such as sepsis or hemorrhagic shock, and then experience irreversible deterioration of renal function, ending in ARF. In recent studies, patients with hepatorenal syndrome have been treated with infusion of vasoconstrictor agents (vasopressin analogues or [alpha]-adrenergic agents) in combination with albumin to expand blood volume. Remarkably, patients with hepatorenal syndrome who have undergone successful liver transplant experience prompt restoration of normal renal function.

THE SURGEON'S RESPONSE TO OLIGURIA

Oliguria is an immediate indication that a hypotensive patient in septic shock is at risk for renal damage. Figure 3 The surgeon follows a systematic process in evaluating a patient who develops oliguria for the purpose of determining the specific cause and implementing proper therapy. The patient with an abrupt cessation of all urine flow should be evaluated for an obstruction. If the urine is dark (4+ positive on orthotolidine test site), the patient should be worked up for

Figure 3 Guideline for evaluation of oliguria (<0.5 cc/kg per hour) in the intensive care unit.

GUIDELINES FOR EVALUATION
OF OLIGURIA (<0.5 ML/KG PER HOUR) IN ICU

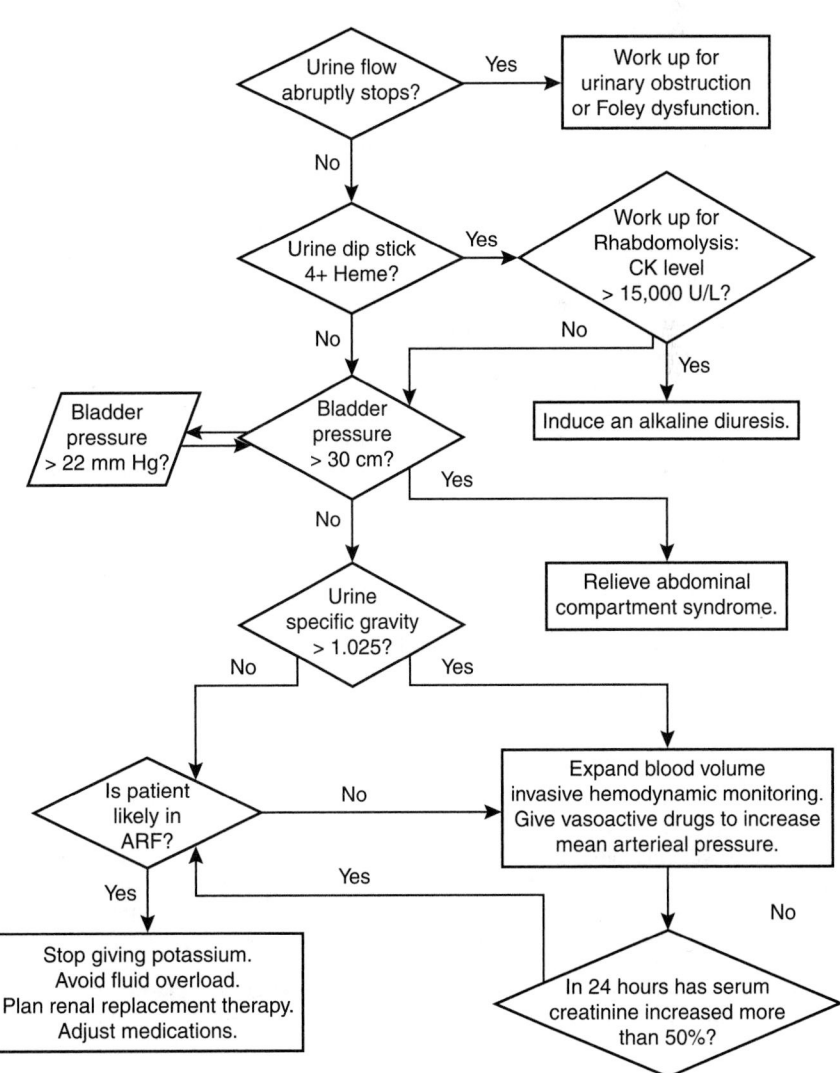

myoglobinuria by checking a serum CK level. Patients with evidence of abdominal compartment syndrome with oliguria require intervention that reduces abdominal pressure. Urine and serum samples from patients with oliguria can be sent to the laboratory for determination of the fractional excretion of sodium (FENa), which is the ratio of sodium clearance to creatine clearance. FENa can be calculated using urine and serum concentrations of sodium (Na) and creatinine (Cr) using the following equation, where U indicates urine concentration and P indicates plasma concentration:

$$FENa = \{(UNa \times PCr)/(UCr \times PNa)\} \times 100.$$

Patients with a FENa less than 1.0% have renal function, whereas the risk of ARF increases the more FENa exceeds 3% in an oliguric patient. Patients given a diuretic can have an elevated FeNa because of the influence of the drug. Patients with hypotension and impaired renal function require interventions that restore renal perfusion. If the surgeon's efforts at resuscitation do not restore urine flow and the patient's serum creatinine is rapidly increasing over 12 to 24 hours, the surgeon should conclude that the patient is likely in ARF and proceed to adjust medications, stop potassium administration, and plan for renal replacement therapy.

SUGGESTED READINGS

Barrett BJ, Parfrey PS: Preventing nephropathy induced by contrast medium, N Engl J Med 354:379, 2006.
Mayberry JC, Burgess EA, Goldman RK, and others: Enterocutaneous fistula and ventral hernia after absorbable mesh prosthesis closure for trauma: the plain truth, J Trauma 57:157, 2004.
Schrier RW, Wang W: Acute renal failure and sepsis, N Engl J Med 351:159, 2004.
Teehan GX, Liangos O, Jaber BL: Update on dialytic management of acute renal failure, J Intensive Care Med 18:130, 2003.
Uchino S, Kellum JA, Bellomo R, and others: Acute renal failure in critically ill patients: a multinational, multicenter study, JAMA 294:813, 2005.

ELECTROLYTE DISORDERS

Brett Waibel, MD, and Anthony Meyer, MD, PhD

Electrolytes play critical roles in all actions of the body. They are necessary messengers in many cellular activation mechanisms, such as muscle contraction, nerve conduction, and hormonal secretion. Electrolyte gradients between cells and interstitial fluid are also essential for maintaining homeostasis of all cell types. Multiple mechanisms (fluid shifts; alterations in absorption, distribution, and excretion; inappropriate administration; and altered homeostatic mechanisms) lead to electrolyte disorders. The potential consequences of an electrolyte disorder depend on the electrolyte involved and the severity of the disorder (see Fig. 1). Those disorders that develop rapidly generally have more severe symptoms, requiring more rapid treatment. However, using sound clinical judgment, the physician should evaluate each patient individually for clinical response to therapy.

SODIUM

Sodium (normal range: 135–145 mEq/L) is the major determinant of tonicity and osmolality in extracellular space, which is kept in a narrow range (275–290 mOsm/kg) by renal sodium and water management. Thus the dysnatremias involve alterations not only in body sodium but in water balance, as well.

Hyponatremia

Hyponatremia (<135 mEq/L) is usually from an excess of body water compared with sodium. The evaluation algorithm for hyponatremia can be seen in Figure 2, A. Serum osmolality is elevated in hypertonic and isotonic hyponatremia (>275 mOsm/L) from plasma volume expansion without changes in sodium. In hypertonic hyponatremia, aqueous solutes (mannitol, glucose) expand plasma volume from solute drag, whereas in isotonic hyponatremia, the nonaqueous phase of plasma (lipids, proteins) is expanded. Treatment involves treating the underlying cause of the hyponatremia.

Hypotonic hyponatremia (<275 mOsm/L) exists when free water excretion is impaired or renal diluting capacity is exceeded. Chronic sodium-retaining diseases, such as liver dysfunction, often lead to hypotonic hyponatremia despite the overall increase in total body sodium. Psychogenic polydipsia and reset osmostat, which have normal renal diluting capacity, can be identified by measurement of urine osmolality and sodium and respond to fluid abstinence.

Hypotonic hyponatremia causes cerebral edema from water shifts into the central nervous system (CNS). Treatment depends on the volume status of the patient, speed at which the disorder developed, and symptoms the patient is experiencing. In hypovolemic patients, volume expansion is the initial therapy. Hypovolemia from dehydration over several days must be managed differently from acute hypovolemia caused by acute intravascular volume loss resulting from blood loss or fluid loss from burn injury. Care should be taken because sodium levels can rise too rapidly with resumption of euvolemia, causing central pontine myonecrosis.

Nonhypovolemic patients require water restrictions and possibly loop diuretics. Symptomatic patients may require hypertonic saline until the symptoms resolve. Vigilant monitoring of the patient and sodium levels during correction of hyponatremia is necessary. Acute hyponatremia (<48 hours) can be corrected more rapidly (1–2 mEq/hr) than chronic hyponatremia (>48 hours, 0.5 mEq/hr). Only 8 to 12 mEq should be corrected in a 24-hour period. If corrected too rapidly, central pontine myelinolysis may occur 1 to 6 days later. It is characterized by pseudobulbar palsy, quadriparesis, seizures, and movement disorders and associated with a high mortality.

Hypernatremia

Hypernatremia (>145 mEq/L), reflecting a water deficit relative to sodium levels, causes cellular dehydration in the CNS. Evaluation of hypernatremia, as seen in Figure 2, B, is mainly performed on the basis of volume status. Treatment depends on patient volume status, degree of the disorder, and presentation of symptoms. Hypovolemic patients require volume expansion with isotonic intravenous fluids before replacement of the free water deficit. Nonhypovolemic patients require replacement of the free water deficit with hypotonic fluids. If the patient is hypervolemic, diuretic therapy may also be necessary to remove excess sodium and volume. Acute hypernatremia (<48 hours) can be corrected rapidly (1–2 mEq/hr) compared with chronic hypernatremia (0.5 mEq/hr).

SIGNS AND SYMPTOMS OF ELECTROLYTE DISORDERS

Hyponatremia	**Hypokalemia**	**Hypomagnesemia**	**Hypocalcemia**	**Hypophosphatemia**
1. Headache	1. Nausea	1. Hyperreflexia	1. Tetany	1. Muscle weakness
2. Lethargy	2. Vomiting	2. Tetany	2. Seizures	2. Respiratory
3. Confusion	3. Weakness	3. Constipation/ileus	3. Weakness	insufficiency
4. Weakness	4. Constipation	4. Vertigo/ataxia	4. Cramps	3. Decreased cardiac
5. Seizure	5. Ileus	5. Nystagmus	5. Confusion	contractility
6. Coma	6. Paralysis	6. Parasthesias	6. Dementia	4. Paralysis
7. Death	7. Respiratory	7. Seizures	7. Heart block	5. Parasthesias
	insufficiency	8. Coma	8. Cardiac arrest	6. Irritability
	8. Tachydysrhythmias	9. Death	9. Laryngospasm	7. Ataxia
		10. Cardiac		8. Tremor
		dysrhythmias		9. Seizures

Hypernatremia	**Hyperkalemia**	**Hypermagnesemia**	**Hypercalcemia**	**Hyperphosphatemia**
1. Lethargy	1. Cramping	1. Nausea	1. Lethargy	1. Metastatic
2. Irritability	2. Paralysis	2. Vomiting	2. Confusion	calcifications
3. Thirst	3. Nausea	3. Hyporeflexia	3. Obtundation	2. Signs and symptoms
4. Hyperreflexia	4. Vomiting	4. Hypotension	4. Seizures	of hypocalcemia
5. Seizures	5. Tachydysrhythmias	5. Respiratory	5. Constipation/ileus	3. Anorexia
6. Coma	6. Cardiac arrest	paralysis	6. Abdominal pain	4. Ileus
7. Death		6. Diplopia	7. Polyuria	
		7. Heart block	8. Polydipsia	
		8. Paralysis	9. Cardiac	
		9. Cardiac arrest	dysrhythmias	

Figure 1 Signs and symptoms of electrolyte disorders.

Only 10 to 12 mEq should be corrected daily to prevent the development of cerebral edema.

POTASSIUM

Potassium (normal range: 3.5–5.0 mEq/L) provides the resting potential of the cellular membrane required for cardiac and nerve function. Potassium homeostasis is primarily controlled through renal function. The normal intracellular concentration of potassium is 120 μmol and serves as a reservoir of potassium, which can soak up large amounts of potassium in replacement strategies and is a source of sudden, potentially fatal hyperkalemia in certain disorders.

Hypokalemia

Hypokalemia (<3.5 mEq/L) causes hyperpolarization of the resting potential of the cell, which interferes with neuromuscular function. In evaluating hypokalemia (Fig. 3, *A*), intracellular shifts of potassium should be excluded first; this can usually be accomplished with review of the medications, history, and acid-base status of the patient. Further workup involves differentiating between renal potassium wasting and extrarenal losses using urine potassium levels or transtubular potassium gradient. Serum aldosterone, renin, and cortisol levels are useful in the evaluation of chronic hypokalemia.

Potassium replacement can be achieved by oral or intravenous routes. Oral supplementation is generally 40 to 100 mEq daily divided between 2 and 4 doses. Intravenous replacement is usually performed at 10 to 20 mEq/hour, but cardiac monitoring is required at rates greater than 10 mEq/hr. Replacement rates as high as 40 mEq/hour have been used in emergency situations. Levels should be checked every 60 to 80 mEq delivered. Patients with reduced renal function should receive lower total doses. Because hypokalemia usually reflects a large intracellular potassium deficit, it often takes several days to replenish

total body potassium levels. Magnesium levels should be checked because hypomagnesemia produces a refractory hypokalemia. A switch to potassium-sparing diuretics should be considered for patients with persistent hypokalemia.

Hyperkalemia

Hyperkalemia (>5.0 mEq/L) causes a depolarization of the resting membrane potential, resulting in neuromuscular excitability. Multiple mechanisms exist to cause hyperkalemia (Fig. 3, *B*). Pseudohyperkalemia, a condition resulting from sample hemolysis or release of potassium from severe thrombocytosis or leukocytosis, is a spurious result. Extracellular potassium shifts occur with metabolic acidosis with nondiffusable anions, medications, or tissue destruction. Life-threatening hyperkalemia is more often due to these sudden shifts in intracellular potassium. Renal failure is the most common cause of hyperkalemia in the hospitalized patient. Finally, dysfunctional renal handling of potassium from mineralocorticoid deficiency or resistance leads to hyperkalemia. Transtubular potassium gradient can help to differentiate between renal and extrarenal etiologies of hyperkalemia. Renal failure is commonly associated with tubular defects in potassium management along with hypoaldosteronism. However, with normal renal function, differentiating between mineralocorticoid deficiency and resistance using aldosterone, renin, and cortisol levels is necessary.

Treatment involves elimination of exogenous sources and potassium-sparing medications, stabilization of the cardiac membrane with calcium in symptomatic patients, and removal of endogenous potassium. An overview of the various treatments can be found in Figure 3, *C*. Intracellular redistribution of potassium with insulin and glucose, sodium bicarbonate, and beta-2 adrenergic agonists (albuterol) can provide time to eliminate potassium from the body. Elimination of endogenous potassium requires increasing renal excretion with diuretics (loop or thiazide), renal replacement therapies, or sodium exchange resins (sodium polystyrene sulfonate). Finally, mineralocorticoids (fludrocortisone) are useful in patients with aldosterone deficiency.

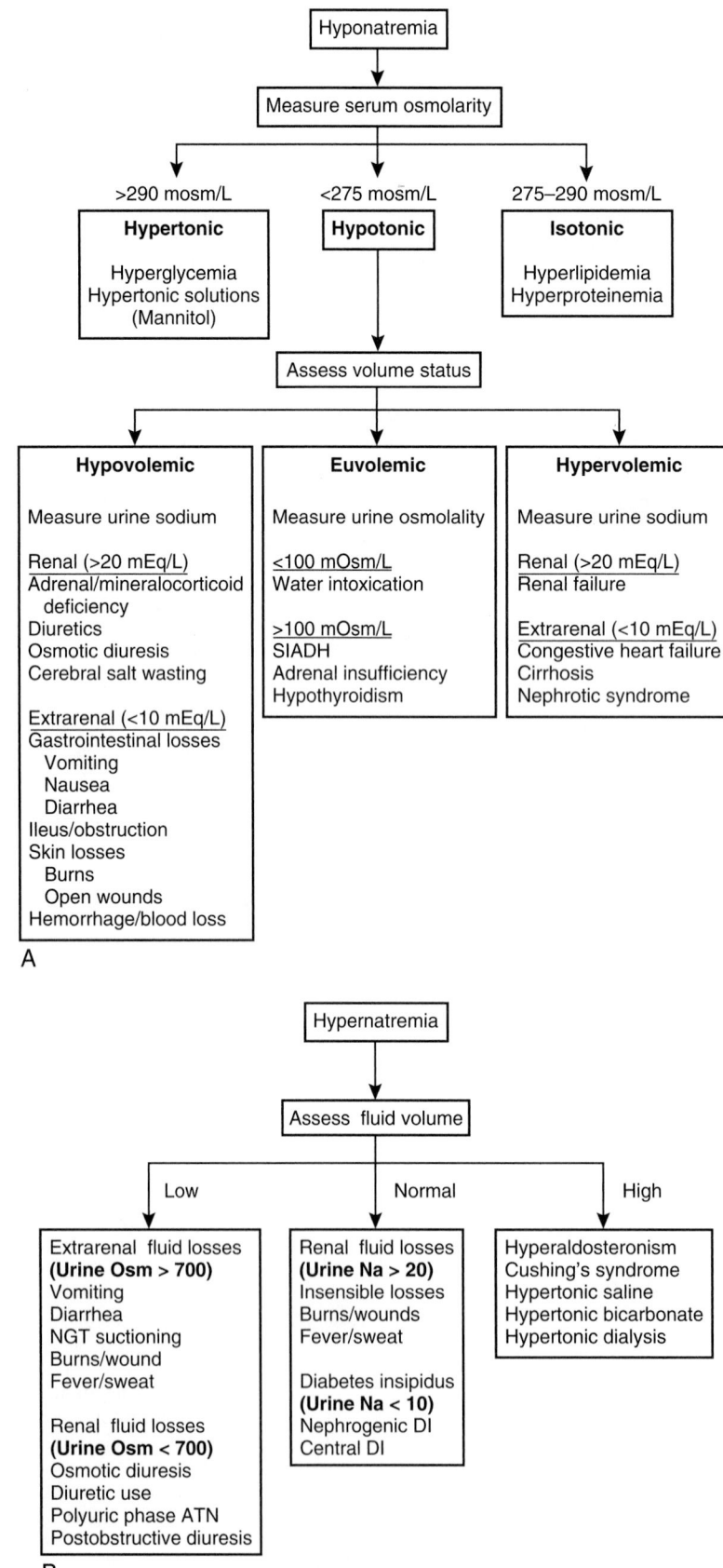

Figure 2 Hyponatremia *ATN*, Acute tubular necrosis; *DI*, diabetes incipitus; *NGT*, nasogastric tube; *SIADH*, syndrome of inappropriate antidiuretic hormone.

MAGNESIUM

Magnesium (normal range: 1.5–2.4 mg/dL) is found as a cofactor in numerous reactions and modulator of calcium fluxes. The extracellular fraction (1% of total) exists as protein bound (33%), complexed (6%), or ionized (61%). Renal reabsorption of the filtered magnesium load (the main regulator of magnesium homeostasis) is mainly passive and dependent on the loop of Henle sodium-potassium-chloride transport. Figure 3, *D* shows the multiple mechanisms causing hypomagnesemia and hypermagnesemia.

HYPOMAGNESEMIA

Hypomagnesemia (<1.5 mg/dL) is associated a mixture of neuro-muscular defects. Differentiating between renal and extrarenal losses (excess gastrointestinal losses, decreased intake/administration, transcellular shift) is achieved with a 24-hour urine collection of magnesium (<12 mg extrarenal, >24 mg renal) or fractional excretion of magnesium (FEMg) (see Fig. 4).

Treatment of hypomagnesemia involves replacement using oral or intravenous formulations. Oral replacement therapy is slower and associated with gastrointestinal disturbances. Intravenous replacement has a slow tissue distribution with significant urine losses. Mild to moderate hypomagnesemia (1.0–1.5 mg/dL) requires 8 to 32 mEq replacement, where more severe cases of hypomagnesemia (<1.0 mg/dL) require larger replacements (32–64 mEq) at a rate of 8 mEq/hour. The dose of magnesium should be reduced for patients with renal failure. Symptomatic and eclampsia patients may require a bolus of 32 mEq magnesium (4 g magnesium sulfate) over 4 to 5 minutes with cardiac monitoring.

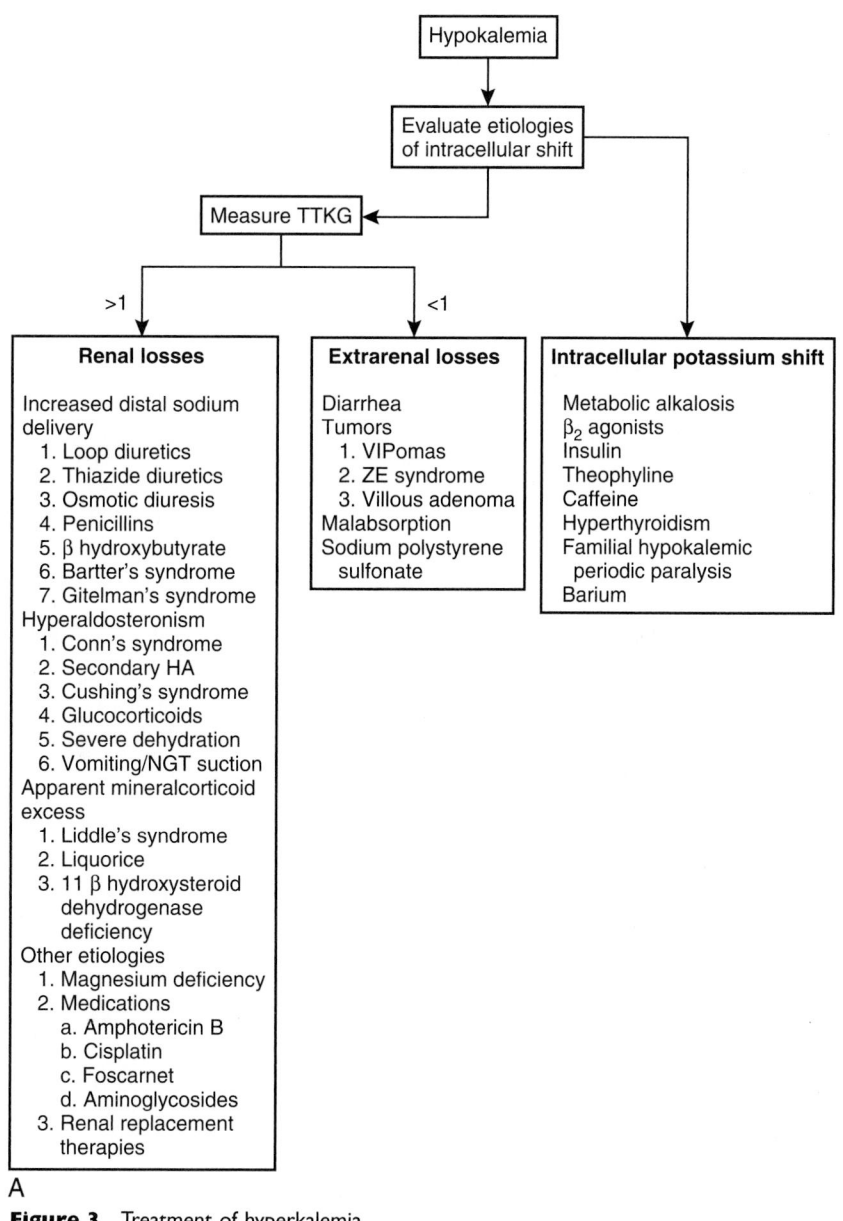

A

Figure 3   Treatment of hyperkalemia.

(continued)

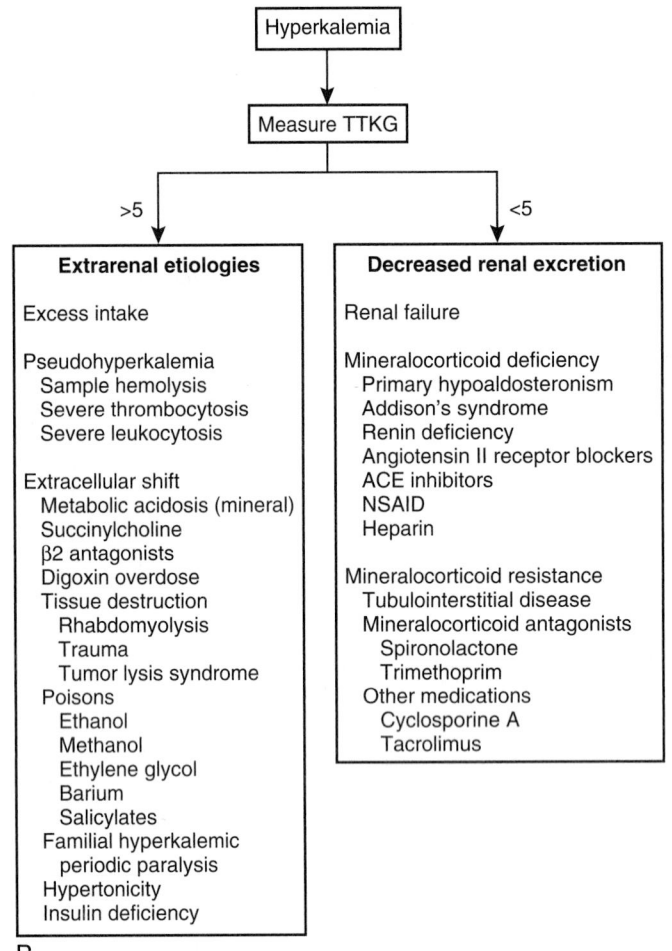

B

TREATMENT OF HYPERKALEMIA				
Mechanism	**Therapy**	**Dose**	**Onset of action**	**Duration of action**
Membrane stabilization	Calcium gluconate	1–2 grams IV over 5–10 minutes	1–2 minutes	30 minutes
Intracellular potassium shift	Sodium bicarbonate	50–100 meq IV over 2–5 minutes	30 minutes	2–6 hours
	Insulin and glucose	5–10 units RHI IV with 50 ml of 50% dextrose (25 g)	15–45 minutes	2–6 hours
	β2 agonists Albuterol	Depends upon drug 10–20 mg nebulized	20–30 minutes	1–2 hours
Potassium removal	Furosemide	20–40 mg IV	5–15 minutes	4–6 hours
	Sodium polystyrene sulfonate	15–60 g PO or PR	4–6 hours	4–6 hours
	Hemodialysis	2–4 hours	Immediate	Duration of dialysis

C

Figure 3 Cont'd—*ACE*, Angiotensin converting enzyme; *HA*, hyperaldosteronism; *IV*, intravenous; *NGT*, nasogastric tube; *NSAID*, nonsteroidal anti-inflammatory drug; *PO*, per os (by mouth); *PR*, by rectum; *RHI*, regular human insulin; *VIP*, vasoactive intestinal peptide; *TTKG*, transtubular potassium gradient; *ZE*, Zollinger-Ellison.

MAGNESIUM DISORDERS ETIOLOGIES

Hypomagnesemia	Hypermagnesemia
Extrarenal (FEMg<2%)	Severe renal failure (GFR<30 ml/minute)
Excess gastrointestinal losses	
Malabsorption	Iatrogenic/Excess intake
Steatorrhea	Parenteral nutrition
Diarrhea	Laxatives
Nasogastric suction	Enemas
Fistulas	Antacids
Decreased intake	Eclampsia therapy
Parenteral nutrition	
Starvation	Adrenal Insufficiency
Malnutrition	
Transcellular shift	Lithium
Digoxin	
Adrenergic agonists	Tissues destruction
Insulin	Rhabdomylosis
Refeeding syndrome	Tumor lysis syndrome
Magnesium binder	Trauma
Citrate (blood transfusion)	
	Familial hypocalciuric hypercalcemia
Renal (FEMg<2%)	
Medications	Near drowning in Dead Sea
Diuretics	
Amphotericin B	
Aminoglycosides	
Alcohol	
Cyclosporine A	
Tacrolimus	
Cisplatin	
Hypercalcemia	
Osmotic diuresis	
Mannitol	
Glucose	
Genetic defects	
Bartter's syndrome	
Gitelman's syndrome	

Figure 4 Magnesium disorders etiologies. *GFR,* Glomerular filtration rate.

Hypermagnesemia

Hypermagnesemia (>2.4 mg/dL) acts to depress the neuromuscular system and is usually related to severe renal failure and exogenous sources. Adrenal insufficiency, lithium toxicity, familial hypocalciuric hypercalcemia, and tissue destruction are other potential causes of hypermagnesemia (Fig. 4).

First, exogenous sources of magnesium should be discontinued, if possible. Second, the cardiac effects of hypermagnesemia can be stabilized with calcium. Finally, maneuvers to decrease the serum magnesium level are performed. An intracellular shift of magnesium can be obtained with intravenous insulin and glucose. Intravenous hydration, loop diuretics, and renal replacement therapy are used to eliminate excess magnesium.

◼ CALCIUM

Calcium (normal range: 8.6–10.2 mg/dL) is important for neuromuscular function, platelet adhesion, coagulation, endocrine and exocrine secretion, and bone metabolism. Approximately 40% to 50% of the serum calcium is protein bound, primarily by albumin. The ionized calcium (normal range: 1.12–1.30 µmol/L) is dependent on the acid-base status of the patient. Metabolic acidosis increases calcium dissociation from albumin leading to a higher ionized fraction, whereas metabolic alkalosis causes the reverse. Therefore albumin levels and the acid-base status are important when evaluating calcium disorders.

Hypocalcemia

Hypocalcemia (<8.6 mg/dL total, <1.1 µmol/L ionized) causes neuromuscular excitability. Etiologies, shown in Figure 5, include increased protein binding, resistance or deficiency in parathyroid hormone and vitamin D, rapid bone accretion, increased urinary losses, and ion precipitation/binding.

Symptomatic patients require aggressive replacement with either calcium gluconate or calcium chloride. Calcium chloride, which has three times the available elemental calcium, is associated with phlebitis and tissue necrosis. In symptomatic patients, 1 g of calcium chloride (12.6 mEq) or 3 g calcium gluconate (13.7 mEq) over 10 minutes intravenously is often used and repeated as needed until the patient is asymptomatic. Often a continuous drip (0.8–1.5 mEq/min maximum) is required with cardiac monitoring and frequent measurement of calcium levels. Asymptomatic patients can receive a slower correction (calcium gluconate 1–2 g in 100 ml D5W/NS over 30–60 minutes) with monitoring of levels or oral calcium replacements. Figure 5 shows multiple calcium replacement formulations to help guide therapy.

Magnesium levels and acid-base status are also important in hypocalcemia. Hypomagnesemia, which impairs PTH release and activity, should be corrected first. Metabolic acidosis should be corrected after the calcium deficit. Finally, citrate binders found in blood transfusions can cause hypocalcemia. Generally this effect is transitory as the citrate is metabolized.

Hypercalcemia

Hypercalcemia (>10.2 mg/dL total, >1.3 µmol/L ionized) produces the well-known complex of "bones, stones, belly groans, and mental status overtones" along with polyuria and polydipsia. The majority of patients have either a malignancy or primary hyperparathyroidism. Other etiologies include medications, familial hypocalciuric hypercalcemia, immobilization, rhabdomyolysis, Paget's disease, vitamin A and D toxicity, adrenal insufficiency, and pheochromocytoma (Fig. 5). The workup involves first differentiation between primary hyperparathyroidism and other etiologies. PTH levels, serum electrolytes, and urine calcium levels help in determining the underlying etiology of the hypercalcemia. PTHrP and vitamin D levels may be necessary in the workup of patients with low PTH levels.

Hypercalcemia requires therapies to increase elimination and inhibit bone turnover. Intravenous hydration with isotonic fluids is the initial treatment for volume contraction. After volume resuscitation, loop diuretics can be used to enhance calcium loss. The combination fluids and loop diuretics can drop the calcium level by 2 to 3 mg/dL over 48 hours. Life-threatening hypercalcemia or patients with renal failure may require renal replacement therapy to treat the hypercalcemia.

Bisphosphonates are used to inhibit bone reabsorption, but these drugs have a slow onset of action (48 hours) and are generally reserved for hypercalcemia from malignancy. Calcitonin (4 mcg/kg subcutaneous) can also be used, but its effect is mild, and tachyphylaxis rapidly develops. Plicamycin and gallium nitrate also inhibit bone reabsorption, but toxicity is too common to permit recommendation of routine usage. Finally, glucocorticoids (hydrocortisone 200 mg/day or prednisone 20–60 mg/day in divided doses for 2–5 days) are used in hypercalcemia associated with granulomatous diseases (tuberculosis, sarcoidosis). Intravenous phosphate should be avoided in hypercalcemic patients because of metastatic calcifications.

ETIOLOGIES OF CALCIUM DISORDERS

Hypocalcemia	**Hypercalcemia**
Metabolic alkalosis	Metabolic acidosis
Hypoalbuminemia	Primary hyperparathyroidism
Hypomagnesemia	Malignancy
Hyperphosphatemia	Vitamin A or D toxicity
Sepsis	Milk alkali syndrome
Pancreatitis	Adrenal insufficiency
Renal insufficiency	Immobilization
Hypoparathyroidism	Paget's disease
Blood transfusion (citrate)	Rhabdomyolysis
Hepatic dysfunction	Granulomatous diseases
Medications	Tuberculosis
Loop diuretics	Sarcoidosis
Bisphosphonates	Pheochromocytoma
Phenytoin	Medications
Heparin	Thiazide diuretics
PTU	Lithium
Radiocontrast agents	Estrogen

A

CALCIUM REPLACEMENT THERAPIES

Calcium formulation	Administration	Elemental calcium (meq/gram)
Calcium gluconate	IV/PO	4.56
Calcium chloride	IV/PO	13.6
Calcium acetate	IV/PO	12.7
Calcium citrate	PO	10.5
Calcium carbonate	PO	20.0

B

Figure 5 Etiologies of calcium disorders. *IV*, Intravenous; *PO*, per os (by mouth); *PTU*, propylthiouracil.

PHOSPHORUS

Phosphorus (normal range: 2.7–4.5 mg/dL) has multiple functions, including bone composition, nerve and muscle function, glucose utilization, 2,3 diphosphoglycerate synthesis, and synthesis of high-energy bonds (adenosine triphosphate). It is tightly regulated with calcium and forms a precipitate with calcium when the calcium-phosphate product is greater than 60 mg^2/dL^2.

Hypophosphatemia

Hypophosphatemia (<2.7 mg/dL) presents with poor neuromuscular function. The etiologies of hyperphosphatemia include decreased gastrointestinal absorption, increased renal losses, intracellular shifts, and hyperparathyroidism and vitamin D deficiency. Mechanisms and etiologies of hypophosphatemia are found in Figure 6.

Treatment involves either oral or intravenous replacement. Oral replacement is generally used in asymptomatic patients, whereas intravenous therapy is necessary in more severely depleted patients. Renal failure patients require lower replacement doses, but those on renal replacement therapy require closer to normal doses to replete phosphorus. Figure 6, *B* shows an empiric phosphorus replacement strategy for patients with normal renal function. The replacement rate should be approximately 7 µmol of phosphorous per hour to prevent precipitation with calcium.

PHOSPHATE DISORDERS ETIOLOGIES

Hypophosphatemia	**Hyperphosphatemia**
Decreased absorption/intake	Increased absorption/intake
Malnutrition	Excessive administration
Malabsorption	Phosphate containing enemas
Inadequate administration	Phosphate containing laxatives
Vomiting	Vitamin D toxicity
Diarrhea	Granulomatous diseases
Vitamin D deficiency	Extracellular shift
Sucralfate	Acidosis
Antacids	Decreased renal elimination
Intracellular shift	Renal failure
Alkalosis	Hypoparathyroidism
Insulin	Hyperthyroidism
DKA (treated)	Tissues destruction
Refeeding syndrome	Trauma
Glucocorticoids	Rhabdomyolysis
Epinephrine	Tumor lysis syndrome
Increased renal elimination	Sepsis
Osmotic diuresis	
Diuretics	
Hyperparathyroidism	
Hyperaldosterone	
Nephrotoxic proteins	
Renal replacement therapies	

A

TREATMENT OF HYPOPHOSPHATEMIA

Serum phosphorus concentration (mg/dL)	Intravenous phosphate replacement (mmole/kg adjusted body weight)
2.3–3.0	0.08–0.16
1.5–2.2	0.16–0.32
<1.5	0.32–0.64

B

Figure 6 Phosphate disorder etiologies. *DKA*, Diabetic ketoacidosis.

Hyperphosphatemia

Hyperphosphatemia (>4.5 mg/dL), when symptomatic, presents with symptoms of hypocalcemia and metastatic calcification. Etiologies include renal failure, excess administration (especially with renal failure), extracellular shifts and tissue damage, hypoparathyroidism, and vitamin D toxicity (Fig. 6, *A*).

Exogenous sources discontinued or reduced in patients with hyperphosphatemia. Protein intake should be reduced in patients with renal failure because of its phosphorus load. Volume expansion increases renal losses in patients with normal renal function. Insulin and glucose cause a transient intracellular shift of phosphorus. However, patients with symptomatic hyperphosphatemia may require renal replacement therapy to control the hyperphosphatemia.

Oral phosphate binders are commonly used in patients with chronic hyperphosphatemia. Calcium is used if the patient is not hypercalcemic. In hypercalcemic patients, magnesium and aluminum can be used but are associated with diarrhea and constipation, respectively, and may accumulate in patients with renal failure. Sevelamer, a nonionic phosphate binder, is used in patients who fail other phosphate binder therapies.

■ SUMMARY

As stated earlier, sound clinical judgment is necessary in the treatment of electrolyte disorders. Although multiple equations are available (Fig. 7, *A*) to assist in the analysis of the various disorders to guide choices of fluid (Fig. 7, *B*) and therapy strategies, individual response to therapy should determine treatment. It is crucial to monitor the patient closely during therapy, and those patients with severe disorders or potentially dangerous therapies should receive closer monitoring.

IMPORTANT EQUATIONS FOR ELECTROLYTE DISORDER

Serum osmolality (calculated)

$$\text{Serum osmolality (mOsm/kg)} = 2 * [Na] + \frac{BUN}{2.8} + \frac{glucose}{18}$$

[Na] in mEq/L
BUN and glucose in mg/dL

Sodium deficit

$$\text{Sodium deficit (mEq)} = ([Na]_{goal} - [Na]_{plasma}) * TBW$$

TBW = total body water

Free water deficit

$$\text{Free water deficit (L)} = \left(\frac{[Na]}{140} - 1\right) * TBW$$

Adrogue-Madias equation

$$\text{Change in sodium after Infusion of 1 L of IVF} = \frac{([Na] + [K])_{infusate} - [Na]_{plasma}}{TBW + 1}$$

Transtubular potassium gradient (TTKG)

$$TTKG = \frac{[K]_{urine} * \text{Plasma osmolality}}{[K]_{plasma} * \text{Urine osmolality}}$$

Assumptions
Urine osmolality > plasma osmolality
[Na] > 20 mEq/L

Hyperkalemia
<5 Renal potassium gain
>5 Extrarenal potassium increases

Hypokalemia
>1 Renal potassium losses
<1 Extrarenal potassium losses

Fractional excretion of sodium

$$FENa = \frac{[Na]_{urine} * creatinine_{plasma}}{[Na]_{plasma} * creatinine_{urine}}$$

<1% Prerenal azotemia
>2% Intrinsic renal disorder

Fractional excretion of magnesium

$$FEMg = \frac{[Mg]_{urine} * creatinine_{plasma}}{0.7 * [Mg]_{plasma} * creatinine_{urine}}$$

>2% Renal magnesium loss
<2% Extrarenal magnesium loss

Corrected calcium (albumin)

$$\text{Calcium (corrected)} = calcium + 0.8 * (4 - albumin)$$

Calcium in mg/dL

A

Figure 7 **(A)** Important equations for electrolyte disorders.

(continued)

COMPOSITION OF INTRAVENOUS FLUIDS

(mEq/L)

Fluid	Sodium	Potassium	Chloride	Calcium	Magnesium	Bicarbonate	Osmolality
Plasma	141	4–5	103	5	2	27	289
LR	130	4	109	3	0	28	273
3% Saline	513	0	513	0	0	0	1026
0.9% Saline	154	0	154	0	0	0	308
0.45% Saline	77	0	77	0	0	0	154
0.2% Saline	34	0	34	0	0	0	68
D5W	0	0	0	0	0	0	253

B

Figure 7 Cont'd—**(B)** Composition of intravenous fluids. *BUN,* Blood urea nitrogen; *D5W,* dextrose 5% in water; *LR,* lactated Ringer's.

SUGGESTED READINGS

Adrogue HJ, Madias NE: Aiding fluid prescription for the dysnatremias, *Inten Care Med* 23:309, 1997.
Elgart HN: Assessment of fluids and electrolytes, *AACN Clinical Issues* 15:607, 2004.
Kapoor M, Chan GZ: Fluid and electrolyte abnormalities, *Crit Care Clin* 17:503, 2001.

Kraft MD, Btaiche IF, Sacks GS, and others: Treatment of electrolyte disorders in adult patients in the intensive care unit, *Am J Health-Syst Pharm* 62:1663, 2005.
Nguyen MK, Kurtz I: A new quantitative approach to the treatment of the dysnatremias, *Clin Exp Nephrol* 7:125, 2003.
Rastergar A, Soleimani M: Hypokalemia and hyperkalemia, *Postgrad Med J* 77:759, 2001.
Topf JM, Murray PT: Hypomagnesemia and hypermagnesemia, *Rev Endo Met Disorders* 4:195, 2003.

ACID-BASE PROBLEMS

Kristen C. Sihler, MD, MS, and
Ronald V. Maier, MD

NORMAL ACID-BASE METABOLISM

Normal cellular function is dependent on tight control of body fluid pH. The normal range is 7.35 to 7.45, which corresponds to the optimal range for most enzyme function. The corresponding concentration of free hydrogen ion in body fluids is approximately 40 nEq/L. The usual North American diet provides 70 mEq of H^+ per day, and daily metabolism produces 15,000 mEq H_2CO_3. Therefore acidosis occurs easily with any failure of buffering and clearance mechanisms, and even slight accumulation of the hydrogen ion produced daily is rapidly fatal. Endogenously produced acid must be immediately buffered such that free hydrogen ions do not accumulate. Alkalosis is more difficult to achieve but can still have detrimental effects on body functions because of numerous alterations in physiologic processes.

Three systems maintain normal H^+ concentration in body fluids: (1) the bicarbonate buffer system, (2) proteins, and (3) bone. The bicarbonate buffer system is the principal buffer in the extracellular fluid compartment and the most physiologically important buffer overall. Clinical evaluation of acid-base status depends on assessment of the concentrations of the key components of this buffering system: H^+, CO_2, and HCO_3, which are related as follows:

$$CO_2 \text{ (gas)} \leftrightarrow CO_2 \text{ (aqueous)} + H_2O \leftrightarrow H_2CO_3 \leftrightarrow H^+ + HCO_3^-$$

Alveolar ventilation controls the concentration of CO_2, whereas the kidney regulates serum bicarbonate concentration. The remarkable buffering capacity of this system is related to the ability to quickly change $PaCO_2$ through respiratory effort. The addition of H^+ to body fluids drives the equilibrium to the left, resulting in the production of CO_2. At the same time, the resultant acidosis stimulates medullary chemoreceptors, resulting in increased alveolar ventilation and elimination of CO_2, further driving the equilibrium to the left. CO_2 diffuses 20 times faster than O_2, making it relatively easy to clear CO_2 as long as gas exchange is unimpaired. The result is a rapid net acid loss and maintenance of a relatively normal pH.

The role of the kidney in this buffering system is to excrete the anions associated with the endogenously produced acid (e.g., phosphates, sulfates) and, more important, to regenerate the 60 to 70 mEq of bicarbonate consumed daily in buffering the endogenous acid load. There are two components of renal regeneration of HCO_3: reabsorption of filtered HCO_3^- and generation of new HCO_3^-. The bulk of filtered HCO_3^- is reabsorbed in an indirect fashion in the proximal convoluted tubule as a result of H^+ excretion. At a normal glomerular filtration rate, approximately 85% of filtered HCO_3^- is reabsorbed. Reabsorption may be increased in the presence of an elevated $PaCO_2$, extracellular fluid volume contraction, hypokalemia, and mineralocorticoid activity. Carbonic anhydrase inhibitors work in the proximal tubule by preventing intraluminal conversion of H_2CO_3 to H_2O and CO_2, thus impeding HCO_3^- reabsorption. Generation of new HCO_3- occurs primarily in the distal tubule, where H^+ is secreted in exchange for a reabsorbed Na^+ under the influence of aldosterone. The secreted hydrogen ion (50–100 mEq/day) is then buffered in the urine by weak acid salts in the glomerular filtrate and by ammonia, which is generated by the renal tubular cells. This secretion of hydrogen ion into the urine is coupled with regeneration of the bicarbonate ion, which is then returned to the extracellular fluid.

Proteins are the principle intracellular buffering system. There are H^+ binding sites on intracellular proteins (e.g., hemoglobin). These binding sites are on histidine moieties. The influence of the protein buffering system is seen in the adjustment that must be made in the anion gap for low albumen.

Bone represents a secondary extracellular buffer reservoir. It can absorb hydrogen ions in exchange for sodium and potassium and, through reabsorption, release alkali stores in the form of bicarbonate and phosphate salts. Although the buffering capacity of bone is enormous, it plays little, if any, role in attenuating acute changes in acid-base status.

Any change in the concentration of hydrogen ions in body fluids results in a compensatory response to restore the pH into the normal range. The Henderson-Hasselbach equation predicts that the hydrogen ion concentration of a solution is dictated by the ratio of the proteinated and unproteinated species of any buffer pair in that solution. A simplification of this relationship in the form of the Henderson equation uses the most important buffer pair in body fluids (i.e., HCO_3^- and CO_2) to predict the hydrogen ion concentration as follows:

$$[H^+] = 24 \times PaCO_2/[HCO_3^-]$$

The pH is the negative of the log of $[H^+]$. The implications of this relationship are twofold. First, pH is dictated by the ratio of CO_2 to HCO_3^- and not by the absolute concentrations of either. Second, this relationship demonstrates mathematically the way

the body has to compensate. To maintain a normal or near-normal pH if CO_2 rises, then HCO_3^- must fall and vice versa.

DISORDERS OF ACID-BASE HOMEOSTASIS

As discussed earlier, diet and metabolic processes produce a significant acid load each day. Thus an acidosis can occur not only by addition of this large amount of acid but also by failure of buffering and clearance mechanisms, whereas alkalosis is less common. Blood can have only one pH, even though several coexistent acid-base disorders may change that pH to different degrees or in different directions. In fact, a normal pH may be present even with marked changes in acid-base status (e.g., a respiratory acidosis combined with a metabolic alkalosis). *Acidemia* is defined as a plasma pH less than 7.35, and *alkalemia* is defined as a plasma pH more than 7.45. These are to be differentiated from acidosis and alkalosis, respectively, which are disorders that tend to alter plasma pH but the effects of which on pH may be modulated by the coexistence of other acid-base alterations.

The first step in interpreting arterial blood gases is to determine whether an acidemia or alkalemia is present and then to assess whether a respiratory or metabolic acid-base disorder is present. If the $PaCO_2$ and the pH are altered in opposite directions from normal, there is a respiratory component to the acid-base disorder. If altered in the same direction, a metabolic disorder is present. Finally, the third step is assessment of whether an appropriate compensatory response to the primary disorder is present (see Fig. 1 and Table 1). If not, a second disorder is present.

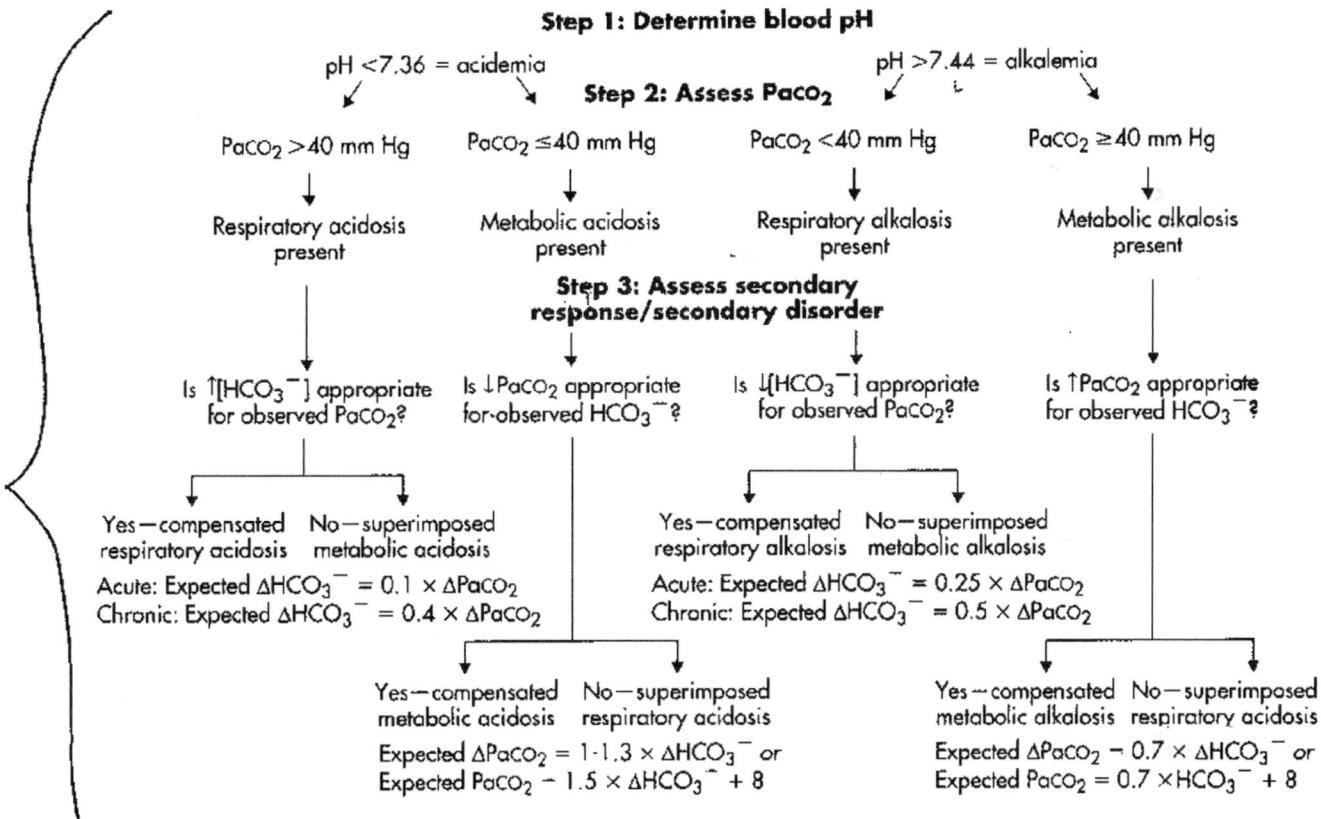

Figure 1 Flowchart for the interpretation of acid-base disorders and arterial blood gases.

ACID-BASE PROBLEMS

Table 1: Expected Changes in Acid-Base Disturbances

Disorder	Primary Disturbance	Compensatory Response	Compensation Formula*
Metabolic acidosis	↓ HCO_3^-	↓ $PaCO_2$	$\Delta PaCO_2 = 1.2 \times \Delta HCO_3^-$
Metabolic alkalosis	↑ HCO_3^-	↑ $PaCO_2$	$\Delta PaCO_2 = 0.6 \times \Delta HCO_3^-$
Acute respiratory acidosis	↑ $PaCO_2$	↑ HCO_3^-	$\Delta HCO_3^- = 0.1 \times \Delta PaCO_2$
Chronic respiratory acidosis	↑ $PaCO_2$	↑↑ HCO_3^-	$\Delta HCO_3^- = 0.35 \times \Delta PaCO_2$
Acute respiratory alkalosis	↓ $PaCO_2$	↓ HCO_3^-	$\Delta HCO_3^- = 0.2 \times \Delta PaCO_2$
Chronic respiratory alkalosis	↓ $PaCO_2$	↓↓ HCO_3^-	$\Delta HCO_3^- = 0.5 \times \Delta PaCO_2$

*$PaCO_2$ (change in $PaCO_2$) is calculated from the normal value of 40. ΔHCO_3^- is calculated from the normal value of 24.

Compensation is never complete, thus a normal pH in the presence of an acid-base disorder implies the presence of another, opposite disorder.

SPECIFIC ACID-BASE DISORDERS

Metabolic Acidosis

Disorders resulting in metabolic acidosis occur through one of two mechanisms: (1) acid production in excess of the ability of the kidneys to excrete the acid and regenerate bicarbonate or (2) loss of bicarbonate from the extracellular fluid either through the kidneys or the gastrointestinal (GI) tract. These two pathophysiologic mechanisms and, in a broader sense, the underlying disease processes critical to their development can be distinguished by the presence or absence of an anion gap. The addition of fixed acids results in an anion gap metabolic acidosis, whereas bicarbonate loss results in a nonanion gap metabolic acidosis

(Table 3). The anion gap (AG) refers to the difference between measured cations (Na^+) and measured anions (Cl^- and HCO_3^-) and represents unmeasured anions, including negatively charged proteins, phosphates, and other weak acids. It is readily calculated as follows:

$$AG = Na^+ - (Cl^- + HCO_3^-)$$

The normal anion gap ranges from 3 to 11 mEq/L. A reduction in the plasma albumin concentration reduces the baseline AG approximately 2.5 mEq for every 1 g/dL fall in the serum albumin. Thus a severely hypoalbuminemic patient may have an AG metabolic acidosis with an apparently "normal" AG if this is not considered. Causes of AG acidosis may be remembered by the mnemonic "MUDPILES" (see Table 2).

Lactic acidosis is the most common cause of acidosis in the hospitalized patient. Lactic acid is produced during anaerobic metabolism and suggests that oxygen delivery is inadequate to meet tissue oxygen demands. This is usually due to hypoperfusion or hypoxia. Tissue O_2 delivery can be compromised by a lack of hemoglobin in

Table 2: Metabolic Acidosis

Cause	Mechanism	Treatment
Anion Gap		
Renal failure	Accumulation of fixed acids (proteins, sulfates, phosphates), impaired bicarbonate reabsorption/regeneration	Low-protein diet, administration of sodium bicarbonate, dialysis
Lactic acidosis	Accumulation of lactic acid caused by anaerobic glycolysis	Restoration of cellular oxygen delivery
Diabetic ketoacidosis, fasting, chronic alcoholism	Increased glucagon-to-insulin ratio leads to enhanced lipolysis and metabolism through ketoacids, dehydration	Administration of insulin (for diabetic ketoacidosis); provision of carbohydrate; rehydration
Toxic ingestions: salicylates, methanol, ethylene glycol, paraldehyde, toluene	Addition of fixed acids	Enhancement of excretion (hydration, dialysis); urine alkalinization for salicylate poisoning; ethanol was used in the past for ethylene glycol and methanol poisoning to block the conversion by alcohol dehydrogenase into toxic metabolites, but now fomepizole is used
Nonanion Gap		
Diarrhea, ileus, fistula, and ureterosigmoidostomy	Gastrointestinal HCO_3^- loss	Replacement of volume and electrolytes
Proximal renal tubular acidosis, acetazolamide	Renal HCO_3^- loss	Discontinuation of acetazolamide
Saline administration (large volumes administered quickly)	Renal HCO_3^- loss	Avoidance
Distal renal tubular acidosis	Failure of renal HCO_3^- production	Alkali administration

Table 3: Causes of Anion Gap Acidosis

M	Methanol, metformin
U	Uremia
D	Diabetic ketoacidosis, other causes of ketoacidosis
P	Paraldehyde
I	Isoniazid, iron
L	Lactic acidosis (including cyanide and carbon monoxide poisoning)
E	Ethylene glycol, ethanol
S	Salicylates

severe anemia or by occupation of O_2 binding sites on hemoglobin as with carbon monoxide poisoning. Cyanide poisoning induces lactic acidosis through uncoupling of oxidative phosphorylation in the mitochondria. Mild lactic acidosis can be seen in liver failure and represents a failure of clearance, sometimes combined with increased production. Diagnosis may be confirmed by the presence of a widened AG and an elevated serum lactate in the appropriate clinical setting. Therapy for lactic acidosis is directed toward restoring cellular oxygenation by restoring normal tissue oxygen delivery. Addition of acids such as ketoacids, as in diabetic ketoacidosis, starvation, and chronic alcoholism, also cause an AG acidosis.

Advanced renal failure may also produce an AG acidosis because of an inability of the kidneys to excrete the daily acid load. However, in uncomplicated renal failure, it is rare to see an AG greater than 23 and a bicarbonate less than 12 mEq/L. If these parameters are exceeded, a coexistent cause of the acidosis should be sought. Depending on the clinical setting, either dialysis or exogenous sodium bicarbonate administration may be necessary to remove fixed acids and correct the base deficit, respectively.

For patients in whom no cause for the AG metabolic acidosis can be ascertained and in whom blood ketone and lactate levels are normal, suspect ingestion of a toxin such as ethylene glycol, methanol, or salicylates. A toxic agent screen may be helpful, but the results may not be available for several hours. A faster evaluation can be obtained by calculating the osmolar gap. This refers to the difference between the calculated and measured plasma osmolarity. Under normal circumstances, plasma osmolarity may be estimated as follows (BUN = blood urea nitrogen):

Osmolarity = $2[Na^+]$ + glucose (mg/dL)/18 + BUN (mg/dL)/2.8

If the plasma osmolarity determined by the laboratory exceeds the estimated plasma osmolarity, an unidentified osmotically active substance is present in the plasma. Typically, metabolic acidoses associated with the greatest increase in the osmolar gap are those associated with methanol or ethylene glycol administration.

Non-AG acidoses are caused by GI or renal HCO_3^- loss. Although the clinical situation may aid in the differential diagnosis of a non-AG acidosis, several urine studies may be diagnostic. If the metabolic acidosis is caused by bicarbonate loss from the GI tract, the normal kidney should compensate by increasing net acid excretion and bicarbonate regeneration, leading to a urine pH less than 5 and an increased (negative) urinary AG, representing ammonium loss. The urinary AG is measured as follows:

Urinary AG = [UNa + UK] − UCl

Patients with renal tubular acidosis have an inability to acidify the urine and a defect in renal ammonium excretion. This leads to an inappropriately high urine pH (>6) and a decrease in urinary ammonium excretion manifested as a positive urinary AG.

The principal early manifestation of metabolic acidosis is an increase in minute ventilation primarily because of an increased tidal volume. The increase in minute ventilation compensates for the metabolic acidosis by eliminating more CO_2. If the patient's respiratory drive is insufficient to maintain a $PaCO_2$ less than 60 mm Hg, ventilatory support should be strongly considered because any further aggravation of the acidosis may lead to rapid decompensation. As the pH drops below 7.2, loss of vasomotor tone and a reduction in myocardial contractility may lead to cardiovascular collapse.

Treatment of metabolic acidosis depends on the underlying cause. Administration of sodium bicarbonate usually is not indicated unless the acidosis is severe (pH <7.15, HCO_3^- less than 12 mEq/L), at which point the buffering capacity is significantly reduced. Furthermore, at a pH less than 7.2, catecholamine resistance develops such that the myocardium and resistance vessels may not respond to either endogenous or exogenous catecholamines. In the setting of myocardial depression or hypotension unresponsive to vasopressors, sodium bicarbonate may be administered as a bolus over several minutes (100 mEq), followed by a continuous infusion (3 ampoules of $NaHCO_3$ in 1 L D5W) to maintain a pH greater than 7.2.

A brief mention should be made of the strong ion difference (SID) because readers may encounter mention of it. This was first proposed by Peter Stewart in 1981 and states that bicarbonate is a dependent variable rather than an independent cause. The SID is the difference between strong cations and strong anions:

$$[SID] = [Na^+] + [K^+] + [Ca^{2+}] + [Mg^{2+}] - [Cl^-] - [\text{other strong anions}]$$

The theory is interesting but does not result in a change in clinical management of acid-base disturbances.

Metabolic Alkalosis

The diagnosis of metabolic alkalosis is made on the basis of an elevated blood pH (>7.44) in the presence of a normal or high $PaCO_2$. Metabolic alkaloses may arise from one of three mechanisms: (1) loss of acid from the GI tract or urine; (2) administration of HCO_3^- or a precursor, such as citrate (e.g., massive blood transfusion); or (3) loss of fluid with higher chloride-to-bicarbonate ratio than that of plasma. The kidney normally defends against an abnormal rise in plasma bicarbonate concentration by limiting reabsorption of filtered bicarbonate in the proximal tubule. Thus the development of a metabolic alkalosis is contingent on there being some impairment of renal HCO_3^- handling. For example, volume contraction, hypokalemia, and increased mineralocorticoid activity may all result in persistent alkalosis. Hypochloremic metabolic alkalosis associated with prolonged vomiting or nasogastric suction illustrates this principle. The loss of hydrogen ion in gastric secretions leads to relative excess plasma HCO_3^-. The key to the persistence of alkalosis relates to the associated volume depletion and chloride depletion. Because the body's normal pH is slightly alkaline, volume contraction exaggerates this and increases Na+ reabsorption from the proximal tubule. In the presence of chloride depletion, Na+ is reabsorbed with HCO_3^- to maintain electroneutrality, leading to aggravation of the alkalosis. The hypokalemia associated with vomiting is caused by renal, rather than GI, potassium loss because of accelerated Na+-K+ exchange (an aldosterone-mediated effect) in the distal tubule. The hypokalemia further accelerates bicarbonate reabsorption in the proximal tubule, as well as hydrogen secretion in the distal tubule, an effect mediated by the elevated levels of aldosterone. The result is paradoxical aciduria in the setting of metabolic alkalosis.

The differential diagnosis and treatment of metabolic alkaloses is simplified by their classification into chloride-sensitive or chloride-resistant forms, reflecting the extent that they are reversed by

Table 4: Metabolic Alkalosis

Cause	Mechanism	Urine Chloride	Treatment
Chloride Responsive			
Vomiting, nasogastric suction	Loss of HCl, leading to relative excess of HCO_3^-, increased renal absorption of Cl- because of depletion	Negligible	Provision of Cl^- (as NaCl or KCl); restoration of intravascular volume
Diuretic therapy	Cl- loss in urine, volume depletion, increased renal HCO_3^- generation, hypokalemia	High during diuretic use, negligible afterward	Provision of Cl^- as NaCl and KCl; restoration of intravascular volume
Posthypercapnia	Renal excretion of acid and generation of HCO_3^- during respiratory acidosis	Negligible	Provision of Cl^-
Chloride Resistant			
Mineralocorticoid excess (Cushing's syndrome, hyperaldosteronism, exogenous steroids)	Direct stimulation of Na^+-H^+ and Na^+-K^+ exchange in distal tubule; increased renal generation and reabsorption of HCO_3^-	High (>15 mEq/L)	Correction of underlying disorder; spironolactone; K^+ replacement
Bartter's syndrome (renal tubular salt wasting)	Increased distal tubular Na^+ delivery increases distal tubular Na^+ reabsorption and exchange with K^+ and H^+	High (>15 mEq/L)	K^+ replacement; nonsteroidal antiinflammatory agents; volume expansion
Excessive alkali administration	Usually associated with renal insufficiency; citrate (from red cell transfusions); hyperalimentation solutions; milk-alkali syndrome	High (>15 mEq/L)	Cessation of alkali administration
Severe potassium depletion	Impaired renal Cl^- reabsorption leading to increased Na^+-H^+ exchange and generation of HCO_3^-	High (>15 mEq/L)	K^+ repletion

the administration of normal saline (Table 4). Low urinary chloride (<15 mEq/L) indicates that the process will be responsive to chloride administration, whereas high urinary chloride (≥15 mEq/L) indicates chloride resistance. Patients who have received diuretics within the prior 24 hours may have a high urinary chloride but a chloride-responsive alkalosis. Chloride-sensitive metabolic alkaloses are treated by the parenteral administration of saline, which corrects the Cl^- deficit and restores intravascular volume, both of which facilitate urinary HCO_3^- excretion. Coexistent hypokalemia, a phenomenon known to perpetuate the alkalosis, should be treated after the intravascular volume has been restored.

Patients with chloride-resistant metabolic alkaloses do not have a chloride deficit and therefore do not respond to chloride-containing solutions. The primary defect is usually an increase in mineralocorticoid activity (e.g., aldosteronoma). Mineralocorticoid-mediated reabsorption of Na+ in the distal tubule leads to extracellular volume expansion and persistent K^+ and H^+ excretion, despite the alkalosis. Treatment is directed toward the underlying cause of mineralocorticoid excess. Spironolactone is of limited use.

Clinical manifestations of metabolic alkaloses are rare but when they do occur are chiefly those of excess neuromuscular excitability, including paresthesias, carpopedal spasm, or lightheadedness. Increased protein binding of ionized calcium can lead to tetany. Hypokalemia often accompanies metabolic alkalosis, so its symptoms of muscle weakness, cramping, ileus, and polyuria may also occur. Ventricular irritability may be present at a pH greater than 7.55. The expected respiratory response is a reduction in minute ventilation (see Table 1). Because the hypoventilatory response to metabolic alkalosis is limited by the development of hypoxemia, the compensatory rise in $PaCO_2$ tends to be limited. The need to

administer exogenous acid is extremely unusual, but if the pH exceeds 7.55, immediate partial correction is best achieved with ammonium chloride or HCl. Be aware that HCl administration can be complicated by hemolysis.

Respiratory Acid-Base Disorders

Although the normal $PaCO_2$ is 38 to 42 mm Hg, alterations in $PaCO_2$ are expected if a coexistent metabolic acidosis or alkalosis exists. Therefore the assessment of $PaCO_2$ and the presence or absence of a respiratory acid-base disorder must be taken in the context of the metabolic acid-base status of the patient (see Table 1). In addition, respiratory disorders are classified as either acute or chronic, depending on the extent of renal compensation in which increased tubular excretion of NH_4^+ or reabsorption of HCO_3^- reverse the pH alterations induced by the primary respiratory disorder. This renal compensatory response typically requires approximately 2 to 3 days to reach equilibrium; thus disorders occurring over this interval are considered chronic.

Alkalosis is more difficult to achieve.

Acute rises in $PaCO_2$ cause a dramatic change in serum pH, reflecting the limited capacity of the nonbicarbonate intracellular buffering systems. Persistent elevation of $PaCO_2$ stimulates renal hydrogen excretion and reabsorption of HCO_3^-, which helps, albeit incompletely, to normalize the pH.

The central chemoreceptors, located on the ventral surface of the medulla, stimulate ventilation primarily in response to decreases in the pH of the cerebrospinal fluid and in response to increases in $PaCO_2$ (mediated by a drop in pH). Normally, the drive to maintain eucapnia is remarkably powerful. Thus CO_2

Table 5: Respiratory Acidosis

Cause	Mechanism	Treatment
Sedatives, hypnotics, narcotics, central nervous system lesions	Suppression of respiratory drive	Discontinuation or reversal of pharmacologic suppression of respiration; mechanical ventilation
Restrictive lung disease Pulmonary fibrosis Pleural effusions Ankylosing spondylitis Severe kyphosis	Increased work of breathing	Treatment of underlying disease; mechanical ventilation as needed
Obstructive lung disease Upper airway obstruction Asthma	Increased work of breathing	Treatment of underlying disease; mechanical ventilation as needed
Myopathies/neuropathies Paralysis Guillain-Barré syndrome	Relative increase in work of breathing	Mechanical ventilation if severe
Fever, seizures	Increased CO_2 production in the presence of a fixed minute ventilation	Control of fever; mechanical ventilation rarely required in cases of excess CO_2 production
Large pulmonary embolus	Increased alveolar dead space in the presence of fixed minute ventilation	Thrombolytic therapy; mechanical ventilation to further increase minute ventilation

accumulation usually implies suppression of the respiratory center by either pharmacologic or other means, or alternatively, normal respiratory drive with failure to maintain adequate alveolar ventilation because of underlying pulmonary dysfunction (Table 5). Patients with fixed minute ventilation (e.g., ventilator dependent) develop increases in $PaCO_2$ if they have an increase in their dead space or an increase in their rate of CO_2 production caused by an accelerated metabolic rate or in overfeeding.

Manifestations of acute increases in $PaCO_2$ consist of the syndrome of CO_2 narcosis: headache, blurred vision, restlessness, and anxiety progressing to tremors, asterixis, and ultimately delirium and coma. These symptoms are due to relatively abrupt changes in cerebrospinal fluid pH, leading to cerebral vasodilation and cerebral edema. Treatment should be directed at reversing the underlying cause leading to inadequate minute ventilation. Administration of bicarbonate is usually not indicated and may further aggravate CO_2 accumulation. However, in the setting of acute lung injury requiring lung-protective ventilation, hypercapnia may be tolerated with its accompanying acidosis to allow the patient to be ventilated with low tidal volumes. Because of the changes that hypercapnia causes in cerebral circulation, permissive hypercapnia should not be used in the setting of acute brain injury.

Respiratory Alkalosis

Respiratory alkalosis presents as a low $PaCO_2$, a variable pH, and a variable HCO_3-. Like other respiratory acid-base disorders, interpretation must take into account the metabolic acid-base status of the patient. For example, both gram-negative sepsis and salicylate poisoning may induce a metabolic acidosis, the former by means of increased lactate production and the latter through the addition of fixed acid. Both salicylates and the circulating inflammatory mediators induced by endotoxemia directly stimulate respiratory drive. As a result, the pH may be low, normal, or high, depending on the relative contribution of acidosis, renal compensation, and degree of stimulation of the medullary respiratory center.

The underlying mechanism leading the development of respiratory alkalosis is the same irrespective of its cause (Table 6): alveolar ventilation in excess of that necessary to eliminate the daily

Table 6: Respiratory Alkalosis

Cause	Mechanism	Therapy
Pain, fever, gram-negative sepsis, cirrhosis, central nervous system lesions, pregnancy (progesterone effect), salicylates, theophylline	Increased respiratory drive	Treatment of underlying cause; discontinuation/increased elimination of pharmacologic stimulation
Hypoxia, hypotension	Peripheral chemoreceptor stimulation	Correction of hypoxia, hypotension
Pneumonia, pulmonary edema, pulmonary embolus	Pulmonary receptor stimulation	Treatment of underlying cause

production of CO_2. Persistent hypocapnia leads to impaired H+ excretion and reduced HCO_3 reabsorption in the proximal tubule, ultimately leading to the renal compensatory response over a 2- to 3-day period.

The degree of respiratory alkalosis is rarely sufficient to produce symptoms. When the alkalosis is acute and severe, the increased pH leads to an increased avidity of calcium for the binding sites on circulating plasma proteins, resulting in a reduction of ionized calcium. As a result, the principal symptoms relate to hypocalcemia and manifest as neuromuscular irritability with circumoral or peripheral paresthesias, cramps, and carpopedal spasm. With an abrupt 20- to 40- mm Hg drop in $PaCO_2$, cerebral blood flow may be impaired, resulting in alterations in the level of consciousness. If the cause of hyperpnea is psychogenic, the decreased level of consciousness may be therapeutic in that it will slow the respiratory rate. Arrhythmias, both supraventricular and ventricular, may result if the increase in pH is rapid and profound. As with many other acid-base disorders, treatment should be directed toward the underlying cause. Administration of acid or respiratory depressants is rarely indicated.

SUGGESTED READINGS

Beers MH, Berkow R, editors: Water, electrolyte, mineral, and acid-base metabolism. In *The Merck manual of diagnosis and therapy*, ed 17, Whitehouse Station, NJ, 1999, Merck.

Fall PJ: A stepwise approach to acid-base disorders: practical patient evaluation for metabolic acidosis and other conditions, *Postgrad Med* 107:249, 2000.

Nathens AB, Maier RV: Fluids and electrolytes. In Norton JA, Bollinger R, Chang AE, and others editors: *Surgery: scientific basis and current practice*, New York, 2000, Springer Verlag.

THE SEPTIC RESPONSE

Badar U. Jan, MD, and Stephen F. Lowry, MD

INTRODUCTION

Sepsis is the leading cause of death in the intensive care unit (ICU) and the tenth leading cause of mortality in the United States. Although the incidence of sepsis is rising, with more than 700,000 cases per year and an estimated mortality of 30% to 40%, recent studies suggest that the mortality from this disease may be slowly declining.

Sepsis is defined as the systemic inflammatory response syndrome (SIRS) accompanied by a documented and clinically relevant infection. SIRS is the physiologic response to significant stressors, including surgery, trauma, toxins, ischemia, burns or sterile inflammation such as pancreatitis (Table 1). A clinical phenotype including various combinations of elevated heart rate, significant deviation in core body temperature, tachypnea, and significant deviation in white blood cell count characterizes this syndrome. Gram-negative and gram-positive bacteria, as well as viruses and fungi, can induce the septic state. Whether these organisms infect the lungs as in pneumonia, peritoneal cavity as in a postsurgical abscess, or the bladder from a urinary tract infection, the resulting dysregulation of systemic inflammation is central to the pathogenic mechanisms and consequences of severe sepsis. A persistent and unregulated proinflammatory response can lead to hypotension and progressive multisystem organ failure (MSOF).

The host immune response to an invasive infection usually generates an exaggerated inflammatory SIRS response resulting in leukocyte accumulation, microvascular permeability, hemodynamic instability, and severe tissue injury. Several proinflammatory cytokines including tumor necrosis factor-alpha, interleukin (IL)-1, IL-6, and IL-8 are released by immune effector cells, including circulating neutrophils, monocytes, and lymphocytes, as well as immunoactive cells in solid organs. Under normal conditions, proinflammatory cytokine production is regulated by numerous feedback mechanisms, including anti-inflammatory cytokines such as soluble IL-10, as well as by sympathetic and parasympathetic nerve traffic. These anti-inflammatory feedback pathways inhibit the production of tissue proinflammatory mediators.

Given the complexity of inflammatory signaling pathways but relatively constrained clinical phenotype resulting from sepsis, it is necessary to have a systematic approach in treating the septic patient (Fig. 1). The surviving sepsis campaign has provided multidisciplinary guidelines designed to optimize the treatment of septic patients. These guidelines are continually updated and are an excellent resource to the practitioner caring for patients with sepsis.

HISTORY AND PHYSICAL EXAMINATION

A complete history often cannot be obtained from the patient because of critical illness. Hence every attempt should be made to confer with all health care professionals involved in the patient's care, as well as previous diagnostic studies and therapeutic maneuvers.

A thorough physical examination is necessary and should evaluate the range of etiologies that can contribute to the inciting infection.

DIAGNOSTICS

Diagnostic testing is performed to confirm a clinical suspicion of infection and to assist in localizing its source. Often the clinical picture is unclear, and one must consider broad differential diagnoses. Obtaining blood and tissue cultures with Gram staining is imperative. The timing of cultures is also relevant because the goal is to collect such cultures before administering antibiotics. All potential sources should be considered and evaluated as indicated, including blood, wounds, catheter tips, urine, and sputum.

Laboratory studies are important adjuncts in clinical evaluation and provide objective trends over the course of management. A complete blood count is useful in recognizing increasing infection or decreasing hemoglobin, and a complete metabolic panel evaluates numerous physiologic parameters, including electrolyte imbalance, as well as liver and kidney dysfunction. Coagulation profiles may be relevant when preparing a patient for surgery or identifying and treating coagulopathy. These studies must be interpreted with respect to the patient's clinical condition, as well as trended from previous values.

RADIOGRAPHIC STUDIES

Radiographic evaluations are often useful to localize the source of infection. An expedient response to testing and subsequent intervention must be applied to these studies. Consideration must be given to the critically ill patient who is too unstable to transport for diagnostic testing. For these patients, it is prudent to use studies that can be performed at the bedside, such as ultrasound and portable x-ray.

Table 1: The Clinical Continuum of Sepsis

SIRS Includes Two of the Following:	
Temperature	$\geq$38 °C or $\leq$36 °C
Heart rate	$\geq$90 beats per minute
Respiratory rate	$\geq$20 breaths per minute
White blood cell count	$\geq$12,000/μL or $\leq$4000/μL or $\geq$10% band form
Sepsis	
Sepsis	Infection + SIRS
Severe sepsis	Infection + SIRS + organ dysfunction
Septic shock	Infection + SIRS + hemodynamic instability

SIRS, Systemic inflammatory response syndrome.

MEDICAL THERAPY

Table 2 provides a summary of recommendations for medical and surgical care of the septic patient.

Antibiotics

Antibiotics are almost uniformly used to treat an infectious focus in septic patients. The antibiotics used should target the most likely pathogenic species or, as directed by culture results, against the specific offending microorganism.

Empiric antibiotic therapy often must be initiated on the basis of preliminary diagnostic testing but without definitive culture results. In cases such as these, it is prudent to use broad-spectrum antibiotics and to adjust therapy toward specific pathogens when culture and sensitivity results return. Neutropenic and immuno-compromised patients represent a notable exception to this rule because broad-spectrum antibiotics should continue to treat the offending organism and opportunistic infections.

A timeline for antimicrobial therapy should be established prior to administration; for example, a 3-to 5-day course of antibiotics should be estimated to treat a urinary tract infection, whereas endocarditis or bacteremia may require several weeks of therapy. The duration of empiric therapy should be limited to a short course of 5 to 7 days and then either discontinued or switched to culture-specific therapy as soon as results are available. The patient must also be monitored for evidence of clinical response during treatment. In addition, the institutional susceptibility pattern of an offending organism to antibiotics should be used to guide treatment.

Antibiotics alone may be insufficient for treating sepsis. One must be cautious not to overlook a potential surgical intervention while relying on antibiotic support. For example, in the case of perforated viscus or a loculated pleural effusion, antibiotics will not clear the infectious source, and a thorough surgical procedure is indicated to repair defects and remove any infectious contaminants.

Activated Protein C

Endothelial cell activation and systemic inflammation may result in a relative deficiency of anticoagulant and fibrinolytic mechanisms, thereby propagating a prothrombotic state. Systemic microvascular thrombosis is hypothesized to contribute to ischemia and solid organ dysfunction. A therapy that has shown mortality outcome improvements in some critically ill septic patients is the anticoagulant activated protein C (APC), which functions by inhibiting procoagulant factors and by exhibiting anti-inflammatory effects. APC is recommended in septic patients with a less favorable predicted outcome, such as those with septic shock, MSOF, or sepsis-induced acute respiratory distress syndrome. The main hazard with APC therapy is a significant potential for bleeding, and thus patients must be selected with consideration of this risk. Specifically, patients who have intracranial hemorrhage, are less than 12 hours postoperative, or thrombocytopenic may be unsuitable for this therapy. Septic patients should also be screened and meet specific physiologic criteria indicating a high risk of mortality prior to initiation of APC therapy.

Table 2: Summary of Recommendations for Care of the Septic Patient

Initial resuscitation	MAP >65, CVP 8–12, UOP >0.5 ml/kg/hr, Hgb >10g/dL
Diagnostics	History and physical examination, cultures, radiographic studies
Antibiotics	Initiate broad-spectrum antibiotics against likely pathogens; adjust therapy when culture results are available
Source control	Surgical repair of abnormality leading to ongoing contamination; debridement and evacuation of infectious material
Vasopressors	Goal is to achieve MAP >65; requires fluid resuscitation and arterial catheter
Inotropes	Goal is to achieve physiologic cardiac output; requires fluid resuscitation and PAC
APC	Initiate in severe sepsis with high likelihood of mortality; use with caution if there is risk of bleeding
Steroids	Useful in septic shock unresponsive to fluid resuscitation and vasopressors; may be beneficial in relative adrenal insufficiency
Blood transfusion	Transfuse to Hgb of 10 g/dl for initial resuscitation, lactic acidosis, hemorrhage, and coronary ischemia; otherwise transfuse if Hgb <7g/dL for a goal of 7–9 g/dL
Ventilation	Maintain tidal volume of 6 ml/kg and plateau pressure <30 for ARDS
Glucose control	Maintain blood sugar between 80 and 110 mg/dL; may require insulin infusion and frequent blood sugar monitoring
Renal replacement	Intermittent hemodialysis for hemodynamically stable patients; consider continuous hemodialysis for hemodynamically unstable patients;
Prophylaxis	VTE—mechanical compression devices and heparin or low-molecular-weight heparin; use cautiously for risk of bleeding; consider inferior vena cava filter when unable to use heparin
	Stress ulcer: histamine blocker or proton pump inhibitor
	VAP—maintain intubated patients in a half sitting position with 45-degree head elevation

ARDS, Acute respiratory distress syndrome; *CVP,* central venous pressure; *Hgb,* hemoglobin; *MAP,* mean arterial pressure; *PAC,* pulmonary artery catheter; *UOP,* urine output; *VAP,* ventilator-associated pneumonia; *VTE,* venous thromboembolism.

Steroids

Cortisol, an endogenous steroid, has a plethora of physiologic effects that include maintaining vascular tone in conjunction with circulating catecholamines. Cortisol is constitutively secreted, and this secretion is increased during times of stress such as surgery, burns, and severe infection. During sepsis, dysregulation of the hypothalamic-pituitary-adrenal (HPA) axis may occur such that the relatively elevated levels of cortisol may be inadequate considering the degree of stress.

There is substantial debate regarding the use of steroids in sepsis. Although earlier studies suggested that high-dose steroid administration did not yield any outcome benefit, recent studies evaluating lower doses of continuously administered steroid have shown some benefit in certain subgroups. Current management guidelines suggest using 100 mg of hydrocortisone every 8 hours for up to 7 days in patients with septic shock who do not respond to adequate fluid resuscitation and vasopressors.

A specific subgroup of septic patients who benefit from steroid therapy is the adrenally insufficient population. One way to determine the presence of relative adrenal insufficiency is to perform a cortisol stimulation test. This test is highly sensitive for diagnosing adrenal insufficiency, which is presently defined as a serum cortisol less than 15 mcg/dl or an inappropriately low response (<9 µg/dL) to cosyntropin injection. Patients diagnosed with adrenal insufficiency in septic shock should be supplemented with 50 mg of hydrocortisone every 6 hours for a period of up to 7 days.

SURGICAL THERAPY

Source control is the guiding philosophy behind surgical therapies in sepsis. The goal is to completely remove any infectious material. Damage control surgery may be necessary in some critically ill septic patients. Damage control implies a rapid correction of life-threatening processes such as bleeding or severe contamination. Often these patients are temporarily closed, with a planned return to the operating room for thorough exploration after resuscitation in the ICU. Care must also be taken to medically optimize these patients before operation and ensure adequate hemodynamic monitoring intraoperatively.

SUPPORT

Pulmonary Artery Catheter

Although there is controversy over the efficacy of the pulmonary artery catheter, when properly interpreted the data may be clinically helpful. This balloon-tipped catheter provides several critical pieces of information, including the pulmonary artery occlusion pressure (PAOP), which estimates intravascular volume status, and cardiac output. This information is extremely important because it guides therapy. For example, a tachycardic, hypotensive patient who has a low PAOP requires fluid rather than vasopressors. A patient who is tachycardic, hypotensive with a high PAOP, and has adequate cardiac output may suffer pulmonary edema and cardiac dysfunction from additional fluid and may instead benefit from vasopressors. Also, a patient with a low cardiac output and high PAOP may require inotropes to combat systemic hypoperfusion. Thus pulmonary artery catheters may have value in managing the hypotensive septic patient.

Resuscitation

Studies have shown a mortality benefit in septic patients with expedient (within 6 hours), goal-directed fluid resuscitation. This initial resuscitation may require a combination of treatments including

Table 3: Endpoints of Initial Resuscitation

Central venous pressure	8–10
Urine output	≥0.5 ml/kg/hr
Heart rate	<100
Pulmonary artery occlusion pressure	15–20
Hemoglobin	>10 g/dL
Mean arterial pressure	65–70

intravenous (IV) fluids, packed red blood cells (PRBCs), vasopressors, and inotropes to achieve normal hemodynamic parameters and thus prevent systemic ischemia. The endpoints of resuscitation can be measured in several ways (Table 3). Either crystalloid or colloid solutions may be used, and current evidence suggests that these solutions provide equal clinical outcomes.

Vasopressors

Vasopressors are used to maintain perfusion in patients who are hypotensive or are in shock and have been adequately volume resuscitated. Also, vasopressors may be required during the initial phase of resuscitation, while IV fluid is being infused in a hypotensive patient. When initiating vasopressors, it is important to have an arterial catheter in place to determine blood pressure, as well to provide continuous data regarding the effects of therapy on blood pressure.

Because of the HPA axis dysfunction, there may also be an insufficient amount of vasopressin secretion. This relative deficiency may contribute to hypotension in septic patients; and, although not a first-line vasoactive agent, an IV vasopressin infusion at 0.01 to 0.04 units/minute may benefit some septic patients.

Inotropes

Although cardiac output is initially increased during sepsis, some patients may not respond to fluid resuscitation and cardiac output may decline to subphysiologic levels. In these cases, it is often necessary to start an inotrope to increase cardiac output and maintain perfusion. Great care must be exercised when using inotropes because they increase myocardial oxygen demand and consequently should be used to target normal hemodynamic parameters.

Blood Transfusion

Blood transfusion is recommended during initial resuscitation, acute hemorrhage, lactic acidosis, and coronary ischemia to achieve a hemoglobin (Hgb) of 10g/dL. Critically ill patients who do not meet these criteria can maintain adequate perfusion with an Hgb of 7 to 9 g/dL. Thus critically ill patients without signs of hypoperfusion or coronary ischemia should receive PRBC transfusion only when the Hgb is less than 7 g/dL because it remains to be determined whether septic patients achieve benefit with higher Hgb levels.

Ventilation

Ventilator support is often required in septic patients. Current evidence suggests a mortality benefit consequent to the use of low tidal volumes (6 ml/kg) and by maintenance of plateau pressures less than 30 cm H_2O. Using low tidal volumes, mild hypercapnia may be tolerated in order to minimize the mechanical stress on the lungs. Also, the lowest permissible level of positive end expiratory pressure should be used in septic patients to maintain adequate oxygenation and cardiac output.

Endotracheal intubation presents a constant and noxious stimulus to intubated patients. This often requires sedatives to improve compliance with mechanical ventilation and to reduce anxiety. Patients who are difficult to ventilate despite adequate sedation may require paralytic agents in order to optimize respiration. It is beneficial to use sedation and paralytic protocols, which include either intermittent dosing or daily lightening, to provide a clinical assessment and to adjust therapy. In particular, intermittent lightening of sedation has been shown to decrease the duration of mechanical ventilation.

Renal

Renal failure may present early during the septic response or may develop as part of the constellation with MSOF. Renal replacement therapy is required when kidney dysfunction has progressed to failure, as determined by clinical parameters such as anuria, uremia, and electrolyte imbalance. The two most common modalities of renal replacement therapy are continuous and intermittent hemodialysis. No clear benefit of one therapy over the other has been documented in hemodynamically stable patients. However, continuous hemodialysis results in less hemodynamic fluctuation and thus may be better tolerated in patients who are unstable or may require vasopressors for support.

Glucose Control

Attention to control of blood glucose levels has been shown to improve outcome including reduced risk of infection, as well as improved mortality in some critically ill patients. The goal of this therapy is to maintain a blood sugar between 80 and 110 mg/dL. At times, this may require a continuous insulin infusion and frequent blood sugar monitoring. However, the degree to which the benefits of tight glucose control influences outcome in patients with established sepsis remains to be determined.

Nutrition

The basal metabolic rate for a healthy person is estimated at 20 to 22 kcal/kg/day. This may increase to 30 to 35 kcal/kg/day during sepsis, and endogenous stores of glycogen can be quickly dissipated in a hypermetabolic state. Consequently, efforts to provide adequate levels of readily available substitutes are warranted at an early stage. Nutritional supplementation in septic patients is critical to prevent starvation and resulting organ and immune dysfunction.

There are two modes of nutritional supplementation, enteral and parenteral. When feasible, the enteral route is usually preferred, and recent data suggest that enteral feeding may exert some anti-inflammatory effects. Parenteral nutrition is acceptable when gastrointestinal (GI) access is unavailable, such as during prolonged ileus. The clinician must judge the relative risks and benefits of nutritional support route in patients who may remain critically ill for extended periods of time. It remains to be determined whether parenteral supplementation is beneficial in cases where only partial nutritional support can be provided enterally.

Prophylaxis

Venous thromboembolism, or deep venous thrombosis (DVT), is a significant cause of morbidity in septic patients, and therapy to reduce the risk of this complication is prudent. Mechanical compression devices and low-dose unfractionated heparin or low-molecular-weight heparin should be used in septic patients. Heparin therapy should be used cautiously in patients with a high risk

of bleeding. Thus inferior vena cava filters may be required in patients who cannot receive heparin, and although this may not prevent a DVT, it can reduce the risk of its potentially lethal complication, which is pulmonary embolism.

Critically ill patients have a significantly greater risk of developing ulceration in the upper GI tract and should thus receive either H2 (histamine) blockers or proton pump inhibitors to decrease the likelihood of complications such as ulcer bleeding and perforation.

One major risk to mechanical ventilation is ventilator-associated pneumonia. This can be reduced by maintaining the patient in a half-sitting position with 45-degree head elevation.

CONCLUSION

The treatment of septic patients is a challenging task, and a standardized, evidence-based approach to sepsis has played a role in decreasing the mortality rate of this process. These guidelines should be supplemented with attention to clinical detail and vigilance to the myriad complications that may accompany this condition (Fig. 1). There are many ongoing research activities in the field of sepsis, and practitioners should stay current with developing innovations in this dynamic field.

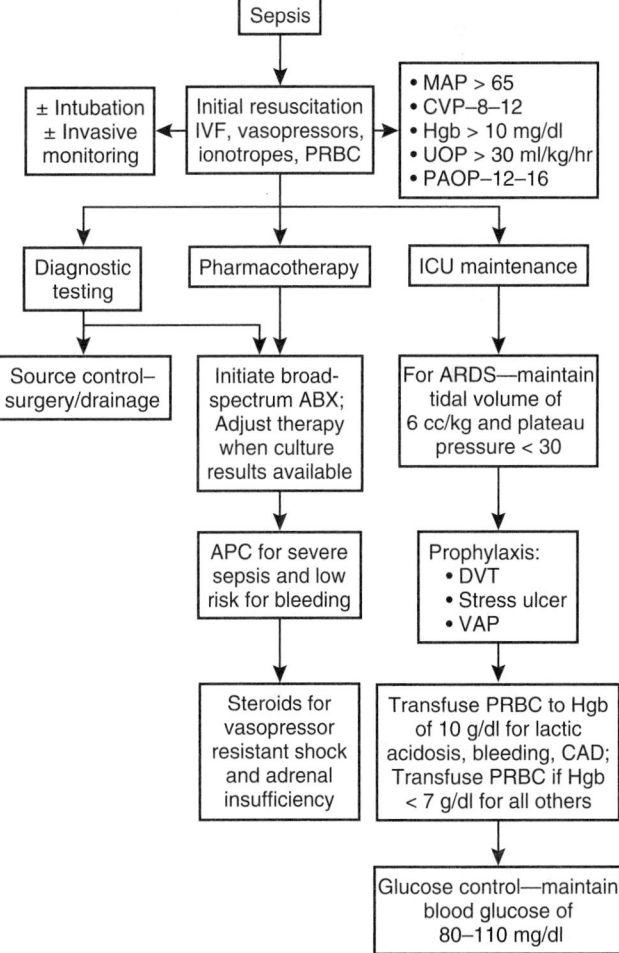

Figure 1 Algorithm for the treatment of sepsis. *ABX*, Antibiotics; *APC*, activated protein C; *ARDS*, acute respiratory syndrome; *CAD*, coronary artery disease; *CVP*, central venous pressure; *DVT*, deep venous thrombosis; *Hgb*, hemoglobin; *ICU*, intensive care unit; *IVF*, intravenous fluids; *MAP*, mean arterial pressure; *PRBC*, packed red blood cells; *UOP*, urine output; *VAP*, ventilator-associated pneumonia.

SUGGESTED READINGS

Cooper SM, Stewart PM: Corticosteroid insufficiency in acutely ill patients, *N Engl J Med* 348:727, 2003.

Dellinger RP, Carlet JM, Masur H, and others: Surviving Sepsis Campaign guidelines for management of severe sepsis and septic shock, *Crit Care Med* 32:858, 2004.

Rivers E, Nguen B, Havstad S, and others: Early goal-directed therapy in the treatment of severe sepsis and septic shock, *N Engl J Med* 345:1368, 2001.

ANTIBIOTICS FOR CRITICALLY ILL PATIENTS

John M.A. Bohnen, MD

GENERAL PRINCIPLES

Patients with critical conditions, mainly those in intensive care units (ICUs), harbor infections acquired either before hospitalization or, more often, in hospital ("nosocomial") under pressures of antibiotics, invasive procedures, and suppression of host defenses. Antibiotic use, patient density, and patient-provider contact promote rapid transmission of antimicrobial resistance. The prevalence and outbreaks of resistant pathogens demand infection control and rational antibiotic use and challenge effective treatment of individual patients, which may include agents that predispose to antibiotic resistance. The inexorable increase in drug resistance leads to obsolescence of recent knowledge, expansion of pharmacopoeias, and difficulty remembering new therapies.

To satisfy these competing needs, the provider should treat infection rather than mere colonization, limit the use of agents that promote bacterial resistance (e.g., piperacillin alone, ceftazidime), and use the narrowest possible antimicrobial spectrum, in adequate dosages, for the shortest duration possible, often only until the patient recovers clinically. Exceptions include bacteremias with *Staphylococcus aureus* and *Enterococcus* spp., which require generally 2 weeks of therapy to prevent endocarditis and metastatic infections, and deep *S. aureus* and serious fungal infections, which require at least 4 weeks. My recommendations for specific pathogens apply generally, but local sensitivity patterns, which vary widely among ICUs, should be heeded.

Clinicians use antibiotics prophylactically or, more commonly in ICUs, therapeutically. Therapy in ICU is most commonly given empirically while awaiting culture and sensitivity tests, which may lead to changes in treatment that had been initiated. This chapter provides recommendations for empiric and subsequent therapy of nine important conditions, eight listed by anatomic region, followed by a section on fungal infections.

Please consult a pharmacopoeia for dosages. Critically ill patients often have expanded extracellular fluid volumes and require high doses for drug benefit and to diminish antibiotic resistance. Generally, intravenous (IV) therapy is used. Suggested readings at the end of the chapter will help the reader to stay current on rapid changes in antibiotic activity spectra, new agents, dosing (e.g., use in renal or hepatic failure), and how patient factors such as age and concurrent illnesses influence therapeutic decisions.

IMPORTANT PATHOGENS AND THE ANTIBIOTICS THAT COVER THEM

A complete list of microbial pathogens in ICU patients is beyond the scope of this chapter. Any community-acquired microbe, such as *Streptococcus pyogenes*, sensitive to penicillin, can bring a patient to the ICU.

For brevity, drug class names (e.g., "carbapenems") are used, and examples (e.g., "imipenem") are sometimes added as reminders. "Carbapenems" refers to imipenem, meropenem, and ertapenem; "antistaphylococcal penicillins" refers to methicillin (laboratory use only), cloxacillin, oxacillin, and nafcillin. Cefazolin is a first-generation cephalosporin, cefuroxime is second generation, and the numerous third- and fourth-generation cephalosporins include ceftazidime, cefepime, ceftriaxone, and cefotaxime. Fluoroquinolones, or "quinolones" include several drugs that end in "floxacin," such as ciprofloxacin. "Beta-lactam/beta-lactamase" refers to piperacillin/tazobactam, ampicillin/sulbactam, and ticarcillin/clavulanic acid. "Aminoglycoside" refers to gentamicin, tobramycin, netilmicin, and amikacin. Trimethoprim/sulfamethoxazole is written "TMP/SMZ." The following sections discuss the important microbial offenders that plague ICU patients, in particular, and the antibiotics that cover them.

Gram-Positive Cocci

The *Staphylococci S. aureus* and *S. epidermidis* are most important. *S. aureus* causes infections at any anatomic site and foreign bodies; bacteremia is dangerous. *S. epidermidis* causes foreign-body infections, especially vascular catheters; bacteremia is less dangerous. *S. epidermidis* infections often respond to foreign-body removal without antibiotics. Treat methicillin-sensitive *Staphylococci,* predominantly *S. aureus*, with an antistaphylococcal penicillin, cefazolin, or cefuroxime; treat methicillin-resistant staphylococci (MRSA and MRSE) generally with vancomycin or a new agent: linezolid, quinupristin/dalfopristin, tigecycline, or daptomycin. Failure of vancomycin treatment of MRSA infections is a growing problem; high vancomycin serum levels are necessary (trough >10 and peak >25 µg/ml). Linezolid may be superior to vancomycin for MRSA bacteremia and pneumonia. Carbapenems, beta-lactam/beta-lactamases, TMP/SMZ, and clindamycin cover MRSA and MRSE unevenly. Aminoglycosides add synergistic therapy for methicillin-sensitive *Staphylococci*.

Enterococcus spp. are usually copathogens in abdominal and biliary infections and cause urinary infections and endocarditis. Enterococcal bacteremia may signify endocarditis (rule out with echocardiogram) and requires at least 2 weeks of antibiotic therapy. Controversy surrounds the necessity of treating *Enterococcus* spp. when it is a copathogen. For unimicrobial enterococcal infections, penicillin, ampicillin, or vancomycin plus an aminoglycoside is first-line therapy, but resistant strains (VRE) call for one of several regimens, such as linezolid, quinupristin/dalfopristin, tigecycline, or daptomycin. The foregoing simplifies a complex problem for which local sensitivity patterns and experts should be consulted.

Streptococcus pyogenes causes soft-tissue infections and sometimes streptococcal toxic shock; penicillin, antistaphylococcal penicillins, cefazolin, carbapenems, and clindamycin provide coverage; for toxic shock, the addition of clindamycin to penicillin adds synergy and toxin neutralization.

Gram-Negative Rods

Facultative and aerobic gram-negative rods, such as *Escherichia coli*, *Klebsiella* spp., *Pseudomonas* spp., and *Enterobacter* spp., act as copathogens in abdominal infections, pneumonia, and incisional infections and as sole pathogens in urinary and other anatomic sites, including cannulas and implants. They acquire resistance to multiple antibiotics. A continuum of antibiotics runs from generally older agents that have lost some activity to newer, expensive agents that cover broader spectra of resistant pathogens. Older agents include aminoglycosides, first- and second-generation cephalosporins, aztreonam, TMP/SMZ, and ampicillin. Generally these agents are not often used in ICUs because of toxicity (aminoglycosides) and resistance. Their use has been superseded by beta-lactam/beta-lactamase combinations, third- and fourth-generation cephalosporins, new tetracyclines (i.e., tigecycline), and carbapenems (except for ertapenem, with its narrower antibacterial spectrum).

Gram-Negative Anaerobic Rods

Bacteroides spp. and others act as copathogens in abdominal and incisional infections, and pneumonia in particular if secondary to aspiration. Inadequately treated anaerobic bacteremia is associated with increased mortality rates. Metronidazole is the most popular agent. Second-generation cephalosporins (e.g., cefoxitin) are increasingly subject to resistance and no longer recommended. Carbapenems, beta-lactam/beta-lactamases and clindamycin are alternatives.

Gram-Positive Rods

Clostridia spp., the most important gram-positive rods, emit toxins. *C. difficile* toxin causes antibiotic-associated colitis; the pathogen is sensitive to metronidazole and vancomycin. Other community-acquired *Clostridia*, such as *C. perfringens*, cause soft-tissue infections, treated by penicillin, metronidazole, clindamycin, or a carbapenem.

Fungi

Although *Candida* spp., especially *C. albicans*, remain the most common pathogens in critical care, *Aspergillus* spp. have achieved prominence for patients with transplants and hematologic cancers. *C. albicans* accounts for approximately half of *Candida* infections, with the other half composed of non-*Albicans* species, especially *C. glabrata*, *C. parapsilosis*, and *C. tropicalis*.

Amphotericin B targets the key fungal pathogens but is toxic; the toxicity is attenuated in expensive amphotericin-lipid formulations. Fluconazole, a safe alternative, works well against *C. albicans* but not some non-*Albicans Candida* (mainly *C. krusei* and *C. glabrata*) or *Aspergillus* spp. Pathogens resistant to fluconazole require more toxic (amphotericin) or expensive (amphotericin/lipid, voriconazole, caspofungin) agents.

ADVERSE EFFECTS OF ANTIBIOTICS

Patients in ICU suffer numerous effects of medical conditions and therapies. Antibiotics cause adverse effects frequently—consider

Table 1: Adverse Effects of Important Agents in Critical Care Surgery

Adverse Effects	Antimicrobial Agent
Nephrotoxicity	Aminoglycosides, amphotericin, vancomycin
Rigors, dysrhythmias	Amphotericin
Red person syndrome	Vancomycin
Biliary sludge/gallstones	Ceftriaxone
Seizure	Imipenem, especially high-dose, renal insufficiency
Coombs positive anemia	Cefepime
Prolonged QT interval	Quinolones

them when explaining clinical findings and minimize them with avoidance and cessation of therapy, when possible. Most antibiotics can cause fever, hypersensitivity reactions including anaphylaxis, antibiotic-associated colitis, coagulopathy, anemia, and other superinfections, and a variety of lab test (e.g., liver) abnormalities. Table 1 lists some important side effects associated with particular agents. Antibiotics interact commonly with other drugs. Check the pharmacopoeia when adding or changing agents.

ANTIBIOTICS FOR SPECIFIC CONDITIONS

Pneumonia

Background

The indication and selection of antibiotics for critically ill patients with pneumonia, especially those on ventilators, continue to evolve. Decades ago, clinicians treated on the basis of the same signs as community-acquired pneumonia: fever, leukocytosis, cough, lung infiltrate, and respiratory deterioration. This approach was unreliable because ventilated patients with pneumonia may not have sputum, and other conditions, such as acute respiratory distress syndrome, pulmonary embolus, and heart failure, cause lung infiltrates. To avoid antibiotic overtreatment of lung infiltrates, studies in the 1980s and 1990s established more specific criteria for treatment, such as quantitative cultures of protected brush specimens taken at bronchoscopy. This narrowing of the indication to treat with antibiotics suffered sampling error, the need for invasive procedures, and findings that delayed or inappropriate treatment of pathogens was associated with worse outcomes. More recently, the emphasis has shifted back to early (as possible) empiric treatment with short courses (3–7 days) of therapy with broad-spectrum agents. This approach may lead to "unnecessary" treatment of some patients but has the advantage of early cessation of unneeded antibiotics, early targeting of pathogens, and minimization of antibiotic resistance.

Aminoglycosides are controversial because of poor bronchial fluid penetration (which mandates pairing with another agent) and toxicity, but they provide good coverage, are less prone to resistance in many centers, and are inexpensive.

Key Pathogens

Key pathogens are often multiresistant. Gram-negative rods include *P. aeruginosa* and enteric bacteria (e.g., *E. coli*); gram-positive cocci include *S. pneumoniae* and *S. aureus*. Anaerobes include anaerobic streptococci and *Bacteroides* spp.

Antimicrobial Therapy

Start empiric therapy with imipenem or meropenem, beta-lactam/beta-lactamase, a quinolone, or a third- or fourth-generation cephalosporin. Use narrow coverage if possible according to culture results, especially for unimicrobial infection (e.g., *S. aureus*). Discontinue treatment after the patient has recovered clinically except for 1-month treatment of *S. aureus* pneumonia.

Vascular Catheter–Related Infections

Background

Vascular catheter-associated infections occur at the catheter or in the bloodstream. If the catheter can be removed, antibiotics may not be necessary. Treat with antibiotics for the following conditions: unstable patient; cellulitis; suppurative thrombophlebitis; metastatic infection such as cerebral or renal abscess; immunosuppression; remote endovascular prosthesis; recent foreign-body implant; and bacteremia with *S. aureus*, *Enterococcus* spp., or *S. pyogenes* (also search for endocarditis). Except for fungal infections, the catheter can often be preserved in situ with antibiotic therapy that covers cultured microorganisms.

Key Pathogens

The key pathogens are *S. epidermidis*, *S. aureus*, *Enterococcus* spp., and gram-negative rods. Fungal infection is increasing in frequency.

Antimicrobial Therapy

If indicated, start empiric therapy with vancomycin because most offending pathogens are gram positive and methicillin resistant. Discontinue treatment after the patient has recovered clinically. Treat fungemia attributed to a vascular catheter with 2 weeks of fluconazole for *C. albicans*. For non-*Albicans* species, therapy is controversial; caspofungin is surpassing amphotericin as first-line therapy.

Abdominal Infections: Peritonitis and Abscess

Background

Peritonitis and abdominal abscess secondary to gastrointestinal inflammation, perforation, or ischemia commonly bring patients to ICUs and may complicate the condition of a patient who is already there. Treat for no more than 5 to 7 days for generalized peritonitis and 1 to 2 days to support local abscess drainage or for peritonitis with minimal contamination (e.g., colonoscopic perforation, nonoperative treatment of perforated ulcer). For persistent or recurrent signs of infection 5 days after a first procedure for abdominal infection, rule out a drainable abdominal collection or extra-abdominal infection (e.g., vascular catheter infection) before simply changing or prolonging antibiotics.

Multiply recurrent abdominal infections, termed "tertiary peritonitis," may not have discrete, drainable abdominal collections. Infected tissue or fluid usually carries multiply resistant bacteria and fungi. Therapy is controversial because broader-spectrum agents may promote more resistance, yet failure to target the pathogens is associated with treatment failure.

Key Pathogens

Peritonitis from a gastrointestinal source is polymicrobial. Gram-negative facultative/aerobic rods (e.g., *E. coli*), gram-negative anaerobes (e.g., *Bacteroides* spp.), *Enterococci*, and numerous others species are present. Treatment must cover *E. coli* and *Bacteroides*

spp. The need for broader coverage than that is unproved but generally accepted.

Antimicrobial Therapy

Treat empirically with imipenem or meropenem, beta-lactam/beta-lactamase, quinolone, or third- or fourth-generation cephalosporin plus metronidazole.

Surgical Site Infections

Background

Patients in intensive care may require antibiotics for surgical site infection prophylaxis or therapy. Prophylactic antibiotics should be given within 60 minutes before the incision as a single dose to be repeated intraoperatively for long cases (2.5 hours or more).

Key Pathogens

Infections may be unimicrobial or polymicrobial. Clean operations such as cardiovascular and orthopedic implants, craniotomy, cerebrospinal fluid shunt insertion, vascular groin incisions, open heart operations, internal fracture fixation, and lower limb amputations are vulnerable to gram-positive skin organisms such as *S. aureus* and *S. epidermidis*. Gastrointestinal operations risk infection with intestinal organisms including *E. coli*, *Bacteroides* spp., and hospital-acquired, multiresistant gram-negative rods.

Antimicrobial Prophylaxis

For the clean operations just listed, use an antistaphylococcal penicillin or vancomycin (if MRSA is endemic). Patients undergoing gastrointestinal procedures should receive a quinolone or third- or fourth-generation cephalosporin (agents not used in a non-ICU setting) plus metronidazole or clindamycin; a carbapenem; or a beta-lactam/beta-lactamase. Other agents might be appropriate, depending on local flora and resistance patterns.

Antimicrobial Therapy

Incision and drainage without antibiotic treatment may suffice. Antibiotics should be given if there is regional spread, such as cellulitis; an endovascular prosthesis or recent prosthetic implant; immunosuppression; or *S. aureus* infection, which can cause bacteremia. The empiric choice of drug depends on whether the operation was clean or enteric as for prophylaxis. Modify according to culture and sensitivity. Discontinue treatment after the patient has recovered clinically.

Antibiotic-Associated Colitis

Background and Pathogen

Virulent, toxin-producing strains of *C. difficile* have turned antibiotic-associated colitis into a killer complication of antibiotics, especially clindamycin, cephalosporins, and, recently, quinolones.

Antimicrobial Therapy

Although metronidazole is inexpensive and usually curative, relapses are common (≈30%). Vancomycin has similar success and relapse rates; although it is more expensive and risks vancomycin-resistant enterococcus, some experts believe it is more effective than metronidazole and should be used from the start in serious cases. Treat orally, but if a patient has paralytic ileus, use IV metronidazole, which is secreted into the colon lumen. New agents are being studied, including antibiotics, nonantibiotic polymers, and probiotics.

Urinary Tract Infections

Background

Urinary infections arise from a combination of catheterization and urinary bacterial or fungal colonization. Antimicrobial prophylaxis at catheterization is not effective, and attempts to "sterilize" catheterized urine with antibiotics will fail. Therefore accept colonization without infection in a critically ill, catheterized patient, and remove the catheter at the earliest opportunity. Treat with antibiotics for systemic signs, such as fever, chills, flank pain, and tenderness; remote endoprosthesis; or infected or colonized obstructed urinary tract. Obstruction with infection is a surgical emergency; septic shock is common, and antibiotics will fail without relief of the obstruction (get imaging and consult with urology specialist).

S. aureus in the urine may be associated with preexisting and subsequent *S. aureus* bacteremia, which in turn mandates a search for a source, such as a vascular catheter, and diagnostic imaging to rule out endocarditis.

Key Pathogens

Urinary infections are unimicrobial. Multiple organisms indicate specimen contamination or intestinal-urinary fistula. Gram-negative aerobic and facultative rods such as *P. aeruginosa* and *E. coli*, enterococcal spp., and coagulase negative (i.e., non–*S. aureus*) *Staphylococci* predominate among bacteria. Fungi such as *C. albicans* can colonize or infect the urinary system and, at worst, can cause a fungus ball that may require drainage or excision.

Antimicrobial Therapy

For empiric therapy of community-acquired pathogens, TMP/SMZ will generally work, but for hospital-acquired infections, which comprise the majority, start treatment with broad-spectrum gram-negative coverage. This includes imipenem or meropenem; beta-lactam/beta-lactamase; quinolone (except moxifloxacin or gemifloxacin, which do not enter urine well); third- or fourth-generation cephalosporin; or ampicillin plus an aminoglycoside. Switch agents if indicated from the culture and sensitivity result and treat for 2 to 3 weeks if the catheter must stay in.

Spreading Soft-Tissue Infections

Background

Cellulitis and more serious spreading soft-tissue infections such as fasciitis and myositis/myonecrosis generally start outside the hospital, sometimes causing such physiologic mayhem that they bring patients to ICU, usually following surgical excision and debridement. For simple cellulitis, antibiotic therapy suffices; for necrotizing cellulitis and deeper infections, antibiotics support surgical debridement.

Key Pathogens

Community-acquired infections can be unimicrobial, commonly caused by *S. pyogenes*, *S. aureus*, *Clostridia*, or, less commonly, gram-negative aerobic pathogens, or they may be polymicrobial from any combination but usually from enteric pathogens. Patients who acquire these infections in the hospital, after therapeutic immunosuppression, or following traumatic encounters with environments harboring unusual bacterial flora, such as earthquakes, mudslides, animal bites, or marine exposure, may harbor exotic pathogens not usually seen in critical care settings. Providers should acquire cultures of infected tissue before starting antibiotic therapy.

Antimicrobial Therapy

Treat generally until clinical resolution (exception for cases of actinomycosis, which requires 6 months of therapy). Antibiotic failure may indicate failure to target the offending organism; inadequate duration; poor circulation (may require revascularization); or, most commonly, devitalized tissue that requires drainage.

Biliary Infections and Acalculous Cholecystitis

Background

Biliary tract infections arise from combinations of bactibilia (common by age 60), gallstones, parasites, neoplasm, obstruction, and biliary procedures. Cholecystitis, whether calculous or acalculous, is treated by gallbladder excision or drainage. Antibiotics diminish surgical site infections at cholecystectomy and therapeutically treat peritoneal infection following gallbladder perforation. Diabetes predisposes to rapidly lethal emphysematous cholecystitis with *Clostridia*; urgent cholecystectomy and penicillin are necessary.

Common bile duct obstruction with infection (cholangitis) may cause septic shock and requires urgent antimicrobial therapy. With the possible exception of quinolones, antibiotics do not penetrate an obstructed biliary tract and will fail without biliary drainage.

Liver abscesses may complicate biliary infections, arise through portal bacteremia from other enterogenic abdominal sources, or from systemic hematogenous spread.

Key Pathogens

Biliary tract and liver infections are commonly polymicrobial. Cholecystitis and cholangitis are caused by gram-negative enteric bacteria such as *E. coli* and *Klebsiella* spp., *Enterococci* spp., and *Clostridia*. Anaerobes are not common except in elderly and individuals with vascular pathology. Biligenic liver abscesses harbor similar pathogens; enterogenic liver abscesses harbor the same pathogens as abdominal infections; liver abscesses from systemic bacteremia are more commonly gram positive (e.g., *Streptococci*) but can involve any bacteremic pathogen. Fungal liver abscess occurs generally in the setting of fungemia, as well as multisite colonization and infection. Diagnosis of amebic abscess requires serology.

Antimicrobial Therapy

For empiric therapy of infections originating in the biliary tree, use a quinolone such as ciprofloxacin, beta-lactam/beta-lactamase, carbapenem, or ampicillin plus an aminoglycoside. Similar regimens apply to biligenic or enterogenic liver abscess; if bacteremic origin is suspected, therapy should target any pathogen detected in the bloodstream. Although advanced-generation cephalosporins are commonly used, they do not cover *Enterococci* spp. Amebic liver abscess responds to metronidazole without drainage.

Fungal Infections

The diagnosis and indications for treatment of fungal infections challenge clinicians because of the blurred continuum among colonization, foreign–body-related infection (usually in vascular catheters), and deep site infections, which generally require, respectively, no therapy, short-course therapy, and more protracted treatment (e.g., 1 month or more).

Growth in culture and histologic findings of tissue invasion establish fungal infection that requires therapy, but these may be hard to obtain. Always treat fungemia, and remove a vascular catheter source, if possible. Antifungal susceptibility tests are controversial: they are generally not necessary for amphotericin B; are helpful for fluconazole, which does not cover all *Candida* spp.; and are still being determined for the echinocandins (e.g., caspofungin).

For *Candida* infections, fluconazole is generally the first-line agent unless resistant (assume for *C. krusei* and, commonly, for *C. glabrata*) or for empiric treatment of immediately life-threatening infections in which amphotericin B, caspofungin, or voriconazole are used. The patient's clinical course and culture results determine whether therapy should be changed. Voriconazole is the agent of choice for *Aspergillus* infections.

SUGGESTED READINGS

Gilbert DN, Moellering RC, Eliopoulos GM, and others: *The Sanford guide to antimicrobial therapy 2006*, ed 36, Sperryville, VA, 2006, Antimicrobial Therapy.

Kollef MH: The intensive care unit as a research laboratory: developing strategies to prevent antimicrobial resistance, *Surg Infect* 7:85, 2006.

Muder RR, Brennen C, Rihs JD, and others: Isolation of *Staphylococcus aureus* from the urinary tract: association of isolation with symptomatic urinary tract infection and subsequent staphylococcal bacteremia, *Clin Infect Dis* 42:46, 2006.

Singh N, Rogers P, Atwood CW, and others: Short-course empiric antibiotic therapy for patients with pulmonary infiltrates in the intensive care unit. A proposed solution for indiscriminate antibiotic prescription, *Am J Respir Crit Care Med* 162:505, 2000.

Spellberg BJ, Filler SG, Edwards JE Jr: Current treatment strategies for disseminated candidiasis, *Clin Infect Dis* 42:244, 2006.

Stevens DL: The role of vancomycin in the treatment paradigm, *Clin Infect Dis* 42:S51, 2006.

ENDOCRINE CHANGES WITH CRITICAL ILLNESS

Frank Rosemeier, MD, MRCP, and Sean Berenholtz, MD, MHS

INTRODUCTION

Critical illness attributable to any cause, including surgery, sepsis, trauma, or burns, can result in profound and interlinked alterations of the endocrine system. The endocrine system response may be largely adaptive in the early stages of critical illness. Sustained hormonal and metabolic changes with prolonged or severe critical illness, however, can be maladaptive and contribute to multisystem organ dysfunction and death. This chapter first describes the impact of critical illness on the endocrine system response along each of the main axes and then reviews several evidence-based therapies that attempt to modify the endocrine system response to critical illness.

RESPONSE TO CRITICAL ILLNESS

The endocrine system response to critical illness is commonly divided into two phases, an early acute phase and a prolonged phase (Table 1). The acute phase is largely an adaptive response to critical illness, with an overall goal to improve survival, characterized by a release of hormones to sustain substrate and oxygen delivery to vital tissue, delay of unwanted anabolism, and modulation of the immune response. The prolonged or chronic phase response to critical illness is characterized by persistent hypercatabolism; a loss of lean body mass; and, often, concomitant fatty infiltration of vital organs. The prolonged and maladaptive response of the endocrine system to critical illness may contribute to further organ dysfunction and the development of polymyoneuropathy of critical illness and can substantially delay or impede organ recovery.

Sympathomimetic System

Critical illness activates the sympathetic nervous system with secretion of catecholamines from the adrenal medulla as part of the "fight or flight" response. Increased norepinephrine, epinephrine, and dopamine secretion lead to complex changes in the cardiovascular, metabolic, immunologic, and endocrine systems. Most plasma norepinephrine is derived from synaptic nerve clefts and functions as a neurotransmitter, whereas circulating epinephrine is produced largely in the adrenal gland and secreted as a circulating hormone. The enteric nervous system is also capable of contributing a previously unrecognized proportion of total sympathetic

Table 1: Overview of the Endocrine System Response to Acute and Prolonged Phase of Critical Illness and Potential Interventions

Hormone	Acute Phase	Prolonged Phase	Potential Intervention
Sympathomimetic System			
Norepinephrine	++	+/=	May need vasopressor therapy if endogenous stores inadequate
Epinephrine	++	+/=	
Somatotropic axis			
Pulsatile GH release	+	-	Exogenous GH administration associated with increased mortality
GHBP		+	
IGF-1	-	--	
ALS	-	--	
IGFBP-3	-	--	
Hypothalamic-Pituitary-Thyroid Axis			
Pulsatile TSH release	+/=	-	No benefit of replacement and may prolong recovery to euthyroid state.
T4	+/=	-	
T3	-	--	
rT3	+	+/=	
Hypothalamic-Pituitary-Gonadal and Lacto tropic Axis			
Pulsatile LH release	+/=	-	No benefit of replacement
Testosterone	-	--	
Dehydroepiandrosterone	--	--	
Pulsatile prolactin release	+	-	
Hypothalamic-Pituitary-Adrenal Axis			
ACTH	+	-	Replace if biochemical evidence of relative insufficiency in septic shock
Cortisol	++	+/=	

Modified from Vanhorebeek I, Van den Berghe G: Crit Care Clin 22:1, 2006, Table 1.) "+" Increase from baseline; "-" decrease from baseline; "=" no change from baseline; *ACTH,* adrenocorticotropic hormone; *ALS,* acid-labile subunit; *GH,* growth hormone; *GHBP,* growth hormone binding protein; *IGF-1,* insulin like growth factor-1; *IGFBP-3,* insulin-like growth factor binding protein-3; *LH,* luteinizing hormone; *rT3,* reverse triiodothyronine; *T3,* triiodothyronine; *T4,* thyroxine; *TSH,* thyroid stimulating hormone.

outflow. Mesenteric organs, for example, have been shown to produce considerable amounts of norepinephrine and dopamine, which accounts for 37% and more than 50%, respectively, of the total amount of these catecholamines formed in the body.

Activation of the sympathetic nervous system and elevated catecholamines often manifest as vasoconstriction, tachycardia, and tachypnea. Usually, the elevated catecholamine levels are sufficient to maintain adequate end organ perfusion and typically decrease within 3 to 5 days. Systemic inflammatory response syndrome (SIRS) in the postoperative period, for example, is a common self-limited response to stress and critical illness. However, in severe stress, such as septic shock, the administration of exogenous vasoactive amines and inotropes may be necessary to meet requirements for oxygen and substrate delivery.

Hypothalamic-Pituitary-Adrenal Axis

Appropriate activation of the hypothalamic-pituitary-adrenal (HPA) axis and increased cortisol secretion in response to critical illness is essential for survival. Several mechanisms have been proposed to explain the etiology of increased cortisol level in critical illness. The net effect is a shift in hormone secretion, favoring glucocorticoid over mineralocorticoid production with up to a sixfold increase in free cortisol levels. The vast majority of circulating cortisol is subsequently bound by corticosteroid binding globulin (CBG), and only free, biologically active, circulating cortisol is available to bind to intracellular steroid receptors. Corticosteroids such as cortisol have complex effects on a variety of metabolic and inflammatory processes. Corticosteroid-induced catabolism of carbohydrate, fat, and protein provides energy acutely and protects against excessive inflammation by suppressing the inflammatory response. Hemodynamic stability is improved further by corticosteroid-induced increases in alpha-receptors and beta-receptors, reduces production of nitric oxide, causes fluid retention, and leads to sensitization of adrenergic receptors to catecholamines.

Cortisol levels increase transiently, proportional in magnitude and duration to the degree of stress and critical illness, and generally subside within 48 hours in the absence of ongoing stress. During prolonged periods of stress, however, a dissociation between high plasma cortisol and low adrenocorticotropic hormone (ACTH) levels is observed. Differentiation between normal adrenal responses to critical illness and adrenal insufficiency is further complicated by wide interindividual variation in cortisol response. We discuss the clinical diagnosis of adrenal insufficiency later.

Somatropic Axis

Physiologic secretion of growth hormone (GH) by the somatotrope cells in the anterior pituitary occurs in a pulsatile fashion. GH has direct lipolytic effects, whereas its anabolic effect is indirectly mediated by insulin-like growth factor-1 (IGF-1). IGF-1 combines with various IGF binding proteins (IGFBP), particularly the larger IGFBP-3, and its associated acid-labile subunit (ALS), which reduces the bioavailability of IGF-1 but prolongs its half-life in the circulation.

Critical illness is associated with complex alterations in the GH/IGF-1 axis. The pulsatile release of GH is attenuated, and basal GH levels are elevated, whereas levels of IGF-1 and IGFBP-3 are reduced. A state of peripheral GH resistance develops, in part triggered by cytokine release in response to stress and critical illness. The indirect anabolic action of GH is reduced, whereas the direct effects of raised basal GH concentrations promote lipolysis and insulin antagonism, thus providing metabolic energy at the expense of muscle protein loss. Clinically this protein-wasting syndrome may delay wound healing, attenuate immune function, and contribute to respiratory muscle dysfunction. In the chronic phase of

critical illness, GH resistance associated with acute illness is partially reversed, whereas the levels of IGF-1, IGFBP-3, and ALS are even lower in prolonged critically ill patients (see Table 1).

Insulin

Hyperglycemia is a common metabolic derangement in critical illness and not limited to patients with known diabetes mellitus. Typically blood glucose levels are maintained in a narrow range of 70 mg/dL to 110 mg/dL (3.9–6.1 μmol/L) with the exception of short and temporary postprandial surges. Glucose uptake and metabolism is tightly regulated by insulin, which binds to its cellular membrane receptor and activates several protein cascades, including translocation of Glut-4 transporter to the plasma membrane; influx of glucose; and increased glycogen, glycolysis, and fatty acid synthesis. Several mechanisms contribute to the metabolic syndrome of acute hyperglycemia in response to critical illness, such as norepinephrine-mediated inhibition of insulin release, increased synthesis of glucose-generating hormones such as glucocorticoids, proinflammatory cytokines, pancreatic beta-cell dysfunction, dysregulation of hepatic glucose production, and increased peripheral insulin-resistance. Hyperglycemia in turn results in escalated oxidative burden on cell membrane and intracellular processes and augments stress-signaling pathways. In addition, lack of muscular activity, use of dextrose solutions, and drugs may contribute to hyperglycemia.

Poorly controlled hyperglycemia during critical illness is associated with increased mortality in surgery, trauma, head injury, shock, and an increased risk for perioperative myocardial infarctions. Hyperglycemia may also lead to abnormal immune function, including neutrophil dysfunction, and is associated with increased wound infection rates.

Hypothalamic-Pituitary-Thyroid Axis

With the onset of critical illness, conversion of thyroxine (T4) to the bioactive thyroid hormone triiodothyronine (T3) is inhibited. As a result, total serum T3 levels are frequently decreased and inactive metabolite reverse T3 (rT3) serum levels are increased (Fig. 1) during critical illness.

This low T3 syndrome may be part of an adaptive process in an attempt to reduce energy expenditure and protein wasting during stress and critical illness. In severely ill patients, serum T4 levels decrease as well (low T4 syndrome). Although thyroid-stimulating hormone (TSH) levels may increase briefly with the onset of critical illness, serum TSH levels usually remain within the low-normal range, despite the decreased levels of total serum T3. The nocturnal surge of TSH that occurs in the normal physiologic state is absent in the acute phase of critical illness, and response to thyrotropin-releasing hormone from the hypothalamus is blunted. Administration of dopamine and steroids can also lead to decreased serum TSH levels. With prolonged critical illness, decreased serum TSH, total serum T3 and T4 levels, and absence of pulsatility have been associated with increasing mortality. Conversely, survival from critical illness is associated with increased serum TSH levels, which often precedes increases in total serum T3, T4 levels, and the T3/rT3 ratio.

Clinically, patients with decreased total serum T3 levels, increased serum rT3 levels, normal or decreased total serum T4 levels, and decreased TSH levels are diagnosed as having euthyroid sick syndrome. Patients with euthyroid sick syndrome behave neither overtly hypothyroid nor hyperthyroid. Patients with primary hypothyroidism typically have TSH levels greater than 10 mU/L, decreased T4 and, at an advanced stage, decreased T3 levels. Patients with primary hypothyroidism can present with hypothermia, bradycardia, hypotension, and respiratory failure. Although

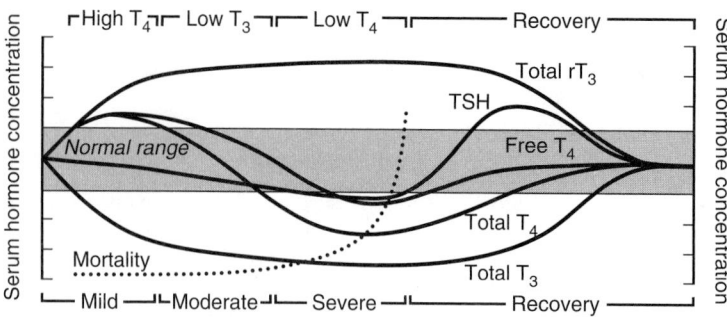

rT₃ = reverse triiodothyronine (3,3',5'–triiodothyronine); T₃ = triiodothyronine (3,5,3'–triiodothyronine); T4 = thyroxine; TSH = thyroid-stimulating hormone.

Figure 1 Alterations in thyroid hormone concentrations with critical illness. *rT3*, Reverse triiodothyronine (3,3',5'-triiodothyronine); *T3*, triiodothyronine (3,5,3'-triiodothyronine); *T4*, thyroxine; *TSH*, thyroid-stimulating hormone. *Adapted with permission from Farwell AF: Sick euthyroid syndrome in the intensive care unit. In Irwin RS, Rippe JM, editors:* Intensive care medicine, *ed 5, Philadelphia, 2003, Lippincott Williams & Wilkins.*

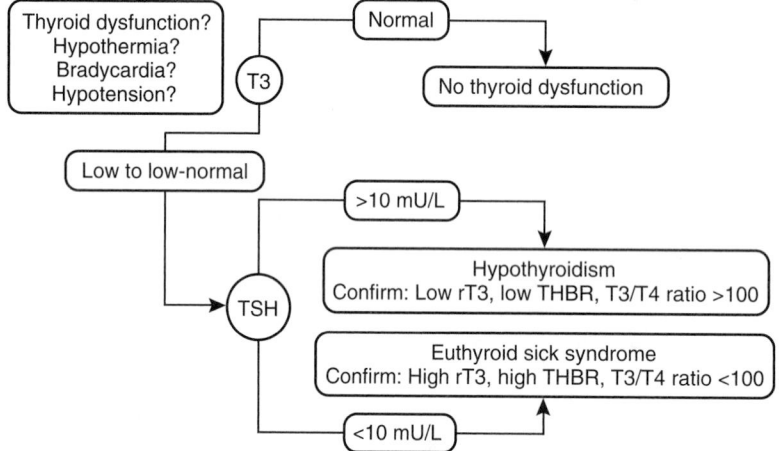

TSH = thyroid stimulating hormone; THBR = thyroid hormone binding ratio; rT₃ = reverse triiodothyronine (3,3',5'–triiodothyronine).

Figure 2 Flow chart for the identification of thyroid abnormalities in critical illness. TSH, *Thyroid stimulating hormone;* THBR, *thyroid hormone binding ratio;* rT3, *reverse triiodothyronine (3,3',5'-triiodothyronine)*

TSH elevation can also be seen in the recovery phase of critical illness, these values rarely exceed 10 mU/L. A flow chart for the identification of thyroid abnormalities in critical illness is provided in Figure 2.

Hypothalamic-Pituitary-Gonadal Axis

In males, critical illness is associated with a progressive fall of testosterone levels in the continuum of acute phase to prolonged phase of critical illness. The severity of hypotestosteronemia is directly correlated to mortality among critically ill men. Dehydroepiandrosterone levels correlate inversely with APACHE (Acute Physiology And Chronic Health Evaluation) score with low levels found in septic shock and nonsurvivors. Critically ill women demonstrate the "hypothalamic amenorrhea of stress," which results from complex immunoneural events between the HPA axis, corticotrophin-releasing hormone (CRH) in particular, and the hypothalamic-pituitary-gonadal (HPG) axis.

ENDOCRINE INTERVENTIONS IN CRITICAL ILLNESS

Several evidence-based therapies attempt to modify the endocrine system response to critical illness and have been shown to improve

outcomes among critically ill patients. Therapies that target the acute phase of hypercatabolism are unlikely to be of clinical benefit because the aim of the endocrine system response is to optimize the chance for survival. Pharmacologic modulation of the prolonged or maladaptive phase, on the other hand, may decrease the loss of lean body mass, decrease fatty infiltration of organ systems, and accelerate organ function recovery. Nevertheless, there is no obvious delineation between the acute and prolonged phases; rather, a continuum exists between the acute and chronic phase, with considerable interindividual divergence in terms of clinical, pathophysiologic, and hormonal response. This dilemma may be complicated further by preexisting endocrine abnormalities, which may be unmasked or exacerbated by critical illness. In this section, we review the current evidence to support therapies that attempt to modify the endocrine system response to critical illness. It is beyond the scope of this chapter to discuss management of common medical endocrine emergencies, including thyrotoxicosis, diabetic ketoacidosis, and hyperglycemic coma.

Exogenous Catecholamines in Circulatory Failure

Although sepsis and the systemic inflammatory response syndrome (SIRS) can cause circulatory failure in the surgical patient, the final common pathway of late-phase shock of any etiology is vasodilatory shock. Three major pathways appear to contribute to the development of vasodilatory shock: (1) overproduction of nitric oxide (NO) by inducible NO synthase (iNOS), (2) hyperpolarization of the vascular smooth muscle membrane potential through opening ATP-sensitive potassium channels (KATP channels), and (3) relative deficiency of vasopressin mediated through an inhibitory role of NO on vasopressin release during endotoxemia.

Surprisingly, there is little evidence to guide the optimal pharmacologic management of vasodilatory shock, and the exact blood pressure goal in these patients remains unclear. A meta-analysis by the Cochrane Database concluded that no firm proof exists that any one catecholamine is more effective or safer than any other in the treatment of circulatory failure. Comprehensive recommendations by the "Surviving Sepsis Campaign" and the recently revised practice parameters for hemodynamic support of patients with sepsis are largely based on nonrandomized, observational studies and expert opinion. As such, dopamine and the more potent vasoactive medication norepinephrine are both endorsed as first-choice agents when an appropriate fluid challenge fails to restore adequate blood pressure and organ perfusion in patients with vasodilatory shock. Use of epinephrine is recommended in patients who do not respond adequately to volume replacement and either dopamine or norepinephrine. Data on the microcirculatory effect of vasoactive medications in humans are sparse, likely reflecting the complexity and heterogeneity of interactions and pathophysiologic changes in vasodilatory shock.

Two multicenter trials comparing epinephrine with combined dobutamine and norepinephrine, and dopamine versus norepinephrine, are ongoing and may guide clinical practice in the future. In the meantime, the choice of vasoactive medications should be individualized on the basis of sound clinical principles with an appreciation of the underlying pathology and patient-specific characteristics, and providers should evaluate the response to empiric therapy.

Role of Vasopressin

Arginine vasopressin, an endogenous peptide hormone, generates its effect predominantly via vascular smooth muscle cell V1 and renal tubular V2 receptors through a G-protein receptor pathway. This results in antidiuresis, hemostasis, and arterial vasoconstriction. Vasopressin deficiency and down-regulation of V1 receptors mediated by proinflammatory cytokines may be responsible for the loss of vasomuscular tone in vasodilatory shock. As a result, endogenous and exogenous catecholamines may be ineffective in some forms of vasodilatory shock (sepsis, postcardiotomy).

In a number of small, randomized, controlled trials (RCTs), V1 agonist administration increased mean arterial pressure and reduced norepinephrine requirements with variable results on cardiac output and microcirculatory blood flow. Studies evaluating the hemodynamic effects of low-dose V1 agonist administration on splanchnic circulation in patients with vasodilatory shock, however, have produced conflicting results, highlighting the complexity and heterogeneity of the population group and their disease process.

Although evidence for the beneficial effect of low-dose V1 agonist administration on global hemodynamics is accumulating, V1 agonist administration is not presently recommended over norepinephrine or dopamine administration as a first-line agent in patients with vasodilatory shock. Major concerns exist related to the deleterious effects on platelet count and reductions in splanchnic perfusion and cardiac output associated with V1 agonist administration. As a result, V1 agonist administration should be reserved for critically ill patients with refractory vasodilatory states, ideally in the setting of clinical investigation protocols. The Surviving Sepsis Campaign guideline endorses the use of low-dose, or "physiologic" (0.01–0.04 U/min) dose continuous vasopressin infusions as an adjuvant in the treatment of vasodilatory shock refractory

to fluid replacement and high-dose conventional vasopressors until more data are available.

Steroids Replacement in Adrenal Insufficiency

The classic presentation of adrenal insufficiency (AI) includes abdominal pain, mental changes, gastrointestinal alterations, hypoglycemia, hyponatremia, hyperkalemia, neutropenia, eosinophilia, and fever. The clinical diagnosis of AI is often unreliable during critical illness and may be masked by the pathologic process underlying the critical illness, fluid resuscitation, diuretic administration, electrolyte repletion, intensive insulin therapy, and mixed forms of shock caused by hypovolemia and vasodilatation. Steroid replacement may be indicated, however, in the setting of hemodynamic instability and suspected AI.

ABSOLUTE ADRENAL INSUFFICIENCY

Causes of adrenal insufficiency are listed in Table 2, yet absolute adrenal insufficiency (AAI) is rare in critically ill patients with an incidence of up to 3%. Random cortisol levels ranging from less than 3.6 mcg/dL (100 nmol/L) to less than 34 mcg/dL (938 nmol/L) have been proposed to be an adequate response of the endocrine system during critical illness. Several studies suggest a cortisol threshold of less than 15 mcg/dL (414 nmol/L), a value that is widely quoted, to have reasonable specificity but poor sensitivity for the diagnosis of AAI during critical illness. Of note, patients with critical illness are often hypoproteinemic, with low levels of CBG and corresponding low total serum glucocorticoid concentrations, yet these patients may have normal levels of bioactive, free cortisol. In a recent study, for example, nearly 40% of critically ill patients had normal free cortisol levels despite a low total cortisol. Measurement of free cortisol levels, however, is not routinely available in clinical practice, and the interpretation of free cortisol levels in critically ill patients remains unclear. Thus steroid replacement is recommended in the setting of hypotension and random cortisol levels less than 15 mcg/dL (414 nmol/L).

RELATIVE ADRENAL INSUFFICIENCY

Relative adrenal insufficiency (RAI) has been proposed to describe critically ill patients with volume and catecholamine refractory vasodilatory shock but who improve hemodynamically with the coadministration of corticosteroids in the absence of other factors influencing the HPA axis. The prevalence of RAI among critically ill patients may be as high as 50% to 75%. In this patient population, a normal or even high total cortisol level may be inadequate for the degree of pathophysiological stress.

An ACTH (or corticotropin) stimulation test is often performed to evaluate patients with clinically suspected adrenal insufficiency. The test consists of measuring a total cortisol level before, 30 and 60 minutes after stimulation with a 250-mcg intravenous (IV) bolus of synthetic corticotropin. Interpretation of ACTH stimulation test results remains controversial in critically ill patients. Studies have evaluated random baseline cortisol values, incremental changes in cortisol values with ACTH stimulation, and absolute cortisol values after stimulation (Fig. 3). In a prospective, observational cohort study of patients with septic shock, mortality was lowest in patients with basal cortisol levels less than 34 mcg/dL (938 nmol/L) and a greater than 9 mcg/dL (>250 nmol/L) increase after cosyntropin stimulation. Conversely, patients with a highest basal cortisol level greater than 34 mcg/dL (938 nmol/L) and an incremental cortisol increase less than 9 mcg/dL (>250 nmol/L) were at the highest risk of death. The latter group likely represents patients under the most severe stress and patients who are unable to respond hormonally to an additional or protracted insult. In addition, an absolute incremental cortisol increase less than 9 mcg/dL (<250 nmol/L),

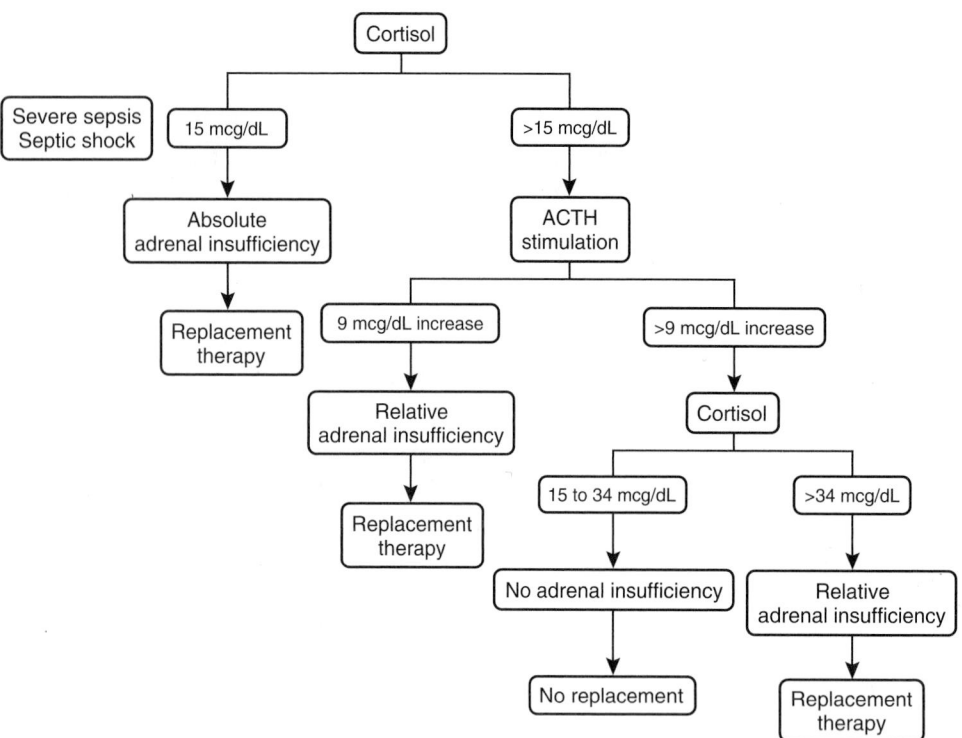

Figure 3 Flow chart for the identification of adrenal insufficiency in critical illness. *Adapted with permission from Gonzalez H, Nardi O, Annane D Crit Care Clin 22:105, 2006, Figure 2.*

independent of basal cortisol levels, was associated with increased mortality.

On the basis of these "best fit" prognostic cutoff values, a large, multicenter RCT involving 300 patients with severe volume and catecholamine refractory septic shock was conducted. Responders, defined as an incremental cortisol increase greater than 9 mcg/dL, and nonresponders, defined as an incremental cortisol increase less than 9 mcg/dL, were randomized to receive both 50 mg of hydrocortisone IV every 6 hours and 50 mcg fludrocortisone or placebo orally daily for 7 days. Nonresponders in the active treatment group had significantly higher 28-day all-cause mortality rates (63% vs. 53%, p = .02, risk ratio: 0.67; 95% confidence interval: 0.47–0.95). This RCT demonstrated for the first time that low doses of hydrocortisone reduced mortality in septic shock patients with RAI. These results are supported by a subgroup analysis of five trials with low-dose corticosteroids, which were included in a Cochrane meta-analysis of 15 RCT of low- and high-dose corticosteroids. This meta-analysis also identified systematic differences in study design and conduct, in terms of dose and duration of corticosteroids and time to corticosteroid administration, that help to explain why earlier trials found a detrimental effect of corticosteroid administration and more recent trials found a beneficial effect. Empiric treatment of patients with septic shock with hydrocortisone 50 mg IV every 6 hours for 7 days is also embraced by the Surviving Sepsis Campaign guidelines. Nevertheless, additional large randomized trials are currently under way and their results may influence these recommendations.

Importantly, clinicians should not wait for ACTH stimulation results to administer corticosteroids inpatients with septic shock. Dexamethasone can be administered until such time that an ACTH stimulation test can be performed because dexamethasone, unlike hydrocortisone and other steroids, does not interfere with the cortisol assay. Available data do not currently support empiric corticosteroid use in other nonseptic critically ill patients, including trauma and burn patients, especially in the absence of corticotropin stimulation testing. It remains unclear whether patients with recurrent episodes of septic shock benefit from repeated steroid administration, and the optimal duration of the steroid replacement remains controversial. It is also unknown whether tapering

Table 2: Etiology of Adrenal Insufficiency in Critical Illness

Adrenal Insufficiency	Etiology
Primary	Bilateral adrenal necrosis and hemorrhage caused by sepsis, hypotension, and hemorrhage Unmasking of chronic known or latent primary insufficiency Autoimmune adrenalitis in developed countries Tuberculous adrenalitis in developing countries Infectious diseases (fungal, viral, HIV)
Secondary	Irreversible anatomic damage to the hypothalamus or the pituitary gland Necrosis or hemorrhage in sepsis as a result of prolonged hypotension or coagulopathy Unmasking of chronic known or latent secondary AI caused by sepsis Hypothalamic or pituitary tumors Chronic inflammation Congenital adrenocorticotropic hormone deficiency Drug therapy Inhibition of early increase in adrenocorticotropic hormone caused by high-dose diazepam and fentanyl administration Previous treatments with glucocorticoids including topical administration Inhibition of steroid genesis with a single dose of etomidate Accelerated metabolism of cortisol by ketoconazole and cyclosporine, clarithromycin, rifampicin, and antiepileptic drugs, such as phenytoin and phenobarbital

AI, Adrenal insufficiency; *HIV,* human immunodeficiency virus.

corticosteroids is necessary after completing a 7-day course versus an abrupt termination. These controversies remain important because inappropriate use of potent corticosteroids may contribute to increased morbidity, including prolonged hospital length of stay, increased risk for wound infections, and hyperglycemia.

PERIOPERATIVE STEROID COVERAGE

Despite common practice, no practice advisory or professional guidelines exist with regard to the perioperative management of patients who use glucocorticoids. To date, no prospective RCT has demonstrated an advantage to treating patients on long-term steroid therapy with stress-dose steroids to prevent the development of AI during the perioperative period. In contrast, there is growing consensus that patients should be maintained on their preoperative steroid dose, or equivalent dose of intravenous steroids, during the perioperative period. This strategy effectively prevents hypotensive crisis and may avoid the potential complications associated with higher-dose steroids, such as protein catabolism, immunosuppression, and hyperglycemia.

A multidisciplinary group of authors recommends steroid supplementation, as outlined in Table 3, on the basis of the following assumptions: (1) steroid supplementation should reflect the amount of cortisol necessary to cover the physiologic response to surgery and (2) the risk of anesthesia and surgery in glucocorticoid-treated patients, who undergo surgery without coverage, is a function of the duration and severity of the surgical procedure. Despite supplementation, steroid-dependent patients should be carefully monitored in the perioperative period for development of AI.

Stress Hyperglycemia

Hyperglycemia is common during stress and critical illness. Hyperglycemia has long been associated with increased morbidity, including increased risk for surgical site infections and worse outcomes for patients with acute myocardial infarction and stroke. Several mechanisms for this association have been proposed (Table 4). Two recent RCTs have contributed substantially to this body of literature. The first RCT found that intensive insulin therapy (target glucose 80–110 mg/dL; 4.4–6.1 mmol/L) was associated with a significant reduction in 1-year mortality among mechanically ventilated patients in a predominantly cardiac surgical intensive care unit (ICU). The results were consistent for patients with and without a history of diabetes. The greatest reduction in mortality occurred in patients with sepsis-induced multiple-organ failure and ICU stay for 5 days or more. Intensive insulin therapy was also associated with significant reductions in morbidity, including reductions in nosocomial infections, new-onset renal failure requiring dialysis, critical illness polymyoneuropathy, and proportion of patients with prolonged mechanical ventilation and ICU length of stay.

Table 3: Recommended Perioperative Hydrocortisone Coverage for Patients Who Use Glucocorticoids

Degree of Surgical Stress	Hydrocortisone or Equivalent Dose	Duration
Minor (e.g., inguinal herniorrhaphy)	25 mg/day	1 day
Moderate (e.g., total knee replacement)	50–75 mg/day	1–2 days
Major (e.g., cardiopulmonary bypass)	100–150 mg/day	2–3 days

Table 4: Effects of Blood Glucose Control with Intensive Insulin Therapy

Biological Marker or Process	Metabolic or Nonmetabolic Effect
Lipid profile	Reversal of hypertriglyceridemia Elevation of high-density and low-density lipoproteins Decrease free fatty acids
Nutritional status	Prevention of weight loss in prolonged critical illness Increased total protein content in skeletal muscle
Inflammatory process	Decreased C-reactive protein Increased phagocytosis Reduction if proinflammatory cytokines and proteins Stimulation of the anti-inflammatory cascade Prevention of hyperglycemia-induced inactivation of immunoglobulins by glycosylation Neutrophil dysfunction Impairment of intracellular bactericidal and opsonic activity
Endothelial function	Inhibition of excessive inducible nitric oxide synthetase–induced nitric oxide release Reduced production of nitric oxide by inhibition of constitutive endothelial nitric oxide synthetase

A second large RCT found that intensive insulin therapy was associated with reductions in mortality for medical patients who were in the ICU for 3 or more days. Similar to the previous trial, intensive insulin therapy was also associated with significant reductions in a variety of clinically important morbidities. In both of these trials, intensive insulin therapy was initiated at the time of ICU admission, and rates of hypoglycemia were low.

Informed by the results of these two RCTs, the American Association of Clinical Endocrinologists recently published guidelines recommending a target glucose of 80 to 110 mg/dL (4.4–6.1 mmol/L) for all critically ill patients and a target glucose of less than 180 mg/dL (9.9 mmol/L) for all hospitalized patients. Evidence to support specific glucose targets, especially in critically ill patients, continues to emerge, and it remains likely that the results from several large randomized trials that are currently under way may influence these recommendations.

Thyroid Hormone Replacement

Although the low serum levels of total T4, T3, and low T3-to-rT3 ratio in protracted critical illness is associated with higher mortality, it is not clear whether this is an adaptive process protecting against hypercatabolism or a maladaptive process contributing to the pathologic process. One small RCT found no difference in mortality associated with administration of T4 versus placebo, despite normalization of thyroid hormone levels. In addition, return of normal thyroid function was delayed in the intervention group. Another small, nonrandomized, observational cohort study found no difference in clinical outcomes among critically ill patients associated with continuous thyrotropin releasing hormone infusions combined with a growth hormone (GH) secretagogue, although physiologic parameters such as pulsatile pituitary hormone, physiologic levels of thyroid hormone, and decreased urea production and bone degradation as markers of catabolism were restored. There is currently no evidence to support interventions in patients with euthyroid sick syndrome. The diagnosis of true thyroid dysfunction, however, remains challenging in critically ill patients, and the constellation of a high TSH level in the setting of refractory hypotension and low total serum T3 levels may indicate hypothyroidism, warranting thyroid hormone replacement (Fig. 2).

Growth Hormone Replacement

The hypothesis of sustained GH resistance in the prolonged phase of critical illness and an enthusiasm for potential reversal of the catabolic state during critical illness led to two large clinical trials to evaluate the impact of pharmacologic GH administration in critically ill patients. These trials found an increased risk for infection and subsequent death associated with pharmacologic GH administration. The deleterious effects of GH in critically ill patients are probably multifactorial, complex, and interlinked and depend on the timing of treatment, the patient's condition, and the dose of GH. However, any beneficial effect might have been diminished by detrimental effect of hyperglycemia because GH worsens stress hyperglycemia and insulin resistance.

Alternative approaches focused on restoring the pulsatile nature of GH and TSH secretion through secretagogue administration may better restore normal physiology. To date, the role of exogenous IGF-1 alone and in conjunction with administration of other mediators within the somatotropic axis is not well defined. In addition, critically ill patients with the best anabolic profile have not been shown to have a survival benefit, underscoring our incomplete understanding of these complex interactions.

Gonadal Therapy

Low levels of sex hormones likely represent a marker of severity of illness. Current evidence does not support the routine use of anabolic steroids or androgens during the acute or prolonged phase of critical illness. Although estrogen supplementation has been shown to be beneficial in critical illness, the current body of evidence precludes a recommendation for routine use at this time. In addition, the role of hormone supplementation during the recovery phase of critical illness is not well defined.

SUMMARY

Critical illness can result in profound and interlinked alterations of the endocrine system. In the early stages of critical illness, this response may be largely adaptive, but sustained hormonal and metabolic changes with prolonged or severe critical illness can be maladaptive, leading to multisystem organ dysfunction and death. As a result, most endocrine system abnormalities serve as surrogate markers of severity of illness and prognosis in critical illness. The active replacement of low levels of hormones has proved to be too simplistic of an approach given the complex impact of critical illness on the endocrine system. Currently, only two evidence-based therapies that modify the endocrine system response to critical illness can be endorsed: intensive insulin therapy to maintain a target glucose of 80 to 110 mg/dL (4.4–6.1 mmol/L) and a 7-day course of low-dose physiologic steroid replacement for patients with relative adrenal insufficiency in the setting of fluid and catecholamine refractory septic shock.

SUGGESTED READINGS

Annane D, Bellissant E, Bollaert PE, and others: Corticosteroids for treating severe sepsis and septic shock [review], Cochrane Library 1.

Annane D, Sebille V, Charpentier C, and others: Effect of treatment with low doses of hydrocortisone and fludrocortisone on mortality in patients with septic shock, JAMA 288: 862, 2002.

Beishuizen A, Thijs LG: The immunoneuroendocrine axis in critical illness: beneficial adaptation or neuroendocrine exhaustion? Curr Opin Crit Care 10:461, 2004.

Dellinger RP, Carlet JM, Masur H, and others: Surviving Sepsis Campaign guidelines for management of severe sepsis and septic shock, Crit Care Med 32:858, 2004.

Nylen ES, Muller B: Endocrine changes in critical illness, J Intensive Care Med 19:67, 2004.

Singer M, De Santis V, Vitale D, and others: Multiorgan failure is an adaptive, endocrine-mediated, metabolic response to overwhelming systemic inflammation, Lancet 364:545, 2004.

Takala J, Ruokonen E, Webster NR, and others: Increased mortality associated with growth hormone treatment in critically ill adults, N Engl J Med 341:785, 1999.

Van den Berghe G: Endocrinology of critical illness, Crit Care Clin 22:1, 2006.

Van den Berghe G, Wilmer A, Milants I, and others: Intensive insulin therapy in the medical ICU, N Engl J Med 354:449, 2006.

Van den Berghe G, Wouters P, Weekers F, and others: Intensive insulin therapy in the critically ill patients, N Engl J Med 345:1359, 2001.

NUTRITIONAL SUPPORT IN THE CRITICALLY ILL

William B. Norbury, Esther Situ and David N. Herndon, MD

INTRODUCTION

Patients who will return to a normal diet less than 7 days following an intervention rarely require any specialized nutritional support. However, those with a critical illness are less likely to be able to return to normal diet within this timeframe and therefore may require the introduction of a diet tailored to their needs. Whether this is enteral or parenteral, the diet must be started at an early stage to prevent a deficit from forming in an already precipitous condition. Various factors associated with chronic severe illness such as increased proteolysis, gluconeogenesis, glycogenolysis, peripheral lipolysis, and metabolic rate contribute to reduced constitutive proteins and impaired immunity. Together with any preexisting comorbid states such as malnutrition, diabetes, heart failure, or renal failure, there is an increase in morbidity and mortality when the nutritional requirements of the patient are not met. This chapter concentrates on the indications for the introduction of various feeding programs, the techniques involved, and the results of such treatments.

METABOLIC RESPONSE TO STRESS AND INJURY IN CRITICAL ILLNESS

Specific conditions often require specific diets; however, what remains relatively constant among critically ill patients is a state of increased metabolic rate. The initial stress reaction following the initiation of severe illness is an attempt by the body to restore homeostasis; if limited both in time and severity, this response is beneficial in restoring normal organ function. However, when this response is severe and unrelenting, a period of hypermetabolism is created, resulting in a catabolic state. It has long been known that traumatic injury results in increased consumption of energy and loss of body nitrogen. Further studies have shown that when the patient was placed on a ventilator, these energy requirements increased to between 30% and 70% above normal. Burn patients show an amplification of this response to injury above and beyond that seen in any other state.

The exact pathways that drive this condition are poorly understood. Increased production of catecholamines and glucocorticoids lead to increased gluconeogenesis, glycogenolysis, peripheral lipolysis, and proteolysis of skeletal muscle. Other systems implicated in regulating this deleterious response are endotoxin, platelet-activating factor, tumor necrosis factor, interleukins 1 and 6, arachidonic acid metabolites using the cyclooxygenase and lipo-oxygenase pathways, neutrophil-adherence complexes, reactive oxygen species, nitric oxide, and the coagulation and complement cascades.

INDICATIONS

Any condition that results in a net negative balance in protein for more than 5 to 7 days following intervention requires a feeding regimen to prevent deleterious effects. Preexisting illnesses resulting in nutritional deficits should be addressed in patients preparing to undergo elective surgery. These include Crohn's disease, neoplasia, alcoholism, chronic diarrhea, and drug abuse. In those patients with a nutritional deficit a course of 7 to 10 days, preoperative feeding has been shown to be of benefit by reducing postoperative complications. A recent study from Milan, Italy, by Brag and colleagues showed that preoperatively loading elective surgery patients with immune-enhancing substrates in an oral formula for 5 days and continuing therapy by jejunal infusion for 7 days after surgery results in significant reductions in postoperative infections and length of hospital stay in patients undergoing gastrointestinal surgery for cancer.

NUTRITIONAL REQUIREMENTS

Exact nutritional requirements differ among patients and conditions. However, the following recommendations were recently made on the basis of several studies and clinical trials:

- Enteral nutrition as opposed to parenteral nutrition results in a decrease in infectious complications in critically ill patients.
- Enteral feeding should commence within 24 to 48 hours following admission to the intensive care unit.
- Diets supplemented with arginine and other select nutrients should not be used for critically ill patients.
- Enteral glutamine should be considered for burn and trauma patients but not for routine critical care patients.
- Although probably of benefit, there are insufficient data to recommend probiotics in critically ill patients.
- Parenteral glutamine supplementation is recommended for those patients who are requiring total parenteral nutrition.
- An intensive insulin protocol to ensure tight glycemic control throughout nutritional support is required in trauma and surgical critical care patients.

Table 1: Commonly Used Equations for Calculating Energy Requirements in the Absence of Indirect Calorimetry

Equation	Age and Gender	Formula
Harris Benedict	Male	$66.5 + (13.75 \times W) + (5.003 \times H) - (6.775 \times A)$
	Female	$655.1 + (9.563 \times W) + (1.850 \times H) - (4.676 \times A)$
WHO	Male <3 years	$(60.9 \times W) - 54$
	Male 3–10 years	$(22.7 \times W) + 495$
	Female <3 years	$(61 \times W) - 51$
	Female 3–10 yrs	$(22.5 \times W) + 499$

A, Age in years; *H*, height in cm; *W*, weight in kg; *WHO*, World Health Organization.

ENERGY REQUIREMENTS

In the absence of access to indirect calorimetry to measure resting energy expenditure (REE) in the intensive care unit, several equations are available for calculating patient requirements. The most common are illustrated in Table 1.

Indirect calorimetry is carried out at the bedside using a metabolic cart that measures CO_2 production and oxygen consumption; from these and using the Weir equation, one can calculate the REE of the patient. Of significant use in burns acute care, this technique requires dedicated teams who know the limitations of its use and are able to limit any confusing factors such as high flow oxygen (greater than 60%) and air leaks in the respiratory circuit and to identify possible confounding factors such as high positive end expiratory pressure.

The REE calculated can then be increased by a factor appropriate for the patient, such as 1.4 for burn patients, and caloric intake adjusted accordingly. If, for instance, the caloric intake is too large in a burn patient, the body does not increase protein synthesis further, but rather the body mass increases because of fat being laid down. Recommendations for caloric intake for most patients in critical care are 25 to 30 kcal/kg/24 hours; this allows 90% of patients to reach the required intake, and only 20% will be overfed.

PROTEIN REQUIREMENTS

Sufficient protein intake is vital to maintain lean body mass because the rate of oxidation of most amino acids is raised in patients in critical care and can reach 50% higher than normal in burn patients. Therefore raising protein intake by more than 50% from 1g/kg/day to between 1.5 and 2 g/kg/day ensures adequate supply in adults. The same cannot be said for children, however, who may increase urea production without any beneficial anabolic effect. One study by Wolfe and colleagues in burn patients showed a balance between protein synthesis and catabolism could be achieved with a protein intake of 1.4 g protein/kg/day. Patterson and colleagues found that additional delivery of protein above 1.5 g/kg/day has been shown to only increase urinary excretion of urea. The relative concentrations of certain amino acids can be modified for certain disease states. Essential amino acid–enriched solutions are often used for renal failure patients, and branched chain amino acids, although more expensive, may be used in hepatic failure.

TECHNIQUES

In most cases, enteral feeding is possible; parenteral feeding is principally reserved for the presence of mitigating circumstances in which enteral feeding is not feasible, such as Ogilvie's syndrome, bowel obstruction, ischemic enterocolitis, protracted ileus, or high output intestinal fistula in which there is less than 1 m of functioning jejunum. Even in cases of proximal small bowel obstruction, a feeding stoma can be placed distal to the occlusion, resulting in a beneficial outcome for the patient.

Enteral Feeding

The most cost-efficient method of tube feeding is nasogastric (NG); the main risk of this method is gastroparesis, resulting in large gastric residuals. If, however, the hourly residuals remain below 50 ml, this method may be employed without significant problem for patient or caregiver as long as the head of the bed is kept raised. Feeding the patient distal to the stomach also has benefits. In patients with severe acute burn injuries, nasojejunal feeding is the method of choice because such patients remain obtunded for a protracted period of time and require multiple operations, precluding NG feeding within 6 hours of each operation. Generally, if distal to the stomach, the feeding tube should be advanced into the third or fourth part of the duodenum and preferably to beyond the ligament of Treitz. This can be performed blind, under fluoroscopy, or with the help of an endoscope, if problematic. Percutaneous endoscopic gastrostomy (PEG) feeding should be considered when it is expected that the patient's nutritional intake is likely to be inadequate for a period exceeding 2 to 3 weeks. Comparisons between PEG feeding and NG feeding have shown a higher rate of discomfort and complications (see Table 2) in those fed via the nasal route in the long term. PEG feeding was found to be more socially acceptable and had

reduced rates of esophageal reflux and aspiration pneumonia. Therefore if nutritional intake is likely to be deficient for more than 3 weeks, a patient may tolerate a PEG feed better.

Indications for Percutaneous Endoscopic Gastrostomy Feeding

- Oncologic disorders (stenosing tumors in the ear, nose, and throat region or the upper gastrointestinal tract; PEG tubes may be used palliatively in inoperable cases or placed before surgery, radiotherapy, or chemotherapy and removed when the patient has recovered and has a reliable and adequate oral intake)
- Neurologic disorders (dysphagic states after cerebrovascular stroke or craniocerebral trauma and in patients with cerebral tumors, bulbar paralysis, Parkinson's disease, amyotrophic lateral sclerosis, cerebral palsy)
- Other clinical conditions (wasting in acquired immunodeficiency syndrome, short bowel syndrome, reconstructive facial surgery, prolonged coma, polytrauma, Crohn's disease, cystic fibrosis, chronic renal failure, congenital abnormalities, e.g., tracheoesophageal fistula)

Transgastric (TGJ) and direct jejunostomy are also beneficial routes of feeding if gastroparesis is anticipated. The advantage of TGJ is decompression of the stomach during jejunal feeding.

Table 2 reviews the available modes of enteral feeding, and Table 3 describes methods for monitoring it. Table 4 lists potential complications of the technique.

Table 2: Modes of Enteral Feeding

Feeding Route	Considerations	Insertion Methods	Benefits	Complications
Nasogastric	Short-term Smaller tubes clog more easily Requires fully functional gastrointestinal tract Can be inserted orally	Blindly at bedside Endoscopically or radiologically in usual cases	Easily inserted and replaced Can use bolus feeding	Sinusitis Aspiration Aspiration-associated pneumonia Airway obstruction (postcricoid ulceration) Nasal necrosis Pneumothorax from inadvertent tracheal insertion Displacement Occlusion
Nasoenteric	Short term Use in patients with aspiration Poor gastric emptying (postoperative ileus gastroparesis) Can insert but do not use if patient is not volume resuscitated or is hemodynamically unstable Cannot check residuals to determine tolerance Requires continuous infusion	Blindly at bedside Directed in operating room Endoscopically Radiologically	Reduces aspiration risk Some tubes allow suction of the stomach while feeding into small bowel	Sinusitis Aspiration (gastroesophageal reflux) Airway obstruction (postcricoid ulceration) Nasal necrosis Pneumothorax from inadvertent tracheal insertion Displacement (end may reflux back into stomach) Occlusion Pneumatosis, intestinal ischemia, or infarction Mechanical (e.g., tube blockage, malposition or removal)

Gastrostomy	Long term Requires well-emptying stomach Not a good choice for patients with significant reflux and aspiration May be difficult to replace early after insertion	Surgically Endoscopically Radiologically	Allows bolus feeding Can be placed at the bedside Low-profile tubes available, which may decrease dislodgement	Bleeding Retching Infection of abdominal wall Perforation of other abdominal organs may cause dehiscence Migration of internal bolster though pylorus or through gastric wall into abdominal wall Aspiration Dislodgement (contamination of peritoneum) Bowel obstruction Occlusion Pneumoperitoneum Mechanical (e.g., tube blockage, malposition or removal, granulation around tube site)
Transgastric jejunostomy	Long term Requires continuous infusion Use in patients with aspiration, poor gastric emptying (postoperative ileus, gastroparesis) Can insert but do not use if patient is not volume resuscitated or is hemodynamically unstable (determine tolerance)	Surgically Endoscopically Radiologically	Reduces aspiration risk Allows suction of the stomach while feeding small bowel May be used immediately after placement Can be converted later to a gastric tube	Bleeding Infection of abdominal wall Perforation of other abdominal organs, wound dehiscence Migration of internal bolster though pylorus or through gastric wall into abdominal wall Aspiration Dislodgement (contamination of peritoneum) Occlusion Bowl obstruction Pneumatosis, intestinal ischemia or infarction
Jejunostomy	Short or long term Requires continuous infusion Use in patients with aspiration, poor gastric emptying (postoperative ileus, gastroparesis) Can insert but do not use if patient is not volume resuscitated or is hemodynamically unstable Cannot check residuals to determine tolerance Very difficult to replace	Surgically Endoscopically Radiologically	Reduces aspiration risk May be used immediately after placement Low-profile tubes available, which may decrease dislodgment	Bleeding Infection of abdominal wall Wound dehiscence Dislodgement (contamination of peritoneum) Pneumatosis, intestinal ischemia or infarction Bowel obstruction Occlusion Gastrointestinal (e.g., vomiting and diarrhea) Mechanical (e.g., tube blockage, malposition or removal Aspiration

Table 3: Monitoring Enteral Feeding

	Acute Patient	Stable Patient
Electrolytes	Daily	Weekly or biweekly
Glucose	Three times per day or more often until reading is consistently <200	Three times per day or more often until reading is consistently <200
Weight	Daily	2–3 times per week
Intake/output	Daily	Daily
BUN/creatinine	Daily until reach to normal limit	Weekly or biweekly
Urine specific gravity	Daily	Weekly or biweekly
Blood count	Weekly	Weekly

BUN, Blood urea nitrogen.

Table 4: Potential Complications of Enteral Feeding

Problem	Cause	Treatment
Hyponatremia	Overhydration	Restrict fluids Change formula (avoid low sodium intake)
Hypernatremia	Inadequate fluid intake	Increase free water
Dehydration	Diarrhea	Determine etiology of diarrhea Increase fluid intake
Hyperglycemia	High concentration of carbohydrate intake Insulin insensitivity	Evaluate total carbohydrate intake Adjust insulin level
Hypokalemia, hypomagnium, and hypophosphate	Refeeding syndrome	Replace K, Mg, P Decrease the rate of the feed
Hyperkalemia	Excess K intake Renal insufficiency	Change formula

K, Potassium; *Mg,* magnesium; *P,* phosphate.
Table adapted from Skipper A, Marian MA: Parenteral nutrition. In Gottschlich MM, Matarese LE, Shronts EP, editors: Nutrition support dietetics core curriculum, *1993, ed 2, Silver Spring, MD: Aspen.*

Parenteral Feeding

Reserved for those patients who are unable to consume adequate nutrition via the oral or enteral route, parenteral nutrition (PN) may be given by a central or peripheral route. It may also be total (TPN) or partial (PPN). PN has been shown to increase the rate of infectious complications when used routinely in well-nourished patients. One of the main problems is hyperglycemia, leading to a multitude of pathologies including immune function derangements in leukocytes, glycosylation of circulating immunoglobulin, increases in inflammatory cytokines, and aggravating cardiac disease. The use of TPN has also been associated with increases in rates of bacterial translocation, although evidence of any subsequent sepsis being due to an intestinal organism is questionable.

Absolute indications for TPN are as follows:

1. Short bowel syndrome with less than 1 m of small intestine
2. Radiation enteritis
3. High-output gastrointestinal fistula
4. Persistent ileus
5. Persistent pseudo-obstruction
6. Nonoperative obstruction such as desmoid tumor

Parenteral nutrition is usually given via a central venous catheter, the tip of which is normally in the superior vena cava. Most complications arise from improper placement and include pneumothorax, hematoma, damage to local structures, and air embolism. Placement must be checked with a chest x-ray before commencing feeds. Line-sepsis and thromboembolic events are the most serious complications during parenteral therapy. Organisms isolated may be related to the disease process; common ones include *Klebsiella, Candida, Staphylococcus, Pseudomonas,* and *Enterobacter* species.

Monitoring in parenteral feeding is described in Table 5 and complications in Table 6.

Table 5: Monitoring in Parenteral Feeding

Parameter	Acute Patient	Stable Patient
Body temperature	Every shift	Daily
Intake/output	Daily	Daily
Serum or urinary glucose	Every 8 hours	Every 6 hours
Electrolytes (Na, K, Cl, HCO₃, BUN, Cr, Ca, Mg, phosphorus)	First 3 days	3 times/week
Glucose	QID until <180 mg/dl then daily	QID until <180 mg/dl then daily
Magnesium	1–2 times/week	Weekly
Calcium/phosphorus	1–2 timesweek	Weekly
BUN/creatinine	3 times/week	Biweekly
Albumin/total protein	Baseline	Weekly
Cholesterol	Baseline	Weekly
Triglycerides	Baseline	As clinically indicated
Liver enzymes: SGPT, SGOT, LDH, alkaline	Baseline	Weekly
PT/PTT	Baseline	Weekly
Platelet count*	Baseline	As needed
Zinc/copper	Baseline	As needed
Fe/TIBC	Baseline	As needed
Nitrogen balance (24-hour UUN)	24–48 hours after full rate achieved	As clinically indicated
AST, ALT, GGT, ALP	Weekly	Monthly
Weight	Daily	2–3 times weekly
Vital signs	Daily	Daily
Prealbumin, C-reactive protein	Weekly	Weekly

*Necessary initially for catheter insertion.
BUN, Blood urea nitrogen; *LDH,* lactate dehydrogenase; *PT,* prothrombin time; *PTT,* partial thromboplastin time; *QID,* four times daily; *SGOT,* serum glutamic-oxaloacetic transaminase; *SGPT,* serum glutamic-pyruvic transaminase; *TIBC,* total iron-binding capacity; *UUN,* urinary urea nitrogen.

Table 6: Metabolic Complications of Parenteral Feeding

Problem	Cause	Treatment
Hypoglycemia	Sudden cessation of concentrated dextrose infusion	Peripheral IV of 5%–10% dextrose for 24 hours before resuming central-line feeding
Hyperglycemia	Highly concentrated dextrose infusion	Insulin infusion/long acting
Serum electrolyte and mineral abnormalities	Inadequate monitoring	Modification of subsequent infusions
Elevation of BUN	Hyperosmolar dehydration	Free water given as 5% dextrose via a peripheral vein
Metabolic bone disease	Low serum calcitriol	Temporary or permanent discontinuance of TPN
Increases in transaminases, bilirubin, and alkaline phosphatase	Common following initiation; usually temporary	If persistent, usually due to amino acid load; reduce protein delivery
Temporary hyperlipidemia	Common in renal and hepatic failure	Temporary or permanent discontinuance of lipid infusion

BUN, Blood urea nitrogen; *IV,* intravenous; *TPN,* total parenteral nutrition.

SPECIFIC MACRONUTRIENTS AND MICRONUTRIENTS

Specific macronutrients and micronutrients are often necessary in specific quantities during an admission to intensive care. This topic would require an entire chapter to itself; however, Table 7 outlines the main vitamins and trace elements required for enhanced nutrition. Table 8 shows the main food groups necessary to sustain life, together with information outlining advantages and disadvantages of various types of preparation.

CONCLUSION

Nutritional support in critical care patients has continued to change over the years, and yet some features are consistent. If possible, enteral nutrition should be given in almost all cases of nutritional deficit. Early and aggressive use of nutritional support increases the chances of a successful outcome. Specific dietary requirements differ among patients and disease processes. A comprehensive protocol-driven framework of decision making that allows ongoing assessment of the patient provides optimal care and supports patient needs.

Table 7: Main Vitamins and Trace Elements Required for Enhanced Nutrition

Micronutrient	Function in Critical Care	General Deficiency Problems	Inadequacy Associated with Critical Care
Vitamin A	Enhances tissue regeneration by aiding in glycoprotein synthesis; cofactor for collagen synthesis and cross linkage	Xerophthalmia (night blindness, conjunctival xerosis, Bitot's spots) Respiratory ailments (pneumonia, bronchopulmonary dysplasia) Affects epithelial tissues of the gut	Diminish activity of helper T-cells and weaken mucus secretion
Thiamin (B1)	Cofactor in collagen crosslinking	Beriberi, anorexia, fatigue, peripheral neuropathy, foot and wrist drop Cardiomegaly, hyperlactatemia	N/A
Riboflavin (B2)	Cofactor in collagen crosslinking May repair DNA and calcium mobilization	Cheilosis, angular stomatitis, glossitis, scrotal dermatitis, cessation of growth, photophobia	N/A
Pyridoxine (B6)	Coenzyme that activates protein synthesis	Irritability, depression, stomatitis, glossitis, cheilosis, seborrhea of the nasal labial folds, normochromic, microcytic or sideroblastic anemia	Anemia
Pantothenic acid	A component of coenzymes that participate in energy release from macronutrients and synthesis of heme and fat	Fatigue, sleep disturbances, nausea, abdominal cramps, vomiting, diarrhea, muscle cramps, mental depression, hypoglycemia	Poor wound healing and diminished graft taking
Cobalamin (B12)	Coenzyme for protein and DNA synthesis	Megaloblastic anemia, loss of appetite, weight loss, fatigue, glossitis, leucopenia, thrombocytopenia, achlorhydria	Megaloblastic anemia, constipation, diarrhea, and neurologic defect

(continued)

Table 7: Main Vitamins and Trace Elements Required for Enhanced Nutrition—Cont'd

Micronutrient	Function in Critical Care	General Deficiency Problems	Inadequacy Associated with Critical Care
Vitamin C	Necessary for hydroxylation of lysine and praline in collagen formation, as well as crosslinking; protects tissue from superoxide damage; enhances tissue regeneration Immune-mediated and antibacterial functions of white blood cells	Fatigue, anorexia; muscular pain, scurvy (characterized by anemia, hemorrhagic disorders, weakening of collagenous structures in bone cartilage, teeth, and connective tissue, degeneration of muscle, gingivitis, gingivitis, capillary weakness, and rheumatic leg pain)	Impaired wound healing, weakened collagen in bone, teeth, and connective tissue Sudden death
Vitamin D	Regulates the synthesis of several structural proteins, including collagen type I	Bone demineralization	Susceptible to osteoporosis and osteomalacia, low serum circulation of Ca and P, increase alkaline phosphatase
Vitamin E	Antioxidant properties promote cell membrane integrity	Increased platelet aggregation, decreased red blood cell survival, hemolytic anemia, neurologic abnormalities, decreased serum creatinine levels, excessive creatinuria	Prolonged steatorrhea and neuronal degeneration
Vitamin K	Essential for coagulation, which is a prerequisite for wound healing	Hemorrhage	Mild bruising or hemorrhage
Magnesium	Cofactor for enzymes involved in protein and collagen synthesis	Nausea, muscle weakness, irritability, mental derangement	Cardiac arrhythmia, increased irritable nervous system with tetany
Calcium	Both the remodeling process and the degradation of collagen are accomplished through the action of various collagenases, all of which require calcium	Osteoporosis	Cardiovascular collapse, hypotension unresponsive to fluids and vasopressors, end-organ resistance to PTH, dysrhythmias
Copper	Promotes the crosslinking reactions of collagen and elastin synthesis scavenges free radicals	Skeletal demineralization, impaired glucose tolerance, anemia, neutropenia, leucopenia, changes in hair and skip pigmentation	Increase erythrocyte turnover, abnormal electrocardiographic patterns
Iron	Necessary for hydroxylation of lysine and praline in collagen synthesis, as well as transportation of oxygen to the wound bed	Anemia, cheilosis, glossitis, atrophy of the tongue, hair loss, brittle fingernails, koilonychias, pallor, tissue hypoxia, exertional dyspnea, heart enlargement	Decreased resistance to infections and reduce ability to maintain body temperature in cold environment
Selenium	Reduces intracellular hydroperoxides, thereby protecting membrane lipids from oxidant damage May reduce the rate of mortality in critical ill patients	Growth retardation, muscle pain and weakness, myopathy, cardiomyopathy	Alter thyroid hormone metabolism, increase plasma glutathione levels
Zinc	A cofactor in more than 100 enzyme systems that promote protein synthesis, cellular replication, and collagen formation	Hair loss, dermatitis, growth retardation, delayed sexual maturation, testicular atrophy, decreased appetite, depressed smell and taste acuity, depression, diarrhea, decreased dark adaptation	Impaired wound healing
Folic acid	Synthesis of DNA	Megaloblastic or macrocytic anemia	Gastrointestinal disturbances (diarrhea), weight loss, depression of cell-mediated immunity

CA, Calcium; *DNA*, dioxyribonucleic acid; *N/A*, not available; *P*, phosphate; *PTH*, parathyroid hormone.

Table 8: Main Food Groups Necessary to Sustain Life

Macronutrient	Controversy	Types	Advantage	Disadvantage
Carbohydrate (28%*–82% of Total Calories)				
		Monosaccharide, disaccharide, and oligosaccharides	Elemental carbohydrate; does not require pancreatic enzyme digestion	High osmolality may cause intolerance in digestion.[1]
		Oligosaccharides (3–10 glucose units) or polysaccharides (>10 glucose units)	Lower osmolality Provides more calories per unit of glucose	Require digestion from pancreatic enzyme May decrease tolerance for lower gastrointestinal enteral feed
		Lactose	May increase calcium absorption[2,3]	Decreased gastrointestinal tolerance for lactose intolerance patients Allergen
		Fiber	Promote gut health May prevent diarrhea	Require excessive water to prevent constipation High fiber can cause abdominal gas, bloating, and distention
Protein (6%–25% of Total Calories)				
	There are contradictory studies about small-peptide-based formulas. Debates concern whether there is a benefit and whether it is superior to free amino acid–based formulas. Both are well tolerated in lower GI with minimum stimulation of pancreatic secretion.[3]	Whey-based formula:	Increased gastric emptying[4,5] Lower gastric residuals[6] Cysteine, in the presence of is conditional essential nutrient for neonates and critical ill patients[7] High biological value of protein has higher nitrogen absorption rate for tissue replenishing and growth	N/A
		Small peptide (3–10 linkage of amino acids)	Well tolerated and absorbed in midgut[3,8–10] May improve nitrogen retention and maintenance of visceral protein status[9]	N/A

(continued)

Table 8: Main Food Groups Necessary to Sustain Life—Cont'd

Macronutrient	Controversy	Types	Advantage	Disadvantage
		Free amino acid	Well tolerated and absorbed without the need of digestion[3]	Hypertonicity (500–919 mOsm/kg) that may increase diarrhea
		Glutamine	A conditional essential amino acid in burns[11,12] Reduces infections and improves visceral protein status in burn patients[13-15] Maintains the physiologic intestinal barrier and reduces rates of infections[16]	An excess of any particular amino acid is likely to result in reduced absorption of other amino acids.
	Questions have been raised as to the benefits of arginine in trauma, elective surgery, and burns[11,17-19]	Arginine	Stimulates T-lymphocytes and stimulates synthesis of nitric oxide[20,21]	N/A
		Gluten	A source of protein from wheat and other cereal products.	Decrease GI tolerance Allergen
Fat (1%-55% of Total Calories; Provides Concentrated Source of Energy)				
Essential fatty acid (linoleic and linolenic acids—required 4% of total calories to meet[8])		Long-chain triglyceride (LCT)	Provide the densest calories among the macronutrients May be a source of essential fatty acid when derived from plants	May decrease tolerance of feed overall High concentrations of LCT are not well tolerated in critically ill patients[22-24]
		Medium-chain triglyceride (MCT) (6-12 carbon chains)	Easy to be absorb because there is little requirement for digestion by bile salts or pancreatic lipase[25] Readily used as fuel because of direct transfer into portal system[25] Deleterious effects are reduced by decreasing dose[26]	High quantities of MCT lead to ketosis[25,27] Pure MCT infusion can cause hyperketonemia, narcotic effects, and raised lactic acid[28,29] High quantity of intravenous MCT can cause central nervous system toxicity Does not provide essential fatty acid

Some studies have shown beneficial effects of n-3 fat over n-6 fat in critical care; however, the evidence is not yet clear as to the level of benefit imparted[30]		
n-3 fat: alpha-linolenic, eicosapentaenoic acid and docosahexaenoic acid	Improve immune response Reduce incidence of hyperglycemia[32]	Excess n-3 fatty acid (>3 g/day) may increase risk of hemorrhagic stroke,[31] nose bleed, or hematuria[32]
n-6 fat: linoleic acid, arachidonic acid from corn, sunflower, and safflower oil	The most common plant source of lipid Prevents essential fatty acids deficiency	Precursor to leukotrienes, a proinflammatory and immunosuppressive[19]

N/A, Not available.

1. Fussell ST: Enteral nutrition: a comprehensive overview. In Matarese LE, Gottschlich MM, editors: Contemporary nutrition support practice: a clinical guide, ed 2, Philadelphia, 2003, WB Saunders, pp. 188–200.
2. Schuette SA, Knowles JB, Ford HE: Am J Clin Nutr 50:1084, 1989.
3. Rodriguez DJ, Clevenger FW: West J Med 159:192, 1993.
4. Billeaud C, Guillet J, Sandler B: Euro J Clin Nutr 44:577, 1990.
5. Tolia V, Lin C-H, Kuhns LR: J Ped Gastr Nutr 15:297, 1992.
6. Fried MD, Khoshoo V, Secker DJ: Pediatrics 120: 569, 1992.
7. White AC, Thannickal VJ, Fan burg BL: J Nutr Bichem 5:218, 1994.
8. Zaloga GP: Nutr Clin Pract 5:235, 1990.
9. Brinson RR, Hanumanthu SK, Pitts WM: Nutr Clin Pract 4:211, 1989.
10. Donald P, Miller E, Schirmer B: Nutr Res 14:3, 1994.
11. Saffle J, Wiebke G, Jennings K, and others: J Trauma 42:793, 1997.
12. Huschak G, Zur Nieden K, Hoell T, and others: Intensive Care Med 31:1202, 2005.
13. Wischmeyer PE, Lynch J, Liedel J, and others: Crit Care Med 29:2075, 2001.
14. Zhou YP, Jiang ZM, Sun YH, and others: J Ped Gastr Nutr 27:241, 2003.
15. Garrel D: J Ped Gastr Nutr 28:123; 2004.
16. De-Souza DA, Greene LJ: Crit Care Med 33:1125, 2005.
17. Dietscher IE, Foulks CJ, Smith RW: J Am Diet Assoc 98:335, 1998.
18. Moore FA, Moore EE, Kudsk KA, and others: J Trauma 37:607, 1994.
19. Daly JM, Lieberman MD, Goldfine J, and others: Surgery 112:56, 1992.
20. Hishikawa K, Nakaki T, Tsuda M, and others: Japan Heart J 33:41, 1992.
21. Kirk S, Barbul A: J Ped Gastr Nutr 14:226S, 1990.
22. Nanni G, Pittiruti M, Castagneto M: Am J Clin Nutr 38:339, 1983.
23. Nanni G, Pittiruti M, Snoswell AM, and others: J Ped Gastr Nutr 9:483, 1985.
24. Worthley LIG, Fishlock RC, Snoswell AM: J Ped Gastr Nutr 7:176, 1983.
25. Michele M: Gottschlich: 7:152, 1992.
26. Jensen GL, Mascioli EA, Seidner DL, and others: J Ped Gastr Nutr 14:467, 1990.
27. Bell SJ, Mascioli EA, Bistrian BR, and others: J Am Diet Assoc 91:701, 1991.
28. Ruppin DC, Middleton WRJ: Drugs 20:216, 1980.
29. Bach A, Guisard D, Debry G, and others: Arch Physiol Biochim 82:705, 1974.
30. Garcia-de-Lorenzo A, Denia RA, Martinez-Ratero S, and others: Br J Nutr 94:221, 2005.
31. Kromann N, Green A: Acta Med Scand 208:401, 1980.
32. Stacpoole PW, Alig J, Ammon L, and others: Metabolism 38:946, 1989.

*Lower percentage of CHO may be used in cases of respiratory failure.

Suggested Readings

Akkersdijk WL, Roukema JA, van der Werken C: Percutaneous endoscopic gastrostomy for patients with severe cerebral injury, *Injury* 29:11, 1998.

Akobeng AK, Miller V, Thomas A: Percutaneous endoscopic gastrostomy feeding improves nutritional status and stabilizes pulmonary function in patients with cystic fibrosis, *J Pediatr Gastroenterol Nutr* 29:485, 1999.

Bach A, Guisard D, Debry G, and others: Metabolic effects following a medium chain triglyceride load in dogs. V. Influence of the perfusion rate, *Arch Physiol Biochim* 82:705, 1974.

Bell SJ, Mascioli EA, Bistrian BR, and others: Alternative lipid sources for enteral and parental nutrition: long and medium-chain triglycerides, structured triglycerides, and fish oils, *J Am Diet Assoc* 91:701, 1991.

Billeaud C, Guillet J, Sandler B: Gastric emptying in infants with or without gastro-oesophageal reflux according to the type of milk, *Eur J Clin Nutr* 44:577, 1990.

Black CT, Hennessey PJ, Andrassy RJ: Short-term hyperglycemia depresses immunity through nonenzymatic glycosylation of circulating immunoglobulin, *J Trauma* 30:830; discussion 832, 1990.

Braga M, Gianotti L, Radaelli G, and others: Perioperative immunonutrition in patients undergoing cancer surgery: results of a randomized double-blind phase 3 trial, *Arch Surg* 134:428, 1999.

Brinson RR, Hanumanthu SK, Pitts WM: A reappraisal of the peptidebased enteral formulas: Clinical applications, *Nutr Clin Pract* 4:211, 1989.

Calon B, Pottecher T, Frey A, and others: Long-chain versus medium and long-chain triglyceride-based fat emulsion in parental nutrition of severe head trauma patients, *Infusionstherapie* 17(5): 246, 1990.

Chuntrasakul C, Siltham S, Sarasombath S, and others: Comparison of a immunonutrition formula enriched arginine, glutamine and omega-3 fatty acid, with a currently high-enriched enteral nutrition for trauma patients, *J Med Assoc Thai* 86:552, 2003.

Cosgrove M, Jenkins HR: Experience of percutaneous endoscopic gastrostomy in children with Crohn's disease, *Arch Dis Child* 76:141, 1997.

Cuthbertson D: Historical perspectives in hospital nutrition. CXXXVIII. The disturbance of metabolism produced by bony and non-bony injury, with notes on certain abnormal conditions of bone. David Paton Cuthbertson. May 18, 1930, *J Parenter Enteral Nutr* 2:31, 1978.

Daly JM, Lieberman MD, Goldfine J, and others: Enteral nutrition with supplemental arginine, RNA and omega-3 fatty acids in patients after operation: Immunologic, metabolic, and clinical outcome, *Surgery* 112(1): 56, 1992.

De-Souza DA, Greene LJ: Intestinal permeability and systemic infections in critically ill patients: effect of glutamine, *Crit Care Med* 33:5: 1125, 2005.

Dietscher JE, Foulks CJ, Smith RW: Nutritional response of patients in an intensive care unit to an elemental formula vs a standard enteral formula, *J Am Diet Assoc* 98:335, 1998.

Donald P, Miller E, Schirmer B: Repletion of nutrition parameters in surgincal patients receiving peptide versus amino acid elemental feeds, *Nutr Res* 14:3, 1994.

Esposito K, Nappo F, Marfella R, and others: Inflammatory cytokine concentrations are acutely increased by hyperglycemia in humans: role of oxidative stress, *Circulation* 106:2067, 2002.

Favus MJ, Angeid-Backman E: Effects of lactose on calcium absorption and secretion by rat ileum, *Am J Physiol* 246(3 Pt 1): G281, 1984.

Fietkau R, Iro H, Sailer D, and others: Percutaneous endoscopically guided gastrostomy in patients with head and neck cancer, *Recent Results Cancer Res* 121:269, 1991.

Fired MD, Khoshoo V, Secker DJ, and others: Decrease in gastric emptying time and episodes of regurgitation in children with spastic quadriplegia fed a whey-based formula, *Pediatrics* 120:569, 1992.

Fuentes-Orozco C, Anaya-Prado R, Gonzalez-Ojeda A, and others: L-alanyl-Lglutamine-supplemented parenteral nutrition improves infectious morbidity in secondary peritonitis, *Clin Nutr* 23:13, 2004.

Fussell St: Enteral nutrition: a comprehensive overview. In: Matarese LE, Gottschlich MM, editors: *Contemporary nutrition support practice: A clinical guide*, ed 2, Philadelphia, 2003, WB Saunders, p. 188.

Garcia-de-Lorenzo A, Denia RS, Martinez-Ratero S, and others: Parenteral nutrition providing a restricted amount of linoleic acid in severely burned patients: a randomized double-blind study of an olive oil-based lipid emulsion v. medium/long-chain triacylglycerols, *Br J Nutr* 94:221, 2005.

Garrel D: The effect of supplemental enteral glutamine on plasma levels, gut function, and outcome in severe burns, *J Parenteral Enteral Nutr* 28(2):123; 2004, author reply.

Goodall M, Stone C, Haynes BW, Jr: Urinary output of adrenaline and noradrenaline in severe thermal burns, *Ann Surg* 145:479, 1957.

Gottschlich MM: Selection of optimal lipid sources in enteral and parental nutrition, *Nutr Clin Pract* 7:152, 133, 1992.

Gramlich LKK, Pinilla J, Rodych NJ, and others: Does enteral nutrition compared to parenteral nutrition result in better outcomes in critically ill adult patients? A systematic review of the literature, *Nutrition* 20:843, 2004.

Grey NJ, Perdrizet GA: Reduction of nosocomial infections in the surgical intensive-care unit by strict glycemic control, *Endocr Pract* 10(suppl 2): 46, 2004.

Hishikawa K, Nakaki T, Tsuda M, and others: Effect of systemic L-arginine administration on hemodynamics and nitric oxide release in man, *Japan Heart J* 33:41, 1992.

Huschak G, Zur Nieden K, Hoell T, and others: Olive oil based nutrition in multiple trauma patients: a pilot study, *Intensive Care Med* 31(9):1202, 2005. Epub Aug 17, 2005.

Jain PK, McNaught CE, Anderson AD, and others: Influence of symbiotic containing *Lactobacillus acidophilus* La5, *Bifidobacterium lactis* Bb 12, *Streptococcus thermophilus*, *Lactobacillus bulgaricus* and oligofructose on gut barrier function and sepsis in critically ill patients: a randomised controlled trial, *Clin Nutr* 23:467, 2004.

Jeejeebhoy KN: Management of short bowel syndrome: avoidance of total parenteral nutrition, *Gastroenterology* 130:S60, 2006.

Jensen GL, Mascioli EA, Seidner DL, and others: Parenteral infusion of long- and medium chain triglycerides and reticuloendothelial system function in man, *J Parenteral Enteral Nutr* 14:(5): 467, 1990.

Kieft H, Roos AN, van Drunen JD, and others: Clinical outcome of immunonutrition in a heterogeneous intensive care population, *Intensive Care Med* 31:524, 2005.

Kirk S, Barbul A: Role of arginine in trauma, sepsis, and immunity, *J Parenteral Enteral Nutr* 14:226S, 1990.

Koehler J, Buhl K: Percutaneous endoscopic gastrostomy for postoperative rehabilitation after maxillofacial tumor surgery, *Int J Oral Maxillofac Surg* 20:38, 1991.

Kinney JM, Long CL, Gump FE, and others: Tissue composition of weight loss in surgical patients. I. Elective operation, *Ann Surg* 168:459, 1968.

Kromann N, Green A: Epidemiological studies in the Upernavik district, Greenland. Incidence of some chronic diseases 1950–1974, *Acta Med Scand* 208:5: 401, 1980.

Lee JH, Machtay M, Unger LD, and others: Prophylactic gastrostomy tubes in patients undergoing intensive irradiation for cancer of the head and neck, *Arch Otolaryngol Head Neck Surg* 124:871, 1998.

Long CL, Spencer JL, Kinney JM, and others: Carbohydrate metabolism in man: effect of elective operations and major injury, *J Appl Physiol* 31:110, 1971.

Malhotra A, Mathur AK, Gupta S: Early enteral nutrition after surgical treatment of gut perforations: a prospective randomised study, *J Postgrad Med* 50:102, 2004.

McNaught CE, Woodcock NP, Anderson AD, and others: A prospective randomised trial of probiotics in critically ill patients, *Clin Nutr* 24:211, 2005.

Miller TL, Awnetwant EL, Evans S, and others: Gastrostomy tube supplementation for HIV-infected children, *Pediatrics* 96:696, 1995.

Moore FA, Moore EE, Kudsk KA, and others: Clinical benefits of an immune-enhancing diet for early postinjury enteral feeding, *J Trauma* 37(4): 607, 1994.

Nanni G, Pittiruti M, Castagneto M: Carnitine plasma levels during total parental nutrition, *Am J Clin Nutr* 38:339, 1983.

Nanni G, Pittiruti M, Snoswell AM, and others: Plasma carnitine levels and urinary carnitine excretion during sepsis, *J Parenteral Enteral Nutr* 9:483, 1985.

Nielson CP, Hindson DA: Inhibition of polymorphonuclear leukocyte respiratory burst by elevated glucose concentrations in vitro, *Diabetes* 38:1031, 1989.

Nightingale JM: The medical management of intestinal failure: methods to reduce the severity, *Proc Nutr Soc* 62:703, 2003.

Ockenga J, Suttmann U, Selberg O, and others: Percutaneous endoscopic gastrostomy in AIDS and control patients: risks and outcome, *Am J Gastroenterol* 91:1817, 1996.

Patterson BW, Nguyen T, Pierre E, and others: Urea and protein metabolism in burned children: effect of dietary protein intake, *Metabolism* 46:573, 1997.

Peck MD, Kessler M, Cairns BA, and others: Early enteral nutrition does not decrease hypermetabolism associated with burn injury, *J Trauma* 57:1143, 2004.

Peng X, Yan H, You Z, and others: Effects of enteral supplementation with glutamine granules on intestinal mucosal barrier function in severe burned patients, *Burns* 30:135, 2004.

Rodriguez DJ, Clevenger FW: Successful enteral refeeding after massive small bowel resection, *West J Med* 159:192, 1993.

Ruppin DC, Middleton WRJ: Clinical use of medium-chain triglycerides, *Drugs* 20:216, 1980.

Saffle J, Wiebke G, Jennings K, and others: Randomized trial of immune-enhancing enteral nutrition in burn patients, *J Trauma* 42:793, 1997.

Schuette SA, Knowles JB, Ford HE: Effect of lactose or its component sugars on jejunal calcium absorption in adult man, *Am J Clin Nutr* 50:5: 1084, 1989.

Scolapio JS: A review of the trends in the use of enteral and parenteral nutrition support, *J Clin Gastroenterol* 38:403, 2005.

Sheridan RL: A great constitutional disturbance, *N Engl J Med* 345:1271, 2001.

Skipper A, Marian MA: Parenteral nutrition. In: Gottschlich MM, Matarese LE, Shronts EP, editors: *Nutrition support dietetics core curriculum*, ed 2, Silver Spring, MD, 1993, Aspen.

Stacpoole PW, Alig J, Ammon L, and others: Dose-response effects of dietary marine oil on carbohydrate and lipid metabolism in normal subjects and patients with hypertriglyceridemia, *Metabolism* 38(10): 946, 1989.

Tolia V, Lin C-H, Kuhns LR: Gastric emptying using three different formulas in infants with gastroesophageal reflux, *J Ped Gastr Nutr* 15:297, 1992.

Tsuei BJ, Bernard AC, Barksdale AR, and others: Supplemental enteral arginine is metabolized to ornithine in injured patients, *J Surg Res* 123:17, 2005.

Wah N, Cheung B, Zaccaria C, and others: Hyperglycemia is associated with adverse outcomes in patients receiving total parenteral nutrition, *Diabetes Care* 28:2367, 2004.

White AC, Thannickal VJ, Fanburg BL: Glutathione in human disease, *J Nutr Bichem* 5:218, 1994.

Wischmeyer PE, Lynch J, Liedel J, and others: Glutamine administration reduces Gram-negative bacteremia in severely burned patients: a prospective, randomized, double-blind trial versus isonitrogenous control, *Crit Care Med* 29(11): 2075, 2001.

Wolfe RR, Goodenough RD, Burke JF, and others: Response of protein and urea kinetics in burn patients to different levels of protein intake, *Ann Surg* 197:163, 1983.

Worthley LIG, Fishlock RC, Snoswell AM: Carnitine deficiency with hyperbilirubinemia, generalized skeletal muscle weakness and reactive hypoglycemia in a patient on long-term parenteral nutrition: treatment with intravenous L-carnitine, *J Parenteral Enteral Nutr* 7:176, 1983.

Xian-Li H Q-JM, Jiang-guo L: Effect of total parenteral nutrition (TPN) with and without glutamine dipeptide supplementation on outcome in severe acute pancreatitis (SAP), *Clin Nutr Suppl* 1(43), 2004.

Zaloga GP: Physiologic effects of peptide-based enteral formulas, *Nutr Clin Pract* 5:235, 1990.

Zeigler TR F-EC, Griffth P: Parenteral nutrition supplemented with alanyl-glutamine dipeptide decreases infectious morbidity and improves organ function in critically ill post-operative patients: results of a double-blind, randomized, controlled pilot study, *Nutr Clin Pract* 28, 2004.

Zhou YP, Jiang ZM, Sun YH, and others: The effect of supplemental enteral glutamine on plasma levels, gut function, and outcome in severe burns: a randomized, double-blind, controlled clinical trial, *J Parenter Enteral Nutr* 27:241, 2003.

Zhou YJZ, Sun Y: The effects of supplemental glutamine dipeptide on gut integrity and clinical outcomes after major escharectomy in severe burns: a randomized, double blind, controlled clinical trial, *Clin Nutr* 1, 2004.

COAGULOPATHY IN THE CRITICALLY ILL PATIENT

Michael B. Streiff, MD

Hemostatic defects are a common problem among critically ill patients. One recent prospective observational study found that almost 14% of patients in a combined medical/surgical intensive care unit had abnormal hemostasis. Consequently, a working knowledge of the diagnostic evaluation and management of patients with hemostatic disorders is essential for physicians caring for critically ill patients. The purpose of this chapter is to review (1) a brief description of the hemostatic system; (2) a common-sense approach to critically ill patients with abnormal bleeding; and (3) an approach to the diagnosis and management of platelet, coagulation, and vascular disorders.

A MODEL OF HEMOSTASIS

Hemostasis is the end result of the coordinated and cooperative efforts of the endogenous procoagulant and anticoagulant proteins, the fibrinolytic proteins, platelets, and the vessel wall. Defects in any one of these elements can predispose the affected individual to pathologic hemorrhage or thrombosis. Hemostasis is initiated by vascular damage that exposes subendothelial collagen and tissue factor. Platelets avidly bind to collagen via platelet membrane glycoproteins and von Willebrand factor to form a platelet monolayer at the site of injury. This event triggers platelet activation and the release of platelet granule components that activate surrounding platelets, promoting platelet aggregation, formation of a multilayer platelet plug, and vasoconstriction.

Although it is now known that the classical concept of the coagulation cascade does not accurately represent the true sequence of chemical reactions that occurs during coagulation in vivo, this model, although imperfect, remains useful for clinically assessing patients for coagulation defects. Therefore I use the model to describe coagulation in vivo and as a basis for the approach to patients with coagulation disorders (Fig. 1). Simultaneous to the platelet activation events just described, exposed tissue factor complexes with circulating activated factor VII to initiate clot formation through activation of factor X, the first serine protease in the classical common pathway. Activated factor X subsequently activates small amounts of prothrombin to form thrombin that initiates fibrin clot formation and, importantly, activates factor XI

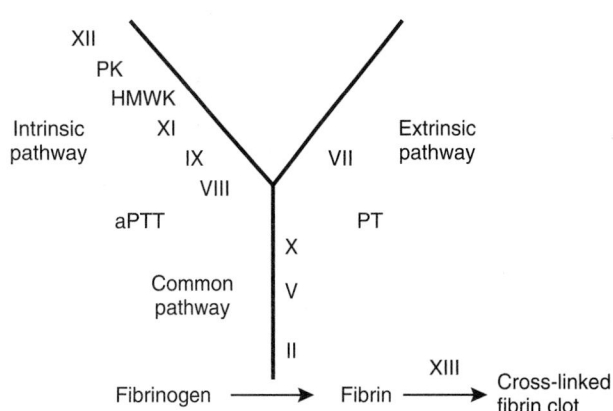

Figure I The coagulation cascade. *APTT,* Activated partial thromboplastin time; *HMWK,* high-molecular-weight kininogen; *PK,* prekallikrein; *PT,* prothrombin time.

and the cofactor protein factor VIII in the intrinsic pathway, as well as the common pathway cofactor protein factor V and platelets. The potent amplification of factor X activation provided by the intrinsic pathway "tenase" complex (activated factors IX and VIII) leads to an exponential increase in thrombin generation that is essential to production of sufficient fibrin clot and activated platelets to reinforce the accumulating platelet plug. The prothrombotic components of the hemostatic mechanism are balanced by endogenous antithrombotic proteins such as antithrombin (III) (which inhibits serine proteases such as thrombin—a reaction accelerated several-thousand-fold by heparin), and the vitamin K–dependent protein C and protein S complex that inactivates the critical cofactor proteins, factor VIII and factor V. The fibrinolytic proteins provide additional balance to the hemostatic mechanism by digesting and remodeling existing fibrin clot to focus clot formation at the site of vascular injury and maintain vascular patency.

AN INITIAL APPROACH TO THE CRITICALLY ILL PATIENT WITH A COAGULOPATHY

Optimal management of the critically ill patient with bleeding requires that the clinician determine the answer to one question: what is the etiology of this patient's bleeding disorder—a coagulation factor deficiency, a disorder of platelet function, a vascular defect, or a disorder of platelets and coagulation factors? After the answer to this question is known, the physician can initiate rational therapy (Table 1). Helpful information regarding the etiology of bleeding can come from the patient's presentation. Bleeding from one location (the surgical site, the site of a recent invasive procedure) is usually due to an anatomic vascular defect and not from a systemic disorder of hemostasis. Sudden-onset bleeding, large-volume blood loss over short time intervals, and bright red blood also characterize surgical bleeding. Conversely, bleeding from multiple locations, slow and persistent oozing, and temporally delayed

Table 1: Evaluation of the Bleeding Patient

1. Assess character of bleeding—rapid, single location, multifocal, persistent oozing:
   Surgical bleeding—rapid blood loss, localized to surgical site, bright red blood or pulsatile blood loss;
   Coagulopathic bleeding—multifocal, persistent slow blood loss

2. Send blood for hemoglobin, platelet count, activated partial thromboplastin time, prothrombin time, thrombin time, fibrinogen, D-dimer, mixing studies, heparin contamination

3. Review preoperative laboratory results (including liver and renal function)

4. Review patient's perioperative medications: antiplatelet agents (aspirin, ticlopidine, clopidogrel, ketorolac, IIb/IIIa inhibitors); anticoagulants (unfractionated heparin, low-molecular-weight heparin, fondaparinux, lepirudin, argatroban, bivalirudin, warfarin); vitamins/dietary supplements/herbal remedies (vitamin E, omega 3 fatty acids, garlic, ginkgo biloba, ginger, willow bark, etc.)

5. Review patients medical/surgical and family history:
   Platelet type bleeding—epistaxis, easy bruising, menorrhagia, dental bleeding;
   Coagulation factor bleeding—hemarthrosis, hematomas, soft-tissue bleeds;
   Vessel wall disorder—easy bruisability, joint laxity, poor wound healing

6. Review compatibility of any intraoperative transfusions

hemorrhage (from invasive procedures) generally indicate the presence of a systemic coagulopathy. Petechiae (small red spots, usually <3 mm in diameter, that do not blanch with pressure) indicate a defect in the number or function of platelets. Large hematomas or ecchymoses that elevated the skin surface or blood collections in deep tissue locations are characteristic of a coagulation factor defect.

If the patient has recently undergone a surgical procedure, the type of procedure should be considered in the evaluation. The presence of residual heparin following protamine reversal in patients returning from a cardiac bypass procedure can cause bleeding and abnormal coagulation test results. These patients can also develop quantitative or qualitative defects in platelets resulting from the cardiac bypass procedure. Therefore the approach to these patients should focus on assessing the character of the bleeding (surgical versus coagulopathic) and the results of tests evaluating the patient for the presence of residual heparin or coagulation factor deficiencies (activated partial thromboplastin time, thrombin time, heparin neutralized thrombin time, Hepzyme), thrombocytopenia (complete blood count), and, perhaps, platelet dysfunction (Platelet Function Analyzer 100, PFA-100; Dade Behring, Deerfield, IL).

It is also important to review the patient's medical and surgical history for disorders that can affect hemostasis or bleeding difficulties after invasive procedures. Patients with renal or hepatic disorders often have abnormal hemostasis because of the impact of these disease processes on platelet function and numbers and coagulation factor levels. Patients with platelet disorders typically suffer from bleeding that affects mucosal sites (history of menorrhagia, epistaxis, gum bleeding), whereas coagulation defects such as hemophilia typically trigger deep-tissue bleeding or hemarthroses. It is also important to get an accurate list of a patient's prescription and nonprescription medications including vitamins, supplements and herbal remedies because these can significantly influence hemostasis. If these details are not available in the medical record, interviewing patients (if possible) or family members can be revealing.

Simultaneous with this evaluation, basic screening tests of coagulation factor; platelet; and, if appropriate on the basis of the history and physical examination, fibrinolytic function, should be ordered. The basic tests of coagulation factor function include the activated partial thromboplastin time (aPTT), the prothrombin time (PT), the thrombin time (TT), and a fibrinogen level. Platelet testing includes the platelet count (usually available as part of a complete blood count) and the bleeding time or platelet function analyzer test (PFA-100). Thromboelastography is increasingly being used in some patient settings (liver transplantation, cardiac bypass) to assess patients for hyperfibrinolysis. Patient blood samples for hemostatic testing should be obtained, whenever possible, by a peripheral blood stick rather than through a central venous catheter to avoid the common pitfall of heparin contamination that can confuse diagnosis and lead to unnecessary blood product use. In the next sections, I review the commonly used tests to assess hemostasis and then the clinical presentation and management of platelet, coagulation factor, and vascular wall disorders.

HEMOSTATIC TESTING FOR THE CRITICALLY ILL PATIENT

Coagulation Tests

The most commonly used tests of hemostasis are the aPTT, PT, the TT, and a fibrinogen level. More specialized yet important coagulation tests to understand include the D-dimer assay, mixing studies, coagulation factor levels, heparin contamination (Hepzyme; Dade Behring) testing, and von Willebrand factor testing (Table 2). The aPTT measures the function of factors in the intrinsic pathway

Table 2: Laboratory Tests of Hemostasis

Activated Partial Thromboplastin Time (aPTT)

Used to identify deficiencies or inhibitors of factors in the intrinsic pathway (factors XII, XI, IX and VIII, HMWK and PK) and common pathway (factors X, V, II [prothrombin] and fibrinogen)

Used to monitor unfractionated heparin and direct thrombin inhibitors (lepirudin, argatroban, and bivalirudin)

Used to identify lupus inhibitors (antiphospholipid antibodies)

Prothrombin Time (PT)

Used to identify deficiencies or inhibitors of factors in the extrinsic pathway (factor VII) and common pathway (factors X, V, II [prothrombin] and fibrinogen)

Used to monitor warfarin (use the INR)

Thrombin Time (TT)

Used to identify deficiency or dysfunction of fibrinogen or thrombin inhibitors

Used to identify the presence of unfractionated heparin

Fibrinogen

A sensitive test of fibrinogen function
Insensitive to heparin

Heparin Contamination (Hepzyme, Dade Behring, Deerfield, IL)

Used to identify the presence of heparin by measuring an aPTT before and after heparinase treatment of patient sample

Mixing Studies

Used to discriminate between deficiency states and inhibitors by assessing the correction of a prolonged PT or aPTT after addition of one part or four parts patient plasma to one part normal pooled plasma

Correction of abnormal assay = deficiency state
Failure to correct = factor inhibitor or lupus inhibitor

Factor Activity Assays

Use to determine the activity level of a specific factor using plasma deficient in the factor of interest and the PT or aPTT

D-Dimer Assays

Used to detect D-dimers, fragments of crosslinked fibrin that have been digested by plasmin, a marker of disseminated intravascular coagulation or active thrombus formation

Template Bleeding Time

Rough in vivo assessment of platelet function

Platelet Function Analyzer 100 (Dade Behring)
An in vitro assay of platelet function

Platelet Aggregometry

Used to assess platelet aggregation and secretion in response to platelet agonists

Von Willebrand Antigen assay

Used to measure the amount of von Willebrand protein

Ristocetin Cofactor Assay

Used to measure von Willebrand factor function

Thromboelastography

A global test of coagulation, platelet, and fibrinolytic function that is particularly useful for identifying patients with hyperfibrinolysis

INR, International normalized ratio.

(factors XII, XI, IX and VIII, as well as prekallikrein and high-molecular-weight kininogen) and the common pathway (see Fig. 1). The aPTT is performed by adding phospholipid (an in vitro surrogate for activated platelet membranes) and an activator of factor XII, as well as calcium (to reverse the sodium citrate anticoagulant in the blood collection tube) and measuring the time to clot formation. Unfractionated heparin and direct thrombin inhibitors are measured using the aPTT.

The PT measures the function of the extrinsic pathway (factor VII) and the common pathway (factors X and V, prothrombin, and fibrinogen) (see Fig. 1). The PT is performed by adding a source of tissue factor and phospholipids (an in vitro surrogate for activated platelet membranes), also called thromboplastin, and calcium and then measuring the time required for clot formation to occur. In addition to assessing disorders of the extrinsic and common pathway factors, the PT is also used to measure warfarin anticoagulation. For patients on warfarin, the results of the PT are usually expressed as an international normalized ratio (INR) value, which normalizes PT results for the sensitivity of the laboratory's thromboplastin to reductions in factor levels compared with an international reference standard. The INR should not be used to express the results of the PT for patients not on warfarin.

The TT is useful for assessing the functional status of fibrinogen, which is not as sensitively measured by the PT or the aPTT. The TT is performed by adding thrombin and calcium to the citrated patient plasma sample and measuring the time to clot formation. The TT is exquisitely sensitive to heparin contamination. Rare antibodies directed against thrombin (thrombin inhibitors) can also result in an abnormal thrombin time. The results of the TT can be confirmed by obtaining a fibrinogen assay. This functional test of fibrinogen is performed by adding a large amount of thrombin to the patient plasma sample and measuring the time to clot formation. There is a linear relationship in this assay between the time to clot formation and the concentration of clottable fibrinogen. Fibrinogen assays are significantly less sensitive to the presence of heparin because of the increased amount of thrombin used in the test.

When a patient's aPTT, PT or TT is prolonged, it is important to determine whether the abnormal result is due to a deficiency state (such as hemophilia A) or an inhibitor (such as a factor VIII inhibitor). Deficiency states will respond to factor replacement therapy (factor concentrates, fresh frozen plasma, cryoprecipitate), whereas inhibitors will not respond. This distinction can be made by mixing the patient's plasma sample with normal pooled plasma. If a factor deficiency is responsible, then a 1:1 mix with normal pooled plasma will correct the abnormal clotting time. Conversely, if a specific factor inhibitor or a lupus inhibitor is present, the addition of normal plasma will not correct the clotting time. Coagulation laboratories often perform 4:1 mixes of patient plasma and normal pooled plasma to detect low-titer inhibitors.

Specific factor levels are performed to identify the presence of particular factor deficiency states such as hemophilia A (factor VIII deficiency). These assays are performed by adding patient plasma to factor-deficient plasma. Consequently, the clotting time of such a mix is dependent on the patient sample's contribution of the particular factor of interest. Heparin contamination is assessed by measuring the aPTT of a plasma sample before and after addition of heparinase, an enzyme that digests heparin. In the presence of significant heparin contamination, the aPTT after heparinase addition is significantly shorter than the baseline sample. D-dimers are a fragment of cross-linked fibrin that is produced by lysis of fibrin clot. It is a marker of clot formation that has been used as a sensitive test for the presence of disseminated intravascular coagulation and acute thrombosis. D-dimer assays generally use antibodies directed against this fragment to measure its concentration in plasma by enzyme-linked immunosorbent assays or antibody-coated bead agglutination.

Platelet Tests

Common tests of platelet function include platelet numbers as assessed in a complete blood count, the template bleeding time, the PFA-100, and platelet aggregation studies (see Table 2). Blood cell analyzers such as the Coulter counter can accurately assess the number and size of platelets in a volume of blood. In addition to the absolute number of platelets, the mean platelet volume is useful because a large mean platelet volume suggests the presence of a large number of immature platelets (young platelets are larger), such as might be seen in thrombocytopenic disorders associated with excessive platelet destruction. The template bleeding time (TBT) is a rough guide of platelet function reflecting the importance of platelet function to primary hemostasis. The TBT is performed by making a standardized incision in the forearm with a razor-blade-containing template device with a blood pressure cuff inflated proximally to 40 mm Hg and measuring the time required for hemostasis to occur. Unfortunately this result can be influenced by many factors other than platelet function, including operator technique and tissue vascularity.

The shortcomings of the TBT led to the development of more standardized and convenient tests of platelet function such as the PFA-100. The PFA-100 assesses platelet function by aspirating whole blood at high shear rates through perforated membranes coated with the platelet agonists collagen and epinephrine or collagen and adenosine diphosphate (ADP). The time required for the aperture in the membrane to occlude correlates with platelet function. Both the TBT and the PFA-100 will be abnormal in patients with thrombocytopenia (platelet count <80–100,000/μl); therefore the results of these tests cannot be used to assess platelet function in patients with platelet counts at or below this level. The PFA-100 appears to be more sensitive and reproducible than the TBT, but neither test has proved useful in predicting surgical blood loss.

Platelet aggregation studies assess platelet function by exposing platelet-rich plasma or whole blood to different platelet agonists such as thrombin, epinephrine, ADP, and ristocetin. Platelet aggregation is assessed by measuring the change in electrical impedance or light transmission through the sample after agonist addition. Platelet granule release can be assessed by measuring the amount of granule constituents such as ATP released into the test solution on platelet activation. Thrombocytopenia (platelets <80,000/μl) yields abnormal test results. Because platelet aggregation studies require considerable expertise to perform and interpret, they are not available at all medical centers or on an emergent basis. Nevertheless, platelet aggregation studies remain an invaluable test in the assessment of platelet function disorders.

Fibrinolytic Tests

The fibrinolytic system can be measured by assessing the amount and function of fibrinolytic proteins such as plasminogen, alpha-2-antiplasmin and plasminogen activator inhibitor 1 (PAI-1). In recent years, there has been a resurgence of interest in the use of thromboelastography in the assessment of the total hemostatic mechanism. This test can assess global function of clotting proteins, platelets and the fibrinolytic system. It has found use as a point-of-care test to identify patients with decreased coagulation of platelet function or hyperfibrinolysis in liver transplantation and cardiac surgery.

PLATELET DISORDERS

Platelet disorders can be categorized as being quantitative (characterized by a reduced number of normally functioning platelets) or qualitative (characterized by the presence of dysfunctional platelets) (Table 3). Because platelets play an essential role in primary hemostasis, patients with platelet disorders often bleed during or soon after invasive procedures. Findings typical of platelet dysfunction include a history of mucosal bleeding (epistaxis, gingival bleeding, menorrhagia) or easy bruising and petechiae or purpura on physical examination. For most surgical procedures, a platelet count above 50,000/μl is adequate for hemostasis. For neurosurgery or cardiac surgery, platelet counts in excess of 100,000/μl are often preferred. In a patient without bleeding and no invasive procedure planned, a platelet count transfusion trigger of 10,000/μl is often used to guide transfusion therapy. A higher target of 20,000/μl is used for febrile patients, given their more rapid platelet turnover. In the typical 70-kg patient, an increment of 5000/μl is expected for each random donor unit transfused. In platelet disorders characterized by platelet destruction, platelet increments in response to transfusion are negligible or short-lived (or both). Nevertheless, platelet transfusions should never be withheld for this reason in

Table 3: Platelet Disorders

Quantitative (Thrombocytopenia)	Qualitative (Platelet Dysfunction)
Decreased production	**Congenital platelet dysfunction**
Vitamin deficiencies (vitamin B12, folate deficiency)	Bernard-Soulier syndrome
Bone marrow disease (aplastic anemia, leukemia, myelodysplastic syndrome, etc.)	Glanzmann's thrombasthenia
Drugs (ethanol, chemotherapy)	Storage pool diseases (e.g., gray platelet syndrome)
Infection (HIV, tuberculosis) Liver failure	Platelet-type von Willebrand disease
Increased destruction	**Acquired platelet dysfunction**
Immune thrombocytopenic purpura	Drugs (acetylsalicylic acid, ticlopidine, clopidogrel, nonsteroidal anti-inflammatory drug)
Infection	Uremia
Disseminated intravascular coagulation	Liver disease
Drugs (heparin, quinine, glycoprotein IIb/IIIa inhibitors, etc.)	Postcardiopulmonary bypass
Thrombotic thrombocytopenic purpura/hemolytic uremic syndrome (TTP/HUS)	Primary thrombocytosis (polycythemia rubra vera, essential thrombocythemia)
Posttransfusion purpura	
Catastrophic antiphospholipid syndrome	
Dilutional (massive transfusions)	
Sequestration (hypersplenism)	
"Pseudo-thrombocytopenia"	

HIV, Human immunodeficiency virus.

urgent situations associated with significant bleeding caused by thrombocytopenia.

Quantitative Platelet Disorders

Acquired Quantitative Platelet Disorders

Quantitative platelet disorders can be rapidly identified with a complete blood cell count. These disorders can result from decreased production, increased destruction, splenic sequestration, or dilution associated with massive transfusions (see Table 3). Although most laboratories confirm low platelet counts (platelets <50,000/μl) by visual inspection of a peripheral smear, it is essential for the clinician to make sure this procedure has been performed to avoid being misled by the entity of "pseudo-thrombocytopenia." Pseudo-thrombocytopenia is caused by antibodies that aggregate platelets in the presence of sodium ethylenediaminetetraacetic acid (the anticoagulant used in blood collection tubes for blood count measurement), resulting in significant platelet undercounting. Review of the peripheral blood smear and measurement of platelet counts in blood collected in sodium citrate or sodium heparin are diagnostic.

If true thrombocytopenia has been established, identification of the primary etiology of the thrombocytopenia is essential to selection of the appropriate therapy. Decreased platelet production is often associated with abnormalities in other counts (anemia or leukopenia), reflecting a diffuse disruption of normal marrow function. Disorders associated with decreased platelet production include acute leukemia, aplastic anemia, myelodysplastic syndrome, myelofibrosis, vitamin B_{12} or folate deficiency, liver disease, and exposure to myelotoxic substances such as chemotherapeutic agents and alcohol (see Table 3). A hematologist should be called if thrombocytopenia caused by decreased production is suspected to assist in management. Treatment consists of platelet transfusions until definitive therapy targeted at the underlying defect can be initiated.

Dilutional thrombocytopenia can result when patients receive large volumes of blood during resuscitation. Thrombocytopenia and abnormal coagulation tests result because packed red cell units retain only small volumes of plasma (25-50 ml/U) and platelets. This syndrome is most commonly seen in patients with massive gastrointestinal bleeding or trauma. One study found that 75% of patients who received 20 or more units of red cells within a 24-hour period developed significant thrombocytopenia (platelet counts less than 50,000/μl). No patients receiving less than 20 U of red cells developed platelet counts in this range. However, the use of prespecified triggers (e.g., six to eight random donor platelet units or one plate-letpheresis unit and 4 U of fresh frozen plasma [FFP] for every 10 U of blood transfused) for platelet and FFP transfusion should be avoided. Bone marrow and hepatic function differ substantially among patients. Therefore transfusion practice should be guided by regular measurement of platelet counts and screening coagulation studies and not formulas. Patients with platelet counts less than 50,000/μl and recent surgery or bleeding should be transfused with one to two pheresis (or six to twelve random donor) units of platelets. Routine measurement of the platelet count to assess response to transfusions and determine the need for additional blood products is essential because many patients with dilutional thrombocytopenia caused by massive bleeding also have reduced platelet survival.

Consumptive thrombocytopenia is a much more common reason for thrombocytopenia in the critically ill patient. Common causes of consumptive thrombocytopenia are sepsis, drug-induced immune thrombocytopenia, disseminated intravascular coagulation (DIC), and immune thrombocytopenic purpura (ITP). Review of the patient's medical history, medication lists, microbiology, and coagulation test results are frequently useful in pinpointing the cause. Sepsis can be associated with rapid (within hours) dramatic reductions in platelet numbers that are coincident with clinical manifestations of bacteremia. Therapy should focus on identification of the

bacteria responsible, provision of broad-spectrum antibiotics directed at the most likely and serious pathogens, and blood product support. In severe cases of sepsis, particularly cases associated with gram-negative organisms and large amounts of lipopolysaccharide release, DIC can occur, heralded by consumptive thrombocytopenia and coagulopathy accompanied by thrombocytopenia and abnormalities in screening coagulation tests (PT, aPTT, fibrinogen), as well as elevations of D-dimer levels. Therapy should be multidimensional, directed at the proximate cause of DIC and supportive to correct the thrombocytopenia and coagulopathy.

Drug-induced thrombocytopenia is an increasingly common cause of thrombocytopenia that must be considered in any critically ill patient developing thrombocytopenia. In general, drug-induced thrombocytopenia usually occurs within the first 2 weeks of drug exposure. Therefore identification of possible agents should focus on drugs started within the last 14 days. However, given the large number of medications to which critically ill patients are exposed, the list of potential suspects can be large. Although laboratory testing to identify causative agents is available, it is generally time consuming and available only through reference laboratories. A list of medications commonly associated with thrombocytopenia is given in Table 4. The best approach to drug-induced thrombocytopenia is to eliminate potential suspects promptly. In severe cases, intravenous immunoglobulin (IVIG), anti-D immunoglobulin (Winrho SDF; Baxter Healthcare, Deerfield, IL), and to a lesser extent, corticosteroids, can be useful therapeutic maneuvers in severely affected patients. When using IVIG, it is important to use low-osmolality products, particularly in patients at heightened risk for renal toxicity (preexisting renal dysfunction, diabetic and elderly patients). Anti-D should be avoided in patients with concomitant autoimmune hemolytic anemia or positive direct antiglobulin testing.

Among causes of medication associated thrombocytopenia, identification of heparin-induced thrombocytopenia (HIT) is particularly important. HIT is an antibody-mediated consumptive form of thrombocytopenia that occurs in 1% to 5% of patients, most commonly after 4 to 14 days of heparin therapy, and is associated with a substantial risk of thromboembolism (50% risk at 30 days). The diagnosis can be confirmed with laboratory testing for

Table 4: Drug Associated Thrombocytopenia

Drug-Associated Immune Thrombocytopenia	Drug-Associated TTP/HUS
Unfractionated heparin	Ticlopidine
Low-molecular-weight heparin	Mitomycin C
Quinine/quinidine	Cyclosporin
Rifampin	Tacrolimus
Trimethoprim/sulfamethoxazole	Cisplatin
Acetaminophen	Gemcitabine
Digoxin	Quinine
Danazol	
Vancomycin	
Abciximab	
Eptifibatide	
Amiodarone	
Clopidogrel	
Ticlopidine	

TTP/HUS, Thrombotic thrombocytopenic-purpura/hemolytic uremic syndrome.

Note: This list includes common causes of drug-associated thrombocytopenia but is by no means all inclusive.

HIT antibodies. Any patient suspected to have HIT should avoid all heparin (and low-molecular-weight heparin [LMWH]) exposure and be treated with a direct thrombin inhibitor. Platelet transfusions should be avoided because they are ineffective and may precipitate thrombotic complications. The presence of subclinical thrombosis should be sought with routine screening duplex ultrasound on diagnosis because half of patients diagnosed with HIT have asymptomatic thrombosis, and the presence of thrombosis changes the duration of warfarin therapy. Because HIT is associated with a high incidence of thrombosis within 30 days of diagnosis, warfarin therapy for at least a month is recommended for patients diagnosed with HIT. Warfarin should not be initiated until platelet counts have recovered to normal levels because early warfarin therapy has been associated with extensive venous thrombosis and gangrene.

Immune thrombocytopenic purpura (ITP) is caused by antibodies directed at platelet surface glycoproteins, such as glycoprotein IIb/IIIa or Ib/IX. These antibodies precipitate platelet destruction in the reticuloendothelial system (spleen, liver, bone marrow). Patients with autoimmune disorders such as systemic lupus erythematosus or viral infections such as human immunodeficiency virus (HIV) or hepatitis C are at higher risk for ITP. Typical ITP patients have significant thrombocytopenia (platelet counts <20,000/μl) but a normal hematocrit and white blood cell count. Direct platelet antibody testing demonstrates the presence of antiplatelet antibodies, and bone marrow examinations reveal normal numbers of platelet progenitor cells (megakaryocytes). Not surprisingly, platelet transfusions are generally ineffective but should not be withheld in the setting of life-threatening bleeding. Active therapies include intravenous immunoglobulin, anti-D immunoglobulin (Winrho SDF) or corticosteroids. Rituximab (Rituxan; Genentech, South San Francisco, CA) and splenectomy are highly active chronic therapy for persistent disease.

Rare consumptive causes of thrombocytopenia are thrombotic thrombocytopenic purpura/hemolytic uremic syndrome (TTP/HUS), posttransfusion purpura, and catastrophic antiphospholipid syndrome. The most common form of TTP results from an autoantibody directed at the von Willebrand factor (VWF) cleaving protease, a protein that normally degrades larger, more adhesive von Willebrand factor multimers into smaller, less active fragments. In its absence, large von Willebrand factor multimers accumulate, triggering the spontaneous formation of platelet aggregates that cause consumptive thrombocytopenia, a mechanical hemolytic anemia (from the physical cleavage of red cells as they traverse the microcirculation), as well as microvascular plugging, ischemia–induced renal and neurological dysfunction. Diagnosis rests on clinical recognition of these features, confirmation of a microangiopathic picture on the peripheral smear, and laboratory testing confirming the absence of the vWF cleaving protease in the patient's plasma. Plasmapheresis is the most effective form of treatment. Immunosuppression in the form of corticosteroids or Rituxan is also likely beneficial. Platelet transfusions should be avoided except in the setting of life-threatening bleeding because they can precipitate a dramatic worsening of the patient's clinical condition. Other causes of TTP/HUS that should be considered in the critically ill patient are drug-induced TTP/HUS, associated most commonly with calcineurin inhibitors (cyclosporine, tacrolimus) used for organ transplantation immunosuppression and less commonly with chemotherapeutic agents such as mitomycin C and gemcitabine (see Table 4). Calcineurin inhibitor TTP/HUS usually responds to discontinuation of the offending agent and employment of non-cross-reactive immunosuppressive agents. Chemotherapy-associated TTP/HUS is often treated with plasmapheresis and Staphylococcal protein A columns, although results are less satisfactory.

Posttransfusion purpura is a rare, antibody-mediated, consumptive form of thrombocytopenia that occurs in patients after transfusion with blood products. This rare, consumptive thrombocytopenia in the vast majority of cases affects women because they are exposed to the causative antigen during childbirth. A typical presentation is the development of sudden, dramatic, and severe thrombocytopenia overnight approximately 1 week after a blood product transfusion. Identification of antibodies directed against the causal antigen and typing the affected patient's platelets are diagnostic. Platelet transfusions are ineffective and can cause severe allergic reactions in affected individuals. IVIG has proven effective in shortening the course of thrombocytopenia.

Catastrophic antiphospholipid syndrome (CAS) is another uncommon cause of thrombocytopenia that can have devastating consequences. Affected patients typically have systemic lupus erythematosus or another autoimmune disorder associated with antiphospholipid antibodies or the primary form of antiphospholipid syndrome unassociated with another rheumatologic condition. Antiphospholipid syndrome is a hypercoagulable disorder associated with recurrent venous or arterial thromboembolism (or both), recurrent pregnancy losses, and thrombocytopenia. CAS is typically triggered by discontinuation of immunosuppressive medications for associated autoimmune disorders, severe infections, discontinuation of anticoagulation, or major surgery. Clinical manifestations include disseminated microvascular thrombosis with evidence of peripheral ischemia, multiorgan dysfunction (including renal and neurologic dysfunction), and consumptive thrombocytopenia. Diagnosis is made on the basis of the characteristic clinical presentation and laboratory testing demonstrating the presence of a lupus inhibitor or anticardiolipin antibodies. Multimodality treatment is essential for optimal outcomes and includes anticoagulation, immunosuppression with high-dose corticosteroids, and plasmapheresis.

Splenic Sequestration

Thrombocytopenia may also result from splenic sequestration of platelets in patients with significantly enlarged spleens. Normally, approximately one third of the circulating platelet mass resides in the spleen. This proportion may grow substantially in patients with significant splenomegaly and result in moderately reduced platelet counts, as well as lower than expected responses to platelet transfusions. Splenic sequestration is commonly seen in patients with liver cirrhosis and hypersplenism caused by hematologic disorders such as myelofibrosis. Although splenectomy or operative portosystemic shunting may result in a reduction in the severity of thrombocytopenia, production defects also contribute to thrombocytopenia in these patients; therefore such major surgical procedures are rarely considered solely for treatment of thrombocytopenia due to splenic sequestration.

Inherited Quantitative Platelet Disorders

Inherited platelet disorders are a rare cause of bleeding in critically ill patients because these conditions are often identified before surgical procedures. Inherited aplastic anemia syndromes, such as Fanconi's anemia and inherited disorders affecting platelet production, such as inherited amegakaryocytic thrombocytopenia, the thrombocytopenia with absent radius (TAR) syndrome, and Wiskott-Aldrich syndrome (WAS), result in chronic thrombocytopenia of varying severity. These patients can be identified by the presence of reduced peripheral blood counts and abnormal bone marrow examinations showing reductions in all three progenitor cell lines and hypersensitivity to DNA-damaging agents (Fanconi's anemia) or selective reductions in megakaryocytes, the platelet progenitor cells (inherited amegakaryocytic thrombocytopenia, TAR syndrome). The WAS is an X-linked disorder characterized by microthrombocytopenia, for example, the production of reduced numbers of small platelets, eczema, and immunodeficiency. Any boy with thrombocytopenia and a small mean platelet volume on his complete blood count should be suspected as having WAS.

Qualitative Platelet Disorders

Acquired Platelet Dysfunction—Drug-Induced Platelet Dysfunction

Platelet dysfunction can also contribute to bleeding in critically ill patients. The most common qualitative disorders of platelet function are acquired (see Table 3). Use of medications or supplements with antiplatelet effects are a common cause of unanticipated surgical bleeding. Medications such as aspirin, clopidogrel, or ticlopidine should be discontinued at least 10 to 14 days before surgical procedures in most instances. This rule also applies to all supplements and herbal remedies, particularly vitamin E and omega-3 fatty acids, which are known to have antiplatelet effects. Exposure to these medications should be considered in any critically ill patient with bleeding. Although the TBT and the PFA-100 can measure the effects of antiplatelet medications, these tests should not be relied on to identify patients at increased risk of bleeding with an invasive procedures because these tests are not sensitive or specific enough for this purpose. In patients with significant bleeding, platelet transfusions, desmopressin (1-desamino-8-D-arginine vasopressin, or DDAVP), an arginine vasopressin analogue that induces factor VIII and von Willebrand factor secretion, or both these agents can be used to improve hemostasis in the setting of antiplatelet therapy. In life-threatening bleeding, recombinant human factor VIIa (NovoSeven; Novo Nordisk, Princeton, NJ) has been used successfully to treat patients with acquired platelet dysfunction. Given the expense of this agent, it should be used for this purpose only when conventional therapy has been ineffective.

Uremia/Myeloproliferative Disorders

Uremia is a common cause of platelet dysfunction among critically ill patients. The bleeding tendency in patients with renal insufficiency is multifactorial. Some contributing factors include increased production of platelet inhibitory factors prostacyclin and nitric oxide by the endothelium, acquired defects in von Willebrand factor activity, decreases in platelet adhesive glycoprotein quantities on the platelet surface, anemia (red cells serve as a sink for nitric oxide), and altered clearance of antithrombotic medications (heparin, LMWH, aspirin, etc.). The TBT, the PFA-100, or both are usually prolonged in patients with uremic platelet dysfunction. Screening coagulation testing including a PT and aPTT should be included in any investigation of bleeding in a uremic patient to exclude the possibility of persistent heparinization associated with hemodialysis or acquired vitamin K deficiency. Bleeding in uremic patients can be improved by regular dialysis and increasing the hematocrit to 30% to 35% with transfusions or erythropoietin supplementation. Administration of DDAVP can also improve hemostasis caused by platelet dysfunction in dialysis patients transiently by increasing the amount of von Willebrand factor available to assist in platelet adhesion and aggregation. Cryoprecipitate is also effective but carries a risk of transfusion-borne infectious illnesses and therefore should be avoided for this purpose. Conjugated estrogens produce slower but more durable responses at the cost of hormonal side effects.

Acquired platelet dysfunction is also common among patients with chronic myeloproliferative disorders such as polycythemia vera and essential thrombocythemia in association with markedly elevated platelet counts (often exceeding 1,000,000/μl). Von Willebrand antigen levels (measures the amount of von Willebrand factor protein) and ristocetin cofactor activity (measures the function of von Willebrand factor), as well as TBT and the PFA-100, can be used to confirm the presence of this entity. Acute therapy for symptomatic patients includes administration of DDAVP or use of von Willebrand factor containing factor VIII concentrates or platelet transfusions. Cryoprecipitate should be avoided. Reduction of platelet counts with chemotherapeutic agents is often beneficial for long-term treatment.

Inherited Qualitative Platelet Disorders

Inherited qualitative platelet disorders include the Bernard-Soulier syndrome, Glanzmann's thrombasthenia, and the platelet storage pool diseases such as gray platelet syndrome. Patients with these conditions have platelet dysfunction that can vary from mild to severe. Common historical complaints include chronic epistaxis, gum bleeding, menorrhagia, easy bruisability, and excessive bleeding with invasive procedures, including dental extractions and minor surgery. The TBT and the PFA-100 are usually abnormal in these patients. In patients with severe Bernard-Soulier syndrome or Glanzmann's thrombasthenia, a TBT should probably be avoided if the diagnosis has been previously documented because TBT can be extremely prolonged and lead to significant bleeding. Platelet aggregometry and platelet flow cytometry are invaluable in the diagnosis of inherited qualitative platelet disorders and thus should be ordered for definitive diagnosis. Platelet transfusions, DDAVP, and antifibrinolytic medications such as epsilon-amino caproic acid (Amicar; Wyeth-Ayerst, Collegeville, PA) or aprotinin (Trasylol; Bayer Healthcare Pharmaceuticals, West Haven, CT) have all been used to achieve hemostasis in patients with these disorders. In general, platelet transfusions should be reserved for major surgery or serious bleeding in patients with platelet receptor disorders (Bernard-Soulier syndrome, Glanzmann's thrombasthenia) because these patients have a propensity to develop platelet alloantibodies, which can make them unresponsive to platelet transfusions in the future. Whenever possible, adjuvant hemostatic agents (epsilon aminocaproic acid, aprotinin, fibrin sealants) should be employed.

COAGULATION DISORDERS

Five Basic Patterns of Coagulation Test Results

Coagulation factor disorders are a common cause of bleeding in the critically ill patient. Similar to platelet disorders, inherited and acquired coagulation factor disorders must be considered in the differential when approaching a bleeding patient. Rapid, accurate interpretation of screening coagulation tests is key to identifying coagulation disorders. Five basic patterns of coagulation test results can be identified: (1) prolonged PT, (2) prolonged aPTT, (3) prolonged TT, (4) prolonged PT and aPTT, and (5) prolongation of all three screening tests. An isolated prolonged PT occurs only in the presence of factor VII deficiency or a factor VII inhibitor. A factor VII activity assay can be used to confirm the presence of factor VII deficiency. Factor VII inhibitors are rarely seen except in patients with inherited factor VII deficiency. The presence of an inhibitor can be identified using mixing studies that demonstrate the failure of the PT to correct after the addition of normal pooled plasma.

An isolated prolonged aPTT can be seen in association with any deficiency state or factor inhibitor affecting one of the intrinsic pathway coagulation proteins (factors XII, XI, IX, VIII, prekallikrein, and high-molecular-weight kininogen). Specific factor assays can confirm the identity of the responsible factor. Knowledge of the incidence and clinical manifestations of coagulation disorders can help to prioritize factor testing. Factor VIII deficiency (hemophilia A) is the most common intrinsic factor deficiency disorder, followed by factor IX deficiency (hemophilia B) and factor XI deficiency (hemophilia C). Therefore factor testing should proceed in this order in most patient populations. One exception is when caring for patients of Ashkenazi Jewish ethnicity, among whom the prevalence of heterozygous factor XI deficiency can be as high as 8%. Deficiency of factor XII, prekallikrein, or high-molecular-weight kininogen are not associated with a clinical bleeding disorder; therefore factor assays for these coagulation disorders should be performed later.

The only deficiency state associated with a prolonged TT is a deficiency of fibrinogen. Confirmation of this result can be obtained by ordering a fibrinogen assay. Combined prolongation of both the aPTT and the PT in the presence of a normal TT generally indicates that there is a deficiency of a common pathway factor (factor X, factor V, or prothrombin). Less commonly, this result is a consequence of factor deficiencies affecting both the extrinsic (factor VII) and intrinsic pathways (factors XII, XI, IX, VIII, prekallikrein, and high-molecular-weight kininogen). Vitamin K deficiency is an example. Likewise, prolongation of the PT, aPTT, and the TT generally represents severe fibrinogen deficiency or an inhibitor of thrombin (factor II inhibitor, heparin, etc.), although abnormalities in multiple factors could also generate this result.

Inherited Coagulation Disorders

The most common inherited factor deficiency states are the hemophilias and von Willebrand disease (Table 5). Hemophilia A (factor VIII deficiency) is an X-linked recessive trait that affects 1 in 5000 male births. Disease severity correlates closely with factor levels. The normal range for factor VIII levels is generally 50% to 150%. Severe hemophilia A is characterized by factor VIII levels less than 1% and places affected individuals at high risk for spontaneous joint and soft-tissue bleeds. People with moderate hemophilia have factor VIII levels between 1% and 5% and usually bleed after trauma or invasive procedures. Minor hemophilia patients have factor levels greater than 5% and usually bleed only after significant trauma or surgical procedures. The diagnosis of hemophilia A can be confirmed with a factor VIII assay. Factor VIII inhibitors occur in approximately 15% to 25% of severe hemophiliacs, thus mixing studies and factor VIII inhibitor assays should be assessed before surgical procedures and whenever a patient does not appear to respond appropriately to factor VIII replacement therapy. Plasma-derived and recombinant factor VIII concentrates are the principal treatment for patients with hemophilia (Tables 6 and 7). Although cryoprecipitate contains factor VIII, this product should not be used for treatment of hemophilia because it is a less concentrated source of factor VIII and is associated with a risk of transmitting bloodborne infectious diseases. Recombinant factor concentrates are generally preferred over plasma-derived concentrates for most patients because they are associated with a lower risk of transfusion-associated infections. DDAVP, which induces release of factor VIII and Von Willebrand factor, can be used for hemostasis in patients with mild hemophilia undergoing minor surgical procedures. Antifibrinolytic medications such as epsilon aminocaproic acid (Amicar) are useful adjuvant hemostatic agents for hemophilia. For major surgery, factor VIII levels should be raised to 80% to 100% preoperatively, maintained there for the first 3 days, and then maintained at 50% or more for 10 to 14 days. Daily trough factor VIII activity assays should be obtained to ensure that minimal factor VIII levels for hemostasis are maintained. For cardiac surgery and neurosurgery, trough levels should be maintained at 100% for the first 72 hours and then at 80% to 100% for the first week. Trough levels of 50% to 80% are adequate for days 8 through 14.

Factor IX deficiency (hemophilia B) is inherited in an X-linked recessive fashion and is approximately sevenfold less common than hemophilia A. Factor levels correlate with clinical severity similar to hemophilia A. Laboratory diagnosis relies on factor IX assays, and plasma-derived and recombinant factor IX concentrates are used for therapy. The duration of therapy for surgery is similar to that for patients with factor VIII deficiency. Factor IX inhibitors are much less common, affecting only 2% of patients. Allergic reactions to factor IX concentrates often herald the development of a factor IX inhibitor.

Factor XI deficiency (hemophilia C) is an uncommon disorder except in patients of Ashkenazi Jewish descent, in whom as many

Table 5: Coagulation Disorders

Inherited Coagulation Disorder	Acquired Coagulation Disorders
Von Willebrand Disease	Vitamin K deficiency
Hemophilia A (factor VIII deficiency)	Liver disease
Hemophilia B (factor IX deficiency)	Anticoagulation-associated coagulopathy
Hemophilia C (factor XI deficiency)	Unfractionated heparin
Factor VII deficiency	Low-molecular-weight heparin
Factor X deficiency	Fondaparinux
A-, hypofibrinogenemia	Direct thrombin inhibitors
Factor V deficiency	Disseminated intravascular coagulation
Factor II deficiency	Acquired factor inhibitors
Factor XII deficiency*	Factor V/thrombin inhibitors associated with bovine thrombin exposure
Factor XIII deficiency	Factor VIII inhibitors
High-molecular-weight kininogen deficiency*	Cardiac bypass coagulopathy
Prekallikrein deficiency*	Dilutional coagulopathy (massive transfusions)

*Indicates disorders that can cause a markedly prolonged activated partial thromboplastin time but do not cause clinical bleeding.

as 8% carry one mutated allele. Fortunately, most individuals have mild to moderate deficiencies of factor XI and mild bleeding symptoms. Consequently, many individuals with factor XI deficiency are first identified on preoperative testing or after developing bleeding with invasive procedures. Unlike hemophilia A and B, low factor XI levels do not always correlate with a bleeding tendency. Those patients who do bleed do so after significant trauma or major surgery. Factor XI inhibitors are rare except in patients with severe factor XI deficiency (<1%) who have been exposed to previous replacement therapy. Diagnosis is made by factor XI activity assays. Although factor XI concentrates are used in Europe, FFP is the only replacement product available in the United States. Generally, 15 ml/kg of plasma are transfused before invasive procedures. Factor XI levels of 20% to 25% are typically adequate for hemostasis. Daily assessment of factor XI levels and plasma replacement to maintain adequate factor levels for at least 3 to 5 days and 10 to 14 days are used to treat patients undergoing minor surgery and major surgery, respectively.

Von Willebrand disease (vWD) is caused by inherited autosomal deficiency of von Willebrand factor (vWF), a protein that plays a key role in platelet adhesion and serves as a carrier protein for factor VIII, protecting it from degradation by activated protein C. Reflecting its primary role in platelet function, vWD patients generally suffer mucosal bleeding (epistaxis, gum bleeding, menorrhagia, bleeding with dental surgery). The best laboratory assays for diagnosis of von Willebrand disease are the von Willebrand antigen assay, which measures the amount of von Willebrand factor protein, and the ristocetin cofactor assay or the collagen-binding assay, both of which measure vWF function. Factor VIII levels are generally normal or only mildly reduced. Thus the aPTT is not a useful screening test for vWD. Most patients with mild disease can be treated with DDAVP; however, confirmation of DDAVP response

Table 6: Treatment of Coagulation Factor Disorders

Bleeding Disorder	Target Factor Level	Plasma Product
Hemophilia A		
Minor surgery	>50% for 3–7 days	Recombinant (preferred) or plasma-derived monoclonal factor VIII concentrates
Major surgery	>80%-100% for 3 days then >50% for next 7–11 days	
Cardiovascular, prostate, and neurosurgery	>100% for 3 days then 80%-100% for day 4–7 and >50% for days 8–14	
Hemophilia B		
Minor surgery	> 50% for 3–7 days	Recombinant or monoclonal plasma derived factor IX concentrates
Major surgery	>80%-100% for 3 days then > 50% for next 7–11 days	
Cardiovascular, prostate, and neurosurgery	>100% for 3 days then 80%-100% for day 4–7 and >50% for days 8–14	
Von Willebrand Disease		
Minor surgery	>50% for 1–3 days	DDAVP or Von Willebrand factor-containing factor VIII concentrates (e.g., Humate P)
Major surgery	Keep 50%-100% for 7–14 days	
Factor XI Deficiency		
Minor surgery	>30% for 3–4 days	FFP
Major surgery	>45% for 7–10 days	
Factor VII Deficiency		
Minor surgery	>15%	FFP or recombinant human factor VIIa
Major surgery	>25%	
Factor X Deficiency		
Minor surgery	>15%	FFP or prothrombin complex concentrates
Major surgery	>50% perioperatively, then >30%	
Factor V Deficiency		
Minor surgery	>25%	FFP
Major surgery	>50% perioperatively, then >25%	
Prothrombin deficiency		
Minor surgery	20%-40%	FFP or prothrombin complex concentrates
Major surgery	20%-40%	
Afibrinogenemia or Hypofibrinogenemia		
Minor surgery	>50%-100 mg/dL for 3 days	Cryoprecipitate
Major surgery	>50%-100mg/dL for 2 weeks	
Factor XIII Deficiency		
Minor surgery	>5%	FFP or cryoprecipitate
Major surgery	>5%	

DDAVP, 1-Desamino-8-D-arginine vasopressin; *FFP,* fresh frozen plasma.

preoperatively is important to avoid bleeding complications in nonresponders. In addition, it is important to remember that DDAVP cannot be used for extended replacement therapy (>72 hours) because of tachyphylaxis. For extended therapy or treatment of patients with severe disease, vWF-containing factor VIII concentrates therefore should be used. Cryoprecipitate should not be used for treatment of vWD because of its greater risk of transfusion-transmitted infectious diseases. A functional measure of vWF such as the ristocetin cofactor assay should be used to monitor therapy.

Inherited deficiency states involving other factors are rare, affecting in general fewer than 1 in 500,000. Except for factor VII deficiency, for which recombinant human factor VIIa (Novo-Seven) can be used, and fibrinogen deficiency, for which cryoprecipitate is available, FFP is the only available replacement product for these deficiency states. The available plasma products for treatment of coagulation disorders and the appropriate doses and durations of therapy for bleeding and surgical procedures are listed in Table 6.

Table 7: Hemostatic Agents

Fresh frozen plasma

Contains all coagulation factors in low concentrations (1 U/ml)
Used for treatment of factor deficiency states without available factor concentrates
Used for treatment of coagulopathies associated with deficiency of multiple factors (e.g., liver disease, cardiac surgery, dilutional coagulopathy)

Cryoprecipitate

Contains factor VIII, von Willebrand factor, fibrinogen, factor XIII
Used for treatment of fibrinogen and factor XIII deficiency
Should *not* be used for treatment of factor VIII deficiency or von Willebrand disease *unless* factor VIII/von Willebrand containing concentrates are not available

Factor VIII Concentrates (Recombinant, Plasma Derived)

Used for treatment of hemophilia A (factor VIII deficiency) and von Willebrand disease (e.g., Humate P and other von Willebrand factor containing factor VIII concentrates)

Factor IX Concentrates (Recombinant, Plasma Derived)

Used for treatment of hemophilia B (factor IX deficiency)

Prothrombin Complex Concentrate

Contains vitamin K–dependent factors II, IX, and X
Used for reversal of warfarin anticoagulation in patients with serious bleeding

Activated Prothrombin Complex Concentrates

Contain activated factors II, VII, IX, and X
Used for treatment for factor VIII inhibitors

Recombinant Human Factor VIIa (NovoSeven; NovoNordisk, Princeton, NJ)

Licensed for treatment of factor VIII inhibitors (e.g., used off-label for treatment of bleeding in patients with inherited platelet dysfunction, cardiac surgery coagulopathy)

Fibrin Sealants (e.g., Tisseel; Baxter Healthcare, Deerfield, IL)

Contains fibrinogen, thrombin, factor XIII
Used as a local hemostatic agent

Antifibrinolytic agents (epsilon aminocaproic acid, aprotinin)
Inhibit the fibrinolysis by inhibiting plasmin activity or generation

Desmopressin

Induces release of von Willebrand factor and factor VIII
Used for treatment of mild von Willebrand disease and factor VIII deficiency

Fibrin sealants are a useful hemostatic adjunct to traditional blood products for critically ill patients with bleeding. Although fibrin sealants have traditionally been made in the operating room by adding bovine thrombin to cryoprecipitate, these "bedside" products are associated with the development of inhibitors against factor V and thrombin. Commercial fibrin sealants such as Tisseel VH (Baxter Healthcare) have been shown to be more efficacious than homemade fibrin glue and have not been associated with coagulation inhibitors. In addition, commercial fibrin sealants are pathogen-inactivated, and thus they are associated with a lower risk of transfusion-associated infections.

Acquired Coagulation Disorders

Acquired coagulation disorders are a common cause of coagulopathy in the critically ill patient (see Table 5). Of acquired coagulopathies, DIC is among the most common and difficult to treat.

Although there are a large number of stimuli that can trigger it (e.g., sepsis, snake venom, trauma, cancer, heparin-induced thrombocytopenia), DIC ultimately is a syndrome of excessive thrombin production. The end result is diffuse fibrin clot and platelet plug formation, consumption of fibrinogen, platelets and coagulation factors, and activation of the fibrinolytic system. Clinically, DIC has at least three presentations: (1) diffuse microvascular thrombosis characterized by cool, cyanotic, or necrotic digits or extremities; (2) diffuse hemorrhage manifested by diffuse bleeding from sites of previous invasive procedures; or (3) asymptomatic. Clinical manifestations are dictated by the degree of activation of the coagulation cascade and the balance between clot formation and fibrinolysis. Laboratory markers of DIC include thrombocytopenia; a prolonged aPTT, PT, or TT; elevations of D-dimers or fibrin degradation products, and hypofibrinogenemia. Although rarely measured, antithrombin, protein C, and protein S levels are often reduced in DIC as well. Although aPTT and PT are the most commonly ordered tests when investigating patients for DIC, D-dimer levels are the most sensitive assay for this entity. Therapy for DIC should be directed principally against the underlying cause. Antibiotics and supportive therapy (intravenous fluids, vasoactive medications, blood products, etc.) should be used in DIC associated with infections. Recombinant activated protein C concentrate (Drotrecogin alpha, Xigris; Eli Lilly, Indianapolis, IN) has been useful for some patients with purpura fulminans, a severe form of DIC associated with infections such as meningococcemia and postsplenectomy pneumococcal sepsis, which is characterized by diffuse microvascular thrombosis. Because recombinant activated protein C concentrate results in reductions in factor VIII and V levels and prolongation of the aPTT, blood product support to maintain the platelet count above 50,000/μl and aPTT and PT ratio below 1.5 are necessary. Aggressive blood product support is also reasonable for patients with DIC and bleeding. Although anticoagulation has generally not improved outcomes for most patients with thrombotic forms of DIC, it is essential for patients with HIT and DIC or catastrophic antiphospholipid syndrome and DIC because anticoagulation is essential to suppress the prothrombotic stimulus responsible for these forms of DIC.

Vitamin K deficiency is a common cause of acquired coagulopathy in the intensive care unit because critically ill patients often have limited vitamin K intake, exposure to broad-spectrum antibiotics, and disrupted hepatobiliary recirculation of vitamin K. The primary sources of vitamin K are green vegetables such as broccoli and spinach and supplemental vitamin K produced by intestinal flora. Therefore patients who are not eating well and are being treated with broad-spectrum antibiotics are at high risk for this acquired coagulopathy. Several antibiotics containing the N-methyl-thiotetrazole side chain (e.g., cefamandole, cefotetan, cefoperazone) that inhibits vitamin K epoxide reductase, an enzyme in the vitamin K recycling pathway, place patients at particularly high risk of this complication. Vitamin K is essential to the production of functional forms of the coagulation factors prothrombin (factor II), factor VII, factor IX, and factor X, as well as the anticoagulant proteins, protein C, and protein S. Because factors such as factor VII have a half-life of 6 hours, prolongation of the PT can occur rapidly after vitamin K stores are depleted. Clinically, vitamin K deficiency is manifested by the development of ecchymoses and bleeding from the site of blood draws or invasive procedures. Because factor VII has the shortest half-life of the vitamin K–dependent coagulation factors, the PT is the first test to become abnormal, followed by prolongation of the aPTT. Mixing studies demonstrate complete correction of the laboratory abnormalities. Administration of vitamin K results in rapid correction of the coagulopathy. Because oral vitamin K1 is as effective as subcutaneous vitamin K1 in patients without biliary disease and poses no risk of anaphylaxis, this route should be used in patients without serious bleeding or biliary disease. Patients with serious or life-threatening bleeding should be treated with intravenous vitamin K1 because it can result in substantial correction of the PT within 4 to 8 hours. Whenever intravenous vitamin K1 is administered to a patient, it should be given slowly (no more rapidly than 1 mg/minute) with close monitoring for evidence of anaphylaxis (estimated absolute risk 1/3000). FFP should be used for treatment of vitamin K deficiency only in situations of life-threatening bleeding when rapid correction is necessary.

Anticoagulant-Associated Bleeding

Anticoagulants are an important cause of bleeding that should be investigated in any patient presenting with bleeding after anticoagulation. The most common anticoagulants in the inpatient environment are unfractionated heparin, LMWH, and warfarin. Newer anticoagulants that are being used increasingly in inpatients are direct thrombin inhibitors such as lepirudin (Refludan; Berlex

Laboratories, Wayne, NJ) and argatroban (Novastan; GlaxoSmithKline, Research Triangle Park, NC), which are used for treatment of HIT, and fondaparinux (Arixtra; GlaxoSmithKline,) which is used in the treatment and prevention of venous thromboembolism and acute coronary syndromes.

Unfractionated Heparin

Unfractionated heparin results in anticoagulation by virtue of its interaction with the endogenous anticoagulant protein antithrombin (III), which results in a several-thousand-fold acceleration of its inhibitory interaction with thrombin and activated factors X and IX and factor XI. Because of its broad spectrum of activity, unfractionated heparin results in a prolongation of the aPTT. The TT is also exquisitely sensitive to its effects. Definitive demonstration that heparin is responsible for a coagulopathy can be obtained by repeating the aPTT after exposing the patient's plasma to heparinase. A dramatic correction of the aPTT is conclusive evidence of heparin contamination. The most frequent clinical situations in which heparin is associated with clinical bleeding include patients immediately postcardiac bypass surgery, patients undergoing hemodialysis, and patients receiving heparin for DVT prophylaxis or treatment. Protamine-administered intravenously in a dose of 1 mg per 100 units of heparin can be used to reverse heparin-associated coagulopathy.

Low-Molecular-Weight Heparin

LMWH can also precipitate bleeding complications. The three LMWH available in the United States are dalteparin (Fragmin; Pfizer, New York, NY), enoxaparin (Lovenox; Sanofi-Aventis, Bridgewater, NJ), and tinzaparin (Innohep; Pharmion, Boulder, CO). LMWH-associated bleeding most commonly develops in patients receiving LMWH for treatment or prevention of venous thromboembolism (VTE) who develop worsening renal function or undergo unanticipated invasive procedures. LMWH exerts its anticoagulant effects through accelerating the antithrombotic effects of antithrombin (III) against factor Xa. Because it has significantly less inhibitory activity toward thrombin, LMWH does not prolong the aPTT. LMWH concentrations can be measured using specialized assays measuring the activity of factor Xa. However, these assays are generally less rapidly available than routine assays such as the aPTT. Protamine can reverse a variable amount of LMWH activity (between 60% and 80%) depending on the agent used. The intravenous dose of protamine should be 1 mg per 100 U (of dalteparin or tinzaparin) or 1 mg per mg of enoxaparin if the LMWH dose was given within 8 hours. If the LMWH was given earlier, 0.5 mg of protamine should be given for each 100 U (of dalteparin or tinzaparin) or each milligram of enoxaparin. If life-threatening bleeding is occurring and incomplete protamine reversal is a concern, recombinant human factor VIIa (NovoSeven) has been used successfully in this situation. However, the potential for prothrombotic effects associated with rhFVIIa should be weighed against the severity of bleeding when using this product in such situations.

Warfarin

Millions of Americans are treated with warfarin each year for chronic anticoagulation. Warfarin results in anticoagulation by virtue of its inhibition of two enzymes in the vitamin K recycling pathway, vitamin K epoxide reductase, and vitamin K reductase. The result is acquired vitamin K deficiency and significant reductions in the functional levels of the vitamin K–dependent coagulation factors prothrombin, factor VII, factor IX, and factor X. The impact of warfarin on the coagulation cascade can be assessed using the PT. In situations in which rapid reversal is not necessary, oral vitamin K can be used to reverse warfarin within 24 hours. If rapid reversal is necessary, combined modality therapy with intravenous vitamin K and FFP should be used. RhFVIIa or prothrombin complex concentrates and IV vitamin K should be used for treatment of life-threatening hemorrhage (e.g., intracranial bleeding).

Direct Thrombin Inhibitors and Fondaparinux

Direct thrombin inhibitors (DTIs) such as lepirudin (Refludan) and Argatroban (Novastan) are used for treatment of HIT. Another DTI, bivalirudin (Angiomax; The Medicines Co., Parsippany, NJ), is used for percutaneous coronary interventions in patients with and without HIT. Each of these agents directly binds and inhibits thrombin. Their anticoagulant effects can be assessed using the aPTT and the activated clotting time (ACT). No reversal agent is available for any of the DTIs, although rhFVIIa has been used in the event of life-threatening hemorrhage with these agents. Fondaparinux (Arixtra) is used in the prevention and treatment of VTE and acute coronary syndromes. Fondaparinux is an indirect factor Xa inhibitor that functions by accelerating the inactivation of factor X by antithrombin. It is cleared renally and has a half-life of 17 to 21 hours in patients with normal renal function. It cannot be measured using the aPTT or PT. It should not be used in patients with compromised renal function (creatinine clearance less than 30 ml/min). There is no reversal agent available for fondaparinux, although rhFVIIa has been demonstrated to partially reverse its anticoagulant activity.

Liver Disease

The liver is the principal synthetic organ for all of the coagulation factors, except for von Willebrand factor and factor VIII, and the main source of thrombopoietin, the platelet growth factor. In addition, the liver is responsible for clearance of activated coagulation factors, plasmin, fibrin split products, and D-dimers and produces fibrinolytic inhibitors such as alpha2-antiplasmin and plasminogen activator inhibitor-1. Consequently, patients with significant liver disease are at high risk for bleeding caused by multiple acquired factor deficiencies, thrombocytopenia, platelet dysfunction resulting from the inhibitory effects of fibrin split products and a tendency toward hyperfibrinolysis. PT, aPTT, and TT, as well as fibrinogen level and platelet count, are useful parameters to assess the bleeding risk associated with liver disease. The thromboelastogram or euglobulin lysis time can help to identify excessive fibrinolytic activity. D-dimer levels will often be moderately elevated but do not indicate DIC unless markedly elevated because the liver plays an important role in clearance of D-dimers and fibrin split products. Factor deficiencies associated with liver disease are amenable to FFP replacement. Factor replacement should be guided by clinical findings and coagulation test results. Generally, 15 ml of FFP per kg body weight is an adequate dose. It is important not to strive to normalize the results of coagulation studies, particularly the PT, because factor VII has a short half-life, and attempting to achieve normal levels often precipitates fluid overload. Generally factor VII levels of 10% to 15% are adequate to stop bleeding. Factor VII levels of 15% to 20% are sufficient for surgical procedures. Often reducing the PT and aPTT ratio to less than 1.5 is sufficient for most procedures. If the fibrinogen level is less than 100 mg/dL, transfusion of cryoprecipitate is a more efficient product to achieve correction. In a 70-kg patient, each bag of cryoprecipitate will result in a 10-mg/dL increment in the fibrinogen level. On average 3 U of cryoprecipitate must be transfused on a daily basis to maintain fibrinogen levels, but transfusions should be guided by fibrinogen levels. Platelet transfusions should be given to any afebrile patient with a platelet count less than 10,000/μl or a febrile patient with platelets less than 20,000/μl. Patients with active bleeding or planned surgery should have platelet counts increased to 50,000/μl. To ensure that unsuspected vitamin K

deficiency is not contributing to a patient's coagulopathy, all liver patients with bleeding who do not have contraindications should be treated with vitamin K. Use of antifibrinolytic agents should be considered in any patient suspected to have primary fibrinolysis as a cause of bleeding. The presence of DIC should be ruled out before initiating antifibrinolytic therapy because these medications can precipitate widespread microvascular thrombosis in this situation. The dose of epsilon aminocaproic acid is a 5-g intravenous loading dose followed by 1 g per hour for 8 hours. The maximal daily dose is 30 g.

Acquired Factor Inhibitors

Factor V and Thrombin Inhibitors

Inhibitors to factor V and, less commonly, thrombin can develop in patients exposed to bovine thrombin. Most commonly this exposure occurs during cardiac surgery or neurosurgery when bovine thrombin is mixed with cryoprecipitate to make fibrin glue for topical hemostasis. Bovine thrombin is commonly contaminated with factor V. Exposure, particularly repeated exposure, is associated with development of antibodies to bovine thrombin and factor V, which occasionally cross-react with human factor V and, less commonly, thrombin. These antibodies typically arise approximately 1 week postoperatively and occasionally have been associated with significant hemorrhagic consequences. Factor V and thrombin inhibitors should be considered in any patient who develops an abnormal PT and aPTT in the postoperative period. Thrombin times will be markedly prolonged in these patients, and mixing studies will demonstrate the presence of an inhibitor. Factor V levels or prothrombin levels, or both will be reduced. Many patients do not have bleeding symptoms, perhaps because platelet granule–derived factor V that is not accessible to the inhibitor is sufficient for hemostasis. In the absence of symptoms, patients should not be treated with blood products or immunosuppressant agents. In patients with bleeding, IVIG and corticosteroids have demonstrated utility in eliminating the inhibitor and reducing bleeding symptoms. Patients with life-threatening bleeding should receive multimodality therapy including immunosuppression and plasmapheresis. Fortunately, bovine thrombin–associated factor inhibitors are transient, persisting for a mean of 2.3 months.

Cardiac Surgery–Associated Bleeding

Cardiac bypass is associated with significant perturbations of the hemostatic mechanism. Excessive bleeding, defined as a blood loss of greater than 1 liter, occurs in 5% of cardiac surgery patients. The reasons for postcardiac surgery bleeding are multifactorial. Large doses of heparin are used to prevent thrombosis of the bypass circuit. Platelet number and function decline during and after cardiac bypass because of activation and consumption. Coagulation protein levels drop, and activation of the fibrinolytic system also occurs. Each of these abnormalities contributes to an increased risk of bleeding after cardiac surgery. The approach to bleeding in the postcardiac surgery patient depends on the rate of bleeding and the clinical status of the patient. Unstable patients with rapid blood loss (≥500 ml/hour) should be resuscitated and surgically explored for a bleeding vessel. Because residual heparin may contribute to excessive bleeding, a second dose of protamine can be given to reverse any residual heparin present. If rapid access to point of care or conventional laboratory testing is available, the presence of residual heparin can be measured using an aPTT, TT, or heparin-neutralized TT.

In stable patients with excessive bleeding, use of laboratory testing to guide therapy is appropriate. A heparin-neutralized TT, PT, aPTT, complete blood count including platelet count, and fibrinogen level should be measured. Patients with evidence of residual heparin (elevated thrombin time, aPTT, reversal with heparinase) should receive a second dose of protamine. Patients with platelet counts less than 50,000/μl should be transfused with platelets. Platelet counts in excess of 50,000/μl are generally not associated with excessive bleeding in the absence of platelet dysfunction. If other laboratory testing does not reveal an abnormality, platelet transfusions should be considered for patients with platelet counts less than 100,000/μl because cardiac bypass can result in dysfunctional spent platelets. Platelet function tests such as the PFA-100 may help to identify affected patients. Patients with hypofibrinogenemia (fibrinogen <100 mg/dl) should be treated with cryoprecipitate (each bag of cryoprecipitate will raise the fibrinogen level 10 mg/dL in a 70-kg patient), whereas patients with abnormal aPTT and PT test results unassociated with heparin or hypofibrinogenemia should be transfused with FFP (initial dose 10–15 ml/kg). Because hyperfibrinolysis can result postcardiac bypass, use of antifibrinolytic agents such as epsilon-amino caproic acid or aprotinin should be considered for patients without significant thrombocytopenia (platelets >100,000/μl) and normal or minimally impaired PT and aPTT test results (PT and/or aPTT ratio <1.4). Thromboelastography can be useful in identifying patients with hyperfibrinolysis, although studies demonstrating superior outcomes with thromboelastography-guided management are lacking.

DDAVP and rhFVIIa have been used to improve hemostasis in cardiac surgery patients. DDAVP, an analogue of arginine vasopressin, is most useful as a hemostatic agent when applied to patients with platelet dysfunction. Case series of patients with critical bleeding after cardiac surgery suggest rhFVIIa has great utility in selected patients. Because it is expensive and can be associated with thrombotic complications, rhFVIIa should be reserved for patients with excessive or critical postcardiac surgical bleeding who are not responding to conventional hemostatic measures.

Vessel Wall Disorders

Disorders of vascular function are unusual causes for excessive surgical bleeding. Nevertheless, awareness of these disorders can be invaluable for the management of the occasional patient with a vessel wall disorder. A listing of some inherited and acquired disorders of vascular function is presented in Table 8. Among the inherited disorders of vascular function, Ehlers-Danlos syndrome is the most common to cause hemostatic difficulties. These patients have an inherited defect in collagen synthesis that results in a propensity to easy bruisability, skin and joint tissue laxity, arterial aneurysm formation, and poor wound healing. Occasionally, patients display evidence of abnormal platelet function. A history of platelet type bleeding in addition to the characteristic clinical findings is useful to identify affected individuals. Generally, coagulation testing is normal. In patients with abnormal bleeding associated with surgical procedures, DDAVP has proven useful for improving hemostasis. Because patients with Ehlers-Danlos syndrome have poor wound healing, surgery should be undertaken only when absolutely necessary.

Table 8: Vascular Disorders

Inherited Disorders	Acquired Disorders
Hereditary hemorrhagic telangiectasia (Osler-Weber-Rendu syndrome)	Amyloidosis
Congenital hemangiomas	Hypercorticosteroidism (Cushing's syndrome, Cushing's disease)
Connective tissue disorders Ehlers-Danlos syndrome Marfan syndrome Osteogenesis imperfecta Pseudo-xanthoma elasticum	Vitamin C deficiency (Scurvy)

An unusual but important acquired cause of excessive surgical bleeding is amyloidosis. Amyloidosis is most often caused by a monoclonal proliferation of plasma cells that produce light chains, a fragment of immunoglobulin that can collect in vessel walls and organs such as the kidney, liver, spleen, heart, and tongue. In addition to causing organ dysfunction, infiltration of the amyloid protein can vascular fragility and acquired factor X deficiency as a consequence of adsorption of factor X by exposed vessel wall amyloid fibrils. Patients with acquired factor X deficiency typically have a prolonged PT and aPTT and reduced factor X levels. Treatment with FFP is often associated only with transient increases in factor X levels because the amyloid fibrils avidly adsorb the transfused factor. RhFVIIa has also been used anecdotally to achieve hemostasis in these individuals. Patients with amyloidosis can be diagnosed by the presence of urinary monoclonal light chain proteins on urine protein electrophoresis and biopsy evidence of amyloid fibrils in skin or affected organs (kidney, heart, liver, bone marrow). Reduction of the amyloid protein with chemotherapy or, occasionally, splenectomy, in patients with massive splenic amyloid deposits has been associated with amelioration of bleeding manifestations. Some additional acquired vascular disorders are listed in Table 8.

SUGGESTED READINGS

DeLoughery TG: Hemorrhagic and thrombotic disorders in the intensive care setting. In: Kitchens CS, Alving BM, Kessler CM, editors: *Consultative hemostasis and thrombosis*, Philadelphia, 2002, WB Saunders, p. 493.

George JN, Raskob GE, Shah SR, and others: Drug-induced thrombocytopenia: a systematic review of published case reports, *Ann Intern Med* 129:886, 1998.

Kitchens CS: Surgery and hemostasis. In: Kitchens CS, Alving BM, Kessler CM, editors: *Consultative hemostasis and thrombosis*, Philadelphia, 2002, WB Saunders, p. 463.

Whitlock R, Crowther MA, Ng HJ: Bleeding in cardiac surgery: its prevention and treatment—an evidence-based review, *Crit Care Clin* 21:589, 2005.

EXTRACORPOREAL LIFE SUPPORT FOR RESPIRATORY FAILURE

Jonathan Haft, MD, and Robert Bartlett, MD

Extracorporeal life support (ECLS) refers to the use of a modified heart-lung machine to sustain life during critical cardiac or pulmonary failure. Because the use of a membrane oxygenator was essential in the development of ECLS, the technique is often referred to as *extracorporeal membrane oxygenation* (ECMO).

The first successful case was reported by Hill in 1972, in which a 20-year-old man with posttraumatic respiratory failure was supported for 3 days and survived. Bartlett reported the first successful neonate with persistent fetal circulation in 1976, and a series of 45 babies supported with ECMO was reported by the same group in 1982. ECMO became standard treatment for newborn infants with respiratory failure unresponsive to conventional management by 1986. ECLS is now used for severe cardiac or pulmonary failure in newborn infants, children, and adults. This report describes the use of ECLS in severe respiratory failure in adult patients.

INDICATIONS

ECLS is indicated in acute severe reversible heart or lung failure in which organ recovery or replacement can be expected in 4 weeks.

Acute respiratory distress syndrome (ARDS) is defined as severe hypoxia ($Pa/FIO2 <200$), bilateral pulmonary infiltrates, and the absence of cardiogenic pulmonary edema, requiring intubation and mechanical ventilation. It can result from primary pulmonary processes, such as pneumonia or vasculitis, or from extrapulmonary sources such as shock, pancreatitis, trauma, or sepsis. The incidence is approximately 150,000 annually in the United States. The overall mortality rate is nearly 50% and 30% in good-risk patients selected for interventional studies. There have been few advances in the treatment of this syndrome aside from elimination of iatrogenic causes of lung damage such as high airway pressure, high oxygen in inspired oxygen concentration, and fluid overload. Severe ARDS (defined as $Pa O2/FI O2 <70$ on 100% O_2 for more than 2 days) has a 90% mortality.

ECLS is also indicated for high-risk mortality respiratory failure from other causes, such as massive pulmonary embolism and combined cardiopulmonary failure with pulmonary edema.

In severe hypercarbic respiratory failure (such as status asthmaticus or acute airway occlusion), extracorporeal support is effective in removing carbon dioxide. In this circumstance, low blood flow is required, and gas exchange can be achieved through a small arteriovenous connection or low flow venovenous connection.

CONTRAINDICATIONS

ECLS is supportive in nature, providing the necessary exchange of oxygen and carbon dioxide without directly affecting the course of lung injury, except by reducing further lung damage with elevated inspired oxygen concentrations or airway pressures. Therefore ECLS is considered if the primary injury is believed to be reversible. Chronic lung disease in exacerbation and acute lung disease requiring mechanical ventilation for more than 7 days are relative contraindications because of the small likelihood of healthy recovery. Ongoing bleeding or any condition that would prevent systemic anticoagulation, advanced age, premorbid neurological dysfunction, and morbid obesity are relative contraindications. Sepsis is not a contraindication for extracorporeal life support.

TECHNIQUE

ECLS for ARDS is accomplished by circulation of venous blood by a mechanical pump through an artificial membrane lung (oxygenator) and heat exchanger followed by return to the native vascular system. In isolated respiratory failure, oxygenated blood is returned to the venous circulation, placing the artificial lung in series with the native lungs (venovenous [VV] ECLS). If both respiratory and cardiac support are required, the oxygenated blood is returned to the systemic circulation, placing the artificial lung in parallel with the native lungs (venoarterial [VA] ECLS). Vascular catheters are placed for blood access; the maximal blood flow is determined by the resistance in the venous drainage catheter. Because the amount of oxygen that can be delivered to the patient is dependent on the amount of blood flow, the largest possible venous drainage catheter is placed. Each membrane lung (oxygenator) has a gas exchange limit based on the surface area of the gas transfer membrane. The relationship between the surface area and blood flow is defined as the" rated flow," which is the amount of venous blood that can be fully oxygenated by the device per minute. The extracorporeal circuit is designed to use the largest possible vascular access catheters and a membrane lung with rated flow higher than the maximal possible flow expected for the patient. For adults this is 60 ml/kg/min, or 4.2 L/min for a 70-kg adult. At an outlet-inlet difference of 5 ml O_2/dL, 4.2 L/minute supplies 210 ml O_2/minute (normal O_2 consumption for a 70-kg adult is 210 ml/min).

CANNULATION

The majority of adult patients can be cannulated percutaneously, whether support is intended for VV or VA ECLS. Before cannula placement, the patient is systemically anticoagulated with 100 IU/kg intravenous (IV) heparin. Argatroban (GlaxoSmithKline, Triangle Research Park, NC) has been used for patients with known heparin-induced thrombocytopenia.

For VV ECLS, a 24- to 28-F venous drainage cannula is inserted into the common femoral vein and advanced approximately 50 cm from the skin level. This positions the tip near the junction of the inferior vena cava and right atrium. Hypoxic blood draining from the inferior vena cava and hepatic and renal veins drains into the ECMO circuit. Oxygenated blood is reinfused into the right internal jugular vein via a 23-F ECMO cannula advanced into the upper right atrium. We use thin-walled catheters made by Medtronic (Minneapolis, MN). Newborn infants and children are supported with a double-lumen catheter inserted into the right atrium via the jugular. Within the next year, double-lumen catheters large enough for adults will be available.

For VA ECLS, venous cannulation for drainage is identical to that for VV ECLS support, using 24- to 28-F catheters. For arterial infusion, a 17-F (female) or 19-F (male) cannula is used. This may result in femoral artery occlusion resulting in distal ischemia. At our institution, after a patient has been placed on VA ECLS using the femoral artery, the ipsilateral posterior tibial artery is exposed and cannulated retrograde with an 8-F cannula and perfused at 100 ml/minute, providing retrograde blood flow to the leg.

If the femoral artery is unsuitable for cannulation, the right common carotid artery is used, exposed directly by the cutdown technique. The distal common carotid artery is ligated during cannulation. Although this is well tolerated in neonates and children, carotid cannulation in adults carries a 5% to 10% risk of stroke. Because of this risk, as well as the additional time and equipment required for cervical exposure, the carotid is rarely used for ECLS cannulation in adults.

PATIENT MANAGEMENT

ECLS support is titrated to provide adequate gas exchange; normalization of arterial blood gases; reduction in mechanical ventilator settings; and, in the case of VA ECLS, to provide adequate systemic perfusion. Extracorporeal blood flow is increased until the maximal level is determined, then decreased to the lowest level that will totally support gas exchange at low or no mechanical ventilation. To prevent thrombosis within the extracorporeal circuit, heparin is continuously infused to maintain an activated clotting time (ACT) 1.5 times normal (180–220 seconds, depending on the device used to measure the ACT). ACT is the preferred measure over plasma partial thromboplastin time because results can be obtained immediately at the bedside and because platelets, red blood cells, and white blood cells in whole blood affect the level of anticoagulation achieved by heparin. Target ACT levels are lowered during bleeding complications or invasive procedures. The lowest tolerable ACT range to avoid circuit thrombosis is 150 seconds. Platelet consumption occurs from contact with the plastic surfaces. To avoid bleeding complications, platelet counts are maintained greater than 100,000, often requiring daily platelet transfusion.

Mechanical ventilator settings are immediately adjusted to avoid further lung injury from barotrauma and oxygen toxicity. We use pressure-controlled ventilation at a rate of five breaths per minute, plateau inspiratory airway pressure of 30 cm of water, positive end expiratory pressure of 10 cm of water, inspired-to-expired ratio 2:1, and inspired oxygen concentrations less than 0.5. Tracheostomy is performed after the patient has been stabilized on ECLS to facilitate therapeutic and diagnostic bronchoscopy and to improve patient comfort. Patients are turned prone at regular intervals (i.e., every 6 hours), with particular attention paid to avoiding kinking or dislodgement of the ECLS tubing. Hemodynamics typically improves rapidly after initiation of VV ECLS as pH normalizes and intrathoracic airway pressure is reduced, dramatically increasing cardiac output. Inotropes and vasoconstrictors can be rapidly weaned. Aggressive diuresis to return patients to dry weight is begun, and if acute renal failure has already set in, continuous hemofiltration can be easily added to the ECLS circuit.

All aspects of patient management are controlled according to protocol by the intensive care unit (ICU) nurse or ECLS specialist; management includes adjustments in heparin dose, ECLS flow rates, sweep gas, and transfusions to meet specified parameters. Patients remain lightly sedated, allowing rapid awakening during daily drug holidays. Full parenteral nutrition is supplied. Prolonged use of neuromuscular blocking agents is avoided.

Weaning is considered when the native lungs have recovered, as measured by improved pulmonary compliance and native lung gas exchange. When the requirement for extracorporeal support is minimal, the patient is trialed off of ECLS. During a trial off of VV ECLS, the sweep gas through the oxygenator is discontinued, allowing continuous extracorporeal flow but without gas exchange. The patient can be observed for many hours to determine the status of native lung function. Patients are decannulated when adequate oxygenation can be obtained with moderate ventilator settings and FiO$_2$ of less than 50%. A trial off of VA ECLS requires clamping of the arterial and venous lines. To avoid thrombosis of stagnant blood within the circuit, a bridge between the two limbs is opened, allowing continuous circulation. The cannulae are flushed intermittently with heparin or heparinized blood to prevent cannula thrombosis. When the patient is stable on low ventilator settings, percutaneous cannulae are removed, and hemostasis is achieved with prolonged direct pressure.

RESULTS

ECLS is used when the risk of dying from acute respiratory failure is greater than 80%. The Extracorporeal Life Support Organization (ELSO) maintains a voluntary registry of ECLS cases, now totaling more than 30,000. Of these, 1292 are adult patients with severe respiratory failure. The overall survival in the ELSO registry is 51%. Several groups have reported their single-series results of ECLS for adult respiratory failure. Most groups report discharge survival rates of approximately 50%. The University of Michigan recently published a 14-year experience, with 255 consecutive patients. Seventy-seven percent were weaned from ECLS, and overall discharge survival was 52%. Multivariate predictors of death included severe pre-ECLS acidosis and prolonged mechanical ventilation before ECLS. Long-term function of survivors was excellent. Although most survivors demonstrate a mild restrictive pattern on pulmonary function testing, exercise performance was mostly limited by overall debility from prolonged hospitalization.

In the modern era, complications of ECLS are frequent but rarely serious. The most common is bleeding related to anticoagulation. The cause of death in patients who do not recover is usually progressive irreversible pulmonary fibrosis from days of high-stretch ventilation pre-ECLS. The next most common cause of mortality is multiple organ failure related to the condition that initially caused ARDS.

There have been two prospective randomized trials of ECLS in adult ARDS. A multicenter trial of VA ECLS was sponsored by the National Institutes of Health from 1975 to 1979. In 90 randomized patients, the survival for both conventional therapy and VA ECMO was 10%. This study was conducted in inexperienced centers with primitive extracorporeal devices and techniques and (in retrospect) damaging ventilator management. The results of this trial do not apply to modern management of ARDS. However, the trial provided a valuable lesson concerning premature evaluation and conclusions regarding complex artificial organ technology. Morris and colleagues conducted a prospective randomized trial of low-flow extracorporeal CO$_2$ removal in 1994, with approximately 40% survival in both conventional and extracorporeal treatment groups. The number of patients was small, and the technique and devices are not used today.

In the modern era, there have been four prospective randomized trials of ECLS in neonatal respiratory failure, all demonstrating the value of extracorporeal support. The most recent of these trials was conducted in the United Kingdom. Currently there is a prospective randomized trial of ECLS for adult ARDS being conducted in United Kingdom (the CESAR trial: Conventional versus Extracorporeal Support in Acute Respiratory Failure). The results of this trial will be published soon.

We expect that the CESAR trial will show a major survival advantage to the use of ECLS in severe ARDS. On the basis of this evidence, ECLS will be used frequently in the management of salvageable patients with severe ARDS. In the next 5 years, the pumps, membrane lungs, and catheters will be simplified and improved so that ECLS can be conducted easily in any ICU, similar to the way that mechanical ventilators are used today. Currently the survival rate in salvageable patients with ARDS is approximately 70%. Assuming that the 30% of patients who die today will survive with ECLS in the future, the overall survival of ARDS in salvageable patients will increase to 85% to 90% in the next decade.

CONCLUSIONS

Extracorporeal life support can sustain life in the absence of native lung function for periods up to 1 month, with minimal complications. The use of ECLS in ARDS allows elimination of iatrogenic lung injury from the mechanical ventilator and time for diagnosis, treatment, and lung recovery. Currently, 50% of patients who would die from severe ARDS can be salvaged with ECLS.

SUGGESTED READINGS

All aspects of ECLS history, physiology, methods, and results are available from the Extracorporeal Life Support Organization (ELSO) and are published in Van Meurs K, Lally K, Peek G, and others, editors: *ECMO: cardiopulmonary support in critical care,* ed 3, Ann Arbor, MI: ELSO (www.elso.med.umich.edu).

MULTIPLE ORGAN DYSFUNCTION AND FAILURE

Lena M. Napolitano, MD

MULTIPLE ORGAN DYSFUNCTION AND FAILURE: DEFINITIONS

Advances in intensive care have allowed many critically ill patients to survive their initial insult. These patients may later demonstrate multiple organ dysfunction and failure, the genesis of which appears to be the body's reaction to critical illness, manifested by an imbalance and failure of inflammatory and immune system homeostasis, dysregulation of coagulation, mitochondrial dysfunction and consequent cellular energetic failure, and dysregulated apoptosis (programmed cell death). The manifestation of multiple organ dysfunction in the critically ill has been termed *multiple organ dysfunction syndrome* (MODS) and *multiple organ failure* (MOF).

MODS mortality is high, is directly related to the number of failing organs (Fig. 1), and remains a leading cause of death in intensive care units (ICUs). The understanding of the pathophysiology of severe sepsis and MODS has moved from a focus on inflammation to include an understanding of the associated anti-inflammatory responses. Loss of homeostasis can manifest as malignant inflammation or immune paralysis. Increased emphasis

is emerging on the role of loss of immune homeostasis and disordered coagulation as a cause of organ injury and dysfunction.

A MODS severity score is used for standardization to improve the understanding of the course of disease. Whereas MOF was once described as an all-or-nothing phenomenon, organ dysfunction actually occurs in gradations. Scoring systems for MODS that measure organ dysfunction by the severity of the dysfunction, rather than whether the organ has or has not failed, have enabled better predictability of whether MOF and mortality will occur. Furthermore, a MODS scoring systems allow scientific evaluation of the impact of new treatments on outcome other than mortality, including organ failure. Two MODS severity scores are commonly used, including the Marshall MODS score (Table 1), and the Sequential Organ Failure Assessment (SOFA) score (Table 2).

Table 1: The Multiple Organ Dysfunction Score (Marshall MODS Score)

Variables	MODS Score				
	0	**1**	**2**	**3**	**4**
Respiratory PaO_2/FiO_2 ratio	>300	226–300	151–225	76–150	≤75
Renal Serum creatinine	≤100	101–200	210–350	351–500	>500
Hepatic Serum bilirubin	≤20	21–60	61–120	121–240	>240
Cardiovascular Pulse-adjusted HR	≤10.0	10.1–15.0	15.1–20.0	20.1–30.0	>30.0
Hematologic Platelet count	>120	81–120	51–80	21–50	≤20
Neurologic Glasgow Coma Score	15	13–14	10–12	7–9	≤6

PaO_2/FiO_2 ratio is calculated with reference to the use or mode of mechanical ventilation and without reference to the use or level of positive end-expiratory pressure the serum creatinine concentration is measured in μmol/L, without reference to the use of dialysis. The serum bilirubin concentration is measured in μmol/L. The pressure-adjusted heart rate *(PAR)* is calculated as the product of the heart rate *(HR)* multiplied by the ratio of the right atrial (central venous) pressure *(RAP)* to the mean arterial pressure *(MAP)*: PAR = HR × RAP / MAP. The platelet count is measured in platelets/ml 10–3. The Glasgow Coma Score is preferably calculated by the patient's nurse and is scored conservatively (for the patient receiving sedation or muscle relaxants, normal function is assumed unless there is evidence of intrinsically altered mentation).
From Marshall JC: Crit Care Med 23:1638, 1995.

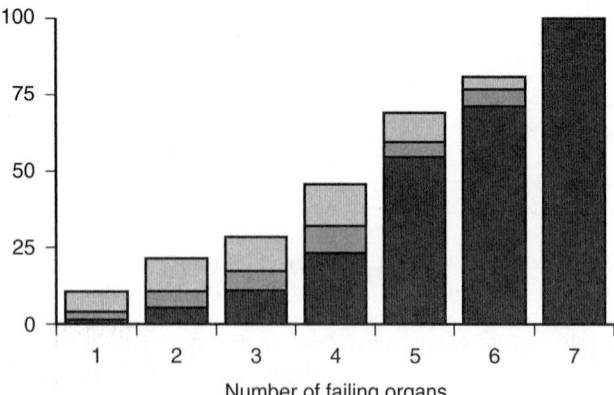

Figure 1 Mortality and organ failure. Mortality (percentage) of critically ill patients with different numbers of failing organs at intensive care unit discharge *(black),* hospital discharge *(black + dark grey),* and 1 year after intensive care unit admission *(black + dark grey + light grey). From Mayr VD and others: Crit Care 10:R154, 2006.*

Table 2: The Sequential Organ Failure Assessment (SOFA) Score

Variables	SOFA Score			
	1	2	3	4
Respiration				
PaO$_2$/FiO$_2$ ratio	<400	300	<200*†	< 100*†
Coagulation				
Platelets, 10^3/µL	<150	<100	<50	<20
Liver				
Bilirubin	1.2–1.9	2.0–5.9	6.0–11.9	>12.0
mg/dL µmol/L	20–32	33–101	102–204	>204
Cardiovascular				
Hypotension	MAP <70 mm Hg	Dopamine ≤5, or dobutamine any dose†‡	Dopamine >5, or epinephrine ≤0.1, or norepinephrine ≤0.1†‡	Dopamine >15, or epinephrine >0.1, or norepinephrine >0.1†‡
CNS				
Glasgow coma scale	13–14	10–12	6–9	<6
Renal				
Creatinine	1.2–1.9	2.0–3.4	3.5–4.9	>5
mg/dL	110–170	171–299	300–440	>440
µmol/L				

*With respiratory support.
†Adrenergic agents administered for at least 1 hour (dosages are in µg/kg/min).
CNS, Central nervous system; *MAP*, mean arterial pressure.
From Vincent JL, Moreno R, Takala J, and others: Intensive Care Med, 22:707, 1996.

▓ INCIDENCE AND OUTCOME

Critically ill patients who develop MODS (one or more organ system failures) have increased mortality compared with critically ill patients without MODS (Fig. 2). This has been documented for medical, surgical, and trauma critically ill patients. A number of studies have identified, however, that there has been a significant improvement in survival in patients with MODS over the past 3 decades. However, acute, refractory MODS is still the most frequent cause of death in the ICU (47%), and central nervous system failure and cardiovascular failure are the two most important risk factors for death in the ICU.

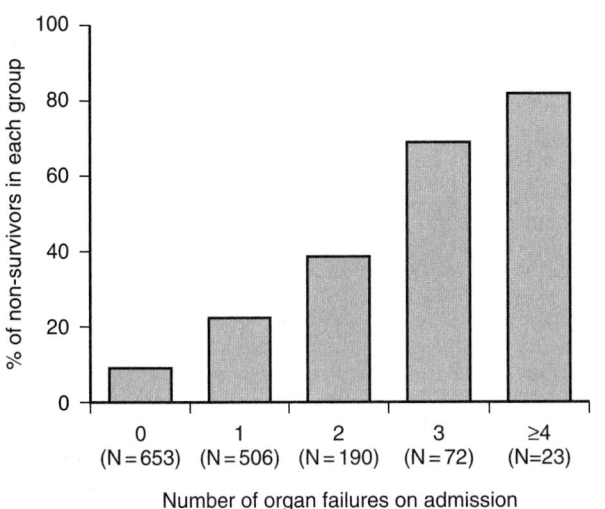
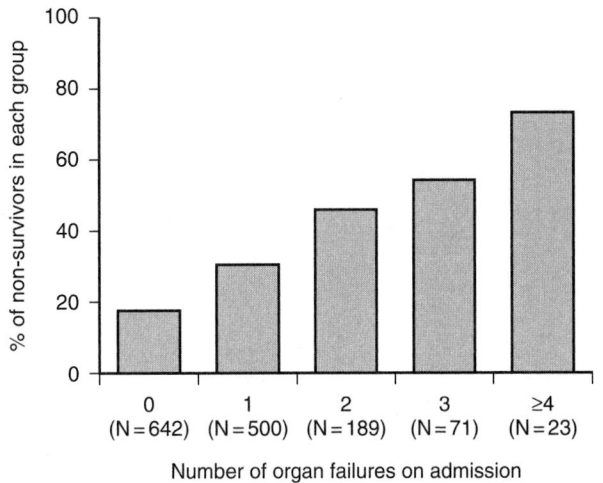

Figure 2 Organ failure and mortality. **(A)** Number of failing organs on admission versus mortality. The mortality rate was 9% in patients with no organ failure, 22% in patients with one failing organ, 38% in patients with two failing organs, 69% in patients with three failing organs, and 83% in patients with four or more failing organs (chi-square test for trend = 229, p < .00001). **(B)** Number of failing organs on admission versus presence of infection: 17% of patients with no organ failure were infected, 31% of patients with one failing organ were infected, 47% of patients with two failing organs were infected, 55% of patients with three failing organs were infected, and 74% of patients with four or more failing organs were infected (chi-square test for trend = 121, p < .00001). *From Vincent JL and others: Crit Care Med 26:1793, 1998.*

In trauma, the incidence of postinjury MOF has been reported to be between 7% and 66%, with an associated mortality rate between 30% and 80%. Previously identified risk factors for postinjury MOF were increased age, Injury Severity Score (ISS), and receiving a blood transfusion within 12 hours of injury. A recent prospective 12-year study documented that MOF was diagnosed in 25% of patients with ISS greater than 15, representing a decreased incidence of MOF over the study period. Overall, the incidence, severity, and attendant mortality of postinjury MOF decreased over the past 12 years despite an increased MOF risk. Improvements in MOF outcomes can be attributed to improvements in trauma and critical care and are associated with decreased use of blood transfusion during resuscitation.

Mortality for single organ failure is low and appears to be related primarily to the patient's underlying injuries and not to organ failure. Mortality for two or three organ system failures is lower than reported 15 to 20 years ago. Mortality for patients with four or more organ system failures remains high, approaching 100%.

The incidence and outcome of acute respiratory failure, the most common early organ failure, is dependent on dysfunction in other organs. ICU, hospital, and 3-month mortality rates are lowest in single-organ acute respiratory failure. Mortality increases with each additional organ failure. When acute respiratory failure occurs with four or five additional organ failures, the mortality rate approaches 75%. The prognosis for ICU patients with single-organ respiratory failure is good, both in the short and long term, but the high overall mortality rate observed is caused by dysfunction in other organs. Organ dysfunction is also an independent risk factor for increased mortality related to acute lung injury or acute respiratory distress syndrome.

Longitudinal analyses of MODS in surgical ICU patients have documented that 54% of patients develop some degree of MODS during their ICU stay. The most common risk factor for the development of MODS is hypoperfusion/ischemia without shock, although sepsis and shock are also notable risk factors. MODS is also associated with increased ICU length of stay and thus has an important impact on the use of resources.

TIME COURSE

The time course of MODS and MOF is variable, with some patients developing early versus late MOF (Fig. 3). Early MOF is related to an excessive inflammatory response (systemic inflammatory

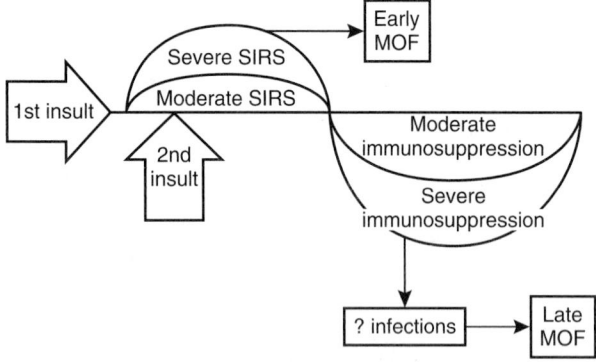

Figure 3 Progression from systemic inflammatory response syndrome *(SIRS)* to multiple organ dysfunction syndrome *(MODS)* and multiple organ failure *(MOF)*. Following major trauma, patients develop an early physiologic state of hyperinflammation (i.e., SIRS) because of a dysfunctional inflammatory response. This can lead to *early* MODS or MOF. Subsequently, the compensatory anti-inflammatory response is associated with significant immunosuppression and risk for infectious complications that is the most common cause of *late* MODS and MOF. *From Partrick DA, Moore FA, Moore EE: New Horizons 4:194, 1996.*

response syndrome [SIRS]). This is commonly seen in patients with traumatic injury or noninfectious inflammatory states, such as severe acute pancreatitis. Late MOF occurs later in the course of critical illness, is related to an excessive anti-inflammatory response, and is commonly related to the development of hospital-acquired or nosocomial infections. For instance, a trauma patient survives the initial hemorrhagic shock but develops a ventilator-associated pneumonia in the ICU with subsequent MOF. Therefore preventive strategies for MODS and MOF include all attempts at prevention of hospital-acquired infections.

PATHOPHYSIOLOGY

MODS is thought to be caused by an overwhelming, uncontrolled systemic inflammatory response that is activated by a number of hostile stimuli, including infection, sepsis, shock, and trauma. The indiscriminate activation of the inflammatory response resulting from these insults causes loss of the host's ability to localize the inflammation to the focus of the problem, leading to systemic inflammation and severe host tissue damage. Neutrophils, macrophages, endothelial cells, endotoxin, cytokines, and oxidants can all play a role in this inflammatory response. Cellular dysfunction in MODS is the final outcome of a process with multiple stimuli. Prominent mechanisms include cellular ischemia, disruption of cellular metabolism by the effects of inflammatory mediators, and toxic effects of free radicals.

Additionally, apoptosis (programmed cell death) may play a major role in MODS. Organs from patients who died from sepsis-induced MODS had extensive evidence of apoptosis. Furthermore, apoptosis of lymphocytes and intestinal epithelial cells was detected more often in septic patients that in nonseptic controls. Activation of caspases and induction of heat shock proteins may lead to apoptotic cell death in patients with MODS. This accelerated cell death was associated with marked depletion of lymphocyte populations in spleens and samples of peripheral blood. Likewise, trauma complicated by shock also increased apoptosis in intestinal epithelial cells and lymphocytes.

It has also been suggested that the gut plays a significant role in the development of MODS (Fig. 4). The role of the gut may be an indirect one. It may be that the oxidants generated during gut ischemia-reperfusion injury rather than the bacteria actually serve as priming molecules for the subsequent inflammatory response. It has been documented that oxidants generated in the gut are able to induce translocation of the transcription factor NF-κB into the nucleus in distant organs, initiating cytokine expression and subsequent neutrophil chemotaxis and damage to those organs. Furthermore, proinflammatory molecules from the gastrointestinal tract may reach the circulation through the mesenteric lymph. Resuscitation strategies to maintain the gastrointestinal mucosal barrier and minimize the effects of gut-derived mediator injury (such as early enteral nutritional support and antioxidant administration) may be critically important for the reduction of MODS.

Mechanisms by which sepsis induces organ dysfunction have not been fully elucidated. The coexisting findings of metabolic acidosis yet increased tissue oxygen tensions that are unique to sepsis suggest cellular availability but decreased use of oxygen, that is, tissue dysoxia. Because mitochondria use more than 90% of total body oxygen consumption for adenosine triphosphate (ATP) generation, a bioenergetic abnormality is implied. Cell and animal data have shown that nitric oxide (and its metabolites), produced in considerable excess in patients with sepsis, can affect oxidative phosphorylation by inhibiting several of its component respiratory enzymes. Human data are scarce. However, in skeletal muscle biopsies taken from patients with sepsis, a relationship between increased nitric oxide production, antioxidant depletion, reduced respiratory chain complex I activity, and low ATP levels was recently demonstrated. These findings correlated with severity of disease and outcome and support the notion that mitochondrial dysfunction resulting in bioenergetic

Figure 4 Gut-liver-lung axis in response to shock and hemorrhage. The gut-liver-lung axis in response to hemorrhagic shock injury. These organs seem to be the major target organs of systemic inflammatory response syndrome. Initiation of the inflammatory state can occur in any of these organs following trauma or shock. The gut can leak inflammatory mediators into the portal circulation, causing a response in the liver. Inflammatory mediators then travel in the hepatic vein to the inferior vena cava and to the lungs. The lungs may become injured, may inactivate some substances (not shown), or can release inflammatory substances themselves, which travel systemically to distant organs (including the gut). *LPS,* Lipopolysaccharide. *From Martinez-Mier G, Toledo-Pereyra LH, Ward PA: J Trauma 51:408, 2001.*

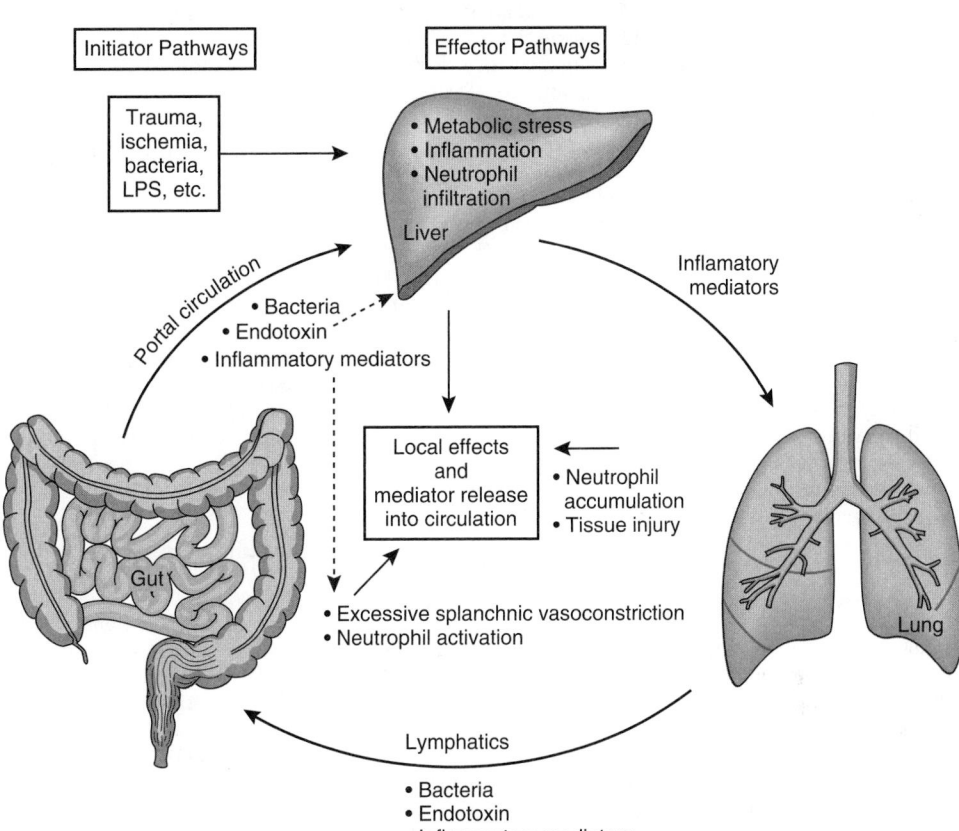

PROPOSED EVENTS IN MULTIORGAN FAILURE

failure may be an important factor in the pathophysiology of sepsis-associated multiorgan failure. However, a reasonable argument can be made that the reduction in energy supply could represent a final attempt at an adaptive response to ongoing inflammation, resulting in a cellular shutdown analogous to hibernation that allows eventual restoration of organ function and long-term survival in patients who are sufficiently fit to survive the acute phase.

EARLY IDENTIFICATION

Early identification of failing organs is critical. As each organ fails, the average risk of death increased 11 to 23 percentage points, with up to 75% mortality in patients having at least two-organ failure. The organ system that most commonly fails is the pulmonary system, followed by the cardiovascular, renal, and hematologic systems. Respiratory failure often presents with hypoxemia, and nearly 80% of patients require mechanical ventilation for 7 to 14 days. Cardiovascular failure manifests as hypotension that is unresponsive to adequate fluid resuscitation and requires vasopressors. Renal dysfunction often manifests as diminished urine output or increased serum creatinine, related to renal hypoperfusion. Hematologic failure commonly presents as disseminated intravascular coagulation, thrombocytopenia, and anemia. Additional organ failures include gastrointestinal, hepatic, and central nervous system. Identification of patients with early organ dysfunction or failure is critical because timely therapeutic interventions may substantially improve outcome.

RISK FACTORS

In all critically ill patients, hypoperfusion, shock, and sepsis are the leading causes of MODS. MODS is commonly associated with

nosocomial infectious complications. About half of the patients who succumb to septic shock die of MODS and MOF. In trauma patients, injury severity, degree of hemorrhagic shock, and amount of blood transfused within 12 hours of injury have been confirmed as independent risk factors for MOF. Obesity has also been confirmed as an independent risk factor of postinjury MOF, after adjusting for patient age, injury severity, and amount of blood transfused during resuscitation.

TREATMENT STRATEGIES FOR PREVENTION OR REDUCTION

Adequate resuscitation for the treatment of hypoperfusion and shock is the initial priority for prevention and reduction of MODS. Because infection and sepsis are common etiologies of MODS, a number of the treatment strategies focused on reducing septic complications in the ICU are therefore effective in reducing MODS.

Early Resuscitation and Hemodynamic Support

Because hypoperfusion is a common etiology of MODS and MOF, early aggressive resuscitation to prevent or treat hypoperfusion is a mainstay of therapy. The administration of intravenous fluids to increase intravascular volume is necessary. Early aggressive fluid resuscitation should be the initial step in hemodynamic support of patients with shock of any etiology. The goal of fluid resuscitation is restoration of tissue perfusion and normalization of oxidative metabolism. Increasing cardiac output and oxygen delivery is dependent on expansion of blood and plasma volume.

Intravascular volume can be repleted through the use of packed red cells, crystalloid solutions, and colloid solutions. Fluid resuscitation with isotonic crystalloid solutions is recommended for treatment of shock, and blood transfusion is reserved for the treatment of severe hemorrhagic shock. Multiple studies have documented that the use of albumin for fluid resuscitation in ICU patients had no effect on mortality or the development of organ failure, MODS, or MOF. Fluid infusion is best initiated with crystalloid boluses titrated to clinical endpoints of heart rate, urine output, and blood pressure. Patients who do not respond rapidly to initial fluid boluses or those with poor physiologic reserve should be considered for invasive hemodynamic monitoring.

If fluid therapy alone fails to restore adequate arterial pressure and organ perfusion, therapy with vasopressor agents should be initiated to maintain mean arterial pressure over 60 mm Hg. Potential vasopressor agents include dopamine, norepinephrine, epinephrine, or phenylephrine. Dopamine, norepinephrine, and epinephrine are all effective for increasing arterial blood pressure, although norepinephrine may be a more effective vasopressor in some patients, particularly those with septic shock. Norepinephrine is also preferred in patients with preexisting tachycardia because dopamine and epinephrine are associated with increased tachycardia and tachyarrhythmias. Vasopressors, however, should not be used instead of adequate, aggressive fluid resuscitation.

Prevention of Ventilator-Associated Pneumonia

Ventilator-associated pneumonia (VAP) is the most common nosocomial infection encountered in the ICU setting and is associated with increased mortality. A number of strategies are recommended for reduction of VAP in the ICU (Table 3). All strategies aimed to reduce the duration of mechanical ventilation are potentially beneficial because risk of VAP is directly related to the duration of mechanical ventilation. Many institutions have adopted the "ventilator bundle" (Table 4) approach to reduce VAP, which includes aggressive infection control education, and respiratory–therapist-driven ventilator-weaning protocols. The ventilator bundle is a series of interventions related to ventilator care that, when implemented together, will achieve significantly better outcomes

Table 3: Strategies to Prevent Ventilator-Associated Pneumonia

Oral endotracheal tube as preferred route of intubation
Semirecumbent positioning, with a goal of 45 degrees
Endotracheal tube with drainage of subglottic secretions
Ventilator weaning protocol
Daily interruption of sedation
Early tracheostomy
No scheduled ventilator circuit changes unless soiled
Heat and moisture exchangers for airway humidification with weekly changes
Closed endotracheal suction systems

Table 4: Ventilator Bundle for Prevention of Ventilator-Associated Pneumonia

Elevate the head of the patient's bed (semirecumbent positioning)
Interrupt sedation daily
Assess for weaning and readiness to extubate daily
Apply prophylaxis for deep venous thrombosis and peptic ulcer disease

Adapted from Institute for Healthcare Improvement, "Implement the Ventilator Bundle," www.ihi.org/IHI/Topics/CriticalCare/IntensiveCare/Changes/ ImplementtheVentilatorBundle.htm.

than when implemented individually. A number of institutions have documented a significant reduction in VAP with the use of ventilator bundles, but continuing education regarding this effort is an important component of this strategy.

Prevention of Catheter-Related Bacteremia

ICU patients are at increased risk for catheter-related bacteremia because 50% of patients have indwelling central venous catheters, accounting for 15 million catheter days per year in the United States. Assuming an average rate of catheter-related bacteremia of 5.3 per 1000 catheter days and an attributable mortality of 18%, as many as 28,000 ICU patients die annually, with MODS and MOF a frequent cause of death. Therefore efforts to decrease catheter-related bacteremia rates can improve outcome in critically ill patients. A number of interventions have been documented to be effective in reducing catheter-related bacteremia (Table 5) and should be implemented.

Insulin and Glycemic Control

Hyperglycemia and insulin resistance are common in critically ill patients, even without prior history of diabetes. A number of studies have documented that mortality is significantly reduced by maintenance of normoglycemia using intensive insulin therapy in critical care. Intensive insulin therapy (defined as maintenance of blood glucose between 80 and 110 mg/dL) reduced mortality from 8.0% to 4.6% ($p < .04$) compared with conventional treatment (insulin infusion only if blood glucose >215 mg/dL and maintenance of glucose between 180 and 200 mg/dL). The benefit of intensive insulin therapy was attributable to its effect on reducing mortality among patients with ICU length of stay of more than 5 days (mortality 20.2% in conventional group versus 10.6% with intensive insulin therapy, $p = .005$). The greatest reduction in mortality involved deaths attributable to MODS with a proven septic focus. Intensive insulin therapy also reduced overall in-hospital mortality by 34%, bloodstream infections by 46%, and acute renal failure requiring dialysis or hemofiltration by 50%. The majority of patients included in this surgical study were cardiac surgical patients (63%).

A subsequent analysis of this study cohort, using multivariate logistic regression analysis, determined that the lowered blood glucose level rather than the insulin dose was related to reduced

Table 5: Strategies to Prevent Catheter-Related Bacteremia

Create a catheter-insertion cart with all appropriate supplies
Educate the staff regarding evidence-based infection control practices
Ask providers daily whether catheters can be removed
Implement a checklist to ensure adherence to evidence-based guidelines for catheter insertion
Cleaned hands
Sterilized procedure site
Draped patient in sterile fashion
Used hat, mask, and sterile gown
Used sterile gloves
Applied sterile dressing
Empower nurses to stop the catheter-insertion procedure if there is a violation of the guidelines

From Berenholtz SM, Pronovost PJ, Lipsett PA, and others: Crit Care Med *32:2014, 2004.*

mortality ($p < .0001$), critical illness polyneuropathy ($p < .0001$), bacteremia ($p = .02$), and inflammation ($p = .0006$) but not to prevention of acute renal failure, for which the insulin dose was an independent determinant ($p = .03$). As compared with normoglycemia, an intermediate blood glucose level (110–150 mg/dL) was associated with worse outcome. Metabolic control, as reflected by normoglycemia, rather than the infused insulin dose, was related to the beneficial effects of intensive insulin therapy in these surgical critical care patients. Glycemic control is therefore emerging as a strategy for prevention of MODS in critically ill patients.

Other studies have documented an associated between hyperglycemia and worse outcome in trauma and burn victims. Hyperglycemia is a risk marker of morbidity and mortality in acute, critical illness, and insulin therapy seems to be beneficial in this patient group. These findings suggest that aggressive normalization of plasma glucose in critically ill and injured patients may be beneficial.

The mechanisms underlying the beneficial effects of aggressive glycemic control in critical illness are myriad. Intensive insulin therapy is associated with increased serum levels of low-density lipoprotein and high-density lipoprotein, whereas it suppressed the elevated serum triglyceride concentrations. In postmortem biopsies obtained from patients who died in the ICU, intensive insulin therapy increased mRNA levels of skeletal muscle glucose transporter 4 and hexokinase. These data suggest that intensive insulin therapy normalizes blood glucose levels through stimulation of peripheral glucose uptake and concomitantly partially restores the abnormalities in the serum lipid profile, possibly contributing significantly to the improved outcome of protracted critical illness.

Recent studies suggest that intensive insulin therapy may also exert anti-inflammatory effects and result in decreased apoptosis, a mechanism associated with organ failure in severe sepsis. Acute hyperglycemia induces hyperinsulinemia and increases circulating cytokine concentrations, and these effects are more pronounced in sepsis. This suggests a potential modulation of immunoinflammatory responses in human sepsis by hyperglycemia. A prominent component of the hypermetabolism in sepsis is impaired glucose tolerance and hyperglycemia. Elevations in plasma glucose concentration impair immune function, in part, by altering cytokine production from macrophages. The finding that high insulin serum concentrations induce a more prolonged increase in the anti-inflammatory cytokine interleukin-6 and suppress the levels of free fatty acids (FFA) in normal volunteers receiving intravenous endotoxin suggests that insulin treatment of patients with sepsis may exert beneficial effects by inducing anti-inflammation and protection against FFA toxicity and inhibiting FFA-induced insulin resistance.

The protective mechanism of insulin in critical care is not fully known. The phagocytic function of neutrophils is impaired in patients with hyperglycemia, and correcting hyperglycemia may improve bacterial phagocytosis. Another potential mechanism involves the antiapoptotic effect of insulin. Insulin prevents apoptotic cell death from numerous stimuli, and the antiapoptotic effects of insulin are mediated via tyrosine kinase and PI3-kinase signalling pathways.

Regardless of mechanism, it seems reasonable to control blood glucose more tightly in critically ill patients. Frequent monitoring of blood glucose is imperative to avoid potential detrimental effects related to hypoglycemia. Studies are necessary to determine whether less tight control of blood glucose —for example, a blood glucose level of 120 to 160 mg/dL — provides similar benefits. Additional studies to determine whether tight glycemic control results in improved outcomes in patients with established MODS and MOF are necessary.

Reduction in Allogeneic Blood Transfusion

Numerous studies have documented an association between blood transfusion and risk for infection, SIRS, MODS, and worse outcome after traumatic injury and in critical illness. Furthermore,

two recent, large, prospective studies have documented the high use of blood transfusion in critically ill patients, including the Anemia and Blood Transfusion in Critical Care (ABC) trial in Western Europe and the CRIT (anemia and blood transfusion in the critically ill) study in the United States. These studies documented that approximately 40% of ICU patients are transfused, with a mean of approximately 5 U of blood during their ICU stay. The number of blood transfusions a patient received during both studies was independently associated with longer ICU and hospital lengths of stay and an increase in mortality.

The TRICC Trial (Transfusion Requirements in Critical Care Trial) by the Canadian Critical Care Trials Group documented that a restrictive transfusion strategy (hemoglobin maintained between 7 and 9 g/dL) was as effective as a liberal transfusion strategy (hemoglobin maintained between 10 and 12 g/dL) in critically ill patients and the hospital mortality rate was significantly lower in the restrictive-strategy group (22.3% vs. 28.1%, $p = .05$). This study documented that a restrictive strategy of red blood cell transfusion in critically ill patients was at least as effective as and possibly superior to a liberal transfusion strategy, with the possible exception of patients with acute myocardial infarction and unstable angina. Continued efforts to reduce blood transfusion rates in the ICU are warranted, and blood transfusion should be reserved for physiologic indications and hemorrhagic shock.

The incidence, severity, and attendant mortality of postinjury MOF has decreased over the past 12 years, despite an increased MOF risk, and improvement in MOF outcomes can be attributed to improvements in critical care and are associated with decreased use of blood transfusion during resuscitation. Alternatives to allogeneic blood transfusion are currently undergoing preclinical and clinical investigation. These include the use of the new generation of hemoglobin-based oxygen carriers from both human (PolyHeme; Northfield Laboratories, Evanston, IL) and bovine source (Bovine Polymerized Hemoglobin, HBOC-201, Hemopure; Biopure, Cambridge, MA).

SEPSIS AND MULTIPLE ORGAN DYSFUNCTION SYNDROME

Sepsis is recognized as the systemic response to infection. Sepsis connotes a clinical syndrome that may occur in any age group, in markedly different patient populations, and in response to a multitude of microbial pathogens from multiple anatomical sites within the human body. Sepsis may range in severity from mild systemic inflammation without significant clinical consequences to multisystem organ failure in septic shock with an exceedingly high mortality rate. In sepsis, the lung is the most common site of infection, followed by the abdomen.

Systemic inflammatory response syndrome is defined as a clinical response arising from a nonspecific insult such as infection, trauma, thermal injury, or sterile inflammatory processes such as pancreatitis. This clinical response includes fever or hypothermia, tachycardia, tachypnea, and leukocytosis or leukopenia (Table 6). SIRS is characterized by two or more of these clinical manifestations. *Sepsis* is defined as SIRS with a presumed or confirmed infectious process. Sepsis can progress to *severe sepsis*, which is defined as sepsis with organ dysfunction or evidence of hypoperfusion or hypotension. *Septic shock* is defined as sepsis-induced hypotension, persisting despite adequate fluid resuscitation, along with the presence of hypoperfusion abnormalities or organ dysfunction.

More than 750,000 cases of severe sepsis occur in the United States annually, with 215,000 deaths. In this country, more than 500 patients die of severe sepsis daily. The mortality rate associated with severe sepsis is greater than the mortality rates for acquired immunodeficiency syndrome (AIDS) and breast cancer,

Table 6: Definitions of SIRS, Sepsis, and Severe Sepsis

Term	Definition
Systemic inflammatory response syndrome (SIRS)	A clinical response arising from a nonspecific insult, including two or more of the following: Temperature ≥38 °C or ≤36 °C Heart rate ≥90 beats/min Respirations ≥20/min White blood cell count ≥12,000/mm³ or ≤4000/mm³ or >10% neutrophils
Sepsis	SIRS with a presumed or confirmed infectious process
Severe sepsis	Sepsis with one or more sign of organ failure: Cardiovascular (refractory hypotension) Renal Respiratory Hepatic Hematologic Central nervous system Metabolic acidosis
Septic shock	Sepsis-induced hypotension, despite adequate fluid resuscitation, with presence of perfusion abnormalities

From Bone RC, Balk RA, Cerra FB and others: Chest *101:1644, 1992.*

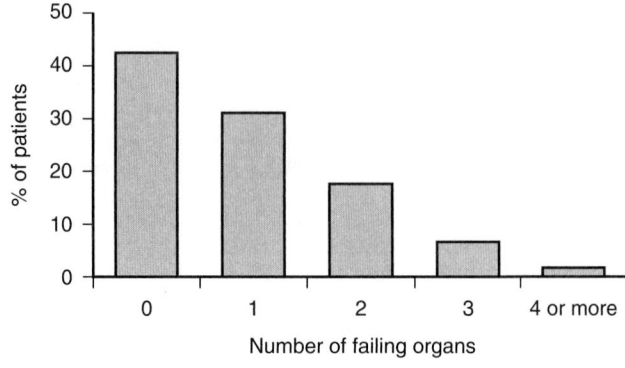

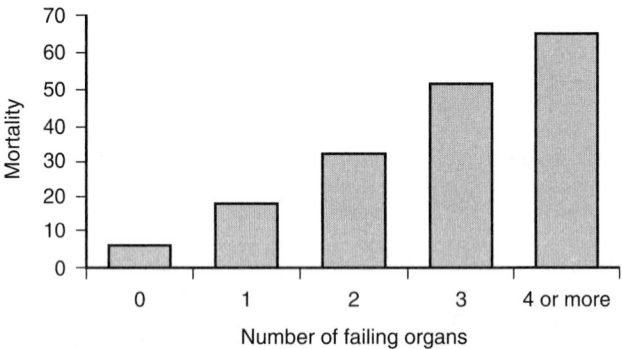

Figure 5 Frequency of organ failure in septic patients on intensive care unit admission and corresponding ICU. *From Vincent JL, Sakr Y, Sprung C and others, for the Sepsis Occurrence in Acutely Ill Patients (SOAP) Investigators:* Crit Care Med *34:344, 2006.*

and similar to mortality rates for patients with acute myocardial infarction. Sepsis is a leading cause of death in noncoronary ICUs in the United States; severe sepsis is the tenth leading cause of death overall. In sepsis, there is a direct relationship between the number of organs failed and ICU mortality (Fig. 5). It has been clearly documented that patients with severe sepsis who experience organ failure (single or multiple) have significantly higher ICU and hospital mortality rates compared with nonseptic ICU patients.

In October 2002, the Centers for Medicare and Medicaid Services (CMS) established new International Classification of Diseases (ICD-9) codes for sepsis that included specific delineation regarding whether organ dysfunction was present (Table 7). Before this, the only ICD-9 code for sepsis was "Septicemia". As medical practitioners caring for SIRS and sepsis patients use these new codes, additional information will be captured regarding the accurate incidence and outcome of patients with sepsis and organ dysfunction in the U.S.

Table 7: New ICD-9 Codes for Sepsis with or without Organ Dysfunction

ICD-9 Code	Diagnosis
995.90	SIRS, unspecified
995.91	SIRS caused by infectious process without organ dysfunction
995.92	SIRS caused by infectious process with organ dysfunction (severe sepsis)
995.93	SIRS caused by noninfectious process without organ dysfunction
995.94	SIRS caused by noninfectious process with organ dysfunction

ICD-9, International Classification of Disease, ed 9; SIRS, systemic inflammatory response syndrome.

TREATMENT STRATEGIES FOR PREVENTION OR REDUCTION OF MULTIPLE ORGAN DYSFUNCTION SYNDROME IN SEPSIS

Standard therapy for sepsis and severe sepsis includes source control, antibiotics, aggressive resuscitation and hemodynamic support, and nutrition and supportive therapy for other organ dysfunctions.

Source Control

Optimal management of infection and sepsis encompasses the important concept of source control, that is, control of the source of the infection. Decisive implementation of optimal source control measures includes the drainage of abscesses and collections of infected fluid, the debridement of necrotic infected tissue, and the use of definitive measures to prevent further contamination. Source control in pneumonia, for example, may require endotracheal intubation for adequate clearance of purulent tracheal secretions. In complicated pneumonia, source control may require tube thoracostomy for a parapneumonia empyema.

Source control is a particularly important concept in the treatment of abdominal sepsis and surgical sepsis. Outcome in abdominal sepsis is dependent on timely and accurate diagnosis, early adequate source control, and vigorous resuscitation and antibiotic support. Source control is critical to therapeutic success; antimicrobial therapy and other adjunctive interventions will fail if the source of infection is not controlled by resection, exteriorization, or other means. Adequacy of source control can be determined by radiographic evidence (i.e., drainage of an abscess, resolution of pneumonia infiltrate); repeated surgical evaluation (i.e., adequacy of debridement of necrotizing soft-tissue infections until there is evidence of healthy granulation tissue throughout the wound); and microbiologic eradication of infection (i.e., blood cultures negative after episode of bacteremia). The appropriate interventions to determine the adequacy of source control are dictated by the clinical circumstances and the site and source of infection. The general principles that guide the use of source control techniques in the management of the patient with severe sepsis or septic shock are fundamental to effective sepsis treatment.

Systemic Antibiotics

Systemic antibiotic therapy is a fundamental component of the standard therapy of sepsis. Antibiotics are essential to the treatment of bacterial sepsis because they reduce the bacterial burden. The adequacy of initial empirical antimicrobial treatment is therefore crucial in terms of successful outcome. Unfortunately, many studies have documented high rates of inadequate initial antibiotic therapy in infection and sepsis, ranging from 20% to 70%. These studies have also confirmed increased mortality associated with inadequate antimicrobial therapy in the treatment of nosocomial infections, including pneumonia and bacteremia. In patients admitted to the ICU for sepsis, the adequacy of initial empirical antimicrobial treatment is an independent predictor of in-hospital mortality.

One important factor contributing to the high incidence of inadequate initial antimicrobial therapy in sepsis is the increasing incidence of antibiotic-resistant organisms as the etiology of infection and sepsis. In critical care, particularly problem pathogens include methicillin-resistant *Staphylococcus aureus* and multidrug-resistant *Pseudomonas* species. There is now convincing evidence and consensus that initiation of empiric broad-spectrum antimicrobial therapy to cover the likely pathogens and their resistances pending culture results is mandatory in sepsis to minimize adverse outcomes. De-escalation of this therapy from broad-spectrum initial coverage to targeted antimicrobial therapy after results of cultures and susceptibility tests become available is a necessary component of this strategy to minimize unnecessary use of broad-spectrum antibiotics and possibly promote further bacterial resistance.

Resuscitation and Hemodynamic Support

Severe sepsis is often complicated by hypotension as a result of failure of vascular smooth muscle to constrict (vasodilatory shock) and maldistribution of blood flow in microcirculation (distributive shock). The foremost priority in managing patients with septic shock is to maintain acceptable mean arterial pressure to sustain tissue and cellular perfusion. These patients have large fluid deficits, and early, aggressive intravascular volume repletion should be the first maneuver in an attempt to restore tissue homeostasis. Meta-analyses comparing crystalloid with colloid resuscitation in all critically ill patients did not establish a difference in clinical outcomes. Consequently, the American College of Chest Physicians and the

Society of Critical Care Medicine recommend repleting intravascular volume with crystalloid solutions, administered as bolus infusions. Appropriate resuscitation endpoints are heart rate of 80 to 110 beats/minute, urine output greater than 0.5 ml/kg/hour, and targeted mean arterial pressure of 60 mm Hg or greater. When noninvasive endpoint measures fail to respond to volume challenges, invasive hemodynamic monitoring is recommended, with resuscitation titrated to endpoints of oxygen delivery and organ function.

Vasopressors are indicated for patients with persistent hypotension despite adequate fluid resuscitation. After they are adequately fluid resuscitated, most septic patients are hyperdynamic, but myocardial contractility, as assessed by ejection fraction, is impaired. Dobutamine is the first choice for patients with low cardiac index or low mixed venous oxygen saturation and an adequate mean arterial blood pressure following fluid resuscitation. Early goal-directed therapy has been used for severe sepsis and septic shock in the ICU. This approach (Fig. 6) involves aggressive resuscitation in septic patients to be initiated before admission to the ICU and is associated with significantly improved outcomes.

The practice guidelines published by the Surviving Sepsis Campaign have been distilled into two practical bundles that facilitate implementation in all hospital settings (emergency department and ICU), including the "Sepsis Resuscitation Bundle" and the "Sepsis Management Bundle" (Table 8).

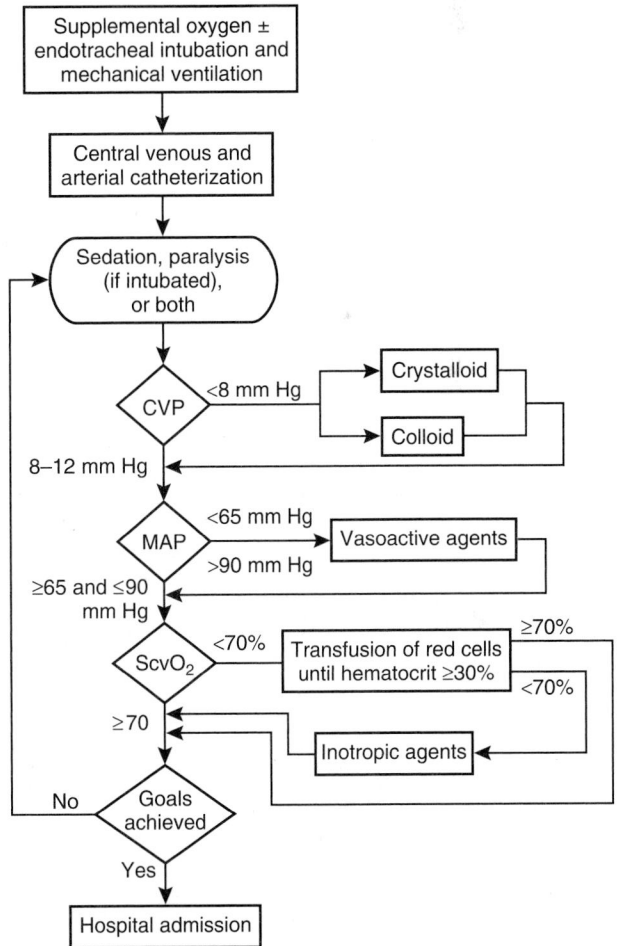

Figure 6 Protocol for Early Goal-Directed Therapy in Severe Sepsis and Septic Shock. *CVP,* Central venous pressure; *MAP,* mean arterial pressure; *ScvO₂,* central venous oxygen saturation. *From Rivers E, Nguyen B, Havstad S, and others, for the Early Goal-Directed Therapy Collaborative Group: N Engl J Med 345:1368, 2001.*

Table 8: Severe Sepsis Bundles

Sepsis Resuscitation Bundle

Should begin immediately but must be accomplished within the first 6 hours of presentation for patients with severe sepsis or septic shock.

Serum lactate measured

Blood cultures obtained before antibiotic administration

From the time of presentation, broad-spectrum antibiotics administered within 3 hours for ED admissions and 1 hour for non-ED ICU admissions

In the event of hypotension and/or lactate >4 mmol/L (36 mg/dL):
- deliver an initial minimum of 20 ml/kg of crystalloid (or colloid equivalent)
- apply vasopressors for hypotension not responding to initial fluid resuscitation to maintain mean arterial pressure ≥65 mm Hg

In the event of persistent hypotension despite fluid resuscitation (septic shock) and/or lactate >4 mmol/L (36 mg/dL):
- achieve central venous pressure of >8 mm Hg
- achieve central venous oxygen saturation of >70%

Sepsis Management Bundle

Should begin immediately but may be completed within 24 hours of presentation for patients with severe sepsis or septic shock

Low-dose steroids administered for septic shock in accordance with a standardized ICU policy

Drotrecogin alfa (activated) administered in accordance with a standardized ICU policy

Glucose control maintained over lower limit of normal, but <150 mg/dL (8.3 mmol/L)

Inspiratory plateau pressures maintained <30 cm H_2O for mechanically ventilated patients

ED, Emergency department; *ICU,* intensive care unit.
From Institute for Healthcare Improvement, "Sepsis," www.ihi.org/ihi/topics/criticalcare/sepsis.

▮ NEW STRATEGIES FOR THE TREATMENT OF SEPSIS

Considerable progress has been made in the past few years in the development of therapeutic interventions that can reduce mortality in sepsis. The supportive evidence regarding a number of new strategies for treatment of sepsis will be reviewed.

Adrenal Insufficiency and Steroids

The hypothalamic-pituitary-adrenal (HPA) axis is a major determinant of the host response to stress. During sepsis the HPA axis is rapidly activated through a systemic pathway, that is, by circulating proinflammatory cytokines and through the vagus nerve. Subsequently, the adrenal glands release cortisol, a hormone that will likely counteract the inflammatory process and restore cardiovascular homeostasis. Both experimental models and studies in humans suggest that inadequate HPA axis response to stress accounts, at least partly, for the genesis of shock and organ dysfunction in sepsis.

Adrenal insufficiency has been documented in a significant portion of patients with severe sepsis and septic shock. Subnormal adrenal corticosteroid production during acute severe illness has been termed *functional adrenal insufficiency* to reflect the notion that hypoadrenalism can occur without obvious structural defects in the HPA axis. A related concept is that of *relative adrenal insufficiency* in which cortisol levels, although high in absolute terms, are insufficient to control the inflammatory response. Inability to mount an adequate cortisol response, as seen in patients with structural disease of the HPA axis, adrenal suppression by corticosteroids, or prolonged treatment with offending drugs, increases the risk of death during acute illness. Thus if functional adrenal insufficiency can be identified, treatment with supplemental corticosteroids may be of significant benefit. However, the correct method to diagnose adrenal insufficiency in a septic shock patient remains controversial.

A recent meta-analysis of five trials revealed a consistent and beneficial effect of physiologic hydrocortisone dosages (200–300 mg daily) for short course (5–7 days) on survival and shock reversal in septic patients with vasopressor-dependent shock. The effects of physiologic steroid doses did not differ between responders and nonresponders to corticotrophin stimulation testing for adrenal insufficiency. Steroids were beneficial at lower doses and were harmful as the dose increased. Therefore in patients requiring vasopressors for septic shock, steroids can be considered as a potential treatment strategy.

Vasopressin Therapy for Septic Shock

Vasopressin is emerging as a rational therapy for the hemodynamic support of septic shock and vasodilatory shock due to SIRS. Both hemorrhagic and septic shock are associated with a biphasic response in vasopressin levels. In early shock, appropriately high levels of vasopressin are produced to support organ perfusion. As the shock state progresses, plasma vasopressin levels fall for reasons that are not entirely clear. Importantly, vasopressin levels in established septic and vasodilatory shock are low. Several mechanisms for this vasopressin deficiency have been proposed. The potential mechanisms of vasopressin deficiency include (1) depletion of pituitary stores of vasopressin resulting from excessive baroreceptor firing or exhaustive release in early septic shock; (2) autonomic dysfunction, citing lack of baroreflex-mediated bradycardia after vasopressin infusion as evidence; (3) elevated norepinephrine levels (endogenous or exogenous) that have a central inhibitory effect on vasopressin release; and (4) increased nitric oxide release by vascular endothelium within the posterior pituitary during sepsis that may inhibit vasopressin production.

In addition to the deficiency of vasopressin identified in septic shock patients, these patients are exquisitely sensitive to low-dose vasopressin. Vasopressin deficiency may contribute to the refractory hypotension of late septic shock, resulting in the continued requirement of vasopressor therapy. In physiologic dosages (0.01–0.04 U/min), low-dose vasopressin infusion causes a pressor response in septic shock and a sparing of conventional exogenous catecholamines, with no evidence of organ hypoperfusion. Vasopressin mediates vasoconstriction via V1-receptors, coupled to phospholipase C, and increases intracellular calcium concentration. This action is not impaired during sepsis, and thus vasopressin has been shown effective in reversal of catecholamine-resistant hypotension in septic shock patients. The use of higher doses of vasopressin in septic shock may be associated with potentially deleterious vasoconstriction of mesenteric, renal, pulmonary, and coronary vasculature. On the basis of these limited data, it does not appear beneficial, and may be potentially harmful, to use high-dose vasopressin in septic shock.

On the basis of the results of studies to date, clinicians should consider the addition of low-dosage (up to 0.04 U/min) continuous infusion vasopressin in individual septic shock patients who are adequately resuscitated and still requiring high dosages of vasopressors. Whether the use of low-dosage vasopressin in septic shock, with the goal of restoring vasopressin levels to a physiologic level, will translate to improved clinical outcomes (i.e., improved organ dysfunction or improved survival) awaits the conduct of future large, prospective, randomized clinical trials.

Activated Protein C for Severe Sepsis

Dysregulation of coagulation and inflammation is common in sepsis and is thought to be fundamental to the pathogenesis of MODS.

Severe infection and inflammation almost invariably lead to hemostatic abnormalities, ranging from insignificant laboratory changes to severe disseminated intravascular coagulation (DIC). Systemic inflammation results in activation of coagulation because of tissue factor-mediated thrombin generation, downregulation of physiologic anticoagulant mechanisms, and inhibition of fibrinolysis. Proinflammatory cytokines play a central role in the differential effects on the coagulation and fibrinolysis pathways. In contrast, activation of the coagulation system may importantly affect inflammatory responses by direct and indirect mechanisms. The relevance of the cross-talk between inflammation and coagulation is underlined by the promising results in the treatment of severe systemic infection with modulators of coagulation and inflammation.

Increased D-dimers and decreased protein C blood concentrations are common in patients with sepsis and organ dysfunction. Decreased protein C concentrations play an active role in the development of the hypercoagulable state in patients with severe sepsis and are linked to the development of organ dysfunction and increased mortality. Activated protein C, an endogenous protein that promotes fibrinolysis and inhibits thrombosis and inflammation, is an important modulator of the coagulation and inflammation associated with severe sepsis (Fig. 7). The properties of activated protein C include (1) antithrombotic activity, by inhibition of thrombin formation and inhibition of factors V and VIII; (2) profibrinolytic activity, enhancing the body's ability to lyse fibrin, via inhibition of PAI-1; and (3) anti-inflammatory activity, indirectly through reduced thrombin resulting in less tumor

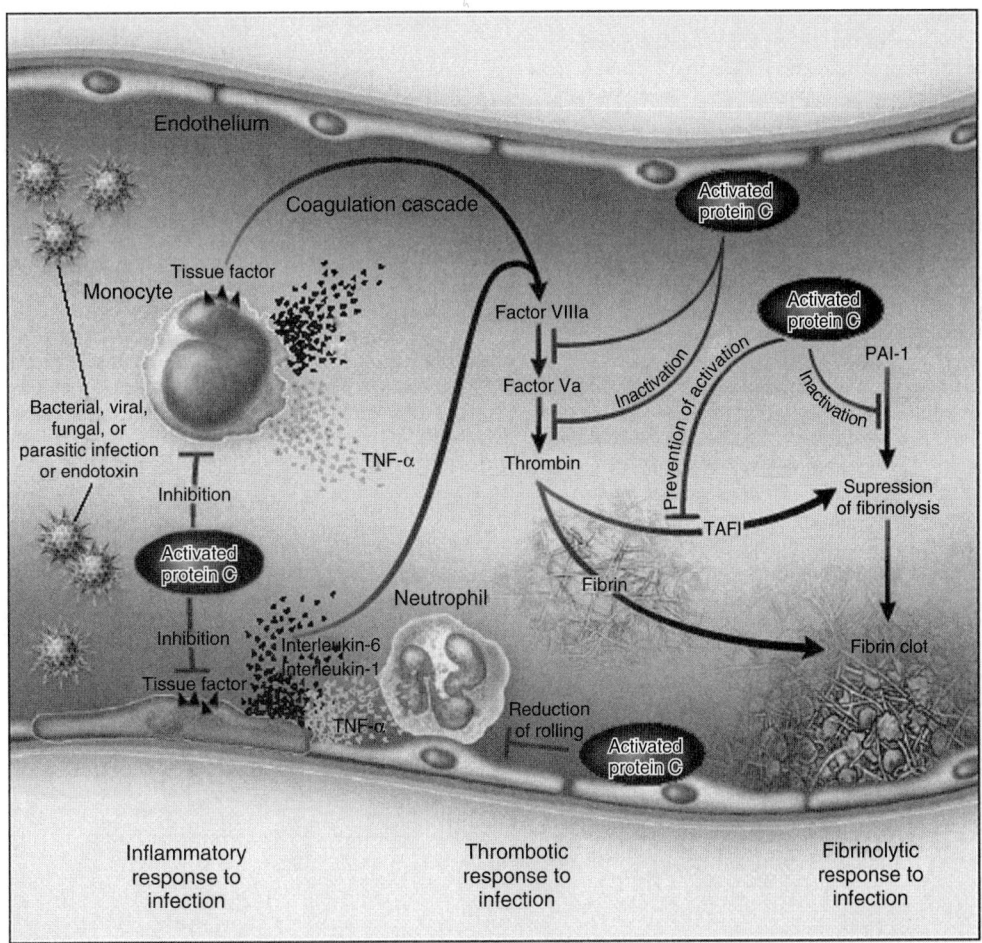

Figure 7 Proposed actions of activated protein C in modulating the systemic inflammatory, procoagulant, and fibrinolytic host responses to infection. *From Bernard GR, Vincent JL, Laterre PF and others:* N Engl J Med *344:699, 2001.*

necrosis factor and interleukin-1 production, and via a direct effect on monocytes and endothelial cells through an NFκB mechanism.

The conversion of protein C to activated protein C may be impaired during sepsis as a result of the down-regulation of thrombomodulin by inflammatory cytokines. Reduced levels of protein C are found in the majority of patients with sepsis and are associated with an increased risk of death. In fact, protein C deficiency was documented in approximately 80% of all severe sepsis patients studied.

The administration of a 96-hour continuous infusion of drotrecogin alfa (activated) or recombinant human activated protein C in the Recombinant Human Activated protein C Worldwide Evaluation in Severe Sepsis (PROWESS) trial was associated with a significant reduction in 28-day mortality (31% vs. 44%) in patients with severe sepsis who have a high risk of death (assessed by Acute Physiology and Chronic Health Evaluation [APACHE] II score >25). This survival advantage in septic patients who were randomized to activated protein C treatment was confirmed to persist for 2.5 years after conclusion of the PROWESS trial. PROWESS is the first successful trial of a biological modifying agent in the treatment of severe sepsis, and bleeding is the only notable side effect. In surgical patients, a careful assessment of risk for bleeding must be completed when considering the use of activated protein C in the treatment of severe sepsis and septic shock. Furthermore, the conduct of invasive procedures in patients receiving activated protein C treatment requires transient discontinuation of the drug infusion. Because of the anticoagulant properties of activated protein C, caution must be exercised with its use in those patients who meet the contraindications for its use or who have risk factors for increased bleeding complications.

Two additional analyses of the PROWESS trial documented significant improvements in organ function measured by SOFA scores for 28 days, and significantly faster resolution of cardiovascular (p = .009) and respiratory (p = .009) dysfunction, and significantly slower onset of hematologic organ dysfunction (p = .041) compared with placebo patients for days 1 to 7. Treatment with activated protein C represents an important advance in the care of selected patients with sepsis and was associated with more prompt resolution of MODS.

Early Enteral Nutrition and Immunonutrition

Multiple studies have confirmed that the administration of early enteral nutrition in trauma is associated with improved outcome. Furthermore, clinical evidence suggests that enteral feeding supplemented with specific immunonutrients (glutamine, arginine, omega-3 polyunsaturated fatty acids, or nucleotides) may further improve clinical outcome in trauma. Several clinical studies in trauma patients with significant injury (ISS >20, abdominal trauma index >25) show reduced septic complications, significant

reduction in MODS, and reduced use of resources in patients randomized to the immune-enhancing diets. One comprehensive review of clinical studies of immune-enhancing diets concluded that immune-enhancing enteral formulas should be used in all patients sustaining major torso trauma. Enteral diets enriched with eicosapentaenoic acid, gamma-linolenic acid, and antioxidants have also been documented to reduce mortality and reduce the development of new organ dysfunction in patients with severe sepsis and septic shock.

SUGGESTED READINGS

Baue AE: MOF, MODS and SIRS: What is in a name or an acronym? *Shock* 26:438, 2006.

Berenholtz SM, Pronovost PJ, Lipsett PA, and others: Eliminating catheter-related bloodstream infections in the intensive care unit, *Crit Care Med* 32:2014, 2004.

Ciesla DJ, Moore EE, Johnson JL, and others: A 12-year prospective study of postinjury multiple organ failure: has anything changed? *Arch Surg* 140:432, 2005.

Dellinger RP, Carlet JM, Masur H, and others: For the Surviving Sepsis Campaign Management Guidelines Committee. Surviving Sepsis Campaign guidelines for management of severe sepsis and septic shock, *Crit Care Med* 32:858, 2004.

Dodek P, Keenan S, Cook Dothers for the Canadian Critical Care Trials Group and the Canadian Critical Care Society.: Evidence-based clinical practice guideline for the prevention of ventilator-associated pneumonia, *Ann Intern Med* 141:305, 2004.

Finfer S, Bellomo R, Boyce Nothers for the Saline versus Albumin Fluid Evaluation (SAFE) Study Investigators.: A comparison of albumin and saline for fluid resuscitation in the intensive care unit, *N Engl J Med* 350:2247, 2004.

Hebert PC, Wells G, Blajchman MA, and others: A multicenter, randomized, controlled clinical trial of transfusion requirements in critical care. *N Engl J Med* 340:409..

Malone DL, Dunne J, Tracy JK, and other: Blood transfusion, independent of shock severity, is associated with worse outcome in trauma, *J Trauma* 54:898, 2003.

Mayr VD, Dunser MW, Greil V, and others: Causes of death and determinants of outcome in critically ill patients, *Crit Care* 10:R154, 2006.

Minneci PC, Deans K, Banks SM, and others: Meta-analysis: the effect of steroids on survival and shock during sepsis depends on the dose, *Ann Intern Med* 14:47, 2004.

Napolitano LM, Faist E, Wichmann MW, and others: Immune dysfunction in trauma, *Surg Clin North Am* 79:1385, 1999.

Protti A, Singer M: Bench-to-bedside review: potential strategies to protect or reverse mitochondrial dysfunction in sepsis-induced organ failure, *Crit Care* 10:228, 2006.

Singer M, DeSantis V, Vitale D: Multiorgan failure is an adaptive, endocrine-mediated, metabolic response to overwhelming systemic inflammation, *Lancet* 364:545, 2004.

Van den Berghe G, Wouters P, Weekers F, and others: Intensive insulin therapy in critically ill patients, *N Engl J Med* 345:1359, 2001.

MINIMALLY INVASIVE SURGERY

LAPAROSCOPIC CHOLECYSTECTOMY

Kimberly Steele, MD, and Anne Lidor, MD, MPH

INTRODUCTION

Introduced in the United States by Reddick in 1988, laparoscopic cholecystectomy was rapidly adopted by general surgeons, to the point where it is now the second most commonly performed general surgical procedure in the United States. Within just 4 years of its introduction, a National Institutes of Health Consensus Statement, published in 1992, concluded that laparoscopic cholecystectomy "provides safe and effective treatment for most patients with symptomatic gallstones" and "appears to have become the treatment of choice." Since then, laparoscopic cholecystectomy has essentially supplanted open procedures, so that approximately three quarters of the more than 600,000 cholecystectomies performed in the United States in 2001 were conducted laparoscopically. Advantages of the laparoscopic technique include decreased pain, smaller incisions, and shorter length of hospital stay, which in turn lead to decreased costs and improved patient satisfaction. Despite the advantages of the approach, meticulous technique is required to avoid complications.

INDICATIONS

The indications for laparoscopic cholecystectomy do not differ from open cholecystectomy and can be classified according to the clinical status of the patient at the time of presentation. Patients may present with asymptomatic, symptomatic, or complicated gallbladder disease.

Asymptomatic Gallbladder Disease (Cholelithiasis or Polyps)

Approximately 20 million Americans have gallstones, and the majority of them remain asymptomatic over their life span. It has long been well established that the incidence of gallstones is associated with increasing age and a high-fat diet and that heredity is also influential. The incidence of gallstones is highest among women, those who are obese or have diabetes, and those aged between 40 and 60 years. Additional risk factors include inflammatory bowel disease,

pregnancy, some hematologic disorders, and rapid weight loss after bariatric surgery. Because only 2% to 3% of generally healthy persons with asymptomatic gallstones will become symptomatic per year, prophylactic cholecystectomy is not justified. However, patients who are immunocompromised, awaiting organ allotransplantation, or who have sickle cell disease are at higher risk of developing complications and should be treated irrespective of the presence or absence of symptoms. The presence of diabetes mellitus, in and of itself, does not confer sufficient risk to warrant prophylactic cholecystectomy in asymptomatic individuals.

Certain findings on imaging of the gallbladder increase the likelihood that gallbladder cancer is present. The finding of a calcified or "porcelain" gallbladder or of gallbladder polyps larger than 1 cm or gallstones larger than 3 cm necessitates removal of the gallbladder unless metastatic disease or other contraindications are present.

Symptomatic Gallbladder Disease

Symptomatic gallstone disease, also termed *biliary colic*, is characterized by the presence of intermittent, colicky, right upper quadrant or epigastric abdominal pain, sometimes radiating to the right upper back and shoulder, which may be accompanied by bloating, nausea, and vomiting and is triggered by a fatty or high-protein meal. Patients who experience such symptoms are 25% more likely to develop complications within 10 to 20 years compared with patients with asymptomatic cholelithiasis. This increased risk is the rationale behind the treatment of symptomatic gallbladder disease. However, patients who present with typical biliary colic symptoms must first be ruled out for other disease processes, including myocardial infarction, pneumonia, peptic ulcer disease, and inflammatory bowel disease. Occasionally, patients present with biliary colic in the absence of sonographically identifiable gallstones. In such cases, biliary dyskinesia should be considered and a hepatobiliary iminodiacetic acid scan obtained. The finding of a gallbladder ejection fraction less than 35% at 20 minutes is considered abnormal and constitutes another indication for laparoscopic cholecystectomy.

Acute cholecystitis, when diagnosed within 72 hours from the onset of symptoms, can and usually should be treated laparoscopically. The challenge arises, however, when patients present more than 72 hours after the onset of symptoms, at which point inflammatory changes in the surrounding tissues render dissection planes difficult, significantly increasing the likelihood of complications. Under such circumstances, the rate of conversion to an open procedure may increase to 20% to 25%. An acceptable approach is to pursue conservative management with bowel rest, intravenous antibiotics, and hydration. Patients responding to this treatment can be discharged home, with instructions to follow a low-fat diet until interval cholecystectomy can be performed in 4 to 6 weeks.

Complicated Gallbladder Disease

Patients hospitalized with gallstone pancreatitis should undergo cholecystectomy before discharge after they are clinically stable and the pancreatitis has resolved. Additional delay in surgery has been shown to increase the risk of recurrent pancreatitis by 32% to 57%. Patients diagnosed with gallstone pancreatitis should undergo imaging to determine the presence of choledocholithiasis. This can be achieved either by preoperative magnetic resonance cholangiopancreatography (MRCP) or endoscopic retrograde cholangiopancreatography (ERCP) intraoperative cholangiography. In an institution with skilled gastroenterologists, ERCP has the advantage of being not only diagnostic but also therapeutic while still affording the surgeon the opportunity to perform common bile duct exploration if endoscopic therapy proves unsuccessful.

Patients with documented choledocholithiasis and concomitant cholangitis likewise should have cholectectomy performed after appropriate management of the common bile duct stones with decompression of the biliary tract, appropriate resuscitation of the patient, and antibiotic therapy.

CONTRAINDICATIONS TO LAPAROSCOPIC CHOLECYSTECTOMY

The absolute contraindications to laparoscopic cholecystectomy are identical to those for open cholecystectomy: inability to tolerate general anesthesia and uncorrectable coagulopathy. Conditions that favor use of an open rather than laparoscopic approach to cholecystectomy include acute pancreatitis, cholangitis with sepsis, end-stage liver disease (cirrhosis and portal hypertension), cholecystenteric fistulae (e.g., gallstone ileus), Mirizzi's syndrome, and suspicion of gallbladder cancer. Previous abdominal surgery does not preclude attempt at a laparoscopic approach, although good surgical judgment should be used when laparoscopic adhesiolysis proves to be treacherous.

All women of childbearing potential should undergo a pregnancy test before any surgical procedure, including laparoscopic cholecystectomy. The safest approach to the pregnant woman with gallbladder disease is conservative management followed by elective laparoscopic cholecystectomy. For those who fail conservative management, operation in the second trimester confers the lowest risk of complications. First-trimester risks include teratogenesis and miscarriage, and third-trimester risks include technical difficulties and poor visualization because of the gravid uterus, as well as increased chance of preterm labor and delivery.

PREOPERATIVE PREPARATION

Preoperative evaluation should include a complete blood count, renal function and electrolytes, hepatic enzymes, and coagulation parameters; amylase and lipase may be obtained if pancreatitis is suspected. An electrocardiogram is usually performed in patients older than age 50. Additional investigations such as echocardiography and exercise treadmill testing should be performed only if the patient's history or symptoms suggest the presence of cardiac disease.

Imaging of the gallbladder and biliary tract with ultrasound is routinely performed to confirm the presence of gallstones and to identify biliary tract dilatation or anomalous anatomy. Patients with biliary dilatation or anomalous anatomy should undergo additional imaging with ERCP, MRCP, or computed tomography (CT). If common bile duct stones are present, the surgeon may elect to perform an intraoperative cholangiogram and common bile duct exploration or to clear the duct preoperatively or postoperatively via ERCP and sphincterotomy. Intraoperative cholangiogram has not been found to prevent injury of the biliary system but does help to identify important structures and discover unsuspected duct injury when it has occurred.

The use of preoperative antibiotics has long been debated; however, a substantial body of literature, including a meta-analysis, a systematic review, and a recent prospective randomized study, has found no value to the use of prophylactic antibiotics for elective cholecystectomy. Thus this practice should be discouraged. Nevertheless, the use of prophylactic antibiotics may be warranted for a patient presenting emergently with acute cholecystitis.

PATIENT PREPARATION, POSITIONING, AND OPERATING ROOM SETUP

The patient should be placed in the supine position. A footboard may be used to prevent the patient from slipping off the end of the bed during the procedure. Venous thromboembolic prophylaxis should be instituted. Our approach includes thromboembolytic device (TED) hose and sequential compression devices (SCDs) to bilateral lower extremities, placed before induction of anesthesia. In high-risk patients, the use of anticoagulants should be considered. A Foley catheter may be placed at the discretion of the operating surgeon. The arms are extended and padded. If an intraoperative cholangiogram is performed, the patient should be placed on a fluoroscopy-compatible table, with the one arm tucked to allow for easier manipulation of the fluoroscopy machine.

The main viewing monitor should be positioned on the patient's right at the level of the shoulder. The second monitor is placed to the patient's left at the same level as the main monitor. The operating surgeon stands on the left side of the patient, and the assistant stands to the right. After the trocars are placed and the operation initiated, the patient should be placed in reverse Trendelenburg with a slight tilt to the patient's left to improve exposure of the gallbladder.

When the patient is pregnant, adequate hydration should be provided before, during, and after surgery. The patient should be placed in the supine position with a padded bump tilting the patient slightly to her left side to increase venous return.

Trocar Placement

The optimal approach for insertion of the first trocar remains controversial. We favor the Hasson technique because it is derived from the same safe general surgical principles used to enter the abdomen during traditional laparotomy. Most commonly, a small incision is made at, just above, or just below the umbilicus (the thinnest part of the abdomen) and visualization of each tissue layer is attempted. The fascia is grasped and divided, and anchoring sutures are secured. The peritoneum is grasped and entered sharply, and the blunt Hasson trocar is inserted. This first trocar site becomes the camera port. Three accessory ports (5 mm) are then inserted under direct vision. The position of these accessory ports may vary on the basis of the patient's body habitus and anatomy and the individual surgeon's preference. In general, two 5-mm ports are placed approximately two fingerbreadths below the right costal margin, one in the anterior axillary line and the other in the midclavicular line. Should it be necessary to convert to an open procedure, these incisions can be joined. The position of the fourth trocar is important because it is the site for the dissection instrument. To help determine the optimal placement for the fourth trocar, it is best to elevate the gallbladder using two graspers placed through the two 5-mm trocar sites already placed. The fourth trocar is generally placed subxiphoid to the right or through the falciform ligament. If the cystic duct is too large for a 5-mm clip applier, we use a 5-mm camera through the subxiphoid port and the 10-mm clip applier through the umbilical port (see Fig. 1).

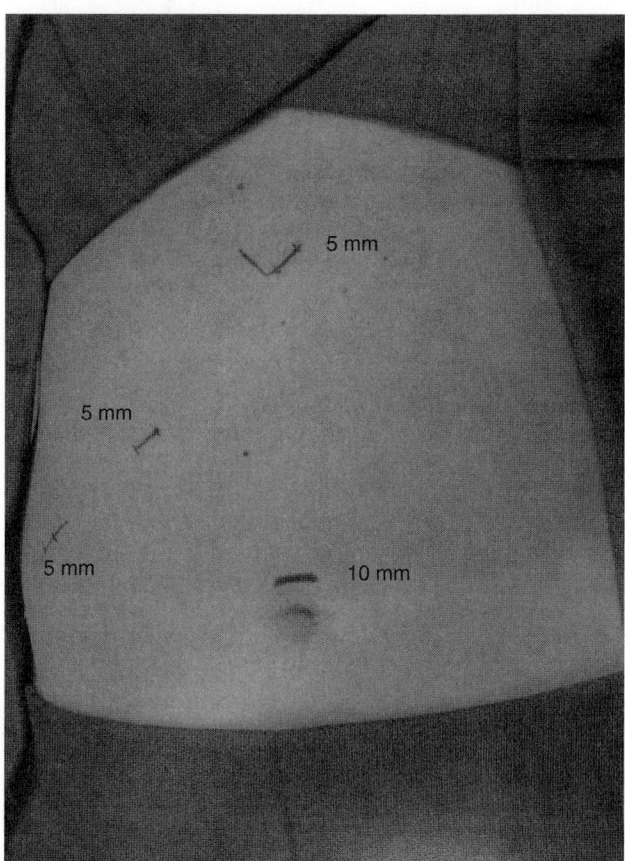

Figure I Common trocar size and placement for laparoscopic cholecystectomy. The umbilical trocar is almost always 10 mm, whereas the size and location of the remaining trocars may vary (2–10 mm), depending on surgeon preference and the availability of smaller instrumentation. (*See color insert Figure 55.*)

Depending on the surgeon's experience with laparoscopes, a 0-, 30-, or 45-degree scope may be used. The 30- or 45-degree scope provides better visualization of the ductal anatomy, helping to avoid bile duct injury.

Various authors have advocated the use of 5- or 2-mm trocars. One prospective study compared various trocar sizes, including the use of only 2-mm and 5-mm trocars for the procedure. The study concluded that there was no overall difference in cosmetic satisfaction, the incidence of complications, or postoperative pain score. It is also worth noting that, irrespective of the use of small trocars, the gallbladder must be delivered through one of the trocar sites, and this may frequently necessitate wound extension to retrieve the gallbladder.

In the pregnant patient, the Hasson blunt technique in the supraumbilical position is the best option for safe access to the abdomen. The use of low pressures (10–12 mm Hg) to create pneumoperitoneum is important in the pregnant patient but is desirable in all patients because it will also improve venous return and renal perfusion and decrease the risk of vagal overstimulation.

TECHNIQUES OF LAPAROSCOPIC CHOLECYSTECTOMY

Adhesiolysis

Laparoscopic cholecystectomy can be difficult when right upper quadrant adhesions obscure visualization and access to the gallbladder; however, careful, sharp dissection using Metzenbaum scissors

and countertraction is usually successful in overcoming this problem. After the gallbladder fundus has been identified, the dissection can then continue by remaining close to the gallbladder wall, locating the gallbladder neck and cystic duct junction, the cystic duct and cystic artery. Electrocautery should be minimized to decrease the risk of thermal injury to surrounding bowel or ductal structures.

Decompression of a Tense Gallbladder

Occasionally, the gallbladder may be tense and difficult to grasp because of acute cholecystitis or hydrops. To manage this and to improve exposure, the gallbladder can be decompressed under direct visualization using a 14- or 16-gauge needle, or an opening can be made in the gallbladder and its contents aspirated using a suction irrigator. To prevent further leakage of gallbladder contents, an atraumatic grasper can be used to retract the gallbladder and occlude the opening.

One-Handed or Two-Handed Technique

The key to a safe and successful operative dissection is exposure of the critical view. Several anatomic landmarks have been described that help to attain this view, including the gallbladder neck, the cystic lymph node, the gallbladder-cystic duct junction, Calot's triangle, and Rouviere's sulcus.

An atraumatic grasper is placed through the lateral-most right-sided port, and the fundus of the gallbladder is retracted in a superior and lateral position over the right lobe of the liver. In the one-handed technique, the assistant grasps the infundibulum with a second atraumatic grasper through the remaining right-sided 5-mm port and provides traction in an inferolateral direction, thereby opening the angle between the cystic duct and the common bile duct. The surgeon then operates the camera with the left hand while performing a meticulous circumferential dissection of the cystic duct and cystic artery through the epigastric port with the right hand. Staying close to the gallbladder during exposure of the gallbladder neck will help to define the cystic artery, which at this level invariably terminates on the gallbladder. Similarly, identifying the cystic lymph node and dissecting lateral to it provides a signpost for the cystic duct and artery. After the gallbladder-cystic duct junction has been identified, Calot's triangle (the inferior border of the liver superiorly, the cystic duct inferolaterally and the common hepatic duct medially) may be dissected out (see photos of Calot's triangle and the critical view in Fig. 2). When fibrosis, a contracted gallbladder, edema, or adhesions preclude the identification of the gallbladder-cystic duct junction, identification of Rouviere's sulcus can be an invaluable aid in directing the operative dissection. This sulcus, found in 70% to 80% of livers, was described by Henri Rouviere in 1924. Located to the right of the hepatic hilum and anterior to the caudate lobe, this 2- to 5-cm sulcus defines the right portal triad and consistently defines the plane of the common bile duct. If the biliary anatomy remains unclear despite the aforementioned maneuvers, intraoperative cholangiography is indispensable in resolving any ambiguities.

In contrast, the two-handed technique requires the surgeon to use the left hand to grasp the infundibulum and provide traction inferolaterally to expose the critical view. Dissection begins high on the gallbladder, and the loose areolar tissue is gently teased away to expose both the cystic duct at its point of entry into the gallbladder and the liver bed behind it, creating the critical view. Identifying the gallbladder-cystic duct junction provides essential anatomic confirmation, which allows attention to be safely turned to the careful placement of metallic clips.

In either technique, one clip is placed as close to the gallbladder as possible and two clips are placed distally on the cystic duct, leaving enough space between the clips to divide the duct safely. An Endo-loop (Ethicon Endosurgery, Somerville, NJ) can also be used for

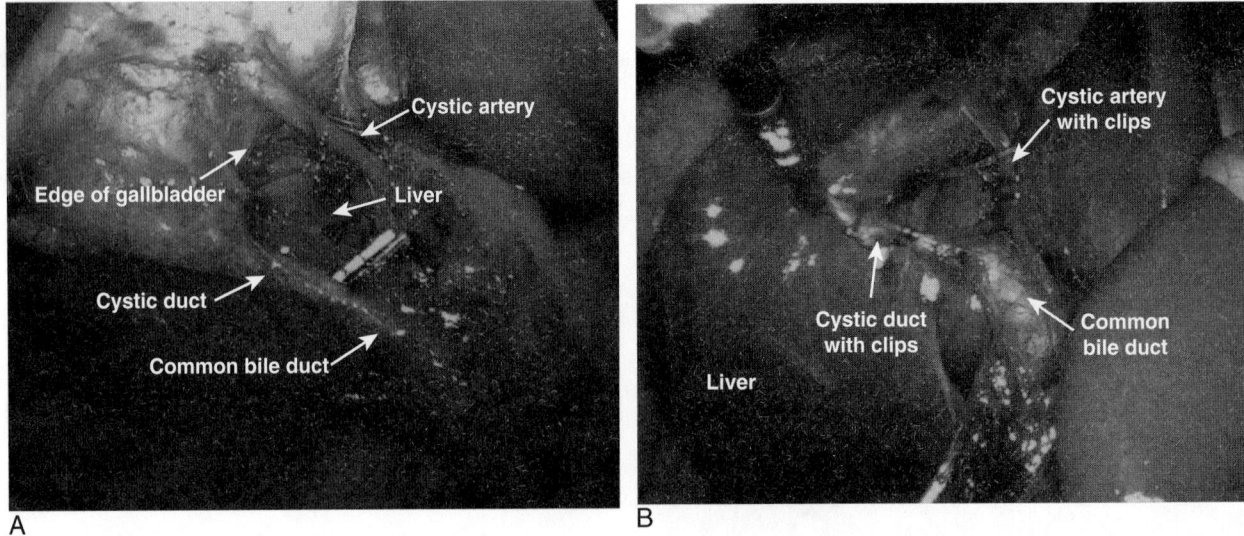

A B

Figure 2 **(A)** Calot's triangle, defined superiorly by the inferior border of the liver, inferolaterally by the cystic duct, and medially by the common hepatic duct, is clearly identified. **(B)** The "critical view" affords unobstructed visualization of the liver posterior to the structures in Calot's Triangle, allowing the surgeon to safely place clips proximally and distal on the cystic duct and cystic artery before transaction. Failure to achieve this critical view risks potential injury to the common bile duct. (*See color insert Figure 56.*)

ligation of the cystic duct for additional security as in the case of a dilated duct. The cystic artery is then ligated and divided, and the gallbladder is dissected away from the liver bed using electrocautery. The camera is then moved to the epigastric port (5 mm), an Endo-catch bag (US Surgical, Norwalk, CT) is inserted through the umbilical port (10 mm), and the gallbladder is removed under direct visualization. The umbilical trocar is then replaced and pneumoperitoneum recreated to visualize the operative field and confirm hemostasis. After removing the remaining ports, the abdomen is then desufflated, and standard fascial closure is performed.

Dome Down Technique

This technique essentially reproduces the approach taken during traditional open cholecystectomy in that the dissection is initiated at the dome of the gallbladder and is carried down toward the triangle of Calot. Dissection of the gallbladder away from the liver bed

affords circumferential exposure of the infundibulum and readily allows identification of the cystic duct and artery. This technique is especially helpful for thick cystic ducts or in cases in which fibrosis or scarring within Calot's triangle renders dissection especially hazardous (see Fig. 3).

Conversion to Open Procedure

The surgeon's main objective is to remove the gallbladder safely and avoid injury to adjacent vital structures. Consequently, it is imperative that the surgeon recognize the circumstances under which conversion to open cholecystectomy is warranted. It is important to emphasize here that conversion to open cholecystectomy should never be considered a complication or a failure of the laparoscopic technique. Livingston and colleagues reviewed data from the National Hospital Discharge database from 1998 to 2001 and found that three quarters of all cholecystectomies were completed

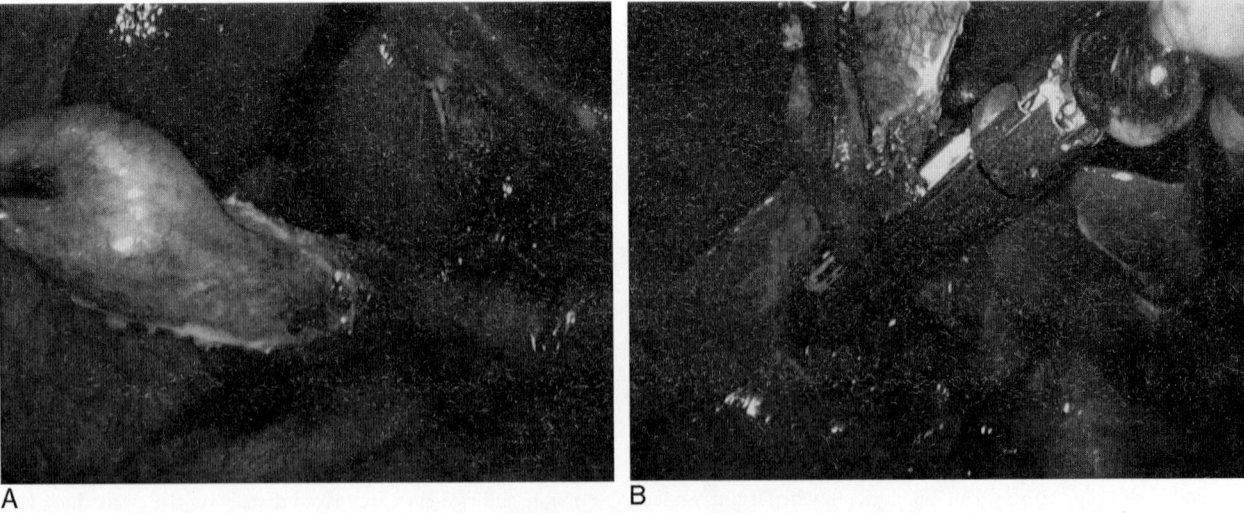

A B

Figure 3 **(A)** "Dome down technique." Note that the gallbladder has been dissected free from the liver bed and is attached only to the cystic duct. **(B)** The thickened, inflamed cystic duct is transected with the use of an endostapler. (*See color insert Figure 57.*)

Table 1: Risks Factors Influencing the Conversion from Laparoscopic to Open Cholecystectomy

Acute cholecystitis
Chronic cholecystitis
Male sex
Obesity
Cancer
Hypertension
Psychoses
Rheumatoid arthritis
Collagen vascular disease
Acquired immunodeficiency syndrome (AIDS)

laparoscopically, with a conversion rate of 5% to 10%. Risk factors for conversion included acute or chronic cholecystitis, male sex, obesity, acquired immunodeficiency syndrome (AIDS), arthritis, psychosis, cancer, and hypertension (Table 1). However, the authors concluded that, even in patients with multiple risk factors (but without clear contraindications), there is benefit in attempting laparoscopic cholecystectomy. More than two thirds of such high-risk patients underwent laparoscopic procedures successfully and thus benefited from a reduction in length of stay and postoperative complications.

Nevertheless, it is essential that all patients undergoing laparoscopic cholecystectomy be fully informed of the possibility that conversion to open cholecystectomy may be necessary and also receive a thorough description of the specific risks of the procedure.

COMPLICATIONS

Bleeding

Bleeding may arise from several sources during laparoscopic cholecystectomy, including abdominal wall and trocar sites, the cystic artery or its branches, the liver bed, or omental adhesions. During initial trocar insertion, transillumination of the abdominal wall is helpful in identifying and avoiding small superficial and epigastric vessels. Similarly, removal of the trocars should always be performed under direct visualization. If trocar removal is met with significant bleeding, the use of electrocautery or a suture (Carter Thompson approach) is usually sufficient to achieve hemostasis. During the dissection of Calot's triangle, care should be taken to identify posterior cystic artery branches and ligate them as needed. Any bleeding arising from the lysis of omental adhesions from the gallbladder during initial dissection may be treated with judiciously applied electrocautery, taking care to avoid injury to the nearby duodenum and hepatic flexure. Bleeding from the liver bed is common and is usually well treated with electrocautery as well. If such bleeding proves refractory to electrocautery, additional modalities may be required, such as the use of fibrin glue, prothrombotic agents (e.g., Gelfoam [Pfizer, New York, NY], Surgicel [Johnson & Johnson, New Brunswick, NJ]), or argon beam coagulation. In cases in which hemorrhage cannot be controlled, conversion to an open procedure may become necessary.

Bile Duct Injuries

The incidence of bile duct injuries remains higher with laparoscopic cholecystectomy (0.3%-1.0%) than during open cholecystectomy (0.1%-0.2%). Essential to minimizing the incidence of these injuries during either technique is a keen awareness of the local anatomy and its variations and the use of exacting surgical technique. Bile duct injury, when it occurs, is identified intraoperatively in only 40% to 80% of cases. It should go without saying that such detection is desirable because immediate repair of the injury can be performed only when it is correctly identified. Any such bile duct injury should be repaired as an open procedure and should not be attempted laparoscopically. A small choledochotomy may be managed by reconstruction over a T-tube. Most bile duct injuries are more extensive than can be managed in this manner and require formal hepaticojejunostomy for definitive management. In cases of delayed recognition of bile duct injury, management principles include immediate percutaneous drainage of any biloma, transhepatic biliary decompression, and formal biliary tract reconstruction after a period of at least 6 weeks.

Other Complications

Several other complications to consider include trocar hernias and bowel injuries. Care should be taken to close the umbilical port site, taking good bites of the fascia. In an obese patient, one option is to close the defect using a Carter Thompson technique. Bowel injuries can be avoided by ensuring careful and meticulous dissection.

CONCLUSION

In 1991, the National Institutes of Health concluded that laparoscopic cholecystectomy was a safe and acceptable alternative treatment modality in the management of gallbladder disease. During the years that have followed this pronouncement, dramatic advances in both the technology of surgical endoscopy and technical skills of practitioners have led to laparoscopic cholecystectomy's supplanting traditional open surgery as the gold standard for treating gallbladder disease. Advantages of the procedure include improved cosmesis, decreased incisional pain, and faster recovery time and quicker return to work; several recent series suggest that laparoscopic cholecystectomy can be performed safely and effectively as an outpatient procedure.

SUGGESTED READINGS

Calland JF, Tanaka K, Foley E, and others: Outpatient laparoscopic cholecystectomy: patient outcomes after implementation of a clinical pathway, *Ann Surg* 233:704, 2001.

Chang WT, Lee KT, Chuang SC, and others: The impact of prophylactic antibiotics on postoperative infection complication in elective laparoscopic cholecystectomy: a prospective randomized study, *Am J Surg* 191:721, 2006.

Debru E, Dawson A, Leibman S, and others, Department of Upper Gastrointestinal Surgery, Concord Repatriation General Hospital: Does routine intraoperative cholangiography prevent bile duct transaction? *Surg Endosc* 20:176, 2006.

Gallstones and Laparoscopic Cholecystectomy, NIH Consensus Statement, 10(3), September 14-16, 1992.

Lillemoe KD, Lin JW, Talamini MA, and others: Laparoscopic cholecystectomy as a "true outpatient procedure; intial experience in 130 consecutive patients", *J Gastrointest Surg* 3:44, 1999.

MacFadyen BV Jr, Vecchio R, Ricardo AE, and others: Bile duct injury after laparoscopic cholecystectomy. The United States experience, *Surg Endosc* 12:315, 1998.

Novitsky YW, Kercher KW, Czerniach DR, and others: Advantages of mini-laparoscopic vs conventional laparoscopic cholecystectomy, *Arch Surg* 140:1178, 2005.

LAPAROSCOPIC COMMON BILE DUCT EXPLORATION

John D. Mellinger, MD, and Bruce V. MacFadyen, MD

For decades before the advent of laparoscopic cholecystectomy (LC) in the late 1980s, surgeons had perfected their skills in open surgical techniques for the management of choledocholithiasis. Common duct stones (CBDS) were recognized in 5%-15% of patients undergoing routine operative cholangiography, and endoscopic retrograde cholangiopancreatography (ERCP) was already established as a tool in the parasurgical management of such pathology. As gastrointestinal surgeons developed laparoscopic skill and tools that expanded their therapeutic armamentarium, attempts to achieve laparoscopic clearance of choledocholithiasis were reported and developed. These techniques provided the potential for simultaneous therapy of concomitant choledocholithiasis at the time of laparoscopic cholecystectomy. Randomized trials have now documented the potential of such procedures to achieve common duct clearance with similar efficacy, morbidity, and mortality, as well as decreased cost and hospitalization time, compared with other approaches such as LC in concert with preoperative or postoperative ERCP. This review highlights the various therapeutic options the surgeon may employ in approaching CBDS laparoscopically and details the equipment necessities, technique, and appropriate use of each in the spectrum of management options for choledocholithiasis.

THERAPEUTIC OPTIONS

Choledocholithiasis can occur without any associated historical, laboratory, or radiologic abnormalities. Frequently, however, there may be preoperative clues that should increase the suspicion of CBDS. These include a history of jaundice, cholangitis, or pancreatitis or abnormal serum liver function studies such as elevated alkaline phosphatase or gamma glutamyl transferase levels. Radiologic evidence, including a dilatated common bile duct on ultrasound or computed tomography (>6 mm in younger patients, >8 mm at any age), or evidence of visible choledocholithiasis on transabdominal or endoscopic ultrasound or magnetic resonance cholangiopancreatography (MRCP) may also heighten suspicion. In settings in which these indicators are present, preoperative techniques may be considered if the expertise and equipment to allow laparoscopic common bile duct exploration (LCBDE) is not available. Techniques for managing common bile duct stones preoperatively or postoperatively should be within the surgeon's purview to guide patient care. Conversely, single-session diagnosis and therapy can be facilitated by operative cholangiography with concomitant LCBDE when dictated by cholangiographic findings. A detailed listing of all therapeutic options is outlined in Table 1.

Preoperative ERCP is an appropriate consideration in patients with rapidly progressing biliary pancreatitis or cholangitis or in patients who are poor candidates for general anesthesia. It may also be considered in elderly patients with presentations specific for complications of CBDS because the majority of these patients do not require cholecystectomy for other symptoms or complications during their remaining longevity, provided that the choledocholithiasis is cleared at the time of ERCP. Dissolution therapy is of primarily research interest because oral agents (ursodeoxycholic acid) require a prolonged period of time to work, and infusible agents (methyl-*tert*-butyl ether [MTBE] or mono-octanoin) require

Table 1: Therapeutic Options for Managing Common Bile Duct Stones

Preoperative

ERCP/ES

PTC and balloon dilatation of papilla or extraction

Extracorporeal lithotripsy

Chemical dissolution agents

Intraoperative

Laparoscopic/open CBDE, with or without choledochoscopy

ERCP/ES

Antegrade sphincterotomy

Intracorporeal lithotripsy

Laparoscopic/open choledochoduodenostomy or transduodenal sphincteroplasty

Postoperative

ERCP/ES

PTC

T-tube tract stone extraction

Choledochoscopy via transhepatic (post-PTC) or T-tube tract

Extracorporeal or intracorporeal lithotripsy

Chemical dissolution agents

CBDE, Common bile duct exploration; *ERCP,* endoscopic retrograde cholangiopancreatography; *ES,* endoscopic sphincterotomy; *PTC,* percutaneous transhepatic cholangiography;

invasive biliary access and associated significant complication (MTBE) or poor success rates (mono-octanoin). Extracorporeal lithotripsy may be a consideration in patients who are not operative candidates but often requires ERCP or other drainage procedures to allow uncomplicated clearance of stone fragments and is seldom considered an independent, primary, therapeutic maneuver. Percutaneous transhepatic cholangiographic (PTC) access is an alternative to ERCP and may be considered in similar settings such as cholangitis, particularly when ERCP is unsuccessful or rendered difficult by surgically altered anatomy such as prior Roux-en-Y reconstruction of the gastric outlet.

Intraoperative options include LCBDE via a transcystic method or via choledochotomy, intraoperative ERCP with endoscopic sphincterotomy, antegrade sphincterotomy, and intracorporeal lithotripsy. LCBDE technique is detailed later and is the preferred method when expertise and equipment capabilities allow. Intraoperative ERCP is more difficult with supine patient positioning but may be successfully employed with good results in experienced hands. Antegrade sphincterotomy as described by DePaula may be employed via a transcystic approach. In this technique, the surgeon passes a standard endoscopic sphincterotome over a guidewire passed via the cystic duct into the duodenal lumen. A duodenoscope is passed perorally and used to observe the orientation of the sphincterotome as it traverses the papilla, so that a sphincterotomy can be safely performed and facilitate common duct stone clearance (Fig. 1). The sphincter may also be balloon dilated, although both endoscopic and laparoscopic reports with this approach document an associated risk of pancreatitis. Intracorporeal lithotripsy can be performed with a variety of laser tools, electrohydraulic lithotripters, or simple mechanical agents such as crushing baskets. Lithotripsy techniques are particularly worthy of

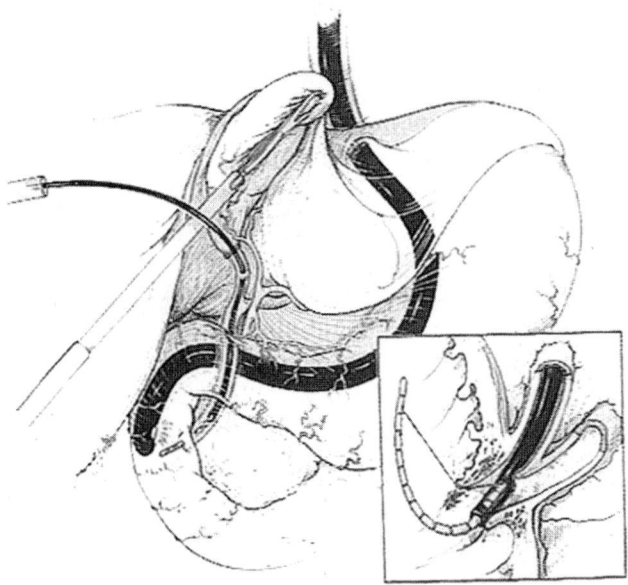

Figure 1 Technique of antegrade sphincterotomy.

Table 2: Supplies for Laparoscopic Common Bile Duct Exploration Cart

Medications: glucagon, lidocaine
3- to 5-F Fogarty catheter
Segura-type baskets (2.4- or 3-F, spiral, flat, 3 and 4 wire)
0.035-inch guidewire
Balloon (8-mm outer diameter) and/or mechanical (7- to 12-F) over the wire dilatators
3-mm or smaller choledochoscope with 1.1-mm or larger working channel
Additional choledochoscopic equipment: light source, saline tubing, adapter to allow simultaneous irrigation and instrumentation via biopsy channel, second camera, second monitor or picture-in-picture display with video switcher
Atraumatic grasping forceps (if not already in laparoscopic tray)
Pretied loop ligatures
Cystic duct drainage tube of choice
T-tubes, or other suitable common bile duct drainage catheter or stent
Lithotripter probes (if desired or necessary)
Sphincterotome (if antegrade sphincterotomy necessary)
Sleeve for choledochoscope passage via trocar (if desired)

consideration with impacted stones, although a concomitant drainage procedure to facilitate fragment clearance is often required.

Postoperative options include ERCP, PTC, dissolution, and lithotripsy as described earlier. T-tube stone extraction after tube placement at the time of operative CBDE and choledochoscopic extraction via transhepatic or T-tube access tracts are additional postoperative options. Such methods may be particularly helpful when expeditious decompression without definitive clearance of CBDS is dictated by the patient's comorbid status intraoperatively or when CBDE is unsuccessful. The surgeon is wise to have all these options in mind as the patient's care is executed.

TECHNIQUE

Preparation and Equipment

It is helpful to have all potentially necessary equipment available on a cart. General requirements include fluoroscopy with digital storage capacity and video playback capability. The supplies necessary for transcystic and choledochotomy approaches are detailed in Table 2. As with any technically complex, multiple-device procedure, it is wise for the surgeon and entire operating team to have had troubleshooting, dry laboratory, and intraoperative rehearsals with the equipment before using them in direct patient care.

Operating room setup can be as for standard LC. It may be helpful for the patient's arms to be tucked to optimize options in positioning the surgical team and the fluoroscope, and this can also facilitate later placement of a table-held retractor, if required. Being able to rotate the table so that the patient is in reverse Trendelenburg position and has the right side elevated may help to allow exposure of the porta hepatis. Use of a footboard, beanbag cushion, and securing straps or tape may be helpful and should be strongly considered for obese patients. Lead protection for members of the operating team should be used and standard radiation safety measures followed. Total fluoroscopic averages 5 minutes for LCBDE when performed by experienced surgeons.

A typical four-trocar technique as used most commonly for LC is typically employed. The initial steps of the operation, with elevation of the gallbladder via the fundus, lateral retraction of the infundibulum, and dissection of the structures within the

hepatoduodenal ligament are as per usual LC conduct. After the anatomy of the gallbladder/cystic duct junction is clearly delineated, a clip is placed on the gallbladder side of the junction, and a small ductotomy made to allow performance of an operative cholangiogram. It is true that laparoscopic ultrasound may be reliably used in experienced hands to identify the anatomy and presence of CBDS, but real-time imaging during common duct manipulation for identified choledocholithiasis is best accomplished under fluoroscopic guidance.

A variety of tools may be used to perform the cholangiogram. Typically a 4- or 5-F ureteral or cholangiographic catheter is employed and is positioned through the right subcostal trocar either via direct advancement or with the use of a specially designed clamp such as the Olsen-Berci clamp. Cholangiogram catheters may also be positioned via separate sleeves or intravenous cannulae (typically 14 gauge), which can provide adequate access for all maneuvers of transcystic CBDE up to choledochoscopy. Catheters may be secured by a clamp with laparoscopic clips or via balloon inflation if a balloon-type catheter is employed. Careful performance and interpretation of the cholangiogram by the surgeon is the prerequisite of any laparoscopic approach to the CBD. Care should be taken to visualize the entire biliary tree, including the major intrahepatic radicals, the cystic duct–common duct junction, and the distal common duct–papillary area. Incomplete visualization proximally, if not related to stone, stricture, or neoplastic obstruction, can often be addressed by intravenous narcotic administration to induce sphincter of Oddi spasm, change to a Trendelenburg position, or allow distal extrinsic compression of the biliary system by a laparoscopic instrument with continued contrast injection. Inadequate proximal filling may also be due to incorrect identification of the anatomy and inadvertent cannulation of the CBD, which must always be considered, or it may be secondary to balloon occlusion of the common duct if a balloon catheter is used and advanced beyond the cystic duct–common duct junction. The latter circumstance is readily recognized and relieved by gradual balloon deflation under continued fluoroscopic injection and inspection. Inadequate flow into the duodenum can be relieved by intravenous glucagon administration if it is due simply to sphincter spasm.

Common features suggesting the presence of CBDS include a dilatated system, filling defects that are fixed, irregular, or obstructive to flow or failure of contrast to flow into the duodenum or to fill one of the hepatic radicals. In the setting of such abnormalities, the surgeon may appropriately commence with laparoscopic exploration of the biliary system.

Transcystic Approach

Transcystic manipulation of the CBD is the simplest technique and is suitable, using one or more of the techniques subsequently outlined, for settings in which stones are less than 10 mm in size, distal to the cystic duct junction, and fewer than 10 in number. The simplest initial maneuver is the flushing technique. This technique works in 50% to 60% of cases for stones in the 2- to 3-mm size range and requires no other special preparation. In this technique 10 ml of 1% lidocaine without epinephrine is instilled via the cholangiogram catheter, and 1 mg of glucagon is given intravenously by the anesthesiologist. The surgeon then irrigates the bile duct with approximately 20 ml of saline or dilute contrast. Under fluoroscopic guidance, the stones can often be seen flushing through the papilla, and completion cholangiography can then be performed to document the absence of persistent filling defects or obstruction to flow. Pressurized systems for irrigation other than manual control by the surgeon are not advised because reflux into the pancreatic duct is common and, if performed with excessive pressure, may increase the risk of postoperative pancreatitis.

If flushing does not work or the stones are too large to expect success with this approach, transcystic duct manipulation is performed. The surgeon should initially assess the size of the stones in relation to the size and course of the cystic duct. If the duct is long or tortuous or if choledochoscopy is believed likely to be required, repositioning the ductotomy closer to the cystic duct/ CBD junction may be mechanically advantageous. Dilatation of the cystic duct with either over-the-wire serial mechanical dilators (e.g., ureteral dilatation bougies) or a balloon dilatator (preferred) may be required for larger stones, although it is useful to remember that most CBDS originate from the gallbladder and have thus demonstrated the ability to traverse the cystic duct at some point to reach the CBD. If required, dilatating maneuvers should be performed with care because tearing of the duct onto its junction with the common duct can occur.

After assessing and, if necessary, performing the described preparatory maneuvers, the simplest next step is to perform balloon or basket extraction. These techniques may be employed under fluoroscopic guidance without choledochoscopy or with choledochoscopic guidance. The latter is usually necessary for proximal or distal stones that cannot be captured under simple fluoroscopic guidance. With the balloon technique, the cholangiogram catheter is exchanged for a 4-F Fogarty catheter, which is advanced into the duodenum—typically a distance of approximately 10 cm from the cystic ductotomy site. This may be performed as a freehand technique or may be accomplished as an over-the-wire maneuver by passing a 0.035-inch hydrophilic wire through the cholangiogram catheter, which is then exchanged for the balloon catheter. Duodenal entry of the balloon catheter is confirmed fluoroscopically by inflating the balloon and gently tugging it back until resistance is felt at the papillary level. Positioning may be further confirmed by observing duodenal wall motion with gentle traction at the papilla by the balloon under fluoroscopy. At this point, the balloon is deflated and the catheter withdrawn slightly to place it in the distal-most CBD, where it is reinflated and then gently withdrawn (Fig. 2). The maneuver can be repeated until no stones or debris are retrieved at the cystic ductotomy site with further passes, at which point a completion cholangiogram is obtained to document CBDS clearance. One problem with this technique is that stones are trolled rather than grasped in the duct, and they may

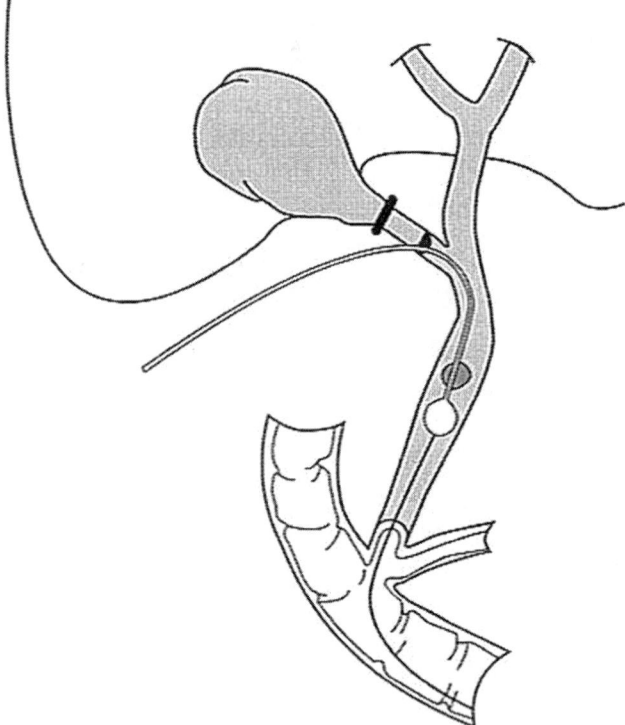

Figure 2 Transcystic removal of stone with balloon catheter under fluoroscopic guidance.

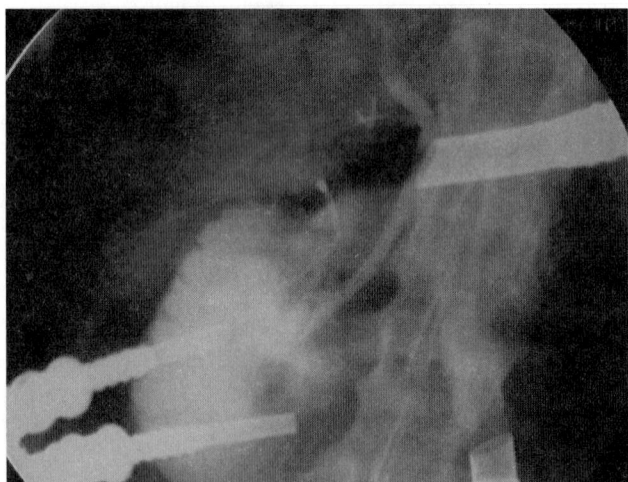

Figure 3 Operative cholangiogram demonstrating extravasation at ampulla after attempted transcystic laparoscopic common bile duct exploration with balloon catheter.

be displaced into the common hepatic duct rather than retrieved via the cystic duct by these manipulations; accordingly they may become more difficult to clear thereafter. Balloon damage to the papilla may also occur, although rarely, with these maneuvers (Fig. 3).

The basket technique may also be performed freehand but, given the metal-tipped nature of the device, may be more safely accomplished via catheter-guided placement. This is accomplished by advancing the 0.035-inch hydrophilic guidewire through the cholangiocatheter (CC) into the duodenum under fluoroscopic guidance. This is most facile if the CC is of 5-F size. The catheter is then advanced over the wire into the duodenum, and the wire is removed and exchanged for a 2.4-F basket. Baskets with straight and spiral, three- and four-wire designs should be available. Larger stones may require spiral or three-wire baskets (or both), which allow larger spaces between the wires for stone capture. The basket is advanced through the CC into the duodenal lumen, and then the CC and basket are withdrawn until the basket is in the lumen of the CBD distal to the stone. The basket is then opened and rapidly moved back and forth in the area of the stone to facilitate capture. If adequate contrast is still present, it may be possible to see the stone begin to move with the basket when it is captured. If not, capture may be inferred by closing the basket gently and noting resistance or incomplete closure of the basket handle. The basket is then withdrawn and the stone deposited on the omentum for subsequent removal, with further passes being made if required. Basket techniques are reported to be successful in 85% to 95% of cases.

Transcystic choledochoscopy is more technically demanding than the techniques just described but can improve success rates in experienced hands. After initial cholangiography and placement of the cystic ductotomy close to the CBD junction to overcome the resistance of the valves of Heister, a guidewire is passed into the duct and dilatation performed with one of the techniques mentioned earlier; this is typically necessary. Ureteral bougie-type dilatators are placed over a guidewire typically introduced through the midclavicular port. Dilatation to a 12-F size is typically required to allow subsequent passage of a 3-mm (9-F) or smaller choledochoscope with a 1.1 mm or greater working channel. A 5- to 8-mm balloon dilatator is typically employed for balloon dilatation (Fig. 4). Ducts smaller than 2.5 mm in size at outset are often not adequately dilatable to allow transcystic choledochoscopy. Once dilatation is achieved, the choledochoscope is advanced through the midclavicular port and manipulated into the duct with atraumatic grasping forceps positioned via the epigastric trocar. A sleeve may be used to facilitate the manipulation of the scope into the duct. A combination of external scope rotation and manipulation of the scope shaft by the atraumatic forceps intracorporeally (or

both) with deflection of the scope tip within its 180-degree range of motion, are used to position the scope. Warm saline irrigation is employed via the scope biopsy channel, and a special adapter is employed to allow simultaneous passage of a stone basket and pressurized irrigation via the biopsy channel. After the stone is visualized, a 2.4-F basket is passed via the biopsy channel to allow endoscopically visualized stone capture and withdrawal (Fig. 5). If multiple stones are present, it is wise to progress from proximal to distal in removal so that stones are not displaced in the process of extraction. Gravity may sometimes be used to reposition stones distally if they migrate proximally in the manipulation process. Stones that cannot be captured with a basket may be captured with a balloon and trapped against the endoscope to allow removal of the stone, balloon, and scope as a combined unit. Following successful stone removal, suture closure of the dilatated cystic ductotomy site is typically performed with a laparoscopic loop ligature because clip closure may not adequately secure the dilatated duct.

Stones that fail to respond to this measure may be dealt with in several ways. Direct laparoscopic choledochotomy (discussed later), intraoperative or postoperative ERCP, antegrade sphincterotomy (as described earlier), laparoscopic or open biliary bypass such as choledochoduodenostomy, simple biliary drainage with delayed endoscopic or radiologic management of residual choledocholithiasis, and lithotripsy may all be used. It is sometimes wise in such settings simply to leave a tube in place via the cystic duct that assures postoperative access by either the endoscopist or interventional radiologist and use a staged approach to complete common duct clearance while ensuring biliary drainage in the interim. Novel tubes such as those described by Fanelli and Cuschieri may be useful in achieving such transcystic access for subsequent ERCP or other interventions. We have used an 8-F red rubber catheter, which is inexpensive and readily available, in some such settings in the past; others have described using ureteral catheters in a similar fashion. Such transcystic tubes can be secured with absorbable suture at the cystic duct entry site and later removed

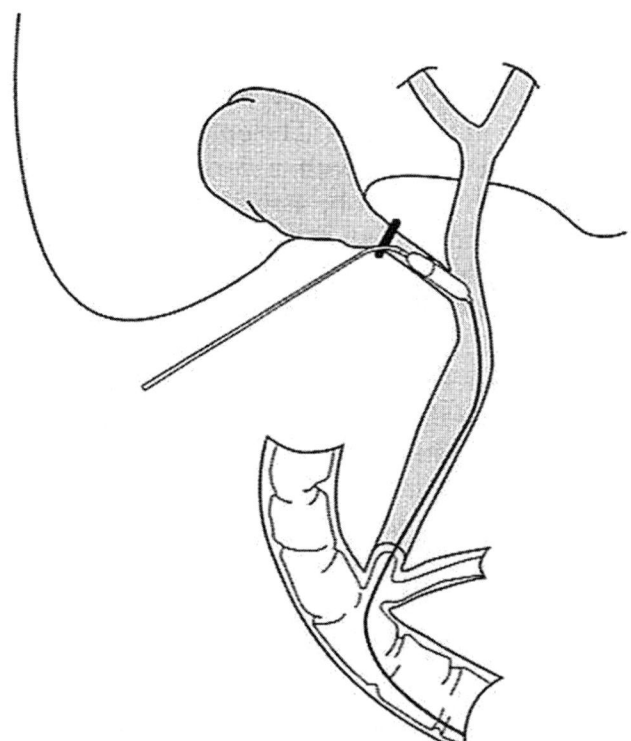

Figure 4 Balloon dilatation of cystic duct in preparation for choledochoscopy.

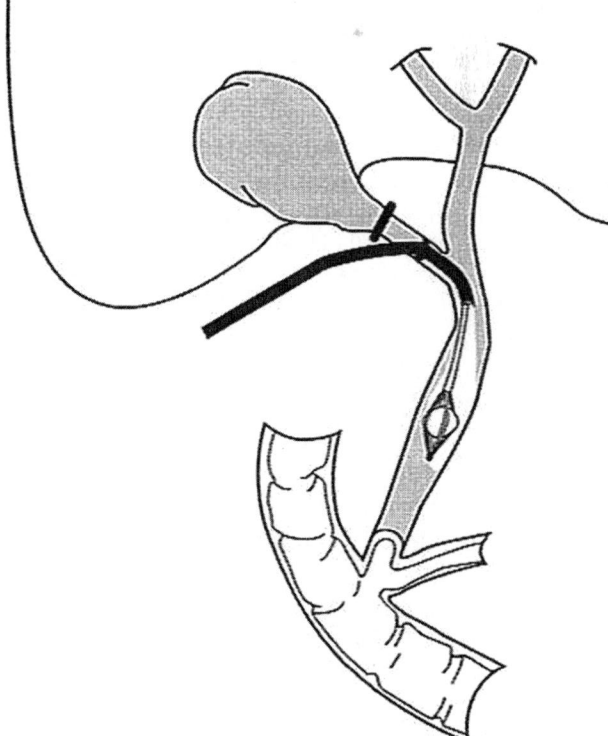

Figure 5 Basket stone extraction under choledochoscopic guidance via transcystic approach.

at the bedside. Lithotripsy may be performed mechanically if basket capture is achievable, but the stone will not deliver via the cystic duct by using one of the over-the-basket sheath devices not uncommonly employed with challenging stones during ERCP. These devices, although useful and relatively low cost, are somewhat stiff and may be difficult to maneuver via a transcystic approach. Laser and electrohydraulic (EHL) lithotripters may also be used under choledochoscopic guidance if care is taken to avoid damage to the adjacent duct and impacted or otherwise unclearable stones are encountered. EHL is less costly than laser and requires careful application of the lithotripsy probe against the stone itself. Lithotripsy techniques may be a helpful way to avoid more complex approaches for impacted stones, such as choledochoduodenostomy or transduodenal sphincteroplasty, and may also be a means for dealing with the problem of a trapped basket, should this occur in the process of LCBDE. We have found these techniques useful in truly rare situations that fail the other measures outlined or when alternative postoperative measures are made more challenging by anatomic constraints or knowledge of failed preoperative attempts at ERCP.

Transductal Choledochotomy Approach

Laparoscopic choledochotomy is considered when cystic duct insertion anatomy renders transcystic exploration difficult (Fig. 6), when the cystic duct is small (<2–2.5 mm), when CBDS are large (>6–8 mm), when proximal CBDS are present, or when transcystic or other measures fail and CBD diameter is at least 8 mm. Choledochotomy should not be used if the CBD is less than 6 mm in diameter. If the bile duct is grossly dilatated (>2.5 cm) or multiple stones are present (>10), consideration should be given to a definitive biliary drainage procedure such as choledochoduodenostomy. The laparoscopic skill level required for laparoscopic choledochotomy is greater than that necessary for transcystic CBDE, particularly with regard to suturing skill, and this should be weighed in decision making, depending on the experience of the surgeon and surgical team.

Room setup and preparation are as for laparoscopic cholecystectomy. The gallbladder is left attached following cholangiography to assist in exposure, and use of a table-held retractor may facilitate a stable operative field. A 30- or 45-degree laparoscope, which is used for all laparoscopic procedures routinely, is necessary to give an adequate view of the supraduodenal CBD. The CBD itself must be cleared anteriorly by dividing the overlying peritoneal and investing fascial tissues. The dissection should be kept on the anterior aspect of the duct to avoid injury to the blood supply, which runs longitudinally along the medial and lateral aspects of the duct. By clearing the duct and performing the ductotomy in a supraduodenal location, the surgeon is well prepared for choledochoduodenostomy

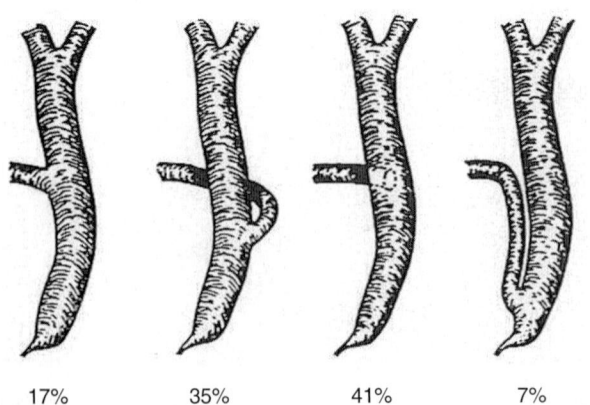

Figure 6   Variants in cystic duct insertion anatomy.

17%   35%   41%   7%

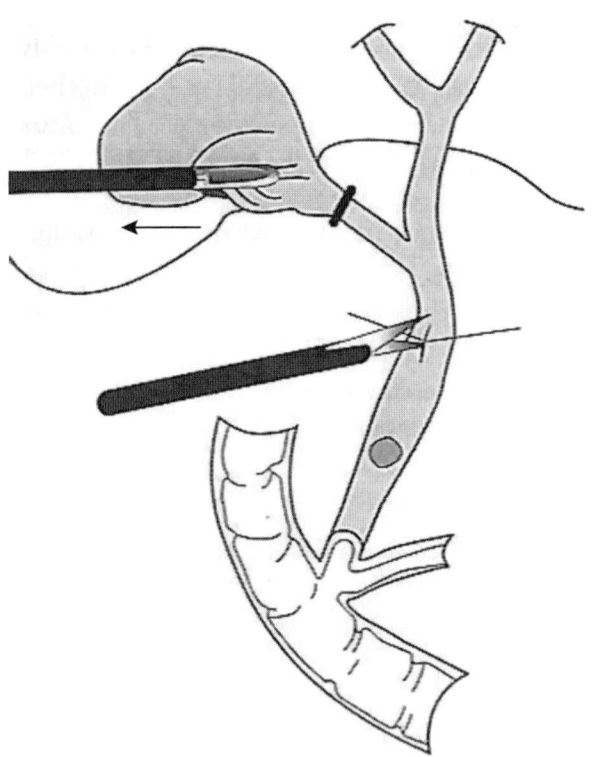

Figure 7   Choledochotomy with stay sutures to elevate anterior duct.

should it become necessary. At least 2 cm of duct are cleared, but excessive stripping beyond the area necessary for ductotomy and closure is avoided. A 1-cm ductotomy may be marked out with limited application of coagulating current and then made with the scissors and oriented vertically. By keeping the ductotomy on the small side, suturing requirement is minimized and most stones are still readily retrieved. Stay sutures may be used on the medial and lateral aspects of the ductotomy if desired (Fig. 7).

Initial maneuvers such as irrigating and balloon catheter sweeping of the duct may be employed with laparoscopic visualization and fluoroscopic guidance without choledochoscopy. If these methods fail, choledochoscopic guided extraction is performed. The choledochoscope may be inserted through the epigastric trocar or via a separately placed trocar positioned over the choledochotomy site. For difficult stones, use of a 10-mm accessory trocar and larger-caliber choledochoscope may improve maneuvering capabilities and accessory options for stone removal. The use of catheters, baskets, and lithotripsy devices is otherwise as outlined earlier in the chapter for transcystic choledochoscopy.

Tube drainage of the CBD via T-tube or specially designed biliary drainage catheters is advised following choledochotomy. This allows decompression of the duct in settings where postoperative edema resulting from manipulation is likely and may reduce the attendant risk of bile leakage with simple primary closure. Such drainage also can provide postoperative access for cholangiography and further therapy if retained stones are found. T-tube placement is performed by advancing a tube sized appropriately for CBD diameter (commonly 12–14 F) into the abdomen and manipulating the "T" ends into the duct proximal and distal to the choledochotomy. The latter maneuver may be facilitated by use of a guidewire or by grasping the two ends of the "T" with an atraumatic grasper and advancing into the choledochotomy before releasing. Monofilament fine suture (4.0–5.0) closure of the ductotomy is then performed by pushing the tube cephalad and placing the first suture adjacent to the tube to hold it in a stable position as the more distal sutures are placed (Fig. 8). Placement of an additional trocar to facilitate suturing

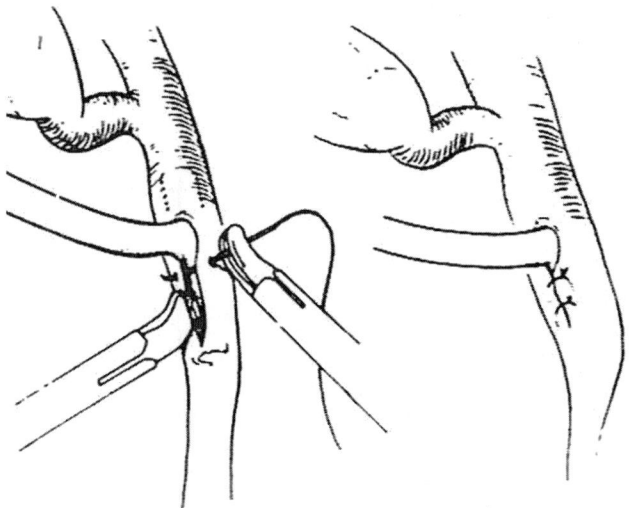

Figure 8   Closure of choledochotomy after T-tube placement.

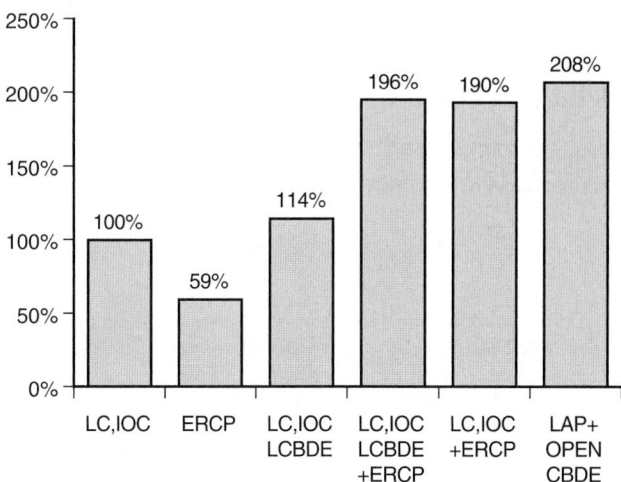

PERCENT OF LC/IOC CHARGES

Figure 9   Cost comparisons of various approaches to common duct stones with laparoscopic cholecystectomy.

OUTCOMES

The techniques outlined are well attested as providing CBD clearance in 85% to 96% of cases, with attendant morbidity in the range of 1.6% to 13%. Postoperative ERCP or conversion to an open procedure is required in 5% of cases in published series. Prospective randomized trials have shown overall success, and complication rates are comparable when LC combined with perioperative ERCP is compared with single-session LC/LCBDE. Cost analyses have shown that the latter approach is much more cost effective than a variety of other options (Fig. 9). Mean operative times for combined LC/transcystic LCBDE are in the 2- to 3-hour range, and in the 3- to 4-hour range for LC/LCBDE via choledochotomy. Higher morbidity and mortality rates with laparoscopic choledochotomy, compared with transcystic LCBDE, have been reported in several nonrandomized studies, reflecting the more challenging nature of both the pathology and surgery when this technique is required.

may be required, particularly if the epigastric trocar is high in the epigastrium, as is commonly done for laparoscopic cholecystectomy. Lower placement of the epigastric trocar in settings in which LCBDE via choledochotomy is anticipated may obviate the need for additional trocar placement. The external end of the tube is brought out through the abdominal wall in as straight a line as possible from the choledochotomy site and secured at the skin level. A closed suction drain is placed in the subhepatic space.

In summary, LCBDE is well attested as an outcome-equivalent and cost-containment-superior method for single-session therapy of choledocholithiasis in concert with LC. Team rehearsal, availability of all potentially necessary equipment in the operating suite or on a mobile cart, and awareness of other available management options for complex situations facilitate appropriate use of these techniques in the surgeon's practice.

SUGGESTED READINGS

Cuschieri A, Lezoche E, Morino M, and others: EAES multicenter prospective randomized trial comparing two-stage vs. single-stage management of patients with gallstone disease and ductal calculi, *Surg Endosc* 13:952, 1999.

DePaula AL, Hashiba K, Bafutto M, and others: Laparoscopic antegrade sphincterotomy, *Surg Laparosc Endosc* 3:157, 1993.

Petelin JB: Laparoscopic common bile duct exploration, *Surg Endosc* 17:1705, 2003.

Rhodes M, Sussman L, Cohen L, and others: Randomised trial of laparoscopic exploration of common bile duct versus postoperative endoscopic retrograde cholangiography for common bile duct stones, *Lancet* 351:159, 1998.

Traverso LW: A cost analysis of the treatment of common bile duct stones discovered during laparoscopic cholecystectomy, *Semin Laparosc Surg* 7:302, 2000.

Vecchio R, MacFadyen BV: Laparoscopic common bile duct exploration, *Arch Surg* 387:45, 2002.

Wood T, MacFadyen BV: Diagnostic and therapeutic choledochoscopy, *Semin Laparosc Surg* 7:288, 2000.

LAPAROSCOPIC APPENDECTOMY

Avraham Belizon, MD, Daniel L. Feingold, MD, and Richard L. Whelan, MD

Appendicitis is the most common surgical emergency in the United States, with an incidence of 1.1 cases per 1000 people per year. Since its introduction in 1894, appendectomy has been the treatment of choice for acute appendicitis. Open appendectomy, as described by McBurney, is typically a simple and effective treatment for appendicitis and has remained nearly unchanged for more than a century because of its low morbidity and high success rate.

Laparoscopic appendectomy was first reported by Dr. K. Semm in 1983; it did not gain immediate acceptance because the potential advantages over the open procedure were unclear. Over time it became evident that laparoscopic appendectomy offers advantages beyond the traditional open procedure by providing superior exposure, decreasing the rate of wound complications, and improving cosmesis. These factors have influenced many surgeons to adopt laparoscopy as their preferred approach to the patient with acute appendicitis.

OPERATIVE TECHNIQUE

The patient is placed in the supine position. After the induction of general endotracheal anesthesia, a urinary catheter is placed and the left arm is positioned at the patient's side, padded, and then secured with a draw sheet. Perioperative antibiotics and deep venous thrombosis prophylaxis are administered per routine before the incision. The surgeon and first assistant stand on the left side of the patient facing a single video monitor located on the right side of the patient (Fig. 1). The skin is appropriately prepared and draped, and a 12-mm port is placed via cutdown technique in the supraumbilical ridge. This site will serve as the main camera port, accommodate the laparoscopic linear stapler, and be the incision through which the specimen is extracted. A figure-of-eight suture is placed across the fascial defect, after which a blunt port with a grip is placed in the abdomen. After securing the fascial sutures to the port, pneumoperitoneum is established via CO$_2$ insufflation to 12 to 15 mm Hg. A 5-mm angled laparoscope is then introduced, and the abdomen is inspected immediately adjacent to the port to rule out an iatrogenic injury. Two 5-mm working ports are then placed under direct laparoscopic visualization in the midline, at least 4 fingerbreadths below the camera port, and in the left lower quadrant, lateral to the rectus sheath and equidistant from the pubis and the umbilicus. Reusable ports are used, when available, to help contain costs, per routine.

Although there are several adequate, alternative port configurations, this port setup places the surgeon opposite from the pathology, optimizes tissue triangulation, and allows successful completion of the operation laparoscopically in the vast majority of cases. Laparoscopic appendectomy is best accomplished by two-handed dissection, with the surgeon standing at the patient's left hip and the camera-holder standing on the same side in a more cephalad position.

First the diagnosis must be confirmed. Atraumatic bowel graspers are used to survey the abdomen, paying particular attention

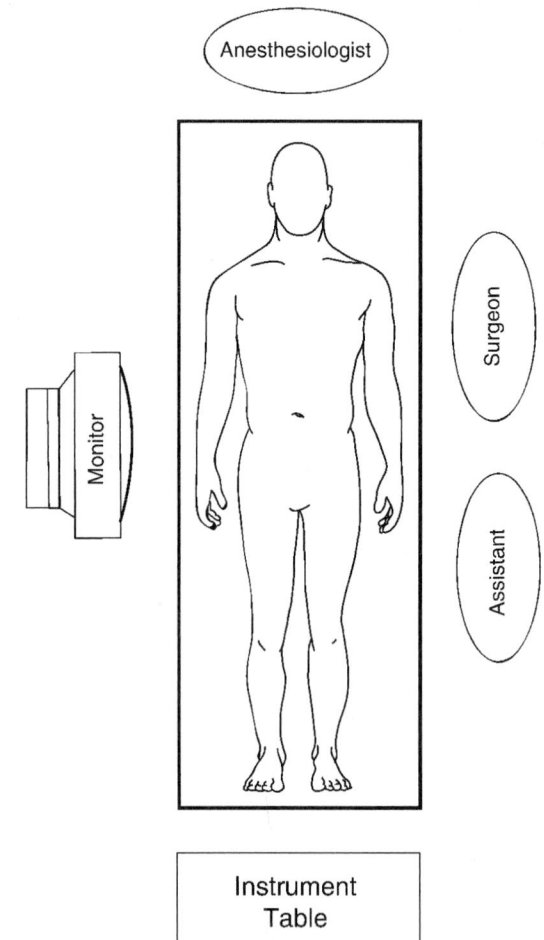

Figure 1   Room setup for laparoscopic appendectomy.

to the right lower quadrant. If the appendix is found to be normal and not inflamed, then a thorough search of the abdomen and pelvis with consideration of the adnexa, uterus, ileum, colon, gallbladder, and other viscera must be carried out in an effort to find an explanation for the patient's signs and symptoms. Regardless of the findings, a thorough examination of the uterus, adnexa, and terminal ileum should be carried out. Assuming that the diagnosis of appendicitis is confirmed, the patient is positioned in a slight Trendelenburg position with the table tilted to the left side. This position encourages the small bowel to fall away from the right lower quadrant and improves exposure. The bowel can usually be carefully manipulated using closed instruments; if possible, direct grasping of the bowel should be avoided. The acutely inflamed appendix is typically edematous, distended, and indurated and may not allow for retraction with an atraumatic grasper. In this situation, a heavier grasping instrument may be used, taking care not to avulse or perforate the diseased appendix.

Depending on the degree of inflammation, the position of the appendix and factors such as adhesions from prior surgery and the amount of intra-abdominal fat, the surgeon often must rely on local anatomic landmarks to guide the dissection. In particular, the terminal ileum is followed, moving toward the cecum until the antimesenteric, ileal fat pad is observed, marking the most terminal ileum (Fig. 2). In addition, the taenia libera of the ascending colon is followed toward the cecum to help identify the base of the appendix.

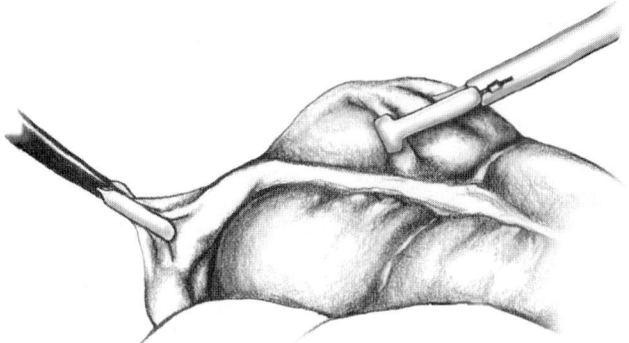

Figure 2 Exposure of the appendix.

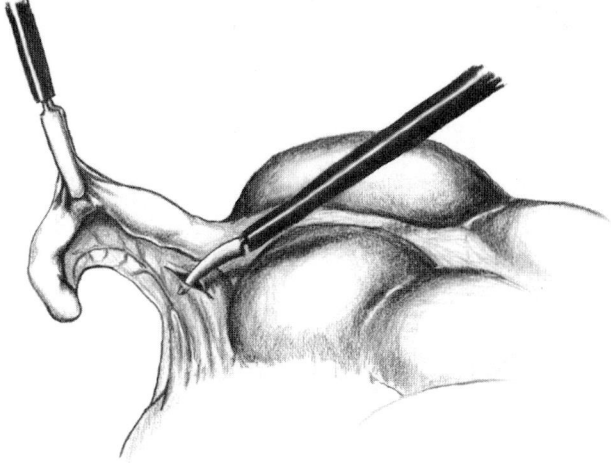

Figure 3 Dissection of the mesoappendix to create a window near the base of the appendix.

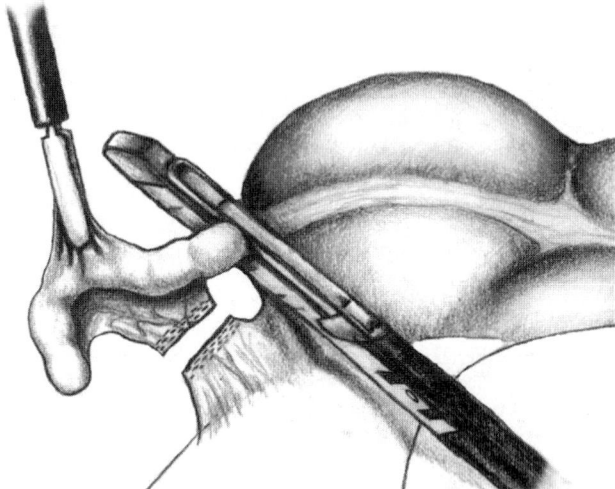

Figure 4 Transection of the appendix with a linear stapling device.

It is helpful to begin the dissection of the acutely inflamed appendix by mobilizing the appendix from the associated inflammatory process. This is usually accomplished by peeling the appendix off of the secondarily inflamed tissues in a fashion similar to the blunt, finger-fracture technique used in the open approach to appendectomy. The inflammatory process often involves the ileal fat pad, the terminal ileum, the cecum, the right iliac fossa, and the abdominal sidewall. On occasion the sigmoid colon or the right adnexa may also be involved.

In the event of a retrocecal appendix, the cecum and terminal ileum must be mobilized medially and in a cephalad direction to access the appendix. By retracting through the lateral port and using the shears through the suprapubic port, the lateral wall attachments of the cecum are divided with a combination of sharp and blunt dissection. As with the other portions of the case, minimal, if any, electrocautery is required. Care should be taken to avoid dissecting laterally into the abdominal wall or posteriorly into the retroperitoneum. As mentioned earlier, to mobilize the cecum fully and to expose a retrocecal appendix, the terminal ileum must be mobilized. This is accomplished by retracting the ileal fat pad anteriorly and medially and incising the peritoneum at the base of the terminal ileum mesentery at the level of the pelvic inlet. Structures in jeopardy with this dissection are the right iliac vessels and ureter. The plane of dissection typically has a dark blue hue, and the peritoneum need only be incised superficially to begin the mobilization.

After the appendix is freed and the cecum adequately mobilized, attention is directed toward developing a mesenteric window at the base of the appendix using a blunt straight or curved dissector. Using the suprapubic port, the surgeon's left hand retracts the appendix anteriorly and medially. The best angle with which to make the window is usually achieved by placing the right-handed dissector through the umbilical port and using the lateral port for the camera. This approach helps to prevent the technical misadventure of carrying the dissection through the mesoappendix and into the caput of the cecum and sets up the field to allow easy placement of the laparoscopic stapler through the umbilical port. The window is created bluntly and requires that the surgeon maintain adequate tension on the tissues using the left-handed retraction (Fig. 3). Insufficient tension may be remedied by replacing the retracting instrument closer to the base of the appendix. The dissection should stay close to the appendix and is usually bloodless. After the window is fully through the mesentery and wide enough to accommodate the stapler, the dissector is replaced with an appropriate laparoscopic, linear stapler with a bowel cartridge. This is most easily accomplished by rotating the stapler so that the thinner arm of the stapler is fed through the window (Fig. 4). The stapler is closed over the healthy-appearing base of the appendix flush with the cecum while care is taken to avoid catching the surrounding bowel within the staple line. This critical view is best accomplished by gently rotating the stapler along its long axis. The device is then fired, and the appendiceal stump is inspected.

Attention is then turned to the mesoappendix. The stapler is reloaded with an appropriate vascular cartridge and is placed across the mesoappendix, staying close to the wall of the appendix (Fig. 5). Proper positioning of the stapler requires adequate left-handed retraction. Keeping the stapler high on the mesentery is helpful in the event of bleeding from the staple line. Although typically a single firing is sufficient, sequential loads of the stapler may be used until the mesentery is completely transected.

On occasion, the base of the appendix is involved in the inflammatory process and may not be suitable for laparoscopic stapling. In these situations, it is usually helpful to transect the mesentery first. The mobility gained by addressing the mesoappendix first, rather than the base of the appendix, allows the surgeon to more easily manipulate the appendix and the caput of the cecum. This allows for proper positioning of the stapler across healthy-appearing cecum to perform a partial cecectomy. Typically, the appendix along with a cuff of cecum is wedged out with sequential firings of the stapler.

After the specimen is free, a containment bag is deployed through the umbilical port and the appendix is placed inside; however, the bag is not yet delivered through the umbilical port site. Delaying extraction until the end of the operation obviates the need for replacing the umbilical port and reinsufflating the abdomen. The laparoscope is placed through the umbilical port, and the operative field is inspected

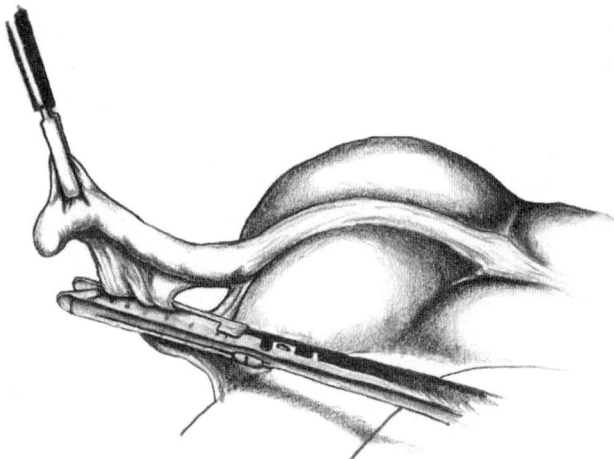

Figure 5 Transection of the mesoappendix with a linear stapling device.

while maintaining pneumoperitoneum. In the case of bleeding at the staple line, applying manual pressure for a few minutes with a grasping instrument usually results in hemostasis. Occasionally, a clip, electrocautery, a loop tie, or a suture may be required to achieve hemostasis. Alternatives to stapling the appendix and mesoappendix include using a variety of energy sources in conjunction with pretied looped sutures, suture ligatures, and clips.

The laparoscopic suction-irrigator is used to irrigate and aspirate the fluid from the right paracolic gutter, the operative field, and the pelvis. In particular, the uterus is reflected anteriorly to allow access to the cul-de-sac. The two working ports are removed under laparoscopic visualization, and the pneumoperitoneum is evacuated to confirm hemostasis. The umbilical port is then removed along with the bagged specimen and the port-site fascia is closed as usual.

As with other laparoscopic operations, conversion to an open operation is warranted in certain situations. Confounding anatomy because of the acute inflammatory process, failure of the laparoscopic operation to progress, and inadequate exposure of critical structures are common causes for converting from the laparoscopic approach to appendectomy. Before converting, consideration should be given to placing a third 5-mm working port in the right upper quadrant to assist in the laparoscopic effort. In the event of conversion, approaching the operative field away from the inflammatory process through a midline laparotomy may be preferable to a right lower-quadrant incision.

ADVANTAGES

The utility and advantages of the laparoscopic approach to appendectomy in the setting of acute appendicitis remain controversial. Understandably, surgeons may be reluctant to adopt this technique because the conventional, open approach is effective and may be more familiar. There is much literature regarding open and closed appendectomy; however, there is no clear consensus regarding the superiority of laparoscopic appendectomy. The results of several randomized, controlled trials comparing laparoscopic to open appendectomy are reviewed in Table 1 and do not clearly support one method over another. In general, laparoscopic appendectomy is associated with less postoperative pain and improved cosmesis, and some studies have demonstrated lower wound infection and intra-abdominal abscess formation rates compared with open appendectomy. The length of stay in most studies is shorter after laparoscopic appendectomy but the differences are, typically, not significant. Although the data remain subjective, return to normal activity appears to be quicker following laparoscopy. Although most trials report shorter operative times in patients randomized to open surgery, the differences are usually small and the clinical impact remains unclear. Finally, most series report higher operative costs for laparoscopy; however, the health economics are unique to different regions and may be offset by the speedier convalescence associated with laparoscopy.

The results of a Cochrane evidence-based review and meta-analysis by Sauerland and others help to explain why controversy persists regarding the ideal approach to appendectomy. This review noted that wound infections were approximately half as likely following laparoscopic appendectomy when compared with open appendectomy. The routine use of a specimen bag for extraction may be one explanation for the decreased wound morbidity. However, the same review noted nearly a threefold increase in the formation of intra-abdominal abscesses after laparoscopic appendectomy when compared with the open approach, especially in the setting of perforated or gangrenous appendicitis. In fact, the Cochrane review generally does not recommend the laparoscopic approach in the setting of perforated or gangrenous appendicitis to reduce the risk of abscess formation inherent in these situations.

The reluctance to embrace minimally invasive methods that was widely prevalent during the first decade after the introduction of laparoscopic methods into the general surgery arena is now past. The current generation of surgical residents largely has a laparoscopic mindset. It is our opinion that the vast majority of appendectomies being performed in teaching hospitals in the United States are achieved via closed methods. It is the responsibility of

Table 1: Selected Randomized Trials of Laparoscopic (L) versus Open (O) Appendectomy

Reference	n L	n O	OR Time L	OR Time O	Conv. Rate (%)	LOS (days) L	LOS (days) O	RTNA L	RTNA O	Wound Infection (%) L	Wound Infection (%) O	Complications (%) L	Complications (%) O
Long (2002)	93	105	107	91	16	2.6	3.4	14	21	18.2	16.2	28	28
Pedersen (2001)	282	301	60	40	23	2	2	7	10	2.8	6.9	10.3	9.0
Ozmen (1999)	35	35	28	28	—	1.6	3.7	—	—	5.7	8.6	18	52
Hellberg (1999)	244	256	60	35	12	2	2	13	21	—	—	4.9	6.2
Heikkinen (1998)	19	21	31	41	5.3	2	2	10	19	0	4.8	—	—
Klinger (1998)	87	82	35	31	0	3	4	14	15	6	7	—	—
Reiertsen (1997)	42	42	51	25	0	3.5	3.2	15.0	19.7	2.4	0	40.5	28.6
Minne (1997)	27	23	82	67	7.4	1.1	1.2	14	14	—	—	18.5	4.3
Macarulla (1997)	106	104	55	45	8.3	3.4	4.8	—	—	0.9	4.8	5.6	7.7
Ortega (1995)	167	86	68	58	6.5	2.6	2.8	9	14	2.4	12.8	4.2	20.9

Conv., Conversion; *LOS*, length of hospital stay; *OR*, operating room; *RTNA*, return to normal activities.

the attending surgeon to ensure that conversion is carried out when appropriate.

In conclusion, laparoscopic appendectomy is associated with a decreased rate of wound infection, improved cosmesis, and shorter convalescence. Additionally, the diagnostic utility of laparoscopy in the setting of suspected appendicitis is undisputed. Minimal-access methods are therefore an excellent alternative to open appendectomy for the treatment of uncomplicated acute appendicitis. It is unclear, however, on the basis of the available data whether the laparoscopic approach is advisable in the setting of gross perforation or a gangrenous appendix. Further prospective studies are necessary to better address these questions; in the meantime, judicious conversion to open methods is appropriate when indicated.

SUGGESTED READINGS

Chung RS, Rowland DY, Li P, and others: A meta analysis of randomized controlled trials of laparoscopic versus conventional appendectomy, *Am J Surg* 177:250, 1999.

Long KH, Bannon MP, Zietlow SP, and others: A prospective randomized comparison of laparoscopic appendectomy with open appendectomy; clinical and economic analysis, *Surgery* 129:390, 2001.

Pederson AG, Petersen OB, Wara P, and others: Randomized controlled trial of laparoscopic versus open appendectomy, *Br J Surg* 88:200, 2001.

Sauerland S, Lefering R, Neugebauer EAM: Laparoscopic versus open surgery for suspected appendicitis, *Cochrane Database Syst Rev* 2004; Issue 4.

Wullstein C, Barkhausen S, Gross E, and others: Results of laparoscopic vs. conventional appendectomy in complicated appendicitis, *Dis Colon Rectum* 44:1700, 2001.

LAPAROSCOPIC INGUINAL HERNIA

Jonathan Pearl, MD, Michael Rosen, MD, and Raymond P. Onders, MD

The technique of laparoscopic inguinal hernia repair was developed in the early 1990s and builds on the methods originally championed by Rene Stoppa. Despite the theoretical advantages of placing a large piece of prosthetic mesh into the preperitoneal space using minimally invasive techniques, today less than 15% of all hernia repairs in the United States are performed laparoscopically. The reasons for the modest penetrance are manifold: favorable results with anterior mesh repair, a steep learning curve with laparoscopic repair, and the need for general anesthesia, among others. Despite this, laparoscopic inguinal herniorrhaphy should continue to gain momentum as surgeons amass experience with the technique.

The issue of whether to repair inguinal hernias laparoscopically has historically been embroiled in controversy. Recently the results of a multicenter Veterans Affairs trial suggested that recurrence rates were doubled with the laparoscopic method compared with anterior mesh herniorrhaphy, and some authors have suggested abandoning the procedure. However, close inspection of the aforementioned data indicates that surgeons with expertise in laparoscopic inguinal herniorrhapy have recurrence rates comparable with open repairs. This finding emphasizes the need to understand the anatomic and technical aspects of laparoscopic inguinal hernia repair to achieve salutary results.

Despite the controversy, most surgeons accept that laparoscopic inguinal herniorrhaphy has clear indications. Laparoscopic repair of bilateral inguinal hernias results in less postoperative pain with a speedier return to normal activities. Additionally, repair of recurrent hernias is facilitated by access to the unadulterated preperitoneal space in the laparoscopic repair. To those ends, all contemporary general surgeons should be comfortable with the laparoscopic approach to inguinal herniorrhaphy.

ANATOMIC CONSIDERATIONS

Inguinal anatomy can be disorienting when viewed from a posterior-to-anterior perspective, as in the laparoscopic approach; therefore clear understanding of the anatomy is imperative. Figure 1 outlines the anatomic landmarks as seen laparoscopically. The medial umbilical ligament envelopes the obliterated umbilical artery, and

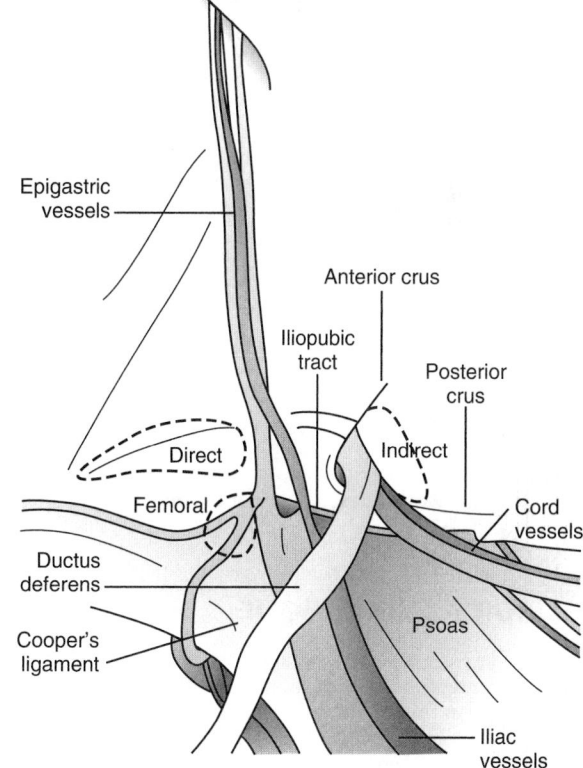

Figure 1 Laparoscopic view of preperitoneal anatomy.

the lateral umbilical ligament contains the inferior epigastric vessels. The space of Bogros is situated lateral to the space of Retzius between the peritoneum and the anterior lamina of the transversalis fascia. After this extraperitoneal space is entered, the surgeon has access to the myopectineal orifice of Fruchaud, which contains the direct, indirect, and femoral spaces. The key structures to identifying these spaces are the iliopubic tract, the inferior epigastric vessels, and the pectineal (Cooper's) ligament. The iliopubic tract divides the myopectineal orifice into a superior and inferior portion, and the inferior epigastric vessels divide medial from lateral. The direct and indirect spaces are located medial and lateral to the inferior epigastric vessels, respectively, and above the iliopubic tract. The femoral canal lies in the area bounded by the iliopubic tract superiorly, Cooper's ligament inferiorly, and the origin of the inferior epigastric vessels medially.

The potential for neurovascular injuries is harrowing, but these complications can be minimized by awareness of two danger areas in laparoscopic inguinal hernia repair. The external iliac artery and vein course deep to the iliopubic tract in an area bounded medially by the vas deferens and laterally by the spermatic vessels, which has been deemed the "triangle of doom." The lateral femoral cutaneous, femoral, and genitofemoral nerves traverse the "quadrangle of pain," bounded by the iliopubic tract, the lateral aspect of the spermatic vessels, and the pelvic sidewall. Although the iliopubic tract often is not visualized during laparoscopic repair, taking care to ensure the tip of the spiral tacking device can be palpated with the nondominant hand on the anterior abdominal wall will avoid nerve entrapment.

PATIENT SELECTION

There are no clear guidelines stating which patients are best approached laparoscopically. Perhaps the most important factor is the surgeon's expertise with the laparoscopic approach and command of the inguinal anatomy. If one possesses the appropriate skill level, any patient with an inguinal hernia who can tolerate general anesthesia may be considered for laparoscopic hernia repair. Learning curves for the laparoscopic repair have been reported to be from as few as 30 cases to as many as 250 and likely have more to do with the surgeon's comfort level with laparoscopy and inguinal anatomy than with any particular number of cases. Absolute contraindications for laparoscopic inguinal herniorrhaphy include active intra-abdominal infection or coagulopathy. A relative contraindication includes pelvic irradiation; previous operations in the space of Retzius, such as a retropubic prostatectomy; or extensive prior lower-abdominal surgery. Large scrotal hernias and incarcerated hernias can be particularly challenging laparoscopic cases and should be avoided during one's early experience with this operation. It is important to present each patient with the available options for inguinal hernia repair, including both laparoscopic and open approaches. The unilateral primary hernia in an elderly patient with multiple comorbidities is probably best approached anteriorly under local anesthesia. We view laparoscopic inguinal hernia as another technique that all surgeons should be able to offer the appropriately selected patient and not the only way to fix inguinal hernias.

SURGICAL TECHNIQUE

When considering a laparoscopic approach for repairing inguinal hernias, the surgeon has several options. Initially, laparoscopic repairs involved an intraperitoneal onlay mesh (IPOM). Using this technique, the surgeon placed a large piece of mesh in an intraperitoneal position, similar to a laparoscopic ventral hernia repair. This approach has largely been abandoned secondary to high recurrence rates and the drawbacks of intraperitoneal mesh. The remaining two techniques include a totally extraperitoneal (TEP) and a transabdominal preperitoneal (TAPP) approach. The main difference between these two techniques is the sequence of gaining access to the preperitoneal space. In the TEP approach, the dissection begins in the preperitoneal space with a balloon dissector. In the TAPP approach, the preperitoneal space is accessed after initially entering the peritoneal cavity. Each approach has its own merits. Using the TEP approach, the preperitoneal dissection is quicker, and the potential risks of intraperitoneal visceral damage are minimized. However, the use of dissection balloons can be costly, the working space is more limited, and in the case of prior preperitoneal surgery or mesh the space may be impossible to create. Additionally, if large tears in the peritoneal flap are created during a TEP, the potential working space can become obliterated, necessitating conversion to a transabdominal approach. For these reasons, knowledge of a transabdominal technique is essential when performing laparoscopic inguinal hernia repairs. The transabdominal approach allows

immediate identification of the groin anatomy before extensive dissection and disruption of natural planes. The larger working space of the peritoneal cavity can make early experience with the laparoscopic approach safer and easier.

TRANSABDOMINAL PREPERITONEAL HERNIA REPAIR

Routine use of Foley catheterization is not performed. The patients are instructed to empty their bladders before entering the operating room. A single dose of a first-generation cephalosporin is given, and sequential compression devices are applied. The patient is placed under general anesthesia, with both arms tucked at the side, and the abdomen and groin are sterilely prepared. The surgeon stands on the side opposite the hernia, and the first assistant stands on the ipsilateral side of the hernia along with the scrub nurse. The laparoscopic tower is positioned at the foot of the table.

The abdominal cavity is entered through an infraumbilical skin incision with a 10-mm trocar, and a 0- or 30-degree camera is used at this site. Two 5-mm trocars are then placed just lateral to either inferior epigastric vessels.

The patient is placed in a slight Trendelenburg position. The dissection begins at the ipsilateral medial umbilical fold. The preperitoneal flap is raised from a medial to lateral direction using the curved scissors, with minimal cautery. It is important to begin this dissection rather cephalad on the abdominal wall to leave enough space for reduction of the hernia and placement of an appropriately sized piece of mesh. Additionally, as the initial incision is carried laterally, one should avoid the temptation to drift inferiorly toward the inguinal canal, again compromising the eventual space necessary for mesh placement. The proper incision carries transversely across the abdominal wall toward the anterior superior iliac spine. Achieving the appropriate dissection plane is critical to the success of the operation. The first structure identified is Cooper's ligament. By sweeping down the bladder, staying high on the anterior abdominal wall, one eventually encounters this white, firm ligament. Even in unilateral hernias, I routinely sweep the bladder far medially past the midline to provide adequate mesh overlap. Cooper's ligament is cleared off laterally until a fairly constant crossing vessel is identified. This so-called aberrant obturator vessel is present in more than 75% of patients. Next, the lateral dissection is begun by clearing the peritoneum until the spermatic vessels and then the vas deferens are encountered.

At this point, the hernia sac should be reduced. If a direct defect is encountered, the hernia contents are grasped, and the attenuated transversalis fascia is gently teased away. If an indirect hernia is identified, the sac is likewise grasped and retracted while attachments to the cord structures are bluntly swept off. Large, chronic, indirect sacs can be particularly challenging. In cases in which the hernia sac cannot be completely reduced, it can be transected and either sutured or closed with an Endoloop (Ethicon Endosurgery, Somerville, NJ), leaving the distal end open. Any cord lipoma typically located inferior and lateral to the cord structures should be completely reduced to avoid potential confusion as a recurrence. After reduction of the hernia sac, the peritoneal flap should be dissected at least 3 cm off the vessels and cord structures to prevent any peritoneum from sneaking under the mesh, predisposing to recurrence. The upper flap of peritoneum is then grasped and retracted cephalad to develop a larger pocket for the mesh.

At least a 10 × 15 cm piece of polypropylene mesh is used. We do not place a slit for wrapping around the cord structures because recurrences have occurred through these defects. Although some groups advocate no mesh fixation, we currently believe that some form of mesh fixation is important to prevent migration. After the mesh is situated, we place one tack in Cooper's ligament. Because only one tack is placed, the mesh can still be rotated to obtain ideal lateral placement. However, the mesh will not migrate during lateral retraction. We then place a spiral tack at the superior lateral aspect of the mesh. It is critical that the tip of the tacker can be palpated with the nondominant hand of the surgeon through the anterior abdominal wall before deploying any tacks. If the tacker cannot be palpated, it indicates that it is likely below the iliopubic tract, and therefore the lateral femoral cutaneous, genitalfemoral, or femoral nerve could be entrapped. We then place one tack just lateral to the inferior epigastric and one at the superior medial border of the mesh. Finally, another tack may be placed in Cooper's ligament. At the conclusion, the peritoneum is reexamined, with particular attention paid to the vessels to ensure that the peritoneum is not encroaching underneath the mesh.

The peritoneal flap is then secured to the anterior abdominal wall. This can be completed with spiral tacks, staples, or suturing. Any defects in the peritoneum should be closed. Occasionally, the reduced hernia sac can be used to close these defects. If a large hole in the peritoneum is created, several maneuvers can aid closure. The peritoneal flap dissection should be extended inferiorly to gain laxity for closure, the pneumoperitoneum pressures can be reduced to 8 to 10 mm Hg to decrease tension, and the patient can be taken out of the Trendelenburg position. For left-sided defects, the sigmoid colon can be released from its peritoneal attachments.

TOTALLY EXTRAPERITONEAL HERNIA REPAIR

An infraumbilical skin incision is made, and the anterior rectus sheath is incised horizontally. The rectus muscle is retracted upward and laterally to gain access to the preperitoneal space, and a dissecting balloon is inserted to the level of the pubic symphysis. The balloon is inflated while the inferior epigastric vessels coursing along the posterior bellies of the rectus muscles are visualized. The dissection is between the peritoneum and the transversalis fascia. The balloon should be kept inflated for a few moments to allow tamponading of small capillary vessels. The dissecting balloon is subsequently replaced with a 10-mm structural trocar, and the space is insufflated to 12 mm Hg, creating a pneumoextraperitoneum. Two 5-mm trocars are then placed in the midline: one just above the pubic symphysis and the other midway between the symphysis and the umbilicus, avoiding the structural balloon. Various fixation devices are available to secure the trocars in the small working space. We prefer short, reusable spikes with threads on the shafts to prevent migration during instrument exchanges.

With the surgeon standing opposite the hernia, the dissection proceeds. Often a small direct hernia is reduced with the dissecting balloon; if not, it is reduced using blunt graspers. Cooper's ligament is exposed and the inferior epigastric vessels are visualized along the anterior abdominal wall. The lateral space is then dissected by using one grasper to suspend the inferior epigastric vessels and the other grasper to open the space by bluntly retracting inferiorly. The spermatic cord and vas deferens are identified, and an indirect hernia is sought in the anterolateral position of the cord, as opposed to the anteromedial location during the open repair. The hernia sac is dissected in a perpendicular fashion to the cord structures with blunt graspers. The peritoneum comprising the indirect sac is completely dissected away from the cord, and the vas deferens is parietalized. Large, indirect sacs can be adherent to the cord structures and can be divided and ligated as previously mentioned. A large piece of mesh (10 × 15 cm) is then inserted through the umbilical trocar and positioned to cover all potential hernia spaces. It is fixed at Cooper's ligament, in the superior midline, and laterally above the iliopubic tract. At this point, the contralateral side should be assessed for another hernia. At the completion of the procedure, the carbon dioxide is evacuated under direct vision while holding down the lateral aspect of the mesh, ensuring that the peritoneum does not encroach under the mesh. The trocars are removed and the incisions closed.

POSTOPERATIVE CARE

The patients are typically discharged home from the recovery room. The patients must void before discharge because urinary retention can be a problem, especially in bilateral hernias. The patients are instructed to avoid heavy lifting for several weeks postoperatively. Patients are followed up in the office in 2 to 3 weeks.

RESULTS

Two large clinical trials comparing laparoscopic and open inguinal hernia repair have recently been published. In the Veterans Affairs Cooperative Study, 1695 patients were followed for 2 years after either laparoscopic repair or open anterior mesh repair. For primary hernias, recurrence rates were reported as 10.1% for the laparoscopic group and 4.0% for the open group. Among those surgeons who reported performing more than 250 laparoscopic inguinal herniorrhaphies, overall recurrence rates were less than 5% and comparable with anterior and laparoscopic repair. Recurrent hernias demonstrated similar recurrence rates regardless of level of experience. In another study, a Swedish group followed 1184 patients for 5 years after either TAPP repair or anterior Shouldice repair. Recurrence rates were similar for both groups, approximately 6%, but those surgeons deemed proficient using a standardized scoring method demonstrated a lower recurrence rate. Both of these powerful studies emphasize that favorable results accompany proficiency with the laparoscopic techniques.

AVOIDING PITFALLS IN LAPAROSCOPIC INGUINAL HERNIA REPAIRS

Recurrence

Minimizing recurrence is crucial for laparoscopic hernia repair to gain widespread acceptance. Some maneuvers aid in preventing recurrences: the mesh must be large enough to overlap the entire myopectineal orifice, including the indirect, direct, and femoral spaces. Because the mesh may migrate or shrink over time, we recommend that it be fixed, as detailed earlier. Additionally, when using the TEP repair, the peritoneum must be adequately dissected off the cord structures to prevent slippage underneath the mesh when desufflating. As surgeons gain experience with the laparoscopic approach, the dissection plane enlarges, larger pieces of mesh can be placed, and recurrence rates are minimized. Early in one's experience, a clue of an inadequate preperitoneal dissection occurs when the surgeon cannot place an appropriately sized piece of mesh in the working space created.

Hemorrhage

Life-threatening hemorrhage can occur if the external iliac vessels are injured. This can be avoided by restricting dissection to the area above the iliopubic tract near the spermatic cord. In addition, an aberrant obturator artery, present in up to 40% of the population, may be encountered during the lateral dissection of Cooper's ligament. The aberrant obturator artery arises from the inferior epigastric or external iliac arteries and crosses Cooper's ligament in the vicinity of the femoral space. It may anastomose with a normal obturator artery, thereby completing the corona mortis. This anomaly should be recognized and its injury should be avoided during initial dissection and eventual placement of spiral tacks.

Meddlesome bleeding may occur from the inferior epigastric vessels or the iliopubic vein. The epigastrics could be torn by the dissecting balloon during the TEP repair. This can be averted through visualizing the balloon dissection with the laparoscope. If the vessels are being dissected posteriorly, inflation should immediately stop, the balloon should be removed, and dissection should continue using graspers rather than the balloon. Should bleeding occur from the inferior epigastrics, it can be readily stopped by applying a hemostatic clip. The iliopubic vein lies adjacent to Cooper's ligament just lateral to the symphysis pubis. Its injury can be avoided by being cognizant of its location and using gentle dissection in the region.

Nerve Injury

Disabling postoperative pain may result from entrapment of the femoral, genitofemoral, or lateral femoral cutaneous nerves. The risk is alleviated through familiarity with the anatomy and avoiding tack placement below the iliopubic tract laterally, as previously mentioned. If nerve entrapment pain is noted in the immediate postoperative period, the patient should be returned to the operating room for removal of the offending tack.

Bowel Obstruction

The potential for small bowel obstruction exists in two scenarios. In the TAPP repair, incomplete closure of the peritoneum may permit a loop of small bowel to slip into the preperitoneal space (shower curtain effect). This is averted by placing the staples, tacks, or sutures at 5-mm intervals. In TEP repair, an unrecognized rent in the peritoneum might permit passage of a loop of small bowel. All holes in the peritoneum must be closed, and rents must be actively sought before desufflating. Patients presenting with bowel obstructions early after laparoscopic inguinal hernia repair should be reexplored early.

Visceral Injury

The specter for bowel injury is higher in the TAPP repair because the abdominal cavity is entered. In patients with numerous previous intra-abdominal operations, TAPP should not be performed.

Also, the urinary bladder could be injured during either a TEP or TAPP repair. To minimize the risk of such an occurrence, the patient should void just before entering the operating room. Bladder injuries should be repaired when discovered, and an indwelling catheter should remain in place for 7 to 10 days.

CONCLUSIONS

Laparoscopic repair of inguinal hernias can be rewarding for both patient and surgeon. When it is meticulously performed, patients may benefit from less postoperative pain, quicker return to regular activities, and a low rate of recurrence. For the surgeon, the laparoscopic repair offers an alternative approach for recurrent and bilateral hernias and could be offered to any patient who can tolerate general anesthesia after the surgeon becomes expert in the operation. Mastering the familiar inguinal anatomy from an alternative perspective can also be intellectually fulfilling.

Thorough knowledge of the anatomy and rigorous attention to technical detail can minimize the potential risks of laparoscopic inguinal herniorrhaphy. As more surgeons gain an understanding of this procedure, it should gain widespread acceptance.

Suggested Readings

Arvidsson D, Berndsen FH, Larsson LG, and others: Randomized clinical trial comparing 5-year recurrence rate after laparoscopic versus Shouldice repair of primary inguinal hernia, *Br J Surg* 92:1085, 2005.

Colburn GL, Skandalakis JE: Laparoscopic inguinal anatomy, *Hernia* 2:179, 1998.

Neumayer L, Giobbie-Hurder A, Jonasson O, and others, for the Veterans Affairs Cooperative Studies Program 456 Investigators: Open mesh versus laparoscopic mesh repair of inguinal hernia, *N Engl J Med* 350:1819, 2004.

Neumayer LA, Gawande AA, Wang J for the CSP #456 Investigators: Proficiency of surgeons in inguinal hernia repair: effect of experience and age, *Ann Surg* 242:344; discussion 348, 2005.

LAPAROSCOPIC REPAIR OF RECURRENT INGUINAL HERNIAS

Robert Fang, MD, and Thomas Vargish, MD

INTRODUCTION

Inguinal hernia repair is one of the most common operations in the United States, with approximately 800,000 performed each year. Up to 15% of these procedures are reported as repairs for recurrence. The current generation of open, tension-free repairs appears to have narrowed the role for laparoscopic inguinal hernia repair. However, in experienced hands, this approach still remains an attractive option.

Recurrence is often secondary to a technical failure, such as wound infection, excessive tension, missed defect, inadequate mesh coverage, or mesh migration. Nevertheless, one should remember that undiagnosed or untreated medical illnesses may also contribute

to recurrence, particularly if the time between the original repair and the recurrence is long. Patients must be assessed for medical conditions that may predispose them to recurrence. All abnormalities that are uncovered should be corrected, when possible, before initiating therapy.

RATIONALE

The rationale underlying the laparoscopic approach to recurrent inguinal hernias is based on several concepts. First, the dissection proceeds through a previously unoperated and unscarred field. Second, the vantage point from this exposure provides an excellent view of the defect and anatomy. These advantages allow the surgeon the opportunity to delineate the exact nature of the recurrence and to identify all the critical structures in the surrounding region. Thus the risk of injury to the cord structures and nerves within the inguinal canal may be diminished. Third, the space created by this approach allows the placement of a generous-sized mesh over the entire myopectineal orifice. Finally, the positioning of mesh behind the abdominal wall in the preperitoneal space is hypothesized to be mechanically advantageous to that of an anterior repair. The same intra-abdominal pressure that may be a factor in hernia recurrence after an anterior approach is harnessed in the fixation of a posterior "buttress" to the abdominal wall. The laparoscopic approach provides the same benefits that Nyhus, Stoppa, and Wantz have

Table 1: Indications and Contraindications for Laparoscopic Recurrent Inguinal Hernia Repair

Indications	Contraindications
Recurrent inguinal hernia	**Absolute** Inability to tolerate general anesthesia History of irradiation to pelvis Irreducible incarcerated hernia after induction of anesthesia Uncontrolled coagulopathy **Relative** Surgeon inexperience Previous preperitoneal surgery Cirrhosis

described in their open preperitoneal approaches but without large abdominal wall incisions.

INDICATIONS AND CONTRAINDICATIONS

The indications for laparoscopic recurrent inguinal hernia repair are similar to those for open repair (Table 1). These include all enlarging, symptomatic, and incarcerated hernias. Specific contraindications include (1) the patient's inability to tolerate general anesthesia or laparoscopy, (2) history of radiation therapy to the pelvis, (3) an irreducible incarcerated hernia after induction of anesthesia, and (4) uncontrolled coagulopathy. Relative contraindications include (1) cirrhosis with portal hypertension, (2) surgeon inexperience with the totally extraperitoneal (TEP) or transabdominal preperitoneal (TAPP) repairs, and (3) a previous laparoscopic repair or other retroperitoneal surgery that has violated the preperitoneal space, especially in the area of the hernia.

Inguinal pain after a previous open hernia repair is not an indication to perform a laparoscopic procedure. This subset of patients requires a careful, open groin exploration to discover the cause of the pain, remove foreign material, or repair the potential recurrent hernia.

ADVANTAGES AND DISADVANTAGES

The advantages parallel those aspects mentioned for the rationale of a laparoscopic approach (Table 2). In particular, the peritoneum is not violated with the TEP approach, minimizing the risk of bowel injury and adhesions to the mesh. Decreased postoperative pain and faster recovery have also been demonstrated in multiple studies.

Table 2: Advantages and Disadvantages for Laparoscopic Recurrent Inguinal Hernia Repair

Advantages	Disadvantages
Exposure through an unoperated field	Technically difficult
Excellent visualization of the pelvic floor	Increased costs (equipment, operating time)
Allows placement of mesh over the entire myopectineal orifice	Potential for significant injury to bowel or vasculature
Mechanically advantageous to the anterior approach	
Reduced postoperative pain and recovery time	

The advantages of the laparoscopic approach are countered by distinct disadvantages. Greater laparoscopic skill is essential to performing these operations successfully and safely. Until a level of proficiency is attained, there is an increased risk of neurologic or vascular injury because preperitoneal anatomy is not familiar territory to most surgeons (especially with the TEP approach). The approach becomes even more challenging with the distorted anatomy after a previous repair. There are increased costs associated with equipment requirements and longer operating times. This disadvantage is offset by increasing experience with the laparoscopic approaches and by performing the procedure safely in centers specializing in laparoscopy.

TECHNIQUE

The two current methods of performing laparoscopic repairs for recurrent inguinal hernias are the TAPP and TEP approaches. In our experience, we favor the TEP approach because it avoids potential visceral injury and minimizes the risk of adhesions and future bowel obstruction. However, the TAPP repair may be preferable in selected cases, such as the patient who has had prior pelvic surgery and requests the laparoscopic approach.

For the TEP approach, the procedure is begun by administering local anesthesia at each incision site after appropriate general anesthesia induction and Foley catheter placement. A small transverse incision is made just below the umbilicus on the side with the hernia. Dissection is carried down to the fascia overlying the rectus abdominus muscle. The fascia is incised, and the muscle is reflected away from the midline. As the muscle is separated from the posterior fascia and then from the peritoneum (inferior to the arcuate line), care must be taken not to enter the peritoneal cavity. A dissecting balloon is then placed into this preperitoneal space, directed caudally until the pubis is reached, and inflated under direct vision with a 10-mm 0-degree scope. After the balloon has been inflated completely (all wrinkles in balloon will disappear), 2 to 3 minutes are given for the small vessels in the preperitoneal fat to tamponade.

The balloon is deflated and replaced with a "structural" balloon port before the preperitoneal space is insufflated with carbon dioxide gas to 10 to 12 mm Hg. Two additional 5-ml working ports are placed under direct vision. If only one hernia is being repaired, the superior port should be placed in the midline just inferior to the structural balloon. The inferior port should then be placed midway between the superior port and the pubic symphysis, 2 to 3 cm off the midline toward the side that is contralateral to the hernia. When bilateral hernias are being repaired, both working ports should be placed in the midline (Fig. 1).

Starting just posterior to the inferior epigastric vessels (elevating them with a grasper if necessary), the surgeon uses blunt graspers to "sweep" the peritoneum and preperitoneal fat downward and cephalad off the abdominal wall. The blunt dissection continues just under the rectus muscle until the lateral pelvic wall muscles are encountered. This portion of the dissection is completed when the peritoneum has been swept cephalad to the anterior iliac crest. After the lateral pelvis is cleared, the remaining peritoneum is swept cephalad, proceeding in a lateral-to-medial direction and staying anterior to the cord structures. The dissection continues until the midline is reached, exposing the entire floor of the inguinal canal. Direct hernia defects will become obvious, and indirect hernias will appear as a thickened cord with intimately adherent peritoneum and preperitoneal fat.

The fat and peritoneum are slowly pulled out of the internal ring in a "hand-over-hand" fashion until they no longer retract back when released. Then the surgeon gently strips the fat and peritoneum from the cord structures, being vigilant for the vas deferens on the medial side of the cord. After the cord is freed, the blunt dissection is continued cephalad for several more centimeters, staying

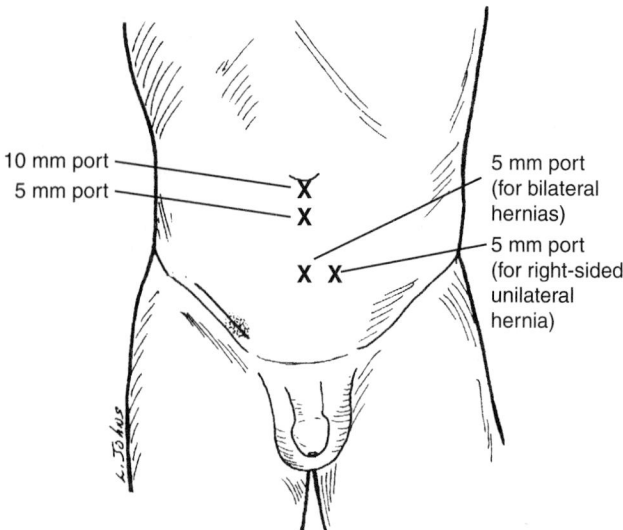

Figure 1 Port placement for the totally extraperitoneal (TEP) approach.

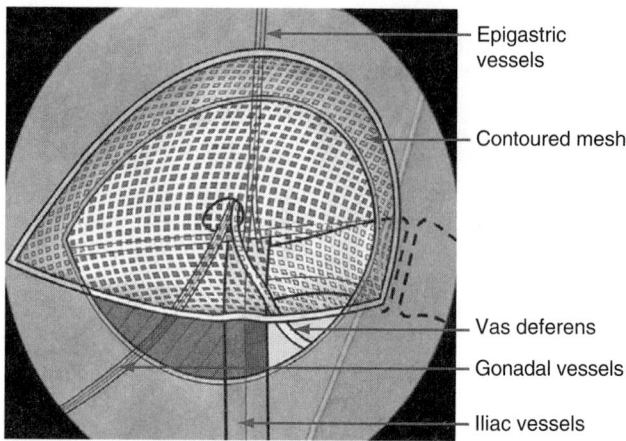

Figure 3 Placement of the contoured mesh (left-sided). *From Davol/CR Bard, Inc. Used with permission.*

just anterior to the gonadal vessels. Because the peritoneum may be adherent to the previous hernia repair, this gentle separation of the recurrent hernia sac from cord structures can be tedious and time-consuming.

Although it is important to avoid perforating the peritoneum, an injury should be repaired immediately using intracoporeal suturing. By keeping a lower pressure in the preperitoneal space, the risk of intraabdominal insufflation is minimized. The completed dissection should appear as shown in Figure 2.

We have switched from using a flat polypropylene mesh to using a preformed contoured mesh (3D Max; Davol/CR Bard, Cranston, RI) because it conforms well to the pelvic floor and requires almost no fixation. The shape of the mesh also reduces buckling and makes placement easier for the surgeon. It is important to use an adequately large-sized mesh (sizes M, L, XL; we use size L for almost all patients) and to position it high enough superomedially to cover the direct space. The appropriate mesh (right or left) is rolled, inserted blindly through the camera port, and directed to the appropriate location. Under direct vision, the mesh is unrolled and

positioned with the pointed tail toward the anterior iliac spine, the notch over the cord structures, and the broad medial segment just over the floor, reaching the midline (Fig. 3). When bilateral repairs are being performed, the two pieces of mesh should overlap each other in the midline by 1 or 2 cm. Two technical points are helpful: (1) it is important to make sure that the peritoneum is swept cephalad so that the lower edge of the mesh is clearly caudad to the peritoneum as it crosses the cord structures (the peritoneum can be placed on top of the mesh); (2) it is not necessary to tack the mesh in place. If we have concerns about mesh migration (usually only with bilateral repairs), we will place one tack medially into Cooper's ligament for each piece of mesh. If lateral fixation is deemed necessary, the tack must be placed anterior to the iliac crest to minimize the risk of nerve injury (only one tack is usually sufficient).

After hemostasis is confirmed, the preperitoneal space is desufflated under direct vision. Holding the bottom of the mesh down with a grasper during this process may help to keep the peritoneum anterior to the lower edge of the mesh. We generally wait approximately 2 minutes before reinsufflating to confirm that the mesh and peritoneum have remained appropriately positioned. At this point, the preperitoneal space is desufflated again, and the ports are removed. The rectus muscle fascia of the larger incision is reapproximated, and the skin is closed for all incisions. Patients can be discharged the day of surgery.

Some authors have recommended the TAPP approach for recurrent inguinal hernias, especially for those patients who have had the preperitoneal space violated (e.g., previous laparoscopic inguinal hernia repair or previous retroperitoneal surgery). However, we do not use this approach for either primary or recurrent hernia repairs. We have been dissatisfied with our ability to dissect enough peritoneum off the abdominal wall to permit sufficient exposure for adequate mesh placement and subsequent closure of the peritoneal flap. Nevertheless, others have had success with the TAPP approach, and the technique is well described in the 8th edition of this text.

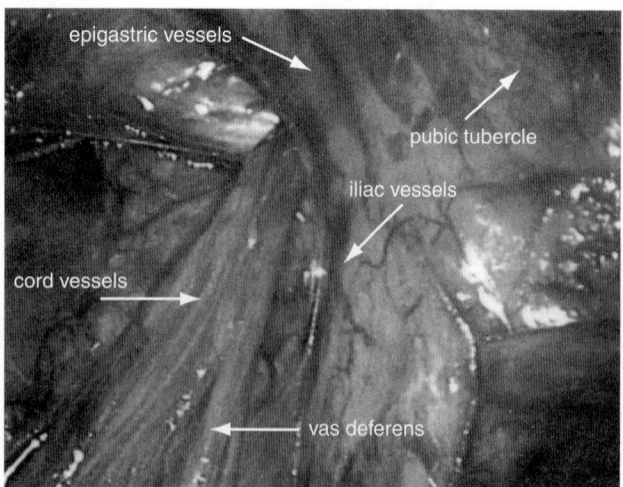

Figure 2 Completed dissection during the totally extraperitoneal (TEP) approach (left sided). (*See color insert Figure 58.*)

COMPLICATIONS

One of the major obstacles with the TEP approach to recurrent inguinal hernia repairs is surgeon experience. Until a certain level of proficiency is attained in identifying the correct planes of dissection laparoscopically, there may be an increased risk of injuring the

Table 3: Randomized Control Trials Comparing Open and Laparoscopic Approaches to Recurrent Inguinal Hernias

Author	Study Type	Repair	Hernias (REC)	Findings
Beets 1999	PRCT/SI REC	GPRVS TAPP	41 52	TAPP: less pain, earlier return to activity Significantly higher recurrence rate for TAPP
Mahon 2003	PRCT/SI REC/BIL	Lichtenstein repair TAPP	60 60	TAPP: less pain, earlier return to work, decreased operating time No significant difference in recurrence rate
McCormack 2003	MA/MC REC/BIL/ PRIM	Open repair TEP/TAPP	125–232 143–216	TEP/TAPP: decreased length of stay, earlier return to activity, less pain, increased operating time No significant difference in recurrence rate
Neumayer 2004	PRCT/MC REC/BIL/ PRIM	Lichtenstein repair TEP/TAPP	88 96	TEP/TAPP: less early postoperative pain, earlier return to work No significant difference in recurrence rate (for recurrent hernias only)

BIL, Bilateral inguinal hernias; *GPRVS*, giant prosthetic reinforcement of the visceral sac; *MA*, meta-analysis; *MC*, multicenter; *PRCT*, prospective randomized controlled trial; *PRIM*, primary inguinal hernia; *REC*, recurrent inguinal hernia; *SI*, single-institution; *TAPP*, transabdominal preperitoneal approach; *TEP*, totally extraperitoneal approach.

cord structures and iliac vessels. Postoperative neurologic complaints have been reported, but we believe that the minimal use of tacks makes this complication a rare occurrence. An unrepaired hole in the peritoneum is a concern because it can lead to adhesions and postoperative bowel obstruction. Bleeding and wound infections are rare.

DISCUSSION

We prefer to repair recurrent inguinal hernias using the TEP approach when possible. Although a more technically challenging procedure, the benefits of decreased postoperative pain and rapid recovery with successful operations are significant.

Despite their theoretical advantages, laparoscopic repairs of recurrent inguinal hernias have not gained increasing popularity. A major factor may be the steep learning curve of these procedures, even when performed for primary groin hernias. Thus the benefits are realized only by those with extensive experience.

No clearly convincing evidence showing the superiority of the laparoscopic approach over an open approach exists in the current literature. Several retrospective series analyzing personal or single-institution experiences have been reported. These data support the assertion that those with adequate experience have been able to provide the benefits of a laparoscopic repair.

Three randomized control trials comparing open and laparoscopic approaches to recurrent inguinal hernias have been published (Table 3). The first study was performed in the Netherlands and compared the TAPP approach versus an open preperitoneal repair (see Beets 1999). The patients experienced significantly less pain in the TAPP group and had a more rapid return to full activity. However, the recurrence rate was significantly higher in the TAPP patients than in those undergoing an open procedure. The authors acknowledged that they had minimal experience with the TAPP repair before initiation of the study. The second trial compared TAPP with the Lichtenstein repair for bilateral and recurrent inguinal hernias in the United Kingdom (see Mahon 2003). The investigators found that the TAPP repair resulted in less operating time, decreased postoperative pain, and earlier return to work. The recurrence rates were similar between the two approaches and were comparable to previously published results for open repairs. The most recent trial

was a multicenter study comparing the Lichtenstein procedure with the laparoscopic procedure (TEP and TAPP) for all inguinal hernias (see Neumayer 2004). Among the 1983 patients studied, the recurrent hernia subset comprised approximately 9% in each arm. The investigators found that recurrence was significantly higher after laparoscopic repair of primary hernias but not recurrent hernias. In addition, the results suggested that the higher recurrence rate decreased only among surgeons who have performed more than 250 procedures. Regarding postoperative pain and return to activity, the results showed a significant advantage for the laparoscopic approach in the early postoperative period only. A large meta-analysis published in 2003 reviewed 41 trials comparing open and laparoscopic approaches to inguinal hernia repair (see McCormack 2003). A subgroup analysis of patients with recurrent hernias (11% of 7161 patients) was performed in this study. The reviewers found that the laparoscopic approach resulted in less pain, earlier return to activity, and longer operating times. The recurrence rates did not differ between the two approaches. Furthermore these results for the recurrent hernia subgroup were consistent with the overall results of the study.

As long as inguinal hernia repairs continue to be common procedures for the general surgeon, the management of recurrences must be a routine part of his armamentarium. The skill set of some will afford them the ability to provide patients the benefits of a laparoscopic repair. However, a high level of proficiency with the laparoscopic approach seems necessary for the benefits to outweigh the risks and costs. The two laparoscopic options, TEP and TAPP, appear to have similar results in experienced hands. Therefore the best repair for recurrent inguinal hernias still remains the approach that the surgeon can perform most confidently and safely.

SUGGESTED READINGS

Beets GL, Dirksen CD, Go PM, and others: Open or laparoscopic preperitoneal mesh repair for recurrent inguinal hernia? *Surg Endosc* 13:323, 1999.

Bell RC, Price JG: Laparoscopic inguinal hernia repair using an anatomically contoured three-dimensional mesh, *Surg Endosc* 17:1784, 2003.

Mahon D, Decadt B, Rhoades M, and others: Prospective randomized trial of laparoscopic (transabdominal preperitoneal) vs open (mesh) repair for bilateral and recurrent inguinal hernia, *Surg Endosc* 17:1386, 2003.

McCormack K, Scott NW, Go PM, and others: Laparoscopic techniques versus open techniques for inguinal hernia repair, *Cochrane Database Syst Rev* (1):CD001785, 2003.

Neumayer M, Giobbie-Hurder A, Jonasson O, and others: Open mesh versus laparoscopic mesh repair of inguinal hernia, *N Engl J Med* 350:1819, 2004.

Pajotin P: Laparoscopic groin hernia repair using a curved prosthesis without fixation: A report on 500 cases, *J Celio-Chir* 28:64, 1998.

LAPAROSCOPIC VENTRAL AND INCISION HERNIA REPAIR

Adrian Park, MD, and Stephen M. Kavic, MD

INTRODUCTION

Abdominal wall hernias remain a common and serious health care issue because as many as one in five patients who undergo a laparotomy develop an incisional hernia. Although such hernias can be small and relatively asymptomatic, most cause significant discomfort and affect the patient's quality of life. Furthermore, a small proportion of these hernias progress to incarceration and even strangulation of bowel and other viscera, which may be life threatening.

The surgical shift since the 1990s from primary suture repair (initially under tension) to a tension-free repair with placement of a prosthetic mesh has been one of the most important trends in herniorrhaphy. We have learned that when ventral and incisional hernias are repaired primarily, they have recurred, historically, at an alarming rate (up to or even exceeding 50%). The minimally invasive, or laparoscopic, approach to ventral hernias provides a durable, tension-free repair that avoids some of the complications of open surgery. First described in the early 1990s, it is a procedure being increasingly adopted by surgeons around the world.

INDICATIONS

There are in general three reasons to repair an incisional hernia. First, symptomatic hernias, most commonly presenting with pain or discomfort, should be repaired. Second, patients who have a hernia that results in an "unsightly bulge" that affects their quality of life should be offered surgery. Last, and most difficult to define, hernia surgery should be considered in those patients for whom the hernia poses a "significant" risk of bowel strangulation in the estimation of the surgeon.

Virtually any patient with an incisional hernia is a candidate for laparoscopic ventral hernia repair, but there are several considerations in patient selection. First, the experience of the surgeon must be taken into account, selecting cases of increasing difficulty as laparoscopic skills are developed and refined. Patients with compromised cardiopulmonary function should be approached cautiously. Similarly, patients presenting with acute obstruction should not be attempted by the novice surgeon. Patients with hernias in less accessible locations, such as the high epigastrium or immediate suprapubic region may also be deferred. Finally, those patients with large, long-standing hernias may suffer some loss of domain, and reduction of the hernia contents may lead to a degree of abdominal compartment syndrome. Even when the laparoscopic approach is not possible to complete, it must be remembered that conversion to an open procedure is not a complication when performed for the patient's safety and well-being.

PREOPERATIVE PREPARATION

All patients, as part of the informed consent process, should be counseled regarding their expectations. These patients do have pain, particularly in the area of the mesh suture fixation sites. Those caught unaware by such discomfort may experience anxiety or fear that something was amiss with their surgery. Also emphasized is that such mesh suture fixation is indispensable to the long-term durability of the repair.

The second point that we routinely discuss relates to the formation of a seroma postoperatively. Following laparoscopic ventral and incision hernia (LVIH) repair, a seroma commonly develops between the mesh and hernia sac. This is a practically unavoidable sequela of the operation because, despite efforts over the years either to scarify the sac or raise peritoneal flaps including the sac to cover the mesh, the sac is left in situ. Such seroma formation is almost invariably a transient, self-limited phenomenon.

Probably the most important issue to discuss preoperatively with the patient is the possibility of inadvertent enterotomy or colotomy, whether observed or "missed." One of the most lethal complications of LVIH repair has proved to be the missed bowel injury. Obviously, the surgeon must make every effort to avoid such an injury during surgery and remain vigilant postoperatively for the possibility that such a complication may have occurred. Preoperatively, the patient must have a clear appreciation of the risk involved. In the event of an enterotomy (and of any suspicion of spillage of succus), the adhesiolysis portion of the operation is completed, but the ventral hernia repair is staged a few days or several weeks later. For this reason, our patients understand preoperatively that they may awake from their surgery without having had their hernia repair completed.

EQUIPMENT AND MATERIALS

The most important consideration is the prosthetic material used in the ventral hernia repair. Although no ideal prosthetic agent exists, the unique properties of each biomaterial make all more or less suitable. In our practice, we use expanded polytetrafluoroethylene (ePTFE) prosthetics. Current formulations of ePTFE have been developed that may be safely placed adjacent to the abdominal viscera without risk of intestinal fistula formation. The ePTFE patches have a microporous surface formulated with porosity less than 3 microns to minimize intra-abdominal adhesion formation. The opposite surface of ePTFE patches has larger porosity to allow for rapid ingrowth into abdominal wall tissues. ePTFE patches have little memory and require more manipulation when the graft is positioned, but experienced surgeons may quickly master the required technical skills.

Innovative bilayer prosthetic materials may be used in both open and laparoscopic ventral hernia repair. These combine a prosthetic with favorable ingrowth characteristics with a prosthetic that minimizes adhesion formation. The most commonly used bilayer prosthetics are created with polypropylene and PTFE.

Despite ingrowth from the abdominal wall into a prosthetic, permanent sutures are a necessity to prevent hernia recurrence by providing long-term stabilization of the prosthetic. Monofilament sutures are optimal to minimize interstices, which may harbor bacteria that could result in latent prosthetic infections.

STANDARD SETUP

- Light source and cord
- Insufflator and tubing
- Camera
- Laparoscope (5-mm, 30-degree)
  - Ports
  - 5-mm (2)
- 10–12 mm (1)
- Mesh
- Dualmesh (W.L. Gore, Newark, DE), varying sizes
- Tacking device
- 5-mm ProTack (Autosuture, Norwalk, CT)
- Suture
- Gore CV-0, CV-2 (W.L. Gore)

TECHNIQUES

Although there is some variation in the techniques of tension-free LVIH repair reported in the literature and in practice, several elements are common to such procedures. The technique of LVIH repair we practice follows.

Under general anesthesia the patient is placed supine on the operating room (OR) table with arms tucked by the sides (Fig. 1). An orogastric tube is inserted, as is a Foley catheter. In addition to a standard surgical scrub, we place a protective barrier, such as an Ioban (3M, St. Paul, MN) film, over the patient's abdomen.

Our practice is to establish pneumoperitoneum by introducing a Veress needle through a small (1- or 2-mm) incision in the subcostal region. Many surgeons prefer to employ an open or Hasson technique of initial port placement and insufflation. However, it is our preference to use a Veress needle because the contour of the insufflated abdomen often differs significantly from the native state. This "preinsufflation" allows the surgeon to optimize trocar placement as far lateral from the closest hernia

defect as comfortably possible. Otherwise an initial trocar placed into a flat abdomen may "migrate" too medially following insufflation. As with most advanced laparoscopic procedures, port placement for LVIH repair can facilitate or substantially hinder the operation.

Each trocar must be inserted under direct visualization either via cutdown or by means of a direct view trocar. It is our practice to array three trocars (one 12-mm and two 5-mm) between the iliac crest and costal margin on the side of the patient farthest from the closest hernia defect, whether midline, upper, or lower abdomen (Fig. 2). Such trocar locations, with the patient's arms tucked by the sides, allow low displacement of instrument handles to gain "end effector" access to the anterior abdominal wall. We have found it possible to repair all shapes and sizes of hernia using this trocar configuration with only occasional insertion of an extra 5-mm trocar on the contralateral side to aid in adhesiolysis or mesh fixation. A 5-mm, 30-degree laparoscope is used and can be moved among all trocars as needed.

Adhesiolysis is first performed to achieve exposure of the hernia (Fig. 3). The goal is not to remove all adhesions, but rather to clear a margin of at least 5 cm around the defect. Great care must be taken to avoid excessive traction on adhesions, particularly those involving bowel. Meticulous sharp dissection is the preferred method of adhesiolysis, seizing on the advantages of enhanced

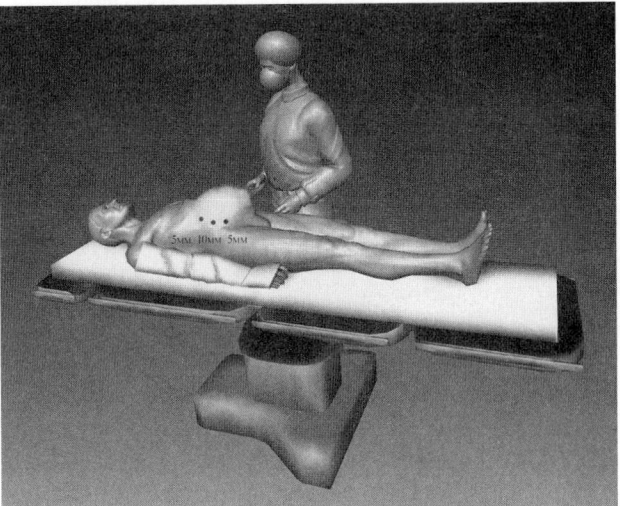

Figure 2 Trocar placement for laparoscopic ventral or incisional hernia repair.

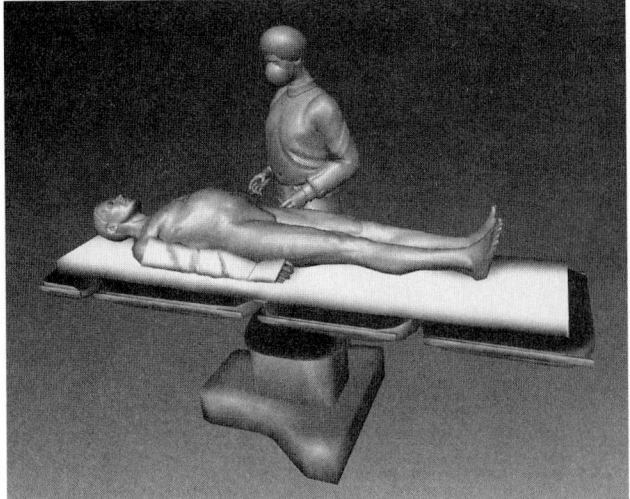

Figure 1 Patient positioning for laparoscopic ventral or incisional hernia repair.

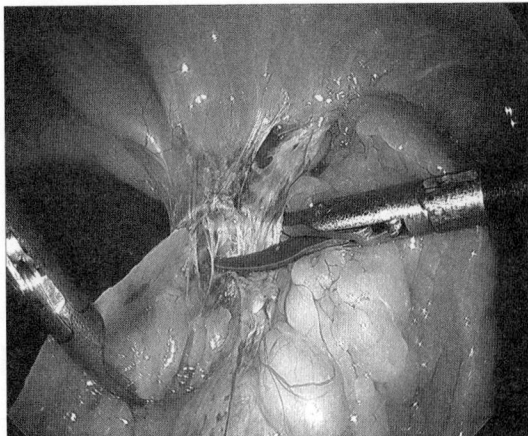

Figure 3 Adhesiolysis, performed with sharp dissection and judicious use of electrocautery. (*See color insert Figure 59.*)

laparoscopic visualization of the planes of dissection and the suspension (by pneumoperitoneum) of structures adherent to the abdominal wall. Limited and judicious use of energy sources during initial dissection is recommended because bowel may be hidden by innocuous-appearing adhesive bands.

After the hernia has been adequately exposed, it is measured either intracorporeally or by external palpation, depending on abdominal wall thickness (Fig. 4). A mesh is then selected to overlap all defect margins by at least 5 cm. In our practice, we use Dualmesh Plus, an antimicrobial-impregnated biomaterial made of expanded polytetrafluoroethylene. It is oriented and marked with symbols or letters to correspond with similar marks on the abdominal wall (Fig. 5). These serve to orient the mesh appropriately after it is introduced into the abdomen. This is particularly helpful in the case of large hernias that require the exact placement of large meshes. Before the mesh is introduced into the abdomen, four anchoring sutures are placed equidistant around its periphery. If the mesh is particularly large, six or eight sutures may be placed in this fashion. The mesh and sutures are then furled around a laparoscopic grasper and inserted through the 12-mm trocar. After the mesh is inside the abdomen, it is unfurled, and the anchor sutures are retrieved with a suture passer. The device is passed through a small incision that has been marked by one of the orienting symbols on the anterior abdominal wall (Fig. 6). Each pair of sutures is picked up by a separate pass of the suture passer, resulting in a wedge of abdominal wall muscle and fascia encompassed by the suture. The knot is tied and buried subcutaneously. It is helpful to tie opposite ends of the mesh first, to ensure the appropriate amount of tension on the patch.

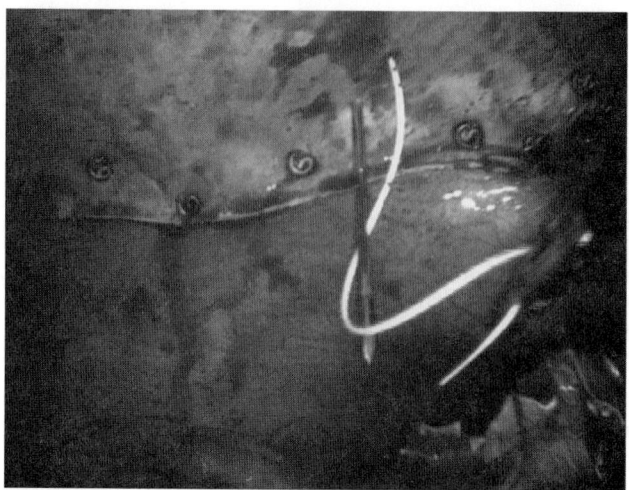

Figure 6 Use of the suture passer device to retrieve the ends of the transfascial sutures. (*See color insert Figure 61.*)

Further sutures are then placed every 5 to 6 cm around the periphery of the patch. As mentioned previously, these contribute significantly to the long-term durability of the repair. Here the suture passer is loaded extracorporeally and passed via a small incision through all layers of the abdominal wall and the mesh. The free end is left in place and retrieved by a separate pass of the instrument through the same skin incision but from a slightly different position on the mesh.

An alternative technique to placing transfascial sutures involves the use of a Keith needle and a spinal needle cannula. The straight Keith needle is passed with a clamp externally through the abdominal wall and mesh through a 1- to 2-mm skin puncture. The needle is grasped intracorporeally. Although direct passage of the needle back through the mesh and abdominal wall would be conceptually easiest, in practice this is not readily accomplished. Therefore through the same skin site, a spinal needle and cannula are passed through the abdominal wall and mesh a few millimeters away from the initial suture. The spinal needle is withdrawn, and the Keith needle passed into the spinal cannula (Fig. 7). The combination of the cannula and Keith needle is pulled through the abdominal wall, and the suture is tied externally as usual.

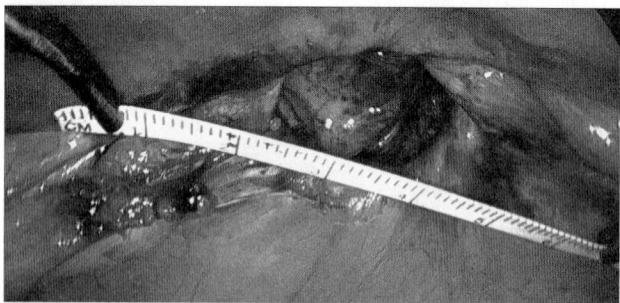

Figure 4 Measurement of the exposed hernia defect. (*See color insert Figure 60.*)

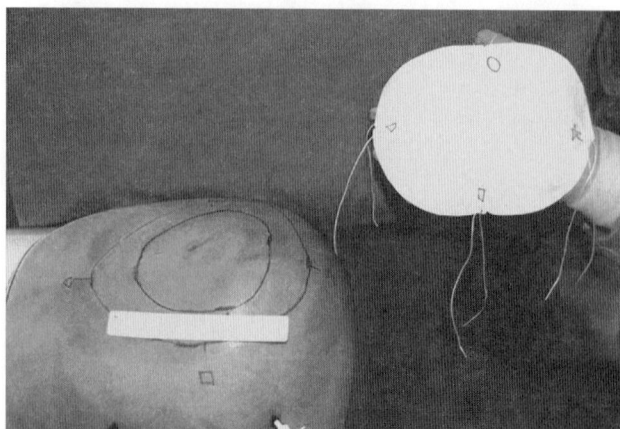

Figure 5 Orientation of the mesh before introduction into the abdomen.

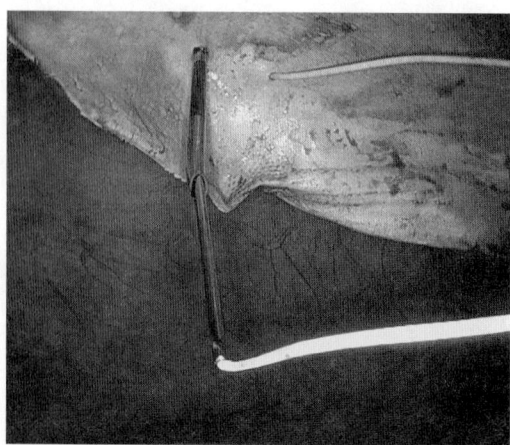

Figure 7 Use of the Keith needle and spinal cannula as an alternate means of placing transfascial sutures. (*See color insert Figure 62.*)

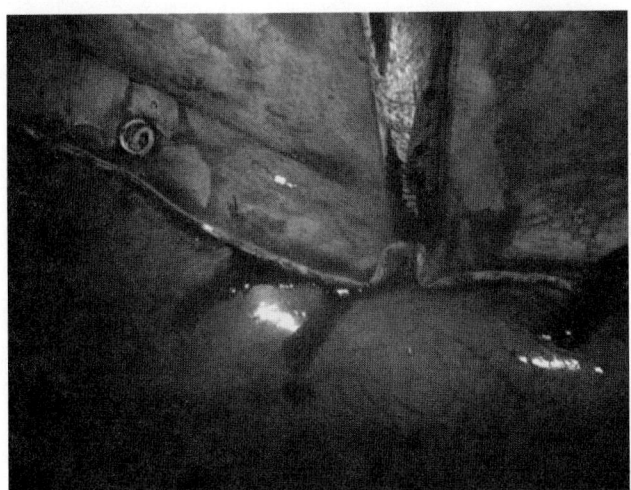

Figure 8 The mesh is secured by means of stapling device. (*See color insert Figure 63.*)

A stapler or tacker is used to secure the edge of the mesh at approximately 1-cm intervals (Fig. 8). This ensures that while the process of mesh incorporation into the host tissue is under way, no bowel or other abdominal contents are trapped above the patch. A final survey is then performed to ensure that hemostasis is secure and that there is no evidence of bowel injury. The trocars are then removed, and fascia at the 12-mm port site is closed, either externally or with the aid of a fascial closure device. Local anesthesia is then injected into all trocar and suture sites. The skin at each suture site is also inspected and released as needed to ensure that no permanent puckering results. The orogastric tube and Foley catheter are removed in the OR.

Postoperative care is based on surgical tradition more than rigorous evidence. Patients are permitted a gradual return to full activity. We counsel our patients to avoid lifting objects heavier than 10 pounds for 1 month postoperatively.

All patients undergoing repair of significant abdominal wall hernia should be given an abdominal binder during the immediate postoperative period. There is minimal evidence-based literature to guide the duration that a binder should remain in place. Most clinicians recommend maintaining the binder from 2 to 4 weeks postoperatively.

The natural history of seromas is resorption over time. Accordingly, a seroma discovered incidentally may be best managed expectantly. In the event that the seroma must be drained, there exists a real risk of introducing infection into an otherwise sterile fluid collection. Therefore aspiration of routine seromas is contraindicated. Similarly, the routine placement of drains intraoperatively may decrease the incidence of early seroma formation at the expense of increased wound and mesh infections.

Anatomic Variants

High epigastric hernias provide a challenge to even the most experienced surgeons. The repair must not impinge on the normal mobility of the diaphragm, and the mesh cannot be secured in

any location that will potentially puncture the pericardium. In this case, it may be necessary for sutures to be anchored to the posterior rib, which is best achieved through intracorporeal suturing. As a further measure to ensure adequate cephalad overlap of the defect, the falciform ligament is taken down, and the mesh is laid under the anterior abdominal wall in a retrosternal location. As pneumoperitoneum is evacuated, the liver rises to hold the mesh in position. These hernias may be technically complex and require conversion to an open procedure.

Suprapubic hernias may result from Pfannenstiel incisions (at a rate of 2% to 5%), lower midline defects, or even suprapubic tube catheter placement. The bony prominence of the symphysis pubis and the complex anatomy of the inguinal region provide most of the constraints in either laparoscopic or open repair. Because transfascial suturing is not always possible in the lower midline, the pubic periosteum has been used for successful repair of these low hernias. To access these structures for mesh fixation from a laparoscopic approach, the suspensory ligaments of the bladder are divided and the bladder is brought down. Following placement of the mesh, the peritoneal flap attached to the bladder and ligaments are tacked over the mesh.

RESULTS OF TREATMENT

Laparoscopic repair of ventral hernia is now a mature procedure, having been the subject of numerous trials and variations since the early 1990s. Numerous studies have compared laparoscopic and open approaches to ventral hernia, with the majority favoring the laparoscopic technique from the standpoint of length of stay, complications, and recurrence. Laparoscopic ventral hernia repair is undoubtedly a safe and effective procedure.

The largest single series of laparoscopic ventral hernia repair remains a four-surgeon experience of 850 cases. The authors of this study averaged an operative time of 120 minutes and had excellent results. Thirteen percent of patients experienced some complication, most of these being minor. Over 20-month follow-up, the recurrence rate was 4.7%, comparing favorably with historical controls of open ventral hernia repair.

Currently there are seven major reports in the literature of laparoscopic ventral hernia repair employing transfascial sutures in more than 100 patients. Aggregate data from these series suggest that the length of stay is approximately 3 days and that surgeons should anticipate a recurrence rate of 6% or less at 20-month follow-up. Laparoscopic ventral herniorrhaphy not only offers patients the prospect of low recurrence rates but also the significant benefit (and advantage over open repairs) of markedly diminished wound infection and complication rates.

Suggested Readings

Heniford BT, Park A, Ramshaw BJ, and others: Laparoscopic repair of ventral hernias. Nine years' experience with 850 consecutive hernias, *Ann Surg* 238:391, 2003.

LeBlanc KA, Booth WV: Laparoscopic repair of incisional abdominal hernias using expanded polytetrafluoroethylene: preliminary findings, *Surg Laparosc Endosc* 3:39, 1993.

Park A, Birch DW, Lovrics P: Laparoscopic and open incisional hernia repair: a comparison study, *Surgery* 124:816, 1998.

LAPAROSCOPIC GASTRIC SURGERY

B. Todd Heniford, MD

INTRODUCTION

Operative treatment of gastric pathology has changed dramatically since Theodore Billroth performed the first successful gastrectomy in the 1880s. Its evolution includes dramatic surgical and mechanical progress, such as the description of various types of anastomoses, the development of surgical staplers, use of nasoenteric sump tubes, and, as important as any advancement, the invention of the flexible endoscope and the skills set necessary to perform diagnostic and therapeutic upper endoscopy. Medical progress has also had an impact on gastric surgery; the advent of selective histamine-receptor blocker medications, proton pump inhibitors, and the description and treatment strategies for *Helicobacter pylori* all contributed to dramatically reducing the surgical management of peptic ulcer disease.

However, with the technical innovations of minimally invasive surgery, surgeons have generated renewed interest in upper gastrointestinal surgery. There is little doubt that laparoscopy, with its resultant reduction in morbidity and time necessary for patient recovery, has been responsible for a dramatic growth in gastric surgery since the early 1990s. Patients who were previously palliated with medications or were being observed for a variety of reasons are now seeking definitive surgical therapy. Few areas in all of surgery have seen growth as that which has been documented in the area of the lower esophagus and stomach. The numbers of antireflux procedures and bariatric operations performed have grown exponentially since the nearly systematic conversion to a laparoscopic approach. The applicability of laparoscopic gastric resection and other procedures stems from the accessibility of the stomach both laparoscopically and endoscopically, the abundance of experience with other gastric operations (e.g., antireflux surgery), the availability and reliability of laparoscopic staplers, and the fact that many gastric tumors require only simple negative margins without lymphadenectomy for curative resection. Although the indications and the expected end result for laparoscopic gastric surgery are the same as those performed via a laparotomy, the stepwise performance of the procedure and the skill set are somewhat different.

INDICATIONS

Peptic Ulcer Disease

With the improved medical agents to control gastric acid secretion and eradicate *H. pylori* infection, few patients require surgical intervention for peptic ulcer disease today. More often, surgical therapy is relegated to those patients with failure of medical therapy such as pain, obstruction, perforation, or concern for malignancy. Medical therapy has even affected the operations performed. Omental patch closure followed by medical therapy to eradicate *H. pylori* and reduce acid production is considered by many to be the standard of care for perforations caused by peptic ulcer disease. Common minimally invasive anti-ulcer procedures include truncal vagotomy and antrectomy with Billroth I or Billroth II reconstruction, vagotomy and pyloroplasty, and proximal gastric vagotomy. Several series from

Europe report success with posterior truncal vagotomy combined with either an anterior seromyotomy or anterior linear gastrectomy. For patients with gastric outlet obstruction, a laparoscopic truncal vagotomy with pyloroplasty or vagotomy with antrectomy are both valid surgical options. In the setting of an acute perforation, a laparoscopic omental (Graham) patch with simple closure followed by peritoneal lavage is often straightforward and frequently preferred. A more definitive antiulcer procedure with or without resection may be performed if there is minimal contamination, the patient has chronic symptoms or has failed medical management, and the condition of the patient allows it.

Gastric Masses

Many gastric tumors can be managed with local resections only. Given that a minimal negative margin without formal lymphadenectomy is all that is required, these tumors are especially amenable to a laparoscopic wedge resection. Gastrointestinal stromal tumors (GISTs), most carcinoids, pancreatic rests, and adenomyomas all fall into this category. They had previously been described as rare. However, with the rise in the number of upper endoscopies, we have seen a remarkable increase in referrals for what is often an asymptomatic tumor.

The cellular origin of GISTs was previously recognized to be smooth muscle, and benign tumors were characterized as leiomyomas, malignant tumors as leiomyosarcomas. Identification of the interstitial cell of Cajal as the cell of origin of smooth muscle tumors led to the change in nomenclature to GISTs. The interstitial cell of Cajal is a pacemaker cell of the gastrointestinal tract and is found within the myenteric plexus, submucosa, and muscularis propria. Immunohistochemistry established the derivation of GISTs from the interstitial cell of Cajal by demonstrating the expression of cellular markers such as CD-117, a marker of the c-kit gene product, and CD 34, a human progenitor cell antigen.

Significant effort has been put forth with regard to predicting the biologic nature of GISTs. Unfortunately, distant metastasis or local invasion may not present until many years after diagnosis of the primary tumor and is not affected by the extent of the resection. A combination of prognostic factors (patient age, histologic grade, mitotic rate, tumor size, and DNA analysis) has been used to predict the biologic behavior of GISTs. The most significant clinical predictors of malignant behavior are tumor size (>5 cm) and mitotic activity (five or more mitoses per 50 high-power fields). However, GISTs with completely benign characteristics have recurred or metastasized (or both). The only absolute signs of malignancy are metastasis or invasion into adjacent organs.

Gastric carcinoid (neuroendocrine) tumors are typically divided into three main categories, classified on the basis of pathogenesis and histomorphologic characteristics, which differ in biologic behavior and prognosis. Type I, such as found in pernicious anemia (type I) or gastrin-producing neoplasms as in Zollinger-Ellison's syndrome, and type II (multiple endocrine neoplasia I) are characteristically localized to the gastric body or fundus and are usually considered benign with a low risk of malignancy. Treatment of these lesions is simple excision. Type III gastric carcinoids are composed of poorly differentiated endocrine and exocrine cells that grow sporadically, irrespective of gastrin hypersecretion. Most of these tumors show a low- to high-grade malignant transformation and are treated much more aggressively, as for an adenocarcinoma.

Gastric Cancer

Surgical resection is the only cure for gastric cancer. In North America, most patients present with an advanced stage of disease at the time of diagnosis, precluding a curative resection. The surgical objectives for treating patients with gastric cancer include maximizing the probability for cure in patients with localized tumor and to provide safe and effective palliation to patients with metastatic disease.

The crucial point in the decision for or against limited surgery for gastric cancer is the preoperative differentiation between mucosal and submucosal extension of the carcinoma. Endoscopic ultrasound is essential to make this decision. Lymphatic spread from early gastric cancer occurs at variable rates and appears most reliant on the grade of the tumor, its size, and its depth of invasion. Gastric cancers that measure less than 3 cm, are limited to the mucosa, and are nonscirrhous can be treated by local, full-thickness resection with a negative margin. This is true because lymph node metastasis is rare (1%-3%) in these cases. Essentially, all other lesions should be treated with an extended resection. Although resections of virtually any extent can be performed using minimally invasive techniques, the more extensive resections are difficult and lengthy when performed laparoscopically. The time/cost versus benefit conundrum that surgeons face must be carefully examined when a procedure of this extent is to be undertaken. The gastric resections described in this chapter are limited to nonmetastatic lesions or those intended for palliation.

OPERATIVE TECHNIQUES

The operative approach to gastric resection depends on the indication for surgery (ulcer disease vs. tumor), tumor size, location, and growth morphology. Laparoscopic wedge, transgastric, intragastric, and limited segmental resections have all been used to treat a variety of gastric lesions. Before the resection, a formal abdominal exploration is performed to rule out peritoneal seeding or hepatic metastasis. The diaphragm, peritoneum, and surface of the liver are examined. Intraoperative ultrasound provides distinctive anatomic detail of the liver for evaluation of metastatic deposits. During a laparoscopic procedure in which tactile feedback is not available, a concomitant gastric endoscopy allows for a coordinated examination both inside and outside the stomach, which I find remarkably valuable.

The operating room setup is the same for most foregut surgeries. The patient is placed in the supine position with arms abducted on armboards or tucked at the patient's side. We use a split-leg table in nearly all circumstances, allowing the surgeon to stand between the patient's legs and directly face the epigastrium. Monitors are placed over each of the patient's shoulders (Fig. 1). The typical size and locations of the ports are demonstrated in Figure 2. The upper midline and left midabdominal ports are two main operative ports used by the operating surgeon. The camera is placed through the lower midline port. A liver retractor is placed via the right abdominal port. The assistant on the patient's left side uses the left lateral accessory port to provide retraction. An endoscopic linear stapler is usually introduced through the surgeon's right-hand port, although any port can be replaced with a 12-mm sleeve to allow for a better angle for gastric transection. The first port placed is usually in the midline, one quarter to one third of the distance between the umbilicus and the xiphoid, and is used for the camera. Periumbilical placement of the camera may be appropriate for the lesions in the distal half of the stomach. In our experience, an umbilical port tends to be too low when the dissection is focused on the proximal stomach. Similarly, when the lesion is in the distal portion of the stomach, all of the trocar positions can be moved slightly inferiorly to keep the ports from being directly over the operative site.

After insertion of the initial ports and peritoneal exploration, the patient is placed in a steep reverse Trendelenburg position.

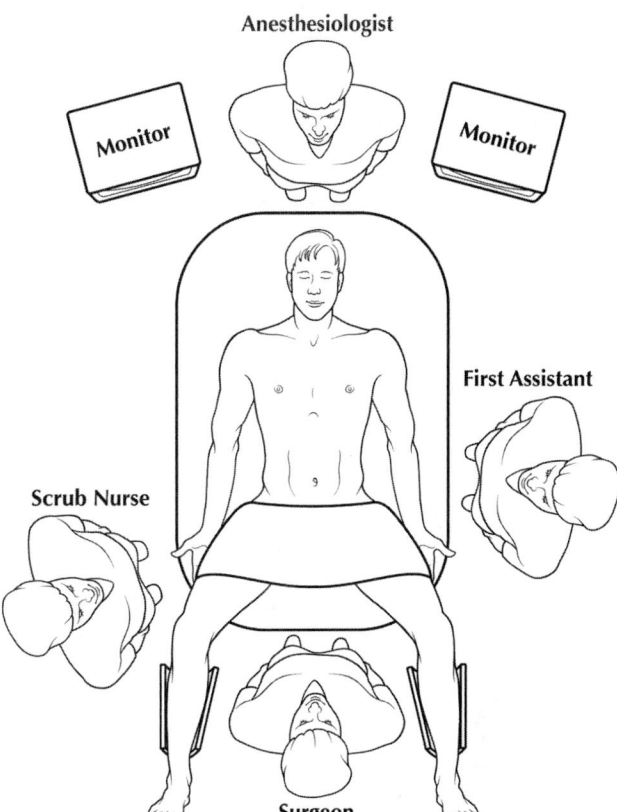

Figure 1 Operative positioning for gastric resection.

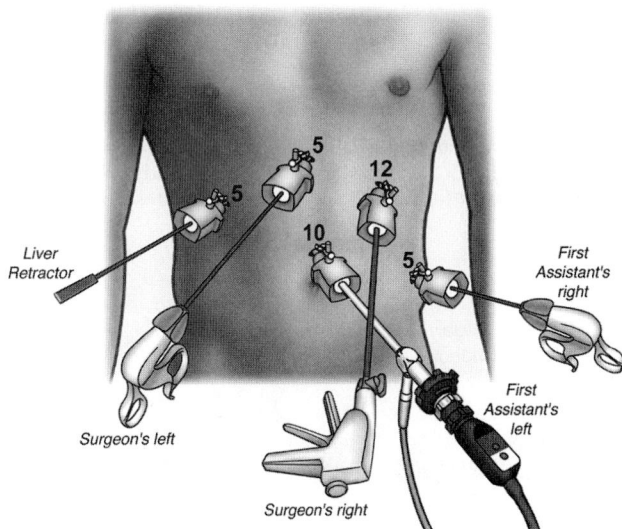

Figure 2 Port placement for laparoscopic gastric resection.

Intraoperative endoscopy is crucial to facilitate the localization of small lesions and assist in the evaluation of both the extent of resection and the integrity of the staple/suture lines. An experienced endoscopist and the judicious use of air insufflation are important in avoiding troublesome insufflation of the small intestine with a resultant loss of an intra-abdominal working space. In all cases, specimens are placed in an impervious retrieval bag before extraction. I believe this technique may help to prevent tumor spread within the abdomen and trocar sites and may decrease bacterial contamination of the abdomen and the extraction site.

Laparoscopic Treatment of Gastric Perforation

Several techniques have been described for laparoscopic treatment of perforated peptic ulcer. Following the principle of conventional open repair, ulcer closure may be performed by simple or running suture techniques incorporating omental patches. Gastroscopic-guided techniques for creating plugs of omentum of the ligamentum teres hepatic have been described. Sutureless techniques including plugs of gelatin sponges or fibrin glue have been used but are associated with higher leak rates, particularly if the perforation is larger than 5 mm in diameter. I prefer a simple, interrupted suture technique incorporating an omental patch based on Graham's closure and not using any additional foreign body.

Laparoscopic Highly Selective Vagotomy

Denervation of the parietal cell mass via a true highly selective vagotomy is an exigent operation. When performed laparoscopically, it is most often performed by combining a posterior truncal vagotomy with an anterior seromyotomy. Following the truncal vagotomy, the seromyotomy is started at the level of the first branch of the crow's foot, which is usually found approximately 6 cm from the pylorus. The superficial gastric incision proceeds along the lesser curve, crosses over the anterior aspect of the cardia to the angle of His and as far posteriorly as the lateral aspect of the left crus (Fig. 3). The seromyotomy is closed with a running stitch of 2–0 silk or Vicryl (Ethicon Endosurgery, Somerville, NJ) (Fig. 4). Essentially, the same anterior disruption of the vagus nerve can be carried out with an endomechanical stapler as seen in Fig. 5. The outcomes of this procedure are not well documented; however, although a few series have demonstrated a 5% failure rate, the majority of reports show a 15% to 20% rate of recidivism.

Laparoscopic Wedge Resections

Anterior Gastric Wall Lesions

Masses within the anterior wall of the stomach are amenable to wedge resection with a linear endoscopic gastrointestinal anastomosis (GIA) stapler. After identifying the lesion laparoscopically and

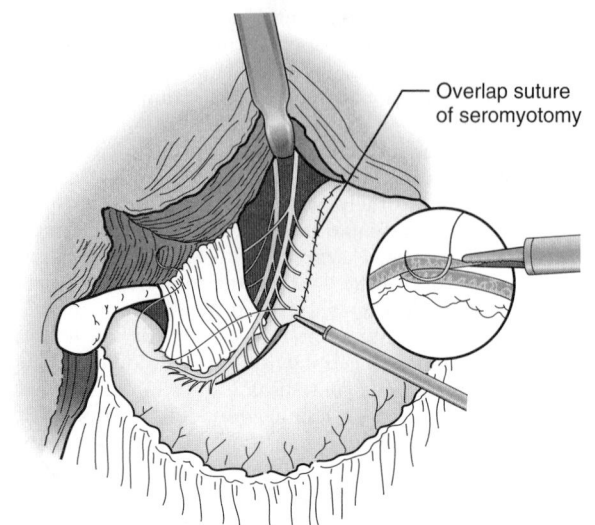

Figure 4 Oversewing of lesser curve seromyotomy. *From Kathouda N, Mouiel J: Laparoscopic vagotomy for treatment of peptic ulcer. In Zucker KA, editor: Surgical laparoscopy, ed 2, Philadelphia, 2001, Lippincott Williams & Wilkins. Used with permission.*

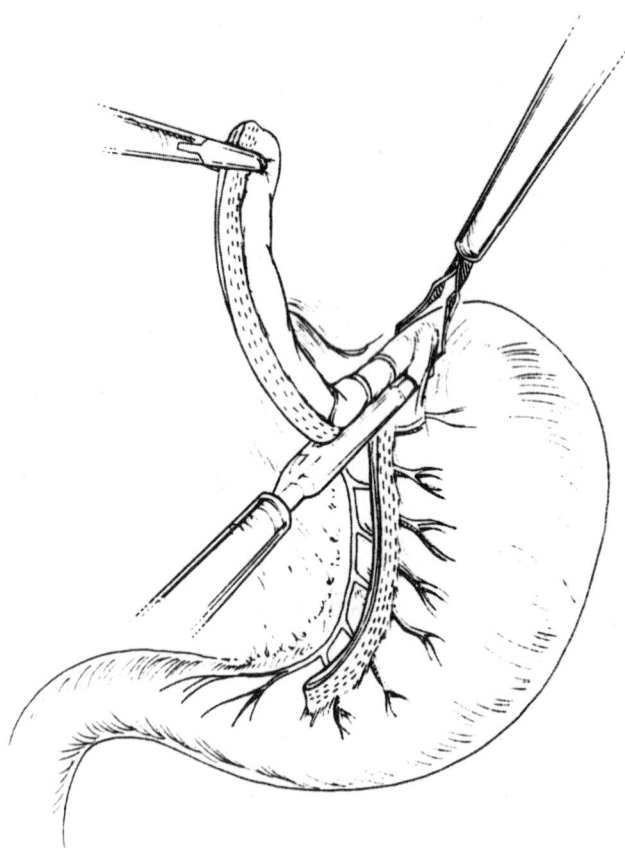

Figure 5 Linear gastrectomy is carried up lesser curve. *From Bailey RW: Abdominal vagotomy, In MacFadyen BV, Ponsky JL, editors: Operative laparoscopy and thoracoscopy, Philadelphia, 1996, Lippincott-Raven. Used with permission.*

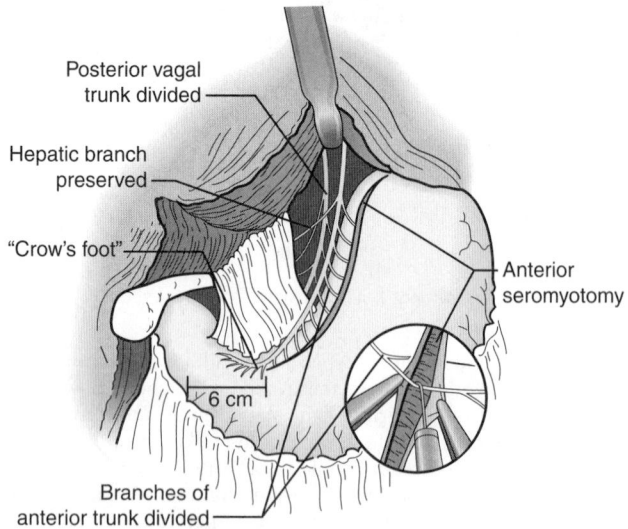

Figure 3 Anterior lesser curve seromyotomy. *From Kathouda N, Mouiel J: Laparoscopic vagotomy for treatment of peptic ulcer. In Zucker KA, editor: Surgical laparoscopy, ed 2, Philadelphia, 2001, Lippincott Williams & Wilkins. Used with permission.*

endoscopically, the short gastric and gastroepiploic vessels are ligated and divided as needed. Typically this maneuver is performed with the assistant on the left retracting the omentum and gastro-splenic ligament toward the patient's left side while the surgeon retracts the stomach medially or superiorly and transects the vessels with ultrasonic coagulating shears (Harmonic Scalpel; Johnson & Johnson Gateway, Piscataway, NJ). Laparoscopic gastric wedge resection is accomplished by elevating the gastric wall by two seromuscular sutures placed opposite each other 1 to 2 cm beyond a mass or an ulcer. The lesion and a small cuff of the normal stomach are then divided by an endoscopic linear stapler placed just under the sutures (Fig. 6) with intraluminal guidance of the endoscope. Alternatively, a lesion and surrounding rim of normal tissue may be excised using ultrasonic coagulating shears. The latter technique allows for a more precise excision of the normal tissue at the margin. The gastrotomy can be closed by laparoscopic intracorporeal suturing or by placing two to four full-thickness traction sutures along the cut edge of the gastrotomy to elevate the cut edges of the stomach so that it can be closed effectively using an endoscopic linear stapler (Fig. 7).

Posterior Gastric Wall Lesions

Subserosal posterior wall lesions can be approached through the lesser sac. Following the division of the gastrocolic omentum, the greater curvature is grasped to expose the posterior surface of the stomach. The lesion is then resected similar to the technique described earlier. I commonly perform two alternative approaches to intraluminal posterior wall ulcers or larger posterior gastric wall tumors. One method entails a creation of an anterior gastrotomy over the lesion after it is endoscopically localized within the stomach. Normal gastric tissue adjacent to the lesion is grasped with laparoscopic bowel graspers or, alternatively, traction sutures are placed 1 to 2 cm from the lesion or ulcer on opposite sides, and the lesion is elevated through the gastrotomy (Fig. 8). A margin of normal tissue is also resected with the lesion using an endoscopic linear stapler. The staple line is examined for bleeding through the gastrotomy using the laparoscope, and any bleeding points are oversewn. The anterior gastrotomy is closed as previously described.

Intraluminal posterior wall lesions that are not amenable to endoscopic treatment can be approached via a percutaneous intragastric resection. Laparoscopic intragastric or "endoluminal" surgery involves the placement of balloon-tipped laparoscopic trocars (2, 5, or 10 mm) percutaneously into the stomach (insufflated by a flexible endoscope) similar to the placement of a percutaneous endoscopic gastrostomy tube (Figs. 9 and 10). My preference is to perform transperitoneal laparoscopy via a single port at the umbilicus before inserting transgastric ports. This allows for assessment of the peritoneal cavity and the serosal surface of the stomach and provides for visualization of the stomach and adjacent organs during placement of percutaneous, transgastric ports. The laparoscope is directed through one of the trocars and into the insufflated stomach. A dilute epinephrine solution (1:100,000) is injected circumferentially around the stromal tumor as a tumescent to aid in dissection of the submucosal plane and to limit bleeding or oozing. The lesion is enucleated from the submucosal-muscular junction using an electrocautery hook. The mucosal defect is left

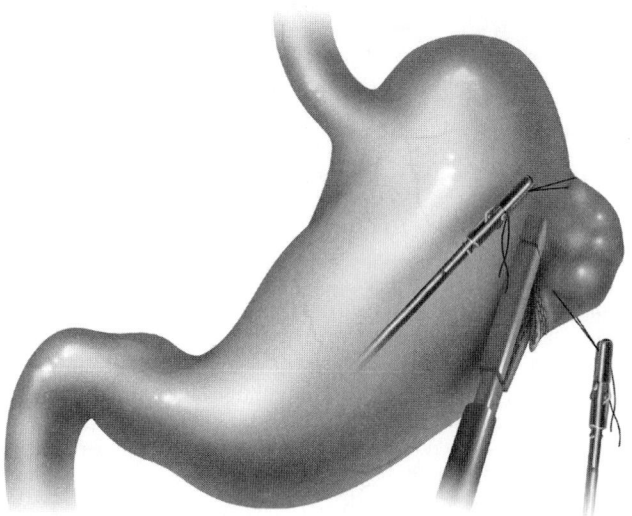

Figure 6   Laparoscopic anterior wall gastric wedge resection with linear stapler.

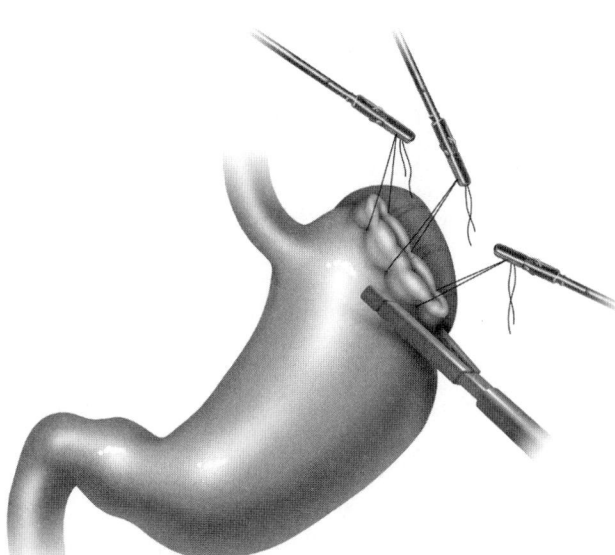

Figure 7   Linear stapler closure after laparoscopic anterior wall gastric wedge resection with Harmonic Scalpel (Johnson & Johnson Gateway, Piscataway, NJ).

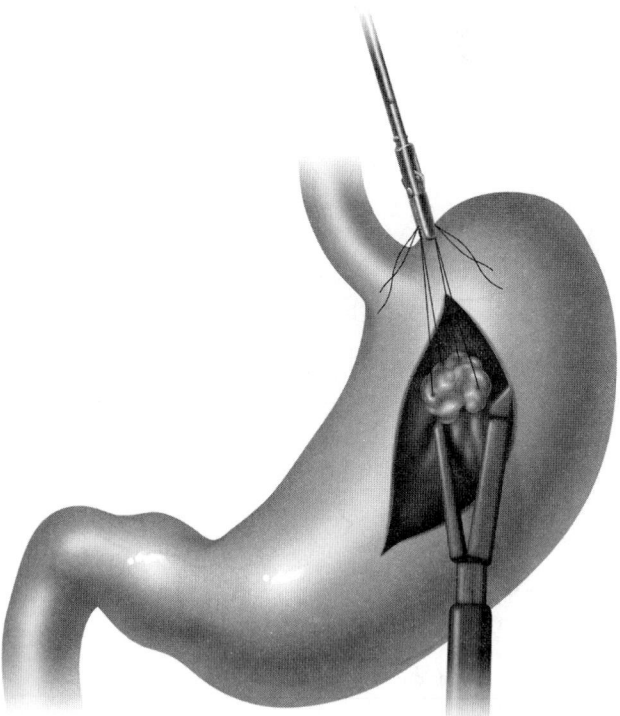

Figure 8   Laparoscopic posterior wall gastric wedge resection with linear stapler.

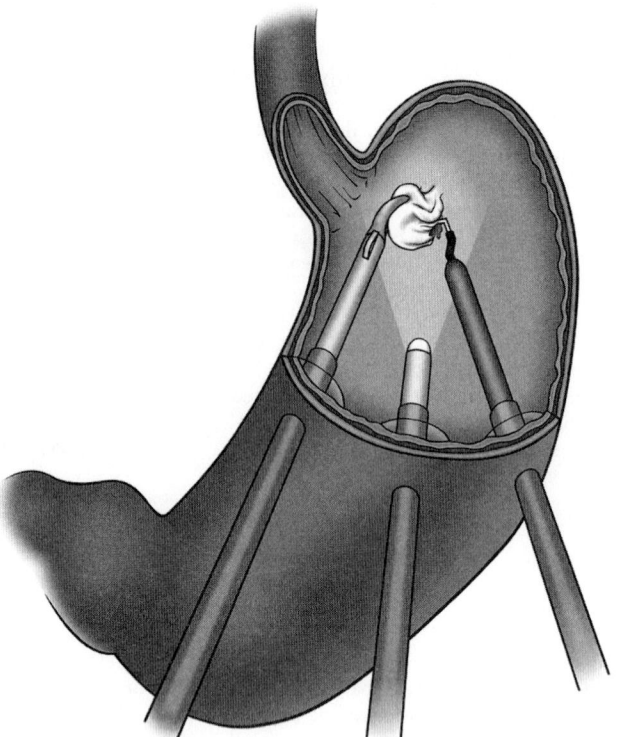

Figure 9 Transgastric laparoscopic resection of posterior gastric tumor.

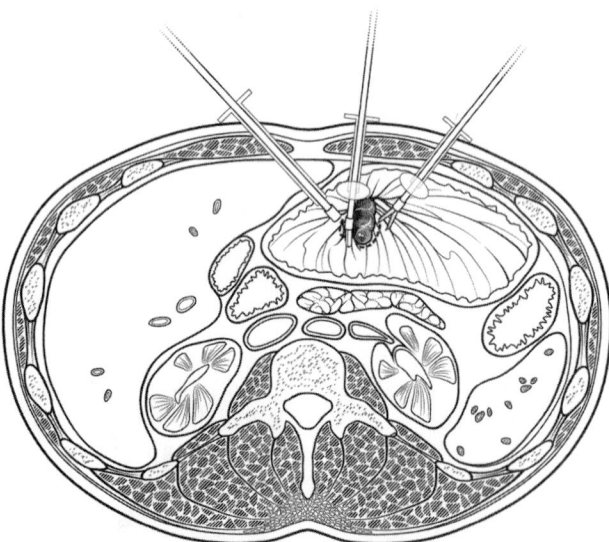

Figure 10 Sagittal view of transgastric laparoscopic resection of posterior gastric tumor.

open to heal or can be closed with intragastric suturing. The tumor is placed in a retrieval bag and removed transorally with the flexible endoscope. Despite the novelty of this technique, there is some concern about the adequacy of the resection. To date, we have noted no local or systemic recurrence.

Lesions of the Greater and Lesser Curves

Lesions of the greater and lesser curvatures are typically amenable to simple wedge resection with an endoscopic linear stapler. The greater omentum is mobilized for greater curvature tumors and

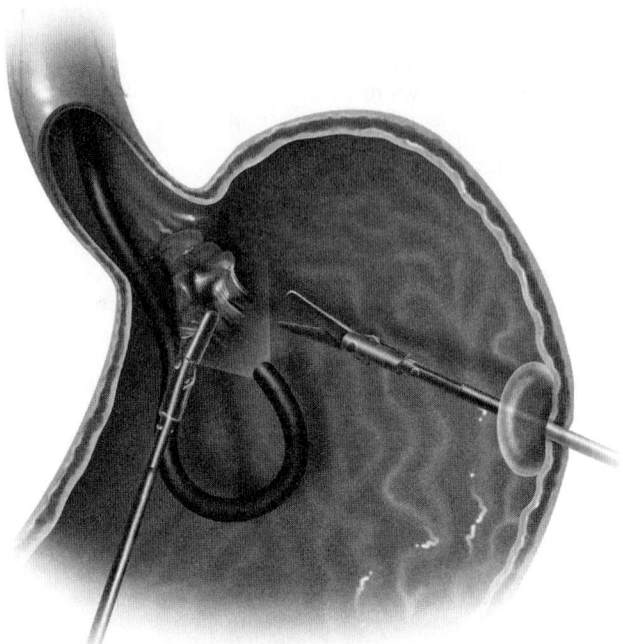

Figure 11 Endoscopic-assisted transgastric laparoscopic resection of gastroesophageal junction tumor.

the lesser omentum/gastrohepatic ligament for those lesions located on the lesser curve. The Harmonic Scalpel, LigaSure (ValleyLab, Boulder, CO), or laparoscopic clip ligation (or a combination of these) allows for a safe division of the short gastric vessels on the greater curvature and branches of the left gastric artery and coronary vein on the lesser curvature. Rotating the stomach so that the lesion faces anteriorly facilitates the resection. Lesions are resected using an endoscopic linear stapler and removed in an impermeable extraction bag through an enlarged 12-mm trocar site.

Lesions Near the Gastroesophageal Junction

We have previously described the technique for minilaparoscopic intragastric resection for gastroesophageal junction stromal tumors using a flexible endoscope as the "camera" and insufflator. Working ports are provided by two 2-mm mushroom-tipped trocars or 5-mm trocars placed percutaneously into the gastric lumen as described above (Fig. 11). Hook electrocautery is used to enucleate the gastroesophageal junction tumor following a submucosal injection of dilute epinephrine. To avoid directly handling the tumor and possibly fracturing it, we frequently endoloop the lesion after the dissection is begun. The mass is removed transorally with the flexible endoscope with the aid of an endoscopic snare.

Gastrectomy

Partial Gastrectomy

The trocar strategy used for the laparoscopic local resection of anterior, posterior, and greater/lesser curvature gastric masses is essentially the same for minimally invasive techniques to perform a subtotal gastrectomy. We frequently move our trocars just slightly inferior while maintaining their position in a medial-to-lateral location. For a gastric adenocarcinoma in particular, examination of the peritoneal surfaces, visual (laparoscopic and intra-abdominal ultrasound) inspection of the liver, and exploration of the lesser sac are critical when the resection is going to be performed for curative intent. In approximately 25% of patients, laparoscopic exploration detects metastasis that precludes curative resection despite the tumor's appearing to be resectable with standard preoperative radiographic examinations.

The first steps in performing a gastric resection are initiated during the general exploration. The gastrocolic omentum—or when the procedure is performed for curative resection, the omentum–is taken off the transverse colon to the end of the lesser sac. The assistant, on the patient's left side, elevates the omentum and reflects it up and over the stomach. The surgeon, retracting downward on the colon with the left hand, can divide the thin attachments between the omentum and colon using ultrasonic coagulating shears. When the resection is for palliation, the surgeon holds the stomach with his or her left hand while the assistant retracts the colon inferiorly to "tent up" the gastrocolic ligament. The gastrocolic ligament is divided, and the lesser sac is entered as the dissection proceeds from the midstomach up along the greater curve of the stomach toward the spleen. The gastroepiploic vessel branches are then ligated by the Harmonic Scalpel or LigaSure. Distal mobilization of the stomach is continued beyond the pylorus, which is identified by its muscular rings or the vein of Mayo. The small vessels surrounding the duodenum are coagulated and transected with a 45- or 60-mm endoscopic stapler (3.5-mm staple load). The duodenal staple line is frequently fortified with a staple line reinforcement (Seamguard, W.L. Gore, Newark, DE) or imbricated with 2–0 silk sutures. After transecting the duodenum, the distal part of the stomach can be rotated toward the patient's left flank, significantly facilitating transection of the posterior attachments of the stomach. The plane between the stomach and the liver can also be transected with the LigaSure or Harmonic Scalpel. After deciding the level at which the stomach will be transected, additional short, gastric vessels or branches of the descending left gastric artery can be divided as needed. If there is any concern regarding the level of transection of the stomach, an intraoperative endoscopy, as well as laparoscopic visual and palpable cues, should be able to plot the course of the gastric transection. Depending on the level of the stomach to be transected, the endoscopic stapler can be placed through the left subcostal port or through a 12-mm port in the left lateral subcostal support. The stomach is placed on some stretch as the stapler is applied. Three or four staple loads (3.5- or 4.8-mm cartridges) of a 45- to 60-mm stapler are usually required, depending on the level of the stomach to be transected. In the more proximal stomach, we have found a 3.5-mm stapler to work well and to reduce bleeding. The more distal and thicker portions of the stomach require a 4.8-mm staple cartridge.

Several techniques are used for reconstruction following a subtotal gastrectomy. I typically prefer a standard loop jejunostomy or, if the gastric pouch is small, a Roux-en-Y gastrojejunostomy. This portion of the operation is initiated by taking the patient out of Trendelenburg position and maintaining him or her in a more neutral orientation. The omentum is rolled upward and over the colon, and a colonic epiploica is grasped and pulled upward to expose the full undersurface of the transverse colon mesentery and to identify the ligament of Treitz. I measure approximately 20 to 35 cm distal to the ligament of Treitz and roll this portion of the jejunum upward to the gastric remnant. If the intestine easily reaches the gastric remnant, an anticolic route is chosen. To facilitate the anticolic positioning of the jejunal limb, one can split the omentum midline in a caudal-cranial fashion using the ultrasonic coagulating shears. Otherwise a small window can be made in the avascular area of the transverse mesocolon just above and lateral to the ligament of Treitz. The loop of the jejunum can be brought through the mesocolon easily in a retrocolic, retrogastric fashion. The anastomosis can be performed in an isoperistaltic or antiperistaltic manner. I typically choose an antiperistaltic anastomosis, which allows placement of a stapler from the cut edge of the stomach angling slightly upward on the stomach and distally on the small intestine (Fig. 12).

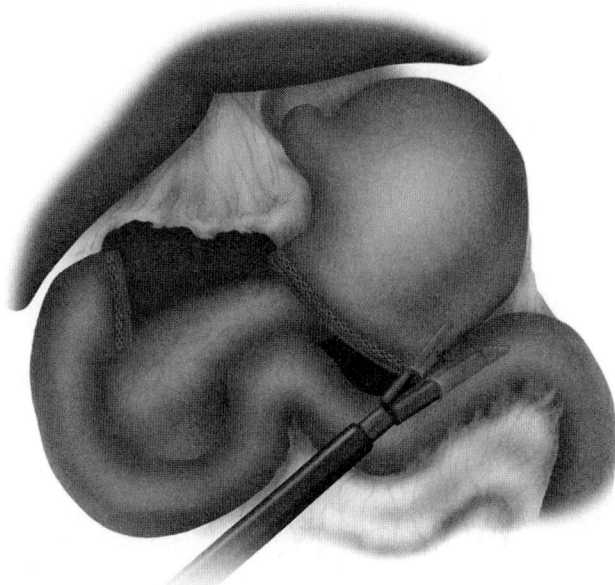

Figure 12 Gastrojejunal anastomosis performed with laparoscopic gastrointestinal anastomosis stapler.

Total Gastrectomy

Laparoscopic total gastrectomy is performed in a method comparable with partial or subtotal gastrectomy, except for the more proximal mobilization and division of the esophagus and a more complex intestinal reconstruction. Several 12-mm ports are placed to allow for versatility in employing the endoscopic linear stapler from many angles. The short gastric vessels, posterior lesser curve attachments, and phrenoesophageal ligament are divided with ultrasonic coagulating shears, and the distal esophagus is mobilized well into the mediastinum. The division of the phrenoesophageal ligament, as well as the mediastinal dissection, is facilitated by an assistant who retracts the stomach in a caudal direction with a Penrose drain placed around the gastroesophageal junction. The posterior dissection of the stomach and anterolateral dissection of the esophageal hiatus is relatively avascular and can be performed with blunt techniques. The distal esophagus is mobilized by "pushing" the left and right crura away from the esophagus. In general, any tubes in the esophagus (orogastric, nasogastric, bougie, esophageal stethoscope) are removed before initiating the hiatal dissection. Posterior to the esophagus, segmental arteries from the aorta are divided with the ultrasonic coagulating shears. After the esophagus is mobilized, the anterior and posterior vagal trunks are identified and divided between clips. The left gastric artery is isolated and divided using an endoscopic linear staler and vascular load (2.0–2.5 mm). After complete mobilization and vascular division from the celiac trunk (left gastric artery), the esophagus is transected with an endoscopic linear stapler or LigaSure. The distal stomach is divided with an endoscopic linear stapler beyond the pylorus, as previously described for subtotal gastrectomy.

The circular, flip-top EEA stapler (US Surgical, Norwalk, CT) or endoscopic linear stapling device can be used to complete the esophagojejunostomy. The technique of using a 25-mm flip-top EEA stapler to perform a Roux-en-Y gastrojejunostomy for laparoscopic gastric bypass is the same technique for reconstruction by a Roux-en-Y esophagojejunostomy after laparoscopic total gastrectomy. Before performing an esophagojejunostomy, the ligament of Treitz is identified and the proximal jejunum is divided approximately 30 to 45 cm distal to the ligament of Treitz with the endoscopic linear stapler. The biliary (proximal) limb is subsequently anastomosed to the more distal jejunum, approximately 30 to 40 cm distal to the staple line on the proximal Roux limb.

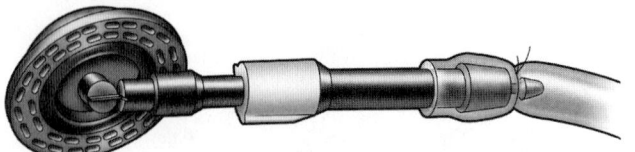

Figure 13 Orogastric tube secured to a flipped, 25-mm anvil.

To complete a circular-stapled anastomosis, the anvil has to be brought out of the distal esophagus. This is facilitated by securing (suture) a flipped, 25-mm anvil to the distal end of a 16-F orogastric tube that has previously been transected proximal to the sump airport (Fig. 13). The proximal end of the orogastric tube with the flipped anvil secured to the distal end is passed transorally and guided down the esophagus, and the proximal end of the orogastric tube is gently pulled into the abdomen and out one of the trocar sites. As the tube is pulled through the enterotomy in the esophagus, the anvil is guided through the oropharynx by the anesthesiologist. After the anvil tip emerges from the esophagotomy, the orogastric tube is cut free of the anvil and removed. The EEA stapler is placed directly through the abdominal wall via an enlarged trocar site in the left upper quadrant and advanced into an enterotomy created along the staple line on the proximal Roux (jejunum) limb. The EEA stapler is advanced antegrade through the Roux limb, and the spike of the EEA is advanced through the antimesenteric border of the jejunum. The anvil protruding through the esophagotomy is united with EEA stapler, and the stapler is tightened and fired. The enterotomy in the proximal Roux limb is closed with an endoscopic linear stapler.

CONTRAINDICATIONS

There are few absolute contraindications to laparoscopy; most often surgeon experience and disease state dictate the relative feasibility and possible advantages of laparoscopic therapy. Several of these might include uncorrected coagulopathy, a patient who is unable to tolerate a laparotomy, and a surgeon's true lack of experience with this or similar procedures. Relative contraindications would include extensive previous surgery, previous peritonitis, severe cardiopulmonary disease, and a tumor of a size that would preclude safe handling.

SUGGESTED READINGS

Cuschieri A: Laparoscopic gastric resection, *Surg Clin North Am* 80:1269, viii, 2001.

Kitano S, Shiraishi N, Fujii K, and others: A randomized controlled trial comparing open vs laparoscopy-assisted distal gastrectomy for the treatment of early gastric cancer: an interim report, *Surgery* 131:S306, 2002.

Novitsky YW, Kercher KW, Sing RF, and others: Long-term outcomes of laparoscopic resection of gastric gastrointestinal stromal tumors, *Ann Surg* 243:738, 2006.

Uyama I, Sugioka A, Sakurai Y, and others: Hand-assisted laparoscopic function- preserving and radical gastrectomies for advanced-stage proximal gastric cancer, *J Am Coll Surg* 199:508, 2004.

LAPAROSCOPIC COLON SURGERY

Deborah Nagle, MD

INTRODUCTION

Laparoscopic colectomy is a complex surgical procedure requiring advanced laparoscopic techniques. The reported benefits to patients of minimally invasive colon resection include quicker return of gastrointestinal (GI) tract function, less postoperative pain and narcotic use, shorter postoperative hospitalization, lower incidence of wound infection and small bowel obstruction, and better cosmesis. However, adoption of laparoscopic colectomy in surgical practice has been relatively slow. No doubt the technical difficulty of the surgery and time commitment for skill acquisition has deterred many. Controversy over the advantages to patients and institutional costs stirred skepticism. Real concern about unfavorable oncologic implications with laparoscopic colectomy was expressed. A growing body of surgical literature has now substantiated time and cost effectiveness and some postoperative benefits. The 2003 publication of the COST (Clinical Outcomes of Surgical Therapy) study, a randomized, prospective trial of open versus laparoscopic colon resection, quelled many concerns. In essence, this large study documented that in experienced hands, laparoscopic and open colectomy were equivalent techniques with no oncologic disadvantage to patients.

BASIC PRINCIPLES

The most fundamental principle of laparoscopic colectomy is that no case should be approached without adequate training and self-study. The surgeon's learning curve can be steep, given the multiple advanced tasks required. Technical issues differ for surgeons with extensive laparoscopic experience versus surgeons with extensive open colectomy experience. For surgeons beyond the residency years, training may include instruction in cadaver courses, video review, reading, and mentor support. The learning curve is approximately 50 cases for comfort and competence.

Learning progress is thought to be facilitated by mimicking the operative steps the surgeon uses in open colectomy. The key steps of bowel mobilization, vascular division and bowel resection, and anastomosis must be accomplished with either approach. Setting a time limit or a technical benchmark, such as bowel mobilization, for laparoscopic cases can be helpful to prevent unduly long cases and mishaps resulting from frustration. Good judgment is essential for successful open or laparoscopic surgeries.

PATIENT SELECTION AND SURGICAL APPROACH

Most open colectomy procedures can be performed laparoscopically. However, the degree of technical difficulty in laparoscopic colectomy is increased in patients with previous abdominal surgery, left-sided or pelvic dissection and complex disease processes. During the surgeon's early laparoscopic colectomy experience, it is advisable to select patients without previous abdominal surgery, close to ideal body weight, and with straightforward pathology. Cases that are most amenable to a straightforward laparoscopic approach are right colectomy for polyp and sigmoid colectomy for uncomplicated diverticulitis.

Laparoscopic colectomy may be performed with or without hand assistance. The advantages of hand-assisted laparoscopic (HALS) technique include restoration of three-dimensional depth perception and tactile feedback and dissection. These benefits can help the novice laparoscopic colon surgeon move up the learning curve more rapidly. Hand-assisted technique can also facilitate more difficult cases by restoring manual dissection of complex tissue planes or anatomy. HALS can help surgeons teach by allowing presentation of the target structure to the laparoscopic learner. The reported patient benefits of shortened hospital stay and quicker recovery are the same for pure laparoscopic and hand-assisted technique.

The challenge of hand-assisted technique is placing the hand-port device, and thereby the surgeon's hand, so that it facilitates rather than obstructs visualization and dissection. Hand fatigue can be significant in cases of longer operative time. Hand-port devices can leak and drain pneumoperitoneum, and incisions to accommodate larger surgeon hands can approximate small open incisions.

Again, surgeons should use whichever technique they are trained in and comfortable with.

OPERATING ROOM

A moveable operating table is essential for positioning the patient for optimal exposure of the target organ. Patients are uniformly placed on the table in the low lithotomy position. For left-sided and pelvic anastomoses, this position allows for transanal stapling. For all procedures, lithotomy positioning allows free access to the abdominal wall. The surgeon or assistant can stand between the patient's legs. In lithotomy position, it is important that the patient's thighs be at or below the plane of the anterior-superior iliac spine to allow for free movement of the laparoscopic instruments in the field. Both of the patient's arms should be tucked at the sides, again to facilitate surgeon movement, with protection for the patient's hands. The patient is prepared and draped, with the entire abdominal wall exposed (Fig. 1). For surgeries with left-sided anastomosis, the perineum is prepared and access through the drapes available.

Laparoscopic colectomy requires specific equipment. In addition to a video tower system, laparoscopic instruments that allow for atraumatic handling of the bowel are important. The most basic form of laparoscopic colectomy involves laparoscopic mobilization

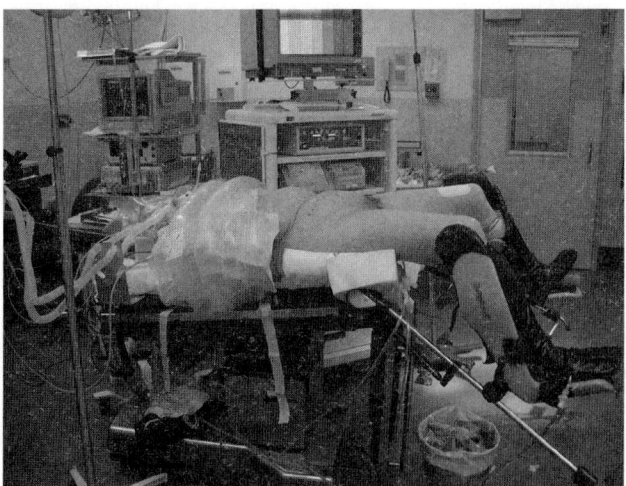

Figure 1 Patient positioning for laparoscopic colectomy.

of the bowel, followed by exteriorization of the specimen. Division of the mesentery, bowel, and anastomosis is performed extracorporeally. For all other permutations of laparoscopic colectomy, a device for vascular control and division is necessary. Endoscopic staplers for bowel division and vascular division are essential. Standard transanal stapling devices are used for left-sided anastomoses.

A consistent operating room team of nurses and technicians familiar with laparoscopic surgery and open colectomy greatly facilitates flow and ease of operation.

SURGICAL FIELD TECHNIQUES

The placement of laparoscopic ports on the abdominal wall varies significantly among surgeons, planned technique, and the surgical procedure. A consistent principle is triangulating the ports to minimize clashing instruments within the abdomen. In general, a periumbilical camera port is used. A diamond pattern of trocars, with a suprapubic port, a periumbilical port, and one port in each hemiabdomen is an adaptable arrangement. Five-millimeter ports can be used for most access points; 10-mm trocars are required for endoscopic staplers. Some surgeons favor using 10-mm ports because they are most versatile. Trocars should be inserted through the abdominal wall in the direction of the target organ for ergonomic advantage while operating.

In every case, a specimen extraction incision is created. In many cases, the periumbilical port incision is extended around the umbilicus; a protective sleeve or hand port is placed and the operation continues. For left-sided and pelvic anastomoses, a Pfannenstiel extraction site can be used, as well as an incision directly over the left lower quadrant.

If a hand port is placed for use during the laparoscopic colectomy, the incision created should be large enough to accommodate the palm of the hand with the thumb tucked under it. An alternative measurement is 1 to 2 cm smaller than the surgeon's glove size. Because the abdominal wall is compliant, the port should be placed with pneumoperitoneum already established to yield the smallest effective incision. The hand port is placed in the midline or paramedian toward the target organ. A Pfannenstiel incision can also be used for left-side or pelvic surgery.

The fundamental surgical principles of traction and countertraction are equally important for laparoscopic colon surgery as for open surgery. For accurate identification and exposure, the bowel or adjacent mesentery is grasped in two points opposite the intended point of dissection. Tension is applied to expose the area of interest. Sequential, not simultaneous, movements by the surgeon and assistant are important to maintain the field of focus and avoid wasting time.

SURGICAL PROCEDURES

Right Colectomy

Right hemicolectomy is considered to be the simplest laparoscopic colon resection; it is commonly the first operation undertaken by novice laparoscopists. There are three distinct approaches to right colectomy. Pure laparoscopic or hand-assisted technique may be used. Any small mucosal lesion should be marked by colonoscopic tattooing before surgery. The localization of lesions by colonoscopy is not reliable, except in areas of anatomic landmarks such as the cecum and the rectum. The preoperative tattoo should not immediately precede the surgery because the air-filled colon will fill the abdominal cavity.

Port placement typically includes three ports, either all midline or two midline and one to left of center (Fig. 2). Five-millimeter ports can be used, or a 10/12 port is placed in one of the two lower

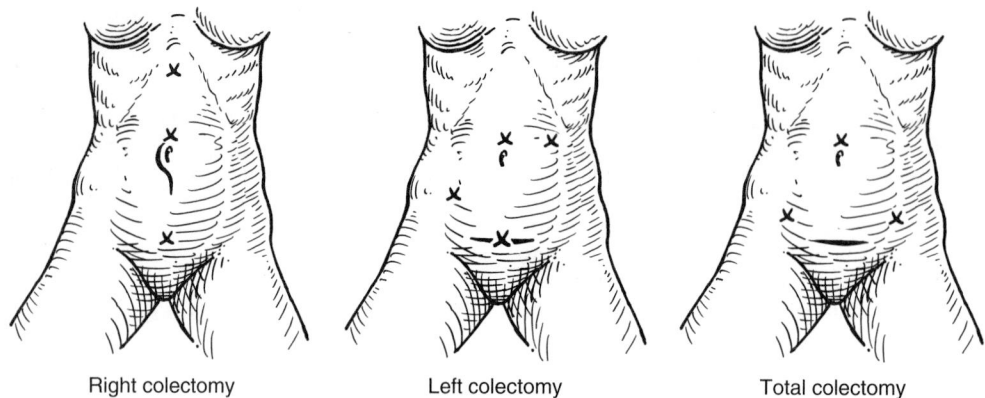

Figure 2 Suggested placement of ports. Vertical or transverse line indicates specimen extraction site or hand-port site.

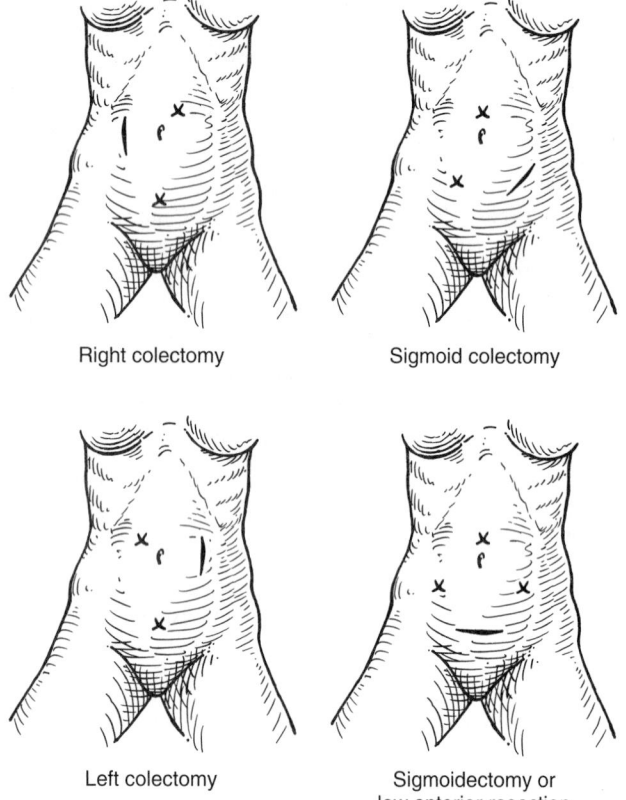

Figure 3 Suggested port placement for hand-assisted laparoscopic colectomy with the hand port near the target organ and ports placed opposite the target.

abdominal ports to allow stapler access. For HALS approach, the hand port is placed in the midline or in a right paramedian position. If the midline hand-port position is used, the camera and dissecting ports are shifted off midline (Fig. 3).

It is possible to place the patient in supine position for right hemicolectomy because no access to the perineum is required. However, in the interest of standardizing practice within the operating room and ease of access to the abdomen, low lithotomy position is to be recommended.

The lateral-to-medial approach approximates the technique familiar to so many surgeons. The patient is positioned with the right side elevated. The camera is placed through the supraumbilical port, and the dissection commences at the white line of Toldt at the cecum. Grasping the cecum and retracting toward the midline, the suprapubic port is used for scissors or Harmonic Scalpel (Johnson & Johnson Gateway, Piscataway, NJ) or similar device to mobilize the cecum. Each dissection move to separate the colon from its attachments has a corresponding increase in tension on the traction instrument. When the limit of retraction is reached in one position, the grasper is moved up the bowel. In this manner, the right colon is mobilized up out of the right gutter toward the midline. A common error is to work too laterally on the abdominal wall and hence dissect toward or around the kidney. The dissection plane should be monitored and brought medially as the colon is mobilized (Fig. 4). The hepatic flexure is taken down by shifting the patient to reverse Trendelenburg position. Elevating the gallbladder over the liver may facilitate this maneuver as well. The plane is separated by retracting the gastrocolic ligament cephalad or toward the anterior abdominal wall and the transverse colon inferiorly. The duodenum should be carefully identified. Downward traction on the colon toward the pelvis aids in peeling the specimen from the retroperitoneum. At completion of mobilization, the right colon is now a midline structure that can be exteriorized through a midline incision for division and anastomosis. In contrast to traditional teaching, the colonic mesentery is not closed. Although there are no randomized studies on the benefit of mesenteric closure, most laparoscopic surgeons do not close mesentery on patients in open or laparoscopic procedures.

With hand-assisted technique, the surgeon's hand (either dominant or nondominant) is used through the hand port to grasp, elevate, and retract the colon as in an open procedure. Operating ports must be placed away from the hand port to facilitate dissection. The surgeon's hand provides constant traction and can gently dissect tissue planes. The extracorporeal hand operates an instrument to cut attachments. Mesentery may be divided intracorporeally or extracorporeally.

The medial-to-lateral approach to laparoscopic colectomy prioritizes vascular isolation and division as the first operative step. The lateral attachments of the colon to the sidewall serve as a fixation point for the colon, and traction is applied to the mesentery adjacent to the bowel wall. The ileocolic artery is thus identified, isolated, and divided by clips or staplers (Fig. 5). The thin mesentery between the ileocolic and middle colic vessels is divided, and then the colon is freed along the lateral attachments in the method described earlier. The bowel is divided intracorporeally with endoscopic staplers. The specimen is exteriorized, and only the anastomosis must be accomplished exteriorly.

The inferior approach to laparoscopic right colectomy is so named because it begins at the ileal peritoneal attachments at the pelvic brim. This approach is useful for large or inflammatory tumors of the cecum in which identification of the ureter is especially important. It can also be helpful when the medial, vascular

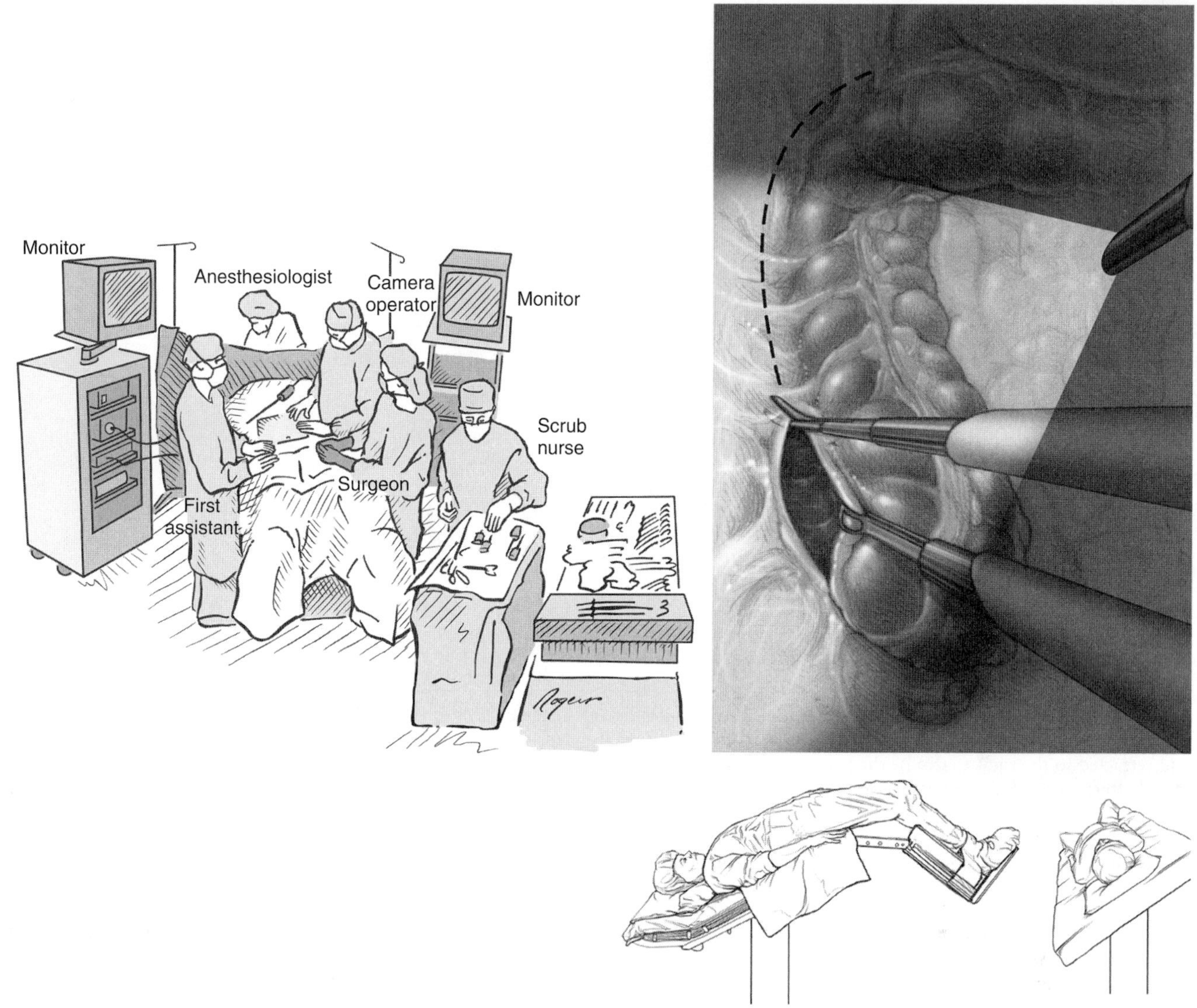

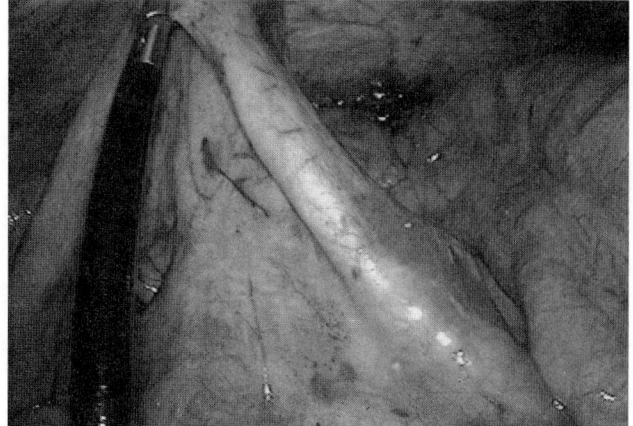

Figure 4 Room setup and operator positioning for laparoscopic right hemicolectomy. Division of the lateral attachments to the right abdominal sidewall.

Figure 5 The ileocolic artery is identified by elevating the cecum at the junction of the bowel and the mesentery. (*See color insert Figure 64.*)

anatomy is unclear. The terminal ileum is elevated, and dissection commences at the base of the ileal mesentery along the pelvic brim (Fig. 6). Dissection continues cephalad, elevating the colon and

mesentery off of the retroperitoneum. The duodenum is visualized directly as one proceeds cephalad. The vessels are divided, and the operation is completed as described previously.

Sigmoid and Left Colectomy

Patient positioning for laparoscopic sigmoid and left colectomy is always in the low lithotomy position to allow access to the perineum. The patient's arms are tucked at the sides. The primary video monitor is placed adjacent to the left hip, and the surgeon stands at the patient's right side. A supraumbilical port is placed for the camera, and a 10- to 12-mm port is placed in the right lower quadrant. A 5-mm port is placed in the suprapubic midline; a 5-mm port may be used in the left upper hemiabdomen as well. As in right colectomy, most lesions that are not large should be tattooed in advance of surgery.

The lateral-to-medial approach mobilizes the sigmoid and left colon along the white line of Toldt. If a sigmoid colectomy is planned, it can be helpful to mark the junction of the descending and sigmoid colon with clips before dissection. This allows accurate identification of the anatomic margins when the colon is divided. The patient is placed in the Trendelenburg position with the left side

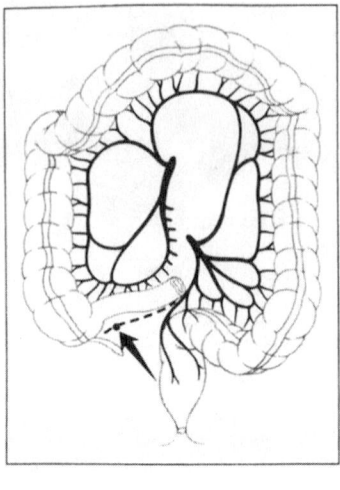

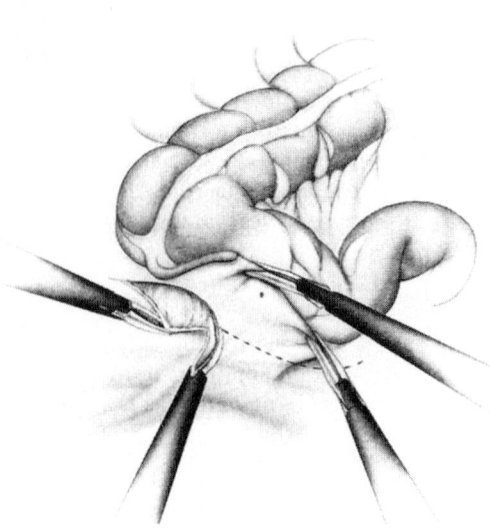

Figure 6 The peritoneum is incised at the base of the ileal attachments in the inferior approach to laparoscopic right hemicolectomy.

up. The small bowel is brought out of the pelvis and swept into the right upper quadrant of the abdomen. The sigmoid colon is grasped and retracted to the right to expose the pelvic brim and lateral peritoneal attachments. Using a scissors or a cautery device through the suprapubic port, the surgeon mobilizes the colon toward the splenic flexure. Appropriate traction and countertraction are placed as dissection moves cephalad. As the splenic flexure is approached, the table position should be changed to reverse Trendelenburg position to facilitate visualization. It is important to dissect in the plane just lateral to the colon. Failure to stay close to the colon can violate retroperitoneal planes, the kidney, and the spleen (Fig. 7).

Splenic flexure mobilization is required in left colectomy and may be necessary for sigmoid colectomy. This maneuver may be a less arduous process laparoscopically than in open surgery because visualization is enhanced with a 30-degree scope or flexible-tip camera. The colon should be retracted inferiorly with two graspers that are on opposite lateral aspects of the plane of dissection to create tension. The distal transverse colon is freed from the omentum by upward traction on the omentum, downward traction on the colon, and division in the bloodless plane between that is used in open surgery.

The medial-to-lateral approach requires identification of the left ureter before vascular division because of the proximity of the left ureter to the inferior mesenteric artery at the pelvic brim. The sigmoid colon is elevated to identify the inferior mesenteric artery. The peritoneum on the medial aspect of the sigmoid mesentery is opened, and a window created at the level of the sacral promontory. At this point, the left ureter can be visualized on the left sidewall. The inferior mesenteric artery is then isolated and divided while protection of the ureter is ensured. After mesenteric division, the colon is mobilized laterally (Fig. 8).

Pelvic dissection is best accomplished with the patient in Trendelenburg position. The peritoneum on either side of the rectosigmoid is scored down to and across the anterior reflection. The presacral space is identified and dissected while the rectosigmoid is elevated toward the bladder. A window is created between the rectosigmoid and the mesentery. The colon is divided by an endoscopic stapler passed through the right lower quadrant port. The mesentery, if substantial, is divided by a vascular stapler or cautery. Before exteriorization of the specimen, it is helpful to verify that adequate length of descending or transverse colon is available for tension-free anastomosis.

The specimen can be exteriorized through a variety of incisions: extension of the supraumbilical port, a small Pfannenstiel, a small left lower quadrant, or lower midline incision. The proximal end of the colon is prepared for anastomosis precisely as in the open setting, with purse-string suture closure of the end of the colon and placement of the anvil. The proximal end is returned to the abdomen, and pneumoperitoneum is reestablished.

Circular stapled anastomosis is performed by placing the camera through the right lower quadrant port. The stapler is passed transanally, and the spear extruded under direct visualization. The anvil is coupled to the stapler, taking care to prevent twisting of the mesentery. The anastomosis is tested by instilling air per rectum, with the anastomosis under water.

Hand-assisted technique can be particularly helpful for left colectomy. The specimen can often be easily retracted and controlled by the operator's hand. This technique can also be useful while instructing a learner because the surgeon's hand controls the exposure and presents the operative target. Hand technique can allow for more rapid dissection of tissue planes that are so familiar in the open setting. Placement of the hand port on the abdominal wall is variable. Most surgeons use a lower abdominal (midline or Pfannenstiel) or muscle-splitting left lower quadrant incision. An important point is that the hand must be deployed in a peripheral plane of the field of dissection to avoid obscuring the visual field.

Anastomotic options are broadened with the use of a hand port. The hand can be used to facilitate stapler placement in the rectal stump and deliver the anvil to the pelvis. The anastomosis can be performed under direct visualization through the hand port with any midline incision.

Transverse Colectomy

Transverse colectomy is infrequently performed, given the low incidence of neoplasm localized to this anatomic segment. The patient is placed in reverse Trendelenburg position. Mobilization of the hepatic or splenic flexure is usually required, depending on the site

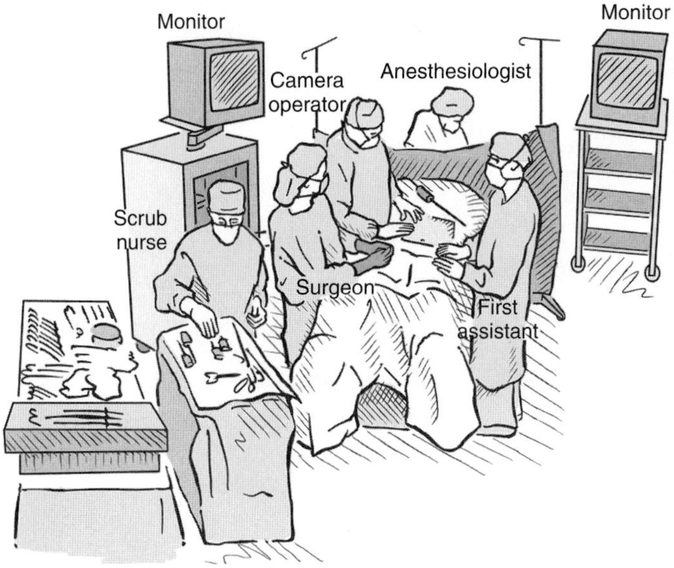

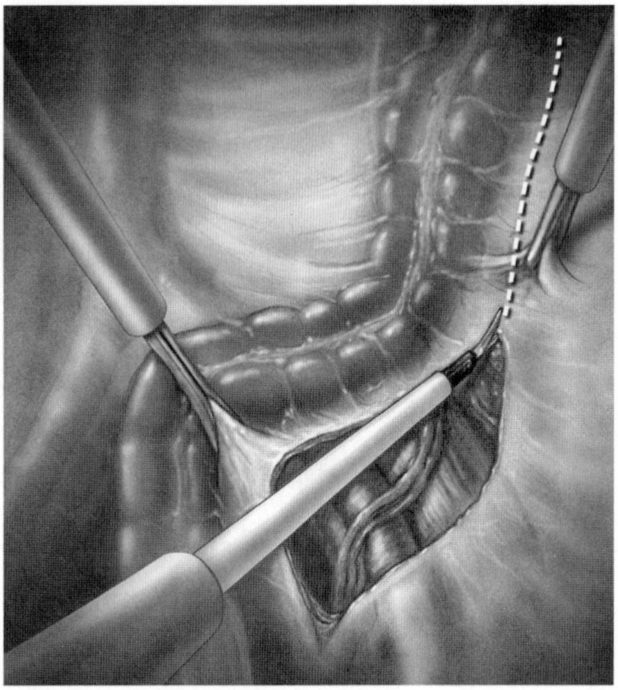

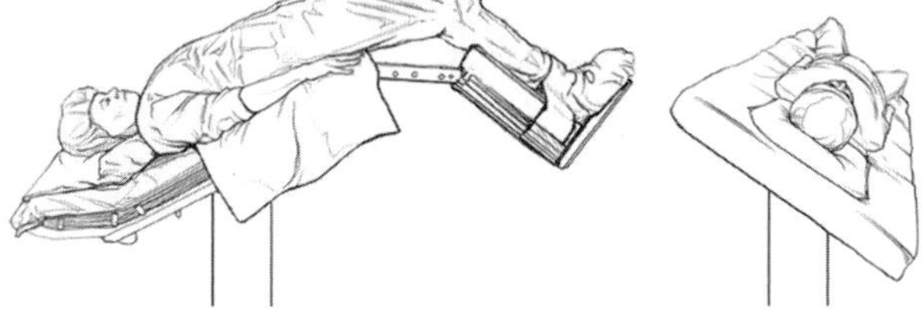

Figure 7 Laparoscopic left colectomy room setup.

of the lesion. The key step in this procedure is adequate mobilization of the colon to allow for tension-free side-to-side anastomosis. The bowel can be exteriorized through an upper midline, periumbilical, or transverse incision. Anastomosis is performed as for right colectomy.

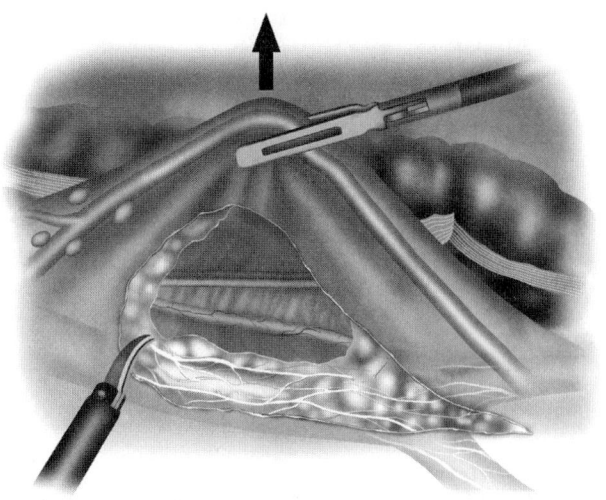

Figure 8 Medial dissection of the rectosigmoid mesentery with view through the mesentery of the left ureter.

Total Abdominal Colectomy

Total abdominal colectomy is a compilation of the techniques and skills outlined in right, left, and transverse colectomy. The specimen is exteriorized, and the ileum or ileal pouch is prepared for anastomosis in the usual fashion. A Pfannenstiel incision is advantageous in these cases for specimen extraction, anastomosis, and cosmesis. Suggested port placement is seen in Figures 2 and 3.

Low Anterior Resection and Proctectomy

Low anterior resection is accomplished by applying laparoscopic principles to pelvic dissection of the rectum. Port sites are placed similarly to left colectomy. It is important to use a sufficient number of ports because retraction of the target organ can be especially challenging in the confined pelvis. For straight laparoscopic cases, four to five ports are used. When a hand port is chosen, usually three additional ports are necessary. The patient is placed in Trendelenburg position.

The small bowel is retracted out of the pelvis. In female patients, it can be helpful to suspend or retract the uterus, especially if it is large. An instrument such as a suction device may simply deflect the uterus if it is smaller. Meticulous hemostasis is key to successful completion of laparoscopic pelvic surgery.

The rectosigmoid junction is retracted to the right, and the left pararectal peritoneum is scored (the left ureter is lateral to the incision) in the usual manner by scissors or cautery. The presacral space is entered. While the mesorectum is elevated up and to the

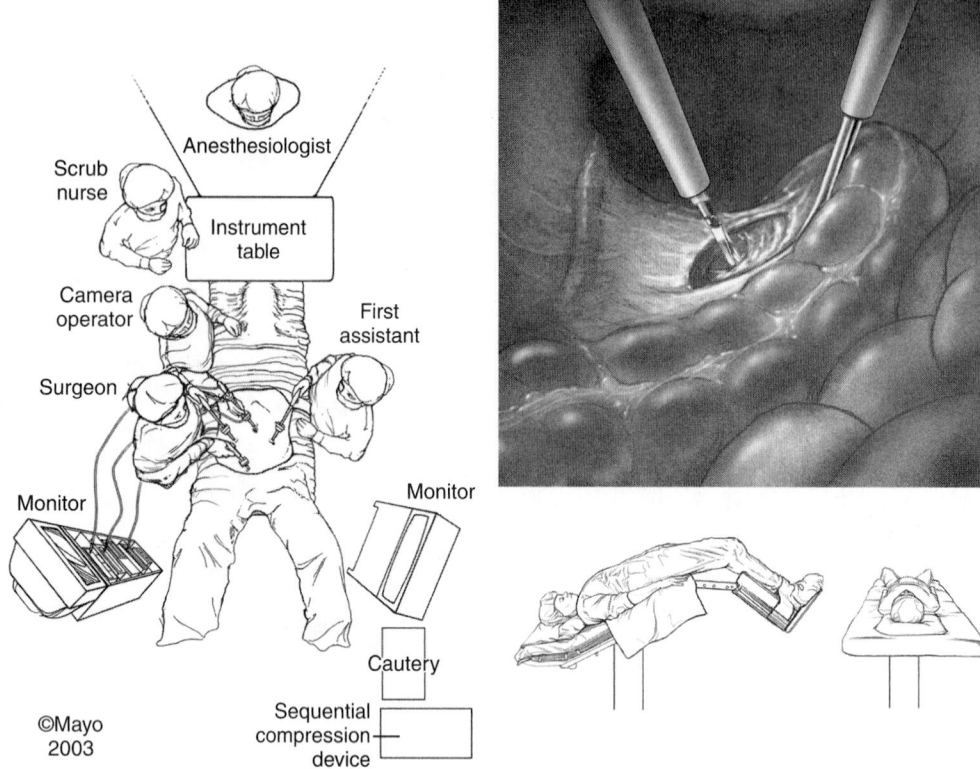

Figure 9 Mobilization of the rectum. The patient is level on the horizontal axis and in the Trendelenburg position. The left pararectal peritoneum is scored, and the presacral space entered.

right, the presacral space is developed inferiorly. The presacral nerves should be preserved as far as possible. Care is taken to follow the natural curve of the sacrum. The right pararectal peritoneum is scored, and the incisions are joined at the anterior reflection. The right side of the presacral space is dissected to join with the left (Fig. 9).

Separation of the rectovaginal septum can be facilitated by transvaginal digital or instrument retraction of the vagina toward the anterior abdominal wall. The rectum is mobilized circumferentially to the pelvic floor or to the desired site of bowel division. A window is created between the rectum and the mesorectum, and both are divided with staplers. It is sometimes advantageous to divide the mesorectum first to allow for optimal visualization of the rectal division. Careful placement of the stapler—and often, upward pressure on the perineum—is required to ensure accurate transverse division of the rectum (Fig. 10).

Hand-assisted technique for pelvic surgery again uses a lower abdominal hand port. The intracorporeal hand can retract, dissect, and facilitate stapling. Anastomosis options are the same as those described for left colectomy.

POSTOPERATIVE CARE AND HOSPITAL COURSE

The operative advantage of minimally invasive surgery is extended with appropriate postoperative care. The use of nasogastric tubes is avoided postoperatively. Pain management is multimodality, emphasizing local therapy such as fascial injection or implanted pain pumps. Parenteral nonsteroidal anti-inflammatory medication can be used for pain control. Systemic narcotic infusion or injection is an adjunctive measure, not primary pain management. Early mobilization and early feeding are safe and appropriate.

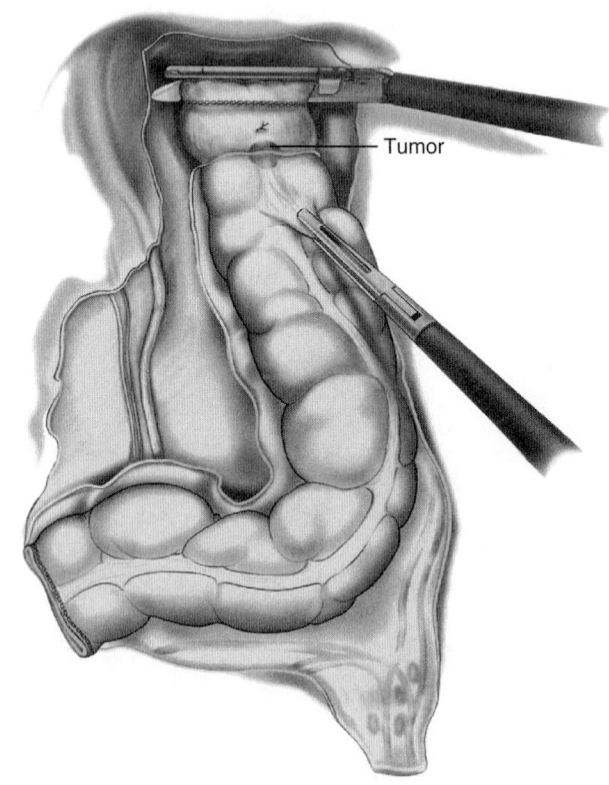

Figure 10 Laparoscopic division of the rectum low in the pelvis.

Multiple studies suggest that with principles of early mobilization, feeding, and minimal narcotics, laparoscopic colectomy patients can be discharged from the hospital approximately 24 hours earlier, on average, than patients undergoing open colectomy.

COMPLICATIONS OF LAPAROSCOPIC COLECTOMY

The well-known complications of open colectomy are also seen in laparoscopic colectomy. However, the incidence of wound infection, incisional hernia, and postoperative small bowel obstruction are reduced in laparoscopic colectomy, with statistical significance. The anastomotic leak rate for laparoscopic colectomy is, as would be expected, the same as in open technique because the procedure of anastomosis is precisely the same.

Earlier in laparoscopic colectomy experience, there was great concern over the possibility of tumor cell implantation in port sites and incisions. The risk of this complication was thought to be heightened by the dissemination of tumor cells via gas flow in the peritoneal cavity. The COST Study Group prospective trial of open versus laparoscopic colectomy clearly demonstrated that risk of tumor implantation at port site or any incision was the same in both techniques and low.

Ureteral injury is a recognized, rare complication of colectomy, both open and laparoscopic. Literature on this complication specific to laparoscopic colectomy is sparse. It is not known whether the incidence of injury is higher in laparoscopic than open cases. There is no conclusive evidence that the use of ureteral catheters decreases the low risk of ureteral injury; they are currently used selectively.

Inadvertent bowel injury is most often due to trocar placement. Management of abdominal entry—use of optical trocars, establishment of pneumoperitoneum before trocar placement or open insertion (Hassan) technique—should obviate this rare complication. Lysis of adhesions may also injure the bowel. Careful inspection is key to intraoperative identification and primary repair of any injury.

CONCLUSIONS

Techniques of laparoscopic colectomy continue to evolve. The ongoing challenge is to develop techniques and equipment that surgeons can adopt easily and safely while minimizing time away from practice for learning. The key precept remains that sufficient training and experience are gained before independent practice.

Suggested Readings

Clinical Outcomes of Surgical Therapy Study Group: A comparison of laparscopically assisted and open colectomy for colon cancer, *N Engl J Med* 350:2050, 2004.

Lee SW, Yoo J, Dujovny N, and others: Laparoscopic vs. hand-assisted laparoscopic sigmoidectomy for diverticulitis, *Dis Colon Rectum* 49:464, 2006.

Milsom J, Bohm B, Nakajima K, editors: *Laparoscopic colorectal surgery*, ed 2, New York, 2006, Springer.

Senagore AJ, Delaney CP: A critical analysis of laparoscopic colectomy at a single institution: lesions learned after 1000 cases, *Am J Surg* 191:377, 2006.

Tekkis PP, Senagore AJ, Delaney CP, and others: Evaluation of the learning curve in laparoscopic colorectal surgery: comparison of right-sided and left-sided resections, *Ann Surg* 242:83, 2005.

Laparoscopic Management of Crohn's Disease

Thomas E. Read, MD

The adoption of laparoscopic approaches to the management of patients suffering from intestinal Crohn's disease has been relatively slow. Crohn's patients requiring operation may have extensive or recurrent disease, fragile tissue because of disease severity or steroid use, and thickened mesentery that bleeds easily. Surgeons have had concerns regarding the loss of tactile control in these situations. Nevertheless, these patients may be faced with the prospect of repeated abdominal operations, may be immunocompromised, and may be highly motivated to undergo a procedure that limits trauma to the abdominal wall and peritoneal cavity. As this chapter outlines, accumulating data suggest that the application of laparoscopic techniques to patients with Crohn's disease results in quicker recovery, fewer complications, less trauma, and reduced adhesion formation compared with open laparotomy. I review the rationale for the laparoscopic approach, technical considerations, and reported outcomes for patients undergoing fecal diversion for severe anal Crohn's disease, ileocolic resection for simple and complicated Crohn's ileitis, and total colectomy for Crohn's colitis.

LAPAROSCOPIC FECAL DIVERSION FOR SEVERE ANORECTAL CROHN'S DISEASE

One of the first laparoscopic procedures used to treat patients with Crohn's disease was creation of a diverting intestinal stoma, usually a diverting loop ileostomy or colostomy for patients suffering from severe anorectal sepsis. Laparoscopic stoma creation can be accomplished using one or two 5-mm ports and a port at the stoma extraction site, which limits postoperative morbidity. Loop stoma creation requires neither division of the bowel nor anastomosis; thus the full benefits of the totally laparoscopic approach can be realized.

Some authors have argued that trephine stoma creation is an easier, quicker, and less expensive method of stoma creation than the laparoscopic technique. For the thin patient with a virgin abdomen who will not benefit from abdominal exploration, the trephine method of stoma creation may be appropriate. However, for patients who are obese, who have had multiple prior laparotomies, who would benefit from abdominal exploration, or who require mobilization of the intestine from its retroperitoneal attachments, the laparoscopic approach offers significant advantages.

Technical Considerations

If the patient requiring fecal diversion is thin and would not necessarily benefit from laparoscopic exploration of the peritoneal cavity, I selectively use a method that combines the advantages of both trephine and laparoscopic stoma creation. The patient is approached initially with the intention of creating a trephine stoma, with the laparoscopic equipment held in reserve. The patient is positioned for a laparoscopic procedure, the stoma incision is made; and, if the bowel can be delivered in correct orientation to the skin level, the stoma is created, and the laparoscopic equipment remains unopened. However, if trephine creation of the stoma is not possible, a Hasson trocar is placed through the stoma incision; and the procedure proceeds laparoscopically. If the patient is obese or would benefit from exploration of the peritoneal cavity, the procedure is performed laparoscopically from the outset.

Patients undergoing diverting colostomy should be placed in dorsal lithotomy position to provide access to the anorectum; patients undergoing ileostomy may be placed in the supine position. The preselected stoma site is opened, a purse-string suture is placed in the posterior rectus sheath, and a Hasson trocar is placed. A 5-mm trocar is placed, and the abdomen explored. If the bowel to be used for the stoma is mobile, it is not necessary to place other trocars. If mobilization is required, additional 5-mm trocars can be placed to facilitate the dissection. Mobility is usually adequate when the bowel reaches the peritoneal surface at the stoma site because the distance to the skin level decreases when pneumoperitoneum is released. A 5-mm camera is then placed through one of the 5-mm port sites, and the bowel is grasped in correct orientation using an instrument through the Hasson trocar at the stoma site. It is often helpful to mark the bowel for orientation of proximal and distal with suture or clips before delivery through the stoma site; this is especially true when creating an ileostomy. The pneumoperitoneum is then released, and the posterior rectus sheath is opened over the trocar, allowing the bowel to be delivered through the stoma opening. If an end stoma is to be fashioned, it is critical that orientation be confirmed. Left-sided colostomy orientation can be confirmed by insufflation of air through a proctoscope, instillation of povidone iodine or dye through a small opening in the distal limb of stoma with confirmation of dye passage to the rectum via a proctoscope, or passage of a flexible sigmoidoscope to the stoma site.

The rapidity with which postoperative ileus resolves following laparoscopic creation of intestinal stomas may allow patients to return home within 1 or 2 days. This may create a problem for the patient and the enterostomal therapist, who has little time to perform in-hospital stoma-care training. Therefore it is advantageous to have the patient meet with the enterostomal therapist preoperatively—not only for stoma-site marking but also for stoma-care teaching as well.

Outcomes

There have been several case series reported in the literature demonstrating the safety and efficacy of laparoscopic fecal diversion, and case-controlled series have shown reduced duration of postoperative ileus and reduced length of hospital stay with the laparoscopic approach to stoma creation compared with the open approach. Because of the virtual absence of postoperative adhesions, reoperation is made easier. The readily apparent benefits of this technique obviate a randomized, prospective trial to evaluate the differences between open and laparoscopic colostomy or ileostomy creation.

LAPAROSCOPIC ILEOCOLIC RESECTION

Patients with uncomplicated terminal ileal Crohn's disease are often ideal candidates for the application of laparoscopic techniques to the treatment of their disease. Patients are typically young and interested in procedures that minimize incision size, both for cosmetic concerns and to minimize postoperative morbidity.

Technical Considerations

My favored approach to ileocolic resection is to place a 12-mm port at the umbilicus and three additional 5-mm trocars, two in the left abdomen and one in the suprapubic position. The abdomen is explored and the bowel inspected from ligament of Treitz to rectum. The mobilization required to perform laparoscopic ileocolic resection is essentially that of a right colectomy. The ileocolic vessels are isolated at their origin adjacent to the duodenum and divided. Although the mesentery adjacent to the diseased bowel is often thickened, the root of the mesentery is usually thinner, allowing for safe intracorporeal division of these vessels. However, if the root of the mesentery is severely diseased, division of the vasculature can be performed extracorporeally after mobilization is complete. The mesocolon is then separated from the retroperitoneum, working from medial to lateral, staying anterior to the duodenum and pancreas. Working in retrograde fashion, the surgeon then separates the omentum from the transverse colon, divides the last attachments of hepatic flexure, and divides the lateral attachments of the colon to the level of the pelvic brim. The terminal ileal mesentery is then mobilized to the midline, returning the right colon to its embryologic midline position. The specimen is exteriorized through a 4- to 5-cm umbilical incision that incorporates the 12-mm port site, and resection and anastomosis are completed using conventional techniques. Remote areas of possible small-bowel involvement with Crohn's can be reevaluated by exteriorizing and palpating the proximal small bowel if necessary.

Outcomes

As one might expect, the short-term outcomes following laparoscopic ileocolic resection for Crohn's disease mirror those of other studies of laparoscopic colectomy for benign and malignant disease. In comparative studies, including a few prospective, randomized controlled trials, laparoscopic ileocolic resection is associated with a quicker return of bowel function, earlier tolerance of oral diet, reduced postoperative pain, shorter length of stay, and improvement in postoperative pulmonary function versus open resection. Analyses of costs have had mixed results, with some studies showing that increased operative costs are more than offset by the reduction in postoperative care requirements and length of stay. The real benefit of the laparoscopic approach for Crohn's patients may be in the long term because of the paucity of adhesions created after laparoscopic surgery in a group of patients that frequently require reoperation. A recently published meta-analysis identified six trials with adequate long-term follow-up; the authors found that the incidence of small-bowel obstruction was reduced after laparoscopic resection compared with open surgery. There has been no evidence that the laparoscopic approach leads to missed areas of disease or earlier recurrence, suggesting that operative principles for dealing with Crohn's disease have been preserved by surgeons who use the laparoscopic approach.

COMPLICATED ILEOCOLIC DISEASE

Patients with recurrent terminal ileal disease or those with abscess, phlegmon, or fistula can be approached laparoscopically, but appropriate preoperative treatment and careful operative planning are necessary to ensure the best possible outcome. Abscesses should be drained percutaneously, nutritional support maximized, and disease thoroughly investigated by endoscopic and radiographic methods. After inflammation is minimal, many patients may be candidates for laparoscopic management of their disease (Fig. 1). We have previously demonstrated the efficacy of this approach for the management of patients with complicated terminal ileal Crohn's disease, comparing outcomes of patients undergoing laparoscopic

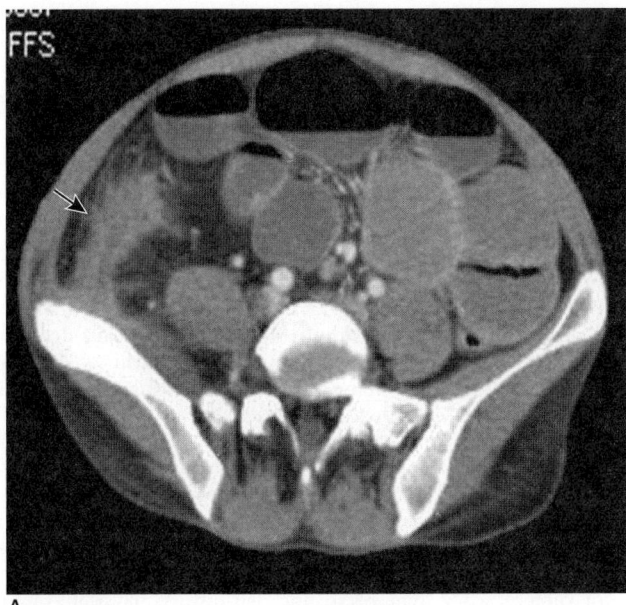

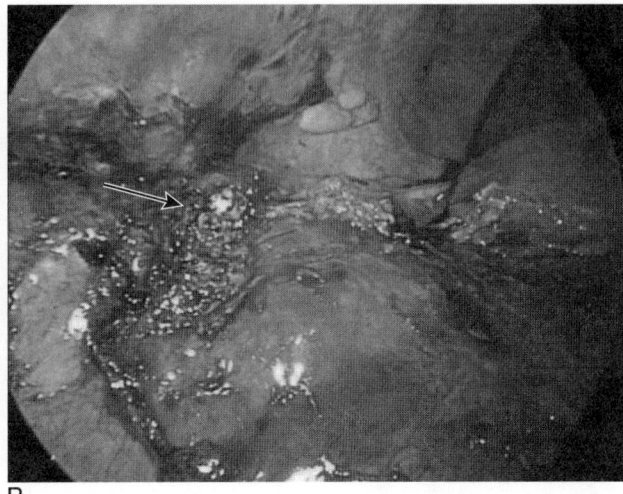

Figure 1 Complicated ileocolic Crohn's with fistula through retroperitoneum. **(A)** Computed tomography demonstrating inflammation and fistula. **(B)** Retroperitoneum after laparoscopic mobilization of terminal ileum and right colon demonstrating fistula. (*See color insert Figure 65*.)

ileocolic resection who suffered from abscess/phlegmon, recurrent disease, or first-time disease with patients undergoing open resection. It may sometimes be helpful to use a hand-assist device for management of patients with complex disease, although the site of the incision must be carefully planned to maximize effect and maintain laparoscopic visualization.

LAPAROSCOPIC TOTAL COLECTOMY

Laparoscopic total abdominal colectomy or proctocolectomy for severe colonic Crohn's disease can be extremely challenging because of the thickness of the mesentery and inflammation in the surrounding retroperitoneum and pelvis. It is often helpful to make a 7- to 8-cm Pfannenstiel or lower midline incision at the onset of the procedure and place a hand-assist device to facilitate retraction, exposure, and control of thickened mesentery (Fig. 2). This

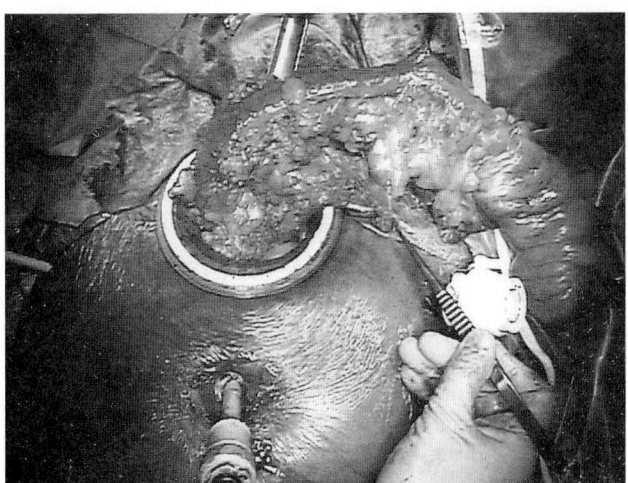

Figure 2 Extraction of the colon via the base of the Gelport hand-assist device (*Applied Medical Resources, Rancho Santo Margarita, CA*). (*See color insert Figure 66*.)

incision also allows direct access to the pelvis to assist with pelvic dissection and rectal transection. The Pfannenstiel incision is cosmetically appealing to many patients, especially to women. There have been few well-designed trials of hand-assisted laparoscopic colectomy versus open colectomy or "standard laparoscopic" colectomy (however that is defined). In sum, published studies have demonstrated that short-term outcomes after hand-assisted laparoscopic colectomy are similar to those following laparoscopic colectomy, with similar incision size, similar reduction in duration of ileus when compared with open colectomy, with the advantage of reduced conversion rates, and shorter operative times in the hand-assisted groups. The reduction in operative time is most notable during total abdominal colectomy and proctocolectomy in which the use of a hand-assist method can save approximately 1 hour in the operating room.

CONCLUSIONS

Patients suffering from Crohn's disease remain plagued by our lack of understanding of disease mechanism and, in many cases, the failure of medical therapy alone to control their disease. Facing the possibility of multiple abdominal operations during their lifetime, patients are justified in their apprehension regarding the morbidity associated with repeated laparotomy. It is thus paramount that we continually strive to minimize the short- and long-term morbidity associated with the surgical act itself. The application of laparoscopic methods to treat patients with Crohn's disease should be strongly considered as one of the current methods available to limit this morbidity.

Suggested Readings

Maartense S, Dunker MS, Slors JF, and others: Laparoscopic-assisted versus open ileocolic resection for Crohn's disease: a randomized trial, *Ann Surg* 243:143, 2006.

Marcello PW, Milsom JW, Wong SK, and others: Laparoscopic total colectomy for acute colitis: a case-control study, *Dis Colon Rectum* 44:1441, 2001.

Milsom JW, Hammerhofer KA, Böhm B, and others: Prospective, randomized trial comparing laparoscopic vs. conventional surgery for refractory ileocolic Crohn's disease, *Dis Colon Rectum* 44:1, 2001.

Rivadeneira DE, Marcello PW, Roberts PL, and others: Benefits of hand-assisted laparoscopic restorative proctocolectomy: a comparative study, *Dis Colon Rectum* 47:1371, 2004.

Rosman AS, Melis M, Fichera A: Metaanalysis of trials comparing laparoscopic and open surgery for Crohn's disease, *Surg Endosc* 19:1549, 2005.

Wu JS, Birnbaum EH, Kodner IJ, and others: Laparoscopic-assisted ileocolic resections in patients with Crohn's disease: are abscesses, phlegmons, or recurrent disease contraindications? *Surgery* 122:682, 1997.

LAPAROSCOPIC NISSEN FUNDOPLICATION

David Hazzan, MD, Edward H. Chin, MD, and Barry A. Salky, MD

INTRODUCTION

Over the past 50 years, gastroesophageal reflux disease (GERD) has become progressively more common throughout the developed world. In the United States, more than 40% of the adult population experiences at least occasional reflux symptoms (Table 1). Preventing and treating the sequelae of GERD, particularly Barrett's metaplasia and adenocarcinoma of the esophagus, are also important health care issues.

Proton pump inhibitors (PPIs) are currently the most effective medications for symptomatic GERD and, for many, represent adequate treatment. Since the introduction of laparoscopy, however, the number of patients choosing antireflux surgery has greatly increased.

Laparoscopic Nissen fundoplication (LNF) is the most commonly performed procedure for GERD. Despite the rapid recovery and low morbidity of this operation, careful selection of patients is critical for successful results. Of great controversy is the use of antireflux surgery in patients with Barrett's metaplasia, particularly those who have progressed to low-grade dysplasia. Although many surgeons have supported this indication, it remains a topic of great debate. This chapter focuses on the widely accepted indications and the technical details of LNF.

PATIENT SELECTION

The best candidate for LNF is a young, healthy individual with the classic symptoms of GERD (heartburn, regurgitation) that respond

Table 1: Symptoms of Gastroesophageal Reflux Disease

Typical Symptoms
Heartburn (retrosternal pain)
Regurgitation
Dysphagia

Atypical Symptoms
Asthma
Pneumonitis
Recurrent pneumonia
Hoarseness
Chronic cough
Dental erosion

well to PPIs but recur after medication cessation. In these patients, LNF with a short, floppy wrap has a success rate greater than 90%. During history taking, heartburn should be specifically defined as substernal pain that improves with food or antacids and is worsened at night or lying supine. Dynamic pH testing should confirm acid reflux that correlates with onset of GERD symptoms. The majority of patients with GERD have normal esophageal motility by manometry testing but a lower esophageal sphincter (LES) with a short length and below-normal resting pressure.

Unfortunately the presentation and diagnostic findings for many patients referred for LNF is less clear. This all-too-frequent scenario underscores the importance of fulfilling the indications for surgery, which requires a thorough history, physical examination, appropriate diagnostic studies, and finally a discussion with the patient regarding the expectations of surgery.

A complete history should distinguish true symptoms attributable to GERD from those suggestive of other processes. Extraesophageal symptoms such as laryngitis and hoarseness require careful evaluation; although often consistent with GERD, malignancy and infectious etiologies must be considered, especially with significant smoking history. Although healthy patients with classic GERD symptoms require minimal diagnostic studies before surgery, the presence of atypical symptoms of GERD (cough, hoarseness, or asthma) mandates objective documentation of acid reflux. It is more difficult to predict symptom relief after surgery in these patients, with an overall success rate of 60% to 70%.

The presence of abdominal pain with GERD requires further evaluation, which is best begun with an ultrasound to rule out cholelithiasis. When GERD occurs in the presence of symptomatic gallstones, a cholecystectomy can be performed in the same setting as LNF.

Complaints of bloating or severe postprandial distention should raise the suspicion of delayed gastric emptying coinciding with GERD. If suspected, a gastric emptying study will confirm this diagnosis, and these patients carry the risk of gas bloat after LNF. Paradoxically, in mild to moderate cases of GERD, fundoplication may actually improve gastric emptying, but in severely atonic patients, it can lead to dangerous gastric dilatation. A simultaneous gastric emptying procedure or partial fundoplication should be considered with these patients.

Nearly everyone referred for LNF will have "failed" medical therapy. Treatment failure must be carefully defined, however (Table 2). At the minimum, 3 months of PPI therapy followed by endoscopic evaluation constitutes an adequate trial of medical management.

PREOPERATIVE EVALUATION

Although a history of frequent heartburn is adequate to begin antacid therapy, candidates for antireflux surgery require confirmation of acid reflux by one or more of the following modalities (Table 3):

- upper endoscopy
- 24-hour pH probe monitoring
- esophageal manometry
- barium swallow study
- radioscintigraphy

Each test is useful for specific circumstances and unnecessary in others. Patients with classic GERD symptoms that have an excellent response to PPIs should first undergo upper endoscopy. If moderate

Table 2: Indications for Laparoscopic Nissen Fundoplication

1. Complications of GERD not responding to medical therapy
   - Barrett's metaplasia
   - Esophageal stricture
   - Severe esophagitis
2. Persistent symptoms requiring increased medication
3. Atypical symptoms with objective evidence of GERD
   - Asthma
   - Recurrent pneumonia or pneumonitis
   - Hoarseness
4. Paraesophageal hernia with GERD
5. Significant patient circumstances
   - Noncompliance with medication
   - Financial burden
   - Lifestyle choice
   - Age younger than 50

GERD, Gastroesophageal reflux disease.

Table 3: Diagnostic Modalities for Gastroesophageal Reflux Disease

- Esophagogastroduodenoscopy (with or without biopsy)
- Esophagography with barium
- 24-hour pH test or Bravo test (Medtronic, Minneapolis, MN)
- Esophageal manometry
- Radioscintigraphy

or severe esophagitis is found that is consistent with chronic GERD, no further invasive testing is necessary unless dysphagia is present. If the esophagus shows no reflux changes, however, a 24-hour pH test should follow after PPIs have been discontinued to confirm abnormal acid exposure in the esophagus. A positive study requires exposure to a pH less than 4 more than 4% of time in the distal esophagus, or more than 1% of time in the proximal esophagus. Standard 24-hour pH testing by nasogastric probe can be poorly tolerated; if available, a Bravo study (Medtronic, Minneapolis, MN), which employs an endoscopically placed capsule, can be performed.

At our institution, barium esophagography is considered mandatory for the following reasons: (1) to define the location of the gastroesophageal junction to the esophageal hiatus, (2) to measure the intra-abdominal length of esophagus, and (3) to rule out paraesophageal hernia.

In the presence of dysphagia or chest pain, esophageal manometry is necessary to exclude a primary esophageal motility disorder. If present, an esophageal myotomy or partial fundoplication may be indicated, depending on the degree of dysmotility.

For patients with atypical symptoms or minimal symptom relief with medical therapy, a complete preoperative evaluation consisting of upper endoscopy, manometry, 24-hour pH testing, and barium esophagography is necessary before surgery.

SURGICAL TECHNIQUE

We favor a right crus approach, which allows for early identification and preservation of the anterior and posterior vagus nerves. The principles of this operation consist of

- circumferential mobilization of the distal esophagus,
- division of the short gastric vessels,
- closure of the esophageal hiatus, and
- creation of a short, floppy, 360-degree fundoplication.

Positioning

The patient is placed in modified lithotomy position. Both knees should be flexed sufficiently to allow the legs to be perpendicular to the floor when the operating table is in reverse Trendelenburg position, thereby providing support for the patient's weight.

The right arm is tucked alongside the patient, and the left arm is abducted 90 degrees. The monitor is placed at the head of the table. The surgeon stands between the patient's legs and the assistant at the left side of the patient. If a self-retaining retractor (e.g., Iron Intern; Automated Medical Products, Edison, NJ) is used, it is mounted at the patient's right side.

Access

Access to the peritoneal cavity is achieved by an open or closed technique on the basis of the patient's previous abdominal surgery. Five trocars are used (Fig. 1): (1) right subcostal, midclavicular line (surgeon's left hand); (2) subxiphoid, for retraction of the lateral segment of left liver; (3) left subcostal, midclavicular line (surgeon's right hand); (4) left anterior axillary line (assistant's port); and (5) midline, between xiphoid and umbilicus (camera port). All trocars are 5 mm except the camera port, which is 10 mm. All cases are performed with a 10-mm, 45-degree telescope. Rarely an extra 5-mm trocar is required to retract a large amount of intra-abdominal fat.

Right Crus Exposure

Using a Nathanson retractor or 5-mm probe, the surgeon elevates the left lateral segment of the liver to expose the esophageal hiatus. The assistant retracts the gastric fundus to the left, and after inspecting for a large replaced left hepatic artery, the surgeon incises the gastrohepatic ligament with the ultrasonic shears. The gastrohepatic ligament is widely opened to expose the right crus of the diaphragm (Fig. 2). The phrenoesophageal ligament is then incised near the right crux, with care being taken to preserve its overlying fascia. After the phrenoesophageal ligament is divided, the esophagus is identified. Throughout the dissection, care is taken never to grasp the esophagus itself. The dissection continues anteriorly across the esophagus until the left crus of the diaphragm is identified (Fig. 3). The anterior vagal trunk will be encountered

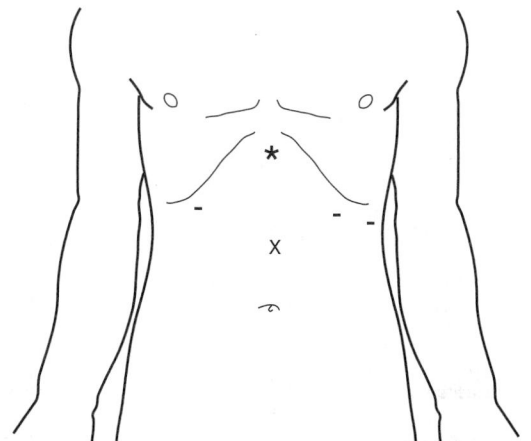

Figure 1 Five trocars are used: (-) right subcostal, midclavicular line (surgeon's left hand); (*) subxiphoid, for retraction of the lateral segment of left liver; (-) left subcostal, midclavicular line (surgeon's right hand); (-) left anterior axillary line (assistant's port); (x) midline, between xiphoid and umbilicus (camera port).

(Fig. 4). The groove between the esophagus and the left crus is bluntly dissected, beginning superiorly and continuing inferiorly toward the junction with the right crus. There is frequently a prominent anterior fat pad that is removed to completely expose the left crus.

Next the dissection returns to the right crus, as the phrenoesophageal ligament is dissected inferiorly until the junction of right and left crus is identified, this time from the right side. The posterior vagal trunk is seen at this point (Fig. 5). The posterior aspect of the phrenoesophageal ligament is dissected from the inferior aspect of the left crus, with care being taken to stay on the abdominal side of the left crus to avoid injury to the left pleura. The posterior esophagus is mobilized away from the left crus to open the posterior space; this is performed under direct vision. This maneuver is greatly facilitated by dissecting the left crus as inferiorly as possible from the left side of the esophagus. After an adequate window is created behind the esophagus, a medium Penrose drain is used to encircle the distal esophagus and both vagal trunks (Fig. 6). This permits atraumatic manipulation of the esophagus for the remainder of the procedure. The posterior window is enlarged to accommodate the fundus. This requires dissection of the posterior fat pad away from the stomach. Vascular structures in this area should be carefully identified, with all tissue divided using the ultrasonic shears.

Next additional esophageal length is obtained by mobilizing the intrathoracic esophagus. Again, any visible blood vessels are divided with the ultrasonic shears. Care is taken to avoid contact between the active blade of the shears and either vagal trunks or esophagus. On completion, 4 to 5 cm of esophagus should lie below the diaphragmatic crus without tension.

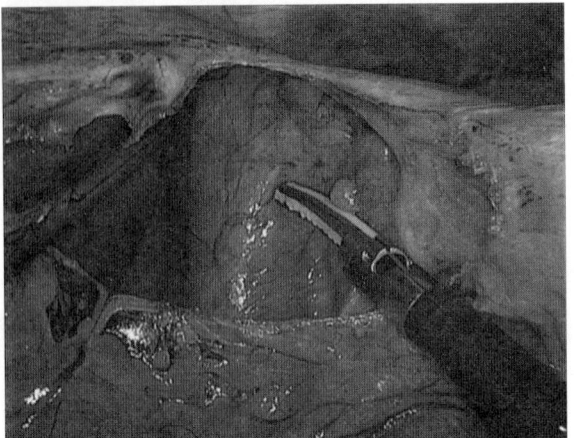

Figure 2 The gastrohepatic ligament is widely opened to expose the right crus of the diaphragm. (See *color insert Figure 67*.)

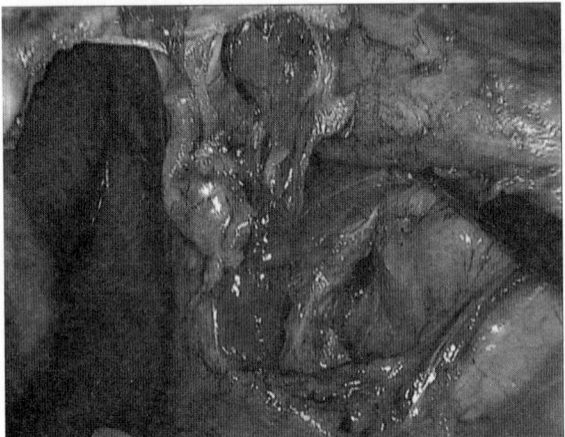

Figure 3 The dissection continues anteriorly across the esophagus until the left crus of the diaphragm is identified. (See *color insert Figure 68*.)

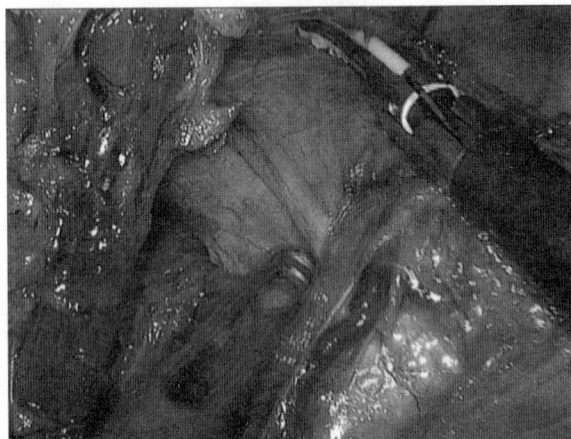

Figure 5 The posterior vagal trunk is identified. (See *color insert Figure 70*.)

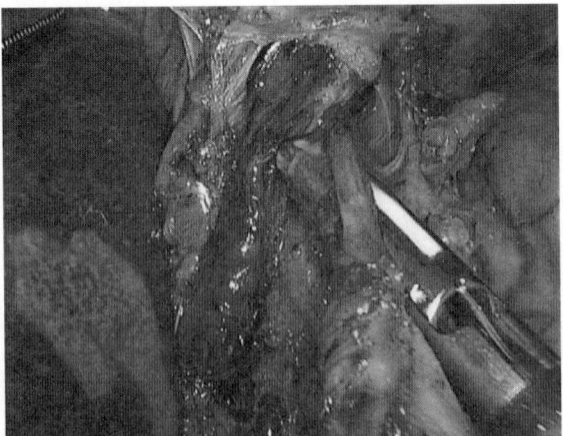

Figure 4 The anterior vagal trunk is identified and preserved. (See *color insert Figure 69*.)

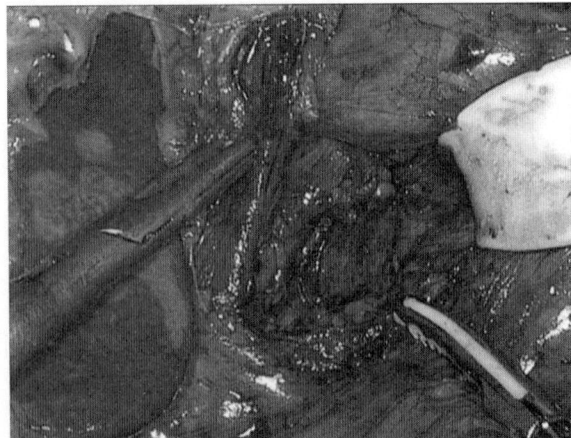

Figure 6 After an adequate window is created behind the esophagus, a Penrose drain is used to encircle the distal esophagus and both vagal trunks. (See *color insert Figure 71*.)

Short Gastric Vessels

After the esophagus is completely mobilized and the right and left crus have been fully exposed, the short gastric vessels are divided. We begin inferiorly on the greater curvature of the stomach and continue proximally (Fig. 7). The assistant retracts the greater omentum to the left, and the surgeon retracts the stomach to the right. The lesser sac is initially entered close to the stomach. Rapid progress can be made using ultrasonic shears for coagulation. Invariably there is a posterior short gastric vessel that must be divided to mobilize the fundus fully away from the pancreas and spleen. The posterior gastric dissection is continued until the left crus is reached.

Crural Closure and Fundoplication

After the short gastric vessels are divided, the fundus is passed behind the esophagus to test the planned wrap. If sufficiently mobile, the fundus is returned to its anatomic location to enable reapproximation of the right and left crus. Multiple U stitches of 0-Ethibond (Ethicon, Somerville, NJ) buttressed with pledgets are used. Because these sutures are long, they are tied extracorporeally and cinched down with a knot pusher. The size of the hiatal defect dictates the number of sutures placed, typically two or three (Fig. 8). Excessive narrowing of the hiatus will lead to postoperative dysphagia. A 5-mm telescope is used for this portion of the operation as sutures are passed through the 10-mm port. After the crural closure is complete, the fundus is again passed behind the esophagus. A 56-F Maloney dilatator is then carefully passed into the stomach. This is a potentially dangerous maneuver and must be performed by an experienced anesthesiologist. If significant resistance is encountered, passage of the dilatator is aborted.

A short, floppy fundoplication is then performed with two sutures of 2-0 silk, placed 3 to 4 cm apart. Each suture incorporates the left gastric wrap, esophagus, and right gastric wrap, and care must be taken to avoid the anterior vagal trunk. To facilitate intracorporeal tying, these sutures are measured to 20-cm length (Figs. 9 and 10).

Final Step

The Penrose drain and all needles are removed. Appropriate hemostasis, especially in the left upper quadrant, is confirmed. All trocars are removed under direct vision and inspected for bleeding. The fascia of the 10-mm trocar site is closed.

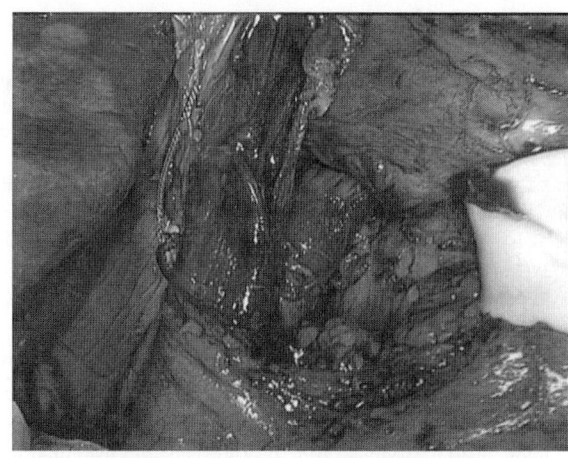

Figure 8   The size of the hiatal defect dictates the number of sutures placed, typically two or three. Excessive narrowing of the hiatus leads to postoperative dysphagia. A 5-mm telescope is used for this portion of the operation, as sutures are passed through the 10-mm port. (*See color insert Figure 73.*)

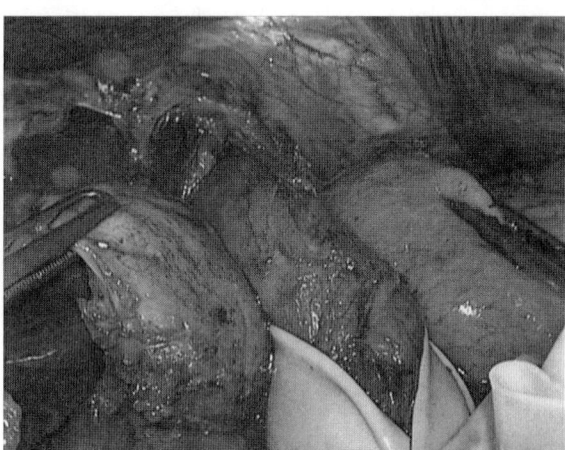

Figure 9   A short, floppy fundoplication is then performed with two sutures of 2-0 silk, placed 3 to 4 cm apart. See also Fig. 10. (*See color insert Figure 74.*)

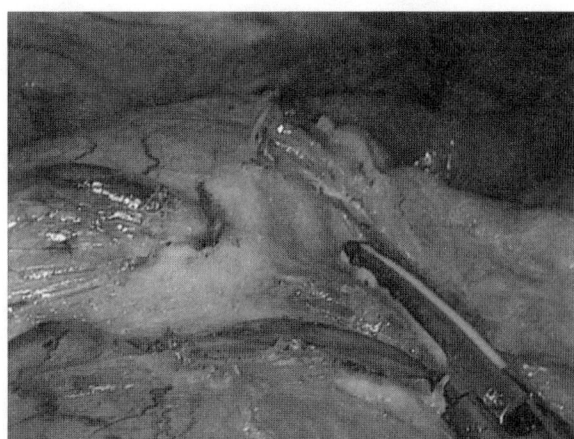

Figure 7   After the esophagus is completely mobilized and the right and left crus have been fully exposed, the short gastric vessels are divided completely. (*See color insert Figure 72.*)

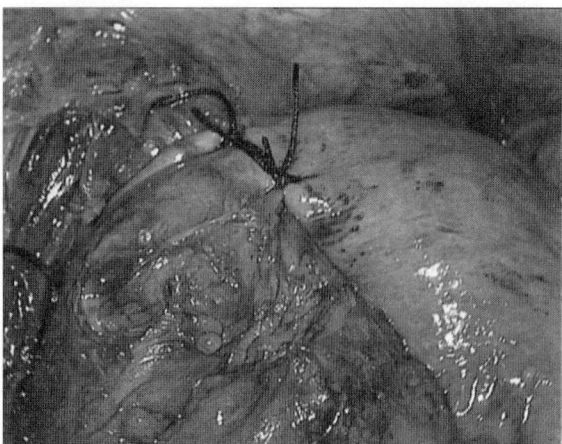

Figure 10   (*See color insert Figure 75.*)

POSTOPERATIVE CARE

Intravenous ketorolac and ondansetron are administered before extubation. Clear liquids are begun 4 hours postsurgery. A barium esophagogram is performed the first day postsurgery to evaluate the repair. Ninety percent of patients are discharged within 24 hours of surgery. Ketorolac minimizes the use of narcotics and potential nausea. We have found that early postoperative emesis can lead to disruption of the crural closure and migration of the wrap into the chest. After discharge, the patient is maintained on a soft diet for 3 weeks.

COMPLICATIONS

The safety of laparoscopic Nissen fundoplication has been well established, with extremely low mortality. Complications have occurred in 4% to 15% of our patients, most of these minor (urinary retention, wound infection, ileus). Major complications are rare but occur during the dissection and repair (splenic injury, esophageal or stomach perforation). Postoperative dysphagia can be minimized by routine use of a 56-F dilatator during fundoplication and avoidance of an excessively tight crural closure. Atraumatic dissection also minimizes tissue edema.

Splenic injury requiring splenorrhaphy or splenectomy has been reduced dramatically with laparoscopy. Pneumothorax remains one of the most common complications, but only 3% to 6% are of clinical significance. Many cases of asymptomatic pneumothorax go undetected unless routine chest x-rays are obtained. If incidentally discovered, only observation is required because the pneumothorax consists of carbon dioxide and is rapidly absorbed from the pleural space. Unless an underlying lung injury is present, the lung will reexpand quickly.

Gastric and esophageal injuries are far less common (<1%) and result from aggressive tissue handling or during passage of the Maloney dilatator. If detected intraoperatively, these injuries can be repaired laparoscopically with minimal sequelae.

Immediate recurrence is rare and usually caused by postoperative emesis during the first 24 hours. This should prompt immediate reoperation and repair. During 461 cases of LNF at Mount Sinai Medical Center in New York, only five patients required immediate reoperation (Table 4).

OUTCOMES

With long-term follow-up of more than 5 years, LNF has been shown to resolve typical GERD symptoms completely in 80% to 85% of patients. Atypical symptoms resolve in 60% to 75% of cases.

Table 4: Reoperations in 461 Laparoscopic Nissen Fundoplications

Immediate recurrence	2 (0.4%)
Hemorrhage	1 (0.2%)
Severe dysphagia	1 (0.2%)
Esophageal perforation	1 (0.2%)

Mild dysphagia is reported by up to 40% of patients within the first 30 days after surgery. Diet modification is usually effective, and only 4% of patients continue to complain of any degree of dysphagia at 3 months. Similarly, gas bloat and diarrhea may be reported by some patients during the early postoperative period but improve with time.

The use of LNF versus PPIs as optimal treatment for GERD is continually debated; a recent randomized study showed that LNF led to significantly less acid exposure of the lower esophagus at 3 months and greater improvements in gastrointestinal function and general well-being after 12 months. Although promising, longer follow-up and increased statistical power studies are required to validate these potential benefits of LNF.

Suggested Readings

Allen CJ, Anvari M: Does laparoscopic fundoplication provide long-term control of gastroesophageal reflux related cough? *Surg Endosc* 18:633, 2004.

Cookson R, Flood C, Koo B, and others: Short-term cost-effectiveness and long-term cost analysis comparing laparoscopic Nissen fundoplication with proton pump inhibitor maintenance for gastroesophageal reflux, *Br J Surg* 92:700, 2005.

Mahon D, Rhodes M, Decadt B, and others: Randomized clinical trial of laparoscopic Nissen fundoplication compared with proton pump inhibitors for the treatment of chronic gastroesophageal reflux, *Br J Surg* 92:695, 2005.

Papasavas P: Functional problems following esophageal surgery, *Surg Clin N Am* 85:525, 2005.

Patterson EJ, Herron DM, Hansen PD, and others: Effect of an esophageal bougie on the incidence of dysphagia following laparoscopic Nissen fundoplication, *Arch Surg* 135:1055, 2000.

Pessauz P, Arnaud JP, Dellatre JF, and others: Laparoscopic antireflux surgery—five year result and beyond in 1340 patients, *Arch Surg* 140:946, 2005.

Rossi M, Barreca M, de Bortoli N, and others: Efficacy of Nissen fundoplication versus medical therapy in the regression of low-grade dysplasia in patients with Barrett esophagus, *Ann Surg* 243:58, 2006.

Tran T, Spechler SJ, Richardson P, and others: Fundoplication and the risk of esophageal cancer in gastroesophageal reflux disease: a veterans affairs cohort study, *Am J Gastroenterol* 100:1002, 2005.

LAPAROSCOPIC REPAIR OF PARAESOPHAGEAL HERNIAS

Sarah M. Cowgill, MD, and Alexander S. Rosemurgy II, MD

INTRODUCTION

In the 1950s, the term "hiatal hernia" was introduced into the American lexicon. Although the diagnosis seems to be of note to patients, inasmuch as they greatly overstate its significance, hiatal hernias are common among Americans as they age and are usually asymptomatic.

Hiatal hernias are classified according to the position of the gastroesophageal junction and stomach in relation to the diaphragm and the esophageal hiatus. Type I hiatal hernias are the most common. They are also called *sliding hiatal hernias*. With type I hiatal hernias, the gastroesophageal junction and proximal stomach migrate above the diaphragm (Fig. 1). With type II hiatal hernias, the gastric fundus migrates cephalad into the mediastinum alongside the esophagus, but the gastroesophageal junction remains in its normal subdiaphragmatic position (Fig. 1). Type II hiatal hernias are also called *paraesophageal hernias*. More frequent than type II hiatal hernias are type III hiatal hernias, which are a combination of type I and type II hernias. With type III hernias both the fundus and lower esophageal sphincter herniate into the thorax, and the fundus herniates cephalad above the gastroesophageal junction (Fig. 1). Type III hiatal hernias are combined sliding and paraesophageal hiatal hernias. In chronic, giant hernias, the hernia sacs can contain the spleen, colon, omentum, small bowel, or a combination of these. These chronic, giant hiatal hernias are classified as type IV hiatal hernias. This chapter focuses on laparoscopic repair of type II, III, and IV hiatal hernias.

Paraesophageal hernias generally occur in older patients, and they are generally asymptomatic. Thus paraesophageal hernias are often initially detected by studies undertaken for reasons not directly attributable to paraesophageal hernias or that are unrelated to them.

Paraesophageal hernias, particularly when large, can cause displacement of the lower esophagus and thereby result in delayed esophageal emptying and obstructive symptoms. Delayed esophageal emptying is usually perceived as a sensation of the delayed passage of a food bolus (i.e., dysphagia). Regurgitation, chest pain, and a host of other symptoms can occur. Symptoms of gastroesophageal acid reflux can occur, but reflux is generally limited by the paraesophageal hernia's deviating the course of the lower esophagus and causing relative lower esophageal obstruction. However, type III or IV hernias may be associated with gastroesophageal reflux because the large size of the hernias denotes significant stretching and disruption of phrenoesophageal membranes that are physiologically important in preventing and limiting reflux. For patients with symptoms of dysphagia, regurgitation, chest pain, chronic cough, or heartburn (or any combination of these), paraesophageal hernias are documented through studies undertaken to determine the etiology of the symptoms.

The natural history of paraesophageal hernias is somewhat controversial. The phrenoesophageal membranes, which tether the esophagus in place at the diaphragmatic esophageal hiatus, fatigue with age. Although the rate and degree of fatigue are dependent on many factors (e.g. body mass index, chronic cough, pregnancy, etc.), it can generally be said that the membranes will fatigue to varying degrees in all and thus, given enough time, allow a "sliding" (type I) hiatal hernia. The development of a paraesophageal hernia is not so clear or common. As opposed to a general weakness in the phrenoesophageal membranes, a paraesophageal hernia requires a more specific defect in the phrenoesophageal membranes that allows the fundus of the stomach to migrate cephalad to the gastroesophageal junction. In time, given the negative pressure in the thorax, a paraesophageal hernia will increase in size and may presage migration of the gastroesophageal junction into the mediastinum and consequently the development of a type III or IV hernia. With increases in hernia size, symptoms generally attributable to distal esophageal obstruction are more likely to increase in frequency and severity.

The traditional fear with paraesophageal hernias is that they will incarcerate and strangulate, possibly as a consequence of twisting of the fundus with compromise of venous outflow or arterial inflow. Early reports by Belsey and Hill suggested that elective repair of paraesophageal hernias was mandatory because the risks of gastric perforation, bleeding, and infarction were significant. Many recent studies indicate that acute, catastrophic events are notably less frequent than originally believed. These studies and current "conventional wisdom" question the necessity for urgent repair of these hernias, advising repair primarily for patients who are notably symptomatic, younger than 60 years of age, or who present with a hernia of impressive size. However, the triad of a sudden inability

Figure 1 Hiatal hernias are classified as type I (the gastroesophageal junction is above the diaphragm), type II (the gastroesophageal junction is in an intra-abdominal location, but the gastric fundus has herniated above the diaphragm into the mediastinum), type III (both the gastroesophageal junction and the gastric fundus have herniated above the diaphragm into the mediastinum), or type IV (type III hiatal hernias that include other viscera, such as small bowel or colon, in the hernia sac in addition to the stomach).

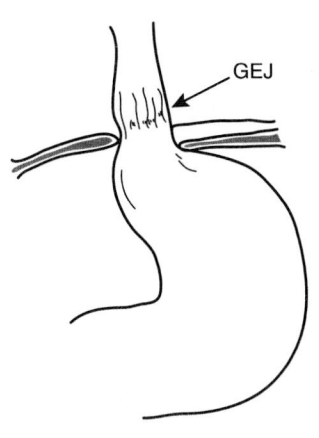
Type I

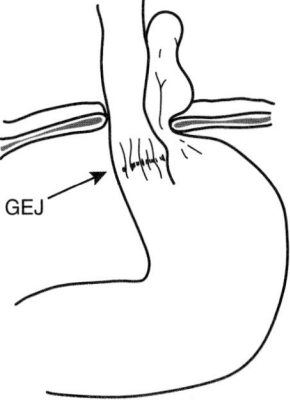
Type II

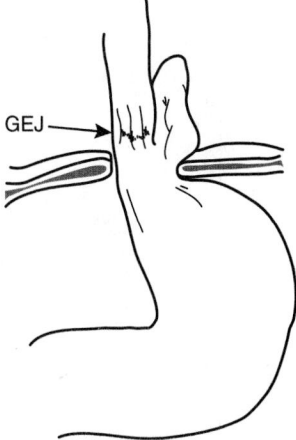
Type III

to vomit, intense epigastric pain, and an inability to pass a nasogastric tube may be a harbinger of gastric infarction and should initiate an immediate evaluation and, if indicated, a prompt operation.

Some controversy has been generated regarding the best manner of repairing paraesophageal hernias. In the past, some advocated a transthoracic or thoracoscopic approach for repair because there was a perceived advantage in mobilizing the hernia sac and its contents, as well as the lower esophagus, from the thorax into the abdominal cavity. However, the consensus now is that laparoscopic repair of paraesophageal hernias provides better operative exposure and offers results that are durable and efficacious. Although laparoscopic repair of a paraesophageal hernia requires advanced laparoscopic skills, it offers improved cosmesis, more rapid patient recovery, less patient pain, and shorter hospital stay than an "open" approach.

The addition of a concomitant antireflux procedure to the reduction and repair of a paraesophageal hernia has been historically debated. It is now accepted that before repair of paraesophageal hernias, 24-hour pH monitoring generally documents excessive gastroesophageal reflux, nearly identical in severity to the acid exposure seen with symptomatic "sliding" (type I) hiatal hernias. This excessive acid exposure promotes concomitant application of an antireflux procedure. Furthermore, necessary aggressive mobilization of paraesophageal hernia during its correction includes division of phrenoesophageal membranes and mobilization of the cardia. This dissection renders the lower esophageal sphincter mechanism incompetent, necessitating a concomitant antireflux procedure. Thus before undertaking operative repair of a paraesophageal hernia, it must be anticipated that a concomitant antireflux "valve" will be constructed at the gastroesophageal junction, and it is imperative that the strength and quality of esophageal motility is known to guide construction of the antireflux mechanism.

DIAGNOSIS AND PATIENT SELECTION

Fiberoptic endoscopy should be undertaken on patients with symptoms attributable to a hiatal hernia. These symptoms include but are not limited to dysphagia, heartburn, and noncardiac chest pain. A paraesophageal hernia, if present, can be identified on retroflexed view (Fig. 2). Fiberoptic endoscopy can identify esophageal and gastric pathology, if present, and also serves to rule out other causes of dysphagia. Endoscopy can detect esophagitis and the consequences of gastroesophageal reflux, as well as other "unexpected" pathology such as strictures and cancer.

Before any considerations for operative intervention for a paraesophageal hernia, patients should undergo an upper gastrointestinal (GI) barium contrast study. This is an underrated and underappreciated study that can yield much important information. First, an upper GI contrast study delineates anatomy, thereby documenting the paraesophageal hernia and defining its extent (Figs. 3 and 4). Second, this study can document other pathology of the esophagus, stomach, and duodenum. Third, it can define the gastric outlet, and, albeit poorly, it can subjectively measure gastric contractility and emptying. Fourth, and importantly, an upper GI contrast study, when properly undertaken, can be a worthwhile measure of clinically relevant esophageal motility. In essence, to determine the ability of the esophagus to handle a food bolus, test esophageal motility with a food bolus. The upper GI contrast (barium esophagogram) motility study is undertaken with the patient in a 15-degree Trendelenburg position with the patient swallowing a barium-laden food bolus, such as a bite of a bagel or a marshmallow. In this position, the patient should clear the food bolus from the esophagus with one or two stripping motions of the esophagus. If this is the case, the patient will tolerate concomitant construction of a Nissen fundoplication without excessive risks of postoperative dysphagia.

A manometric study to measure and document esophageal motility and strength is the gold standard measure of esophageal function before operative intervention. It is recommended. However, it may not be available at all surgical centers, and it might be excessively sensitive, suggesting inadequate esophageal contractility in a patient without clinically apparent problems with esophageal emptying. The upper GI study described previously may be more clinically relevant or more readily available. However, there is one caveat: the upper GI contrast study to determine esophageal motility requires an interested and engaged radiologist.

A pH study before operative intervention should be considered, but is not essential if dominant symptoms are not consistent with gastroesophageal reflux. With symptoms of gastroesophageal reflux, an ambulatory, 24-hour or 48-hour pH study before operative

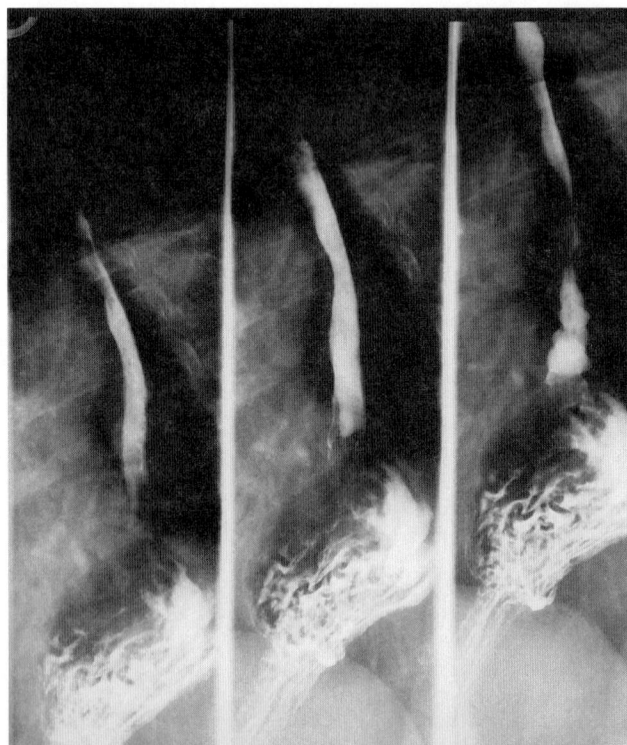

Figure 3 Contrast esophagography documents a large paraesophageal hernia with the gastroesophageal junction above the diaphragm (type III hiatal hernia). Note the esophageal dysmotility in the far right image.

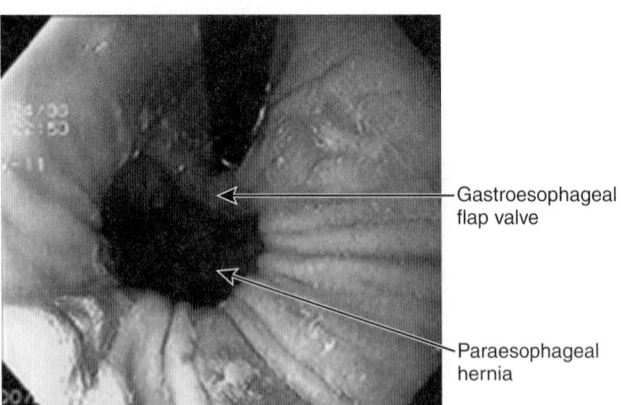

Gastroesophageal flap valve

Paraesophageal hernia

Figure 2 Retroflexed view of the gastroesophageal junction on endoscopy demonstrates an intact gastroesophageal flap valve and a large paraesophageal hernia.

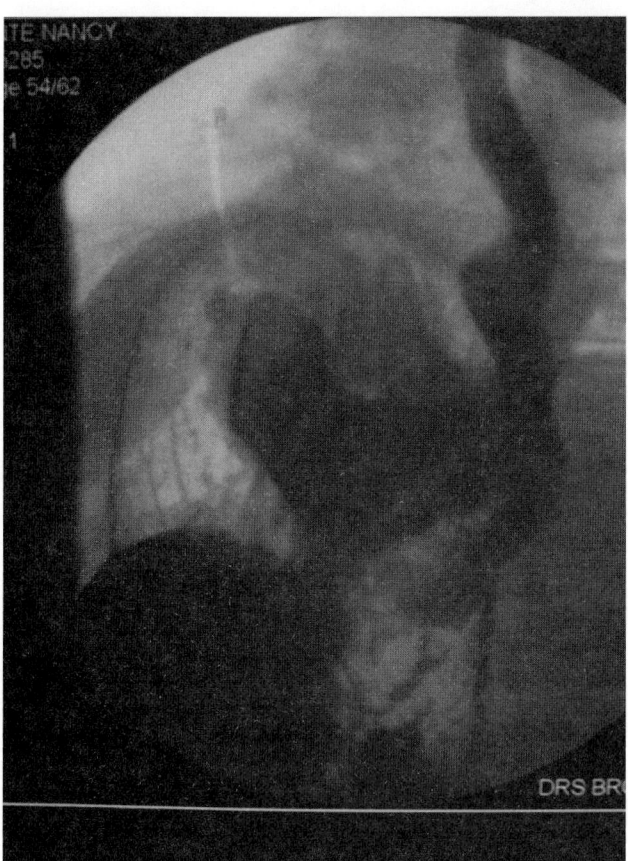

Figure 4 Contrast esophagography documents a large paraesophageal hernia with displacement of the lower esophagus (a type II hiatal hernia).

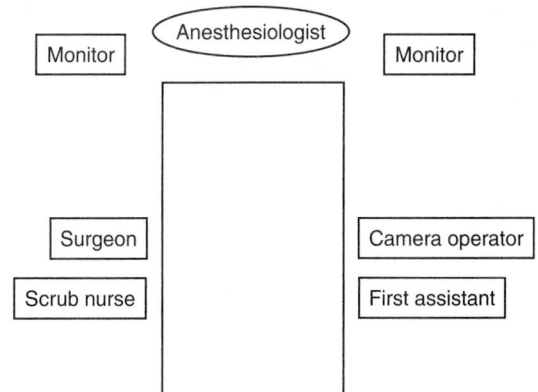

Figure 5 Operative setup for laparoscopic paraesophageal hernia repair.

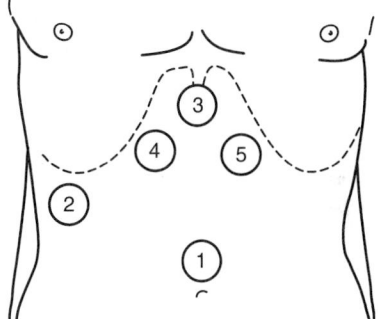

Figure 6 Trocar location for laparoscopic repair of a paraesophageal hernia. Numbers refer to the order in which the trocars are placed.

intervention is helpful to document the frequency and severity of acid reflux and is a useful baseline for postoperative follow-up.

OPERATIVE TECHNIQUE

Patients with paraesophageal hernias are usually electively admitted the day of their operation. In the operative suite, they are positioned in a flat, supine position with both arms extended. Although others have described using a bed that allows the operating surgeon to stand between the patient's legs, we prefer to use a standard bed. The surgeon stands on the patient's right with the first assistant standing on the patient's left (Fig. 5). In addition, the camera operator ultimately stands cephalad to the first assistant on the left.

The initial camera port is placed using a cutdown technique at the umbilicus (site 1). A 0-degree camera is used. After placing the camera site, four more port sites are placed (Fig. 6). Through the farthest right-side port, a fan retractor is placed to retract the liver (site 2). The surgeon's working port is a 5- to 11-mm trocar just to the right of the falciform ligament (site 4), through which an ultrasonic dissector and, ultimately, an Endo Stitch (Autosuture, Norwalk, CT) can pass. The first assistant works through the most left-side (5-mm) port (site 5) and the umbilical port (site 1), allowing for the use of a Babcock grasper. The camera is placed through the 5- to 11-mm port at the subxiphoid position (site 3).

Grasped with an atraumatic grasper (e.g., Babcock clamp), the stomach is retracted toward the spleen, and the avascular gastrohepatic ligament is opened in a stellate fashion. Care is taken to avoid an aberrant left gastric artery, if present. The dissection is carried to the right crus, up and down the right crus, and into

the mediastinum. Care is taken not to enter the right pleural space. Mobilization and reduction of the hiatal hernia begins. Next the dissection is carried up and over the top of the esophagus and stomach at the esophageal hiatus as the first assistant elevates overlying tissues. With the stomach rolled to the patient's right using the Babcock clamp, the short gastric vessels are divided and the dissection is carried to the left crus, up and down the left crus, and into the mediastinum. Progressively, the entire hiatal hernia is reduced. The hernia sac is excised, as is the gastroesophageal fat pad. Special care is taken to avoid vagal nerve injury and violation of the left pleural space. The esophagus is sufficiently mobilized to bring 8 cm of distal esophagus into the intra-abdominal cavity. Notably, several centimeters of esophageal length will be gained with crural reconstruction (i.e., reconstruction of the esophageal hiatus), which occurs next.

As the first assistant uses a blunt laparoscopic dissector, passed through port site 5, to elevate the esophagus, the surgeon uses a laparoscopic suturing technique of choice to approximate the cura. As many permanent sutures as necessary are used to close the wide hiatus snugly but not tightly about the esophagus. Large "bites" of the crura with overlying peritoneum are taken to ensure that stitches do not pull through. The surgeon should avoid sawing the crura when placing and tying the sutures.

Occasionally, prosthetic material is used as an adjunct in hiatal reconstruction, almost always as an onlay patch over the cruroplasty. Recent reports indicate that recurrent hiatal disruption may be lower with prosthetic, buttressed repairs. Those who support hiatal reconstruction with adjunctive prosthetic material report a 20% to 40% recurrence rate after primary repair of hiatal defects. This seems excessively high. As yet, the rate of failure of hiatal reconstruction with or without adjunctive prosthetic material is unestablished, and the safety profile and efficacy of prosthetic mesh repair has not been determined in studies of long-term outcome.

All of our laparoscopic paraesophageal hernia repairs are undertaken with a concomitant antireflux procedure. Depending on esophageal motility, the patient undergoes either a partial posterior (e.g., Toupet fundoplication) or complete 360-degree (e.g., Nissen) fundoplication. Most patients have normal esophageal motility and undergo a Nissen fundoplication. We now briefly describe our method of laparoscopic Nissen fundoplication.

After the crural repair, the posterior fundus is brought behind the esophagus, and a 52- to 60-F bougie is passed per os into the stomach. With smaller women, we use a 52- to 54-F bougie and with men, a 56- to 60-F bougie. After passing the bougie with appropriate laparoscopic guidance, the first assistant grasps the gastroesophageal junction and retracts it to the patient's right, creating a "collar" along the cardia and anterior fundus through which the initial suture of the fundoplication is placed. Care should be taken to avoid placing this stitch in the body of the stomach. Next the surgeon passes the suture through the cephalad-most aspect of the anterior intraabdominal esophagus. Finally, the posterior fundus, grasped to the right of the esophagus by the assistant with a Babcock clamp, is incorporated into the repair. As the knot is tied, care is taken not to displace the tissues and saw through the delicate muscular fibers of the esophagus. Two more successive stitches are taken to complete the fundoplication. The second stitch also incorporates the esophagus with the fundoplication, but the final caudad stitch of the wrap simply approximates the anterior fundus and the posterior fundus at the level of the gastroesophageal junction. The bougie is removed, and a final stitch secures the lateral aspect of the wrap to the right crus and esophagus to augment the angle of His and to prevent twisting of the esophagus and relieve tension on the wrap, which would otherwise promote its coming undone.

We close all but the 5-mm port sites using absorbable suture and an Endo Close (Autosuture). The skin edges are reapproximated with absorbable suture and Steri-Strips (3M, St. Paul, MN), and sterile dressings are applied.

Postoperatively, the patient is advanced to a full liquid diet. Generally patients are discharged the following morning with instructions to continue the full liquid diet until seen again in our outpatient clinic.

RESULTS OF TREATMENT

For 3 to 4 weeks following the laparoscopic repair of hiatal hernias, patients complain, to varying degrees, of dysphagia, bloating, flatulence, defecatory frequency, early satiety, shoulder pain, nausea, and trocar-site pain, particularly at the right-most trocar incision where the liver retractor was used. The shoulder pain is a residual effect of referred pain from the CO_2 insufflation and should last only days.

Bloating, flatulence, and defecatory frequency can be attributed to the excessive aerophagia that occurs as a learned behavior in patients with prolonged histories of gastroesophageal reflux disease. Complaints and symptoms should be expected to subside after 3 to 4 weeks postoperatively. Bothersome symptoms lasting beyond 1 month after fundoplication should be evaluated as indicated with an upper gastrointestinal contrast study using a 13-mm barium tablet or an ambulatory pH study (or both).

Studies of patients undergoing laparoscopic paraesophageal hernia repairs are encouraging. Laparoscopic repairs can be undertaken with relatively little morbidity and promising efficacy. Some studies do report failure of the hiatal reconstruction and recurrence of the paraesophageal hernia. Further application of laparoscopy in repair of paraesophageal hernias is encouraged. Several key points should be emphasized:

- Patient selection is important. Avoid significantly obese patients, those with a chronic cough, or those in generally poor health.
- Document esophageal motility before repair. Base the nature of the concomitantly constructed antireflux repair on documented esophageal motility.
- Reduce the entire hiatal hernia and establish 8 cm of intraabdominal esophagus. Excise the hernia sac.
- Reconstruct the esophageal hiatus snugly, but not tightly, about the esophagus. Use prosthetic material when necessary, particularly soft products such as Surgisis (Cook Medical, Bloomington, IN), to accomplish a tension-free reconstruction.

CONCLUSIONS

Laparoscopic paraesophageal hernia repair can be accomplished with minimal morbidity; however, the operation requires advanced minimally invasive surgical skills. Clinical outcomes after laparoscopic paraesophageal hernia repairs encourage further application.

SUGGESTED READINGS

D'Alessio MJ, Rakita S, Bloomston M, and others: Esophagography predicts favorable outcome after laparoscopic Nissen fundoplication for patients with esophageal dysmotility, *J Am Coll Surg* 201:335, 2005.

Draaisma WA, Gooszen HG, Tournoij E, and others: Controversies in paraesophageal hernia repair. A review of the literature, *Surg Endosc* 19:1300, 2005.

Luketich JD, Raja S, Fernando HC, and others: Laparoscopic repair of giant paraesophageal hernia: 100 consecutive cases, *Ann Surg* 232:608, 2000.

Rosemurgy AS, Arnaoutakis DJ, Thometz DP, and others: Reoperative fundoplications are effective treatment for dysphagia and recurrent gastroesophageal reflux, *Am Surg* 70:1061, 2004.

Skinner DB, Belsey RH: Surgical management of esophageal reflux and hiatus hernia. Long-term results with 1030 patients, *J Thorac Cardiovasc Surg* 53:33, 1967.

View a video of our technique of laparoscopic Nissen fundoplication at www.or-live.com/tgh/1332/.

Laparoscopic Treatment of Esophageal Motility Disorders

Robert W. O'Rourke, MD, and Blair A. Jobe, MD

INTRODUCTION

Esophageal motility disorders (EMDs) comprise a spectrum of disease that includes achalasia, as well as spastic and nonspastic disorders of the esophagus. The spastic disorders include hypertensive lower esophageal sphincter (HTN-LES), diffuse esophageal spasm (DES), and nutcracker esophagus and are characterized by elevated esophageal body or LES pressures that may or may not be accompanied by disordered esophageal body peristalsis. Ineffective esophageal motility is the primary nonspastic EMD and is characterized by ineffective esophageal peristalsis without elevated body or lower esophageal sphincter (LES) pressures. Disorders of esophageal motility that do not fit strict definitions for these named motility disorders are categorized as nonspecific EMDs.

PATHOPHYSIOLOGY

The primary causes of most EMDs are unknown. Infection with the parasite *Trypanosoma cruzi* is the primary cause of achalasia in the southern hemisphere. Data support a potential autoimmune etiology for nontrypanosomal achalasia, the dominant form of disease in the northern hemisphere, but definitive causal proof is lacking. Anecdotal cases document progression of DES to achalasia over many years. Similarly, an absence of ganglion cells in the LES similar to that seen in achalasia has been demonstrated in HTN-LES. Some speculate that these disorders may therefore represent variable manifestations of achalasia. Gastroesophageal reflux disease (GERD) leading to chronic damage of esophageal musculature is a known cause of ineffective esophageal motility, as well as some cases of nonspecific EMDs, and may also be the underlying cause of HTN-LES and nutcracker esophagus in some cases. Other disease processes, such as scleroderma and mixed connective tissue disease, may also lead to EMD. The precise causes of most EMDs remain unknown and thus represent an important area of research.

EPIDEMIOLOGY

Achalasia is the most common EMD, with an annual incidence of approximately 0.5 to 1 case per 100,000 in the United States. Of note, the incidence of achalasia caused by infection with *T. cruzi* in some areas in the southern hemisphere may be significantly higher, correlating with a high local prevalence of parasitic disease. Ineffective esophageal motility (IEM) or other nonspecific EMDs secondary to GERD are the second most common EMDs. Spastic disorders of the esophagus, including DES, HTN-LES, and nutcracker esophagus are relatively rare.

CLINICAL PRESENTATION

All EMDs share common clinical characteristics, and diagnosis based on symptoms alone is therefore not reliable. Achalasia is characterized by the classic triad of dysphagia, regurgitation, and weight loss. The specificity of these symptoms is poor, however. Dysphagia is the most common symptom in achalasia, seen in more than 90% of patients. Regurgitation is present in up to 70% of patients with achalasia. Weight loss is less common and is usually seen in patients who seek care late in the course of their disease. Dysphagia and chest pain are the dominant presenting symptoms in spastic disorders of the esophagus, and it is important to rule out ischemic coronary disease in such patients. Of note, although generally considered to be typical of spastic disorders of the esophagus, chest pain is by no means pathognomonic. One series demonstrated chest pain in 100%, 50%, and 80% of patients eventually diagnosed with HTN-LES, DES, and nutcracker esophagus, respectively, but of note, 50% of patients with achalasia also complain of chest pain. Furthermore, heartburn and regurgitation may be dominant symptoms in up to 50% of patients with achalasia, as well as in patients with spastic disorders of the esophagus, and distinguishing these entities from GERD may be difficult.

DIAGNOSTIC TESTING

The lack of specificity of symptoms mandates esophageal physiology testing for diagnosis of EMDs. Tools in the diagnostic armamentarium include esophagogastroduodenoscopy (EGD); contrast esophagram; esophageal manometry; 24-hour ambulatory esophageal pH monitoring; and most recently, esophageal impedance monitoring.

Although often not useful in the specific diagnosis of most EMDs, EGD and contrast esophagram are mandatory in all patients to identify coexisting pathology, such as a dilatated or sigmoid esophagus, esophageal diverticula (Fig. 1, *A*), hiatal or paraesophageal hernia, esophagitis, or tumor. Contrast esophagram is not a sensitive or specific test for most EMDs, but may be helpful in some cases. In cases of achalasia in which manometric results are equivocal, such as in patients with partially preserved LES relaxation or esophageal body peristalsis, contrast esophagram may demonstrate a classic "bird's beak" tapering of the distal esophagus despite the absence of clear manometric evidence of achalasia (Fig. 1, *B*). Contrast esophagram may also be useful in the diagnosis of other spastic disorders of the esophagus, most notably DES, which shows a "corkscrew" appearance of the esophageal body during episodes of spasm (Fig. 1, *C*). An obvious limitation of this test in such patients is that a spasm event must occur during the study. Contrast esophagram is less useful in the diagnosis of other disorders of esophageal motility and often is not associated with specific findings.

Manometry is the mainstay of diagnosis for EMDs, and specific manometric features define the various disorders of esophageal motility. Of note, many abnormal manometric findings are nonspecific and common to many EMDs. For example, increased intrabolus pressure is common among the spastic EMDs, a result of outflow obstruction associated with the elevated LES pressure often associated with these disorders. Abnormal esophageal body peristaltic wave morphology is another relatively nonspecific manometric finding evident in many EMDs. It is important to be familiar with the pathognomonic manometric features that define the various EMDs, as well as common nonspecific features that may confuse diagnosis.

The manometric sine qua non of achalasia consists of a non-relaxing LES and aperistalsis of the esophageal body (Fig. 2, *A*). These findings are variable, however, complicating diagnosis in some patients. LES relaxation may be present but incomplete. Resting LES pressures in achalasia are often normal but may be elevated in more than 40% of cases. Esophageal body peristalsis

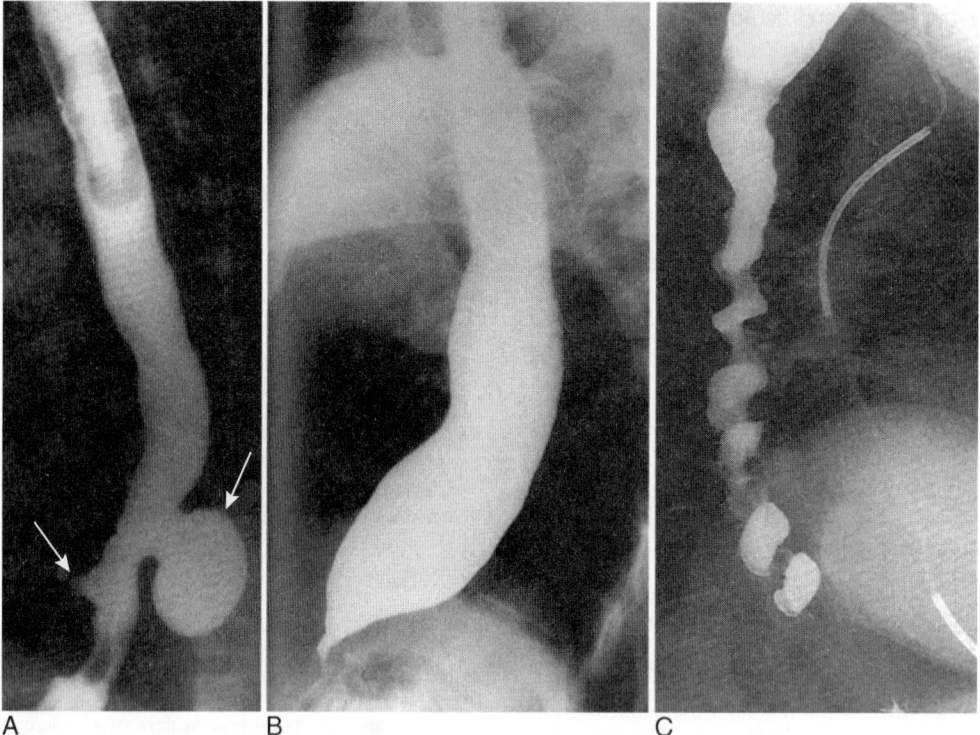

Figure 1 Contrast esophagograms demonstrating distal esophageal diverticula (**A**); achalasia, with "bird's beak" tapering of the distal esophagus (**B**); and DES, demonstrating a corkscrew appearance of the esophageal body (**C**). *(A) and (C) reprinted from Bremner CG, DeMeester TR, Huprich JE, and others: Esophageal disease and testing, New York, 2005, Taylor & Francis, pp 27–28; (B) reprinted with permission from Eubanks WS, Swanstrom LL, Soper NJ, editors: Mastery of endoscopic and laparoscopic surgery, ed 1, Philadelphia, 2000, Lippincott Williams & Wilkins p. 175.*

likewise may be preserved proximally but absent distally. A subset of patients present with manometric findings of "vigorous" achalasia, characterized by simultaneous esophageal body peristalses with elevated amplitudes accompanied by partial or complete failure of LES relaxation. Vigorous achalasia may represent an early form of disease.

HTN-LES is characterized by elevated resting LES pressures and normal LES relaxation. By definition, a diagnosis of HTN-LES alone requires the presence of normal esophageal body function. It is important to recognize, however, that a hypertensive LES may be present in up to 40% of patients with achalasia or nutcracker esophagus and in more than 20% of patients with DES. Elevated resting LES pressure is therefore a common finding in all spastic disorders of the esophagus.

DES is characterized by intermittent simultaneous esophageal body contractions, which may be increased in amplitude or duration, and abnormal in morphology, typically with multiple peaks (Fig. 2, *B*). These contractions are often associated with chest pain and may be increased in amplitude, although not to the same degree as in nutcracker esophagus, and usually are approximately 150 mm Hg. LES relaxation may be incomplete, and resting LES pressures may be elevated in more than 20% of cases, features that DES shares with achalasia and HTN-LES.

The defining manometric feature of nutcracker esophagus is spontaneous esophageal body contractions of increased amplitude, often greater than 180 mm Hg. Unlike DES, in which abnormal contractions are simultaneous, nutcracker esophagus demonstrates progressive peristaltic waveforms (Fig. 2, *C*). Contractions may be prolonged, and LES pressures may be elevated in more than 40% of cases. Of note, correlation of elevated intraesophageal pressures with chest pain in patients with nutcracker esophagus is often poor.

Confusion regarding the precise manometric definition of IEM affects interpretation of the literature, much of which includes nonspecific disorders of esophageal motility with IEM. A diagnosis of IEM requires average distal esophageal peristaltic amplitudes less than 30 mm Hg, nontransmitted waveforms in more than 30% of wet swallows, or both. IEM may also be associated with other manometric signs of abnormal esophageal body function, including multipeaked, low-amplitude, prolonged, nonprogressive or retrograde waveforms. The presence of these or other manometric findings in the absence of the aforementioned defining characteristics of IEM or other named EMDs defines the nonspecific EMDs.

Monitoring of ambulatory esophageal pH over a 24-hour period provides valuable information in the patient with EMD. GERD may be present in up to 25% of patients with achalasia, and the presence of acid reflux affects treatment decisions: dilatation will likely worsen GERD in a patient with achalasia, whereas a myotomy with partial fundoplication generally provides excellent relief of symptoms. GERD may be the underlying cause of HTN-LES and DES in 10% to 25% of cases, and 24-hour pH monitoring is necessary to identify these subgroups of patients. In addition to identifying coexisting GERD, EMDs may affect the results of pH monitoring. For example, achalasia may be associated with frank LES incompetence and acid reflux, but alternatively, fermentation of retained food in the distal esophagus may cause acidification in the absence of gastroesophageal acid reflux, so-called pseudo-reflux. A pattern of prolonged acid exposure as opposed to intermittent exposure associated with reflux events distinguishes true reflux from pseudo-reflux. Impedance monitoring, which measures electrical impedance within the esophageal lumen, may also aid in distinguishing between these entities, and as a new diagnostic tool, it holds promise for enhancing understanding of EMDs.

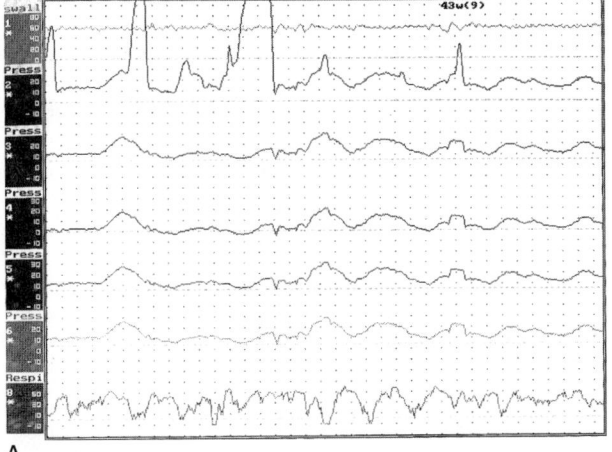

A

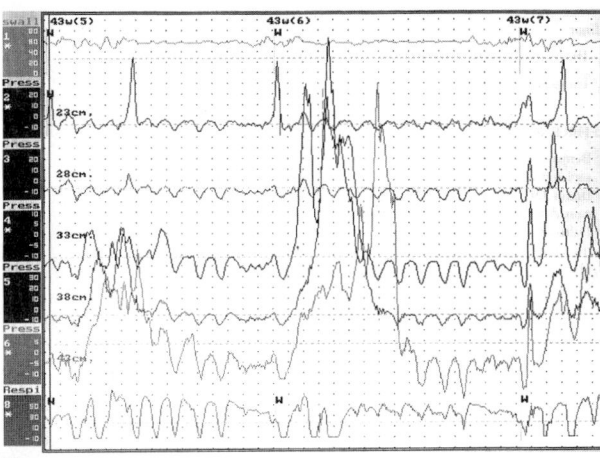

B

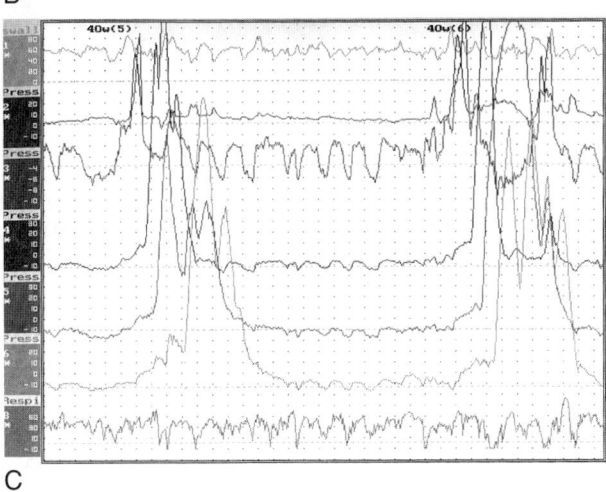

C

Figure 2 Esophageal body manometry tracings for achalasia, demonstrating aperistalsis (**A**); diffuse esophageal spasm, demonstrating high-amplitude, nonprogressive peristaltic waveforms (**B**); and nutcracker esophagus, demonstrating high-amplitude, progressive peristaltic waveforms (**C**). *Reprinted with permission from Bremner CG: Esophageal motility testing made easy, St. Louis, 2001, Marcel Dekker, pp. 75, 83, 85.*

▊ TREATMENT

Few prospective randomized trials compare therapeutic options for EMDs; treatment recommendations must therefore be inferred from

small series and noncomparative trials. As a result, consensus treatment recommendations for EMDs remain elusive, and practice patterns are variable. Despite continuing debate, the importance of appropriate treatment in this frequently vexing group of patients cannot be overemphasized. Improperly treated EMD can culminate in significant morbidity and the need for total esophagectomy. Careful consideration of primary treatment is essential to avoid this outcome.

Best Treatment for Achalasia

Surgical myotomy is a highly effective therapy for achalasia, and the majority of patients will eventually undergo operation for their disease. The introduction of a laparoscopic approach to surgery for achalasia has reduced morbidity to low levels, reinforcing its dominant role in treatment. Nevertheless, other treatment options are available, most notably pneumatic balloon dilatation and botulinum toxin injection of the LES, and debate persists regarding the optimal choice of initial therapy. In addition, not all patients are operative candidates, necessitating consideration of alternative therapies. Currently, no effective pharmacologic treatment exists for achalasia. Nitrates and calcium channel antagonists are the most commonly used pharmacologic agents, and their efficacy is poor.

Pneumatic balloon dilatation of the LES was the earliest described treatment for achalasia. The first esophageal dilatation for what was likely achalasia was reported in 1674 by Sir Thomas Willis, who used a whale bone with a piece of sponge fixed to its tip. Modern dilatation involves delivery of a balloon dilatator via EGD, followed by graded dilatations of the LES with balloon dilatators ranging from 3 to 4 cm in diameter for 15 to 60 seconds. Balloon dilatation as a treatment for achalasia suffers from two primary drawbacks: a risk of iatrogenic perforation and a high rate of recurrent dysphagia. Perforation rates range from 2% to 5%, with modern estimates of approximately 4% to 5%. Of note, these injuries are usually detected during the procedure, and with expeditious operative repair, associated morbidity and mortality are low. Operative repair in such cases is performed via a laparoscopic approach; myotomy opposite the perforation and partial fundoplication are performed concomitant with repair. Recurrence of dysphagia is the other primary drawback of dilatation and may occur in more than 60% to 70% of patients over long-term follow-up. For this reason, dilatation is generally reserved for elderly or otherwise poor operative candidates. Nevertheless, preparations should be made for urgent operative therapy in case of perforation during dilatation procedures. Another important consideration is the presence of GERD: dilatation will likely significantly worsen acid reflux in patients with achalasia and coexisting GERD because of partial disruption of the antireflux mechanism. Consideration should be given to primary surgical therapy in such patients.

Given its relatively low morbidity, dilatation has been suggested as the best initial therapy for achalasia. Decision analyses suggest, however, that surgical therapy is more expeditious and effective in most patients. It is important to note that these analyses report only a slight advantage for primary surgical therapy when compared with initial dilatation therapy. Depending on local practice patterns and expertise, dilatation is not an unreasonable choice for initial therapy, as long as both patient and clinician understand that a high percentage of patients will eventually require operative therapy.

In contrast to the long history of dilatation in the treatment of achalasia, endoscopic botulinum toxin injection of the LES is a relatively recent development, introduced in the early 1990s. Botulinum toxin inhibits presynaptic acetylcholine release in the myenteric plexus, thus reducing LES smooth muscle tone. Similar to dilatation, the primary limitation of botulinum toxin therapy is long-term recurrence of dysphagia. Although botulinum toxin injection provides immediate relief from dysphagia in up to 90% of patients, with longer follow-up more than 70% of patients may suffer recurrent dysphagia. Another important consideration is that botulinum toxin injection may complicate subsequent surgical therapy. Botulinum toxin generates an inflammatory response, which may make subsequent surgical therapy difficult, and may be associated with a higher rate of esophageal perforation during myotomy. For these reasons, interest in botulinum toxin therapy as primary therapy for achalasia is waning.

Surgical Therapy for Achalasia

Heller first described bilateral esophageal myotomy for the treatment of achalasia in 1913. This was subsequently modified to a unilateral esophagogastric myotomy, usually combined with an antireflux procedure. Surgical myotomy provides long-term relief from dysphagia for more than 90% of patients with achalasia. With advances in minimally invasive approaches for the treatment of achalasia over the past decade, morbidity and mortality have been reduced to low levels. A number of studies have demonstrated that a laparoscopic approach to achalasia provides equivalent results to an open approach, but with lower morbidity and faster recovery. Currently, an open approach to the surgical treatment of achalasia is therefore reserved for patients with a history of foregut surgery that would make a laparoscopic approach untenable or when surgeon experience with a minimally invasive approach is limited.

The most commonly performed operation for the treatment of achalasia consists of a laparoscopic Heller myotomy combined with a partial (≈270-degree) fundoplication. Laparoscopic access to the hiatus is obtained with 5 or 6 trocars placed in the upper abdomen (Fig. 3). Depending on preference, the operating surgeon may stand to the patient's right or left or between the legs, with the latter position most commonly used (Fig. 4). Preparations should be made for intraoperative EGD, which may be useful in identifying the location of the LES, and testing the myotomized esophagus for leaks. A retractor elevates the left hepatic lobe away from the operative field. A limited anterior hiatal dissection is performed, exposing at least 8 cm of anterior esophagus. A posterior hiatal dissection is necessary only if a posterior fundoplication is planned. The proximal short gastric vessels are divided. The anterior vagus nerve must be dissected free and elevated from the esophagus before myotomy is performed. The gastroesophageal fat pad is mobilized and rotated

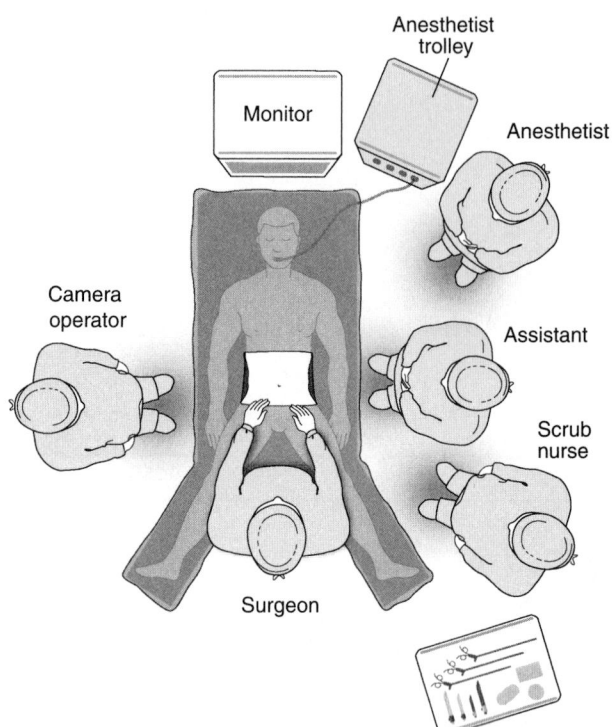

Figure 4 Typical operating room arrangement. *Reprinted with permission from Toouli J, Gossot D, Hunter J: Endosurgery, New York, 1996, Churchill Livingstone, p. 307.*

to the patient's right, thereby exposing the entire esophagogastric junction and collar sling musculature. A 7-cm esophageal myotomy is then created over the anterior esophagus and carried across the LES and onto the stomach for 2 or 3 cm. The myotomy may be created with standard hook cautery, Harmonic Scalpel (Johnson & Johnson Gateway, Piscataway, NJ), bipolar scissors, or blunt dissection with fine graspers. Our preference is to use a combination of the latter two methods. Placement of an esophageal bougie may aid in performance of the myotomy. The exposed esophageal mucosa may be tested for integrity with instillation of air or methylene blue via an orogastric tube or an endoscope. A partial fundoplication is then performed over a bougie (52F–56F).

The length of the myotomy is an important determinant of success. Failure to create at least a 7-cm esophageal myotomy or at least a 2-cm gastric myotomy has been shown to be the primary cause of recurrent dysphagia. Myotomy without fundoplication is associated with significant acid reflux in more than 50% of patients. Myotomy accompanied by a 360-degree (Nissen) fundoplication is associated with high rates of recurrent dysphagia in most series. Partial fundoplication is therefore considered by most to be the appropriate procedure to accompany myotomy for achalasia, and it relieves dysphagia in 90% to 96% of patients, with postoperative acid reflux occurring in less than 10%. The posterior Toupet and the anterior Dor fundoplications are most often used. Although no prospective randomized trials compare these antireflux procedures, existing data suggest that long-term results are equivalent. A Dor fundoplication is often simpler to construct (Fig. 5). A Toupet fundoplication may not be technically feasible in patients with a dilatated (sigmoid) distal esophagus (Fig. 6).

Proponents of a thoracoscopic approach argue that myotomy may be performed with less disruption of the native antireflux mechanism. Although thoracoscopy is an accepted technique, recent data suggest that the ability to obtain an adequate gastric myotomy may be compromised with a thoracoscopic approach and that failure rates may

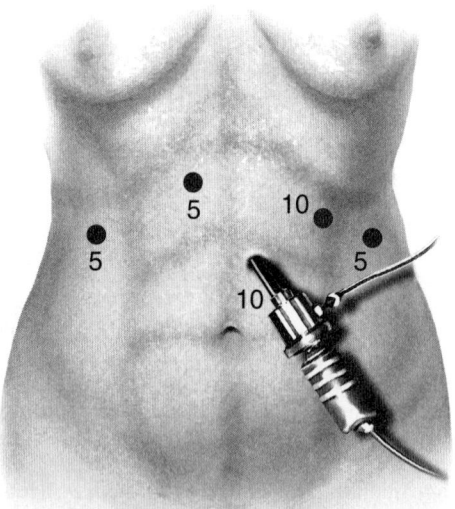

Figure 3 Typical trocar arrangement for surgical therapy of esophageal motility disorders. *Reprinted with permission from Toouli J, Gossot D, Hunter J: Endosurgery, New York, 1996, Churchill Livingstone, p. 307.*

Figure 5   Myotomy with Dor fundoplication. **(A)** First suture line; **(B)** completed Dor fundoplication.   *Reprinted with permission from Soper NJ, Swanstrom, LL, Eubanks WS, editors: Mastery of endoscopic and laparoscopic surgery, ed 2, Philadelphia, 2005, Lippincott Williams & Wilkins, p. 219.*

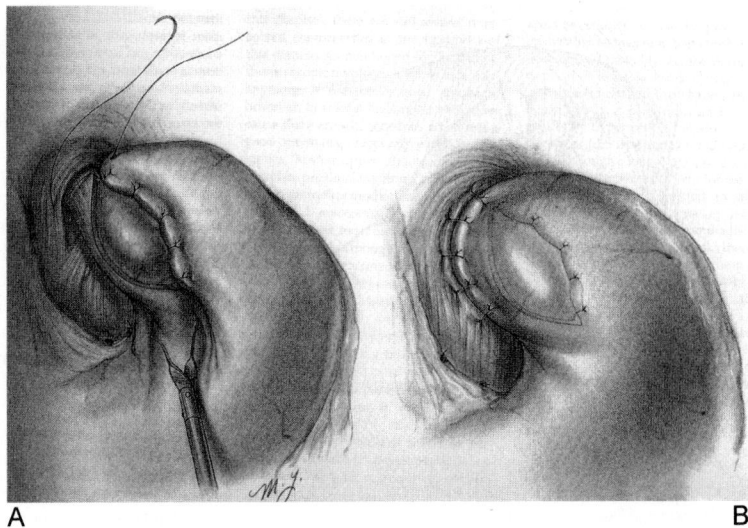

A   B

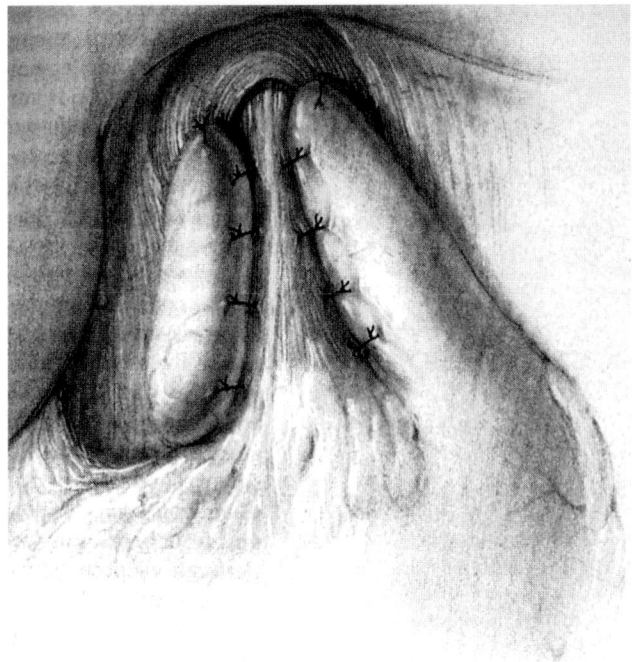

Figure 6   Toupet fundoplication.   *Reprinted with permission from Soper NJ, Swanstrom, LL, Eubanks WS, editors: Mastery of endoscopic and laparoscopic surgery, ed 2, Philadelphia, 2005, Lippincott Williams & Wilkins, p. 209.*

therefore be higher than with a laparoscopic approach. In addition, such an approach affords less flexibility in choice of fundoplication. For these reasons, a laparoscopic approach is the dominant mode of access for the surgical treatment of achalasia.

Treatment of Spastic Disorders of the Esophagus

Interpretation of results of treatment for spastic disorders of the esophagus is difficult because of their infrequency and variable response to therapy. Treatment recommendations are therefore based on small series and expert opinions. An important principle of management of these disorders is that current treatment, both medical and surgical, should be considered palliative. Current therapies do not correct underlying motility disorders; rather, their primary purpose is relief of symptoms. Patient selection based on an understanding of this concept will optimize results.

Just as in achalasia, the most common pharmacologic agents used in the treatment of spastic disorders of the esophagus are calcium channel antagonists and nitrates. Although some patients may experience a transient response, most studies demonstrate poor long-term efficacy of these agents and many show no difference when compared with placebo. Dilatation and botulinum toxin therapies likewise are less efficacious for these disorders than for achalasia, with short-term success in less than 25% of patients. In contrast, modern surgical therapy, aided by advances in the understanding of these disorders, provides effective treatment for carefully selected patients with spastic disorders of the esophagus.

An important observation underlying surgical management is that a hypertensive LES is a common finding among the spastic disorders of the esophagus. In fact, some have suggested that this observation supports the hypothesis that HTN-LES, DES, and perhaps nutcracker esophagus, are related and represent early or variant forms of achalasia. Although the true etiology of these disorders remains unknown, a hypertensive LES is the sine qua non of HTN-LES and also occurs in more than 20% of patients with DES and more than 40% of patients with nutcracker esophagus. Furthermore, surgical therapy directed toward this unequivocal manometric finding, especially when associated with dysphagia, appears to be more effective in the treatment of spastic disorders of the esophagus than when applied to patients without a hypertensive LES. Consistent with this observation, surgery is more effective in relieving dysphagia than chest pain for all spastic disorders of the esophagus. This realization has allowed for better patient selection and improved results.

Appropriate operative therapy for most patients with DES is esophagogastric myotomy with partial fundoplication, as described earlier for achalasia. Some argue for extended myotomy to as high as the aortic arch in these patients; this modification generally requires a thoracoscopic approach. Others have reported excellent results with a laparoscopic approach and a standard myotomy as performed for achalasia. Proponents of this latter approach report only rare failures requiring treatment with extended myotomy and report a higher failure rate associated with a thoracoscopic approach secondary to failure or inability to perform an adequate gastric myotomy. For these reasons, the dominant approach for the surgical treatment of DES is laparoscopic esophagogastric myotomy with partial fundoplication, just as in achalasia. Extension of the myotomy as proximally as possible may prevent failures in the rare patient who requires extended myotomy, but as in achalasia, at least a 7-cm esophageal myotomy is necessary and is adequate in the majority of cases. Results with this approach are good, with dysphagia and chest pain relieved in approximately 85% and 80% of patients, respectively.

Debate surrounding the appropriate operative therapy for HTN-LES is focused on the length of the myotomy required to effectively treat symptoms. Some argue for tailoring the myotomy to manometric findings, performing only a limited myotomy over the area of the manometric hypertensive LES, combined with partial fundoplication. It is unknown whether this approach provides better results than standard esophagogastric myotomy. Regardless of the length of the myotomy, a laparoscopic approach is appropriate for the treatment of HTN-LES and provides excellent relief of both dysphagia and chest pain in the vast majority of patients.

Nutcracker esophagus, in contrast to HTN-LES and DES, continues to pose a therapeutic dilemma. Results of myotomy are poor, with less than one third of patients experiencing relief of symptoms. An important exception is patients who have coexisting hypertensive LES and dysphagia, who may comprise up to 40% of patients with nutcracker esophagus. Such patients may experience relief of dysphagia after esophagogastric myotomy with partial fundoplication. Some have suggested that surgical therapy be restricted to this subgroup of patients with nutcracker esophagus.

An important caveat to the aforementioned operative recommendations are the subgroups of patients in whom GERD is the primary cause of nutcracker esophagus or HTN-LES, estimated to be between 15% and 25% of cases. These patients will respond to fundoplication without myotomy and can be identified with 24-hour ambulatory esophageal pH monitoring.

Treatment of Nonspastic Esophageal Motility Disorders: Ineffective Esophageal Motility

IEM is most often the result of GERD, and treatment must address this underlying problem. As a result, fundoplication remains the primary therapy. In fact, elimination of esophageal reflux by fundoplication often leads to improvement in motility in these patients and resolution of reflux. Partial fundoplication has been applied to patients with GERD and IEM in the past because of concerns of postoperative dysphagia. Recent data suggest that this practice is accompanied by high rates of persistent acid reflux, however, and furthermore, that a 360-degree fundoplication does not lead to higher rates of dysphagia when compared with partial fundoplication. Although still debated, there has been a general trend over the past decade toward the application of 360-degree fundoplication for all but the most severe forms of IEM (i.e., aperistalsis) or when dysphagia is the dominant presenting symptom. This latter group of patients must, of course, undergo thorough manometric evaluation to rule out a coexisting spastic disorder of the esophagus.

Complicated Esophageal Motility Disorders

A markedly dilatated, or "sigmoid" esophagus is found in more than 10% of patients with achalasia. These patients appear to respond as well to myotomy as do patients with a nondilatated esophagus, but operative difficultly is increased. An anterior Dor-type fundoplication is usually required in these patients because

a posterior fundoplication may not be possible in the face of significant distal esophageal dilatation.

Approximately 80% of esophageal diverticula are associated with EMDs and are of the pulsion type. Myotomy alone may be effective treatment for small distal esophageal diverticula. If, on the basis of visual inspection after myotomy, a small diverticulum resolves, then no resection is required. Large diverticula require resection, which may be quite challenging because of adhesions to surrounding mediastinal tissues. Peridiverticular dissection followed by resection with a linear cutting stapler is performed. If possible, the staple line should be covered with a partial fundoplication to minimize the risk of leak.

A subset of patients may have advanced disease unresponsive to standard surgical therapy or disease that has been complicated by previous inappropriate operations secondary to misdiagnosis. The patient with achalasia who initially showed symptoms of coexisting GERD and in whom Nissen fundoplication was performed is a common example of this latter group. In such cases, esophageal function may be so compromised that total esophagectomy becomes necessary. Morbidity from untreated EMD in such cases may be significant, and these issues must be weighed against the inherent risks of esophagectomy. Operative morbidity aside, long-term functional results for esophagectomy for end-stage EMD are good.

Esophageal disease is the most common gastrointestinal manifestation of scleroderma. Experience with these rare patients is limited, and recommendations by necessity are made on the basis of anecdotal experience. Scleroderma may result in impairment of esophageal body peristalsis, LES function, or both, and may be associated with dysphagia or GERD. The general approach to these patients should be conservative because this is often a progressive disease. Nonsurgical therapy should be exhausted before surgical intervention is considered.

CONCLUSION

Surgery is the mainstay of treatment for EMDs and is effective in relieving symptoms in carefully selected patients. Our understanding of the natural history and pathogenesis of these disorders has increased greatly over the past decade, accompanied by advances in minimally invasive surgical therapy. Modern surgical therapy now provides effective treatment with minimal morbidity to most patients with EMDs. Nevertheless, little is known about the precise cause of disease in most cases. An improved understanding of disease pathogenesis at the cellular and molecular levels has the potential to further improve on modern therapy for these disorders and eventually provide effective pharmacologic interventions.

Suggested Readings

Hunter JG, Trus TL, Branum GD, and others: Laparoscopic Heller myotomy and fundoplication for achalasia, *Ann Surg* 225(6): 655, 1997.

Patti MG, Gorodner MV, Galvani C, and others: Spectrum of esophageal motility disorders: implications for diagnosis and treatment, *Arch Surg* 140:442, 2005.

Tamhankar AP, Almogy G, Arain MA, and others: Surgical management of hypertensive lower esophageal sphincter with dysphagia or chest pain, *J Gastrointest Surg* 7(8): 990, 2003.

ESOPHAGEAL ACHALASIA

Colleen B. Gaughan, MD, and Jeffrey A. Hagen, MD

Esophageal achalasia is a motor disorder characterized by absent peristalsis in the smooth muscle portion of the esophageal body and incomplete relaxation of the lower esophageal sphincter (LES) in response to swallowing. Achalasia has been classified as primary or secondary, depending on whether or not it occurs in association with other systemic diseases (Table 1). The most common forms of secondary achalasia include Chagas's disease in South America and cancer in the United States. Chagas's disease is caused by chronic infection by the parasite *Trypanosoma cruzi,* which is endemic in South America and which causes destruction of the parasympathetic ganglion cells throughout the body, resulting in a condition indistinguishable from primary achalasia, as well as a cardiomyopathy and cardiac arrhythmias, and dilatation of the gastrointestinal, urinary, and respiratory tracts. Therapy for patients with secondary forms of achalasia is focused on treatment of the underlying condition, with the exception of Chagas's disease, the management of which follows the principles outlined in this chapter for primary achalasia.

Primary esophageal achalasia occurs in 0.4 to 0.6 per 100,000 population. No predisposition for either gender seems to exist, and it is most common in adults between ages 20 and 50. Achalasia may also occur in association with adrenal insufficiency and alacrima, in a condition termed the *triple-A syndrome.* Whereas there is general agreement that esophageal achalasia is a neurogenic disorder involving the myenteric plexus, the details of the pathogenesis of this condition are poorly understood. Most authorities consider it to be an autoimmune condition, with histopathologic studies consistently showing inflammatory cell infiltration of the myenteric plexus, along with fibrosis and depletion or total loss of ganglion

Table 1: Classification of Achalasia

I. Primary (idiopathic) achalasia
   A. Classic achalasia
   B. Vigorous achalasia

II. Secondary achalasia
   A. *Trypanosoma cruzi* infection (Chagas's disease)
   B. Cancer
      1. Obstructing LES (pseudoachalasia)
      2. Remote from LES (paraneoplastic)
   C. Infiltrating disorders of the LES
      1. Amyloidosis
      2. Fabry's disease
      3. Sarcoidosis
      4. Eosinophilic infiltration
   D. Systemic disease
      1. Diabetes mellitus
      2. Familial adrenal insufficiency with alacrima (triple-A syndrome)
      3. Sicca syndrome with gastric hyposecretion
   E. Generalized GI dysmotility
      1. Intestinal pseudo-obstruction
   F. Neuromuscular disorders
      1. Parkinson's disease

GI, Gastrointestinal; *LES,* lower esophageal sphincter.

cells. Degenerative changes have also been described in the vagus nerve and its dorsal motor nucleus in the brainstem, leading to speculation that a neurotropic infectious agent may be involved. This hypothesis is supported by the demonstrated increase in serum antibodies to Varicella-Zoster virus in achalasia patients as compared with controls and by DNA hybridization studies that have localized the virus to the myenteric plexus. Increased serum antibody titers against the measles virus have also been reported in achalasia patients. Whatever the cause, the result is impairment of the nonadrenergic, noncholinergic inhibitory nerves of the LES with intact cholinergic excitatory nerves. Other manifestations of this neurotropic injury have been observed, including impaired acid secretion and pancreatic polypeptide release with sham meals, and prolonged gastrointestinal transit in patients with achalasia, suggesting a more global vagal nerve dysfunction.

DIAGNOSIS

Patients with achalasia often suffer with severe symptoms for prolonged periods before the correct diagnosis is established. The most common initial symptom is progressive dysphagia to both solids and liquids, which is present in nearly all patients. Regurgitation of recently ingested or undigested food is also common. Chest pain may be present in up to 75% of patients and tends to be more severe early in the course of the disease. As the esophagus dilatates, the chest pain often subsides with the development of prominent symptoms of nocturnal regurgitation and aspiration. Whereas true gastroesophageal reflux is rare because of the nonrelaxing hypertensive LES, patients may experience the sensation of heartburn caused by dilatation of the esophagus or irritation of the esophagus caused by retained food.

Characteristic findings on radiography, endoscopy, and esophageal manometry serve to confirm the diagnosis. Plain chest radiographs may suggest the diagnosis of achalasia, particularly late in the course of disease when the dilatated esophagus containing an air-fluid level can be seen in the absence of a gastric air bubble. The characteristic findings on upper gastrointestinal (GI) radiography include dilatation of the esophagus with a tapered narrowing distally, the so-called *bird's beak deformity* (Fig. 1). Endoscopy should be performed in all patients suspected of having achalasia to exclude the presence of malignancy. In the absence of a mass, endoscopy is often normal, especially in early achalasia. In more advanced cases, a dilatated esophagus with retained food may be seen. Esophagitis with a cobblestone appearance may also be seen because of stasis and fermentation of the swallowed food.

Esophageal manometry is considered the gold standard for the diagnosis of achalasia. There are four characteristic findings on manometry: (1) a high pressure LES (>26 mm Hg), (2) failure of or incomplete LES relaxation, (3) absence of peristaltic contractions in the body of the esophagus and (4) elevation of the resting pressure in the body of the esophagus (esophageal pressurization) (Fig. 2). Not all of these manometric findings are required for the diagnosis of achalasia, but the diagnosis of achalasia should be restricted to patients with incomplete relaxation of the LES and absent peristalsis in the esophageal body. A vigorous form of achalasia has been described that has the typical LES findings of achalasia but with high-amplitude (>50 mm Hg) simultaneous pressure waves in the esophageal body. These findings may be difficult to distinguish from diffuse esophageal spasm (DES), with the latter condition suggested by the presence of a normally relaxing LES.

MANAGEMENT

Achalasia typically follows an indolent course, with patients complaining of several years of gradually progressive dysphagia.

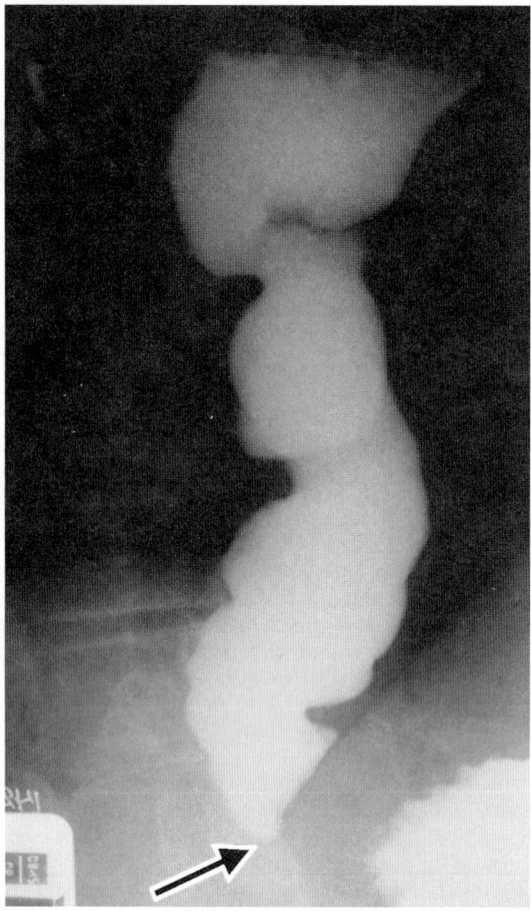

Figure 1 Characteristic findings on upper gastrointestinal radiography in achalasia, including dilatation of the esophagus with a tapered narrowing distally, the so-called bird's beak deformity *(arrow)*.

Untreated, it may progress to the development of complications such as airway obstruction and pulmonary infection caused by aspiration. It has been estimated that approximately 10% of patients with achalasia will develop a lower esophageal diverticulum, and a fourteenfold to sixteenfold increased risk of squamous cell cancer has been described. Because these cancers develop in the dilatated midesophagus, dysphagia is not experienced until late, and the prognosis is typically poor. Long-term retention of food with inflammation and chronic esophagitis is believed to be responsible for the increased risk of cancer.

The primary goal of therapy in achalasia is the relief of outflow obstruction at the LES. This can be accomplished by medical therapy, pneumatic dilatation, Botox (Allergan, Irvine, CA) injection, and surgical myotomy. Despite controversy, the increased patient acceptance and reduced morbidity of laparoscopic myotomy and partial fundoplication have resulted in surgical therapy being considered by most medical professionals to be the ideal therapy, especially in patients younger than 40 years of age.

Medical Therapy

Several pharmacologic agents are known to lower the resting pressure of the LES, including calcium channel blockers, nitrates, beta-agonists, and anticholinergic agents. Although each of these classes of drugs has been shown to improve symptoms to a degree, clinical improvement in patients with achalasia is usually modest at best. Side effects are also common, especially with anticholinergic

agents, and headaches and hypotension limit the long-term usefulness of nitrate therapy. As a result, medical treatment is generally reserved for use in high-risk elderly patients and those who refuse other forms of therapy. Recent studies in small groups of patients have suggested a role for phosphodiesterase inhibitors, such as sildenafil in lowering LES pressure in patients with achalasia. Long-term studies in larger numbers of patients will be necessary to assess the role of these agents in the medical treatment of achalasia.

Pneumatic Dilatation

Pneumatic dilatation has replaced early techniques of rigid or semirigid dilatation in the treatment of achalasia. The dilatating balloon is positioned across the gastroesophageal junction (GEJ), usually under fluoroscopy, and it is inflated to a diameter of 30 to 40 mm. Good to excellent results are reported in approximately 70% of patients following balloon dilatation, with 17% requiring repeat dilatations. Perforations occur in 3%, with an overall mortality rate of approximately 0.3%. In addition, the uncontrolled destruction of the LES by pneumatic dilatation may result in the development of reflux, which has been reported in up to 22% of patients.

Botox Injection

Endoscopic injection of botulinum toxin (80–100 U) in the LES has been proposed as a safe alternative to dilatation and surgical myotomy. Recent series have shown initial injections to be effective in approximately 65% of patients. The results, however, are usually temporary, with most patients requiring a second injection within 1 year. Mild to moderate postprocedure pain is the only common side effect of this procedure, although esophageal ulceration and hemorrhage have been reported. Long-term studies of the efficacy, safety, and cost effectiveness of repeat Botox injections require further review because the temporary nature of the benefit is likely to limit its applicability.

Surgical Myotomy

Although the best initial treatment for patients with achalasia is still debated, esophago-cardiomyotomy is considered by many to be the most definitive treatment for achalasia. The goal of surgery is to relieve the outflow obstruction at the LES without destroying the normal mechanisms responsible for the prevention of reflux. Historically, the most common operation performed for achalasia has been the transthoracic modified Heller myotomy, with a partial antireflux operation. An alternative approach, advocated by Ellis, used limited dissection of the cardia, eliminating the need for the addition of an antireflux procedure, which he believed may impart resistance to emptying, a situation that over time can lead to progressive dilatation of the esophagus and ultimately esophageal failure. Opponents to the limited myotomy approach argue that extending the myotomy precisely 5 mm onto the cardia is difficult. An error in either direction leads to either dysphagia from incomplete myotomy or reflux from an overly generous myotomy. To circumvent these complications, most centers, including our own, now recommend a complete LES myotomy, most often by the laparoscopic approach, with the addition of an antireflux procedure.

OPERATIVE TECHNIQUE

The laparoscopic myotomy and partial antireflux procedure is performed with the patient in a modified lithotomy position and the surgeon standing between the patient's legs. The laparoscopic ports are placed as for other laparoscopic upper GI procedures, such as the laparoscopic Nissen. The camera port is placed one third of the distance between the umbilicus and the xyphoid, either at the midline or in the left paramedian position. A self-retaining liver retractor is placed through a 5-mm port site just below the xyphoid. A retracting port is placed in the left lower quadrant, through which a Babcock clamp is inserted to allow retraction of the GEJ. The left-hand working port is placed in the epigastric region at or slightly to the right of the patient's midline. Finally, the surgeon's right-hand working port is placed in the left subcostal region.

The myotomy should be performed on the left anterolateral aspect of the GEJ to prevent injury to the anterior vagus nerve. In most patients, this requires little dissection of the hiatus, but it does require mobilization of the fat pad off of the GEJ, reflecting this tissue to the patient's right side. Placing the myotomy on the greater curvature side results in destruction only of the oblique fibers of the LES (Fig. 3). It has been suggested that preservation of the clasp fibers may result in less reflux, which is the most common problem long term after surgical treatment for achalasia. The myotomy should be started on the stomach, 1 to 2 cm below the GEJ, extending approximately 6 cm up the esophageal body.

After the myotomy has been completed, the edges of the divided muscle should be dissected off of the mucosa on each side of the myotomy to prevent rehealing of the myotomy and to facilitate

the performance of the partial fundoplication. This is best accomplished by grasping the muscle edge and gently separating the muscle from the mucosa by blunt dissection using a Kitner.

There are two options for performing a partial fundoplication laparoscopically. Debate persists with regard to the relative benefits of each. Our preferred approach is to perform a modified Dor anterior fundoplication in most patients. We reserve the more complicated Toupet posterior fundoplication for patients who need more extensive mobilization of the cardia region, such as the reoperative setting or in the presence of a hiatal hernia. The Dor fundoplication is performed by suturing a tongue of fundus to the left margin of the myotomy beginning at the GEJ, with four or five 2–0 silk sutures placed sequentially upward along on the myotomy. In most patients, there is sufficient mobility of the gastric fundus, but if tension exists, the short gastric vessels should be divided. At the apex of the tongue of fundus, a suture is placed between the tip of the stomach and the margin of the esophageal hiatus anteriorly. The tongue of fundus is then sutured to the esophageal muscle along the right margin of the myotomy, with these sutures placed parallel to and approximately 2 to 3 cm from the previous row of sutures.

In the setting of a hiatal hernia, which is present in approximately 5% of patients with achalasia, the hiatal region should be fully mobilized to allow reduction of the hernia and crural repair.

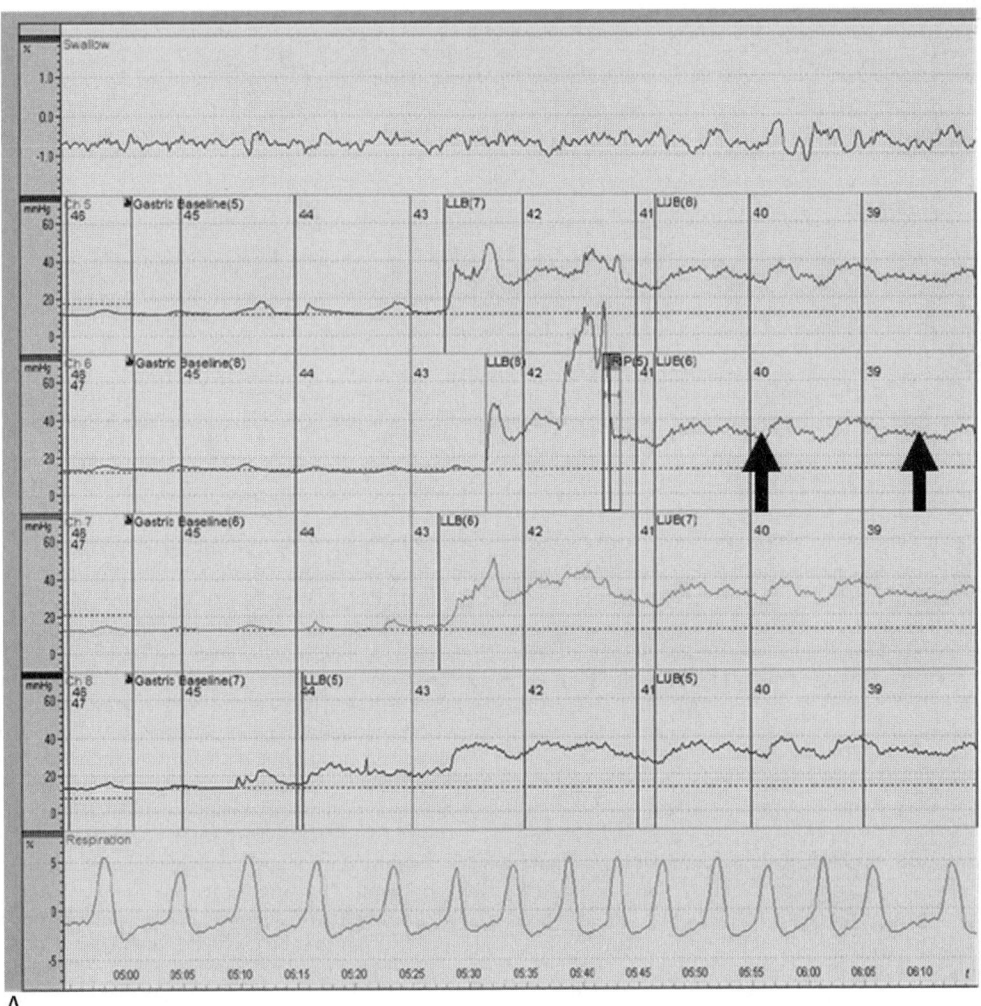

A

Figure 2 Manometric features in achalasia. **(A)** Motorized pull-through of the lower esophageal sphincter (LES) demonstrating a hypertensive LES and pressurization of the esophagus (*bold arrows*).

(continued)

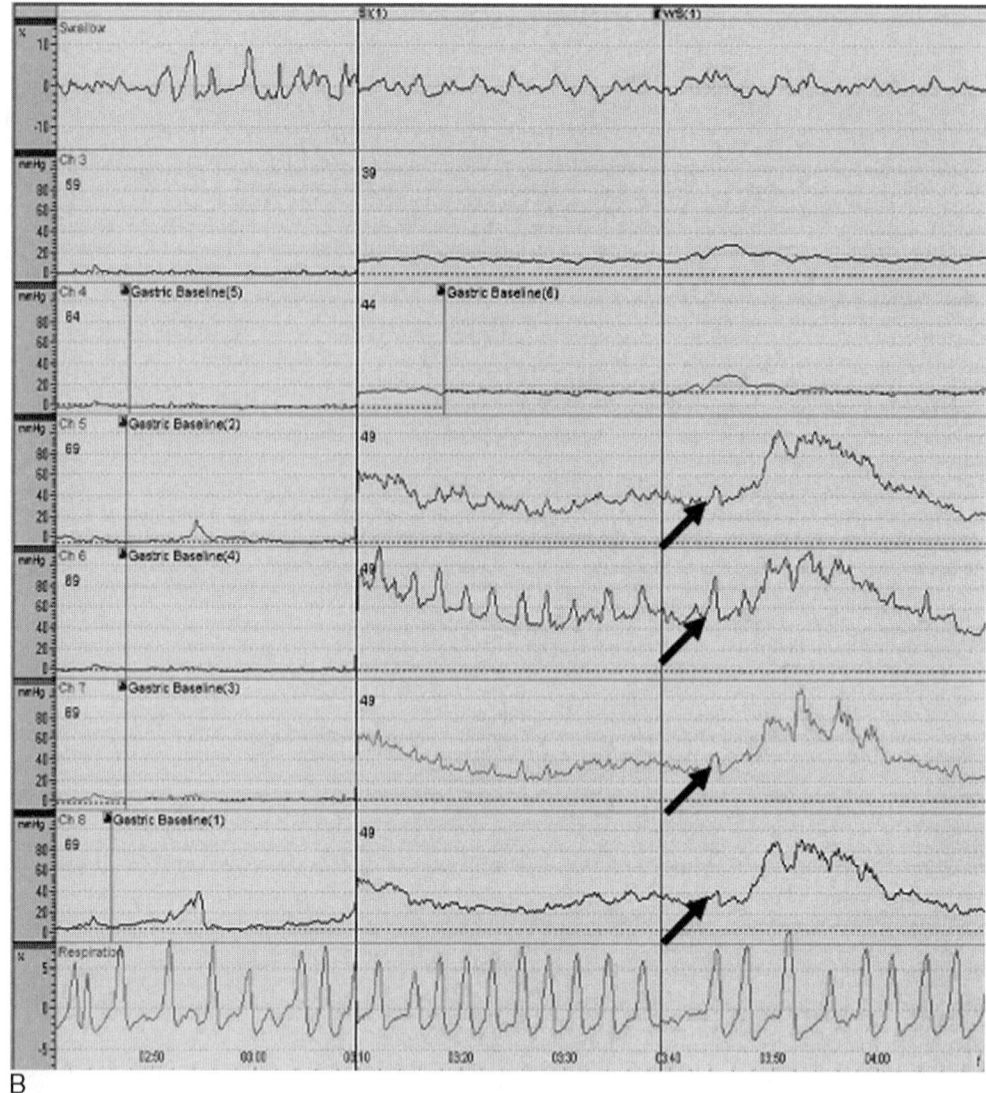

B

Figure 2 Cont'd—(B) LES relaxation study using four circumferential transducers showing failure of LES relaxation *(arrows)*. Note the simultaneous contractions in the esophageal body 5 and 10 cm above the LES.

These steps are identical to those used for a laparoscopic Nissen. Because of an increased tendency to reflux after such extensive dissection of the hiatal region, we recommend a Toupet posterior fundoplication. After division of the short gastric vessels, the fundus is delivered behind the GEJ, and the partial fundoplication is completed by suturing the anterior fundus to the left margin of the myotomy and the posterior fundus to the right margin along the length of the myotomy.

RESULTS

Despite the fact that both a randomized, prospective study by Csendes and retrospective studies by Okike and Donahue have demonstrated superior long-term results of myotomy compared with dilatation, many gastroenterologists still argue that the low cost, short recovery time, efficacy, and safety of pneumatic dilatation are reasons to consider it as first-line therapy for achalasia. However, these recommendations were made on the basis of experience before the advent of laparoscopic surgery, when the morbidity and recovery time associated with surgical therapy was considerably higher. Modern series reporting the results of pneumatic dilatation suggest that long-term success can be expected in approximately 70% of patients, even when repeated dilatations are performed. A number of risk factors for failure of pneumatic dilatation have been described. These include age older than 40 years and a residual LES pressure after dilatation of less than 20 mm Hg.

In comparison, 90% of patients treated by laparoscopic myotomy and partial antireflux procedures experience relief of dysphagia. These results appear to be independent of the age of the patient; however, like balloon dilatation, they depend on achieving a low resting LES pressure. The major late complications of myotomy are the development of gastroesophageal reflux with resulting esophagitis and peptic stricture formation. Reflux-induced Barrett's esophagus and esophageal adenocarcinoma have also been described.

Caution should be exercised in patients with a dilatated and tortuous esophagus. The sigmoid nature of the distal esophagus in these patients prevents gravity clearance after either dilatation or

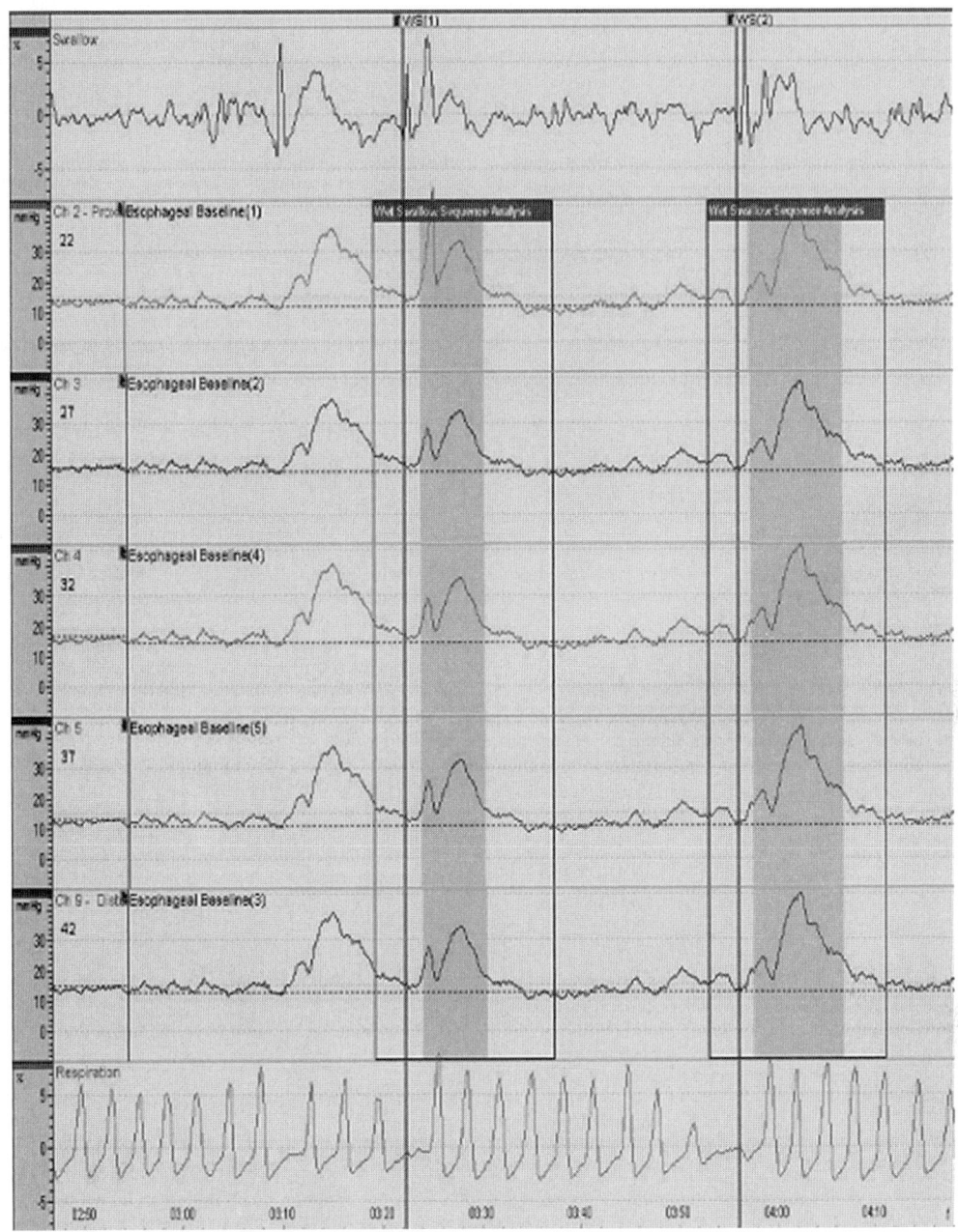

Figure 2 Cont'd—**(C)** Esophageal body study demonstrating absence of peristalsis, with isobaric simultaneous contractions in response to two wet swallows.

surgical myotomy. Esophageal resection should be considered in these patients. Esophagectomy should also be considered in patients who have failed multiple previous attempts at myotomy. Common causes of failure include an incomplete myotomy (usually on the gastric side), increased outflow resistance at the fundoplication, or a stricture as the result of reflux injury. The final circumstance for which esophagectomy should be considered is in patients with significant reflux following myotomy or dilatation. In this setting, poor esophageal clearance makes medical therapy difficult, and an operation to perform an effective antireflux procedure is likely to result in dysphagia. When resection is to be performed, we recommend a vagus-sparing esophagectomy as described by Akiyama, in which the esophagus is removed using a vein stripper. The excellent upper GI function associated with vagal nerve preservation makes this an attractive option when esophagectomy is considered for benign diseases such as achalasia.

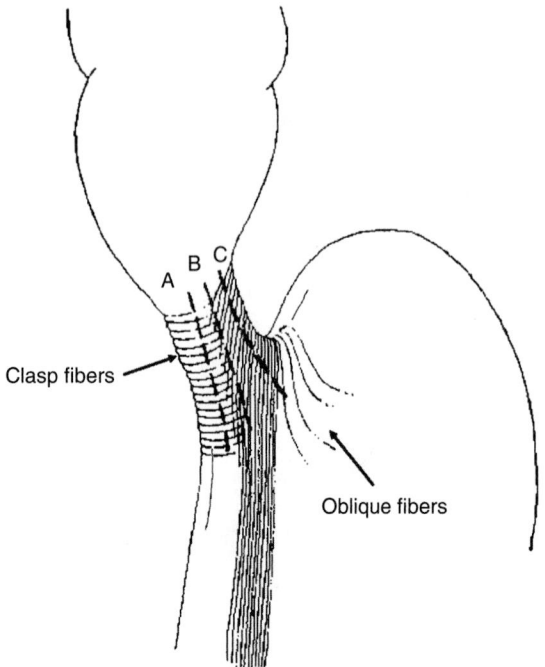

Figure 3 Possible sites for location of the myotomy. Myotomy performed at *A* results in division of the clasp fibers alone and may result in incomplete relief of outflow obstruction. *Line B* traverses both the clasp and oblique fibers and may result in total destruction of the lower esophageal sphincter (LES) mechanism, resulting in difficult-to-manage reflux. Performing the myotomy on the greater curvature side, *line C*, results in destruction of the oblique fibers alone, leaving some protection against reflux by the clasp fibers on the lesser curvature side of the LES.

SUGGESTED READINGS

Akiyama H, Tsurumaru M, Ono Y, and others: Esophagectomy without thoracotomy with vagal preservation, *J Am Coll Surg* 178:83, 1994.

Bonavina L, Nosadini A, Bardini R, and others: Primary treatment of esophageal achalasia. Long-term results of myotomy and Dor fundoplication, *Arch Surg* 127:222, 1992.

Csendes A, Braghetto I, Henríquez A, and others: Late results of a prospective randomized study comparing forceful dilatation and oesophagomyotomy in patients with achalasia, *Gut* 30:299, 1989.

Cuillière C, Ducrotté P, Zerbib F, and others: Achalasia: outcome of patients treated with intrasphincteric injection of botulinum toxin, *Gut* 41:87, 1997.

Donahue PE, Samelson S, Schlesinger PK, and others: Achalasia of the esophagus: treatment controversies and the method of choice, *Ann Surg* 203:505, 1986.

Eckardt VF, Aignherr C, Bernhard G: Predictors of outcome in patients with achalasia treated by pneumatic dilation, *Gastroenterology* 103:1732, 1992.

Eckhardt VF, Gockel I, Bernhard G: Pneumatic dilatation for achalasia: late results of a prospective follow-up investigation, *Gut* 53:629, 2004.

Ellis FH Jr., Watkins E Jr., Gibb SP, and others: Ten to 20-year clinical results after short esophagomyotomy without an antireflux procedure (modified Heller operation) for esophageal achalasia, *Eur J Cardiothorac Surg* 6:86, 1992.

Ferguson MK: Achalasia: current evaluation and therapy, *Ann Thorac Surg* 52:336, 1991.

Hunter JG, Trus TL, Branum GD, and others: Laparoscopic Heller myotomy and fundoplication for achalasia, *Ann Surg* 225:655, 1997.

Okike N, Payne SW, Neufeld DM, and others: Esophagomyotomy versus forceful dilation for achalasia of the esophagus: results in 899 patients, *Ann Thorac Surg* 28:119, 1979.

Patti MG, Pellegrini CA, Horgan S, and others: Minimally invasive surgery for achalasia: an 8-year experience with 168 patients, *Ann Surg* 230:587, 1999.

Peters JH, Werner KH, Crookes PF, and others: Esophageal resection with colon interposition for end-stage achalasia, *Arch Surg* 130:632, 1995.

Speiss AE, Kahrilas PJ: Treating achalasia: From whalebone to laparoscope, *JAMA* 280:638, 1998.

Wehrmann T, Jacobi V, Jung M, and others: Pneumatic dilation in achalasia with a low-compliance balloon: results of a 5-year prospective evaluation, *Gastrointest Endosc* 42:31, 1995.

MINIMALLY INVASIVE ESOPHAGECTOMY

Lee L. Swanstrom, MD, and Christy Dunst, MD

BACKGROUND

Esophagectomy has been identified by governing and advisory bodies as one of the current crop of "volume-sensitive" procedures. This is because of its relative rarity as a procedure (<14,000 per year in the United States), complexity as a surgical procedure, and high morbidity and mortality even in the best of hands. Like Whipple procedures and coronary artery bypass, esophagectomy outcomes are best when performed by highly experienced surgeons in high-volume centers. Esophagectomy numbers have been further reduced because of competitive, less invasive, alternative treatments that, although not curative, offer an escape from the perceived "fate-worse-than-death" status of open esophagectomy. Application of laparoscopic and thoracoscopic techniques therefore makes supreme sense because they offer the patient the best chance of a cure while sparing some of the morbidity of large incisions. Totally endoscopic esophagectomy was first described by DePaula in 1995 as a laparoscopic transhiatal approach. Subsequently, the combined laparoscopic/thoracoscopic approaches, with anastomosis in either the chest or neck, became more popular, with more and more esophageal centers offering minimally invasive approaches.

Table 1: Indications for Minimally Invasive Esophagectomy

- Benign disease
  - End-stage achalasia
  - Refractory strictures
  - Failed motor function
- Multiple redo antireflux surgery
- Scleroderma or profound dysmotility
- Acute problems
  - Perforations
- Premalignant disease
  - Dysplastic Barrett's esophagus
- Malignant disease
  - Barrett's adenocarcinoma
  - Squamous cell carcinoma

INDICATIONS

Although rare, end-stage, benign esophageal disorders represent an ideal patient population for a less invasive surgical approach (Table 1). Another rare indication for palliative esophagectomy is incurable cancers not amenable to palliative treatments. By far the most common indication for any esophagectomy is curative cancer resection. There are few data to support or refute the appropriateness of minimally invasive esophagectomy as a curative cancer surgery. The overall number of esophageal cancer surgeries is so low, in fact, that it has proved difficult to define the indications for and technical impacts of any open surgical approaches. Oncologic data from laparoscopic colon cancer surgery seem to support the equivalence, if not the superiority, of minimally invasive cancer treatments, and there is no doubt that the overall poor cure rates with esophageal cancer make a less invasive approach appealing.

PATIENT PREPARATION

There is little difference between the preparation and counseling of a minimally invasive esophagectomy patient and a patient who will undergo an open resection. Maximizing pulmonary function is critical, as is deep vein thrombosis prophylaxis. Patients should be cautioned about the possibility of conversion to an open procedure, should that become necessary; standard complications; and expected course of recovery. Cancer patients should be informed that laparoscopy offers the potential for an improved recovery but that its long-term efficacy has yet to be proved. The surgeon should have blood products and an intensive care unit (ICU) bed available regardless of whether they seem necessary. Invasive monitoring is indicated as well. Even for thoracoscopic procedures, we no longer use a double-lumen endotracheal tube, preferring instead to use standard laparoscopic ports and low-pressure CO_2 insufflation.

TECHNIQUES

Each of the three different open esophagectomy techniques (transhiatal, thoracic/abdominal [Ivor Lewis], and "three hole") has been replicated with an endoscopic or endoscopically assisted technique. Laparoscopic reconstruction, however, has so far been limited to gastric pull-up procedures, and there are as yet no reports of a colon or jejunal interposition being performed endoscopically. A combination approach with thoracoscopic mobilization, laparoscopic creation of the gastric interposition, and a cervical anastomosis is currently the most popular procedure, with totally laparoscopic approaches being the next most popular. The

availability of flexible, circular, anastomotic staplers may make the laparoscopic/thoracoscopic Ivor Lewis procedure more popular, as well. We favor the use of a narrow (3-cm) gastric tube because of its superior, long-term function (better clearance and bolus transport) and lack of dilatation over time. A pyloroplasty is not routinely used because it contributes to bile reflux. On rare occasions, patients will experience delayed gastric emptying for more than a few months after surgery; for these cases we perform endoscopic pyloric dilatation with or without Botox (Allergan, Irvine, CA) injections.

Laparoscopic Transhiatal Esophagectomy

For benign disease and smaller distal esophageal cancers, we prefer the laparoscopic transhiatal approach. Although the upper mediastinal dissection is more difficult, anesthesia is less complex and there is no requirement to undrape and reposition the patient mid-procedure. The magnification and precision of the laparoscope permit both an upper abdominal lymphadenectomy and a lower mediastinal clean-out; the inability to perform either of these functions remains a criticism of the open transhiatal approach.

The patient is anesthetized, lines are placed, and the patient is positioned on a split-leg operating table with legs spread. Care is taken to carefully pad and protect all extremities to prevent neuropraxia or pressure ulcers during these long procedures. The head is placed on a donut pad and turned to the patient's right to allow access to the left neck for the proximal dissection and anastomosis. Instrumentation needed is listed in Table 2, and operating room setup is illustrated in Figure 1.

Five abdominal ports (2 10-mm and 3 5-mm) are placed, as shown in Figure 2. Careful staging laparoscopy is performed,

Table 2: Instruments Required for Minimally Invasive Esophagectomy

Laparoscopic Tools

10-mm ports × 2, 5-mm ports × 3
30-degree laparoscope
Bariatric length 30-degree scope
Atraumatic graspers
Standard length
Bariatric length (45 cm)
Maryland grasper
Laparoscopic needle holders
5-mm ultrasonic coagulating shears
Scissors

Open Instruments

Emergency conversion laparotomy set
Minor instrument set for neck dissection
Atraumatic deep self-retaining retractors
Suction
Electrocautery
Long curved aortic clamp
Kitner-type dissectors
Other
Specimen retrieval bags
Drains
Flexible upper endoscope

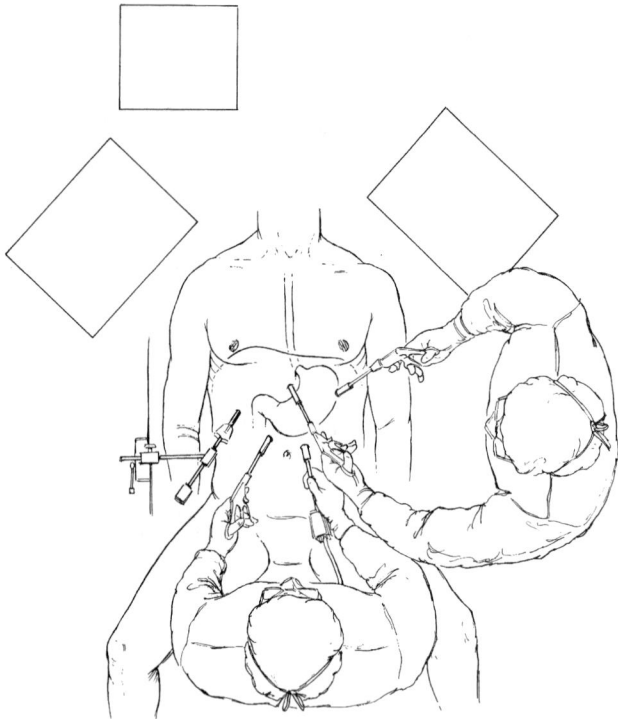

Figure 1   Typical operating room setup for a totally laparoscopic transhiatal esophagectomy.   *From Soper NJ, Swanstrom LL, editors: Mastery of endoscopic and laparoscopic surgery, ed 2, Philadelphia, 2005, Lippincott Williams & Wilkins, p. 206, with permission.*

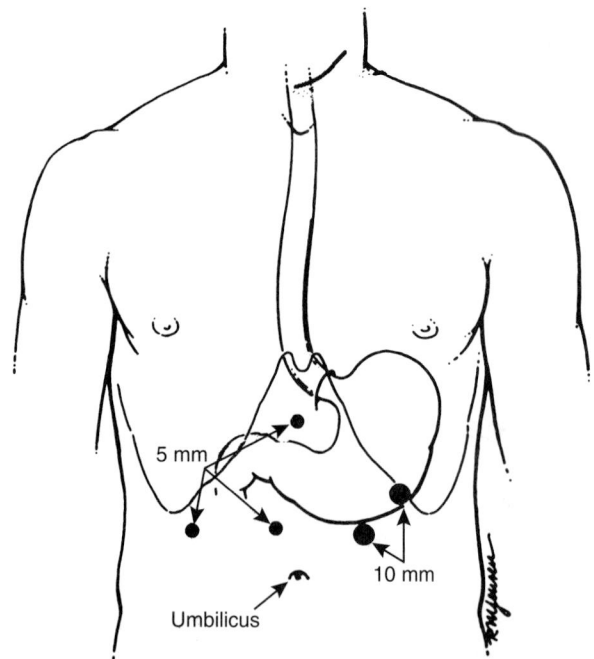

Figure 2   Port placement for the laparoscopic transhiatal approach.

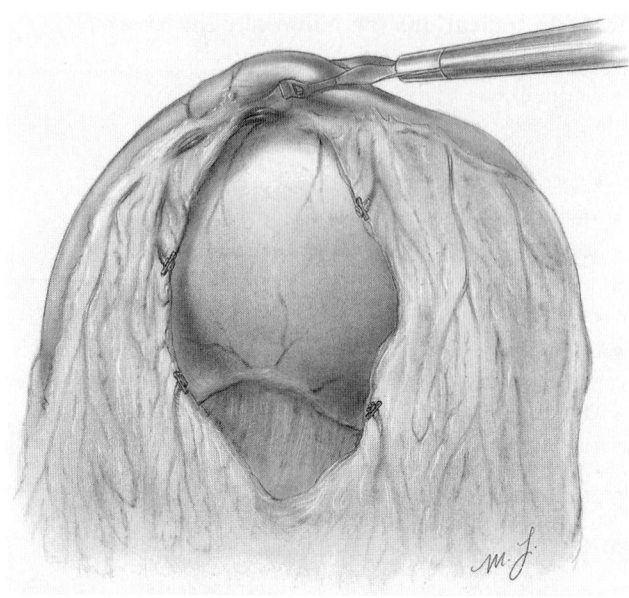

Figure 3   The greater curve of the stomach is mobilized, staying well away from the epiploic vascular arcade.   *From Soper NJ, Swanstrom LL, Eubanks WS, editors: Mastery of endoscopic and laparoscopic surgery, ed 2, Philadelphia, 2005, Lippincott Williams & Wilkins, p. 253, with permission.*

and any suspicious lesions are biopsied and sent for frozen section analysis. The gastroepiploic arcade is identified along the greater gastric curvature, and the gastrocolic omentum is divided, opening into the lesser sack. With a "no touch" technique, the stomach is gently elevated and the greater curve is mobilized with the

ultrasonic shears; care is taken to stay away from the vascular arcade (Fig. 3). This dissection is taken cephalad to the left crus and inferiorly to the point at which the gastroepiploic vessels pass behind the duodenum. Retrogastric adhesions to the pancreas and retroperitoneum are divided, and the surgeon checks again for evidence of tumor invasion. Division of these adhesions exposes the left gastric pedicle as it arises from the celiac axis. The origin of the left gastric artery is dissected free, and a removable clip is placed across it to document the vascularity of the gastric replacement. Attention is now directed to the lesser curvature, where the duodenum is Kocherized and the hepatogastric ligament is widely resected (Fig. 4), exposing the primary lymphatic basin and the celiac trunk. For distal esophageal or cardiac cancers, an en bloc lymphadenectomy is performed; all nodes and lymph tissue superior to the portal vein, lateral to the hepatic artery, medial to the vena cava, and inferior to the diaphragm (station 16, 17, 18 and 20 nodes) are removed. With a vascular stapler the left gastric artery and vein are divided at their origin, exposing the suprapancreatic nodes (station 19 nodes) along the left crus, which can be removed, labeled, and sent to the pathology laboratory. A narrow, 3–cm-diameter gastric conduit is created using multiple firings of an endoscopic linear stapler (Fig. 5). The first firing is immediately below the crow's foot vessels on the lesser curve in a transverse fashion. Subsequent firings follow the greater curve up to the cardia of the stomach, where the neoesophagus is then transected. Next, the mediastinum is opened by excising a rim of hiatus while pulling downward on the gastric remnant. Mediastinal dissection is performed by staying directly on the aorta, mediastinal pleura, and pericardium. This effectively leaves all lymph nodes and lymphatics with the surgical specimen. Two methods are available for the mediastinal mobilization. The first is simply to continue the transhiatal dissection by advancing the scope and instruments into the mediastinum while the assistant continues to pull downward on the esophagus (Fig. 6). This will usually allow dissection up to the carina, where the subcarinal nodes can be removed and sent separately for staging. The retrotracheal esophagus is usually mobilized by a second team from the neck incision using a gentle finger and Kitner dissection. The last bit of upper mediastinum is mobilized under laparoscopic visualization using the long bariatric

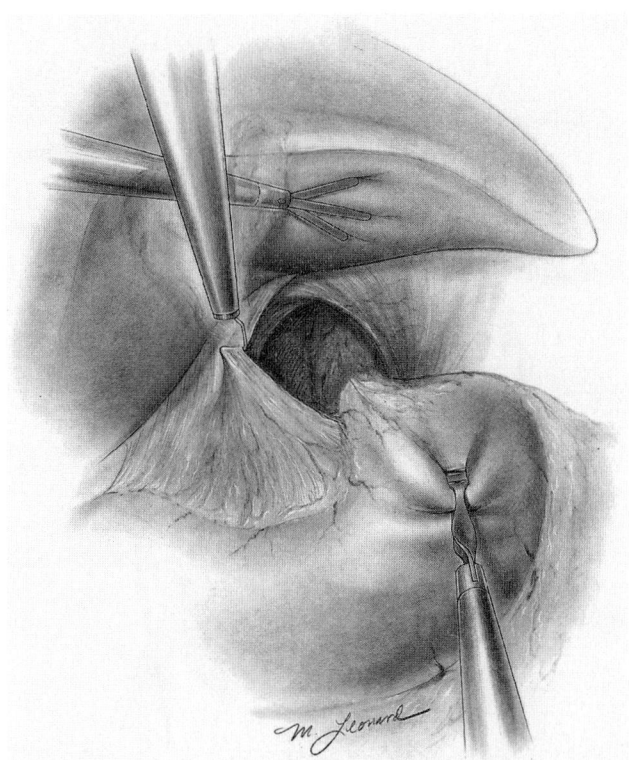

Figure 4 Mobilization of the lesser curve of the stomach. *From Soper NJ, Swanstrom LL, Eubanks WS, editors: Mastery of endoscopic and laparoscopic surgery, ed 2, Philadelphia, 2005, Lippincott Williams & Wilkins, p. 225, with permission.*

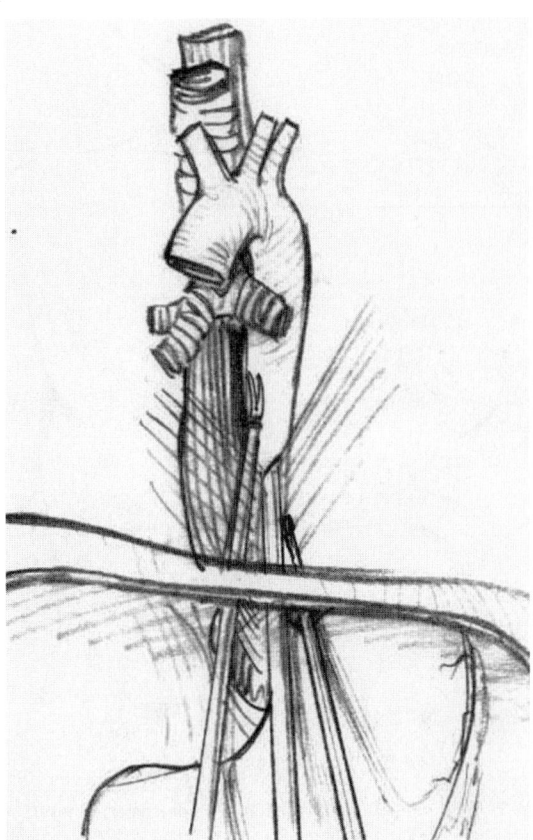

Figure 6 Transhiatal dissection of the esophagus proceeds by moving the laparoscope and dissecting instruments progressively into the mediastinum.

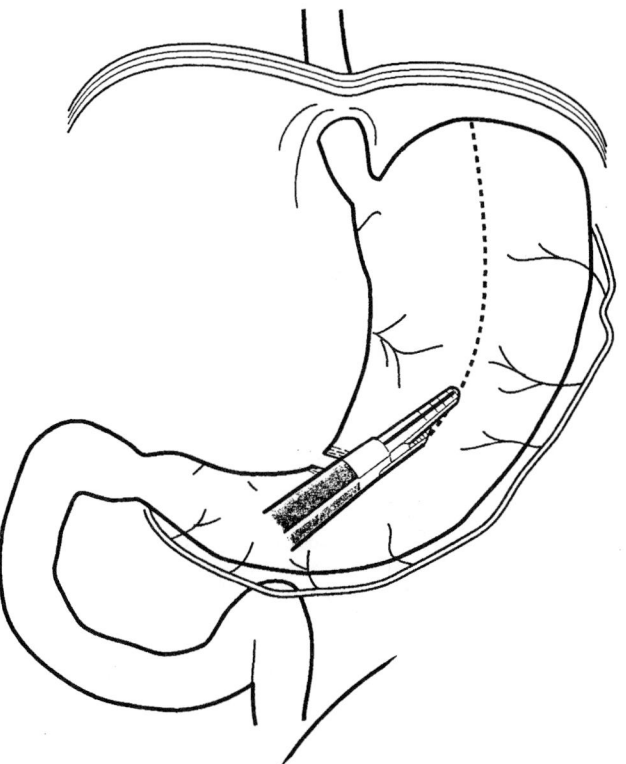

Figure 5 A 3-cm gastric conduit is created with multiple firings of the articulating endoscopic linear stapler. *From Soper NJ, Swanstrom LL, Eubanks WS, editors: Mastery of endoscopic and laparoscopic surgery, ed 2, Philadelphia, 2005, Lippincott Williams & Wilkins, p. 241, with permission.*

laparoscope and a sponge stick made with the long curved aortic clamp and folded gauze. A standard, 15-cm laparoscopic specimen bag is placed over the nodes, and the cancerous part of the gastro-esophageal remnant and the purse string are tightened. The specimen can then be removed from the neck incision.

The other technique is the "inversion" method. This is useful for small cancers and benign disease. An esophagotomy is made in the cervical esophagus, and a nasogastric tube or a vein stripper is passed down to the blind pouch. It is advanced out through a nick in the stomach and sutured, or the largest vein-stripper "olive" is placed. The team at the cervical incision then starts to pull on the stripper, which imbricates the stomach into the esophagus (Fig. 7). The laparoscopic team can then follow the inverting esophagus into the mediastinum and divide tissues shown to be still holding it in place. The esophagus therefore serves as its own specimen bag to prevent tumor contamination. After dividing the cervical esophagus, a 28-F chest tube is then passed from the neck into the abdomen, where the gastric tube can be sewn to its end. The chest tube is withdrawn, pulling the neoesophagus along with it. Care must be taken to prevent the narrow tube from twisting and to keep the gastric mesentery from tearing as it advances into the mediastinum. The proximal tube can be resected back to freely bleeding tissue and an anastomosis performed using either a stapler technique or suturing in a two-layer fashion. The hiatus is loosely closed with permanent sutures, and a slight antireflux valve is created by suturing the anterior antrum to the rim of the hiatus, creating a right-sided Dor-type repair. The narrow tube and antireflux mechanism obviate the need for a pyloroplasty. A laparoscopic feeding jejunostomy is routinely added. A closed-suction drain is inserted through a port site and placed partly across the mediastinum after the area is irrigated well and hemostasis has been confirmed. A drain is likewise

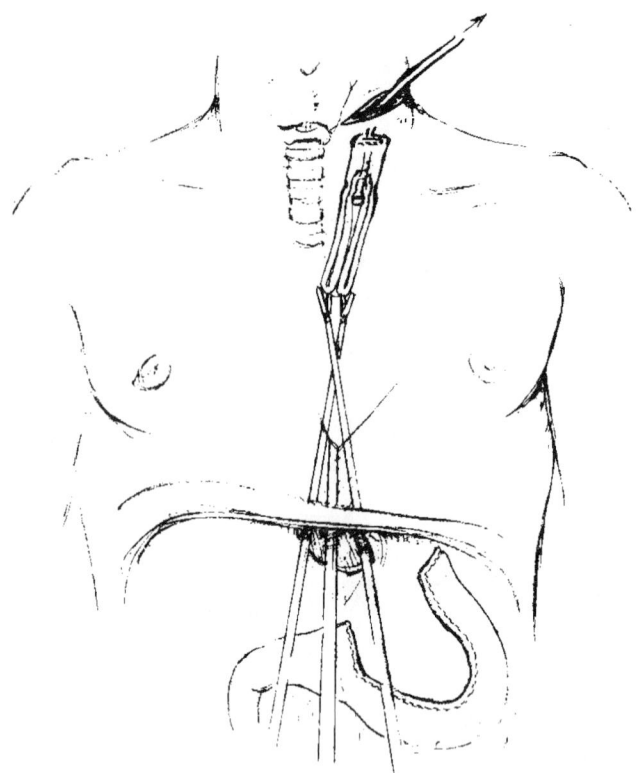

Figure 7   The mediastinal dissection is made easier by inverting the esophagus into itself.   *From Arch Surg 141(9):857, 2006, with permission.*

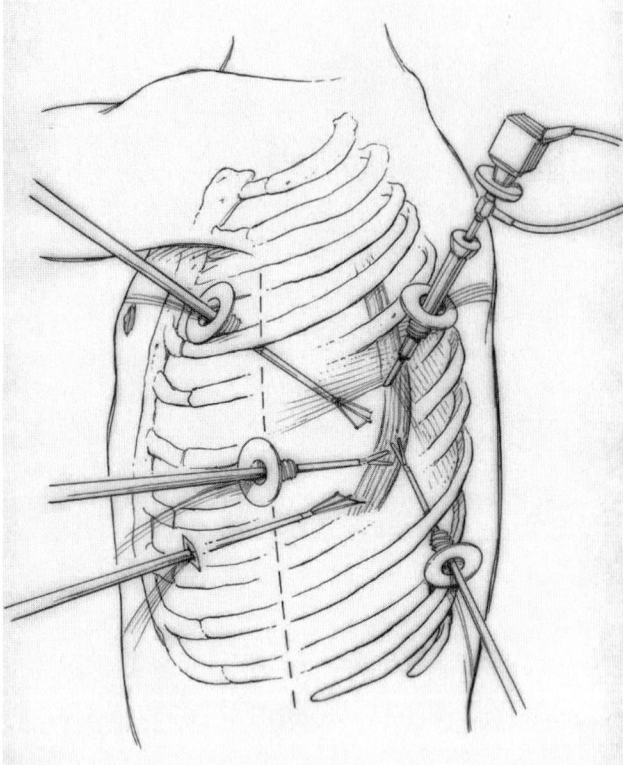

Figure 8   The lateral decubitus position and port placement for thoracoscopic esophageal mobilization.   *From Arch Surg 141(9): 857, 2006, with permission.*

placed in the neck wound, with the tip directed slightly into the upper mediastinum, before the neck is closed.

Thoracoscopic/Laparoscopic Esophagectomy

Many prefer a combination thoracoscopic/laparoscopic approach for minimally invasive esophagectomy. Arguments in favor of this approach include the ability to stage and perform wide nodal dissections of the mediastinal esophagus and to operate more quickly by avoiding the tedious transhiatal dissection. Arguments against this approach include the more complex anesthesia required with thoracoscopy and the added time of repositioning and repreparing the patient midway through the procedure.

There are two combined approaches: the first replicates the traditional Ivor Lewis approach with an intrathoracic anastomosis. The second involves thoracoscopic mobilization first with subsequent laparoscopic gastric mobilization and a cervical anastomosis. With either choice, the gastric mobilization and tailoring are the same as described for the transhiatal approach. Choice of the laparoscopic/thoracoscopic Ivor Lewis or three-hole approach depends on tumor location and the surgeon's comfort with an intrathoracic anastomosis. For distal small tumors we prefer the Ivor Lewis approach because of the resulting larger gastric reservoir and lower stricture rates.

Laparoscopic/Thoracoscopic Ivor Lewis

Laparoscopic/thoracoscopic Ivor Lewis procedures begin in the standard split-leg position with five laparoscopic ports placed as in a laparoscopic transhiatal resection (LTHR)(Fig. 2). The abdomen is explored, the stomach is mobilized, and a 20-cm

gastric conduit is created from the greater curvature of the proximal stomach. A D-2 node dissection is carried out when indicated, and the lower mediastinum is opened by widely excising the phrenoesophageal ligament. The mediastinal esophagus is mobilized transhiatally for 5 to 10 cm, staying wide to keep the lymphatics in continuity with the esophagus. The right mediastinal pleura is then opened, and the transected stomach and neoesophagus are pushed up into the right chest. The gastric antrum is then sutured to the rim of the hiatus, or, alternatively, the hiatus can be closed with sutures around the narrow neoesophagus approximately 2 cm above the junction of the neoesophagus and antrum. This allows the surgeon to tack the anterior gastric wall to the hiatal rim to form a type of antireflux mechanism.

The patient is then repositioned on a beanbag cushion in the left lateral decubitus position, with the usual precautions being taken to prevent any pressure points. Two 10-mm and three 5-mm ports are placed in a diamond configuration (Fig. 8). The lung is swept anteriorly and held, and the mediastinum is opened from above the azygous vein to the hiatus. The azygous is routinely divided with a vascular staple load to allow adequate dissection. Once again, wide dissection is performed, removing all paraesophageal lymphatics including the thoracic duct, which should be carefully ligated. The subcarinal nodes are removed as a packet and sent separately for staging. The esophagus is divided at the level of the azygous, and the gastric conduit is brought up to it. The anastomosis can be performed in any of several ways: hand sewn, with a circular stapler, or with a linear stapler. Use of a flexible-shaft, circular stapler is a new possibility that permits the per-oral insertion of a circular stapler; this makes intrathoracic anastomosis fairly straightforward (Fig. 9). Finally, one of the port sites is widened, and the specimen is removed and sent to the pathology laboratory to confirm clear margins. A chest tube is inserted through one of the port sites. Recently we have begun to place a removable covered esophageal

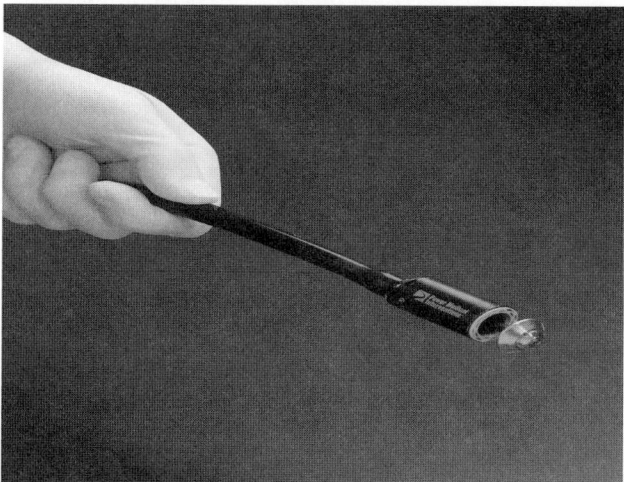

Figure 9 Newer flexible shafted staplers permit per-oral insertion for an easier thoracic anastomosis. *Courtesy Power Medical Interventions, Langhorne, PA.*

stent (PolyFlex, Boston Scientific, Natick, MA) across the anastomosis, fixing it with a transmural absorbable suture. This serves to prophylactically protect the high-risk anastomosis and prevent strictures during healing.

"Three-Hole" Laparoscopic/Thoracoscopic Esophagectomy

The same dissection, resection, and anastomosis are performed in a three-hole procedure (as popularized by Luketich and colleagues) as in the techniques described previously, but the order is changed. The patient starts with a right thoracoscopy. The esophagus is mobilized as described earlier, except that the dissection is continued to the proximal thoracic outlet. After this has been accomplished and the node dissection has been performed, a chest tube is placed and the patient is repositioned in the supine split-leg position. The abdominal portion of the procedure is performed in the standard fashion, while at the same time a left cervical incision is made and the cervical esophagus is mobilized. Typically the stomach and tumor are placed in a specimen bag and withdrawn through the neck wound following transection of the cervical esophagus. A chest tube is then passed from the neck incision through the mediastinum and into the abdomen. The gastric tube is then sutured to the end of the chest tube and carefully pulled up into the neck, where an anastomosis can be performed. This can be a sutured or stapled anastomosis. A feeding jejunostomy is created by suturing a section of proximal jejunum to the anterior abdominal wall. A needle is inserted into the lumen of the jejunum, a guidewire is placed, and a 14-F peel-away sheath is inserted. A 14-F red rubber catheter is inserted, and the peel-away sheath removed. Finally, closed-suction drains are placed in the neck and via one of the port sites across the hiatus (Fig. 10).

POSTOPERATIVE CARE

Depending on the patient's underlying comorbidities and anesthesia factors, a decision is made regarding postoperative disposition. Effort is made to extubate the patient immediately after surgery. Patients are usually observed overnight in the ICU. Tube feedings are started on postoperative day 1, and a Gastrografin (Bracco diagnostics, Princeton, NJ) swallow is ordered for day 3. Patients are started on a thickened liquid diet and sent home on a pureed diet for 2 weeks, along with nighttime tube feeding supplements.

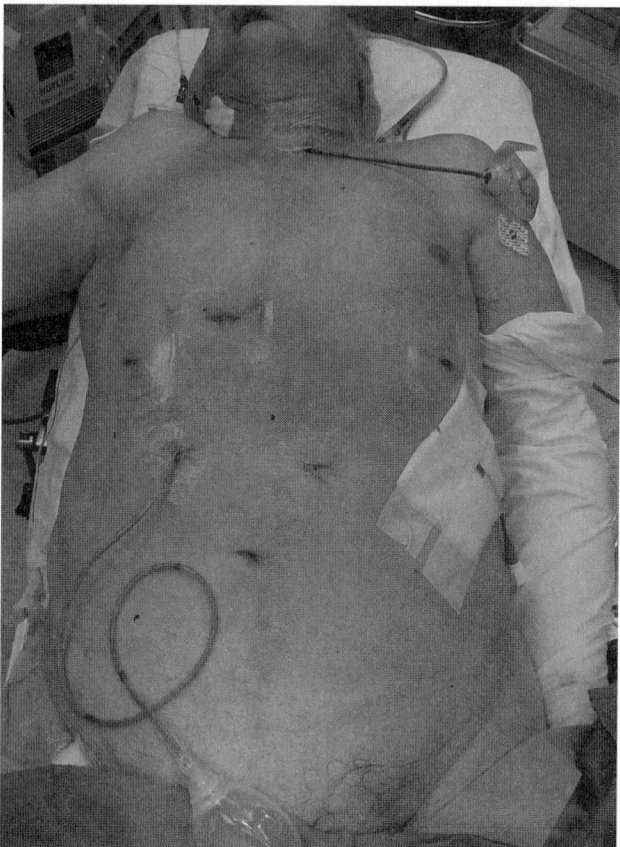

Figure 10 Final view after minimally invasive esophagectomy, with drains and feeding jejunostomy in place.

RESULTS

Overall results of the various minimally invasive techniques are good, showing promise of reduced patient morbidity; speedier recovery; and, for selected patients, equivalent oncologic results. Table 3 shows our institutional results with regard to operative outcomes. Figure 11 describes our survival results for cancer cases.

Table 3: Operative Outcomes for Minimally Invasive Esophagectomy at Legacy Health System (1994–2005)

$N = 128$ (45 female, 83 male); mean age = 67 (range 32–84) Indication	12 benign
	33 Barrett's high-grade dysplasia
	83 cancer resection
Procedure	103 laparoscopic transhiatal
	19 thoracoscopic/ laparoscopic with cervical anastomosis
	6 laparoscopic/thoracoscopic with thoracic anastomosis Conversion 5 (4%)
Operative time	382 min (235–525)
Blood loss	280 ml (120–780)

(continued)

Table 3: Operative Outcomes for Minimally Invasive Esophagectomy at Legacy Health System (1994–2005)—Cont'd

Operative complications	
Bleeding	6
Splenectomy	2
Bowel injury	1
Gastric interposition ischemia	2
Tracheal injury	1
Perioperative complications	
MI	
PE	
Pneumonia	
Anastomotic leak	
Neoesophagus ischemia	
Stroke	
Bleeding	
Wound infection	
Chylothorax	
Mortality	
In hospital	2
30 days	1
LOS	6 days (4–31)

LOS, Length of (hospital) stay; *MI,* myocardial infarction; *PE,* pulmonary embolism.

CONCLUSION

Minimally invasive esophagectomy is a necessary development if surgery is going to remain an option for treatment of end-stage benign disease and cancers. Experiences to date support this as an effective treatment, but the learning curve is long and difficult. The best surgical approach remains subject to debate, and it will probably be some time before a consensus on the optimal technique is reached.

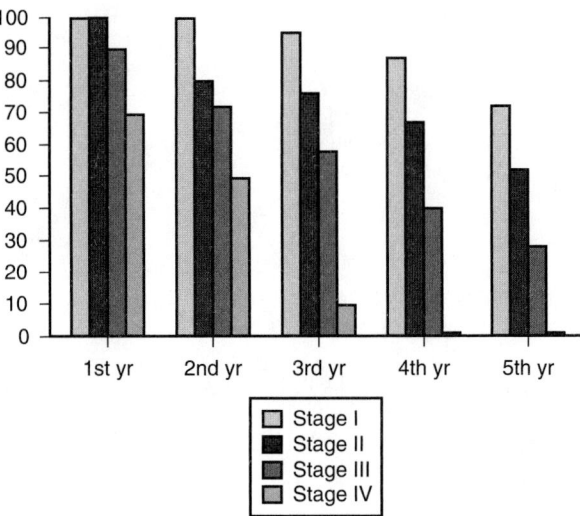

Figure 11 Cancer survival rates by stage following laparoscopic esophagectomy.

SUGGESTED READINGS

Avital S, Zundel N, Szomstein S, and others: Laparoscopic transhiatal esophagectomy for esophageal cancer, *Am J Surg* 190(1):69, 2005.

Cuesta MA, van den Broek WT, van der Peet DL, and others: Minimally invasive esophageal resection, *Semin Laparosc Surg* 11(3):147, 2004.

Huscher CG, Mingoli A, Sgarzini G, and others: Laparoscopic approach for the treatment of type II gastroesophageal junction tumors, *J Am Coll Surg* 200(6):983, 2005.

Jobe BA, Reavis KM, Davis JJ, and others: Laparoscopic inversion esophagectomy: simplifying a daunting operation, *Dis Esophagus* 17(1):95, 2004.

Luketich JD, Alvelo-Rivera M, Buenaventura PO, and others: Minimally invasive esophagectomy: outcomes in 222 patients, *Ann Surg* 238(4):486, 2003.

McConkey PP, Moore PG, Nguyen NT: Haemodynamic compromise during thoracoscopic/laparoscopic oesophagectomy, *Anaesth Intensive Care* 29(6):631, 2001.

Nguyen NT, Follette DM, Lemoine PH, and others: Minimally invasive Ivor Lewis esophagectomy, *Ann Thorac Surg* 72(2):593, 2001.

LAPAROSCOPIC HEPATECTOMY

Edward C.S. Lai, MS

Over the past two decades, surgical outcome following liver resection has improved dramatically as technologies have advanced. Surgeons are now able to select their patients for the appropriate procedure by localizing the target lesion with greater accuracy, especially its relationship with the neighboring key anatomic structures. The availability of different instruments allows meticulous and precise transection of the liver tissue along the plane desired, minimizing the risk of biliary and vascular injury and the amount of intraoperative blood loss. At the same time, surgeons take great care not only to evaluate the functional reserve of the proposed liver remnant but also to keep the duration of temporary hepatic blood flow interruption to the necessary minimum to protect the liver function. Depending on the degree of underlying cirrhosis and extent of surgery, the accepted mortality rates following conventional open hepatectomy have dropped precipitously, to ≤6%. In addition, liver surgeons are now able to spare the majority of their patients from perioperative blood transfusion. In the absence of severe cirrhosis, most patients can be discharged from hospital approximately 1 week after surgery. It is against these developments that the worth of any new procedure should be measured.

Despite technical advances, liver surgery is still a complicated and high-risk operation. Nonetheless, committed surgeons are able to broaden the scope of laparoscopic surgery to include liver resection. Over the past decade, laparoscopic hepatectomy has gained acceptance by the medical community as a viable therapeutic alternative to traditional open hepatectomy. At the end of the twentieth century, when laparoscopic liver resection first became popular, the literature was filled primarily with isolated case reports or summaries of limited early experiences. More recently prospective or retrospective comparative studies on cohorts of larger case numbers, and even major anatomic liver resection of three or more Couinaud segments, have been reported. To date, most surgeons agree that small lesions of less than 5 cm in diameter and located close to the edge of liver, namely, segments 5, 6, 4b, and the left lateral segment (segments 2 and 3) can be considered for laparoscopic resection, especially if they are pedunculated. Major anatomic resection, however, remains a great technical challenge, with no general consensus on its role as a routine procedure.

PATIENT PREPARATION AND POSITION

The necessary preoperative preparation for a laparoscopic liver resection is no different from that of open liver surgery. All potential candidates for liver resection are evaluated on the basis of anatomic location, lateralization of the tumor, and functional reserve of the liver remnant. An estimation of the risk of posthepatectomy liver failure depends on a combination of liver volumetry, with the help of computed tomography, and hepatic functional reserve using standard liver function tests with focus on the serum total bilirubin titer, serum albumin level, prothrombin time, and in many Asian centers, indocyanine green retention rate. The cardiopulmonary status of the patient must be considered carefully. When a pneumoperitoneum was established with carbon dioxide, repeated episodes of subclinical gas embolism, resulting in occasional runs of arrhythmia, had been documented with transesophageal echocardiography in a porcine model. A clear informed consent for open resection must be obtained because, even in experienced centers, a conversion rate of 15% is anticipated for major liver resection. After induction of anesthesia, a large-bore central line is placed for monitoring purposes, a nasogastric tube is passed to keep the stomach deflated, and a urinary catheter is inserted to observe closely the urinary output. Compressive stockings with sequential compressive devices are routinely used to guard against deep vein thrombosis. The body temperature is kept normothermic throughout the operation with the help of a warm-air pneumatic bag covering the upper extremity.

Patient position is dictated primarily by the location of the liver tumor and the preference of the surgical team. As a general guideline, and if the lesion can be resected with the usual standard abdominal incision, the patient is placed supine with legs separated in a modified lithotomy position (fully extended hip joints and 90-degree flexed knees). The operating surgeon stands between the legs of the patient for lesions located at segments 2 to 5 and peripheral aspect for lesions at segment 6. For lesions located at the back of the right hepatic lobe (segments 6 and 7), the patient is tilted right-side up at a 45-degree angle from the table. The right arm of the patient is supported across the chest. The operating surgeon stands at the left of the table. In selected cases, a hand port can offer much better retraction of the mobilized right hepatic lobe.

A 30-degree laparoscope is introduced via a supraumbilical or infraumbilical incision, depending on the build of the patient. In case of a difficult tumor with a considerable chance of conversion, the planned abdominal incision is marked first on the abdominal wall before the abdomen is inflated. Pneumoperitoneum is established by keeping the intra-abdominal pressure at approximately 12 mm Hg. As the central venous pressure is preferably kept low to reduce bleeding from the hepatic veins during major anatomic liver resection, a mechanical abdominal lifting device is often used (especially in Japan) to prevent gas embolism. On the basis of the information gathered from the preoperative computed tomography and the visual assessment of the liver through the laparoscope, two 12-mm trocars are placed on each side and slightly proximal to the camera to accommodate the laparoscopic ultrasound probe and ultrasonic dissector. An additional one or two 5-mm trocars are placed further laterally. Laparoscopic ultrasound is then used for further intraoperative evaluation, as in open surgery.

LAPAROSCOPIC WEDGE RESECTIONS

Of the various types of laparoscopic liver resection procedures performed, laparoscopic wedge liver resection is the most common. If the lesion is smaller than 5 cm and located at one or more of the so-called laparoscopic segments, which include the inferior edge of segments 4 through 6 and the left lateral segment, laparoscopic resection is probably the procedure of choice. In open liver resection, parenchymal transection can be accomplished in a number of ways. Crushing of the hepatic parenchyma with an artery forceps to expose the bile duct and blood vessels before individual ligation is seldom practiced in the laparoscopic approach, and various electrocautery and ultrasonic devices are used instead. After the tumor is located, the liver capsule is cauterized to mark the proposed line of transection, providing a 1-cm or larger resection margin whenever feasible. The immediate underlying liver tissue is divided with one of the commercially available ultrasonic coagulation devices, for example, AutoSonix (US Surgical, Norwalk, CT), Harmonic Scalpel (Johnson & Johnson Gateway, Piscataway, NJ), or SonoSurg (Olympus, Tokyo, Japan), for a short distance of approximately 4 to 5 mm deep. Further division of the hepatic parenchyma depends on its thickness. If the thickness to be transected is less than 3 cm, the entire procedure can be completed safely using the same ultrasonic devices because most of the terminal branches of vascular and biliary structures are small enough to be sealed satisfactorily. A small bite of the hepatic parenchyma is taken with the jaws of the hand piece along the proposed line of transection, and the blood vessels are secured with clips if they are larger than 3 mm. If thicker liver tissue must be divided, the cavitronic ultrasonic aspirator (CUSA EXcel; Integra Radionics, Burlington, MA)—using its modified laparoscopic hand piece (23 kHz) together with its monopolar electrocautery attachment—is preferred. With the help of the vibration of ultrasound, the hepatic parenchyma is fragmented, and coupled with the continuous aspiration and irrigation via the hand piece, the underlying structures are exposed clearly and dealt with accordingly. A 5-mm or 10-mm laparoscopic argon beam coagulator helps stop any minor oozing from the raw surface, and the usual flow rate of the argon gas is set at approximately 120 ml per second. Extreme caution must be exercised during its application, however, because the intra-abdominal pressure could rapidly exceed the safety limit and result in air embolism. In fact, the air vent of one or more of the trocars should be turned to the open position when the argon beam is used. After complete resection, the specimen is put into a specimen bag and retrieved via the paraumbilical port after enlargement, if necessary.

LAPAROSCOPIC SEGMENTECTOMY

Among the different types of anatomic segmentectomy that can be performed, left lateral segmentectomy has perhaps gained the widest acceptance. On the other hand, an accurate anatomic segmental resection of segments 5 and 6 is difficult because the anatomic boundary cannot be defined without the help of a colored dye injection under ultrasound-guided portal vein branch puncture. As a result, a subsegmentectomy, which includes the tumor and a layer of normal hepatic parenchyma surrounding it, is often performed when the lesions are located in these segments.

In a left lateral segmentectomy the camera and 12-mm ports are placed as described earlier. After initial exploratory laparoscopy and ultrasound examination have confirmed the resectability, the omentum to the left of the hepatoduodenal ligament is divided, and cotton tape is passed to encircle the inflow vascular structures in preparation for the use of Pringle's maneuver when the need arises. The ends of the cotton tape are then brought outside the abdomen, guided through the lumen of a 16-F plastic catheter, and returned together with the plastic catheter back to the abdomen. When temporary hepatic vascular inflow control becomes necessary, both ends are tightened above the far end of the plastic tube with the help of a grasper, and a large metal clip is placed to maintain the necessary pressure to occlude the hepatic inflow. A complete mobilization of the left lateral segment is not necessary at the early stage of surgery, but the round ligament is usually divided first with an ultrasonic coagulation device, then grasped and pulled toward the right to open up the plane for parenchymal transection as the liver tissue is gradually divided. A large, laparoscopic intestinal forceps is usually used to compress gently on the divided liver tissue on the left and, at the same time, open up the liver toward its left. With the help of the CUSA EXcel, the hepatic parenchyma is reduced to a thickness amenable to the application of articulating laparoscopic stapling devices. Because the blood vessels and bile ducts feeding the left lateral segment are end structures with no clinically significant anatomic variation, clear skeletonization of these structures before division is not always necessary. With the parenchymal transection carried toward the left hepatic vein, a laparoscopic vascular stapler is used to control and divide the vessel within the liver. After mobilization from the diaphragm, the specimen can be retrieved via an extension of the paraumbilical incision or a horizontal suprapubic incision.

Occasionally, technical modifications might be required for patients with intrahepatic calculi. These patients often have an atrophic left lateral segment that adheres to adjacent structures and the diaphragm. The bile ducts are usually markedly thickened; dilatated with strictures of various lengths at different levels from the recurrent attacks of cholangitis; and packed with multiple, soft, bilirubinate stones inside the lumen. Furthermore, the anatomic relationship to the segment-4 ducts (left medial segment) is often distorted and tightly tethered to its neighboring portal vein branches. Under such circumstances, the left hepatic duct is best divided under visual guidance to allow stone removal and insertion of a flexible choledochoscopy through the cut end of the left hepatic duct to verify complete ductal clearance. Liberal use of a hand port is recommended. Incision is made to the right abdomen at a site that does not interfere with the other operating ports and allows the operating surgeon to insert his or her left hand into the abdomen. The length of the incision correlates approximately to the size of the glove in centimeters, that is, a 7-cm incision for a size 7 glove. After the conclusion of the choledochoscopy, the bile duct remnant is closed with continuous monofilament suture, and the raw surface is covered with the detached falciform ligament; these procedures are facilitated by an indwelling hand through the hand port. The resected specimen is then extracted via the incision for the hand port after a thorough lavage.

LAPAROSCOPIC MAJOR HEPATECTOMY

The more complicated laparoscopic endeavor should be performed only after a surgeon has mastered the basic skills of minor liver resection. The larger transection area and anatomic variation of the biliary tract and the vascular structures make a safe parenchymal transection crucial to achieving a satisfactory operative outcome. A left hepatectomy is perhaps technically easier when compared with a right lobe resection. Nonetheless, extreme caution must be exercised to define the origin of the right posterior segmental duct before dividing the left hepatic duct in case of a left lobe resection. In the event that the anatomic variant is present, as in approximately 15% of the normal population, the integrity of the right segmental duct must be verified by an intraoperative cholangiogram. The proposed line of bile duct division can be marked with a metal clip or by closing the mechanical stapler without firing, followed by another cholangiogram.

After a laparoscopic evaluation, the first step of a major laparoscopic hepatectomy is usually the isolation and cannulation of the cystic duct with a 3.5-F cannula. The cystic duct is then divided, and the gallbladder is left in situ, grasped and pushed cephalically to expose the hilar structures. The ipsilateral hepatic artery and portal vein branch are dissected free and divided between ligatures. In the case of a right or extended right hepatectomy, the usual

practice of complete mobilization of the liver lobe, allowing control of the small caval venous branches and hepatic veins extra-hepatically, as in the case of open hepatectomy, is rarely done. Some investigators advocated a trial of dissection by first dividing the peritoneum distal to the border of the caudate lobe. The posterior surface of the liver is then mobilized anteriorly away from the inferior vena cava to expose its anterior surface. The small caval branches encountered are then individually isolated and divided with metal clips. Through the retrohepatic tunnel thus created, the right hepatic vein can then be accessed and secured with a mechanical endovascular stapler. (As reported in the literature, this step has been successfully performed in select patients who underwent laparoscopic right hepatectomy.) Establishing a retrohepatic tunnel, a concept comparable to the "liver-hanging" technique, is theoretically sound because it also allows better identification of the transection plane; and in case of minor venous oozing, lifting the liver forward might slow down the bleeding, making it easier to obtain hemostasis. In the event that there is a large right inferior hepatic vein (as in approximately 15% of the population), the use of an endovascular stapler is preferred for a more secure closure because the venous stump is usually short. The liver parenchyma is then divided with instruments selected by the operating surgeon, and any luminal structure exposed is managed with an instrument appropriate to its nature and size. A hand port is used liberally, particularly when the lesion is located at the right posterior segment.

CONCLUSION

Laparoscopic hepatectomy of one or two Couinaud segments has earned its place in the armamentarium for the surgical resection of liver tumors. Similar to our experience when laparoscopic cholecystectomy was first introduced, the benefits from the complicated laparoscopic intervention are marginal if not comparable to conventional surgery. If the size and location of the lesion were favorable, few would deny the minimally invasive procedure of limited hepatectomy and left lateral segmentectomy as a serious option. On the other hand, the advantage of major laparoscopic hepatectomy of three or more Couinaud segments is still debatable. Only a few centers have published enthusiastic support for the procedure. The laparoscopic techniques used by these pioneers vary, and the methods chosen to transect the hepatic parenchyma are less accurate and potentially more hazardous than the techniques routinely used in open liver resection. Early results reported by these experienced centers—which focused on the amount of intraoperative blood loss, morbidity, and mortality rates—are respectable. One should bear in mind that the patients reported on were cautiously selected for the major laparoscopic undertaking and therefore do not represent results that might be obtained from the majority of patients who require similar surgical liver resection. In addition, the published literature on the long-term outcome of patients undergoing laparoscopic liver resection for malignancy was sparse. Given all these limitations, the available data support, at best, the belief that the laparoscopic endeavor is technically feasible in the hands of a team of skilled laparoscopic and liver surgeons. More experience is necessary to show whether the use of major laparoscopic hepatectomy can reproduce the current perioperative outcome and long-term results accomplished with open surgery.

SUGGESTED READINGS

Buell JF, Koffron AJ, Thomas MJ, and others: Laparoscopic liver resection, *J Am Coll Surg* 200:472, 2005.
Cherqui D: Laparoscopic liver resection, *Br J Surg* 90:644, 2003.
Cherqui D, Laurent A, Tayar C, and others: Laparoscopic liver resection for peripheral hepatocellular carcinoma in patients with chronic liver disease. Midterm results and perspectives, *Ann Surg* 243:499, 2006.
Cherqui D, Soubrane O, Husson E, and others: Laparoscopic living donor hepatectomy for liver transplantation in children, *Lancet* 359:392, 2002.

Huang MT, Lee WJ, Wang W, and others: Hand-assisted laparoscopic hepatectomy for solid tumor in the posterior portion of the right lobe: initial experience, *Ann Surg* 238:674, 2003.

Lesurtel M, Cherqui D, Laurent A, and others: Laparoscopic versus open left lateral lobectomy: a case-control study, *J Am Coll Surg* 196:236, 2003.

O'Rourke N, Fielding G: Laparoscopic right hepatectomy, *J Gastrointest Surg* 8:213, 2004.

Tang CN, Li MKW: Laparoscopic-assisted liver resection, *J Hepatobiliary Pancreat Surg* 9:105, 2002.

LAPAROSCOPIC SPLENECTOMY

David Maccabee, MD, and John G. Hunter, MD

Since its initial description in 1992, laparoscopic splenectomy has become the preferred method for elective splenectomy in all patients except those with massive splenomegaly. The benefits of laparoscopy include minimal abdominal wall trauma, small incisions, minimal pain, and minimal blood loss; these result in rapid recovery and return to preoperative functional status. Consequently, surgeons who have training in advanced laparoscopic procedures have adopted this technique enthusiastically.

INDICATIONS

Indications for laparoscopic splenectomy (LS) are limited to elective and urgent situations in relatively stable patients. The most common indication is immune thrombocytopenic purpura (ITP), which usually manifests as easy bruising in women aged 20 to 40 years. For this indication, complete response to splenectomy (as evidenced by maintenance of normal platelet count) can be expected in approximately 65% to 85% of adult patients, and the majority of published case series demonstrate persistent response to splenectomy through 5 years. Other indications are noted in Table 1 and are well described in the Section 9 of this book

Although LS was initially restricted to benign conditions, the spleen harboring malignancy may be removed intact in a bag with the use of a hand port or a limited incision (midline, Pfannenstiel, or subcostal) to allow pathologic examination.

Table 1: Indications for Laparoscopic Splenectomy by Frequency

Idiopathic thrombocytopenic purpura

Myeloproliferative disorder (chronic and acute myeloid leukemia)

Malignancy (leukemia, lymphoma, Hodgkin's disease, metastases)

Autoimmune hemolytic anemia

Thrombotic thrombocytopenic purpura

Splenomegaly

Splenic cyst

Splenic abscess

Hereditary spherocytosis

Sickle cell disease

Splenic artery aneurysm

Felty's syndrome

Myelofibrosis

In general, the laparoscopic approach is contraindicated in emergent situations, effectively eliminating splenic trauma with associated hemorrhagic shock (the most common indication for splenectomy) and spontaneous splenic rupture. The extra time required to set up most laparoscopy suites and to position the patient and the inability to effectively pack the abdomen make this approach impractical.

Relative contraindications to LS include massive splenomegaly (>25 cm in length), portal hypertension, pregnancy, and morbid obesity, although LS has been reported in all of these conditions with increasing frequency in the past decade.

TECHNIQUES

Preoperative preparation of the ITP patient includes the administration of pneumococcal and haemophilus influenza vaccine at least 2 weeks before operation. Preoperative treatment of thrombocytopenia with gamma globulin directed at antiplatelet antibody may temporarily restore a normal platelet count at the time of operation and serve as an indicator of response to splenectomy. Alternatively, platelets may be administered at the time of the operation, after the splenic artery has been ligated, to minimize "first pass" clearance by the antibody-rich splenic pulp (Table 2). Furthermore "neoadjuvant" chemotherapy for patients with hematologic malignancy, such as chronic myeloid leukemia, can reduce spleen size and increase the safety and success rate of this procedure. We do not recommend preoperative splenic artery embolization. Coils placed in the splenic artery will impede the use of laparoscopic staplers, the principal method of securing the splenic hilar vessels.

Table 2: Preparation for Splenectomy

2 weeks preoperative	Pneumococcal & haemophilus influenza vaccine	All patients
	Consideration of plasmapheresis	TTP
	Consideration of Chemotherapy	CML & other malignancy
48 hours preoperative	For platelet count <150,000	2 g per kg body weight IV immune globulin divided into 2 doses
Preoperative	IV antibiotic prophylaxis	First-generation cephalosporin
	DVT prophylaxis	TED hose & SCD pump
Intraoperative	For platelet count <50,000	Platelet transfusion following ligation of splenic artery

CML, Chronic myeloid leukemia; *DVT,* deep vein thrombosis; *IV,* intravenous; *SCD,* sequential compression device; *TED,* thromboembolism deterrent; *TTP,* thrombotic thrombocytopenic purpura.

The operating room requires two video monitors positioned on either side of the patient and reliable or redundant insufflation and video imaging systems. We routinely use a 30-degree angled 10-mm laparoscope, having found the light transmission and durability superior to the 5-mm laparoscopes. A 45-degree angled scope also is often used. Surgeons should be skilled in bimanual laparoscopic technique, including intracorporeal knot tying, which is helpful but not crucial to the procedure.

Although use of a dynamic nonautomated or robotic laparoscope holder is now standard for many laparoscopic surgical procedures, LS does not lend itself well to using these devices because of patient positioning, and the camera remains the primary responsibility of the surgical assistant.

Right Lateral Approach (the "Leaning Spleen")

Initial descriptions of LS placed the patient in a supine position. Extending the experience of laparoscopic adrenalectomy, surgeons in France and Canada adopted a lateral approach, the "hanging spleen" technique. Noting the benefits of both positions, most surgeons have evolved to using a 45-degree tilt, the "leaning spleen." Pivotal to success is the positioning of the patient, which gives adequate exposure for both laparoscopic and open procedures.

After establishing general anesthesia and securely taping the endotracheal tube, a Foley catheter, orogastric tube, and sequential compression devices are applied to the lower extremities. The patient is rolled halfway toward a right lateral decubitus position (45-degree tilt—the "lean") and then moved up or down the bed to put the space between the costal margin and superior iliac spine directly over the break in the table. We find it helpful to mark the center of this space in the patient's left midaxillary line and also to mark the break on the bed; these two marks can then be lined up easily. After the patient has been correctly positioned, arms are protected with an axillary roll under the right axilla and the right arm out on an armboard. The left arm is suspended on a sling with the elbow flexed. Legs are flexed and protected with pillows between the knees and ankles (Fig. 1). We have found that using an inflatable beanbag cushion holds the patient in the leaning position well (Fig. 2). The beanbag should not be deflated until the operating table is flexed. Some surgeons use a "jelly roll" positioning pad on either side of the torso to keep the patient in this semilateral position. These are secured best by rolling them into a sheet placed under the patient. The table is flexed maximally to open the space between the costal margin and iliac crest. If available, an elevated "kidney rest" accentuates the flex of the torso. The beanbag is inflated at this point, and the patient is secured in this position with padded adhesive tape at the hips, shoulders, and knees. Potential pressure points are assessed and further padded as needed. The table is tilted fully left, right, and into Trendelenburg and reverse Trendelenburg positions to ensure that the patient will not shift after being draped. The table is then optimally and ergonomically positioned.

Sterile preparation extends from nipples to pubis and beyond the midline anteriorly and posteriorly. The surgeon and camera operator stand in front of the patient; the first assistant stands at the opposite side. The operation begins with the table tilted to the left to approximate a supine position. The pneumoperitoneum is established using a Veress needle in the umbilicus followed by a 10-mm trocar in the left upper quadrant, approximately 15 cm from the surface projection of the splenic hilum in a line toward the umbilicus. Depending on the size of the patient, this port may be quite close to or quite a distance from the costal margin. Three additional trocars are placed: one 12-mm trocar for the surgeon's dominant hand to admit the stapling device and two 5-mm trocars for the surgeon's nondominant hand and assistant's right hand (see Fig. 1). These latter three trocars are placed close to the costal margin unless there is significant splenomegaly.

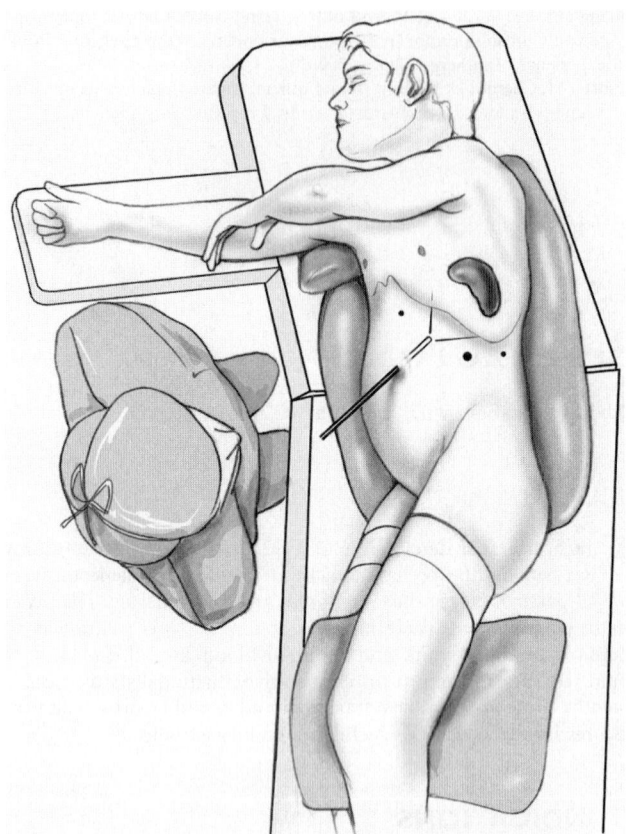

Figure 1   Patient, port, and telescope positions for the leaning spleen technique.   *Reprinted with permission from Hunter JG, editor: The atlas of minimally invasive surgical operations, New York, McGraw-Hill, (in press).*

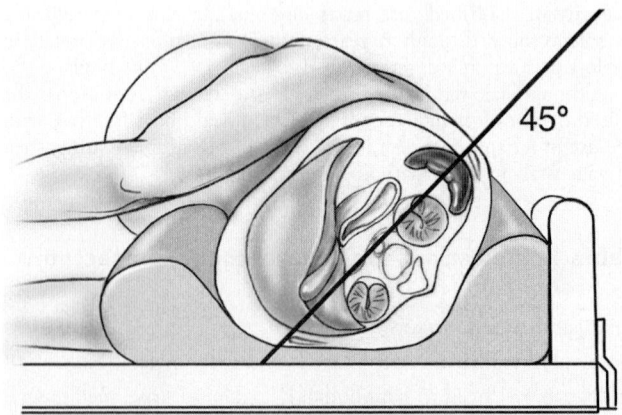

Figure 2   The leaning spleen requires a 45-degree tilt, using a beanbag or jelly roll positioning pad.   *Reprinted with permission from Hunter JG, editor: The atlas of minimally invasive surgical operations, New York, McGraw-Hill, (in press).*

Initial inspection of both sides of the greater omentum and left upper quadrant is conducted, searching for accessory spleens. If encountered, these are usually easily removed with ultrasonic shears (e.g., Harmonic Scalpel, Johnson & Johnson Gateway, Piscataway, NJ) or a similar device. We avoid using a clip application device during this procedure, especially in the vicinity of the splenic hilum, because the clips can interfere later with stapler placement and function. The splenocolic ligament is taken down, with care to prevent heat or conductive injury to the bowel. Frequently, exposure of the lower pole of the spleen demonstrates inferior polar arteries, which are easily taken with the Harmonic Scalpel without jeopardizing the main hilar vasculature. The spleen is gently and bluntly elevated by the assistant with either the suction device or a blunt elevator. This is best accomplished by passing the blunt instrument all the way under the spleen along either axis, with the tip of the instrument past the parenchyma of the spleen and elevating it with the shaft of the instrument. This creates tension, which allows medial and cranial dissection anteriorly of the short gastric vessels, which are taken with the Harmonic Scalpel. Use of a blunt retractor or suction device by the assistant and two-handed surgical technique (with a Harmonic Scalpel in the dominant hand and grasper in the nondominant hand of the surgeon) is extremely helpful. As the greater curve of the stomach falls away and the lesser sac is entered, the superior-most short gastric vessels (which are occasionally so short that the stomach appears adherent to the superior pole of the spleen) are carefully taken individually with the Harmonic Scalpel, similar to laparoscopic fundoplication. If a greater curve of stomach injury is created, this is easily repaired with an intracorporeally or extracorporeally tied simple suture.

After the lesser sac has been opened, the splenic artery and vein are relatively easily visualized and dissected proximal to the splenic hilum, over the tail of the pancreas in thin patients. It is our practice to ligate these individually with 10-cm lengths of braided suture, using an intracorporeal knotting technique (Fig. 3). Preligation allows the administration of platelets in a thrombocytopenic patient before the retroperitoneal and splenic hilar dissection is started. Also, preligation acts as an "insurance policy" against major hemorrhage during the dissection of the splenic vessels in the hilum of the spleen. When these vessels are not easily visualized in the lesser sac, we do not attempt preligation and move directly to the next step. Frequently we judge the artery worthy of preligation but decide to leave the more deeply embedded splenic vein alone.

The operating room table is tilted in the opposite direction to approximate the right lateral decubitus position. The posterior

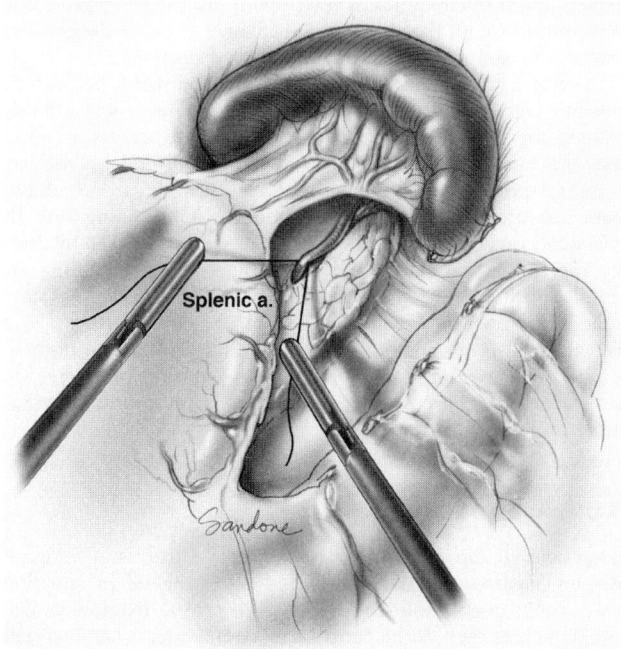

Figure 3 The splenic artery is preligated if platelets are to be administered. *Reprinted with permission from Hunter JG, editor. The atlas of minimally invasive surgical operations, New York, McGraw-Hill, (in press).*

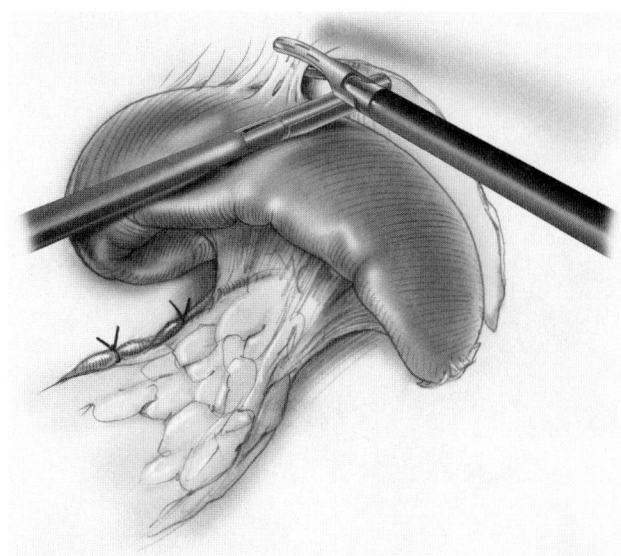

Figure 4 The spleen is released by dividing the peritoneal reflection with the Harmonic Scalpel (Johnson & Johnson Gateway, Piscataway, NJ). *Reprinted with permission from Hunter JG, editor. The atlas of minimally invasive surgical operations, New York, McGraw-Hill, (in press).*

aspect of the spleen is then freed from the lateral abdominal wall and diaphragm by dividing the peritoneal reflection with the ultrasonic shears, beginning at the lower pole and working cephalad (Fig. 4). With this maneuver the spleen will roll anteriorly to expose the dorsal surface of the tail of the pancreas, and the hilar vessels will be seen from the posterior or dorsal exposure. As the dissection reaches the superior pole, some surgeons will leave a small strip of splenophrenic ligament to maintain fixation of the spleen to the diaphragm until later in the operation.

After the spleen has become free anteriorly and posteriorly, the hilar vessels are addressed. Sometimes, these vessels may be easy to separate into an inferior and superior bundle, in which case each bundle is ligated and divided separately with an articulated stapling device (2.8-mm staple length, 45-mm cartridge length). More commonly, surgeons do not carefully define the anatomy of the hilar structures and elect to divide the hilar vessels en masse with several firings of the stapler (Fig. 5).

After it has been devascularized, the spleen is manipulated into a tough nylon sac introduced into the abdomen through the largest trocar. This can be the most difficult part of the operation. Two techniques are available for "bagging" and removing the spleen. In the first technique, the spleen is left attached to the diaphragm at the superior pole. The free inferior pole of the spleen is introduced into a large specimen bag (15-mm LapSac; Cook Medical, Bloomington, IN), and then the splenophrenic ligament is divided to complete the separation of the spleen from all attachments. Many authors have reported using sterilized freezer bags as a cost-saving technique. We prefer to use a ripstop nylon specimen bag (Cook Surgical, Bloomington, IN), which is opened in the left upper quadrant after the detached spleen has been pulled inferomedially. The mouth of the bag faces the spleen and is held open with two graspers. The surgeon, grasping the detached spleen by the hilar structures, pushes the spleen back toward its native position and into the specimen sac (Fig. 6). The bag is then pulled up to the trocar incision, which is enlarged, and the spleen is morcellized using ring forceps and pulled out piecemeal. If the organ is required intact, this incision can be enlarged; however, we find it preferable to use a midline incision or Pfannenstiel incision when preservation of splenic architecture is important.

Any enlarged incisions are temporarily closed with towel clips, and pneumoperitoneum is reestablished. The surgical field is closely

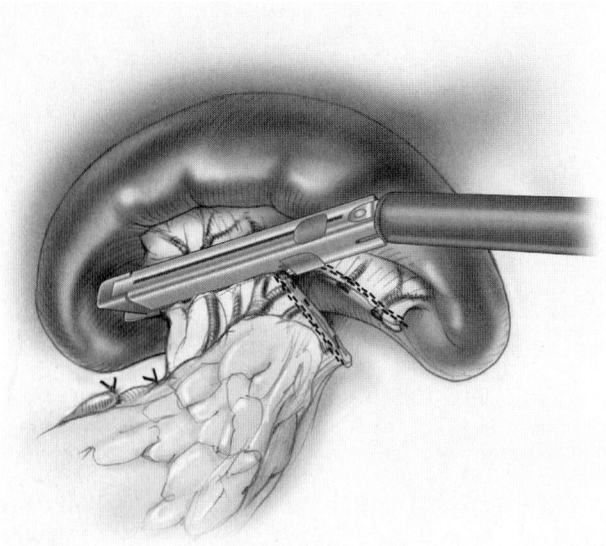

Figure 5 The splenic blood supply is controlled in the splenic hilum with a linear cutting stapler. *Reprinted with permission from Hunter JG, editor. The atlas of minimally invasive surgical operations, New York, McGraw-Hill, (in press).*

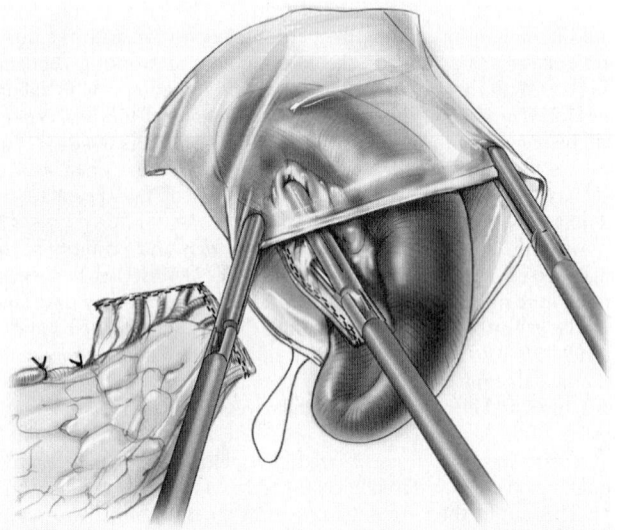

Figure 6 The spleen is pushed into a sturdy specimen bag opened in the left upper quadrant. *Reprinted with permission from Hunter JG, editor. The atlas of minimally invasive surgical operations, New York, McGraw-Hill, (in press).*

inspected for hemostasis, and a second search for accessory spleens is conducted. The 10- and 12-mm trocar sites are closed at the fascial level with interrupted absorbable sutures, and all skin incisions are closed with absorbable suture.

Supine Approach

The supine approach, described earlier, has largely been supplanted by the lateral approach described in the previous section. Its setup is similar to that required for a laparoscopic Nissen fundoplication, with the patient in the split-leg or lithotomy position and tilted into the head-up, reverse Trendelenburg, and left–side-up position (Fig. 7). This approach affords reasonable visualization of the

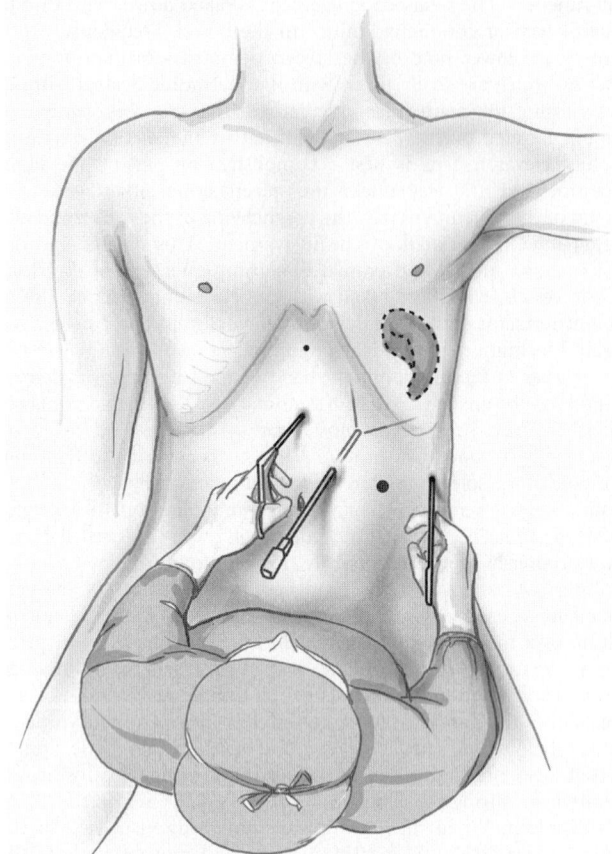

Figure 7 Patient and port locations for supine positioning. *Reprinted with permission from Hunter JG, editor. The atlas of minimally invasive surgical operations, New York, McGraw-Hill, (in press).*

splenic hilum but requires at least one more trocar to allow adequate retraction on the stomach and colon. The tail of the pancreas may not be well exposed during posterior dissection.

As with a Nissen fundoplication, the surgeon stands between the patient's legs, with the first assistant or automated scope holder holding the camera on the patient's right. Five trocars are used, and the laparoscope alternates between the midepigastric and umbilical ports. Dissection and vascular ligation are conducted from the inferior pole in a cranial direction, beginning with the splenocolic ligament. Short gastric vessels are easily taken by drawing the stomach medially and inferiorly while gently lifting and bluntly pushing the spleen laterally. After the hilum has been isolated anteriorly, it is carefully dissected posteriorly using a blunt instrument. An articulating device such as an esophageal dissector or 10-mm "lap band" passing instrument can be helpful here. This is followed by transection of the hilum, as previously described, either individually or en masse.

Hand-Assisted Approach

Hand-assisted laparoscopy has found acceptance as a bridge to learning laparoscopic techniques and is often used in situations when doubt exists about the ability to control or manipulate delicate structures such as the pancreas or vasculature. A hand (usually the surgeon's left) can be inserted through an upper midline incision with either the right lateral or supine approach. We have used this method for laparoscopic distal pancreatectomy or when doubtful about the security of the splenic hilar vascular ligation (Figs. 8 and 9).

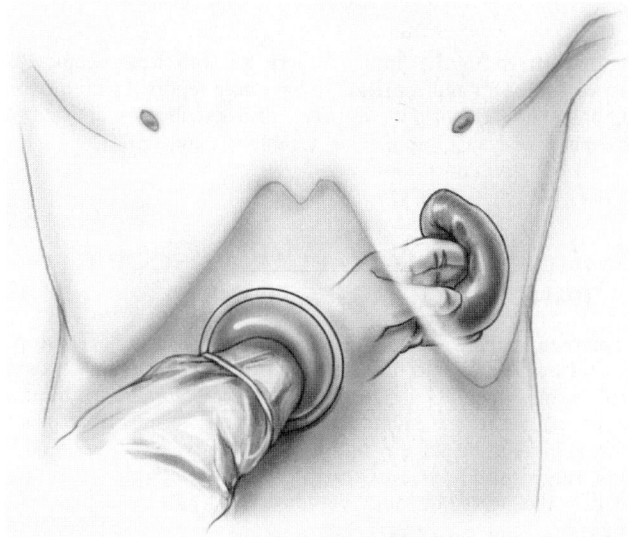

Figure 8 A hand port may be used if it is necessary to remove the spleen intact. *Reprinted with permission from Hunter JG, editor: The atlas of minimally invasive surgical operations, New York, McGraw-Hill, (in press).*

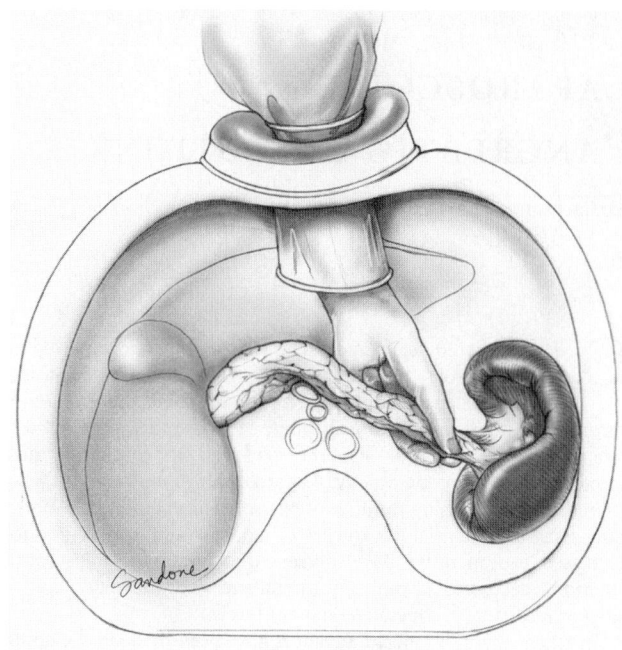

Figure 9 With the hand port it is possible to control the splenic artery and vein with one's fingers by encircling the tail of the pancreas during dissection and stapling of the hilum. *Reprinted with permission from Hunter JG, editor: The atlas of minimally invasive surgical operations, New York, McGraw-Hill, (in press).*

Table 3: Results of Laparoscopic versus Open Splenectomy

Author	Patient Population	Operative Time (Minutes)	Length of Stay (Days)	Complication Rate	Complete Response	Mortality
Kojouri and others (Meta-analysis of 135 case series)	ITP only N = 2623	NR	NR	LS– 9.6% OS–12.9%	66%	LS–0.2% OS–1.0%
Winslow & Brunt (Meta-analysis of 51 case series)	Elective splenectomy N = 2940	LS–180 OS – 114	LS–3.6 OS–7.2	LS–15.5% OS–26.6%	NR	LS–0.6% OS–1.1%

ITP, Immune thrombocytopenic purpura; *LS,* laparoscopic splenectomy; *N,* total number of patients; *NR,* not reported; *OS,* open splenectomy.

RESULTS

Recent meta-analyses published in the medical and surgical literature are shown in Table 3. No prospective randomized trials comparing LS to open splenectomy (OS) have been published. Evaluation shows most authors report longer operative times for LS compared with OS; however, significantly shorter hospital stays and postoperative recovery times are also consistently reported with LS as compared with OS. Identification of accessory spleens has been comparable and occurs in approximately 10% of cases.

Perhaps most importantly, the two meta-analyses in Table 3 show that over the past 20 years, complication and mortality rates have been significantly lower with LS than with OS. In these reviews of published series totaling nearly 3000 patients, LS complications occurred in 10% to 15% of cases, whereas for OS, complications occurred in 13% to 27%. When specifically evaluated, these studies show significantly fewer pulmonary and infectious complications and the near elimination of wound complications and hernias with LS. Mortality rates show a similar pattern.

The evolution of surgical technology, most significantly the rapid improvement of optical systems and devices that ligate and seal blood vessels, has led to the improvement and acceptance of LS for most splenectomies. For these reasons LS has become the standard for surgical treatment of hematologic disorders affecting the spleen.

SELECTED READINGS

Kojouri, K, Vesely, S, Terrell D, and others: Splenectomy for adult patients with ITP, *Blood* 104:9, 2004.

Park A, Gagner M, Pomp A: The lateral approach to laparoscopic splenectomy, *Am J Surg* 173:126, 1997.

Poulin EC: Laparoscopic splenectomy. In Eubanks WS, Swanstrom LL, Soper NJ, editors: *Mastery of endoscopic and laparoscopic surgery,* Philadelphia, 2000, Lippincott Williams & Wilkins.

Richardson WS, Smith CD, Branum GD, and others: Leaning spleen: a new approach to laparoscopic splenectomy, *J Am Coll Surg* 185:412, 1997.

Rosen M, Brody F, Ponsky J, and others: Outcome of laparoscopic splenectomy based on hematologic indication, *Surg Endosc* 16(2):272, 2002.

Winslow ER, Brunt LM: Perioperative outcomes of laparoscopic versus open splenectomy: a meta-analysis with an emphasis on complications, *Surgery* 134(4):647, 2003.

LAPAROSCOPIC PANCREATIC RESECTIONS

Attila Nakeeb, MD

Over the past 20 years laparoscopic procedures have played an increasing role in the management of intra-abdominal pathology. Laparoscopic surgery has become the gold standard for the management of gallstones, gastroesophageal reflux disease, and achalasia. It is also the preferred approach for most adrenal and splenic pathology. Laparoscopic colectomy is being offered to an increasing number of patients with benign and malignant diseases. Potential advantages of laparoscopic surgery include decreased postoperative pain, decreased ileus, preserved immune function, decreased complications, shorter hospital stay, and a quicker return to preoperative activity levels.

In recent years significant advances have been made in the application of minimally invasive techniques to the management of both benign and malignant pancreatic disorders. Initially, laparoscopic pancreatic surgery was limited to diagnostic staging in patients with pancreatic cancer before resection. More recently minimally invasive techniques have been used to manage inflammatory disorders of the pancreas, including necrotizing pancreatitis and pancreatic pseudocysts. With increasing frequency, surgeons have applied laparoscopic techniques to resect benign and malignant lesions of the pancreas. Laparoscopic pancreaticoduodenectomies (PDs), enucleations, and distal pancreatectomies (DPs) have all been described in the literature.

LAPAROSCOPIC PANCREATICODUODENECTOMY

Laparoscopic PD is performed only in a handful of specialized centers (Table 1). Hand-assisted or laparoscopic-assisted procedures are used with laparoscopic resection, and the reconstruction is completed via a "mini-laparotomy" or through the hand port. In the largest series reported in the literature, Dulucq and colleagues describe 25 patients who underwent an attempted laparoscopic PD with a conversion rate of 12%. Thirteen patients had a laparoscopic reconstruction, and nine patients had a mini-laparotomy for reconstruction. The complication rate was 32%, and the average length of stay was 16.2 days. These results are comparable to those of open PD. Although PD can be performed laparoscopically, it still must be considered an experimental procedure. Its performance should be limited to specialized centers with significant expertise in pancreatic and advanced laparoscopic surgery.

In contrast to the limited experience with laparoscopic PD, laparoscopic DPs and enucleations have been reported with increasing frequency. The balance of this chapter describes the indications, preoperative evaluation, surgical techniques, and results of laparoscopic DPs and enucleations.

INDICATIONS FOR LAPAROSCOPIC PANCREATIC RESECTIONS

Laparoscopic pancreatic resections are complicated laparoscopic procedures and should be undertaken by surgeons with advanced laparoscopic skill sets. Surgeons should be comfortable with intracorporeal suturing, endomechanical staplers, and laparoscopic ultrasound and be able to control intraoperative bleeding. In addition, surgeons should have experience with open pancreatic surgery in case the procedure must be converted to an open pancreatic resection.

Factors important in selecting appropriate patients for laparoscopic resections include the size of the lesion, location of the lesion within the pancreas, involvement of surrounding structures, and the suspected pathology of the lesion.

Conditions that are potentially amenable to a laparoscopic pancreatic resection include benign or premalignant cystic neoplasms, neuroendocrine (islet cell) tumors of the pancreas, chronic pancreatitis with symptomatic ductal obstruction, and pancreatic pseudocysts localized to the distal body and tail of the pancreas (Table 2). Although there have been a small number of patients with malignant pancreatic tumors that have been resected laparoscopically, it is unclear whether it is prudent to attempt a laparoscopic resection in patients with a confirmed malignancy.

Cystic neoplasms of the pancreas that are potentially amenable to laparoscopic pancreatic resections include serous cyst adenomas (SCAs), mucinous cystic neoplasms (MCNs), and benign intraductal papillary mucinous neoplasms (IPMNs). SCAs are benign tumors of the pancreas that occur in twice as many females as males. They have a characteristic microcystic appearance on imaging that often resembles a honeycomb and can have a starburst pattern with a centrally located calcified scar. Most patients are asymptomatic and tend to have large lesions. Surgical treatment is indicated in symptomatic patients (vague abdominal pain likely related to the mass effect of the cyst).

MCNs occur predominantly in the body and tail of the pancreas, have a 2:1 female-to-male ratio, occur in a younger age group (40–50 years), do not communicate with the pancreatic duct, and microscopically are associated with an ovarian-type stroma. Conversely, IPMNs occur more commonly in the head and uncinate process, have a slight male predominance, occur in an older age group (60–80 years), communicate with the pancreatic duct, and do not have an ovarian-like stroma. MCNs and IPMNs have malignant potential, and therefore resection of these lesions is recommended.

Table 1: Results of Laparoscopic Pancreaticoduodenectomy

Author	Year	N	Conversion (%)	LR	Operative Time (Min.)	Comp (%)	LOS (days)	Pancreatic Cancer
Gagner	1997	10	40	6	510	30	22.3	4
Dulucq	2005	11	9	6	268	33	13.4	4
Staudacher	2005	7	43	0	416	—	12	1
Dulucq	2006	25	12	13	287	32	16.2	11

LOS, Length of stay; *LR*, laparoscopic reconstruction; *N*, total number of patients; *min.*, minutes.

Table 2: Indications for Laparoscopic Pancreatic Resection

Solid pancreatic tumors
Functional neuroendocrine tumors
Nonfunctional neuroendocrine tumors
Adenocarcinoma
Cystic pancreatic tumors
Congenital cysts
Serous cystadenoma (SCA)
Mucinous cystadenoma (MCN)
Intraductal papillary mucinous neoplasms (IPMNs)
Chronic pancreatitis
Symptomatic ductal obstruction
Persistent pancreatic pseudocyst

Neuroendocrine tumors (NETs) of the pancreas may be functional (associated with a clinical syndrome related to hormones secreted by the tumor) or nonfunctional (lacking symptoms or hormone production by the tumor). Insulinomas are the most common NETs of the pancreas. These tumors secrete insulin, resulting in hypoglycemic symptoms. The vast majority of insulinomas are benign, making them ideally suited for laparoscopic enucleation.

Patients with chronic pancreatitis and isolated strictures of the pancreatic duct limited to the distal body and tail of the pancreas may also be treated with laparoscopic DP. There is often a dense inflammatory reaction involving the peripancreatic tissues and the splenic vessels in these patients, making a splenectomy more likely.

PREOPERATIVE EVALUATION

Currently, helical (spiral) computed tomography (CT) is the preferred noninvasive imaging test for pancreatic diseases. Helical CT can delineate the anatomy of the pancreas and the surrounding organs in considerable detail and can easily define pancreatic calcifications, inflammation, necrosis, and masses. A triple-phase intravenous (IV) contrast study is ideal for the assessment of pancreatic lesions. Thin cuts are obtained through the pancreas and the liver during both the arterial phase and the venous phase after the IV contrast material has been injected. In addition to being used to determine the primary tumor size, CT is used to look for and evaluate invasion into local structures or metastatic disease. Magnetic resonance imaging scanning provides information similar to that provided by CT. The addition of magnetic resonance cholangiopancreatography can be useful for defining the anatomy and pathology of the bile ducts and the pancreatic duct noninvasively.

Endoscopic retrograde cholangiopancreatography (ERCP) allows direct imaging of the pancreatic and bile ducts and is the gold standard for diagnosing chronic pancreatitis. The sensitivity of ERCP for the diagnosis of pancreatic cancer approaches 90%. The presence of a long, irregular stricture in an otherwise normal pancreatic duct is highly suggestive of a pancreatic malignancy. The identification of mucin in the pancreatic duct or the communication of a cystic lesion with the pancreatic duct suggests the presence of an IPMN.

Endoscopic ultrasonography (EUS) has begun to play an important role in the evaluation of pancreatic diseases. EUS can diagnose the most common causes of extrahepatic biliary obstruction (e.g., choledocholithiasis and pancreaticobiliary malignancies) with a degree of accuracy equaling or exceeding that of direct cholangiography or ERCP, and it is the most sensitive modality for the diagnosis of pancreatic carcinoma. EUS can be combined with fine needle aspiration biopsy of lesions to obtain a tissue diagnosis. The aspiration of cyst fluid and determination of cyst carcinoembryonic antigen (CEA) and mucin levels can help to differentiate serous from mucinous cysts.

Serum tumor markers, including CEA and carbohydrate antigen (CA19-9), are usually measured in patients with both solid and cystic tumors. If a neuroendocrine tumor is suspected by history (symptomatic), imaging (hypervascular on CT scan), or on preoperative biopsy, then serum levels of chromogranins A, insulin, proinsulin, glucagon, gastrin, vasoactive intestinal peptide, or pancreatic peptide can be measured.

PATIENT PREPARATION

Every patient considered for a pancreatic resection must undergo a full evaluation of cardiac, pulmonary, and renal function. A full array of laboratory tests must be obtained, including a complete blood count, renal panel, and liver panel. A nutritional assessment must be made to ensure that the patient can undergo surgery safely. If patient has severe weight loss or has an albumin of less than 3 g/dL, strong consideration for supplemental nutrition is indicated.

Patients undergoing DP or enucleation of lesions in the body or tail of the pancreas should receive vaccinations against encapsulated organisms in case a splenectomy is required. These include *Streptococcus pneumoniae*, *Neisseria meningitidis*, and *Haemophilus influenzae* vaccines. The vaccines should be administered 1 or 2 weeks before the operation.

INSTRUMENTATION

In addition to standard laparoscopic equipment available in most operating rooms, certain specialized equipment is necessary to safely carry out laparoscopic pancreatic surgery (Table 3). Intraoperative ultrasound is an invaluable tool during laparoscopic pancreatic resections. Ultrasound can be used to help localize lesions in the pancreas, define the relationship between the lesion and the pancreatic duct, assess for vascular invasion by the lesion, assess resection margins, and rule out metastatic disease.

POSITIONING AND ROOM SETUP

Following endotracheal intubation and general anesthesia, an orogastric tube and Foley catheter are placed. Sequential compression devices, subcutaneous heparin, or both are used for deep venous thrombosis prophylaxis, and a first-generation cephalosporin is used for infectious prophylaxis.

For lesions in the head, uncinate, or neck of the pancreas the patient is positioned supine on a split-leg table or in a low lithotomy position. The surgeon stands between the legs and the first assistant to the patient's left. For lesions located in the body and tail

Table 3: Equipment for Laparoscopic Pancreatic Resection

30-degree laparoscope
Flexible laparoscopic ultrasound probe
Ultrasonic dissector
Endo GIA stapler
5-mm and 10-mm clip appliers
Laparoscopic needle holders
Atraumatic graspers
Table mounted retractor

GIA, Gastrointestinal anastomosis.

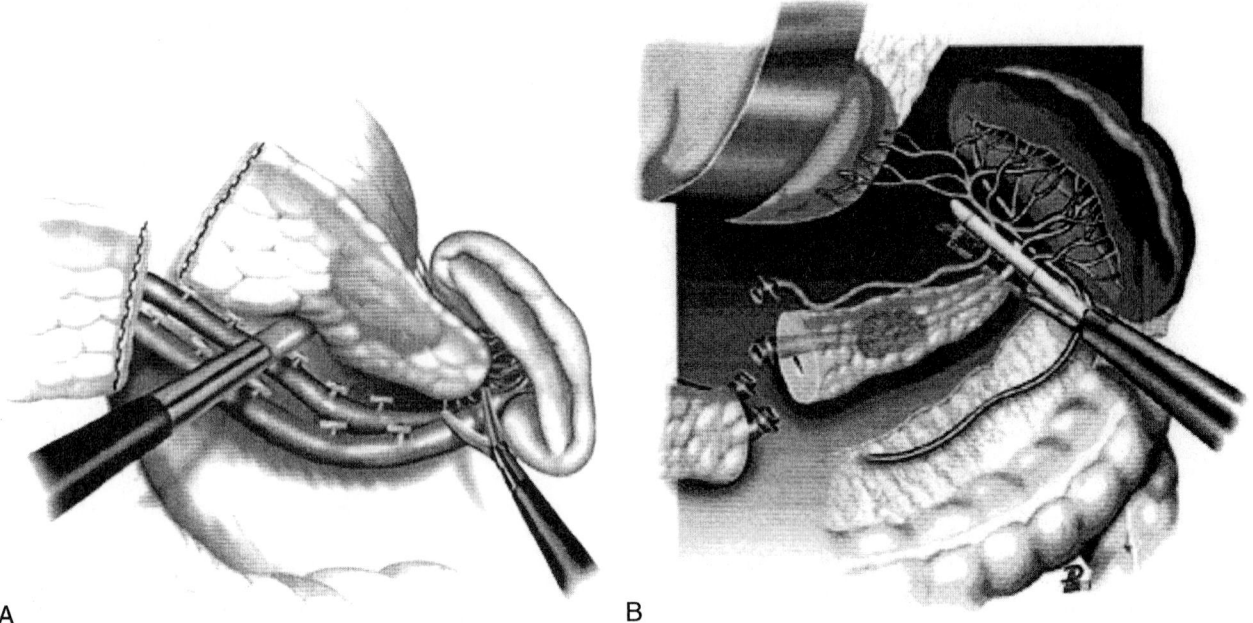

A   **B**

Figure 1 **(A)** Laparoscopic splenic-preserving distal pancreatectomy with preservation of the splenic vessels. **(B)** Laparoscopic splenic-preserving distal pancreatectomy with ligation of the splenic vessels. The spleen is vascularized by the short gastric vessels and the left gastroepiploic vessel. *From Fernández-Cruz L, Martínez I, Gilabert R, and others: Laparoscopic distal pancreatectomy combined with preservation of the spleen for cystic neoplasms of the pancreas, J Gastrointest Surg 8:493, 2004.*

of the pancreas, we prefer to position the patient in a semilateral position (30-45 degrees) with the left side up. The surgeon and the camera operator stand at the patient's right side, while the first assistant and the scrub nurse stand at the patient's left side. Video monitors are placed over both shoulders, and the laparoscopic ultrasound monitor is placed at the patient's left side near the video monitor.

LAPAROSCOPIC DISTAL PANCREATECTOMY WITH OR WITHOUT SPLENECTOMY

Laparoscopic DP may be performed as a splenic-preserving DP (SPDP) or an en bloc DP plus splenectomy. Two techniques for splenic preservation have been described. The first involves preservation of the splenic artery and vein and requires a careful dissection and ligation of the small branches from the splenic artery and vein to the pancreas. The second technique involves the division of the splenic artery and vein proximally, followed by a second division of the vessels as they emerge from the tail of the pancreas (Fig. 1). The spleen is vascularized by the short gastric vessels and the left gastroepiploic vessels. Attempts at splenic preservation are appropriate for benign cystic neoplasms and neuroendocrine tumors. Splenectomy is often necessary if the tail of the pancreas extends well into the splenic hilum or if there is significant peripancreatic inflammation that makes dissection of the pancreas off of the splenic vessels hazardous. Splenectomy should be performed if the procedure is being undertaken for malignancy or if there is left-sided portal hypertension secondary to splenic vein thrombosis.

Access to the peritoneal cavity is achieved by either an open technique or via an Optiview technique. Five ports are placed (Fig. 2), and a 10-mm, 30-degree laparoscope is used. As in all pancreatic procedures, the peritoneal surfaces, the omentum, the mesentery, and the viscera should be carefully inspected to rule out metastatic disease. Intraoperative ultrasonography may be used to evaluate the liver and locate the lesion in the pancreas.

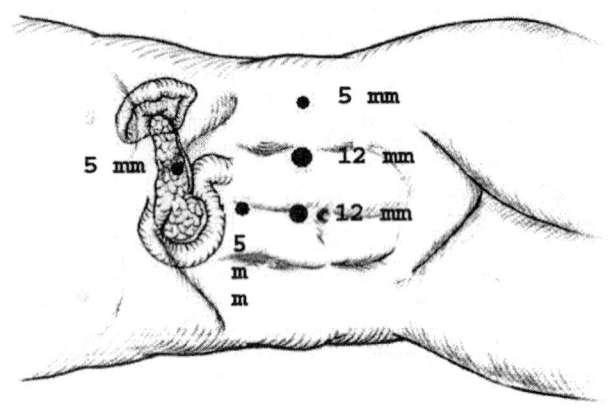

Figure 2 Positioning and port placement for laparoscopic distal pancreatectomy.

The body and tail of the pancreas are exposed by opening the lesser sac. The gastrocolic omentum is divided and widely mobilized with an ultrasonic dissector (e.g., Harmonic Scalpel; Johnson & Johnson Gateway, Piscataway, NJ), with care taken to stay outside the gastroepiploic vessels. The short gastric vessels usually do not need to be divided, and every effort should be made to preserve them if a splenic-preserving procedure is being attempted. A retractor is advanced into the lesser sac through the subxiphoid port and used to elevate the stomach anteromedially. The splenocolic ligament is divided, and the splenic flexure of the colon is reflected inferiorly.

After these maneuvers have been accomplished, the inferior pancreatic margin should be exposed. The peritoneum is then incised along the inferior pancreatic border, and the pancreatic body is separated from the retroperitoneum by means of sharp and blunt dissection along its inferior border. Laparoscopic ultrasonography and direct visual inspection, combined with the findings

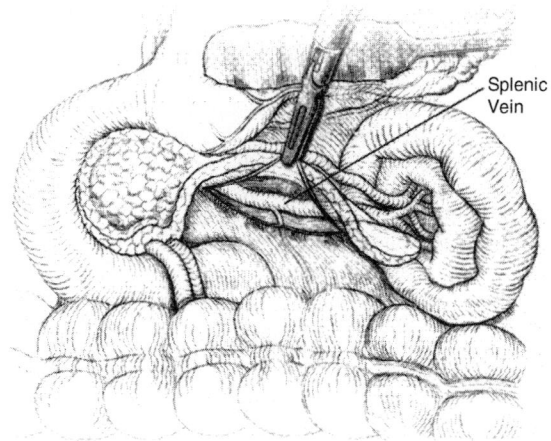

Figure 3 Identification of the splenic vein following mobilization of the pancreatic body from the retroperitoneum.

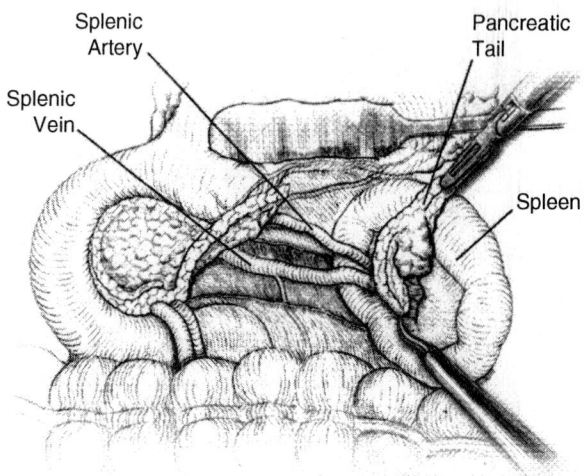

Figure 5 Medial-to-lateral dissection of the pancreas off of the splenic vessels.

from preoperative imaging, may be used to determine the extent of the dissection. Initially, the dissection should be directed so that it is medial to the pancreatic lesion. The pancreatic body is elevated by means of blunt and sharp dissection, after which the splenic vein should be easily identifiable (Fig. 3). Care must be exercised to prevent inadvertent injury to this vessel. After the splenic vein has been identified, a careful circumferential dissection around the splenic vein is performed, and a vessel loop is placed around the vein. The splenic artery can be identified from the under surface of the pancreas by retracting on the vessel loop around the splenic vein, or it can be identified along the superior border of the pancreas anteriorly. After it has been dissected circumferentially, it is controlled with a vessel loop. These precautionary measures allow quick control of bleeding should a vascular tear occur later in the procedure.

After the pancreatic body has been adequately mobilized from the splenic vessels, the pancreatic parenchyma is divided with the ultrasonic scalpel. Alternatively, an endoscopic stapler can be placed across the pancreas, sparing the main splenic vessels (Fig. 4). After the proximal pancreatic tissue has been divided, the specimen is grasped and gently retracted anteriorly to allow further dissection of the vessels. The dissection proceeds toward the splenic hilum in a medial-to-lateral direction. The pancreatic branches of the splenic vein are sequentially identified, dissected free with laparoscopic Metzenbaum scissors, and divided with the ultrasonic scalpel

(Fig. 5). The branches of the splenic artery, which runs just superior to the vein, are treated similarly. Special care must be taken because the dissection approaches the hilum of the spleen.

At the completion of an SPDP, the specimen is placed and removed in a standard endoscopic retrieval bag. The pancreatic remnant is then oversewn with a series of interrupted absorbable horizontal mattress sutures. A single round Jackson-Pratt drain is placed near the pancreatic transection line and brought out through one of the 5-mm lateral ports.

An alternative approach to SPDP involves dividing the splenic vessels proximally and distally while preserving the short gastric and left gastroepiploic vessels to maintain splenic perfusion (see Fig. 1). The initial steps of this technique are essentially the same as those described earlier, up to the division of the pancreas. In the alternative approach to SPDP, after pancreatic transection the splenic artery and vein are divided with an endovascular stapler. The left portion of the pancreas is lifted up and mobilized posteriorly along with the splenic artery and vein, and the vessels are again divided as they emerge from the pancreatic tail to enter the hilum of the spleen. The spleen is then supplied solely by the short gastric vessels and the left gastroepiploic vessels.

If an en bloc DP with splenectomy is performed, the splenic artery and vein are divided after the pancreas is transected. The distal pancreas is dissected free in a medial-to-lateral direction. The short gastric vessels are divided with the ultrasonic scalpel, with care taken not to injure the stomach wall. The retroperitoneal attachments of the spleen and the tail of the pancreas are divided with the ultrasonic scalpel. The specimen is then placed in a specimen retrieval bag and extracted from a port site that has been enlarged to a size of 3 to 6 cm. To facilitate extraction of the specimen, the spleen may be morcellated within the bag.

LAPAROSCOPIC PANCREATIC ENUCLEATION

Recently, laparoscopic techniques have been applied to the enucleation of benign neuroendocrine tumors of the pancreas. This approach is indicated for tumors located in the body and tail of the pancreas that do not appear to involve the pancreatic duct on preoperative imaging. Patient positioning and trocar placement are similar to the procedures for laparoscopic DP (see previous section). The body and tail of the pancreas are widely exposed by entering the lesser sac through the gastrocolic omentum. Intraoperative ultrasound is useful for the identification of the tumor

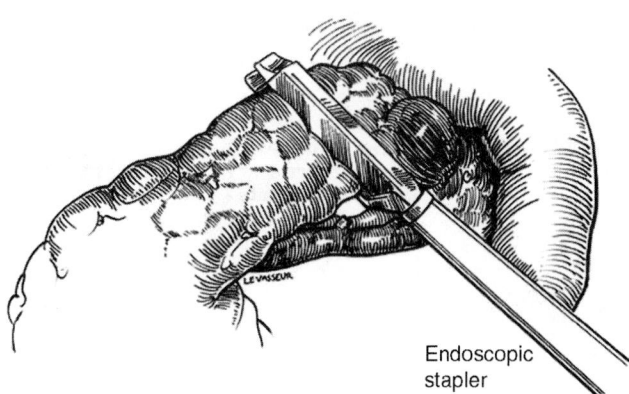

Figure 4 Transection of the body of the pancreas sparing the main splenic vessels.

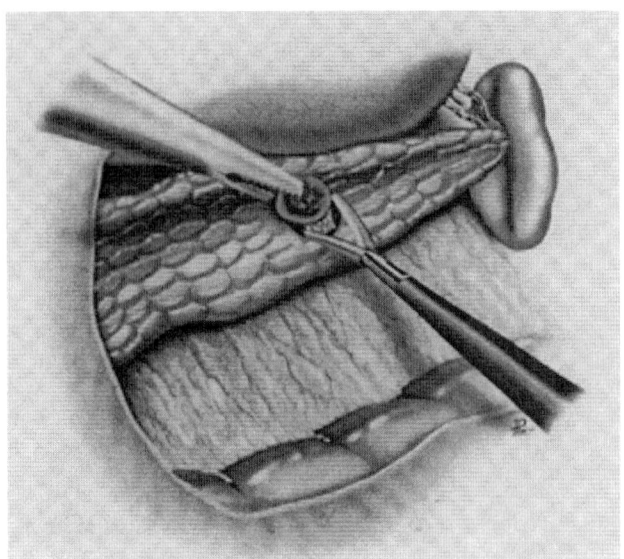

Figure 6 Laparoscopic pancreatic enucleation. *From Fernández-Cruz L, Saenz A, Astudillo E, and others: Outcome of laparoscopic pancreatic surgery: endocrine and nonendocrine tumors, World J Surg 26:1057, 2002.*

and to further delineate the relationship to the splenic vessels and the pancreatic duct. The lesion can then be dissected out of the pancreatic parenchyma using the ultrasonic shears and electrocautery (Fig. 6). The specimen is placed in a specimen retrieval bag and removed. The enucleation bed is then inspected for hemostasis, and a closed-suction drain is placed to control any potential pancreatic leak.

RESULTS

In the past 5 years it has become clear that laparoscopic DP can be performed safely by surgeons experienced in both advanced laparoscopic techniques and pancreatic surgery. One large, multi-institutional series and several smaller, single-institution series have been published (Table 4). In these series the operative time ranged from 3 to 5 hours, the complication rate was between 17% and 41%, the pancreatic fistula rate was between 4% and 38%, and the length of stay between 4 and 11 days. In comparison, in a large series of open DP reported by Lillemoe and colleagues, the mean operative time was 4.7 hours, and the overall morbidity was 31%. The pancreatic fistula rate and abdominal abscess rate were 5% and 4%, respectively. The safety of laparoscopic splenic-preserving DP was demonstrated by Fernández-Cruz and colleagues. In a series of 19 patients with cystic neoplasms of the pancreas, they showed that splenic preservation can be accomplished safely with or without splenic artery and vein ligation (Table 5). In their series, the overall conversion rate was 0%; the mean operative time was 222 minutes, and the overall morbidity 31%. Splenic vessel preservation was associated with a longer operative time and a greater amount of blood loss.

Although there has not been a prospective randomized comparison of laparoscopic and open DP, it appears that laparoscopic DP can be accomplished with a similar mortality, morbidity, and pancreatic fistula rate as open pancreatic surgery. However, laparoscopic surgery may be associated with a shorter hospital stay, a smaller amount of blood loss, and a higher likelihood of splenic preservation.

The largest report of laparoscopic pancreatic enucleations comes from a multicenter European study (Table 6). The authors report on successfully completing laparoscopic enucleations in 21 of 22 patients (95%). The mean operative time was 120 minutes and the mean length of stay 7 days. The pancreatic-related

Table 4: Results of Laparoscopic Distal Pancreatectomy

Author	Year	Procedure	N	Spleen Preservation (%)	Operative Time (hr)	Pancreatic Fistula/ Abscess (%)	Morbidity (%)	LOS (days)
Marbut and others	2005	Lap	82	71	3.3	27–38	41	7.0
Park	2002	Lap	23	41	3.7	4	17	4.1
Dulucq	2005	Lap	21	76	4.6	14	23	10.8
Fernández-Cruz and others	2004	Lap	19	100	3.7	15	31	5.7
Patterson	2001	Lap	19	37	4.4	16	26	6.0
Edwin	2004	Lap	17	29	4.0	—	38	5.5
Lillemoe	1999	Open	235	16	4.7	9	31	10

Lap, Laparoscopic; *LOS,* length of stay.

Table 5: Spleen-Preserving Distal Pancreatectomy for Cystic Neoplasms of the Pancreas

	N	Size (cm)	Operative Time (min.)	EBL (ml)	Complication Rate (%)	LOS (days)
Splenic vessel Preservation	11	5.3	222	496	27	5.5
Splenic vessel Ligation	8	5.1	165	275	38	5.6

EBL, Estimated blood loss; *LOS,* length of stay; *min.,* minutes; *N,* total number of patients.
Adapted from Fernández-Cruz L, Martínez I, Gilabert R, and others: J Gastrointest Surg 8:493, 2004.

Table 6: Results of Laparoscopic Pancreatic Enucleation

Author	Year	N	Operative Time (min.)	Complication Rate (%)	LOS (days)
Marbut	2005	21	120	29	7
Fernández-Cruz	2005	7	180	42	5
Edwin	2004	6	120	—	5.5
Berends	2000	5	180	40	7

LOS, length of stay; *min.*, minutes; *N*, total number of patients.

(pancreatic fistula, fluid collection, or both) complication rate was 29%, which is comparable to that reported for open pancreatic enucleation.

It has become clear that laparoscopic DP and laparoscopic pancreatic enucleation can be accomplished with acceptable morbidity and a shorter length of stay as compared with open procedures. However, laparoscopic pancreatic resections are advanced minimally invasive procedures and should be performed in carefully selected patients by surgeons with extensive experience in pancreatic surgery and advanced laparoscopic skills.

SUGGESTED READINGS

Dulucq JL, Wintringer P, Mahajna A: Laparoscopic pancreaticoduodenectomy for benign and malignant diseases, *Surg Endosc* 20:1045, 2006.

Fernández-Cruz L, Martínez I, Gilabert R, and others: Laparoscopic distal pancreatectomy combined with preservation of the spleen for cystic neoplasms of the pancreas, *J Gastrointest Surg* 8:493, 2004.

Mabrut JY, Fernández-Cruz L, Azagra JS, and others: Laparoscopic pancreatic resection: results of a multicenter European study of 127 patients, *Surgery* 137:597, 2005.

Nakeeb A: The role of minimally invasive surgery for pancreatic pathology, *Adv Surg* 39:455, 2005.

LAPAROSCOPIC MANAGEMENT OF PANCREATIC PSEUDOCYST

Swee H. Teh, MD, and Brett C. Sheppard, MD

INTRODUCTION

Pancreatic pseudocysts are found in 10% to 15% of patients following acute pancreatitis, and they are a sequela in 20% to 40% of patients with chronic pancreatitis. Pancreatic pseudocysts may be managed with a range of therapeutic modalities depending on the clinical context. For the majority of patients, nonoperative management is appropriate because most pseudocysts will resolve spontaneously within 6 to 8 weeks. Persistent pancreatic pseudocysts usually require intervention. Management options include percutaneous, endoscopic, and surgical drainage. Percutaneous and endoscopic drainage procedures have been shown to have a higher failure rate than surgical approaches. Laparoscopic approaches are attractive because they combine the benefit of a less invasive approach with the outcome of a more traditional surgical procedure. However, a minimally invasive approach for the management of pancreatic pseudocyst must have long-term outcomes equivalent to those of open series to be accepted. Laparoscopic approaches to pancreatic pseudocysts have been described by several groups. Currently there is a paucity of level I data to support the laparoscopic approach over open operative conduct for the management of pancreatic pseudocysts. There are, however, level II and III data that demonstrate that minimally invasive drainage procedures for pancreatic pseudocysts are technically feasible, safe, and associated with less perioperative morbidity and a shorter hospital stay when compared with open procedures. Mature, long-term outcomes are not yet available for laparoscopic approaches to pancreatic pseudocysts.

INDICATIONS

Indications for the laparoscopic approach to pancreatic pseudocysts are identical to those for an open approach: that is, persistence of a 6-cm pseudocyst beyond 4 to 6 weeks from diagnosis or persistence of symptoms. An understanding of pancreatic ductal anatomy may help to guide therapeutic decisions. Most pseudocysts are found within the body and tail of the pancreas. Pseudocysts may be found less commonly in the head of the pancreas. Surgical options include laparoscopic cystogastrostomy, cystojejunostomy, cystoduodenostomy, or external drainage. In patients with ductal disruption within the body of the pancreas associated with a distal pancreatic pseudocyst, laparoscopic distal pancreatic resection may be the procedure of choice. Laparoscopic splenic preservation with distal pancreatic resection is often technically challenging secondary to the significant amount of inflammation and fibrosis around the splenic vein. Splenic preservation rates are generally lower for this indication than for other indications of laparoscopic distal pancreatic resection.

PREOPERATIVE INVESTIGATION AND PREPARATION

A standardized preoperative evaluation should be performed independent of the operative approach. The essential investigation is a contrast-enhanced, spiral computed tomography (CT) scan with a pancreatic protocol that includes both arterial and venous phases. This will provide detailed anatomic information of the size, location, number of pseudocysts, and the important relationship to adjacent structures. In patients who have suspicious cystic lesions on CT or for those who do not have a clear clinical history of pancreatitis, endoscopic ultrasound (EUS) with fine needle aspiration and cyst fluid sampling are indicated. Magnetic resonance cholangiopancreatography may be useful to help define pancreatic ductal anatomy and may obviate the need for an endoscopic retrograde cholangiopancreatography (ERCP). In selected patients who have a dilatated pancreatic duct, it is appropriate to obtain an ERCP to ensure a normal papilla and normal ductal anatomy in the head of the pancreas.

The optimal interval to internally drain pancreatic pseudocysts is usually 6 to 8 weeks following diagnosis. By this time, the pseudocyst wall is sufficiently strong for a surgical anastomosis: the surrounding inflammation is quiescent and the secondary fibrosis promotes close adhesion of the pseudocyst to surrounding structures. For patients with pseudocysts caused by biliary pancreatitis, laparoscopic cholecystectomy is often concurrently performed. Preoperative medical evaluation for cardiopulmonary disease and overall fitness for surgery are essential. Adequate hydration, preoperative antibiotics, and deep vein thrombosis prophylaxis are indicated.

The list of essential laparoscopic equipment includes either a 5-or 10-mm, 30- and 45-degree laparoscope, a flexible or rigid laparoscopic US probe, an ultrasonic dissector, a 10-mm clip applier, blunt-tipped atraumatic bowel graspers, fine-tipped needle drivers, and an articulating endo-GIA stapler (US Surgical, Norwalk, CT) (with 2.5- and 3.5-mm staple height loads). A hand port should be available because some of these procedures may be facilitated and may be safer with the use of a hand port. Fibrin glue application may also be useful in some settings and should be available.

OPERATION

Operative principles are delineated in Table 1. Positioning and setup for patients undergoing laparoscopic cystoenteric drainage are similar to those for patients undergoing distal pancreatic resection. General anesthesia with endotracheal intubation and complete neuromuscular blockade are required for this operation. Whenever possible, all trocar sites larger than 5 mm should be closed on completion of the procedure. Additional infiltration of local anesthetic into the trocar site at the end of the procedure will promote patient comfort.

POSITION

The patient is placed in supine position with the upper and lower extremities well padded and comfortably secured. This prevents adverse loads while the operating table is tilted during the procedure. The surgeon stands at the right, and the assistant stands at the left of the patient. An alternative approach is for the operating surgeon to stand between the legs while the assistant remains at the left side of the patient. At times during the course of the operative conduct for pseudocyst drainage, it will be useful for both the surgeon and the assistant to be at the left side of the patient. This is most helpful during creation of the cyst gastrostomy because it allows positioning of the ultrasonic dissector and the stapler in the same vector as the camera image. Trocar placement will depend on body habitus and operative intent. Operative principles of triangulation of instruments relative to the laparoscope are followed in all cases (Fig. 1). Pneumoperitoneum is achieved by either a Veress needle placed through the

Table 1: Operative Principles of Laparoscopic Management of Pancreatic Pseudocysts

Laparoscopic cystoenteric drainage (cystogastrostomy, cystojejunostomy, cystoduodenostomy)
a. Pseudocyst localization, fluid aspiration, and wall biopsy
b. Cystoenteric anastomosis (suture or staple)

Laparoscopic distal pancreatic resection
a. Lesser sac exposure, splenic flexure, and mesocolon mobilization
b. Pancreatic mobilization, splenic artery, and vein isolation and ligation
c. Pancreatic transaction and pancreatic stump management

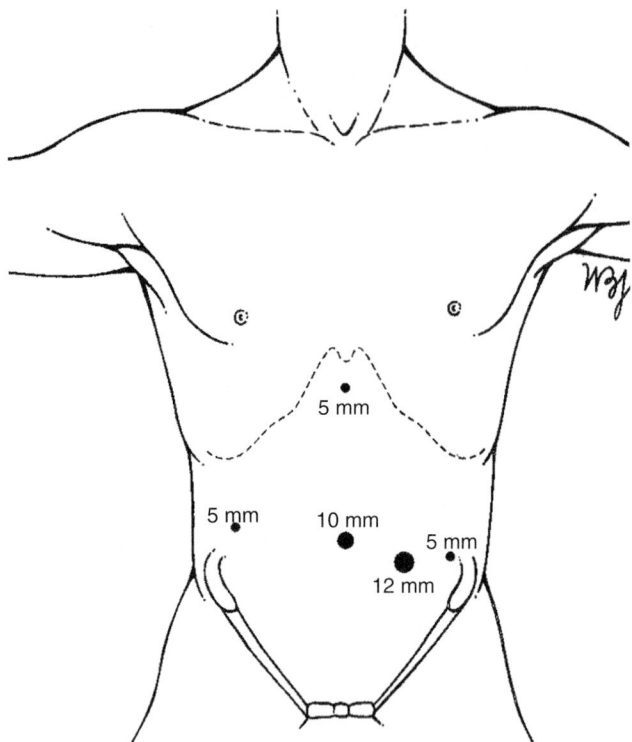

Figure I   Trocar position: Triangulation of trocars.

umbilicus or a cutdown Hasson technique at the site of the operating laparoscope. All subsequent trocars are inserted under direct vision.

ENDOLUMINAL LAPAROSCOPIC CYSTOGASTROSTOMY

Method with Esophagogastroduodenoscopy

After the patient is prepped and draped, an esophagogastroduodenoscope (EGD) is advanced into the stomach, and pneumoperitoneum is achieved. A 5-mm trocar is placed through the umbilicus, and a 5-mm 30-degree ***is inserted and the abdomen explored. A 5-mm trocar is placed 6 to 8 cm below the right costal margin in the midclavicular line, and a 10-mm trocar is placed in a similar position below the left costal margin. The stomach is now insufflated using the eEGD. Under direct exoluminal and endoluminal vision, the first T-piece is placed near the greater curve of the stomach across from the incisura, and the stomach wall brought up to the abdominal wall. If T-pieces are not available, a 2–0 Prolene (Ethicon, Somerville, NJ) suture on a Keith needle can be placed through the abdominal wall into the stomach and brought back out through the abdominal wall. Decreasing the pneumoperitoneum to 10 mm Hg will facilitate this maneuver. Next, a 5-mm trocar is placed through the abdominal wall directly through the gastric wall and into the lumen of the stomach. A 5-mm 30-degree camera is inserted and after a secure image has been obtained, the eEGD is withdrawn back to near the gastroesophageal junction. Two additional endoluminal trocars must be placed: a 12-mm trocar to support the use of the endo-GIA stapler and laparoscopic US and an additional 5-mm port for additional instrumentation. Usually two additional T-pieces are required to control the gastric wall before placing the next trocars.

We prefer to place the 5-mm endoluminal trocar next to maintain principles of triangulation. This allows for use of 5-mm instruments to explore the stomach and "feel" for the pseudocyst if it is not readily apparent on visual inspection. We place the 12-mm trocar close to the greater curve oriented toward the pylorus. This provides the correct angle for US examination and later use of the stapler. When all the endoluminal trocars are in place, we desufflate the abdomen and switch the insufflation tubing to the endoluminal trocar. Endogastric insufflation can be set to 10 to 15 mm Hg. The laparoscopic US probe is inserted, the pseudocyst is imaged, and its configuration and relation to the posterior gastric wall are evaluated. If there is close apposition without significant intervening vasculature, we proceed. The ultrasonic dissector is used to create a posterior gastrotomy and enter the pseudocyst. A small jet of cyst fluid confirms entry. This area is enlarged, and the cyst fluid aspirated. Atypical fluid should be sent to the pathology laboratory for cytology or Gram stain and culture (or both). After the fluid has been drained, the entry site into the pseudocyst is enlarged to accommodate a stapler load. Before stapling, we explore the pseudocyst to ensure an absence of both suspicious septae and exposed cyst wall vessels. If encountered, the septae are biopsied and the vessels oversewn. Otherwise we place a 3.5-mm staple height (blue) articulating load, usually 30 mm or 45 mm in length, for the initial stapler application. Subsequent staple applications are used to create a 5- to 7-cm cystogastrostomy and to obtain a portion of the pseudocyst wall for biopsy. Following this, additional necrotic debris can be removed as needed. Hemostasis along the staple line is evaluated. Isolated "bleeders" may require interrupted 2–0 silk sutures. If there is any question of staple line integrity, it is oversewn using a running 3–0 monofilament absorbable suture.

Trocars are then withdrawn from the stomach but remain in the abdominal cavity, and the abdomen is reinsufflated. The three trocar defects in the stomach wall can then be closed under direct vision by interrupted 2–0 silk suture.

Method without Esophagogastroduodenoscopy

Following preparation and draping, pneumoperitoneum is obtained and a 5-mm trocar is placed at the umbilical site. Trocars are placed as previously described. The abdomen is explored with a 5-mm, 30-degree laparoscope. The stomach is insufflated through an oral gastric tube. Under direct vision the stomach is then elevated and fixed to the abdominal wall using T fasteners or Keith needles passed through the abdominal wall and placed into the seromuscular layer of the gastric wall. Generally, 2–3 sutures are placed to provide fixation and some degree of tension. A 5-mm trocar is then placed directly through the gastric wall. A 5-mm, 30-degree laparoscope is then used to explore the stomach and to guide the next series of trocars (Fig. 2). The remainder of the cystogastrostomy procedure is similar to that described for endoluminal laparoscopic cystogastrostomy with EGD.

EXTRALUMINAL LAPAROSCOPIC CYSTOGASTROSTOMY

For a pseudocyst that is located more on the inferior aspect of the stomach, an extraluminal cystogastrostomy approach may be reasonable. The greater omentum is dissected off the greater curvature of the stomach below the epiploic arch. The pseudocyst is usually easily identified and is confirmed with laparoscopic US. Color Doppler US may also be useful to ensure the intended cystogastrostomy site does not contain significant vascular structures. The cystostomy site is created using the ultrasonic dissector. Pseudocyst contents are suctioned, and the cystostomy is enlarged to

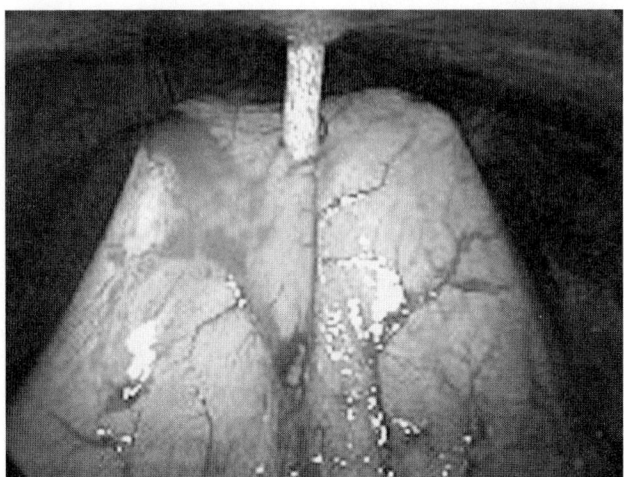

Figure 2 Two T-pieces are placed near the greater curvature of the stomach from the incisura, and the stomach wall is brought up to the abdominal wall.

approximately 1 cm. A portion of the pseudocyst wall is sent to the pathology laboratory, and the cystic cavity is inspected with the laparoscope. Next, a 1-cm gastrotomy is similarly created in juxtaposition to the cystotomy site. A 6-cm cystogastrostomy is then fashioned with an articulated endo-GIA stapler with multiple blue loads. The remaining defect is closed with interrupted 2–0 silk sutures or an absorbable running monofilament suture.

LAPAROSCOPIC CYSTOJEJUNOSTOMY (LOOP OR ROUX-EN-Y)

Following laparoscopic exploration, two additional 5-mm trocars are inserted, one on the right approximately 10 cm lateral and above the umbilicus and the other on the left approximately 10 cm from the umbilicus. Using atraumatic graspers, the greater omentum is reflected in the cephalad direction to expose the transverse mesocolon. A large bulge is usually appreciated near the base of the transverse mesocolon, and the wall of the pseudocyst can usually be located here. A 12-mm trocar is then inserted on the far left of the abdominal wall for use of the laparoscopic ultrasound and the articulated endo-GIA stapler. The location of the pseudocyst is confirmed by US. The middle colic vessels may be adherent to the pseudocyst and may be difficult to identify because of inflammation and fibrosis. The most dependent portion of the pseudocyst, usually located superior and lateral to the ligament of Treitz, is chosen for the initial cystotomy. Following the cystotomy, the contents of the pseudocyst are aspirated, and a portion of the cyst wall is resected for pathology. The laparoscope is then advanced into the pseudocyst to inspect the lining, and irrigation is performed.

The cystojejunostomy can be created with a simple loop of jejunum or a Roux-en-Y. For a loop cystojejunostomy, the small bowel is run distally from the ligament of Treitz, and the most proximal loop of jejunum that can be easily brought up to the location of the pseudocyst without tension is chosen. Two silk stay sutures are placed, approximately 5 cm apart, to approximate the pseudocyst and the jejunum. Placement of suture on the antimesenteric side of the jejunum minimizes the chance that the small bowel mesentery will be caught in the endo-GIA stapler. A 1-cm jejunotomy is created with ultrasonic dissector. An articulated, blue load, endo-GIA staple is inserted into the cystostomy and jejunotomy from the left lateral 12-mm trocar. Stapling of these two defects will create a cystojejunostomy. The enterotomy is then closed with interrupted 2–0 silk sutures or a running absorbable monofilament suture.

For a Roux-en-Y cystojejunostomy, the small bowel is again run from the ligament of Treitz. A Roux limb of 45 cm is created with a blue staple load of appropriate length. The end of the Roux limb is brought up to the cystotomy site, and two silk sutures are placed, approximately 5 cm apart, to approximate the pseudocyst and the jejunum. The cystojejunostomy is then created in fashion similar to that of the loop cystojejunostomy. It is critical to ensure that the mesentery of the Roux limb is not injured by the stapler. A functional end-to-side jejunojejunostomy is performed, and the mesenteric defect is closed with interrupted 3–0 silk sutures.

LAPAROSCOPIC CYSTODUODENOSTOMY

Laparoscopic cystoduodenostomy is rarely indicated because it requires the pseudocyst to be located at the head of the pancreas and to be sufficiently large to impinge on to the duodenum. Both of these conditions are clinically uncommon. Clinical symptoms from this rare entity may be best treated with a pancreatic ductal drainage procedure or pancreatic resection. Therefore before laparoscopic cystoduodenostomy is considered, the etiology of the clinical symptoms should be fully investigated and understood.

If cystoduodenostomy is to be performed, the preferred site to drain the pseudocyst is into the second portion of the duodenum. To begin, the greater omentum is dissected off the inferior aspect of the stomach. The origin of the right epiploic and arch can be preserved. Taking the time to fully Kocherize the duodenum will facilitate the subsequent cystoduodenostomy. The pseudocyst is localized visually and confirmed by US. The sites for duodenotomy and cystotomy are critical to creating a tension-free anastomosis and preventing injury to the ampulla of Vater. Full Kocherization will usually allow use of the anterior duodenal wall and prevent injury to the Vaterian complex. A small cystotomy is created, and the contents of the pseudocyst are aspirated. A portion of the pseudocyst wall is sent to the pathology laboratory. A 1-cm cystostomy is then created, and the laparoscope is inserted inside the pseudocyst to inspect the lining. A transverse duodenostomy less than 1 cm is created at the distal end of the second part of duodenum at least 0.5 cm away from the duodenopancreatic groove. The endo-GIA staple is then inserted into these two defects. The distal end of the staple is articulated to aim away from the ampulla of Vater. The enterostomy is then closed with interrupted 3–0 silk. If a cystoduodenostomy is to be created with suture only, then a 2- to 3-cm duodenostomy should be created in the vertical axis. Care is exercised to avoid taking large "bites" of tissue with each suture and thereby injuring the ampulla. Suturing of the posterior and the anterior aspect of the anastomosis is accomplished with interrupted 3–0 silk.

LAPAROSCOPIC DISTAL PANCREATIC RESECTION

The lesser sac exposure can be achieved by mobilizing the omentum from the greater curvature of the stomach below the right epiploic arch. This mobilization is continued up the greater curvature by dividing the short gastric vessels up to the left crura. The fibrous bands between the posterior wall of the stomach and the pancreas are divided. To further enhance exposure, the posterior wall of the stomach at the greater curvature can be brought up to the anterior abdominal wall using a Keith needle technique as previously described. The splenic flexure of the colon is then extensively mobilized, but the splenophrenic attachment is intentionally left intact to provide lateral retraction. Laparoscopic ultrasound is used to provide information on the location of the pseudocyst and its relationship with the splenic vessels and to help determine the feasibility of splenic preservation. The surgical resection line for distal

pancreas resection is chosen on the basis of the information obtained from the intraoperative US.

It is usually easier to perform pancreatic dissection from the neck/body toward the tail. In patients with a pseudocyst at the tail and also significant fibrosis from chronic inflammation, the tail-to-neck approach may be safer and easier. A hand port can be used in difficult cases. Pancreatic mobilization starts with dissection of the visceral peritoneum along the inferior border of the pancreas and extends laterally. It is important to first create a superficial plane along this margin before advancing too posteriorly. Next, the dissection drops down to below the level of the splenic vein. The tissue plane below the pancreas but above the kidney and adrenal gland is generally easy to separate. The splenic vein is mobilized while still adherent to the posterior pancreatic surface for distal pancreatic resection and splenectomy. The inferior mesenteric vein (IMV) located just lateral to ligament of Treitz should be identified. An attempt to save the IMV if it courses superiorly to join the splenic vein is not unreasonable. Some venous tributaries from the splenic vein into the retroperitoneum may be encountered and must be dissected and divided with the use of the ultrasonic dissector or endoclips.

Next, the superior margin of the pancreas should be dissected. The splenic artery is often identified during this part of the dissection, although it may lie deeper and close to the splenic vein. With use of a hand port, the thumb and index finger of the surgeon's left hand can facilitate this part of the dissection. The splenic artery, vein, and pancreatic parenchyma should be dissected separately. A dissection length of at least 1.5 cm is necessary for the application of an articulated endo-GIA 2.5-mm staple height (white) load. Alternatively, endoclips can be used. However, the use of endoclips on one vessel may impede the use of the endo-GIA stapler for the other vessel. The dissection of the splenic vein is challenging because of its thin wall and it branches. Venous branches should be divided with ultrasonic dissection or 5-mm clips. Splenic preservation requires gentle dissection of the splenic vein off the underside of the pancreas. A hand port can also facilitate this dissection. If no hand port is used, an umbilical tape or vessel loop can be placed around the splenic vein to provide the necessary counter-traction for dissection. Dissection of the splenic artery is generally straightforward. If splenic preservation is not possible, then the splenic artery and vein can be divided with a white stapler load. The choice of staple size for pancreatic transaction varies depending on the thickness of the pancreas. We commonly use blue loads and less commonly 4.8-mm green loads. White or gray loads should not be used because the staples are not deep enough to provide a secure stable line. It is important to visualize the distal end of the stapler to ensure it does not injure adjacent structures. It is also important to ensure that none of the endoclips are within the path of the endo stapler application. Gentle and slow application of the staples may help hemostasis and prevent unnecessary traumatic injury to the pancreas parenchyma. The pancreatic dissection is continued laterally, and the splenic mobilization is completed. The specimen is then removed via the hand port or with a retrieval Endobag (Autosuture, Norwalk, CT).

The main pancreatic duct is routinely identified and oversewn with 3–0 Prolene suture in a figure-of-eight pattern. If the pancreatic duct cannot be identified, a running 3–0 Prolene suture is placed along the entire staple line. Fibrin glue may be used to cover the staple line. A surgical drain is placed.

POSTOPERATIVE CARE

Patients are cared for on the regular surgical ward unless otherwise indicated. We routinely provide 24 hours of antibiotics and remove the nasogastric tube the following day. Sips of liquid are then initiated as tolerated. We found that postoperative ileus and pain are not significant issues in most patients who undergo laparoscopic management of pancreatic pseudocysts. Patients are typically

Table 2: Published Series (*n* > 10) for Laparoscopic Management of Pancreatic Pseudocyst

Authors	N	Conversion	LOS (Days)	OR Time (Minutes)	Morbidity	Mortality	Follow-up (Months)	Pseudocyst Recurrence
Hindmarsh, Lewis, Rhodes (2005)	15	3/15 (20%)	7	82	33%	0%	37	0
Davila-Cervantes, Gomez, Chan, and others (2004)	10	0	7	240	20%	0%	22	0
Hauters, Weerts, Navez, and others (2004)	17	0	6	100	11%	0%	12	0
Park, Heniford (2002)	28	1/29 (3%)	4.4	162	3%	0%	15.8	0

LOS, Length of stay; *N,* total number of patients; *OR,* operating room.

discharged home on postoperative day 3 to 5 without dietary restriction and with the surgical drain removed.

Pancreatic leak remains a vexing issue for distal pancreatic resection regardless of the approach. We do not routinely send drain fluid for amylase unless indicated by high-volume output or persistent intra-abdominal irritation manifested commonly as fever, ileus, or lack of clinical improvement.

Laparoscopic management of pancreatic pseudocyst is safe and technically feasible with an overall perioperative mortality of 0% and morbidity of 5% to 30% (Table 2). It is also associated with a shorter hospital stay. The frequency of pancreatic ductal leaks in patients with laparoscopic distal pancreatic resection (8%) is approximately equivalent to that of patients with open surgical resection. The perioperative morbidity of laparoscopic management of pancreatic pseudocysts is significantly improved from the results seen with open approach. In the open approach, most of the morbidity is related to ileus, wound infection, and cardiopulmonary complications. These are typically not seen in patients with a laparoscopic approach and are a distinct advantage of the minimally invasive approach.

The long-term durability of the laparoscopic management of pancreatic pseudocyst is yet to be established. The intermediate-term results are encouraging and seem to be comparable with those of open approach.

Suggested Readings

Davila-Cervantes A, Gomez F, Chan C, and others: Laparoscopic drainage of pancreatic pseudocysts, *Surg Endosc* 18(10):1420, 2004.

Hauters P, Weerts J, Navez B, and others: Laparoscopic treatment of pancreatic pseudocysts, *Surg Endosc* 18(11):1645, 2004.

Hindmarsh A, Lewis MP, Rhodes M: Stapled laparoscopic cystgastrostomy: a series with 15 cases, *Surg Endosc* 19(1):143, 2005.

Park AE, Heniford BT: Therapeutic laparoscopy of the pancreas, *Ann Surg* 236(2):149, 2002.

Video-Assisted Thoracic Surgery

Sunil Singhal, MD, and Larry R. Kaiser, MD

The hemithorax is arguably the best body cavity for minimal access surgery. The rib cage provides a fixed space within which to work, and the ability to collapse the lung using a double-lumen endotracheal tube allows maximal exposure and visualization. Thoracoscopy was first performed in 1910 by a Swedish internist, Hans Christian Jacobaeus, to deal with the problem of pleural adhesions complicating the creation of an artificial pneumothorax. Thoracoscopy was at one time a first-line treatment for pulmonary tuberculosis. In the 1940s, the advent of streptomycin caused pneumothorax therapy to be abandoned, except at some European centers. Technological advances in the 1990s, in particular the development of the charged coupled device video camera, and percutaneous endoscopic instruments gave birth to the use of video-assisted techniques, known as video-assisted thoracic surgery (VATS), which could be applicable for both diagnostic and therapeutic procedures in the thoracic cavity. Specifically the use of these techniques in the chest quickly followed the development of laparoscopic cholecystectomy and other procedures being performed in the abdominal cavity.

Currently VATS is being used to perform virtually all thoracic procedures, including complex anatomic pulmonary resections, lung volume reduction surgery, antireflux procedures, and esophagectomies. The central goal of VATS approaches is to reduce postoperative pain and other postthoracotomy-related morbidity that follows thoracic surgery without compromising the therapeutic principles of an open approach. In this chapter, we discuss the general principles of performing a VATS procedure and describe the most common indications for this approach.

GENERAL PRINCIPLES

Proper patient selection is key to the use of any minimally invasive technique, and this certainly applies to VATS procedures. Indications and contraindications for VATS are listed in Table 1. A careful assessment of the patient's physiologic reserve is mandatory. The anesthesia personnel must be experienced in open thoracic procedures and be well versed in the principles of selective "one-lung" ventilation, as well as the use of double-lumen endotracheal tubes and bronchial blockers. VATS instruments that should

Table 1: Indications and Contraindications for Video-Assisted Thoracic Surgery

Diagnostic

Pleural effusions (benign vs. malignant)

Tissue diagnosis

    Pleural-based masses

    Indeterminate pulmonary nodules

    Diffuse parenchymal lung disease

    Anterior and posterior mediastinal masses

Staging for esophageal and pulmonary malignancies

Therapeutic

Pleural

    Trauma: retained hemothorax, suspicion of diaphragmatic injury

    Infections: early empyema

    Pneumothorax: persistent, recurrent

Pulmonary

    Neoplasms: wedge resection, VATS lobectomy

    Lung volume reduction surgery

Mediastinal

    Resection of mediastinal masses

    Pericardial diseases

    Sympathectomy

    Thymectomy

Esophageal

    Transthoracic vagotomy

    Esophageal motility disorders: myotomy, fundoplication

    Benign esophageal neoplasms: enteric cysts, leiomyoma

    Malignant esophageal neoplasms: VATS esophagectomy

Contraindications

Dense pleural adhesions

Unable to tolerate one-lung ventilation

Severe emphysema

Pulmonary hilar lesions or lesions located deep within the lung parenchyma

    Large pulmonary masses (>3 cm)

    Chest wall invasion

    Noncompliant lung or inability to achieve pulmonary atelectasis

VATS, Video-assisted thoracic surgery.

be available include 0- and 30-degree thoracoscopes, 12- to 15-mm ports, coaxially designed thoracoscopic graspers and scissors, tissue retractors, suction devices, and endoscopic stapling devices.

The patient is positioned in a full lateral decubitus position (Fig. 1), and the operating surgeon and assistant must have an unobstructed view of the monitors. After the double-lumen endotracheal tube position is confirmed in the left main bronchus, the operative site can be prepared and draped with adequate exposure in case the procedure must be converted to an open thoracotomy.

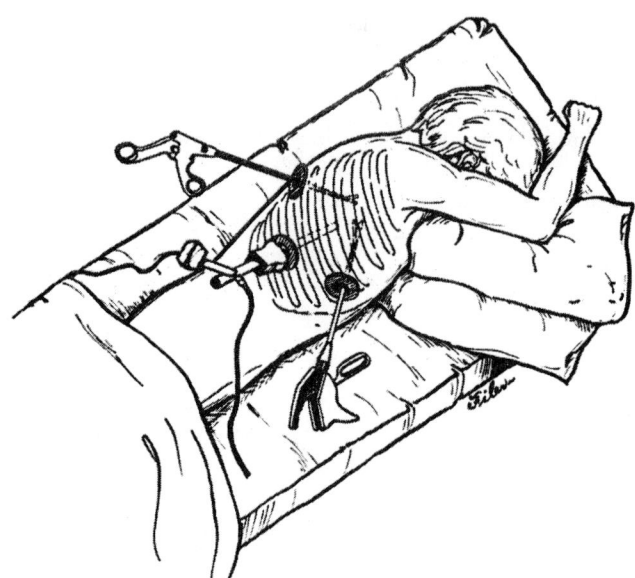

Figure 1 Generalized port placement for VATS. *From Dowling RD, Landreneau RJ, Magee MJ, and others: Thoracoscopic wedge resection of the lung,* Surg Rounds *16:341, 1993.*

The most important step in the operation is careful port placement. The computed tomography (CT) scan should be reviewed to formulate a plan for the proper port placement for the thoracoscopic instruments. The first port should be based at a site that will allow for optimal visualization of the pleural space and not interfere with the other instruments. The thoracoscope should be placed at a distance across from the lesion to achieve a panoramic view of the operative field. For most procedures, a second port should be placed over the pathology of interest. This permits better manipulation of the object, if necessary, and digital palpation for disease confirmation. Additional sites should allow instruments to be placed without crowding the operative space. Ideally the location of the lesion on the CT scan should be conceptualized in three dimensions, and the location of the trocars or incisions placed to form a triangulated setup that allows for the best use of the instruments and the best visualization. The camera and two instrument ports should face the lesion in question (Fig. 2).

For most routine procedures, we place the first port in the seventh or eighth intercostal space aligned with the anterior superior iliac spine. For operations that will require significant hilar dissection, we may place this incision slightly more anteriorly. At the end of the procedure, we can convert this port to the chest tube insertion site. We often plan the second port along the axillary line through the fourth intercostal space. The advantage of this site is it allows us to convert this incision to a muscle-sparing vertical axillary thoracotomy, if necessary, while reducing any excessive incision. Finally, we plan the third port slightly inferior and anterior to the tip of the scapula and enter through the sixth intercostal space. If it becomes necessary to convert to a posterolateral thoracotomy, this incision can be incorporated into the operation. In our practice we have evolved a scheme for port placement that essentially does not vary from case to case. The locations are "generic" and thus easier to use, and the position of the incisions allows for any procedure to be performed. Rarely have we found it necessary to use more than three incisions and, for that matter, not all operations require three ports. Routine diagnostic pleural procedures can often be performed through one port site. Two instruments (a thoracoscope and dissector) can fit through a 3-cm single incision.

After the initial port strategy is planned, the skin incision is made directly over the intercostal space where entry is planned.

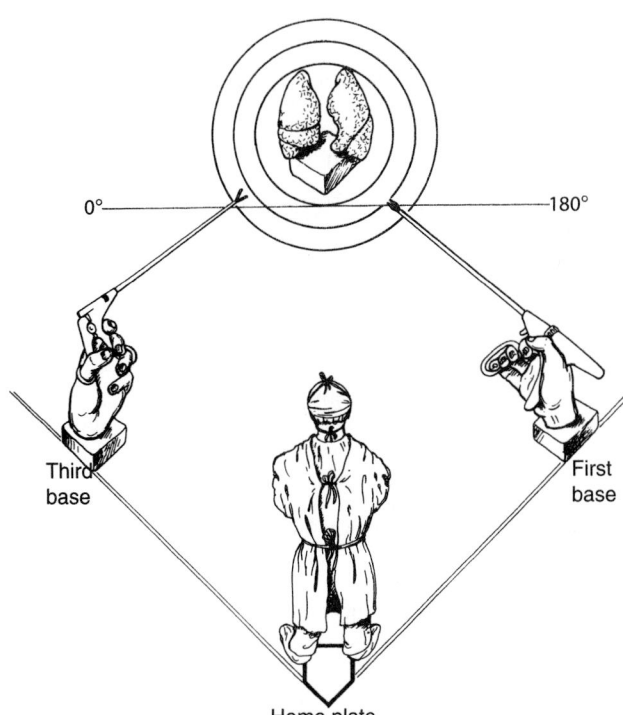

Figure 2 Baseball diamond: concept for triangulation of the instruments and the thoracoscope for strategic visibility and manipulation of the target pathology. *Reprinted from Landreneau RJ, Mack MJ, Hazelrigg RD, and others: Ann Thorac Surg 54:800, 1992.*

Electrocautery is used to dissect to the pleura, and the pleura is then entered either with a curved Kelly clamp or, more commonly, with the index finger. Carbon dioxide insufflation to 5 to 8 mm Hg occasionally is used to gently compress the lung to permit better access to esophageal and mediastinal diseases. Direct digital exploration is followed by trocar placement and initial thoracoscopic examination. The entire hemithorax should be examined. No opportunity should be allowed to pass without obtaining photo documentation of all pathologies.

VATS implies that no rib spreading is required throughout the entire procedure. If the operation requires placement of a rib spreader, the correct description of the procedure is minithoracotomy with VATS assistance.

Following completion of the operation, hemostasis should be ensured, and a chest tube should be inserted to monitor air leaks and hemorrhage overnight. In situations in which there has been minimal lung manipulation and thus no chance for an air leak, air can be cleared from the pleural space with a rubber catheter and no chest tube must remain. VATS ports should be closed in two layers; lung tissue has been reported to herniate through small, unclosed port sites, with resulting local abscess and tissue loss. Often a single, 2-cm bandage can be used to cover the wound. Pain should be well controlled with nonsteroidal anti-inflammatory agents and oral narcotics, particularly after the chest tube has been removed. Patients rarely require more than 24 to 48 hours in the hospital following these procedures.

PLEURAL PATHOLOGY

For presumed pleural pathology, VATS is primarily used for the diagnosis of pleural effusions and pleural-based masses. VATS can be also be used to manage empyemas, chest trauma with hemopneumothorax, spontaneous pneumothorax, and abdominal trauma with concerns of diaphragmatic rupture.

The most common presentation of a patient with pleural disease is pleural effusion. Needle thoracentesis is the first step in determining the etiology of an unknown pleural effusion; however, following thoracentesis 50% of patients remain without a known etiology or diagnosis. Particularly in pleural effusions for which the differential diagnosis is between adenocarcinoma and pleural malignant mesothelioma or simply reactive mesothelial cells, the fluid cytology yield is less than 20% accurate. VATS is used to sample the effusion as well as to visualize the entire pleural space to look for metastatic implants on either the visceral or parietal pleura, or both.

Obliteration of the pleural space or pleurodesis may be required to prevent reaccumulation of the fluid, depending on the etiology of the effusion. The majority of malignant pleural effusions require pleurodesis unless they have a high likelihood of clinical response to further therapy (e.g., lymphoma). Pleurodesis can be performed at the time of evacuation of the pleural fluid. The mechanism of action is to produce an inflammatory pleuritis, resulting in an obliteration of the pleural space by fusion of the parietal and visceral pleurae. The pleurodesis can be performed mechanically by disrupting the parietal pleura by mechanical abrasion. The main complication from this procedure includes inadvertent injury to the thoracic duct, sympathetic ganglion, or the esophagus. Alternatively, talc can be insufflated to effect a chemical pleuritis, with the resultant formation of dense adhesions. Two ports may be required: one for the telescope and one for suction and administration of the talc.

VATS is useful also in the management of early empyema. An empyema is a collection of pus or infected pleural effusion that evolves in three stages: exudative phase, fibropurulent phase, and chronically organized phase. Most commonly, empyema is postpneumonic in origin; that is, it results from an underlying pneumonia (65%). Diagnosis usually is made on clinical grounds, according to etiology, radiographic signs, and demonstration of infected fluid via thoracentesis. CT scan should be used to determine whether the pleural collection is free or loculated. Empyemas should be surgically drained as soon as suspected. Mortality increases rapidly as the infection remains trapped in the pleural space. During the early phase of an empyema, VATS can be used to explore the pleural space; drain and evacuate all infected fluid and debris; disrupt loculations; confirm good reexpansion of the lung; and, at times, correct the etiologic factor that caused the empyema. At the time of operation, if these goals cannot be achieved, the procedure should be converted to an open thoracotomy and pleurectomy and formal decortication performed as needed.

VATS is an ideal approach to diagnose pleural-based mass lesions. The sensitivity of thoracoscopic diagnosis of pleural-based lesions approaches 100%. Benign lesions can be completely removed by VATS. Malignant lesions usually are metastatic in origin, but VATS commonly is used for the initial diagnosis or confirmation of a diagnosis of primary malignancy of the pleura, malignant mesothelioma. Intraoperative frozen section should be performed to confirm adequate tissue sampling before terminating the procedure. Talc pleurodesis should be considered if recurrent pleural effusion is a concern.

VATS plays an important role in the management of chest trauma. Following an initial chest injury managed with tube thoracostomy, undrained blood and organized fibrinous material and clot can be removed from the thoracic cavity by VATS, thereby circumventing a formal thoracotomy. Early evacuation of blood from the chest cavity is critical to prevent the complications of empyema and fibrothorax. For blunt and penetrating trauma, VATS can be used to rule out a diaphragmatic injury, particularly for left-sided injuries. Small diaphragmatic perforations may be present with few signs or symptoms; however, they can result in bowel strangulation if not closed.

Chylothorax is an uncommon condition that arises from a broad range of etiologies, including cancer, trauma, and congenital abnormalities. A diagnosis of chylothorax is usually suspected on the basis of excess volume from the chest tube, often milky white, with chemical analysis that confirms an elevated triglyceride level.

Initially, a chylothorax should be treated by complete drainage of the pleural space, reexpansion of the lung, nutritional support, and decreased oral intake. Surgical intervention should be considered within 1 week of diagnosis if the leak does not resolve to prevent severe protein depletion and immunosuppression.

VATS can be used to drain the pleural space, identify and ligate the source of a chyle leak, and perform a pleurodesis. The thoracic duct arises from the cisterna chyli and ascends into the chest on the anterior surface of the vertebral column via the aortic hiatus. It continues posterior to the esophagus, the azygous vein, and the aorta to the level of the fifth or sixth vertebral body, where it crosses to the left and ascends posterior to the aortic arch. The duct continues along the left lateral wall of the esophagus and crosses the thoracic inlet posterior to the subclavian artery, where it joins the venous system near the confluence of the subclavian vein and left internal jugular vein. Unless the exact location of the chyle leak can be ascertained, the right side of the chest is the optimal approach to ligate the duct as close as possible to the point at which it enters the chest through the aortic hiatus.

The patient can be given a fatty enteral load; this will help the surgeon to identify the site of the leak. At the time of operation, it usually is difficult to identify the exact site of chyle leakage, but on occasion this is possible, and a clip can be applied to the leaking branch of the thoracic duct. More commonly the duct is simply ligated as low in the chest as possible by placing a ligature around all of the tissue on the vertebral column between the azygous vein and the aorta without attempting specific identification of the thoracic duct. Postoperatively, the patient is given a fatty diet, and if no additional chest drainage occurs and the chest radiograph remains clear, the chest tube can be removed. This approach is successful in more than 95% of cases.

Spontaneous pneumothorax is due to the rupture of small blebs or bullae, usually at the lung apices. The typical patient with small blebs is a young, tall, asthenic man with what appears to be normal lung parenchyma who experiences sudden onset of chest pain and shortness of breath, especially with exertion. This is referred to as *primary spontaneous pneumothorax*. The second group of patients is older individuals with known obstructive lung disease, usually with a bullous component. These patients are said to have a *secondary spontaneous pneumothorax*. The general goal of treatment includes elimination of the source of the leak, full lung reexpansion, and minimization of the risk of recurrence. Surgical indications for primary spontaneous pneumothorax include recurrent pneumothorax, prolonged air leak, associated complications, and unique sociogeographic reasons (type of employment, access to medical care). VATS permits excellent visualization of the lung apex for stapling of apical blebs as definitive management of this process. Apical blebs and bullae are resected with the endoscopic stapler. A concurrent mechanical pleurodesis can be performed to prevent recurrence. Overall this procedure has a less than 5% recurrence rate. For primary pneumothorax, a single port and a small transaxillary incision are all that is required to complete the procedure. Older patients with bullous parenchymal lung disease usually require standard port placement for access to the leaking bulla and often require thoracotomy with muscle mobilization and transposition to obliterate a residual space.

PARENCHYMAL PATHOLOGY

Diagnostic

VATS has an important role in many parenchymal processes from both a diagnostic and a therapeutic standpoint. Thoracic surgeons often are called on to establish a diagnosis in patients with diffuse interstitial lung disease. VATS allows the thoracic surgeon to obtain a substantial sample of lung parenchyma for analysis through a small incision in the chest wall. For patients with minimal oxygen requirements, the procedure can be performed quickly, safely, and with minimal morbidity. Often, however, these patients are referred while requiring ventilator support, being treated with high-dose steroids or other immunosuppressive agents, and failing conventional therapies. CT scan should be performed to confirm specific areas of involvement or sparing of certain areas. If both lungs are equally involved, we prefer to use the right side because there is somewhat more room to work without the heart in the way. At least two distinct areas should be sampled, ideally from two separate lobes. After a specimen is obtained, it should be sent for frozen section to confirm that diagnostic material has been obtained. In addition, a portion of the specimen should be sent to the microbiology laboratory for cultures, including acid-fast bacilli, fungi, aerobic and anaerobic bacteria. Both sensitivity and specificity for this procedure approach 100%. Although the operation has minimal complications, the patient's underlying pulmonary status can be the source of significant postoperative morbidity.

Another use of VATS is to perform lung volume reduction surgery for end-stage emphysema. Emphysema is caused by parenchymal lung tissue destruction that results in destruction of the alveolar walls and abnormal, permanent enlargement of the air spaces distal to terminal bronchioles. Lung volume reduction surgery has been proposed to help patients with emphysema by removing hypofunctioning apical segments of the lung, thereby permitting reexpansion of the remainder lung to improve physiologic recoil. The indications for lung volume reduction surgery have been well described in the National Emphysema Treatment Trial.

Following a thorough preoperative preparation that is required before surgery is conducted, a bilateral VATS approach can be taken to resect the apical segments. To resect emphysematous lung tissue, staple lines should be buttressed with either expanded polytetrafluoroethylene or glutaraldehyde-fixed bovine pericardium. The postoperative care is the most challenging aspect of this procedure. The most common complications are prolonged air leak and respiratory infections. Most series report 80% of patients have significant improvement with regard to their pulmonary status. Spirometric indices such as forced expiratory volume at 1 second and forced vital capacity continue to improve following surgery. This operation remains controversial, and the pulmonary community remains skeptical of its benefit to patients with end-stage emphysema.

VATS has assumed an important role in establishing the diagnosis of pulmonary nodules. In a patient with multiple nodules, a VATS wedge excision of one of the nodules establishes a tissue diagnosis allowing for the appropriate treatment to be prescribed. In the patient with a solitary pulmonary nodule, a diagnosis of primary lung cancer may be established before definitive anatomic resection is performed. In the event that the solitary nodule represents metastatic disease or benign disease, the patient may be spared a thoracotomy. The CT scan is useful to assess whether the lesion is accessible for VATS wedge excision. A lesion deep in the center of a lobe, for instance, proves to be difficult to excise with a wedge-type excision, even via open thoracotomy. Large (>3 cm) tumors usually are not approached by thoracoscopy because of the risks of inadequate resection and technical difficulties in accomplishing this resection endoscopically. If a nodule appears to be difficult to localize by digital palpation because of its small size or deep location, radiographic localization can be performed with wire or injection with methylene blue, but in our experience rarely, if ever, have we used these adjuncts. Lesions can always be palpated by the probing index finger inserted through one of the VATS incisions with a portion of the lung grasped with a ring forceps (Kaiser-Pilling Thoracoscopy Instruments, Pilling Co., Fort Washington, PA) and moved to the examining finger.

Port placement is the most important step for a successful operation. For almost every case, no matter the pathology, we have used a standard technique for port placement. Other than for the camera port we do not routinely use trocars but place the instruments or the examining finger directly through the incision into the chest. The first port is placed in alignment with the inferior superior iliac spine, usually in the seventh or eighth intercostal space. The videothoracoscope is placed through this port. The second port most commonly is placed one fingerbreadth inferior and slightly anterior to the scapular tip. The third port is placed just posterior to the lateral border of the pectoralis major muscle, usually in the third or fourth interspace. We make the third incision in a vertical direction so that it can be converted to a vertical axillary muscle-sparing incision. The result is a triangular configuration of the port placement that allows enough space so that the instruments are not "fighting" with each other within the pleural cavity. These three port sites have proved versatile in our hands, allowing parenchymal and mediastinal procedures to be performed. Pleural procedures, especially pleural biopsy with pleurodesis, most commonly may be performed via the single incision made for placement of the videothoracoscope. Because the intercostal spaces are widest anteriorly, usually the examining finger is placed through the anterior incision to permit digital palpation and location of a lesion prior to wedge excision. After the lesion has been located, the nodule should not be grasped directly. Instead the lung parenchyma just adjacent to the lesion should be grasped, and keeping in mind the location of the nodule, a wedge-type resection should be performed to completely encompass the lesion. At times, depending on the location of the lesion, the lesion itself may be grasped and elevated and the linear endoscopic stapler placed beneath the lesion to allow it to be resected. Before removal from the chest, the nodule should be placed in a specimen bag specifically designed for this purpose, although a rubber glove can also be used. This is simply to prevent implantation of tumor in the port site—an unlikely complication, but one that has been known to occur. If the nodule cannot be successfully located or is in a location where wedge excision would be difficult, the procedure should be converted to an open thoracotomy, using at least one of the incisions that have already been made.

Therapeutic

VATS has proved useful not just for removal of pulmonary nodules for diagnosis but also for staging of lung cancer. The superior mediastinum, specifically right and left levels II and IV and level VII, may be sampled adequately and preferentially by mediastinoscopy. For left-sided tumors (particularly left upper lobe lesions), VATS permits excellent exposure to the aortopulmonary window for sampling of nodal stations level V and VI, should this information be wanted before pulmonary resection. After the chest has been entered with the videothoracoscope, the pleural cavity is explored to rule out visceral or parietal pleural involvement. With counter-traction on the apical portion of the lung, the aortopulmonary window lymph nodes can be easily visualized and resected. Because of the proximity of the recurrent laryngeal nerve, electrocautery use should be minimized. If necessary, subcarinal lymph nodes can also be sampled to aid in planning the appropriate therapy. Thoracoscopy is also useful in ruling out unresectable T4 invasion in primary lung cancer and T3 invasion in high-risk patients. CT scanning may suggest aortic or chest wall involvement, but it is only 50% accurate in distinguishing abutment from invasion. This approach has been proven to reduce the necessity for thoracotomy for previously undiagnosed advanced lung cancer. Whether VATS ultimately permits an adequate lymph node dissection is debated. However, it is unclear whether there is any difference in patient survival by performing a complete mediastinal lymph node dissection versus a sampling of nodal tissue. This issue is currently being addressed in a prospective randomized clinical trial by the American College of Surgeons Oncology Group.

VATS anatomic lung resection for early-stage lung cancer remains a debated topic even though it has been widely accepted and adopted by a number of surgeons. Although there is no well-defined set of standards, VATS lobectomy probably should be limited to stage I lesions or some stage II lesions without extensive nodal involvement, although a number of surgeons have extended these indications. Proponents of this approach argue that VATS lobectomy permits adequate visualization for a complete resection of the tumor-containing lobe, as well as allowing for a standard mediastinal lymph node dissection, and is safe, in experienced hands, with equivalent short- and long-term outcomes. Opponents believe that VATS lobectomy violates oncologic principles and increases the risk of recurrence. Three ports are needed in the standard positions, discussed earlier. Typically an anterior-placed utility thoracotomy is performed to allow for the use of standard thoracotomy instruments to complete the dissection. The operation follows the standard open approach, with visualization provided indirectly by the video camera and the procedure guided by the magnified appearance on the video monitor. There are at present substantial data demonstrating that this operation can be performed safely with results equal to those of the open approach, although it remains debatable as to whether VATS lobectomy offers any significant advantages. VATS has reduced hospital stay by, at most, 1 day in most series; the limiting factors in discharge are typically pain control and removal of the chest tube, a decision based on cessation of air leaks and discontinuation of drainage. Overall costs may be equal for the two procedures even though patients may be discharged a day earlier using the VATS approach; intraoperative equipment costs cancel out any gains obtained by the shorter length of stay. Most of the costs associated with a surgical stay are accumulated during the first day or two of the stay. Pain may be less with the VATS approach, but it is naive to think that because these patients have smaller incisions they will have less pain than patients who have undergone open surgery. Often the pain experienced by VATS patients is as significant as if they had undergone an open procedure. There is no question that the prevention of rib spreading should result in fewer long-term pain problems. Long-term patient satisfaction is no different when the two procedures are compared and is more related to the disease stage and patient outcome. Until a randomized controlled study is performed with long-term follow-up, the controversy will continue.

Under certain circumstances VATS may be used for pulmonary metastasectomy. Resection of pulmonary metastases currently is the standard of care for multiple epithelial and mesenchymal primary neoplasms when the only site of metastatic disease is the lung, especially if there is a solitary nodule. Most metastatic lesions are peripherally located and appear well circumscribed. Often, they are discovered incidentally during follow-up for a known previous extra-thoracic malignancy. Surgical resection of all visible and palpable metastases is indicated when there is control of the primary tumor and metastases are confined to the lung. Preoperative pulmonary function tests must confirm whether a patient can tolerate multiple wedge resections that may be required for complete resection. A common concern voiced is that the VATS approach does not permit adequate palpation of the lung parenchyma for small lesions that cannot be seen by CT scan. Complete resection of all metastatic pulmonary lesions is the major determinant of long-term survival for patients with lung lesions as their only metastatic site. For the patient with a limited number of pulmonary nodules a VATS resection is a reasonable option.

MEDIASTINAL PATHOLOGY

The indications for VATS for mediastinal pathology include the diagnosis of mediastinal masses, excision of certain cysts and masses, sympathectomy, and thymectomy.

The most frequently encountered cysts in the middle and posterior mediastinum are bronchogenic, pericardial, esophageal duplication cysts, and neuroenteric cysts. Indications for resection vary, but if the patient is symptomatic, usually because of mass effect, or if there is suspicion of malignancy, resection clearly is indicated. The natural history of incidentally found asymptomatic mediastinal cysts is not known. Although it is possible to thoracoscopically drain these cysts, inadequate removal of the cyst wall has been associated with a high recurrence rate. VATS provides excellent access and visualization of all compartments of the mediastinum. Dissection of posterior mediastinal cysts begins by incising the overlying pleura, taking care to prevent injury to the cyst wall. If the cyst wall is inadvertently entered, the contents should be suctioned and the chest cavity copiously irrigated at the termination of the procedure. If the cysts are large and unresectable, controlled thoracoscopic-guided needle aspiration for decompressing the cyst may facilitate subsequent dissection and mobilization. If a small portion of the cyst wall cannot be resected because of adherence to adjacent structures, it should be destroyed by electrocautery.

Posterior mediastinal masses can be accessed easily by a VATS approach. The vast majority of posterior mediastinal tumors in adults are benign, whereas these tumors in children are often malignant. Schwannomas comprise half of all posterior mediastinal tumors, and ganglioneuromas and ganglioneuroblastomas account for one third of cases. These tumors usually are found incidentally and, for the most part, are asymptomatic. A computerized axial tomography scan can usually define whether a posterior mediastinal mass is a cyst or tumor. If there are concerns of a neuroendocrine origin of the tumor, a metaiodobenzylguanidine scan should be performed to detect a neuroblastoma or pheochromocytoma. Solid posterior mediastinal masses are circumferentially dissected to remove the mass in its entirety, and the nerve root from which the tumor arises must be clipped. Blood supply to neurogenic tumors should be clipped or divided as vessels are encountered. An endoscopic specimen bag should be used to remove the tumor from the chest.

One of the most common indications for VATS is dorsal sympathectomy for palmar hyperhidrosis, a common problem that results in hand sweating so excessive that social interactions become difficult and often embarrassing. This bilateral procedure does not require an inpatient stay and is designed to divide the sympathetic chain at the T2 level. The patient is positioned supine and placed in reverse Trendelenburg position. Two needle ports using Veress needles as trocars are placed in alignment with the mid-axillary line in the second and third intercostal spaces. A 2-mm zero-degree thoracoscope is more than adequate for the visualization required to complete this procedure. We use limited carbon dioxide insufflation to drop the lung away from the apex of the hemithorax. The sympathetic chain is identified along the vertebral bodies, and electrocautery is used to divide the sympathetic chain at the T2 level. Excision of a portion of the chain or a ganglion is not required for a successful outcome. Positive pressure ventilation via a single-lumen endotracheal tube is used to reinflate the lung, and no chest tubes are required because there is no air leak. The same procedure then is used on the contralateral side. Intraoperative finger temperature should rise by a degree or two if the sympathetic chain has been interrupted at the correct level. The success rate of bilateral dorsal sympathectomy for palmar hyperhidrosis approximates 100%, with the main morbidity being compensatory sweating that occurs in almost one third of patients. Common areas of compensatory sweating include the axilla, lower back, buttocks, and inner thighs, but in almost all patients this is found to be preferable to the hand sweating that interferes with social interactions. Most compensatory sweating is mild and well tolerated, but in the rare patient it can be severe and debilitating.

VATS thymectomy may be indicated to remove an encapsulated thymoma or to remove the thymus gland in patients with myasthenia gravis. For patients with other than Masaoka stage I disease, that is, any tumor that is not well encapsulated without violation of the capsule, the VATS approach currently is not considered the standard of care, and the procedure should be performed via a median sternotomy. In patients with myasthenia gravis, removal of the thymus gland has been associated with symptom improvement or remission in a majority of cases. A significant number of patients with myasthenia gravis have thymic hyperplasia and thus an enlarged gland. Although the exact relationship of thymic hyperplasia and myasthenia gravis is not understood, the pathology of the gland has not been predictive of outcome from thymectomy. The VATS approach, usually performed from the right side of the chest, can be used to remove the thymus gland, although we prefer a transcervical approach in almost all cases because it is both easier on the patient and significantly less invasive. The VATS procedure entails removing all mediastinal tissue located anterior to the phrenic nerve and superior vena cava. Using blunt dissection, the gland is lifted off the innominate vein, with thymic venous branches clipped and divided as they are encountered. Unless a bilateral approach is taken, it is difficult to visualize the contralateral phrenic nerve by this approach. No direct comparisons of long-term outcome comparing the VATS approach with other approaches for either thymoma excision or thymectomy for myasthenia gravis are available. Most surgeons continue to prefer a median sternotomy or limited sternotomy for thymectomy, especially for excision of even well-encapsulated thymomas.

■ ESOPHAGEAL PATHOLOGY

With technologic advances, including better optics and more versatile thoracoscopic dissectors, VATS has developed an important role in the management of esophageal diseases. It can be used to treat esophageal motility disorders (vagotomy, myotomy, fundoplication), remove benign esophageal neoplasms (enteric cysts, leiomyoma), and resect malignant esophageal neoplasms (esophagectomy).

VATS provides a minimally invasive approach to treat motility disorders quickly and with minimal dissection, preventing the morbidity of a large thoracotomy incision. Patients are often referred to a thoracic surgeon after a complex abdominal procedure that requires a vagotomy but that would be a technically challenging abdominal dissection. Approached from the left side of the chest, the mediastinal pleura is dissected off the esophagus slightly above the diaphragmatic hiatus. The esophagus is visualized, and circumferential dissection reveals the left and right vagus nerves. The nerves are clipped and divided, and a section removed for histologic confirmation.

VATS is a useful approach to perform a myotomy in achalasia refractory to medical management or previous laparoscopic myotomy. However, laparoscopic myotomy with a fundoplication has become the procedure of choice for patients with achalasia. If performed via a VATS procedure, a 50-F Maloney bougie is placed in the esophagus, and the distal esophagus is approached via the left side of the chest. The inferior pulmonary ligament is divided, and the mediastinal pleura overlying the esophagus is incised. Starting at the diaphragmatic hiatus, we extend the myotomy to the aortic arch by using a hook cautery to excise the outer longitudinal muscle and inner circular muscle. Because of the high incidence of postoperative reflux, we usually perform a simultaneous antireflux procedure at the time of surgery. If a perforation occurs, primary repair can be performed via the thoracoscope, without extending to an open procedure.

In patients with gastroesophageal reflux disease, insufficient resting lower esophageal sphincter pressures are frequently the cause. A fundoplication re-creates a barrier to limit the exposure of the esophagus to the refluxate. After the appropriate diagnostic evaluations (upper gastrointestinal series, 24-hour esophageal pH monitor, manometry) are completed, the laparoscopic Nissen fundoplication is usually performed. It remains the standard of care by which other antireflux operations are measured. This technique provides results comparable with the open procedure with respect to patient satisfaction, postoperative dysphagia, gas blot, and recurrent symptoms. Partial fundoplications (i.e., Toupet) are indicated if the patient's esophageal motility is abnormal. Thoracoscopic repair (Collis-Belsey procedure) is an appropriate alternative in patients with previous abdominal surgery or a foreshortened esophagus. This procedure has many advantages over the traditional approach. It permits lengthening of the esophagus and provides easy access in obese patients. It also is useful in patients undergoing reoperative surgery.

VATS can be used to remove benign esophageal lesions, such as leiomyomas and esophageal duplication cysts. After an intraoperative esophagoscopy has been performed and a nasogastric tube has been placed, the esophageal pathology can be approached from either side of the chest, depending on whether the lesion is in the upper two thirds (right side) or lower one third (left side) of the chest. Operative ports should be placed posteriorly along the fourth and seventh intercostal spaces; ports for retraction and the camera should be placed closer to the posterior axillary line. The lung is retracted anteriorly, and the pleura is opened overlying the esophageal leiomyoma or duplication cyst. The tumor can be dissected away from the esophagus while care is taken to prevent injury to the esophageal mucosa. Small perforating vessels are managed with endoscopic clip appliers. This minimally invasive approach lends itself well to managing benign esophageal lesions.

The incidence of esophageal cancer is increasing, and methods of management also have evolved. Depending on depth of tumor invasion and lymph node metastasis, patients are candidates for esophagectomy or neoadjuvant therapy before surgery. Accurate staging of esophageal cancer has remained a challenge, although the use of positron emission tomography and endoscopic ultrasound has improved accuracy.

One use of VATS has been to assess the depth of invasion and lymph node metastasis. Right thoracoscopy is performed to mobilize the tissues adjacent to the tumor and to sample peritracheal, periesophageal, and inferior pulmonary ligament lymph nodes. For definitive management of esophageal cancer, VATS has two roles in an esophagectomy: to mobilize the intrathoracic esophagus for a transhiatal approach or as part of a laparoscopic abdominal approach. To date, the survival rate for patients undergoing the thoracoscopic esophagectomy appears to be identical to that for patients undergoing an open procedure.

COMPLICATIONS

Major complications from VATS are uncommon. Typical complications, although infrequent, include persistent air leak (<2%), hemorrhage, empyema, intercostal neurovascular bundle injury, tumor implantation, injury to intrathoracic structures (sympathetic ganglion, recurrent nerve, thoracic duct, esophagus), and

abdominal organ trauma from inadvertent abdominal entry with a trocar.

Persistent air leak is the most common problem and can be minimized by preventing traumatic entry into the chest cavity with sharp instruments, performing minimal lung manipulation in patients with severe emphysema, and using endoscopic staplers with care to prevent tearing lung parenchyma. Pleural symphysis or adhesions are most commonly responsible for parenchymal tears that cause air leaks. The most morbid complication that can occur during a VATS procedure is injury to a great vessel with uncontrollable hemorrhage. Most bleeding can be temporarily controlled with a sponge placed on a ring forceps and pressure applied over the torn vessel site. While the assistant holds the bleeding in check, the surgeon should rapidly perform a thoracotomy and repair the injury.

Intercostal neurovascular injury can occur at the port sites from compression by instruments. Many patients get paresthesias over the dermatome of the damaged intercostal nerve. This complication is usually self-limiting. Long-term neurapraxia does occur on occasion and may require management with intercostal nerve ablation. An additional source of bleeding can occur because of injury to intercostal vessels at the site of the intercostal access used for the VATS procedure.

Tumor implantation has been reported after VATS resection for cancer. Implantation can be prevented by refraining from tumor manipulation, using wound protectors, irrigating the chest cavity and port site before closure, and placing the specimen in a plastic bag before removing it from the chest cavity. Finally, any chest surgery may result in injury to intrathoracic structures. Right-sided procedures may cause injury to the thoracic duct, azygous vein, esophagus, or sympathetic chain. Left-sided procedures can potentially injure the recurrent laryngeal nerve, esophagus, sympathetic chain, or aorta. Injuries to any of these structures should occur infrequently.

CONCLUSIONS

VATS is a safe alternative to conventional open surgery for the management of a host of diagnostic and therapeutic indications in thoracic surgery. This approach minimizes pain while permitting the surgeon to achieve the objectives of the operation. Improvements in equipment make it possible to perform almost any procedure in a minimally invasive fashion. The key is to recognize the appropriate indications and carry out a procedure that is equivalent to the analogous open procedure.

SUGGESTED READINGS

Sedrakyan A, van der Meulen J, Lewsey J, and others: Video assisted thoracic surgery for treatment of pneumothorax and lung resections: systematic review of randomised clinical trials, *BMJ* 329(7473):1008, 2004.

Yim A, Hazelrigg S, Izzat MB, and others: *Minimal access cardiothoracic surgery*, Philadelphia, 2000, WB Saunders.

Video-assisted thoracic surgery. In Yang SC, Cameron DE, editors: *Current therapy in thoracic and cardiovascular surgery*, Philadelphia, 2004, Mosby.

LAPAROSCOPIC ADRENALECTOMY

Vimal K. Narula, MD, and W. Scott Melvin, MD

INTRODUCTION

The surgical approach to the adrenal gland has undergone quite a transition in the past decade. With the advent of laparoscopic surgery, the preferred technique has gone from the open approach to minimally invasive. The first laparoscopic adrenalectomy was performed in 1992; since then, it has become the method of choice for adrenal pathology. Morbidity for the open technique can be as high as 40% and mortality approximately 2% to 4%. In 1995 the benefits of the laparoscopic approach were presented by Prinz in a retrospective review. The advantages included decreased postoperative length of stay, decreased postoperative pain, and decreased narcotic usage. Other studies have reaffirmed these results over the past decade. This chapter focuses on the operative technique and the preoperative and postoperative care of patients with adrenal pathology.

INDICATIONS AND CONTRAINDICATIONS

Adrenalectomy is indicated in any patient with a hormonally active or suspected malignancy. Most adrenal masses can be labeled as functional or nonfunctional. Most functional tumors are less than 6 cm in size and are good candidates for the laparoscopic approach (Fig. 1, *A*). These include aldosteronoma, pheochromocytoma, and Cushing's syndrome patients with cortisol-producing adenoma, primary adrenal hyperplasia, and failed treatment of adenocorticotrophin hormone (ACTH)-dependent Cushing's. The second group that meets the criteria for resection is nonfunctional tumors greater than 6 cm. These include nonfunctional cortical adenoma, adrenal metastasis, and other miscellaneous tumors such as myelolipoma, adrenal cyst, ganglioneuroma, and enlarging adenomas or lesions of uncertain behavior or etiology.

The main reason for performing an open approach is the size of the tumor mass in the adrenal gland. There are reports in the literature that show the technical feasibility of removal of larger adrenal masses, that is, greater than 8 to 10 cm and even as large as 13 to 14 cm. However, size greater than 8 to 10 cm is a relative contraindication (Fig. 1, *B*). It has been found that the dissection planes are not as well defined and the tumor is most likely adherent to the surrounding structures, causing an inflammatory reaction. This makes laparoscopic removal difficult. Large masses are hard to manipulate laparoscopically, and mobilization can be difficult. The increased risk of significant hemorrhage may outweigh the potential benefits of laparoscopy.

Malignant tumors such as adrenocortical carcinomas, especially the large ones (>5–6 cm), should be removed with the open approach. The rationale behind this is to prevent any tumor spillage and the increased risk of inadequate resection margin. Complete resection may be possible via the laparoscopic approach; however, oncologic principles should not be compromised. Finally, any contraindication to laparoscopic surgery obviously precludes the minimally invasive approach. Technical difficulty may be encountered in the case of reoperative surgery or morbid obesity, but these are not contraindications.

PREOPERATIVE PREPARATION

Medical management of patients with hormonally active tumors is essential. Patients with aldosterone-producing tumors must have their electrolytes monitored before surgery. For patients with Cushing's disease, exogenous steroid dose should be administered before the induction of anesthesia. The medical management of a pheochromocytoma is the most important. These patients must be treated for 3 to 4 weeks preceding surgery. The medical treatment consists of alpha-blockade with either phenoxybenzamine or phentolamine, in conjunction with a beta-blocker if necessary to treat the hypertension. These patients should also be admitted to the hospital the day before their surgery to adequately volume-resuscitate them to prevent hypotension during or after the operation.

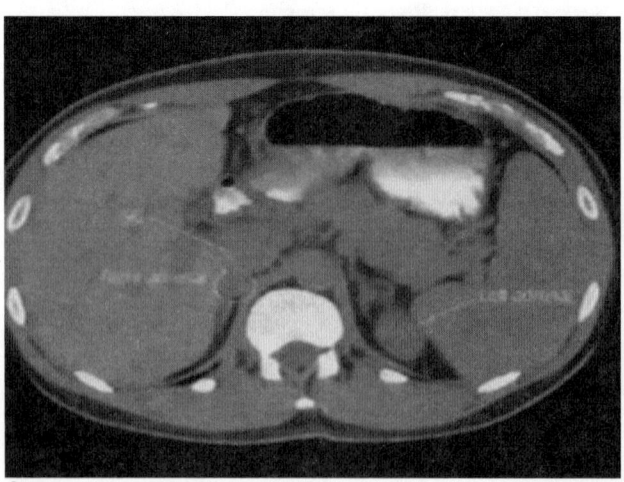
A

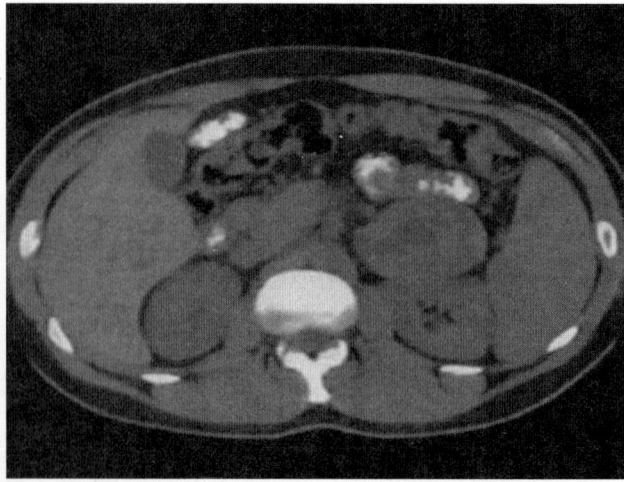
B

Figure 1 Computed tomography scan. **(A)** Bilateral adrenal masses. **(B)** Left adrenal mass.

OPERATIVE TECHNIQUE

Transabdominal Lateral Flank Approach

In the operating room the patient is positioned in the lateral decubitus position with the operative side positioned superiorly. Before the patient is positioned, the orogastric tube, urinary catheter, and the sequential compression devices are placed. Appropriate padding is placed on the pressure points, such as the arms and legs, and an axillary roll is placed to prevent neurapraxia. The patient is positioned using a gel-padded beanbag cushion. A break in the table coinciding with the anterior superior iliac spine allows the table to be flexed to further open the area of operation (Fig. 2, A).

Access to the abdomen is gained via the Veress needle placed at a site 2 cm below the costal margin and just medial to the anterior axillary line. Using the muscle-splitting technique, a 10-mm trocar is placed in the abdomen. A 30-degree, 5-mm laparoscopic camera is used throughout the operation. Pneumoperitoneum is established, and three additional 5-mm trocars are placed along the costal margin, one of which is placed in supraumbilical midline, depending on the side of the lesion. The trocars are placed at least 6 cm apart to prevent interference with the instruments.

The first step is to perform a diagnostic laparoscopy to rule out any metastatic disease. Ultrasound may also be helpful in identifying the exact location of the lesion, as well as other structures including vascular anatomy, especially in the morbidly obese patient. The camera is placed in the midline trocar. The working instruments are placed in the medial trocars. Both the surgeon and the first assistant start the operation opposite each other, but they both can choose to stand facing the anterior aspect of the patient (Fig. 2, B).

Left Adrenalectomy

The lienocolic ligament is divided to allow for medial and inferior retraction of the splenic flexure of the colon. This dissection is carried out from the left paracolic gutter to the inferior pole of the spleen (Fig. 3, A). Care should be taken not to dissect posterior to the left kidney because this will cause the kidney to fall medially over the adrenal gland. The splenorenal ligament is divided from the inferior pole of the spleen to the diaphragm, allowing for the medial rotation of the spleen and the tail of the pancreas and exposing the retroperitoneum. At this point the adrenal gland should be visible below the pancreas and the superior pole of the kidney (Fig. 3, B). It may be difficult to identify the adrenal gland if there is a large amount of retroperitoneal fat or if the gland contains a small tumor or is hyperplastic. The adrenal gland is identified by its characteristic bright yellow color. The tail of the pancreas should be identified and is not to be mistaken for the gland. Gentle retraction should be used around the pancreas to prevent unnecessary bleeding and injury.

The dissection of the gland is started in the inferomedial aspect of the gland to expose and ligate the adrenal vein initially. If the exposure to this area is difficult, then the superior, medial, and the lateral aspects are dissected off first. All the dissection should be close to the gland to prevent injury or ligation of the renal vessels. The gland itself should not be grasped because it can fragment. The best way to mobilize the adrenal gland is to manipulate the adjacent tissues. The adrenal vein measures approximately 5 to 10 mm and is often controlled with a medium or large clip. If the vein is too large for a clip, an endoscopic vascular stapler may be required. For this, the 5-mm port must be exchanged for the 12-mm port. Also of note is the inferior phrenic vein, which frequently joins the adrenal vein just above the junction of the left renal vein. After the vein has been traced to make sure it is not an accessory renal vein, it should be ligated and divided. The remaining attachments and the small arterial vessels can be controlled with the ultrasonic coagulator. Other structures at risk of injury are the colon, spleen, tail of the pancreas, and the diaphragm. When the gland is completely free, it should be placed in an impermeable bag and removed via the 10-mm port (Fig. 4). If there is any suspicion of a pancreatic injury, a drain should be placed in the retroperitoneum.

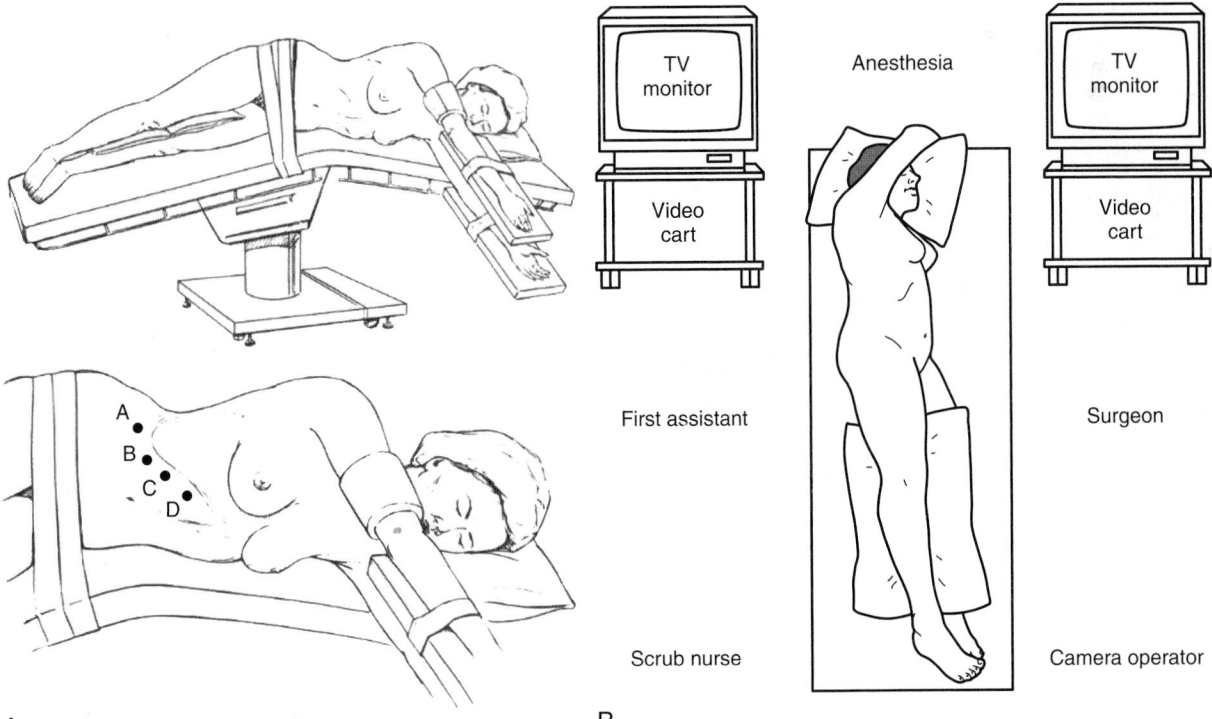

A   B

Figure 2   Transabdominal approach. **(A)** Patient positioning and port placement for right adrenalectomy. **(B)** Operating room setup for laparoscopic right adrenalectomy.

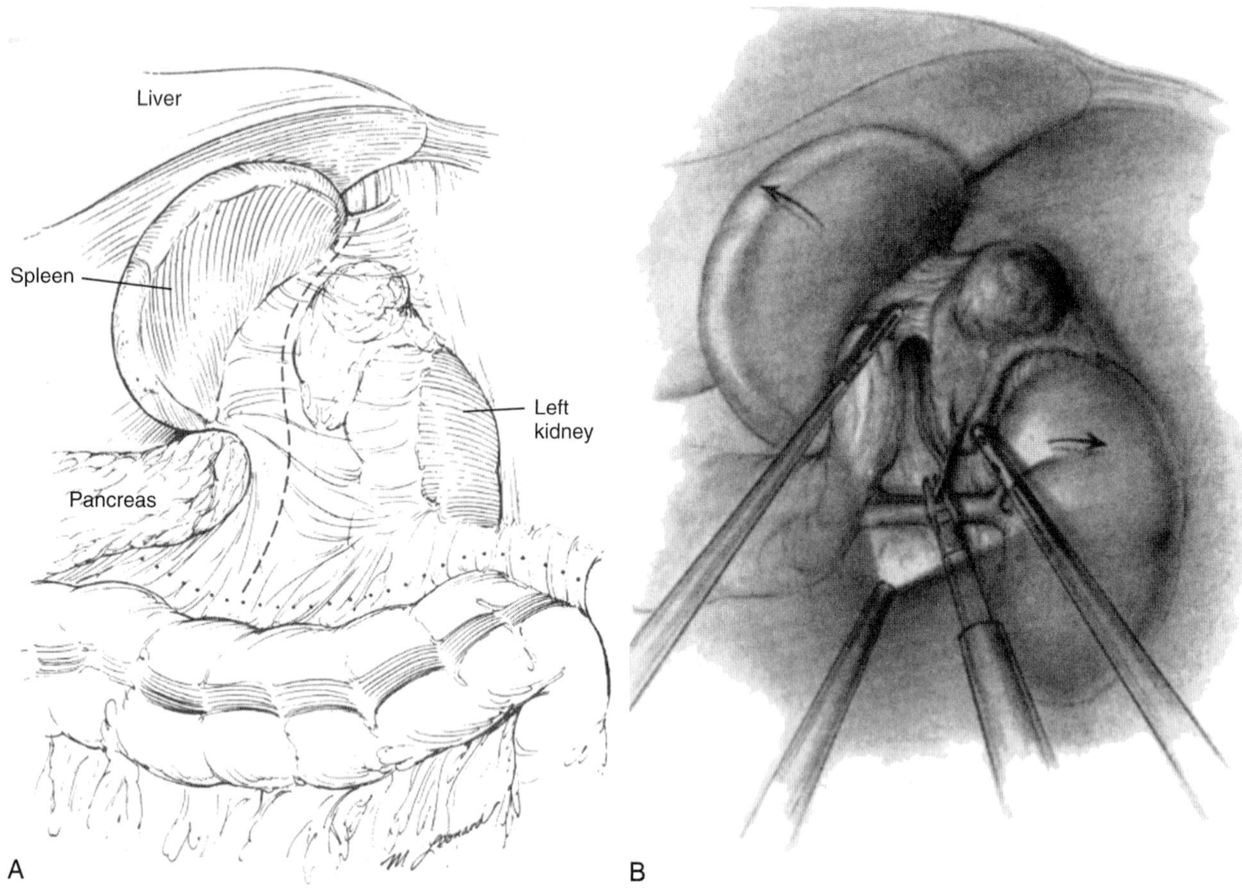

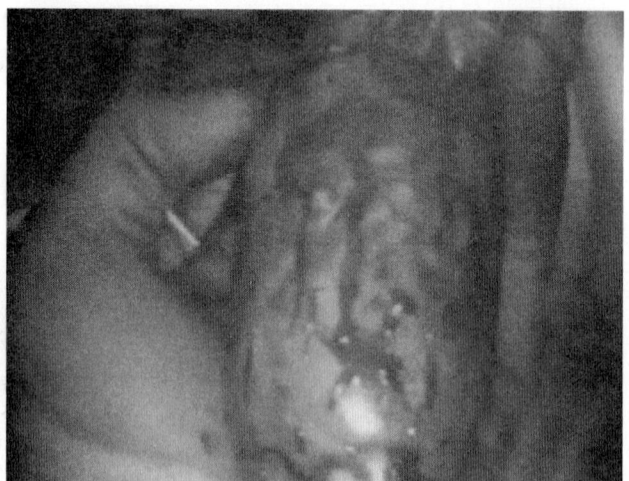

Figure 3 **(A)** Operative exposure and dissection of the left adrenal gland. The splenocolic is divided first followed by the splenorenal ligaments. **(B)** Laparoscopic view of the exposed left adrenal gland.

Figure 4 Extraction of the adrenal gland in an impermeable bag. (*See color insert Figure 76.*)

Right Adrenalectomy

The first step of the dissection for the right adrenal involves the division of the right triangular ligament and the right hepatic attachments to the retroperitoneum (Fig. 5). Following this, the most medial port is used to place a liver retractor to expose the medial aspect of the adrenal gland as it abuts the inferior vena cava. The right hepatic lobe must be completely mobilized to expose the

junction of the inferior vena cava and the adrenal gland (Fig. 6). It is rare that the surgeons will have to mobilize the duodenum or the colon when using this approach.

The Gerota's fascia overlying the gland is opened, and the dissection is carried along the lateral border of the inferior vena cava from the right adrenal vein superiorly to the right renal vein inferiorly. After complete dissection and control of the vein has been accomplished, the rest of the gland is mobilized with ease. The dissection begins in the inferomedial fashion similar to that of the left side. This right adrenal vein is dissected as it comes off the inferior vena cava; it is short, broad, and oriented transversely. The vein is ligated with medium-to-large clips or an endo-GIA vascular stapler. There is often a right accessory adrenal vein, which is ligated in similar fashion. The dissection continues superiorly, and if the branches off the inferior phrenic vessels are identified, they are either clipped or coagulated with the ultrasonic coagulator. After the posterior attachments (which are generally avascular) are taken down, the plane between the right kidney and the adrenal gland is developed (Fig. 7). Staying right in the fat just off the gland to prevent inadvertent fragmentation of the adrenal gland, the surgeon divides these attachments. The last step is the division of the lateral areolar attachments of the gland to completely free it. The specimen is then placed in the impermeable bag and retrieved from the 10-mm port site.

Anterior Abdominal Approach

In the anterior approach, the patient is in the supine or hemilateral position. The number of ports may vary between four and six, depending on the patient's body habitus (Fig. 8). Peritoneal access is

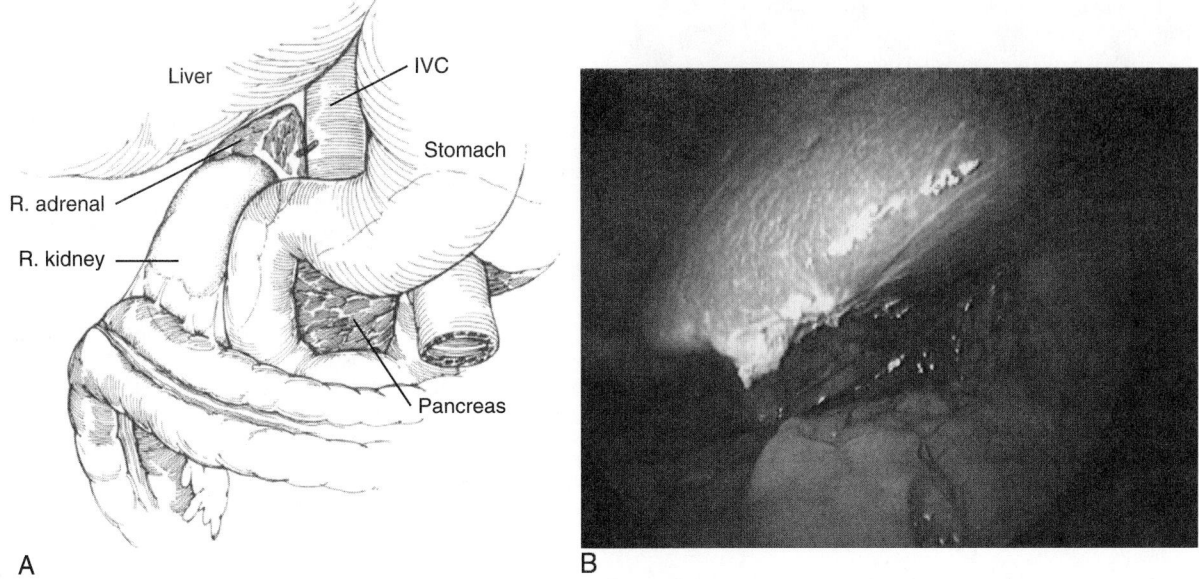

Figure 5 Right adrenal gland. **(A)** Anatomic relationships (*IVC*, inferior vena cava). **(B)** Laparoscopic view. (*See color insert Figure 77*.)

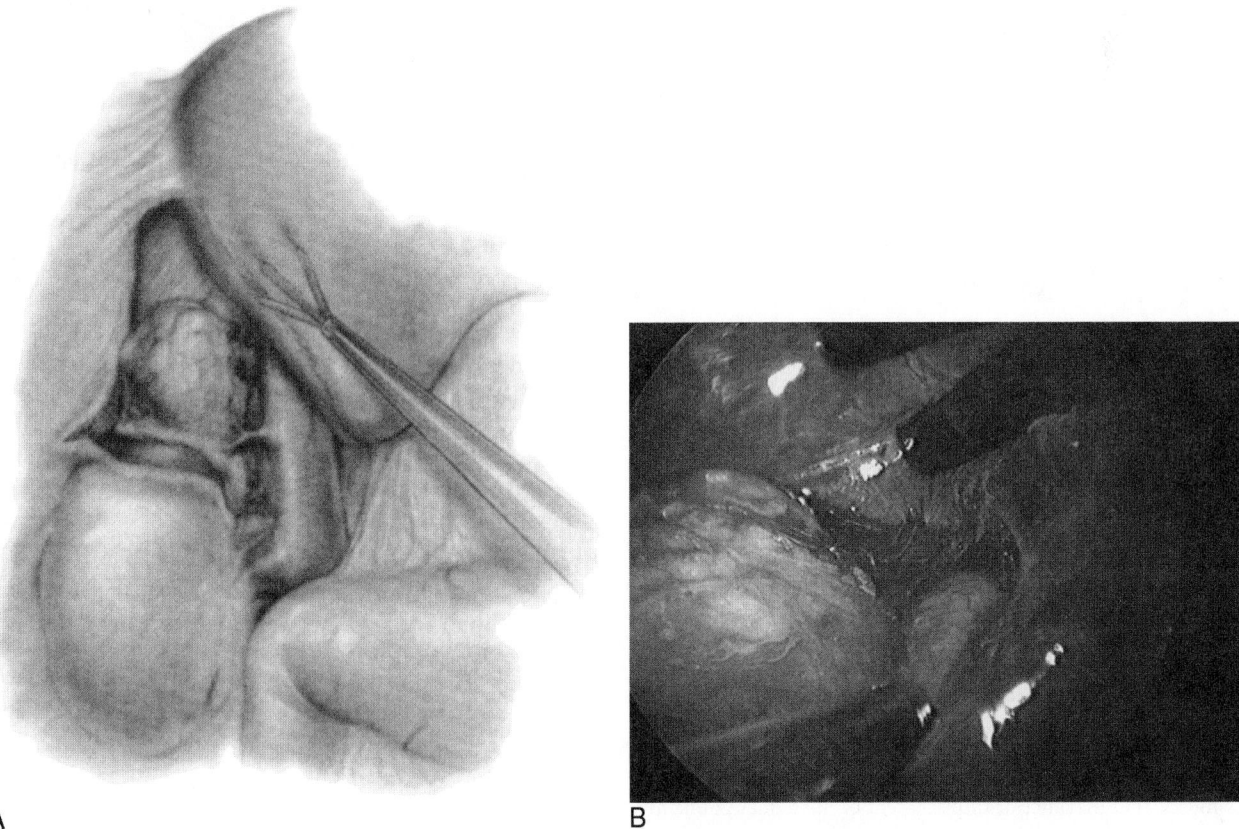

Figure 6 Dissection of the right adrenal gland. **(A)** Operative view. **(B)** Laparoscopic view. (*See color insert Figure 78*.)

established at the umbilicus. For right adrenalectomy, in addition to the liver retraction, mobilization of the hepatic flexure and transverse colon is sometimes necessary. The surgeon may have to Kocherize the duodenum if the gland is large and visualization is an issue. The rest of the procedure is the same as the lateral transabdominal approach. For the left adrenal gland, the splenic flexure is mobilized, with superior retraction of the tail of the pancreas and spleen. After Gerota's fascia has been entered and the adrenal gland exposed, the rest of the dissection is the same as for the lateral approach.

Retroperitoneal Approach

For the retroperitoneal approach, the patient is positioned in the dorsal or lateral manner. The posterior lumbar/dorsal approach requires the patient to be in the prone or semi-jackknife position with the hips flexed. Incision is made at the inferior aspect of the twelfth rib, and this is carried down in a muscle-splitting fashion to enter the anterior thoracolumbar fascia. After the retroperitoneal space has been reached, balloon dissection is carried out and the

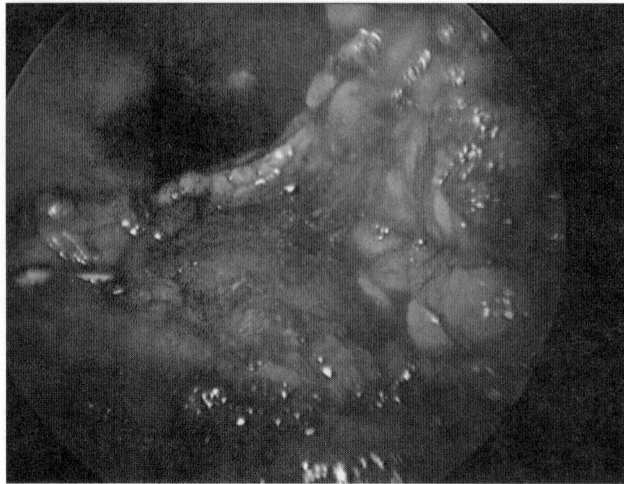

Figure 7 Laparoscopic view of the inferomedial dissection of the right adrenal gland. (*See color insert Figure 79.*)

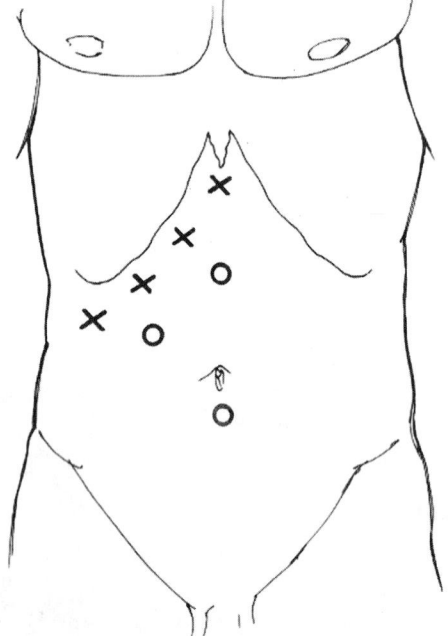

Figure 8 Port placement for anterior transabdominal approach. Initial access via the umbilical site o, Accessory port site; *x*, port site.

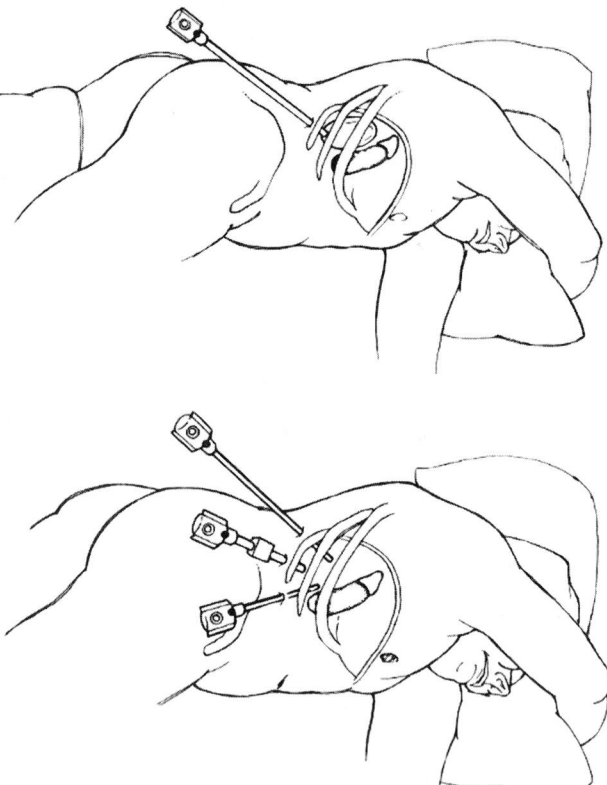

Figure 9 Port placement for retroperitoneal approach. Initial port is inferior to the twelfth rib.

space is then insufflated with CO_2 to an initial pressure of 12 mm Hg up to 20 mm Hg if necessary for operating. A 30- or 45-degree, 5-mm laparoscope is then inserted (Fig. 9). Visualization of the psoas muscle and the anterior displacement of the kidney confirms proper balloon placement of the retroperitoneum. Two or three additional ports are placed in the posterior axillary line and at the lateral border of the psoas (Fig. 10). Identifying the adrenal gland can be a challenge if the patient is obese; the laparoscopic ultrasound may be helpful in these cases. This is more of an issue with the left adrenal gland than with the right side.

For a left adrenalectomy, the dissection begins with the opening of Gerota's fascia at the renal hilum. The adrenal arteries that arise from the aorta are divided first, with the dissection extending laterally into the avascular plane between the superior pole of the kidney and the adrenal gland. Complete retroperitoneal dissection of the upper pole allows the adrenal gland to fall posterior onto the psoas

muscle. The adrenal vein off the left renal vein is identified and dissected toward the hilum. It is then ligated and divided. Clips or a vascular endo-GIA stapler is used, depending on the size of the vessel. Circumferential dissection with the ultrasonic coagulator then completes the mobilization of the gland. The inferior phrenic branches to the adrenal gland may be located along the superior edge of the gland. The adrenal gland is then placed in the impermeable bag and delivered from the patient.

The difference in the dissection of the right adrenal gland is twofold. First the identification of the right adrenal gland is easier than that of the left side because the surgeon can follow the inferior vena cava to the gland. The second difference is the steps involved in controlling the adrenal vein. The right adrenal gland may have two to three smaller branches as opposed to one main vein, which is generally short and located in a posteromedial location. Thus the vein is encountered before the arterial branches. After the vein has been taken care of, the rest of the operation is the same as it is for the left side. An advantage of this retroperitoneal approach is that if the dissection is difficult, conversion to the transperitoneal approach is easily accomplished.

POTENTIAL COMPLICATIONS

There are several complications that can occur during a laparoscopic adrenalectomy. Because of the lateral decubitus positioning of the patients, they can have nerve and soft-tissue compression injuries. To prevent these injuries, proper padding should be placed at the extremities, an axillary roll should be placed, potential pressure points should be inspected, and the beanbag should be used. During a right adrenalectomy, two specific aspects of the dissection can lead to complications. Diaphragmatic perforation or injury to the extrahepatic bile ducts can be prevented if, while performing the lateral dissection, the surgeon takes care in performing the to adequately remove the gland without undue traction. With the adrenal located in the retroperitoneum, bleeding in this area can be difficult to control laparoscopically. Meticulous dissection should be carried out with good hemostasis, especially after the division of the adrenal vein. If the vein is large in diameter, a vascular endo-GIA stapler should be used. Careful inspection of the operative bed should be performed before loss of pneumoperitoneum. Finally, in the case of a pheochromocytoma, even though the patient has been adequately blocked preoperatively, excessive manipulation of the gland can cause wide shifts in the hemodynamics. Control of the adrenal vein early is key to preventing this complication.

POSTOPERATIVE CARE

The majority of the patients stay overnight on a regular surgical unit after a laparoscopic adrenalectomy. Following resection of pheochromocytomas, patients may become hypotensive and require large amounts of intravenous fluids because of the loss of the alpha-mediated sympathetic tone and the expansion of the intravascular volume. These patients require monitoring in an advanced care unit. Hypoglycemia may be secondary to rebound hyperinsulinemia from the loss of inhibitory control by the circulating catecholamines. These patients are placed on telemetry units and resuscitated and treated symptomatically for 24 to 36 hours.

Patients with Cushing's syndrome, especially those who undergo bilateral adrenalectomies, require a perioperative stress dose of steroids. Oral hydrocortisone is then started at a maintenance dose after the steroid taper. In patients with Cushing's syndrome caused by an adenoma, replacement steroid therapy should be continued until the hypothalamic-pituitary axis shows recovery. This can be followed by ACTH stimulation testing. The axis may take up to 2 years for complete recovery. Patients with bilateral adrenalectomies also require lifelong mineral corticoid replacement in addition to the steroids. After discharge, patients require minimal pain medications, and they return to work and normal activity earlier than patients with an open operation.

In summary, laparoscopic adrenalectomy, like other minimally invasive procedures, has reduced the operative trauma to patients requiring adrenalectomy. Although technically demanding, laparoscopic adrenalectomy is a satisfying operation associated with generally good outcomes.

SUGGESTED READINGS

de Canniere L, Michel L, Hamoir E, and others: Multicentric experience of the Belgium Group for Endoscopic Surgery (BGES) with endoscopic adrenalectomy, Surg Endosc 11:1065, 1997.

Deodhar SD, Mehendale VG, Bhave GG: Renal cell carcinoma with unusual metastases: a case report, J Postgrad Med 24:54A, 1978.

Duh Q-Y, Siperstein AE, Clark OH, and others: Laparoscopic adrenalectomy: comparison of lateral and posterior approaches, Arch Surg 131:870, 1996.

Fillipони S, Guerrieri M, Arnaldi GGM, and others: Laparoscopic adrenalectomy: a report on 50 operations, Eur J Endocrinol 138:548, 1998.

Gagner M, Laroix A, Bolte E: Laparoscopic adrenalectomy in Cushing's syndrome and pheochromocytoma, N Engl J Med 327:1033, 1992.

Gagner M, Pomp A, Heniford BT, and others: Laparoscopic adrenalectomy: lessons learned from 100 consecutive procedures, Ann Surg 226:238, 1997.

Prinz RA: A comparison of laparoscopic and open adrenalectomies, Arch Surg 130:489, 1995.

Staren ED, Prinz RA: Adrenalectomy in the era of laparoscopy, Surgery 120:706, 1996.

Terachi T, Kawakita M, Yoshiyuka K: Laparoscopic adrenalectomy: results of 47 cases, J Urol 153:513, 1995.

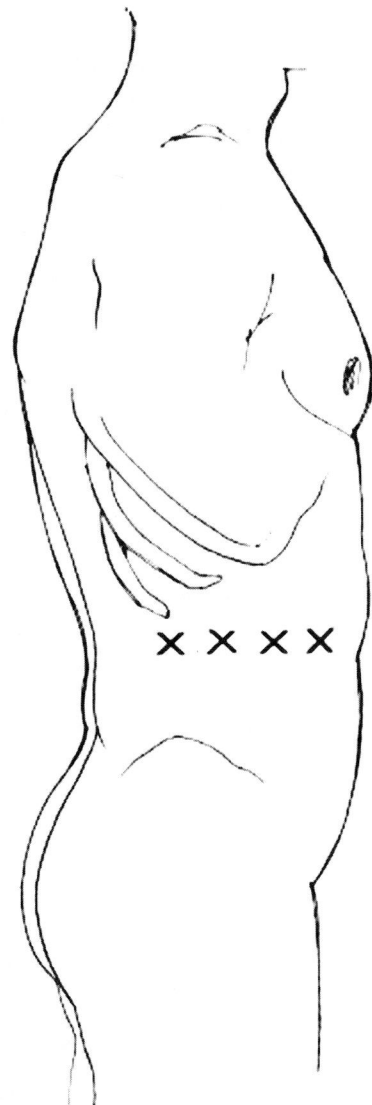

Figure 10 Port placement for lateral retroperitoneal approach. These can be sites of accessory ports as well.

cephalad dissection over the bare surface of the liver. Occasionally during this part of the mobilization the gallbladder will be injured; this can easily be managed by a cholecystectomy. Patients undergoing a right adrenalectomy should be made aware of risk for cholecystectomy; although uncommon, cholecystectomy may be necessary. The other area of concern is the vena cava. Injury to this vessel occurs if the vena cava is obscured during the lateral dissection of the gland before the adrenal vein has been controlled. Also, the surgeon should not put too much traction on the gland or kidney during dissection.

Injury to the pancreatic tail, splenic vessels, or both, can occur during a left adrenalectomy. This can be avoided by mobilizing the spleen early in the operation by dividing the splenocolic ligaments and using gentle, blunt retraction. Complications universal to all adrenalectomy patients include injury to the adrenal gland with spillage that can lead to peritoneal seeding. Care must be taken to prevent excessive manipulation of the gland by grasping it with the stump of the divided vein. Furthermore, the retrieved tissue should be secured in an impermeable bag, and the fascia should be opened

LAPAROSCOPIC SURGERY FOR MORBID OBESITY

Michael Schweitzer, MD, and Thomas Magnuson, MD

The morbid obesity epidemic continues to spread throughout industrialized nations. Prevention methods have failed to halt the further spread of this disease. Medical therapy that can cause sustained significant weight loss may be years away. Bariatric surgery continues to be the only proven method to achieve sustained weight loss in the majority of patients. Currently, the three most common bariatric operations in the United States are Roux-en-Y gastric bypass, adjustable gastric band, and duodenal switch with biliopancreatic diversion. These operations are now performed laparoscopically at most bariatric centers in the United States.

INDICATIONS

The National Institutes of Health Consensus Development Conference Statement for Gastrointestinal Surgery for Severe Obesity was issued in 1991 and is still regarded as the starting point for criteria to accept patients in a surgical weight loss program. Patients are considered morbidly obese and candidates for surgery if they have a body mass index of at least 35 kg/m^2 with an obesity-related comorbidity of greater than 40 kg/m^2. It is recommended that patients should have tried dieting in the past before surgical therapy is considered as a treatment option (Table 1).

When evaluating a potential patient for bariatric surgery, a multidisciplinary team should be used. This team should include a dietitian and a mental health professional who are familiar with bariatric surgery. Their purpose is to obtain a past dietary and behavioral eating history, discuss postoperative dietary expectations, and decide whether the individual is an appropriate patient for the type of surgery he or she has chosen. Patients who currently have known drug or alcohol addictions are not considered for surgical therapy. Support for the surgery from family members and friends is important. A spouse who is adamantly opposed to the surgery should be counseled along with the patient and may be a relative contraindication to the procedure. If the team believes that the patient is not appropriate for surgery, then consideration should be given to nonoperative medical management with appropriate counseling.

Table 1: Indications for Laparoscopic Bariatric Surgery for Morbid Obesity

1. Individuals with a body mass index (BMI) of 40 kg/m^2 or greater are potential candidates for bariatric surgery.
2. Individuals with a BMI of 35 to 40 kg/m^2 with significant obesity-related comorbidity are also potential candidates for bariatric surgery.
3. Weight loss by nonoperative means should be attempted before surgery.
4. Patients should be evaluated by a multidisciplinary team that includes a dietitian and a mental health professional before surgery.

At this time there is not enough evidence to support surgery in patients who cannot ambulate and are bedridden. These patients are also at greater risk for postoperative complications, and therefore the benefits may not outweigh the risks. Patients with end-stage heart failure or respiratory failure are also at high risk for morbidity and mortality. Surgery is not necessarily contraindicated for them, but weight loss may not be the solution to their attempt to correct fatal heart or lung disease. Cirrhotic patients may be at higher risk for surgery but certainly may benefit from weight loss. Patients who are morbidly obese may be rejected as liver or kidney transplant candidates, and therefore patients with early-stage cirrhosis or chronic renal insufficiency may benefit from bariatric–surgery-induced weight loss. There are currently not enough data concerning cirrhotic and renal failure patients to determine who is an appropriate candidate for weight loss surgery and who is too late in their disease course for surgery.

TECHNIQUES

Preparing the Patient in the Operating Room

On the morning of surgery the patient is injected subcutaneously with low-molecular-weight heparin to prevent venous thromboembolic complications. A peripheral intravenous (IV) line is placed, and a second-generation cephalosporin is administered intravenously. The patient is placed on the operating room table in the supine position with a footboard. Sequential compression devices are placed on the lower extremities. General anesthesia is administered and a urinary catheter is inserted. The anesthetist inserts, applies suction to, and then immediately removes the orogastric tube before starting the operation. We do not allow esophageal temperature probes because these can migrate into the stomach during stapling. The operating surgeon stands at the patient's right side and the assistant at the left (Fig. 1). We have found that the safest way to enter the abdomen in morbidly obese patients is under direct vision using a device that allows visualization of the abdominal wall layers sequentially with a zero-degree laparoscope (12-mm Visiport; Autosuture, Norwalk, CT) inserted inside of it. Initial access is in the left upper quadrant. Pneumoperitoneum is created with a high-flow insufflator with air warmer (Stryker Endoscopy, Kalamazoo, MI).

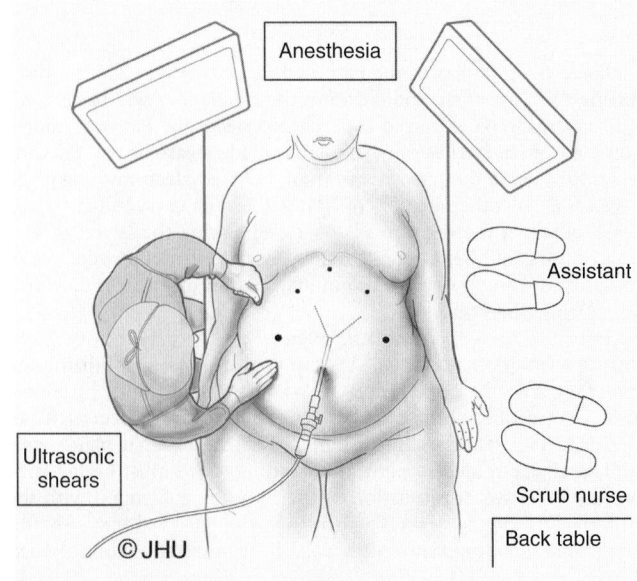

Figure 1 Positioning for laparoscopic gastric bypass.

Laparoscopic Antecolic Gastric Bypass Operative Technique

The 45-degree angled viewing laparoscope is inserted, and four additional four trocars (two 12-mm trocars and two 5-mm trocars) (VersaStep Plus, Autosuture, Norwalk, CT) are placed under direct vision. The omentum and transverse colon are retracted cephalad until the transverse colon mesentery is visualized. Anterior retraction of the mesentery allows visualization of the jejunum at the ligament of Treitz. The jejunum is then transected with a 60-mm white cartridge of 2.5-mm staples (Endo GIA Universal XL, Autosuture, Norwalk, CT) approximately 40 to 75 cm distal to the ligament of Treitz. The mesentery usually has a section here that is sufficiently long to enable the Roux limb to be connected antecolic to the gastric pouch without any significant tension. The mesentery is divided with a 2.0-mm gray staple cartridge, and the ultrasonic shears (AutoSonix XL, US Surgical, Norwalk, CT) are then used to extend this division. A stay suture is placed on the proximal Roux limb and then is measured 60 to 75 cm distal, where the stapled, side-to-side jejunojejunostomy will be constructed. If the patient's body mass index is greater than 50 kg/m^2, the length of the Roux is extended to 150 cm. The 60-cm mark of the Roux limb is then sutured to the proximal jejunum (biliopancreatic end) using a stay suture. The anastomosis is performed with the EndoGIA, loaded with a 60-mm white cartridge and inserted through small enterotomies made with the ultrasonic shears below the stay suture. The enterotomy opening is then closed by firing a 60-mm length blue cartridge of 3.5-mm staples that have been placed under two stay sutures, one at each end of the opening (Fig. 2). An unzippering stitch is placed in the crotch of the stapled anastomosis, and an antiobstruction stitch is placed to keep the Roux limb from kinking at the jejunojejunostomy. The mesenteric defect is then closed with a running suture. Clips or sutures are placed on the staple line if there is any bleeding.

Next we place the patient into steep reverse Trendelenburg position. The legs and feet are checked to make sure they are still straight and on the footboard. The left lateral segment of the liver is retracted using a Nathanson retractor through a subxiphoid 4-mm puncture, which is then held in position with a movable arm that attaches to the operating room table (Iron Intern with Nathanson liver retractors, Automated Medical Products, Edison, NJ). We then begin by dissecting the peritoneal attachments at the angle of His to expose the left crus, followed by the bare area of the

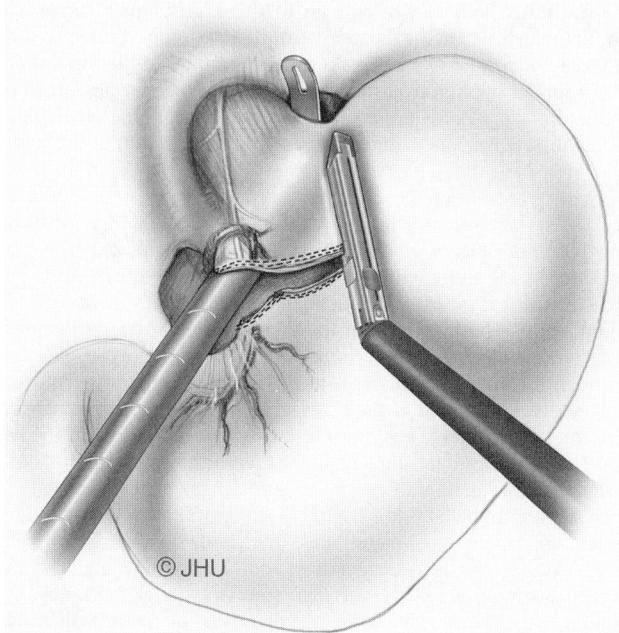

Figure 3 Stapled division of stomach.

gastrohepatic omentum to enter the lesser sac. Division of the neurovascular bundle on the lesser-curved side of the stomach just distal to the left gastric vein is accomplished using a vascular gray staple 2.0-mm cartridge. Multiple 60-mm blue staple cartridges are used in the extra-long Endo GIA to transect the stomach into a small, 15- to 20-ml, proximal gastric pouch. The first gastric staple transection is started on the lesser curved side just below the left gastric vein and is then followed by sequential stapling until completion at the angle of His (Fig. 3). It is important to retract the posterior fundus downward and bring the stapler around the tissue at the angle of His to avoid making a large fundal pouch. This is prevented by entering the open space of the lesser sac after the first division of the stomach with a blue cartridge and dissecting through to the angle of His by using an articulating dissector instrument (Richard Wolf Medical Instruments, Vernon Hills, IL) that can then lock in place after forming a right angle. The articulating dissector can then be used to retract the fundus inferiorly while stapling sequentially with blue cartridges to the angle of His. The stomach staple lines on both sides should be inspected for adequate staple formation, bleeding, and ischemia. Bleeding staple lines are usually easily taken care of with a clip or direct suture ligation. In 5% to 10% of patients, the left lateral segment of the liver is so large that the angle of His cannot be visualized before gastric transaction. In these cases we insert a bougie transorally into the stomach along the lesser curve and then staple alongside it. After each stapled transaction we dissect posterior until we reach the angle of His.

The Roux limb is brought up antecolic with care to prevent a twist in the mesentery. It is occasionally necessary to use the retrocolic retrogastric approach when a short mesentery would put too much tension on the anastomosis. A window is then made in the transverse mesocolon just above and slightly to the left of the ligament of Treitz using the ultrasonic shears. After entering the lesser sac, the stomach is grasped and retracted inferiorly and anteriorly. A red rubber tube attached to the Roux limb (which is removed after the Roux is attached to the gastric pouch) is placed into the lesser sac through this window. The patient is then placed back in steep reverse Trendelenburg position, and the omentum and transverse colon are retracted inferiorly to visualize the lesser sac. The drain with attached Roux limb is retrieved from the lesser sac posterior to the distal stomach.

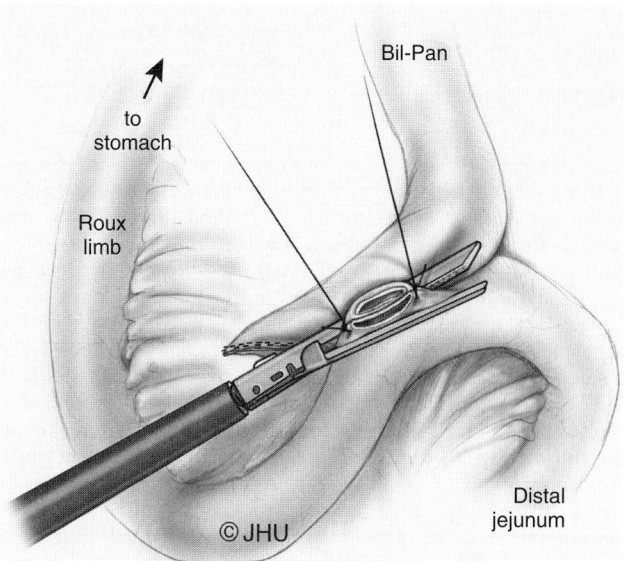

Figure 2 Closure of jejunojejunostomy opening.

The Roux limb is then sutured to the gastric pouch staple line approximately where the first and second gastric staple lines intersect. A small enterotomy is made below the stay suture in the Roux limb, and a similar sized gastrotomy is made in the pouch for placement of the Endo GIA. The stapler is loaded with a 45-mm blue cartridge to create the gastrojejunostomy using only the first 30 mm of the staple cartridge. After the stapler is fired, a stay suture is placed on the lesser curve (right) side of the opening, and the suture is then used to retract the anastomosis to the left and anterior, thereby exposing the posterior side. A running 2–0 suture is then placed posterior on the left side and continuously run to the stay suture on the right side to which it is tied. The anesthesia team carefully passes a 32-F, blunt, round-end bougie from the mouth through the gastrojejunal anastomosis and into the Roux limb. The bougie can be seen through the opening that was formed after the stapler was removed. A stay suture is placed at the halfway point of the opening between the end stay sutures. This stay suture and the stay suture on the left (angle of His side) are used again, just as in the jejunojejunostomy, to elevate the tissue so that the 60-mm length cartridge with 3.5-mm staples can be used to close the openings. The stapler is brought down on top of the bougie while the tissue to be transected is retracted. This firing will then close most of the opening, and the small remaining defect on the right side is easily closed with a 2–0 suture. Alternatively, the entire opening could be closed with a running 2–0 suture. The gastrojejunal anastomosis is then completed by running 2–0 suture to cover the entire anterior portion in a second layer. The resultant anastomosis is approximately 12 mm in diameter and has been completely encircled in multiple, continuous, running 2–0 suture (Fig. 4). An air leak test can be performed, if desired, to test the gastrojejunal anastomosis. The Roux limb distal to the anastomosis is clamped, and air is insufflated either with an endoscope or an orogastric tube while the gastric pouch and anastomosis are submerged in saline.

The mesenteric defect is then closed between the Roux limb mesentery and the transverse mesocolon, up to the transverse colon. The remaining jejunojejunostomy mesenteric defect is closed with a purse-string or running suture. A drain is placed in the left upper quadrant, and the trocars are removed. Long-acting local anesthetic is placed in the wound, and the sites are closed with subcuticular suture.

Laparoscopic Adjustable Gastric Band

The 45-degree angled viewing laparoscope is then inserted, and three trocars (two 12-mm trocars and one 5-mm trocar; VersaStep Plus) are then placed under direct vision (Fig. 6; the black dots are trocars, so the figure shows the port). The angle of His attachment is taken down with blunt dissection, and the gastrohepatic omentum in the bare area is divided with a hook electrocautery. The right crus is identified, and after the hook cautery has been used to divide peritoneal tissue, two graspers are used to carefully dissect over to the angle of His. An articulating dissector is placed from the right crus side to the angle of His; it is then flexed into a right angle and locked. The 12-mm left upper quadrant trocar is removed, and a 15-mm trocar is placed. The adjustable band is placed into the abdomen through the 15-mm trocar. Alternatively, instead of using a 15-mm trocar, the 12-mm trocar is removed, the band is placed directly through the trocar site, and the 12-mm trocar is replaced. The band tubing is then placed through the opening in the articulating dissector and brought over to the right crus side (Fig. 5). The tubing is removed from the dissector and placed through the buckle of the band, which is then locked. Next, three to four interrupted 2–0 nonabsorbable sutures are placed from the fundus to the proximal stomach (superior to the band). It is easier to work closer to the angle of His side of the stomach and then sew to the patient's right side. It is important to get the superior fundus in this anterior wrap to prevent a herniation of the stomach through the band, which can lead to strangulation. The last two interrupted sutures are placed with a 40-F

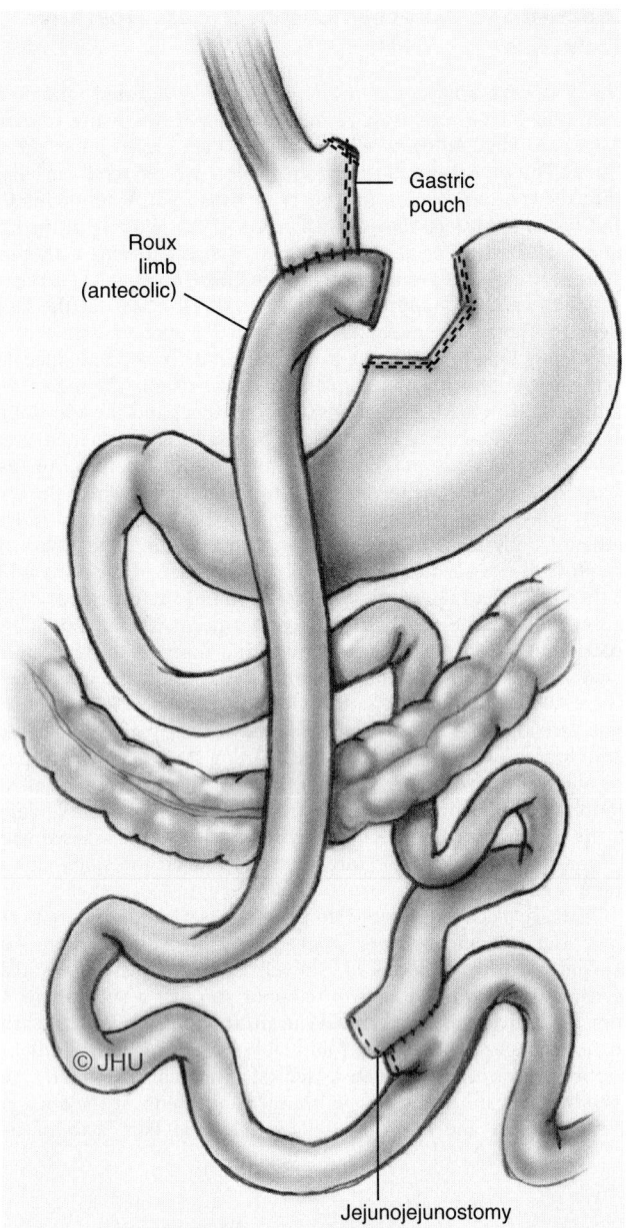

Figure 4 Antecolic Roux-en-Y gastric bypass.

bougie inside the stomach to prevent a complete gastric obstruction from the wrap. The buckle of the band should not be covered because of the increased risk of erosion. The band should lie inside the wrap without tension. The 15-mm left upper quadrant fascia is then closed with an absorbable suture. A Kelly clamp is placed in the left upper quadrant trocar site and is used to puncture the peritoneal cavity more medial and superior than the previous trocar fascial entry site so that a less acute angle is formed with the tubing of the port where it enters the abdomen. The tubing of the band is placed in the clamp and brought out of the wound. A subcutaneous pocket is formed on superior side of the fascia, and four interrupted, nonabsorbable fascial sutures are placed. A small amount of band tubing is cut to size and connected to the port tubing. The port is then tied down to the fascia. It is extremely important to check the tubing to ensure that it has no kinks as it enters the fascia. The port is injected using a side port needle with 4 ml of normal saline to test resistance to flow, and then it is removed. The site is irrigated, and all the trocar sites are closed with subcuticular suture (Fig. 6).

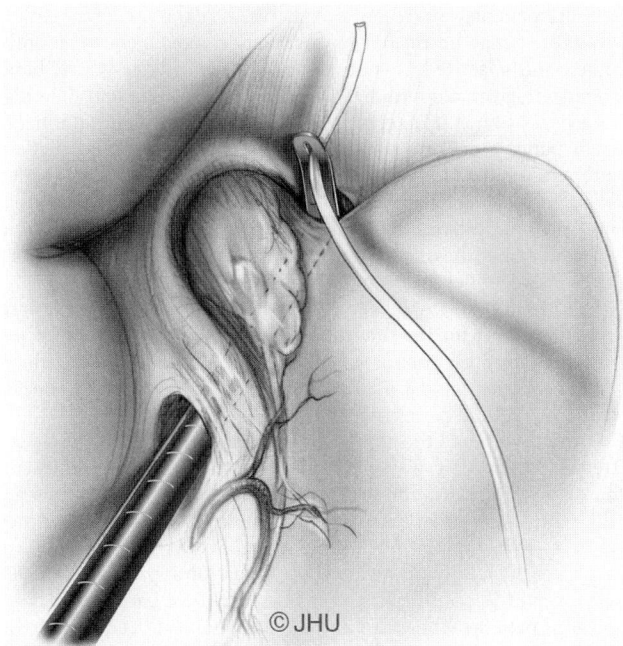

Figure 5 Band tubing about to be brought under stomach, superior to left crura, and over to right crura side.

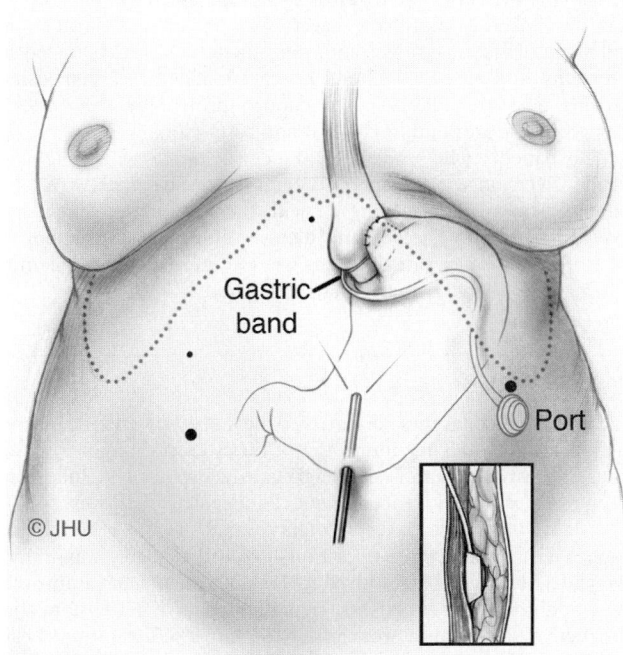

Figure 6 Adjustable gastric band with port placement in left upper quadrant.

Laparoscopic Duodenal Switch with Biliopancreatic Diversion

The 45-degree angled viewing laparoscope is inserted, and an additional five trocars (three additional 12-mm trocars and two 5-mm trocars, VersaStep Plus) are placed under direct vision.

The operating surgeon stands at the patient's left side, and the assistant at the right. The left upper quadrant trocar is used as the camera port for the small bowel anastomosis. The left mid quadrant 12-mm port and left lower 5-mm port are the surgeon's operating ports for the ileoileostomy. The operating room table is placed flat, and the omentum and transverse colon are retracted cephalad. The cecum and ileocecal valve are identified, and the ileum is measured back 100 cm proximal to the cecum. A stay suture is placed, and another 150 cm of ileum is measured proximal from the suture. This is where the ileum is transected using a 60-mm cartridge of 2.5-mm (white) staples. The mesentery is divided with the ultrasonic shears, and a stay suture is placed on the distal transected bowel to mark the Roux end that will connect to the duodenum. The proximal divided bowel is the biliopancreatic limb, which is brought down to the previous stay suture marking the ileum at 100 cm from the cecum. A stapled, side-to-side ileoileostomy is then constructed. Care should be taken to prevent a twist or misalignment of the bowel at this point. The anastomosis is performed with the Endo GIA stapler loaded with a 60-mm cartridge of 2.5-mm staples (white) inserted through small enterotomies made with the ultrasonic shears below the stay suture. The enterotomy opening is then closed using a 60-mm cartridge of 3.5-mm staples (blue cartridge). It helps to place a second stay suture to elevate the enterotomy site while placing the stapler in position. The mesenteric defect is then closed with a running suture.

Next the patient is placed in steep reverse Trendelenburg position, and a liver retractor is placed in the epigastric position to retract the left lateral segment of the liver. The short gastric vessels are divided all the way up to the angle of His. A 48-F bougie is placed in the stomach, and blue (or green) stapler cartridges are used to divide the stomach starting at a point 7 cm from the pyloric valve on the greater curved side. The stomach is divided all the way up to the angle of His, and the lateral stomach that is now disconnected will be removed (Fig. 7). The duodenum is freed from its lateral attachments, taking great care to not injure any of the structures in the hepatoduodenal ligament. The duodenum is then divided approximately 3 to 4 cm distal to the pylorus with a blue stapler cartridge. The Roux limb is brought antecolic up to the proximal

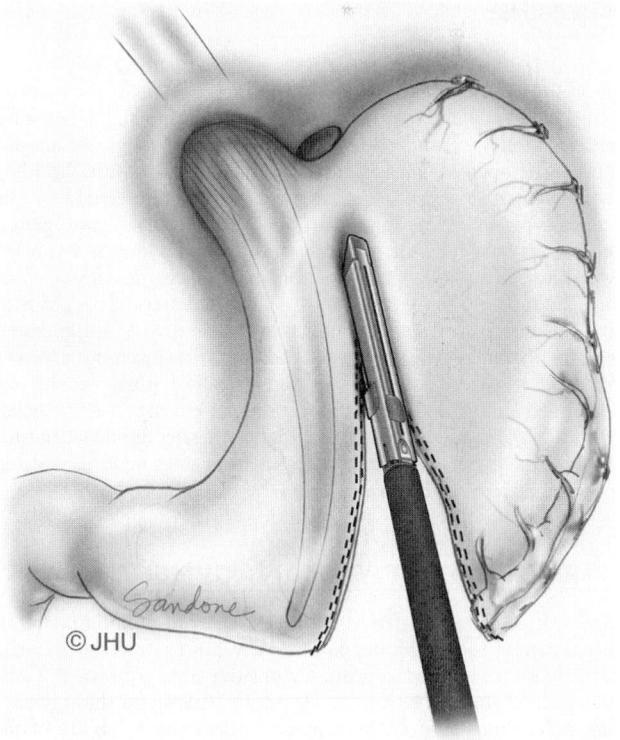

Figure 7 Sleeve gastrectomy.

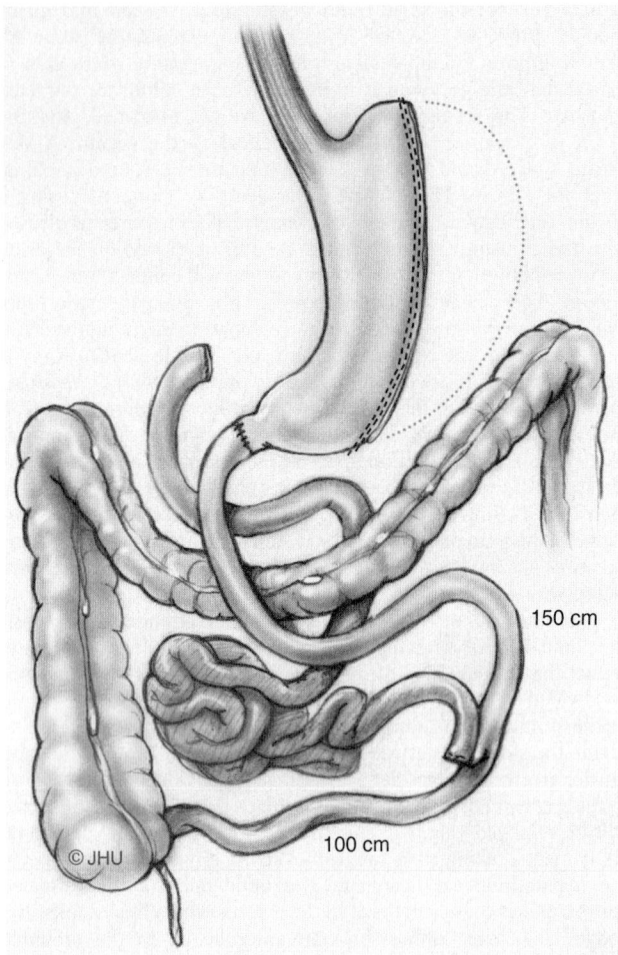

Figure 8 Antecolic duodenal switch with biliopancreatic diversion.

duodenal end, and two stay sutures are placed for a side-to-side anastomosis. Under the inferior stay suture, both ends are opened, and a blue cartridge is placed for 2.5 to 3 cm and fired. The 48-F bougie is removed, and a 40-F bougie is placed through the anastomosis. The opening is now closed with a running suture. Multiple seromuscular interrupted sutures are placed circumferentially. The bougie is removed, and the Roux limb is clamped off. An orogastric tube is inserted into the stomach, and any old blood is removed. An air leak or liquid dye test is performed on the stomach staple line and ileoduodenostomy anastomosis. The mesenteric defect is then closed between the Roux limb mesentery and the transverse mesocolon, up to the transverse colon. The lateral stomach specimen is removed from the midline superior umbilical port, which may require widening, and its fascia may require closing. A drain is left by the stomach, and another drain is left by the ileoduodenal anastomosis. The trocars are removed, and local anesthetic is injected followed by a subcuticular closure of the trocar sites (Fig. 8).

POSTOPERATIVE MANAGEMENT

Most patients are transferred to floor after routine monitoring in the recovery room. Moderate-to-severe obstructive sleep apnea patients are prescribed continuous positive airway pressure while they are sleeping. Occasionally, we admit patients to the intensive care unit if their respiratory demands exceed the capability of the floor staff. IV antibiotics are continued for 24 hours in most cases. Low-molecular-weight heparin is continued during hospitalization

for most patients, whereas the higher risk venous thromboembolism patient may be treated up to an entire postoperative month. Ambulation is started as soon as possible. Adjustable gastric band patients are given a liquid diet the following morning and then discharged to home if tolerating it. Gastric bypass and duodenal switch patients are started on a limited, nonsugar liquid diet on postoperative day 1 and then advanced to a pureed diet on day 2 (day 3 for duodenal switch patients) with discharge planned that day. We use selective upper gastrointestinal series in patients who have a sustained heart rate over 120 beats per minute, respiratory distress, anxiety, fever, or abdominal pain.

Follow-up is in 2 weeks for all patients. All patients are placed on a pureed diet for the first month. They are strongly encouraged to attend a monthly support group meeting and see the dietitian on a routine basis, as well as a mental health professional if one is needed or requested.

Patients who had the adjustable gastric band procedure are evaluated for their first fill at a 6-week postoperative appointment. Those with no restriction and who are hungry between meals get a fill. Patients are then asked to follow up in 2 months unless they feel no restriction, continued hunger, and no weight loss. They are then asked to follow up in 2 weeks. A goal of approximately 40% excess weight loss in the first year is set for most band patients.

Those patients who had gastric bypass and duodenal switch are placed on multivitamin, calcium, and vitamin B12 supplements. All menstruating women are placed on iron to prevent anemia. Patients whose gallbladders were not previously removed are placed on ursodiol 300 mg twice a day for 6 months to reduce the risk of symptomatic cholelithiasis.

Patients who underwent gastric bypass are asked to follow up at 3, 6, 12, 18, and 24 months and every year thereafter. An iron panel and hematologic, electrolyte, and liver function tests are obtained at 3 months, and vitamin B12 and D1,25 are added at 1-year visits. Patients who are not taking in enough protein by diet history may require a prealbumin checked and counseling.

The patients who underwent duodenal switch with biliopancreatic diversion are seen every 3 months for the first two years. Patients who are not keeping up with their protein requirements have a prealbumin checked and dietary counseling. Hematologic, electrolyte, and liver function tests are routinely checked. Vitamin D1,25, B12, A, E, and K also may be requested.

RESULTS

Buchwald and colleagues conducted a meta-analysis of the bariatric literature in 2003. They found that a mean excess weight loss for adjustable gastric band, Roux-en-Y gastric bypass, and biliopancreatic diversion with or without duodenal switch were 48%, 62%, and 70%, respectively. Mortality was 0.1%, 0.5% and 1.1%, respectively, for the three operations. Type II diabetes was found overall to be completely resolved in 77% of patients and improved in an additional 9% of patients. Hyperlipidemia, hypertension, and obstructive sleep apnea were improved in 70%, 79%, and 84%, respectively. In an observational, two-cohort study comparing bariatric surgery patients who were matched with morbidly obese patients who did not undergo surgery, Christou and colleagues found a mortality rate of 0.68% with surgery versus 6.17% without surgery over 5 years. This meant a mortality relative risk reduction of 89% with surgery where 80% were gastric bypass operations.

Pulmonary embolism or sepsis secondary to a leak are the two leading causes of death in the postoperative period after bariatric surgery. Both complications are less than 1% at many major bariatric surgery centers. Despite inconclusive data, some centers are going beyond the routine prophylaxis against venous thromboembolism (VTE) by using a combination of mechanical devices, fractionated or unfractionated heparin, and inferior vena cava filter placement for patients whom they believe to be at higher risk.

Table 2: Gastric Bypass

Advantages

Proven weight loss over 5 years

Better weight loss than restrictive (stomach only) operations

Proven improvement in medical comorbidities

Mortality less than 1% at most centers

Disadvantages

Malabsorption

Marginal ulcer

Stomal stenosis

Inability to easily access distal stomach

Internal hernia

Iron deficiency anemia

Calcium and vitamin B12 deficiencies

Table 3: Adjustable Gastric Band

Advantages

Reversible

Least invasive

Lowest risk of death

No malabsorption

Disadvantages

Erosion

Esophageal dilation

Break

Slippage

Failure to lose weight

Lower average weight loss

Table 4: Duodenal Switch with Biliopancreatic Diversion

Advantages

Excellent weight loss

Increased food intake

Preserved pylorus = less dumping

Less risk of marginal ulcers

Disadvantages

Increased risk of protein malabsorption

Increased risk of fat-soluble vitamin malabsorption (A, D, E, K)

Iron deficiency anemia

Diarrhea and excess gas more common

Internal hernia

Higher complication rate

Higher risk of osteoporosis

These may include patients who have a history of pulmonary embolism or deep venous thrombosis, poor ambulation, severe venous stasis disease, and a body mass index greater than 70 kg/m². Extended prophylaxis with low-molecular-weight heparin after the

Table 5: Complications for 251 Cases

Stomal stenosis 10 (4%)

Marginal ulcer 11 (4%)

Symptomatic gallstones 8 (3%)

Internal hernia 4 (2%)

Postoperative bleeding 5 (2%)

Stroke (minor) 1 (0.4%)

Trocar hernia 0 (0%)

Deep venous thrombosis 0 (0%)

Pulmonary emboli 0 (0%)

Wound infection 0 (0%)

Leaks 0 (0%)

Death 1 (0.4%)

patient has left the hospital can also be employed in higher-risk patients. It is unclear to date whether these extra measures used to prevent VTE are helpful because we do not have any randomized trials that specifically address the morbidly obese patients, whose medication doses tend to be higher than those for patients who are not obese.

Preventing a leak is one of the primary ways to decrease mortality after bariatric surgery. The most common area for a leak to occur after gastric bypass is at the gastrojejunostomy. However, a leak may also occur at the distal stomach staple line or the jejunojejunostomy. There are several ways of performing the upper anastomosis of a gastric bypass or duodenal switch, including circular stapler, linear stapler, handsewn, or combination of stapling with an outer layer of suturing. This may account for variation in the reported rates of a leak, stomal stenosis, and marginal ulcer. At Johns Hopkins, we have performed more than 500 laparoscopic Roux-en-Y gastric bypass operations using the previously described technique that has an inner stapled layer and outer running suture layer with no reported leaks.

Table 5 shows our published complication rate following laparoscopic gastric bypass. We have been using an antecolic antegastric technique for the past 2 years with an internal hernia rate of less than 1%. We continue to close the defect between the transverse mesocolon and Roux limb mesentery up to the transverse colon, believing that without closing it a future hernia may occur because it is a large defect. Stomal stenosis most commonly occurs between 2 and 6 weeks but occasionally may be seen late and in conjunction with a marginal ulcer. All cases have responded to balloon dilatation(s) and, to date, we have not had to reoperate. Marginal ulcers occur on the jejunal side of the gastrojejunal anastomosis and, to date, have all healed with proton pump inhibitor therapy. Patients should be asked if they are smoking, using nonsteroidal anti-inflammatory drugs, or drinking mass quantities of caffeinated drinks (coffee, tea, etc.), because all of these have been associated with marginal ulceration.

COMMENTS

Bariatric surgery continues to be the only effective means of producing weight loss in the majority of patients. Mortality rates less than 1% and leak rates less than 2% have been published by several leading surgical centers committed to bariatric surgery. Center of excellence certification programs will begin to collect outcome data that will not only help to document the beneficial long-term effects of bariatric surgery but also define acceptable outcomes and complication rates.

Suggested Readings

Buchwald H, Avidor Y, Braunwald E, and others: Bariatric surgery: a systemic review and meta-analysis, *JAMA* 292:1724, 2004.

Christou NV, Sampalis JS, Liberman M, and others: Surgery decreases long-term mortality, morbidity, and health care use in morbidly obese patients, *Ann Surg* 240:416, 2004.

Fernandez AZ Jr, DeMaria EJ, Tichansky DS, and others: Experience with over 3,000 open and laparoscopic bariatric procedures: multivariate analysis of factors related to leak and resultant mortality, *Surg Endosc* 18:193, 2004.

Schweitzer MA, Lidor A, Magnuson TH: 251 consecutive laparoscopic gastric bypass operations using a 2 layer gastrojejunostomy technique with a zero leak rate, *J Laparoendosc Adv Surg Tech A* 16:83, 2006.

Wittgrove AC, Clark GW: Laparoscopic gastric bypass Roux-en-Y: 500 patients: technique and results, with 3–60 month follow-up, *Obes Surg* 10:233, 2000.

Note: Page numbers followed by *f* indicate figures; *t*, tables.